MW00339585

Cardiovascular Medicine and Surgery

Cardiovascular Medicine and Surgery

SENIOR EDITORS

Debabrata Mukherjee, MD, MS

Professor and Chair
Department of Internal Medicine
Texas Tech University Health Sciences Center El Paso
El Paso, Texas

Richard A. Lange, MD, MBA

President
Texas Tech University Health Sciences Center El Paso
Rick and Ginger Francis Endowed Professor
Dean, Paul L. Foster School of Medicine
El Paso, Texas

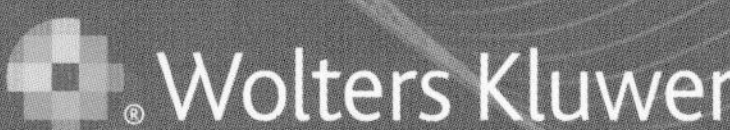

Philadelphia • Baltimore • New York • London
Buenos Aires • Hong Kong • Sydney • Tokyo

SECTION EDITORS

Steven R. Bailey, MD, MSCAI, MACP, FACC, FAHA
Professor and Chairman, Department of Internal Medicine
Malcolm Feist Chair of Interventional Cardiology
Professor Emeritus, UT Health San Antonio
LSU Health School of Medicine
Shreveport, Louisiana

Ragavendra R. Baliga, MBBS, MBA
Professor of Internal Medicine
Inaugural Director, Cardio-Oncology Center of Excellence
The Ohio State University College of Medicine
The Ohio State University Wexner Medical Center
Columbus, Ohio
Editor-in-Chief, *Heart Failure Clinics of North America*

Michael J. Blaha, MD, MPH
Professor of Medicine, Division of Cardiology
Director of Clinical Research
The Johns Hopkins Ciccarone Center for the Prevention of Cardiovascular Disease
The Johns Hopkins University School of Medicine
Baltimore, Maryland

Biykem Bozkurt, MD, PhD, FHFSA, FACC, FAHA, FACP
The Mary and Gordon Cain Chair and Professor of Medicine
Associate Provost of Faculty Affairs, Senior Associate Dean of Faculty Development
Director, Winters Center for Heart Failure Research
Associate Director, Cardiovascular Research Institute
Vice-Chair of Medicine, Baylor College of Medicine
Medicine Chief, Michael E. DeBakey VA Medical Center
Houston, Texas
Immediate Past President, Heart Failure Society of America
Senior Associate Editor, *Circulation*

Joaquin E. Cigarroa, MD, FSCAI
Professor of Medicine
Clinical Chief, Knight Cardiovascular Institute
Chief of Cardiology
Oregon Health & Sciences University
Portland, Oregon

Mario J. Garcia, MD, FACC
Professor of Medicine and Radiology
Chief, Division of Cardiology
Co-Director, Montefiore-Einstein Center for Heart and Vascular Care
Montefiore University Hospital/Albert Einstein College of Medicine
Bronx, New York

Michael E. Jessen, MD
Professor and Chair, Department of Cardiovascular and Thoracic Surgery
Frank M. Ryburn Jr. Distinguished Chair in Cardiothoracic Surgery and Transplantation
University of Texas Southwestern Medical School
University of Texas Southwestern Medical Center
Dallas, Texas

Kalyanam Shivkumar, MD, PhD
Professor of Medicine (Cardiology), Radiology and Bioengineering
Director, UCLA Cardiac Arrhythmia Center and Electrophysiology Programs
Director and Chief, UCLA Interventional Cardiovascular Programs and Catheterization Laboratories
David Geffen School of Medicine at UCLA
UCLA Health System
Los Angeles, California

Karen K. Stout, MD, FACC
Professor of Medicine, Adjunct Professor of Pediatrics
Associate Division Head, Cardiology
University of Washington School of Medicine
Seattle, Washington

Senior Acquisitions Editor: Sharon Zinner, Keith Donnellan
Freelance Development Editor: Carole Wonsiewicz
Senior Development Editor: Ashley Fischer
Editorial Coordinator: Sean Hanrahan
Marketing Manager: Kirsten Waturd
Production Project Manager: Barton Dudlick
Design Coordinator: Stephen Druding
Manufacturing Coordinator: Beth Welsh
Prepress Vendor: S4Carlisle Publishing Services

9 8 7 6 5 4 3 2 1

Printed in Mexico

Library of Congress Cataloging-in-Publication Data

Names: Mukherjee, Debabrata, editor. | Lange, Richard A, editor.
Title: Cardiovascular medicine and surgery/[edited by] Debabrata Mukherjee, Richard A. Lange.
Description: First edition. | Philadelphia : Wolters Kluwer Health/ Lippincott Williams & Wilkins, [2022] | Includes bibliographical references and index.
Identifiers: LCCN 2021017774 | ISBN 9781975148218 (hardcover)
Subjects: MESH: Cardiovascular Diseases--diagnosis | Cardiovascular Diseases--therapy | Cardiovascular Surgical Procedures—methods | Diagnostic Techniques, Cardiovascular
Classification: LCC RC667 | NLM WG 120 | DDC 616.1—dc23
LC record available at https://lccn.loc.gov/2021017774

shop.lww.com

QUADM1021

For our families.

To the cardiology fellows, cardiologists, cardiovascular nurses, pharmacists, and colleagues everywhere for their hard work and dedication to patient care and from whom I have learned so much; to my parents for their infinite patience, love, and understanding; to my nephew Rohin; and to Suchandra, for her love and support.

—Debabrata Mukherjee

To the many mentors, colleagues, fellows, and medical residents who have instructed, inspired, and encouraged me over the years; to my parents whose love and support was unending; and to my sweetheart of over 40 years, Bobette, and our three sons—David, Jonathan, and Brian—who have sacrificially allowed me to pursue my dreams. But for all of you, this book would not have been possible.

—Richard A. Lange

CONTENTS

CONTRIBUTORS

Amal Abdellatif, MD
Instructor in Clinical Medicine
Researcher
Division of Cardiology
Weill Cornell Medicine in Qatar
Hamad Medical Corporation
Ar-Rayyan, Qatar

Dmitry Abramov, MD
Assistant Professor, Medicine
Loma Linda University School of Medicine
Loma Linda University Medical Center
Loma Linda, California

Daniel Addison, MD
Cardiologist
Department of Internal Medicine
The Ohio State University College of Medicine
Columbus, Ohio

Olujimi A. Ajijola, MD, PhD
Associate Professor of Medicine
Director, Neurocardiology Research Program
UCLA Cardiac Arrhythmia Center
David Geffen School of Medicine at UCLA
Los Angeles, California

Olabisi Akanbi, MD
Fellow, Interventional Cardiology
Division of Cardiovascular Medicine
Stanford University School of Medicine
Stanford, California

Jonathan Alis, MD
Director of Cardiothoracic Imaging
Jacobi Medical Center
Bronx, New York

Nicholas S. Amoroso, MD
Assistant Professor of Medicine
Division of Cardiology
The Medical University of South Carolina
Charleston, South Carolina

Lauren Andrade, MD
Adult Congenital Heart Disease Fellow
Division of Cardiology
Hospital of the University of Pennsylvania
Philadelphia, Pennsylvania

Panagiotis Antiochos, MD
Cardiology and Cardiovascular Imaging Fellow
Cardiovascular Division, Department of Medicine
Harvard Medical School
Brigham and Women's Hospital
Boston, Massachusetts

Ehrin J. Armstrong, MD, MSc
Director, Adventist Heart and Vascular Institute
Adventist St. Helena Hospital
St. Helena, California

Zain Ul Abideen Asad, MD, MS
Assistant Professor of Medicine
Department of Internal Medicine, Cardiovascular Disease Section
University of Oklahoma College of Medicine
University of Oklahoma Health Science Center
Oklahoma City, Oklahoma

Federico Asch, MD
Professor of Medicine
Georgetown University School of Medicine
Director, Cardiovascular Core Labs
MedStar Health Research Institute
Washington, District of Columbia

Jessica Atkins, MD
Cardiovascular Disease Fellow
Division of Cardiology
The Medical University of South Carolina
Charleston, South Carolina

Talal T. Attar, MD, MBA
Associate Professor
Department of Internal Medicine, Cardiovascular Disease Section
The Ohio State University College of Medicine
Columbus, Ohio

Ralph Augostini, MD
Professor of Medicine
Bob & Corrine Frick Chair in Cardiac Electrophysiology
Co-Director, Electrophysiology Fellowship Program
The Ohio State University College of Medicine
The Ohio State University Wexner Medical Center
Columbus, Ohio

Vinay Badhwar, MD
Gordon F. Murray Professor and Chairman
Department of Cardiovascular and Thoracic Surgery
West Virginia University School of Medicine
Morgantown, West Virginia

Steven R. Bailey, MD
Professor and Chairman, Department of Internal Medicine
Malcolm Feist Chair of Interventional Cardiology
Professor Emeritus, UT Health San Antonio
Louisiana State University School of Medicine - Shreveport
Shreveport, Louisiana

Retesh Bajaj, MBBS, BSc, MRCP (Lond)
Interventional Cardiology Research Fellow
Barts Heart Centre
London, United Kingdom

Ragavendra R. Baliga, MBBS, MBA
Professor of Internal Medicine
Inaugural Director, Cardio-Oncology Center of Excellence
The Ohio State University College of Medicine
The Ohio State University Wexner Medical Center
Columbus, Ohio
Editor-in-Chief, *Heart Failure Clinics of North America*

Gary S. Beasley, MD
Assistant Professor of Pediatrics
University of Tennessee College of Medicine
University of Tennessee Health Science Center
The Heart Institute at Le Bonheur Children's Hospital
St. Jude Children's Research Hospital
Memphis, Tennessee

Craig J. Beavers, PharmD
Adjunct Assistant Professor
Cardiovascular Clinical Pharmacist
University of Kentucky College of Pharmacy
Lexington, Kentucky

Aron Bender, MD
Cardiac Electrophysiologist
UCLA Cardiac Arrhythmia Center
David Geffen School of Medicine at UCLA
Los Angeles, California

Peyman Benharash, MD, MS
Associate Professor of Surgery and Bioengineering
Director of Cardiovascular Outcomes Research Laboratories
David Geffen School of Medicine at UCLA
Los Angeles, California

Anju Bhardwaj, MD
Assistant Professor
Advanced Cardiopulmonary Therapies and Transplantation
The John P. and Kathrine G. McGovern Medical School
The University of Texas Health Science Center at Houston
Houston, Texas

Sukhdeep Bhogal, MBBS, MD
Interventional Cardiology Fellow
Medstar Washington Hospital Center
Washington, District of Columbia

Katrina A. E. L. Bidwell, MD
Interventional Cardiology Fellow
The Medical University of South Carolina
Charleston, South Carolina

Edo Y. Birati, MD
Chief, Division of Cardiovascular Medicine
Padeh-Poriya Medical Centre
Tiberias, Israel

Marcio Sommer Bittencourt, MD, MPH, PhD
Attending Cardiologist
University Hospital
University of São Paulo School of Medicine
São Paulo, Brazil

Michael J. Blaha, MD, MPH
Professor of Medicine, Division of Cardiology
Director of Clinical Research
The Johns Hopkins Ciccarone Center for the Prevention of Cardiovascular Disease
The Johns Hopkins University School of Medicine
Baltimore, Maryland

James C. Blankenship, MD, MHCM, MSCAI, MACC
Professor of Medicine
Director of Cardiac Catheterization Laboratory
Interim Director of Cardiology
The University of New Mexico School of Medicine
University of New Mexico Health Sciences Center
Albuquerque, New Mexico

Ron Blankstein, MD
Professor of Medicine and Radiology
Harvard Medical School
Associate Director, Cardiovascular Imaging Program
Director, Cardiac Computed Tomography
Co-Director, Cardiovascular Imaging Training Program
Associate Physician, Preventive Cardiology
Brigham and Women's Hospital
Boston, Massachusetts

Lori A. Blauwet, MD, MA
Physician
Olmsted Medical Center
Rochester, Minnesota

Roger S. Blumenthal, MD
Professor of Medicine
The Johns Hopkins University School of Medicine
Director
The Johns Hopkins Ciccarone Center for the Prevention of Cardiovascular Disease
The Johns Hopkins Medicine
Baltimore, Maryland

Josiah Bote, MD
Fellow, Noninvasive Cardiology
Hartford Hospital
Hartford, Connecticut

Konstantinos Dean Boudoulas, MD
Professor of Medicine
Section Head, Interventional Cardiology
Director, Cardiac Catheterization Laboratories
The Ohio State University College of Medicine
The Ohio State University Wexner Medical Center
Columbus, Ohio

Noel G. Boyle, MD, PhD
Professor of Medicine
Director of Cardiac EP Fellowship Program
UCLA Cardiac Arrhythmia Center
David Geffen School of Medicine at UCLA
Los Angeles, California

Jason S. Bradfield, MD
Associate Professor of Medicine
Director, Specialized Program for Ventricular Tachycardia
UCLA Cardiac Arrhythmia Center
David Geffen School of Medicine at UCLA
Los Angeles, California

Elisa A. Bradley, MD
Associate Professor of Internal Medicine and Cardiovascular Medicine
Department of Internal Medicine, Cardiovascular Disease Section
The Ohio State University College of Medicine
Columbus, Ohio

Yonatan Buber, MD
Associate Professor of Medicine
Department of Internal Medicine
University of Washington School of Medicine
University of Washington Medical Center
Seattle, Washington

Eric Buch, MD, MS
Associate Professor of Medicine
Director, Electrophysiology Labs and Specialized Program for AF
UCLA Cardiac Arrhythmia Center
David Geffen School of Medicine at UCLA
Los Angeles, California

Christine Bui, MD
Pediatric Cardiology Fellow
Stanford University School of Medicine
Stanford Health – Lucile Packard Children's Hospital
Stanford, California

Miguel Cainzos-Achirica, MD, MPH, PhD
Research Fellow
Division of Cardiology
Johns Hopkins University School of Medicine
Johns Hopkins Bloomberg School of Public Health
Baltimore, Maryland

Courtney M. Campbell, MD, PhD
Fellow
Department of Cardio-Oncology and Amyloidosis
Washington University School of Medicine
St. Louis, Missouri

Andrea J. Carpenter, MD, PhD
Professor, Cardiothoracic Surgery
Program Director, Thoracic Surgery Residency
The Joe R. and Teresa Lozano Long School of Medicine
UT Health San Antonio
San Antonio, Texas

Frank Cecchin, MD
Professor of Pediatrics and Internal Medicine
New York University Grossman School of Medicine
New York, New York

Khalil Chamseddin, MD
General Surgery Resident
University of Texas Southwestern Medical School
University of Texas Southwestern Medical Center
Dallas, Texas

Alice Chan, DMP, MSN, RN
Clinical Program Manager
Adult Congenital Heart Disease Center
The Mount Sinai Hospital
New York, New York

Hugo Quinny Cheng, MD
Clinical Professor of Medicine
University of California, San Francisco School of Medicine
San Francisco, California

Maureen E. Cheung, DO
Cardiothoracic Surgery Fellow
Department of Internal Medicine, Cardiovascular Disease Section
The Ohio State University College of Medicine
The Ohio State University Wexner Medical Center
Columbus, Ohio

Ricardo Cigarroa, MD
Interventional Cardiology Specialist
Cigarroa Heart and Vascular Institute
Laredo Medical Center
Laredo, Texas

Andrew Civitello, MD
Associate Professor
Department of Medicine, Section of Cardiology
Baylor College of Medicine
Medical Director
Advanced Heart Failure Program
Baylor St. Luke's Medical Center
Texas Heart Institute
Houston, Texas

Suparna C. Clasen, MD
Assistant Professor of Clinical Medicine
Medical Director of Cardio-Oncology
Krannert Institute of Cardiology
Indiana University School of Medicine
Indianapolis, Indiana

Monica Mechele Colvin, MD, MS
Professor of Medicine
Cardiovascular Division
University of Michigan Medical School
Ann Arbor, Michigan

Heidi M. Connolly, MD
Professor of Medicine
Consultant
Division of Structural Heart Disease, Department of Cardiovascular Medicine
Department of Cardiovascular Medicine
Mayo Clinic College of Medicine and Science
Mayo Clinic
Rochester, Minnesota

Chris C. Cook, MD
Associate Professor
Program Director, Thoracic Surgery Residency
Department of Cardiovascular and Thoracic Surgery, Division of Cardiac Surgery
West Virginia University School of Medicine
Morgantown, West Virginia

Leslie T. Cooper, Jr, MD
Professor of Medicine
Chair
Department of Cardiovascular Medicine
Mayo Clinic College of Medicine and Science
Mayo Clinic
Jacksonville, Florida

Lorraine Cornwell, MD
Assistant Professor
Cardiothoracic Surgery
Department of Surgery
Baylor College of Medicine
Michael E. DeBakey Veterans Affairs Medical Center
Houston, Texas

Ranjan Dahal, MD
Cardiology Fellow
Department of Internal Medicine
Paul L. Foster School of Medicine
Texas Tech University Health Sciences Center El Paso
El Paso, Texas

V. Vivian Dimas, MD
Associate Professor
Department of Pediatrics
University of Texas Southwestern Medical School
University of Texas Southwestern Medical Center
Dallas, Texas

Louis-Philippe David, MD
Cardiologist
University of Montreal
Montreal, Quebec, Canada

Ryan R. Davies, MD
Associate Professor
Department of Cardiovascular and Thoracic Surgery
Director of Pediatric Heart Transplantation and Mechanical Circulatory Support
University of Texas Southwestern Medical School
University of Texas Southwestern Medical Center
Dallas, Texas

Jennifer DeSalvo, MD
Clinical Instructor
Departments of Internal Medicine and Pediatrics
The Ohio State University Medical Center
Nationwide Children's Hospital
Columbus, Ohio

Anita Deswal, MD, MPH
Professor of Medicine
Department of Cardiology
Ting Tsung and Wei Fong Chao Distinguished Chair
University of Texas MD Anderson Cancer Center
Houston, Texas

Thomas A. Dewland, MD
Associate Professor of Medicine
University of California, San Francisco School of Medicine
San Francisco, California

Punag Divanji, MD
Associate Professor, Interventional Cardiology
Division of Cardiology
Knight Cardiovascular Institute
Oregon Health & Science University
Portland, Oregon

Jeffrey A. Dixson, MD
Fellow, Cardiology and Critical Care Medicine
Duke University School of Medicine
Durham, North Carolina

Duc H. Do, MD, MS
Clinical Instructor
UCLA Cardiac Arrhythmia Center
David Geffen School of Medicine at UCLA
Los Angeles, California

Mark H. Drazner, MD, MSc
Professor of Internal Medicine
Clinical Chief of Cardiology, James M. Wooten Chair in Cardiology
University of Texas Southwestern Medical School
University of Texas Southwestern Medical Center
Dallas, Texas

Steven P. Dunn, PharmD
Lead Pharmacist
Heart & Vascular, UVA Health
University of Virginia School of Medicine
Charlottesville, Virginia

William Lane Duvall, MD
Professor of Medicine
University of Connecticut School of Medicine
Director, Nuclear Cardiology
Hartford Hospital
Hartford, Connecticut

Omar Dzaye, MD, PhD
Senior Research Fellow
The Johns Hopkins Ciccarone Center for the Prevention of Cardiovascular Disease
The Johns Hopkins University School of Medicine
Baltimore, Maryland

Mohamed B. Elshazly, MD
Adjunct Assistant Professor of Medicine
The Johns Hopkins University School of Medicine
The Johns Hopkins Ciccarone Center for the Prevention of Cardiovascular Disease
The Johns Hopkins Hospital
Baltimore, Maryland

Anthony L. Estrera, MD
Professor and Chair
Department of Cardiothoracic and Vascular Surgery
The John P. and Kathrine G. McGovern Medical School
The University of Texas Health Science Center at Houston
Memorial Hermann Health System
Houston, Texas

Justin Ezekowitz, MBBCh, MSc
Professor of Medicine
University of Alberta
Edmonton, Alberta, Canada

Oluwaseun E. Fashanu, MD
Resident
Department of Medicine
The Johns Hopkins Ciccarone Center for the Prevention of Cardiovascular Disease
The Johns Hopkins University School of Medicine
Saint Agnes Hospital
Baltimore, Maryland

Savitri E. Fedson, MD, MA
Professor of Medicine and Medical Ethics
Department of Medicine, Section of Cardiology
Baylor College of Medicine
Michael E. DeBakey VA Medical Center
Houston, Texas

William H. Fennell, MD
Adjunct Professor of Medicine
University College Cork
Cardiologist (retired), Cork University Hospital
Cork, Ireland
Research Associate, Cardiology
Paris, France

Valerian Fernandes, MD
Professor of Medicine
The Medical University of South Carolina
Director of Cardiac Catheterization Laboratory
Ralph H Johnson VA Medical Center
Charleston, South Carolina

Matt Finn, MD, MSc
Assistant Professor of Medicine
Department of Cardiology
Columbia University Vagelos College of Physicians and Surgeons
Columbia University Irving Medical Center
New York, New York

Jeff Fowler, DO
Assistant Professor of Medicine
University of Pittsburgh School of Medicine
Heart and Vascular Institute
University of Pittsburgh Medical Center
Pittsburgh, Pennsylvania

Camille L. Hancock Friesen, MD
Professor
Department of Surgery
University of Nebraska Medical Center College of Medicine
Pediatric Cardiothoracic Surgery
Children's Hospital & Medical Center
Omaha, Nebraska

Margaret M. Fuchs, MD
Fellow
Department of Cardiovascular Diseases
Mayo Clinic College of Medicine and Science
Mayo Clinic
Rochester, Minnesota

Kana Fujikura, MD, PhD, MPH
Division of Cardiology
Department of Internal Medicine
Montefiore Medical Center
Bronx, New York
Staff Clinician
NIH - Advanced Cardiovascular Imaging Laboratory
National Heart, Lung and Blood Institute
Bethesda, Maryland

Osamu Fujimura, MD[‡]
Professor of Medicine
David Geffen School of Medicine at UCLA
Los Angeles, California

[‡]Deceased

Jeffrey Gaca, MD
Associate Professor of Surgery
Duke University School of Medicine
Durham, North Carolina

Roberto G. Gallotti, MD
Assistant Professor
Division of Pediatric Cardiology
David Geffen School of Medicine at UCLA
Ronald Regan UCLA Medical Center
Los Angeles, California

Mario J. Garcia, MD
Professor of Medicine and Radiology
Chief, Division of Cardiology
Co-Director, Montefiore-Einstein Center for Heart and Vascular Care
Montefiore University Hospital/Albert Einstein College of Medicine
Bronx, New York

Zachary Garrett, MD
Cardiology Fellow
Department of Cardiovascular Medicine
The Ohio State University School of Medicine
The Ohio State University Wexner Medical Center
Columbus, Ohio

Giuliano Generoso, MD, PhD
Center for Clinical and Epidemiological Research
University Hospital
Critical Cardiology Unit
Hospital Sirio Libanes
São Paulo, Brazil

Arjun K. Ghosh, MBBS, MSc, PhD
Honorary Clinical Senior Lecturer
University College London
Queen Mary University of London
Consultant Cardiologist (Cardio-oncology)
Barts Heart Centre
St Bartholomew's Hospital
London, United Kingdom

Stefanos Giannopoulos, MD
Postdoctoral Research Fellow in Vascular Medicine
University of Colorado Anschutz Medical Campus
Aurora, Colorado

Irakli Giorgberidze, MD
Associate Professor
Department of Internal Medicine, Section of Cardiology
Baylor College of Medicine
Director, Cardiac Electrophysiology Service
Michael E. DeBakey VA Medical Center
Houston, Texas

Laurie Bossory Goike, MD
Cardiology Fellow
The Ohio State University School of Medicine
The Ohio State University Wexner Medical Center
Columbus, Ohio

Lee R. Goldberg, MD, MPH
Professor of Medicine
Vice Chair of Medicine
Department of Medicine
Perelman School of Medicine at the University of Pennsylvania
Philadelphia, Pennsylvania

Gerardo Gonzalez-Guardiola, MD
Assistant Professor Vascular and Endovascular Surgery
University of Texas Southwestern Medical School
University of Texas Southwestern Medical Center
Dallas, Texas

Gowtham R. Grandhi, MD, MPH
Resident
Department of Medicine
MedStar Union Memorial Hospital
Baltimore, Maryland

Justin L. Grodin, MD, MPH
Assistant Professor of Medicine
Division of Cardiology, Department of Internal Medicine
University of Texas Southwestern Medical School
University of Texas Southwestern Medical Center
Dallas, Texas

Maya Guglin, MD, PhD
Professor of Clinical Medicine
Director, Heart Failure
Indiana University School of Medicine
Indianapolis, Indiana

Avirup Guha, MBBS, MPH
Assistant Professor of Medicine
Division of Cardiology
Case Western Reserve University School of Medicine
Cleveland, Ohio

Amy E. Hackmann, MD
Associate Professor
Department of Cardiovascular and Thoracic Surgery
University of Texas Southwestern Medical School
Surgical Director, ECMO Program
University of Texas Southwestern Medical Center
Dallas, Texas

Joseph Hadaya, MD
Resident
David Geffen School of Medicine at UCLA
Los Angeles, California

Dan G. Halpern, MD
Assistant Professor of Medicine
Director, Adult Congenital Heart Disease
Leon H. Charney Division of Cardiology
New York University Grossman School of Medicine
NYU Langone Health
New York, New York

Peter Hanna, MD, PhD
Cardiac Electrophysiology Fellow
David Geffen School of Medicine at UCLA
Los Angeles, California

Linda B. Haramati, MD, MS
Professor of Radiology and Medicine
Division Lead, Cardiothoracic Imaging
Department of Radiology
Albert Einstein College of Medicine
Montefiore Medical Center
Bronx, New York

Reema Hasan, MD, FACC
Clinical Assistant Professor,
Advanced Heart Failure and Transplant Cardiology, Cardiovascular Disease, Internal Medicine
University of Michigan Medical School
Ann Arbor, Michigan

Justin Hayase, MD
Clinical Instructor
UCLA Cardiac Arrhythmia Center
David Geffen School of Medicine at UCLA
Los Angeles, California

Nicholas S. Hendren, MD
Fellow
Division of Cardiology
Department of Internal Medicine
University of Texas Southwestern Medical School
University of Texas Southwestern Medical Center
Dallas, Texas

Benjamin S. Hendrickson, MD
Assistant Professor
Division of Cardiology
Department of Pediatrics
University of Tennessee College of Medicine
University of Tennessee Health Science Center
Le Bonheur Children's Hospital
Memphis, Tennessee

Carrie Herbert, MD
Assistant Professor
Department of Pediatrics
University of Texas Southwestern Medical School
University of Texas Southwestern Medical Center
Dallas, Texas

Edwin Ho, MD
Assistant Professor of Medicine
Director, Interventional Echocardiography
Co-Director, Heart Valve/Structural Heart Center
Attending Cardiologist, Department of Cardiology
Montefiore Medical Center
Bronx, New York

Luise Holzhauser, MD
Assistant Professor of Clinical Medicine
Department of Medicine, Division of Cardiovascular Medicine
Advanced Heart Failure, Transplantation and Mechanical Circulatory Support Section
Perelman School of Medicine at the University of Pennsylvania
Philadelphia, Pennsylvania

Tamara Beth Horwich, MD, MS
Professor of Medicine and Cardiology
Medical Director, UCLA Cardiac Rehabilitation Program
Co-Director, UCLA Women's Cardiovascular Center
David Geffen School of Medicine at UCLA
Los Angeles, California

Ray Hu, MD
Fellow
Division of Cardiovascular Medicine
Department of Medicine
Perelman School of Medicine at the University of Pennsylvania
Philadelphia, Pennsylvania

Dawn S. Hui, MD
Associate Professor of Cardiothoracic Surgery
The Joe R. and Teresa Lozano Long School of Medicine
University of Texas Health San Antonio
San Antonio, Texas

Zeeshan Hussain, MD
Assistant Professor of Medicine
Case Western Reserve University School of Medicine
University Hospitals
Cleveland, Ohio

Ahmed Ibrahim, MD, MSc
Assistant Professor
Division of Cardiology
Department of Internal Medicine
Paul L. Foster School of Medicine
Texas Tech University Health Science Center El Paso
El Paso, Texas

Yuki Ikeno, MD, PhD
Research Fellow
Department of Cardiovascular Surgery
The John P. and Kathrine G. McGovern Medical School
The University of Texas Health Science Center at Houston
Houston, Texas

Ignacio Inglessis, MD
Assistant Professor in Medicine
Director of Structural Heart Disease Program
Department of Cardiology
Massachusetts General Hospital
Boston, Massachusetts

Joseph J. Ingrassia, MD
Director
Vascular Medicine and Endovascular Intervention
Interventional Cardiologist
Department of Cardiology
Hartford Healthcare Heart and Vascular Institute
Hartford, Utah

Dana Irrer, MD
Fellow, Pediatric and Adult Congenital Cardiology
Division of Cardiology
University of Colorado School of Medicine
Aurora, Colorado

Ijeoma Isiadinso, MD, MPH
Associate Professor
Department of Medicine
Emory University School of Medicine
Emory Heart and Vascular Center
Atlanta, Georgia

Dipti Itchhaporia, MD
Associate Professor
Eric & Sheila Samson Endowed Chair in Cardiovascular Health
Director of Disease Management, Hoag Heart and Vascular Institute
Newport Beach, California
University of California, Irvine School of Medicine
Irvine, California
President, American College of Cardiology

C. Charles Jain, MD
Clinical Fellow
Department of Cardiovascular Medicine
Mayo Clinic College of Medicine and Science
Mayo Clinic
Rochester, Minnesota

Robert D. B. Jaquiss, MD
Professor of Cardiovascular and Thoracic Surgery and Pediatrics
Chief of Pediatric and Congenital Heart Surgery
University of Texas Southwestern Medical Center
Children's Health System of Texas
Dallas, Texas

Gharibyan Rosie Jasper, DO
Cardiology Fellow
Department of Cardiology
Geisinger Commonwealth School of Medicine
Geisinger Medical Center
Danville, Pennsylvania

Omar Jawaid, MD, MS
Cardiology Fellow
Division of Cardiology
Department of Medicine
Indiana University School of Medicine
Indianapolis, Indiana

Lalithapriya Jayakumar, MD
Vascular Surgeon
Community Care Physicians-Vascular Health Partners
Latham, New York

J. Stephen Jenkins, MD
Associate Professor of Medicine
Section Head, Interventional Cardiology
Director, Interventional Cardiology Research
John Ochsner Heart and Vascular Institute
Ochsner Medical Center
The Ochsner Clinical School (University of Queensland)
New Orleans, Louisiana

Michael E. Jessen, MD
Professor and Chair, Department of Cardiovascular and Thoracic Surgery
Frank M. Ryburn Jr., Distinguished Chair in Cardiothoracic Surgery and Transplantation
University of Texas Southwestern Medical School
University of Texas Southwestern Medical Center
Dallas, Texas

Parag H. Joshi, MD, MHS
Associate Professor
Departments of Medicine and Cardiology
University of Texas Southwestern Medical School
University of Texas Southwestern Medical Center
Dallas, Texas

Rami Kahwash, MD
Professor in Internal Medicine
Department of Internal Medicine, Cardiovascular Disease Section
The Ohio State University College of Medicine
Columbus, Ohio

Yaquta Kaka, MD
Cardiovascular Medicine Fellow
Clinical Instructor
The Ohio State University Wexner Medical Center
Columbus, Ohio

Jahnavi Kakuturu, MD
Fellow
Department of Cardiovascular and Thoracic Surgery
West Virginia University School of Medicine
Morgantown, West Virginia

Munish Kannabhiran, MD
Physician
Department of Cardiology-Electrophysiology
David Geffen School of Medicine at UCLA
Los Angeles, California

Karan Kapoor, MD
Fellow in Cardiovascular Medicine
The Johns Hopkins University School of Medicine
The Johns Hopkins Hospital
Baltimore, Maryland

Risheek Kaul, MD
Chief Cardiology Fellow
Department of Cardiology
Westchester Medical Center
Valhalla, New York

Joseph D. Kay, MD
Associate Professor, Pediatrics-Cardiology
University of Colorado School of Medicine
University of Colorado Hospital
Children's Hospital Colorado
Aurora, Colorado

Toshinobu Kazui, MD, PhD
Associate Professor
Department of Surgery
University of Arizona College of Medicine
Barnes University Medical Center
Tucson, Arizona

Houman Khakpour, MD
Assistant Professor of Medicine
UCLA Cardiac Arrhythmia Center
David Geffen School of Medicine at UCLA
Los Angeles, California

Abigail D. Khan, MD
Associate Professor of Medicine
Oregon Health & Science University
Portland, Oregon

Abhishek Khemka, MD, MBA
Assistant Professor of Clinical Medicine
Division of Cardiology, Department of Medicine
Indiana University School of Medicine
Indiana University Health
Indianapolis, Indiana

Todd L. Kiefer, MD
Associate Professor
Division of Cardiology
Duke University School of Medicine
Duke University Medical Center
Durham, North Carolina

Sooyeon Kim, MD
Department of Vascular Surgery
University of Texas Southwestern Medical School
University of Texas Southwestern Medical Center
Dallas, Texas

Yuli Y. Kim, MD
Associate Professor of Medicine
Department of Medicine, Division of Cardiovascular Medicine
Perelman School of Medicine at the University of Pennsylvania
Medical Director
Philadelphia Adult Congenital Heart Center
Penn Medicine
Children's Hospital of Philadelphia
Philadelphia, Pennsylvania

Melissa L. Kirkwood, MD
Associate Professor
Division Chief of Vascular Surgery
University of Texas Southwestern Medical School
University of Texas Southwestern Medical Center
Dallas, Texas

Richard A. Krasuski, MD
Professor of Medicine and Pediatrics (Cardiology)
Adult Congenital Heart Disease Specialist
Duke University School of Medicine
Durham, North Carolina

Joseph M. Krepp, MD
Assistant Professor of Medicine
Department of Medicine
Division of Cardiology
The George Washington University School of Medicine and Health Sciences
Washington, District of Columbia

Darshan Krishnappa, MD
Assistant Professor, Cardiac Electrophysiology
Sri Jeyadeva Institute of Cardiovascular Sciences and Research
Bangalore, India

Yuliya Krokhaleva, MD
Assistant Clinical Professor
UCLA Cardiac Arrhythmia Center
David Geffen School of Medicine at UCLA
Los Angeles, California

Raymond Y. Kwong, MD, MPH
Professor of Medicine
Director of Cardiovascular Magnetic Resonance Imaging
Cardiovascular Division of the Department of Medicine
Brigham and Women's Hospital
Harvard Medical School
Boston, Massachusetts

Brent C. Lampert, DO
Associate Professor
Department of Clinical Medicine
The Ohio State University College of Medicine
The Ohio State University Wexner Medical Center
Columbus, Ohio

Richard A. Lange, MD, MBA
President
Texas Tech University Health Sciences Center El Paso
Rick and Ginger Francis Endowed Professor
Dean, Paul L. Foster School of Medicine
El Paso, Texas

Gurion Lantz, MD
Assistant Professor of Surgery
Division of Cardiothoracic Surgery
Oregon Health & Science University
Portland, Oregon

Taylor Alexander Lebeis, MD
Clinical Assistant Professor
Division of Cardiovascular Medicine
University of Michigan Medical School
University of Michigan Health
Ann Arbor, Michigan

David Lee, MD
Professor of Medicine
Department of Medicine, Cardiovascular Medicine
Stanford University School of Medicine
Stanford, California

James S. Lee, MD
Assistant Clinical Professor
Associate Regional Director of Interventional Cardiology
David Geffen School of Medicine at UCLA
Los Angeles, California

Marc V. Lee, MD
Clinical Assistant Professor
Section of Cardiology
Department of Pediatrics
Nationwide Children's Hospital
Columbus, Ohio

Randall J. Lee, MD, PhD
Professor of Medicine
Deparment of Medicine
University of California, San Francisco School of Medicine
Cardiac Electrophysiology and Arrhythmia Service
UCSF Health
San Francisco, California

Jonathan Lerner, MD
Fellow
Division of Cardiology
Harbor-UCLA Medical Center
Torrance, California

Jeannette Lin, MD
Associate Clinical Professor
Department of Medicine
David Geffen School of Medicine at UCLA
Ronald Reagen UCLA Medical Center
Los Angeles, California

Gina P. Lundberg, MD
Associate Professor
Emory University School of Medicine
Clinical Director
Emory Women's Cardiovascular Health Center
Atlanta, Georgia

Melissa A. Lyle, MD
Senior Associate Consultant
Department of Cardiovascular Medicine
Mayo Clinic College of Medicine and Science
Mayo Clinic
Jacksonville, Florida

Janet Ma, MD
Physician
Massachusetts General Hospital
Boston, Massachusetts

Carlos Macias, MD
Cardiac Electophysiologist
UCLA Health Systems
Valencia, California

Nidhi Madan, MD, MPH
Structural Heart Disease Fellow
Rush University Medical Center
Chicago, Illinois

Stephanie M. Madonis, MD
Fellow, Interventional Cardiology
John Ochsner Heart and Vascular Institute
New Orleans, Louisiana

David S. Majdalany, MD
Assistant Professor of Medicine
Cardiologist
Department of Cardiovascular Medicine
Mayo Clinic College of Medicine and Science
Mayo Clinic
Scottsdale, Arizona

Fatemeh Malekpour, MD
Assistant Professor, Vascular Surgery
University of Texas Southwestern Medical School
University of Texas Southwestern Medical Center
Dallas, Texas

Anbukararasi Maran, MD
Associate Professor, Cardiology
The Medical University of South Carolina
Charleston, South Carolina

Francois Marcotte, MD
Associate Professor of Medicine
Chair, Subspecialty Clinics
Director, Adult Congenital Heart Disease Clinic
Department of Cardiovascular Medicine
Mayo Clinic College of Medicine and Science
Mayo Clinic
Scottsdale, Arizona

Ali J. Marian, MD
Professor and Director
Center for Cardiovascular Genetic Research
The Brown Foundation Institute of Molecular Medicine
The John P. and Kathrine G. McGovern Medical School
The University of Texas Health Science Center at Houston
Houston, Texas

William H. Marshall V, MD
Fellow, Adult Congenital Heart Disease and Pulmonary Hypertension
The Ohio State University Wexner Medical Center
Nationwide Children's Hospital
Columbus, Ohio

Seth S. Martin, MD, MHS
Associate Professor of Medicine
Department of Cardiology
The Johns Hopkins University School of Medicine
Baltimore, Maryland

Hugo Martinez, MD
Assistant Professor
Division of Pediatric Cardiology and Genetics
University of Tennessee College of Medicine
University of Tennessee Health Science Center
Director, Cardiovascular Genetics Service
Co-Director, Hypertrophic Cardiomyopathy Program
The Heart Institute at Le Bonheur Children's Hospital
Consulting Cardio-Oncologist, Department of Pediatric Medicine
St. Jude Children's Research Hospital
Memphis, Tennessee

Paul J. Mather, MD
Professor of Clinical Medicine
Heart Failure and Transplant Program
Department of Medicine, Division of Cardiovascular Medicine
Advanced Heart Failure, Transplantation and Mechanical Circulatory Support Section
Perelman School of Medicine at the University of Pennsylvania
Philadelphia, Pennsylvania

John W. McEvoy, MB, BCh, MEd, MHS
Professor of Preventive Cardiology
National University of Ireland Galway
Galway, Ireland

Sean R. McMahon, MD
Assistant Professor of Medicine,
Associate Director of Echocardiography Laboratory
Director of Quality, Division of Cardiology
University of Connecticut School of Medicine
Hartford Healthcare
Hartford, Connecticut

Andres Samayoa Mendez, MD
Cardiothoracic Surgery Fellow
Department of Cardiovascular and Thoracic Surgery
University of Texas Southwestern Medical School
University of Texas Southwestern Medical Center
Dallas, Texas

Erin D. Michos, MD
Associate Professor of Medicine
Director of Women's Cardiovascular Health
Associate Director of Preventive Cardiology
Division of Cardiology
The Johns Hopkins University School of Medicine
Baltimore, Maryland

Rebecca Miller, PharmD, BCPS
Specialty Practice Pharmacist
Departments of Internal Medicine and Surgery
Ohio State University East Hospital
Columbus, Ohio

Arunima Misra, MD
Associate Professor
Department of Medicine
Baylor College of Medicine
Cardiology and Director of Echocardiography Lab
Michael E. DeBakey VA Medical Center
Houston, Texas

Jeremy P. Moore, MD, MS
Associate Professor of Pediatrics
Director of Adult Congenital Electrophysiology Program
David Geffen School of Medicine at UCLA
Ronald Reagen UCLA Medical Center
Los Angeles, California

Tyler Moran, MD, PhD
Assistant Professor of Medicine/Cardiology
Department of Medicine, Section of Cardiology
Baylor College of Medicine
Baylor St. Luke's Medical Center
Houston, Texas

Humberto Butzke da Motta, MD
Cardiology Fellow
Hospital de Clinicas de Porto Alegre
Porto Alegre, Brazil

Abdallah Mughrabi, MD
Medical Resident
Department of Internal Medicine–Transitional Residency
King Hussein Cancer Center
Amman, Jordan

Debabrata Mukherjee, MD, MS
Professor and Chair
Department of Internal Medicine
Texas Tech University Health Sciences Center El Paso
El Paso, Texas

Srihari S. Naidu, MD
Professor of Medicine
Director, Cardiac Catheterization Laboratory
Director, Hypertrophic Cardiomyopathy Center
Westchester Medical Center and WMC Health Network
New York Medical College
Valhalla, New York

Ajith Nair, MD
Assistant Professor
Department of Medicine, Section of Cardiology
Baylor College of Medicine
Houston, Texas

Shuktika Nandkeolyar, MD
Cardiology Fellow
Loma Linda University Medical Center
Loma Linda, California

Arash B. Nayeri, MD
Clinical Instructor
Department of Medicine
David Geffen School of Medicine at UCLA
Los Angeles, California

Nils Patrick Nickel, MD
Assistant Professor–Pulmonary and Critical Care Medicine
Department of Internal Medicine
Texas Tech University Health Sciences Center El Paso
El Paso, Texas

Timothy J. O'Connor, MB, BCH, BAO, BA, MSc
Specialist Registrar in Cardiology
University Hospital Galway
County Galway, Ireland

Kazue Okajima, MD, PhD
Assistant Professor of Medicine
Division of Cardiology
Department of Internal Medicine
Texas Tech University Health Science Centre EI Paso
EI Paso, Texas

Gurusher Panjrath, MD
Associate Professor of Medicine
Director, Heart Failure and Mechanical Circulatory Support Program
George Washington University School of Medicine and Health Sciences
George Washington University Hospital
Washington, District of Columbia

Sahil Parikh, MD
Associate Professor of Medicine
Columbia University Vagelos College of Physicians and Surgeons
Director, Endovascular Services
Columbia University Irving Medical Center
NY Presbyterian Hospital
Division of Cardiology, Department of Medicine
Center for Interventional Vascular Therapy
New York, New York

Purvi Parwani, MBBS, MPH
Assistant Professor of Medicine
Director of Women's Health Clinic
Loma Linda University School of Medicine
Loma Linda University Health
Loma Linda, California

Kelly Paschke, DO
Fellow, Cardiovascular Medicine
Department of Internal Medicine, Cardiovascular Disease Section
The Ohio State University College of Medicine
The Ohio State University Wexner Medical Center
Columbus, Ohio

Timir K. Paul, MD, PhD, MPH
Associate Professor, Division of Cardiology
Director, Interventional Cardiology
Associate Program Director, Cardiology Fellowship
Director, Cardiovascular Research
Quillen College of Medicine, East Tennessee State University
Johnson City, Tennessee

Matthias Peltz, MD
Surgical Director of Cardiac Transplantation and Mechanical Circulatory Support
Department of Cardiovascular and Thoracic Surgery
University of Texas Southwestern Medical School
University of Texas Southwestern Medical Center
Dallas, Texas

Rebecca Pinnelas, MD
Cardiovascular Fellow
New York University Langone Health
New York, New York

Timothy J. Pirolli, MD
Assistant Professor of Pediatric Cardiothoracic Surgery
Department of Cardiovascular and Thoracic Surgery
University of Texas Southwestern Medical School
University of Texas Southwestern Medical Center
Children's Medical Center of Dallas
Dallas, Texas

Andrew R. Pistner, MD
Fellow, Adult Congenital Heart Disease
Division of Cardiology
Department of Medicine
University of Washington School of Medicine
Seattle, Washington

Antonios Pitsis, MD, PhD
Head of Cardiac Surgery
Thessaloniki Heart Institute
Interbalkan Medical Center
Thessaloniki, Greece

Mathias Possner, MD
ACHD Fellow, Internal Medicine
University of Washington Medical Center
Seattle, Washington

Renato Quispe, MD, MHS
Clinical and Research Postdoctoral Fellow
The Johns Hopkins Ciccarone Center for the Prevention of Cardiovascular Disease
Baltimore, Maryland

Amir Behzad Rabbani, MD
Assistant Clinical Professor
Department of Medicine (Interventional Cardiology)
Clinical Instructor
David Geffen School of Medicine at UCLA
University of California Los Angeles Health System
Los Angeles, California

Tanuja Rajan, MD, MPH
Postdoctoral Fellow
The Johns Hopkins Ciccarone Center for the Prevention of Cardiovascular Disease
The Johns Hopkins University School of Medicine
Baltimore, Maryland

Saurabh Rajpal, MBBS, MD
Assistant Professor
Department of Internal Medicine, Cardiovascular Disease Section
The Ohio State University College of Medicine
Nationwide Children's Hospital
Columbus, Ohio

Anantharaman Ramasamy, MBChB, MRCP
Specialist Registrar in Interventional Cardiology
Barts Heart Centre
St Bartholomew's Hospital
London, United Kingdom

Sunil V. Rao, MD
Professor of Medicine
Duke University School of Medicine
Duke University Health System
Durham, North Carolina

Surendranath Veeram Reddy, MD
Associate Professor
Department of Pediatrics
University of Texas Southwestern Medical School
University of Texas Southwestern Medical Center
Dallas, Texas

Cara Reiter-Brennan, MD
Fellow
Department of Radiology and Neuroradiology
Charite Universitatsmedizin Berlin
Berlin, Germany

Anitra W. Romfh, MD
Clinical Associate Professor
Stanford University School of Medicine
Stanford, California

Jennifer A. Rymer, MD, MBA, MHS
Assistant Professor of Medicine
Duke University School of Medicine
Duke University Medical Center
Durham, North Carolina

Ayesha Salahuddin, MD
Assistant Professor of Medicine
Department of Cardiology
Rutgers Robert Wood Johnson Medical School
New Brunswick, New Jersey

Raul D. Santos, MD, PhD, MSc
Lipid Clinic Heart Institute (InCor)
University of São Paulo Medical School Hospital
Academic Research Organization Hospital
Israelita Albert Einstein
São Paulo, Brazil

Salvatore Savona, MD
Clinical Cardiac Electrophysiology Fellow
Department of Internal Medicine, Cardiovascular Disease Section
The Ohio State University College of Medicine
The Ohio State University Wexner Medical Center
Columbus, Ohio

Alexis Shafii, MD
Associate Professor of Surgery
Surgical Director, Heart Transplantation and Cardiothoracic Transplant
Baylor College of Medicine
Baylor St. Luke's Medical Center
Houston, Texas

Evan F. Shalen, MD
Assistant Professor of Medicine
Division of Cardiovascular Medicine
Oregon Health & Science University
Portland, Oregon

Madhan Shanmugasundaram, MD
Associate Professor of Medicine
Director of Cardiac Cath Labs and Endovascular Services
University of Arizona College of Medicine
Banner University Medical Center
Tucson, Arizona

Kevin M. Shannon, MD
Professor
Department of Pediatrics
David Geffen School of Medicine at UCLA
Los Angeles, California

Richard J. Shemin, MD
Professor and Chief
Division of Cardiac Surgery
David Geffen School of Medicine at UCLA
Los Angeles, California

Kalyanam Shivkumar, MD, PhD
Professor of Medicine (Cardiology), Radiology and Bioengineering
Director, UCLA Cardiac Arrhythmia Center and Electrophysiology Programs
Director and Chief, UCLA Interventional Cardiovascular Programs and Catheterization Laboratories
David Geffen School of Medicine at UCLA
UCLA Health System
Los Angeles, California

Supriya Shore, MBBS
Clinical Lecturer, Advanced Heart Failure and Transplant Cardiology, Cardiovascular Disease, Internal Medicine
Cardiology Clinic
Brighton Center for Specialty Care
Brighton, Michigan

Michael C. Siah, MD
Assistant Professor of Surgery
Department of Vascular Surgery
University of Texas Southwestern Medical School
University of Texas Southwestern Medical Center
Dallas, Texas

Helme Silvet, MD, MPH
Assistant Professor of Medicine
Loma Linda University School of Medicine
Chief of Cardiology
VA Loma Linda Health Care System
Loma Linda, California

Toniya Singh, MBBS
Managing Partner, St. Louis Heart and Vascular
Chair, National Women in Cardiology Council for the American College of Cardiology
St. Louis, Missouri

Vasvi Singh, MD
Advanced Cardiovascular Imaging Fellow
Harvard Medical School
Brigham and Women's Hospital
Boston, Massachusetts

Albert J. Sinusas, MD, BS
Professor of Medicine, Radiology, and Biomedical Imaging, and Biomedical Engineering
Director, Yale Translational Research Imaging Center
Yale School of Medicine
New Haven, Connecticut

Chittur A. Sivaram, MD
David Ross Boyd Professor
Department of Medicine, Cardiovascular Section,
Associate Dean for Continuing Professional Development
University of Oklahoma College of Medicine
University of Oklahoma Health Sciences Center
Oklahoma City, Oklahoma

Jeremy Slivnick, MD
Clinical Fellow
Department of Internal Medicine, Cardiovascular Disease Section
The Ohio State University College of Medicine
The Ohio State University Wexner Medical Center
Columbus, Ohio

Gbemiga Sofowora, MBChB, MSc
Associate Professor
Department of Clinical Internal Medicine
The Ohio State University College of Medicine
The Ohio State University Wexner Medical Center
Columbus, Ohio

Aadhavi Sridharan, MD, PhD
Clinical Cardiac Electrophysiology Fellow
UCLA Cardiac Arrhythmia Center
David Geffen School of Medicine at UCLA
Los Angeles, California

Zachary L. Steinberg, MD
Assistant Professor of Medicine
University of Washington School of Medicine
Seattle, Washington

John M. Suffredini, DO
Cardiology Fellow
Department of Medicine, Section of Cardiology
Baylor College of Medicine
Houston, Texas

Kevin Sung, MD, MS
Resident
Department of Medicine
University of California, San Diego School of Medicine
San Diego, California

Rajesh V. Swaminathan, MD
Associate Professor of Medicine
Duke University School of Medicine
Duke University Medical Center
Duke Clinical Research Institute
Director, Cardiac Catheterization Laboratories
Durham VA Medical Center
Durham, North Carolina

Jose D. Tafur, MD
Associate Professor of Medicine
Program Director, Cardiovascular Disease Fellowship
Ochsner Clinic Foundation
New Orleans, Louisiana

Weiyi Tan, MD, MPH
Adult Congenital Cardiology Fellow
Department of Medicine, Division of Cardiology
David Geffen School of Medicine at UCLA
Los Angeles, California

Akiko Tanaka, MD, PhD
Resident
Department of Cardiothoracic and Vascular Surgery
University of Texas Health Science Center
Houston, Texas

Cynthia Taub, MD, MBA
Professor of Medicine
Chief, Section of Cardiovascular Medicine
Dartmouth-Hitchcock Medical Center
Lebanon, New Hampshire

Isac C. Thomas, MD, MPH
Assistant Clinical Professor of Medicine
Division of Cardiovascular Medicine
University of California, San Diego School of Medicine
San Diego, California

Catalin Toma, MD
Assistant Professor of Medicine
Director, Interventional Cardiology Heart and Vascular Institute
University of Pittsburgh School of Medicine
University of Pittsburgh Medical Center
Pittsburgh, Pennsylvania

Jeffrey A. Towbin, MD
Professor of Medicine
Executive Co-Director, The Heart Institute
Chief, Pediatric Cardiology
University of Tennessee Health Science Center
Le Bonheur Children's Hospital
St. Jude Children's
Research Hospital
Memphis, Tennessee

Vincenzo Tufaro, MD
Medicine and Surgery, Specialization in Cardiology
Clinical Fellow in Interventional Cardiology
Barts Heart Centre
St Bartholomew's Hospital
London, United Kingdom

Ajay Vallakati, MD, MPH
Assistant Professor
Department of Internal Medicine, Cardiovascular Disease Section
The Ohio State University College of Medicine
Columbus, Ohio

Bibin Varghese, MD
Fellow, Cardiovascular Disease
Vanderbilt University
Nashville, Tennessee

Marmar Vaseghi, MD, PhD
Associate Professor of Medicine
Director of Clinical and Translational Research
UCLA Cardiac Arrhythmia Center
David Geffen School of Medicine at UCLA
Los Angeles, California

Ryan J. Vela, MD, MS
Research Fellow
University of Texas Southwestern Medical School
University of Texas Southwestern Medical Center
Dallas, Texas

Prashanth Venkatesh, MD
Adult Congenital Heart Disease Fellow
Department of Medicine, Division of Cardiology
David Geffen School of Medicine at UCLA
Los Angeles, California

Michael A. Wait, MD
Professor
Department of Thoracic and Cardiovascular Surgery
University of Texas Southwestern Medical School
University of Texas Southwestern Medical Center
William Clements University Hospital
Dallas, Texas

James A. Walker, MD
General Surgery Resident
University of Texas Southwestern Medical Center
Dallas, Texas

James N. Weiss, MD
Distinguished Professor (Emeritus) of Medicine (Cardiology) and Physiology
David Geffen School of Medicine at UCLA
Los Angeles, California

Christopher J. White, MD, MACC, MSCAI
Professor and Chairman of Medicine and Cardiology
The Ochsner Clinical School, University of Queensland
Queensland, Australia
System Chairman for Cardiology
Ochsner Health
New Orleans, Louisiana

Bryan A. Whitson, MD, PhD
The Jewel and Frank Benson Family Research Professor
Professor and Vice Chair of Innovation and Translational Research
Director, Section of Thoracic Transplantation and Mechanical Circulatory Support
Co-Director, COPPER Laboratory
Division of Cardiac Surgery, Department of Surgery
The Ohio State University College of Medicine
Columbus, Ohio

Diana Wolfe, MD, MPH
Associate Professor Obstetrics & Gynecology and Women's Health
Associate Professor of Medicine, Cardiology
Division of Maternal Fetal Medicine
Albert Einstein College of Medicine
Bronx, New York

Srikanth Yandrapalli, MD
Fellow
Division of Cardiology
Harvard Medical School
Massachusetts General Hospital
Boston, Massachusetts

Joseph Yang, MD
Assistant Professor
Division of Cardiology
Department of Medicine
University of California, San Francisco School of Medicine
San Francisco Veterans Affairs Health Care System
San Francisco, California

Yang Yang, MD
Cardiac Electrophysiology Fellow
University of California, San Diego School of Medicine
San Diego, California

Firas Zahr, MD
Director
Department of Interventional Cardiology
Oregon Health & Science University
Portland, Oregon

Ali N. Zaidi, MD
Associate Professor
Internal Medicine and Pediatrics
Icahn School of Medicine at Mount Sinai
Director
Mount Sinai Adult Congenital Heart Disease Center
Mount Sinai Cardiovascular Institute
The Children's Heart Center
Mount Sinai Kravis Children's Hospital
New York, New York

Thomas M. Zellers, MD, MScMM
Professor of Pediatrics
Director of the Heart Center at Children's Health Dallas
Interventional Pediatric Cardiology
University of Texas Southwestern Medical School
University of Texas Southwestern Medical Center
Children's Health Dallas and Plano
Clements University Hospital
Parkland Hospital
Dallas, Texas

PREFACE

The field of cardiovascular medicine continues to rapidly evolve in both diagnostic and therapeutic arenas. Over the past decade, substantial advances have been made on many fronts including cardiovascular imaging, electrophysiology mapping and ablation techniques, heart failure diagnosis and management, percutaneous hemodynamic support, drug-eluting stents, drug-coated balloons, and structural heart endovascular techniques. Concurrent with advances in percutaneous techniques, cardiovascular surgery has also evolved with minimally invasive and robotic techniques. The evolution of newer drugs, devices, and improvements in both percutaneous and surgical techniques challenges providers to stay abreast of cutting-edge pharmacologic, endovascular, and surgical strategies for optimal patient care. The *Cardiovascular Medicine and Surgery* textbook aims to provide clinicians with comprehensive guidance on the topics of clinical cardiology, cardiovascular imaging, cardiac catheterization and intervention, electrophysiology, heart failure, vascular medicine, cardiovascular surgery, and importantly the field of preventative cardiology. The text features evidence-based guidance on physical examination, diagnosis, and general principles of management of patients with cardiovascular diseases and serves as a comprehensive, easily accessible reference for busy practitioners and cardiovascular trainees.

Of foremost importance, the topic areas covered are relevant to the daily practice of cardiovascular medicine. The content of this textbook reflects the rapidly changing field of cardiovascular medicine and surgery. Moreover, all of this content as well as additional online-only tables, figures, and videos will be available through the eBook associated with this text. In addition to the basic cardiovascular concepts, we have included advanced concepts and new technologies, including chapters on percutaneous mitral valve repair, mechanical circulatory support, hybrid and robotic-assisted coronary bypass surgery, and surgical approaches for congenital heart disease. A large number of algorithms and high-quality illustrations make this textbook particularly attractive to the practitioner.

Essential to the quality and appropriateness of the text is the expertise of the chapter authors. We are fortunate to have assembled a stellar roster of cardiovascular specialists as section editors and authors for this text from leading medical centers around the world who have published thousands of peer-reviewed manuscripts. We are greatly indebted to them. The practice of cardiovascular medicine is exciting, rewarding, and a privilege each of us enjoys. Likewise, it has been our personal honor to work with these superb contributors, our colleagues in cardiovascular medicine, as well as the editorial team at Wolters Kluwer. It is our hope that you will enjoy this book and that it will be a valuable resource to you in providing the highest quality care to your patients.

Debabrata Mukherjee, MD, MS
Richard A. Lange, MD, MBA

ABBREVIATIONS

^{18}F-FDG	F-18-fluorodeoxyglucose
^{123}I-*m*IBG	^{123}Iodine-metaiodobenzylguanidine
AAA	abdominal aortic aneurysm
AAD	antiarrhythmic drug
AARCC	Alliance for Adult Research in Congenital Cardiology
AAV	ANCA-associated small-vessel vasculitides
ABC	ATP-binding cassette
ABI	ankle-brachial index
ABPM	ambulatory blood pressure monitoring
ACA	anterior cerebral arteries
ACC	American College of Cardiology
ACCF	American College of Cardiology Foundation
ACE	angiotensin-converting enzyme
ACEP	American College of Emergency Physicians
ACHD	adult congenital heart disease
ACLS	advanced cardiovascular life support
ACM	arrhythmogenic cardiomyopathy
ACP	American College of Chest Physicians
ACR	American College of Radiology
ACS	acute coronary syndrome
ACT	activated clotting time
ADA	American Diabetes Association
ADE	adverse drug events
ADH	antidiuretic hormone
ADHF	acute decompensated heart failure
ADT	androgen deprivation therapy
AED	automatic external defibrillator
AEPC	Association for European Paediatric and Congenital Cardiology
AF	atrial fibrillation
AFD	Anderson-Fabry disease
AGE	advanced glycation end product
AH	atrial-His
AHA	American Heart Association
AHI	apnea-hypopnea index
AHRQ	Agency for Healthcare Research Quality
AI	artificial intelligence
AICD	automatic implantable cardioverter defibrillator
AIS	acute ischemic stroke
AIUM	American Institute of Ultrasound in Medicine
AIVR	accelerated idioventricular rhythm
AKI	acute kidney injury
AL	amyloidosis light-chain
ALARA	as low as reasonably achievable
ALCAPA	anomalous left coronary artery from the pulmonary artery
ALVD	acute left ventricular dysplasia
AMI	acute myocardial infarction
AMPK	adenosine monophosphate protein kinase
AMS	atrial mode switch
ANA	antinuclear antibody
ANCA	antineutrophil cytoplasmic antibody
AnkB	ankyrin-B
ANP	atrial natriuretic peptide
ANS	autonomic nervous system
AoV	aortic valve
AP	accessory pathway
APD	action potential duration
ApoB	apolipoprotein B
APS	antiphospholipid syndrome
AR	aortic regurgitation
ARAS	atherosclerotic renal artery stenosis
ARB	angiotensin receptor blocker
ARDS	acute respiratory distress syndrome
ARNI	angiotensin receptor-neprilysin inhibitors
ART	antiretroviral therapy
ARVC	arrhythmogenic right ventricular cardiomyopathy
ARVD	arrhythmogenic right ventricular cardiomyopathy/dysplasia
AS	aortic stenosis
ASA	atrial septal aneurysm/aspirin
ASCO	American Society of Clinical Oncology
ASCVD	atherosclerotic cardiovascular disease
ASD	atrial septal defect
ASE	American Society of Echocardiography
ASH	asymmetric septal hypertrophy
ASO	antisense oligonucleotide
ASPECTS	Alberta Stroke Program Early CT Score
ASV	adaptive servoventilation
AT	atrial tachycardia
ATG	antithymocyte globulin
ATP	adenosine triphosphate
ATTR	transthyretin amyloidosis
AUC	appropriate use criteria
AV	aortic valve/atrioventricular
AVA	aortic valve area
AVB	atrioventricular block
AVCD	atrioventricular canal defect
AVM	arteriovenous malformation
AVN	atrioventricular node
AVNRT	atrioventricular nodal reentrant tachycardia
AVP	arginine vasopressin
AVR	aortic valve replacement
AVRT	atrioventricular reentrant tachycardia
AVSD	atrioventricular septal defect
BAS	bile acid sequestrants
BAV	bicuspid aortic valve
BB	beta-blocker
BBB	bundle branch block
BIB	balloon-in-balloon
BIVAD	biventricular assist device
BMI	body mass index
BMD	Becker muscular dystrophy
BMS	bare metal stent
BNP	B-type natriuretic peptide

BP	blood pressure
BPA	bisphenol A
BRS	Brugada syndrome
BSA	body surface area
BTK	Bruton tyrosine kinase
BTT	Blalock-Thomas-Taussig
BVH	biventricular hypertrophy
CABG	coronary artery bypass graft
CAC	coronary artery calcium
CAD	coronary artery disease
CAN	cardiovascular autonomic neuropathy
CBC	complete blood count
CBF	coronary blood flow
CCB	calcium channel blockers
CCS	Canadian Cardiovascular Society
CCT	cardiac computed tomography
CCTA	cardiac computed tomography angiography
CCTGA	congenitally corrected transposition of the great arteries
CCU	coronary care unit
CDC	Centers for Disease Control and Prevention
CDT	catheter-directed thrombolysis
CDUS	color Doppler ultrasound
CE	Conformitè Europëenne
CEID	cardiac electronic implantable device
CETP	cholesterol ester transfer protein
CFA	common femoral artery
CFR	coronary flow reserve
CFU	colony-forming units
CHB	complete heart block
CHD	congenital heart disease
CHF	congestive heart failure
CHRS	Canadian Heart Rhythm Society
CI	confidence interval
CIED	cardiovascular implantable electrical device
CIMT	carotid intima-media thickness
CIN	contrast-induced nephropathy
CKD	chronic kidney disease
CK-MB	creatine kinase myocardial band
CL	contralateral
CLI	critical limb ischemia
CLTI	chronic limb-threatening ischemia
CMB	cerebral microbleed
CM	cardiomyopathy
CMD	coronary microvascular dysfunction
CMP	cardiomyopathy
CMR	cardiac magnetic resonance
CMRA	cardiac magnetic resonance angiography
CMRI	cardiac magnetic resonance imaging
CMS	Centers for Medicare & Medicaid Services
CNS	central nervous system
CO	cardiac output
CoA	coarctation of the aorta
COPD	chronic obstructive pulmonary disease
COR	class of recommendation
COVID-19	coronavirus disease 2019
COX	cyclooxygenase
CP	constrictive pericarditis/chest pain
CPAP	continuous positive airway pulmonary pressure
CPB	cardiopulmonary bypass
CPET	cardiopulmonary exercise test
CPO	cardiac power output
CPR	cardiopulmonary resuscitation
CPT	current procedural terminology
CPVT	catecholaminergic polymorphic ventricular tachycardia
CR	cardiac rehabilitation
CrCL	creatinine clearance
CRP	C-reactive protein
CRS	cytokine release syndrome
CRT	cardiac resynchronization therapy
CS	coronary sinus/cardiogenic shock
CSD	cardiac sympathetic denervation
CSM	carotid sinus massage
CT	computed tomography
CTA	computed tomography angiography
CTEPH	chronic thromboembolic pulmonary hypertension
CTI	cavotricuspid isthmus
CTO	chronic total occlusion
CTPA	computed tomographic pulmonary angiography
CV	conduction velocity/cardiovascular
CVA	cerebrovascular accident
CVD	cardiovascular disease
CVI	cardiovascular imaging
CVIS	cardiovascular information system
CVP	central venous pressure
CW	continuous wave
CXR	chest x-ray
CZT	cadmium-zinc-telluride
DALY	disability-adjusted life years
DAP	dose area product
DAPT	dual antiplatelet therapy
DASH	Dietary Approach to Stop Hypertension
DBP	diastolic blood pressure
DCB	drug-coated balloons
DCM	dilated cardiomyopathy
DCRV	double-chambered right ventricle
DCS	decompression sickness
DD	Danon disease
DES	drug-eluting stent
DFNA	autosomal dominant late-onset progressive nonsyndromic deafness
DFT	defibrillation threshold testing
DICOM	Digital Imaging and Communications in Medicine
DILV	double-inlet left ventricle
DIR	double inversion recovery
DKA	diabetic ketoacidosis
DL	deep learning
DLCO	diffusing capacity of the lung for carbon monoxide
DM	diabetes mellitus
DMD	Duchenne muscular dystrophy
DOAC	direct oral anticoagulation
DORV	double outlet right ventricle
DPAH	drug-induced pulmonary arterial hypertension
DPG	diastolic pressure gradient
DSA	digital subtraction angiography
DSE	dobutamine stress echocardiography
DSP	desmoplakin
DSS	decision support systems

DSWI	deep sternotomy wound infection
DTPA	diethylamine triamine pentaacetic acid
DUS	duplex ultrasonography
DVI	Doppler velocity index
DVT	deep vein thrombosis
DWI	diffusion-weighted imaging
EACVI	European Association of Cardiovascular Imaging
EAD	early afterdepolarization
EAE	European Association of Echocardiography
EAM	electroanatomic mapping
EAR	ectopic atrial rhythm
EAS	European Atherosclerosis Society
EAST	Eastern Association for the Surgery of Trauma
EAT	ectopic atrial tachycardia
ECG	electrocardiogram
ECHO	echocardiogram
EchoCRT	Echocardiography-guided Cardiac Resynchronization Therapy
ECM	extracellular matrix
ECMO	extracorporeal membrane oxygenation
ECV	extracellular volume
ED	emergency department
EDD	end-diastolic dimension
EDMD	Emery-Dreifuss muscular dystrophy
EDP	end-diastolic pressure
EDPVR	end-diastolic pressure-volume relationship
EDTA	ethylene diamine tetraacetic acid
EDV	end-diastolic volume
EECP	enhanced external counterpulsation
EF	ejection fraction
EGCG	epigallocatechin 3-gallate
EGD	esophagogastroduodenoscopy
EGM	electrogram
EGPA	eosinophilic granulomatosis with polyangiitis
EHM	extended Holter monitor
EHR	electronic health record
EHRA	European Heart Rhythm Association
EKG	electrocardiogram
EMB	endomyocardial biopsy
EMF	endomyocardial fibrosis
EMR	electronic medical records
ENDS	electronic nicotine delivery systems
EOA	effective orifice area
EOMFC	early-onset myopathy with fatal cardiomyopathy
EP	electrophysiology
EPS	electrophysiologic study
ERA	endothelin receptor antagonists
ERASE	endovascular revascularization and supervised exercise
ERNA	equilibrium radionuclide angiography
ERO	effective regurgitant orifice
EROA	effective regurgitant orifice area
ERP	effective refractory period
ERS	European Respiratory Society
ES	electrical storm
ESC	European Society of Cardiology
ESD	end-systolic dimension
ESH	European Society of Hypertension
ESMO	European Society for Molecular Oncology
ESPVR	end-systolic pressure-volume relationship
ESR	erythrocyte sedimentation rate
ESRD	end-stage renal disease
ESV	end-systolic volume
ET	ejection time
ETRA	endothelin receptor antagonist
ETT	exercise treadmill test
FAERS	FDA's Adverse Reporting System
FALD	Fontan-associated liver disease
FAST	focused assessment with sonography for trauma
FAT	focal atrial tachycardia
FC	flow convergence
FCH	familial combined hypercholesterolemia
FCMD	Fukuyama congenital muscular dystrophy
FCNCG	fatal congenital nonlysosomal cardiac glycogenosis
FDA	Food and Drug Administration
FDG	fluorodeoxyglucose
FFA	free fatty acid
FFR	fractional flow reserve
FGF	fibroblast growth factor
FH	familial hypercholesterolemia
FHS	Framingham Heart Study
FHT	familial hypertriglyceridemia
FLAIR	fluid-attenuated inversion recovery
FMC	first medical contact
FMD	fibromuscular dysplasia
FOCUS	Formation of Optimal Cardiovascular Utilization Strategies
FOV	field of view
FPG	fasting plasma glucose
FPLD2	familial partial lipodystrophy of the Dunnigan type
FPRA	first-pass radionuclide angiography
FPS	frames per second
FSH	follicle-stimulating hormone
GAD	glutamic acid decarboxylase
GAS	group A streptococcal infection
GBCA	gadolinium-based contrast agent
GBD	Global Burden of Disease
GCM	giant cell myocarditis
GDM	gestational diabetes mellitus
GDMT	guideline-directed medical therapy
GERD	gastroesophageal reflux disease
GFR	glomerular filtration rate
GH	growth hormone
GI	gastrointestinal
GLP	glucagonlike peptide
GLS	global longitudinal strain
GLSEF	global longitudinal strain ejection fraction
GnRH	gonadotropin-releasing hormone
GPA	granulomatosis with polyangiitis
GRACE	Global Registry of Acute Coronary Events
GRE	gradient recalled echo

GRK G protein–coupled receptor kinase
GSV greater saphenous vein
GTP guanosine triphosphate
GvHD graft-versus-host disease
H&E hematoxylin and eosin
HAART highly active antiretroviral therapy
HAC hospital-acquired conditions
HAMP hepcidin antimicrobial peptide
HBPM home BP monitoring
HCM hypertrophic cardiomyopathy
HCN hyperpolarization-activated cyclic nucleotide gated
HCT hematologic stem cell transplant/hematocrit
HDL high-density lipoprotein
HERA herceptin adjuvant
HF heart failure
HFA Heart Failure Association
HFmrEF heart failure with mid-range ejection fraction
HFpEF heart failure with preserved ejection fraction
HFrEF heart failure with reduced ejection fraction
HGPS Hutchinson-Gilford progeria syndrome
HIS His bundle
HIT heparin-induced thrombocytopenia
HIV human immunodeficiency virus
HLA human leukocyte antigen
HLD hyperlipidemia
HLHS hypoplastic left heart syndrome
HMERF hereditary myopathy with early respiratory failure
HMR heart-to-mediastinum ratio
HOCM hypertrophic obstructive cardiomyopathy
HPAH heritable pulmonary arterial hypertension
HR heart rate
HRA high right atrium
HRCT high resolution CT
HRS Heart Rhythm Society
HRV heart rate variability
HSFA Heart Failure Society of America
HSR hyperemic stenosis resistance
HTN hypertension
HV His-ventricular
HVAD HeartWare ventricular assist device
HYVET HYpertension in the Very Elderly Trial
IABP intra-aortic balloon pump counterpulsation
IAC Intersocietal Accreditation Commission
IART intraatrial reentrant tachycardia
IASD interatrial shunt device
IBD Inflammatory bowel disease
IC intermittent claudication/intracoronary
ICA invasive coronary angiography/internal carotid artery
ICAM intercellular adhesion molecule
ICD implantable cardioverter defibrillator
ICE intracardiac echo
ICH intracranial hemorrhage
ICI immune checkpoint inhibitors
ICM ischemic cardiomyopathy
ICP intracranial pressure
ICU intensive care unit
IDL intermediate-density lipoprotein
IE infective endocarditis
IGF insulin-like growth factor
IgG immunoglobulin G
IHD ischemic heart disease
IL interleukin
ILD interstitial lung disease
ILR implantable loop recorders
IM internal mammary
IMA internal mammary artery
INR international normalized ratio
INOCA ischemia with non-obstructive coronary arteries
INTER-MACS Interagency Registry for Mechanically Assisted Circulatory Support
IPAH idiopathic pulmonary arterial hypertension
IR insulin resistance
IRAD International Registry of Acute Aortic Dissection
ISACHD International Society for Adult Congenital Heart Disease
ISHLT International Society for Heart and Lung Transplantation
ISR in-stent restenosis
IT intrathoracic pressure
ITA internal thoracic artery
IUD intrauterine devices
IV intravenous
IVA idiopathic ventricular arrhythmias
IVC inferior vena cava
IVDU intravenous drug use
IVIG intravenous immune globulin
IVUS intravascular ultrasound
JL Judkins left
JR Judkins right
JVD jugular venous distention
JVP jugular venous pressure
KERMA kinetic energy released per unit mass
LA left atrium
LAA left atrial appendage
LAD left anterior descending
LAE left atrial enlargement
LAHB left anterior hemiblock
LAI left atrial isomerism
LAO left anterior oblique
LAP left atrial pressure
LAVI left atrial volume index
LBBB left bundle branch block
LBD Lewy bodies dementia
LBP lipopolysaccharide binding protein
LCA left coronary artery
LDL low-density lipoprotein
LE Lambl excrescences/lower extremity
LGE late gadolinium enhancement
LGMD limb-girdle muscular dystrophy
LH luteinizing hormone
LHC left heart catheterization
LIMA left internal mammary artery
LISH lipomatous interatrial septal hypertrophy
LMCA left main coronary artery
LMIC low- and middle-income countries

LMWH low-molecular-weight heparin
LOE level of evidence
LPA left pulmonary artery
LPL lipoprotein lipase
LQTS long QT syndrome
LR likelihood ratio
LUPV left upper pulmonary vein
LV left ventricle
LVAD left ventricular assist device
LVED left ventricular end diastole
LVEDD left ventricular end-diastolic dimension
LVEDP left ventricular end-diastolic pressure
LVEDVI left ventricular end-diastolic volume index
LVEF left ventricular ejection fraction
LVES left ventricular end systole
LVESD left ventricular end-systolic dimension
LVH left ventricular hypertrophy
LVHF left ventricular heart failure
LVMI left ventricular mass index
LVNC left ventricular non-compaction cardiomyopathy
LVOT left ventricular outflow tract
LVOTO left ventricular outflow tract obstruction
LVT left ventricular thrombus
MAC mitral annular calcification
MACCE major adverse cardiac and cerebrovascular event
MACE major adverse cardiac events
MADA mandibuloacral dysplasia type A with partial lipodystrophy
MAE major adverse event
MAGIC Myoblast Autologous Grafting in Ischemic Cardiomyopathy
MAP mean arterial pressure
MAPK mitogen-activated protein kinase
MAT multifocal atrial tachycardia
MCA middle cerebral artery
MDCT multidetector computed tomography
MELAS mitochondrial encephalopathy with lactic acidosis and stroke-like
MERRF myoclonic epilepsy with ragged red muscle fibers
MESA Multi-Ethnic Study of Atherosclerosis
MET metabolic equivalent
MFM myofibrillar myopathy
MFR myocardial flow reserve
MG mean gradient
MGUS monoclonal gammopathy of uncertain significance
MHC myosin heavy chain
MI myocardial infarction
MIBG meta-iodobenzylguanidine
ML machine learning
MMP matrix metalloproteinase
MODY maturity-onset diabetes of the young
MPI myocardial perfusion imaging
MR mitral regurgitation
MRA magnetic resonance angiography
MRAT macroreentrant atrial tachycardia
MRCA magnetic resonance coronary angiography
MRI magnetic resonance imaging
MRSA methicillin-resistant *Staphylococcus aureus*
MS mitral stenosis
MSA multiple system atrophy
MUGA multigated acquisition
MV mitral valve
MVA mitral valve area
MVD multivessel disease
MVDT mitral valve deceleration time
MVP mitral valve prolapse
MVR mitral valve replacement
NAPA *N*-acetyl procainamide
NCDR National Cardiovascular Data Registry
NCSI National Cardiogenic Shock Initiative
NCX Na^+/Ca^{2+} exchanger
ND Naxos disease
NEP neutral endopeptidase
NGAL neutrophil gelatinase-associated lipocalin
NHANES National Health and Nutrition Examination Survey
NHLBI National Heart, Lung and Blood Institute
NICE National Institute of Health and Care Excellence
NICM nonischemic cardiomyopathy
NIHSS National Institutes of Health Stroke Scale
NM nuclear medicine
NNIS National Nosocomial Infection Surveillance
NNRTI nonnucleoside reverse transcriptase inhibitor
NOAC non-vitamin K oral anticoagulants
NP natriuretic peptide
NPH neutral protamine Hagedorn
NPV negative predictive value
NRT nicotine replacement therapies
NRTI nucleoside reverse transcriptase inhibitor
NSAID nonsteroidal anti-inflammatory drug
NSF nephrogenic systemic fibrosis
NSQIP National Surgical Quality Improvement Program
NSR normal sinus rhythm
NSTEMI non-ST segment elevation myocardial infarctions
NSVT nonsustained ventricular tachycardia
NT-proBNP N-terminal-proBNP
NVE native valve endocarditis
NYHA New York Heart Association
OAC oral anticoagulation
OCT optical coherence tomography
OGTT oral glucose tolerance test
OHT orthotopic heart transplant
OM obtuse marginal
OMT optimal medical therapy
OPCAB off-pump coronary artery bypass
OR odds ratio
OSA obstructive sleep apnea
PA pulmonary artery
PAC premature atrial complexes
PACES Pediatric and Congenital Electrophysiology Society
PACS picture archiving and communication system (radiology)
PAD peripheral arterial disease
PADP pulmonary artery diastolic pressure
PAF pure autonomic failure/paroxysmal atrial fibrillation

PAH pulmonary arterial hypertension
PAN polyarteritis nodosa
PAOP pulmonary artery occlusion pressure
PAP pulmonary artery pressure
PAPVC partial anomalous pulmonary venous connection
PAPVR partial anomalous pulmonary venous return
PASP pulmonary artery systolic pressure
PAWP pulmonary arterial wedge pressure
PBF pulmonary blood flow
PBMV percutaneous balloon mitral valvulotomy
PC pericardial cyst
PCA posterior cerebral artery
PCCD progressive cardiac conduction disease
PCE pooled cohort equation
PCH pulmonary capillary hemangiomatosis
PCI percutaneous coronary intervention
PCIS postcardiac injury syndrome
PCR polymerase chain reaction
PCT primary cardiac tumors
PCW pulmonary capillary wedge
PCWP pulmonary capillary wedge pressure
PDA posterior descending artery
PDE phosphodiesterase
PDGF platelet-derived growth factor
PE pulmonary embolism
PEA pulseless electrical activity
PERC Pulmonary Embolism Rule-out Criteria
PERT Pulmonary Embolism Response Teams
PESI Pulmonary Embolism Severity Index
PET positron emission tomography
PF papillary fibroelastoma
PFO patent foramen ovale
PFOA perfluorooctanoic acid
PFT pulmonary function testing
PG plasma glucose/pressure gradient
PGE prostaglandin E
PH pulmonary hypertension
PHT pressure half-times
PHV prosthetic heart valve
PI protease inhibitor
PISA proximal isovelocity surface area
PJRT permanent junctional reciprocating tachycardia
PKA protein kinase A
PLN phospholamban
PM particulate matter
PMBC percutaneous mitral balloon commissurotomy
PMI point of maximal impulse
PMIP postmyocardial infarction pericarditis
PMT pacemaker-mediated tachycardia
PO oral
POCUS point-of-care ultrasound
POTS postural orthostatic tachycardia syndrome
PP pericardial pressure
PPCM peripartum cardiomyopathy
PPG photoplethysmograph
PPI proton pump inhibitor
PPM patient-prosthesis mismatch
PPP proportional pulse pressure
PPS postpericardiotomy syndrome
PPT primary pericardial tumors
PPV positive predictive value
PR pulmonary regurgitation
PREVEND Prevention of Renal and Vascular End-Stage Disease
PRF pulse repetition frequency
PROM predictive risk of mortality
PS pulmonary valve stenosis
PSIR phase-sensitive inversion recovery
PSV peak systolic velocity
PSVT paroxysmal supraventricular tachycardia
PTA percutaneous transluminal angioplasty
PTCA percutaneous transcatheter coronary angioplasty
PTFE polytetrafluoroethylene
PTMC percutaneous transvenous mitral commissurotomy
PTT partial thromboplastin time
PVARP postventricular atrial refractory period
PVC premature ventricular contractions
PVD peripheral vascular disease
PVE prosthetic valve endocarditis
PVH pulmonary venous hypertension
PVL paravalvular leak
PVLP polyoma virus–like particles
PVML paravalvular mitral leak
PVOD pulmonary vascular obstructive disease
PVR pulmonary vascular resistance
PVT prosthetic valve thrombosis
PW pulsed-wave
PWD pulsed-wave Doppler
PYP pyrophosphate
QALY quality-adjusted life-years
QoL quality of life
QSART quantitative sudomotor axon reflex test
RA refractory angina/right atrium
RAA right atrial appendage
RAAS renin-angiotensin-aldosterone system
RAD right-axis deviation
RAE right atrial enlargement
RAO right anterior oblique
RAP right atrial pressure
RAR renal to aortic
RAS renal artery stenosis
RBBB right bundle branch block
RBC red blood cells
RCA right coronary artery
RCC right coronary cusp
RCM restrictive cardiomyopathy
RCRI Revised Cardiac Risk Index
RCT randomized controlled trial
RDG relative diagnostic gain
REMS Risk Evaluation and Mitigation Strategies
RF regurgitant fraction
RFA radiofrequency ablation
RFFR renal fractional flow reserve
RHC right heart catheterization
RHD rheumatic heart disease
RI resistive index
RIMA right internal mammary artery
RiskMAP Risk Minimization Action Plans
RLQ right lower quadrant
RNA ribonucleic acid
ROC receiver-operating characteristic
ROPAC Registry of Pregnancy and Cardiac
ROS reactive oxygen species

ROSC	return of spontaneous circulation
ROSE	Renal Optimization Strategies Evaluation
RPA	right pulmonary artery
RPG	random plasma glucose
RR	relative risk
RUPV	right upper pulmonary vein
RUQ	right upper quadrant
RV	right ventricle
RVE	right ventricular enlargement
RVEDP	right ventricular end-diastolic pressure
RVEF	right ventricular ejection fraction
RVG	radionuclide ventriculography
RVH	right ventricular hypertrophy
RVHF	right ventricular heart failure
RVOT	right ventricular outflow tract
RVP	right ventricular pressure
RVSP	right ventricular systolic pressure
RVT	right ventricular thrombus
RWT	relative wall thickness
RyR	ryanodine receptor
SA	sinoatrial
SAM	systolic anterior motion
SAPT	single antiplatelet therapy
SAQ	Seattle Angina Questionnaire
SAVI	surgical aortic valve implantation
SAVR	surgical aortic valve replacement
SBP	systolic blood pressure
SC	subcutaneous
SCA	sudden cardiac arrest
SCAD	spontaneous coronary artery dissection
SCAI	Society for Cardiovascular Angiography and Interventions
SCD	sudden cardiac death
SCORE	Systematic Coronary Risk Evaluation
SCS	spinal cord stimulation
SCT	secondary cardiac tumors
SDS	summed difference score
SENS	subcutaneous electrical nerve stimulation
SERCA	sarcoplasmic/endoplasmic reticulum calcium ATPase
SFA	superficial femoral artery
sGC	soluble guanylate cyclase
SGLT	sodium-glucose cotransporter
SHD	structural heart disease
SHEP	Systolic Hypertension in the Elderly Program
SI	signal intensity
SIHD	stable ischemic heart disease
SL	septal leaflet
SLE	systemic lupus erythematosus
SMART	Strategies for Management of Antiretroviral Therapy
SMC	smooth muscle cell
SND	sinus node dysfunction
SNP	single nucleotide polymorphism
SNRT	sinus node recovery time
SNS	sympathetic nervous system
SOLVD	Studies on Left Ventricular Dysfunction
SPECT	single-photon emission computed tomography
SPEI	serum protein electrophoresis and immunofixation
SPEP	serum protein electrophoresis
SPERRI	shortest preexcited R-R interval
SPP	skin perfusion pressure
SPT	secondary pericardial tumors
SQ	subcutaneous
SQTS	short QT syndrome
SR	sarcoplasmic reticulum
SRS	summed rest score
SSFP	steady-state free-precession
SSS	summed stress score
STEMI	ST-elevation myocardial infarction
STS	Society of Thoracic Surgeons
SUVmax	maximum standardized uptake value
SV	stroke volume
SVC	superior vena cava
SVD	structural valve degeneration
SVG	saphenous vein graft
SVR	systemic vascular resistance
SVS	Society of Vascular Surgery
SVT	supraventricular tachycardias
SWI	superficial wound infections
TA	truncus arteriosus
TAA	thoracic aortic aneurysm
TAP	target arterial path
TAPSE	tricuspid annular plane systolic excursion
TAPVC	total anomalous pulmonary venous connection
TASC	Trans-Atlantic Inter-Society Consensus
TAV	transcatheter aortic valve
TAVI	transcatheter aortic valve implantation
TAVR	transcatheter aortic valve replacement
TBI	toe brachial index
TC	total cholesterol
TCD	transcranial Doppler
TdP	torsades de pointes
TEA	thoracic epidural anesthesia
TEAVR	totally endoscopic aortic valve replacement
TEE	transesophageal echocardiography
TEER	transcatheter edge-to-edge repair
TENS	transcutaneous electrical nerve stimulation
TEVAR	thoracic endovascular aortic repair
TG	triglyceride
TGA	transposition of the great arteries
TGRL	triglyceride-rich lipoprotein
THC	Δ9-tetrahydrocannabinol
TIA	transient ischemic attack
TID	transient ischemic dilation/three times daily
TIMACS	Timing of Intervention in Acute Coronary Syndromes
TIMI	thrombolysis in myocardial infarction
TKI	tyrosine kinase inhibitors
TLE	transvenous lead extraction
TLOC	transient loss of consciousness
TLR	target lesion revascularization
TMD	tibial muscular dystrophy
TMLR	transmyocardial laser revascularization
TMR	transmyocardial revascularization

TMVR transcatheter mitral valve replacement
TNF tumor necrosis factor
TOD target organ damage
TOF tetralogy of Fallot
TP threshold potential
TPG transvalvular pressure gradient
TR tricuspid regurgitation
TRV tricuspid regurgitation velocity
TSH thyroid stimulating hormone
TSM trabecula septomarginalis
TST thermoregulatory sweat test
TTE transthoracic echocardiography
TTVR transcatheter tricuspid valve-in-valve replacement
TUDCA tauroursodeoxycholic acid
TV tricuspid valve
TVI tissue velocity integral
TVP transvenous pacemaker
TVR target vessel revascularization
TZD thiazolidinedione
UA unstable angina
UFH unfractionated heparin
UPEI urine protein electrophoresis and immunofixation
UPEP urine protein electrophoresis
UPS undifferentiated pleomorphic sarcomas
USB universal serial bus
VA Veterans Administration
VAD ventricular assist device
VC vena contracta
VCAM vascular cell adhesion molecule
VCFS velocardiofacial syndrome
VEGF vascular endothelial growth factor
VF ventricular fibrillation
VFO valve of the fossa ovalis
VHD valvular heart disease
VKA vitamin K antagonist
VLDL very-low-density lipoprotein
VOC volatile organic chemicals
VPC ventricular premature complexes
VQI Vascular Quality Initiative
VSD ventricular septal defect
VT ventricular tachycardia
VTE venous thromboembolism
VTI velocity time integral
VUS venous ultrasonography
VVS vasovagal syncope
WHF World Heart Federation
WHO World Health Organization
WMI wall motion imaging
WPW Wolff-Parkinson-White
WSPH World Society of Pulmonary Hypertension
WT wild-type
wtATTR wild-type amyloidosis
WU Wood units

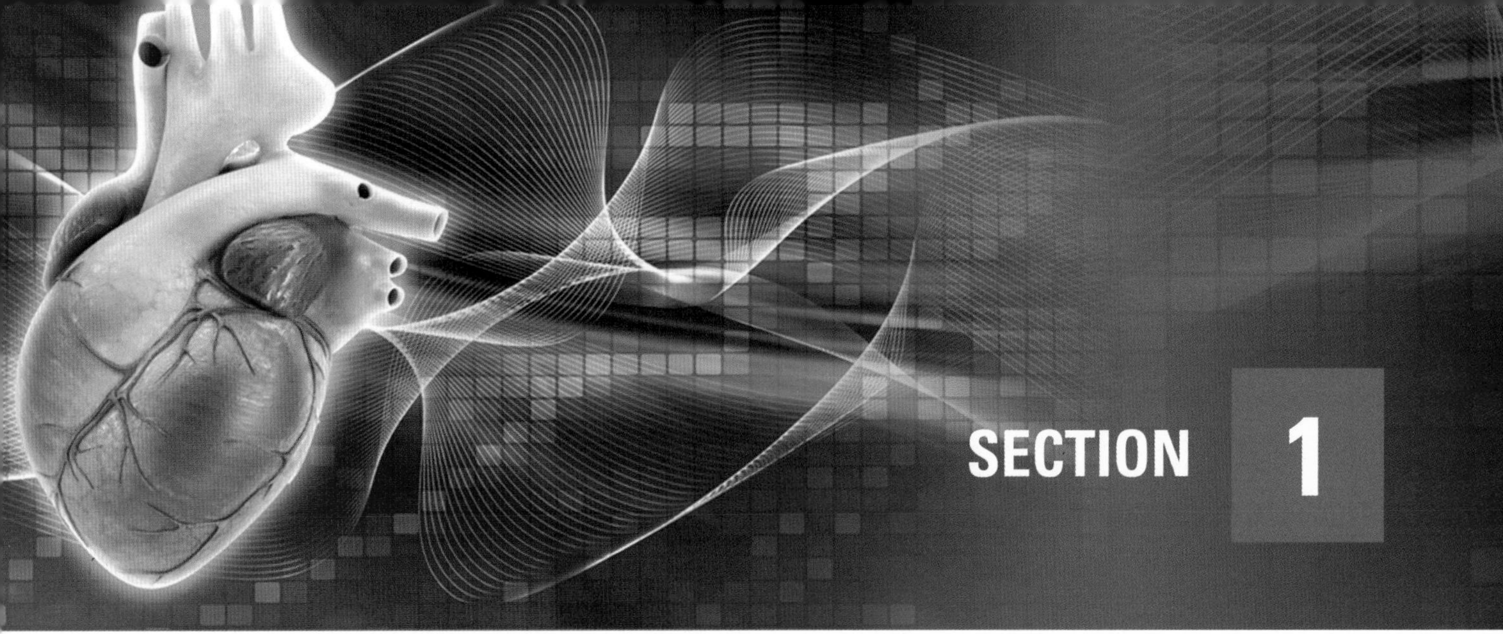

CLINICAL CARDIOLOGY

SECTION EDITOR: Ragavendra R. Baliga

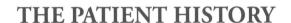

CHAPTER 1

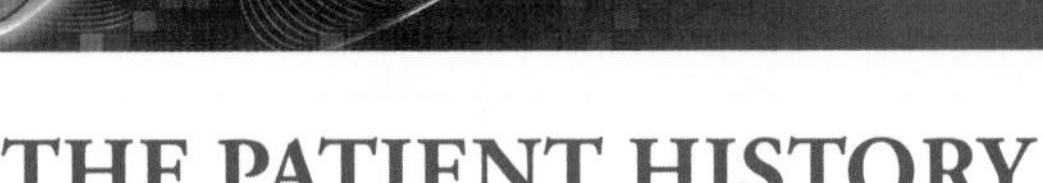

THE PATIENT HISTORY

Kazue Okajima and Richard A. Lange

HISTORY: KEY STEP IN DIAGNOSIS

Obtaining a detailed history is crucial to the proper evaluation of the patient with suspected cardiovascular disease and the first step in establishing the provider-patient relationship. The time spent with the patient, the attitude the provider displays, and the listening skills exhibited by the provider set the tone for the relationship. In addition to gaining information about the patient's health condition(s), obtaining the history is an opportunity to display to the patient that the provider is a compassionate person who cares about the individual's condition and genuinely wants to help. The relationship that is built on strong communication skills with attention to details during the interview is more likely to lead to a complete and candid history that may avert unnecessary, expensive, and potentially hazardous diagnostic testing.

Studies show that physicians are able to collect 60% to 80% of the information relevant for a diagnosis by taking a detailed medical history, which leads to a final diagnosis in more than 70% of cases.[1-4] Conversely, inaccurate and/or incomplete patient histories are among the leading causes for diagnostic errors.[5]

In the era of extensive testing, the "art" of history taking is often neglected. Additionally, patient overload, multitasking, time constraints, and lack of available interpreters may interfere with taking a complete history. However, taking the time to listen to patients improves rapport with and trust from patients, patient recall of information, patient and physician satisfaction, adherence to therapy, and patient health outcomes.[6-8]

The history is not only an opportunity to elicit symptoms, but it may also reveal the influences of other medical conditions, identify risk factors that increase the likelihood of cardiovascular disease, and provide insight into the patient's compliance with prescribed treatment. The history should be obtained directly by the health care provider caring for the patient rather than being delegated to another individual or collected from the medical record, in order for the provider to assess the patient's medical knowledge, comprehension of their condition, attitudes, desires, trust, and treatment preferences.

Although certain elements of the social history are routinely obtained to ascertain if the individual is at risk of cardiovascular disease (ie, diet, exercise, alcohol intake, smoking history), other valuable aspects are often ignored. Illicit drug use is associated with myocardial infarction (MI), cardiomyopathy, and endocarditis; however, patients are often not questioned about it. Identifying the patient's exposure to areas where Lyme disease, Chagas disease, rheumatic fever, or tuberculosis is endemic may provide insight into the etiology of conduction system disease, cardiomyopathy, valvular disease, and pericarditis. Finally, the socioeconomic status of the patient is known to be a risk factor for heart disease and predictive of the patient's access to care and compliance with treatment.

Obtaining a detailed family history is also important, because many cardiovascular disorders are heritable, including arrhythmias (atrial fibrillation, Brugada syndrome, catecholaminergic polymorphic ventricular tachycardia, long QT syndrome, short QT syndrome), congenital heart disease (Holt-Oram syndrome, supravalvular aortic stenosis, bicuspid aortic valve), coronary artery disease (CAD), cardiomyopathy (hypertrophic, dilated, restrictive, left ventricular noncompaction, and arrhythmic right ventricular dysplasia), cardiac tumors (Carney complex), vascular disease (Marfan syndrome, Ehlers-Danlos syndrome, familial thoracic aortic aneurysm, Loeys-Dietz syndrome), and lipid abnormalities (autosomal dominant [PCSK9] hypercholesterolemia, familial hypercholesterolemia).

Tools are available for patients and health professionals (www.hhs.gov/familyhistory) that (1) facilitate the procurement and organization of a detailed family history in the form of a pedigree and (2) provide the basis for appropriate diagnostic testing in family members of patients with suspected heritable cardiovascular disease. An up-to-date listing of health (including cardiac) conditions with genetic inheritance patterns is available at https://ghr.nlm.nih.gov/condition

CARDIAC DISEASE SYMPTOMS

The major symptoms associated with cardiac disease (ie, myocardial ischemia, heart failure, arrhythmias) include chest discomfort, dyspnea, edema, fatigue, palpitations, and syncope. Assessment of symptom severity is useful for assessing functional limitation, documenting improvement (or worsening) of the condition, and assessing response to therapy. Accordingly, clinicians and researchers often use semiquantitative activity scales—the New York Heart Association (NYHA) or Canadian Cardiovascular Society (CCS) functional classification systems—to assess symptom severity (**Table 1.1**).[9]

TABLE 1.1 Activity Scales Used to Assess Functional Capacity

Class	New York Heart Association (NYHA)	Canadian Cardiovascular Society (CCS)	Specific Activity Scale
I	Patients with cardiac disease but without resulting limitations of physical activity. Ordinary physical activity does not cause undue fatigue, palpitation, dyspnea, or anginal pain.	Ordinary physical activity does not cause angina, such as walking and climbing stairs. Angina with strenuous or rapid or prolonged exertion at work or recreation	Patient can perform to completion any activity requiring ≥7 metabolic equivalents.
II	Patients with cardiac disease resulting in slight limitation of physical activity. They are comfortable at rest. Ordinary physical activity results in fatigue, palpitation, dyspnea, or anginal pain.	Slight limitation of ordinary activity. Walking or climbing stairs rapidly, walking uphill, walking or stair climbing after meals, or in cold, or in wind, or under emotional stress, or only during the few hours after awakening. Walking more than two blocks on the level and climbing more than one flight of ordinary stairs at a normal pace and in normal conditions	Patient can perform to completion any activity requiring ≥5 metabolic equivalents but cannot or does not perform to completion activities requiring ≥7 metabolic equivalents.
III	Patients with cardiac disease resulting in marked limitation of physical activity. They are comfortable at rest. Less than ordinary physical activity causes fatigue, palpitation, dyspnea, or anginal pain.	Marked limitation of ordinary physical activity. Walking one to two blocks on the level and climbing one flight of stairs in normal conditions and at normal pace	Patient can perform to completion any activity requiring ≥2 metabolic equivalents but cannot or does not perform to completion any activities requiring ≥5 metabolic equivalents.
IV	Patients with cardiac disease resulting in inability to carry on any physical activity without discomfort. Symptoms of cardiac insufficiency or of the anginal syndrome may be present even at rest. If any physical activity is undertaken, discomfort is increased.	Inability to carry on any physical activity without discomfort—anginal syndrome may be present at rest.	Patient cannot or does not perform to completion activities requiring ≥2 metabolic equivalents.

Data from Goldman L, Hashimoto B, Cook EF, Loscalzo A, et al. Comparative reproducibility and validity of systems for assessing cardiovascular functional class: advantages of a new specific activity scale. *Circulation.* 1981;64(6):1227-1234.

Chest Discomfort

Chest discomfort may be the primary symptom in a number of cardiac and noncardiac conditions. A careful history that pays attention to specific characteristics of the chest discomfort—location, quality, duration, inciting events, radiation, alleviating factors, and associated symptoms—is often sufficient to recognize noncardiac etiologies of chest pain (**Table 1.2**). This is important because less than 10% of patients with chest pain in the primary care setting are ultimately identified as having a coronary cause for their symptoms.[10]

Angina is typically a retrosternal, pressure-like discomfort that may radiate to the jaw, neck, left shoulder, left arm, back, or epigastrium. Various adjectives are often used by patients to describe the pain, including "crushing," "squeezing," "pressure-like," "gripping," and "suffocating," or they may refer to it as "heaviness" or "fullness." Not uncommonly, they insist that it is a "discomfort," rather than a "pain." Angina is almost never sharp or stabbing in quality, and it usually does not change with position or respiration. Atypical presentations of angina may include indigestion, belching, and dyspnea and are more common in women, older patients, and patients with diabetes.

Stable Angina

Angina is also characterized as stable or unstable. Stable angina usually is precipitated by physical exertion, emotional stress, eating a meal, or exposure to cold, and it is readily relieved by rest or nitroglycerin. The anginal episode typically lasts only a few minutes; fleeting discomfort for a few seconds or a dull ache lasting for hours is rarely angina. The term "chronic stable angina" refers to angina that has been stable in frequency and severity for at least 2 months. Chronic stable angina is the initial manifestation of coronary heart disease (CHD) in about half of the patients; the other half initially experience unstable angina, MI, or sudden death.

Chest Pain in Risk Assessment of Patients With Stable Angina. In individuals with stable chest discomfort, U.S. and European guidelines recommend using a diagnostic strategy based on the individual's pretest probability of obstructive CAD.[11-13] For example, individuals with chest discomfort who are determined to have a low probability of obstructive CAD

TABLE 1.2 Differential Diagnosis of Chest Pain

Diagnosis	Characteristics	Comments
Ischemic heart disease	Typical or atypical angina	Caused by diminished coronary blood flow and/or increased myocardial oxygen demand
Nonischemic heart disease	Palpitations or typical angina	Tachycardia
Arrhythmias	Typical angina, often exertional	Heart murmur present
Valvular heart disease	"Tearing" pain, often abrupt onset	Widened mediastinum, often with hypertension
Aortic dissection	Pleuritic pain, relieved by sitting up and leaning forward	Friction rub may be present; diffuse ST segment elevation (PR segment depression) on electrocardiogram
Pericarditis		
Pulmonary disease		
Pulmonary embolus	Pleuritic pain (sharp, worse with inspiration), associated dyspnea	Hypoxia/hypoxemia, pulsus paradoxus, and risk factors for thromboembolic disease
Pneumothorax	Acute onset, pleuritic pain, associated dyspnea	Hyperresonance; tension pneumothorax associated with distended neck veins, hypotension, and tachycardia
Pneumonia	Pleuritic pain, associated fever and cough	Associated with fever and productive cough
Gastrointestinal disease		
Esophageal disease	May be indistinguishable from angina (ie, relieved with nitroglycerin), may note regurgitation of food and relief with antacids	Often diagnosed following a negative evaluation for ischemic heart disease
Gastritis, peptic ulcer disease	May be indistinguishable from angina	May be exacerbated by alcohol and aspirin and relieved by food and antacids
Biliary disease	Right upper quadrant pain that radiates to the back or scapula	Exacerbated by fatty foods
Pancreatitis	"Boring" epigastric pain, may radiate to the back	Typically worse following meals
Chest wall or dermatologic pain		
Costochondritis	Reproduced with palpation or movement	
Rib fracture	Point tenderness	
Herpes zoster	Point tenderness	
Fibrositis	Follows a nerve distribution/dermatome	Pain may precede rash
	Characteristic point tenderness	
Psychiatric disorders	Nonexertional, often associated with anxiety, hyperventilation, perioral paresthesia, and "panic attacks"	Often diagnosed following a negative evaluation for angina Often associated with palpitations, sweating, and anxiety
Anxiety disorders		
Affective disorders (eg, depression)		
Somatoform disorders		
Thought disorders (eg, fixed delusions)		
Factitious disorders (eg, Munchausen syndrome)		

usually do not need further cardiac investigation, those with an extremely high pretest probability may proceed directly to invasive angiography, and individuals with an intermediate probability are recommended to undergo evaluation with noninvasive cardiovascular imaging. Determining whether or not the patient has "typical" angina is an integral feature of all clinical risk assessments that are currently used to predict the likelihood of obstructive CAD.

Typical angina has three characteristic features (Table 1.3): the chest discomfort is (1) substernal; (2) initiated by exertion or stress; and (3) relieved with rest or sublingual nitroglycerin. Chest discomfort with only two of these characteristics is considered atypical angina. If none or only

TABLE 1.3 Traditional Classification of Chest Pain

Typical angina (definite)	Meets all three of the following characteristics: • substernal chest discomfort of characteristic quality and duration • provoked by exertion or emotional stress • relieved by rest and/or nitrates within minutes
Atypical angina (probable)	Meets two of the above-mentioned characteristics
Nonanginal chest pain	Lacks or meets only one or none of the above-mentioned characteristics

one of the characteristics is present, it is considered nonanginal chest discomfort.

The first score to calculate the pretest probability of obstructive CAD introduced more than three decades ago by Diamond and Forrester (the DF score) was calculated on the basis of the chest pain type (typical, atypical, or nonanginal chest pain), sex, and age. Subsequent studies demonstrated that the predictors selected by Diamond and Forrester are robust; however, their calibration was not adequate for the modern population of patients investigated for CAD. Accordingly, many centers in the United States utilize the Duke Clinical Score instead (**Table 1.4**), which includes modifiable cardiovascular risk factors. The most recent European Society of Cardiology (ESC) guidelines for stable CAD have replaced the DF score with two new revised scores, the CAD Consortium Basic and Clinical scores (Table 1.4).

The DF score results in a significant overestimation of the prevalence of obstructive CAD compared with the Duke Clinical Score and the two models recommended by the ESC. Accordingly, the use of the DF risk score may result in the overuse of noninvasive and invasive diagnostic testing in individuals with a low prevalence of disease. The Duke Clinical Score and the ESC-recommended CAD Consortium pretest probability scores more accurately predict coronary disease and cardiovascular events than the DF score. Importantly, all scoring systems used are based on clinically available information.

Three distinct approaches have been independently adopted by the American College of Cardiology/American Heart Association (ACC/AHA), the ESC, and the U.K. National Institute of Health and Care Excellence (NICE) to assess the probability of CAD in patients with chest pain.[11-14] Both the ACC/AHA and ESC guidelines adopt the concept of Bayesian probability (ie, initial estimation of probability is updated based on diagnostic test results to determine the posttest probability of obstructive CAD), with pretest probability determined from clinical risk scores (ie, DF, Duke Clinical Score, or CAD Consortium) that incorporate age, sex, and chest pain typicality with or without modifiable risk factors.

In contrast, the recently updated NICE guidelines[14] has abandoned this probabilistic approach in favor of a symptom-focused assessment. Patients found to have (1) typical or atypical symptoms or (2) an abnormal resting electrocardiogram are categorized into a possible angina group for whom additional noninvasive imaging is recommended. The remainder are classified as nonanginal, with no further testing indicated.

Compared with risk-based guidelines (ie, DF, CAD Consortium), symptom-focused assessment identifies a larger group of low-risk chest pain patients potentially deriving limited benefit from noninvasive testing; the use of a symptom-focused strategy endorsed by NICE, in contrast with the Bayesian risk–based approach endorsed by ACC/AHA and ESC, resulted in a three- to fourfold increase in the number of patients for whom no further investigation for the presence of CAD was recommended. This strongly supports the use of the characterization of patient symptoms as central in the assessment of suspected stable angina.

Unstable Angina

Unstable angina—which usually results from plaque rupture with subsequent platelet aggregation and thrombus formation—is typified by prolonged chest discomfort at rest; new-onset angina that is severe, prolonged, or frequent; or previously stable angina that has become more frequent, longer in duration, more easily provoked, and more difficult to relieve.

Chest Pain in Risk Assessment of Patients With Unstable Angina. About 10% of patients with acute chest pain are ultimately diagnosed with acute coronary syndrome (ACS). Although characteristics of chest pain may increase or decrease the likelihood of ACS,

TABLE 1.4 Commonly Used Clinical Risk Scores for Determining Pretest Probability of Obstructive Coronary Artery Disease

	Risk Scores			
	Diamond-Forrester	**Duke Clinical Score**	**CAD Consortium Basic**	**CAD Consortium Clinical**
Recommended by	ACC/AHA	ACC/AHA	ESC	ESC
Clinical Variables Included	Age Sex Angina typicality	Age Sex Angina typicality DM Smoking status Previous MI Dyslipidemia ECG changes	Age Sex Angina typicality	Age Sex Angina typicality DM Smoking status HTN Dyslipidemia
Validation	Patients referred to invasive angiography during the 1970s	Patients referred to invasive angiography during the 1970s	Contemporary patients referred to invasive angiography or coronary CTA	Contemporary patients referred to invasive angiography or coronary CTA

ACC/AHA, American College of Cardiology/American Heart Association; CAD, coronary artery disease; CTA, computed tomography angiography; ESC, European Society of Cardiology; DM, diabetes mellitus; ECG, electrocardiogram; HTN, hypertension; MI, myocardial infarction.

the accuracy of symptoms for the diagnosis of ACS is weak.[15] For example, chest pain that is sharp, pleuritic, or reproducible with palpation is usually noncardiac (positive likelihood ratio <0.3 for all). Conversely, ACS is more likely if the patients note chest pain with radiation to both arms, pain similar to prior ischemia, change in pattern over the prior 24 hours, "typical" chest pain or pain that is precipitated by exertion (positive likelihood ratio 1.5-2.6 for all). To improve diagnostic accuracy for identifying ACS, providers should utilize clinical prediction tools that incorporate aspects of the history and examination with electrocardiographic findings (Q waves, ST changes) and serum biomarkers of cardiac injury (troponin).

Dyspnea

Dyspnea is a term used to characterize a subjective experience of breathing discomfort. Cardiopulmonary conditions are among the most common causes of acute dyspnea, with other etiologies including anemia, obesity, pregnancy, neuromuscular diseases, and deconditioning. Typical cardiac causes include heart or valvular disease, which results in pulmonary edema and/or low cardiac output.

Dyspnea can occur at rest or with exertion. When it is due to chronic heart disease, it is typically exacerbated by exertion. During exercise, patients may describe their dyspnea as "feeling of suffocating," "breaths feel too small," "hunger for air," or "cannot get enough air."[16] The NYHA functional classification (**Table 1.1**) is widely used to obtain a semiquantitative assessment of symptom severity.

The patient with heart disease may also experience dyspnea at rest, including orthopnea and paroxysmal nocturnal dyspnea. Orthopnea is the sensation of breathlessness in the recumbent position because of redistribution of fluid from dependent parts of the circulation to the thorax causing the person to sleep propped up in bed or sitting in a chair. The number of pillows used by the patient to obtain relief is a way to semi-quantify orthopnea. Paroxysmal nocturnal dyspnea is an extreme form of orthopnea that usually occurs 2 to 4 hours after the onset of sleep in the recumbent position, with the patient waking with a sense of severe breathlessness and suffocation. The dyspnea is severe enough to compel the patient to sit upright or stand.

Cardiac and noncardiac etiologies of dyspnea may share the same patient descriptors, thereby making it difficult to distinguish the cause based solely on the patient's symptoms.[17,18] Hence, additional investigations—such as imaging studies (chest radiograph, chest computed tomography, or echocardiogram) or bioassays (B-type natriuretic peptide [BNP] or its N-terminal prohormone precursor [NT-proBNP])—may be useful in determining the cause.[19] Obstructive sleep apnea and obesity hypoventilation syndrome have emerged as important causes of cardiopulmonary diseases reflecting the increase in obesity rates in developed countries.[20,21] Individuals with these may note nocturnal choking/air gasping, daytime somnolence, and morning headache. Additionally, the patient's partner may observe signs of sleep-disordered breathing at night such as loud snoring or periods of apnea.

Cough and hemoptysis associated with dyspnea may be due to cardiac or pulmonary causes. Hemoptysis with pink frothy sputum may suggest pulmonary edema from cardiac causes, although other cardiovascular causes (ie, mitral stenosis, pulmonary embolism, arteriovenous malformation, pulmonary artery rupture) may also present with frank hemoptysis. Other heart failure–related symptoms include peripheral edema, general fatigue/weakness, abdominal swelling, right upper quadrant discomfort, and gastrointestinal symptoms because of right-sided heart failure.

Syncope

The lifetime prevalence of syncope in the population is estimated at nearly 40%, accounting for 1% to 3% of emergency department visits and 6% of hospital admissions. A comprehensive and detailed history is essential to differentiate life-threatening syncope from benign forms with an avoidance of unnecessary extensive studies.

Syncope is an abrupt, transient, complete loss of consciousness, associated with inability to maintain postural tone, with subsequent rapid and spontaneous recovery. The presumed mechanism is cerebral hypoperfusion, excluding other forms of transient loss of consciousness, such as seizure, antecedent head trauma, and pseudosyncope.[22]

To determine the cause of syncope, the patient should be questioned about the details of the event including presence of an aura or warning sign before the loss of consciousness, triggers, duration of symptoms, and recovery symptoms. Obtaining a history of coexisting medical conditions—particularly the existence of preexisting cardiovascular disease—is also important in guiding the evaluation of syncope. Comorbidities and medication use are particularly important factors in older patients. A family history should be obtained, with particular emphasis on histories of syncope or sudden unexplained death (or drowning). Obtaining information from any witnesses of the syncopal event is helpful because it is not uncommon that patients may not remember the events well. Historical characteristics associated with, though not diagnostic of, cardiac and noncardiac syncope are summarized in **Table 1.5**.[22]

The causes of syncope can be broadly categorized as cardiac, reflex (neurally mediated), and orthostatic.[23-25] In over one-third of individuals with syncope, the cause is not determined; in the remainder, reflex syncope is the most common identifiable cause (21%), which includes vasovagal, situational, and carotid sinus syndrome. The next most common cause is cardiac syncope (9.5%) that carries a significantly worse prognosis than does reflex syncope and orthostatic syncope (9.4%).

Cardiac syncope includes (1) tachyarrhythmias (ventricular fibrillation, ventricular tachycardia); (2) bradyarrhythmias (advanced atrioventricular block, sinus node dysfunction); and (3) structural heart abnormalities (aortic stenosis, hypertrophic obstructive cardiomyopathy, atrial myxoma, cardiac tamponade, and great vessel disorders such as pulmonary embolus, acute aortic dissection, and pulmonary hypertension).

TABLE 1.5 Historical Features Associated With Increased Probability of Cardiac or Noncardiac Causes of Syncope

More Often Associated With Cardiac Causes of Syncope
- Older age (>60 years)
- Male sex
- Presence of known ischemic heart disease, structural heart disease, previous arrhythmias, or reduced ventricular function
- Brief prodrome, such as palpitations, or sudden loss of consciousness without prodrome
- Syncope during exertion
- Syncope in the supine position
- Low number of syncope episodes (one or two)
- Abnormal cardiac examination
- Family history of inheritable conditions or premature sudden cardiac death (<50 years of age)
- Presence of known congenital heart disease

More Often Associated With Noncardiac Causes of Syncope
- Younger age
- No known cardiac disease
- Syncope only in the standing position
- Positional change from supine or sitting to standing
- Presence of prodrome (ie, nausea, vomiting, feeling warmth)
- Presence of specific triggers (ie, dehydration, pain, distressful stimulus, medical environment)
- Situational triggers (i.e., cough, laugh, micturition, defecation, deglutition)
- Frequent recurrence and prolonged history of syncope with similar characteristics

Reprinted from Shen W-K, Sheldon RS, Benditt DG, et al. 2017 ACC/AHA/HRS Guideline for the Evaluation and Management of Patients With Syncope: A Report of the American College of Cardiology/American Heart Association Task Force on Clinical Practice Guidelines and the Heart Rhythm Society; *J Am Coll Cardiol*. 2017;70:e39-e110.

The most common form of reflex syncope is vasovagal syncope and typically occurs in persons undergoing emotional or physical stress. It can be preceded by dim vision, sweating, nausea, light-headedness, giddiness, or yawning—reflecting autonomic nervous system hyperactivity—and is fully alleviated by lying down. After the episode, the patient is often pale and complains of fatigue on recovery. Carotid sinus hypersensitivity—another form of reflex syncope—is manifested as fainting spells after slight pressure to the neck (sudden head motion, tight collar, or shaving) and occurs more frequently in older individuals. Studies comparing characteristics of cardiac and reflex syncope found that a longer duration of warning signs, recovery symptoms, and fatigue following syncope were more often associated with reflex syncope than a cardiac source.[26]

Orthostatic hypotension is another important cause of syncope, especially in the elderly population. Patients with hypovolemia or autonomic dysfunction experience fainting while standing because of decline in blood pressure. A history of positional (standing/sitting) syncope and orthostatic vital signs on physical are crucial to establishing this diagnosis.

Seizures may cause transient loss of consciousness, mimicking syncope. Alternatively, myoclonic jerks and incontinence may occur with syncope (so-called convulsive syncope), and the episode may be mistaken for a seizure. Neurogenic causes with subsequent seizure activity often have an aura and early warning sign (nausea, yawning); prolonged convulsions and marked postictal confusion are uncommon in patients with syncope associated with convulsive movements. Fatigue is frequent after reflex syncope and may be confused with a postictal state.

Metabolic causes (ie, hypoglycemia hyperventilation) can also lead to transient loss of consciousness, which typically occurs gradually.

Palpitations

Palpitations are an unpleasant awareness of forceful heart beats. Palpitations may result from a variety of arrhythmias, such as premature atrial or ventricular contractions, sustained or nonsustained supraventricular or ventricular tachycardia, and less commonly from bradyarrhythmia with sinus node dysfunction or advanced atrioventricular block.[27,28] Patients may describe the sensation as "skipping," "pounding," "racing," or "fluttering." The "skipping" is often attributed to the post-extrasystolic pause in the rhythm, whereas the "pounding" or "racing" is due to forceful ventricular contraction following the pause. A feeling of rapid fluttering in the chest may result from atrial or ventricular arrhythmias, including sinus tachycardia.

Palpitations that last for an "instant" or are described as an "occasional skipped beat" are more likely to represent premature atrial or ventricular contractions; those that are sustained and last for minutes or longer are more consistent with supraventricular or ventricular arrhythmias. Abrupt onset is common for these palpitations secondary to a pathologic arrhythmia as opposed to a gradual onset that occurs with sinus tachycardia. The sensation of rapid and regular pounding in the neck is most typical of reentrant supraventricular arrhythmias—especially atrioventricular nodal tachycardia—and is due to dissociation of atrial and ventricular contractions (ie, atria contract against closed tricuspid and mitral valves). Electrocardiographic documentation of rhythm disorder during spontaneous symptoms provides strongest evidence of causality.

It is important to inquire about associated symptoms, such as dizziness, syncope, and chest discomfort, in order to determine the seriousness and causes of palpitation. The presence of any underlying cardiac disease may help to narrow the differential diagnosis. Other less common cardiac causes of palpitations include valvular heart disease (mitral valve prolapse), atrial myxoma, pacemaker syndrome (atrioventricular dyssynchrony because of single-chamber ventricular pacing), and high-output cardiac states.

Noncardiac causes of palpitation include endocrine and metabolic abnormalities, psychiatric disorders, and medications or substance use effects. Palpitations are also remarkably common in healthy individuals and can simply occur with anxiety.

TABLE 1.6 Differential Diagnosis of Claudication

Condition	Location	Pain Description	How Affected By Various Conditions: Exercise	Rest	Position	Other Features
Spinal stenosis	Often bilateral buttocks, posterior leg	Pain and weakness	May mimic claudication ("pseudoclaudication")	Variable relief, but may take a long time to recover	Relief by lumbar spinal flexion	Worse with standing and extending spine, sometimes worse with sitting
Nerve root compression	Radiates down leg	Sharp "electric" pain	May be induced by sitting, standing, or walking	Often present at rest	Relief when supine or sitting	History of back problems; not intermittent
Symptomatic Baker's cyst	Behind knee, down calf	Swelling, tenderness	Worse with ambulation	Present at rest	Unchanged	History of knee problems; not intermittent
Compartment syndrome, chronic	Calf muscles	Tight, bursting pain	Provoked by vigorous exercise (ie, jogging)	Subsides very slowly	Relief with elevation	Typically in heavily muscled athletes
Venous claudication	Entire leg (worse in calf)	Tight, bursting pain	Worse after walking	Subsides slowly	Relief with elevation	History of DVT (iliofemoral), edema, venous congestion signs
Hip arthritis	Thigh, lateral hip	Aching	Occurs with variable degrees of exercise	Not quickly resolved	Improved with non–weight bearing	History of degenerative arthritis

DVT, deep vein thrombosis.

Claudication

Individuals with peripheral arterial disease (PAD) are more likely to have atherosclerosis in the coronary and carotid arteries than those without PAD. The symptoms of PAD are variable. Intermittent claudication is the hallmark of PAD and is characterized as fatigue, discomfort, cramping, or pain of vascular origin in the calf muscles of the lower extremities that is consistently induced by exercise and consistently relieved within 10 minutes by rest.[29] However, only about 10% of persons with known PAD have classic intermittent claudication. Approximately 40% do not complain of leg symptoms at all, and 50% have atypical symptoms, such as pain or discomfort that begins at rest but worsens with exertion, exertional pain that does not stop the individual from walking, does not involve the calves, or does not resolve within 10 minutes of rest.[30]

Many conditions can result in leg pain or claudication-like symptoms (**Table 1.6**). Clinical findings suggestive of lower extremity PAD include abnormal lower extremity pulse examination, vascular bruits, nonhealing lower extremity wound, and arterial ulcerations that are characterized by well-demarcated, "punched-out" lesions. Other common lower extremity findings include hair loss, shiny skin, and muscle atrophy. Dependent rubor and elevation pallor may be present in advanced disease and result from impaired autoregulation in the dermal microvasculature.

KEY POINTS

- ✔ A detailed medical history leads to a final diagnosis in more than 70% of cases.
- ✔ The time spent with the patient, the attitude the provider displays, and the listening skills exhibited by the provider set the tone for the physician-patient relationship.
- ✔ Tools are available (www.hhs.gov/familyhistory) that facilitate the procurement and organization of a detailed family history in the form of a pedigree.
- ✔ Less than 10% of patients with chest pain in the primary care setting are ultimately identified as having a coronary cause for their symptoms. The individual's pretest probability of obstructive CAD dictates the diagnostic strategy.
- ✔ In over one-third of individuals with syncope, the cause is not determined; in the remainder, reflex (neurally mediated) syncope is the most common identifiable cause, which includes vasovagal, situational, and carotid sinus syndrome.
- ✔ Only 10% of persons with known PAD have classic intermittent claudication; approximately 40% do not complain of leg symptoms, and 50% have atypical symptoms.

REFERENCES

1. Hampton JR, Harrison MJ, Mitchell JR, Prichard JS, Seymour C. Relative contributions of history-taking, physical examination, and laboratory investigation to diagnosis and management of medical outpatients. *Br Med J.* 1975;2(5969):486-489.
2. Peterson MC, Holbrook JH, Von Hales D, Smith NL, Staker LV. Contributions of the history, physical examination, and laboratory investigation in making medical diagnoses. *West J Med.* 1992;156(2):163-165.
3. Roshan M, Rao AP. A study on relative contributions of the history, physical examination and investigations in making medical diagnosis. *J Assoc Physicians India.* 2000;48(8):771-775.
4. Sandler G. The importance of the history in the medical clinic and the cost of unnecessary tests. *Am Heart J.* 1980;100(6 Pt 1):928-931.
5. Faustinella F, Jacobs RJ. The decline of clinical skills: a challenge for medical schools. *Int J Med Educ.* 2018;9:195-197.
6. Lazare A, Putnam SM, Lipkin M Jr. Three functions of the medical interview. In: Lipkin M Jr, Putnam SM, Lasare A, et al., eds. *The Medical Interview.* Springer; 1995.
7. Novack DH, Dube C, Goldstein MG. Teaching medical interviewing. A basic course on interviewing and the physician-patient relationship. *Arch Intern Med.* 1992;152(9):1814-1820.
8. Rosenberg EE, Lussier MT, Beaudoin C. Lessons for clinicians from physician-patient communication literature. *Arch Fam Med.* 1997;6(3):279-283.
9. Goldman L, Hashimoto B, Cook EF, Loscalzo A. Comparative reproducibility and validity of systems for assessing cardiovascular functional class: advantages of a new specific activity scale. *Circulation.* 1981;64(6):1227-1234.
10. Bösner S, Becker A, Haasenritter J. Chest pain in primary care: epidemiology and pre-work-up probabilities. *Eur J Gen Pract.* 2009;15(3):141-146.
11. Fihn SD, Blankenship JC, Alexander KP, et al. 2014 ACC/AHA/AATS/PCNA/SCAI/STS focused update of the guideline for the diagnosis and management of patients with stable ischemic heart disease: a report of the American College of Cardiology/American Heart Association Task Force on Practice Guidelines, and the American Association for Thoracic Surgery, Preventive Cardiovascular Nurses Association, Society for Cardiovascular Angiography and Interventions, and Society of Thoracic Surgeons. *J Am Coll Cardiol.* 2014;64(18):1929-1949.
12. Fihn SD, Gardin JM, Abrams J, et al. 2012 ACCF/AHA/ACP/AATS/PCNA/SCAI/STS Guideline for the diagnosis and management of patients with stable ischemic heart disease: a report of the American College of Cardiology Foundation/American Heart Association Task Force on Practice Guidelines, and the American College of Physicians, American Association for Thoracic Surgery, Preventive Cardiovascular Nurses Association, Society for Cardiovascular Angiography and Interventions, and Society of Thoracic Surgeons. *J Am Coll Cardiol.* 2012;60(24):e44-e164.
13. Task Force Members; Montalescot G, Sechtem U, Achenbach S, et al. 2013 ESC guidelines on the management of stable coronary artery disease: the Task Force on the management of stable coronary artery disease of the European Society of Cardiology. *Eur Heart J.* 2013;34(38):2949-3003.
14. National Clinical Guideline Centre for Acute and Chronic Conditions (UK). Chest Pain of Recent Onset: Assessment and Diagnosis of Recent Onset Chest Pain or Discomfort of Suspected Cardiac Origin. Royal College of Physicians; 2010.
15. Fanaroff AC, Rymer JA, Goldstein SA, Simel DL, Newby LK. Does this patient with chest pain have acute coronary syndrome?: the rational clinical examination systematic review. *JAMA.* 2015;314(18):1955-1965.
16. Scano G, Stendardi L, Grazzini M. Understanding dyspnoea by its language. *Eur Respir J.* 2005;25(2):380-385.
17. Caroci Ade S, Lareau SC. Descriptors of dyspnea by patients with chronic obstructive pulmonary disease versus congestive heart failure. *Heart Lung.* 2004;33(2):102-110.
18. Simon PM, Schwartzstein RM, Weiss JW, Fencl V, Teghtsoonian M, Weinberger SE. Distinguishable types of dyspnea in patients with shortness of breath. *Am Rev Respir Dis.* 1990;142(5):1009-1014.
19. Ambrosino N, Serradori M. Determining the cause of dyspnoea: linguistic and biological descriptors. *Chron Respir Dis.* 2006;3(3):117-122.
20. Bradley TD, Floras JS. Obstructive sleep apnoea and its cardiovascular consequences. *Lancet.* 2009;373(9657):82-93.
21. Myers KA, Mrkobrada M, Simel DL. Does this patient have obstructive sleep apnea?: the Rational Clinical Examination systematic review. *JAMA.* 2013;310(7):731-741.
22. Writing Committee Members; Shen WK, Sheldon RS, Benditt DG, et al. 2017 ACC/AHA/HRS guideline for the evaluation and management of patients with syncope: A report of the American College of Cardiology/American Heart Association Task Force on Clinical Practice Guidelines and the Heart Rhythm Society. *Heart Rhythm.* 2017;14(8):e155-e217.
23. Benditt DG, Adkisson WO. Approach to the patient with syncope: venues, presentations, diagnoses. *Cardiol Clin.* 2013;31(1):9-25.
24. Hanna EB. Syncope: etiology and diagnostic approach. *Cleve Clin J Med.* 2014;81(12):755-766.
25. Parry SW, Tan MP. An approach to the evaluation and management of syncope in adults. *BMJ.* 2010;340:c880.
26. Calkins H, Shyr Y, Frumin H, Schork A, Morady F. The value of the clinical history in the differentiation of syncope due to ventricular tachycardia, atrioventricular block, and neurocardiogenic syncope. *Am J Med.* 1995;98(4):365-373.
27. Giada F, Raviele A. Clinical approach to patients with palpitations. *Card Electrophysiol Clin.* 2018;10(2):387-396.
28. Zimetbaum P, Josephson ME. Evaluation of patients with palpitations. *N Engl J Med.* 1998;338(19):1369-1373.
29. Gerhard-Herman MD, Gornik HL, Barrett C, et al. 2016 AHA/ACC guideline on the management of patients with lower extremity peripheral artery disease: a report of the American College of Cardiology/American Heart Association Task Force on Clinical Practice Guidelines. *Circulation.* 2017;135(12):e726-e779.
30. McDermott MM, Kerwin DR, Liu K, et al. Prevalence and significance of unrecognized lower extremity peripheral arterial disease in general medicine practice. *J Gen Intern Med.* 2001;16(6):384-390.

CHAPTER 2

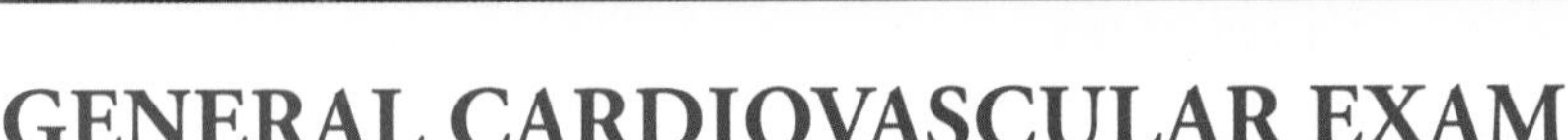

GENERAL CARDIOVASCULAR EXAM

Timothy J. O'Connor, William H. Fennell, and John W. McEvoy

INTRODUCTION

Physical examination of the cardiovascular system remains central to the contemporary practice of clinical medicine, despite technologic advances. The physical examination is an immediately available, rapid, repeatable, and noninvasive tool to not only identify the presence, nature, and severity of cardiovascular disease but also assess response of medical therapy and guide future therapy. The diagnostic value of the physical examination is user dependent. It relies on a thorough and accurate recording of the patient's presenting complaint and prior medical history, demands a thorough understanding of the concepts on which the physical examination is based, and requires the adoption of a standardized and systematic approach to the examination.

INDICATIONS

Whether performed by a cardiologist or noncardiologist, the physical examination is a critical skill that must be utilized in every aspect of patient contact and care. In the symptomatic patient presenting to the emergency department or outpatient setting, the physical examination can identify possible underlying diagnoses, determine the choice of investigations, and dictate initial treatment. Once a diagnosis is established, repeating the physical examination is important to assess response to therapy and guide future management. In the asymptomatic patient, the physical examination also provides an opportunity to identify important underlying diseases such as atrial fibrillation that have the potential to adversely affect health prior to the development of symptoms.

FUNDAMENTALS AND CLINICAL APPLICATION OF THE PHYSICAL EXAMINATION

Before focusing on the examination of the heart itself, pertinent "extracardiac" aspects of the physical examination that are important in the comprehensive assessment of the cardiovascular patient are described. These include the general appearance of the patient; assessment of the skin, extremities, head, and neck; as well as examination of the chest wall and the abdomen.

The Extracardiac Examination

General Appearance

The starting point of the cardiovascular examination begins with an assessment of the general appearance of the patient. An overall appraisal of the patient's status can aid quick identification of the acutely unwell patient and provide vital clues to underlying cardiac conditions. Is the patient in obvious pain? What is their posture, demeanor, level of consciousness, and breathing pattern? Is the patient cyanotic, pale, or diaphoretic (sweaty)? In addition, a number of syndromes with important cardiovascular associations may be evident from the patient's appearance, such as Marfan syndrome, Turner syndrome, and Down syndrome (**Table 2.1**).

With respect to posture, patients with acute pericarditis often find relief of their chest pain with sitting forward and with short shallow breathing. In the acute heart failure patient, lying supine may cause significant distress and indicate pulmonary edema. Sitting forward with hands supported on knees and breathing through pursed lips (tripod position) may direct suspicion toward a pulmonary etiology of dyspnea rather than a cardiac one.

The patient's breathing pattern should be routinely assessed. Inspection can identify abnormal patterns of breathing such as Kussmaul breathing or Cheyne-Stokes breathing. Kussmaul breathing is rapid, deep, and labored breathing associated with underlying metabolic acidosis. Cheyne-Stokes breathing is a pattern of crescendo-decrescendo breathing with periods of apnea, which is well recognized in congestive heart failure and is associated with increased mortality.[1]

Early identification of the acutely unwell patient is critically important. Besides general inspection, assessment of vital signs, such as respiratory rate, peripheral oxygen saturation, heart rate, blood pressure, and temperature, can help dictate the pace of assessment and any therapeutic actions that may be required. For example, a speedy bedside hemodynamic assessment of perfusion (warm vs cold) and congestion (wet vs dry) (**Figure 2.1**) helps guide initial management in acute heart failure. Determination of the patient's level of consciousness contributes to assessment of cerebral and systemic perfusion.

Inspection of the patient's nutritional status and degree of frailty can also help direct their cardiovascular care. The

TABLE 2.1 Syndromes and Cardiac/Physical Manifestations

Syndrome	Cardiac Associations	Physical Features
Noonan syndrome	Dysplastic/stenotic pulmonary valve Hypertrophic cardiomyopathy Atrial septal defect (ASD) Ventricular septal defect (VSD) Tetralogy of Fallot	Short stature *Face:* widely set eyes (ocular hypertelorism), ptosis, micrognathia, short nose with broad base, low-set ears, short webbed neck *Body:* pectus carinatum/excavatum, scoliosis, joint laxity
Turner syndrome	Aortic isthmus stenosis Bicuspid aortic valve Pulmonary valve stenosis Coarctation of the aorta	Short stature *Face:* short neck with webbed appearance and low hairline at the back of the head *Face:* receding jaw (retrognathia), strabismus, amblyopia, drooping eyelids *Body:* short bones of the hands (particularly 4th metacarpal)
Down syndrome	ASD VSD Patent ductus arteriosus Tetralogy of Fallot	*Face:* flattened facial profile and nose; small ears and mouth; eyelids slant up and out *Body:* wide, short hands with short fingers, single transverse palmar crease
Marfan syndrome	Structural disease: aortic regurgitation and mitral valve prolapse with mitral regurgitation Aortic dilatation	*Face:* narrow and long cranium (dolichocephaly), exophthalmos, malar hypoplasia, micro- or retrognathia *Body:* tall and thin with long limbs and elongated digits (arachnodactyly), curvature of the spine (scoliosis/kyphosis), pectus excavatum/pectus carinatum
Myotonic dystrophy	Conduction abnormalities and tachyarrhythmias	*Face:* frontal baldness, expressionless triangular face, atrophy of temporal muscles, neck muscle atrophy *Body:* myotonia and weakness—delayed release of handshake
Holt-Oram syndrome	ASD VSD	*Body:* unequal arm length due to aplasia, hypoplasia, or anomalous development of radial, carpel, and thenar bones. Triphalangeal or absent thumb
Wolf-Hirschhorn syndrome	ASD VSD Persistent left superior vena cava Pulmonary stenosis/aortic insufficiency	Short stature *Face:* microcephaly, hypertelorism; eyelids that slant down, broad nose, small jaw
Edward syndrome	ASD VSD Patent ductus arteriosus Pulmonary and aortic valve abnormalities Coarctation of the aorta Tetralogy of Fallot Transposition of great arteries	Short stature *Cranial:* microcephaly, elongated skull, prominent occiput *Facial:* microphthalmia, ocular hypertelorism, short nose with upturned nares, malformed ears *Body:* overlying fingers

presence of cachexia may indicate an underlying systemic disorder or malignancy but may also be present in advanced chronic heart failure. Frailty has been shown to be a strong risk factor for adverse outcomes in cardiovascular disease, and quantitative frailty assessments are increasingly used in advanced heart failure as well as in the assessment of heart valve disease and determining a patient's suitability for intervention. Examples of such frailty assessments include both individual measures (handgrip strength, 5-meter gait speed) and multi-item frailty scales such as the Fried scale.[2]

Skin

A detailed examination of the skin may draw attention toward abnormalities that are manifestations of underlying cardiac disease or other disorders (inherited or systemic) with important cardiovascular sequelae.

Bluish discoloration of the skin and/or mucous membranes can indicate cyanosis. Approximately 2 g/dL or more of deoxyhemoglobin in subpapillary capillaries is required for cyanosis to manifest. Central cyanosis causes bluish discoloration of both the skin and mucous membranes (including the tongue) and is typically seen in disorders with right-to-left shunting of blood such as in congenital heart disease with pulmonary hypertension. Peripheral cyanosis, seen in disorders such as severe heart failure, spares the mucous membranes and is indicative of diminished blood flow and increased oxygen extraction in the peripheral circulation. Blue-gray cutaneous discoloration of sun-exposed skin infrequently occurs in patients on long-term amiodarone therapy.

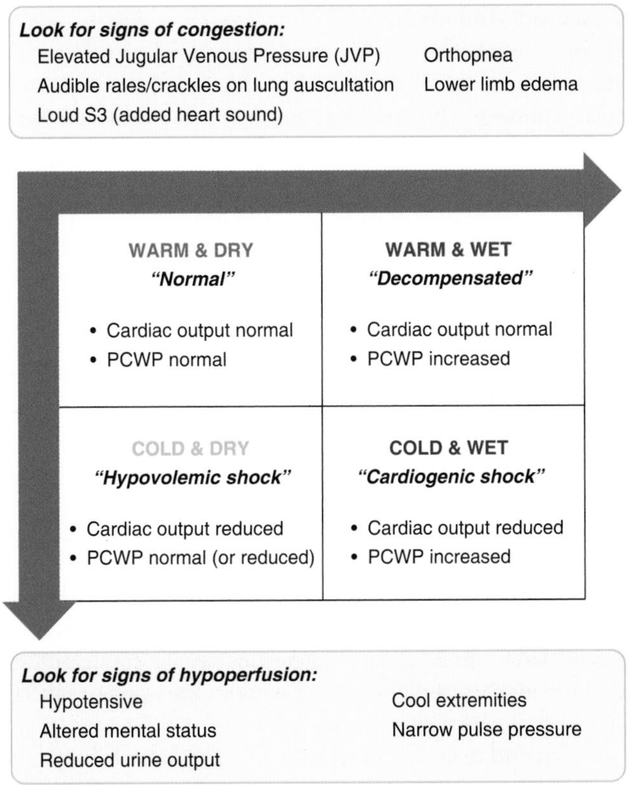

Look for signs of congestion:		
	Elevated Jugular Venous Pressure (JVP)	Orthopnea
	Audible rales/crackles on lung auscultation	Lower limb edema
	Loud S3 (added heart sound)	

WARM & DRY "Normal"	WARM & WET "Decompensated"
• Cardiac output normal • PCWP normal	• Cardiac output normal • PCWP increased
COLD & DRY "Hypovolemic shock"	**COLD & WET "Cardiogenic shock"**
• Cardiac output reduced • PCWP normal (or reduced)	• Cardiac output reduced • PCWP increased

Look for signs of hypoperfusion:		
	Hypotensive	Cool extremities
	Altered mental status	Narrow pulse pressure
	Reduced urine output	

FIGURE 2.1 Basic hemodynamic assessment at bedside. Rapid assessment of hemodynamic status at the bedside. Quickly classify patient's hemodynamic status by looking for typical signs of hypoperfusion and increasing congestion. PCWP, pulmonary capillary wedge pressure; S3, third heart sound.

Tanned or bronzed hyperpigmentation of the skin on the face, dorsal hands, and extensor forearms may indicate hemochromatosis, a disorder of iron storage that can result in diabetes and dilated cardiomyopathy. A plum or red discoloration of the cheeks with a butterfly pattern (i.e., malar flush) is a known manifestation of mitral stenosis. Systemic disorders such as systemic lupus erythematosus (SLE) can also present with malar erythema and provide clues to a systemic cause of cardiac disease (eg, Libman-Sacks endocarditis in SLE).

Disorders of lipid metabolism resulting from genetic disease or secondary etiologies can present with yellow cutaneous lesions (termed xanthomas) at various body sites. Xanthomas can be seen on the eyelids (where they are termed xanthelasmas), neck, palms, chest, or along extensor tendons of the extremities. Tendonous xanthomata typically indicate type IIa hyperlipoproteinemia (otherwise known as familial hypercholesterolemia or FH). Xanthelasmas involve soft yellow plaques on the upper and lower eyelids. Discrete yellow macules/papules along the creases of the palms (palmar xanthomata) are associated with type III familial hyperlipoproteinemia (defined by the Fredrickson-Levy classification). Tuberous and tuberoeruptive xanthomata are painless yellow nodules that are not attached to tendons and can be located on the buttocks, hands, and knees and are associated with types IIa and III familial hyperlipoproteinemias. Eruptive xanthomata are crops of small erythematous yellow papules that suddenly appear on extensor surfaces and are linked with types I and V hyperlipoproteinemias. Cholesterol embolization syndrome resulting from disruption of atheromatous plaques of the aorta and other arteries can manifest with ulceration, purpura, painful nodules, or livedo reticularis (particularly in the lower extremities).

Nontender red or hemorrhagic macules of the palms and soles (Janeway lesions) and painful, raised, erythematous nodules involving the pulp of the fingers and toes (Osler nodes) are well-known manifestations of infective endocarditis. Telangiectasia are seen in patients with systemic disorders such as scleroderma (associated with pulmonary hypertension, right heart failure, and nonischemic cardiomyopathy) or SLE (associated with pericarditis and Libman-Sacks endocarditis, among other cardiac sequelae), whereas hereditary telangiectasia of the lips, tongue, and mucous membranes is a finding of Osler-Weber-Rendu syndrome (associated with pulmonary arteriovenous malformations causing right-to-left intracardiac shunting).

Extensive freckle-like brown spots (lentigines) on the face, neck, and trunk can be cutaneous manifestations of rare inherited cardiovascular syndromes such as Carney syndrome (associated with cardiac myxomas) and LEOPARD syndrome (*L*entigines, *E*lectrocardiographic conduction abnormalities, *O*cular hypertelorism, *P*ulmonary stenosis, *A*bnormal genitalia, *R*etardation of growth, and *D*eafness). Pseudoxanthoma elasticum (associated with premature coronary artery disease) is a genetic disorder of connective tissue resulting in leathery, inelastic "plucked chicken" skin appearance of the flexural areas of the neck, axilla, and inguinal regions.

Head and Neck

A stepwise review of the face should begin with an examination of the eyes. For example, yellow discoloration of the sclera (scleral icterus) may be seen in severe heart failure with hepatic congestion, whereas patients with osteogenesis imperfecta have blue sclera and may potentially manifest mitral regurgitation or aortic regurgitation. As highlighted earlier, disorders of lipid metabolism can result in yellow deposits around the eyelids (xanthelasmas) or a gray circle around the outer rim of the pupil (arcus senilis). Bilateral periorbital ecchymosis is a characteristic sign of amyloidosis, a condition with major cardiac manifestations (most notably heart failure with preserved ejection fraction).

A thorough examination of the dentition is important in ruling out active infection, which has implications for the likelihood of infectious endocarditis. The oral cavity may also expose a high-arched palate (Marfan syndrome), palatal petechiae (infective endocarditis), or macroglossia (amyloidosis, most typically of the light chain [AL] subtype). A bifid uvula is a recognized sign of Loeys-Dietz syndrome (which is a similar condition to Marfan syndrome in that it is also associated with aortopathy and aneurysmal changes of the aorta). As noted earlier malar rash involving the facial cheeks and nasal bridge with sparing of the nasolabial folds is indicative of SLE, whereas the mitral facies of rheumatic mitral valve stenosis produces flushed plethoric cheeks with pink-purplish patches.

Dysmorphic facial features are a common sign of many inherited syndromes with associated congenital heart defects. Micrognathia, ocular hypertelorism, a short philtrum, and low-set ears can point toward underlying disorders, such as Noonan, Edwards, Turner, or Down syndrome. A webbed neck is a classical sign of Turner syndrome (Table 2.1). Individuals with myotonic dystrophy may have a long, thin face with drooping eyelids and a swanlike neck.

Although the examination of jugular venous pressure (JVP) is anatomically part of the head and neck examination, it is discussed in detail later in the "Cardiac examination" section.

Extremities

Inspection of the hands can provide valuable clues to underlying cardiovascular disorders, and the initial examination should focus on abnormalities of the digits and nail beds. Longitudinal red-brown hemorrhages under the nail suggest splinter hemorrhages, which have a wide etiology including infective endocarditis and systemic disorders, such as cutaneous vasculitis. Visible pulsation of the nail bed capillaries can suggest Quincke sign, a sign of severe aortic regurgitation. Abnormalities in the shape of the nail, such as koilonychia (spooning of the nail), are associated with a variety of conditions, such as iron deficiency anemia, hemochromatosis, and coronary disease. Skeletal abnormalities of the hands, such as arachnodactyly, are seen in Marfan syndrome. The absence of a thumb or a finger-sized thumb are manifestations seen in Holt-Oram syndrome. Clubbing is an increase in the soft tissue of the distal phalanx, which has a large differential but includes underlying cardiovascular etiologies like infective endocarditis, left atrial myxoma, or congenital heart disease with right-to-left shunting.

In the lower extremities, bilateral pitting edema is seen in many volume overload states, including heart failure, particularly if accompanied by a raised JVP. A clear identification of the extent of edema is important to guide and evaluate medical therapy, remembering that bedbound patients tend to manifest dependent edema in their sacrum and buttocks rather than their legs. Bilateral lower limb edema without a raised JVP makes the diagnosis of heart failure less likely and is seen in disorders such as chronic venous insufficiency; it is supported by signs such as varicose veins, venous ulceration, hyperpigmentation, stasis dermatitis, and lipodermatosclerosis. Unilateral swelling can suggest a localized venous thrombosis, lymphatic obstruction, or previous vein graft harvesting in the company of a medial longitudinal scar. Cold extremities with muscle wasting and loss of body hair may suggest underlying arterial disease. Cold extremities more generally may also reflect poor cardiac output if accompanied by other signs of poor organ perfusion. It is important to examine distal pulsations including the dorsal pedis, posterior tibial, and popliteal pulses. Differential clubbing and cyanosis of the toes (ie, without similar abnormalities noted in the fingers) can be a sign of patent ductus arteriosus with Eisenmenger syndrome.

Chest and Abdomen

Deformities of the chest wall can be acquired or congenital, and their presence can be associated with underlying cardiovascular pathology. Emphysema can cause a barrel-shaped chest and is associated with cor pulmonale and right heart failure. A pigeon chest (pectus carinatum) manifests with an outward bowing of the sternum, whereas a funnel chest (pectus excavatum) creates a localized depression of the sternum, and both are associated with connective tissue disorders. Severe kyphosis is a recognized sign of ankylosing spondylitis and may raise suspicion of coexisting aortic regurgitation.

Careful examination of the entire chest wall should be carried out to identify any scars. A central sternotomy scar for coronary artery bypass or open cardiac valve surgery may be obvious; however, be sure to inspect for a "J" sternotomy (mini-sternotomy) or right mini-thoracotomy, seen in minimally invasive valve surgery. The scar of an indwelling cardiac implantable electronic device (CIED) can be located on either side of the upper chest wall but typically on the left. The presence of a CIED can be associated with rare complications, such as unilateral arm swelling or cutaneous venous congestion of the anterior chest wall, because of superior vena cava or subclavian vein obstruction.

Hepatomegaly can be present in right heart failure, and prominent or palpable systolic hepatic pulsations can indicate severe tricuspid regurgitation (TR). Ascites has a broad spectrum of etiologies but can be the result of chronic right heart failure (most notable in cases of constrictive pericarditis or restrictive cardiomyopathy). Splenomegaly is a well-recognized sign of subacute infective endocarditis. Careful and gentle palpation and auscultation of the abdomen should be done to rule out an abdominal aortic aneurysm or aortic or renal bruits.

Cardiac Examination

Jugular Venous Pressure

Assessment of the JVP remains a fundamental element of the cardiovascular examination and provides clinically useful information that allows estimation of the patient's volume status, ventricular filling pressures, and response to medical therapy. This is because a distended internal jugular vein can discriminate between a high and low central venous pressure (CVP). Consequently, an increased JVP can be used to infer the presence of an increased pulmonary capillary wedge pressure (PCWP) among patients with advanced left heart failure.[3]

Evaluation of the JVP is difficult to master. The initial starting point begins with correct positioning of the patient. Full exposure of the neck and chest is essential to allow the physician to observe the venous pulse. The patient should be lying down at 45° to the horizontal with the head turned slightly to the left and chin extended. It is important not to overrotate the neck because doing so will cause contraction of the sternocleidomastoid muscle with resulting compression of the external and internal jugular veins and obstruction of view. Next, identify the internal jugular vein that lies lateral to the carotid artery and descends deep to the sternocleidomastoid

TABLE 2.2 Differentiating Jugular Venous Pulse and Carotid Pulse

Feature	Jugular Venous Pulse	Carotid Pulse
Waveform	Biphasic (2 waveforms per cardiac cycle)	Monophasic (single upstroke)
Palpability	Not palpable (except possibly in severe tricuspid regurgitation)	Palpable
Breathing	Decreases on inspiration	No change with respiration
Pressure	Obliterated with gentle pressure at base of neck	Not obliterated with gentle pressure

muscle (the external jugular vein descends anteriorly to the sternocleidomastoid muscle, traveling in a posterior and inferior direction). Differentiating the JVP pulsation from that of the carotid pulse requires observation of the pulse appearance, response to inspiration, and palpation (**Table 2.2**).

The next step is to determine the mean height of the JVP, which is an indicator of right atrial pressure (or right heart filling pressure). The units of measurement for JVP are in centimeters of water. The JVP is measured as the vertical distance in centimeters from the top of the venous pulsation down to the anterior angle formed by the junction of the manubrium and the body of the sternum (the so-called angle of Louis) (**Figure 2.2A,B**). A height of more than 3 cm (ie, anything visible above the clavicle) at 45° is considered an abnormal JVP and infers elevated right heart filling pressures. If an approximate estimation of CVP is also desired, the measured height of the JVP is then added to the distance from the sternal angle to the mid-right atrium. In the supine position at 45° to the horizontal, this distance is estimated at 5 cm. Thus, an appropriately measured JVP of 3 cm above the sternal angle can be estimated to reflect a CVP of 8 cm of water (note that cm of water can be converted to approximate millimeters of mercury for comparison with catheterization values [1.36 cm of water = 1 mm Hg]). A caveat is that this 5-cm value is an approximation of the distance between the sternal angle and the right atrium and can vary with such patient factors as increased age, smoking status, height, obesity, and increased anteroposterior chest wall diameter. Thus, it is our view that the primary utility in measuring the height of the JVP is in identifying a raised right heart filling pressure, rather than quantifying a specific value for CVP.

In addition to using JVP as a surrogate for elevation in right heart filling pressure, the morphology of the JVP waveform should be observed to inform the clinical assessment of the patient. The waveform of the JVP includes a number of distinct peaks and troughs that correspond with changes in the cardiac cycle and can be correlated with intervals on the electrocardiogram (**Figure 2.3**). The "a" wave is the first positive deflection in the JVP morphology and reflects atrial contraction. It occurs just after the electrocardiographic P wave and before the first heart sound (mitral valve closure). The "a" wave is absent in atrial fibrillation and is prominent in conditions of reduced right ventricular compliance. A cannon "a" wave occurs when the atria contracts against a closed tricuspid valve in atrioventricular dissociation. The "x" descent follows the "a" wave and reflects the fall in right atrial pressure normally seen during early ventricular systole (descent of the tricuspid valve annulus with ventricular contraction is thought to increase the volume in the right atrium, thereby reducing the pressure of the blood present in the atrium).

The "c" wave can interrupt this descent and occurs because of the closed tricuspid valve leaflets (not annulus) being pushed back up toward the right atrium during early ventricular systole. The "c" wave is extremely difficult to discern and is not of much, if any, clinical significance; therefore, for most intents and purposes, it can be ignored. After the "c" wave, the "x" descent then continues as the tricuspid valve annulus continues to be pulled downward by ventricular systole. The "v" wave represents passive atrial filling against the closed tricuspid valve (ie, in mid- to late ventricular systole). The "y" descent then occurs as the tricuspid valve opens, allowing diastolic ventricular filling with a drop in right atrial pressure. A heuristic to aid understanding of the JVP waveform is provided in **Table 2.3**.

In the normal heart, the "v" wave is smaller than the "a" wave because of low right atrial compliance, but can be of equal size in the presence of an atrial septal defect (ASD) and even larger in severe TR. In severe TR, the "v" wave starts right after the "c" deflection (thus, some call this specific abnormality the "c-v" wave) and can produce a single large waveform because of simultaneous retrograde regurgitation of blood into the right atrium and antegrade atrial filling. In severe TR, the diastolic "y" descent is particularly steep and brief in duration because of more rapid right ventricular filling than normal, caused by the excess volume in the right atrium as a consequence of regurgitation during systole.

In the dyspneic patient, the abdominojugular (so-called hepatojugular) reflex is a useful maneuver to help the clinician predict the presence of elevated JVP because of heart failure with elevated right heart filling pressures or reduced right ventricular compliance. With patient consent, persistent gentle and firm pressure is exerted over the upper abdomen for a period of 10 seconds, which will result in increased venous return to the right atrium from the hepatic veins and inferior vena cava. The JVP normally rises transiently during this maneuver. A positive abdominojugular reflex is defined as a rise in the venous pressure of 3 cm or more for at least 15 seconds. It is important that the patient breathes normally throughout because holding one's breath or performing a Valsalva maneuver will falsely elevate the venous pressure.

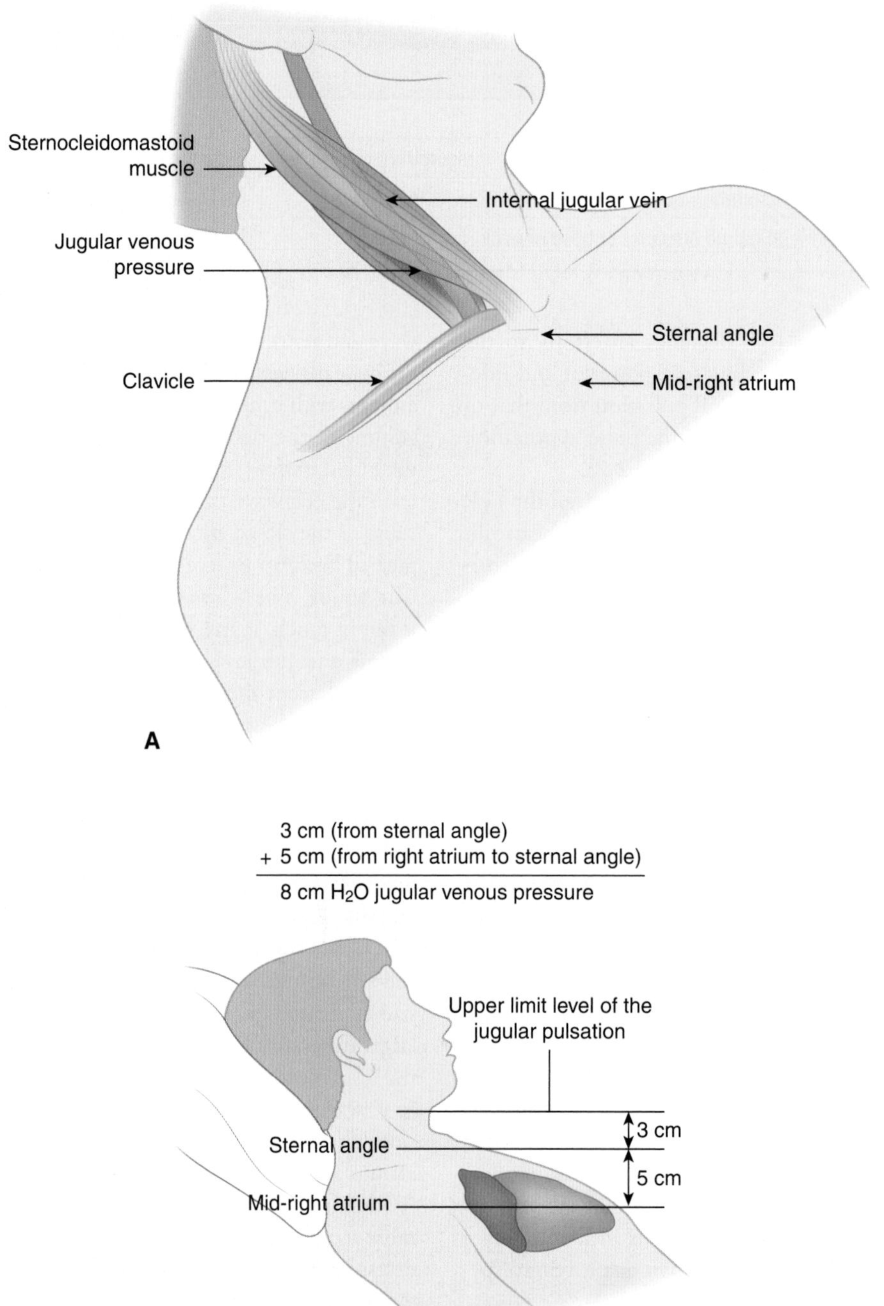

FIGURE 2.2 Locating and assessing jugular venous pressure. **A:** With the patient lying at 45° and the head slightly turned to the left, look for a distended jugular vein and its relationship to surrounding surface anatomy. The internal jugular vein descends from the ear lobe to the medial end of the clavicle, deep to the medial aspect of the sternal head of the sternocleidomastoid muscle. **B:** The jugular venous pressure is determined by measuring the height of the jugular pulsation above the sternal angle in centimeters of water (cm of H_2O) and then assuming the sternal angle is 5cm above the mid-right atrium. Normally this is 8 cm or lower in height.

The impact of inspiration on the JVP is also important to consider during the examination. In the normal state, inspiration reduces intrathoracic pressure, which increases right-sided venous return that is in turn then facilitated by increased right ventricular ejection. This results in a normal drop of approximately 3 mm Hg of CVP transiently, with a consequent transient drop in the level of JVP. This normal transient drop in JVP may be blunted in conditions where right ventricular filling is restricted (eg, constrictive pericarditis, restrictive cardiomyopathy, severe right ventricular failure or infarction, tricuspid stenosis, or massive pulmonary embolism). Indeed, because of the restriction of right ventricular filling induced by these conditions, the right ventricle is unable to accommodate the increased venous return that occurs with inspiration and, in contrast to the normal pattern, the JVP may rise

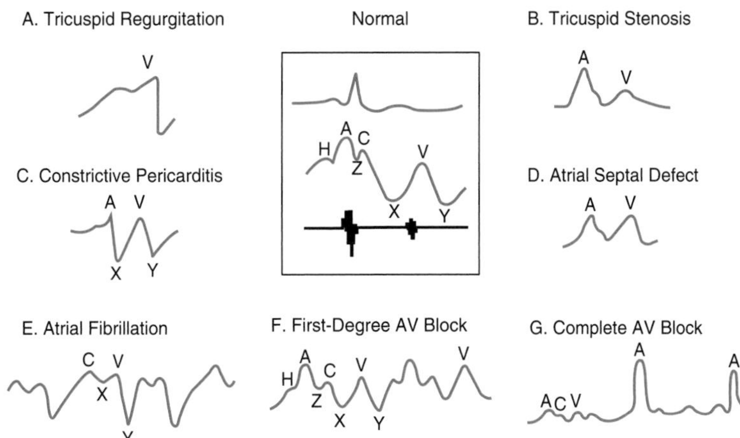

FIGURE 2.3 Pathologic jugular venous waveforms. Normal. **A:** Tricuspid regurgitation (TR, *with severe TR, "ventricularization" of the jugular venous waveform can be seen, with an absent x descent, prominent v wave, and rapid Y descent*). **B:** Tricuspid stenosis. **C:** Constrictive pericarditis (*note the prominent "x" and "y" descents, note also by contrast that the "x" descent is blunted in restrictive cardiomyopathy*). **D:** Atrial septal defect *(note prominent v wave though not as prominent as that seen with TR.* **E:** Atrial fibrillation (*note that there is no "a" wave present*). **F:** First-degree atrioventricular (AV) block. **G:** Complete AV block (*note cannon "a" waves*). (Reprinted with permission from Cuculich, PS Kates AM. *Washington Manual of Cardiology Subspecialty Consult.* Figure 2.2. © Wolters Kluwer.)

with inspiration. This is known as Kussmaul sign. Contrary to common belief, Kussmaul sign is not typically seen in cardiac tamponade until perhaps the most extreme cases. This is because, until late in the process, the increase in negative intrathoracic pressure with inspiration may still be transmitted to the right side of the heart in tamponade, despite the fact that the increase in pericardial pressure exerts an inward force compressing the entire heart throughout the full cardiac cycle.

Measuring Blood Pressure

In the modern health care setting, blood pressure measurement is increasingly carried out with the use of digital devices that do not require mercury. Nonetheless, indirect measurement of systolic and diastolic pressure with manual sphygmomanometer remains an essential bedside skill. The correct technique requires the patient to be in a seated position with the arm at the level of the heart using an appropriately sized arm cuff. The bladder of the cuff is then sited over the brachial artery, and the diaphragm of the stethoscope is placed under the distal end of the cuff overlying the brachial artery. If the arm is positioned too high, the blood pressure reading will be lower than the true value. Positioning the arm lower than the level of the heart will result in a falsely raised reading. Utilization of an undersized cuff will result in an overestimation of true blood pressure and is a frequent occurrence in obese patients.

First, the cuff is fully inflated (typically to approximately 200 mm Hg). With slow deflation of the inflated cuff, five different phases, known as Korotkoff sounds, can usually be heard (**Table 2.4**). The systolic pressure is the pressure at which the

TABLE 2.3 The Jugular Venous Pressure Waveform

Wave/Descent	Physiology
A wave	Atrial contraction = atrial systole
X descent	Ventricular contraction = ventricular systole
V wave	Atrial filling = atrial diastole
Y descent	Ventricular filling = ventricular diastole

TABLE 2.4 Korotkoff Sounds

Phase	Korotkoff Sounds	Typical Cuff Pressure/mm Hg
Phase 1	Tapping sound. *Faint tapping sound increasing in intensity—systolic pressure*	120 mm Hg systolic
Phase 2	A blowing noise. *Tapping softens and acquires a swishing quality*	110 mm Hg
Phase 3	Crisp tapping sound. *Return of sharper sounds*	100 mm Hg
Phase 4	A disappearing blowing noise. *Muffling of sounds that gain a soft blowing quality*	90 mm Hg
Phase 5	Nothing. *All sounds disappear—this is diastolic pressure*	80 mm Hg

first sound (Korotkoff I) is heard, whereas diastolic pressure is recorded at the point when this sound disappears (Korotkoff V). In some cases of severe vascular calcification of the brachial artery (eg, in chronic kidney disease), the cuff may have difficulty compressing the artery, resulting in a falsely elevated Korotkoff 1 and thereby a falsely elevated systolic blood pressure reading (this phenomenon is termed "pseudohypertension"). In addition, in some children, pregnant patients, and patients with chronic severe aortic regurgitation or a large arteriovenous fistula, Korotkoff sounds may be heard all the way down to 0 mm Hg with the cuff fully deflated (ie, Korotkoff V never occurs). In this case, Korotkoff IV sound (a muffled sound) can be utilized as the diastolic pressure.

Systolic blood pressure measurement can vary between the arms by up to 10 mm Hg. Although interarm differences larger than this can be normal, they should raise concern for subclavian artery disease, supravalvular aortic stenosis, aortic coarctation, or aortic dissection. Systolic blood pressures in the legs can be up to 20 mm Hg higher, when compared to arm measurements, under normal conditions. However, larger blood pressure differences between the legs and arms can be seen in patients with extensive lower extremity calcified peripheral vascular disease (akin to the process described for pseudohypertension) and in patients with severe aortic regurgitation (ie, Hill sign). With coarctation of the aorta, systolic pressures in the legs are lower than those in the upper limbs. Measurement of blood pressure in the legs should utilize a large cuff placed over the mid-thigh and the stethoscope placed in the popliteal fossa behind the knee.

Brachial blood pressure should routinely be taken with the patient in both the standing and supine positions, in order to identify orthostatic hypotension. This condition is defined as a fall in blood pressure of more than 20 mm Hg systolic and 10 mm Hg diastolic occurring 1 to 5 minutes after moving from a supine to standing position. Orthostatic changes should preferably not be recorded prior to 1 minute from the change in position because blood pressure can normally fluctuate during this period. Note also that orthostatic blood pressure drops are typically accompanied with compensatory increases in heart rate. Orthostatic hypotension associated with a lack of compensatory tachycardia is indicative of possible autonomic dysfunction that is seen in such conditions as Parkinson disease and diabetes.

Pulsus paradoxus is a marked fall in systolic blood pressure (>10 mm Hg) during inspiration and is a sign of pericardial tamponade, massive pulmonary embolus, or tension pneumothorax, among others. To assess for this phenomenon, the blood pressure cuff is inflated (typically to ~200 mm Hg) and slowly deflated. Pulsus paradoxus is identified by the degree of difference between the systolic blood pressure at which the Korotkoff 1 sounds are first heard intermittently (ie, just during expiration) and the point at which all Korotkoff 1 sounds are no longer intermittent and are heard consistently during both phases of respiration. It is critically important that the patient breathes normally during this maneuver. Any fall of 10 mm Hg or more is considered abnormal. When the blood pressure difference exceeds 15 mm Hg, the pulsus paradoxus may be palpable (best felt for at the carotid pulse location). Beck triad is another related sign of tamponade and comprises hypotension, venous distention, and diminished heart sounds.

Assessing the Pulse

The bedside assessment of arterial pulses involves a stepwise assessment of the arterial tree including the radial, carotid, abdominal aorta, femoral, and pedal pulses. The nature and character of the arterial pulsation are dependent on left ventricular stroke volume, ejection velocity, vascular capacity and compliance, and systemic resistance. Palpation of the pulse is carried out to determine the rate, rhythm, volume, amplitude, and contour (or character) of the pulsation.

Assessment of the rate and rhythm of the pulse is derived from the radial pulse. The pulse rate is calculated by counting the arterial pulse for 15 seconds and multiplying by 4 to obtain the heart rate. The normal pulse occurs at a regular rate and rhythm. The heart rate can quicken slightly with inspiration and slow slightly with expiration, a normal phenomenon called sinus arrhythmia. An irregularly irregular pulsation can be due to atrial fibrillation or frequent ectopic beats. In these states, a pulse deficit may exist where the auscultated heart rate varies from the palpated radial pulse. This is due to inadequate diastolic filling during some heart beats with resulting cardiac output that is of too low a volume to be felt peripherally at the radial site. For similar reasons, automated blood pressure machines may report an alarmingly low heart rate in patients with frequent ventricular ectopic beats.

The character and volume of the pulse is assessed by palpation of the carotid pulse. As the arterial pulse travels from the central aorta, the elastic properties and caliber of the peripheral arteries can distort and dampen the pulsation, and thus, carotid pulsation is the most useful. Correct interpretation of the character of the pulse requires an understanding of the physiology of the arterial waveform. The arterial waveform has early systolic, mid-to-late systolic, and diastolic components (**Figure 2.4**). The rapid upstroke in early systole (percussion wave) is the predominant monophasic pulse felt at the bedside. It provides useful information regarding ventricular contraction and antegrade flow. The mid- and late systolic components consist of the anacrotic notch and tidal wave (also called pre-dicrotic wave), often have a rounded peak, and are due to propagation of blood from the central aorta to the peripheral circulation and the subsequent reflection of these waves from the extremities back to the central aorta. Thereafter, the dicrotic notch and subsequent post-dicrotic wave identify aortic valve closure and diastole, respectively. The tidal (pre-dicrotic) and post-dicrotic waves provide useful information regarding the arterial system. In a poorly compliant, diseased vascular system, the reflected wave (which represents a retrograde reflection from the distal vessels of the anterograde systolic pressure wave) returns very early in the cardiac cycle, leading to an augmented tidal wave with pressures after the anacrotic notch that abnormally exceed the pressures seen during the percussion wave (because the reflected wave returns early, it also does not

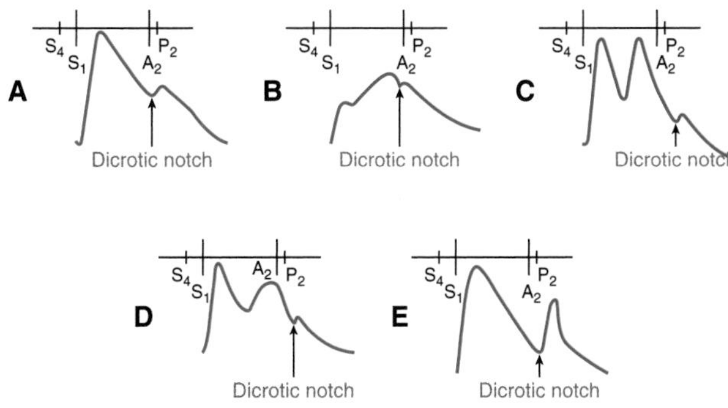

FIGURE 2.4 Carotid pulse waveforms and heart sounds. **A:** Normal. **B:** Aortic stenosis. Anacrotic pulse with slow upstroke and peak near S2. **C:** Severe aortic regurgitation: bifid pulse with two systolic peaks. **D:** Hypertrophic obstructive cardiomyopathy (HOCM): bifid pulse with two systolic peaks. The second peak (tidal or reflected wave) is of lower amplitude than the initial percussion wave. **E:** Dicrotic pulse with systolic and diastolic peaks in the setting of an accentuated dicrotic notch may occur with sepsis, hypovolemia, severe heart failure, or tamponade. A2, aortic component of S2; P2, pulmonic component of S2. (Reprinted with permission from Topol EJ, Califf RM, Prystowsky EN, et al. *Textbook of Cardiovascular Medicine.* 3rd ed. Figure 16.8. © Wolters Kluwer.)

contribute to the post-dicrotic wave and, therefore, results in a low diastolic blood pressure). In contrast, the reflected wave comes later in a normally compliant arterial system and contributes to the post-dicrotic wave during diastole.

A hypokinetic pulse is of low volume and amplitude is due to low cardiac output with reduced left ventricular stroke volume, shorter left ventricular ejection time, or intense vasoconstriction. A slow rising pulse of small volume suggests valvular obstruction. Severe aortic stenosis produces a weak and slow rising pulse with delayed upstroke called "pulsus parvus et tardus" (Figure 2.4, View B). The delay is assessed during simultaneous auscultation of the heart sounds and palpation of the pulse. A hyperkinetic or bounding pulse is a large-amplitude pulsation, which is due to increases in left ventricular ejection, stroke volume, sympathetic drive, or elevated arterial pressure. Thus, it can be seen in hyperkinetic states, such as anxiety, pregnancy, anemia, fever, and thyrotoxicosis or in other pathologic states, such as patent ductus arteriosus, aortic regurgitation, or arteriovenous fistula. The pulse of severe aortic regurgitation is described as a water hammer (or Corrigan) pulse. It produces a rapid upstroke with swift descent without dicrotic notch, which produces a collapsing sensation (View C).

A bifid pulse is created by two distinct pressure peaks. Hypertrophic obstructive cardiomyopathy (HOCM) can rarely produce a bifid pulse with separate percussion and tidal waves (View D). Diastolic augmentation of pressure with an intra-aortic balloon pump also results in a bifid pulse, although the two components are separated by the aortic valve closure. Pulsus alternans describes the beat-to-beat variability of peak systolic arterial blood pressure and pulse volume in a patient with normal sinus rhythm and severe ventricular dysfunction. It is present only when every other phase 1 Korotkoff sound is audible as the pressure cuff is released (irrespective and independent of respiration) and is a sign of severe heart failure. Thus, it may be present with other signs of severe heart failure such as an S3 gallop rhythm.

Palpation of the Heart

Palpation of the heart is performed with the patient in a spine position at 30° elevation. The apex beat is typically located at the fifth intercostal space at the midclavicular line, but successful palpation may require repositioning the patient into the lateral decubitus position with their left arm raised above the head, or in the seated position with the patient leaning forward. Use firm pressure with the tips of the fingers in the rib interspace as the area over the apex beat is smaller than 2 cm. In 50% of normal adults as well as in obese or muscular patients or those with chest deformities, the apex beat may not be palpable. Enlargement of the left ventricle displaces the apex downward and to the left.

The character of the palpated apex beat can provide vital clues to diagnosis. A forceful and sustained impulse is seen in aortic stenosis and hypertension and is evidence of pressure overload (also termed a "heaving or hyperdynamic apex beat"). The volume-loaded apex beat is a displaced, diffuse, and nonsustained impulse that can occur in severe mitral regurgitation and dilated cardiomyopathy. A large ventricular aneurysm may yield a double impulse with a palpable ectopic pulsation, which is discrete from the apex beat. Rarely, HOCM may cause a triple cadence apex beat, with contributions from a palpable S4 and the two components of the systolic pulse.

A parasternal lift is a sign of volume overload or elevated right ventricular pressure and may be felt with the heel of the hand rested just to the left of the sternum and with the fingers lifted off the chest. When present, the physician should look for other relevant signs, such as a jugular venous c-v wave (indicating TR) or a loud or palpable P2 (suggestive of pulmonary arterial hypertension).

A palpable murmur, also called a thrill, can be identified with the flat of the hand, first over the apex and left sternal border, and then over the base of the heart. Thrills are best felt with the patient sitting up and leaning forward and in full expiration. A thrill that coincides in time with the apex beat is a systolic thrill, whereas a diastolic thrill does not.

Cardiac Auscultation

A critical part of the cardiovascular examination is auscultation of the heart. This requires a stepwise approach. Initial auscultation begins in the mitral area (midclavicular left fifth intercostal space), first utilizing the diaphragm of the stethoscope and then the bell. The stethoscope is then placed in the tricuspid area (parasternal left fifth intercostal space) and moved up the left sternal edge to the pulmonary area (second left intercostal space) and finally the aortic area (second right intercostal space). The diaphragm of the stethoscope helps reproduce higher pitched sounds such as the systolic murmur of mitral regurgitation, whereas the bell acts as a resonating chamber and amplifies low-pitched sounds such as the diastolic murmur of mitral stenosis.

Heart Sounds. Begin with palpating the carotid (or radial) pulse to identify the timing of systole and thereby accurately differentiate the heart sounds within the cardiac cycle. The normal first heart sound (S1) comprises mitral and tricuspid valve closure at the beginning of ventricular systole. The second heart sound, resulting from aortic and pulmonary valve closure at the end of systole, is softer, shorter, and with a slightly higher pitch than the first heart sound. A splitting of the second heart sound (A2-P2) may be audible and can be a normal variant. Although right and left ventricular systole occur at the same time, the lower pressure in the pulmonary circulation compared to the aorta means that flow continues into the pulmonary artery after the end of left ventricular systole, resulting in slightly delayed closure of the pulmonary valve (P2) compared to the aortic valve (A2). This physiologic splitting of the heart sound is best heard at the second left intercostal space with the patient in the supine position. With normal breathing, the A2-P2 interval widens with inspiration (because of a further delay in P2 from the increased venous return seen to the right ventricle on inspiration) and shortens with expiration.

The intensity or loudness of the heart sounds should be assessed. A loud S1 is heard in the early stages of rheumatic mitral stenosis and in states of reduced diastolic filling time, such as tachycardia or any cause of a short atrioventricular conduction time. S1 becomes softer with prolonged diastolic filling (first-degree heart block), contractile dysfunction (left bundle branch block), or failure of the leaflets to coapt normally (mitral regurgitation). The aortic component of the second heart sound (A2) can be loud in systemic hypertension, whereas a loud P2 may be present in pulmonary hypertension. The intensity of A2 and P2 decreases with aortic and pulmonary stenosis. Although splitting of the second heart sound is a normal variant, it is accentuated with right bundle branch block (delayed right ventricular depolarization), mitral regurgitation (early aortic valve closure because of rapid left ventricular emptying), pulmonary stenosis (delayed right ventricular ejection), and ventricular septal defects (increased right ventricular volume load). With fixed splitting of S2 (ie, splitting that does not change with respiration), the A2-P2 interval is consistently widened and can indicate an ASD. Reverse, or paradoxical, splitting occurs because of pathologic delay in closure of the aortic valve and can be due to left bundle branch block, severe aortic stenosis/HOCM (delayed left ventricle emptying), TR (early pulmonic valve closure because of rapid right ventricular emptying), or large patent ductus arteriosus (increased left ventricle volume load).

Systolic Sounds. An ejection systolic click is a high-pitched, early systolic sound that is heard over the aortic or pulmonary areas and is usually associated with congenital bicuspid aortic or pulmonic valve stenosis. It is due to the abrupt doming of the abnormal valve early in systole and often disappears as the culprit valve loses its pliability over time. A nonejection click heard over the mitral area is related to mitral valve prolapse. This high-pitched click, which occurs after S1 and which may be followed by a systolic murmur, can be affected by positioning. Specifically, with standing, ventricular preload and afterload decrease, resulting in the click (and murmur) moving closer to S1. With squatting, ventricular preload and afterload increase, and the click (and murmur) move away from S1.

Diastolic Sounds. An opening snap is a high-pitched sound that occurs in mitral stenosis shortly after S2. It is due to the sudden opening of the thickened mitral valve and is followed by the diastolic murmur of mitral stenosis. A diastolic pericardial knock is another high-pitched early diastolic sound that occurs when there is sudden cessation of diastolic filling as seen in constrictive pericarditis (unlike the opening snap, the pericardial knock is not accompanied by a diastolic murmur). A tumor plop is a low-pitched early diastolic sound caused by an atrial myxoma. Diastolic prolapse of the tumor across the mitral valve generates this sound, but it is rarely heard, even in patients with large myxomas.

A third heart sound (S3) is a low-pitched mid-diastolic sound that is best appreciated when listening for a triple rhythm with the bell of the stethoscope. It occurs during the rapid filling phase of ventricular diastole and can be a normal variant in children or young adults. In older patients, it is due to reduced ventricular compliance and is strongly associated with increased atrial and ventricular end-diastolic pressure. A right ventricular S3 is louder at the left sternal border on inspiration and with the patient in supine position. It occurs in right ventricular failure secondary to pulmonary embolus and constrictive pericarditis. A left ventricular S3 is louder at the apex with the patient in the left lateral decubitus position. It is a sign of left ventricular failure. A fourth heart sound (S4) is a late diastolic sound that occurs during the atrial filling phase of ventricular diastole (ie, during atrial contraction). It is due to a high-pressure atrial wave reflected back from an abnormally noncompliant ventricle (like in left ventricular hypertrophy). It is absent in the setting of atrial fibrillation.

Murmurs of the Heart. Murmurs result from the audible vibrations caused by turbulent blood flow. Some turbulence is inevitable as blood accelerates through the aortic and pulmonary valves in ventricular systole. In hyperdynamic states—such as pregnancy, thyrotoxicosis, and anemia—increased turbulence over normal valves may produce a benign functional systolic murmur. However, very often, an audible murmur is secondary to valvular or structural heart disease. Correct identification and determination of the origin of a cardiac murmur require a standard approach that includes determining the location of the murmur, the timing within the cardiac cycle (systolic or diastolic), the impact of respiration (inspiration/expiration), the radiation of the murmur, its intensity, and response to dynamic maneuvers.

Area of Greatest Intensity. The first step in characterizing an audible murmur is to identify the place on the precordium where the murmur is of greatest intensity. This will allow the clinician to optimally examine the murmur, but it is important to note that this is not a completely reliable sign as to the location of the valvular abnormality. For example, the murmur of mitral regurgitation is typically loudest over the apex with radiation to the axilla; however, a very loud mitral murmur may be audible throughout the precordium.

Systolic Murmurs. Systolic murmurs may be early, mid-systolic, late, or pansystolic in their timing (**Figure 2.5**). Acute severe mitral regurgitation produces a decrescendo, early systolic murmur (eg, begins with S1) that does not continue throughout systole because of the steep rise in pressure within the noncompliant atrium. In acute TR with normal pulmonary artery pressures, an early systolic murmur that increases in intensity with inspiration (Rivero-Carvallo sign) may be heard over the left sternal border, and regurgitant "c-v" waves may be visible on inspection of the JVP. A mid-systolic murmur begins after S1 and ends before S2 (in other words, there is a distinct separation between S1, the murmur, and S2). The intensity is greatest in mid-systole or later and is described as a crescendo-decrescendo murmur. The most common cause of such a murmur is aortic stenosis, but other causes of mid-systolic murmurs include HOCM, pulmonary stenosis, and a large ASD with left-to-right shunting. When there is a distinguishable gap between the first heart sound and the murmur, which then continues up until and includes the second heart sound, the murmur is defined as late systolic. This is typical of mitral valve prolapse or papillary muscle dysfunction where mitral regurgitation begins in mid-systole. A pansystolic (or holosystolic) murmur extends throughout systole and is continuous in its loudness and pitch (**Table 2.5**). It is associated with chronic mitral regurgitation, chronic TR, and ventricular septal defects. Mitral regurgitation is best heard over the cardiac apex and is typically conducted to the axilla, TR over the left sternal border, and a ventricular septal defect murmur at the mid-left sternal border where a thrill may be palpable. Variability in intensity with respiration can help aid differentiation of tricuspid and mitral regurgitation, with the former being louder on inspiration (also known as Rivero-Carvallo sign).

Diastolic Murmurs. Diastolic murmurs are always abnormal and can be classified as early or mid-diastole in timing (Table 2.5). The early diastolic murmurs of aortic and pulmonary regurgitation begin immediately after the second heart sound, are high pitched, and have a decrescendo quality. With primary aortic regurgitation, the murmur is often best heard along the left sternal border with the patient sitting forward and on full expiration. With secondary aortic regurgitation (because of aortic root enlargement), the murmur may radiate along the right sternal border. The murmur of pulmonary regurgitation is heard along the left sternal border and is often caused by annular enlargement from chronic pulmonary artery hypertension (Graham Steell murmur). A mid-diastolic murmur is classic of mitral stenosis and has a much lower pitch quality compared to early diastolic murmurs. The murmur is best heard over the apex with the patient in the left lateral decubitus position. Less common causes of a mid-diastolic murmur include atrial myxoma, complete heart block, aortic regurgitation causing reverberation of the anterior mitral valve

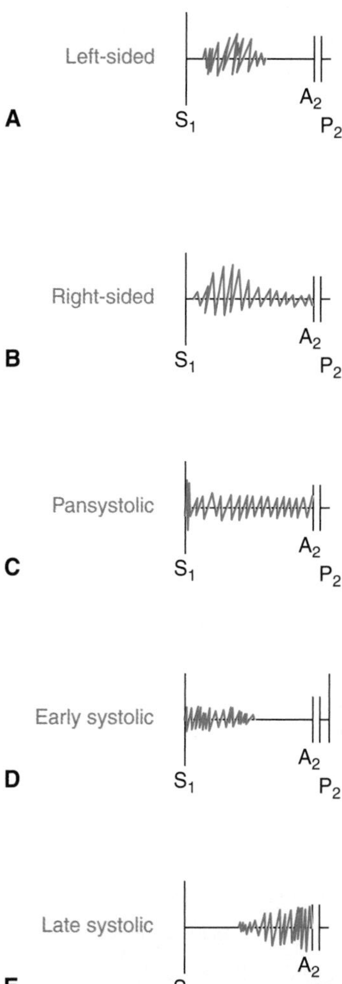

FIGURE 2.5 Heart sounds and systolic murmurs. A left-sided ejection systolic murmur starts after the first heart sound (S1) and terminates before the aortic component of the second heart sound (A2). A right-sided ejection systolic murmur starts after S1 and terminates before the pulmonary component of the second heart sound (P2). A pansystolic murmur starts with S1 and extends to second heart sound. An early systolic murmur starts with the S1 and terminates before the second heart sound. A late systolic murmur starts after the S1 and extends up to second heart sound. **A:** Aortic stenosis, aortic sclerosis, flow murmur, innocent murmur, hypertrophic cardiomyopathy, and bicuspid aortic valve. **B:** Pulmonary stenosis, infundibular stenosis, flow murmur (atrial septal defect), idiopathic dilatation of the pulmonary artery, and innocent murmurs. **C:** Mitral regurgitation, tricuspid regurgitation, and ventricular septal defect. **D:** Mitral regurgitation, tricuspid regurgitation, and ventricular septal defect. **E:** Mitral regurgitation and tricuspid regurgitation. (Reprinted with permission from Topol EJ, Califf RM, Prystowsky EN, et al. *Textbook of Cardiovascular Medicine.* 3rd ed. Philadelphia, PA: Lippincott Williams & Wilkins; 2006. Figure 16.10.)

TABLE 2.5 Cardiac Murmurs and How to Differentiate Them

Timing and Lesion	Site	Radiation/Dynamic Maneuvers	Helpful Hints
		SYSTOLIC MURMURS	
Early systolic			
Acute mitral regurgitation (MR)	Apex	Radiates to the axilla when the regurgitant leaflet is the anterior mitral valve leaflet but may radiate to the cardiac base with posterior leaflet disease	• Loud early systolic murmur that increases with expiration and diminishes as the pressure gradient between the left ventricle and left atrium decreases in late systole
Acute tricuspid regurgitation	Left lower sternal border		• Increases in intensity during inspiration with a prominent "v" wave (or "c-v" wave) in jugular venous pressure (JVP)
Mid-systolic			
Aortic stenosis	Upper right sternal border (second intercostal space)	Radiates to carotids	• High-pitched murmur that is louder on expiration. • Intensity is greatest in mid-systole and wanes in late systole—crescendo-decrescendo pattern. • Murmur preceded by an ejection click in young patients • S2 variable and can be absent in severely calcified valve • Reverse splitting in severe aortic stenosis (P2-A2)
Pulmonary stenosis	Upper left sternal border (second intercostal space)	Can radiate slightly toward the neck and back	• Harsh and high-pitched murmur louder on inspiration • Similar crescendo-decrescendo pattern • Ejection click, delayed P2 may be soft
Hypertrophic obstructive cardiomyopathy	Left lower sternal border	Louder and longer on standing and Valsalva maneuver	• Ejection crescendo-decrescendo murmur that can mimic aortic stenosis —differentiate with dynamic maneuvers (ie, Valsalva, squat) • A pansystolic murmur at the apex and radiating to axilla may occur in the presence of systolic anterior motion of the mitral valve • Patients may present with an S4 gallop and a reverse splitting of S2.
Atrial septal defect	Left upper sternal border	Can radiate to the back	• Fixed splitting of A2-P2—interval is wide and remains constant throughout respiration.
Innocent murmur	All areas		• Soft murmur that can appear when cardiac output is high.
Late systolic			
Mitral valve prolapse	Apex	Radiates to the axilla but also may go to the neck or back. Enhanced by Valsalva maneuvers and decreased by squatting	• Following a normal S1, the valve prolapses resulting in a mid-systolic click. Immediately after the click, a brief crescendo-decrescendo murmur is heard.
Pansystolic			
Chronic MR	Apex	Radiates to the axilla	• Mild MR is characterized by a systolic murmur plateau louder on expiration while moderate MR is accompanied by an S3 gallop. Severe MR has an associated diastolic flow rumble.
Chronic tricuspid regurgitation	Left sternal border	Has a blowing quality and often associated with an S3	• Increases in intensity during inspiration with a prominent "v" wave in JVP. Left parasternal heave may be present.

DIASTOLIC MURMURS			
Early diastolic			
Aortic regurgitation	Mid-left sternal border (third intercostal space)	Louder over left sternal border with patient sitting up and leaning forward on full expiration	• Begins directly after S2 and has a blowing decrescendo quality.
Mid-diastolic			
Mitral stenosis	Apex	Maximal intensity with patient in lateral decubitus position	• Soft rumbling diastolic murmur preceded by an opening snap and best heard with the bell of the stethoscope and patient in the lateral decubitus position • Useful mnemonic, "*Rup-t-t-eee.*" *Rup* (loud S1)— *t* (S2)—*t* (opening snap)—*eee* (diastolic murmur)
Atrial tumors	Apex		Rarely present Low-pitched sound that fluctuates with patient positioning as the tumor moves toward or away from mitral valve

leaflet (Austin Flint murmur), and rheumatic mitral valvulitis (Carey Coombs murmur).

Continuous Murmurs. As the name implies, continuous murmurs extend throughout systole and diastole. They are produced when a communication exists between two chambers or vessels that produce a permanent pressure gradient. Examples include a patent ductus arteriosus, an aortopulmonary window, a ruptured sinus of Valsalva aneurysm, or arteriovenous fistulas. They can be difficult to differentiate from combined systolic and diastolic murmurs in patients with mixed aortic valve disease.

Dynamic Movements. For all newly diagnosed murmurs, a series of dynamic maneuvers should be carried out to help identify and characterize their significance. Changes in murmur intensity with respiration should be noted. Right-sided cardiac murmurs increase in intensity with inspiration and decrease with expiration (100% sensitivity, 88% specificity).4 The opposite occurs with left-sided cardiac murmurs. Sustained hand grip (isometric exercises) increases left ventricular afterload and results in an increase in intensity of aortic regurgitation, mitral regurgitation, and the murmur of a ventricular septal defect. Changes in patient positioning are a useful exercise to help the clinician differentiate the murmur of HOCM from aortic stenosis. When a patient squats from a standing position, venous return and systemic resistance increase, causing a rise in left ventricular diastolic volume and arterial pressure. Murmurs such as aortic stenosis will become louder with squatting, but the intensity of the systolic murmur of HOCM will diminish as left ventricular diastolic volume increases and reduces the obstruction of outflow. Thus, the murmur of HOCM becomes shorter and softer with squatting (95% sensitivity, 85% specificity) and longer and louder with standing rapidly (95% sensitivity, 84% specificity).4 The Valsalva maneuver is a forceful expiration against a closed glottis. With Valsalva, left ventricular diastolic volume, stroke volume, and arterial blood pressure fall, and most cardiac murmurs become softer. However, the reduction of left ventricular diastolic volume increases the burden of obstruction in HOCM, resulting in an increase in the systolic murmur (65% sensitivity, 95% specificity). The late systolic murmur of mitral valve prolapse occurs earlier and becomes longer and louder with Valsalva.

Loudness or Intensity. The loudness of a murmur can be helpful in defining the severity of the valve lesion. A grading system such as the Levine grading system can be utilized to classify the intensity of a systolic murmur from grade 1 to 6. The presence of a thrill automatically corresponds to a grade 4 or higher murmur. The intensity of diastolic murmurs is graded on a scale of 1 to 4. This grading is particularly useful as a change in the intensity of the murmur can be of great significance—as, for example, after a myocardial infarction. In primary mitral and aortic regurgitation, the intensity of the audible murmur can correlate with the severity of regurgitation.[5] However, the correlation is weak in functional mitral regurgitation, and the murmur intensity is a not a reliable clinical indicator of regurgitation severity. Similarly, murmur intensity is not a reliable indicator of aortic stenosis severity; at the latter most extreme phase of stenosis, as stroke volume decreases, intensity may fall.

LIMITATIONS OF TECHNIQUE

The cardiovascular physical examination remains central to the practice of modern cardiovascular medicine. Evidence about the value of the physical examination is typically based on its diagnostic accuracy and varies widely in methodologic quality and statistical power.[6] Because of its historical evolution, the physical examination is not well supported by randomized controlled trials or other modern forms of assessment typically seen in evidence-based medicine. Nonetheless, the absence of high-quality evidence-based trials on the physical examination should not be considered a weakness of the examination, because the virtues of the physical examination are self-evident and based on years of experience; not everything needs to be proven within the confines of a clinical trial.[7] Unfortunately, the dependence of modern medicine on technology has resulted in a diminishing opportunity and incentive for direct physician-patient interaction and, as a result, diminishing use of the physical examination in everyday medicine. The increased reliance on technologic aids and the reduced reliance on clinical skills in modern medicine have a potential detrimental effect on the diagnostic accuracy of physical examination.

RESEARCH AND FUTURE DIRECTIONS—COVID-19

Since its introduction in 1816 by Laennec, the stethoscope has become the symbolic tool of the cardiovascular physical examination.[8] With advancements in technology, new devices such as miniaturized handheld ultrasound machines are increasingly utilized at the point of care to aid in the diagnosis and management of cardiovascular disease.[9] Such devices can provide a direct visual assessment of cardiac structures and function as well as provide information on cardiac abnormalities that cannot be assessed by the physical examination such as left ventricular dysfunction or thrombus. The pragmatic clinical value of these devices remains to be determined, despite their clear potential.

The coronavirus disease 2019 (COVID-19) global pandemic has altered our economy, society, and health care systems since December 2019. In many nonacute settings, the traditional model of patient-physician interaction fundamentally changed, given the requirements for physical distancing measures that alters every aspect of the delivery of patient care. The physical examination, while remaining the cornerstone of patient-physician interaction, has had to adapt in order to provide effective care from a distance in many clinical scenarios.

As a result of the COVID-19 pandemic, technology is rapidly transforming the health care environment in order to allow delivery of care without the need for direct physical contact. Cloud-based video conferencing is increasingly replacing the traditional face-to-face interactions in outpatient and community settings. However, the inability to physically examine a patient is a limitation of this platform. A number of telehealth solutions exist, and these will no doubt grow in importance in the post-COVID environment, particularly as remote monitoring devices advance. Digital devices such as digital stethoscopes and handheld/smartphone electrocardiographic monitors that can aid in the physician's virtual physical examination are increasingly becoming available to patients. In addition, the insertion of pulmonary artery pressure sensors and digital heart failure management systems is transforming the management of remote heart failure care from a distance.

KEY POINTS

- ✔ General inspection: Do not underestimate the value of the "end of bed" assessment, it provides valuable important information as to a patient's overall status and dictates the urgency and direction of assessment.
- ✔ Hemodynamic status: Every physical examination should begin with an assessment of overall hemodynamic assessment and take time to assess perfusion and the presence of congestion.
- ✔ Holistic assessment: Complete a full cardiovascular examination every time a patient is examined, and evaluate the relevance and association of all physical signs in order to identify differential diagnosis. Beware focusing attention and relying too heavily on a single physical sign.
- ✔ Evaluation of a murmur: Once a murmur is heard, a standardized approach to evaluation is required to accurately classify it, including the site of greatest intensity, timing in cardiac cycle, response to respiration, response to dynamic maneuvers, and overall intensity.
- ✔ Examine the JVP: The JVP is a sensitive physical sign as to patient's volume status, ventricular filling pressures, and response to medical therapy. It is difficult to master, so take time to position the patient correctly, carry out the abdominojugular reflex, assess the impact of inspiration, and interpret the JVP waveform (summarized in **Table 2.3**).

REFERENCES

1. Emdin M, Mirizzi G, Giannoni A, et al. Prognostic significance of central apneas throughout a 24-hour period in patients with heart failure. *J Am Coll Cardiol.* 2017;70(11):1351-1364. doi:10.1016/j.jacc.2017.07.740
2. Afilalo J, Alexander KP, Mack MJ, et al. Frailty assessment in the cardiovascular care of older adults. *J Am Coll Cardiol.* 2014;63(8):747-762. doi:10.1016/j.jacc.2013.09.070
3. Drazner MH, Hellkamp AS, Leier CV, et al. Value of clinician assessment of hemodynamics in advanced heart failure: the ESCAPE trial. *Circ Heart Fail.* 2008;1(3):170-177. doi:10.1161/circheartfailure.108.769778
4. Lembo NJ, Dell'Italia LJ, Crawford MH, O'Rourke RA. Bedside diagnosis of systolic murmurs. *N Engl J Med.* 1988;318(24):1572-1578. doi:10.1056/nejm198806163182404
5. Desjardins VA, Enriquez-Sarano M, Jamil Tajik A, Bailey KR, Seward JB. Intensity of murmurs correlates with severity of valvular regurgitation. *Am J Med.* 1996;100(2):149-156. doi:10.1016/s0002-9343(97)89452-1
6. Elder A, Japp A, Verghese A. How valuable is physical examination of the cardiovascular system? *BMJ.* 2016;354:i3309. doi:10.1136/bmj.i3309
7. Smith GCS, Pell JP. Parachute use to prevent death and major trauma related to gravitational challenge: systematic review of randomised controlled trials. *BMJ.* 2003;327(7429):1459-1461. doi:10.1136/bmj.327.7429.1459
8. Bank I, Vliegen HW, Bruschke AV. The 200th anniversary of the stethoscope: can this low-tech device survive in the high-tech 21st century? *Eur Heart J.* 2016;37:3536-3543. doi:10.1093/eurheartj/ehw034
9. Chamsi-Pasha MA, Sengupta PP, Zoghbi WA. Handheld echocardiography. *Circulation.* 2017;136(22):2178-2188. doi:10.1161/circulationaha.117.026622

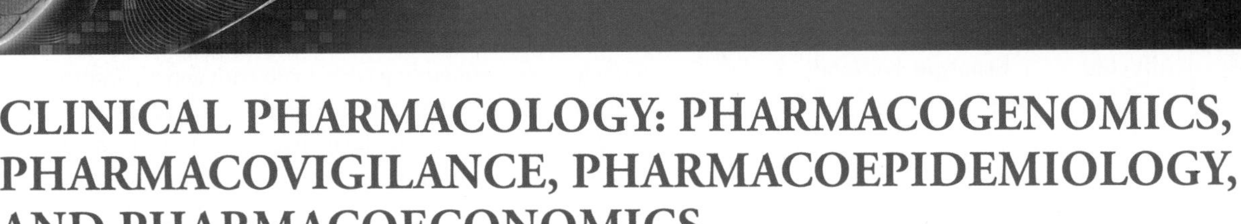

CLINICAL PHARMACOLOGY: PHARMACOGENOMICS, PHARMACOVIGILANCE, PHARMACOEPIDEMIOLOGY, AND PHARMACOECONOMICS

Steven P. Dunn and Craig J. Beavers

INTRODUCTION

In order to achieve comprehensive pharmacotherapy management of the patient with cardiovascular disease, it is critical to appreciate various concepts in pharmacology beyond the traditional pharmacokinetic and therapeutic principles widely taught. These concepts include pharmacogenomics, pharmacoeconomics, pharmacovigilance, and pharmacoepidemiology. These principles can directly impact a single patient at the time of treatment while also leading to population-level changes to potentially optimize cardiovascular medication use. This chapter focuses on the four aforementioned topics in efforts to provide an overview and examples of each.

PHARMACOGENOMICS

Pharmacogenomics is defined as the genome in the drug response.[1] This encompasses pharmacogenetics, a subcategory of pharmacogenomics, which refers to single genetic variation in response to a medication.[1] Pharmacogenetics has largely been used to study the inherited genetic differences in drug metabolic pathways.[1] The impact from genetic differences on pharmacotherapy is typically categorized into four influences: (1) the effect on a drug's pharmacokinetics; (2) the effect on a drug's pharmacodynamics; (3) the effect on idiosyncratic reactions; and (4) the effect on disease pathogenesis or severity and response to specific therapy.[2,3] The central concept is the interindividual response to drug therapy with aims to maximize efficacy while minimizing adverse drug events as opposed to the "one-size-fits-all" approach.[2] The detailed overview of genetic principles is beyond the scope of this chapter.

Since the mid-2000s, regulatory agencies, such as the Food and Drug Administration (FDA), have increased the focus on the impact of pharmacogenetics on drug efficacy and safety.[4] From the FDA perspective, this voluntary effort has led to over 300 medications having pharmacogenetic information included in the labeling.[5] Although the vast majority are medications used for oncologic indications, close to 30 medications are cardiovascular specific. Well-known examples include clopidogrel and the *CYP2C19* genotype, warfarin with both *CYP2C9 and VKORC1* genotypes, and simvastatin and the *SLCO1B1* genotype (**Table 3.1**). As cardio-oncology has emerged as a subspecialty, the pharmacogenomics of anticancer agents are also increasingly relevant to cardiovascular practice.[6] An example of this is ongoing efforts and partial successes in identifying genetic polymorphisms that may help predict the risk of cardiotoxicity with doxorubicin.[7]

Despite the continued efforts to identify genetic ties to medication response, widespread incorporation of pharmacogenetic data into clinical practice currently remains a challenge. The reasons behind this is multifactorial and include availability and timing of testing, education about or ability to interpret the results, and real or perceived cost.[8] In terms of timing, genotype testing can be done preemptively or reactively. Preemptive genotyping is completed through a multigene, chip-based approach that leads to several genes and/or genetic polymorphisms being tested simultaneously and leads to availability of information when needed in the future.[9] The advantages of this include reduced cost and more compressive profiling, whereas, the disadvantages may include denial of reimbursement. Outside of this limited disadvantage, preemptive genetic testing allows the clinician to be proactive during therapy selection. In contrast, reactive genotyping typically tests a single gene or a few selected genes at the time the information is needed.[9] Third-party reimbursement is more likely with reactive testing; however, since the results are not usually available at the time of treatment assignment or dosing, it may delay and increase the cost of optimal care.

Other considerations of pharmacogenetic testing include analytic validity, clinical validity, and clinical utility.[10] Analytic validity refers to the ability of a test to accurately detect the presence or absence of a genetic variant. Clinical validity is the relevance of the variant to the drug's response. An example of this, as noted above, is the *CYP2C19* genetic variation's impact on the bioactivation of clopidogrel. Finally, clinical utility is the test's usefulness in guiding the prevention, diagnosis, treatment, and management of therapy. It is critical for the selected test to be highly accurate and clinically valid for use; however, the biggest determinate of a test's value is its clinical utility. For example, in regard to simvastatin therapy, since most statins are now generic (ie, widely available and inexpensive), the utility of *SLCO1B1* genotype testing to avoid simvastatin-induced myopathy is of questionable value, as clinicians can readily

TABLE 3.1 Common Cardiovascular Pharmacogenetic Variants

Gene	Major Drug Affected	Genotype	Functional Effect
CYP2C19	Clopidogrel	*1/*1	Normal metabolizer
		*1/*2	Intermediate metabolizer
		*1/*3	Intermediate metabolizer
		*1/*17	Rapid metabolizer
		*2/*17	Intermediate metabolizer
		*2/*2	Poor metabolizer
		*2/*3	Poor metabolizer
		*3/*3	Poor metabolizer
		*17/*17	Ultra-rapid metabolizer
SLCO1B1	Simvastatin	*1a/*1a *1a/*1b *1b/*1b	Normal function= Expected statin effect and normal myopathy risk
		*1a/*5 *1a/*15 *1a/*17 *1b/*5 *1b/*15 *1b/*17	Decreased function= Increased risk of myopathy
		*5/*5 *5/*15 *5/*17 *15/*15 *15/*17 *17/*17	Low function= High risk of myopathy
CYP2C9 (*VKORC1* abnormalities not presented)	Warfarin	*1/*1	Normal metabolizer
		*1/*2 *1/*3	Intermediate metabolizer
		*2/*2 *2/*3	Poor metabolizer

prescribe alternative generic statins that are unaffected by this gene. In this example, if suddenly all other statins became unavailable, the clinical utility of testing for the *SLCO1B1* genotype to guide simvastatin therapy would change. In contrast, experts have generally outlined a significant number of scenarios where genetic testing may be utilized in personalizing $P2Y_{12}$ inhibitor therapy for patients receiving dual antiplatelet therapy,[11] despite the availability of newer agents that circumvent this concern.

As described previously, understanding how to interpret the results of genetic tests is critical for successful clinical implementation of pharmacogenetics. In order to assist with this, the Clinical Pharmacogenetic Implementation Consortium (CPIC) was established in 2009.[12] Consisting of experts in pharmacogenomics and laboratory medicine, the CPIC devises guidelines recommending what to do with genetic information that has been obtained. For example, several of the aforementioned cardiovascular drug gene pairs have robust evidence regarding use in clinical practice. It is important that providers using this information have full understanding of the results or know how to consult someone who can assist. In terms of implementation, several programs at the forefront of the adoption of cardiovascular pharmacogenomics have outlined how to initiate and develop this service.[13] The central elements for implementation include engaging all key stakeholders, prioritizing gene-drug pairs to include informed test selection, establishing an electronic health record infrastructure, demonstrating value, and maintaining sustainability. These challenges need to be addressed on both a national and health-system level in order to facilitate widespread adoption.

PHARMACOECONOMICS

As health care moves toward a value-based care system, it is imperative to understand the efficacy and safety of our therapies in the context of their cost. Pharmacoeconomics is a type of outcomes research that can be used to quantify the value of pharmacotherapy. It is the description and analysis of the costs of medications and pharmaceutical services and their effects on individuals, health care systems, and society.[14] The means through which value is determined is by way of economic evaluations, which identify, measure, and compare the costs and consequences of a pharmaceutical product or service. The four common types of economic evaluations utilized in pharmacoeconomics are (1) cost-minimization analysis; (2) cost–benefit analysis; (3) cost-effectiveness analysis; and (4) cost–utility analysis.[15]

Before one can elucidate the differences between these analyses, one must have a general grasp on what constitutes cost. In economics, costs are the combination of losses of any goods that have value attached to them by any one individual.[12] Cost can be broken down into direct, indirect, intangible, and incremental.[15] In health care, direct costs are resources consumed in the prevention, detection, or treatment of disease or illness. This can be further divided into cost associated with medical care and nonmedical cost. Within medical cost, there can be fixed cost, which remains constant, and variable cost. Fixed costs include items like electricity or lighting and are not routinely included in an analysis. Variable costs include items like medications, hospitalization, and laboratory costs. Examples of nonmedical costs are costs as a result of the disease or illness, like transportation to appointments. The aforementioned indirect costs are costs that occur as a result of morbidity or mortality, such as income lost because of premature death. Intangible costs are cost that represent nonfinancial outcomes of the disease and medical care. Examples of this cost include costs from pain and suffering; assigning value to these is challenging. The final cost, incremental cost, is the extra cost needed to purchase an additional benefit or effect of the medical care. For example, in heart failure it would be additional medications beyond the standard of care to control the disease state.

The above mentioned costs create the backbone of the economic evaluations previously outlined. Understanding the difference between analyses helps clinicians answer pharmacoeconomic questions and interpret results published in the literature.[11] The first evaluation tool is the cost-minimization analysis.[15] In this analysis, costs are expressed in monetary terms, and outcomes are considered equivalent. In this design, investigators can compare the cost of two or more treatment alternatives, treatments, or services that are determined to be equal in efficacy. This type of analysis provides results in terms of cost savings and provides information on the least expensive alternative. The advantage of this type of analysis is that it is relatively simple, but the disadvantage is the need for the intervention(s) to be equivalent.

One of the most common analyses is the cost–benefit analysis.[15] In this evaluation, outcomes of the treatment are expressed in monetary terms with the cost of resources consumed. The resources consumed by the intervention are measured in dollars. Benefits are also converted to a dollar amount. Results are expressed as either a cost–benefit ratio or a net cost/net benefit. The advantage of this analysis is that one can compare alternatives with different outcomes; however, the disadvantage is the difficulty in assigning monetary value to health benefits or consequences.

The third evaluation is the cost-effectiveness analysis in which two or more treatment alternatives or programs in which resources used are measured in monetary terms and outcomes in natural health units (eg, blood pressure).[15] The aim of cost-effectiveness analysis is to determine which alternative can either produce the desired effect or demonstrate the most optimal alternative which may (or may not) be the least expensive. The advantage of this analysis is that outcomes are readily understood by providers and need not be converted to monetary values; the disadvantage is that alternatives used in comparison must have outcomes measured in the same units.

The final evaluation, which is a form of a cost-effectiveness analysis, is the cost–utility analysis in which two or more treatment alternatives or programs in which resources are measured in monetary terms and outcomes are expressed in patient preferences or quality of life or quality-adjusted life-years (QALYs).[15] The outcomes of this type of analysis determine the life-years gained and then multiplied by the utility of that life-year. A great example of the use of a cost–utility analysis can be found in the 2018 American College of Cardiology Guidelines on the Management of Blood Cholesterol.[16] In this guideline, the authors suggested, based on mid-2018 medication list prices in the simulations, that proprotein convertase subtilisin/kexin type 9 (PCSK9) inhibitors had an incremental cost-effectiveness ratio from $141,700 to $450,000 per QALY added when used in secondary-prevention patients with atherosclerotic cardiovascular disease. For perspective, most experts consider less than $50,000 per QALY added to be of "good" value and $150,000 or more per QALY to be added cost. The advantage of this analysis is that different outcomes are compared using a common unit (eg, QALY) without requiring a monetary value. The challenge of this analysis is the difficulty in determining an accurate QALY and it is less precise than natural health units.

PHARMACOVIGILANCE AND PHARMACOEPIDEMIOLOGY

Within the regulatory environment, it is critical that medication therapy demonstrates its efficacy within the confines of clinical trials prior to approval. These trials are the foundation for approval of their release into the market for treatment in patients. All these trials include safety analyses in order to also assure harm is limited and/or to determine any unforeseen adverse effects. However, preapproval trials have many limitations including populations limited by size or demographics, narrow indications of use, and boundaries on duration.[17] These limitations may not provide a complete prolife of adverse drug events (ADE) or their true severity. In order to evaluate medication safety beyond the confines of the clinical trial or post approval, the use of pharmacovigilance is instituted.

Pharmacovigilance, as defined by the World Health Organization, is the science and activities related to the detection, assessment, understanding, and prevention of adverse effects or any other drug-related problem.[18] The scope of pharmacovigilance is broad and includes, but is not limited to, rare and expected adverse events, adverse events in high-risk groups, adverse events in long-term use, drug–drug interactions, drug–food interactions, misuse or abuse of product, manufacturing issues, and medication errors.[19] In addition, pharmacovigilance activities include mechanisms to address safety during studies in the preapproval process in addition to post-marketing actions.

The United States Code of Federal Regulations, which guides the FDA, classifies an adverse drug event/experience as any undesirable event that is associated with the use of a drug in humans, whether or not considered drug related, and occurs in the course of the use of a drug product in professional practice.[19] Thus, pharmacovigilance efforts devise systems to monitor these events, evaluate them, and communicate them to medical professionals and the public. A general overview of pharmacovigilance activities in relation to pre- and post-market approval are detailed in **Figure 3.1**.

The process and science of monitoring the safety of medications and taking action to reduce risk and increase benefit within pharmacovigilance is called risk management.[17] Through risk management, a systematic approach is implemented given the numerous sources and locations through which adverse drug information is collected.[20] These sources can include voluntary reporting systems, clinical trials, meta-analysis, and registry data. Having a systematic approach allows investigators and regulators to efficiently perform risk identification via monitoring for a safety signal. A safety signal is established with any new reported information on a possible causal relationship between an adverse event and a drug, with the relationship being unknown or incompletely documented, an increased occurrence of a known labeled event, a labeled event at a greater severity, or an event in a new at-risk population. Furthermore, a safety signal is usually supported by multiple case reports either in the literature or via an agency's adverse event reporting system, such as the FDA's Adverse Reporting System (FAERS).

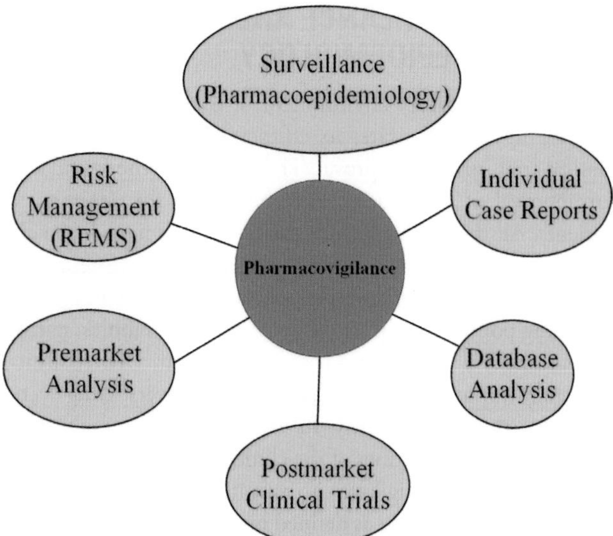

FIGURE 3.1 An overview of pharmacovigilance activities and methods. Regulators work to ensure the ongoing safety of medications approved for use through a variety of methods, collectively known as pharmacovigilance. These can range from premarket activities, such as risk mitigation programs, to identifying unanticipated risk via case reporting or database analysis. In some cases, postmarket clinical trials may be required to assess safety.

Cardiovascular pharmacovigilance activities have been strongly supported by the FDA in recent decades. These largely stemmed from the unanticipated detection of excess cardiovascular events with noncardiovascular therapies, such as rofecoxib and rosiglitazone.[21,22] In both cases, these medications were approved for use for substantial intervals of time before phase IV clinical trials gradually revealed adverse cardiovascular events when pooled together.[22,23] The withdrawal of rofecoxib subsequently led to substantial reevaluation of the risk versus benefits of FDA-approved cyclooxygenase-2 (COX-2) inhibitors. In the case of rosiglitazone, the FDA determined in 2008 that all newly approved diabetes medications must undergo Phase IV evaluation to determine cardiovascular safety.[24] Ironically, this may have led to the serendipitous discovery of the benefits of dapagliflozin in treating patients with heart failure, where it appears that those with and without diabetes benefit substantially from the drug in addition to standard heart failure medical therapy.[25] Another example where pharmacovigilance activities needed to be applied was in the discovery of the p-glycoprotein (P-gp) system in drug transport and clearance.[26] Many cardiovascular drugs (eg, amiodarone, diltiazem, colchicine, etc) were substrates of this transporter, and clinical events related to coadministration with P-gp inhibitors were linked to significant adverse events and toxicities through the FAERS system. This led to significant revision of product labeling to provide guidance to clinicians on the management of this new drug–drug interaction.

Premarket pharmacovigilance activities are also increasingly used by regulators on a case-by-case basis upon drug approval. In 2002, the Prescription Drug User Fee Act III led to the creation of Risk Minimization Action Plans (RiskMAPs) that allowed some drugs with significant safety concerns to be used in patients under a structured management program.[27] Examples of cardiovascular medications approved with RiskMAPs include endothelin antagonists used in pulmonary hypertension that confer significant fetal teratogenicity, and the antiarrhythmic dofetilide that may potentially cause sudden cardiac death via QT prolongation. Legislation changes in 2008 allowed the FDA to more broadly require various actions by a company to mitigate risk to patients; these have become collectively known as Risk Evaluation and Mitigation Strategies (REMS) and can be used when the FDA determines a risk to safety is present that is not sufficiently minimized by the standard product labeling.[28] Previous RiskMAPs programs have been recategorized under this new initiative. REMS programs vary from drug to drug but include activities such as pharmacist and provider certification, restricted dispensing, patient registries, and simpler plans such as mandatory medication guide provision or communication plan development with a patient regarding the risks versus benefits of a given therapy. Cardiovascular therapies under current REMS programs are detailed in **Table 3.2**.

Once a safety signal is identified, investigators or regulators may use principles of pharmacoepidemiology to further characterize the benefits and risk of a medication. Pharmacoepidemiology is the study of the use and effects of drugs in large, defined populations and may be used extensively in pharmacovigilance programs.[29] Pharmacoepidemiologic studies have many benefits, including the ability to detect adverse events that are rare or not detected in clinical trials, the ability to detect efficacy and safety over longer durations of time, and the ability to review use of therapy in a real-world setting beyond the controlled population and monitoring of a trial. For example, geriatric patients are often excluded from many cardiovascular trials, and thus data regarding medication use in this population can be explored via these mechanisms. Pharmacoepidemiologic approaches have also increasingly been used by regulators as technology has developed and data analytic capabilities improve; this may be considered the "big picture" monitoring of drug safety as opposed to the specific scrutiny applied to REMS programs. A classic example in the cardiovascular literature to demonstrate the use of pharmacoepidemiology to perform pharmacovigilance is the study reporting the rates of hyperkalemia associated with spironolactone use after the publication of the Randomized Aldactone Evaluation Study (RALES) trial.[30] The authors performed a population-based, time-series analysis to examine trends in the rate of spironolactone prescriptions and rates of hospitalization for hyperkalemia in ambulatory heart failure patients with reduced ejection fraction after the publication of RALES. They were able to demonstrate an abrupt increase in the rate of both spironolactone prescriptions and hyperkalemia-associated morbidity and mortality. The authors suspected this was owing to indiscriminate patient selection in the real-world setting.

TABLE 3.2 Cardiovascular Medications with Risk Evaluation and Mitigation Strategies (REMS) by the U.S. Food and Drug Administration (FDA)

Drug	Mechanism of Action	Use in Cardiovascular Disease	Rationale	Mitigation Strategies
Ambrisentan Bosentan Macitentan	Endothelin receptor antagonist (ETRA)	Pulmonary hypertension	Teratogenicity	• Mandatory provider certification and education • Mandatory pharmacy certification and education • Mandatory patient education and annual assessment of contraception • Documentation of negative pregnancy status
Riociguat	Soluble guanylate cyclase (sGC) stimulator	Pulmonary hypertension	Teratogenicity	• Mandatory provider certification and education • Mandatory pharmacy certification and education • Mandatory patient education and annual assessment of contraception • Documentation of negative pregnancy status
Tolvaptan	Vasopressin antagonist	Heart failure with hyponatremia	Hepatotoxicity	• Mandatory provider certification and education • Mandatory pharmacy certification and education • Mandatory patient education • Mandatory liver function monitoring

This study also highlights potential limitations of these studies that can include confounding and bias.

One of the biggest challenges with any identified risk is to assure that there is some causality from the suspected medication.[18,19] Investigators and regulators will assure the adverse event(s) happen at an expected timeframe that are consistent with the medication's pharmacokinetics. They will also attempt to assure absence of symptoms, when able, prior to exposure. In a case report/series, they will attempt to rechallenge or dechallenge patients to determine if the adverse effect re-occurs. They will also try to determine a potential biologic mechanism as well as confirm that there are no alternative explanations. Importantly, the FDA relies on public reporting of adverse effects via FAERS. In many cases, a pooling of rare case events or reports has led to labeling changes by regulators prior to substantial knowledge of the risk in the medical community.

Once a risk is identified and confirmed, investigators or regulators must establish a risk–benefit profile of efficacy versus safety in order to determine appropriate next steps.[20] It may be deemed that the drug should be avoided in the population at risk or additional monitoring may need to occur in order to change the risk–benefit profile. In some cases, the risk may so significantly outweigh the benefit that the medication should be removed from the market. If regulatory agencies determine a drug is safe to remain on the market, then they must provide a means of communicating any changes to the label as well and establish risk management plans when needed. Common risk management plans include required documented prescriber training in order to use, pharmacist certification to dispense, restricted dispensing to certain populations, recommended/required additional patient testing, and patient registries. Overall, these activities help make new and existing medications demonstrate value to the global public while also lowering unintended risk of adverse effects.

KEY POINTS

- ✔ Pharmacogenomics is increasingly being applied to cardiovascular pharmacotherapy with several commercially available pathways designed to individualize therapy on the basis of genetic polymorphisms.
- ✔ Pharmacoeconomic analyses are commonly used to assess cost-effectiveness of new therapies, especially those that only incrementally improve disease processes.
- ✔ Pharmacovigilence activities are widely used by regulatory agencies to mitigate known risk (e.g, dofetilide) or to monitor for unexpected safety concerns that arise (e.g., rosiglitazone).

REFERENCES

1. Cavallari LH, Weitzel K. Pharmacogenomics in cardiology—genetics and drug response: 10 years of progress. *Future Cardiol.* 2015;11:281-286.
2. Johnson JA. Pharmacogenetics: potential for individualized drug therapy through genetics. *Trends Genet.* 2003;19:660-666.
3. Roden DM, Van Driest SL, Wells QS, Mosley JD, Denny JC, Peterson JF. Opportunities and challenges in cardiovascular pharmacogenomics: from discovery to implementation. *Circ Res.* 2018;122:1176-1190.
4. Johnson JA, Cavallari LH. Pharmacogenetics and cardiovascular disease—implications for personalized medicine. *Pharmacol Rev.* 2013; 65:987-1009.
5. U.S. Food and Drug Administration. Table of pharmacogenomics biomarkers in drug labeling. Accessed February 21, 2020. https://www.fda.gov/drugs/science-and-research-drugs/table-pharmacogenomic-biomarkers-drug-labeling
6. Magdy T, Burridge PW. Pharmacogenomics in cardio-oncology. *American College of Cardiology.* Published May 07, 2017. Accessed January 25, 2021. https://www.acc.org/latest-in-cardiology/articles/2017/02/20/09/27/pharmacogenomics-in-cardio-oncology

7. Magdy T, Burmeister BT, Burridge PW. Validating the pharmacogenomics of chemotherapy-induced cardiotoxicity: what is missing? *Pharmacol Ther.* 2016;168:113-125.
8. Cavallari LH, Lee CR, Duarte JD, et al. Implementation of inpatient models of pharmacogenetics programs. *Am J Health Syst Pharm.* 2016;73:1944-1954.
9. Weitzel KW, Cavallari LH, Lesko LJ. Preemptive panel-based pharmacogenetic testing: the time is now. *Pharm Res.* 2017;34:1551-1555.
10. Constable S, Johnson MR, Pirmohamed M. Pharmacogenetics in clinical practice: considerations for testing. *Expert Rev Mol Diagn.* 2006;6:193-205.
11. Sibbing D, Aradi D, Alexopoulos D, et al. Updated expert consensus statement on platelet function and genetic testing for guiding P2Y12 receptor inhibitor treatment in percutaneous coronary intervention. *JACC Cardiovasc Interv.* 2019;12:1521-1537.
12. Relling MV, Klein TE, Gammal RS, Whirl-Carrillo M, Hoffman JM, Caudle KE. The clinical pharmacogenetics implementation consortium: 10 years later. *Clin Pharmacol Ther.* 2020;107:171-175.
13. Valgus J, Weitzel KW, Peterson JF, Crona DJ, Formea CM. Current practices in the delivery of pharmacogenomics: impact of the recommendations of the Pharmacy Practice Model Summit. *Am J Health Syst Pharm.* 2019;76:521-529.
14. Grauer DW, Lee T, Odom T, et al. *Pharmacoeconomics & Outcomes: Applications for Patient Care.* Amer College of Clinical Pharmacy; 2003.
15. Drummond MF, ed. *Methods for the Economic Evaluation of health Care Programmes.* 3rd ed., reprint. Oxford University Press; 2007.
16. Grundy SM, Stone NJ, Bailey AL, et al. 2018 AHA/ACC/AACVPR/AAPA/ABC/ACPM/ADA/AGS/APhA/ASPC/NLA/PCNA guideline on the management of blood cholesterol: executive summary: a report of the American College of Cardiology/American Heart Association Task Force on Clinical Practice Guidelines. *J Am Coll Cardiol.* 2019;73:3168-3209.
17. Beninger P. Pharmacovigilance: an overview. *Clin Ther.* 2018;40:1991-2004.
18. World Health Organization. Pharmacovigilance. Accessed April 1, 2021. https://www.who.int/teams/regulation-prequalification/regulation-and-safety/pharmacovigilance
19. Tobenkin A. An introduction to drug safety surveillance and the FDA adverse event reporting system. Accessed February 27, 2020. https://www.fda.gov/files/about%20fda/published/Drug-Safety-Surveillance-and-the-FDA-Adverse-Event-Reporting-System-%28PDF—1.31MB%29.pdf
20. Jalali R. Risk management in pharmacovigilance. In: Vohora D, Singh G, eds. *Pharmaceutical Medicine and Translational Clinical Research.* Elsevier/Academic Press; 2018.
21. Mukherjee D, Nissen SE, Topol EJ. Risk of cardiovascular events associated with selective COX-2 inhibitors. *JAMA.* 2001;286:954-9.
22. Nissen SE, Wolski K. Effect of rosiglitazone on the risk of myocardial infarction and death from cardiovascular causes. *N Engl J Med.* 2007;356:2457-2471.
23. Jüni P, Nartey L, Reichenbach S, Sterchi R, Dieppe PA, Egger M. Risk of cardiovascular events and rofecoxib: cumulative meta-analysis. *Lancet.* 2004;364:2021-2029.
24. U.S. Food and Drug Administration. Guidance for industry: diabetes mellitus—evaluating cardiovascular risk in new antidiabetic therapies to treat type 2 diabetes. Published 2008. Accessed April 1, 2021 https://www.fda.gov/media/71297/download
25. McMurray JJV, Solomon SD, Inzucchi SE, et al. Dapagliflozin in patients with heart failure and reduced ejection fraction. *N Engl J Med.* 2019;381:1995-2008.
26. Wessler JD, Grip LT, Mendell J, Giugliano RP. The P-glycoprotein transport system and cardiovascular drugs. *J Am Coll Cardiol.* 2013;61:2495-2502.
27. Balian JD, Wherry JC, Malhotra R, Perentesis V. Roadmap to risk evaluation and mitigation strategies (REMS) success. *Ther Adv Drug Saf.* 2010;1:21-38.
28. Nelson LS, Loh M, Perrone J. Assuring safety of inherently unsafe medications: the FDA risk evaluation and mitigation strategies. *J Med Toxicol.* 2014;10:165-172.
29. West-Strum D. Introduction to pharmacoepidemiology. In: Yang Y, West-Strum D, eds. *Understanding Pharmacoepidemiology.* McGraw-Hill Education/Medical; 2010.
30. Juurlink DN, Mamdani MM, Lee DS, et al. Rates of hyperkalemia after publication of the Randomized Aldactone Evaluation Study. *N Engl J Med.* 2004;351:543-551.

CHAPTER 4

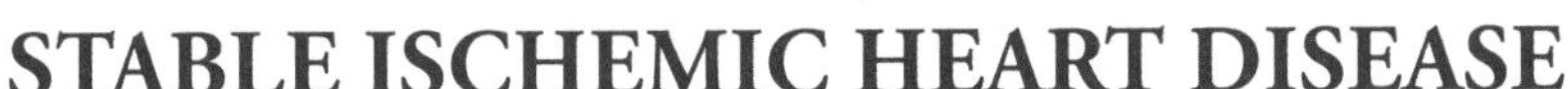

STABLE ISCHEMIC HEART DISEASE

Gharibyan Rosie Jasper and James C. Blankenship

INTRODUCTION

Epidemiology

Coronary artery disease (CAD) remains the leading cause of death and morbidity worldwide. Cardiovascular disease (CVD) remains the number one cause of death in the United States, accounting for one in three deaths, and it claims more lives than all cancers and pulmonary diseases combined.[1] The overall CAD prevalence is 6.7% (18.2 million) in US adults over 20 years of age and is higher in men (7.4%) than in women (6.2%). Over the past two decades, the incidence of CAD declined from 3.9 to 2.2 per 1000 person-years in people without diabetes and from 11.1 to 5.4 per 1000 person-years among those with diabetes.[2] The lifetime risk of developing CAD in 40-year-old persons is greater than 40% in men and greater than 30% in women. Of note, the incidence of angina rises continuously with age in women. Stable angina or stable ischemic heart disease (SIHD) is the most common presentation of CAD in women, compared to acute myocardial infarction (MI) and sudden coronary death in men. The direct and indirect costs of heart disease in 2014 to 2015 were estimated at $219 billion in the United States, 42% of which was spent on persons over 60 years of age. Chronic CAD and MI were two of the 10 most expensive conditions treated in US hospitals and accounted for 14% of total health expenditures in 2014 to 2015.[2]

Risk Factors

The traditional risk factors for atherosclerosis include age, sex, smoking, hypertension, hyperlipidemia, obesity, metabolic syndrome, diabetes mellitus, sedentary lifestyle, and family history. Nontraditional risk factors include socioeconomic and psychosocial stress, autoimmune diseases, malignancy and its therapies, infections, sleep apnea, and pregnancy-related complications.

PATHOGENESIS

Angina pectoris is the result of myocardial ischemia caused by an imbalance between myocardial blood supply and oxygen demand. Myocardial ischemia typically results from a reduction of coronary blood flow caused by fixed and/or dynamic epicardial coronary artery stenosis. Less commonly, it may be due to abnormal constriction (or deficient relaxation) of coronary microcirculation, markedly increased myocardial oxygen demands (ie, malignant hypertension, severe aortic stenosis), or reduced oxygen-carrying capacity of the blood (ie, severe anemia, carboxyhemoglobin).

Coronary stenosis is typically caused by atherosclerosis, affecting large and medium size arteries. Atherosclerosis begins in young adulthood, as demonstrated by an incidence of coronary atherosclerosis of 45% to 75% in soldiers killed in combat.[3] The disease progresses in an indolent fashion and is usually clinically silent for many decades.

CLINICAL PRESENTATION

Common Signs and Symptoms

Identifying individuals with cardiac chest pain or SIHD requires careful evaluation of the patient's history, examination, testing, and risk. Traditionally, "typical angina" is described as substernal chest discomfort with: (1) ischemic quality and duration; (2) exacerbation by exercise and/or emotional stress; and (3) relief by rest and/or nitrates. "Atypical angina" meets two of the above three characteristics, whereas "non-anginal chest pain" meets only one or none. It is generally safe to assume symptoms are noncardiac if the symptoms meet criteria for "non-anginal" and an alternative diagnosis is readily apparent (eg, chest pain reproducible by palpation in a trauma patient). A diagnosis of "non-anginal chest pain," with only one of the three characteristics present, carries intermediate risk for CAD in women older than 60 years and men older than 40 years.

Angina pectoris is characterized by pain in the retrosternal and/or surrounding areas, often radiating to the jaw, epigastrium, and left shoulder and arm. It is often described as a pressure-like, constricting, burning, or squeezing sensation. It may be accompanied by dyspnea, fatigue, and nausea. The Canadian Cardiovascular Society classification is widely used to grade the severity of typical angina (**Table 4.1**).[4]

Diabetic patients with coronary disease are more likely to have "noncardiac" chest pain compared to nondiabetics. However, diabetics and nondiabetics have similar ratios of "typical" to "atypical" angina, and most diabetics have typical angina when they present with symptomatic SIHD.

Physical Examination Findings

The physical examination is often unremarkable in stable CAD. Physical examination findings, which are nonspecific, but may accompany CAD, include the presence of S4, S3, mitral regurgitation murmur, rales, carotid bruit, diminished pedal pulse,

TABLE 4.1 Grading of Angina Severity by the Canadian Cardiovascular Society

Class I	Ordinary physical activity does not cause angina, such as walking, climbing stairs, etc. Angina with strenuous or rapid or prolonged exertion at work or with recreation
Class II	Slight limitation of ordinary activity such as walking uphill, walking rapidly, climbing stairs after meals, or cold, or in wind, or under emotional stress or upon first hours after awakening.
Class III	Marked limitation of ordinary physical activity. Angina on walking one or two blocks or one flight of stairs.
Class IV	Inability to carry on any physical activity without discomfort; and may be present at rest

retinal exudates, and xanthomas. Reproducible chest wall pain/pressure in two studies of nontrauma patients significantly correlated with a noncardiac etiology of chest pain. Chest pain that is reproduced by coughing, deep inspiration, lying supine, moving arms and shoulders, rotating the torso, or swallowing is usually not due to myocardial ischemia

Differential Diagnosis

The majority of patients presenting with chest pain in an outpatient setting have noncardiac etiologies, and these conditions should be considered in the differential diagnosis of chest pain or SIHD (**Table 4.2**).

DIAGNOSIS

Patient Risk and Recommendations for Further Testing

The diagnosis of CAD starts with the clinical history including assessment of risk factors and comorbidities, physical examination, and the electrocardiogram (ECG). Patient-specific risk can be assessed using probability estimate models, which are derived from basic variables including age, gender, symptom characteristics, presence of risk factors, and ECG findings (Q waves, ST/T waves).[5] The factors most consistently associated with CAD are the patient's age and gender.

The limitations of probability estimate models include the following: (1) underrepresentation of the elderly and specific populations; (2) tendency to overestimate risk; (3) poor performance in women because of the lower prevalence of obstructive CAD; and (4) their performance is compared to prevalence of obstructive CAD on imaging (ie, cardiac computed tomography angiography [CCTA] or coronary angiography) and may not necessarily reflect clinical outcomes. The 2014 ACC/AHA/AATS/PCNA/SCAI/STS Focused Update of the Guideline for the Diagnosis and Management of Patients with SIHD references the Diamond-Forrester and Updated Diamond-Forrester estimate models for the determination of pretest probability.[6] Critical concepts for assessing pretest likelihood include the following:

(a) If the probability of disease is less than 5%, additional testing is not recommended, as false-positive test results are more likely than true-positive test results.
(b) Patients with intermediate probability for CAD (15%-85%) benefit the most from further testing and warrant noninvasive functional or anatomic cardiac evaluation, the results of which should be interpreted with a Bayesian approach. The type of noninvasive stress test employed depends upon patient characteristics, baseline ECG, ability to exercise, physician preference, and test availability. Stress testing with exercise or pharmacologic stress testing is the "gold standard" for provoking cardiac ischemia and for detecting effects of ischemia by ECG changes, perfusion abnormality, or regional wall motion abnormality. In comparison to functional stress testing, CCTA and cardiac magnetic resonance angiography (CMRA) allow anatomic analysis of coronary obstruction similar to invasive coronary angiography. **Algorithm 4.1** provides guidance on choice of noninvasive study for the evaluation of newly suspected SIHD or change in clinical status in a patient with SIHD.
(c) If the probability of disease or risk of mortality is high, then early angiography without stress testing is recommended because stress testing has an unacceptably high rate of false-negative results and will not alter the need for invasive evaluation.

Noninvasive Stress (Functional) Testing

Stress testing involves either exercise testing or pharmacologic stress testing with the use of dobutamine or vasodilators (ie, adenosine, regadenoson, or dipyridamole). Exercise testing is preferred. Exercise testing without imaging provides information about prognosis based on threshold for ischemia, reproduction of and correlation with symptoms, and exercise tolerance. Imaging (ie, echocardiography, radionuclide scintigraphy, or magnetic resonance imaging) provides additional sensitivity.

Table 4.3 summarizes the sensitivity and specificity of different stress modalities, including guideline-graded recommendations and specific benefits and pitfalls of each modality. In summary, the guidelines give a Class I recommendation for exercise as an initial stress modality if the patient is able to perform moderate exercise and has an interpretable ECG. For patients with baseline ECG abnormalities, exercise with imaging should be performed. If patients are unable to exercise, then pharmacologic stress testing with imaging is recommended.

Noninvasive Anatomic Imaging

Cardiac Computed Tomography Angiography

The role of CCTA as an initial diagnostic test for CAD has been validated in randomized controlled trials (RCTs).[7] CT imaging

TABLE 4.2 Differential Diagnosis of Chest Pain

Diagnosis	Characteristics of Chest Pain	Typical Physical Findings, if Present
Cardiac		
Stable ischemic heart disease	Chronic typical or atypical angina	None
Acute coronary syndrome	Unstable angina (progressive, new onset, or new occurrence of rest angina)	None
Arrhythmias	Palpitations	Irregular heart sounds
Aortic dissection	Sharp or *tearing*, sudden onset radiating from substernal to intrascapular	Loss of carotid or upper extremity pulses, stroke
Pericarditis	Pleuritic pain relieved by sitting up	Friction rub
Pulmonary		
Pulmonary embolus	Pleuritic pain with dyspnea	Pleural friction rub
Pneumothorax	Acute onset, pleuritic, with dyspnea	Diminished breath sounds unilaterally
Pleuritis	Pleuritic pain	Pleural friction rub
Gastrointestinal		
Esophageal disease	Substernal pain or pressure, sharp or dull	None
Gastroesophageal reflux	Substernal and/or epigastric burning	None
Biliary	Right upper quadrant pain radiating to back or scapula	Right upper quadrant tenderness
Pancreatitis	Epigastric pain, may be boring, radiating to back	Epigastric tenderness
Musculoskeletal		
Costochondritis	Chest wall tenderness	Pain to palpation
Chest trauma	Inspiratory pain, chest wall tenderness	Pain to palpation or with motion of torso and shoulders
Fibrositis	Chest wall pain	Pain to palpation
Dermatologic		
Herpes zoster	Radicular pain	Rash
Psychiatric		
Anxiety, depression	Nonexertional, related to emotion or stress, may be accompanied by acute anxiety, hyperventilation, palpitations, diaphoresis	Physical signs of anxiety (eg, pressured speech) or depression (eg, flat affect)
Schizophrenia	Atypical pattern	Schizophrenic affect
Factitious (ie, Munchausen)	Atypical pattern	None

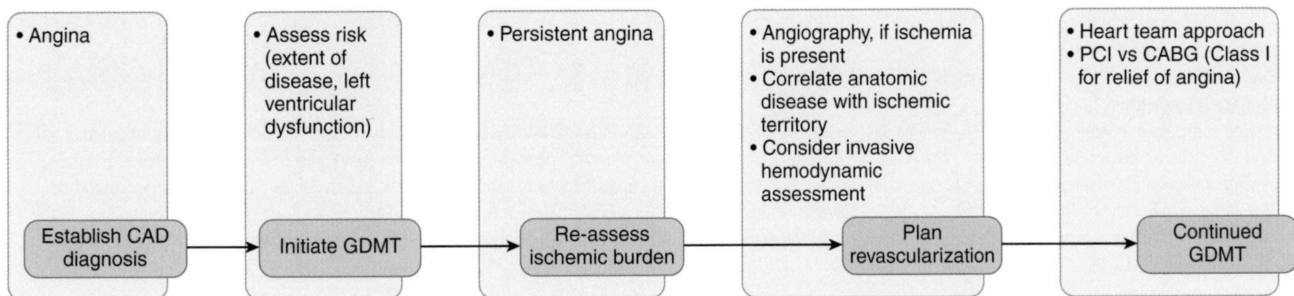

ALGORITHM 4.1 Guidelines on noninvasive versus invasive therapy in suspected disease or established disease with new clinical change. CABG, coronary artery bypass graft; CAD, coronary artery disease; GDMT, guideline-directed medical therapy; PCI, percutaneous coronary intervention.

TABLE 4.3 Noninvasive Functional Stress Testing Modalities and Guideline Recommendations

Testing Modality	Sensitivity and Specificity for Obstructive CAD	Benefits and Pitfalls	Guideline Recommendations ACCF/AHA 2012 and ESC 2013
Exercise electrocardiography	Sensitivity: 61%[a] Specificity: 70%-77%[b] *Performs well in low- to intermediate-risk group (risk 10%-60%)*	Prognostic findings: exercise duration chronotropic incompetence, HR recovery angina arrhythmias blood pressure drop with exercise extent and duration of ST changes	**Class I** for intermediate-risk patients **Class IIa** for low-risk patients **Class III**—patients unable to exercise, using digitalis or have uninterpretable ECG *Rated the same for ACCF and ESC guidelines*
Exercise echocardiography	Sensitivity: 70%-85% Specificity: 77%-89%	Assessment of systolic and diastolic left ventricular function and response to stress	**Class Ib** for intermediate- to high-risk patients and uninterpretable ECG **Class IIa** (ESC) symptomatic patients with prior revascularization and to assess functional severity of intermediate coronary lesions
Dobutamine echocardiography	Sensitivity: 85%-90% Specificity: 79%-90%	Assesses viability better than exercise, favorable when there is resting wall motion abnormality	**Class Ia**—intermediate- to high-risk patients and unable to exercise **Class III**—not recommended if patient is able to exercise and has interpretable ECG
Exercise myocardial perfusion imaging	Sensitivity: 82%-88% Specificity: 70%-88%	Balanced flow reduction may lead to underestimation of extent of ischemia in multivessel or left main coronary disease. Transient ischemic dilation, reduced poststress ejection fraction, and increased uptake in lung field can help identify severe coronary artery disease.	**Class Ib** for intermediate- to high-risk patients **Class IIa** for intermediate- to high-risk patients and interpretable ECG **Class III**—in low-risk patients
Vasodilator[c] myocardial perfusion imaging	Sensitivity: 88%-91% Specificity: 75%-90%	Balanced flow reduction may lead to underestimation of extent of ischemia in multivessel or left main coronary disease.	**Class Ia**—intermediate- to high risk and unable to exercise **Class III**—not recommended if patient is able to exercise and has interpretable ECG
Cardiac magnetic resonance imaging with dobutamine or perfusion stress	Sensitivity: 88% Specificity: 72% Cardiac magnetic resonance angiography has shown good correlation with FFR measurements.	Not widely used	No recommendations

ACCF, American College of Cardiology Foundation; AHA, American Heart Association; CAD, coronary artery disease; ECG, electrocardiogram; ESC, European Society for Cardiology; FFR, fractional flow reserve; HR, heart rate.

[a]Valid in patients with normal ECG.

[b]Lower in women.

[c]Adenosine, regadenoson, or dipyridamole.

Compiled with data from Fihn SD, Gardin JM, Abrams J, et al. 2012 ACCF/AHA/ACP/AATS/PCNA/SCAI/STS Guideline for the diagnosis and management of patients with stable ischemic heart disease: a report of the American College of Cardiology Foundation/American Heart Association Task Force on Practice Guidelines, and the American College of Physicians, American Association for Thoracic Surgery, Preventive Cardiovascular Nurses Association, Society for Cardiovascular Angiography and Interventions, and Society of Thoracic Surgeons. *J Am Coll Cardiol.* 2012;60(24):e44-e164 and Montalescot G, Sechtem U, Achenbach S, et al. 2013 ESC guidelines on the management of stable coronary artery disease: The Task Force on the management of stable coronary artery disease of the European Society of Cardiology. *Eur Heart J.* 2013;34(38):2949-3003.

of the coronary arteries can be performed with or without intravenous iodinated contrast. With noncontrast CT, coronary calcifications as a reflection of atherosclerosis can be detected and quantified using the Agatston coronary artery calcium score.[8] The extent of coronary calcification correlates with the extent of atherosclerosis but does not imply luminal narrowing of the coronary arteries. Subsequently, the specificity of CCTA decreases with high calcium scores, leading to an overdiagnosis of obstructive CAD if the Agatston score is over 400.

Combined Imaging

Combined anatomic and physiologic imaging applications are currently under investigation. The combination of positron emission tomography (PET) or single-photon emission computed tomography (SPECT) and CT, fractional flow reserve (FFR) with CCTA, PET, and CMRA is available in selected centers. The benefit of combined imaging is the availability of hemodynamic assessment of an anatomic lesion. A drawback to this approach is an increase in radiation dosage. The 2012 and 2014 American College of Cardiology Foundation/American Heart Association (ACCF/AHA) guidelines do not include recommendations for hybrid imaging.[6,9,10]

Coronary Angiography

The role of coronary angiography in diagnosis of suspected CAD is discussed in detail in the 2014 ACCF/AHA guideline update.[6] In the majority of patients with suspected CAD, noninvasive stress testing is the initial diagnostic test. However, in high-risk patients in whom a negative stress test would be suspected of being falsely negative, angiography may be reasonable without prior stress testing. A coronary angiogram is performed to evaluate the severity of obstructive CAD, assess cardiovascular risk, and determine an approach for revascularization if indicated. Angiographic data regarding lesion complexity and vessel involvement are used to generate the SYNTAX score—scored from 0 to 60 with a higher score indicating a higher burden and complexity of CAD—and to formulate appropriate revascularization strategies.

Limitations of angiography include inter- and intraobserver variability in assessment of lesion severity and inability to predict hemodynamic significance of intermediate stenotic lesions. The evaluation of FFR is often necessary as an invasive assessment of physiologic significance of intermediate angiographic lesions (defined as 40%-70% luminal diameter narrowing).

MANAGEMENT OF PATIENTS WITH STABLE ISCHEMIC HEART DISEASE

Medical Approach

The treatment goals in stable CAD are to:

(1) reduce premature cardiovascular death; (2) prevent complications (ie, heart failure and MI); (3) maintain optimal functional capacity; (4) eliminate or decrease ischemic symptoms; and (5) minimize health care costs by eliminating unnecessary tests, procedures, and hospitalizations.[8]

Clinicians are obligated to help patients understand their disease etiology, clinical manifestations, and signals of worsening disease. Patients should be empowered to make shared decisions regarding revascularization options and actively participate in risk reduction, behavioral modification, and medication adherence.[11]

Antianginal Therapies

Nitrates. All patients with stable CAD should be prescribed sublingual nitroglycerin or a nitroglycerin spray for immediate relief of angina (Class Ib).[9] Long-acting formulations are recommended when an initial anginal therapy with maximum tolerated beta-blocker is not effective in preventing angina. Failure of nitrate therapy is often due to nitrate tolerance. Therefore, depending on nitrate formulation used, a 10- to 14-hour nitrate-free interval is indicated.

Beta-blockers. Beta-blockers should be prescribed as a first-line therapy for relief of ischemic symptoms in patients with stable CAD (Class I).[9] In the *Clinical Outcomes Utilizing Revascularization and Aggressive Drug Evaluation* (COURAGE) trial, patients with stable CAD and coronary stenosis greater than 70% on angiography who received a beta-blocker reported a 22% improvement in symptoms of angina, similar to results following percutaneous coronary intervention (PCI).[12] Similarly, in the *Objective Randomized Blinded Investigation with optimal medical Therapy of Angioplasty in stable angina* (ORBITA) trial, PCI did not improve exercise angina after medical therapy with beta-blockers was optimized.[13] All beta-blockers have similar efficacy in patients with angina. The dose of beta-blocker is titrated for a goal heart rate of 55 to 60 beats per minute. An abrupt discontinuation of beta-blockers may be poorly tolerated and is discouraged, as it can worsen angina and precipitate an acute coronary syndrome (ACS) (9).

Calcium Channel Blockers. The calcium channel blockers (CCBs) are as effective as beta-blockers in relieving angina and increasing angina-free exercise time. CCBs can be used alone as antianginal therapy, though their combination with nitrates and beta-blockers exerts a more potent antianginal effect. All CCB classes are equally efficacious in treating angina, and selection of a specific agent should be based on drug interactions and potential side effects. Dihydropyridine (DHP) CCBs or long-acting nitrates should be prescribed in combination with beta-blockers for relief of anginal symptoms (Class Ib).[9] Alternatively, long-acting non-DHP CCBs (ie, diltiazem or verapamil) can be considered instead of beta-blockers as initial therapy (Class IIa).[9]

Ranolazine. Ranolazine is a selective late sodium channel inhibitor that reduces sodium-dependent calcium currents in ischemic myocardium. It is administered orally in doses of 500 to 2000 mg daily to reduce angina and increase symptom-free exercise capacity. Ranolazine has antianginal efficacy when used as a monotherapy or in combination with first- and second-line antianginal agents and shows a more potent effect in diabetic patients with elevated hemoglobin A1C levels. Ranolazine can be useful as a substitute for beta-blockers for relief of angina in stable CAD (Class IIb) or in combination with beta-blockers (Class IIa).[9,10]

Ivabradine. Ivabradine was approved in the United States in 2015 for the treatment of heart failure with reduced ejection fraction (EF). Although it has not been approved in the United States for angina, it has been reported to have antianginal properties. Ivabradine as monotherapy improves treadmill test performance and decreases frequency of angina attacks with efficacy similar to that of beta-blockers and amlodipine.[14]

Other Antianginal Therapies. Nicorandil and trimetazidine are antianginal therapies not available in the United States but are used in Europe and other countries.[10]

Nonpharmacologic Therapies for Refractory Angina in Stable Ischemic Heart Disease

Individuals with refractory angina constitute approximately 10% of stable CAD patients. Refractory angina is defined as angina despite maximal medical therapy because of CAD that is not amenable to revascularization. Nonpharmacologic therapies may be considered in patients to improve quality of life.[6] These new therapies attempt to either (1) improve myocardial perfusion or (2) modulate afferent and efferent pain pathways to change perception of ischemic pain.[15]

Angiogenesis. Intracoronary or transendocardial injection of autologous cells ($CD34^+$, $CD133^+$) that activate myocardial angiogenesis can improve exercise capacity. Their therapeutic use for refractory angina is currently under review.[16]

Enhanced External Counterpulsation. The Food and Drug Administration (FDA) approved the use of enhanced external counterpulsation (EECP) in 1995 for the treatment of refractory angina. The full treatment course consists of 1-hour treatments, 5 days per week, for 35 sessions. Contraindications include heart failure, severe peripheral arterial disease (PAD), and aortic regurgitation. Studies have shown some benefit of EECP for treatment of refractory angina not responsive to conventional antianginal therapies.[15] EECP has a Class IIb (may be considered for refractory angina) indication for angina therapy per the ACCF/AHA 2014 guidelines.[6,15]

Chelation Therapy. Chelation therapy consists of intravenous infusion of disodium ethylene diamine tetraacetic acid. Small RCTs failed to show any benefit of chelation therapy in cardiovascular outcomes. Hence, its use was not endorsed in the 2012 ACCF/AHA SIHD guidelines. However, after the positive results of the *Trial to Assess Chelation Therapy* (TACT)[17] the recommendation for chelation was changed from Class III (harmful) to Class IIb (usefulness of chelation therapy is uncertain) in the 2014 ACCF/AHA guideline update on management and diagnosis of SIHD.[6]

Transmyocardial Revascularization. Transmyocardial revascularization (TMR) utilizes a laser that is surgically applied to the beating heart to drill holes in the epicardial surface of ischemic myocardium. In RCTs, TMR improved angina class and quality of life, but it failed to improve survival. Hence, TMR may be considered for relief of refractory angina in a patient with severe CAD, but it is rarely used in clinical practice in the United States (Class IIb ACCF/AHA 2012).[9] Trials of transcatheter TMR applied to the endocardial surface of ischemic myocardium failed to show significant benefit, and it is not used clinically.

Extracorporeal Shockwave Myocardial Revascularization. This technology uses ultrasound-guided, ECG-synchronized delivery of low acoustic energy waves via a shockwave applicator device applied to the chest wall to trigger vasodilation and angiogenesis in ischemic areas. Adverse side effects have not been reported, but it is contraindicated in patients with left ventricular (LV) mural thrombus. Small controlled studies report improvement in angina class and quality of life. Randomized studies and clear guideline recommendations are lacking.[16]

TENS and SENS. Stimulation of subcutaneous afferent nerves can modulate anginal pain sensation. Transcutaneous electrical nerve stimulation (TENS) uses chest electrodes and subcutaneous electrical nerve stimulation (SENS) uses parasternal subcutaneous electrodes. These procedures seem to be safe, but evidence of efficacy is lacking.[16]

Sympathectomy. Surgical or percutaneous radiofrequency sympathectomy can provide permanent denervation of the cervicothoracic stellate ganglion where sympathetic synaptic modulation occurs. By inhibiting efferent sympathetic myocardial stimulation, incessant arrhythmic and vasospastic myocardial activation can be treated. The use of this therapy is based on small, observational studies and lacks guideline recommendations.[16]

Spinal Cord Stimulation. Spinal cord stimulation at T1 to T2 levels has been studied in small cohorts (<200 patients) and has been found to help control refractory angina. It has a Class IIb indication in the 2012 ACCF/AHA guidelines.[9]

Medical Therapy to Reduce Cardiovascular Risk

Aspirin. Lifelong aspirin in doses of 75 to 162 mg daily is recommended for platelet inhibition in all patients with CAD (Class Ia). Compared to placebo, it reduces vascular events by 37%, unstable angina by 47%, and need for angioplasty by 53% (Antithrombotic Trialists' Collaboration).[18] It should be administered without interruption in patients undergoing PCI or coronary artery bypass graft (CABG) surgery. It can also be continued without interruption in most patients undergoing noncardiac surgery.

P2Y12 Inhibitors. Clopidogrel inhibits platelet aggregation by irreversible and selective P2Y12 receptor blockade. Clopidogrel is considered a reasonable alternative to aspirin (Class Ib)[9] in stable CAD patients. Prasugrel and ticagrelor have not been studied in SIHD patients and are not approved by the FDA for use in them.

Statins. In CAD patients, statin therapy decreases vascular events, rates of MI, CABG, and cardiovascular mortality. High-intensity statin therapy induces plaque regression in some patients.[19] The 2018 ACCF/AHA guideline recommendations for cholesterol management and therapy choices for patients with stable CAD are summarized in **Table 4.4**.[20] Reductions

TABLE 4.4 2018 ACCF/AHA Guideline Recommendations for Cholesterol Management and Therapy Choices for Patients with Stable Coronary Artery Disease

(a) High-intensity or maximally tolerated statin is recommended to reduce serum LDL cholesterol concentration by >50% (Class Ia).
(b) In very high-risk patients,[a] use serum LDL cholesterol threshold of 70 mg/dL to consider the addition of non-statin therapy.
(c) In very high-risk patients who have a serum LDL cholesterol concentration >70 mg/dL despite high-intensity statin therapy, addition of ezetimibe is reasonable (Class IIa) and addition of a PCSK9 inhibitor is reasonable, although long-term safety (>3 years) is uncertain (Class IIa).
(d) In not very high-risk patients who have a serum LDL cholesterol concentration >70 mg/dL despite high-intensity statin therapy, addition of ezetimibe is a Class IIb recommendation.
(e) Fibrate and niacin use is not endorsed in recent guidelines. Instead, statin therapy and lifestyle modifications are recommended for moderate and severe hypertriglyceridemia.

ACCF, American College of Cardiology Foundation; AHA, American Heart Association; CABG, coronary artery bypass graft; LDL, low-density lipoprotein; PCI, percutaneous coronary intervention; PCSK-9, proprotein convertase subtilisin/kexin type 9.
[a]Very high-risk patients are those with multiple major cardiovascular events, or one major event and multiple high-risk conditions (ie, diabetes mellitus, familial hypercholesterolemia, smoking, chronic kidney disease, heart failure, history of CABG or PCI).
Data from Grundy SM, Stone NJ, Bailey AL, et al. 2018 AHA/ACC/AACVPR/AAPA/ABC/ACPM/ADA/AGS/APhA/ASPC/NLA/PCNA guideline on the management of blood cholesterol: a report of the American College of Cardiology/American Heart Association Task Force on Clinical Practice Guidelines. *Circulation.* 2019;139(25):e1082-e1143.

in cardiovascular events and mortality with statins are dose dependent, leading to guideline recommendations to treat CAD patients with high-intensity statin therapy. For example, every 40 mg/dL reduction in low-density lipoprotein (LDL) cholesterol is associated with an additional 10% reduction in all-cause mortality and a 20% reduction in coronary mortality.[21] Proprotein convertase subtilisin/kexin type 9 (PCSK9) inhibitors (evolocumab and alirocumab) are monoclonal antibodies administered subcutaneously every 2 to 4 weeks to block the liver enzyme PCSK9, thereby lowering serum LDL cholesterol levels. They are reserved for patients with established CVD with serum LDL cholesterol greater than 70 mg/dL despite high-intensity statin therapy. Their use is associated with decreased atheroma volumes and cardiovascular events.

Beta-blockers. As noted earlier, beta-blockers reduce death and recurrent MI rates in patients who have suffered an ACS, especially an ST-elevation MI. Beta-blocker therapy started after an ACS should continue into the SIHD phase for a total of at least 3 years (Class Ib)[9,10] and indefinitely in all patients with LV dysfunction (EF <40%), unless contraindicated.

Angiotensin-Converting Enzyme Inhibitor/Angiotensin Receptor Blocker Therapy. In patients with stable CAD, angiotensin-converting enzyme inhibitor (ACE-I) therapy reduces overall mortality, nonfatal MI, and heart failure by 20% to 28%.[22] For adults with stable CAD who have systolic heart failure (EF < 40%), hypertension, or diabetes mellitus, therapy with an ACE-I is a Class Ia recommendation.[9,10] In the absence of heart failure or LV dysfunction, ACE-I use is a Class IIa indication.[23] An ACE-I/angiotensin receptor blocker (ARB) should be avoided in patients with hypotension or potassium levels greater than 5.5 mEq/L. ARB therapy is recommended for patients who are intolerant to ACE-I therapy (Class Ia). Simultaneous use of an ACE-I and an ARB is not recommended because of the high incidence of adverse outcomes.[9]

Patient Risk Factor Management

Lipid Management. Dietary approaches to reduce cholesterol include weight loss, replacing saturated and trans fatty acids with unsaturated fatty acids, adding fiber and plant stanols, and reducing dietary cholesterol intake (<200 mg/day) (Class Ib). Dietary changes can lower the serum LDL cholesterol by 10% to 15%.[24] The 2018 ACCF/AHA guideline recommendations for cholesterol management and therapy choices for patients with stable CAD are summarized in Table 4.4.[20]

Blood Pressure Management. Nonpharmacologic measures to reduce blood pressure should be implemented before starting antihypertensive drugs. These measures include exercise, weight loss, the DASH (Dietary Approach to Stop Hypertension) diet with low sodium intake (<1500 mg/day), high potassium intake (>3500 mg/day), and a restricted alcohol intake (<2 drinks daily for men and <1 drink daily for women).[25] The 2017 ACCF/AHA and 2018 European Society for Cardiology (ESC) guidelines target a blood pressure goal of less than 130/less than 80 mm Hg in patients with stable CAD. Beta-blockers, ACE-Is, and ARBs are Class I antihypertensive therapeutic choices in CAD patients. Further addition of DHP CCBs, thiazide diuretics, and mineralocorticoid receptor antagonists are advised if hypertension is not at goal.[26]

Diabetes Mellitus Management. Diabetes mellitus is a strong independent risk factor for CAD and should be managed diligently to improve cardiovascular risk. Type 1 diabetes mellitus is associated with a 10-fold increase in cardiovascular events, and type 2 diabetes mellitus increases cardiovascular mortality by two to six times.[27]

The 2018 ACC Expert Consensus Report for Cardiovascular Risk Reduction in Patients with Type 2 Diabetes Mellitus and Atherosclerotic Cardiovascular Disease recommends two novel classes of glucose-lowering therapies—sodium-glucose cotransporter 2 (SGLT2) inhibitors and glucagonlike peptide 1 (GLP-1) receptor agonists—that improve cardiovascular outcomes in diabetic patients with stable CAD already on metformin with hemoglobin A1c greater than 7%.[28] In large, well-conducted RCTs, agents in these two classes reduced cardiovascular deaths, acute MIs, and strokes; and SGLT2 inhibitors reduced heart failure hospitalizations.[28] The cardiovascular benefits of these therapies may result from their diuretic effect, weight loss, the ability to lower blood pressure and serum LDL cholesterol levels, and their anti-inflammatory effects.

Diet. A balanced caloric intake and adherence to a high-quality diet (prudent vs. western) reduce cardiovascular risk and improve blood pressure, serum glucose levels, and lipid metabolism. The ideal diet includes abundant fruits, vegetables, fiber, whole grains, nuts, legumes, and marine fish (rich in long chain omega-3 fatty acids) and avoids processed meats, sweetened beverages, refined grains, and dairy. Alcohol intake has a U-shaped effect on cardiac risk, with one to two drinks consumption per day associated with the lowest cardiovascular risk. Three to five cups of coffee or tea daily also reduce cardiovascular risk. A high-quality diet is more important for healthy individuals than supplemental vitamins and nutrients; their value, when added to a high-quality diet, is uncertain.[9,10]

Smoking Cessation. Smoking is an independent and modifiable risk factor for CAD. In the *Atherosclerosis Risk In Communities* (ARIC) study, smoking showed a dose-response relationship between pack-years of smoking and three outcomes—CAD, PAD, and stroke—with the strongest results for PAD. For CAD, the risk persisted up to 20 years after smoking cessation.[29] Behavioral and pharmacologic assistance (nicotine replacement, bupropion, varenicline) is safe and should be offered routinely and repeatedly to patients.

Exercise/Cardiac Rehab and Weight Loss. Guidelines recommend moderate- to vigorous-intensity exercise training five times a week, for 30 minutes per session. Exercise should be offered to CAD patients in the form of a cardiac rehab program to assess capacity and risk.[10] Numerous studies show protective effects of physical activity among cardiovascular patients.[30] Exercise is associated with decreased cardiovascular mortality as well as beneficial effects on comorbid conditions including lipid control, blood pressure, inflammation reduction, and psychological stress. In a large meta-analysis, exercise programs were associated with 28% risk reduction in mortality.[31]

Influenza and Pneumococcal Vaccines. Annual influenza and age-appropriate pneumococcal vaccination is recommended for patients with CAD, especially for those greater than 65 years of age[9,10] to decrease cardiovascular mortality and events.

Percutaneous and Surgical Revascularization

The goals of revascularization are to improve survival and/or relieve symptoms.[6] **Algorithm 4.2** provides guidance for revascularization to improve symptoms in patients with SIHD. Regardless of the revascularization approach, aggressive risk factor management and adherence to guideline-directed medical therapy remain paramount to successful management of CAD.

A Heart Team approach to revascularization and patient-centered decision-making are strongly recommended in all guidelines with collaboration among surgeons, interventionalists, and general cardiologists. Incorporation of the Society of Thoracic Surgeons (STS) risk score and the SYNTAX score (ie, assessments of the risk of mortality and morbidities with cardiac surgery and angiographic grading of the burden and complexity of CAD, respectively) into decisions about revascularization for multivessel and left main CAD is recommended (Class IIa).[9] Potential risks and benefits, such as early and late mortality, stroke, freedom from angina, and role of medical therapies related to PCI and CABG, should be discussed among physicians and with patients.

Clinical factors, in addition to angiographic findings, influence revascularization and are incorporated in the SYNTAX II score[32] that incorporates eight predictors: anatomic SYNTAX score, age, creatinine clearance, left ventricular ejection fraction (LVEF), presence of unprotected left main coronary artery (LMCA) disease, peripheral vascular disease, female sex, and chronic obstructive pulmonary disease. In addition to the SYNTAX II score, patient-specific circumstances that guide collaborative decision-making include: (1) feasibility and benefit from complete revascularization; (2) extent of LV dysfunction; (3) history of previous CABG, patency of internal mammary artery (IMA), and presence of anterior ischemia; (4) lesion complexity; (5) surgical risk; (6) presence of diabetes mellitus; (7) life expectancy; and (8) ability to comply with dual antiplatelet therapy.

Revascularization for Survival

A survival benefit with coronary revascularization (Class 1) is apparent in: (1) patients with left main diameter stenosis greater than or equal to 50%; ([2]) significant (≥70% diameter) stenosis in the proximal left anterior descending (LAD) plus one other major coronary artery; and (3) significant (>70% diameter stenosis) three-vessel disease.[33] Revascularization to improve survival is reasonable (Class IIa) in patients with significant (≥70% diameter) stenoses in two major coronary arteries with severe or extensive myocardial ischemia (eg, high-risk criteria on stress testing, abnormal FFR or >20% perfusion defect by myocardial perfusion stress imaging).[9]

Revascularization to improve survival is not recommended (Class III) for single-vessel disease in left circumflex or right coronary artery, without proximal LAD involvement, with only a small area of viable myocardium, or with a small area of ischemia on stress testing.[9]

Revascularization for Symptoms

CABG and PCI are rated as Class I indications for one or more significant coronary artery stenoses amenable to revascularization and unacceptable angina despite guideline-directed medical therapy.

Coronary Artery Bypass Graft Revascularization

A survival benefit is in favor of CABG in stable CAD with LMCA disease or multivessel disease when compared to medical therapy. In addition, there is a survival benefit with CABG

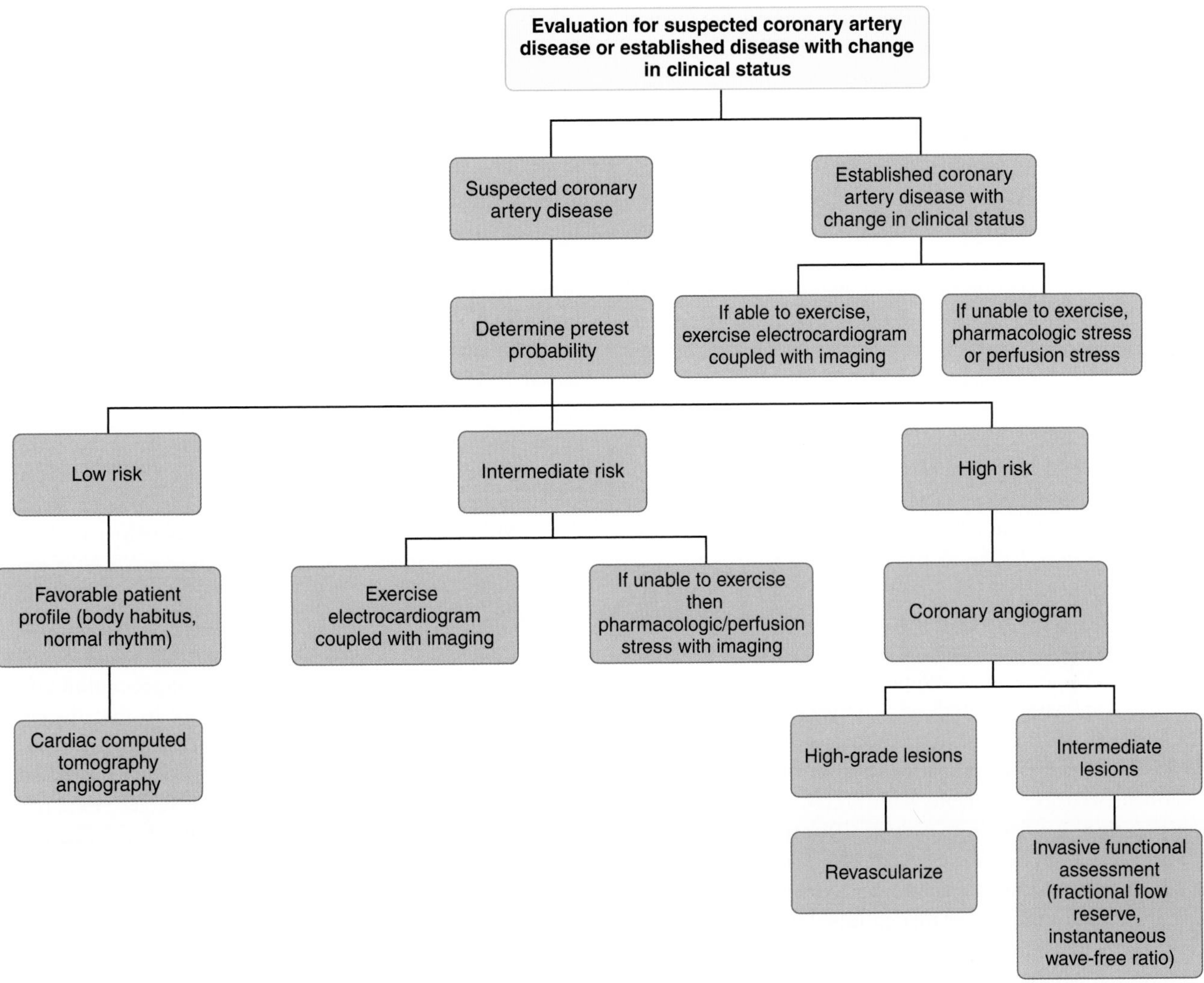

ALGORITHM 4.2 Approach to revascularization in an attempt to relieve angina.

in patients with two-vessel disease with involvement of the proximal LAD, especially with a high SYNTAX score and with diabetes mellitus.[9,33] Yusuf et al[34] noted fluctuating mortality benefits for CABG versus medical therapy, with an early hazard with surgery, followed by superior survival results 2 to 10 years after the surgery, followed by a drop in relative surgical benefit over medical therapy with long-term (>10 years) follow-up. Patients with the highest clinical risk profile had the most benefit from surgical revascularization (ie, LVEF 35% to 50%, evidence of moderate to severe ischemia on stress testing).[34]

Complete arterial revascularization with bilateral IMAs produces a significant survival benefit with a hazard ratio of 0.78 (confidence interval [CI] 0.72-0.84) when compared to patients receiving only a left IMA graft. In practice, bilateral IMA grafts are seldom employed because their use prolongs surgical time and is associated with an increased risk of sternal wound infections, particularly in diabetic and obese patients. Overall, the superiority of CABG compared to PCI relies on the longevity of the IMA graft, the ability to achieve complete revascularization, the improvement of flow in larger coronary beds compared to a focal treatment with stenting, and the prevention of ischemia from new lesions arising in the coronaries.[35]

Percutaneous Coronary Intervention Revascularization

Data are lacking to show improvement in mortality with PCI versus medical therapy in patients with stable CAD, although PCI does improve angina and quality of life.[36] PCI is more efficacious than medical therapy in reducing ACS and the need for urgent revascularization in patients who have a large ischemic burden on functional testing or an abnormal FFR.[37]

In the presence of angina or severe ischemia, PCI is recommended as a first-line revascularization strategy for one- or two-vessel CAD not involving the proximal LAD.[11] PCI is considered as a reasonable alternative to CABG for three-vessel CAD, or one- to two-vessel CAD with involvement of the proximal LAD when the SYNTAX score is low (<22) and in nondiabetics.

The *COURAGE trial* randomized patients to medical therapy with PCI with bare metal stents (BMSs) versus without PCI. Stenting showed no benefit over medical therapy in composite end points of MI and death from any cause at 7 years.[38] The lessons learned from the COURAGE trial include: (1) an initial trial with medical therapy as the first choice for stable CAD is reasonable and does not accrue harm; (2) medical and catheter-based therapies play at least complementary, if not synergistic, roles in the treatment of patients with SIHD; (3) a significantly better angina-free status as well as a reduction in the requirement for subsequent revascularization is associated with PCI compared with medical therapy alone; and (4) incomplete revascularization of patients with a multivessel disease may be associated with lesser degrees of clinical benefit.[34] The COURAGE trial nuclear substudy showed that PCI was more effective than medical therapy in reducing functional ischemia with subsequent improvement in cardiovascular outcomes.[38]

The *Fractional Flow Reserve Versus Angiography for Multivessel Evaluation* (FAME) 2 trial randomized higher risk patients to PCI versus medical therapy and showed a decreased risk of urgent revascularizations and ACS in the PCI group (0.9% vs 5.2%; $P \leq .001$) at 8 months.[37]

The International Study of Comparative Health Effectiveness with Medical and Invasive Approaches (ISCHEMIA) trial is the largest trial comparing invasive versus conservative treatment strategy in patients with SIHD. The trial assessed whether there is a benefit to early cardiac catheterization and, if feasible, early revascularization, in stable patients with at least moderate ischemia on a stress test compared to medical therapy alone. The study shows that an initial invasive strategy as compared with an initial conservative strategy does not reduce the primary endpoint events (cardiovascular death, MI, hospitalization for unstable angina, heart failure, and cardiac arrest) over a median of 3.3 years. Yet, the study demonstrates that patients with stable CAD and moderate to severe ischemia have significant, durable improvements in angina control and quality of life with an invasive strategy. The inclusion and exclusion criteria of the study are notable to better categorize which subgroup of patients can undergo initial conservative approach without higher cardiovascular event risk (ie, the study excluded patients with high-grade left main disease, New York Heart Association [NYHA] III-IV heart failure, recent ACS or revascularization or LV dysfunction).[39]

In conclusion, PCI is more effective in treating severe angina and severe ischemia, assessed by stress testing or by FFR compared to medical therapy alone, but has not shown to prevent future MI or survival in clinical studies.

SPECIAL CONSIDERATIONS

Unprotected Left Main Coronary Artery Revascularization

Overall, CABG for stable LMCA disease (>50% diameter stenosis) is the preferred method of revascularization (Class I), with PCI being an acceptable alternative (Class IIa-b) when the surgical mortality risk is high (>5%), a favorable PCI anatomy is present (ostial or trunk disease, SYNTAX score <22), and operator expertise is available.[40]

Revascularization of the LMCA with CABG provides a significant survival benefit when compared to medical therapy (13 vs 6.6 years, respectively) in symptomatic, as well as in asymptomatic, patients. The *Veterans Administration* (VA) and the *Coronary Artery Surgery Study* (CASS) registries noted an annual mortality of 10% in patients with significant LMCA disease treated with medical therapy, which was reduced to 2% in those who received CABG.[41,42]

The trials that studied PCI versus CABG in an unprotected LMCA in the drug-eluting stent (DES) era include the *Premier of Randomized Comparison of Bypass Surgery versus Angioplasty Using Sirolimus-Eluting Stent in Patients with Left Main Coronary Artery Disease* (PRECOMBAT) trial (sirolimus, first-generation DES), the *Synergy between PCI with Taxus and Cardiac Surgery* (SYNTAS) trial (paclitaxel, first-generation DES), the *Evaluation of XIENCE versus Coronary Artery Bypass Surgery for Effectiveness of Left Main Revascularization* (EXCEL) trial (everolimus, second-generation DES), and the *Nordic Baltic British Left Main Revascularization* (NOBLE) trial (biolimus, second-generation DES). These studies show a relative concordance in that the composite incidence of death, MI, and stroke appears similar in CABG- and DES-treated groups. The patients treated with PCI showed a higher incidence of repeat target vessel revascularization, and those treated with CABG had a higher incidence of stroke. The patients with a high (>32) SYNTAX score had lower rates of major cardiac adverse events and procedural complications including repeat revascularization and lower mortality from surgical revascularization as compared to PCI.[43,44] In conclusion, current data show efficacy and safety of the modern generation DES in the treatment of LMCA CAD in short-term follow-up and in patients with a low-intermediate SYNTAX score.

Revascularization in Multivessel Disease

A Heart Team approach and incorporation of the SYNTAX II score (to assess CAD complexity) and the EuroSCORE or STS score (to assess surgical mortality and morbidity) are used to plan the method of revascularization. Features that may preclude surgery include: (1) a high (>5%) predicted surgical mortality; (2) diffuse small vessel disease with poor distal targets; (3) inability to graft the LAD; (4) poor bypass conduits; (5) severe lung disease; and (6) a history of disabling strokes.

The largest trial to compare PCI and CABG in patients with multivessel CAD is the SYNTAX trial. The SYNTAX trial randomized patients with two, three, and left main disease to CABG (with low use of bilateral IMAs and low use of secondary prevention) versus PCI with a DES (first generation). The CAD complexity was graded using the SYNTAX score. At the 5-year follow-up, the trial showed a relative reduction in mortality (5.4%), revascularization (12.8%), and MI (7.3%) in the CABG group. The major adverse cardiac and cerebrovascular event (MACCE) outcomes depended on the SYNTAX score.[45,46] The patients with intermediate (23-32) and high (>32) SYNTAX scores had improved outcomes with CABG. In comparison, the group with a low SYNTAX score (≤22) had similar rates of death and MI with CABG and PCI, although CABG patients had a higher rate of postoperative stroke. Unlike PCI, CABG outcomes were not affected by the patient's SYNTAX score.[46]

Revascularization and Diabetes Mellitus

Evidence from registries and RCTs supports the use of CABG over PCI in diabetic patients with multivessel CAD.[9,33] A meta-analysis of eight trials—four trials using BMS and four using DES—with 3612 patients and an average 5-year follow-up reported that patients treated with CABG have a 20% to 30% lower all-cause mortality compared to PCI with BMS or DES, although the incidence of stroke is higher in patients treated with CABG.[47] Observational studies in patients with type 1 diabetes mellitus show similar results.

Hybrid Revascularization

Hybrid revascularization is increasingly being considered as an alternative to conventional CABG. With hybrid revascularization, the IMA is grafted to the LAD via a small thoracotomy followed by PCI with DES to other diseased coronaries, with excellent short-term clinical outcomes. This approach may be technically more challenging and suboptimal for diabetic patients, and long-term outcomes are not available.

FOLLOW-UP PATIENT CARE IN STABLE ISCHEMIC HEART DISEASE

After diagnosis and initial treatment, CAD follow-up strategies should focus on: (1) continuing evidence-based medical management; (2) implementing risk factor modifications; (3) assessing adherence and effectiveness of prescribed therapies; and (4) monitoring symptoms, functional capacity, progression of disease, and emergence of its complications.[9,10]

Clinical evaluation is recommended every 4 to 6 months in the first year and at least annually thereafter to monitor for recurrent or new symptoms and change in functional capacity. The Seattle Angina Questionnaire (SAQ) is a patient-centered tool that can effectively assess physical limitations, angina stability and frequency, quality of life, and treatment efficacy. Its routine use in stable CAD patients may identify clinical changes that prompt ischemia testing.[6,9]

An annual evaluation should include an ECG, hemoglobin A1C measurement, lipid panel, basic metabolic panel, hepatic panel, and administration of the annual influenza vaccine. Echocardiography should be considered after CABG and PCI to assess LV function, but routine echocardiography is not recommended for stable patients and for those in whom no therapy change is being considered.[9,10] For patients who have known stable CAD and present with a change in their clinical status, the guidelines are consistent in recommending further evaluation with either invasive or noninvasive testing depending on clinical suspicion and the patient's risk profile. Specific guideline recommendations are summarized in **Algorithm 4.3**.

RESEARCH AND FUTURE DIRECTIONS

Areas of intense research with enormous potential to decrease the disease burden of SIHD include the following:

- Population health. As accountable care organizations take responsibility for populations of patients, they are implementing policies and practices to improve overall health that will help prevent CAD and its complications. Examples include: (1) systematically identifying patients who need influenza or pneumonia vaccines; (2) mining electronic medical records to identify patients who are not on optimal medical therapy for prevention or treatment of CAD; and (3) using behavioral techniques and collaborating with pharmacies to ensure compliance with recommended medications.
- Use of genetic testing to identify patients at risk for developing CAD. CAD is a polygenetic disease, but genome-wide surveys are able to identify patients at increased risk.[48] It is likely the accuracy and use of genetic testing will increase.
- Secondary prevention. PCSK9 inhibitors, GLP-1 receptor agonists, and SGLT2 inhibitors are examples of recently developed medications that prevent cardiovascular events in patients with known CVD and comorbidities such as hypercholesterolemia or diabetes mellitus. Additional therapies are under development.
- Diagnosis. The utility of noninvasive CT-FFR and less invasive FFR_{angio} (FFR derived from routine angiography without an invasive pressure wire) is being tested. Their place in diagnostic algorithms remains to be determined.
- Revascularization therapies. Although both PCI and CABG are mature therapies, new technologies (bioresorbable metallic stents, mechanical support for PCI) and techniques (chronic total occlusion PCI, no-contrast PCI, advanced surgical techniques) are constantly being refined.

Finally, the *2019 ESC guidelines* recommended a new paradigm for categorizing ischemic heart disease as chronic coronary disease syndromes:[49]

(i) patients with suspected CAD and "stable" anginal symptoms and/or dyspnea;
(ii) patients with new-onset heart failure or LV dysfunction and suspected CAD;
(iii) asymptomatic and symptomatic patients with stabilized symptoms less than 1 year after an ACS or patients with recent revascularization;
(iv) asymptomatic and symptomatic patients greater than 1 year after initial diagnosis or revascularization;
(v) patients with angina and suspected vasospastic or microvascular disease;
(vi) asymptomatic subjects in whom CAD is detected at screening.

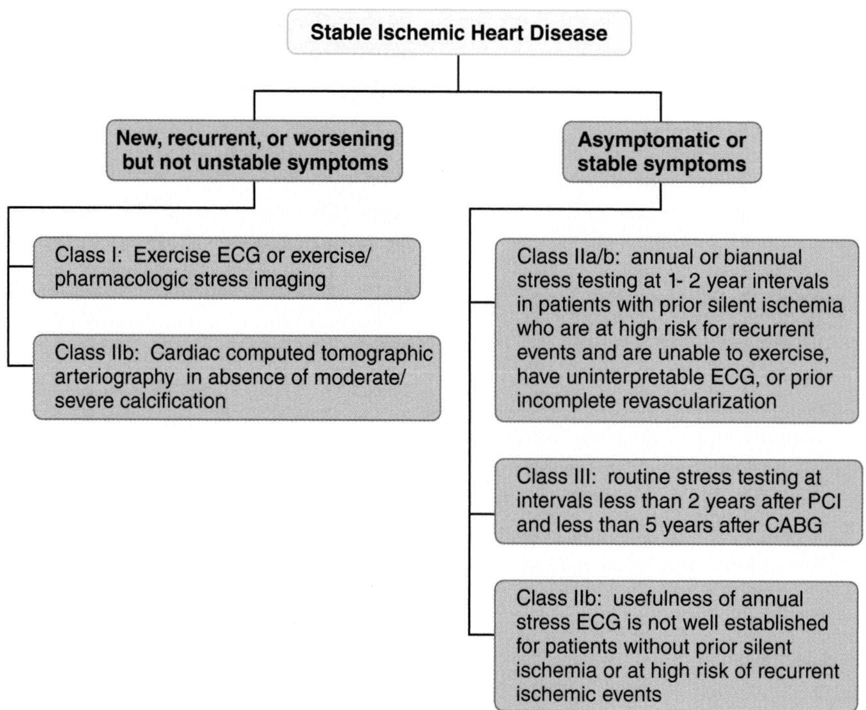

ALGORITHM 4.3 Guidelines for follow-up for patients with stable ischemic heart disease. ECG, electrocardiogram; MV, multivessel.

This paradigm has the advantage of distinguishing distinct chronic coronary syndromes and describing therapies specific to each. It is unclear to what extent this new paradigm will be adopted by clinicians and guideline writing committees in the United States.

KEY POINTS

- ✔ The incidence of coronary disease in the United States has decreased by about half between 1990 and 2010 but is increasing in third world countries with their rise of middle-class populations.
- ✔ Symptoms of stable angina are diverse, but chest "pressure" provoked reliably by "hurrying" or exertion is a relatively specific indicator of myocardial ischemia.
- ✔ All patients with known CAD should be treated with guideline-directed medical therapy including: low-dose aspirin; moderate- to high-intensity statin; sublingual nitroglycerine as needed, antianginal therapy as needed to control symptoms (beta-blockers first, then long-acting nitrates or CCBs, then ranolazine if needed), and an ACE-I in patients with diabetes mellitus, hypertension, or LVEF less than 40%.
- ✔ Extensive guidance regarding CAD revascularization (with PCI or CABG) has been provided by professional society guidelines and appropriate use criteria. These should be familiar to and utilized by cardiologists and cardiac surgeons.
- ✔ For SIHD involving the left main coronary, three vessels, or the proximal LAD and one other major coronary vessel, revascularization may improve survival. For lesser degrees of coronary disease, revascularization improves angina symptoms, but does not prolong life or prevent MI.
- ✔ *The Heart Team approach* to revascularization of complex coronary disease has been universally endorsed by professional societies. This involves an interventional cardiologist, a cardiac surgeon, primary cardiologist, and the patient and family participating in patient-centered decision-making.

REFERENCES

1. Benjamin EJ, Muntner P, Alonso A, et al. Heart disease and stroke statistics—2019 update: a report from the American Heart Association. *Circulation.* 2019;139(10):e56-e528.
2. Quispe R, Elshazly MB, Zhao D, et al. Total cholesterol/HDL-cholesterol ratio discordance with LDL-cholesterol and non-HDL-cholesterol and incidence of atherosclerotic cardiovascular disease in primary prevention: the ARIC study. *Eur J Prev Cardiol.* 2020;27(15):1597-1605.
3. Strong JP. Landmark perspective: coronary atherosclerosis in soldiers. A clue to the natural history of atherosclerosis in the young. *JAMA.* 1986;256(20):2863-2866.
4. Campeau L. Canadian Cardiovascular Society classification. *Can J Cardiol.* 2002;18(4):371-379.
5. Diamond GA, Forrester JS. Analysis of probability as an aid in the clinical diagnosis of coronary-artery disease. *N Engl J Med.* 1979;300(24):1350-1358.
6. Fihn SD, Blankenship JC, Alexander KP, et al. 2014 ACC/AHA/AATS/PCNA/SCAI/STS focused update of the guideline for the diagnosis and

management of patients with stable ischemic heart disease: a report of the American College of Cardiology/American Heart Association Task Force on Practice Guidelines, and the American Association for Thoracic Surgery, Preventive Cardiovascular Nurses Association, Society for Cardiovascular Angiography and Interventions, and Society of Thoracic Surgeons. *J Thorac Cardiovasc Surg*. 2015;149(3):e5-e23.

7. Paech DC, Weston AR. A systematic review of the clinical effectiveness of 64-slice or higher computed tomography angiography as an alternative to invasive coronary angiography in the investigation of suspected coronary artery disease. *BMC Cardiovasc Disord*. 2011;11:32.
8. Agatston AS, Janowitz WR, Hildner FJ, et al. Quantification of coronary artery calcium using ultrafast computed tomography. *J Am Coll Cardiol*. 1990;15(4):827-832.
9. Fihn SD, Gardin JM, Abrams J, et al. 2012 ACCF/AHA/ACP/AATS/PCNA/SCAI/STS guideline for the diagnosis and management of patients with stable ischemic heart disease: a report of the American College of Cardiology Foundation/American Heart Association Task Force on Practice Guidelines, and the American College of Physicians, American Association for Thoracic Surgery, Preventive Cardiovascular Nurses Association, Society for Cardiovascular Angiography and Interventions, and Society of Thoracic Surgeons. *J Am Coll Cardiol*. 2012;60(24):e44-e164.
10. Montalescot G, Sechtem U, Achenbach S, et al. 2013 ESC guidelines on the management of stable coronary artery disease: the Task Force on the management of stable coronary artery disease of the European Society of Cardiology. *Eur Heart J*. 2013;34(38):2949-3003.
11. Patel MR, Calhoon JH, Dehmer GJ, et al. ACC/AATS/AHA/ASE/ASNC/SCAI/SCCT/STS 2017 appropriate use criteria for coronary revascularization in patients with stable ischemic heart disease: a report of the American College of Cardiology Appropriate Use Criteria Task Force, American Association for Thoracic Surgery, American Heart Association, American Society of Echocardiography, American Society of Nuclear Cardiology, Society for Cardiovascular Angiography and Interventions, Society of Cardiovascular Computed Tomography, and Society of Thoracic Surgeons. *J Am Coll Cardiol*. 2017;69(17):2212-2241.
12. Weintraub WS, Spertus JA, Kolm P, et al. Effect of PCI on quality of life in patients with stable coronary disease. *N Engl J Med*. 2008;359(7):677-687.
13. Al-Lamee R, Thompson D, Dehbi HM, et al. Percutaneous coronary intervention in stable angina (ORBITA): a double-blind, randomised controlled trial. *Lancet*. 2018;391(10115):31-40.
14. Giavarini A, de Silva R. The role of ivabradine in the management of angina pectoris. *Cardiovasc Drugs Ther*. 2016;30(4):407-417. doi:10.1007/s10557-016-6678-x
15. Arora RR, Chou TM, Jain D, et al. The multicenter study of enhanced external counterpulsation (MUST-EECP): effect of EECP on exercise-induced myocardial ischemia and anginal episodes. *J Am Coll Cardiol*. 1999;33(7):1833-1840.
16. Gallone G, Baldetti L, Tzanis G, et al. Refractory angina: from pathophysiology to new therapeutic nonpharmacological technologies. *JACC Cardiovasc Interv*. 2020;13(1):1-9.
17. Lamas GA, Boineau R, Goertz C, et al. EDTA chelation therapy alone and in combination with oral high-dose multivitamins and minerals for coronary disease: the factorial group results of the Trial to Assess Chelation Therapy. *Am Heart J*. 2014;168(1):37-44.e5.
18. Antithrombotic Trialists' Collaboration. Collaborative meta-analysis of randomised trials of antiplatelet therapy for prevention of death, myocardial infarction, and stroke in high risk patients. *BMJ*. 2002;324(7329):71-86. doi:10.1136/bmj.324.7329.71
19. Nissen SE, Nicholls SJ, Sipahi I, et al. Effect of very high-intensity statin therapy on regression of coronary atherosclerosis: the ASTEROID trial. *JAMA*. 2006;295(13):1556-1565.
20. Grundy SM, Stone NJ, Bailey AL, et al. 2018 AHA/ACC/AACVPR/AAPA/ABC/ACPM/ADA/AGS/APhA/ASPC/NLA/PCNA guideline on the management of blood cholesterol: a report of the American College of Cardiology/American Heart Association Task Force on Clinical Practice Guidelines. *Circulation*. 2019;139(25):e1082-e1143.
21. Cholesterol Treatment Trialists' (CTT) Collaboration; Baigent C, Blackwell L, Emberson J, et al. Efficacy and safety of more intensive lowering of LDL cholesterol: a meta-analysis of data from 170,000 participants in 26 randomised trials. *Lancet*. 2010;376(9753):1670-1681.
22. Dagenais GR, Pogue J, Fox K, Simoons ML, Yusuf S. Angiotensin-converting-enzyme inhibitors in stable vascular disease without left ventricular systolic dysfunction or heart failure: a combined analysis of three trials. *Lancet*. 2006;368(9535):581-588.
23. Wijns W, Kolh P, Danchin N, et al. Guidelines on myocardial revascularization: the Task Force on Myocardial Revascularization of the European Society of Cardiology (ESC) and the European Association for Cardio-Thoracic Surgery (EACTS). *Eur Heart J*. 2010;31(20):2501-2555.
24. Ginsberg HN, Kris-Etherton P, Dennis B, et al. Effects of reducing dietary saturated fatty acids on plasma lipids and lipoproteins in healthy subjects: the DELTA Study, Protocol 1. *Arterioscler Thromb Vasc Biol*. 1998;18(3):441-449.
25. Bakris G, Ali W, Parati G. ACC/AHA versus ESC/ESH on hypertension guidelines: JACC guideline comparison. *J Am Coll Cardiol*. 2019;73(23):3018-3026.
26. Whelton PK, Carey RM, Aronow WS, et al. 2017 ACC/AHA/AAPA/ABC/ACPM/AGS/APhA/ASH/ASPC/NMA/PCNA guideline for the prevention, detection, evaluation, and management of high blood pressure in adults: executive summary: a report of the American College of Cardiology/American Heart Association Task Force on Clinical Practice Guidelines. *Circulation*. 2018;138(17):e426-e483.
27. Gu K, Cowie CC, Harris MI. Diabetes and decline in heart disease mortality in US adults. *JAMA*. 1999;281(14):1291-1297.
28. Das SR, Everett BM, Birtcher KK, et al. 2018 ACC expert consensus decision pathway on novel therapies for cardiovascular risk reduction in patients with type 2 diabetes and atherosclerotic cardiovascular disease: a report of the American College of Cardiology Task Force on Expert Consensus Decision Pathways. *J Am Coll Cardiol*. 2018;72(24):3200-3223.
29. Ding N, Sang Y, Chen J, et al. Cigarette smoking, smoking cessation, and long-term risk of 3 major atherosclerotic diseases. *J Am Coll Cardiol*. 2019;74(4):498-507.
30. Fletcher GF, Landolfo C, Niebauer J, Ozemek C, Arena R, Lavie CJ. Promoting physical activity and exercise: JACC Health Promotion Series. *J Am Coll Cardiol*. 2018;72(14):1622-1639.
31. Taylor RS, Brown A, Ebrahim S, et al. Exercise-based rehabilitation for patients with coronary heart disease: systematic review and meta-analysis of randomized controlled trials. *Am J Med*. 2004;116(10):682-692.
32. Farooq V, van Klaveren D, Steyerberg EW, et al. Anatomical and clinical characteristics to guide decision making between coronary artery bypass surgery and percutaneous coronary intervention for individual patients: development and validation of SYNTAX score II. *Lancet*. 2013;381(9867):639-650.
33. Windecker S, Stortecky S, Stefanini GG, et al. Revascularisation versus medical treatment in patients with stable coronary artery disease: network meta-analysis. *BMJ*. 2014;348:g3859.
34. Yusuf S, Zucker D, Peduzzi P, et al. Effect of coronary artery bypass graft surgery on survival: overview of 10-year results from randomised trials by the Coronary Artery Bypass Graft Surgery Trialists Collaboration. *Lancet*. 1994;344(8922):563-570.
35. Bypass Angioplasty Revascularization Investigation (BARI) Investigators. Comparison of coronary bypass surgery with angioplasty in patients with multivessel disease. *N Engl J Med*. 1996;335(4):217-225.
36. Boden WE, O'Rourke RA, Teo KK, et al. Optimal medical therapy with or without PCI for stable coronary disease. *N Engl J Med*. 2007;356(15):1503-1516.
37. De Bruyne B, Pijls NH, Kalesan B, et al. Fractional flow reserve-guided PCI versus medical therapy in stable coronary disease. *N Engl J Med*. 2012;367(11):991-1001.
38. Shaw LJ, Berman DS, Maron DJ, et al. Optimal medical therapy with or without percutaneous coronary intervention to reduce ischemic burden: results from the Clinical Outcomes Utilizing Revascularization and Aggressive Drug Evaluation (COURAGE) trial nuclear substudy. *Circulation*. 2008;117(10):1283-1291.
39. Maron DJ, Hochman JS, Reynolds HR, et al. Initial invasive or conservative strategy for stable coronary disease. *N Engl J Med*. 2020;382(15):1395-1407. doi:10.1056/NEJMoa1915922

40. Chieffo A, Park SJ, Valgimigli M, et al. Favorable long-term outcome after drug-eluting stent implantation in nonbifurcation lesions that involve unprotected left main coronary artery: a multicenter registry. *Circulation.* 2007;116(2):158-162.
41. Veterans Administration Coronary Artery Bypass Surgery Cooperative Study Group. Eleven-year survival in the Veterans Administration randomized trial of coronary bypass surgery for stable angina. *N Engl J Med.* 1984;311(21):1333-1339.
42. Mock MB, Ringqvist I, Fisher LD, et al. Survival of medically treated patients in the coronary artery surgery study (CASS) registry. *Circulation.* 1982;66(3):562-568.
43. Ahn JM, Roh JH, Kim YH, et al. Randomized trial of stents versus bypass surgery for left main coronary artery disease: 5-year outcomes of the PRECOMBAT study. *J Am Coll Cardiol.* 2015;65(20):2198-2206.
44. Serruys PW, Morice MC, Kappetein AP, et al. Percutaneous coronary intervention versus coronary-artery bypass grafting for severe coronary artery disease. *N Engl J Med.* 2009;360(10):961-972.
45. Serruys PW, Onuma Y, Garg S, et al. Assessment of the SYNTAX score in the Syntax study. *EuroIntervention.* 2009;5(1):50-56.
46. Mohr FW, Morice MC, Kappetein AP, et al. Coronary artery bypass graft surgery versus percutaneous coronary intervention in patients with three-vessel disease and left main coronary disease: 5-year follow-up of the randomised, clinical SYNTAX trial. *Lancet.* 2013;381(9867):629-638.
47. Hakeem A, Garg N, Bhatti S, Rajpurohit N, Ahmed Z, Uretsky BF. Effectiveness of percutaneous coronary intervention with drug-eluting stents compared with bypass surgery in diabetics with multivessel coronary disease: comprehensive systematic review and meta-analysis of randomized clinical data. *J Am Heart Assoc.* 2013;2(4):e000354.
48. Severance LM, Contijoch FJ, Carter H, et al. Using a genetic risk score to calculate the optimal age for an individual to undergo coronary artery calcium screening. *J Cardiovasc Comput Tomogr.* 2019;13(4):203-210.
49. Knuuti J, Wijns W, Saraste A, et al. 2019 ESC Guidelines for the diagnosis and management of chronic coronary syndromes. *Eur Heart J.* 2020;41(3):407-477.

CHAPTER 5

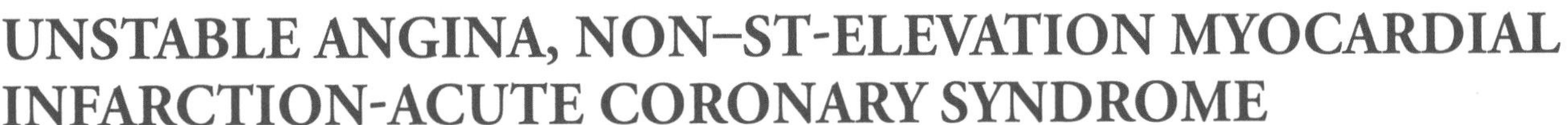

UNSTABLE ANGINA, NON–ST-ELEVATION MYOCARDIAL INFARCTION-ACUTE CORONARY SYNDROME

Talal T. Attar and Rebecca Miller

INTRODUCTION

Epidemiology

The 2020 Heart Disease and Stroke Statistics update of the American Heart Association (AHA) has reported that in the United States the prevalence of coronary heart disease (CHD) is 6.7% in persons 20 years of age or older. The prevalence of myocardial infarction (MI) is 3.0% in that population, with an MI every 40 seconds in the United States.

The median age at acute coronary syndrome (ACS) presentation is 65.6 years in males and 72 years in females.

PATHOGENESIS

ACS is the result of a sudden imbalance between myocardial oxygen consumption (MVO_2) and demand. Coronary artery obstruction caused by atherosclerotic lesions is the most common cause of such imbalance. In the acute phase, the obstruction and the associated myocardial ischemia are caused by plaque rupture with superimposed obstructive thrombus. They can also be caused by hemorrhage inside the plaque core. Distal embolization from the ruptured plaque and the associated thrombus can also cause microvascular obstruction, resulting in myocardial ischemia or necrosis.

CLINICAL PRESENTATION

ACS, usually caused by sudden reduction in coronary blood flow, is a clinical term that encompasses a spectrum of presentations associated with acute myocardial ischemia. The classic presenting symptom of ACS is anginal chest pain. A dull, deep, ill-defined discomfort is felt in the substernal region with common radiation to the left arm. At times, the symptoms could be atypical with either unusual location of the pain (neck, back, epigastric region, etc) or the chest pain is replaced with "angina-equivalent" symptoms. These symptoms could be cardiovascular such as dyspnea, or at times can mimic gastric symptoms such as nausea and epigastric burning.

With clinically suggestive symptoms, electrocardiographic (ECG) findings divide ACS syndromes. With the presence of ST elevation, the presentation is characterized as ST-elevation myocardial infarction (STEMI). In the presence of ST depression, transient ST elevation, or T-wave inversion, the presentation is characterized as unstable angina (UA) or non–ST-elevation myocardial infarction (NSTE-ACS). A key branch point between those two syndromes is the presence of elevated cardiac biomarkers.

A normal ECG and negative cardiac biomarkers do not completely exclude an ischemic etiology if the clinical features of the presentation are highly suggestive. Such a scenario is classified as UA.

DIAGNOSIS

History and Symptoms

A detailed history will help clinicians determine the likelihood that the main complaint and the associated symptoms are suggestive of ischemic presentation. The most common presenting symptom for ACS is chest pain. The typical ischemic pain is usually a deep, poorly defined, pressure-type chest pain in the substernal area with occasional radiation to the left arm. Common associated symptoms are dyspnea, diaphoresis, palpitations, dizziness, and syncope.

Atypical characteristics, location, and associated symptoms will decrease the likelihood of ischemic etiology, but does not completely exclude the diagnosis. Atypical locations of the pain include the neck, the mandible, shoulders, the periscapular area, upper back, and the epigastric region. Atypical characteristics of the pain include pleuritic stabbing pain. Pain localized to the tip of one finger, inducible with movement, palpation, and deep inspiration, or a brief duration of a few seconds is less likely ischemic. Atypical symptoms include nausea, vomiting, indigestion, and increased dyspnea without pain.

Some elements in the history that increase the probability of ACS include older age, male sex, diabetes, peripheral vascular disease, prior history of coronary artery disease (CAD), MI, or prior revascularization.

The relief of symptoms with nitroglycerin or gastrointestinal cocktails is not predictive of likelihood of ACS.[3]

Physical Examination

The physical examination in ACS could be normal. The presence of S4 or paradoxical splitting of S2 are nonspecific potential findings. Physical findings of left ventricular (LV) dysfunction such as S3 gallop, rales, or murmurs suggestive of acute mitral regurgitation also could be present, but nonspecific to the presentation and diagnosis of ACS.

Physical examination is also helpful in identifying findings suggestive of alternative diagnosis for the presenting symptoms. A pericardial rub in pericarditis, a blood pressure and pulse differential between extremities in acute aortic dissection, or a pulsatile mass with abdominal bruit in aortic aneurysm are a few examples.

Occasionally, findings of physical examination can impact therapeutic decisions. A focal neurologic deficit on neurologic examination, or evidence of occult blood on rectal examination, for example, will be implications for anticoagulation decisions in the management of ACS.

Electrocardiogram

A normal ECG at initial presentation with symptoms suggestive of ACS does not completely exclude this diagnosis. Of the patients with normal initial ECG, 1% to 6% will have an MI. Four percent will have UA.[4-6]

Given the fact that ECG changes could be dynamic, ECG should be repeated at 15- to 30- minute intervals during the first hour after presentation, especially if symptoms recur. Having a previous ECG for comparison is also beneficial, especially when the changes are nondynamic or nonspecific.

Diagnostic ECG findings include horizontal ST depression (>1 mm), transient ST elevation, and T-wave inversion. ST depression (<1 mm) and T-wave inversions (<2 mm) are nonspecific findings. Other causes for ECG changes that resemble ischemic abnormalities include LV hypertrophy, pericarditis, and electrolyte imbalances. Repolarization abnormalities, left bundle branch block, and paced rhythm can mask ischemia.

Cardiac Biomarkers

Cardiac biomarkers are essential to the diagnosis and stratification of patients with suspected ACS. As troponin I and T are cardiac-specific biomarkers present in high concentrations in cardiac tissue, but largely absent in nonmyocardial tissues, they are highly sensitive biomarkers for myocardial injury.[7] High-sensitivity cardiac troponin T (hs-cTnT) and high-sensitivity cardiac troponin I (hs-cTnI) have similar diagnostic sensitivity, but hs-cTnT appears to have greater prognostic accuracy.[8]

Troponin levels should be evaluated at the time of presentation as well as 3 to 6 hours after onset of symptoms in patients with suspected UA or NSTE-ACS. Troponin levels greater than the 99th percentile of the upper reference limit in a healthy population are indicative of myocardial necrosis.[7,8]

Additional causes of troponin elevation include hypertension, myocardial trauma, myocarditis, pulmonary embolism, critical illness, renal dysfunction, and burns.[7,8] As such, elevated troponin levels alone are indicative of myocardial necrosis that is the result of a nonthrombotic condition causing an imbalance between coronary oxygen supply and demand (ie, type 2 MI). To meet the definition of type 2 MI, in addition to elevated cardiac biomarkers, at least one of the following must be present:[9]

- Symptoms of acute myocardial ischemia
- New ischemic ECG changes
- Development of pathologic Q waves
- Imaging evidence of new loss of viable myocardium or new regional wall motion abnormality in a pattern consistent with an ischemic etiology

Other biomarkers such as creatine kinase-MB and myoglobin have been previously used in the diagnosis of ACS, but are less sensitive than is troponin in the detection of myocardial necrosis.

Diagnostic Imaging

A chest roentgenogram should be part of the initial evaluation of patients presenting with chest pain and suspected ACS. It can identify potential noncardiac etiology of the symptoms including pulmonary abnormalities. A widening mediastinum can suggest the diagnosis of aortic dissection.

If an intrathoracic etiology of symptoms is suspected, computed tomography is very useful, and could be incorporated with the initial evaluation process.

Transthoracic echocardiography can be helpful in detecting regional wall motion abnormalities. It is also the test of choice in identifying pericardial effusions and potential tamponade physiology.

Coronary computed tomography angiogram (CCTA) may be an option in patients with low-to-moderate clinical likelihood of UA because a normal scan excludes CAD. CCTA has a high negative predictive value (NPV) to exclude ACS.[10]

Risk Stratification

Early risk stratification is helpful in guiding the care path for the patient from the time of presentation. Triage decisions including appropriate placement could be optimized using risk stratification. The risk-benefit balance for early initiation of some therapy with significant potential side effects such as anticoagulation is based on patient risk assessment.

Clinical risk scores are also critical to the decision of pursuing an early invasive strategy versus a more conservative ischemia-guided approach for patients with NSTE-ACS and UA.

The thrombolysis in myocardial infarction (TIMI) risk score is composed of seven 1-point risk indicators rated on presentation.[11] A score of (0-1) is considered low. The composite endpoints increase as the score increases. The TIMI risk score has been validated internally within the TIMI 11B trial and in two separate cohorts of patients from the ESSENCE (Efficacy and Safety of Subcutaneous Enoxaparin in Non–Q-Wave Coronary Event) trial.[12] The TIMI risk score calculator is available at http://www.timi.org/index.php?page=riskUA-NSTEMI

The TIMI risk index is useful in predicting 30-day and 1-year mortality in patients with NSTE-ACS[13] (**Table 5.1**).

The Global Registry of Acute Coronary Events (GRACE) risk model predicts in-hospital and postdischarge mortality or MI (**Table 5.2**).[14-17] The GRACE tool was developed from 11,389 patients in GRACE and validated in subsequent GRACE and GUSTO IIb (Global Utilization of Streptokinase and Tissue Plasminogen Activator for Occluded Coronary

TABLE 5.1 TIMI Risk Score for NSTE-ACS

Present on Admission	Points
Age older than 65	1
Greater than three risk factors for coronary artery disease	1
Prior coronary artery disease	1
ST elevation on ECG	1
Greater than two angina events in the past 24 hours	1
Use of aspirin in the past 7 days	1
Elevated cardiac biomarkers	1
TOTAL POINTS	7 possible

ECG, electrocardiogram; NSTE-ACS, non–ST-elevation myocardial infarction-acute coronary syndrome; TIMI, thrombolysis in myocardial infarction.

Arteries) cohorts. The sum of the scores is applied to a reference nomogram to determine all-cause mortality from hospital discharge to 6 months. A GRACE score of less than 109 is considered low and is available at: https://www.outcomes-umassmed.org/grace/acs_risk2/index.html

MANAGEMENT

Antianginal Therapy

Oxygen

Supplemental oxygen therapy should be administered to patients presenting with possible UA or NSTE-ACS with oxygen saturation below 90% or in respiratory distress.[7,8] There is no evidence to support supplemental oxygen therapy in all patients with UA or NSTE-ACS because it may increase coronary vascular resistance and increase the risk of mortality in those without hypoxemia.[7,18]

Nitrates

Nitroglycerin reduces cardiac oxygen demand by primarily reducing cardiac preload, modestly reducing afterload, dilating coronary arteries, and increasing collateral blood flow to ischemic myocardial tissue. Sublingual nitroglycerin (0.3-0.4 mg) should be administered every 5 minutes for up to three doses in patients with continued ischemic pain.[7] Nitroglycerin infusion is appropriate for patients with refractory ischemic symptoms, heart failure, or hypertension. Nitrate therapy is contraindicated within 24 hours of sildenafil or vardenafil administration or within 48 hours of tadalafil administration because of the risk of severe hypotension.[7,8] Patients with right ventricular infarction may develop severe hypotension following the administration of nitroglycerin or other agents that reduce preload, so its use is contraindicated in such patients.[7]

Analgesics

Morphine is an opioid commonly used to alleviate acute or chronic pain; in the setting of UA or NSTE-ACS, morphine is a venodilator and can modestly reduce systolic blood pressure and heart rate by increasing vagal tone.[7] Morphine (1-5 mg) may be given intravenously every 5 to 30 minutes as needed for chest pain refractory to nitrates and beta-blockers, but empiric use of morphine in all patients with ACS is associated with worse clinical outcomes and impaired absorption of oral antiplatelet medications.[7,19] Nonsteroidal anti-inflammatory drugs (NSAIDs) such as ibuprofen, naproxen, and celecoxib interfere with the antiplatelet activity of aspirin, and are associated with an increased risk of major adverse cardiovascular outcomes and should be avoided in patients with NSTE-ACS.[7,20,21]

TABLE 5.2 Global Registry of Acute Coronary Events (GRACE) Risk Calculator

GRACE Risk Model		
Killip class	I	0
	II	20
	III	39
	IV	59
Systolic blood pressure	<80	58
	80-99	53
	100-119	43
	120-139	34
	140-159	24
	160-199	10
	>200	0
Heart rate	<60	0
	60-69	3
	70-89	9
	90-109	15
	110-149	24
	150-199	38
	>200	46
Age	<30	0
	30-39	8
	40-49	25
	50-59	41
	60-69	53
	70-79	75
	80-89	91
	>90	100
Creatinine level	0-0.39	1
	0.4-0.79	4
	0.8-1.19	7
	1.2-1.59	10
	1.6-1.99	13
	2.00-3.99	21
	>4	28
Cardiac arrest on admission	Present	39
	Absent	0
ST-segment deviation	Present	28
	Absent	0
Elevated cardiac biomarkers	Present	14
	Absent	0
TOTAL POINTS		

Beta-blockers

Beta-blockers prevent sympathetic activation of beta-receptors in the myocardium, thus reducing heart rate, contractility, and blood pressure, and, subsequently, myocardial oxygen consumption. An oral beta-blocker should be initiated within 24 hours of presentation, provided there are no signs of heart failure or reduced cardiac output, increased risk of cardiogenic shock (age older than 70 years, heart rate >110 beats per minute, systolic pressure <120 mm Hg, late presentation after symptom onset), or other contraindications to beta-blocker therapy.[7,8,22] Beta-blocker therapy is associated with reductions in cardiac ischemia, reinfarction, and ventricular arrhythmias, as well as increased long-term survival.[7,8,23]

Calcium Channel Blockers

Verapamil and diltiazem are non-dihydropyridine (non-DHP) calcium channel blockers that relax coronary vascular smooth muscle and reduce heart rate and blood pressure, thus increasing myocardial oxygen delivery and reducing myocardial oxygen demand. Oral non-DHP calcium channel blockers are recommended when beta-blockers are unsuccessful in relieving myocardial ischemia, contraindicated, or cause intolerable side effects.[7]

Ranolazine

Ranolazine reduces ventricular tension and myocardial oxygen consumption with minimal effect on blood pressure and heart rate. Ranolazine is approved for treatment of chronic angina, and the MERLIN-TIMI (Metabolic Efficiency With Ranolazine for Less Ischemia in Non–ST-Elevation Acute Coronary Syndromes-Thrombosis in Myocardial Infarction) 36 trial failed to demonstrate statistically significant reduction in major cardiovascular events in patients with ACS.[24]

Anticoagulant Therapy

Anticoagulants inhibit thrombin generation and activity, and have been shown to reduce ischemic outcomes in NSTE-ACS.[7] Anticoagulation is recommended for all patients presenting with NSTE-ACS, regardless of initial treatment strategy, unless contraindicated.[19]

Unfractionated Heparin

Unfractionated heparin (UFH) enhances the activity of antithrombin III, inactivating thrombin and preventing the conversion of fibrinogen to fibrin. The anticoagulant effect and pharmacokinetics of UFH varies widely between patients.[8] Weight-based dosing provides more consistent anticoagulation than fixed dosing of UFH.[7] UFH is dosed as a 60 IU/kg bolus (up to 4000 IU) followed by 12 IU/kg/hour infusion (up to 1000 IU/hour) for 48 hours or until coronary angiography or percutaneous coronary intervention (PCI) is performed.[7,8]

Low-molecular-weight Heparin

Enoxaparin is a low-molecular-weight heparin (LMWH) that has a more predictable pharmacokinetic profile than does UFH. Enoxaparin is dosed 1 mg/kg subcutaneously twice daily for the duration of hospitalization or until coronary angiography or PCI is performed.[7,8] When compared to UFH in high-risk patients with NSTE-ACS, enoxaparin was comparable to UFH in efficacy, but was associated with increased major bleeding.[25]

Bivalirudin

Bivalirudin is a direct thrombin inhibitor and prevents the conversion of fibrinogen to fibrin. Bivalirudin is administered with a 0.1 mg/kg intravenous (IV) loading dose followed by a 0.25 mg/kg/hour infusion until diagnostic angiography or PCI; if proceeding with PCI, an additional 0.5 mg/kg bolus should be administered with an increased infusion rate of 1.75 mg/kg/hour.[7,8] Bivalirudin in combination with a glycoprotein (GP) IIb/IIIa inhibitor was shown to be comparable to UFH with a GP IIb/IIIa inhibitor with respect to ischemic outcomes, but may be less preferable than is UFH because of increased cost.[26]

Fondaparinux

Fondaparinux inhibits factor Xa to interrupt the clotting cascade. Fondaparinux is dosed 2.5 mg subcutaneously once daily for the duration of hospitalization or until coronary angiography or PCI. When compared to enoxaparin in NSTE-ACS, fondaparinux was noninferior with regard to ischemic outcomes, but associated with significantly less major bleeding.[27] When using fondaparinux, an anticoagulant with anti-IIa activity (eg, 85 IU/kg UFH bolus) should be used to prevent catheter thrombosis in the patient who is referred for PCI.[7,8,27]

Argatroban

Argatroban is a direct thrombin inhibitor indicated as an anticoagulant for PCI in patients with or at risk for developing heparin-induced thrombocytopenia. Argatroban should be initiated at 0.5 to 1 μg/kg/minute IV and titrated to an activated partial thromboplastin time (aPTT) of 1.5 to 3 times the baseline aPTT or to an institution-specific goal.[7]

Antiplatelet Therapy

Aspirin

Aspirin irreversibly inhibits cyclooxygenase-1 and -2 (COX-1, COX-2), leading to inhibition of thromboxane A_2 and platelet aggregation. Aspirin reduces the risk of recurrent MI and death in patients with ACS.[7,8] Non–enteric-coated aspirin 162 to 325 mg should be given to all patients with NSTE-ACS without contraindications immediately after presentation, followed by a maintenance dose of 81 to 100 mg daily.[7,8] Maintenance doses 160 mg and greater are associated with increased risk of bleeding without improved efficacy.[7,28]

$P2Y_{12}$ Inhibitors

$P2Y_{12}$ inhibitors (clopidogrel, prasugrel, ticagrelor, and cangrelor) prevent the binding of adenosine diphosphate to the GP IIb/IIIa receptor, which attenuates platelet aggregation and reaction to stimuli of thrombus aggregation, such as thrombin. In patients with NSTE-ACS, an oral $P2Y_{12}$ inhibitor should be given as a higher one-time dose initially ("loading" dose), followed by a lower maintenance dose for up to 12 months. The duration of dual antiplatelet therapy (DAPT) with aspirin and a $P2Y_{12}$ inhibitor may be shortened depending on individual patient ischemic and bleeding risks, as well as whether PCI with stenting was performed.[8]

Clopidogrel

Clopidogrel is an oral irreversible $P2Y_{12}$ inhibitor that inhibits platelet activity for the duration of their lifespan (7-10 days). DAPT with aspirin and clopidogrel demonstrated greater reduction in the composite endpoint of cardiovascular death, nonfatal MI, or stroke than did aspirin alone in patients with UA or NSTE-ACS, with a slight but significant increase in major bleeding.[29] An initial loading dose of 300 to 600 mg is recommended (600 mg is the preferred loading dose because of greater, faster, and more reliable antiplatelet effect), followed by 75 mg daily.[7,8] Clopidogrel is a prodrug requiring cytochrome P450 oxidation to produce its active metabolite. Significant variability in antiplatelet response has been demonstrated in pharmacokinetic and pharmacodynamic studies, owing largely to genetic polymorphisms in cytochrome P450 function.[8]

Prasugrel

Prasugrel is an oral irreversible $P2Y_{12}$ inhibitor and prodrug with faster and more consistent antiplatelet effects than clopidogrel.[7] Prasugrel is administered with a 60 mg loading dose followed by 10 mg daily. Compared to clopidogrel, prasugrel reduced the composite endpoint of cardiovascular death, nonfatal MI, or nonfatal stroke, largely due to reductions in MI, urgent target-vessel revascularization, and stent thrombosis in patients with ACS. Severe bleeding complications, including spontaneous bleeding, life-threatening bleeds, and fatal bleeds, were significantly increased in patients who received prasugrel compared to those treated with clopidogrel. Net harm was demonstrated in patients with a history of cerebrovascular events, whereas no benefit was shown in patients older than 75 years or who weighed less than 60 kg; therefore, prasugrel therapy should be avoided in patients with these characteristics.[7,8,30] Increased bleeding risk without improvement in efficacy has been demonstrated with "upfront" prasugrel administration (eg, at the time of diagnosis) in patients with NSTE-ACS, so prasugrel should only be given at the time of PCI.[7,31]

Ticagrelor

Ticagrelor is an oral reversible $P2Y_{12}$ inhibitor that, unlike clopidogrel and prasugrel, is supplied as an active metabolite. Ticagrelor has a faster onset and greater degree of platelet inhibition than does clopidogrel, as well as quicker recovery of platelet function.[7,8] Ticagrelor is dosed as a 180 mg load followed by 90 mg twice daily. Compared with clopidogrel in patients with NSTE-ACS, ticagrelor reduced the composite endpoint of death from vascular causes, MI, or stroke with a slight increase in major bleeding and non–procedure-related bleeding (no difference in transfusions or fatal bleeding).[7,8,32] Side effects unique to ticagrelor include dyspnea, bradycardia, and increased uric acid levels. Ticagrelor is recommended as the first-line $P2Y_{12}$ inhibitor for patients with NSTE-ACS in the absence of contraindications.[7,8]

Cangrelor

Cangrelor is an IV reversible $P2Y_{12}$ inhibitor with highly effective platelet inhibition, rapid half-life (3-6 minutes), and recovery of platelet function within 1 hour of drug cessation.[8] Cangrelor is indicated for use in PCI for patients who have not been treated with a $P2Y_{12}$ inhibitor and are not receiving a GP IIb/IIIa inhibitor. Cangrelor is administered as a 30 μg/kg bolus before PCI followed by a 4 μg/kg/minute infusion for at least 2 hours or duration of the PCI, whichever is longer. Compared to clopidogrel, cangrelor reduced the composite outcome of death, MI, ischemia-driven revascularization, or stent thrombosis with a significant increase in mild bleeding.[8,33]

Glycoprotein IIb/IIIa Receptor Inhibitors

GP IIb/IIIa receptor inhibitors (tirofiban and eptifibatide) are IV infusions that bind reversibly to the GP IIb/IIIa receptor, blocking the fibrinogen binding site and preventing platelet aggregation. Owing to limited beneficial impact on ischemic outcomes and increased risk of bleeding complications, tirofiban and eptifibatide are usually only used downstream for "bailout" purposes (eg, thrombotic complications during PCI).[7,8,26] GP IIb/IIIa inhibitors may be appropriate as part of initial antiplatelet therapy in high-risk patients with NSTE-ACS undergoing early invasive management.[7]

Lipid-Lowering Therapy

Statins

In addition to a primary function of reducing low-density lipoprotein cholesterol and increasing high-density lipoprotein cholesterol levels, statins produce a number of pleiotropic effects including improved endothelial function, decreased inflammation in coronary vasculature affected by atherosclerosis, and reduced platelet aggregation. High-intensity statin therapy (atorvastatin 40-80 mg or rosuvastatin 20-40 mg) should be initiated in all patients presenting with NSTE-ACS without contraindications to statin therapy.[7,8,34] Statins have been shown to reduce the composite endpoint of cardiovascular death, MI, admission for UA, need for coronary revascularization, or stroke.[7,8,35]

Renin-Angiotensin-Aldosterone System Inhibition

Angiotensin-converting Enzyme Inhibitors

Angiotensin-converting enzyme (ACE) inhibitors reduce mortality and major adverse cardiovascular events in patients with recent MI, particularly in patients with reduced LV function.[7,8,36,37] ACE inhibitors should be initiated in patients with LV ejection fraction below 40%, hypertension, diabetes mellitus, or stable chronic kidney disease (CKD) in the absence of contraindications.[7,8] Angiotensin II receptor blockers (ARBs) may be substituted for ACE inhibitors with comparable mortality benefits.[7,8,38]

Aldosterone Receptor Antagonists

Aldosterone receptor antagonists (spironolactone and eplerenone) increase sodium and water excretion in the distal renal tubules.[23] When added to ACE inhibitors and beta-blockers, aldosterone receptor antagonists reduce mortality in patients with heart failure and/or LV ejection fraction below 40%.[7,39] Aldosterone receptor antagonists are recommended in all patients after MI on therapeutic doses of ACE inhibitors and beta-blockers with ejection fraction below 40% and diabetes mellitus or heart failure.[7,8] Aldosterone receptor antagonists should be avoided in patients with significant renal dysfunction or hyperkalemia[7,39] (**Table 5.3**).

Invasive Therapy

Ischemia-Guided Strategy Versus Early Invasive Strategies

In conjunction with optimal medical therapy, two treatment pathways have emerged for all patients with NSTE-ACS.

TABLE 5.3 Treatments in the Management of Acute Coronary Syndrome

Therapy/Medication	Medical Therapy without Planned PCI	Medical Therapy with Invasive Strategy
Antianginal Therapy		
Oxygen	+	+
Nitroglycerin	+	+
Morphine	+	+
Beta-blocker	+	+
Calcium channel blocker	+	+
Antiplatelet Therapy		
Aspirin	+	+
Clopidogrel	+	+
Prasugrel		+
Ticagrelor	+	+
Cangrelor		+
Tirofiban		+
Eptifibatide		+
Anticoagulant Therapy		
Enoxaparin	+	+
Unfractionated heparin	+	+
Bivalirudin		+
Argatroban	+	+
Fondaparinux	+	+
Subsequent Medical Management		
Statin	+	+
Angiotensin-converting enzyme inhibitor	+	+
Aldosterone receptor antagonist	+	+

PCI, percutaneous coronary intervention.

The invasive strategy triages patients to an invasive diagnostic evaluation (ie, coronary angiography) with plans for revascularization in suitable anatomy. In contrast, the initial ischemia-guided strategy calls for a more conservative approach with medical management. Invasive evaluation would be considered for those patients who fail medical therapy (refractory angina or angina at rest or with minimal activity despite vigorous medical therapy) or have objective evidence of ischemia (dynamic ECG changes, significant myocardial perfusion defect), as identified on a noninvasive stress test. Also, clinical indicators of very high prognostic risk (eg, TIMI ≥4 or GRACE >140 score) favor an early invasive strategy.

The ischemia-guided strategy seeks to avoid the routine early use of invasive procedures unless patients experience refractory or recurrent ischemic symptoms or develop hemodynamic instability. When the ischemia-guided strategy is chosen, a plan for noninvasive evaluation is required to detect severe ischemia that occurs at a low threshold of stress and to promptly refer these patients for coronary angiography and revascularization as indicated. The major advantage offered by the ischemia-guided strategy is that some patients' conditions stabilize during medical therapy and will not require coronary angiography and revascularization. Consequently, the ischemia-guided strategy may potentially avoid costly and possibly unnecessary invasive procedures.

The optimal timing of angiography has not been conclusively defined. An early invasive procedure is defined as one within 24 hours. A delayed invasive procedure is within 25 to 72 hours of initial presentation. In most studies using the invasive strategy, angiography was deferred for 12 to 72 hours, whereas antithrombotic and anti-ischemic therapies were intensified.[40-45] The concept of deferred angiography espouses that revascularization may be safer once plaque is stabilized with optimal antithrombotic and/or anti-ischemic therapies. Conversely, early angiography facilitates earlier risk stratification and consequently speeds revascularization and discharge.

Although some studies such as the FRISC-II trial and RITA-3[43] showed a benefit of revascularization in men that was not observed in women;[46] other studies and meta-analysis showed more universal benefits.[47] TACTICS-TIMI 18 also showed equal benefits between men and women.[40]

Although both groups benefited from an early invasive strategy, patients with diabetes mellitus is another subgroup that received greater benefit from early invasive strategy when compared to nondiabetics.[48]

Approximately half of all PCI procedures are performed in patients with UA or NSTE-ACS, and approximately 32% to 40% of patients with NSTE-ACS will undergo PCI.[49] In-hospital coronary artery bypass grafting (CABG) is performed in 7% to 13% of patients hospitalized with NSTE-ACS. Approximately one-third of patients with NSTE-ACS undergo CABG within 48 hours of hospital admission. In these patients, CABG was performed at a median time of 73 hours after admission (interquartile range: 42-122 hours). In-hospital mortality in patients with NSTE-ACS undergoing CABG is approximately 3.7%.[50]

As discussed previously, in patients with NSTE-ACS, a strategy of early angiography and revascularization (primarily with PCI) results in lower rates of recurrent UA, recurrent rehospitalization, MI, and death.[51]

Initial revascularization trials focused on the number of lesions, diseased vessels, the presence of left main disease, and the LV systolic function in comparing PCI to CABG. Many other factors influence the choice of revascularization procedure including the extent and complexity of CAD, short-term risk and long-term durability of PCI, operative mortality (which can be estimated by the STS score), diabetes mellitus, CKD, completeness of revascularization, LV systolic dysfunction, previous CABG, and the ability of the patient to tolerate and comply with DAPT. In general, the greater the extent and complexity of the multivessel disease, the more compelling the choice of CABG over multivessel PCI. In patients with NSTE-ACS, PCI of a culprit unprotected left main coronary artery lesion is an option if the patient is not a candidate for CABG.

Given the complexity of the factors influencing the choice between revascularization strategies, "heart team" approach to revascularization decisions, involving an interventional cardiologist and cardiothoracic surgeon is recommended in the approach to patients with complex disease and multiple comorbid conditions. Calculation of SYNTAX (Synergy Between Percutaneous Coronary Intervention With TAXUS and Cardiac Surgery) and Society of Thoracic Surgeons (STS) scores is reasonable in these patients to guide the choice of revascularization[52] (**Algorithm 5.1**).

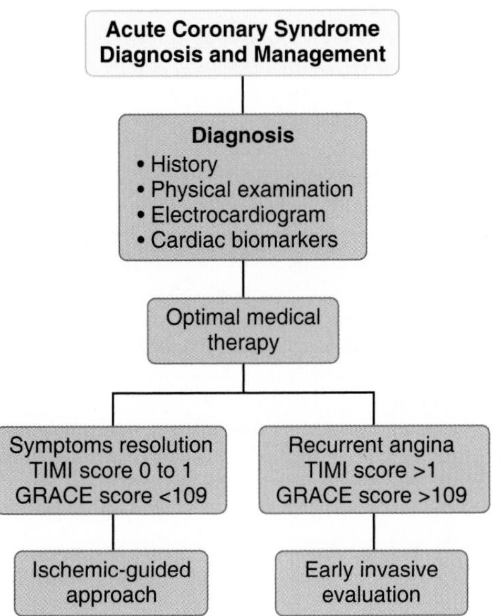

ALGORITHM 5.1 Ischemic-guided versus early invasive management. TIMI, thrombolysis in myocardial infarction.

SPECIAL PATIENT POPULATIONS

Older Patients

Older adults have the highest incidence, prevalence, and adverse outcomes of NSTE-ACS.[53] Older patients more often present with atypical symptoms, less diagnostic ECG changes, higher rate of comorbidities, polypharmacy, and age- and disease-related physiologic changes that adversely impact NSTE-ACS presentation, management, and outcome. Furthermore, older patients are generally underrepresented in randomized trials.

Older patients with NSTE-ACS derive the same benefits from pharmacologic and interventional therapies, and cardiac rehabilitation as younger patients. In a 5-year follow-up meta-analysis of FRISC-II and RITA-3, an early invasive strategy versus an ischemia-guided strategy was associated with a significant reduction in death/MI and MI in patients older than 75 years of age.[54] Despite the benefit, this strategy is still associated with threefold increase in bleeding risk. Special consideration of strategy associated with decreasing bleeding risk should be considered.

Operative mortality rates for CABG in patients older than 80 years of age with NSTE-ACS range from 5% to 8% (11% for urgent cases) and increase to approximately 13% at 90 years of age.[55] Complications occur more frequently in older patients with CABG.[56] Length of stay averages 6 days longer in older patients, and discharge to home is less frequent than in younger patients.[56]

Patients in Cardiogenic Shock

Acute myocardial infarction (AMI) is the leading cause of cardiogenic shock. Early revascularization is the mainstay in the treatment of cardiogenic shock, and it is associated with improved 6-month mortality.[57] Urgent revascularization with CABG may be indicated for failed PCI, coronary anatomy not amenable to PCI, and at the time of surgical repair of a mechanical defect (eg, septal, papillary muscle, free-wall rupture). Age alone is not a contraindication to urgent revascularization for cardiogenic shock.

Patients with NSTE-ACS developed cardiogenic shock later than did patients with STEMI, and had higher risk clinical characteristics, more extensive CAD, and more recurrent ischemia and infarction before developing shock compared with patients with STEMI.[58]

In the SHOCK trial registry, patients with NSTE-ASC were older and had more comorbidities. They constituted 17% of the study population.[59]

FOLLOW-UP PATIENT CARE

The four pillars of follow-up care in patients with UA and NSTE-ACS are follow-up, risk factor modification, lifestyle modification, and patient education.

Follow-up is recommended every 4 to 6 months to monitor for symptoms and to ensure optimal guideline-directed medical therapy (GDMT). Routine testing in asymptomatic patients is not recommended. Ischemic evaluation should be considered for reoccurrence of symptoms, new symptoms, or change in functional capacity.

Risk reduction strategies for secondary prevention are a critical aspect of the management of the survivors of NSTE-ACS. It has been clearly established that in this high-risk cohort, subsequent cardiovascular morbidity and mortality can be reduced by a comprehensive approach to favorably modifying patients' risk profiles.[59] Risk reduction strategies include smoking cessation, blood pressure control, diabetes control, lipid management, diet, and exercise.

Regular physical activity reduces symptoms in patients with cardiovascular disease, enhances functional capacity, improves other risk factors such as insulin resistance and glucose control, and is important in weight control.[59]

Comprehensive cardiac rehabilitation programs provide patient education, enhance regular exercise, monitor risk factors, and address lifestyle modification. Aerobic exercise training can generally begin 1 to 2 weeks after discharge in patients treated with PCI or CABG. Mild-to-moderate resistance training can be considered and started 2 to 4 weeks after aerobic training.[60]

Patient education and awareness is critical in enhancing compliance and achieving lifestyle modification.

RESEARCH AND FUTURE DIRECTIONS

Bleeding is a major adverse effect of NSTE-ACS treatment, especially in the setting of revascularization and long-term use of DAPT. Effort to decrease bleeding risk is ongoing on multiple fronts:

- The wide adoption of radial access in PCI played a significant role in decreasing procedural related bleeding.
- Recent studies suggested that DAPT for 1 month or shorter followed by $P2Y_{12}$ inhibitor as a single agent after PCI might be as effective, with less bleeding complication.
- The management of the patient requiring triple therapy is evolving, with emphasis on shorter duration and earlier transition to dual and monotherapy.
- From the risk factor modification and secondary prevention standpoint, the past few years have seen significant advancement.
- The role of PCSK9 inhibitors is evolving in lipid management.
- Newer diabetes agents such as GLP-1 and SGLT2 inhibitors are demonstrating added cardiac benefit beyond the traditional benefit of glucose control.

KEY POINTS

- ✔ Unstable angina, NSTE-ACS is the most common presentation among the acute coronary syndromes.
- ✔ GDMT is key in the management of this condition.
- ✔ Invasive evaluation and revascularization, when added to GDMT, is shown to improve clinical outcome.
- ✔ Elderly patients benefit from same management approach.
- ✔ Heart team approach to revascularization decision is strongly recommended given the complexity of patients and disease.
- ✔ Appropriate follow-up is an essential part of the long-term care for patients with ACS.

REFERENCES

1. Peterson ED, Roe MT, Mulgand J, et al, Association between hospital process performance and outcomes among patients with acute coronary syndromes. *JAMA.* 2006;295;1912-1920.
2. Heart disease and stroke Statistics-2020 Update: a report from the American Heart Association. *Circulation.* 2020;141:e139-e596.
3. Henrikson CA, Howell EE, Bush DE, et al. Chest pain relief with Nitroglycerin does not predict active coronary disease. *Ann Intern Med.* 2003;139:979-986.
4. Rouan GW, Lee TH, Cook EF, et al. Clinical characteristics and outcome of acute myocardial infarction in patient with initially normal or nonspecific electrocardiograms (a report from the multicenter chest pain study). *Am J Cardiol.* 1989;64:1087-1092.
5. McCarthy BD, Wong JB, Selker HP. Detecting acute cardiac ischemia in the emergency department: a review of the literature. *J Gen Intern Med.* 1990;5:365-373.
6. Slater DK, Hlatky MA, Mark DB, et al. Outcome in suspected myocardial infarction with normal or minimally abnormal admission electrocardiographic findings. *Am J Cardiol.* 1987;60:766-770.
7. Amsterdam EA, Wenger NK, Brindis RG, et al. 2014 AHA/ACC Guideline for the Management of Patients with Non-ST-Elevation Acute Coronary Syndromes: a report of the American College of Cardiology/American Heart Association Task Force on Practice Guidelines. *J Am Coll Cardiol.* 2014;64(24):e139-e228.
8. Roffi M, Patrono C, Collet JP, et al. 2015 ESC Guidelines for the management of acute coronary syndromes in patients presenting without persistent ST-segment elevation: Task Force for the Management of Acute Coronary Syndromes in Patients Presenting without Persistent ST-Segment Elevation of the European Society of Cardiology (ESC). *Eur Heart J.* 2016;37(3):267-315.
9. Thygesan K, Alpert JS, Jaffe AS, et al. Fourth Universal Definition of Myocardial Infarction (2018). *Circulation.* 2018;138:e618-e651.
10. Collet J-P, Thiele H, Barbato E, et al. 2020 ESC Guidelines for the management of acute coronary syndromes in patients presenting without persistent ST-segment elevation. *Eur Heart J.* 2020 Aug 29;ehaa575. doi: 10.1093/eurheartj/ehaa575. Online ahead of print.
11. Antman EM, Cohen M, Bernink PJ, et al. The TIMI risk score for unstable angina/non ST elevation MI: A method for prognostication and therapeutic decision making. *JAMA.* 2000;284:835-842.
12. Cohen M, Demers C, Gurfinkel EP, et al. A comparison of low-molecular-weight heparin with unfractionated heparin for unstable coronary artery disease. Efficacy and Safety of Subcutaneous Enoxaparin in Non-Q-Wave Coronary Event Study Group. *N Engl J Med.* 1997;337:447-452.
13. Morrow DA, Antman EM, Giugliano RP, et al. A simple risk index for rapid initial triage of patients with ST elevation myocardial infarction: an In TIMI II substudy. *Lancet.* 2001;358:1571-1575.
14. Granger CB, Goldberg RJ, Dabbous O, et al. Predictors of hospital mortality in the Global Registry of Acute Coronary Events. *Arch Intern Med.* 2003;163:2345-2353.
15. Eagle KA, Lim MJ, Dabbous OH, et al. A validated prediction model for all forms of acute coronary syndrome: estimating the risk of 6-month post discharge death in an international registry *JAMA.* 2004;291:2727-2733.
16. Abu-Assi E, Ferreira-Gonzalez I, Ribera A et al. "Do Grace (Global Registry of Acute Coronary Events)risk scores still maintain their performance

for predicting mortality in the era of contemporary management of acute coronary syndrome?". *Am Heart J.* 2010;160:826-834.

17. Eggers KM, Kempf T, Venge P, et al. Improving long-term risk prediction in patients with acute chest pain: the Global Registry of Acute Coronary Events (GRACE) risk score is enhanced be selected nonnecrosis biomarkers. *Am Heart J.* 2010;160:88-94.
18. Stub D, Smith K, Bernard S, et al. Air versus oxygen in ST-segment-elevation myocardial infarction. *Circulation.* 2015;131(24):2143-2150.
19. Welsh P, Pressis D, Sattar N. Utility of high-sensitivity troponin T and I: are they the same? *J Am Coll Cardiol.* 2019.
20. Antman EM, Bennett JS, Daugherty A, et al. Use of nonsteroidal anti-inflammatory drugs: an update for clinicians: a scientific statement from the American Heart Association. *Circulation.* 2007;115(12):1634-1642.
21. Nissen SE, Yeomans ND, Solomon DH, et al. Cardiovascular Safety of Celecoxib, Naproxen, or Ibuprofen for Arthritis. *N Engl J Med.* 2016;375(26):2519-2529.
22. Chen ZM, Pan HC, Chen YP, et al. Early intravenous then oral metoprolol in 45,852 patients with acute myocardial infarction: randomised placebo-controlled trial. *Lancet.* 2005;366(9497):1622-1632.
23. Yusuf S, Wittes J, Friedman L. Overview of results of randomized clinical trials in heart disease. I. Treatments following myocardial infarction. *JAMA.* 1988;260(14):2088-2093.
24. Morrow DA, Scirica BM, Karwatowska-Prokopczuk E, et al. Effects of ranolazine on recurrent cardiovascular events in patients with non-ST-elevation acute coronary syndromes: the MERLIN-TIMI 36 randomized trial. *JAMA.* 2007;297(16):1775-1783.
25. Ferguson JJ, Califf RM, Antman EM, et al. Enoxaparin vs unfractionated heparin in high-risk patients with non-ST-segment elevation acute coronary syndromes managed with an intended early invasive strategy: primary results of the SYNERGY randomized trial. *JAMA.* 2004;292(1):45-54.
26. Stone GW, McLaurin BT, Cox DA, et al. Bivalirudin for patients with acute coronary syndromes. *N Engl J Med.* 2006;355(21):2203-2216.
27. Jolly SS, Faxon DP, Fox KA, et al. Efficacy and safety of fondaparinux versus enoxaparin in patients with acute coronary syndromes treated with glycoprotein IIb/IIIa inhibitors or thienopyridines: results from the OASIS 5 (Fifth Organization to Assess Strategies in Ischemic Syndromes) trial. *J Am Coll Cardiol.* 2009;54(5):468-476.
28. Berger JS, Sallum RH, Katona B, et al. Is there an association between aspirin dosing and cardiac and bleeding events after treatment of acute coronary syndrome? A systematic review of the literature. *Am Heart J.* 2012;164(2):153-162.e155.
29. Yusuf S, Zhao F, Mehta SR, et al. Effects of clopidogrel in addition to aspirin in patients with acute coronary syndromes without ST-segment elevation. *N Engl J Med.* 2001;345(7):494-502.
30. Wiviott SD, Braunwald E, McCabe CH, et al. Prasugrel versus clopidogrel in patients with acute coronary syndromes. *N Engl J Med.* 2007;357(20):2001-2015.
31. Montalescot G, Bolognese L, Dudek D, et al. Pretreatment with prasugrel in non-ST-segment elevation acute coronary syndromes. *N Engl J Med.* 2013;369(11):999-1010.
32. Wallentin L, Becker RC, Budaj A, et al. Ticagrelor versus clopidogrel in patients with acute coronary syndromes. *N Engl J Med.* 2009;361(11): 1045-1057.
33. Steg PG, Bhatt DL, Hamm CW, et al. Effect of cangrelor on periprocedural outcomes in percutaneous coronary interventions: a pooled analysis of patient-level data. *Lancet.* 2013;382(9909):1981-1992.
34. Murphy SA, Cannon CP, Wiviott SD, McCabe CH, Braunwald E. Reduction in recurrent cardiovascular events with intensive lipid-lowering statin therapy compared with moderate lipid-lowering statin therapy after acute coronary syndromes from the PROVE IT-TIMI 22 (Pravastatin or Atorvastatin Evaluation and Infection Therapy-Thrombolysis In Myocardial Infarction 22) trial. *J Am Coll Cardiol.* 2009;54(25):2358-2362.
35. Cannon CP, Blazing MA, Giugliano RP, et al. Ezetimibe added to statin therapy after acute coronary syndromes. *N Engl J Med.* 2015;372(25):2387-2397.
36. Indications for ACE inhibitors in the early treatment of acute myocardial infarction: systematic overview of individual data from 100,000 patients in randomized trials. ACE Inhibitor Myocardial Infarction Collaborative Group. *Circulation.* 1998;97(22):2202-2212.
37. Pfeffer MA, Braunwald E, Moye LA, et al. Effect of captopril on mortality and morbidity in patients with left ventricular dysfunction after myocardial infarction. Results of the survival and ventricular enlargement trial. The SAVE Investigators. *N Engl J Med.* 1992;327(10):669-677.
38. Pfeffer MA, McMurray JJ, Velazquez EJ, et al. Valsartan, captopril, or both in myocardial infarction complicated by heart failure, left ventricular dysfunction, or both. *N Engl J Med.* 2003;349(20):1893-1906.
39. Pitt B, Remme W, Zannad F, et al. Eplerenone, a selective aldosterone blocker, in patients with left ventricular dysfunction after myocardial infarction. *N Engl J Med.* 2003;348(14):1309-1321.
40. Cannon CP, Weintraub WS, Demopoulos LA, et al. Comparison of early invasive and conservative strategy in patients with unstable coronary syndromes treated with glycoprotein IIb/IIIa inhibitor tirofiban. *N Engl J Med.* 2001;344:1879-1887.
41. Boden WE, O'Rourke RA, Crawford MH, et al. Outcomes in patients with acute non-Q-wave myocardial infarction randomly assigned to an invasive as compared with a conservative management strategy. Veterans Affairs Non-Q Wave Infarction Strategies in Hospital (VANQWISH) Trial Investigators *N Engl J Med.* 1998;338:1785-1792.
42. De Winter RJ, Windhausen F, Cornel JH, et al. Early invasive versus selectively invasive management for acute coronary syndromes. *N Engl J Med.* 2005;353:1095-1104.
43. Fox KA, Poole-Wilson PA, Henderson RA, et al. Interventional vs conservative treatment for patients with unstable angina or non-ST-elevation myocardial infarction: The British Heart Foundation RITA 3 randomized trial. Randomized Intervention Trial of unstable Angina. *Lancet.* 2002;360:743-751.
44. McCullough PA, O'Neill WW, Graham M, et al. A prospective randomized trial of triage angiography in acute coronary syndromes ineligible for thrombolytic therapy. Results of the medicine versus angiography in thrombolytic exclusion (MATE) trial. *J Am Coll Cardiol.* 1998;32:596-605.
45. Neumann FJ, Kastrati A, Pogastra-Murray G, et al. Evaluation of prolonged antithrombotic pretreatment ("cooling-off" strategy) before intervention in patients with unstable coronary syndromes: a randomized controlled trial. *JAMA.* 2003;290:1593-1599.
46. Lagerqvist B, Safstrom K, Stahle E, et al. Is early invasive treatment of unstable coronary artery disease equally effective for both women and men? FRISC II Study Group Investigators. *J AM Coll Cardiol.* 2001;38:41-48.
47. Glaser R, Herrmann HC, Murphy SA, et al. Benefit of an early invasive management strategy in women with acute coronary syndromes. *JAMA.* 2002;288:3124-3129.
48. O'Donoghue ML, Vaidya A, Afsal R, et al. An invasive or conservative strategy in patients with diabetes mellitus and non-ST-segment elevation acute coronary syndromes: a collaborative meta-analysis of randomized trials. *J Am Coll Cardiol.* 2012;60:106-111.
49. Chan PS, Patel MR, Klein LW, et al. Appropriateness of percutaneous coronary intervention. *JAMA.* 2011;306:53-61.
50. Parikh SV, De Lemos JA, Jessen ME, et al. Timing of in hospital coronary artery bypass graft surgery for non-ST-segment elevation myocardial infarction patients results from the national cardiovascular data registry ACTION registry-GWTG (Acute Coronary Treatment and Intervention Outcomes Network Registry-Get With The Guidelines). *JACC Cardiovasc Interv.* 2010;3:419-427.
51. Bavry AA, Kumbhani DJ, Rassi AN, et al. Benefit of early invasive therapy in acute coronary syndromes: a meta-analysis of contemporary randomized clinical trial. *J Am Coll Cardiol.* 2006;48:1319-1325.
52. Hillis LD, Smith PK, Anderson JL, et al. 2011 ACCF/AHA guidelines for coronary artery bypass graft surgery. A report of the American College of Cardiology Foundation/American Heart Association Task Force on Practice Guidelines. *J Am Coll Cardiol.* 2011;58:e123-e210.
53. Devlin G, Gore JM, Elliott J, et al. Management and 6 month outcomes in elderly and very elderly patients with high-risk non-ST-elevation acute coronary syndromes: The Global Registry of Acute Coronary Events. *Eur Heart J.* 2008;29:1275-1282.

54. Damman P, Clayton T, Wallentin L, et al. Effects of age on long-term outcomes after a routine invasive or selective invasive strategy in patients presenting with non-ST segment elevation acute coronary syndromes: a collaborative analysis of individual data from FRISC II—ICTUS—RITA–3 (FIR) trials. *Heart.* 2012;98:207-213.
55. Krane M, Voss B, Hiebinger A, et al. Twenty years of cardiac surgery in patients aged 80 years and older: risks and benefits. *Ann Thorac Surg.* 2011;91:506-513.
56. Bardakci H, Cheema FH, Topkara VK, et al. Discharge to home rates are significantly lower for octogenarians undergoing coronary artery bypass graft surgery. *Ann Thorac Surg.* 2007;83:483-489.
57. Hockman JS, Sleeper LA, Webb JG, et al. Early revascularization in acute myocardial infarction complicated by cardiogenic shock. SHOCK investigators. Should We Emergently Revascularize Occluded Coronaries for Cardiogenic Shock. *N Engl J Med.* 1999;341:625-634.
58. Holmes DR Jr, Berger PB, Hockman JS, et al. Cardiogenic shock in patients with acute ischemic syndromes with and without ST-segment elevation. *Circulation.* 1999;100:2067-2073.
59. De Luca L, Olivari Z, Farina A, et al. Temporal trends in the epidemiology, management, and outcome of patients with cardiogenic shock complicating acute coronary syndromes: management changes in cardiogenic shock. *Eur J Heart Fail.* 2015;17:1124-1132.
60. Thompson PD, Buchner D, Pina IL, et al. Exercise and physical activity in the prevention and treatment of atherosclerotic cardiovascular disease: a statement from the Council on Clinical Cardiology (Subcommittee on Exercise, Rehabilitation, and Prevention) and the Council on Nutrition, Physical Activity, and Metabolism (Subcommittee on Physical Activity). *Circulation.* 2003;107:3109-3116.

CHAPTER 6

ST-ELEVATION MYOCARDIAL INFARCTION

Ranjan Dahal and Debabrata Mukherjee

INTRODUCTION

Acute myocardial infarction (AMI) is defined as an acute myocardial injury with detection of a rise and/or fall of cardiac troponin (cTn) values with at least one value greater than 99th percentile of the upper reference limit of normal along with symptoms consistent with myocardial ischemia; or new ischemic changes in the electrocardiogram (ECG); or development of pathological Q waves; or imaging evidence of ischemic wall motion abnormalities or new loss of viable myocardium; or identification of a coronary thrombus by angiography or autopsy.[1]

ST-elevation myocardial infarction (STEMI) is defined as a clinical syndrome characterized by symptoms of myocardial ischemia along with persistent ST-segment elevation in ECG and subsequent release of cardiac biomarkers of myocardial injury. The ECG criteria for STEMI are listed in **Table 6.1**. Considering immediate reperfusion strategies and mortality benefit, it is imperative to designate patients with symptoms suggestive of myocardial ischemia and ST elevations in two contiguous ECG leads as STEMI.

Epidemiology

Ischemic heart disease remains a major public health problem with an estimated prevalence of around 153 million globally. Approximately 1.3 million hospital discharges from the US hospitals in 2014 had an acute coronary syndrome (ACS) listed as a primary or secondary diagnosis.[2] There have been changing patterns in the incidence of ischemic heart disease. The overall incidence of STEMI visits has declined significantly whereas non-STEMI has increased. The trends of yearly STEMI incidence of emergency department visits have decreased by more than 60% from 2005-2007 to 2014-2015.[3] Women have a later presentation and longer reperfusion (door-to-balloon and door-to-fibrinolysis) time even without contraindications to reperfusion therapy compared to men.[4] There is a decreasing mortality trend following STEMI, which is likely from increased reperfusion strategy using primary percutaneous coronary intervention (PCI), newer generation stents, potent antiplatelet therapy, and aggressive secondary risk factors reduction.[5] But overall mortality from STEMI is still substantial, accounting for 6.4% of total STEMI cases, with mortality influenced by advanced age, higher Killip class at presentation, time delay to treatment, treatment strategies, left ventricular dysfunction, higher number of diseased coronary arteries, unstable hemodynamics, anterior infarction, and comorbid conditions such as diabetes mellitus and renal failure.[6]

Risk Factors

The traditional modifiable risk factors for coronary artery disease are tobacco exposure, diabetes mellitus, hyperlipidemia, hypertension, metabolic syndrome, obesity, and physical inactivity. Nonmodifiable risk factors include a family history of premature cardiovascular diseases (first cardiovascular event at age <55 years for men and <65 years for women), genetics, and chronic kidney diseases. Nontraditional risk factors include socioeconomic and psychosocial stress, autoimmune diseases, malignancy, and its therapies, infections, sleep apnea, and pregnancy-related complications.

A substantial proportion of STEMI patients without prior cardiovascular diseases are noted to have no history of standard modifiable cardiovascular risk factors. These patients have higher in-hospital mortality compared to patients with traditional modifiable risk factors.[7]

PATHOGENESIS

Coronary artery atherosclerosis, nonatherosclerotic causes, and coronary vasospasm can all lead to coronary artery occlusion and STEMI. The most common cause is acute total or subtotal coronary artery occlusion by thrombus from the rupture or ulceration or erosion of atherosclerotic plaque.[8] Nonatherosclerotic causes of STEMI include air emboli and emboli from the left ventricle, left atrial appendage, atrial myxomas, and infective endocarditis. Chest trauma, thoracic aortic dissection, spontaneous coronary artery dissection, collagen vascular diseases, and arteritis are other nonatherosclerotic causes. Drugs like cocaine or serotonin receptor agonists (triptans) and Prinzmetal angina can cause severe coronary vasospasm and STEMI.

The atherosclerotic plaque rich in lipids with necrotic core and thin fibrous cap are considered vulnerable plaques. The progression of plaques with the expansion of lipid core and macrophage accumulation causes plaques to rupture. Partial occlusion of the blood vessel lumen leads to myocardial ischemia and non-STEMI, whereas complete occlusion leads to transmural infarction and STEMI. The size of infarction depends on the duration of blood vessel occlusion, the presence of collateral blood supply, the level of occlusion, and microvascular circulation. However, the development of Q waves in ECG depends on the infarct size, not on the depth of myocardial involvement.

TABLE 6.1 ECG Criteria for ST-Elevation Myocardial Infarction (STEMI)

• New ST-segment elevation at the J point in two contiguous leads with the cutoff point as >0.1 mV in all leads other than V2 or V3 • In leads V2-V3, the cutoff point is ST-segment elevation >0.2 mV in men older than 40 years and >0.25 in men <40 years old, or >0.15 mV in women
Left bundle branch block: • ST-segment elevation of 1 mm or more that is concordant with (in the same direction as) the QRS complex • ST-segment depression of 1 mm or more in lead V1, V2, or V3 • ST-segment elevation of 5 mm or more that is discordant with (in the opposite direction) the QRS complex
Ventricular-paced rhythm: Left bundle branch block (LBBB) pattern seen during isolated RV pacing. Same diagnostic criteria as LBBB may be helpful.
Isolated posterior myocardial infarction: Isolated ST depression ≥0.5 mm in V1-V3 and ST-segment elevation ≥0.5 mm in posterior leads V7-V9
Ischemia owing to left main coronary artery occlusion or multivessel disease: ST-segment depression ≥1 mm in multiple leads along with ST elevation in aVR
Right ventricular infarction: ST-segment elevation ≥1 mm in right precordial leads V3R and V4R

aVRRV, aVR = augmented Vector Right.

CLINICAL PRESENTATION

The most common symptom is retrosternal chest pain or discomfort radiating to the jaw, neck, left arm, or shoulder. The chest pain is usually diffuse, nonpositional, and dull aching or heavy pressure in nature, lasting more than 20 minutes. Other symptoms may be epigastric pain, neck pain, jaw pain, shortness of breath, nausea, vomiting, fatigue, diaphoresis, and generalized weakness. Occasionally, patients may present with sudden cardiac arrest.

The physical signs at presentation may mostly be unremarkable. It may vary depending on the extent and anatomy of myocardial infarction. Hypotension, tachycardia, cool skin, rales, an S3 gallop, and diminished pedal pulses are signs of left ventricular dysfunction and carry a worse prognosis. A new systolic murmur is indicative of mitral regurgitation or ventricular septal rupture. Thoracic ascending aortic dissection is a life-threatening condition that can involve coronaries and present as a STEMI. Myocarditis, pericarditis, and pneumo-mediastinum may all have STEMI-like presentations. A high index of clinical suspicion is required for the diagnosis of myocardial infarction as some patients may have atypical presentations.

DIAGNOSIS

Emergent Electrocardiogram

An ECG should be performed within 10 minutes of first medical contact (FMC) if an ACS is suspected.[5] ECG criteria for STEMI are defined in Table 6.1, anatomic location of myocardial injury based on ST changes in ECG in **Table 6.2**, and Stillshot 6.1–6.4, showing coronary artery occlusions and respective ECG changes. Standard ECG calibration is 10 mm/mV and 0.1 mV is equal to 1 mm square on the vertical axis.

A new or presumably new left bundle branch block (LBBB) is considered STEMI equivalent but should not be considered AMI in isolation. Inferior myocardial infarction is commonly associated with concomitant right ventricular infarction. However, a paced rhythm, Brugada syndrome, and left ventricular hypertrophy (LVH) make interpretation of ST segments challenging. The ECG should be repeated if the diagnosis is unclear. A complete resolution of the ST-segment elevation and symptoms after nitroglycerine administration is suggestive of coronary spasm. It is imperative to understand other causes of ST-segment elevation to manage accordingly. ST-segment elevations can be present in left ventricular aneurysm, ventricular-paced rhythm, early repolarization pattern, pneumo-mediastinum, LBBB, myocarditis, pericarditis, takotsubo cardiomyopathy, hemorrhagic cerebrovascular accident and can be a normal variant in young patients.

TABLE 6.2 Anatomical Location of Myocardial Injury Based on ECG Lead Changes and Involved Coronaries

Anatomic Location	ECG Lead Changes	Probable Involved Coronary Artery
Septal	V1-V2 ST-segment elevations	Left anterior descending artery
Anterior	V3-V4 ST-segment elevations (Stillshot 1 and Stillshot 3)	Left anterior descending artery
Inferior	II, III, aVF ST-segment elevations (Stillshot 2)	Right coronary artery
Lateral	V5, V6, I, aVL ST-segment elevations (Stillshot 4)	Left circumflex artery
Posterior	V1-V3 ST-segment depression V7-V9 ST-segment elevation in posterior leads	Right coronary artery/left circumflex artery
Right ventricular	V4R V5R V6R ST-segment elevation in right-sided leads	Right coronary artery

ECG, electrocardiogram.

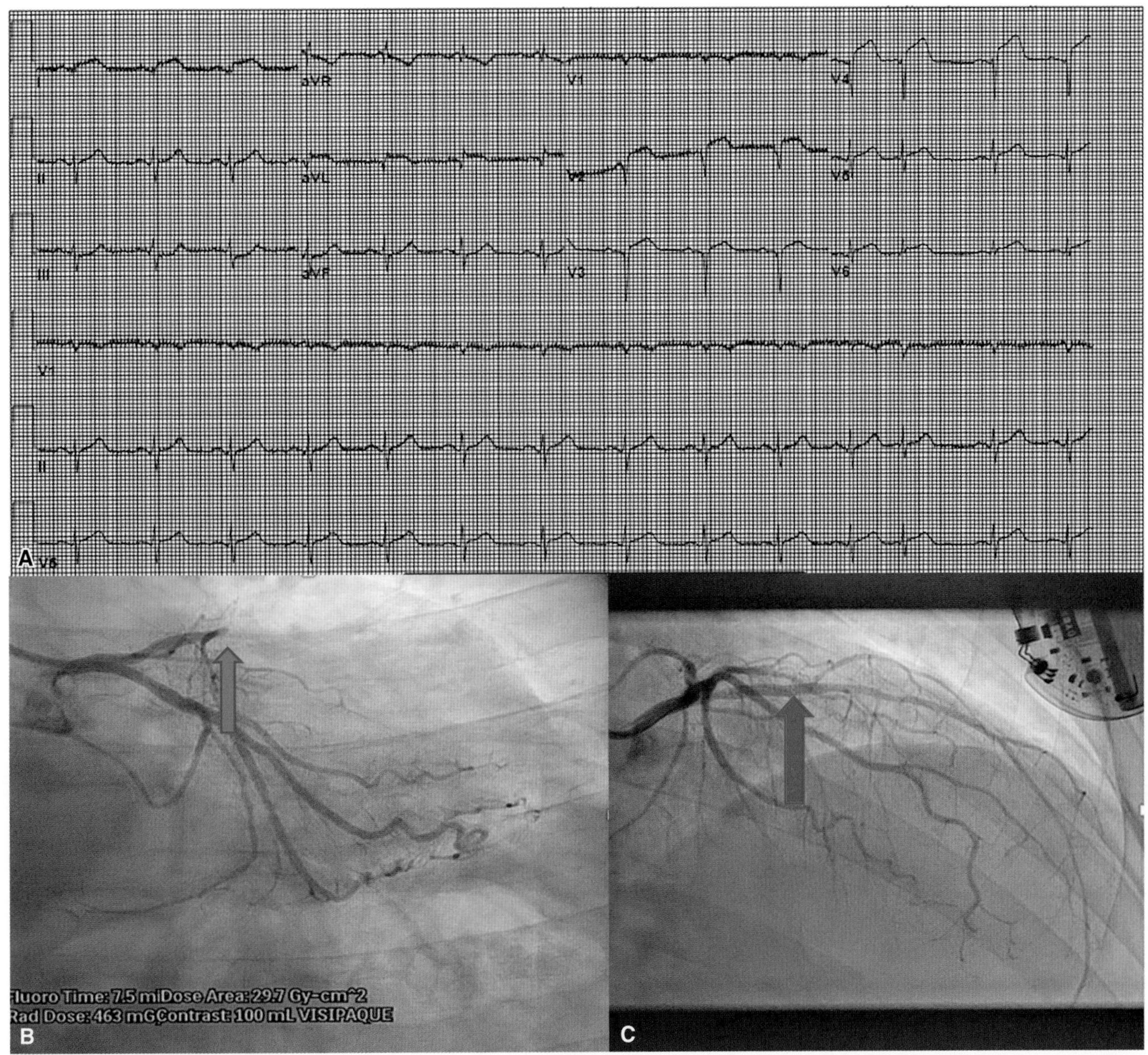

STILLSHOT 6.1 A 63-year old male presented with chest pain for 1 hour. **(A)** 12-lead electrocardiogram showing anteroseptal ST-segment myocardial infarction. **(B)** Coronary angiogram right anterior oblique (RAO) caudal view showing 100% occlusion of mid-LAD (blue arrow). **(C)** Coronary angiogram RAO cranial post-percutaneous coronary intervention (red arrow)

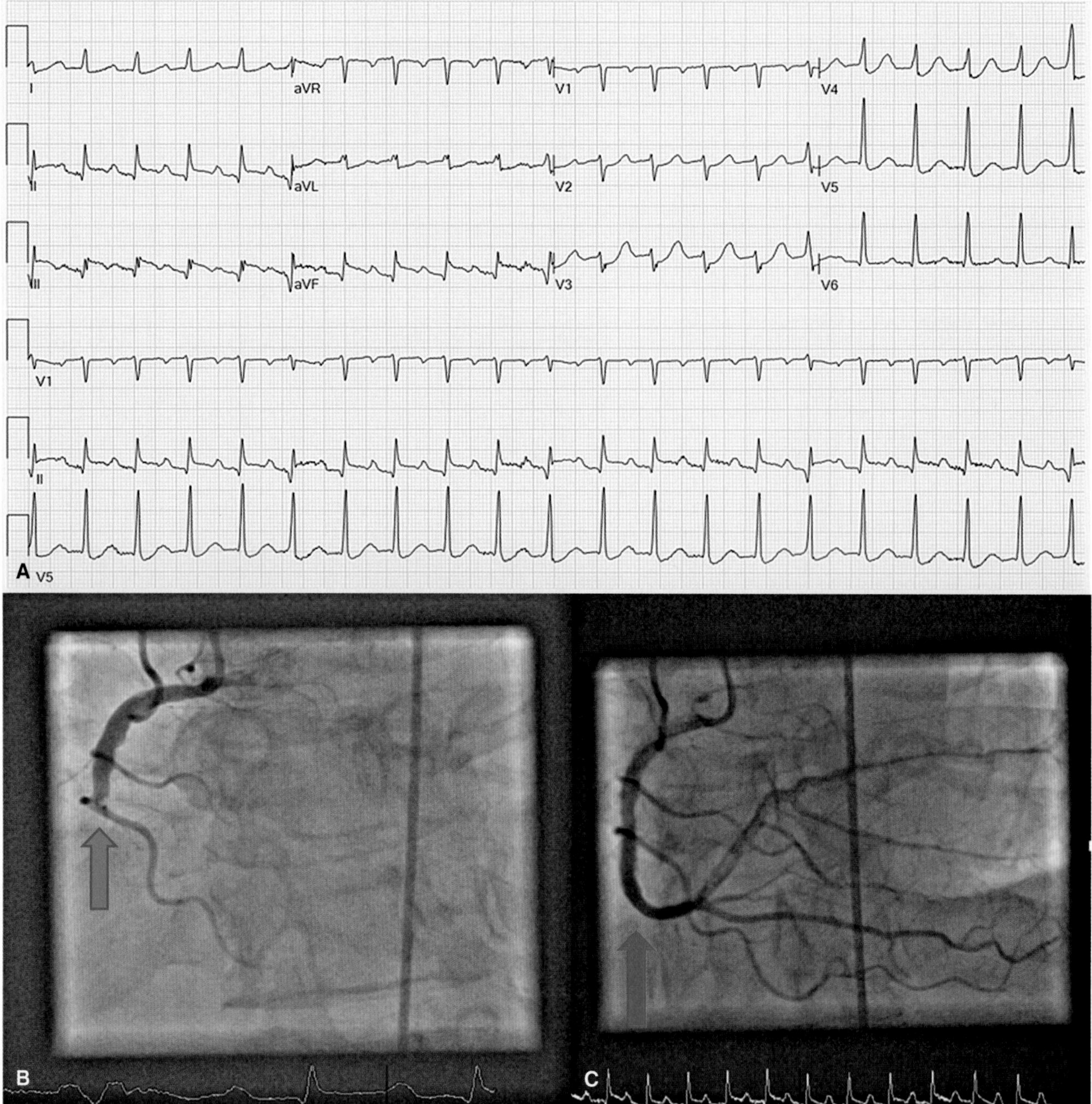

STILLSHOT 6.2 A 53-year-old male admitted with chest pain for 1 hour. **(A)** 12-lead electrocardiogram showing inferior ST-segment myocardial infarction. **(B)** Coronary angiogram showing 100% occlusion of mid-right coronary artery (blue arrow). **(C)** Post-percutaneous coronary intervention (red arrow).

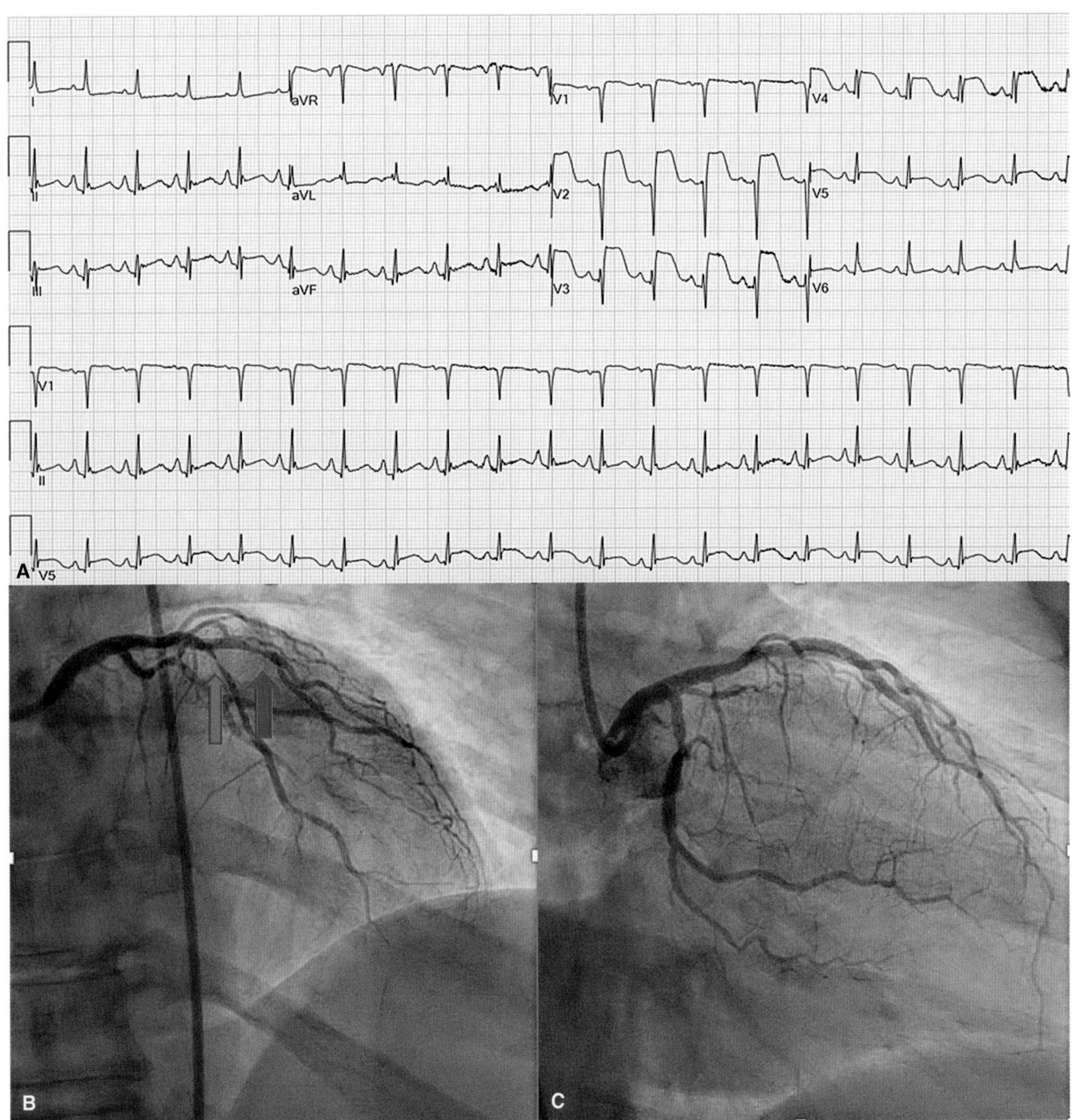

STILLSHOT 6.3 A 60-year-old female presented with chest pain. **(A)** 12-lead electrocardiogram showing anteroseptal ST-segment elevation myocardial infarction. **(B)** Left anterior oblique cranial view showing subtotal occlusion of mid-left anterior descending (LAD) (blue arrow) and subtotal occlusion of mid-left circumflex (red arrow). **(C)** Right anterior oblique caudal view post-percutaneous coronary intervention of LAD and left circumflex

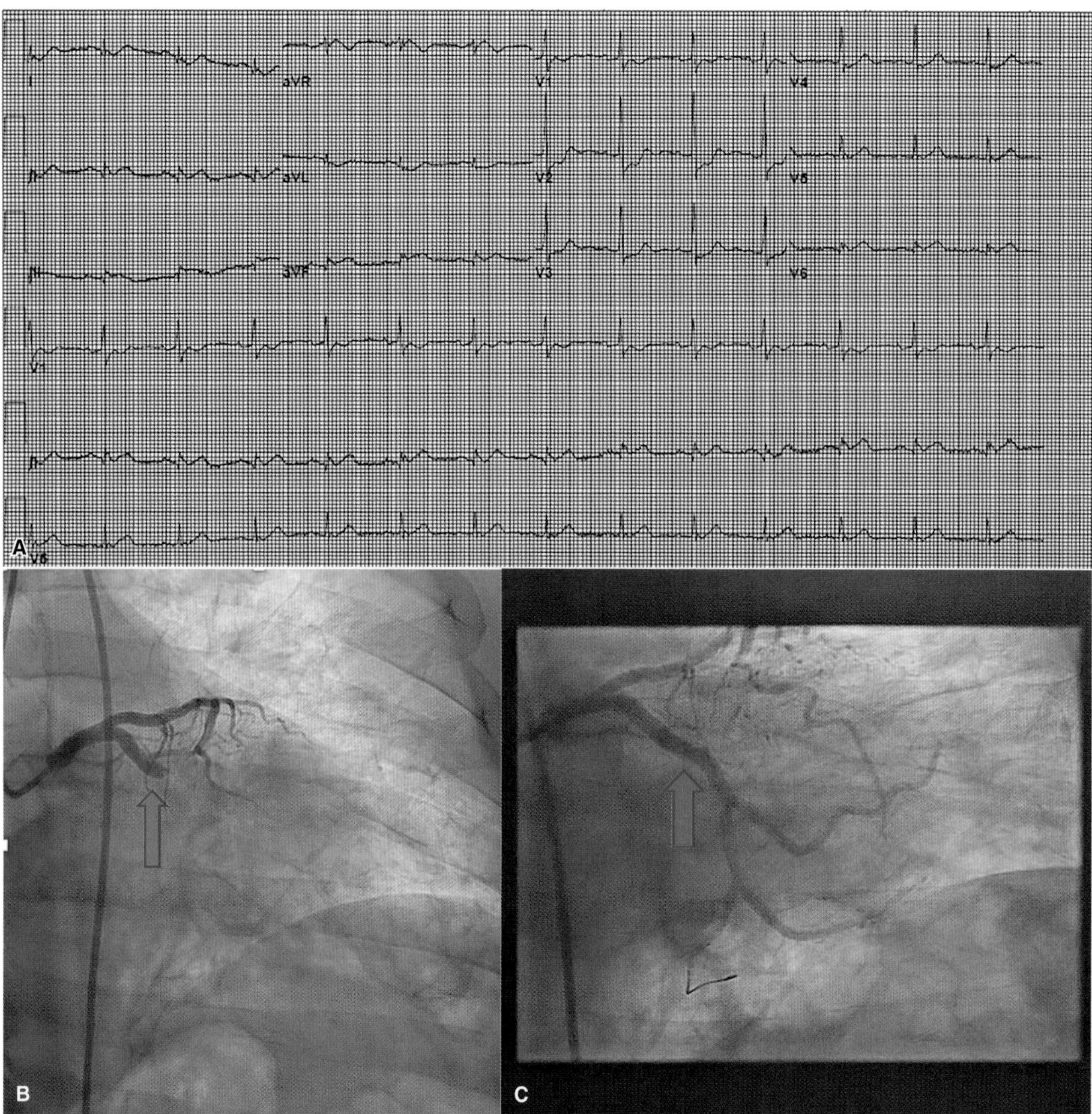

STILLSHOT 6.4 An 88-year-old male presented with chest pain. **(A)** 12-lead electrocardiogram showing infero-posterior ST-segment elevation myocardial infarction. **(B)** Right anterior oblique caudal view showing 100% occlusion of the proximal left circumflex (blue arrow). **(C)** Post-percutaneous coronary intervention of proximal left circumflex (red arrow).

Emergent Bedside Echocardiogram and Other Possible Diagnostic Testing

A bedside echocardiogram can be performed emergently if the diagnosis is uncertain to identify regional wall motion abnormalities and mechanical complications related to STEMI. It may also provide an alternate diagnosis such as ascending aortic dissection, pericardial effusion, and massive pulmonary embolism. A chest x-ray may be useful to detect features of aortic dissection. However, routine echocardiogram and chest x-ray delaying emergent coronary angiography are not recommended. (See **Video 6.1d&e** and **Video 6.2b&c**)

Cardiac magnetic resonance imaging (MRI) and coronary computed tomography (CT) have limited roles in STEMI. Routine blood tests for the cardiac serum marker cTn are indicated but should not delay reperfusion strategy. Other laboratory tests augmenting patient care may include complete blood count, coagulation profile, renal function test, liver function test, serum lipids, hemoglobin A1c, and serum glucose.

Thrombolysis in myocardial infarction (TIMI) and Global Registry of Acute Coronary Events (GRACE) risk scores can be used for early risk assessment of patients presenting with an ACS.[9,10] Risk assessment should be repeated during hospitalization and at the time of discharge. These risk scores will provide an overall estimate of the patient's prognosis, guide the treatment strategy, and inform family members of the potential outcomes.

MANAGEMENT

Appropriate management strategy begins with community awareness about anginal symptoms and preparedness to deliver reperfusion therapy expeditiously and effectively with efforts to make primary PCI the primary reperfusion strategy (**Algorithm 6.1**). Regional systems of STEMI care should be created and maintained for quality checks.

The optimal management begins at the scene before reaching the hospital. Patients with suspected ACS should be transported by ambulance rather than private vehicles owing to the small risk of cardiac arrest en route to the hospital. A prehospital ECG performed by trained personnel facilitates early reperfusion times and improved outcomes.[11] If STEMI is suspected, devices with defibrillator capacity and continuous ECG monitor should be attached to the patient.[5] Aspirin (162-325 mg loading dose) should be given orally en route to the hospital if not contraindicated. Sublingual nitroglycerine can also be given for chest pain if tolerated by hemodynamics. The facility receiving the patient should be alerted so that preparation for reperfusion therapy can be initiated. Some facilities even bypass emergency departments to achieve early reperfusion. Ambulances in European countries are well-equipped to administer prehospital fibrinolytic therapy, but are not currently available in the United States.[12]

Immediate Therapies

Oxygen: Oxygen should be given only if SaO_2 less than 90% or PaO_2 less than 60 mm Hg. Routine oxygen therapy in STEMI patients with normal oxygen saturation is not recommended because it increases the risk of myocardial injury and recurrent myocardial infarction (MI).[13]

Nitroglycerine: Sublingual tablets 0.3 to 0.6 mg and nitro sprays 0.4 to 0.8 mg can be administered every 5 minutes, up to three doses as needed for angina. Intravenous nitroglycerine can be administered for hypertensive and heart failure patients with ongoing ischemia. It should be used cautiously in patients with hypotension, right ventricular infarction, and recent phosphodiesterase inhibitor use.

Analgesics: Intravenous opioids can be used for pain control with dose titration based on symptoms and hemodynamics. However, it should be used cautiously in opioid naive, elderly, and patients with borderline hemodynamics. Nonsteroidal anti-inflammatory drugs other than aspirin should be avoided in STEMI patients.

Reperfusion Strategies

Primary Percutaneous Coronary Intervention

Reperfusion therapy should be administered to all STEMI patients with symptoms onset of fewer than 12 hours and no contraindications. Primary PCI is the preferred reperfusion therapy with the greatest survival benefit in high-risk patients.[4] It has shown superior outcomes in reducing mortality, reinfarction, or stroke compared to fibrinolysis with similar treatment delays in high volume centers with an experienced operator and skilled staff. It also has lower rates of recurrent ischemia, emergency repeat revascularization, and intracranial hemorrhage.[14] Patients should be considered for fibrinolysis therapy if they cannot be transferred to PCI-capable hospital with the goal of FMC to device time of 120 minutes.[4,5] As per the catheterization laboratory registry in 2014, the median door-to-balloon time for primary PCI at presenting hospitals was 59 and 105 minutes if transferred from another facility.[6]

The 2017 European guidelines have started using the term door-to-reperfusion time.[5] Both the American College of Cardiology (ACC) and the European Society of Cardiology (ESC) recommend primary PCI in patients with contraindications to fibrinolytic therapy, cardiogenic shock or acute severe heart failure, or life-threatening arrhythmias from STEMI irrespective of symptoms onset. ACC recommends primary PCI for up to 12 to 24 hours after symptoms onset whereas ESC recommends PCI for up to 48 hours.[4,5] Early angiography within 24 hours is recommended if symptoms are completely relieved along with the complete resolution of ST spontaneously or after nitroglycerine administration. A routine coronary angiography can be performed in patients presenting 48 hours of symptom onset. However, routine PCI of the culprit artery is not recommended in asymptomatic STEMI patients presenting greater than 48 hours after symptom onset.[5]

The Minimizing Adverse hemorrhagic events by TRansradial access site and systemic Implementation of angioX (MATRIX) showed radial access was associated with lower risks of access site bleeding, vascular complications, and need for the blood transfusion compared to femoral access. The radial first

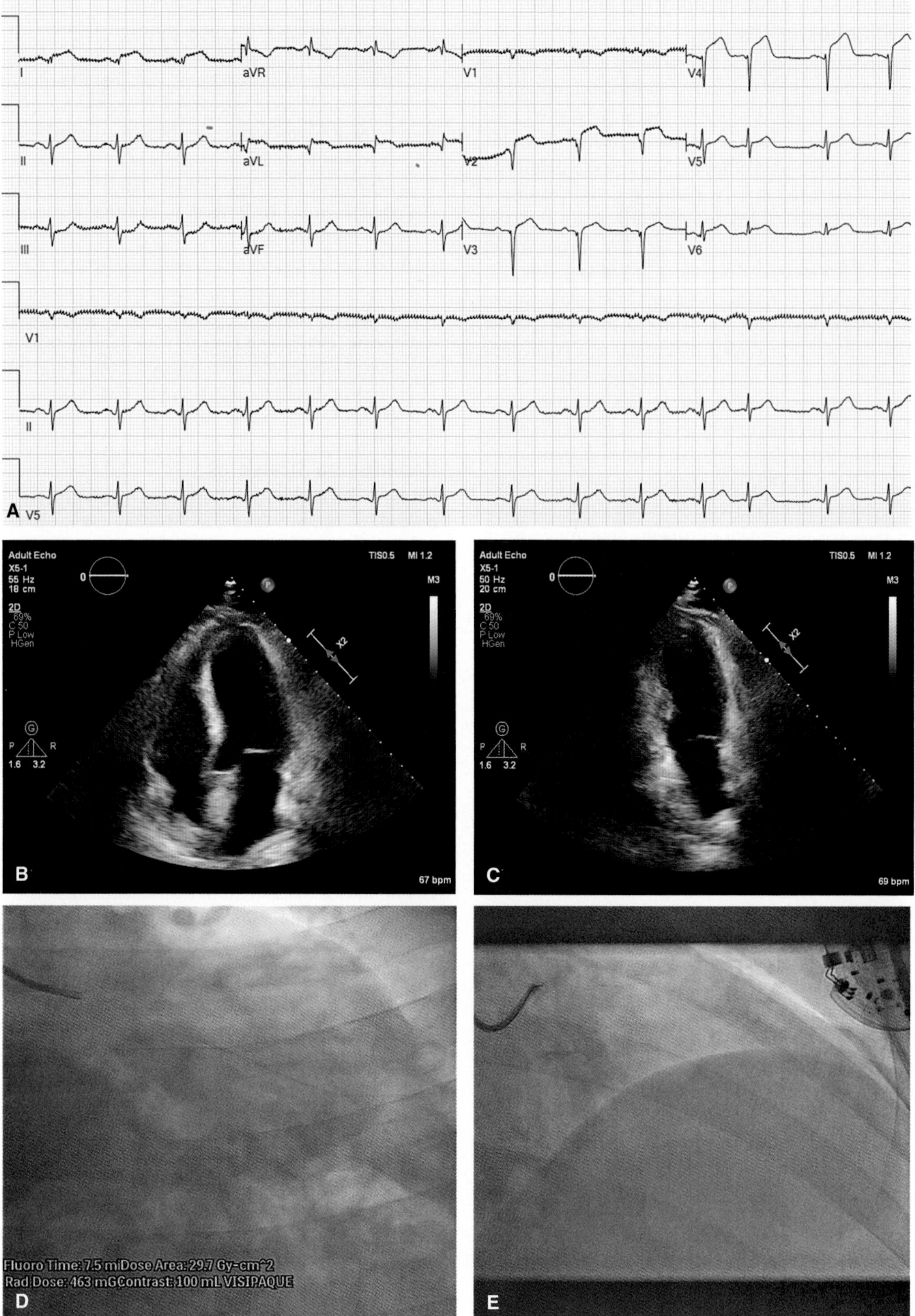

CLINICAL CASE 6.1 A 63-year old male presented with chest pain for 1 hour. **(A)** 12-lead electrocardiogram showing anteroseptal ST-segment myocardial infarction. **(B, C)** Transthoracic echocardiography apical four chambers and apical two chambers showing hypokinesis in left anterior descending (LAD) territory. **(D)** Coronary angiogram right anterior oblique (RAO) caudal view showing 100% occlusion of mid-LAD (▶ VIDEO 6.1d). **(E)** Coronary angiogram RAO cranial post-percutaneous coronary intervention (▶ VIDEO 6.1e).

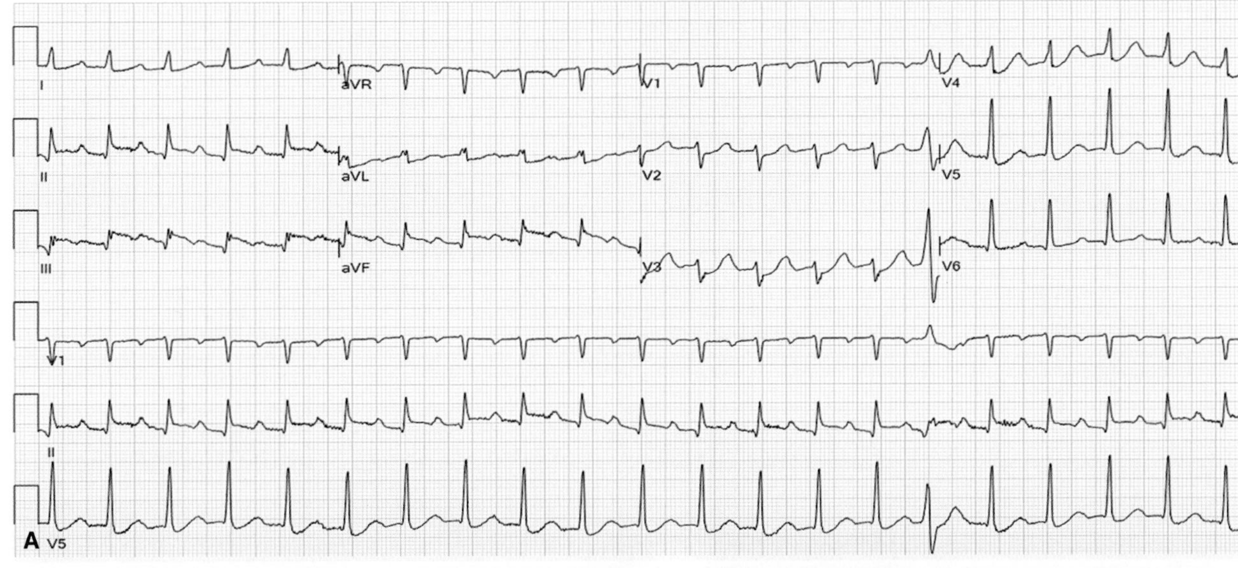

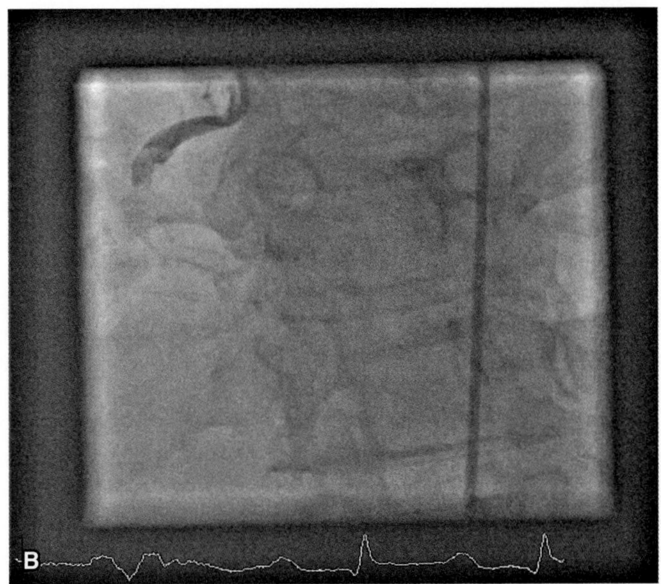

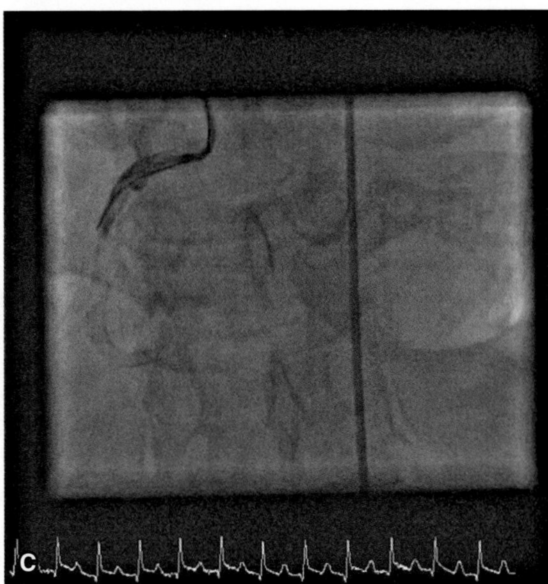

CLINICAL CASE 6.2 A 53-year-old male admitted with chest pain for 1 hour. **(A)** 12-lead electrocardiogram showing inferior ST-segment myocardial infarction. **(B)** Coronary angiogram showing 100% occlusion of mid-right coronary artery (VIDEO 6.2b). **(C)** Post-percutaneous coronary intervention (VIDEO 6.2c).

approach is the preferred technique depending on operator skills.[15] (See **Video 6.3b&c** and **Videos 6.4**)

Compared to PCI alone, routine aspiration thrombectomy with PCI showed no differences in cardiovascular death, recurrent MI, cardiogenic shock, thrombosis, New York Heart Association class IV heart failure or target vessel revascularization at 180 days but increased risk of stroke as per the TOTAL (Trial of Routine Aspiration Thrombectomy with PCI versus PCI Alone in Patients with STEMI) study.[16] Compared to balloon angioplasty, a bare-metal stent was associated with a lower risk of reinfarction and target vessel revascularization with no mortality benefit.[17] The everolimus-eluting stent versus bare-metal stent in ST-segment elevation myocardial infarction (EXAMINATION) study showed a reduced rate of stent thrombosis and target vessel revascularization at 1 year and reduced rate of all-cause mortality at 5 years with drug-eluting stent.[18,19] The time targets for reperfusion as per ACC and ESC guidelines are summarized in **Table 6.3**.

Antiplatelets Used in Primary PCI. Nonenteric coated aspirin—162 to 325 mg orally or 600 mg rectally if the oral route is not feasible—is recommended. Prasugrel 60 mg oral once as a loading dose, then 10 mg/day or ticagrelor 180 mg oral loading dose and 90 mg twice per day maintenance dose are preferred P2Y12 inhibitors. They have a rapid onset of action, greater potency, and better efficacy than clopidogrel.[20,21] Prasugrel is contraindicated in patients with a prior history of stroke or transient ischemic attack because of increased risk of

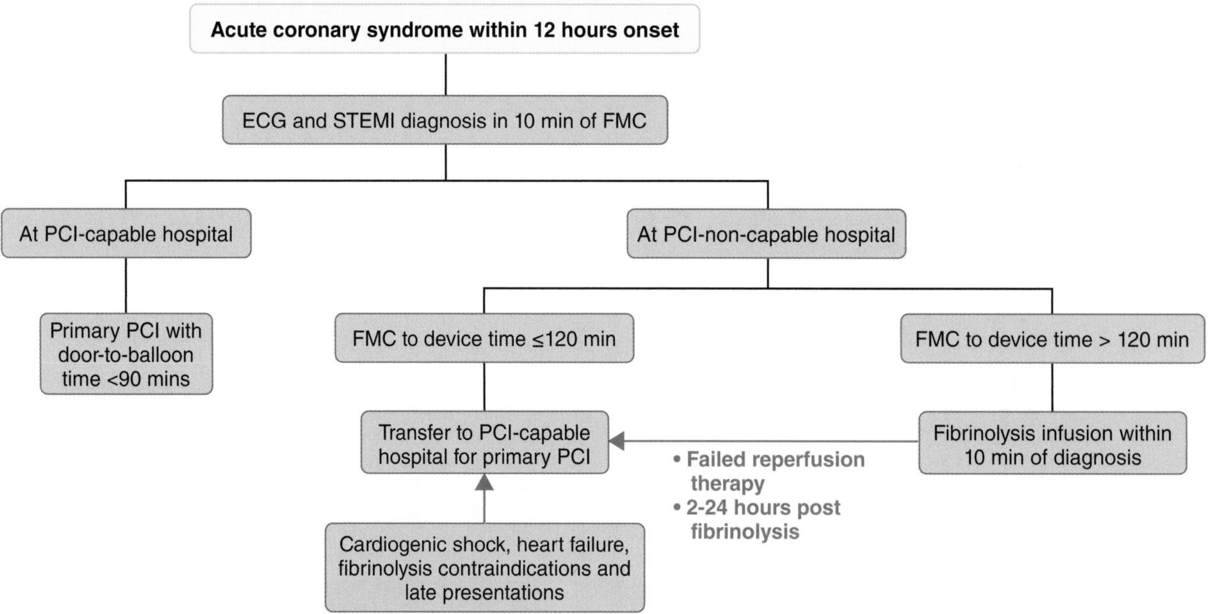

ALGORITHM 6.1 Management strategies for STEMI patients. ECG, electrocardiogram; FMC, first medical contact; PCI, percutaneous coronary intervention; STEMI, ST-elevation myocardial infarction.

intracranial hemorrhage. Prasugrel 5 mg daily maintenance dose should be used in patients with weight less than 60 kg or age greater than or equal to 75 years because of potentially increased bleeding risk. Clopidogrel 600 mg loading dose should be used if prasugrel or ticagrelor is not available.[22] Cangrelor is a potent intravenous antiplatelet that can be used as an adjunct to PCI in patients not treated with P2Y12 platelet inhibitors and glycoprotein (GP) IIb/IIIa inhibitors. It decreases periprocedural ischemia but increases bleeding risk.[23] Patients on cangrelor infusion should be transitioned to oral P2Y12 inhibitors as follows: clopidogrel 600 mg or Prasugrel 60 mg loading dose should be given immediately after discontinuation of cangrelor, whereas ticagrelor 180 mg can be given any time during intravenous (IV) infusion or immediately after discontinuation. The loading dose and maintenance dose of P2Y12 inhibitors are summarized in **Table 6.4**.

GP IIb/IIIa Inhibitors: Intravenous GP IIb/IIIa inhibitors can be used in patients with angiographic evidence of large thrombus burden or slow or no-reflow after angioplasty and inadequate P2Y12 inhibitors loading if there are no contraindications. However, it lacks consistent data in terms of reducing mortality and reinfarction.[5] The bolus dose and maintenance dose of GP IIb/IIIa inhibitors are summarized in **Table 6.5**.

Anticoagulation Used with Primary PCI. Unfractionated heparin (UFH), bivalirudin, or enoxaparin can be used for primary PCI. Bivalirudin is preferred in patients with heparin-induced thrombocytopenia. The Organization for the Assessment of Strategies for Ischemic Syndromes 6 (OASIS 6) trial showed fondaparinux use as a sole anticoagulant in STEMI patients during primary PCI increased catheter-related thrombosis.[24] The recommended dose of anticoagulation used in primary PCI is listed in **Table 6.6**.

Fibrinolytic Therapy

Fibrinolytic therapy can be used for STEMI patients with symptoms onset less than 12 hours if primary PCI cannot be performed within 120 minutes of FMC. Fibrin-specific agents tenecteplase, reteplase, and alteplase are typically used, and all have comparable mortality, reinfarction, and stroke rates. Streptokinase is no longer available in the United States. The Strategic Reperfusion Early after Myocardial Infarction (STREAM) study showed effective reperfusion with prehospital fibrinolysis when coupled with timely PCI in early STEMI patients who could not undergo PCI within 1 hour of FMC. However, a small increased risk of intracranial hemorrhage was noted in the fibrinolytic arm.[25] Ideally, fibrinolytic should be injected within 10 minutes from STEMI diagnosis if the reperfusion strategy chosen is fibrinolysis.[5]

The decision to use fibrinolytic agents is based on the timing of symptoms onset, the time delay of PCI, hemodynamics at presentation, patient comorbidities, risk of bleeding, and any contraindications to fibrinolytic. Fibrinolytic checklist and contraindications should be reviewed as per institutional policy. Fibrinolytic doses and contraindications are listed in **Tables 6.7** and **6.8,** respectively.

Antiplatelets and Anticoagulation with Fibrinolytics. Aspirin, 162 to 325 mg loading dose, should be used followed by a maintenance dose of 81 mg daily. Clopidogrel is the only P2Y12 drug recommended for use with fibrinolytic therapy. For patients less than or equal to 75 years old, a 300-mg loading dose of clopidogrel is recommended. For patients greater than 75 years old, no loading dose of clopidogrel is used. UFH, enoxaparin,

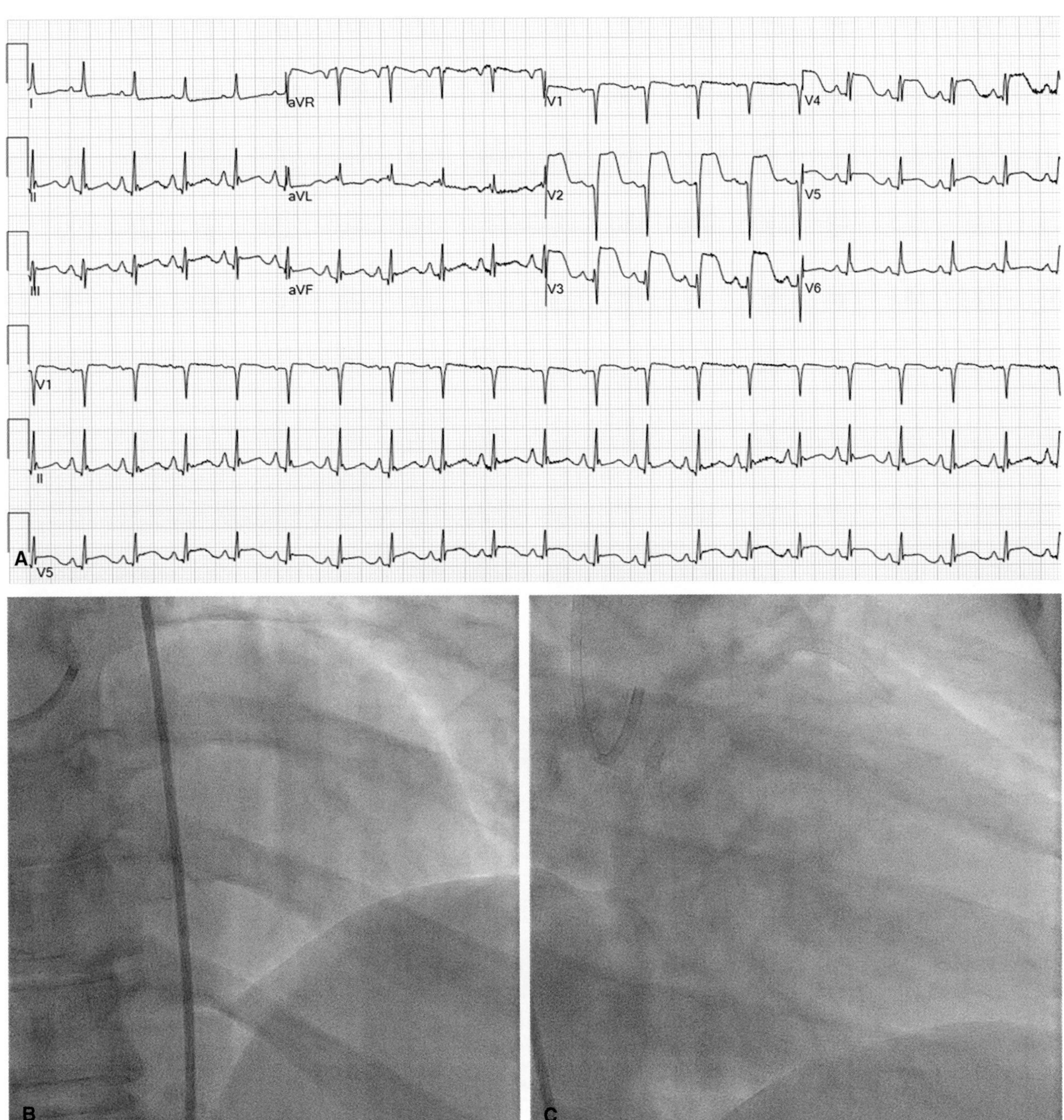

CLINICAL CASE 6.3 A 60-year-old female presented with chest pain. **(A)** 12-lead electrocardiogram showing anteroseptal ST-segment elevation myocardial infarction. **(B)** Left anterior oblique cranial view showing subtotal occlusion of mid-left anterior descending (LAD) and subtotal occlusion of mid-left circumflex (▶ VIDEO 6.3b). **(C)** Right anterior oblique caudal view post-percutaneous coronary intervention of LAD and left circumflex (▶ VIDEO 6.3c).

or fondaparinux are the anticoagulants recommended with fibrinolysis. Administration of GP IIb/IIIa inhibitors along with fibrinolysis may increase bleeding without evidence of improved outcomes.[26] The anticoagulation doses used with fibrinolytic are summarized in **Table 6.9**.

Fondaparinux should not be used as a sole anticoagulant for primary PCI because of the risk of catheter thrombosis. Another anticoagulation with anti-IIa activity like UFH should be used along with fondaparinux. In patients with known Heparin-induced thrombocytopenia (HIT), bivalirudin or argatroban should be used.

Coronary Angiography after Fibrinolytic Therapy. The combination of lack of improvement in chest pain, less than 50% resolution in ST-segment elevation in the ECG lead with the largest elevation within 60 to 90 minutes, and the absence of reperfusion arrhythmia

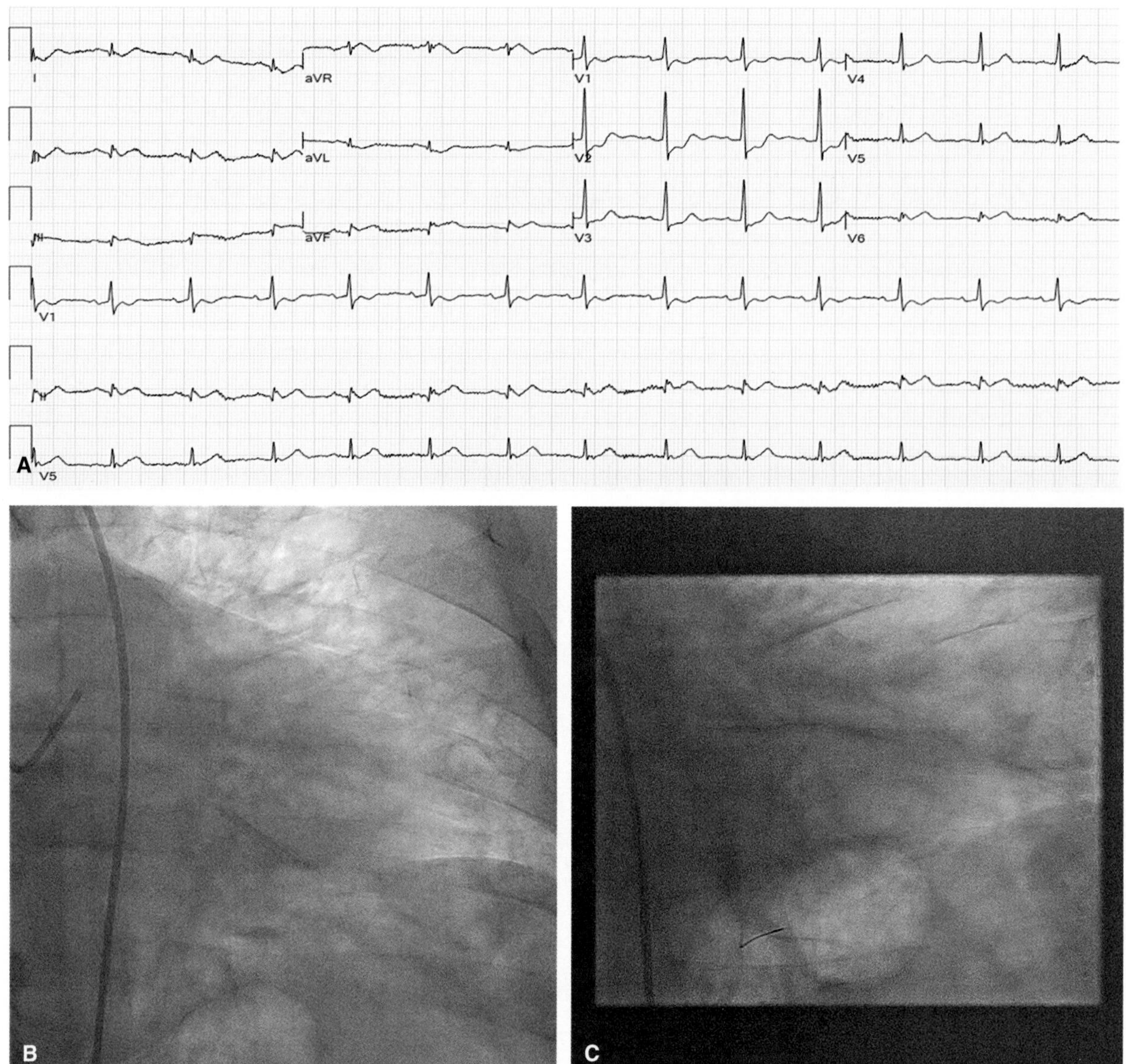

CLINICAL CASE 6.4 An 88-year-old male presented with chest pain. **(A)** 12-lead electrocardiogram showing infero-posterior ST-segment elevation myocardial infarction. **(B)** Right anterior oblique caudal view showing 100% occlusion of the proximal left circumflex (VIDEO 6.4b). **(C)** post-percutaneous coronary intervention of proximal left circumflex (VIDEO 6.4c).

TABLE 6.3 Comparison of Time Targets of ACC and ESC Guidelines Based on Reperfusion Strategy

Intervals	Time Targets per ACC	Time Target per ESC
FMC to ECG diagnosis	As soon as possible	10 minutes
Time for primary PCI at presenting hospital	≤90 minutes FMC to device time	STEMI diagnosis to wire crossing: ≤60 minutes
Transferred patients from another facility	≤120 minutes	≤90 minutes
Consider fibrinolysis if time to primary PCI exceeds	>120 minutes	>120 minutes
Fibrinolysis bolus or infusion	FMC to needle time ≤30 minutes	Within 10 minutes of STEMI diagnosis
Fibrinolysis response evaluation	60-90 minutes	60-90 minutes
Cath timing post fibrinolysis	3-24 hours	2-24 hours

ACC, American College of Cardiology; Cath, Cardiac Catheterization; ECG, electrocardiogram; ESC, European Society of Cardiology; FMC first medical contact; PCI, percutaneous coronary intervention; STEMI, ST-elevation myocardial infarction.

TABLE 6.4 P2Y12 Inhibitors Dose

P2Y12 Inhibitors	Loading Dose	Maintenance Dose
Clopidogrel	600 mg usual dose **With Fibrinolytics:** ≤75 years: 300 mg loading dose >75 years: No loading dose	75 mg daily
Ticagrelor	180 mg	90 mg q12h
Prasugrel	60 mg	10 mg daily 5 mg daily in patients with weight <60 kg or age ≥75 years
Cangrelor[a] (intravenous)	30 μg/kg bolus prior to percutaneous coronary intervention (PCI)	4 μg/kg/minute for at least 2 hours or duration of the PCI, whichever is longer

[a]Cangrelor should be transitioned to oral P2Y12 inhibitor therapy.

TABLE 6.5 Glycoprotein (GP) IIb/IIIa Inhibitors Dosing

GP IIb/IIIa Inhibitors	Bolus Dose	Maintenance Dose
Abciximab	0.25 mg/kg	0.125 μg/kg/minute up to 10 μg/minute for 12 hours
Eptifibatide	180 μg/kg double bolus at 10 minutes interval	2 μg/kg/minute for up to 18 hours
Tirofiban	25 μg/kg over 3 minutes	0.15 μg/kg/minute for up to 18 hours

TABLE 6.6 Anticoagulation Dose Used in Primary Percutaneous Coronary Intervention (PCI)

Unfractionated heparin (UFH):
70-100 units/kg boluses to achieve therapeutic activated clotting time (ACT) of 250-350 seconds

UFH with GP IIb/IIIa inhibitors:
50-70 units/kg IV boluses to achieve therapeutic ACT of 200-250 seconds

Bivalirudin: 0.75 mg/kg IV bolus, then 1.75 mg/kg/hour infusion
Additional 0.3 mg/kg bolus can be given if needed
Reduce infusion to 1 mg/kg/hour with estimated creatinine clearance <30 mL/minute

Enoxaparin: 0.5 mg/kg iv bolus (an additional bolus of 0.25 mg/kg if the procedure is prolonged by more than 2 hours)

IV, intravenous.

TABLE 6.7 Fibrinolytic Dose

Fibrinolytic	Dose
Tenecteplase (TNK-PA)	Single 30-50 mg (weight based) IV bolus; Consider half dose in patients ≥75 years old <60 kg: 30 mg 60-69 kg: 35 mg 70-79 kg: 40 mg 80-89 kg: 45 mg ≥90 kg: 50 mg
Reteplase (rPA)	Two 10-unit IV boluses given 30 minutes apart
Alteplase (tPA, t-PA)	15 mg IV bolus, then 0.75 mg/kg (maximum 50 mg) infused over 30 minutes, then 0.5 mg/kg (maximum 35 mg) infusion over the next 60 minutes; maximum total dose 100 mg

IV, intravenous.

(eg, accelerated idioventricular rhythm) at 2 hours after treatment implies failed reperfusion. Patients should be urgently transferred to PCI-capable hospitals for rescue PCI.[27] Stable patients should also be routinely transferred for PCI preferably between 2 and 24 hours of successful thrombolytic treatment.[28] Cardiogenic shock or severe acute heart failure, hemodynamically and electrically unstable patients should be immediately transferred irrespectively of time delay from STEMI onset for rescue PCI.

Surgical Approach

Early revascularization with coronary artery bypass graft surgery (CABG) is indicated in STEMI patients with coronary anatomy not amenable to PCI and cardiogenic shock, a high risk of ischemia involving a large area of the myocardium, or those with mechanical complications. Early revascularization showed a significant survival advantage after 6 months when compared to initial medical stabilization in such patients.[29] Patients with unstable hemodynamics and a high risk of ongoing recurrent ischemia should proceed to surgery urgently without waiting for platelet function recovery. For elective CABG, clopidogrel and ticagrelor should be discontinued 5 days and prasugrel 7 days before surgery.

Surgical repair is indicated for mechanical complications like acute papillary muscle rupture, ventricular septal, or free wall rupture after STEMI. Coronary revascularization should be performed during surgery for mechanical complications.

TABLE 6.8 Fibrinolytic Contraindications

Absolute Contraindications	Relative Contraindications
• History of spontaneous intracranial hemorrhage • Cerebral vascular lesion like arteriovenous malformations • Malignant intracranial neoplasm • Ischemic stroke within 3 months (except for acute ischemic stroke within 4.5 hours) • Suspected aortic dissection • Active bleeding or bleeding diathesis (except menses) • Significant closed head trauma or facial trauma within 3 months • Intracranial or spinal surgery within 2 months • Severe uncontrolled hypertension (unresponsive to emergency therapy)	• Systolic blood pressure >180 mm Hg or diastolic blood pressure >110 mm Hg • Prior ischemic stroke >3 months ago • Dementia • Known intracranial pathology not covered in contraindications • Prolonged cardiopulmonary resuscitation for >10 minutes • Major surgery within 3 weeks • Internal bleeding within 2-4 weeks • Noncompressible vascular punctures • Pregnancy • Active peptic ulcer • Oral anticoagulant therapy

TABLE 6.9 Anticoagulation Dose Used with Fibrinolytics

Unfractionated heparin: 60 units/kg, maximum 4000 units and infusion, 12 units/kg/hour, maximum 1000 units/hour, adjusted to obtain activated partial thromboplastin time (aPTT) of 1.5-2 times control (about 50-70 seconds) Duration 48 hours or until revascularization
Enoxaparin: For <75 years old—30 mg IV bolus, followed in 15 minutes by 1 mg/kg subcutaneously every 12 hours (maximum 100 mg/dose for first two doses) For >75 years old—0.75 mg/kg subcutaneously every 12 hours (maximum 75 mg/dose for first two doses) For creatinine clearance <30 mL/minute (regardless of age)—1 mg/kg subcutaneously every 24 hours For the duration of index hospitalization, up to 8 days or until revascularization
Fondaparinux: Initial dose 2.5 mg IV, followed in 24 hours by 2.5 mg subcutaneously once daily, if estimated creatinine clearance >30 mL/minute Contraindicated if creatinine clearance <30 mL/minute For the duration of index hospitalization, up to 8 days or until revascularization

IV, intravenous.

SPECIAL CONSIDERATIONS

Cardiogenic Shock

Patients with cardiogenic shock should undergo emergent revascularization with either PCI or CABG irrespective of symptoms onset.[29] Intravenous inotropic support or vasopressors may be required to maintain systolic blood pressure and improve systemic organ perfusion. Norepinephrine is more effective in severe hypotension and cardiogenic shock, but dobutamine can be considered in a low cardiac output state.[30] There are inconsistent data on multivessel PCI versus culprit vessel only PCI in cardiogenic shock patients. The 2017 European guidelines suggest early and complete revascularization during index procedures for cardiogenic shock patients.[5] However, a study showed evidence of higher mortality in STEMI patients with cardiogenic shock treated with multivessel PCI strategy.[31]

Intra-aortic balloon pump counterpulsation (IABP) can be useful in unstable patients despite appropriate pharmacological therapy, but no clear mortality benefit is associated with its use.[32] Percutaneous Impella (Abiomed, Danvers, MA, USA) circulatory support devices showed no 30-day mortality benefit over IABP in AMI and cardiogenic shock patients.[33] Mechanical left ventricular assist devices may provide greater hemodynamic support and can be used as a bridge to the recovery of myocardial function, cardiac transplantation, or even as destination therapy in select patients.[34]

Cardiac Arrest

Ventricular fibrillation (VF) arrest is the common cause of death in many patients with STEMI.[35] All suspected ACS patients should be transported to the hospital by emergency medical service personnel with continuous ECG monitoring and access to defibrillation equipment. Urgent coronary angiography with primary PCI is the treatment strategy of choice for resuscitated cardiac arrest patients with STEMI. High-risk patients with established coronary artery disease, chest pain before an arrest, and high-risk ECG features should also undergo urgent coronary angiography. Resuscitated comatose cardiac arrest patients should be put on therapeutic hypothermia protocol with a targeted core temperature of 32 to 36 °C for at least 24 hours. However, unwitnessed cardiac arrest, prolonged cardiac resuscitation for 30 minutes without return of spontaneous circulation, advanced age greater than 85 years, severe acidemia with pH less than 7.2, lactate greater than 7 mmol/L, and end-stage renal disease suggest an unfavorable outcome with no clear mortality benefit from revascularization.[36]

Nonreperfused Patients

Coronary angiography with primary PCI is recommended in the setting of ongoing myocardial ischemia, heart failure, unstable hemodynamics, or life-threatening arrhythmias irrespective of the time onset of symptoms. Elective coronary angiography can be performed after 48 hours but routine PCI of occluded culprit artery is not recommended. A noninvasive stress test either stress echocardiography, cardiac MRI, single-photon emission computed tomography (SPECT), or positron emission tomography (PET) is recommended for assessing myocardial ischemia/viability to guide late invasive strategy for delayed presentation. Dual antiplatelet therapy (DAPT) with aspirin and clopidogrel, statins, secondary prevention medical therapy, and anticoagulation, preferably fondaparinux, is recommended until reperfusion or discharge.[24]

Patients Taking Oral Anticoagulation

Reperfusion strategy should be primary PCI as fibrinolysis is a relative contraindication for patients in this group. The loading dose of aspirin and clopidogrel should be given as early as possible. Prasugrel and ticagrelor are not recommended. Parenteral anticoagulation should be given regardless of the time of the last dose of oral anticoagulation. Triple therapy (aspirin, clopidogrel, and oral anticoagulation) should be continued for 6 months for most patients. But in cases of very high bleeding risk, triple therapy can be reduced to 1 month after STEMI. After that either aspirin or clopidogrel can be continued with oral anticoagulation for up to 1 year, and then only oral anticoagulation can be continued.[37]

Multivessel Coronary Artery Disease

Complete revascularization of vessels is recommended in STEMI patients with multivessel disease before hospital discharge, but optimal timing has not been investigated adequately. A meta-analysis using 10 randomized controlled trials compared outcomes of multivessel PCI versus culprit vessel only PCI and showed multivessel PCI was associated with a lower risk of reinfarction, cardiovascular mortality, and repeat revascularization without any difference in all-cause mortality.[38]

Microvascular Dysfunction

Microvascular dysfunction is diagnosed by the incomplete resolution of ST segments after revascularization; or less than 3 TIMI flow despite lack of epicardial stenosis; or myocardial blush grade is 0 or 1 in case of TIMI 3 flow. Late gadolinium enhancement (LGE) cardiac MRI, contrast echocardiography, SPECT, and PET can also help diagnose microvascular dysfunction. Aggressive risk reduction along with DAPT and statins are the only available treatment strategies right now.

Myocardial Infarction with Nonobstructive Coronaries

MI with nonobstructive coronary arteries is defined as clinical evidence of AMI but angiographic evidence of nonobstructive coronary artery disease. It is not an uncommon presentation with an estimated prevalence of 5% to 25% of all MIs. Coronary plaque ruptures, coronary artery dissection, microvascular dysfunction, vasospasm, and coronary embolism are the potential etiology of MI with nonobstructive coronaries.[39] The treatment strategy is individualized and targeted based on the etiology. Antiplatelet agents, angiotensin converting enzyme (ACE) inhibitors or angiotensin receptor blockers (ARB), statins, and aggressive risk reductions should be considered for the majority of the patients.[40]

Heart Blocks

Patients may need prophylactic temporary transvenous pacemaker placement for hemodynamically significant bradycardia and atrioventricular (AV) block. A permanent pacemaker may be indicated in patients with second-degree Mobitz type 2 AV block, high-grade AV block, alternating bundle branch block, or third-degree AV block after a waiting period for myocardial recovery.

Other Medications and Devices

Lipid-Lowering Therapy

High-intensity statins atorvastatin 40 to 80 mg or rosuvastatin 20 to 40 mg should be given to patients without contraindications irrespective of cholesterol level. Lipid profile should be obtained during index hospitalization and repeated after 4 to 6 weeks. The goal is to reduce low-density lipoprotein cholesterol (LDL-C) by greater than or equal to 50% if baseline is 1.8 to 3.5 mmol/L (70-135 mg/dL) or achieve target LDL-C less than 1.8 mmol/L (70 mg/dL). Additional therapy is recommended if LDL-C is greater than or equal to 1.8 mmol/L (≥70 mg/dL) despite the maximally tolerated statin. Patients should be monitored for myopathy and hepatotoxicity.

β-Blockers

An oral β-blocker should be started during index hospitalization and preferably within 24 hours if tolerated by hemodynamics. It should be avoided in patients with active heart failure, hypotension, bradycardia, cocaine abuse, or heart block. However, a patient's status should be revisited during the same hospital admission. It should be changed to cardioselective β-blockers on discharge if there is evidence of left ventricular dysfunction.

Angiotensin Converting Enzyme Inhibitors or Angiotensin Receptor Blockers

An ACE inhibitor or ARB should be started in 24 hours in patients with anterior myocardial infarction, heart failure, hypertension, type 2 diabetes mellitus, and left ventricular ejection fraction less than 40% unless contraindicated. It should be avoided in hypotension, acute kidney injury, allergy, and bilateral renal artery stenosis.

Aldosterone Antagonists

An aldosterone antagonist should be added to ACE inhibitors and β-blockers in patients with AMI and left ventricular ejection fraction less than 40% with either symptomatic heart failure or diabetes mellitus and avoided in renal failure (serum creatinine >2.5 mg/dL in men, >2 mg/dL in women) and hyperkalemia (serum potassium ≥5 mEq/L).

Implantable Cardioverter Defibrillator (ICD)

An ICD is indicated in patients with sustained ventricular tachycardia (VT) or VF greater than 48 hours after revascularization.

Reversible causes like ischemia, reinfarction, or metabolic derangement should be corrected before contemplating ICD placement. An ICD or temporary wearable cardioverter defibrillator can be considered in patients with incomplete revascularization of the nonculprit lesion, prior known heart failure with reduced left ventricular ejection fraction, and secondary prophylaxis such as ventricular arrhythmia greater than 48 hours post revascularization and polymorphic VT or VF.[41]

PATIENT RECOVERY AND FOLLOW-UP

All STEMI patients should be monitored in cardiac care/intensive care units for a minimum of 24 hours. Consequently, patients can be transferred to a step-down monitored bed for an additional 24 to 48 hours. Patients with successful primary PCI and without evidence of ongoing myocardial ischemia, arrhythmia, or hemodynamic instability and not needing further early revascularization can be transferred back to a referring non-PCI hospital. However, unstable hemodynamics, arrhythmias, left ventricular ejection fraction less than 40%, failed reperfusion, additional critical stenosis of major vessels, and PCI-related complications mandate longer monitoring. Early ambulation is recommended if tolerated by patients. All patients should have an evaluation of left ventricular ejection fraction by echocardiography, assessment of coronary artery disease severity, residual ischemia and completeness of coronary revascularization, and any complications during hospitalization. Metabolic risk parameters like total cholesterol, LDL-C, high-density lipoprotein cholesterol, fasting triglycerides, plasma glucose, and renal function tests should be evaluated. Blood pressure and serum glucose should be well controlled. Low-risk patients (ie, age <70 years, left ventricular ejection fraction >45%, one- or two-vessel disease, successful primary PCI, hemodynamically stable, and no persistent arrhythmias) can be discharged within 48 to 72 hours.[42]

Follow-up outpatient appointments should be scheduled with the patient's primary care physician and cardiologist before hospital discharge. The medication list, the importance of compliance, and side effects should be reviewed. Appropriate dietary habits (ie, a Mediterranean diet with less saturated fat, salt intake <5 g/day, high fiber), physical activities, smoking cessation counseling, travel, and work restrictions should be discussed on hospital discharge and subsequent office visits. Patients should also be referred to cardiac rehabilitation on discharge. Cardiac rehabilitation focuses on physical activity and lifestyle modifications which include healthy dietary habits, smoking cessation, medication compliance, and psychosocial support.

DAPT should ideally be continued for 12 months irrespective of revascularization status unless the bleeding risk is very high. If the bleeding risk is very high, DAPT can be discontinued in 6 months. Proton pump inhibitors can be added to the DAPT regimen in patients with high gastrointestinal bleeding risk. If patients require long-term anticoagulation, then aspirin or clopidogrel can be discontinued after 1 to 6 months of the triple regimen. Anticoagulant and aspirin or clopidogrel are recommended to continue up to 12 months total. Prolonged ticagrelor 60 mg twice daily in addition to aspirin may be considered in patients with high ischemic risk based on the Prevention of Cardiovascular Events in Patients with Prior Heart Attack Using Ticagrelor Compared to Placebo on a Background of Aspirin-Thrombolysis in MI 54 (PEGASUS-TIMI 54) study.[43] Patients with evidence of heart failure should have a transthoracic echocardiogram to assess for left ventricular ejection fraction greater than or equal to 40 days postdischarge to assess the need for ICD for primary prevention. Noninvasive stress tests can be considered to evaluate the functional significance of non-infarct-related arterial stenosis and assess functional capacity. All patients should receive the annual flu vaccine.

RESEARCH AND FUTURE DIRECTIONS

The leading cause of mortality among females is coronary heart disease, yet when compared to males, it is known that females are late-arriving to the hospital and delayed in receiving appropriate care.[4] There is a dire need for more research to understand the trends of gender and ethnicity disparities and to improve quality care and awareness among health care workers.

The optimal dosing, duration, and loading of the DAPT regimen showing obvious benefit should be clearly defined. More data and studies are needed on triple regimen duration considering newer generation stents being available. Current data do not provide any mortality benefit in the use of mechanical circulatory devices. Considering the increasing popularity of the use of left ventricular assist devices, Impella, and extracorporeal membrane oxygenation in patients with cardiogenic shock, there is a need for randomized controlled clinical trials and clinical guidelines to guide appropriate use. In addition, appropriate guidelines and criteria to guide PCI in cardiogenic shock patients with multivessel coronary artery disease are needed.

Even though the incidence of coronary heart disease is declining, the mortality related to it is still substantial. Many PCI-eligible patients do not receive PCI or meet the desired door-to-perfusion time. More studies are needed to understand the gap and improve quality. Optimal use of secondary preventative therapies remains a challenge. There is a growing need for public awareness to be raised about angina and heart attack symptoms. This will increase the emergency medical services involvement for transport to the hospital as a significant number of deaths related to coronary heart disease occurs outside the hospital. This will also augment early STEMI diagnosis, facilitate transfer to PCI-capable hospitals, and improve door-to-balloon time and overall outcome.

Around 7% of patients who underwent PCI are not discharged on aspirin, P2Y12 inhibitors, and statins.[6] Continuous quality improvement projects are needed at the facility level to improve it. A substantial proportion of STEMI patients are noted to have no prior history of standard modifiable cardiovascular risk factors. These patients also have higher in-hospital mortality compared to patients with traditional modifiable risk factors. More studies are needed to identify the mechanism and chemical markers for coronary artery disease in those populations.[7]

KEY POINTS

- ✔ The incidence and mortality associated with ischemic heart disease have declined significantly worldwide, but it is still the leading cause of death worldwide.
- ✔ Primary PCI is the reperfusion strategy for patients meeting STEMI criteria in ECG along with ongoing ischemia. STEMI patients with chest pain for less than 12 hours should undergo primary PCI with a target door-to-balloon time of 90 minutes. Patients transferred from non-PCI-capable facilities should have a goal door-to-balloon time of 120 minutes.
- ✔ Fibrinolysis should be started within 10 minutes of STEMI diagnosis if the door-to-balloon time cannot be achieved and no contraindications. Patients should be transferred to PCI-capable facilities for failed reperfusion or routine PCI 2 to 24 hours post fibrinolysis.
- ✔ Cardiac arrest patients with post-resuscitation ECG showing STEMI should undergo primary PCI.
- ✔ Radial access is the preferred access site if the operator is trained and comfortable.
- ✔ Evaluation of left ventricular ejection fraction, severity of coronary artery disease, residual ischemia, completeness of coronary revascularization, and any complications during hospitalization should be done before discharge.
- ✔ DAPT is recommended for 1 year as maintenance therapy irrespective of reperfusion strategy unless the bleeding risk is high. Triple regimen (DAPT with aspirin and clopidogrel and anticoagulation) can be continued for 1 to 6 months depending on bleeding risks. Then, single antiplatelet either aspirin or clopidogrel can be continued with oral anticoagulation for the next 6 months.
- ✔ Appropriate follow-up to assess medication adherence and aggressive risk factor reduction with optimal control of hypertension, diabetes mellitus, hyperlipidemia, and smoking cessation is recommended to reduce the recurrent events.
- ✔ Annual flu vaccination is recommended for all individuals after a STEMI.

VIDEO CAPTIONS

VIDEO 6.1 A 63-year old male presented with chest pain for 1 hour. **(A)** 12-lead electrocardiogram showing anteroseptal ST-segment myocardial infarction. **(B, C)** Transthoracic echocardiography apical four chambers and apical two chambers showing hypokinesis in left anterior descending (LAD) territory. **(D)** Coronary angiogram right anterior oblique (RAO) caudal view showing 100% occlusion of mid-LAD (▶ VIDEO 6.1d). **(E)** Coronary angiogram RAO cranial post-percutaneous coronary intervention (▶ VIDEO 6.1e).

VIDEO 6.2 A 53-year-old male admitted with chest pain for 1 hour. **(A)** 12-lead electrocardiogram showing inferior ST-segment myocardial infarction. **(B)** Coronary angiogram showing 100% occlusion of mid-right coronary artery (▶ VIDEO 6.2b). **(C)** Post-percutaneous coronary intervention (▶ VIDEO 6.2c).

VIDEO 6.3 A 60-year-old female presented with chest pain. **(A)** 12-lead electrocardiogram showing anteroseptal ST-segment elevation myocardial infarction. **(B)** Left anterior oblique cranial view showing subtotal occlusion of mid-left anterior descending (LAD) and subtotal occlusion of mid-left circumflex (▶ VIDEO 6.3b). **(C)** Right anterior oblique caudal view post-percutaneous coronary intervention of LAD and left circumflex (▶ VIDEO 6.3c).

VIDEO 6.4 An 88-year-old male presented with chest pain. **(A)** 12-lead electrocardiogram showing infero-posterior ST-segment elevation myocardial infarction. **(B)** Right anterior oblique caudal view showing 100% occlusion of the proximal left circumflex (▶ VIDEO 6.4b). **(C)** post-percutaneous coronary intervention of proximal left circumflex (▶ VIDEO 6.4c).

REFERENCES

1. Thygesen K, Alpert JS, Jaffe AS, et al. Fourth universal definition of myocardial infarction (2018). *J Am Coll Cardiol.* 2018;72(18):2231-2264. doi:10.1016/j.jacc.2018.08.1038
2. Benjamin EJ, Muntner P, Alonso A, et al. Heart disease and stroke statistics-2019 update: a report from the American Heart Association. *Circulation.* 2019;139(10):e56-e528. doi:10.1161/CIR.0000000000000659 [published correction appears in *Circulation.* 2020;141(2):e33].
3. Pendyal A, Rothenberg C, Scofi JE, et al. National trends in emergency department care processes for acute myocardial infarction in the United States, 2005 to 2015. *J Am Heart Assoc.* 2020;9(20):e017208. doi:10.1161/JAHA.120.017208
4. O'Gara PT, Kushner FG, Ascheim DD, et al. 2013 ACCF/AHA guideline for the management of ST-elevation myocardial infarction: a report of the American College of Cardiology Foundation/American Heart Association Task Force on Practice Guidelines. *Circulation.* 2013;127(4):e362-e425. doi:10.1161/CIR.0b013e3182742cf6 [published correction appears in *Circulation.* 2013;128(25):e481].
5. Ibanez B, James S, Agewall S, et al. 2017 ESC Guidelines for the management of acute myocardial infarction in patients presenting with ST-segment elevation: The Task Force for the management of acute myocardial infarction in patients presenting with ST-segment elevation of the European Society of Cardiology (ESC). *Eur Heart J.* 2018;39(2):119-177. doi:10.1093/eurheartj/ehx393
6. Masoudi FA, Ponirakis A, de Lemos JA, et al. Executive summary: trends in U.S. cardiovascular care: 2016 report from 4 ACC NATIONAL CARDIOVASCULAR DATA REGISTRIES. *J Am Coll Cardiol.* 2017;69:1424-1426. doi:10.1016/j.jacc.2016.12.004
7. Vernon ST, Coffey S, D'Souza M, et al. ST-Segment-Elevation Myocardial Infarction (STEMI) patients without standard modifiable cardiovascular risk factors-how common are they, and what are their outcomes? *J Am Heart Assoc.* 2019;8(21):e013296. doi:10.1161/JAHA.119.013296
8. Trost JC, Lange RA. Treatment of acute coronary syndrome: part 2: ST-segment elevation myocardial infarction. *Crit Care Med.* 2012;40(6):1939-1945. doi:10.1097/CCM.0b013e31824e18c2
9. Morrow DA, Antman EM, Charlesworth A, et al. TIMI risk score for ST-elevation myocardial infarction: a convenient, bedside, clinical score for risk assessment at presentation: an intravenous nPA for treatment of infarcting myocardium early II trial substudy. *Circulation.* 2000;102(17):2031-2037. doi:10.1161/01.cir.102.17.2031
10. Fox KA, Fitzgerald G, Puymirat E, et al. Should patients with acute coronary disease be stratified for management according to their risk? Derivation, external validation and outcomes using the updated GRACE risk score. *BMJ Open.* 2014;4(2):e004425. doi:10.1136/bmjopen-2013-004425
11. Garot P, Lefevre T, Eltchaninoff H, et al. Six-month outcome of emergency percutaneous coronary intervention in resuscitated patients after cardiac arrest complicating ST-elevation myocardial infarction. *Circulation.* 2007;115(11):1354-1362. doi:10.1161/CIRCULATIONAHA.106.657619

12. Welsh RC, Chang W, Goldstein P, et al. Time to treatment and the impact of a physician on prehospital management of acute ST elevation myocardial infarction: insights from the ASSENT-3 PLUS trial. *Heart.* 2005;91(11):1400-1406. doi:10.1136/hrt.2004.054510
13. Stub D, Smith K, Bernard S, et al. Air versus oxygen in ST-segment-elevation myocardial infarction. *Circulation.* 2015;131(24):2143-2150. doi:10.1161/CIRCULATIONAHA.114.014494
14. Keeley EC, Boura JA, Grines CL. Primary angioplasty versus intravenous thrombolytic therapy for acute myocardial infarction: a quantitative review of 23 randomised trials. *Lancet.* 2003;361(9351):13-20. doi:10.1016/S0140-6736(03)12113-7
15. Valgimigli M, Gagnor A, Calabró P, et al. Radial versus femoral access in patients with acute coronary syndromes undergoing invasive management: a randomised multicentre trial. *Lancet.* 2015;385(9986):2465-2476. doi:10.1016/S0140-6736(15)60292-6
16. Jolly SS, Cairns JA, Yusuf S, et al. TOTAL Investigators. Stroke in the TOTAL trial: a randomized trial of routine thrombectomy vs. percutaneous coronary intervention alone in ST elevation myocardial infarction. *Eur Heart J.* 2015;36(35):2364-2372. doi:10.1093/eurheartj/ehv296
17. Nordmann AJ, Hengstler P, Harr T, et al. Clinical outcomes of primary stenting versus balloon angioplasty in patients with myocardial infarction: a meta-analysis of randomized controlled trials. *Am J Med.* 2004;116(4):253-262. doi:10.1016/j.amjmed.2003.08.035
18. Sabate M, Cequier A, Iñiguez A, et al. Everolimus-eluting stent versus bare-metal stent in ST-segment elevation myocardial infarction (EXAMINATION): 1 year results of a randomised controlled trial. *Lancet.* 2012;380(9852):1482-1490. doi:10.1016/S0140-6736(12)61223-9
19. Sabaté M, Brugaletta S, Cequier A, et al. Clinical outcomes in patients with ST-segment elevation myocardial infarction treated with everolimus-eluting stents versus bare-metal stents (EXAMINATION): 5-year results of a randomised trial. *Lancet.* 2016;387(10016):357-366. doi:10.1016/S0140-6736(15)00548-6
20. Wiviott SD, Braunwald E, McCabe CH, et al. Prasugrel versus clopidogrel in patients with acute coronary syndromes. *N Engl J Med.* 2007;357(20):2001-2015. doi:10.1056/NEJMoa0706482
21. Wallentin L, Becker RC, Budaj A, et al. Ticagrelor versus clopidogrel in patients with acute coronary syndromes. *N Engl J Med.* 2009;361(11):1045-1057. doi:10.1056/NEJMoa0904327
22. Mehta SR, Tanguay JF, Eikelboom JW, et al. CURRENT-OASIS 7 trial investigators. Double-dose versus standard-dose clopidogrel and high-dose versus low-dose aspirin in individuals undergoing percutaneous coronary intervention for acute coronary syndromes (CURRENT-OASIS 7): a randomised factorial trial. *Lancet.* 2010;376(9748):1233-1243. doi:10.1016/S0140-6736(10)61088-4
23. Steg PG, Bhatt DL, Hamm CW, et al. CHAMPION Investigators. Effect of cangrelor on periprocedural outcomes in percutaneous coronary interventions: a pooled analysis of patient-level data. *Lancet.* 2013;382(9909):1981-1992.
24. Yusuf S, Mehta SR, Chrolavicius S, et al. Effects of fondaparinux on mortality and reinfarction in patients with acute ST-segment elevation myocardial infarction: the OASIS-6 randomized trial. *JAMA.* 2006;295(13):1519-1530. doi:10.1001/jama.295.13.joc60038
25. Armstrong PW, Gershlick AH, Goldstein P, et al. Fibrinolysis or primary PCI in ST-segment elevation myocardial infarction. *N Engl J Med.* 2013;368(15):1379-1387. doi:10.1056/NEJMoa1301092
26. Sánchez PL, Gimeno F, Ancillo P, et al. Role of the paclitaxel-eluting stent and tirofiban in patients with ST-elevation myocardial infarction undergoing postfibrinolysis angioplasty: the GRACIA-3 randomized clinical trial. *Circ Cardiovasc Interv.* 2010;3(4):297-307. doi:10.1161/CIRCINTERVENTIONS.109.920868
27. Gershlick AH, Stephens-Lloyd A, Hughes S, et al. Rescue angioplasty after failed thrombolytic therapy for acute myocardial infarction. *N Engl J Med.* 2005;353(26):2758-2768. doi:10.1056/NEJMoa050849
28. Madan M, Halvorsen S, Di Mario C, et al. Relationship between time to invasive assessment and clinical outcomes of patients undergoing an early invasive strategy after fibrinolysis for ST-segment elevation myocardial infarction: a patient-level analysis of the randomized early routine invasive clinical trials. *JACC Cardiovasc Interv.* 2015;8(1 Pt B):166-174. doi:10.1016/j.jcin.2014.09.005
29. Hochman JS, Sleeper LA, Webb JG, et al. Early revascularization in acute myocardial infarction complicated by cardiogenic shock. SHOCK Investigators. Should We Emergently Revascularize Occluded Coronaries for Cardiogenic Shock. *N Engl J Med.* 1999;341(9):625-634. doi:10.1056/NEJM199908263410901
30. De Backer D, Biston P, Devriendt J, et al. SOAP II Investigators. Comparison of dopamine and norepinephrine in the treatment of shock. *N Engl J Med.* 2010;362(9):779-789. doi:10.1056/NEJMoa0907118
31. Khera R, Secemsky EA, Wang Y, et al. Revascularization practices and outcomes in patients with multivessel coronary artery disease who presented with acute myocardial infarction and cardiogenic shock in the US, 2009-2018. *JAMA Intern Med.* 2020;180(10):1317-1327. doi:10.1001/jamainternmed.2020.3276
32. Thiele H, Zeymer U, Neumann FJ, et al. Intraaortic balloon support for myocardial infarction with cardiogenic shock. *N Engl J Med.* 2012;367(14):1287-1296. doi:10.1056/NEJMoa1208410
33. Alushi B, Douedari A, Froehlig G, et al. Impella versus IABP in acute myocardial infarction complicated by cardiogenic shock *Open Heart.* 2019;6(1):e000987. doi:10.1136/openhrt-2018-000987 [published correction appears in *Open Heart.* 2019;6(1):e000987corr1].
34. Starling RC, Naka Y, Boyle AJ, et al. Results of the post-U.S. Food and Drug Administration-approval study with a continuous flow left ventricular assist device as a bridge to heart transplantation: a prospective study using the INTERMACS (Interagency Registry for Mechanically Assisted Circulatory Support). *J Am Coll Cardiol.* 2011;57(19):1890-1898. doi:10.1016/j.jacc.2010.10.062. [Erratum in: *J Am Coll Cardiol.* 2011;58(20):2142].
35. Larsen JM, Ravkilde J. Acute coronary angiography in patients resuscitated from out-of-hospital cardiac arrest—a systematic review and meta-analysis. *Resuscitation.* 2012;83(12):1427-1433. doi:10.1016/j.resuscitation.2012.08.337
36. Rab T, Kern KB, Tamis-Holland JE, et al. Cardiac arrest: a treatment algorithm for emergent invasive cardiac procedures in the resuscitated comatose patient. *J Am Coll Cardiol.* 2015;66(1):62-73. doi:10.1016/j.jacc.2015.05.009
37. Kirchhof P, Benussi S, Kotecha D, et al. 2016 ESC Guidelines for the management of atrial fibrillation developed in collaboration with EACTS. *Eur Heart J.* 2016;37(38):2893-2962. doi:10.1093/eurheartj/ehw210
38. Atti V, Gwon Y, Narayanan MA, et al. Multivessel versus culprit-only revascularization in STEMI and multivessel coronary artery disease: meta-analysis of randomized trials. *JACC Cardiovasc Interv.* 2020;13(13):1571-1582. doi:10.1016/j.jcin.2020.04.055
39. Scalone G, Niccoli G, Crea F. Editor's Choice-Pathophysiology, diagnosis and management of MINOCA: an update. *Eur Heart J Acute Cardiovasc Care.* 2019;8(1):54-62. doi:10.1177/2048872618782414
40. Mukherjee D. Myocardial infarction with nonobstructive coronary arteries: a call for individualized treatment. *J Am Heart Assoc.* 2019;8(14):e013361. doi:10.1161/JAHA.119.013361
41. Priori SG, Blomström-Lundqvist C, Mazzanti A, et al. 2015 ESC Guidelines for the management of patients with ventricular arrhythmias and the prevention of sudden cardiac death: The Task Force for the Management of Patients with Ventricular Arrhythmias and the Prevention of Sudden Cardiac Death of the European Society of Cardiology (ESC). Endorsed by: Association for European Paediatric and Congenital Cardiology (AEPC). *Eur Heart J.* 2015;36(41):2793-2867. doi:10.1093/eurheartj/ehv316
42. Grines CL, Marsalese DL, Brodie B, et al. Safety and cost-effectiveness of early discharge after primary angioplasty in low risk patients with acute myocardial infarction. PAMI-II Investigators. Primary Angioplasty in Myocardial Infarction. *J Am Coll Cardiol.* 1998;31(5):967-972. doi:10.1016/s0735-1097(98)00031-x
43. Bonaca MP, Bhatt DL, Cohen M, et al. PEGASUS-TIMI 54 Steering Committee and Investigators. Long-term use of ticagrelor in patients with prior myocardial infarction. *N Engl J Med.* 2015;372(19):1791-1800. doi:10.1056/NEJMoa1500857

CHAPTER 7

ACUTE MYOCARDIAL INFARCTION: COMPLICATIONS

Retesh Bajaj, Anantharaman Ramasamy, Vincenzo Tufaro, and Arjun K. Ghosh

INTRODUCTION

The advent of coronary reperfusion therapy has substantially reduced the incidence of complications following acute myocardial infarction (MI). However, their occurrence is still associated with significant morbidity and mortality. Cardiac complications can be broadly divided into mechanical, arrhythmic, and pericardial. A high index of suspicion and vigilance must be maintained to ensure these rare, but important, complications are diagnosed in a timely manner and appropriately managed.

MECHANICAL COMPLICATIONS OF ACUTE MYOCARDIAL INFARCTION

Ischemic injury frequently results in structural and mechanical changes in the myocardium, the magnitude of which is directly related to the amount of muscle affected and, therefore, impacted by extent of infarction. Structural complications and their severity are more common in patients who have sustained a transmural infarction in comparison to a nontransmural infarction. Patients who have not been treated with coronary reperfusion therapy have a significantly higher risk of mechanical cardiac complications. The incidence of mechanical complications has diminished to approximately 1% in the era of reperfusion therapy,[1] but the mortality rate remains high.

These complications can present acutely as life-threatening deteriorations in the immediate aftermath of a MI or more chronically, related to scar formation and remodeling of the heart as its architecture modifies to maintain cardiac output after the injury.

Acute Mechanical Complications

Acute mechanical complications of MI include sequelae from left or right ventricular systolic impairment or a loss of structural integrity that results in cardiac wall rupture, papillary muscle rupture, or ventricular septal rupture. Broadly, the latter share the same pathogenesis: myocyte necrosis, interstitial edema, inflammation, and matrix metalloproteinase secretion and activations that lead to degradation of the extracellular matrix impairing structural integrity.[2-4] Complete coronary occlusion and transmural infarction are the biggest risk factors for acute mechanical complication, with the timing of clinical presentation occurring in a bimodal distribution; most manifest within the first 24 hours of MI and the remainder in the following week.[5] The clinical presentations include an acute deterioration in symptoms that may be nonspecific, new or worse chest pain, cardiogenic shock, and sudden cardiac death. In patients with these presentations, urgent transthoracic echocardiography is critical in establishing the diagnosis. Mechanical complications can also be diagnosed on contrast ventriculography at the time of angiography or by alternative imaging modalities such as computerized tomographic (CT) scanning (if performed to rule out dissection or pulmonary embolus for symptoms) or cardiac magnetic resonance imaging (MRI).

Optimal management of acute mechanical complications involves a multidisciplinary team including cardiologists, cardiothoracic surgeons, intensivists, and advanced imaging specialists, and should ideally occur in specialized cardiac centers equipped to care for these high-risk patients.

Cardiogenic Shock

Cardiogenic shock is defined by persistent hypotension (systolic blood pressure ≤90 mm Hg) despite adequate volume replacement accompanied by signs of hypoperfusion (oliguria, cool peripheries, altered mental status, or end-organ hypoperfusion).[6] Although cardiogenic shock can result from structural complications (ie, septal rupture, papillary muscle rupture, ventricular septal defect, etc), the commonest cause remains depressed left ventricular (LV) function and less commonly right ventricular (RV) infarction. The incidence of cardiogenic shock following acute MI is variably described in registries as between 3% and 13%. Despite a reduction in incidence as a result of coronary reperfusion, it remains a leading cause of death with in-hospital mortality rates of 50% or more. Patients are most likely to develop cardiogenic shock within the first 24 hours of admission after MI. Elevation of serum lactate and creatinine levels is associated with a higher mortality, as is RV dysfunction complicating LV failure. Accordingly, echocardiography is helpful in assessing LV and RV function. The treatment of cardiogenic shock complicating MI is multipronged[7]: early revascularization of the infarct-related artery with percutaneous coronary intervention (PCI) is recommended (or failing that, coronary artery bypass graft surgery [CABG]), followed by hemodynamic monitoring and support in an intensive care environment. Most patients with cardiogenic shock have multivessel coronary disease, and the management strategy of nonculprit vessels has been a subject of recent study. The CULPRIT-SHOCK[8] trial found a reduction in death and renal failure at 30 days in patients undergoing PCI to the culprit-vessel only as compared to complete revascularization. This has been reflected in a recommendation to defer non–infarct-related artery PCI.[7] Mechanical support measures may be considered in individualized cases, but at present there is a lack of evidence for these to be used routinely.

Right Ventricular Infarction

Right ventricular infarction complicates up to 50% of inferior MIs and can be diagnosed by detecting ST elevation in electrocardiographic leads aVR and V1 or the right precordial leads (V3R and V4R). The presence of RV infarction increases the risk of cardiogenic shock, arrhythmia, and death with reported mortality at one year being 18% in those with isolated right coronary artery lesions and 27% in the presence of left and right coronary artery disease. Most RV MIs involve a dominant right coronary artery occluded proximal to the RV branches, but it may be associated with a left-dominant circumflex occlusion, or rarely the left anterior descending (LAD) if it provides collaterals to the RV free wall. As a result of the coronary anatomy involved, RV MI may be complicated by bradyarrhythmia and atrioventricular (AV) nodal block. The classic triad of hypotension, clear lung fields, and elevated jugular venous pressure (JVP) is also associated with RV MI. Between 25% and 50% of affected patients may suffer hemodynamic compromise owing to acute RV dilatation and the effects of ventricular interdependence resulting in decreased LV filling and contributing to systemic hypoperfusion.

Treatment includes restoration of flow in the RV branches and hemodynamic support—specifically intravascular volume infusion and avoiding medications, such as nitrates, that reduce preload. Volume supplementation should be attempted with careful assessment of the patient's fluid status and, if possible, with hemodynamic monitoring. Although RV infarction is a preload-dependent condition, excessive RV dilatation as a result of volume replacement may lead to further hemodynamic compromise as a result of impaired left heart filling caused by ventricular interdependence.[9]

Cardiac Free Wall Rupture

Cardiac rupture is commonest within four days of ST-elevation MI (STEMI) and more likely to affect the LV anteroapical wall (although RV involvement has been reported). Rates of cardiac rupture in acute MI patients who did not receive reperfusion therapy are as high as 6%. The incidence has halved in the last 30 years because of the use of reperfusion therapy,[10] but the mortality rate (>70%) is the highest among all acute mechanical complications and may account for up to 20% of acute mortality associated with MI.[11] Risk factors associated with cardiac free wall rupture include older age, female gender, and first MI.

The presentation is typically dramatic with sudden cardiac tamponade, although individuals with a slow leak of blood into the pericardium may note nonspecific symptoms including chest pain and signs ranging from minimal hemodynamic changes to frank hemodynamic collapse. Electromechanical dissociation on the ECG without preceding cardiac failure in the context of MI has been reported as a very specific sign of cardiac rupture.[12]

Early recognition and treatment are essential. In the unstable patient with cardiac tamponade, emergency pericardiocentesis can be lifesaving, but emergent surgical repair (ie, resecting the infarcted area and applying a patch to the ruptured zone) is the definitive treatment option. Perioperative mortality remains high because surgery on the friable and necrotic myocardium is technically challenging.

Ventricular Septal Rupture

Ventricular septal rupture classically develops 3 to 5 days post MI. It complicates 2 to 3 of every 1000 MIs[13] with a higher incidence among older females. The mortality rate approaches 100% without closure.[14] The anatomic location of the ventricular septal rupture is relevant as it impacts mortality: apicoanterior septal ruptures are associated with an LAD infarction and carry a better prognosis than posterior septal ruptures that are associated with occlusion of the posterior descending artery.[15] The latter are associated with RV dysfunction and are anatomically more challenging to treat (**Figure 7.1**). The dissection plane of the rupture can take a serpiginous route (ie, the LV entry and RV exit sites occur in different locations)[16] and is best assessed using transthoracic echocardiography with color flow imaging.

The acute left-to-right shunt results in hemodynamic compromise and biventricular failure. The presentation can be acute with pulmonary edema, and a new, harsh pansystolic murmur with a thrill may be found at the left sternal border.

Treatment involves surgical closure, which may be complicated by the technical challenges of operating on necrosed myocardial tissue. More recently, percutaneous closure devices have been introduced and may be an option in experienced centers.[17,18] Initial observational studies reported that postoperative survival was better for surgery deferred for a week; however, this was likely owing to survival bias, because early surgery is usually performed on individuals with marked hemodynamic instability and circulatory compromise. Consequently, it is now recommended that surgery or percutaneous treatment not be delayed. Afterload reduction with nitrates (in patients with a blood pressure that allows this) and intra-aortic balloon pump placement may stabilize patients with hemodynamic compromise until definitive surgery can be performed or a closure device is inserted.[17]

Papillary Muscle Rupture

Acute papillary muscle rupture is most commonly associated with inferior MIs and typically occurs 2 and 7 days after infarction. The posteromedial papillary muscle is 10 times more likely to be involved than the anterolateral papillary muscle, because it has a single blood supply from either the right or left circumflex coronary; the anterolateral papillary muscle is typically supplied by both the LAD and the left circumflex arteries. Papillary muscle rupture may be partial or complete and can result in a new pansystolic murmur; however, the murmur may be soft or inaudible in the presence of cardiac failure. The acute mitral regurgitation that results is typically poorly tolerated,

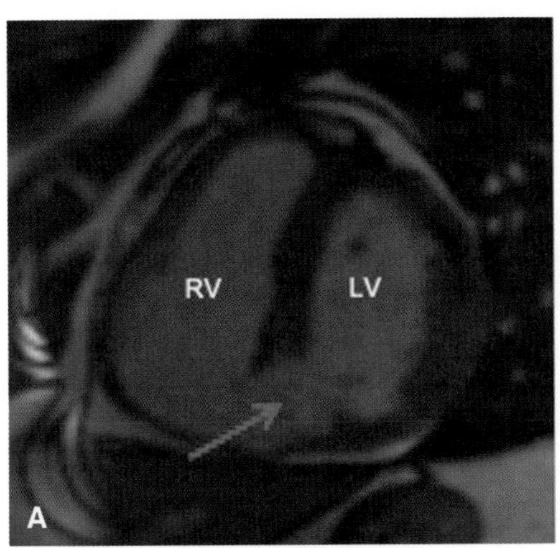

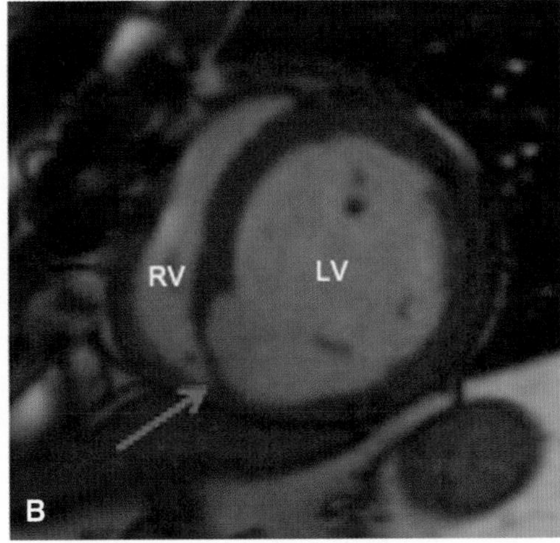

FIGURE 7.1 Inferoseptal VSD following a large inferior myocardial infarction on cardiac magnetic resonance imaging (**A**) before and (**B**) after surgical repair. LV, left ventricular; RV, right ventricular.

resulting in pulmonary edema and a high mortality without treatment in the first 24 hours.

Surgical options include mitral valve repair or replacement depending on anatomy and extent of the rupture. In patients who are deemed to be inoperable, successful treatment with the percutaneous MitraClip (Abbott, Lake Bluff, Illinois, USA) has been reported.[19,20]

MANAGEMENT OF ACUTE MECHANICAL COMPLICATIONS AFTER MYOCARDIAL INFARCTION

Acute mechanical complications after MI represent a collection of life-threatening scenarios that may be difficult to diagnose and effectively treat. Accordingly, early involvement of cardiology and cardiothoracic teams is essential. Mechanical circulatory support devices such as intra-aortic balloon pumps[21] may aid stabilization, improve hemodynamics, and delay deterioration until definitive treatment (ie, surgery or percutaneous) can be provided. More recently, extracorporeal membrane oxygenation in experienced centers has been used as an adjunct[22] to allow time for more definitive surgical management.

CHRONIC MECHANICAL COMPLICATIONS

Ventricular remodeling after MI is common with secondary progression to heart failure. Up to 20% of patients older than 65 years who have survived an MI will develop heart failure.[23] The process of healing that follows an MI leads to thinning of the myocardium and elongation of the infarcted region in response to myocardial wall stress, resulting in topographic changes to the ventricle—a process termed "infarct expansion." Depending on the size and extension of the infarction, this can result in a spectrum of effects—from no impairment of ventricular function to significant remodeling and ventricular aneurysm formation to depression of systolic function owing to loss of myocytes. These architectural changes can result in significant morbidity as well as risk of secondary complications.

Left Ventricular Aneurysms

LV aneurysms are fibrous, noncontractile outpouchings of the myocardial wall and most commonly occur in the anteroapical region. The anteroapical region has a relatively thinner wall anatomically as well as the greatest geometric curvature, predisposing it to aneurysm formation[3,24] in the context of transmural anterior infarction. Posterior and inferior wall aneurysms have been described but are much less common (**Figure 7.2**), and pseudoaneurysms that occur owing to chronic myocardial rupture are rarer still. Pseudoaneurysms are formed when the cardiac rupture is contained by the pericardium, organizing thrombus, and hematoma (ie, no myocardial tissue) and are considered a surgical emergency. Specific risk factors for aneurysm formation include hypertension, the use of steroids, and nonsteroidal anti-inflammatory drugs (NSAIDs).[25]

LV aneurysms may be entirely asymptomatic or the patient may complain of symptoms of heart failure owing to the impaired LV systolic function that would typically accompany significant anterior wall dyskinesia. Clinical signs depend on the size of the aneurysm; however, a diffuse, pansystolic apical thrust with a double impulse because of late systolic expansion of the aneurysmal sac has been detected on palpation of the left chest wall. A third heart sound may be present on auscultation because the aneurysmal sac may contribute to rapid ventricular filling.

A classic finding is the persistence of ST segment elevation in the ECG leads corresponding to the infarct region: ST elevation in V1-V6 in the presence of loss of R wave progression and well-established Q waves signifies a transmural infarction in the anterior region.[26,27] The mechanism for this is unclear but may be caused by traction and mechanical stress affecting the normal myocardium surrounding the aneurysm.

Aneurysms can be diagnosed on transthoracic echocardiography and most may be apparent early, often within days of the infarction. A previous study[28] found that it is rare for new aneurysms to develop beyond 3 months postinfarction.

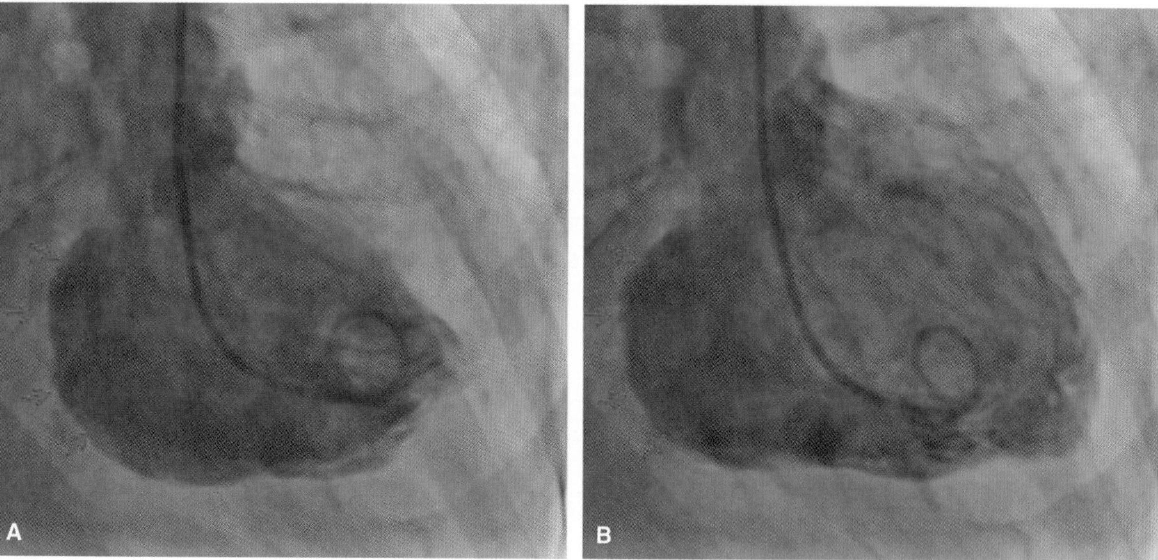

FIGURE 7.2 Left ventricular aneurysm in (**A**) systole and (**B**) diastole following a transmural inferior myocardial infarction on contrast ventriculography.

The aneurysmal LV has a risk of rupture, is a locus of ventricular arrhythmias, and increases the risk of development of intraventricular thrombus that may embolize. Treatment with surgery is an option and is considered for aneurysms to mitigate these risks.

LV pseudoaneurysms have a predilection for the lateral or diaphragmatic wall and are at a higher risk of rupture.[29] They result from quick hematoma formation or pericardial adhesions that limit bleeds from a cardiac rupture. Given the anatomic location, imaging with CT angiography or cardiac MRI is often helpful[30] in delineating the topography.

Left Ventricular Thrombus

LV thrombus formation is an important complication after acute MI that is associated with worse outcomes owing to the risk of systematic embolization. The pathogenesis is related to both blood stasis as a result of regionally depressed myocardial function, hypercoagulability in the aftermath of an MI, and activation of the clotting cascade by necrosed myocardial tissue.[31] Although the risk of thrombus formation has reduced in the PCI era, it can complicate up to 25% of anterior MIs and 15% of all MIs that are not treated with reperfusion therapy.[31] Other causes of myocardial injury that result in regional LV dysfunction—such as Takotsubo cardiomyopathy—may also result in LV thrombus formation. The diagnosis can be made on transthoracic echocardiography, but this imaging modality has a relatively low sensitivity; in suspected cases, a contrast echocardiogram or cardiac MRI is helpful in confirming the diagnosis, The treatment is with oral anticoagulation, most commonly with warfarin in addition to dual antiplatelet therapy for up to 6 months.[32]

Ventricular Failure

Ultimately, loss of myocardial tissue owing to ischemic necrosis can result in depression of systolic function and mechanical change or remodeling as a consequence of a complex interplay of neurohormonal factors and homeostatic mechanisms attempting to maintain cardiac output in the presence of weakened musculature. Chronic heart failure in the long term should be managed broadly as heart failure from other causes and should be treated by a specialist with serial interval imaging to assess ventricular function.

Early revascularization is the only therapy that has been shown to reduce in-hospital mortality in acute MI complicated by heart failure and may be guided by viability imaging studies. Beta blockers should be avoided in the first 24 hours after an MI with heart failure, and patients should be reviewed for reconsideration daily. There is evidence for administration of angiotensin converting enzyme (ACE) inhibitors within the first 24 hours to reduce mortality after hospital discharge (unless contraindicated by hypotension, acute kidney injury, renal failure, or drug allergy), and for administration of aldosterone antagonists in the first 7 days after an MI.[33] Angiotensin receptor blockers may be substituted for ACE inhibitors if contraindicated by drug allergy.

ARRHYTHMIC COMPLICATIONS OF ACUTE MYOCARDIAL INFARCTION

Cardiac arrhythmias are a known complication of acute MI. Myocardial ischemia and infarction often lead to intracellular metabolic derangement and autonomic dysfunction that can lead to cardiac arrhythmias. Clinical characteristics such as infarct size, hemodynamic instability, pre-existing conduction disease, and use of ionotropic support agents may exacerbate myocardial ischemia and provoke cardiac arrhythmias. Although the majority of patients with cardiac arrhythmias post MI may be asymptomatic, patients can present with a variety of symptoms such as palpitations, chest pain, breathlessness, syncope, or cardiac arrest. Timely recognition and management are essential because these arrhythmias—both tachycardic or bradycardic episodes—can provoke hemodynamic instability and lead to life-threatening rhythm disturbances and cardiac death.

Tachyarrhythmias

Atrial Arrhythmias

Sinus Tachycardia. A marked rise in sinus node discharge is common during the acute phase of MI. This is usually associated with the chest pain and anxiety surrounding the presentation, which often resolve following administration of pain relief and revascularization. However, a physiologic tachycardia as a compensatory mechanism for reduced stroke volume may indicate pump failure, which is associated with poor prognosis. Studies have shown that sinus tachycardia in patients with acute MI is associated with larger proportion of anterior infarcts, multiple infarct sites, and higher mean peak biomarker release.[34] These patients are also more likely to suffer from post-MI complications such as peri-infarct pericarditis and an increased risk of in-hospital mortality. Early and cautious administration of beta blockers to lower the sympathetic tone should be considered in these patients.

Premature Atrial Ectopics. Premature atrial ectopics (PACs) are the most of common type of atrial arrhythmias in patients with acute MI. They are characterized by abnormal morphology of the P waves. These may be because of increased sympathetic tone, atrial distensions from either left or right ventricular infarction, or atrial ischemia/infarction. PACs rarely cause symptoms; therefore, suppressive treatment is not required in these patients.[35]

Supraventricular Tachycardias. Paroxysmal or persistent supraventricular tachycardia (SVT) including atrial tachycardia (AT) and atrioventricular nodal ventricular tachycardia (AVNT) are relatively rare in patients with acute MI. Most of these arrhythmias are transient and cause no symptoms.[36] However, when present with rapid ventricular response, patients can be highly symptomatic with associated hemodynamic collapse. Management is directed toward controlling the rapid ventricular rate. This can be attempted by carotid sinus massage or Valsalva maneuver, both of which increase the vagal tone and alter the AV nodal properties. Intravenous adenosine can be useful to terminate these arrhythmias, but resuscitation facilities with an external defibrillator should be available because a small number of patients develop ventricular fibrillation from adenosine. Intravenous beta blockers and calcium channel blockers may also be used to slow the rapid ventricular rate, but this should be done cautiously to avoid hypotension in patients with acute MI. Hemodynamically unstable patients should be treated with urgent, synchronized direct current cardioversion to terminate these arrhythmias.

Atrial Fibrillation. The incidence of atrial fibrillation (AF) in the setting of acute MI has been reported to be 7% to 21%.[37] Rapid and irregular ventricular rates may impair coronary perfusion and LV function, which can lead to symptoms such as chest pain, palpitations, and breathlessness. Coronary ischemia, irregular RR intervals, and enhanced sympathetic nervous system in the presence of atrial fibrillation can lead to life-threatening ventricular arrhythmias. Advanced heart failure (Killip class IV) is the most significant predictor of development of AF in acute MI.[38] In addition, advanced age, male gender, and admission heart rate greater than 100 beats per minute are associated with the development of AF.

AF in the setting of acute MI is associated with increased morbidity and mortality[39] independent of age, diabetes mellitus, hypertension, history of previous MI, cardiac failure, or coronary revascularization status. However, it is unclear if AF is purely a complication of MI or a severity marker of the acute infarction. The TRACE study concluded that the excess mortality in these patients is likely related to sudden and non-sudden cardiac deaths.[40]

Traditional antiplatelet therapy have not reduced the risk of thromboembolism in patients with AF. The addition of oral anticoagulant to antiplatelets increases the absolute risk of major hemorrhage. Accordingly, patients with AF undergoing primary PCI should be treated with newer third-generation drug-eluting stents with shorter duration of antiplatelet therapy, because they will require long-term oral anticoagulation.[41]

The management of AF in acute MI should focus on adequate rate control that can be achieved with administration of beta blockers or calcium channels blockers. However, this should be done cautiously in patients who have suffered large infarcts with LV dysfunction because the negative chronotropic effect of these medications can further compromise their hemodynamic status. Class 1C antiarrhythmic agents such as flecainide and propafenone are contraindicated in patients with coronary artery disease and should be avoided. Prompt treatment with synchronized DC cardioversion should be considered when patients with AF present with hemodynamic instability.

Ventricular Arrhythmias

Premature Ventricular Contractions. Premature ventricular contractions (PVCs) occur frequently in patients with acute MI (**Figure 7.3**). They rarely cause hemodynamic compromise and do not require specific treatments. Frequent PVCs may be related to electrolyte imbalance, so plasma levels of potassium and magnesium should be checked and corrected accordingly.[42] Frequent PVCs persisting longer than 48 hours are associated with increased long-term arrhythmic risk, especially in patients with impaired LV function.[43]

Accelerated Idioventricular Rhythm. Accelerated idioventricular rhythm (AIVR) is defined by three or more ventricular complexes with QRS duration greater than 120 milliseconds and a regular ventricular rate between 50 and 110 beats per

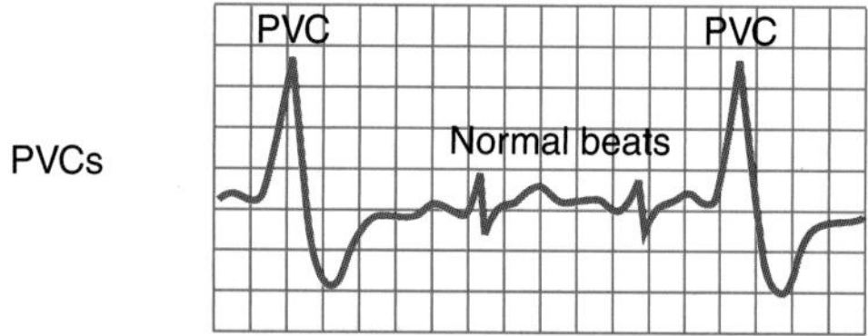

FIGURE 7.3 Electrocardiographic (ECG) tracings of ventricular arrhythmias. Premature ventricular contractions (PVCs) originate from an ectopic focus in the ventricles, causing a distortion of the QRS complex. Because the ventricle usually cannot repolarize sufficiently to respond to the next impulse that arises in the SA node, a PVC is frequently followed by a compensatory pause. (Reprinted with permission from Norris TL. *Porth's Essentials of Pathophysiology*. 5th ed. Philadelphia, PA: Wolters Kluwer; 2019. Figure 28.12.)

minute. AIVR occurs when the rate of an ectopic ventricular pacemaker exceeds that of the sinus node. AIVR is commonly seen during the reperfusion phase of acute MI and is usually a well-tolerated, self-limiting, benign heart rhythm that rarely requires any specific treatment. The administration of antiarrhythmic agents should be avoided because these may precipitate systemic hypotension and hemodynamic collapse.[44]

Ventricular Tachycardia. Ventricular tachycardia (VT) is a wide complex tachycardia on ECG originating from the ventricles (**Figure 7.4**). In general, wide complex tachycardia in acute MI should be treated as VT unless proven otherwise. VT is classified by its duration and onset as (1) sustained (spontaneous termination after more than 30 seconds or requiring intervention) or non-sustained (spontaneously terminating in >30 seconds) and (2) early (occurring within 24 hours of MI) or late (occurring more than 48 hours of MI). Early VT is associated with reversible causes related to the presentation, such as residual or persistent ischemia and electrolyte imbalance, and does not predict the occurrence of VT later. On the other hand, late VT is more common in patients following an extensive, transmural infarct and likely to recur.

Prompt revascularization and initiation of secondary prevention medications have reduced the incidence of VT in

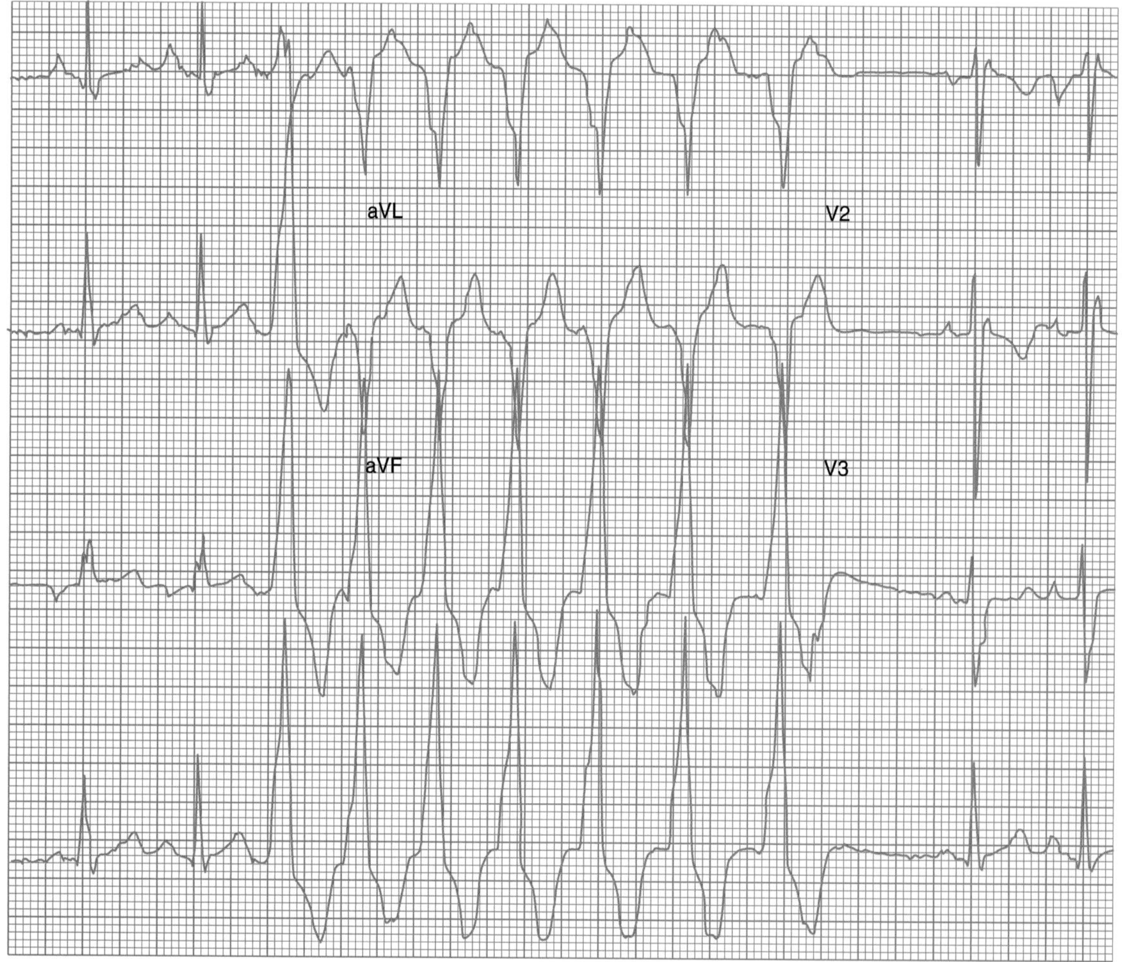

FIGURE 7.4 This rhythm strip demonstrates ventricular tachycardia. There is a sudden onset of a wide QRS tachycardia. No P wave is visible during the tachycardia. The tachycardia ends with a widening of the last two R-R intervals. (Adapted with permission from Kline-Tilford AM, Haut C. © *Lippincott Certification Review: Pediatric Acute Care Nurse Practitioner*. Philadelphia, PA: Wolters Kluwer; 2015. Figure 5.35.)

patients with acute MI. However, patients with no or incomplete revascularization and those that carry arrhythmogenic substrate prior to the acute MI are more likely to suffer from life-threatening ventricular tachyarrhythmias.[45] Patients with VT post MI have a worse prognosis than those without VT. The adjusted risk of 90-day mortality is increased twofold and sixfold in patients with early and late VT, respectively.[46]

The management of VT in acute MI should focus on eliminating ischemia. Prompt reperfusion of the occluded vessel and early use of beta blockers in acute MI reduce in-hospital mortality. Correction of electrolyte abnormalities, specifically hypokalemia and hypomagnesemia, is recommended. Antiarrhythmic drugs (AAD) are widely used but limited data from clinical trials are available supporting their use in acute MI (**Table 7.1**). AAD should be used cautiously given their side effects and potential harmful effects in acute MI patients. Electrical defibrillation is recommended to acutely terminate VT that is sustained or results in hemodynamic compromise in acute MI patients. AAD treatment with amiodarone (class III AAD) should be considered if the VT episodes are frequent and refractory to electrical defibrillation. Pooled analysis from studies showed that amiodarone reduces cardiac and arrhythmic deaths in comparison to placebo when given in combination with beta blockers.[47] However, long-term use of amiodarone is associated with increased mortality, especially in patients with impaired LV function.[48] Intravenous lidocaine (class I AAD) can be considered in patients not responding to beta blockers, amiodarone, or in the case of contraindications to these medications. In patients with intractable, drug-refractory VT, catheter ablation should be considered in specialized cardiac centers with expertise.

Ventricular Fibrillation. Ventricular fibrillation (VF) is characterized by rapid, chaotic irregular deflections of varying amplitude. VF is the leading cause of death during the early course of acute MI, occurring in up to 18% of patients. It is more likely to occur in patients with large infarcts, but no difference has been noted between anterior or inferior infarcts. Primary VF occurs early during the clinical presentation with no other causes whereas secondary VF is usually related to cardiogenic shock during the course of the MI. In patients with VF post MI, myocardial ischemia should be considered as a potential underlying etiology. Prompt recognition and early revascularization is advocated in these patients. Immediate electrical defibrillation should be administered at the point of VF detection. Advanced life support protocols, including cardiopulmonary resuscitation, should be initiated without delay to improve patient outcomes.

Bradyarrhythmia

Sinus Bradycardia. Sinus bradycardia is traditionally described as heart rate of less than 60 beats per minute. It is three times more common in inferoposterior infarction compared to anterolateral MI. Ischemia or infarction of the sinus node (supplied by the atrial branch of right coronary artery in 55%

TABLE 7.1 Common Antiarrhythmic Drugs Used in Acute Myocardial Infarction

Class	Drug	Indications	Primary Mechanism of Action	Side Effects
1A	Procainamide	VT	Na^+ channel blocker that prolongs duration of the action potential	Lupus erythematosus-like syndrome, agranulocytosis, bone marrow suppression
IB	Lidocaine	VT	Na^+ channel blocker with rapid dissociation that shortens the action potential	AV block, hypotension, drowsiness, nystagmus, tremor, blurred vision, abnormal sensation
II	Beta blockers (e.g. carvedilol, metoprolol, atenolol, bisoprolol)	AF, AVNT, AT	β-adrenergic receptor blockers that decrease the sympathetic activity of the heart	Bradycardia, headache, sleep disorders, dyspnea, fatigue, confusion, peripheral coldness, peripheral vascular disease
III	Amiodarone	VT, VF	K^+ channel blocker that prolongs repolarization and refractory period	Bradycardia, hepatic disorders, hyperthyroidism, nausea, pulmonary toxicity, skin rashes
IV	Calcium channel blockers (e.g. verapamil, diltiazem)	AF, AVNT, AT	Ca^{2+} channel blockers that decrease conduction through the AV node	Dizziness, drowsiness, abdominal pain, headache, peripheral edema, skin reactions, angioedema, gingival hyperplasia
V	Digoxin	AF, AVNT	Increases vagal activity and reduces conduction velocity through the AV node	Nausea, dizziness, diarrhea, vomiting, vision disorders, eosinophilia, conduction abnormalities
V	Adenosine	AVNT	Suppresses AV conduction	Chest discomfort, dry mouth, dyspnea, hypotension, flushing, headache

of patients and the left circumflex artery in 45%) and, more commonly, increased vagal tone can lead to sinus bradycardia. In some cases, this may be related to opioid administration. Isolated sinus bradycardia usually does not require any specific treatments. If the heart rate is extremely low and accompanied with hypotension, intravenous atropine or temporary pacing can be considered.

First-Degree Atrioventricular Block. The PR interval measures electrical conduction between the atria and the ventricle and includes atrial depolarization and conduction through the AV node, bundle of His, bundle branches, and fascicles. First-degree AV block is characterized by a prolonged PR interval (>200 msec). This arrhythmia can arise from the occlusion of the artery supplying the AV node, bundle of His, or the bundle branches. AV nodal blocking medications, beta blockers, calcium channel blockers, digoxin, and AAD may also be responsible for a prolonged PR interval. Generally, first-degree AV block is a benign condition and rarely requires treatment. If associated with significant bradycardia and hypotension, intravenous atropine may be considered.

Second-Degree Atrioventricular Block. Type 1 second-degree AV block, also known as Wenckebach or Mobitz type 1 AV block, is characterized by progressively lengthening PR intervals leading to a non-conducted P wave (**Figure 7.5**). This arrhythmia is likely due to ischemia of the AV node and is usually a transient phenomenon. The management is similar to that of a first-degree AV block where specific treatments are rarely needed unless accompanied with significant bradycardia and systemic hypotension.

Type II second-degree AV block is characterized by non-conducted P waves and is usually owing to failure of conduction at the level of the His-Purkinje system. In 25% of cases, this occurs in the setting of inferior or posterior MI where the conduction block is located within the His bundle itself leading to narrow complex rhythms. This is usually transient and can be managed conservatively. However, in patients with anterior MI, the conduction block is located distal to the bundle of His, which produces a wide-complex escape rhythm. These patients are more likely to suffer from hemodynamic instability with higher risk of progression to complete heart block. In this setting, patients should be treated with temporary external or transvenous pacing.[49]

Third-Degree Heart Block (Complete Heart Block.) Complete heart block (CHB) refers to complete absence of AV conduction where the underlying cardiac rhythm is maintained by a junctional or ventricular escape rhythm (**Figure 7.6**). CHB resulting from inferior MI is more common than anterior MI. It generally results from an infranodal lesion and develops gradually, progressing from first to second degree to CHB. Given the location of the ischemia, these patients have a narrow-complex (ie, junctional) escape rhythm with minimal risk of asystole. Patients usually tolerate the rhythm well.

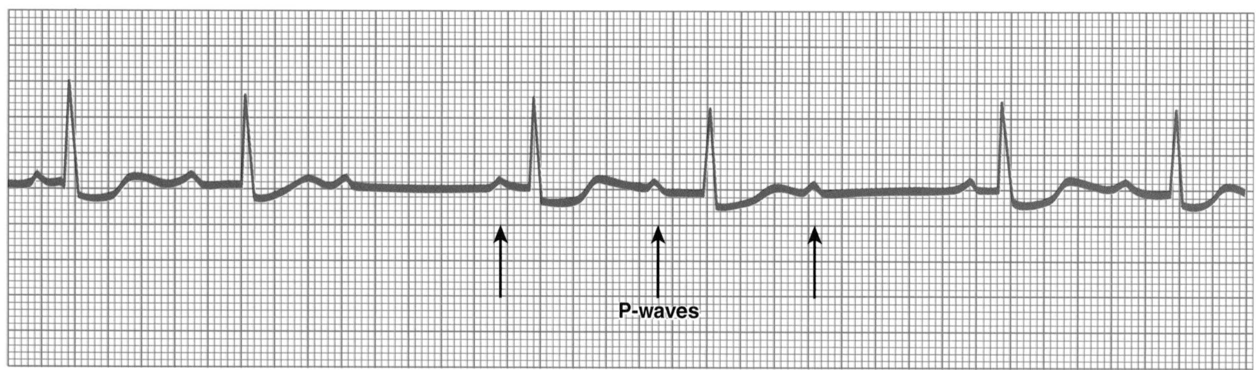

FIGURE 7.5 Second-degree heart block: Mobitz type I. Note prolonging PR interval prior to the dropped beat. (Reprinted with permission from Huff J. *ECG Workout: exercises in arrhythmia interpretation.* 4th ed. Philadelphia, PA: Lippincott Williams & Wilkins; 2002. Figure 8.19.)

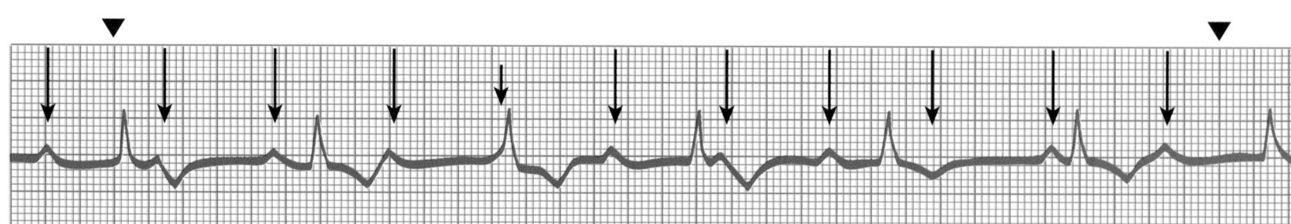

FIGURE 7.6 Third-degree heart block (complete AV block). Arrows denote P waves. Note the lack of relationship between the atria (P wave) and ventricles (QRS). (Adapted with permission from Morton PG, Fontaine DK. *Critical Care Nursing: A holistic approach.* 11th ed. Philadelphia, PA: Wolters Kluwer; 2017. Figure 17.29 View D.)

Pacing is generally not required because CHB in this setting is usually transient, resolving within 5 to 7 days.[45]

On the other hand, CHB in the setting of anterior MI may occur suddenly within 24 hours of infarction, but it can be preceded by Mobitz type II AV block or bifascicular/trifascicular blocks. Because the His-Purkinje system is damaged owing to the extensive septal infarction, these patients present with unstable escape rhythms with wide QRS complexes. The in-hospital and 30-day mortality of these patients is much higher than those with CHB following inferior MI because of the more extensive myocardial necrosis and cardiogenic shock.[50]

Prophylactic temporary pacing is recommended in patients with CHB or new bifascicular bundle branch block following anterior MI to protect against asystole. There is no evidence that temporary transvenous pacing improves outcomes in these patients, but this is likely driven by their poor prognosis following the large MI. Temporary pacemaker placements should be performed by those who are trained and aware of the potential serious complications including infections and cardiac perforations leading to cardiac tamponade. In patients with persistent CHB or high-grade AV block with new bifascicular bundle branch blocks, permanent pacemaker should be considered during the same hospital admission.

PERICARDIAL COMPLICATIONS OF MYOCARDIAL INFARCTION

There are three major types of pericardial complications that may occur following an acute MI:

- Early post-MI pericarditis—also called early infarct-associated pericarditis *or pericarditis epistenocardica*—occurs a few days after an acute MI, typically within the first 2 to 4 days.
- Late post-MI pericarditis (also termed Dressler syndrome) usually occurs after 1 to 2 weeks following an acute MI.
- Post-MI pericardial effusion (**Figure 7.7**).

Postmyocardial Infarction Pericarditis

Early infarct-associated pericarditis and Dressler syndrome are the major pericardial complications after an acute MI. Each of these complications has been related to infarct size and decreased in incidence because of the introduction and widespread use of coronary revascularization therapies. Previous studies reported that early and late postmyocardial infarction pericarditis (PMIP) had an incidence of 10% to 20% and 3% to 4%, respectively, in acute MI patients. In the primary reperfusion era, the incidence of early PMIP declined to less than 5%, mainly related to late or failed coronary reperfusion and transmural extension of the acute MI. Dressler syndrome is rare (<1%) in the era of primary PCI and may reflect a larger size acute MI and/or late reperfusion as well.[51,52]

In addition to infarct size and delayed reperfusion, the development of PMIP has been associated with other factors, such as anterior infarct location, markedly elevated serum cardiac biomarkers, inferior infarction complicated by RV involvement, and more commonly reduced LV ejection fraction.[53]

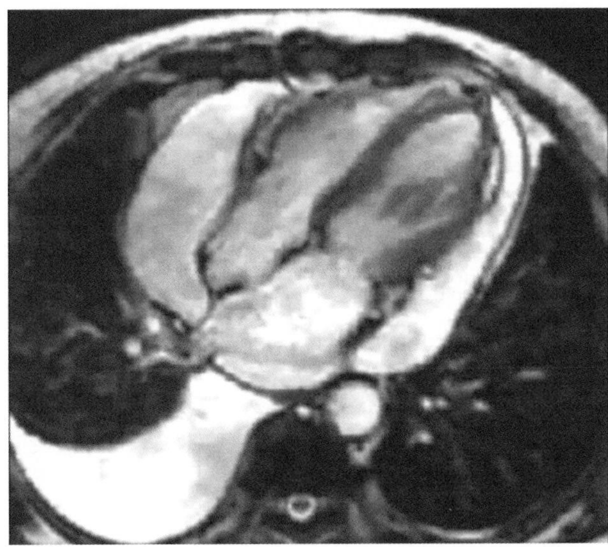

FIGURE 7.7 Global pericardial effusion on cardiac MRI. MRI, magnetic resonance imaging.

The term *postcardiac injury syndrome (PCIS)* is applied to a group of inflammatory pleuropericardial syndromes, including PMIP, postpericardiotomy syndrome (PPS), and post-traumatic pericarditis. With the exception of early PMIP, these syndromes have an autoimmune pathogenesis triggered by a damage to pericardial tissue related to myocardial necrosis (late PMIP), surgical trauma (PPS), accidental thoracic trauma (traumatic pericarditis), or iatrogenic trauma (pericarditis after cardiac procedures).

Early PMIP is caused by an inflammatory process that is mainly related to extension of the acute MI. Indeed, transmural acute MI by definition involves the epicardial surface and may lead to local pericardial inflammation. An acute fibrinous pericarditis occurs frequently after transmural MI, but most patients do not report pericardial symptoms.

By contrast, the exact pathophysiology of late PMIP and other PCIS is thought to be elicited by an insult to pericardial mesothelial cells as well as minor bleeding into the pericardial space and release of cardiac antigens, which lead in turn to an inflammatory and autoimmune response in predisposed patients. This inflammation causes a spectrum of clinical presentations that may include pericarditis, pleuropericarditis, pericardial and/or pleural effusions, pulmonary infiltrates, and cardiac tamponade.[52,54]

The following clinical aspects support the immune-mediated pathogenesis of Dressler syndrome: the latent period of a few weeks till the onset of the disease, concomitant pleural effusion and/or pulmonary infiltrates, and a favorable response to anti-inflammatory therapies (NSAIDs, corticosteroids, colchicine) with relapse after treatment withdrawal.

Patients who develop PMIP typically present with signs and symptoms similar to those experienced by patients with acute pericarditis and/or pericardial effusion. The diagnosis of PMIP is often suspected because of a history of characteristic pleuritic chest pain within days or weeks following an acute MI. The following are the most common clinical signs and symptoms:

- Chest pain (in more than 80% of cases), that is typically sharp, pleuritic, and centrally located; the pain is improved by sitting up and leaning forward
- Dyspnea and/or pleural friction rubs (50%-60%)
- Low-grade fever (>50%)
- Pericardial friction rubs (30%-60%).

Although the physical examination is often unremarkable in patients with PMIP, it may be important in asymptomatic cases with only pericardial friction rubs signaling the occurrence of this syndrome. A superficial scratchy or squeaking sound is best heard with the diaphragm of the stethoscope over the left sternal border. The rub is frequently intermittent and can be difficult to appreciate.[52,53]

Diagnostic criteria of early PMIP do not differ from those for acute pericarditis. At least two of the following criteria are required to make the diagnosis: (1) chest pain; (2) pericardial friction rub; (3) evidence of ECG changes; and/or (4) pericardial effusion (**Algorithm 7.1**).

By contrast, diagnosis of late PMIP is established according to criteria that have been proposed for PPS and more in general for PCIS. In patients presenting with cardiac injury related to acute MI, surgery, or trauma, at least two of the following five criteria should be fulfilled: (1) fever without alternative etiologies; (2) pericarditic or pleuritic chest pain; (3) pericardial or pleural rubs; (4) pericardial effusion; and/or (5) pleural effusion with elevated C-reactive protein (CRP).[55]

Clinical evaluation of patients affected by PMIP typically includes blood tests, chest x-ray, ECG, and echocardiography. Blood tests may reveal leukocytosis and elevated inflammatory markers, (ie, erythrocyte sedimentation rate and CRP) in more than 80% of cases. Moreover, increased troponin levels may suggest myocardial involvement (eg, myopericarditis). Chest radiography is usually normal, but it can show the presence of a new pleural effusion with or without pulmonary infiltrates (>60%) and an enlarged cardiac silhouette. ECG changes are present in 60% to 80% of patients, but the typical ECG abnormalities observed with other presentations of pericarditis (diffuse ST segment elevations in association with PR segment depressions) are often overshadowed by changes owing to the MI. PMIP diagnosis is typically suggested by ST segments that remain elevated after an acute MI with persistence of upright T waves or T waves that become upright after having been inverted.[52,54,56] Transthoracic echocardiography should be performed to evaluate the presence and size of pericardial effusion as well as evidence of cardiac tamponade. In patients with PMIP, most pericardial effusions are small (ie, echo-free space in systole and diastole <10 mm) and not hemodynamically significant in subjects with PMIP. By contrast, patients with a moderate (10-20 mm) or larger effusion are at significantly increased risk of subacute ventricular free wall rupture and should be carefully monitored. Cardiac MRI can be used in selected cases to investigate pericardial inflammation and/or myocardial involvement.[57,58]

A supportive treatment is generally sufficient in patients affected by early PMIP because most cases are self-limited. The recommended approach is to avoid using NSAIDs for the initial 7 to 10 days post MI, with the exception of once-daily aspirin for secondary prevention. However, a minority of cases may have persistent symptoms and medical therapy with high-dose aspirin and colchicine may be considered according to European Society of Cardiology (ESC) guidelines.[55] Aspirin (750-1000 mg orally every 8 hours for 1-2 weeks, followed by gradual tapering of the doses by 250-500 mg every 1-2 weeks) is recommended rather than other NSAIDs or glucocorticoids that are considered harmful in the early period following an MI. The role of colchicine is more controversial in patients with early PMIP compared to those affected by PCIS because there is lack of evidence on its use in this clinical setting, in part reflecting the fact that so few cases persist long enough to warrant consideration of further treatment in addition to aspirin. However, some persistent cases of early PMIP may represent a transition to late PMIP and a combined therapy (aspirin plus colchicine) can be effective in such unusual cases.[49,55]

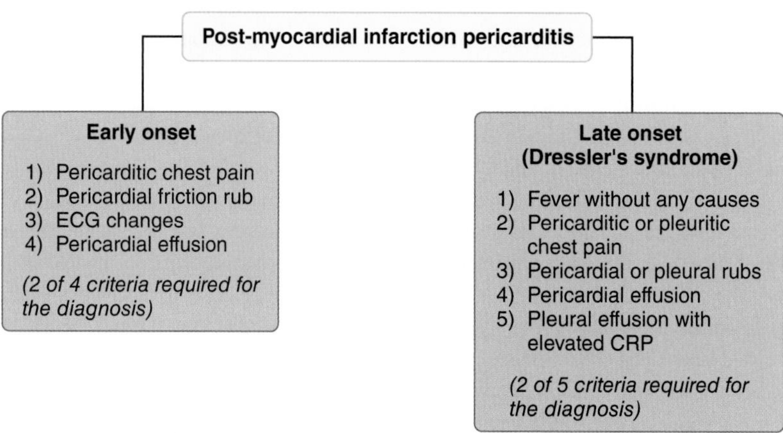

ALGORITHM 7.1 Diagnostic criteria for early and late postmyocardial infarction pericarditis.

On the other hand, treatment for late occurring PMIP is mostly supportive and anti-inflammatory therapy is recommended as first-line therapy to accelerate symptom remission and lower recurrence rate. According to ESC guidelines, colchicine should be added to aspirin as in the treatment plan of acute pericarditis.[55] Regarding NSAIDs, aspirin is the drug of choice for anti-inflammatory therapy of PMIP because it is already needed as antiplatelet treatment after MI. Moreover, anti-inflammatory actions of other NSAIDs may interfere with early myocardial healing and scar formation. High-dose aspirin has been shown to be efficacious for PMIP in several studies. Indomethacin should be avoided because it decreases coronary blood flow. Ibuprofen, which may increase coronary flow, can be used at a dose of 600 mg every 6 hours per 1 to 2 weeks, with tapering of the doses by 200 mg to 400 mg every 1 to 2 weeks. Gastric protection with a proton pump inhibitor should be provided in all patients treated with NSAIDs.

Colchicine (0.5 mg twice daily for patients weighing ≥70 kg or 0.5 mg once daily for patients <70 kg, for 3 months) has been shown to relieve pain and prevent recurrences in the treatment of acute pericarditis, and it is expected to provide similar beneficial effects also in patients with late PMIP, although there is limited data in this setting. However, colchicine should be avoided in subjects at risk for bone marrow suppression and those affected by liver disease, gastrointestinal motility disorders, or renal insufficiency.[51,55,56]

Low doses of corticosteroids (ie, oral prednisone at a starting dose of 0.25-0.50 mg/kg/day) are shown to be effective in patients in whom aspirin/NSAIDs are contraindicated and those who fail to respond to first-line therapy and have refractory symptoms. Unfortunately, recurrent pericarditis is more common following treatment with corticosteroids than with NSAID or colchicine therapy, and its administration early post MI is associated with an increased risk of myocardial rupture. Hence, it is not recommended for first-line therapy. Glucocorticoid therapy is usually adopted, after careful exclusion of infectious causes, in combination with colchicine. In terms of dosages, every decrease in prednisone dose should be done only if the patient is asymptomatic and CRP is normal in order to avoid recurrences.[46,50,54]

Inpatient admission is not necessary for all patients with PMIP, but those who have at least one high-risk feature should be hospitalized. High-risk characteristics include patients with fever greater than 38 °C, immunosuppressed state, elevated troponin levels, subacute onset (symptoms developing over days to weeks), large pericardial effusion (>20 mm) or cardiac tamponade, lack of response to aspirin or NSAIDs after at least 1 week of therapy, and concurrent oral anticoagulant use.[51]

In-hospital and 1-year mortality and major adverse cardiac events were similar in patients with and without pericarditis, even though both early and late PMIP are typically associated with larger infarct size. Although the prognosis of PMIP is relatively good for most patients, late PMIP may have a recurrence rate of 10% to 15%. In addition, a careful follow-up after PCIS should be considered to exclude possible evolution toward constrictive pericarditis that has an estimated risk of 2% to 5% in a long-term follow-up of 72 months.[52,55]

Postmyocardial Infarction Pericardial Effusion

Post-MI pericardial effusion is common in the early course of transmural MI and is minimal or small (<10 mm). In the era of primary PCI, pericardial effusion may be detected by cardiac MRI in around 60% of patients with STEMI because cardiac MRI is more sensitive than echocardiography in identifying effusions. However, clinically significant pericardial effusions causing signs and symptoms of cardiac tamponade are rare post MI; more specifically, isolated cases of cardiac tamponade (without any sign of myocardial rupture) accounted for less than 1% among hospitalized patients with STEMI.[59,60]

The major risk factor for development of a post-MI pericardial effusion is poor hemodynamic LV function, which is mainly associated with a larger infarct size; however, the effusion is typically small. By contrast, potential mechanisms of cardiac tamponade include pericardial involvement with hemorrhagic pericarditis, transmural MI resulting in free wall rupture, or iatrogenic coronary artery perforation during PCI.[61]

The majority of patients with a post-MI pericardial effusion are asymptomatic, with the presence of a pericardial effusion identified incidentally on an echocardiogram performed for other reasons (ie, evaluation of LV function). However, in case of ongoing pericardial fluid accumulation and increased intrapericardial pressure that leads to cardiac tamponade, patients suffer from dyspnea, rapid breathing, chest discomfort, dizziness, palpitations, and, in severe cases, loss of consciousness owing to low cardiac output.

Cardiac tamponade is a life-threatening clinical condition related to elevated intrapericardial pressure that exceeds normal filling pressures of the heart. Physical examination may reveal sinus tachycardia, elevated JVP, paradoxical pulse (>10 mm Hg decrease of systolic blood pressure with inspiration) and hypotension; however, none of these findings is really sensitive or specific to establish the diagnosis. For instance, Beck's triad (i.e., a combination of hypotension, elevated JVP, and muffled heart sounds) can be extremely useful for establishing the diagnosis of cardiac tamponade, but it is detectable in only a small number of cases.[62] Transthoracic echocardiography is the imaging modality of choice in patients with suspected cardiac tamponade to evaluate the presence, size, and hemodynamic impact of a pericardial effusion. The following echocardiographic parameters are consistent with and highly suggestive of cardiac tamponade, and they need to be carefully assessed: evidence of cardiac chamber collapse, reciprocal changes in ventricular volumes and septum motion toward LV with inspiration and toward RV during expiration, dilatation of the inferior vena cava with blunted respiratory changes, and mitral and tricuspid Doppler velocity profiles with respiratory variation exceeding 30%.[63]

The management of post-MI pericardial effusion may be different according to the etiology of the effusion and the presence of symptoms of hemodynamic instability. For patients with a post-MI pericardial effusion that leads to cardiac tamponade and hemodynamic shock, urgent pericardiocentesis, which is almost always accomplished percutaneously, is mandatory. Percutaneous pericardiocentesis may represent a bridge to surgical treatment when a mechanical complication (ie, free wall rupture) is diagnosed and emergency surgical repair is required. For patients with a pericardial effusion and no suspected mechanical complications or findings of cardiac tamponade, a conservative treatment approach is usually sufficient.[64]

The risk of developing a small to moderate post-MI pericardial effusion is not increased with the use of fibrinolytic agents, heparin, oral anticoagulants, aspirin, and other antiplatelet agents. However for patients with large pericardial effusions, there is a lack of evidence on how to properly manage antiplatelet and anticoagulant therapy. Generally, it is not necessary to discontinue antiplatelet therapy, whereas anticoagulation should be immediately withdrawn if a pericardial effusion develops or significantly increases in size (>3 mm). Monitoring the size of a pericardial effusion with serial echocardiograms and the patient's hemodynamic status is mandatory in order to promptly detect signs of cardiac tamponade.[49]

In terms of follow-up, patients who develop a moderate-to-large (>10 mm) post-MI pericardial effusion have a higher 30-day mortality (43%) in comparison to those with small or no effusion (10% and 6%, respectively). However, the complete reabsorption and resolution of a pericardial effusion can be slow with a 10% prevalence of persistent effusion after a 6-month follow-up.[58]

KEY POINTS

- ✔ The mortality rate for patients who suffer complications post MI remains high despite advances in cardiac management, even as the incidence of complications has decreased in the era of reperfusion therapy.
- ✔ Acute deterioration in patients with post-MI complications is common and may only manifest as a general clinical deterioration. Symptoms of chest pain and palpitations are poor discriminators for the presence of post-MI complications, and a high index of suspicion is needed to exclude life-threatening complications.
- ✔ A focused clinical examination, ECG, and bedside echocardiogram should be considered mandatory in the acutely deteriorated patient after MI.
- ✔ Management of complications varies depending on etiology, and a multidisciplinary approach with cardiology and cardiothoracic surgery should be considered.
- ✔ Advanced multimodality imaging with cardiac CT and cardiac MRI should be considered where available in the case of ambiguity or to monitor progression of pericardial or structural complications.

REFERENCES

1. Magalhães P, Mateus P, Carvalho S, et al. Relationship between treatment delay and type of reperfusion therapy and mechanical complications of acute myocardial infarction. *Eur Heart J Acute Cardiovasc Care.* 2016;5:468-474.
2. Sato S. Connective tissue changes in early ischemia of porcine myocardium: an ultrastructural study. *J Mol Cell Cardiol.* 1983;15:261-275.
3. Pfeffer MA, Braunwald E. Ventricular remodeling after myocardial infarction. Experimental observations and clinical implications. *Circulation.* 1990;81:1161-1172.
4. Takahashi S, Barry AC, Factor SM. Collagen degradation in ischaemic rat hearts. *Biochem J.* 1990;265:233-241.
5. Durko AP, Budde RPJ, Geleijnse ML, Kappetein AP. Recognition, assessment and management of the mechanical complications of acute myocardial infarction. *Heart.* 2018;104:1216-1223.
6. Baran DA, Grines CL, Bailey S, et al. SCAI clinical expert consensus statement on the classification of cardiogenic shock: this document was endorsed by the American College of Cardiology (ACC), the American Heart Association (AHA), the Society of Critical Care Medicine (SCCM), and the Society of Thoracic Surgeons (STS) in April 2019. *Catheter Cardiovasc Interv.* 2019;94:29-37.
7. Thiele H, Ohman EM, de Waha-Thiele S, Zeymer U, Desch S. Management of cardiogenic shock complicating myocardial infarction: an update 2019. *Eur Heart J.* 2019;40:2671-2683.
8. Thiele H, Akin I, Sandri M, et al. PCI strategies in patients with acute myocardial infarction and cardiogenic shock. *N Engl J Med.* 2017;377:2419-2432.
9. Konstam MA, Kiernan MS, Bernstein D, et al. Evaluation and management of right-sided heart failure: a scientific statement from the American Heart Association. *Circulation.* 2018;137:e578-e622.
10. Figueras J, Alcalde O, Barrabés JA, et al. Changes in hospital mortality rates in 425 patients with acute ST-elevation myocardial infarction and cardiac rupture over a 30-year period. *Circulation.* 2008;118:2783-2789.
11. Gao X-M, White DA, Dart AM, Du X-J. Post-infarct cardiac rupture: recent insights on pathogenesis and therapeutic interventions. *Pharmacol Ther.* 2012;134:156-179.
12. Figueras J, Curós A, Cortadellas J, Soler-Soler J. Reliability of electromechanical dissociation in the diagnosis of left ventricular free wall rupture in acute myocardial infarction. *Am Heart J.* 1996;131:861-864.
13. Moreyra AE, Huang MS, Wilson AC, Deng Y, Cosgrove NM, Kostis JB. Trends in incidence and mortality rates of ventricular septal rupture during acute myocardial infarction. *Am J Cardiol.* 2010;106:1095-1100.
14. Omar S, Morgan GL, Panchal HB, et al. Management of post-myocardial infarction ventricular septal defects: a critical assessment. *J Interv Cardiol.* 2018;31:939-948.
15. Crenshaw BS, Granger CB, Birnbaum Y, et al. Risk factors, angiographic patterns, and outcomes in patients with ventricular septal defect complicating acute myocardial infarction. *Circulation.* 2000;101:27-32.
16. Vargas-Barrón J, Molina-Carrión M, Romero-Cárdenas Á, et al. Risk factors, echocardiographic patterns, and outcomes in patients with acute ventricular septal rupture during myocardial infarction. *Am J Cardiol.* 2005;95:1153-1158.
17. Jones BM, Kapadia SR, Smedira NG, et al. Ventricular septal rupture complicating acute myocardial infarction: a contemporary review. *Eur Heart J.* 2014;35:2060-2068.
18. Faccini A, Butera G. Techniques, timing, and prognosis of transcatheter post myocardial infarction ventricular septal defect repair. *Curr Cardiol Rep.* 2019;21:59.
19. Estévez-Loureiro R, Arzamendi D, Freixa X, et al. Percutaneous mitral valve repair for acute mitral regurgitation after an acute myocardial infarction. *J Am Coll Cardiol.* 2015;66:91-92.
20. Adamo M, Curello S, Chiari E, et al. Percutaneous edge-to-edge mitral valve repair for the treatment of acute mitral regurgitation complicating myocardial infarction: a single centre experience. *Int J Cardiol.* 2017;234:53-57.
21. Kettner J, Sramko M, Holek M, Pirk J, Kautzner J. Utility of intra-aortic balloon pump support for ventricular septal rupture and acute mitral regurgitation complicating acute myocardial infarction. *Am J Cardiol.* 2013;112:1709-1713.
22. McLaughlin A, McGiffin D, Winearls J, et al. Veno-arterial ECMO in the setting of post-infarct ventricular septal defect: a bridge to surgical repair. *Heart Lung Circ.* 2016;25:1063-1066.

23. Mozaffarian D, Benjamin EJ, Go AS, et al. Heart disease and stroke statistics—2015 update: a report from the American Heart Association. *Circulation.* 2015;131:e29-e322.
24. Ba'Albaki HA, Clements SD. Left ventricular aneurysm: a review. *Clin Cardiol.* 1989;12:5-13.
25. Friedman BM, Dunn MI. Postinfarction ventricular aneurysms. *Clin Cardiol.* 1995;18:505-511.
26. Engel J, Brady WJ, Mattu A, Perron AD. Electrocardiographic ST segment elevation: left ventricular aneurysm. *Am J Emerg Med.* 2002;20:238-242.
27. Rosenberg B, Messinger WJ. The electrocardiogram in ventricular aneurysm. *Am Heart J.* 1949;37:267-277.
28. Visser CA, Kan G, Meltzer RS, Koolen JJ, Dunning AJ. Incidence, timing and prognostic value of left ventricular aneurysm formation after myocardial infarction: a prospective, serial echocardiographic study of 158 patients. *Am J Cardiol.* 1986;57:729-732.
29. Frances C, Romero A, Grady D. Left ventricular pseudoaneurysm. *J Am Coll Cardiol.* 1998;32:557-561.
30. Konen E, Merchant N, Gutierrez C, et al. True versus false left ventricular aneurysm: differentiation with MR imaging—initial experience. *Radiology.* 2005;236:65-75.
31. McCarthy CP, Vaduganathan M, McCarthy KJ, Januzzi JL, Bhatt DL, McEvoy JW. Left ventricular thrombus after acute myocardial infarction: screening, prevention, and treatment. *JAMA Cardiol.* 2018;3:642.
32. Ibanez B, James S, Agewall S, et al. 2017 ESC Guidelines for the management of acute myocardial infarction in patients presenting with ST-segment elevation. *Eur Heart J.* 2018;39:119-177.
33. Bahit MC, Kochar A, Granger CB. Post-myocardial infarction heart failure. *JACC: Heart Failure.* 2018;6:179-186.
34. Crimm A, Severance HW, Coffey K, et al. Prognostic significance of isolated sinus tachycardia during first three days of acute myocardial infarction. *Am J Med.* 1984;76:983-988.
35. Berisso MZ, Carratino L, Ferroni A, et al. Frequency, characteristics and significance of supraventricular tachyarrhythmias detected by 24-hour electrocardiographic recording in the late hospital phase of acute myocardial infarction. *Am J Cardiol.* 1990;65:1064-1070.
36. Serrano CV, Antônio J, Ramires F, Mansur AP, Pileggi F. Importance of the time of onset of supraventricular tachyarrhythmias on prognosis of patients with acute myocardial infarction. *Clin Cardiol.* 1995;18:84-90.
37. Schmitt J, Duray G, Gersh BJ, Hohnloser SH. Atrial fibrillation in acute myocardial infarction: a systematic review of the incidence, clinical features and prognostic implications. *Eur Heart J.* 2009;30:1038-1045.
38. Rathore SS, Berger AK, Weinfurt KP, et al. Acute myocardial infarction complicated by atrial fibrillation in the elderly: prevalence and outcomes. *Circulation.* 2000;101:969-974.
39. Jabre P, Roger VL, Murad MH, et al. Mortality associated with atrial fibrillation in patients with myocardial infarction: a systematic review and meta-analysis. *Circulation.* 2011;123:1587-1593.
40. Pedersen O. The occurrence and prognostic significance of atrial fibrillation/-flutter following acute myocardial infarction. *Eur Heart J.* 1999;20:748-754.
41. Kirchhof P, Benussi S, Kotecha D, et al. 2016 ESC guidelines for the management of atrial fibrillation developed in collaboration with EACTS. *Eur Heart J.* 2016;37:2893-2962.
42. Nordrehaug JE, Johannessen KA, von der Lippe G. Serum potassium concentration as a risk factor of ventricular arrhythmias early in acute myocardial infarction. *Circulation.* 1985;71:645-649.
43. Maggioni AP, Zuanetti G, Franzosi MG, et al. Prevalence and prognostic significance of ventricular arrhythmias after acute myocardial infarction in the fibrinolytic era. GISSI-2 results. *Circulation.* 1993;87:312-322.
44. Terkelsen CJ, Sørensen JT, Kaltoft AK, et al. Prevalence and significance of accelerated idioventricular rhythm in patients with ST-elevation myocardial infarction treated with primary percutaneous coronary intervention. *Am J Cardiol.* 2009;104:1641-1646.
45. Gorenek B, Blomström Lundqvist C, Brugada Terradellas J, et al. Cardiac arrhythmias in acute coronary syndromes: position paper from the joint EHRA, ACCA, and EAPCI task force. *EP Europace.* 2014;16:1655-1673.
46. Newby KH, Thompson T, Stebbins A, Topol EJ, Califf RM, Natale A. Sustained ventricular arrhythmias in patients receiving thrombolytic therapy: incidence and outcomes. *Circulation.* 1998;98:2567-2573.
47. Boutitie F, Boissel J-P, Connolly SJ, et al. Amiodarone interaction with β-blockers: analysis of the merged EMIAT (European Myocardial Infarct Amiodarone Trial) and CAMIAT (Canadian Amiodarone Myocardial Infarction Trial) databases. *Circulation.* 1999;99:2268-2275.
48. Bardy GH, Lee KL, Mark DB, et al. Amiodarone or an implantable cardioverter–defibrillator for congestive heart failure. *N Engl J Med.* 2005; 352:225-237.
49. O'Gara PT, Kushner FG, Ascheim DD, et al. 2013 ACCF/AHA guideline for the management of ST-elevation myocardial infarction: a report of the American College of Cardiology Foundation/American Heart Association Task Force on Practice Guidelines. *Circulation.* 2013;127:e362-e425.
50. Meine TJ, Al-Khatib SM, Alexander JH, et al. Incidence, predictors, and outcomes of high-degree atrioventricular block complicating acute myocardial infarction treated with thrombolytic therapy. *Am Heart J.* 2005;149:670-674.
51. Montrief T, Davis WT, Koyfman A, Long B. Mechanical, inflammatory, and embolic complications of myocardial infarction: an emergency medicine review. *Am J Emerg Med.* 2019;37:1175-1183.
52. Imazio M, Hoit BD. Post-cardiac injury syndromes. An emerging cause of pericardial diseases. *Int J Cardiol.* 2013;168:648-652.
53. Mehrzad R, Spodick DH. Pericardial involvement in diseases of the heart and other contiguous structures: part I: pericardial involvement in infarct pericarditis and pericardial involvement following myocardial infarction. *Cardiology.* 2012;121:164-176.
54. Khandaker MH, Espinosa RE, Nishimura RA, et al. Pericardial disease: diagnosis and management. *Mayo Clin Proc.* 2010;85:572-593.
55. The 2015 ESC Guidelines on the diagnosis and management of pericardial diseases. 'Ten Commandments' of 2015 ESC Guidelines for diagnosis and management of pericardial diseases. The Russian National Congress of Cardiology 2015. Germany's largest heart centre. Professor Christoph Bode. Professor Franz-Josef Neumann. The CHA_2DS_2-VASc score for stroke risk stratification in patients with atrial fibrillation: a brief history. CardioPulse Articles. *Eur Heart J.* 2015;36:2873-2885.
56. Imazio M, Spodick DH, Brucato A, Trinchero R, Adler Y. Controversial issues in the management of pericardial diseases. *Circulation.* 2010;121:916-928.
57. Doulaptsis C, Goetschalckx K, Masci PG, Florian A, Janssens S, Bogaert J. Assessment of early post-infarction pericardial injury by CMR. *JACC: Cardiovasc Imaging.* 2013;6:411-413.
58. Figueras J, Barrabés JA, Serra V, et al. Hospital outcome of moderate to severe pericardial effusion complicating ST-elevation acute myocardial infarction. *Circulation.* 2010;122:1902-1909.
59. Patel MR, Meine TJ, Lindblad L, et al. Cardiac tamponade in the fibrinolytic era: analysis of >100000 patients with ST-segment elevation myocardial infarction. *Am Heart J.* 2006;151:316-322.
60. Bière L, Mateus V, Clerfond G, et al. Predictive factors of pericardial effusion after a first acute myocardial infarction and successful reperfusion. *Am J Cardiol.* 2015;116:497-503.
61. Figueras J, Barrabés JA, Lidón R-M, et al. Predictors of moderate-to-severe pericardial effusion, cardiac tamponade, and electromechanical dissociation in patients with ST-elevation myocardial infarction. *Am J Cardiol.* 2014;113:1291-1296.
62. Imazio M, Adler Y. Management of pericardial effusion. *Eur Heart J.* 2013;34:1186-1197.
63. Neumann F-J, Sousa-Uva M, Ahlsson A, et al. 2018 ESC/EACTS guidelines on myocardial revascularization. *Eur Heart J.* 2019;40:87-165.
64. Risti AD, Imazio M, Adler Y, et al. Triage strategy for urgent management of cardiac tamponade: a position statement of the European Society of Cardiology Working Group on Myocardial and Pericardial Diseases. *Eur Heart J.* 2014;35:2279-2284.

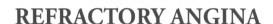

CHAPTER 8

REFRACTORY ANGINA

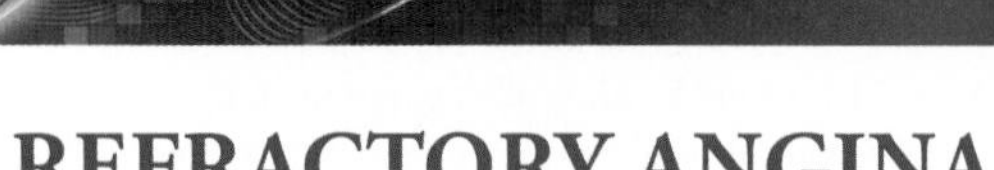

Anbukarasi Maran, Katrina A. E. L. Bidwell, and Valerian Fernandes

INTRODUCTION

Angina pectoris is the symptom complex resulting from mismatch in myocardial oxygen supply and demand. Most commonly, this imbalance occurs in the setting of compromised blood flow to the myocardium as a result of progressive atherosclerotic disease of the coronary arteries. There are several definitions for refractory angina (RA); generally, criteria that must be met include the following:

- Objective evidence of ischemia demonstrated by exercise treadmill testing, stress imaging, or invasive coronary testing such as fractional flow reserve measurement
- Persistent angina despite conventional medical therapy[1]

The European Society of Cardiology (ESC) Joint Study Group further stipulates that RA is a chronic (>3 months), persistent, painful condition characterized by the presence of angina caused by coronary insufficiency in the presence of coronary artery disease (CAD) that cannot be controlled by a combination of medical therapy, angioplasty/percutaneous interventions, and coronary bypass surgery. Although the presence of reversible myocardial ischemia must be clinically established to be the root cause, the pain experienced may arise or persist with or without this ischemia.[2]

Prevalence

The subset of patients with advanced CAD who develop RA represent a substantive and growing population. The exact prevalence and incidence of RA are unknown because of the heterogeneity of patients labeled with a diagnosis of RA. It is estimated that there are 600,000 to 1.8 million patients with RA in the United States, with 50,000 to 100,000 new cases diagnosed per year.[3,4] The Canadian Community Health Survey suggests that approximately 500,000 Canadians are living with RA and 30,000 to 50,000 new cases are diagnosed in Europe annually.[2,5] Many case series did not include patients with nonobstructive CAD or possible microvascular angina.[6,7]

The patient population with RA experiences an impaired quality of life with high utilization of health care resources in the form of recurrent emergency room visits, hospitalizations, repeated stress tests, and, frequently, repeated invasive procedures such as cardiac catheterization. The Joint Study Group estimates that the incidence of RA is from 5% to 10% of patients undergoing cardiac catheterization.[2] In the United Kingdom, evaluation and management of RA accounts for 1.3% of the total National Health Service expenditure, which is around £669,000,000 annually ($865,241,115 in US dollars). In 2008, an Ontario-based study quoted an annualized cost of Canadian dollars of $19,209 per patient.[5] Not uncommonly, these patients also leave the work force secondary to their poor quality of life and limited functional status and subsequently go on disability. Subsequently there is also increased psychological stress and increased levels of depression in this population. Patients are not infrequently labeled being "palliative," "end-stage," having no options or are overlooked by their health care providers, adding yet another layer of stress. One of the most robust prospective studies on RA described a mortality rate of 3.9% at 1 year and 28.4% at 9 years, which is comparable to survival seen in chronic stable CAD.[8] Thus, patients with RA have a long life expectancy coupled with a poor quality of life. The incidence and prevalence of RA will continue to rise as the general population continues to age and the condition is increasingly recognized in clinical practice.

PATHOGENESIS

Deficient myocardial blood flow can occur in the presence of flow-limiting atherosclerotic CAD; however, processes that affect the microvasculature can also be responsible, as can spontaneous coronary artery dissection, infection, vasculitis, and metabolic and genetic diseases. Owing to the infrequency with which some of these are seen, they pose a challenge both from a diagnostic and management standpoint. Delay in diagnosis, possible lack of treatment options for the inciting disease, and absence of targets for revascularization can result in what is ultimately labeled as RA.

The role of coronary microcirculation in the development of anginal symptoms is increasingly recognized. In contrast to the epicardial vessels in which flow is limited by stenosis from obstruction, microvascular impairment stems from abnormal function or remodeling. Abnormal remodeling can occur because of the following[6,9]:

- Medial hypertrophy or intimal proliferation of small arterioles
- Small vessel compression
- Obstruction in the setting of hypertrophic cardiomyopathy
- Microvasculopathy
- Microemboli
- Inflammatory disease
- Idiopathic disease

Pathophysiologic mechanisms of microvascular dysfunction include endothelial dysfunction, decreased coronary perfusion pressure across a stenosis or diffuse epicardial narrowing, increased intercapillary oxygen perfusion distances as a result of hypertrophy, microvasculopathy or microemboli, and differential hyperemic responses of subendocardium versus subepicardium.[6] Microvascular dysfunction can occur both with and without CAD and in the presence or absence of traditional risk factors for CAD.[10]

In patients with CAD, microvascular dysfunction is highly prevalent, being found in anywhere from 39% to 60% of patients with both obstructive and nonobstructive disease; and in 20% or more of patients with CAD, microvascular dysfunction can cause anginal symptoms and occasionally ischemic changes on electrocardiogram. The pain episodes are not rapidly relieved after cessation of activity or sublingual nitroglycerine. Focal, scattered ischemia throughout the myocardium is felt to be caused by prearteriolar dysfunction, and the presence of such defects might explain the paradox of angina and ST-segment depression or elevation in the absence of wall-motion changes.

Increased myocardial oxygen demand can be triggered by increase in physical, emotional, or metabolic activities; the mechanisms that lead to myocardial supply/demand mismatch and the pathways that link the myocardial and neural axes to result in the subjective experience of angina are complex. The relationship between angina and inadequate myocardial oxygen supply encompasses the spectrum of (1) classic angina in the presence of ischemia; (2) lack of symptoms in the setting of myocardial ischemia/infarction or "silent" ischemia; and (3) anginal symptoms in the absence of objective findings of ischemia, mediated in some cases by unobserved subendocardial ischemia and in other cases by aberrant pain mechanisms. The spectrum of presentations illustrates the intricate interplay of coronary circulation on the micro- and macro-level myocyte metabolism, and nociception. The subjectivity of the experience of angina is also reflected in the variety of manifestations from patients and the significant symptomatic improvement observed when RA is treated with placebo.[11]

The patient with RA experiences a cyclic relationship between myocardial hypoxia and the neuropathophysiology of persistent pain.[12] In the presence of noxious stimuli (such as ischemia), bradykinin, adenosine, lactate, and potassium are released into the coronary sinus.[13,14] These substances stimulate the polymodal afferent cardiac sensory neurons. Calcitonin gene–related peptide and substance P are also synthesized and augment adenosine-provoked pain. These noxious inputs enter the upper thoracic spinal cord and synapse with the second-order sensory neurons in the dorsal horn. This information is amplified and ascends via multiple pathways including Lissauer tract, the spinothalamic tract, and spinoamygdaloid and spinohypothalamic pathways to cortical and subcortical areas of the brain with somatic receptive fields in the chest and arm. The parietal cortex and anterior cingulate cortex cognitively apprise these stimuli as threatening, in turn causing activation of the bilateral prefrontal cortex and limbic system and producing an impending sense of doom, anxiety, and further pain[15-18] (**Algorithm 8.1**). Modulation of the neural pathways by which the subjective experience of pain is elaborated and amplified has provided an additional therapeutic target in the treatment of patients with RA.

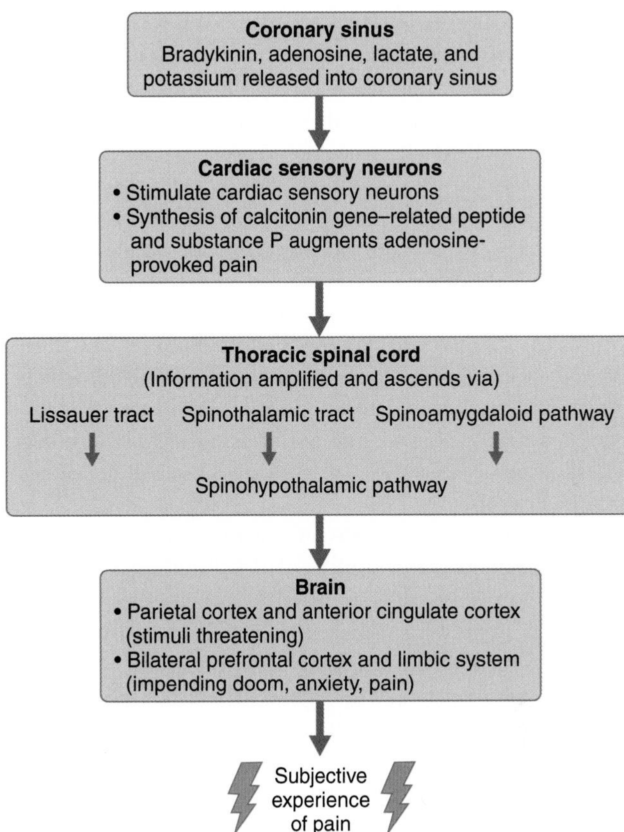

ALGORITHM 8.1 Neuropathophysiology of persistent pain.

MANAGEMENT OF THE PATIENT WITH REFRACTORY ANGINA

Medical Approach

The approach to patients begins with the assumption that optimization of traditional risk factors for CAD and other significant comorbidities have been performed. If not, the patient does not meet criteria for RA; furthermore, addressing poorly controlled comorbidities such as uncontrolled hypertension, severe anemia, or heart failure generally produces the symptomatic relief sought by the patient.[19] Ideally, other lifestyle interventions such as initiation of an exercise program and tobacco cessation will already have been made, and, if not, provide another opportunity for improvement. When seeing a patient in consultation for RA, a detailed history should be obtained, with attention to what symptoms the patient experiences, in what settings, how those symptoms have changed over time, what limitations they experience because of their symptoms, and the effect on their quality of life. A detailed family history for relevant inherited disorders (such as hypertrophic cardiomyopathy and Fabry disease) and less obvious entities that can rarely present initially with angina (such as sickle cell disease) should be obtained. A careful physical examination can suggest suboptimally controlled comorbid conditions that the patient may not identify. Routine laboratory assessment includes complete metabolic panel (including liver function testing), complete blood count, lipid panel, and glycosylated hemoglobin to rule out or assess any comorbid or contributing diseases as well as evaluate the suitability of certain medications.

Gastrointestinal disease is a frequent comorbid condition in the evaluation and treatment of RA. Entities such as gastroesophageal reflux disease, hiatal hernia, presbyesophagus, esophageal dysmotility and spasm, gallbladder disease, and biliary dysfunction are frequently convincing mimics of angina, and are seen frequently in the patient population with known coronary disease or risk factors. Further confounding the clinical picture is the fact that many of these smooth muscle pains may be relieved by nitroglycerine. A careful clinical history may help differentiate these symptoms from angina, particularly in patients who have continued symptoms despite complete revascularization.

Conventional therapy for chronic stable angina due to CAD includes aspirin, statin, beta-blockers, calcium channel blockers, and angiotensin-converting enzyme (ACE) inhibitors or aldosterone receptor blockers (ARBs). Calcium channel blockers and nitrates are mainstays for coronary vasospasm. In the setting of microvascular dysfunction, the data is less robust concerning appropriate therapy. Moderate-quality evidence suggests that ACE inhibitors and ranolazine may improve quality of life. Beta-blockers, calcium channel blockers, and statins each have been shown to produce significant improvements in anginal frequency and ischemia based on lower quality evidence.[20]

When patients are on maximum dose or maximally tolerated conventional therapy and still symptomatic, second-line therapies can be considered. Ivabradine, nicorandil, trimetazidine, long-acting nitrates, and ranolazine are considered second-line therapies in the treatment of RA in the ESC guidelines. Nicorandil and trimetazidine are not yet available in the United States.[21] In the context of microvascular disease, ivabradine and trimetazidine each failed to improve symptoms or objective measures of ischemia.[20] Narcotic analgesics can be considered in a very select group of patients; however, they should be used rarely. See **Table 8.1** for a summary of first- and second-line antianginal medications.

Patients who have continued symptoms on second-line therapies for RA should be considered for repeat angiography. Where available, cardiac magnetic resonance imaging (MRI) and positron emission tomography (PET) can be

TABLE 8.1 First- and Second-line Pharmacotherapy for Angina Pectoris

Medication	Action	Side Effects
Ivabradine	Negative inotropy	Bradycardia, hypertension
Nicorandil	K^+ ATP channel opener, vasodilator, decreases preload and afterload	No tolerance issues Note: not available in the United States
Ranolazine	Partial fatty acid oxidation inhibitor	Acute renal failure in underlying chronic kidney disease, cannot be used in hepatic impairment
Trimetazidine	Reversible 3-ketoacyl-thiolase inhibition, reduced mitochondrial fatty acid oxidation	Gastrointestinal disturbances, vomiting, nausea Note: not available in the United States
Beta-blockers	Decrease heart rate and contractility	Bradycardia
Calcium channel blockers	Decrease heart rate and contractility, arterial vasodilation	Hypotension
Nitrates	Venous and arterial vasodilator	Hypotension
ACE-I, ARB	Improved endothelial function, anti-inflammatory activity	Hypotension
Statins	Improved endothelial function, anti-inflammatory activity	Myopathy
Antiplatelet agents	Anti-inflammatory activity, platelet inhibition	Increased bleeding

ACE-I, angiotensin-converting enzyme 1; ARB, aldosterone receptor blocker; ATP, adenosine triphosphate.

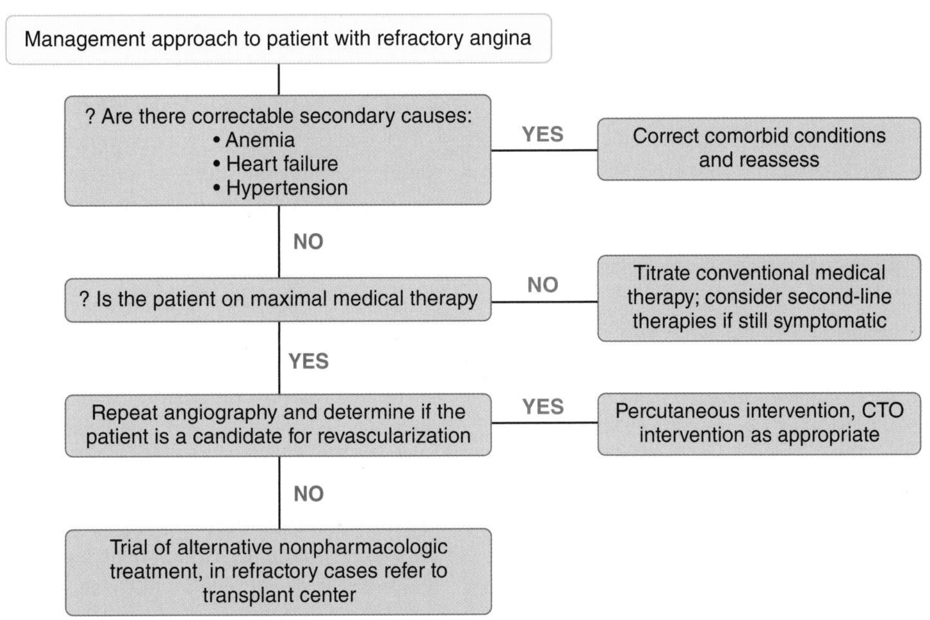

ALGORITHM 8.2 Approach to the patient with refractory angina. CTO, chronic total occlusion.

used in the evaluation of coronary flow reserve and myocardial viability. Other invasive studies for angiographically normal coronaries are discussed later. Most of the time, patients are not candidates for revascularization for multiple reasons[2]:

- Unsuitable coronary anatomy, such as diffuse CAD or severe distal vessel disease that are not amenable to percutaneous coronary intervention (PCI) or coronary artery bypass surgery (CABG)
- Prior history of CABG that precludes further surgical intervention (redo-CABG, unavailable conduits for bypass grafting)
- Severely depressed left ventricular systolic function (especially presence of left ventricular thrombus)
- Severe concurrent comorbid conditions that increase periprocedure mortality and morbidity (chronic kidney disease, severe cerebrovascular disease, severe peripheral arterial disease)
- Advanced age

In such patients, we would consider alternative nonpharmacologic treatments that are discussed in the remaining sections of the chapter or intervention on vessels with chronic total occlusion (CTO), if present (**Algorithm 8.2**)

Percutaneous Coronary Interventions

In patients who have symptoms that are out of proportion to known CAD or are known to have nonobstructive disease, it is reasonable to consider repeat angiography with assessment of coronary flow reserve to evaluate for microvascular disease and/or provocative testing to evaluate for coronary spasm. In the presence of risk factors but no angiographic evidence of CAD, intravascular ultrasound may demonstrate diffuse atherosclerotic disease.[22] Patients with known CTO lesions with persistent symptoms despite maximal guideline-directed medical therapy and no acute coronary lesions can be considered for PCI. With the advent of increasingly complex coronary interventions and many centers performing CTO PCI, a consensus regarding the inappropriateness of revascularization for an individual patient should be established by second or third opinions, because the most common cause of RA in the patient with CAD is incomplete revascularization.[1] This is best achieved with a multidisciplinary team that includes both interventional cardiologists and cardiothoracic surgeons. It is advisable to evaluate myocardial viability when planning CTO interventions. In our practice, we frequently utilize MRI; however, echocardiography, nuclear imaging with single-photon emission tomography and PET imaging and computed tomography are all validated modalities used to assess viability. When discussing the intervention with the patient, particularly if complex or multiple lesions are present, the expectation should be set that they may require more than one procedure to achieve the desired effect.

The following is a case study illustrating appropriate selection and utilization of CTO intervention in a patient with RA:

The patient is a 75-year-old male with a history of CAD status post prior CABG and multiple prior stents and early Parkinson disease with orthostatic hypotension who had repeated hospitalizations for anginal symptoms and progressive functional decline. Previously, he enjoyed a good functional status and was able to complete his activities of daily living in addition to being employed outside of his home. He was also found to be in atrial fibrillation, which was a new diagnosis. He was transferred from an outside hospital to our tertiary referral center for evaluation. He was taken for cardiac catheterization, which demonstrated unchanged anatomy from his last catheterization approximately 18 years prior: CTO of his mid left anterior descending (LAD) artery, CTO of an obtuse marginal branch, a small right coronary artery (RCA) with severe diffuse disease not amenable to stenting and occluded vein grafts to the LAD and diagonal. **Figure 8.1** demonstrates a dual angiogram with CTO segment of the LAD and diffusely diseased RCA giving collaterals to the LAD; **Figure 8.2** is a selective angiogram of the RCA and collaterals to the LAD. He was evaluated by cardiothoracic surgery for redo-CABG and deemed not a candidate because of multiple CTOs and diffuse CAD with poor targets. His baseline hypotension precluded addition of long-acting nitrates for anginal control, and he continued to have symptoms on maximum dose ranolazine. He underwent electrical cardioversion of his atrial fibrillation after appropriate anticoagulation to rule out arrhythmia as the cause of his symptoms, which persisted after restoration of sinus rhythm, and he had several visits to the emergency department for chest pain over this time. Given the refractoriness of his symptoms, he was felt to be appropriate for CTO PCI. The LAD CTO was crossed with antegrade wire escalation technique. Intravascular ultrasound-guided PCI was done in the standard manner with excellent results; **Figure 8.3** demonstrates the final angiogram of the LAD. At subsequent follow-up, the patient reported resolution of his symptoms, and was able to return to work.

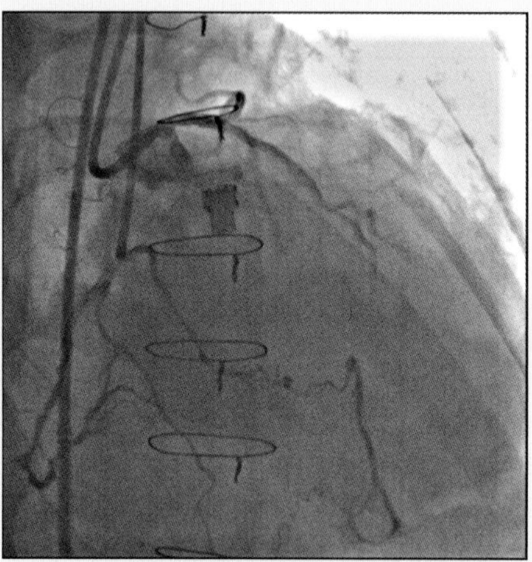

FIGURE 8.1 Dual angiogram with chronic total occlusion (CTO) segment of the left descending artery (LAD) and diffusely diseased right coronary artery (RCA) giving collaterals to the LAD.

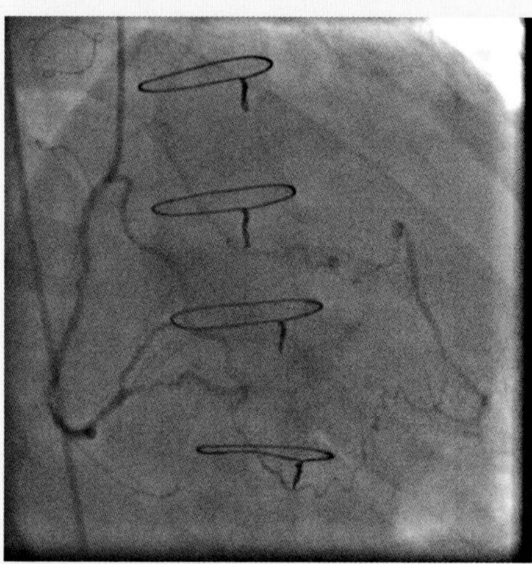

FIGURE 8.2 Selective angiogram of the RCA demonstrating collaterals to the LAD.

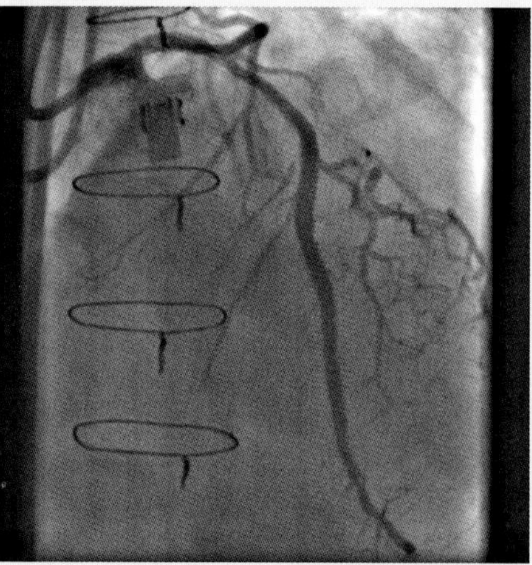

FIGURE 8.3 Final angiogram of the LAD.

Surgical Approach

Transmyocardial laser revascularization (TMLR) involves either surgical or percutaneous application of laser to ablate channels in the ischemic myocardium to improve perfusion. It was initially thought that this procedure's efficacy derived from the creation of tiny conduits for blood; however, these small channels ultimately occlude in the weeks following surgery. Other potential therapeutic mechanisms are promotion of angiogenesis, denervation of the myocardium, and the placebo effect.[23] To date, percutaneous TMLR that has been evaluated in a double-blinded trial showed no benefit over the sham procedure. Similar findings were demonstrated in a meta-analysis of five other trials, with no benefit for subjective (such as angina scoring) or objective (such as left ventricular ejection fraction) findings over time.[23,24] In contrast with surgical TMLR, mortality was not increased.

Trials with surgical TMLR have demonstrated mixed results, with a general improvement in subjective measures such as exercise tolerance testing, angina score, and quality of life but with significant increases in postoperative morbidity and mortality.[23] Perioperative morbidity and mortality have improved with a shift away from open thoracotomy to a thoracoscopic approach for the procedure. However, the lack of control groups in the majority of studies and limited long-term data on morbidity and mortality make the benefit of the procedure on clinical outcomes unclear. The most recent ESC guidelines (2019) advise against use of both forms of TMLR, whereas in the most recent American Heart Association/American College of Cardiology (AHA/ACC) guidelines (2012), TMLR is still considered class IIb/level recommendation of evidence B.[21,25]

Sympathetic blockade has been used in the treatment of RA. Beyond the pain-modulating effect of sympathectomy, the removal of sympathetic input on atrial and ventricular myocardium and vasculature also has an anti-ischemic effect.[26] Left stellate ganglion blockade can be performed with injection of local anesthetic near the C6 vertebra; this usually offers temporary relief of angina. Left stellate ganglion blockade has been tested in a single double-blind, placebo-controlled trial that failed to show a difference in patients treated with bupivacaine or saline injections,[27] showing favorable outcomes in RA due to vasospasm and advanced CAD.[28,29]

When patients continue to have disabling symptoms despite attempts at aggressive conventional, alternative medical therapies and invasive percutaneous therapy (when indicated), orthotopic heart transplant should be considered. The most recent data from the International Society for Heart and Lung Transplantation reports 1-year survival post heart transplant at 83.6% and the median survival post heart transplant at 11.5 years; this stands in contrast with what is likely the most reliable prospective data on RA in which 1-year survival is 96.1% with 10-year survival at 71.6%.[8,30] Because the majority of patients with RA would have a longer life expectancy with their current symptoms than post-transplant, the patient's quality of life should be truly unacceptable, and an extensive risk-benefit discussion should be had, ideally with an advanced heart failure specialist at a center that specializes in transplant.

SPECIAL CONSIDERATIONS AND EMERGING THERAPIES

Coronary sinus augmentation has been utilized in practice since the 1950s, when it was accomplished via surgical approach.[31] Mechanistically, alteration of the coronary sinus is performed to reduce venous outflow, thus increasing backward pressure and redistributing blood flow to the ischemic myocardium and thereby improve global perfusion. Devices that can be implanted percutaneously have since been developed. The supporting body of evidence is limited to one randomized controlled trial and several observational studies; at present, the longest published follow-up period is 2 years.[32-34] Currently, coronary reduction devices are a class IIb/level of evidence B recommendation in the most recent ESC guidelines from 2019.[21] In the United States, coronary sinus reduction is not discussed in the most current AHA/ACC guidelines, and the devices are not commercially available.

Chelation therapy has been proposed as an adjunct therapy for RA. Treatment consists of intravenous infusions of disodium ethylene diamine tetraacetic acid (EDTA) in combination with other substances that combine with polyvalent cations, such as calcium, to form soluble complexes that can be excreted. It is performed under the assumption that this process can result in both regression of atherosclerotic plaques and relief of angina, and that EDTA reduces oxidative stress in the vascular wall.[35] Although conceptually promising, this modality has yet to be shown to have clear benefit in reducing cardiovascular events in this patient population; in the most recent AHA/ACC guidelines, chelation therapy was updated from class III (no benefit) to IIb.[36] Tenuous data in combination with the potential risks associated with disodium EDTA, including hypocalcemia, renal failure, and death have resulted in this modality being used largely only as part of experimental protocols.[37,38] It is not currently approved for use in the treatment or prevention of cardiovascular disease by the U.S. Food and Drug Administration (FDA).

Enhanced external counterpulsation (EECP) is a noninvasive technique that uses inflatable cuffs wrapped around the lower extremities to increase venous return and augment diastolic blood pressure. The cuffs are inflated sequentially from the calves to the thigh muscles during diastole up to 300 mm Hg and are deflated instantaneously during systole. The resultant diastolic augmentation increases coronary perfusion pressure, and the systolic cuff depression decreases peripheral resistance, increasing cardiac output and potentially adding a peripheral training effect.[39] Treatment is associated with improved left ventricular diastolic filling, peripheral flow-mediated vasodilation, and endothelial function. Additional mechanisms of improvement in symptoms include collateral recruitment, attenuation of oxidative stress and proinflammatory cytokines, and the promotion of angiogenesis and vasculogenesis.[40-42] The majority of the data surrounding EECP comes from two relatively small randomized controlled trials and several unrandomized trials, and suggests that this can be a useful therapy for patients with RA. It is a class IIb recommendation in current

AHA/ACC guidelines.[36,42-44] A typical treatment course requires both availability of the modality and a significant time commitment from the patient, generally 35 sessions of 1-hour duration done 5 days per week for 7 weeks, which are the major limitations to its use. EECP is generally well tolerated; however, as many as 55% of patients in the clinical trials experienced side effects including bruising, pain, abrasions, or paresthesia.[44]

Several therapies that act on interruption or modification of afferent neurologic pathways through which the sensation of pain is elaborated are available. Transcutaneous electrical nerve stimulation (TENS), subcutaneous electrical nerve stimulation (SENS), and spinal cord stimulation (SCS) utilize electrical stimuli at varying points along the neural pathway to disrupt the pain signal. TENS units involve external electrodes placed on the chest to apply low-intensity electrical currents to large afferent fibers. TENS is rarely definitive therapy, but can be used to assess response before committing a patient to the more invasive SENS or SCS. The SCS device consists of a subcutaneously placed pulse generator connected to electrode leads that are placed, under local anesthesia, in the epidural space where the afferent myocardial sympathetic fibers synapse with second-order sensory neurons in the area that produces maximal paresthesia where the patient experiences anginal pain. SENS involves the placement of subcutaneous electrodes in the parasternal space where the patient experiences angina and is connected to a pulse generator. Of these, SCS has the most compelling evidence for efficacy in terms of exercise duration, anginal frequency, and nitrate consumption; it may also have positive effects on myocardial perfusion by inhibiting abnormal sympathetic activation.[11,45,46] SENS units have only recently begun to be applied in cardiac pain and have limited clinical data, but they have the advantage of ease of placement over SCS.[47] The effectiveness of neuromodulation is uncertain, given the small body of data supporting its use and the difficulty in effective blinding when they are studied. With all of these therapies, a strong placebo effect may be present.

RESEARCH AND FUTURE DIRECTIONS

Improving myocardial perfusion through the promotion of angiogenesis has been identified as a novel target for the treatment of RA. Therapeutic angiogenesis has most promisingly been investigated in the form of intracoronary or intramyocardial administration of bone marrow–derived CD34$^+$ or CD133$^+$ cells or viral transfer–based vectors encoding DNA for vascular endothelial growth factor (VEGF) and fibroblast growth factor. At present, the availability of both cell-based and viral transfer–based modalities is limited to research trials.

KEY POINTS

- ✔ RA is the presence of chronic (>3 months' duration), persistent anginal symptoms in the setting of demonstrated ischemia despite maximal conventional medical therapy. Although most commonly associated with traditional atherosclerotic CAD, it can occur in the setting of other disease states.
- ✔ Initial evaluation of patients referred for management of RA should include assessment for comorbid conditions that can confound symptoms and confirmation that they have been optimally treated and that conventional pharmacologic therapies have been titrated to maximally tolerated dosages.
- ✔ Consider obtaining a second or third opinion if a patient with CAD is initially deemed inappropriate for revascularization (CABG or CTO PCI) because the most common cause of RA is incomplete revascularization.
- ✔ Consider referral to a center experienced in complex/high-risk percutaneous and surgical interventions and/or which has availability of alternative treatments (such as EECP) or clinical trials. If all other therapies fail, referral to a transplant center is reasonable.

REFERENCES

1. Kim MC, Kini A, Sharma SK. Refractory angina pectoris: mechanism and therapeutic options. *J Am Coll Cardiol.* 2002;39(6):923-934. doi:10.1016/S0735-1097(02)01716-3
2. Mannheimer C, Camici P, Chester MR, et al. The problem of chronic refractory angina: report from the ESC Joint Study Group on the Treatment of Refractory Angina. *Eur Heart J.* 2002;23(5):355-370. doi:10.1053/euhj.2001.2706
3. Sainsbury PA, Fisher M, De Silva R. Alternative interventions for refractory angina. *Heart.* 2017;103(23):1911-1922. doi:10.1136/heartjnl-2015-308564
4. Povsic TJ, Broderick S, Anstrom KJ, et al. Predictors of long-term clinical endpoints in patients with refractory angina. *J Am Heart Assoc.* 2015;4(2):e001287. doi:10.1161/JAHA.114.001287
5. Béland Y. Canadian community health survey—methodological overview. *Health Rep.* 2002;13(3):9-14.
6. Gould KL, Johnson NP. Coronary physiology beyond coronary flow reserve in microvascular angina: JACC state-of-the-art review. *J Am Coll Cardiol.* 2018;72(21):2642-2662. doi:10.1016/j.jacc.2018.07.106
7. Sara JD, Widmer RJ, Matsuzawa Y, Lennon RJ, Lerman LO, Lerman A. Prevalence of coronary microvascular dysfunction among patients with chest pain and nonobstructive coronary artery disease. *JACC Cardiovasc Interv.* 2015;8(11):1445-1453. doi:10.1016/j.jcin.2015.06.017
8. Henry TD, Satran D, Hodges JS, et al. Long-term survival in patients with refractory angina. *Eur Heart J.* 2013;34(34):2683-2688. doi:10.1093/eurheartj/eht165
9. Willis M, Homeister J, Stone J. *Cellular and Molecular Pathobiology of Cardiovascular Disease.* Academic Press; 2014. doi:10.1016/C2012-0-02409-X
10. Camici PG, Crea F. Coronary microvascular dysfunction. *N Engl J Med.* 2007;356:830-840. doi:10.1056/NEJMra061889
11. Gallone G, Baldetti L, Tzanis G, et al. Refractory angina: from pathophysiology to new therapeutic nonpharmacologic technologies. *JACC Cardiovasc Interv.* 2020;13(1):1-32.
12. McGillion M, Arthur HM, Cook A, et al. Management of patients with refractory angina: Canadian Cardiovascular Society/Canadian Pain Society Joint Guidelines. *Can J Cardiol.* 2012;28(suppl 2):S20-S41. doi:10.1016/j.cjca.2011.07.007
13. Meller ST, Gebhart GF. A critical review of the afferent pathways and the potential chemical mediators involved in cardiac pain. *Neuroscience.* 1992;48(3):501-524. doi:10.1016/0306-4522(92)90398-L

14. Wang Y, Zeng X-L, Gao R-R, Wang X-I, Wang XT, Zheng G-Q. Neurogenic hypothesis of cardiac ischemic pain. *Med Hypotheses.* 2009;72(4):402-404. doi:10.1016/j.mehy.2008.12.001
15. Foreman RD, Garrett KM, Blair RW. Mechanisms of cardiac pain. *Compr Physiol.* 2015;5(2):929-960. doi:10.1002/cphy.c140032
16. Foreman RD. Mechanisms of cardiac pain. *Annu Rev Physiol.* 1999;61:143-167. doi:10.1146/annurev.physiol.61.1.143
17. Foreman RD. Neurological mechanisms of chest pain and cardiac disease. *Cleve Clin J Med.* 2007;74(suppl 1):S30-S33. doi:10.3949/ccjm.74.Suppl_1.S30
18. Maran A, Wiggins B. Role of ranolazine in the management of refractory angina. *J Pharmacol Res.* 2018;2(1):1-4.
19. Mukherjee D. Management of refractory angina in the contemporary era. *Eur Heart J.* 2013;34(34):2655-2657. doi:10.1093/eurheartj/eht190
20. Turgeon RD, Pearson GJ, Graham MM. Pharmacologic treatment of patients with myocardial ischemia with no obstructive coronary artery disease. *Am J Cardiol.* 2018;121(7):888-895. doi:10.1016/j.amjcard.2017.12.025
21. Knuuti J, Wijns W, Saraste A, et al. 2019 ESC guidelines for the diagnosis and management of chronic coronary syndromes. *Eur Heart J.* 2020;41(3):407-477. doi:10.1093/eurheartj/ehz425
22. Lee BK, Lim HS, Fearon WF, et al. Invasive evaluation of patients with angina in the absence of obstructive coronary artery disease. *Circulation.* 2015;131(12):1054-1060. doi:10.1161/CIRCULATIONAHA.114.012636
23. Schofield PM, McNab D. NICE evaluation of transmyocardial laser revascularisation and percutaneous laser revascularisation for refractory angina. *Heart.* 2010;96(4):312-313. doi:10.1136/hrt.2009.185769
24. Leon MB, Kornowski R, Downey WE, et al. A blinded, randomized, placebo-controlled trial of percutaneous laser myocardial revascularization to improve angina symptoms in patients with severe coronary disease. *J Am Coll Cardiol.* 2005;46(10):1812-1819. doi:10.1016/j.jacc.2005.06.079
25. Fihn SD, Gardin JM, Abrams J, et al. 2012 ACCF/AHA/ACP/AATS/PCNA/SCAI/STS guideline for the diagnosis and management of patients with stable ischemic heart disease. *J Am Coll Cardiol.* 2012. doi:10.1016/j.jacc.2012.07.013
26. Coveliers HME, Hoexum F, Nederhoed JH, Wisselink W, Rauwerda JA. Thoracic sympathectomy for digital ischemia: a summary of evidence. *J Vasc Surg.* 2011;54(1):273-277. doi:10.1016/j.jvs.2011.01.069
27. Denby C, Groves DG, Eleuteri A, et al. Temporary sympathectomy in chronic refractory angina: a randomised, double-blind, placebo-controlled trial. *Br J Pain.* 2015;9(3):142-148. doi:10.1177/2049463714549775
28. Sharma R, Sharma S, Fuster V. Coronary vasospastic angina: a rare case of ergonovine positivity and curative bilateral cardiac sympathectomy. *EuroIntervention.* 2018;14(12):e1332-e1333. doi:10.4244/EIJ-D-18-00144
29. Stritesky M. Endoscopic thoracic sympathectomy—its effect in the treatment of refractory angina pectoris. *Interact Cardiovasc Thorac Surg.* 2006;5(4):464-468 doi:10.1510/icvts.2005.118976
30. International Thoracic Organ Transplant (TTX) Registry Data. *J Heart Lung Transplant.* 2019;30(10):1015-1066.
31. Beck CS, Leighninger DS. Scientific basis for the surgical treatment of coronary artery disease. *J Am Med Assoc.* 1955;159(13):1264-1271. doi:10.1001/jama.1955.02960300008003
32. Ponticelli F, Tzanis G, Gallone G, et al. Safety and efficacy of Coronary Sinus Reducer implantation at 2-year follow-up. *Int J Cardiol.* 2019;292:87-90. doi:10.1016/j.ijcard.2019.05.026
33. Abawi M, Nijhoff F, Doevendans PA, Agostoni P, Stella PR. Clinical efficacy of the coronary sinus reducer for refractory angina: a single-centre "real-world" experience. *EuroIntervention.* 2015.
34. Giannini F, Baldetti L, Ponticelli F, et al. Coronary sinus reducer implantation for the treatment of chronic refractory angina: a single-center experience. *JACC Cardiovasc Interv.* 2018;11(8):784-792. doi:10.1016/j.jcin.2018.01.251
35. Lamas GA, Goertz C, Boineau R, et al. Effect of disodium EDTA chelation regimen on cardiovascular events in patients with previous myocardial infarction: the TACT randomized trial. *JAMA.* 2013;309(12):1241-1250. doi:10.1001/jama.2013.2107
36. Fihn SD, Blankenship JC, Alexander KP, et al. 2014 ACC/AHA/AATS/PCNA/SCAI/STS focused update of the guideline for the diagnosis and management of patients with stable ischemic heart disease. *Circulation.* 2014;130(19):1749-1767. doi:10.1161/cir.0000000000000095
37. Brown MJ, Willis T, Omalu B, Leiker R. Deaths resulting from hypocalcemia after administration of edetate disodium: 2003-2005. *Pediatrics.* 2006;118(2):e534-e536. doi:10.1542/peds.2006-0858
38. Chyka PA. Book Review: *Goldfrank's Toxicologic Emergencies, 8th edition.* Ann Pharmacother. 2007;41(3):532-532. doi:10.1345/aph.1H26
39. Ahlbom M, Hagerman I, Ståhlberg M, et al. Increases in cardiac output and oxygen consumption during enhanced external counterpulsation. *Heart Lung Circ.* 2016;25(11):1133-1136. doi:10.1016/j.hlc.2016.04.013
40. Akhtar M, Wu GF, Du ZM, Zheng ZS, Michaels AD. Effect of external counterpulsation on plasma nitric oxide and endothelin-1 levels. *Am J Cardiol.* 2006;98(1):28-30. doi:10.1016/j.amjcard.2006.01.053
41. Shechter M, Matetzky S, Feinberg MS, Chouraqui P, Rotstein Z, Hod H. External counterpulsation therapy improves endothelial function in patients with refractory angina pectoris. *J Am Coll Cardiol.* 2003;42(12):2090-2095. doi:10.1016/j.jacc.2003.05.013
42. Shah SA, Shapiro RJ, Mehta R, Snyder JA. Impact of enhanced external counterpulsation on Canadian Cardiovascular Society angina class in patients with chronic stable angina: a meta-analysis. *Pharmacotherapy.* 2010;30(7):639-645. doi:10.1592/phco.30.7.639
43. Braith RW, Conti CR, Nichols WW, et al. Enhanced external counterpulsation improves peripheral artery flow-mediated dilation in patients with chronic angina: a randomized sham-controlled study. *Circulation.* 2010;122(16):1612-1620. doi:10.1161/CIRCULATIONAHA.109.923482
44. Arora RR, Chou TM, Jain D, et al. The multicenter study of enhanced external counterpulsation (MUST-EECP): effect of EECP on exercise-induced myocardial ischemia and anginal episodes. *J Am Coll Cardiol.* 1999;33(7):1833-1840. doi:10.1016/S0735-1097(99)00140-0
45. Eddicks S, Maier-Hauff K, Schenk M, Müller A, Baumann G, Theres H. Thoracic spinal cord stimulation improves functional status and relieves symptoms in patients with refractory angina pectoris: the first placebo-controlled randomised study. *Heart.* 2007;93(5):585-590. doi:10.1136/hrt.2006.100784
46. Southerland EM, Milhorn DM, Foreman RD, et al. Preemptive, but not reactive, spinal cord stimulation mitigates transient ischemia-induced myocardial infarction via cardiac adrenergic neurons. *Am J Physiol Heart Circ Physiol.* 2007;292(1):H311-H317. doi:10.1152/ajpheart.00087.2006
47. Goroszeniuk T, Kothari S, Hamann W. Subcutaneous neuromodulating implant targeted at the site of pain. *Reg Anesth Pain Med.* 2006;31(2):168-171. doi:10.1016/j.rapm.2006.02.001

CHAPTER 9

RHEUMATIC HEART DISEASE

Gbemiga Sofowora

INTRODUCTION

Acute rheumatic fever and rheumatic heart disease remain prevalent in the developing world although their incidence has declined substantially in Western countries, except in certain pockets, because of improved health care services, hygiene, and accommodation.[1,2] Developing countries are cognizant of the need for progress in preventing and treating acute rheumatic fever and its sequelae. In Africa, the Addis Ababa communique was launched to put forth recommendations to assist with the eradication of rheumatic heart disease, particularly in hyperendemic areas.[3] Reports of successful implementation are not yet available, but this may serve as a template for future programs in other similarly hyperendemic areas.[4]

Epidemiology

The global burden of group A streptococcus is estimated to be at least 18.1 million cases with 1.78 million cases yearly,[4] and the greatest burden is due to rheumatic heart disease, with a prevalence of 15.6 million cases and an estimated 282,000 new cases occurring yearly. These cases occur disproportionately in developing countries and among migrants and socioeconomically disadvantaged populations, as well as indigenous populations in high-income countries. Widespread availability of penicillin G, better housing and hygiene, and the health care access that exists in the United States and Western Europe have contributed to the decline in these regions, although variations in population susceptibility to disease have also been proposed.[5]

The mean incidence of first attack of acute rheumatic fever per annum ranged from 5 to 51 per 100,000 with a mean of 19 per 100,000 (95% confidence interval [CI]: 9 to 30 per 100,000) in a study,[6] with the highest mean annual incidences found in India (51 per 100,000) and the Maori community in New Zealand (>80 per 100,000). Low incidence rates (≤10/100,000) were found in the United States and Western Europe and higher rates in Asia, Australasia, and the Middle East. It must be noted that accurate figures are hard to come by in regions of sub-Saharan Africa and Asia.

In 2015, the age-standardized prevalence of rheumatic heart disease was estimated to be approximately 444 per 100,000 in countries that showed an endemic pattern versus 3.4 per 100,000 in countries that did not show an endemic pattern. The endemic pattern in the study was defined as "having a high mortality and prevalence among children" versus the nonendemic pattern with low mortality and prevalence mostly among adults. This prevalence was highest in Oceania, central sub-Saharan Africa, and South Asia.[7] Most epidemiologic estimates of disease come from clinical data. Comparing clinical data with the use of echocardiographic data, Marijon et al.[7] showed that echocardiography was 10 times more sensitive in picking up cases of rheumatic heart disease in Cambodia and Mozambique than clinical data alone. This suggests that our estimates of the global burden of this disease may be grossly underestimated.

More recent figures show the largest numbers of deaths in 2015 because of rheumatic heart disease in India (119,100), China (72,600), and Pakistan (18,900),[8] although statistics are somewhat skewed by such large populations. The highest estimated age-standardized death rates because of rheumatic heart disease occurred in the Central African Republic and Lesotho in Africa, the Solomon Islands, Pakistan, Papua New Guinea, Kiribati, Vanuatu, Fiji, India, the Federated States of Micronesia, and the Marshall Islands.

PATHOGENESIS

Acute rheumatic fever is preceded by infection with rheumatogenic strains of Lancefield group A β-hemolytic streptococci (*Streptococcus pyogenes*) usually in the form of pharyngitis. There is exception in Australia among the aboriginal people who have one of the highest rates of acute rheumatic fever and rheumatic heart disease in the world, and colonization of the throat with group A streptococcus and symptomatic pharyngitis are uncommon. In this community, group A streptococcus infections of the skin (pyoderma) and group C and G streptococci are thought to account for the higher incidence, suggesting that epidemiology may vary from region to region.[9]

In populations exposed to rheumatogenic strains of *S. pyogenes*, the cumulative incidence of acute rheumatic fever is between 3% and 6%, implicating host susceptibility as a factor in the transmission of this disease. That genetic factors may also play a part in the susceptibility to acute rheumatic fever was highlighted by the fact that, in a meta-analysis of 175 monozygotic twins and 260 dizygotic twins,[10] concordance between monozygotic twins was six times that of dizygotic twins. The major histocompatibility complex human leukocyte antigen (HLA) molecules are attractive candidates that may determine susceptibility, and research in this area is still ongoing.[11] Early findings using genome-wide association studies point to HLA-DQA1-HLA-DQB2 regions as well as the immunoglobulin heavy chain locus on chromosome 14.[12]

After pharyngeal infection with Lancefield group A β-hemolytic streptococci, approximately 3% to 6% of the population will develop acute rheumatic fever, which generally occurs 2 to 5 weeks after onset of the pharyngitis and may indicate development of antibodies against host tissues. The antibodies formed are specific to the M moiety on the bacteria, which confer it with the ability to attach to host tissues. These M proteins are similar in structure to cardiac myosin, tropomyosin, actin, and laminin, so that repeated infection leads to development of autoantibodies against these structures on valves. In support of this fact, the vast majority of patients with acute rheumatic fever have elevated titers of antibodies to streptococcal antigens including antistreptolysin O (ASO), anti–DNase B, and anti–group A carbohydrate. Although much is still unknown about its pathogenesis, it is thought that there is ultimately autoantibody-mediated injury, leading to destruction and scarring of the valves. These autoantibodies also lead to inflammation of the joints, brain, and subcutaneous tissues, contributing to the features of acute rheumatic fever. Repeated or ongoing infections possibly drive the inflammation of the heart valves over subsequent years, leading to rheumatic heart disease.

Natural History

Following infection with Lancefield group A streptococcus, 3% to 6% of patients will develop acute rheumatic fever.[13] The most common age group is 5 to 15 years with no gender predominance. Most persons with acute rheumatic fever present with polyarthritis, which is usually migratory, symmetrical, and tends to involve the larger joints, mainly the knees, ankles, wrist, elbows, and shoulders. Carditis occurs in fewer patients than arthritis, whereas Sydenham chorea occurs in only about a quarter of patients with acute rheumatic fever and tends to be predominantly female. The skin features of erythema marginatum (**Figure 9.1**) and subcutaneous nodules occur less frequently than the other symptoms, and the subcutaneous nodules may not be present at all. These cardinal symptoms if left untreated usually resolve within 3 months. Years later, in some cases up to decades, the features of rheumatic heart disease appear with predominant mitral valve involvement.

CLINICAL PRESENTATION

Acute rheumatic fever may present with the following features:

- *Arthritis* occurs in most people with acute rheumatic fever and is usually described as a migratory, symmetric, aseptic polyarthritis, which most commonly affects the knees, ankles, wrists, elbows, and shoulder joints. Symptoms of pain and swelling are generally present and last about 5 to 7 days before affecting another joint. Aspiration of a joint typically does not yield bacteria. In select hyperendemic communities, however, a monoarthritis has been described,[14] and a revision of the Jones Criteria recommends "at present, consideration that monoarthritis may be part of the acute rheumatic fever spectrum should be limited to patients from moderate to high risk populations (Class 1; Level of Evidence C)."[15]
- *Carditis* usually described as a pancarditis affects mainly the valves and is better described as a valvulitis. The mitral valve is the most commonly affected, and mitral regurgitation is the most common valve lesion seen. If severe, the patient may present with signs and symptoms of congestive heart failure with shortness of breath with exertion, paroxysmal nocturnal dyspnea and orthopnea with rales and edema on examination as well as tachycardia, and a third heart sound on auscultation. Murmurs include a holosystolic murmur of mitral regurgitation heard at the apex that radiates to the axilla, an apical mid-diastolic flow murmur (Carey Coombs murmur), and an aortic diastolic murmur heard at the base and radiating down the left sternal border.
- *Pericarditis* with a pericardial rub best heard over the second or third interspace and a pericardial effusion may be noted on echocardiography.

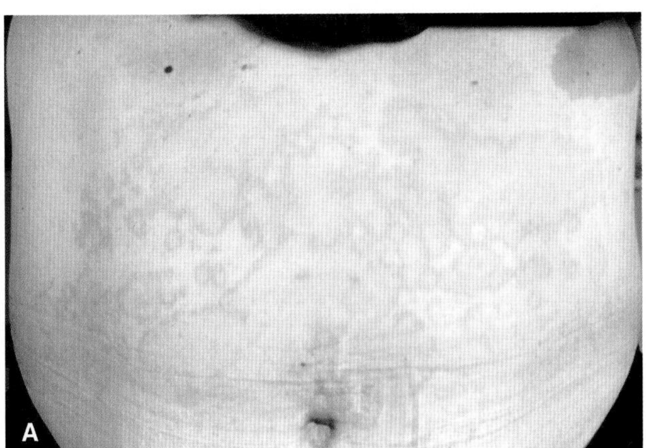

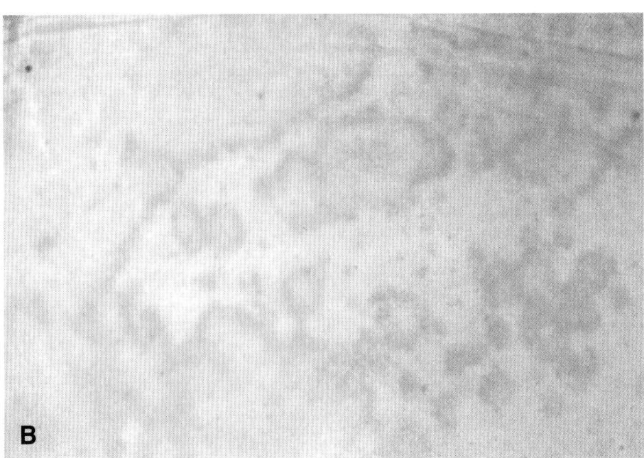

FIGURE 9.1 **A,B**: The rash of erythema marginatum begins as a serpiginous area of erythema, and the margins of the rash progress as the center clears. It primarily occurs over the trunk and proximal extremities. **A**: Erythema marginatum in an adult with rheumatic fever. **B**: Closer view of rash. (Courtesy of P. Witman, Mayo Clinic. Used with permission of Mayo Foundation for Medical Education and Research. All rights reserved.)

- *Sydenham chorea (St Vitus dance, St Johannis' chorea)* may be due to the effect of autoantibodies on the basal ganglia and occurs in 26% of patients with acute rheumatic fever.[16] Patients with Sydenham chorea are usually female and between 5 and 15 years. St Vitus dance is characterized by jerky, involuntary, semi-purposeful movements involving the face and limbs with emotional lability and personality disorders. These movement disorders tend to abate during sleep. The chorea presents as gait changes, a tendency to drop objects, and bursts of dysarthric speech (Sydenham speech).
- Psychological features range from emotional lability and anxiety to frank obsessive compulsive disorder and tend to precede the movement disorders by 2 to 4 weeks.
- *Muscle weakness* typically characterized by the inability of the patient to sustain a muscle contraction (milkmaid's grip) usually resolves within a few months with no permanent sequelae.
- *Erythema marginatum* (**Figure 9.1**) is a nonpruritic, serpiginous rash that is usually located over the trunk and proximal limbs and appears intermittently over weeks to months as transient macules that tend to heal in the center while advancing at the margins. The appearance of this rash may be induced by heat, and the macules blanche with pressure.
- *Subcutaneous nodules* are usually associated with carditis and are painless nodules found over bony prominences or tendons such as the knees, wrist, elbows, Achilles tendon, back of the scalp, and spinous processes of the vertebrae. These nodules are painless and may escape attention and are almost never the only manifestation of acute rheumatic fever.[13]
- *Polyarthralgia, fever (>38.5 °C), erythrocyte sedimentation rate 60 mm/hr or more in the first hour and/or C-reactive protein 3.0 mg/dL or more, and prolonged PR interval* on electrocardiogram. In moderate- to high-risk populations, however, the presence of monoarthralgia, fever 38 °C or more, and erythrocyte sedimentation rate 30 mm/hr or more in the first hour and/or C-reactive protein 3.0 mg/dL or more may be appropriate to make the diagnosis.
- *Tachycardia during sleep* may accompany fever, tachycardia out of proportion to the fever, malaise, anemia, leukocytosis, and abdominal pain.

DIAGNOSIS

The revised Jones Criteria (**Table 9.1**) outline criteria for diagnosis.[15] All patients require evidence of a preceding group A streptococcal infection before diagnosis.

TABLE 9.1 Revised Jones Criteria

A. For all patient populations with evidence of preceding GAS infection	
Diagnosis: initial ARF	Two major manifestations or one major plus two minor manifestations
Diagnosis: recurrent ARF	Two major or one major and two minor or three minor
B. Major criteria	
Low-risk populations[a]	Moderate- and high-risk populations
Carditis[b] (clinical or subclinical)	Carditis (clinical or subclinical)
Arthritis (polyarthritis only)	Arthritis (monoarthritis, polyarthritis or polyarthralgia)[c]
Chorea	Chorea
Erythema marginatum	Erythema marginatum
Subcutaneous nodules	Subcutaneous nodules
C. Minor criteria	
Low-risk populations[a]	Moderate-and high-risk populations
Polyarthralgia	Monoarthralgia
Fever (≥38.5 °C)	Fever (≥38 °C)
ESR ≥60 mm in first hour and/or CRP ≥3.0 mg/dL[d]	ESR ≥30 mm/h and/or CRP ≥3.0 mg/dL[d]
Prolonged PR interval, after accounting for age variability (unless carditis is a major criterion)	Prolonged PR interval, after accounting for age variability (unless carditis is a major criterion)

ARF, acute rheumatic fever; CRP, C-reactive protein; ESR, erythrocyte sedimentation rate; GAS, group A streptococcal infection.

[a]Low-risk populations are those with ARF incidence ≤2 per 100,000 school-aged children or all-age rheumatic heart disease prevalence of ≤1 per 1000 population per year.

[b]Subclinical carditis indicates echocardiographic valvulitis as defined in Table.9.4.

[c]Polyarthralgia should only be considered as a major manifestation in moderate- to high-risk populations after exclusion of other causes. As in past versions of the criteria, erythema marginatum and subcutaneous nodules are rarely "stand-alone" major criteria. Additionally, joint manifestations can only be considered in either the major or minor categories but not both in the same patient.

[d]CRP value must be greater than upper limit of normal for laboratory. Also, because ESR may evolve during the course of ARF, peak ESR values should be used.

Reprinted with permission from Gewitz MH, Baltimore RS, Tani LY, et al; American Heart Association Committee on Rheumatic Fever, Endocarditis, and Kawasaki Disease of the Council on Cardiovascular Disease in the Young. Revision of the Jones Criteria for the diagnosis of acute rheumatic fever in the era of Doppler echocardiography: a scientific statement from the American Heart Association. *Circulation.* 2015;131(20):1806-1818.

TABLE 9.2 Morphologic Features of Rheumatic Heart Disease (RHD)

Morphologic Features of RHD
Features in the MV
• AMVL thickening[a] ≥3 mm (age specific)[b]
• Chordal thickening
• Restricted leaflet motion[c]
• Excessive leaflet tip motion during systole[d]
Features in the AV
• Irregular or focal thickening
• Coaptation defect
• Restricted leaflet motion
• Prolapse

[a]AVML thickness should be measured during diastole at full excursion. Measurement should be taken at the thickest portion of the leaflet, including focal thickening, beading, and nodularity. Measurement should be performed on a frame with maximal separation of chordae from the leaflet tissue. Valve thickness can only be assessed if the images were acquired at optimal gain settings without harmonics and with a frequency ≥2.0 MHz.
[b]Abnormal thickening of the AMVL is age-specific and defined as follows: ≥3 mm for individuals aged ≤20 years; ≥4 mm for individuals aged 21–40 years; ≥5 mm for individuals aged >40 years. Valve thickness measurements obtained using harmonic imaging should be cautiously interpreted and a thickness up to 4 mm should be considered normal in those aged ≤20 years.
[c]Restricted leaflet motion of either the anterior or the posterior MV leaflet is usually the result of chordal shortening or fusion, commissural fusion, or leaflet thickening.
[d]Excessive leaflet tip motion is the result of elongation of the primary chords, and is defined as displacement of the tip or edge of an involved leaflet towards the left atritun resulting in abnormal coaptation and regurgitation. Excessive leaflet tip motion does not need to meet the standard echocardiographic definition of MV prolapse disease, as that refers to a different disease process. This feature applies to only those aged <35 years. In the presence of a flail MV leaflet in the young (≤20 years), this single morphological feature is sufficient to meet the morphological criteria for RHD (that is, where the criteria state "at least two morphological features of RHD of the MV" a flail leaflet in a person aged ≤20 years is sufficient).
AMVL, anterior mitral valve leaflet; AV, aortic valve; MV, mitral valve; RHD, rheumatic heart disease.
Reprinted by permission from Nature: Reményi B, Wilson N, Steer A, et al. World Heart Federation criteria for echocardiographic diagnosis of rheumatic heart disease—an evidence-based guideline. *Nat Rev Cardiol.* 2012;9(5):297-309.

Initial acute rheumatic fever requires two major criteria or one major plus two minor criteria, whereas recurrent acute rheumatic fever requires two major or one major + two minor criteria or three minor criteria.

Major criteria include:

- Carditis (clinical or detected by echocardiography)
- Arthritis
- Chorea
- Erythema marginatum (see **Figure 9.1**)
- Subcutaneous nodules

Minor criteria include:

- Polyarthralgia

TABLE 9.3 Criteria for Pathologic Regurgitation

Pathologic Mitral Regurgitation
(All four Doppler echocardiographic criteria must be met)
• Seen in two views
• In at least one view, jet length ≥2 cm[a]
• Velocity ≥3 m/s for one complete envelope
• Pansystolic jet in at least one envelope
Pathologic Aortic Regurgitation
(All four Doppler echocardiographic criteria must be met)
• Seen in two views
• In at least one view, jet length ≥1 cm[a]
• Velocity ≥3 m/s in early diastole
• Pandiastolic jet in at least one envelope

[a]The length of the regurgitant jet should be measured from the vena contracta to the last pixel of regurgitant color.
Reprinted by permission from Nature: Reményi B, Wilson N, Steer A, et al. World Heart Federation criteria for echocardiographic diagnosis of rheumatic heart disease—an evidence-based guideline. *Nat Rev Cardiol.* 2012;9(5):297-309.

- Fever (≥38.5 °C)
- Erythrocyte sedimentation rate 60 mm or more in the first hour and/or C-reactive protein 3.0 mg/dL or more
- Prolonged PR interval on electrocardiogram after accounting for age variability (unless carditis is a major criterion)

The diagnosis of rheumatic heart disease, on the other hand, does not require demonstration of previous group A streptococcal infection. The findings of characteristic rheumatic damage on echocardiography are sufficient. These include pure mitral stenosis, mixed mitral valve disease, and aortic valve disease in the presence of mitral valve disease. In endemic regions, mitral regurgitation is often the commonest lesion found followed by mixed mitral valve disease or combined aortic and mitral valve disease noted depending on the region.[17–20] Regurgitant lesions appear to be more frequent than stenotic lesions, and the order of valve involvement is mitral > aortic > tricuspid > pulmonic. Rarely are the right-sided valves involved in isolation without mitral valve involvement.

The World Heart Federation has criteria for the diagnosis of rheumatic valvular disease and these involve morphologic criteria, criteria for pathologic regurgitation, and echocardiographic criteria for the diagnosis of rheumatic heart disease (**Tables 9.2 to 9.4**).[21]

MANAGEMENT OF THE PATIENT WITH RHEUMATIC HEART DISEASE

Treatment involves antibiotic treatment of group A streptococcal throat infection, secondary prevention of acute rheumatic fever, and possible surgical valve replacement or repair according to current valve guidelines, as well as treating ancillary issues such as congestive heart failure or complications such as infective endocarditis.

TABLE 9.4 Criteria for Echocardiographic Diagnosis of Rheumatic Heart Disease (RHD)

2012 WHF Criteria for Echocardiographic Diagnosis of RHD

Echocardiographic Criteria for Individuals Aged ≤ 20 Years

Definite RHD (A, B, C, or D):

- A) Pathologic MR and at least two morphologic features of RHD of the MV
- B) MS mean gradient ≥4 mmHg[a]
- C) Pathologic AR and at least two morphologic features of RHD of the AV[b]
- D) Borderline disease of both the AV and MV[c]

Borderline RHD (A, B, or C):

- A) At least two morphologic features of RHD of the MV without pathologic MR or MS
- B) Pathologic MR
- C) Pathologic AR

Normal echocardiographic finding (all of A, B, C, and D):

- A) MR that does not meet all four Doppler echocardiographic criteria (physiologic MR)
- B) AR that does not meet all four Doppler echocardiographic criteria (physiologic AR)
- C) An isolated morphologic feature of RHD of the MV (eg, valvular thickening) without any associated pathologic stenosis or regurgitation
- D) Morphologic features of RHD of the AV (eg, valvular thickening) without any associated pathologic stenosis or regurgitation

Echocardiographic Criteria for Individuals Aged >20 Years

Definite RHD (A, B, C, or D):

- A) Pathologic MR and at least two morphologic features of RHD of the MV
- B) MS mean gradient ≥4 mmHg[a]
- C) Pathologic AR and at least two morphologic features of RHD of the AV, only in individuals aged <35 years[b]
- D) Pathologic AR and at least two morphologic features of RHD of the MV

[a]Congenital MV anomalies must be excluded. Furthermore, inflow obstruction due to nonrheumatic mitral annular clacification must be excluded in adults.
[b]Bicuspid AV, dilated aortic root, and hypertension must be excluded.
[c]Combine AR and MR in high prevalence regions and in the absence of congenital heart disease is regarded as rheumatic.
AR, aortic regurgitation; AV, aortic valve; MR, mitral regurgitation; MS, mitral stenosis; MV, mitral valve; RHD, rheumatic heart disease; WHF, World Heart Federation.
Loading conditions should be accounted for at time of echocardiography/Doppler assessment
Reprinted by permission from Nature: Reményi B, Wilson N, Steer A, et al. World Heart Federation criteria for echocardiographic diagnosis of rheumatic heart disease—an evidence-based guideline. *Nat Rev Cardiol.* 2012;9(5):297-309.

Antibiotic Treatment of Group a Streptococcal Throat Infection

Primary prevention involves eradication of overcrowding and poverty as well as antibiotic treatment of group A streptococcal infection. The World Health Organization (WHO) guidelines for treating group A streptococcal infection are outlined in **Table 9.5** [22]

Secondary prevention of acute rheumatic fever has no effect in preventing the eventual development of rheumatic heart disease (**Table 9.6**). The erythrocyte sedimentation rate also normalizes with both aspirin and steroid therapy.

The course or development of rheumatic heart disease appears to be most dependent on the severity of heart disease at the onset of treatment. Mild disease at onset tends to resolve, but in moderate to severe disease, there appears to be no improvement with either steroid use or acetylsalicylic acid.[23] The Combined Rheumatic Fever Study group recommends that prednisone be given at a dose of 1 mg/lb daily for 1 to 2 weeks or until the acute cardiac features are stable, after which aspirin can be given for 6 to 8 weeks. This regimen minimizes the side effects of steroids while maximizing their suppressive actions.[23]

Treatment of Valvular Heart Disease and Congestive Heart Failure

Treatment of rheumatic heart disease largely involves treatment of the underlying valvular heart disease and management of congestive heart failure as discussed further.

Mitral Stenosis

Treatment of mitral stenosis primarily involves slowing the heart rate to improve the diastolic filling time and optimize left atrial emptying. This has the effect of improving left atrial pressures and ultimately symptoms of shortness of breath. This effect is achieved using beta-blockers, calcium channel blockers, or, in persons with systolic heart failure because of concomitant mitral regurgitation and atrial fibrillation, digoxin. For symptomatic patients with severe mitral stenosis, a mitral balloon valvuloplasty may be performed in the absence of significant mitral regurgitation or left atrial thrombus and if the valve anatomy is favorable. In developing countries without access to balloon therapy, a closed mitral commissurotomy can be performed on the beating heart. Valve replacement with a bioprosthetic or mechanical valve is a definitive treatment.[24]

Mitral Regurgitation

Mitral regurgitation is the most common lesion in acute rheumatic fever and rheumatic heart disease and may progress to being severe. Once symptomatic, medical management of mitral regurgitation involves use of diuretics to reduce preload and eventual mitral valve replacement or repair. Surgery is also a consideration in asymptomatic patients with severe mitral regurgitation and left ventricular dysfunction, atrial fibrillation, and/or pulmonary artery systolic pressure above 50 mmHg.

Aortic Stenosis

Aortic stenosis can be monitored closely until severe and symptomatic. Caution must be exercised when using vasodilators,

TABLE 9.5 Antibiotics Used in Primary Prevention of Group A Streptococcal Infection (World Health Organization Guidelines)

Antibiotic	Route of Administration	Dose
Benzathine benzylpenicillin (benzathine penicillin G)	Intramuscular injection; children should be kept under observation for 30 minutes	Single-dose 1.2 million U; <27 kg, 600,000 U
Phenoxymethylpenicillin (penicillin V)	Oral, two to four times daily for 10 days	Children 250 mg twice or three times daily, adolescents or adults 250 mg three or four times daily or 500 mg twice daily
Amoxicillin	Oral, two to three times daily for 10 days	25-50 mg/kg/d in three doses; total adult dose 750-1500 mg/d
First-generation cephalosporins	Oral, two to three times daily for 10 days	Varies with formulation
Erythromycin if allergic to penicillin	Oral, four times daily for 10 days	Varies with formulation

Reproduced from Cilliers AM. Rheumatic fever and its management. *BMJ.* 2006;333(7579):1153-1156; with permission from BMJ Publishing Group Ltd.

TABLE 9.6 Secondary Prevention of Rheumatic Fever (World Health Organization Guidelines)

Antibiotic	Route of Administration	Does
Benzathine benzylpenicillin (benzathine penicillin G)	Intramuscular injection, every 3-4 weeks	≥30 kg, 1.2 million U; ≤30 kg, 600,000 U
Phenoxymethylpenicillin (penicillin V)	Oral	250 mg twice daily
Erythromycin if allergic to penicillin	Oral	250 mg twice daily

Reproduced from Cilliers AM. Rheumatic fever and its management. *BMJ.* 2006;333(7579):1153-1156; with permission from BMJ Publishing Group Ltd.

which may cause hypotension in the patient unable to increase cardiac output because of severe valve stenosis. Sinus tachycardia or atrial fibrillation should be avoided and treated promptly if detected as this would reduce the left ventricular filling time and ultimately stroke volume across an already narrow valve. Definitive treatment involves valve replacement. The mode of valve replacement may be either surgical or percutaneous depending on valve anatomy and surgical risk. Because severe aortic valve damage in rheumatic heart disease rarely occurs independent of the mitral valve, combined mitral and aortic valve replacement may be required.

Aortic Regurgitation

Aortic regurgitation is usually monitored until the lesion becomes severe and symptomatic. If present with hypertension a reasonable approach is to add an angiotensin receptor blocker for optimal blood pressure control and to maximize forward flow. Valve replacement is required once the lesion is severe with signs and symptoms of congestive heart failure present or evidence of left ventricular systolic dysfunction and ventricular dilation.

Congestive Heart Failure

Treatment of congestive heart failure requires the use of goal-directed medical therapy for systolic heart failure using beta-blockers, angiotensin-converting enzyme inhibitors, angiotensin receptor blockers, or sacubitril/valsartan with or without an aldosterone antagonist. Use of anticoagulation and beta-blockers for the management of accompanying atrial fibrillation may be required.

PREVENTION

Acute rheumatic fever is endemic in developing countries where overcrowding, poor hygiene, and reduced access to health care exist, so it follows that better housing facilities and living conditions should reduce the prevalence of disease. Primary prevention involves early treatment of sore throat caused by Lancefield group A streptococcus to prevent the subsequent development of acute rheumatic fever and rheumatic heart disease. Ideally antibiotics should be commenced within 9 days of the onset of sore throat. Known regimens include single-dose benzathine penicillin G 1.2 million units intramuscularly (IM) or 600,000 units IM if body weight is less than 27 kg, phenoxymethylpenicillin (penicillin V) or amoxicillin 250 mg two to three times daily for 10 days for children and 500 mg for adults.[27] Erythromycin or the cephalosporins may be used if the individual is allergic to penicillin and antibiotic susceptibility testing confirms the strain is not resistant. Effective delivery of these antibiotic regimens should be accompanied by an overall improvement in health care delivery. To date, the only proven strategy is secondary prophylaxis, which involves long-term treatment of people with a history of acute rheumatic fever or rheumatic heart disease. Effective regimens include: benzathine penicillin G 1.2 million units IM every 3 to 4 weeks (600,000 units if weight is <30 kg), penicillin V 250 mg twice daily or erythromycin 250 mg twice daily. The duration is for at least 5 years since the last episode of acute rheumatic fever or till the age of 18 years (whichever is longer). For patients with mild or healed carditis, the duration is 10 years since the last episode or till the age of 25 years (whichever is longer), and for patients who had severe carditis or required surgery, the duration of treatment needs to be lifelong.[25]

FUTURE DIRECTIONS

The use of vaccines remains an attractive strategy, but this has been hampered by the fact that the countries with the most resources to produce these vaccines are the countries with the least incidence of rheumatic fever. Also, serotypes of streptococcus not only vary from region to region but may also change within the same region, so the effectiveness of vaccination may gradually decline. However, using a cluster-based strategy that is based on the distribution of group A streptococcal M proteins in Africa, a 30-valent vaccine currently being developed could theoretically provide coverage to 80.3% of bacterial isolates in Africa. This could be a game changer for the entire continent, and if successful, this strategy may be reproduced in other similarly hyperendemic areas of the world.[26]

KEY POINTS

- ✔ Acute rheumatic fever and rheumatic heart disease are still prevalent in socioeconomically disadvantaged populations of the world.
- ✔ Acute rheumatic fever is generally preceded by pharyngeal infection with Lancefield group A β-hemolytic streptococcus.
- ✔ After infection, 3% to 6% of persons will develop acute rheumatic fever after approximately 2 to 5 weeks.
- ✔ Acute rheumatic fever is an autoimmune phenomenon characterized by autoimmune damage by antibodies to group A streptococci.
- ✔ Diagnosis of acute rheumatic fever involves demonstration of antecedent group A streptococcal infection and the modified Jones Criteria.
- ✔ Primary prevention involves eradication of poverty and overcrowding as well as antibiotic treatment of group A streptococci.
- ✔ Secondary prevention involves use of antibiotics to prevent recurrent episodes of group A streptococci.
- ✔ Treatment of acute rheumatic fever involves the use of aspirin and corticosteroids to ameliorate symptoms.
- ✔ Treatment of rheumatic heart disease ultimately involves management of the underlying valvular heart disease and heart failure, if present.

REFERENCES

1. Bland EF, Jones TD. The natural history of rheumatic fever and rheumatic heart disease. *Trans Am Clin Climatol Assoc.* 1936;52:85-87.
2. Bland EF, Jones TD. Clinical observations on the events preceding the appearance of rheumatic fever. *J Clin Invest.* 1935;14(5):633-648.
3. Watkins D, Zuhlke L, Engel M, et al. Seven key actions to eradicate rheumatic heart disease in Africa: the Addis Ababa communique. *Cardiovasc J Afr.* 2016;27(3):184-187.
4. Carapetis JR, Steer AC, Mulholland EK, Weber M. The global burden of group A streptococcal diseases. *Lancet Infect Dis.* 2005;5(11):685-694.
5. Carapetis JR, Currie BJ, Mathews JD. Cumulative incidence of rheumatic fever in an endemic region: a guide to the susceptibility of the population? *Epidemiol Infect.* 2000;124(2):239-244.
6. Tibazarwa KB, Volmink JA, Mayosi BM. Incidence of acute rheumatic fever in the world: a systematic review of population-based studies. *Heart.* 2008;94(2):1534-1540.
7. Marijon E, Ou P, Celermajer DS, et al. Prevalence of rheumatic heart disease detected by echocardiographic screening. *N Engl J Med.* 2007;357(5):470-476.
8. Watkins DA, Johnson CO, Colquhoun SM, et al. Global, regional, and national burden of rheumatic heart disease, 1990-2015. *N Engl J Med.* 2017;377(8):713-722.
9. McDonald M, Currie BJ, Carapetis JR, Acute rheumatic fever: a chink in the chain that links the heart to the throat? *Lancet Infect Dis.* 2004;4(4):240-245.
10. Engel ME, Stander R, Vogel J, Adeyemo AA, Mayosi BM. Genetic susceptibility to acute rheumatic fever: a systematic review and meta-analysis of twin studies. *PLoS One.* 2011;6(9):1-6.
11. Bryant PA, Robins-Browne R, Carapetis JR, Curtis N, Some of the people, some of the time: susceptibility to acute rheumatic fever. *Circulation.* 2009;119(5):742-753.
12. Muhamed B, Parks T, Sliwa K, Genetics of rheumatic fever and rheumatic heart disease. *Nat Rev Cardiol.* 2020;17(3):145-154.
13. Wallace MR, Lutwick LI, Ravishankar J. Rheumatic fever. *Medscape.* 2019.
14. Carapetis JR, Currie BJ. Rheumatic fever in a high incidence population. *Arch Dis Child.* 2001;85(3):223-227.
15. Gewitz MH, Baltimore RS, Tani LY, et al. Revision of the Jones criteria for the diagnosis of acute rheumatic fever in the era of doppler echocardiography: a scientific statement from the American Heart Association. *Circulation.* 2015;131(20):1806-1818.
16. Cardoso F, E.C., Silva AP, Mota CC. Chorea in fifty consecutive patients with rheumatic fever. *Mov Disord.* 1997;12(5):701-703.
17. Lubega S, Aliku T, Lwabi P. Echocardiographic pattern and severity of valve dysfunction in children with rheumatic heart disease seen at Uganda Heart Institute, Mulago Hospital. *Afr Health Sci.* 2014;14(3):617-625.
18. Essien IO, Onwubere BJC, Anisiuba BC, Ejim EC, Andy JJ, Ike SO. One year echocardiographic study of rheumatic heart disease at Enugu, Nigeria. *Niger Postgrad Med J.* 2008;15(3):175-178.
19. Nkoke C, Lekoubou A, Dzudie A, et al. Echocardiographic pattern of rheumatic valvular disease in a contemporary sub-Saharan African pediatric population: an audit of a major cardiac ultrasound unit in Yaounde, Cameroon. *BMC Pediatr.* 2016;16:1-5.
20. Sani MU, Karaye KM, Borodo MM. Prevalence and pattern of rheumatic heart disease in the Nigerian savannah: an echocardiographic study. *Cardiovasc J Afr.* 2007;18(5):295-299.
21. Remenyi B, Wilson N, Steer A, et al. World Heart Federation criteria for echocardiographic diagnosis of rheumatic heart disease—an evidence-based guideline. *Nat Rev Cardiol.* 2012;9(5):297-309.
22. Cilliers AM. Rheumatic fever and its management. *BMJ.* 2006;333(7579):1153-1156.
23. Segal MS, Dulfano MJ. A comparison of short-term, intensive prednisone and acetylsalicylic acid therapy in the treatment of acute rheumatic fever. Combined Rheumatic Fever Study Group. *N Engl J Med.* 1965;272:63-70.
24. Nishimura RA, Otto CM, Bonow RO, et al. AHA/ACC focused update of the 2014 AHA/ACC guideline for the management of patients with valvular heart disease: a report of the American College of Cardiology/American Heart Association Task Force on Clinical Practice Guidelines. *Circulation.* 2017;135(25):e1159-e1195.
25. World Health Organization. *Rheumatic Fever and Rheumatic Heart Disease: Report of a WHO Expert Consultation, Geneva, November 2001.* WHO Tech Rep Ser. WHO; 2004.
26. Salie, T., et al., Systematic review and meta-analysis of the prevalence of Group A streptococcal emm clusters in Africa to inform vaccine development. *mSphere.* 2020;5(4):e00429-e00520.

CHAPTER 10

MITRAL VALVE DISEASE

Nicholas S. Amoroso, Jessica Atkins, and Valerian Fernandes

INTRODUCTION

The mitral valve (MV) regulates blood flow between the left atrium (LA) and left ventricle (LV) of the heart. It is believed to have been popularly named by Andreas Vesalius, who alluded to the leaflet shape that resembles a bishop's hat: a mitre.[1]

The MV is composed of two leaflets, an annular perimeter and the subvalvular apparatus that functions in the setting of both low central and high systemic circulatory pressures (**see Figure 10.1**). The annulus is a saddle-shaped confluence of several cardiac structures including the LA, LV, mitral leaflets, and aortomitral continuity with heterogeneous consistency with both fibrous and nonfibrous tissue components in its plane of leaflet hinge. The subvalvular apparatus includes the chordae tendinae, the papillary muscles, and the LV, to which they are attached.[1] Accordingly, abnormalities of the valve leaflets or any of the mitral apparatus components can influence valve function, thereby leading to mitral regurgitation (MR) or mitral stenosis (MS).

Epidemiology

The prevalence of MV disease is difficult to determine from available data sources. Studies documenting any presence of MR report prevalence ranging from 40% to 92%. However, the Framingham Offspring Study reported MR equal to or greater than mild in 19% of women and men.[2,3] When focused on moderate to severe MR, the prevalence in Olmstead County, Minnesota was 1.7% in the adult population, and MS affected 0.1% of the population.[4] A study of a Chinese population reported that roughly 3% of 133,729 patients undergoing echocardiogram had moderate to severe MR.[3] These studies imply that millions of people worldwide suffer from MV disease.

MV disease is very rarely congenital (rate of 5/100,000); it is most commonly acquired secondary to other heart disease.[5] MR frequency by etiology varies depending on cohort age, geography, comorbidities, and so on, but degenerative and functional etiologies (see subsequent description) each constitutes 50% of severe MR prevalence.[3,4,6]

Mitral Stenosis

The incidence of MS is much lower than that of MR, and is related to the prevalence of rheumatic heart disease in the population being reported. Rheumatic fever and, thus, rheumatic MS, disproportionately affects developing countries and the low-income groups in developed countries that lack access to health care and treatment for *Streptococcus pyogenes* infections. Although rheumatic heart disease is the primary cause of MS—largely driven by its prevalence in the developing world (ranging from 46 to 2400 cases per 100,000)—the incidence is dropping, and nonrheumatic MV calcification is an increasingly common cause of MS and/or MR.[6] This increase in nonrheumatic mitral calcinosis is most probably related to the older average age of patients, increased frequency of multiple cardiovascular risk factors, and increased prevalence of chronic kidney disease.[7] Other modern disease entities, such as metabolic and autoimmune disorders, also contribute to nonrheumatic MS.[7,8]

PATHOGENESIS

Mitral Regurgitation

MR occurs, chiefly, when there is malcoaptation of the leaflets, allowing for regurgitant flow from the LV to the LA. It has been categorized in several ways, but most useful is the distinction between degenerative and functional MR.

Degenerative Mitral Regurgitation

Degenerative MR (aka primary MR) is due to inherent or acquired pathology of the valve leaflets, chordae tendinae, or papillary muscles. Degenerative MR may be secondary to MV prolapse or myxomatous MV disease, which sometimes progresses to chordae tendinae rupture, as a result of leaflet malcoaptation. Rheumatic heart can also lead to valve leaflet and chordal thickening that decreases leaflet pliability and prevents adequate leaflet coaptation. Valve leaflet degeneration can also be observed with MV endocarditis. In recent decades, infectious endocarditis has become predominantly associated with *Staphylococcus aureus* and coagulase-negative Staphylococcus bacteremia as a result of intravenous drug use and health care–associated infections, respectively.[6] Valve calcinosis is increasingly recognized as a source of degenerative valve disease, whereby calcium deposits collect along the annulus, chordae, and valve leaflets, leading to restriction in leaflet movement, poor coaptation, and regurgitation.[7] Iatrogenic causes of leaflet destruction include radiation-induced and medication-induced (eg, serotonergic appetite suppressants such as fenfluramine or benfluorex and ergot-derived dopamine agonists such as cabergoline or

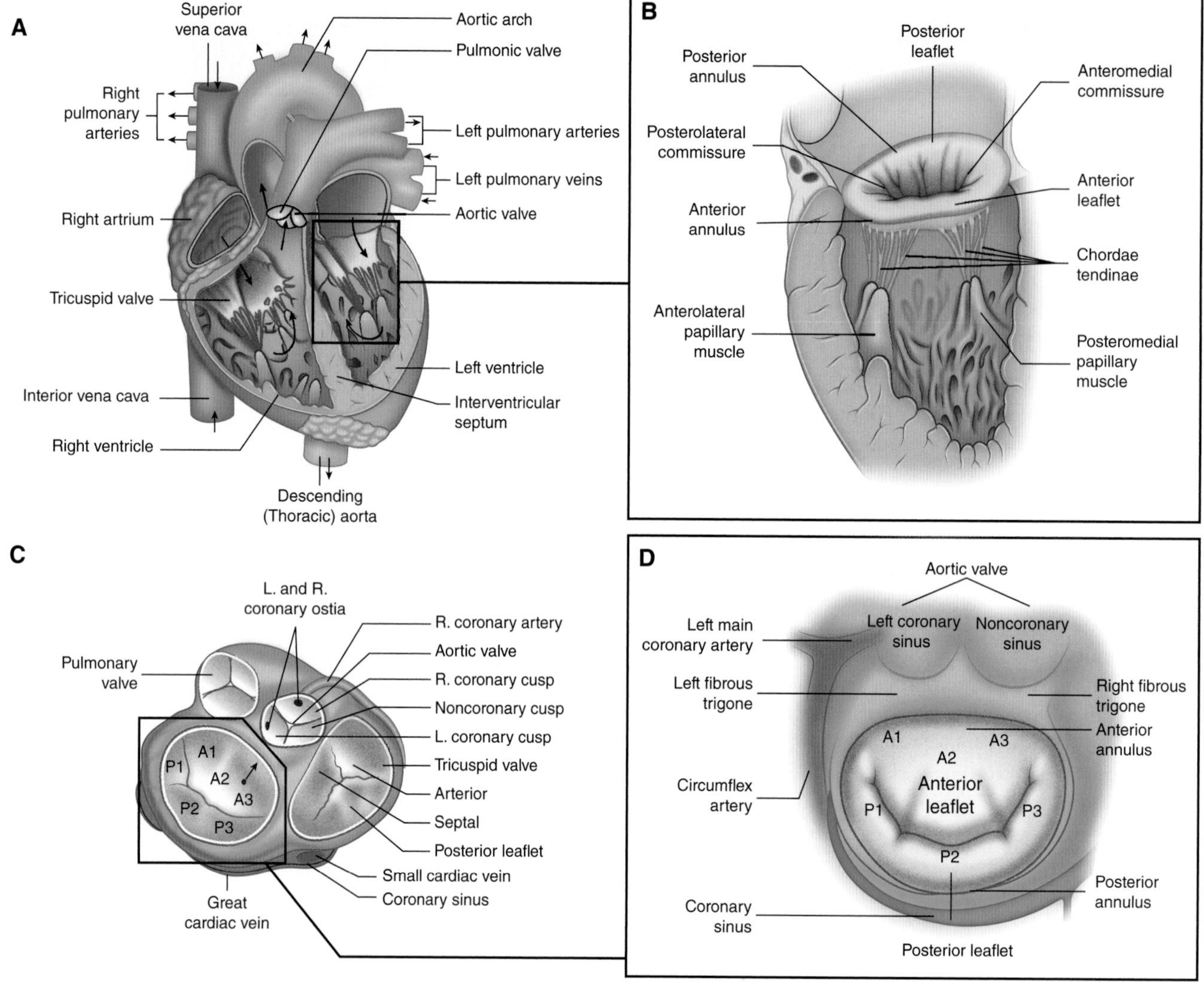

FIGURE 10.1 Highlighted anatomy of the mitral valve.

pergolide, etc) valve disease result in calcified and noncalcified fibrous plaques, respectively, and resultant restrictive valvulopathy.[9-11] Serotonin-receptor–related MV pathology has a characteristic short, stubby appearance of the mitral leaflets, which is pathognomonic.

Regardless of the mechanism of chronic degenerative MR, regurgitant flow into the LA increases LA pressure, which elevates pulmonary venous pressure and, if severe, causes pulmonary edema. Over time, the LA dilates to accommodate the regurgitant volume and decrease LA pressure. The increased LV end-diastolic volume (as a result of retrograde plus antegrade blood flow) precipitates eccentric hypertrophy of the LV to accommodate the larger stroke volumes and preserve antegrade flow (compensated chronic MR).[12] Over time, this LV volume overload results in contractile myofibril loss, reduced LV contractility, and chronic heart failure.[13] Avoiding or halting this natural history is the goal of treatment interventions.

Functional Mitral Regurgitation

Functional MR (eg, secondary MR) is related to disruptions of the supporting valve apparatus despite the presence of normal leaflet and chordae tissue. The most common cause of functional MR is a dilated LV (seen in both nonischemic cardiomyopathy and late compensatory manifestations of ischemic cardiomyopathies) with stretching of the mitral annulus.[4,6] Thus, functional MR can be viewed as a pathologic consequence of heart failure rather than the initial precipitant of heart failure, although they may be coincident or intertwined. Ischemic heart disease that causes focal infarcts of the LV papillary muscles can also lead to functional MR resulting from restriction of this subvalvular mitral component. Papillary muscle dysfunction can occur acutely with myocardial ischemia, leading to acute MR, or as a component of chronic ischemic heart disease and result in chronic MR. Dilated cardiomyopathy of the LA is similarly thought to cause functional MR, although isolated dilated atrial cardiomyopathy is much less common and typically occurs in concert with other left heart structural pathology.[1]

Mitral Stenosis

MS is rarely congenital; but when it occurs, it may be supravalvular, subvalvular, or due to leaflet narrowing in association with other left heart congenital lesions.

Most commonly, MS is due to rheumatic fever, with the reduced orifice area caused by restricted leaflet excursion. Rheumatic carditis manifests with characteristic inflammatory Aschoff nodules and thickening of the valvular and subvalvular components, which subsequently leads to reduced leaflet mobility and fusion of leaflet commissures.[14]

Severe mitral annular calcification (MAC) or subvalvular calcification can also reduce the orifice area of the MV apparatus. Bulky calcific buildup along the circumference of the valve annulus can lead to concentric narrowing of the valve area, whereas calcific deposits of the valve structures can restrict leaflet mobility and excursion, which further reduces the mitral orifice.[7]

CLINICAL PRESENTATION

Common Signs and Symptoms

Mitral Regurgitation

Owing to the pathophysiologic changes described earlier, chronic MR results in LA and LV dilatation, pulmonary venous hypertension, heart failure, and arrhythmias. Patients commonly complain of typical heart failure symptoms: fatigue, dyspnea on exertion, orthopnea, chest discomfort, shortness of breath, and peripheral edema. Arrhythmias can provoke palpitations.

The characteristic blowing, holosystolic murmur is best heard at the LV apex (which may be displaced to the axilla), and may radiate to the axilla or left infrascapular area overlying the LA. Radiation of the murmur to the parasternal region can occur if valve pathology creates an anteriorly directed regurgitant jet. The murmur increases in intensity with maneuvers that increase afterload (eg, handgrip or arterial compression with blood pressure cuff) or preload (such as squatting). Murmur intensity does *not* correspond well to MR severity. The timing of the murmur in systole can vary depending on the MV pathology; with MV prolapse, the murmur is mid-late systolic, whereas an early systolic murmur is observed with functional MR. The mitral component of S1 is soft or absent. An S3 and low-pitch, soft diastolic flow murmur can be present from LA volume overload. Other physical examination findings consistent with heart failure may be present, including rales, jugular venous distension, pitting-dependent edema, and laterally displaced cardiac point of maximal impulse. A parasternal heave may be palpated if pulmonary hypertension is present. As with more advanced heart failure, ascites, hepatosplenomegaly, or cardiac wasting can occur.

Acute MR manifests as pulmonary edema and acute decompensation, and is usually due to valve destruction from endocarditis, ruptured or flail chordae from myxomatous MV prolapse, or papillary muscle dysfunction with active ischemia, or papillary muscle rupture following acute myocardial infarction. Acute MR generates a soft, short, early, systolic murmur as the systolic pressures in the noncompliant LA and LV equalize rapidly, halting regurgitant flow early and making auscultatory diagnosis difficult. Isolated right middle or upper lobe rales and lobar consolidation can be present when the regurgitant jet is directed at the right upper pulmonary vein with acute MR, although bilateral pulmonary edema is more common.[15]

Mitral Stenosis

Owing to the insidious progression of symptoms, patients often do not appreciate their slow decline in functional capacity. Patients may experience symptoms of dyspnea, orthopnea, pulmonary edema, and hemoptysis. With less blood flow across the stenotic valve, the LV is often small and underfilled, and can manifest as symptoms of hypotension or dizziness with exertion or standing up. Atrial arrhythmias, such as atrial fibrillation, from the dilated LA are common and are noted as palpitations or tachycardia. Lastly, thromboembolic phenomenon, including stroke or embolism to the coronary arteries or visceral organs, can be the sentinel event.

In developed countries, MS usually manifests two to three decades after an episode of acute rheumatic fever; hence, pregnancies are generally unaffected. However, in developing countries where rheumatic fever is endemic, individuals may experience multiple episodes of rheumatic fever, which accelerates the development of MS. In this situation, MS can be seen in the second and third decades of life, and often complicates pregnancy with resultant miscarriages, pulmonary edema, or death.

Auscultation for MS is best performed with the patient in the left lateral decubitus position to reveal the "opening snap" of the mitral leaflets, followed by a soft diastolic rumbling murmur and prominent S1 in the apical region. Irregular rhythms are common. Patients with pulmonary hypertension can have a prominent pulmonic component of the second heart sound, a right ventricular heave, and signs of right heart failure such as peripheral edema, hepatosplenomegaly, and ascites frequently in the absence of rales (unless acute decompensation).

Chest radiographs can show prominent pulmonary vasculature and LA enlargement, but pulmonary edema is less common because the pulmonary vessels have remodeled and are "protected" from any elevations in LA pressure unless in the setting of acute hemodynamic decompensation such as paroxysmal rapid atrial fibrillation. Electrocardiogram can reveal LA enlargement and atrial arrhythmias with an absence of LV hypertrophy.

Differential Diagnosis

When considering the differential diagnoses for etiologies of MV disease, special consideration should be paid to the acuity of symptom onset and a focused history of risk factors.

Mitral Regurgitation

Acute MR is most often from sudden rupture of a myxomatous chordae or leaflet segment, acute ischemia of the papillary muscle from coronary artery disease, postinfarction rupture of a papillary muscle, direct trauma, or bacterial endocarditis. Chronic primary MR is associated with myxomatous valve disease or MV prolapse, calcific degeneration, remote rheumatic fever, infectious or autoimmune endocarditis, papillary muscle dysfunction due to nonischemic cardiomyopathy, or prior inferolateral myocardial infarction. Secondary MR is usually due to LV dilation from any cause, mostly from ischemic or nonischemic cardiomyopathy

Mitral Stenosis

MS is predominantly from rheumatic MV disease. Rarely, it could be from lupus or autoimmune inflammation. In the elderly, calcific MV stenosis may be associated with MAC or hemodialysis-dependent end-stage renal disease. Congenital MS or parachute MV causing stenosis is rare. Similar presentations are rarely seen with flow-obstructing cardiac thrombus or cardiac tumor (ie, LA myxoma).

A careful history of rheumatic fever in childhood should be sought from family members who may remember the episode. Prolonged absence from school, frequent sore throats, tonsillectomy/adenoidectomy, multiple family members living in a small cloistered home, family members with frequent sore throats, and history of painful monthly penicillin injections are helpful clues to prior rheumatic fever.

DIAGNOSIS: MITRAL VALVE DISEASE

The diagnosis of MV disease and assessment of severity is now largely based on noninvasive imaging results. Echocardiography, magnetic resonance imaging (MRI), and computed tomography (CT) are used in the assessment of MV disease (see **Table 10.1**). Notably, the imaging criteria for diagnosis should incorporate multiple supportive findings to assess disease severity, not just one, because each measurement has its pitfalls for inaccuracy. For example, the diagnosis of MR should not rely on color Doppler findings alone, and the diagnosis of MS should not be based on planimetry or pressure half-time measurements alone. This approach of multiple complementary measurements is recommended. But, ultimately, clinical judgment utilizing history of present illness, imaging, and physical examination, is critical for providing optimal patient care.

Echocardiography

Echocardiographic imaging is the gold standard for diagnosis of MV disease, because it provides measurements of blood flow, pressure gradients, and anatomic visualization when used properly. It is most commonly performed via transthoracic views. Alternatively, a transesophageal echocardiogram (whereby the probe is advanced into the esophagus) provides an added advantage of imaging in close proximity to the MV given the anatomic approximation of the esophagus to the LA. The improved visualization of the MV with transesophageal echocardiogram is further enhanced by three-dimensional imaging. Exercise echocardiography is recommended when imaging at rest does not adequately assess the significance of a valvular lesion. Imaging with exercise demonstrates the hemodynamic consequences of MR and MS during exertion with elevated heart rate (shortened diastole) and increased flow, when the most symptoms are present.

Diagnostic criteria for MR and MS include qualitative, semiquantitative, and quantitative assessments summarized in **Tables 10.2 and 10.3** adapted from the American Society for Echocardiography and European Association of Echocardiography. The severity of MV disease is predominantly characterized by semiquantitative and quantitative flow measurements, whereas visualization of the MV apparatus and supporting structures is most critical to differentiating between degenerative or functional MR as well as mechanisms of MS. Coexisting pathology and differing hemodynamic states can impact the accuracy of each of these measurements and their assessment of severity of valve disease.[16] For example, reduced blood flow or LV diastolic dysfunction can affect transvalvular gradient assessments and accurate diagnosis. A commonly encountered scenario occurs when patients have severe MR on transthoracic echocardiogram while conscious and then undergo transesophageal echocardiogram for further study, wherein anesthesia decreases cardiac preload and systemic vascular afterload, and the MR severity is less than it is when awake. Another opportunity for underdiagnosis is seen with acute MR at a time where there has not been the progressive increase in pulmonary vascular resistance (seen with chronic MR), and there is unimpeded regurgitant flow such that the pressure gradient between the LV and LA equalizes so rapidly that Doppler and color-flow Doppler assessments appear very brief, thereby making it difficult to appreciate the hemodynamic severity. Owing to the interplay of various patient and technologic limitations, accurate diagnosis requires an experienced echocardiogram interpreter to reconcile multiple diagnostic criteria and comorbidities.

Certain echocardiographic findings are unique to specific mitral disease etiologies. Rheumatic MS classically includes a hockey stick shape to the anterior leaflet when viewed in the parasternal long axis during diastole.[17] This shape is due to the thickening of the leaflet and commissural fusion that creates a less mobile hinge point in the midpoint of the leaflet, creating this characteristic appearance. Ergotamine-induced valve disease, metastatic carcinoid heart disease, and fenfluramine-phentermine–associated heart disease share a common pathway of serotonin-mediated endocardial fibrosis. This creates the classic appearance of short, thick-valve leaflets with regurgitation. Although these three syndromes may not be fully distinguishable by echocardiogram alone, a focused history will establish the diagnosis.

Magnetic Resonance Imaging

Cardiac MRI is a useful additional method for evaluation of mitral disease, particularly for assessment of the severity of MR and mechanism of LV remodeling, myocardial viability, and myocardial scarring.[16] The benefits of MRI include evaluation of the entire heart without limitations in imaging windows or body habitus that occur with echocardiography. Accordingly, cardiac MRI may be more accurate than is echocardiography in quantifying the severity of MR.[17]

LV and right ventricular function, valve structure, and apparatus can be thoroughly evaluated. Regurgitation severity can be assessed via planimetry or, more accurately, via regurgitant volume using either the direct measurement of velocity-encoded sequences of the regurgitant jet or indirectly with easily obtained three-dimensional cardiac volume

TABLE 10.1 Recommended Diagnostic Imaging of Mitral Valve Disease

Imaging Modality	Main Imaging Tasks	Main Imaging Tasks in Specific Mitral Valve (MV) Disease				
		Mitral stenosis (MS)	Primary mitral regurgitation (MR)	Secondary mitral regurgitation (MR)	Paravalvular mitral leak (PVML)	Failed mitral bioprosthesis or annuloplasty (PVML)
TTE	• Primary imaging modality to define MV abnormality • Grading of MR and MS severity • Associated valve/heart disease • LV/A function • Hemodynamic consequences	• Rheumatic/nonrheumatic MS	• AML/PML prolapse	• Ischemic/non-ischemic MR	• Paravalvular vs valvular leak	• Confirm valvular MS or MR
2D/3D TEE	• Detailed assessment of MV pathology • Re-confirmation of MS/MR severity • Exclusion of thrombi/infective endocarditis/pericardial effusion • Exclusion of specific CI for the planned procedure	• Presence of commissural fusion/calcification • Annular dimensions • Exclusion of MR ≥ grade 2	• Exact localization and extent of the lesion(s) • Flail gap and width • Leaflet-to-annulus index • Annular dimensions • Calcification	• Coaptation depth/length • Annular dimensions • Calcification	• Localization, number, size and orientation of the leak(s) to the sewing ring/mechanical prosthesis	• Annular dimensions • Dimension of the bioprosthesis • Exclusion of PVML • Calcification
	Determination of morphological suitability for a specific transcatheter procedure	• PMBV • TMVR	• Edge-to-edge repair • Artificial chord implantation • TMVR	• Edge-to-edge repair • Indirect annuloplasty (CS) • Direct annuloplasty • TMVR	• Transcatheter PVML closure	• TMVR

(contineud)

TABLE 10.1 Recommended Diagnostic Imaging of Mitral Valve Disease (*contineud*)

Imaging Modality	Main Imaging Tasks	Main Imaging Tasks in Specific Mitral Valve (MV) Disease				
		Mitral stenosis (MS)	Primary mitral regurgitation (MR)	Secondary mitral regurgitation (MR)	Paravalvular mitral leak (PVML)	Failed mitral bioprosthesis or annuloplasty (PVML)
3D TEE Imaging Examples						
CT	• Annular dimensions • Localization and extent of calcification of structures of the MV apparatus • Anatomical relationship of target lesions to surrounding cardiac/extracardiac structures	• When a TMVR procedure is planned: • Annular dimensions • Distribution and extent of calcification • Aortomitral angle	When a TMVR procedure is planned: • Annular dimensions • Distribution and extent of calcification • Aortomitral angle	When a direct or indirect annuloplasty is planned: • Annular dimensions • Relationship of mitral annulus and LCx and CS • Distribution and extent of annular calcification	• Localization, number, size and orientation of the leak (s) to the sewing ring/ mechanical prosthesis • Determination of transapical puncture site	• Annular dimensions • Distribution and extent of calcification • Aortomitral angle
MRI	• Evaluation of chamber volumes and ejection fraction • Regurgitant volumes • Regional and global myocardial function		• MR grading when doubtful	• MR grading when doubtful	• MR grading when doubtful	

Reprinted from Wunderlich NC, Beigel R, Ho SY, et al. Imaging for Mitral Interventions: Methods and Efficacy. *JACC Cardiovasc Imaging.* 2018;11(6):872-901.

TABLE 10.2 ASE/EAE Criteria for Echocardiographic Evaluation of Mitral Regurgitation

	Mild	Moderate	Severe	
Structural Evaluation				
Valve morphology	Normal to mild leaflet abnormality	Normal to moderate leaflet abnormality or moderate tenting	Severe valve lesions: (primary: flail/perforation, ruptured papillary muscle, leaflet retraction Secondary: tending, poor coaptation)	
LA and LV size	Usually normal	Normal or mildly dilated	Dilated	
Qualitative Doppler Evaluation				
Color-flow jet area	Small, central, narrow, brief	Variable	Large central jet, eccentric wall-impinging jet	
Flow convergence	Not visible, small, transient	Intermediate in size and duration	Large throughout systole	
CWD jet	Faint, partial, parabolic	Dense but partial/parabolic	Holosystolic, dense, triangular	
Quantitative Evaluation:				
Vena contracta width (cm)	<0.3	Intermediate	>0.7	
Pulmonary vein flow	Systolic dominance	Normal or systolic blunting	Minimal to no systolic flow or systolic flow reversal	
Mitral inflow	A-wave dominant	Variable	E-wave dominant, high E-wave velocity (>1.2 m/s— ASE; >1.5 m/s—EAE)	
PWD TVI mitral/TVI aortic (EAE)	<1	Intermediate	>1.4	
EROA (cm^2)	<0.2	0.2-0.29	0.3-0.39	>0.4
RV (mL)	<30	30-44	45-59	>60
RF (%) (*ASE)	<30	30-39	40-49	>60

ASE, American Society of Echocardiography; CWD, continuous wave Doppler; EAE, European Association of Echocardiography; EROA, effective regurgitant orifice area; LA, left atrium; LV, left ventricle; PWD, pulse wave Doppler; RF, regurgitant fraction; RV, regurgitant volume; TVI, tissue velocity integral

Adapted from Zoghbi WA, Adams D, Bonow RO, et al. Recommendations for noninvasive evaluation of native valvular regurgitation: a report from the American Society of Echocardiography Developed in collaboration with the Society for Cardiovascular Magnetic Resonance. *J Am Soc Echocardiogr.* 2017;30(4):303-371. Copyright © 2017 by the American Society of Echocardiography. With permission.

measurement.[18] The regurgitant volume is calculated from measurements of LV stroke volume—derived from measurements of the LV end-diastolic and end-systolic volumes—crossing the aortic valve and comparison with LA volumes. The difference of LV stroke volume and stroke volume across the aortic valve is computed as the mitral regurgitant volume.[16]

The use of MRI in the evaluation of MS is directed at a thorough evaluation of the MV apparatus and degree of leaflet restriction and mobility. Calcium deposition within the leaflets and annulus can be appreciated, but this is best evaluated and characterized with CT. The degree of stenosis and calculation of valve area can be quantified via two methods using MRI: planimetry and pressure half-time. Pressure half-time has been shown to overestimate valve area when compared to echocardiography, whereas planimetry has a result more comparable to that of echocardiography, and thus is considered a more reliable means of evaluation.[18]

Unfortunately, MRI has its downsides, including less clarity with ferrous-containing devices/implants and measurements averaged over multiple cardiac cycles that can decrease momentary accuracy, especially with irregular arrhythmias or small/chaotic jets due to loss of temporal and spatial resolution.

Computed Tomography

CT provides a semiquantitative measure of flow, assessment of leaflet motion, and quantitation of chamber and annulus dimensions or surrounding structures. CT also plays a role in characterizing valve calcification, which is key in evaluating the appropriateness of transcatheter mitral valve repair (TMVr) or replacement devices. Valve calcification can also be a major hurdle to successful surgical valve intervention. For example, increasing degrees of MAC correlate with worse surgical outcomes, higher degrees of paravalvular leak, more reoperations, and higher incidence of conversion to MV replacement rather than repair.[19] Alternatively, performing transcatheter MV placement in the setting of MAC for patients with too little annular calcification is associated with a high risk of valve

TABLE 10.3 ASE/EAE Criteria for Echocardiographic Assessment of Valve Stenosis

ASE/EAE Criteria for Evaluation of Mitral Stenosis			**Mild**	**Moderate**	**Severe**
	Supportive				
	Mean PG (mm Hg)		<5	5-10	>10
	PAP (mm Hg)		<30	30-50	>50
	Specific				
	MVA (cm^2)		>1.5	1.0-1.5	<1
	MVA (cm^2) by ACC/AHA 2014		>1.5		<1.5
	Via: Planimetry (level I), PHT (level 1), continuity equation (level II), PISA (level II)				
	With HR 60 to 80 bpm in sinus rhythm				
Revised Echo Score for Evaluation of Mitral Balloon Valvuloplasty			**Low Risk**	**Intermediate Risk**	**High Risk**
	MVA <1 cm^2	2 points	0-3	5	6-11
	Maximum leaflet displacement <12 mm	3 points			
	Commissural area ratio >1.25	3 points			
	Subvalvular involvement: absent/mild vs thickened	3 points			
Wilkins Score for Echocardiographic Assessment of Mitral Valve Anatomy		**1**	**2**	**3**	**4**
	Leaflet mobility	Mobile	Mobile mid-base	Restricted	Immobile
	Leaflet thickening	1-4 mm	4-5 mm	5-8 mm	>8-10 mm
	Leaflet calcification	Single area	Scattered, leaflet margins	Extending brightness	Extensive, most of leaflet
	Subvalvular involvement	Minimal, below leaflets	Thickening, 1/3 of chordal length	Thickening extending to distal 1/3 chords	Extensive, all chordal structure
	Scoring: <8: optimal outcome and >12: poor outcome from percutaneous valvuloplasty				

ACC, American College of Cardiology; AHA, American Heart Association; ASE, American Society of Echocardiography; EAE, European Association of Echocardiography; HR, heart rate MVA, mitral valve area; PAP, pulmonary artery pressure; PG, pressure gradient; PHT, pressure half-time; PISA, proximal isovelocity surface area.
Data from Wunderlich NC, Beigel R, Ho SY, et al. Imaging for Mitral Interventions: Methods and Efficacy. JACC Cardiovasc Imaging 2018;11(6):872-901; Baumgartner H, Hung J, Bermejo J, et al. Echocardiographic assessment of valve stenosis: EAE/ASE recommendations for clinical practice. *J Am Soc Echocardiogr.* 2009;22(1): 1-23;quiz 101-102 and Wilkins GT, Weyman AE, Abascal VM, et al. Percutaneous balloon dilatation of the mitral valve: an analysis of echocardiographic variables related to outcome and the mechanism of dilatation. *Br Heart J.* 1988;60(4):299-308.

embolization.[20] Therefore, for both the evaluation of transcatheter and more traditional surgical interventions, CT is particularly valuable in characterizing valvular calcification to evaluate procedural candidacy.[20]

Positron Emission Tomography

Nuclear positron emission tomography (PET) uses fluorodeoxyglucose as a tracer for glucose utilization, which can quantify uptake in the myocardium and assess myocardial viability. Although PET does not have a direct role in the evaluation of MV disease, it can be used as a modality for risk stratification for patients requiring intervention for their mitral disease. PET allows for the evaluation and identification of viable myocardium, giving valuable insight into patients who may benefit from revascularization before MV surgery, leading to improved myocardial function and better opportunity for positive LV remodeling in the postoperative period.[21]

Cardiac Catheterization

Mitral Stenosis

The simultaneous, dual-catheter measurement of an LA-to-LV diastolic pressure difference should be regarded as gold standard for assessing transvalvular gradient. This method classically uses venous access to the right atrium and a transseptal needle to puncture across the interatrial septum to the LA, whereas a pigtail catheter is advanced retrograde to the LV from the arterial system and simultaneous pressure tracings are recorded. A common surrogate for LA pressure is pulmonary artery wedge pressure from venous access with a balloon-tipped catheter to compare to LV pressure because it does not incur the risks of transseptal puncture and provides similar results in most patients. Other configurations of catheter placement have been described, but, in essence, perform the same measurement. It is important to consider that increased diastolic flow across the MV (from high cardiac output or severe MR) can also increase the transvalvular pressure gradient and grading of MS.

One can calculate the MV area using the Gorlin equation, which is the product of diastolic flow, empirical constant, gravity acceleration, and the transvalvular pressure gradient.[22] This is practically simplified to the Hakki equation for quick estimations with close correlations.[23] Significant MR and tachycardia can skew the accuracy of this calculation.

Gorlin Equation[24]:

Mitral valve area = (Cardiac output/heart rate × diastolic filling period) / (37.7 × $\sqrt{\text{mean gradient}}$)

Simplified Gorlin equation (aka Hakki equation)[23]:

Mitral valve area = Cardiac output / $\sqrt{\text{mean gradient}}$

Mitral Regurgitation

During routine hemodynamic catheterization, the V-wave on pulmonary artery wedge pressure or LA pressure tracing provides an indication of MR presence, but cannot be used for direct quantification reliably and is subject to interference from other pathology. The Gorlin equation can also be used to calculate the effective regurgitant orifice area in MR, but rarely ever is in clinical catheterization laboratories, and instead MR is more commonly assessed with contrast ventriculography.[25]

Contrast ventriculogram is typically performed in right anterior oblique projection to best separate atrial, ventricular, and aortic silhouettes. The Sellers' criteria is used to semiquantify the degree of MR, and can be correlated to modern imaging quantification parameters, as given in **Table 10.4.**[26,27] Quantitative contrast ventriculography, whereby volume measurements are calculated from tracing chamber outlines on a ventriculogram, can be used to determine a regurgitant fraction of LV stroke volume, but this is rarely performed in standard cardiac catheterization laboratory procedures in lieu of echocardiography in the present day.

MANAGEMENT OF THE PATIENT WITH MITRAL VALVE DISEASE

Medical Approach: Mitral Regurgitation

Degenerative Mitral Regurgitation

There is minimal role for medical therapy to directly influence degenerative MR long-term outcomes. Negative inotropes can acutely worsen the heart failure of severe primary MR. Hypertension control is helpful with a focus on afterload reduction with medications with peripheral arterial vasodilators (angiotensin-converting enzyme inhibitors [ACEIs], angiotensin receptor blockers [ARBs], hydralazine, etc) because increased afterload worsens the severity of MR. Afterload reduction in normotensive patients is not helpful based on several clinical trials. In the case of MV prolapse, it is important to remember that reductions in LV dimensions (with reducing preload and/or afterload) can closer approximate the mitral annulus, allowing greater prolapse of myxomatous leaflets and worsen MV prolapse–related regurgitation.[28]

Patients with decompensated acute MR are tenuous and at high risk for mortality. Afterload reduction is used in an attempt to bridge patients to emergency surgical intervention. One may utilize peripheral arterial vasodilators if systemic blood pressure allows, but intra-aortic balloon pump may be necessary to lower afterload and maintain adequate mean arterial pressure, especially in hypotensive patients. Once again, careful consideration of the mechanism of MR is vital because afterload reductions can worsen mitral prolapse and MR for some patients.

Functional Mitral Regurgitation

Unlike degenerative MR, medical therapy is paramount to the treatment of patients with functional MR, and can significantly influence outcomes. Given that functional MR is largely due to underlying cardiomyopathy, guideline-directed heart failure therapy is indicated for those with ventricular cardiomyopathy. The mainstays of therapy for heart failure with reduced LV ejection fraction is discussed in more detail

TABLE 10.4 Sellers' Criteria for Mitral Regurgitation Assessment with Contrast Ventriculography

Severity	Contrast Opacification of Left Atrium	Estimated Regurgitant Fraction (%)
1+	Faint opacification of the left atrium with clearing of the contrast during each beat	<30
2+	Opacification of the atrium that does not clear, but is not as dense as the left ventricle	30-39
3+	Opacification of the atrium with the same density as the ventricle	40-49
4+	Immediate, dense, opacification of the atrium with filling of the pulmonary veins	≥50

Data from Sellers RD, Levy MJ, Amplatz K, et al. Left retrograde cardioangiography in acquired cardiac disease: technic, indications and interpretations in 700 Cases. *Am J Cardiol.* 1964;14:437-447.

elsewhere, but focuses on long-term neurohormonal blockade (beta-blockers, ACEIs, ARBs, aldosterone antagonists, and neprilysin inhibition), long-acting nitrates (isosorbide dinitrate), vasodilators (hydralazine), diuretics, and cardiac resynchronization therapy with biventricular pacemakers[28] (see **Table 10.5**). These heart failure therapies frequently reduce the severity of MR and ameliorate symptoms in patients with functional MR, often avoiding the need for valve procedures. Patients with functional MR must be treated with maximally tolerated heart failure therapy, as mentioned earlier (for at least 3 months), and then the severity of their MR should be reassessed before they are considered for surgical or transcatheter intervention.[29,30]

Medical Approach: Mitral Stenosis

Once MS is suspected or diagnosed, these patients should be closely followed up clinically and with transthoracic echocardiography at regular intervals[28,31] (**Algorithm 10.1**). As per the American College of Cardiology/American Heart Association (ACC/AHA) guidelines, for mild MS (MV area >1.5 cm^2), echocardiography should be performed every 3 to 5 years, for moderate MS (MV area 1.0-1.5 cm^2) every 1 to 2 years, and for severe MS (MV area <1.0 cm^2) every year. It should be done more frequently if there is coexistent MR or other valve disease and in pregnancy.[28]

Heart Rate Control/Prevention of Tachycardia

Lower heart rates increase diastolic filling time and decrease mean transmitral gradient, improving hemodynamics and symptoms (**Table 10.4**). Beta-blockers are the drugs of choice for slowing the heart rate in MS. Other atrioventricular nodal blockers such as non-dihydropyridine calcium channel blockers and digoxin can also be used or added to the regimen.

TABLE 10.5 Commonly Used Medications in Mitral Valve Disease

Mitral Stenosis	
Control of Heart Rate	Beta-blockers Non-dihydropyridine calcium channel blockers Digoxin
Treatment of Pulmonary Congestion	Diuretics
	Nitrates
	Morphine
	Oxygen
Management of Thromboembolism	Warfarin
Functional Mitral Regurgitation	
Systolic Heart Failure	Angiotensin-converting enzyme inhibitors
	Angiotensin receptor blockers
	Beta-blockers
	Aldosterone antagonists
	Neprilysin inhibitors
Afterload Reduction	Peripheral arterial vasodilators (eg, hydralazine)

Control of Pulmonary Congestion

Diuretics can relieve edema. Nitrates, oxygen, and morphine cause pulmonary venodilation and rapidly relieve pulmonary congestion.

Management of Thromboembolism

Rheumatic MS with atrial fibrillation makes one highly vulnerable to LA clot formation and embolic events because of the tissue inflammation (if active rheumatism) and blood stasis from obstruction of outflow and lack of atrial contractility. This risk cannot be estimated by the CHADS or CHA$_2$DS$_2$-VASC score, which is used for nonvalvular atrial fibrillation and requires therapeutic anticoagulation for thromboembolic risk reduction. Warfarin for anticoagulation is recommended. Thromboembolism is a common complication in up to a third of patients with MS, and the risk is significantly increased with atrial fibrillation. Warfarin is the only approved oral anticoagulant in "valvular" (rheumatic) MS. Heparin and enoxaparin can be used in acute situations and in pregnancy (see **Table 10.5**). LA appendage closure is not approved for use in valvular MS because the intra-atrial thrombus is thought to be less isolated to the appendage than is nonvalvular atrial fibrillation, and it has not been adequately studied in this population.

Management of Pregnancy

Preconceptual risk stratification and intervention is very important to prevent pulmonary edema and complications of MV disease in pregnancy. In patients with moderate or severe MS, the pregnancy-associated increase in intravascular volume can lead to pulmonary edema, adverse outcome of the pregnancy, or maternal death. Medical management is otherwise similar as in nonpregnant patients except for the avoidance of warfarin anticoagulation during the embryogenetic period. When feasible, percutaneous mitral valvuloplasty is the procedure of choice for relieving intractable symptoms and can be done with adequate radiation protection to the fetus in the second or third trimester of pregnancy.

Percutaneous Transcatheter Interventions

Mitral Regurgitation

Mitral Valve Repair. TMVr has become the second most common percutaneous treatment of valvular heart disease, with the MitraClip now having been used in over 100,000 patients worldwide as of 2020.[32] The MitraClip device was developed in emulation of the Alfieri stitch technique, whereby the anterior and posterior leaflet tips are joined together to create a double-orifice MV.[33]

The MitraClip has been studied in various populations compared to medical therapy with several large randomized trials (see **Table 10.6**) for treatment of both degenerative and functional MR. Trials have shown this device therapy to be a very useful alternative to surgical intervention and superior to medical therapy alone when used in patients with appropriate anatomy.

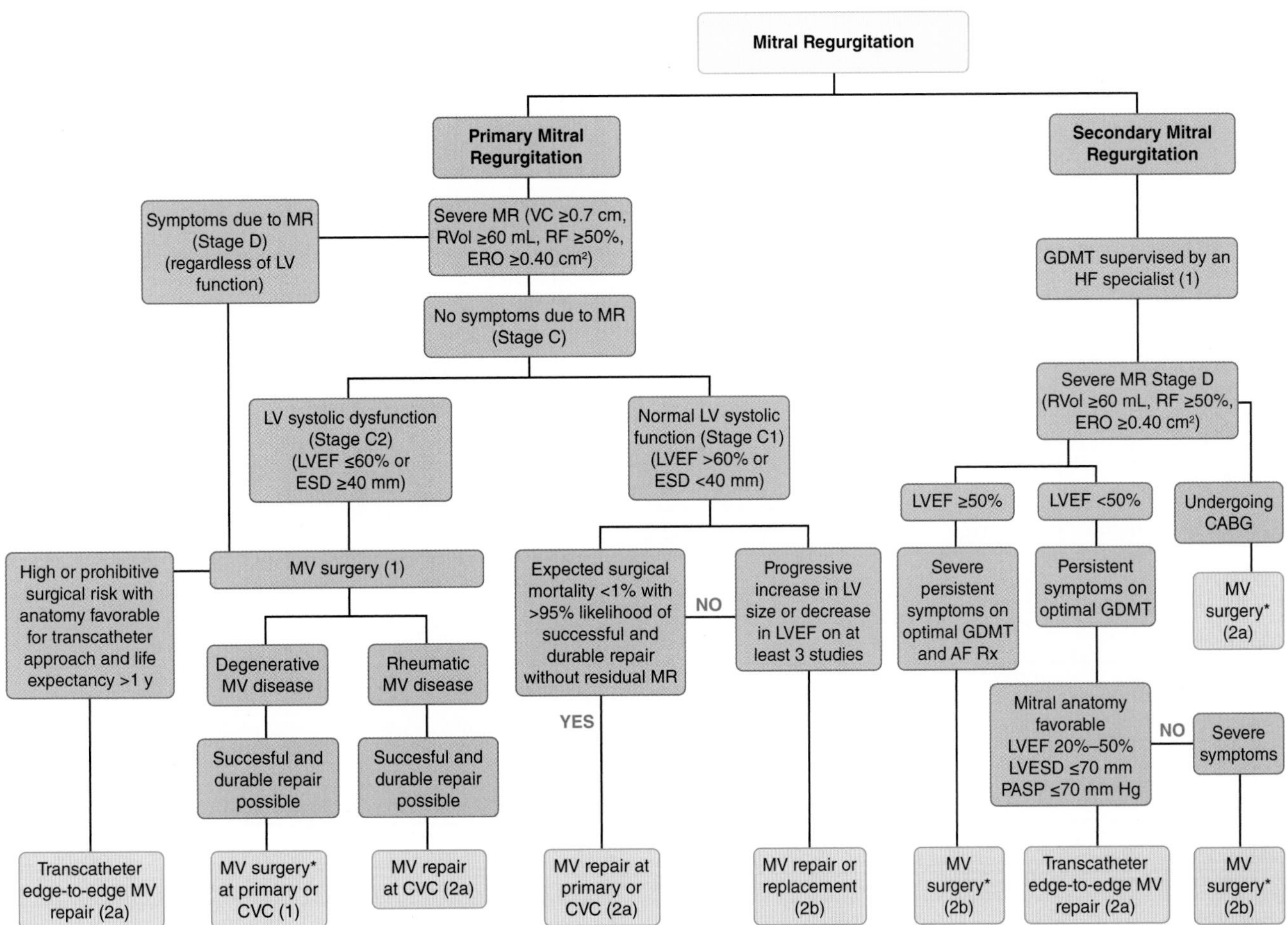

AF, atrial fibrillation; CABG, coronary artery bypass graft; CVC, Comprehensive Valve Center; ERO, effective regurgitant office; ESD, end-systolic dimension; GDMT, guideline-directed medical therapy; HF, heart failure; LVEF, ejection fraction; MR, mitral regurgitation; MV, mitral valve; MVR, mitral valve replacement; PA, pulmonary artery; RF, regurgitant fraction; RVol, regurgitant volume; Rx, treatment; VC, vena contracta

ALGORITHM 10.1 Practical approach to mitral regurgitation treatment. Reprinted from Otto CM, Nishimura RA, Bonow RO, et al. 2021. 2020 ACC/AHA guideline for the management of patients with valvular heart disease: executive summary: a report of the American College of Cardiology/American Heart Association Joint Committee on clinical practice guidelines. *Circulation.* 143(5):e35-e71.

Landmark trials of degenerative MR include the EVEREST (Endovascular Valve Edge-to-Edge REpair STudy) and EVEREST II trials that showed the MitraClip to be a safe and effective device treatment for symptomatic severe or moderate-severe degenerative MR in patients considered to have unfavorable risks for traditional MV surgery.[34-36] Significant and durable reductions in MR and major adverse events were noted compared to surgery.

Arguably, the patient population who could benefit most from a safe, minimally invasive corrective procedure is a group with functional MR, those who have not been shown to derive benefit from surgical repair; this is the population studied in the COAPT (Cardiovascular Outcomes Assessment of the MitraClip Percutaneous Therapy) and MITRA-FR trials (see **Table 10.6**).[29,37] In these trials, patients with disproportionately more severe MR as compared to their degree of LV dysfunction (ie, less dilated LV) were more likely to benefit than were patients with severe LV dilatation,[38,39] with a reduction in heart failure hospitalizations and all-cause death at 24 months compared to goal-directed medical therapy alone (hazard ratios of 0.53 and 0.81, respectively).[29] This major advance for the treatment of MR, particularly functional MR, is the new benchmark for TMVr.

Mitral Valve Replacement. Transcatheter mitral valve replacement (TMVR) is another therapy in the growing armamentarium of minimally invasive transcatheter therapies. Many devices are in development, but currently only two are commercially available: the Tendyne™ (Abbott, Chicago IL) and Sapien (Edwards Lifesciences, Irvine CA) balloon-expandable valve systems, with the latter utilizing the third-generation transcatheter valve approved for aortic use. Both provide valve replacement with bioprosthetic leaflets anchored inside of the patient's preexisting MV annulus, thereby pushing the native mitral leaflets to the perimeter. They are placed with fluoroscopic and echocardiographic guidance and can forgo cardiopulmonary bypass. TMVR systems present more challenges than do

TABLE 10.6 Pivotal Trials in Transcatheter Edge-to-Edge Mitral Valve Repair With MitraClip

	COAPT		MITRA-FR		EVEREST II	
	Device	**GDMT**	**Device**	**GDMT**	**Device**	**Surgery**
Populations						
Total patients (*n*)	302	312	152	152	184	95
Age (years)	71.7	72.8	70.1	70.6	67.3	65.7
Gender, male (%)	66.6	61.5	78.9	77	62	66
AF (%)	57.3	53.2	34.5	32.7	34	39
EF (%)	31.3 ± 9.1	31.3 ± 9.6	33.3	32.9	60	60.6
RV (mL)			45 ± 13	45 ± 14	42 ± 23.3	45.2 ± 26.6
EROA (mm^2)	41 ± 15	40 ± 15	31 ± 10	31 ± 11	56 ± 38	59 ± 35
LVES dimension (cm)	5.3 ± 0.9	5.3 ± 0.9				
LVED volume (mL) / (mL/m^2)[a]	194.4 ± 69.2	191.0 ± 72.9	136.2 ± 37.4	134.5 ± 33.1		
MV dysfunction						
Degenerative %	0	0	0	0	74	72
Functional %	100	100	100	100	27	27
Follow-up						
Duration of follow-up	12, 24 months		12 months		30 days, 12 months, 24 months	
Outcomes (%)						
1-year mortality	19.1	23.2	24.2	22.4	6	6
1-year HF hospitalization	35.8[a]	67.9[a]	48.7	47.4		
1-year mortality + HF hospitalization:	33.9	46.5	54.6[a]	51.3[a]		
12 months MR <2 +	94.8	46.9			82	96
24 months MR <2 +	99.1	43.4			80	78
LVED volume, change (mL)	−1.1 ± 67.4	18.6 ± 74.6	−2	7	−25.3 ± 28.3	−40.2 ± 35.9
12 months efficacy (freedom from death, surgery, >2 + MR)					55[a]	73[a]
24 months efficacy (freedom from death, surgery, >2 + MR)					52[a]	66[a]
30-day MAE					15[a]	48[a]

AF, atrial fibrillation; COAPT, Cardiovascular Outcomes Assessment of the MitraClip Percutaneous Therapy; EF, ejection fraction; EROA, effective regurgitant orifice area; EVEREST, Endovascular Valve Edge-to-Edge REpair Study; GDMT, guideline-directed medical therapy; HF, heart failure; LVES, left ventricular end systolic; LVED, left ventricular end diastolic; MAE, major adverse event; MR, mitral regurgitation; RV, regurgitant volume.
[a]Primary outcome for trial.

transcatheter aortic valve replacement technologies because of differing anatomic and pathologic considerations.

The Tendyne system is a transapical MV replacement system placed via limited thoracotomy access and cardiotomy near the apex of the heart. It is anchored at the mitral annulus and tethered to the LV apical insertion site. It received the CE ("Conformité Européene," which literally means "European Conformity") mark in 2020, is available for commercial use in Europe for the indication of treatment for native valve MR, and is in clinical trials in the United States.

The Sapien valve can perform TMVR either from a transapical approach (similar to Tendyne) or from a transseptal approach, whereby the delivery system is advanced from the femoral vein across the interatrial septum to the LA and mitral annulus for implant. Because the Sapien valve is not designed to anchor to the mitral annulus, it is utilized in patients with a preexisting bioprosthesis (ie, commercially approved for the indication of "valve-in-valve" TMVR). In addition, there is published experience using this system for "valve-in-annuloplasty ring" implantation and "valve-in-mitral annular calcification" TMVR, with success rates highly dependent on the landing zone and patient anatomy.[40]

Paravalvular Leak Closure. One of the challenges seen with TMVR is paravalvular leak. This can occur when the transcatheter valve implant makes irregular contact with the native (or preexisting bioprosthesis) mitral annulus or lands off plane to the native annulus plane, revealing an area of contact gaps. The consequences of paravalvular leak are often similar to those of valvular MR, but also may include intravascular hemolysis due to the shearing forces on blood moving through the small paravalvular orifice with high pressure and velocity.

Transcatheter plugging of these paravalvular leaks can be achieved using self-expanding transcatheter vascular plugs, ductal occluders, and other devices. If a defect is due to active endocarditis or the defect is too large to be securely closed with a transcatheter device, surgical repair should be considered.[41,42]

Mitral Stenosis

See **Algorithm 10.2** Indications for Rheumatic Mitral Stenosis Intervention.

Balloon Valvuloplasty. In appropriate patients with an MV apparatus conducive to commissurotomy, percutaneous mitral valve commissurotomy (PTMC) is the treatment of choice for relieving the MV gradient and symptoms of MS.28,42 Patients with moderate to severe MS, with or without symptoms, may be candidates for PTMC.

Valve structure must be assessed to ensure conduciveness to commissurotomy. The Wilkins score assesses degree of leaflet rigidity, severity of leaflet thickening, amount of leaflet calcification, and extent of subvalvular thickening to predict success of PTMC,[43] with lower scores (<8) generally portending a favorable result with PTMC.[43] In addition, patients should not have any contraindications to commissurotomy, such as the presence of more than mild MR and LA thrombus. If the patient has another clear indication for cardiac surgery (coronary bypass surgery, other valve lesions needing surgery, etc), then PTMC should not be considered.

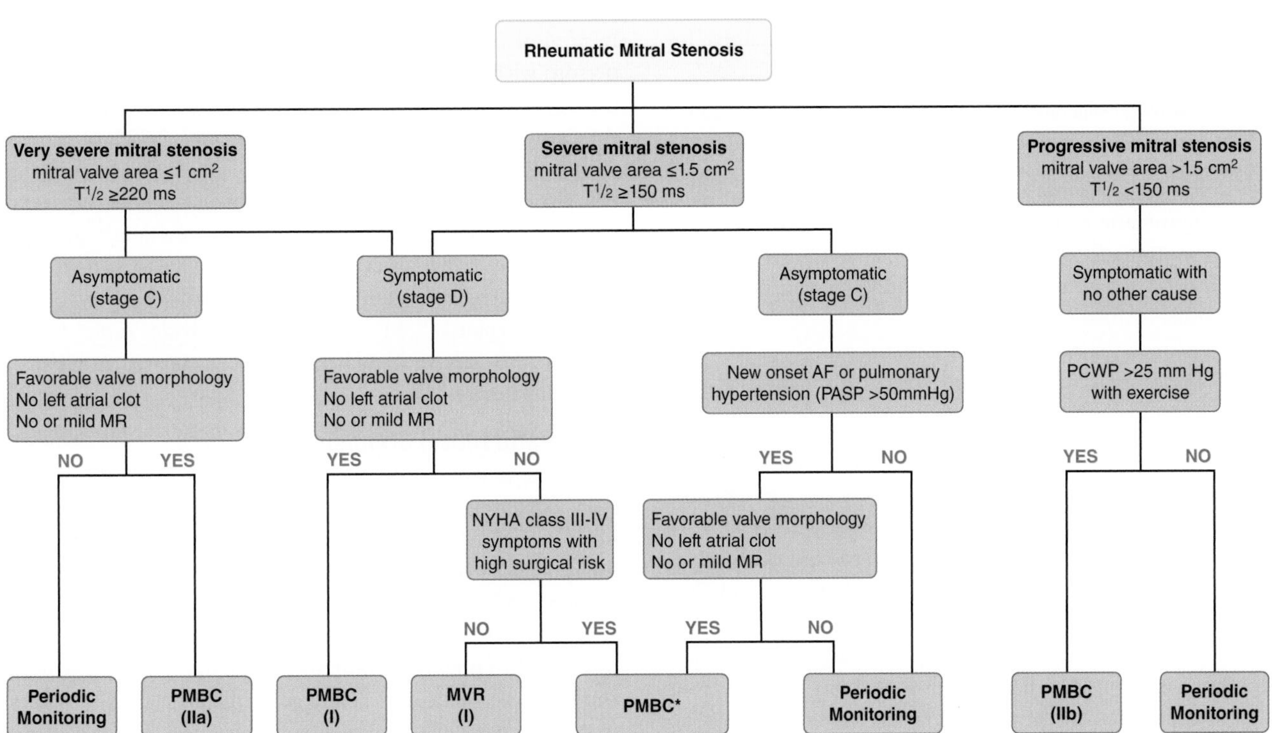

ALGORITHM 10.2 Indications for rheumatic mitral stenosis intervention. Reprinted with permission from Otto CM, Nishimura RA, Bonow RO, et al. 2021. 2020 ACC/AHA guideline for the management of patients with valvular heart disease: executive summary: a report of the American College of Cardiology/American Heart Association Joint Committee on clinical practice guidelines. *Circulation.* 143(5):e35-e71.

PTMC is generally done safely with the Inoue balloon. With experienced operators, a double-balloon technique may also give excellent results.

Mitral Valve Surgery. MV surgery—commissurotomy, repair, or replacement—is the procedure of choice in symptomatic patients with moderate to severe MS who cannot be treated with PTMC, are predicted to have a poor result with PTMC (ie, those with a Wilkins score >12), or have additional conditions (ie, coronary artery disease, aortic stenosis, etc) that would benefit from surgery.

Surgical Approach

The distinction between "surgical" and "percutaneous" treatment of MV disease is blurring progressively as technology advances toward less invasive devices and the personnel (cardiac surgeons and interventional cardiologists) train in hybrid techniques and skills. Certain techniques are performed almost entirely through catheters or endoscopes by surgeons, whereas other catheter-based techniques that involve thoracotomy access are predominantly executed by interventional cardiologists. Accordingly, an MV intervention that can *only* be performed by a trained "cardiac surgeon," and is outside the scope of practice of an interventional cardiologist, is the definition of "surgical" mitral intervention utilized here.

Surgery for Mitral Regurgitation

The success and recommendations for MV surgery differ for degenerative and functional MR.

Degenerative Mitral Regurgitation. Persons primarily indicated for MV surgery include those who have severe MR, besides the following[30,42]:

1. Symptomatic with or without LV systolic dysfunction
2. Asymptomatic with mild or moderate LV systolic dysfunction or dilatation (progressive dilation and/or LV end-systolic diameter ≥40 mm)
3. Due for cardiac surgery for another reason
4. Asymptomatic with new-onset atrial fibrillation or pulmonary hypertension

MV surgery is discouraged in patients with severe, chronic MR and LV ejection fraction <30%—they have a high surgical mortality and are unlikely to experience symptom improvement—unless they are refractory to medical therapy, the pathology is highly amenable to durable repair, and they have low comorbidities.

Alternatively, patients with high surgical risk and appropriate anatomy should be considered for percutaneous edge-to-edge repair (ie, MitraClip) rather than for surgery.[30,42]

Unlike chronic degenerative MR, acute MR almost uniformly is symptomatic, and is poorly tolerated by patients. Compensatory physiologic changes (ie, LA enlargement, LV remodeling, pulmonary vascular remodeling) mount over time in patients with chronic progressive MR, whereas these do not occur with sudden acute MR, and the resultant acute heart failure can be profound. In these cases, patients warrant urgent surgical intervention to halt progressive heart failure and death.

Mitral Valve Repair and Replacement

MV repair is preferred over replacement whenever possible to preserve the valve apparatus' geometric support of LV function.[44] MV repair can commonly involve (1) an annuloplasty ring to concentrically tighten the annular perimeter; (2) quadrangular resection and approximation of leaflet tissue; and/or (3) repair of chordae tendinae attachments. Compared to valve replacement, repair of chronic degenerative MR is associated with better postoperative LV function and mortality.[45] Maintenance of the chordal attachment is recommended over excision to maintain LV function and obtain better postoperative outcomes.[46] It is recommended that patients undergo MV surgery at a heart valve center of excellence—where the expected mortality rate of repair is typically <1% with experienced surgeons—to achieve best outcomes.[28]

When MV replacement is performed, either a mechanical or bioprosthetic valve may be used. Although mechanical valves require lifelong anticoagulation that incurs bleeding risks, their durability is superior—often lasting lifelong—whereas bioprosthetic valves typically degenerate 10 to 20 years post the implant.

Surgery for Functional Mitral Regurgitation

Surgical intervention for functional MR is not viewed as favorably as it is for degenerative MR. Because functional MR is a secondary consequence of cardiomyopathy, goal-directed medical therapy for heart failure is usually more effective than is surgical intervention in treating this condition. Although persons with symptomatic severe MR despite optimal medical therapy for heart failure can be considered for MV surgery, the significant morbidity and overall poor prognosis of patients with heart failure and secondary MR outweighs the potential benefits of surgical MR reduction in most patients.[28,42] In patients with ischemic cardiomyopathy and moderate or severe MR, randomized trials of coronary artery bypass surgery with and without concomitant MV repair did not show benefit with MV repair.[47,48] MV replacement provides more durable reduction in MR and less heart failure compared to repair in secondary severe MR.[47]

Rheumatic Mitral Stenosis

For patients with severe rheumatic MS not amenable to balloon valvuloplasty and acceptable surgical risk, MV replacement is indicated (**Algorithm 10.2**).[39,42] MV repair is not useful in such patients because it leads to poor outcomes. Although surgical commissurotomy was widely used in appropriately selected individuals, percutaneous balloon valvuloplasty was found to provide a similarly good commissurotomy result and durability in those with favorable features (eg, low Wilkins score). Accordingly, surgical commissurotomy is now confined to patients who do not have access to percutaneous balloon valvuloplasty (ie, those living in developing countries).

Degenerative (Nonrheumatic) Mitral Stenosis

The most common manifestation of nonrheumatic degenerative MS is MAC rather than adhesive commissural fusion (as in rheumatic disease). Accordingly, balloon commissurotomy is not an effective treatment: MV replacement is the only available treatment.[42] MV replacement and calcium debridement is often a high-risk surgery given the risk of annular perforation with debridement, difficulty securing the mitral prosthesis into place, and risk of paravalvular leak. There is growing experience with Sapien transcatheter valve replacement in patients with MAC, where the valve is placed percutaneously or with hybrid surgical technique. This may be a reasonable approach in severely symptomatic patients at prohibitive risk for standard MV replacement.[40]

FOLLOW-UP PATIENT CARE

Patients with either MR or MS should undergo routine follow-up with a physician familiar with the treatment of valvular heart disease, particularly when the disease is moderate or severe. The frequency of follow-up before procedural intervention should increase as the severity of MV disease increases for optimization of medical therapy and in anticipation of intervention when appropriate. Follow-up surveillance every couple of years is appropriate for patients with mild MR or MS, whereas patients with severe disease should be seen every few months for serial history, physical examination, and echocardiographic imaging to assess for worsening heart failure, arrhythmia, pulmonary hypertension, and complications.[28,30,42]

RESEARCH AND FUTURE DIRECTIONS

Innovation is predominantly focused on the development and study of transcatheter mitral therapies, and mostly for MR at this time. These therapies include an array of devices tailored to address the different components or mechanisms of MV disease to accomplish annuloplasty, ventriculoplasty, leaflet repair/modifiers, chordae tendinae replacement, and valve replacement devices. They may be delivered via transthoracic access (using thoracotomy) or transvenous (often crossing the interatrial septum similar to a MitraClip system approach). To date, only a handful of these devices have been used in humans or undergone clinical trials. The challenges for these therapies include the relatively large size of the MV, its three-dimensional saddle shape, subvalvular apparati, potential for obstruction of the LV outflow tract, and variations in annular shape/size/calcified surface. Expanded indications for use of existing technologies are also expected. For example, there is ongoing investigation regarding the use of the Tendyne valve system in persons with severe MAC and MR or MS.[49] Overcoming the inherent challenges will require iterative improvements in imaging, engineering, procedural technique, and patient selection.

KEY POINTS

- ✔ Mitral Stenosis
- ✔ The transvalvular gradient in MS is dependent on the heart rate. Slowing the heart rate with medications improves LV diastolic filling and symptoms.
- ✔ Patients with MS have pulmonary edema without LV failure, and they tolerate beta-blockers well.
- ✔ Exercise echocardiogram should be used to assess MV gradients and pulmonary pressure in response to exercise in indeterminate cases.
- ✔ Warfarin is the only approved long-term anticoagulant for atrial fibrillation or systemic thromboembolism with MS/MR.
- ✔ Degenerative MR is a primary valve issue, whereas functional MR is a result of cardiomyopathy.
- ✔ Degenerative MR does not improve without surgical or transcatheter valve intervention, whereas functional MR often improves with guideline-directed heart failure medical therapy.
- ✔ Signs and symptoms of MR vary significantly depending on acuity of onset.
- ✔ Treatment of severe MR is best performed with joint consultation of interventional cardiologists and cardiac surgeons highly experienced in MV intervention.

REFERENCES

1. Ho SY. Anatomy of the mitral valve. *Heart.* 2002;88(suppl 4):iv5-iv10.
2. Singh JP, Evans JC, Levy D, et al. Prevalence and clinical determinants of mitral, tricuspid, and aortic regurgitation (the Framingham Heart Study). *Am J Cardiol.* 1999;83(6):897-902.
3. Li J, Pan W, Yin Y, Cheng L, Shu X. Prevalence and correlates of mitral regurgitation in the current era: an echocardiography study of a Chinese patient population. *Acta Cardiol.* 2016;71(1):55-60.
4. Nkomo VT, Gardin JM, Skelton TN, Gottdiener JS, Scott CG, Enriquez-Sarano M. Burden of valvular heart diseases: a population-based study. *Lancet.* 2006;368(9540):1005-1111.
5. Remenyi B, Gentles TL. Congenital mitral valve lesions: correlation between morphology and imaging. *Ann Pediatr Cardiol.* 2012;5(1):3-12.
6. Coffey S, Cairns BJ, Iung B. The modern epidemiology of heart valve disease. *Heart.* 2016;102(1):75-85.
7. Abramowitz Y, Jilaihawi H, Chakravarty T, Mack MJ, Makkar RR. Mitral annulus calcification. *J Am Coll Cardiol.* 2015;66(17):1934-1941.
8. Zuily S, Regnault V, Selton-Suty C, et al. Increased risk for heart valve disease associated with antiphospholipid antibodies in patients with systemic lupus erythematosus. *Circ J.* 2011;124(2):215-224.
9. Schade R, Andersohn F, Suissa S, Haverkamp W, Garbe E. Dopamine agonists and the risk of cardiac-valve regurgitation. *N Engl J Med.* 2007;356(1):29-38.
10. Zanettini R, Antonini A, Gatto G, Gentile R, Tesei S, Pezzoli G. Valvular heart disease and the use of dopamine agonists for Parkinson's disease. *N Engl J Med.* 2007;356(1):39-46.
11. Nadlonek NA, Weyant MJ, Yu JA, et al. Radiation induces osteogenesis in human aortic valve interstitial cells. *J Thorac Cardiovas Surg.* 2012;144(6):1466-1470.
12. Carabello BA. Mitral valve regurgitation. *Curr Probl Cardiol.* 1998;23(4):202-241.
13. Mulieri LA, Leavitt BJ, Ittleman FP, et al. Forskolin reverses the force-frequency defect in left ventricular subepicardium (EPI) but not in papillary myocardium (PAP) in human mitral regurgitation heart failure. *Circ J.* 1993;88(suppl 1):406.
14. Aschoff L. The Rheumatic nodules in the heart. *Ann Rheum Dis.* 1939;1(3):161-166.
15. Alarcón JJ, Guembe P, De Miguel E, Gordillo I, Abellás A. Localized right upper lobe edema. *Chest J.* 1995;107(1):274-276.
16. Zoghbi WA, Asch FM, Bruce C, et al. Guidelines for the evaluation of valvular regurgitation after percutaneous valve repair or replacement: A report from the American society of echocardiography developed in

collaboration with the Society for Cardiovascular Angiography and interventions, Japanese Society of Echocardiography, and Society for Cardiovascular Magnetic Resonance. *J Am Soc Echocardiogr.* 2019;32(4):431-475.
17. Bach DS. Images in clinical medicine. Rheumatic mitral stenosis. *N Engl J Med.* 1997;337(1):31.
18. Cawley PJ, Maki JH, Otto CM. Cardiovascular magnetic resonance imaging for valvular heart disease: technique and validation. *Circ J.* 2009;119(3):468-478.
19. Tomsic A, Hiemstra YL, van Brakel TJ, et al. Outcomes of valve repair for degenerative disease in patients with mitral annular calcification. *Ann Thorac Surg.* 2019;107(4):1195-1201.
20. Eleid MF, Foley TA, Said SM, Pislaru SV, Rihal CS. Severe mitral annular calcification. *JACC Cardiovasc Imag.* 2016;9(11):1318-1337.
21. Capoulade R, Piriou N, Serfaty JM, Le Tourneau T. Multimodality imaging assessment of mitral valve anatomy in planning for mitral valve repair in secondary mitral regurgitation. *J Thorac Dis.* 2017;9(suppl 7):S640-S660.
22. Gorlin R, Gorlin SG. Hydraulic formula for calculation of the area of the stenotic mitral valve, other cardiac valves, and central circulatory shunts. I. *Am Heart J.* 1951;41(1):1-29.
23. Hakki AH, Iskandrian AS, Bemis CE, et al. A simplified valve formula for the calculation of stenotic cardiac valve areas. *Circ J.* 1981;63(5):1050-1055.
24. Gorlin WB, Gorlin R. A generalized formulation of the Gorlin formula for calculating the area of the stenotic mitral valve and other stenotic cardiac valves. *J Am Coll Cardiol.* 1990;15(1):246-247.
25. Grayburn PA. Vasodilator therapy for chronic aortic and mitral regurgitation. *Am J Med Sci.* 2000;320(3):202-208.
26. Sellers RD, Levy MJ, Amplatz K, Lillehei CW. Left retrograde cardioangiography in acquired cardiac disease: technic, indications and interpretations in 700 cases. *Am J Cardiol.* 1964;14:437-447.
27. Dujardin KS, Enriquez-Sarano M, Bailey KR, Nishimura RA, Seward JB, Tajik AJ. Grading of mitral regurgitation by quantitative Doppler echocardiography: calibration by left ventricular angiography in routine clinical practice. *Circ J.* 1997;96(10):3409-3415.
28. Nishimura RA, Otto CM, Bonow RO, et al. 2014 AHA/ACC guideline for the management of patients with valvular heart disease. *J Am Coll Cardiol.* 2014;63(22):e57-e185.
29. Stone GW, Lindenfeld J, Abraham WT, et al. Transcatheter mitral-valve repair in patients with heart failure. *N Engl J Med.* 2018;379(24):2307-2318.
30. Nishimura RA, Otto CM, Bonow RO, et al. 2017 AHA/ACC Focused update of the 2014 AHA/ACC guideline for the management of patients with valvular heart disease. A report of the American College of Cardiology/American Heart Association task force on clinical practice guidelines. *Circulation.* 2017;70(2):252-289.
31. Vahanian A, Baumgartner H, Bax J, et al. Guidelines on the management of valvular heart disease: the task force on the management of valvular heart disease of the European Society of Cardiology. *Eur Heart J.* 2007;28(2):230-268.
32. MitraClip set for significantly broader use website. Accessed May 10, 2021. https://www.abbott.com/corpnewsroom/strategy-and-strength/mitraclip-set-for-significantly-broader-use.html
33. Fucci C, Sandrelli L, Pardini A, Torracca L, Ferrari M, Alfieri O. Improved results with mitral valve repair using new surgical techniques. *Eur J Cardiothorac Surg.* 1995;9(11):621-626; discussion 626-627.
34. Feldman T, Kar S, Elmariah S, et al. Randomized comparison of percutaneous repair and surgery for mitral regurgitation: 5-Year results of EVEREST II. *J Am Coll Cardiol.* 2015;66(25):2844-2854.
35. Feldman T, Wasserman HS, Herrmann HC, et al. Percutaneous mitral valve repair using the edge-to-edge technique: six-month results of the EVEREST Phase I Clinical Trial. *J Am Coll Cardiol.* 2005;46(11):2134-2140.
36. Whitlow PL, Feldman T, Pedersen WR, et al. Acute and 12-month results with catheter-based mitral valve leaflet repair: the EVEREST II (Endovascular Valve Edge-to-Edge Repair) high risk study. *J Am Coll Cardiol.* 2012;59(2):130-139.
37. Obadia JF, Messika-Zeitoun D, Leurent G, et al. Percutaneous repair or medical treatment for secondary mitral regurgitation. *N Engl J Med.* 2018;379(24):2297-2306.
38. Pibarot P, Delgado V, Bax JJ. MITRA-FR vs. COAPT: lessons from two trials with diametrically opposed results. *Eur Heart J Cardiovasc Imaging.* 2019;20(6):620-624.
39. Nishimura RA, Bonow RO. Percutaneous repair of secondary mitral regurgitation—a tale of two trials. *N Engl J Med.* 2018;379(24):2374-2376.
40. Eleid MF, Whisenant BK, Cabalka AK, et al. Early outcomes of percutaneous transvenous transseptal transcatheter valve implantation in failed bioprosthetic mitral valves, ring annuloplasty, and severe mitral annular calcification. *JACC Cardiovasc Interv.* 2017;10(19):1932-1942.
41. Sorajja P, Bae R, Lesser JA, Pedersen WA. Percutaneous repair of paravalvular prosthetic regurgitation: patient selection, techniques and outcomes. *Heart.* 2015;101(9):665-673.
42. Baumgartner H, Falk V, Bax JJ, et al. 2017 ESC/EACTS guidelines for the management of valvular heart disease. *Eur Heart J.* 2017;38(36):2739-2791.
43. Wilkins GT, Weyman AE, Abascal VM, Block PC, Palacios IF. Percutaneous balloon dilatation of the mitral valve: an analysis of echocardiographic variables related to outcome and the mechanism of dilatation. *Br Heart J.* 1988;60(4):299-308.
44. Hansen DE, Sarris GE, Niczyporuk MA, Derby GC, Cahill PD, Miller DC. Physiologic role of the mitral apparatus in left ventricular regional mechanics, contraction synergy, and global systolic performance. *J Thorac Cardiovasc Surg.* 1989;97(4):521-533.
45. Chikwe J, Goldstone AB, Passage J, et al. A propensity score-adjusted retrospective comparison of early and mid-term results of mitral valve repair versus replacement in octogenarians. *Eur Heart J.* 2010;32(5):618-626.
46. Hennein HA, Swain JA, McIntosh CL, Bonow RO, Stone CD, Clark RE. Comparative assessment of chordal preservation versus chordal resection during mitral valve replacement. *J Thorac Cardiovasc Surg.* 1990;99(5):828-836; discussion 836-837.
47. Goldstein D, Moskowitz AJ, Gelijns AC, et al. Two-year outcomes of surgical treatment of severe ischemic mitral regurgitation. *N Engl J Med.* 2016;374(4):344-353.
48. Michler RE, Smith PK, Parides MK, et al. Two-year outcomes of surgical treatment of moderate ischemic mitral regurgitation. *N Engl J Med.* 2016;374(20):1932-1941.
49. Feasibility study of the tendyne mitral valve system for use in subjects with mitral annular calcification. Published May 29, 2018. Updated January 26, 2021. https://clinicaltrials.gov/ct2/show/NCT03539458

CHAPTER 11

AORTIC VALVE DISEASE

Laurie Bossory Goike, Antonios Pitsis, and Konstantinos Dean Boudoulas

INTRODUCTION

Aortic valvular disease is a major cause of morbidity and mortality worldwide. Although the incidence of aortic regurgitation has decreased over the past half century owing to a dramatic decline in the incidence of syphilis and rheumatic fever, the prevalence of aortic stenosis is increasing because of the aging population. Close monitoring of symptoms and/or the development of left ventricular (LV) remodeling and dysfunction is required to provide timely interventional therapy in patients with aortic stenosis or regurgitation.

The etiology of valvular heart disease (VHD) has changed over the past several decades. Several of the factors contributing to these changes include the advancements of technology, life expectancy of patients, novel prosthetic devices, and underlying cardiomyopathies.[1] Currently, aortic stenosis is the most common valvular disorder that requires interventional therapy in industrialized countries. In the United States, moderate to severe aortic stenosis is present in approximately 2.8% to 3.4% of the population older than age 75 years, and has a prevalence upward of 10% in the eighth decade of life.[2,3] On the contrary, rheumatic fever and syphilis, common causes of aortic regurgitation in the first half of the past century, have almost disappeared in industrialized countries,[1] aortic regurgitation is less prevalent than is aortic stenosis, with moderate and severe aortic regurgitation occurring in 0.5% of the population in the Framingham study; any degree of aortic regurgitation was seen in 5% of the population.[4] This chapter discusses pathophysiology, diagnosis, and management of aortic stenosis and aortic regurgitation.

AORTIC STENOSIS

The aortic valve is composed of three leaflets that have three cusps (right, left, and noncoronary cusps) that are attached to the annulus. The normal aortic valve area (AVA) is 3 cm^2 to 5 cm^2 with complete leaflet separation. The most common causes of aortic stenosis are calcification of an anatomically "normal" (tricuspid) aortic valve that occurs with aging, whereas calcification of a congenital bicuspid aortic valve occurs at a younger age. Bicuspid aortic valve, with a prevalence of approximately 2%, is the most common cause of aortic stenosis in those younger than age 70 years.[3] An overlap in age exists in patients with severe tricuspid and bicuspid aortic stenosis undergoing aortic valve replacement (AVR) (**e-Figure 11.1**).[5] The valvular appearance of the common causes of aortic stenosis is shown in **Figure 11.1**.

EPIDEMIOLOGY AND FACTORS CONTRIBUTING TO THE DEVELOPMENT OF AORTIC STENOSIS

Adjusted mortality rates for coronary artery disease have declined in the United States since the 1960s. Approximately 45% of this decline is attributed to a reduction in risk factors.[6] Trends in the prevalence of aortic stenosis, however, are much less clear and not well defined. Several factors determine the prevalence of calcific aortic stenosis. As the population ages, the prevalence is expected to increase because aortic stenosis increases with advancing age. Improvements in surgical techniques and transcatheter valve replacement are also expected to increase the prevalence of the disease because these patients live longer after these procedures. In contrast, controlling risk factors is expected to decrease the prevalence of aortic stenosis.[7] In a nationwide Swedish study, the mortality rate and age-adjusted mortality in aortic stenosis declined substantially from 1989 to 2009.[8] This decrease in mortality was similar to that observed with heart failure and acute myocardial infarction. Controlling risk factors in a large proportion of the population may have contributed to a decrease in the overall prevalence of aortic stenosis, as was the case with coronary atherosclerosis. This decrease due to risk factor control could offset the increase in the prevalence of aortic stenosis expected from the aging population and better management of the disease. Thus, the age of the population, better risk factor control, and effective management of the disease are the major determinants of the prevalence of calcific aortic stenosis at any particular time and in any specific population.

Traditionally, calcification of the tricuspid aortic valve resulting in aortic stenosis was thought to be secondary to a wear and tear effect on the valve due to the aging process. Newer developments, however, suggested that calcific aortic stenosis is the result of an active inflammatory process in which genetic, anatomic, and environmental risk factors contribute to the development of the disease. Several of these risk factors involved in the development of coronary atherosclerosis, such as arterial hypertension, high cholesterol, and smoking

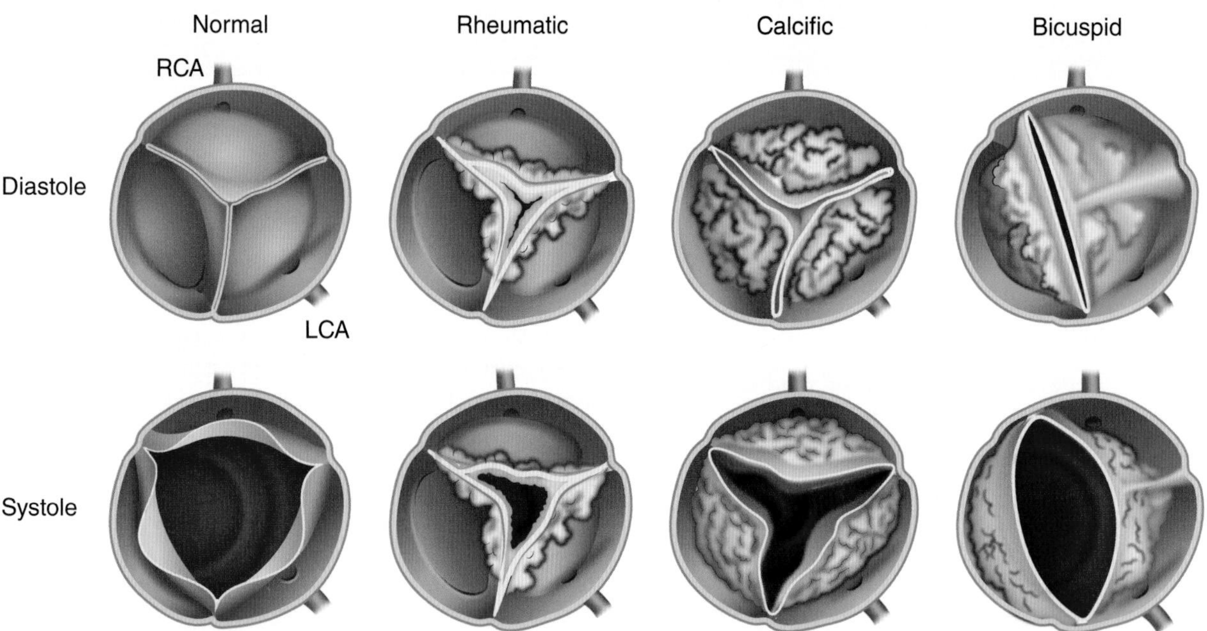

FIGURE 11.1 Different etiologies of aortic stenosis are shown, including rheumatic, calcific, and bicuspid. LCA, left coronary artery; RCA, right coronary artery.

actively contribute to the development and progression of calcific aortic stenosis. Severe hypercholesterolemia in children or adults may be associated with aortic stenosis. Radiation therapy to the chest also increases the risk of aortic stenosis and coronary artery disease. It is speculated that the initial event of calcific aortic stenosis is damage to the endothelium, caused by stress allowing the entry of lipids. This, in turn, initiates an inflammatory process where T cells, myocytes, mast cells, and CD3-positive leucocytes accumulate. Inflammation results in the stimulation of neoangiogenesis with new vessel formation; rupture of the fragile new vessels may occur, which also contribute to the acceleration and progression of the disease. The atherosclerotic process over time may differentiate into various pathways including calcification. Despite the close association, however, between atherosclerosis and calcific aortic stenosis, many patients with risk factors and coronary atherosclerosis do not have aortic stenosis, and conversely many patients with aortic stenosis do not have coronary atherosclerosis.[5,7,9]

A 2015 study of patients undergoing AVR found that 62% of patients with a tricuspid aortic valve and calcific aortic stenosis and 26% of patients with a bicuspid aortic valve and calcific aortic stenosis required concomitant coronary artery bypass surgery (**Figure 11.2**).[5] It seems, therefore, that other parameters in addition to coronary atherosclerosis risk factors contribute to the development of calcific aortic stenosis. Anatomic abnormalities in the aortic valve, more prominent in the bicuspid and less prominent in the tricuspid aortic valve, certainly play an important role. The increased mechanical stress of a bicuspid aortic valve results in increased structural degeneration and calcification at an earlier age. A stiff aorta (related to aging, risk factors, atherosclerosis, etc) may also contribute to the development of calcific aortic stenosis. Studies using magnetic resonance techniques have shown different patterns of blood flow in the root of the aorta in various disorders and diseases and in the elderly. In support of this observation, other studies have shown that the first abnormalities in patients who develop calcific aortic stenosis occur at the site of the aortic valve leaflets where turbulent blood flow is present. It is also known that valvular and vascular calcifications are inversely related to mineral density of the bones. Several disorders and diseases that affect mineral metabolism in the bones, such as osteoporosis, chronic kidney disease, Paget disease, and others, are associated with valvular calcification.[5,7,9] Recent studies have shown that plasma-converting enzyme—angiotensin-converting enzyme 2 (ACE2)—activity is directly related to the severity of calcification in aortic stenosis. Thus, the renin-angiotensin-aldosterone system, and especially tissue ACE2 activity, facilitates the development of calcific aortic stenosis.[9,10] In addition to traditional risk factors, several genetic variants have been associated with the development of aortic stenosis, and one such variant has been described in the lipoprotein(a) locus (rs10455872).[11]

CLINICAL PRESENTATION: AORTIC STENOSIS

The progression of VHD, and especially the progression of aortic stenosis, can be categorized into stages. Stage A are

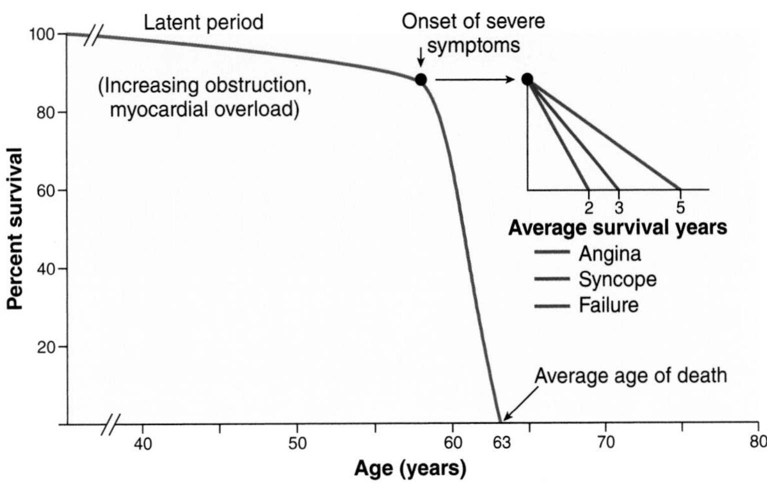

FIGURE 11.2 Aortic stenosis in adults, depicting average survival with the onset of severe symptoms, including angina, syncope, and heart failure. (Reprinted with permission from Ross J Jr, Braunwald E. Aortic stenosis. *Circulation.* 1968;38(1 Suppl5):61-67. Copyright © 1968 American Heart Association, Inc.)

patients at risk for development of valvular disease. Stage B are patients with mild to moderate disease that are asymptomatic. Stage C are patients that have severe disease, but remain asymptomatic: Stage C1 patients have preserved LV function, and stage C2 patients have decompensated LV function. Stage D are patients who are symptomatic because of severe valvular disease.

The classic triad of symptoms associated with aortic stenosis includes lightheadedness and/or syncope, heart failure, and chest pain. The onset of these symptoms is known to reflect advanced disease and correlates with increased mortality. This was elegantly described in 1968 by Ross and Braunwald, who published the well-known "aortic stenosis mortality curve" that displays the rapid decline of survival associated with the onset of symptoms (Figure 11.2).[12]

As aortic stenosis progresses, it results in increased afterload, which if left untreated can cause LV hypertrophy, myocardial fibrosis, and, ultimately, manifest as heart failure. This causes classic symptoms of heart failure; shortness of breath and orthopnea are common and a decrease in exercise tolerance and increased fatigue can also occur. Severe symptoms with end-stage disease include severe dyspnea, orthopnea, pulmonary edema, and paroxysmal nocturnal dyspnea. Angina also presents as a late symptom and reflects, among others, an increase in oxygen consumption due to hypertrophied myocardium.

Clinical Signs of Aortic Stenosis

The murmur of aortic stenosis can easily be identified on clinical examination as a crescendo-decrescendo systolic ejection murmur that is best heard at the base of the heart and radiates to the carotids, and sometimes to the apex of the heart, with a musical quality (so-called Gallavardin phenomenon). The more late peaking the murmur, the more severe the aortic stenosis. The other key features of severe aortic stenosis on clinical examination are diminished intensity or paradoxical splitting of the second heart sound and a weak, delayed, late-peaking carotid impulse (ie, *pulsus parvus et tardus*). The murmur of aortic stenosis is augmented by an increase in stroke volume with maneuvers such as squatting, and decreases with standing or Valsalva that reduces the flow across the valve. See **Table 11.1** for a summary of physical examination findings.

DIAGNOSIS: AORTIC STENOSIS

A thorough history and physical examination are often sufficient to obtain a level of suspicion regarding aortic valve disease.

The most common imaging modality for the diagnosis of aortic stenosis is transthoracic echocardiography (TTE) and Doppler echocardiography. TTE and Doppler echocardiography can be used to diagnose aortic stenosis in a noninvasive, radiation-free, and inexpensive manner. It is also the modality of choice for monitoring the progression of disease.

TABLE 11.1 Physical Examination Findings of Severe Aortic Stenosis

Physical Examination	Description
Systolic murmur	Time to peak murmur intensity (late peaking) correlates with severity of disease; radiates to the carotids and apex of the heart
Pulses parvus et tardus	Weak and delayed carotid upstroke; correlates with severity of disease
Single S2	Severe calcification of the aortic valve results in inaudible closure of the aortic valve
Split S2	Paradoxical splitting of S2 due to delay in closure of the aortic valve
Audible S4	An S4 develops in the setting of severe concentric LV hypertrophy

LV, left ventricular.

TABLE 11.2 Echocardiographic Grading of Severe Aortic Stenosis

Stenosis Severity	Aortic Valve Area (cm^2)	Mean Transvalvular Gradient (mm Hg)	Peak Jet Velocity (m/sec)	Velocity Ratio (LVOT VTI/AV VTI)
Mild	>1.5	<20	2.6-2.9	>0.5
Moderate	1.1-1.5	20-39	3.0-3.9	0.25-0.5
Severe	≤1.0	≥40	≥4	<0.25

AV, aortic valve; LVOT, left ventricular outflow tract; VTI, velocity time integral.

Transesophageal echocardiogram (TEE) can also provide additive information when needing to better visualize valve morphology, vegetations associated with infective endocarditis, leaflet perforation, or flail leaflets.

Using TTE and Doppler echocardiography, current guidelines define severe aortic stenosis as AVA less than or equal to 1.0 cm^2, peak aortic jet velocity greater than or equal to 4 m/sec, and a mean aortic transvalvular gradient greater than or equal to 40 mm Hg (**Table 11.2**).[13] **Figure 11.3** shows the continuous-wave Doppler pattern and peak velocity of severe aortic stenosis.

Discrepant values that confound the diagnosis of severe aortic stenosis may be present and need special consideration. Low-flow, low-gradient severe aortic stenosis (AVA ≤1 cm^2) presents with a nonsevere transvalvular gradient (ie, ≤40 mm Hg). This is often seen in patients with poor LV systolic function (ie, LV ejection fraction <50%), resulting in a reduced forward stroke volume (stroke volume index <35 mL/m^2) and, thus, a low gradient.[14] Dobutamine stress echocardiography (DSE) can be used in this clinical scenario to differentiate patients with true severe aortic stenosis from those with "pseudoaortic stenosis" resulting from a decrease in aortic leaflet excursion due to severe LV systolic dysfunction. In true severe aortic stenosis, as dobutamine is administered stroke volume is augmented, the aortic valve gradient increases, and the AVA remains in the severe range. Conversely, in pseudoaortic stenosis, dobutamine infusion augments stroke volume and the transvalvular gradient, and the AVA increases as aortic valve leaflet excursion improves.

Low-flow, low-gradient severe aortic stenosis can also be seen in patients with preserved LV systolic function (ie, LV ejection fraction >50%). Often referred to as paradoxical low-flow, low-gradient aortic stenosis, patients with this condition are challenging to diagnose because they often have small LV cavities, normal LV ejection fraction, and infusion of dobutamine does little to augment their stroke volume or gradient. These patients are important to identify because intervention has been shown to improve outcomes.[15]

In assessment of aortic stenosis, the most common technical error leading to the misdiagnosis of severe aortic stenosis by echocardiogram is the underestimation of the left ventricular outflow tract (LVOT) diameter. The LVOT diameter is used in the continuity equation to calculate AVA and, when measured incorrectly, can lead to inaccurate assessment of the severity of aortic stenosis. Multidetector computed tomography (MDCT) and cardiac magnetic resonance imaging (MRI) can more accurately measure the LVOT and provide additive information when needed. For example, MDCT can be used to determine aortic valve calcium scoring[16]; an aortic valve calcium score greater than 2000 AU in men and greater than 1200 AU in women can help differentiate severe aortic stenosis from nonsevere aortic stenosis.[17] Cardiac MRI is also used to evaluate the degree of myocardial fibrosis, an important factor that provides prognostic information beyond that provided by LV ejection fraction and LV volumes.

Cardiac catheterization is recommended and relied on only when noninvasive imaging is inconclusive or there are discrepancies between echocardiographic findings and clinical symptoms or findings. In the patient with severe aortic stenosis, coronary angiogram is often performed before aortic valve intervention to evaluate the need for coronary artery revascularization.

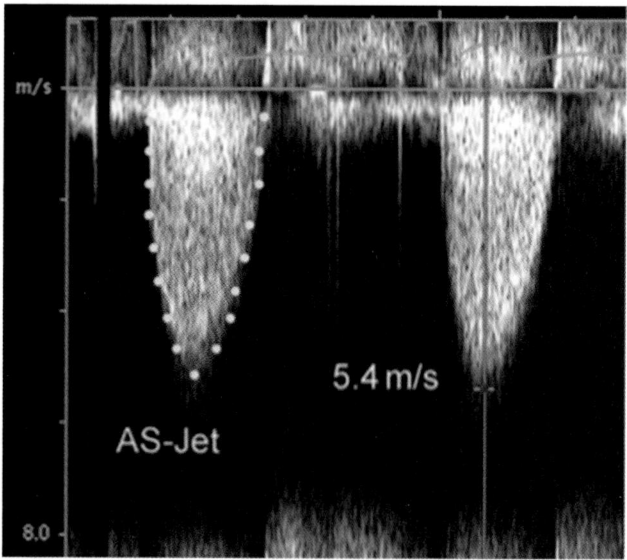

FIGURE 11.3 Continuous-wave Doppler echocardiography of severe aortic stenosis showing maximum velocity and tracing of the velocity curve to calculate aortic valve mean gradient. AS, aortic stenosis. (Reprinted from Baumgartner H, Hung J, Bermejo J, et al. Echocardiographic assessment of valve stenosis: EAE/ASE recommendations for clinical practice. *J Am Soc Echocardiogr*. 2009;22(1):1-23;quiz 101-102. Copyright © 2009 Elsevier. With permission.)

MANAGEMENT: AORTIC STENOSIS

Medical Management

Medical management of advanced aortic stenosis is rather limited. Management of systemic arterial hypertension is a Class I recommendation in patients with asymptomatic aortic stenosis or those at risk for development of aortic stenosis. Hypertension results in increased LV afterload, and is associated with higher rates of cardiovascular events and mortality compared to patients with aortic stenosis without arterial hypertension. Diuretics and vasodilators such as hydralazine, nitroglycerin, and nifedipine should be avoided to prevent hypotension. ACE inhibitors are often first-line agents, initiated at low dose and with slow titration. Beta-blockers can be prescribed if there is concomitant coronary artery disease, but should be avoided if there is concern for decompensated heart failure. Statin therapy in patients with advanced disease has not been proved to prevent progression of aortic stenosis.

Interventional Therapy

Calcific aortic stenosis accounts for approximately 85,000 valve replacement procedures each year in the United States.[16] The most challenging aspect in the management of VHD is choosing the optimal timing of valve replacement. It is prudent not to rush into a therapeutic intervention prematurely to avoid exposing the patient to unnecessary procedural and surgical risk. Further, bioprosthetic valves have a limited life expectancy, and if a mechanical valve is used, there is the risk associated with oral anticoagulation. As a general rule, AVR should be performed when the stenosis is severe and symptoms or LV dysfunction/dilation have developed. **Table 11.3** shows the recommendations for frequency of imaging with echocardiography when monitoring asymptomatic patients with aortic valvular disease.

Class I recommendations for AVR in patients with severe aortic stenosis include LV ejection fraction less than 50%, undergoing CABG or other heart surgery, and/or in the symptomatic patient. **Algorithm 11.1** summarizes indications and level of recommendation for AVR in severe aortic stenosis from the 2017 American Heart Association (AHA) and American College of Cardiology (ACC) updated Guidelines for the Management of Patients With Valvular Heart Disease and the 2014 AHA/ACC Guidelines for the Management of Patients with Valvular Heart Disease.[13,18]

Aortic Valve Replacement

There are several approaches for AVR. Traditionally, extensive sternotomy, cardiopulmonary bypass, aortic cross-clamping, and cardioplegia have been used for more than 50 years for AVR. In the current era, surgical mortality is 1% to 4% in patients without serious comorbidities and normal LV function.[19] Older age, LV dysfunction, myocardial fibrosis, chronic obstructive pulmonary disease, diabetes mellitus, obesity, concomitant coronary artery disease, and atrial fibrillation are all associated with increased mortality risk.[20] Surgery is typically considered in patients with severe aortic stenosis with symptoms and/or LV ejection fraction less than 50%, or if undergoing coronary artery bypass graft (CABG)/other heart surgery.

As a general rule, mechanical aortic valves are often used in younger patients because of their excellent durability, despite the inconvenience and risk of long-term oral anticoagulation with warfarin therapy. Bioprosthetic valves are the valve of choice in patients older than 70 years of age and comprise 80% of surgical AVR because of an aging surgical population. Long-term follow-up of bioprosthetic AVR revealed that at 10 years, approximately 64% of patients had died and 6.6% of patients had clinically relevant structural valve degeneration.[21] The reported durability of surgical aortic bioprosthetic valves is greater than 85% at 10 years, although variability is reported anywhere from 5 to 20 years, often dependent on the bioprosthesis model and age of the patient (ie, less durable in young patients).[22] Certain younger patients, however, especially those who are involved in sports, prefer a bioprosthetic valve to avoid the long-term risks of anticoagulation therapy.

Minimally Invasive Aortic Valve Replacement

Today, most centers are using a mini-sternotomy (**Figure 11.4**) or hemisternotomy approach to replace the diseased aortic valve. This is usually completed through a midline 5- to 8-cm skin incision and a "J"-shaped sternal cut to the third or fourth right intercostal space. Associated aortic pathology can also be treated through this approach.

Another less commonly used minimally invasive AVR approach is through a mini-right anterior thoracotomy approach (**e-Figure 11.2**). This is usually completed parasternally through a 6-cm skin incision above the second or third intercostal space and does not require sternal cutting, although the third costal cartilage is typically cut. This technique is technically more demanding than is the mini-sternotomy approach

TABLE 11.3 Recommended Frequency of Echocardiographic Evaluation in Asymptomatic Patients With Aortic Valve Disease and Normal Left Ventricular Function

Stage	Severity	Aortic Stenosis	Aortic Regurgitation
Progressive (stage B)	Mild	Every 3-5 years	Every 3-5 years
	Moderate	Every 1-2 years	Every 1-2 years
Severe (stage C)	Severe	Every 6-12 months	Every 6-12 months

Note: Stage B—patients with mild to moderate disease who are asymptomatic. Stage C—patients who have severe disease, but remain asymptomatic.

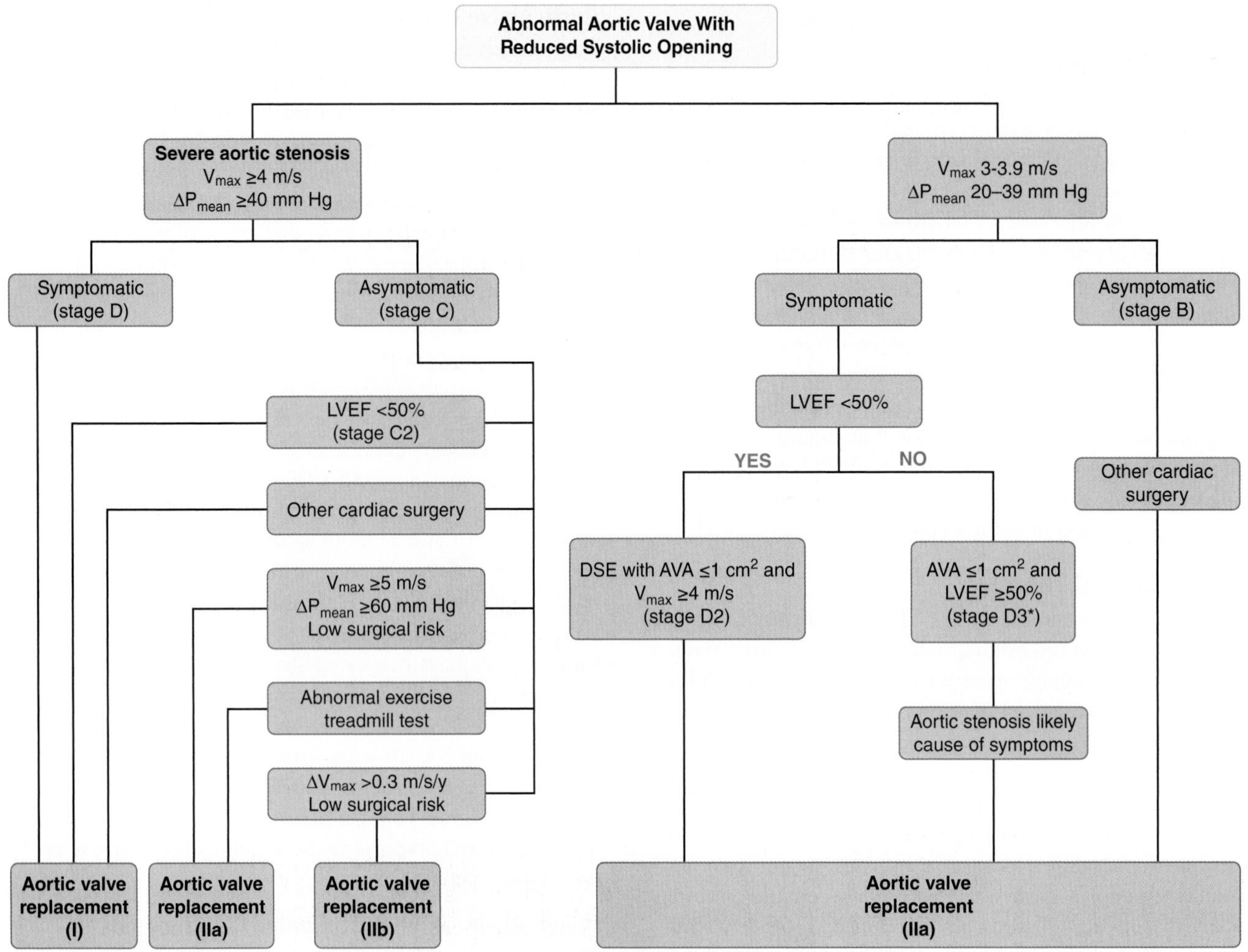

ALGORITHM 11.1 Indication of aortic valve replacement (AVR) in aortic stenosis. Stage B—patients with mild to moderate disease who are asymptomatic. Stage C—patients who have severe disease, but remain asymptomatic. Stage C1—patients have preserved left ventricular (LV) function. Stage C2—patients with decompensated LV function. Stage D—patients who are symptomatic because of severe valvular disease. *In stage D3 aortic stenosis, AVR should be considered if valve obstruction is likely the cause of symptoms, stroke volume index is <35 mL/m² and indexed AVA is 0.6 cm²/m² (obtained when the patient is normotensive with a systolic blood pressure < 140 mmHg). AVA, aortic valve area; DSE, dobutamine stress echocardiography; LVEF, left ventricular ejection fraction; ΔP_{mean}, mean pressure gradient; V_{max}, maximum velocity. (Adapted from Nishimura RA, Otto CM, Bonow RO, et al. 2014 AHA/ACC guideline for the management of patients with valvular heart disease: executive summary: a report of the American College of Cardiology/American Heart Association Task Force on Practice Guidelines. *J Am Coll Cardiol.* 2014;63(22):2438-2488. Copyright © 2014 American Heart Association, Inc., and the American College of Cardiology Foundation. With permission.)

and requires prolonged aorta cross-clamping. Many centers that use the right anterior thoracotomy approach typically use rapid deployment aortic valves (ie, sutureless) in an effort to decrease aorta cross-clamping times. The right anterior thoracotomy approach is usually performed under direct visualization, but it can also be performed with endoscopic video assist.

Totally Endoscopic Aortic Valve Replacement

Totally endoscopic aortic valve replacement (TEAVR) is the least invasive surgical approach and the least commonly used. It is performed through a 3- to 4-cm working incision and two 10-mm ports without sternotomy or rib cutting (**e-Figure 11.3**). Cardiopulmonary bypass, aortic cross-clamping, and cardioplegia are performed. There is a steep learning curve for this procedure that requires special skills. Once learned, however, they can provide a less invasive surgery with shorter intensive care and hospital stay, better quality of life, and faster return to work compared to traditional AVR. Compared to transcatheter aortic valve replacement (TAVR; see next section), TEAVR has the advantage of removing the diseased valve, ability to implant a mechanical or biological valve, precise sizing of prosthesis, and avoidance of paravalvular leak or permanent pacemaker. In our experience, with this approach at St Luke's Hospital in Thessaloniki, Greece, patients with aortic stenosis undergoing TEAVR have excellent results with no short-term mortality, no evidence of paravalvular leak, and no need for a permanent pacemaker. The equipment needed to perform TEAVR is less expensive compared to that used in classic robotic surgery.

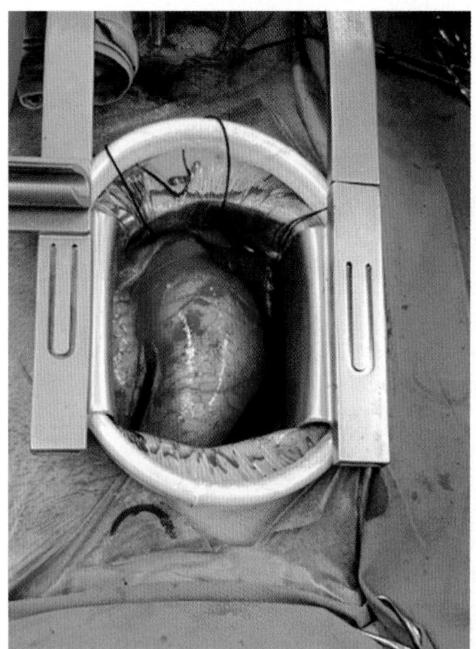

FIGURE 11.4 Aortic valve replacement via a mini-sternotomy is completed through a midline 5- to 8-cm skin incision and a "J"-shaped sternal cut to the third or fourth right intercostal space. (Image provided courtesy of St Luke's Hospital, Thessaloniki, Greece.)

Aortic Valve Disease Associated With Aortic Root Dilation

The Bentall procedure is considered the gold standard for patients who require an aortic root replacement due to aortic root dilation with concomitant AVR primarily due to bicuspid aortic stenosis. The procedure involves replacement of the aortic valve and root, with reimplantation of the coronary arteries into the aortic graft. In a recent meta-analysis, early mortality following a Bentall procedure was 5.6%, whereas surgical mortality from the same procedure several decades ago was 8.9%; the incidence of major bleeding and thrombotic complications was 14.1% at 10 years.[23]

Transcatheter Approaches

The decision regarding surgical or TAVR in patients with severe aortic stenosis should be made by a multidisciplinary heart valve team. The choice of intervention is often determined by a variety of factors including vascular anatomy, risk of surgery, patient frailty, comorbid conditions, and severity of coronary artery disease, among others. In the recent past, surgery was typically considered for low- or intermediate-risk patients with severe aortic stenosis, and TAVR often was the treatment of choice in high surgical risk patients; however, TAVR is now being used more frequently in low- and intermediate-risk patients because studies have consistently proved its safety and efficacy in these patients.

TAVR can be performed with either balloon-expandable or self-expanding valves. The procedure is commonly performed via femoral artery access in the cardiac catheterization laboratory or hybrid cardiovascular operating room under conscious sedation or monitored anesthesia care; general anesthesia is rarely required. Alternatively, access can be performed via the subclavian artery, transapically through the LV, or through direct aortic access via anterior thoracotomy in patients with inadequate lower extremity vessel size. During TAVR, a temporary pacemaker lead is advanced into the right ventricle for rapid pacing during deployment of the valve. The prosthetic valve is positioned across the native aortic valve with confirmation of the valve position with fluoroscopy. Patients typically are on antiplatelet therapy post procedure.

Over the past decade, several trials have demonstrated the safety and efficacy of TAVR in low-, intermediate-, and high-risk surgical patients. Although long-term data are limited, the durability of transcatheter aortic valves has been seen in older patients (ie, mean age older than 80 years), which over 90% of patients remain free from structural valve degeneration between 5 and 10 years after implantation.[24]

The series of Paortic regurgitationTNER trials evaluated the use of balloon-expandable TAVR compared to surgical AVR in low-, moderate-, and high-risk surgical patients. In high-risk surgical patients, the 30-day mortality was 3.4% in the balloon-expandable TAVR group and 6.5% in the surgical AVR group ($P = 0.07$)[25]; respective 1-year mortality rates were 24.2% and 26.8% ($P = 0.44$). Intermediate-risk surgical patients undergoing balloon-expandable TAVR or surgical AVR were found to have similar rates of death from any cause at 2 years, with event rates of 19.3% and 21.1%, respectively.[26] The most recent Paortic regurgitationTNER 3 trial evaluated the use of balloon-expandable TAVR compared to surgical AVR in low-risk surgical patients and found that the primary endpoint—rate of the composite of death, stroke, or rehospitalization at 1 year—was lower with TAVR (8.5%) as compared with surgical AVR (15.1%; $P = 0.001$). The rate of stroke at 30 days was 0.6% and 2.4% in the TAVR and surgical AVR groups, respectively ($P = 0.02$); the rate of death or stroke at 30 days was 1.0% and 3.3% in the TAVR and surgical AVR groups, respectively ($P = 0.01$). Death from any cause at 1 year was 1.0% in the TAVR group and 2.5% in the surgical AVR group.[27]

Additional trials evaluated the use of self-expanding TAVR compared to surgical AVR in low-, moderate-, and high-risk surgical patients. In high-risk surgical patients, the rate of death from any cause at 1 year was 14.2% in the TAVR group and 19.1% in the surgical AVR group ($P = 0.04$ for superiority).[27] At 5 years, all-cause mortality was found to be similar for self-expanding TAVR and surgical AVR, 55.3% and 55.4%, respectively.[28] In intermediate-risk surgical patients, self-expanding TAVR was shown to be noninferior to surgical AVR; the primary endpoint of death from any cause or disabling stroke at 2 years was 12.6% and 14.0% in TAVR and surgical AVR groups, respectively.[29] A more recent trial evaluated the use of self-expanding TAVR compared to surgical AVR in low-risk surgical patients and found that the primary endpoint, composite of death from any cause or disabling stroke at 24 months, was 5.3% and 6.7% in the TAVR and surgical AVR groups, respectively, which met criteria for noninferiority.[30]

In the 2017 AHA/ACC updated guidelines for the management of patients with VHD, TAVR is a Class I recommendation for severe symptomatic aortic stenosis in high surgical risk patients or those with prohibitive surgical risk[18]; there is a Class IIa recommendation for TAVR in patients with intermediate surgical risk. In 2019, the U.S. Food and Drug Administration expanded the indication for TAVR to low surgical risk patients.

Balloon aortic valvuloplasty may be an option for treatment of aortic stenosis in highly select patients because of particular clinical circumstances. It offers only modest and short-term improvement in hemodynamics, survival, and quality of life.[31]

The consensus from experts around the world is that the preferred therapy for patients with aortic stenosis who are not surgical candidates should be TAVR. TAVR should also be considered as a preferred alternative to surgical intervention in high-risk patients, particularly elderly patients.[32] TAVR may often be the preferred strategy for certain intermediate- and low-risk patients as well. The ultimate decision should stem from a multidisciplinary heart valve team approach considering individual characteristics of each patient.

PATIENT FOLLOW-UP: AORTIC STENOSIS

The 2014 AHA/ACC Guidelines for the Management of Patients with Valvular Heart Disease and the 2017 AHA/ACC Focused Update on the 2014 guidelines recommend, regardless of indication (aortic stenosis or aortic regurgutation), continuous anticoagulation of mechanical heart valves with a vitamin K antagonist (VKA), commonly warfarin; this is in addition to aspirin 75 to 100 mg daily, Class I recommendation.[13] International normalized ratio (INR) goal depends on valve type and additional thromboembolic risk factors. It is a Class IIa recommendation for patients with bioprosthetic heart valves to take aspirin 75 to 100 mg daily. It is also a Class IIa recommendation for patients with a bioprosthetic valve to be anticoagulated with a VKA for the first 3 to 6 months post surgery.[18]

It is a Class IIa recommendation to prescribe infective endocarditis prophylaxis for any patient with a prosthetic valve, including transcatheter valves.[18]

All patients with valve replacement should have a baseline echocardiogram following their surgery, ideally within 30 days and at 1 year. Serious complications in patients with prosthetic heart valves, such as thromboembolism, valve obstruction, valve or paravalvular regurgitation, bleeding and infection, occur at a rate of approximately 3% per year.[33] The European 2017 VHD guidelines recommend yearly clinical assessment and echocardiogram, as well as repeat echocardiogram for the development of any new symptoms.[34]

Typically following a TAVR procedure, an echocardiogram is obtained before discharge to evaluate valvular function including mean valve gradient and valvular/paravalvular regurgitation; this is repeated at 30 days and 1 year together with a follow-up clinic appointment. Long-term antiplatelet therapy is prescribed post procedure. Although dual-antiplatelet therapy had often been prescribed for the first 3 to 6 months post procedure,[35] more recent data suggest that single-antiplatelet therapy compared to dual-antiplatelet therapy decreases the risk of bleeding without a significant difference in thrombotic events and cardiovascular mortality.[36,37] Further studies are still needed to determine best practice guidelines including taking into account the patient's bleeding risk, coronary artery disease with recent percutaneous coronary intervention, and need for long-term anticoagulation.[38]

AORTIC REGURGITATION

Aortic regurgitation is less prevalent than is aortic stenosis, and patients often present at a younger age because of the association with congenital bicuspid aortic valve and primary diseases of the aortic root/ascending aorta.[32]

Aortic regurgitation is often caused by aortic root dilatation; much less often it is due to aortic dissection that disrupts the integrity of the aortic root and valve, infective endocarditis that destroys the valve leaflets, bicuspid aortic valve, or rheumatic valve disease. Aortic root dilatation is a common cause of aortic regurgitation in developed countries, with rheumatic fever being a common cause in developing countries and worldwide.[1]

CHRONIC AORTIC REGURGITATION

Etiology

Because aortic regurgitation is often associated with aortic root pathology, several of the causes of aortic regurgitation are related to genetic predispositions for aortic root enlargement including Marfan syndrome, Loeys-Dietz syndrome, polycystic kidney disease, and other heritable connective tissue disorders. Inflammatory conditions, such as psoriatic arthritis, ankylosing spondylitis, Behçet syndrome, and giant cell arthritis, are chronic conditions associated with aortic disease leading to progressive aortic regurgitation. Rarely, syphilitic aortitis may cause aortic aneurysm formation and aortic regurgitation.

Hemodynamics in Chronic Aortic Regurgitation

Aortic regurgitation is a unique condition that results in both an increase in LV preload and afterload. The extra volume that regurgitates into the LV during diastole results in LV volume overload, and the ejected volume into the aorta during systole results in a large stroke volume and systolic hypertension. The pressure overload results in thickening of the LV walls and concentric hypertrophy; this is in addition to an already preceded eccentric hypertrophy due to volume overload. The LV dilatation (eccentric hypertrophy) and concentric hypertrophy present in chronic aortic regurgitation alters LV geometry, which in turn affects LV function. During the compensated phase of aortic regurgitation, concentric hypertrophy (thick LV walls) results in normalization of the LV wall stress (stress $= P \times r/2h$, where P = pressure, r = radius of the LV cavity and h = LV wall thickness). During the compensated phase, the LV ejection fraction may be maintained despite a high afterload. However, as the disease progresses, the afterload increases, and the LV ejection fraction eventually declines. Certain patients with chronic aortic regurgitation may be asymptomatic, even when the LV ejection fraction decreases. Surgery in asymptomatic patients with aortic regurgitation and a reduced LV ejection fraction is associated with a suboptimal outcome. Several indices of LV function have been proposed to predict optimal timing for AVR, including echocardiographic measurements, hemodynamic data, and resting and exercise ejection fraction; however, because changes in preload, afterload, and LV geometry often coexist in patients with chronic aortic regurgitation, none of these indices alone are predictive. For this reason, a combination of different indices should be considered. In the clinical setting, one should be aware of the shortcomings of each technique and select the methods that are least sensitive to the factors that are most altered in a given setting.[38,39]

Clinical Presentation: Chronic Aortic Regurgitation

Chronic aortic regurgitation often remains asymptomatic until the signs and symptoms of heart failure gradually develop. Progression of symptoms occurs over the course of many years, with many patients reporting symptoms in their fourth to fifth decade and rapid decline once symptoms present.[40] Symptoms develop as the disease severity progresses, and the most common symptoms include shortness of breath with exertion, orthopnea, and paroxysmal nocturnal dyspnea. Angina may occur later in the course of the disease. The prognosis of symptomatic patients with chronic aortic regurgitation and abnormal LV function is poor.[41]

Clinical Signs of Chronic Severe Aortic Regurgitation

The physical examination of chronic severe aortic regurgitation is often considered the most impressive in cardiology. The findings of clinical examination in aortic regurgitation are summarized in **Table 11.4**. The pulse pressure is wide, as opposed to acute aortic regurgitation that has a normal or only slightly widened pulse pressure. There may be an Austin Flint murmur, which is a mid-diastolic murmur. There is not a consensus regarding the etiology of the murmur, although several mechanisms are hypothesized including severe aortic regurgitation alone, abutment of the aortic regurgitation jet against the LV epicardium, mitral valve leaflet displacement combined with turbulent mixing of antegrade mitral blood flow, and retrograde aortic blood flow, among others.[42,43]

TABLE 11.4 Peripheral Signs of Severe Aortic Regurgitation

Physical Examination Sign	Description
Becker sign	Visible arterial pulsations in the retinal arteries
Landolfi sign	Alternating systolic constriction and diastolic dilation of the pupil
de Musset sign	Head bobbing with each heartbeat
Duroziez sign	Systolic murmur over the femoral head with compression proximally and diastolic murmur with distal compression
Müller sign	Systolic pulsation of the uvula
Quincke sign	Capillary pulsation visible at the tip of the fingernail
Traube sign	Pistol shot sounds heard over the femoral arteries in both systole and diastole
Water hammer or Corrigan pulse	Rapid upstroke followed by quick collapse of arterial pulse
Hill sign	Increased systolic arterial pressure in lower (popliteal) compared to upper (brachial) limbs

Diagnosis: Chronic Aortic Regurgitation

After the initial clinical evaluation, TTE and Doppler echocardiography should be performed (**Algorithm 11.2**). The severity of aortic regurgitation can be graded using color Doppler parameters. Color flow imaging is used in the assessment of the origin of the aortic regurgitation jet, regurgitant direction, and size of the jet. Color flow Doppler is used to visualize the vena contracta (VC), jet area, and flow convergence. The VC is the narrowest portion of the regurgitant flow beyond the regurgitant orifice, with severe aortic regurgitation defined as a VC greater than 0.6 cm (**Figure 11.5**). Flow convergence proximal to the lesion corresponds to severity of the aortic regurgitation, and is used in calculating the effective regurgitant orifice area (EROA); severe aortic regurgitation is an EROA greater than or equal to 0.3 cm^2. EROA is more often used in the assessment of mitral regurgitation than of aortic regurgitation, because measurement of flow convergence in the latter may be altered with severe valve thickening or calcification. Jet area is a visual estimate of severity, but can be confounded by many factors, so it is never solely relied on for the assessment of aortic regurgitation severity.[44] Using continuous-wave Doppler, pressure half-time (which represents the rapid equilibration of the aortic and LV diastolic pressures) in severe aortic regurgitation is less than 200 msec. Diastolic flow reversal in the aortic arch greater than 40 cm/sec is also consistent with severe aortic regurgitation. Short deceleration of the mitral flow velocity curve and M-mode can also be used to assess early closure of the mitral valve in severe aortic regurgitation.[13] However, cardiac MRI is considered to be the best method for the evaluation of the severity of aortic regurgitation and the status of LV structure and function.

In patients with bicuspid aortic valve, imaging of the aorta should be performed to evaluate the size of the ascending aorta because approximately 25% have concomitant aortic root dilatation. MRI or MDCT can be considered, particularly when the structure and morphology of the aortic sinus, sinotubular junction, or ascending aorta is not fully visualized using echocardiography.

MANAGEMENT: AORTIC REGURGITATION

Medical Management

Similar to aortic stenosis, medical management of advanced aortic regurgitation is also limited. For chronic aortic regurgitation, treatment of systemic arterial hypertension is a Class

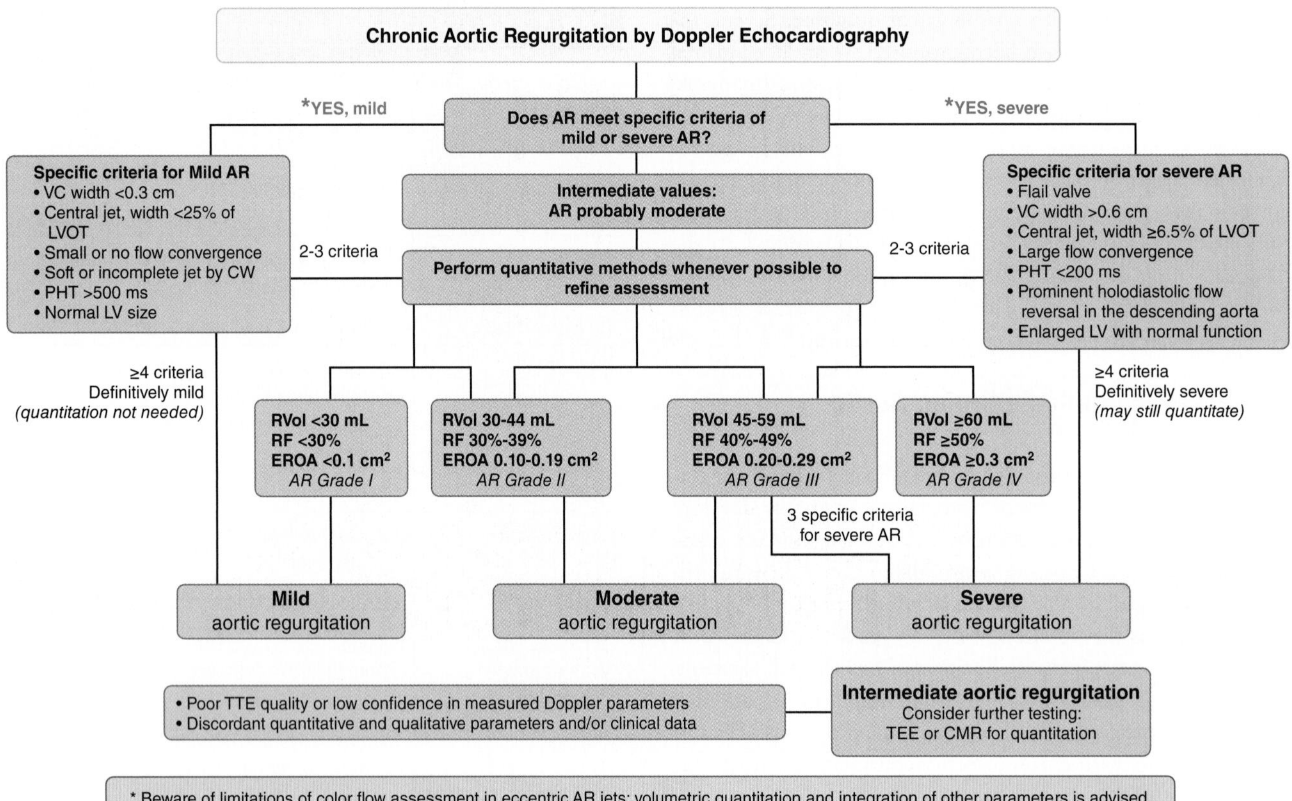

ALGORITHM 11.2 Algorithm to determine severity of chronic aortic regurgitation (aortic regurgitation) by echocardiography and Doppler echocardiography. CMR, cardiac magnetic resonance imaging; CW, continuous wave; EROA, effective regurgitant orifice area; LV, left ventricle; LVOT, left ventricular outflow tract; PHT, pressure half-time; RF, regurgitant fraction; RVol, regurgitant volume; TEE, transesophageal echocardiogram; TTE, transthoracic echocardiogram; VC, vena contracta. (Adapted from Nishimura RA, Otto CM, Bonow RO, et al. 2014 AHA/ACC guideline for the management of patients with valvular heart disease: executive summary: a report of the American College of Cardiology/American Heart Association Task Force on Practice Guidelines. *J Am Coll Cardiol.* 2014;63(22):2438-2488. Copyright © 2014 American Heart Association, Inc., and the American College of Cardiology Foundation. With permission.)

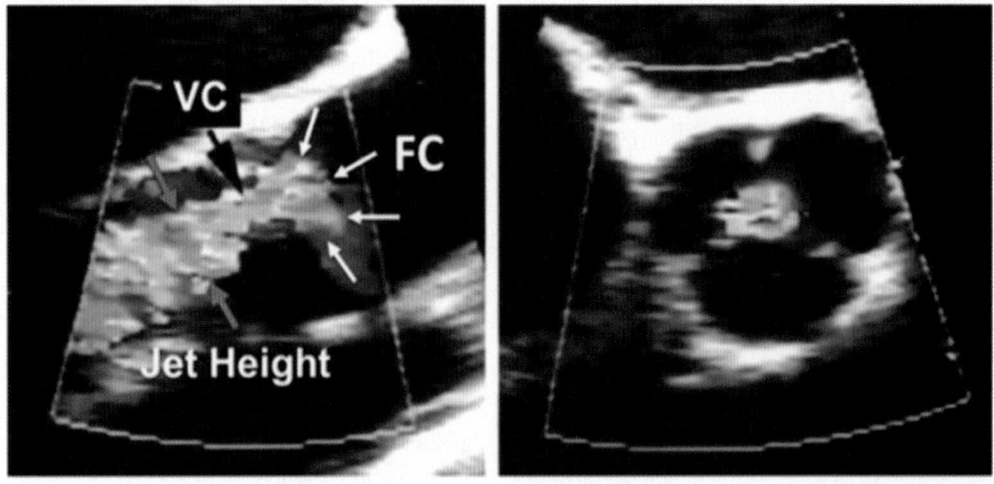

FIGURE 11.5 Color flow Doppler of aortic regurgitation in the parasternal long- and short-axis views (left and right panels, respectively). The three components of the jet are shown with arrows: flow convergence (FC), vena contracta (VC), and jet height (or width) in the left ventricular outflow. VC is the narrowest portion of the regurgitant flow beyond the regurgitant orifice, with severe aortic regurgitation defined as VC greater than 0.6 cm. FC proximal to the lesion corresponds to severity of the aortic regurgitation and is used in calculating the effective regurgitant orifice area. Jet height is a visual estimate of width of the LV outflow tract. (Reprinted from Zoghbi WA, Adams D, Bonow RO, et al. Recommendations for noninvasive evaluation of native valvular regurgitation: a report from the American Society of Echocardiography developed in collaboration with the Society for Cardiovascular Magnetic Resonance. *J Am Soc Echocardiogr.* 2017;30(4):303-371. Copyright © 2017 by the American Society of Echocardiography. With permission.)

I recommendation, preferably with dihydropyridine calcium channel blockers or ACE inhibitors/angiotensin II receptor blockers (aortic regurgitationBs). Although vasodilators can improve hemodynamics and increase cardiac output, they are not routinely recommended in the treatment of chronic aortic regurgitation because they do not delay the need for AVR in patients with normal LV function.

Surgical Approaches for Severe Aortic Regurgitation

AVR is indicated (Class I) in patients with severe aortic regurgitation who are symptomatic, in asymptomatic patients with an LV ejection fraction less than 50%, or in patients undergoing another cardiac surgery. **Algorithm 11.3** summarizes indications and level of recommendation for AVR in severe aortic regurgitation from the 2017 AHA/ACC updated Guidelines for the Management of Patients with Valvular Heart Disease and the 2014 AHA/ACC Guidelines for the Management of Patients with Valvular Heart Disease.[13,18] Surgical aortic valve repair or replacement (when repair is not feasible or durable) is the preferred treatment option for patients with chronic severe aortic regurgitation. Minimally invasive approaches for aortic valve repair or replacement and TEAVR can be used in patients with aortic regurgitation without any added difficulty and with very good results, as is the case with aortic stenosis. See section "Surgical Approaches" within "Aortic Stenosis' for various surgical approaches. Approximately 20% of patients with severe aortic regurgitation with LV ejection fraction of 30% to 50% are actually referred for surgery, and only 3% of patients with an LV ejection fraction less than 30% ultimately undergo AVR.[45]

In addition, there are several surgical approaches for patients with an aortic root dilation with or without concomitant aortic regurgitation including aortic root reimplantation (David technique) and aortic root remodeling (Yacoub technique).

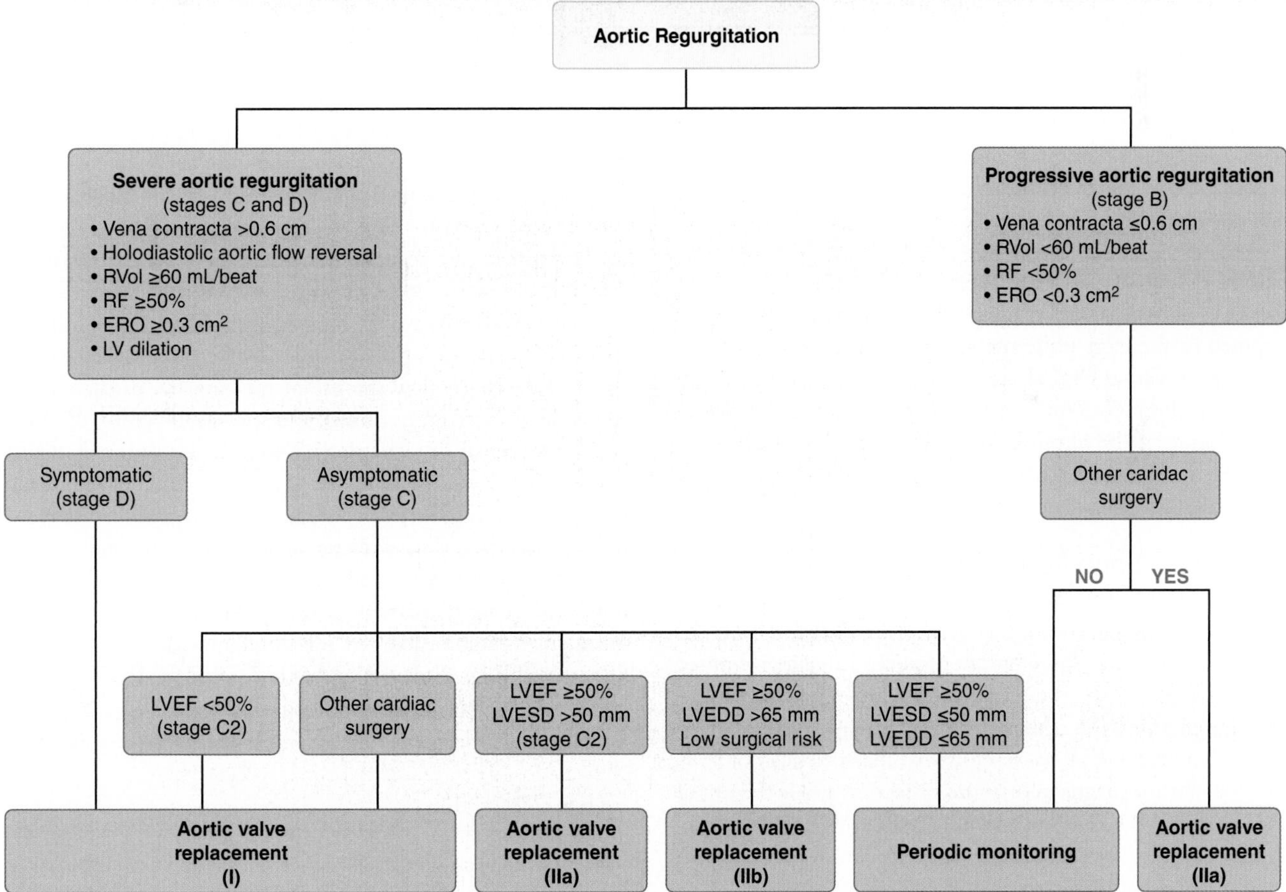

ALGORITHM 11.3 Indication for aortic valve replacement (AVR) in chronic aortic regurgitation (aortic regurgitation). Stage B—patients with mild to moderate disease who are asymptomatic. Stage C—patients who have severe disease, but remain asymptomatic. Stage C1—patients have preserved left ventricular (LV) function. Stage C2—patients with decompensated LV function. Stage D—patients who are symptomatic because of severe valvular disease. ERO, effective regurgitant orifice; EROA, effective regurgitant orifice area; LV, left ventricular; LVEDD, left ventricular end-diastolic dimension; LVEF, left ventricular ejection fraction; LVESD, left ventricular end-systolic dimension; LVOT, left ventricular outflow tract; RF, regurgitant fraction; RVol, regurgitant volume. (Adapted from Nishimura RA, Otto CM, Bonow RO, et al. 2014 AHA/ACC guideline for the management of patients with valvular heart disease: executive summary: a report of the American College of Cardiology/American Heart Association Task Force on Practice Guidelines. *J Am Coll Cardiol.* 2014;63(22):2438-2488. Copyright © 2014 American Heart Association, Inc., and the American College of Cardiology Foundation. With permission.)

Transcatheter Approaches

There are no guidelines for the use of TAVR in patients with pure aortic regurgitation. The development of transcatheter valves to treat pure aortic regurgitation is an emerging area. A recent meta-analysis found that transcatheter valve replacement for pure aortic regurgitation was feasible and safe for patients who were not surgical candidates,[46] although data overall is limited.

ACUTE AORTIC REGURGITATION

Etiology

Acute aortic regurgitation often results from aortic dissection, traumatic injury of the aorta, or infective endocarditis.[47] Because intravenous drug use and addiction have become more prevalent, drug abuse–related endocarditis has become an important risk factor for aortic regurgitation.

Clinical Presentation: Acute Aortic Regurgitation

Acute aortic regurgitation often presents with rapid and progressive hemodynamic instability, resulting in acute onset of shortness of breath. As mentioned previously, this is often associated with an acute structural change, such as aortic dissection or leaflet destruction with infective endocarditis. Symptoms of acute aortic regurgitation include heart failure symptoms such as shortness of breath with exertion, orthopnea, and paroxysmal nocturnal dyspnea.

Clinical Signs

There is normal or only slightly widened pulse pressure, as opposed to the large pulse pressure seen in chronic aortic regurgitation. Other clinical signs of acute aortic regurgitation include a diminished intensity of the first heart sound due to early closure of the mitral valve, and a short, low-pitch, early diastolic murmur because there is rapid equilibration of the LV and aortic diastolic pressures.

Diagnosis: Acute Aortic Regurgitation

The severity of acute aortic regurgitation can be defined by TTE and Doppler echocardiography. TTE is excellent in the evaluation of aortic regurgitation; however, its value is limited when assessing aortic dissection as the etiology of acute aortic regurgitation with a sensitivity and specificity of 60% to 80%. Conversely, TEE has a sensitivity and specificity of 95% to 100% for the diagnosis of aortic dissection and is the test of choice when MDCT is not feasible. Cardiac MRI is also useful in the evaluation of acute aortic regurgitation in patients with suboptimal echocardiographic images.[48]

Management: Acute Aortic Regurgitation

Medical Approach

Management of acute severe aortic regurgitation is surgical, with medical therapy providing a bridge to definitive therapy. Inotropic agents and vasodilators may be useful, while beta-blockers should be avoided because they prolong diastole, which in turn increases regurgitant volume. Intra-aortic balloon pump is contraindicated because it augments pressure in diastole, thereby worsening aortic regurgitation.

Surgical Approach

In patients with acute aortic regurgitation, surgery should not be delayed. Early surgery improves in-hospital and long-term survival, particularly in patients with hypotension, pulmonary edema, or evidence of cardiogenic shock.[49] The 2014 AHA/ACC Guidelines for the Management of Patients with Valvular Heart Disease recommends prompt surgical intervention for acute severe aortic regurgitation. Surgical aortic root and valve repair (eg, type A dissections) or valve replacement (eg, endocarditis cases) is the preferred treatment option for patients with acute severe aortic regurgitation.

PATIENT FOLLOW-UP: AORTIC REGURGITATION

See previous section "Patient Follow-up Aortic Stenosis."

RESEAORTIC REGURGITATIONCH AND FUTURE DIRECTIONS

An important future direction in the treatment of VHD continues to be identifying patients with VHD and improving outcomes of therapeutic intervention through the standardization of care for patients with VHD. This requires an understanding of VHD, including pathophysiology, progression of disease, and appropriate diagnostic testing among all providers. Ideally, patients with VHD will be identified early and referred to a comprehensive valve center where they will participate in shared decision-making with a multidisciplinary team.[50]

An additional area of focus continues to be identifying the optimal timing of therapeutic intervention. Several studies are emerging where the use of imaging (ie, cardiac MRI) can assist in predicting timing and success of AVR.[51-53] With the advancement of technology, TAVR has become a standard therapy for the treatment for aortic stenosis, as likely will be the case in the near future for pure aortic regurgitation. As technology is continuously evolving, new transcatheter and surgical approaches will soon become available. A better understanding of the genetic, anatomic, pathophysiologic, and molecular mechanisms responsible for the development of aortic valve disease will help clinicians optimize current management and eventually prevent the development of disease.

KEY POINTS

- ✔ Patients with symptomatic, severe aortic stenosis or aortic regurgitation, if untreated, have poor outcomes.
- ✔ In certain cases, early intervention should be considered to improve survival and quality of life, because rapid progression may occur even in asymptomatic patients.
- ✔ Echocardiography and Doppler echocardiography are the most commonly used methods for the diagnosis and follow-up of patients with aortic stenosis or aortic regurgitation.
- ✔ Cardiac computed tomography, and especially cardiac MRI, often provide additional useful information.

- ✔ TAVR often is used for the treatment of severe aortic stenosis in low-, intermediate-, and high-risk patients with very satisfactory results. Surgical AVR, however, still remains an important method of management in these patients.
- ✔ Currently, aortic regurgitation is mainly treated surgically; however, transcatheter approaches are emerging, and ongoing trials will assist in determining the safety and efficacy of this approach.
- ✔ TEAVR in patients with aortic stenosis or regurgitation provides an additional vital option.
- ✔ Aortic stenosis in patients with tricuspid aortic valve typically occurs at an older age, whereas manifestations of aortic valve disease (stenosis or regurgitation) in patients with bicuspid aortic valve appear at a younger age.
- ✔ As the population continues to age, the need for surgical and transcatheter aortic valve therapies in these patients will continue to grow.

REFERENCES

1. Boudoulas KD, Borer JS, Boudoulas H. Etiology of valvular heart disease in the 21st century. *Cardiology.* 2013;126(3):139-152.
2. Osnabrugge RL, Mylotte D, Head SJ, et al. Aortic stenosis in the elderly: disease prevalence and number of candidates for transcatheter aortic valve replacement: a meta-analysis and modeling study. *J Am Coll Cardiol.* 2013;62(11):1002-1012.
3. Thaden JJ, Nkomo VT, Enriquez-Sarano M. The global burden of aortic stenosis. *Prog Cardiovasc Dis.* 2014;56(6):565-571.
4. Maurer G. Aortic regurgitation. *Heart.* 2006;92(7):994-1000.
5. Boudoulas KD, Wolfe B, Ravi Y, et al. The aortic stenosis complex: aortic valve, atherosclerosis, aortopathy. *J Cardiol.* 2015;65(5):377-382.
6. Centers for Disease Control and Prevention. Prevalence of coronary heart disease—United States, 2006-2010. *MMWR Morb Mortal Wkly Rep.* 2011;60(40):1377-1381.
7. Boudoulas KD, Triposkiadis F, Boudoulas H. The aortic stenosis complex. *Cardiology.* 2018;140(3):194-198.
8. Martinsson A, Li X, Andersson C, et al. Temporal trends in the incidence and prognosis of aortic stenosis: a nationwide study of the Swedish population. *Circulation.* 2015;131(11):988-994.
9. Boudoulas H, Boudoulas KD. Calcific aortic stenosis: an evolution of thoughts. *JACC Cardiovasc Imaging.* 2020;13(3):665-666.
10. Ramchand J, Patel SK, Kearney LG, et al. Plasma ACE2 activity predicts mortality in aortic stenosis and is associated with severe myocardial fibrosis. *JACC Cardiovasc Imaging.* 2020;13(3):655-664.
11. Thanassoulis G, Campbell CY, Owens DS, et al. Genetic associations with valvular calcification and aortic stenosis. *N Engl J Med.* 2013;368(6):503-512.
12. Ross J Jr, Braunwald E. Aortic stenosis. *Circulation.* 1968;38(suppl 1):61-67.
13. Nishimura RA, Otto CM, Bonow RO, et al. 2014 AHA/ACC guideline for the management of patients with valvular heart disease: executive summary: a report of the American College of Cardiology/American Heart Association Task Force on Practice Guidelines. *J Am Coll Cardiol.* 2014;63(22):2438-2488.
14. Baumgartner H, Hung J, Bermejo J, et al. Recommendations on the echocardiographic assessment of aortic valve stenosis: a focused update from the European Association of Cardiovascular Imaging and the American Society of Echocardiography. *J Am Soc Echocardiogr.* 2017;30(4):372-392.
15. Clavel M-A, Dumesnil JG, Capoulade R, et al. Outcome of patients with aortic stenosis, small valve area, and low-flow, low-gradient despite preserved left ventricular ejection fraction. *J Am Coll Cardiol.* 2012;60(14):1259-1267.
16. Clavel M-A, Burwash IG, Pibarot P. Cardiac imaging for assessing low-gradient severe aortic stenosis. *JACC Cardiovasc Imaging.* 2017;10(2):185-202.
17. Aggarwal SR, Clavel M-A, Messika-Zeitoun D, et al. Sex differences in aortic valve calcification measured by multidetector computed tomography in aortic stenosis. *Circ Cardiovasc Imaging.* 2013;6(1):40-47.
18. Nishimura RA, Otto CM, Bonow RO, et al. 2017 AHA/ACC focused update of the 2014 AHA/ACC guideline for the management of patients with valvular heart disease: a report of the American College of Cardiology/American Heart Association Task Force on Clinical Practice Guidelines. *J Am Coll Cardiol.* 2017;70(2):252-289.
19. Braunwald E. Aortic stenosis: then and now. *Circulation.* 2018;137(20):2099-2100.
20. Hannan EL, Samadashvili Z, Lahey SJ, et al. Aortic valve replacement for patients with severe aortic stenosis: risk factors and their impact on 30-month mortality. *Ann Thorac Surg.* 2009;87(6):1741-1749.
21. Rodriguez-Gabella T, Voisine P, Dagenais F, et al. Long-term outcomes following surgical aortic bioprosthesis implantation. *J Am Coll Cardiol.* 2018;71(13):1401-1412.
22. Rodriguez-Gabella T, Voisine P, Puri R, Pibarot P, Rodés-Cabau J. Aortic bioprosthetic valve durability: incidence, mechanisms, predictors, and management of surgical and transcatheter valve degeneration. *J Am Coll Cardiol.* 2017;70(8):1013-1028.
23. Mookhoek A, Korteland NM, Arabkhani B, et al. Bentall procedure: a systematic review and meta-analysis. *Ann Thorac Surg.* 2016;101(5):1684-1689.
24. Blackman DJ, Saraf S, MacCarthy PA, et al. Long-term durability of transcatheter aortic valve prostheses. *J Am Coll Cardiol.* 2019;73(5):537-545.
25. Smith CR, Leon MB, Mack MJ, et al. Transcatheter versus surgical aortic-valve replacement in high-risk patients. *N Engl J Med.* 2011;364(23):2187-2198.
26. Leon MB, Smith CR, Mack MJ, et al. Transcatheter or surgical aortic-valve replacement in intermediate-risk patients. *N Engl J Med.* 2016;374(17):1609-1620.
27. Adams DH, Popma JJ, Reardon MJ. Transcatheter aortic-valve replacement with a self-expanding prosthesis. *N Engl J Med.* 2014;371(10):967-968.
28. Gleason TG, Reardon MJ, Popma JJ, et al. 5-year outcomes of self-expanding transcatheter versus surgical aortic valve replacement in high-risk patients. *J Am Coll Cardiol.* 2018;72(22):2687-2696.
29. Reardon MJ, Van Mieghem NM, Popma JJ, et al. Surgical or transcatheter aortic-valve replacement in intermediate-risk patients. *N Engl J Med.* 2017;376(14):1321-1331.
30. Popma JJ, Deeb GM, Yakubov SJ, et al. Transcatheter aortic-valve replacement with a self-expanding valve in low-risk patients. *N Engl J Med.* 2019;380(18):1706-1715.
31. Kapadia S, Stewart WJ, Anderson WN, et al. Outcomes of inoperable symptomatic aortic stenosis patients not undergoing aortic valve replacement: insight into the impact of balloon aortic valvuloplasty from the Paortic regurgitationTNER trial (Placement of AoRtic TraNscathetER Valve trial). *JACC Cardiovasc Interv.* 2015;8(2):324-333.
32. Bonow RO, Leon MB, Doshi D, Moat N. Management strategies and future challenges for aortic valve disease. *Lancet.* 2016;387(10025):1312-1323.
33. Pibarot P, Dumesnil JG. Prosthetic heart valves: selection of the optimal prosthesis and long-term management. *Circulation.* 2009;119(7):1034-1048.
34. Baumgartner H, Falk V, Bax JJ, et al. 2017 ESC/EACTS guidelines for the management of valvular heart disease. *Eur Heart J.* 2017;38(36):2739-2791.
35. Guedeney P, Mehran R, Collet J-P, Claessen BE, Berg JT, Dangas GD. Antithrombotic therapy after transcatheter aortic valve replacement. *Circ Cardiovasc Interv.* 2019;12(1):e007411.
36. Vavuranakis M, Siasos G, Zografos T, et al. Dual or single anti-platelet therapy after transcatheter aortic valve implantation? A systematic review and meta-analysis. *Curr Pharm Des.* 2016;22:4596-4603.
37. Eckstein J, Liu S, Toleva O, et al. Antithrombotic therapy after transcatheter aortic valve replacement: current perspective. *Curr Opin Cardiol.* 2021;36(2):117-124.
38. Boudoulas KD, Triposkiadis F, Boudoulas H. Evaluation of left ventricular performance: is there a gold standard? *Cardiology.* 2018;140(4):257-261.

39. Triposkiadis F, et al. Left ventricular geometry as a major determinant of left ventricular ejection fraction: physiological considerations and clinical implications. *Eur J Heart Fail.* 2018;20(3):436-444.
40. Akinseye OA, Pathak A, Ibebuogu UN. Aortic valve regurgitation: a comprehensive review. *Curr Probl Cardiol.* 2018;43(8):315-334.
41. Dujardin KS, Enriquez-Sarano M, Schaff HV, Bailey KR, Seward JB, Tajik AJ. Mortality and morbidity of aortic regurgitation in clinical practice. A long-term follow-up study. *Circulation.* 1999;99(14):1851-1857.
42. Carabello B. How to follow patients with mitral and aortic valve disease. *Med Clin North Am.* 2015;99(4):739-757.
43. Foth C, Nair R, Zeltser R. Austin Flint Murmur. In: StatPearls. Updated April 14, 2020.
44. Zoghbi WA, Adams D, Bonow RO, et al. Recommendations for noninvasive evaluation of native valvular regurgitation: a report from the American Society of Echocardiography developed in collaboration with the Society for Cardiovascular Magnetic Resonance. *J Am Soc Echocardiogr.* 2017;30(4):303-371.
45. Iung B, Baron G, Butchart EG, et al. A prospective survey of patients with valvular heart disease in Europe: The Euro Heart Survey on Valvular Heart Disease. *Eur Heart J.* 2003;24(13):1231-1243.
46. Wernly B, Eder S, Navarese EP, et al. Transcatheter aortic valve replacement for pure aortic valve regurgitation: "on-label" versus "off-label" use of TAVR devices. *Clin Res Cardiol.* 2019;108(8):921-930.
47. Hamirani YS, Dietl CA, Voyles W, Peralta M, Begay D, Raizada V. Acute aortic regurgitation. *Circulation.* 2012;126(9):1121-1126.
48. Myerson SG, d'Arcy J, Mohiaddin R, et al. Aortic regurgitation quantification using cardiovascular magnetic resonance: association with clinical outcome. *Circulation.* 2012;126(12):1452-1460.
49. Lalani T, Cabell CH, Benjamin DK, et al. Analysis of the impact of early surgery on in-hospital mortality of native valve endocarditis: use of propensity score and instrumental variable methods to adjust for treatment-selection bias. *Circulation.* 2010;121(8):1005-1013.
50. Nishimura RA, O'Gara PT, Bavaria JE, et al. 2019 AATS/ACC/ASE/SCAI/STS expert consensus systems of care document: a proposal to optimize care for patients with valvular heart disease: a joint report of the American Association for Thoracic Surgery, American College of Cardiology, American Society of Echocardiography, Society for Cardiovascular Angiography and Interventions, and Society of Thoracic Surgeons. *J Am Coll Cardiol.* 2019;73(20):2609-2635.
51. Herrmann S, Störk S, Niemann M, et al. Low-gradient aortic valve stenosis myocardial fibrosis and its influence on function and outcome. *J Am Coll Cardiol.* 2011;58(4):402-412.
52. Dahou A, Magne J, Clavel M-A, et al. Tricuspid regurgitation is associated with increased risk of mortality in patients with low-flow low-gradient aortic stenosis and reduced ejection fraction: results of the multicenter TOPAS Study (True or Pseudo-Severe Aortic Stenosis). *JACC Cardiovasc Interv.* 2015;8(4):588-596.
53. Cavalcante JL, Rijal S, Althouse AD, et al. Right ventricular function and prognosis in patients with low-flow, low-gradient severe aortic stenosis. *J Am Soc Echocardiogr.* 2016;29(4):325-333.

CHAPTER 12

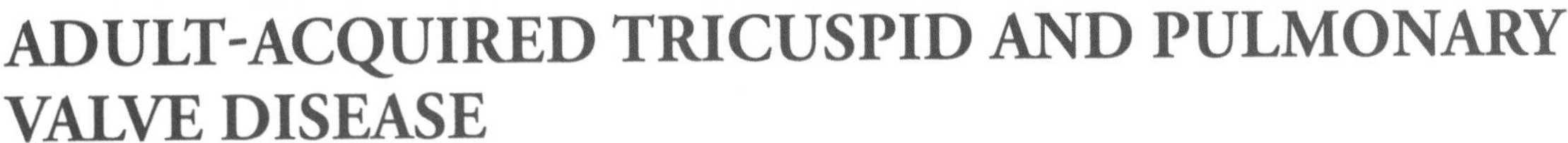

ADULT-ACQUIRED TRICUSPID AND PULMONARY VALVE DISEASE

Maureen E. Cheung and Bryan A. Whitson

INTRODUCTION

Right-sided valve disease can occur from a number of primary and secondary causes. These processes are often associated with an asymptomatic period but have a significant independent effect on morbidity and mortality. To appropriately address these pathologies, a thorough understanding of the unique anatomy and function of each of these valves is necessary.

The tricuspid valve consists of three leaflets connected via chordae tendinea to two papillary muscles. It sits within a fibrous annulus and the junction of the right atrial and ventricular myocardium. Unlike the mitral valve, the tricuspid annulus is not saddle shaped but rather elliptical shaped and is dynamic, changing substantially with variations in loading conditions. For example, during the cardiac cycle, there is an approximately 20% reduction in annular circumference during atrial systole compared to diastole.[1–4]

The pulmonary valve is a semilunar valve; thus, it does not have an annulus in the traditional sense.[1] Instead, it occurs at the intersection of three distinct rings. The first is along the sinotubular ridge of the pulmonary trunk. The second is at the ventriculoarterial junction. And the third is at the basal attachments of the leaflets to the infundibular muscle. The circumferential muscular structure supports the leaflets and the semilunar shape allows for valve competence.

PATHOGENESIS

Tricuspid valve dysfunction can be caused by a number of primary and secondary causes (**Table 12.1**). Primary tricuspid valve dysfunction occurs in up to 25% of patients with tricuspid regurgitation (TR), with the majority of cases related to a congenital abnormality. In the adult population, primary valve etiology is responsible for 10% of TR presentations.[1,5] These are termed acquired primary conditions and include rheumatic disease, carcinoid disease, posttraumatic flail leaflet (chronic presentation), and postendocarditis-related valvular damage.

Secondary causes are responsible for 75% of TR presentations, with the most common overall cause being left-sided valvular pathology, most frequently mitral valve disease.[1] This left-sided disease leads to pulmonary hypertension, right ventricular dilation with subsequent tricuspid annular dilation. Other common secondary causes include other pathologies causing right ventricular dysfunction and dilation, myocardial infarction, or infectious processes.[1,5,6]

In the case of pathologies involving right ventricular dysfunction with dilation, there are two primary sources of tricuspid dysfunction. First, ventricular dilation leads to chordal tethering, causing loss of leaflet apposition and subsequent regurgitation. Second, right ventricular free wall dilation also leads to annular enlargement. This occurs primarily at the anterior and posterior leaflets, with the septal leaflet largely spared because of its origin from the fibrous annulus.[1] The annular enlargement leads to leaflet malcoaptation, contributing to functional TR. Myocardial infarction involving the right ventricle can result in either papillary muscle disruption or regional wall motion abnormalities, which can lead to leaflet malfunction and loss of coaptation. On transthoracic echocardiogram, patients with functional TR will have preferential dilation in the septal-lateral direction, resulting in a more circular and flat shape with a more planar annulus, thus losing the elliptical shape found in healthy subjects.[2]

Another cause of functional TR that is perhaps underrecognized is iatrogenic. These include pacemaker or defibrillator leads and endomyocardial biopsies following orthotopic heart transplants. Pacemaker or defibrillator leads cause tricuspid leaflet dysfunction directly as they pass from the right atrium to the right ventricle. Kim et al. found that of 248 subjects imaged before and after device implantation, 24% had worsened TR by one or more grades.[3,6] Another study examined 5-year outcomes of successful tricuspid valve repairs and found a nearly twofold increase in the incidence of severe TR in patients who had pacemakers implanted compared to those without a pacemaker (42% vs 23%, respectively).[7]

TR following orthotopic heart transplant is exceedingly common with a reported incidence up to 84%, with approximately 34% resulting in decreased quality of life with associated peripheral edema, exertional dyspnea or fatigue, and 6% requiring surgical correction.[8] Although the etiology of TR following orthotopic heart transplant is complex and multifactorial, one recognized correlation is with endomyocardial biopsies.[8] Endomyocardial biopsies are the current standard of care of graft surveillance; however, the number of biopsies performed is correlated with the development of TR. In one single-center study, they found that the incidence of severe TR in patients with more than 31 biopsies was 60% compared to 0% in patients with less than 18 biopsies performed.[8,9] The most common mechanism is direct chordal damage with multiple reports of chordal tissue on pathologic examination.

TABLE 12.1 Etiologies and Pathogenesis of Right-Sided Regurgitant Valve Lesions

Etiology	Pathogenesis
Primary Causes (25%)	
Infectious endocarditis	Leaflet destruction
Trauma	Blunt or penetrating with disruption of structural components
Carcinoid syndrome	Fibrous tissue deposits on valve cusps
Rheumatic disease	Right and/or left-sided valve thickening
Takayasu arteritis	Involvement of pulmonary arteries with pulmonary hypertension
Congenital causes (ie, Ebstein's)	Tricuspid valve regurgitation
Iatrogenic: Pacemaker/defibrillator leads Endomyocardial biopsies	 Direct interference with leaflet coaptation Structural disruption—chordae or papillary muscle destruction/injury
Secondary Causes (75%)	
Left-sided valvular dysfunction	Pulmonary hypertension with progressive right ventricular dilation, tricuspid annular enlargement
Eisenmenger syndrome	Progressive right ventricular dilation, tricuspid annular enlargement
Primary pulmonary hypertension	Progressive right ventricular dilation, tricuspid annular enlargement
Right ventricular infarct	Papillary muscle dysfunction and/or regional wall motion abnormalities
Marfan syndrome and other myxomatous diseases	Mitral and tricuspid valve prolapse and/or chordae elongation or rupture
Dilated cardiomyopathy	Biventricular failure
Drug induced	

Leaflet tissue has also been reported but is relatively uncommon. In one series, Mielniczuk et al. reported that 47% of patients with new acute-onset TR had evidence of chordae tissue in their biopsy.[10]

Tricuspid valve stenosis is more commonly a primary disease process, usually rheumatic related, and is rarely isolated to the tricuspid valve (See **Table 12.2**). These patients frequently have mitral valve disease and occasionally aortic valve involvement as well. Additionally, although the patients will have tricuspid valve stenosis, some degree of regurgitation is also present.[1]

In contrast to tricuspid valve dysfunction, adult-acquired pulmonary valve disease is rare. Nearly all pulmonary valve stenosis is congenital in origin and often occurs as an isolated lesion. There are case reports of isolated pulmonary valve endocarditis, but this is also rare and unlikely to result in need for

TABLE 12.2 Etiologies and Pathogenesis of Right-Sided Stenotic Valve Lesions

Etiology	Pathogenesis
Primary Causes (25%)	
Infectious endocarditis	Leaflet thickening/scaring
Carcinoid syndrome	Fibrous tissue deposits on valve cusps
Rheumatic disease	Leaflet thickening and sclerosis
Congenital anomalies	Ebstein anomaly, congenital tricuspid atresia, congenital tricuspid stenosis
Secondary Causes (75%)	
Systemic lupus erythematosus	Vascular fibroelastic tissue deposition and fibrinoid necrosis
Drug induced (ergot alkaloids, 5-hydroxytryptamine uptake regulators/inhibitors, and ergot-derived dopamine agonists)	Serotonin-related valvular changes, subendothelial plaques with cuspal hyperplasia, and increased collagen synthesis
Right ventricular infarct	Endomyocardial fibrosis

intervention. Serotonin-induced pulmonary valvular pathology has also been described in carcinoid heart disease as well as in patients taking ergot alkaloids, 5-hydroxytryptamine uptake regulators/inhibitors, and ergot-derived dopamine agonists.[11] Additionally, on rare occasion, pulmonary regurgitation may be seen as a late finding of long-standing pulmonary hypertension or even more rarely because of pulmonary artery aneurysms and concomitant annular dilation.

CLINICAL PRESENTATION

Regardless of the underlying etiology, patients with tricuspid valve regurgitation typically present with vague symptoms of fatigue and weakness. This is usually a result of reduced cardiac output and right-sided heart failure.[1] These patients will often have ascites, congestive hepatosplenomegaly, a pulsatile liver, pleural effusion, peripheral edema, jugular vein distention accentuated on inspiration, and atrial fibrillation. In more advanced cases with chronic untreated disease, patients will present with cyanosis, jaundice secondary to cardiac cirrhosis, and cachexia. In the case of secondary functional TR, patients may also exhibit evidence of primary disease progression such as biventricular heart failure.

Tricuspid valve stenosis is usually rheumatic related with concomitant mitral valve and aortic valve involvement. Additionally, some degree of TR is present.[1] The typical patient presentation is a young female with fatigue and malaise who has associated jugular venous distention, pleural effusion, ascites, and peripheral edema. Right upper quadrant tenderness from hepatomegaly with palpable, pulsatile liver may also be present.

With respect to the pulmonary stenosis and/or regurgitation, progressive symptoms of right-sided ventricular dysfunction, dyspnea, and fatigue may occur.

DIAGNOSIS

Echocardiography

The diagnostic modality of choice for valvular disease diagnosis and quantification is transthoracic echocardiography. This examination, when coupled with color Doppler flow imaging, can map the direction, size, and origination of regurgitant jets; provide waveform recordings across the valve; and assess right ventricular function.[1,2,4]

The quantitative echocardiographic diagnostic criteria for severe TR include central jet area more than 10 cm^2, vena contracta diameter more than 0.7 cm, effective regurgitant orifice area 40 mm^2 or more, and regurgitant volume 45 cc or more.[5] Other characteristic echocardiography findings in TR include a "dagger-shaped" Doppler signal, paradoxical septal motion, flow reversal across the valve within the inferior vena cava (IVC) and hepatic veins, and decreased right ventricular function.[1,5] Unlike the left ventricle, right ventricular shape and function can be affected profoundly by both preload and afterload; therefore, interpretations should always consider the clinical condition of the patient. To assess the right ventricular function, a four-chamber view is utilized and the fractional change in area between the end-diastolic and end-systolic areas is calculated. Another measure of right ventricular function is the tricuspid annular peak systolic excursion, which is the apical movement of the annulus during systole.[1]

Echocardiography may also demonstrate findings consistent with the disease process such as in the case of infective endocarditis with vegetations or leaflet destruction or in carcinoid disease with thickened, retracted leaflets fixed in a semi-open position. An investigation for atrial septal defect or patent foramen ovale should also be performed during echocardiography.

In cases of tricuspid stenosis, echocardiography will reveal shortened chordae possibly with fusion and leaflet thickening. In later disease stages, the leaflets will be fused along the free edge with calcification deposits throughout the valve. The diastolic gradient between the right ventricle and atrium will be significantly elevated, which will eventually lead to right atrial wall hypertrophy with chamber dilation. Thickened tricuspid valve leaflets with reduced mobility, diastolic doming, and reduced orifice area with prolonged antegrade flow slope is diagnostic of tricuspid valve stenosis.[1]

Pulmonary valvular regurgitation would be deemed severe with a broad-based color jet filling the right ventricular outflow tract. Severe pulmonary stenosis is identified as a peak Doppler velocity more than 4 m/s and a peak Doppler gradient greater than 64 mmHg.[12]

Magnetic Resonance Imaging

Although echocardiography remains the most common method of assessing valvular disease and ventricular function, magnetic resonance imaging (MRI) is emerging as an alternative method of assessing right ventricular diastolic and systolic volumes and, therefore, function.[1] The utilization of MRI requires cine sequencing as the spin-echo double inversion recovery MRI technique produces dark-blood sequences that make it difficult to discriminate valve from the surrounding blood.[12] In MRI cine sequencing, 20 to 40 images are obtained over a single cardiac cycle in a plane through the heart. These are then replaced with steady-state free-precession (SSFP) sequences that offer higher intrinsic contrast between the cardiac structures and blood. This "bright-blood" sequencing also allows visualization of thin structures such as valve leaflets.[12] With this sequencing, valve morphology, function, and blood flow patterns can be studied. When turbulent flow occurs, it appears as an area of low signal intensity that can be graded as a semiquantitative estimation. In addition to the balanced-SSFP cine MRI technique, phase-contrast or velocity-encoded cine MRI is also being utilized in cardiac imaging.[12] In this technique, flow is visualized and can be quantified, allowing calculations of velocity and volume to measure cardiac output, regurgitant flows, ventricular stroke volumes, and high-velocity jets. This measurement can be made at any point in the cardiac cycle. Additional techniques may be utilized to assess for myocardial infarction, intracavitary thrombi, or coronary artery stenosis at the same imaging setting. By utilizing multiple MRI techniques, a comprehensive evaluation of a diseased valve is possible.[12]

MANAGEMENT OF PATIENT

Medical Approach

Current guidelines regarding management of symptomatic TR focus on treatment of the underlying etiology and management of volume status. Volume status is typically addressed with diuretics with clinical examination, echocardiogram, or central filling pressures. Medical treatment of the underlying etiology is essentially limited to pulmonary hypertension and endocarditis. In the case of endocarditis, a full course of antibiotic therapy should be completed with documented resolution of bacteremia. Follow-up echocardiography will determine the extent of residual tricuspid valve destruction and dictate the need for operative intervention. Medical management of pulmonary hypertension–related tricuspid valve dysfunction consists of volume optimization and addition of pulmonary vasodilators, if appropriate, after determining the etiology of the pulmonary hypertension. In some cases, such as chronic thromboembolic pulmonary hypertension, treatment of the underlying etiology addresses the right ventricular dysfunction and the TR.

In the setting of endocarditis of the tricuspid or pulmonary valves, medical management tends to be initial therapy and evaluation for structural valvular damage and any residual stenosis or regurgitation. In the setting of repeated pulmonary emboli, right ventricular failure, hepatic failure/dysfunction, new-onset arrhythmia, or large vegetation (>3 cm though sometimes smaller in the setting of an atrial septal defect or patent foramen ovale), surgery may be needed.

In cases of aortic or mitral valve dysfunction leading to subsequent TR, if mitral or aortic valve repair or replacement is recommended, concomitant tricuspid repair is often indicated.[1,5] This recommendation is based on findings that the tricuspid valve dysfunction does not consistently resolve despite relief of the right ventricular strain, and subsequent isolated tricuspid valve intervention via redo sternotomy is associated with increased in-hospital mortality.

Surgical Approach

The majority of tricuspid valve interventions occur concomitantly with other cardiac surgical interventions, with over 80% of all tricuspid valve operations associated with left valve surgeries; however, recent guideline updates have expanded the recommendation for isolated tricuspid valve operations.[1,5,13] In the case of concurrent cardiac surgery, surgical treatment of severe TR is a class 1 recommendation, with tricuspid annulus greater than 4 cm and/or right heart failure a class 2a recommendation. Isolated tricuspid valve operations are generally associated with endocarditis, with a minority related to post-traumatic valvular dysfunction. Additionally, isolated tricuspid valve operations for severe primary TR with symptomatic right heart failure is shown to reduce hospitalizations and is now a class 2a guideline recommendation. The operative approach to the tricuspid valve may be dictated by the concurrent operation, and the order of operation should be preoperatively planned. The choice between repair and replacement is typically dictated by anatomic concerns, specifically degree of annular dilation and the presence of an intracardiac pacer/defibrillator lead. When replacement is indicated, bioprosthetic and mechanical valves demonstrate no definitive survival benefit of one over the other. Nevertheless, tissue bioprosthesis is most commonly used. Factors that should be considered when deciding between the two include valve thrombosis rates, need for anticoagulation and compliance, potential need for future pacemaker, and risk of structural deterioration.

In patients with TR and pulmonary hypertension, the right ventricle not only dilates but also increases in length along the superior-inferior axis, leading to valvular tethering and reduced coaptation.[12] TR in these settings is a particularly vexing conundrum as repair or replacement options that fix the regurgitation may do little to influence overall right ventricular function.[8] One option is repair/replacement of the tricuspid valve during left ventricular assist device implantation with the goal of unloading and reversal of pulmonary hypertension in preparation for heart transplantation. In patients who develop severe TR after orthotopic heart transplantation (which often is attributed to iatrogenic injury from endomyocardial biopsy, **Figure 12.1**) and need a tricuspid valve replacement, a tissue bioprosthesis should be used. It has good durability[8] in the low-pressure right heart, does not require anticoagulation, and, as opposed to a mechanical valve, would allow continued cardiac surveillance with endomyocardial biopsies.

It remains unproven if surgical tricuspid valve annuloplasty, in the setting of pulmonary hypertension, alters the natural course of right ventricular dilation and recurrent TR.[1] Recurrent TR (≥3+) following repair occurs in up to 14% of patients within months and the incidence steadily increases over time and affects up to 20% of patients by 5 years.[5] This risk appears to be lower in patients treated with a rigid annuloplasty band. Reoperation for recurrent TR is rare but associated with up to 37% in-hospital mortality.[5,14] Risk factors for recurrence include baseline regurgitant severity, pulmonary hypertension, left ventricular dysfunction, right ventricular device leads, leaflet tenting, and degree of annular dilation.[5,14]

There are multiple advantages to bioprosthetic tricuspid and pulmonic valve replacements including lower risk of valve thrombosis and avoidance of anticoagulation. However, there is an increased risk of severe bioprosthetic degeneration, up to 7% at 7 to 8 years requiring stand-alone redo replacement.[5]

Percutaneous Intervention Approach

At present, there are limited percutaneous approaches to tricuspid and pulmonary valve intervention for regurgitation. In using percutaneous valves in the tricuspid position for TR, particularly with annular dilation, a major limitation is inability to anchor the valve. There are clinical trials around tricuspid valve clipping (eg Edwards PASCAL system CLASP trial) and off-label use of the Abbott Mitraclip. There are case anecdotes around the use of Edwards Sapien valve and Medtronic Melody valves for pulmonic valve interventions. Typically, these are through collaboration with pediatric interventional cardiologists, with most pulmonic valve interventions in the setting of adult congenital heart patients. Creative anecdotal experiences are reported around stented valves being deployed in the

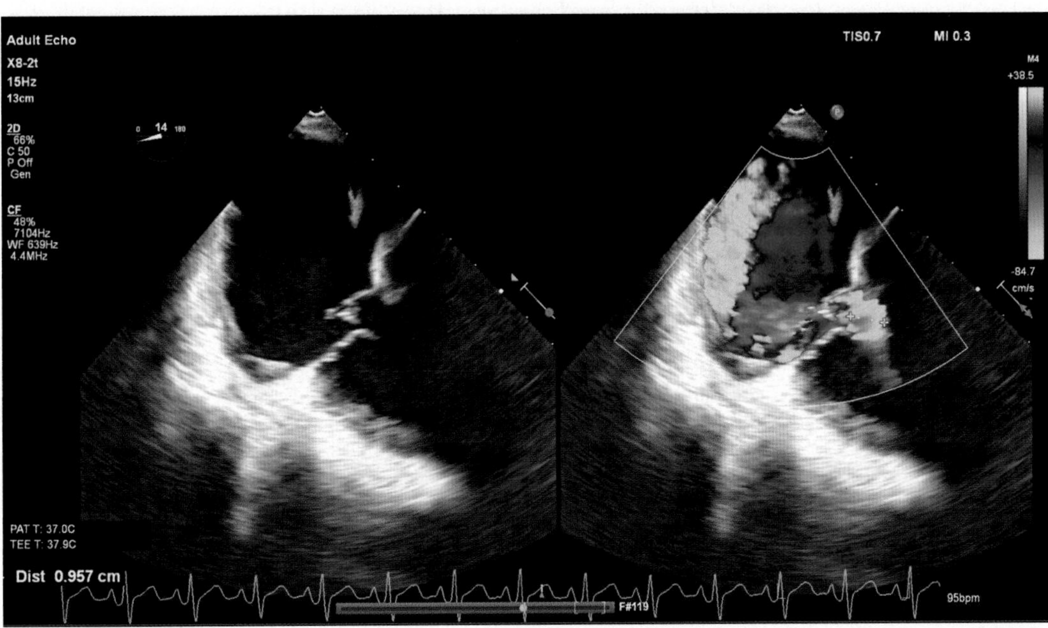

FIGURE 12.1 Transesophageal echocardiographic images of tricuspid regurgitation following endocardial biopsy in an orthotopic heart transplant recipient; an iatrogenic etiology.

suprahepatic IVC, stenting the tricuspid valve and deploying into the tricuspid valve stent, and so on. The trials and off-label indications are beyond the scope of this chapter.

FOLLOW-UP PATIENT CARE

In patients undergoing tricuspid or pulmonic valve replacement, particularly for regurgitation, the postsurgical care is focused on treating exacerbated hepatic and renal insufficiency, managing the right ventricle though meticulous surgical technique, volume management, inotropic support, and addressing any underlying pulmonary hypertension. In patients with bioprosthetic valves, there may be a role for vitamin K antagonist anticoagulation for ~3 months to prevent valvular thrombosis, though the risk needs to be balanced with any underlying hepatic insufficiency. In the setting of a mechanical valve, vitamin K antagonist anticoagulation is initiated rather quickly—often with a heparin bridge—and with goal international normalized ratio (INR) of 2.5 to 3.5. There is an underlying inherent risk of complete heart block and/or bradycardia necessitating a pacemaker because of disruption of the conduction system, particularly with tricuspid valve interventions. Especially with mechanical valves, though often in bioprosthetic valves as well, during valve replacement there should be a low threshold for epicardial lead placement tunneled to a subclavicular location in the event of need for permanent pacemaker placement. Routine echocardiographic follow-up would be per guideline recommendations.[12]

RESEARCH AND FUTURE DIRECTIONS

Industry research and development is focused toward stented percutaneous bioprosthesis development and testing, valve leaflet clipping devices, and right atrial to left atrial shunt devices to improve right-sided heart hemodynamics.

In the surgical setting, the role of isolated[13,15] and concomitant tricuspid valve repair/replacement during left-sided (particularly mitral valve) intervention[16–19] and with coronary artery bypass[20] will continue to evolve.

KEY POINTS

- ✔ For tricuspid repair, sizing is based on base dimension of the septal leaflet because it is relatively spared from annular dilation.
- ✔ Removal of intracardiac pacemaker or defibrillator leads at the time of tricuspid valve surgery with placement of permanent epicardial leads reduces late repair failures.
- ✔ A tethered tricuspid valve because of intracardiac lead placement may be repaired, though progression of disease may recur.
- ✔ Managing the right ventricular function, underlying pulmonary hypertension, and any exacerbated hepatorenal dysfunction is critical to successful outcome of pulmonic or tricuspid valve surgery.
- ✔ There is an evolving literature to support concomitant tricuspid valve intervention with other cardiac surgery, particularly if repair is possible.

REFERENCES

1. Cohn LH, ed. *Cardiac Surgery in the Adult*. 5th ed. McGraw Hill Education; 2016.
2. Fukuda S. Three-dimensional geometry of the tricuspid annulus in healthy subjects and in patients with functional tricuspid regurgitation: a real-time, 3-dimensional echocardiographic study. *Circulation*. 2006;114(1 suppl):I492-I498. doi:10.1161/CIRCULATIONAHA.105.000257

3. Kim JB, Spevack DM, Tunick PA, et al. The effect of transvenous pacemaker and implantable cardioverter defibrillator lead placement on tricuspid valve function: an observational study. *J Am Soc Echocardiogr.* 2008;21(3):284-287. doi:10.1016/j.echo.2007.05.022
4. Ton-Nu T-T, Levine RA, Handschumacher MD, et al. Geometric determinants of functional tricuspid regurgitation: insights from 3-dimensional echocardiography. *Circulation.* 2006;114(2):143-149. doi:10.1161/CIRCULATIONAHA.106.611889
5. Fender EA, Zack CJ, Nishimura RA. Isolated tricuspid regurgitation: outcomes and therapeutic interventions. *Heart.* 2018;104(10):798-806. doi:10.1136/heartjnl-2017-311586
6. Taira K, Suzuki A, Fujino A, Watanabe T, Ogyu A, Ashikawa K. Tricuspid valve stenosis related to subvalvular adhesion of pacemaker lead: a case report. *J Cardiol.* 2006;47(6):301-306.
7. McCarthy PM, Bhudia SK, Rajeswaran J, et al. Tricuspid valve repair: durability and risk factors for failure. *J Thorac Cardiovasc Surg.* 2004;127(3):674-685. doi:10.1016/j.jtcvs.2003.11.019
8. Kwon MH, Shemin RJ. Tricuspid valve regurgitation after heart transplantation. *Ann Cardiothorac Surg.* 2017;6(3):270-274. doi:10.21037/acs.2017.04.02
9. Nguyen V, Cantarovich M, Cecere R, Giannetti N. Tricuspid regurgitation after cardiac transplantation: how many biopsies are too many? *J Heart Lung Transplant.* 2005;24(7):S227-S231. doi:10.1016/j.healun.2004.07.007
10. Mielniczuk L, Haddad H, Davies RA, Veinot JP. Tricuspid valve chordal tissue in endomyocardial biopsy specimens of patients with significant tricuspid regurgitation. *J Heart Lung Transplant.* 2005;24(10):1586-1590. doi:10.1016/j.healun.2004.11.007
11. Masci PG, Dymarkowski S, Bogaert J. Valvular heart disease: what does cardiovascular MRI add? *Eur Radiol.* 2008;18(2):197-208. doi:10.1007/s00330-007-0731-x
12. Nishimura RA, Otto CM, Bonow RO, et al. 2014 AHA/ACC guideline for the management of patients with valvular heart disease: a report of the American College of Cardiology/American Heart Association Task Force on Practice Guidelines. *Circulation.* 2014;129(23):2440-2492.
13. Otto CM, Nishimura RA, Bonow RO, et al. ACC/AHA guideline for the management of patients with valvular heart disease: a report of the American College of Cardiology/American Heart Association Joint Committee on Clinical Practice Guidelines. *J Am Coll Cardiol.* 2021;77(4):e25-e197. doi:10.1016/j.jacc.2020.11.018
14. Hwang HY, Kim KH, Kim KB, Ahn H. Reoperations after tricuspid valve repair: re-repair versus replacement. *J Thorac Dis.* 2016;8(1):133-139. doi:10.3978/j.issn.2072-1439.2016.01.43
15. LaPar DJ, Likosky DS, Zhang M, et al. Development of a risk prediction model and clinical risk score for isolated tricuspid valve surgery. *Ann Thorac Surg.* 2018;106(1):129-136.
16. Rotar E, Lim DS, Ailawadi G. Risk stratification for surgery in tricuspid regurgitation. *Prog Cardiovasc Dis.* 2019;62(6):500-504.
17. Ghoreishi M, Brown JM, Stauffer CE, et al. Undersized tricuspid annuloplasty rings optimally treat functional tricuspid regurgitation. *Ann Thorac Surg.* 2011;92(1):89-95
18. Badhwar V, Rankin JS, He M, et al. Performing concomitant tricuspid valve repair at the time of mitral valve operations is not associated with increased operative mortality. *Ann Thorac Surg.* 2017;103(2):587-593.
19. Chancellor WZ, Mehaffey JH, Beller JP, et al. Impact of tricuspid regurgitation with and without repair during aortic valve replacement. *J Thorac Cardiovasc Surg.* 2020;S0022-5223(20)30424-4.
20. Haywood N, Mehaffey JH, Chancellor WZ, et al. Burden of tricuspid regurgitation in patients undergoing coronary artery bypass grafting. *Ann Thorac Surg.* 2021;111(1):44-50.

CHAPTER 13

PROSTHETIC VALVE DYSFUNCTION

Shuktika Nandkeolyar, Dmitry Abramov, Helme Silvet, and Purvi Parwani

INTRODUCTION

Epidemiology

The prevalence of patients with prosthetic heart valves (PHVs) is growing quickly. With the advent of transcatheter valve implantation, it is estimated that around 850,000 patients will undergo PHV implantation annually by 2050.[1] Although these devices have been effective in treating native heart valve disease, they require continued evaluation and management. PHVs can be categorized as mechanical, bioprosthetic, homograft, or xenograft. Mechanical heart valves are comprised of an occluder, occluder restraint, and a sewing ring. They are bileaflet (most common), single tilting disc, or caged ball.[2] Bioprosthetic valves are stented, stentless, sutureless, or the increasingly common transcatheter valves. The material for bioprosthetic valves are usually either bovine pericardial tissue or porcine valve tissue.[2,3] Finally, homograft and xenograft valves are less commonly used, and typically implanted in the aortic or pulmonic position.[4]

There are several manifestations of PHV dysfunction, with significant implications for patient care. In this chapter, we focus on the most commonly encountered and clinically relevant complications: prosthetic valve thrombosis (PVT), pannus formation, patient-prosthesis mismatch (PPM), structural valve degeneration (SVD), endocarditis, and paravalvular leak (PVL).

Overall, the annual incidence of PHV dysfunction ranges between 0.7% and 3.5%,[2,5-10] although this varies greatly between the type, location, and number of PHVs implanted.[2,5-15] The incidence, risk factors, and pathogenesis of these PHV pathologies are important when considering their evaluation by various imaging modalities and are summarized in **Table 13.1**.

Risk Factors

Risk factors for developing PHV disease vary by the prosthesis used and the disease in question, with specific risk factors for each category of PHV dysfunction summarized in Table 13.1. There are also several common factors: young age, female gender, obesity, elevated calcium in end-stage renal disease or hyperparathyroidism, hypertension, pregnancy, metabolic syndrome, diabetes, and increased lipids.[2,5,9,11,15-18] Valve positioning, particularly for supra-annular transcatheter valve placement of aortic PHV, is a risk factor for PVL. Risk factors for PPM include low ejection fraction, high body surface area, and a small annulus area.

PATHOGENESIS

Acute Prosthetic Heart Valve Dysfunction

There are several types of PHV dysfunction, including thrombosis and infection, which can develop over a short time and present with acute symptoms. PVT in a bioprosthetic valve occurs because of a hypercoagulable state as a reaction to recent tissue injury during surgery or an incompletely endothelialized prosthesis[5]; with a mechanical prosthetic valve, it occurs with inadequate anticoagulation. Slow blood flow (due to low pressure venous flow for right-sided valves, stasis in the setting of atrial fibrillation or atrial dilation for tricuspid and mitral PHV, or low ejection fraction for aortic or pulmonic PHV) can contribute to PVT.[5,19] Finally, valve frame fracture, incomplete apposition, or leaflet injury may cause turbulent flow, promoting acute thrombosis formation.[5]

Infective endocarditis may be caused by perioperative bacterial contamination or may occur any time after valve implantation because of bacterial or fungal bloodstream infection. Endocarditis is often seen at the sewing ring and annulus in addition to valvular leaflet vegetations. It can lead to paravalvular abscess, dehiscence, pseudoaneurysms, fistulae, and conduction system block.[14,19,20] Endocarditis can be a subacute process, but more commonly presents with acute valvular and paravalvular destruction, leading to prominent symptoms.

PVL occurs because of a number of mechanisms, including tissue friability, suture failure, infection, and annular or valvular calcification (for transcatheter procedures), preventing full PHV expansion, malapposition of the PHV, and underexpansion or undersizing of the PHV.[2,3,15] PVLs often are seen immediately after valve implantation and most reduce or resolve over time, although PVLs can also occur from endocarditis.[2,3]

Chronic Prosthetic Heart Valve Dysfunction

Prosthetic valve pathology that manifests over a longer period of time includes pannus formation, valve degeneration, and PPM.

Pannus formation is caused by an autoimmune reaction between the host and prosthesis, creating a fibrous ingrowth (either on mechanical or bioprosthetic PHVs, leading to impaired movement of the PHV leaflets.[2,6]

SVD predominantly affects bioprosthetic PHV. The three primary mechanisms are calcification or degradation of the valve tissue, immune response to residual xenoantigens, or lipid-mediated inflammation.[2,11] Calcification or degradation

TABLE 13.1 Incidence, Risk Factors, Pathogenesis, and Clinical Signs and Symptoms of Prosthetic Heart Valve Disorders[2-15,17-19]

PHV Dysfunction	Incidence	Risk Factors	Pathogenesis	Clinical Presentation
Thrombosis	• Mechanical PHV 0.1%-5.7%/year • Bioprosthetic PHV 0.03-0.74%/year	• Mechanical PHV • Subtherapeutic INR • Atrial fibrillation	• Hypercoagulable state • Slow blood flow • Turbulent blood flow	• Heart failure • Muffled heart sound or absence of "click" • Embolism
Pannus	• 0.7%-1.8% per year	• Young age • Female	• Autoimmune reaction between host and prosthesis	• Heart failure • Progressive dyspnea on exertion
Patient-prosthesis mismatch	• SAVI 20%-70% • TAVI 9.6%-24% • MVR 9%-71%	• Smaller valve annulus • Large BSA • TAVI without post-balloon dilation • Female	• Small EOA	• Heart failure • Incomplete resolution of symptoms
Structural valve degeneration (bioprosthetic valves)	• 2%-10% at 10 years	• Elevated calcium (ESRD or hyperparathyroidism) • Young age • Valve position (mitral) • Diabetes • Hyperlipidemia	• Calcification • Immune response to residual xenoantigens • Lipid-mediated inflammation	• New murmur • Heart failure
Endocarditis	• 1%-6% per year	• Older age • Diabetes • Hypertension • Hyperlipidemia • Poor oral dentition	• Perioperative contamination • Gram-positive infections	• New murmur • Heart failure • Fever • Chills • Embolism • Renal failure
Paravalvular leak	• 5%-18%	• Mechanical mitral PHV • Supra-annular aortic PHV • Calcified annulus • History of endocarditis	• Tissue friability • Endocarditis • Annular/valvular calcification	• New murmur • Heart failure • Hemolytic anemia

BSA, body surface area; EOA, effective orifice area; ESRD, end-stage renal disease; INR, international normalized ratio; MVR, mitral valve replacement; PHV, prosthetic heart valve; SAVI, surgical aortic valve implantation; TAVI, transcatheter aortic valve implantation.

is thought to occur because of a coating of glutaraldehyde on the bioprosthetic valves. Although the coating decreases thromboembolic risk and decreases immune response against porcine and bovine tissues, it also attracts calcium deposits that ultimately lead to stenosis from limitation of leaflet motion or regurgitation from disruption of the connective tissue matrix.[2,11]

PPM is caused by a valve size or effective orifice area (EOA) that is too small to accommodate unimpeded blood flow across the valve, thereby causing a functional obstruction despite a normally functioning valve.[2,18]

CLINICAL PRESENTATION

Common Signs and Symptoms

The clinical presentation of acute PHV diseases includes a new murmur, embolic phenomena, or decompensated heart failure including cardiogenic shock. Chronic PHV pathology can present with more indolent symptoms that can be difficult to recognize, such as progressive dyspnea and fatigue. Development of new symptoms in a patient with a PHV requires a high index of suspicion on the part of the clinician to recognize, diagnose, and treat PHV diseases in a timely manner.

Symptoms commonly seen with each type of PHV disorder are summarized in Table 13.1.[19] PVT is suggested when a patient with known mechanical PHV presents with interruption in anticoagulation and new acute heart failure, thromboembolism, and absence or diminution of the "click" on routine examination of the valve.[5,19] PPM or pannus may present with progressive shortness of breath and fatigue, or incomplete resolution of symptoms post initial PHV placement.[2,19] In addition to these symptoms common to all PHV diseases, endocarditis can present with fatigue, fever, conduction disease, chills, and cutaneous immunologic or septic thrombotic signs (ie, Osler nodes, splinter hemorrhages, petechiae, and Janeway lesions),[15,19] whereas PVL can present with pallor, fatigue, petechiae, or jaundice consistent with hemolytic anemia.

Differential Diagnosis

The differential diagnosis of PHV dysfunction can be categorized by obstruction and regurgitation. Although manifestations of various etiologies of PHV dysfunction can overlap, typical causes of obstruction include SVD, PVT, pannus, and PPM, whereas typical causes of regurgitation include PVL, SVD, and endocarditis. Symptoms mimicking valve dysfunction also need to be differentiated from other cardiac or noncardiac conditions that can have similar presentations.

DIAGNOSIS

Initial Evaluation of Suspected Prosthetic Heart Valve Dysfunction

PHV dysfunction can be suspected on the basis of the signs and symptoms, as shown in Table 13.1. Typical first-line evaluation modality is transthoracic echocardiogram (TTE) or transesophageal echocardiogram (TEE), although other modalities including fluoroscopy, cardiac computed tomography (CCT), cardiac magnetic resonance (CMR) imaging, and positron emission tomography/computed tomography (PET/CT) may play an important role in the diagnosis depending on the patient presentation and clinical suspicion (**Algorithms 13.1 and 13.2**). Although PHV dysfunction can present with a wide range of pathologic findings on imaging, the presentation commonly includes imaging findings of valve flow obstruction, flow regurgitation, or endocarditis-related changes.

Echocardiography (Transthoracic Echocardiogram and Transesophageal Echocardiogram)

Two-Dimensional Imaging/Three-Dimensional Visual Appearance

Stenotic Lesions: Use of echocardiography (TTE and/or TEE) is a class I indication if there is suspicion of PHV dysfunction, and is generally the first diagnostic study ordered.[21,22] TEE may be required for PHV evaluations, especially those in the mitral position, because of acoustic shadowing.[2,4] A complete echocardiographic assessment of suspected PHV disease should include visualization of leaflet mobility, calcification, thickening, or vegetation, as well as thrombus and pannus. Thrombus generally begins at the valve ring and expands inward, obstructing leaflet mobility, with a soft echogenicity and smooth contour (**Case Studies 13.1 and 13.2**).[5] Pannus generally appears more dense than does thrombus on echocardiography, although the differentiation between the two by echocardiography can be

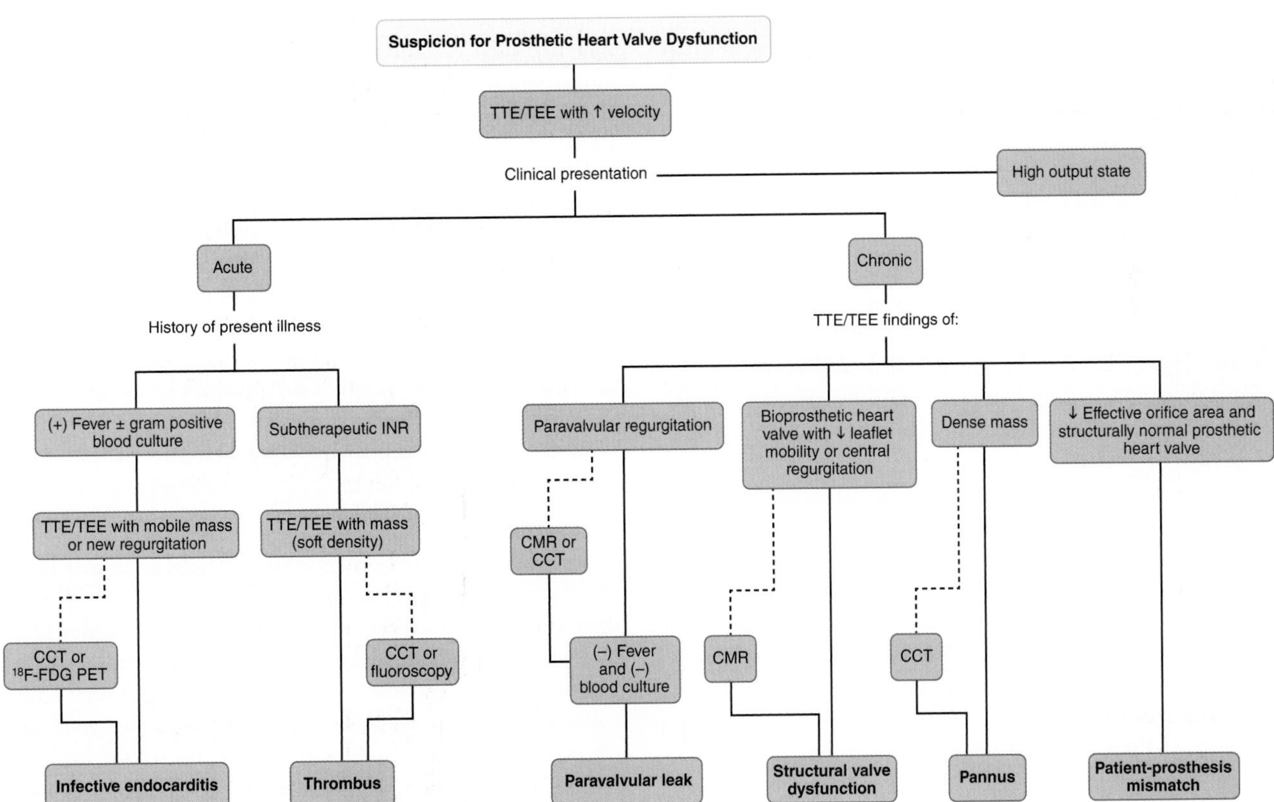

ALGORITHM 13.1 Diagnosis of prosthetic heart valve dysfunction*

*References 2-4

CCT, cardiac computed tomography; CMR, cardiac magnetic resonance imaging; ^{18}F-FDG PET, ^{18}F-fluorodeoxyglucose positron emission tomography; INR, international normalized ratio; PPM, patient prosthesis mismatch; PVL, paravalvular leak; SVD, structural valve dysfunction; TEE, transesophageal echocardiography; TTE, transthoracic echocardiography.

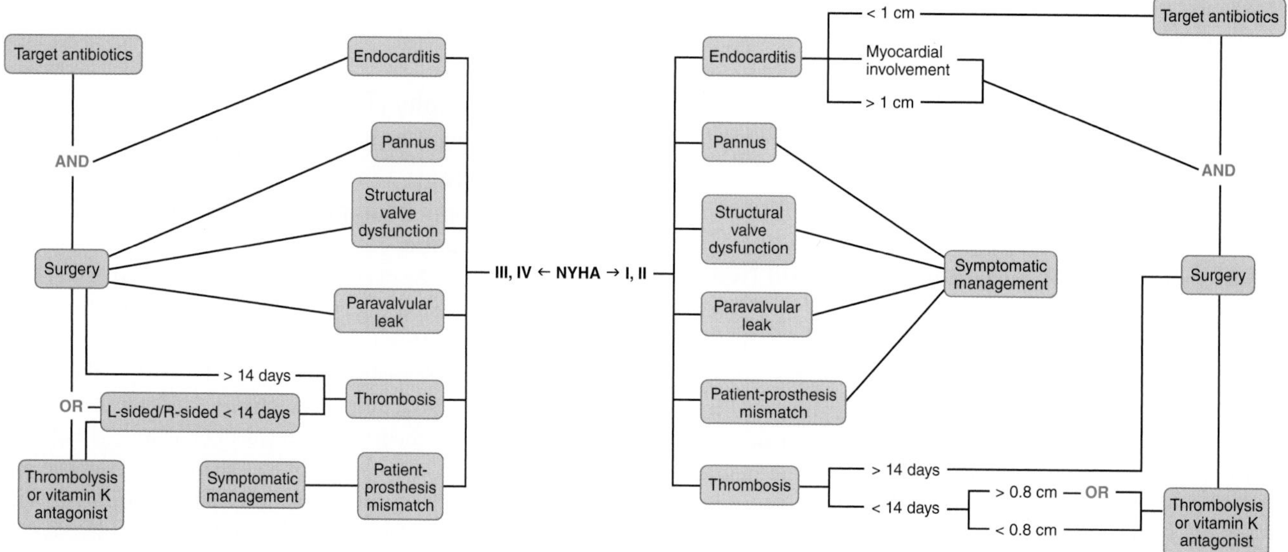

ALGORITHM 13.2 Management of prosthetic heart valve dysfunction.(19, 21, 37) AR, aortic regurgitation; AS, aortic stenosis; CCT, cardiac computed tomography; CMR, cardiac magnetic resonance; ^{18}F-FDG PET, ^{18}F-fluorodeoxyglucose positron emission tomography; LA, left atrium; LVOT, left ventricular outflow tract; NYHA, New York Heart Association; PHV, prosthetic heart valve; TEE, transesophageal echocardiogram; TTE, transthoacic echocardiogram.

challenging in clinical practice.[2] SVD-related stenosis is diagnosed by visualization of decreased leaflet mobility with calcification and/or fusion of the valve leaflets (**Case Studies 13.3 and 13.4, Video 13.3**).[2,19] In addition to two-dimensional (2D) imaging, three-dimensional (3D) echocardiography is helpful in visualizing components of the PHV and presence of pannus or thrombus that are not well seen on 2D imaging because of acoustic shadowing.[4]

Regurgitant Lesions: A complete 2D or 3D echocardiographic study evaluates for the presence of perivalvular abscess, abnormal rocking motion of the valve, and dehiscence at the sewing ring. SVD-related regurgitation is caused by torn or flail leaflets, and usually causes central or eccentric valvular regurgitation.[2,3] Infective endocarditis can cause paravalvular or valvular regurgitation depending on the site, and can lead to destruction of the surrounding paravalvular areas, including abscess formation. Vegetations are generally irregularly shaped, independently mobile structures of low echogenicity, although imaging cannot easily distinguish infected vegetations from noninfected echodensities such as thrombi.[2] Idiopathic PVL due to malposition or malapposition of the PHV may not be immediately evident on 2D or 3D imaging, and may require the addition of color Doppler.

Patient-Prosthesis Mismatch (PPM): The 2D appearance of the valve in the case of PPM may be normal because PPM is a functional obstruction without mechanical dysfunction of the valve itself.[2] The physiologic relationship between the flow, valve area, and transvalvular gradient can be explained by the formula: gradient $= Q^2/K \times EOA^2$, where $Q =$ flow, K is a constant, and $EOA =$ effective orifice area.[2] For the gradient to remain normal, the EOA must be proportionate to flow. The flow can be disproportionately increased (leading to an elevated gradient) in patients with high cardiac output states such as anemia, thyrotoxicosis, pregnancy, and infection; hence, these etiologies must be ruled out before a diagnosis of PPM is made.[19] If no other etiology for an elevated gradient is discovered, then PPM can be diagnosed,[2,19] implying that valve area is too small for the patient's body size during normal flow conditions.

Chamber Quantification and Volumes

Chamber quantification of all chambers and both left ventricular outflow tract (LVOT) and right ventricular outflow tract (RVOT) measurements should be obtained to diagnose PHV dysfunction optimally.[2] Dilation of atrial or ventricular chambers may indicate or support the presence or progression of PHV dysfunction. Accurate outflow tract measurements are important in calculations including Doppler velocity index (DVI) or regurgitant volume.

Color Doppler

Color Doppler should be used to visualize and accurately locate and quantify regurgitation (paravalvular or valvular) within the context of what is expected for the specific PHV. Color Doppler may reveal a narrowed color inflow jet and areas of turbulent or high-velocity flow with regurgitation (**Video 13.2**). Color Doppler assesses inflow and regurgitant jets, vena contracta (VC), proximal isovelocity surface area (PISA), and flow reversal in the hepatic vein and aorta. If significant acoustic shadowing is present, 3D color Doppler can define the presence, origin, direction, and extension of regurgitant jets.[4] Mechanical PHVs all have some degree of physiologic regurgitation with valve closure, and at the hinges of the occluder, stentless valves frequently have minor paravalvular regurgitant jets.[2] It is important to differentiate such physiologic findings from pathologic regurgitation.

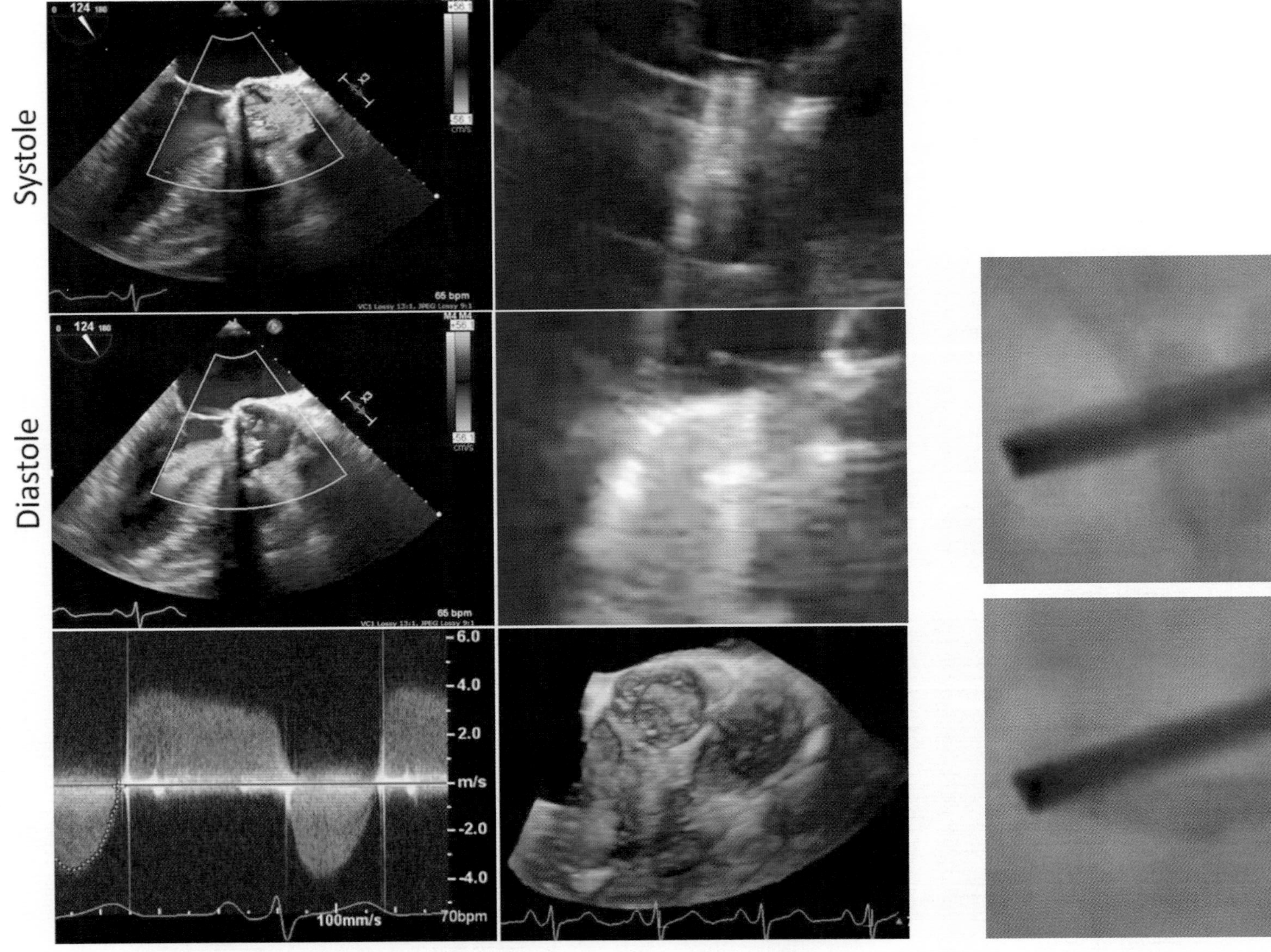

THROMBOSIS CASE 13.1 (ECHOCARDIOGRAPHY AND FLUORSCOPY): A 70-year-old male with mechanical aortic PHV who held warfarin without bridging anticoagulation therapy before prostate cancer surgery presented 2 weeks later with dyspnea on exertion. Fluoroscopy images show a St. Jude bileaflet mechanical disk aortic valve with the posterolateral leaflet stuck in the open position. 2D and 3D TEE images show thrombus on the posterolateral leaflet along with 3.8 m/s velocity during systole with a mean gradient of 31 mm Hg and mild-moderate aortic regurgitation seen on continuous-wave Doppler. PHV, prosthetic heart valve; TEE transesophageal echocardiogram.

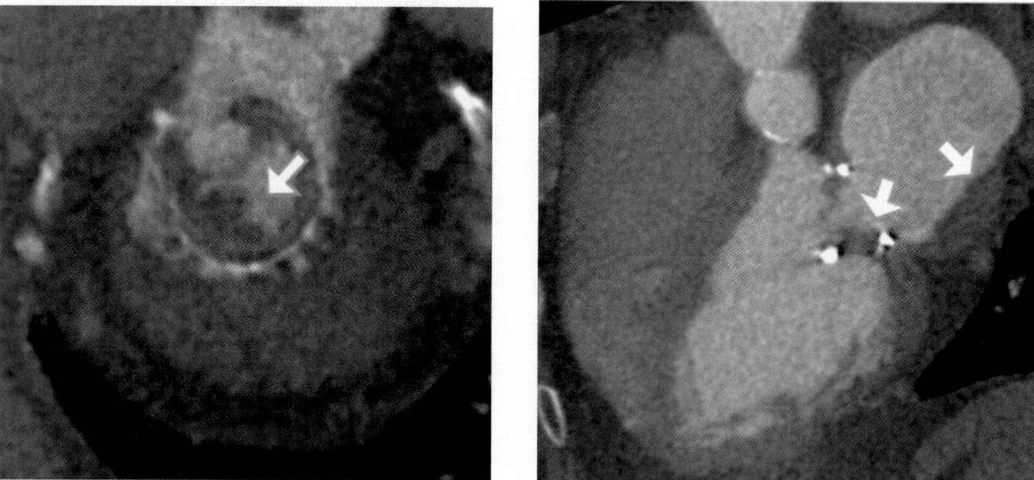

THROMBOSIS CASE 13.2: A 65-year-old female with bioprosthetic mitral PHV and atrial fibrillation presents with a stroke and an INR of 1.0. CCT images show a left atrial thrombus extending to the mechanical mitral valve. CCT, cardiac computed tomography; INR, international normalized ratio; PHV, prosthetic heart valve.

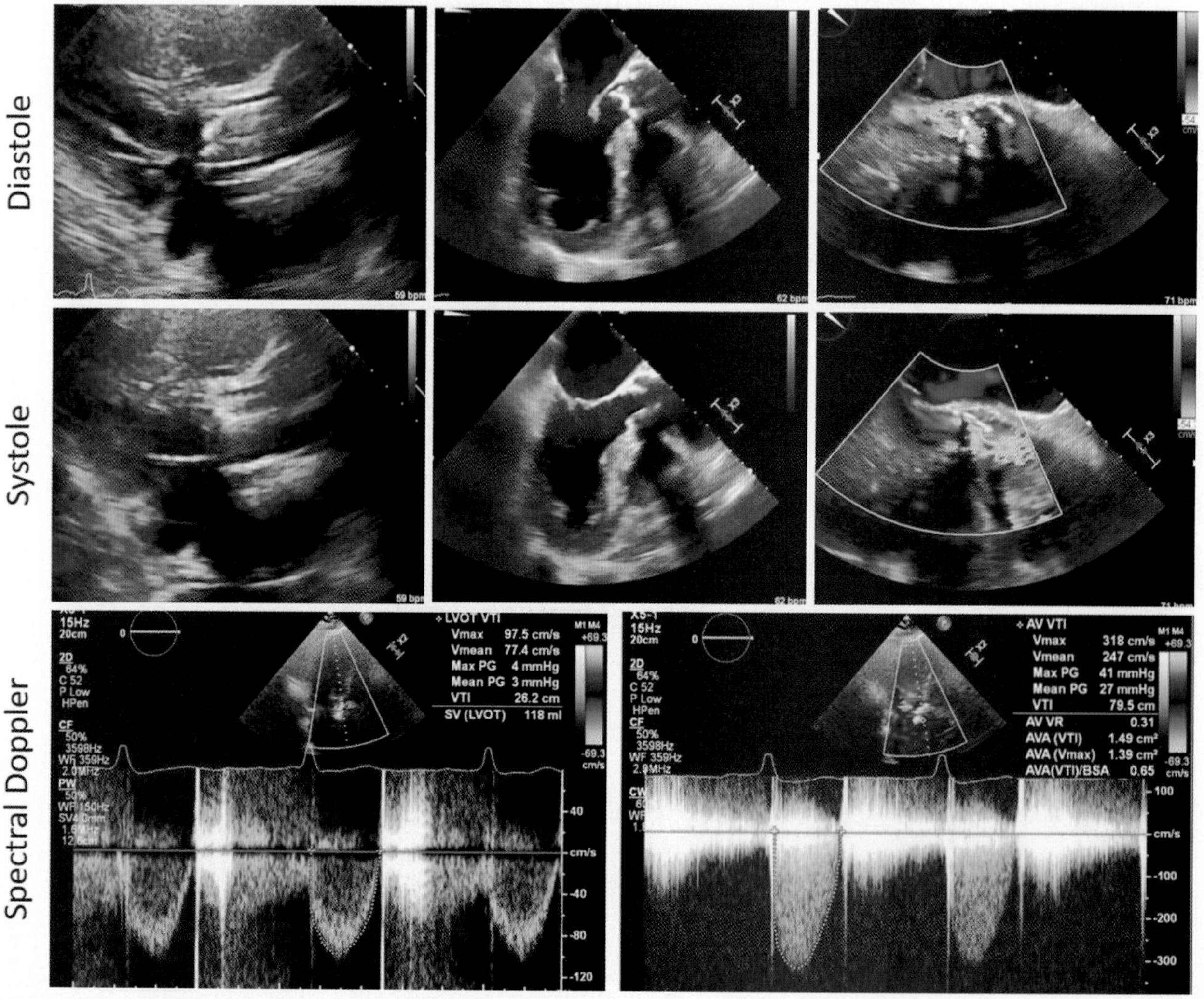

STRUCTURAL VALVE DEGENERATION CASE 13.3: An 80-year-old male with bioprosthetic aortic PHV presented with slowly progressive dyspnea on exertion, orthopnea, and peripheral edema. A #25 Medtronic Porcine Mosaic Aortic Bioprosthesis is visualized with 2D echocardiographic images demonstrating severe calcification. Color Doppler images show mild AR and moderate-severe AS in diastole and systole. The LVOT velocity (0.96 m/s) and aortic valve velocity (3.2 m/s) estimate an aortic valve area of 1.4 cm^2. AR, aortic regurgitation; AS, aortic stenosis. LVOT, left ventricular outflow; PHV, prosthetic heart valve.

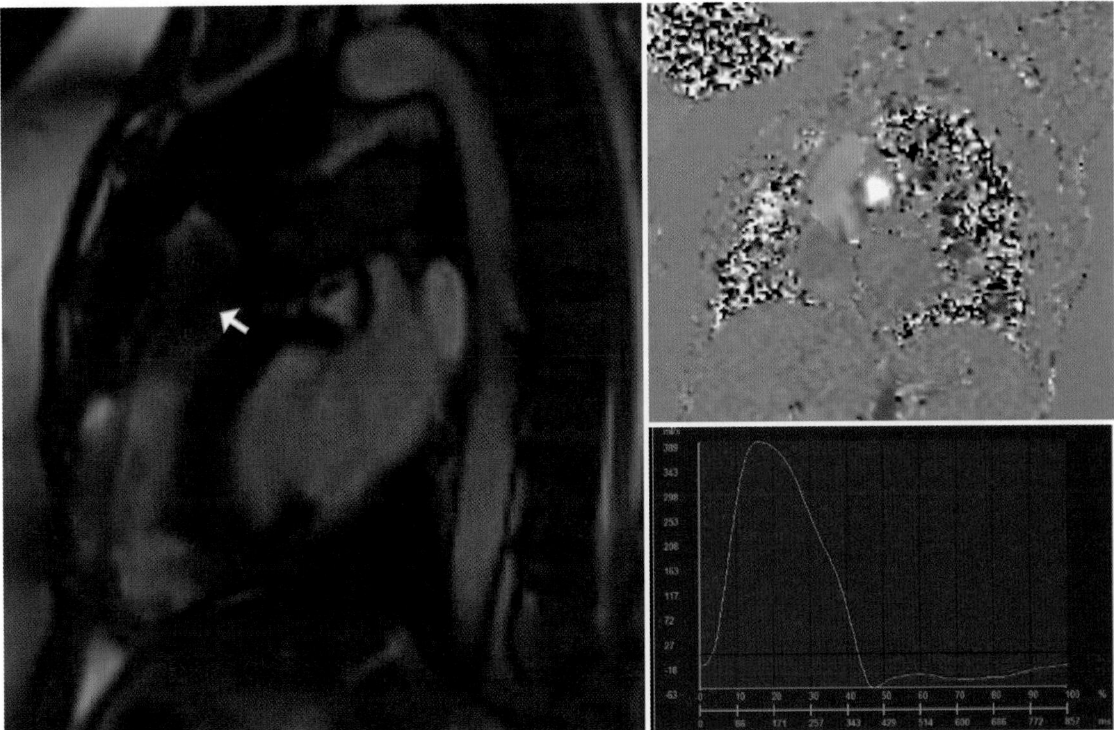

STRUCTURAL VALVE DEGENERATION CASE 13.4: A 24-year-old female with pulmonic valve xenograft presents with progressive dyspnea on exertion and a holodiastolic murmur. CMR SSFP images show pulmonic regurgitation of the 27-mm Carpentier-Edwards Perimount Magna Ease bioprosthetic pulmonary valve implanted 4 years ago for treatment of pulmonic regurgitation following tetralogy of Fallot repair. Phase-contrast images of the bioprosthetic pulmonic valve reveal a regurgitant fraction of 24%, consistent with moderate pulmonary regurgitation. CMR, cardiac magnetic resonance; SSFP, steady-state free precession.

Spectral Doppler

Stenotic Lesions: Spectral Doppler should be used to calculate acceleration time, ejection time, and pressure half-times (PHTs), velocity time integral (VTI), stroke volume (SV), mean pressure gradient, EOA, and the DVI (VTI_{PHV}/VTI_{LVOT}). The $EOA = SV/VTI_{PHV}$, with pulsed-wave (PW) Doppler used to calculate the SV ($Area_{LVOT}/VTI_{LVOT}$) and continuous-wave (CW) Doppler used to determine VTI_{PHV} (**Case Studies 13.1, 13.3, and 13.5, and Videos 13.2 and 13.3**).[2] In general, 1 to 3 heart beats are needed for each measurement in sinus rhythm, and 5 to 15 heart beats are needed in atrial fibrillation because of variation in SV, PHT, and other Doppler parameters.[2] Spectral Doppler findings concerning for PHV stenosis are listed in **Table 13.2**. Note that these measurements and calculations are impacted by body surface area, hemoglobin, heart rate, and type and size of the specific type of PHV.

Regurgitant Lesions: Spectral Doppler with either CW or PW is used to calculate velocity, regurgitant volume (Rvol), effective regurgitant orifice area (EROA), VTI, PHT, and flow reversal in the hepatic veins, pulmonary artery (PA), pulmonic veins, and aorta (**Case Studies 13.2 and 13.7**). A summary of Doppler findings for PHV regurgitation is provided in **Table 13.3**. Doppler findings indirectly related to valve flow can also be important in raising suspicion for PHV pathology—for example, development of new pulmonary hypertension can be seen in prosthetic mitral regurgitation that would otherwise be masked by valve shadowing.

Comparison to Baseline Findings

When evaluating possible PHV dysfunction, it is useful to compare imaging to prior studies, and this is the reason for guideline recommendations to obtain baseline echocardiographic evaluation within a few weeks to months of PHV implantation.[2,19] Postsurgical findings, including sutures, ruptured cords and paravalvular thickening, may mimic pathologic changes, and make evaluation of concerning findings more difficult to interpret in the absence of a baseline study. In addition, baseline gradients are useful to gauge whether follow-up gradients represent a true pathologic change. Finally, if a patient's symptoms and hemodynamics are discordant, either exercise or dobutamine stress echocardiography can be used to further evaluate PHV function.[2,4,23]

Limitations of Echocardiography

There are several limitations of echocardiographic evaluation of PHV that require the clinician to modify the standard echocardiographic imaging views of a PHV, correct for assumptions typically made in hemodynamic calculations, or utilize additional imaging modalities. Etiologies of an elevated transvalvular gradient include PHV obstruction, high SV, and PPM. Differentiating pathologic valve findings from these other conditions can be challenging. Etiologies of high SV include high cardiac output states—such as anemia, fever, thyrotoxicosis, pregnancy, arteriovenous shunts, and bradycardia—and paravalvular or valvular regurgitation from SVD, endocarditis,

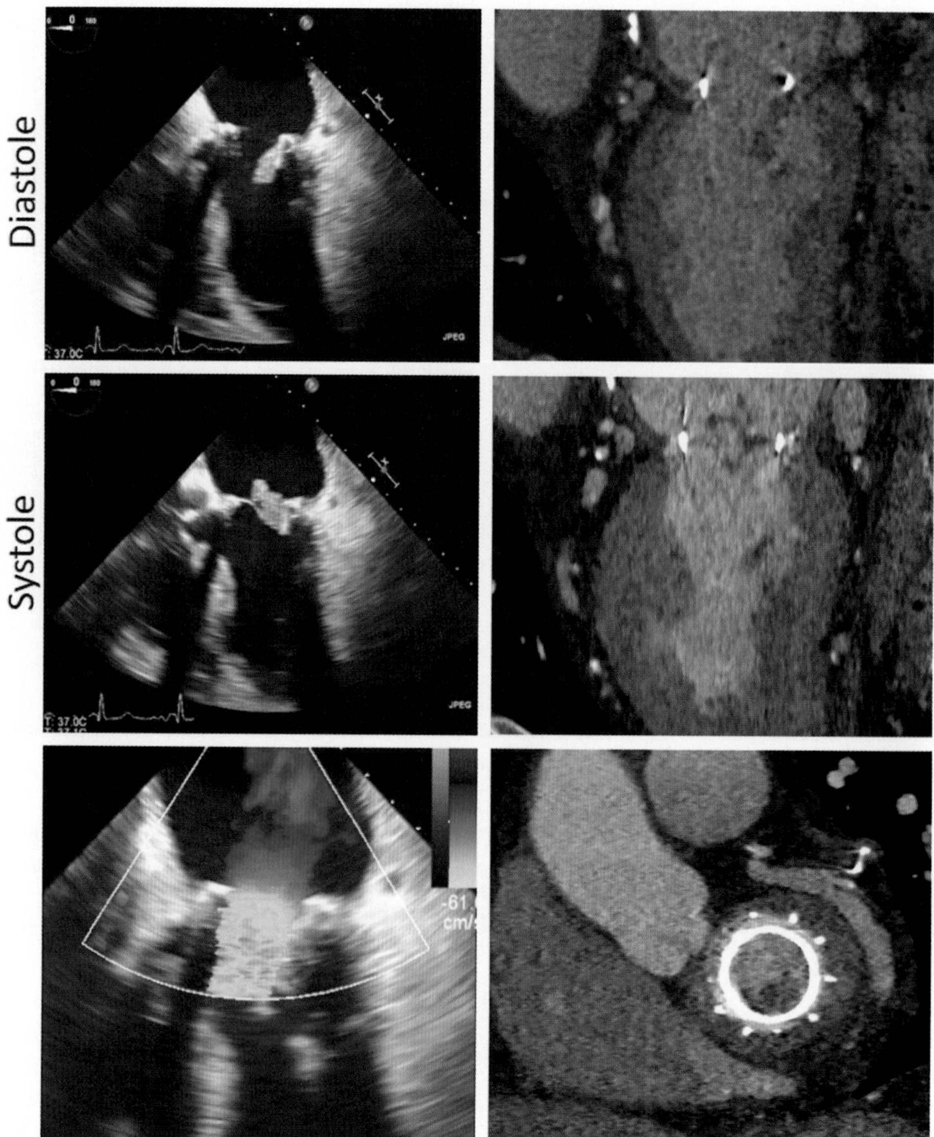

INFECTIVE ENDOCARDITIS CASE 13.5: A 42-year-old male with a history of bioprosthetic mitral PHV with fatigue, fever, brain abscess, and splinter hemorrhages was found to have *Staphylococcus aureus* bacteremia. Side-by-side TEE and CCT images in systole and diastole identify a bioprosthetic mitral PHV endocarditis vegetation. Severely turbulent flow demonstrated on TEE color Doppler studies is consistent with moderate mitral stenosis and mild mitral regurgitation. CCT, cardiac computed tomography; PHV, prosthetic heart valve; TEE, transthoacic echocardiogram.

or valve dehiscence. High cardiac output states or obstruction at the level of LVOT (as evidenced by an LVOT velocity >1.5 m/s) means that the LVOT velocity is not negligible and the mean pressure gradient is more accurately predicted by $\Delta P = 4(v^2_{APHV} - v^2_{LVOT})$.[2] Pressure recovery, which is a focal area of elevated pressure often detected by CW Doppler with little physiologic significance, often leads to overestimation of gradients and an underestimation of EOA compared to invasive measurements.[2] Acoustic shadowing, mirror artifacts, refraction, or reverberation frequently limits visualization of prosthetic disk and leaflets and other areas of interest on or around the valve, and therefore may require off-axis views, additional views on multiplanar TEE, or multimodality imaging.[4] CCT and CMR have been proposed as new methodologies to differentiate between pannus and thrombus, but their use in this area has not yet been widely validated.[24] Evaluation of PVT in cases where the leaflets are difficult to visualize because of acoustic reverberations can be accomplished with cine-fluoroscopy or CCT to visualize leaflet opening.[19,21]

Cine-fluoroscopy

Cine-fluoroscopy is a readily available, easy-to-use noninvasive technique to evaluate the type and functionality of mechanical PHVs (**Case Study 13.1**, ▶ **Video 13.1**).[2,4,25] It is indicated as an adjunct to echocardiography for evaluation of mechanical PHVs with abnormally elevated gradients.[4,21,22] This technique

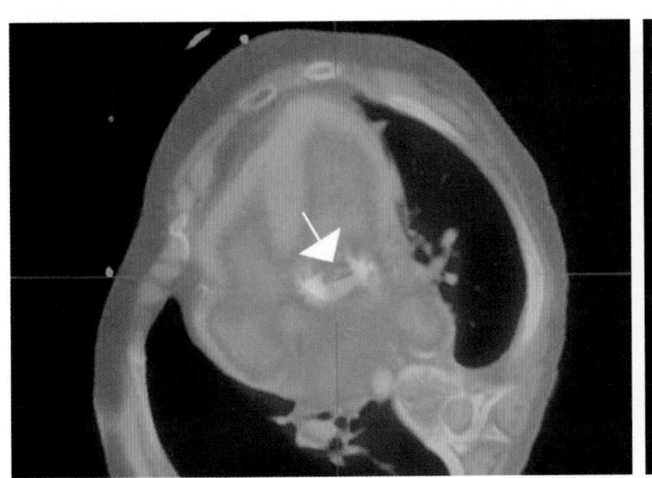

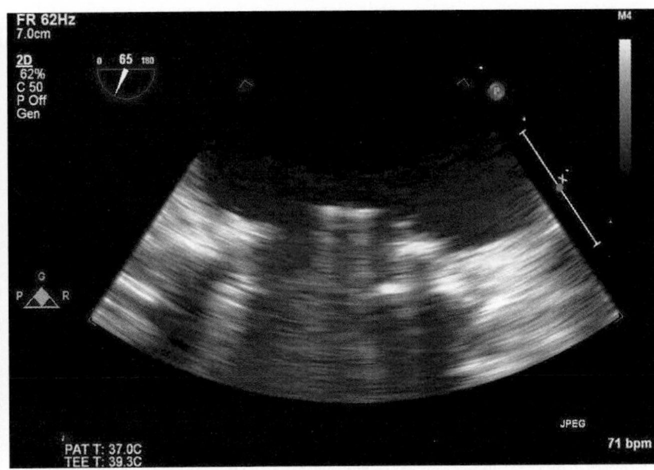

INFECTIVE ENDOCARDITIS CASE 13.6: A 56-year-old female with a history of mechanical mitral PHV with unexplained leukocytosis, fever, and embolic events. Mechanical mitral valve seen in systole and diastole with an unremarkable TEE, and paravalvular ring uptake consistent with abscess seen on ^{18}F-FDG PET. ^{18}F-FDG PET, ^{18}F-fluorodeoxyglucose positron emission tomography; PHV, prosthetic heart valve; TEE, transthoacic echocardiogram. (Image courtesy of Dr. Venkatesh L. Murthy, Rubenfire Professor of Preventive Cardiology, University of Michigan Frankel Cardiovascular Center.)

TABLE 13.2 Doppler Parameters for Prosthetic Heart Valve Stenosis in Different Positions[2,3]

PHV Stenosis	Peak Velocity	Mean Gradient	PHT	DVI	EOA (cm^2)	Other
Tricuspid	>1.7 m/s	>6 mm Hg	>230 msec			
Pulmonic	>3 m/s (xenograft) >2 m/s (homograft)					
Mitral	>2.5 m/s	>10 mm Hg	>200 msec	>2.5	<1	
Aortic	>3 m/s			<0.25		AT >100 ms
Moderate					0.65-0.85	AT:ET <0.4
Severe					<0.65	

AT, acceleration time; DVI, Doppler velocity index; EOA, effective orifice area; ET, ejection time; m, meter; msec, milliseconds; PHT, pressure half-time; PHV, prosthetic heart valve; s, seconds.

TABLE 13.3 Doppler Parameters for Prosthetic Heart Valve Regurgitation in Different Positions[2,3]

PHV Regurgitation	VC	Regurgitant Jet Width/Area	PISA Radius (cm)	Rvol (mL/beat)	EROA (cm^2)	PHT (ms)	Other
Tricuspid	0.3-0.69 cm		0.6-0.89	>45	>0.4		Dense, early peaking, triangular CW signal; holodiastolic flow reversal in hepatic vein
Moderate	VC >0.7 cm (or two moderate jets)		>0.9				
Severe							
Pulmonic[a]							
Mild		<25%		<30			
Moderate		25%-50%		30-60			Flow reversal in PA
Severe		>50%		>60		<100	

(*Continued*)

TABLE 13.3 Doppler Parameters for Prosthetic Heart Valve Regurgitation in Different Positions[2,3] (*Continued*)

PHV Regurgitation	VC	Regurgitant Jet Width/Area	PISA Radius (cm)	Rvol (mL/beat)	EROA (cm^2)	PHT (ms)	Other
Mitral[b]							Peak velocity > 1.9 m/s
Mild	1-2 mm	<4 cm^2			<0.2		DVI >2.5
Moderate	3-6 mm	4-8 cm^2			0.2-0.50		Mean gradient > 5 mm Hg
Severe	>6 mm	>8 cm^2			>0.5		
Aortic							
Mild		<25%		<30		<500	
Moderate		25%-64%		30-59		200-500	
Severe		≥65%		≥60		>500	Holodiastolic reversal in aorta

CW, continuous wave; DVI, Doppler velocity index; EROA, effective regurgitant orifice area; PA: pulmonary artery. PHV, prosthetic heart valve; PHT: pressure half time; PISA, proximal isovelocity surface area; Rvol, regurgitant volume;VC, vena contracta. Pulmonica, paravalvular leak (PVL) better predicted with flow reversal, intravalvular regurgitation better predicted with regurgitant jet width. Mitralb, VC more accurate for PVL, regurgitant jet area more accurate for intravalvular regurgitation.

can be used to diagnose abnormalities in leaflet mobility, valvular ring motion or migration of valve parts. Impaired excursion or incomplete seating of the moving parts (the ball, disk, or leaflet) suggests the presence of tissue growth or thrombus.[2] Two basic views are required: first, the orientation of the PHV is noted in the anterior-posterior (0 degree) and lateral position (90 degree). Second, the radiation beam should be aligned parallel to the valve ring plane and to the tilting axis of the disk or leaflet to allow calculation of the opening and closing angles. For the mitral valve, a view parallel to the outflow tract should be obtained as well.[4] About 10 beats can be captured in each cine-fluoroscopy, after which the best frames can be used to calculate the leaflet opening and closing radius. For single-leaflet or tilting-disk models, the distance between the housing and the position of the disk when fully open is the opening radius. For bileaflet models, the distance between the two leaflets when fully open and fully closed are the opening and closing radii, respectively.[4] Although cine-fluoroscopy shows valve opening more clearly than does echocardiography, particularly in the aortic position, it provides neither hemodynamic assessment nor the etiology of reduced disk mobility.[4,26]

Cardiac Computed Tomography

CCT is a rapidly expanding imaging modality for evaluating PHVs (**Case Studies 13.2, 13.5, 13.7, and 13.8 and Video 13.4**). It is indicated for adjunct imaging for bioprosthetic and mechanical PHV dysfunction if TTE or TEE is nondiagnostic.[22] In addition, for patients undergoing repeat surgery due to PHV disease, CCT can be used to evaluate bypass graft patency, coronary arteries, and the distance from the heart to the sternum for surgical planning.[4] Ensuring the patient has a low heart rate and has practiced breath-holding will optimize CCT image quality.[27] For proper evaluation of PHV dysfunction, visualization of leaflet motion in both systolic and diastolic phases is required, making retrospective electrocardiogram (ECG)-gated acquisition a better choice compared to prospective gating. If full 4D imaging is needed for functional data, dose modulation should not be used. CCT with contrast is preferred to visualize paravalvular structure, differentiate pannus from thrombus and vegetation; and obtain additional information about left and right ventricular function, SV, and coronaries, if applicable. However, if contrast is contraindicated, then a non–contrast-gated study can be used to visualize mechanical leaflet motion if thrombosis is suspected.

3D volumetric reconstruction allows accurate calculation of opening and closing angles of mechanical leaflets, for which there are published proposed norms based on a cohort study.[28] Similarly, there are published data on the usefulness of CCT in differentiating thrombus and pannus in bioprosthetic valves.[29,30]

Cardiac Magnetic Resonance Imaging

CMR is safe in patients with bioprosthetic and mechanical PHVs, and can be used for volumetric assessment of cardiac chambers and flows, and bioprosthetic valve function (**Case Study 13.2, Video 13.5**).[4,22,31] CMR sequences for PHV assessment include T_1-weighted spin echo, gradient-echo sequences (steady-state free precession [SSFP] and fast gradient echo), and phase-contrast sequences. T_1-weighted spin echo sequences are less susceptible to artifacts from metallic structures, but only provide static images.[32] These may be useful to identify structural defects such as fracture of a PHV. Acquisition of SSFP images, which discriminate blood from tissue, can clearly identify turbulent flow and provide accurate, reproducible ventricular volumes and mass as compared to echocardiography.[32,33] Most bioprosthetic PHV anatomy is amenable to SSFP imaging in the standard two-, three-, and four-chamber long-axis views, as well as oblique long-axis cine sequences orthogonal to the line of coaptation. Conversely, visualization of mechanical PHV is limited because of artifact.[4] In addition, the geometric orifice area can be measured in bioprosthetic valves.[4] SSFP sequences are particularly useful

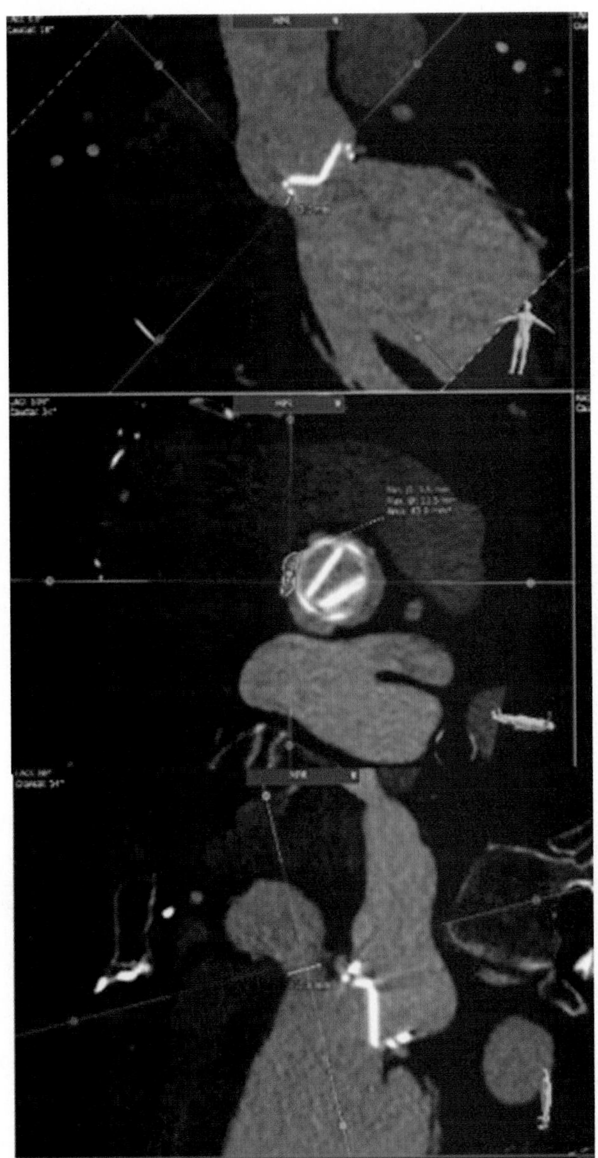

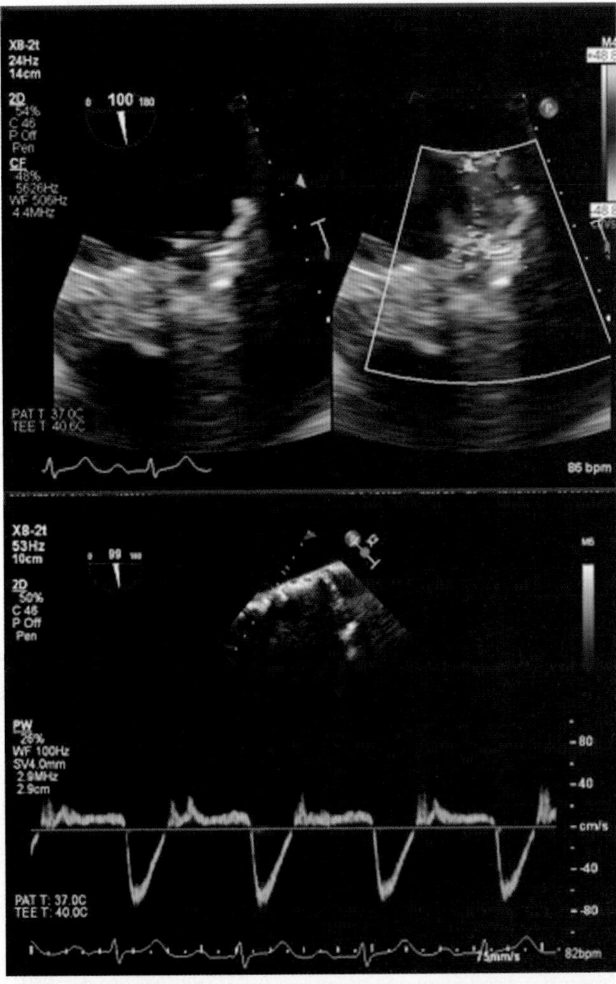

PARAVALVULAR LEAK CASE 13.7: A 68-year-old female who underwent surgery for mechanical AVR 15 years prior in the setting of endocarditis was found to have a dilated left ventricle and reduced ejection fraction on surveillance echo. The mechanical aortic PHV with abdominal aorta flow reversal is seen on pulsed-wave Doppler, and the paravalvular leak is evident on color Doppler. The CCT reveals areas of valve malapposition. AVR, aortic valve replacement; CCT, cardiac computed tomography; PHV, prosthetic heart valve.

when assessing right-sided PHV, which are otherwise difficult to evaluate with an echocardiogram.[32,33]

Acquisition of blood flow and velocity obtained by phase-contrast velocity mapping is performed for para- or valvular regurgitation, particularly in the congenital population. This technique relies on phase shift imaging from altered rotational spin of protons as compared with stationary protons within a magnetic field gradient. Flow is derived by integrating the velocity of each pixel over a single cardiac cycle from through-plane velocity maps, which has correlated well with in vivo hemodynamic measurements.[33] For PHV, this is best acquired above the valve in "through-plane" sequences due to artifacts.

CMR is emerging as an important imaging modality for right-sided PHV and in patients with congenital heart disease with pulmonary conduit dysfunction. For pulmonic (and tricuspid) regurgitation, quantification of flow and volume in the main PA (or right ventricle) as compared to the left ventricle provides regurgitant volume, although artifacts from the stent may limit this determination.[3,31] Furthermore, after percutaneous pulmonic valve insertion into the conduit, CMR is used to monitor hemodynamic changes in the right ventricle that provide important prognostic information.[34]

Although CMR provides complementary diagnostic information of PHV disease, it has a few limitations. SSFP can

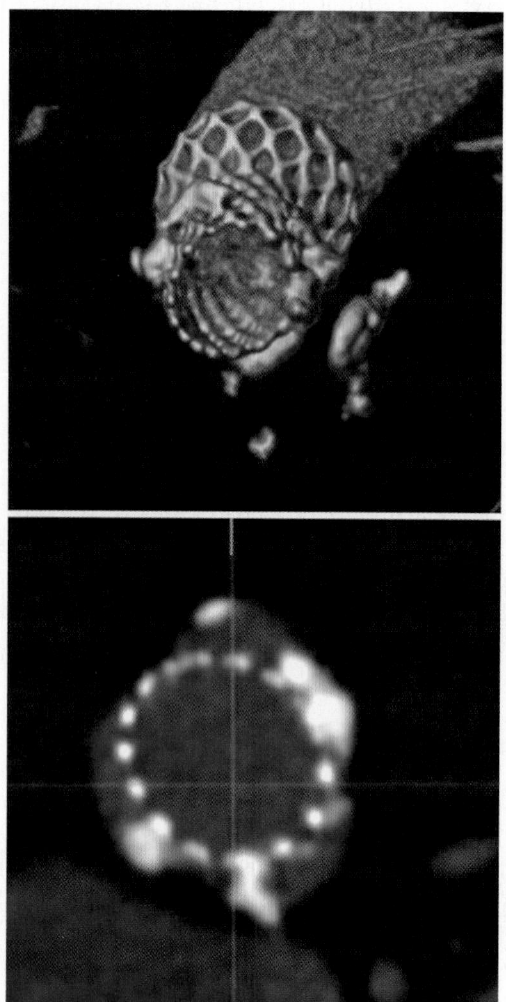

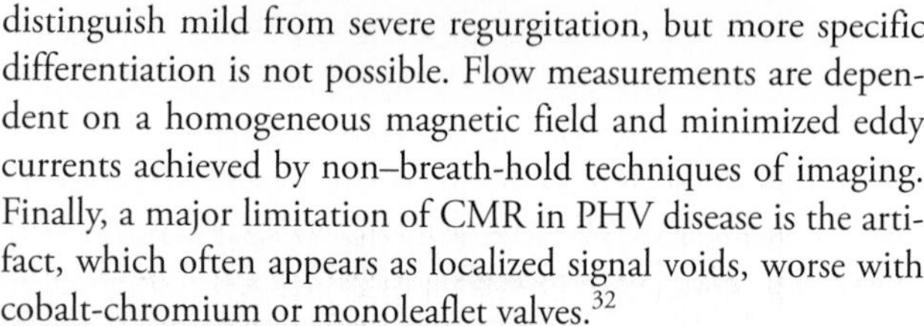

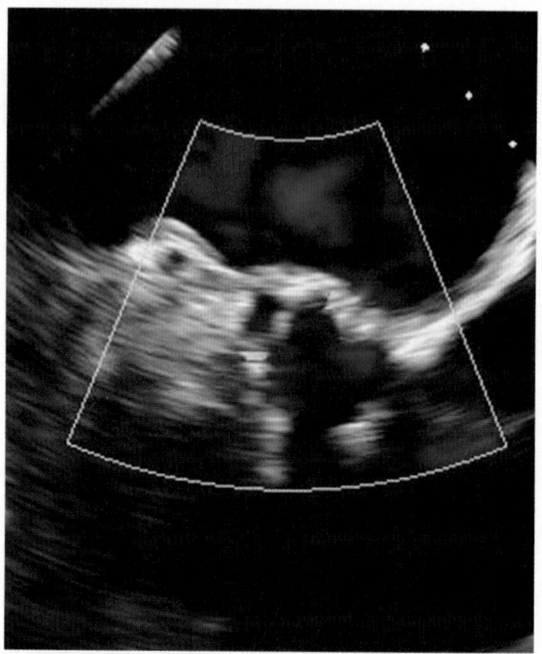

PARAVALVULAR LEAK CASE 13.8: An 86-year-old female with multiple comorbidities, who underwent TAVI 9 months prior, presented with respiratory distress and volume overload and was found to have significant aortic PVL. The PVL after TAVI is visualized on CCT and with Doppler echocardiography. CCT, cardiac computed tomography; PVL, paravalvular leak; TAVI, transcatheter aortic valve implantation. (Image courtesy of Dr. Omar Khalique, Associate Professor of Medicine (Radiology) at Columbia University Medical Center.)

distinguish mild from severe regurgitation, but more specific differentiation is not possible. Flow measurements are dependent on a homogeneous magnetic field and minimized eddy currents achieved by non–breath-hold techniques of imaging. Finally, a major limitation of CMR in PHV disease is the artifact, which often appears as localized signal voids, worse with cobalt-chromium or monoleaflet valves.[32]

Positron Emission Tomography/Computed Tomography

^{18}F-fluorodeoxyglucose (^{18}F-FDG) PET/CT has been shown in numerous small studies to improve the diagnosis of paravalvular infective endocarditis in patients with PHV if the valve was placed more than 3 months prior (**Case Study 13.6**).[14,35,36] Although still in its nascence, this mode of imaging exploits ^{18}F-FDG that is actively taken up by leukocytes, monocytes, macrophages, and CD4 T lymphocytes at sites of infection. As noted in the European Society of Cardiology Infective Endocarditis Guidelines of 2015, this technique is most useful to reduce the rate of misdiagnosed infective endocarditis by Duke's criteria.[14] It can also locate embolic metastatic foci of infection as a complication of PHV endocarditis.[14]

MANAGEMENT OF PROSTHETIC HEART VALVE DISEASE

Pannus

Pannus that causes severe prosthetic dysfunction requires surgical excision and sometimes replacement of the PHV (Class I if symptomatic, class IIa if asymptomatic; **Table 13.4**).[19] There is no known medication to prevent or treat pannus formation, but standard medical therapy such as diuretics, rate-controlling medications, and pressor or inotropic support may stabilize patients before reoperation.[19,37] For a bioprosthetic aortic valve, a percutaneous approach with valve-in-valve transcatheter aortic valve implantation (TAVI) may be considered if the risk of reoperation is too high.[21,37-39] Transcatheter mitral valve replacement (TMVR) for bioprosthetic mitral valve stenosis or regurgitation is not yet approved by the U.S. food and Drug Administration (FDA), although a number of clinical trials studying TMVR for mitral valve stenosis and regurgitation are currently under way.[40]

Prosthetic Heart Valve Thrombosis

Choice of fibrinolysis, anticoagulation, or surgical therapy for PHV thrombosis depends on whether the thrombosis

TABLE 13.4 Summary of Management of Prosthetic Heart Valve Disease[19,21,37,39,43]

	Medical	Surgical	Percutaneous
Thrombosis	• Thrombolysis: streptokinase or tissue plasminogen activator • Anticoagulation: warfarin (target INR: Aortic 3.0-4.0, Mitral: 3.5-4.5)	• Removal of thrombus ± valve replacement	• N/A
Pannus	• N/A	• Resection ± valve replacement	• Reported valve-in-valve TAVI
Structural valve degeneration	• N/A	• Valve replacement	• Valve-in-valve approaches, established for TAVI and pulmonary homo/xenografts, upcoming in TMVR and TTVR
Infective endocarditis	• Organism/sensitivity-guided antibiotic therapy	• Valve replacement and debridement/patch of surrounding tissues if concurrent abscess	• N/A
Paravalvular leak	• N/A	• Valve replacement • Additional stitches in sewing ring	• Plug • Postdilation (if immediately after transcatheter PHV placement)
Patient-prosthesis mismatch	• N/A	• Valve replacement only if larger valve can be placed	• N/A

N/A, not applicable; PHV, prosthetic heart valve; TAVI, transcatheter aortic valve implantation; TMVR, transcatheter mitral valve replacement; TTVR, Transcatheter tricuspid valve-in-valve replacement.

is right- or left sided, the suspected duration, the size of the thrombus, and the severity of the symptoms. Medical therapy with fibrinolytic therapy is reasonable for left-sided mechanical prosthetic valves with a suspected recent onset of thrombosis of less than 14 days in mildly symptomatic patients (New York Heart Association [NYHA] Class I or II) with a nonmobile thrombus less than 0.8 cm^2 in area.[19] Fibrinolytic therapy is also reasonable for all right-sided thrombosed PHVs, because resultant pulmonary emboli appear to be small and well tolerated.[19] Fibrinolysis can be achieved with (1) intravenous recombinant tissue plasminogen activator (TPA) 10 mg bolus followed by 90 mg over 90 minutes with unfractionated heparin or (2) streptokinase 1,500,000 units in 60 minutes without unfractionated heparin.[19,37] Stable patients with bioprosthetic PHV thrombosis can be managed with vitamin K antagonists (VKAs) or unfractionated heparin before considering intervention.[21,37] Fibrinolysis is favored if there is no contraindication to fibrinolysis, first-time episode of valve thrombosis, no left atrial thrombus, no other known valve disease, and no surgical expertise available.[21]

Surgical therapy is reasonable in asymptomatic patients with thrombosis greater than 0.8 cm^2 in area and is emergently recommended for unstable patients with thrombosed left-sided PHVs, or those in whom the thrombus is suspected to be present for more than 14 days.[19] Factors favoring surgical intervention include readily available surgical expertise, low surgical risk, contraindication to fibrinolysis, recurrent valve thrombosis, left atrial thrombus, mobile thrombus, concomitant coronary artery disease requiring revascularization, other valve disease requiring intervention, evidence of embolization or if pannus may also be present.[21,37] The decision between surgical and fibrinolytic therapy should involve shared decision-making with the patient. There are no current percutaneous options for PHV thrombosis.

Structural Valve Degeneration

SVD typically affects bioprosthetic valves, and can present as either stenosis or regurgitation (**Case Studies 13.3 and 13.4, and Videos 13.3 and 13.5**). There is no known medical therapy to prevent SVD. Surgical replacement of the valve is recommended if the patient develops hemolysis or heart failure due to severe prosthetic valve stenosis or regurgitation.[19,37] Surgery is also reasonable in asymptomatic patients with severe bioprosthetic regurgitation if there is acceptable operative risk.[21] Transcatheter aortic valve-in-valve replacement is reasonable in symptomatic, high-surgical-risk patients with severe aortic PHV stenosis or regurgitation and if improvement in hemodynamics is expected.[21,37,39] This should be performed by an experienced operator and only in select patients with a larger PHV because a smaller valve will always be placed within the malfunctioning valve, raising the possibility of future PPM.[21]

Paravalvular Leak

There is no effective medical therapy for significant PVL; only surgical or percutaneous options exist (**Case Studies 13.7 and 13.8**). Surgery is recommended for bioprosthetic or mechanical heart valves if patients have heart failure (NYHA Class III/IV) or intractable hemolysis due to severe PVL.[19]

For bioprosthetic valves, percutaneous repair of PVL can also be considered if there are suitable anatomic features for catheter-based repair.[19,37] Of note, if a new PVL is discovered, infective endocarditis should be ruled out as a potential cause of the regurgitation.[19]

Infective Endocarditis

Therapy for PHV complicated by infective endocarditis varies depending on the organism, the size of the vegetation, the presence and severity of valvular regurgitation or stenosis, the patient's surgical risk, and thromboembolic events (Table 13.4). Initial therapy with broad-spectrum antibiotics should be narrowed depending on antibiotic sensitivity and infectious disease consultation recommendations.[19] Patients with PHV are more likely to benefit from medical therapy when there is a non-Staphylococcal infection and no evidence of embolism or PHV dysfunction.[19] For patients who develop embolism or stroke, anticoagulation should be held even in patients with mechanical PHV, because hemorrhagic conversion can occur up to 11 days after an embolic or stroke event.[19]

Early surgery is indicated in patients presenting with symptomatic PHV dysfunction or left-sided infectious endocarditis caused by *Staphylococcus aureus*, fungal or other highly resistant organisms, heart block, annular or aortic abscess or destructive penetrating lesions, or a vegetation greater than 10 mm in size.[19,41] In addition, patients with PHV and either relapsing infection or persistent positive blood cultures despite appropriate antibiotic therapy[19,41] should undergo surgery.[19] Early surgery is also reasonable in patients who have recurrent emboli or persistent vegetations despite appropriate antibiotic therapy.[19] Percutaneous options should not be considered for patients with infective endocarditis.

Patient-Prosthesis Mismatch

There is no known medical management for PPM. Surgery should only be attempted if a larger valve or a different valve with improved hemodynamics can be implanted.[19] Prevention of PPM can occur by enlarging the aortic root (for aortic PHV) or using stentless valves.[7] There is no percutaneous therapy for PPM.

SPECIAL CONSIDERATIONS AND EMERGING THERAPIES

Subclinical Prosthetic Heart Valve Thrombosis

Subclinical leaflet thrombosis on bioprosthetic aortic valves (transcatheter and surgical) have been noted on subsequent CCT imaging and are associated with increased risk of transient ischemic attack (TIA) and stroke. These have been successfully managed with direct oral anticoagulants (DOACs) or VKAs.[42]

Transcatheter Mitral Valve-in-Valve Replacement

Initially performed in 2009, the valve-in-valve TMVR has been performed via a transapical or antegrade transfemoral approach in patients deemed at high surgical risk.[43] Transcatheter mitral valve-in-valve replacement is being performed for mitral PHV dysfunction from SVD or pannus. Although currently performed with valves initially intended for the aortic (Edwards) and pulmonic (Melody) positions, dedicated mitral valve systems are being tested currently.[38,40,43]

Transcatheter Tricuspid Valve-in-Valve Replacement

Transcatheter tricuspid valve-in-valve replacement (TTVR) was first described in 2011, and has since been performed via the transfemoral, transjugular, and transatrial approach in patients at high surgical risk for repeat cardiac surgery.[44] Multimodality imaging with CCT is necessary to select the appropriately sized valve. Of note, pacemaker leads have been reportedly jailed during this procedure; although this is generally well tolerated, impedance and thresholds should be checked after the procedure. Furthermore, jailing the pacemaker leads can lead to significant PVL.[44]

FOLLOW-UP PATIENT CARE

After Repeat Valve Surgery

Patients should be followed up routinely after repeat PHV surgery, with at least one echocardiogram within the first 2 to 12 weeks to assess the function of the new PHV.[19,22] Thereafter, the patient should be seen yearly for a cardiac history and physical, unless other complications arise.[19]

Prosthetic Heart Valve Infective Endocarditis

In patients treated medically, repeat echocardiography is only recommended for deterioration of symptoms or lack of improvement.[19] If surgery is performed, intraoperative TEE provides an essential postoperative baseline.[19] The remaining antibiotic therapy is continued after surgery, in addition to the abovementioned recommendations for surveillance after redo surgery.[19]

RESEARCH AND FUTURE DIRECTIONS

Transcatheter valve replacement options and cardiac imaging (particularly CCT, CMR, and PET/CT) are rapidly expanding to provide multimodality imaging to better diagnose PHV dysfunction.[24,34,36,40,44]

KEY POINTS

- ✔ Diagnosis of PHV disease requires a high index of suspicion, requiring a detailed history including specifics of the valve implanted, severity and acuity of symptoms, and reviewing prior imaging or functional assessments.
- ✔ The most common symptom of PHV disease is decompensated heart failure or shortness of breath. Initial evaluation should include basic vitals including heart rate, blood pressure, and temperature. Initial laboratory diagnostics should include complete blood count, international normalized ratio (INR; for those on

anticoagulation), basic metabolic panel, and blood cultures (for febrile patients).

- ✔ Echocardiography is generally the first diagnostic imaging modality used to evaluate the PHV, although it can be limited by artifact or location of the valve.
- ✔ For right-sided PHV disease, CMR provides more accurate evaluation as compared with echocardiography.
- ✔ In patients with PVL or infective endocarditis where the extent of disease cannot be clearly evaluated on echocardiography, CCT may better clarify anatomy and severity of disease.
- ✔ For patients without clear infective endocarditis by Duke criteria, ^{18}F-FDG PET/CT may prevent overdiagnosis and unnecessary treatment of infective endocarditis.
- ✔ Unless causing NYHA Class III or IV heart failure, the management of pannus, SVD, and PVL is focused on symptom alleviation.
- ✔ Management of PVT on right-sided valves is either thrombolysis or anticoagulation with VKA. Management of PVT on left-sided valves can be achieved by thrombolysis, anticoagulation with VKA or surgery, depending on size and duration of thrombus, and severity of heart failure symptoms.
- ✔ Management of endocarditis in PHV patients usually includes surgery and antibiotic therapy, unless the vegetation is quite small and only on the valve itself, and the patient is free of peripheral metastatic lesions and major heart failure symptoms.
- ✔ Valve-in-valve replacement of the tricuspid, mitral, pulmonic, and aortic valves have all been reported, although pulmonic and aortic valves are the only two valve-in-valve procedures currently approved.

VIDEO CAPTION

VIDEO 13.1 Echocardiography and fluoroscopy video of prosthetic heart valve (PHV) thrombus.

VIDEO 13.2 Echocardiographic video of endocarditis.

VIDEO 13.3 Echocardiography of structural valve degeneration (SVD)

VIDEO 13.4 Computed tomography (CT) cine of thrombus.

VIDEO 13.5 Cardiac magnetic resonance (CMR) imaging of pulmonic xenograft structural valve degeneration (SVD).

REFERENCES

1. Yacoub MH, Takkenberg JJM. Will heart valve tissue engineering change the world? *Nat Clin Pract Cardiovasc Med.* 2005;2:60-61.
2. Zoghbi WA, Chambers JB, Dumesnil JG, et al. Recommendations for evaluation of prosthetic valves with echocardiography and doppler ultrasound. *J Am Soc Echocardiogr.* 2009;22:975-1014.
3. Zoghbi WA, Asch FM, Bruce C, et al. Guidelines for the evaluation of valvular regurgitation after percutaneous valve repair or replacement. *J Am Soc Echocardiogr.* 2019;32:431-475.
4. Lancellotti P, Pibarot P, Chambers J, et al. Recommendations for the imaging assessment of prosthetic heart valves: a report from the European Association of Cardiovascular Imaging endorsed by the Chinese Society of Echocardiography, the Inter-American Society of Echocardiography, and the Brazilian Department of Cardiovascular Imaging. *Eur Heart J Cardiovasc Imaging.* 2016;17:589-590.
5. Dangas GD, Weitz JI, Giustino G, Makkar R, Mehran R. Prosthetic heart valve thrombosis. *J Am Coll Cardiol.* 2016;68:2670-2689.
6. Darwazah AK. Recurrent pannus formation causing prosthetic aortic valve dysfunction: Is excision without valve re-replacement applicable? *J Cardiothorac Surg.* 2012;7:62.
7. Fallon JM, DeSimone JP, Brennan JM, et al. The incidence and consequence of prosthesis-patient mismatch after surgical aortic valve replacement. *Ann Thorac Surg.* 2018;106:14-22.
8. León del Pino MDC, Ruíz Ortiz M, Delgado Ortega M, et al. Prosthesis-patient mismatch after transcatheter aortic valve replacement: prevalence and medium term prognostic impact. *Int J Cardiovasc Imaging.* 2019;35:827-836.
9. Miyasaka M, Tada N, Taguri M, et al. Incidence, predictors, and clinical impact of prosthesis–patient mismatch following transcatheter aortic valve replacement in Asian patients: the OCEAN-TAVI Registry. *JACC Cardiovasc Interv.* 2018;11:771-780.
10. Hwang HY, Kim YH, Kim K-H, Kim K-B, Ahn H. Patient-prosthesis mismatch after mitral valve replacement: a propensity score analysis. *Ann Thorac Surg.* 2016;101:1796-1802.
11. Côté N, Pibarot P, Clavel M-A. Incidence, risk factors, clinical impact, and management of bioprosthesis structural valve degeneration. *Curr Opin Cardiol.* 2017;32:123.
12. McElhinney DB, Sondergaard L, Armstrong AK, et al. Endocarditis after transcatheter pulmonary valve replacement. *J Am Coll Cardiol.* 2018;72:2717-2728.
13. Amat-Santos IJ, Ribeiro HB, Urena M, et al. Prosthetic valve endocarditis after transcatheter valve replacement: a systematic review. *JACC Cardiovasc Interv.* 2015;8:334-346.
14. Habib G, Lancellotti P, Antunes MJ, et al. 2015 ESC guidelines for the management of infective endocarditis. The Task Force for the Management of Infective Endocarditis of the European Society of Cardiology (ESC)Endorsed by: European Association for Cardio-Thoracic Surgery (EACTS), the European Association of Nuclear Medicine (EANM). *Eur Heart J.* 2015;36:3075-3128.
15. Bernard S, Yucel E. Paravalvular leaks—from diagnosis to management. *Curr Treat Option Cardiovasc Med.* 2019;21:67.
16. Rodriguez-Gabella T, Voisine P, Puri R, Pibarot P, Rodés-Cabau J. Aortic bioprosthetic valve durability: incidence, mechanisms, predictors, and management of surgical and transcatheter valve degeneration. *J Am Coll Cardiol.* 2017;70:1013-1028.
17. Liao Y, Li Y, Jun-li L, et al. Incidence, predictors and outcome of prosthesis-patient mismatch after transcatheter aortic valve replacement: a systematic review and meta-analysis. *Sci Rep.* 2017;7:1-8.
18. Bonderman D, Graf A, Kammerlander AA, et al. Factors determining patient-prosthesis mismatch after aortic valve replacement—a prospective cohort study. *PLoS One.* 2013;8:e81940.
19. Nishimura RA, Otto CM, Bonow RO, et al. 2014 AHA/ACC guideline for the management of patients with valvular heart disease. *J Am Coll Cardiol.* 2014;63:e57-e185.
20. Pettersson GB, Coselli JS, Pettersson GB, et al. 2016 The American Association for Thoracic Surgery (AATS) consensus guidelines: surgical treatment of infective endocarditis: executive summary. *J Thorac Cardiovasc Surg.* 2017;153:1241-1258.e29.
21. Nishimura RA, Otto CM, Bonow RO, et al. 2017 AHA/ACC focused update of the 2014 AHA/ACC guideline for the management of patients with valvular heart disease: a report of the American College of Cardiology/American Heart Association Task Force on Clinical Practice Guidelines. *Circulation.* 2017;135:e1159-e1195. Accessed November 9, 2019. https://www.ahajournals.org/doi/10.1161/CIR.0000000000000503
22. Doherty JU, Kort S, Mehran R, et al. ACC/AATS/AHA/ASE/ASNC/HRS/SCAI/SCCT/SCMR/STS 2017 appropriate use criteria for multimodality imaging in valvular heart disease. *J Am Soc Echocardiogr.* 2018;31:381-404.

23. Bonow RO, O'Gara PT, Adams DH, et al. 2020 focused update of the 2017 ACC expert consensus decision pathway on the management of mitral regurgitation. *J Am Coll Cardiol.* 2020;75(17):2236-2270. Accessed April 9, 2020. http://www.onlinejacc.org/content/early/2020/02/19/j.jacc.2020.02.005
24. Gündüz S, Özkan M, Kalçik M, et al. Sixty-four–section cardiac computed tomography in mechanical prosthetic heart valve dysfunction. *Circ Cardiovasc Imaging.* 2015;8:e003246.
25. Kalçık M, Güner A, Yesin M, et al. Identification of mechanical prosthetic heart valves based on distinctive cinefluoroscopic and echocardiographic markers. *Int J Artif Organs.* 2019;42:603-610.
26. Muratori M, Montorsi P, Maffessanti F, et al. Dysfunction of bileaflet aortic prosthesis: accuracy of echocardiography versus fluoroscopy. JACC *Cardiovasc Imaging.* 2013;6:196-205.
27. Abbara S, Blanke P, Maroules CD, et al. SCCT guidelines for the performance and acquisition of coronary computed tomographic angiography: a report of the Society of Cardiovascular Computed Tomography Guidelines Committee. *J Cardiovasc Comput Tomogr.* 2016;10:435-449.
28. Suh YJ, Kim YJ, Hong YJ, et al. Measurement of opening and closing angles of aortic valve prostheses in vivo using dual-source computed tomography: comparison with those of manufacturers' in 10 different types. *Korean J Radiol.* 2015;16:1012-1023.
29. Symersky P, Budde RPJ, de Mol BAJM, Prokop M. Comparison of multidetector-row computed tomography to echocardiography and fluoroscopy for evaluation of patients with mechanical prosthetic valve obstruction. *Am J Cardiol.* 2009;104:1128-1134.
30. Makkar RR, Fontana G, Jilaihawi H, et al. Possible subclinical leaflet thrombosis in bioprosthetic aortic valves. *N Engl J Med.* 2015;373:2015-2024.
31. Hundley WG, Bluemke DA, Finn JP, et al. ACCF/ACR/AHA/NASCI/SCMR 2010 expert consensus document on cardiovascular magnetic resonance. *J Am Coll Cardiol.* 2010;55:2614-2662.
32. Suchá D, Symersky P, Tanis W, et al. Multimodality imaging assessment of prosthetic heart valves. *Circ Cardiovasc Imaging.* 2015;8:e003703. Accessed December 2, 2019. https://www.ahajournals.org/doi/10.1161/CIRCIMAGING.115.003703
33. Myerson SG. Heart valve disease: investigation by cardiovascular magnetic resonance. *J Cardiovasc Magn Reson.* 2012;14:7.
34. Secchi F, Resta EC, Cannaò PM, et al. Four-year cardiac magnetic resonance (CMR) follow-up of patients treated with percutaneous pulmonary valve stent implantation. *Eur Radiol.* 2015;25:3606-3613.
35. Saby L, Laas O, Habib G, et al. Positron emission tomography/computed tomography for diagnosis of prosthetic valve endocarditis: increased valvular ^{18}F-fluorodeoxyglucose uptake as a novel major criterion. *J Am Coll Cardiol.* 2013;61:2374-2382.
36. Pizzi María N., Roque A, Fernández-Hidalgo N, et al. Improving the diagnosis of infective endocarditis in prosthetic valves and intracardiac devices with ^{18}F-fluordeoxyglucose positron emission tomography/computed tomography angiography. *Circulation.* 2015;132:1113-1126.
37. Baumgartner H, Falk V, Bax JJ, et al. 2017 ESC/EACTS guidelines for the management of valvular heart disease. *Eur Heart J.* 2017;38:2739-2791.
38. Paradis J-M, Trigo MD, Puri R, Rodés-Cabau J. Transcatheter valve-in-valve and valve-in-ring for treating aortic and mitral surgical prosthetic dysfunction. *J Am Coll Cardiol.* 2015;66:2019-2037.
39. Webb JG, Murdoch DJ, Alu MC, et al. 3-year outcomes after valve-in-valve transcatheter aortic valve replacement for degenerated bioprostheses: the PARTNER 2 Registry. *J Am Coll Cardiol.* 2019;73:2647-2655.
40. Testa L, Rubbio AP, Casenghi M, Pero G, Latib A, Bedogni F. Transcatheter mitral valve replacement in the transcatheter aortic valve replacement era. *J Am Heart Assoc.* 2019;8:e013352.
41. Baddour LM, Wilson WR, Bayer AS, et al. Infective endocarditis in adults: diagnosis, antimicrobial therapy, and management of complications. *Circulation.* 2015;132(15):1435-1486.
42. Chakravarty T, Søndergaard L, Friedman J, et al. Subclinical leaflet thrombosis in surgical and transcatheter bioprosthetic aortic valves: an observational study. *Lancet.* 2017;389:2383-2392.
43. Sorajja P, Moat N, Badhwar V, et al. Initial feasibility study of a new transcatheter mitral prosthesis: the first 100 patients. *J Am Coll Cardiol.* 2019;73:1250-1260.
44. Sanon S, Cabalka AK, Babaliaros V, et al. Transcatheter tricuspid valve-in-valve and valve-in-ring implantation for degenerated surgical prosthesis. *J Am Coll Cardiovasc Interv.* 2019;12:1403-1412.

CHAPTER 14

INFECTIVE ENDOCARDITIS

Jeffrey A. Dixson, Jeffrey Gaca, and Todd L. Kiefer

INTRODUCTION

Since its early descriptions by Osler in 1885, infective endocarditis (IE) has been recognized as a "vexing" problem, challenging to recognize, and associated with high morbidity and mortality. Beginning in the 1940s, two major advances—the development of penicillin, and in subsequent decades, advances in cardiac surgical therapy—have substantially reduced mortality from endocarditis. Early reports of endocarditis therapy for susceptible organisms using various forms and routes of penicillin with heparin for 10 to 62 days of therapy resulted in 70% cure rates. In 1965, Wallace et al. offered one of the first descriptions of surgery for antibiotic refractory endocarditis, ushering in the modern era of surgical management for complicated endocarditis.

Shifting Epidemiology

Several clinically important shifts in IE epidemiology warrant attention. In developed countries, the proportion of IE cases related to rheumatic heart disease has decreased, whereas cases related to indwelling vascular access, cardiac implantable electronic devices (CIEDs), prosthetic valves, other prosthetic implants, and health care contact have increased.[1] Prosthetic valve infections now account for up to 20% of IE cases, and CIED infections comprise 4% to 8% of cases. As many as 25% of cases in one series had recent health care exposure.[2] Patients with comorbidities requiring indwelling catheters, immunosuppression, or frequent health care contact (specifically human immunodeficiency virus [HIV], cancer, hemodialysis, and older patients) are at increased risk for IE as a result of immunosuppression and frequent transient bacteremia. Patients who use intravenous (IV) drugs similarly represent a growing proportion of endocarditis cases, particularly in the United States with the ongoing opioid epidemic. A recent analysis of claims data in Pennsylvania showed a 20% increase in the overall incidence of endocarditis between 2013 and 2017, but a 238% increase in endocarditis related to intravenous drug use (IVDU).[3]

Concurrent with the shift in risk factors toward an older population with more comorbidities and indwelling prosthetic implants has been a shift in microbiology toward more virulent organisms. Several studies have found an increase in the percentage of cases due to *Staphylococcus aureus*, both in the United States and in Europe, making it the most common microorganism isolated.[1,4] In a nationwide inpatient cohort in the United States, a steady increase in the percentage of endocarditis cases due to *S. aureus* was reported: from 33% in 2000 to 40% in 2011.[1] The same study reported increases in *Streptococcus*, fungal, and gram-negative endocarditis over the study period, with an increase in the percentage of cases due to *Streptococcus* after 2007 IE guidelines restricted the populations for whom endocarditis prophylaxis was recommended. Others have questioned the finding of increased *Streptococcus* endocarditis after guidelines were updated.[5]

Incidence

Overall, the incidence of IE is at least stable, if not increasing, and is generally reported between 3 and 10 cases per 100,000 population.[6] Among certain subgroups, however, the incidence is higher. The incidence in areas with high IVDU has been reported at 16 per 100,000[1] and among older individuals 20 per 100,000.[7] In a U.S. hospital database, rates of hospitalization for endocarditis increased from 11 per 100,000 to 15 per 100,000 between 2001 and 2012.[1] Increasing incidence is generally attributed to high rates of IVDU, increasing use of implantable cardiac devices and prosthetic valves, higher rates of indwelling or repeated vascular access for chemotherapy and hemodialysis, and an aging population with more immunocompromising comorbidities.[1] A male predominance is consistently observed, with an estimated ratio of 1.2 to 2.7:1 in comparison to females.

With respect to the sites of valve involvement, the most common valve affected is the aortic valve (38% of cases).[8] This is followed closely by the mitral valve, which is involved in 34% of cases. Isolated tricuspid valve endocarditis is less common, but is linked to IVDU, chronic hemodialysis, or the presence of pacemaker or implantable cardioverter defibrillator (ICD) leads.[9]

PATHOGENESIS

IE develops when a platelet-fibrin matrix deposits at the site of endothelial disruption in the heart or great vessels, providing a suitable milieu for bacteria or fungal attachment and reproduction. Complications result from primary tissue destruction, local extension of the infection, embolization of vegetative material, or immune complex activation and deposition. A variety of microorganism-specific factors interact with the host substrate to determine the clinical manifestations of the infection. Understanding these processes helps explain several clinical entities associated with IE.

Intact valvular endothelium effectively resists bacterial adhesion and colonization despite experimental intravascular inoculation.[10] Endothelial disruption, therefore, is a necessary precursor to IE, and may result from a variety of mechanisms: systemic disease (eg, rheumatic carditis), turbulent blood flow (eg, regurgitant valve lesions), mechanical injury (eg, from catheters or electrodes), or repeated insult from foreign material (eg, from particles injected during IV drug use).[11] Vegetations classically form in the line of closure of valve leaflets, on the "low-flow" side of the valves (ie, atrial side of atrioventricular valves and ventricular side of the semilunar valves).[12] Endothelial damage promotes sterile platelet-fibrin deposition and interstitial edema at the damaged site, thereby providing the substrate for capable bacteria to colonize an otherwise sterile thrombus.[11]

Although adhesion to platelet-fibrin matrix on damaged endothelium appears to be held in common between microorganisms causing IE, the mechanisms vary considerably between species. *S. aureus* may bind directly to damaged endothelial cells via species-specific clumping factors and coagulase interactions with fibrinogen. *S. aureus* also binds and activates platelets via the von Willebrand receptor. Other organisms bind to components of damaged endothelium or platelet-fibrin matrix, such as fibronectin, laminin, or collagen.[13,14] Streptococcal species may use dextran and other virulence factors to adhere to the platelet-fibrin matrix.[15]

Once microorganisms establish residence in the sterile thrombus, complex interactions determine the subsequent progression of the vegetation. Bacteria proliferate and promote additional platelet aggregation and activation. Species such as *S. aureus* resist the inherent bactericidal activity of platelet microbicidal proteins and interact with monocytes to promote release of tissue factor and the procoagulant cascade that facilitate bacterial and vegetation proliferation, respectively.[11] Deep inside a vegetation, some bacteria exhibit reduced metabolic activity that promotes survival against some antibiotics. *S. aureus*—and methicillin-resistant *Staphylococcus aureus* (MRSA) in particular—produce a biofilm, although the clinical relevance of this has been questioned.[11] IE related to CIEDs has been more directly linked to biofilm formation and contributes to the clinical challenges managing these infections.

Transient bacteremia is a necessary, but not sufficient, event to promote endocarditis. Although bacteremia is common after mild mucosal disruption following dental, gynecologic, urologic, or gastrointestinal procedures,[16] this rarely leads to the development of IE. The minimal magnitude of bacteremia necessary to cause IE is unknown, but it is likely that values above 10^4 colony-forming units (CFUs) per milliliter of blood are required.[16,17] In addition, bacteria-specific factors help determine whether transient bacteremia establishes IE. Gram-negative pathogens are usually eliminated by complement-mediated bactericidal activity in the blood, protecting against IE from gastrointestinal sources of bacteremia.[11] Organisms well suited to adhere to valve leaflets, on the other hand, such as *Staphylococcus, Streptococcus species*, and *Pseudomonas*, are more likely to cause IE.

The immunologic response of the host accounts for several clinical manifestations of IE. In response to infection, a variety of circulating antibodies are produced, including rheumatoid factor in up to half of patients with IE for more than 6 weeks, and antinuclear antibodies that may contribute to musculoskeletal manifestations, fever, and pleurisy.[18,19] Circulating immune complexes can be found in high titers in patients with IE, and are implicated in the development of IE-associated glomerulonephritis, tenosynovitis, Osler nodes, splinter hemorrhages, Roth spots, and mycotic aneurysms of blood vessels.[20]

Complications are the rule rather than the exception in IE, and can affect nearly any organ via a variety of mechanisms. Large emboli can occlude vessels in any downstream organ. Most notably, cerebral emboli are clinically apparent in 20% to 30% of patients with IE and present in the majority of asymptomatic patients undergoing magnetic resonance imaging (MRI), a risk that declines precipitously with appropriate antibiotic therapy.[21-23] Splenic infarcts are common, and myocardial infarction can occur with aortic valve vegetations, in particular.[24] If the emboli are infected, bacteria can directly invade adjacent tissues, leading to abscess formation (commonly in the kidney and spleen) or mycotic aneurysm (commonly at the branch points of cerebral vessels). Bacterial seeding in the absence of emboli can similarly lead to tissue infection and abscess formation. Within the heart, infections can lead to perforation of a leaflet, rupture of chordae tendinae, erosion of the interventricular septum, valve ring abscess with fistulae, myocardial infarction, and conduction system block. Right-sided endocarditis commonly leads to septic pulmonary emboli, which in turn are associated with pneumonia, abscesses, pleural effusions, and empyema. In the skin, immune-mediated perivascular inflammation can cause Osler nodes, and septic emboli lead to Janeway lesions. Ocular manifestations include immune-mediated micro hemorrhages (Roth spots) or, less commonly, direct bacterial seeding causing endophthalmitis.

Microbiology

Microbiology of IE can be divided broadly between native and prosthetic valve infections, with native valve endocarditis (NVE) further characterized according to predisposing heart conditions and comorbidities. *Staphylococcus, Streptococcus, or Enterococcus* species account for the vast majority (80%-90%) of native valve infections.[6] *S. aureus* now accounts for up to 30% of cases in high-income countries and affects patients across risk groups, including those with no identifiable predisposing valve lesions.[6] Coagulase-negative staphylococci (eg, *S. epidermidis* and *S. lugdunensis*) are ubiquitous skin commensals and are associated with health care–acquired NVE. In low-income countries, *Streptococcus viridans* species are the most common causes of IE and are common commensal organisms of the oral, gastrointestinal, and genitourinary tracts. Enterococci account for about 10% of cases overall, but particularly affect elderly and immunocompromised hosts.[6] Gram-negative (eg, *Acinetobacter* and *Pseudomonas* species) and HACEK organisms (*Haemophilus, Actinobacillus, Cardiobacterium, Eikenella, and Kingella* species) that are slow-growing colonizers of the oropharynx are rare offenders, accounting for fewer than 3% of cases.[6] Other rare causes of IE with particular exposures include zoonotic infections such as *Brucella* (livestock), *Bartonella* (cats), *Chlamydia* (birds), and fungal infections (esp. *Candida* and *Aspergillus*) after cardiac surgery and in immunocompromised hosts.[6] Viral endocarditis is essentially nonexistent.[12] Endocarditis associated with IVDU (IVDU-IE) can be either right- or left-sided, and the vast majority (>80%) of IVDU-associated tricuspid valve infections are caused by *S. aureus.*[8]

The microbiology of prosthetic valve endocarditis (PVE) is characterized by the time interval since valve surgery. Early infections (<2 months from the time of surgery) are usually due to nosocomial infections with coagulase-negative Staphylococci or *S. aureus.*[6] Late infections (>12 months after surgery) have a microbiology similar to that of NVE, with gram-positive Staphylococci, Streptococci, and Enterococci species predominating. Mid-term IE (2-12 months after surgery) is a mixture of the nosocomial infections and the usual native valve organisms. Although rare, fungal infections carry a high mortality and predominantly affect prosthetic valves.[6] Intracardiac device-related IE (CIED-IE) occurs in up to 2% of implanted devices, and can occur at the device pocket, on the leads, or in adjacent areas of disturbed endocardium.[6] Staphylococcal skin commensal organisms predominate as pathogens in CIED-IE, including coagulase-negative species and *S. aureus.*[25]

Risk Factors

IE develops as a result of transient bacteremia in the setting of endothelial damage and platelet-fibrin matrix deposition. Therefore, conditions that increase transient bacteremia or are associated with endothelial disruption predispose to endocarditis.

Historically, the most common predisposing cardiac condition was rheumatic heart disease. Although this remains true in developing countries,[26] rheumatic disease accounts for less than 5% of IE cases in developed countries in the modern era.[27]

In developed countries, the dramatic increase in implantable cardiac devices—including prosthetic valves, pacemakers, and defibrillators—now makes prosthetic device implantation one of the most important risk factors for IE. A recent report of more than 2000 IE cases from 25 countries found that 20% had a prosthetic valve and 7% had an implantable cardiac device.[27] Mitral valve prolapse (MVP) is the most common predisposing native valve abnormality, accounting for between 8% and 30% of NVE cases,[12] and has been reported to carry an odds ratio (OR) for IE of 8.2 (95% CI 2.4-38.4)[28] in comparison to individuals without MVP. As the population ages, degenerative valve lesions also become important risk factors. In autopsy studies, mitral annular calcification has been found more commonly among those with endocarditis than among the general population, suggesting this may represent an important substrate for the development of IE.[29] Finally, as more children with congenital heart disease reach adulthood—often after multiple surgeries and some with implantable devices—they are at increased lifetime risk for developing IE.[30]

Factors that increase the risk of transient bacteremia or alter the immune response also increase the risk of IE. In the United States, the proliferation of IVDU has contributed particularly to the development of tricuspid valve endocarditis. This is likely the result of increases in transient bacteremia and endothelial damage caused by injection of solid particle contaminants.[11] Increased frequency of health care contact—itself associated with more indwelling vascular access catheters, repeated procedures, and exposure to virulent organisms—is also an increasingly important risk factor for IE. A recent, prospective, multinational series of NVE found that health care exposure accounted for up to 30% of cases.[31] Some of the associated risk of health care exposure may also be related to the underlying disease state and altered immune response, as can be the case for HIV, malignancy, and patients on hemodialysis.[32] Finally, although endocarditis was formerly a disease of young patients with rheumatic heart disease, the highest risk in modern cohorts appears to be among older patients (aged 58-77 years) with other predisposing comorbidities.[32]

Clinical Outcomes

Despite advances in diagnosis and management, mortality remains high. In-hospital mortality in the contemporary era is 20%,[33] although it varies substantially by age, risk factors, and microorganism. For example, right-sided endocarditis is generally reported to have less than 10% early mortality;[34] adults with congenital heart disease were recently reported to have a similarly low early mortality of 6.9%.[35] In contrast, 30-day mortality was 27.5% in patients on dialysis and 27.7% among older (58-77 years old) patients in a single-center study.[36] In the International Collaboration on Endocarditis Prospective Cohort Study, the strongest risk factor for in-hospital mortality is paravalvular complications (OR 2.25, 95% CI: 1.64-3.09), followed by pulmonary edema (OR 1.79, 1.39-2.3), *S. aureus* infection (OR 1.54, 1.14-2.08), coagulase-negative Staphylococcal infection (OR 1.50, 1.07-2.10), prosthetic valve involvement (OR 1.47, 1.13-1.90), mitral valve vegetation (OR 1.34, 1.06-1.68), and increasing age (OR 1.30, 1.17-1.46 per 10-year interval).[27] *S. viridans* infection (OR 0.52, 0.33-0.81) and surgery (OR 0.61, 0.44-0.83) were associated with lower mortality.[27]

Although short-term mortality from endocarditis remains around 20%, longer term (up to 1 year) mortality is substantially higher at 30% to 40%.[37] This too, however, varies substantially by age and comorbidities, suggesting that some of the late mortality reflects the substrate more than the disease. For instance, a small study of octogenarians with IE reported 1-year mortality of 37.3% compared to 13% among those younger than 65 years of age,[38] and 6-month mortality among patients on dialysis was 38.5% versus 29.2% in the cohort overall in a single tertiary-care teaching hospital.[36]

DIAGNOSIS

Because the clinical manifestations of IE are most commonly vague and nonspecific and many patients lack the classic textbook findings, combined clinical, microbiologic, imaging, and pathologic criteria as defined in the modified Duke criteria remain the cornerstone of diagnosis (**Table 14.1**). After an initial set of investigations, a diagnosis of IE is characterized as definite, possible, or rejected.[39] For a definite diagnosis, two major, one major, and three minor, or five minor clinical criteria must be met. Alternatively, pathologic criteria may be met by culture or histologic examination of in situ valve tissue, embolized vegetations, or an intracardiac abscess. The diagnosis is rejected when there is a clear alternative diagnosis, the IE syndrome resolves with less than or equal to 4 days of antibiotic therapy, there is no pathologic evidence of IE after surgery or autopsy despite less than or equal to 4 days of antibiotic therapy, or criteria for possible IE are not met. Possible endocarditis is defined as the presence of one major plus one minor criterion or three minor criteria.

Despite well-documented sensitivity and specificity in several thousand diverse patients, the modified Duke criteria have important limitations.[40] First, the criteria were originally developed to facilitate epidemiologic and clinical research: Extending the criteria into the clinical arena has been more challenging. Secondly, IE is a highly heterogeneous disorder that relies on detailed microbiologic, imaging, and clinical investigations, each with their own limitations. For example, echocardiography can be negative or inconclusive in up to

TABLE 14.1 Summary of Modified Duke Criteria for Infective Endocarditis

Modified Duke Criteria for Infective Endocarditis	
Major Criteria	
Positive blood cultures	Typical microorganism isolated from two separate blood cultures • Viridans streptococci • *Streptococcus bovis* • HACEK group • *Staphylococcus aureus* • Community-acquired enterococci
	Persistently positive blood culture from microorganisms consistent with IE • ≥2 cultures drawn >12 h apart • ≥3 cultures *or* a majority of ≥4 cultures with first and last drawn at least 1 h apart
	Single culture positive for *Coxiella burnetii* or IgG Ab titer >1:800
Endocardial involvement (echocardiogram)	Vegetation (oscillating mass in the path of regurgitant jets without an alternative anatomic explanation) • TEE if prosthetic valve, "possible" IE, or complicated IE (eg, paravalvular abscess)
	Intracardiac abscess
	New prosthetic valve dehiscence
	New valve regurgitation
Minor Criteria	
Predisposition	Predisposing heart condition or IVDU
Fever	>38 °C
Vascular phenomena	Emboli, mycotic aneurysm, ICH, conjunctival hemorrhage
Immunologic phenomena	Glomerulonephritis, Osler nodes, Roth spots, rheumatoid factor
Microbiology *not* meeting major criteria	Positive blood cultures not meeting major criteria or serological evidence of infection
Interpretation	
Definite endocarditis	• 2 major criteria • 1 major + 3 minor • 5 minor
Possible	• 1 major + 1 minor criterion • 3 minor
Rejected	• Firm alternative diagnosis • Resolution of IE syndrome with ≤4 days of antibiotics • Lack of pathologic evidence of IE with antibiotic therapy for ≤4 days • Does not meet "possible" criteria

ICH, intracranial hemorrhage; IE, infective endocarditis; IgG, immunoglobulin G; IVDU, intravenous drug abuse; TEE, transesophageal echocardiogram.

30% of cases of prosthetic valve or CIED lead infections.[41,42] As such, the Duke criteria have limited sensitivity in detecting infections of prosthetic valves and CIEDs.[6] Finally, guidelines recognize that criteria are intended as a guideline and cannot supplant clinical judgment in any individual patient.[40,43]

Echocardiography

Echocardiography remains the initial and primary diagnostic imaging modality for IE. The goals of initial imaging include establishing the diagnosis, identification of complications, and risk stratification. As a general principle, transthoracic echocardiography (TTE) is noninvasive and readily available, but has lower sensitivity for detecting IE than does transesophageal echocardiography (TEE). This is particularly true in prosthetic valve or implantable cardiac device infections and for detecting complications such as abscess, where TTE has sensitivity of approximately 50% versus greater than 90% for TEE.[43] Regardless of modality, echocardiography has to be interpreted with caution, because alternative valve pathologies (degenerative calcified lesions, chordal rupture, Lambl excrescences, valvular fibroelastomas, etc) can be difficult to distinguish from IE.[43]

Despite the lower sensitivity of TTE relative to TEE for detecting IE, TTE is commonly the first imaging modality employed in suspected cases of IE based on availability, noninvasive nature, better ability to interrogate right-sided structures, and greater accuracy in defining hemodynamic consequences of valve lesions. Guidelines recommend prompt evaluation with TEE in cases of suspected prosthetic valve/CIED infection, where TTE is inconclusive or negative; yet clinical suspicion remains high and in cases where TTE is diagnostic to detect complications.[40,43] Guidelines also encourage repeat imaging as a patient's clinical course evolves, either with the development of new clinical features to suggest complications or with ongoing clinical suspicion for disease despite initial negative imaging.[40,43]

Multimodality Imaging

More recently, multimodality imaging has emerged as an effective adjunct to echocardiography. Although guidelines have yet to define a precise role for these modalities, they have demonstrated particular utility in select situations, most notably in prosthetic valve infections, early detection of paravalvular extension, and in cases where echocardiography is particularly limited (myxomatous or calcific valve degeneration) or inconclusive. Specifically, ^{18}F-fluorodeoxyglucose (^{18}F-FDG) positron emission tomography and computed tomography (PET/CT) has been shown to be more sensitive than is echocardiography in patients with possible NVE by modified Duke criteria and in prosthetic and intracardiac device infections.[44,45] Radiolabeled leukocyte scintigraphy has a higher specificity for the diagnosis of IE than does PET but lower spatial resolution.[46] Cardiac computed tomography angiography (CCTA) is useful in cases of right-sided infection, and is more sensitive for identification and definition of paravalvular extension, including paravalvular abscess and pseudoaneurysm.[32] CCTA can also define the coronary anatomy before surgery in select patients where cardiac catheterization is not performed and identify pulmonary complications such as abscess and embolism. Cardiac MRI has similarly shown greater sensitivity relative to echocardiography in the early stages of intracardiac spread of infection. In rare cases, it can help distinguish tumor from infection.[47] However, the temporal resolution of MRI is inferior to echocardiography and may not detect a vegetation. Brain MRI is also very sensitive for the detection of cerebral emboli and mycotic aneurysm. Finally, three-dimensional (3D) echocardiography can help identify leaflet perforation and is particularly helpful for surgical planning.[48]

MANAGEMENT OF THE PATIENT WITH INFECTIOUS ENDOCARDITIS

Effective management of IE revolves around two critical decisions: choice and duration of antimicrobial therapy and whether to perform surgery (**Algorithm 14.1**). These decisions, in turn, are influenced by the size and location of infection, development of complications, presence of prosthetic material, and particular microorganism strain and resistance profile. A multidisciplinary team from cardiology, cardiac surgery, and infectious diseases should collaborate on each case of IE to achieve optimal patient outcomes.

Antimicrobial Therapy

The goal of antibiotic treatment is to completely eradicate infection, including sterilizing vegetations. Early and effective antimicrobial therapy is critical to effective management and reduces the risk of developing complications, particularly embolization.[21] Unfortunately, infected vegetations pose a variety of challenges to sterilization, including high bacterial density, slow rate of bacterial growth with reduced metabolic activity, presence of biofilms, and a fibrin-platelet matrix that is relatively resistant to antibiotic penetration.[40] Antimicrobial agents have variable penetration into the vegetation and differ in their bactericidal activity. Achieving concentrations effective against the high bacterial load within the protected milieu is challenging and usually requires prolonged courses of IV antibiotic combinations.

The choice of antimicrobial therapy is principally determined by the infecting organism and associated resistance profile and influence by the presence of prosthetic material. Before the infecting organism is known, empiric antibiotic therapy should be directed toward gram-positive organisms and is determined by patient demographics, risk factors, and local epidemiology.[40,43] PVE with *S. aureus* usually necessitates the addition of rifampin and gentamicin for biofilm penetration,[40] whereas these agents are largely ineffective and have potential associated toxicity in NVE. Highly susceptible, uncomplicated infections may be treated successfully with oral therapy and/or for shorter durations. For example, uncomplicated right-sided *S. aureus* has been successfully treated with a combination of oral ciprofloxacin plus rifampin in IV drug users.[49] More recently, a randomized Danish trial demonstrated equivalent outcomes for patients with uncomplicated left-sided IE

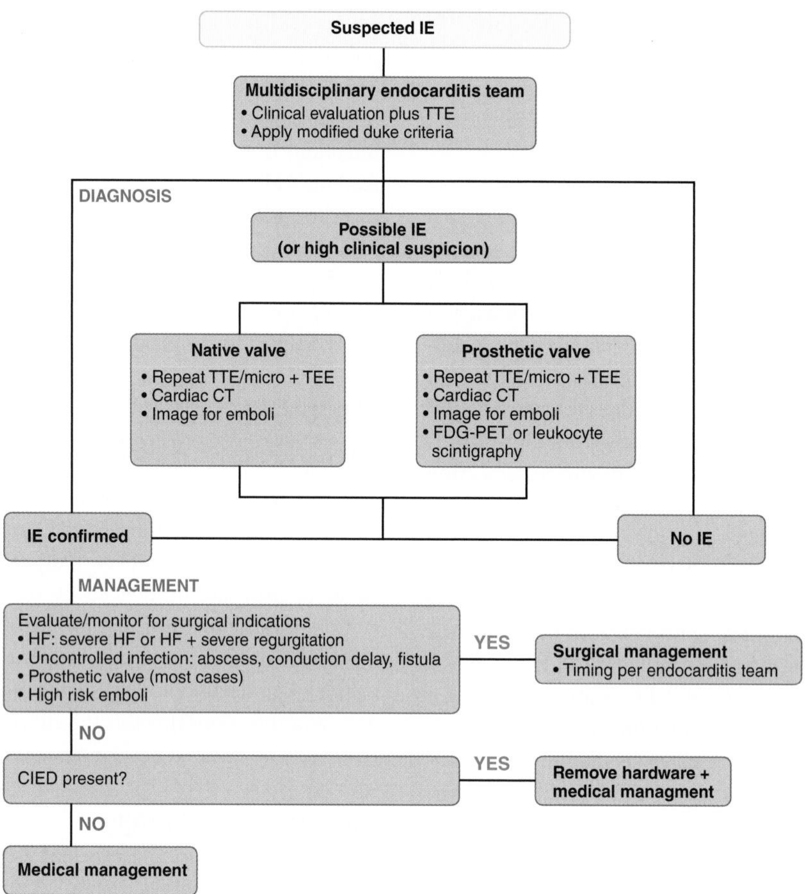

ALGORITHM 14.1 Simplified diagnostic and management algorithm for infective endocarditis. CIED, cardiac implantable electronic device; CT, computed tomography; FDG-PET, fluorodeoxyglucose-positron emission tomography; IE, infective endocarditis; HF, heart failure; TEE, transesophageal echocardiogram; TTE, transthoracic echocardiogram.

treated with oral versus IV antibiotics after an initial 2-week course of IV antibiotics, although no patients with MRSA were included.[50]

The duration of antimicrobial therapy depends on the location of infection, presence of complications, timing of surgical intervention, presence of prosthetic or implanted material, and particular organism. NVE is typically treated with 2 to 6 weeks of therapy, whereas prosthetic valve or device infections typically require 4 to 6 weeks of therapy, with the "clock" beginning at the time of first negative blood culture finding.[40,43] Blood cultures should be drawn every 24 to 72 hours during therapy until they return negative findings, and patients must be monitored closely for development of complications. Uncomplicated IE with susceptible organisms such as viridans group streptococci can be treated successfully with 2 weeks of combination therapy,[51] whereas MRSA infections treated with vancomycin will require longer courses of therapy.[11] After surgery, antibiotics were traditionally extended if cultures grew from excised material, but more recent data suggests that 2 weeks of therapy following surgical intervention may be sufficient, irrespective of the presence of positive cultures from excised tissues.[52] Again, expert consultation with infectious disease colleagues is critical to select the optimal antibiotic regimen and duration of treatment to achieve optimal patient outcomes.

There is an interest in moving toward shorter courses of therapy and transition to oral antibiotics to reduce the risks of prolonged hospitalization, indwelling catheters, misuse of IV catheters in the IVDU population, and toxicity of prolonged IV therapy, although more research is required.[53] Longer acting depot injections of antibiotics that would avoid some of the complications of long-term IV antibiotic therapy may also become available in the future.[54]

Surgery

Surgical management of IE is ultimately required in 50% to 60% of patients,[55] making it a cornerstone of therapy. Several studies have shown a mortality benefit with surgical intervention in selected patients. Indications for surgery fall into four categories: heart failure, presence of fungal infection, presence of intracardiac abscess, and conduction abnormalities such as heart block. U.S.[40,56] and European[43] guidelines differ subtly in how these are defined, but heart failure is generally defined as valve dysfunction or mechanical complication leading to signs and symptoms of heart failure. Uncontrolled infection involves paravalvular extension such as abscess or destructive penetrating lesions, fistulae from one cardiac chamber to another, infection with highly resistant organisms such as fungi, or failure of medical therapy despite appropriate antibiotics for greater than 5 to 7 days. Prevention of embolization is indicated in the event of large vegetations associated with recurrent emboli or severe valve dysfunction, with additional consideration given to very large (>3 cm) vegetations and vegetations on the anterior leaflet of the mitral valve.[40,43,56] PVE is most effectively treated with prompt surgical therapy with few exceptions. Select cases of PVE due to viridans group streptococci can be treated with medical therapy.[57]

Once surgical criteria are met, prompt surgical intervention is associated with improved outcomes in IE. This appears to be particularly true in patients with heart failure, paravalvular invasion, and prosthetic valve dysfunction or dehiscence. A randomized trial of surgery within 48 hours of diagnosis in patients with NVE and large vegetations with severe valve regurgitation showed a reduction in the combined endpoint of in-hospital death or embolism following surgery.[58] In addition, greater than 90% of patients in the conventional care group ultimately required surgery, validating the appropriateness of current surgical indications. An analysis of the *International Collaboration on Endocarditis-Prospective Cohort Study (ICE-PCS)* of patients with endocarditis and heart failure found that valvular surgery was associated with roughly 50% reduction in in-hospital and 1-year mortality compared to medical therapy alone.[59] A meta-analysis of studies comparing outcomes of surgical versus medical management in PVE similarly showed reduced 30-day mortality and improved survival at follow-up with no difference in PVE recurrence.[60] Another retrospective analysis of PVE suggested lower in-hospital and 1-year mortality, although this effect disappeared when survivor bias (whereby patients who survive are more likely to get surgery) was taken into account.[61]

Despite evidence that surgery reduces mortality in patients meeting surgical indications, a significant portion of patients meeting surgical criteria do not undergo surgery. In the ICE-PCS study, 24% of patients with left-sided endocarditis meeting guideline indications for surgery did not undergo the procedure.[62] This is likely for a variety of reasons, but most commonly because patients are deemed "too sick" to undergo a major operation. Among 181 patients in the ICE-PCS study who did not undergo surgery, 34% were deemed to have a poor prognosis regardless of surgery, 20% were hemodynamically unstable, 23% died before they could undergo surgery, and 21% had sepsis. Thus, a central challenge in determining who will benefit from surgery is that critically ill patients face higher risks at surgery, yet evidence suggests that sicker patients are more likely to benefit from surgical intervention.[54] Ultimately, the decision to proceed to surgery has to balance the risks and benefits of surgical intervention for individual patients and should be a consensus decision by a multidisciplinary team.[63] Various risk scores have been developed to assist clinicians in making decisions around surgical intervention in IE.[53] Referral of patients to surgical centers experienced in the operative management of IE should be considered early once the diagnosis of IE is confirmed.

Timing of surgical intervention should also be a joint decision by the multidisciplinary endocarditis team. Generally, the most recent surgical guidelines for the management of IE suggest that surgery should be performed "within days" once an indication for surgery has been established.[63] There is no evidence that delaying an indicated surgery improves outcomes. Patients with intracardiac abscesses, conduction abnormalities, and fistula formation are at highest risk for decompensation and should be operated on in an emergent or urgent manner. Although each day of appropriate antimicrobial therapy dramatically reduces the risk of embolism during the first 2 weeks of therapy,[21] this is also the period of highest risk for embolization, particularly with large (>1 cm) vegetations or those on the anterior leaflet of the mitral valve. Urgent (<48 hours) or even emergent surgery is reasonable in these patients deemed at imminent risk for embolization.[63] An additional consideration in surgical timing is the presence of symptomatic stroke that increases the risk of undergoing full anticoagulation during cardiac surgery and hemorrhagic conversion or extension. Traditionally, cardiac surgery has been delayed for 6 weeks after a stroke; however, recent evidence supports reducing the waiting period to 1 to 2 weeks for stroke without evidence of hemorrhage, and 3 to 4 weeks with evidence of hemorrhage.[63]

Adjunctive Therapy

Dental Evaluation

Indices of oral hygiene and gingival disease correlate with incidence of bacteremia from IE-related species, and evidence suggests that it may be oral hygiene and periodontal disease—not dental procedures per se—that are responsible for IE originating from the mouth.[40] Guidelines recommend inpatient dental evaluation for patients IE with subsequent attention to oral hygiene and dental care in follow-up to prevent recurrence.[40,43] In addition, guidelines recommend lifelong antibiotic endocarditis prophylaxis before dental visits for survivors of prior IE.

Anticoagulation

Generally, the indications for anticoagulation and antiplatelet therapy are the same for patients with IE as for those without. There is no proven benefit to anticoagulation to prevent embolic phenomena, and aspirin use for this purpose has been associated with increased bleeding.[40,43] Therefore, the routine use of antiplatelet agents is not recommended. For patients with mechanical valves and evidence of a central nervous system embolic event, guidelines recommend holding anticoagulation for 2 weeks, then cautiously reintroducing anticoagulation with a closely monitored heparin infusion.[40]

Endocarditis Team

Caring effectively for patients with IE is complex, and all current society guidelines emphasize the importance of a multidisciplinary endocarditis team.[40,43,63] The team should involve cardiology, cardiac surgery, and infectious disease at a minimum, but may also require involvement from neurologists, pharmacists, radiologists, pathologists, and addiction specialists in the case of IVDU.[54] Implementation of endocarditis teams has been associated with reduced in-hospital, 1-year, and 3-year mortality, higher rates of adherence to guideline therapy, and lower rates of complications from renal failure and embolic events.[64]

SPECIAL CONSIDERATIONS AND FUTURE DIRECTIONS

Transcatheter Aortic Valve Replacement Infective Endocarditis

An increasingly important subset of PVE is that associated with transcatheter aortic valve replacement (TAVR). As a result of increasing indications, the number of patients with transcatheter aortic valves is expected to rise substantially.[65] IE associated with TAVR is uncommon and is usually caused by *S. aureus*, coagulase-negative *Staphylococci*, and *Enterococci*.[65] One-year incidence varies from 0.2% in recent TAVR trials to 3.1% in an earlier real-world Danish registry,[66-68] and 5-year cumulative incidence is reported to be 2% to 6%.[69-71] Mortality from TAVR-associated IE is exceedingly high, from 36% to 64%.[72,73] Management is generally the same as for PVE, although there are no data to support surgical intervention in this particular subset of patients.[65] Registry data also show that patients with TAVR IE are less likely to be operated on than are other patients with PVE (15% vs 50%, respectively), likely related to the fact that many TAVR patients underwent the procedure because they were considered to be at high surgical risk.[65] Future research will need to define optimal diagnostic imaging modalities, clarify patient and procedural risk factors, and identify which patients will benefit from surgery versus antimicrobial therapy alone.[65]

Cardiac Implantable Electronic Device Infection

The increased rate of CIED implantation, particularly among elderly patients with comorbidities, has set the stage for increasing rates of CIED-related IE (CIED-IE). The incidence is roughly 2 per 1000 device-years, and (1) higher among patients with defibrillators than with pacemakers and (2) higher with cardiac resynchronization devices compared with dual-chamber pacemakers.[43] The predominant organism in CIED-IE is coagulase-negative *Staphylococci* species, with other organisms rarely reported. Management is with prolonged antimicrobial therapy and complete removal of implanted hardware often requiring laser lead extraction. Antimicrobial therapy alone without hardware removal has been associated with higher mortality and risk of recurrence.[74] Although the duration of antibiotic therapy is not well established, guidelines recommend 4 to 6 weeks of antibiotics, including at least 2 weeks of parenteral therapy after hardware removal or 4 weeks if blood cultures remain positive for more than 24 hours after hardware removal. Device reimplantation can be considered after critically reassessing the need for CIED therapy, but should not occur before blood cultures are negative for at least 72 hours.[43] In the event of ongoing valvular infection after hardware removal, device reimplantation may need to be delayed by up to 14 days.[43] Temporary pacing is a risk factor for subsequent device infection, so it should be avoided if possible.[76] In the event that temporary pacing is required as a bridge to reimplantation of a permanent device, active fixation leads attached to an external generator allow for early mobility.

Intravenous Drug Use–Associated Infective Endocarditis

Patients with IVDU-associated IE represent a significant and increasing portion of IE cases, now estimated between 8% and 37.8% of all IE cases,[76] but more than 50% of IE cases in one tertiary care center serving a rural southeastern U.S. population were more affected by the opioid epidemic.[77] Similar to non-IVDU IE, the majority of cases are caused by *S. aureus*, although the proportion of cases from *S. aureus* is higher than in the non-IVDU population (64% for IVDU-IE vs 28% for non-IVDU IE).[76,78] Patients with IVDU also have a higher proportion of polymicrobial, *Pseudomonas*, and fungal infections as well as infection with typically nonpathologic bacteria found in saliva.[76] Unique mechanisms for IE in these patients include direct mechanical damage due to impurities in the injected substances (especially talcum powder), high bacterial load inoculated directly into the venous circulation, and IVDU-induced vasospasm that can cause intimal damage and thrombus formation, providing a nidus for infection.[78] Consequently, up to 76% of IVDU-IE is right-sided, compared to only 10% to 13% of non-IVDU IE.[79] There are important management considerations unique to the IVDU population, driven principally by the high rates of recidivism and reinfection. Readmission within 90 days is reported in 22% and 49% of patients with IVDU-IE, with 28% of patients reporting injection drug use again at readmission. Among those reinfected and requiring repeat surgery, operative mortality is roughly double that of first-time intervention,[80] and risk of reoperation and mortality within 3 to 6 months of initial intervention are roughly 10-fold higher than in non-IVDU populations.[81] Aggressive addiction counseling and treatment can reduce mortality, health care utilization, and cost, but up to half of patients may not receive appropriate addiction counseling and referral during their index hospitalization for IE.[82] Long-acting depot antibiotic formulations, shorter IV antibiotic courses, and oral regimens may avoid the need for indwelling IV catheters and associated risks of misuse, but further research is needed.

FOLLOW-UP PATIENT CARE

At the completion of therapy, guidelines recommend repeating an echocardiogram to establish a new baseline. Any indwelling IV catheters should be promptly removed. The patient should be educated about signs and symptoms of endocarditis and the need for antibiotic prophylaxis with dental procedures. Routine dental hygiene and regular dental follow-up should be emphasized. Patients with IVDU should be referred for addiction counseling and drug rehabilitation, if not already done. In the event of any febrile illness, three sets of blood cultures should be drawn before the initiation of antibiotics.[40]

KEY POINTS

- ✔ Despite advances in medical and surgical therapy, IE continues to be associated with high mortality.
- ✔ Older patients with comorbidities, and particularly those with prosthetic valves, are at highest risk of mortality from IE.
- ✔ IE results from transient bacteremia in the setting of endothelial disruption and platelet-fibrin matrix deposition.
- ✔ Patients with IVDU and aging populations with more implantable cardiac devices represent increasingly important high-risk populations for developing IE.
- ✔ Management of endocarditis centers on appropriate antimicrobial therapy, with close attention to the development of complications necessitating a surgical approach.
- ✔ The management of patients with IE is complicated and requires a multidisciplinary approach to achieve optimal patient outcomes.

REFERENCES

1. Pant S, Patel NJ, Deshmukh A,et al. Trends in infective endocarditis incidence, microbiology, and valve replacement in the United States from 2000 to 2011. *J Am Coll Cardiol.* 2015;65(19):2070-2076.
2. Fernández-Hidalgo N, Almirante B, Tornos P, et al. Contemporary epidemiology and prognosis of health care-associated infective endocarditis. *Clin Infect Dis.* 2008;47(10):1287-1297. doi:10.1086/592576
3. Meisner JA, Aseni J, Chen X, Grande D. Changes in infective endocarditis admissions in Pennsylvania during the opioid epidemic. *Clin Infect Dis.* 2020;71(7):1664-1670.
4. Vogkou CT, Vlachogiannis NI, Palaiodimos L, Kousoulis AA. The causative agents in infective endocarditis: a systematic review comprising 33,214 cases. *Eur J Clin Microbiol Infect Dis.* 2016;35(8):1227-1245.
5. Khan O, Shafi AMA, Timmis A. International guideline changes and the incidence of infective endocarditis: a systematic review. *Open Heart.* 2016;3(2):e000498.
6. Cahill TJ, Prendergast BD. Infective endocarditis. *Lancet.* 2016; 387(10021):882-893.
7. Cabell C, Fowler VG Jr, Engemann JJ, et al. Endocarditis in the elderly: incidence, surgery, and survival in 16,921 patients over 12 years. *Circulation.* 2002;106:547. ©Lippincott Williams & Wilkins
8. Kiefer TL, Wang A. Infective endocarditis. In: Stergiopoulos K, Brown DL, eds. *Evidence-Based Cardiology Consult.* 2014; Springer-Verlag London:71-78.
9. Stuesse DC, Vlessis A. Epidemiology of native valve endocarditis. In: Vlessis A, Bolling S, eds. *Endocarditis: A Multidisciplinary Approach to Modern Treatment.* 1999; Futura Publishing Company:77-84.
10. Durack DT, Beeson PB, Petersdorf RG. Experimental bacterial endocarditis. 3. Production and progress of the disease in rabbits. *Br J Exp Pathol.* 1973;54(2):142-151.
11. Holland TL, Baddour LM, Bayer AS, Hoen B, Miro JM, Fowler VG Jr. Infective endocarditis. *Nat Rev Dis Primers.* 2016;2:16059.
12. Thiene G, Basso C. Pathology and pathogenesis of infective endocarditis in native heart valves. *Cardiovasc Pathol.* 2006;15(5):256-263.
13. Lowrance JH, Baddour LM, Simpson WA. The role of fibronectin binding in the rat model of experimental endocarditis caused by Streptococcus sanguis. *J Clin Invest.* 1990;86(1):7-13.
14. Scheld WM, Strunk RW, Balian G, Calderone RA. Microbial adhesion to fibronectin in vitro correlates with production of endocarditis in rabbits. *Proc Soc Exp Biol Med.* 1985;180(3):474-482.
15. Scheld WM, Valone JA. Sande MA. Bacterial adherence in the pathogenesis of endocarditis. Interaction of bacterial dextran, platelets, and fibrin. *J Clin Invest.* 1978;61(5):1394-1404.
16. Forner L, Larsen T, Kilian M, Holmstrup P. Incidence of bacteremia after chewing, tooth brushing and scaling in individuals with periodontal inflammation. *J Clin Periodontol.* 2006;33(6):401-407.
17. Veloso TR, Chaouch A, Roger T, et al. Use of a human-like low-grade bacteremia model of experimental endocarditis to study the role of Staphylococcus aureus adhesins and platelet aggregation in early endocarditis. *Infect Immun.* 2013;81(3):697-703.
18. Bacon PA, Davidson C, Smith B. Antibodies to candida and autoantibodies in sub-acute bacterial endocarditis. *Q J Med.* 1974;43(172):537-550.
19. Williams R, Kunkel H. Rheumatoid factors and their disappearance following therapy in patients with subacute bacterial endocarditis. *Arthritis Rheumatism.* 1962; Lippincott Williams & Wilkins:19106.
20. Deck CR, Guarda ES, Bianchi CC, et al. [Circulating immune complexes in infective endocarditis]. *Rev Med Chil.* 1988;116(11):1101-1104.
21. Dickerman SA, Abrutyn E, Barsic B, et al. The relationship between the initiation of antimicrobial therapy and the incidence of stroke in infective endocarditis: an analysis from the ICE Prospective Cohort Study (ICE-PCS). *Am Heart J.* 2007;154(6):1086-1094.
22. Duval X, lung B, Klein I, et al. Effect of early cerebral magnetic resonance imaging on clinical decisions in infective endocarditis: a prospective study. *Ann Intern Med.* 2010;152(8):497-504, W175.
23. Snygg-Martin U, Gustafsson L, Rosengren L, et al. Cerebrovascular complications in patients with left-sided infective endocarditis are common: a prospective study using magnetic resonance imaging and neurochemical brain damage markers. *Clin Infect Dis.* 2008;47(1):23-30.
24. Weinstein L, Schlesinger JJ. Pathoanatomic, pathophysiologic and clinical correlations in endocarditis (second of two parts). *N Engl J Med.* 1974;291(21):1122-1126.
25. Sohail MR, Uslan DZ, Khan AH, et al. Management and outcome of permanent pacemaker and implantable cardioverter-defibrillator infections. *J Am Coll Cardiol.* 2007;49(18):1851-1859.
26. Watt G, Lacroix A, Pachirat O, et al. Prospective comparison of infective endocarditis in Khon Kaen, Thailand and Rennes, France. *Am J Trop Med Hyg.* 2015;92(4):871-874.
27. Murdoch DR, Corey GR, Hoen B, et al. Clinical presentation, etiology, and outcome of infective endocarditis in the 21st century: the International Collaboration on Endocarditis–Prospective Cohort Study. *Arch Intern Med.* 2009;169(5):463-473.
28. Clemens JD, Horwitz RI, Jaffe CC, et al. A controlled evaluation of the risk of bacterial endocarditis in persons with mitral-valve prolapse. *N Engl J Med.* 1982;307(13):776-781.
29. Movahed M-R, Saito Y, Ahmadi-Kashani M, Ebrahimi R. Mitral annulus calcification is associated with valvular and cardiac structural abnormalities. *Cardiovasc Ultrasound.* 2007;5(1):14.
30. Benziger CP, Stout K, Zaragoza-Macias E, Bertozzi-Villa A, Flaxman AD. Projected growth of the adult congenital heart disease population in the United States to 2050: an integrative systems modeling approach. *Popul Health Metr.* 2015;13:29.
31. Benito N, Miro JM, de Lazzari E, et al. Health care-associated native valve endocarditis: importance of non-nosocomial acquisition. *Ann Intern Med.* 2009;150(9):586-594.
32. Vincent LL, Otto CM. Infective endocarditis: update on epidemiology, outcomes, and management. *Curr Cardiol Rep.* 2018;20(10):86.
33. Slipczuk L, Codolosa JN, Davila CD, et al. Infective endocarditis epidemiology over five decades: a systematic review. *PLoS One.* 2013;8(12):e82665.
34. Moss R, Munt B. Injection drug use and right sided endocarditis. *Heart.* 2003;89(5):577-581.
35. Tutarel O, Alonso-Gonzalez R, Montanaro C, et al. Infective endocarditis in adults with congenital heart disease remains a lethal disease. *Heart.* 2018;104(2):161-165.
36. Mostaghim AS, Lo HYA, Khardori N. A retrospective epidemiologic study to define risk factors, microbiology, and clinical outcomes of infective endocarditis in a large tertiary-care teaching hospital. *SAGE Open Med.* 2017;5:2050312117741772.
37. Bashore TM, Cabell C, Fowler V Jr, Update on infective endocarditis. *Curr Probl Cardiol.* 2006;31(4):274-352.
38. Oliver L, Lavoute C, Giorgi R, et al. Infective endocarditis in octogenarians. *Heart.* 2017;103(20):1602-1609.

39. Li JS, Sexton DJ, Mick N, et al. Proposed modifications to the Duke criteria for the diagnosis of infective endocarditis. *Clin Infect Dis.* 2000;30(4):633-638.
40. Baddour LM, Wilson WR, Bayer AS, et al. Infective endocarditis in adults: diagnosis, antimicrobial therapy, and management of complications: a scientific statement for healthcare professionals from the American Heart Association. *Circulation.* 2015;132(15):1435-1486.
41. Hill EE, Herijgers P, Claus P, Vanderschueren S, Peetermans WE, Herregods M-C. Abscess in infective endocarditis: the value of transesophageal echocardiography and outcome: a 5-year study. *Am Heart J.* 2007;154(5):923-928.
42. Vieira ML, Grinberg M, Pomerantzeff PMA, Andrade JL, Mansur AJ. Repeated echocardiographic examinations of patients with suspected infective endocarditis. *Heart.* 2004;90(9):1020-1024.
43. Habib G, Lancellotti P, Antunes MJ, et al. 2015 ESC Guidelines for the management of infective endocarditis: The Task Force for the Management of Infective Endocarditis of the European Society of Cardiology (ESC). Endorsed by: European Association for Cardio-Thoracic Surgery (EACTS), the European Association of Nuclear Medicine (EANM). *Eur Heart J.* 2015;36(44):3075-3128.
44. Cautela J, Alessandrini S, Cammilleri S, et al. Diagnostic yield of FDG positron-emission tomography/computed tomography in patients with CEID infection: a pilot study. *Europace.* 2013;15(2):252-257.
45. Pizzi MN, Roque A, Fernández-Hidalgo N, et al. Improving the diagnosis of infective endocarditis in prosthetic valves and intracardiac devices with ^{18}F-fluordeoxyglucose positron emission tomography/computed tomography angiography: initial results at an infective endocarditis referral center. *Circulation.* 2015;132(12):1113-1126.
46. Rouzet F, Chequer R, Benali K, et al. Respective performance of ^{18}F-FDG PET and radiolabeled leukocyte scintigraphy for the diagnosis of prosthetic valve endocarditis. *J Nucl Med.* 2014;55(12):1980-1985.
47. Pazos-López P, Pozo E, Siqueira ME, et al. Value of CMR for the differential diagnosis of cardiac masses. *JACC Cardiovasc Imaging.* 2014;7(9):896-905.
48. Thompson KA, Shiota T, Tolstrup K, Gurudevan SV, Siegel RJ. Utility of three-dimensional transesophageal echocardiography in the diagnosis of valvular perforations. *Am J Cardiol.* 2011;107(1):100-102.
49. Heldman AW, Hartert TV, Ray SC, et al. Oral antibiotic treatment of right-sided staphylococcal endocarditis in injection drug users: prospective randomized comparison with parenteral therapy. *Am J Med.* 1996;101(1):68-76.
50. Iversen K, Ihlemann N, Gill SU, et al. Partial oral versus intravenous antibiotic treatment of endocarditis. *N Engl J Med.* 2019;380(5):415-424.
51. Francioli P, Ruch W, Stamboulian D, et al. Treatment of streptococcal endocarditis with a single daily dose of ceftriaxone and netilmicin for 14 days: a prospective multicenter study. *Clin Infect Dis.* 1995;21(6):1406-1410.
52. Morris AJ, Drinkovic D, Pottumarthy S, et al. Bacteriological outcome after valve surgery for active infective endocarditis: implications for duration of treatment after surgery. *Clin Infect Dis.* 2005;41(2):187-194.
53. Cahill TJ, Baddour LM, Habib G, et al. Challenges in infective endocarditis. *J Am Coll Cardiol.* 2017;69(3):325-344.
54. El-Dalati S, Cronin D, Shea M, et al. Clinical practice update on infectious endocarditis. *Am J Med.* 2020;133(1):44-49.
55. Prendergast BD, Tornos P. Surgery for infective endocarditis: who and when? *Circulation.* 2010;121(9):1141-1152.
56. Nishimura RA, Otto CM, Bonow RO, et al. 2017 AHA/ACC focused update of the 2014 AHA/ACC guideline for the management of patients with valvular heart disease: a report of the American College of Cardiology/American Heart Association Task Force on Clinical Practice Guidelines. *J Am Coll Cardiol.* 2017;70(2):252-289.
57. Truninger K, Jost C, Seifert B, et al. Long term follow up of prosthetic valve endocarditis: what characteristics identify patients who were treated successfully with antibiotics alone? *Heart.* 1999;82(6):714-720.
58. Kang DH, Kim Y-J, Kim S-H, et al. Early surgery versus conventional treatment for infective endocarditis. *N Engl J Med.* 2012;366(26):2466-2473.
59. Kiefer T, Park L, Tribouilloy C, et al. Association between valvular surgery and mortality among patients with infective endocarditis complicated by heart failure. *JAMA.* 2011;306(20):2239-2247.
60. Mihos CG, Capoulade R, Yucel E, Picard MH, Santana O. Surgical versus medical therapy for prosthetic valve endocarditis: a meta-analysis of 32 studies. *Ann Thorac Surg.* 2017;103(3):991-1004.
61. Lalani T, Chu VH, Park LP, et al. In-hospital and 1-year mortality in patients undergoing early surgery for prosthetic valve endocarditis. *JAMA Intern Med.* 2013;173(16):1495-1504.
62. Chu VH, Park LP, Athan E, et al. Association between surgical indications, operative risk, and clinical outcome in infective endocarditis: a prospective study from the International Collaboration on Endocarditis. *Circulation.* 2015;131(2):131-140.
63. Pettersson GB, Hussain ST. Current AATS guidelines on surgical treatment of infective endocarditis. *Ann Cardiothorac Surg.* 2019;8(6):630-644.
64. Davierwala PM, Marin-Caurtas M, Misfeld M, Borger MA. The value of an "Endocarditis Team". *Ann Cardiothorac Surg.* 2019;8(6):621-629.
65. Harding D, Cahil TJ, Redwood SR, Prendergast BD. Infective endocarditis complicating transcatheter aortic valve implantation. *Heart.* 2020;106(7):493-498.
66. Mack MJ, Leon MB, Thourani VH, et al. Transcatheter aortic-valve replacement with a balloon-expandable valve in low-risk patients. *N Engl J Med.* 2019;380(18):1695-1705.
67. Olsen NT, Backer OD, Tyregod HGH, et al. Prosthetic valve endocarditis after transcatheter aortic valve implantation. *Circ Cardiovasc Interv.* 2015;8(4):e001939.
68. Popma JJ, Deeb GM, Yakubov SJ, et al. Transcatheter aortic-valve replacement with a self-expanding valve in low-risk patients. *N Engl J Med.* 2019;380(18):1706-1715.
69. Butt JH, Ihlemann N, Backer OD, et al. Long-term risk of infective endocarditis after transcatheter aortic valve replacement. *J Am Coll Cardiol.* 2019;73(13):1646-1655.
70. Mack MJ, Leon MB, Smith CR, et al. 5-year outcomes of transcatheter aortic valve replacement or surgical aortic valve replacement for high surgical risk patients with aortic stenosis (PARTNER 1): a randomised controlled trial. *Lancet.* 2015;385(9986):2477-2484.
71. Thyregod HGH, Ihlemann N, Jorgensen TH, et al. Five-year clinical and echocardiographic outcomes from the Nordic Aortic Valve Intervention (NOTION) randomized clinical trial in lower surgical risk patients. *Circulation.* 2019;139(4):2714-2723.
72. Mangner N, Woitek F, Haussig S, et al. Incidence, predictors, and outcome of patients developing infective endocarditis following transfemoral transcatheter aortic valve replacement. *J Am Coll Cardiol.* 2016;67(24):2907-2908.
73. Regueiro A, Linke A, Latib A, et al. Association between transcatheter aortic valve replacement and subsequent infective endocarditis and in-hospital death. *JAMA.* 2016;316(10):1083-1092.
74. Baddour LM, Bettmann MA, Bolger AF, et al. Nonvalvular cardiovascular device–related infections. *Circulation.* 2003;108(16):2015-2031.
75. Klug D, Balde M, Pavin D, et al. Clinical perspective. *Circulation.* 2007;116(12):1349-1355.
76. Sanaiha Y, Lyons R, Benharash P. Infective endocarditis in intravenous drug users. *Trends Cardiovasc Med.* 2020;30(8):491-497.
77. Hartman L, Barnes E, Bachmann L, Schafer K, Lovato J, Files DC. Opiate injection-associated infective endocarditis in the southeastern United States. *Am J Med Sci.* 2016;352(6):603-608.
78. Frontera JA, Gradon JD. Right-side endocarditis in injection drug users: review of proposed mechanisms of pathogenesis. *Clin Infect Dis.* 2000;30(2):374-379.
79. Chambers HF, Korzeniowski OM, Sande MA. Staphylococcus aureus endocarditis: clinical manifestations in addicts and nonaddicts. *Medicine (Baltimore).* 1983;62(3):170-177.
80. Mori M, Mahmood SUB, Schranz AJ, et al. Risk of reoperative valve surgery for endocarditis associated with drug use. *J Thorac Cardiovasc Surg.* 2019;159(4):1262-1268.e2.
81. Shrestha NK, Jue J, Hussain ST, et al. Injection drug use and outcomes after surgical intervention for infective endocarditis. *Ann Thorac Surg.* 2015;100(3):875-882.
82. Gray ME, McQuade ETR, Scheld WM, Dillingham RA. Rising rates of injection drug use associated infective endocarditis in Virginia with missed opportunities for addiction treatment referral: a retrospective cohort study. *BMC Infect Dis.* 2018;18(1):532.

CHAPTER 15

PERICARDIAL DISEASE

Yaquta Kaka and Brent C. Lampert

INTRODUCTION

The pericardium is the site of many cardiac diseases that display classic physical examination signs and symptoms, imaging findings, and hemodynamic changes. These diseases include pericardial effusion, tamponade, pericarditis, and constrictive and effusive-constrictive pericarditis.

Anatomy and Physiology of the Pericardium

The pericardium (**Figure 15.1**) consists of two layers—a serous inner membrane and a fibrous outer sac—that surround the heart. The serous membrane forms the outer covering of the heart and is referred to as the visceral pericardium, whereas the thick fibrous sac covers the atria, ventricles, and proximal great vessels and is referred to as the parietal pericardium.[1] As a mesothelial monolayer, the visceral pericardium adheres firmly to the epicardium and blends over the great vessels joining the parietal pericardium.[2] The space between the parietal and visceral pericardium contains fluid and is called the pericardial cavity or sac. The pericardial space is defined by its attachment to the great vessels anteriorly, manubrium and xiphoid process ventrally, diaphragm caudally, and vertebral column dorsally.[1] The space generally contains 50 cc of serous fluid that reduces the friction on the epicardium.[1,2]

The pericardial nerve fibers arise from the vagus, left recurrent laryngeal, and esophageal plexus along with the first dorsal ganglion and the stellate ganglion. Lymphatics are present on the parietal surface of the epicardium and drain into lymph nodes at the base of the heart,[1] with the pericardial lymph having immunologic properties.[3] Furthermore, the

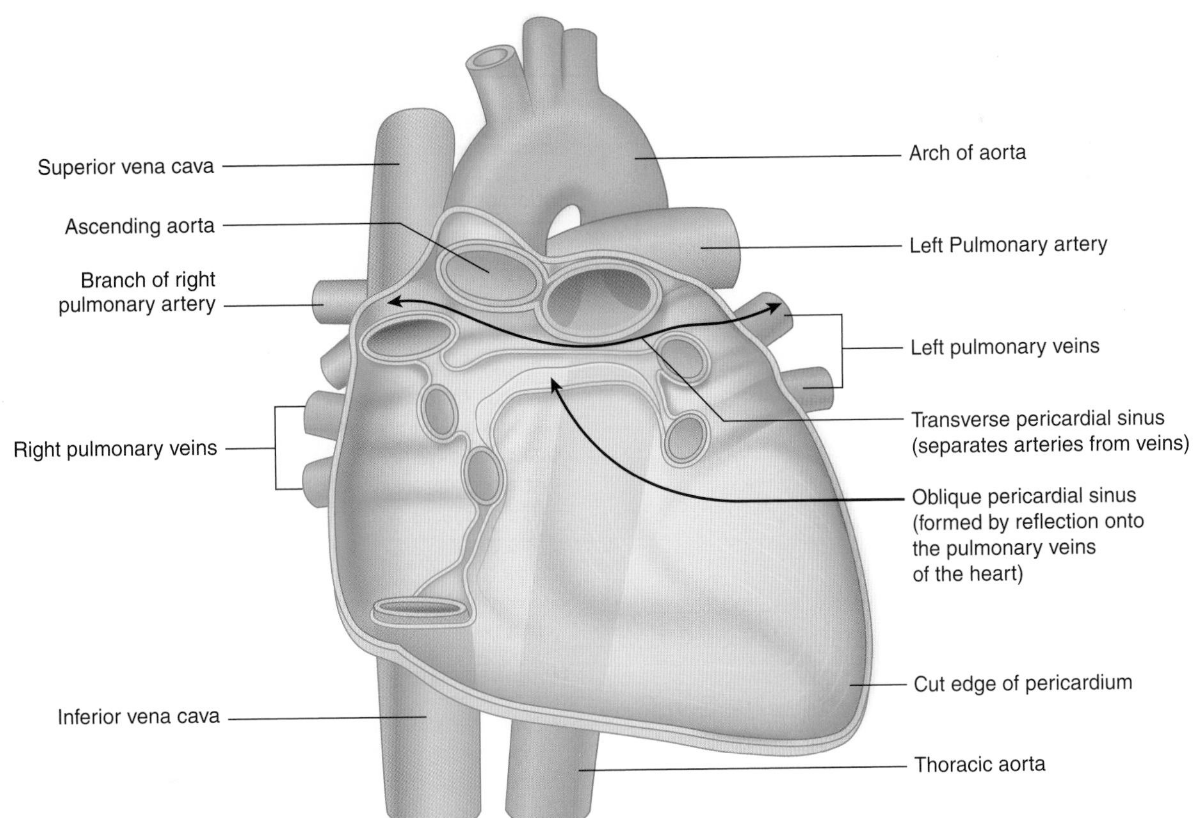

FIGURE 15.1 Structures of the pericardium with the great vessels.

pericardial membrane is active and assists with the transfer of water, electrolytes, and small molecules.

Two important functions of the pericardium include preventing displacement of the heart within the thorax and serving as a barrier to infection.[1,3] It also helps with maintaining pressure differences within the different cardiac chambers. Mechanistically, the pericardium at times exhibits a restrictive function on the heart. At low stress, the pericardial tissue is flexible and can be easily stretched, and at the upper range of physiologic cardiac volumes, it becomes stiff. This is called the pericardial reserve volume. Once the pericardium reaches its reserve volume, further distention of the sac causes an increase in intrapericardial pressure, which is easily transmitted to the cardiac chambers resulting in coupling of the ventricles and atria.[1,3,4] The pressure-volume curve of the pericardium is nonlinear: once the pericardial reserve is exhausted, small volume changes in the acute setting can cause dramatic increases in pressure and cardiac dysfunction (**Figure 15.2**).

PERICARDIAL EFFUSIONS

Pericardial effusions can occur because of a variety of causes, including excess production from an inflammatory state, damage to the cardiac chambers resulting in bleeding, decreased reabsorption because of increased systemic venous pressures in conditions such as decompensated heart failure, decreased lymphatic drainage from tumors or cancers, and lastly because of surgical manipulation of the area such as post–heart transplant.[5-7]

Most patients with pericardial effusions are asymptomatic, being discovered either on routine chest x-ray showing a globular shape to the heart or on transthoracic echocardiogram done for unrelated reasons.[5] Pericardial effusions can be classified according to onset, location, hemodynamic effects, size, and composition (**Table 15.1**).[5] Onset is defined as acute, subacute, or chronic. Location is circumferential, posterior, or loculated. Size is defined by echocardiographic measurement: small (<10 mm), medium (10-20 mm), and large (>20 mm) based on linear measurements of the largest echo-free space between the two layers of the pericardium at end diastole, and composition is transudative, exudative, chylous, pyopericardium, or hemopericardium.[7]

The etiology of pericardial effusions in developed countries is most often idiopathic (up to 50%) and in developing countries is tuberculosis, which has a mortality rate up to 40% in 6 months if untreated (**Table 15.2**).[5,7] If suspected,

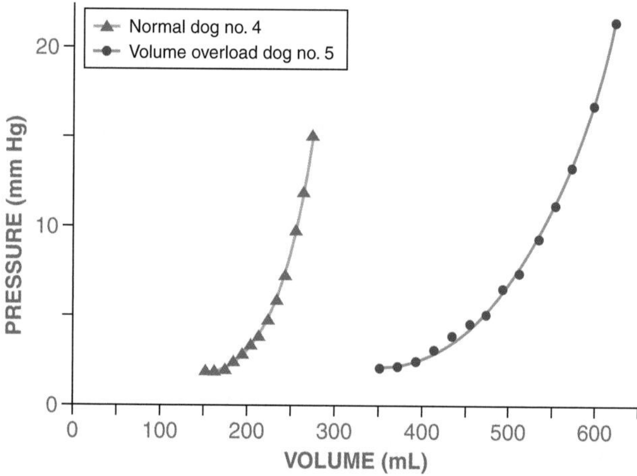

FIGURE 15.2 Pressure-volume curves (normal canine heart) of a pericardium after 4 weeks of chronic dilation because of volume. (Reprinted from LeWinter MM, Kabbani S. Pericardial diseases. In: Zipes DP, Libby P, Bonow RO, Braunwald E, eds. *Braunwald's Heart Disease: A textbook of cardiovascular medicine.* 7th ed. Philadelphia, PA: Elsevier Saunders; 2005:1757–1780. Copyright © 2005 Elsevier. With permission.)

TABLE 15.1 Classification of Pericardial Effusion

Onset	Acute (<1 week) Subacute (1 week to 3 months) Chronic (>3 months)
Size (echo-free space on echocardiography)	Mild <10 mm Moderate 10-20 mm Large >20 mm
Location	Circumferential Loculated Posterior
Composition	Transudate Exudate Chylous Pyopericardium Hemopericardium

TABLE 15.2 Causes of Pericardial Effusion

Inflammatory

Infections:
- Viral: *Enterococcus*, adenovirus, herpesviruses, parvovirus B19, human immunodeficiency virus, hepatitis C, coronavirus
- Bacterial: *Mycobacterium* (tuberculosis, avium-intracellulare), mycoplasma, *Neisseria*
- Fungal: *Histoplasma, Candida*
- Protozoan: *Toxoplasma* species

Autoimmune: Systemic lupus erythematosus, rheumatoid arthritis, scleroderma, eosinophilic granulomatosis with polyangiitis (Churg-Strauss syndrome), Dressler syndrome (postmyocardial infarction)

Uremic

Cardiac injury: Postmyocardial infarction, post-pericardiotomy, post-percutaneous interventions, postcardiac surgery, postablation

Noninflammatory

Neoplastic: Primary tumors (mesothelioma, sarcoma), secondary (lung, breast, lymphoma, ovarian)

Traumatic: Iatrogenic, blunt chest wall trauma

Metabolic: Hypothyroidism

Reduced lymphatic drainage: Congestive heart failure, cirrhosis, thoracic duct occlusion extracardiac screening should be performed, the pericardial effusion should be drained and analyzed, and a pericardial biopsy for culture and polymerase chain reaction (PCR) should be pursued.[7] Other causes include cancer (10%-25%), infections (15%-30%), iatrogenic (15%-20%), and rheumatologic (5%-15%).

Pericardial effusions because of infections are usually exudative and, in some cases, present as pyopericardium. If infection is suspected, the pericardial effusion should be drained and sent for culture. In certain high-risk individuals, human immunodeficiency virus (HIV) and hepatitis C screening should also be pursued.[7]

Systemic diseases and metabolic changes can also lead to pericardial effusions. Uremia can cause an inflammatory effusion with fibrinous material in the pericardial sac. If uremic effusion results in pericarditis, the classic uremic pericardial rub may be audible. Primary treatment for this is hemodialysis.

Other systemic conditions such as hypothyroidism, severe malnutrition, and rheumatologic diseases can also lead to pericardial effusions. Primary treatment focuses on addressing the underlying condition.[1,6,7]

Hemopericardium can result from injury to cardiac structures or the great vessels from either blunt force/trauma or from systemic causes. Type A aortic dissection extending to the aortic root is one example.

Lastly, new-onset symptomatic large pericardial effusions can in some cases be the first manifestation of an underlying malignancy. Malignant effusions are usually transudative and hemorrhagic and more commonly associated with extracardiac cancers (lung, breast, lymphoma) as opposed to primary cardiac tumors. Patients with chest radiation and bone marrow transplant can also have pericardial effusions.[1,7]

Chylous effusions result from obstruction of pericardial lymphatic drainage. Hence, they may occur after cardiothoracic surgery or in association with congenital lymphangiomatosis. Other causes include chest trauma, mediastinal radiation, malignant neoplasm of the mediastinum, and thrombosis of the subclavian vein or superior vena cava.

Clinical features of a pericardial effusion vary based on the acuity and rapidity of fluid accumulation. With slow accumulation, the patient may have no symptoms. Classic symptoms of rapid accumulation or large effusions include dyspnea on exertion, chest fullness or tightness, and orthopnea. Additional symptoms include nausea, hoarseness, dysphagia from compression of surrounding structures, fatigue, palpitations, and fever. On physical examination, patients may be without findings unless there is pericarditis or hemodynamic compromise from tamponade.[8,9]

When a pericardial effusion is suspected, a transthoracic echocardiogram should be performed. An echocardiogram provides semiquantitative information regarding the hemodynamic effects of the effusion, size, and location. Generally, for uncomplicated effusions, echocardiogram is sufficient for diagnosis, and rarely other imaging modalities such as cardiac computed tomography (CT) or magnetic resonance imaging (MRI) are needed. Gated CT can be useful for delineating the effusion for surgical planning and estimating the composition based on Hounsfield units. Cardiac MRI like echocardiography has the ability to provide both hemodynamic and anatomic assessment of the fluid. However, unlike echocardiography it can also give insight into pericardial thickening and inflammation. Therefore, MRI can be useful in complicated cases or cases with inconclusive evidence via echocardiography.[5,7,9]

Management of pericardial effusion without hemodynamic compromise usually depends on the underlying etiology. Most cases (up to 60%) of pericardial effusion are associated with a known disease and the treatment is aimed at the underlying disease instead of the effusion itself. In idiopathic cases where there is concern for pericarditis, the patient should be treated as such with anti-inflammatory agents (see Acute Pericarditis, Treatment). In cases where there is no evidence of inflammation, aspirin, nonsteroidal anti-inflammatory drugs (NSAIDs), or colchicine has not shown to be effective.

Pericardial effusions contributing to hemodynamic compromise (ie, cardiac tamponade, see below) should undergo urgent drainage for therapeutic (and possibly diagnostic) reasons. However, hemodynamically stable patients with a pericardial effusion do not require routine drainage or immediate drainage. Diagnostic sampling may be indicated if there is no clear etiology or when the results may alter subsequent management. The choice between percutaneous pericardiocentesis and surgical drainage depends on individual experience and specific clinical indications. Pericardiocentesis is the most common method and can be performed with echocardiographic or fluoroscopic guidance. Surgical drainage may be preferred for recurrent or loculated effusions or in cases where pericardial biopsy is needed for diagnosis.

Following pericardiocentesis, pericardial catheter is typically left in place for 24 to 48 hours or until the volume of drainage is less than 25 mL/day. Careful follow-up over days to weeks is important following pericardiocentesis to monitor for recurrence. For patients in whom pericardial fluid reaccumulates despite repeated pericardiocentesis, pericardiectomy can be considered.

Cardiac Tamponade

Cardiac tamponade is a life-threatening condition occurring when a pericardial effusion causes hemodynamic changes resulting in cardiac collapse. It is not necessarily dependent on the size of an effusion, as the rapidity of fluid accumulation also plays a role. If an effusion accumulates acutely, it can result in tamponade with only 200 cc of fluid. Conversely, a large effusion (>2 L) may result in no or minimal hemodynamic changes if it accumulates slowly, thereby allowing time for the pericardial sac to enlarge.

Under physiologic conditions, ventricular filling occurs with little interventricular dependence because of low pericardial pressures. Inspiration decreases pericardial pressure (because of reduced intrathoracic pressure) and increases system venous return to the right atrium (**Figure 15.3**). However, the decrease in intrathoracic pressure also causes decreased pulmonary venous pressure, resulting in a slight decrease in the

NORMAL PATIENT

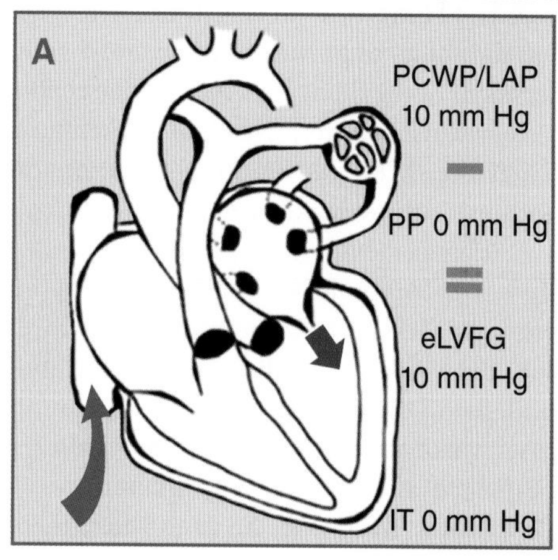

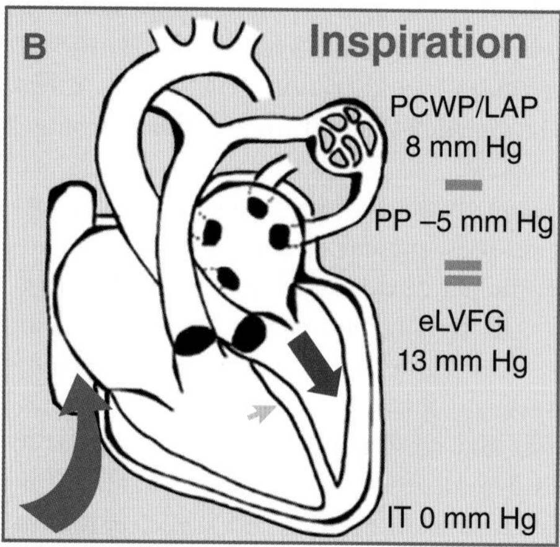

CARDIAC TAMPONADE

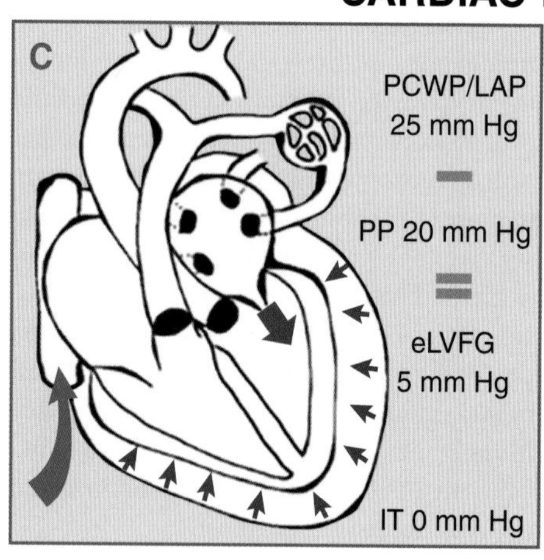

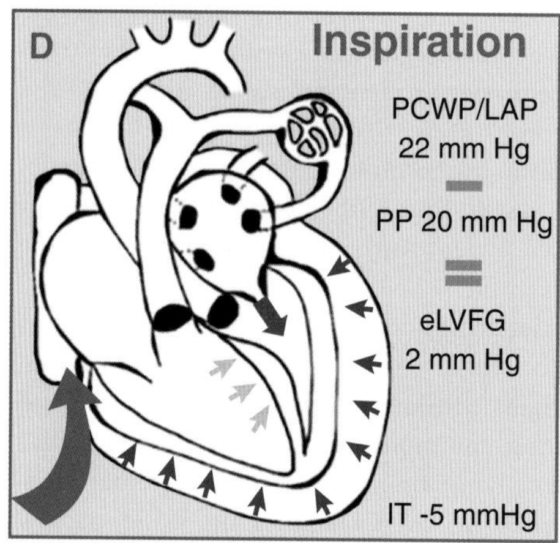

FIGURE 15.3 Respiratory variation in left ventricular filling. Effective left ventricular filling pressure (eLVFP) in normal patients at baseline (**A**) and with inspiration (**B**) and with cardiac tamponade at baseline (**C**) and with inspiration (**D**). The eLVFP is the difference between the pulmonary capillary wedge pressure (PCWP) or left atrial pressure (LAP) and the pericardial pressure (PP). In normal patients, the PP is low and equal to the intrathoracic pressure (IT). With inspiration, the PCWP/LAP decreases and the PP becomes negative, resulting in a net increase in the eLVFP (**B**). In patients with cardiac tamponade, both the PCWP/LAP are elevated because of the high PP (orange arrows), resulting in a lower eLVFP. With inspiration, there is increased venous return to the right side (blue arrow) and a drop in PCWP/LAP (which lies external to the pericardium) relative to the PP, thus decreasing the eLVFP (D). The LV is consequently restrained both by pressure externally from the pericardium (orange arrows) and internally from interventricular interaction (green arrows). (Adapted from Vakamudi S, Ho N, Cremer PC. Pericardial effusions: causes, diagnosis, and management. *Prog Cardiovasc Dis*. 2017;59(4):380-388. Copyright © 2017 Elsevier. With permission.)

left ventricular (LV) preload and filling pressures. This in turn causes a slight decrease in LV stroke volume and systolic blood pressure (<10 mm Hg). In tamponade there is a substantial increase in pericardial pressure, which is directly transmitted to the cardiac chambers resulting in equalization of right ventricular (RV) and LV diastolic pressures. Therefore, during inspiration, the normal physiologic changes (such as a decrease in systolic blood pressure) are magnified resulting in substantial decreases in LV stroke volume. Furthermore, as the RV volume increases in inspiration, the interventricular septum bulges toward the left ventricle. This phenomenon is exaggerated in tamponade, further reducing LV stroke volume.[7,10]

Clinical features of a patient in tamponade include tachycardia, hypotension, muffled heart sounds, pulsus paradoxus, and increased jugular venous pressure. Electrocardiographic (ECG) signs of tamponade can include decreased QRS voltage with electrical alternans. These clinical features correlate with the hemodynamic changes. For example, the pulsus paradoxus results from the exaggerated decrease (>10 mmHg) of systolic blood pressure during inspiration, with the magnitude of the decrease correlating with the intrapericardial pressure.[5,10]

Echocardiography is the most useful diagnostic tool in a patient with suspicion for clinical tamponade. Echocardiogram can identify the size of the effusion, location, and assess for hemodynamic effects. Echocardiographic features of tamponade include: swinging or rocking of the heart within the pericardium, right atrial late diastolic collapse, RV early diastolic collapse, exaggerated respiratory variation with tricuspid and mitral inflow on Doppler, and abnormal ventricular septal motion.[5,6,10]

The hemodynamic effects of tamponade are reversed by decreasing the pericardial pressure by draining the fluid via pericardiocentesis. Elective pericardiocentesis can be done with echocardiographic or fluoroscopic guidance. In an emergency, pericardiocentesis can be accomplished via a subxiphoid approach without imaging guidance. Pericardial fluid can also be drained surgically via a pericardial window or pericardiectomy. Surgical drainage is usually reserved for effusions that are more likely to reaccumulate, such as malignant effusions or in cases with localized effusions that are difficult to drain percutaneously. Following drainage of the effusion in tamponade, patients should have continuous telemetry monitoring and frequent vital sign measures for at least 48 hours. Echocardiogram should be done prior to hospital discharge to assess for any reaccumulation of fluid. Furthermore, follow-up echocardiograms should be considered within 1 to 2 weeks following discharge and again at 6 to 12 months to evaluate for recurrence or diagnose early constriction.

ACUTE PERICARDITIS

Pathogenesis and Epidemiology

Pericarditis is an inflammatory condition of the pericardium that can occur with or without an effusion. It can occur in isolation or because of systemic inflammatory conditions such as rheumatologic, metabolic, or secondary to cardiac injury. Acute pericarditis is the most common condition related to the pericardium. It accounts for ~5% of emergency room visits for nonischemic chest pain and has been reported in ~0.1% of admitted patients. The incidence of pericarditis is not completely known because of the lack of a gold standard way to diagnose pericarditis.[11,12]

The average age of patients with pericarditis is 40 to 60 years, with men having a twofold increased incidence compared to women. There are many different etiologies for pericarditis and the causes can be broadly divided into three categories: (1) infectious; (2) noninfectious; and (3) immune mediated.[6]

In general, pericardial inflammation occurs with thickening of parietal pericardium, causing edema with or without an exudative effusion and an increase in friction between the two layers.[4] A small pericardial effusion is present in ~60% of cases of pericarditis as seen on echocardiography, and approximately 15% of cases also have epicardial involvement as characterized by elevation in cardiac biomarkers.[6,12]

History and Physical

Patients with acute pericarditis usually present with sharp, severe chest pain that is generally substernal or retrosternal and may radiate to the neck and shoulders. The pain is pleuritic in nature and, therefore, worse with inspiration and lying down. Because of phrenic nerve involvement, the pain can also be located posteriorly along the trapezius ridge.[3,12] Other associated symptoms of fatigue, malaise, cough, and rhinorrhea can also be present.

The pericardial friction rub is pathognomonic for pericarditis, with the prevalence varying widely among studies and is anywhere between 35% and 85%.[13] The friction rub is thought to occur because of friction between the inflamed parietal and visceral pericardium, resulting in a high-pitched "scratchy" sound. The friction rub is best heard with the patient leaning forward, at the end of expiration, with the diaphragm of the stethoscope placed over the left sternal border. The pericardial friction is heard throughout the respiratory cycle with varying intensity unlike a pleural rub that is only heard in inspiration. The pericardial friction rub is also dynamic and therefore can vary in intensity throughout the day.[6,11,12] The classic pericardial rub usually consists of three components—atrial systole, ventricular systole, and ventricular filling. Only half of all patients with a pericardial rub have all three components, with one-third having two components and the remainder a single component.

ECG analysis is a critical part of assessing any patient with suspected pericarditis. The classic findings include diffuse ST elevation with PR segment depression and ST depression in aVR. The ST elevation generally occurs secondary to an injury current from epicardial inflammation because the pericardium is technically not innervated. However, the classic ECG changes may not be present at the time of diagnosis as the ECG findings evolve over time. The ECG changes associated with pericarditis occur in four stages that may progress over a few to 10 days. The four stages include: (1) Stage 1 (hours to days)—diffuse concave ST segment elevation with associated PR segment depression; (2) Stage 2 (within the first week)—normalization of ST and PR segments; (3) Stage 3—ST segments are isoelectric with diffuse T-wave inversion; (4) Stage 4—normalization of ECG (**Figure 15.4**).[4,6,11,12] The ST segment elevation does not usually exceed 5 mm and there are no reciprocal changes, no QRS widening or q waves, which helps to distinguish it from acute myocardial infarction.

Diagnosis

Patients with suspected pericarditis should have routine lab work including complete blood count, comprehensive metabolic panel, inflammatory markers such as erythrocyte sedimentation rate and C-reactive protein (CRP), and cardiac biomarkers.

A mild nonspecific leukocytosis and elevation of the inflammatory markers is common and can help support the diagnosis. These markers can be useful to monitor clinical course and response to treatment. If there is epicardial involvement, cardiac biomarkers such as troponin will also be elevated.

Every patient with suspected pericarditis should get a routine echocardiogram. An echocardiogram can help evaluate for pericardial fluid, pericardial thickening, assess ventricular function, and provide hemodynamic assessment. It can also help

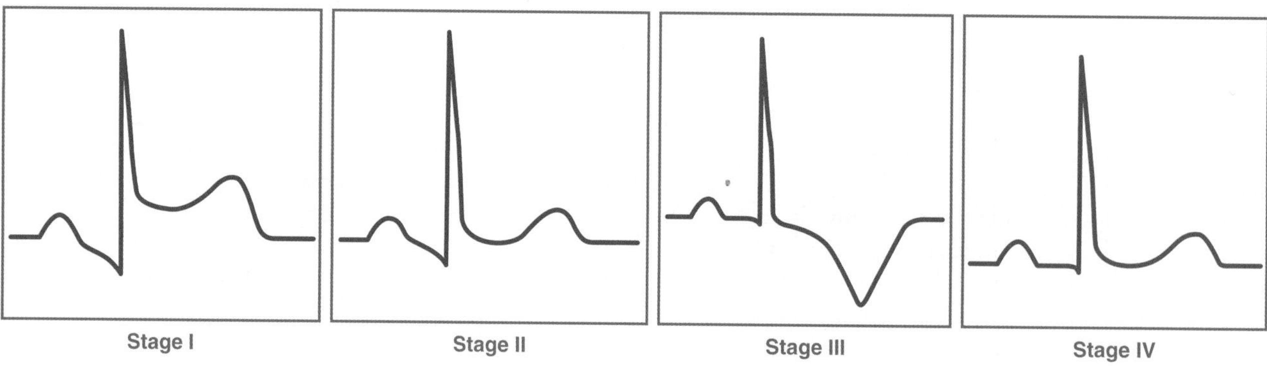

FIGURE 15.4 Classical four stages of electrocardiographic (ECG) evolution in acute pericarditis. Stage I: diffuse ST elevation with PR depression, Stage II: normalization of ST and PR segments, Stage III: diffuse deep T-wave inversions, Stage IV: normalization of the ECG. (Reprinted by permission from Springer: Imazio M. Diagnosis: History, Physical Examination and ECG. In: Imazio M., ed. *Myopericardial Diseases*. Cham: Springer; 2016:15-26. Copyright © 2016 Springer International Publishing Switzerland.)

distinguish the acute presentation from myocardial ischemia. In certain cases, additional imaging with CT and MRI will also be needed.

Additional advanced imaging is particularly important in cases that are atypical with uncertain diagnosis and also to help determine the etiology. An MRI can show late gadolinium enhancement, supporting a diagnosis of myopericarditis.

Given all these features, the clinical diagnosis can be made with two of the following criteria: (1) typical sharp, pleuritic chest pain; (2) pericardial friction rub—a harsh scratchy sound heard with the diaphragm of the stethoscope; (3) ECG changes—widespread ST elevation with PR segment depression; and (4) new or worsening pericardial effusion. Elevated biomarkers and pericardial inflammation seen on CT or MRI is considered additional supportive information.

Management of Pericarditis

Most cases of pericarditis may be managed in the outpatient setting. However, persons with any of the high-risk features associated with worse outcomes should be admitted to the hospital. These high-risk features include: fever greater than 38 °C, subacute onset, large pericardial effusion (>20 mm) or tamponade, and failure to respond within 7 days of initiation of anti-inflammatory medications. Other concerning findings include myocardial involvement, trauma, being on oral anticoagulation, and immunosuppression (**Algorithm 15.1**). Accordingly, the European Society of Cardiology (ESC) has proposed triage based on these clinical features.

Based on clinical findings and presentation, there should be an attempt to identify the specific etiology. For young women, rheumatologic disorders such as systemic lupus erythematosus should be considered and additional evaluation with antinuclear antibodies should be pursued. Bacterial causes should be ruled out in patients with recent bacteremia, instrumentation, or based on geographic location (tuberculosis in endemic places). If bacterial infection is suspected, pericardial fluid should be obtained for analysis, as purulent pericarditis is a potentially life-threatening condition that requires specific antimicrobial treatment according to the causative etiologic agent along with pericardial drainage. When no underlying cause can be identified for pericarditis, it is presumed to be viral and/or idiopathic in origin. Routine viral testing is not done because of its low diagnostic yield.

Medical Therapy

Treatment for pericarditis is based on the underlying etiology.[14] For viral or idiopathic or inflammatory pericarditis, the general approach is medical therapy with NSAIDs, primarily ibuprofen or aspirin and colchicine. Steroids are not generally recommended unless there is a specific rheumatologic indication, pregnancy, or contraindication to aspirin or NSAID. Corticosteroids have been shown to cause recurrences with pericarditis and, therefore, should only be used as second line or when there are no other options.

Ibuprofen (600-800 mg every 8 hours) or high-dose aspirin (750-1000 mg every 8 hours) should be used until symptom resolution and reduction in inflammatory markers and then should be tapered. Low-dose colchicine (0.5 mg twice daily for patients weighing >70 kg or 0.5 mg once daily for patients weighing ≤70 kg) is used to prevent recurrence and relapses and can be used initially in combination with NSAIDs or added later if the individual is not responding to NSAIDs or aspirin. Colchicine is continued for at least 3 months and then slowly tapered. If steroids are used as an alternative agent, a low dose should be administered (prednisone, 0.2-0.5 mg/kg/day), continued until symptom resolution and normalization of inflammatory markers, and then tapered very slowly over months.[5,11,12] Other immunosuppressive medications such as azathioprine, intravenous immunoglobulin, or biologics may be considered in specific cases.[11]

Other nonpharmacologic interventions include limitation of activity to only generalized day-day sedentary work until symptoms improve and inflammatory markers are negative. Competitive athletes should not participate in competitive sports for at least 3 months following symptom resolution.

Only 15%-30% of cases of acute idiopathic pericarditis have recurrence and the risk of major complication is low, including developing constrictive pericarditis (CP).

Follow-Up Patient Care

Patients should be evaluated closely throughout treatment to assess response. In patients not responding to aspirin or

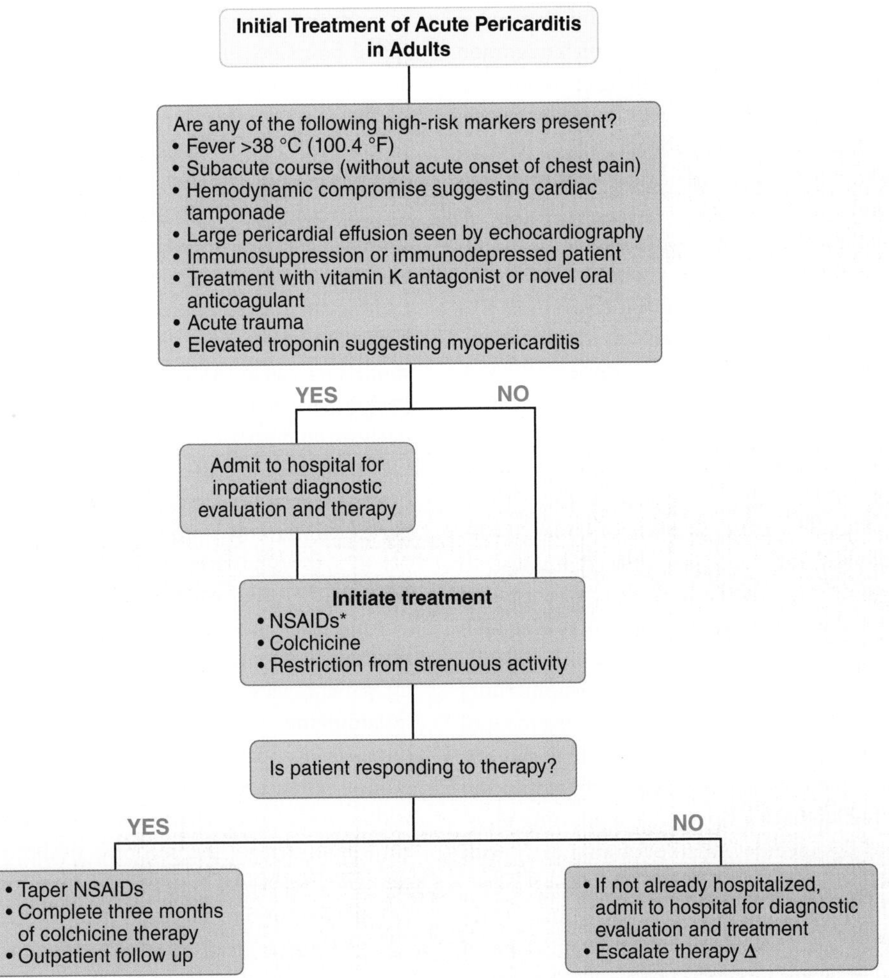

ALGORITHM 15.1 Initial treatment of acute pericarditis in adults.
*NSAIDs are the preferred antiinflammatory for nearly all patients with acute idiopathic or viral pericarditis. Glucocorticoids should be used for initial treatment of acute pericarditis only in patients with contraindications to NSAIDs or for specific indications (i.e., systemic inflammatory diseases, pregnancy, renal failure),and should be used at the lowest effective dose. (Reproduced with permission from Imazio M. *Acute pericarditis: Treatment and prognosis.* In: UpToDate, Post TW (Ed), UpToDate, Waltham, MA. (Accessed on Aug 10, 2020.) Copyright © 2020 UpToDate, Inc. For more information visit www.uptodate.com.)

colchicine, corticosteroids may be used. If corticosteroids are used, a slow taper should be completed after symptom resolution. Serum CRP can be followed to guide treatment length and assess treatment response.

CONSTRICTIVE PERICARDITIS

Pathophysiology and Etiology

CP is a consequence of a thick and inelastic pericardium that can present as severe diastolic dysfunction. Long-standing pericardial inflammation can lead to pericardial scarring from thickening, fibrosis, and calcification. The scarred or inflamed pericardium is inelastic, limiting distention of the cardiac chambers resulting in impaired diastolic filling.[6,15] The timing of initial pericardial insult to the development of constriction varies.

CP can occur after any pericardial disease, with the common etiologies varying widely depending on geography. In developed countries, idiopathic or postoperative and postradiation are the most common causes. Infectious etiologies are more frequent in the developing world. Tuberculosis should be considered as a cause in endemic areas and in patients with HIV. The classic form of CP is chronic constructive, but other forms such as acute-subacute, transient, and effusive-constrictive also exist.[4,6,15] CP can be primary or secondary based on whether there is an underlying superimposed myocardial process.[16]

The hallmark of CP is enhanced ventricular dependence and dissociation of intrathoracic and intracardiac pressures. The inelastic pericardium leads to equalization of all cardiac pressures at the end of diastole and also isolates the cardiac chambers from the negative intrathoracic pressures, similar to the physiology previously described for cardiac tamponade.[16,17] Further hemodynamic changes can occur if there is myocardial involvement, which is overall rare.[6,16]

History and Physical: Constrictive Pericarditis

Patients with CP predominantly present with right-sided heart failure symptoms but can also have low-output symptoms and at times pulmonary congestion. Patients will usually complain of peripheral edema, abdominal distention, fatigue, nausea, and shortness of breath. They can also get hepatic congestion causing liver dysfunction and develop pleural effusions and recurrent ascites requiring paracentesis. Because of the gastrointestinal and pulmonary symptoms, patients may be referred to these providers and, therefore, a high degree of suspicion is required.[6,15,16]

The physical examination is an important step in the diagnosis of constriction and can provide important clues. The classic physical examination findings include increase or lack of decrease in central venous pressure during inspiration, which is referred to as Kussmaul sign. This occurs because of the lack of association of the intrathoracic and intracardiac pressures. Observation of the jugular venous pressures will reveal a steep X and Y descent, which occurs because of limited distention of the cardiac chambers in diastole.[15,16] Palpation of the pericardium should reveal a normal apical impulse in patients with primary constriction but can reveal a displaced impulse in secondary constriction. Furthermore, if there is a parasternal heave—suggestive RV dilation or hypertrophy—the diagnosis of constriction should be questioned. The classic and typically end-stage finding of CP is the pericardial knock—sometimes mistaken as a loud S3—that is thought to occur because of rapid cessation of RV filling in diastole.[15,16] This is a high-pitched sound, heard best via the diaphragm of the stethoscope over the apex and/or the left sternal border. Other supporting physical examination findings include pulsatile hepatomegaly with or without ascites and jaundice.

ECG analysis in constriction can reveal low-voltage QRS with nonspecific ST-T changes. Because of the presence of pericardial calcification, atrioventricular block and atrial fibrillation are common manifestations as a result of pericardial irritation.

Diagnostic Laboratory Tests and Imaging: Constrictive Pericarditis

There are no specific diagnostic labs, but abnormal liver function tests can be seen because of the hepatic congestion and cardiac cirrhosis. Brain natriuretic peptide levels can also be elevated but less so than with restrictive cardiomyopathy (RCM). Pericardial calcifications may be present in ~20%-25% of patients and can be visualized on the lateral projection of a chest x-ray. Pericardial thickening can be diagnosed via transthoracic echocardiography (TTE), but CT and MRI provide better resolution and measurement. Of note, CP can be present without pericardial thickening in ~20% of cases.[17]

TTE is the mainstay to diagnose constriction and should be done with Doppler imaging during inspiratory flow measurements. It can provide noninvasive hemodynamic measurements of constrictive physiology and also help rule out mimics of CP. A full detailed examination for the diagnosis of constriction should include careful examination of the ventricular septum, pulse-wave Doppler of the mitral and tricuspid inflows, tissue Doppler of the mitral annulus, assessment of the inferior vena cava, and pulse-wave Doppler of the hepatic veins.[16]

Abnormal ventricular septal motion is characterized by a septal bounce visualized in early diastole. Another finding of abnormal ventricular septal motion is the geometrical change of the septum with the respiratory cycle. In inspiration, the septum will bow toward the left ventricle and in expiration it will be seen bowing to the right ventricle.

Assessment of mitral and tricuspid inflow via pulse-wave Doppler is useful to demonstrate dissociation of intrathoracic and intracardiac pressures. If the initial echocardiogram is technically limited or yields indeterminate findings, suspected CP should be further evaluated by CT scan or MRI. Both modalities can provide additional details about the extent of pericardial calcification and thickening, which may impact the decision and surgical planning for possible pericardiectomy. CT is superior to MRI in detecting calcification, but MRI can better identify pericardial inflammation and adherence of the pericardium to myocardium.

Management: Constrictive Pericarditis

For most patients with CP, surgical pericardiectomy is the definitive treatment. A trial of medical therapy can be considered for patients with transient CP or CP associated with elevated inflammatory markers, recent surgery, or pericardial trauma. Furthermore, patients with cardiac MRI showing late gadolinium enhancement have been shown to have better success with a trial of anti-inflammatory medications. Treatment with anti-inflammatory medications, similar to that of acute pericarditis with NSAIDs or corticosteroid and colchicine, is recommended for 8 to 12 weeks before reassessing.

Definitive treatment with surgery should be the next step if anti-inflammatory medications do not provide resolution of constrictive physiology (Table 15.3). Pericardiectomy can potentially be curative if done in a timely manner.[18] Radiation-related CP has a poor prognosis overall compared to idiopathic cases, in part because myocardial involvement

TABLE 15.3 Indications and Contraindications for Pericardiectomy in Constrictive Pericarditis

Clinical features supporting referral for pericardiectomy:
- Presence of increasing JVP
- Need for diuretics
- Evidence of hepatic dysfunction
- Reduced exercise tolerance

Contraindications for pericardiectomy
- Very early constriction (asymptomatic)
- Transient constriction
- Extensive myocardial fibrosis and/or atrophy on CT/MRI
- Severe, advanced symptoms (NYHA Class IV).

CT, computed tomography; JVP, jugular venous pressure; MRI, magnetic resonance imaging; NYHA, New York Heart Association.
Adapted with data from Seferović PM, Ristić AD, Maksimović R, et al. Pericardial syndromes: an update after the ESC guidelines 2004. *Heart Fail Rev.* 2013;18(3):255-266.

is usually also present. Two- and 5-year mortality following pericardiectomy for all patients has been shown to be approximately 78% and 57%, respectively, with symptomatic improvement noted in the majority of patients. Furthermore, at times (~20%) echocardiographic features of CP persist after pericardiectomy despite a decrease in RV filling pressures.[18]

EFFUSIVE-CONSTRICTIVE PERICARDITIS

Pathophysiology and Epidemiology

Effusive-constrictive pericarditis is a phenomenon in which there is a pericardial effusion with features of constrictive physiology. Effusive-constrictive pericarditis is considered a clinical spectrum between true effusive tamponade and chronic CP.[20] Patients with effusive-constrictive physiology have different right atrial pressure wave contours compared to tamponade or CP.[20] The development of an effusion in patients with an already scarred and inelastic pericardium not only can cause constriction of the cardiac chambers but also exerts increased pressure from the pericardial effusion, resulting in tamponade physiology.

Classically, effusive-constrictive pericarditis is diagnosed in patients who present with initial tamponade physiology but continue to have elevated intracardiac pressures post-pericardiocentesis. It is defined as a failure of the right atrial pressure to decrease by at least 50% or below 10 mm Hg when the intrapericardial pressure is reduced to 0 mm Hg.

The prevalence of effusive-constrictive pericarditis in patients with pericarditis is ~1%-2%. In patients with chronic effusion, it may be diagnosed in 3.6% of patients.[20,21] The most common causes of effusive-constrictive pericarditis are idiopathic (58%) and tuberculosis (38%), with postradiation and postsurgery occasionally identified.[19]

Clinical Presentation

The clinical presentation is generally similar to pericardial effusion and CP, with most patients complaining of shortness of breath, lower extremity edema, and chest discomfort. Kussmaul sign and pulsus paradoxus can both be present, but the classic jugular venous X and Y descent of constrictive physiology will not be identified initially.

Diagnosis and Management of Effusive-Constrictive Pericarditis

Invasive hemodynamic assessment is usually required to confirm the diagnosis of effusive-constrictive pericarditis. Invasive hemodynamic measurements provide a real-time assessment of increased intracardiac pressures causing compression even in the setting of decreased intrapleural pressure post-pericardiocentesis. Noninvasive modalities such as echocardiogram and MRI/CT can also provide useful clues. The epicardial layer of the pericardium is responsible for the constrictive component of the process and does not always appear thickened on echocardiography. Cardiac MRI, in this case, can show visceral pericardial thickening and can provide real-time hemodynamics showing ventricular interdependence. Cardiac MRI can also provide information on myocardial involvement.[5,20] Treatment for effusive-constrictive pericarditis is tailored to the underlying etiology. It usually requires visceral pericardiectomy, which can be very challenging and should be done at tertiary centers.[5,19,20]

HEMODYNAMIC ASSESSMENT OF CONSTRICTIVE PERICARDITIS, RESTRICTIVE CARDIOMYOPATHY, AND TAMPONADE

CP is a disease of the pericardium secondary to thickening and scarring of the sac, resulting in impaired cardiac filling during late diastole, whereas RCM occurs because of intrinsic myocardial dysfunction causing restriction of filling and impaired ventricular diastolic filling. CP and RCM can appear similar and cause confusion for clinicians (**Table 15.4**). Because CP can be treated with surgery, whereas RCM has no definitive treatment except for cardiac transplantation, differentiating these entities has important therapeutic consequences.

In RCM, ventricular pressure rises significantly even with a small increase in volume because of the stiff myocardium. The impaired diastolic filling occurs in both early and late diastole, whereas in CP diastolic filling is impaired mainly in late diastole.[21] In CP, there is ventricular interdependence and changes in intrathoracic pressures are not transmitted to the cardiac chambers, whereas in RCM there is no ventricular

TABLE 15.4 Constrictive Pericarditis versus Restrictive Cardiomyopathy

	Constrictive Pericarditis	Restrictive Cardiomyopathy
Mechanism of disease	Inelastic pericardium impairs filling	Impaired ventricular diastolic filling impairs filling
Physiologic response	Changes in intrathoracic pressure not transmitted to cardiac chambers (space obliteration)	Normal respiratory variations and they are normally transmitted to cardiac chambers
Ventricular interaction	Enhanced	Unchanged
Intrinsic myocardial function	Normal	Abnormal

Adapted with data from Mookadam F, Jiamsripong P, Raslan SF, et al. Constrictive pericarditis and restrictive cardiomyopathy in the modern era. *Future Cardiol.* 2011;7(4):471-483.

interdependence and an association between intrathoracic and intracardiac pressures is present.[20]

CP and RCM should both be considered in patients with symptoms of diastolic heart failure. CP is more likely to be present in patients with a history of pericarditis, whereas RCM is more likely in patients suspected to have infiltrative cardiomyopathy. Patients with CP or RCM will —both have distended neck veins, rapid X and Y descent, and prominent a-wave in the jugular venous pulse because of ventricular non-compliance. On physical examination, RCM patients can have prominent mitral and tricuspid valve regurgitation murmurs and a prominent P2, whereas these features are not typically present in CP.

Noninvasive imaging modalities—mainly echocardiography—can help distinguish between CP and RCM (**Table 15.5**). In RCM, echocardiography will show normal sized ventricles with marked atrial dilation. Both CP and RCM have similar Doppler mitral inflow velocities showing a small or absent a-wave and a short rapid early diastolic deceleration in the form of an E-wave. In order to distinguish between CP and RCM, the mitral and tricuspid valve inflows need to be measured during inspiration and expiration. In CP because there is ventricular interdependence, during inspiration when the RV systolic pressure increases, the LV systolic pressure decreases. The dissociation of the intrathoracic and intracardiac pressures in patients with CP leads to a lower LV preload because of decrease in forward flow during inspiration.[21] With CP, mitral inflow Doppler assessment during the first beat of inspiration will show a decrease in initial velocity of the transmitral flow (E-wave) followed by a greater than 25% increase in the initial E-velocity at expiration. Reciprocal changes occur in the RV when measuring the inflow Doppler across the tricuspid valve, with the E-wave increasing during inspiration by greater than 40% and decreasing during expiration. In RCM there is no change in inflow variation within the respiratory cycle. Furthermore, analysis of hepatic vein flow velocity shows that there is significant diastolic flow reversal in both CP and RCM, but in CP this occurs during expiration, whereas in RCM it occurs during inspiration.[20] Mitral annular velocities also vary in CP and RCM, with the peak early diastolic mitral annular velocity being reduced in RCM but normal to elevated in CP patients.

Invasive hemodynamic measurement in the cardiac catheterization also distinguishes CP from RCM. The classic invasive hemodynamic finding of CP includes the dip and plateau (or square root) phenomenon on the ventricular pressure tracing at end diastole. Ventricular filling during early diastole from the atria to the ventricles is rapid and once the pericardial constraining limit is reached, the diastolic filling comes to a halt producing the classic dip and plateau (or square root) pressure tracing (**Figure 15.5**). During cardiac catheterization, both CP and RCM have elevated filling pressures, but in CP the LV and RV filling pressure are almost equal (ie, rarely differ by more than 3-5 mm Hg), whereas in RCM the LV diastolic pressure is higher than the RV. Extremely high diastolic pressures and severe pulmonary hypertension are common in RCM, but not in CP. The systolic area index, which is defined as the ratio of the RV to LV pressure-time area during inspiration and expiration and is calculated using the area under the ventricular pressure curves, of greater than 1.1 is suggestive of CP with a high sensitivity and specificity.[22]

Cardiac tamponade on the other hand occurs because of increased intrapericardial pressure that impedes atrial relaxation and therefore ventricular filling. The concept of cardiac transmural pressure becomes important in differentiating cardiac tamponade from CP and RCM. Cardiac transmural pressure is the pressure difference between the intracardiac and pericardial pressures and is the true cardiac filling pressure. As the ventricles attempt to fill against higher intrapericardial pressure

TABLE 15.5 Echocardiographic Parameters of Constrictive Pericarditis and Restrictive Cardiomyopathy

Septal bounce	Yes	No
MV inflow respiratory variation	≥25%	None
TV inflow respiratory variation	>40%	None
MVDT	≤160 ms	<160 ms
Hepatic vein reversal	Diastolic reversal with expiration	None
IVRT	Decrease with expiration Increase with inspiration	Unchanged
TR duration	Increased	Normal
Mitral annulus velocity (i.e., early diastolic Doppler tissue velocity e' at mitral annulus)	Normal or increased (≥8 cm/second)	Normal or decreased (<8 cm/second)
Strain analysis (absolute global longitudinal strain)	>16%	≤10%

IVRT, isovolumic relaxation time; MV, mitral valve; MVDT, mitral valve deceleration time; TR, tricuspid regurgitation; TV, tricuspid valve.

Adapted with data from Mookadam F, Jiamsripong P, Raslan SF, et al. Constrictive pericarditis and restrictive cardiomyopathy in the modern era. *Future Cardiol.* 2011;7(4):471-483.

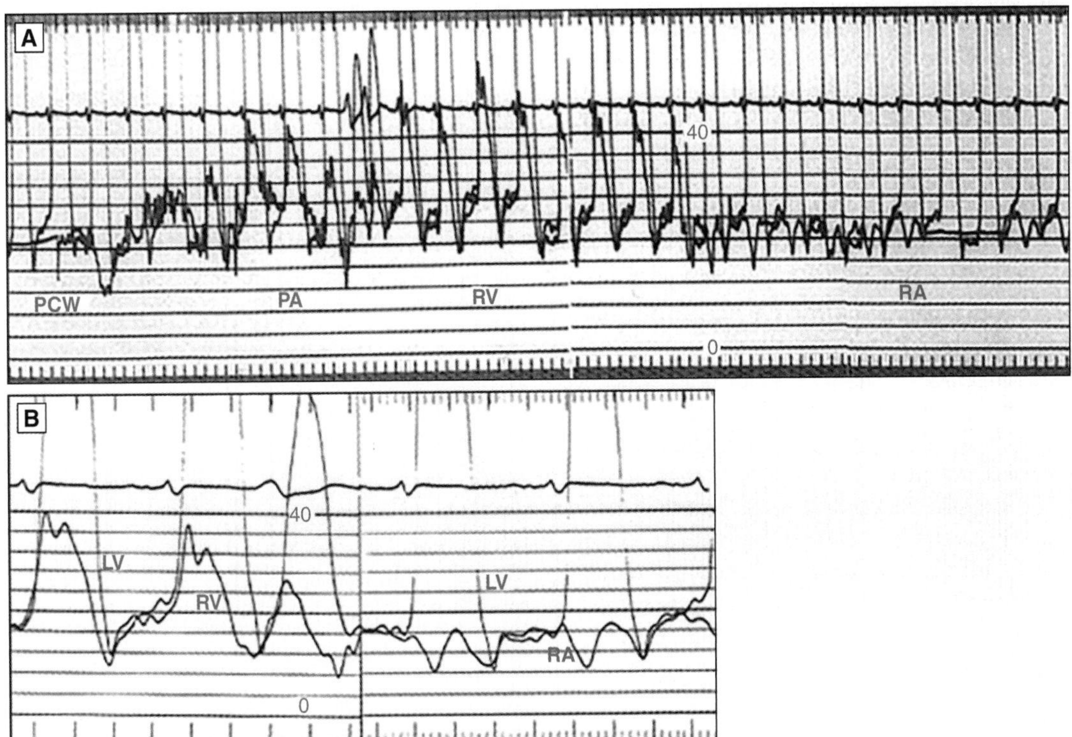

FIGURE 15.5 Dip and plateau in constrictive pericarditis. Hemodynamic record of a patient with surgically proven constrictive pericarditis. (**A**) Slow-paper-speed recording of high-gain left ventricular (LV) pressure and simultaneous right heart pullback from pulmonary capillary wedge (PCW) to pulmonary artery (PA), right ventricle (RV), and right atrium (RA). (**B**) Fast-paper-speed recording of LV and simultaneous RV and RA pressure tracings. Note the increased and equal atrial and diastolic pressures, the prominent X and Y descents on the RA tracing, and the dip and plateau on the RV and LV tracings during longer diastoles. (Reprinted from Hoit BD. *Pericardial disease and pericardial heart disease.* In: O'Rourke RA, ed. Stein's Internal Medicine. 5th ed. St. Louis: Mosby-Year Book; 1998. Copyright © 1998 Elsevier. With permission.)

(because of the effusion), the left and right atrial pressures increase, causing an effective decrease in transmural pressure. The rapid increase in pericardial pressure during early diastole exceeds the atrial pressure, which results in ventricular diastolic expansion in a limited area (because of a tight pericardium) and therefore impedes atrial emptying. When the right atrium is exposed to the increased pericardial pressure, it collapses in late diastole and isovolumetric systole, further compromising the hemodynamic effects.[21]

Cardiac catheterization findings during tamponade include elevated and equalization of RV and LV pressures. The left atrial pressure or pulmonary capillary wedge pressure (PCWP) is also elevated as is the intrapericardial pressure that causes a decrease in the transmural pressure. During inspiration, there is increased venous return to the right side causing increased right atrial pressures and a decrease of the left atrial pressure or PCWP relative to the pericardial pressure, therefore causing a further decrease in the transmural pressure. However, LV diastolic pressure remains elevated because of a leftward shift of the interventricular septum, which occurs to accommodate the increased venous return. The leftward shift of the septum results in a decreased LV filling pressure gradient and therefore leads to a lower effective stroke volume.[7,10,23]

KEY POINTS

- ✔ The pericardium consists of two layers, a serous inner membrane (visceral pericardium) and fibrous outer sac (parietal pericardium), that surround the heart. The space between the parietal and visceral pericardium contains a small amount of fluid and is called the pericardial cavity.
- ✔ The pericardium functions to prevent displacement of the heart within the pericardium, maintain pressure differences within cardiac chambers, and serve as a barrier to infection.
- ✔ Pericardial effusion occurs from excess fluid accumulation in the pericardial cavity and can occur because of a variety of causes. Most patients with pericardial effusions are asymptomatic and treatment should be directed at the underlying cause.
- ✔ Cardiac tamponade is a life-threatening condition that occurs when a pericardial effusion causes hemodynamic collapse. Treatment of cardiac tamponade requires emergent drainage of the pericardial fluid by pericardiocentesis.
- ✔ Acute pericarditis is an inflammatory condition of the pericardium that can occur in isolation or because of

other systemic inflammatory conditions. Treatment is directed at the underlying etiology. For idiopathic cases, medical therapy with NSAIDs is the first-line treatment.

- ✔ CP results from inelastic pericardium causing impaired diastolic filling, with the hallmark hemodynamic change being ventricular dependence and equalization of all cardiac pressures at end diastole. Surgical pericardiectomy is the definitive treatment for CP.
- ✔ Effusive-constrictive pericarditis occurs when there is a pericardial effusion with features of constrictive physiology. It is diagnosed in patients who present with initial tamponade physiology that continue to have elevated intracardiac pressures despite pericardial fluid drainage. Treatment is focused on the underlying etiology and may require visceral pericardiectomy.
- ✔ CP is a disease of the pericardium resulting in impaired cardiac filling in late diastole, whereas RCM occurs because of intrinsic myocardial dysfunction causing impaired filling. Echocardiography and invasive hemodynamic measurements can help distinguish between the two.

REFERENCES

1. Holt JP. The normal pericardium. *Am J Cardiol.* 1970;26(5):455-465.
2. Hoit BD. Pathophysiology of the pericardium. *Prog Cardiovasc Dis.* 2017;59(4):341-348.
3. Shabetai R, Mangiardi L, Bhargava V, Ross J Jr, Higgins CB. The pericardium and cardiac function. *Prog Cardiovasc Dis.* 1979;22(2):107-134.
4. LeWinter MM, Kabban S. Pericardial disease. In: Mann D, Zipes D, Libby P, et al., eds. *Braunwald's Heart Disease: A Textbook of Cardiovascular Medicine.* 10th ed. ©Elsevier Inc.; 2018.
5. Adler Y, Charron P, Imazio M, et al. 2015 ESC Guidelines for the diagnosis and management of pericardial diseases: the Task Force for the Diagnosis and Management of Pericardial Diseases of the European Society of Cardiology (ESC) Endorsed by: The European Association for CardioThoracic Surgery (EACTS). *Eur Heart J.* 2015;36(42):2921-2964.
6. Seferović PM, Ristić AD, Maksimović R, et al. Pericardial syndromes: an update after the ESC guidelines 2004. *Heart Fail Rev.* 2013;18(3):255-266.
7. Vakamudi S, Ho N, Cremer PC. Pericardial effusions: causes, diagnosis, and management. *Prog Cardiovasc Dis.* 2017;59(4):380-388.
8. Ristić AD, Imazio M, Adler Y, et al. Triage strategy for urgent management of cardiac tamponade: a position statement of the European Society of Cardiology Working Group on Myocardial and Pericardial Diseases. *Eur Heart J.* 2014;35(34):2279-2284.
9. Imazio M, Mayosi BM, Brucato A, et al. Triage and management of pericardial effusion. *J Cardiovasc Med.* 2010;11(12):928-935.
10. Shabetai R, Oh JK. Pericardial effusion and compressive disorders of the heart: influence of new technology on unraveling its pathophysiology and hemodynamics. *Cardiol Clin.* 2017;35(4):467-479.
11. Imazio M, Gaita, F. Diagnosis and treatment of pericarditis. *Heart.* 2015;101(14):1159-1168.
12. Doctor NS, Shah AB, Coplan N, Kronzon I. Acute pericarditis. *Prog Cardiovasc Dis.* 2017;59(4):349-359.
13. Chahine J, Siddiqui WJ. Pericardial friction rub. In: *StatPearls.* StatPearls Publishing; 2020. Updated September 5, 2020. https://www.ncbi.nlm.nih.gov/books/NBK542284/
14. Chiabrando JG, Bonaventura A, Vecchié A, et al. Management of acute and recurrent pericarditis JACC state-of-the-art review. *J Am Coll Cardiol.* 2020;75:76-92.
15. Mookadam F, Jiamsripong P, Oh JK, Khandheria BK. Spectrum of pericardial disease: Part I and II. *Expert Rev Cardiovasc Ther.* 2009;7(9):1149-1157.
16. Miranda WR, Oh JK. Constrictive pericarditis: a practical clinical approach. *Prog Cardiovasc Dis.* 2017;59(4):369-379.
17. Talreja DR, Edwards WD, Danielson GK, et al. Constrictive pericarditis in 26 patients with histologically normal pericardial thickness. *Circulation.* 2003;108(15):1852-1857.
18. Kim KH, Miranda WR, Sinak, LJ, et al. Effusive-constrictive pericarditis after pericardiocentesis: incidence, associated findings, and natural history. *JACC Cardiovasc Imaging.* 2018;11(4):534-541.
19. Syed FF, Ntsekhe M, Mayosi, BM, Oh JK. Effusive-constrictive pericarditis. *Heart Fail Rev.* 2013;18(3):277-287.
20. Miranda WR, Oh JK. Effusive-constrictive pericarditis. *Cardiol Clin.* 2017;35(4):551-558.
21. Mookadam F, Jiamsripong P, Raslan SF, et al. Constrictive pericarditis and restrictive cardiomyopathy in the modern era. *Future Cardiol.* 2011;7(4):471-483.
22. Sorajja P. Invasive hemodynamics of constrictive pericarditis, restrictive cardiomyopathy, and cardiac tamponade. *Cardiol Clin.* 2011;29(2):191-199.
23. Spodick DH. Pericarditis, pericardial effusion, cardiac tamponade, and constriction. *Crit Care Clin.* 1989;5(3):455-476.

CHAPTER 16

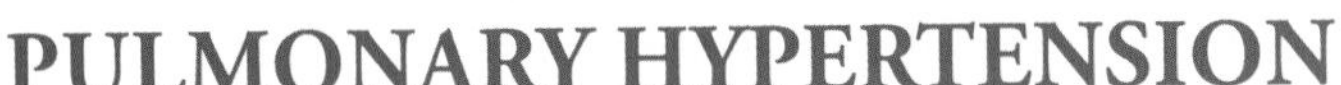

PULMONARY HYPERTENSION

Saurabh Rajpal, Jeremy Slivnick, William H. Marshall V, and Zachary Garrett

INTRODUCTION

Rapid growth in understanding the pathophysiology of pulmonary hypertension (PH) and introduction of new medications in the past few decades have improved the life and longevity of patients with PH previously considered untreatable. In the next few sections, the pathophysiology, classification, diagnosis, risk stratification, and management of PH will be discussed in light of these recent developments.

The classification system and definition of PH have changed over time as there has been increased recognition of outcomes and options for treatment through efforts by the National Institutes of Health and the World Society of Pulmonary Hypertension (WSPH). The first WSPH conference was held in 1973, and PH was defined as a mean pulmonary artery (PA) pressure of 25 mm Hg or more. In the sixth WSPH held in 2018, this definition was updated as a mean PA pressure greater than 20 mm Hg.[1]

Normal Growth and Development of Pulmonary Vasculature

The PAs start to develop in the fifth week of human development along with development of lung buds. The proximal sixth aortic arches sprout the future PAs, which grow toward the capillary plexus surrounding the lung buds. Several growth factors and vasoactive molecules regulate development of the pulmonary vasculature, including endothelin, nitric oxide, and prostacyclin.[2]

During fetal life, pulmonary vascular resistance (PVR) is increased, PA pressures are high, and blood flow through the pulmonary vasculature is minimal. Accordingly, blood flow is directed right-to-left through the foramen ovale and ductus arteriosus. In the newborn period when respiration begins and placental blood flow ceases, the PVR decreases, the ductus arteriosus closes, and the right-sided chamber pressures decrease, whereas left-sided pressures increase. By 2 to 3 months of life, the PVR is near normal.[2]

PATHOGENESIS

PA pressures may be elevated for numerous reasons: an increase in PVR, pulmonary blood flow, and/or pulmonary capillary wedge pressure (PCWP). Elevated PA pressure may eventually lead to progressive right ventricular (RV) dysfunction and failure.

The progressive increase in PVR is due to obstructive remodeling and loss of the pulmonary vascular bed, which occurs because of accumulation of PA smooth muscle cells, endothelial cells, pericytes, and fibroblasts. This leads to endothelial dysfunction with altered secretion of pulmonary vasodilator and vasoconstrictor molecules and mesenchymal smooth muscle hypertrophy. Bronchopulmonary vascular anastomoses occur with the bronchial vessels to bypass PA occlusive lesions, causing increased flow and further muscular hyperplasia in the distal vessels. Dysregulation of the innate immune system with increased expression of inflammatory cytokines and cell adhesion molecules also occurs.

Approximately 10% to 20% of patients with pulmonary arterial hypertension (PAH) have mutations in the gene encoding bone morphogenetic protein receptor type 2, and other genes have been identified. Molecular mechanisms such as transcription factor modulation, altered DNA methylation, and mitochondrial dysfunction are implicated, causing altered gene expression in the pulmonary vascular cells.[3]

Hypoxia, pain, and sympathetic activation can also increase PVR. Table 16.1 outlines vasoactive mediators that act on the pulmonary vasculature and affect PVR. The endothelin pathway mediates vasoconstriction, whereas nitric oxide and prostacyclin pathways mediate vasodilation.

The outcome of patients with PH depends on the function of the right ventricle. The right ventricle is thin walled, crescent shaped, and has smaller myocytes in a more circumferential arrangement as compared to the left ventricle. Under normal physiologic conditions, the right ventricle facilitates venous return into the low-impedance pulmonary vasculature, with one-fourth of the stroke work of the left ventricle. PH leads to RV pressure overload, causing RV hypertrophy, flattening of the interventricular septum, and eventually progressive RV dilation and dysfunction.[4]

TABLE 16.1 Factors Affecting Pulmonary Vasculature

	Vasodilation	Vasoconstriction
Molecular/hormonal mediators	Prostacyclin Nitric oxide Atrial natriuretic peptide Adrenomedullin Vasopressin	Endothelin-1 Angiotensin II Thromboxane A2 5-Hydroxytryptamine Catecholamines

DIAGNOSIS

Hemodynamic Definitions and Clinical Definitions

In the sixth WSPH, PH was defined by a mean PA pressure greater than 20 mm Hg. This decrease from the previous cutoff of 25 mm Hg or more is based on evidence demonstrating increased mortality and disease progression in patients with mean PA pressure of 21 to 24 mm Hg.[1] Precapillary PH is contrasted from postcapillary PH by the presence of elevated PVR and normal PCWP in the former (**Table 16.2**).[1] A subset of patients with precapillary PH are further categorized by a positive response to invasive vasoreactivity testing (eg, nitric oxide), defined as a decrease in mean PA pressure 10 mm Hg or more to 40 mm Hg or less[1,5] with vasodilator administration. As described further, these patients have more improved survival when treated with high-dose calcium channel blockers.[5]

The clinical PH groups and subgroups are displayed in **Table 16.3**.[1] There are five clinical groups of PH: group I is PAH, group II is PH because of left heart disease, group III is PH because of lung disease, group IV is PH because of PA obstruction, and group V is PH because of unclear or multifactorial mechanisms. In addition to including chronic thromboembolic PH, group IV was recently reclassified to also include PH secondary to other causes of pulmonary obstruction such as tumors, PA stenosis, and arteritis. Additionally, hemolytic anemias were added to group V because of increasing recognition of their causal relationship.

Group I: Pulmonary Arterial Hypertension

Group I PH or PAH is composed of precapillary PAH subtypes including idiopathic PAH, heritable PAH, connective tissue disease–associated PAH, human immunodeficiency virus (HIV), portopulmonary hypertension, and drug/toxin-associated PAH. Idiopathic PAH refers to sporadic PAH occurring in the absence of family history or risk factors. Heritable PAH generally occurs as a result of growth factor mutations, mostly with an autosomal dominant inheritance pattern.[3]

Drugs/toxins with definitive association with PAH include methamphetamine, anorexigens, and dasatinib.[6,7] Drugs with possible association with PAH include cocaine, St. John's wort, amphetamine, and certain Chinese herbs.[1] Of the connective tissue diseases, scleroderma has the strongest association with PAH and may be prevalent in as many as 10% of afflicted patients.[8] Unfortunately, these patients have poorer survival when compared with idiopathic PAH.[8] Portopulmonary hypertension is present in 2% to 6% of cirrhotic patients and is associated with high mortality when undergoing liver transplantation.[9] Congenital heart diseases that result in precapillary PH are also classified as group I; this generally occurs from chronic left-to-right shunts such as atrial or ventricular septal defects and patent ductus arteriosus.

Pulmonary veno-occlusive disease is also categorized as group I PH, but it has a different pathophysiology compared with other group I subtypes: it is characterized by vascular remodeling of the pulmonary venules and septal veins.[10] This leads to focal areas of pulmonary venous congestion in involved regions. It is most commonly associated with mutations in the EIF2AK4 gene,[10] but it may also be seen in association with connective tissue diseases such as scleroderma or with certain drug/toxin exposures. Pulmonary veno-occlusive disease should be suspected in patients with markedly reduced diffusing capacity of the lung for carbon monoxide (DLCO) or in those who develop pulmonary edema in response to vasoreactivity testing. Additionally, the presence of centrilobular ground glass opacities, increased septal line thickness, and mediastinal lymphadenopathy on high-resolution computerized tomography is also suggestive of the diagnosis. These patients have a poor prognosis and frequently develop pulmonary edema in response to pulmonary vasodilators.[10]

Group II: Pulmonary Hypertension as a Result of Left Heart Disease

PH because of left heart disease is the most common of the five clinical groups of PH and is associated with a high morbidity and mortality. Left heart disorders—including heart failure with reduced ejection fraction (HFrEF), heart failure with preserved ejection fraction (HFpEF), valvular heart disease, or congenital heart disease—increase left atrial filling pressures that are subsequently transmitted to the pulmonary circuit resulting in PH.[11] High-output heart failure, because of morbid obesity, arteriovenous shunts, or liver disease, is also associated with higher filling pressures and PA pressures.[12]

TABLE 16.2 Sixth WSPH Hemodynamic Definitions of Pulmonary Hypertension

Pulmonary Hypertension Etiology	Mean Pulmonary Artery Pressure (mm Hg)	Pulmonary Capillary Wedge Pressure (mm Hg)	Pulmonary Vascular Resistance (Wood Units)
Precapillary	>20	≤15	≥3
Postcapillary	>20	>15	<3
Combined	>20	>15	≥3

WSPH, World Society of Pulmonary Hypertension.

From Simonneau G, Montani D, Celermajer DS, et al. Haemodynamic definitions and updated clinical classification of pulmonary hypertension. *Eur Respir J*. 2019;53(1):1801913. doi: 10.1183/13993003.01913-2018. Reproduced with permission of the © ERS 2021.

TABLE 16.3 Sixth WSPH Clinical Classifications of Pulmonary Hypertension

PH Groups	Subgroups
Group I: PAH	1.1 Idiopathic PAH 1.2 Heritable PAH 1.3 Drug or toxin-induced PAH 1.4 PAH associated with: Connective tissue disease HIV Portal hypertension Congenital heart disease Schistosomiasis 1.5 PAH responsive to calcium channel blockers 1.6 Pulmonary veno-occlusive disorder 1.7 Persistent PH of the newborn syndrome
Group II: PH due to left heart disease	2.1 With preserved LVEF 2.2 With reduced LVEF 2.3 Due to valvular heart disease 2.4 Left-sided due to congenital heart disease
Group III: PH due to lung disease	3.1 Obstructive lung disease 3.2 Restrictive lung disease 3.3 Mixed obstructive/restrictive lung disease 3.4 Hypoxemia without lung disease 3.5 Congenital lung disorders
Group IV: PH due to pulmonary artery obstruction	4.1 Chronic thromboembolic PH 4.2 Other chronic pulmonary obstructions, for example, tumors, congenital (Alagille syndrome)
Group V: PH of unclear or multifactorial mechanism	5.1 Hematologic disorders 5.2 Systemic and metabolic disorders 5.3 Others 5.4 Complex congenital heart disease

HIV, human immunodeficiency virus; LVEF, left ventricular ejection fraction; PAH, pulmonary arterial hypertension; PH, pulmonary hypertension; WSPH, World Society of Pulmonary Hypertension.

From Simonneau G, Montani D, Celermajer DS, et al. Haemodynamic definitions and updated clinical classification of pulmonary hypertension. *Eur Respir J.* 2019;53(1):1801913. doi: 10.1183/13993003.01913-2018. Reproduced with permission of the © ERS 2021.

The transpulmonary gradient (TPG) is the difference between mean PA and PCWP pressures. Traditionally, a TPG greater than 12 mm Hg is used to identify patients with PH out of proportion to left heart disease. The diastolic pulmonary gradient is the difference between PA diastolic pressure and mean PCWP.

In the sixth WSPH recommendations, PH because of left heart disease is defined hemodynamically by right heart catheterization as a mean PA pressure greater than 20 mm Hg and a PCWP greater than 15 mm Hg. It can be further classified as isolated postcapillary PH or combined postcapillary and precapillary PH.[13] The term "isolated postcapillary PH" describes those patients whose PH is merely because of passive pulmonary venous congestion. A minority of patients subject to long-standing elevated left-sided heart filling pressures undergo structural and functional pathophysiologic changes in the precapillary vasculature, including remodeling and vasoconstriction, resulting in mean PA pressure disproportionately elevated relative to the PCWP. Such patients are described as having combined postcapillary and precapillary PH. Isolated postcapillary PAH is defined as a PVR less than 3 Wood units or diastolic pulmonary gradient less than 7 Wood units and combined post- and precapillary PH as PVR greater than 3 Wood units or diastolic pulmonary gradient greater than 7 Wood units. Combined precapillary PAH is associated with reduced exercise capacity compared to isolated postcapillary PH and a phenotype similar to PAH[14] but may have a different genetic profile from isolated postcapillary PAH.[15]

Mortality and morbidity with PH because of left heart disease is associated with increasing PA pressures, mean PA pressures, PVR, and TPG. PH because of left heart failure is also associated with an increased 30-day mortality after orthotopic heart transplant in patients with a TPG greater than 15 mm Hg and PVR greater than 5 Wood units.[14,15]

The treatment of PH because of left heart disease is primarily focused on management of the underlying heart disease itself, as no PAH therapies have been shown to be beneficial in this condition.[16,17] The placement of a left ventricular assist device decreases pulmonary pressures by ventricular unloading.[18] PH because of left heart disease also improves with heart transplantation with the greater decrease in PVR 1 month after transplantation.[19]

Group III: Pulmonary Hypertension because of Lung Disease or Hypoxia

PH in chronic lung disease may be associated with chronic obstructive pulmonary disease (COPD), interstitial lung disease (ILD), cystic fibrosis, and bronchopulmonary dysplasia. In COPD, the destruction of lung parenchyma, decreased vascular dispensability, and decreased ability to recruit additional vasculature contribute to the development of PH.[20]

PH because of chronic lung disease should be considered and right heart catheterization pursued when symptoms or DLCO is out of proportion to the underlying lung disease; in those suspected to have concomitant PAH or chronic thromboembolic disease and when RV failure is present; and prior to undergoing lung transplantation or lung reduction surgery.[20]

PH because of chronic lung disease may be difficult to differentiate from PAH; however, significant lung disease (forced expiratory volume in one second [FEV1] <60% in COPD or forced vital capacity [FVC] <70 in ILD), characteristic lung parenchymal changes, absence of risk factors for PAH, and mild to moderate PH are more consistent with PH because of chronic lung disease. Severe PH is uncommon in isolated COPD or ILD alone but may be seen in mixed diseases.[20,21]

Treatment of PH-CLD is targeted toward the underlying lung disease. The use of PAH therapies is generally not recommended and may worsen outcomes.[22,23] Some recent studies have shown benefit of inhaled treprostinil in ILD-associated PH.[24] Oxygen therapy may improve or potentially slow the progression of PH in COPD.[25] Obstructive sleep apnea alone is rarely a cause of severe PH unless there is concomitant lung disease, such as COPD or obesity hypoventilation syndrome, and therapy is nocturnal noninvasive ventilation. When present, treatment of obstructive sleep apnea is of great importance whatever the subtype of PH: improved outcome has been shown in all types of PH with concomitant treatment of obstructive sleep apnea.[20]

Group IV: Pulmonary Hypertension because of Pulmonary Artery Obstructions

Although chronic thromboembolic PH is the predominant etiology, group IV PH can also be caused by pulmonary obstruction from PA sarcoma, congenital or acquired PA stenosis, foreign body or tumor embolism, and parasitic infections.[1] The incidence of chronic thromboembolic PH after acute pulmonary embolism is approximated to be 0.5% to 2%.[26] Despite a relatively low incidence after an acute pulmonary embolism (PE), nearly 74% of patients with chronic thromboembolic PH have a prior history of a pulmonary embolism, with 33% having recurrent pulmonary embolism, 31% with a known thrombophilic disorder and 3.4% with a prior splenectomy.[27]

The pathophysiology of chronic thromboembolic PH is not entirely elucidated, but occlusion because of thromboembolism alone is unlikely to result in PH. Rather, it is likely a combination of endothelial dysfunction, deficient thrombolysis, and inappropriate angiogenesis triggered by an embolic event.[27,28]

Routine screening for chronic thromboembolic PH with imaging after a PE is not recommended. Exertional dyspnea after pulmonary embolism should raise concern for chronic thromboembolic PH; however, symptoms normally do not begin until the disease is advanced with right heart dysfunction. Ventilation-perfusion (VQ) imaging remains the gold standard screening modality with 97% sensitivity and 95% specificity.[29] The diagnosis of chronic thromboembolic PH requires a perfusion mismatch on a VQ scan in addition to elevated pulmonary pressures with a normal PCWP by right heart catheterization. Computerized tomography pulmonary angiography and magnetic resonance angiography also may provide evidence of chronic thromboembolic PH.

Patients diagnosed with chronic thromboembolic PH should be evaluated in a multidisciplinary center that includes a surgeon experienced in pulmonary endarterectomy, PH specialist, and radiologist. These patients should be treated with lifelong anticoagulation and be evaluated for PA endarterectomy. A multicenter, retrospective study found a higher incidence of recurrent PE with the use of directly acting oral anticoagulants in comparison to vitamin K antagonists.[30] Endarterectomy with removal of the medial layer of the PA under circulatory arrest and hypothermia improves 3-year mortality from 70% to 90%. Patient suitability, preoperative functional capacity, and surgical accessibility of thrombi should be considered, as there are no established PVR thresholds or markers of right heart dysfunction that exclude surgical candidacy.[31,32]

Symptomatic patients with disease too distal to undergo endarterectomy can be considered for balloon pulmonary angioplasty to improve symptoms, hemodynamics, and RV function.[33] Riociguat and macitentan have been used in nonoperable patients or those with PH after endarterectomy in multicenter trials, respectively.[34,35] Insertion of an inferior vena caval filter does not improve outcomes and is not recommended.

Group V: Pulmonary Hypertension with Unclear and/or Multifactorial Mechanisms

Group V is a heterogeneous group of conditions with variable mechanisms resulting in PH. Several chronic myeloproliferative diseases including polycythemia, essential thrombocythemia, and primary myelofibrosis may result in PH because of vascular remodeling, tumor microembolism, pulmonary venous occlusion, and drug-induced PH.[1] Dasatinib is commonly used for the treatment of chronic myeloproliferative disease and has been associated with drug-induced PH.[6] There are no known therapies for PH associated with myeloproliferative diseases: treatment is directed at the underlying hematologic disease. Splenectomy has been associated with thrombotic and thromboembolic phenomena that may result in chronic thromboembolic PH and PAH[27] and should be managed by the predominant mechanism. Sickle cell disease–associated PH is discussed in the section on special populations.

The incidence of PH in sarcoidosis is 5% to 28% and is associated with increased morbidity and mortality. The cause of PH in sarcoidosis is often multifactorial and may include fibrotic lung disease, vasculitis, and pulmonary venous occlusion. Cardiac involvement can result in postcapillary PH because of left heart disease and has a more favorable prognosis compared to other forms of sarcoid-associated PH. The efficacy of treating sarcoid-associated PH with PAH therapies is unclear, but several studies have shown some advantageous outcomes with inhaled nitric oxide and prostacyclin therapy.[36]

Thyroid disease and chronic renal failure on dialysis are also associated with PH. PH in chronic renal disease may be due to concomitant left heart disease, hypervolemia, and high output from either anemia or an arteriovenous fistula.[1,37] Patients on dialysis with RV dysfunction or an estimated PA systolic pressure greater than 50 mm Hg on echocardiography, hypotension with hemodialysis, or being evaluated for transplantation should undergo right heart catheterization to evaluate for underlying PH. Treatment is targeted toward fluid balance, managing left heart disease, and avoiding anemia.[37]

CLINICAL PRESENTATION

Symptoms associated with PH are often nonspecific and include fatigue, dizziness, syncope, angina, exertional dyspnea, progressive limitation of exercise capacity, and exertional nausea or vomiting. Additional symptoms related to comorbid conditions may also be present, such as those associated with common cardiac and pulmonary conditions, connective tissue disease, congenital heart disease, HIV, or portal hypertension.

Physical examination findings may include the holosystolic murmur of tricuspid regurgitation, the diastolic murmur of pulmonic regurgitation, a right-sided third heart sound, a left parasternal lift, or an accentuated component of the pulmonic component of the second heart sound. With disease progression, there may be findings of RV failure including elevated jugular venous pressure, edema, ascites, and hepatomegaly.

Diagnostic Testing Findings

Common findings associated with PH by testing modality (electrocardiography, chest x-ray, and pulmonary function testing and blood gases) are summarized in **Table 16.4**. It is important to note that in most modalities, electrocardiography and chest x-ray for example, a normal result does not exclude PH.

TABLE 16.4 Testing Modalities in Pulmonary Hypertension

Testing Modality	Common Findings
Electrocardiography	Right axis deviation, right ventricular strain or hypertrophy, right bundle branch block, P-pulmonale, and QTc prolongation. Findings are more commonly found in the setting of severe disease.
Chest X-ray	Central pulmonary arterial dilation with pruning of peripheral vessels. Right atrial and ventricular enlargement in advanced disease. Concomitant lung disease may be seen.
Pulmonary function testing and blood gases	Evaluates for underlying airway and parenchymal lung disease including emphysema and interstitial lung disease. Most patients with PAH have a low DLCO and include pulmonary veno-occlusive disease, scleroderma-associated PAH, and parenchymal lung disease. A DLCO <45% predicted is associated with poor outcomes. Combined emphysema and interstitial disease may present with normal spirometry (pseudonormalization) but a low DLCO and decreased lung volumes.
Echocardiography	Echocardiography is used for screening, differential diagnosis, follow-up, and prognostication of patients with PH. It can estimate portions of the PVR including PA systolic pressure using the tricuspid regurgitant velocity and estimated right atrial pressure, PCWP using the transmitral Doppler inflow velocity (E) to mitral annular tissue Doppler velocity (e′) ratio, and cardiac output using the aortic velocity time integral and left ventricular outflow tract dimensions. Mean PA pressure can also be estimated from the right ventricular outflow tract acceleration time and pulmonary valve regurgitant velocity. These parameters can also help in initial differentiation of precapillary versus postcapillary forms of PH. Echocardiogram can also show further evidence of PH including right atrial or ventricular dilation, right ventricular systolic dysfunction, a flattened interventricular septum, dilation of the IVC, and notching of the spectral pulse wave Doppler of the right ventricular outflow tract. Echocardiography can also evaluate for left heart disease, intracardiac shunts, and congenital heart disease. Several echocardiographic parameters like right atrial size and presence of pericardial effusion are important prognostic factors for pulmonary hypertension.
Ventilation-perfusion scan	Gold standard imaging modality for the evaluation of chronic thromboembolic PH due to its high sensitivity (90%-100%) and specificity (94%-100%). A normal or low-probability VQ scan essentially excludes chronic thromboembolic PH.
Computed tomography	CT can reveal indirect evidence of PH, such as PA enlargement or right ventricular dilation, and help detect underlying causes, such as pulmonary or vascular disease. A PA diameter >29 mm or ratio to the ascending aorta diameter greater than 1 should raise concern for PH in symptomatic patients. Evidence of pulmonary veno-occlusive disease can also be seen on CT including diffuse ground glass opacities, pulmonary edema, and thickened interlobar septa. Nonspecific ground glass opacities might also be seen in up to one-third of patients with PAH. With angiography, CT can also show evidence of chronic thromboembolism with complete pulmonary obstruction of arteries, bands, webs, and intimal irregularities. CT pulmonary angiography can also be used to assess vasculitis and arteriovenous fistulas.
Cardiac magnetic resonance	CMR can accurately assess right ventricular size, mass, and function as well as hemodynamics including cardiac output and stroke volume. CMR may also be useful if underlying congenital heart disease is suspected but not well evaluated with echocardiography. MR angiography provides an accurate assessment of pulmonary vasculature, which is particularly useful in suspected chronic thromboembolic PH when CT angiography is precluded due to either pregnancy or the presence of contraindications to iodinated contrast.
Blood testing	Chemistry, hematology, and thyroid function testing should be obtained in all patients with confirmed or suspected PH. Liver function tests and hepatitis serologies should also be considered in patients with PH to evaluate for underlying liver disease related to high central venous pressures and in cases where endothelin receptor antagonist therapy is considered. Thyroid disease is commonly associated with PAH or may develop during disease and should be considered if there is an abrupt clinical worsening. Markers for connective tissue disease, systemic scleroderma, hepatitis serologies, and HIV should also be assessed. Limited scleroderma may have a positive ANA, anticentromere, dsDNA, anti-Ro, U3-RNP, B23, Th/To, and U1-RNP, whereas diffuse scleroderma is usually associated with U3-RNP. All patients with chronic thromboembolic PH should be evaluated for hypercoagulability disorders including antiphospholipid antibodies, anticardiolipin antibodies, and lupus anticoagulant. BNP and NT pro-BNP are useful markers for diagnosis and prognostication of PH.

(*continued*)

TABLE 16.4 Testing Modalities in Pulmonary Hypertension (*continued*)

Testing Modality	Common Findings
Ultrasonography	Abdominal ultrasonography can be used to evaluate for portal hypertension.
Six-minute walk test	Useful for assessing disease progression and response to treatment. A 6-minute walk distance over 500 m indicates good prognosis, whereas less than 300 m indicates poor prognosis.
Cardiopulmonary exercise testing	Cardiopulmonary exercise testing should be used after diagnosis of PH to assess the severity of exercise limitation related to PH and response to therapies. It can also be utilized to better define the predominant cardiopulmonary pathophysiology resulting in symptoms and PH.
Right heart catheterization	RHC is required to confirm the diagnosis and assess the severity of PH. Left heart catheterization should also be considered in select patients when there are risk factors for coronary disease or HFpEF. RHC may also be considered to assess treatment effect of drugs, evaluate congenital cardiac shunts to support decisions on correction, and in patients planning to undergo transplantation. If the accuracy of measurements obtained during RHC is in question, then a left ventricular end-diastolic pressure should be directly measured. RHC for the evaluation of PH should be performed in expert centers. Pressures should be zeroed at the midthoracic line halfway between sternum and bed at the level of the left atrium. The PCWP should be measured as the mean of three measurements at the end of normal expiration. Full oximetry testing—in all right heart chambers, both vena cava and the PAs—should be done if PA oxygen saturation is >75% or if a left-to-right shunt is suspected. Vasoreactivity testing is used to evaluate the response of pulmonary pressures to calcium channel blocker therapy but should only be performed in expert centers. A positive response is a reduction in mean PA pressure ≥10 mm Hg to reach an absolute mean PA pressure <40 with increased or unchanged cardiac output. The PCWP can be reduced <15 mm Hg with diuretics, and some institutions have administered a 500 mL saline bolus to help distinguish PAH from left ventricular dysfunction; however, this is not routine practice. A transpulmonary gradient and PVR should be calculated. PVR is sensitive to changes in flow and filling pressures and may not represent the pulmonary circulation at rest. The diastolic pulmonary gradient (ie, difference between diastolic PA diastolic and mean PCWP pressures) is less affected by flow and filling pressures. Hemodynamic sensors implanted during RHC may be used for long-term monitoring of PA pressures to guide management.

ANA, antinuclear antibody; BNP, brain natriuretic peptide; CMR, cardiac magnetic resonance; CT, computed tomography; DLCO, diffusing capacity of the lung for carbon monoxide; HFpEF, heart failure with preserved ejection fraction; HIV, human immunodeficiency virus; IVC, inferior vena cava; MR, magnetic resonance; PA, pulmonary artery; PAH, pulmonary arterial hypertension; PCWP, pulmonary capillary wedge pressure; PH, pulmonary hypertension; PVR, pulmonary vascular resistance; RHC, right heart catheterization; VQ, ventilation-perfusion.

MANAGEMENT

Risk Stratification

Appropriate risk stratification is crucial in order to assess prognosis and guide therapies in PAH. In the REVEAL registry, the presence of high-risk PH subtype (ie, familial, connective tissue disease, and portopulmonary hypertension), World Health Organization (WHO) functional class III/IV symptoms, poor 6-minute walk test distance, renal dysfunction, elevated plasma brain natriuretic protein (BNP) level, low DLCO, pericardial effusion on echocardiogram, or high-risk right heart catheterization hemodynamics were all associated with worse survival. Based on this, the REVEAL 1.0 risk score was developed. The REVEAL 2.0 risk score was later developed to reflect the contribution of estimated glomerular filtration rate and hospitalization on survival.[38] This score has excellent value in predicting survival and adverse PH events. One drawback of the REVEAL 2.0 risk score is its numerous variables. Accordingly, several simpler risk prediction tools have been developed including the 2015 European Society of Cardiology (ESC)/European Respiratory Society (ERS) PH score.[38,39]

Treatment

Treatments of group I PAH generally target three main biochemical pathways: endothelin, prostacyclin, and nitric oxide (**Figure 16.1**)[40] and are discussed below. Management of group II and III PH largely focuses on treatment of underlying condition and is discussed in the appropriate sections earlier. Treatment of group IV PAH, as noted previously, is centered on anticoagulation therapy and consideration of pulmonary endarterectomy. Management of a few entities in group V PH is discussed in the section on special populations.

Vasoreactivity testing with inhaled nitric oxide, intravenous adenosine, or intravenous prostacyclin is recommended in all group I patients with precapillary PH, with a positive response defined as a decrease in mean PA pressure by 10 mm Hg or more to 40 mm Hg or less. High-dose calcium channel blockers are the treatment of choice in patients with a positive response, called *super responders*, and are associated with improved survival.[1,5] These super responders are, however, only a minority of group I PAH patients.

In nonvasoreactive PH, numerous oral agents have demonstrated benefits in 6-minute walk test distance, quality

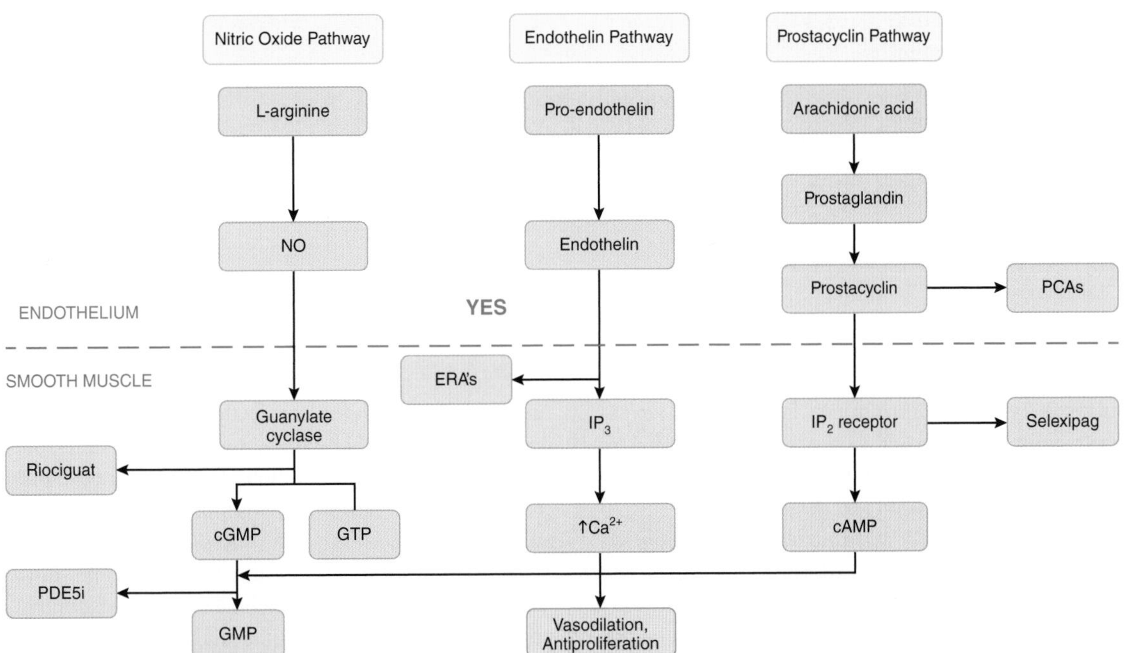

FIGURE 16.1 Diagram of biochemical pathways and drug targets in the nitric oxide, endothelin, and prostacyclin pathways. Drugs that act as agonists are indicated in green, whereas inhibitors are denoted with red.
Ca^{2+}, calcium; cAMP, cyclic adenosine monophosphate; cGMP, cyclic guanosine monophosphate; ERA, endothelin receptor antagonist; GTP, guanosine triphosphate; IP_2, inositol biphosphate; IP_3, inositol triphosphate; NO, nitric oxide; PCA, prostacyclin antagonists; PDE5i, phosphodiesterase-5 inhibitor. (Adapted from Benza RL, Park MH, Keogh A, et al. Management of pulmonary arterial hypertension with a focus on combination therapies. *J Heart Lung Transplant.* 2007;26(5):437-446. Copyright © 2007 International Society for Heart and Lung Transplantation. With permission.)

of life, disease progression rates, or reduction in PH-related events in randomized studies[41–45] (**Table 16.5**). However, no oral monotherapeutic agent has currently demonstrated mortality benefit. Because no comparison trials are available, there is no preferred initial oral agent, and the choice of agent should be based on the side-effect profile and patient preference.

Compared with monotherapy, dual oral therapy with oral agents is associated with a reduction in PH-related events and improvement in 6-minute walk test distances.[46] In the 500-patient AMBITION[47] trial, the initial use of a combination of ambrisentan and tadalafil resulted in lower PH event rates than monotherapy. Based on this trial, the WSPH recommends initial dual oral therapy with an endothelin receptor antagonist and phosphodiesterase-5 inhibitor in patients with PAH at low-to-intermediate risk by either the ESC/ERS or REVEAL 2.0 assessment tools. Initial monotherapy may be considered in older patients, those with milder disease, or those in whom there is concern for pulmonary veno-occlusive disease.[48] Patients who progress on monotherapy should be escalated to dual oral therapy. The combination of sildenafil and riociguat should be avoided because of the risk of hypotension.[49] Patients with persistent intermediate-/high-risk disease despite dual/triple therapy should be considered for inhaled or intravenous prostacyclin therapy.

In patients with high-risk disease—defined as 1-year mortality of 10% or more—or persistent intermediate- to high-risk symptoms despite dual oral therapy, treatment with intravenous prostacyclin or its analogues should be considered. To date, intravenous epoprostenol—a synthetic analogue of prostacyclin—is the only PH medication with a demonstrated survival benefit. Treprostinil, another form of parenteral prostacyclin therapy, is also commonly used because of its stability at room temperature, longer half-life (~4 hrs), and its ability to be administered by subcutaneous infusion. Deescalation of therapy in responders is generally not recommended given the progressive nature of PH. Given the poor survival and risk for progression, PH patients with intermediate/high risk should generally be referred to a tertiary facility with experience treating these patients.[48]

Although classified in group I, PAH patients with pulmonary venous occlusive disease may respond poorly to pulmonary vasodilators. In this subgroup, pulmonary vasodilator medications should be used with extreme caution because of the risk of life-threatening pulmonary edema.[1]

Advanced Therapies/Transplant

For select patients with advanced PH, lung transplantation may be an option. The perioperative mortality following lung transplant is around 10% (although lower at some experienced centers); therefore, appropriate patient selection is crucial. Lung transplant should be reserved for patients with 1-year survival of 90% or less such as those with persistent high-risk disease despite optimal

TABLE 16.5 List of Drugs Available Classified by Mechanism of Action

PDE5 Inhibitors	Guanyl Cyclase Stimulators	Endothelin Receptor Antagonists	Prostacyclin Agonists	Prostaglandin Receptor Agonists
Sildenafil (PO) Tadalafil (PO)	Riociguat (PO)	Bosentan (PO) Ambrisentan (PO) Macitentan (PO)	Epoprostenol (IV) Treprostinil (IV/SQ/PO) Iloprost (INH)	Selexipag (PO)

INH, inhaled; IV, intravenous; PDE, phosphodiesterase; PO, oral; SQ, subcutaneous.

medical therapy including parenteral prostacyclin therapies.[50] Other populations in whom transplant may be considered are patients with refractory hypoxemia or progressive end organ failure (ie, renal, hepatic) because of PH. Early referral is important prior to significant end organ dysfunction and debility.

In patients with severe RV dysfunction and cardiogenic shock, the use of ventriculoarterial extracorporeal membrane oxygenation has been reported as a bridge to transplantation.[50] Mechanical circulatory support is generally reserved as a bridge to transplantation and avoided in patients who are not candidates for lung transplantation. The use of long-term surgical assist devices is currently investigational.

Investigational Therapies

Several nonpharmacologic therapies have been utilized in the care of PH patients. One procedure is balloon atrial septostomy, in which an iatrogenic atrial septal defect is created, allowing right-to-left shunting that decreases RV volume and preserves cardiac output.[51] Retrospective studies have demonstrated safety and improved quality of life with this procedure. Although not commonly used in the United States, it has gained popularity elsewhere worldwide. Other potential therapies include the Potts shunt (ie, a side-to-side anastomosis is created from the left PA to the descending aorta, resulting in a right-to-left shunt) for end-stage PH patients for palliation and pulmonary angioplasty in patients with chronic thromboembolic PH.[52] These interventional strategies have yet to reach widespread use.

PULMONARY HYPERTENSION IN SPECIAL POPULATIONS

Pediatric Pulmonary Hypertension and Congenital Heart Disease

PH in children has varied distribution of etiologies as compared to adults, with a predominance of idiopathic PAH and PAH associated with congenital heart disease and some types of transient PAH.[53] The most common form of transient PAH in children is persistent PH in the newborn, with the incidence inversely related to gestational age and associated with other conditions such as Down syndrome, meconium aspiration syndrome, and respiratory distress syndrome.

Eisenmenger Syndrome

Eisenmenger syndrome (see Chapter 110) occurs when a long-standing left-to-right cardiac shunt caused by a congenital heart defect (ie, ventricular septal defect, patent ductus arteriosus, atrial septal defect, or, less commonly, patent ductus arteriosus) results in PH with systemic-level PA pressure because of high PVR (>10 Wood units) and reversal of the shunt into a cyanotic right-to-left shunt. Bosentan—an endothelin receptor antagonist—is currently the only pulmonary vasodilator with a class I indication for Eisenmenger syndrome; however, experiences with other endothelin receptor antagonists and the phosphodiesterase-5 inhibitors sildenafil and tadalafil show favorable functional and hemodynamic results.[54] Intravenous epoprostenol (a prostacyclin analogue) has been used, but is generally avoided because of the risk of paradoxical embolism associated with indwelling central lines.

Survival among patients with Eisenmenger is better than for patients with idiopathic PAH, possibly because of the ability to maintain cardiac output at the expense of systemic hypoxemia with the former. Treatment-naïve patients with Eisenmenger syndrome had a 34% 10-year survival, which was improved to 57% with pulmonary vasodilators in one cohort.[53] Combined heart-lung or lung transplant with cardiac repair is an alternative treatment, with an 84% 1-year posttransplant survival and, of those alive at 1 year, a median survival of 14.8 years posttransplant.[55]

Although large, unrepaired posttricuspid shunts (ie, ventricular septal defect and patent ductus arteriosus) generally lead to Eisenmenger syndrome, patients with pretricuspid shunts such as atrial septal defects can develop concomitant elevated PVR and PAH (Table 16.6). Although closure of the atrial septal defect early in life with normal PVR has an excellent prognosis, the decision to close is more difficult for those with any evidence of elevated PVR as there is a risk of developing PAH after closure. The current guidelines do not recommend closure if the PVR is more than 4.6 Wood units, and if between 2.3 and 4.6 Wood units the decision should be made on an individualized basis.[56] There is some evidence for a "treat to close" strategy where pulmonary vasodilators can be used to improve PVR followed by closure of the shunt,[57] but this is not yet supported by the guidelines.

Sickle Cell Disease

PH is present in 6% to 11% of patients with sickle cell disease and is associated with increased mortality.[58] Although the etiology for PH in sickle cell disease appears to be multifactorial, decreased bioavailability of nitric oxide because of hemolysis and oxidative stress likely contributes.[59]

TABLE 16.6 Congenital Heart Disease Patients in Sixth WSPH Clinical Classification Scheme

PH Group	Examples
Group 1.4.4 PAH and congenital heart disease	• Eisenmenger physiology • PAH and left-to-right shunts • PAH with incidental congenital heart disease • PAH with closed/repaired congenital heart disease defects
Group 2.4 Left-sided obstructive lesions (postcapillary)	• Pulmonary vein stenosis • Cor triatriatum • Obstructive total anomalous pulmonary venous return • Mitral or aortic stenosis (including supra- and subvalvar)
Group 5.4 Complex congenital heart disease	• Segmental PH (eg, pulmonary atresia with ventricular septal defect and major aortopulmonary collaterals) • Single ventricle • Scimitar syndrome

PAH, pulmonary arterial hypertension; PH, pulmonary hypertension; WSPH, World Society of Pulmonary Hypertension.
From Rosenzweig EB, Abman SH, Adatia I, et al. Paediatric pulmonary arterial hypertension: updates on definition, classification, diagnostics and management. *Eur Respir J.* 2019;53(1):1801916. doi: 10.1183/13993003.01916-2018. Reproduced with permission of the © ERS 2021.

PH because of sickle cell disease is categorized as group V, as the etiology can be precapillary, postcapillary or mixed. Anemia increases cardiac output and decreases blood viscosity. Consequently, an elevated PVR in precapillary PH (PAH) associated with sickle cell disease is lower (≥2 Wood units) compared to group I PAH patient (≥3 Wood units).

Sickle cell patients should be screened with Doppler echocardiography every 1 to 3 years. If the tricuspid regurgitant velocity is 3 m/s or more, then right heart catheterization is recommended. Alternatively, N-terminal prohormone BNP can also be used as a screening test: plasma levels of 160 pg/mL or more are also associated with increased mortality. Escalation therapy is recommended for sickle cell patients considered at high risk, which includes hydroxyurea, chronic transfusion therapy, consideration of anticoagulation, and oxygen therapy. If precapillary PH is present (PVR ≥2 Wood units, PCWP <15 mm Hg), select patients can be treated with a prostacyclin agonist or endothelial receptor antagonist. Phosphodiesterase-5 inhibitors are contraindicated in this population because of an increased risk of vaso-occlusive crisis.[59]

Elderly

Of individuals with PH, 9% to 13% are diagnosed at an age greater than 70 years.[59] The majority of elderly patients with PH have group II or PH of mixed etiology. Those patients with group I PH (PAH) are more likely to have concomitant connective tissue disease.[60] Age-related changes to the systemic and pulmonary circulation can make accurate diagnosis of PH challenging in this population. Decreased lung elastic recoil, increased chest wall thickness, vascular stiffening, and decreased left heart compliance can alter PVR. PAH-specific treatments have not been studied in elderly populations. This population may be at higher risk for adverse effects of therapies, making referral to an expert center for accurate diagnosis and initiation of therapy essential.[60,61]

Pregnancy

Pregnancy in patients with PH has been associated with high maternal mortality and is contraindicated based on the modified WHO classification system.[11] Historically, the maternal mortality was 30% to 56%, although recent data from Europe have suggested that maternal mortality may be less, but still significant. Women determined to be at moderate or high risk for pregnancy complications based on modified WHO classification are recommended to have care at an expert center that utilizes a multidisciplinary team.[62]

PROGNOSIS

Historically, the prognosis was poor for patients with PH. However, with improvements in diagnosis and treatment, outcomes have improved. In 1991, the estimated 5-year survival for patients with PAH was 34%.[63] Recent outcomes for patients with PAH on intravenous or subcutaneous pulmonary vasodilators report a 67% survival 5 years from initiation of therapy.[64] In children with idiopathic PAH, survival is 72% at 5 years, which is much improved compared historically to untreated patients.[65]

In all types of PH, one recent report of survival at 1, 5, and 10 years was 88%, 73%, and 63%, respectively. After stratifying by age and sex, those younger than 50 years and female patients had a higher risk of mortality.[66] Other reports have demonstrated higher mortality in connective tissue disease–associated PAH as compared with idiopathic PAH.[64] Although there have been few comparative studies, survival appears similarly poor in group II PH, with only 48% of patients alive at 5 years in one report.[67]

RESEARCH AND FUTURE DIRECTIONS

Although there has been considerable improvement in the outlook of patients with PH, it remains a challenging disease to treat with high morbidity, mortality, and cost and the most effective medication being a continuous intravenous infusion. With improvement in therapy and emphasis on early diagnosis and discovery of novel therapeutic options, it is likely that outcome in these patients will continue to improve over time. Future research is focused on early recognition of disease in high-risk subsets such as those with connective tissue and sickle cell disease, noninvasive modalities and algorithms for diagnosis and prognosis, and development of novel drug delivery systems like long-acting subcutaneous drug delivery system, implantable pumps, and metered dose inhalers.[68]

KEY POINTS

- ✔ A mean PA pressure greater than 20 mm Hg is used to diagnose PH.
- ✔ Right heart catheterization is the gold standard for diagnosis of PH. Echocardiogram is an excellent tool for screening and follow-up.
- ✔ There are five clinical groups of PH: Group I is PAH, group II is PH because of left heart disease, group III is PH because of lung disease, group IV is PH because of PA obstruction, and group V is PH because of unclear or multifactorial mechanisms.
- ✔ A mean PA pressure greater than 20 mm Hg with a PCWP less than 15 mm Hg is diagnostic of group I PH or PAH in the absence of chronic thromboembolic disease or chronic lung disease.
- ✔ Group IV PH because of chronic thromboembolic disease should be excluded by VQ scan in all patients with PH because surgical treatment is potentially curable for this form of disease.
- ✔ Idiopathic and connective tissue PAH respond well to pulmonary vasodilator therapy.
- ✔ Treatment of PAH is based on risk stratification using tools like the REVEAL 2.0 score. Low-risk patients can be treated with combination oral therapy, whereas high-risk patients can be started on a combination of oral and parenteral pulmonary vasodilator therapy.

REFERENCES

1. Simonneau G, Montani D, Celermajer DS, et al. Haemodynamic definitions and updated clinical classification of pulmonary hypertension. *Eur Respir J.* 2019;53(1):1801913. doi:10.1183/13993003.01913-2018
2. Allen HD, Shaddy RE, Penny DJ, Feltes TF, Cetta F. *Moss and Adams' Heart Disease in Infants, Children, and Adolescents: Including the Fetus and Young Adult.* 9th ed. Wolters Kluwer; 2016.
3. Morrell NW, Aldred MA, Chung WK, et al. Genetics and genomics of pulmonary arterial hypertension. *Eur Respir J.* 2019;53(1):1801899. doi:10.1183/13993003.01899-2018
4. Sanz J, Sánchez-Quintana D, Bossone E, Bogaard HJ, Naeije R. Anatomy, function, and dysfunction of the right ventricle: JACC state-of-the-art review. *J Am Coll Cardiol.* 2019;73(12):1463-1482. doi:10.1016/j.jacc.2018.12.076
5. Sitbon O, Humbert M, Jaïs X, et al. Long-term response to calcium channel blockers in idiopathic pulmonary arterial hypertension. *Circulation.* 2005;111(23):3105-3111. doi:10.1161/CIRCULATIONAHA.104.488486
6. Weatherald J, Chaumais MC, Savale L, et al. Long-term outcomes of dasatinib-induced pulmonary arterial hypertension: a population-based study. *Eur Respir J.* 2017;50(1):1700217. doi:10.1183/13993003.00217-2017
7. Zamanian RT, Hedlin H, Greuenwald P, et al. Features and outcomes of methamphetamine-associated pulmonary arterial hypertension. *Am J Respir Crit Care Med.* 2018;197(6):788-800. doi:10.1164/rccm.201705-0943OC
8. Launay D, Sobanski V, Hachulla E, Humbert M. Pulmonary hypertension in systemic sclerosis: different phenotypes. *Eur Respir Rev.* 2017;26(145):170056. doi:10.1183/16000617.0056-2017
9. Krowka MJ, Miller DP, Barst RJ, et al. Portopulmonary hypertension: a report from the US-based REVEAL registry. *Chest.* 2012;141(4):906-915. doi:10.1378/chest.11-0160
10. Montani D, Lau EM, Dorfmüller P, et al. Pulmonary veno-occlusive disease. *Eur Respir J.* 2016;47(5):1518-1534. doi:10.1183/13993003.00026-2016
11. Galiè N, Humbert M, Vachiery JL, et al. 2015 ESC/ERS guidelines for the diagnosis and treatment of pulmonary hypertension: the Joint Task Force for the Diagnosis and Treatment of Pulmonary Hypertension of the European Society of Cardiology (ESC) and the European Respiratory Society (ERS): Endorsed by: Association for European Paediatric and Congenital Cardiology (AEPC), International Society for Heart and Lung Transplantation (ISHLT). *Eur Heart J.* 2016;37(1):67-119. doi:10.1093/eurheartj/ehv317
12. Reddy YNV, Melenovsky V, Redfield MM, Nishimura RA, Borlaug BA. High-output heart failure: a 15-year experience. *J Am Coll Cardiol.* 2016;68(5):473-482. doi:10.1016/j.jacc.2016.05.043
13. Vachiéry JL, Tedford RJ, Rosenkranz S, et al. Pulmonary hypertension due to left heart disease. *Eur Respir J.* 2019;53(1):1801897. doi:10.1183/13993003.01897-2018
14. Dragu R, Rispler S, Habib M, et al. Pulmonary arterial capacitance in patients with heart failure and reactive pulmonary hypertension. *Eur J Heart Fail.* 2015;17(1):74-80. doi:10.1002/ejhf.192
15. Miller WL, Grill DE, Borlaug BA. Clinical features, hemodynamics, and outcomes of pulmonary hypertension due to chronic heart failure with reduced ejection fraction: pulmonary hypertension and heart failure. *JACC Heart Fail.* 2013;1(4):290-299. doi:10.1016/j.jchf.2013.05.001
16. Liu LC, Hummel YM, van der Meer P, et al. Effects of sildenafil on cardiac structure and function, cardiopulmonary exercise testing and health-related quality of life measures in heart failure patients with preserved ejection fraction and pulmonary hypertension. *Eur J Heart Fail.* 2017;19(1):116-125. doi:10.1002/ejhf.662
17. Vachiéry JL, Delcroix M, Al-Hiti H, et al. Macitentan in pulmonary hypertension due to left ventricular dysfunction. *Eur Respir J.* 2018;51(2):1701886. doi:10.1183/13993003.01886-2017
18. Masri SC, Tedford RJ, Colvin MM, Leary PJ, Cogswell R. Pulmonary arterial compliance improves rapidly after left ventricular assist device implantation. *ASAIO J.* 2017;63(2):139-143. doi:10.1097/MAT.0000000000000467
19. Goland S, Czer LS, Kass RM, et al. Pre-existing pulmonary hypertension in patients with end-stage heart failure: impact on clinical outcome and hemodynamic follow-up after orthotopic heart transplantation. *J Heart Lung Transplant.* 2007;26(4):312-318. doi:10.1016/j.healun.2006.12.012
20. Nathan SD, Barbera JA, Gaine SP, et al. Pulmonary hypertension in chronic lung disease and hypoxia. *Eur Respir J.* 2019;53(1):1801914. doi:10.1183/13993003.01914-2018
21. Hurdman J, Condliffe R, Elliot CA, et al. Pulmonary hypertension in COPD: results from the ASPIRE registry. *Eur Respir J.* 2013;41(6):1292-1301. doi:10.1183/09031936.00079512
22. Vitulo P, Stanziola A, Confalonieri M, et al. Sildenafil in severe pulmonary hypertension associated with chronic obstructive pulmonary disease: a randomized controlled multicenter clinical trial. *J Heart Lung Transplant.* 2017;36(2):166-174. doi:10.1016/j.healun.2016.04.010
23. Nathan SD, Behr J, Collard HR, et al. Riociguat for idiopathic interstitial pneumonia-associated pulmonary hypertension (RISE-IIP): a randomised, placebo-controlled phase 2b study. *Lancet Respir Med.* 2019;7(9):780-790. doi:10.1016/S2213-2600(19)30250-4

24. Waxman A, Restrepo-Jaramillo R, Thenappan T, et al. Inhaled treprostinil in pulmonary hypertension due to interstitial lung disease. *N Engl J Med.* 2021;384(4):325-334. doi:10.1056/NEJMoa2008470
25. Timms RM, Khaja FU, Williams GW. Hemodynamic response to oxygen therapy in chronic obstructive pulmonary disease. *Ann Intern Med.* 1985;102(1):29-36. doi:10.7326/0003-4819-102-1-29
26. Pengo V, Lensing AW, Prins MH, et al. Incidence of chronic thromboembolic pulmonary hypertension after pulmonary embolism. *N Engl J Med.* 2004;350(22):2257-2264. doi:10.1056/NEJMoa032274
27. Pepke-Zaba J, Delcroix M, Lang I, et al. Chronic thromboembolic pulmonary hypertension (CTEPH): results from an international prospective registry. *Circulation.* 2011;124(18):1973-1981. doi:10.1161/CIRCULATIONAHA.110.015008
28. Coquoz N, Weilenmann D, Stolz D, et al. Multicentre observational screening survey for the detection of CTEPH following pulmonary embolism. *Eur Respir J.* 2018;51(4):1702505. doi:10.1183/13993003.02505-2017
29. Tunariu N, Gibbs SJ, Win Z, et al. Ventilation-perfusion scintigraphy is more sensitive than multidetector CTPA in detecting chronic thromboembolic pulmonary disease as a treatable cause of pulmonary hypertension. *J Nucl Med.* 2007;48(5):680-684. doi:10.2967/jnumed.106.039438
30. Bunclark K, Newnham M, Chiu YD, et al. A multicenter study of anticoagulation in operable chronic thromboembolic pulmonary hypertension. *J Thromb Haemost.* 2020;18(1):114-122. doi:10.1111/jth.14649
31. Madani MM, Auger WR, Pretorius V, et al. Pulmonary endarterectomy: recent changes in a single institution's experience of more than 2,700 patients. *Ann Thorac Surg.* 2012;94(1):97-103; discussion 103. doi:10.1016/j.athoracsur.2012.04.004
32. Delcroix M, Lang I, Pepke-Zaba J, et al. Long-term outcome of patients with chronic thromboembolic pulmonary hypertension: results from an international prospective registry. *Circulation.* 2016;133(9):859-871. doi:10.1161/CIRCULATIONAHA.115.016522
33. Fukui S, Ogo T, Morita Y, et al. Right ventricular reverse remodelling after balloon pulmonary angioplasty. *Eur Respir J.* 2014;43(5):1394-1402. doi:10.1183/09031936.00012914
34. Ghofrani HA, D'Armini AM, Grimminger F, et al. Riociguat for the treatment of chronic thromboembolic pulmonary hypertension. *N Engl J Med.* 2013;369(4):319-329. doi:10.1056/NEJMoa1209657
35. Ghofrani HA, Simonneau G, D'Armini AM, et al. Macitentan for the treatment of inoperable chronic thromboembolic pulmonary hypertension (MERIT-1): results from the multicentre, phase 2, randomised, double-blind, placebo-controlled study. *Lancet Respir Med.* 2017;5(10):785-794. doi:10.1016/S2213-2600(17)30305-3
36. Bonham CA, Oldham JM, Gomberg-Maitland M, Vij R. Prostacyclin and oral vasodilator therapy in sarcoidosis-associated pulmonary hypertension: a retrospective case series. *Chest.* 2015;148(4):1055-1062. doi:10.1378/chest.14-2546
37. Sise ME, Courtwright AM, Channick RN. Pulmonary hypertension in patients with chronic and end-stage kidney disease. *Kidney Int.* 2013;84(4):682-692. doi:10.1038/ki.2013.186
38. Benza RL, Gomberg-Maitland M, Elliott CG, et al. Predicting survival in patients with pulmonary arterial hypertension: the REVEAL risk score calculator 2.0 and comparison with ESC/ERS-based risk assessment strategies. *Chest.* 2019;156(2):323-337. doi:10.1016/j.chest.2019.02.004
39. Kylhammar D, Kjellström B, Hjalmarsson C, et al. A comprehensive risk stratification at early follow-up determines prognosis in pulmonary arterial hypertension. *Eur Heart J.* 2018;39(47):4175-4181. doi:10.1093/eurheartj/ehx257
40. Benza RL, Park MH, Keogh A, Girgis RE. Management of pulmonary arterial hypertension with a focus on combination therapies. *J Heart Lung Transplant.* 2007;26(5):437-446. doi:10.1016/j.healun.2007.01.035
41. Pulido T, Adzerikho I, Channick RN, et al. Macitentan and morbidity and mortality in pulmonary arterial hypertension. *N Engl J Med.* 2013;369(9):809-818. doi:10.1056/NEJMoa1213917
42. Sitbon O, Channick R, Chin KM, et al. Selexipag for the treatment of pulmonary arterial hypertension. *N Engl J Med.* 2015;373(26):2522-2533. doi:10.1056/NEJMoa1503184
43. Galiè N, Brundage BH, Ghofrani HA, et al. Tadalafil therapy for pulmonary arterial hypertension. *Circulation.* 2009;119(22):2894-2903. doi:10.1161/CIRCULATIONAHA.108.839274
44. Barst RJ, Rubin LJ, Long WA, et al. A comparison of continuous intravenous epoprostenol (prostacyclin) with conventional therapy for primary pulmonary hypertension. *N Engl J Med.* Feb 1996;334(5):296-301. doi:10.1056/NEJM199602013340504
45. Tapson VF, Jing ZC, Xu KF, et al. Oral treprostinil for the treatment of pulmonary arterial hypertension in patients receiving background endothelin receptor antagonist and phosphodiesterase type 5 inhibitor therapy (the FREEDOM-C2 study): a randomized controlled trial. *Chest.* 2013;144(3):952-958. doi:10.1378/chest.12-2875
46. Lajoie AC, Lauzière G, Lega JC, et al. Combination therapy versus monotherapy for pulmonary arterial hypertension: a meta-analysis. *Lancet Respir Med.* 2016;4(4):291-305. doi:10.1016/S2213-2600(16)00027-8
47. Frost AE, Hoeper MM, Barberá JA, et al. Risk-stratified outcomes with initial combination therapy in pulmonary arterial hypertension: application of the reveal risk score. *J Heart Lung Transplant.* 2018;37(12):1410-1417. doi:10.1016/j.healun.2018.07.001
48. Galiè N, Channick RN, Frantz RP, et al. Risk stratification and medical therapy of pulmonary arterial hypertension. *Eur Respir J.* 2019;53(1):1801889. doi:10.1183/13993003.01889-2018
49. Galiè N, Müller K, Scalise AV, Grünig E. PATENT PLUS: a blinded, randomised and extension study of riociguat plus sildenafil in pulmonary arterial hypertension. *Eur Respir J.* 2015;45(5):1314-1322. doi:10.1183/09031936.00105914
50. Hoeper MM, Benza RL, Corris P, et al. Intensive care, right ventricular support and lung transplantation in patients with pulmonary hypertension. *Eur Respir J.* 2019;53(1):1801906. doi:10.1183/13993003.01906-2018
51. Sandoval J, Gaspar J, Peña H, et al. Effect of atrial septostomy on the survival of patients with severe pulmonary arterial hypertension. *Eur Respir J.* 2011;38(6):1343-1348. doi:10.1183/09031936.00072210
52. Esch JJ, Shah PB, Cockrill BA, et al. Transcatheter Potts shunt creation in patients with severe pulmonary arterial hypertension: initial clinical experience. *J Heart Lung Transplant.* 2013;32(4):381-387. doi:10.1016/j.healun.2013.01.1049
53. Rosenzweig EB, Abman SH, Adatia I, et al. Paediatric pulmonary arterial hypertension: updates on definition, classification, diagnostics and management. *Eur Respir J.* 2019;53(1):1801916. doi:10.1183/13993003.01916-2018
54. Diller GP, Körten MA, Bauer UM, et al. Current therapy and outcome of Eisenmenger syndrome: data of the German National Register for congenital heart defects. *Eur Heart J.* 2016;37(18):1449-1455. doi:10.1093/eurheartj/ehv743
55. Hjortshøj CS, Gilljam T, Dellgren G, et al. Outcome after heart-lung or lung transplantation in patients with Eisenmenger syndrome. *Heart.* 2019;106(2):127-132. doi:10.1136/heartjnl-2019-315345
56. Stout KK, Daniels CJ, Aboulhosn JA, et al. 2018 AHA/ACC guideline for the management of adults with congenital heart disease: executive summary: a report of the American College of Cardiology/American Heart Association Task Force on Clinical Practice Guidelines. *Circulation.* 2019;139(14):e637-e697. doi:10.1161/CIR.0000000000000602. Erratum in: *Circulation.* 2019;139(14):e831-e832.
57. Bradley EA, Ammash N, Martinez SC, et al. "Treat-to-close": non-repairable ASD-PAH in the adult: results from the North American ASD-PAH (NAAP) Multicenter Registry. *Int J Cardiol.* 2019;291:127-133. doi:10.1016/j.ijcard.2019.03.056
58. Klings ES, Machado RF, Barst RJ, et al. An official American Thoracic Society clinical practice guideline: diagnosis, risk stratification, and management of pulmonary hypertension of sickle cell disease. *Am J Respir Crit Care Med.* 2014;189(6):727-740. doi:10.1164/rccm.201401-0065ST
59. Akinsheye I, Klings ES. Sickle cell anemia and vascular dysfunction: the nitric oxide connection. *J Cell Physiol.* 2010;224(3):620-625. doi:10.1002/jcp.22195
60. Hoeper MM, Huscher D, Ghofrani HA, et al. Elderly patients diagnosed with idiopathic pulmonary arterial hypertension: results from the COMPERA registry. *Int J Cardiol.* 2013;168(2):871-880. doi:10.1016/j.ijcard.2012.10.026

61. Pugh ME, Sivarajan L, Wang L, Robbins IM, Newman JH, Hemnes AR. Causes of pulmonary hypertension in the elderly. *Chest.* 2014;146(1):159-166. doi:10.1378/chest.13-1900
62. Sliwa K, van Hagen IM, Budts W, et al. Pulmonary hypertension and pregnancy outcomes: data from the Registry Of Pregnancy and Cardiac Disease (ROPAC) of the European Society of Cardiology. *Eur J Heart Fail.* 2016;18(9):1119-1128. doi:10.1002/ejhf.594. Epub 2016 Jul 7. Erratum in: *Eur J Heart Fail.* 2017;19(3):439.
63. D'Alonzo GE, Barst RJ, Ayres SM, et al. Survival in patients with primary pulmonary hypertension. Results from a national prospective registry. *Ann Intern Med.* 1991;115(5):343-349. doi:10.7326/0003-4819-115-5-343
64. Bartolome SD, Sood N, Shah TG, Styrvoky K, Torres F, Chin KM. Mortality in patients with pulmonary arterial hypertension treated with continuous prostanoids. *Chest.* 2018;154(3):532-540. doi:10.1016/j.chest.2018.03.050
65. Haworth SG, Hislop AA. Treatment and survival in children with pulmonary arterial hypertension: the UK pulmonary hypertension service for children 2001-2006. *Heart.* 2009;95(4):312-317. doi:10.1136/hrt.2008.150086
66. Chang WT, Weng SF, Hsu CH, et al. Prognostic factors in patients with pulmonary Hypertension-A Nationwide Cohort Study. *J Am Heart Assoc.* 2016;5(9):e003579. doi:10.1161/JAHA.116.003579
67. Salamon JN, Kelesidis I, Msaouel P, et al. Outcomes in World Health Organization group II pulmonary hypertension: mortality and readmission trends with systolic and preserved ejection fraction-induced pulmonary hypertension. *J Card Fail.* 2014;20(7):467-475. doi:10.1016/j.cardfail.2014.05.003
68. Keshavarz A, Kadry H, Alobaida A, Ahsan F. Newer approaches and novel drugs for inhalational therapy for pulmonary arterial hypertension. *Expert Opin Drug Deliv.* 2020;17(4):439-461. doi:10.1080/17425247.2020.1729119

CHAPTER 17

ADULT CONGENITAL HEART DISEASE

Benjamin S. Hendrickson, Marc V. Lee, Jennifer DeSalvo, and Elisa A. Bradley

INTRODUCTION

Surgical and medical advances have touched fewer fields more profoundly than congenital heart disease (CHD). As a result, there are now more adults surviving with CHD (ACHD) than there are children.[1] Current data suggest that approximately 4 to 10 in every 1000 live births in the United States is affected by CHD, and that the number surviving into and throughout adulthood will continue to rise.[2-6] Given the increased size of the adult population with CHD, there has been increased focus in how to best care for these patients. This has resulted in the establishment and development of a subspecialty field within cardiology dedicated to the care of ACHD patients. As recent as the past decade, there has been evidence that supports that this specialized ACHD care has led to improved survival.[7] However, the field is complex in that there is significant heterogeneity in the spectrum of CHD diagnoses and treatment options available. Therefore, the goal here is to provide a general overview of the types of CHD that can be seen in the adult population, clinical presentation, management, and discussion of ongoing lifelong care.

PATHOGENESIS

CHD arises from abnormal cardiovascular development during embryogenesis or in the transition to postnatal circulation. Therefore, an understanding of cardiac morphogenesis is necessary to understand the anatomic and pathophysiologic consequences of individual defects and corrective or palliative treatment options.

Cardiac morphogenesis begins during the third week of embryogenesis with the formation of the primitive heart tube. It develops from paired clusters of mesodermal cells that proliferate longitudinally, canalize, and fuse in the ventral midline to form a single heart tube (**Figure 17.1A,B**).[8] This consists of an inner endocardium, gelatinous connective tissue, and outer myocardium. The heart tube also conducts action potentials, resulting in cardiac contraction during the third week. As it elongates during the fourth week, primitive chambers develop and looping occurs to establish polarity. This leads to the sinus venosus, connected to the venous system caudally, and primitive atrium, to move above and behind the primitive ventricle (**Figure 17.1B**). The bulbus cordis and truncus arteriosus, on the other hand, are connected to the aortic arches cranially.[8] Septation of the chambers occurs between 4 and 6 weeks (**Figure 17.1C,D**). The ventricular outflow tracts derive from migration of neural crest cells that proliferate within the bulbus cordis and truncus arteriosus to form ridges, which fuse and spiral to form an aorticopulmonary septum divided into the pulmonary artery and aorta, respectively (**Figure 17.1E**). The aortic and pulmonic valves are derived from endocardial cushions of the ventricular outflow tracts, whereas mitral and tricuspid valves are derived from that of the atrioventricular canal. Throughout cardiac morphogenesis, fetal circulation allows for oxygenated blood from the placenta to be shunted from the umbilical vein to the inferior vena cava via the ductus venosus bypassing hepatic circulation, from the right to left atria via the foramen ovale, and from the pulmonary artery to the aorta to the systemic circulation via the ductus arteriosus bypassing the lungs. The anatomic and physiologic transition to postnatal circulation after delivery lead to shunt closure, as pulmonary vascular resistance decreases.

CHD is felt to arise from the interaction of multiple complex factors, and approximately only 15% has been linked to inherited or de novo genetic mutations. Environmental and maternal factors are also important, and risk factors for CHD in the offspring include: maternal chronic or gestational diseases, maternal medical illness, exposure to teratogenic medications or toxins in utero, and exposure to various environmental factors.[9] As a child with CHD progresses into adulthood, the development of sequelae from their native CHD or surgical intervention, in addition to acquired comorbidities, including hypertension, hyperlipidemia, obesity, and coronary disease, may exacerbate the physiologic regulatory mechanisms of CHD, ultimately affecting overall health and quality of life.[9]

The AHA/ACC have proposed comprehensive guidelines that highlight both the anatomic abnormalities and physiologic consequences of CHD.[10] This classification system is used to help define appropriate evaluation, management, and follow-up care in the disparate ACHD population. The anatomic portion of classification is divided into the complexity of CHD: simple, moderate, and severely complex. The physiologic stage encompasses hemodynamic and anatomic sequelae, which vary from valvular involvement, pulmonary vascular disease, ventricular

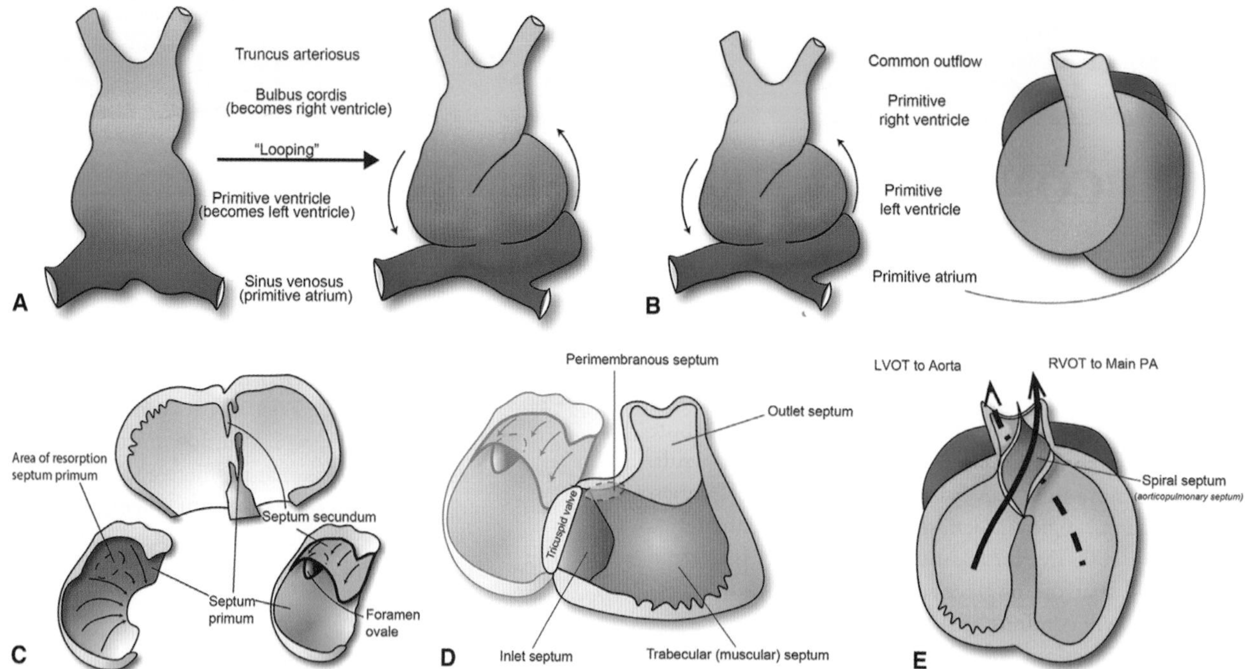

FIGURE 17.1 Embryologic cardiac development. The primitive heart tube develops in week 3 of gestation when paired clusters of mesodermal cells canalize and fuse in the ventral midline to form the heart tube **(A,B)**. The primitive heart chambers develop and looping establishes polarity during the fourth week of gestation **(B)**. Septation of the chambers occurs next **(C,D)** followed by neural crest cell migration to the bulbus cordis and truncus arteriosus to form ridges that fuse and spiral, leading to formation of the aorticopulmonary septum that later divides into the aorta and pulmonary artery **(E)**. LVOT, left ventricular outflow tract; PA, pulmonary artery; RVOT, right ventricular outflow tract.

dysfunction, and arrhythmia, among others. A diagrammatic representation of the Anatomic/Physiologic ACHD Classification system is represented in **Algorithm 17.1**.

CLINICAL PRESENTATION

It is important to understand that the heterogenous nature of CHD impacts the clinical presentation of this population. In general, the clinical presentation may be affected by the type, number, or magnitude of the underlying defect and repair. Some examples of common congenital defects/patterns and consequences are outlined in **Table 17.1**.

The most anatomically severe or hemodynamically significant derangements generally present soon after birth with cyanosis, heart failure, or cardiovascular collapse and require percutaneous or surgical intervention to remain compatible with life. Initial stabilization may require prostaglandin E to maintain patency of the fetal ductus arteriosus to provide pulmonary blood flow. Critical cardiac lesions palliated by early surgery include: transposition of the great arteries (TGA), aortic coarctation (CoA), hypoplastic ventricles, and obstructed total anomalous pulmonary venous connections (TAPVCs). Modern transcatheter approaches with balloon valvuloplasty can delay or eliminate neonatal surgery for many conditions.

Less severe or small defects may present in adolescent or adulthood without obvious symptoms. Physiologic adaptation to the progressive effects of smaller shunts or slow valve deterioration may go unnoticed until hemodynamic compromise occurs. Patients may present with fatigue, mild exertional complaints, or a new murmur. There are several examples of CHD that may present later in life. For instance, atrial septal defects (ASDs) and partial anomalous pulmonary venous connections (PAPVCs) can evade detection for years and are forms of CHD frequently diagnosed in adulthood. Common auscultatory findings with pre–tricuspid valve shunts, such as an ASD, are wide splitting of the second heart sound and a murmur of pulmonary stenosis, because of the increased flow across the pulmonary valve. Another example of late CHD presentation may include Ebstein anomaly of the tricuspid valve, which is associated with accessory pathways, and may present for evaluation of an abnormal electrocardiogram. Yet another example is the bicuspid aortic valve, which is one of the most common congenital malformations yet if normal function is present and may go undetected. Severe cardiac disease arising from undiagnosed CHD in adulthood is less common, but when present often is a result of inattention to symptoms, avoidance of medical care, or lack of access to health care.

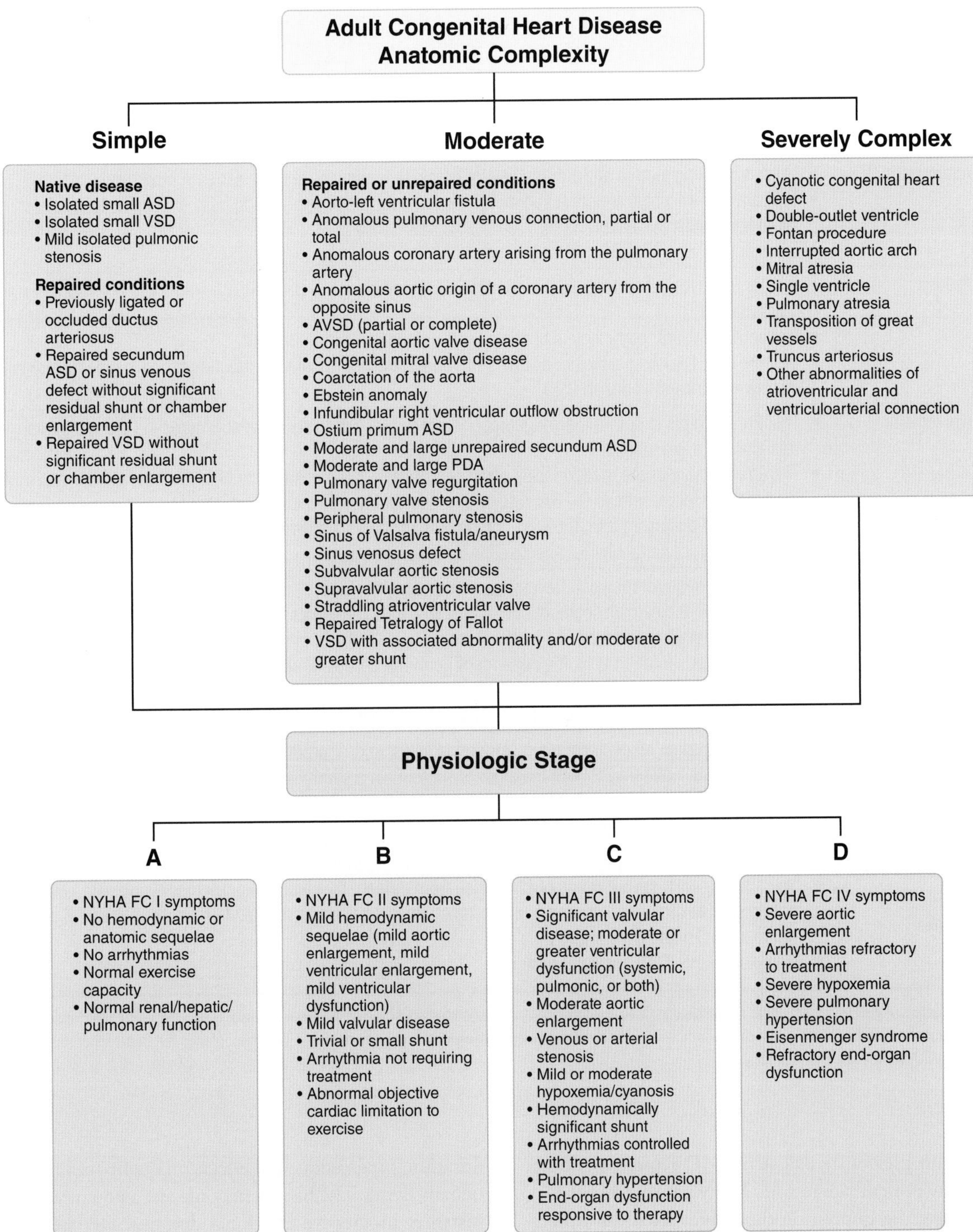

ALGORITHM 17.1 Anatomic and physiologic classification of ACHD disease severity. The most recent guidelines propose both anatomic and physiologic classification of ACHD. ASD, atrial septal defect; AVSD, atrioventricular septal defect; NYHA FC, New York Heart Association functional class; PDA, patent ductus arteriosus; VSD, ventricular septal defect. (From Stout KK, Daniels CJ, Aboulhosn JA, et al. 2018 AHA/ACC guideline for the management of adults with congenital heart disease: executive summary: a report of the American College of Cardiology/American Heart Association Task Force on Clinical Practice Guidelines. *Circulation*. 2019;139:e637-e697.)

TABLE 17.1 Common CHD Patterns and Clinical Presentation

Congenital Defect/Pattern	Consequence
Septal defects Patent communications	• Permits blood flow between structures not normally connected. • Leads to overcirculation and volume and/or pressure loading of the downstream structures. • Typically pre–tricuspid shunts result in right-sided heart enlargement and post–tricuspid shunts result in left-sided heart enlargement. • Examples: ASD, VSD, PDA
Valvular disease	• Similar to valvular structures in the normal heart, valves in CHD patients are subject to both stenosis and regurgitation. • Frequently, valvular pathology is observed in combination with other CHD. • In some cases, such as a bicuspid valve with unrepaired ventricular septal defect, there may be higher risk of infective endocarditis due to CHD.
Arterial involvement	• There are defects in both the arrangement of and patency of the arterial structures in CHD (pulmonary arterial tree and aorta/branches). • The arrangement of the great vessels often contributes to the complexity of CHD observed (ie, malrotation of the great vessels results in D-TGA, a form of moderate–severely complex CHD). • Stenosis and aneurysm formation are common abnormalities observed in CHD. These findings may be isolated or a part of serial obstructive disease (ie, Shone complex).
Rearrangement cardiac segments	• Abnormal cardiac rotation and development may result in CHD. • In such cases, the cardiac segments (ie, ventricles, atria, great vessels) may result in parallel postnatal circulation or systemic positioning of the morphologic right ventricle and tricuspid valve. • The clinical presentation is highly dependent upon the particular anatomy and cardiac/extracardiac connections. • Examples of rearrangements include: D-TGA, CCTGA, DORV.
Aberrant septation	• Aberrant septation leads to common cambers, valves, and/or great vessels. • These patients may present with the signs/symptoms of a shunt, valvular disease, and/or vascular obstruction or heart failure. • Examples: ASD, AVSD, truncus arteriosus, VSD
Ventricular hypoplasia	• In the most severe form, this is not a survivable lesion without early neonatal intervention. • Typically, the most severe forms of CHD arise from defects that lead to ventricular hypoplasia, and patients that do survive often are left with a single-functioning systemic ventricle via a series of surgical palliations that result in Fontan circulation. • Examples: HLHS, DILV, tricuspid atresia

ASD, atrial septal defect; AVSD, atrioventricular septal defect; CCTGA, congenitally corrected transposition of the great arteries; CHD, congenital heart disease; DILV, double-inlet left ventricle; DORV, double-outlet right ventricle; D-TGA, **dextro-transposition of the great arteries**; HLHS, hypoplastic left heart syndrome; PDA, patent ductus arteriosus; VSD, ventricular septal defect.

Adults with previously palliated CHD represent another group that may present late to care. Many patients report feeling well or have the impression they were "fixed" and therefore did not seek follow-up. Unfortunately, CHD specialists discover hemodynamically significant lesions in approximately 60% of patients with CHD who have been lost to follow-up. In this group, there is a threefold increase in the need for late intervention/surgery.[11]

DIAGNOSIS

The clinical workup of ACHD patients, both repaired and unrepaired, should begin with a thorough history and physical examination (**Algorithms 17.2** and **17.3**). The medical history should focus on symptoms and associated features such as duration, progression, and effects on quality of life or activities of daily living. The history may suggest a potential etiology, for instance, progressive exertional dyspnea, exercise intolerance, and fatigue are common among patients with right ventricular volume overload (ie, ASD, Ebstein anomaly, pulmonary insufficiency from transannular patch repair in Tetralogy of Fallot, etc.) or pressure overload (ie, pulmonary stenosis, pulmonary hypertension). Lower extremity claudication or cramping suggests limitation of lower extremity blood flow, such as in coarctation of the aorta, and chest pain may be due to subendocardial ischemia from obstructive left-sided lesions (aortic stenosis) or coronary anomalies.

Physical examination, in turn, should also focus on generating a differential diagnosis. To start, it is important to take note of dysmorphic features, which often suggests a genetic

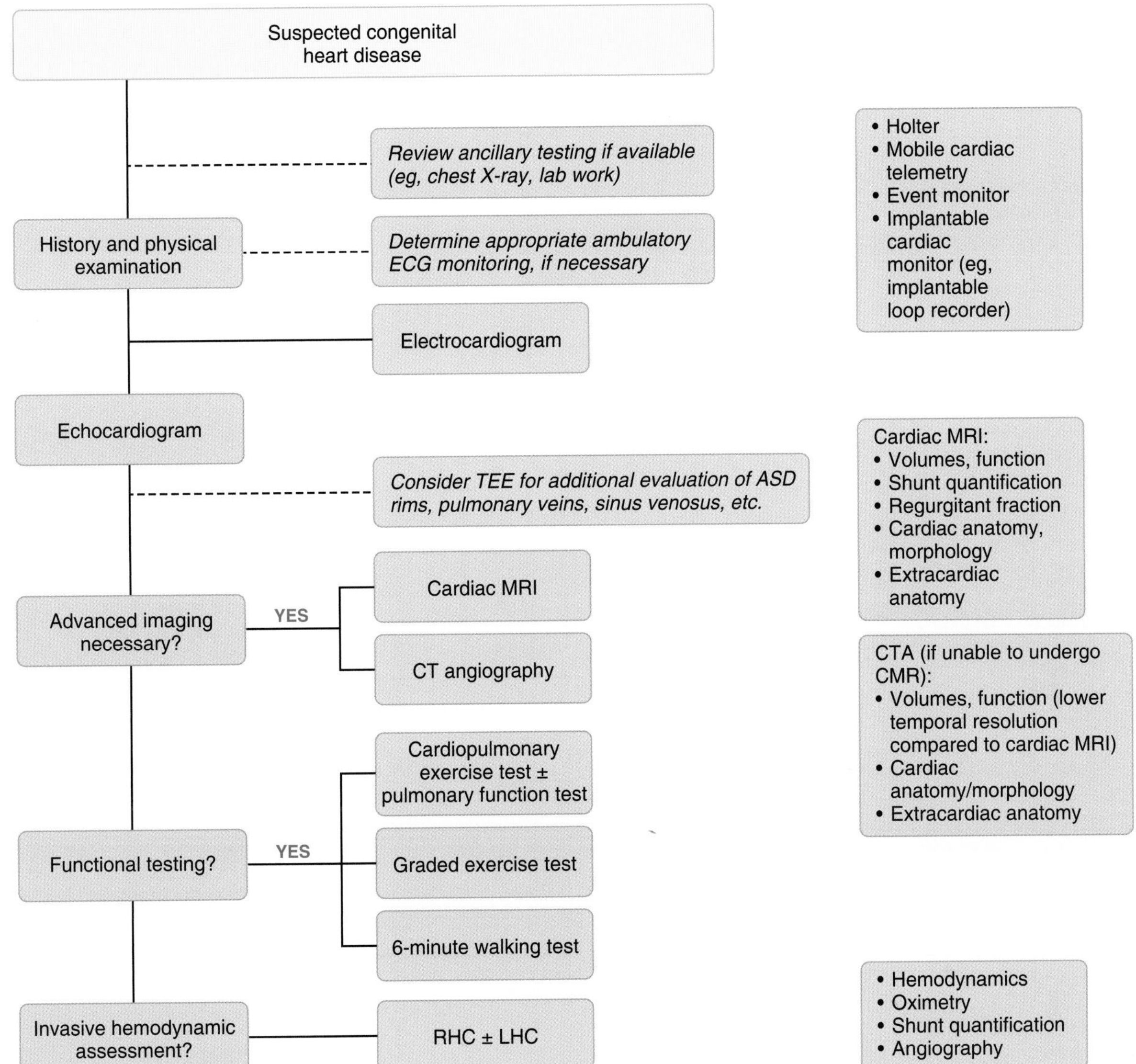

ALGORITHM 17.2 Approach to suspected congenital heart disease in the adult. Evaluation of an adult with suspected congenital heart disease. Diagnostic algorithm typically starts with history and physical examination, followed by appropriate diagnostic testing. Cardiac catheterization is typically reserved for cases in which invasive hemodynamic assessment is necessary. ASD, atrial septal defect; CMR, cardiac magnetic resonance; CT, computed tomography; ECG, electrocardiogram; LHC, left heart catheterization; MRI, magnetic resonance imaging; RHC, right heart catheterization; TEE, transesophageal echocardiogram.

diagnosis that may be associated with specific types of CHD. A list of common genetic syndromes seen in the ACHD population is outlined in **Table 17.2**.

Assessment of the resting vital signs is particularly useful in CHD. Resting pulse oximetry reveals hypoxemia in patients with bidirectional shunting across an intracardiac defect, total admixing lesions as seen in single-ventricle physiology, or right-to-left shunting seen in Eisenmenger syndrome. Blood pressure evaluation may often reveal hypertension, which is highly prevalent in coarctation of the aorta where patients will often have a differential arm/leg gradient as well. Heart rate too may reveal a cause of what is going on, as many patients with CHD are at increased risk of arrhythmia, and often an elevated heart rate is the first clue to this problem.

In the patient with CHD, cardiac auscultation may reveal findings that are similar to the non-congenital population, in that regurgitant and stenotic murmurs are common and not vastly different. However, murmurs should also prompt the clinician to consider a shunt and/or problems with the central or peripheral arterial systems. On full examination, a unique finding that many congenital patients may have is clubbing and/or acrocyanosis. Clubbing or cyanotic discoloration of lips

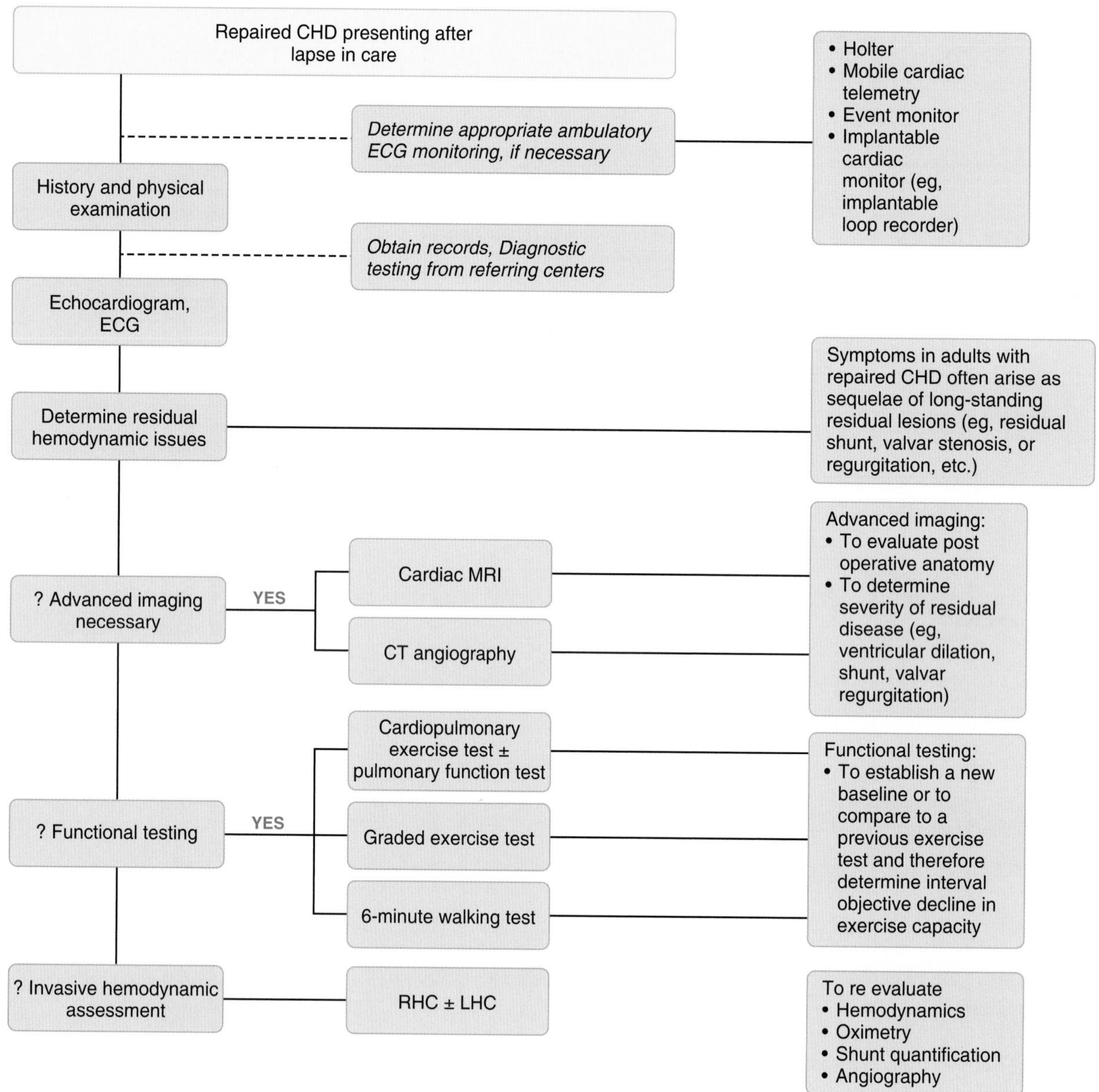

ALGORITHM 17.3 Approach to repaired congenital heart disease in the adult. Evaluation of an adult with repaired congenital heart disease. An important consideration is that symptoms usually arise from residual hemodynamic lesions. Cardiac catheterization is typically reserved for cases in which invasive hemodynamic assessment is necessary. CHD, congenital heart disease; CT, computed tomography; ECG, electrocardiogram; LHC, left heart catheterization; MRI, magnetic resonance imaging; RHC, right heart catheterization.

TABLE 17.2 Common Syndromes Associated with Congenital Heart Disease

Syndrome	Genetic Mutation	Dysmorphic/Associated Features	Associated CHD
22q11.2 deletion (spectrum of conditions including velocardiofacial and DiGeorge syndromes)	Microdeletions in region of 22q11.2	Cleft palate, long face with small mouth and chin, short palpebral fissures, low-set ears, thymic hypoplasia, abnormal immune system with T-cell deficiency, hypocalcemia	Conotruncal defects (eg, ToF, DORV, truncus arteriosus, interrupted aortic arch type B, other aortic arch anomalies)
Alagille	*JAG1, NOTCH2*	Broad forehead, narrow face, small pointed chin, butterfly vertebrae, bile duct paucity	Supravalvular PS (typically peripheral), pulmonary valve stenosis, ToF

TABLE 17.2 Common Syndromes Associated with Congenital Heart Disease (*Continued*)

Syndrome	Genetic Mutation	Dysmorphic/Associated Features	Associated CHD
CHARGE	*CHD7*	**C**oloboma, **H**eart defects, choanal **A**tresia, **G**enital abnormalities and growth retardation, **E**ar abnormalities	Conotruncal defects, aortic arch anomalies, AVSD, VSD
Ehlers-Danlos (type IV)	*COL3A1*	Hypermobility and extensibility (fingers, toes, including easy dislocation), fragile skin (easy bruising, thin skin), pneumothorax	Aortopathy including thoracic aortic aneurysm, vasculopathy with risk for arterial aneurysms and dissection
Ellis-Van Creveld	*EVC, EVC2*	Polydactyly, short limbs, short stature, abnormal teeth	Common atrium (lack of atrial septation), ASD
Goldenhar	*Unknown*	Craniofacial abnormalities (typically affecting one side), cleft palate, deafness	ToF, VSD
Heterotaxy	*Heterogeneous, genes determining laterality, ciliary function*	Abnormal situs or sidedness of visceral organs and lungs, absence or duplication of unilateral structures (eg, asplenia vs polysplenia) bronchiectasis (ie, Kartagener syndrome)	Complex congenital heart disease including univentricular hearts, AVSD, intracardiac situs inversus
Holt-Oram	*TBX5*	Limb anomalies, typically abnormalities with thumbs	ASD
Kabuki	*KMT2D, KDM6A*	Long palpebral fissures, arched eyebrows, long broadened nose, high palate	ASD, VSD
Loeys-Dietz	*TGFBR1-TGFBR2, TGFB2, TGFB3 SMAD3*	Skeletal abnormalities (pectus deformities, pes planus, scoliosis), thin and stretched skin, bifid uvula	Aortopathy including aneurysms of aorta, vasculopathy with aneurysms and tortuosity of large arterial vessels including intracranial arteries
Marfan	*FBN1*	Tall body habitus with long limbs, fingers, and toes, ectopia lentis, myopia, skeletal abnormalities including pectus deformity, pes planus, scoliosis/kyphosis, long face, pneumothorax, skin striae	Aortopathy including aortic root and thoracic aortic aneurysm, MVP, aortic valve dysplasia including BAV
Noonan	*PTPN11, SOS1, RAF1, RIT1*	Down-slanting palpebral fissures, ptosis, hypertelorism, broad forehead, webbed neck	Subvalvar, valvar, and supravalvular PS can all occur, ASD, VSD, ToF
Trisomy 21 (Down syndrome)	Aneuploidy—extra copy of chromosome 21	Upslanting palpebral fissures, epicanthal folds, short stature, endocrine (eg, thyroid) and hematologic (eg, leukemia) dyscrasias	AVSD, ASD, VSD, ToF, PDA
Turner	*45X*—aneuploidy with absence of second X chromosome	Webbed neck, short stature, widely spaced nipples, lymphedema, ovarian dysplasia (variable fertility in mosaic Turner syndrome)	Left-sided obstructive lesions including CoA, BAV, aortopathy/vasculopathy with increased risk for dissection, PAPVR
VACTERL association	Unknown, likely multifactorial	**V**ertebral anomalies, anal **A**tresia, **C**ardiac defects, **T**racheo-**E**sophageal fistula, **R**enal anomalies, **L**imb anomalies	VSD, ASD, ToF
Williams	Microdeletions in region of 7q11.23	"Elfin" facies with broad forehead, short face, sharp chin, and wide mouth, friendly personalities in childhood, with psychiatric issues prevalent in adulthood	Supravalvular aortic stenosis that progresses, coronary ostial stenosis, supravalvular/peripheral PS that may regress or improve

ASD, atrial septal defect; AVSD, atrioventricular septal defect; BAV, bicuspid aortic valve; CHD, congenital heart disease; CoA, coarctation of the aorta; DORV, double-outlet right ventricle; MVP, mitral valve prolapse; PAPVR, partial anomalous pulmonary venous return; PDA, patent ductus arteriosus; PS, pulmonary stenosis; ToF, Tetralogy of Fallot; VSD, ventricular septal defect.

and nail beds suggests the presence of long-standing cyanosis. Differential clubbing with higher oxygen saturations in the right hand compared to the lower extremities, on the other hand, is consistent with right-to-left shunting across a patent ductus arteriosus.

Advanced testing options for the ACHD patient are frequently included in both acute and long-term cardiovascular care. Although the review of individual tests is beyond the scope of this chapter, general principles for various types of testing in the ACHD patient are outlined in **Table 17.3**.

TABLE 17.3 Common Diagnostic Testing in Adult Congenital Heart Disease

Diagnostic Test	Common Findings	Examples
Echocardiogram	Often initial imaging test to evaluate for septal defects, valvular heart disease, aortic arch obstruction, aortic aneurysm, aortic arch anomalies, and complex CHD	• ASD, AVSD, VSD • CoA • Ebstein anomaly • LVOTO • PS • Univentricular heart • CCTGA
Transesophageal echocardiogram	Typically reserved after initial surface echocardiogram to further characterize septal defects, pulmonary veins, ventricular outflow tract obstruction, or valvular heart disease	• Sinus venosus ASD • Ebstein anomaly • LVOTO such as subaortic membrane
Electrocardiogram (ECG)	Useful to establish baseline ECG abnormalities, assess for arrhythmia during clinical encounter, screen for cardiac chamber enlargement, conduction systemic abnormalities	• RBBB in repaired ToF • LAD (eg, in AVSD) • Massive right atrial enlargement (eg, Ebstein anomaly)
Ambulatory ECG monitor	Such as Holter, mobile cardiac telemetry, event monitors, and implantable cardiac monitors used to evaluate for arrhythmias and ectopy, which can be correlated with patient symptoms on corresponding patient diaries or triggers	• Ectopy • AF, AFL/IART • SVT • VT
Exercise testing	With CPET: physiologic parameters or indices of exercise capacity (peak VO_2, VE/VCO_2, etc.). With CPET and other forms of exercise testing: exercise-induced symptoms, ECG changes, arrhythmias, heart rate response, blood pressure response	• Evaluate exercise capacity in various repaired and unrepaired forms of CHD
Pulmonary function test	Spirometric measures of pulmonary function to characterize various lung disease patterns including obstruction or restriction	• Restrictive lung disease pattern in patients with history of sternotomy (and multiple sternotomies), scoliosis
Cardiac magnetic resonance imaging (CMRI)	Noninvasive gold standard for quantification of ventricular volumes and function, quantification of valve regurgitation, tissue characterization (eg, myocardial fibrosis), anatomic assessment	• Repaired ToF with pulmonary insufficiency and progressive RVE • Quantification of shunt in ASD • Quantification of aortic regurgitation in BAV • Aortopathies
Computed tomography angiography (CTA)	Advanced imaging using contrast-enhanced CT for anatomic assessment with highest spatial resolution	• Anomalous coronary arteries • PAPVR • Aortopathies • CoA • Peripheral PS
Cardiac catheterization	Invasive method of assessment to measure oximetry (and thereby calculate shunts and cardiac output by Fick equation), pressure gradients across stenosis, intracardiac filling pressures, and PVR	• Baffle stenosis or leak in D-TGA s/p atrial switch • ASD, VSD • CoA • PAPVR • Fontan • Conduit stenosis in ToF or other CHD repaired with use of RV-PA conduit

AF, atrial fibrillation; AFL, atrial flutter; ASD, atrial septal defect; AVSD, atrioventricular septal defect; BAV, bicuspid aortic valve; CCTGA, congenitally corrected transposition of the great arteries; CHD, congenital heart disease; CoA, coarctation of the aorta; CPET, cardiopulmonary exercise test; D-TGA, **D-TRANSPOSITION OF THE GREAT ARTERIES**; IART, intra-atrial reentrant tachycardia; LAD, left anterior descending artery; LVOTO, left ventricular outflow tract obstruction; PAPVR, partial anomalous pulmonary venous return; PS, pulmonary stenosis; PVR, pulmonary vascular resistance; RVE, right ventricular enlargement; RV-PA, right ventricle to pulmonary artery; SVT, supraventricular tachycardia; ToF, Tetralogy of Fallot; VE/VCO_2, ventilatory efficiency; VO_2, oxygen consumption; VSD, ventricular septal defect; VT, ventricular tachycardia.

MANAGEMENT AND SPECIAL CONSIDERATIONS

Management for CHD requires individualized planning based on the specific lesion, interventional history, and clinical presentation. Ambulatory patients may not present overtly with symptoms that expose the underlying problem. Surveillance for complications of native defects and/or surgical repair is often performed using multiple modalities. A comprehensive approach includes patient education, family planning, and access to noncardiovascular specialists familiar with CHD. Acute presentations commonly include heart failure and arrhythmia, which are generally managed, first by ruling out a new hemodynamically significant lesion and offering correction, followed by traditional therapies similar to that in non-CHD populations. However, the pharmacologic armamentarium may be limited or without clear benefit in certain forms of complex CHD. With disease recurrence or progression, repeat intervention or consideration for transplant may be necessary.

Medical Approach

General recommendations for healthy lifestyles in patients with CHD include healthy diet and exercise. Specifically in CHD, better exercise capacity is associated with improved outcomes including quality of life. Higher levels of physical activity are associated with better patient-reported quality of mental health, physical health, and exercise capacity, independent of patient heterogeneity.[12] That said, exercise capacity is reduced in CHD compared to the general population and varies greatly across different congenital diagnoses.[13] Additionally, performance on exercise testing has been shown to correlate with rate of hospitalization and survival in ACHD.[14] For all of these reasons, it is important to emphasize healthy choices and active lifestyle in the adult CHD patient.

ACHD patients are at risk not only for cardiac issues related to their original defect or repair. They may also develop acquired conditions such as coronary artery disease, hyperlipidemia, or other conditions that portend increased cardiovascular risk (obesity, diabetes mellitus).[15] This is especially true as the ACHD population continues to increase and grow in age. As in the general population, prevalence of risk factors for acquired heart disease increases with age, and providers should continue to screen patients for modifiable risk factors so that they may provide appropriate counseling or intervention. Current guidelines in the management of lipid disorders may be applied in ACHD patients, and good control of hypertension, treatment of obstructive sleep apnea, and smoking cessation are all necessary.

Medication prescription is generally recommended based upon individualized assessment and whether or not there are comorbid conditions associated with CHD. In CHD patients with arrhythmia and heart failure, standard cardiovascular medications are often prescribed similarly to the same disease in patients with normal cardiac anatomy. Common medications and their indication in the ACHD population are outlined in **Table 17.4**.

TABLE 17.4 Common Medications Prescribed in the ACHD Population

Medication Class	CHD Use	Considerations
Beta-blocker	• LVHF • Arrhythmia, rate control	• Minimal data in RVHF
Calcium channel blocker	• Arrhythmia, rate control	• Use caution in heart failure
RAAS inhibition	• LVHF • Fontan circulation	• Minimal data in RVHF, Fontan failure
Mineralocorticoid receptor antagonist	• LVHF • Fontan circulation	• Minimal data in RVHF, Fontan failure
Diuretic	• LVHF/RVHF • Fontan circulation	• Reduce symptoms and congestion, caution with preload-dependent physiology (ie, Fontan)
Corticosteroid (oral budesonide, prednisone)	• Fontan circulation	• Budesonide first choice for protein-losing enteropathy (caution use with hepatic dysfunction or malignancy)
Pulmonary vasodilators (PDE5i, ERA, prostacyclin)	• Pulmonary arterial hypertension • Eisenmenger physiology • Fontan circulation	• Caution with reproductive potential (ERAs are teratogenic and contraindicated in pregnancy)
Antiarrhythmic therapy (flecainide, propafenone, sotalol, amiodarone, dofetilide)	• SVT/IART • VT	• Complex CHD with any dysfunctional ventricle (amiodarone or dofetilide) • Simple CHD without ventricular hypertrophy or dysfunction (any listed)

ACHD, adult congenital heart disease; CHD, congenital heart disease; ERA, endothelin receptor antagonist; IART, intraatrial reentrant tachycardia; LVHF, left ventricular heart failure; PDE5i, phosphodiesterase inhibitor type 5; RAAS, renin-angiotensin-aldosterone system; RVHF, right ventricular heart failure; SVT, supraventricular tachycardia; VT, ventricular tachycardia.

Percutaneous Interventions

Modern catheter-based approaches and technology have led to percutaneous treatment options for both native and postoperative CHD. Many patients who require a surgical intervention to correct an anatomic or physiologic abnormality will require subsequent intervention. Transcatheter procedures avoid many of the risks associated with cardiothoracic surgery and result in shorter hospitalization while either eliminating or delaying the need for (re)operation. Indications for percutaneous treatments are well described and vary based on the specific type of defect.[10] In unoperated CHD, angioplasty of stenotic valves, arterial stenoses, and device closure of shunts may be accomplished percutaneously. However, it is important that these patients be evaluated by a team with expertise and experience in the care of the ACHD patient, as there are many nuances, such as concomitant pulmonary arterial hypertension, that may require medical therapy prior to consideration for percutaneous intervention. Currently available transcatheter devices in the United States are outlined in **Table 17.5**.

Surgical Approach

Cardiothoracic surgery forms the foundation of definitive palliation and/or repair for most forms of CHD. Contemporary surgical techniques have evolved for even the most complex anatomy including transposition of cardiac segments, complex atrioventricular septal malformations, and the functionally univentricular heart. In the present era, initial operation on adults is commonly for late diagnosis of congenital defects (ie, anomalous pulmonary venous connections, ASDs, bicuspid aortic valve). Repeat surgery occurs in one-third of CHD patients, most commonly for pulmonary valve replacement, conduit reoperations, arrhythmia management or device placement, and Fontan palliation.[16]

Surgeons and operative teams with experience in congenital heart surgery are generally recommended to perform procedures on ACHD patients. Predictors of early surgical morbidity include: prior sternotomy, prolonged aortic cross-clamp time, cyanosis, and emergent indication.[17] Risk factors for surgical mortality or major adverse events include: cerebrovascular disease, advanced New York Heart Association class, left heart surgery, and multiple concomitant major operations.[18] Therefore, surgical assessment in adults with CHD involve consideration of the underlying diagnosis, comorbidity, and prior interventional history in conjunction with an experienced team in the care of adults with CHD, in particular, as many of these patients go on to require late consideration for advanced heart failure and transplantation options.

FOLLOW-UP PATIENT CARE

Adults with CHD require lifelong care, and despite surgical interventions, their CHD is not considered "fixed" or "cured." Residual hemodynamic lesions may progress over years and manifest as new symptoms in previously well patients. An appropriate surveillance strategy in many patients is to establish a baseline and then monitor with serial testing over time to detect late manifestations prior to symptomatology. Multiple

TABLE 17.5 Common Transcatheter Occlusion Devices and Pulmonary Valves Used in ACHD

	Device	Description	Sizes
Septal defect closure devices	Amplatzer™ Atrial Septal Occluder (Abbott, Co.)	Differently sized disks of nitinol metal wire mesh connected by a wide waist	Designed for 3-38 mm defects
	Amplatzer™ Cribriform Multifenestrated Septal Occluder (Abbott, Co.)	Equally sized disks of nitinol metal wire mesh connected by a thin waist	Designed with disk diameters from 18 to 40 mm
	Amplatzer™ Muscular VSD Occluder (Abbott, Co.)	Double disk device of nitinol wire mesh connected by a waist corresponding to the size of the defect (Humanitarian Device Exemption for postinfarction VSDs)	Muscular defect sizes 4-18 mm (16-24 mm sizes for postinfarct VSDs)
	GORE® CARDIOFORM Septal Occluder (Gore and Associates, Inc.)	Two corkscrew-like disks of nitinol wire frame covered by an expanded polytetrafluoroethylene coating	Three sizes available, designed to close ASD or PFO up to 17 mm in diameter
	GORE® CARDIOFORM ASD Occluder (Gore and Associates, Inc.)	Hourglass-like shape from a nitinol wire frame covered by an expanded polytetrafluoroethylene coating	Five sizes designed to close 8-35 mm defects
Prosthetic pulmonary valves	Melody™ valve (Medtronic, Inc.)	Bovine jugular vein Platinum iridium stent	Two sizes: expandable to 20 and 22 mm diameters
	SAPIEN® XT (Edwards Lifesciences, Corp.)	Bovine pericardial valve Cobalt chromium frame	Three sizes: expandable to 23, 26, and 29 mm diameters

ACHD, adult congenital heart disease; ASD, atrial septal defect; PFO, patent foramen ovale; VSD, ventricular septal defect.

surgical or transcatheter interventions may be necessary in the course of a patient's life, and newer techniques or devices may become available by the time a patient requires a repeat intervention. In addition, additional comorbidities affecting other systems, such as neuropsychiatric issues or respiratory comorbidities like restrictive lung disease, require specialized care and coordination of services.

Emphasis on lifelong care should begin in childhood and continue throughout visits and the transition process with the pediatric cardiology clinic. Many patients are lost to follow-up because of various reasons, including feeling well, loss of insurance, and inability to find an ACHD provider to whom he or she can transition care.[19] It is important to educate about the need for lifelong follow-up, so that appropriate steps can be taken by both the pediatric cardiologist and families to identify potential obstacles to continuation of care and therefore ensure a smooth transition.

KEY POINTS

- ✔ ACHD patients require specialized lifelong CHD care by an experienced and specialized team.
- ✔ CHD in the adult is a diverse group of disease that should be stratified based upon underlying anatomy and physiology.
- ✔ The clinical presentation in ACHD patients is as diverse given the heterogeneity in the underlying defect and prior repair.
- ✔ Adults with CHD are at risk for late cardiovascular and extracardiac disease and should be monitored to determine if and when further intervention or therapy is indicated.
- ✔ Medical care for the ACHD patient is highly specialized and requires the integration of understanding nuances of CHD and the natural history of these defects and prior repairs, which may result in the need for evaluation of percutaneous or surgical intervention into adulthood.

REFERENCES

1. Marelli AJ, Ionescu-Ittu R, Mackie AS, Guo L, Dendukuri N, Kaouache M. Lifetime prevalence of congenital heart disease in the general population from 2000 to 2010. *Circulation.* 2014;130:749-756.
2. Warnes CA, Liberthson R, Danielson GK, et al. Task Force 1: the changing profile of congenital heart disease in adult life. *J Am Coll Cardiol.* 2001;37:1170-1175.
3. Hoffman JI, Kaplan S. The incidence of congenital heart disease. *J Am Coll Cardiol.* 2002;39:1890-1900.
4. Botto LD, Correa A, Erickson JD. Racial and temporal variations in the prevalence of heart defects. *Pediatrics.* 2001;107:E32.
5. Talner CN. Report of the New England Regional Infant Cardiac Program, by Donald C. Fyler, MD, *Pediatrics*, 1980;65(suppl):375–461. *Pediatrics.* 1998;102:258-259.
6. Ferencz C, Rubin JD, McCarter RJ, et al. Congenital heart disease: prevalence at livebirth. The Baltimore-Washington Infant Study. *Am J Epidemiol.* 1985;121:31-36.
7. Mylotte D, Pilote L, Ionescu-Ittu R, et al. Specialized adult congenital heart disease care: the impact of policy on mortality. *Circulation.* 2014;129:1804-1812.
8. Lilly LS; Harvard Medical School. *Pathophysiology of Heart Disease: A Collaborative Project of Medical Students and Faculty.* 5th ed. Wolters Kluwer/ Lippincott Williams & Wilkins; 2011.
9. Bouma BJ, Mulder BJ. Changing landscape of congenital heart disease. *Circ Res.* 2017;120:908-922.
10. Stout KK, Daniels CJ, Aboulhosn JA, et al. 2018 AHA/ACC guideline for the management of adults with congenital heart disease: executive summary: a report of the American College of Cardiology/American Heart Association Task Force on Clinical Practice Guidelines. *Circulation.* 2019;139:e637-e697.
11. Yeung E, Kay J, Roosevelt GE, Brandon M, Yetman AT. Lapse of care as a predictor for morbidity in adults with congenital heart disease. *Int J Cardiol.* 2008;125:62-65.
12. Muller J, Amberger T, Berg A, et al. Physical activity in adults with congenital heart disease and associations with functional outcomes. *Heart.* 2017;103:1117-1121.
13. Kempny A, Dimopoulos K, Uebing A, et al. Reference values for exercise limitations among adults with congenital heart disease. Relation to activities of daily life—single centre experience and review of published data. *Eur Heart J.* 2012;33:1386-1396.
14. Diller GP, Dimopoulos K, Okonko D, et al. Exercise intolerance in adult congenital heart disease: comparative severity, correlates, and prognostic implication. *Circulation.* 2005;112:828-835.
15. Lui GK, Fernandes S, McElhinney DB. Management of cardiovascular risk factors in adults with congenital heart disease. *J Am Heart Assoc.* 2014;3:e001076.
16. Jacobs JP, Mavroudis C, Quintessenza JA, et al. Reoperations for pediatric and congenital heart disease: an analysis of the Society of Thoracic Surgeons (STS) Congenital Heart Surgery Database. *Semin Thorac Cardiovasc Surg Pediatr Card Surg Annu.* 2014;17:2-8.
17. Talwar S, Kumar MV, Sreenivas V, Choudhary SK, Sahu M, Airan B. Factors determining outcomes in grown up patients operated for congenital heart diseases. *Ann Pediatr Cardiol.* 2016;9:222-228.
18. Kogon B, Grudziak J, Sahu A, et al. Surgery in adults with congenital heart disease: risk factors for morbidity and mortality. *Ann Thorac Surg.* 2013;95:1377-1382; discussion 1382.
19. Gurvitz M, Valente AM, Broberg C, et al; Alliance for Adult Research in Congenital Cardiology and Adult Congenital Heart Association. Prevalence and predictors of gaps in care among adult congenital heart disease patients: HEART-ACHD (The Health, Education, and Access Research Trial). *J Am Coll Cardiol.* 2013;61:2180-2184.

CHAPTER 18

PREGNANCY AND HEART DISEASE

Alice Chan, Ayesha Salahuddin, Diana Wolfe, and Ali N. Zaidi

INTRODUCTION

Cardiac disease is a leading cause of morbidity and mortality in pregnant women.[1] An increased prevalence of cardiovascular disease (CVD) has been found in women of childbearing age, in which the responsibility of the treating physician extends to the unborn fetus. As a result, care of these high-risk patients often requires a team approach including specialists in maternal-fetal medicine, cardiology, and obstetric anesthesiology. The body undergoes significant amounts of physiologic changes during this period of time, and the underlying cardiac disease can affect both the mother and the fetus. Cardiac medications are usually needed for one out of three women with CVD and may have side effects that lead to additional fetal risks. This chapter will review the epidemiology and risk factors of cardiac disease in pregnancy, the physiologic cardiovascular changes that occur with pregnancy, and the management of pregnant women with various cardiovascular conditions.

Epidemiology

Historically, rheumatic heart disease was the most common form of cardiac disease encountered in pregnant women. It continues to be prevalent in developing countries, but more recently, congenital heart disease has become the most common form of heart disease complicating pregnancy in the United States. Mortality has been increasing throughout the years for women in pregnancy, with a maternal mortality of approximately 1%-2% of pregnancies.[2,3] It increased from 9.1 deaths per 100,000 live births in 1987-1990 to 11.5 deaths in 1991-1997 to 14.5 deaths in 1998-2005 and to 16.0 deaths per 100,000 live births in 2006-2010. According to national data from 2006 to 2010, cardiovascular conditions and cardiomyopathy resulted in 15.5% and 11.0% of these deaths, respectively. In 2011 to 2013, the mortality further increased to approximately 17.0 deaths per 100,000 live births in women with pregnancies,[4] with 43.5 deaths in black women, 12.7 deaths in white women, and 14.4 deaths in women of other races per 100,000 live births.

Approximately 40.5% of deaths from pregnancy are from cardiac-related conditions such as cardiomyopathy, CVD, and hypertensive disorders. Some of the adverse events seen in pregnant women with hypertension include fetal growth restriction (4%), placental abruption (1%), and preterm delivery (26%).[5] For women with known cardiomyopathy with symptomatic heart failure from congenital heart disease, primary cardiac events occurred in 13%, fetuses small for gestational age in 20%, and fetal and neonatal death in 2% of the pregnancies.[6]

Cardiac disease complicates about 1%-4% of all pregnancies in the developed world and is a major cause of nonobstetric morbidity and mortality.[7] Because of advances in medical care, increasing numbers of women with congenital and acquired heart disease are becoming pregnant and delivering safely. Hypertensive disease is the most common cardiovascular disorder in pregnancy occurring in 5%-10% cases. With the development of advanced medical and surgical therapies, more than 85% of children with congenital heart disease are expected to reach adulthood. Naturally, a greater number of women with underlying congenital heart disease are becoming pregnant. However, in the developing world, rheumatic heart disease is still a significant contributor to maternal morbidity and mortality in pregnant women.[8]

Risk Factors

Women with cardiac disease are at a higher risk of cardiovascular and neonatal complications during their pregnancy.[9,10] The morbidity and mortality risks of the mother and the neonate will depend on the severity of the cardiac condition.[11,12] Some of these complications include preterm labor, preeclampsia, miscarriage, intrauterine fetal death, and postpartum hemorrhage[1,13] Arrhythmias and heart failure may also manifest during pregnancy in women with cardiac disease.[11]

In the Western world, women are increasingly having children later in life. With advanced maternal age, the incidence of acquired cardiovascular risk factors increases, including diabetes, hypertension, hyperlipidemia, coronary artery disease, and obesity. These comorbidities can complicate pregnancy and lead to poor maternal and neonatal outcomes.[1]

For healthy women without a history of cardiovascular or congenital heart disease, the chance of their offspring having congenital heart disease is 1 in 100. However, if either of the parents has congenital heart disease, then the risk of them passing it to their children ranges from 3% to 50% depending on their particular cardiac defect.[1,14] For first-degree relatives of individuals with CHD, the prevalence of congenital heart disease in their children is approximately 1%-5%. Hence, pregnant women who have family members with congenital heart disease are often referred for a fetal echocardiogram.

Risk factors for coronary artery disease, such as drug use, alcohol use, smoking, diabetes, and hypertension, also increase the risk of cardiac morbidity and mortality in pregnancy.

Additional risk factors for peripartum cardiomyopathy have been identified: African race, preeclampsia, and a family history of cardiomyopathy.[15] Studies have suggested that there may be a genetic predisposition to developing peripartum cardiomyopathy. A genetic study of 172 patients with postpartum cardiomyopathy showed mutations in common with dilated cardiomyopathy.[16]

RISK ASSESSMENT

It is important to have a proper risk assessment for women of childbearing age with known CVD.[17] Preconception counseling can help inform patients of their risk of pregnancy. In some cases, the individual's cardiac status requires optimization before pregnancy. Additionally, teratogenic medications have to be exchanged for safer options. For women considering fertility treatments, the risk and benefits of these treatments with regard to cardiac disease can be evaluated during prepregnancy counseling. Women with congenital heart disease and an identified genetic mutation may consider preimplantation genetic screening. In women who choose not to become pregnant, safe contraception is an important consideration.[18]

Risk assessment includes a detailed history and physical examination, a 12-lead electrocardiogram, and transthoracic echocardiogram. When needed, advanced imaging including cardiac computerized tomography and magnetic resonance imaging can provide valuable additional details. Certain valvular conditions, cardiomyopathies, and complex congenital heart disease might require exercise testing or cardiopulmonary testing to complete risk assessment.

Different risk estimation scores and algorithm have been developed based on large population-based studies. The CARPREG (CARdiac disease in PREGnancy) risk score includes four predictors[7,19] (**Table 18.1**). Women with a score of zero and no lesion-specific risks are considered low risk, whereas women with a risk score of one or more require a comprehensive evaluation. The CARPREG II risk index added more predictors[20] (**Table 18.2**). ZAHARA (Zwangerschap bij vrouwen met een Aangeboren HARtAfwijking-II) investigators assessed pregnancy-related complications in women with congenital heart disease[21] (**Table 18.3**) and developed a weighted risk score, which includes eight predictors with each quintile of score assigning a maternal risk of cardiovascular complications during pregnancy ranging from 2.9% to 70%. The most widely used risk classification system, which is recommended by the European Society of Cardiology, is the modified World Health Organization (mWHO) classification (**Table 18.4**).[1,22] The mWHO classification categorizes patients into four pregnancy

TABLE 18.1 CARPREG Risk Score

Predictors of Adverse Cardiovascular Events	Points
• Prior cardiac event (heart failure, transient ischemic attack) • Infarction prior to pregnancy or arrhythmia	1
• NYHA functional class at baseline > II or cyanosis	1
• Left heart obstruction (mitral valve area <2.0 cm²) • Aortic valve area <1.5 cm² • Left ventricular outflow tract gradient >30 mm Hg	1
• Reduced systolic ventricular function (ejection fraction <40%)	1

CARPREG, Cardiac Disease in Pregnancy; NYHA, New York Heart Association

TABLE 18.2 CARPREG II Risk Score

Predictors of Adverse Cardiovascular Events	Weighted Score
History of arrhythmias	1.5
Cardiac medications before pregnancy	1.5
NYHA functional class prior to pregnancy ≥II	0.75
Left heart obstruction (PG >50 mmHg or AVA <1 cm²)	2.5
Systemic atrioventricular valve regurgitation (moderate/severe)	0.75
Pulmonary atrioventricular valve regurgitation (moderate/severe)	0.75
Mechanical valve prosthesis	4.25
Cyanotic heart disease (corrected/uncorrected)	1.0

AVA, aortic valve area; LVEF, left ventricular ejection fraction; NYHA, New York Heart Association; PG, pressure gradient;

TABLE 18.3 ZAHARA Risk Score

Predictors of Adverse Cardiovascular Events	Points
• Prior cardiac events or arrhythmias	3
• Baseline NYHA III-IV or cyanosis	3
• Mechanical valve	3
• Systemic ventricular dysfunction (LVEF <55%)	2
• High-risk valve disease or • LVOTO (AVA <1.5 cm², subaortic gradient >30 mm Hg or moderate to severe mitral regurgitation, mitral stenosis <2.0 cm²)	2
• Pulmonary hypertension • RVSP >49 mm Hg	2
• Coronary artery disease	2
• High-risk aortopathy	2
• No prior cardiac intervention	1
• Late pregnancy assessment	1

AVA, aortic valve area; LVEF, left ventricular ejection fraction; LVOTO, left ventricular outflow tract obstruction; NYHA, New York Heart Association; RVSP, right ventricular systolic pressure; ZAHARA, Zwangerschap bij vrouwen met een Aangeboren HARtAfwijking.

TABLE 18.4 Modified World Health Organization (mWHO) Classification

WHO Classification		
I	Uncomplicated small or mild PS PDA Mitral valve prolapse Successfully repaired simple lesions (ASD, VSD, PDA, PAPVC)	No detectable increased risk of maternal mortality and no/mild increase in morbidity.
II	Unrepaired ASD or VSD Unrepaired tetralogy of Fallot	Small increase in maternal risk mortality or moderate increase in morbidity.
II-III	Mild left ventricular impairment Hypertrophic cardiomyopathy Native or tissue valvular heart disease not considered WHO I or IV Marfan syndrome without aortic dilation Aorta <45 mm in association with BAV Repaired coarctation	Small to moderate increase in maternal risk mortality or moderate increase in morbidity.
III	Mechanical valve Systemic right ventricle Fontan circulation Unrepaired cyanotic heart disease Other complex congenital heart disease Aortic dilation 40-45 mm in Marfan syndrome Aortic dilation 45-50 mm in BAV	Significantly increased risk of maternal mortality or severe morbidity. Expert counseling required. If pregnancy is decided upon, intensive specialist cardiac and obstetric monitoring needed throughout pregnancy, childbirth, and the puerperium.
IV (Conditions in which pregnancy contraindicated)	PAH of any cause Severe systemic ventricular dysfunction (LVEF <30%, NYHA functional class III-IV) Previous peripartum cardiomyopathy with any residual impairment of left ventricular function Severe MS, severe asymptomatic AS Marfan syndrome with aorta dilated >45 mm Aortic dilation of >50 mm in aortic disease associated with BAV Native severe coarctation	

AS, aortic stenosis; ASD, atrial septal defect; BAV, bicuspid aortic valve; LVEF, left ventricular ejection fraction; LVOTO, left ventricular outflow tract obstruction; MS, mitral stenosis; NYHA, New York Heart Association; PAH, pulmonary arterial hypertension; PAPVC, partial anomalous pulmonary venous connection; PDA, patent ductus arteriosus; PS, pulmonary stenosis; VSD, ventricular septal defect; WHO, World Health Organization.

Data compiled from Regitz-Zagrosek V, Roos-Hesselink JW, Bauersachs J, et al. 2018 ESC Guidelines for the management of cardiovascular diseases during pregnancy: The Task Force for the Management of Cardiovascular Diseases during Pregnancy of the European Society of Cardiology (ESC). *Eur Heart J.* 2018;39:3165-3241; Thorne S, MacGregor A, Nelson-Piercy C. Risks of contraception and pregnancy in heart disease. *Heart.* 2006;92:1520-1525.

risk classes, class I-IV.[22] When compared with the mWHO classification, both CARPREG and ZAHARA underestimate the cardiac risk for low-risk pregnancies.[10,23]

Women with cardiac disease are also at a higher risk of obstetric complications including miscarriage, preterm delivery, premature rupture of membranes, and postpartum hemorrhage. There is also an increased risk of adverse neonatal outcomes in women with cardiac disease. Cardiomyopathy and pulmonary hypertension portend the highest risk of obstetric and neonatal complications. Based on the risk assessment, the frequency of antenatal visits and the site and mode of delivery are established. In most cases, vaginal delivery is recommended and is the preferred choice, but some exceptions exist. High-risk patients should be managed at expert centers by a multidisciplinary team that includes cardiologists, obstetricians, maternal-fetal medicine specialists, and cardiac anesthesiologists.

PATHOGENESIS

Physiologic Changes During Pregnancy and Puerperium

Pregnancy has a profound effect on the circulatory system. The major hemodynamic changes induced by pregnancy include an increase in cardiac output, sodium and water retention leading to blood volume expansion, and reductions in systemic vascular resistance and subsequently systemic blood pressure. These changes begin early in pregnancy, reach their peak during the second trimester, and then remain relatively constant until delivery. Cardiac output rises 30%-50% above baseline during normal pregnancy: half occurring as early as 8 weeks' gestation.[24,25] Blood pressure decreases by 10 to 15 mm Hg owing to a decrease in systemic vascular resistance caused by the creation of a low-resistance circuit by the placenta and vasodilation. Additionally, heart rate normally increases by 10 to 15 beats per minute.[25]

The hematocrit level decreases because of a disproportionate increase in plasma volume that exceeds the rise in red cell mass.

Maternal and fetal metabolic requirements increase as pregnancy progresses. This results in a change in the magnitude and distribution of cardiac output during pregnancy to meet these demands. The elevation in cardiac output primarily results from changes in three important factors: increased preload because of the associated rise in blood volume; reduced afterload because of the decline in systemic vascular resistance (see later); and a 15 to 20 beats per minute rise in maternal heart rate. Stroke volume normally increases in the first and second trimester and decreases in the third trimester. This decrease is due to partial vena cava obstruction. During the third trimester, cardiac output is further influenced by body position, where the supine position causes caval compression by the gravid uterus. This leads to a decrease in venous return, which can cause supine hypotension of pregnancy.

Systolic and diastolic blood pressure typically fall early in gestation and continue into the second trimester. In the third trimester, blood pressure gradually increases and may normalize to nonpregnant values by term. The fall in blood pressure is attributed to a reduction in systemic vascular resistance, which in pregnancy appears to parallel changes in afterload.[26] Both creation of a high-flow, low-resistance circuit in the uteroplacental circulation and vasodilation contribute to the decline in systemic vascular resistance. The factors responsible for vasodilation during pregnancy are not well-understood, but one of the major findings is decreased vascular responsiveness to the vasopressor effects of angiotensin II and norepinephrine. Increased responsiveness to endothelial prostacyclin and nitric oxide production is also seen.

Although changes in blood volume during pregnancy affect right ventricular preload, central venous pressure remains unchanged throughout pregnancy. This is due to the reduction in cardiac afterload induced by substantial decreases in both systemic vascular resistance and pulmonary vascular resistance.

Pregnancy is associated with important changes in several coagulation factors. Activated proteins C and S plasma levels decrease, whereas plasma levels of factors I, II, V, VII, VIII, X, and XII increase. Activity of the fibrinolytic inhibitors plasminogen activator inhibitor (PAI)-1 and PAI-2 also increases, though total fibrinolytic activity may not be impaired. The net effect of these pregnancy-induced changes is to produce a hypercoagulable state with increased prothrombin and partial thromboplastin times. As a result, venous thrombosis in pregnancy rarely occurs though it is three- to fourfold higher in the puerperium period: the time from delivery of the placenta through the first few weeks after the delivery. The risk is also increased in women with an underlying inherited thrombophilia, such as factor V Leiden deficiency or prothrombin gene mutation.[27]

Intrapartum Hemodynamic Changes

Normal labor and delivery are associated with significant hemodynamic changes because of anxiety, exertion, pain, uterine contractions, uterine involution, and bleeding. Cardiovascular effects can also occur because of the effects of infection, hemorrhage, or administration of anesthesia or analgesia.

During delivery, cardiac output, heart rate, blood pressure, and systemic vascular resistance increase with each uterine contraction.[38,39] Delivery-related pain and anxiety accentuate the increase in heart rate and blood pressure. During delivery, blood from the uterine sinusoids is forced into the systemic circulation with each uterine contraction, which increases preload. Cardiac output, therefore, increases by 15% above prelabor levels in early labor and by ~25% during the active phase. The additional exertion associated with pushing in the second stage results in a 50% rise in cardiac output. These changes can place an intolerable strain on an abnormal heart, necessitating invasive hemodynamic monitoring and aggressive medical management.[39]

Postpartum Hemodynamic Changes

The postpartum period is marked by significant hemodynamic fluctuations in cardiac output, stroke volume, and heart rate. Within the first 10 minutes following a term vaginal delivery, the cardiac output and stroke volume increase and continue to remain increased up to 1 hour postpartum. The maternal heart rate, however, decreases. The increases in stroke volume and cardiac output most likely result from autotransfusion of uteroplacental blood into the intravascular space, a process associated with uterine involution that is more pronounced than the normal blood loss of delivery (ie, blood loss is typically 300-400 mL during vaginal delivery and 500-800 mL during cesarean [CD] delivery). As the uterus decompresses, a reduction in the mechanical compression of the vena cava further allows for increased preload. Delivery of the placenta increases afterload by removing the low-resistance circulation, and a significant amount of intravascular fluid shift is seen during the postpartum period, especially in the first 24 to 48 hours after birth.[1] Following this, cardiac output and systemic vascular resistance gradually return to nonpregnant levels over a period of 3 months or more.

CLINICAL PRESENTATION

The circulatory and respiratory changes during normal pregnancy are sometimes erroneously attributed to heart disease. As a result, the clinician should be aware of the normal maternal cardiovascular adaptations to pregnancy. Shortness of breath, easy fatigability, decreased exercise tolerance, basal rales that disappear with cough or deep breathing, and peripheral edema commonly occur during normal pregnancy. The jugular venous pulse is more conspicuous after the 20th week, though the mean jugular venous pressure, as estimated from the superficial jugular vein, remains normal in most cases. The pregnant woman's heart is shifted to the left, anterior, and rotated toward a transverse position as the uterus enlarges. The apical impulse is shifted cephalad to the fourth intercostal space and lateral to the midclavicular line. The right ventricle may be palpable because—like the left ventricle—it handles a larger volume of blood that is ejected against a relatively low resistance.

Auscultatory changes accompanying normal gestation begin in the late first trimester and generally disappear within the first week after delivery. A higher basal heart rate, louder heart sounds, wide splitting of S1, splitting of S2 in the third trimester, and a systolic ejection murmur over the pulmonary and tricuspid areas are regularly appreciated. In addition, a third heart sound is present in most pregnant women. The fourth heart sound, however, is rarely heard and its presence may indicate cardiac dysfunction. A venous hum, appreciated best along the sternal border in the second intercostal space, is almost universal in healthy women during gestation. The mammary soufflé (systolic or continuous) heard over the breasts in late gestation is especially common postpartum in lactating women. Diastolic murmurs are uncommon and, like an S4, more often represent a pathologic condition requiring further diagnostic evaluation.

MANAGEMENT OF CARDIOVASCULAR CONDITIONS DURING PREGNANCY

Hypertension

One of the most common cardiac disorders is hypertension, affecting 5%-10% of all pregnancies.[1] High blood pressure in pregnancy is associated with both maternal and fetal morbidity and mortality. Associated complications include organ failure, stroke, placental abruption, intrauterine growth restriction, preterm delivery, and fetal death.[28] Pregnant women with a systolic blood pressure 140 mm Hg or more and/or diastolic blood pressure 90 mm Hg or more are considered hypertensive.[1] Patients with elevated blood pressure may have chronic hypertension or newly diagnosed preeclampsia, which is sometimes difficult to differentiate. There are different classifications of hypertension in pregnancy, which include unclassifiable hypertension, preexisting hypertension, preexisting hypertension with gestational hypertension and proteinuria, preeclampsia, and gestational hypertension.[14,17,28] Medications should be administered to lower the blood pressure in pregnant patients who are hypertensive. The condition of the patient and the potential side effects of the medication on the fetus will determine which medication is ultimately selected for treatment.[1] Research shows that nifedipine, labetalol, and methyldopa are all safe during pregnancy.[2,29]

Congenital Heart Disease

In the United States, congenital heart disease is the most common form of heart disease complicating pregnancy and the largest group of women with underlying cardiac disease presenting with pregnancy have this condition. Some of these defects include atrial septal defect, ventricular septal defect, atrioventricular septal defect, coarctation of the aorta, tetralogy of Fallot, transposition of the great arteries, Ebstein anomaly, and hypoplastic right or left heart syndrome. With advancement in surgery, more and more women with congenital heart disease are surviving and reaching childbearing years. International surveys have shown that approximately two-thirds of pregnant women with cardiac disease have congenital heart disease.

Although the management of individual congenital heart lesions is outside the scope of this chapter, the principles outlined earlier for assessing the presence and severity of valvular heart disease, ventricular dysfunction, arrhythmias, or coronary artery disease still apply. The care of these high-risk patients often requires a multidisciplinary approach including specialists in maternal-fetal medicine, cardiology, and obstetric anesthesiology to optimize outcomes in the peripartum and even late postpartum periods. Nevertheless, most can tolerate the pregnancy and their cardiac defect is rarely the cause of maternal death.[1]

The overall pregnancy risk will depend on not only the mother's congenital heart defect but also their comorbidities and cardiac function. Women with more complex congenital heart defects have a higher risk of maternal and fetal complications, which can include preeclampsia, miscarriage, neonatal death, and maternal death.[1] In women with congenital heart disease, fetal echocardiograms should be performed between 18 and 22 weeks of gestation to assess the cardiac anatomy of the fetus.[30] If there is a major fetal cardiac defect, an ultrasound at 12 weeks' gestation is 85% sensitive and 99% specific in detecting it.[14] However, in smaller fetal cardiac defects, the fetal echocardiogram may not detect the actual lesion until after delivery.

Arrhythmias

Arrhythmias and conduction disturbances can be present prior to or originate during pregnancy.[17] Recurrence of arrhythmias in women with preexisting rhythm disorders is common and usually increases the risk of adverse fetal complications. Factors related to pregnancy that may promote or exacerbate arrhythmias include the hyperdynamic state associated with increased cardiac output and contractility, the altered hormonal milieu, and the presence of underlying heart disease (acquired or congenital). Additionally, some women may need to discontinue certain teratogenic antiarrhythmic medications. **Table 18.5** shows a list of cardiac medications and their safety in pregnancy. Most beta-blockers can be continued during the course of the pregnancy.

Pregnant women with a history of congenital heart disease are more likely to experience tachyarrhythmias compared to those without congenital heart disease. Two of the most common arrhythmias seen are paroxysmal supraventricular tachycardia (PSVT) and atrial fibrillation (AF)[1]: bradyarrhythmias and dangerous rhythms such as ventricular fibrillation and ventricular tachycardia are rare. Percutaneous ablation procedures are infrequently needed during pregnancies for rhythm concerns but should be considered prior to pregnancy if a history of arrhythmias is present. If a tachyarrhythmia develops during pregnancy, medical management can be considered.

The *ESC Guidelines for the Management of Cardiovascular Diseases During Pregnancy* provides recommendations for the treatment of common arrhythmias seen in pregnancy.[1]

- To convert PSVT, first use vagal maneuvers and adenosine.
- Verapamil and beta-blockers are the drugs of choice to prevent PSVT.

TABLE 18.5 Cardiac Medications in Pregnancy

Medications	FDA Category	Pregnancy	Lactation
Adenosine	C	Safe	Use with caution
Alpha-methyldopa	B	Safe	Safe
Amiodarone	D	Contraindicated	Contraindicated
Amlodipine	C	Use with caution	Use with caution
Argatroban	B	Use with caution	Unknown
Aspirin	C	Use with caution	Use with caution
Atenolol	D	Contraindicated	Use with caution
Carvedilol	C	Safe	Unknown
Clonidine	C	Use with caution	Unknown
Clopidogrel	B	Use with caution	Use with caution
Digoxin	C	Safe	Safe
Diltiazem	C	Use with caution	Unknown
Dobutamine	B	Safe	Unknown
Dopamine	C	Safe	Unknown
Enoxaparin	B	Safe	Safe
Epoprostenol	B	Use with caution	Unknown
Flecainide	C	Use with caution	Use with caution
Furosemide	C	Safe	Use with caution
Heparin	C	Safe	Safe
Hydralazine	C	Use with caution	Safe
Hydrochlorothiazide	B	Use with caution	Safe
Isosorbide dinitrate	C	Use with caution	Unknown
Labetalol	C	Safe	Use with caution
Lidocaine	B	Safe	Safe
Metolazone	B	Use with caution	Unknown
Metoprolol	C	Safe	Use with caution
Nifedipine	C	Safe	Safe
Nitroglycerin	C	Use with caution	Unknown
Nitroprusside	C	Use with caution	Use with caution
Norepinephrine	C	Safe	Unknown
Procainamide	C	Use with caution	Use with caution
Propranolol	C	Safe	Use with caution
Sildenafil	B	Use with caution	Use with caution
Sotalol	B	Use with caution	Unknown
Ticagrelor	C	Use with caution	Unknown
Torsemide	B	Use with caution	Unknown
Treprostinil	C	Unknown	Unknown
Verapamil	C	Safe	Safe
Warfarin	D	Use with caution	Safe

Food and Drug Administration (FDA) Categories:
A) Human studies have not shown fetal risk; B) Animal studies have not shown fetal risk; C) Animal studies have shown fetal side effects (no human studies); D) Human studies have shown side effects on the fetus, but medication can be used if there are potential benefits.

- In AF and atrial flutter, atrioventricular nodal blocking agents such as beta-blockers are the preferred choice for rate control.
- In stable women with atrial flutter or AF, ibutilide or flecainide may be administered if the heart is structurally normal.
- In women with Wolff-Parkinson-White syndrome, flecainide or propafenone is recommended for the prevention of supraventricular tachycardia.
- In women with atrial flutter or AF who are not stable, electrical cardioversion is recommended for conversion to sinus rhythm.
- Beta-blockers should be used with caution in women with systemic ventricular dysfunction.
- If a catheter ablation is necessary during the pregnancy, performing it in the second trimester is preferable.

Coronary Artery Disease

Pregnant women have three to four times the risk of nonpregnant women of developing an acute myocardial infarction (MI). Some of the risk factors that contribute to coronary artery disease include hypertension, maternal age, smoking, diabetes, dyslipidemia, and obesity. Although it is not very common for pregnancies to be complicated by acute MI, it contributes to approximately 20% of the cardiac deaths in pregnant women.[1] Nevertheless, women with a history of prior MI, percutaneous coronary interventions (PCIs), coronary artery bypass surgery, or coronary artery disease may still contemplate pregnancy. Baseline left ventricular function should be determined and stress testing should be considered to rule out active ischemia prior to pregnancy. Medications—including certain lipid-lowering therapies, angiotensin-converting enzyme inhibitors, and antiplatelet agents—should be discontinued as these have been shown to have teratogenic effects. Because cessation of medications may have a negative impact on prior coronary interventions or cardiac function, the desire for pregnancy must be weighed carefully with the potential risks.[31] Although MI is a rare event in women of childbearing age, studies have suggested an increased risk during pregnancy and in the early postpartum period. Management of an acute MI in the setting of concurrent pregnancy is guided by the same principles as in the general population. Low-dose aspirin (75-162 mg/day), beta-blockers, and nitrates have been used without apparent harmful effects. Heparin can also be used because it does not cross the placenta and will not affect the fetus directly.[2,32] Complications related to bleeding, however, can become more problematic.[33]

Spontaneous coronary artery dissection (SCAD) is a rare cause of acute coronary syndrome, particularly seen in women during pregnancy or in the puerperium, but it has a high acute mortality rate. Hormonal changes during pregnancy, hemodynamic stress, and changes in the autoimmune status have been considered as possible etiologic factors. In most SCAD patients, conservative therapy is the preferred initial strategy after diagnosis is established. Patients presenting with acute MI with symptoms of ongoing ischemia or hemodynamic compromise should be considered for revascularization with PCI or coronary artery bypass grafting as appropriate.

Cardiomyopathy

Cardiomyopathies may be inherited or acquired and include diagnoses such as peripartum cardiomyopathy, dilated cardiomyopathy, hypertrophic cardiomyopathy, toxic cardiomyopathy, and Takotsubo cardiomyopathy.[34]

In women with hypertrophic cardiomyopathy, pregnancy is generally well tolerated with a mortality rate of 0.5%. The risk of premature birth in these women is increased, but stillbirth and spontaneous abortion rates are similar to the general population.

Women with peripartum cardiomyopathy have impaired left ventricular function (ie, ejection fraction <45%) that typically occurs in late pregnancy or within 6 months of delivery. Dilated cardiomyopathy, on the other hand, not only affects left ventricular function but also results in left ventricular dilation.[34] Dilated cardiomyopathy can be a result of many etiologies including prior drug or alcohol use, ischemia, viral infections, and genetics. Women with dilated cardiomyopathy often do not tolerate pregnancy well and may have worsening ventricular function. Counseling and management with a multidisciplinary team are important because these women are at a higher risk for maternal mortality, fetal loss, and ventricular function deterioration that may not be reversible. Left ventricular ejection fraction less than 40% and New York Heart Association Class III and IV symptoms are predictors of mortality in pregnant women.[35] Heart failure medications (ie, angiotensin-converting enzyme inhibitors and angiotensin receptor blockers) may need to be discontinued to prevent fetal harm for women who are actively trying to conceive and stopped immediately in pregnant women.[36]

Anticoagulation in Pregnancy

Women who are pregnant have hormonal changes that cause an increase in clotting activity, and venous thromboembolism is a major cause of maternal death. For some, their comorbidities and surgical history—such as AF or flutter, mechanical valve replacement, Fontan palliation for single ventricle—can further increase their thrombotic risk[37] and anticoagulation should be considered.[38] However, managing pregnant women who require ongoing anticoagulation for the prophylaxis or treatment of thrombotic complications during the duration of pregnancy can be a challenging dilemma.

There are different modalities for anticoagulation that can be used during pregnancy including warfarin, unfractionated heparin (UFH), and low-molecular-weight heparin (LMWH).[2] Warfarin is the long-term anticoagulant of choice in many nonpregnant patients, but it freely crosses the placental barrier in pregnant women because of its low molecular weight and can cause fetal embryopathy in ~10% of unborn children. The bones and cartilage may be affected in the first trimester, whereas fetal warfarin exposure after the first trimester increases the risk of central nervous system defects. A dose-dependent effect of warfarin on fetal embryopathy has been reported, with warfarin 5 mg per day or less having lower rates of fetal complications than warfarin more than 5 mg per day.[35,36] In a systematic review and meta-analysis of almost 500 patients, warfarin 5 mg or less daily results in minimal fetal and maternal complications and can be used in pregnant women who achieve adequate anticoagulation with this low dose.[39] UFH does not cross the placenta in pregnant women because of its large molecular size and, therefore, does not carry the same risk of embryopathy as warfarin. There are limited data on the use of UFH throughout pregnancy in women with mechanical valves, though some have advocated for the use of UFH in the first trimester, followed by oral anticoagulants during the remainder of pregnancy until closer to delivery.[2]

Studies show that LMWH—such as enoxaparin—is not harmful to the fetus and can be used for the prevention of thromboembolism during pregnancy. It has several advantages over UFH including more predictable therapeutic levels for anticoagulation, less bone demineralization, and less bleeding and thrombocytopenia. Like UFH, LMWH does not cross the placenta.[2] Overall, anticoagulation should be considered for patients with an increased risk of cerebral vascular accident and thromboembolism. However, because there can be major complications with these medications (ie, hemorrhage, premature deliveries, and miscarriages), the risks and benefits should be reviewed carefully and recommendations should come from specialists in the field.[38]

POSTPARTUM MANAGEMENT

Delivery is associated with hemodynamic changes that can lead to heart failure in women with preexisting CVD. In the immediate postpartum period, there are significant changes in the cardiac output and heart rate. Therefore, patients considered to be at high risk for cardiovascular complications require hemodynamic monitoring for at least 24 hours after delivery. In some of the highest risk groups, such as patients with pulmonary hypertension, monitoring could be required for 2 to 4 days. Overall, early ambulation, meticulous leg care, and elastic support stockings are important preventive measures that reduce the risk of thromboembolism postpartum. After expulsion of the placenta, some patients may have prolonged uterine bleeding that can be reduced by uterine massage or intravenous oxytocin administration. Breastfeeding also promotes uterine contraction and is important to initiate. Prostaglandin F analogs and methylergonovine can be used in the event of postpartum hemorrhage but should not be used routinely because of resultant elevation in pulmonary artery and/or systemic blood pressures.[40,41]

Percutaneous Interventions in Pregnancy

Both acute coronary syndromes and classic congenital valve disorders are increasingly being treated successfully with invasive catheterization laboratory techniques even though such procedures carry some degree of risk to the pregnancy. In the general population, PCI is the first-line interventional therapy for acute coronary syndrome. However, PCI in pregnancy exposes the fetus to higher radiation levels compared to a diagnostic angiogram alone. High doses of radiation place the fetus at risk of spontaneous abortion, organ deformation, mental retardation, and childhood cancer. Accordingly, the decision to recommend PCI can present a challenge to obstetricians and interventional cardiologists who are concerned about radiation risk to the developing fetus.[42]

Published data show that physicians who commonly care for pregnant patients may be unfamiliar with the magnitude of radiation risks in pregnancy.[42] Radiation that scatters from the directly irradiated area reaches the fetus, which is only a small fraction of the radiation delivered to the thorax. Chest radiography during PCI results in a mean fetal exposure of 0.02 mSv with a maximum of 0.1 mSv in difficult PCI procedures. Shielding the abdomen and pelvis will not intercept the scattered irradiation. Accordingly, radiation exposure of the fetus before completion of major organogenesis (15 weeks after menses) must be avoided whenever possible. Doses in excess of 50-100 mSv increase the incidence of fetal malformation.

In general, catheterization through the radial artery will keep fetal radiation exposure to a minimum. PCI in pregnancy can be relatively safe given the minimal radiation exposure. However, the use of drug-eluting stents during PCI implies the use of dual antiplatelet agents (ie, aspirin and clopidogrel) in the post-PCI period. Currently, there is no information available about the effects of clopidogrel on the fetus, although animal experiments have not demonstrated teratogenic effects. Because there are no studies in pregnant women, clopidogrel should only be used in pregnancy if clearly needed.

Cardiac Surgical Interventions in Pregnancy

Any cardiac surgery during pregnancy represents a major challenge as it comprises a single operation but two survivors. The presence of valve pathology may result in cardiac decompensation that threatens the lives of both mother and fetus, and unavoidably calls for surgical intervention that might require cardiopulmonary bypass (CPB). Unfortunately, CPB has many potential adverse effects on uteroplacental perfusion and fetal development. In patients with mitral stenosis, which is the case in most scenarios, closed mitral valvulotomy, which is accomplished without CPB, is life saving and offers low feto-maternal risk. It is a viable, efficient, and practical alternative to percutaneous mitral balloon commissurotomy, when the latter cannot be performed. When CPB becomes mandatory, the shortest possible periods of mildly hypothermic or normothermic CPB with a strategy of high-flow, high-pressure perfusion should be followed. There has consistently been a low maternal mortality of approximately 3%, but a fetal mortality up to 30% with such strategy.

The most frequent reason a cardiac intervention is performed during pregnancy is for treatment of severe rheumatic mitral stenosis. This is a major health problem in developing countries. Although the best option is to address severe valvular disease before pregnancy, the symptoms may remain subtle or be masked until late in gestation and manifest only when precipitated by the physiologic changes associated with pregnancy. Hemodynamic decompensation often occurs immediately after delivery, partly because of the relief of caval vein compression resulting in increased venous return. The pulmonary capillary wedge pressure usually increases by 20%-40% during this period. In the presence of mitral stenosis, these elevations in preload can lead to maternal pulmonary edema during the early postnatal period. In such cases, mechanical relief of the stenosis should be considered to treat or prevent pulmonary edema. This can be achieved by percutaneous balloon mitral valvulotomy (PBMV), closed mitral valvulotomy, or open-heart surgery (open mitral valvulotomy or prosthetic valve replacement), although CPB is required with the latter, which is not desirable for the mother or fetus. PBMV is less invasive and carries the risk of radiation exposure that is of particular concern in a pregnant patient. Compared to PBMV, closed mitral valvotomy provides a higher primary success rate, greater valve area augmentation, and better technical control during the procedure.

SPECIAL CONSIDERATIONS

Few cardiac conditions in pregnant women require delivery by CD. There are, on the contrary, many obstetric indications for CD. The major consideration is whether a woman can Valsalva during the second stage of labor, the time period from full cervical dilation to delivery of the fetal head. This can correspond with changes in heart rate and blood pressure, and therefore regional anesthesia is recommended early in the labor process. For many pregnant patients with complex cardiac conditions, application of epidural or spinal anesthesia will require multidisciplinary planning. Siu et al outlined a risk assessment tool, CARPREG I, that incorporates the type of cardiac lesion and may influence and/or inform the mode of delivery.[40,41] For example, Marfan syndrome patients with a dilated aorta 45 mm or more are not recommended to labor because of the risk of aortic dissection. Patients with a cardiac condition that could decompensate during a prolonged labor and delivery may need to expedite delivery with a CD. In addition, a woman with pulmonary hypertension on intravenous medications who needs cardiac anesthesia and extracorporeal membrane oxygenation at bedside may have a better outcome with a controlled delivery in the operating room and CD. Because women can labor spontaneously any time of day and any day of the week, including when members of the multidisciplinary team are not in the hospital, an organized planned delivery in the operating room with a multidisciplinary team may be safer for patients with complex cardiac disease. Compared to a vaginal delivery, CD imposes risks to the pregnant cardiac patient such as a higher risk of thromboembolism, bleeding, infection, and damage to internal organs including both the bladder and the bowel. Furthermore, there are greater fluid shifts during CD than other methods of delivery.

Regional anesthesia is preferable, but there are situations where general anesthesia is necessary.[43] For example, patients who are on therapeutic anticoagulation and planning to have regional anesthesia have to time delivery according to when their medication has been discontinued because of the risk of a spinal hematoma in anticoagulated patients. The goal is to avoid regional anesthesia during delivery because it increases the release of catecholamines, which then raises heart rate and blood pressure. It also poses a higher risk of postpartum hemorrhage because of uterine atony.

FOLLOW-UP PATIENT CARE

Pregnant women who are at higher risk of cardiovascular complications need to be seen by a multidisciplinary team that includes obstetrics, maternal-fetal medicine, anesthesia, cardiologists, pharmacists, and primary care providers.[5,44] In general, the pregnancy and delivery process is safe when managed by the appropriate team.[45] Postdelivery, women with cardiac disease who have been identified as higher risk should continue to have long-term follow-up care by a cardiologist. This multidisciplinary approach can prevent complications and improve pregnancy outcomes overall.[11,46] Contraception and preconception counseling are also important topics to discuss so that women make informed decisions for future pregnancies. They should understand the maternal and fetal risk, prognosis, risk of passing their diagnosis to their offspring, and future needs for care management.[47]

FUTURE DIRECTIONS

A recent position paper was published by the American Heart Association (AHA) to bolster understanding and foster the collaboration between subspecialists caring for pregnant women with cardiac conditions.[17] However, clinicians caring for cardio-obstetric patients need additional guidelines on how to appropriately manage these individuals. There also needs to be a directed consensus toward women with chronic medical conditions with a focus on contraception and life planning during their reproductive years. Prior studies on women with cardiac disease showed that contraception counseling is needed during all reproductive years of life including pregnancy.[48,49] Focus groups including women with acquired or congenital cardiac conditions describing their experiences during their prenatal, peripartum, and postpartum care would add qualitative data to further describe patient perspectives on their own reproductive life plan. Ultimately, an understanding of patients' needs will allow physicians to better provide directed and appropriate health services.

KEY POINTS

- ✔ Risk assessment for maternal mortality and morbidity should begin preconception, particularly for women with underlying acquired or congenital cardiac conditions.
- ✔ Pregnant patients with known cardiac disease should have expedited, streamlined evaluation by cardiologists experienced in cardio-obstetrics and maternal-fetal medicine specialists.
- ✔ Obstetricians should know the warning signs of cardiac disease in their pregnant and postpartum patients including abnormal symptoms, vital signs, physical examination, laboratory, or imaging findings that might point to high-risk disease.

- ✔ Institutions and departments should support multidisciplinary team work such that maternal-fetal medicine specialists and cardiologists can see patients simultaneously.
- ✔ Clinical and research teams should be constructed to include a multidisciplinary team of cardiology, maternal-fetal medicine, obstetric anesthesia, public health, social work, and nursing to address all aspects of the pregnant cardiac patient including the psychosocial component.

REFERENCES

1. Regitz-Zagrosek V, Roos-Hesselink JW, Bauersachs J, et al. 2018 ESC Guidelines for the management of cardiovascular diseases during pregnancy: The Task Force for the Management of Cardiovascular Diseases during Pregnancy of the European Society of Cardiology (ESC). *Eur Heart J.* 2018;39:3165-3241.
2. Halpern DG, Weinberg CR, Pinnelas R, Mehta-Lee S, Economy KE, Valente AM. Use of medication for cardiovascular disease during pregnancy: JACC state-of-the-art review. *J Am Coll Cardiol.* 2019;73:457-476.
3. Pieper PG. Use of medication for cardiovascular disease during pregnancy. *Nat Rev Cardiol.* 2015;12:718-729.
4. Creanga AA, Syverson C, Seed K, Callaghan WM. Pregnancy-related mortality in the United States, 2011-2013. *Obstet Gynecol.* 2017;130:366-373.
5. Kaye AB, Bhakta A, Moseley AD, et al. Review of cardiovascular drugs in pregnancy. *J Womens Health (Larchmt).* 2019;28:686-697.
6. Stout KK, Broberg CS, Book WM, et al. Chronic heart failure in congenital heart disease: a scientific statement from the American Heart Association. *Circulation.* 2016;133:770-801.
7. Siu SC, Sermer M, Colman JM, et al. Prospective multicenter study of pregnancy outcomes in women with heart disease. *Circulation.* 2001; 104:515-521.
8. van Hagen IM, Thorne SA, Taha N, et al. Pregnancy outcomes in women with rheumatic mitral valve disease: results from the registry of pregnancy and cardiac disease. *Circulation.* 2018;137:806-816.
9. Pieper PG, Balci A, Aarnoudse JG, et al. Uteroplacental blood flow, cardiac function, and pregnancy outcome in women with congenital heart disease. *Circulation.* 2013;128:2478-2487.
10. Balci A, Sollie-Szarynska KM, van der Bijl AG, et al. Prospective validation and assessment of cardiovascular and offspring risk models for pregnant women with congenital heart disease. *Heart.* 2014;100:1373-1381.
11. Elkayam U, Goland S, Pieper PG, Silversides CK. High-risk cardiac disease in pregnancy: part II. *J Am Coll Cardiol.* 2016;68:502-516.
12. Elkayam U, Goland S, Pieper PG, Silverside CK. High-risk cardiac disease in pregnancy: part I. *J Am Coll Cardiol.* 2016;68:396-410.
13. Regitz-Zagrosek V. 'Ten Commandments' of the 2018 ESC Guidelines for the management of cardiovascular diseases during pregnancy. *Eur Heart J.* 2018;39:3269.
14. Regitz-Zagrosek V, Roos-Hesselink JW, Bauersachs J, et al. 2018 ESC Guidelines for the management of cardiovascular diseases during pregnancy. *Kardiol Pol.* 2019;77:245-326.
15. Irizarry OC, Levine LD, Lewey J, et al. Comparison of clinical characteristics and outcomes of peripartum cardiomyopathy between African American and Non-African American Women. *JAMA Cardiol.* 2017;2:1256-1260.
16. Stergiopoulos K, Lima FV, Yang J. Shared genetic predisposition in peripartum and dilated cardiomyopathies. *N Engl J Med.* 2016;374:2601.
17. Mehta LS, Warnes CA, Bradley E, et al. Cardiovascular considerations in caring for pregnant patients: a scientific statement from the American Heart Association. *Circulation.* 2020;141(23):e884-e903.
18. Haberer K, Silversides CK. Congenital heart disease and women's health across the life span: focus on reproductive issues. *Can J Cardiol.* 2019;35:1652-1663.
19. Siu SC, Colman JM, Sorensen S, et al. Adverse neonatal and cardiac outcomes are more common in pregnant women with cardiac disease. *Circulation.* 2002;105:2179-2184.
20. Silversides CK, Grewal J, Mason J, et al. Pregnancy outcomes in women with heart disease: The CARPREG II Study. *J Am Coll Cardiol.* 2018;71:2419-2430.
21. Drenthen W, Boersma E, Balci A, et al. Predictors of pregnancy complications in women with congenital heart disease. *Eur Heart J.* 2010;31:2124-2132.
22. Thorne S, MacGregor A, Nelson-Piercy C. Risks of contraception and pregnancy in heart disease. *Heart.* 2006;92:1520-1525.
23. Kim YY, Goldberg LA, Awh K, et al. Accuracy of risk prediction scores in pregnant women with congenital heart disease. *Congenit Heart Dis.* 2019;14:470-478.
24. Masini G, Foo LF, Cornette J, et al. Cardiac output changes from prior to pregnancy to post partum using two non-invasive techniques. *Heart.* 2019;105:715-720.
25. van Mook WN, Peeters L. Severe cardiac disease in pregnancy, part I: hemodynamic changes and complaints during pregnancy, and general management of cardiac disease in pregnancy. *Curr Opin Crit Care.* 2005;11:430-434.
26. Grindheim G, Estensen ME, Langesaeter E, Rosseland LA, Toska K. Changes in blood pressure during healthy pregnancy: a longitudinal cohort study. *J Hypertens.* 2012;30:342-350.
27. Kevane B, Donnelly J, D'Alton M, Cooley S, Preston RJ, Ni Ainle F. Risk factors for pregnancy-associated venous thromboembolism: a review. *J Perinat Med.* 2014;42:417-425.
28. American College of Obstetricians and Gynecologists, Task Force on Hypertension in Pregnancy. Hypertension in pregnancy. Report of the American College of Obstetricians and Gynecologists' Task Force on Hypertension in Pregnancy. *Obstet Gynecol.* 2013;122:1122-1131.
29. Firoz T, Magee LA, MacDonell K, et al. Oral antihypertensive therapy for severe hypertension in pregnancy and postpartum: a systematic review. *BJOG.* 2014;121:1210-1218; discussion 1220.
30. Zhang YF, Zeng XL, Zhao EF, Lu HW. Diagnostic value of fetal echocardiography for congenital heart disease: a systematic review and meta-analysis. *Medicine (Baltimore).* 2015;94:e1759.
31. Burchill LJ, Lameijer H, Roos-Hesselink JW, et al. Pregnancy risks in women with pre-existing coronary artery disease, or following acute coronary syndrome. *Heart.* 2015;101:525-529.
32. Dey M, Sahoo I, Chawla S, Rajput M. Pregnancy with prior coronary artery disease: Specific concerns. *Med J Armed Forces India.* 2020;76:109-111.
33. Roos-Hesselink JW, Duvekot JJ, Thorne SA. Pregnancy in high risk cardiac conditions. *Heart.* 2009;95:680-686.
34. Dodeja A, Urbina F, Dodd K, et al. Cardiomyopathy in pregnancy—risk in the era of goal-directed medical therapy: a tertiary care center experience & systematic review. *J Am Coll Cardiol.* 2020;75:889-889.
35. Boyle S, Nicolae M, Kostner K, et al. Dilated cardiomyopathy in pregnancy: outcomes from an Australian Tertiary Centre for Maternal Medicine and Review of the Current Literature. *Heart Lung Circ.* 2019;28:591-597.
36. Halpern DG. Use of medication for cardiovascular disease during pregnancy: JACC state-of-the-art review. *J Am Coll Cardiol.* 2020;75:780.
37. Moe TG, Abrich VA, Rhee EK. Atrial fibrillation in patients with congenital heart disease. *J Atr Fibrillation.* 2017;10:1612.
38. Karbassi A, Nair K, Harris L, Wald RM, Roche SL. Atrial tachyarrhythmia in adult congenital heart disease. *World J Cardiol.* 2017;9:496-507.
39. Wang J, Li K, Li H, Zhu W, Sun H, Lu C. Comparison of anticoagulation regimens for pregnant women with prosthetic heart valves: a meta-analysis of prospective studies. *Cardiovasc Ther.* 2017;35.
40. Elkayam U, Bitar F. Valvular heart disease and pregnancy: part II: prosthetic valves. *J Am Coll Cardiol.* 2005;46:403-410.
41. Elkayam U, Bitar F. Valvular heart disease and pregnancy part I: native valves. *J Am Coll Cardiol.* 2005;46:223-230.
42. Kuba K, Wolfe D, Schoenfeld AH, Bortnick AE. Percutaneous coronary intervention in pregnancy: modeling of the fetal absorbed dose. *Case Rep Obstet Gynecol.* 2019;2019:8410203.

43. Ankichetty SP, Chin KJ, Chan VW, et al. Regional anesthesia in patients with pregnancy induced hypertension. *J Anaesthesiol Clin Pharmacol.* 2013;29:435-444.
44. Swan L. Congenital heart disease in pregnancy. *Best Pract Res Clin Obstet Gynaecol.* 2014;28:495-506.
45. Roos-Hesselink JW, Ruys TP, Stein JI, et al. Outcome of pregnancy in patients with structural or ischaemic heart disease: results of a registry of the European Society of Cardiology. *Eur Heart J.* 2013;34:657-665.
46. Burgess APH, Dongarwar D, Spigel Z, et al. Pregnancy-related mortality in the United States, 2003-2016: age, race, and place of death. *Am J Obstet Gynecol.* 2020;222:489.e1-489.e8.
47. Moussa HN, Rajapreyar I. ACOG Practice Bulletin No. 212: pregnancy and heart disease. *Obstet Gynecol.* 2019;134:881-882.
48. Ladouceur M, Calderon J, Traore M, et al. Educational needs of adolescents with congenital heart disease: Impact of a transition intervention programme. *Arch Cardiovasc Dis.* 2017;110:317-324.
49. Roos-Hesselink JW, Cornette J, Sliwa K, Pieper PG, Veldtman GR, Johnson MR. Contraception and cardiovascular disease. *Eur Heart J.* 2015;36:1728-1734, 1734a-1734b.

CHAPTER 19

WOMEN AND HEART DISEASE

Kelly Paschke and Dipti Itchhaporia

INTRODUCTION

Cardiovascular disease (CVD) remains the leading cause of death in the United States and accounts for one in five deaths in women.[1] The risk of mortality from CVD increases with age in women, accounting for one in four deaths after the age of 85 years.[1] Despite declining cardiovascular mortality rates in the past three decades, CVD continues to be a significant source of morbidity and mortality especially in younger women (<55 years of age).[2] To reduce future CVD morbidity and mortality, it is important to recognize traditional as well as emerging, nontraditional risk factors unique to or more common in women that contribute to the understanding of mechanisms and risk profiles.

In spite of public awareness campaigns, recognition of CVD as a leading cause of death in women remains low, improving in the last decade from 30% to 56%, particularly in women of younger age, lower education, ethnic minorities, and lower socioeconomic status. The awareness remains most suboptimal in regard to recognition of atypical symptoms of myocardial infarction and symptoms of acute coronary syndrome (ACS).[3] Improving awareness of the mortality and morbidity associated with CVD in women remains critical to help guide prevention and treatment in the future.

Many clinical trials that have provided the basis for guidelines and recommendations for the prevention of CVD have enrolled low percentages of women in their study populations. This underrepresentation raises concern for the generalizability of these data to women in the general population. Many recommendations in the 2019 American College of Cardiology/American Heart Association (ACC/AHA) Guidelines on the Primary Prevention of Cardiovascular Disease are not gender specific and may not support the unique differences of women within the practice of cardiovascular medicine.[4]

Risk factor stratification specific for women that includes traditional risk factors—such as age, physical inactivity, tobacco use, hypertension, diabetes mellitus, and obesity—and nontraditional risk factors—such as rheumatologic disorders, depression, and pregnancy-associated complications—is important to improve prevention and treatment strategies in women.

This chapter will examine the latest clinical perspectives on CVD in women, as they relate to the prevention, diagnosis, and treatment of CVD (**Figure 19.1**).

TRADITIONAL RISK FACTORS FOR CARDIOVASCULAR DISEASE

Age

Advanced age is a major risk factor for mortality from CVD, in particular for women over the age of 85 years who have coexisting risk factors, reduced physical activity, and other comorbidities. CVD accounts for 27% of deaths in women over the age of 85 years.[1] CVD appears to have a later onset in

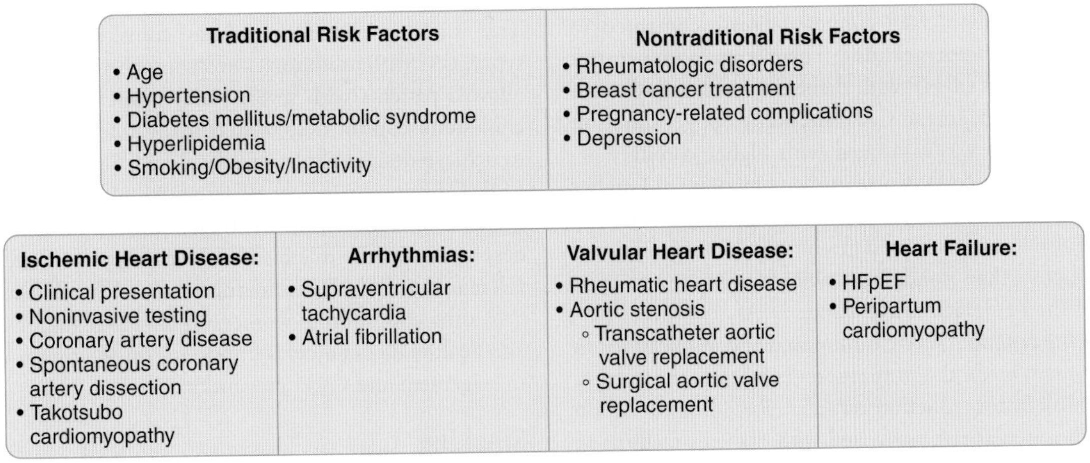

Traditional Risk Factors	Nontraditional Risk Factors
• Age • Hypertension • Diabetes mellitus/metabolic syndrome • Hyperlipidemia • Smoking/Obesity/Inactivity	• Rheumatologic disorders • Breast cancer treatment • Pregnancy-related complications • Depression

Ischemic Heart Disease:	Arrhythmias:	Valvular Heart Disease:	Heart Failure:
• Clinical presentation • Noninvasive testing • Coronary artery disease • Spontaneous coronary artery dissection • Takotsubo cardiomyopathy	• Supraventricular tachycardia • Atrial fibrillation	• Rheumatic heart disease • Aortic stenosis ◦ Transcatheter aortic valve replacement ◦ Surgical aortic valve replacement	• HFpEF • Peripartum cardiomyopathy

FIGURE 19.1 Cardiovascular disease in women: chapter overview. HFpEF, heart failure with preserved ejection fraction.

women as compared to men, with estrogen hypothesized to be protective in their early years and CVD more prevalent after menopause—natural or surgical—when the circulating levels of estrogen are decreased.[4] Estrogen is thought to have a role in vasodilation, inhibition of smooth muscle cellular proliferation, and regulation of blood pressure control. Nevertheless, postmenopausal estrogen replacement therapy is not recommended for prevention of CVD, as it has failed to demonstrate a protective benefit in clinical studies.

Hypertension

Hypertension affects more men than premenopausal women. It is believed that endogenous estrogens help maintain vasodilation and contribute to blood pressure control in premenopausal women. However, after the age of 65 years, the incidence of hypertension increases in women and the associated mortality is higher than at younger years.[2,5] This is due to the increased risk of CVD, heart failure (HF), and stroke with hypertension as well as the confounded risk with advancing age.

Despite modern advancements in antihypertensive agents, mortality associated with hypertension has increased over the past decade.[6] Nearly one-third of individuals with hypertension are unaware of their diagnosis. However, women tend to have better awareness of their hypertension diagnosis, receive treatment, and have better blood pressure control compared to men.[7] It is estimated that with improvement in hypertension, cardiovascular mortality may be improved by 38% in women.[6] Based on the SPRINT trial, the blood pressure targets should be less than 130 mm Hg systolic and less than 80 mm Hg diastolic in both men and women.

Diabetes Mellitus

Diabetes mellitus is a well-recognized risk factor for the development of CVD and affects at least 10% of the population.[8] The prevalence of diabetes mellitus in women is lower compared to men (8.4% vs 9.5%, respectively) and has a lower associated overall mortality.[2,8,9]

Interestingly, diabetes is more common in younger women (18-54 years) and associated with a greater risk for CVD compared to similarly aged men.[10] Women with diabetes mellitus have a threefold risk of fatal coronary disease compared to women without diabetes mellitus.[11] There is also a known risk for the development of HF with diabetes, which is higher in women than in men. In the CARDIA study, longer duration of diabetes mellitus was associated with higher coronary artery calcium (CAC) scores, worse cardiac function, and higher diastolic filling pressures and diastolic dysfunction.[12] Diabetic women are also known to have a greater number of traditional CVD risk factors than nondiabetic women, with poorer optimization of their risk factors over time.

Given the potential severe cardiovascular complications in diabetic women, medical optimization of glycemic control and concurrent risk factor reduction is crucial. Providing education on the cardiovascular risk associated with diabetes mellitus in women is recommended. Women should have dietary education to optimize glycemic control and target weight loss if they are overweight or obese. Additionally, the addition of diabetic agents that confer a cardiovascular benefit, such as sodium glucose cotransporter-2 inhibitor or glucagon-like peptide-1 receptor agonists, should be considered. In general, the presence of diabetes mellitus is an imperative for aggressive CVD risk prevention in women.

Metabolic syndrome is also a significant risk factor for CVD given its known association with diabetes mellitus, myocardial infarction, stroke, and increased all-cause mortality. Metabolic syndrome confers an increased risk of CVD in women compared to men. This may be due to subclinical atherosclerosis, which is a consequence of metabolic syndrome and demonstrated by the higher CAC scores in women with metabolic syndrome compared to those without it. The pathophysiology of associated risk for CVD is thought to be related to microvascular (ie, endothelial) and macrovascular dysfunction, leading to atherosclerotic plaques at high risk of progression and thrombosis, impairment in coronary blood flow reserve, and both systolic and diastolic left ventricular dysfunction. In women, metabolic syndrome is also associated with a number of comorbid autoimmune and inflammatory diseases such as systemic lupus erythematosus (SLE) and rheumatoid arthritis (RA). Gestational diabetes and hypertension, which confer a high risk of CVD progression, are also associated with metabolic syndrome in women.[13,14]

Hyperlipidemia

Hyperlipidemia is a recognized modifiable risk factor for CVD. Women typically have higher total cholesterol and high-density lipoprotein cholesterol (HDL-C) levels compared to men; however, they have lower low-density lipoprotein cholesterol (LDL-C) and triglyceride levels compared to men. The advent of cholesterol-lowering agents, especially statins, has resulted in a significant reduction in hypercholesterolemia within the population. Despite baseline gender differences in cholesterol and triglycerides, treatment recommendations remain the same for both women and men. The 2019 AHA/ACC Guidelines on the Primary Prevention of Cardiovascular Disease includes recommendations for statin therapy based on atherosclerotic CVD (ASCVD) risk scoring and associated risk factor consideration.[4] The introduction of proprotein convertase subtilisin/kexin type 9 (PCSK9) inhibitors—evolocumab and alirocumab—has allowed patients with severe statin intolerance or suboptimal cholesterol control despite maximally tolerated statin therapy to achieve desired cholesterol levels. PCSK9 inhibitors reduce LDL-C by approximately 40% to 50% and the risk of ASCVD events by 15%.[15] Women with suboptimal cholesterol control despite maximally tolerated statin therapy or severe statin intolerances are ideal candidates for PCSK9 inhibitor therapy. Providing education to women on target ranges for cholesterol and healthy diet choices is important for long-term cholesterol management and CVD prevention.

Smoking

Tobacco use remains the most significant cause of preventable death worldwide. Approximately 13.5% of women are tobacco users but represent a smaller proportion of the population of smokers compared to men.[16] Additionally, up to 7.2% of women continue to smoke during pregnancy, which may increase the overall risk of pregnancy-associated hypertension and preterm birth. Although overall rates for smoking continue to decline, the use of e-cigarettes has substantially risen in recent years, in particular, in younger individuals. The cardiovascular implications of e-cigarette use have not been studied and the long-term CVD effects are not yet known.[2]

Tobacco is a recognized independent risk factor for CVD and also increases the risk for the development of hypertension, hyperlipidemia, and diabetes mellitus, which further increases the risk for CVD. Women tobacco users are thought to be at a greater risk for CVD compared to men. In a recent meta-analysis of over 75 studies, women had a 25% increased risk for coronary artery disease (CAD) conferred by cigarette smoking compared with men.[17] It is also important to note that the combination of smoking with oral contraceptive use has a synergistic effect on the risk of acute myocardial infarction, stroke, and thromboembolism. Hence, counseling concerning smoking cessation and the risks of CVD with tobacco use should be provided to women. Complete tobacco cessation is important given the increased risk of CVD even with reduced tobacco use: women who smoke one cigarette per day have a 57% higher risk of heart disease and a 31% higher risk of stroke (or 119% and 46% when allowing for multiple confounders) compared with never smokers.[18] In female patients, the risk of smoking with pregnancy should be strongly discouraged. Additionally, education on the increased risk of myocardial infarction, thromboembolism, and stroke associated with tobacco use and oral contraceptive use should be provided to women of childbearing years. Younger tobacco users and e-cigarette users should be warned about the unknown cardiovascular side effects of newer nicotine and tobacco agents.

Obesity and Physical Inactivity

Obesity is a significant risk factor for CAD, HF, and atrial fibrillation, and its impact on the development of CAD appears to be greater in women than in men. More than two in three adults in the United States are considered to be overweight or obese, and the prevalence of obesity is higher among women than men. According to National Health and Nutrition Examination Survey (NHANES) data, the prevalence of obesity in the United States is 42% in women and 43% in men.[19] The prevalence of obesity in women has continued to rise over the past 15 years and class III obesity (ie, severe or extreme, with body mass index [BMI] of 40 kg/m^2 or higher) in particular. Conversely, this upward trend in class III obesity is not seen in the male population. Class III obesity rates are highest in women, accounting for 9.7% of the female population versus 5.6% of males. CVD risk is increased in class III obesity compared to classes I or II, which is concerning given the higher prevalence in women.[20,21] Numerous studies, including data from the Framingham Heart Study, associate a higher risk of CVD in obese women compared to obese men: obesity increased the relative risk of CAD by 64% in women, as opposed to 46% in men.[22]

Additionally, obesity has an important role in the development of other risk factors for CVD such as hypertension, diabetes mellitus, and dyslipidemia.[21,23] Subclinical atherosclerosis has also been implicated in the obese population, with this group having higher CAC and carotid intima-media thickness compared with patients with normal body size, even after adjustment for traditional CVD risk factors.[24] Furthermore, there are data showing obese women who present with ACS have worse outcomes. For patients with ST elevation myocardial infarction, in-hospital mortality rates are highest for individuals with class III obesity, which is of concern given a higher prevalence of class III obesity in women.[25]

The CVD risk associated with obesity is underappreciated by women. When asked to categorize their weight status, nearly 23% of obese women categorized themselves in a healthier weight status. This behavior has been associated with less weight loss over time.[26] Aggressive weight reduction to a normal BMI range of 18.5 to 24 kg/m^2 in women is important for the reduction of CVD and associated risk factors. Given the increased risk of CVD in women with class III obesity, this subset of patients should be referred for weight management and appropriately counseled on their increased risk for CVD over time.

Physical inactivity is an independent risk factor for CVD and stroke. The AHA guidelines currently recommend at least 150 minutes of moderate-intensity exercise or 75 minutes of vigorous aerobic exercise per week for both men and women.[27] Interestingly, only one-third of the population is aware of current physical activity guidelines. Multiple studies have shown all-cause mortality reduction with increased physical activity levels. Physical activity is thought to reduce the incidence and severity of associated CVD risk factors including hypertension, hyperlipidemia, CAD, HF, stroke, and diabetes mellitus. Physical activity declines after the age of 50 years and further at 60 years of age when reportedly only 2% of the female population achieves target physical activity goals: women in the highest risk group for CVD are achieving the lowest physical activity. Hence, patients should be counseled on current AHA recommendations for physical activity on a routine basis to improve adherence.

NONTRADITIONAL RISK FACTORS FOR CARDIOVASCULAR DISEASE

Rheumatologic Disorders

Numerous population studies have demonstrated an association between inflammatory diseases and increased mortality, in both men and women, mainly as a consequence of CVD. For most systemic autoimmune disorders, there is a clear sex difference in prevalence, making this a more common CVD risk factor in women.

Autoimmune conditions are prevalent in women and are associated with an increased risk of numerous CVDs. CAD is known to be a major source of morbidity and mortality in women with SLE, RA, or psoriatic arthritis.[28] However, despite the prevalence of these autoimmune diseases, their association with CVD is frequently underrecognized. RA is more than twice more common in women than in men and is associated with a twofold increase in risk for myocardial infarction. SLE is nearly nine times more common in women than in men and is associated with a tenfold increased risk for myocardial infarction. CVD is the leading cause for reduced life expectancy in patients with SLE.[29] CVD risk in women with SLE is underestimated by traditional risk assessments tools such as the Framingham risk model. The etiology for increased cardiovascular risk with rheumatologic diseases is not well understood. However, it is likely multifactorial due, at least in part, to chronic inflammation in the setting of autoimmune disease. Women with rheumatologic disease should have a thorough cardiovascular risk assessment and aggressive risk factor management given their increased risk of accelerated atherosclerosis and complications of CAD.[30]

Breast Cancer Treatment

Breast cancer is primarily a disease of women. Although treatment strategies, including anthracycline-based chemotherapy agents and trastuzumab, are associated with improved survival in breast cancer patients, they also carry the highest risk for the development of HF. Women treated with these agents have a threefold increased risk of HF. Women undergoing treatment for breast cancer should undergo further cardiovascular risk factor assessment. Individuals with preexisting risk factors for CVD and those with previous chemotherapy and radiation of the left side of the chest are at the highest risk for HF. These individuals should be monitored closely during and after breast cancer treatment for the development of HF.[31]

Pregnancy-Related Complications

Many hemodynamic changes occur with pregnancy (**Table 19.1**). Pregnancy-related complications such as gestational hypertension, preeclampsia, gestational diabetes, and preterm delivery confer a higher risk of CVD and should be considered as nontraditional risk factors. Thirty percent of pregnant women experience gestational complications. Women with pregnancy-related complications should be considered as an at-risk population that would benefit from primary prevention of CVD. Additionally, women with preexisting risk factors for CVD have an elevated risk of pregnancy-related complications and should be monitored closely (**Figure 19.2**).[32] Women who are diagnosed with gestational hypertension and preeclampsia are at risk for developing chronic hypertension and CVD later in life. The risk of CVD is higher in women exposed to early preeclampsia than in women who develop preeclampsia later in pregnancy. Additionally, the severity of preeclampsia is correlated with the severity of CVD later in life. Hypertensive disorders of pregnancy also confer an increased risk of HF development in the future, even when adjusting for numerous other contributory factors.[33]

Another complication of pregnancy is preterm delivery, which is defined as birth at less than 37 weeks' gestation. A recent study concluded that preterm delivery is an independent risk factor for subsequent long-term cardiovascular morbidity and cardiovascular-related hospitalizations. The risk for ASCVD is further increased with a history of early preterm delivery (<34 weeks' gestation).[34]

Gestational diabetes is a risk factor for CVD development and confers a sevenfold increased risk of diabetes mellitus later in life, which further raises the risk for CVD. However, gestational diabetes is also known to be an independent risk factor for CVD and women should be educated of such at the time of diagnosis.[35,36]

TABLE 19.1 Common Hemodynamic Changes in Pregnancy

Hemodynamic Parameter	Direction	Change
Cardiac Output	↑	30%-50% increase
Stroke Volume	↑↓	40% increase by week 26, then decreases
Heart Rate	↑	10-15 bpm increase
Blood Volume	↑	40%-50% increase
Oxygen Consumption	↑	20% increase
Systemic Vascular Resistance	↑	30%-40% decrease
Blood Pressure	↓	5%-15% decrease

Depression

Depression is a prevalent and well-recognized nontraditional risk factor for CVD in women.

Depression and other psychosocial risk factors may be more important risk factors in younger than older individuals, especially young women. CVD mortality rates have declined in older women in recent years, but not to the same degree as in younger women. This coincides with a time period when rates of depression have continued to increase in women.[36]

CLINICAL PRESENTATION

Although chest pain is the most common symptom of ischemic heart disease (IHD) in both genders—31% in women and 42% in men—, women are more likely to report non–chest pain symptoms such as dyspnea, weakness, arm, back or jaw pain, nausea, palpitations, and light-headedness.[37,38] Hence, atypical symptoms should always be thoroughly investigated in women with risk factors for CVD.

DIAGNOSIS

Noninvasive Testing for Ischemic Heart Disease

Noninvasive testing for the diagnosis of IHD may be accomplished with exercise stress testing, stress echocardiography, nuclear stress testing, or computerized tomographic (CT) angiography. The choice of test is based in part on the pretest probability of IHD and appropriate use criteria. Exercise stress testing is the initial recommended stress testing modality in

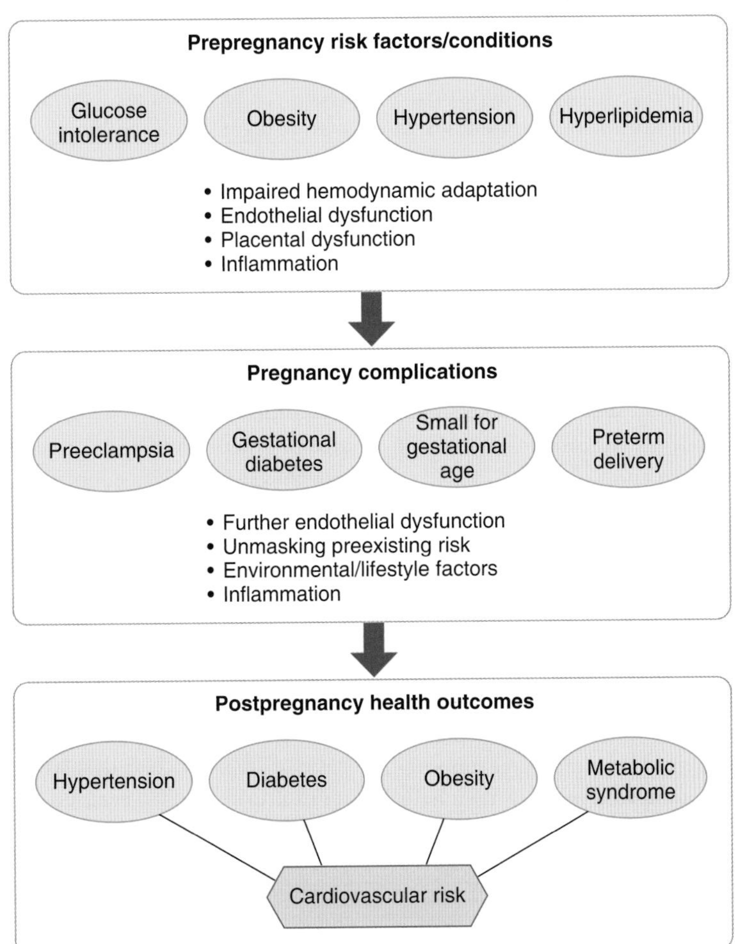

FIGURE 19.2 Risk factors and conditions associated with pregnancy complications and future cardiovascular risk.

women of intermediate risk who are able to exercise and have a normal resting electrocardiogram (ECG). It is postulated that the higher false-positive rate in women compared to men may be due to ECG effects from estrogen, reduced exercise capacity given older age at the onset of CAD, and paucity of women in the studies that established the test's specificity.[39] Exercise treadmill testing can provide important information with regard to exercise capacity and response to exercise and recovery.[36]

Stress testing with imaging can give additional information about wall motion or perfusion abnormalities and provide assessment of ventricular function. Stress testing with imaging is recommended for women with a pretest probability that is intermediate to high with baseline ECG changes or when an exercise ECG stress test is abnormal. A stress echocardiogram is particularly advantageous in women because it can give additional information about left ventricular systolic function, wall motion abnormalities, and valvular disease. Diagnostic accuracy of stress echocardiography is similar in both men and women.

In patients unable to exercise, pharmacologic stress testing with single-photon emission computed tomography (SPECT) or positron emission tomography (PET) should be considered. SPECT imaging of the anterior wall may be affected by breast attenuation in women. Additionally, the small left ventricular size in women may affect the accuracy of imaging. The use of gating and attenuation correction has helped improve SPECT imaging in both men and women. PET myocardial perfusion imaging is less affected by breast attenuation and may provide superior imaging in women. Additionally, PET has the ability to better identify microvascular disease and ischemia that can be seen in women.[39]

Anatomic assessment with coronary CT angiography (CCTA), with its improved imaging accuracy, provides another diagnostic option. The Prospective Multicenter Imaging Study for Evaluation of Chest Pain (PROMISE) trial compared anatomic assessment by CCTA with functional assessment (exercise ECG, nuclear stress testing, or stress echocardiography) and showed similar outcomes (death, myocardial infarction, hospitalization for unstable angina, or major procedural complication) for both over the 2-year follow-up.[40] Additionally, the Rule Out Myocardial Infarction using Computer Assisted Tomography (ROMICAT) trial showed that in patients admitted to the hospital with acute chest pain, CCTA can predict ACSs independent of cardiovascular risk factors or TIMI (Thrombolysis in Myocardial Infarction) risk score.[41] Furthermore,

The ROMICAT II trial found that women had a lower hospital admission rate and greater reduction in length of stay than men when early CCTA was used in the emergency department evaluation of chest pain suggestive of ACS.[42] Limitations to CCTA include radiation exposure, and given the smaller size of coronary arteries in women, mid- to distal lesions may be more difficult to identify.

Calcium scoring is a method to help aid in the prediction of obstructive CAD; however, it may underestimate plaque deposition. It is not recommended for low-risk and asymptomatic patients or in high-risk and symptomatic patients. However, in the intermediate-risk patient population, CAC scoring can be helpful in guiding treatment. Women typically have lower CAC scores than men; however, the prognostic value of CAC remains the same in both men and women.[39]

Ischemic Heart Disease in Women

IHD is characterized by narrowing or obstruction of the epicardial coronary arteries. However, IHD in women typically differs from that in men and frequently involves microvascular and endothelial dysfunction. At cardiac catheterization, women more commonly have nonobstructive CAD; however, they may also have a higher predisposition for acute plaque rupture and thrombus formation. There are three important features of IHD in women compared to men: they have a higher prevalence of angina, a lower burden of obstructive CAD on angiography, and a worse prognosis in comparison.

IHD in women involves atherosclerosis that obstructs epicardial coronary vessels as well as atherosclerosis in the microvasculature with resultant fibrosis of the vessels. IHD in women also includes coronary microvascular dysfunction (CMD), which is characterized by coronary endothelial dysfunction, vasomotor abnormalities, and decreased microvascular coronary blood flow, which are not detected during routine cardiac catheterization. If suspected, detection of microvascular dysfunction requires special vasomotor testing such as vasoreactivity testing with intracoronary acetylcholine, which should be done by an experienced interventional cardiologist using a standardized protocol. In recent years, PET and cardiac magnetic resonance (CMR) detection of subendocardial disease has improved and may be an option for screening for microvascular disease. N-13 ammonia PET imaging can assess coronary flow reserve (CFR): a CFR less than 2.5 is considered to be abnormal, and a CFR less than 2.0 is associated with adverse cardiac outcomes. Women with symptoms of angina twice as often have ischemia with nonobstructive coronary arteries (ie, coronary stenosis of $<50\%$ at angiography with a fractional flow reserve [FFR] ≥ 0.80), so-called "INOCA," compared with men. In more than 60% of patients with INOCA, concomitant CMD is present, which is defined as limited CFR and coronary vasomotor disorders, such as spasm and endothelial dysfunction of the larger and smaller branches of the coronary tree. INOCA is associated with major adverse cardiovascular events in both symptomatic women and men.[43] Women with INOCA represent a very heterogeneous group because of their extent of atherosclerosis, risk factors, and symptoms.[44]

In women with suspected CMD, it important to treat them with aggressive risk factor modification and medical therapy that includes beta-blockers, nitrates, angiotensin-converting enzyme inhibitors, calcium channel blockers, and statins. For women with refractory angina despite maximal medical therapy, modern nonpharmacologic therapies should be explored.[45]

Spontaneous Coronary Artery Dissection

Spontaneous coronary artery dissection (SCAD) is characterized by dissection of the coronary artery wall creating a false lumen and subsequent intramural hematoma leading to acute myocardial ischemia. The presentation of SCAD varies in degree of severity and may present with acute HF and/or cardiogenic shock. The majority of SCAD cases occur in young women; however, more recent data suggest increasing numbers of postmenopausal women and men presenting with SCAD. Nearly one-quarter of SCAD cases occur during pregnancy and the peripartum period, which is likely the result of hormonal changes involving the coronary vessels and hemodynamic stress during labor. There is a strong association with fibromuscular dysplasia, occurring in up to half of women presenting with SCAD. Most women have a predisposing risk for SCAD because of fibromuscular dysplasia, connective tissue disease, or are multiparous. However, up to 20% of cases are idiopathic and patients do not have traditional risk factors associated with CAD.[46] It is important to screen women with SCAD for fibromuscular dysplasia with CT imaging of the brain, chest, abdomen, and pelvis.

The diagnosis of SCAD requires a high degree of suspicion and careful angiographic analysis. It is important to differentiate ACS resulting from SCAD versus ACS as a result of atherosclerosis because acute and long-term management vary. Percutaneous coronary intervention success rates are lower for SCAD than atherosclerotic lesions, so generally conservative management for SCAD is favored given more spontaneous vascular healing that leads to better outcomes with this approach. Treatment of SCAD with percutaneous coronary intervention can be challenging and is not recommended in most cases given the propensity to worsen the coronary dissection. Treatment with beta-blockers and aspirin, and referral to cardiac rehabilitation are recommended. Statin therapy is recommended if hyperlipidemia is also present. Long-term surveillance is also recommended given the recurrence of SCAD in up to 10% of individuals.[47]

Takotsubo or Stress-Induced Cardiomyopathy

Takotsubo cardiomyopathy—also called broken heart syndrome or stress-induced cardiomyopathy—is a rare but recognized nonischemic cause of ACS. It is characterized by transient left ventricular dysfunction most classically with mid- to apical dyskinesis and basal hyperdynamic function. Eighty percent of the cases occur in postmenopausal women, and it is typically preceded by extreme physical or emotional stress. The clinical presentation, ECG findings, and cardiac enzymes can be consistent with ACS, but the coronary arteries are without significant obstructive disease at coronary angiography. The pathophysiology is thought to be catecholamine mediated with resultant microvascular dysfunction, spasm, and myocardial stunning, which is typically reversible. Treatment is supportive and typically involves beta-blockers, especially if left ventricular outflow tract obstruction is present. Up to 10% of patients develop cardiogenic shock and require more supportive treatment for acute HF and potentially inotropic support.[48]

Coronary Artery Disease

CAD affects nearly 150 million individuals with a higher prevalence in men compared to women. The incidence of myocardial infarction has decreased over the past decade, in particular with the decline of prehospital fatal myocardial infarction. Nevertheless, a majority of the mortality associated with myocardial infarction occurs prior to hospitalization, with women experiencing a lower incidence than men. CAD and myocardial infarction are more prevalent in males in nearly all age groups. The average age for first myocardial infarction is higher in women than in men (72 years vs 65 years, respectively).[2] Women are more likely to die within 1 year and at 5 years post–myocardial infarction compared to men. This may be due to several factors: compared to men, women are older at initial presentation of CAD; more likely to develop HF post–myocardial infarction; and less likely to participate in cardiac rehabilitation,[49] all of which are associated with higher hospital readmissions and mortality.

Arrhythmias

Supraventricular tachycardia (SVT) is an arrhythmia that is more predominant in women than in men, particularly those over the age of 65 years.[50] Atrioventricular (AV) nodal reentrant tachycardia, a form of SVT, is also more common in women compared to men. A Swedish study found that women with SVT had a longer history of symptomatic arrhythmia, were less likely to have been taken seriously regarding their symptom burden, and continued to have persistent symptoms even after ablation compared to men.[51] SVT during pregnancy is associated with a higher rate of poor fetal and maternal outcomes such as cesarean delivery, low birth weight, fetal distress, and preterm labor.[52]

Atrial fibrillation is a common atrial arrhythmia and is slightly more prevalent in women compared to men and has an association with hypertension and HF. Mortality is increased with atrial fibrillation in all patients; however, it is higher in women compared to men.[53] Mortality with atrial fibrillation is strongly associated with HF, hypertension, hyperthyroidism, obesity, heavy alcohol use, smoking, diabetes mellitus, and obstructive sleep apnea. Systemic embolization is a more common complication of atrial fibrillation in women than in men and is associated with an increased risk of death. Additionally, the risk of myocardial infarction is higher in women with atrial fibrillation compared to men.

Sudden cardiac death, unrelated to structural heart disease, is less frequent in women than in men. Torsades de pointes, a form of polymorphic ventricular tachycardia, is more common in women, given that they are two to three times more likely to have drug-induced QT prolongation.[54]

Valvular Heart Disease in Women

Valvular heart disease incidence is similar among men and women in the general population; however, women have a higher incidence of mitral stenosis. Rheumatic heart disease is uncommon in the developed world but remains endemic in numerous countries. Rheumatic heart disease is twice as common in women, and the resulting mortality risk is twice as high in women compared to men.[55]

Aortic stenosis is prevalent in both men and women. In the setting of aortic stenosis, women tend to have concurrent left ventricular hypertrophy, preservation in systolic function, and lower concurrent CAD, which may be the reason for older age at symptom onset than in men. Women are less likely to undergo surgical aortic valve replacement (SAVR) and have worse outcomes with SAVR, to include increased hospital mortality, compared to men. With regard to transcatheter aortic valve replacement (TAVR), women have a lower 12-month mortality compared to men. Additionally, women have a lower mortality rate with TAVR compared to SAVR at 2 years, a finding that does not occur in men. Women who undergo TAVR have less postprocedural complication risk of acute kidney injury and postprocedural aortic regurgitation, a well-known risk factor for cardiovascular mortality post-TAVR. However, there is an increased risk of postprocedural bleeding and vascular complications with TAVR, including stroke, in women versus men. These should be kept in mind when exploring treatment options in women with severe aortic stenosis.[56]

Heart Failure in Women

The incidence of HF has continued to rise in recent years in the setting of improved myocardial infarction and HF survival. Approximately 50% of patients living with HF are women, with older age and less commonly an ischemic cause. The prevalence of HF with preserved ejection fraction (HFpEF) is nearly two times more common in women compared to men. In the presence of hemodynamic stress, the myocardium in women is more likely to remodel in a concentric pattern compared to men who experience eccentric hypertrophy. Risk factors for developing HFpEF include hypertension, obesity, and atrial fibrillation.[57] Female patients should be educated on risk reduction and undergo aggressive blood pressure and weight control to prevent HFpEF.[58]

Hypertension is a significant important modifiable risk factor for HF with nearly a twofold increased risk with uncontrolled blood pressure. Obesity is also another important modifiable risk factor and also carries a twofold increased risk of HF. This is particularly important with regard to the female population because, as previously mentioned, they have a higher prevalence of severe obesity. Biomarker levels may be different in women with a 1.6-fold increase in baseline circulating plasma brain natriuretic protein (BNP) levels and a 1.3-fold increase in N-terminal pro b-type natriuretic peptide (NT-proBNP) levels when compared to men.[59] As with many other aspects of CVD treatment, treatment guidelines for HF are not gender specific and women continue to be underrepresented in clinical HF trials.

Peripartum Cardiomyopathy

Peripartum cardiomyopathy (PPCM) is a rare but recognized syndrome during pregnancy and/or the postpartum period, typically affecting women without a history of CVD. It is characterized by global left ventricular systolic dysfunction with left ventricular ejection fraction below 45%. The incidence of this condition in the United States is 1 in 3000 deliveries, typically affecting mothers over the age of 30 years, with a significantly higher incidence in African Americans, and those with a history of pregnancy-associated hypertension.[60] The majority of women show a partial or complete recovery within 2 to 6 months after the diagnosis of PPCM and after initiation of goal-directed medical therapy for HF, although approximately 10% will have major complications including the need for advanced therapies, transplantation, or death. There is a potential for recurrence with subsequent pregnancies even if the left ventricular function has recovered to normal.

RESEARCH AND FUTURE DIRECTIONS

CVD continues to be the leading cause of death for women in the United States. Identification of risk factors, including the emerging risk factors such as SLE, RA, pregnancy-related complications, and depression, with a primary focus on primary prevention, especially in younger women where there is an increase in prevalence and severity, is necessary to reduce overall CVD burden and mortality. Supporting research with adequate power for sex-specific analysis is crucial to improving our understanding about mechanism and developing more effective treatment and management.

KEY POINTS

- ✔ CVD is a significant source of morbidity and mortality, especially in younger women (<55 years of age). Yet awareness of CVD as a leading cause of death in women remains low.
- ✔ Conventional risk factors for CVD, such as age, hypertension, diabetes, hyperlipidemia, smoking, and obesity, should be addressed by the clinician, in addition to female-specific risk factors, such as rheumatologic disorders, breast cancer treatment, pregnancy-related complications, and depression.
- ✔ Although chest pain is the most common symptom of IHD, women are more likely to report non–chest pain symptoms. Clinicians should develop a high index of suspicion for IHD in women with cardiac risk factors.
- ✔ Presentation of IHD in women includes obstructive CAD, CMD, SCAD, and INOCA. Compared to men, women have a higher prevalence of angina, a lower burden of obstructive CAD on angiography, and a worse overall prognosis.
- ✔ The prevalence of HFpEF is nearly two times more common in women compared to men.
- ✔ More research is needed to better understand CVD in women and to direct appropriate management options.

REFERENCES

1. Centers for Disease Control and Prevention. Leading causes of death—females—all races and origins—United States, 2017. Accessed November 20, 2019. https://www.cdc.gov/women/lcod/2017/all-races-origins/index.htm
2. Benjamin EJ, Muntner P, Alonso A, et al. Heart disease and stroke statistics-2019 update: a report from the American Heart Association. *Circulation.* 2019;139(10):e56-e528. doi:10.1161/CIR.0000000000000659
3. Mosca L, Hammond G, Mochari-Greenberger H, et al. Fifteen-year trends in awareness of heart disease in women: results of a 2012 American Heart Association national survey. *Circulation.* 2013;127(11):1254-1263. e1-29. doi:10.1161/CIR.0b013e318287cf2f
4. Arnett DK, Blumenthal RS, Albert MA, et al. 2019 ACC/AHA Guideline on the primary prevention of cardiovascular disease: executive summary: a report of the American College of Cardiology/American Heart Association Task Force on Clinical Practice Guidelines. *J Am Coll Cardiol.* 2019;74(10):1376-1414. doi:10.1016/j.jacc.2019.03.009
5. National Center for Health Statistics and National Heart Lung, and Blood Institute. Prevalence of hypertension in adults>20 years of age by sex and age.
6. Patel SA, Winkel M, Ali MK, Narayan KM, Mehta NK. Cardiovascular mortality associated with 5 leading risk factors: national and state preventable fractions estimated from survey data. *Ann Intern Med.* 2015;163(4):245-253. doi:10.7326/M14-1753
7. National Center for Health Statistics and National Heart Lung, and Blood Institute. Heart disease and stroke statistics-2019 update: a report from the American Heart Association 2013-2016. Extent of awareness, treatment, and control of high blood pressure by race/ethnicity and sex.
8. Loop MS, Howard G, de Los Campos G, et al. Heat maps of hypertension, diabetes mellitus, and smoking in the continental United States. *Circ Cardiovasc Qual Outcomes.* 2017;10(1):e003350. doi:10.1161/CIRCOUTCOMES.116.003350
9. Kochanek KD, Murphy SL, Xu J, Arias E. Deaths: final data for 2017. *Natl Vital Stat Rep.* 2019;68(9):1-77.
10. Centers for Disease Control and Prevention. Diabetes data and statistics. Accessed May 30, 2019. https://www.cdc.gov/diabetes/data
11. Huxley R, Barzi F, Woodward M. Excess risk of fatal coronary heart disease associated with diabetes in men and women: meta-analysis of 37 prospective cohort studies. *BMJ.* 2006;332(7533):73-78. doi:10.1136/bmj.38678.389583.7C
12. Reis JP, Allen NB, Bancks MP, et al. Duration of diabetes and prediabetes during adulthood and subclinical atherosclerosis and cardiac dysfunction in middle age: the CARDIA Study. *Diabetes Care.* 2018;41(4):731-738. doi:10.2337/dc17-2233
13. Noctor E, Crowe C, Carmody LA, et al. ATLANTIC-DIP: prevalence of metabolic syndrome and insulin resistance in women with previous gestational diabetes mellitus by International Association of Diabetes in Pregnancy Study Groups criteria. *Acta Diabetol.* 2015;52(1): 153-160. doi:10.1007/s00592-014-0621-z
14. Facca TA, Mastroianni-Kirsztajn G, Sabino ARP, et al. Pregnancy as an early stress test for cardiovascular and kidney disease diagnosis. *Pregnancy Hypertens.* Apr 2018;12:169-173. doi:10.1016/j.preghy.2017.11.008
15. Lloyd-Jones DM, Morris PB, Ballantyne CM, et al. 2017 Focused Update of the 2016 ACC Expert Consensus Decision Pathway on the role of non-statin therapies for LDL-cholesterol lowering in the management of atherosclerotic cardiovascular disease risk: a report of the American College of Cardiology Task Force on Expert Consensus Decision Pathways. *J Am Coll Cardiol.* 2017;70(14):1785-1822. doi:10.1016/j.jacc.2017.07.745

16. Jamal A, King BA, Neff LJ, Whitmill J, Babb SD, Graffunder CM. Current cigarette smoking among adults—United States, 2005-2015. *MMWR Morb Mortal Wkly Rep*. 2016;65(44):1205-1211. doi:10.15585/mmwr.mm6544a2
17. Huxley RR, Woodward M. Cigarette smoking as a risk factor for coronary heart disease in women compared with men: a systematic review and meta-analysis of prospective cohort studies. *Lancet*. 2011;378(9799):1297-1305. doi:10.1016/S0140-6736(11)60781-2
18. Hackshaw A, Morris JK, Boniface S, Tang JL, Milenković D. Low cigarette consumption and risk of coronary heart disease and stroke: meta-analysis of 141 cohort studies in 55 study reports. *BMJ*. 2018;360:j5855. doi:10.1136/bmj.j5855
19. Centers for Disease Control and Prevention. National Center for Health Statistics (NCHS). National Health and Nutrition Examination Survey Data. U.S. Department of Health and Human Services. https://www.cdc.gov/nchs/data/hestat/obesity-adult-17-18/overweight-obesity-adults-H.pdf
20. Flegal KM, Kruszon-Moran D, Carroll MD, Fryar CD, Ogden CL. Trends in obesity among adults in the United States, 2005 to 2014. *JAMA*. 2016;315(21):2284-2291. doi:10.1001/jama.2016.6458
21. Khan SS, Ning H, Wilkins JT, et al. Association of body mass index with lifetime risk of cardiovascular disease and compression of morbidity. *JAMA Cardiol*. 2018;3(4):280-287. doi:10.1001/jamacardio.2018.0022
22. Wilson PW, D'Agostino RB, Sullivan L, Parise H, Kannel WB. Overweight and obesity as determinants of cardiovascular risk: the Framingham experience. *Arch Intern Med*. 2002;162(16):1867-1872. doi:10.1001/archinte.162.16.1867
23. Eckel N, Meidtner K, Kalle-Uhlmann T, Stefan N, Schulze MB. Metabolically healthy obesity and cardiovascular events: A systematic review and meta-analysis. *Eur J Prev Cardiol*. 2016;23(9):956-966. doi:10.1177/2047487315623884
24. Burke GL, Bertoni AG, Shea S, et al. The impact of obesity on cardiovascular disease risk factors and subclinical vascular disease: the Multi-Ethnic Study of Atherosclerosis. *Arch Intern Med*. 2008;168(9):928-935. doi:10.1001/archinte.168.9.928
25. Das SR, Alexander KP, Chen AY, et al. Impact of body weight and extreme obesity on the presentation, treatment, and in-hospital outcomes of 50,149 patients with ST-segment elevation myocardial infarction results from the NCDR (National Cardiovascular Data Registry). *J Am Coll Cardiol*. 2011;58(25):2642-2650. doi:10.1016/j.jacc.2011.09.030
26. Duncan DT, Wolin KY, Scharoun-Lee M, Ding EL, Warner ET, Bennett GG. Does perception equal reality? Weight misperception in relation to weight-related attitudes and behaviors among overweight and obese US adults. *Int J Behav Nutr Phys Act*. 2011;8:20. doi:10.1186/1479-5868-8-20
27. American Heart Association. American Heart Association recommendations for physical activity in adults and kids. 2020. https://www.heart.org/en/healthy-living/fitness/fitness-basics/aha-recs-for-physical-activity-in-adults
28. Gianturco L, Bodini BD, Atzeni F, et al. Cardiovascular and autoimmune diseases in females: the role of microvasculature and dysfunctional endothelium. *Atherosclerosis*. 2015;241(1):259-263. doi:10.1016/j.atherosclerosis.2015.03.044
29. Zhang J, Chen L, Delzell E, et al. The association between inflammatory markers, serum lipids and the risk of cardiovascular events in patients with rheumatoid arthritis. *Ann Rheum Dis*. 2014;73(7):1301-1308. doi:10.1136/annrheumdis-2013-204715
30. Durante A, Bronzato S. The increased cardiovascular risk in patients affected by autoimmune diseases: review of the various manifestations. *J Clin Med Res*. 2015;7(6):379-384. doi:10.14740/jocmr2122w
31. Mavrogeni SI, Sfendouraki E, Markousis-Mavrogenis G, et al. Cardio-oncology, the myth of Sisyphus, and cardiovascular disease in breast cancer survivors. *Heart Fail Rev*. 2019;24(6):977-987. doi:10.1007/s10741-019-09805-1
32. Hauspurg A, Ying W, Hubel CA, Michos ED, Ouyang P. Adverse pregnancy outcomes and future maternal cardiovascular disease. *Clin Cardiol*. 2018;41(2):239-246. doi:10.1002/clc.22887
33. Chen SN, Cheng CC, Tsui KH, et al. Hypertensive disorders of pregnancy and future heart failure risk: a nationwide population-based retrospective cohort study. *Pregnancy Hypertens*. 2018;13:110-115. doi:10.1016/j.preghy.2018.05.010
34. Gotsch F, Romero R, Erez O, et al. The preterm parturition syndrome and its implications for understanding the biology, risk assessment, diagnosis, treatment and prevention of preterm birth. *J Matern Fetal Neonatal Med*. 2009;22(suppl 2):5-23. doi:10.1080/14767050902860690
35. Vrachnis N, Augoulea A, Iliodromiti Z, Lambrinoudaki I, Sifakis S, Creatsas G. Previous gestational diabetes mellitus and markers of cardiovascular risk. *Int J Endocrinol*. 2012;2012:458610. doi:10.1155/2012/458610
36. Garcia M, Mulvagh SL, Merz CN, Buring JE, Manson JE. Cardiovascular Disease in Women: Clinical Perspectives. *Circ Res*. 2016;118(8):1273-1293. doi:10.1161/CIRCRESAHA.116.307547
37. Aggarwal NR, Patel HN, Mehta LS, et al. Sex differences in ischemic heart disease: advances, obstacles, and next steps. *Circ Cardiovasc Qual Outcomes*. 2018;11(2):e004437. doi:10.1161/CIRCOUTCOMES.117.004437
38. Gudnadottir GS, Andersen K, Thrainsdottir IS, James SK, Lagerqvist B, Gudnason T. Gender differences in coronary angiography, subsequent interventions, and outcomes among patients with acute coronary syndromes. *Am Heart J*. 2017;191:65-74. doi:10.1016/j.ahj.2017.06.014
39. Brewer LC, Svatikova A, Mulvagh SL. The challenges of prevention, diagnosis and treatment of ischemic heart disease in women. *Cardiovasc Drugs Ther*. 2015;29(4):355-368. doi:10.1007/s10557-015-6607-4
40. Douglas PS, Hoffmann U, Patel MR, et al. Outcomes of anatomical versus functional testing for coronary artery disease. *N Engl J Med*. 2015;372(14):1291-1300. doi:10.1056/NEJMoa1415516
41. Hoffmann U, Bamberg F, Chae CU, et al. Coronary computed tomography angiography for early triage of patients with acute chest pain: the ROMICAT (Rule Out Myocardial Infarction using Computer Assisted Tomography) trial. *J Am Coll Cardiol*. 2009;53(18):1642-1650. doi:10.1016/j.jacc.2009.01.052
42. Truong QA, Hayden D, Woodard PK, et al. Sex differences in the effectiveness of early coronary computed tomographic angiography compared with standard emergency department evaluation for acute chest pain: the rule-out myocardial infarction with Computer-Assisted Tomography (ROMICAT)-II Trial. *Circulation*. 2013;127(25):2494-2502. doi:10.1161/CIRCULATIONAHA.113.001736
43. Murthy VL, Naya M, Taqueti VR, et al. Effects of sex on coronary microvascular dysfunction and cardiac outcomes. *Circulation*. 2014;129(24):2518-2517. doi:10.1161/CIRCULATIONAHA.113.008507
44. Maas A. Characteristic symptoms in women with ischemic heart disease. *Curr Cardiovasc Risk Rep*. 2019;13(17). https://doi.org/10.1007/s12170-019-0611-3
45. Gallone G, Baldetti L, Tzanis G, et al. Refractory angina: from pathophysiology to new therapeutic nonpharmacological technologies. *JACC Cardiovasc Interv*. 2020;13(1):1-19. doi:10.1016/j.jcin.2019.08.055
46. Saw J, Aymong E, Sedlak T, et al. Spontaneous coronary artery dissection: association with predisposing arteriopathies and precipitating stressors and cardiovascular outcomes. *Circ Cardiovasc Interv*. 2014;7(5):645-655. doi:10.1161/CIRCINTERVENTIONS.114.001760
47. Clare R, Duan L, Phan D, et al. Characteristics and clinical outcomes of patients with spontaneous coronary artery dissection. *J Am Heart Assoc*. 2019;8(10):e012570. doi:10.1161/JAHA.119.012570
48. Gianni M, Dentali F, Grandi AM, Sumner G, Hiralal R, Lonn E. Apical ballooning syndrome or takotsubo cardiomyopathy: a systematic review. *Eur Heart J*. 2006;27(13):1523-1529. doi:10.1093/eurheartj/ehl032
49. Dunlay SM, Pack QR, Thomas RJ, Killian JM, Roger VL. Participation in cardiac rehabilitation, readmissions, and death after acute myocardial infarction. *Am J Med*. 2014;127(6):538-546. doi:10.1016/j.amjmed.2014.02.008
50. Orejarena LA, Vidaillet H, DeStefano F, et al. Paroxysmal supraventricular tachycardia in the general population. *J Am Coll Cardiol*. 1998;31(1):150-157. doi:10.1016/s0735-1097(97)00422-1
51. Carnlöf C, Iwarzon M, Jensen-Urstad M, Gadler F, Insulander P. Women with PSVT are often misdiagnosed, referred later than men, and have more symptoms after ablation. *Scand Cardiovasc J*. 2017;51(6):299-307. doi:10.1080/14017431.2017.1385837

52. Chang SH, Kuo CF, Chou IJ, et al. Outcomes associated with paroxysmal supraventricular tachycardia during pregnancy. *Circulation.* 2017;135(6):616-618. doi:10.1161/CIRCULATIONAHA.116.025064
53. Piccini JP, Hammill BG, Sinner MF, et al. Incidence and prevalence of atrial fibrillation and associated mortality among Medicare beneficiaries, 1993-2007. *Circ Cardiovasc Qual Outcomes.* 2012;5(1):85-93. doi:10.1161/CIRCOUTCOMES.111.962688
54. Makkar RR, Fromm BS, Steinman RT, Meissner MD, Lehmann MH. Female gender as a risk factor for torsades de pointes associated with cardiovascular drugs. *JAMA.* 1993;270(21):2590-2597. doi:10.1001/jama.270.21.2590
55. Andell P, Li X, Martinsson A, et al. Epidemiology of valvular heart disease in a Swedish nationwide hospital-based register study. *Heart.* 2017;103(21):1696-1703. doi:10.1136/heartjnl-2016-310894
56. Itchhaporia D. Transcatheter aortic valve replacement in women. *Clin Cardiol.* 2018;41(2):228-231. doi:10.1002/clc.22912
57. Stock EO, Redberg R. Cardiovascular disease in women. *Curr Probl Cardiol.* 2012;37(11):450-526. doi:10.1016/j.cpcardiol.2012.07.001
58. Ballard-Hernandez J, Itchhaporia D. Heart Failure in Women Due to Hypertensive Heart Disease. *Heart Fail Clin.* 2019;15(4):497-507. doi:10.1016/j.hfc.2019.06.002
59. Eisenberg E, Di Palo KE, Piña IL. Sex differences in heart failure. *Clin Cardiol.* 2018;41(2):211-216. doi:10.1002/clc.22917
60. Elkayam U. Clinical characteristics of peripartum cardiomyopathy in the United States: diagnosis, prognosis, and management. *J Am Coll Cardiol.* 2011;58(7):659-670. doi:10.1016/j.jacc.2011.03.047

CHAPTER 20

ELDERLY AND HEART DISEASE

Madhan Shanmugasundaram and Toshinobu Kazui

INTRODUCTION

Heart disease is common in the elderly, and health care providers are often met with unique therapeutic challenges in this group. The elderly are often excluded from trials; hence, generalizing various treatment strategies becomes difficult. Health care providers should understand the physiology of cardiovascular changes that occurs with aging. Age should not be the only factor used in making therapeutic decisions. It is critical to individualize treatment to elderly patients. Although prolonging survival is a goal of many cardiovascular therapies, older adults may prioritize quality of life over reduction in mortality.

EPIDEMIOLOGY

Older adults or the elderly (>65 years of age) are a rapidly growing population. In the United States, 12% of the population in 2000 was older than 65 years, and it is estimated that this will increase to 20% by 2030 with the very elderly (>85 years of age) constituting almost one-third of this population.

Coronary artery disease (CAD), congestive heart failure (CHF), and atrial fibrillation (AF) are the most common cardiac diseases seen in the elderly, and cardiovascular disease is the most common cause of death in the elderly. Heart disease in the elderly is different from that in younger patients because of physiologic changes that occur with aging and an increased prevalence of comorbidities. Even though the elderly appear to have high morbidity and mortality from heart disease, therapies have shown to be more beneficial in this group than that in younger patients. Unfortunately, a treatment risk paradox exists in that even though the elderly are considered to be a high-risk population in whom treatments would have more benefit, they do not receive guideline-directed therapies. This chapter presents an overview of various heart diseases pertaining to the elderly and available evidence supporting various therapeutic strategies.

AGING AND THE HEART

Various physiologic changes occur in the cardiovascular system with age. Understanding these physiologic changes and differentiating them from various pathologic conditions is critical. These physiologic changes also form the basis of some of the pathologic changes in the elderly. Increased arterial stiffness and decreased compliance, especially in the central arteries, is one of the most important changes seen in the elderly. A combination of increased collagen and elastase—that, in turn, results in decreased elastin in the arteries—results in stiff noncompliant arteries with poor distensibility. There are other biologic changes such as increase in levels of matrix metalloproteinase, angiotensin II, and transforming growth factor that lead to endothelial dysfunction, with decreased nitric oxide production and impaired vasodilatation. These changes result in isolated systolic hypertension in the elderly, which is characterized by increased systolic pressure, decreased diastolic pressure, and widened pulse pressure.

In the heart, there is loss of myocytes, but the remaining myocytes hypertrophy resulting in concentric left ventricular (LV) hypertrophy. Excess fibroblast activity has been demonstrated in the aging heart, which causes fibrosis and ventricular noncompliance (stiffness). This results in diastolic dysfunction that, when advanced, can result in heart failure (HF) symptoms. Even though the LV ejection fraction remains normal with age, there are other structural changes such as "sigmoid" septum (ie, isolated hypertrophy [>15 mm] of the basal LV septum without hypertrophy elsewhere) that may cause LV outflow tract obstruction in the setting of hypovolemia or tachycardia. A decrease in sinoatrial nodal cells and fibrosis in the conduction system may result in bradyarrhythmia. Aortic and mitral valve (MV) thickening (sclerosis) are noted in the aging heart. Although this is not linearly associated with development of stenotic valve disease,[1] it is considered to be a marker of increased cardiovascular outcomes.

TREATMENT GOALS IN ELDERLY WITH HEART DISEASE

Most therapeutic strategies in cardiology are associated with a reduction in mortality and improved survival. Although these are very important objectives, elderly patients may prefer a better quality of life over extended survival. Some treatment strategies that improve survival in the elderly may adversely impact the quality of life. Elderly patients being treated for chronic diseases report that independence in activities of daily living is their primary goal.[2] Other equally important goals in elderly include decreased hospitalization and symptom-free living.[3] The elderly patients also consider psychosocial and financial burden of the disease and its treatments before making therapeutic decisions. In addition to estimating the potential gain in life expectancy achievable in elderly patients with various treatment options, health care providers should thus account for all these variables before offering treatments in elderly patients.

Hypertension

Hypertension has been well established as an important risk factor for cardiovascular disease in the elderly. Initially thought to be a physiologic response to aging because of increased arterial stiffness, it is now known to be associated with stroke, myocardial infarction (MI), peripheral artery disease, and cognitive impairment that increases the risk of dementia. The Joint National Committee 8 (JNC 8) guidelines for management of hypertension defines hypertension in the elderly (60 years or older) as blood pressure (BP) greater than or equal to 150 mm Hg systolic and/or greater than or equal to 90 mm Hg diastolic. The treatment goal in the elderly is BP less than 150/90 mm Hg; however, if the patient is on well-tolerated medications with a BP less than 140/80 mm Hg, then the guidelines recommend no changes to therapy or treatment goal.[4] However, based on more recent results from the Systolic Blood Pressure Intervention Trial (SPRINT, see later), for most adults 65 years or older, a more aggressive systolic BP target less than 130 mm Hg is recommended **(see Table 20.1)**.[5]

The Systolic Hypertension in the Elderly Program (SHEP) study that randomized elderly patients (average age 72 years) with isolated *systolic hypertension* to pharmacotherapy versus placebo, demonstrated a significant reduction in hemorrhagic and ischemic strokes in patients in the treatment arm. A significant reduction in the nonfatal MI, coronary deaths, and all-cause mortality was also reported.[6] In the HYpertension in the Very Elderly Trial (HYVET) that randomized over 3000 patients older than 80 years (mean age 84 years) to treatment or placebo, a significant reduction in fatal and nonfatal stroke, all-cause mortality and cardiovascular death occurred with treatment, thus confirming the benefits of antihypertensive therapy even in the very elderly patients.[7] SPRINT randomized over 9000 patients with hypertension (≥130 mm Hg systolic BP) to intensive treatment (<120 mm Hg) or standard therapy (<140 mm Hg) and demonstrated a significant reduction in the composite outcome of MI, stroke, HF, and cardiovascular death in the intensive treatment arm, with the benefits of intensive BP lowering seen in the elderly patient (≥75 years) subgroup as well **(Table 20.2)**.

Dyslipidemia

Dyslipidemia is common in elderly patients, but is undertreated because of the perceived lack of "benefit" and theoretical increased risk of adverse effects from statin therapy. The PROSPER (PROspective Study of Pravastatin in the Elderly at Risk) study randomized approximately 6000 patients older than 70 years of age at risk for vascular disease to pravastatin or placebo and demonstrated a significant reduction in the composite end point of death, nonfatal MI, and fatal or nonfatal stroke in the pravastatin arm.[9] The Heart Protection Study (HPS) randomized more than 20,000 patients with known history of vascular disease or diabetes to either simvastatin or placebo, and demonstrated a significant reduction in all-cause mortality and fatal and nonfatal vascular events in the simvastatin arm. A subgroup analysis of this study showed that the benefit was preserved in the elderly patients.[10] A post hoc analysis of the TNT (Treatment to New Targets) trial that included over 3000 patients older than 65 years of age, showed a significant reduction in first major cardiovascular event (death from CAD, nonfatal non–procedure-related MI, resuscitated cardiac arrest, or fatal or nonfatal stroke) in patients treated with high-dose (80 mg/day) versus low-dose (10 mg/day) atorvastatin. A large primary prevention trial (Justification for the Use of Statins in Prevention: an Intervention Trial Evaluating Rosuvastatin, JUPITER) randomized approximately 17,000 patients with no prior cardiovascular disease and low-density lipoprotein cholesterol (<130 mg/dL, high-sensitive C-reactive protein > 2 mg/L) to either rosuvastatin or placebo and showed a significant reduction in the combined primary end point of MI, stroke, arterial revascularization, hospitalization for unstable angina, or death from cardiovascular causes with rosuvastatin.[11] A secondary analysis of this study showed that in elderly patients (70 years or older), there was a greater benefit with rosuvastatin than with that in younger patients, thus confirming the benefits of statin therapy for primary prevention in the elderly patients.

A population-based study in France showed that statin cessation in elderly patients (older than 75 years of age) for primary prevention was associated with a 33% increased risk of admission for cardiovascular event. Consequently, the

TABLE 20.1 A Comparison of Blood Pressure Thresholds and Targets Between ACC/AHA, ACP/AAFP, and ESC/ESH Guidelines

	ACC/AHA 2017	ACP/AAFP 2017	ESC/ESH 2018
Definition of older patients	≥65 years	≥60 years	Elderly 65-79 years Very old ≥ 80 years
BP threshold for initiation of pharmacotherapy	≥130/80 mm Hg	SBP ≥ 150 mm Hg	Elderly ≥ 140/90 mm Hg Very old ≥ 160/90 mm Hg
Blood pressure target	<130/80 mm Hg	SBP < 150 mm Hg	SBP 130-139 mm Hg DBP 70-79 mm Hg

ACC/AHA, American College of Cardiology/American Heart Association; ACP/AAFP, American College of Physicians/American Academy of Family Physicians; BP, blood pressure; DBP, diastolic blood pressure; ESC/ESH, European Society of Cardiology/European Society of Hypertension; SBP, systolic blood pressure.

TABLE 20.2 Cardiovascular Conditions and Therapies in Elderly With Strength of Evidence

Condition	Therapy	Strength of Evidence
Dyslipidemia	Statins	Strong
Coronary artery disease	Aspirin Beta-blockers ACEI/ARB PCI	Strong Strong Strong Strong
HFrEF	Beta-blockers ACEI/ARB ARNI Aldosterone antagonists	Strong Strong Strong Weak

ACEI/ARB, angiotensin-converting enzyme inhibitor/angiotensin receptor blocker; ARNI, angiotensin receptor neprilysin inhibitor; HFrEF, heart failure with reduced ejection fraction; PCI, percutaneous coronary intervention.

American Heart Association/American College of Cardiology (AHA/ACC) lipid guidelines assign a Class II level A recommendation for statin therapy in elderly patients for secondary prevention of cardiovascular disease and a Class II level B recommendation for primary prevention.

Coronary Artery Disease

The prevalence of CAD increases with age, and the elderly with CAD have high morbidity and mortality. About 20% of men and 13% of women aged 60 to 79 years in the United States have CAD. In those older than 80 years, over 30% of men and 25% of women have established CAD, with the majority of them presenting with acute MI. In 2014, about 50% of percutaneous coronary intervention (PCI) procedures were performed in the elderly (65 years or older). The financial burden of this disease is significant as well. CAD in the elderly is more advanced than it is in younger patients, with multivessel involvement, a higher incidence of left main coronary stenosis, more calcified lesions, diffuse critical disease, and impaired LV function. The elderly with stable CAD also have a different presentation compared to that in the younger patients, with only a minority reporting angina. Most elderly patients present with atypical symptoms such as fatigue, exertional dyspnea, and lack of energy.

DIAGNOSIS

Owing to the high prevalence of baseline electrocardiogram abnormalities, exercise treadmill testing (ETT) alone is often not sufficient to evaluate the presence of CAD. Also, many elderly have orthopedic issues or limited functional status that precludes them from performing adequate levels of exercise needed for traditional ETT. That said, there are several modified ETT protocols that provide valuable information with good diagnostic accuracy. The rationale for stress testing in the elderly is very similar to that in the younger population, which is to diagnose CAD, but these tests should only be used in patients with intermediate pretest probability for CAD; these tests do not add prognostic value in patients with either low or high pretest probability. Adding an imaging modality—either nuclear perfusion or echocardiography—increases the sensitivity and specificity of stress testing. A meta-analysis of different stress test modalities in elderly patients (65 years of age or older) concluded that imaging-based stress testing improved the diagnostic yield compared to ETT alone.[12] For elderly patients with poor exercise capacity, pharmacologic stress testing could be considered. Owing to the high prevalence of calcific CAD in the elderly, coronary calcium score and coronary computed tomography angiography are not usually recommended. Invasive angiography is typically reserved for elderly patients with markedly abnormal noninvasive stress tests or medically refractory symptoms.

MANAGEMENT OF THE OLDER PATIENT WITH CORONARY ARTERY DISEASE

Medical Management

Antianginal medications work in a similar manner and are as effective in the elderly as in the non-elderly patients, although one should be cognizant of their side effects such as hypotension and bradycardia, which may be more pronounced in the elderly. The goals of medical therapy in stable CAD include improvement of symptoms, decreased risk of future cardiovascular events, and reduction in mortality.

Aspirin (low dose, 81 mg) in combination with beta-blocker (sotalol) was shown to reduce the risk of death and MI in patients with stable angina compared to sotalol alone.[13] A meta-analysis of over 140 trials confirms the benefit of aspirin therapy in both primary and secondary prevention of cardiovascular events.[14]

Beta-blockers decrease heart rate, thereby lowering the myocardial oxygen demand in patients with angina, and they are currently indicated as first-line therapy for these patients because of their negative inotropic and chronotropic properties. However, beta-blockers need to be carefully administered in the elderly because of their potential to cause bradyarrhythmias and heart block.

Angiotensin-converting enzyme inhibitors (ACEIs) are indicated in patients with stable CAD to reduce major adverse cardiovascular events. This was studied in three major trials: (1) Heart Outcomes Prevention Evaluation (HOPE)[15]; (2) EUropean trial on Reduction Of cardiac events with Perindopril in patients with stable coronary Artery disease (EUROPA)[16]; and (3) Prevention of Events with Angiotensin-Converting Enzyme inhibition trial (PEACE).[17] A meta-analysis of these trials concluded that ACEI use in patients with stable CAD is associated with significant reduction in all-cause mortality, cardiovascular mortality, nonfatal MI, and stroke.

Nitrates and calcium channel blockers are also indicated for treatment of angina in patients with stable CAD, but these drugs do not reduce cardiovascular events. Ranolazine is another antianginal medication that has been shown in a subgroup analysis to provide anginal relief in elderly patients without causing hemodynamic compromise.

PCI is a well-established treatment strategy for angina relief in patients with stable CAD; however, PCI is associated with a greater risk of complications in the elderly than in younger patients, including acute kidney injury, bleeding, stroke, death, and periprocedural MI. In recent years, the role of PCI in patients with stable CAD has been debated since the publication of Clinical Outcomes Utilizing Revascularization and Aggressive druG Evaluation (COURAGE) trial that showed no significant difference in outcomes among patients with stable CAD treated with optimal medical therapy (OMT) versus those treated with PCI and OMT.[18] Analysis of the elderly (older than 65 years) subgroup in this study showed no difference in major cardiac events or angina-free rates between the OMT and PCI plus OMT-treated patients.[19] The randomized Trial of Invasive versus Medical therapy in Elderly patients (TIME) study reported an early benefit for PCI with OMT compared to OMT alone in elderly patients with stable CAD; however, after 1 year of follow-up, there was no difference in the symptoms, quality of life, and death or nonfatal MI with PCI between the groups.[20] Hence, PCI should be reserved for patients who have refractory symptoms despite maximal tolerated medical therapy in patients with stable CAD.

Acute Coronary Syndromes

It is estimated that 60% of patients admitted for acute coronary syndrome (ACS) are older than 65 years of age, and they account for about 80% of deaths from ACS. Chest pain is reported only in a minority of elderly patients presenting with ACS, thus delaying the diagnosis. They present with atypical symptoms including dyspnea, diaphoresis, nausea, vomiting, syncope, presyncope, fatigue, altered mental status, or confusion. Compared to the non-elderly patients, elderly patients with ACS are typically sicker, have more multivessel CAD, and have more comorbidities that present unique therapeutic challenges.

Antiplatelet agents are indicated in all patients with ACS to improve cardiovascular outcomes. Aspirin has been shown to reduce death and vascular events in elderly patients with ACS.[14] The addition of clopidogrel, a P2Y12 inhibitor, to aspirin is associated with a significant reduction in nonfatal MI, cardiac death, and stroke compared to aspirin alone in elderly patients. Administration of newer antiplatelet drugs (prasugrel and ticagrelor[21]) with aspirin is also beneficial in elderly patients compared to aspirin alone, although the bleeding risks need to be considered before initiating these medications in this cohort. Prasugrel is contraindicated in patients older than 75 years of age because of an increased risk of intracranial bleeding. The current standard of care is dual antiplatelet therapy (aspirin plus a P2Y12 inhibitor) for at least 12 months for patients with ACS.[22] Intravenous (IV) glycoprotein IIb/IIIa inhibitors (GPIs) have been advocated to improve short-term outcomes in patients presenting with ACS, especially in those undergoing an early invasive approach with angiography followed by revascularization. However, there is a significant increase in nonfatal bleeding with these agents, which is concerning in the elderly. The evidence supporting the use of GPI in the elderly is mixed with the PRISM-PLUS (Platelet Receptor inhibition in Ischemic Syndrome Management in Patients Limited by Unstable Signs and symptoms) study showing a significant reduction in death, MI, or ischemia with IV tirofiban in both elderly and younger patients.[23] Conversely, another study of IV eptifibatide in patients with ACS was unable to show a benefit in death and MI in the elderly subgroup.[24] Two other studies examining early or upfront GPI use in patients with ACS also failed to show a benefit in the elderly.[25,26] A meta-analysis of six GPI trials showed no benefit with these agents in elderly (older than 59 years) patients.[27] Heparin and low-molecular-weight heparin (LMWH) are indicated in elderly patients with ACS, with no clear superiority of one agent over the other.

Percutaneous Coronary Intervention for Acute Coronary Syndrome

PCI is effective in reducing death and recurrent MI in patients with ACS, including the elderly. The Treat angina with Aggrastat and determine Cost of Therapy with an Invasive or Conservative Strategy–Thrombolysis In Myocardial Infarction-18 (TACTICS-TIMI 18) trial showed significant reduction in death, MI, and hospitalization at 6 months in patients randomized to early invasive strategy (angiogram followed by revascularization within 48 hours) compared to conservative strategy, with the benefit primarily seen in high-risk patients. A prespecified subgroup analysis confirmed this benefit in the elderly, but with a significant increase in bleeding risk.[28] The Invasive versus Conservative Treatment in Unstable coronary Syndromes (ICTUS) study did not show a superiority of early invasive strategy in elderly patients with ACS over conservative strategy after 1-year follow-up.[29] However, a meta-analysis of three randomized trials demonstrated a significant reduction in death and MI with early invasive strategy in elderly patients.[30] The American College of Cardiology/American Heart Association (ACC/AHA) guidelines recommend an early invasive approach in patients with ACS with high- or intermediate-risk features.[31]

In patients with ST-segment elevation myocardial infarction (STEMI), use of fibrinolytic therapy or PCI is recommended to reperfuse the occluded coronary artery to improve cardiovascular outcomes. Because fibrinolytic therapy in the elderly is associated with increased bleeding risk, including intracranial hemorrhage, it is reserved for those who do not have access to expeditious PCI. PCI was compared to thrombolytic therapy in a study with primarily elderly (older than 75 years) patients, but was stopped prematurely because there was a significant reduction in death, MI, or stroke with PCI.[32] A pooled analysis (Primary Coronary Angioplasty Trialists [PCAT]) of 11 randomized trials that included over 800 elderly (70 years or older) demonstrated a significant reduction in mortality with PCI over fibrinolytic therapy in elderly patients.[33]

Optimal Revascularization Strategy for Elderly Patients With Multivessel Coronary Artery Disease

The optimal revascularization strategy for elderly patients with multivessel CAD remains controversial: Whether the survival benefit from coronary artery bypass graft (CABG) compared with PCI in patients with multivessel CAD extends to the elderly remains unclear. PCI is often the preferred strategy in elderly patients, because of the perceived increased early risk with CABG. However, a meta-analysis that evaluated the long-term outcomes of CABG versus PCI with drug-eluting stents in older adults with left main or multivessel CAD showed that CABG was associated with approximately 50% fewer MIs and repeat revascularizations than was PCI, but had no effect on all-cause mortality or stroke.[34]

Congestive Heart Failure

CHF is common in the elderly, with increasing incidence and prevalence with age. It is associated with significant morbidity and mortality in the elderly. Both heart failure with reduced ejection fraction (HFrEF) and heart failure with preserved ejection fraction (HFpEF) are common in the elderly. Hypertension and CAD are common risk factors for development of HFrEF, whereas hypertension, diabetes, and AF increase susceptibility to HFpEF. Compared to younger patients, the elderly patients with HFpEF have more comorbidities (AF, chronic kidney disease, and hypertension), are more commonly white women and are more likely to die from noncardiovascular causes.

Similar to other cardiovascular diseases, the guideline-directed medical therapies that demonstrate improvement in cardiovascular outcomes in patients with CHF are less studied in elderly patients. Several classes of medications that are indicated in systolic HF include beta-blockers, ACEIs, angiotensin receptor blockers (ARBs), aldosterone antagonists, and diuretics.

Beta-blockers are indicated in patients with HFrEF to reduce mortality and decrease HF-related hospitalizations. A meta-analysis of five studies showed significant reduction in mortality in elderly patients with HFrEF treated with beta-blockers compared to those not receiving them, thus confirming their efficacy in this population.[35] The Study of the Effects of Nebivolol Intervention on Outcomes and Rehospitalization in Seniors with heart failure (SENIORS) trial also showed significant reductions in mortality and HF hospitalizations in elderly patients treated with a beta-blocker.[36]

ACEIs significantly reduced mortality and HF hospitalization in the elderly patients (older than 60 years) in a meta-analysis of 27 trials.[37] Although the goal is to achieve maximally tolerated dose of an ACEI, in elderly patients this may not be achievable because of hypotension and renal insufficiency.

Subgroup analysis of large randomized, controlled ARB trials confirms significant reduction in cardiovascular outcomes in elderly patients with HFrEF treated with ARB compared to placebo. ARBs were evaluated in elderly patients with HFrEF and shown to be equally effective compared to ACEI in preventing HF-related hospitalizations and mortality. ARBs can be safely used in ACEI-intolerant elderly patients, but the two should not be administered concomitantly because patients receiving both have increased risk of mortality and morbidity. The sacubitril-valsartan combination (ie, a neprilysin inhibitor and ARB combination) was shown to be superior to an ACEI in preventing all-cause mortality, cardiovascular mortality, and HF-related hospitalization in patients with HFrEF, with these benefits extending to the elderly subgroup.[38]

Aldosterone antagonists were evaluated in three trials including the Randomized ALdactone Evaluation Study (RALES),[39] Eplerenone Post-acute myocardial infarction Heart failure Efficacy and Survival Study (EPHESUS),[40] and Eplerenone in Mild Patients Hospitalization And SurvIval Study in Heart Failure (EMPHASIS-HF).[41] Subgroup analysis of the RALES and EMPHASIS studies showed significant reduction in death or HF hospitalization in elderly patients treated with an aldosterone antagonist compared to placebo, whereas the EPHESUS subgroup analysis failed to show this benefit. It should, however, be noted that hyperkalemia was common, and patients with significant renal insufficiency were excluded from these studies. The African American Heart Failure Trial (A-HeFT) showed a significant reduction in mortality with vasodilators compared to placebo, including in the elderly patients.[42] Diuretics are indicated to reduce symptoms; however, they not been shown to improve outcomes.

In patients with HFpEF, none of these medications (BBs, ACEIs, ARBs, or aldosterone antagonists) have shown to improve outcomes compared to placebo, which makes the management of these patients incredibly frustrating and difficult. Recently, the U.S. Food and Drug Administration (FDA) approved the use of sacubitril-valsartan in patients with HFpEF to improve cardiovascular outcomes based on the results of the The Prospective comparison of ARNI [angiotensin receptor–neprilysin inhibitor] with ARB [angiotensin-receptor blockers] Global Outcomes in HF with Preserved Ejection Fraction (PARAGON-HF) PARAGON HF study, making it the only drug that is approved for these patients.[43] Diuretics are used to improve symptoms in these patients.

Cardiac resynchronization therapy (CRT) in combination with implantable cardioverter-defibrillator (ICD) improves mortality, symptoms, and HF hospitalizations in patients with HFrEF. These devices were shown to be beneficial in elderly patients as well.

An aging HF population together with improvements in mechanical circulatory support technology have led to increasing left ventricular assist device (LVAD) implantations in older adults. According to the Interagency Registry for Mechanically Assisted Circulatory Support, the number of patients who required durable LVAD between 2008 and 2017 was 20,939. Of that, 4.9% of patients were 75 years of age or older. These patients had increased mortality post-LVAD implantation compared to younger patients: only 47% of adults 75 years of age or older were discharged home following LVAD implantation. Age remains a significant predictor of mortality.[44] On the other hand, orthotopic heart transplant recipients in their 70s had similar outcomes to recipients in other age groups: 5-year mortality was 27% for recipients aged 18 to 59 years, 29% for age 60 to 69 years, and 31% for age 70 or older. Therefore, selected elderly patients should not be routinely excluded from consideration for heart transplantation.[45]

Aortic Valve Disorders

Aortic Stenosis

Aortic stenosis is the most common valvular heart disease in the elderly, with an estimated prevalence of 4% in those older than 70 years. In the elderly, calcific degeneration of the trileaflet aortic valve is the most common etiology; bicuspid valves present a decade earlier. Generally, patients are asymptomatic, with a steep decline in functional status at the onset of symptoms. Echocardiography is the gold standard diagnostic test that shows restricted opening of aortic valve, peak velocity of 4 m per s, and mean gradient of 40 mm Hg in patients with severe aortic stenosis. However, low-flow (stroke volume <35 mL/m^2), low-gradient severe aortic stenosis is common in the elderly, and is associated with similar morbidity and mortality as in those with normal-flow, high-gradient disease. These patients benefit from treatment of their aortic valve disease similar to normal-flow, high-gradient severe aortic stenosis. Traditionally, surgical aortic valve replacement was considered standard of care, but minimally invasive transcatheter aortic valve replacement (TAVR) has emerged as the treatment of choice for elderly patients with aortic stenosis. Initially, TAVR was limited to inoperable patients or those with high surgical risk, but more recent studies demonstrate similar outcomes in intermediate- and low-risk patients as compared to surgical valve replacement.[46,47] It is predicted that the majority of patients with aortic stenosis will be treated by TAVR in the future given the durability of these percutaneous valves and comparable, if not superior, outcomes to surgical valve replacement.

Aortic Regurgitation

Aortic regurgitation is either due to valvular (degenerative) or aortic root pathologies, and its prevalence increases with age. Although chronic aortic regurgitation is well tolerated for years, eventually LV dilatation results in systolic dysfunction. Hence, it is critical to follow up these patients by assessing clinical and echocardiographic findings to decide on optimal time of intervention. Once symptoms develop, there is a rapid decline in functional status and increased mortality. Surgical aortic valve replacement is the treatment of choice, although TAVR with self-expanding valves has reported reasonable outcomes in patients with high surgical risk.

Mitral Valve Disorders

Mitral Regurgitation

Because rheumatic heart disease has rapidly decreased in the United States, MV prolapse resulting in mitral regurgitation (MR) is the most common MV disease in the elderly. Other etiologies of MR include endocarditis, papillary muscle rupture following MI, and functional MR due to either annular dilatation or ischemic papillary muscle dysfunction. Chronic regurgitant lesions are well tolerated, and hence patients, especially the elderly, are asymptomatic for a long time until they develop CHF or pulmonary hypertension. Echocardiography is the gold standard for diagnosing MR and assessing its severity. Patients with untreated severe MR and LV systolic dysfunction have high morbidity and mortality. These patients have to be optimized initially via ACEIs or ARBs followed by referral for definitive therapy, which is surgery for most patients. The ACC/AHA guidelines for management of valve disease recommend MV surgery for symptomatic severe MR and LV decompensation (end-systolic dimension > 45 mm or LV ejection fraction < 60%) or pulmonary hypertension.[48] MV surgery in elderly patients is associated with significant morbidity and mortality. A study that compared MV repair to MV replacement in elderly patients with MR demonstrated higher mortality in patients undergoing MV replacement at 90 days.[49] In recent years, percutaneous MV repair with the MitraClip device has been shown to reduce MR severity, improve symptoms and quality of life, and decrease LV dimensions compared to medical therapy in patients with high surgical risk.[50] Newer therapies, including percutaneous MV replacement, that promise to change therapeutic options available to frail elderly patients are being studied.

Mitral Stenosis

Mitral stenosis (MS) due to rheumatic heart disease is rare in the United States. Most patients with MS are functional in nature because of mitral annular calcification. These patients are treated surgically with MV replacement when severe and symptomatic. However, MV surgery can be technically challenging in the presence of severe mitral annular calcification. Extensive decalcification during surgery can lead to nonrepairable atrioventricular (AV) disconnection. Owing to this concern, implantation of a transcatheter valve via open surgical or a percutaneous transvenous transseptal approach has been reported.

Arrhythmias

Bradyarrhythmias

Bradyarrhythmias increase in frequency with age because of changes in the conduction system: A reduction in pacemaker cells in the sinoatrial node may result in bradycardia, and fibrosis or calcification of the conduction system may result in AV block.

Patients with bradyarrhythmias often present with symptoms or signs of low cardiac output, such as presyncope or syncope, but other symptoms such as fatigue, poor exercise tolerance, or dyspnea may be seen as well. Diagnosis begins with a 12-lead electrocardiogram, but many patients need prolonged outpatient monitoring with Holter, event monitor, or loop recorders. Assessment of chronotropic competence with a simple exercise treadmill test may be needed in some patients. After cessation of potential medications that can cause or exacerbate bradyarrhythmias, pacemaker implantation is indicated for symptomatic sinus node dysfunction or high-grade AV block.

Tachyarrhythmias

Supraventricular tachycardias in the elderly include atrial tachycardia, AV nodal reentry tachycardia, AV reciprocating tachycardia, multifocal atrial tachycardia, atrial flutter, and

AF. The management of these arrhythmias is similar to that in younger patients.

AF is the most common arrhythmia in the elderly, and its prevalence increases with age. It is associated with a significant increase in the risk of stroke, which is estimated by the CHA_2DS_2-VASc score, with 1 point for age between 65 and 74 years and 2 points for age older than 75 years. The HAS-BLED score predicts the risk of bleeding in these patients. One should weigh the risks and benefits of anticoagulation for stroke prophylaxis in the elderly before recommending a therapy.

Warfarin with an international normalized ratio (INR) goal of 2 to 3.0 or direct oral anticoagulants (DOACs) are used for stroke prophylaxis. Unlike warfarin, DOACs do not need regular monitoring, nor do they interact with food and other medications. In addition, DOACs have been well established to be safe and effective in the elderly compared to warfarin.[51]

In regard to therapies for AF, rate control or rhythm control strategies are options. Several trials comparing rhythm control to rate control strategy in AF and a meta-analysis of five trials showed no difference in outcomes with either approach.[52] Because antiarrhythmics have more drug interactions and side effects in the elderly than in younger patients, generally rate control is the preferred strategy in the elderly. This was confirmed in the Atrial Fibrillation Follow-up Investigation of Rhythm Management (AFFIRM) trial that showed increased mortality in elderly patients with AF with rhythm control when compared to rate control.[53] Intensive (ventricular rate < 80 bpm) versus lenient (<110 bpm) rate control strategy was compared in the RAte Control Efficacy in permanent atrial fibrillation (RACE) II trial, which concluded that a lenient rate control was noninferior in the elderly.[54] Catheter-based ablation therapies are recommended to improve symptoms, but their benefit in the elderly is not well established.

Ventricular arrhythmias increase in incidence with age, and their medical management is similar to what is offered to younger patients. ICDs are recommended for both primary and secondary prevention in patients with ventricular arrhythmias. However, their benefit is less well established in the elderly: A meta-analysis of three major trials failed to show a significant benefit with ICDs in the elderly for secondary prevention.[55] Conversely, the Multicenter Automatic Defibrillator Implantation Trial (MADIT II) showed a significant reduction in mortality in elderly patients who received an ICD for primary prevention.[56] Although age by itself should not be used to decide whether one gets an ICD or not, it should be recognized that older adults (older than 80 years) were poorly represented in ICD trials. The decision should be individualized, and guidelines recommend not implanting an ICD in patients with poor expected 1-year survival.

Critically Ill Elderly With Cardiovascular Disease

Elderly patients with heart disease are often admitted to the intensive care units (ICU) where common geriatric conditions such as delirium, dementia, frailty, immobility, polypharmacy, and multiple comorbidities may be exacerbated, thus affecting overall care. These patients present unique therapeutic challenges given associated comorbidities and lack of literature supporting treatment decisions. It is recommended that instead of an algorithmic approach, a thoughtful approach with careful consideration of geriatric syndromes be applied to elderly patients in the ICU.[57]

RESEARCH AND FUTURE DIRECTIONS

There are well-established risk factors causing heart disease in the elderly, but what remains poorly studied is how aging affects the interplay of these risk factors. Another area that requires significant advancement is the design of animal model of aging to aid in the development and testing of newer therapies. Also, there needs to be a conscious effort from the investigators to design studies for the elderly or to include a significant proportion of the elderly in contemporary clinical trials.

KEY POINTS

- ✔ Older adults are a rapidly increasing subset of the U.S. population.
- ✔ Cardiovascular disease is the most common cause of morbidity and mortality in the elderly.
- ✔ Managing heart disease in the elderly is challenging owing to physiologic changes that occur with aging and the increased prevalence of comorbidities.
- ✔ CAD, CHF, and AF are the most common cardiac diseases in the elderly.
- ✔ Treatment goals in the elderly consider quality of life, reduction in hospitalizations, and symptom-free living more important than prolonging survival.
- ✔ Elderly are often excluded from clinical trials; hence, literature supporting various therapies is often extrapolated from younger patients.
- ✔ Age alone should not limit treatment options in the elderly.

REFERENCES

1. Lindroos M, Kupari M, Heikkilä J, Tilvis R. Prevalence of aortic valve abnormalities in the elderly: an echocardiographic study of a random population sample. *J Am Coll Cardiol.* 1993;21(5):1220-1225.
2. Huang ES, Gorawara-Bhat R, Chin MH. Self-reported goals of older patients with type 2 diabetes mellitus. *J Am Geriatr Soc.* 2005;53(2):306-311.
3. Morrow AS, Haidet P, Skinner J, Naik AD. Integrating diabetes self-management with the health goals of older adults: a qualitative exploration. *Patient Educ Couns.* 2008;72(3):418-423.
4. James PA, Oparil S, Carter BL, et al. 2014 evidence-based guideline for the management of high blood pressure in adults: report from the panel members appointed to the Eighth Joint National Committee (JNC 8). *JAMA.* 2014;311(5):507-520.
5. Agarwala A, Yang E, Parapid B. Older adults and hypertension: beyond the 2017 Guideline for prevention, detection, evaluation, and management of high blood pressure in adults. Published 2020. Accessed March 12, 2021. https://www.acc.org/latest-in-cardiology/articles/2020/02/26/06/24/older-adults-and-hypertension

6. Prevention of stroke by antihypertensive drug treatment in older persons with isolated systolic hypertension. Final results of the Systolic Hypertension in the Elderly Program (SHEP). SHEP Cooperative Research Group. *JAMA.* 1991;265(24):3255-3264.
7. Beckett NS, Peters R, Fletcher AE, et al. Treatment of hypertension in patients 80 years of age or older. *N Engl J Med.* 2008;358(18):1887-1898.
8. Wright JT Jr, Williamson JD, Whelton PK, et al. A randomized trial of intensive versus standard blood-pressure control. *N Engl J Med.* 2015;373(22):2103-2116.
9. Shepherd J, Blauw GJ, Murphy MB, et al. Pravastatin in elderly individuals at risk of vascular disease (PROSPER): a randomised controlled trial. *Lancet.* 2002;360(9346):1623-1630.
10. Heart Protection Study Collaborative Group. MRC/BHF Heart Protection Study of cholesterol lowering with simvastatin in 20,536 high-risk individuals: a randomised placebo-controlled trial. *Lancet.* 2002;360(9326):7-22.
11. Ridker PM, Danielson E, Fonseca FAH, et al. Rosuvastatin to prevent vascular events in men and women with elevated C-reactive protein. *N Engl J Med.* 2008;359(21):2195-2207.
12. Rai M, Baker WL, Parker MW, Heller GV. Meta-analysis of optimal risk stratification in patients >65 years of age. *Am J Cardiol.* 2012;110(8):1092-1099.
13. Juul-Moller S, Edvardsson N, Jahnmatz B, Rosén A, Sørensen S, Omblus R. Double-blind trial of aspirin in primary prevention of myocardial infarction in patients with stable chronic angina pectoris. The Swedish Angina Pectoris Aspirin Trial (SAPAT) Group. *Lancet.* 1992;340(8833):1421-1425.
14. Collaborative overview of randomised trials of antiplatelet therapy—I: prevention of death, myocardial infarction, and stroke by prolonged antiplatelet therapy in various categories of patients. Antiplatelet Trialists' Collaboration. *BMJ.* 1994;308(6921):81-106.
15. Yusuf S, Sleight P, Pogue J, Bosch J, Davies R, Dagenais G. Effects of an angiotensin-converting-enzyme inhibitor, ramipril, on cardiovascular events in high-risk patients. *N Engl J Med.* 2000;342(3):145-153.
16. Fox KM, EURopean trial On reduction of cardiac events with Perindopril in stable coronary Artery disease Investigators. Efficacy of perindopril in reduction of cardiovascular events among patients with stable coronary artery disease: randomised, double-blind, placebo-controlled, multicentre trial (the EUROPA study). *Lancet.* 2003;362(9386):782-788.
17. Braunwald E, Domanski MJ, Fowler SE, et al. Angiotensin-converting-enzyme inhibition in stable coronary artery disease. *N Engl J Med.* 2004;351(20):2058-2068.
18. Boden WE, O'Rourke RA, Teo KK, et al. Optimal medical therapy with or without PCI for stable coronary disease. *N Engl J Med.* 2007;356(15):1503-1516.
19. Teo KK, Sedlis SP, Boden WE, et al. Optimal medical therapy with or without percutaneous coronary intervention in older patients with stable coronary disease: a pre-specified subset analysis of the COURAGE (Clinical Outcomes Utilizing Revascularization and Aggressive druG Evaluation) trial. *J Am Coll Cardiol.* 2009;54(14):1303-1308.
20. Pfisterer M, Buser P, Osswald S, et al. Outcome of elderly patients with chronic symptomatic coronary artery disease with an invasive vs optimized medical treatment strategy: one-year results of the randomized TIME trial. *JAMA.* 2003;289(9):1117-1123.
21. Wallentin L, Becker RC, Budaj A, et al. Ticagrelor versus clopidogrel in patients with acute coronary syndromes. *N Engl J Med.* 2009;361(11):1045-1057.
22. Levine GN, Bates ER, Bitti JA, et al. 2016 ACC/AHA Guideline focused update on duration of dual antiplatelet therapy in patients with coronary artery disease: a report of the American College of Cardiology/American Heart Association Task Force on Clinical Practice Guidelines: an update of the 2011 ACCF/AHA/SCAI Guideline for Percutaneous Coronary Intervention, 2011 ACCF/AHA Guideline for coronary artery bypass graft surgery, 2012 ACC/AHA/ACP/AATS/PCNA/SCAI/STS Guideline for the diagnosis and management of patients with stable ischemic heart disease, 2013 ACCF/AHA Guideline for the management of ST-elevation myocardial infarction, 2014 AHA/ACC Guideline for the management of patients with non-ST-elevation acute coronary syndromes, and 2014 ACC/AHA Guideline on perioperative cardiovascular evaluation and management of patients undergoing noncardiac surgery. *Circulation.* 2016;134(10):e123-e155.
23. Platelet Receptor Inhibition in Ischemic Syndrome Management in Patients Limited by Unstable Signs and Symptoms (PRISM-PLUS) Study Investigators. Inhibition of the platelet glycoprotein IIb/IIIa receptor with tirofiban in unstable angina and non-Q-wave myocardial infarction. *N Engl J Med.* 1998;338(21):1488-1497.
24. Platelet Glycoprotein IIb/IIIa in Unstable Angina: Receptor Suppression Using Integrilin Therapy (PURSUIT) Trial Investigators. Inhibition of platelet glycoprotein IIb/IIIa with eptifibatide in patients with acute coronary syndromes. *N Engl J Med.* 1998;339(7):436-443.
25. Giugliano RP, White JA, Bode C, et al. Early versus delayed, provisional eptifibatide in acute coronary syndromes. *N Engl J Med.* 2009;360(21):2176-2190.
26. Lopes RD, Alexander KP, Manoukian SV, et al. Advanced age, antithrombotic strategy, and bleeding in non-ST-segment elevation acute coronary syndromes: results from the ACUITY (Acute Catheterization and Urgent Intervention Triage Strategy) trial. *J Am Coll Cardiol.* 2009;53(12):1021-1030.
27. Boersma E, Harrington RA, Moliterno DJ, et al. Platelet glycoprotein IIb/IIIa inhibitors in acute coronary syndromes: a meta-analysis of all major randomised clinical trials. *Lancet.* 2002;359(9302):189-198.
28. Cannon CP, Weintraub WS, Demopoulos LA, et al. Comparison of early invasive and conservative strategies in patients with unstable coronary syndromes treated with the glycoprotein IIb/IIIa inhibitor tirofiban. *N Engl J Med.* 2001;344(25):1879-1887.
29. de Winter RJ, Windhausen F, Cornel JH, et al. Early invasive versus selectively invasive management for acute coronary syndromes. *N Engl J Med.* 2005;353(11):1095-1104.
30. Fox KA, Clayton TC, Damman P, et al. Long-term outcome of a routine versus selective invasive strategy in patients with non-ST-segment elevation acute coronary syndrome a meta-analysis of individual patient data. *J Am Coll Cardiol.* 2010;55(22):2435-2445.
31. Amsterdam EA, Wenger NK, Brindis RG, et al. 2014 AHA/ACC Guideline for the management of patients with non-ST-elevation acute coronary syndromes: a report of the American College of Cardiology/American Heart Association Task Force on Practice Guidelines. *J Am Coll Cardiol.* 2014;64(24):e139-e228.
32. de Boer MJ, Ottervanger J-P, van't Hof AWJ, et al. Reperfusion therapy in elderly patients with acute myocardial infarction: a randomized comparison of primary angioplasty and thrombolytic therapy. *J Am Coll Cardiol.* 2002;39(11):1723-1728.
33. Grines C, Patel A, Zijlstra F, et al. Primary coronary angioplasty compared with intravenous thrombolytic therapy for acute myocardial infarction: six-month follow up and analysis of individual patient data from randomized trials. *Am Heart J.* 2003;145(1):47-57.
34. Chang M, Lee CW, Ahn J-M, et al. Outcomes of coronary artery bypass graft surgery versus drug-eluting stents in older adults. *J Am Geriatr Soc.* 2017;65(3):625-630.
35. Dulin BR, Haas SJ, Abraham WT, Krum H. Do elderly systolic heart failure patients benefit from beta blockers to the same extent as the non-elderly? Meta-analysis of >12,000 patients in large-scale clinical trials. *Am J Cardiol.* 2005;95(7):896-898.
36. Flather MD, Shibata MC, Coats AJS, et al. Randomized trial to determine the effect of nebivolol on mortality and cardiovascular hospital admission in elderly patients with heart failure (SENIORS). *Eur Heart J.* 2005;26(3):215-225.
37. Garg R, Yusuf S. Overview of randomized trials of angiotensin-converting enzyme inhibitors on mortality and morbidity in patients with heart failure. Collaborative Group on ACE Inhibitor Trials. *JAMA.* 1995;273(18):1450-1456.
38. Jhund PS, Fu M, Bayram E, et al. Efficacy and safety of LCZ696 (sacubitril-valsartan) according to age: insights from PARADIGM-HF. *Eur Heart J.* 2015;36(38):2576-2584.
39. Pitt B, Zannad F, Remme WJ, et al. The effect of spironolactone on morbidity and mortality in patients with severe heart failure.

Randomized Aldactone Evaluation Study Investigators. *N Engl J Med.* 1999;341(10):709-717.

40. Pitt B, Remme W, Zannad F, et al. Eplerenone, a selective aldosterone blocker, in patients with left ventricular dysfunction after myocardial infarction. *N Engl J Med.* 2003;348(14):1309-1321.
41. Zannad F, McMurray JJV, Krum H, et al. Eplerenone in patients with systolic heart failure and mild symptoms. *N Engl J Med.* 2011;364(1):11-21.
42. Taylor AL, Ziesche S, Yancy C, et al. Combination of isosorbide dinitrate and hydralazine in blacks with heart failure. *N Engl J Med.* 2004;351(20):2049-2057.
43. Solomon SD, McMurray JJV, Anand IS, et al. Angiotensin-neprilysin inhibition in heart failure with preserved ejection fraction. *N Engl J Med.* 2019;381(17):1609-1620.
44. Caraballo C, DeFilippis EM, Nakagawa S, et al. Clinical outcomes after left ventricular assist device implantation in older adults: an INTERMACS analysis. *JACC Heart Fail.* 2019;7(12):1069-1078.
45. Cooper LB, Lu D, Mentz RJ, et al. Cardiac transplantation for older patients: Characteristics and outcomes in the septuagenarian population. *J Heart Lung Transplant.* 2016;35(3):362-369.
46. Mack MJ, Leon MB, Thourani VH, et al. Transcatheter aortic-valve replacement with a balloon-expandable valve in low-risk patients. *N Engl J Med.* 2019;380(18):1695-1705.
47. Popma JJ, Deeb GM, Yakubov SJ, et al. Transcatheter aortic-valve replacement with a self-expanding valve in low-risk patients. *N Engl J Med.* 2019;380(18):1706-1715.
48. Nishimura RA, Otto CM, Bonow RO, et al. 2017 AHA/ACC Focused Update of the 2014 AHA/ACC Guideline for the management of patients with valvular heart disease: a report of the American College of Cardiology/American Heart Association Task Force on Clinical Practice Guidelines. *Circulation.* 2017;135(25):e1159-e1195.
49. Chikwe J, Goldstone AB, Passage J, et al. A propensity score-adjusted retrospective comparison of early and mid-term results of mitral valve repair versus replacement in octogenarians. *Eur Heart J.* 2011;32(5):618-626.
50. Glower DD, Kar S, Trento A, et al. Percutaneous mitral valve repair for mitral regurgitation in high-risk patients: results of the EVEREST II study. *J Am Coll Cardiol.* 2014;64(2):172-181.
51. Sharma M, Cornelius VR, Patel JP, Davies JG, Molokhia M. Efficacy and harms of direct oral anticoagulants in the elderly for stroke prevention in atrial fibrillation and secondary prevention of venous thromboembolism: systematic review and meta-analysis. *Circulation.* 2015;132(3):194-204.
52. Wyse DG. Rate control vs rhythm control strategies in atrial fibrillation. *Prog Cardiovasc Dis.* 2005;48(2):125-138.
53. Shariff N, Desai RV, Patel K, et al. Rate-control versus rhythm-control strategies and outcomes in septuagenarians with atrial fibrillation. *Am J Med.* 2013;126(10):887-893.
54. Van Gelder IC, Groenveld HF, Crijns HJGM, et al. Lenient versus strict rate control in patients with atrial fibrillation. *N Engl J Med.* 2010;362(15):1363-1373.
55. Healey JS, Hallstrom AP, Kuck K-H, et al. Role of the implantable defibrillator among elderly patients with a history of life-threatening ventricular arrhythmias. *Eur Heart J.* 2007;28(14):1746-1749.
56. Huang DT, Sesselberg HW, McNitt S, et al. Improved survival associated with prophylactic implantable defibrillators in elderly patients with prior myocardial infarction and depressed ventricular function: a MADIT-II substudy. *J Cardiovasc Electrophysiol.* 2007;18(8):833-838.
57. Damluji AA, Forman DE, van Diepen S, et al. Older Adults in the cardiac intensive care unit: factoring geriatric syndromes in the management, prognosis, and process of care: a scientific statement from the American Heart Association. *Circulation.* 2020;141(2):e6-e32.

CHAPTER 21

CARDIAC MANIFESTATIONS OF SYSTEMIC DISEASES

Toniya Singh, Ijeoma Isiadinso, Gina P. Lundberg, and Nidhi Madan

INTRODUCTION

The cardiovascular (CV) system is a common target for systemic diseases. Effects can range from cellular changes in the myocardium to altering the risk for developing coronary artery disease (CAD). Understanding the cardiac manifestations of commonly encountered diseases is critical to appropriate patient assessment and management.

AUTOIMMUNE/INFLAMMATORY SYSTEMIC DISEASES

Systemic Lupus Erythematosus

Systemic lupus erythematosus (SLE) is a chronic, multisystem inflammatory disease (**Table 21.1**). It is estimated that 50% of SLE patients have cardiac abnormalities.[1] Although deaths because of SLE have decreased as a result of advances in medical therapies, cardiovascular disease (CVD) remains the leading cause of mortality accounting for more than one-third of deaths in these patients.

Premature atherosclerosis is a major contributing factor for the increased rate of ischemic heart disease in patients with SLE (**Figure 21.1**). The risk of myocardial infarction (MI) in SLE patients ranges from 2- to 10-fold higher than in the general population.[2] Studies have shown a higher prevalence of traditional risk factors, such as hypertension, among SLE patients. However, even after adjusting for traditional CV risk factors, the risk of CVD is greater among SLE patients compared with the general population, suggesting that additional factors are also playing a role. SLE-specific risk factors, such as immune-complex factors, circulating inflammatory cytokines, antiphospholipid antibodies, and lupus nephritis, are also associated with an increased risk of CVD and mortality. Although corticosteroids are central to controlling systemic inflammation, they also contribute to the progression of atherosclerosis in SLE patients. Both higher doses and longer duration of steroid use are associated with accelerated atherosclerosis. Coronary artery calcification, which is a marker of subclinical atherosclerosis, is more common in patients with SLE[3] than in unaffected individuals. Patients with SLE also have a proatherogenic lipid profile consisting of elevated total cholesterol (TC), triglycerides (TG), and low-density lipoprotein cholesterol (LDL-C), whereas high-density lipoprotein cholesterol (HDL-C) is reduced. Additionally, a dysfunctional, proinflammatory form of HDL (piHDL) is more prevalent in SLE patients. Unlike normal HDL, piHDL promotes oxidation of HDL and inhibits cholesterol efflux from foam cells. Studies have reported that up to 45% of SLE patients have piHDL.[4]

Nonbacterial endocarditis (Libman-Sacks endocarditis), valvular thickening, and mitral valve prolapse (MVP) occur with increased frequency in patients with SLE. Heart failure, with or without systolic dysfunction, can occur from ischemia, hypertension, valvular disease, or immune-mediated injury in SLE. Myocarditis is a rare but serious complication of SLE. Echocardiography and cardiac magnetic resonance imaging (CMR) may demonstrate systolic dysfunction and regional wall motion abnormalities. Areas of necrosis or scar can be detected on CMR as late gadolinium enhancement (LGE). Pericardial effusion and pericarditis are the most commonly recognized and presenting cardiac complications of SLE. Cardiac arrhythmias ranging from sinus tachycardia to atrial fibrillation may also be seen in SLE patients.

Rheumatoid Arthritis

Patients with rheumatoid arthritis (RA) have a higher morbidity and mortality from CVD compared to control populations. The risk of CVD is higher in patients with RA compared with the general population by nearly two-fold, similar to that of diabetes.[5] Premature atherosclerosis in RA patients is one factor that leads to an increased risk of CAD. Additionally, studies have demonstrated underdiagnosis and undertreatment of traditional CVD risk factors in RA patients. There is a paradoxical relationship between body mass index (BMI) and CV risk in RA patients, such that low BMI is associated with increased CV risk. It is hypothesized that the low BMI is a reflection of a heightened inflammatory state. Conversely, RA patients who are rheumatoid factor negative or on steroid doses less than 7.5 do not appear to have an increased risk of CV events.[6]

Chronic inflammation may result in pericarditis, dyslipidemia, and heart failure in RA patients, with the latter primarily because of diastolic dysfunction rather than ischemic heart disease.[7] Elevated interleukin-6 (IL-6) levels confer an increased risk of diastolic dysfunction and atherosclerosis in RA patients.[8] Mitral regurgitation is the most common valvular disease in patients with RA.

Antirheumatic drugs can also negatively impact CV risk in RA patients. High-dose corticosteroids increase the risk of

TABLE 21.1 Cardiovascular Manifestations of Autoimmune/Inflammatory Systemic Diseases

Disease/Disorder	Coronary Arteries	Myocardium	Valves	Conduction	Pericardium
Systemic lupus erythematosus	Coronary artery disease Coronary microvascular dysfunction	Heart failure Myocarditis	Libman-Sacks endocarditis Valvular thickening and nodules	Atrioventricular block Sinus tachycardia Atrial fibrillation Supraventricular tachycardia Prolonged QT	Pericardial effusion Pericarditis
Rheumatoid arthritis	Coronary artery disease	Heart failure Myocardial dysfunction	Valvular regurgitation	Ventricular arrhythmias	Pericardial effusion Pericarditis
Psoriatic arthritis	Coronary artery disease	Heart failure			
Scleroderma/systemic sclerosis	Coronary artery disease Coronary vasospasm Coronary microvascular dysfunction	Myocardial fibrosis		Atrial fibrillation Atrial flutter Paroxysmal supraventricular tachycardia Ventricular tachycardia Premature ventricular contractions	Pericardial effusion Pericarditis
Ankylosing spondylitis			Aortic regurgitation	First-degree atrioventricular block	
Inflammatory bowel disease	Coronary artery disease	Heart failure Myocarditis	Mitral and aortic regurgitation	Atrial and ventricular arrhythmias	Pericarditis
Human immunodeficiency virus	Coronary artery disease	Heart failure Myocardial fibrosis	Myxomatous degeneration		Pericarditis

dyslipidemia, insulin resistance, atherosclerosis, and hypertension. Nonsteroidal anti-inflammatory drugs can precipitate new-onset hypertension and worsen blood pressure in those with an established diagnosis of hypertension.

Psoriatic Arthritis

Psoriatic arthritis is a multisystem, autoinflammatory, seronegative arthritis affecting 20% of patients with psoriasis. Patients with psoriatic arthritis have an increased prevalence of

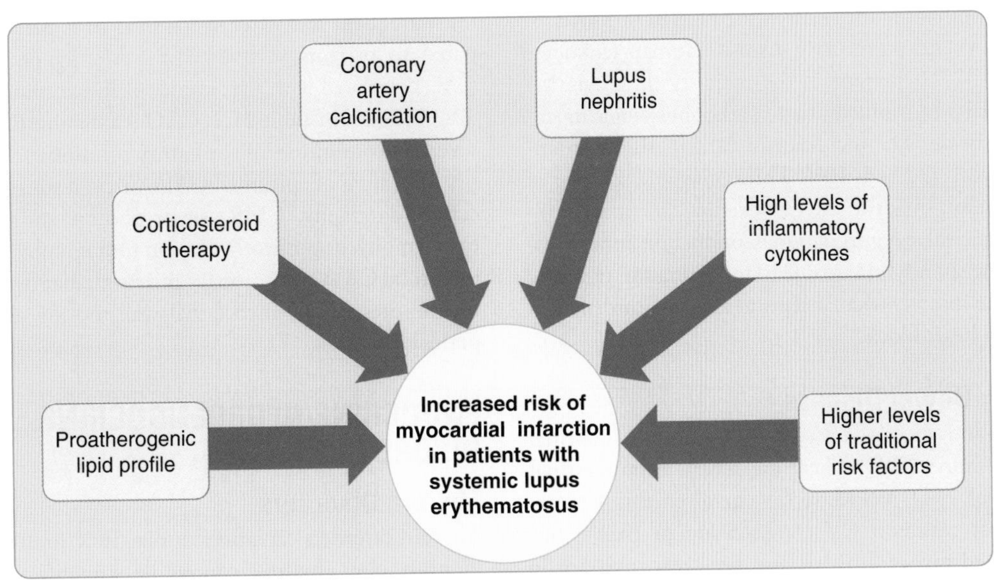

FIGURE 21.1 Increased risk of myocardial infarction among patients with systemic lupus erythematosus.

traditional CV risk factors.[9] In addition, cyclosporine, which is used to treat psoriatic arthritis, can cause hypertension and dyslipidemia. However, the increased risk of CVD cannot be fully explained by the greater prevalence of CV risk factors. An important finding has been a common pathway of psoriatic plaque formation and atherosclerosis.[10] T-helper cells are integral in the formation of plaque and inflammation in both disorders. Once activated, the T-helper cells secrete proinflammatory cytokines, including IL-2, tumor necrosis factor-alpha, and interferon-gamma, promoting the inflammatory cascade and atherosclerotic plaque formation.

Systemic Sclerosis

Systemic sclerosis is a diffuse, multisystem connective tissue disorder of unknown etiology characterized by systemic inflammation, fibrosis of organs and skin, and vascular dysfunction. Fibrosis can be caused by profibrotic cytokines, including transforming growth factor-beta (TGF-β), IL-4, platelet-derived growth factor, and connective tissue growth factor, and lead to left ventricular (LV) systolic and diastolic dysfunction. Coronary microvascular disease is common in systemic sclerosis and is mediated by TGF-β, reactive oxygen species, and inflammatory mediators. Patients with systemic sclerosis have an increased risk of atherosclerosis because of endothelial dysfunction and inflammation resulting in the release of proinflammatory markers, including C-reactive protein and homocysteine, with hyperhomocysteinemia associated with increased risk of CVD. Systemic sclerosis is also responsible for a wide range of conduction abnormalities including supraventricular arrhythmias (including atrial fibrillation or flutter), premature ventricular contraction, and heart block.[11]

Ankylosing Spondylitis

Ankylosing spondylitis is a chronic, multisystem inflammatory disorder primarily affecting the sacroiliac joint and spine that occurs predominantly in males. Extra-articular involvement includes uveitis, inflammatory bowel disease (IBD), psoriasis, arthritis, and CV and pulmonary disease. Human leukocyte antigen (HLA)-B27 is present in the majority of ankylosing spondylitis patients and contributes to pathophysiologic mechanisms of the disease. The incidence of cardiac disease in ankylosing spondylitis is 2% to 10%. Thickening and scarring of the aortic wall result in aortic valve thickening, aortic root dilatation, and aortic valve regurgitation. Conduction abnormalities in ankylosing spondylitis are due to inflammation resulting in damage to the interventricular septum and myocardial scarring resulting in heart block.[12]

Inflammatory Bowel Disease

Crohn disease and ulcerative colitis are chronic, intestinal diseases that comprise IBD. There are several extraintestinal manifestations of IBD including CV involvement. Pericarditis is the most common CV complication of IBD,[13] but immune-mediated myocarditis has also been reported. Aortic and mitral valve regurgitation are the most common valvulopathies seen in IBD patients. The valvular disease occurs due to systemic inflammation resulting in thickening and shortening of the valve leaflets. Atrioventricular conduction disorders may occur due to infliximab therapy, inflammation-related ischemia in the conduction system, vasculitis, or microvascular endothelial dysfunction.

Human Immunodeficiency Virus

Human immunodeficiency virus (HIV) is now considered a chronic disease as a result of effective antiviral therapy. HIV patients commonly have other comorbidities, including hypertension, dyslipidemia, atherosclerosis, diabetes, and obesity. One of the leading causes of non–HIV-related mortality is CVD. HIV infection can cause pericardial effusion, with most being asymptomatic. HIV may also result in cardiomyopathy because of the dysregulated immune response, atherosclerosis, and myocarditis. Antiretroviral therapy can also cause dyslipidemia and heart failure.

ROLE OF IMAGING IN EVALUATION OF CARDIAC MANIFESTATIONS OF INFLAMMATORY SYSTEMIC DISEASES

Echocardiography, cardiac computed tomography (CCT), and CMR are excellent noninvasive diagnostic imaging tools for the evaluation of CV complications of multisystem inflammatory diseases. Echocardiography can detect evidence of subclinical LV systolic and diastolic dysfunction in RA, pericardial effusion (in RA or SLE), valvular heart disease, and pericardial thickening.[14-16] Valvular complications of systemic inflammatory diseases, including valvular thickening or regurgitation, can be easily seen on echocardiography.

In RA and SLE, CMR demonstrates LGE that reflects inflammation because of myocarditis.[16] In addition to estimating ejection fraction and assessing wall motion abnormalities, CMR can also identify areas of inflammation, fibrosis, and edema. Coronary artery calcification, as measured by CCT, is more frequent and extensive among SLE patients when compared to patients without SLE.[3] Among patients with RA, CAC correlated with the severity of inflammation.[17]

As noted in Table 21.1, CAD is a manifestation of CVD in several autoimmune inflammatory conditions. CCT can quantify the extent of epicardial CAD. Stress testing combined with echocardiography, CMR, single-photon emission computed tomography, or positron emission tomography can detect both epicardial CAD and coronary microvascular dysfunction based on the presence of myocardial wall motion abnormalities or perfusion defects.

ENDOCRINE/NEUROENDOCRINE DISORDERS

Thyroid Disorders

Thyroid disorders can affect cardiac function through changes in heart rate, rhythm, contractile strength, and the risk of CAD via their effects on blood pressure and inflammatory and lipid profiles (**Table 21.2**). Patients with either hypo- or

TABLE 21.2 Cardiac Manifestations of Endocrine Disorders

Disorder	Coronary Arteries	Myocardium	Valves	Conduction	Pericardium
Hypothyroidism	Hypercholesterolemia Hyperlipidemia	Decreased contractility and cardiac output Heart failure		Sinus bradycardia	Pericardial effusion
Hyperthyroidism	Systolic hypertension	LVH secondary to increased cardiac output Heart family		SVT Atrial fibrillation	
Acromegaly	Endothelial changes Increased arterial stiffness Atherosclerosis	Ventricular dilatation LVH Heart failure	Aortic regurgitation Mitral regurgitation	Atrial fibrillation Ectopic beats SVT	
Pheochromocytoma	Catecholamine-induced vasospasm Vascular wall thickening	LVH Cardiomyopathy Ischemic heart disease Heart failure		Sinus tachycardia SVT VT Sick sinus syndrome	
Carcinoid		Plaque-like, fibrous endocardial thickening Heart failure	Tricuspid and pulmonary regurgitation		Pericardial effusions
Neurofibromatosis		Hypertrophic cardiomyopathy	Pulmonary stenosis Mitral regurgitation		

LVH, left ventricular hypertrophy; SVT, supraventricular tachycardia; VT, ventricular tachycardia.

hyperthyroidism are at increased risk for CVD, even with subclinical disease.

Hyperthyroidism is associated with increased risk of CAD, atrial fibrillation, heart failure, and cardiac-related mortality. The hemodynamic effects of excess thyroid hormone include increased heart rate and cardiac output, decreased systemic vascular resistance (SVR) secondary to arterial smooth muscle relaxation, and increased nitrous oxide production (**Figure 21.2**). The decreased SVR activates the renin-angiotensin-aldosterone system, which leads to increases in blood volume. Thyroid hormone also regulates intracellular calcium levels, and increases in thyroid hormone lead to enhanced myocyte calcium cycling and contractility. These alterations lead to an increase in cardiac output, which can be 50% to 300% higher than normal in patients with symptomatic hyperthyroidism. This increased cardiac workload may eventually lead to LV hypertrophy and heart failure. In fact, the leading cause of CV-related death in both overt and subclinical hyperthyroidism is heart failure. Both subclinical and overt hyperthyroidism are also associated with an increased risk of atrial fibrillation.[18] Increased levels of the mediators of thrombogenesis, including fibrinogen, factor X, and von Willebrand factor, may be tied to an increase in CV events observed in patients with hyperthyroidism.[19]

Hypothyroidism is associated with increased SVR and decreased heart rate and contractility. As a result, cardiac output may be reduced by 30% to 40% in patients with overt hypothyroidism.[20] The increased vascular resistance is due to a reduction in nitrous oxide production and smooth muscle relaxation. Decreased contractility is a result of diminished myocyte calcium cycling (**Figure 21.3**). These changes can lead to heart failure in patients predisposed either by age or underlying cardiac disease. Hypothyroidism is also associated with an increased risk of CAD, in part, because of an increased incidence of diastolic hypertension and altered lipid metabolism resulting in elevated levels of TC and LDLs. Pericardial effusions, as a result of increased capillary permeability, are seen in nearly a quarter of hypothyroid patients but rarely have clinical implications.[21]

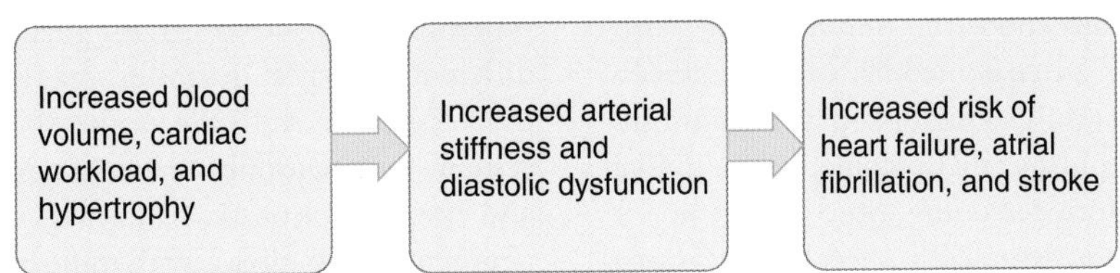

FIGURE 21.2 Hemodynamic effects of hyperthyroidism.

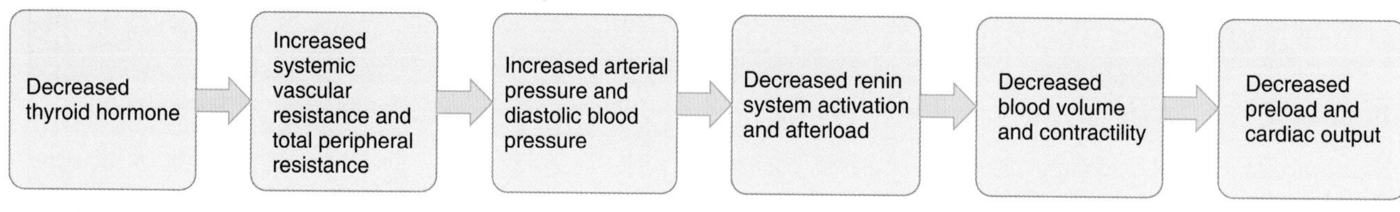

FIGURE 21.3 Cardiac effects of hypothyroidism.

Acromegaly

Acromegaly is caused by excess growth hormone secreted by a pituitary adenoma. The increased mortality rate seen among patients with acromegaly is often attributable to CVD, which accounts for nearly 60% of deaths among these patients.[22] Excess growth hormone triggers release of supranormal levels of insulin-like growth factor-1 (IGF-1) by the liver. Both growth hormone and IGF-1 have direct effects on the CV system by increasing contractility, stimulating cardiac myocyte growth, and reducing SVR.

Hypertension is the most common cardiac manifestation of acromegaly, occurring in 20% to 50% of these patients, and has been tied to increased mortality and an increased risk of cardiac hypertrophy and heart failure. Although the mechanism of acromegaly-induced hypertension has not been fully explained, it appears connected to increased plasma volume as a result of sodium and water retention, possibly because of secondary effects on the renin-angiotensin network, insulin resistance, increased arterial wall stiffness, and increased cardiac output.[23] Patients with acromegaly are at increased risk of CAD because of the presence of acromegaly-associated risk factors, including hypertension, dyslipidemia, sleep apnea, and diabetes, but it is unclear if these additional disease processes contribute.

Acromegaly is associated with cardiomyopathy, as a direct result of the effects of growth hormone and IGF-1 on myocytes. These effects—including increased contractile gene expression, increased intracellular calcium levels, and fibrosis—can lead to cardiac hypertrophy, diastolic and/or systolic dysfunction, decreased cardiac output, and, eventually, heart failure. The remodeling effects of growth hormone and IGF-1 also result in up to 75% of acromegalic patients having cardiac valvulopathy, including mitral, aortic, and tricuspid regurgitation.[24] Growth hormone and IGF-1 increase the risk for arrhythmias, ectopic beats, paroxysmal atrial fibrillation, paroxysmal supraventricular tachycardia, sick sinus syndrome, ventricular tachycardia, and bundle branch blocks.[23]

Pheochromocytoma

Pheochromocytomas are rare endocrine tumors of the chromaffin cells found in the adrenal medulla or extra-adrenal paraganglia. These tumors result in high plasma levels of catecholamines—mainly epinephrine and norepinephrine—which stimulate adrenergic receptors, including those within the CV system. In the majority of patients with pheochromocytoma, sustained or paroxysmal hypertension is present. Catecholamine excess can also manifest as arrhythmias, hypotension, shock, myocardial ischemia, cardiomyopathy (including Takotsubo), aortic dissection, and peripheral ischemia.[25] Although the most life-threatening CV complication is hypertensive crisis, increased risk of cardiac-related death can also be attributed to stroke, aortic dissection, MI, arrhythmia, and heart failure. Sinus tachycardia is the most prevalent arrhythmia, but ventricular arrhythmias have also been reported.

Increased levels of catecholamines and their metabolites have a direct effect on myocardial tissue, including alpha-receptor-mediated vasoconstriction and oxygen-derived free radial injury resulting in myocyte injury and death, with subsequent cardiac remodeling and fibrosis, decreased LV contractility, lower peak systolic circumferential strain, lower diastolic strain rate, and global LV dysfunction.[26] Pheochromocytoma can also lead to dilated or hypertrophic cardiomyopathy, which can be found in approximately 10% of patients with this tumor.[27]

Carcinoid

Carcinoid heart disease affects more than half of patients with carcinoid tumors, which are rare, slow-growing tumors derived from neuroectoderm in the gastrointestinal or respiratory tract. Carcinoid tumors secrete vasoactive substances, including serotonin, kallikrein, prostaglandins, and histamines. Carcinoid heart disease is responsible for significant morbidity and mortality among patients with carcinoid tumors.[28] Although the etiology of carcinoid heart disease is unknown, chronic exposure to excessive circulating serotonin is considered an important etiologic factor. Carcinoid heart disease is most often characterized by the development of plaque-like, fibrous thickening of valve leaflets, chordae, papillary muscles, and endocardium of the heart chambers. Carcinoid heart disease almost always involves the tricuspid valve, although pulmonary valvular involvement is seen in two-thirds of patients. Valve involvement leads to regurgitation and can progress to right heart failure. Additional cardiac manifestations include myocardial metastasis and pericardial effusions.

Neurofibromatosis

Neurofibromatosis is a rare neurocutaneous genetic disorder inherited in an autosomal dominant pattern. It comprises two different subtypes: neurofibromatosis type 1 (NF1), which is more common and affects the skin and peripheral nervous system, and neurofibromatosis type 2 (NF2), which is rare and results in acoustic neuromas. NF1 is the most common neurocutaneous disease with multisystem involvement, including CV manifestations. The prevalence of CV complications in NF1 ranges from 2% to 28%.[29] Vascular changes are the hallmark of NF1 and can affect any vessels by producing stenosis, occlusion, and aneurysm, although the pathophysiology of these abnormalities is unknown. Renal arteries are the most common site of vascular changes and lead to the predominant cardiac manifestation of NF1, which is hypertension. Additional CV manifestations of NF1 may include congenital heart disease, hypertrophic cardiomyopathy, and, less frequently, valvular pulmonary stenosis, branch peripheral pulmonary stenosis, atrial and ventricular septal defects, coarctation of the aorta, and hypertrophic cardiomyopathy.[29]

Antiphospholipid Syndrome

Antiphospholipid syndrome (APS) is a complex systemic autoimmune disorder characterized by the presence of antiphospholipid antibodies, recurrent venous and arterial thrombosis, and obstetric complications including recurrent fetal loss and placental insufficiency.[30,31] It can occur as a primary disorder or as a secondary manifestation to another autoimmune disease, most commonly seen with SLE. Cardiac involvement in APS includes valvular disorders, accelerated atherosclerosis, CAD, MI, myocardial dysfunction, pulmonary hypertension, and intracardiac thrombi formation.[32] Of these, valvular abnormalities are the most common and can occur in the form of valve thickening or valve lesions (such as Libman-Sacks endocarditis) or valvular dysfunction in the absence of a history of rheumatic fever or infective endocarditis. The valve lesions typically involve the mitral valve followed by aortic valve and are characterized by valve thickening of more than 3 mm involving the proximal or middle portions of the valve leaflets or as irregular nodules on the atrial side of mitral valve or vascular surface of the aortic valve.[30] In about 4% to 6% of APS patients with valvular abnormalities, severe valvular regurgitation can occur requiring surgical intervention.[33] Acute MI is another known manifestation and can sometimes be the first presentation of APS. It is thought to be a consequence of accelerated atherosclerosis (caused by inflammatory and immune-mediated mechanisms), microvascular injury, or coronary embolism. Coronary embolism occurs as a more frequent cause of MI in young individuals. Myocardial dysfunction can also occur in APS. LV dysfunction is seen more frequently with APS secondary to SLE,[34] whereas right ventricle (RV) is more commonly involved in primary APS.[35] Venous thromboembolism is a common phenomenon in APS, and APS-associated pulmonary embolism often results in chronic thromboembolic pulmonary hypertension (CTEPH), which over time can lead to RV dysfunction and right-sided heart failure. Furthermore, APS is also associated with intracardiac thrombi formation that is rare; however, it can be potentially life threatening. There are reports ranging from LV thrombus associated with LV systolic dysfunction causing stroke to thrombi in all four cardiac chambers.[36,37]

LIPID DISEASES

Familial Hypercholesterolemia

Familial hypercholesterolemia is an autosomal dominant disorder that has been associated with a 20-fold increase in risk for CVD events (**Table 21.3**). Familial hypercholesterolemia can either be homozygous, with a reported prevalence from 1 in 160,000 to 1 in 1,000,000, or heterozygous, which is more frequent with prevalence of 1 in 200 to 1 in 500.[38] Cardiac manifestations of familial hypercholesterolemia include premature atherosclerosis and coronary stenosis, which develop in men

TABLE 21.3 Cardiac Manifestations of Lipid Disorders

	Arterial Disease	Myocardium	Valves	Conduction	Pericardium
Familial hypercholesterolemia	Premature coronary atherosclerosis Peripheral artery disease		Aortic stenosis		
Familial combined hypercholesterolemia	Premature coronary atherosclerosis Peripheral artery disease		Aortic valve disease		
Familial dysbetalipoproteinemia	Premature coronary atherosclerosis Peripheral artery disease				
Sitosterol	Premature coronary atherosclerosis	Left ventricle dysfunction Cardiac interstitial fibrosis			
Elevated Lp(a)	Advanced coronary atherosclerosis Peripheral artery disease		Aortic stenosis		
Lysosomal storage disorders		Left ventricular hypertrophy Cardiomyopathy	Mitral and aortic regurgitation	Second-degree atrioventricular block	

during the fourth or fifth decade and in women approximately 10 years later. Systemic manifestations include arcus cornealis, xanthelasma, tendon xanthomas, and peripheral artery atherosclerotic disease including aortic aneurysm and claudication. Genetically confirmed familial hypercholesterolemia is reported in 8.7% of acute coronary syndrome patients under age 65 with LDL-C over 160 mg/dL.[39] Familial hypercholesterolemia is also associated with stroke, peripheral artery disease, carotid artery disease, and chronic kidney disease.

Familial Combined Hypercholesterolemia

Familial combined hypercholesterolemia is associated with a 24-fold increase in CVD events.[40] It is found in 1% to 2% of the population and in up to 38% patients with MI before the age of 40 years.[40] Familial combined hypercholesterolemia includes very high TG, in addition to high levels of LDL-C. In familial combined hypercholesterolemia patients with MI before age 40 years, elevated very-low-density lipoprotein cholesterol (VLDL-C) and elevated non–HDL-C plasma levels were most strongly associated with MI.[40] Central obesity and metabolic syndrome are components of the variable familial combined hypercholesterolemia phenotype. Familial combined hypercholesterolemia is thought to be oligogenetic with a high incidence of CVD, type 2 diabetes, metabolic syndrome, nonalcoholic fatty liver disease, and steatohepatitis.[41]

Familial Dysbetalipoproteinemia or Type III Hyperlipoproteinemia

Familial dysbetalipoproteinemia, or type III hyperlipoproteinemia, is a chylomicron and VLDL-C remnant removal disease and is associated with premature CVD.[42] Most patients are homozygous for a mutation in the apoprotein E2 (apoE2) gene, which results in impaired hepatic uptake of apoE-containing lipoproteins (ie, chylomicrons and VLDL remnants). This disorder is generally autosomal recessive, but up to 10% is caused by autosomal dominant mutations.[42] Approximately 15% of apoE2/E2 patients will develop familial dysbetalipoproteinemia because of additional risk factors including obesity, metabolic syndrome, insulin resistance, and diabetes. In addition to premature CAD, patients with familial dysbetalipoproteinemia have xanthomas and mixed hyperlipidemia with high TG and non–HDL-C plasma levels.[42]

Sitosterolemia

Sitosterolemia is a genetic disorder associated with ATP-binding cassette (ABC) gene mutations, specifically subfamily G member 5 or 8 (ABCG5 or ABCG8). Occurring in 1 in 200,000 individuals in the general population, it is characterized by increased absorption and decreased biliary excretion of plant sterols and cholesterol, thus resulting in prominently elevated serum concentrations of plant sterols, such as sitosterol and campesterol. Patients with this mutation have tendinous and tuberous xanthomas and premature atherosclerosis, with the elevation of LDL-C the major cause of development of atherosclerosis and not the elevation of sitosterol.[43]

Elevated Lipoprotein (a)

Elevated lipoprotein (a) [Lp(a)] is an inherited genetic disorder that is associated with CVD and calcific aortic valve stenosis. Lp(a) is known to be proatherogenic, proinflammatory, and prothrombotic.[44] People with elevated Lp(a) have advanced CAD, carotid atherosclerosis, peripheral artery disease, and renal artery disease.[45] In North America, it is estimated that 20% of the population has an elevated Lp(a) (ie, >50 mg/dL). Elevated Lp(a) is considered an atherosclerotic cardiovascular disease (ASCVD) "risk enhancer," and guidelines recommend that patients with elevated plasma levels of Lp(a) be considered for lipid-lowering therapy with a statin.[46]

Lysosomal Storage Disorders

Lysosomal storage disorders are classified according to the type of material that is accumulated; for example, lipid storage disorders, mucopolysaccharidoses, and glycoproteinoses. Cardiac disease is particularly important in lysosomal glycogen storage diseases (Pompe and Danon diseases), mucopolysaccharidoses (Hurler and Hunter syndrome), and glycosphingolipidoses (Anderson-Fabry disease). Cardiac manifestations of these systemic diseases include hypertrophic cardiomyopathy, dilated cardiomyopathy, CAD, valvular dysfunction, and arrhythmias.[47]

INFILTRATIVE DISORDERS

Amyloidosis

Amyloidosis refers to a group of protein-folding disorders characterized by deposition of these proteins in tissues throughout the body (**Table 21.4**). The deposition of these proteins in the heart carries a worse prognosis than the involvement of any other organ. The two subtypes of amyloid that account for 95% of all cardiac amyloidosis include light-chain amyloidosis (AL), which is the most common subtype, and transthyretin amyloidosis (ATTR). There are two subtypes of ATTR, a noninherited wild-type ATTR and an inherited mutant ATTR. Both these types result from a misfolding of the protein transthyretin, which is produced in the liver. These misfolded proteins combine to form amyloid fibers, which deposit in the interstitial space of the myocardium. Cardiac manifestations of amyloidosis include heart failure and arrhythmias. AL, also known as primary amyloidosis, is the most serious form of the disease, with an untreated survival rate of less than 6 months in patients who present with heart failure.[48]

The deposition of amyloid proteins throughout the myocardial tissue leads to ventricular hypertrophy, decreased cardiac output, atrial dilatation, and atrial fibrillation. Hence, cardiac amyloidosis can present with diastolic heart failure with preserved ejection fraction, dilated cardiomyopathy, or atrial fibrillation.

Hemochromatosis

Hemochromatosis is an inherited disorder that causes excessive iron absorption from the gastrointestinal system, leading to abnormal accumulation of iron in organs, manifested as organ

TABLE 21.4 Cardiac Manifestations of Infiltrative Disorders

	Coronary Arteries	Myocardium	Valves	Conduction	Pericardium
Amyloidosis	Angina without coronary artery disease	Ventricular hypertrophy Heart failure	Valvular regurgitation	Atrial fibrillation Bundle branch block Complete heart block	Pericardial effusion
Hemochromatosis		Congestive cardiomyopathy Restrictive cardiomyopathy Heart failure		Atrioventricular block Atrial and ventricular tachyarrhythmias Atrial fibrillation	Pericardial constriction or tamponade
Sarcoidosis		Dilated cardiomyopathy Restrictive cardiomyopathy Heart failure	Mitral regurgitation	Atrioventricular block Ventricular arrhythmias	Pericarditis

toxicity and failure. Deposition of iron may occur in the cardiac conduction system, especially in the atrioventricular node, and lead to arrhythmias.[49]

Cardiac hemochromatosis results in a dilated cardiomyopathy, with dilated ventricles, diastolic dysfunction, and a reduced ejection fraction. Subsequent pulmonary congestion and peripheral edema can signal worsening disease and the development of heart failure. Once heart failure develops, the prognosis is poor.

Sarcoidosis

Sarcoidosis is a multisystem disease of unknown etiology characterized by the formation of granulomas in many organs, predominantly the lungs and intrathoracic lymph nodes. Approximately 5% of sarcoid patients will exhibit symptoms of cardiac involvement, with an additional 20% to 25% having asymptomatic cardiac involvement. Clinical symptoms of cardiac sarcoidosis are commonly the disease's presenting symptoms, as two-thirds of patients with cardiac sarcoidosis have no other systemic signs of the disease.[50] Cardiac sarcoidosis can present with ventricular arrhythmias, conduction abnormalities, or heart failure.

Sarcoid infiltrations are common at the base of the septum, which can lead to heart block, ventricular tachyarrhythmias, and an increased risk of sudden death. Infiltrations can also affect the mitral valve, leading to regurgitation. Dilated cardiomyopathy, pericarditis, and LV aneurysms can also be seen in cardiac sarcoidosis.

VASCULAR DISORDERS

Fibromuscular Dysplasia

Fibromuscular dysplasia (FMD) is an arteriopathy that predominantly affects middle-aged women; however, it can occur at any age in both sexes (**Table 21.5**). Most commonly, it involves the renal, carotid, and vertebral arteries; less commonly, coronary arteries are affected. It is important to recognize coronary artery involvement of FMD, as it can result in significant morbidity and mortality from consequent coronary dissection, acute coronary syndrome, or LV dysfunction.

FMD is typically characterized by a "string of beads" appearance on angiography. This appearance is considered to be diagnostic of FMD in the renal, carotid, and other arterial beds; however, it rarely occurs in the coronary arteries. Most FMD patients with coronary artery involvement present with spontaneous coronary artery dissection, smooth narrowing, intramural hematoma, or coronary spasm and are subsequently found to have typical FMD findings in the noncoronary arteries. FMD with coronary artery involvement should be considered in a patient presenting with acute coronary syndrome or new LV dysfunction, particularly in middle-aged women who are found to have mid- to distal coronary artery involvement with otherwise normal coronary arteries. Furthermore, there are reported cases of histopathologic findings consistent with FMD of the sinoatrial and atrioventricular nodal arteries identified on postmortem examination in individuals with sudden cardiac death.[51]

Vasculitis

Primary systemic vasculitis is a group of autoimmune disorders characterized by occlusion, stenosis, or aneurysmal dilatation of blood vessels secondary to intramural inflammation. These are classified depending on the predominant type of vessel involved into small-vessel, medium-vessel, large-vessel, and variable-vessel vasculitis. Cardiac involvement in vasculitis can occur as a direct consequence of the disease process or because of drugs such as corticosteroids that are used for its treatment.

Granulomatosis with polyangiitis, microscopic polyangiitis, and eosinophilic granulomatosis with polyangiitis or Churg-Strauss syndrome are the antineutrophil cytoplasmic antibody (ANCA)–associated *small-vessel vasculitides* (AAV). Valvular involvement including aortic insufficiency (most common), mitral regurgitation, and aortic stenosis is described in patients with AAV, as are pericardial effusion, cardiomyopathy, endomyocardial fibrosis, and small-vessel disease leading to coronary ischemia with normal coronary angiography or

TABLE 21.5 Cardiac Manifestations of Vascular Disorders

Disorder	Coronary Arteries	Myocardium	Valves	Conduction	Pericardium
Fibromuscular dysplasia	Coronary artery dissection Coronary spasm	Left ventricular dysfunction		Pathology in sinoatrial and atrioventricular nodal arteries	
Small-vessel vasculitis	Coronary artery inflammation	Cardiomyopathy	Aortic regurgitation Mitral regurgitation Aortic stenosis		Pericarditis
Medium-vessel vasculitis	Coronary artery inflammation Coronary artery aneurysm			Prolonged PR and QT intervals Ventricular arrhythmias	
Large-vessel vasculitis	Coronary artery inflammation		Aortic regurgitation		
Marfan syndrome	Dilated cardiomyopathy	Aortic dissection	Aortic regurgitation Mitral valve prolapse		
Ehlers-Danlos syndrome		Aortic aneurysm Atrial septal defect	Mitral valve disease	Incomplete right bundle branch block Sinus bradycardia Complete heart block	

involvement of the conduction system resulting in arrhythmia. Of the three types of AAV, cardiac abnormalities are more commonly seen with eosinophilic granulomatosis with polyangiitis. A study showed a correlation between the degree of peripheral blood eosinophilia at baseline with higher prevalence of rhythm disturbances and lower ejection fraction.[52] In a cohort of 517 patients with granulomatosis with polyangiitis, only 3.3% were found to have cardiac involvement, with pericarditis being the most common followed by cardiomyopathy, conduction defects, ischemic heart disease, and valvular involvement.[53]

Polyarteritis nodosa and Kawasaki disease are classified as *medium-vessel vasculitides*. Coronary artery involvement is a well-known feature of Kawasaki disease. Conversely, clinically overt cardiac involvement is rare in polyarteritis nodosa—seen in about 4% to 18% of patients—and associated with poor prognosis.[54] It includes coronary arteritis, typically involving small subepicardial vessels with resultant necrosis and occlusion. Kawasaki disease is recognized as an important cause of acquired pediatric CVD.[55] It is typically characterized by coronary artery aneurysms that can result in coronary artery stenoses or thrombosis. Electrocardiographic abnormalities, such as prolonged PR interval and QT interval, have also been described in children with Kawasaki disease. Patients with increased dispersion of the QTc interval in the absence of coronary artery involvement have a propensity to ventricular arrhythmias.[56]

Giant cell arteritis and Takayasu arteritis are *large-vessel vasculitides* that predominantly affect the aorta and its branches. Giant cell arteritis is common in people of Northern European and Scandinavian descent and is typically seen in patients older than 50 years. It involves aneurysm formation in the thoracic or abdominal aorta that can result in dissection. Aneurysm of the ascending aorta with consequent aortic valve regurgitation is also described. The risk of CAD is increased in patients with giant cell arteritis when compared with healthy controls. Takayasu arteritis also involves the proximal branches of the aorta with an incidence of 0.4 to 2/million/year in Northern Europe.[57] Aortic involvement predominantly results in stenosis that can cause a discrepancy in arm blood pressures on physical examination. Aneurysms can also form in a minority of the patients (10%) and can affect the entire length of the aorta and its branches. Functional aortic valve regurgitation can occur in cases of ascending aortic aneurysms. Takayasu arteritis can also affect the coronary arteries and is typically seen in young women (similar to FMD) presenting with angina. Severe, focal stenosis of the left main trunk is common. Patients with Takayasu arteritis have also been shown to have accelerated carotid atherosclerosis.[58]

Marfan Syndrome

Marfan syndrome is an autosomal dominant inherited connective tissue disorder that is caused by mutations in the extracellular matrix protein fibrillin (*FBN1*). Its systemic manifestations include involvement of the CV, ocular, and skeletal organ systems. The common CV manifestations involve aortic aneurysm, aortic valve regurgitation, aortic dissection, MVP, and dilated cardiomyopathy. The CV manifestations form a large proportion of the morbidity and mortality in patients with Marfan syndrome.

The most prominent CV finding in the majority of these patients is dilatation of the aortic root, at the level of the sinus of Valsalva. This aortic dilatation can further evolve into an aneurysm, dissection, or rupture. Aortic regurgitation has also been observed to occur as a consequence of the dilatation at the aortic root. In about 10% to 20% of patients with Marfan syndrome, dilatation of the descending and abdominal aorta can also occur and lead to a type B aortic dissection.[59] MVP is another important CV feature of Marfan syndrome. However, surgical intervention for MVP is required in only a small number of patients. MVP can cause severe mitral regurgitation that can, in turn, result in heart failure and pulmonary hypertension. Marfan syndrome can also involve other cardiac valves, such as tricuspid valve prolapse, tricuspid regurgitation, and bicuspid aortic valve. Dilatation of the main pulmonary artery has also been reported in these patients; however, dissection or rupture is very rare. Marfan syndrome can also result in dilated cardiomyopathy that is commonly thought to be a consequence of valvular insufficiency and volume overload; however, it has also been noted to occur in the absence of valvular abnormalities. Additionally, arrhythmias have also been reported in a minority of patients, both in the presence and absence of ventricular dysfunction.[60]

Ehlers-Danlos Syndrome

Ehlers-Danlos syndrome is a group of rare familial connective tissue disorders inherited as an autosomal dominant trait or through an X-linked form. It is caused by mutations in genes coding collagen fibrils or proteins involved in the processing of collagen. It is characterized by abnormalities of skin, ligaments and joints, blood vessels, and internal organs, with features such as joint hypermobility, skin hyperextensibility, and tissue fragility. Aortic aneurysmal disease is seen in about 25% of these patients.[61] Few reports describe cardiac abnormalities in patients with Ehlers-Danlos syndrome. Beighton studied 100 patients with Ehlers-Danlos syndrome and described 29 patients with cardiac abnormalities. In this study, 24 patients had a systolic murmur that was either attributed to a thoracic wall deformity or benign.[62] Previous reports have described mitral valvular disease, atrial septal defect, and incomplete right bundle branch block with pulmonary ejection murmur. Other abnormal electrocardiogram (ECG) findings reported include sinus bradycardia, complete heart block, wandering pacemaker, low-voltage flat T waves, and abnormal T waves. Other CV manifestations with Ehlers-Danlos syndrome include aortic arch abnormalities, rupture of the great vessels, arteriovenous malformations, tetralogy of Fallot, tricuspid stenosis, aneurysm of the right sinus of Valsalva, which was associated with aortic incompetence and pulmonary hypertension, and tricuspid valve with two leaflets.

From RA to hypothyroidism, the CV system is a common target for systemic diseases. Understanding the cardiac manifestations of commonly encountered diseases is essential to assessing and managing patients with systemic diseases.

REFERENCES

1. Jain D, Halushka MK. Cardiac pathology of systemic lupus erythematosus. *J Clin Pathol.* 2009;62(7):584-592.
2. Hak AE, Karlson EW, Feskanich D, Stampfer MJ, Costenbader KH. Systemic lupus erythematosus and the risk of cardiovascular disease: results from the nurses' health study. *Arthritis Rheum.* 2009;61(10):1396-1402.
3. Asanuma Y, Oeser A, Shintani AK, et al. Premature coronary-artery atherosclerosis in systemic lupus erythematosus. *N Engl J Med.* 2003; 349(25):2407-2415.
4. McMahon M, Grossman J, Skaggs B, et al. Dysfunctional proinflammatory high-density lipoproteins confer increased risk of atherosclerosis in women with systemic lupus erythematosus. *Arthritis Rheum.* 2009;60(8):2428-2437.
5. Peters MJ, van Halm VP, Voskuyl AE, et al. Does rheumatoid arthritis equal diabetes mellitus as an independent risk factor for cardiovascular disease? A prospective study. *Arthritis Rheum.* 2009;61(11):1571-1579.
6. Davis JM 3rd, Kremers HM, Crowson CS, et al. Glucocorticoids and cardiovascular events in rheumatoid arthritis: a population-based cohort study. *Arthritis Rheum.* 2007;56(3):820-830.
7. Bruce IN, Urowitz MB, Gladman DD, Ibañez D, Steiner G. Risk factors for coronary heart disease in women with systemic lupus erythematosus: the Toronto Risk Factor Study. *Arthritis Rheum.* 2003;48(11):3159-3167.
8. Liang KP, Myasoedova E, Crowson CS, et al. Increased prevalence of diastolic dysfunction in rheumatoid arthritis. *Ann Rheum Dis.* 2010; 69(9):1665-1670.
9. Radner H, Lesperance T, Accortt NA, Solomon DH. Incidence and prevalence of cardiovascular risk factors among patients with rheumatoid arthritis, psoriasis, or psoriatic arthritis. *Arthritis Care Res.* 2017;69(10):1510-1518.
10. Coumbe AG, Pritzker MR, Duprez DA. Cardiovascular risk and psoriasis: beyond the traditional risk factors. *Am J Med.* 2014;127(1):12-18.
11. Champion HC. The heart in scleroderma. *Rheum Dis Clin North Am.* 2008;34(1):181-190; viii.
12. Ozkan Y. Cardiac involvement in ankylosing spondylitis. *J Clin Med Res.* 2016;8(6):427-430.
13. Aarestrup J, Jess T, Kobylecki CJ, Nordestgaard BG, Allin KH. Cardiovascular risk profile among patients with inflammatory bowel disease: a population-based study of more than 100 000 individuals. *J Crohns Colitis.* 2019;13(3):319-323.
14. Lang RM, Badano LP, Mor-Avi V, et al. Recommendations for cardiac chamber quantification by echocardiography in adults: an update from the American Society of Echocardiography and the European Association of Cardiovascular Imaging. *J Am Soc Echocardiogr.* 2015;28(1):1-39.e14.
15. Nagueh SF, Smiseth OA, Appleton CP, et al. Recommendations for the evaluation of left ventricular diastolic function by echocardiography: an update from the American Society of Echocardiography and the European Association of Cardiovascular Imaging. *J Am Soc Echocardiogr.* 2016;29(4):277-314.
16. Ikonomidis I, Makavos G, Katsimbri P, Boumpas DT, Parissis J, Iliodromitis E. Imaging risk in multisystem inflammatory diseases. *JACC Cardiovasc Imaging.* 2019;12(12):2517-2537.
17. Wahlin B, Meedt T, Jonsson F, Henein MY, Wållberg-Jonsson S. Coronary artery calcification is related to inflammation in rheumatoid arthritis: a long-term follow-up study. *Biomed Res Int.* 2016;2016:1261582.
18. Rhee SS, Pearce EN. Update: systemic diseases and the cardiovascular system (II). The endocrine system and the heart: a review. *Rev Esp Cardiol.* 2011;64(3):220-231.
19. Razvi S, Jabbar A, Pingitore A, et al. Thyroid hormones and cardiovascular function and diseases. *J Am Coll Cardiol.* 2018;71(16): 1781-1796.
20. Udovcic M, Pena RH, Patham B, Tabatabai L, Kansara A. Hypothyroidism and the heart. *Methodist Debakey Cardiovasc J.* 2017;13(2):55-59.
21. Chahine J, Ala CK, Gentry JL, Pantalone KM, Klein AL. Pericardial diseases in patients with hypothyroidism. *Heart.* 2019;105(13):1027-1033.
22. Mizera Ł, Elbaum M, Daroszewski J, Bolanowski M. Cardiovascular complications of acromegaly. *Acta Endocrinol (Buchar).* 2018;14(3):365-374.
23. Ramos-Leví AM, Marazuela M. Bringing cardiovascular comorbidities in acromegaly to an update. how should we diagnose and manage them? *Front Endocrinol.* 2019;10:120.
24. Pereira AM, van Thiel SW, Lindner JR, et al. Increased prevalence of regurgitant valvular heart disease in acromegaly. *J Clin Endocrinol Metab.* 2004;89(1):71-75.
25. Gu YW, Poste J, Kunal M, Schwarcz M, Weiss I. Cardiovascular manifestations of pheochromocytoma. *Cardiol Rev.* 2017;25(5):215-222.

26. Higuchi S, Ota H, Ueda T, et al. 3T MRI evaluation of regional catecholamine-producing tumor-induced myocardial injury. *Endocr Connect.* 2019;8(5):454-461.
27. Ferreira VM, Marcelino M, Piechnik SK, et al. Pheochromocytoma is characterized by catecholamine-mediated myocarditis, focal and diffuse myocardial fibrosis, and myocardial dysfunction. *J Am Coll Cardiol.* 2016;67(20):2364-2374.
28. Davar J, Connolly HM, Caplin ME, et al. Diagnosing and managing carcinoid heart disease in patients with neuroendocrine tumors. An expert statement. *J Am Coll Cardiol.* 2017;69(10):1288-1304.
29. Ýncecik F, Herguner OM, Erdem SA, et al. Neurofibromatosis type 1 and cardiac manifestations. *Turk Kardiyol Dern Ars.* 2015;43(8):714-716.
30. Garcia D, Erkan D. Diagnosis and management of the antiphospholipid syndrome. *N Engl J Med.* 2018;378(21):2010-2021.
31. Miyakis S, Lockshin MD, Atsumi T, et al. International consensus statement on an update of the classification criteria for definite antiphospholipid syndrome (APS). *J Thromb Haemost.* 2006;4(2):295-306.
32. Tenedios F, Erkan D, Lockshin MD. Cardiac involvement in the antiphospholipid syndrome. *Lupus.* 2005;14(9):691-696.
33. Cervera R, Tektonidou MG, Espinosa G, et al. Task Force on Catastrophic Antiphospholipid Syndrome (APS) and Non-criteria APS Manifestations (I): catastrophic APS, APS nephropathy and heart valve lesions. *Lupus.* 2011;20(2):165-173.
34. Paran D, Caspi D, Levartovsky D, et al. Cardiac dysfunction in patients with systemic lupus erythematosus and antiphospholipid syndrome. *Ann Rheum Dis.* 2007;66(4):506-510.
35. Kampolis C, Tektonidou M, Moyssakis I, et al. Evolution of cardiac dysfunction in patients with antiphospholipid antibodies and/or antiphospholipid syndrome: a 10-year follow-up study. *Semin Arthritis Rheum.* 2014;43(4):558-565.
36. Martinuzzo ME, Pombo G, Forastiero RR, et al. Lupus anticoagulant, high levels of anticardiolipin, and anti-beta2-glycoprotein I antibodies are associated with chronic thromboembolic pulmonary hypertension. *J Rheumatol.* 1998;25(7):1313-1319.
37. Bruce D, Bateman D, Thomas R. Left ventricular thrombi in a patient with the antiphospholipid syndrome. *Br Heart J.* 1995;74(2):202-203.
38. Singh S, Bittner V. Familial hypercholesterolemia—epidemiology, diagnosis, and screening. *Curr Atheroscler Rep.* 2015;17(2):482.
39. Amor-Salamanca A, Castillo S, Gonzalez-Vioque E, et al. Genetically confirmed familial hypercholesterolemia in patients with acute coronary syndrome. *J Am Coll Cardiol.* 2017;70(14):1732-1740.
40. Wiesbauer F, Blessberger H, Azar D, et al. Familial-combined hyperlipidaemia in very young myocardial infarction survivors (<or =40 years of age). *Eur Heart J.* 2009;30(9):1073-1079.
41. Bello-Chavolla OY, Kuri-García A, Ríos-Ríos M, et al. Familial combined hyperlipidemia: current knowledge, perspectives, and controversies. *Rev Invest Clin.* 2018;70(5):224-236.
42. Koopal C, Marais AD, Visseren FL. Familial dysbetalipoproteinemia: an underdiagnosed lipid disorder. *Curr Opin Endocrinol Diabetes Obes.* 2017;24(2):133-139.
43. Tada H, Nohara A, Inazu A, et al. Sitosterolemia, hypercholesterolemia, and coronary artery disease. *J Atheroscler Thromb.* 2018;25(9):783-789.
44. Tsimikas S, Fazio S, Ferdinand KC, et al. NHLBI working group recommendations to reduce lipoprotein(a)-mediated risk of cardiovascular disease and aortic stenosis. *J Am Coll Cardiol.* 2018;71(2):177-192.
45. Tsimikas S. A test in context: lipoprotein(a): diagnosis, prognosis, controversies, and emerging therapies. *J Am Coll Cardiol.* 2017;69(6):692-711.
46. Grundy SM, Stone NJ, Bailey AL, et al. 2018 AHA/ACC/AACVPR/AAPA/ABC/ACPM/ADA/AGS/APhA/ASPC/NLA/PCNA guideline on the management of blood cholesterol: a report of the American College of Cardiology/American Heart Association Task Force on Clinical Practice Guidelines. *J Am Coll Cardiol.* 2019;73(24):3168-3209.
47. Nair V, Belanger EC, Veinot JP. Lysosomal storage disorders affecting the heart: a review. *Cardiovasc Pathol.* 2019;39:12-24.
48. Donnelly JP, Hanna M. Cardiac amyloidosis: an update on diagnosis and treatment. *Cleve Clin J Med.* 2017;84:12-26.
49. Aronow WS. Management of cardiac hemochromatosis. *Arch Med Sci.* 2018;14(3):560-568.
50. Birnie DH, Kandolin R, Nery PB, et al. Cardiac manifestations of sarcoidosis: diagnosis and management. *Eur Heart J.* 2017;38(35):2663-2670.
51. Cohle SD, Suarez-Mier MP, Aguilera B. Sudden death resulting from lesions of the cardiac conduction system. *Am J Forensic Med Pathol.* 2002;23(1):83-89.
52. Szczeklik W, Miszalski-Jamka T, Mastalerz L, et al. Multimodality assessment of cardiac involvement in Churg-Strauss syndrome patients in clinical remission. *Circ J.* 2011;75(3):649-655.
53. McGeoch L, Carette S, Cuthbertson D, et al. Cardiac involvement in granulomatosis with polyangiitis. *J Rheumatol.* 2015;42(7):1209-1212.
54. Bae YD, Choi HJ, Lee JC, et al. Clinical features of polyarteritis nodosa in Korea. *J Korean Med Sci.* 2006;21(4):591-595.
55. Singh S, Vignesh P, Burgner D. The epidemiology of Kawasaki disease: a global update. *Arch Dis Child.* 2015;100(11):1084-1088.
56. Ghelani SJ, Singh S, Manojkumar R. QT interval dispersion in North Indian children with Kawasaki disease without overt coronary artery abnormalities. *Rheumatol Int.* 2011;31(3):301-305.
57. Reinhold-Keller E, Herlyn K, Wagner-Bastmeyer R, et al. Stable incidence of primary systemic vasculitides over five years: results from the German vasculitis register. *Arthritis Rheum.* 2005;53(1):93-99.
58. Seyahi E, Ugurlu S, Cumali R, et al. Atherosclerosis in Takayasu arteritis. *Ann Rheum Dis.* 2006;65(9):1202-1207.
59. Bradley TJ, Bowdin SC, Morel CFJ, Pyeritz RE. The expanding clinical spectrum of extracardiovascular and cardiovascular manifestations of heritable thoracic aortic aneurysm and dissection. *Can J Cardiol.* 2016;32(1):86-99.
60. Judge DP, Dietz HC. Marfan's syndrome. *Lancet.* 2005;366(9501):1965-1976.
61. Verstraeten A, Alaerts M, Van Laer L, Loeys B. Marfan syndrome and related disorders: 25 years of gene discovery. *Hum Mutat.* 2016;37(6):524-531.
62. Beighton P. Cardiac abnormalities in the Ehlers-Danlos syndrome. *Br Heart J.* 1969;31(2):227-232.

CHAPTER 22

SUBSTANCE ABUSE AND THE HEART

Janet Ma and Isac C. Thomas

INTRODUCTION

Substance abuse is a growing public health concern. In 2017, an estimated 271 million individuals worldwide abused a substance, an increase of nearly 30% from 2009.[1] Of those who abused a substance, 35 million have an ongoing substance abuse disorder requiring treatment.[1] In the United States (US), 10.6% of the population aged 12 or older used an illicit drug in the past 30 days.[2] Complex patterns of global substance abuse have developed, including regional differences in substance abuse patterns and trafficking of illicit substances across borders.

New challenges in substance abuse prevention and treatment have emerged. Electronic cigarettes and vaporizers ("vaping") have grown in popularity, particularly among adolescents, threatening to erode global tobacco cessation efforts. Moreover, an epidemic of a severe form of acute lung injury recently emerged, linked to the inhalation of the vaping additive vitamin E acetate.[3] Opium (a non-synthetic opiate) has been abused globally for centuries but, in the past two decades, a sharp rise in opioid-related mortality has been traced to the prescription of synthetic opioids.[4] Fentanyl abuse has become widespread in the US and much of Europe; in contrast, non-prescription tramadol is at the center of the opioid crisis in West, Central, and North Africa.[1] The global manufacture of cocaine reached an all-time high in 2017, with rates of cocaine seizure by law enforcement increasing by 74% in the past decade.[1] Amphetamine-type stimulants, chief among them methamphetamine, have increased in potency, with global rates of abuse now trailing only marijuana and opioids.[1]

When evaluating patients with substance abuse, it is important to recognize the potential short-term and long-term cardiovascular impact these drugs may have (**Table 22.1**). This chapter aims to discuss the latest evidence to guide the clinician in screening, monitoring, and treating patients with substance abuse disorders. The most widely used substances will be discussed, including alcohol, tobacco, marijuana, opioids, cocaine, and methamphetamine.

PATHOGENESIS AND CLINICAL PRESENTATION

Effects of Alcohol Abuse

Over half of American adults regularly consume alcohol, and 44% of those who drink regularly (61 million) report engaging in at least one episode of binge drinking (defined as five or more drinks in one setting) in the past month.[5] According to the 2015 National Survey on Drug Use and Health, 15.1 million adults aged 18 years or older met criteria for an alcohol use disorder.[6] These US findings are reflected worldwide, with an overall increase in global per-capita consumption of alcohol between 1990 and 2017 and a decrease in prevalence of lifetime abstinence during that time.[7] Cardiac effects of alcohol have been extensively studied and include alcoholic cardiomyopathy, atrial fibrillation, and hypertension.

Cardiomyopathy

Alcoholic cardiomyopathy is a result of direct cardiotoxic effects from heavy alcohol consumption resulting in left ventricular (LV) systolic dysfunction.[8] Up to 40% of dilated cardiomyopathy in western countries has been attributed to excess alcohol use, although what constitutes excess alcohol consumption varies among studies.[8,9] Few clinical or histological characteristics are specific to alcoholic cardiomyopathy, but it shares characteristics with other forms of dilated cardiomyopathy including a dilated left ventricle and a reduced LV ejection fraction (EF).[8] In a cohort study of 52 patients with alcohol abuse, Urbano-Márquez et al found a significant decrease in the LVEF that was directly proportional to the patients' lifelong cumulative alcohol intake.[10] Some studies suggest worse outcomes in alcoholic cardiomyopathy compared with other forms of dilated cardiomyopathy. Fauchier et al studied 50 patients with alcoholic cardiomyopathy and 84 patients with dilated cardiomyopathy over a follow-up period of 47 months, finding a significantly higher survival rate in patients with dilated cardiomyopathy compared to their counterparts with alcoholic cardiomyopathy.[11] Gavazzi et al studied 79 patients with alcoholic cardiomyopathy and 259 patients with dilated cardiomyopathy over a mean follow-up period of 59 months and found that transplant-free survival was significantly worse among patients with alcoholic cardiomyopathy than among those with dilated cardiomyopathy (41% vs 53%, respectively).[12] Guzzo-Merello et al examined alcoholic cardiomyopathy in a cohort study, finding that one-third of these patients had a poor prognosis while two-thirds remained clinically stable.[9] Out of the clinically stable patients, one-half recovered LV systolic function (ie, an absolute increase in LVEF >10% to a final value of >40%). In contrast, no significant difference in clinical outcomes was identified between patients with alcoholic cardiomyopathy who completely abstained from alcohol compared with those who reduced their intake to moderate.

TABLE 22.1 Suggested Considerations for Specific Substances and Associated Cardiovascular Effects

Substance	Cardiovascular Effects	Special Considerations
Tobacco smoking/e-cigarettes	Atherosclerotic disease	Preliminary data shows that vaping and e-cigarette use have less harm compared with traditional cigarettes but still confer risk of myocardial infarction and lung disease
Alcohol	Dilated cardiomyopathy Atrial fibrillation Hypertension	Moderate consumption has traditionally been thought to confer a cardioprotective effect, however recent data challenge this notion
Methamphetamine	Dilated cardiomyopathy Pulmonary hypertension	The incidence of methamphetamine-associated cardiomyopathy has grown in the last decade and should be considered in anyone with nonischemic cardiomyopathy and history of methamphetamine use
Cocaine	Acute coronary syndrome Stroke Dilated cardiomyopathy	Avoid beta-blockers acutely in cocaine-associated myocardial infarction. Consider using bare mental stents due to increased risk of stent thrombosis
Marijuana	Acute coronary syndrome	Abstinence from marijuana smoking is advisable for patients with pre-existing cardiac disease
Opioids	None established	More research is needed

Arrhythmias

Alcohol is a well-known trigger of atrial fibrillation, so much so that patients who present with atrial fibrillation after alcohol consumption are commonly referred to as having 'holiday heart syndrome'. Heavy alcohol consumption may be a stronger risk factor for atrial fibrillation than hypertension or obesity.[13] Multiple meta-analyses suggest that even moderate alcohol consumption increases the risk of atrial fibrillation.[14,15] Infrequent binge drinking has also been implicated in the development of atrial fibrillation. Atrial fibrillation has been shown to occur even in infrequent and nondrinkers after a binge. Even though atrial fibrillation typically terminates after 24 hours, it will recur in about a quarter of patients with subsequent binges. Liang et al found that binge drinking among individuals who consumed a moderate amount of alcohol conferred a risk of atrial fibrillation similar to habitual heavy consumption.[16]

It has been postulated that alcohol may increase the risk of arrhythmias by inducing electrical atrial remodeling.[17] Patients who drink alcohol have a higher recurrence of atrial fibrillation after ablation. In one study, 1-year arrhythmia-free survival post circumferential pulmonary vein isolation was found in 81% of patients who abstained from alcohol, 69% patients with light-moderate consumption, and only 35% in patient with heavy consumption.[18] Patients with heavy alcohol consumption were also more likely to have adverse outcomes such as thromboembolism, even after adjusting for anticoagulation use and the CHA_2DS_2Vasc score.[18] Importantly, abstinence from alcohol appears to reduce the risk of atrial fibrillation recurrence, with a recent randomized controlled trial showing that patients with a history of atrial fibrillation who previously consumed more than 10 drinks per week and subsequently abstained from alcohol significantly reduced their risk of arrhythmia recurrence and overall burden.[19]

Atherosclerotic Cardiovascular Disease

Alcohol abuse and/or heavy alcohol use, including binge drinking, have been associated with an increased risk of myocardial infarction.[20] The effects of habitual light to moderate alcohol consumption on the risk of atherosclerotic cardiovascular disease (CVD) are not clear. Several epidemiological studies have suggested that light to moderate alcohol consumption confers a protective effect compared to both abstinence and heavy alcohol consumption. In the Physician's Health Study, a prospective cohort of 89,299 US men, alcohol consumption appeared to be inversely associated with CVD mortality at any level of consumption, although at the highest consumptions levels the benefit seemed to be balanced by an increased risk of non-CVD mortality.[21] However, the conclusions regarding cardioprotective effects arise from cohort studies and observational data rather than randomized, controlled trials. These studies tend to recruit populations that are more likely to be health conscious, have stable access to care, and may therefore have confounding characteristics.[22] Results from Mendelian randomization studies ("nature's randomized trials"), suggest higher CVD risk due to alcohol consumption. In a study of a large cohort of European descent, the presence of a variant in the gene for alcohol dehydrogenase was associated with lower alcohol consumption and lower odds of both coronary heart disease and ischemic stroke.[23] Given inherent challenges in performing traditional randomized trials of alcohol consumption—such as participant recruitment and blinding, long- term adherence to assigned intervention, and ethical considerations,—the effects of light to moderate alcohol consumption on atherosclerotic CVD are likely to remain uncertain.

Hypertension

There is a long-established link between alcohol and hypertension.[24] Up to 16% of hypertension cases may be attributed to alcohol consumption. A meta-analysis of 15 randomized controlled trials showed that alcohol reduction significantly lowered systolic and diastolic blood pressures in a dose-dependent fashion.[25] Notably, blood pressure does not appear to acutely rise after alcohol exposure, and has been shown to decrease for up to 8 hours after heavy evening drinking.[26] Rather, hypertension related to alcohol consumption develops subacutely over days to weeks.[27]

Effects of Tobacco and Electronic Cigarettes

Cigarettes smoking is a well-known public health hazard, yet the prevalence remains high with almost 14% of adults in the US reported as current smokers in 2018.[28] Moreover, e-cigarette use is now on the rise. Since entering the US marketplace in 2007, e-cigarettes have quickly gained traction as an alternative to smoking tobacco cigarettes. The popularity of e-cigarettes has also increased among youth who do not regularly smoke cigarettes. The prevalence of e-cigarette use is estimated to be around 6%, with half of users citing its perceived lower risk compared with smoking regular cigarettes.[29]

Atherosclerotic Cardiovascular Disease

Tobacco has been a leading cause of CVD for decades.[30] One large prospective study by Banks et al looked at 188,167 CVD- and cancer-free individuals aged greater than or equal to ≥45 years in Australia and examined cardiovascular effects associated with cigarette smoking.[31] The study demonstrated that tobacco abuse increases the risk of all CVD subtypes, with current tobacco smokers having at least double the risk of developing the most significant types of CVD, including over five times the risk of developing peripheral arterial disease, and three times the risk of mortality from CVD compared to people who have never smoked.[31]

Complete smoking cessation has been shown to substantially reduce the excess risk of tobacco-related CVD, and should be reinforced in every clinical encounter. Banks et al showed that former smokers aged greater than 45 years reduced their excess smoking-related risk by 90% if they had quit by age 35 to 44 years.[31] These findings are consistent with other studies, such as a prospective study conducted by Pirie et al who found a risk reduction of over 90% for patients who quit by the age of 40 years and 97% for those who quit by the age of 30 years.[32]

Younger recreational smokers may be prone to incorrectly assuming that light smoking carries low harm. One study surveying 24,658 adolescents showed that a tenth of them thought light smoking was not harmful, and that 65% of light smokers did not associate this behavior with significant harm.[33] However, a meta-analysis of 141 cohort studies and 55 case reports that examined low cigarette consumption and the risk of CVD found that reduction in cigarette smoking did not proportionally correlate to a reduction in cardiovascular risk; even smoking only one cigarette a day still carried half the risk of smoking 20 cigarettes a day.[34]

E-cigarette use has exponentially risen in recent years, in part due to its marketing as a healthier alternative or bridge to smoking cessation. With the growing popularity of e-cigarettes, one question more and more patients may ask is whether switching to e-cigarettes may reduce cardiovascular risk. One randomized trial found that the use of e-cigarettes resulted in a 1-year rate of abstinence from cigarettes of only 18%, though this was significantly higher than those randomized to other nicotine replacement products.[35]

A prospective, randomized control trial by George et al with chronic smokers without known coronary artery disease who switched to e-cigarettes compared with those who continued traditional cigarettes found a significant improvement in endothelial function within one month of switching to e-cigarettes, especially for female participants, suggesting a potential in risk reduction for select patients.[36] While the use of e-cigarettes may be a useful harm reduction strategy among select adults who abuse cigarettes, the increasing penetration of e-cigarette use among adolescents is a public health concern, made all the more pressing by widespread reports of e-cigarette related acute lung injury in the US associated with vitamin E acetate.[3]

Growing evidence also suggests that e-cigarette use may confer cardiovascular risk. One study showed exposure of human-induced pluripotent stem cell–derived endothelial cells to flavored e-cigarettes exacerbated endothelial dysfunction.[37] Another study found that daily e-cigarette use, adjusted for smoking conventional cigarettes as well as other risk factors, was associated with increased risk of myocardial infarction.[38]

Effects of Opioid Abuse

Opioid abuse has increased in the national awareness with widespread abuse of both prescription opioid medication and illegal opioids such as heroin and synthetic fentanyl. The abuse of prescription opioid medications increased greatly in the two decades leading up to 2010. From 2010 to 2013, the prescription of opioid medications decreased; unfortunately, illegal heroin abuse increased over the same period.[4]

The opioid epidemic has also been associated with increasing rates of infective endocarditis due to the associated intravenous heroin use. Rudasill et al found that the incidence of intravenous drug-related infective endocarditis almost doubled from 2010 to 2015.[39] Cardiac arrest is also more common in patients with opioid overdoses compared with non-opioid overdoses due to respiratory depression, with the rate of cardiac arrest increasing disproportionately in patients with opioid overdoses.[40] However, opioids generally have been considered to have a benign cardiovascular profile since they do not have a direct effect on cardiac contractility or atherosclerotic disease. A few retrospective studies evaluated the association of chronic opioid use with cardiovascular outcomes. Carman et al found that the risk for myocardial infarction was 2.7 times higher in patients with chronic opioid use compared with matched controls.[41] Another study by Nishimura et al examined the burden of substance abuse among patients with heart failure and its association with hospital encounters.[42] They found that out of 11,268 patients with heart failure, 8.2% had concomitant opioid use or abuse which was associated with a greater number of hospital encounters for heart failure with an incidence risk ratio of 1.57, which was comparable to patients with concomitant heart failure and chronic kidney disease.[42] Although these studies merely suggest a possible association, they do highlight the need for further research regarding the relationship between opioid use and abuse and CVD.

Effects of Abuse of Marijuana and Synthetic Cannabinoids

Marijuana abuse has been steadily rising in the US over the past several years with recent legalization and decriminalization in several states. In addition, synthetic cannabinoids (K2, spice) have also grown in popularity in the US since 2009; their abuse may even be underestimated given an inability to detect them by standard toxicology screens.[2]

Marijuana and its synthetic counterparts are now the most widely used psychoactive substances after tobacco and alcohol. An increasing number of adverse cardiovascular effects have been reported in association with cannabis use, including myocardial infarction, vascular events including stroke, arrhythmias, and stress cardiomyopathy.[43] The immediate effects of marijuana and its psychoactive compound Δ9-tetrahydrocannabinol (THC) on the cardiovascular system are well-documented, including transient tachycardia and slight increase in blood pressure.[44] These effects appear to be due to the complex interactions within the endocannabinoid system. THC effects are mediated by the G-protein-coupled cannabinoid receptors 1 and 2 (CB_1R and CB_2R). While CB_1R are the most abundant G-protein-coupled receptors in the mammalian brain, low levels of CB_1R are also present in most peripheral tissues, including the myocardium, vascular endothelial and smooth muscle cells, and blood cells. CB_1R activation has been shown to exert complex hemodynamic effects that ultimately lead to decreased myocardial contractility. In contrast, CB_2R do not seem to affect the cardiovascular system.[45]

Atherosclerotic Cardiovascular Disease

Mittleman et al conducted a study showing a 4.8-fold increase in risk of myocardial infarction within the first 60 minutes after marijuana use, which rapidly decreased thereafter.[46] The study suggested that marijuana's acute physiological changes may result in a transiently increased risk of adverse cardiovascular events.[46] A retrospective analysis by Patel et al found a higher prevalence of acute myocardial infarction among patients aged 15 to 22 years with cannabis abuse compared with the general population.[47]

Evidence is still lacking regarding the long-term consequences of marijuana abuse on CVD risk. In a prospective study with 3.8 years of follow-up, Mukamal et al found that patients who smoked marijuana less than weekly were at a 2.5-fold increased risk of mortality following myocardial infarction with a graded increase in risk with more frequent use.[48] However, continued follow-up for up to 18 years found that this apparent increased mortality rate did not reach statistical significance.[49]

There is conflicting evidence that marijuana may lead to an increased risk of stroke. Rumalla et al found that marijuana abuse was independently associated with an increased risk of hospitalization for ischemic stroke as well as subarachnoid hemorrhage in younger adults aged 25 to 34 years.[50,51] However, other studies refute these findings. One population-based cohort study examined 45,000 men to investigate the association between cannabis abuse and early-onset stroke; the study found almost twice the risk of ischemic stroke in men with increased cannabis use, but this risk was not significant after adjusting for tobacco usage.[52]

As the medical marijuana industry gains traction, public opinion has become increasingly favorable and its cardiovascular risk may be overlooked. Based on the current literature, patients with pre-existing CVD disease should be discouraged from using marijuana either for medical or recreational use. Additionally, patients of younger age and without traditional risk factors should be counseled on the risks that using marijuana recreationally may confer for acute coronary syndrome.[47]

Effects of Methamphetamine

Amphetamine-type stimulants, in particular methamphetamine, are one of the most commonly abused illegal drug classes in the US. In the 2014 National Survey on Drug Abuse and Health, 4.9% of Americans aged 12 and older reported having used methamphetamine in their lifetimes.[6] There is stark geographical variability, with the western and Midwestern US most affected by methamphetamine abuse.[53] Worldwide data show that amphetamine-type stimulants are the second most widely used illicit drug in the world after cannabis.[1] Following overdose and accidents, the leading cause of death in methamphetamine abusers is CVD, in particular methamphetamine-associated cardiomyopathy and pulmonary arterial hypertension.[54]

Cardiomyopathy

Given the high prevalence of methamphetamine abuse, an increasing number of methamphetamine-associated cardiomyopathy and heart failure cases have emerged in the literature. Multiple theories have been proposed about the mechanism of methamphetamine-associated cardiomyopathy, including catecholamine surge, increased free radical formation, mitochondrial injury, and direct toxicity to cardiomyocytes.[55] Associated pathologic findings have been reported to include ventricular dilatation, interstitial fibrosis, contraction band necrosis, and inflammatory cellular infiltrate.[56,57] Another retrospective study by Neeki et al found similar results with a larger cohort of 591 patients (age < 50 years), further suggesting methamphetamine abuse as an independent risk factor for an increase in the severity of cardiomyopathy and heart failure.[58] Nishimura et al further characterized armed-services veterans with methamphetamine-associated heart failure, finding these patients were younger, with more frequent co-morbid psychiatric disorders and social issues such as homelessness and unemployment than their heart failure counterparts who did not abuse methamphetamine.[59] The results of this study were further corroborated by Thomas et al, who found that predictors of poor outcome among patients with methamphetamine-associated heart failure included mood/anxiety disorders and opioid use.[60] Additionally, Thomas et al found that these patients had higher 5-year heart failure readmission rate but a lower 10-year total mortality than their heart failure counterparts who did not abuse methamphetamine. However, after age adjustment, the risk of total mortality was not significantly different.[60]

Currently, little is known about the effects of methamphetamine cessation and the time window for potential reversibility of methamphetamine-associated cardiomyopathy. A study by Schürer et al examined 30 patients with methamphetamine abuse and LVEF less than 40% using endomyocardial biopsy; the investigators found that the extent of myocardial fibrosis appeared to predict at least partial reversibility of LV function with cessation.[56] The results of this study suggest that complete cessation of methamphetamine abuse along with medical therapy may be able to improve function and symptoms for some patients with methamphetamine-associated cardiomyopathy.

Pulmonary Arterial Hypertension

Methamphetamine abuse has also been implicated in the development of pulmonary arterial hypertension.[61] The mechanism for this association remains unclear. One nuclear medicine study using radiolabeled methamphetamine analogues demonstrated that methamphetamine concentrations accumulate highest within lung tissue.[62] A retrospective study by Zhao et al found that the only clinical factor shown to be significantly associated with pulmonary arterial hypertension among patients who abuse methamphetamine was female sex.[63]

Effects of Cocaine Abuse

Although the prevalence of cocaine abuse in the US peaked in the 1980s, it remains a widespread public health concern. In recent years, there has been a resurgence in cocaine abuse, with the prevalence increasing 20% from 2011 to 2015, and the number of cocaine-related deaths increasing from 2012 to 2015.[64] Cocaine abuse has a number of deleterious CVD associations, including myocardial infarction and stroke.

Atherosclerotic Cardiovascular Disease

In the US, cocaine is among the most commonly abused illicit substances associated with a visit to the emergency department, with chest pain being the most common presenting symptom.[65-67] In one study, the risk of myocardial infarction was found to acutely increase by 24-fold in the first hour of abusing cocaine.[65] However, it is also worth noting that only 6% of these cocaine-abusing patients presenting with chest pain were found to have myocardial infarction as the etiology.[66,67] Identifying acute coronary syndrome as an etiology for chest pain may be difficult in cocaine-abusing patients, given many of them will have an abnormal electrocardiogram even in the absence of a myocardial infraction.[68] Cardiac biomarkers including troponin I and CK-MB, however, do not seem to be affected by cocaine abuse and maintain their accuracy in determining myocardial infarction.[69]

There is uncertainty surrounding the benefits and risks of beta-blockers for the treatment of acute coronary syndromes and ischemic heart disease in patients who are actively abusing cocaine. Multiple studies found that many patients who received beta-blockers after using cocaine had a neutral or even mildly beneficial cardiovascular outcome compared with their cocaine-using counterparts who did not receive beta-blockers.[70,71] However, the 2014 ACC/AHA guidelines reissued a class III recommendation against the use of beta-blockers in patients with myocardial infarction and active cocaine use, a reversal of previous recommendations.[72] A class IIa recommendation was issued on using benzodiazepines alone or in combination with nitroglycerin for management in hypertension and tachycardia in these patients. Regarding stent use in cocaine-associated myocardial infarction, attention must be paid to the increased risk of stent thrombosis in patients persistently using cocaine.[73] The 2012 ACC/AHA guidelines therefore recommended implantation of bare metal stents in patients with myocardial infarction who abuse cocaine.

Cocaine may increase the risk of both ischemic and hemorrhagic stroke, though the precise mechanism remains unclear.[74] One study examined underlying stroke etiologies in 96 patients who had been hospitalized and actively or formerly abusing cocaine.[74] Among the 45 patients with ischemic stroke, the most likely common etiology was due to underlying atherosclerosis rather than acute vasospasm. For the 25 patients who had a hemorrhagic stroke, the majority of cocaine abuse was active/current, as opposed to former, suggesting that acute elevations in blood pressure associated with cocaine intake may have played a causal role. Although data are limited regarding the use of thrombolytic therapy in ischemic stroke associated with cocaine exposure, one small study showed that 29 cocaine-positive patients received tissue plasminogen activator without complications.[75]

Cardiomyopathy

There have been multiple case reports on acute heart failure in the setting of cocaine abuse. Little is known about its incidence or pathophysiology, although in some cases it has been described as a takotsubo-like (stress-induced cardiomyopathy) presentation. There are several postulated mechanisms contributing to cocaine-associated cardiomyopathy, including acute catecholamine surge, increased oxidative stress, and increased prothrombotic risk leading to coronary thrombus development.[76] Overall, cocaine should be considered among the potential etiologies of heart failure in any cocaine-abusing patient. Limited available data suggest patients with heart failure may benefit from guideline-directed medical therapy, including beta-blocker therapy. A retrospective study of 72 patients with heart failure with reduced ejection and active cocaine abuse found that beta-blocker therapy was associated with improvements in both exercise tolerance and LVEF.[77]

DIAGNOSIS AND MANAGEMENT

For the clinician, a number of factors should be considered in the diagnostic and management approaches to patients with known or suspected substance abuse-associated CVD (see **Algorithm 22.1**). A comprehensive substance abuse history should be taken, including drug abuse frequency, amount,

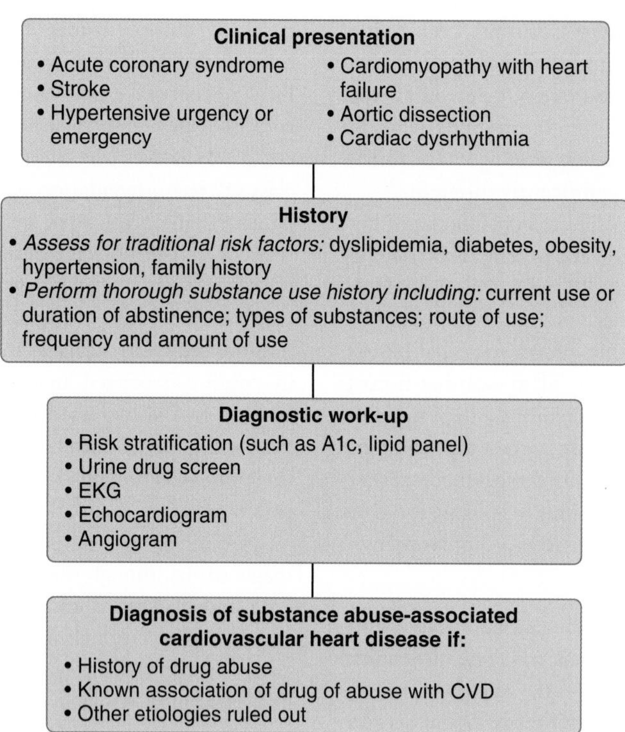

ALGORITHM 22.1 Suggested diagnostic approach to substance abuse-related cardiovascular disease. A1c, hemoglobin A1c; CVD, cardiovascular disease; EKG, electrocardiogram.

and route of abuse (eg, smoking, snorting, vaping, ingestion, and intravenous administration). Patients may endorse abusing more than one type of substance. Duration of abstinence in those who report a prior history of drug abuse should be determined. Urine or serum drug screening should be considered for any patient with a reported history of substance abuse, even if purportedly remote, as patients may not be willing to admit relapse. However, the duration of time that metabolites are detectable on drug screening tests varies by substance, and a negative result, therefore, does not rule out recent abuse.[78] CVD disease. For patients with cardiomyopathy or acute coronary syndrome, for instance, atherosclerotic coronary artery disease should be evaluated as there is no gold-standard for the diagnosis of substance abuse-associated CVD. There has not been an established role for routine advanced work-up such as cardiac magnetic resonance imaging or endomyocardial biopsy, and the diagnosis of substance abuse-associated CVD is largely made on clinical suspicion in the absence of other identifiable etiologies.

A frequently encountered patient with substance abuse-associated CVD is a younger adult without traditional risk factors, but with a clear history of recent or chronic ongoing substance abuse or a positive urine drug screen. Furthermore, patients with substance abuse-associated CVD have been linked to an increased rate of psychiatric co-morbidities, homelessness, and unemployment compared with patients who have other etiologies of CVD.[59] However, the role that substance abuse plays in the clinical presentation of any patient should be considered regardless of demographics and co-morbidities, especially if in an area with a high prevalence of substance abuse, or if the etiology of the patient's CVD is unclear.

The primary goal in treating substance-associated CVD is simple in theory, yet often frustratingly difficult in practice: cessation of the offending substance. There has been evidence, such as in methamphetamine-associated cardiomyopathy or alcoholic cardiomyopathy, that complete cessation may result in recovery of EF.[9,56] Clinicians who are treating these patients may find benefit by involving an interdisciplinary team of social workers, counselors, addiction specialists, and psychiatrists to work toward achieving cessation of the offending substance.

While evidence is limited regarding the use of traditional therapies for CVD in substance-abuse populations, these therapies should be pursued absent compelling evidence of a lack of effectiveness. For instance, in patients with substance abuse-associated heart failure with reduced EF, guideline-directed medical therapy should be prescribed. Similarly, it would be reasonable to treat patients with myocardial infarction or stroke with standard therapy, including aspirin, beta-blockers, angiotensin converting enzyme inhibitors, statins, and percutaneous intervention if indicated, especially if there may be concomitant atherosclerosis. Contributing traditional risk factors should also be addressed, as the etiology of CVD among patients who abuse illicit substances may be multifactorial.

Unfortunately, in the face of drug addiction, adherence to medical therapy and clinical follow up is frequently suboptimal, and can be frustrating for the cardiovascular clinician. It has been our experience that these considerations play a role in treatment decisions, particularly for higher-risk interventions such as percutaneous coronary and valvular interventions, and cardiac surgeries. Consequently, the early and frequent involvement of members of the aforementioned interdisciplinary team may be essential to a successful treatment plan for these patients.

RESEARCH AND FUTURE DIRECTIONS

As the global epidemiology of substance abuse continues to evolve, it has become increasingly apparent that CVD is an important cause of morbidity and mortality in patients with substance abuse. The need for further research is increased by the potential reversibility of some cardiovascular disorders with cessation of the offending substance. Opportunities for future patient-centered research include focus on the incidence and prevalence of CVD among substance abusers, pathophysiology and natural history of cardiac manifestations, and optimal management of these patients. The research focus should also extend beyond illicit substances to elucidating the relationship between legal substances and adverse cardiovascular effects, including e-cigarettes and opioids, to improve risk stratification and counseling. However, certain limitations inherent to researching cardiovascular complications of substance abuse should be acknowledged. The patient population presents a challenge given psychosocial and economic barriers to care. The ability to conduct randomized, controlled trials is also limited by difficulties in implementing an effective intervention to achieve cessation. It seems likely that similar to the management of substance abuse-related CVD, successful research will also rely on an interdisciplinary, team-based approach.

KEY POINTS

- ✔ Substance abuse has been implicated in all forms of CVD
- ✔ A comprehensive substance abuse history should be taken, including drug abuse frequency, amount, and route of abuse (eg, smoking, snorting, vaping, ingestions, and intravenous administration).
- ✔ A frequently encountered patient with substance abuse-associated CVD is a younger adult without traditional risk factors, but with a clear history of recent or chronic ongoing substance abuse or a positive urine drug screen. However, substance abuse in any patient residing in an area with a high prevalence of substance abuse should be considered, especially if the etiology of the patient's CVD is unclear.
- ✔ Patients with substance abuse-associated CVD have been linked to an increased rate of psychiatric co-morbidities, homelessness, and unemployment compared with patients who have other etiologies of CVD. An interdisciplinary approach should therefore be considered in the management of substance abuse-associated CVD.
- ✔ Further research is needed to better elucidate the relationship between substance abuse and its adverse cardiovascular effects, although many challenges exist in implementing large-scale, high-quality clinical studies.

REFERENCES

1. United Nations Office on Drugs and Crime. World Drug Report 2019. Sales No: E.19.XI.8, 2019.
2. National Institute on Drug Abuse. Drug facts: emerging trends and alerts. 2019. Accessed November 3, 2019. https://www.drugabuse.gov/drugs-abuse/emerging-trends-alerts
3. Blount BC, Karwowski MP, Shields PG, et al. Vitamin E acetate in bronchoalveolar-lavage fluid associated with EVALI. *N Engl J Med.* 2020;382:697-705.
4. Cicero TJ, Ellis MS, Harney J. Shifting patterns of prescription opioid and heroin abuse in the united states. *N Engl J Med.* 2015;373:1789-1790.
5. Centers for Disease Control and Prevention. Alcohol use and youth health. 2018. Accessed October 24, 2019. https://www.cdc.gov/alcohol/fact-sheets/alcohol-use.htm
6. Substance Abuse and Mental Health Services Administration. Behavioral health trends in the United States: Results from the 2014 National Survey on Drug Use and Health. Center for Behavioral Health Statistics and Quality. Accessed October 24, 2019. https://www.samhsa.gov/data/sites/default/files/NSDUH-FRR1-2014/NSDUH-FRR1-2014.pdf
7. Burton R, Sheron N. No level of alcohol consumption improves health. *Lancet.* 2018;392:987-988.
8. Piano MR. Alcoholic cardiomyopathy: incidence, clinical characteristics, and pathophysiology. *Chest.* 2002;121:1638-1650.
9. Guzzo-Merello G, Segovia J, Dominguez F, et al. Natural history and prognostic factors in alcoholic cardiomyopathy. *JACC Heart Fail.* 2015;3:78-86.
10. Urbano-Márquez A, Estruch R, Navarro-Lopez F, Grau JM, Mont L, Rubin E. The effects of alcoholism on skeletal and cardiac muscle. *N Engl J Med.* 1989;320:409-415.
11. Fauchier L, Babuty D, Poret P, et al. Comparison of long-term outcome of alcoholic and idiopathic dilated cardiomyopathy. *Eur Heart J.* 2000;21:306-314.
12. Gavazzi A, De Maria R, Parolini M, Porcu M. Alcohol abuse and dilated cardiomyopathy in men. *Am J Cardiol.* 2000;85:1114-1118.
13. Sano F, Ohira T, Kitamura A, et al. Heavy alcohol consumption and risk of atrial fibrillation. The Circulatory Risk in Communities Study (CIRCS). *Circ J.* 2014;78:955-961.
14. Di Castelnuovo A, Costanzo S, Bonaccio M, et al. Moderate alcohol consumption is associated with lower risk for heart failure but not atrial fibrillation. *JACC Heart Fail.* 2017;5:837-844.
15. Larsson SC, Drca N, Wolk A. Alcohol consumption and risk of atrial fibrillation: a prospective study and dose-response meta-analysis. *J Am Coll Cardiol.* 2014;64:281-289.
16. Liang Y, Mente A, Yusuf S, et al. Alcohol consumption and the risk of incident atrial fibrillation among people with cardiovascular disease. *CMAJ.* 2012;184:E857-E866.
17. Voskoboinik A, Wong G, Lee G, et al. Moderate alcohol consumption is associated with atrial electrical and structural changes: insights from high-density left atrial electroanatomic mapping. *Heart Rhythm.* 2019;16:251-259.
18. Qiao Y, Shi R, Hou B, et al. Impact of alcohol consumption on substrate remodeling and ablation outcome of paroxysmal atrial fibrillation. *J Am Heart Assoc.* 2015;4:e002349.
19. Voskoboinik A, Kalman JM, De Silva A, et al. Alcohol abstinence in drinkers with atrial fibrillation. *N Engl J Med.* 2020;382:20-28.
20. Whitman IR, Agarwal V, Nah G, et al. Alcohol abuse and cardiac disease. *J Am Coll Cardiol.* 2017;69:13-24.
21. Gaziano JM, Gaziano TA, Glynn RJ, et al. Light-to-moderate alcohol consumption and mortality in the Physicians' Health Study enrollment cohort. *J Am Coll Cardiol.* 2000;35:96-105.
22. Criqui MH, Thomas IC. Alcohol consumption and cardiac disease: where are we now? *J Am Coll Cardiol.* 2017;69:25-27.
23. Holmes MV, Dale CE, Zuccolo L, et al. Association between alcohol and cardiovascular disease: Mendelian andomization analysis based on individual participant data. *BMJ.* 2014;349:g4164.
24. Kodavali L, Townsend RR. Alcohol and its relationship to blood pressure. *Curr Hypertens Rep.* 2006;8:338-344.
25. Xin X, He J, Frontini MG, Ogden LG, Motsamai OI, Whelton PK. Effects of alcohol reduction on blood pressure: a meta-analysis of randomized controlled trials. *Hypertension.* 2001;38:1112-1127.
26. Klatsky AL, Gunderson EP. Alcohol and hypertension. In: Mohler ER, Townsend RR, eds. *Advanced Therapy in Hypertension and Vascular Disease.* BC Decker Press; 2006:108-117.

27. Puddey IB, Beilin LJ. Alcohol is bad for blood pressure. *Clin Exp Pharmacol Physiol.* 2006;33:847-852.
28. Centers for Disease Control and Prevention. Tobacco use. 2019. Accessed December 5, 2019. https://www.cdc.gov/alcohol/fact-sheets/alcohol-use.htm
29. E-cigarettes: an emerging category. Ernst & Young; 2016.
30. Thun MJ, Carter BD, Feskanich D, et al. 50-year trends in smoking-related mortality in the United States. *N Engl J Med.* 2013;368:351-364.
31. Banks E, Joshy G, Korda RJ, et al. Tobacco smoking and risk of 36 cardiovascular disease subtypes: fatal and non-fatal outcomes in a large prospective Australian study. *BMC Med.* 2019;17:128.
32. Pirie K, Peto R, Reeves GK, Green J, Beral V. The 21st century hazards of smoking and benefits of stopping: a prospective study of one million women in the UK. *Lancet.* 2013;381:133-141.
33. Amrock SM, Weitzman M. Adolescents' perceptions of light and intermittent smoking in the United States. *Pediatrics.* 2015;135:246-254.
34. Hackshaw A, Morris JK, Boniface S, Tang JL, Milenkovic D. Low cigarette consumption and risk of coronary heart disease and stroke: meta-analysis of 141 cohort studies in 55 study reports. *BMJ.* 2018;360:j5855.
35. Hajek P, Phillips-Waller A, Przulj D, et al. A randomized trial of e-cigarettes versus nicotine-replacement therapy. *N Engl J Med.* 2019;380:629-637.
36. George J, Hussain M, Vadiveloo T, et al. Cardiovascular effects of switching from tobacco cigarettes to electronic cigarettes. *J Am Coll Cardiol.* 2019;74:3112-3120.
37. Lee WH, Ong SG, Zhou Y, et al. Modeling cardiovascular risks of e-cigarettes with human-induced pluripotent stem cell-derived endothelial cells. *J Am Coll Cardiol.* 2019;73:2722-2737.
38. Alzahrani T, Pena I, Temesgen N, Glantz SA. Association between electronic cigarette use and myocardial infarction. *Am J Prev Med.* 2018; 55:455-461.
39. Rudasill SE, Sanaiha Y, Mardock AL, et al. Clinical outcomes of infective endocarditis in injection drug users. *J Am Coll Cardiol.* 2019;73:559-570.
40. Sakhuja A, Sztajnkrycer M, Vallabhajosyula S, Cheungpasitporn W, Patch R 3rd, Jentzer J. National trends and outcomes of cardiac arrest in opioid overdose. *Resuscitation.* 2017;121:84-89.
41. Carman WJ, Su S, Cook SF, Wurzelmann JI, McAfee A. Coronary heart disease outcomes among chronic opioid and cyclooxygenase-2 users compared with a general population cohort. *Pharmacoepidemiol Drug Saf.* 2011;20:754-762.
42. Nishimura M, Bhatia H, Ma J, et al. The Impact of Substance Abuse on Heart Failure Hospitalizations. *Am J Med.* 2020;133:207-213.e1.
43. Mir A, Obafemi A, Young A, Kane C. Myocardial infarction associated with use of the synthetic cannabinoid K2. *Pediatrics.* 2011;128:e1622-e1627.
44. Beaconsfield P, Ginsburg J, Rainsbury R. Marihuana smoking. Cardiovascular effects in man and possible mechanisms. *N Engl J Med.* 1972;287:209-212.
45. Pacher P, Steffens S, Hasko G, Schindler TH, Kunos G. Cardiovascular effects of marijuana and synthetic cannabinoids: the good, the bad, and the ugly. *Nat Rev Cardiol.* 2018;15:151-166.
46. Mittleman MA, Lewis RA, Maclure M, Sherwood JB, Muller JE. Triggering myocardial infarction by marijuana. *Circulation.* 2001;103:2805-2809.
47. Patel RS, Manocha P, Patel J, Patel R, Tankersley WE. Cannabis use is an independent predictor for acute myocardial infarction related hospitalization in younger population. *J Adolesc Health.* 2020;66:79-85.
48. Mukamal KJ, Maclure M, Muller JE, Mittleman MA. An exploratory prospective study of marijuana use and mortality following acute myocardial infarction. *Am Heart J.* 2008;155:465-470.
49. Frost L, Mostofsky E, Rosenbloom JI, Mukamal KJ, Mittleman MA. Marijuana use and long-term mortality among survivors of acute myocardial infarction. *Am Heart J.* 2013;165:170-175.
50. Rumalla K, Reddy AY, Mittal MK. Recreational marijuana use and acute ischemic stroke: a population-based analysis of hospitalized patients in the United States. *J Neurol Sci.* 2016;364:191-196.
51. Rumalla K, Reddy AY, Mittal MK. Association of recreational marijuana use with aneurysmal subarachnoid hemorrhage. *J Stroke Cerebrovasc Dis.* 2016;25:452-460.
52. Barber PA, Pridmore HM, Krishnamurthy V, et al. Cannabis, ischemic stroke, and transient ischemic attack: a case-control study. *Stroke.* 2013;44:2327-2329.
53. McKetin R, Lubman DI, Baker AL, Dawe S, Ali RL. Dose-related psychotic symptoms in chronic methamphetamine users: evidence from a prospective longitudinal study. *JAMA Psychiatry.* 2013;70:319-324.
54. Darke S, Duflou J, Kaye S. Prevalence and nature of cardiovascular disease in methamphetamine-related death: a national study. *Drug Alcohol Depend.* 2017;179:174-179.
55. Lord KC, Shenouda SK, McIlwain E, Charalampidis D, Lucchesi PA, Varner KJ. Oxidative stress contributes to methamphetamine-induced left ventricular dysfunction. *Cardiovasc Res.* 2010;87:111-118.
56. Schürer S, Klingel K, Sandri M, et al. Clinical characteristics, histopathological features, and clinical outcome of methamphetamine-associated cardiomyopathy. *JACC Heart Fail.* 2017;5:435-445.
57. Voskoboinik A, Ihle JF, Bloom JE, Kaye DM. Methamphetamine-associated cardiomyopathy: patterns and predictors of recovery. *Intern Med J.* 2016;46:723-727.
58. Neeki MM, Kulczycki M, Toy J, et al. Frequency of methamphetamine use as a major contributor toward the severity of cardiomyopathy in adults ≤50 years. *Am J Cardiol.* 2016;118:585-589.
59. Nishimura M, Ma J, Fox S, et al. Characteristics and outcomes of methamphetamine abuse among veterans with heart failure. *Am J Cardiol.* 2019;124:907-911.
60. Thomas IC, Nishimura M, Ma J, et al. Clinical characteristics and outcomes of patients with heart failure and methamphetamine abuse. *J Card Fail.* 2020;26:202-209.
61. Zamanian RT, Hedlin H, Greuenwald P, et al. Features and outcomes of methamphetamine-associated pulmonary arterial hypertension. *Am J Respir Crit Care Med.* 2018;197:788-800.
62. Volkow ND, Fowler JS, Wang GJ, et al. Distribution and pharmacokinetics of methamphetamine in the human body: clinical implications. *PLoS One.* 2010;5:e15269.
63. Zhao SX, Kwong C, Swaminathan A, Gohil A, Crawford MH. Clinical characteristics and outcome of methamphetamine-associated pulmonary arterial hypertension and dilated cardiomyopathy. *JACC Heart Fail.* 2018;6:209-218.
64. John WS, Wu LT. Trends and correlates of cocaine use and cocaine use disorder in the United States from 2011 to 2015. *Drug Alcohol Depend.* 2017;180:376-384.
65. Mittleman MA, Mintzer D, Maclure M, Tofler GH, Sherwood JB, Muller JE. Triggering of myocardial infarction by cocaine. *Circulation.* 1999;99:2737-2741.
66. Hollander JE, Hoffman RS, Gennis P, et al. Prospective multicenter evaluation of cocaine-associated chest pain. Cocaine Associated Chest Pain (COCHPA) Study Group. *Acad Emerg Med.* 1994;1:330-339.
67. Weber JE, Chudnofsky CR, Boczar M, Boyer EW, Wilkerson MD, Hollander JE. Cocaine-associated chest pain: how common is myocardial infarction? *Acad Emerg Med.* 2000;7:873-877.
68. Weber JE, Shofer FS, Larkin GL, Kalaria AS, Hollander JE. Validation of a brief observation period for patients with cocaine-associated chest pain. *N Engl J Med.* 2003;348:510-517.
69. Hollander JE, Levitt MA, Young GP, Briglia E, Wetli CV, Gawad Y. Effect of recent cocaine use on the specificity of cardiac markers for diagnosis of acute myocardial infarction. *Am Heart J.* 1998;135:245-252.
70. Rangel C, Shu RG, Lazar LD, Vittinghoff E, Hsue PY, Marcus GM. Beta-blockers for chest pain associated with recent cocaine use. *Arch Intern Med.* 2010;170:874-879.
71. Ibrahim M, Maselli DJ, Hasan R, Hamilton A. Safety of beta-blockers in the acute management of cocaine-associated chest pain. *Am J Emerg Med.* 2013;31:613-616.
72. Amsterdam EA, Wenger NK, Brindis RG, et al. 2014 AHA/ACC Guideline for the Management of Patients with Non-ST-Elevation Acute Coronary Syndromes: a report of the American College of Cardiology/American Heart Association Task Force on Practice Guidelines. *J Am Coll Cardiol.* 2014;64:e139-e228.

73. McKee SA, Applegate RJ, Hoyle JR, Sacrinty MT, Kutcher MA, Sane DC. Cocaine use is associated with an increased risk of stent thrombosis after percutaneous coronary intervention. *Am Heart J.* 2007;154:159-164.
74. Toossi S, Hess CP, Hills NK, Josephson SA. Neurovascular complications of cocaine use at a tertiary stroke center. *J Stroke Cerebrovasc Dis.* 2010;19:273-278.
75. Martin-Schild S, Albright KC, Misra V, et al. Intravenous tissue plasminogen activator in patients with cocaine-associated acute ischemic stroke. *Stroke.* 2009;40:3635-3637.
76. Figueredo VM. Chemical cardiomyopathies: the negative effects of medications and nonprescribed drugs on the heart. *Am J Med.* 2011; 124:480-488.
77. Lopez PD, Akinlonu A, Mene-Afejuku TO, et al. Clinical outcomes of beta-blocker therapy in cocaine-associated heart failure. *Int J Cardiol.* 2019;277:153-158.
78. Hammett-Stabler CA, Pesce AJ, Cannon DJ. Urine drug screening in the medical setting. *Clin Chim Acta.* 2002;315:125-135.

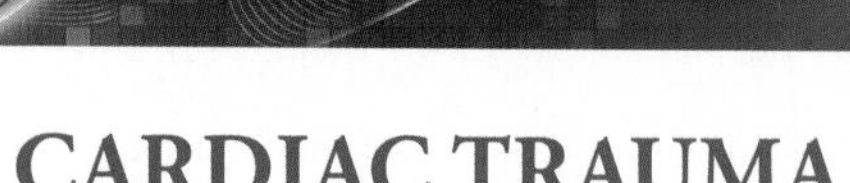

CHAPTER 23

CARDIAC TRAUMA

Debabrata Mukherjee

INTRODUCTION

Trauma is the leading cause of death among Americans between the ages of 1 and 46 years, according to the Coalition for National Trauma Research[1,2] and the third leading overall cause of death in the United States. Of all trauma-related deaths, at least a quarter of them are related to cardiothoracic injuries.[1] The most common cause of significant blunt chest and cardiac trauma is motor vehicle collision, followed by crush or blast injury.[3] On the other hand, the most common cause of penetrating chest trauma is gunshot or stab wound. In general, cardiac trauma is associated with a very high mortality rate. As a result, its diagnosis and management must be done expediently and in a timely manner. Some of the complications related to cardiac trauma may not be detected on initial examination, and a high degree of suspicion is warranted because complications may present later and be life-threatening.

PATHOGENESIS

Blunt cardiac trauma and penetrating cardiac trauma are the two main mechanisms of cardiac trauma, and both of these can also result in aortic injury.

Blunt Cardiac Injuries

Blunt chest trauma commonly results in chest wall injuries, but may also be associated with significant cardiac and great vessel injuries. Blunt trauma to the chest primarily occurs from abrupt deceleration such as in motor vehicle crashes. Because of inertia of motion, the internal organs remain in motion and get compressed between the sternum and the spine, with the abrupt stoppage of the motor vehicle.[4] The second most common cause of blunt chest trauma is an explosion, in which cardiac injury can be from multiple sources. The primary cause is the blast that creates a pressure wave which can result in tissue disruption and lead to a tear in a major blood vessel.[5] In addition, penetrating injuries from nearby objects flying from the area of the blast may also cause cardiac injury.

Blunt chest trauma results in five major injuries that occur either in isolation or in conjunction with each other: myocardial contusions, traumatic aortic dissection or tear, flail chest, tracheobronchial disruption, and sternal fractures.[6] The severity of cardiac injury may range from minor, asymptomatic myocardial concussion to ventricular rupture. Cardiac concussion represents segmental wall-motion abnormality without evidence of myocardial injury in the form of elevated plasma cardiac enzymes.[7] On the other hand, cardiac contusions represent actual myocardial cell injury, leading to myocardial necrosis and hemorrhage with elevated plasma cardiac biomarkers.[5] Extensive myocardial contusion with hemopericardium may develop in the absence of external thoracic injuries, and thus appropriate testing should be performed depending on the impact of the injury.[8] Because the right ventricular free wall is located anteriorly, it is the most common site of ventricular injury with blunt chest trauma. Patients with ventricular free wall rupture present with severe hypotension and rapid diagnosis, and early operative intervention is lifesaving.[9] Occasionally, relatively minor impact injuries may lead to contained ventricular rupture and ventricular pseudoaneurysm.[10] Atrial rupture occurs less often, with right atrial rupture occurring more frequently than does left atrial rupture because of its relative anterior location.[11] Cardiac tamponade due to atrial rupture occurs more slowly than with ventricular rupture because of lower pressures in the atria. Despite the anterior location of the tricuspid and pulmonary valves, the aortic and mitral valves are affected more commonly in trauma because of high mural pressures.[12] Valve rupture as a result of trauma can cause rapid heart failure and is usually manifested with sudden onset of shortness of breath, severe orthopnea, and a murmur (**Figure 23.1**). Ventricular septal rupture can be associated with myocardial contusion and initially may not cause any symptoms, but present later with heart failure.[13] A rare complication of blunt cardiac injury is myocardial infarction secondary to coronary artery injury, leading to dissection, laceration, and thrombosis.[14] The left anterior descending artery is the coronary artery most commonly affected vessel because of its anterior location.[15]

Pericardial injury and effusion may occur from direct high-energy impact or secondary to a significant increase in intra-abdominal pressure (**Figure 23.2**). A pericardial tear typically involves either the pleuropericardium or diaphragmatic pericardium. Clark et al. reported that the left pleuropericardium was involved in 50% of cases, followed by diaphragmatic pericardium, right pleuropericardium, and the superior pericardium.[16] Cardiac evisceration or herniation is a serious complication from pericardial rupture, and is associated with a high mortality rate. It can lead to torsion of the great vessels along with strangulation of the heart and impaired cardiac output.[17]

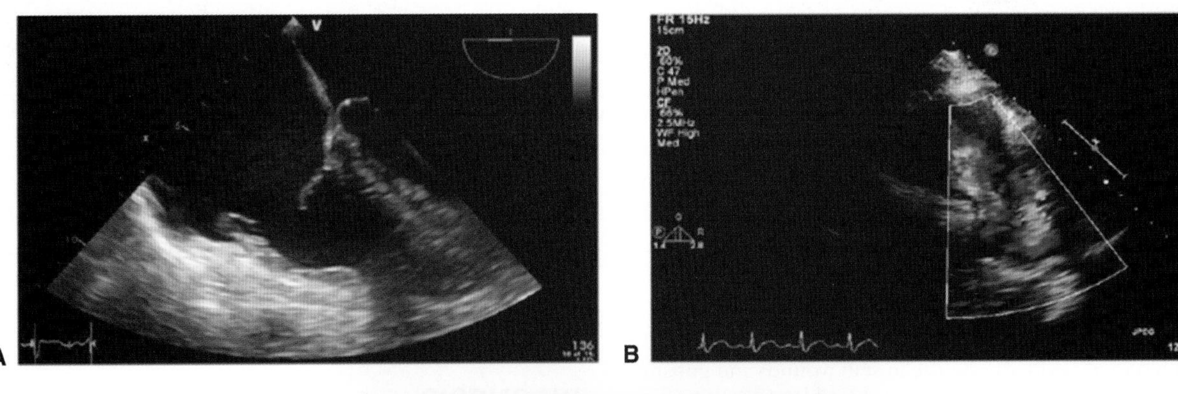

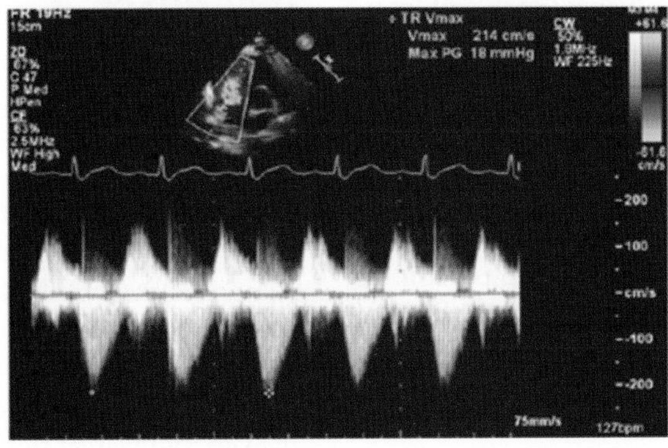

FIGURE 23.1 **(A)** Two-dimensional (2D) transesophageal echocardiogram showing avulsion of anterior tricuspid leaflet and flail posterior leaflet in a patient after a motor vehicle crash. **(B)** Two-dimensional transthoracic echocardiogram with color Doppler showing severe tricuspid regurgitation in a patient after a motor vehicle crash. **(C)** Two-dimensional transthoracic echocardiogram with continuous-wave Doppler showing acute tricuspid regurgitation in a patient after a motor vehicle crash. (From Gosavi S, Tyroch AH, Mukherjee D. Cardiac Trauma. *Angiology.* 2016;67(10):896-901. Copyright © 2016 SAGE Publications. Reprinted by permission of SAGE Publications, Inc.)

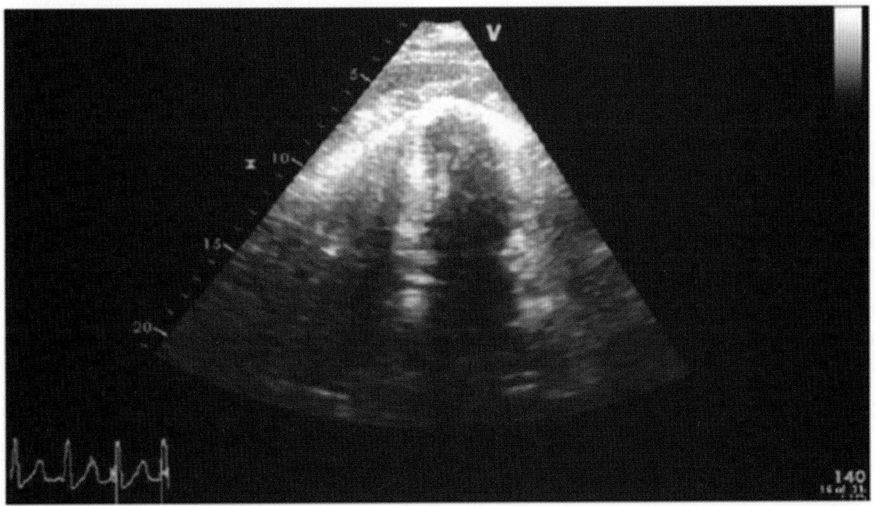

FIGURE 23.2 Two-dimensional (2D) transthoracic echocardiogram showing pericardial effusion with fibrinous strands in a patient after a motor vehicle collision. (From Gosavi S, Tyroch AH, Mukherjee D. Cardiac Trauma. *Angiology.* 2016;67(10):896-901. Copyright © 2016 SAGE Publications. Reprinted by permission of SAGE Publications, Inc.)

Commotio cordis is a fairly low-impact blunt trauma to the chest. This usually occurs in athletes with a projectile object such as a baseball, lacrosse ball, or hockey puck that strikes the chest at a certain time of the cardiac cycle and triggers ventricular fibrillation. It has frequently been noted in males and in individuals without underlying structural heart disease.[18] Even though the injury is a mechanical event, the cause of death is secondary to an electrical event or arrhythmia. The timing of the impact in relation to the cardiac cycle has a direct relation to the generation of ventricular fibrillation. When the impact happens to fall in the early ventricular repolarization phase, within 20 to 40 ms of the upslope of the T-wave, it can trigger ventricular fibrillation with sudden cardiac arrest and death.[19] The velocity of the projectile also seems to have a relation to the onset of ventricular fibrillation. If the impact is less than 40 miles per hour, there is an increased chance of developing ventricular fibrillation, whereas if the velocity is more than 40 miles per hour, it may cause myocardial contusion instead.[20]

Penetrating Cardiac Injuries

Over the past several years, the incidence of penetrating cardiac trauma has increased with the rise in stab wounds and gunshot injuries. Penetrating cardiac injury is highly lethal, with mortality rates of about 70% to 80%.[21] In the past, stab wounds were more common; however, recently, gunshot wounds have been noted to be more frequent—even in the civilian setting—and carry a higher mortality than do stab wounds.[22] The right ventricle is the most common site of entry—62% of penetrating cardiac injuries—because of its anterior location. Even though the left ventricle is less affected with penetrating injuries, the mortality is significantly higher at 98%.[23] The two most common causes of death in individuals with penetrating cardiac trauma are hemorrhagic shock (77.5%) and cardiac tamponade (22.5%).[24]

Aortic Injuries

Thoracic aortic injuries can result from either blunt or penetrating trauma (ie, stab wounds or gunshot injuries). Aortic injuries are more commonly caused by blunt trauma, typically deceleration injuries from a motor vehicle crash or from a fall from height. Most blunt aortic injuries occur because of head-on motor vehicle crash (72%), followed by side impact (24%), and then by rear impact crashes (4%).[25] Trauma to the aorta occurs most commonly at the isthmus, approximately 90% of the time.[26] This is the portion of the proximal descending thoracic aorta that lies between the origin of the left subclavian artery and the ligamentum arteriosum, which tethers the aorta. With deceleration injuries, shearing forces and luminal compression against this fixed portion of the aorta may lead to a tear and transection of the aorta.[26] Blunt trauma to the aorta may also result in aortic laceration that is typically a transverse intimal tear or an aortic transection where the injury traverses through the three layers of the vessel wall. Occasionally, aortic rupture is contained by the adventitia or periaortic tissue leading to an aortic pseudoaneurysm or may cause a hematoma in the wall of the aorta leading to an aortic intramural hematoma.[27] Aortic dissection, which is a longitudinal tear in the aortic wall, may also occur secondary to blunt trauma. Penetrating aortic injuries secondary to either a stab wound or a gunshot wound has a very high mortality rate despite contemporary improvement in trauma care in recent years.[28]

CLINICAL FEATURES

The clinical features of cardiac trauma, either blunt injury or penetrating trauma, vary widely, and clinical presentation may range from being asymptomatic to cardiogenic shock. Concomitant injuries often affect clinical presentation, and it may be difficult to determine whether symptoms are from the cardiac injury. Mortality from major structural injuries, such as cardiac chamber rupture or perforation, remains high, and most such patients die in the field before making it to the hospital. Clinical presentations may include chest pain, myocardial infarction, heart failure, hypotension, and atrial and ventricular arrhythmias depending on the type and location of cardiac injury. On physical examination, chest wall bruising may be seen in a third of the patients, and new murmurs or pericardial rubs may suggest cardiac involvement.

DIAGNOSIS

Because time is of essence in almost all of the traumatic injuries, early yet focused and careful evaluation is the key to early intervention and can improve mortality and morbidity.

Cardiac Biomarkers

Initial evaluation should start with a complete blood count, comprehensive metabolic panel, blood type and cross match, coagulation profile, an arterial blood gas, and cardiac enzymes. Swaanenburg et al. found that plasma creatine kinase myocardial band (CK-MB) levels were not diagnostic of myocardial damage, but plasma troponin I and troponin T concentrations were noted to be more reliable.[29] The study reported that in the presence of thoracic injury, if initial values of plasma troponin levels are negative, repeat values at 24 hours are indicated to rule out myocardial damage. Although sustained increase in plasma troponin I levels suggests likelihood of myocardial injury, these elevated troponins do not have prognostic value.[30,31] For the patient whose initial plasma troponin level is elevated, the 2012 practice management guideline from the Eastern Association for the Surgery of Trauma (EAST) recommends hospital admission in a monitored setting and obtaining serial troponins, although the optimal timings for such serial troponin is not well established.[32]

Electrocardiography

Electrocardiography (ECG) is a very useful screening tool for hemodynamically stable patients with blunt cardiac or aortic injury. The most commonly noted rhythm is sinus tachycardia, followed by atrial fibrillation in cardiac injuries. ST depressions or elevations may occur with blunt cardiac injuries, and it is often difficult to ascertain whether ST abnormalities are secondary to a primary cardiac event (ie, infarction or ischemia) or a result of direct myocardial injury. Comparison with a prior ECG is of significant benefit in such cases. The EAST guidelines recommend that all patients with suspected cardiac injury have an ECG and plasma troponin levels measured. Cardiac injury can be ruled out if both ECG and troponin return negative values (level 2 of evidence).[32]

Echocardiography

The American Institute of Ultrasound in Medicine (AIUM) and the American College of Emergency Physicians (ACEP) have collaboratively developed guidelines for a rapid and early screening of trauma patients with ultrasound. This is called a focused assessment with sonography for trauma patients (FAST). The FAST examination can identify post-traumatic hemorrhage around the heart and lungs as well as in the abdominal cavity. FOCUS (focused cardiac ultrasound) is a part of the FAST examination, and is helpful in evaluating pericardial effusion as well as in detecting obvious cardiac injury that may need immediate surgical intervention.[33] This is a screening test, and hence has the potential of false negatives. False positives may also be noted occasionally in patients with ascites. However, the sensitivity and specificity of detecting pericardial effusion is high.[33] The FOCUS examination can evaluate the size and location of the pericardial effusion as well as right ventricular collapse and determine whether it is the cause of hemodynamic instability. Left and right ventricular size along with systolic function can also be assessed. FOCUS has made improvement in overall outcomes because it leads to early diagnosis and timely management.[34] In both blunt and penetrating trauma, FOCUS has become the standard of care in trauma centers.

As mentioned, FOCUS and FAST examinations are screening examinations and can have false negative results. Hence, when time permits, a complete transthoracic echocardiogram should be performed. An echocardiogram can show focal myocardial contusions and can assess wall-motion abnormalities more precisely. It can detect valvular injuries with color and spectral Doppler. Tricuspid valve injuries can be well assessed with transthoracic echocardiogram because of its anterior location. Echocardiography also plays a vital role in assessing ventricular septal defects that develop as a result of traumatic injury. The ventricular septal defect sometimes occurs immediately after a traumatic injury or sometimes later because of necrosis occurring as a result of septal injury.[35] A follow-up echocardiogram is useful in such cases. Echocardiogram has also been able to detect cardiac thrombus and cardiac aneurysm that develop secondary to trauma.[36]

Transesophageal echocardiography (TEE) has increased sensitivity and specificity in comparison to a transthoracic echocardiogram in detecting cardiac contusions, atrial lacerations, valve injuries, rupture of the interatrial or interventricular septum, and for detecting pericardial effusions.[37] However, TEE may not be safely performed in unstable patients, specifically in hypotensive patients and in patients with trauma to the head or neck. Similarly, even though TEE has a role to play in blunt or penetrating aortic injuries and can detect aortic transections and tears, it may not be feasible in unstable patients.

Chest X-ray

A chest radiograph (CXR) is often used as a primary screening study because of its easy availability and ease of performing. Despite its low sensitivity, it provides important information. It gives information about the bony thorax and detects pneumothorax and hemothorax that often accompany cardiac trauma. A widened mediastinum often suggests an aortic disruption, and a CXR has about 53% sensitivity and 59% specificity for detecting it.[38] A widened mediastinum always prompts further testing with computed tomography (CT) or TEE. A normal CXR, on the other hand, has a nearly 90% negative predictive value.

Computed Tomography

CT, especially multidetector CT with intravenous contrast, is one of the most valuable imaging tools in patients with cardiac and thoracic injuries. It can be performed in an expedited manner and yet provide good spatial contrast and temporal resolution. CT has a valuable role in detecting hemopericardium in patients with blunt aortic injury or cardiac injury resulting in ventricular free wall rupture, aortic root injuries, and myocardial contusions.

Depending on its availability, ECG-gated multidetector CT is an excellent tool for blunt and penetrating cardiac trauma, and can detect coronary artery laceration in addition to other cardiac and aortic injuries.[39] Pericardial rupture resulting from blunt cardiac trauma is detected on CT, and is represented with focal pericardial dimpling and discontinuity, with pneumopericardium, empty pericardial sac, or a dislocated ventricular silhouette.[40]

Invasive Aortography

Aortography had been the gold standard in the past before the introduction of the multidetector CT. However, after the introduction of multidetector CT scans, it is rarely used (ie, when the results of the CT scan are equivocal). Invasive aortography is superior to CT in detecting injuries of the great vessel and injuries of the thoracic great vessels.

Magnetic Resonance Imaging

Magnetic resonance imaging has little role to play in acute traumatic injuries because of its extended time of testing. In addition, with traumatic injuries, the feasibility is often unknown, because metallic objects are sometimes part of the blunt cardiac injuries. Delayed enhancement cardiac magnetic resonance imaging can detect myocardial infarction that occurs as a fairly uncommon complication of blunt cardiac injury.[41]

MANAGEMENT OF THE PATIENT WITH CARDIAC TRAUMA

Appropriate cardiac imaging plays a critical role in the diagnosis and characterization of cardiac trauma in patients with abnormal ECG and/or plasma troponin I levels, and helps guide the management of these patients. **Algorithm 23.1** provides a clinical algorithm for management of patients presenting with cardiac trauma.[44] Overall, presentation and clinical findings determine management. Cardiology consultation is needed for any patient with a new arrhythmia (including persistent tachycardia), signs of heart failure, or hemodynamic instability likely due to cardiac dysfunction. Cardiovascular surgery consult is indicated in hemodynamically unstable patients or in those individuals who need emergent surgery (ie, those with aortic dissection, valvular rupture, myocardial free wall, and septal rupture).

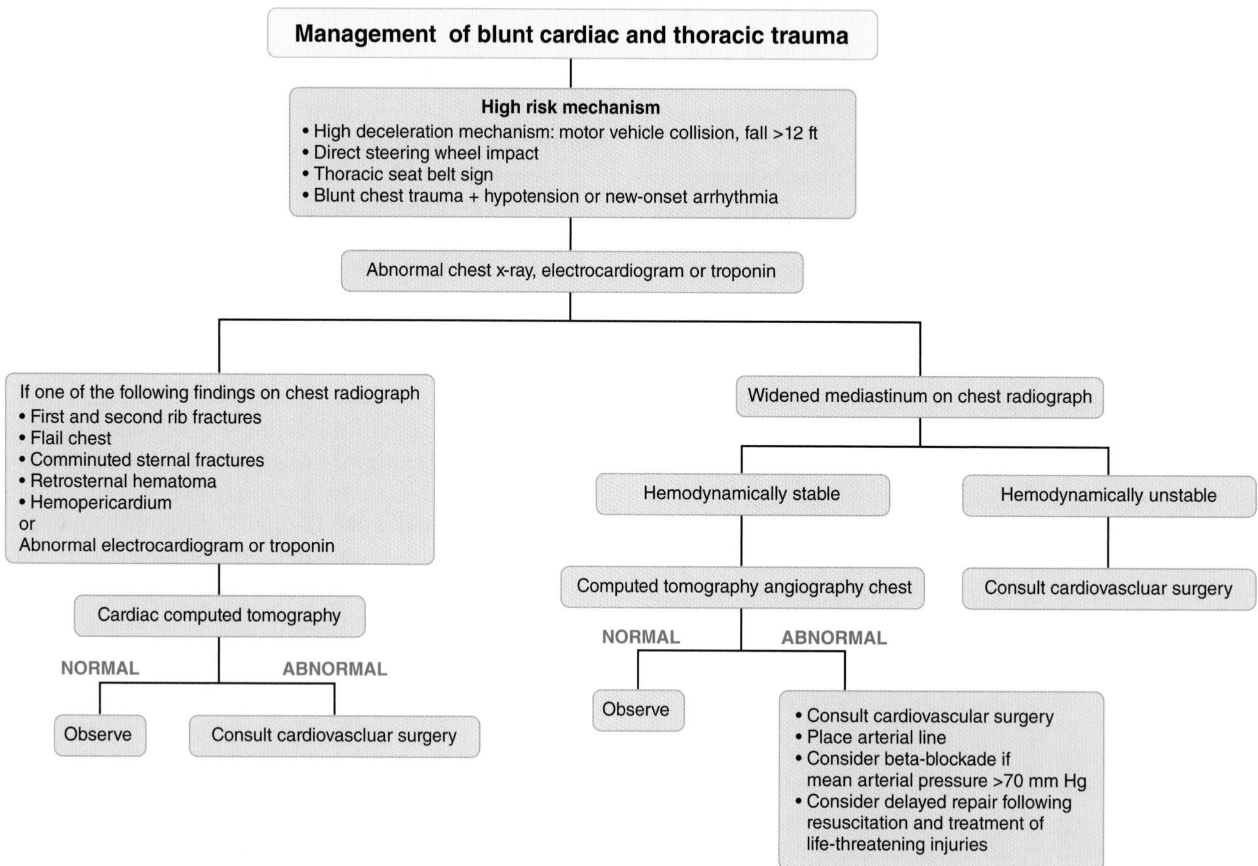

ALGORITHM 23.1 Clinical algorithm for management of patients presenting with cardiac trauma. (Adapted from Wu Y, Qamar SR, Murray N, et al. Imaging of Cardiac Trauma. *Radiol Clin North Am.* 2019;57(4):795-808. Copyright © 2019 Elsevier. With permission.)

SPECIAL CONSIDERATIONS AND GUIDELINES

The 2015 practice management EAST guidelines provide recommendations regarding an evidence-based approach to patient selection for emergency department (ED) thoracotomy after cardiac trauma.[42] The recommendations are as follows:

- In patients who present pulseless to the ED with signs of life after penetrating thoracic injury, the guidelines committee strongly recommends that patients undergo ED thoracotomy.
- In patients who present pulseless to the ED without signs of life after penetrating thoracic injury, the guidelines committee conditionally recommends that patients undergo ED thoracotomy. This recommendation is based on a moderate quality of evidence and places emphasis on patient preference for improved survival and neurologically intact survival after ED thoracotomy, but also acknowledges that elapsed time without signs of life is an important component.
- In patients who present pulseless to the ED with signs of life after penetrating extrathoracic injury, the guidelines committee conditionally recommends that patients undergo ED thoracotomy. This recommendation does not pertain to patients with isolated cranial injuries. This recommendation is based on a moderate quality of evidence and places emphasis on patient preference for improved survival and neurologically intact survival after ED thoracotomy, but also acknowledges that penetrating injuries to all extrathoracic anatomic areas will not have equivalent salvage rates after ED thoracotomy.
- In patients who present pulseless to the ED without signs of life after penetrating extrathoracic injury, the guidelines committee conditionally recommends that patients undergo ED thoracotomy. This recommendation does not pertain to patients with isolated cranial injuries and is based on a low quality of evidence.
- In patients who present pulseless to the ED with signs of life after blunt injury, the guidelines committee conditionally recommends that patients undergo ED thoracotomy. This recommendation is based on a moderate quality of evidence and places emphasis on patient preference for improved survival and neurologically intact survival after EDT.
- In patients who present pulseless to the ED without signs of life after blunt injury, the guidelines committee conditionally recommends *against* the performance of ED thoracotomy. This recommendation is based on a low quality of evidence and reflects subcommittee group disagreement regarding the strength of the unanimous recommendation against ED thoracotomy.

The 2015 practice management EAST guidelines also made recommendations regarding the evaluation and management of blunt traumatic aortic injury.[43] The recommendations are as follows:

- In patients with suspected blunt traumatic aortic injury, the guidelines committee strongly recommends that patients undergo a CT scan of the chest with intravenous contrast for the diagnosis of clinically significant blunt traumatic aortic injury.
- In patients diagnosed with blunt traumatic aortic injury, the guidelines committee strongly recommends the use of endovascular repair unless contraindicated.
- In patients diagnosed with blunt traumatic aortic injury, the guidelines committee recommend delayed repair for those with other major injuries. It is critical that effective blood pressure control with antihypertensive medication be used in these patients. The patients who benefit most from delayed repair are those who have major associated injuries. These patients clearly require resuscitation and treatment of immediate life-threatening injuries before aortic repair. The data are not as clear for patients without associated injuries who have no reason to undergo delayed repair. The guidelines do not advocate delaying repair of blunt traumatic aortic injury (eg, until the following weekday morning) merely for surgeon convenience.

PATIENT FOLLOW-UP

Clinical follow-up will depend on the particular cardiac injury sustained, but, in general, patients need a follow-up cardiology clinical evaluation. Select patients may need repeat cardiac imaging.

FUTURE DIRECTIONS

Mortality secondary to blunt or penetrating cardiac trauma remains high despite improvements in diagnostic technologies. Assessing cardiac injury is often challenging and needs prompt recognition and treatment. There is a need for refinements in current diagnostic modalities to make them more point of care and rapidly available. Extracorporeal membrane oxygenation (ECMO) is being used more often in cardiac trauma patients using both venovenous and venoarterial ECMO. In addition to ECMO, there is a need for additional data on the role of ventricular assist devices in individuals with cardiac injury complicated by acute severe heart failure.

KEY POINTS

- ✔ All patients with suspected cardiac trauma should have an ECG and measurement of plasma troponin I level.
- ✔ Only after the exclusion of more common etiologies for hemodynamic instability (eg, hemorrhage, pneumothorax, and pericardial tamponade) should hemodynamic compromise be viewed as cardiac in origin.
- ✔ For those patients who have persistent hemodynamic instability without alternative explanations, an echocardiographic study should be considered to evaluate for structural cardiovascular injuries, such as septal or free wall rupture, aortic dissection, or acute valvular regurgitation.
- ✔ CT, especially multidetector CT with intravenous contrast, is a valuable imaging tool in patients with cardiac and thoracic injuries. It can be performed expediently and provides good spatial, contrast, and temporal resolution.

REFERENCES

1. Gosavi S, Tyroch AH, Mukherjee D. Cardiac trauma. *Angiology*. 2016;67:896-901.
2. Coalition for National Trauma Research. Trauma Statistics & Facts. 2020. Accessed on June 6, 2021. https://www.nattrauma.org/trauma-statistics-facts/
3. van Wijngaarden MH, Karmy-Jones R, Talwar MK, Simonetti V. Blunt cardiac injury: a 10 year institutional review. *Injury*. 1997;28:51-55.
4. Orliaguet G, Ferjani M, Riou B. The heart in blunt trauma. *Anesthesiology*. 2001;95:544-548.
5. Tenzer ML. The spectrum of myocardial contusion: a review. *J Trauma*. 1985;25:620-627.
6. Emet M, Akoz A, Aslan S, Saritas A, Cakir Z, Acemoglu H. Assessment of cardiac injury in patients with blunt chest trauma. *Eur J Trauma Emerg Surg*. 2010;36:441-447.
7. El-Chami MF, Nicholson W, Helmy T. Blunt cardiac trauma. *J Emerg Med*. 2008;35:127-133.
8. Gonin J, de la Grandmaison GL, Durigon M, Paraire F. Cardiac contusion and hemopericardium in the absence of external thoracic trauma: case report and review of the literature. *Am J Forensic Med Pathol*. 2009;30:373-375.
9. Roxburgh JC. Myocardial contusion. *Injury*. 1996;27:603-605.
10. Namai A, Sakurai M, Fujiwara H. Five cases of blunt traumatic cardiac rupture: success and failure in surgical management. *Gen Thorac Cardiovasc Surg*. 2007;55:200-204.
11. De Maria E, Gaddi O, Navazio A, Monducci I, Tirabassi G, Guiducci U. Right atrial free wall rupture after blunt chest trauma. *J Cardiovasc Med (Hagerstown)*. 2007;8:946-949.
12. Baxter BT, Moore EE, Synhorst DP, Reiter MJ, Harken AH. Graded experimental myocardial contusion: impact on cardiac rhythm, coronary artery flow, ventricular function, and myocardial oxygen consumption. *J Trauma*. 1988;28:1411-1417.
13. Hiatt JR, Yeatman LA Jr, Child JS. The value of echocardiography in blunt chest trauma. *J Trauma*. 1988;28:914-922.
14. Plautz CU, Perron AD, Brady WJ. Electrocardiographic ST-segment elevation in the trauma patient: acute myocardial infarction vs myocardial contusion. *Am J Emerg Med*. 2005;23:510-516.
15. Christensen MD, Nielsen PE, Sleight P. Prior blunt chest trauma may be a cause of single vessel coronary disease; hypothesis and review. *Int J Cardiol*. 2006;108:1-5.
16. Clark DE, Wiles CS 3rd, Lim MK, Dunham CM, Rodriguez A. Traumatic rupture of the pericardium. *Surgery*. 1983;93:495-503.
17. Wall MJ Jr, Mattox KL, Wolf DA. The cardiac pendulum: blunt rupture of the pericardium with strangulation of the heart. *J Trauma*. 2005;59:136-141; discussion 141-142.
18. Maron BJ, Estes NA 3rd. Commotio cordis. *N Engl J Med*. 2010;362:917-927.
19. Madias C, Maron BJ, Weinstock J, Estes NA 3rd, Link MS. Commotio cordis—sudden cardiac death with chest wall impact. *J Cardiovasc Electrophysiol*. 2007;18:115-122.

20. Link MS, Maron BJ, Wang PJ, VanderBrink BA, Zhu W, Estes NA 3rd. Upper and lower limits of vulnerability to sudden arrhythmic death with chest-wall impact (commotio cordis). *J Am Coll Cardiol.* 2003;41:99-104.
21. Carr JA, Buterakos R, Bowling WM, et al. Long-term functional and echocardiographic assessment after penetrating cardiac injury: 5-year follow-up results. *J Trauma.* 2011;70:701-704.
22. Karrel R, Shaffer MA, Franaszek JB. Emergency diagnosis, resuscitation, and treatment of acute penetrating cardiac trauma. *Ann Emerg Med.* 1982; 11:504-517.
23. Sugg WL, Rea WJ, Ecker RR, Webb WR, Rose EF, Shaw RR. Penetrating wounds of the heart. An analysis of 459 cases. *J Thorac Cardiovasc Surg.* 1968;56:531-545.
24. Altun G, Altun A, Yilmaz A. Hemopericardium-related fatalities: a 10-year medicolegal autopsy experience. *Cardiology.* 2005;104:133-137.
25. Fabian TC, Richardson JD, Croce MA, et al. Prospective study of blunt aortic injury: multicenter trial of the American Association for the Surgery of Trauma. *J Trauma.* 1997;42:374-380; discussion 380-383.
26. Fabian TC, Davis KA, Gavant ML, et al. Prospective study of blunt aortic injury: helical CT is diagnostic and antihypertensive therapy reduces rupture. *Ann Surg.* 1998;227:666-676; discussion 676-677.
27. Malhotra AK, Fabian TC, Croce MA, et al. Minimal aortic injury: a lesion associated with advancing diagnostic techniques. *J Trauma.* 2001; 51:1042-1048.
28. Demetriades D, Theodorou D, Murray J, et al. Mortality and prognostic factors in penetrating injuries of the aorta. *J Trauma.* 1996;40:761-763.
29. Swaanenburg JC, Klaase JM, DeJongste MJ, Zimmerman KW, ten Duis HJ. Troponin I, troponin T, CKMB-activity and CKMB-mass as markers for the detection of myocardial contusion in patients who experienced blunt trauma. *Clin Chim Acta.* 1998;272:171-181.
30. Salim A, Velmahos GC, Jindal A, et al. Clinically significant blunt cardiac trauma: role of serum troponin levels combined with electrocardiographic findings. *J Trauma.* 2001;50:237-243.
31. Velmahos GC, Karaiskakis M, Salim A, et al. Normal electrocardiography and serum troponin I levels preclude the presence of clinically significant blunt cardiac injury. *J Trauma.* 2003;54:45-50; discussion 50-51.
32. Clancy K, Velopulos C, Bilaniuk JW, et al. Screening for blunt cardiac injury: an Eastern Association for the Surgery of Trauma practice management guideline. *J Trauma Acute Care Surg.* 2012;73:S301-S306.
33. Mandavia DP, Hoffner RJ, Mahaney K, Henderson SO. Bedside echocardiography by emergency physicians. *Ann Emerg Med.* 2001;38:377-382.
34. Plummer D, Brunette D, Asinger R, Ruiz E. Emergency department echocardiography improves outcome in penetrating cardiac injury. *Ann Emerg Med.* 1992;21:709-712.
35. Rollins MD, Koehler RP, Stevens MH, et al. Traumatic ventricular septal defect: case report and review of the English literature since 1970. *J Trauma.* 2005;58:175-180.
36. Chirillo F, Totis O, Cavarzerani A, et al. Usefulness of transthoracic and transoesophageal echocardiography in recognition and management of cardiovascular injuries after blunt chest trauma. *Heart.* 1996;75:301-306.
37. Karalis DG, Victor MF, Davis GA, et al. The role of echocardiography in blunt chest trauma: a transthoracic and transesophageal echocardiographic study. *J Trauma.* 1994;36:53-58.
38. Mirvis SE, Bidwell JK, Buddemeyer EU, et al. Value of chest radiography in excluding traumatic aortic rupture. *Radiology.* 1987;163:487-493.
39. Co SJ, Yong-Hing CJ, Galea-Soler S, et al. Role of imaging in penetrating and blunt traumatic injury to the heart. *Radiographics.* 2011; 31:E101-E115.
40. Schir F, Thony F, Chavanon O, et al. Blunt traumatic rupture of the pericardium with cardiac herniation: two cases diagnosed using computed tomography. *Eur Radiol.* 2001;11:995-999.
41. Southam S, Jutila C, Ketai L. Contrast-enhanced cardiac MRI in blunt chest trauma: differentiating cardiac contusion from acute peri-traumatic myocardial infarction. *J Thorac Imaging.* 2006;21:176-178.
42. Seamon MJ, Haut ER, Van Arendonk K, et al. An evidence-based approach to patient selection for emergency department thoracotomy: a practice management guideline from the Eastern Association for the Surgery of Trauma. *J Trauma Acute Care Surg.* 2015;79:159-173.
43. Fox N, Schwartz D, Salazar JH, et al. Evaluation and management of blunt traumatic aortic injury: a practice management guideline from the Eastern Association for the Surgery of Trauma. *J Trauma Acute Care Surg.* 2015;78:136-146.
44. Wu Y, Qamar SR, Murray N, Nicolaou S. Imaging of cardiac trauma. *Radiol Clin North Am.* 2019;57:795-808.

CHAPTER 24

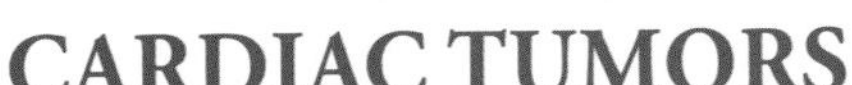

CARDIAC TUMORS

Avirup Guha, Abdallah Mughrabi, and Zeeshan Hussain

INTRODUCTION

Cardiac masses are rare but critical entities that may involve the endocardium, myocardium, epicardium, and/or pericardium. These include benign tumors, malignant tumors (primary and secondary), and tumor-like conditions (eg, thrombus, Lambl excrescences [LEs], pericardial cyst [PCs]). Similarities in clinical and radiologic features often result in confusion and misdiagnosis. In an effort to help the clinician develop a reliable approach to such entities, this chapter reviews the epidemiology, clinical presentation, imaging, diagnosis, management, and outcome of cardiac masses.

Cardiac tumors are rare neoplasms involving the heart classified into primary and secondary tumors (ie, metastasis to the heart). Primary cardiac tumors (PCTs) are extremely rare and originate from the pericardium, myocardium, or endocardium. The incidence of clinically diagnosed PCTs is 1380 per 100 million individuals, of which 5% to 6% are malignant.[1,2] Compared to PCTs, secondary cardiac tumors (SCTs) are 132 times more common.[3] Over the past few decades, a notable increase in the incidence of PCTs was shown.[1,4]

PCTs are classified into three main classes: benign, malignant, and intermediate with uncertain biologic behavior.[5] The latter class was newly featured in the 2015 World Health Organization (WHO) classification **(Table 24.1)**.[6] Benign etiologies comprise the majority of all primary tumors (more than 90%), whereas less than 10% are malignant and only 1% are intermediate.[4,7,8] It is shown that different pathologic subtypes have anatomic predilection for specific cardiac locations **(Figure 24.1)**, with most cases to be found in the left atrium.[8]

BENIGN PRIMARY CARDIAC TUMORS

Benign PCTs are relatively more prevalent among all PCTs and have a predilection for older females.[7,8] Histopathologic subtypes include myxoma, rhabdomyoma, papillary fibroelastoma, fibroma, hemangioma, lipoma, and leiomyoma. Myxoma is by far the predominant pathologic subtype.[7] Non-myxoma subtypes, which mostly occur in children and adolescents, are less reported.[4,7,8] Benign tumors exhibit favorable prognosis, with 30-day mortality of only 1%.[7]

Clinical Presentation of Benign Primary Cardiac Tumors

According to their size and location, benign PCTs manifest with a wide array of symptoms. Blood flow obstruction can result in dyspnea, chest pain, and palpitations. Thromboembolic complications, mostly cerebral, are found in approximately 10% of patients. Incidental detection is in 13.3% to 27.7% of cases. Affected individuals may also remain asymptomatic.[4,7]

Cardiac Myxoma

Cardiac myxoma is the most common PCT.[7] Myxoma is primarily a left atrial mass arising from the septum. Atrial free wall and mitral valve leaflets are less likely anatomic origins.[4] Association with Carney complex is well established.[9] Nonetheless, most cardiac myxomas are sporadic.[10]

Myxomas are morphologically classified into polypoid and papillary (Figure 24.1). The former, when large, may present with obstructive symptoms, with a "tumor plop" being occasionally heard on auscultation. By contrast, papillary myxoma tends to cause embolic events. In both variants, constitutional symptoms like fatigue, fever, and weight loss are also reported.[10]

Papillary Fibroelastoma

Papillary fibroelastoma (PF) is a rarer tumor comprising only 11.5% of PCTs.[7] Patients are typically middle-aged presenting with embolic complications, particularly cerebral. This is due to the tumor's predilection for left-sided valves.[11]

Rhabdomyoma and Fibroma

Rhabdomyoma is the most prevalent pediatric PCT and typically presents during the first year of life.[12] Rhabdomyomas are arrhythmogenic, but cavitary protrusion with resulting flow obstruction is also seen.[12] Association with tuberous sclerosis is well established.[12] Cardiac fibroma is the second most common PCT in infants.[12] Similarly, involvement of the interventricular septum and left ventricular free wall is typical.[9] Consequently, arrhythmias and flow obstruction result.[12]

Rare Primary Cardiac Tumors—Hemangiomas, Lipomas, Leiomyomas

Rarer PCTs include hemangiomas, lipomas, and leiomyomas. Hemangioma may involve any chamber.[4] When larger than a few centimeters, it can cause obstructive symptoms. Cardiac lipomas are often seen in individuals between their fourth and seventh decade.[4] These tumors may also involve any chamber and are mostly asymptomatic. When large, they may impede blood flow.[4] Primary cardiac leiomyomas

TABLE 24.1 The 2015 WHO Classification of Cardiac Tumors with Associated Incidence, Survival and Outcome

Class	Subtype and References	Subtype (%) of Class[a]	Outcome/Survival
Benign tumors (and tumor-like conditions) Incidence rate/year: 1.24/100,000 individuals[e] Mean survival (months): 187.2 ± 2.7	Cardiac myxoma[4,7,10,12,18,19]	76.5%-93%[b]	Surgical therapy is definitive with low likelihood of recurrence (1%-5.4%).
	Papillary fibroelastoma[7,20]	13%[b]	Surgical resection is curative with minimal risk/recurrence.
	Rhabdomyoma[5,12]	Most common in children	Spontaneous regression in most cases. Postresection relapse: 2.6%.
	Cardiac fibroma[12,19]	Second most common in children	Surgical resection is curative. Postresection relapse: 1.6%.
	Hemangioma, NOS Capillary hemangioma Cavernous hemangioma Arteriovenous malformation Intramuscular hemangioma[7,19]	2%[b]	In patients with resectable tumors, surgery is recommended and results in good prognosis.
	Lipoma[4,7,63]	1%-2%[b]	Surgical resection is curative but carries risk, particularly in cases with hemodynamic complications.
	Hamartoma of mature cardiac myocytes[7]	2%[b]	Mean survival: 68.5 ± 48.4 months
	Schwannoma[4]	0.5%[b]	–
Tumors of uncertain biologic behavior	Inflammatory myofibroblastic tumor	–	–
	Paraganglioma[4,7]	0.5%-1%[b]	–
Germ cell tumors	Teratoma, mature[14,50,53]	1%[b]	Postresection relapse in 3.4% of cases.
	Teratoma, immature[4,12]		
	Yolk sac tumor	–	–
Malignant tumor Incidence rate[c]/year: 0.000894[d]-0.24[e]/100,000 Mean survival (months): 26.2 ± 9.8 Median survival (months): 10 (25th, 75th percentiles, 1, 29 months)	Angiosarcoma[1,4,7,31,36]	8%-29%[f]	Median overall survival for all sarcomas: 17.2 months (95% confidence interval 13.5-22.3) Angiosarcoma: • Median overall survival: 13 months • 5-year survival rate: 8% Leiomyosarcoma: • 5-year overall survival is 25.4%. Synovial sarcoma: • Median overall survival: 24 months. • 5-year overall survival is 29.9%.
	Leiomyosarcoma[1,38]	7%[f]	
	Rhabdomyosarcoma[1]	4%[f]	
	Undifferentiated pleomorphic sarcoma[1,4,7]	9%-25%[f]	
	Myxofibrosarcoma[4,7]	17%-18%[f]	
	Synovial sarcoma[1,7,39,68]	2%-9% [f]	
	Osteosarcoma	–	
	Miscellaneous sarcomas[1,4,7]	8%-9%[f]	
	Cardiac lymphomas[1,4,7]	9%-42%[f]	Median survival: 23 months (25th, 75th percentiles, 5, 120 months) 5-year survival is 38% in the past decade.
	Metastatic tumors[4,46]	1%-3.5% of all autopsies	Poor survival, determined by the primary malignancy.
Tumors of the pericardium	Malignant mesothelioma[g],[1,50,51,55]	2%-8%[f]	Median survival: 2-6 months 5-year survival rates: 9%
	Angiosarcoma[g],[31,36]	See above	See above
	Synovial sarcoma[1,7,39,68]	See above	See above

Class	Subtype and References	Subtype (%) of Class[a]	Outcome/Survival
	Solitary fibrous tumor • Malignant	–	–
	Germ cell tumors[14,50,53] • Teratoma, mature • Teratoma, immature • Yolk sac tumor	See above	See above

NOS: Not Otherwise Specified
[a]Rounded number for simplicity.
[b]Calculated percentage is among all benign tumors including germ cell tumors and paragangliomas.
[c]Excluding metastatic tumors, but including pericardial tumors.
[d]Calculated incidence rate derived from a population study from 1973 through 2011.[1]
[e]Population study from 1998 through 2011.[2]
[f]Calculated percentage includes pericardial and intracardiac malignant tumors and is among malignant masses including pericardial and intracardial tumors. Metastatic cardiac tumors are excluded.
[g]Mesotheliomas comprise most of the cases of malignant pericardial tumors followed by pericardial angiosarcomas.[51,52,56]
Non-exhaustive list.
Adapted with permission from Burke A, Tavora F. The 2015 WHO Classification of Tumors of the Heart and Pericardium. *J Thorac Oncol.* 2016;11(4):441-452. Copyright © 2016 Elsevier and Travis WD, Brambilla E, Burke A, et al. *WHO classification of tumours of the lung, pleura, thymus and heart. International Agency for Research on Cancer,* 2015.

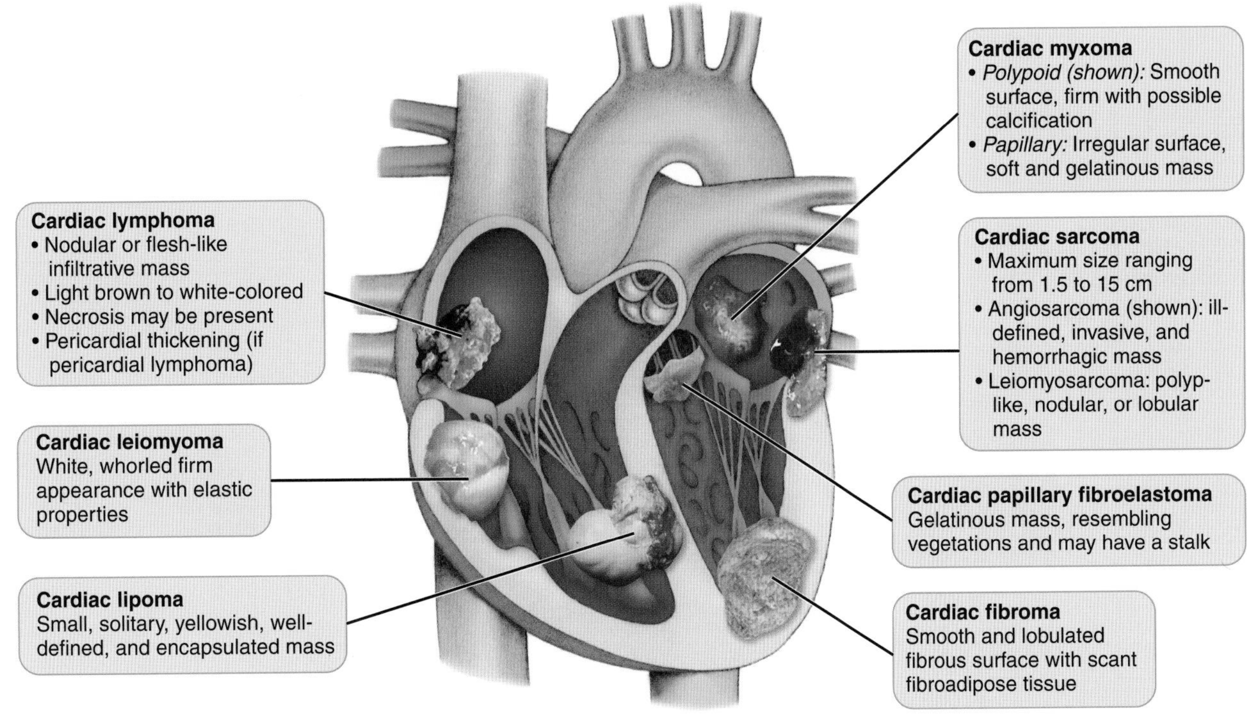
Cardiac myxoma
• Polypoid (shown): Smooth surface, firm with possible calcification
• Papillary: Irregular surface, soft and gelatinous mass
Cardiac lymphoma
• Nodular or flesh-like infiltrative mass
• Light brown to white-colored
• Necrosis may be present
• Pericardial thickening (if pericardial lymphoma)
Cardiac sarcoma
• Maximum size ranging from 1.5 to 15 cm
• Angiosarcoma (shown): ill-defined, invasive, and hemorrhagic mass
• Leiomyosarcoma: polyp-like, nodular, or lobular mass
Cardiac leiomyoma
White, whorled firm appearance with elastic properties
Cardiac papillary fibroelastoma
Gelatinous mass, resembling vegetations and may have a stalk
Cardiac lipoma
Small, solitary, yellowish, well-defined, and encapsulated mass
Cardiac fibroma
Smooth and lobulated fibrous surface with scant fibroadipose tissue

FIGURE 24.1 Gross appearance of different pathologic subtypes of primary cardiac tumors. Note the predilection for specific anatomic locations. Cardiac myxoma and sarcoma predominantly affect the left atrium. Papillary fibroelastoma affects valve leaflets and papillary muscles. Lipoma may involve any chamber and arises from subendocardium or intramyocardium. Cardiac lymphoma affects the right heart predominantly. Mesothelioma and paraganglioma (not shown) affect the pericardium.

are exceedingly rare tumors, described only in a handful of cases.[13] Consequently, this entity is not listed in the WHO classification.[6] Those tumors are derived from smooth muscles and exhibit white, whorled, and firm appearance (Figure 24.1).[13]

Diagnosis and Imaging of Benign Primary Cardiac Tumors

Echocardiography is a ubiquitous diagnostic tool utilized in several cardiologic settings. Certainly, it remains a cornerstone in the evaluation of a suspected cardiac mass. A cardiac mass detected on echocardiography requires a vigilant clinician. Simultaneously, awareness of the rarity of cardiac tumors is key in averting overdiagnosis. A mass on echocardiography is predominantly a thrombus or a vegetation. Upon exclusion, a tumor diagnosis may then be pursued.[14] A comprehensive diagnostic approach for cardiac masses has been presented in the review of Mankad and Herrmann [14] and adapted in **Algorithm 24.1.**

Imaging is often sufficient for presumptive diagnosis (**Table 24.2**). Individual subtypes of benign PCTs exhibit imaging characteristics that aid in their differentiation by multimodality imaging such as echocardiography, cardiac computed tomography (CCT), and cardiac magnetic resonance (CMR) (**Figures 24.2 to 24.4** and **e-Figures 24.1 to 24.5**). Challenges, however, arise when certain mass-like conditions need

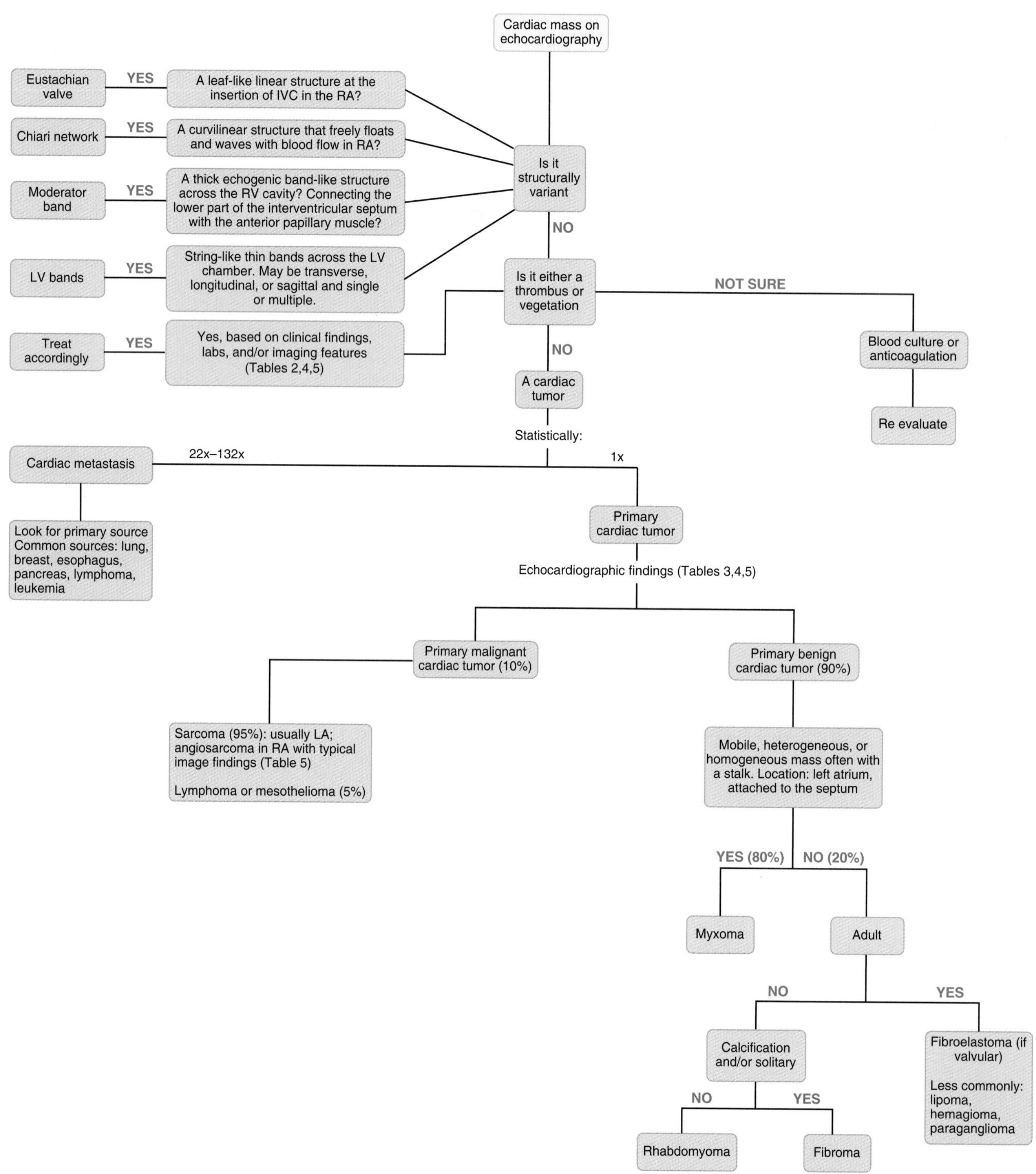

ALGORITHM 24.1 Diagnostic approach to cardiac masses. IVC, inferior vena cava; LA, left atrium; LV, left ventricle; RA, right atrium; RV, right ventricle.

TABLE 24.2 Radiologic Findings for Benign Primary Cardiac Tumors

	Echocardiography	Cardiac Computed Tomography (CCT)	Cardiac Magnetic Resonance (CMR)
Myxoma[9,14,17]	A mobile, heterogeneous or homogeneous mass often with a stalk (Figure 24.2) Two subtypes: Polypoid: Larger, smooth surface, rough cystic core due to hemorrhage or necrosis Papillary: Smaller with villi	Hypodense, possible calcifications. With contrast: filling defects with heterogeneous enhancement (based on presence of necrosis or hemorrhage)	On T1: variable; hemorrhage (increased signal), calcification (decreased signal) On T2: hypointense, especially if the myxoma contains iron With gadolinium: core may be enhanced due to high vascularity, unless thrombosed
Fibroelastoma[14,17]	A small mass, with "shimmering or stippled borders." Attached to the endocardium. Mobile, not in sync with other cardiac structures (Figure 24.3).	Identification is challenging.	On T1: isointense On T2: hyperintense With late gadolinium study: possible enhancement
Rhabdomyoma[9,14,17]	Small, homogeneously echogenic, well-demarcated, pedunculated, or nodular mass. May be multiple (e-Figure 24.1)	Homogeneous, density similar to myocardium	Solid and homogeneous appearance. On T1: similar intensity to myocardium, may be slightly less On T2: hyperintense On GRE: Very low signal contrasting it from surrounding myocardium
Fibroma4,[14,16,17]	Well-demarcated, non-contractile, hyperechogenic mass in the myocardial wall.	Hypervascular. With contrast: homogeneous or heterogeneous enhancement Central calcifications are common (vs rhabdomyoma).	On T1: similar intensity when compared to skeletal muscles. Hemorrhage (increased signal), calcification (decreased signal) On T2: intensity decreases relative to myocardium With gadolinium: late enhancement is present (e-Figure 24.2)
Hemangioma[9,14,17]	Echogenic mass with some echolucencies	Intense enhancement is seen with contrast administration.	On T1 and T2: hyperintense compared to myocardium. First-pass perfusion study with gadolinium: rapid centripetal heterogeneous enhancement (e-Figure 24.3)
Lipoma[9,14,17]	Well-circumscribed mass with a wide base limiting its mobility. Intracardiac: hyperechogenic Pericardial: hypoechogenic	Smooth, well-defined, with fat attenuation With contrast: no enhancement	On T1: hyperintense (as subcutaneous fat). Decrease in intensity on "fat presaturation" technique verifies diagnosis. On T2: mild decrease in intensity With gadolinium contrast: no enhancement. (Figure 24.4)
Cardiac leiomyoma[13,17]	Hyperechogenic mass (e-Figure 24.4)	A well-defined mass with possible calcifications.	Similar signal intensity to myocardium
Mitral annular calcification with caseous necrosis[22,64]	Large, echogenic and round mass with a central echolucency (e-Figure 24.7)	Calcified ring surrounding a less dense core	On T1: hyperintense center with hypointense periphery On gadolinium study: late enhancement at core and periphery
Intracardiac thrombus[14,17]	Nonenhancing mass on contrast echocardiography and possible wall motion abnormalities	Hypodense (e-Figure 24.5)	On T1: hyperintense On T2: hyperintense Upon aging of thrombus: intensity decreases On gradient recalled echo: lowest intensity compared to surrounding structures. With gadolinium contrast: no enhancement, unless mature organized thrombus
Lambl excrescences[15,28,29]	Multiple mobile echogenicities with very thin lint-like appearance often arising from the aortic valvular leaflets (**Figure 24.5**)	Identification is challenging.	Identification is challenging.

GRE, Gradient Echo Sequences.

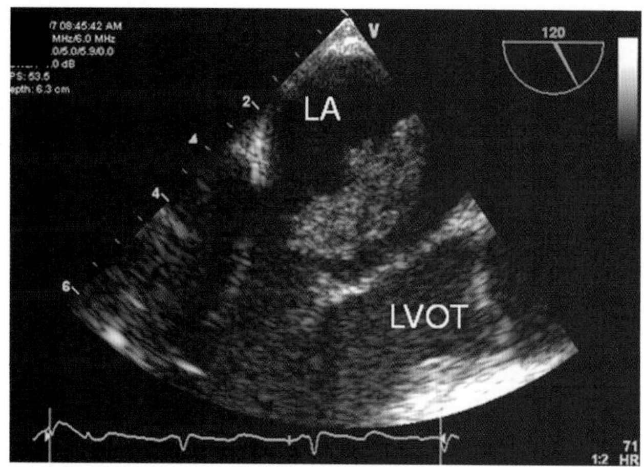

FIGURE 24.2 A Transesophageal echocardiogram (TEE) (midesophageal long axis view) revealing a Left atrial (LA) myxoma. (Reprinted with permission from Barash PG, Cullen BF, Stoelting RK, et al. *Clinical Anesthesia*. 6th ed. Philadelphia, PA: Wolters Kluwer Health/Lippincott Williams & Wilkins; 2009. Figure 28.47 View A.)

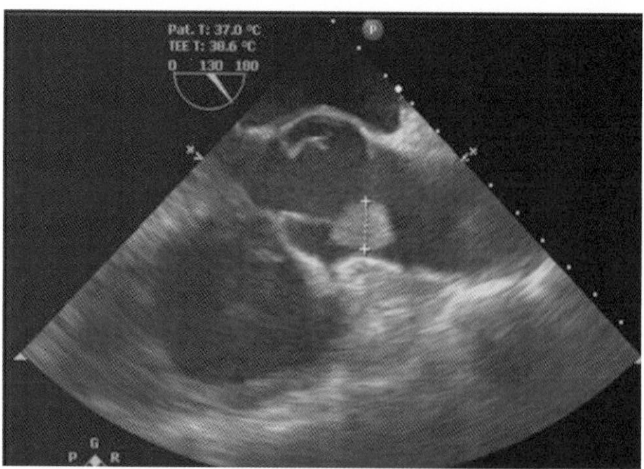

FIGURE 24.3 Transesophageal echocardiogram showing a homogeneously echogenic pedunculated mass, measuring 1.5 cm and arising from the aortic valve (papillary fibroelastoma). (Reprinted with permission from Vimalesvaran K, Lumley M, Child N, et al. Recurrent right coronary artery occlusion caused by cardiac fibroelastoma attached to the aortic valve. *Circulation*. 2015;131(6):593-595. Copyright © 2015 American Heart Association, Inc.)

to be discerned from benign PCTs. Atrial septal aneurysm (ASA) and lipomatous interatrial septal hypertrophy (LISH) both mimic myxomas and—in the case of LISH—lipomas.[14] On echocardiography, ASA exhibits a redundant septal bulging, beyond the interatrial septal plane with synchronous oscillation through the cardiac cycle.[15] LISH spares fossa ovalis and exhibits a bilobed "dumbbell" echocardiographic appearance[15] (**e-Figure 24.6**). PF may be confused with a thrombus, vegetation, or LEs. On echocardiography, a solitary mass in the middle part of the valve's leaflet, with a characteristic shimmering border vibrating independently from neighboring structures, make PF a more likely diagnosis.[14]

Pediatric PCTs, namely rhabdomyomas and fibromas, are challenging to distinguish through imaging. Nonetheless, unlike the former, fibroma is typically solitary and centrally calcified.[16] Hemangiomas appear echogenic with interspersed lucencies on echocardiography.[14] Lipomas characteristically demonstrate a decrease in signal intensity after fat presaturation on T1 CMR sequence.[17]

Management and Outcome of Benign Primary Cardiac Tumors

Definitive management of benign PCTs is surgical (**Table 24.3**). Myxomas, hemangiomas, and fibromas should be resected because of the risk of complications including sudden cardiac death.[18,19] Unlike fibromas, most

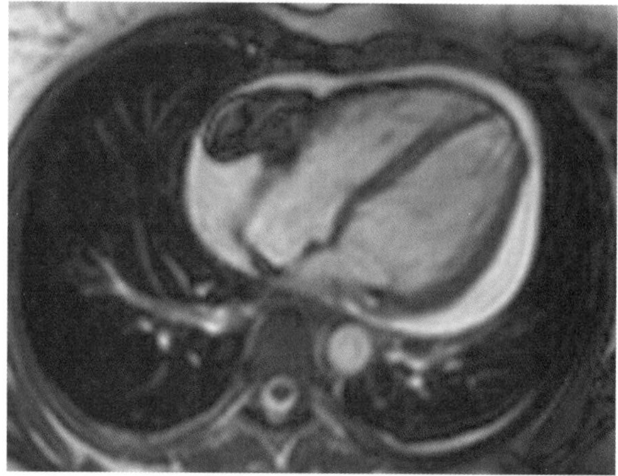

FIGURE 24.4 Cardiac magnetic resonance (CMR) imaging of a cardiac lipoma. Note the infarcted mass (white arrow) and the associated pericarditis. (Reprinted with permission from Bezuidenhout AF, Ridge CA, Litmanovich D. Lung. In: Lee EY, Hunsaker A, Siewert B, eds. *Computed Body Tomography with MRI Correlation*. 5th ed. Philadelphia, PA: Wolters Kluwer; 2020:253-398. Figure 6.6.)

TABLE 24.3 Treatment of Benign Primary Cardiac Tumors

Benign Primary Cardiac Tumors	Treatment
Myxoma	Resection is indicated due to risk of complications.[18]
Fibroelastoma	Nonmobile, small, and asymptomatic: anticoagulants + follow-up Symptomatic: excision. Asymptomatic but large (>1 cm) or mobile: excision is considered.[19-21]
Rhabdomyoma	Spontaneous regression. If significant cardiac flow limitation or electrophysiologic complications: surgical removal should be considered.[5]
Fibroma	Excision[19]
Hemangioma	Complete resection. Partial resection in complex cases.[19]
Lipoma	Symptomatic or large: excision[19]
Cardiac leiomyoma	Surgical excision to relieve hemodynamic obstructive complications[13]
Mitral annular calcification with caseous necrosis	Surgical intervention is needed in select cases with hemodynamic or embolic complications[22]
Intracardiac thrombus	Anticoagulation with vitamin K antagonists (target INR: 2-3).[26]
Lambl excrescences	It is suggested that asymptomatic patients should be monitored, whereas patients who develop cerebral complications may be managed with antiplatelet or anticoagulation therapy. If cerebral events persist despite maximal medical management, surgical excision is warranted.[29,30]

INR, international normalized ratio.

rhabdomyomas regress spontaneously, but surgical removal should be considered once complications arise.[5] Large or symptomatic lipomas and leiomyomas require excision.[13,19] Similarly, symptomatic PFs require surgical intervention.[19-21] Asymptomatic patients with large (>1 cm) or mobile PFs may also be surgical candidates whereas nonmobile, small, and asymptomatic lesions are managed with anticoagulants and followed up.[20,21]

Surgical outcome for most benign PCTs is excellent. In myxomas, unless associated with Carney complex, surgical therapy is definitive with low recurrence (1%-5.4%).[10,18,19] The 2015 WHO classification of cardiac tumors with associated incidence, survival, and outcome is listed in Table 24.1.

Masses Mimicking Benign PCTs

Mitral Annular Calcification with Caseous Necrosis

Mitral annular calcification (MAC) is a progressive condition often associated with atherosclerosis. It may get complicated by caseous necrosis, producing a radiologic picture mimicking a tumor. An echogenic mass with echolucent core is characteristic on echocardiography (**e-Figure 24.7**). Surgical intervention is needed in select cases with hemodynamic or embolic complications.[22]

Intracardiac Thrombus

Intracardiac thrombi can develop in any chamber.

Left ventricular thrombus (LVT) is commonly secondary to acute myocardial infarction with ventricular dysfunction, particularly in the apical segment. These thrombi are highly embolic and have been associated with acute ischemic stroke in 11.8% of patients with mortality as high as 31.8%.[23] A right ventricular thrombus (RVT) is often seen in a migrating deep venous thrombus transiently residing in the right ventricle. Mortality is estimated to be 27.1% [24].

Clinical Presentation and Imaging. Cardiac thrombi are discovered during radiologic evaluation of the precipitating event. Echocardiography can readily detect thrombi. When needed, adding contrast can differentiate the nonenhancing thrombus from a tumor.[14] CMR is highly specific and sensitive and may be alternatively used. Embolic risk is high and typically seen in thrombi that are mobile, protruding, or with central echolucency.[25] In severe cases, a thrombus may result in cardiogenic shock.[25]

Management. Anticoagulation with vitamin K antagonists is recommended with a target international normalized ratio (INR) of 2 to 3 and duration tailored according to patient's bleeding risk and precipitating event.[26] Use of direct oral anticoagulants (DOACs) for LVT is off-label and should be undertaken with caution because clinical studies have reported higher risk of stroke or systemic embolism with DOACs compared with warfarin use.[27]

Lambl Excrescences

LEs are rare valvular growths, typically involving the aortic valve leaflets. They may remain asymptomatic or, less commonly, embolize to the brain. Echocardiography is the main diagnostic tool showing mobile echogenicities on valvular leaflets, which are more linear and smaller than fibroelastomas (Figure 24.5).[14,28,29]

It is suggested that asymptomatic patients should be monitored, whereas patients who develop cerebral complications may be managed with antiplatelet or anticoagulation therapy.

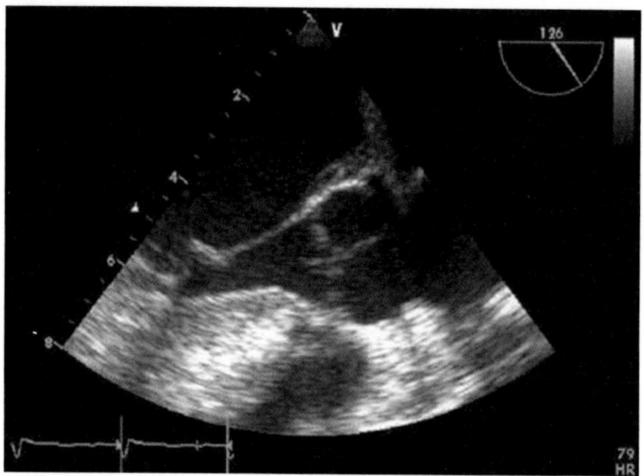

FIGURE 24.5 A case of Lambl excrescences seen on transesophageal echocardiogram (TEE) imaging as mobile echogenic densities, linear in shape, residing on the aortic leaflets. (Reprinted with permission from Aziz F, Baciewicz FA Jr. Lambl's excrescences: review and recommendations. *Tex Heart Inst J.* 2007;34(3):366-368.)

If cerebral events persist despite maximal medical management, surgical excision is warranted.[29,30]

MALIGNANT PRIMARY CARDIAC TUMORS

Malignant tumors are extremely rare and represent only 5% to 6% of PCTs.[1,2] Sarcomas are most common (64.8%), followed by lymphomas (27%) and then mesotheliomas (8%).[1] Compared to benign PCTs, cardiac malignancies present with more serious and even catastrophic symptoms. In addition to the obstructive and embolic complications seen with benign PCTs, patients may present with syncope and cardiac arrest.[7]

Clinical Presentation of Malignant Primary Cardiac Tumors

Clinical presentation is determined by the site of tumoral involvement. Right-sided malignancies tend to grow outward and present only when the mass is large, with heart failure occurring at later stage.[31] Metastasis on presentation is seen in over half of the cases.[32] Left-sided malignancies tend to present with early hemodynamic complications of systemic outflow obstruction and heart failure.[33] Other clinical findings include malignant effusions and tamponade.

Diagnosis and Imaging of Malignant Primary Cardiac Tumors

Similar to benign tumors, cardiovascular imaging is paramount in the evaluation of malignant PCTs. After excluding common entities (ie, thrombus and vegetation), the differentiation between benign and malignant masses is a key step. Echocardiography and CMR findings may guide this process (**Table 24.4**).[14,34] Although contrast echocardiography continues to be utilized in various applications, there are not enough data to support its role in differentiating malignant (eg, angiosarcomas) from benign tumors. Although angiosarcomas are known for their increased vascularity, not all exhibit enhancement on contrast echocardiography.[14,34,35]

Compared to its role in benign tumor evaluation, CMR is less reliable in further subclassification of malignant tumors. This is because of the differences malignant tumors exhibit in terms of vascularity, water content, and differentiation among patients.[17] CCT is useful in the localization of the mass and determining its relationship with adjacent structures. Positron emission tomography (PET) with computed tomography (CT) remains very sensitive in differentiating malignancies from benign entities, estimating the grade of tumor and screening for metastasis.[34]

Upon imaging-based suspicion of malignancy, definitive histologic diagnosis and subtyping should follow.[34] Radiologic findings and specific treatment regimens of individual malignant PCT are summarized in **Tables 24.5 and 24.6** and illustrated in **e-Figures 24.8 to 24.12**.

Primary Cardiac Sarcomas

Cardiac sarcomas represent more than two-thirds of all malignant primary tumors.[1] Compared to extracardiac soft tissue sarcomas (STSs), cardiac sarcomas are seen in younger patients in their forties who have worse prognosis with a 5-year survival rate of 14%.[1] Cardiac sarcomas tend to arise from either atria.[1,36]

TABLE 24.4 Role of Echocardiography and Cardiac Magnetic Resonance in Distinguishing Benign and Malignant Primary Cardiac Tumors

Modality and References	Benign Cardiac Tumors	Malignant Cardiac Tumors
Echocardiography[14,33]	• Arises from left atrial septal wall or valves • Narrow base	• Arises from right side (50% chance of malignancy) or pericardium • Wide base, absent stalk • Invasive
Cardiac magnetic resonance[17,65,66]	Smaller (<5 cm) Less associated with late gadolinium enhancement (41% of tumors) Less associated with contrast first-pass perfusion (47% of tumors)	• Larger (>5 cm) • More associated with late gadolinium enhancement (92% of tumors) • More associated with contrast first-pass perfusion (84% of tumors) Other characteristics: multiple, infiltration of adjacent tissues, necrosis, calcification, high vascularity, peritumorous edema, pleural/pericardial effusions

TABLE 24.5 Radiologic Findings of Malignant Primary Cardiac Tumors

Subtype	Echocardiography	Cardiac Computed Tomography (CCT)	Cardiac Magnetic Resonance (CMR)
Angiosarcoma[5,9,14,17]	Lobulated, distinctly heterogeneous mass. Areas of necrosis or hemorrhage are present. Even though vascular, contrast echocardiography may not always reveal significant enhancement. Tends to involve the pericardium, resulting in pericardial effusions or tamponade.	Hypodense mass with broad base and hematogenous continuity with the chamber. On contrast: Late enhancement with scattered areas of nonenhancing necrosis. Invades adjacent structures. Pericardial involvement appears as "sheet-like" thickening (vs rhabdomyosarcoma: nodular) (e-Figure 24.8)	Heterogeneous, nodular mass with polymorphic appearance. Typically, appearance is a "cauliflower" on black-blood images. Central hyperintense area (necrosis, hemorrhage, or blood vessels). Moderate signal intensity (SI) in peripheral regions in T1- and T2-weighted images. With gadolinium contrast: strong signal enhancement with "sunray" aspect
Leiomyosarcoma[17,39]	Echogenic mass with a well-defined border Rarely originates from the interatrial septum or has a stalk (vs myxoma).	Irregular mass with nonspecific malignant findings.	On T1: SI is slightly higher than liver parenchyma, but lower than the adjacent mediastinal fat. On T2: SI is high. With gadolinium contrast: slight enhancement. Intravascular tumor extension into the superior major veins and chambers may be appreciated.
Rhabdomyosarcoma[9,17,39]	Thickened myocardial wall with an isoechoic mass within (e-Figure 24.9)	Irregular mass with nonspecific malignant findings	On T1: isointense to the myocardium. With gadolinium contrast: homogeneous enhancement (unless necrosis is present)
Undifferentiated pleomorphic sarcoma[14,17]	Broad-based, heterogeneous echogenicity typically in the left atrium. Necrotic (hypoechogenic) areas may be present.	Irregular mass with nonspecific malignant findings	On T1: irregular mass, with heterogeneous signal. On T2: high to intermediate signal. With gadolinium contrast: heterogeneous enhancement (e-Figure 24.10)
Myxofibrosarcoma[9,46,67]	Homogeneous, echogenic, lobulated mass	Irregular mass with nonspecific malignant findings	Fibrosarcoma: On T1: heterogeneous or isointense. On T2: hyperintense. With gadolinium contrast: mild contrast enhancement
Synovial sarcoma[39,68]	Pericardial mass: pericardial effusion may limit visibility Intracardiac mass: Nonspecific malignant findings	With contrast: slightly enhanced mass with possible calcifications and cysts. Pericardial mass: pericardial effusion with an intrapericardial heterogeneous mass (e-Figure 24.11).	Pericardial mass: mass within the pericardial space associated with effusion
Liposarcoma[9,17,46]	Heterogenous hypoechogenic mass	Large infiltrative mass with fat and soft tissue attenuation. On contrast: mild enhancement	Bright SI equal to subcutaneous fat. (Liposarcomas rarely contain significant amounts of macroscopic fat, making diagnosis challenging.) On fat presaturation technique: Decrease in SI. With gadolinium contrast: slight enhancement (e-Figure 24.12)
Lymphoma[4,17,45]	Homogeneously echogenic lobular or nodular mass. Infiltrates the wall resulting in apparent thickening. May protrude into the chamber.	Nonspecific findings	On T1 and T2: large polypoid or infiltrative lesion that is isointense or hypointense relative to myocardium. With gadolinium contrast: heterogeneous (necrotic center: relatively less enhancing) (**e-Figure 24.13**)

TABLE 24.6 Treatment of Malignant Primary Cardiac Tumors

Subtype	Treatment
Angiosarcoma[5,9,14,17] Leiomyosarcoma[17,39] Rhabdomyosarcoma[9,17] Undifferentiated pleomorphic sarcoma[14,17] Myxofibrosarcoma[9,46,67] Synovial sarcoma[39,68] Liposarcoma[9,17,46]	**Right-sided cardiac sarcomas:** • Less than half of surgeries result in complete resection.[36] • To reduce tumor size, a trial of neoadjuvant chemotherapy should be attempted before surgical intervention.[19,33,36] • After chemotherapy, candidacy for resection is evaluated. Surgical intervention should be deterred if tumor is widely metastatic, new metastasis occurs during therapy, or if existing metastasis was unresponsive to chemotherapy.[19] **Left-sided cardiac and pulmonary artery sarcomas:** • Present early with hemodynamic compromise. This precludes neoadjuvant therapy and may even render preoperative biopsy infeasible.[31] • To relieve symptoms, surgical excision should take place. • Complete excision may be challenging due to anatomic complexities inherent to the left side.[33] • Autotransplantation (ie, ex vivo tumor resection, reconstruction, and then reimplantation) may be employed.[19] **Chemotherapy regimens (if indicated):** • Anthracycline (eg, doxorubicin) with ifosfamide. Gemcitabine with docetaxel are less commonly used.[19,31] • Agents aimed for specific entities have been studied; paclitaxel (with or without gemcitabine) is suggested in angiosarcoma,[19] whereas trabectedin is approved as second-line therapy for leiomyosarcomas and liposarcomas.[34] **Radiotherapy:** Limited role **Adjuvant chemotherapy:** No beneficial impact on survival in extracardiac soft tissue sarcomas[34]
Lymphoma[4,17,45]	• R-CHOP (Rituximab added to cyclophosphamide, doxorubicin, vincristine and prednisolone) regimen is the most used, especially in non–T-cell lymphomas.[34,42] • Surgical resection or debulking may be reserved in cases with hemodynamic impairment.[34]

Under microscopic evaluation, cardiac sarcomas are further classified into various histopathologic subtypes, which exhibit predilection for different cardiac regions (e-Table 24.1). Histopathologic subtypes of primary cardiac sarcomas include angiosarcomas, leiomyosarcomas, liposarcomas, rhabdomyosarcomas, synovial sarcomas, myxofibrosarcomas, and undifferentiated pleomorphic sarcomas (UPS). Angiosarcoma followed by leiomyosarcoma are the most common differentiated sarcomas.[1,36]

Cardiac angiosarcomas preferentially affect males.[32] These tumors often present late as a large mass that already invaded neighboring critical structures.[32] Metastasis is seen on presentation in more than half of the patients, with the lung being the commonest site because of the tumor's right-sided location.[14,32] Cardiac leiomyosarcomas represent 7% to 15% of cardiac sarcomas.[36-38] Cardiac leiomyosarcomas present with obstructive symptoms and are more aggressive than their extracardiac counterparts.[39] Rhabdomyosarcomas are rare cardiac sarcomas primarily diagnosed in children and adolescents.[5,17] These skeletal muscle tumors typically involve the myocardium.[9]

Less differentiated tumors include cardiac UPS and myxofibrosarcomas. UPS are a group of sarcomas lacking histopathologic and/or immunohistochemical characteristics, pointing to a specific tissue of origin. In the previous WHO classification, this entity was termed malignant fibrous histiocytoma. UPS are typically invasive with diffuse wall involvement.[4] Myxofibrosarcoma are relatively less common and represent 12% of all cardiac sarcomas.[38] This new term is coined by merging the old classes of fibrosarcoma and myxosarcoma.[5]

Synovial sarcomas are extremely rare tumors often diagnosed in younger males.[40] They represent only 3% to 7% of primary cardiac sarcomas.[36-38] These tumors commonly present with dyspnea and may cause effusions.[40] Similarly, cardiac liposarcomas are exceedingly rare.[38,41] These locally aggressive tumors may not present until symptoms of cardiac constriction arise.[41]

Management and Outcome. The scientific literature on primary cardiac sarcomas remains limited because of the rarity of the disease; consequently, disease-specific guidelines are not established. Management is guided by extracardiac STS guidelines modified through accumulating institutional experience.[34] Cardiac sarcoma presentation is determined by their anatomic location. Right- and left-sided sarcomas present differently and management is tailored accordingly.[33] Regardless of the location, however, complete surgical excision with non-infiltrated margins (R0) is the aim of management.

This is because R0 resection was shown to be the major determinant of overall survival.[32,34]

Malignant PCTs have poor prognosis. It is estimated that more than 80% of patients die within 20 months of diagnosis. The 1-year survival in patients with cardiac sarcomas is 47%, with angiosarcomas carrying the worst prognosis.[1]

Primary Cardiac Lymphoma

Lymphomas may arise from any organ harboring lymphatic tissue. Only 3 out of 10,000 lymphomas arise from the heart.[1] Comprising 27.2% of malignant PCTs, cardiac lymphomas are relatively less common than sarcomas.[1] Cardiac lymphomas are typically diagnosed in older adults in their sixth and seventh decade.[1,4,42] Nearly half of patients are immunocompromised.[42]

Clinical Presentation. Although right atrial involvement is classical, the pericardium may also be affected.[4,42] Dyspnea, arrhythmia, and congestive heart failure are common presentations.[4,42] Pericardial effusion develops in two-thirds of cases.[42]

Imaging and Diagnosis. Cardiac imaging modalities vary according to their ability in detecting lymphomas. Transesophageal echocardiography (TEE) and CMR are most sensitive, followed by transthoracic echocardiography (TTE) and CCT[43] (e-Figure 24.13). Multimodality imaging findings are listed in Table 24.5. Histopathologic evaluation is paramount in establishing the diagnosis. The most common histologic subtype is diffuse large B-cell lymphoma (DLBCL).[42] Follicular and Burkitt lymphomas are also seen.[1,4,5] When biopsy is infeasible, cytologic analysis of pleural or pericardial fluid is sufficient in some cases and shows abnormal lymphocytes.[43]

Management and Outcome. There is significant contrast between management of primary cardiac lymphoma and that of sarcoma (Table 24.6). Because of documented good response, the former's treatment is centered around chemotherapy.[42,43] R-CHOP (Rituximab added to cyclophosphamide, doxorubicin, vincristine, and prednisolone) regimen is the most used, especially in non–T-cell lymphomas.[34,42] Overall survival was shown to increase in patients treated with chemotherapy, whereas radiotherapy is of no additional benefit.[42] Surgical resection or debulking is reserved for cases with hemodynamic impairment.[34]

With a 1-year survival of 62%, cardiac lymphomas exhibit relatively better prognosis than sarcomas.[1] Survival is negatively impacted by immunologic deterioration, concomitant extracardiac disease, left ventricular location, and, interestingly, absence of arrhythmia.[42]

SECONDARY CARDIAC TUMORS

SCTs are more common than primary tumors. In autopsy cases, 0.7% to 3.5% harbor cardiac metastases.[14] Although any malignant tumor may spread to the heart, certain tumors are common culprits. Lung (36%-39%), breast (10%-12%), and hematologic malignancies (ie, lymphomas and leukemias) (10%-21%) are the majority of cases.[6,44]

Routes of Metastasis

Malignant tumors utilize one of four routes to reach the heart: (1) hematogenous, (2) lymphatic, (3) transvenous, and (4) direct invasion.[44,45] **Figure 24.6** illustrates that different tumors have predilection for different metastatic routes.[31,45-47] Additionally, metastatic route significantly determines the target tissue. For instance, masses spreading through lymphatics often seed the pericardium or epicardium.[44] Conversely, hematogenous spread results in myocardial or endocardial tumoral implantation.[44]

Clinical Presentation of Secondary Cardiac Tumors

Patients with SCTs are often in a late stage of their primary disease and are usually terminal.[45] Subsequently, cardiac metastasis is often detected after death.[45] When cardiac symptoms are prominent, however, they are variable and determined by the involved tissue.[44] Pericardial involvement may give rise to pericardial effusion and tamponade.[44,47] Myocardial metastasis can result in conduction disturbances triggering arrhythmias.[47] Myocardial replacement with neoplastic cells may eventually lead to congestive heart failure.[44] Intracavitary masses impede blood flow and cause valvular dysfunction.[47]

Diagnosis and Imaging of Secondary Cardiac Tumors

Imaging aids in both the detection and evaluation of metastatic heart disease. Echocardiography is often the first modality to detect SCTs. Lesions are often small and multiple, although a single large mass may also be seen.[47] Echocardiography can also assess anatomic characteristics and complications of the lesions.[14,45] CCT is more accurate in determining the tumor's location, extension, and tissue invasion. SCTs often enhance during contrast study.[9,48] According to the tissue involved, pericardial or myocardial thickening, nodularity, and disruption may be demonstrated.[9] Hemorrhagic effusion may also be seen.[9]

CMR provides additional image resolution, aiding in further characterization of the mass. On T1-weighted sequence, metastatic tumors are hypointense to isointense while hyperintense on T2-weighted sequence[46] (**e-Figure 24.14**). An exception is melanomas; these tumors are typically, unless amelanocytic, hyperintense on T1 and hyperintense/hypointense on T2.[46,48,49] Dense pericardial bands indicative of inflammation or infiltration may also be seen.[48]

Fluorodeoxyglucose (FDG)-PET/CT imaging is commonly utilized to evaluate the body for metastatic lesions. In most extracardiac tissues, delineation of an FDG-avid focus is relatively simple. In cardiac metastases, this task is more challenging. The myocardium, owing to its high metabolic activity, exhibits FDG uptake similar to a tumor.[48] Patients should therefore fast 4 to 6 hours prior to imaging.[47,48]

Definitive diagnosis, when warranted, is established by histopathologic or cytologic analysis. A cytologic sample is acquired by pericardiocentesis when effusion is present. Cytologic

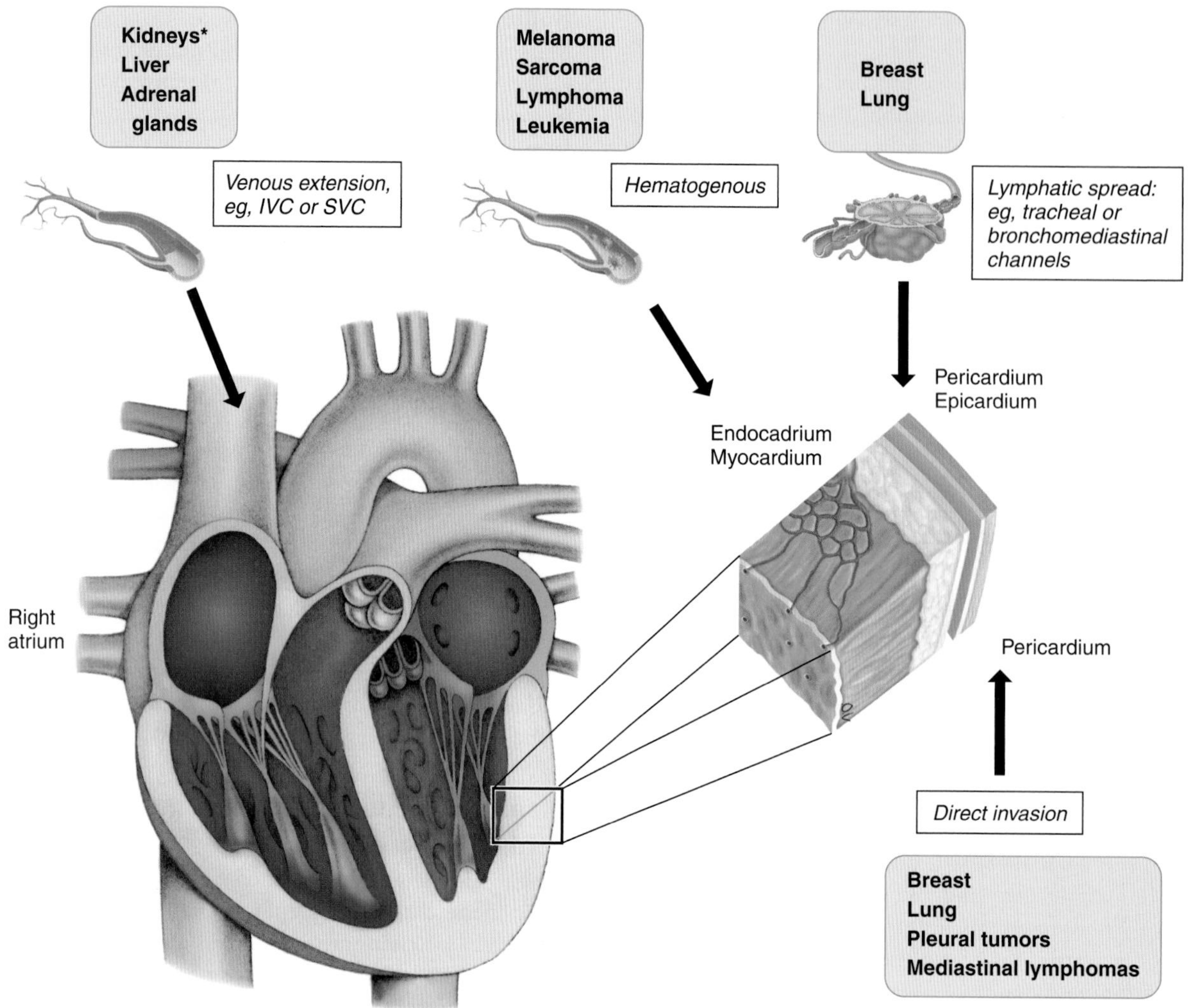

FIGURE 24.6 Different primary tumors utilize different routes for cardiac metastasis. *Cases of RCC that don't use the direct IVC route are also documented. IVC, inferior vena cava; RCC, renal cell carcinoma; SVC, superior vena cava.

analysis was shown to offer high correlation with pathologic diagnosis.[44] However, in metastatic melanoma, sensitivity of cytologic detection is low (44%-65%).[48] Percutaneous biopsy can be achieved in right-sided lesions.[44] However, open biopsy is sometimes necessary.[44] Pericardioscopy may aid in pericardial inspection and tissue harvest.[45]

Management and Outcome of Secondary Cardiac Tumors

Cardiac metastasis usually occurs in the late stages of the primary disease.[44,48] Management is individualized and directed toward the primary tumor.[47] Radiotherapy may have a palliative role.[47] Resection is usually not indicated, except in select conditions[31]: (1) patients with intracavitary metastases resulting in significant hemodynamic complications progressing to cardiac decompensation,[19,48] (2) patients with solitary cardiac disease when the primary tumor is controlled and good prognosis is expected.[47] Furthermore, in certain cases of renal cell carcinoma, it was shown that surgical resection of the "tumor thrombus" improves survival.[19,31] A general rule remains that the lesion should be surgically resectable while maintaining adequate myocardial function.[19]

PERICARDIAL MASSES

The pericardium is a flask-shaped sac composed of fibrous and serous layers that enclose the heart.[50] Pericardial masses include primary and secondary tumors, PCs, and diverticula. Additionally, conditions presenting as masses include hematomas, fibrosis, and abscesses.[51]

Primary pericardial tumors (PPTs) are rare and represent 7% to 13% of PCTs.[17,51] They may be benign or malignant. Benign tumors include lipomas, teratomas, fibromas, hemangiomas, neuromas, leiomyomas, lipoblastomas, and paragangliomas.[17,51,52] Malignant tumors include mesotheliomas, sarcomas (eg, angiosarcoma, synovial sarcoma, and fibrosarcoma), primary lymphomas, and thymomas.[17,51] Secondary pericardial tumors (SPTs) are more common than PPTs, with most frequent primary etiologies being lung and breast carcinomas, melanomas, and lymphomas.[53]

Benign Primary Pericardial Tumors

Benign PPTs are extremely rare entities as less than 1% of benign PCTs arise from the pericardium.[4] Lipoma is the most common.[51] Cardiac teratomas are less diagnosed but have a strong predilection for the pericardium, with 90% of teratomas arising from there.[54]

Clinical Presentation of Benign Primary Pericardial Tumors

Benign PPTs manifest in various presentations. Factors determining presentation include size, location of the mass, and age of patient. Smaller lesions are discovered incidentally on imaging.[50] Larger masses present in nonspecific compressive symptoms including chest pain and discomfort, cough, dyspnea, palpitations, and possible hemodynamic compromise.[14,50,51,54] Pericardial teratomas most commonly present in neonates and infants.[14,51,54] Adults with pericardial teratomas are often asymptomatic, while affected fetuses may critically present with hemodynamic complications.[54] Pericardial effusions resulting in decreased cardiac output with hydrops fetalis may ensue, with eventual death.[51,55]

Diagnosis and Imaging of Benign Primary Pericardial Tumors

Imaging is often sufficient in diagnosing benign PPTs. On echocardiography, benign tumors show mixed echogenicities. In cases of teratomas and hemangiomas, cystic components may be seen.[50] Pericardial lipomas are hypoechogenic and ill-circumscribed, in contrast to their echogenic and well-circumscribed intracardiac counterparts.[31,51] Although echocardiography remains the initial study to detect a pericardial mass, further multimodality evaluation is recommended to better characterize the lesion and assess its relationship with adjacent structures.[50] On CCT and CMR, benign teratomas are well-defined, multicystic masses with fat and calcifications.[9,51] Specific imaging findings of other benign tumors are listed in Table 24.2.

Management of Benign Primary Pericardial Tumors

Complete excision of benign PPTs is recommended.[50] In case of hydrops fetalis because of teratoma, temporizing measures include intrauterine pericardiocentesis or thoracoamniotic shunts.[55]

Malignant Primary Pericardial Tumors

Malignant PPTs are exceedingly rare entities. It is estimated that only 16% of malignant PCTs arise from the pericardium.[4] Although mesotheliomas comprise most of the cases, pericardial angiosarcomas are also seen.[51,52,56]

The pericardium is a rare primary site for mesotheliomas representing less than 1% of all sites.[1,57] This pericardial malignancy more commonly affects males in their sixth decade.[57] Asbestos exposure is not an established risk factor for the pericardial variant of mesothelioma,[56] whereas radiation exposure is shown to increase risk.[56]

Clinical Presentation of Malignant Primary Pericardial Tumors

In contrast to benign PPTs, malignant tumors are often symptomatic, presenting with dyspnea, chest pain, nonproductive cough, and palpitations.[50,56,57] These are usually a manifestation of underlying pericardial effusions, myocardial invasion, or cardiac constriction.[50,57] Mesotheliomas are aggressive and may present as pericarditis, effusion, and cardiac tamponade.[56] Because of their vascular nature, angiosarcomas may cause hemopericardium.[51] Complications include recurrent pericardial effusions, constrictive pericarditis, heart failure, and metastasis.[51,56] The latter is seen in nearly half of pericardial mesotheliomas.[58]

Diagnosis and Imaging of Malignant Primary Pericardial Tumors

Echocardiographic evaluation has a limited role, and it shows similar findings across different subtypes of malignant PPTs. Pericardial effusions and diffuse pericardial thickening may be seen.[14] A defined mass is not always appreciated.[50] Upon further imaging by computed tomography, findings include enhancing, thickened pericardium with irregular appearance, and possible nodular formations[9,50] (**e-Figure 24.15**). On CMR, pericardial mesotheliomas are isointense to myocardium on T1-weighted sequence, while on T2 they exhibit a heterogenous appearance.[17] Imaging findings of individual malignant tumors are listed in Table 24.5.

Microscopic evaluation is needed to establish the diagnosis. A cytologic sample may be obtained by pericardiocentesis but is commonly unrevealing and only clues of hemorrhage and/or inflammation are found.[35,56,57] Histopathologic analysis is therefore required.[50] Tissue sample can be obtained through open biopsy, after pericardiectomy or after mass resection.[50] Histologically, mesotheliomas can be epithelial, sarcomatous, or biphasic.[57] Angiosarcoma's pathologic appearance is elusive and may be mislabeled as mesothelioma or mesothelial hyperplasia (e-Table 24.1).[51]

Management and Outcome of Malignant Primary Pericardial Tumors

Management is palliative, as most cases are unresectable on diagnosis.[50] Palliative measures include pericardial fluid removal, pericardiectomy, and partial resection.[56] Chemotherapy and radiotherapy may be offered, although rarely results in survival benefit.[50,59] Nonetheless, observational evidence has suggested that combination chemotherapy prolongs survival in patients with pericardial mesothelioma.[57] Prognosis of malignant PPTs is poor. The median postdiagnosis survival is 6 months in patients with pericardial mesothelioma.[51] A similar survival is seen in angiosarcomas ranging from 6 to 11 months.[59]

Secondary Pericardial Tumors

SPTs are far more common than PPTs.[51] The source of metastases is commonly lung or breast carcinomas, lymphomas, or melanomas.[50,58] Such tumors spread to the pericardium by blood, lymphatics, or directly from nearby organs[52] (Figure 24.6).

Clinical Presentation of Secondary Pericardial Tumors

Neoplastic involvement of the pericardium often remains masked by symptoms of the primary malignancy. Although postpartum diagnosis is more common, patients may present with pericarditis or pericardial fluid collection.[52] The latter, however, is more commonly secondary to nonmetastatic etiologies (eg, irradiation, opportunistic infections) in patients with known malignancies.[60] Metastatic pericardial effusions are often hemorrhagic and disproportionally larger than the underlying lesion.[50]

Imaging and Diagnosis of Secondary Pericardial Tumors

Cardiac imaging modalities may demonstrate mediastinal widening, masses, or effusions.[60] On CCT, pericardial thickening or disruption can be seen.[9] Upon contrast administration, pericardial metastases exhibit enhancement.[53] On CMR, a normal pericardium appears as a hypointense, curvilinear structure.[53] With metastatic infiltration, disruption of the pericardial line will be evident.[50] Diagnosis is established by demonstrating malignant infiltration in the pericardial cavity.[60] With the exception of metastatic lymphoma, pericardiocentesis is reliable for diagnosing pericardial metastases.[50] Equivocal cases may require obtaining a tissue biopsy.[60]

Management of Secondary Pericardial Tumors

As patients present in advanced stages, treatment is often palliative. Managing pericardial effusion is critical and achieved with chemotherapy or pericardiocentesis. To prevent recurrence, extended pericardial drainage with intrapericardial cytostatic or sclerotherapy may be required.[60]

Pericardial Cysts

PCs are single-layered, fluid-filled cavities arising from the outer layer of the heart.[51] PCs are seen in 1 per 100,000 individuals and represent 6% and 2.8% of all mediastinal and primary cardiac masses, respectively.[4,60,61] PCs are mostly congenital but may also be acquired.[17] Congenital cysts are secondary to failure of pericardial lacunae fusion during embryologic development.[61] Acquired PCs may be iatrogenic (ie, postsurgery) or infectious (eg, echinococcosis or tuberculosis).[52,61]

Clinical Presentation of Pericardial Cysts

Patients are most commonly females with a mean age of 49 ± 16.[61] Most patients are asymptomatic and diagnosed incidentally on imaging.[50,61] Symptoms include fever, chest pain, dyspnea, cough, and palpitations.[51,62] Cysts may get infected, compress adjacent structures, or rupture, leading to tamponade or sudden death.[51,53,62,63]

Imaging and Diagnosis of Pericardial Cysts

Chest radiography and echocardiography are often the first modalities to detect a PC.[52] On chest x-ray, a PC appears as a well-demarcated, smooth radiopacity, possibly with calcifications indicating an infection[51,63] (**e-Figure 24.16A-F**). Although PCs are typically seen in the right anterior cardiophrenic angle, they may be found anywhere in the mediastinum.[61,63] On echocardiography, a PC appears as a nonechogenic space with thin walls alongside the heart.[61] Because the sensitivity of echocardiography is only 38%, further imaging is needed.[61] CCT or CMR is the recommended modality to confirm the diagnosis.[50] On CCT, PCs appear homogeneous and nonenhancing, with sharp demarcations and water-like attenuation that varies according to content[53,63] (**Figure 24.7**). On CMR, PCs are hypointense on T1 and nonenhancing upon gadolinium administration.[50] Various pericardial masses may mimic cysts on imaging. Certain imaging features that aid in the discrimination between those entities are listed in **Table 24.7**.

Management and Outcome of Pericardial Cysts

PCs are managed according to the clinical presentation. Asymptomatic lesions are to be followed by CCT or CMR every 1 to 2 years.[50] Intervention by percutaneous aspiration with possible ethanol sclerosis is recommended in symptomatic cysts.[60] However, observational evidence suggests that this strategy is associated with high recurrence rates.[61] Surgical resection may be necessary if the cyst is large or recurring, when imaging is insufficient for definitive diagnosis and malignancy is suspected, or in cysts with high propensity for rupture.[50,60] On follow-up, it is estimated that the size of PCs is not significantly changed in 48% of cases, decreases in 34%, while increases in the remainder.[61] Echinococcal cysts are managed by albendazole, followed by aspiration and subsequent silver nitrate or ethanol therapy.[60]

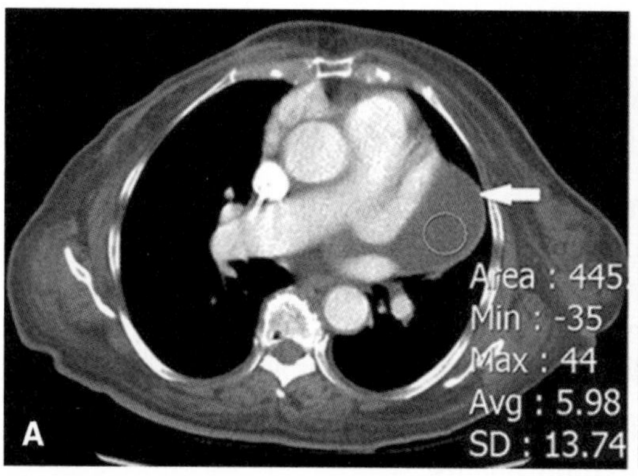

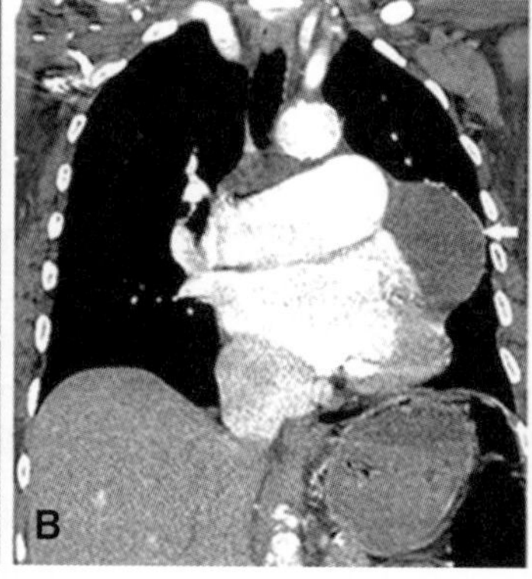

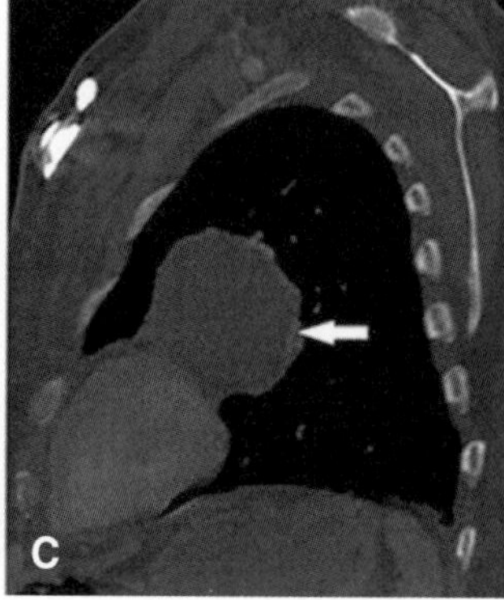

FIGURE 24.7 A pericardial cyst as it appears on different views of contrast computed tomography (CT) angiography of the chest. Images demonstrate a well-defined, low-attenuating (−20 and 20 Hounsfield Unit), nonenhancing mass (arrow). Cross-sectional view **(A)**, coronal view **(B)**, and sagittal view **(C)**. (Reproduced with permission from Lin AN, Lin S, Lin K, et al. Pericardial incidentaloma: benign pericardial cyst. *BMJ Case Rep.* 2017; 2017:bcr-2017-220097.)

TABLE 24.7 Imaging Findings That Aid in Differentiating Pericardial Cysts and Other Pericardial Masses

Pericardial cyst differentials	Appearance of the Differential Diagnosis	Appearance of Pericardial Cysts
Fat pads[60]	Echogenic on echocardiography (e-Figure 24.17)	Nonechogenic on echocardiography
Venous anomalies[52]	Enhancing on contrast echocardiography	Nonenhancing on contrast echocardiography
Pericardial diverticula[49,52]	Connected to pericardial space. Pericardial connection results in positional changes of the mass's size and shape.	No pericardial connection
Bronchogenic or thymic cysts[49,62]	Location in the right anterior cardiophrenic angle is atypical.	Typical anatomic location is in the right anterior cardiophrenic angle.
Cystic teratomas[49]	Fat and calcium components are apparent on CCT.	No fat components. May be calcified if infected.

KEY POINTS

- ✔ Cardiac tumors may present with symptoms of organ invasion, valvular obstruction, thromboembolism, and/or nonspecific constitutional complaints. Clinical presentation is often determined by the location of the tumor.
- ✔ Unlike other tumors, diagnosis is possible without obtaining a biopsy/tissue sample.
- ✔ Different tumors exhibit specific imaging characteristics that aid in diagnosis. Echocardiography is the initial modality of choice; and CCT and CMR provide further characterization.
- ✔ PCTs are very rare, with 90% of them being benign. Different pathologic subtypes have a predilection for specific cardiac locations, with the left atrium being most common. Treatment is surgical, when feasible.
- ✔ SCTs are more common than PCTs. Metastatic spread from lung, breast, and hematologic malignancies (ie, lymphomas and leukemias) are commonly culpable. They should be suspected if a patient with a known malignancy develops cardiac symptoms.
- ✔ Prognosis is contingent on type and location, but early diagnosis is usually associated with a favorable outcome.

REFERENCES

1. Oliveira GH, Al-Kindi SG, Hoimes C, Park SJ. Characteristics and survival of malignant cardiac tumors. *Circulation*. 2015;132(25):2395-2402.
2. Cresti A, Chiavarelli M, Glauber M, et al. Incidence rate of primary cardiac tumors: a 14-year population study. *J Cardiovasc Med*. 2016;17(1):37-43.
3. Butany J, Leong SW, Carmichael K, Komeda M. A 30-year analysis of cardiac neoplasms at autopsy. *Can J Cardiol*. 2005;21(8):675-680.
4. Wang J-G, Wang B, Hu Y, et al. Clinicopathologic features and outcomes of primary cardiac tumors: a 16-year-experience with 212 patients at a Chinese medical center. *Cardiovasc Pathol*. 2018;33:45-54.
5. Burke A, Tavora F. The 2015 WHO classification of tumors of the heart and pericardium. *J Thorac Oncol*. 2016;11(4):441-452.
6. Travis WD, Brambilla E, Burke A, Marx A, Nicholson AG. *WHO Classification of Tumours of the Lung, Pleura, Thymus and Heart*. International Agency for Research on Cancer; 2015.
7. Habertheuer A, Laufer G, Wiedemann D, et al. Primary cardiac tumors on the verge of oblivion: a European experience over 15 years. *J Cardiothorac Surg*. 2015;10(1):56.
8. Wu HM, Chen Y, Zhang F, et al. Clinical and pathological characteristics of cardiac tumors: analyses of 689 cases at a single medical center. *Chinese J Pathol*. 2019;48(4):293-297.
9. Kassop D, Donovan MS, Cheezum MK, et al. Cardiac masses on cardiac CT: a review. *Curr Cardiovasc Imaging Rep*. 2014;7(8):9281.
10. Garatti A, Nano G, Canziani A, et al. Surgical excision of cardiac myxomas: twenty years experience at a single institution. *Ann Thorac Surg*. 2012;93(3):825-831.
11. Cianciulli TF, Soumoulou JB, Lax JA, et al. Papillary fibroelastoma: clinical and echocardiographic features and initial approach in 54 cases. *Echocardiography*. 2016;33(12):1811-1817.
12. Tzani A, Doulamis IP, Mylonas KS, Avgerinos DV, Nasioudis D. Cardiac tumors in pediatric patients: a systematic review. *World J Pediatr Congenit Heart Surg*. 2017;8(5):624-632.
13. Careddu L, Foà A, Leone O, et al. Primary cardiac leiomyoma causing right ventricular obstruction and tricuspid regurgitation. *Ann Thorac Surg*. 2017;104(3):e231-e233.
14. Mankad R, Herrmann J. Cardiac tumors: echo assessment. *Echo Res Pract*. 2016;3(4):R65-R77.
15. Kim M-J, Jung HO. Anatomic variants mimicking pathology on echocardiography: differential diagnosis. *J Cardiovasc Ultrasound*. 2013;21(3):103-112.
16. Tao TY, Yahyavi-Firouz-Abadi N, Singh GK, Bhalla S. Pediatric cardiac tumors: clinical and imaging features. *RadioGraphics*. 2014;34(4):1031-1046.
17. Frank H, Sykora T, Alpendurada F. Cardiac and paracardiac masses. In: Manning WJ, Pennell DJ, eds. *Cardiovascular Magnetic Resonance*. 3rd ed. Elsevier; 2019:440-453.e3.
18. Wang Z, Chen S, Zhu M, et al. Risk prediction for emboli and recurrence of primary cardiac myxomas after resection. *J Cardiothorac Surg*. 2016;11:22.
19. Yanagawa B, Chan EY, Cusimano RJ, Reardon MJ. Approach to surgery for cardiac tumors: primary simple, primary complex, and secondary. *Cardiol Clin*. 2019;37(4):525-531.
20. Mariscalco G, Bruno VD, Borsani P, Dominici C, Sala A. Papillary fibroelastoma: insight to a primary cardiac valve tumor. *J Card Surg*. 2010;25(2):198-205.
21. Gowda RM, Khan IA, Nair CK, Mehta NJ, Vasavada BC, Sacchi TJ. Cardiac papillary fibroelastoma: a comprehensive analysis of 725 cases. *Am Heart J*. 2003;146(3):404-410.
22. Akram M, Hasanin AM. Caseous mitral annular calcification: is it a benign condition? *J Saudi Heart Assoc*. 2012;24(3):205-208.
23. Leow AS-T, Sia C-H, Tan BY-Q, et al. Characterisation of acute ischemic stroke in patients with left ventricular thrombi after myocardial infarction. *J Thromb Thrombolysis*. 2019;48(1):158-166.
24. Rose PS, Punjabi NM, Pearse DB. Treatment of right heart thromboemboli. *Chest*. 2002;121(3):806-814.
25. Egolum UO, Stover DG, Anthony R, Wasserman AM, Lenihan D, Damp JB. Intracardiac thrombus: diagnosis, complications and management. *Am J Med Sci*. 2013;345(5):391-395.

26. O'Gara PT, Kushner FG, Ascheim DD, et al. 2013 ACCF/AHA guideline for the management of ST-elevation myocardial infarction. *Circulation.* 2013;127(4):e362-e425.
27. Robinson AA, Trankle CR, Eubanks G, et al. Off-label use of direct oral anticoagulants compared with warfarin for left ventricular thrombi. *JAMA Cardiol.* 2020;5(6):685-692.
28. Chong-lei R, Sheng-li J, Rong W, Cang-song X, Yao W, Chang-qing G. Diagnosis and treatment of Lambl's excrescence on the aortic valve. *Heart Surg Forum.* 2018;21(3):E148-E150.
29. Aziz F, Baciewicz FA Jr. Lambl's excrescences: review and recommendations. *Tex Heart Inst J.* 2007;34(3):366-368.
30. Ammannaya GKK. Lambl's excrescences: current diagnosis and management. *Cardiol Res.* 2019;10(4):207-210.
31. Palaskas N, Thompson K, Gladish G, et al. Evaluation and management of cardiac tumors. *Curr Treat Options Cardiovasc Med.* 2018;20:29.
32. Hong NJL, Pandalai PK, Hornick JL, et al. Cardiac angiosarcoma management and outcomes: 20-year single-institution experience. *Ann Surg Oncol.* 2012;19(8):2707-2715.
33. Blackmon SH, Reardon MJ. Surgical treatment of primary cardiac sarcomas. *Tex Heart Inst J.* 2009;36(5):451-452.
34. Lestuzzi C, De Paoli A, Baresic T, Miolo G, Buonadonna A. Malignant cardiac tumors: diagnosis and treatment. *Future Cardiol.* 2015;11(4):485-500.
35. Kupsky DF, Newman DB, Kumar G, Maleszewski JJ, Edwards WD, Klarich KW. Echocardiographic features of cardiac angiosarcomas: the Mayo Clinic experience (1976-2013). *Echocardiography.* 2016;33(2):186-192.
36. Ramlawi B, Leja MJ, Abu Saleh WK, et al. Surgical treatment of primary cardiac sarcomas: review of a single-institution experience. *Ann Thorac Surg.* 2016;101(2):698-702.
37. Isambert N, Ray-Coquard I, Italiano A, et al. Primary cardiac sarcomas: a retrospective study of the French Sarcoma Group. *Eur J Cancer.* 2014;50(1):128-136.
38. Simpson L, Kumar SK, Okuno SH, et al. Malignant primary cardiac tumors. *Cancer.* 2008;112(11):2440-2446.
39. Wang J-G, Cui L, Jiang T, Li Y-J, Wei Z-M. Primary cardiac leiomyosarcoma: an analysis of clinical characteristics and outcome patterns. *Asian Cardiovasc Thorac Ann.* 2015;23(5):623-630.
40. Wang J-G, Li N-N. Primary cardiac synovial sarcoma. *Ann Thorac Surg.* 2013;95(6):2202-2209.
41. Papavdi A, Agapitos E. Undiagnosed primary cardiac liposarcoma in an adult: a case report and review of the literature. *Am J Forensic Med Pathol.* 2013;34(4):299-301.
42. Petrich A, Cho SI, Billett H. Primary cardiac lymphoma. *Cancer.* 2011;117(3):581-589.
43. Miguel CE, Bestetti RB. Primary cardiac lymphoma. *Int J Cardiol.* 2011;149(3):358-363.
44. Goldberg AD, Blankstein R, Padera RF. Tumors metastatic to the heart. *Circulation.* 2013;128(16):1790-1794.
45. Burazor I, Aviel-Ronen S, Imazio M, et al. Metastatic cardiac tumors: from clinical presentation through diagnosis to treatment. *BMC Cancer.* 2018;18(1):202.
46. Aghayev A, Steigner ML. CMR assessment of cardiac masses. In: Kwong RY, Jerosch-Herold M, Heydari B, eds. *Cardiovascular Magnetic Resonance Imaging.* Springer-Verlag New York; 2019:273-307.
47. Katalinic D, Stern-Padovan R, Ivanac I, et al. Symptomatic cardiac metastases of breast cancer 27 years after mastectomy: a case report with literature review—pathophysiology of molecular mechanisms and metastatic pathways, clinical aspects, diagnostic procedures and treatment modalities. *World J Surg Oncol.* 2013;11(1):14.
48. Allen BC, Mohammed TL, Tan CD, Miller DV, Williamson EE, Kirsch JS. Metastatic melanoma to the heart. *Curr Probl Diagn Radiol.* 2012;41(5):159-164.
49. Judge JM, Tillou JD, Slingluff CL Jr, Kern JA, Kron IL, Weiss GR. Surgical management of the patient with metastatic melanoma to the heart. *J Card Surg.* 2013;28(2):124-128.
50. Klein AL, Abbara S, Agler DA, et al. American Society of Echocardiography clinical recommendations for multimodality cardiovascular imaging of patients with pericardial disease: endorsed by the Society for Cardiovascular Magnetic Resonance and Society of Cardiovascular Computed Tomography. *J Am Soc Echocardiogr.* 2013;26(9):965-1012.e15.
51. Restrepo CS, Vargas D, Ocazionez D, Martínez-Jiménez S, Betancourt Cuellar SL, Gutierrez FR. Primary pericardial tumors. *RadioGraphics.* 2013;33(6):1613-1630.
52. Verhaert D, Gabriel RS, Johnston D, Lytle BW, Desai MY, Klein AL. The role of multimodality imaging in the management of pericardial disease. *Circ Cardiovasc Imaging.* 2010;3(3):333-343.
53. Yared K, Baggish AL, Picard MH, Hoffmann U, Hung J. Multimodality imaging of pericardial diseases. *JACC Cardiovasc Imaging.* 2010;3(6):650-660.
54. Cohen R, Mirrer B, Loarte P, Navarro V. Intrapericardial mature cystic teratoma in an adult: case presentation. *Clin Cardiol.* 2013;36(1):6-9.
55. Yuan S-M. Fetal primary cardiac tumors during perinatal period. *Pediatr Neonatol.* 2017;58(3):205-210.
56. Mezei G, Chang ET, Mowat FS, Moolgavkar SH. Epidemiology of mesothelioma of the pericardium and tunica vaginalis testis. *Ann Epidemiol.* 2017;27(5):348-359.e11.
57. McGehee E, Gerber DE, Reisch J, Dowell JE. Treatment and outcomes of primary pericardial mesothelioma: a contemporary review of 103 published cases. *Clin Lung Cancer.* 2019;20(2):e152-e157.
58. Dawson D, Mohiaddin R. Assessment of pericardial diseases and cardiac masses with cardiovascular magnetic resonance. *Prog Cardiovasc Dis.* 2011;54(3):305-319.
59. Timóteo A, Branco LM, Bravio I, et al. Primary angiosarcoma of the pericardium: case report and review of the literature. *Kardiol Pol.* 2010;68(7):802-805.
60. Adler Y, Charron P, Imazio M, et al. 2015 ESC Guidelines for the diagnosis and management of pericardial diseases: The Task Force for the Diagnosis and Management of Pericardial Diseases of the European Society of Cardiology (ESC) Endorsed by: The European Association for Cardio-Thoracic Surgery (EACTS). *Eur Heart J.* 2015;36(42):2921-2964.
61. Alkharabsheh S, Gentry lii JL, Khayata M, et al. Clinical features, natural history, and management of pericardial cysts. *Am J Cardiol.* 2019;123(1):159-163.
62. Najib M, Chaliki H, Raizada A, Ganji J, Panse P, Click R. Symptomatic pericardial cyst: a case series. *Eur J Echocardiogr.* 2011;12(11):E43.
63. Vargas D, Suby-Long T, Restrepo CS. Cystic lesions of the mediastinum. *Semin Ultrasound CT MR.* 2016;37(3):212-222.
64. Gianluca DB, Giorgi MP, Javier G, Steven D, Jan B. Liquefaction necrosis of mitral annulus calcification. *Circulation.* 2008;117(12):e292-e294.
65. Lopez-Mattei J, Iliescu C, Durand JB, et al. The role of cardiac MRI in cardio-oncology. *Future Cardiol.* 2017;13(4):311-316.
66. Pazos-López P, Pozo E, Siqueira ME, et al. Value of CMR for the differential diagnosis of cardiac masses. *JACC Cardiovasc Imaging.* 2014;7(9):896-905.
67. Sun D, Wu Y, Liu Y, Yang J. Primary cardiac myxofibrosarcoma: case report, literature review and pooled analysis. *BMC Cancer.* 2018;18(1):512.
68. Carpino F, Pezzoli F, Petrozza V, et al. Angiosarcoma of the heart: structural and ultrastructural study. *Eur Rev Med Pharmacol Sci.* 2005;9(4):231-240.
69. Suehiro S, Matsuda M, Hirata T, et al. Primary cardiac rhabdomyosarcoma developed after receiving radiotherapy for left breast cancer 18 years prior. *J Cardiol Cases.* 2017;15(6):181-183.
70. Kimura A, Tsuji M, Isogai T, et al. A mass filling the right atrium: primary cardiac rhabdomyosarcoma. *Intern Med.* 2018;57(24):3575-3580.
71. Seo G-W, Seol S-H, Song P-L, et al. Right ventricle inflow obstructing mass proven to be a synovial sarcoma. *J Thorac Dis.* 2014;6(10):E226-E229.
72. Yoshino M, Sekino Y, Koh E, et al. Pericardial synovial sarcoma: a case report and review of the literature. *Surg Today.* 2014;44(11):2167-2173.
73. Deppe A, Adler C, Madershahian N, et al. Cardiac liposarcoma—a review of outcome after surgical resection. *Thorac Cardiovasc Surg.* 2013;62(4):324-331.

CHAPTER 25

CARDIAC EVALUATION FOR NONCARDIAC SURGERY

Hugo Quinny Cheng

INTRODUCTION

Epidemiology

The annual worldwide surgical volume may exceed 300 million cases.[1] Because intraoperative techniques and postoperative care and monitoring have improved, the surgical population has expanded to include patients who once would have been considered too sick to undergo surgery because of their cardiovascular disease (CVD). However, although these patients are now receiving surgery, they remain at increased risk for perioperative cardiac complications. In the Perioperative Ischemia Evaluation (POISE) and POISE 2 trials examining over 18,000 patients with established CVD or other high-risk features undergoing major surgery, the incidence of cardiac-related death or nonfatal myocardial infarction (MI) was approximately 7%.[2,3]

Risk Factors

The risk of perioperative cardiac complications depends on both patient-related risk factors and the risk of the operation. The presence of end-organ CVD or its equivalents is the main patient-related risk factor. This includes coronary artery disease (CAD), heart failure (HF), severe valvular heart disease, and serious arrhythmias. In addition, disease in other organ systems resulting from atherosclerotic vascular disease or chronic hypertension, such as chronic kidney disease or stroke, is also associated with higher risk of perioperative cardiac complications.[4] Diabetes has also been shown to be an independent predictor, especially if it requires insulin to treat, is long standing, or has been poorly controlled. In contrast, many traditional atherosclerotic risk factors such as hyperlipidemia, tobacco smoking, family history of premature heart disease, and mild-moderate hypertension add little to risk prediction in the absence of identifiable end-organ disease. Advanced age likely increases risk independently of comorbidity. Severe systemic disease, even if unrelated to the cardiovascular system, also increases cardiac risk.

High-risk noncardiac operations are typically prolonged cases involving extensive blood loss, large-volume fluid shifts, or abrupt changes in afterload. Major vascular surgery involving the aorta (eg, abdominal aortic aneurysm repair) is often considered the epitome of a high-risk operation. A major operation performed on an emergency basis can have a much higher risk of cardiac complications than does the same surgery done electively. In contrast, minimally invasive operations, endoscopic cases, or procedures performed on the skin or eye have a very low risk of cardiac complications. Patients undergoing low-risk procedures generally do not require an in-depth preoperative cardiac evaluation.

Outcome Definitions

Death from cardiac causes (cardiac arrest) and nonfatal MI are the most important complications, and are often combined as a composite endpoint termed *major adverse cardiac events* or MACE.[5] The definition sometimes also includes other events such as stroke, need for urgent coronary artery revascularization, or overall mortality. In some cases, the definition of perioperative cardiac complication is expanded to include pulmonary edema, angina, and non–life-threatening arrhythmia. Although the risks of these less serious complications cannot be ignored, their impact on the decision on whether to perform surgery is substantially lower. Thus, when contemplating or communicating risk estimates, it is important to understand what outcomes are included.

APPROACH TO CARDIAC EVALUATION FOR NONCARDIAC SURGERY

When evaluating a patient's cardiovascular status before noncardiac surgery, the clinician must identify patients at increased risk for cardiac complications to implement appropriate diagnostic and prophylactic strategies. However, it is equally important to avoid unnecessary tests or interventions that delay surgery, increase costs, and potentially harm the patient. On a fundamental level, the preoperative cardiac evaluation addresses these goals by asking three questions:

1. What is the patient's risk for perioperative cardiac complications based on clinical assessment?
2. Is diagnostic testing needed to supplement clinical assessment to better define and manage risk?
3. On the basis of clinical assessment and diagnostic testing (if done), what management strategies should be implemented to reduce risk?

PATHOGENESIS

One proposed mechanism for postoperative ischemia and MI centers on the increase in sympathetic nervous system activity that is triggered by perioperative stressors such as blood loss, tissue injury, and pain.[6] Catecholamines and stress hormone

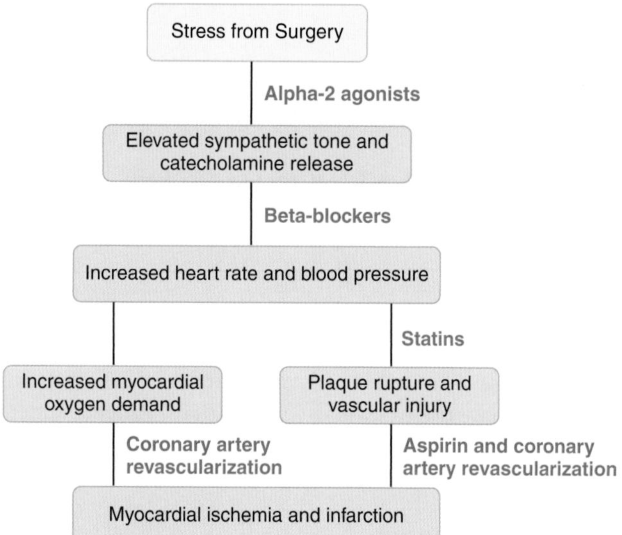

ALGORITHM 25.1 Mechanisms leading to postoperative myocardial ischemia and infarction and possible interventions.

levels rise acutely with surgery, leading to elevated myocardial oxygen demand as heart rate and contractility increase. Patients unable to accommodate the greater need for myocardial oxygen because of coronary artery obstruction can suffer myocardial ischemia and injury. Blood loss anemia and perioperative hypotension can further potentiate ischemia. Most postoperative MIs are demand-mediated (type 2) MIs. It is also possible that elevated sympathetic tone causing hypertension and tachycardia, perioperative hypercoagulability, and other factors may cause vascular injury or destabilization of coronary artery plaques, leading to acute coronary artery thrombosis and type 1 MI (**Algorithm 25.1**).

CLINICAL RISK ASSESSMENT

Preoperative cardiac evaluation begins with a detailed history. For patients without an established cardiac diagnosis, it is important to elicit a history of suggestive symptoms such as exertional chest pain, dyspnea, edema, or syncope. For patients with known CVD, the clinician should ask about complications, current symptom severity, prior diagnostic test results, and the timing and nature of prior invasive procedures such as percutaneous coronary intervention (PCI) or coronary artery bypass graft (CABG) surgery. In addition, the patient's functional status and exercise capacity should be assessed. Independent patients who are able to perform at least moderate physical activity without symptoms have a lower risk of cardiac complications, whereas patients who require assistance with activities of daily living or have limited exercise capacity are at increased risk. It is also easy to overlook CVD in patients with poor function because they may never perform activities strenuous enough to provoke symptoms. A threshold of four metabolic equivalents (METs) is often used to define adequate exercise capacity, which corresponds to the ability to walk several blocks at a normal pace or climb one or two flights of stairs.[7]

Physical examination should focus on looking for signs that confirm a clinical suspicion of undiagnosed or decompensated CVD, such as elevated jugular venous pressure, a third heart sound, and pulmonary crackles pointing to acute HF or a murmur suggestive of severe aortic stenosis. An electrocardiogram (ECG) is not routinely needed for all preoperative cardiac evaluations. However, an ECG should be done in patients with known or suspected CVD and considered for other patients undergoing major surgery. Patients undergoing low-risk surgery do not benefit from receiving an ECG or other cardiac testing unless indicated for reasons other than the operation.[8]

Patients with severe chronic CVD may be reasonable candidates for noncardiac surgery if benefits are felt to outweigh risks, but some conditions warrant delaying or canceling elective noncardiac surgery because of excessive risk. Patients with severe or decompensated heart disease that require urgent or emergent evaluation or treatment regardless of upcoming surgery should have their cardiac problem thoroughly addressed before elective noncardiac surgery. Examples include acute coronary syndrome, new or decompensated HF, symptomatic valvular heart disease, symptomatic ventricular arrhythmia, and supraventricular arrhythmia with uncontrolled ventricular rate. Conversely, emergency noncardiac surgery should not be delayed to perform a detailed cardiac evaluation. The clinician assessing a patient undergoing emergency noncardiac surgery should quickly identify conditions that affect the risk of MACE; discuss risk, monitoring, and postoperative care with the rest of the perioperative care team; and pursue a more thorough cardiac evaluation after surgery.

Prediction Tools

Owing to the complex interaction between patient-related risk factors and risk that is intrinsic to the operation, clinical risk assessment has long relied on formal multivariate prediction tools. The most widely used tool is the Revised Cardiac Risk Index (RCRI).[9] The RCRI uses six predictive variables: history of ischemic heart disease; HF; stroke or transient ischemic attack; serum creatinine greater than 2.0 mg/dL (177 μmol/L); diabetes treated with insulin; and high-risk surgery defined as major vascular surgery or an open abdominal or thoracic operation (see **Table 25.1**). The risk for MACE (defined as MI, primary cardiac arrest, pulmonary edema, and complete heart block) increases with the number of predictors present. More recently, a cardiac risk calculator was derived from the American College of Surgeons' National Surgical Quality Improvement Program (NSQIP) database.[10] The NSQIP calculator (available online or through a mobile device application at https://qxmd.com/calculate/calculator_245/gupta-perioperative-cardiac-risk) uses five variables: type or location of surgery; age; serum creatinine; ability to perform activities of daily living; and the American Society of Anesthesiology (ASA) physical status classification. The ASA classification is an overall subjective assessment of the severity of systemic disease in a surgical patient (see **Table 25.2**). The outcome predicted by the NSQIP tool is

TABLE 25.1 Revised Cardiac Risk Index

Predictors	Number of Predictors	Risk of Cardiac Death, Nonfatal Cardiac Arrest, or Myocardial Infarction (%)
• Ischemic heart disease • Heart failure • Stroke or transient ischemic attack • Creatinine >2 mg/dL (177 µmol/L) • Diabetes treated with insulin • Elevated-risk surgery (major intraperitoneal, intrathoracic, or suprainguinal vascular)	0 1 2 ≥3	0.4 1.0 2.4 5.4

Data from Lee TH, Marcantonio ER, Mangione CM, et al. Derivation and prospective validation of a simple index for prediction of cardiac risk of major noncardiac surgery. *Circulation*. 1999;100(10):1043-1049; Devereaux PJ, Goldman L, Cook DJ, et al. Perioperative cardiac events in patients undergoing noncardiac surgery: a review of the magnitude of the problem, the pathophysiology of the events and methods to estimate and communicate risk. *CMAJ*. 2005;173(6):627-634.

the 30-day incidence of *m*yocardial *i*nfarction or *c*ardiac *a*rrest, leading to it being called the MICA calculator.

When assessing the risks predicted by these two tools, only the risk of MI, cardiac death, and nonfatal cardiac arrest outcomes from the RCRI should be used for comparison.[11] The NSQIP calculator has greater external validity, because it was derived and validated in a large database that included patients and hospitals across the United States, whereas the RCRI originated from a single tertiary care hospital. Routine postoperative surveillance ECG and cardiac enzyme levels were obtained in many of the patients who were evaluated to derive the RCRI, whereas screening for MI was not part of the NSQIP study.

Although other prediction models and tools exist and may perform better in specific populations, the RCRI and NSQIP MICA calculator are broadly applicable, easy to use, and incorporated into clinical practice guidelines from North America and Europe. The 2014 American College of Cardiology (ACC) and American Heart Association (AHA) guideline on cardiac evaluation for noncardiac surgery endorses both the RCRI and NSQIP MICA tool for clinical risk assessment.[12] Patients with two or more RCRI predictors or an estimated complication risk greater than or equal to 1%, as calculated by the NSQIP tool, are defined as being at elevated risk.

PREOPERATIVE DIAGNOSTIC TESTING

Most surgical patients can be adequately evaluated using clinical assessment alone. The ACC/AHA guideline recommends no further testing for patients with less than two RCRI predictors or an NSQIP-derived risk of less than 1%. In addition, some patients with increased clinical risk have good exercise capacity and may be able to forego formal diagnostic testing. Finally, in many cases, the results of diagnostic testing will not influence treatment or the decision to proceed to surgery. This situation frequently occurs in acutely ill, hospitalized patients where the patient and surgeon are willing to accept a relatively high risk of cardiac complications to treat life- or limb-threatening disease. **Algorithm 25.2** provides a stepwise approach to preoperative cardiac evaluation in patients with stable CVD undergoing major, nonemergency surgery, based on the ACC/AHA guideline.

Noninvasive Stress Testing

Preoperative noninvasive stress testing is sometimes performed to improve risk stratification in patients with known or suspected ischemic heart disease. Most studies on the predictive utility of stress testing have been conducted in patients undergoing major vascular surgery and utilized radionuclide

TABLE 25.2 American Society of Anesthesiology (ASA) Physical Classification

ASA Class I	**Normal, healthy patient** Example: nonsmoking without systemic disease
ASA Class II	**Patient with mild systemic disease** Examples: mild lung disease, well-controlled hypertension
ASA Class III	**Patient with severe systemic disease** Examples: stable coronary artery disease, poorly controlled diabetes
ASA Class IV	**Patient with severe systemic disease that is a constant threat to life** Examples: recent acute coronary syndrome, sepsis
ASA Class V	**Moribund patient not expected to survive without surgery** Examples: ruptured aortic aneurysm, intracranial hemorrhage with mass effect

Data from Hurwitz EE, Simon M, Vinta SR, et al. Adding examples to the ASA-Physical Status classification improves correct assignments to patients. *Anesthesiology*. 2017;126:614-622.

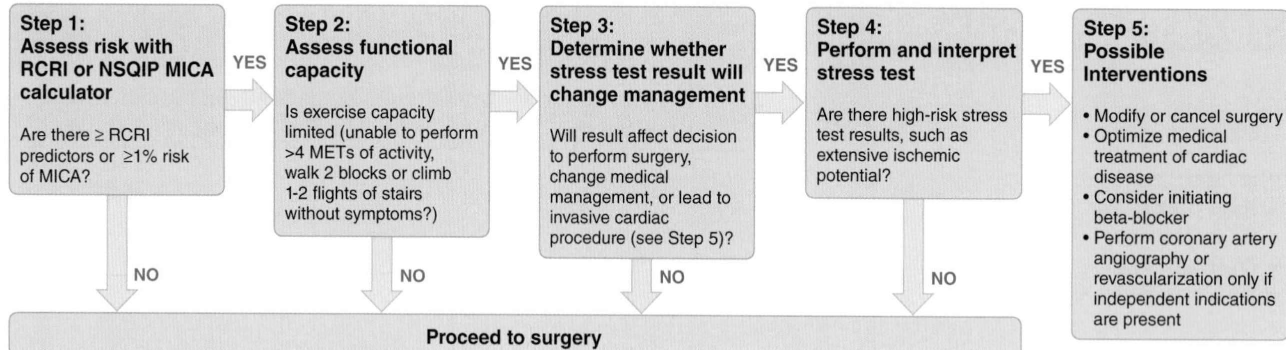

Notes

Step 1: RCRI, Revised Cardiac Risk Index; NSQIP MICA, National Surgical Quality Improvement Program Myocardial Infarction and Cardiac Arrest.
Step 2: METs, metabolic equivalents; reasonable to avoid stress test in patients with excellent functional capacity (>10 METs) and not unreasonable to avoid stress test in patients with moderate or good functional capacity (4-10 METs); patients with unknown functional capacity should be considered unable to perform 4 METs.
Step 3: Regardless of decision to perform stress test, patients should receive optimal guideline-concordant medical therapy.
Step 4: Pharmacologic stress test preferred because of assumption of poor exercise capacity.
Step 5: Possible indications for beta-blockers include three RCRI predictors, ischemia on stress test, or indications independent of surgery.

ALGORITHM 25.2 Stepwise approach to preoperative cardiac evaluation in patients with stable cardiovascular disease undergoing major, nonemergency surgery. (Based on the Fleisher LA, Fleischmann KE, Auerbach AD, et al. 2014 ACC/AHA guideline on perioperative cardiovascular evaluation and management of patients undergoing noncardiac surgery: a report of the American College of Cardiology/American Heart Association Task Force on practice guidelines. *J Am Coll* Cardiol. 2014;64:e77-e137.)

myocardial perfusion imaging or echocardiography. It remains unclear how well the conclusions from these studies apply to patients undergoing nonvascular operations, especially where the baseline risk for MACE is much lower than that with vascular surgery. In patients undergoing vascular surgery (and presumably other surgical populations), stress testing has strong negative predictive value. Patients without demonstrated ischemic potential typically have a very low risk of cardiac death or MI and can proceed to surgery without further cardiac testing. The positive predictive value of a stress test is limited. Evidence of ischemic potential on a stress test predicts increased risk in major vascular surgery; however, the large majority of patients with a positive stress test will not suffer a serious perioperative cardiac complication.[13,14] The complication rate correlates with the amount of myocardium at risk. In a meta-analysis, stress tests showing only fixed abnormalities or very limited ischemic potential (<20% of myocardium at risk) had no predictive value.[15] Tests results showing 20% to 29% reversibility were associated with a borderline significant increase in pretest probability of adverse events (positive likelihood ratio of 1.6). In patients with 30% to 49% of myocardium at risk, the posttest probability of complications increased by roughly threefold (positive likelihood ratio of 2.9), and those showing greater than or equal to 50% reversibility had an 11-fold increase in risk.

Because a positive test result generally does not increase the probability of complications by a large margin, stress testing should only be reserved for patients determined to have a high pretest probability of MACE based on clinical assessment or who have indications for the test independent of the surgery. Guidelines from the ACC/AHA and European Society of Cardiology and European Society of Anesthesiology (ESC/ESA) identify patients who have both multiple RCRI predictors and poor functional capacity (<4 METs) who are undergoing major surgery as the most appropriate population for noninvasive stress testing.[16] A pharmacologic stress test (pharmacologic myocardial perfusion imaging or dobutamine stress echocardiography) is generally preferred because these modalities have been better studied, and many stress testing candidates will have limited exercise capacity.

Echocardiography

The indications for preoperative resting transthoracic echocardiography (TTE) are similar to those for nonsurgical patients. Patients with a new or suspected HF diagnosis without a prior TTE should undergo the study before surgery, if possible. Similarly, patients with worsening HF symptoms should have a reassessment of left ventricular function with TTE. Patients with a murmur or other findings that raise concern for serious valvular heart disease (particularly aortic stenosis) should be evaluated with TTE. Patients with established moderate to severe valvular disease should undergo surveillance echocardiography if not performed in the prior year or if cardiovascular symptoms have worsened. Similarly, TTE should be considered when there is concern for other undiagnosed structural heart disease that can assessed by echocardiography (eg, hypertrophic obstructive cardiomyopathy, severe pulmonary hypertension).

Cardiac Biomarkers

Elevated preoperative levels of B-type natriuretic peptide (BNP) or N-terminal-proBNP (NT-proBNP) are associated with increased risk of postoperative MI and overall mortality. A meta-analysis including 2179 patients found that elevated levels of these biomarkers (BNP ≥92 mg/L or NT-proBNP ≥300 ng/L) before noncardiac surgery were associated with a fourfold increase in 30-day incidence of mortality and MI.[17] The guidelines from the AHA/ACC and ESC/ESA are ambivalent about the utility of measuring preoperative biomarker levels. The Canadian Cardiovascular Society (CCS) strongly recommends measuring BNP or NT-proBNP levels before major noncardiac surgery in all patients older than age 65 years and younger patients with CVD or a RCRI score greater than or equal to 1 to enhance risk prediction.[18] Biomarker measurement replaces preoperative noninvasive stress testing in the CCS guideline.

Coronary Angiography

In general, the indications for coronary angiography before noncardiac surgery are the same as those for patients who are not having surgery. In fact, left heart catheterization is rarely performed before noncardiac surgery because of the procedural risks, costs, associated delay in surgery, and lack of evidence that it improves outcomes. The role of noninvasive coronary computed tomographic angiography (CCTA) remains speculative. A prospective cohort study found that adding CCTA results to the RCRI score improved sensitivity by classifying more patients who suffered MACE as high risk. However, CCTA also impaired specificity by misclassifying more patients who did not suffer MACE as high risk.[19]

MANAGEMENT OF THE PATIENT

With a few exceptions, the management of CVD in a surgical patient is the same as that for patients not undergoing surgery. It is uncommon to initiate treatment with a new medication just because the patient will have an operation (see **Table 25.3**). Invasive interventions before noncardiac surgery generally should be performed for the same guideline-concordant indications as for the general population.

Medical Approach

On the basis of the pathophysiologic model of perioperative myocardial ischemia and injury (see Algorithm 25.1), several medication classes could hypothetically interrupt the cascade of events that begins with surgery-related stress and culminates in MACE. However, after an earlier period of excitement about the potential of medical prophylaxis, enthusiasm has waned because large trials failed to demonstrate meaningful benefit and revealed significant risks.

Beta-blockers

Beta-adrenergic blockade decreases myocardial oxygen demand by reducing heart rate and contractility, and can prevent ischemia in patients with limited coronary flow reserve. Beginning

TABLE 25.3 Perioperative Management of Cardiovascular Medications

Medication	Initiation to Reduce Risk	Continuation of Chronic Use	Notes
Alpha-2 agonist	No	Yes	
Angiotensin-converting enzyme inhibitor or angiotensin receptor blocker	No	Uncertain	ACC/AHA: continue on day of surgery ESC/ESA: continue on day of surgery only if HF CCS: hold on day of surgery
Anti-arrhythmia agent	No	Yes	
Antiplatelet agents (aspirin and $P2Y_{12}$ platelet receptor-inhibitor)	No	Yes, if prior PCI	Individualize management of antiplatelet agents based on risks of bleeding and MACE Benefit of continuation is greater in patients with prior PCI Continuing DAPT is strongly indicated within 4-6 weeks of BMS and 3 months of DES implantation
Beta-blocker	Consider in high-risk patients	Yes	Initiation can be considered in patients with >3 RCRI predictors, ischemia on preoperative stress test, or if independent indications. Do not initiate on day of surgery
Calcium channel blocker	No	Yes	
Diuretic	No	Uncertain	Likely safe to continue on day of surgery in stable patients
Nitrate	No	Yes	
Statin	Yes	Yes	Initiation reasonable in patients undergoing vascular surgery and considered in patients at elevated risk undergoing major surgery

ACC/AHA, American College of Cardiology/American Heart Association; BMS, bare metal stent; CCS, Canadian Cardiovascular Society; DAPT, dual antiplatelet therapy; DES, drug-eluting stent; ECS/ESA, European Society of Cardiology/European Society of Anaesthesiology; HF, heart failure; MACE, major adverse cardiac events PCI, percutaneous coronary intervention; RCRI, Revised Cardiac Risk Index.

in the mid-1990s, several small trials found that prophylactic beta-blockers started before surgery prevented postoperative MI and cardiac death. The number of patients needed to treat to prevent MACE was small, and side effects were minimal in these studies. As a result, perioperative beta-blockade was widely endorsed and practiced. Subsequent larger studies, however, failed to confirm the early positive results and found substantial risks related to hypotension and bradycardia.[20] In the POISE trial, metoprolol succinate started immediately before major surgery in high-risk patients only reduced the primary endpoint (cardiac death, nonfatal cardiac arrest, or MI) from 6.9% to 5.8%. Moreover, patients receiving metoprolol had higher all-cause mortality, in part due to a greater risk of stroke. Shortly thereafter, some of the influential studies supporting beta-blockade were discredited because of concerns about scientific misconduct, further calling into question the evidence for this practice.[21,22] Presently, indications for beta-blockers in the perioperative periods are limited. Patients taking beta-blockers chronically should continue to do so before and after surgery if they are hemodynamically stable. The ACC/AHA guideline gives a weak recommendation to consider initiating beta-blockers before major surgery in patients with an RCRI score greater than or equal to 3, evidence of ischemia on a preoperative stress test, or compelling indications outside of the surgery. If used, beta-blockers should not be initiated on the day of surgery.

Alpha-2 Agonists

Alpha-2 agonists are centrally acting sympatholytic agents. The rationale for their use to prevent cardiac complications is similar to that for beta-blockers—reducing myocardial oxygen demand in the setting of surgical stress. The most widely used agent, clonidine, was studied in the POISE 2 trial. Clonidine given orally immediately before surgery and through a transdermal patch postoperatively had no effect on the primary endpoint of 30-day mortality or MI. Clonidine increased the risk of clinically important hypotension and bradycardia. Presently, guidelines recommend against using clonidine to prevent postoperative adverse cardiac events.

Statins

Beta-hydroxy beta-methylbutyryl-*c*oenzyme A (HMG-CoA) reductase inhibitors or "statins" are effective for primary and secondary prevention against cardiovascular complications in nonsurgical populations. In patients undergoing surgery, it is hypothesized that statins stabilize coronary plaques and prevent their rupture and vascular injury that would lead to postoperative MI. Retrospective studies have shown that patients who received a statin perioperatively (although not specifically for perioperative cardiac risk reduction) had lower overall mortality, fewer postoperative MIs, and lower rates of noncardiac complications.[23] A randomized trial found that high-dose extended release fluvastatin started approximately 1 month before vascular surgery reduced the risk of postoperative MI.[24] Studies so far have not demonstrated an increased risk of liver injury or rhabdomyolysis from perioperative statin use. Although the evidence remains limited, the AHA/ACC and ESC/ESA guidelines recommend initiating statin therapy in patients undergoing vascular surgery and considering initiation in patients at increased risk for cardiac complications based on preoperative clinical evaluation when undergoing major nonvascular surgery. The CCS does not endorse the use of statins for this indication. Lipid levels should not affect the decision to start perioperative statin therapy. It is not known how far in advance of surgery a statin needs to be initiated to be beneficial or how long it should be continued. However, many candidates for perioperative statins have independent, long-term indications for the drug. Similarly, the optimal dose is unknown, but trials have used moderate- to high-intensity treatment, and observational studies suggest the presence of a dose effect.

Antiplatelet Therapy

The role of aspirin in secondary prophylaxis against cardiovascular complications in nonsurgical patients is clear. However, in surgical patients, its potential benefit must be weighed against the risk of intra- and postoperative bleeding. In the POISE 2 trial, patients at increased risk for cardiac complications were randomized to aspirin or placebo started immediately before surgery and continued postoperatively.[25] The study included both aspirin-naive patients and those who were chronic users. In the overall population, aspirin had no effect on cardiac outcomes or mortality. Bleeding (particularly at the surgical site) was more common in aspirin-treated patients. Results were similar whether the patient was initiated on aspirin or was using it chronically; there was no increase in MACE in chronic aspirin users randomized to placebo. For patients without prior PCI, the ACC/AHA guideline recommends against starting aspirin for the purpose of reducing perioperative cardiac complications in noncardiac surgery; continuation of aspirin in chronic users should be decided on a case-by-case basis.

Anticoagulants

Patients receiving long-term anticoagulation frequently need to temporarily discontinue the oral anticoagulant when undergoing an invasive procedure. Because this can increase the risk of thromboembolic complications, some clinicians "bridge" these patients with unfractionated or low-molecular-weight heparin (LMWH) while the oral anticoagulant is held. A placebo-controlled trial of perioperative bridging with LMWH in patients taking warfarin for atrial fibrillation demonstrated no effect on thromboembolism[26]; however, bleeding complications occurred twice as often in bridged patients. Thus, most patients with atrial fibrillation do not require bridging when their oral anticoagulant is held. Patients with very high thromboembolic risk from atrial fibrillation (see Chapter 56) may be candidates for bridging if the thromboembolic risk is felt to outweigh the increased bleeding risk.[27] The relative risks and benefits of bridging in patients taking warfarin for a prosthetic valve remain uncertain, but bridging is more likely to be beneficial for mitral valve prostheses (vs aortic) and older valve designs (vs modern bileaflet designs) because of the higher thrombotic risk associated with these features. Patients who are treated with direct-acting oral anticoagulants (DOACs) generally do not require bridging. A cohort study found that these patients could be safely managed using a protocol where the DOAC is withheld several days before surgery, based on the bleeding risk of the procedure and the patient's kidney function, and restarted 24 to 48 hours after surgery if hemostasis appears adequate[28] (see **Table 25.4**).

Other Medications

Most other cardiac medications should be continued perioperatively in hemodynamically stable patients, but not initiated prophylactically without an independent indication. Angiotensin-converting enzyme inhibitors and angiotensin receptor blockers increase the risk of intra- and postoperative hypotension when administered on the day of surgery. Conversely, holding them on the day of surgery increases the risk of postoperative hypertension.[29] The ACC/AHA guideline recommends their continuation, whereas the CCS recommends holding them on the day of surgery. Some clinicians hold diuretics on the day of surgery because of concern for causing hypovolemia or electrolyte disturbances, but there is no compelling evidence that this practice is beneficial or harmful in stable patients.

Percutaneous and Surgical Approach

Prophylactic coronary artery revascularization, whether through PCI or CABG, has not been demonstrated to prevent cardiac complications or mortality in patients undergoing noncardiac surgery. The Coronary Artery Revascularization Prophylaxis (CARP) trial randomized vascular surgery patients with obstructive CAD to coronary revascularization (using PCI or CABG) or medical management alone.[30] Patients randomized to invasive management had a 5.8% incidence of MI and 1.7% mortality rate complicating their coronary procedure, and there was no difference in mortality or risk of MI after the noncardiac vascular surgery. Guidelines from the ACC/AHA, ESC/ESA, and CCS agree that coronary revascularization should only be performed for independent indications and not merely because of an upcoming noncardiac operation.

SPECIAL CONSIDERATIONS

Coronary Stents

Patients with a history of PCI are at increased risk for acute stent thrombosis if they undergo surgery shortly after the coronary procedure, especially if dual antiplatelet therapy (DAPT) must be temporarily stopped.[31] The period of highest risk is longer with a drug-eluting stent (DES) than with a bare metal stent (BMS). The ACC/AHA guideline recommends delaying elective surgery at least 30 days after BMS implantation. For patients with DES, a delay of 6 months is recommended, but if the operation is time sensitive (such as surgery for cancer), a delay of 3 months after implantation could be considered. PCI should not be performed in patients anticipated to require surgery within these time frames, and elective surgery should not be performed within 30 days of BMS and 3 months of DES implantation if DAPT will be withheld.

Although the overall populations studied in POISE 2 did not benefit from continuing chronic aspirin therapy, a non-prespecified analysis of the subset of patients who had prior PCI found a reduction in the primary endpoint of death or nonfatal MI from 11% to 5.1% if given aspirin.[32] Major bleeding was again more common in aspirin-treated patients. The management of antiplatelet drugs in patients with history of PCI should be decided on an individual patient basis after considering the risks of stent thrombosis and bleeding. The following general recommendations are based on the ACC/AHA guideline for management of DAPT[33]:

- Patients who had very recent PCI (within 4-6 weeks) with either BMS or DES should continue DAPT if at all possible because of the very high risk of stent thrombosis.
- If a patient on DAPT must stop the $P2Y_{12}$ platelet receptor-inhibitor before surgery, aspirin should be continued if possible, and the $P2Y_{12}$ platelet receptor-inhibitor should be restarted as soon as possible after surgery.
- The surgeon, anesthesiologist, cardiologist who performed the PCI, and the patient should collaborate and discuss risks and benefits of delaying surgery and management options for DAPT to develop a consensus plan.

Valvular Heart Disease

Patients with independent indications for percutaneous or surgical treatment of valvular heart disease should have the procedure performed before elective noncardiac surgery, if possible. However, some patients are poor candidates for valve

TABLE 25.4 Perioperative Management of Direct-Acting Oral Anticoagulants

Drug and Renal Function	When to Administer Last Dose Before Procedure	When to Resume Drug After Procedure
Dabigatran with normal creatinine clearance (>50 mL/min/1.73 m² [0.83 mL/s/m²]) **Rivaroxaban** **Apixaban** **Edoxaban**	2 days before low–bleeding-risk procedure 3 days before high–bleeding-risk procedure	If hemostasis adequate: 24 hours after low–bleeding-risk procedure 48-72 hours after high–bleeding-risk procedure
Dabigatran with impaired creatinine clearance (30-50 mL/min/1.73 m² [0.5-0.83mL/s/m²])	3 days before low–bleeding-risk procedure 5 days before high–bleeding-risk procedure	

Data from Douketis JD, Spyropoulos AC, Duncan J, et al. Perioperative management of patients with atrial fibrillation receiving a direct oral anticoagulant. *JAMA Intern Med.* 2019;179(11):1469-1478.

procedures, and others may have urgent need for a noncardiac operation that cannot be delayed. Patients with stenotic valvular disease (especially critical or symptomatic aortic stenosis) are at particularly high risk of cardiovascular complications from noncardiac surgery. Patients with asymptomatic moderate or severe aortic stenosis, however, have generally acceptable mortality rates with surgery performed at tertiary care hospitals.[34] The ACC/AHA guideline recommends proceeding to surgery in patients with asymptomatic severe aortic stenosis if appropriate perioperative hemodynamic monitoring and experience are available. Similarly, severe but asymptomatic mitral stenosis does not preclude noncardiac surgery with appropriate care and monitoring. Mitral regurgitation (MR) and aortic regurgitation (AR) are better tolerated in the operating room than are stenotic lesions because systemic vasodilatation from anesthetic agents can promote forward flow. However, patients with MR or AR are at increased risk for postoperative volume overload. Complication rates are higher in patients with AR if they have reduced left ventricular ejection fraction (LVEF). The ACC/AHA guideline states that noncardiac surgery is reasonable in patients with asymptomatic severe AR and normal LVEF, as well as in patients with asymptomatic severe MR.

Arrhythmias and Conduction Disease

Patients with supraventricular arrhythmia with uncontrolled rate or symptomatic ventricular arrhythmia should have their cardiac disease addressed before elective surgery. Patients with life-threatening arrhythmia or conduction disease who meet independent criteria for placement of a permanent pacemaker or implanted cardiac defibrillator should generally receive their device before their noncardiac operation. Asymptomatic ventricular arrhythmia in the absence of structural heart disease does not predict a higher risk of MACE and does not require treatment.[35] If the patient is taking medications to suppress arrhythmia and control heart rate, they should be continued perioperatively. Electromagnetic interference in the operating room (typically from electrocautery devices) can disrupt the function of cardiac implanted electronic devices (CIEDs). This may impair antibradycardia pacing, cause inappropriate defibrillation shocks, or damage the device itself. It is crucial that the operating room team be made aware that a CIED is present so that appropriate evaluation and precautions are taken.[36]

The Older Patient

Age is not a component of the RCRI, but is one of the five variables in the NSQIP risk prediction tool. Closer analysis of the NSQIP cohort found that risk increased nonlinearly with age after controlling for other studied variables.[37] Among older patients in this cohort, history of stroke, HF, or diabetes predicted a higher risk of perioperative MI and cardiac arrest. These variables were included in a "geriatric-sensitive" version of the NSQIP tool, available at https://qxmd.com/calculate/calculator_448/geriatric-sensitive-perioperative-cardiac-risk-index-gscri. As an illustration of the effect of age, consider a functionally independent patient with stable CAD (ASA class 3) and normal creatinine clearance undergoing surgery for peripheral vascular disease. According to the standard NSQIP calculator, the risk of postoperative MI or cardiac arrest would be 0.5% at age 50 years, whereas the geriatric-sensitive NSQIP risk index predicts 1% risk of these complications at age 80 years.

Emergency Surgery

Patients who require emergency surgery are at much higher risk for cardiac and noncardiac complications than are patients undergoing similar operations performed electively. Neither the RCRI nor NSQIP MICA calculator includes emergency status as a variable, and these tools will therefore underestimate risk for emergency cases. Moreover, the type of preoperative cardiac evaluation described previously often has little clinical relevance in emergencies. There is usually inadequate time to perform a thorough assessment, and even a finding of high cardiac risk may not deter a plan to perform a life-saving operation. Lack of trials and wide variation in clinical presentation mean that management in these situations is often driven by clinical judgment rather than by evidence. The ACC/AHA guideline recommends that preoperative assessment focus on identifying conditions that may influence perioperative management, such as whether to withhold or continue a medication, rather than on risk stratification.

FOLLOW-UP PATIENT CARE

Patients who suffer a postoperative MI have an elevated mortality rate. In the first POISE trial, the mortality rate was fivefold higher among patients who suffered a postoperative MI as defined by ECG abnormality combined with elevated cardiac enzyme level. Two-thirds of these MIs were asymptomatic, and the absence of symptoms was not associated with better outcomes. In fact, studies have shown that elevated postoperative levels of biomarkers, even in the absence of ECG abnormalities or other clinical features of MI, are associated with higher all-cause mortality. In the Vascular Events in Noncardiac Surgery Patients Cohort Evaluation (VISION) study, patients with an elevated postoperative troponin-T level had a fourfold increase in mortality compared to those without troponin-T elevation, with higher levels associated with greater risk.[38] The CCS guideline recommends measuring daily troponin levels for 48 to 72 hours after surgery in patients with an elevated preoperative BNP or NT-proBNP level or when a preoperative biomarker level is unavailable, who have an RCRI score greater than or equal to 1, age 65 years or older, or age 45 to 64 years with significant CVD. The AHA/ACC and ESC/ESA guidelines do not make a strong recommendation for or against screening for asymptomatic postoperative myocardial injury or infarction.

RESEARCH AND FUTURE DIRECTIONS

The CCS guideline stands apart from its American and European counterparts in its broad use of biomarker measurement before and after surgery and its rejection of preoperative stress testing. A randomized trial comparing these different strategies would clarify how to best identify patients who will suffer MACE while minimizing costs, harm, and delays in care. The utility of measuring postoperative troponin levels depends largely on whether studies can show there are practical strategies to reduce mortality in patients with myocardial injury. Medical prophylaxis against MACE has proved disappointing, but there may be subsets of patients who will benefit from beta-blockers. Determining who these patients are and how to use beta-blockers safely and effectively in them requires further research. Despite the gaps in knowledge, much is already known about how to improve cardiac evaluation in surgical patients. Disseminating existing evidence-based practices for which there is broad consensus (such as avoiding cardiac testing in low-risk patients or low-risk operations) can yield as much benefit as new discovery.

KEY POINTS

- ✔ Preoperative cardiac evaluation should include clinical risk assessment, consideration of whether additional risk stratification testing is indicated, and identifying management strategies to reduce the risk of cardiovascular complications.
- ✔ Clinical assessment of perioperative cardiac risk should include use of a risk prediction tool such as the RCRI or NSQIP MICA calculator.
- ✔ Stress testing should only be considered for high-risk patients (based on clinical assessment) with poor functional capacity when test results will influence important management decisions.
- ✔ The indications and management of cardiac medications in surgical patients are generally the same as for nonsurgical patients.
- ✔ Coronary artery revascularization should not be performed preoperatively unless there are independent, guideline-concordant indications.
- ✔ Elective surgery should be delayed at least 30 days after BMS implantation and 6 months (or 3 months if operation is time sensitive) after DES implantation.

REFERENCES

1. Weiser TG, Haynes AB, Molina G, et al. Size and distribution of the global volume of surgery in 2012. *Bull World Health Organ.* 2016;94:201-209F.
2. Devereaux PJ, Yang H, Yusuf S, et al. Effects of extended release metoprolol succinate in patients undergoing non-cardiac surgery (POISE trial): a randomised controlled trial. *Lancet.* 2008;371:1839-1847.
3. Devereaux PJ, Sessler DI, Leslie K, et al. Clonidine in patients undergoing noncardiac surgery. *N Engl J Med.* 2014;370:1504-1513.
4. Jørgensen ME, Torp-Pedersen C, Gislason GH, et al. Time elapsed after ischemic stroke and risk of adverse cardiovascular events and mortality following elective noncardiac surgery. *JAMA.* 2014;312(3):269-277.
5. Kip KE, Hollabaugh K, Marroquin OC, Williams DO. The problem with composite end points in cardiovascular studies: the story of major adverse cardiac events and percutaneous coronary intervention. *J Am Coll Cardiol.* 2008;51(7):701-707.
6. Landesberg G, Beattie WS, Mosseri M, et al. Perioperative myocardial infarction. *Circulation.* 2009;119:2936-2944.
7. Wijeysundera DN, Pearse RM, Shulman MA, et al. Assessment of functional capacity before major non-cardiac surgery: an international, prospective cohort study. *Lancet.* 2018;391:2631-2640.
8. Keay L, Lindsley K, Tielsch J, et al. Routine preoperative medical testing for cataract surgery. *Cochrane Database Syst Rev.* 2019;(1):CD007293. doi:10.1002/14651858.CD007293.pub4
9. Lee TH, Marcantonio ER, Mangione CM, et al. Derivation and prospective validation of a simple index for prediction of cardiac risk of major noncardiac surgery. *Circulation.* 1999;100(10):1043-1049.
10. Gupta PK, Gupta H, Sundaram A, et al. Development and validation of a risk calculator for prediction of cardiac risk after surgery. *Circulation.* 2011;124(4):381-387.
11. Devereaux PJ, Goldman L, Cook DJ, et al. Perioperative cardiac events in patients undergoing noncardiac surgery: a review of the magnitude of the problem, the pathophysiology of the events and methods to estimate and communicate risk. *CMAJ.* 2005;173(6):627-634.
12. Fleisher LA, Fleischmann KE, Auerbach AD, et al. 2014 ACC/AHA guideline on perioperative cardiovascular evaluation and management of patients undergoing noncardiac surgery: a report of the American College of Cardiology/American Heart Association Task Force on practice guidelines. *J Am Coll Cardiol.* 2014;64:e77-e137.
13. Boucher CA, Brewster DC, Darling RC, et al. Determination of cardiac risk by dipyridamole-thallium imaging before peripheral vascular surgery. *N Engl J Med.* 1985;312:389-394.
14. Cutler BS, Leppo JA. Dipyridamole thallium 201 scintigraphy to detect coronary artery disease before abdominal aortic surgery. *J Vasc Surg.* 1987;5:91-100.
15. Etchells E, Meade M, Tomlinson G, Cook D. Semiquantitative dipyridamole myocardial stress perfusion imaging for cardiac risk assessment before noncardiac vascular surgery: a meta-analysis. *J Vasc Surg.* 2002;36(3):534-540.
16. Kristensen SD, Knuuti J, Saraste A, et al. 2014 ESC/ESA Guidelines on non-cardiac surgery: cardiovascular assessment and management: The Joint Task Force on non-cardiac surgery: cardiovascular assessment and management of the European Society of Cardiology (ESC) and the European Society of Anaesthesiology (ESA). *Eur Heart J.* 2014;35:2383-2431.
17. Rodseth RN, Biccard BM, Le Manach Y, et al. The prognostic value of pre-operative and post-operative B-type natriuretic peptides in patients undergoing noncardiac surgery: B-type natriuretic peptide and N-terminal fragment of pro-B-type natriuretic peptide: a systematic review and individual patient data meta-analysis. *J Am Coll Cardiol.* 2014;63:170-180.
18. Duceppe E, Parlow J, MacDonald P, et al. Canadian Cardiovascular Society guidelines on perioperative cardiac risk assessment and management for patients who undergo noncardiac surgery. *Can J Cardiol.* 2017;33:17-32.
19. Sheth T, Chan M, Butler C, et al. Prognostic capabilities of coronary computed tomographic angiography before non-cardiac surgery: prospective cohort study. *BMJ.* 2015;350:h1907.
20. Yang H, Raymer K, Butler R, et al. The effects of perioperative beta-blockade: results of the Metoprolol after Vascular Surgery (MaVS) study, a randomized controlled trial. *Am Heart J.* 2006;152(5):983-990.
21. Bouri S, Shun-Shin MJ, Cole GD, et al. Meta-analysis of secure randomised controlled trials of β-blockade to prevent perioperative death in non-cardiac surgery. *Heart.* 2014;100:456-464.
22. Blessberger H, Kammler J, Domanovits H, et al. Perioperative beta-blockers for preventing surgery-related mortality and morbidity. *Cochrane Database of Syst Rev.* 2018;3(3):CD004476. doi:10.1002/14651858.CD004476.pub3.
23. London MJ, Schwartz GG, Hur K, Henderson WG. Association of perioperative statin use with mortality and morbidity. *JAMA Intern Med.* 2017;177(2):231-242.
24. Schouten O, Boersma E, Hoeks SE, et al. Fluvastatin and perioperative events in patients undergoing vascular surgery. *N Engl J Med.* 2009;361:980-989.

25. Devereaux PJ, Mrkobrada M, Sessler DI, et al. Aspirin in patients undergoing noncardiac surgery. *N Engl J Med.* 2014;370:1494-1503.
26. Douketis JD, Spyropoulos AC, Kaatz S, et al. BRIDGE Investigators. Perioperative bridging anticoagulation in patients with atrial fibrillation. *N Engl J Med.* 2015;373:823-833.
27. Doherty JU, Gluckman TJ, Hucker WJ, et al. 2017 ACC expert consensus decision pathway for periprocedural management of anticoagulation in patients with nonvalvular atrial fibrillation: a report of the American College of Cardiology Clinical Expert Consensus Document Task Force. *J Am Coll Cardiol.* 2017;69:871-898.
28. Douketis JD, Spyropoulos AC, Duncan J, et al. Perioperative management of patients with atrial fibrillation receiving a direct oral anticoagulant. *JAMA Intern Med.* 2019;179(11):1469-1478.
29. Shiffermiller JF, Monson BJ, Vokoun CW, et al. Prospective randomized evaluation of preoperative angiotensin-converting enzyme inhibition (PREOP-ACEI). *J Hosp Med.* 2018;10:661-667.
30. McFalls EO, Ward HB, Moritz TE, et al. Coronary-artery revascularization before elective major vascular surgery. *N Engl J Med.* 2004; 351:2795-2804.
31. Schouten O, van Domburg RT, Bax JJ, et al. Noncardiac surgery after coronary stenting: early surgery and interruption of antiplatelet therapy are associated with an increase in major adverse cardiac events. *J Am Coll Cardiol.* 2007;49(1):122-124.
32. Graham MM, Sessler DI, Parlow JL, et al. Aspirin in patients with previous percutaneous coronary intervention undergoing noncardiac surgery. *Ann Intern Med.* 2018;168(4):237-244.
33. Levine GN, Bates ER, Bittl JA, et al. 2016 ACC/AHA guideline focused update on duration of dual antiplatelet therapy in patients with coronary artery disease: a report of the American College of Cardiology/American Heart Association task force on clinical practice guidelines. *J Am Coll Cardiol.* 2016;68(10):1082-1115.
34. Agarwal S, Rajamanickam A, Bajaj NS, et al. Impact of aortic stenosis on postoperative outcomes after noncardiac surgeries. *Circ Cardiovasc Qual Outcomes.* 2013;6:193-200.
35. O'Kelly B, Browner WS, Massie B, et al. Ventricular arrhythmias in patients undergoing noncardiac surgery. The Study of Perioperative Ischemia Research Group. *JAMA.* 1992;268:217-221.
36. Crossley GH, Poole JE, Rozner MA, et al. The Heart Rhythm Society (HRS)/American Society of Anesthesiologists (ASA) Expert Consensus Statement on the perioperative management of patients with implantable defibrillators, pacemakers and arrhythmia monitors: facilities and patient management. This document was developed as a joint project with the American Society of Anesthesiologists (ASA), and in collaboration with the American Heart Association (AHA), and the Society of Thoracic Surgeons (STS). *Heart Rhythm.* 2011;8:1114-1154.
37. Alrezk R, Jackson N, Al Rezk M, et al. Derivation and validation of a geriatric-sensitive perioperative cardiac risk index. *J Am Heart Assoc.* 2017;6(11):e006648. doi:10.1161/JAHA.117.006648
38. Devereaux PJ, Chan MT, Alonso-Coello P, et al. Association between postoperative troponin levels and 30-day mortality among patients undergoing noncardiac surgery. *JAMA.* 2012;307:2295-2304.

CHAPTER 26

CARDIO-ONCOLOGY

Courtney M. Campbell, Ajay Vallakati, Daniel Addison, and Ragavendra R. Baliga

INTRODUCTION

Cardio-oncology is an emerging discipline that encompasses the cardiovascular care of the oncology patient.[1-5] The discipline also includes cardiac amyloidosis, addressed in Chapter 30. Cardio-oncology patients can present in a variety of settings including (1) prior to initiation of cancer therapy for cardiovascular optimization, (2) acutely with complications directly related to ongoing or recent cancer therapy initiation, (3) prior to intervention or surgery for risk assessment, and (4) during survivorship, years to decades later with complications related to prior oncology therapy. If oncology patients do not already follow with cardiology, ideally they would present to cardiology at the time of initial cancer diagnosis. Patients could then be followed closely by cardiology throughout and after oncology treatment (**Algorithm 26.1**). This chapter's focus is on management of a patient throughout cardiotoxic oncology therapy.

PREVENTATIVE CARDIO-ONCOLOGY

Regardless of oncology treatment modality, primary prevention is paramount. The current approach for cardiotoxicity risk assessment and optimization uses the ABCDE model (**Algorithm 26.2**) that encompasses Awareness, Aspirin (acetylsalicylic acid, ASA), Blood pressure, Cholesterol, Cigarettes, Diet, Diabetes, and Exercise.[6,7] Prior to initiation of oncology therapy, patients should be aware of cardiovascular disease signs and symptoms to allow for prompt recognition of potential cardiovascular complications. Aspirin should be initiated in select patients, if indicated for preexisting cardiovascular disease. Blood pressure should be controlled. Patients should cease all tobacco use. Cholesterol lowering statins should be initiated if indicated. Diabetes mellitus control should be optimized and aggressively treated, if it occurs as a consequence of oncology therapy. Patients should maintain good diet and weight management. Exercise is encouraged throughout oncology treatment.[8]

In addition to improving cardiovascular risk factor management and initiation of guideline-directed medical therapy (GDMT), baseline cardiovascular testing often should be obtained prior to initiation of oncology therapy. This testing can include electrocardiogram (ECG), echocardiogram, biomarkers of troponin (Tn) and brain natriuretic peptide (BNP), and ankle-brachial index (ABI) measurement. If any specific cardioprotective therapies are indicated, these medications should be initiated at this time.

CARDIOTOXICITIES OF CANCER THERAPIES

Many oncologic therapies can cause acute and chronic cardiovascular events including left ventricular (LV) dysfunction leading to heart failure, diastolic dysfunction, fibrosis, cardiac conduction abnormalities and arrhythmias, vascular dysfunction, thrombosis, and metabolic changes. The most common classes of oncology therapy with cardiovascular toxicities as summarized in **Table 26.1** will be discussed in this section.

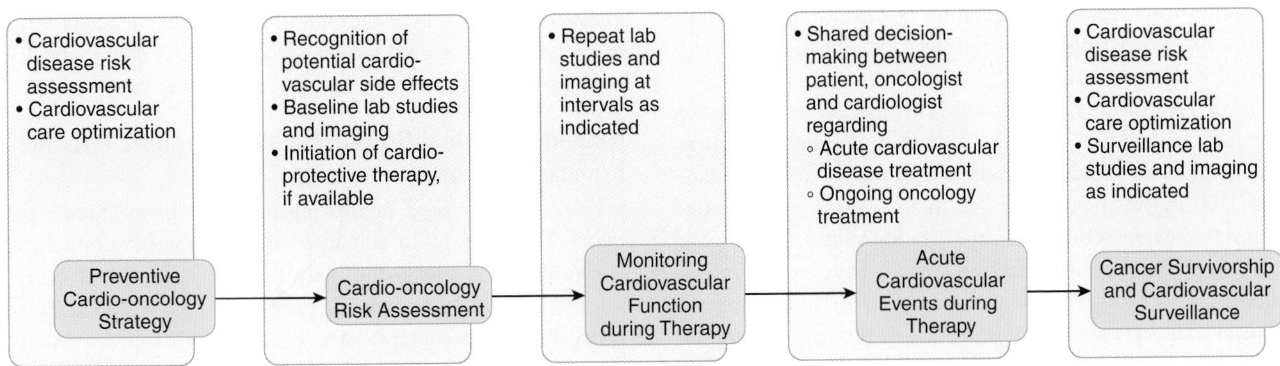

ALGORITHM 26.1 Cardiovascular management strategies throughout oncology therapy.

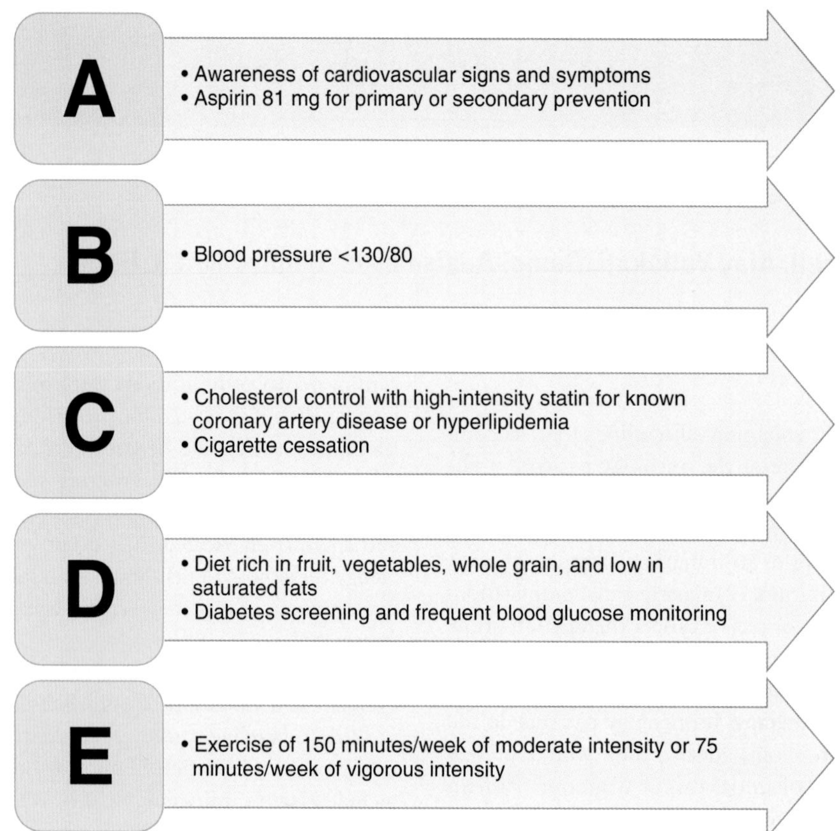

ALGORITHM 26.2 The ABCDE model approach for cardiovascular risk assessment in the oncology patient.

Anthracyclines

Anthracyclines are topoisomerase II inhibitors commonly used to treat multiple malignancies including breast cancer, urothelial cancers, gynecologic cancer, gastroesophageal cancer, acute lymphoblastic/myeloid leukemias, lymphoma, and sarcoma. Cumulative exposure is associated with permanent myocardial damage and carries a U.S. Food and Drug Association (FDA) black box warning for cardiomyopathy. There is no safe dose of anthracycline, and cardiotoxicity occurs at doses below some suggested maximum thresholds.[9] Patient-specific risk factors can increase risk of cardiomyopathy. These risk factors include the extremes of age, female sex, underlying cardiovascular disease, and history of prior irradiation of mediastinum. A heart failure risk prediction model has been developed for patients treated with anthracyclines.[10]

For patients at high risk, dexrazoxane, an iron chelation therapy, can be used. It is FDA indicated to reduce cardiomyopathy in those patients with breast cancer who receive greater than 300 mg/m^2 doxorubicin. A meta-analysis demonstrated that dexrazoxane reduced the risk of clinical heart failure and cardiac events without affecting oncologic response, overall survival, and progression-free survival.[11-13] In addition, small clinical trials have shown some efficacy in mitigating anthracycline-induced cardiotoxicity with the initiation of beta-blockers (BBs), angiotensin-converting enzyme inhibitors (ACEi), angiotensin receptor blockade, mineralocorticoid antagonism, and combinations of the preceding agents.[14-19] Larger trials of cardioprotective strategies are needed.

Tyrosine Kinase Inhibitors

Tyrosine kinase inhibitors (TKIs) are broad class of oncology medications. Tyrosine kinases are enzymes that catalyze protein phosphorylation and are important in cell growth, proliferation, and angiogenesis. Abnormal function of tyrosine kinases is implicated in many cancers. Specific oncologic TKI targets include human epidermal growth factor receptor 2 (HER-2), vascular endothelial growth factor (VEGF), BCR-ABL (formed by the Philadelphia chromosome t(9;22)), and Bruton tyrosine kinase inhibitor (BTK). Although TKIs are categorized by their primary specific targets, most TKIs are active against many different targets resulting in a range of cardiovascular toxicities.

Human Epidermal Growth Factor Receptor 2 Tyrosine Kinase Inhibitors

HER-2 target is used in treating primarily breast cancer patients. Medications in this class are humanized monoclonal antibodies that block the activation of HER-2/neu receptor resulting in impaired cell growth and survival.[20] Not all HER-2 targeted therapies are associated with cardiotoxicity. Trastuzumab and possibly pertuzumab are associated with cardiotoxicity. Cardiotoxicity typically presents as an asymptomatic decrease in left ventricular ejection fraction (LVEF),

TABLE 26.1 Common Classes of Oncology Therapy and Associated Cardiovascular Toxicities

Class	Oncology Therapy	Primary Target	Cardiovascular Risk	Patient Risk Factors
Anthracyclines	Daunorubicin, doxorubicin, liposomal doxorubicin, epirubicin, idarubicin	Topoisomerase II inhibitor	Cardiomyopathy	Extremes of age (young/old) Cumulative dose Female Underlying cardiovascular disease History of prior mediastinal irradiation
Tyrosine Kinase Inhibitors	*HER-2* Small molecules: – Neratinib, Lapatinib Monoclonal antibodies: – Pertuzumab, Trastuzumab	Inhibits human epidermal growth factor receptor 2 (HER-2)	Trastuzumab and pertuzumab specific: –Cardiomyopathy	Age >60 years Past or concomitant use of anthracyclines Underlying cardiovascular disease Diabetes Obesity Renal failure Black race
	VEGF Small molecules: – axitinib, cabozantinib, lenvatinib, pazopanib, regorafenib, sorafenib, sunitinib, vandetanib	Inhibits vascular endothelial growth factor (VEGF)	Hypertension Cardiomyopathy Ischemia Vandetanib specific: –QT prolongation –Torsades de pointes –Sudden death	Hypertension Coronary artery disease Cardiomyopathy Aortic stenosis Pulmonary hypertension
	BCR-ABL Small molecules: – bosutinib, dasatinib, imatinib, nilotinib, and ponatinib	Inhibits activity of BCR-ABL kinase, Philadelphia chromosome	Nilotinib and ponatinib specific: – Peripheral artery disease – Ischemic heart disease – Stroke Ponatinib specific: – Venous thromboembolism – Hypertension	Age >65 years Cardiovascular disease Peripheral vascular disease Cardiomyopathy Diabetes
	BTK Small molecules: – ibrutinib, acalabrutinib, and zanubrutinib	Inhibits activity of Bruton tyrosine kinase	Atrial fibrillation Hypertension Peripheral edema Bleeding	Age >65 years Male Valvular heart disease Hypertension
Immune Checkpoint Inhibitors (ICIs)	Monoclonal antibodies: –atezolizumab, avelumab cemiplimab, durvalumab, ipilimumab, nivolumab, and pembrolizumab	Inhibits programmed cell death protein 1 (PD-1), programmed death-ligand 1 (PD-L1), and cytotoxic T-lymphocyte-associated protein 4 (CTLA-4) receptors	Myocarditis Pericarditis Left ventricular dysfunction Takotsubo-like syndrome Coronary vasospasm Arrhythmias Myocardial infarction	Combination ICI Underlying autoimmune disease Underlying cardiovascular disease Diabetes Concurrent immune-related adverse events (such as myositis, hepatitis, or myasthenia gravis)
Chimeric Antigen Receptor T cells	Tisagenlecleucel, Axicabtagene ciloleucel	Anti-CD19	Cytokine release syndrome – Cardiomyopathy – Arrhythmia –Myocarditis	Age >60 years Cardiovascular disease
Proteasome Inhibitor	Small molecules: –Bortezomib, Carfilzomib, and Ixazomib	Inhibit peptide degradation by the proteasome	Venous thromboembolism Carfilzomib specific: –Hypertension –Arrhythmias –Heart failure	Age >60 years Previous cardiotoxic oncology therapies Carfilzomib dose >45 mg/m^2

(*Continued*)

TABLE 26.1 Common Classes of Oncology Therapy and Associated Cardiovascular Toxicities (*Continued*)

Class	Oncology Therapy	Primary Target	Cardiovascular Risk	Patient Risk Factors
Androgen Deprivation Therapy	Leuprolide, Goserelin, Triptorelin, Histrelin	Gonadotropin-releasing hormone antagonist	Metabolic syndrome Diabetes Cardiovascular events	Prior cardiovascular disease
	Degarelix	Gonadotropin-releasing hormone agonist		
	Abiraterone, flutamide, nilutamide	Antiandrogen		
Radiation Therapy		Direct ablative action on DNA Indirect DNA damage via oxygen free radicals	Cardiomyopathy Coronary artery disease Valvular disease Arrhythmia	Total heart radiation dose (for every 1 Gy 7.4% increase in coronary artery disease) Hodgkin lymphoma treatment (9-25 years posttreatment for cardiac events) Lung cancer treatment (11-26 months posttreatment for cardiac events)

is not related to cumulative dose, and usually is reversible.[21] Patient-specific risk factors that increase the risk of cardiomyopathy include past or concomitant use of anthracyclines, underlying cardiovascular disease, diabetes, obesity, renal failure, age older than 60 years, and black race.

Vascular Endothelial Growth Factor Tyrosine Kinase Inhibitors

VEGF TKIs are used to treat a range of cancers including renal cell carcinoma, hepatocellular carcinoma, thyroid cancers, endometrial cancers, and sarcomas. Drugs in this class are small-molecule inhibitors and include axitinib, cabozantinib, lenvatinib, pazopanib, regorafenib, sorafenib, sunitinib, and vandetanib. TKIs impair angiogenesis, lymphangiogenesis, vascular permeability, and vascular homeostasis.[3] Liver toxicity is the primary major side effect in this class. One drug, vandetanib, carries a black box warning for QT prolongation, torsades de pointes, and sudden death.

Cardiotoxicity with VEGF TKIs most often manifests as hypertension, which is directly related to its mechanism of action. VEGF inhibition decreases nitric oxide production, prostacyclin levels, and increases endothelin resulting in increased systemic vascular resistance. Depending on the specific drug, first-time VEGF TKI use can result in 21% to 80% patients experiencing significant increases in blood pressure as early as the first day of treatment.[22] This response is dose dependent and reversible upon therapy discontinuation. The rise in blood pressure can occur within days of treatment and fall just as quickly. Patients should be empowered to change blood pressure medications based on predefined instructions and home blood pressure monitoring. Other cardiotoxic side effects include LV dysfunction (estimated at 1%-2.5%) and ischemia (1.4%-3%). Appropriately treating blood pressure decreases the risk of LV dysfunction and lowers the risk of vascular events.[23,24] In one retrospective study, the best blood pressure control was observed in patients on calcium channel blockers.[22]

Bcr-Abl Tyrosine Kinase Inhibitors

BCR-ABL TKIs are used in hematologic malignancies, chronic myeloid leukemia, and acute lymphoblastic leukemia, with positive Philadelphia chromosome. Drugs in this class are small-molecule inhibitors and include bosutinib, dasatinib, imatinib, nilotinib, and ponatinib. Imatinib is also used to treat gastrointestinal (GI) stromal tumors, myelodysplastic syndrome, dermatofibrosarcoma protuberans, and hypereosinophilic syndrome. Cardiotoxicity is not class wide and primarily is vasculature related.[25] Nilotinib and ponatinib are significantly associated with peripheral arterial occlusive disease, ischemic heart disease, and stroke. Ponatinib is also associated with venous thromboembolism, platelet dysfunction, and hypertension. Dasatinib is associated with pulmonary hypertension and platelet dysfunction. Baseline testing and monitoring of ABI is recommended for patients on nilotinib and ponatinib.

Bruton Tyrosine Kinase Inhibitors

BTKs are used to treat B-cell malignancies (chronic lymphocytic leukemia, lymphoma) and chronic graft-versus-host disease (GvHD). Drugs in this class include ibrutinib, acalabrutinib, and zanubrutinib. The most common cardiotoxicities are arrhythmia, hypertension, peripheral edema, and bleeding because of abnormal platelet aggregation. Ibrutinib increases the risk of acute hypertension by 10% to 14%. Development of hypertension is associated with double the incidence of cardiovascular events for 2 years after initiation of ibrutinib.[26] Ibrutinib is also significantly associated with atrial fibrillation.[27]

Immune Checkpoint Inhibitors

Immune checkpoint inhibitors (ICIs) are monoclonal antibodies directed at PD-1, PD-L1, and CTLA-4 receptors. ICIs remove the brakes placed on T cell–mediated response and increase the immune system's ability to scavenge for and identify foreign cells. Drugs in this class are monoclonal antibodies and include atezolizumab, avelumab, cemiplimab, durvalumab, ipilimumab, nivolumab, and pembrolizumab. ICIs are used to treat a range of cancers including urothelial carcinoma, non–small cell lung cancer, small cell lung cancer, renal cell carcinoma, melanoma, hepatocellular carcinoma, gastric cancer, and endometrial cancer.

Initial studies of ICIs did not observe a high amount of cardiotoxicity (0.9%-0.27%). Postmarketing studies and meta-analyses have reported a cardiotoxic incidence as high as 1.14% with a 27% to 46% fatality rate.[28] ICI-associated cardiotoxicity is likely related to an autoimmune reaction. ICI-associated cardiotoxicity can result in myocarditis, pericarditis, LV dysfunction, Takotsubo-like syndrome, coronary vasospasm, arrhythmias, and myocardial infarction.

Cardiotoxicity can develop after a single ICI dose. Further, 76% of myocarditis cases occurred within 6 weeks of ICI initiation.[29] Potential risk factors for ICI cardiotoxicity include combination ICI, underlying autoimmune disease, underlying cardiovascular disease, diabetes, and concurrent immune-related adverse events (such as myositis, hepatitis, or myasthenia gravis). Symptoms such as chest pain, dyspnea, fatigue, orthopnea, myalgia, syncope, palpitations, or peripheral edema should prompt cardiovascular investigation. High-dose steroids are the first line of treatment and do not appear to affect malignancy response.[30] Infliximab can be given if myocarditis persists. Unstable patients may benefit from antithymocyte globulin (ATG) or intravenous immunoglobulin (IVIG) and plasma exchange. If there is clinical improvement and patients are able to be tapered off of steroids, one can consider restarting ICI with close monitoring. Otherwise, avoid restarting ICI.

Chimeric Antigen Receptor T Cells

Chimeric antigen receptor T cells (CAR T cells) are genetically modified autologous T cells. Two therapies were FDA approved in 2017. Tisagenlecleucel (Kymriah) is used in acute lymphoblastic leukemia and diffuse large B-cell lymphoma.[31] Axicabtagene ciloleucel (Yescarta) is used for diffuse large B-cell lymphoma.[32] Both therapies target anti-CD19. This therapy is delivered as a one-time infusion 2 to 14 days after lymphocyte-depleting chemotherapy. Current research trials are expanding the use of CAR T cells to multiple myeloma, Hodgkin acute myeloid leukemia (AML), and chronic myelogenous leukemia (CML). Further, researchers are developing allogenic CAR T cells. This therapy could be used "off-the-shelf" with decreased costs, but does have the risk of GvHD and rapid elimination. Cardiotoxicities associated with CAR T cells are primarily related to cytokine release syndrome (CRS).[33] CRS occurred a median of 5 days after CAR T infusion. Registry data revealed that 54% of patients had an elevated troponin, and of these, 28% had a decrease in LVEF. Cardiovascular events, including death, decompensated heart failure, and arrhythmia, occurred in 12% of patients with a median time to event of 21 days.

Proteasome Inhibitors

Proteasome inhibitors (PIs) block the degradation of peptides leading to cell cycle arrest and apoptosis. Drugs in this class are small molecules and include bortezomib, carfilzomib, and ixazomib. PIs are used to treat multiple myeloma and mantle cell lymphoma.[34] Cardiotoxic adverse events have been reported with carfilzomib.[35] These events often occur 2 to 3 months from treatment initiation and include hypertension, arrhythmias, heart failure, and venous thromboembolism (VTE).[36] Potential risk factors include age, comorbidities, previous cardiotoxic therapies, and carfilzomib doses greater than 45 mg/m^2. If cardiotoxicity is recognized promptly and treatment is initiated, myocardial injury often can be reversed, and patients can be rechallenged with PI.

Androgen Deprivation Therapy

Prostate cancer is a hormone-sensitive malignancy. Androgen deprivation therapy (ADT) has been the cornerstone of prostate cancer therapy. The goal of ADT is to induce hypogonadism through disruption of the hypothalamic-pituitary-gonadal axis. ADT can be achieved surgically with bilateral orchiectomy or medically with either a gonadotropin-releasing hormone (GnRH) agonist or antagonist.[37] GnRH agonists include leuprolide, goserelin, triptorelin, and histrelin. These medications result in a surge of follicle-stimulating hormone (FSH), luteinizing hormone (LH), and testosterone before suppression followed by microsurges in LH and testosterone on repeat injection. FSH suppression is not maintained long term. GnRH antagonist is degarelix. This medication had immediate suppression of FSH, LH, and testosterone with FSH suppression long term. Antiandrogen therapy with abiraterone, flutamide, and nilutamide can also be used. The resultant low testosterone, which controls prostate cancer growth, is implicated in the development of metabolic syndrome.[38,39] Patients on this therapy have decreases in lean body mass, increases in subcutaneous abdominal fat, increases in hemoglobin A1C, and elevation in total cholesterol. Studies have shown an increase in diabetes and cardiovascular events.[40] The effects may appear after the first 6 months of treatment. Patients with prior cardiovascular disease are at the highest risk of having a cardiovascular event.

Radiation Therapy

Radiation therapy is a frequently used modality in oncology therapy. The primary cancers treated with radiation therapy in the chest are Hodgkin lymphoma, breast cancer, and lung cancer. Radiation works in cancer through direct ablative action on DNA and indirect action inducing DNA damage via oxygen free radicals. Double-stranded DNA breaks lead to cell killing, mutagenesis, and carcinogenesis. DNA damage occurs in cancer and noncancer tissues. Tumor cells typically die, whereas normal cells often repair. Early complications of radiation therapy occur days to weeks posttreatment. These complications occur most often in rapidly proliferating tissues, such as skin, GI tract, and hematopoietic system. Often the damage can be reversible. Direct targeting of the heart may result in inflammation such as pericarditis. Late complications of radiation therapy occur months to years after therapy and most often in slowly proliferating tissues such as lung, brain, heart, liver, and kidney. Small blood vessels are most often damaged, and it is not reversible. In the heart, cell loss and fibrosis can lead to atherosclerosis, cardiomyopathy, cardiac fibrosis, valvular fibrosis, pericarditis, pericardial effusions, constriction, and arrhythmias. Currently, radiation to the heart is reported as mean heart dose. However, this reporting can mean high dose to a small volume of the heart or a low dose to a large volume of the heart.[41]

In a study of Hodgkin lymphoma patients, cumulative incidence of coronary artery disease was associated with rising mean heart dose.[42] In a study of breast cancer patients who underwent radiotherapy, there was a significant increase in major coronary events within the first 5 years of radiotherapy.[43] Overall, there is a 7.4% increased risk of coronary artery disease for every 1 Gy mean heart dose. In a larger longitudinal study of Hodgkin lymphoma patients treated with radiation therapy, coronary artery disease was seen at 9 years, carotid/subclavian disease at 17 years, and valvular disease at 22 to 25 years posttreatment.[44] In lung cancer, studies have demonstrated a median time to cardiac events as 11 to 26 months. The majority of cardiac events were coronary artery disease, cardiac arrest, cardiomyopathy, and arrhythmia.[45]

In modern era of radiation oncology, we anticipate that these historical cardiac complication rates will decrease with improved techniques to minimize cardiac irradiation. These techniques include computed tomography (CT) planning, breath-holding, prone treatments for breast cancer, reducing treatment target volumes and dose, and emergence of proton therapy.

SPECIAL CONSIDERATIONS AND MANAGEMENT DURING ONCOLOGY THERAPY

Cardiac Surveillance

The American Society of Clinical Oncology (ASCO) guidelines recommend imaging for patients at elevated risk of cardiomyopathy.[1] These patients include those with planned high anthracycline doses (such as doxorubicin $\geq$250 mg/m^2), thoracic radiation dose greater than or equal to 30 Gy, and trastuzumab therapy. There are no clear guidelines for monitoring with cardiovascular imaging for patients on PIs, ICIs, MEK inhibitors, TKIs, VEGF, or alkylating agents. The general recommendation is that any patient planning to undergo therapy with a potentially cardiotoxic agent should have a baseline echocardiogram. The role of repeat echocardiogram imaging during treatment varies per study. For patients at high risk of cardiotoxicity, recommendations range from every 3 (trastuzumab) to 6 months (anthracyclines) to monitor for asymptomatic decreases in LVEF. Otherwise, ASCO recommends symptom-driven cardiac imaging.

The value of global longitudinal strain in conjunction with echocardiogram for cardio-oncology monitoring is not well established. In adjusted meta-analysis, the results are inconsistent.[46] In an expert consensus statement (Plana, Galderisi, and Barac), they recommended treating greater than 15% decrease in global longitudinal strain from baseline with an ejection fraction (EF) greater than 53% as subclinical LV dysfunction.[47] The SUCCOUR randomized control trial is testing this approach.

Cardiac biomarkers, including troponin and BNP, can be used as ancillary measures in conjunction with imaging for asymptomatic cardiotoxicity.[1,2,5,48] Alternations from baseline should prompt further cardiovascular investigation and consideration of cardioprotective medication initiation. In the HERA substudy, Tn and N-terminal B-type natriuretic peptide (NT-proBNP) were significantly associated with LVEF decline, but the discrimination was poor.[49] The value of biomarkers may be in providing a negative predictive value.

Evidence of asymptomatic cardiotoxicity with a drop in EF should prompt initiation of BB and angiotensin blockade. A discussion about holding and when or if to resume the possible cardiotoxic agent should ensue. Repeat echocardiography is often obtained prior to therapy reinitiation. Recent Phase I studies provide evidence for continuing HER-2 targeted therapy during mild cardiotoxicity with BB and ACEi treatment.[50,51] These trials enrolled patients with low LVEF (40%-49%) at initiation. About 90% of patients completed HER-2 targeted therapy without cardiovascular adverse event or asymptomatic LVEF decline.

Interventions and Procedures

Reasons for cardiac interventions for oncology patients include acute coronary syndrome, structural heart disease needing transcatheter aortic valve or mitral clip, pericardial effusion, pericardial constriction, symptomatic bradycardia, and atrial fibrillation needing ablation or Watchman placement. Patients at increased risk of cardiac intervention include mediastinal radiation, previous structural heart disease, previous coronary artery disease, new Phase I study drugs, TKIs, and immunotherapy. In the setting of acute cardiovascular adverse events, differential diagnosis should remain broad with cardio-oncology patients. A thorough history should include a clear oncologic timeline of therapies, dosages, and durations. Cardiovascular disease unrelated to prior chemotherapy should always be considered.

When evaluating an oncology patient with a new cardiomyopathy, it is paramount to always exclude ischemic and other treatable cause of cardiomyopathy. Initiation of GDMT is critical for any patient with a drop in LVEF. In addition, one should consider prognosis, goal of intervention, metastasis status, platelet count, access site, and risk of bleeding. If a patient has acute coronary syndrome, one should discuss with the primary oncologist whether the patient can tolerate at least

3 months of dual antiplatelet therapy. Thrombocytopenia is a common complication of patients receiving cancer therapy. There are little evidence-based data to guide decisions on when it is safe to take a patient to a cardiac catheterization lab. In cancer, low platelets lead to increased risk of bleeding and low risk of thrombosis.[52] This phenomenon is likely linked to increased platelet activation despite low overall platelet count. Patients with thrombocytopenia developed acute myocardial infarctions, pulmonary embolisms (PEs), and strokes. General guidelines are to keep dual antiplatelet therapy for platelet counts greater than 30,000 and keep aspirin for platelet counts greater than 10,000. Overall, the benefits outweigh the risks in performing catheter-based procedures in patients with thrombocytopenia.

Oncology patients are largely undertreated for their cardiovascular disease. In one study, oncology patients with acute coronary syndrome had significantly reduced use of aspirin (46.3%), BB (48.3%), statins (20.6%), and catheter-based revascularization (3.3%).[53] Patients who did not receive appropriate therapy had significantly worse survival outcomes.

Venous Thromboembolism

VTE, including deep vein thrombosis (DVT) and PE, is a frequent complication during the course of malignancy. Patients with cancer have a four- to sevenfold increased risk of developing VTE. In the CASSINI trial, cancer patients with high VTE risk in the ambulatory setting were randomized to rivaroxaban versus placebo.[54] At 6-month endpoint, there was decreased risk of DVT, PE, and VTE-related death with a decreased risk of major bleeding. Per ASCO guidelines, high-risk outpatients should be offered thromboprophylaxis with apixaban, rivaroxaban, or low-molecular-weight heparin (LMWH) provided there are no significant bleeding risk factors or drug-drug interactions.[55] In patients who develop VTE, LMWH monotherapy is the preferred treatment per all major consensus guidelines based on the CLOT and CATCH trials.[56,57] Direct oral anticoagulants (DOACs) can be considered for VTE treatment in cancer patients with a low risk of bleeding and no drug-drug interactions with current systemic therapy. GI and urothelial cancers have higher bleeding risks. The recommended duration of treatment is at least 6 months.[55] Further studies are exploring the role of DOACs in cancer patients.

CARDIAC SURVEILLANCE AND PREVENTATIVE CARE DURING CANCER SURVIVORSHIP

In the United States, there are an estimated 15.5 million cancer survivors, and nearly 40% of Americans will be diagnosed with cancer at some point in their lifetime. With advances in cancer therapy, most patients will die from cardiovascular disease or stroke—not their cancer. Unfortunately, common comorbidities such as hypertension are not closely managed during or soon after cancer therapy. Moreover, undergoing oncologic treatment places a patient at increased lifetime risk of cardiovascular disease. Studies have evaluated cardiovascular reserve of cancer survivors by measuring peak VO_2. In one study, a breast cancer survivor with a 30% reduction in cardiorespiratory fitness was similar to a sedentary woman without cancer at age 70.[58] Hematopoietic stem cell transplant (HSCT) survivors also performed significantly worse than model prediction.[59] Increased vigilance and aggressive risk factor modification beyond standard guideline treatments are essential to reducing cardiovascular morbidity and mortality in this population. Modified risk calculators are being developed. Evidence-based guidelines are needed. Preventative cardiovascular care is the cornerstone of caring for the cancer survivor (**Algorithm 26.3**).

Cardiomyopathy

Asymptomatic high-risk patients should be screened at least once in the 6 to 12 months after completion of treatment.[1] The European Society for Molecular Oncology (ESMO) further recommends high-risk patients also have an echocardiogram at 4 and 10 years posttreatment.[2] High-risk cardiomyopathy cohorts include patients who received greater than or equal to 250 mg/m^2 anthracyclines, chest radiation greater than 30 Gy,

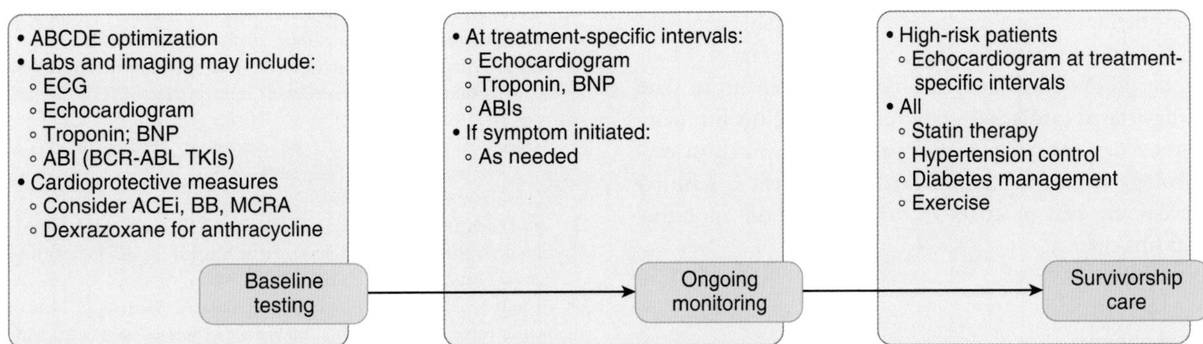

ALGORITHM 26.3 Management of oncology patient on cardiotoxic therapy: baseline testing, ongoing monitoring, and survivorship care. ABI, ankle-brachial index; ACEi, angiotensin-converting enzyme inhibitor; BB, beta-blocker; BCR-ABL TKIs, Bcr-Abl tyrosine kinase inhibitors; BNP, brain natriuretic peptide; MCRA, mineralocorticoid receptor antagonist.

or combination of anthracycline and chest radiation. Anthracycline cardiotoxicity typically occurs within 1 to 2 years of chemotherapy exposure. Patients who received chest radiation greater than 30 Gy are also at high risk of valvular disease. If cardiomyopathy is identified, GDMT should be initiated. Otherwise, ASCO recommends symptom-driven imaging for oncology survivors.

Coronary Artery Disease

Standard atherosclerotic cardiovascular disease (ASCVD) risk calculator underestimates cancer survivor cardiovascular risks. The Childhood Cancer Survivor Study developed a Cardiovascular Risk Calculator that incorporates increased risk for late cardiac effects related to prior cancer.[60,61] For hematopoietic stem cell transplantation survivors, a risk prediction model for cardiovascular disease has also been developed.[62] Statin therapy should be initiated based on this elevated risk. Underlying hyperlipidemia in cancer survivors should be treated with a statin.

Hypertension

The optimal blood pressure control is important to reduce the risk of cardiovascular complications of oncology therapy. In cancer survivors, hypertension significantly increases the risk for coronary artery disease (relative risk [RR] 6.1), heart failure (RR 19.4), valvular disease (RR 13.6), and arrhythmia (RR 6.0).[63]

Exercise Training

Exercise training is important for all cancer survivors. Vigorous exercise was associated with lower risk of cardiovascular events in survivors of Hodgkin lymphoma. Greater than 9 metabolic equivalents (METs) hours/week was associated with a 51% decrease in cardiovascular events.[58] Increasing by 6 MET hours/week was associated with a 13% reduction in rate of death from any cause. Vigorous exercise over 8 years was associated with a 40% reduction in the risk of death from any cause.[8]

RESEARCH AND FUTURE DIRECTIONS

The landscape of oncology therapies is ever changing, and cardiotoxicities are often underreported in oncology therapy trials.[64] It is important to remain up to date with current oncology therapies' cardiovascular risk and evaluate potential cardiac impact of emerging oncologic therapies. Monitoring the FDA's Medwatch can help one keep up to date with drug-related cardiac adverse events. Guidelines for many cardio-oncology scenarios do not yet exist. Research in cardio-oncology is growing exponentially. The field is refining and developing best practices in cardioprotection, monitoring, and surveillance.

KEY POINTS

- ✔ Aggressive cardiac risk factor modification is critical at all stages of caring for the cardio-oncology patient.
- ✔ Cardio-oncology guidelines are specific to the cancer treatment type and address cardiac care pretreatment, during treatment, and posttreatment.
- ✔ In the setting of acute cardiovascular adverse events, differential diagnosis should remain broad with cardio-oncology patients considering both cancer therapy–related and noncancer therapy–related etiologies.
- ✔ Oncology patients are largely undertreated for their acute cardiovascular events and suffer poor outcomes. Benefits of treating cardiovascular disease typically outweigh risks.
- ✔ Consider referring to a cardio-oncology specialty program at any point during cancer therapy for cardiac risk assessment and optimization.
- ✔ Cardio-oncology is an emerging field. Guidelines and best practices are continuously being updated.

REFERENCES

1. Armenian SH, Lacchetti C, Barac A, et al. Prevention and monitoring of cardiac dysfunction in survivors of adult cancers: American Society of Clinical Oncology clinical practice guideline. *J Clin Oncol.* 2017;35:893-911.
2. Curigliano G, Lenihan D, Fradley M, et al. Management of cardiac disease in cancer patients throughout oncological treatment: ESMO consensus recommendations. *Ann Oncol.* 2020;31:171-190.
3. Lenneman CG, Sawyer DB. Cardio-oncology: an update on cardiotoxicity of cancer-related treatment. *Circ Res.* 2016;118:1008-1020.
4. Cardinale D, Biasillo G, Cipolla CM. Curing cancer, saving the heart: a challenge that cardiooncology should not miss. *Curr Cardiol Rep.* 2016;18:51.
5. Zamorano JL, Lancellotti P, Rodriguez Munoz D, et al. 2016 ESC Position Paper on cancer treatments and cardiovascular toxicity developed under the auspices of the ESC Committee for Practice Guidelines: The Task Force for cancer treatments and cardiovascular toxicity of the European Society of Cardiology (ESC). *Eur Heart J.* 2016;37:2768-2801.
6. Guan J, Khambhati J, Jones LW, et al. Cardiology patient page. ABCDE steps for heart and vascular wellness following a prostate cancer diagnosis. *Circulation.* 2015;132:e218-e220.
7. Arnett DK, Blumenthal RS, Albert MA, et al. 2019 ACC/AHA guideline on the primary prevention of cardiovascular disease: executive summary: a report of the American College of Cardiology/American Heart Association Task Force on clinical practice guidelines. *J Am Coll Cardiol.* 2019;74:1376-1414.
8. Scott JM, Li N, Liu Q, et al. Association of exercise with mortality in adult survivors of childhood cancer. *JAMA Oncol.* 2018;4:1352-1358.
9. Henriksen PA. Anthracycline cardiotoxicity: an update on mechanisms, monitoring and prevention. *Heart.* 2018;104:971-977.
10. Kang Y, Assuncao BL, Denduluri S, et al. Symptomatic heart failure in acute leukemia patients treated with anthracyclines. *JACC: CardioOncology.* 2019;1:208-217.
11. Macedo AVS, Hajjar LA, Lyon AR, et al. Efficacy of dexrazoxane in preventing anthracycline cardiotoxicity in breast cancer. *JACC: CardioOncology.* 2019;1:68-79.
12. van Dalen EC, van den Berg H, Raphael MF, Caron HN, Kremer LC. Should anthracyclines and dexrazoxane be used for children with cancer? *Lancet Oncol.* 2011;12:12-13.
13. Shaikh F, Dupuis LL, Alexander S, Gupta A, Mertens L, Nathan PC. Cardioprotection and second malignant neoplasms associated with dexrazoxane in children receiving anthracycline chemotherapy: a systematic review and meta-analysis. *J Natl Cancer Inst.* 2016;108:djv357.
14. Avila MS, Ayub-Ferreira SM, de Barros Wanderley MR Jr, et al. Carvedilol for prevention of chemotherapy-related cardiotoxicity: the CECCY trial. *J Am Coll Cardiol.* 2018;71:2281-2290.

15. Cardinale D, Ciceri F, Latini R, et al. Anthracycline-induced cardiotoxicity: a multicenter randomised trial comparing two strategies for guiding prevention with enalapril: The International CardioOncology Society-one trial. *Eur J Cancer.* 2018;94:126-137.
16. Nakamae H, Tsumura K, Terada Y, et al. Notable effects of angiotensin II receptor blocker, valsartan, on acute cardiotoxic changes after standard chemotherapy with cyclophosphamide, doxorubicin, vincristine, and prednisolone. *Cancer.* 2005;104:2492-2498.
17. Guglin M, Krischer J, Tamura R, et al. Randomized trial of lisinopril versus carvedilol to prevent trastuzumab cardiotoxicity in patients with breast cancer. *J Am Coll Cardiol.* 2019;73:2859-2868.
18. Akpek M, Ozdogru I, Sahin O, et al. Protective effects of spironolactone against anthracycline-induced cardiomyopathy. *Eur J Heart Fail.* 2015;17:81-89.
19. Vaduganathan M, Hirji SA, Qamar A, et al. Efficacy of neurohormonal therapies in preventing cardiotoxicity in patients with cancer undergoing chemotherapy. *JACC: CardioOncology.* 2019;1:54-65.
20. Singh JC, Jhaveri K, Esteva FJ. HER2-positive advanced breast cancer: optimizing patient outcomes and opportunities for drug development. *Br J Cancer.* 2014;111:1888-1198.
21. Florido R, Smith KL, Cuomo KK, Russell SD. Cardiotoxicity from Human Epidermal Growth Factor Receptor-2 (HER2) targeted therapies. *J Am Heart Assoc.* 2017;6:e006915.
22. Waliany S, Sainani KL, Park LS, Zhang CA, Srinivas S, Witteles RM. Increase in blood pressure associated with tyrosine kinase inhibitors targeting vascular endothelial growth factor. *JACC: CardioOncology.* 2019;1:24-36.
23. Hall PS, Harshman LC, Srinivas S, Witteles RM. The frequency and severity of cardiovascular toxicity from targeted therapy in advanced renal cell carcinoma patients. *JACC Heart Fail.* 2013;1:72-78.
24. McKay RR, Rodriguez GE, Lin X, et al. Angiotensin system inhibitors and survival outcomes in patients with metastatic renal cell carcinoma. *Clin Cancer Res.* 2015;21:2471-2479.
25. Moslehi JJ, Deininger M. Tyrosine kinase inhibitor-associated cardiovascular toxicity in chronic myeloid leukemia. *J Clin Oncol.* 2015;33:4210-4218.
26. Dickerson T, Wiczer T, Waller A, et al. Hypertension and incident cardiovascular events following ibrutinib initiation. *Blood.* 2019;134:1919-1928.
27. Leong DP, Caron F, Hillis C, et al. The risk of atrial fibrillation with ibrutinib use: a systematic review and meta-analysis. *Blood.* 2016;128(1):138-140.
28. Zhang L, Jones-O'Connor M, Awadalla M, et al. Cardiotoxicity of immune checkpoint inhibitors. *Curr Treat Options Cardiovasc Med.* 2019;21:32.
29. Mahmood SS, Fradley MG, Cohen JV, et al. Myocarditis in patients treated with immune checkpoint inhibitors. *J Am Coll Cardiol.* 2018;71:1755-1764.
30. Emens LA, Ascierto PA, Darcy PK, et al. Cancer immunotherapy: opportunities and challenges in the rapidly evolving clinical landscape. *Eur J Cancer.* 2017;81:116-129.
31. Schuster SJ, Bishop MR, Tam CS, et al. Tisagenlecleucel in adult relapsed or refractory diffuse large B-cell lymphoma. *N Engl J Med.* 2019;380:45-56.
32. Neelapu SS, Locke FL, Bartlett NL, et al. Axicabtagene ciloleucel CAR T-Cell therapy in refractory large B-cell lymphoma. *N Engl J Med.* 2017;377:2531-2544.
33. Alvi RM, Frigault MJ, Fradley MG, et al. Cardiovascular events among adults treated with Chimeric Antigen Receptor T-Cells (CAR-T). *J Am Coll Cardiol.* 2019;74:3099-3108.
34. Gandolfi S, Laubach JP, Hideshima T, Chauhan D, Anderson KC, Richardson PG. The proteasome and proteasome inhibitors in multiple myeloma. *Cancer Metastasis Rev.* 2017;36:561-584.
35. Waxman AJ, Clasen S, Hwang WT, et al. Carfilzomib-associated cardiovascular adverse events: a systematic review and meta-analysis. *JAMA Oncol.* 2018;4:e174519.
36. Cornell RF, Ky B, Weiss BM, et al. Prospective study of cardiac events during proteasome inhibitor therapy for relapsed multiple myeloma. *J Clin Oncol.* 2019;37:1946-1955.
37. Levine GN, D'Amico AV, Berger P, et al. Androgen-deprivation therapy in prostate cancer and cardiovascular risk: a science advisory from the American Heart Association, American Cancer Society, and American Urological Association: endorsed by the American Society for Radiation Oncology. *Circulation.* 2010;121:833-840.
38. Gupta D, Lee Chuy K, Yang JC, Bates M, Lombardo M, Steingart RM. Cardiovascular and metabolic effects of androgen-deprivation therapy for prostate cancer. *J Oncol Pract.* 2018;14:580-587.
39. Melloni C, Nelson A. Effect of androgen deprivation therapy on metabolic complications and cardiovascular risk. *J Cardiovasc Transl Res.* 2019;13(3):451-462.
40. Keating NL, O'Malley AJ, Smith MR. Diabetes and cardiovascular disease during androgen deprivation therapy for prostate cancer. *J Clin Oncol.* 2006;24:4448-4456.
41. Desai MY, Jellis CL, Kotecha R, Johnston DR, Griffin BP. Radiation-associated cardiac disease: a practical approach to diagnosis and management. *JACC Cardiovasc Imaging.* 2018;11:1132-1149.
42. van Nimwegen FA, Schaapveld M, Cutter DJ, et al. Radiation dose-response relationship for risk of coronary heart disease in survivors of Hodgkin lymphoma. *J Clin Oncol.* 2016;34:235-243.
43. Darby SC, Ewertz M, McGale P, et al. Risk of ischemic heart disease in women after radiotherapy for breast cancer. *N Engl J Med.* 2013;368:987-998.
44. Hull MC, Morris CG, Pepine CJ, Mendenhall NP. Valvular dysfunction and carotid, subclavian, and coronary artery disease in survivors of Hodgkin lymphoma treated with radiation therapy. *JAMA.* 2003;290:2831-2837.
45. Atkins KM, Rawal B, Chaunzwa TL, et al. Cardiac radiation dose, cardiac disease, and mortality in patients with lung cancer. *J Am Coll Cardiol.* 2019;73:2976-2987.
46. Oikonomou EK, Kokkinidis DG, Kampaktsis PN, et al. Assessment of prognostic value of left ventricular global longitudinal strain for early prediction of chemotherapy-induced cardiotoxicity: a systematic review and meta-analysis. *JAMA Cardiol.* 2019;4(10):1007-1018.
47. Plana JC, Galderisi M, Barac A, et al. Expert consensus for multimodality imaging evaluation of adult patients during and after cancer therapy: a report from the American Society of Echocardiography and the European Association of Cardiovascular Imaging. *J Am Soc Echocardiogr.* 2014;27:911-939.
48. Demissei BG, Hubbard RA, Zhang L, et al. Changes in cardiovascular biomarkers with breast cancer therapy and associations with cardiac dysfunction. *J Am Heart Assoc.* 2020;9:e014708.
49. Zardavas D, Suter TM, Van Veldhuisen DJ, et al. Role of Troponins I and T and N-terminal prohormone of brain natriuretic peptide in monitoring cardiac safety of patients with early-stage human epidermal growth factor receptor 2-positive breast cancer receiving trastuzumab: a herceptin adjuvant study cardiac marker substudy. *J Clin Oncol.* 2017;35:878-884.
50. Lynce F, Barac A, Geng X, et al. Prospective evaluation of the cardiac safety of HER2-targeted therapies in patients with HER2-positive breast cancer and compromised heart function: the SAFE-HEaRt study. *Breast Cancer Res Treat.* 2019;175:595-603.
51. Leong DP, Cosman T, Alhussein MM, et al. Safety of continuing trastuzumab despite mild cardiotoxicity. A Phase I Trial. *JACC: CardioOncology.* 2019;1:1-10.
52. Iliescu C, Durand JB, Kroll M. Cardiovascular interventions in thrombocytopenic cancer patients. *Tex Heart Inst J.* 2011;38:259-260.
53. Yusuf SW, Daraban N, Abbasi N, Lei X, Durand JB, Daher IN. Treatment and outcomes of acute coronary syndrome in the cancer population. *Clin Cardiol.* 2012;35:443-450.
54. Khorana AA, Soff GA, Kakkar AK, et al. Rivaroxaban for thromboprophylaxis in high-risk ambulatory patients with cancer. *N Engl J Med.* 2019;380:720-728.
55. Key NS, Bohlke K, Falanga A. Venous thromboembolism prophylaxis and treatment in patients with cancer: ASCO clinical practice guideline update summary. *J Oncol Pract.* 2019;15:661-664.
56. Lee AYY, Levine MN, Baker RI, et al. Low-molecular-weight heparin versus a coumarin for the prevention of recurrent venous thromboembolism in patients with cancer. *N Engl J Med.* 2003;349:146-153.
57. Lee AYY, Kamphuisen PW, Meyer G, et al. Tinzaparin vs warfarin for treatment of acute venous thromboembolism in patients with active cancer: a randomized clinical trial. *JAMA.* 2015;314:677-686.

58. Jones LW, Courneya KS, Mackey JR, et al. Cardiopulmonary function and age-related decline across the breast cancer survivorship continuum. *J Clin Oncol.* 2012;30:2530-2537.
59. Armenian SH, Horak D, Scott JM, et al. Cardiovascular function in long-term hematopoietic cell transplantation survivors. *Biol Blood Marrow Transplant.* 2017;23:700-705.
60. Chow EJ, Chen Y, Hudson MM, et al. Prediction of ischemic heart disease and stroke in survivors of childhood cancer. *J Clin Oncol.* 2018;36:44-52.
61. Armenian SH, Hudson MM, Mulder RL, et al. Recommendations for cardiomyopathy surveillance for survivors of childhood cancer: a report from the International Late Effects of Childhood Cancer Guideline Harmonization Group. *Lancet Oncol.* 2015;16:e123-e136.
62. Armenian SH, Yang D, Teh JB, et al. Prediction of cardiovascular disease among hematopoietic cell transplantation survivors. *Blood Adv.* 2018;2:1756-1764.
63. Armstrong GT, Oeffinger KC, Chen Y, et al. Modifiable risk factors and major cardiac events among adult survivors of childhood cancer. *J Clin Oncol.* 2013;31:3673-3680.
64. Bonsu JM, Guha A, Charles L, et al. Reporting of cardiovascular events in clinical trials supporting FDA approval of contemporary cancer therapies. *J Am Coll Cardiol.* 2020;75:620-628.

CHAPTER 27

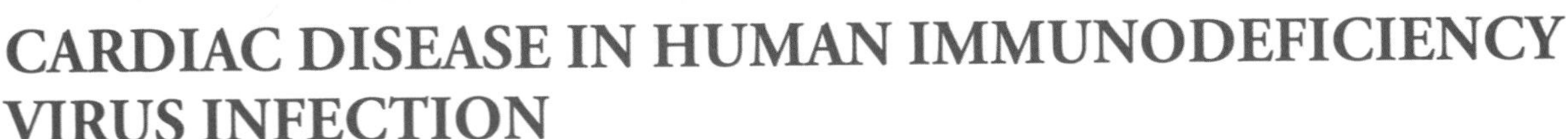

CARDIAC DISEASE IN HUMAN IMMUNODEFICIENCY VIRUS INFECTION

Timir K. Paul and Sukhdeep Bhogal

INTRODUCTION

Since the introduction of antiretroviral therapy (ART) in the mid-1990s, human immunodeficiency virus (HIV) has transformed into a chronic disease with decreased mortality rates. With improved life expectancy, these patients are constantly at risk of being exposed to long-term non–acquired immunodeficiency syndrome (AIDS)-related chronic comorbid diseases such as cardiovascular disease (CVD). Studies have shown that HIV infection poses the increased risk of myocardial infarction (MI), heart failure, and stroke.[1-3] The recent data show the rates of death because of non–HIV attributable causes, such as CVD, have increased in comparison to HIV attributable causes.[4] The underlying mechanism for augmented HIV-associated CVD risk is not clear; however, it extends beyond the traditional risk factors for atherosclerosis. So far, our understanding of this high-risk group is principally based on the observational data, and the randomized controlled studies have largely been underpowered to identify clinical CVD outcomes. This chapter summarizes the epidemiology, pathophysiology, clinical signs and symptoms, angiographic findings, management including ART, and prevention of CVD in HIV-infected patients.

Epidemiology

Latest data from the Joint United Nations Programme on HIV/AIDS (UNAIDS) report that approximately 2.4 million patients are living with HIV in United States and Europe, and it has contributed to about 1.1 million deaths globally in 2015.[5] Studies investigating HIV-infected patients showed they are at increased risk of CVD when compared to controls. A cohort analysis has shown that cumulative CVD risk was estimated to be at 20.5% in persons infected with HIV versus 12.8% in the general U.S. population.[6] Another observational study by Kaiser Permanente California Medical group showed HIV-positive patients are at high risk for coronary heart disease (adjusted relative risk [RR] 1.2 [95% confidence interval [CI] 1.1-1.4; $P < 0.001$]) and MI (adjusted RR 1.4 [95% CI 1.3-1.7; $P < 0.001$]) as compared to HIV-negative population.[7] Similarly, another data on 28,000 Veterans Administration (VA) patients showed significantly increased risk of acute MI in HIV-infected patients with an adjusted hazard ratio (HR) of 1.94 (95% CI 1.58-2.37) as compared to non–HIV-infected patients.[8] Thus, the data suggest that HIV status confers increased risk of CVD independent of traditional risk factors.

Potential Mechanistic Factors

Conventional risk factors, such as smoking, hypertension, obesity, dyslipidemia, insulin resistance, and diabetes, are more prevalent in HIV-infected patients than in noninfected patients and is related to increased CVD risk in this population.[9] The additional risk factors, such as HIV-related immune dysfunction, systemic inflammation, disruption of lipid metabolism, and antiretroviral drug effects, further increase the risk of atherosclerosis in these patients.[10] Besides these, hepatitis C coinfection, low $CD4^+$ T-cell counts, high viral ribonucleic acid (RNA) levels, renal disease, and anemia may also contribute to increased CVD risk.[11] Thus, the presence of multiple risk factors that synergistically escalate the risk of CVD makes it difficult to discern the impact of individual risk factor (**Algorithm 27.1**).

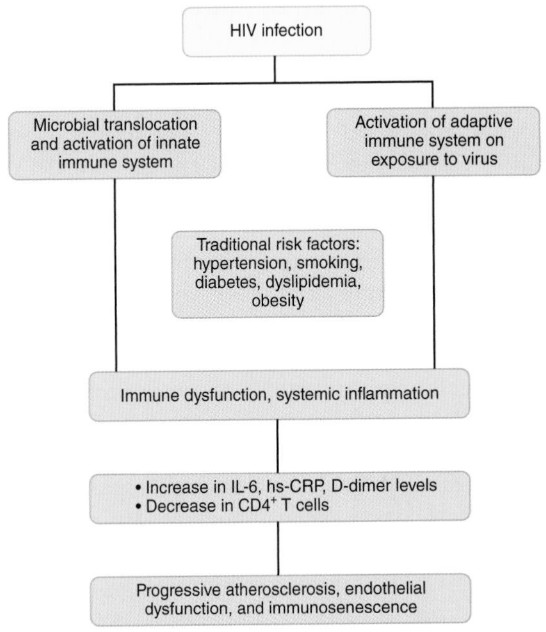

ALGORITHM 27.1 HIV and cardiovascular risk factors. HIV, human immunodeficiency virus; IL-6, interleukin-6; hs-CRP, high-sensitivity C-reactive protein.

PATHOGENESIS: HUMAN IMMUNODEFICIENCY VIRUS–RELATED IMMUNE ACTIVATION AND CARDIOVASCULAR DISEASE

Although the mechanism of increased CVD in HIV-infected patients is incompletely understood and is likely multifactorial, its core is thought to be progressive atherosclerosis. The evidence suggests that onset of atherosclerosis is driven by activation of innate immune system that plays an important role in the pathogenesis. One of the underlying mechanisms is believed to be aberration of intestinal barrier allowing lipopolysaccharide to enter systemic circulation leading to immune system activation.[12] Lipopolysaccharide, a microbial product, is considered as an essential marker of microbial translocation, which binds with lipopolysaccharide binding protein (LBP) and transfers into soluble CD14, leading to nuclear factor-kappa B (NF-κB) activation and cytokine production.[12,13] Soluble CD163, another circulating marker expressed on monocytes and macrophages and has been independently associated with noncalcified plaques among asymptomatic young men in previous studies, is meaningfully correlated to the extent of arterial inflammation in HIV infection.[14] Both microbial translocation and macrophage activation (soluble CD14 and soluble CD163) are associated with subclinical atherosclerosis progression in HIV patients.[15] Furthermore, the activation of adaptive immune system occurs early during acute HIV infection through the T-cell receptors on both CD4 and CD8 after the initial exposure to the virus.[16] Persistent T-cell activation leads to exhaustion and senescence of the immune system leading to declined naive CD4 and CD8 T-cell numbers. This eventually leads to a gradual depletion of total CD4 counts that has been independently linked to increased risk of atherosclerosis.[17]

Systemic Inflammation

The role of inflammation as a central pathophysiologic factor for atherosclerosis is well established.[18] The analysis of Strategies for Management of Antiretroviral Therapy (SMART) trial confirmed that interleukin (IL)-6 and D-dimer are strong predictors of mortality in these patients.[19] Chronic upregulation of inflammatory pathways leads to excess cytokines, such as IL-1β, IL-6, and tumor necrosis factor (TNF)-α; endothelial dysfunction and infiltration of immune cells foster more progressive atherosclerosis.[20] Moreover, increased platelet activation and coagulopathy in these patients further promote vascular thrombosis.[18] Studies have revealed that the level of certain inflammatory markers, including high-sensitivity C-reactive protein (hs-CRP), IL-6, D-dimer, and cystatin C, remains high despite ART.[21] The inflammatory response is observed from the very initial stage of infection and persists throughout its course even on ART and plays a major role in the pathogenesis.

Human Immunodeficiency Virus and Subclinical Atherosclerosis

HIV patients are at increased risk of atherosclerosis compared to the general population. A systematic review in 2009 found that HIV patients have increased carotid intima–media thickness (CIMT, a surrogate marker of atherosclerosis), but no association with carotid plaque and coronary artery calcium (CAC) was observed.[22] A longitudinal cohort study showed CIMT and CAC progressed over 6 years follow-up in HIV patients.[23] However, a 96-week prospective cohort study found that CIMT progressed significantly but similarly in both ART-naive HIV-infected patients and matched healthy controls.[24]

Although several studies showed no higher prevalence of CAC in HIV patients compared to controls, computed tomography angiography (CTA) has shed new insights on this topic. Observational studies have shown more prevalence of noncalcified plaques in HIV status compared to controls.[25] Another meta-analysis of nine studies also showed similar burden of coronary artery stenosis and calcified plaques compared to controls but higher rates of noncalcified plaques among HIV-infected individuals.[26] These noncalcified plaques have a lipid-rich, inflammatory core and are prone to rupture that may be an explanation for younger age of presentation with acute coronary syndrome (ACS) among HIV patients compared to the general population. The detection of arterial inflammation via 18-fluorodeoxyglucose (^{18}FDG) uptake can be used as a marker of early atheroma formation. One study using Framingham risk score (FRS) did show higher aortic inflammation in HIV-infected patients in comparison to matched controls.[14]

Taking together, HIV status does seem to confer increased risk of CIMT and noncalcified plaques based on observational data but larger studies are needed, and the data on the effect of ART on their progression remain unclear. However, one randomized controlled trial did show slow progression of CIMT in atazanavir/ritonavir group compared to darunavir/ritonavir group.[27]

CLINICAL PRESENTATION

The clinical presentation of CVD in HIV-infected patients could range from silent ischemia to ACS. Based on published data, the most common presentation was ST-elevation MI, followed by non–ST-elevation MI and unstable angina.[28,29] HIV patients tend to be on average a decade younger than the uninfected individuals and are more likely to be young men (<50 years), smoker, having dyslipidemia, with lengthier duration (>8 years) of HIV, and taking ART.[28]

HIV also poses increased risk of heart failure independent of MI. A cohort study in VA population of approximately 98,000 patients showed HIV-infected patients are at increased risk of heart failure with persevered ejection fraction (HFpEF), borderline HFpEF, and heart failure with reduced ejection fraction (HFrEF).[1] HFrEF in these patients could manifest even decades earlier than would be expected in the general population.[1] A recent retrospective Veterans Affairs cohort study demonstrated a higher risk of hospitalization and mortality in HIV-positive patients, and worse outcomes were seen in individuals with higher viral count, lower CD4 count, and decreased ejection fraction.[30] A systematic review and meta-analysis showed these patients are at increased risk of both ischemic (HR 1.27, 1.15-1.39) and hemorrhagic stroke (HR 2.20, 1.61-3.02).[2] Immunosuppression and high viral load are considered as independent risks for ischemic stroke and peripheral arterial disease in this population.[31] Taken together, presence of HIV infection itself should be considered as a vascular risk factor, and future strategies should be tailored to reduce the risk and prevention of vascular events in this population.[2]

Angiographic Findings

Angiographically, HIV patients are more likely to have single-vessel disease than three-vessel disease and primarily underwent percutaneous coronary intervention (PCI) followed by coronary artery bypass grafting.[28,32] A meta-analysis of six studies showed that these patients have similar recurrent MI, target vessel revascularization, target lesion revascularization, major adverse cardiac events (MACE), cardiac death, all-cause mortality, and stroke over a follow-up of 1 to 3 years.[33] Also, PCI is considered as a safe treatment strategy for revascularization in HIV-positive patients in comparison to control population without significant differences in terms of restenosis.[34] A retrospective study showed that after multivariate adjustment, drug-eluting stents (DESs) have lower rate of MACE compared to bare metal stents (BMSs) over a mean follow-up of 3.1 years.[35] Similar results were seen in another post hoc analysis, demonstrating the superiority of DES in these patients.[34] Of note, HIV patients who had higher rate of restenosis were found to have excessive levels of hs-CRP and $CD8^+$ T cells[36] as well, which should be monitored carefully in patients undergoing PCI.

MANAGEMENT OF HUMAN IMMUNODEFICIENCY VIRUS PATIENTS

Antiretroviral Therapy

The ART is the combination of any three antiretroviral drugs that usually consist of two nucleoside reverse transcriptase inhibitor (NRTI) and a protease inhibitor (PI) or nonnucleoside reverse transcriptase inhibitor (NNRTI) and/or an integrase inhibitor. The use of ART has been associated with increased life expectancy at the expense of morbidity in HIV patients.[37] Initially, a prospective observational study revealed an increased risk of MI in patients with HIV with longer exposure to combination ART.[38] There is a consensus that the risk of cardiovascular events increases with increased duration of ART. However, SMART, a randomized controlled trial that examined $CD4^+$ guided interruption versus continuous ART in HIV patients, clearly validated that the use of episodic ART was deleterious and associated with significantly increased risk of opportunistic diseases/infections or death from any cause and adverse events including CVD compared to continuous ART.[37] A systematic review also demonstrated that the use of ART in the HIV population was a consistent risk for cardiovascular outcomes,[2] but overall benefits seem to supersede the risks and improve mortality. Thus, HIV infection itself seems to increase the risk of CVD but to what extent is a topic of debate.

ART has been linked with various metabolic disorders in HIV patients. These metabolic abnormalities resemble those seen in metabolic syndrome, namely dyslipidemia, insulin resistance, and lipodystrophy, and it is a growing concern that metabolic derangements associated with HIV and ART lead to increased risk of CVD events.[19] Treatment with stavudine, lamivudine, zidovudine, didanosine, and PIs (indinavir, lopinavir/ritonavir, and efavirenz) has been allied to alteration of glucose metabolism, insulin resistance, and diabetes mellitus.[39,40] Strategic Timing of Antiretroviral Treatment (START) trial showed that immediate ART in patients with $CD4^+$ greater than 500 cells/mm^3 led to increased total cholesterol, high-density lipoprotein cholesterol, and low-density lipoprotein cholesterol (LDL-C) at 3-year follow-up[41]; however, long-term results are awaited.

Data Collection on Adverse Events on anti-HIV Drugs (DAD)[42] and French Hospital Database on HIV (FHDH)[43] are two observational studies with sufficient exposure to PIs, which showed that indinavir and lopinavir/ritonavir in DAD study and amprenavir/fosamprenavir in FHDH study except saquinavir were associated with increased risk of MI. This finding remained significant even after adjustment of lipid abnormalities in subgroup analysis, revealing the independent impact of PIs on MI.[42] However, VA population analysis revealed that ART was not associated with MI after adjustment for other risk factors.[8] Similarly, the risk of MI with abacavir use remains controversial, and recent guidelines recommend to use it with caution or use alternative tenofovir-containing regimen in patients with established CVD.[44] These discrepancies remain inexplicable, and further studies are warranted for better understanding of the underlying mechanism to elucidate the role of ART in increased risk of CVD in this population. The degree to which HIV patients derive benefit from ART to reduce CVD risk remains elusive; however, initiation of ART is warranted as soon as diagnosis of HIV is established.[44] Antiretroviral drugs and their associated cardiovascular risk are summarized in **Table 27.1**.

Management of Cardiovascular Risk Factors

Statins should be considered because they significantly reduce MACE in patients even with low levels of LDL-C (<130 mg/dL) and elevated markers of inflammation such as hs-CRP.[45] One of the largest trials of statins in HIV patients, INTREPID (HIV-Infected Patients and Treatment With Pitavastatin vs Pravastatin for Dyslipidemia), included 252 patients randomized to pitavastatin 4 mg and pravastatin 40 mg daily and demonstrated pitavastatin led to greater reduction in markers of arterial inflammation (soluble CD14 and oxidized LDL-C).[46] However, the use of statins in HIV is usually complicated by potential drug-drug interactions, and they are being underused. Recent data suggest more benign interactions with newer statins and ART.[47] Statins that metabolized through cytochrome P-450 system (CYP3A4 pathway), such as simvastatin and lovastatin, should be avoided in HIV patients as PIs inhibit CYP3A4 system, whereas NNRTIs induce it.[48] Low-dose atorvastatin, pitavastatin, pravastatin, and

TABLE 27.1 Antiretroviral Drugs and Their Associated Cardiovascular Risk

Drugs	Cardiovascular Risk Based on Available Data (Observational)
Protease inhibitors Lopinavir	Increased CVD risk based on DAD and FHDH study
Indinavir	Increased CVD risk based on DAD study
Amprenavir	Increased CVD risk based on FHDH study, although it was underpowered
Fosamprenavir	Increased CVD risk based on FHDH study, although it was underpowered
Saquinavir	Not associated with MI
Darunavir	Increased risk of CVD based on 2018 DAD data
Atazanavir	Not associated with increased risk of CVD based on 2018 DAD data
Ritonavir	Not used alone, used as a booster with other PIs
Nelfinavir	Not associated with MI
Nonnucleoside reverse transcriptase inhibitor (NNRTI) Efavirenz, nevirapine	Not associated with MI
Nucleoside reverse transcriptase inhibitors (NRTIs)	Abacavir and didanosine have been linked with an increased risk for MI based on DAD data but discrepant results based on other studies

CVD, cardiovascular; DAD, Data Collection on Adverse Events on Anti-HIV Drugs; FHDH, French Hospital Database on HIV; MI: myocardial infarction; PIs, protease inhibitors.

TABLE 27.2 Preventive Measures to Mitigate the Increased Risk of Cardiovascular Disease in HIV

Antiretroviral Therapy	Start as Soon as the Diagnosis Is Established
Risk assessment tool	No risk assessment tool is available, currently available ASCVD risk score likely to underestimate the CVD risk
Lifestyle modifications	Physical exercise Smoking cessation Weight loss
Diet	ACC/AHA dietary guidelines—Mediterranean diet rich in vegetables, nuts, fruits, whole grains, fish, and vegetable fiber
Statins	Recent expert consensus gives recommendations of starting statins if ASCVD risk score ≥5% Avoid statins that metabolize through CYP3A4 pathway, such as simvastatin and lovastatin (low-dose atorvastatin 10 mg can be used).
PCSK9 inhibitors	Favorable risk profile, under investigation in new trials
Diabetes and hypertension	Current ACC/AHA guidelines on HbA1c goal of 6.5%-7% and blood pressure goal of <130/80 mm Hg should be considered

ACC/AHA, American College of Cardiology/American Heart Association; ASCVD: atherosclerotic cardiovascular disease; CVD, cardiovascular disease; CYP3A4, cytochrome P-450 3A4; HbA1c: hemoglobin A1c; PCSK9, proprotein convertase subtilisin/kexin type 9.

rosuvastatin are generally considered safe in these patients. As the 2013 American College of Cardiology/American Heart Association (ACC/AHA) guidelines based on pooled cohort equation do not specifically address HIV patients, it is likely to underestimate the risk as these patients are in general considered high risk given multiple risk factors.[47] Recent expert panel of ACC recommend to start statins with an estimated 10-year atherosclerotic cardiovascular disease (ASCVD) risk score greater than or equal to 5%.[47]

PCSK9 (proprotein convertase subtilisin/kexin type 9) are monoclonal antibodies with minimal drug interactions with ART that have shown favorable risk profile in HIV-infected patients.[49] A recent randomized, double-blind controlled trial (BEIJERINCK) comparing monthly subcutaneous evolocumab with placebo showed that it is a safe and an effective therapy for lowering atherogenic lipoproteins in HIV-infected individuals taking maximally tolerated statin therapy.[50]

Another clinical trial investigating the impact of PCSK9 on vascular inflammation, endothelial dysfunction, and noncalcified plaque using alirocumab is under phase 3 of investigation (ClinicalTrials.gov Identifier: NCT03207945; EPIC-HIV study [Effect of PCSK9 Inhibition on Cardiovascular Risk in Treated HIV Infection]). REPRIEVE is also an ongoing prospective, randomized, placebo-controlled trial with pitavastatin for primary prevention of MACE in low-to-moderate conventional risk HIV patients (ClinicalTrials.gov Identifier: NCT02344290). A low threshold to start statin therapy should be considered in HIV-infected patients while paying careful attention to drug-drug interactions in this high-risk group. More vigilance among clinicians would certainly be required for earlier detection and better management of chronic comorbid diseases related to HIV. The strategies of risk factor management and primary prevention are summarized in **Table 27.2**.

Prevention

Even without major cardiovascular risk factors, HIV status is still associated with twice the risk of acute MI compared to uninfected controls.[51] These patients should be evaluated for cardiac risk factors as soon as the diagnosis is established. The primary intervention starts with adherence to lifestyle changes with regular physical activity. A randomized trial on sedentary HIV patients who are at high risk for CVD demonstrated standardized group sessions focusing on behavioral lifestyle modification and was successful in reducing body weight and carbohydrate consumption, although it did not increase physical activity[52] and no consensus on diet in HIV patients and adherence to ACC/AHA dietary guidelines is recommended. Additionally, given smoking is more prevalent in this group, counseling on smoking cessation should be an early step to reduce the risk of future complications. Patient education regarding their disease, better management of concomitant comorbid diseases including diabetes and hypertension, and weight loss in obese patients should be encouraged. There is lack of data on the use of aspirin in reducing CVD. One randomized trial showed no difference in reducing soluble CD14, D-dimer, and T-cell or monocyte activation after 12 weeks of 100 and 300 mg aspirin compared to placebo.[53] Based on ACC/AHA guidelines in the general population, aspirin is not recommended for primary prevention of CVD in these patients.

RESEARCH AND FUTURE DIRECTIONS

We have made considerable progression in understanding HIV-associated CVD over the last two decades. However, the most evidence on these patients is from observational studies, so larger randomized studies are needed for better understanding of their risk profile and management options. Despite effective viral suppression with ART, continued inflammation tends to increase the risk of MI, stroke, and heart failure in these patients. Future studies should also focus on better understanding of pathophysiology of diseases, assessment of biomarkers, and prevention of heart failure and MI in these patients. We should also consider improved CVD risk assessment screening tools that incorporate HIV status for superior decision-making in this high-risk population.

KEY POINTS

- ✔ HIV has become a chronic disease with the advent of ART and is associated with increased risk of chronic diseases including CVD.
- ✔ The underlying mechanism is believed to be immune system dysregulation, systemic inflammation, and ART itself. Traditional risk factors, such as smoking, hypertension, obesity, dyslipidemia, insulin resistance, and diabetes, are more prevalent in HIV-infected patients than in uninfected patients.
- ✔ These patients should be evaluated for cardiac risk factors as soon as the diagnosis is established. The currently available tools for risk assessment underestimate the risk of CVD in these patients. CAC with CTA for assessing soft plaque may be helpful in risk stratification of intermediate risk group patients.
- ✔ Substantial importance to lifestyle changes, including smoking cessation, weight loss, dietary changes, control of hypertension, and diabetes, should be given as a part of initial management strategy.
- ✔ ART should be started as soon as diagnosis is made. Statins play an invaluable role in reducing the risk of CVD in these patients, and clinicians should have low threshold to start them after careful review of drug-drug interactions with ART. Better understanding and vigilance are required on the part of clinicians to prevent the long-term comorbid complications of HIV including CVD.
- ✔ There is no study that directly evaluated the effect of aspirin in reducing CVD in HIV patients. Based on ACC/AHA guidelines in the general population, aspirin is not recommended in these patients for primary CVD prevention.

REFERENCES

1. Freiberg MS, Chang C-CH, Skanderson M, et al. Association between HIV infection and the risk of heart failure with reduced ejection fraction and preserved ejection fraction in the antiretroviral therapy era: results from the veterans aging cohort study. *JAMA Cardiol.* 2017;2(5):536-546.
2. Gutierrez J, Albuquerque ALA, Falzon L. HIV infection as vascular risk: a systematic review of the literature and meta-analysis. *PLoS One.* 2017;12(5):e0176686.
3. Garg H, Joshi A, Mukherjee D, et al. Cardiovascular complications of HIV infection and treatment. *Cardiovasc Hematol Agents Med Chem.* 2013;11(1):58-66. doi:10.2174/1871525711311010010
4. Adih WK, Selik RM, Hall HI, Babu AS, Song R. Associations and trends in cause-specific rates of death among persons reported with HIV infection, 23 U.S. jurisdictions, through 2011. *Open AIDS J.* 2016;10:144-157.
5. UNAIDS. Global AIDS update 2016. https://www.unaids.org/sites/default/files/media_asset/global-AIDS-update-2016_en.pdf
6. Losina E, Hyle EP, Borre ED, et al. Projecting 10-year, 20-year, and lifetime risks of cardiovascular disease in persons living with human immunodeficiency virus in the United States. *Clin Infect Dis.* 2017;65(8):1266-1271.
7. Klein D, Leyden WA, Xu L, et al. Contribution of immunodeficiency to CHD: cohort study of HIV+ and HIV− Kaiser Permanente members. Program and Abstracts of the 18th Conference on Retroviruses and Opportunistic Infections; February 27-March 2, 2011; Boston, MA.
8. Freiberg MS, McGinnis K, Butt A, et al. HIV is associated with clinically confirmed myocardial infarction after adjustment for smoking and other risk factors. Program and Abstracts of the 18th Conference on Retroviruses and Opportunistic Infections; February 27-March 2, 2011; Boston, MA.
9. Saves M, Chene G, Ducimetiere P, et al. Risk factors for coronary heart disease in patients treated for human immunodeficiency virus infection compared with the general population. *Clin Infect Dis.* 2003;37(2):292-298.
10. McGettrick PMC, Mallon PWG. HIV and cardiovascular disease: defining the unmeasured risk. *Lancet HIV.* 2018;5(6):e267-e269.
11. Freiberg MS, Chang C-C H, Kuller LH, et al. HIV infection and the risk of acute myocardial infarction. *JAMA Intern Med.* 2013;173(8):614-622.
12. Brenchley JM, Price DA, Schacker TW, et al. Microbial translocation is a cause of systemic immune activation in chronic HIV infection. *Nat Med.* 2006;12(12):1365-1371.
13. Anderson KV. Toll signaling pathways in the innate immune response. *Curr Opin Immunol.* 2000;12(1):13-19.
14. Subramanian S, Tawakol A, Burdo TH, et al. Arterial inflammation in patients with HIV. *JAMA.* 2012;308(4):379-386
15. Kelesidis T, Kendall MA, Yang OO, Hodis HN, Currier JS. Biomarkers of microbial translocation and macrophage activation: association with

progression of subclinical atherosclerosis in HIV-1 infection. *J Infect Dis.* 2012;206(10):1558-1567.
16. McMichael AJ, Borrow P, Tomaras GD, Goonetilleke N, Haynes BF. The immune response during acute HIV-1 infection: clues for vaccine development. *Nat Rev Immunol.* 2010;10(1):11-23.
17. Lichtenstein KA, Armon C, Buchacz K, et al. Low CD4$^+$ T cell count is a risk factor for cardiovascular disease events in the HIV outpatient study. *Clin Infect Dis.* 2010;51(4):435-447.
18. Rahman F, Martin SS, Whelton SP, Mody FV, Vaishnav J, McEvoy JW. Inflammation and cardiovascular disease risk: a case study of HIV and inflammatory joint disease. *Am J Med.* 2018;131(4):442.e1-e8.
19. Kuller LH, Tracy R, Belloso W, et al. Inflammatory and coagulation biomarkers and mortality in patients with HIV infection. *PLoS Med.* 2008;5(10):e203.
20. Nasi M, De Biasi S, Gibellini L, et al. Ageing and inflammation in patients with HIV infection. *Clin Exp Immunol.* 2017;187(1):44-52.
21. Neuhaus J, Jacobs DR Jr, Baker JV, et al. Markers of inflammation, coagulation, and renal function are elevated in adults with HIV infection. *J Infect Dis.* 2010;201(12):1788-1795.
22. Hulten E, Mitchell J, Scally J, Gibbs B, Villines TC. HIV positivity, protease inhibitor exposure and subclinical atherosclerosis: a systematic review and meta-analysis of observational studies. *Heart.* 2009;95(22):1826-1835.
23. Volpe GE, Tang AM, Polak JF, Mangili A, Skinner SC, Wanke CA. Progression of carotid intima-media thickness and coronary artery calcium over 6 years in an HIV-infected cohort. *J Acquir Immune Defic Syndr.* 2013;64(1):51-57.
24. Hileman CO, Longenecker CT, Carman TL, McComsey GA. C-reactive protein predicts 96-week carotid intima media thickness progression in HIV-infected adults naive to antiretroviral therapy. *J Acquir Immune Defic Syndr.* 2014;65(3):340-344.
25. Fitch KV, Lo J, Abbara S, et al. Increased coronary artery calcium score and noncalcified plaque among HIV-infected men: relationship to metabolic syndrome and cardiac risk parameters. *J Acquir Immune Defic Syndr.* 2010;55(4):495-499.
26. D'Ascenzo F, Cerrato E, Calcagno A, et al. High prevalence at computed coronary tomography of non-calcified plaques in asymptomatic HIV patients treated with HAART: a meta-analysis. *Atherosclerosis.* 2015;240(1):197-204.
27. Stein JH, Ribaudo HJ, Hodis HN, et al. A prospective, randomized clinical trial of antiretroviral therapies on carotid wall thickness. *AIDS.* 2015;29(14):1775-1783.
28. Boccara F, Lang S, Meuleman C, et al. HIV and coronary heart disease: time for a better understanding. *J Am Coll Cardiol.* 2013;61(5):511-523.
29. Varriale P, Saravi G, Hernandez E, Carbon F. Acute myocardial infarction in patients infected with human immunodeficiency virus. *Am Heart J.* 2004;147(1):55-59.
30. Erqou S, Jiang L, Choudhary G, et al. Heart failure outcomes and associated factors among veterans with human immunodeficiency virus infection. *JACC Heart Fail.* 2020;8(6):501-511.
31. Ye Y, Zeng Y, Li X, et al. HIV infection: an independent risk factor of peripheral arterial disease. *J Acquir Immune Defic Syndr.* 2010;53(2):276-278.
32. Ambrose JA, Gould RB, Kurian DC, et al. Frequency of and outcome of acute coronary syndromes in patients with human immunodeficiency virus infection. *Am J Cardiol.* 2003;92(3):301-303.
33. Bundhun PK, Pursun M, Huang W-Q. Does infection with human immunodeficiency virus have any impact on the cardiovascular outcomes following percutaneous coronary intervention: a systematic review and meta-analysis. *BMC Cardiovasc Disord.* 2017;17(1):190.
34. Badr S, Minha Sa, Kitabata H, et al. Safety and long-term outcomes after percutaneous coronary intervention in patients with human immunodeficiency virus. *Catheter Cardiovasc Interv.* 2015;85(2):192-198.
35. Ren X, Trilesskaya M, Kwan DM, Nguyen K, Shaw RE, Hui PY. Comparison of outcomes using bare metal versus drug-eluting stents in coronary artery disease patients with and without human immunodeficiency virus infection. *Am J Cardiol.* 2009;104(2):216-222.
36. Schneider S, Spinner CD, Cassese S, et al. Association of increased CD8$^+$ and persisting C-reactive protein levels with restenosis in HIV patients after coronary stenting. *AIDS.* 2016;30(9):1413-1421.
37. Strategies for Management of Antiretroviral Therapy (SMART) Study Group; El-Sadr WM, Lundgren JD, Neaton JD, et al. CD4$^+$ count–guided interruption of antiretroviral treatment. *N Engl J Med.* 2006;355(22):2283-2296.
38. Friis-Møller N, Sabin CA, Weber R, et al. Combination antiretroviral therapy and the risk of myocardial infarction. *N Engl J Med.* 2003;349(21):1993-2003.
39. van Vonderen MG, Blumer RM, Hassink EA, et al. Insulin sensitivity in multiple pathways is differently affected during zidovudine/lamivudine-containing compared with NRTI-sparing combination antiretroviral therapy. *J Acquir Immune Defic Syndr.* 2010;53(2):186-193.
40. Paula AA, Falcão MC, Pacheco AG. Metabolic syndrome in HIV-infected individuals: underlying mechanisms and epidemiological aspects. *AIDS Res Ther.* 2013;10(1):32.
41. Baker Jason V, Sharma S, Achhra Amit C, et al. Changes in cardiovascular disease risk factors with immediate versus deferred antiretroviral therapy initiation among HIV-positive participants in the START (Strategic Timing of Antiretroviral Treatment) trial. *J Am Heart Assoc.* 2017;6(5):e004987.
42. Worm SW, Sabin C, Weber R, et al. Risk of myocardial infarction in patients with HIV infection exposed to specific individual antiretroviral drugs from the 3 major drug classes: the Data Collection on Adverse Events of Anti-HIV Drugs (D:A:D) study. *J Infect Dis.* 2010;201(3):318-330.
43. Lang S, Mary-Krause M, Cotte L, et al. Impact of individual antiretroviral drugs on the risk of myocardial infarction in human immunodeficiency virus–infected patients: a case-control study nested within the French hospital database on HIV ANRS Cohort CO4. *Arch Intern Med.* 2010;170(14):1228-1238.
44. Saag MS, Benson CA, Gandhi RT, et al. Antiretroviral drugs for treatment and prevention of HIV infection in adults: 2018 recommendations of the International Antiviral Society-USA Panel. *JAMA.* 2018;320(4):379-396.
45. Ridker PM, Danielson E, Fonseca FAH, et al. Rosuvastatin to prevent vascular events in men and women with elevated C-reactive protein. *N Engl J Med.* 2008;359(21):2195-2207.
46. Toribio M, Fitch KV, Sanchez L, et al. Effects of pitavastatin and pravastatin on markers of immune activation and arterial inflammation in HIV. *AIDS.* 2017;31(6):797-806.
47. Hiremath PG, Cardoso R, Blumenthal RS, Martin SS. Evidence-based review of statin use in patients with HIV on antiretroviral therapy. *ACC Expert Anal.* 2018;13(2).
48. Chastain DB, Stover KR, Riche DM. Evidence-based review of statin use in patients with HIV on antiretroviral therapy. *J Clin Transl Endocrinol.* 2017;8:6-14.
49. Kohli M, Patel K, MacMahon Z, et al. Pro-protein subtilisin kexin-9 (PCSK9) inhibition in practice: lipid clinic experience in 2 contrasting UK centres. *Int J Clin Pract.* 2017;71(11).
50. Boccara F, Kumar PN, Caramelli B, et al. Evolocumab use in HIV-infected patients with dyslipidemia: primary results of the randomized, double-blind BEIJERINCK study. *J Am Coll Cardiol.* 2020;75(20):2570-2584.
51. Paisible A-L, Chang C-CH, So-Armah KA, et al. HIV infection, cardiovascular disease risk factor profile, and risk for acute myocardial infarction. *J Acquir Immune Defic Syndr.* 2015;68(2):209-216.
52. Webel AR, Moore SM, Longenecker CT, et al. Randomized controlled trial of the SystemCHANGE intervention on behaviors related to cardiovascular risk in HIV+ adults. *J Acquir Immune Defic Syndr.* 2018;78(1):23-33.
53. O'Brien MP, Hunt PW, Kitch DW, et al. A randomized placebo controlled trial of aspirin effects on immune activation in chronically human immunodeficiency virus-infected adults on virologically suppressive antiretroviral therapy. *Open Forum Infect Dis.* 2017;4(1):ofw278.

CHAPTER 28

DYSAUTONOMIA

Salvatore Savona and Ralph Augostini

INTRODUCTION

The autonomic nervous system is essential for maintaining homeostasis and impacts nearly all organ systems. Dysautonomia can present in a myriad of diseases and be a result of pathology at various levels of the autonomic nervous system. Most frequently, it manifests with abnormal responses of blood pressure and heart rate to positional changes or stress. However, in more advanced diseases, such as heart failure and cardiac arrhythmias, derangements in the autonomic nervous system can play an integral role in disease progression. Many clinical tests are available to interrogate the autonomic nervous system and assess the level of pathology. This review outlines the basic anatomy of the autonomic nervous system, tests available to assess its function, frequently encountered disease states that affect the autonomic function, and current and emerging therapies.

AUTONOMIC NERVOUS SYSTEM ANATOMY

The autonomic nervous system is divided into the sympathetic and parasympathetic nervous systems. The sympathetic nervous system affects the cardiovascular system primarily through arterial vasoconstriction and increased heart rate via release of catecholamines. The parasympathetic nervous system has the opposite effect, causing vasodilation and a decrease in heart rate. The sympathetic nervous system has primarily cervical and upper thoracic afferent and efferent fibers to the heart and lungs via the upper sympathetic chain. The parasympathetic nervous system primarily interacts with the cardiopulmonary system via the vagal nerve (cranial nerve X).

Baroreflex is an essential component of the autonomic nervous system. It maintains circulatory integrity, modulating blood pressure and heart rate. Arterial baroreceptors are located in the carotid sinus and aortic arch and are sensitive to changes in blood pressure. The cardiopulmonary baroreceptors are located in the venous system in the thorax and are sensitive to changes in blood volume. For example, when standing from a seated position, a decrease in blood pressure and venous return to the heart normally stimulates the sympathetic nervous system to promote vasoconstriction and tachycardia to maintain cardiac output. Inputs to the central nervous system in the medulla are supplied peripherally by the vagus and glossopharyngeal nerves.

The heart is richly innervated by the autonomic nervous system. Cardiac extrinsic sympathetic autonomic innervation arises from the superior and middle cervical ganglia, the stellate ganglia, and thoracic ganglia.[1,2] The stellate ganglion is a major contributor to sympathetic innervation of the heart.[2] Parasympathetic innervation arises from the recurrent laryngeal nerves and vagal connections just distal to the recurrent laryngeal nerves. The ventral and dorsal cardiopulmonary plexus are located anterior and posterior to the main pulmonary artery and are formed by connections with the sympathetic and parasympathetic nerves.[1] In addition to extrinsic innervation, the heart is intimately innervated by intrinsic nerves, with the greatest density at the connection between the pulmonary vein and left atrium. However, sympathetic and parasympathetic intrinsic innervation in the pulmonary vein and left atrial junction are in close proximity, limiting isolation of the separate intrinsic nerves from a therapeutic perspective.[3]

CLINICAL EVALUATION

The main goal during evaluation of the autonomic nervous system is differentiating which part of the nervous system is affected. The main portions evaluated include sympathetic/adrenergic function, cardiovagal parasympathetic function, and sudomotor function.[4] Many tests are available to evaluate the autonomic nervous system, but the most commonly used studies are *heart rate variability, Valsalva maneuver, tilt-table test, carotid sinus massage (CSM), radiotracer iodine-123 meta-iodobenzylguanidine (MIBG), quantitative sudomotor axon reflex test (QSART),* and *thermoregulatory sweat test (TST).*

DIAGNOSTIC TESTS

Heart Rate Variability

Heart rate variability is defined as beat-to-beat variation in the heart rate or R-R interval on the electrocardiogram (ECG).[5] In order to assess heart rate variability, standardized breathing techniques are of paramount importance as heart rate changes often occur in concert with the cycle of breathing: so-called "respiratory sinus arrhythmia" in which the heart rate increases with respiration and decreases with expiration.[6] This can be achieved by nine cycles of maximal effort deep breathing when 5 seconds is allowed for both inspiration and expiration, or "paced breathing." Maximal effort must be provided in order to accurately interpret changes in heart rate. These changes are compared to standardized data that account for age and gender. Variability in heart rate declines with age, though diminished variability may also be seen in parasympathetic dysfunction, such as in Parkinson disease (PD).[4] Variability is also reduced in cardiac disease states with sympathetic overdrive, such as congestive heart failure (CHF).[7]

Additionally, variability in the R-R interval on ECG can be evaluated with the "30:15" ratio. Originally studied in diabetic patients with autonomic neuropathy, the 30:15 ratio evaluates the R-R interval at 15 seconds and 30 seconds after standing.[8] Normal ratios are greater than 1.05, and high values are seen as a normal vagal response.[9] This test can also be useful in the evaluation of patients with orthostatic hypotension or postural orthostatic tachycardia syndrome (POTS).[4]

Valsalva Maneuver

The Valsalva maneuver (ie, forced expiration against a closed glottis) evaluates both the sympathetic and parasympathetic response of the baroreflex in four unique phases. In phase I during forced expiration (~40 mm Hg), an increase in blood pressure is noted because of increased intrathoracic pressure compressing the aorta and inferior vena cava. Phase II occurs during the later component of expiration and has a distinct early and late profile. In early phase II, there is decreased cardiac output and blood pressure because of continued compression of the inferior vena cava causing reduced preload and venous return. Heart rate increases reflexively during early phase II. In late phase II, systemic vascular resistance increases as a result of baroreflex activation and increased adrenergic tone. The onset of phase III occurs at end expiration (ie, with cessation of forced expiration), producing an abrupt decrease in blood pressure related to reduced intrathoracic pressure. In phase IV, there is an increase in blood pressure because of sustained vasocontriction and increased cardiac output from restoration of venous return, reflecting elevated adrenergic tone. Additionally, there is a decrease in heart rate as a result of the baroreflex.[4,9,10] The Vasalva maneuver and associated hemodynamic changes are depicted in **Figure 28.1**.

The parasympathetic nervous system is evaluated by the Valsalva ratio, which is defined as the maximum heart rate achieved during the study divided by the lowest heart rate recorded within 30 seconds of the maximum value.[11] A higher Valsalva ratio is indicative of a healthy parasympathetic response, implying intact heart rate variability.[4] Typically, a value below 1.2 is considered abnormal.[12]

In order to assess the sympathetic nervous system, the blood pressure response to late phase II and IV is analyzed. Normal sympathetic responses would include recovery of blood pressure in late phase II (4-7 seconds after phase I) to the baseline value and an increase in blood pressure over the baseline value in phase IV.[4] Patients with mild disease have an absent or reduced late phase II response and reduced phase IV

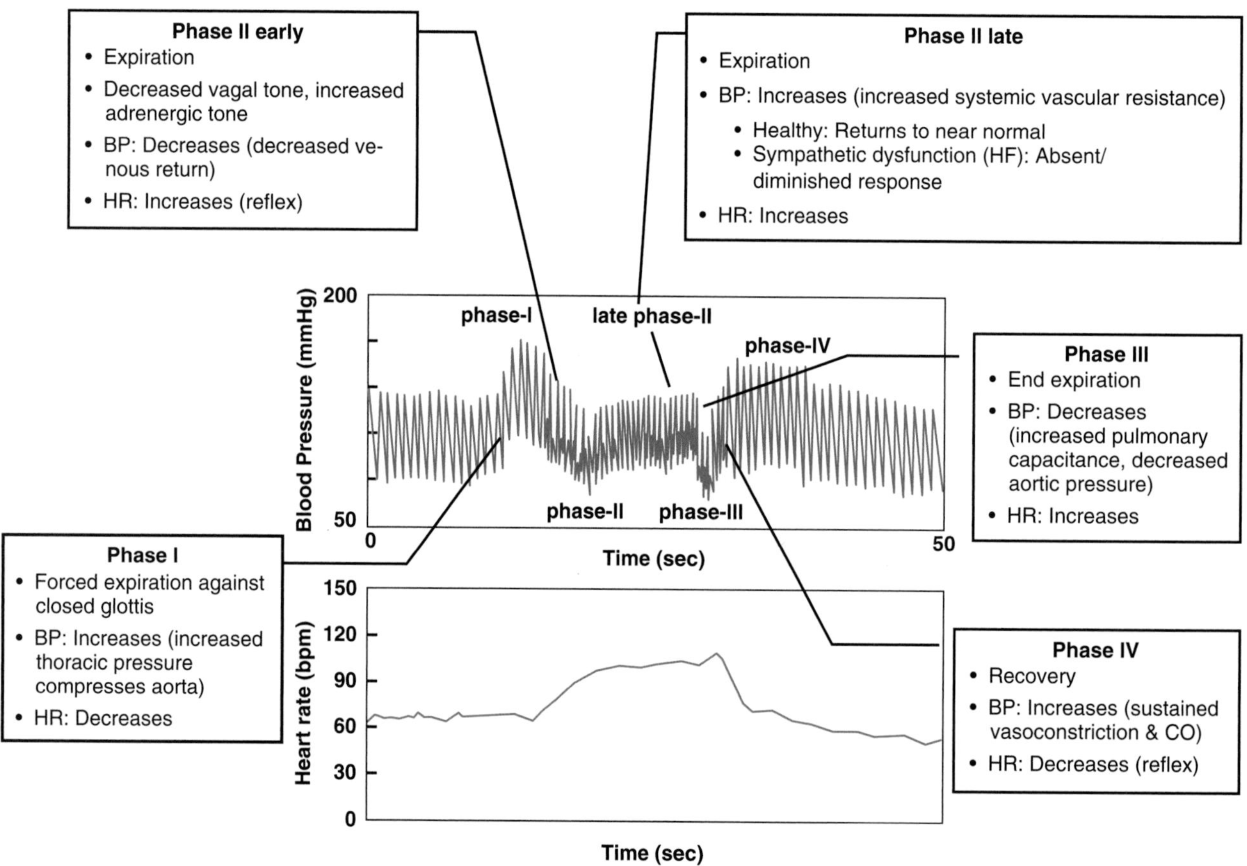

FIGURE 28.1 Phases of the Valsalva Maneuver. Blood pressure and heart rate responses are outlined during each phase. BP, blood pressure; CO, cardiac output; HF, heart failure; HR, heart rate.

TABLE 28.1 Degree of Sympathetic Dysfunction Evaluated During the Valsalva Maneuver, as Seen by the Blood Pressure Recovery in Late Phase II and Phase IV

Degree of Sympathetic Dysfunction	Late Phase II	Phase IV
Mild	Absent or reduced	Reduced
Moderate	Absent	Reduced
Severe	Absent	Blocked

Adapted from Sandroni P, Benarroch EE, Low PA. Pharmacological dissection of components of the Valsalva maneuver in adrenergic failure. *J Appl Physiol (1985)*. 1991;71(4):1563-1567.

hypertensive response. Moderate sympathetic dysfunction causes absent late phase II and reduced phase IV responses and typically mild orthostatic hypotension. In patients with severe sympathetic failure, there is an exaggerated phase II hypotensive response with absent late phase II and phase IV hypertensive responses.[13] The degree of sympathetic dysfunction as defined by blood pressure responses to late phase II and phase IV of the Valsalva maneuver is summarized in **Table 28.1**.

Variations in the results of the Valsalva maneuver can be useful in differentiating various disorders. Neurogenic orthostatic hypotension creates a "V" blood pressure response pattern as a prolonged and exaggerated decrease in blood pressure in phase II with a reduced to absent response in phase III. Inappropriate sinus tachycardia produces an "M" blood pressure response pattern with two systolic peaks (phase II and IV). In POTS, there is an "N" pattern with a sustained overshoot in blood pressure of more than or equal to 10 mm Hg during phase IV.[14]

Cardiovascular autonomic neuropathy (CAN) in patients with diabetes has historically been evaluated with five cardiovascular reflex tests, including deep breathing testing, Valsalva maneuver, 30/15 test, handgrip test, and orthostatic hypotension test. However, the utility of the handgrip test has been questioned, as its result is more likely to be abnormal with an elevated resting diastolic blood pressure (DBP). Additionally, it is unlikely to be positive in the setting of baseline hypertension.[15]

Combining the Valsalva maneuver with lying to standing deep breathing testing has been suggested as an initial screening test for early autonomic neuropathy, with a sensitivity of 85%.[16] Additionally, in a study of patients with type 1 diabetes, combining at least two cardiovascular autonomic reflex tests had a sensitivity of 100% in detecting autonomic dysfunction, when using radiotracer iodine-123 MIBG testing as a reference standard.[17]

Tilt-Table Test

Tilt-table test is a commonly used tool to evaluate the sympathetic and parasympathetic system and is useful in the diagnosis of diseases such as orthostatic hypotension, POTS, and neurocardiogenic syncope.[18,19] The role of the tilt-table test is to evaluate the neurocardiovascular system response to shifts in blood volume. Changes in posture from lying to standing result in 400 to 600 mL of blood shifting from the thorax into the lower extremities by gravitational stress.[20] Hypotension and syncope are prevented by venous contraction by skeletal muscles in the lower extremities and neurocardiogenic baroreflex responses. In active standing, both of these mechanisms are engaged; however, tilt-table test isolates the neurocardiogenic response by removing the active phase of standing.[4]

Patients are initially secured to the table in the supine position and should be attached to an automated external defibrillator with pacing capabilities. The patient is kept in the supine position for approximately 20 minutes to obtain a baseline blood pressure and heart rate. Once the patient is in a supine steady state, the table angle is rapidly increased to a head-up position of 60 to 80 degrees. In order to effectively assess the baroreceptors, patients should stay as still as possible and avoid moving their legs to prevent skeletal muscle–mediated vasoconstriction. The environment should be calm and quiet to avoid central neurologic effects. Patients remain in the head-up position for at least 10 minutes, with continuous heart rhythm monitoring and frequent blood pressure assessments every 2 to 3 minutes. The test may need to be discontinued prematurely if the patient develops severe discomfort, sustained hypotensive response, or syncope.[4]

In adults, a normal response to tilt-table test includes a mild heart rate increase of no more than 30 bpm, systolic blood pressure (SBP) decrease of no more than 20 mm Hg, and a DBP decrease of no more than 10 mm Hg.[18] Patients with orthostatic hypotension exhibit a fall in blood pressure (ie, SBP >20 mm Hg or DBP >10 mm Hg) with a blunted heart rate response. In POTS, patients will have an exaggerated heart rate response (sustained increase of heart rate by at least 30 bpm) with a normal blood pressure response. Neurocardiogenic syncope exhibits an abrupt fall in blood pressure without a compensatory heart rate response and may exhibit asystole. This response may occur late (up to 20 minutes) into the head-up maneuver.[4,10,18] **Figure 28.2** provides examples of the various hemodynamic responses expected during tilt-table test. **Table 28.2** outlines the classification of responses to a positive tilt-table test.

Tilt-table test is time consuming and may take at least 45 minutes to complete the study. In order to facilitate a vasovagal response, isoproterenol may be infused at a rate of 0.05 μg/kg/min with a maximum dose of 5 μg/min, spending 10 minutes at the 70-degree head-up position. When compared to standard tilt-table test, the specificity is slightly reduced from 91% to 83% with isoproterenol infusion, though it had a significantly higher ability to induce a vasovagal response (9% in passive tilt table vs. 17% with isoproterenol).[21]

The "Italian Protocol" is an alternative approach that utilizes sublingual nitroglycerin during tilt-table test and has a reported sensitivity of 62% and specificity of 92%. This protocol has a stabilization phase, passive phase, provocation phase, and finally

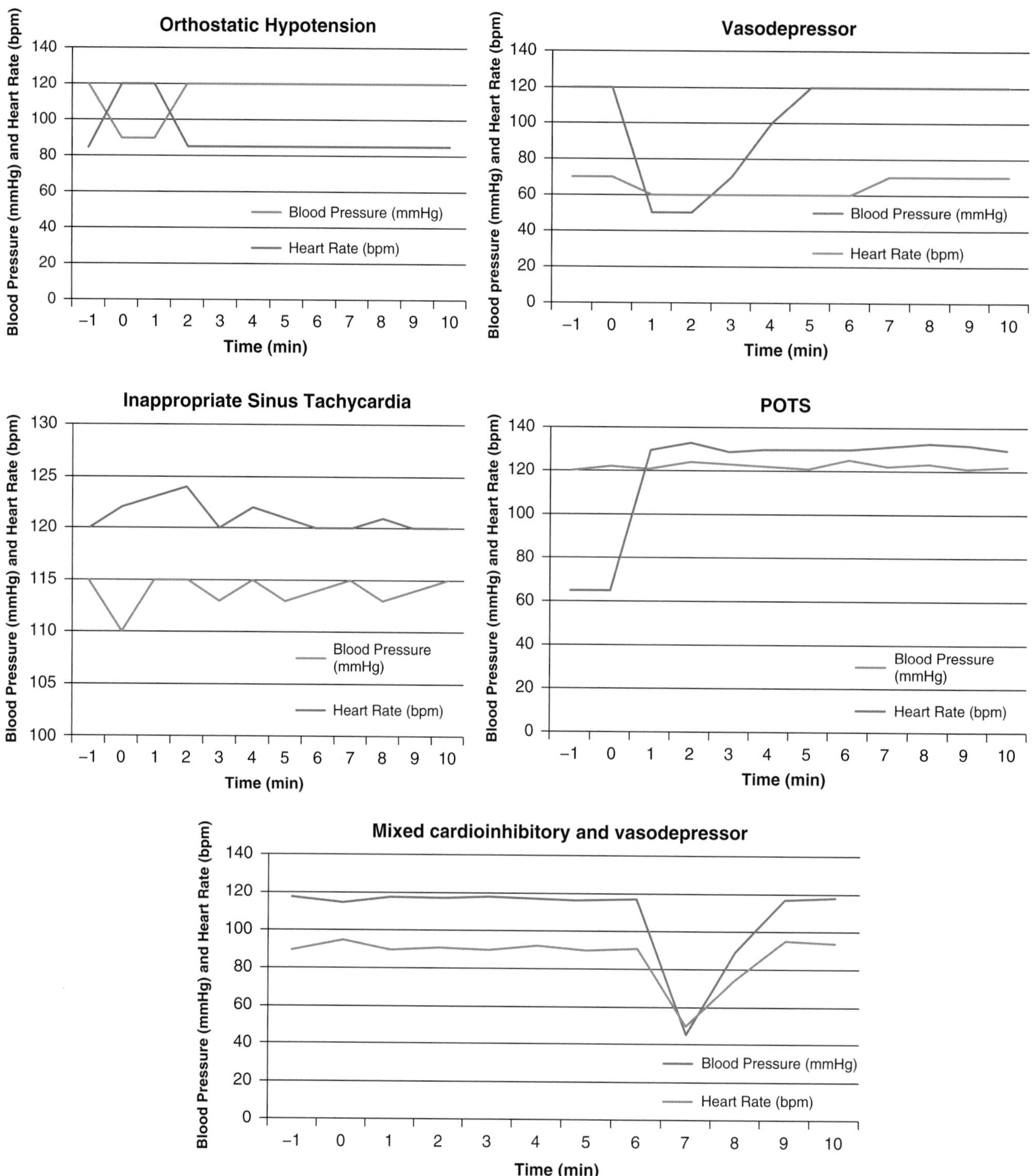

FIGURE 28.2 Expected Hemodynamic Responses to Tilt-Table Test. Each graph plots the blood pressure and heart rate response against time during tilt-table test for orthostatic hypotension, vasodepressor syncope, inappropriate sinus tachycardia, postural orthostatic tachycardia syndrome (POTS), and mixed cardioinhibitory and vasodepressor syncope. Tilt-table test is initiation at time 0 minutes.

completion of the study with test interruption. In the stabilization phase, the patient is kept in the supine position for 5 minutes. During the passive phase, the patient is kept at 60 degree for 20 minutes. In the provocation phase, the patient is administered 400 μg of sublingual nitroglycerin spray and monitored for 15 minutes. The test is completed or interrupted if there is syncope, the development of progressive orthostatic hypotension lasting more than 5 minutes, or if no symptoms are reproduced.[22]

TABLE 28.2 Type and Classification of Positive Tilt-Table Test with Associated Hemodynamic Responses

Type of Response	Hemodynamic Response
POTS	Increase HR ≥30 bpm within 20 seconds of head-up tilt HR ≥120 bpm during head-up tilt No orthostatic hypotension (Δ BP <15 mm Hg)
Inappropriate Sinus Tachycardia	Resting daytime HR >100 bpm Mean 24-hour HR >90 bpm Increases in HR typically not postural
Neurocardiogenic	Hypotension, typically acute, ± bradycardia
Autonomic Dysfunction	Parallel fall in systolic and diastolic BP
Cerebral	Cerebral vasoconstriction
Psychogenic	No objective changes
Classification of Response	**Hemodynamic Response**
Mixed Cardioinhibitory and Vasodepressor (Type 1)	BP falls before HR HR falls during syncope Ventricular rate does not fall below 40 bpm for more than 10 seconds
Cardioinhibitory (Type 2)	Type A: cardio-inhibition without asystole. Ventricular rate <40 bpm for >10 seconds, but asystole does not occur for >3 seconds BP decrease before HR Type B: cardio-inhibition with asystole (at least 3 seconds). BP decrease with or before HR
Vasodepressor (Type 3)	HR does not decrease by >10% during syncope. Exceptions: Chronotropic incompetence or excessive HR increase >130 bpm

BP, blood pressure; bpm, beats per minute, HR, heart rate; POTS, postural orthostatic tachycardia syndrome.
Adapted from Sheldon RS, Grubb BP 2nd, Olshansky B, et al. 2015 heart rhythm society expert consensus statement on the diagnosis and treatment of postural tachycardia syndrome, inappropriate sinus tachycardia, and vasovagal syncope. *Heart Rhythm.* 2015;12(6):e41-e63; Baron-Esquivias G, Martinez-Rubio A. Tilt table test: state of the art. *Indian Pacing Electrophysiol J.* 2003;3(4):239-252; Grubb BP. Neurocardiogenic syncope and related disorders of orthostatic intolerance. *Circulation.* 2005;111(22):2997-3006; Brignole M, Menozzi C, Del Rosso A, et al. New classification of haemodynamics of vasovagal syncope: beyond the VASIS classification: analysis of the pre-syncopal phase of the tilt test without and with nitroglycerin challenge. *Europace.* 2000;2(1):66-76.

Carotid Sinus Massage

The CSM is useful in evaluating the parasympathetic nervous system and carotid sinus baroreceptors. The study should not be performed in patients with carotid stenosis, and patients should undergo continuous ECG recording to assess for heart block or asystole. It is performed by unilateral compression of the carotid sinus for 20 to 30 seconds, followed by releasing compression for a few minutes and repeating compression on the contralateral carotid sinus.[9] The diagnosis of carotid sinus hypersensitivity can be made if asystole occurs for more than 3 seconds, atrioventricular block occurs, a 50 mm Hg or more drop in SBP consistent with a vasodepressor response occurs, or a mixed cardioinhibitory or vasodepressor response occurs.[23] The effect of CSM may also be helpful in delineating the level of atrioventricular block in the setting of second-degree atrioventricular block. Right CSM has a preferential effect on the sinus node, whereas left CSM has a great effect on the atrioventricular node.

Radiotracer Iodine-123 Meta-iodobenzylguanidine

The adrenergic system is able to be evaluated utilizing single-photon emission computed tomography (SPECT) via the radiotracer iodine-123 MIBG, which is an analog for norepinephrine. This study can provide insight into the sympathetic innervation of the heart, specifically presynaptic postganglionic functionality.[10] This study is useful in the assessment of dysautonomia in patients with PD and multiple system atrophy (MSA) (Shy-Drager syndrome).[24]

Quantitative Sudomotor Axon Reflex Test

The QSART is a technically challenging test that evaluates postganglionic sympathetic cholinergic function.[25] The study evaluates axon reflexes via stimulation with a cholinergic agent, typically acetylcholine. Once applied to the skin, acetylcholine binds to nicotinic and muscarinic receptors, creating an impulse that travels proximally along the postganglionic sudomotor axon. The signal reflexively returns distally after reaching a branch point and releases acetylcholine in the nerve terminal, which activates sweat glands. Results of the test are quantified by a change in relative humidity from at least four different sites, typically the forearm, proximal leg, distal leg, and foot.[10] In patients with reduced postganglionic sympathetic cholinergic function, such as diabetics with peripheral neuropathy, there is a reduced density of sweat volume as well as innervated sweat glands.[26]

Thermoregulatory Sweat Test

In order to assess for central versus peripheral sudomotor lesions, the QSART is combined with the TST. Both the QSART and TST will be abnormal in peripheral lesions, though an abnormal TST with a normal QSART represents central preganglionic lesions.[11,27] The test itself is technically challenging and involves the patient laying supine in a temperature- and humidity-controlled room. The patient is covered in an indicator solution that identifies the presence and degree of sweat production during controlled body temperature elevation. Normally, a diffuse equally distributed sweat response is present. However, abnormal responses include an attenuated distal sweat response in length-dependent polyneuropathy, lack of response below the level of a spinal cord injury, focal responses in radiculopathy and lateral femoral cutaneous nerve syndrome, and diffuse anhidrosis.[27]

CLINICAL PRESENTATION AND MANAGEMENT IN VARIOUS DISORDERS

Autonomic derangements are present in a myriad of diseases with diverse clinical presentation, with a significant overlap in the cardiovascular and neurologic diseases that can present with dysautonomia. Outlined below are common disorders/diseases that exhibit dysautonomia.

Vasovagal Syncope

Vasovagal syncope is a transient loss of consciousness that is typically associated with diaphoresis, warmth, and nausea in the setting of emotional stress or unsettling situations. Patients experience hypotension with relative bradycardia following these events and then fatigue. The diagnosis is almost universally made through history, though as previously noted, tilt-table test may be utilized.[28] In these patients, there is a reduction in venous return upon standing, with pooling of blood in the periphery and abdominal viscera. There is a blunted barometric reflex, and instead of experiencing an increased sympathetic response to hypotension, an ineffective heart rate response (vagal-mediated) results in decreased cardiac output and vasodilation.[29,30]

Vasovagal syncope can generally be managed conservatively, especially for patients with infrequent symptoms. These include lifestyle modifications with avoidance of triggers, increased salt/fluid intake, and counterpressure maneuvers/compression stockings.[28,30] Recognition of triggers and prodromal symptoms with subsequent positioning to lying down with elevation of legs may be helpful. Medical therapy may be utilized for patients with more frequent or intolerable symptoms. Regarding beta-blocker therapy, metoprolol is a reasonable initial therapy in patients over 40 years of age, though atenolol should be avoided as it was found to be no better than placebo.[31,32] Other therapies such as midodrine may also be utilized, though there is a lack of strong evidence for its use in this population.[28] Pacing therapy has been evaluated in patients with vasovagal syncope and has primarily shown benefit in patients above 40 years with frequent severe symptoms, including injury from syncope, who have 3 seconds or more of asystole with syncope or 6 seconds or more of asystole in the absence of symptoms. When appropriately selected, this patient population has been shown to have a 32% absolute and 57% relative risk reduction in syncope with dual-chamber pacing.[33]

Postural Orthostatic Tachycardia Syndrome

The diagnosis of POTS and vasovagal syncope is not mutually exclusive, though patients with POTS are frequently symptomatic with standing, experience an increase in heart rate of 30 bpm or more from lying to standing for more than 30 seconds, and do not demonstrate orthostatic hypotension.[28,30] However, any offending drug potentiating symptoms or potential underlying disease process causing symptoms must be excluded.[34] Patients with POTS may be subdivided into neuropathic and non-neuropathic. Previous studies have stratified patients based on the results of skin biopsy results for intraepidermal nerve fiber density to differentiate those with neuropathic versus non-neuropathic POTS. Those with neuropathic POTS had lower rates of anxiety and depression with higher perceived health-related quality of life scores. Additionally, neuropathic POTS was seen to have reduced parasympathetic function, lower Valsalva phase 4 overshoot, and lower resting and tilt-related heart rates when compared to those with non-neuropathic POTS. These findings suggest that skin biopsy may play an important role in the care for these patients.[35]

Both POTS and orthostatic intolerance exhibit high rates of deconditioning. Previous studies have shown reduced VO_2max in those with POTS (95%) and orthostatic intolerance (91%).[36] Though overlap exists between POTS and orthostatic intolerance, dysautonomia is more prevalent in POTS. When compared to patients with orthostatic intolerance, patients with POTS exhibit mild vasomotor derangements and an excessive increase in orthostatic heart rate.[37]

The management of POTS is challenging because of heterogeneous symptomatology and typically requires a multidisciplinary approach. Initially, nonpharmacologic lifestyle modifications should be utilized, including nonupright exercise, psychological treatment, and recreational therapy. Additionally, patients should consume 2 to 3 L of water per day and 10 to 12 g/day of salt. Midodrine may be used during daytime to increase venous return. Propranolol in low doses (10-20 mg orally) may be used to reduce tachycardia during standing. Acetylcholinesterase inhibitors and central sympatholytic agents have been used in complex cases, though their use is typically limited by side effects. There is no invasive therapy currently recommended for the treatment of POTS.[28] Patients with severe refractory POTS may benefit from erythropoietin subcutaneously, because of the vasoconstrictive effects of this agent.[34]

Synucleinopathies

The synucleinopathies are a spectrum of disorders with dysautonomia including MSA, PD, dementia with Lewy bodies (LBD), and pure autonomic failure (PAF). These are neurodegenerative disorders primarily because of abnormal intracellular deposition of alpha-synuclein. Neurogenic orthostatic hypotension is a cardinal feature of these diseases, but patients also frequently experience gastrointestinal and urologic dysfunction.[38] MSA is a rapidly progressive disease with severe autonomic failure.[39] PAF has a slower disease process and is isolated to peripheral autonomic dysfunction.[40]

Cardiac MIBG scintigraphy has been evaluated in patients with PD and has been correlated with clinical cardiac autonomic impairment, especially in male patients.[41,42] Additionally, cardiac MIBG is useful in differentiating MSA from the other synucleinopathies, as the test is typically normal in patients with MSA.[43] Though autonomic denervation in the heart occurs early in PD, it appears to manifest independent of orthostatic hypotension, impaired heart rate variability, and impaired baroreflex.[44] Additionally, in MSA, the QSART testing is typically normal and the TST testing is abnormal, indicating a central preganglionic lesion with preserved postganglionic function.[45] In contrast, PD, LBD, and PAF results are typically consistent with postganglionic lesions.[40]

Dysautonomia associated with PD is debilitating. Additionally, treatment with levodopa typically worsens dysautonomia.[46] However, pedunculopontine nucleus stimulation has been shown to have benefits aside from improvements in gait disorders. A small study showed significant amelioration of SBP fall during tilt-table test, improvements in the Valsalva ratio, and improvements in baroreflex sensitivity.[47]

Diabetes

CAN is seen early in children with type 1 diabetes at a mean age of 15 years and is associated with the duration of diabetes (>5 years), disease-specific microvascular complications, and poor disease control.[48] Cardiovascular autonomic dysfunction in patients with type 2 diabetes is independently associated with older age, hypertension, poor glycemic control (A1c >9.0%), and microvascular complications including diabetic retinopathy and microalbuminuria.[49]

Patients with type 1 diabetes and CAN exhibit increased left ventricular mass and concentric remodeling, when compared to those without CAN. This finding suggests that the presence of CAN may provoke left ventricular structural and functional changes.[50]

Sudomotor dysfunction follows a peripheral distribution, initially with distal abnormalities on testing, which can progress to involve the abdomen.[51] The development of CAN is a strong marker for excess mortality in this population, from 27% to 56% over 5 to 10 years, which stresses the importance of early treatment of diabetes to prevent neuropathy.[52]

Atrial and Ventricular Arrhythmias

Atrial and ventricular arrhythmias are influenced by the autonomic nervous system. Additionally, the neuroplasticity of the autonomic nervous system may promote ventricular and atrial arrhythmias: previous animal models showed increased sympathetic innervation of the atria following myocardial infarction causing ventricular injury.[53] The genesis of atrial fibrillation has been attributed to an imbalance of the autonomic nervous system, primarily through excess sympathetic activity. In patients with structural heart disease, studies have shown increased heart rate variability prior to the initiation of atrial fibrillation, suggestive of an autonomic trigger.[54] Additionally, sympathetic activity may also play a role in sustaining atrial fibrillation, as patients with chronic atrial fibrillation have an increased density of sympathetic innervation in the pulmonary vein-left atrial junction and right atrial appendage.[55]

Vagal-mediated atrial fibrillation is an entity that occurs primarily in younger patients without structural heart disease, and it is initiated during activities with higher vagal tone, such as after eating or during rest, and tends to recover with increased sympathetic tone. It is commonly observed with esophageal stimulation with intake of a cold beverage or large bolus of food. Nocturnal onset is also observed. Clinically, the episodes may be preceded by sinus bradycardia and with lower heart rates during episodes of atrial fibrillation.[56,57]

Comprehensive management of atrial fibrillation is outside the scope of this review (see Chapter 56, Atrial Flutter and Fibrillation), though current established management strategies for atrial fibrillation, such as beta-blockers, reduce sympathetic tone and assist in rate control. Potential autonomic nervous system modifications have been suggested for the management of atrial fibrillation through neuromodulation, including sympathetic and vagal denervation, vagal nerve stimulation, baroreflex stimulation, ganglion plexus ablation, and renal sympathetic denervation.[53]

Ventricular arrhythmias are also intimately influenced by the autonomic nervous system, particularly the sympathetic nervous system. Interventional techniques utilized to modify the cardiac autonomic nervous system in atrial fibrillation are also being applied in the management of ventricular arrhythmias. In patients with structural heart disease and refractory ventricular arrhythmias, thoracic epidural anesthesia and surgical left cardiac sympathetic denervation have resulted in a reduction in ventricular arrhythmia burden by 75% and 56%, respectively.[58] Renal sympathetic denervation reduces central sympathetic tone by inhibition of the renin-angiotensin-aldosterone system and in small studies has resulted in a significant reduction in ventricular arrhythmia burden with a relatively low rate of complications.[59,60]

Cardiomyopathy

Central sleep apnea occurs with high frequency in patients with cardiac disease, and observational studies have detected a 30% to 50% prevalence in heart failure.[61] Additionally, the presence of central sleep apnea in heart failure has been shown to represent more advanced heart failure because of elevated cardiac sympathetic nerve activity.[62] Additionally, these patients exhibit impaired heart rate variability and elevated risk for nonsustained ventricular tachycardia.[63]

Though the management of obstructive sleep apnea has been applied to this population through positive airway pressure, improvement in sleep apnea may be due to patients having mixed central and obstructive sleep apnea. The SERVE-HF trial, which evaluated adaptive servoventilation (ASV) in this population, showed increased cardiac mortality despite improvements in the apnea-hypopnea index (AHI).[64] Therefore, continuous positive airway pressure ventilation with ASV is contraindicated in patients with a left ventricular ejection fraction less than 45%. Transvenous phrenic nerve stimulation has been evaluated in this population and has shown significant improvements in AHI (50% reduction from baseline), improved rapid eye movement sleep, and reduction of hypoxia during sleep (defined by <90% oxygen saturation), which is an independent predictor of all-cause mortality in this population.[65,66]

Additionally, neurostimulation of the vagal nerve has been evaluated in three small studies of heart failure patients, as parasympathetic (vagal nerve) stimulation previously showed reduced mortality in an animal model for CHF.[67] Though the use of such devices in these trials was safe from a procedural perspective, improvements in left ventricular function were not consistent. Further studies are needed to assess the efficacy of these devices.[68]

Patients with pulmonary arterial hypertension are said to be "preload" dependent, and maneuvers such as Valsalva that reduce intrathoracic venous return are avoided because of hemodynamic concerns. However, syncope during Valsalva in this population appears to be related to autonomic dysfunction, similar to patients with intermediate autonomic failure.[69]

Autonomic derangements have been implicated as a potential underlying mechanism in Takotsubo cardiomyopathy as elevated levels of catecholamines are seen in the acute phase of the disease. In follow-up testing at a mean of 37 months after presentation, patients had reduced parasympathetic control of heart rate, with increased responsiveness by the sympathetic nervous system. These results were seen in the setting of similar baseline catecholamine levels with controls, suggesting a role of impaired baroreflex control in the disease.[70] Guideline-directed medical therapy remains the recommended treatment for this entity.

Cancer Survivors

As the population of cancer survivors increases, an emerging field of cardio-oncology has expanded to provide longitudinal care. The autonomic nervous system is not spared in the treatment of cancer. A recent retrospective review of patients treated for primarily hematologic malignancies with vinca alkaloids (54.2%), alkylating agents (66.7%), anthracyclines (54.2%), and radiation therapy to the thorax (66.7%) and neck (53.3%) provides insight into the prevalence of autonomic dysfunction. Eight of these patients had undergone hematopoietic stem cell transplantation, with five developing graft-versus-host disease. Of the 282 patients referred for suspected autonomic dysfunction based on symptoms, 24 underwent comprehensive autonomic testing, including heart rate deep breathing test, Valsalva maneuver, tilt-table test, and sudomotor testing. Within this population, 92% had some degree of autonomic dysfunction, most commonly orthostatic hypotension (50%), inappropriate sinus tachycardia (20.8%), and POTS (12.5%). There should be a low threshold for evaluating cancer survivors for autonomic dysfunction based on presenting symptoms of dizziness, tachycardia, palpitations, and syncope in order to provide appropriate therapy.[71]

RESEARCH AND FUTURE DIRECTIONS

Though medical therapy is available to assist with symptom management, future directions in the management of dysautonomia include device-based therapies through neuromodulation, which has and is currently being studied in heart failure (Chapter 75), arrhythmias (Chapter 50 Cardiac Arrhythmias Mechanisms), syncope (Chapter 61), and movement disorders (Chapter 51).

KEY POINTS

- ✔ The cardiovascular system is richly innervated by the autonomic nervous system, which is subdivided into the sympathetic and parasympathetic systems.
- ✔ Careful attention to bedside and noninvasive evaluation of the autonomic nervous system, including the Valsalva maneuver, CSM, and tilt-table test, can provide a diagnosis of dysautonomia.
- ✔ Comprehensive testing of the autonomic nervous system through MIBG, SPECT, QSART, and TST can provide detailed evaluation when clinically warranted.
- ✔ There is a spectrum of clinical disease including orthostatic hypotension, vasovagal syncope, and POTS, which require a comprehensive patient-centered management plan.
- ✔ Atrial and ventricular arrhythmias can be triggered and exacerbated by the autonomic nervous system, with emerging pharmacologic and interventional management techniques including sympathetic and renal denervation.
- ✔ Many patients with cardiomyopathies have comorbidities, such as central sleep apnea, which increase adrenergic tone. Novel interventional therapies, such as transvenous phrenic nerve stimulation, are evolving for the management of these comorbidities.

REFERENCES

1. Janes RD, Brandys JC, Hopkins DA, Johnstone DE, Murphy DA, Armour JA. Anatomy of human extrinsic cardiac nerves and ganglia. *Am J Cardiol.* 1986;57(4):299-309.
2. Kawashima T. The autonomic nervous system of the human heart with special reference to its origin, course, and peripheral distribution. *Anat Embryol.* 2005;209(6):425-438.
3. Tan AY, Li H, Wachsmann-Hogiu S, Chen LS, Chen P, Fishbein MC. Autonomic innervation and segmental muscular disconnections at the human pulmonary vein-atrial junction: implications for catheter ablation of atrial-pulmonary vein junction. *J Am Coll Cardiol.* 2006;48(1):132-143.
4. Illigens BM, Gibbons CH. Autonomic testing, methods and techniques. In: Levin K, Chauvel P, eds. *Handbook of Clinical Neurology.* Vol 160: Clinical Neurophysiology: Basis and Technical Aspects. Elsevier; 2019:419-433.
5. Billman GE. Heart rate variability–a historical perspective. *Front Physiol.* 2011;2:86.

6. Angelone A, Coulter NA Jr. Respiratory sinus arrhythmia: a frequency dependent phenomenon. *J Appl Physiol.* 1964;19:479-482.
7. Kienzle MG, Ferguson DW, Birkett CL, Myers GA, Berg WJ, Mariano DJ. Clinical, hemodynamic and sympathetic neural correlates of heart rate variability in congestive heart failure. *Am J Cardiol.* 1992;69(8):761-767.
8. Ewing DJ, Campbell IW, Murray A, Neilson JM, Clarke BF. Immediate heart-rate response to standing: simple test for autonomic neuropathy in diabetes. *Br Med J.* 1978;1(6106):145-147.
9. Ziemssen T, Siepmann T. The investigation of the cardiovascular and sudomotor autonomic nervous system—a review. *Front Neurol.* 2019;10:53.
10. Low PA, Tomalia VA, Park K. Autonomic function tests: some clinical applications. *J Clin Neurol.* 2013;9(1):1-8.
11. Low PA. Testing the autonomic nervous system. *Semin Neurol.* 2003;23(04):407-422.
12. Hilz MJ, Dütsch M. Quantitative studies of autonomic function. *Muscle Nerve.* 2006;33(1):6-20.
13. Sandroni P, Benarroch EE, Low PA. Pharmacological dissection of components of the Valsalva maneuver in adrenergic failure. *J Appl Physiol (1985).* 1991;71(4):1563-1567.
14. Palamarchuk IS, Baker J, Kimpinski K. The utility of Valsalva maneuver in the diagnoses of orthostatic disorders. *Am J Physiol Regul Integr Comp Physiol.* 2015;310(3):R243-R252.
15. E Körei A, Kempler M, Istenes I, et al. Why not to use the handgrip test in the assessment of cardiovascular autonomic neuropathy among patients with diabetes mellitus? *Curr Vasc Pharmacol.* 2017;15(1):66-73.
16. Bellavere F, Ragazzi E, Chilelli NC, Lapolla A, Bax G. Autonomic testing: which value for each cardiovascular test? An observational study. *Acta Diabetol.* 2019;56(1):39-43.
17. Didangelos T, Moralidis E, Karlafti E, et al. A comparative assessment of cardiovascular autonomic reflex testing and cardiac 123I-metaiodobenzylguanidine imaging in patients with type 1 diabetes mellitus without complications or cardiovascular risk factors. *Int J Endocrinol.* 2018;2018.
18. Freeman R, Wieling W, Axelrod FB, et al. Consensus statement on the definition of orthostatic hypotension, neurally mediated syncope and the postural tachycardia syndrome. *Auton Neurosci.* 2011;161(1-2):46-48.
19. Benditt DG, Ferguson DW, Grubb BP, et al. Tilt table testing for assessing syncope. *J Am Coll Cardiol.* 1996;28(1):263-275.
20. Florian JP, Simmons EE, Chon KH, Faes L, Shykoff BE. Cardiovascular and autonomic responses to physiological stressors before and after six hours of water immersion. *J Appl Physiol.* 2013;115(9):1275-1289.
21. Shen W, Jahangir A, Beinborn D, et al. Utility of a single-stage isoproterenol tilt table test in adults: a randomized comparison with passive head-up tilt. *J Am Coll Cardiol.* 1999;33(4):985-990.
22. Bartoletti A, Alboni P, Ammirati F, et al. 'The Italian protocol': a simplified head-up tilt testing potentiated with oral nitroglycerin to assess patients with unexplained syncope. *Europace.* 2000;2(4):339-342.
23. Thomas JE. Hyperactive carotid sinus reflex and carotid sinus syncope. *Mayo Clin Proc.* 1969;44(2):127-139.
24. Kimpinski K, Iodice V, Burton DD, et al. The role of autonomic testing in the differentiation of Parkinson's disease from multiple system atrophy. *J Neurol Sci.* 2012;317(1-2):92-96.
25. Low PA, Caskey P, Tuck R, Fealey R, Dyck PJ. Quantitative sudomotor axon reflex test in normal and neuropathic subjects. *Ann Neurol.* 1983;14(5):573-580.
26. Kennedy WR, Sakuta M, Sutherland D, Goetz FC. Quantitation of the sweating deficiency in diabetes mellitus. *Ann Neurol.* 1984;15(5):482-488.
27. Illigens BM, Gibbons CH. Sweat testing to evaluate autonomic function. *Clin Auton Res.* 2009;19(2):79.
28. Al-Khatib SM, Stevenson WG, Ackerman MJ, et al. 2017 AHA/ACC/HRS guideline for management of patients with ventricular arrhythmias and the prevention of sudden cardiac death: a report of the American College of Cardiology/American Heart Association Task Force on Clinical Practice Guidelines and the Heart Rhythm Society. *J Am Coll Cardiol.* 2017;24390.
29. Mosqueda-Garcia R, Furlan R, Fernandez-Violante R. The elusive pathophysiology of neurally mediated syncope. *Circulation.* 2000;102(23):2898-2906.
30. Sheldon RS, Grubb BP 2nd, Olshansky B, et al. 2015 heart rhythm society expert consensus statement on the diagnosis and treatment of postural tachycardia syndrome, inappropriate sinus tachycardia, and vasovagal syncope. *Heart Rhythm.* 2015;12(6):e41-e63.
31. Madrid AH, Ortega J, Rebollo JG, et al. Lack of efficacy of atenolol for the prevention of neurally mediated syncope in a highly symptomatic population: a prospective, double-blind, randomized and placebo-controlled study. *J Am Coll Cardiol.* 2001;37(2):554-559.
32. Sheldon RS, Morillo CA, Klingenheben T, Krahn AD, Sheldon A, Rose MS. Age-dependent effect of β-blockers in preventing vasovagal syncope. *Circ Arrhythm Electrophysiol.* 2012;5(5):920-926.
33. Brignole M, Menozzi C, Moya A, et al. Pacemaker therapy in patients with neurally mediated syncope and documented asystole: third international study on syncope of uncertain etiology (ISSUE-3): a randomized trial. *Circulation.* 2012;125(21):2566-2571.
34. Grubb BP. Postural tachycardia syndrome. *Circulation.* 2008;117(21): 2814-2817.
35. Gibbons CH, Bonyhay I, Benson A, Wang N, Freeman R. Structural and functional small fiber abnormalities in the neuropathic postural tachycardia syndrome. *PLoS One.* 2013;8(12):e84716.
36. Parsaik A, Allison TG, Singer W, et al. Deconditioning in patients with orthostatic intolerance. *Neurology.* 2012;79(14):1435-1439.
37. Parsaik AK, Singer W, Allison TG, et al. Orthostatic intolerance without postural tachycardia: how much dysautonomia? *Clin Auton Res.* 2013;23(4):181-188.
38. Freeman R, Abuzinadah AR, Gibbons C, Jones P, Miglis MG, Sinn DI. Orthostatic hypotension: JACC state-of-the-art review. *J Am Coll Cardiol.* 2018;72(11):1294-1309.
39. Low PA, Reich SG, Jankovic J, et al. Natural history of multiple system atrophy in the USA: a prospective cohort study. *Lancet Neurol.* 2015;14(7):710-719.
40. Garland EM, Hooper WB, Robertson D. Pure autonomic failure. In: Buijs R, Swaab D, eds. *Handbook of Clinical Neurology.* Vol 117: Autonomic Nervous System. Elsevier; 2013:243-257.
41. Guidez D, Behnke S, Halmer R, et al. Is reduced myocardial sympathetic innervation associated with clinical symptoms of autonomic impairment in idiopathic Parkinson's disease? *J Neurol.* 2014;261(1):45-51.
42. Oka H, Toyoda C, Yogo M, Mochio S. Reduced cardiac 123 I-MIBG uptake reflects cardiac sympathetic dysfunction in de novo Parkinson's disease. *J Neural Transm.* 2011;118(9):1323-1327.
43. Braune S, Reinhardt M, Schnitzer R, Riedel A, Lucking CH. Cardiac uptake of [123I]MIBG separates Parkinson's disease from multiple system atrophy. *Neurology.* 1999;53(5):1020-1025.
44. Haensch C, Lerch H, Jörg J, Isenmann S. Cardiac denervation occurs independent of orthostatic hypotension and impaired heart rate variability in Parkinson's disease. *Parkinsonism Relat Disord.* 2009;15(2):134-137.
45. Iodice V, Lipp A, Ahlskog JE, et al. Autopsy confirmed multiple system atrophy cases: Mayo experience and role of autonomic function tests. *J Neurol Neurosurg Psychiatry.* 2012;83(4):453-459.
46. Kujawa K, Leurgans S, Raman R, Blasucci L, Goetz CG. Acute orthostatic hypotension when starting dopamine agonists in Parkinson's disease. *Arch Neurol.* 2000;57(10):1461-1463.
47. Hyam JA, Roy HA, Huang Y, et al. Cardiovascular autonomic responses in patients with Parkinson disease to pedunculopontine deep brain stimulation. *Clin Auton Res.* 2019;29(6):615-624.
48. Metwalley KA, Hamed SA, Farghaly HS. Cardiac autonomic function in children with type 1 diabetes. *Eur J Pediatr.* 2018;177(6):805-813.
49. Ko SH, Park SA, Cho JH, et al. Progression of cardiovascular autonomic dysfunction in patients with type 2 diabetes: a 7-year follow-up study. *Diabetes Care.* 2008;31(9):1832-1836.
50. Pop-Busui R, Cleary PA, Braffett BH, et al. Association between cardiovascular autonomic neuropathy and left ventricular dysfunction: DCCT/EDIC study (diabetes control and complications trial/epidemiology of diabetes interventions and complications). *J Am Coll Cardiol.* 2013;61(4):447-454.
51. Fealey RD, Low PA, Thomas JE. Thermoregulatory sweating abnormalities in diabetes mellitus. *Mayo Clin Proc.* 1989;64(6):617-628.
52. Maser RE, Mitchell BD, Vinik AI, Freeman R. The association between cardiovascular autonomic neuropathy and mortality in individuals with diabetes: a meta-analysis. *Diabetes Care.* 2003;26(6):1895-1901.

53. Chen P, Chen LS, Fishbein MC, Lin S, Nattel S. Role of the autonomic nervous system in atrial fibrillation: pathophysiology and therapy. *Circ Res.* 2014;114(9):1500-1515.
54. Huang J, Wen Z, Lee W, Chang M, Chen S. Changes of autonomic tone before the onset of paroxysmal atrial fibrillation. *Int J Cardiol.* 1998;66(3):275-283.
55. Nguyen BL, Fishbein MC, Chen LS, Chen P, Masroor S. Histopathological substrate for chronic atrial fibrillation in humans. *Heart Rhythm.* 2009;6(4):454-460.
56. Coumel P, Attuel P, Lavallée J, Flammang D, Leclercq JF, Slama R. Syndrome d'arythmie auriculaire d'origine vagale [The atrial arrhythmia syndrome of vagal origin]. *Arch Mal Coeur Vaiss.* 1978;71(6): 645-656.
57. Nemirovsky D, Hutter R, Gomes JA. The electrical substrate of vagal atrial fibrillation as assessed by the signal-averaged electrocardiogram of the P wave. *Pacing Clin Electrophysiol.* 2008;31(3):308-313.
58. Bourke T, Vaseghi M, Michowitz Y, et al. Neuraxial modulation for refractory ventricular arrhythmias in humans: value of thoracic epidural anesthesia and left cardiac sympathetic denervation. *Circulation.* 2009;121(21):2255-2262.
59. Armaganijan LV, Staico R, Moreira DA, et al. 6-month outcomes in patients with implantable cardioverter-defibrillators undergoing renal sympathetic denervation for the treatment of refractory ventricular arrhythmias. *JACC Cardiovasc Interv.* 2015;8(7):984-990.
60. Ukena C, Mahfoud F, Ewen S, et al. Renal denervation for treatment of ventricular arrhythmias: data from an international multicenter registry. *Clin Res Cardiol.* 2016;105(10):873-879.
61. Coats AJ, Abraham WT. Central sleep apnoea in heart failure—an important issue for the modern heart failure cardiologist. *Int J Cardiol.* 2016;206(suppl):S1-S3.
62. Mansfield D, Kaye DM, Brunner La Rocca H, Solin P, Esler MD, Naughton MT. Raised sympathetic nerve activity in heart failure and central sleep apnea is due to heart failure severity. *Circulation.* 2003;107(10):1396-1400.
63. Lanfranchi PA, Somers VK, Braghiroli A, Corra U, Eleuteri E, Giannuzzi P. Central sleep apnea in left ventricular dysfunction: prevalence and implications for arrhythmic risk. *Circulation.* 2003;107(5):727-732.
64. Cowie MR, Woehrle H, Wegscheider K, et al. Adaptive servo-ventilation for central sleep apnea in systolic heart failure. *N Engl J Med.* 2015;373(12):1095-1105.
65. Fox H, Oldenburg O, Javaheri S, et al. Long-term efficacy and safety of phrenic nerve stimulation for the treatment of central sleep apnea. *Sleep.* 2019;42(11):zsz158.
66. Costanzo MR, Ponikowski P, Javaheri S, et al. Transvenous neurostimulation for central sleep apnoea: a randomised controlled trial. *Lancet.* 2016;388(10048):974-982.
67. Li M, Zheng C, Sato T, Kawada T, Sugimachi M, Sunagawa K. Vagal nerve stimulation markedly improves long-term survival after chronic heart failure in rats. *Circulation.* 2004;109(1):120-124.
68. Shivkumar K, Ajijola OA, Anand I, et al. Clinical neurocardiology defining the value of neuroscience-based cardiovascular therapeutics. *J Physiol (Lond).* 2016;594(14):3911-3954.
69. Mar PL, Nwazue V, Black BK, et al. Valsalva maneuver in pulmonary arterial hypertension: susceptibility to syncope and autonomic dysfunction. *Chest.* 2016;149(5):1252-1260.
70. Norcliffe-Kaufmann L, Kaufmann H, Martinez J, Katz SD, Tully L, Reynolds HR. Autonomic findings in Takotsubo cardiomyopathy. *Am J Cardiol.* 2016;117(2):206-213.
71. Noor B, Akhavan S, Leuchter M, Yang EH, Ajijola OA. Quantitative assessment of cardiovascular autonomic impairment in cancer survivors: a single center experience. *Circulation.* 2020;142(suppl 3):A12919.
72. Baron-Esquivias G, Martinez-Rubio A. Tilt table test: state of the art. *Indian Pacing Electrophysiol J.* 2003;3(4):239-252.
73. Grubb BP. Neurocardiogenic syncope and related disorders of orthostatic intolerance. *Circulation.* 2005;111(22):2997-3006.
74. Brignole M, Menozzi C, Del Rosso A, et al. New classification of haemodynamics of vasovagal syncope: beyond the VASIS classification: analysis of the pre-syncopal phase of the tilt test without and with nitroglycerin challenge. *Europace.* 2000;2(1):66-76.

CHAPTER 29

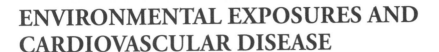

ENVIRONMENTAL EXPOSURES AND CARDIOVASCULAR DISEASE

Ahmed Ibrahim and Richard A. Lange

INTRODUCTION

Cardiovascular diseases (CVDs) are largely preventable but may have increased globally because of a mismatch between slowly adapting human genes and rapidly changing environmental factors.[1] Successful prevention or treatment of environmental cardiac toxins (**Table 29.1**) necessitates recognition of their effects, removal of the toxic agent, and, in some cases, treatment with a known antidote.

AIRBORNE POLLUTANTS

Nonchemical Pollutants: Noise

Industrialization, urbanization, and globalization have led to increased exposure to different sources of noise including road traffic, aircraft, railway, industrial, and crowded neighborhoods.

Stress and annoyance caused by noise lead to endocrine and autonomic effects causing CVD including coronary artery disease (CAD), hypertension, heart failure, atrial fibrillation, and stroke. Noise exerts pathophysiologic effects related to the duration of exposure. Noise-induced stress increases blood pressure, blood sugar, cholesterol, and blood viscosity and can lead to oxidative stress with endothelial dysfunction and activation of prothrombotic and inflammatory pathways, triggering or worsening CVD.[2]

Chemical Pollutants

Air Pollutants

Fossil fuel combustion results in particulate matter (PM) and volatile organic chemicals (VOCs). Particles of varying chemical composition suspended in the air can be separated by particle size: coarse PM less than 10 μm in diameter (PM10), fine PM less than 2.5 μm in diameter (PM2.5), and ultrafine PM less than 0.1 μm in diameter (PM0.1). Ultrafine PM can enter directly into the blood stream, whereas PM2.5 induces systemic inflammation through penetration of pulmonary interstitium.[3] About 70% to 80% of premature deaths resulting from exposure to PM—especially PM2.5—are due to cardiovascular (CV) causes. The World Health Organization (WHO) estimated that 58% of outdoor air pollution–related premature deaths were due to ischemic heart disease and stroke.[4]

Chronic, acute, and even brief exposure to polluted air is associated with myocardial infarction (MI), stroke, arrhythmias, atrial fibrillation, and hospitalization for exacerbation of congestive heart failure (CHF) in susceptible individuals. These are attributed to progression of atherosclerotic lesions and effects on blood pressure regulation, peripheral thrombosis, endothelial function, and insulin sensitivity. These effects, except for the incidence of stroke in response to acute exposure, appear to be less pronounced in healthy subjects.[5]

A Japanese study showed an independent association between the increase in daily PM2.5 concentration— even at lower levels than regulation-recommended standards and guidelines—and out-of-hospital cardiac arrest, especially in older individuals.[6]

In addition to PM, VOC air pollutants like acrolein, benzene, and butadiene contribute to cardiac toxicity. Acute exposure to acrolein, in particular, can cause dyslipidemia, vascular injury, endothelial dysfunction, and platelet activation; chronic exposure accelerates atherogenesis and may induce a dilated cardiomyopathy.[7]

Carbon Monoxide

Carbon monoxide (CO) is an odorless, colorless, and tasteless gas that is produced mainly by incomplete combustion of fossil fuel. Other sources include gas heaters, old appliances, wall ovens, stoves, tobacco smoking, fireplaces, chimneys, and charcoal grills. Accordingly, it is recommended to install a CO detector for all rooms that contain a fuel burning appliance.[8]

Even low exposure to CO can raise blood carboxyhemoglobin concentrations by binding to hemoglobin and exacerbate myocardial ischemia through reducing delivery of oxygen to tissue, because the affinity of hemoglobin for CO is more than 200 times that of oxygen. Other mechanisms for adverse health responses included cardiac dysfunction, impaired myoglobin function, generation of reactive oxygen species, and interruption of the electron transport chain.[9] CO exposure is also associated with out-of-hospital cardiac arrest.[6]

Treatment includes providing maximal oxygenation to facilitate the association of oxygen with hemoglobin. This can be accomplished by delivering 100% high-flow oxygen to the patient through a non-rebreather mask, which reduces the half-life of carboxyhemoglobin from 4 to 6 hours to 40 to 80 minutes.

Inhalants

Individuals use inhalants to obtain an immediate rush, or high. These inhalants have gained popularity for abuse because they are cheap and available without legal restriction. Toluene is the most

TABLE 29.1 Environmental Cardiovascular Toxins

Category	Specific Cardiovascular Toxins
Airborne	Pollutants (noise, chemical) Carbon monoxide Inhalants Solid fuel
Plants	Aconite Cardenolides Mad honey Areca nut Herbal supplements
Household chemicals	Camphor Detergents Skin cleansers Dettol
Industrial exposure	Fluoride Hydrogen sulfide Volatile organic compounds
Fumigants and pesticide	Aluminum phosphide Endosulfan Organophosphates Pyrethroid insecticides Sulfur fluoride
Heavy metals	Antimony Arsenic Bismuth Cadmium Chromium Cobalt Copper Gold Iron Lead Manganese Mercury Molybdenum Nickel Thallium Zinc

widely inhaled organic solvent and is available in glues, paint thinners, dry cleaning fluids, felt-tip marker fluid, hair spray, deodorants, spray paint, and whipped cream dispensers. It is also heavily used in dyes, varnishes, rubber, and the cleaning and cosmetics industries.[10] Acute effects include sinus bradycardia, atrioventricular block, asystole, ventricular arrhythmias, dilated cardiomyopathy, CHF, MI, and sudden cardiac death through direct effects on sodium and calcium voltage-gated channels.[11] Chronic occupational exposure to toluene, trichloroethane, xylene, trichloroethylene, and trichlorotrifluoroethane is associated with autonomic dysfunction,[11] arrhythmias, P wave, and QRS changes.[12]

Solid Fuel

More than half the world's population use solid fuel for cooking and heating. Sources include wood, crop residues, cow dung, and coal. Like fossil fuel combustion, solid fuel produces an amount of fine PM that exceeds the standards for outdoor concentration applied in the United States and European Union.

A study among rural Pakistani nonsmoking women demonstrated an independent significant association between the use of solid fuel and acute coronary syndromes.[13] In rural China, almost 100,000 solid fuel users were followed for 7 years and found to have more CV and all-cause mortality than clean fuel (electricity, natural gas, and liquefied petroleum) users and those with appropriate ventilation.[14] This was confirmed in a multinational study in more than 30,000 solid fuel users from middle- to low-income countries who experienced more fatal and nonfatal CV events (CHF, stroke, and MI) as compared to nonusers over a follow-up period of 9 years.[15] Additional prospective studies on the acute and chronic CV response to household air pollution from solid fuel combustion are needed to better understand how the effects of this exposure differ from ambient air pollution.[3]

PLANT-BASED POLLUTANTS

Aconite

Aconite is derived from the plant *Aconitum*, which is ubiquitous in Europe, North America, and Asia and known by the common names of monkshood, wolfsbane, and "the devil's helmet" (**Figure 29.1**). Aconite poisoning is more common in Asia where dried rootstocks of the *Aconitum* plants are used in Chinese herbal medicine (caowu, chuanwu, and fuzi). Toxicity may occur from ingestion following improper processing of the plant for use in complementary medicines, mistaking the plant for an edible species, and intentional suicide and homicide attempts. Aconite causes persistent activation of voltage-gated sodium and calcium channels, leading to sustained depolarization and resistance to excitation. It is toxic to the neurologic system (causing descending paresthesias, numbness, and mild weakness), gastrointestinal tract (inducing nausea, vomiting,

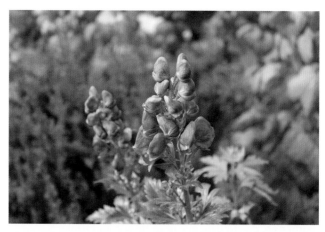

FIGURE 29.1 Aconite is known by the common names of monkshood, wolfsbane, and the devil's helmet. (Martina Unbehauen/Shutterstock.)

and diarrhea), and the CV system (causing malignant ventricular rhythms, hypotension, and shock).

Aconite poisoning is usually established clinically, but it can be confirmed with chromatographic and mass spectrometric analysis of serum and urine alkaloids and metabolites. The treatment of aconite poisoning is supportive.[16] Because of the persistent activation of the voltage-gated sodium channels, class I antiarrhythmic agents (ie, sodium channel blocking agents) have been used to treat aconite-induced ventricular arrhythmias; additionally, high-dose magnesium sulfate therapy has been recommended based on in vitro and animal experiments as well as limited clinical case reports. When arrhythmias are resistant to pharmacologic therapy or direct cardioversion, mechanical support with cardiopulmonary extracorporeal bypass or a left ventricular assist device has been suggested as salvage therapy.

Cardenolides

Cardenolides are naturally occurring cardiac glycosides found in plant species throughout the world. Their CV toxicity results from inhibition of the Na^+/K^+ ATPase channel. Accordingly, ingestion of cardenolides may lead to serious dysrhythmias, including second- or third-degree heart block, and cardiac arrest.

In South Asia, cardenolide poisoning from yellow (*Thevetia peruviana*), pink, or white oleander (*Nerium oleander*) (**Figure 29.2**) and fruits from the *Cerbera manghas* family (sea mango, pink-eyed cerbera, odollam tree, "suicide" tree) (**Figure 29.3**) is a leading cause of attempted suicide, with thousands of cases a year and a 5% to 10% case fatality ratio. Yellow oleander seed (or "codo de fraile") is sold in some markets in Mexico and Central America, as well as on the Internet, as a "safe" and "natural" treatment for obesity.[17] However, all parts of the plant are toxic no matter how it is prepared (fresh, dried, or boiled). Fatality may occur after ingestion of one leaf by children and in adults after eating 8 to 10 seeds, 15 to 20 g of the root, or 5 to 15 leaves. Accidental poisoning occurs in children who mistakenly consume the fruit—either in confusion for water chestnut or out of curiosity; and mixing the dried plant parts in herbal tea has resulted in accidental poisoning in adults.

Although the initial symptoms (headaches, intense abdominal pain, vomiting, diarrhea, and bradycardia) may show up within minutes after ingestion, prolonged hospitalization and observation are recommended after cardenolide ingestion, because the occurrence of dangerous dysrhythmias may be delayed up to 72 hours after ingestion. Patients who develop bradyarrhythmias may be medicated with atropine and isoprenaline or require a temporary pacemaker. A meta-analysis concluded that multiple doses of activated charcoal within 24 hours of toxin ingestion and administration of antidigoxin Fab antitoxin reduce the risk of cardiac dysrhythmias. Hemodialysis or hemoperfusion is ineffective in preventing toxicity because of the large volume of distribution of the toxin.

Mad Honey

Grayanotoxin is a natural compound found in the leaves of various rhododendron species and in the honey derived from the nectar of these plants (so-called "mad honey"). The rhododendrons associated with mad honey are found in the Black Sea region of Eastern Turkey (where mad honey intoxication has been described most often) as well as in North America, Europe, and Asia. Mad honey has been used as a herbal medicine for the treatment of diabetes mellitus, gastrointestinal disorders, heart disease, hypertension, and sexual dysfunction; such usage has contributed to episodes of accidental poisoning.

Grayanotoxin binds with the voltage-dependent sodium channels in their active state, thereby preventing inactivation

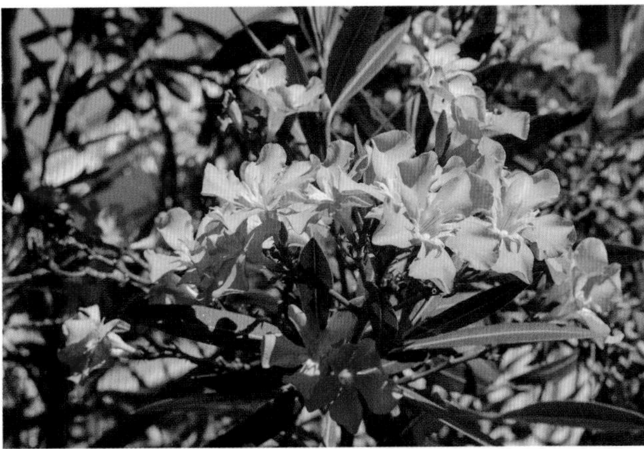

FIGURE 29.2 Pink oleander (*Nerium oleander*) is a source of cardenolides. (Zoran Milosavljevic/Shutterstock.)

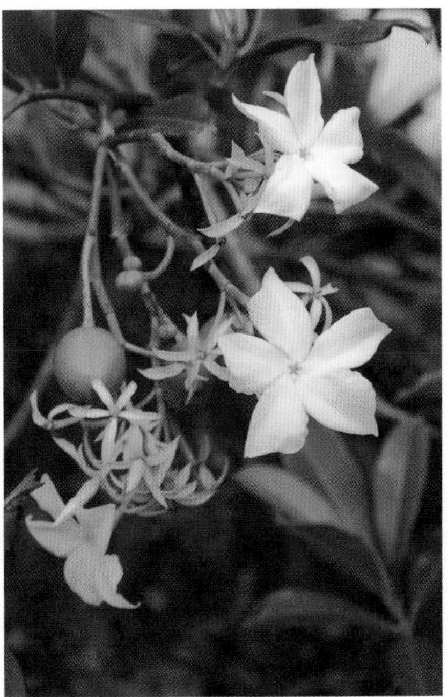

FIGURE 29.3 *Cerbera odollam* (commonly known as suicide tree) is a plant source of cardenolides. (SAM THOMAS A/Shutterstock.)

(ie, the channels remain in a state of depolarization). This effect on the vagus nerve leads to increased parasympathetic tone, causing bradycardia, hypotension, and various degrees of atrioventricular block. Atrial fibrillation, asystole, and MI have also been observed following mad honey ingestion. In a review of ~1200 cases of mad honey intoxication,[18] the most common complaints were dizziness, nausea, and presyncope, and the electrocardiographic (ECG) findings were sinus bradycardia (80%), complete atrioventricular block (46%), atrioventricular block (31%), ST-segment elevation (23%), and nodal rhythm (11%).

The diagnosis of mad honey intoxication is usually based on the clinical history, but grayanotoxin levels from urine and blood of patients with mad honey intoxication—and in the honey consumed—can be measured with liquid chromatography/mass spectrometry for confirmation.[19]

The cardiac and general cholinergic symptoms of grayanotoxin poisoning generally occur within minutes to a few hours of mad honey ingestion and dissipate within 24 hours. If treatment is necessary, intravenous fluids, atropine sulfate, vasopressors, and temporary pacing all have been used successfully until the toxic effects of grayanotoxin resolve.[20]

ARECA (BETEL) NUT

The areca (betel) nut is the seed of the areca palm (*Areca catechu*), which grows in much of the Tropical Pacific, Asia, and parts of East Africa; it is often chewed wrapped in betel leaves (**Figure 29.4**). Betel nut is the fourth most widely used addictive substance in the world—behind alcohol, nicotine, and caffeine—with betel nut chewers making up 10% of the world's population (mostly in Asia and South Asia). Its users describe the stimulating symptoms of betel as similar to tobacco or cocaine, and it has also been used as a diuretic, laxative, and sexual stimulant. The active ingredients—arecoline, arecaidine, guvacine, and guvacoline—are alkaloids that produce parasympathetic effects as an agonist of nicotinic and muscarinic receptors.

Betel nut use can induce hypertension, sinus and supraventricular tachycardia, and acute MI. Compared to nonusers, individuals who chew betel nuts have a higher incidence of CV mortality, which may be attributable to the increased incidence of comorbidities (such as diabetes mellitus, hypertension, and obesity), contamination of trace heavy metals (such as arsenic and manganese), and periodontal disease, a known risk factor for CVD.

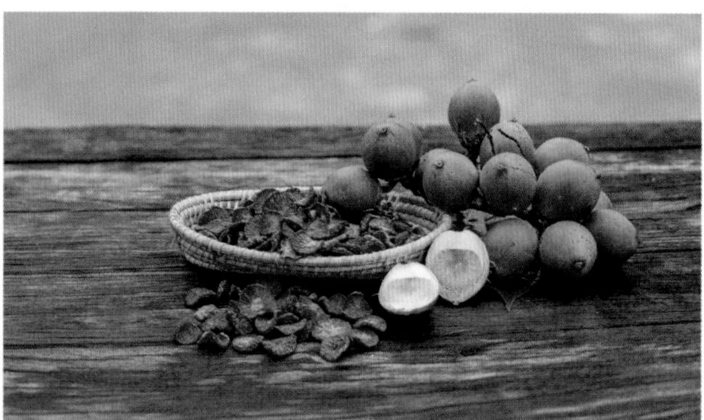

FIGURE 29.4 The areca (betel) nut grows in much of the Tropical Pacific, Southeast and South Asia, and East Africa. (Nirundon/Shutterstock.)

Herbal Supplements

Although the majority of botanical products appear inherently safe, case reports have implicated several herbal supplements with cardiac toxicity risk (**Table 29.2**).[21] Although case reports do not always demonstrate causation or association, reoccurrences raise concerns that the herbal supplements listed may be cardiotoxic for some individuals.

HOUSEHOLD CHEMICALS

Camphor

Camphor is a pleasant smelling terpene used in skin lotions and in many ayurvedic medicines intended for oral use as an abortifacient/contraceptive, analgesic, antipruritic, antiseptic, and aphrodisiac. Ingestion of 2 g of camphor is sufficient to produce toxic effects in adults. Initial symptoms may occur within 5 to 15 minutes of ingestion and include nausea and vomiting, oral and epigastric burning, a feeling of warmth, and headache. These symptoms may progress to altered mental status, convulsions, coma, and death, usually because of respiratory failure or neurologic complications. Clinical toxicity typically resolves within 24 hours in survivors.

CV toxicities include tachycardia, prolonged QTc and QRS intervals, atrioventricular conduction block, and ST-segment changes. Myocarditis and depressed ventricular systolic function may occur following camphor ingestion.[22] Treatment is largely supportive; hemodialysis has not shown to be of benefit.

Detergents

Suicidal intoxication with detergents has been associated with hypotension, refractory ventricular fibrillation, depressed ventricular systolic function, myocarditis, and pulmonary edema. Treatment is supportive.

Skin Cleansers

Topical chlorhexidine application has been implicated in coronary artery vasospasm and MI in angiographically normal arteries. Alcohol-based hand sanitizers usually contain ethanol and isopropyl alcohol. CV complications reported following oral ingestion of these sanitizers include ST-segment and T-wave changes, ventricular fibrillation, and cardiac arrest.

Dettol

Dettol is a liquid household disinfectant containing 4.8% chloroxylenol, pine oil, and isopropyl alcohol. Most toxicity is related to its central nervous system suppressant effects, local corrosion to the gastrointestinal tract, as well as acute respiratory distress syndrome. Hypotension and tachy- and bradyarrhythmias have been described with Dettol poisoning.

TABLE 29.2 Reported Cases of Heart Toxicity Related to Herbal Plant Consumption

Common Name	Scientific Name	Active Compounds	Uses	Side Effects (Cardiac)
Foxglove	*Digitalis lanata* *Digitalis purpurea*	Cardiac glycosides	Congestive heart failure	Tachycardia, bradyarrhythmia, ventricular fibrillation, and death
Henbane	*Hyoscyamus niger*	Tropane alkaloids—atropine (hyoscyamine) and scopolamine (hyoscine)	Herbal therapy in most traditional medicines, stomach complaints, toothaches, ulcers, and tumors	Tachycardia, arrhythmia
Jin Bu Huan	*Lycopodium serratum*	*Levo*-tetrahydropalmatine; pyrrolizidine alkaloids	Traditional Chinese medicine used as a sedative, analgesic, and indigestion aid	Life-threatening bradycardia
Lily of the valley	*Convallaria majalis*	Cardiac glycosides	Arrhythmia, cardiac insufficiency, and "nervous heart" complaints	Arrhythmia, cardiac shock
Squill	*Urginea maritima*	Cardiac glycosides	Cardiac insufficiency, arrhythmia, "nervous heart" complaints. Also bronchitis, asthma, whooping cough, and wounds	Arrhythmias, atrioventricular block, death
Yohimbe	*Pausinystalia yohimbe*	Yohimbine alkaloid	Erectile dysfunction and sports enhancement	Hypertension, tachycardia

Perfluorooctanoic Acid

Perfluorooctanoic acid (PFOA) is a manmade chemical used in the manufacture of common household consumer products and levels are detectable in the serum of more than 98% of the U.S. population. The chemical is widely used in industrial and consumer products, including stain- and water-resistant coatings for carpets and fabrics, fast-food packaging, fire-resistant foams, paints, and hydraulic fluids. Studies have suggested that exposure to PFOA is associated with CVD and peripheral vascular disease (PAD), independent of traditional CV risk factors.[23]

INDUSTRIAL EXPOSURE

Fluoride

Most fluoride toxicity results from accidental exposure. Hydrofluoric acid is used in glass etching, and electronic and chemical industries; toxicity can occur after inhalation or skin absorption. Fluoride salts are found in insecticides, oil refineries, and many household and commercial rust removers. Systemic toxicity is directly related to the amount of fluoride that is absorbed systemically. Systemic toxicity can occur with exposure of ~1% of the body surface area (ie, the size of the palm of a hand) to concentrated hydrofluoride.

Systemic toxicity results in electrolyte abnormalities and direct myocardial toxicity. CV toxicity most often causes QT interval prolongation, tachy- or bradyarrhythmias, and refractory ventricular fibrillation. The therapy for fluoride toxicity has included milk ingestion (to dilute the acid and to bind the fluoride in the gastrointestinal tract), gastric lavage with fluoride binders, parenteral calcium and magnesium administration, and hemodialysis.

High levels of fluoride in the environment (ie, drinking water) have also been associated with CV conditions.[24] Fluorosis—identified by mottled enamel on the teeth of the local population—is endemic in some areas (ie, India, China, and Africa) where fluoride content is high in drinking water. In humans, sinus bradycardia, low voltage, ST- and T-wave changes, increased QT and QTc intervals, and left ventricular diastolic dysfunction have been reported in patients living in fluorosis-endemic areas.[24]

Hydrogen Sulfide

Hydrogen sulfide (H_2S) is a water-soluble, colorless gas with the distinct odor of rotten eggs. It remains a significant chemical hazard in the gas and oil industry, industrial processing (ie, wood pulp processing, manure processing, sugar-beet processing, rayon manufacturing), and various farming and fishing activities. It is also used as a method of suicide accomplished by mixing a source of sulfide and various types of acidic solutions, which are readily available in most household chemicals.

The mechanism of H_2S toxicity is inactivation of mitochondrial cytochrome oxidase. The consequences of an acute exposure to H_2S are usually benign as long as the level of exposure remains low, but when exposure reaches levels greater than 500 ppm, cardiac toxicity can lead to rapid death.

MI, myocarditis, and dilated cardiomyopathy have all been described following H_2S exposure.[25] In patients suspected of exposure, H_2S can be detected with measurement of thiosulfate levels via chromatography of the blood or tissue.

Inhaled amyl nitrite and intravenous sodium nitrite have been used as antidotes to H_2S toxicity and are effective if administered within minutes of H_2S exposure. They induce methemoglobin that competitively binds the sulfide ion, thereby liberating the cytochrome oxidase. The resultant compound—sulfmethemoglobin—can be metabolized and excreted. Close monitoring is recommended because nitrates can induce hypotension, and methemoglobin may reduce oxygen delivery.

Volatile Organic Compounds

Health assessment of volatile organic compound exposures near industrial complexes has shown that the prevalence of CV diseases is higher in these areas than in controlled areas.[26] Dry cleaning workers are commonly exposed to tetrachloroethylene and other volatile organic solvents. Recent studies have shown that these solvent exposure levels are associated with increases in mortality owing to heart disease (hazard ratio 1.6).[27]

FUMIGANTS AND PESTICIDES

Aluminum Phosphide

Aluminum phosphide is an inexpensive rodenticide that can be ingested, absorbed through skin, or inhaled in its gaseous form. Toxic cardiac effects through oxidative stress include myocarditis, MI, CHF, and arrhythmias exacerbated by hypokalemia. Treatment is by gastric lavage, neutralization of gastric contents with dilute potassium permanganate, intravenous magnesium, and *N*-acetyl cysteine.[10]

Endosulfan

Endosulfan is used as an insecticide that can be toxic through ingestion, inhalation, or skin contact and manifests through inhibition of calcium, sodium, and chloride channels leading to MI, CHF, QTc interval prolongation, atrial fibrillation, and ventricular arrhythmias.[10]

Organophosphates

Organophosphates are lipid soluble, and exposure can occur through skin or eye contact, ingestion, and inhalation. They are used as pesticides and irreversibly inhibit anticholinesterase, leading to high parasympathetic surge. Proven CV effects are mainly acute, causing tachycardia and hypertension initially through stimulation of nicotinic receptors followed by a hypercholinergic state manifested by bradycardia and hypotension ending with long QTc interval predisposing to lethal arrhythmias. Treatment includes atropine, pralidoxime, and benzodiazepines for seizures.[10]

Pyrethroid Insecticides

Pyrethroid insecticides are mainly directed against household insects, such as mosquitoes, flies, and cockroaches. They exhibit acute CV toxic effect through inhibiting voltage-gated sodium and chloride channels, leading to sinus tachycardia, sinus arrest, and cardiomyopathy. Long-term exposure has been independently associated with three times the rate of death from CVD, but the mechanism remains unclear.[28]

Sulfur Fluoride

Sulfur fluoride is used as an odorless and tasteless fumigant against wood-boring insects such as termites. Exposure occurs through inhalation, and acute toxicity can cause hypokalemia, hypocalcemia, and hypomagnesemia, leading to arrhythmias that may be lethal. Treatment of sulfuryl fluoride is similar to other manners of intoxication with systemic fluoride: oral administration of dilute calcium hydroxide or calcium chloride to prevent further absorption and injection of calcium gluconate to increase the calcium level in the blood.[10] Chronic exposure to fluoride has been shown to increase oxidative stress and insulin resistance in animal studies and is associated with hypertension and cardiometabolic risk factors in peripubertal Mexican girls.[29]

HEAVY METALS

Antimony

Antimony (Sb) and its compounds are found in the natural environment, including minerals, air, soil, and water. It is also used in metal alloys, storage batteries, bearings, castings, paints, fire-retardant textiles, plastics, and antiparasitic medications. Depending on dose and duration of exposure to antimony, its effect can range from ECG changes to lethal arrhythmias. Other effects include hypertension, peripheral artery disease, CVD, and stroke. Elevated urine antimony levels are associated with CVD mortality, MI, and CHF.[30] The mechanism of its CV effects remains unclear.

Arsenic

Arsenic (AS) is listed as the number one hazardous substance on the Agency of Toxic Substances and Disease Registry (ATSDR) 2017 priority list based on a combination of toxicity, frequency of occurrence, and potential for human exposure.[31] It is mainly ingested in water from wells frequently found in developing countries and American Indians reservations or by ingestion of food—especially rice—contaminated by naturally occurring arsenic, industrial sources, or mineral deposits. After absorption, inorganic forms of arsenic (arsenate and arsenite) are metabolized into monomethylated (MMA) and dimethylated (DMA) compounds that are excreted in the urine together with unmetabolized inorganic arsenic. High proportions of MMA and low proportions of DMA in urine are related to risks of cancer and CVD, whereas low levels of MMA and high levels of DMA are linked to adiposity and diabetes.[31] Even at low-dose exposure, arsenic affects pathways for oxidative stress and inflammation and alters ion channel activity, leading to diabetes, endothelial dysfunction, hypertension, kidney injury, peripheral arterial disease, and CAD.[32,33,34] The Strong Heart Study showed that arsenic exposure was associated with left ventricular hypertrophy in young American Indians without CVD, and its effects were more pronounced in those with hypertension or prehypertension.[35]

Bismuth

Approximately 65% of bismuth (Bi) is consumed in the United States in low-melting alloys and metallurgical additives, including electronic and thermoelectric applications. The remainder is used for catalysts, pearlescent pigments in cosmetics, pharmaceuticals, and industrial chemicals. Bismuth compounds have been used as dusting powders, bullets, astringents, antiseptics, antacids, and radiopaque agents in radiographic diagnosis (now replaced by barium sulfate). Bismuth shielding is used to reduce radiation dosages during radiographic or computed tomography evaluations.[36] In recent years, bismuth salts have been increasingly used for the treatment of *Helicobacter pylori* infections of the gastrointestinal tract. An obsolete use is the treatment of syphilis, where bismuth compounds have been replaced by penicillin. Case reports from the 1940s on the effects of parenteral bismuth used for treatment of syphilis showed that its use was associated with CHF and lower heart rate and blood pressure.[10]

Cadmium

Cadmium (Cd) is a by-product from the mining, smelting, and refining of zinc, lead, and copper ores. Use of cadmium markedly increased throughout the 20th century in applications such as nickel-cadmium batteries, metal coatings, paints, pigments, and plastic stabilizers. Soil is contaminated with cadmium from industrial releases, fuel combustion, and cadmium-containing phosphate fertilizers. Leafy and root vegetables and grains bioconcentrate cadmium that is bound to organic matter in soil, resulting in a major cadmium-exposure pathway through diet and tobacco smoking. Other dietary sources include shellfish and organ meats (liver and kidney). Smoking (direct and secondhand) is the dominant source of inhaled cadmium, but ambient air can also contribute to exposure, particularly in the vicinity of industrial sources (such as incinerator plants). Although only 1% to 5% of ingested and 25% to 50% of inhaled cadmium is absorbed, its biologic half-life in the human body is exceptionally long (15-45 years). Cadmium accumulates predominately in the kidneys, and levels in blood and urine are established biomarkers of recent and total body exposure. CV effects include hypertension, oxidative stress, inflammation, and endothelial cell damage, which can result in atherosclerosis leading to peripheral arterial disease, MI, and stroke.[3]

Chromium

Trivalent chromium (Cr^3) is in the air, water, and soil and is widely found in the food supply. Like other trace minerals, the amount in foods is minute and varies depending on exposure to chromium in the environment and during manufacturing. In general, meat, shellfish, fish, eggs, whole grain cereals, nuts, and some fruits and vegetables are dietary sources of chromium.

Lower plasma chromium levels are associated with hyperglycemia, hyperinsulinemia, hypertension, insulin resistance, and inflammation, whereas high levels are associated with favorable fat distribution.

Chromium enhances glucose and lipid metabolism, thereby reducing CV risk. It functions as a secondary messenger to insulin, thereby improving insulin sensitivity and facilitating glucose utilization by insulin-targeted tissues. Chromium also improves insulin affinity to its receptors, activates insulin receptor kinases, and inhibits insulin receptor phosphatases. Chromodulin, the chromium-binding protein, promotes tyrosine kinase activity of insulin receptor during response to insulin.[37]

Cobalt

Cobalt (Co) is a relatively rare element with properties similar to those of iron and nickel. Occupational contact with cobalt may occur in processing plants, hard-metal industry, diamond polishing, and the manufacture of ceramics.[38] Acute exposure is usually rapid onset and can be associated with polycythemia, pericardial effusion, and goiter.[30] Cobalt is rarely used in medicine anymore, and protective measures to avoid occupational exposure have decreased the incidence of cobalt-induced cardiomyopathy. An echocardiography study among workers at a cobalt production plant followed for 6 years found no evidence of myocardial dysfunction.[39] Nonoccupational exposure to cobalt may occur in athletes who ingest it to increase red blood cell volume to improve exercise performance. Cobalt alloy can also diffuse from degenerated hip prostheses into the blood. Predisposing factors to cobalt-induced cardiomyopathy include low-protein diet, thiamine deficiency, alcoholism, and hypothyroidism. Diagnostic features of cobalt-induced cardiomyopathy include a dilated left ventricle and reduced ejection fraction in the setting of increased blood and tissue cobalt levels with reversal of these changes once cobalt level normalizes.

Copper

Copper (Cu) is a micronutrient that is present in oysters, nuts, whole grains, and dietary supplements. Exposure to copper occurs from diet, supplements, environmental exposures (ie, when copper is released into the air from volcanoes and forest fires), medical treatments (ie, dialysis via copper tubing and prolonged intravenous total parenteral nutrition), and industrial sources (ie, copper smelters, iron and steel production, municipal incinerators, and pesticide production). Excessively low and high levels of copper are deleterious. Increased levels lead to oxidative stress, atherosclerosis, hypertension, diabetes, MI, stroke, and microvascular disease. Increased copper/zinc ratio has been observed in patients with CHF.[40] Copper overload is treated with high-dose zinc, ascorbic acid, and even D-penicillamine.

Low copper levels are also linked to atherosclerosis, dyslipidemia, and hypertension through reduced antioxidant activity and impaired endothelium-dependent relaxation.[10,41] Human subjects fed a diet low in copper may experience severe tachycardia, heart block, and MI.

Gold

Gold-coated coronary stents have been associated with allergic in-stent restenosis and thrombosis. Gold (Au) therapy for rheumatoid arthritis is associated with CHF, MI, and ventricular arrhythmias.

Iron

Iron (Fe) is an essential mineral that is present in dried fruits and vegetables, egg yolk, and red meat. Iron plays a catalytic role for production of reactive oxygen species that might increase atherosclerosis and arterial stiffness. Iron-dependent cell death (ferroptosis) and myocardial hemorrhage releasing free iron are potential other mechanisms for its myocardial toxic effect.

Iron overload states occur in hereditary hemochromatosis, cirrhosis, sickle cell anemia, myelodysplastic syndrome, and severe thalassemia, leading to restrictive and then dilated cardiomyopathies and arrhythmias. T2-weighted cardiac magnetic resonance imaging can early detect myocardial iron deposition that might allow for chelation and reversing iron toxic effects. Iron deficiency anemia increases ischemia and risk of stroke by creating a hypercoagulable state and an oxygen demand-supply mismatch.[10,42] Intravenous ferric carboxymaltose in iron-deficient CHF patients improves 6-minute walk test distance, peak oxygen consumption, quality of life, and New York Heart Association functional class. Meta-analysis also suggests such treatment reduces hospitalizations and mortality in these patients.[43]

Lead

Despite effort for banning its use, lead (Pb) remains an attractive choice for use in multiple products, such as pipes, paints, weights, cables, batteries, and insulation shields because of its low melting temperature and easy malleability. Some developing countries use leaded petroleum that pollutes both the air and soil. Another major source of lead exposure is inhalation by occupational workers in recycling and battery factories. In experimental models, lead increases oxidative stress, decreases nitric oxide, and promotes atherosclerosis, vascular remodeling, and platelet activation. Lead exposure is associated with hypertension, ECG abnormalities, heart rate variability, cardiometabolic syndrome, peripheral arterial disease, left ventricular hypertrophy, CAD, decreased ventricular systolic function, stroke, and CVD mortality, even with low-level exposure.[3,44]

Manganese

Manganese (Mn) is an essential mineral that, if consumed excessively, can be toxic. The mineral can be found in abundance in leafy vegetables, such as spinach and kale, as well as in tea, pineapple, and nuts. Occupational exposure occurs with welding, alloys, and cell batteries. Rarely, it can happen with exposure to contrast material for magnetic resonance imaging, manganese-containing fungicide, or cocaine. In animals, manganese has caused negative inotropy as a calcium antagonist, although it precipitated tachycardia, vasodilatation, and hypertension by releasing catecholamines. Arrhythmias and myonecrosis were also observed.

Intravenous manganese-containing contrast materials may cause transient tachycardia and hypertension that resolves with cessation of the infusion. Occupational exposure can cause arrhythmias and ST-T changes. Toxicity can cause orthostatic hypotension and decreased heart rate variability.[10] Some of these effects can be explained by the accumulation of malondialdehyde in the heart increasing the oxidative stress, especially if combined with other heavy metals like lead or cadmium.[45]

MERCURY

Mercury (Hg) can be found in thermometers, sphygmomanometers, barometers, incandescent lights, batteries, dental amalgams, germicidal soaps, and skin creams. It has been used in small amount in medicines and vaccines as a preservative. The most toxic form of mercury is methylmercury (MeHg) produced by sulfate-producing aquatic bacteria polluting lakes, rivers, and oceans; hence, exposure is through eating seafood. Proposed mechanisms of CV effects are inducing oxidative stress and mitochondrial dysfunction. Effects include hypertension, decreased sympathetic low-frequency and parasympathetic high-frequency modulation heart rate variability, increased risk of MI, atherosclerosis, and coronary dysfunction through producing oxidized low-density lipoprotein and defective high-density lipoprotein cholesterol.[46]

Molybdenum

Molybdenum (Mo) has been used in stainless steel stents and, like nickel (Nickel section), can cause an inflammatory hypersensitivity reaction leading to in-stent restenosis and acute coronary syndrome in patients allergic to molybdenum.[10]

Nickel

Nickel (Ni) is a main component of first-generation stents and atrial septal occluder devices. Subsequently, the nickel in stents has been replaced by cobalt and chromium because of the association between contact dermatitis because of nickel allergy (prevalent in 16% of Americans and up to 25% of Europeans) and "allergic" in-stent restenosis and thrombosis.[10] Maternal and fetal nickel exposure has been linked to congenital heart disease.[47]

Thallium

Thallium (Tl) has been banned from use as a rodenticide in United States since the 1960s, but it is used in the manufacture of electronic components, optical lenses, semiconductor materials, alloys, gamma radiation detection equipment, imitation jewelry, artists' paints, low-temperature thermometers, and green fireworks. It can be inhaled, ingested, or absorbed through the skin. Its toxic CV effects include myocarditis and arrhythmias (eg, sudden cardiac death has been noted up to 2 months after acute intoxication) owing to impaired glucose metabolism, Na-K ATPase inhibition, mitochondrial damage, and accumulation of lipid peroxides with inhibition of electron transport and protein synthesis. Treatment includes early forced diuresis, Prussian blue, and hemodialysis.[10]

Zinc

Zinc (Zn) is an important trace element and is present in red meat, shellfish, legumes, and nuts. It plays an important role in maintaining cellular structure and functions. Zinc homeostasis has been closely linked to copper levels and a decreased zinc/copper ratio has been associated with heart failure. Zinc deficiency has been also linked to increased oxidative stress, hypertension, and diabetes.[40]

DIAGNOSIS AND MANAGEMENT OF A PATIENT WITH SUSPECTED OR KNOWN ENVIRONMENTAL TOXICITY

The principles of diagnosis and management of individuals with suspected or known environmental toxicity include the following:

- Identifying the likely environmental causes of the adverse health outcomes.
- Confirming and (if possible) quantifying the magnitude of exposure and route of exposure, taking into account processes that may have changed the intensity of exposure, such as dispersion or dilution.
- Defining the potentially exposed population.
- Determining whether exposure is sufficient to result in adverse health effects (including assessment of inherent toxicity of the exposure, suspected dose, and pathway and duration of exposure).
- Determining whether exposure has in fact resulted in symptoms or disease in the exposed population, if sufficient time has elapsed for occurrence.
- Recommending or taking actions to prevent further exposure and additional cases of disease.
- Management of toxicity will be related to particular exposure.

RESEARCH AND FUTURE DIRECTIONS

- Further refinements of the Computational Toxicology Chemicals Dashboard (CompTox Chemicals Dashboard) that provides one-stop access to chemistry, toxicity, and exposure information to help make decisions about the safety of chemicals.
- Development of new online tools such as the Chemical and Products Database (CPDat), available in the CompTox Chemicals Dashboard.

KEY POINTS

- ✔ Immediate actions are warranted to stop exposure to a known toxicant.
- ✔ Biologic monitoring can be an important tool to assess exposure and to track the reduction in body burden once interventions to stop exposure have been implemented.
- ✔ Environmental toxicity investigations usually require assembly of multidisciplinary teams whose makeup will depend on the exposure and health concern.

REFERENCES

1. Bhatnagar A. Environmental determinants of cardiovascular disease. *Circ Res.* 2017;121(2):162-180.
2. Munzel T, Schmidt FP, Steven S, Herzog J, Daiber A, Sorensen M. Environmental noise and the cardiovascular system. *J Am Coll Cardiol.* 2018;71(6):688-697.
3. Burroughs Pena MS, Rollins A. Environmental exposures and cardiovascular disease: a challenge for health and development in low-and middle-income countries. *Cardiol Clin.* 2017;35(1):71-86.
4. World Health Organization. Ambient (outdoor) air quality and health, Published May 2, 2018. https://www.who.int/en/news-room/fact-sheets/detail/ambient-(outdoor)-air-quality-and-health.
5. Rajagopalan S, Al-Kindi SG, Brook RD. Air pollution and cardiovascular disease: JACC state-of-the-art review. *J Am Coll Cardiol.* 2018; 72(17):2054-2070.
6. Zhao B, Johnston FH, Salimi F, Kurabayashi M, Negishi K. Short-term exposure to ambient fine particulate matter and out-of-hospital cardiac arrest: a nationwide case-crossover study in Japan. *Lancet Planet Health.* 2020;4(1):e15-e23.
7. Zirak MR, Mehri S, Karimani A, Zeinali M, Hayes AW, Karimi G. Mechanisms behind the atherothrombotic effects of acrolein, a review. *Food Chem Toxicol.* 2019;129:38-53.
8. Ashcroft J, Fraser E, Krishnamoorthy S, Westwood-Ruttledge S. Carbon monoxide poisoning. *BMJ.* 2019;365:12299.
9. Liu C, Yin P, Chen R, et al. Ambient carbon monoxide and cardiovascular mortality: a nationwide time-series analysis in 272 cities in China. *Lancet Planet Health.* 2018;2(1):e12-e18.
10. Ramachandran MS, Thirumalaikolundusubramanian P. *The Heart and Toxins.* Elsevier/AP, Academic Press is an imprint of Elsevier; 2015.
11. Carreon-Garciduenas M, Godinez-Hernandez D, Alvarado-Gomez N, Ortega-Varela LF, Cervantes-Duran C, Gauthereau-Torres MY. Participation of voltage-gated sodium and calcium channels in the acute cardiac effects of toluene. *Toxicol Mech Methods.* 2018;28(9):670-677.
12. Assadi SN. Electrocardiographic changes and exposure to solvents. *J Arrhythm.* 2018;34(1):65-70.
13. Fatmi Z, Coggon D, Kazi A, Naeem I, Kadir MM, Sathiakumar N. Solid fuel use is a major risk factor for acute coronary syndromes among rural women: a matched case control study. *Public Health.* 2014;128(1):77-82.
14. Yu K, Qiu G, Chan KH, et al. Association of solid fuel use with risk of cardiovascular and all-cause mortality in rural China. *JAMA.* 2018; 319(13):1351-1361.
15. Hystad P, Duong M, Brauer M, et al. Health effects of household solid fuel use: findings from 11 countries within the prospective urban and rural epidemiology study. *Environ Health Perspect.* 2019;127(5):57003.
16. Coulson JM, Caparrotta TM, Thompson JP. The management of ventricular dysrhythmia in aconite poisoning. *Clin Toxicol (Phila).* 2017;55(5):313-321.
17. Gonzalez-Stuart A, Rivera JO. Yellow Oleander seed, or "Codo de Fraile" (Thevetia spp.): a review of its potential toxicity as a purported weight-loss supplement. *J Diet Suppl.* 2018;15(3):352-364.
18. Silici S, Atayoglu AT. Mad honey intoxication: a systematic review on the 1199 cases. *Food Chem Toxicol.* 2015;86:282-290.
19. Aygun A, Sahin A, Karaca Y, et al. Grayanotoxin levels in blood, urine and honey and their association with clinical status in patients with mad honey intoxication. *Turk J Emerg Med.* 2018;18(1):29-33.
20. Erenler AK. Cardiac effects of mad honey poisoning and its management in emergency department: a review from Turkey. *Cardiovasc Toxicol.* 2016;16(1):1-4.
21. Brown AC. Heart toxicity related to herbs and dietary supplements: online table of case reports. Part 4 of 5. *J Diet Suppl.* 2018;15(4):516-555.
22. Rahimi M, Shokri F, Hassanian-Moghaddam H, Zamani N, Pajoumand A, Shadnia S. Severe camphor poisoning, a seven-year observational study. *Environ Toxicol Pharmacol.* 2017;52:8-13.
23. Mukherjee D. Perfluorooctanoic acid exposure and cardiovascular disease: potential role and preventive measures: comment on

"Perfluorooctanoic acid and cardiovascular disease in US adults." *Arch Intern Med.* 2012;172(18):1403-1405.

24. Varol E, Akcay S, Ersoy IH, Koroglu BK, Varol S. Impact of chronic fluorosis on left ventricular diastolic and global functions. *Sci Total Environ.* 2010;408(11):2295-2298.
25. Yang Y, Hu D, Peng D. Diffuse ST-segment elevation after hydrogen sulfide intoxication. *J Emerg Med.* 2018;54(2):241-243.
26. Shuai J, Kim S, Ryu H, et al. Health risk assessment of volatile organic compounds exposure near Daegu dyeing industrial complex in South Korea. *BMC Public Health.* 2018;18(1):528.
27. Callahan CL, Stewart PA, Blair A, Purdue MP. Extended mortality follow-up of a cohort of dry cleaners. *Epidemiology.* 2019;30(2):285-290.
28. Bao W, Liu B, Simonsen DW, Lehmler H-J. Association between exposure to pyrethroid insecticides and risk of all-cause and cause-specific mortality in the general US adult population. *JAMA Intern Med.* 2020;180(3):367-374.
29. Liu Y, Tellez-Rojo M, Sanchez BN, et al. Association between fluoride exposure and cardiometabolic risk in peripubertal Mexican children. *Environ Int.* 2020;134:105302.
30. Guo J, Su L, Zhao X, Xu Z, Chen G. Relationships between urinary antimony levels and both mortalities and prevalence of cancers and heart diseases in general US population, NHANES 1999-2010. *Sci Total Environ.* 2016;571:452-460.
31. Agency for Toxic Substances & Disease Registry. ATSDR's substance priority list. 2019. http://www.atsdr.cdc.gov/spl/
32. Kuo CC, Moon KA, Wang SL, Silbergeld E, Navas-Acien A. The association of arsenic metabolism with cancer, cardiovascular disease, and diabetes: a systematic review of the epidemiological evidence. *Environ Health Perspect.* 2017;125(8):087001.
33. Cosselman KE, Navas-Acien A, Kaufman JD. Environmental factors in cardiovascular disease. *Nat Rev Cardiol.* 2015;12(11):627-642.
34. Moon KA, Oberoi S, Barchowsky A, et al. A dose-response meta-analysis of chronic arsenic exposure and incident cardiovascular disease. *Int J Epidemiol.* 2017;46(6):1924-1939.
35. Pichler G, Grau-Perez M, Tellez-Plaza M, et al. Association of arsenic exposure with cardiac geometry and left ventricular function in young adults. *Circ Cardiovasc Imaging.* 2019;12(5):e009018.
36. Nordberg M, Fowler BA, Nordberg GF. *Nordberg. Handbook on the Toxicology of Metals.* 4th ed. Academic Press; 2015:655-666.
37. Ngala RA, Awe MA, Nsiah P. The effects of plasma chromium on lipid profile, glucose metabolism and cardiovascular risk in type 2 diabetes mellitus. A case-control study. *PLoS One.* 2018;13(7):e0197977.
38. Packer M. Cobalt cardiomyopathy: a critical reappraisal in light of a recent resurgence. *Circ Heart Fail.* 2016;9(12):e003604.
39. Linna A, Uitti J, Oksa P, et al. Effects of occupational cobalt exposure on the heart in the production of cobalt and cobalt compounds: a 6-year follow-up. *Int Arch Occup Environ Health.* 2020;93(3):365-374.
40. Yu X, Huang L, Zhao J, et al. The relationship between serum zinc level and heart failure: a meta-analysis. *Biomed Res Int.* 2018;2018;2739014.
41. DiNicolantonio JJ, Mangan D, O'Keefe JH. Copper deficiency may be a leading cause of ischaemic heart disease. Open *Heart.* 2018;5(2):e000784.
42. Kobayashi M, Suhara T, Baba Y, Kawasaki NK, Higa JK, Matsui T. Pathological roles of iron in cardiovascular disease. *Curr Drug Targets.* 2018;19(9):1068-1076.
43. von Haehling S, Ebner N, Evertz R, Ponikowski P, Anker SD. Iron deficiency in heart failure: an overview. *JACC Heart Fail.* 2019;7(1):36-46.
44. Lanphear BP, Rauch S, Auinger P, Allen RW, Hornung RW. Low-level lead exposure and mortality in US adults: a population-based cohort study. *Lancet Public Health.* 2018;3(4):e177-e184.
45. Markiewicz-Gorka I, Januszewska L, Michalak A, et al. Effects of chronic exposure to lead, cadmium, and manganese mixtures on oxidative stress in rat liver and heart. *Arh Hig Rada Toksikol.* 2015;66(1):51-62.
46. Genchi G, Sinicropi MS, Carocci A, Lauria G, Catalano A. Mercury exposure and heart diseases. *Int J Environ Res Public Health.* 2017;14(1):74.
47. Zhang N, Chen M, Li J, et al. Metal nickel exposure increase the risk of congenital heart defects occurrence in offspring: a case-control study in China. *Medicine (Baltimore).* 2019;98(18):e15352.

CHAPTER 30

AMYLOID CARDIOMYOPATHY

Courtney M. Campbell, Rami Kahwash, and Ajay Vallakati

INTRODUCTION

Amyloid cardiomyopathy is increasingly recognized as an underdiagnosed cause of heart failure. Amyloidosis occurs when proteins misfold, form amyloid fibrils, and then deposit in the body resulting in organ dysfunction. Although many proteins can form amyloid fibrils, two proteins are primarily responsible for amyloid cardiomyopathy: light chains and transthyretin. Amyloid deposition of these proteins results in light chain amyloidosis (AL) and transthyretin amyloidosis (ATTR), with the latter due to a wild-type (ATTRwt) or an inherited form (ATTRv) caused by pathogenic variants in the transthyretin gene. The amyloid fibrils have variable organ tropism that results in a range of initial presentations. Most often amyloidosis is a multisystem disease. The extent of cardiac involvement is most closely associated with overall survival. Recent advances in the treatment of AL and ATTR have substantially improved morbidity and mortality, but early diagnosis of amyloidosis is key to achieving maximal benefits.

Epidemiology

Amyloidosis is considered a rare disease. However, the true prevalence of amyloid cardiomyopathy is not known because it is underdiagnosed. Based on 2012 data from billing codes in Medicare beneficiaries, the prevalence of amyloid cardiomyopathy is estimated at 17 per 100,000 person-years with an incidence of 55 per 100,000 person-years.[1] In a study of amyloidosis-related mortality based on U.S. death certificates, the average reported mortality was calculated at 4.95 per 1 million people.[2] Significant geographic differences were noted, with the counties surrounding Mayo Clinic in Minnesota reporting rates of 31.73 and 25.43 per 1 million people. Specific demographics and epidemiology for AL, ATTRv, and ATTRwt are considered in **Table 30.1**.

AL is slightly more common in men compared to women, and the majority of patients with AL are over the age of 65 years.[3] Based on 2015 claims data, the prevalence is estimated at 40.5 cases per million and incidence at 14.0 cases per million person-years.[4] Extrapolated from this data, at least 12,000 adults in the United States are estimated to be living with AL amyloidosis.

ATTRwt has a strong male predominance, and most patients are diagnosed with ATTR in their 60s and 70s,[5] although cases have been reported in patients in their 40s.[6] Autopsy data suggest a high prevalence of ATTRwt in older individuals of Northern European descent: 25% of 85 consecutive Swedish patients older than 80 years,[7] 25% of 256 Finnish patients older than 85 years,[8] and 37% of 63 Finnish patients older than 95 years.[9] A high prevalence of ATTRwt has also been seen in recent studies screening specific patient populations: 13.3% of 120 hospitalized patients admitted with heart failure with preserved ejection fraction (EF), left ventricular hypertrophy, and age older than 60 years[10]; 16% of 151 patients with severe aortic stenosis undergoing transcatheter aortic valve replacement[11]; 5% of patients with presumed hypertrophic cardiomyopathy[12]; and 10% of older patients undergoing bilateral carpal tunnel release.[13]

ATTRv is an inherited autosomal dominant disease and affects an estimated 50,000 people worldwide.[14] Onset is earlier than ATTRwt with a significant male predominance in amyloid cardiomyopathy. The most common mutations in the United States are Val122Ile (p.Val142Ile), Thr60Ala (p.Thr80Ala), and Val30Met (p.Val50Met); the "p" notation is indicative of the 20 amino acid precursor protein inclusion. Val122Ile is primarily found in patients of African Caribbean descent older than 65 years. Among African Americans, 3% to 4% are estimated to carry the Val122Ile mutation,[15] but the penetrance is not known. Thr60Ala occurs in an estimated 1% of a Northwest Ireland population and with an onset older than 45 years.[16] Overall, it is most common in the United Kingdom and Ireland. Thr60Ala can also be found in U.S. descendants, many located in the Appalachia region. Val30Met is the most prevalent ATTRv mutation worldwide with a predominance in Japan, Sweden, and Portugal.[17] In those populations, the prevalence is estimated at 1:1000. The onset is older than 50 years, but there is variable gene penetrance and clinical presentation.

Risk Factors

Populations at higher risk of amyloidosis include the following:

- Age: Most common in those older than 60 years, but earlier onset occurs.
- Sex: The majority of patients are male.
- Family history: Hereditary amyloidosis has an autosomal dominant inheritance pattern.
- Race: 3% to 4% of African Americans may carry a mutation that predisposes them to amyloidosis.

TABLE 30.1 Comparison of AL, ATTRwt, and ATTRv Epidemiology, Clinical Findings, and Prognosis

	AL	ATTRwt	ATTRv
Sex	M > F	M >> F	M > F
Age	• >65 years	• 60-70 years	• V122I: >65 years • T60A: >45 years • V30M: >50 years
Prevalence and incidence	• 40.5 cases per million • 14.0 cases per million person-years	• Uncertain • 13.3% of HFpEF patients age >60 years • 16% of patients undergoing TAVR	• V122I—3-4% African Caribbean descent • T60A—1% Northwest Irish descent • V30M—0.1%, with Japan, Sweden, and Portugal predominance
Cardiac involvement	Yes, in many patients	Yes, in almost all patients	Yes, in many patients, variant dependent
Extracardiac signs and symptoms	• Periorbital purpura (AL, rare) • Carpal tunnel syndrome, lumbar spinal stenosis, knee and hip replacement (ATTR > AL) • Indigestion, GERD, constipation, diarrhea (AL, ATTRv-T60A) • Nephrotic syndrome and kidney dysfunction (all) • Peripheral and autonomic neuropathy (AL, ATTRv > ATTRwt)		
Cardiac signs and symptoms	• Dyspnea on exertion, fatigue, exercise intolerance • Atrial fibrillation, bundle branch block, sinoatrial disease • Heart failure (preserved EF > mildly reduced EF >> severely reduced EF)		
Cardiac study findings	• *ECG:* Low voltage in limb leads, no evidence of LVH • *Echocardiogram:* Concentric remodeling and LVH, apical sparing on global longitudinal strain ("cherry on top") • *CMR*: diffuse late gadolinium enhancement, increased extracellular volume, elevated native T1 with difficulty nulling the myocardium		
Prognosis	• Stage 1: 118 months • Stage 2: 76 months • Stage 3: 64 months • Stage 4: 27 months	• Stage 1: 55 months • Stage 2: 42 months • Stage 3: 20 months	• Variable, variant, and organ system involvement dependent
Amyloid-specific therapies	• Steroids (ie, dexamethasone) • Alkylators (ie, cyclophosphamide) • Proteasome inhibitors (ie, bortezomib) • Autologous stem cell transplant • Heart transplant	• Tafamidis (cardiomyopathy) • Diflunisal (off-label) • Heart transplant	• Tafamidis (cardiomyopathy) • Patisiran (neuropathy) • Inotersen (neuropathy) • Liver and/or heart transplant

AL, light chain amyloidosis; ATTR, transthyretin amyloidosis inherited form; ATTRv, transthyretin amyloidosis variant; ATTRwt, transthyretin amyloidosis wild-type; CMR, cardiac magnetic resonance imaging; ECG, electrocardiogram; EF, ejection fraction; GERD, gastroesophageal reflux disease; HFpEF, heart failure with preserved ejection fraction; LVH, left ventricular hypertrophy; TAVR, transcatheter aortic valve replacement.

PATHOGENESIS

In amyloidosis, proteins misfold, aggregate into beta-sheets, and form amyloid fibrils that are deposited extracellularly, leading to organ dysfunction. When the amyloid is deposited in the heart, the patient initially develops a nonischemic, restrictive cardiomyopathy. Later systolic dysfunction occurs. Over 100 proteins in the body can misfold and result in amyloid deposition. However, only two precursor proteins are primarily involved in amyloid cardiomyopathy: immunoglobulin light chain and transthyretin protein.

In AL, clonal immunoglobulin light chains are secreted by aberrant monoclonal plasma cells or B-cell dyscrasia from the bone marrow. These light chains form insoluble amyloid fibrils that are then deposited in tissue. The fibrils tend to be highly inflammatory. Cardiac impairment can occur prior to significant accumulation and is rapidly progressive.

In ATTR, the tetrameric transthyretin protein, primarily synthesized in the liver, dissociates and misassembles, resulting in amyloid fibrils that deposit in tissue. Functional transthyretin transports thyroxine and retinol-binding protein. ATTRwt is linked to advanced age and occurs when native transthyretin protein misfolds. In hereditary ATTRv, the transthyretin misfolding is linked to a destabilizing transthyretin mutation. Over 120 pathogenic mutations have been identified.[18] Compared to AL amyloidosis, ATTR fibrils are less inflammatory. Disease progression relates more highly to cumulative fibril deposition over a longer period of time.

CLINICAL PRESENTATION

Common Signs and Symptoms

Amyloidosis can smolder subclinically for years to over a decade. Some amyloidosis manifestations reach clinical significance but often are attributed to other causes and are not investigated for amyloidosis. Restrictive cardiomyopathy with diastolic heart failure and dilated cardiomyopathy with systolic heart failure are some of the final amyloidosis manifestations in the disease cascade. The progression of symptoms and involved organs varies by the subtype of amyloidosis. Generally, AL symptoms are more varied and are specific to the organ systems involved. ATTRwt tends to have primarily musculoskeletal and cardiac involvement. In ATTRv, the phenotype can range from neuropathy predominant, cardiac predominant, or a mixed phenotype.

Skin: Easy bruising can accompany amyloidosis. In AL amyloidosis, periorbital purpura is a pathognomonic sign that should prompt diagnostic testing.

Musculoskeletal: The earliest initial symptoms of amyloidosis are often musculoskeletal. Amyloid deposits can build up in the transverse carpal ligament and impinge on the median nerve, resulting in carpal tunnel syndrome. If these deposits build up in the ligamentum flavum of the spine, patients can present with back pain and radiculopathy from lumbar spinal stenosis. Biceps tendon rupture can also occur with amyloid deposition. A high rate of knee and hip replacements has been noted in amyloidosis.[19] ATTR seems to have high rates of musculoskeletal complaints, and these can present 5 to 15 years prior to cardiac manifestations.

Gastrointestinal: Indigestion, gastroesophageal reflux, gastrointestinal immobility, constipation, and diarrhea can all be related to amyloid deposition. An enlarged tongue can also be present. These symptoms are seen most commonly in patients with AL and some variants of ATTRv (specifically T60A, G89Q). When these symptoms are present, they can be prominent and significantly affect quality of life. Patients often seek gastrointestinal specialty care and undergo endoscopy or colonoscopy, at which time tissue from these procedures can be screened for amyloid deposits.

Renal: The kidneys are frequently affected by systemic amyloidosis. Patients with AL can initially present with nephrotic syndrome with or without renal dysfunction. Amyloidosis frequently is diagnosed after renal biopsy. Other patients with less severe deposition may have an elevated creatinine because of reduced glomerular filtration rate.

Nervous system: In addition to nerve compression from thickened ligaments, patients can develop peripheral and autonomic neuropathy. Often the etiology of peripheral neuropathy is not investigated. Some patients with amyloidosis have been on gabapentin for years, but are not diagnosed with amyloidosis until cardiac symptoms develop. If a patient has underlying diabetes, the degree of neuropathy is often out of proportion and more rapidly progressive than otherwise anticipated. Neuropathy can also manifest as erectile dysfunction and sweating abnormalities. For patients that develop autonomic neuropathy, the most prominent symptom is orthostatic hypotension. The first sign of autonomic neuropathy may be improvement of their baseline hypertension that may no longer require antihypertensive medications. For many amyloidosis patients, neuropathy is the most prominent symptom. Neuropathy is common in AL and certain variants of ATTRv (Val-30Met). Peripheral neuropathy is less common in ATTRwt.

Cardiac: Early progression of amyloid heart disease is subclinical and subtle. Amyloid cardiomyopathy becomes more prominent as the disease progresses. Patients can present with mild dyspnea on exertion, fatigue, and exercise intolerance. These symptoms can be accompanied by angina, likely related to coronary microvascular dysfunction. Almost all patients with cardiac amyloidosis (>95%) had significantly reduced peak stress myocardial blood flow (<1.3 mL/g/min).[20] When the conduction system is involved, arrhythmias, bundle branch block, and sinoatrial disease are common. Patients can also present at later stages with heart failure. Most often, patients have heart failure with preserved EF. Yet many patients can present with mildly reduced ejected fraction. In end-stage amyloid cardiomyopathy, severely reduced EF with dilated cardiomyopathy can be seen. Common cardiac tests can reveal signs of amyloidosis and should prompt diagnostic testing. A single normal cardiac test should not stop pursuit of diagnostic testing if clinical suspicion is otherwise present.

Echocardiogram: In the early stages of the disease, a patient may have no obvious abnormalities on echocardiogram—particularly for AL. Subsequently, the heart develops concentric remodeling or mild left ventricular hypertrophy (**Figures 30.1A** and **B**). As the disease progresses, the walls become thicker and the patient develops diastolic dysfunction. On longitudinal strain imaging, apical sparing can be present ("cherry red spot") (**Figures 30.2A-C**). Next, the patient develops an infiltrative phenotype with biventricular concentric hypertrophy, valve thickening, interatrial septal thickening, and pericardial effusion. The left ventricle is often described as having a granular sparkling pattern, although this is neither sensitive nor specific for cardiac amyloidosis and is dependent on the imaging technique. Severe diastolic dysfunction with restrictive physiology ensues. Eventually, the patient develops systolic dysfunction with a nondilated left ventricle. Special attention should also be paid to patients with paradoxical low-flow/low-gradient aortic stenosis that is accompanied by a right ventricular thickening.

Electrocardiogram (ECG): In early stages of amyloidosis, the ECG is unremarkable (Figure 30.1B). Even in patients with amyloid cardiomyopathy, the ECG can be unremarkable, particularly in those with ATTRwt. When they do occur, the initial changes can be a mild first-degree atrioventricular block. As the left ventricle thickens, there is no commensurate increase in voltage on ECG; the voltage remains normal. A pseudo-infarct pattern of Q waves unrelated to prior myocardial infarction is common. Only in late stages of the disease is the classic sign of low QRS voltages in the limb leads sometimes present (**Figure 30.3**). Atrial fibrillation is common in amyloid cardiomyopathy and can present in early or late stages of the disease. Complete heart block and the need for a pacemaker can also occur at late stages.

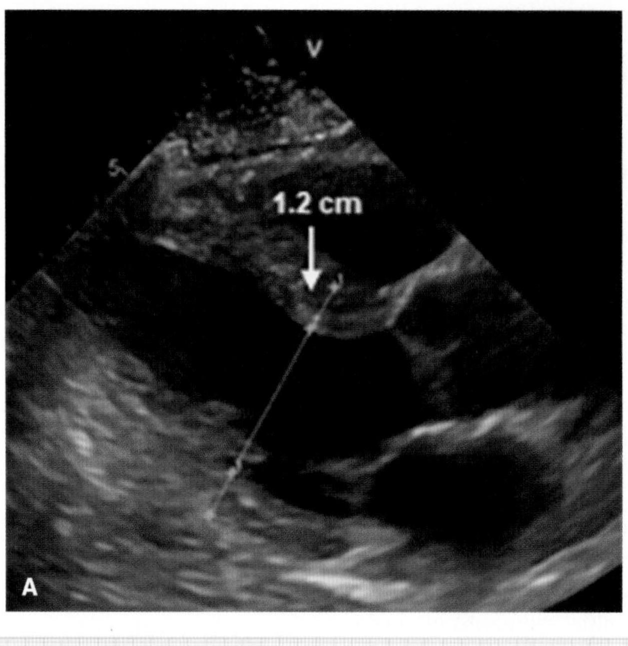

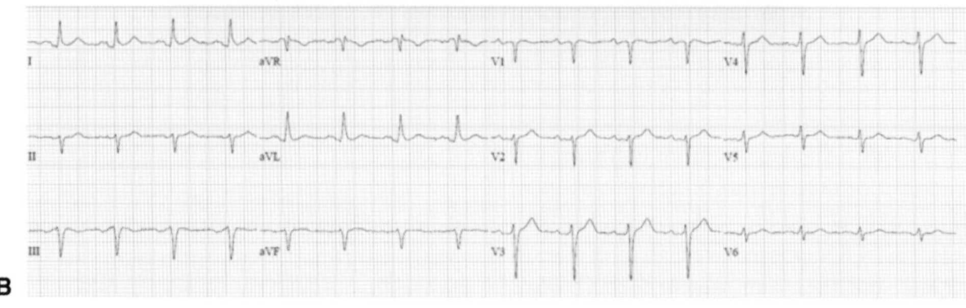

FIGURE 30.1 Cardiac tests in early amyloid cardiomyopathy. **A:** Transthoracic echocardiogram showing concentric remodeling on the parasternal long axis view. **B:** Normal electrocardiogram in a patient with biopsy proven amyloid cardiomyopathy with no evidence of low voltages, a classic amyloidosis red flag.

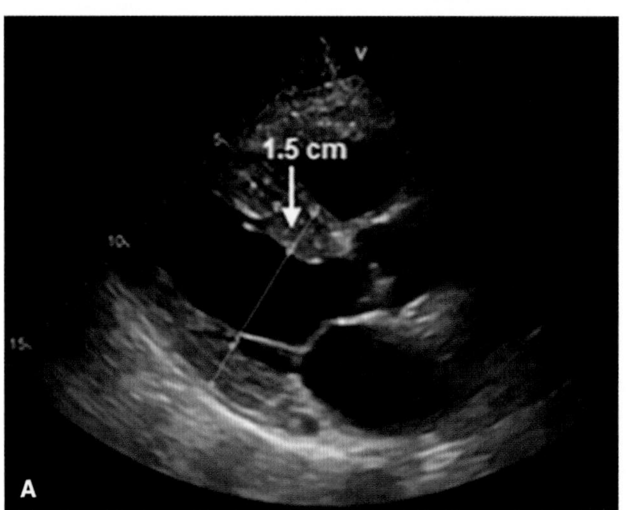

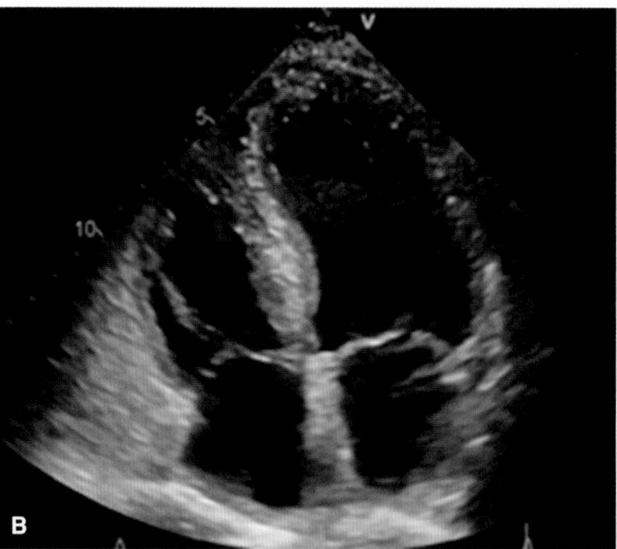

FIGURE 30.2 Transthoracic echocardiogram red flags in late amyloid cardiomyopathy. **A:** Parasternal long axis view demonstrating thick right ventricular walls, thick left ventricular walls (1.5 cm), and granular sparkling appearance of the myocardium. **B:** Four chamber view demonstrating thick mitral and tricuspid valves and thick interatrial septum. Pericardial effusion, another red flag, is not seen in this example.

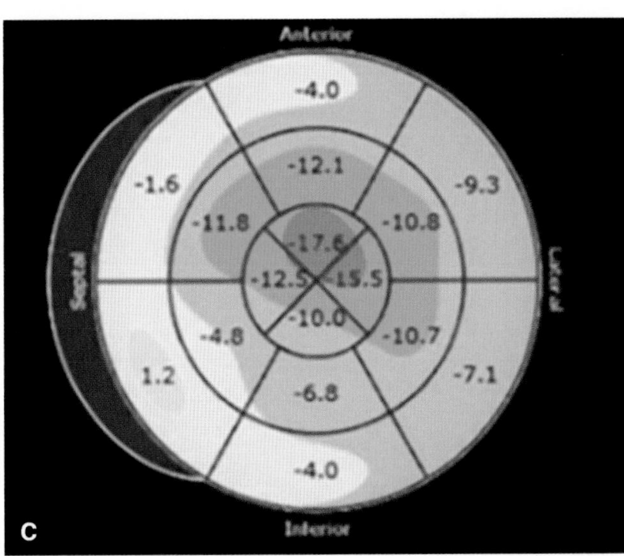

FIGURE 30.2 (*continued*) **C:** Global longitudinal strain demonstrating apical sparing, also known as "cherry on top" sign.

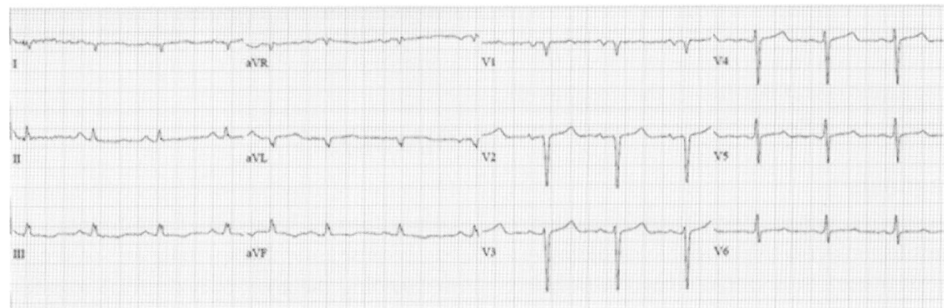

FIGURE 30.3 Electrocardiogram red flags in late amyloid cardiomyopathy. Electrocardiogram demonstrating low voltage in limb leads and normal voltage in the lateral leads despite known left ventricular hypertrophy.

Cardiac magnetic resonance imaging (CMR): On CMR, amyloidosis in the heart is seen as diffuse subendocardial or transmural late gadolinium enhancement. The extracellular volume is increased (typically >0.4). The native T1 can be elevated greater than 1100 ms with difficulty, nulling the myocardium (**Figure 30.4A-C**).

Labs: Troponin and N-terminal pro–B-type natriuretic peptide (NT-proBNP) are useful biomarkers in amyloid cardiomyopathy.

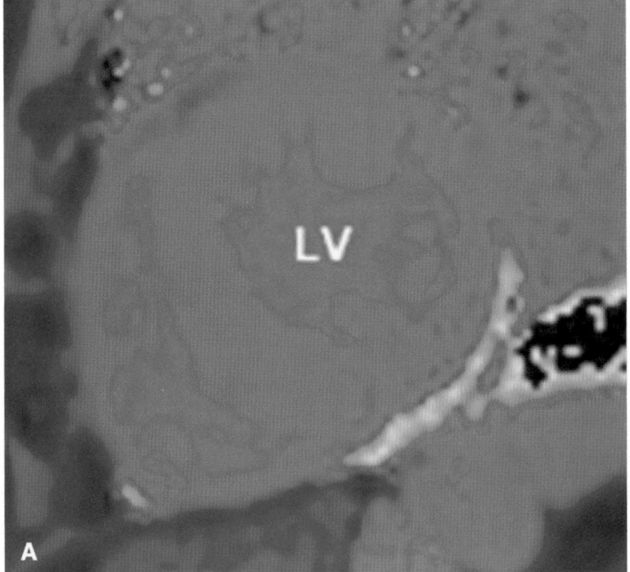

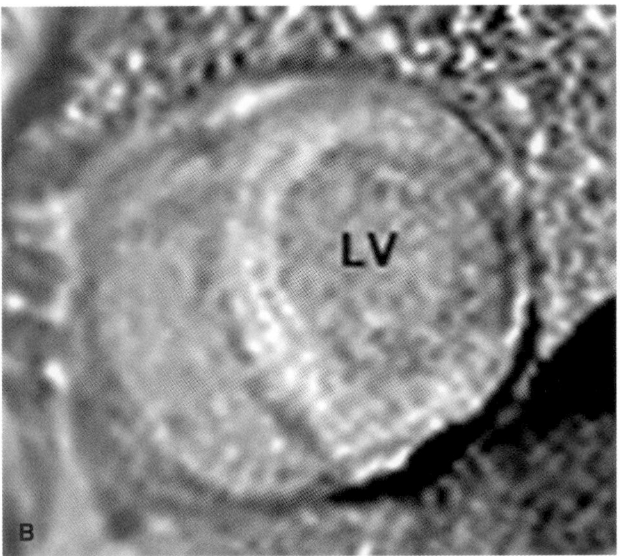

FIGURE 30.4 Cardiac MRI red flags in late amyloid cardiomyopathy. **A:** Native T1 is >1100 ms. **B:** Diffuse late gadolinium enhancement.

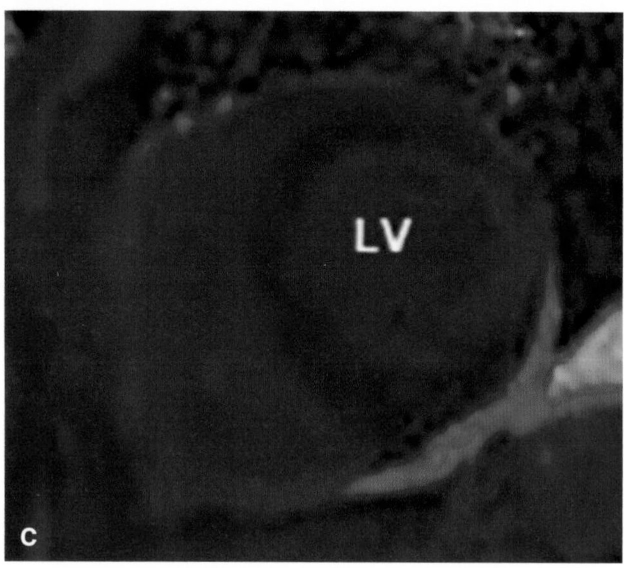

FIGURE 30.4 (*continued*) **C:** Extracellular volume >27% in the short axis view. LV, left ventricle.

In early stages, both tests are normal. As diastolic dysfunction develops, the NT-proBNP elevates commensurate with heart failure with preserved EF. In later stages of the disease, the troponin can be persistently, mildly elevated with little change on repeat testing.

Differential Diagnosis

From a cardiac perspective, patients with amyloid cardiomyopathy are often misdiagnosed as hypertrophic cardiomyopathy, hypertensive heart disease, or undifferentiated heart failure with preserved EF. They may also carry an undifferentiated peripheral neuropathy diagnosis.

DIAGNOSIS

Diagnosis of amyloidosis begins with a high index of suspicion (**Algorithm 30.1A** and **B**). Early diagnosis of amyloidosis is critical because early therapy translates to decreased mortality. Understanding the array of noncardiac manifestations in addition

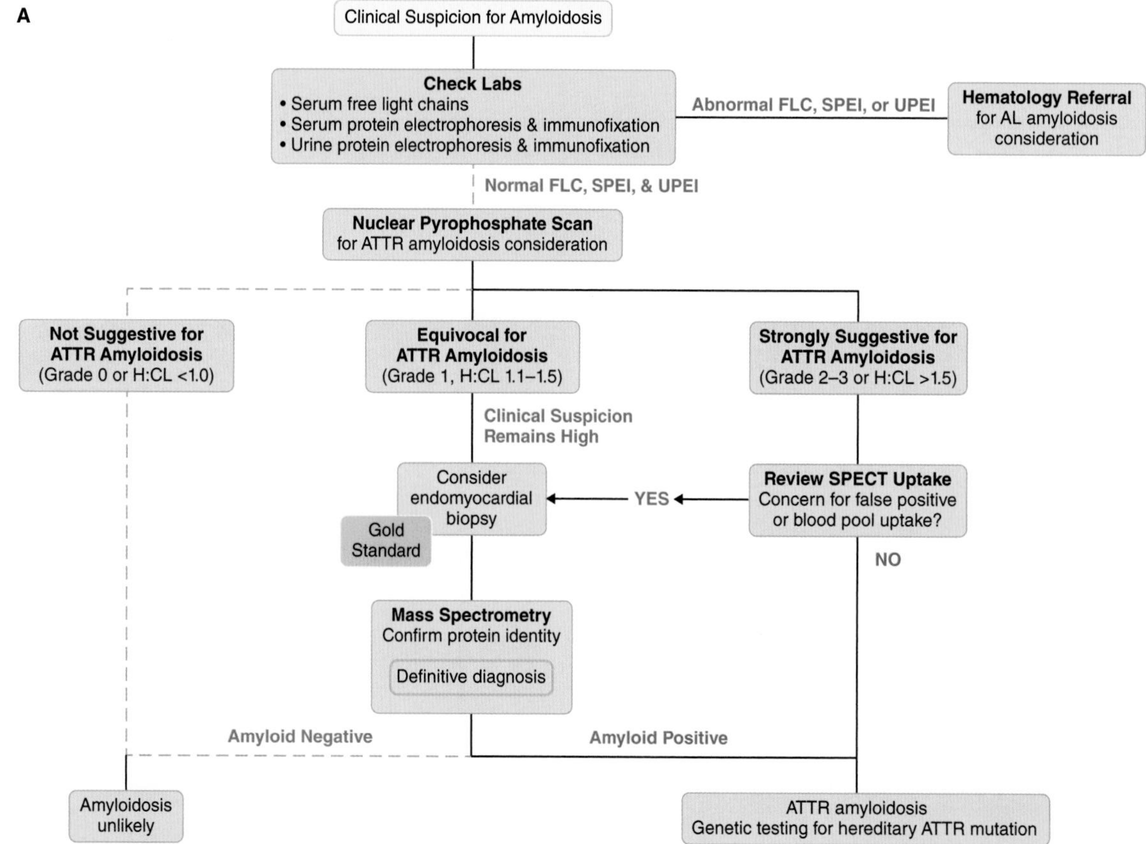

ALGORITHM 30.1 **Part A:** Clinical suspicion for amyloidosis.

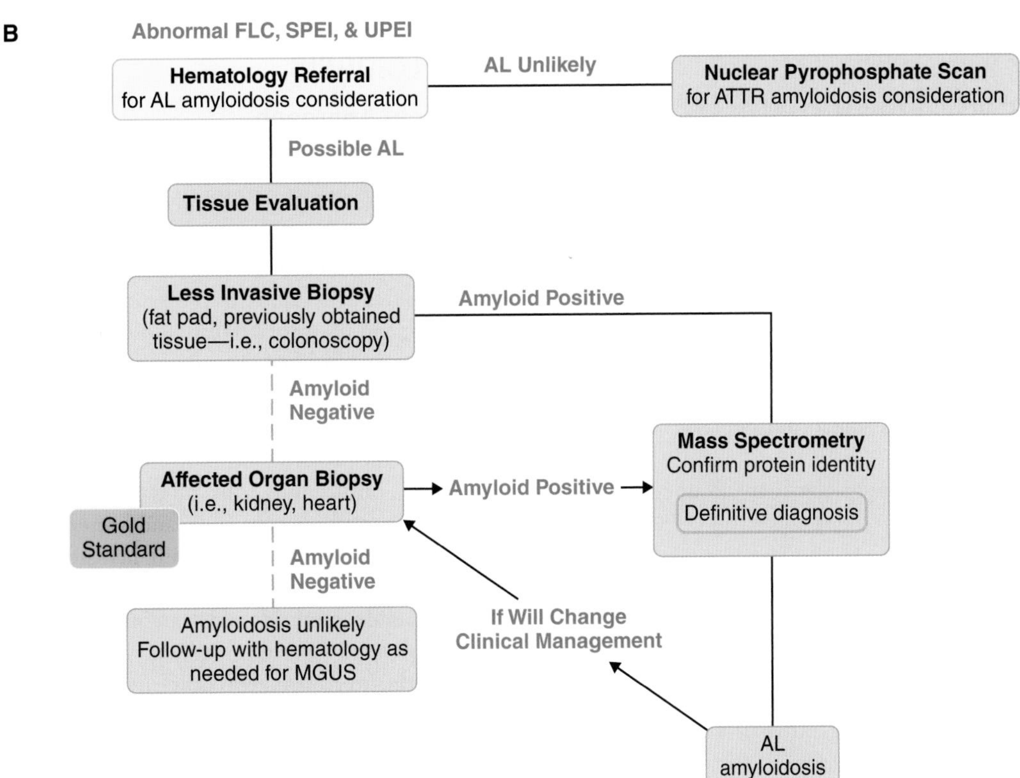

ALGORITHM 30.1 (*continued*) **Part B:** Clinical suspicion for amyloidosis. AL, AL, light chain amyloidosis ATTR, transthyretin amyloidosis; FLC, free light chain; H:CL, heart-to-contralateral lung MGUS, monoclonal gammopathy of uncertain significance; SPECT, single-photon emission computed tomography SPEI, serum protein electrophoresis and immunofixation; UPEI, urine protein electrophoresis and immunofixation.

to cardiac "red flags" can help identify patients who should be screened for amyloidosis. In all suspected cases of amyloidosis, AL must be ruled out first before consideration of ATTR. Once cardiomyopathy develops in AL, the median survival is 6 months if left untreated; therefore, early diagnosis is critical (Table 30.1).

Diagnosis of Light Chain Amyloidosis

Laboratory tests: For AL, initial laboratory tests of choice are serum free light chain quantification, serum protein electrophoresis and immunofixation (SPEI), and urine protein electrophoresis and immunofixation (UPEI). Generally, a kappa–lambda ratio greater than 1.7 with evidence of a monoclonal protein on SPEI or UPEI can be indicative of AL; in the absence of monoclonal protein, a kappa–lambda ratio of up to 2.5 can be considered normal. With chronic kidney disease, mild kappa predominance can occur with a ratio of approximately 2:1. Up to 40% of patients may have monoclonal gammopathy of uncertain significance (MGUS) on immunofixation,[21] and the demographics of MGUS and amyloidosis overlap. In addition, an estimated 10% of patients with multiple myeloma can develop AL.[22] Abnormal results of any of these tests must be discussed with a hematologist.

Tissue diagnosis: With suggestive laboratory or clinical findings, the final diagnostic step is to obtain tissue for analysis of amyloid deposits with Congo red staining. This may include reevaluating any recent tissue biopsy, such as procured during colonoscopy or endoscopy. A fat pad biopsy or bone marrow biopsy can be obtained in an outpatient clinic. However, these biopsies have a high false-negative rate. If the diagnosis cannot be otherwise established, the affected organ—likely heart or kidney—must be biopsied. Congo red staining with apple-green birefringence is specific for amyloid material. Because false positives can occur with any dense aggregates, such as hyaline deposits,[23] positive Congo red staining should be followed with mass spectrometry to identify the specific protein involved. After an initial negative cardiac biopsy, surveillance is important with consideration of repeat biopsy if the index of suspicion remains high or clinical findings progress.[24]

AL amyloid deposits can be found incidentally on biopsies obtained for other medical reasons, commonly in the skin, larynx, or sites of chronic inflammation.[25] If there is no evidence of circulating free light chains or immunoglobulins on serum testing, these localized deposits typically require no treatment.

Diagnosis of Transthyretin Amyloidosis

Nuclear scintigraphy: Once AL is ruled out, screening for ATTR can be done with a nuclear technetium-99m pyrophosphate (PYP) scan, preferably in combination with single-photon emission computerized tomography (SPECT) imaging.[26] Planar imaging is graded with a quantitative score at 1 hour and semiquantitative score at 3 hours. First, the cardiac uptake pattern is categorized as absent, focal, diffuse, or focal on diffuse. Then, planar imaging is used to calculate the heart/contralateral (H:CL) ratio by comparing the mean counts in the respective regions of interest in the heart to the mean counts in contralateral bone (ie, the ribs).

H:CL less than 1 is not suggestive of ATTR.
H:CL 1 to 1.5 is equivocal for ATTR.
H:CL greater than 1.5 is strongly suggestive of ATTR.

At 3 hours, a planar and/or SPECT visual score is reported based on comparison between cardiac uptake and rib uptake on a scale of 0 to 3:

Grade 0: Absent cardiac uptake, not suggestive of ATTR
Grade 1: Cardiac uptake less than rib uptake, equivocal for ATTR
Grade 2: Cardiac uptake equal to rib uptake, strongly suggestive of ATTR
Grade 3: Cardiac uptake greater than rib uptake, strongly suggestive of ATTR

In a positive scan, the cardiac uptake pattern is diffuse. A H:CL ratio greater than 1.5 at 1 hour and/or a visual grade of 2 to 3 is classified as ATTR positive. A H:CL ratio less than 1 and/or a visual grade 0 is classified as ATTR negative. Recommended overall interpretation categories are "not suggestive of TTR amyloidosis," "strongly suggestive of TTR amyloidosis," and "equivocal for TTR amyloidosis."

Certain clinical scenarios can generate false-positive or equivocal results. Positive planar uptake (grade 2-3) in the absence of SPECT uptake (grade 0) indicates blood pool and should be considered a nondiagnostic test. For this reason, both planar and SPECT should be obtained. Patients taking hydroxychloroquine may have a false-positive PYP scan. Focal uptake in the rib may represent a rib fracture and, in the heart, a recent myocardial infarction. AL can have any degree of PYP uptake; hence, PYP scans cannot be used to assess for AL.

An equivocal PYP scan or concern for false-positive PYP should prompt further investigation. For equivocal PYP scans, there are no best practice guidelines for the next steps. These results can be indicative of early-stage ATTR or AL cardiac amyloidosis. One can consider repeat imaging at a later interval or obtaining a tissue biopsy.

Cardiac biopsy: For definitive diagnosis, a referral for cardiac biopsy is appropriate and is the gold standard for diagnosis. Because amyloid cardiomyopathy is a diffuse disease, the sensitivity of endomyocardial biopsy for establishing the diagnosis is estimated at 100%, as long as a sufficient number of biopsies and tissue are obtained.[27] Endomyocardial samples are stained with Congo red. If positive, samples should be sent for mass spectrometry to identify the protein present.

Genetic testing: If ATTR is diagnosed, the patient should undergo genetic testing to determine whether there is a mutation in the transthyretin gene. In the United States, different treatment options are available for ATTRv compared to ATTRwt. In addition, identification of a hereditary mutation can prompt screening of family members. Identified ATTRv carriers can be closely monitored and receive prompt treatment when clinical evidence of amyloidosis emerges. Genetic counseling is highly recommended.

MANAGEMENT OF THE PATIENT WITH AMYLOIDOSIS

Medical Approach

Light Chain Amyloidosis Therapy

Treatment for AL is typically managed by hematologists with therapy aimed at suppression of light chain synthesis (**Figure 30.5A**). Response to treatment is monitored by analysis of serum free light chains. Improvement in cardiac biomarkers of troponin and NT-proBNP can also signal good response. Most AL therapies were initially approved for treatment of multiple myeloma. Currently, first-line therapy includes a combination of steroids (dexamethasone, prednisone), alkylators (cyclophosphamide, melphalan), and proteasome inhibitors (bortezomib, ixazomib, carfilzomib). The most common regimen is dexamethasone, cyclophosphamide, and bortezomib (aka CyBorD) infused on a monthly basis with hematologic response rates ranging from 60% to 94%.[25] Thalidomide-related medications (lenalidomide, pomalidomide) are used as second-line therapy but are poorly tolerated in patients with amyloid cardiomyopathy.[28] Other treatment approaches are emerging.[25] In small studies, venetoclax, a BCL-2 inhibitor, has had a good response in patients with AL and (11;14) translocation. Daratumumab, an antibody against CD38, has shown promising results with an overall response rate of 76% in patients with otherwise refractory AL. The ANDROMEDA trial, a phase 3 randomized trial comparing CyBorD with CyBorD plus daratumumab, is underway.

Transthyretin Amyloidosis Therapy

Until recently, treatments available for ATTR were limited to supportive care of symptoms and organ-specific dysfunction. In 2018, three clinical trials of drugs that successfully targeted the transthyretin protein were published (**Figure 30.5B**). The drugs were subsequently approved by the U.S. Food and Drug Administration (FDA) (**Table 30.2**).

Transthyretin RNA Silencers

Patisiran. Patisiran is a small interfering RNA (siRNA) therapeutic agent. Patisiran binds and promotes the degradation of transthyretin mRNA within the cytoplasm, stopping transthyretin protein production. It is infused intravenously every 3 weeks. It is FDA approved for the treatment of hereditary amyloidosis polyneuropathy based on the results of the APOLLO trial that showed patisiran improved multiple clinical manifestations of ATTRv.[29] In a subgroup analysis, patisiran decreased left ventricular wall thickness, global longitudinal strain, and NT-proBNP.[30] These studies suggest that patisiran may reverse some effects of amyloid deposition.

Inotersen. Inotersen is an antisense oligonucleotide (ASO) therapeutic agent. Inotersen binds and promotes the degradation of transthyretin mRNA within the nucleus, stopping transthyretin protein production. It is administered subcutaneously weekly. Inotersen is FDA approved for the treatment of hereditary amyloidosis polyneuropathy based on the results of the NEURO-TTR trial,[31] which showed that it improved the course of neurologic disease and quality of life. A subsequent study of

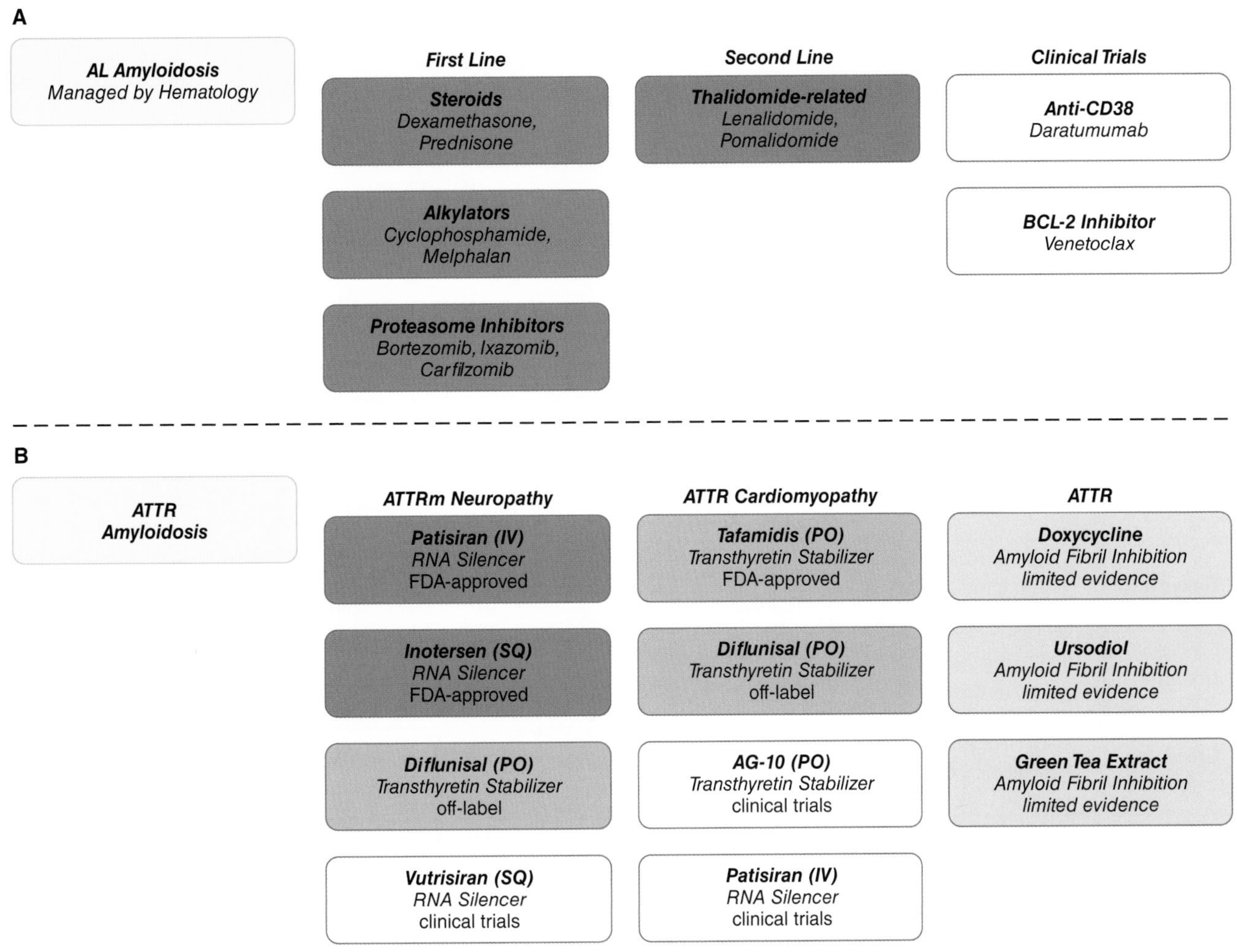

FIGURE 30.5 **A:** Medical treatments available for AL amyloidosis. **B:** Medical treatments available for ATTR amyloidosis. AL, amyloidosis; AL, light chain amyloidosis; ATTR, transthyretin amyloidosis; IV, intravenous; PO, oral SQ, subcutaneous injection

patients with ATTR treated with inotersen demonstrated efficacy in halting disease progression and evidence of cardiomyopathy reversal with decreased left ventricular mass.[32]

Transthyretin Stabilizers

Tafamidis. Tafamidis stabilizes the transthyretin tetramer preventing destabilization and misfolding into the amyloid fibrils. Tafamidis is taken as an oral medication once daily. It is FDA approved for the treatment of both ATTRwt and ATTRv cardiomyopathy. In a randomized placebo-controlled trial (ATTR-ACT),[33] ATTR patients treated with tafamidis had lower all-cause mortality, fewer cardiovascular-related hospitalizations, and less decline in functional capacity/quality of life than placebo-treated patients. Improvements in biomarkers were noted starting at 9 months, and survival benefit was observed after 18 months.

Diflunisal (Off-Label). Diflunisal is a generic nonsteroidal anti-inflammatory drug (NSAID) that stabilizes transthyretin protein. A randomized placebo-controlled trial demonstrated efficacy of diflunisal in reducing the rate of progression of ATTR polyneuropathy.[34] Observational studies of ATTR cardiomyopathy patients demonstrated stabilization of cardiac function with diflunisal.[35] As with other NSAIDs, caution should be used when prescribing to patients with baseline renal dysfunction or patients on systemic anticoagulation. A small number of patients cannot tolerate the gastrointestinal side effects. To date, no studies have compared the efficacy of diflunisal to tafamidis.

Amyloid Fibril Inhibition

Doxycycline and Ursodiol (Off-Label). In in vitro studies, doxycycline appears to disaggregate formed fibrils.[36] Small trials in AL have shown improved response rates in patients on doxycycline.[37] A mouse model of ATTR had improvement in amyloid fibril removal with the combination of doxycycline and ursodiol.[38] In a phase 2 trial, no disease progression was observed in patients on this combined therapy, but some patients discontinued the therapy because of dermatologic and gastrointestinal side effects.[39] In a retrospective study of 53 ATTR patients, treatment with doxycycline and ursodiol was associated with stabilized disease progression.[40] Nevertheless, high-quality evidence supporting treatment of ATTR with doxycycline and ursodiol is needed.

Green Tea Extract (Off-Label). In vitro and animal studies have demonstrated disruption of amyloid fibrils with epigallocatechin 3-gallate (EGCG), the most abundant catechin in green tea.

TABLE 30.2 Transthyretin Amyloidosis Therapy Details

Drug	Dose	Side Effects	Indication	Class	Status
Patisiran (Onpattro)	30 mg infused intravenously over 80 minutes every 3 weeks	• Infusion reaction • Low serum vitamin A levels - supplement recommended	ATTRv neuropathy	RNA silencer	FDA-approved
Inotersen (Tegsedi)	284 mg in 1.5 mL subcutaneous injection weekly	• Infusion reaction • Required monitoring for glomerulonephritis, thrombocytopenia	ATTRv neuropathy	RNA silencer	FDA-approved
Tafamidis (Vyndaqel)	80 mg daily	• No significant effects seen in clinical trials	ATTR cardiomyopathy	Transthyretin stabilizer	FDA-approved
Diflunisal	250 mg twice daily	• GI upset • Drowsiness • Dizziness	ATTR	Transthyretin stabilizer	Off-label; RCT supports use in ATTR neuropathy
Doxycycline	100 mg twice daily	• GI upset • Sun photosensitivity	AL or ATTR	Amyloid fibril inhibition	Off-label; ATTR phase II & observational studies
Ursodiol	250 mg up to three times daily	• GI upset • Dysuria • Itching	ATTR	Amyloid fibril inhibition	Off label; ATTR phase II
Green Tea Extract	1200 mg daily - containing 600 mg EGCG	• Headache • GI upset • Dizziness	ATTRwt	Amyloid Fibril Inhibition	Off-label; Single arm ATTRwt prospective study

AL, light chain amyloidosis; ATTR, transthyretin amyloidosis; ATTRv, transthyretin amyloidosis variant; ATTRwt, transthyretin amyloidosis wild type; EGCG, epigallocatechin gallate; FDA, Food and Drug Administration; GI, gastrointestinal; RCT, randomized controlled trial; RNA, ribonucleic acid

One study in patients with amyloidosis supports the use of green tea extract; 25 patients with ATTRwt cardiomyopathy were given 1200 mg green tea extract capsules (containing 600 mg EGCG) daily for 1 year.[41] CMR showed a decrease in left ventricular mass without a change in left ventricular wall thickness. Further studies are needed to confirm these initial observations.

Transplant Approach

Prior to the current era of new pharmacologic treatments for both AL and ATTR, the mainstay of amyloidosis treatment was transplantation of the organ producing the amyloid protein (bone marrow, liver) or affected organ (heart). With earlier diagnosis and new pharmacotherapies, the use of transplantation may diminish for the treatment of amyloidosis. Transplantation remains a viable approach for properly selected patients.

Autologous Stem Cell Transplant

For AL, appropriately selected patients can be treated with autologous stem cell transplant (ASCT), eliminating the production of light chains. In initial studies of ASCT, high treatment-related mortality (13%-43%) was reported, particularly with advanced amyloid cardiomyopathy.[42] Selection criteria that exclude patients with severe cardiac involvement now limit ASCT as an option for most patients. Induction chemotherapy treatment with good cardiac response can render some ineligible patients eligible. Patients treated with ASCT in a recent cohort (2010-2016) had a treatment-related mortality of only 2.4%, suggesting improved safety of ASCT in a properly selected population.[43] The effectiveness of ASCT remains controversial. The only randomized clinical trial comparing ASCT to standard treatment, completed in 2007, found no difference in outcomes, and ASCT treatment-related mortality was 24%.[44] Yet large retrospective studies suggest superiority of ASCT versus standard chemotherapy, with survival of 30% of patients at 20 years and sustained organ response rates.[45]

Liver Transplant

In patients with ATTRv, liver transplantation is an option because it halts the production of circulating mutant transthyretin. The first liver transplant for amyloidosis was performed in 1990. Good candidates include patients younger than 50 years, symptom duration less than 7 years, low polyneuropathy disability score, no severe autonomic neuropathy, no cardiomyopathy, and no significant renal dysfunction.[46] In the international registry of patients with primarily ATTRv neuropathy, the estimated 10-year survival was ~100% for liver transplant patients compared to 56% for nontransplant patients.[46] However, pretransplant symptoms do not regress significantly after transplant; peripheral neuropathy does not progress, some improvement in autonomic neuropathy can be seen, amyloid cardiomyopathy can progress, and renal recovery is variable. Patients with amyloid cardiomyopathy generally are excluded from liver transplant. A small number of joint liver-heart transplants have been done for patients with significant cardiomyopathy. In a Mayo Clinic cohort, the 5-year survival was 85% for liver-heart transplant patients and 52% for liver-only transplant patients.[47]

Heart Transplant

In patients with refractory heart failure due to advanced cardiac amyloid deposition, orthotopic heart transplantation should be considered for appropriate candidates. Although left ventricular assist device (LVAD) implantation is technically feasible in amyloid cardiomyopathy, it is associated with high short-term mortality and worse outcomes than in dilated cardiomyopathy.[48] Cardiopulmonary testing with peak VO_2 measurement can be useful in monitoring potential candidates. For amyloid cardiomyopathy, few heart transplants have been described in the literature, but the outcomes have been good. The 3-year survival of seven ATTRwt cardiac transplant recipients was 100%[49]; however, five of these patients experienced extracardiac amyloidosis symptoms (peripheral neuropathy, dysautonomia, and carpal tunnel syndrome) during their posttransplant course. In other studies, grouped ATTRwt and ATTRv cardiac transplant survival has been reported as 74% at 1 year in a 10-patient series,[50] 86% at 2 years in a 7-patient series,[51] and 75% 5-year survival in a 8-patient series.[52] For AL patients, 77% 5-year survival was reported for a 16-patient series.[52] The largest series of amyloid cardiomyopathy patients that underwent heart transplants included a total of 31 patients—13 AL and 18 ATTR. Despite older age and worse baseline renal function, there was no significant difference in mortality between patients who underwent heart transplants for amyloid cardiomyopathy compared to all other indications.[53]

SPECIAL CONSIDERATIONS

Hypotension

When the autonomic nervous system is affected by amyloid depositions, patients often present with profound hypotension and orthostatic symptoms including dizziness and syncope. Nonpharmacotherapy approaches such as compression stockings, positional/physical therapy adjustments, and good hydration are important. If a patient has diastolic heart failure, then volume balance is particularly difficult to maintain. Treatment requires close communication between physician and patient. For pharmacologic therapy of autonomic dysfunction, midodrine is the treatment of choice, titrated to the patient's needs. Direct treatment of underlying amyloidosis can mitigate and even improve autonomic dysfunction over the course of months to years. AL patients receiving effective light chain suppression treatment and ATTRv patients on RNA silencers can sometimes reduce or discontinue midodrine therapy.

Heart Failure

Medications

Heart failure management approaches depend on when a patient is diagnosed with amyloid cardiomyopathy. In earlier stages of the disease, most patients have heart failure with preserved EF and diastolic dysfunction. Volume control with diuretics and salt restriction is the primary management. For advanced amyloid cardiomyopathy with systolic dysfunction, guideline-directed medical therapy (GDMT) can be used, if tolerated. Because of hypotension, patients often are intolerant and can only take small doses of angiotensin-converting enzyme inhibitors, angiotensin receptor blockers, and beta-blockers. Mineralocorticoid receptor antagonists are better tolerated. Given the previously poor prognosis of amyloid cardiomyopathy, GDMT has limited utility. With novel amyloidosis therapies, the role of GDMT remains to be determined.

Intracardiac Defibrillators

Intracardiac defibrillators (ICDs) were traditionally considered contraindicated in amyloid cardiomyopathy because of the poor prognosis and perceived lack of successful defibrillation. With significant improvements in treatment and prognosis, ICDs are considered reasonable and favored by experts.[54] In addition to their placement in amyloidosis patients that meet traditional heart failure guidelines (ie, left ventricular EF < 35%), ICDs should be considered for patients with likely arrhythmia-associated syncope or ventricular arrhythmias on ambulatory telemetry.

Atrial Fibrillation

Atrial fibrillation is common in amyloid cardiomyopathy, especially in the later stages of the disease. With underlying restrictive cardiomyopathy, atrial fibrillation is poorly tolerated and can lead to decompensated heart failure. Rate or rhythm control can be pursued. Depending on the degree of cardiac involvement, beta-blockers may be poorly tolerated. Antiarrhythmics can be employed. In one study, 24% ATTR patients with atrial fibrillation were managed successfully with amiodarone and 10% were managed with another class of antiarrhythmic (ie, sotalol or dofetilide).[55] Digoxin has been considered contraindicated because of the potential for toxicity from its direct binding to amyloid fibrils. Yet given the limited effects on blood pressure, digoxin can be a reasonable choice for rate control in carefully selected patients with no other options. Two case series of patients with amyloid cardiomyopathy demonstrated good tolerance of digoxin, with only 11% to 12% developing a digoxin-related adverse event.[56,57] Conflicting results have been reported for atrial fibrillation ablation outcomes in amyloidosis patients: 60% recurrence-free survival at 3 years in one study[58] and 83% recurrence at 1 year in another study.[59]

Multiple studies have demonstrated that amyloid cardiomyopathy patients are more likely to develop an intracardiac thrombus than other patient groups with atrial fibrillation.[60] All amyloid cardiomyopathy patients with atrial fibrillation should be on long-term anticoagulation, regardless of their CHA2DS2-VASc score. If planning to perform a cardioversion for atrial fibrillation, all amyloid cardiomyopathy patients should undergo a transesophageal echocardiogram to rule out atrial thrombus regardless of whether they have been on therapeutic anticoagulation.[60] In addition, anticoagulation bridging with heparin or enoxaparin should be highly considered if systemic anticoagulation needs to be held.

Heart Block

In later stages of amyloid cardiomyopathy, heart block and electrophysiologic disruption are common. Physicians should have a low threshold to place a pacemaker for any qualifying indication such as symptomatic bradycardia.

FOLLOW-UP PATIENT CARE

Prognosis

The prognosis of amyloidosis is rapidly changing with evolving treatment modalities. Yet untreated amyloidosis has a very poor prognosis. Although amyloid can deposit in different organ systems, mortality is most directly correlated to the degree of cardiac involvement. The median survival of AL is 6 months when heart failure symptoms are present. The median survival of ATTR amyloidosis with significant cardiac involvement is 20 months.

For AL, the Mayo staging system is used for assessing prognosis. With the 2004 Mayo Staging system, prognosis was based on two criteria: troponin I 0.1 ng/mL or greater and NT-proBNP greater than 332 pg/mL. Patients who met no criteria were stage 1; those with one criterion were stage 2; and those with two criteria were stage 3. The median survival was 26.4, 10.5, and 3.5 months for stages 1 to 3, respectively. The updated 2012 Mayo system included three criteria: troponin T greater than 0.025 ng/mL, NT-proBNP greater than 1800 pg/mL, and free light chain difference 18 mg/dL or greater. The median survival was 94.1, 40.3, 14, and 5.8 months for stages 1 to 4, respectively.[61] With advancements in AL therapy, a 2019 single-center study demonstrated that survival for patients at each stage has improved[62]; survival was 118, 76, 64, and 27 months, for stages 1 to 4, respectively.

For ATTR amyloidosis, prognostic data are derived from untreated patients. The Boston University 2016 staging for ATTRwt is based on two criteria: NT-proBNP 3000 ng/L or greater and cardiac troponin T 0.05 ng/dL or greater. The median overall survival was 55, 42, and 20 months for individuals who met none, one, or both criteria, respectively.[63] Prognosis for ATTRv is not as well defined given the mutation-specific variability in disease presentation and affected organ systems. With the new FDA-approved therapies, prognosis for ATTR will most likely improve.

RESEARCH AND FUTURE DIRECTIONS

Advancements in early diagnosis and screening are critical to improving outcome and survival. Imaging studies will become more sophisticated for the diagnosis of amyloidosis.[64] If amyloidosis is diagnosed or strongly suspected, referral to an Amyloidosis Center of Excellence is highly recommended. Patients benefit from multidisciplinary care with knowledgeable specialists in cardiology, hematology, neurology, nephrology, and gastroenterology. Furthermore, these centers are hubs for the latest clinical trials. Ongoing trials are exploring additional transthyretin stabilizer medications, evolving regimens for AL treatment, expanding RNA silencer therapy to ATTRwt population, and comparing subcutaneous to infusion delivery of RNA silencer therapy. Future studies will target breakdown of existing amyloid fibrils and plaques.

KEY POINTS

- ✔ If one does not consider amyloidosis, one cannot diagnosis it.
- ✔ Be inquisitive. Inquire about the underlying cause for the patient's diagnoses. Could amyloid be responsible for your patient's peripheral neuropathy, mild left ventricular "hypertrophy," or concentric remodeling on echocardiogram or new-onset atrial fibrillation?
- ✔ Be familiar with amyloidosis "red flags" on common cardiac tests (such as echocardiogram or ECG). The absence of certain red flags should not stop diagnostic amyloidosis testing, if clinical suspicion is otherwise present.
- ✔ Always rule out AL before pursuing diagnostic testing for ATTR.
- ✔ If considering cardioversion for atrial fibrillation in a patient with amyloidosis, a transesophageal echocardiogram should always be done to rule out left atrial thrombus regardless of anticoagulation status.
- ✔ Prognosis for amyloid cardiomyopathy has significantly improved. If a clinical indication emerges, most amyloidosis patients are good candidates for standard cardiac care including ICDs, pacemakers, stents, cardiac surgery, and, in selected patients, cardiac transplant.
- ✔ Consider referral to an Amyloidosis Center of Excellence. Amyloidosis is a systemic disease and care should be multidisciplinary, particularly in collaboration with hematology and neurology.

REFERENCES

1. Gilstrap LG, Dominici F, Wang Y, et al. Epidemiology of cardiac amyloidosis-associated heart failure hospitalizations among fee-for-service Medicare beneficiaries in the United States. *Circ Heart Fail.* 2019;12:e005407.
2. Alexander KM, Orav J, Singh A, et al. Geographic disparities in reported US amyloidosis mortality from 1979 to 2015: potential underdetection of cardiac amyloidosis. *JAMA Cardiol.* 2018;3:865-870.
3. Kyle RA, Linos A, Beard CM, et al. Incidence and natural history of primary systemic amyloidosis in Olmsted County, Minnesota, 1950 through 1989. *Blood.* 1992;79:1817-1822.
4. Quock TP, Yan T, Chang E, Guthrie S, Broder MS. Epidemiology of AL amyloidosis: a real-world study using US claims data. *Blood Adv.* 2018;2:1046-1053.
5. Grogan M, Scott CG, Kyle RA, et al. Natural history of wild-type transthyretin cardiac amyloidosis and risk stratification using a novel staging system. *J Am Coll Cardiol.* 2016;68:1014-1020.
6. Kodaira M, Sekijima Y, Tojo K et al. Non-senile wild-type transthyretin systemic amyloidosis presenting as bilateral carpal tunnel syndrome. *J Peripher Nerv Syst.* 2008;13(2):148-150.
7. Cornwell GG 3rd, Murdoch WL, Kyle RA, Westermark P, Pitkanen P. Frequency and distribution of senile cardiovascular amyloid. A clinicopathologic correlation. *Am J Med.* 1983;75:618-623.
8. Tanskanen M, Peuralinna T, Polvikoski T, et al. Senile systemic amyloidosis affects 25% of the very aged and associates with genetic variation in

alpha2-macroglobulin and tau: a population-based autopsy study. *Ann Med.* 2008;40:232-239.

9. Tanskanen M, Kiuru-Enari S, Tienari P, et al. Senile systemic amyloidosis, cerebral amyloid angiopathy, and dementia in a very old Finnish population. *Amyloid.* 2006;13:164-169.
10. Gonzalez-Lopez E, Gallego-Delgado M, Guzzo-Merello G, et al. Wild-type transthyretin amyloidosis as a cause of heart failure with preserved ejection fraction. *Eur Heart J.* 2015;36:2585-2594.
11. Castano A, Narotsky DL, Hamid N, et al. Unveiling transthyretin cardiac amyloidosis and its predictors among elderly patients with severe aortic stenosis undergoing transcatheter aortic valve replacement. *Eur Heart J.* 2017;38:2879-2887.
12. Damy T, Costes B, Hagege AA, et al. Prevalence and clinical phenotype of hereditary transthyretin amyloid cardiomyopathy in patients with increased left ventricular wall thickness. *Eur Heart J.* 2016;37:1826-1834.
13. Sperry BW, Reyes BA, Ikram A, et al. Tenosynovial and cardiac amyloidosis in patients undergoing carpal tunnel release. *J Am Coll Cardiol.* 2018;72:2040-2050.
14. Hawkins PN, Ando Y, Dispenzeri A, Gonzalez-Duarte A, Adams D, Suhr OB. Evolving landscape in the management of transthyretin amyloidosis. *Ann Med.* 2015;47:625-638.
15. Quarta CC, Buxbaum JN, Shah AM, et al. The amyloidogenic V122I transthyretin variant in elderly black Americans. *N Engl J Med.* 2015;372:21-29.
16. Reilly MM, Staunton H, Harding AE. Familial amyloid polyneuropathy (TTR ala 60) in north west Ireland: a clinical, genetic, and epidemiological study. *J Neurol Neurosurg Psychiatry.* 1995;59:45-49.
17. Rapezzi C, Quarta CC, Riva L, et al. Transthyretin-related amyloidoses and the heart: a clinical overview. *Nat Rev Cardiol.* 2010;7:398-408.
18. Maurer MS, Hanna M, Grogan M, et al. Genotype and phenotype of transthyretin cardiac amyloidosis: THAOS (Transthyretin Amyloid Outcome Survey). *J Am Coll Cardiol.* 2016;68:161-172.
19. Rubin J, Alvarez J, Teruya S, et al. Hip and knee arthroplasty are common among patients with transthyretin cardiac amyloidosis, occurring years before cardiac amyloid diagnosis: can we identify affected patients earlier? *Amyloid.* 2017;24:226-230.
20. Dorbala S, Vangala D, Bruyere J Jr, et al. Coronary microvascular dysfunction is related to abnormalities in myocardial structure and function in cardiac amyloidosis. *JACC Heart Fail.* 2014;2:358-367.
21. Phull P, Sanchorawala V, Connors LH, et al. Monoclonal gammopathy of undetermined significance in systemic transthyretin amyloidosis (ATTR). *Amyloid.* 2018;25:62-67.
22. Rajkumar SV, Gertz MA, Kyle RA. Primary systemic amyloidosis with delayed progression to multiple myeloma. *Cancer.* 1998;82:1501-1505.
23. Yakupova EI, Bobyleva LG, Vikhlyantsev IM, Bobylev AG. Congo Red and amyloids: history and relationship. *Biosci Rep.* 2019;39(1):BSR20181415.
24. Ananthakrishna R, Lloyd R, Kuss Bryone J, Selvanayagam Joseph B. Cardiac Amyloidosis. *JACC: Case Reports.* 2020;2:282-285.
25. Witteles RM, Liedtke M. AL amyloidosis for the cardiologist and oncologist. *Epidemiol Diagn Manage.* 2019;1:117-130.
26. Gillmore JD, Maurer MS, Falk RH, et al. Nonbiopsy diagnosis of cardiac transthyretin amyloidosis. *Circulation.* 2016;133:2404-2412.
27. Adams D, Suhr OB, Hund E, et al. First European consensus for diagnosis, management, and treatment of transthyretin familial amyloid polyneuropathy. *Curr Opin Neurol.* 2016;29(suppl 1):S14-S26.
28. Gertz MA. Immunoglobulin light chain amyloidosis: 2018 Update on diagnosis, prognosis, and treatment. *Am J Hematol.* 2018;93:1169-1180.
29. Adams D, Gonzalez-Duarte A, O'Riordan WD, et al. Patisiran, an RNAi therapeutic, for hereditary transthyretin amyloidosis. *N Engl J Med.* 2018;379:11-21.
30. Solomon SD, Adams D, Kristen A, et al. Effects of patisiran, an RNA interference therapeutic, on cardiac parameters in patients with hereditary transthyretin-mediated amyloidosis. *Circulation.* 2019;139:431-443.
31. Benson MD, Waddington-Cruz M, Berk JL, et al. Inotersen treatment for patients with hereditary transthyretin amyloidosis. *N Engl J Med.* 2018;379:22-31.
32. Dasgupta NR, Rissing SM, Smith J, Jung J, Benson MD. Inotersen therapy of transthyretin amyloid cardiomyopathy. *Amyloid.* 2020;27:52-58.
33. Maurer MS, Schwartz JH, Gundapaneni B, et al. Tafamidis treatment for patients with transthyretin amyloid cardiomyopathy. *N Engl J Med.* 2018;379:1007-1016.
34. Berk JL, Suhr OB, Obici L, et al. Repurposing diflunisal for familial amyloid polyneuropathy: a randomized clinical trial. *JAMA.* 2013;310:2658-2667.
35. Lohrmann G, Pipilas A, Mussinelli R, et al. Stabilization of cardiac function with diflunisal in transthyretin (ATTR) cardiac amyloidosis. *J Card Fail.* 2020;26(9):753-759.
36. Ward JE, Ren R, Toraldo G, et al. Doxycycline reduces fibril formation in a transgenic mouse model of AL amyloidosis. *Blood.* 2011;118:6610-6617.
37. Wechalekar AD, Whelan C. Encouraging impact of doxycycline on early mortality in cardiac light chain (AL) amyloidosis. *Blood Cancer J.* 2017;7(3):e546.
38. Cardoso I, Martins D, Ribeiro T, Merlini G, Saraiva MJ. Synergy of combined doxycycline/TUDCA treatment in lowering Transthyretin deposition and associated biomarkers: studies in FAP mouse models. *J Transl Med.* 2010;8:74.
39. Obici L, Cortese A, Lozza A, et al. Doxycycline plus tauroursodeoxycholic acid for transthyretin amyloidosis: a phase II study. *Amyloid.* 2012;19(suppl 1):34-36.
40. Karlstedt E, Jimenez-Zepeda V, Howlett JG, White JA, Fine NM.
41. aus dem Siepen F, Bauer R, Aurich M, et al. Green tea extract as a treatment for patients with wild-type transthyretin amyloidosis: an observational study. *Drug Des Devel Ther.* 2015;9:6319-6325.
42. Comenzo RL, Vosburgh E, Falk RH, et al. Dose-intensive melphalan with blood stem-cell support for the treatment of AL (amyloid light-chain) amyloidosis: survival and responses in 25 patients. *Blood.* 1998;91:3662-3670.
43. Sidiqi MH, Aljama MA, Buadi FK, et al. Stem cell transplantation for light chain amyloidosis: decreased early mortality over time. *J Clin Oncol.* 2018;36:1323-1329.
44. Jaccard A, Moreau P, Leblond V, et al. High-dose melphalan versus melphalan plus dexamethasone for AL amyloidosis. *N Engl J Med.* 2007;357:1083-1093.
45. Sanchorawala V, Sun F, Quillen K, Sloan JM, Berk JL, Seldin DC. Long-term outcome of patients with AL amyloidosis treated with high-dose melphalan and stem cell transplantation: 20-year experience *Blood* United States; 2015(126):2345-2347.
46. Carvalho A, Rocha A, Lobato L. Liver transplantation in transthyretin amyloidosis: issues and challenges. *Liver Transpl.* 2015;21:282-292.
47. Banerjee D, Roeker LE, Grogan M, et al. Outcomes of patients with familial transthyretin amyloidosis after liver transplantation. *Prog Transplant.* 2017;27:246-250.
48. Swiecicki PL, Edwards BS, Kushwaha SS, Dispenzieri A, Park SJ, Gertz MA. Left ventricular device implantation for advanced cardiac amyloidosis. *J Heart Lung Transplant.* 2013;32:563-568.
49. Rosenbaum AN, AbouEzzeddine OF, Grogan M, et al. Outcomes after cardiac transplant for wild type transthyretin amyloidosis. *Transplantation.* 2018;102:1909-1913.
50. Davis MK, Kale P, Liedtke M, et al. Outcomes after heart transplantation for amyloid cardiomyopathy in the modern era. *Am J Transplant.* 2015;15:650-658.
51. Dubrey SW, Burke MM, Hawkins PN, Banner NR. Cardiac transplantation for amyloid heart disease: the United Kingdom experience. *J Heart Lung Transplant.* 2004;23:1142-1153.
52. Kristen AV, Kreusser MM, Blum P, et al. Improved outcomes after heart transplantation for cardiac amyloidosis in the modern era. *J Heart Lung Transplant.* 2018;37:611-618.
53. Barrett CD, Alexander Kevin M, Zhao H, et al. Outcomes in patients with cardiac amyloidosis undergoing heart transplantation. *JACC: Heart Fail.* 2020;8:461-468.
54. Varr BC, Zarafshar S, Coakley T, et al. Implantable cardioverter-defibrillator placement in patients with cardiac amyloidosis. *Heart Rhythm.* 2014;11:158-162.

55. Mints YY, Doros G, Berk JL, Connors LH, Ruberg FL. Features of atrial fibrillation in wild-type transthyretin cardiac amyloidosis: a systematic review and clinical experience. *ESC Heart Fail.* 2018;5:772-779.
56. Donnelly JP, Sperry BW, Gabrovsek A, et al. Digoxin use in cardiac amyloidosis. *Am J Cardiol.* 2020;133:134-138.
57. Muchtar E, Gertz MA, Kumar SK, et al. Digoxin use in systemic light-chain (AL) amyloidosis: contra-indicated or cautious use? *Amyloid.* 2018;25:86-92.
58. Tan NY, Mohsin Y, Hodge DO, et al. Catheter ablation for atrial arrhythmias in patients with cardiac amyloidosis. *J Cardiovasc Electrophysiol.* 2016;27:1167-1173.
59. Barbhaiya CR, Kumar S, Baldinger SH, et al. Electrophysiologic assessment of conduction abnormalities and atrial arrhythmias associated with amyloid cardiomyopathy. *Heart Rhythm.* 2016;13:383-390.
60. El-Am EA, Dispenzieri A, Melduni RM, et al. Direct current cardioversion of atrial arrhythmias in adults with cardiac amyloidosis. *J Am Coll Cardiol.* 2019;73:589-597.
61. Kumar S, Dispenzieri A, Lacy MQ, et al. Revised prognostic staging system for light chain amyloidosis incorporating cardiac biomarkers and serum free light chain measurements. *J Clin Oncol.* 2012;30:989-995.
62. Barrett CD, Dobos K, Liedtke M, et al. A changing landscape of mortality for systemic light chain amyloidosis. *JACC Heart Fail.* 2019;7:958-966.
63. Connors LH, Sam F, Skinner M, et al. Heart failure resulting from age-related cardiac amyloid disease associated with wild-type transthyretin: a prospective, observational cohort study. *Circulation.* 2016;133:282-290.
64. Dorbala S, Kijewski MF, Park MA. Quantitative molecular imaging of cardiac amyloidosis: the journey has begun. *J Nucl Cardiol.* 2016;23(4):751-753.

SECTION 2

CARDIOVASCULAR IMAGING

SECTION EDITOR: Mario J. Garcia

CHAPTER 31

PRINCIPLES OF IMAGING TECHNIQUES

Mario J. Garcia and Kana Fujikura

INTRODUCTION

The American Heart Association estimates that approximately 17.6 million deaths were attributed to cardiovascular disease (CVD) in the United States, which is 14.5% increase in 10 years.[1] By 2030, CVD deaths are estimated over 23.6 million. Many patients are asymptomatic until they present at a late stage. In most cases, early risk assessment and appropriate interventions are essential to lower CVD morbidity and mortality. Novel acquisition schemes and technological improvements have made coronary artery calcium (CAC) scoring, computed tomography (CT), coronary CT angiography (CCTA), and cardiac magnetic resonance imaging (CMR) more readily available and practical for routine clinical practice. Reductions in CT radiation dose, rapid imaging techniques in CMR, and increased awareness have promoted CT and CMR use for detection and surveillance of CVD. In order to fully utilize multimodality approach and properly stratify risk assessment and management of patients with known or suspected CVD, it is critical for ordering physicians and providers to be aware of the fundamentals for each of the imaging techniques, unique imaging challenges, and appropriate use criteria (AUC).

INDICATIONS

Evaluation of Symptoms

In 1979, Diamond and Forrester introduced the idea of using pretest probability to select an optimum test to diagnose obstructive coronary artery disease (CAD) in stable symptomatic patients.[2] Since then, analysis of pretest probability has been a standard practice in cardiology. Consequently, the analysis of pretest probability of CAD has served as an effective gatekeeper for noninvasive testing and has been used to define its appropriateness of use in guidelines (**Figures 31.1, 31.2, and Table 31.1**).[3,4] For example, noninvasive imaging testing for obstructive CAD is most cost-effective when it is applied to patients with an intermediate likelihood of CAD. Recent technological advances have extended the ability of noninvasive imaging methods to diagnose obstructive CAD reducing the need for invasive diagnostic catheterization. Because of this development, analysis of pretest probability requires appropriate adjustments. Multiple studies in contemporary era have shown that the traditional Diamond and Forrester model overestimates pretest probability of obstructive CAD, which potentially leads to selection of too many low-risk patients for testing. Recent efforts have focused on developing newer risk scores to estimate pretest probability of obstructive CAD suitable for contemporary noninvasive diagnosing tests.

Prognosis and Risk Assessment

Screening is very important to diagnose CAD and assess the prognosis to provide an appropriate treatment. Within the context of screening tests, it is important to avoid misconceptions about sensitivity, specificity, and predictive values.[4] The sensitivity of a screening test can be described as the ability of a screening test to detect a true positive. A definition of sensitivity would be a screening test's probability of correctly identifying, *solely from among people who are known to have a condition.* A definition of positive predictive value (PPV) would be a screening test's probability, when returning a positive result, *from among people who might or might not have a condition.* On the other hand, the specificity of a test can be described as the ability of a screening test to detect a true negative. A definition of specificity would be a screening test's probability of correctly identifying, *solely from among people who are known not to have a condition.* A clear definition of negative predictive value (NPV) would be a screening test's probability, when returning a negative result, *from among people who might or might not have a condition.* By summarizing these definitions, sensitivity and specificity indicate the concordance of a test with respect to a chosen referent, PPV and NPV, respectively, that indicate the likelihood that a test can successfully identify whether people do or do not have a target condition, based on their test results.

Despite the above reservations concerning sensitivity and specificity in a screening situation, sensitivity and specificity can be useful in two circumstances but only if they are extremely high. A highly sensitive screening test is unlikely to produce false-negative outcomes, people who test negative on a screening test with high sensitivity are very unlikely to have the target condition. This statement can also be applied to a highly specific test. In fact, for many screening tests, unfortunately, either sensitivity or specificity is low despite the other being high, or neither sensitivity nor specificity is high.[5] As a consequence, predictive values are more relevant than are sensitivity and specificity when people are being screened. Of note, predictive values also need caution to be adopted because PPVs and NPVs are directly related to the prevalence of the disease in the population. Assuming all other factors remain constant,

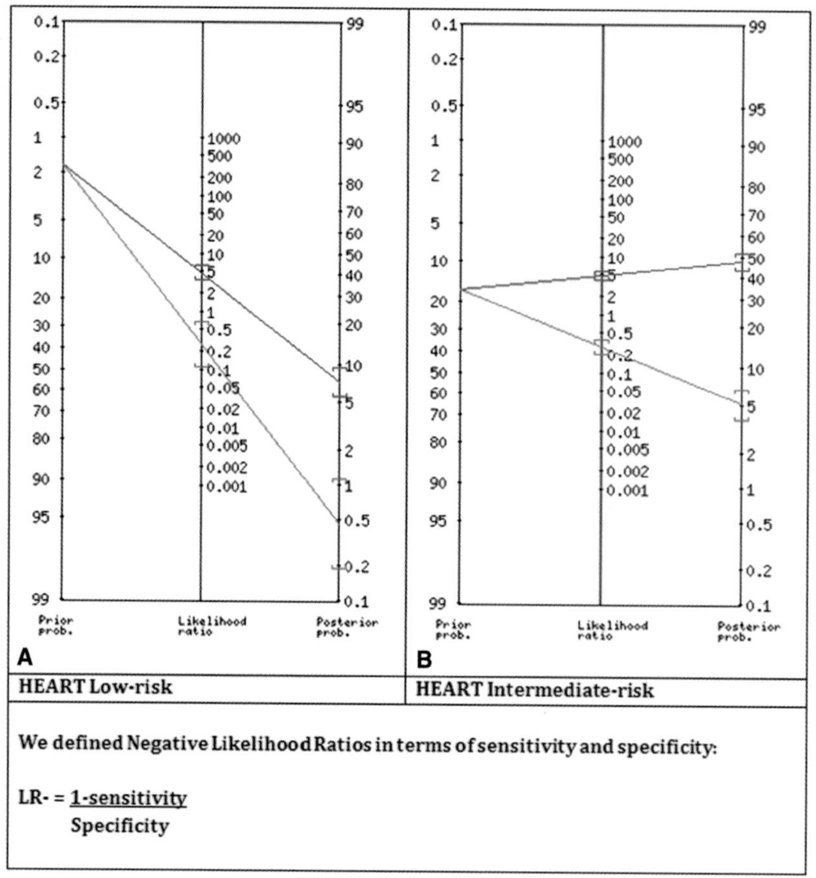

FIGURE 31.1 An example of converting the pretest probability (HEART score) to posttest probability of the event using Bayesian methodology in subjects with (**A**) low-risk and (**B**) intermediate-risk pretest probabilities. Blue lines represent positive LR, and red lines represent negative LR. LR, likelihood ratio; prob., probability. (Reprinted from Farook N, Cochon L, Bode AD, et al. HEART score and stress test emergency department Bayesian decision scheme: Results from the acute care diagnostic collaboration. *J Emerg Med.* 2018;54(2):147-155. Copyright © 2017 Elsevier. With permission.)

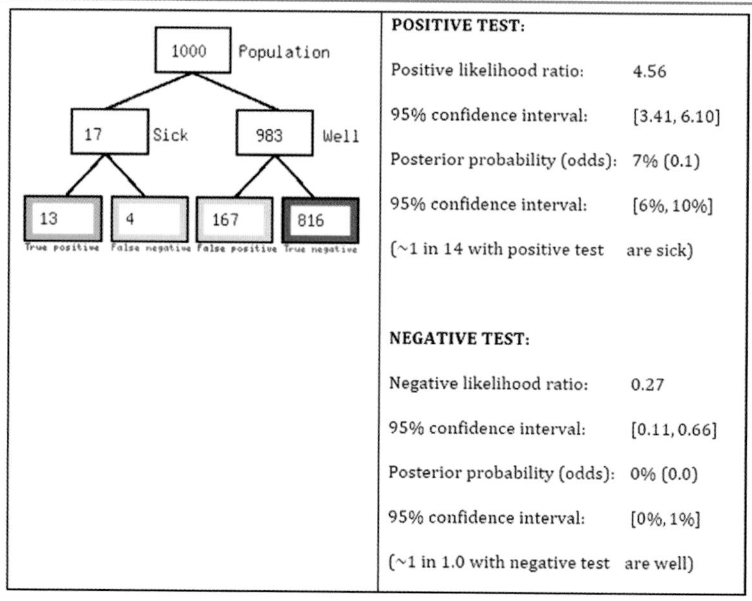

FIGURE 31.2 An example of case distribution scheme for hypothetical low-risk pretest probability. LR, likelihood ratio. (Reprinted from Farook N, Cochon L, Bode AD, et al. HEART score and stress test emergency department Bayesian decision scheme: Results from the acute care diagnostic collaboration. *J Emerg Med.* 2018;54(2):147-155. Copyright © 2017 Elsevier. With permission.)

TABLE 31.1 Analysis of Diagnostic Gain Using Likelihood Ratios

		HEART Score Risk					
Diagnostic Test	**LR$^+$**		**Points**	**%**	**Posttest Probability, %**	**ADG (%)[a]**	**RDG (%)[b]**
Treadmill stress	4.56	Low	0-3	1.7	7.75	6.05	356.0
		Intermediate	4-6	16.6	47.62	31.02	186.87
Stress ECHO	5.65	Low	0-3	1.7	9.09	7.39	434.71
		Intermediate	4-6	16.6	52.63	36.03	217.06

ADG, absolute diagnostic gain; ECHO, echocardiogram; HEART, history, electrocardiogram, age, risk factors, and troponin; LR$^+$, positive likelihood ratio; RDG, relative diagnostic gain.
[a]ADG = post − pre.
[b]RDG = 100 × ADG/pre.
Reprinted from Farook N, Cochon L, Bode AD, et al. HEART score and stress test emergency department Bayesian decision scheme: Results from the acute care diagnostic collaboration. *J Emerg Med.* 2018;54(2):147-155. Copyright © 2017 Elsevier. With permission.

the PPV will increase with increasing prevalence; and NPV decreases with increase in prevalence.[6]

Therapy Guidance

Overuse of low-value clinical services has received greater attention in recent years in response to a report of waste in US health care that estimated over 20% of total expenditure are spent on services that do not improve patient care. Ordering an appropriate diagnostic test is fundamental in providing high-quality cardiovascular care, efficiently guiding to an appropriate therapy, and evaluating the treatment effect. Cardiovascular imaging (CVI) must be used only when the test contributes in improving clinical outcomes and values. Since 2005, the American College of Cardiology (ACC) has been publishing multiple AUC documents and their updates covering CVI tests in common clinical scenarios in partnership with specialty and subspecialty societies. However, "rarely appropriate" imaging tests are still ordered in significant numbers. According to a meta-analysis, percentage of appropriate indications for transthoracic echocardiography (TTE) is 85%, transesophageal echocardiography (TEE) is 95%, stress echocardiography is 52%, CT angiography (CTA) is 55%, and single-photon emission CT is 68%.[7] Educational interventions have been proposed and shown to be effective in reducing inappropriate ordering of tests.[8] National and international educational systems may need to be organized to promote global level of consistent appropriate utilization. To make things complicated, a preferred imaging test for a given clinical scenario varies with each practice setting. Important considerations in modality choice are diagnostic performance, availability of the technology, and physician expertise. Safety considerations including radiation dose and cost should also be considered in relationship to these benefits when determining net value.

ANATOMIC CONSIDERATIONS

Cardiac Chambers

The quantification of cardiac chamber size and function is the cornerstone of cardiac imaging. TTE is most often the first-choice imaging modality in the daily practice of cardiology because it is noninvasive, low-cost, easily available, provides real-time images of the beating heart, portable, and radiation free.[9] However, there are disadvantages of TTE such as operator dependency, difficulties in performing optimal evaluation because of suboptimal image quality associated with body structure, obesity, or chronic lung diseases. CMR provides images with less operator dependency and allows evaluation of the structure and function of the heart more accurately and with greater reproducibly. CMR is now considered to be the gold standard method for the volumetric assessment of ventricular function, mass measurement, and detection of myocardial scarring.[10]

Valves

Etiologies of primary valve regurgitation are numerous and include degeneration, inflammation, infection, trauma, tissue disruption, iatrogenic, or congenital. Doppler techniques are very sensitive, and thus, detect trivial or physiologic valve regurgitation, even in a structurally normal valve. Although echocardiography remains the first-line modality for assessment of valvular regurgitation, in some situations, it may be suboptimal. In addition, volumetric assessment by CMR has been shown to have high reproducibility and, therefore, may be ideal for serial assessments. CMR is generally indicated when (1) echocardiographic images are suboptimal, (2) there is discordance between 2D echocardiographic features and Doppler findings (eg, ventricular enlargement greater than expected on the basis of Doppler measures of valvular regurgitation), or (3) there is discordance between clinical assessment and severity of valvular regurgitation by echocardiography.

Calcific aortic stenosis (AS) is the most prevalent valvular heart disease in the United States and Europe.[11] AS often has a long latency period before symptom onset; however, when symptoms develop and severe AS is present, the average survival is reduced to 2 to 3 years in the absence of treatment. Standard Doppler echocardiography is the cornerstone of the evaluation of AS and is sufficient to guide therapeutic management in almost 65% to 70% of the patients. However, in almost 25%

to 30% of the patients, there are some uncertainties about AS severity at Doppler echocardiographic examination, and these patients may, thus, require multimodality imaging to confirm disease stage and guide therapeutic decision making.

The number of patients requiring heart valve replacement is increasing rapidly as the population is aging. Monitoring and follow-up of patients with prosthetic heart valves (PHVs) are important because of the numerous and potentially life-threatening complications. Echocardiography is the mainstay for evaluation of PHV. However, visual assessment of PHV function and morphology is fundamentally limited by echocardiography because of extensive acoustic shadowing and limited viewing windows. CMR and more prominently cardiac CT are new imaging techniques for PHV assessment to complement echocardiography.[12]

Pericardium

Pericardial conditions ranging from acute pericarditis and constrictive pericarditis to cardiac tamponade represent an important group of cardiovascular disorders. Multimodality CVI is critical in the diagnosis and management of pericardial conditions, providing structural, functional, and hemodynamic information.[13] Imaging should follow a careful history and physical examination, electrocardiogram (ECG), and chest x-ray and then be focused toward the clinical working diagnosis. This stepwise approach is important to avoid unnecessary testing with its potential risk for side effects, false-positive diagnoses, and inappropriate allocation of resources, thus avoiding excessive costs. Among multimodality imaging tests, TTE is most often the first-line test, followed by CMR and/or cardiac CT. Each of the tests can be useful in the evaluation of the structure and hemodynamic and/or functional disturbances of pericardial diseases. For example, TTE with respirometric recording would be considered the first-line modality to evaluate the anatomic and physiologic features of constrictive pericarditis. CMR and cardiac CT would be second-line tests to further assess the degree of increased pericardial thickness, functional effects of the constrictive process, inflammation, as well as the distribution of calcium in the pericardium. It is important to note that all three tests are rarely necessary in the diagnosis of constrictive pericarditis unless there are technically poor or diagnostically uncertain TTE studies; there is a mixed constrictive pericarditis and restriction, being evaluated for pericardiectomy, or there is a concern for transient constriction with ongoing inflammation.

Coronary Vessels

All the noninvasive CVI modalities play an important role in the diagnosis of CAD.[14] Contemporary stress imaging techniques, with stress nuclear myocardial perfusion imaging (MPI) and stress echocardiography, provide a high sensitivity and specificity in the detection and risk assessment of CAD and have incremental value over exercise stress test (ECG) and clinical variables. CAC scoring has emerged as the most predictive single cardiovascular risk marker in asymptomatic subjects, capable of adding predictive information beyond the traditional cardiovascular risk factors.[15] Many studies show that CAC testing is cost-effective compared with alternative approaches when factoring in patient preferences about taking preventive medications, such as statin and aspirin. Among all available noninvasive imaging tests, CCTA has the highest diagnostic accuracy for the detection of obstructive CAD defined as greater than 50% luminal narrowing in major epicardial vessels. CCTA detects CAD, including plaque characteristics and extent of stenosis, and is a strong predictor for future major adverse cardiovascular events. CMR is useful in the assessment of myocardial perfusion and viability, as well as cardiac function. Recently, stress CMR is shown to be excellent in selecting patients who benefit from invasive coronary revascularization. Among patients with stable angina and risk factors for CAD, stress CMR was associated with a lower incidence of coronary revascularization than fractional flow reserve (FFR) and was noninferior to FFR with respect to major adverse cardiac events (MACE).[16]

Great Vessels

Imaging plays a crucial role in treatment planning and postsurgical surveillance of aortic pathology.[17] CTA with intravenous iodinated contrast material is the most widely used diagnostic modality to assess the morphology of aorta. CTA has many advantages including wide availability, rapid acquisition, sub-millimeter spatial resolution, and high value in guiding patient management. Disadvantages include the need for iodinated contrast material and ionizing radiation exposure. CT technology has gone through continuous evolution from its inception and recent advances including dual energy capabilities, rapid gantry rotation, fast table movement, and high output tubes have allowed reduction in both iodinated contrast dose and radiation exposure. MR angiography (MRA) also provides morphologic information of the aorta. The advantage of MRA is free of radiation exposure; however, the disadvantage is longer scanning time. Advancements in MR technology now allow scanning the aorta without intravenous contrast material as well as more rapid image acquisition than in the past. 18F-fluorodeoxyglucose positron emission tomography/computed tomography (18F-FDG-PET/CT) imaging is useful for the evaluation of vascular graft-related infections, large vessel vasculitis, and atherosclerotic plaque inflammation. Contrast-enhanced ultrasound is also emerging as a method of surveillance for the postsurgical abdominal aorta and has a potential to curb the costs and radiation exposure related to aortic imaging.

FUNDAMENTALS OF CARDIAC IMAGING

Image Quality Considerations

Currently, quality in laboratory structure is assessed primarily by accreditation.[18] Laboratory accreditation can be obtained for ultrasound, nuclear, CT, and magnetic resonance imaging (MRI) laboratories through either the American College of Radiology (ACR) or the Intersocietal Accreditation Commission (IAC). Under the umbrella of the IAC, laboratory accreditation is available for noninvasive vascular imaging (ICAVL), echocardiography (ICAEL), nuclear cardiology (ICANL), CT (ICACTL), and MRI (ICAMRL). Accreditation standards of both organizations emphasize physician and technologist training, equipment performance, imaging protocols, report content, and timeliness. In addition, accreditation bodies mandate periodic submission of sample studies to monitor the quality of imaging acquisition. Ongoing quality improvement initiatives and continuing medical education also are required.

Determination of Accuracy

The overarching goal of noninvasive testing is to assess the risk for future cardiovascular events and guide clinical care.[19] For example, in symptomatic patients with an intermediate probability of CAD, the ideal noninvasive test should be capable of both accurately diagnosing and excluding significant disease.[20] Historically, significant CAD has been synonymous with obstructive CAD (≥70% stenosis), as determined by angiographic appearance during invasive coronary angiography (ICA). However, the Fractional Flow Reserve versus Angiography for Multivessel Evaluation (FAME) trial revealed that anatomically obstructive lesions do not always equate to functionally significant lesions as assessed by FFR, an index of the physiologic significance of a coronary stenosis. Furthermore, patients revascularized for lesions that were both anatomically and functionally significant had a 28% lower rate of death, nonfatal myocardial infraction, and repeat revascularization than those patients revascularized on the basis of anatomic stenosis alone. Therefore, if revascularization of stenotic coronary lesions that induce ischemia can improve patient outcomes, then the question is: Can this be accurately identified with noninvasive testing so that only patients with clinically significant CAD are sent for invasive evaluation? Currently, noninvasive testing is capable of evaluating either anatomic or functional significance. Test selection requires choosing either an anatomic or functional evaluation. CCTA is capable of noninvasively assessing the anatomic severity of CAD, whereas stress MPI by single-photon computed emission tomography, positron emission tomography (PET), and CMR, or stress wall motion imaging (WMI) with stress echocardiography (stress echo) or CMR, detects myocardial ischemia and indicates the presence of functional CAD. The recent development of noninvasive FFR by CT (FFR_{CT}) used in conjunction with CCTA may have a potential of the highest accuracy for identifying or excluding anatomically and physiologically significant CAD, and therefore, positively influencing patient management, particularly referrals for ICA.

Benefit and Risk Considerations

The rapid increase in the use of imaging procedures and new imaging modalities has triggered increased scrutiny about indications for noninvasive CVI studies. The various procedures have several risks: stressors, contrast agents, invasiveness, radiation, and so on. Even more importantly, the benefit of performing or not performing the test needs to be balanced with the risk and drawbacks associated with the disease remaining undetected. Knuuti et al[21] evaluated immediate, short-, and long-term risks associated with CVI in relation to the natural course of CAD and to therapeutic interventions. They analyzed (1) the risk of MACE for each component of imaging test; (2) the upper limit for each risk, in order to avoid underestimation of a risk; (3) composite risks calculated for selected common diagnostic tests for CAD; (4) the risks compared with the risk of the disease itself, to assess the potential benefits of tests; and (5) comparison with risks in regular life activities and that associated with long-term prophylactic interventions, such as aspirin use. The study showed that pharmacologic stress agents are relatively major contributors to acute risks related to CVI. However, in absolute figures, the risk is small. In invasive tests, the procedure itself is the most important risk factor. For long-term risks of fatal events, the risks of contrast agents and the radiation risk have high impact on the composite risk of the procedure. It is to be noted that the lifetime risk of imaging procedures for fatal events is small as compared with the general risk of fatal cardiac events by CAD both in asymptomatic and symptomatic populations.

Outcome Analysis

The performance of a CVI procedure provides largely an indirect link to improved clinical outcomes.[21] Improvements in patient outcomes may be realized when postimaging care is prompt and consistent with guideline-directed care. Thus, the intervening treatment initiation or modification is the rate-limiting link to improving the lives of patients after an imaging procedure. This link between imager and referring physician is critical to achieve optimal patient outcomes and communication about the recommended treatment.

Cost/Benefit Analysis

In general, CVI technologies, when implemented for appropriate indications, have shown to provide favorable cost-utility profiles, in keeping with many current clinical evaluation strategies.[22] The increment in number and positive cost-utility profiles may be due to advances in CT, CMR, and other advanced imaging technologies that facilitate an accurate diagnosis. These modalities have begun to replace invasive procedures, such as diagnostic angiography while minimizing patient risks and discomfort.[23] When considering the added value per CVI dollar, we must recognize that each test represents a cost and a risk. However, very small individual costs and risks could become significant when multiplied by the large number of tests performed worldwide annually. Given those considerations, professional societies have made efforts to develop guidelines for appropriate utilization in a variety of clinical scenarios.

CLINICAL APPLICATIONS

Methodology

Image Acquisition and Storage

CVI and data management can be challenging. Procedures are diverse, and many facilities operate multiple decentralized information systems. Multimodality cardiology environments including echocardiography, nuclear cardiology, cardiac CT, CMR, cardiac catheterization, and ECG data management to create a single, integrated cardiovascular image and information solution are useful. Cardiovascular information system (CVIS), also called cardiac picture archiving and communication system (PACS) has been innovated to achieve this goal. The cardiac PACS system stores CVI and reports of all modalities, and now has been expanding to aggregate all cardiac patient data including electronic medical records (EMR), ECG, and cardiac catheterization laboratory information, such as images and hemodynamical wave forms (**Figure 31.3**). The cardiology PACS market is moving beyond just image storage and distribution, focusing on gathering relevant patient data to provide more data points to work with and help physicians make better decisions for patient care.

Digital Imaging and Communications in Medicine

Digital Imaging and Communications in Medicine (DICOM) is a standard for handling, storing, printing, and transmitting information in medical imaging.[24] The goal of DICOM is to achieve compatibility and improve workflow efficiency between imaging systems and other information systems in health care environments worldwide. With hundreds of thousands of medical imaging devices in use, DICOM is one of the most widely deployed health care messaging standards in the world.

Report Distribution

The IAC provides accreditation to set standards and methods for the evaluation of the quality of care delivered including all the modalities of CVI: echocardiography, nuclear/PET, CMR, and cardiac CT.[25-28] IAC requires all physicians interpreting CVI in the facility to agree on uniform diagnostic criteria and a standardized report format. In order to create consistent and structured reporting in busy daily clinical practice, various vendors provide customizable software to create cardiovascular reports fast and efficiently. Using specialized software, measurements can be automatically transferred into a report without retyping, as well as text of the report can be autophrased and completed based on clinical quantifications.

Cardiology Electronic Health Record Integration

As of 2017, nearly 9 in 10 (86%) of office-based physicians had adopted any electronic health record (EHR).[29] Integration of CVI into EHR system allows providers to automatically send report back to referring physicians as well as allows them to access images through a link in the record. Immediate access to CVI provides full-view of the patient to support clinical decision in timely manner.

LIMITATIONS OF NONINVASIVE IMAGING

Health Hazards of Cardiac Imaging

Ionizing Radiation

Along with the benefits patients have received from medical imaging, various imaging procedures expose patients to ionizing radiation (**Table 31.2**).[30] High utilization of CT and nuclear medicine imaging have increased concerns over cumulative dose of ionizing radiation and lifetime risks of cancer (**Figure 31.4**).[31,32] Einstein et al reported that more than 30% of patients who underwent MPI received a cumulative estimated effective dose of more than 100 mSv, a level at which there is little controversy over the potential for increased cancer risks.[33] In 2010, U.S. Food and Drug Administration (FDA) launched an initiative to reduce unnecessary radiation exposure from medical imaging to promote patient safety through two principles[34]: (1) Justification: The imaging procedure should be judged to do more good than do harm to the individual patient. Therefore, all examinations using ionizing radiation should be performed only when necessary to answer a medical question, help treat a disease, or guide a procedure; (2) Dose optimization: Medical imaging examinations should use techniques that are adjusted to administer the lowest radiation dose that yields an image quality adequate for diagnosis or intervention (ie, radiation doses should be "As Low as Reasonably Achievable [ALARA]"). However, a recent study showed CT protocols and radiation doses still vary greatly across countries and are primarily attributable to local choices regarding technical parameters that require worldwide standardization.[35] A more detailed discussion of the specific approaches that can be taken to reduce radiation exposure and improve benefit:risk ratio is provided in Chapters 34 and 35 of this book.

Contrast Agents

It is now over a half century that iodinated radio-contrast materials have been considered as a significant risk of nephrotoxicity.[36] Old generation high-osmolarity contrast media have been replaced by newer generation low-osmolarity contrast media that clearly reduced the incidence of generalized contrast reactions including nephrotoxicity. Very low risk of contrast-induced nephropathy (CIN) has altered practice by clinicians ordering contrast-enhanced studies on more patients with elevated serum creatinine; however, contrast is still frequently withheld for fear of CIN.[37] The consequence of restraining contrast reduces the accuracy of examinations and limits effective management of diseases. In high-risk populations, such as in those with chronic kidney disease (CKD), CIN risk may be higher, and thus, caution should be exerted with contrast exposure. The volumes of contrast should be minimized as much as possible, and hemodynamic status should be optimized before contrast administration.[38]

Nephrogenic systemic fibrosis (NSF) is a rare disease of fibrosis of the skin and internal organs that can be caused by exposure to gadolinium-based contrast agent (GBCA). NSF is noted to occur predominantly in patient with end-stage CKD, particularly in patients on dialysis. All GBCAs share a common structure of an organic ligand that tightly binds to and improves the stability, solubility, and safety of the central gadolinium heavy metal ion. In general a macrocyclic structure confers greater stability than a linear structure, and to a lesser extent ionic GBCAs have greater stability than those with nonionic structure.[39] The incidence of NSF using newer linear and macrocyclic agents has decreased considerably, which is generally cited to be much lesser than 1%; therefore, use of GBCAs is

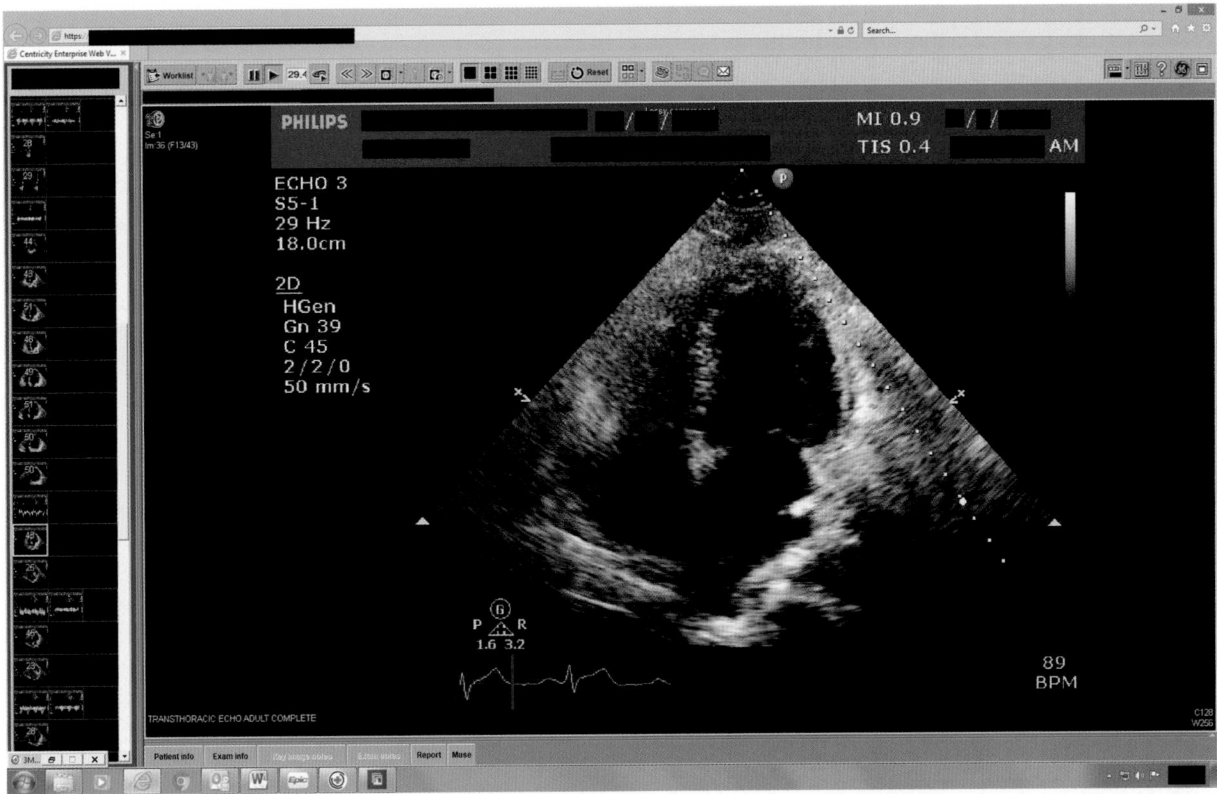

A

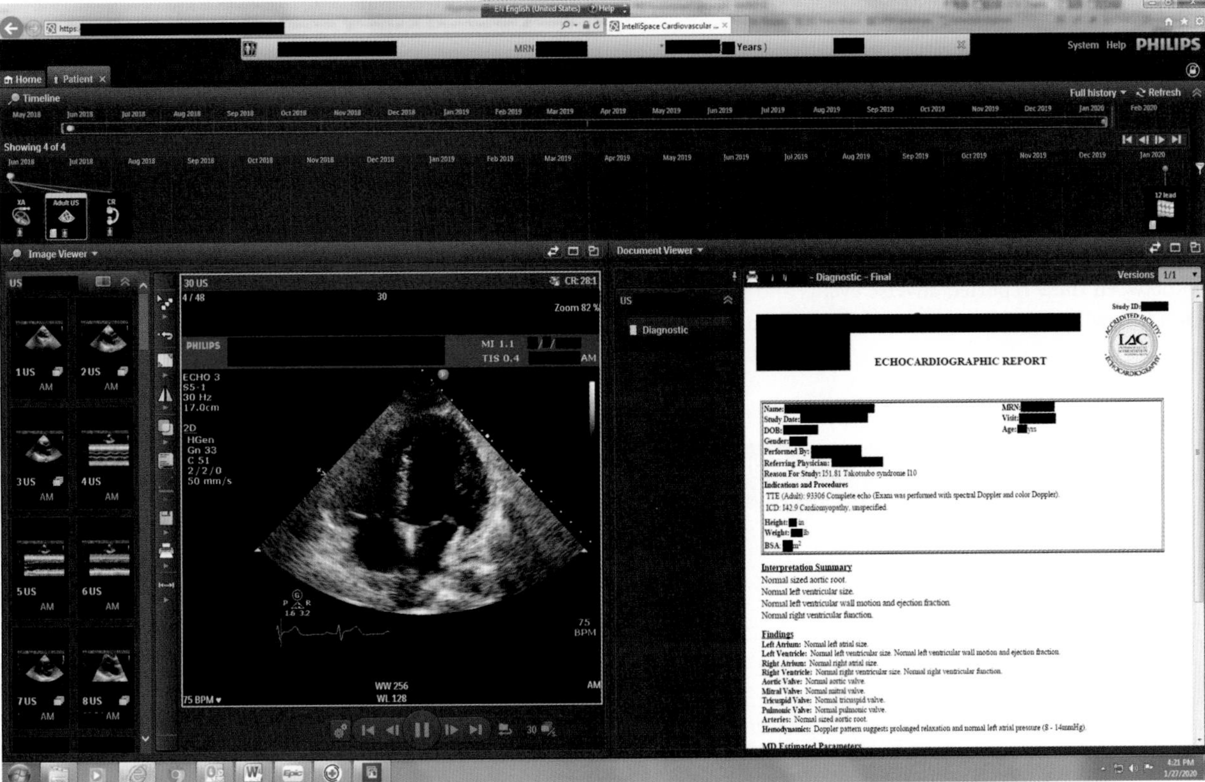

B

FIGURE 31.3 The integration of EMR and PACS and imaging software. (**A**) Echocardiography images, (**B**) cardiac catheterization fluoroscopy, echocardiography, and CT images and reports are all stored in one PACS system, and (**C**) images can be accessed directly from EMR. CT, computed tomography; EMR, electronic medical records; PACS,.

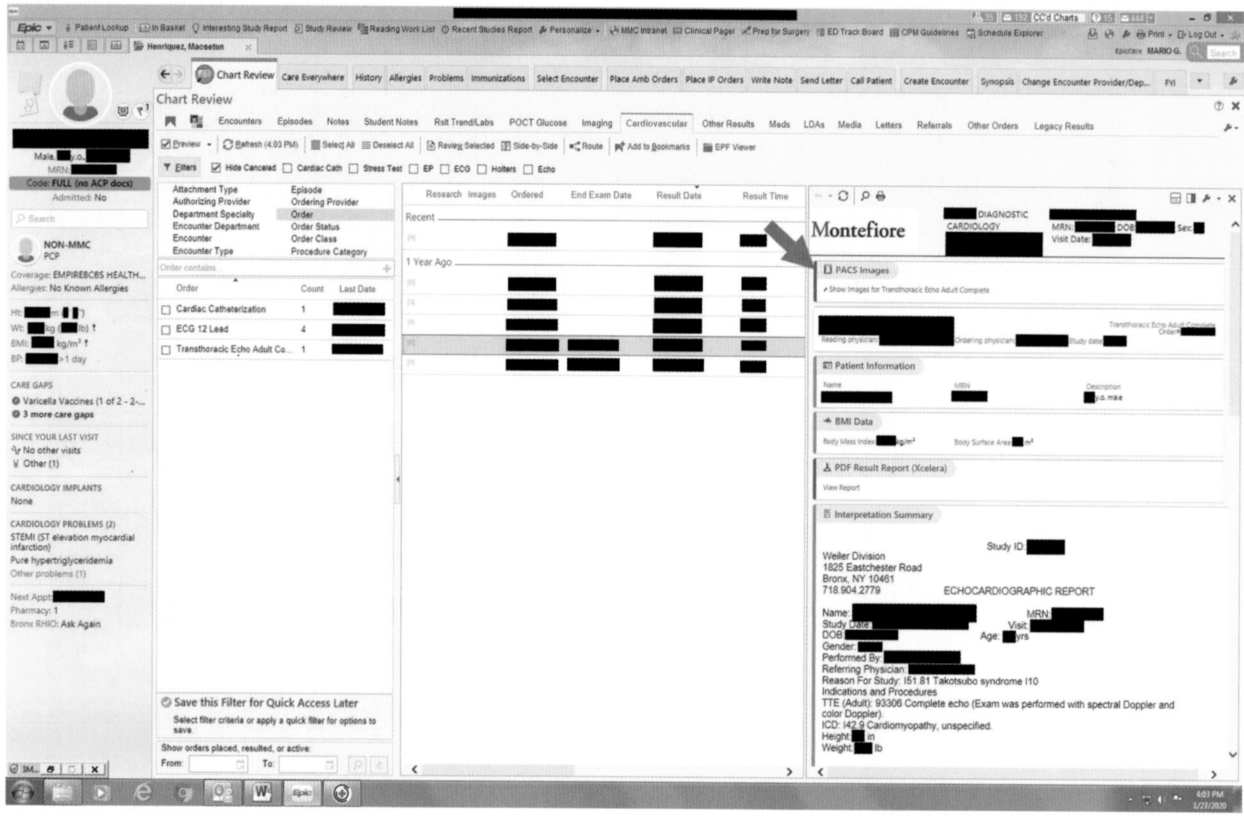

C

FIGURE 31.3 (*Continued*)

currently only restricted for patients with AKI or on hemodialysis.[40] However, a concern remains about gadolinium retention in brain nuclei of subjects exposed, even with preserved kidney function. Based on currently available data in the FDA Adverse Event Reporting System and medical literature, a causal association between these reported adverse events and gadolinium retention following GBCA exposure cannot be established.[41]

Limitations Associated With Noncontrast Cardiac Magnetic Resonance Imaging

There is no ionized radiation with CMR, instead CMR uses a powerful magnetic field, applying radiofrequency waves, and rapidly changing magnetic fields to create images. It is mandatory to perform safety screening of metallic objects as well as confirming MRI compatibility of medical devices and

TABLE 31.2 Effective Dose for Adults From Cardiovascular Imaging

Procedure	Modality	Average Effective Dose (mSv)	Values Reported in Literature (mSv)
Chest x-ray posteroanterior and lateral	X-ray	0.1	0.05-0.24
CT coronary calcium score	CT	3	1.0-12
CT coronary angiogram	CT	16	5.0-32
Cardiac rest-stress test (99mTc-sestamibi 1-day protocol)	PET	6.4	
Cardiac rest-stress test (99mTc-sestamibi 2-day protocol)	PET	13	
Cardiac rest-stress test (82Rb-chloride 2D PET)	PET	4	
Cardiac rest-stress test (13N-chloride 2D PET)	PET	4	
Cardiac (18F-FDG)	PET	14.1	

CT, computed tomography; 18F-FDG, F-18-fluorodeoxyglucose; PET, positron emission tomography.

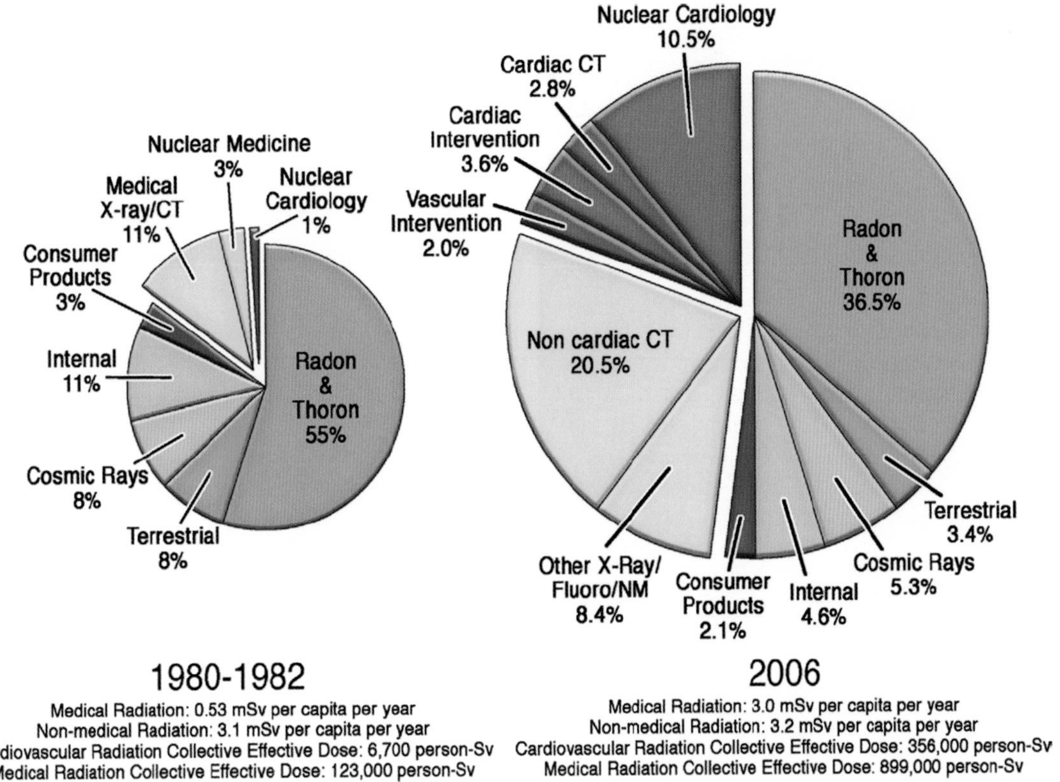

FIGURE 31.4 Radiation burden in United States except radiation therapy. Comparing 2006 to early 1980s, the overall collective effective dose of medical radiation increased over sevenfold. Especially in cardiovascular radiation, the collective effective dose increased over 53-fold. CT, computed tomography; Fluoro, fluoroscopy; NM, nuclear medicine. (Reprinted from Einstein AJ. Effects of radiation exposure from cardiac imaging: how good are the data? *J Am Coll Cardiol*. 2012;59(6):553-565. Copyright © 2012 American College of Cardiology Foundation. With permission.)

implants prior to CMR study. Potential adverse effects of MRI on implanted cardiac devices include radiofrequency-induced heating of the lead tips, pacing inhibition/dysfunction, asynchronous pacing with the possibility of induction of atrial or ventricular tachyarrhythmias, transient reed switch activation, change or loss of programmed data, and changes in capture threshold. In addition, it is important to prescreen subjects for claustrophobia and anxiety, because their related symptoms are the leading causes of inability to undergo or failure in completing CMR studies.

Imaging Artifacts and Misdiagnosis

Traditionally, TTE is one of the first-line imaging modalities used in the evaluation of cardiac function and disease owing to its low cost, portability, widespread availability, and lack of ionizing radiation.[42] It is important to keep in mind that ultrasound artifacts are common in TTE because of the physical properties of ultrasound and may lead to an inaccurate diagnosis. Artifacts include the appearance of structures that do not correspond with anatomic tissue structure (at least not at that location) or the creation of an image with clearly different characteristics than its corresponding anatomic structure (different size and shape) (**Figure 31.5A**, **Video 31.1**). It also includes failure to visualize structures (missing images) because of acoustic interference. TEE, CT, and MRI often reveal these common pitfalls and limitations of TTE and are, therefore, used as rescue modalities. It is important to highlight the fact that artifacts can also appear with both CT and MRI (**Figure 31.5B,C**). Despite the advantages of CVI, numerous categories of artifacts and suboptimal image quality are limitations that we may encounter with any imaging modality. These artifacts may be related to limited hardware or software functionalities, environmental factors, or the human body itself. The operator should understand the bases of these artifacts and be aware of a correct image interpretation for pursuing the final clinical diagnosis.

Hemodynamic Assessment

Accurate assessment of hemodynamics is the key to understanding the heart function. Invasive catheterization measures intracardiac pressure, O_2 saturation, and temperature directly from a desired location; therefore, catheter-based pressure measurements and cardiac output calculations are considered the most accurate assessment of cardiac hemodynamics. However, noninvasive estimation of hemodynamics is often used in daily practice for easy accessibility without procedure risk.

Echocardiography and CMR provide different approaches to measure hemodynamics. Noninvasive CVI tests are often done without sedation; therefore, their hemodynamic estimates are more indicative of "real life" conditions. Doppler

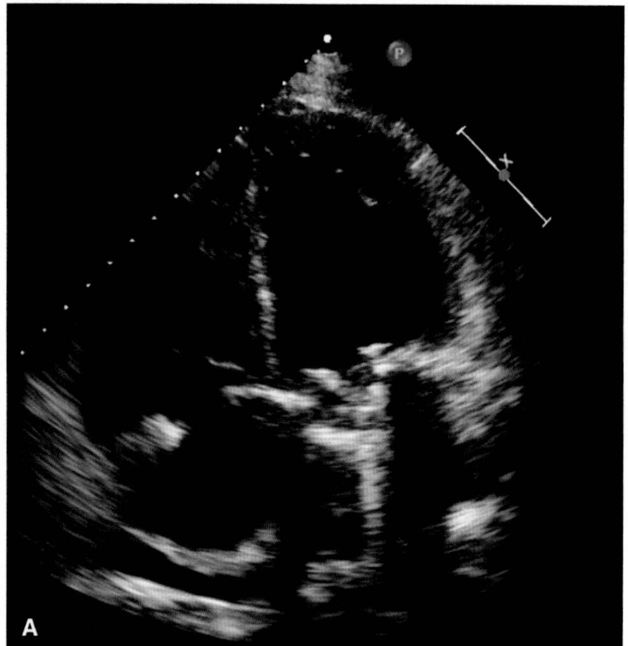

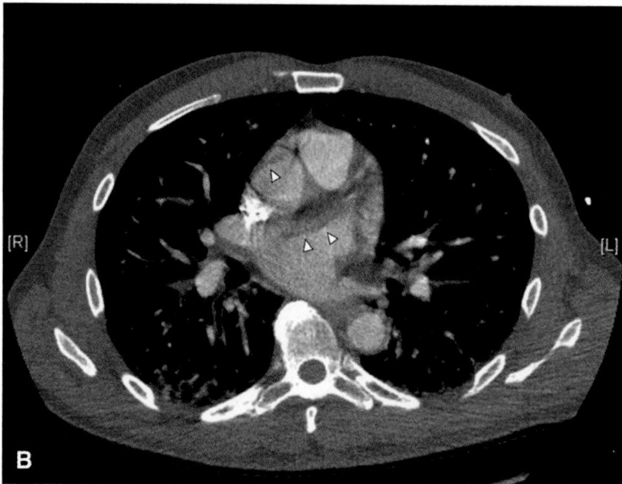

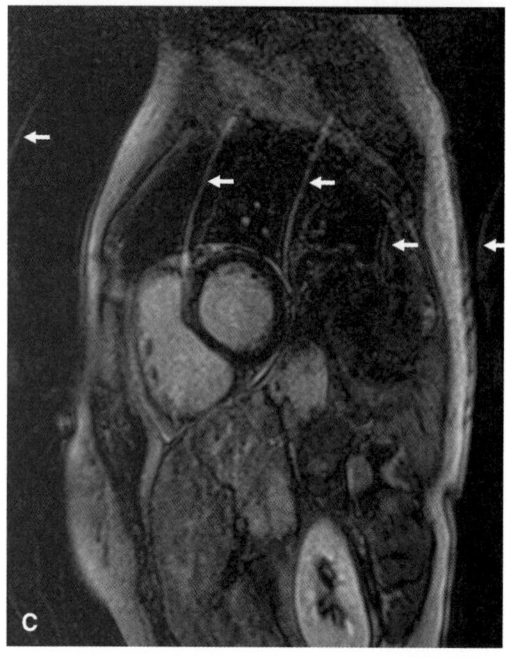

FIGURE 31.5 Artifacts of (**A**) echocardiography, complex reverberation (comet tail) artifact originating from a St. Jude mechanical mitral prosthesis; (**B**) cardiac CT, streak artifact produced by bolus of iodine contrast in the superior vena cava, motion artifact causing blurring of ascending aorta and left atrial walls (arrow heads); and (**C**) CMR, breathing motion artifacts (short arrows) on late gadolinium enhancement imaging. CT, computed tomography; CMR, cardiac magnetic resonance imaging.

echocardiography measures flow velocity, and it is commonly used to evaluate valvular stenosis and regurgitation, intracavitary flow acceleration, and function of prosthetic valves. Doppler echocardiography is considered a robust method because fine adjustments of ultrasound beam angle is rather easy. Combining Doppler echocardiography with 2D dimensional measurements, cardiac output can be calculated, and subsequently valve area as well as flow parameters such as systemic and pulmonic flow volumes (Qs, Qp). Because 2D calculations are based on geometric assumption that the structure is symmetrical, 3D volumetric measurements are more accurate.

CMR is highly reproducible and less operator dependent, and therefore, considered as a gold standard for volumetric assessment. CMR also allows accurate quantification of Qs and Qp using phase-contrast imaging technique. Combining volumetric and flow assessment, CMR provides accurate calculation of regurgitation volume of the valves as well as intracardiac shunt. In addition, phase-contrast imaging technique also provides maximum blood flow velocity; therefore, valvular stenosis or intracardiac obstruction can also be evaluated. However, adjustment of CMR imaging plane is done based on already acquired images, rather than adjusting imaging planes while observing images in real-time like echocardiography; it can be challenging to align the imaging plane with the axis of the blood flow, thus making it difficult to obtain the true maximum velocity.

Economic Considerations

New technologies allow the noninvasive description of cardiac function, perfusion, and metabolism in a polychrome, three-dimensional, often overwhelming fashion. According to many experts, the explosion of technological development in cardiology paradoxically has not brought a parallel increase in the quality of care but rather an exponential increase in cost.[43] The increased burden of cardiac imaging costs is driven by a number of factors, including high patient demand for the newest diagnostic tests, physicians eager to use the most effective technologies, and the financial pressure on providers who may boost utilization to help pay off investments in high-tech equipment. With accelerating health care costs and the desire to achieve the best value (health benefit for every dollar spent), there is growing recognition of the need for more explicit and transparent assessment of the value of health care.

Consideration of cost-effective utilization as an outcome presents special challenges.[44] Costs may vary widely by practice setting, locality, nationality, and over time. Biohazards and downstream long-term costs, such as radiation-induced oncogenesis, should also be considered. Moreover, individuals bear the burden of adverse health outcomes, yet costs typically are shared by society (eg, by families, employers, government, premium payers, fellow employees, taxpayers). Finally, attitudes differ among stakeholders about the extent to which cost should influence treatment decisions for individual patients and who should bear these costs. Consequently, resource utilization debates often become highly politicized, and significant conflicts of interest among individuals impaneled to formulate resource-based guidelines may be difficult to avoid.[44]

SPECIAL CONSIDERATIONS AND CONTRAINDICATIONS

Age Considerations

There are unique considerations of age-specific approaches to the use of specific noninvasive tests for evaluation of cardiac symptoms.[45] For example, noninvasive testing of CAD in older adults may present unique challenges owing to exercise limitations or uninterpretable ECGs. Furthermore, the pretest probability of CAD varies with age and affects interpretation of both positive and negative test results. Among patients with stable symptoms undergoing evaluation for CAD, important differences exist in patient presentation, test results, and prognostic capabilities of noninvasive testing based on the patient's age. In general, CCTA provides additional risk stratification information for patients younger than 65 years, whereas stress testing results are associated with improved risk stratification in patients age 65 years and older.

Pregnancy

In pregnant women, all organs exposed to diagnostic radiation as part of cardiovascular assessment are at risk for carcinogenesis. In the context of female individuals of child-bearing age, there is approximately a 2.8-fold increase in cancer risk for a 20-year-old woman undergoing CCTA compared to a 60-year-old woman.[46]

All the imaging techniques—echocardiography, CT, nuclear imaging, and CMR—are advised to be performed efficiently and only when clinically indicated to minimize fetal exposure risk under ALARA principle.[47] Echocardiography is considered safe for the fetus at all gestational ages and is, therefore, a reasonable initial imaging study in patients with signs or symptoms concerning for cardiac pathology. An understanding of both hemodynamic alterations and anatomic changes that occur during pregnancy is key to interpretation of echocardiograms in pregnant patients.[48] Radiation exposure to the fetus has stochastic and deterministic effects. Stochastic effect indicates the risk of the exposed fetus for carcinogenesis in childhood.[49] MRI is not associated with ionizing radiation exposure. Although use of MRI has not been shown to have any deleterious effects on the fetus, the safety of MRI during pregnancy has yet to be definitively established.

Both iodine and GBCAs are low-molecular weight water soluble extracellular substances that can cross the placenta by passive diffusion to be eventually excreted by the kidneys of the fetus. Their effects on the human embryo or fetus are incompletely understood.[39] Owing to the lack of sufficient evidence that contrast material poses no risk to the fetus, iodine and GBCAs may be given to the pregnant patient only if absolutely necessary.

FOLLOW-UP PATIENT CARE

AUC is a part of ACC's missions to promote standardized patient care to promote cost-effective health outcomes. It is often important to follow-up patients using noninvasive imaging test(s) so that physicians can determine appropriate timing for interventions. Most of the AUC for serial imaging have been developed by expert opinion, taking into consideration the natural history of chronic cardiac conditions. For example, degenerative mitral regurgitation (MR) is a slowly progressing disease where most patients remain asymptomatic for several years. Over time, the increase in preload induces left ventricular (LV) remodeling. Several outcome studies have demonstrated that asymptomatic patients with increased LV systolic dimensions have decreased survival even following mitral valve repair. Thus, serial imaging is appropriate in this setting.[50] In general, serial testing is most valuable in cardiac conditions in which (1) there is a poor correlation between development of symptoms and progression of disease and (2) therapeutic interventions guided by imaging findings have shown to improve outcomes.

RESEARCH AND FUTURE DIRECTIONS

Imaging has become an essential component for the diagnosis and management of patients with CVD. The increasing demand for cardiac imaging has started to exceed the number of available interpreting physicians, reducing the amount of time available to interpret and report studies.

Artificial intelligence (AI) and machine learning (ML) are rapidly gaining importance in medicine, including in the field of medical imaging, and are likely to fundamentally transform clinical practice in the coming years.[51] AI refers to the wider application of machines that perform tasks that are characteristic of human intelligence, for example, infer conclusions from deduction or induction, whereas ML is a more restricted form of computational processing, which uses mathematical modeling together with training data to learn how to make predictions. The most advanced ML techniques, also called deep learning (DL), are especially well suited for this purpose.

In echocardiography and CMR, manual tracing of endocardial borders has been widely used to quantify chamber volume, mass, and global and regional parameters of cardiac function. This process is not only time consuming, but also its accuracy and reproducibility are limited by inter- and intraobserver variabilities. DL has been on creating systems to process measurements in very short amount of time with high reproducibility. Fully automated analysis has recently become available to assess cardiac structure, function, and myocardial strain analysis in 8 ± 1 seconds/patient, without variability.[52-54] In CMR, active research areas in AI also include reduction of image acquisition and reconstruction time, improving spatial and temporal resolution, and analysis of perfusion, myocardial scar quantification, extracellular volume quantification, and T1 and T2 mapping.[51]

In cardiac CT, AI has been used for various applications. Several automated methods have been used to reduce radiation exposure, such as intelligent tube current modulation where the degree of radiation exposure is determined and changed according to tissue attenuation.[55] AI can also play a useful role in image localization, segmentation, and classification.[56] For example, DL may be used to automatically label segments in the coronary artery tree. ML in volumetric models of the coronary artery tree has been demonstrated to be able to identify reduced FFR.

In nuclear cardiology, DL has enabled automated quantitative analysis of MPI that can outperform visual analysis with higher reproducibility.[57] In addition, applying automated algorithms for motion correction leads to improved accuracy. Analysis of dynamic data (ECG-gated images) enables the detection of the endocardial and epicardial walls throughout the cardiac cycle and, thus, calculation of cardiac volumes, function, and wall thickening. The use of software standardizes the image display, analysis, and reporting, which eventually leads to lower inter- and intraobserver variation.

Other important clinical applications of AI are biomedical decision support systems' (DSS) technologies that translate important knowledge to clinical care by enhancing gathering of information and communication. The principal task of clinical DSS is to recognize important key features for the classification or prediction of a problem, and by combining these features, formulate an output that assists the clinician to make clinical decisions or a diagnosis.[57] The Imaging in Formation of Optimal Cardiovascular Utilization Strategies (FOCUS), an initiative of the ACC for the reduction of inappropriate use of imaging, has been adopted for implementing AUC for radionuclide imaging ordering.[58] Wider adoption of DSS in clinical practice will likely improve cost-effectiveness and contribute to reducing waste in US health care expenditure.

There are a number of important challenges associated with AI, such as patient and public support, transparency over the legal basis for health care data use, privacy preservation, and technical challenges related to accessing large-scale and expertly labeled data from health care systems not designed for Big Data analysis.[59] These challenges are substantial and only if addressed proactively will prevent slowing down of development and adoption of AI in cardiac imaging.

KEY POINTS

- ✔ In order to fully utilize multimodality approach and properly stratify risk assessment and management of patients with known or suspected CVD, it is critical for ordering physicians to be aware of the fundamentals for each of the imaging techniques, unique imaging challenges, and AUC.
- ✔ Because of technological advances and gained expertise, noninvasive imaging modalities have been gradually reducing the need for invasive diagnostic testing.
- ✔ Ordering appropriate imaging diagnostic tests can help in providing high-quality cardiovascular care, cost-efficiently guiding to an appropriate therapy, and evaluating the treatment effect. However, rarely appropriate imaging tests are still frequently ordered in the clinical setting.
- ✔ Optimal selection of an imaging test is based on pretest probability; this analysis requires frequent and appropriate adjustments given the constant evolution of technology and therapies, and their application to broader, lower risk populations.
- ✔ CVI tests must be used only when they contribute to improving clinical outcomes and values. Ordering physicians must balance the benefit of performing or not performing the test with the risks and drawbacks associated with none or alternative testing.
- ✔ Cardiac PACS system has been innovated to integrate multimodality cardiology images and reports. Now the cardiology PACS system is expanding beyond imaging, focusing on gathering relevant patient data to provide more data points to work with and help physicians make better decisions for patient care.
- ✔ AI is rapidly gaining importance in medicine. Fully automated analysis of cardiac structure and function analysis is now available, compensating the shortage of interpreting physicians and the amount of time spent to interpret and report studies. In addition, disease detection by AI can be sensitive with high accuracy and reproducibility; therefore, AI can be used as an aid in the interpretation of complex cases and can also act as a "second opinion."

VIDEO CAPTION

VIDEO 31.1 Artifact of echocardiography. Complex reverberation (comet tail) artifact originating from a St. Jude mechanical mitral prosthesis.

REFERENCES

1. Benjamin EJ, Muntner P, Alonso A, et al. Heart disease and stroke statistics-2019 update: a report from the American Heart Association. *Circulation.* 2019;139:e257-e280.
2. Diamond G, Forrester J. Analysis of probability as an aid in the clinical diagnosis of coronary-artery disease. *N Engl J Med.* 1978;299:690-694.
3. Di Carli MF, Gupta A. Estimating pre-test probability of coronary artery disease: battle of the scores in an evolving CAD landscape. *JACC Cardiovasc Imaging.* 2019;12:1401-1404.
4. Farook N, Cochon L, Bode AD, et al. HEART score and stress test emergency department Bayesian decision scheme: results from the acute care diagnostic collaboration. *J Emerg Med.* 2018;54(2):147-155.
5. Trevethan R. Sensitivity, specificity, and predictive values: foundations, pliabilities, and pitfalls in research and practice. *Front Public Health.* 2017;5:307.
6. Pewsner D, Battaglia M, Minder C, et al. Ruling a diagnosis in or out with "SpPIn" and "SnNOut": a note of caution. *Br Med J.* 2004;329:209-213.
7. Berwick DM, Hackbarth AD. Eliminating waste in US health care. *JAMA.* 2012;307:1513-1516.
8. Fonseca R, Negishi K, Otahal P, et al. Temporal changes in appropriateness of cardiac imaging. *J Am Coll Cardiol.* 2015;65:763-773.
9. Bhatia RS, Ivers NM, Yin XC, et al. Improving the appropriate use of transthoracic echocardiography: the echo WISELY trial. *J Am Coll Cardiol.* 2017;70:1135-1144.
10. Lang RM, Badano LP, Mor-Avi V, et al. Recommendations for cardiac chamber quantification by echocardiography in adults: an update from the American Society of Echocardiography and the European Association of Cardiovascular Imaging. *Eur Heart J Cardiovasc Imaging.* 2015;16:233-271.
11. Zoghbi WA, Adams D, Bonow RO, et al. Recommendations for noninvasive evaluation of native valvular regurgitation: a report from the American Society of Echocardiography developed in collaboration with the Society for Cardiovascular Magnetic Resonance. *J Am Soc Echocardiogr.* 2017;30:303-371.
12. Dulgheru R, Pibarot P, Sengupta PP, et al. Multimodality imaging strategies for the assessment of aortic stenosis: viewpoint of the heart valve clinic international database (HAVEC) group. *Circ Cardiovasc Imaging.* 2016;9:e004352.
13. Suchβ D, Symersky P, Tanis W, et al. Multimodality imaging assessment of prosthetic heart valves. *Circ Cardiovasc Imaging.* 2015;8:e003703.
14. Klein AL, Abbara S, Agler DA, et al. American Society of Echocardiography clinical recommendations for multimodality cardiovascular imaging of patients with pericardial disease: endorsed by the Society for Cardiovascular Magnetic Resonance and Society of Cardiovascular Computed Tomography. *J Am Soc Echocardiogr.* 2013;26:965-1012.
15. Greenland P, Blaha MJ, Budoff MJ, et al. Coronary calcium score and cardiovascular risk. *J Am Coll Cardiol.* 2018;72:434-447.
16. Lowenstern A, Alexander KP, Hill CL, et al. Age-related differences in the noninvasive evaluation for possible coronary artery disease: insights from the prospective multicenter imaging study for evaluation of chest pain (PROMISE) trial. *JAMA Cardiol.* 2020;5(2):193-201.
17. Nagel E, Greenwood JP, McCann GP, et al. Magnetic resonance perfusion or fractional flow reserve in coronary disease. *N Engl J Med.* 2019;380:2418-2428.
18. Baliyan V, Verdini D, Meyersohn NM. Noninvasive aortic imaging. *Cardiovasc Diagn Ther.* 2018;8:S3-S18.
19. Douglas PS, Chen J, Gillam L, et al. Achieving quality in cardiovascular imaging II. Proceedings from the second American College of Cardiology-Duke University Medical Center Think Tank on quality in cardiovascular imaging. *JACC Cardiovasc Imaging.* 2009;2:231-240.
20. Douglas PS, Daubert MA. Diagnostic accuracy of noninvasive testing: necessary but insufficient. *Circ Cardiovasc Imaging.* 2015;8(3):e003138.
21. Knuuti J, Bengel F, Bax JJ, et al. Risks and benefits of cardiac imaging: an analysis of risks related to imaging for coronary artery disease. *Eur Heart J.* 2014;35:633-638.
22. Shaw LJ, Blankstein R, Jacobs JE, et al. Defining quality in cardiovascular imaging: a scientific statement from the American Heart Association. *Circ Cardiovasc Imaging.* 2017;10:1-16.
23. Otero HJ, Rybicki FJ, Greenberg D, et al. Cost-effective diagnostic cardiovascular imaging: when does it provide good value for the money? *Int J Cardiovasc Imaging.* 2010;26:605-612.
24. Lamberti S. CVIS, cardiology PACS widening image access. *Health Imaging.* Published March 11, 2019. https://www.healthimaging.com/topics/cardiovascular-imaging/cvis-cardiology-pacs-widening-image-access
25. Digital Imaging and Communications in Medicine. About DICOM: overview. https://www.dicomstandard.org/about/
26. The Intersocietal Accreditation Commission. IAC Standards and Guidelines for Adult Echocardiography Accreditation. Revised April 27, 2018. https://www.intersocietal.org/echo/standards/IACAdultEchocardiographyStandards2017.pdf
27. Intersocietal Accreditation Commission. The IAC Standards and Guidelines for Nuclear/PET Accreditation. Published September 15, 2016. https://www.intersocietal.org/nuclear/standards/IACNuclearPETStandards2016.pdf May 15, 2020
28. Intersocietal Accreditation Commission. The IAC Standards and Guidelines for MRI Accreditation. 2017. https://www.intersocietal.org/mri/standards/IACMRIStandards2017.pdf
29. Intersocietal Accreditation Commission. The IAC Standards and Guidelines for CT Accreditation. 2018. https://www.intersocietal.org/ct/standards/IACCTStandards2018.pdf
30. Mettler FA, Huda W, Yoshizumi TT, et al. Effective doses in radiology and diagnostic nuclear medicine: a catalog. *Radiology.* 2008;248:254-263.
31. Einstein AJ, Berman DS, Min JK, et al. Patient-centered imaging: shared decision making for cardiac imaging procedures with exposure to ionizing radiation. *J Am Coll Cardiol.* 2014;63:1480-1489.
32. Chen J, Einstein AJ, Fazel R, et al. Cumulative exposure to ionizing radiation from diagnostic and therapeutic cardiac imaging procedures: a population-based analysis. *J Am Coll Cardiol.* 2010;56:702-711.
33. Einstein AJ, Weiner SD, Bernheim A, et al. Multiple testing, cumulative radiation dose, and clinical indications in patients undergoing myocardial perfusion imaging. *JAMA.* 2010;304:2137-2144.
34. U.S. Food & Drug Administration. Initiative to reduce unnecessary radiation exposure from medical imaging. Accessed April 29, 2019. https://www.fda.gov/radiation-emitting-products/radiation-safety/initiative-reduce-unnecessary-radiation-exposure-medical-imaging
35. Smith-Bindman R, Wang Y, Chu P, et al. International variation in radiation dose for computed tomography examinations: prospective cohort study. *BMJ.* 2019;364:k4931.
36. Ansell G. A national survey of radiological complications: interim report. *Clin Radiol.* 1968;19:175-191.
37. Luk L, Steinman J, Newhouse JH. Intravenous contrast-induced nephropathy—The rise and fall of a threatening idea. *Adv Chronic Kidney Dis.* 2017;24:169-175.
38. Do C. Intravenous contrast: friend or foe? A review on contrast-induced nephropathy. *Adv Chronic Kidney Dis.* 2017;24:147-149.
39. ACR Committee on Drugs and Contrast Media. ACR Manual on Contrast Media. vol. 105. 2018. https://www.acr.org/Clinical-Resources/Contrast-Manual
40. Schieda N, Blaichman JI, Costa AF, et al. Gadolinium-based contrast agents in kidney disease: comprehensive review and clinical practice guideline issued by the Canadian association of radiologists. *Can Assoc Radiol J.* 2018;69:136-150.

41. US Food & Drug Administration. FDA drug safety communication: FDA warns that gadolinium-based contrast agents (GBCAs) are retained in the body; requires new class warnings. Updated May 16, 2018. https://www.fda.gov/drugs/drug-safety-and-availability/fda-drug-safety-communication-fda-warns-gadolinium-based-contrast-agents-gbcas-are-retained-body
42. Malik SB, Chen N, Parker RA, et al. Transthoracic echocardiography: pitfalls and limitations as delineated at cardiac CT and MR imaging. *Radiographics.* 2017;37:383-406.
43. Picano E. Economic and biological costs of cardiac imaging. *Cardiovasc Ultrasound.* 2005;3:13.
44. Anderson JL, Heidenreich PA, Barnett PG, et al. ACC/AHA statement on cost/value methodology in clinical practice guidelines and performance measures: a report of the American college of cardiology/American heart association task force on performance measures and task force on practice guidelines. *Circulation.* 2014;129:2329-2345.
45. Yingchoncharoen T, Agarwal S, Popović ZB, et al. Normal ranges of left ventricular strain: a meta-analysis. *J Am Soc Echocardiogr.* 2013;26:185-191.
46. Smith-Bindman R, Lipson L, Marcus R, et al. Radiation dose associated with common computed tomography examinations and the associated lifetime attributable risk of cancer. *Arch Intern Med.* 2009;169:2078-2086.
47. Committee on Obstetric Practice. Committee opinion No. 723: guidelines for diagnostic imaging during pregnancy and lactation. *Obstet Gynecol.* 2017;130:e210-216.
48. Ain DL, Narula J, Sengupta PP. Cardiovascular imaging and diagnostic procedures in pregnancy. *Cardiol Clin.* 2012;30:331-341.
49. Litmanovich DE, Tack D, Lee KS, et al. Cardiothoracic imaging in the pregnant patient. *J Thorac Imaging.* 2014;29:38-49.
50. Doherty JU, Kort S, Mehran R, et al. ACC/AATS/AHA/ASE/ASNC/HRS/SCAI/SCCT/SCMR/STS 2017 appropriate use criteria for multimodality imaging in valvular heart disease. *J Am Coll Cardiol.* 2017;70:1647-1672.
51. Leiner T, Rueckert D, Suinesiaputra A, et al. Machine learning in cardiovascular magnetic resonance: basic concepts and applications. *J Cardiovasc Magn Reson.* 2019;21:61.
52. Zhang J, Gajjala S, Agrawal P, et al. Fully automated echocardiogram interpretation in clinical practice. *Circulation.* 2018;138:1623-1635.
53. Knackstedt C, Bekkers SC, Schummers G, et al. Fully automated versus standard tracking of left ventricular ejection fraction and longitudinal strain the FAST-EFs multicenter study. *J Am Coll Cardiol.* 2015;66:1456-1466.
54. Bai W, Sinclair M, Tarroni G, et al. Automated cardiovascular magnetic resonance image analysis with fully convolutional networks. *J Cardiovasc Magn Reson.* 2018;20:65.
55. Alibek S, Brand M, Suess C, et al. Dose reduction in pediatric computed tomography with automated exposure control. *Acad Radiol.* 2011;18:690-693.
56. Litjens G, Ciompi F, Wolterink JM, et al. State-of-the-art deep learning in cardiovascular image analysis. *JACC Cardiovasc Imaging.* 2019;12:1549-1565.
57. Massalha S, Clarkin O, Thornhill R, et al. Decision support tools, systems, and artificial intelligence in cardiac imaging. *Can J Cardiol.* 2018;34:827-838.
58. Saifi S, Taylor AJ, Allen J, et al. The use of a learning community and online evaluation of utilization for spect myocardial perfusion imaging. *JACC Cardiovasc Imaging.* 2013;6:823-829.
59. Petersen SE, Abdulkareem M, Leiner T. Artificial intelligence will transform cardiac imaging—opportunities and challenges. *Front Cardiovasc Med.* 2019;6:133.

CHAPTER 32

CHEST RADIOGRAPHY

Jonathan Alis and Linda B. Haramati

INTRODUCTION

The chest radiograph is one of the most frequently performed imaging tests. Its wide availability, relative low cost, and minimal radiation exposure (0.01-0.02 mSv) result in it being the most common initial imaging test in a patient presenting with chest pain or dyspnea with a suspected cardiac origin. More sensitive modalities such as echocardiogram, computed tomography (CT) and magnetic resonance imaging (MRI) have changed the role of the radiograph to a gateway to further appropriate diagnostic imaging. Guidelines almost exclusively recommend chest radiography as the initial imaging test in a symptomatic patient, while acknowledging that radiographs cannot exclude cardiovascular disease.[1] This chapter focuses on the chest radiograph's dual roles in either supporting a cardiac diagnosis and providing information regarding cardiac function or identifying alternative pathology as the cause of the patient's symptoms.

INDICATIONS

The American College of Radiology's appropriateness criteria recommend chest radiography in patients with acute chest pain from suspected acute coronary syndrome, aortic dissection, or pulmonary embolism. Similarly, in patients with suspected new-onset or unstable heart failure or dyspnea of suspected cardiac origin, a chest radiograph is considered appropriate as initial imaging.[1]

ANATOMIC CONSIDERATIONS

General Anatomy

The right lung has three lobes, and is slightly larger compared to the two-lobed left lung. The right major fissure divides the right upper and middle lobes from the lower lobe, and the left major fissure divides the left upper lobe from the left lower lobe. Typically, the major fissures are only seen on lateral radiographs. The right lung has a minor fissure that separates the right middle lobe from the right upper lobe, and can be seen on a frontal radiograph as a horizontal linear opacity at the level of the fourth anterior rib. The tracheal air column is seen both on the frontal and lateral radiographs. The right- and left-sided bronchi vary by laterality and are visible centrally on a frontal chest radiograph.

The hila comprise a composite of pulmonary arteries, veins, central bronchi, and lymph nodes, with the radiographic appearance predominantly attributed to the pulmonary arteries and superior pulmonary veins. The right and left hila differ depending on pulmonary artery anatomy, which varies by laterality, and the relationship between the vasculature and bronchi. The left hilum is normally cephalad compared to the right hilum, and should never be inferior, relative to the right. On a lateral radiograph, the right pulmonary artery courses anterior to the bronchus, which is eparterial, whereas the left pulmonary artery arches over the hyparterial left main bronchus and courses posteriorly.

On the frontal view, the right mediastinal border is created by, from superior to inferior, the superior vena cava (SVC), paratracheal stripe, azygous vein, right atrium, and the inferior vena cava (IVC). The left mediastinal border is created by, from superior to inferior, the left subclavian vein, aortic arch and descending aorta, pulmonary artery, left atrial appendage (when enlarged), and the left ventricle. On the lateral radiograph, the mediastinal border is formed anteriorly, from superior to inferior, by the ascending aorta, pulmonary artery, and right ventricle; and posteriorly, aortic arch, descending aorta, left atrium, left ventricle, and IVC[2] (**Figure 32.1**).

Cardiac Position/Visceroatrial Situs

The heart is normally positioned to the left of the sternum, with the cardiac apex pointing toward the left, termed *levocardia*. Malpositioning of the heart can be either dextrocardia (within the right hemithorax) or mesocardia (midline), and can be either primary or secondary. Primary malpositioning is a congenital cardiac anomaly affecting both the positioning and the axis, often associated with other congenital cardiac anomalies. Extracardiac causes, such as hypoplastic lung, or bony abnormalities, such as scoliosis or pectus excavatum, can secondarily impact cardiac position, termed *dextroposition* or *mesoposition*. In dextrocardia, the position of the heart and the direction of the cardiac apex do not correspond to the expected radiographic anatomy.[3] The Van Praagh segmental approach, used in classifying congenital heart disease, takes into account the visceroatrial situs, ventricular looping, and great arteries' position.[3] The pulmonary artery and bronchial anatomy on chest radiographs provide information regarding visceroatrial situs, which, in combination with cardiac position, can suggest the possibility of congenital heart disease.[4,5] Abdominal situs is often described by the position of the stomach bubble on the radiograph. The severity and incidence of congenital heart

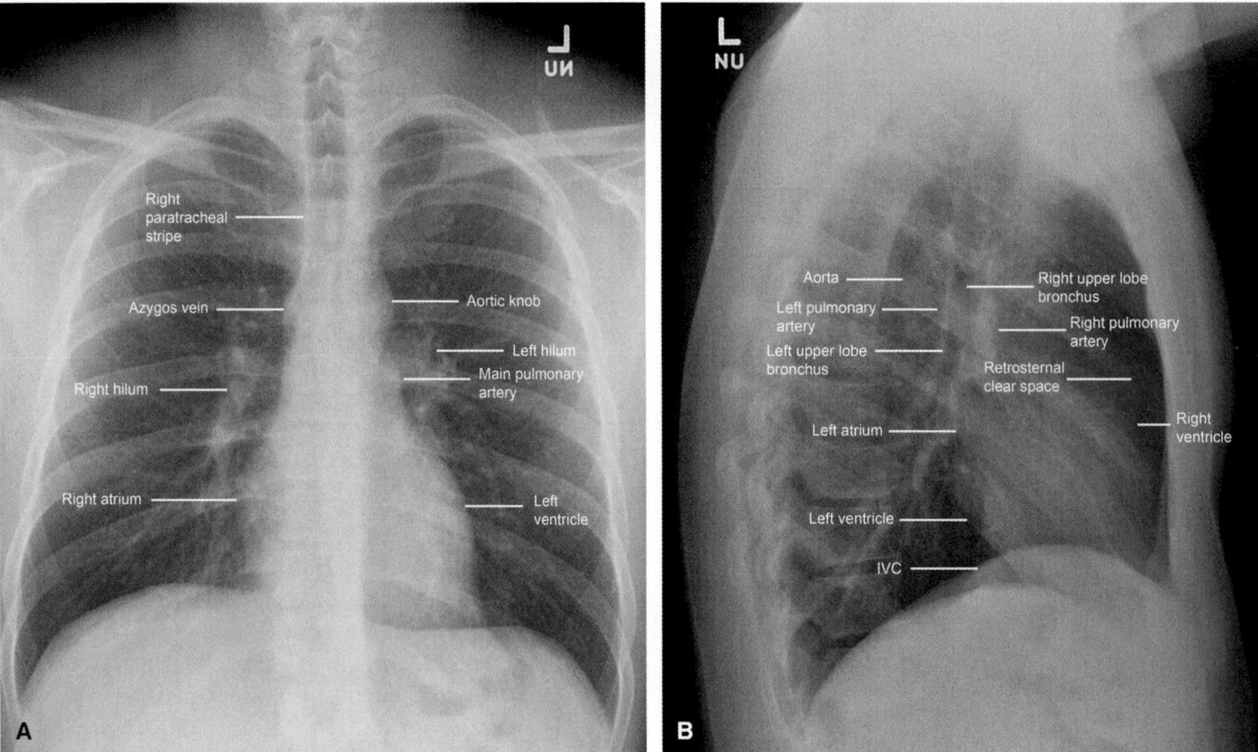

FIGURE 32.1 Mediastinal contours are demonstrated in the frontal posteroanterior (PA) radiograph **(A)** and the lateral radiograph **(B)**. IVC, inferior vena cava.

disease is associated with situs and cardiac position. Situs solitus with levocardia, the normal configuration, has a congenital heart disease incidence of less than 1% (excluding bicuspid aortic valve), whereas situs inversus with dextrocardia has a 3% to 5% incidence. Situs solitus with dextrocardia and situs inversus with levocardia have a congenital heart disease incidence greater than 90%.[4]

Aortic Arch

The aortic knob corresponds to the distal most aspect of the aortic arch as it courses downward to become the descending aorta. At this point, the arch is tangential to the x-ray beam on the frontal view, projecting as a circle that is obscured on the right side by the mediastinum and delineated along its left border by the lucent lung.[6]

The normal arch courses to the left and displaces the trachea to the right, with the aortic knob positioned on the left side of the mediastinum. In a right aortic arch, the aortic knob is seen in the right paratracheal region, and there is displacement of the trachea to the left (**Figure 32.2**). There are two types of right aortic arch, which can be determined by the branching pattern of the great vessels.[7,8] The right arch with mirror image branching is highly associated with congenital heart disease. In contrast, a right arch with an aberrant left subclavian artery is usually an incidental and benign finding, although the left-sided ligamentum arteriosum typically results in a loose vascular ring.

Valves

In a patient with limited clinical history, understanding cardiac implants and support devices and determining valvular position is extremely important. Using the lateral radiograph, a line is drawn from the hilum to the apex, parallel to the long axis of the heart. The aortic valve is above this line and the mitral valve below. On a frontal radiograph, an imaginary line will be drawn from the right cardiophrenic angle to the inferior of left hilum, perpendicular to the long axis of the heart. The aortic valve is above the line and the mitral valve below. On both views, the pulmonic valve is the most superior valve, and, on the lateral radiograph, the tricuspid is the most anterior and inferior on the frontal radiograph[9] (**Figure 32.3 A,B**). Utilizing this technique on supine anteroposterior (AP) radiographs can be inaccurate, and other methods are recommended. The valve orifice method can be utilized, where an aortic valve will be in profile on the frontal radiograph (visualized as a line) while the mitral will be en face (visualize as the whole ring). The perceived direction of flow is useful, with aortic valves being toward the arch and mitral valves toward the apex.[10] The radiographic appearance of prosthetic valves is beyond the scope of this chapter. However, there are multiple online resources with pictorial demonstrations of the appearance of mechanic, bioprosthetic, and transcatheter valves.[11]

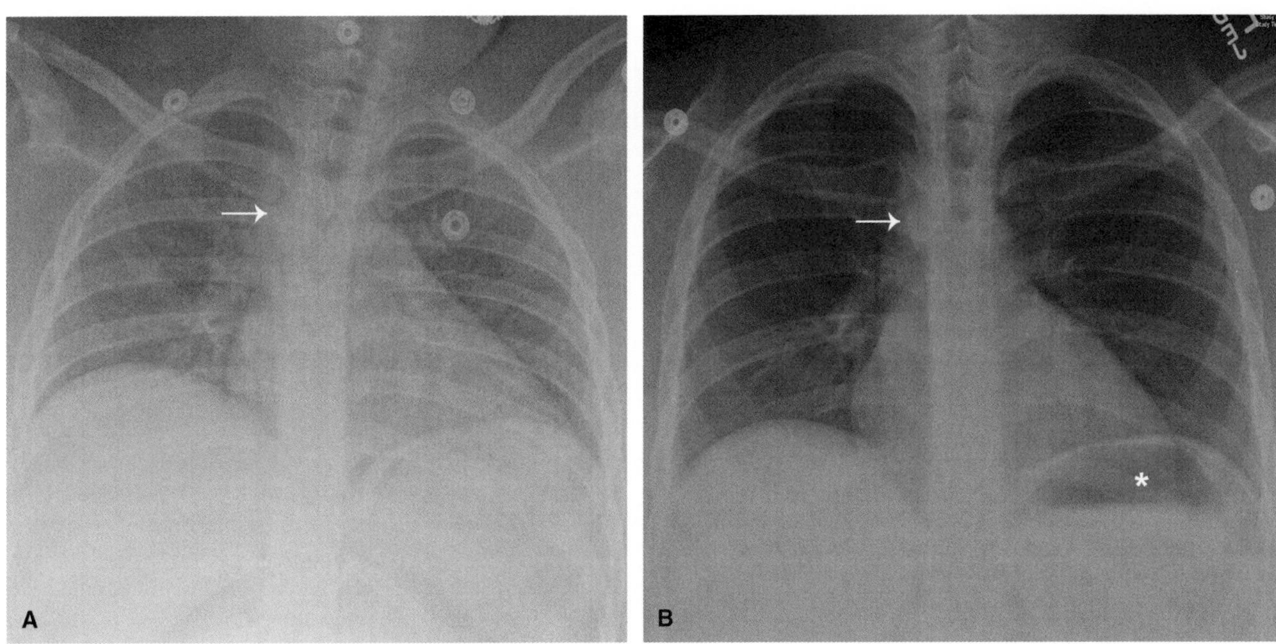

FIGURE 32.2 Differences in techniques can be appreciated in this anteroposterior (AP) portable radiograph taken with poor inspiratory effort **(A)** and posteroanterior (PA) radiograph on the same patient in full inspiration a few hours later **(B)**. The heart is magnified in **(A)** and the low lung volumes appear denser with crowding of the vessels, which can be mistaken for pulmonary edema. The stomach bubble is appreciated on the erect radiograph (asterisk). Incidentally noted is a right aortic arch (white arrows).

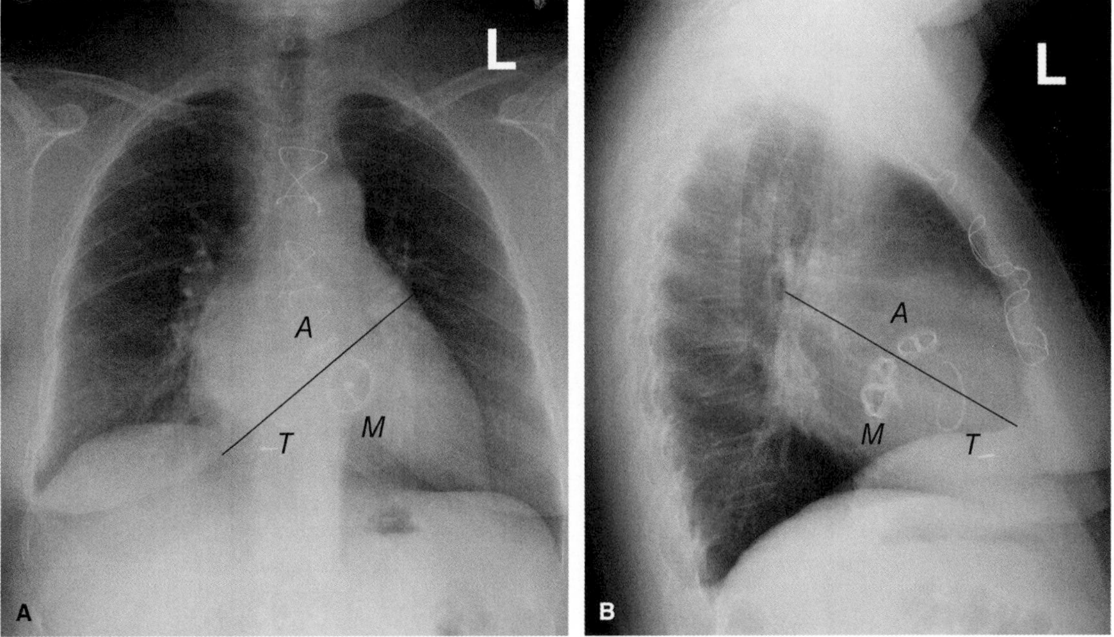

FIGURE 32.3 **(A)** On a frontal radiograph, an imaginary line is drawn from the right cardiophrenic angle to the inferior of left hilum, perpendicular to the long axis of the heart. **(B)** On the lateral radiograph, a line is drawn from the hilum to the apex, parallel to the long axis of the heart. The aortic valve (*A*) is above the line and the mitral valve (*M*) below on both views. The tricuspid valve (*T*) is anteriorly and inferiorly positioned. The pulmonic valve is not seen on this radiograph, and is the most superior positioned valve.

SECTION 2

FUNDAMENTALS OF RADIOGRAPHY

Approach to Interpreting Radiographs

There are varied approaches to interpreting chest radiographs, and each individual should determine what suits his/her needs. The common denominator for accurate interpretation is a systematic approach. One should also be vigilant to avoid a common error in diagnostic radiology termed *satisfaction of search*, defined by prematurely ceasing to search for abnormalities once an abnormality has been identified.[12] Following a systematic interpretation scheme ensures that all aspects of the radiograph have been interpreted. The clinical value achieved from comparison with old studies cannot be overemphasized. When interpreting a chest radiograph from a cardiac standpoint, the findings have a dual purpose. One should not only attempt to identify findings associated with cardiac disease but, in addition, noncardiac thoracic pathology, if identified, may explain the patient's symptoms.

Radiographic Technique

The standard views in chest radiography are posteroanterior (PA), lateral, and AP radiographs. A PA radiograph is obtained with the patient standing up against the detector with the x-ray tube posterior to the patient, at a 6-foot distance, by convention; such that the patient is exposed to the x-ray beam, posterior to anterior. The scapulae are cleared from the lung field by the patient placing their hands on their iliac crests and shoulders rotated forward. The patient's chin should be raised to ensure the apices are not obscured. The radiograph is obtained while the patient is in breath hold at full inspiration, permitting visualization of the 10th posterior rib above the diaphragm. The patient is positioned so that there is no rotation, with the medial ends of the clavicles equidistant from spinous processes. The entire lungs should be demonstrated including the costophrenic angles and apices. There should be adequate exposure so that the thoracic spine and intervertebral disc spaces are visualized in the retrocardiac region. For a lateral radiograph, the patient is erect, seating or standing, with the left side touching the detector. Careful attention is made to ensure the humeri and the chin are excluded from the field of view. Correct positioning is determined by the sternum being seen in profile, the costophrenic angles included, the intervertebral foramina open, and the bilateral anterior ribs and bilateral posterior ribs are nearly superimposed. Adequate exposure should demonstrate the hemidiaphragms clearly, and the ribs should be visualized through the heart and lung markings. When a patient is unable to perform a PA radiograph, a portable radiograph can be obtained. This is particularly useful for patients who are bed bound and/or immobile, because this can be performed supine or semi-recumbent. Typically, these are performed in an AP projection, with the detector positioned behind the patient's back and the x-ray tube anterior to the patient. Therefore, the x-ray beam travels from anterior to posterior, usually at a distance of 3 feet.[13,14]

There are additional chest radiographic views, which were previously used more commonly, but still have a role in troubleshooting. The apical lordotic view is used to visualize the lung apices by projecting the clavicles above the lungs, by either having the patient lean back or angling the x-ray tube cranially if the patient is upright. The lateral decubitus view is useful for evaluation of layering pleural effusion and exclusion of loculation, as well as being useful for demonstration of a small pneumothorax in the nondependent lung. In this view, the patient lies on their side and the radiograph is taken using a horizontal beam.[13]

CLINICAL APPLICATIONS

Pulmonary Vasculature

Congestive Heart Failure

There is extensive literature that supports the use of chest radiography in the diagnosis of congestive heart failure (CHF) in the emergency setting.[15] Chest radiographic findings have been shown to correlate with pulmonary wedge pressures. However, radiographic findings may lag behind the clinical onset of heart failure. Conversely, the radiographic findings can persist after normalization of the pulmonary wedge pressure.[16]

In the upright position, the lower lungs normally have increased blood flow relative to the upper, mainly due to gravity. This can be appreciated on erect radiographs as increased diameter and number of vessels in the inferior lungs. To compensate for varied cardiac output, the pulmonary vascular bed has the capability to recruit when the cardiac output is increased.[17] In acute left-heart failure, there is progressive increase of the pulmonary venous pressure. As a result of increased flow or pressure to the pulmonary vasculature, vascular recruitment takes place with concomitant increase in the diameter and number of vessels in the upper aspects of the lungs. This is termed *pulmonary vascular redistribution*, which is the earliest sign of physiologic changes that can be seen with pulmonary wedge pressure of greater than 12 mm Hg.

During progression of the increasing flow/pressure to 17 to 20 mm Hg, the plasma oncotic pressure will be overcome, resulting in fluid leaking out of the vessels into the interstitium. This is the first phase of pulmonary edema, termed *interstitial edema*. The radiographic correlation for interstitial edema is thickening of the interlobular septa, which is called *Kerley B lines*. Kerley B lines can be seen on the frontal radiograph as peripheral thin (1-2 mm), 1- to 2-cm long, horizontal lines that abut the pleura. Edema involving other pulmonary interstitial structures such as the peribronchovascular and subpleural interstitium results in the chest radiographic findings of peribronchial cuffing and thickening of the fissures. Small pleural effusions are often present[18] (**Figure 32.4A**).

When the pulmonary wedge pressure exceeds 25 mm Hg, the fluid buildup in the interstitium exceeds the capabilities of lymphatic drainage, resulting in fluid seeping into the alveolar spaces, causing *alveolar edema*. During alveolar edema, there is impairment in gas exchange resulting in hypoxia and dyspnea. Radiographically, alveolar edema appears as nodular opacities that coalesce to form patchy, fluffy consolidations in a bilateral, central distribution with sparing of the periphery (**Figure 32.4 B**).

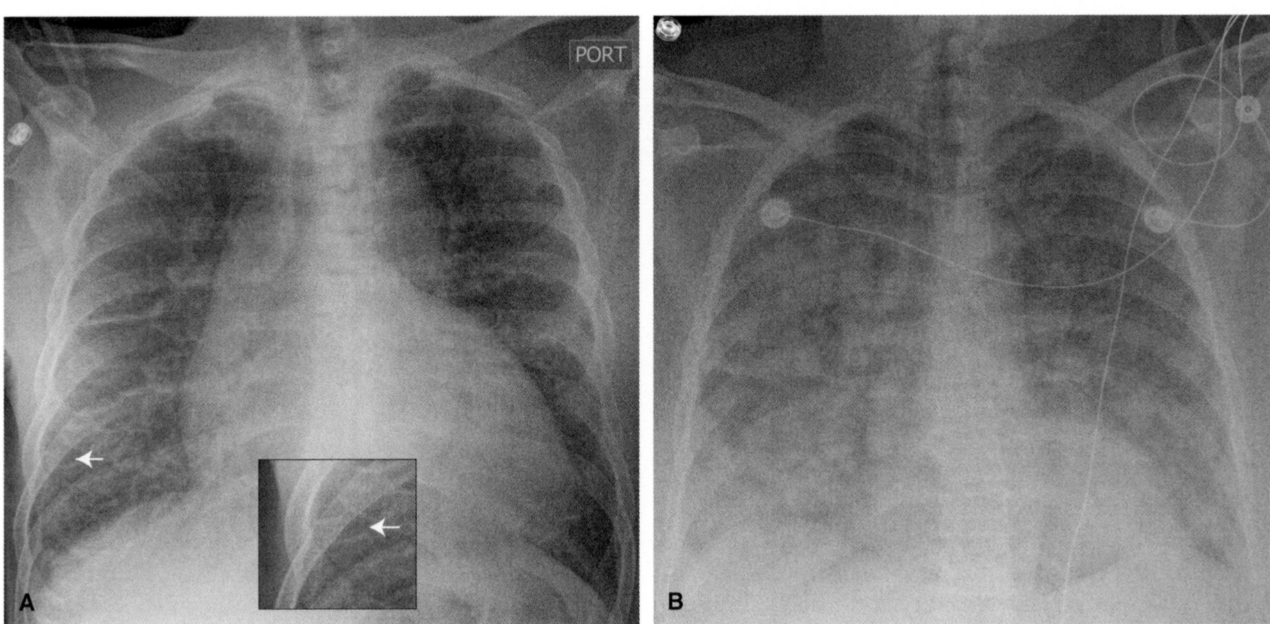

FIGURE 32.4 **(A)** Frontal radiograph demonstrating interstitial edema. Thickening of the interlobular septa called Kerley B lines, can be seen as peripheral thin (1-2 mm), 1- to 2-cm long, horizontal lines that abut the pleura (white arrow; magnified view). **(B)** Frontal radiograph demonstrating alveolar edema. Patchy, fluffy consolidations in a bilateral, central distribution can be seen.

These findings are often accompanied by moderate-sized pleural effusions, which are typically bilateral but can sometimes be unilateral, commonly on the right. Evaluation for pleural effusions is more sensitive on the lateral radiograph because blunting of the posterior costophrenic angle requires less than 75 mL pleural fluid, whereas blunting of the lateral costophrenic angles on the front radiographs requires at least 250 mL of pleural fluid.[18]

When pulmonary wedge pressures are chronically elevated, the lymphatic vessels expand significantly, increasing their drainage capabilities, and the lungs become more resistant to pulmonary edema. Conversely, in cases of sudden high pressures, such as from hypertensive urgency, acute myocardial infarction, or new-onset tachyarrhythmia, flash pulmonary edema can occur. During flash pulmonary edema, interstitial edema is followed in quick succession by alveolar edema.[19]

Although left-heart failure and fluid overload are hard to differentiate radiographically,[16] certain findings can help differentiate between cardiogenic and noncardiogenic causes of pulmonary edema, such as seen in acute respiratory distress syndrome (ARDS).[19-21] Clinical history and clinical presentation are obviously crucial. However, radiographic findings can provide additional information. In ARDS, the alveolar-capillary barrier is compromised, resulting in an immediate alveolar edema phase. Therefore, *interstitial edema*, with septal and peribronchovascular thickening, is more suggestive of cardiogenic edema. ARDS is also less likely to have pleural effusions and more likely to have a peripheral distribution of alveolar edema. Indirect signs such as increased volume prominence of the vascular pedicle and azygos vein, pulmonary vascular redistribution, and cardiomegaly are suggestive of cardiogenic edema.[20,21] Of note, absence of cardiomegaly can be seen in diastolic dysfunction and acute myocardial infarction.

Although pulmonary edema is usually bilateral and symmetric, there are various factors that can result in a nonuniform distribution. Concomitant parenchymal disease can result, with edema occurring predominantly within the normal parenchyma. Patients who are bed bound or nonmobile will often be recumbent on a favored side, resulting in edema occurring on the dependent side owing to gravity. In addition, underlying hemodynamic factors can cause asymmetric pulmonary edema. Classically, right upper lobe edema is associated with mitral regurgitation due to the regurgitant jet pointing toward the right upper pulmonary vein.

Pulmonary Hypertension

Classic radiographic findings of pulmonary hypertension include increased caliber of the central pulmonary arteries in combination with a reduced caliber in the peripheral pulmonary vessels, which is termed *pruning*. The enlarged central pulmonary arteries can be seen as dilatation of the main pulmonary segment and/or an increased diameter of the right interlobar artery (>16 mm in men and >15 mm in women). In addition, right heart chamber enlargement is often seen. However, a normal radiograph does not exclude pulmonary hypertension, especially in mild cases. Additional findings may be present, depending on the etiology, such as emphysema, fibrosis, chest wall deformities, and left-heart disease.[22]

Shunt Vascularity

Shunt vascularity is seen when there is increased pulmonary flow caused by a left-to-right shunt, for example, atrial septal defect (ASD). In this case, there will be enlarged main pulmonary arteries, similar to pulmonary hypertension. However, the peripheral pulmonary arteries are also enlarged because of overcirculation, differing from the decreased caliber peripheral pulmonary arteries seen in pulmonary hypertension (*pruning*). An ASD can present initially in adulthood, and should be suggested when shunt vascularity is seen in the setting of right chamber predominance cardiomegaly.[5] Ventricular septal defects rarely initially present in adults, typically with irreversible pulmonary hypertension (Eisenmenger syndrome).[5,23]

Cardiomegaly

Evaluating the cardiac size is most commonly done subjectively with visual inspection of the frontal radiograph. Objectively, it can be determined by calculating the cardiothoracic ratio (CT ratio). The thoracic width is measured at the widest diameter of the rib cage from the inner aspect of the ribs and the cardiac silhouette is measured at the level of its maximum width. When the CT ratio is calculated on a PA radiograph, a ratio of greater than 0.5 is consistent with an enlarged heart. On a lateral radiograph, if the posterior heart border overlaps with the spine, this is consistent with an enlarged heart. Of note, an enlarged cardiac silhouette can be artificially enlarged in patients with prominent epicardial fat pads, pectus excavatum, and because of technical factors, such as rotated positioning, suboptimal inspiration, or frontal radiographs.

Although echocardiography provides accurate evaluation of specific cardiac chamber enlargement, familiarity with the appearance of chest radiography is useful.

Right atrial enlargement: The right atrium forms the right heart border on the frontal radiograph and enlargement will cause bulging or elongation of the right heart border.

Left atrial enlargement: The left atrium is the most posterior chamber of the heart and does not contribute to the cardiac border on the frontal radiograph, with the exception of an enlarged left atrial appendage. On a frontal radiograph, enlargement may be seen as a convexity/bulge of the appendage, along the left-heart border, just inferior to the main pulmonary artery. Because the atrium enlarges superiorly, splaying of the carina and elevation of the left main stem bronchus occurs. In cases of severe enlargement, the left atrium can extend to the right, projecting over or beyond the right atrial border, which is termed the *double density sign*. On a lateral radiograph, the enlargement of the left atrium results in a posterior bulge of the upper cardiac border with posterior displacement of the left main bronchus (**Figure 32.5**).

Right ventricular enlargement: The right ventricle is anterior and not border forming on the frontal radiograph. Enlargement will cause the cardiac apex to be displaced laterally to

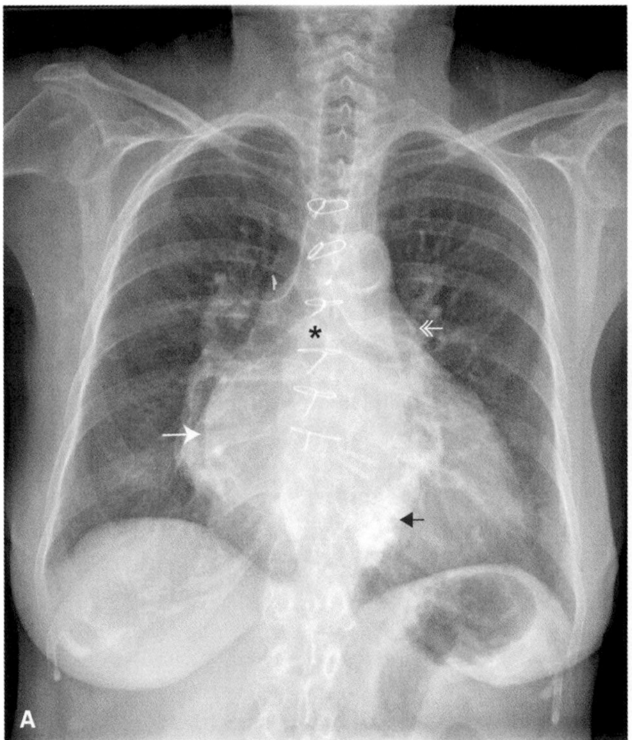

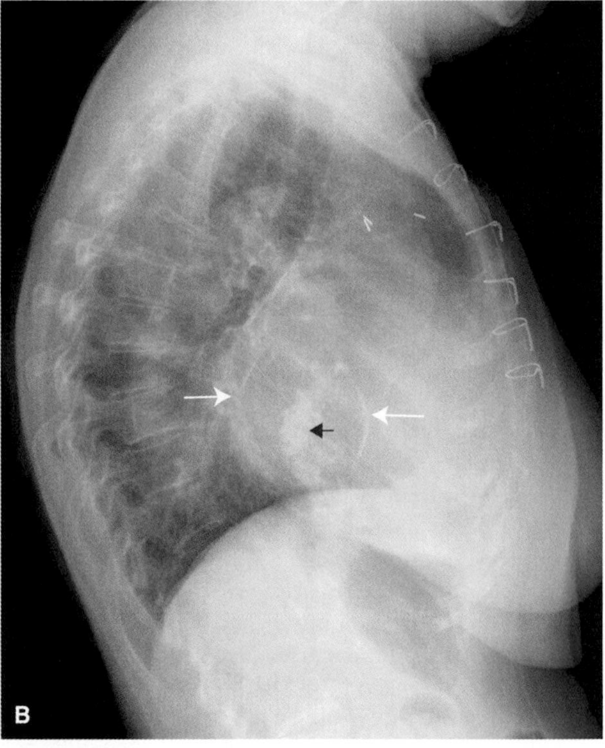

FIGURE 32.5 In this patient with rheumatic heart disease, a calcified enlarged left atrium can be seen. On the frontal radiograph **(A)**, there is a prominent left atrial appendage (white double arrowhead), splaying of the carina (asterisk), and projecting beyond the right atrial border. Left atrial calcification can be appreciated on both the frontal and lateral **(B)** radiographs (white arrows). In addition, mitral annulus calcifications are demonstrated (black arrows).

the left and superiorly. In some cases, the apex can be displaced solely superiorly. On the lateral radiograph, right ventricular enlargement results in filling in of the retrosternal clear space.

Left ventricular enlargement: The left ventricle is border forming on the frontal radiograph; and enlargement will result in a leftward inferior displacement of the left ventricular apex. This is in contrast to right ventricular enlargement, which is either just left or left superior. On a lateral radiograph, a bulging of the posterior cardiac border is expected.

Pericardial Effusion

Radiographs are not sensitive to detection of pericardial effusions, with greater than 200 mL of pericardial fluid required before visualization on the chest radiograph.[24] Differentiating a pericardial effusion from cardiac chamber enlargement is challenging. Pericardial effusion should be favored rather than cardiac chamber enlargement if there is a rapid increase in cardiac size in comparison to recent radiographs; an increase in transverse cardiac diameter of greater than 1.5 cm, compared to a radiograph taken within 30 days, and has a reported 80% sensitivity but only 46% specificity.[25] A globular/water bottle appearance of the heart with a normal-sized superior mediastinum can be seen with large pericardial effusions. On the lateral radiograph, the effusion can sometimes be visualized as a soft-tissue density between the epicardial and pericardial fat, both of which are radiolucent. This has been termed *the pericardial fat stripe, sandwich, or Oreo cookie sign.* This is a specific, but not sensitive, sign that is usually only seen with large pericardial effusions, most commonly on lateral radiographs anterior to the right ventricle[26] (**Figure 32.6 A,B,C**). Unilateral left-sided pleural effusions have been shown to be seen more commonly in pericardial effusions.[25]

Calcifications

Multiple cardiac calcifications can be seen on radiographs from different etiologies; being familiar with location and shape of calcifications can guide interpretation.

Coronary Artery Calcifications. Coronary artery calcifications appear as tram track, curvilinear calcifications. These calcifications are found on the frontal PA radiograph in the "coronary artery calcification triangle," which is created laterally by the left mid-heart border below the level of the left main bronchus, medially by the vertebral column, diagonally by the cardiac margin, and inferiorly by a horizontal line.[27] Mimickers of coronary artery calcifications can be calcification of the left lower bronchial wall or other structures superimposing on this triangle. Often coronary artery stents can be seen, and are more radiopaque than are coronary artery calcifications.

Myocardial Calcifications. Myocardial calcifications are a sign of pathology, and have been broadly categorized into two subgroups—dystrophic and metastatic calcifications.[28] CT is the most sensitive modality for identification of these calcifications, which can also be detected on radiographs. This is particularly relevant because myocardial calcifications can be a cause of arrhythmias and heart dysfunction. Dystrophic calcifications are a consequence of tissue damage and necrosis, and myocardial infarction is the most common cause. They are focal and curvilinear calcifications, located at the edge of an infarct of the left ventricular apex, typically associated with ventricular aneurysm (**Figure 32.7 A,B**). Metastatic calcifications are associated with an imbalance in the calcium homeostasis, most commonly due to renal failure. Metastatic calcifications have varied appearance, and are more often diffuse, amorphous, and globular. The presence of left atrial

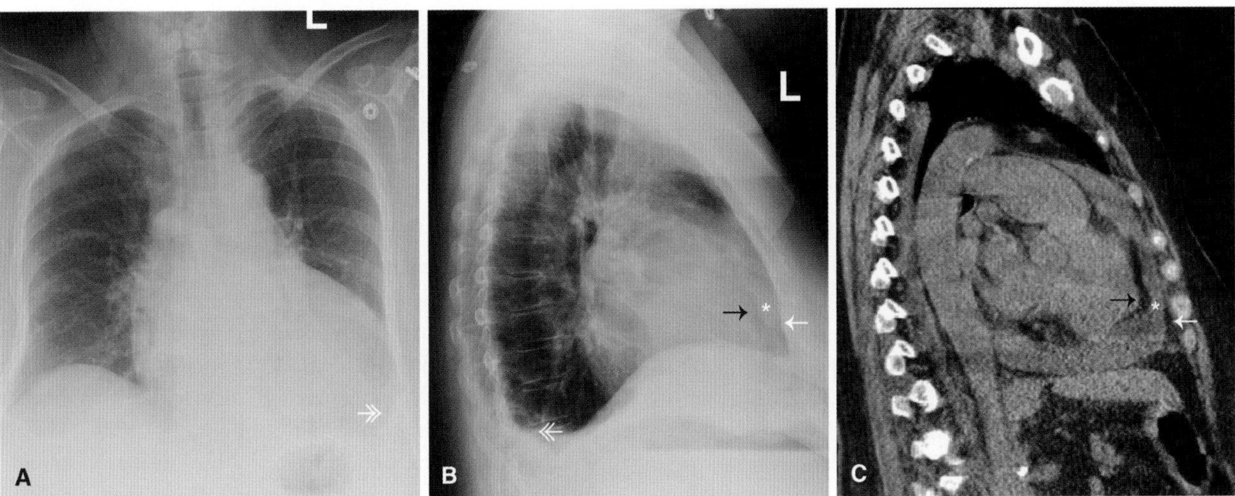

FIGURE 32.6 An enlarged globular cardiac silhouette is seen on the frontal radiograph **(A)**. On the lateral radiograph **(B)** and correlate sagittal image on subsequently performed computed tomography CT **(C)**, the pericardial effusion can be seen as a soft-tissue density (asterisk) between the epicardial fat (black arrows) and the pericardial fat (white arrows), termed *the pericardial fat stripe, sandwich, or Oreo cookie sign.* A left-sided pleural effusion is also seen (white double arrowhead).

SECTION 2

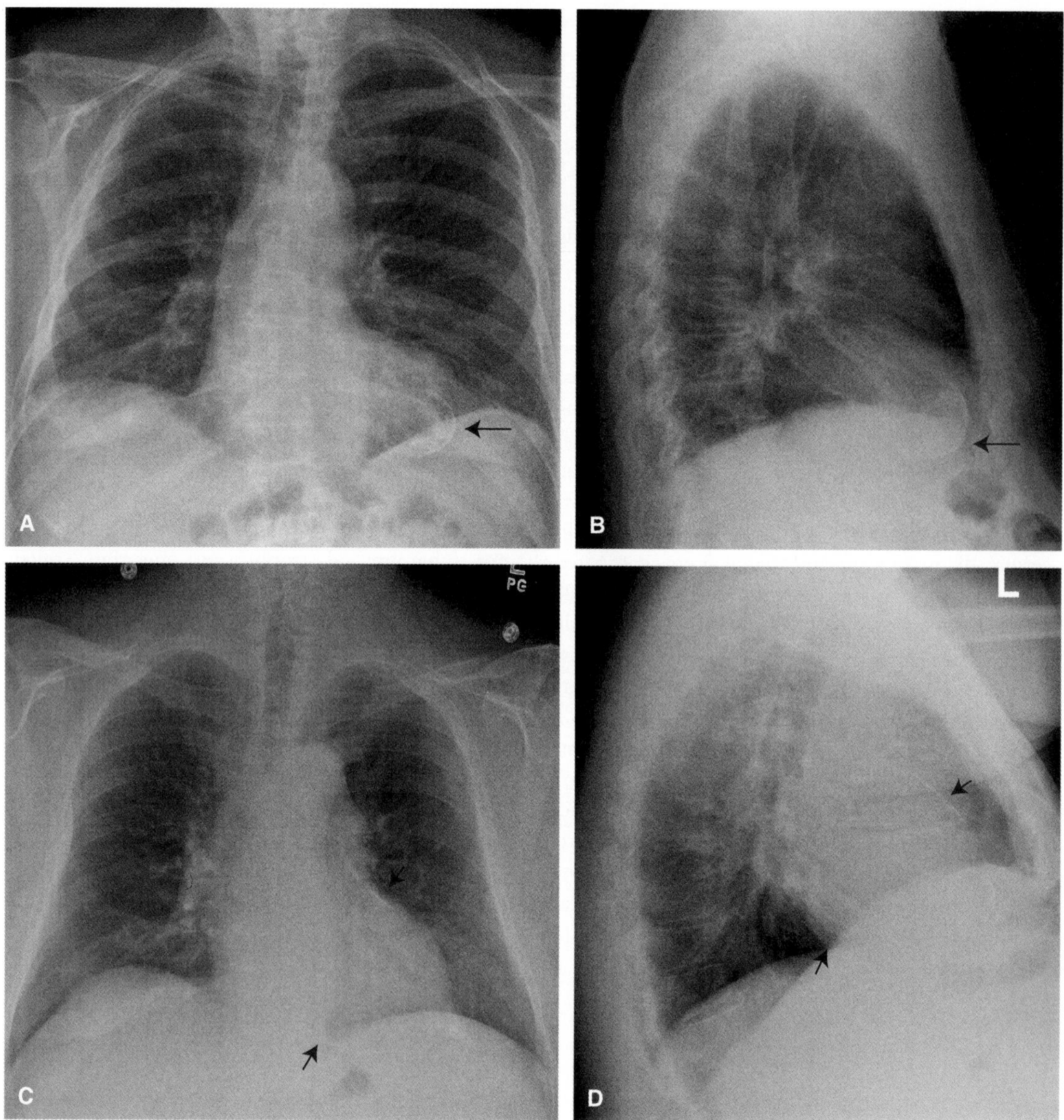

FIGURE 32.7 Frontal and lateral radiographs demonstrate a calcified left ventricular aneurysm (**A, B**, black arrows) and, in a different patient, near-circumferential pericardial calcifications (**C, D**, short black arrows).

calcifications is synonymous with rheumatic heart disease[29] (**Figure 32.5**). Myocardial calcifications in heart transplant patients can be multifactorial.[28]

Pericardial Calcifications. Pericardial calcifications are caused by end-stage disease from prior injury to the pericardium. There are multiple etiologies including prior infections (tuberculosis, viral), trauma, cardiac surgery, radiation, and uremic pericarditis. As with myocardial calcifications, pericardial calcifications appear as curvilinear calcifications at the margin of the cardiac silhouette (**Figure 32.7 C,D**). Location of the calcifications helps differentiate between pericardial and myocardial calcifications. Pericardial calcification more often involves the less pulsatile right chambers, along the anterior and diaphragmatic surfaces, and typically involves the atrioventricular grooves. Pericardial calcifications rarely involve the left ventricular apex, and if involvement of the LV apex is noted, this is part of a more diffuse involvement of the entire heart, as opposed to myocardial calcifications that often focally involve the LV apex. In addition, on the lateral radiograph, the extension of calcification above the pulmonic valve involving the pulmonary outflow flow tract is consistent with pericardial calcifications, as opposed to myocardial calcifications that occur inferior to the pulmonic valve. The left atrium is classically spared from pericardial calcifications.[29,30] The presence of left atrial pericardial calcification should suggest the diagnosis of constrictive pericarditis, although only present in half of the cases. Potential signs of constrictive pericarditis should be assessed for, such as left atrial enlargement, flattening of the cardiac contours, and pulmonary venous hypertension.[29]

Aortic Calcifications. The vast majority of aortic calcifications are degenerative, resulting from atherosclerosis, and have a dense and irregular radiographic appearance. They are commonly seen involving the aortic arch and descending aorta; initially deposited at the site of the ligamentum arteriosum and the origin of the left subclavian artery. The ascending aorta is classically spared. If ascending aortic calcifications are seen, especially in the absence of descending aorta calcifications, alternative etiologies can be considered such as aortic aneurysm, Marfan syndrome, syphilis, or prior radiation.[29]

Valvular Calcifications. Aortic valve calcifications are the most commonly seen valvular calcifications. Three patterns are described as commissure, complete/partial ring, or plaquelike calcifications. In the majority of patients older than 70 years, the calcifications are due to degenerative disease. If seen in a younger patient, bicuspid aortic valve should be considered or prior rheumatic heart disease. Mitral valve calcifications are less commonly seen, and are usually secondary to rheumatic heart disease. This is in contrast to mitral annulus calcifications, which are quite often seen on radiograph with a reverse C configuration (Figure 32.5). Both tricuspid and pulmonic valve calcifications are rare.[29]

Aortic Dissection

Various radiographic findings have been described to suggest a diagnosis of aortic dissection, despite poor specificity. The global finding of an "abnormal" radiograph is the most common finding, with a 90% sensitivity.[31] The most common abnormality in aortic dissection is a widened mediastinum, as defined as a greater than 8-cm mediastinal width at the aortic knob on a PA radiograph (64% sensitivity).[31] However, care should be taken when interpreting AP, supine, or rotated radiographs for mediastinal widening, because the width can be artificially magnified.[32] In addition, mediastinal widening can be seen with chronic vascular ectasia, excessive mediastinal fat, enlarged thyroid, mediastinal mass, or lymphadenopathy. If priors are available, interval progressive widening or change in mediastinal contour has a higher predictive value. Another classically described finding is displacement of intimal aortic calcification from the outer contour of the aortic knob by 6 to 10 mm, which has a poor sensitivity (9%). Additional supportive signs include a pleural cap (apical opacity in a supine radiograph secondary to hemothorax), blurring of the aortic knob, tracheal shift to the right, depression of the left main stem bronchus below 40 degrees, and pleural effusion.[33] However, if aortic dissection is clinically suspected, further imaging is recommended, with CT the most common modality.[1] The primary role of the radiograph remains to exclude other thoracic pathology; however, recognition of abnormal radiographic findings can decrease "time to diagnosis" and improve survival.[33]

Pulmonary Embolism

The classic findings of pulmonary embolism on radiographs discussed subsequently are unfortunately rarely useful because of their lack of sensitivity and specificity. The *Fleischner sign* is an enlarged central pulmonary artery secondary to a distal clot causing proximal increased pressure. The *Westermark sign* occurs when a compromised pulmonary artery causes regional oligemia and increased lung lucency. A pulmonary infarct can occur secondary to a pulmonary embolus, which is seen as peripheral wedge-shaped opacity often in the lower lungs, termed *Hampton's hump*. More commonly, nonspecific findings of pulmonary embolus are a unilateral pleural effusion or focal atelectasis, which should raise concern in the appropriate clinical settings and trigger consideration for further workup.[34]

Noncardiac Pathology

Lobar consolidation is rare in pulmonary edema, and pneumonia should be considered. Alveolar opacities without pleural effusions suggest alternative pathologies such as infection and inflammatory lung diseases. Although alveolar edema can have an appearance similar to viral or atypical pneumonia, more patchy consolidations or nodular opacities in a peripheral distribution with lack of signs of fluid overload should favor infection. A unilateral left-sided pleural effusion is also uncommon in CHF. As is often the case in critical care settings, however, two or more conditions frequently coexist.

Pneumothorax is another cause of dyspnea and chest pain that should be considered on the chest radiograph, particularly in the postprocedure patient (**Figure 32.8**). On erect radiographs, an apical lucency with visualization of the visceral pleural line is typical for pneumothorax. On a supine radiograph,

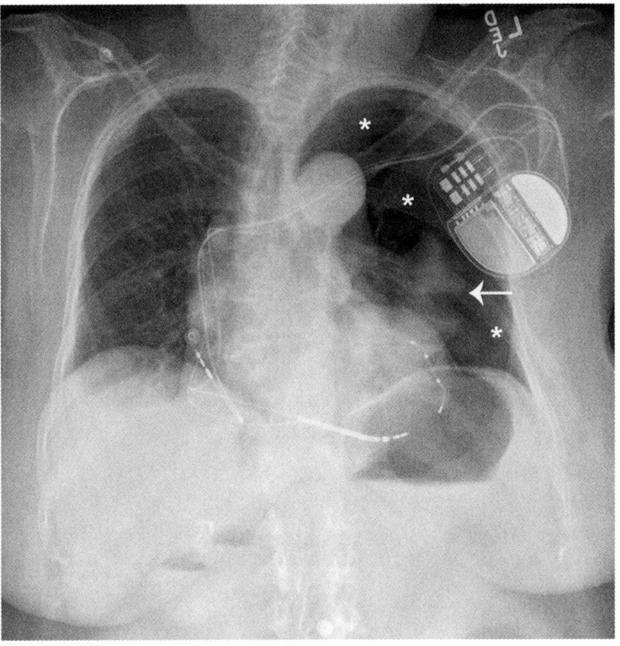

FIGURE 32.8 A routine radiograph taken after placement of a biventricular cardioverter defibrillator in an asymptomatic patient demonstrates a large left pneumothorax with near collapse of the entire left lung (white arrow) and absent lung markings in the near-entire left hemithorax (asterisks).

SECTION 2

pneumothorax is often more subtle and can be seen as a hyperlucent deep costophrenic angle termed the *deep sulcus sign*, or hyperlucency along the mediastinal border. Lung cancer can commonly present as chest pain with dyspnea; therefore, focal nodular or masslike pulmonary opacities should prompt further imaging, especially absent a clinical history suggesting infection. Musculoskeletal causes of chest pain such as rib fractures (seen best on rib series) and sternal fractures or thoracic spine pathology (best on the lateral view) can be demonstrated on chest radiographs. However, costochondritis, which is the cause of up to 30% of emergent chest pain visits, does not have radiographic findings.[35]

Intensive Care Unit Recommendations and Device Complications

Controversy regarding the role of daily intensive care unit (ICU) radiographs has been longstanding. Current recommendations state that placement of an endotracheal or enteric tube, Swan–Ganz catheters, central venous catheters, or other life support devices is an indication for a chest radiograph as is any change in clinical condition in a critical care patient.[1] It is prudent to become familiar with postprocedural complications and appearance of malpositioned devices, which are often clinically unapparent. In addition, evaluating permanent pacemaker leads on both a frontal and lateral radiograph is recommended to determine lead positioning and identify postprocedural complications, such as pneumothorax.[36] The full plethora of devices and their radiographic appearance are beyond the scope of this chapter, and referral to more complete references is recommended.[37-39]

LIMITATIONS OF CHEST RADIOGRAPHY

Comparison Between Posteroanterior and Anteroposterior Techniques

When comparing a PA to an AP radiograph, it is important to be aware of fundamental physics. In an AP view, the heart is magnified by 15% to 20% because there is a decreased distance between the x-ray tube and the detector (3 feet vs 6 feet) and the heart is an anterior structure, and hence more distant from the detector on an AP view. AP radiographs are often obtained when the patient is supine, which decreases lung volumes, and obviates the gravitational gradient between the upper and lower pulmonary vasculature simulating. Awareness of the radiographic projection and positioning is fundamental in evaluation of pleural effusion, because pleural fluid will not be dependent in the lower lungs, but layer posteriorly on a supine radiograph, resulting in subtle increased opacity, which is diagnostically more difficult. Similarly, a pneumothorax is much more inconspicuous on the AP radiograph, because the free air localizes to nondependent locations on a supine radiograph.

If a patient is not positioned well, which often occurs in critically ill patients, an unintentional lordotic projection can be obtained. This can lead to artifactual distortion of thoracic structures, with the most common findings being artificial widening of the superior mediastinum, obscuration of the lower lobes, apparent elevation of the hemidiaphragms, cardiomegaly, and prominence of the upper pulmonary vessels, simulating pulmonary venous hypertension.[40]

Inspiration Versus Expiration

Ideally, the chest radiograph should be taken in full inspiration. If the inspiration is shallow, the lungs appear denser with crowding of the vessels, which can be mistaken for pulmonary edema.

Rotation

If the radiograph is rotated to the left, the heart size will be overestimated, whereas rightward rotation results in underestimation of cardiac size. Similarly, the superior mediastinum can be artifactually enlarged with rotation. Therefore, proper evaluation for interval mediastinal enlargement includes careful examination for rotation.[14]

Exposure

Despite image manipulation on workstations, underexposure or overexposure cannot be compensated for on postprocessing. This may be a technical error; however, underexposure can occur in obese patients because the lungs appear less lucent owing to attenuation of the x-ray beam by increased subcutaneous tissue. This increased lung attenuation can mimic pulmonary edema and limit sensitivity of radiographs to detect pathology. Of note, careful attention to the caliber of the pulmonary vessels can provide differentiation. Similarly, overlying dense breast tissues and breast implants can simulate increased density in the bilateral lower lobes, and can be mistaken for pulmonary edema.[15]

Research and Future Directions

With recent advances in artificial intelligence (AI), particularly deep learning models, emerging studies are demonstrating AI's equivalent performance to radiologists in interpreting various chest radiograph findings. The clinical integration of AI in chest radiograph interpretation promises improved worklist prioritization and improving worldwide access to prompt and accurate radiograph interpretation.[41-43]

KEY POINTS

- ✔ Guidelines almost exclusively recommend chest radiography as the initial imaging test in a patient with chest pain or dyspnea with a suspected cardiac origin, while acknowledging that radiographs cannot exclude cardiovascular disease.
- ✔ The chest radiograph can support a cardiac diagnosis and provide information regarding cardiac function or identify alternative pathology as the cause of the patient's symptoms.

- ✔ Accurate interpretation of chest radiographs requires use of a reproducible, systematic approach, in which comparison with prior studies is highly valued.
- ✔ In CHF, chest radiographic findings have been shown to correlate with pulmonary wedge pressures; the earliest sign is pulmonary vascular redistribution, followed by interstitial edema and alveolar edema.
- ✔ Differentiating between noncardiogenic and cardiogenic edema is important, with interstitial edema and indirect signs of fluid overload more suggestive of cardiogenic edema; the absence of pleural effusion is often seen in ARDS.
- ✔ Familiarity with basic physics and radiographic technique is important in interpreting the chest radiograph, awareness of the differences between PA, and AP portable radiographs.

REFERENCES

1. American College of Radiology. ACR appropriateness criteria. https://www.acr.org/Clinical-Resources/ACR-Appropriateness-Criteria
2. Federle MP, Rosado de Christenson ML, Raman SP, et al. *Imaging Anatomy: Chest, Abdomen and Pelvis.* 2nd ed. Elsevier; 2017.
3. Schallert EK, Danton GH, Kardon R, et al. Describing congenital heart disease by using three-part segmental notation. *Radiographics.* 2013;33(2):E33-E46.
4. Ghosh S, Yarmish G, Godelman A, et al. Anomalies of visceroatrial situs. *Am J Roentgenol.* 2009;193(4):1107-1117.
5. Latson L Jr, Levsky JM, Haramati LB. Adult congenital heart disease: a practical approach. *J Thorac Imaging.* 2013;28(6):332-346.
6. Baron MG. Radiologic notes in cardiology: obscuration of the aortic knob in coarctation of the aorta. *Circulation.* 1971;43(2):311-316.
7. Kanne JP, Godwin JD. Right aortic arch and its variants. *J Cardiovasc Comput Tomogr.* 2010;4(5):293-300.
8. Felson B, Palayew MJ. The two types of right aortic arch. *Radiology.* 1963:81(5):745-759.
9. Cressman S, Rheinboldt M, Klochko C, et al. Chest radiographic appearance of minimally invasive cardiac implants and support devices: what the radiologist needs to know. *Curr Probl Diagn Radiol.* 2019;48.3:274-288.
10. Mundy J, Stickley M, Venkatesh B, et al. The imaginary line method is not reliable for identification of prosthetic heart valves on AP chest radiographs. *Crit Care Resusc.* 2006;8(1):15-18.
11. Dipoce J, Bernheim A, Spindola-Franco H. Radiology of cardiac devices and their complications. *Br J Radiol.* 2015;88(1046):20140540.
12. Berbaum KS, Krupinski EA, Schartz KM, et al. Satisfaction of search in chest radiography 2015. *Acad Radiol.* 2015;22(11):1457-1465.
13. Baruah D, Shahir K, Goodman LR. Radiographic techniques. In: Digumarthy SR, ed. *Problem Solving in Chest Imaging.* 1st ed. Elsevier; 2020.
14. Broder J. Imaging the chest: the chest radiograph. In: Broder J, ed. *Diagnostic Imaging for the Emergency Physician.* 1st ed. Elsevier; 2011.
15. Feldmann EJ, Jain VR, Rakoff S, et al. Radiology residents' on-call interpretation of chest radiographs for congestive heart failure. *Acad Radiol.* 2007;14(10):1264-1270.
16. Gluecker T, Capasso P, Schnyder P, et al. Clinical and radiologic features of pulmonary edema. *Radiographics.* 1999;19(6):1507-1531.
17. Ravin CE. Radiographic analysis of pulmonary vascular distribution: a review. *Bull N Y Acad Med.* 1983;59(8):728-743.
18. Herring W. *Learning Radiology: Recognizing the Basics.* 4th ed. Elsevier; 2019.
19. Tsuchiya N, Griffin L, Yabuuchi H, et al. Imaging findings of pulmonary edema: part 1. Cardiogenic pulmonary edema and acute respiratory distress syndrome. *Acta Radiol.* 2020;61(2):184-194.
20. Milne EN, Pistolesi M, Miniati M, et al. The radiologic distinction of cardiogenic and noncardiogenic edema. *Am J Roentgenol.* 1985;144(5):879-894.
21. Dobbe L, Rahman R, Elmassry M, et al. Cardiogenic pulmonary edema. *Am J Med Sci.* 2019;358(6):389-397.
22. Goerne H, Batra K, Rajiah P. Imaging of pulmonary hypertension: an update. *Cardiovasc Diagn Ther.* 2018;8(3):279-296.
23. Baron MG. Plain film diagnosis of common cardiac anomalies in the adult. *Radiol Clin North Am.* 1999;37(2):401-420.
24. Ridley L. Chest radiograph signs suggestive of pericardial disease. *Am Coll Cardiol.* https://www.acc.org/latest-in-cardiology/articles/2019/09/09/10/46/chest-radiograph-signs-suggestive-of-pericardial-disease
25. Eisenberg MJ, Dunn MM, Kanth N, et al. Diagnostic value of chest radiography for pericardial effusion. *J Am Coll Cardial.* 1993;22(2):588-593.
26. Carsky EW, Azimi F, Mauceri R. Epicardial fat sign in the diagnosis of pericardial effusion. *JAMA.* 1980;244(24):2762-2764.
27. Souza AS Jr, Bream PR, Elliot LP. Chest film detection of coronary artery calcification. The value of the CAC triangle. *Radiology.* 1978;129(1):7-10.
28. Nance JW Jr, Crane GM, Halushka MK, et al. Myocardial calcifications: pathophysiology, etiologies, differential diagnoses, and imaging findings. *J Cardiovasc Comput Tomogr.* 2015;9(1):58-67.
29. Ferguson EC, Berkowitz EA. Cardiac and pericardial calcifications on chest radiographs. *Clin Radiol.* 2010;65(9):685-694.
30. MacGregor JH, Chen JT, Chiles C. The radiographic distinction between pericardial and myocardial calcifications. *Am J Roentgenol.* 1987;148(4):675-677.
31. Klompas M. Does this patient have an acute thoracic aortic dissection? *JAMA.* 2002;287(17):2262-2272.
32. Lai V, Tsang WK, Chan WC, et al. Diagnostic accuracy of mediastinal width measurement on posteroanterior and anteroposterior chest radiographs in the depiction of acute nontraumatic thoracic aortic dissection. *Emerg Radiol.* 2012;19(4):309-315.
33. Chawla A, Rajendran S, Yung WH et al. Chest radiography in acute aortic syndrome: pearls and pitfalls. *Emerg Radiol.* 2016;23(4):405-412.
34. Worsley DF, Alavi A, Aronchick JM, et al. Chest radiographic findings in patients with acute pulmonary embolism: observations from the PIOPED Study. *Radiology.* 1993;189(1):133-136.
35. Habib PA, Huang GS, Mendiola JA, Joseph S. Anterior chest pain: musculoskeletal considerations. *Emerg Radiol.* 2004;11(1):37-45.
36. Belvin D, Hirschl D, Jain VR, et al. Chest radiographs are valuable in demonstrating clinically significant pacemaker complications that require reoperation. *Can Assoc Radiol J.* 2011;62(4):288-295.
37. Godoy MC, Leitman BS, de Groot PM, et al. Chest radiography in the ICU: part 2, evaluation of cardiovascular lines and other devices. *Am J Roentgenol.* 2012;198(3):572-581.
38. Lee S, Chaturvedi A. Imaging adults on extracorporeal membrane oxygenation (ECMO). *Insights Imaging.* 2014;5(6):731-742.
39. Kligerman S, Horowitz M, Jacobs K, et al. Imaging of cardiac support devices. *Radiol Clin North Am.* 2020;58(1):151-165.
40. Hollman AS, Adams FG. The influence of the lordotic projection on the interpretation of the chest radiograph. *Clin Radiol.* 1989;40(4):360-364.
41. Majkowska A, Mittal S, Steiner DF, et al. Chest radiograph interpretation with deep learning models: assessment with radiologist-adjudicated reference standards and population-adjusted evaluation. *Radiology.* 2020; 294(2):421-431.
42. Annarumma M, Withey SJ, Bakewell RJ, et al. Automated triaging of adult chest radiographs with deep artificial neural networks. *Radiology.* 2019;291(1):196-202.
43. Rajpurkar P, Irvin J, Ball RL, et al. Deep learning for chest radiograph diagnosis: a retrospective comparison of the CheXNeXt algorithm to practicing radiologists. *PLoS Med.* 2018;15(11):e1002686.

CHAPTER 33

ELECTROCARDIOGRAPHIC EXERCISE TESTING

Zain Ul Abideen Asad and Chittur A. Sivaram

INTRODUCTION

Diagnosis of myocardial ischemia remains an important clinical challenge in patients presenting with chest pain in the ambulatory clinic. After the initial evaluation, stress testing is frequently employed in such patients to confirm the presence of ischemic heart disease. An array of tests, such as electrocardiographic (ECG) exercise testing, stress echocardiography, and myocardial perfusion imaging (MPI), are currently available to the clinician for this purpose. Although the cost, diagnostic accuracy, and complexities differ between various stress tests, unmasking of a mismatch between myocardial oxygen (O_2) supply and myocardial O_2 demand during stress remains the foundational principle for all the tests. Despite the growth of competing diagnostic tests, ECG exercise testing continues to have a robust, guideline-recommended role in the diagnosis of myocardial ischemia in carefully selected patients with suspected ischemic heart disease.[1]

INDICATIONS

ECG exercise testing is useful in patients with suspected ischemic heart disease for the confirmation of diagnosis as well as obtaining prognostic information. Diagnosis of myocardial ischemia is based on the appearance of significant ST segment deviation (depression or elevation) seen either during or immediately after termination of exercise. In order to maximize the diagnostic accuracy of ECG exercise testing, patients with intermediate pretest probability (15%-65%) for coronary artery disease and normal resting ECG are the most appropriate candidates for this test. Current guidelines also recommend exercise ECG stress test as the initial diagnostic test rather than other modalities of stress tests in patients with suspected ischemic heart disease and normal resting ECG.[1]

PHYSIOLOGIC CONSIDERATIONS

A basic understanding of exercise-related changes in cardiovascular physiology is essential for safe performance of exercise stress test, accurate interpretation of test results, and analysis of the implications of abnormalities observed.

Functional Capacity

During exercise, augmentation of cardiac output occurs, driven by an increase in heart rate (HR) and an increase in venous return and stroke volume through the Frank-Starling mechanism. In addition, increased O_2 utilization by the exercising muscles results in an increase in the peripheral arteriovenous O_2 difference. The O_2 uptake value (VO_2) is obtained by multiplying cardiac output by the arteriovenous O_2 difference and serves as a reliable measure of the energy requirement of the body for a given amount of physical activity. The resting O_2 requirement of 3.5 mL O_2/kg body weight/minute is termed 1 metabolic equivalent (1 MET). Maximal O_2 uptake (VO_2 max) obtained during peak exercise is influenced by the patient's age, sex, exercise conditioning, and other factors. Women have lower VO_2 max compared to men, and VO_2 max values progressively decline with aging, notably with a sharp decline after the 70s.[2,3] The average VO_2 max for healthy young men is approximately 12 METs and could be as high as 18 to 24 METs in long-distance runners.[4]

VO_2 max is considered the best surrogate measure for fitness and functional capacity. This is due to the fact that arteriovenous O_2 difference remains approximately constant at 15 to 17 mL/dL, and any increase in VO_2 max during exercise will have to be attributed to changes in cardiac output. Cardiac output increases four to five times even with modest intensity of exercise because of a two- to threefold rise in HR; at continued higher intensity of exercise, the primary determinant of further augmentation in cardiac output is increased HR because the stroke volume plateaus at 50% to 60% of VO_2 max.

Myocardial Oxygen Demand

The amount of O_2 used by the myocardium, that is, myocardial O_2 uptake, is determined by HR, contractility, and the left ventricular (LV) wall stress. The determinants of LV wall stress are LV end diastolic pressure and volume, wall thickness, and cavity size. Of these variables influencing myocardial O_2 demand, HR and blood pressure (BP) remain the most practical and reliable parameters that could be monitored during exercise. Consequently, the product of HR and systolic BP, referred to as double product or rate pressure product, is commonly used to obtain an estimate of myocardial O_2 consumption. The normal value of double product ranges from 25,000 (10th percentile) to 40,000 (90th percentile) during peak exercise.[5] Higher values of double product correspond to improved myocardial perfusion. Double product has an important role in predicting cardiovascular prognosis.[6-8]

Myocardial Oxygen Supply

Normally, the myocardial O_2 supply increases during exercise. This is driven largely by neurohormonal stimulation during exercise that releases vasodilators, such as nitric oxide, and leads to coronary vasodilation.[9] Approximately a four- to fivefold augmentation of myocardial blood flow occurs during exercise as a result of coronary vasodilation. In patients with coronary artery disease, myocardial blood flow is compromised. A coronary stenosis of 50% to 70% owing to an atherosclerotic plaque will lead to impairment of this reactive hyperemia during exercise, and a 90% or more stenosis would impair myocardial blood flow even at rest. As a result of the reduced myocardial O_2 supply in patients with atherosclerotic coronary artery disease, clinical symptoms of angina pectoris and various ECG changes can occur during exercise.

FUNDAMENTALS OF EXERCISE TESTING

Aerobic Exercise Effects on Cardiovascular Physiology

Heart Rate Response

A decrease in parasympathetic activity and an increase in sympathetic activity lead to a rise in HR immediately after aerobic exercise is started.[10] There is a linear increase in HR with continued exercise. The most widely used equation for maximum predicted HR is 220 minus age in years for men and 80% of the above for women.[11,12] Wide variability exists among subjects when the formula to predict maximum HR is used. Increase in HR rather than increase in stroke volume is responsible for a far greater augmentation in cardiac output during strenuous exercise. Stroke volume increases by about 50% with exercise, whereas the HR increase is more than 250%.[13] Although a resting cardiac output is about 5.5 L/min, an increase of cardiac output up to 30 L/min can be seen in long-distance runners and other well-conditioned athletes. However, the behavior of HR response during exercise could be variable in patients. An exaggerated HR response to exercise is seen in deconditioning, anemia, or LV dysfunction, whereas an inadequate HR response to exercise ("chronotropic incompetence") is seen with sinus node dysfunction. Multiple determinants, such as blood volume, peripheral vascular resistance, medications (beta-blockers), and body position, can also affect HR response to exercise.

HR response after termination of exercise can offer prognostic clues in heart disease. A delayed HR recovery, that is, a slow return of HR back to normal after exercise is terminated, suggests decreased vagal activity, an important predictor of mortality in patients with and without angiographic coronary artery disease.[14-16] Despite some variability, most studies define an abnormal HR recovery as the inability to drop the HR by 12 to 21 bpm, 1 minute after the termination of exercise.[17-19]

Blood Pressure Response

On average, the systolic BP rises by 10 mm Hg/MET during exercise, whereas the diastolic pressure remains unchanged or decreases slightly.[5] Return of BP to the baseline preexercise level within about 6 minutes after termination of exercise is expected in healthy individuals.[20]

Resistance (Isometric) Exercise Effects on Cardiovascular Physiology

There are clear differences between the cardiovascular physiology of aerobic exercise and resistance (isometric) exercise. The small increase in cardiac output occurring during resistance exercise is primarily mediated by an increase in HR. A decrease in venous return owing to increased intrathoracic pressure is common during resistance exercise. An increase in peripheral vascular resistance seen in resistance exercise limits increases in cardiac output. Increase in both systolic and diastolic BP occurs during resistance exercise.

The net result of both aerobic and resistance types of exercise is an increase in myocardial O_2 demand because of increase in HR, BP, and LV wall tension.

CLINICAL APPLICATIONS

Electrocardiographic Exercise Stress Test Procedure

The protocol for exercise ECG stress test involves preprocedural assessment of the patient, recording of baseline ECG and vital signs (including pulse and BP), selection of the appropriate exercise protocol, performance of the test, and interpretation of test findings.

Patient Assessment Preprocedure

In preparation for the exercise ECG test, it is important to perform a thorough clinical assessment of the patient with emphasis on the presence of an appropriate indication and absence of any contraindications. Evaluation of preexisting symptoms particularly those attributable to relevant comorbidities is warranted.

A brief history focused on risk factors and symptoms leading to stress testing should be obtained from the patient and supplemented by chart review. Symptom review allows for identification of symptoms to monitor during the test, especially in patients who present with atypical symptoms of ischemia. Evaluation of a patient's functional capacity is important for the appropriate selection of exercise protocol, reducing the risk of physical injuries during exercise, and improving the overall safety of the test. Assessment of pretest probability of ischemic heart disease is essential for confirming the appropriateness of ECG exercise testing rather than another type of stress modality. The ideal candidate for ECG exercise testing has a predicted intermediate pretest probability (15%-65%) for ischemic heart disease test, based on the type of chest pain (typical angina, atypical angina, or noncardiac chest pain) and sex of the patient.[1] False-positive exercise ECG tests are frequent in those with lower pretest probability, and false-negative tests are of concern in those with higher than 65% pretest probability. Physical examination should be performed with particular attention to the presence of murmurs and orthopedic or neurologic conditions that limit physical activity. Precordial murmurs including late peaking aortic systolic murmurs should warrant echocardiography to exclude severe aortic stenosis prior to the test. Exercise ECG test is of high value for the diagnosis of ischemia only when the resting ECG is normal.[1] In the presence of ST depression, LV hypertrophy, left bundle branch block (LBBB), pre-excitation, or continuously paced rhythm on the resting ECG, exercise ECG becomes uninterpretable for the presence of ischemia.

Patient should be kept fasting for at least 3 hours before the test. Informed consent should be obtained with clear explanation of the procedure, indication, end points, alternatives, and complications of the test. Patients should be encouraged to report symptoms during the test on a rating scale of 1 to 10. When stress testing is performed to establish diagnosis of coronary artery disease, beta-blockers should be stopped 24 hours before the procedure.

Special planning is needed prior to stress testing in patients with implanted cardiac devices such as cardiac pacemakers and implantable cardioverter defibrillators (ICDs). Detailed chart review should be done to determine the indication for pacing, number of device leads implanted, the programmed mode, thresholds, and pacing limits. In pacemaker-dependent patients who are being paced at a fixed rate, HR cannot be used to estimate the intensity or adequacy of exertion and as such an alternate surrogate marker such as the Borg scale of perceived exertion will need to be used.[21] Most patients with continuous pacing would be candidates for MPI rather than ECG exercise testing when myocardial ischemia is suspected. In patients with ICDs, it is important to know the programmed thresholds for defibrillation prior to exercise testing. Maintaining the maximum HR during exercise stress test at 10 to 15 bpm below the device threshold for antitachycardia pacing or defibrillation is recommended for prevention of inappropriate device therapy. With adequate precautions, exercise testing is safe in patients with ICDs, and the rate of ICD firing remains very low during exercise.[22]

Electrocardiogram

A resting supine 12-lead ECG should be obtained before starting exercise and compared with prior ECGs to assess for any progression of changes. Supine and standing ECG findings could show important differences because of relative changes in the position of the heart and ECG electrodes. Therefore, a baseline standing ECG should be done for comparison with subsequent standing exercise ECG tracings. Similarly, baseline BP recordings should be done in the standing position.

To obtain high-quality ECGs free of artifacts, good skin-electrode contact is essential. Shaving and cleansing of skin to remove oils before application of electrodes are helpful in ensuring adequate contact. Use of an elastic bandage wrapped around the torso also improves electrode contact and reduces movement of ECG cables. The arm leads are applied on the upper part of torso lateral to the clavicles and the leg leads under the rib cage. Because this type of limb lead positioning may either mask or mimic inferior Q waves, verification of Q waves with a supine ECG with limb leads in the standard position is recommended.

Exercise Protocols

Treadmill walking and supine bicycle exercise are the two potential methods for ECG exercise testing. Majority of the laboratories utilize a treadmill exercise protocol. Various treadmill exercise protocols (eg, Bruce, Balke, and Naughton) are available for use in clinical practice. All protocols start with a period of low-intensity exercise for warm-up, followed by graded increase in exercise intensity typically at 3-minute intervals till the target HRs are reached and a recovery period. Bruce protocol, the most commonly used protocol, uses a treadmill speed of 1.7 mph with a 10% grade (which is equivalent to 5 METs) for stage I. An estimate of functional capacity can be obtained from the stage of Bruce protocol reached at peak symptom-limited exercise. A limitation of the standard Bruce protocol is the relatively huge increments in workloads between stages that can lead to occasional premature termination of the test because of fatigue. A modified Bruce protocol that incorporates two warm-up stages of 3 minutes each (1.7 mph at 0% grade, 1.7 mph at 5% grade) might be more suitable for such patients. Details on Bruce and other protocols used in clinical practice are available in the literature.[5]

Patient Monitoring

During each stage of the exercise protocol, a 12-lead ECG and BP are recorded, and the patient is asked about symptoms. During recovery, a period of slow walking should be used for active recovery in order to minimize the risk of excessive venous pooling in the limbs and to prevent hypotension.[5] Patient monitoring should continue as long as they are symptomatic or until symptoms return to baseline. Generally, a period of 6 to 8 minutes of monitoring after stopping exercise is sufficient. Occasionally, new ST segment abnormalities appear during the recovery phase. The implication of persistent ECG changes during recovery regarding the extent of residual ischemia independent of the ischemic changes during exercise has been described.[23] Moreover, the patterns of ST segment depression during both exercise and recovery can increase the overall accuracy of exercise ECG to detect ischemia.[24]

The absolute and relative indications for stopping the exercise stress test have been specified in the guidelines (**Table 33.1**).[5]

Test Supervision

The degree of required supervision for an exercise stress test is influenced by several factors, including the patient's age, complexity of comorbidities, indication for test, and experience of staff members. Appropriately trained advance practice providers (nurse, physician assistant, nurse practitioner) trained in cardiopulmonary resuscitation can supervise the test in patients with stable chest pain syndromes.[5] A physician qualified to supervise exercise stress testing should be immediately available.[25] Equipment and medications for cardiopulmonary resuscitation including a defibrillator should be readily available. In-depth recommendations about the necessary equipment and other standards for exercise testing

TABLE 33.1 Indications for Stopping Exercise Stress Test

Absolute Indications

- ST segment elevation (>1.0 mm) in leads without preexisting Q waves because of prior MI (other than aVR, aVL, and V1)
- Drop in systolic blood pressure >10 mm Hg, despite an increase in workload, when accompanied by any other evidence of ischemia
- Moderate-to-severe angina
- Central nervous system symptoms (eg, ataxia, dizziness, near syncope)
- Signs of poor perfusion (cyanosis or pallor)
- Sustained VT or other arrhythmia, including second- or third-degree atrioventricular block, that interferes with normal maintenance of cardiac output during exercise
- Technical difficulties in monitoring the ECG or systolic blood pressure
- The subject's request to stop

Relative Indications

- Marked ST segment displacement (horizontal or downsloping of >2 mm, measured 60 to 80 msec after the J point [the end of the QRS complex]) in a patient with suspected ischemia
- Drop in systolic blood pressure >10 mm Hg (persistently below baseline) despite an increase in workload, in the absence of other evidence of ischemia
- Increasing chest pain
- Fatigue, shortness of breath, wheezing, leg cramps, or claudication
- Arrhythmias other than sustained VT, including multifocal ventricular ectopy, ventricular triplets, supraventricular tachycardia, and bradyarrhythmias that have the potential to become more complex or to interfere with hemodynamic stability
- Exaggerated hypertensive response (systolic blood pressure >250 mm Hg or diastolic blood pressure >115 mm Hg)
- Development of bundle branch block that cannot immediately be distinguished from VT

ECG, electrocardiograph; MI, myocardial infarction; VT, ventricular tachycardia.
Reprinted with permission from Fletcher GF, Ades PA, Kligfield P, et al. Exercise standards for testing and training: a scientific statement from the American Heart Association. *Circulation*. 2013;128(8):873-934. Copyright © 2013 American Heart Association, Inc.

laboratories are available through guidelines.[25] Details of the role of allied health professionals in exercise testing procedure can be found in the guidelines by the American Heart Association.[26]

Complications

Exercise stress test is a relatively safe procedure with only six adverse reported cardiac events per 10,000 tests.[27-30] The complication rates appear to be similar when exercise tests are supervised by physicians or appropriately trained nonphysicians.[31] The most serious complications during the procedure include death, cardiac arrest, cardiac arrhythmias, acute coronary syndromes, syncope, or shock. Other noncardiac complications include soft tissue injury and trauma.

Interpretation of Electrocardiographic Exercise Test

Diagnosis of Myocardial Ischemia

ST Depression. Development of ST segment depression more than 1 mm (0.1 mV), measured 60 to 80 msec from the J point, is the most commonly accepted criterion for the diagnosis of myocardial ischemia during exercise ECG test **(Figure 33.1)**. Correct identification of the baseline (at the end of the PR segment, ie, the PQ junction) is critical for this evaluation. ST depression can be upsloping, horizontal, or downsloping. Both horizontal and downsloping ST depression are indicative of myocardial ischemia, whereas upsloping ST depression may be related to rapid HRs during exercise. In patients with resting ST elevation because of early repolarization changes, ST depression should be measured relative to the PQ junction. When ST segment depression is less than 1 mm, the test is considered equivocal.[5]

ST Elevation. Compared to ST depression, ST elevation is much less frequent during an exercise test. ST elevation occurring during exercise in leads without preexisting Q waves signifies the presence of severe proximal coronary stenosis.[5] Coronary vasospasm is a less common etiology for exercise-induced ST elevation.

Other Markers of Ischemia. Inversion of u waves during exercise and an increase in R wave amplitude (resulting from LV cavity dilation during exercise) in the precordial leads have been described as signs of ischemia.[5]

Equivocal Test. A nondiagnostic or equivocal test is characterized by less than 1 mm ST depression at peak exercise. Both patients with underlying ischemic heart disease or some normal subjects might show an equivocal exercise ECG test. Additional stress testing using more expensive modalities such as stress echocardiography or MPI may be necessary for further work-up of such patients.

Prognostic Information

In addition to establishing the diagnosis of myocardial ischemia, exercise ECG test can provide prognostic information regarding future risk for adverse cardiac events. A short duration of exercise in a symptom-limited exercise test is a powerful predictor of adverse prognosis. Inability to complete stage I of a standard Bruce protocol (which corresponds to a functional capacity of <5 METs) often accompanied by a drop in systolic BP is highly correlated with left main or severe proximal three-vessel coronary artery disease. The degree of ST depression, number of leads showing ST depression, early appearance of significant ST depression during exercise, and a slow resolution of ST depression after exercise portend poor prognosis. Such features help identify patients in need of early invasive therapy. Development of nonsustained or sustained ventricular ectopy during or immediately after exercise has been cited as a marker of adverse prognosis, but ectopy may also be seen in patients with nonischemic conditions, such as catecholaminergic polymorphic

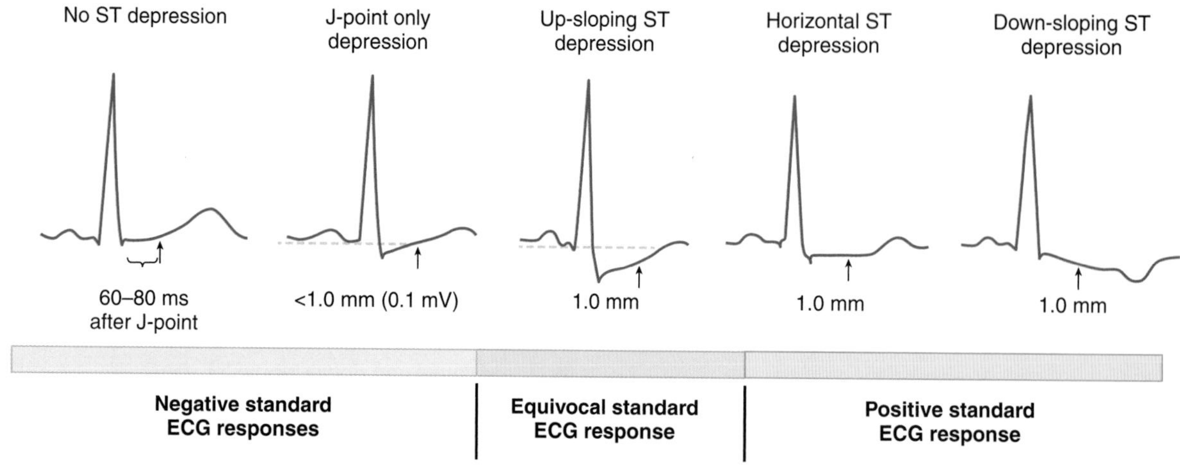

FIGURE 33.1 The definition of ST segment depression changes during exercise. Positive standard test responses include horizontal or downsloping depression of 1.0 mm (0.1 mV) or greater, whereas upsloping ST depression of 1.0 or greater is considered equivocal (a change that does not usefully separate normal from abnormal). All ST depression less than 1.0 mm from baseline is defined as negative. ECG, electrocardiograph. (Reprinted with permission from Fletcher GF, Ades PA, Kligfield P, et al. Exercise standards for testing and training: a scientific statement from the American Heart Association. *Circulation.* 2013;128(8):873-934. Copyright © 2013 American Heart Association, Inc.)

ventricular tachycardia and arrhythmogenic right ventricular cardiomyopathy.[5] The Duke treadmill score that utilizes simple parameters from ECG exercise testing (the duration of exercise, anginal severity during the exercise test, and degree of ST depression) has also been shown be a reliable predictor of prognosis.[32]

LIMITATIONS OF ELECTROCARDIOGRAPHIC EXERCISE TEST

The accuracy (positive and negative predictive values) of all diagnostic tests depends not only on the intrinsic strengths of the test but also on the characteristics of the population in which they are applied (pretest probability). The overall sensitivity of ECG exercise testing has been reported as 45% to 50% and specificity 85% to 90%.[1] Stress echocardiography (sensitivity 80%-85%, specificity 80%-88%) and MPI (sensitivity 73%-92% for exercise MPI and 90%-91% for vasodilator MPI, specificity 63%-87% for exercise MPI and 75%-84% for vasodilator MPI) have higher sensitivity and specificity, but both are limited by greater cost and lesser availability.[1] Repeated MPIs also expose the patient to significant radiation unlike exercise ECG or stress echocardiography. Equivocal exercise ECG tests are not uncommon, and they result from premature termination of exercise because of fatigue and/or noncardiac comorbid conditions, or when only milder degrees of coronary artery disease are present. Although the sensitivity and specificity of ECG exercise testing may be lower in women compared to men, some studies have failed to demonstrate an added value of MPI over symptom-limited ECG exercise testing in women with suspected ischemic heart disease.[1] Lastly, although ST depression seen during exercise test is diagnostic of myocardial ischemia, it has very limited ability to localize the coronary artery involved in the ischemic process.

CONTRAINDICATIONS

Careful screening for contraindications to ECG exercise testing is helpful in improving the diagnostic accuracy of the test as well as to ensuring safe performance of the test. Presence of resting ST depression on ECG, LBBB, pre-excitation pattern, and LV hypertrophy reduces significantly the diagnostic yield of exercise ECG test and indicates the need for another stress modality such as stress echocardiography or MPI. The absolute and relative contraindications for exercise ECG stress test have been outlined in detail by the American Heart Association guidelines (**Table 33.2**).[5]

KEY POINTS

- ✔ ECG exercise testing is helpful in the initial diagnostic work-up of patients presenting with symptoms suggestive of ischemic heart disease.
- ✔ In patients with an intermediate pretest probability for ischemic heart disease (based on patient's sex and the characteristics of chest pain) and a normal resting ECG, exercise ECG is recommended as the preferred initial diagnostic test with a class I recommendation for both men and women.
- ✔ More than 1 mm (0.1 mV) ST depression measured at 60 to 80 msec from the J point constitutes an abnormal test indicative of myocardial ischemia.
- ✔ The overall sensitivity and specificity of exercise ECG test is 45% to 50% and 85% to 90%, respectively, in patients selected appropriately for the test (ie, resting normal ECG).
- ✔ Equivocal tests (<1 mm or 0.1 mV ST depression) may require additional tests using stress echocardiography or MPI.

In addition to the diagnosis of myocardial ischemia, exercise tests can provide prognostic information.

TABLE 33.2 Contraindications to Exercise Stress Testing

Absolute Contraindications

- Acute myocardial infarction within 2 days
- Ongoing unstable angina
- Uncontrolled cardiac arrhythmia with hemodynamic compromise
- Active endocarditis
- Severe aortic stenosis
- Decompensated heart failure
- Acute pulmonary embolism, pulmonary infarction, or deep vein thrombosis
- Acute myocarditis or pericarditis
- Acute aortic dissection
- Physical disability that precludes safe and adequate testing

Relative Contraindications

- Known obstructive left main coronary artery stenosis
- Moderate-to-severe aortic stenosis with uncertain relation to symptoms
- Tachyarrhythmias with uncontrolled ventricular rates
- Acquired advanced or complete heart block
- Hypertrophic obstructive cardiomyopathy with severe resting gradient
- Recent stroke or transient ischemic attack
- Mental impairment with limited ability to cooperate
- Resting hypertension with systolic or diastolic blood pressure >200/110 mm Hg
- Uncorrected medical conditions such as significant anemia, important electrolyte imbalance, and hyperthyroidism

Reprinted with permission from Fletcher GF, Ades PA, Kligfield P, et al. Exercise standards for testing and training: a scientific statement from the American Heart Association. *Circulation.* 2013;128(8):873-934. Copyright © 2013 American Heart Association, Inc.

REFERENCES

1. Montalescot G, Sechtem U, Achenbach S, et al. 2013 ESC guidelines on the management of stable coronary artery disease. *Eur Heart J.* 2013;34:2949-3003.
2. Gulati M, Black HR, Shaw LJ, et al. The prognostic value of a nomogram for exercise capacity in women. *N Engl J Med.* 2005;353:468-475.
3. Fleg JL, Morrell CH, Bos AG, et al. Accelerated longitudinal decline of aerobic capacity in healthy older adults. *Circulation.* 2005;112:674-682.
4. Fletcher GF, Balady GJ, Amsterdam EA, et al. Exercise standards for testing and training: a statement for healthcare professionals from the American Heart Association. *Circulation.* 2001;104:1694-1740.
5. Fletcher GF, Ades PA, Kligfield P, et al. Exercise standards for testing and training: a scientific statement from the American Heart Association. *Circulation.* 2013;128:873-934.
6. Sadrzadeh Rafie AH, Sungar GW, Dewey FE, Hadley D, Myers J, Froelicher VF. Prognostic value of double product reserve. *Eur J Cardiovasc Prev Rehabil.* 2008;15:541-547.
7. Sadrzadeh Rafie AH, Dewey FE, Sungar GW, et al. Age and double product (systolic blood pressure x heart rate) reserve-adjusted modification of the Duke Treadmill Score nomogram in men. *Am J Cardiol.* 2008;102:1407-1412.
8. Villella M, Villella A, Barlera S, Franzosi MG, Maggioni AP. Prognostic significance of double product and inadequate double product response to maximal symptom-limited exercise stress testing after myocardial infarction in 6296 patients treated with thrombolytic agents. GISSI-2 Investigators. Grupo Italiano per lo Studio della Sopravvivenza nell-Infarto Miocardico. *Am Heart J.* 1999;137:443-452.
9. Duncker DJ, Bache RJ. Regulation of coronary blood flow during exercise. *Physiol Rev.* 2008;88:1009-1086.
10. Arai Y, Saul JP, Albrecht P, et al. Modulation of cardiac autonomic activity during and immediately after exercise. *Am J Physiol.* 1989;256:H132-H141.
11. Gulati M, Shaw LJ, Thisted RA, Black HR, Bairey Merz CN, Arnsdorf MF. Heart rate response to exercise stress testing in asymptomatic women: the St. James women take heart project. *Circulation.* 2010;122:130-137.
12. Tanaka H, Monahan KD, Seals DR. Age-predicted maximal heart rate revisited. *J Am Coll Cardiol.* 2001;37:153-156.
13. Anon. *Guyton and Hall Textbook of Medical Physiology.* R2 Digital Library. Accessed December 17, 2019. https://www-r2library-com.webproxy2.ouhsc.edu/resource/detail/1455770051/ch0085s1555
14. Lachman S, Terbraak MS, Limpens J, et al. The prognostic value of heart rate recovery in patients with coronary artery disease: a systematic review and meta-analysis. *Am Heart J.* 2018;199:163-169.
15. Lipinski MJ, Vetrovec GW, Froelicher VF. Importance of the first two minutes of heart rate recovery after exercise treadmill testing in predicting mortality and the presence of coronary artery disease in men. *Am J Cardiol.* 2004;93:445-449.
16. Lauer MS, Froelicher V. Abnormal heart-rate recovery after exercise. *Lancet.* 2002;360:1176-1177.
17. Vivekananthan DP, Blackstone EH, Pothier CE, et al. Heart rate recovery after exercise is a predictor of mortality, independent of the angiographic severity of coronary disease. *J Am Coll Cardiol* 2003;42:831-838.
18. Nishime EO, Cole CR, Blackstone EH, et al. Heart rate recovery and treadmill exercise score as predictors of mortality in patients referred for exercise ECG. *JAMA.* 2000;284:1392-1398.
19. Cole CR, Blackstone EH, Pashkow FJ, et al. Heart-rate recovery immediately after exercise as a predictor of mortality. *N. Engl J Med.* 1999;341:1351-1357.
20. Syme AN, Blanchard BE, Guidry MA, et al. Peak systolic blood pressure on a graded maximal exercise test and the blood pressure response to an acute bout of submaximal exercise. *Am J Cardiol.* 2006;98:938-943.
21. Borg G. Ratings of perceived exertion and heart rates during short-term cycle exercise and their use in a new cycling strength test. *Int J Sports Med.* 1982;3:153-158.
22. Fan S, Lyon CE, Savage PD, et al. Outcomes and adverse events among patients with implantable cardiac defibrillators in cardiac rehabilitation: a case-controlled study. *J Cardiopulm Rehabil Prev.* 2009;29:40-43.
23. Akutsu Y, Shinozuka A, Nishimura H, et al. Significance of ST-segment morphology noted on electrocardiography during the recovery phase after exercise in patients with ischemic heart disease as analyzed with simultaneous dual-isotope single photon emission tomography. Am. *Heart J.* 2002;144:335-342.
24. Okin PM, Ameisen O, Kligfield P. Recovery-phase patterns of ST segment depression in the heart rate domain. Identification of coronary artery disease by the rate-recovery loop. *Circulation.* 1989;80:533-541.
25. Myers J, Arena R, Franklin B, et al. Recommendations for clinical exercise laboratories: a scientific statement from the American heart association. *Circulation.* 2009;119:3144-3161.
26. Myers J, Bellin D. Ramp exercise protocols for clinical and cardiopulmonary exercise testing. *Sports Med.* 2000;30:23-29.
27. Ferguson B. ACSM's Guidelines for Exercise Testing and Prescription. 9th ed. 2014. *J Can Chiropr Assoc.* 2014;58:328.
28. Atterhög JH, Jonsson B, Samuelsson R. Exercise testing: a prospective study of complication rates. *Am Heart J.* 1979;98:572-579.
29. Rochmis P, Blackburn H. Exercise tests. A survey of procedures, safety, and litigation experience in approximately 170,000 tests. *JAMA.* 1971;217:1061-1066.
30. Stuart RJ, Ellestad MH. National survey of exercise stress testing facilities. *Chest.* 1980;77:94-97.
31. Knight JA, Laubach CA, Butcher RJ, et al. Supervision of clinical exercise testing by exercise physiologists. *Am J Cardiol.* 1995;75:390-391
32. Shaw LJ, Peterson ED, Shaw LK, et al. The use of a prognostic treadmill score in identifying diagnostic coronary disease subgroups. *Circulation.* 1998;98:1622-1630.

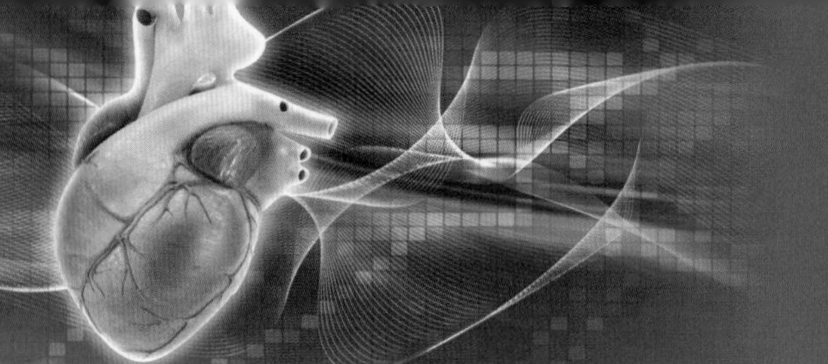

CHAPTER 34

ECHOCARDIOGRAPHY

Edwin Ho and Cynthia Taub

INTRODUCTION

Echocardiography is an imaging modality that utilizes ultrasound to visualize cardiac structure and function. It is the most commonly used imaging technique in cardiology because of the detailed information that can be obtained in a relatively short time, its widespread availability and portability, minimal inconvenience and discomfort for patients, and the lack of ionizing radiation exposure. Over time, the technology and techniques used for echocardiography have evolved to provide more detailed anatomic and cardiac functional assessment than ever before. In addition to two-dimensional and Doppler-based imaging, three-dimensional imaging and strain echocardiography are now integrated into routine clinical practice in certain settings.

Transthoracic echocardiography (TTE) involves image acquisition from outside the body through well-defined standard imaging windows and planes.[1] Transesophageal echocardiography (TEE) provides complementary information by allowing greater spatial resolution in the assessment of certain cardiac structures, such as the atrioventricular valves, because of the proximity of the imaging probe to these structures within the heart. Image acquisition, in this case, involves a transducer that is introduced into the esophagus and stomach through the mouth or nasal cavity.[2,3]

INDICATIONS

Transthoracic Imaging

TTE is the most common echocardiographic modality and has a large number of indications. These can be categorized on the basis of the cardiac structure of interest and associated disease states: left ventricle, right ventricle, atria and the interatrial septum, valves, pericardium, aortic root, aorta, and pulmonary trunk.[4,5] Alternatively, indications can also be categorized on the basis of symptoms and the potential cardiac causes within the differential diagnosis, such as chest pain, exertional dyspnea, or syncope. Special indications also include titration of device therapy, such as temporary or long-term left ventricular assist devices or for guidance of minimally invasive cardiac procedures.[6-8]

Transesophageal Imaging

TEE provides greater spatial resolution of the cardiac structures deeper within the thoracic cavity, because of closer proximity to the esophagus compared to the chest wall. Common indications include more detailed assessment of native or prosthetic valvular structure and function, evaluation for intracardiac masses, atrial and atrial appendage pathology including masses and thrombi, and assessment of the interatrial septum for atrial septal defects or a patent foramen ovale.[9-13] This technique is also being used more and more to guide transcatheter cardiac procedures, such as those performed for valve repair or replacement.[7]

Stress Echocardiography

Stress echocardiography is most commonly indicated to assess for inducible ischemia in the setting of suspected or known ischemic heart disease.[14,15] This can be performed using exercise stress with either a treadmill or supine bicycle according to standard exercise protocols. Alternatively, pharmacologic stressors such as dobutamine can also be used when exercise cannot be performed to reach a target heart rate. Dobutamine stress echocardiography can also be used to assess for myocardial viability when it is unclear if there is viable hibernating myocardium within a coronary territory.

In addition to coronary artery disease, stress echocardiography can provide clinically relevant information in nonischemic heart disease.[16] This is often used to evaluate valvular heart disease such as mitral stenosis, and exercise-induced diastolic dysfunction as well. Exercise stress echocardiography can objectively reveal exercise tolerance and assess hemodynamic changes with exercise in patients with hypertrophic cardiomyopathy, pulmonary hypertension, and nonischemic cardiomyopathy. Low-dose dobutamine stress echocardiography plays a role in clarifying the degree of aortic stenosis in low-flow, low-gradient aortic stenosis with decreased left ventricular ejection fraction (EF).[17-19] Lastly, exercise capacity and myocardial performance augmentation may also be relevant in the diagnosis and risk stratification of cardiomyopathy such as peripartum cardiomyopathy.

Point-of-Care Ultrasound

Point-of-care ultrasound (POCUS) is becoming more commonly used with the miniaturization of echocardiography hardware and advancements in portable computing ability. It is used to provide additional diagnostic information or to monitor response to therapy during the assessment of acute illness, such as in the emergency department or intensive care unit. Examples of the utility of POCUS include assessment of volume status, pericardial or pleural effusions, evaluation of left ventricular function and wall motion, assessment for right ventricular dysfunction associated with pulmonary embolism, or screening for mechanical complications of acute myocardial infarction.[20]

ANATOMIC CONSIDERATIONS

Acoustic Windows

Transthoracic

Imaging windows and views for TTE have been well defined and described (**Figure 34.1**).[1] Study protocols often begin in the left lateral decubitus position with parasternal images, taken from the anterior chest just lateral to the left side of the sternum. This imaging window is found in the third intercostal space, but higher or lower windows can be used in certain situations. Next, apical images are taken by moving the transducer to the apex of the heart, typically near the left anterior axillary line in the fifth or sixth intercostal space. Subcostal images are taken from the upper abdomen just inferior to the xiphoid process and angulating the transducer head cranially, with the patient supine and abdominal muscles relaxed. The suprasternal window is located above the sternal notch at the lower part of the anterior neck, with the transducer head angled caudally. Additional imaging windows can be used in special circumstances. For example, a right parasternal window on the right side of the sternum can provide better visualization of the proximal ascending aorta.

In each acoustic window, the imaging plane can be adjusted to visualize specific cardiac structures by manual rotation of the transducer, or electronically through the control console if using a three-dimensional matrix transducer. Standard imaging planes are outlined in Figure 34.1.

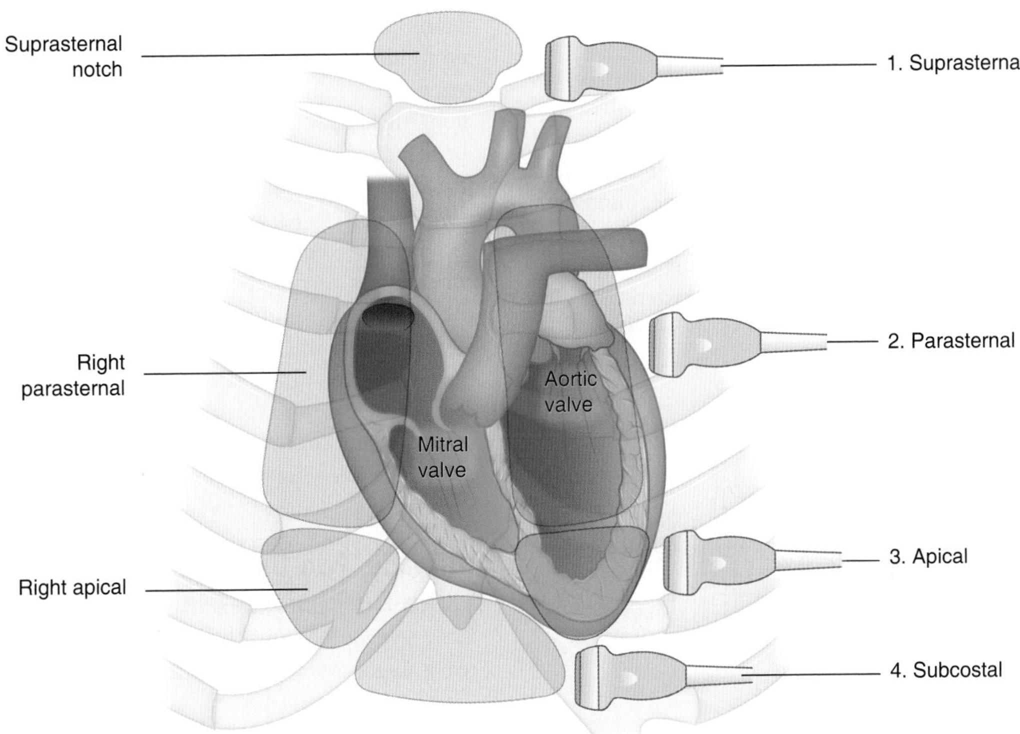

1. Suprasternal: above sternal notch, lower part of anterior neck

2. Parasternal: usual window left third intercostal space (left, unless otherwise stated)

3. Apical: near left anterior axillary line in fifth or sixth intercostal space (left, unless otherwise stated)

4. Subcostal: upper abdomen just inferior to xiphoid process (patient supine, relaxed)

FIGURE 34.1 Standard acoustic windows for transthoracic echocardiography.

Transesophageal

Typical imaging windows for TEE have also been well described (**Figure 34.2B**).[2] Most images are taken from the mid-esophageal position, when the transducer head is located directly behind the left atrium and faces the apex of the heart. From this position, cardiac structures can be seen in different planes by rotating the imaging plane angle on a three-dimensional matrix transducer, adjustment of the probe deeper or shallower in the esophagus, rotating the entire probe, and by gentle adjustments of the distal probe position through ante-, retro-, left-, and right flexion (**Figure 34.2A**). Additional images are also taken from the transgastric window, when the transducer head is passed through the gastroesophageal junction into the stomach. Modified windows higher or lower in the esophagus can also be used for more detailed assessment of specific cardiac structures.

FUNDAMENTALS OF ECHOCARDIOGRAPHY

Physical Principles, Instrumentation, and Basic Ultrasound Physics

Echocardiography is based on the physical principles of ultrasound imaging. Piezoelectric crystals are arranged in a linear or matrix orientation inside a transducer and emit high-frequency (1-10 MHz) sound waves. These waves travel into the body through direct contact, often also assisted using viscous gel that facilitates sound wave transmission. When these sound waves travel through the body, they interact with tissues and reflect back toward the transducer in a variable manner depending on the depth of the structure and reflecting characteristics. Once received at the transducer, the reflected signal is processed into visual images to allow for interpretation. This is possible because the speed of sound can be used to calculate the depth of a structure that is reflecting the signal. The intensity of a reflection is also processed when an image is created. Because sound waves travel poorly through air and bone, the lungs and bony structures can cause significant shadowing where structures cannot be seen.

The axial spatial resolution of a single ultrasound beam is related to the wavelength of the emitted waves. Wavelength (λ) is inversely proportional to frequency (f) when the velocity of ultrasound propagation (c) is constant. In soft tissues, $c \approx 1540$ m/s, and therefore $f \approx c/\lambda$. Accordingly, higher frequency sound waves will produce shorter wavelengths and better resolution. Unfortunately, higher frequency waves are not able to penetrate tissue as effectively and may not be usable if the target structure is deeper. Harmonic imaging (as opposed to fundamental imaging) is based on the principle that tissue which is insonified by ultrasound beams can vibrate at twice the frequency of the source ultrasound waves. These second-order harmonics are received by the transducer and greatly increase signal-to-noise ratio because they are less prone to acoustic interference.

Overall image quality depends on several factors. Lateral resolution is affected by the number of scan lines used to generate an image frame, and is often maximized when the scan sector width is minimized. Ultrasound beams also vary in width along their path depending on the timing of the piezoelectric elements that emit the beam. This narrowest point can be adjusted and defines a depth where lateral resolution is further optimized.

Because sequential frames of a two-dimensional ultrasound image are created by repeated pulses that create scan lines, the temporal resolution, or time required between one frame and the next, will vary depending on the number of pulses needed (related to the scan sector width) and time needed for reflected pulses to be received (related to the scan sector depth). Narrower and shallower scan sectors will increase the temporal resolution, allowing fast-moving cardiac structures to be better visualized.

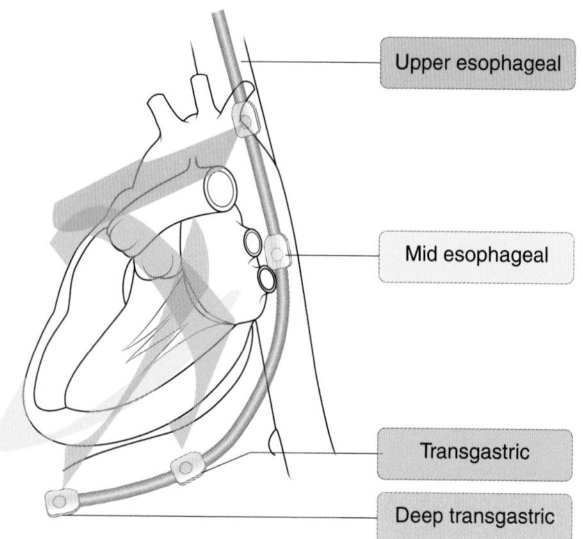

FIGURE 34.2 Probe manipulation options used to obtain transesophageal echocardiographic views.

M-Mode, Two-Dimensional, and Three-Dimensional Imaging

Early generations of echocardiography equipment transmitted a single sound beam only, resulting in a single scan line. This could be displayed in "A-mode" (amplitude), where amplitude of reflections was depicted as spikes from a baseline. "B-mode" maps the amplitude of reflections into a grayscale depiction and represents the ultrasound images we are familiar with currently (**Figure 34.3A**). Two-dimensional B-mode imaging with a wider field of view than a single scan line is possible because modern transducers contain numerous piezoelectric elements that will electronically steer the sound beam to sweep the scan line and reconstruct an image based on the signal received from each scan line position. "M-mode" (motion) maintains a single scan line only, but maps the reflected signal using a grayscale map over time on the horizontal axis (**Figure 34.3B**). The advantage of M-mode imaging is its superior temporal resolution.

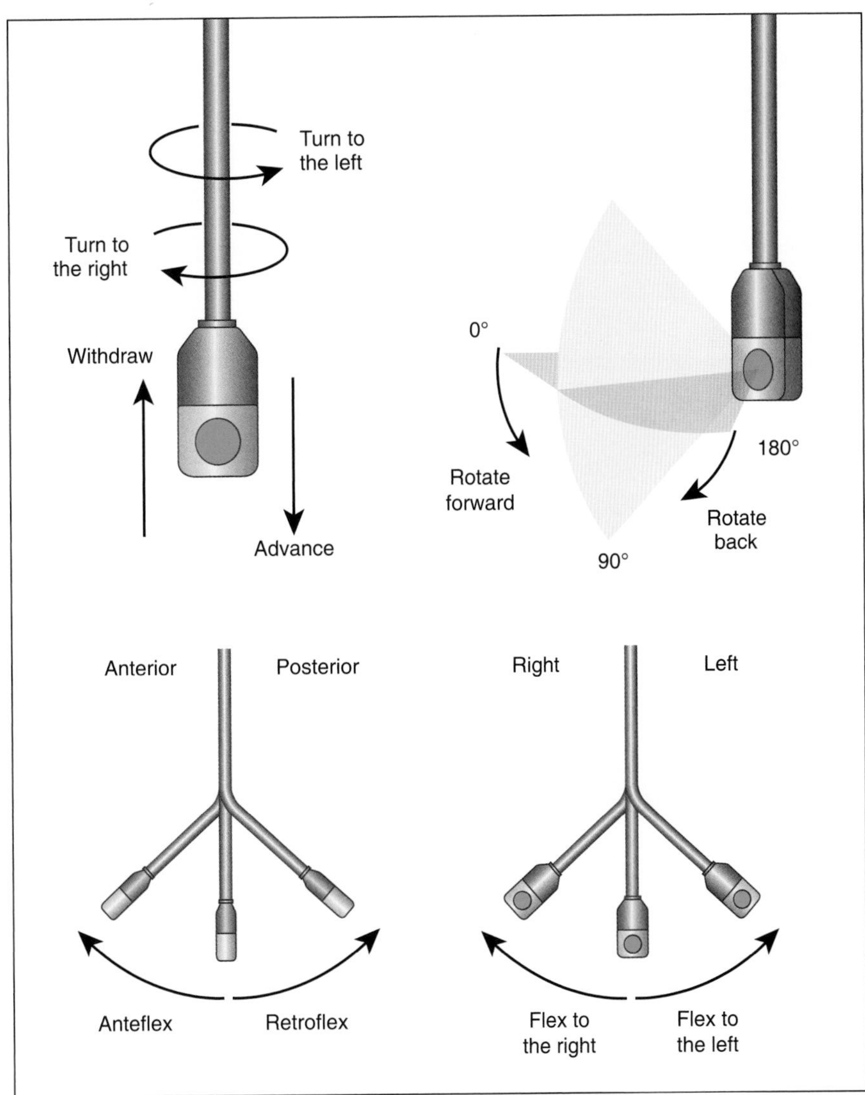

FIGURE 34.3 Standard imaging windows for transesophageal echocardiography.

Modern ultrasound equipment uses transducers containing a large number of emitting and receiving elements that emit and receive ultrasound pulses in an ordered sequence, rather than in a continuous manner. This sequential pulse emission repeats over and over to create moving images, and, therefore, the maximum temporal resolution has an upper limit. The speed of sound in tissue and desired depth of visualization both affect the "pulse repetition frequency (PRF)," or pulse generation rate, because adequate time is required to receive reflected sound waves.

Three-dimensional echocardiography has been made possible because of the modification of transducer crystals into a matrix array (gridlike arrangement) so that sequential pulse emission can occur in a two-dimensional plane instead of only in a linear manner (**Figure 34.3C,D**). Temporal resolution is described as a volume rate because three-dimensional ultrasound volumes are generated instead of two-dimensional image frames.

Doppler Ultrasound

Doppler echocardiography is based on the Doppler principle: $f = \frac{2vf_0 \times \cos\theta}{c}$, where f = Doppler shift frequency, v = velocity of target, f_0 = frequency of transmitted ultrasound beam, θ = angle between the ultrasound beam and direction of flow, and c is velocity of ultrasound in blood. In other words, motion will modify the perceived frequency of a sound wave from that object. This is due to compression of the waves if the object is moving toward the receiver and stretching if moving away. In echocardiography, this principle is commonly applied to sound reflections coming from moving red blood cells. The observed frequency shift can be converted into a velocity using the Doppler equation, and this information can then be displayed two-dimensionally using a color map (**Figure 34.4A**) or as a plot of velocity versus time at one specific sampling location (**Figure 34.4B**) or along an entire line of interrogation (**Figure 34.4C**).

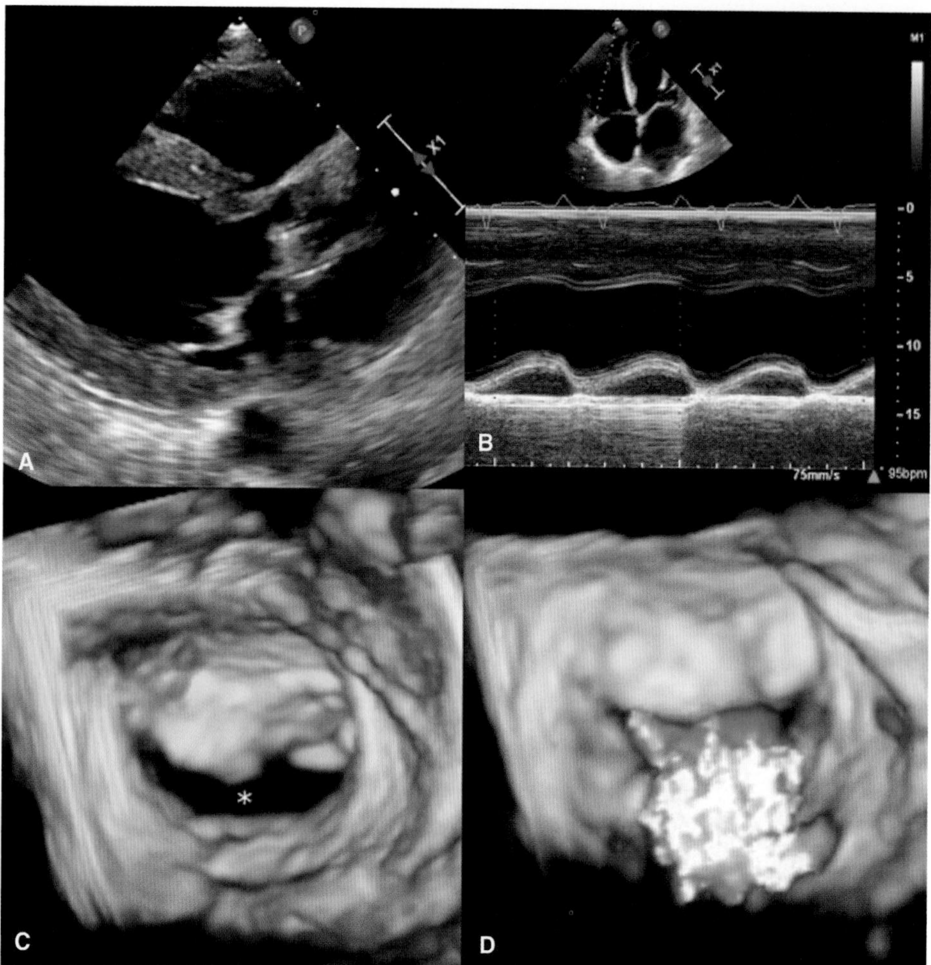

FIGURE 34.4 **(A)** Grayscale B-mode echocardiographic image of the parasternal long-axis view of the heart; **(B)** M-mode echocardiography showing a single scan line over time; **(C)** three-dimensional echocardiography of the mitral valve (asterisk) viewed from the left atrium looking down at the valve (anterior toward the top of the image); **(D)** three-dimensional color Doppler echocardiography of the mitral valve with a large central jet of mitral regurgitation viewed from the left atrium looking down at the valve (anterior toward the top of the image)

Pulsed-Wave Doppler Echocardiography

Pulsed-wave Doppler utilizes separated pulses of ultrasound waves with an adequate time window to receive reflections (PRF) to define velocity at a specified depth and location within the heart. This is typically used to assess blood velocity at the sample volume (location of interest) defined by the operator. Because the PRF has an upper limit based on the depth of the sample volume, the maximum velocity that can be interrogated is also limited. This is due to the fact that the degree of Doppler frequency shift is greater for faster objects and needs to be sampled faster than the PRF may allow. The Nyquist limit is the maximum velocity that can be accurately determined using pulsed-wave Doppler, and is typically around 1.5 m/s. Beyond this velocity, the specific velocity of the reflection is uncertain.

Continuous-Wave Doppler echocardiography

Continuous-wave Doppler is performed by continuous emission and reception of ultrasound waves along a single line. Depth of reflections cannot be determined in this case because continuous ultrasound emission means the timing of a received reflected signal cannot be used to determine the depth of origin. However, this technique removes the Nyquist limit restriction of pulsed-wave Doppler, allowing essentially the maximum velocity across a path to be determined.

Color Doppler Echocardiography

Color Doppler imaging is based on the same principles of pulsed-wave Doppler, except that an entire region of interest is assessed instead of a specific small sample volume. This means the temporal resolution must be lower. Average velocities and direction of movement are displayed using a color map superimposed on grayscale two-dimensional imaging (**Figure 34.4A**) or three-dimensional imaging (**Figure 34.3D**).

As with pulsed-wave Doppler, this technique is subject to a Nyquist limit. Velocities are often depicted on a color map as gradations of red and blue, the colors typically used to demonstrate blood movement toward and away from the transducer, respectively.

Tissue Doppler Echocardiography

Tissue Doppler is another pulsed-wave Doppler–based technique, but limits the velocities interrogated to much lower values than with typical pulse or color Doppler. Using this technique allows for velocity of the myocardium to be assessed at specific locations of cardiac structures (more often at the base of the left ventricle and right ventricle).

Strain Echocardiography

Strain imaging monitors tissue deformation over time to assess myocardial function of the different cardiac chambers. In echocardiography, this is typically done using speckle tracking, where bright points within the myocardium are tracked using specialized software to calculate the change in distance between the two points over time.[21,22]

Strain of the left ventricle can be evaluated in the multiple axes of cardiac motion, including longitudinal (base to apex), circumferential (clockwise or counterclockwise twisting in the short axis), and radial (movement relative to the center of the left ventricle in short axis). Strain imaging can also be performed on other myocardial walls, including the right ventricle, left atrium, and right atrium.

Ultrasound-Enhancing Agents

Echocardiography using ultrasound-enhancing agents is based on the principle that strong ultrasound reflectors can be injected into the blood pool to allow for better visualization of cardiac structures or to more easily evaluate flow patterns.

On the right side of the heart, agitated saline containing small air bubbles is injected through the venous system. When the small air bubbles reach the right side of the heart, a high-intensity signal fills the chambers and appears bright on the echocardiogram. The air bubbles are normally filtered in the pulmonary capillaries and do not appear in the left side of the heart. Presence of bubbles in left-sided chambers raises the possibility of right-to-left shunting, which may be intracardiac or intrapulmonary.

To introduce reflectors into the blood pool on the left side of the heart, microbubbles that are smaller than the pulmonary capillaries must be used to allow entry to the left atrium and ventricle. Several commercial products that consist of small inert gas microbubbles are available. These are imaged using specialized settings (low power) compared to conventional two-dimensional echocardiography because the microbubbles are fragile and are rapidly destroyed by ultrasound waves. Echocardiography with ultrasound-enhancing agents of the left ventricle has allowed for improved visualization of the left ventricular wall motion and EF assessment when imaging windows are difficult, improved detection of apical aneurysms and thrombus, and may be useful in assessing myocardial perfusion.[23]

CLINICAL APPLICATIONS

Methodology

Ischemic Heart Disease

Ischemic heart disease can be assessed by echocardiography to evaluate abnormalities in wall motion and overall left ventricular EF.[24] Cardiac ischemia or infarction may create a regional wall motion, abnormality reflecting the perfusion pattern of the coronary artery. For example, the left anterior descending (LAD) artery typically supplies the anterior wall, apex, and anterior septum with blood. The right coronary artery typically supplies the inferior septum and inferior wall. The left circumflex artery typically supplies the lateral wall. The inferolateral wall can be supplied by either the right coronary or the left circumflex artery.

It is ideal to evaluate wall motion of the left ventricular wall segments in both short-axis (parasternal windows) and long-axis (apical windows) planes to allow assessment in two orthogonal planes. To facilitate standardized communication of wall motion abnormalities, a 16-segment model of the left ventricle can be used and includes six basal and mid segments corresponding to the walls (anterior, anterolateral, inferolateral, inferior, inferoseptal, and anteroseptal) and four apical segments (anterior, lateral, inferior, and septal). A 17-segment model includes the addition of an apical cap representing the tip of the left ventricular apex. Ultrasound-enhancing agents can be used in the setting of difficult imaging to increase the accuracy of wall motion assessment.[23]

Depending on the degree and pattern of wall motion abnormalities, the overall left ventricular EF may be affected variably (the adult normal has been defined as ≥53%). This parameter is defined as the difference between end-diastolic volume (EDV) and end-systolic volume (ESV) divided by the EDV: $EF = \frac{EDV - ESV}{EDV}$ and can be estimated through multiple techniques by echocardiography. In the past, formulae with associated significant geometric assumptions of the left ventricular cavity were used, such as the Teichholz method that estimates EF using only end-diastolic and end-systolic short-axis diameter measurements of the left ventricular cavity. It is now more common to use techniques that make fewer geometric assumptions, most commonly by the Simpson's method of stacked discs. Simpson's method requires the endocardial border to be traced in end diastole and end systole in either two orthogonal planes or in three planes. This information is used to mathematically generate a series of stacked disks that roughly follow the true contour of the left ventricular chamber and provide a more accurate estimated volume. Three-dimensional echocardiographic assessment of left ventricular volumes and EF has the advantage of avoiding geometric assumptions about the shape of the left ventricular cavity.[25] However, because this technique requires accurate tracking of the endocardium, adequate image quality is mandatory. Abnormalities in the left ventricular EF are typically divided between mild (EF 40%-52%), moderate (30%-39%), and severe (<30%).

Aneurysm formation within the LV can occur following infarction, and is defined as a shape deformity that persists throughout the cardiac cycle, in contrast to wall motion abnormalities that are only visible during systole because of abnormal contractility. Apical aneurysms are best assessed using contrast echocardiography, which also increases the sensitivity for detection of associated intracardiac thrombus.

SECTION 2

Ischemic myocardium before infarction follows the ischemic cascade, which describes a series of abnormalities and findings that occur in sequential order with myocardial ischemia. The initial stages of metabolic dysfunction cannot be assessed by echocardiography, but another early sign before systolic dysfunction is diastolic dysfunction. This is because myocardial relaxation is an active process that requires energy. Although there are limits to the accuracy of diastolic function assessment by echocardiography, it is an important consideration in the assessment of ischemic heart disease. Various Doppler parameters, including early diastolic tissue Doppler velocities (e′) of the septal and lateral left ventricular base, the ratio of these tissue velocities relative to the mitral inflow velocity (E/e′), left atrial size, and evidence of pulmonary hypertension (eg, elevated tricuspid regurgitation velocity) are used to estimate left ventricular filling pressures and associated grades of diastolic dysfunction.[26]

Both left ventricular systolic and diastolic dysfunction can be assessed at rest and for inducible abnormalities during stress with stress echocardiography. The standard target heart rate to achieve a diagnostic test for inducible ischemia is 85% of maximum predicted heart rate based on age.[14]

Associated functional mitral regurgitation with ischemic heart disease should be noted and quantified.[10] This is especially clinically relevant because significant functional mitral regurgitation is being increasingly recognized as being prognostically relevant and potentially modifiable.[27]

Valvular Heart Disease

Valvular heart disease represents a common indication for echocardiography.[5] In this case, both detailed morphologic evaluation of the structure and assessment of valve function are important.[1,10,28]

Morphologic evaluation begins by assessing whether the structure of the valve leaflets and associated valvular apparatus is normal or abnormal. Abnormalities may be congenital and present since birth or acquired through the patient's lifetime. Abnormal valve motion is important to note, and can vary from excessive leaflet motion or restricted motion in diastole, systole, or both phases of the cardiac cycle.

Functional evaluation of the valve is then performed using the various modes of Doppler echocardiography. Color Doppler reveals whether there is flow acceleration and turbulence across a valve in the forward or backward directions, which is usually associated with stenosis or regurgitation, respectively. Pulsed-wave and continuous-wave Doppler interrogations confirm the presence of valvular stenosis or regurgitation and establish disease severity. Doppler assessment of valve dysfunction includes qualitative, semiquantitative, and quantitative parameters.

Aortic stenosis is a common valvular pathology assessed well by echocardiography.[28] An underlying tricuspid (normal) or bicuspid (congenital abnormality) morphology should be noted if visible, and is best seen in the parasternal short-axis view of the aortic valve (AV). Other structural abnormalities that are visible include the degree of leaflet thickening and calcification, as well as associated leaflet mobility restriction in systole. Flow acceleration across the valve is demonstrated using color Doppler. Continuous-wave Doppler can identify the blood flow velocity across the narrowed valve and calculate the peak gradient, ΔP, from the maximum velocity and the mean gradient using the integral of velocity over time, based on the modified Bernoulli's equation: $\Delta P = 4(V_2^2 - V_1^2)$, where V_1 is velocity preorifice and V_2 is velocity postorifice. In most clinical scenarios, V_1^2 is significantly less than V_2^2 and can be ignored; thus, $\Delta P = 4V^2$. AV area can then be calculated using the continuity equation, which is based on the principle of conservation of mass, in that flow or volume through the left ventricular outflow tract (LVOT) in systole must equal that through the AV in the same cardiac cycle: $AVA_{AREA} = \frac{LVOT_{AREA} \times LVOT_{VTI}}{AV_{VTI}}$, whereas $LVOT_{VTI}$ and AV_{VTI} are the instantaneous velocities integrated over the ejection time obtained at the LVOT by pulsed-wave Doppler and across the AV orifice by continuous-wave Doppler, respectively.

Cutoffs for severe aortic stenosis can be found in the American College of Cardiology (ACC) and American Heart Association (AHA) valvular heart disease guidelines as well as imaging guidelines published jointly by the European Association of Cardiovascular Imaging (EACVI) and American Society of Echocardiography (ASE).[17,28] Each measure should be interpreted carefully, especially in isolation, because each has its own caveats when the cutoffs may not apply because of factors such as flow state.

The approach to mitral stenosis is similar. Valve morphology is particularly important because leaflet tip thickening, commissural fusion, and anterior leaflet doming in diastole are classic findings for rheumatic mitral stenosis. This is in comparison to mitral inflow restriction due to mitral annular calcification, where calcium deposition is predominantly at the annulus and leaflet base to mid body with relative sparing of the leaflet tips. An inflow gradient can be visually assessed with color Doppler, but then is best evaluated using continuous-wave Doppler. This provides a mean gradient when the velocity-time integral of diastolic flow is traced. Valve area can be assessed through multiple methods. Direct planimetry (tracing) can be performed if the imaging plane is accurately placed at the leaflet tips. The area can also be calculated using the inflow velocity change over time in early diastole (pressure half-time method) or by the proximal isovelocity surface area (PISA) method, which calculates the orifice area using the continuity equation. Echocardiographic criteria for severe mitral stenosis has also been defined in the ACC/AHA valvular heart disease guidelines and EACVI/ASE guidelines.[17,29]

Mitral regurgitation is again assessed by structure followed by function. Morphologic leaflet abnormalities such as excess tissue or rupture chordae in myxomatous disease or calcification should be noted. Leaflet motion evaluation is very important in evaluation of mitral regurgitation, because it differentiates causes of primary mitral regurgitation related to excessive motion, such as flail leaflet or prolapse, from causes of functional mitral regurgitation due to restricted motion, such as apical tethering related to left ventricular dilation or dysfunction. Color Doppler can identify the presence, size, and location of the regurgitant jet. Pulsed-wave and continuous-wave Doppler can then be used to quantify the degree of regurgitation using various quantitative techniques, such as the PISA method, that calculates the effective regurgitant orifice area (ERO_{area}) as $EROA = \frac{2\pi r^2 \times V_n}{V_{max}}$; whereas $2\pi r^2$ represents the surface area of the hemispheric-shaped flow convergence color Doppler shell located in the LV proximal to the regurgitant orifice, derived from the measured flow convergence radius (R) in cm^2; V_N = velocity at the radius of hemispheric shell (color aliased velocity or Nyquist limit) (cm/s); V_{MAX} = peak velocity across the stenotic orifice.[10]

Prosthetic valve evaluation follows a similar structure and function evaluation strategy. The valve leaflets may be difficult to visualize because of shadowing from other parts of the prosthesis and may require TEE to best assess structure and function. Color Doppler, pulsed-wave Doppler, and continuous-wave Doppler are used to evaluate hemodynamic performance and to detect prosthetic valve dysfunction. The effective orifice area can be calculated using the continuity equation similar to native valves, and is an important parameter in helping distinguish between elevated valve gradients with normal valve function, typically related to high flow through the prosthesis, or elevated valve gradients due to abnormal valve function.[11]

Infective endocarditis and associated mechanical complications in both native and prosthetic valves may be visible with TTE if the vegetations or complications are obvious. In many cases, they are not visible or image quality is inadequate; TEE is needed for improved diagnostic accuracy. Careful evaluation of the entire valve structure by performing sweeps of the valve through any available method is important to maximize sensitivity for detecting vegetations.

Heart Failure and Cardiomyopathies

Dilated nonischemic cardiomyopathy is assessed by echocardiography with a focus on left ventricular systolic and diastolic function, including wall motion pattern and left ventricular EF. Typically, there is diffuse hypokinesis compared to the regionality associated with coronary perfusion territories seen in ischemic cardiomyopathy. Contrast echocardiography can similarly increase the accuracy of wall motion assessment and left ventricular volume calculation. Stress echocardiography is used to rule out inducible ischemia and assess for augmentation of contractility in response to exercise. Associated functional mitral regurgitation is important to note, including quantification if it is suspected to be severe.

Hypertrophic cardiomyopathy is well assessed by echocardiography, which is able to evaluate the pattern of left ventricular hypertrophy and assess for associated intracavitary obstruction or dynamic LVOT obstruction caused by systolic anterior motion of the mitral valve leaflets.[30] LVOT obstruction may be present at rest in some cases, but may need to be provoked during the Valsalva strain phase. The pattern seen by continuous wave Doppler is a late systolic peaking "dagger"-shaped signal and provides the peak gradient from the maximum velocity. Care must be taken to avoid contamination of the signal from mitral regurgitation, which can cause overestimation of the degree of obstruction. Exercise stress echocardiography, ideally using a supine bicycle, can evaluate for provoked or increased obstruction and blood pressure response to exercise.[16]

Restrictive cardiomyopathies will typically have the pattern of marked biatrial enlargement, low left ventricular tissue Doppler velocities, and marked diastolic dysfunction including a restrictive Doppler filling pattern.[26]

Arrhythmogenic right ventricular cardiomyopathy has specific echocardiographic criteria including right ventricular dilation on various views and presence of focal right ventricular free wall aneurysms.[31] These can be seen with TTE if imaging windows are adequate and focused right ventricular views are obtained.

Pericardial Disease

Pericardial effusions appear as a dark, echolucent space consistent with the pericardial space. Echogenic fibrin deposition, hematoma, or mass may also be seen. Depending on the intrapericardial pressure and cardiac chamber pressures, varying degrees of compression of the lower pressure right-sided chambers may be observed.

Signs of tamponade physiology by echocardiography include sustained right atrial compression/inversion, right ventricular free wall and/or left ventricular compression, significant early diastolic inflow velocity variation across the mitral and tricuspid valves relative to respiration, and significant change in LVOT flow relative to respiration, usually in the context of inferior vena cava plethora.[32] These signs must also be assessed in the context of the estimated right atrial and pulmonary pressures, which may mask signs of tamponade if significantly elevated.

TTE is commonly used to guide percutaneous pericardiocentesis, by identifying the optimal window, providing live guidance at the time of the procedure, confirming location of the catheter with injection of agitated saline, and allowing immediate reassessment of effusion size and tamponade physiology as drainage is occurring.

Pericardial constriction hemodynamics can be similarly evaluated through Doppler echocardiography with some important differences. The relative septal and lateral tissue Doppler velocity pattern is often reversed from normal ("annulus reversus," where the septal velocity is higher than the lateral) because the typically more mobile lateral annulus has reduced motion due to the thickened adjacent pericardium while the septum is not affected. As in tamponade, there is also mitral and tricuspid inflow velocity variability relative to respiration due to increased ventricular interdependence and reduced transmission of intrathoracic pressure changes to the cardiac chambers from the thickened pericardial sac, but they are smaller in magnitude.

Effusive-constrictive disease is typically seen in the setting of chronic pericardial effusion or disease, and will demonstrate similar Doppler findings of constrictive physiology in the presence of a pericardial effusion.

Cardiac Masses

Intracardiac and valvular masses can be assessed with TTE, but are often better visualized using TEE. Compared to computed tomography and cardiac magnetic resonance imaging, echocardiography has the advantage of higher temporal resolution to detect small, highly mobile valvular masses such as papillary fibroelastomas. Microbubble contrast echocardiography may provide additional information about mass vascularity.

Congenital Heart Disease

Congenital heart disease is often well evaluated by echocardiography. Common pathologies such as a bicuspid AV or atrial septal defect are readily assessed using standard transthoracic imaging protocols. Complex congenital heart disease, however, may require additional imaging views, specialized protocols, and trained readers to properly evaluate unrepaired or repaired disease.[33–36]

Evaluation of Mechanical Assist Devices and Transplant

Echocardiography can play an important role in evaluation and titration of mechanical assist devices.[8] Short-term ventricular assist devices are commonly used for left ventricular and, occasionally, for right ventricular support. Device positioning and interference with normal valve function are typically easily assessed using transthoracic imaging.

Long-term ventricular assist is routinely followed using TTE. Underlying left or right ventricular systolic function and serial changes over time are important to assess. The degree of AV opening in left ventricular assist devices can also be evaluated because this may have implications on formation of left ventricular thrombus or loss of normal AV function over time. Flow parameters of the left ventricular assist device can be adjusted with echocardiographic assistance using specialized ramp study protocols, which evaluate cardiac size and function at various flow rates, to identify optimal device settings based on left ventricular size and AV opening.

Posttransplant heart evaluation by echocardiography is similar to comprehensive evaluation of cardiac structure and function of a native heart. Particular attention is given to left ventricular systolic and diastolic function as well as valvular heart disease. The atria may be enlarged compared to native hearts because of the anastomosis between native and graft tissue.

Acute and Chronic Aortic Syndromes

Aortic disease including dilatation and aneurysms can be evaluated by echocardiography, but often requires additional imaging windows and potentially a combination of transthoracic and transesophageal imaging.[37] TTE is limited to evaluation of the proximal ascending aorta, aortic arch, proximal descending aorta, and limited segments of the descending thoracic and abdominal aorta. Care must be taken to avoid imaging the aorta obliquely in short axis, which may overestimate the size, or imaging off the center of the vessel in long axis, which may underestimate the size. Additional imaging windows, such as the right parasternal window, should also be added to image more of the aorta. TEE can be complementary, but in the stable setting of dilation alone, provides less complete evaluation compared to computed tomography.

Aortic dissection is visualized in echocardiography as a linear dissection flap, but care must be taken to ensure that the structure is not a linear artifact because of the limitations of ultrasound imaging. Color Doppler can be used to distinguish a true flap from artifact because aortic dissections often result in differential flow between the true and false lumens. Because TEE provides higher spatial resolution, more complete imaging of the thoracic aorta, and the esophagus is in very close proximity to most of the aorta, it is an ideal imaging modality to assess for dissection if urgent computed tomography imaging is not available or possible. Simultaneous biplane imaging is very helpful when assessing the aorta because of the orthogonal imaging planes, which allows for more comprehensive and faster assessment. Penetrating aortic ulcers and aortic wall hematomas are usually best seen by TEE because of the higher spatial resolution, and appear as a disruption to the aortic intima and media without an overt visible flap.

Evaluation of the Stroke Patient

Stroke is a common indication of echocardiography. Specifically, it is clinically relevant to exclude a cardioembolic cause.[12] In these situations, a complete evaluation of cardiac structure and function is indicated. Specific etiologies that should be ruled out include left ventricular aneurysm and associated thrombus, valvular masses, right-to-left shunting due to an atrial septal defect or patent foramen ovale, as well as left atrial masses or thrombus. If clinical suspicion is high for a cardioembolic cause or there are questionable findings by TTE, TEE is more sensitive for many of these abnormalities. Left atrial appendage thrombus is generally not well assessed by TTE, and is therefore best assessed using TEE.[2] However, because anticoagulation is often clinically indicated regardless of imaging evaluation for thrombus, it is usually only performed if cardioversion is being attempted without an established period of anticoagulation.

Evaluation for a patent foramen ovale or atrial septal defect should be performed using agitated saline contrast echocardiography for both transthoracic and transesophageal studies. If a resting bubble injection is negative, then the injection should be repeated with a Valsalva maneuver because there may be only transient right-to-left shunting that occurs in the release phase in the presence of a patent foramen ovale.[13]

Clinical Case Examples

Case 1: Coronary artery disease (left anterior descending [LAD] territory wall motion abnormalities)—**Figure 34.5**
Case 2: Dilated cardiomyopathy (spherical remodeling of the left ventricle [LV] with severe systolic dysfunction)—**Figure 34.6**
Case 3: Aortic stenosis (severe calcific aortic stenosis)—**Figure 34.7**
Case 4: Primary mitral regurgitation (flail P2 segment with severe eccentric regurgitation)—**Figure 34.8**
Case 5: Flail P2 segment of the mitral valve—**Figure 34.9**

LIMITATIONS OF ECHOCARDIOGRAPHY

The major limitation of echocardiography is related to imaging windows, because it is ultrasound based and requires adequate transmission of sound waves to the cardiac structures and adequate reflection back to the transducer. An obese body habitus, musculoskeletal abnormalities affecting the chest wall, and barriers to sound transmission such as bone, air (lungs), and prosthetic material (cosmetic implants) can all result in technically difficult studies with suboptimal images or even nondiagnostic imaging. This can be partially overcome using contrast echocardiography, but this generally only improves visualization of left ventricular wall motion and still requires an adequate imaging window. TEE is generally more consistent with respect to image quality, but variability still exists depending on the relative position of the esophagus to the cardiac structures, shadowing from intracardiac structures, and the size of the left atrium. Various head, neck, and esophageal pathologies may be prohibitive for the performance of TEE, as described subsequently.

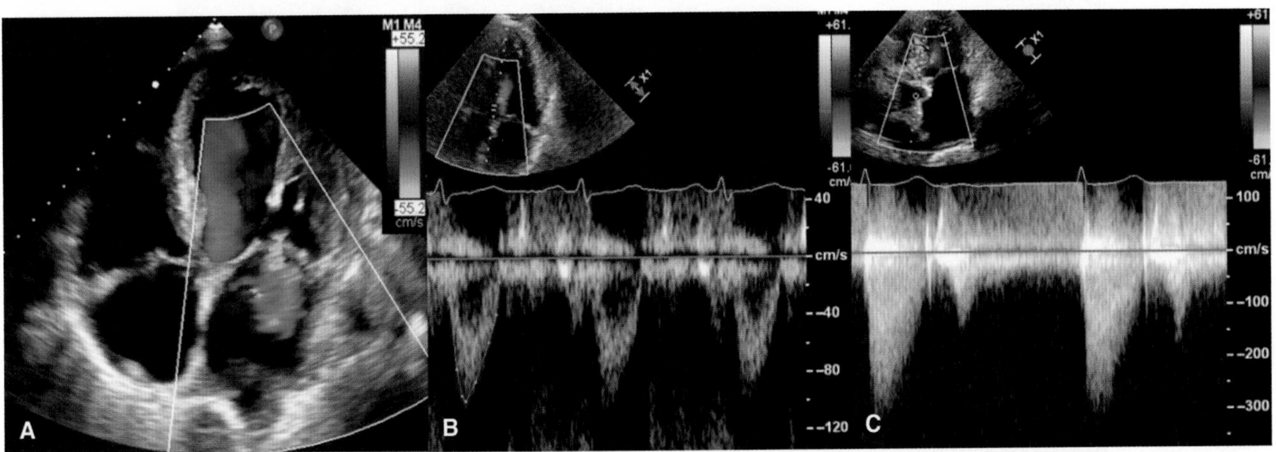

FIGURE 34.5 **(A)** Color Doppler imaging of the apical four-chamber view of the heart superimposing calculated velocities of blood pool regions on top of a grayscale two-dimensional image of the cardiac structures; **(B)** spectral Doppler plot of velocity over time using pulsed-wave Doppler, where velocities at a specific sampling region are evaluated; **(C)** spectral Doppler plot of velocity over time using continuous-wave Doppler, where velocities along a line of interrogation are evaluated.

Imaging artifacts are an important limitation in all ultrasound-based imaging modalities including echocardiography and are related to the physics of sound transmission that can result in misinterpreted signals that return to the receiver.[38] Common artifacts include reverberation, mirror, refraction, side lobe, and beam width. Reverberation and mirror artifacts produce the appearance of false objects at a different distance relative to the transducer compared to the source of the artifact because they are related to the reflection of sound waves in tissues. Refraction artifacts are located at the same distance from the transducer as the source of the artifact. Side lobe and beam width artifacts are properties of the ultrasound beam itself and are also located at the same depth as the source.

SPECIAL CONSIDERATIONS AND CONTRAINDICATIONS

Echocardiography is predominantly limited by the quality of imaging windows, as previously mentioned. TTE, in particular, does not have any specific contraindications outside of lack of patient consent or skin and soft-tissue abnormalities at the location of imaging windows. Even in the latter situation, modified imaging windows or a limited study allow TTE to be used.

TEE contraindications are most commonly related to pathologies in the upper gastrointestinal tract where the transducer is placed. Esophageal pathologies such as strictures, active bleeding, ulcers, varices, and diverticula are examples of absolute and relative contraindications. Because TEE is also typically performed with some degree of sedation, any barriers to safety, such as lack of monitoring, lack of intravenous access, high risk of respiratory compromise or hemodynamic instability may require involvement of anesthesiologists or gastroenterologists before TEE can be performed.

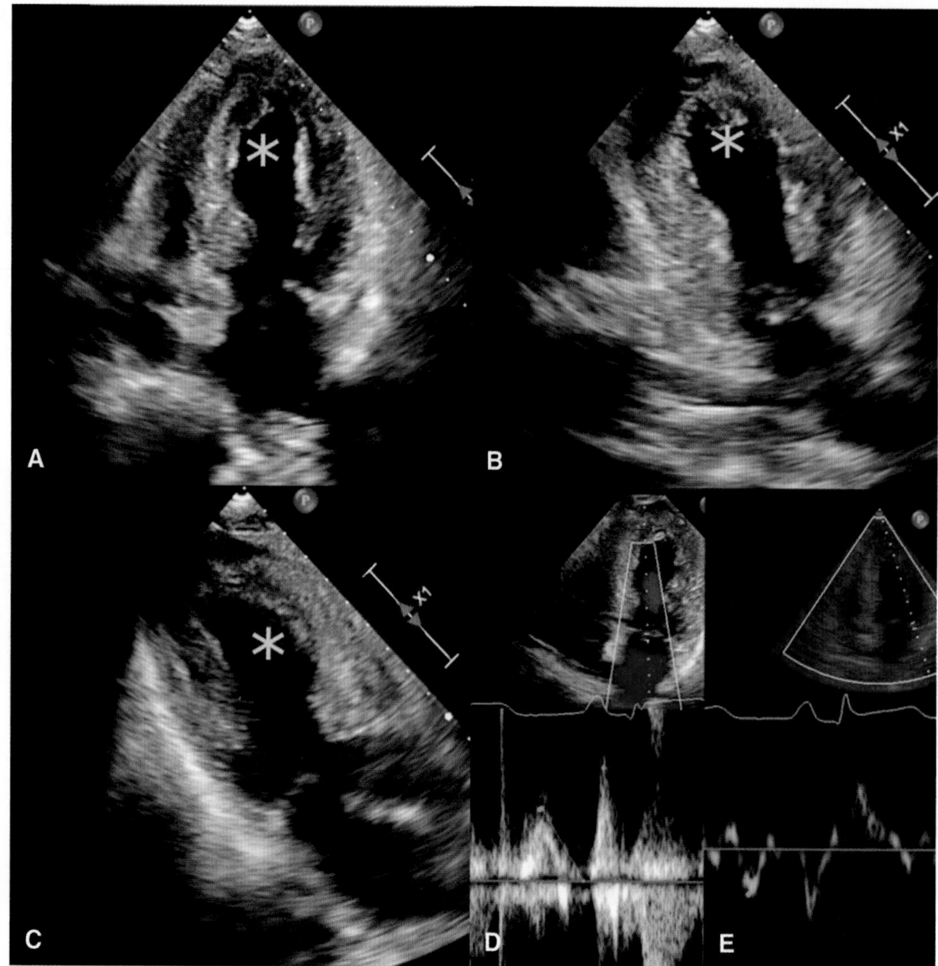

FIGURE 34.6 End systolic images of apical four-chamber **(A)**, two-chamber **(B)**, and three-chamber **(C)** views showing a mid-to-distal septal and apical wall motion abnormality resulting in the left ventricular cavity shape deformity (asterisks); left atrial pressure and diastolic function assessment using pulsed-wave Doppler of the mitral inflow **(D)**, and tissue Doppler of the lateral base of the left ventricle **(E)**.

FOLLOW-UP PATIENT CARE

Echocardiography plays an important role in patient follow-up for a number of cardiac conditions, especially if there is a change in the clinical condition or if the specific disease state is expected to progress on the basis of its natural history.[5] Examples include the development of new or recurrent chest pain in a patient with known coronary artery disease, where new wall motion abnormalities or new inducible ischemia may suggest disease progression. Another example is monitoring the progression of aortic stenosis over time, the rate of which can vary depending on the degree of disease severity, underlying valve anatomy, and other patient-related factors. Serial echocardiographic examinations are indicated to follow up patients who undergo chemotherapy to assess cardiotoxicity during and after treatment.[39]

RESEARCH AND FUTURE DIRECTIONS

Strain echocardiography is a sensitive modality to detect subclinical myocardial mechanical changes. Its clinical applications may be particularly relevant in the evaluation of cardiomyopathy, serial examination of patients undergoing oncologic treatment for cancer, and in the setting of valvular heart disease. Advances in technology and software algorithms have increased the reliability of strain assessment and is reducing the degree of vendor-to-vendor variability.

Artificial intelligence is likely to have a large impact on the field of echocardiography in the future and will likely impact all aspects of the imaging process. This includes assisted or automatic scanning, view recognition and sorting, automated measurements and preliminary report generation. It is also possible that raw data output from an ultrasound transducer may be more sensitive to pathology compared to data that has been converted into a form that is visually interpretable to human beings, such as the commonly used B-mode imaging.

In addition, the use of machine learning to apply computer modeling techniques of cardiac chambers and devices is also very promising. Automated chamber modeling may allow for more accurate volumes and motion to be assessed. In the area of interventional echocardiography, modeling of difficult

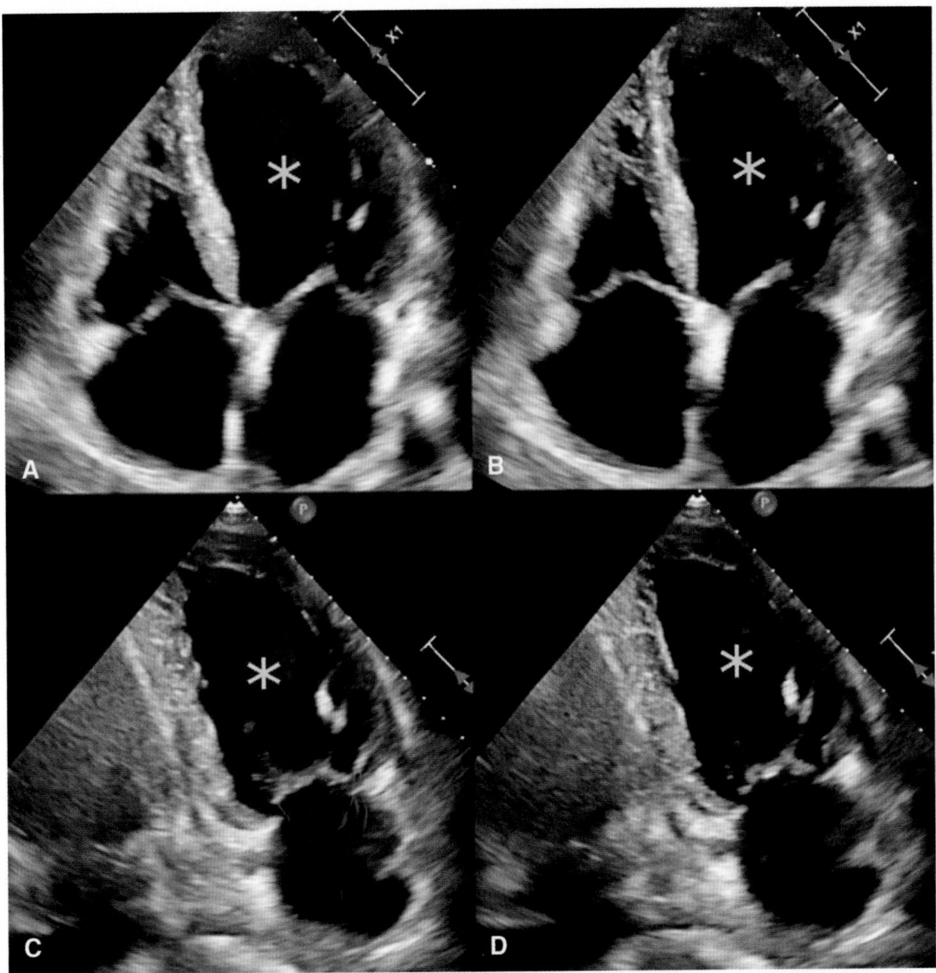

FIGURE 34.7 End diastolic **(A,C)** and end systolic **(B,D)** frames of apical four-chamber **(A, B)** and two-chamber **(C, D)** views in dilated cardiomyopathy showing spherical remodeling of the left ventricle (asterisks) as well as reduced ejection fraction (volume change between end diastole and end systole).

to visualize wires and device components may assist in more accurate assessment of these instruments during procedural guidance and in follow-up.

KEY POINTS

- ✔ An echocardiogram evaluates cardiac structure and function using multiple views of each structure and complementary techniques—individual images/views are generally not enough.
- ✔ Always first check for errors when discordant or inconsistent findings are noted, especially those involving calculations.
- ✔ Irregular rhythms (such as atrial fibrillation) complicate the assessment of several components of an echocardiogram—left ventricular EF, diastolic function, valvular gradients, and pulmonary pressures.
- ✔ Common strategies to improve spatial and temporal resolution include reducing depth and reducing sector width in two-dimensional imaging.
- ✔ Strategies to improve temporal resolution in color Doppler imaging include reducing the size of the region of interest being evaluated.
- ✔ A systematic approach to cardiac disease by echocardiography should include structure, function, and associated abnormalities.

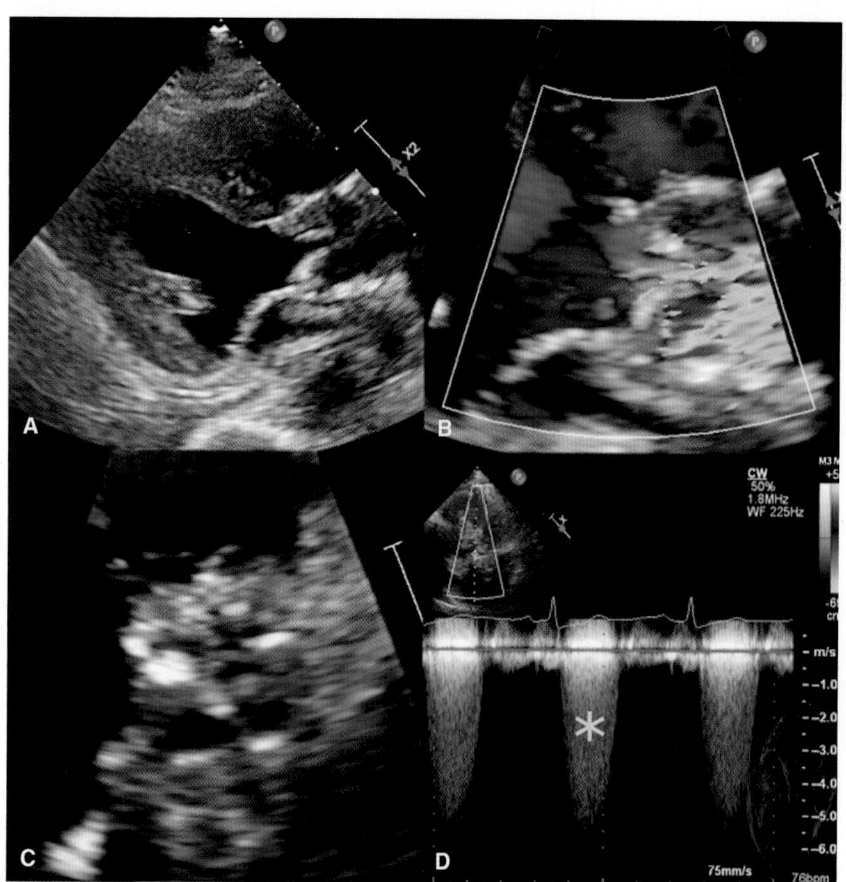

FIGURE 34.8 Severe aortic stenosis findings including thickened and restricted leaflets (**A**, asterisk), aliasing on color Doppler suggesting flow acceleration across the valve in the zoomed parasternal long-axis view **(B)**, severely calcified and restricted leaflets in the zoomed parasternal short axis view **(C)**, and continuous-wave Doppler demonstrating high flow velocities across the valve orifice during systole (**D**, asterisk)

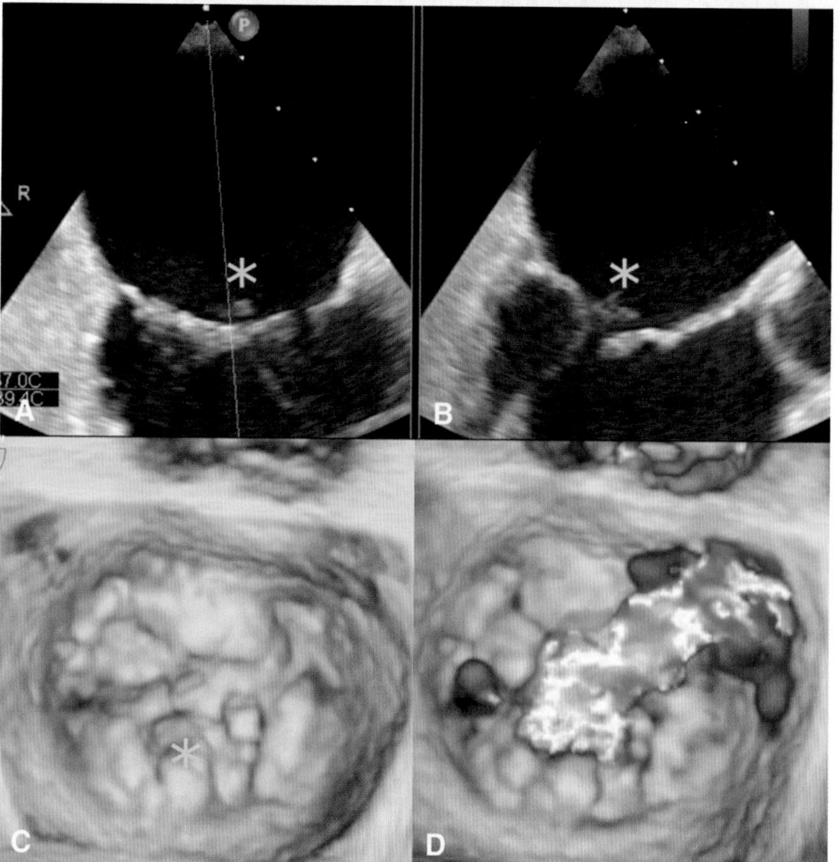

FIGURE 34.9 Flail P2 segment (asterisks) of the mitral valve in systole seen by transesophageal biplane imaging of the intercommissural **(A)** and long-axis **(B)** mid-esophageal views, three-dimensional echocardiography **(C)**, and three-dimensional color Doppler echocardiography revealing a large anteriorly directed regurgitation jet **(D)**.

REFERENCES

1. Mitchell C, Rahko PS, Blauwet LA, et al. Guidelines for performing a comprehensive transthoracic echocardiographic examination in adults: recommendations from the American Society of Echocardiography. *J Am Soc Echocardiogr.* 2019;32(1):1-64. doi:10.1016/j.echo.2018.06.004
2. Hahn RT, Abraham T, Adams MS, et al. Guidelines for performing a comprehensive transesophageal echocardiographic examination. *Anesth Analg.* 2014;118(1):21-68. doi:10.1213/ANE.0000000000000016
3. Lancellotti P, Flachskampf FA, Evangelista A, et al. Recommendations for transoesophageal echocardiography: EACVI update 2014. *Eur Heart J Cardiovasc Imaging.* 2014;15(4):353-365. doi:10.1093/ehjci/jeu015
4. Douglas PS, Garcia MJ, Haines DE, et al. ACCF/ASE/AHA/ASNC /HFSA/HRS/SCAI/SCCM/SCCT/SCMR 2011 Appropriate use criteria for echocardiography. *J Am Soc Echocardiogr.* 2011;24(3):229-267. doi:10.1016/j.echo.2010.12.008
5. Doherty JU, Kort S, Mehran R, et al. ACC/AATS/AHA/ASE/ASNC/HRS/SCAI/SCCT/SCMR/STS 2019 Appropriate use criteria for multimodality imaging in the assessment of cardiac structure and function in nonvalvular heart disease: a report of the American College of Cardiology Appropriate Use Criteria Task Force, American Association for Thoracic Surgery, American Heart Association, American Society of Echocardiography, American Society of Nuclear Cardiology, Heart Rhythm Society, Society for Cardiovascular Angiography and Interventions, Society of Cardiovascular Computed Tomography, Society for Cardiovascular Magnetic Resonance, and the Society of Thoracic Surgeons. *J Am Soc Echocardiogr.* 2019;32(5):553-579. doi:10.1016/j.echo.2019.01.008
6. Bouchez S, Van Belleghem Y, De Somer F, De Pauw M, Stroobandt R, Wouters P. Haemodynamic management of patients with left ventricular assist devices using echocardiography: the essentials. *Eur Heart J Cardiovasc Imaging.* 2019;20(4):373-382. doi:10.1093/ehjci/jez003
7. Zamorano JL, Badano LP, Bruce C, et al. EAE/ASE recommendations for the use of echocardiography in new transcatheter interventions for valvular heart disease. *Eur Heart J.* 2011;32(17):2189-2214. doi:10.1093/eurheartj/ehr259
8. Stainback RF, Estep JD, Agler DA, et al. Echocardiography in the management of patients with left ventricular assist devices: recommendations from the American Society of Echocardiography. *J Am Soc Echocardiogr.* 2015;28(8):853-909. doi:10.1016/j.echo.2015.05.008
9. Lancellotti P, Tribouilloy C, Hagendorff A, et al. Recommendations for the echocardiographic assessment of native valvular regurgitation: an executive summary from the European Association of Cardiovascular Imaging. *Eur Heart J Cardiovasc Imaging.* 2013;14(7):611-644. doi:10.1093/ehjci/jet105
10. Zoghbi WA, Adams D, Bonow RO, et al. Recommendations for noninvasive evaluation of native valvular regurgitation. *J Am Soc Echocardiogr.* 2017;30(4):303-371. doi:10.1016/j.echo.2017.01.007
11. Zoghbi WA, Chambers JB, Dumesnil JG, et al. Recommendations for evaluation of prosthetic valves with echocardiography and doppler ultrasound. *J Am Soc Echocardiogr.* 2009;22(9):975-1014. doi:10.1016/j.echo.2009.07.013
12. Saric M, Maganti K, Tolstrup K, et al. Guidelines for the use of echocardiography in the evaluation of a cardiac source of embolism. *J Am Soc Echocardiogr.* 2016;29(1):1-42. doi:10.1016/j.echo.2015.09.011
13. Silvestry FE, Cohen MS, Armsby LB, et al. Guidelines for the echocardiographic assessment of atrial septal defect and patent foramen ovale: from the American Society of Echocardiography and Society for Cardiac Angiography and Interventions. *J Am Soc Echocardiogr.* 2015;28(8):910-958. doi:10.1016/j.echo.2015.05.015
14. Pellikka PA, Arruda-Olson A, Chaudhry FA, et al. Guidelines for performance, interpretation, and application of stress echocardiography in ischemic heart disease: from the American Society of Echocardiography. *J Am Soc Echocardiogr.* 2019;33(1):1-41.e8. doi:10.1016/j.echo.2019.07.001
15. Sicari R, Nihoyannopoulos P, Evangelista A, et al. Stress echocardiography expert consensus statement—executive summary: European Association of Echocardiography (EAE) (a registered branch of the ESC). *Eur Heart J.* 2009;30(3):278-289. doi:10.1093/eurheartj/ehn492
16. Lancellotti P, Pellikka PA, Budts W, et al. The clinical use of stress echocardiography in non-ischaemic heart disease: recommendations from the European Association of Cardiovascular Imaging and the American Society of Echocardiography. *Eur Heart J Cardiovasc Imaging.* 2016;17(11):1191-1229. doi:10.1093/ehjci/jew190
17. Nishimura RA, Otto CM. 2017 AHA/ACC focused update of the 2014 AHA/ACC guideline for the management of patients with valvular heart disease: a report of the American College of Cardiology/American Heart Association Task Force on Clinical Practice Guidelines. *Circulation.* 2017;135(25):e1159-e1195. doi:10.1161/CIR.0000000000000503.
18. Nishimura RA, Otto CM, Bonow RO, et al. 2014 AHA/ACC guideline for the management of patients with valvular heart disease. *J Am Coll Cardiol.* 2014;63(22):e57-e185. doi:10.1016/j.jacc.2014.02.536
19. Baumgartner H, Falk V, Bax JJ, et al. 2017 ESC/EACTS guidelines for the management of valvular heart disease. *Eur Heart J.* 2017;38(36):2739-2791. doi:10.1093/eurheartj/ehx391
20. Spencer KT, Kimura BJ, Korcarz CE, Pellikka PA, Rahko PS, Siegel RJ. Focused cardiac ultrasound: recommendations from the American Society of Echocardiography. *J Am Soc Echocardiogr.* 2013;26(6):567-581. doi:10.1016/j.echo.2013.04.001
21. Thomas JD, Abe Y, Badano LP, et al. Definitions for a common standard for 2D speckle tracking echocardiography: consensus document of the EACVI/ASE/Industry Task Force to standardize deformation imaging. *Eur Heart J Cardiovasc Imaging.* 2014;16(1):1-11. doi:10.1093/ehjci/jeu184
22. Badano LP, Kolias TJ, Muraru D, et al. Standardization of left atrial, right ventricular, and right atrial deformation imaging using two-dimensional speckle tracking echocardiography: a consensus document of the EACVI/ASE/Industry Task Force to standardize deformation imaging. *Eur Heart J Cardiovasc Imaging.* 2018;19(6):591-600. doi:10.1093/ehjci/jey042
23. Porter TR, Mulvagh SL, Abdelmoneim SS, et al. Clinical applications of ultrasonic enhancing agents in echocardiography: 2018 American Society of Echocardiography guidelines update. *J Am Soc Echocardiogr.* 2018;31(3):241-274. doi:10.1016/j.echo.2017.11.013
24. Lang RM, Badano LP, Mor-Avi V, et al. Recommendations for cardiac chamber quantification by echocardiography in adults: an update from the American Society of Echocardiography and the European Association of Cardiovascular Imaging. *Eur Heart J Cardiovasc Imaging.* 2015;16(3):233-271. doi:10.1093/ehjci/jev014
25. Dorosz JL, Lezotte DC, Weitzenkamp DA, Allen LA, Salcedo EE. Performance of 3-dimensional echocardiography in measuring left ventricular volumes and ejection fraction. *J Am Coll Cardiol.* 2012;59(20):1799-1808. doi:10.1016/j.jacc.2012.01.037
26. Nagueh SF, Smiseth OA, Appleton CP, et al. Recommendations for the evaluation of left ventricular diastolic function by echocardiography: an update from the American Society of Echocardiography and the European Association of Cardiovascular Imaging. *Eur Heart J Cardiovasc Imaging.* 2016;17(12):1321-1360. doi:10.1093/ehjci/jew082
27. Stone GW, Lindenfeld J, Abraham WT, et al. Transcatheter mitral-valve repair in patients with heart failure. *N Engl J Med.* 2018;379(24):2307-2318. doi:10.1056/NEJMoa1806640
28. Baumgartner H, Hung J, Bermejo J, et al. Recommendations on the echocardiographic assessment of aortic valve stenosis: a focused update from the European Association of Cardiovascular Imaging and the American Society of Echocardiography. *Eur Heart J Cardiovasc Imaging.* 2017;18(3):254-275. doi:10.1093/ehjci/jew335
29. Baumgartner H, Hung J, Bermejo J, et al. Echocardiographic assessment of valve stenosis: EAE/ASE recommendations for clinical practice. *J Am Soc Echocardiogr.* 2009;22(1):1-23. doi:10.1016/j.echo.2008.11.029
30. Nagueh SF, Bierig SM, Budoff MJ, et al. American Society of Echocardiography clinical recommendations for multimodality cardiovascular imaging of patients with hypertrophic cardiomyopathy: Endorsed by the American Society of Nuclear Cardiology, Society for Cardiovascular Magnetic Resonance, and Society of Cardiovascular Computed Tomography. *J Am Soc Echocardiogr.* 2011;24(5):473-498. doi:10.1016/j.echo.2011.03.006
31. Marcus FI, McKenna WJ, Sherrill D, et al. Diagnosis of arrhythmogenic right ventricular cardiomyopathy/Dysplasia: proposed modification of the

task force criteria. *Circulation.* 2010;121(13):1533-1541. doi:10.1161/CIRCULATIONAHA.108.840827

32. Klein AL, Abbara S, Agler DA, et al. American Society of Echocardiography clinical recommendations for multimodality cardiovascular imaging of patients with pericardial disease: Endorsed by the Society for Cardiovascular Magnetic Resonance and Society of Cardiovascular Computed Tomography. *J Am Soc Echocardiogr.* 2013;26(9):965-1012.e15. doi:10.1016/j.echo.2013.06.023
33. Puchalski MD, Lui GK, Miller-Hance WC, et al. Guidelines for performing a comprehensive transesophageal echocardiographic: examination in children and all patients with congenital heart disease: recommendations from the American Society of Echocardiography. *J Am Soc Echocardiogr.* 2019;32(2):173-215. doi:10.1016/j.echo.2018.08.016
34. Simpson J, Lopez L, Acar P, et al. Three-dimensional echocardiography in congenital heart disease: an expert consensus document from the European Association of Cardiovascular Imaging and the American Society of Echocardiography. *J Am Soc Echocardiogr.* 2017;30(1):1-27. doi:10.1016/j.echo.2016.08.022
35. Valente AM, Cook S, Festa P, et al. Multimodality imaging guidelines for patients with repaired Tetralogy of fallot: a report from the American Society of Echocardiography: Developed in collaboration with the Society for Cardiovascular Magnetic Resonance and the Society for Pediatric Radiology. *J Am Soc Echocardiogr.* 2014;27(2):111-141. doi:10.1016/j.echo.2013.11.009
36. Cohen MS, Eidem BW, Cetta F, et al. Multimodality imaging guidelines of patients with transposition of the great arteries: a report from the American Society of Echocardiography developed in collaboration with the Society for Cardiovascular Magnetic Resonance and the Society of Cardiovascular Computed Tomography. *J Am Soc Echocardiogr.* 2016;29(7):571-621. doi:10.1016/j.echo.2016.04.002
37. Goldstein SA, Evangelista A, Abbara S, et al. Multimodality imaging of diseases of the thoracic aorta in adults: From the American Society of Echocardiography and the European Association of Cardiovascular Imaging: Endorsed by the Society of Cardiovascular Computed Tomography and Society for Cardiovascular Magnetic Resonance. *J Am Soc Echocardiogr.* 2015;28(2):119-182. doi:10.1016/j.echo.2014.11.015
38. Bertrand PB, Levine RA, Isselbacher EM, Vandervoort PM. Fact or artifact in two-dimensional echocardiography: avoiding misdiagnosis and missed diagnosis. *J Am Soc Echocardiogr.* 2016;29(5):381-391. doi:10.1016/j.echo.2016.01.009
39. Plana JC, Galderisi M, Barac A, et al. Expert consensus for multimodality imaging evaluation of adult patients during and after cancer therapy: a report from the American Society of Echocardiography and the European Association of Cardiovascular Imaging. *J Am Soc Echocardiogr.* 2014;27(9):911-939. doi:10.1016/j.echo.2014.07.012

CHAPTER 35

NUCLEAR CARDIOLOGY AND MOLECULAR IMAGING

Sean R. McMahon, Josiah Bote, and William Lane Duvall

INTRODUCTION

Nuclear cardiology plays a fundamental role in the noninvasive diagnosis and management of cardiovascular disease, which is the leading cause of death in the Western world. It employs radiolabeled tracers, predominantly technetium-99m (^{99m}Tc), in the performance of cardiovascular imaging studies, which include myocardial perfusion imaging (MPI), metabolic imaging, ventricular function assessment, cardiac amyloid studies, and myocardial innervation imaging. Single-photon emission computed tomography (SPECT) and positron emission tomography (PET) used for MPI in the evaluation of coronary artery disease (CAD) are the mainstays of nuclear cardiology imaging. However, nuclear cardiology has also expanded beyond the assessment of obstructive CAD to targeted metabolic imaging with F-18-flourodeoxyglucose (^{18}F-FDG) used in the evaluation of myocardial viability and in the diagnosis of sarcoidosis, to technetium-99m-pyrophosphate (^{99m}Tc-PYP) used for diagnosis of cardiac amyloidosis, and to iodine-123-metaiodobenzylguanidine (^{123}I-*m*IBG) for the identification of cardiac neuronal dysfunction. With millions of nuclear cardiology imaging procedures performed annually, the diagnostic information gained from these studies allows physicians to cost-effectively manage their patients with known or suspected cardiovascular disease. The role of nuclear cardiology and molecular imaging in patient management continues to evolve, and its clinical use continues to expand.

FUNDAMENTALS OF CARDIAC NUCLEAR SCINTIGRAPHY

Physical Principles and Instrumentation

Nuclear cardiology is based on imaging the radioactive decay of isotopes. To become more stable, unstable isotopes undergo radioactive decay, which emits energy that can be collected and used for image construction. Gamma decay emits photons, also known as gamma rays, which are used in SPECT, and positron decay creates an annihilation event that produces two high-energy photons used in PET.

Isotopes for medical imaging are produced from their parent nuclei via four methods, which are fission, neutron activation, cyclotron bombardment, and generator elution.[1] Fission and neutron activation occur in a nuclear reactor. A cyclotron is a linear accelerator that bombards stable nuclei with high-energy charged particles to create new elements. Generators are used to store a mother isotope produced in a nuclear reactor, and, when needed, the daughter isotope is eluted and combined into a radiopharmaceutical.

Thallium-201 (^{201}Tl) was the first radioactive isotope used in widespread SPECT MPI. It is a potassium analog with a half-life of 73 hours, and emits several gamma rays with different energy spectra (69-80 keV, 135 keV, and 167 keV). ^{201}Tl is produced in a cyclotron. Owing to the limitations of thallium, the long half-life resulting in greater radiation exposure and low-energy photons resulting in suboptimal gated images, ^{99m}Tc was introduced as an alternative agent. ^{99m}Tc emits a higher energy photon of 140 keV and has a shorter half-life of 6 hours, resulting in superior image quality and lower effective dose to the patient. ^{99m}Tc is commercially acquired from a molybdenum-99 (^{99}Mo) generator.

Radionuclides used in PET imaging decay by emitting positrons. When a positron interacts with an electron, an annihilation event ensues, and two 511 keV photons are emitted at a 180-degree angle to each other and detected by the PET camera system. The two isotopes used for PET MPI are Rb-82, which has a half-life of 75 seconds and is produced from a strontium-82 (^{82}Sr) generator, and N-13 ammonia (^{13}N) with a half-life of 10 minutes, which is produced in a cyclotron. ^{18}F-FDG, which is produced in a cyclotron, has a half-life of 110 minutes, and is the principal radiopharmaceutical for PET metabolic imaging. Oxygen-15–labeled water (^{15}O water) can also be used as a radiotracer for quantifying myocardial blood flow, but is not routinely used clinically.

Current SPECT cameras employ either traditional sodium-iodide (Na-I) crystals or newer high-efficiency cadmium-zinc-telluride (CZT) crystals.[2] Conventional, dual-head SPECT cameras have two camera heads attached to a gantry that rotates around the patient in a step-and-shoot or continuous manner while acquiring images over a 180-degree arc. The camera heads are composed of a collimator, Na-I crystal, and photomultiplier tubes. The crystals produce visible light photons when struck by gamma rays that are converted into electronic signals, allowing for localization of the origin of the activity. High-efficiency cameras have improved sensitivity, superior energy resolution, and finer spatial resolution through the utilization of cardiocentric collimation and camera geometry along with CZT crystals.

PET cameras differ from SPECT cameras because the scintillation detectors surround a patient in a 360-degree

TABLE 35.1 Pretest Probability of Coronary Artery Disease

Age (years)	Gender	Typical/Definite Angina Pectoris	Atypical/Probable Angina Pectoris	Nonanginal Chest Pain	Asymptomatic
<39	Men	Intermediate	Intermediate	Low	Very low
	Women	Intermediate	Very low	Very low	Very low
40-49	Men	High	Intermediate	Intermediate	Low
	Women	Intermediate	Low	Very low	Very low
50-59	Men	High	Intermediate	Intermediate	Low
	Women	Intermediate	Intermediate	Low	Very low
>60	Men	High	Intermediate	Intermediate	Low
	Women	High	Intermediate	Intermediate	Low

High: Greater than 90% pretest probability. **Intermediate:** Between 10% and 90% pretest probability. **Low:** Between 5% and 10% pretest probability. **Very Low:** Less than 5% pretest probability.

Adapted from Hendel RC, Berman DS, Di Carli MF, et al. ACCF/ASNC/ACR/AHA/ASE/SCCT/SCMR/SNM 2009 appropriate use criteria for cardiac radionuclide imaging: a report of the American College of Cardiology Foundation Appropriate Use Criteria Task Force, the American Society of Nuclear Cardiology, the American College of Radiology, the American Heart Association, the American Society of Echocardiography, the Society of Cardiovascular Computed Tomography, the Society for Cardiovascular Magnetic Resonance, and the Society of Nuclear Medicine. *J Am Coll Cardiol.* 2009;53:2201-2229(5).

circumferential ring.[3] This camera geometry is needed because PET radioisotopes decay by positron emission, which results in two photon pairs that strike opposing detectors at a 180-degree angle from each other. The simultaneous coincidence detection of the two photons is made possible by the detectors completely surrounding the area being imaged. Coincidence events are recorded and reconstruction algorithms used to create the projections of the acquired myocardial or extracardiac activity.[3]

Myocardial Perfusion Imaging

Indications

MPI is a widely available and frequently employed modality in the assessment of known or suspected CAD, providing both diagnostic and prognostic information. Both SPECT and PET MPI can accurately determine the presence, location, and severity of ischemia or infarction, thus indirectly establishing the diagnosis of obstructive CAD. Furthermore, their results provide useful prognostic information that correlates with future risk of adverse cardiovascular events. Most SPECT or PET MPI studies are performed with the intent to evaluate symptoms, provide risk assessment, or to guide therapy.

Evaluation of Symptoms With Single-Photon Emission Computed Tomography and Positron Emission Tomography Myocardial Perfusion Imaging. Both SPECT and PET MPI are frequently performed to evaluate for underlying obstructive CAD in patients with symptoms suggestive of angina. The sensitivity of SPECT MPI to detect obstructive CAD has been reported as 88% with a specificity of 76%, whereas PET MPI has a reported sensitivity and specificity of 93% and 81%, respectively.[4] When evaluating chest pain syndromes, careful patient selection for MPI is needed. Applying concepts of Bayesian probability, a positive result is less likely to be a true positive in low-risk individuals and very likely to be true positive in high-risk individuals (**Table 35.1**). Hence, in patients with very low pretest probability defined as less than 10% probability for CAD, with interpretable electrocardiograms (ECGs) and who are able to exercise, recommendations are to avoid MPI in favor of treadmill exercise ECG testing (see Chapter 32).[5] Similarly, in patients with very high pretest probability (>90%), MPI will not significantly alter posttest probability. Accordingly, stress MPI is best suited for evaluation of symptoms in intermediate-risk patients.

Risk Assessment: Prognostic Implications With Single-Photon Emission Computed Tomography and *Positron Emission Tomography* Myocardial Perfusion Imaging. Assessment of prognosis and risk is well established with SPECT and PET MPI. Patients with normal perfusion and left ventricular (LV) function have an excellent prognosis with a combined death or nonfatal myocardial infarction (MI) rate of less than 1% per year.[6] This, however, is increased in higher risk subsets such as patients with diabetes, reduced ejection fraction, or increased end-diastolic volume.[7,8] Furthermore, in patients who are able to exercise, the ability to achieve at least 10 metabolic equivalents (METs) has been shown to correlate with a low prevalence of underlying ischemia and very low rates of cardiac events.[9] Strong negative predictive value is also seen in patients who have normal stress-only imaging.[10] Conversely, risk has been shown to increase with the extent of myocardial perfusion abnormalities. In patients with LV perfusion defects of less than 10%, 10% to 20%, and greater than 20%, the risk of death, MI, or revascularization was 27%, 31%, and 43% over a 46-month follow-up time, respectively.[11] Regardless of perfusion abnormalities, depressed LV function has been associated with a 7.4% rate of nonfatal MI or cardiac death versus 1.8 in normal individuals.[12] Transient ischemic dilation (TID) of the LV postexercise is a marker of extensive CAD. One large meta-analysis found TID to have a sensitivity of 44% and specificity of 88% for the detection of extensive CAD, and important prognostic implications with up to a 6% annual mortality rate if TID is accompanied by ischemia.[13]

The prognostic abilities of SPECT and PET have further been amplified by the use of attenuation correction (AC) and myocardial blood flow quantification techniques, respectively.[14-16] The incorporation of AC has been shown to decrease the total interpreted burden of ischemia or infarct as measured by the summed stress score (SSS), and has demonstrated superior prognostic availability, likely due to decreased contamination by false-positive results.[14] Another modality useful in risk assessment is myocardial flow reserve (MFR), a quantitative measurement of blood flow derived from PET MPI dynamic acquisitions that has validated prognostic utility independently or when added to perfusion images. In a study with 2783 patients with known or suspected CAD, an MFR less than 1.5 was associated independently with a sixfold increased risk of death. Conversely, with an MFR of greater than 2, prognosis was excellent. A low MFR was associated with poor outcomes even in the setting of normal PET MPI.[16,17]

Therapy Guidance. Stress testing with or without MPI is commonly used for evaluation of acute chest pain in the emergency department (ED), and is useful for decision-making when applied to the appropriate patient population.[18] Clinically derived risk scores may aid in the identification of the appropriate patients who can be safely discharged from the ED without stress testing versus those who benefit from further evaluation.[19]

In those with stable CAD who undergo angiography, MPI may provide further information regarding the hemodynamic impact of indeterminate lesions to aid in the decision about revascularization (**Figure 35.1**).[20] In asymptomatic patients, MPI is reasonable to assess risk and guide therapy after acute coronary syndromes, with incomplete revascularization where further revascularization is feasible or if primary angiography was not performed initially.[5,21]

Myocardial ischemia is understood to contribute to perioperative morbidity and mortality. Hence, in the preoperative evaluation of patients undergoing noncardiac surgery, MPI plays a role in risk stratification. MPI is deemed inappropriate for assessment before low-risk procedures; however, it is appropriate before intermediate or high-risk procedures in patients with cardiac risk factors and poor functional capacity.[22]

The additive value of coronary artery calcification (CAC), which is available from combined SPECT/computed tomography (CT) and PET/CT systems, is particularly useful in those patients with normal myocardial perfusion.[23] In patients with a paucity of CAC, there is an associated excellent prognosis and little utility for primary prevention outside of traditional guidelines. However, in patients with normal MPI but significant CAC, aggressive risk factor modification may be pursued. Furthermore, the incorporation of CT has been shown to add to diagnostic accuracy and yields independent prognostic information regardless of the MPI results. In patients with a positive MPI, the presence of CAC is associated with a 70% true-positive result compared to only 16% in those with no CAC.[24,25]

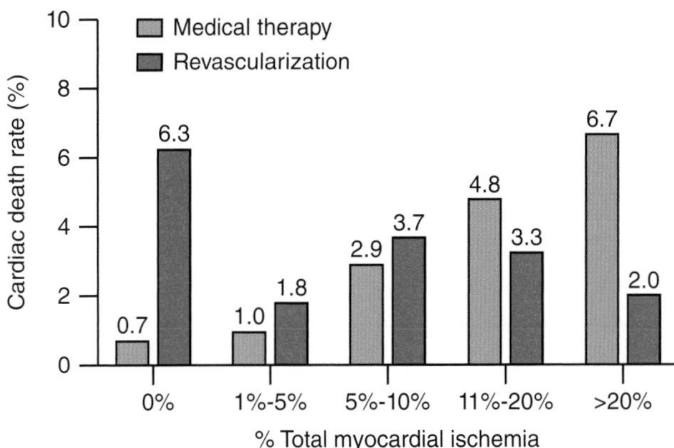

FIGURE 35.1 Observed cardiac death rates over the follow-up period in patients undergoing revascularization versus medical therapy as a function of the amount of inducible ischemia. As the amount of ischemic myocardium increases beyond 10%, the benefit of revascularization increases as well. (Reprinted with permission from Hachamovitch R, Hayes SW, Friedman JD, et al. Comparison of the short-term survival benefit associated with revascularization compared with medical therapy in patients with no prior coronary artery disease undergoing stress myocardial perfusion single photon emission computed tomography. *Circulation.* 2003;107(23):2900-2907.)

Stress Modality Selection

Once the decision is made to pursue MPI, choosing the appropriate modality is determined by a number of patient factors. Typically, in patients who can exercise, treadmill testing is done with injection of radioisotope at peak exercise, ensuring that the patient has achieved 85% of maximal age-predicted heart rate and adequately increased myocardial work. In patients unable to exercise adequately or those who fail to achieve target heart rate, pharmacologic stress testing is an appropriate alternative. Most patients undergoing pharmacologic stress testing do so with administration of a coronary vasodilator. Coronary vasodilators such as dipyridamole, adenosine, and regadenoson activate the adenosine receptors, resulting in coronary vasodilatation and hyperemia. In diseased arteries, the vasodilation is minimal, resulting in less radiotracer uptake than in healthy myocardium. Both adenosine and dipyridamole are nonselective adenosine agonists activating A_1, A_{2B}, and A_3 in addition to A_{2A} receptors. However, regadenoson is a selective A_{2A} receptor agonist, resulting in fewer side effects associated with nonspecific adenosine receptor activation.[26]

Less frequently, dobutamine is used to increase myocardial work by stimulating beta-1 and beta-2 receptors. The result is similar to exercise stress with increased myocardial blood flow in nonobstructed coronary arteries and the ability to detect regional variation of radioisotope uptake. Dobutamine stress protocols utilize incremental increases of dobutamine to target 85% of maximum age-predicted heart rate response. Atropine may be used as an adjunct to increase response to achieve target heart rate.

IMAGING PROTOCOLS

Single-Photon Emission Computed Tomography Imaging Protocol

SPECT imaging protocols may vary depending on clinical factors, equipment, and workflow capabilities. Facilities with newer high-efficiency SPECT cameras benefit from lower radiation exposure and decreased imaging time. The most frequently employed SPECT MPI protocol is a single-day, rest-stress (low-dose/high-dose ^{99m}Tc) study. This protocol involves injection of ^{99m}Tc at rest followed by rest imaging, then proceeding to stress with repeat isotope injection while undergoing stress (exercise, dobutamine, or vasodilator), followed by stress imaging. However, in obese patients, a 2-day, high-radiotracer-dose stress followed by high-dose rest imaging protocol is often used to allow for diagnostic quality images. In selected patients with low to intermediate risk, a stress-first approach may allow for a reduction in radiation exposure, patient testing time, and an increase in laboratory throughput by proceeding to rest images only if stress perfusion images are abnormal. Patients with a normal stress-only MPI have demonstrated low event rates similar to those who have undergone a full rest-stress SPECT,[10] but the use of AC is necessary to increase the yield of the protocol.

Attenuation artifacts have the potential to degrade accuracy of SPECT MPI. Several methods have been implemented to overcome attenuation artifacts including prone imaging, scanning line sources, and CT AC. In a large meta-analysis, the pooled sensitivities for non-AC versus line source or CT AC were 80% and 84%, respectively, with a sensitivity of 68% and 80%, respectively.[27] Furthermore, the CT used for application of AC may provide both prognostic and diagnostic information when evaluated for the burden of CAC. The addition of a formal CAC score has been shown to increase the sensitivity of SPECT from 76% to 86% for detection of CAD.[28]

Acute rest-only MPI is a less commonly used technique that has been found to be accurate and useful in the evaluation of acute chest pain in the ED. This strategy has been useful to expedite diagnosis of MI and safely triage patients with normal results to discharge, resulting in significant hospital cost savings.[29] However, coronary CTA has been shown to be highly reliable and with rapid turnaround time paired with cost-effectiveness; thus, CTA has largely supplanted acute rest MPI studies in the ED setting.[18]

PET MPI utilizes either ^{82}Rb or ^{13}N ammonia tracers that have relatively rapid uptake, clearance, and short half-life (75 seconds and 10 minutes, respectively). Owing to these properties, vasodilator MPI has been adopted as the standard stress modality for ^{82}Rb, whereas pharmacologic or exercise stress may be used with ^{13}N ammonia. Generally, rest images are obtained before stress images, with image acquisition following immediately after injection of the radioisotope.[3] Although stress-first PET MPI is feasible, implementing this protocol is cumbersome and labor intense given the short time for protocol completion.[30] PET imaging is performed with AC via CT or line source AC.

Interpretation: Myocardial Perfusion Images

Interpretation of myocardial perfusion images involves review of raw projected images, perfusion images, and gated images. Facilities with advanced equipment benefit from the addition of reviewing AC images, CT images, and with PET assessment of myocardial blood flow.

Interpretation of the raw projected images should include visual assessment of soft-tissue attenuation, motion artifacts, or abnormal extracardiac uptake. Perfusion images should be assessed for homogeneous or heterogeneous uptake and described using the 17-segment model comparing stress to rest images. Perfusion defects are visually classified by intensity, size, location, and reversibility, and further quantified by the SSS, summed rest score (SRS), and the summed difference score (SDS) (**Figure 35.2**). The use of automated software to quantify perfusion complements standard visual assessment, and has been a reliable tool in research.[31] Perfusion images and gated images should be assessed for high-risk findings such as TID or stress-induced decrease in left ventricular ejection fraction (LVEF), which may be indicative of multivessel CAD. An assessment of LV and right ventricular function, regional wall motion, and LV chamber size is reported in patients where gated images have been acquired. In those with CT used for AC, the interpretation should include a visual assessment of CAC or formal CAC quantification. Apparent extracardiac findings should be commented upon.

SPECIAL CONSIDERATIONS AND CONTRAINDICATIONS: SINGLE-PHOTON EMISSION COMPUTED TOMOGRAPHY AND POSITRON EMISSION TOMOGRAPHY MYOCARDIAL PERFUSION IMAGING

Although the radiation dose of both SPECT and PET MPI are low, caution should be advised with younger patients, and alternative testing should be considered. Pregnancy testing in women of childbearing age is necessary, and if pregnant, alternative imaging modalities should be pursued.

Stress MPI is contraindicated in acute coronary syndromes. However, vasodilator stress has been shown to be safe in patients who are greater than 48 hours post MI.[32,33] Contraindications for the use of vasodilator stressors include advanced conduction disease, hypotension, uncontrolled hypertension, use of dipyridamole-containing medications, and known hypersensitivity to the vasodilator agent. Caution is advised administering to patients with reactive airway disease, and administration should be avoided in patients with active bronchospasm (absolute contraindication). Should side effects occur, reversal agents such as aminophylline, theophylline, or caffeine should be administered. Accordingly, patients should refrain from taking theophylline or caffeine before pharmacologic stress testing. Relative contraindications include profound sinus bradycardia, second-degree Mobitz 1–type heart block, severe aortic stenosis, or seizure disorders.[26]

Dobutamine stress testing is contraindicated in patients with acute coronary syndrome, hypertrophic cardiomyopathy,

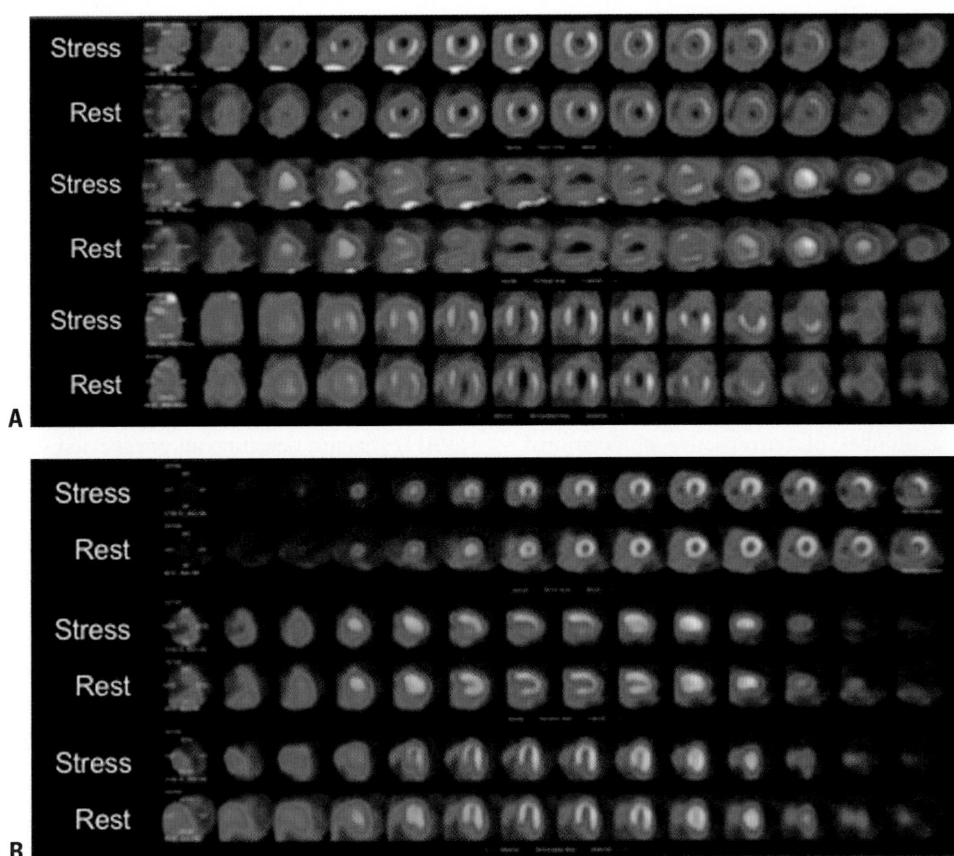

FIGURE 35.2 (**A**) Rest-stress technetium-99m (^{99m}Tc) single-photon emission computed tomography (SPECT) myocardial perfusion imaging showing a large area of severe intensity scar in the mid to distal left anterior descending artery distribution. (**B**) Rest-stress ^{99m}Tc SPECT myocardial perfusion imaging showing a medium sized area of moderate intensity ischemia in the right coronary artery territory.

dynamic outflow obstruction, uncontrolled hypertension, aortic dissection, uncontrolled atrial tachyarrhythmias, or significant ventricular arrhythmias. Relative contraindications include beta blocker use, severe aortic stenosis, left bundle branch block or paced ventricular rhythm, and aortic aneurysms.[26] Patients scheduled for dobutamine stress testing should be advised to hold their beta blockers for 48 hours before testing.

Indications, contraindications, and protocols for exercise stress testing are found in Chapter 33.

LIMITATIONS: SINGLE-PHOTON EMISSION COMPUTED TOMOGRAPHY AND POSITRON EMISSION TOMOGRAPHY MYOCARDIAL PERFUSION IMAGING

SPECT and PET MPI perform well in the diagnosis of obstructive CAD; however, they cannot detect nonobstructive or preclinical disease. Although the effective dose for MPI is low, radiation exposure remains a significant concern, especially in sensitive populations. Performing MPI is labor- and time-consuming, with involvement of specialized nuclear technologist, cardiac nursing, and physician oversight. Typically, several hours are required, especially with SPECT MPI. Unfortunately, cost has prohibited the widespread utilization of AC and PET MPI, which is particularly relevant in larger patients with significant soft-tissue attenuation artifacts.

Metabolic Imaging With ^{18}F-Fluorodeoxyglucose Positron Emission Tomography

Indications of Fluorodeoxyglucose Positron Emission Tomography

Cardiac PET metabolic imaging with ^{18}F-FDG is used for imaging the initial steps of glucose metabolism in cardiac tissue. It takes advantage of the glucose analog (deoxyglucose) that, after initial phosphorylation, becomes trapped intracellularly and allows for identification of metabolically active or hyperactive cells.[3]

Viability. Detection of viable myocardium by demonstration of preserved glucose metabolism in patients with CAD with known or suspected previous MI can play an important role in their management. This is especially true in patients with LV dysfunction, because some of the dysfunction may be reversible if attributable to myocardial hibernation or stunning, as opposed to myocardial scarring. And, therefore, the identification of viable myocardium and its distinction from irreversibly damaged myocardium signifies a different prognosis and suggests different treatment options.

The literature on the use of viability testing to improve outcomes in patients with ischemic cardiomyopathies remains incomplete. The STICH (Surgical Treatment for Ischemic Heart Failure) trial, did not explicitly evaluate viability testing, but it did compare coronary artery bypass grafting (CABG) versus medical therapy in patients with reduced LVEF (<35%), showing no improvement in all-cause mortality with revascularization in the initial assessment.[34] However, in the longer term follow-up, patients who underwent CABG had significantly lower rates of all-cause mortality, cardiovascular death, and hospitalization than did medically treated patients alone.[35] Although a number of retrospective observational studies, meta-analyses, and post hoc analyses of randomized data suggest a benefit to the use of viability testing, they are all limited by retrospective and selection biases.[36] Substudies of the PARR-2 (PET and Recovery Following Revascularization) trial, which evaluated the use of PET viability imaging in the management of patients with ischemic cardiomyopathies, showed that patients whose management adhered to imaging recommendations and those imaged at institutions with local expertise in PET demonstrated a significant reduction in events.[37,38] In the STICH viability substudy, however, SPECT imaging or dobutamine echocardiography did not add value to the management of these patients.[39]

Cardiac Sarcoidosis. Cardiac sarcoidosis is clinically symptomatic in less than 10% of patients with systemic sarcoidosis, but autopsy and imaging studies have suggested a prevalence of 20% to 50%, and cardiac involvement may be responsible for 25% of the deaths from sarcoid.[40] ^{18}F-FDG can be used to image inflammation in sarcoidosis because glucose metabolism is increased in inflammatory cells such as the macrophages in sarcoid granulomas.

FDG PET imaging may be clinically useful for the investigation of suspected cardiac sarcoidosis or as a method of monitoring response to therapy in patients with known cardiac sarcoidosis.[41] The diagnosis of cardiac involvement, however, involves the integration of multiple sources of data including clinical history, laboratory findings, and other diagnostic modalities, including echocardiography and cardiac magnetic resonance imaging (MRI). Patients without known systemic sarcoid who have a new, unexplained nonischemic cardiomyopathy, ventricular arrhythmia, or significant conduction system disease could be considered for diagnostic imaging with FDG PET. In patients with known systemic sarcoid, abnormal cardiac screening studies such as ECG, echocardiography, Holter monitor, cardiac MRI, or complaints of palpitations or syncope would prompt evaluation by FDG PET. Serial assessment by FDG PET in patients undergoing immunosuppressive therapy have suggested an association with improvement of LVEF and reduction in ventricular arrhythmia with reduction in ^{18}F-FDG uptake.[42]

Endocarditis and Cardiac Device Infections. FDG PET has been used for imaging infection because both activated immune cells and bacteria at the site of infection utilize large quantities of glucose, allowing for noninvasive localization. FDG PET has shown the greatest promise in the diagnosis of prosthetic valve endocarditis with sensitivities between 73% and 100% and specificity of 71% to 100% based on a systematic review of the literature.[43] It is in the setting of identifying endocarditis, especially involving prosthetic valves when findings on echocardiography are inconclusive, that FDG PET has been recommended by European Society Guidelines.[44] Additional advantages of FDG PET for the evaluation of cardiac infection include early detection before morphologic valve damage occurs, when compared to transesophageal echocardiography or cardiac CT, diagnosis of infection involving the extracardiac components of a pacemaker or left ventricular assist device (LVAD) systems, detecting an unexpected source of a primary infection, and diagnosing embolic sequelae of endocarditis.[45] In several studies, the use of FDG PET for the diagnosis of endocarditis has improved the sensitivity of modified Duke criteria, and in another, resulted in a change in therapy in a significant proportion of patients.[46]

Imaging Protocols for Fluorodeoxyglucose Positron Emission Tomography

Following the appropriate dietary preparation and blood glucose management, ^{18}F-FDG is administered in an appropriate uptake room, and imaging is started 45 to 90 minutes after injection.[3] A dedicated cardiac scan is performed for viability and sarcoid studies. For sarcoid studies, a partial whole-body scan including the lungs and mediastinum is also performed; whereas for infection studies, a whole-body scan is indicated to see extracardiac sites of uptake. Viability and sarcoid studies also require the acquisition of resting PET (^{82}Rb or ^{13}N-ammonia) perfusion or ^{99m}Tc SPECT resting perfusion studies.

Interpretation: Fluorodeoxyglucose Positron Emission Tomography

Viability. Cardiac PET viability studies require the evaluation of myocardial perfusion, assessed by ^{82}Rb, ^{13}N ammonia, or even ^{99m}Tc, along with ^{18}F-FDG metabolism images. Hibernating myocardium is defined as territories with preserved glucose metabolism with hypoperfusion, the prototypical perfusion-metabolism mismatch (**Figure 35.3**). Territories with preserved myocardial perfusion or glucose metabolism are viable, whereas those with reduced perfusion and glucose metabolism represent nonviable or scarred myocardium. Gated images should be reviewed and overall LV size and function reported along with regional wall motion abnormalities.

Cardiac Sarcoidosis. PET cardiac sarcoidosis studies also require the evaluation of myocardial perfusion along with hot spot ^{18}F-FDG metabolism images. Resting myocardial perfusion defects may be due to scarring/fibrosis or compression of the microvasculature by inflammation. FDG images may display a normal or negative pattern with completely suppressed uptake, a diffuse pattern that is nonspecific and consistent with viable myocardium, or a focal or focal-on-diffuse pattern consistent with active inflammation (**Figure 35.4**). The presence of ^{18}F FDG in the myocardium alone is not specific for

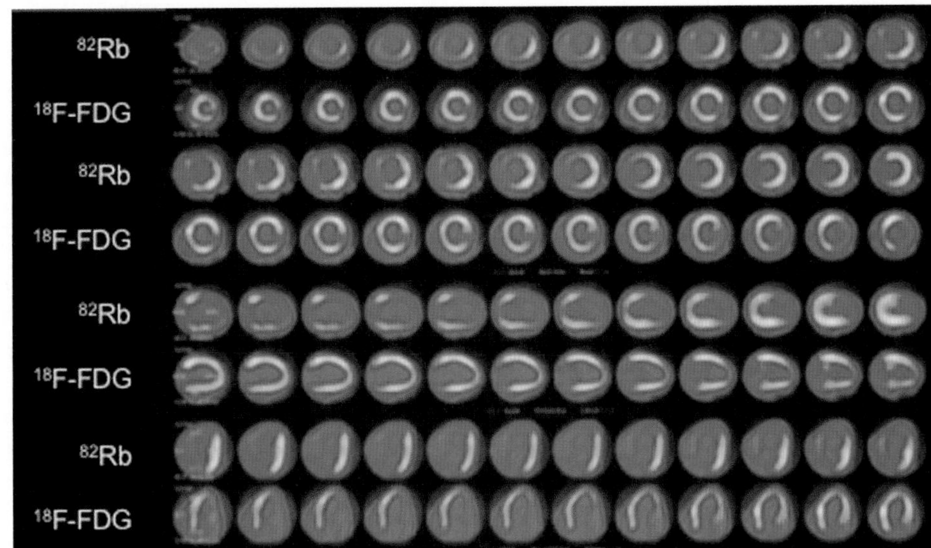

FIGURE 35.3 F-18-flourodeoxyglucose (18F-FDG) positron emission tomography viability study. Rest ^{82}Rb perfusion imaging (top row) shows a large sized, moderate to severe intensity defect in the proximal left anterior descending artery territory distribution. metabolic imaging (bottom row) shows significant radiotracer uptake in the affected segments in a classic perfusion-metabolism mismatch pattern characteristic of hibernating myocardium.

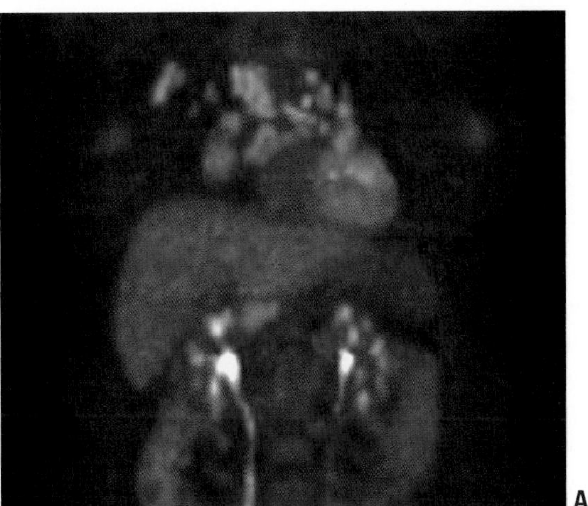

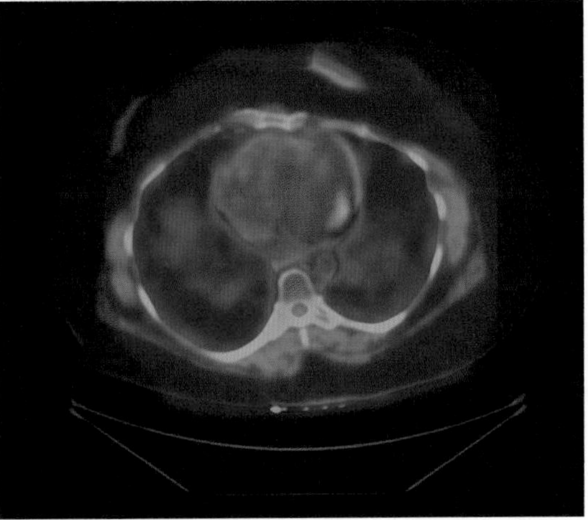

FIGURE 35.4 This F-18-flourodeoxyglucose (^{18}F-FDG) positron emission tomography (PET) cardiac sarcoidosis study demonstrates abnormal, focal cardiac uptake in the mid to basal lateral wall consistent with an inflammatory process such as sarcoidosis. (**A**) represents the chest and upper abdomen acquisition, and **(B)** is a representative fused computed tomography (CT) and PET axial slice through the heart.

cardiac sarcoid because hibernating myocardium, lateral wall artifacts, inflammatory myopathies, and myocarditis may result in focal uptake. ^{18}F FDG uptake can be quantified using the maximum standardized uptake value (SUV_{max}), which is the concentration of tracer corrected for injected activity and the patient's weight. These measurements can be used when comparisons to previous studies are needed to more accurately assess changes compared to visual analysis alone. Gated images should be reviewed and overall LV size and function reported along with regional wall motion abnormalities. Finally, extracardiac ^{18}F FDG uptake should be evaluated for evidence of systemic sarcoidosis or malignancy.

Infection. PET infection studies are assessed visually, with regions of abnormal ^{18}F FDG uptake identified as areas of increased tracer uptake. The CT scan acquired as part of the PET/CT study can then be used to anatomically localize the areas of increased tracer uptake. Prosthetic valves, pacemaker wires and generators, and LVAD components can be identified on the CT images as a site of infection or extracardiac locations of injection or embolization can be seen.

Special Considerations and Contraindications: FDG Positron Emission Tomography

Dietary preparation is essential for the performance of diagnostic FDG PET metabolic studies because cardiac myocytes utilize free fatty acids or glucose in different proportions depending on the prevailing metabolic conditions. Healthy myocardium is able to shift rapidly from predominantly fatty acid metabolism to more or less glucose metabolism depending on environmental factors, whereas diseased myocardium subjected to chronic reductions in perfusion adapts to predominant glucose metabolism. Dietary preparation to standardize the substrate environment for myocytes varies depending on the study indication: myocardial viability or inflammation. For PET viability studies, myocyte metabolism of glucose over fatty acids is preferred to maximize ^{18}F FDG uptake in the myocardium. This is typically accomplished by loading the patient with glucose (by mouth [PO] or intravenous [IV]) after a prolonged fast of over 6 hours.[3] For PET sarcoid or infection studies, myocyte metabolism of fatty acids is preferred, with suppression of carbohydrate metabolism to limit ^{18}F FDG uptake to active inflammatory cells. This is typically accomplished by avoiding carbohydrate-containing foods, eating high-fat and high-protein foods for 24 hours, followed by a prolonged fast and, optionally, IV heparin.[3,40,41]

Limitations: FDG Positron Emission Tomography

Dietary preparation is routinely difficult in all patients, but especially in diabetics referred for viability studies because they have a reduced ability to produce insulin and their cells respond less to exogenous insulin. This often requires more involved glucose-loading protocols and/or delayed PET imaging to allow for minimization of blood pool ^{18}F FDG counts. ^{18}F FDG hot spot imaging for sarcoidosis or infection can identify processes other than sarcoidosis, and can image immune cells at a noninfectious inflammatory site. Data supporting the use of FDG PET imaging is typically limited to single-center experiences or meta-analysis, and comprehensive data from randomized clinical trials is lacking.

Technetium-99m-Pyrophosphate Amyloid

Indications: Technetium-99m-Pyrophosphate Amyloid

Systemic amyloidosis is an infiltrative disease with three main subtypes: light chain amyloidosis (AL), wild-type transthyretin amyloidosis (wtATTR), and hereditary transthyretin amyloidosis (mATTR). ATTR amyloidosis is caused by infiltration of mutant or wild-type transthyretin protein, and cardiac involvement can lead to the development of heart failure and arrhythmias. Recent literature suggests that cardiac amyloid may be more common than was previously thought, and the recent development of new therapies for ATTR hold the promise of improving outcomes.[47] The diagnosis of cardiac amyloidosis is complex in that multiple modalities can be used to aid in the identification of patients with suspected cardiac amyloidosis. The clinical history, echocardiography, cardiac MRI, and endomyocardial biopsy all play a role. However, it is radionuclide imaging with bone-avid tracers (^{99m}Tc-PYP, ^{99m}Tc-DPC, and ^{99m}Tc-HMDP) that has been shown to be 100% specific in identifying ATTR amyloid, and has replaced the need for invasive biopsy once monoclonal disease has been excluded.[48] Formal appropriate use criteria for the performance of cardiac amyloid studies have been recently released.[49]

Imaging Protocols: Technetium-99m-Pyrophosphate Amyloid

No specific preparation or fasting is required for this imaging study. Initially, 10 to 20 mCi of ^{99m}Tc-PYP is injected at rest and imaging performed 1 hour later, and, optionally, additionally at 3 hours if excess blood pool activity is noted on the 1-hour images. Planar acquisition of the chest, or whole body if desired, is performed for approximately 5 minutes for a minimum of 750,000 counts. This is followed by a standard 180-degree, nongated SPECT acquisition using 20 to 25 seconds per stop and 32 stops per detector.[50]

Interpretation: Technetium-99m-Pyrophosphate Amyloid

Interpretation of Tc-PYP amyloid studies relies on the ability to identify diffuse myocardial tracer uptake and differentiate this activity from residual blood pool activity or overlying bony uptake. If planar images suggest myocardial uptake, SPECT images must be reviewed to confirm myocardial uptake because they provide better spatial resolution.

Planar images can be graded using a semiquantitative visual score: grade 0, no myocardial uptake and normal bone

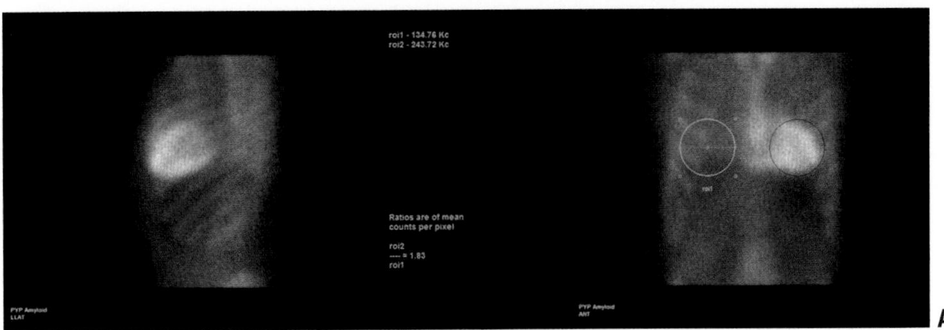

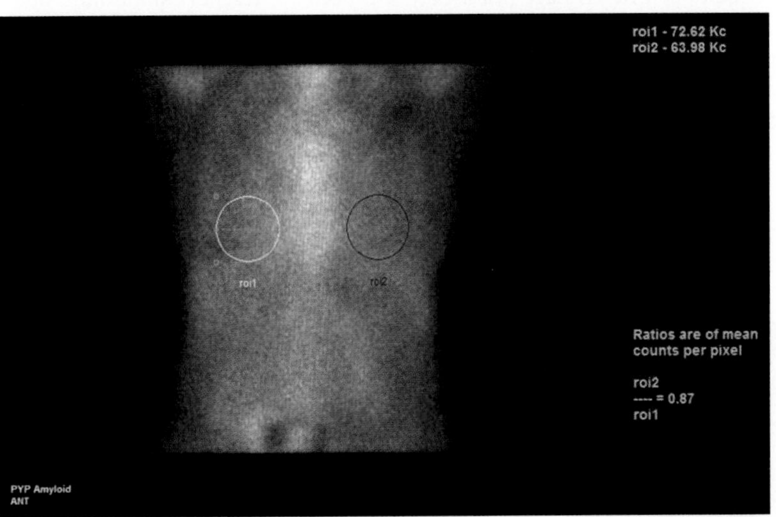

FIGURE 35.5 **(A)** A positive technetium-99m-pyrophosphate (^{99m}Tc-PYP) study with a quantitative visual score of 3 and heart-to-contralateral ratio of 1.83 strongly suggestive of ATTR cardiac amyloidosis. **(B)** A negative ^{99m}Tc-PYP study with a quantitative visual score of 0 and heart-to-contralateral ratio of 0.87 not suggestive of ATTR cardiac amyloidosis. ANT, anterior; ATTR, transthyretin; LLAT, left lateral; PYP, pyrophosphate; ROI, region of interest.

uptake; grade 1, myocardial uptake less than rib uptake; grade 2, myocardial uptake equal to rib uptake; and grade 3, myocardial uptake exceeds rib uptake. A heart-to-contralateral lung (H/CL) ratio is calculated using the mean counts in the heart region of interest (ROI) and the contralateral chest ROI mean counts. A circular or elliptical ROI is created over the heart on the anterior planar images, avoiding the sternum and excess lung or ribs. The same size ROI should be created over the contralateral chest to control for background counts (**Figure 35.5**). A grade 2 or 3 visually assessed semiquantitative uptake score and an H/CL ratio of greater than or equal to 1.5 at 1 hour can accurately differentiate ATTR cardiac amyloid from AL cardiac amyloid once a monoclonal gammopathy has been excluded.[51]

Special Considerations and Contraindications: Technetium-99m-Pyrophosphate Amyloid

A distinction should be made between diffuse and focal myocardial uptake during study interpretation because they may represent different processes. Diffuse uptake is typical for cardiac amyloid, whereas focal uptake may represent early amyloid, but has been described following MI as well. In addition, previous MI may confound image interpretation by resulting in falsely low H/CL ratios due to poor tracer uptake in the infarct zone. Image acquisition should not be limited to planar only for the calculation of the H/CL ratio and visual score, because SPECT imaging is essential for distinguishing blood pool counts from myocardial uptake and for resolving overlying bony uptake.

Limitations: Technetium-99m-Pyrophosphate Amyloid

The appearance of blood pool counts is a particularly problematic issue because it easily confounds the interpretation of images, making the identification of myocardial uptake difficult. Repeat imaging at 3 hours is recommended, but this adds considerable time to the study, and the H/CL ratio at 3 hours has not yet been definitively established. AL amyloid should always be excluded by performing the appropriate laboratory studies to exclude a monoclonal gammopathy and avoid incorrectly diagnosing ATTR amyloid.

Equilibrium Radionuclide Angiography

Indications: Equilibrium Radionuclide Angiography

Gated blood pool scans, equilibrium radionuclide angiography (ERNA), or radionuclide ventriculography (RVG), as it is commonly referred to, is performed by labeling red blood cells with ^{99m}Tc and uses a gamma camera to visualize the cardiac chambers. Image acquisition is routinely done with planar imaging and occasionally with SPECT imaging.[52] The counts obtained at end systole and end diastole are then used to assess chamber size and calculate the LVEF, which is the major use of ERNA (**Figure 35.6**). Before cardiovascular MRI became the preferred technique for ventricular function and volume assessment, ERNA was the gold standard. Because of its favorable reproducibility, ERNA is currently used in patients who need serial assessments of their LV function such as in patients receiving chemotherapy to monitor for cardiotoxicity.[53] Although its role in this setting has been largely supplanted by echocardiography, it continues to play a role in LV function assessment in patients with technically difficult acoustic echocardiographic windows or claustrophobia preventing imaging by cardiac MRI. In addition, ERNAs have historically also been used to assess cardiac shunts, wall motion, valvular disease, and ventricular filling and emptying rates.

Imaging Protocols: Equilibrium Radionuclide Angiography

There are two types of radionuclide angiography protocols: first-pass radionuclide angiography (FPRA) and ERNA. FPRA is used to assess LV and right ventricular function at rest or stress, wall motion, and other systolic and diastolic parameters, and can evaluate left-to-right shunts.[54] The first-pass technique is a method where the radiopharmaceutical is injected rapidly through a large bore, preferably central IV, and imaging is acquired as the tracer initially passes through the cardiac chambers before reaching equilibrium. It utilizes ^{99m}Tc diethylamine triamine pentaacetic acid (DTPA) or ^{99m}Tc pertechnetate (Tc-PYP) with a standard dose of 25 mCi. For shunt evaluation, the protocol is the same as for a standard study, but both lungs should be included in the field of view.

The acquisition of ERNA is done when the radioisotope reaches equilibrium, not during the initial injection.[52] Patients are injected with 20 to 25 mCi of ^{99m}Tc-labeled red blood cells for resting studies and 25 to 35 mCi for exercise studies. The radiotracer can be introduced to the patient in vitro, in vivo, or in a combination of the two methods. In all methods, stannous pyrophosphate is used as a reducing agent to facilitate binding of Tc-PYP to the red cells. The in vitro method involves withdrawing blood from the patient and adding stannous pyrophosphate to the drawn blood. Tc-PYP is then added to the

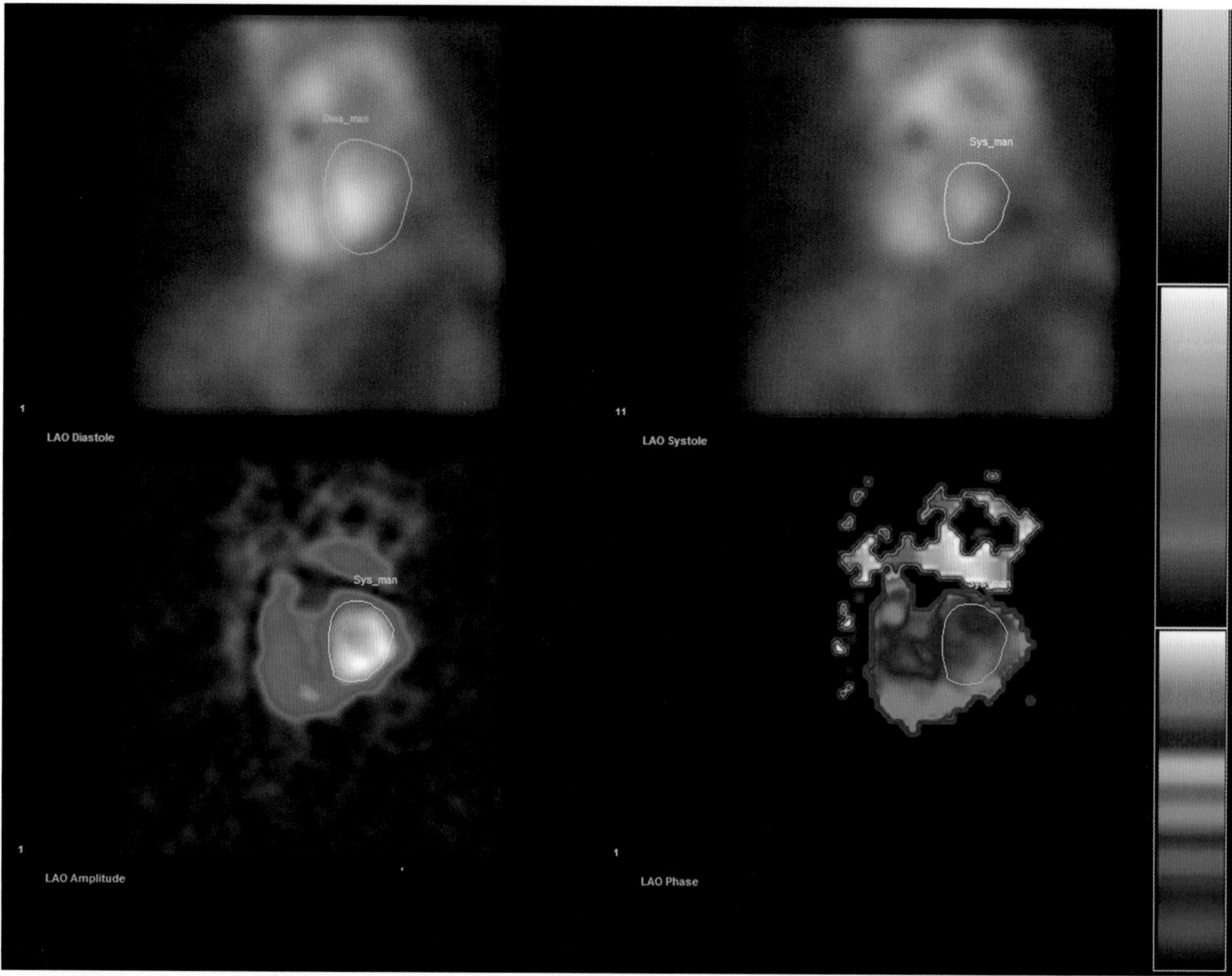

FIGURE 35.6 Left anterior oblique view of an equilibrium radionuclide angiography with manual tracing of the myocardial region of interest at end diastole (left) and end systole (right). EF, ejection fraction; LAO, left anterior oblique.

RBC sample for labeling. This method has the highest labeling efficiency. The in vivo method involves injecting stannous pyrophosphate 15 to 30 minutes before injecting Tc-PYP into the patient. This method is faster, but has lower labeling efficiency compared to the in vitro method. The modified in vivo method involves injecting the patient with stannous pyrophosphate 15 to 30 minutes before labeling with Tc-PYP. The patient's blood is then drawn into a syringe containing anticoagulant and incubated with Tc-PYP at room temperature for at least 10 minutes before being reinjected into the patient. Modified in vivo labeling efficiency is higher than the in vivo method.

With the gated equilibrium technique, data is collected over hundreds of cardiac cycles using ECG gating to assess cardiac function. Both planar acquisition and SPECT imaging can be used as the imaging modality. Planar acquisition should be obtained in view of the best septal separation (typically left anterior oblique [LAO]) projection to allow for isolation of the LV counts for accurate measurement. With three-dimensional (3D) volumetric assessment by SPECT acquisition, the left ventricle can be separated from the left atrium, and assessment of right ventricular size and function is more feasible. RVG studies are routinely performed at rest to provide assessment of resting ventricular function, but can be performed at stress to allow for assessment of ventricular response to exercise, although stress echocardiography has largely taken over this role.

Interpretation: Equilibrium Radionuclide Angiography

With FPRA, the final representation cycle should be displayed in a cinematic, endless loop format. The image should be normalized to peak activity in the ventricle because having higher aortic or left atrial activity can make it difficult to appreciate count changes in the ventricles. Cinematic displays of the bolus transit through the heart and great vessels can show abnormalities of tracer transit, possibly from congenital anomalies. Initial assessment of planar ERNA studies includes size, position, and rotation of the cardiac blood pool and proximal great arteries. A time activity curve is derived from an ROI drawn at end diastole and end systole, demonstrating the change in counts over time in the left ventricle that is proportional to chamber volumes. Reporting of planar ERNA includes chamber sizes, LV volumes and LVEF, regional wall motion, right ventricular size and function, and, optionally, LV emptying and filling parameters. SPECT ERNA includes measurement of right ventricular volumes and ejection fraction as well.

Special Considerations and Contraindications: Equilibrium Radionuclide Angiography

Red blood cell labeling can be affected by factors such as administration method of the radiopharmaceutical, medications, immune disorders, and decreased hematocrit.[52] These factors can cause poor labeling by mechanisms that include oxidation of stannous pyrophosphate, inducing antibodies complexes with ^{99m}Tc, among others. Image acquisition is ECG-gated; therefore, arrhythmias will affect the accuracy of acquired data. The risks and benefits of this study, which involves radiation exposure, are necessary to consider given the potential alternative of echocardiography. Because ERNA studies are performed less frequently than in the past, the expertise needed for the performance and interpretation of the study, especially first-pass studies, has become limited.

Limitations: Equilibrium Radionuclide Angiography

The study quality can be affected by adequacy of injection bolus, number, and type of beats used for inclusion, the count rate, the manner in which back ground activity is determined, and patient motion. There is also an element of interobserver variability in processing, even for laboratories with extensive experience and well-executed acquisition and processing techniques. The overlap of different cardiac structures (right and left ventricle in the anterior projection, left ventricle and left atrium in the "best septal" view) limits planar imaging and precise interpretation.

Cardiac Innervation/Metaiodobenzylguanidine

Indications: Cardiac Innervation/ Metaiodobenzylguanidine

Cardiac innervation imaging is designed to detect neuronal dysfunction even in the absence of structural abnormalities.[55] The sympathetic function of the heart is adversely altered in many conditions such as myocardial ischemia, congestive heart failure, and diabetes.[56] ^{123}I-*m*IBG, a radiopharmaceutical with a structure similar to norepinephrine, is used for scintigraphic imaging in the evaluation of cardiac neurotransmission.^{123}I-*m*IBG was first used for imaging neuroendocrine tumors and later was found to have significant cardiac uptake.[57]

^{123}I-*m*IBG is indicated for the assessment of sympathetic innervation of myocardium in patients with New York Heart Association (NYHA) class II or class III heart failure with an LVEF less than 35% to identify patients with lower 1- and 2-year mortality risks based on the heart-to-mediastinum ratio (HMR).[26] Beyond these indications, it can also be used to monitor cardiac toxicity from chemotherapy, identify patients with increased risk of cardiac arrhythmias, evaluate primary cardioneuropathies, assess pre- and postcardiac transplant patients, investigate diabetics for autonomic dysfunction, and assess the risk of ischemic heart disease.[57] A potential emerging indication is to help with clinical decision-making for patients who need implantable cardioverter-defibrillator (ICD) reimplantation after removal.[58]

Imaging Protocols: Cardiac Innervation/ Metaiodobenzylguanidine

^{123}I-*m*IBG is performed at rest in a fasting state. Medications that can interfere with mechanisms of norepinephrine uptake and granule storage such as opioids, cocaine, tramadol, tricyclic antidepressants, and sympathomimetics should be temporarily discontinued for at least a week before the study. These can also include some antihypertensives, cardiovascular agents, and antipsychotics.[26] Pretreatment with the oral administration of 130 mg potassium iodide or 500 mg potassium perchlorate at least 30 minutes before ^{123}I-*m*IBG injection to prevent thyroid uptake of ^{123}I is a decision made on a patient-by-patient basis, and might be considered more strongly in younger patients. A dose of 3 to 5 mCi of ^{123}I-MIBG administered over 1 minute can be used, but up to 10 mCi can be used for more optimal SPECT images. Planar scintigraphic images and SPECT images are acquired at 20 minutes (early) and 4 hours (delayed image) after injection. Planar images are acquired in the anterior and 45-degree LAO views.

Interpretation: Cardiac Innervation/ Metaiodobenzylguanidine

Planar and SPECT images are visually reviewed. The HMR is used to quantify ^{123}I-*m*IBG uptake by the heart (HMR >1.8 is considered normal). The standard process of deriving the HMR is by manually drawing the cardiac and mediastinal ROIs. The cardiac ROI counts are derived by creating an irregular ROI defining the epicardial border of the heart. Mediastinal ROI counts are derived from a square ROI in the upper mediastinum below the lung apices and midway between the lungs. The HMR is then calculated by dividing the mean counts/pixel in the total myocardium ROI by the mean counts/pixel in the mediastinal ROI.[26] The washout rate is also calculated, and a washout rate less than 10% is considered normal. SPECT images are also obtained for and data reconstructed into short axis, horizontal long axis, vertical long axis, as well as polar plots. These images are used for viewing myocardial ^{123}I-*m*IBG patterns.

Special Considerations and Contraindications: Cardiac Innervation/Metaiodobenzylguanidine

^{123}I-*m*IBG is contraindicated in patients with known hypersensitivity to iobenguane or iobenguane sulfate. This imaging can also be affected by several medications, so a careful history must be obtained.[59] Renal dysfunction is a relative contraindication because ^{123}I-*m*IBG is cleared through the kidneys. Adverse reactions are uncommon, but if ^{123}I-*m*IBG is administered too rapidly, patients can experience palpitations, shortness of breath, heat sensations, transient hypertension, and abdominal cramps.

Limitations: Cardiac Innervation/ Metaiodobenzylguanidine

Noncardiac structures such as the lung and mediastinum can affect visualization of the images. Occasionally, the myocardium is not well visualized, and the ROI should be based on the presumed location of the heart. Adjacent organs such as the lung and liver may also be included in myocardial counts affecting the HMR. Many commonly used medications interfere with ^{123}I-*m*IBG uptake, and this can affect the HMR results. Most importantly, the imaging technique has not found a useful clinical indication or found a routine use in the care of the patient with heart failure.

FUTURE DIRECTIONS

Future directions in nuclear cardiology will focus on novel technologic advances and expanding applications of existing technology. Owing to its relatively recent introduction and limited use, the utilization of SPECT MFR warrants further study assessing its validity, reproducibility, and clinical application as it expands more into mainstream clinical use. Further trials are needed to determine the clinical utility of PET and SPECT MFR's utility in patient care and clinical effectiveness. The role of FDG PET imaging for cardiac infection, including early identification of endocarditis, prosthetic valve endocarditis, or device-related infections is likely to grow as the technique reaches more widespread utilization. With new therapeutic options in the treatment of ATTR amyloid emerging, the future of the imaging technique will address appropriate populations to screen and the utility of follow-up imaging to assess therapeutic response.

KEY POINTS

- ✔ SPECT and PET MPI can accurately diagnose CAD, and plays an active role in patient management in providing useful prognostic information that correlates with future risk of adverse cardiovascular events.
- ✔ MFR derived from PET MPI dynamic acquisitions improves diagnostic accuracy and prognostic utility independently or when added to perfusion images.
- ✔ Cardiac PET metabolic imaging can be used for the assessment of cardiac viability, cardiac sarcoidosis, and cardiac infections.
- ✔ Radionuclide imaging with bone-avid tracers has been shown to be 100% specific in identifying ATTR amyloid and has replaced the need for invasive biopsy once monoclonal disease has been excluded.
- ✔ Equilibrium radionuclide angiography and cardiac innervation imaging have a niche role in the assessment of LV function and cardiomyopathies.

REFERENCES

1. Currie GM, Wheat JM, Davidson R, JKiat H. Radionuclide production. *Radiographer.* 2011;58:46-52.
2. Dorbala S, Ananthasubramaniam K, Armstrong IS, et al. Single Photon Emission Computed Tomography (SPECT) myocardial perfusion imaging guidelines: instrumentation, acquisition, processing, and interpretation. *J Nucl Cardiol.* 2018;25:1784-1846.
3. Dilsizian V, Bacharach SL, Beanlands RS, et al. ASNC imaging guidelines/SNMMI procedure standard for positron emission tomography (PET) nuclear cardiology procedures. *J Nucl Cardiol.* 2016;23:1187-1226.
4. Parker MW, Iskandar A, Limone B, et al. Diagnostic accuracy of cardiac positron emission tomography versus single photon emission computed tomography for coronary artery disease: a bivariate meta-analysis. *Circ Cardiovasc Imaging.* 2012;5:700-707.
5. Hendel RC, Berman DS, Di Carli MF, et al. ACCF/ASNC/ACR/AHA/ASE/SCCT/SCMR/SNM 2009 appropriate use criteria for cardiac radionuclide imaging: a report of the American College of Cardiology Foundation Appropriate Use Criteria Task Force, the American Society of Nuclear Cardiology, the American College of Radiology, the American Heart Association, the American Society of Echocardiography, the Society of Cardiovascular Computed Tomography, the Society for Cardiovascular

Magnetic Resonance, and the Society of Nuclear Medicine. *J Am Coll Cardiol.* 2009;53:2201-2229.
6. Bourque JM, Beller GA. Stress myocardial perfusion imaging for assessing prognosis: an update. *JACC Cardiovasc Imaging.* 2011;4:1305-1319.
7. Kang X, Berman DS, Lewin HC, et al. Incremental prognostic value of myocardial perfusion single photon emission computed tomography in patients with diabetes mellitus. *Am Heart J.* 1999;138:1025-1032.
8. Cremer P, Hachamovitch R, Tamarappoo B. Clinical decision making with myocardial perfusion imaging in patients with known or suspected coronary artery disease. *Semin Nucl Med.* 2014;44:320-329.
9. Bourque JM, Charlton GT, Holland BH, Belyea CM, Watson DD, Beller GA. Prognosis in patients achieving ≥10 METS on exercise stress testing: was SPECT imaging useful? *J Nucl Cardiol.* 2011;18:230-237.
10. Chang SM, Nabi F, Xu J, Raza U, Mahmarian JJ. Normal stress-only versus standard stress/rest myocardial perfusion imaging: similar patient mortality with reduced radiation exposure. *J Am Coll Cardiol.* 2010;55:221-230.
11. Hage FG, Ghimire G, Lester D, et al. The prognostic value of regadenoson myocardial perfusion imaging. *J Nucl Cardiol.* 2015;22:1214-1221.
12. Travin MI, Heller GV, Johnson LL, et al. The prognostic value of ECG-gated SPECT imaging in patients undergoing stress Tc-99m sestamibi myocardial perfusion imaging. *J Nucl Cardiol.* 2004;11:253-262.
13. Alama M, Labos C, Emery H, et al. Diagnostic and prognostic significance of transient ischemic dilation (TID) in myocardial perfusion imaging: a systematic review and meta-analysis. *J Nucl Cardiol.* 2018;25:724-737.
14. Pazhenkottil AP, Ghadri JR, Nkoulou RN, et al. Improved outcome prediction by SPECT myocardial perfusion imaging after CT attenuation correction. *J Nucl Med.* 2011;52:196-200.
15. Ardestani A, Ahlberg AW, Katten DM, et al. Risk stratification using line source attenuation correction with rest/stress Tc-99m sestamibi SPECT myocardial perfusion imaging. *J Nucl Cardiol.* 2014;21:118-126.
16. Murthy VL, Naya M, Foster CR, et al. Improved cardiac risk assessment with noninvasive measures of coronary flow reserve. *Circulation.* 2011;124:2215-2224.
17. Naya M, Murthy VL, Taqueti VR, et al. Preserved coronary flow reserve effectively excludes high-risk coronary artery disease on angiography. *J Nucl Med.* 2014;55:248-255.
18. Raff GL, Hoffmann U, Udelson JE. Trials of imaging use in the emergency department for acute chest pain. *JACC Cardiovasc Imaging.* 2017;10:338-349.
19. Mahler SA, Riley RF, Hiestand BC, et al. The HEART pathway randomized trial: identifying emergency department patients with acute chest pain for early discharge. *Circ Cardiovasc Qual Outcomes.* 2015;8:195-203.
20. Hachamovitch R, Hayes SW, Friedman JD, Cohen I, Berman DS. Comparison of the short-term survival benefit associated with revascularization compared with medical therapy in patients with no prior coronary artery disease undergoing stress myocardial perfusion single photon emission computed tomography. *Circulation.* 2003;107:2900-2907.
21. Neumann FJ, Sousa-Uva M, Ahlsson A, et al. 2018 ESC/EACTS guidelines on myocardial revascularization. *Eur Heart J.* 2019;40:87-165.
22. Fleisher LA, Fleischmann KE, Auerbach AD, et al. 2014 ACC/AHA guideline on perioperative cardiovascular evaluation and management of patients undergoing noncardiac surgery: a report of the American College of Cardiology/American Heart Association Task Force on practice guidelines. *J Am Coll Cardiol.* 2014;64:e77-e137.
23. Thompson RC, McGhie AI, Moser KW, et al. Clinical utility of coronary calcium scoring after nonischemic myocardial perfusion imaging. *J Nucl Cardiol.* 2005;12:392-400.
24. Patchett ND, Pawar S, Miller EJ. Visual identification of coronary calcifications on attenuation correction CT improves diagnostic accuracy of SPECT/CT myocardial perfusion imaging. *J Nucl Cardiol.* 2017;24:711-720.
25. Chang SM, Nabi F, Xu J, et al. The coronary artery calcium score and stress myocardial perfusion imaging provide independent and complementary prediction of cardiac risk. *J Am Coll Cardiol.* 2009;54:1872-1882.
26. Henzlova MJ, Duvall WL, Einstein AJ, Travin MI, Verberne HJ. ASNC imaging guidelines for SPECT nuclear cardiology procedures: stress, protocols, and tracers. *J Nucl Cardiol.* 2016;23:606-639.
27. Huang JY, Huang CK, Yen RF, et al. Diagnostic performance of attenuation-corrected myocardial perfusion imaging for coronary artery disease: a systematic review and meta-analysis. *J Nucl Med.* 2016;57:1893-1898.
28. Schepis T, Gaemperli O, Koepfli P, et al. Added value of coronary artery calcium score as an adjunct to gated SPECT for the evaluation of coronary artery disease in an intermediate-risk population. *J Nucl Med.* 2007;48:1424-1430.
29. Udelson JE, Beshansky JR, Ballin DS, et al. Myocardial perfusion imaging for evaluation and triage of patients with suspected acute cardiac ischemia: a randomized controlled trial. *JAMA.* 2002;288:2693-2700.
30. McMahon SR, Kikut J, Pinckney RG, Keating FK. Feasibility of stress only rubidium-82 PET myocardial perfusion imaging. *J Nucl Cardiol.* 2013;20:1069-1075.
31. Leslie WD, Tully SA, Yogendran MS, Ward LM, Nour KA, Metge CJ. Prognostic value of automated quantification of 99mTc-sestamibi myocardial perfusion imaging. *J Nucl Med.* 2005;46:204-211.
32. Mahmarian JJ, Shaw LJ, Filipchuk NG, et al. A multinational study to establish the value of early adenosine technetium-99m sestamibi myocardial perfusion imaging in identifying a low-risk group for early hospital discharge after acute myocardial infarction. *J Am Coll Cardiol.* 2006;48:2448-2457.
33. Rai M, Ahlberg AW, Marwell J, et al. Safety of vasodilator stress myocardial perfusion imaging in patients with elevated cardiac biomarkers. *J Nucl Cardiol.* 2017;24:724-734.
34. Velazquez EJ, Lee KL, Deja MA, et al. Coronary-artery bypass surgery in patients with left ventricular dysfunction. *N Engl J Med.* 2011;364:1607-1616.
35. Velazquez EJ, Lee KL, Jones RH, et al. Coronary-artery bypass surgery in patients with ischemic cardiomyopathy. *N Engl J Med.* 2016;374:1511-1520.
36. Kandolin RM, Wiefels CC, Mesquita CT, et al. The current role of viability imaging to guide revascularization and therapy decisions in patients with heart failure and reduced left ventricular function. *Can J Cardiol.* 2019;35:1015-1029.
37. Beanlands RS, Nichol G, Huszti E, et al. F-18-fluorodeoxyglucose positron emission tomography imaging-assisted management of patients with severe left ventricular dysfunction and suspected coronary disease: a randomized, controlled trial (PARR-2). *J Am Coll Cardiol.* 2007;50:2002-2012.
38. Abraham A, Nichol G, Williams KA, et al. ^{18}F-FDG PET imaging of myocardial viability in an experienced center with access to ^{18}F-FDG and integration with clinical management teams: the Ottawa-FIVE substudy of the PARR 2 trial. *J Nucl Med.* 2010;51:567-574.
39. Bonow RO, Maurer G, Lee KL, et al. Myocardial viability and survival in ischemic left ventricular dysfunction. *N Engl J Med.* 2011;364:1617-1625.
40. Chareonthaitawee P, Beanlands RS, Chen W, et al. Joint SNMMI-ASNC expert consensus document on the role of (18)F-FDG PET/CT in cardiac sarcoid detection and therapy monitoring. *J Nucl Cardiol.* 2017;24:1741-1758.
41. Slart R, Glaudemans A, Lancellotti P, et al. A joint procedural position statement on imaging in cardiac sarcoidosis: from the Cardiovascular and Inflammation & Infection Committees of the European Association of Nuclear Medicine, the European Association of Cardiovascular Imaging, and the American Society of Nuclear Cardiology. *J Nucl Cardiol.* 2018;25:298-319.
42. Bois JP, Muser D, Chareonthaitawee P. PET/CT evaluation of cardiac sarcoidosis. *PET Clin.* 2019;14:223-232.
43. Gomes A, Glaudemans A, Touw DJ, et al. Diagnostic value of imaging in infective endocarditis: a systematic review. *Lancet Infect Dis.* 2017;17:e1-e14.
44. Habib G, Lancellotti P, Antunes MJ, et al. 2015 ESC guidelines for the management of infective endocarditis: The Task Force for the Management of Infective Endocarditis of the European Society of Cardiology (ESC). Endorsed by: European Association for Cardio-Thoracic Surgery

(EACTS), the European Association of Nuclear Medicine (EANM). *Eur Heart J.* 2015;36:3075-3128.
45. Chen W, Sajadi MM, Dilsizian V. Merits of FDG PET/CT and functional molecular imaging over anatomic imaging with echocardiography and CT angiography for the diagnosis of cardiac device infections. *JACC Cardiovasc Imaging.* 2018;11:1679-1691.
46. Swart LE, Scholtens AM, Tanis W, et al. 18F-fluorodeoxyglucose positron emission/computed tomography and computed tomography angiography in prosthetic heart valve endocarditis: from guidelines to clinical practice. *Eur Heart J.* 2018;39:3739-3749.
47. Ruberg FL, Grogan M, Hanna M, Kelly JW, Maurer MS. Transthyretin amyloid cardiomyopathy: JACC state-of-the-art review. *J Am Coll Cardiol.* 2019;73:2872-2891.
48. Gillmore JD, Maurer MS, Falk RH, et al. Nonbiopsy diagnosis of cardiac transthyretin amyloidosis. *Circulation.* 2016;133:2404-2412.
49. Dorbala S, Ando Y, Bokhari S, et al. ASNC/AHA/ASE/EANM/HFSA/ISA/SCMR/SNMMI expert consensus recommendations for multimodality imaging in cardiac amyloidosis: part 2 of 2-Diagnostic criteria and appropriate utilization. *J Nucl Cardiol.* 2020;27(2):659-673.
50. Dorbala S, Ando Y, Bokhari S, et al. ASNC/AHA/ASE/EANM/HFSA/ISA/SCMR/SNMMI expert consensus recommendations for multimodality imaging in cardiac amyloidosis: part 1 of 2-evidence base and standardized methods of imaging. *J Nucl Cardiol.* 2020;26(6):2065-2123.
51. Maurer MS, Bokhari S, Damy T, et al. Expert consensus recommendations for the suspicion and diagnosis of transthyretin cardiac amyloidosis. *Circ Heart Fail.* 2019;12:e006075.
52. Corbett JR, Akinboboye OO, Bacharach SL, et al. Equilibrium radionuclide angiocardiography. *J Nucl Cardiol.* 2006;13:e56-e79.
53. Schwartz RG, Jain D, Storozynsky E. Traditional and novel methods to assess and prevent chemotherapy-related cardiac dysfunction noninvasively. *J Nucl Cardiol.* 2013;20:443-464.
54. Friedman JD, Berman DS, Borges-Neto S, et al. First-pass radionuclide angiography. *J Nucl Cardiol.* 2006;13:e42-e55.
55. Carrio I. Cardiac neurotransmission imaging. *J Nucl Med.* 2001;42:1062-1076.
56. Chirumamilla A, Travin MI. Cardiac applications of 123I-mIBG imaging. *Semin Nucl Med.* 2011;41:374-387.
57. Travin MI. Current clinical applications and next steps for cardiac innervation imaging. *Curr Cardiol Rep.* 2017;19:1.
58. Sciammarella MG, Gerson M, Buxton AE, et al. ASNC/SNMMI model coverage policy: myocardial sympathetic innervation imaging: Iodine-123 meta-iodobenzylguanidine ((123)I-mIBG). *J Nucl Cardiol.* 2015;22:804-811.
59. Van Vickle SS, Thompson RC. 123I-MIBG imaging: patient preparation and technologist's role. *J Nucl Med Technol.* 2015;43:82-86.

CHAPTER 36

CARDIAC COMPUTED TOMOGRAPHY

Ron Blankstein and Vasvi Singh

INTRODUCTION

Cardiac computed tomography (CCT) has evolved considerably over the past 15 years and now serves an essential role in the practice of cardiology and cardiac surgery. The growth in CCT has been due to both technical advances in the field and clinical effectiveness studies showing how CCT can be useful in diagnosis and patient management. As a result, CCT now provides an opportunity to image many forms of cardiovascular diseases ranging from coronary artery disease (CAD) and myocardial disease to valvular and pericardial heart disease (**Table 36.1**).

CCT—whether with or without contrast—utilizes x-rays to obtain high-resolution three-dimensional (3D) data sets that then allow users to view various parts of the heart. A fundamental advancement that enables computed tomography (CT) imaging of the heart is the use of electrocardiographic (ECG) gating, whereby image acquisition is performed during predetermined phases of the cardiac cycle, thus "freezing" the motion of the heart. There are various protocols and applications of CCT, among them:

- Coronary artery calcium (CAC) scan—non–contrast-enhanced ECG-gated images that are performed to identify the presence and amount of coronary calcium, which is quantified as an Agatston score.
- Coronary computed tomography angiography (CCTA)—contrast-enhanced ECG-gated images that are performed to identify the presence of both calcified and noncalcified plaque, as well as estimate the severity of stenoses.

TABLE 36.1 Examples of Cardiac Pathology That Can Be Evaluated Using Different Cardiac Computed Tomography Applications

Type of Cardiac Pathology	Type of Test	Example of Indications/Data Provided
Coronary plaque	CAC	Presence and amount of calcified coronary plaque
	Coronary CT angiography	Presence, extent, and severity of coronary plaque and stenosis Patency of coronary bypass grafts
	Stress CT perfusion	Evaluate hemodynamic significance of coronary stenosis by assessing for stress-induced myocardial perfusion defects[a]
	CT-FFR	Evaluate hemodynamic significance of coronary stenosis by estimating fractional flow reserve
Pericardial disease	CCT	Pericardial thickness and calcifications Pericardial enhancement[a]
Myocardial disease	Cine-CCT	Evaluate wall thickness and wall motion abnormalities May evaluate some forms of infiltrative heart disease[a] Evaluate for known or suspected cardiac masses
Valvular heart disease	Cine-CCT	Evaluate valvular structure and function[a] Evaluate for endocarditis in native or prosthetic valves Evaluate before TAVR/TMVR Evaluate post TAVR/TMVR
Structural heart disease	Cine-CCT	Evaluate feasibility of repair of various shunts, fistulas, or perivalvular regurgitation. Evaluate pre- and post-left atrial appendage occlusion device placement
Congenital heart disease	Cine-CCT	Evaluate for simple or complex congenital heart disease, including shunts, anomalous coronary arteries, s/p corrective procedures

CAC, coronary artery calcium; CCT, cardiac computed tomography; CT, computed tomography; CT-FFR, computed tomography fractional flow reserve; TAVR, transcatheter aortic valve replacement; TMVR, transcatheter mitral valve replacement.

[a]May require specialized protocol.

- Cine-CCT—contrast-enhanced ECG-gated images that are obtained throughout multiple phases of the cardiac cycle, thus allowing for the reconstruction of cine images. The ability to view the heart throughout the cardiac cycle can be used to determine left ventricular (LV) or right ventricular systolic function and to assess valvular heart disease.

This chapter provides readers with an overview of the various uses of CCT and how to utilize this test in clinical practice.

PHYSICAL PRINCIPLES AND INSTRUMENTATION

Cardiac imaging with CT requires high temporal resolution to limit cardiac motion artifacts, high spatial resolution to visualize small cardiac anatomy, fast anatomic coverage allowing scanning of the heart during a breath-hold to reduce respiratory motion artifacts, and synchronization of data acquisition or reconstruction to the cardiac cycle to ensure imaging during a desired cardiac phase.

In a CT system, an x-ray source rotates continuously in a gantry, emitting a beam that is attenuated by the target (patient's chest) and detected by an array of sensors opposite the x-ray source. Modern scanners permit the simultaneous acquisition of multiple (64, 128, and 320 submillimeter thin) slices at rotation times as short as 270 ms. In the source, x-rays are produced when highly energetic electrons interact with matter. Electrons are accelerated toward a target to gain kinetic energy. For most diagnostic imaging applications, the electrons gain a maximum kinetic energy between 80 and 140 keV. The attenuation, or removal, of photons from x-rays passing through tissue is dependent on both the energy of the x-rays and density of the tissue within the scanned region. Attenuated x-rays are detected opposite the image source by multiple rows of detectors. An 180-degree rotation of the x-ray tube/detector system is required to generate an image.

Data covering the entire heart are acquired using either axial or helical modes within a single breath-hold. Images are reconstructed with thicknesses ranging from 0.5 to 3 mm depending on the specific cardiac application. An ECG signal is used to reference data to the cardiac cycle. The ECG signal may be used to either prospectively trigger data acquisition or retrospectively gate data reconstruction. For static morphologic evaluation of most cardiac structures, data is usually selected from the diastolic phase of the cardiac cycle where heart motion is minimized. During axial mode acquisition (step-and-shoot), data acquisition is prospectively triggered by the ECG signal during the desired cardiac phase. The patient table moves at incremental steps between periods of data acquisition. The number of steps depends on the coverage width of specific scanner models (typically 4 cm/64 slices, 8 cm/128 slices, and 16 cm/320 slices). In the helical mode of operation, data are acquired continuously with simultaneous recording of the ECG signal. Data are then retrospectively gated to the ECG signal after acquisition and reconstructed during one or more cardiac phases.

ANATOMIC CONSIDERATIONS

CCT enables detailed visualization of all cardiac structures, including pericardium, pericardial and epicardial fat, myocardium, coronary arteries and veins, and valves. The strength of CCT is the ability to obtain high spatial resolution images. Accordingly, CCT can provide detailed visualization of coronary artery plaque and stenoses. On the other hand, CCT has lower contrast resolution than do other techniques such as cardiac magnetic resonance (CMR) imaging. Thus CMR—particularly using late gadolinium enhancement imaging—is better suited for evaluating infiltrative disease of the myocardium, or certain types of cardiac masses.

FUNDAMENTALS OF CARDIAC COMPUTED TOMOGRAPHY IMAGING

CAC scan—CAC assessment does not require administration of radiographic contrast agent or premedication. The scan consists of an ECG-gated, limited field-of-view 3D image of the heart during a single phase of the cardiac cycle. The radiation dose of a CAC study is usually approximately 1 mSV, which is similar to that for a mammogram.

Coronary computed tomography angiography—CCTA requires a large-bore (18-gauge) intravenous (IV) catheter for the delivery of contrast material at a rate of 5 to 6 cc/second. To achieve good image quality, patients are often administered beta-blockers (to lower the heart rate) and nitroglycerin (to dilate the coronary arteries). The radiation dose of CCTA using contemporary techniques is usually approximately 2 to 5 mSv,[1] but can be higher when older techniques/scanners are employed, especially if data are acquired throughout multiple phases of the cardiac cycle using a helical acquisition mode. The presence of arrhythmias can also increase the radiation dose.[2]

Cine-CCT—Cine-CCT is acquired in a way similar to that for CCTA scans, except that data from multiple cardiac phases are acquired, and thus the radiation dose may be higher. When detailed anatomy of the coronary arteries is not needed, nitroglycerin is not required. Also, contrast agent administration may differ, particularly when there is a need to image right-sided heart structures.

CLINICAL APPLICATION AND INDICATIONS

Coronary Artery Calcium Scan

CAC testing can quantify the amount of calcified coronary plaque (**Figure 36.1**). There is considerable data showing that among patients who do not have established CAD, there is increased risk of atherosclerotic cardiovascular disease (ASCVD) events with increasing CAC scores. Conversely, patients who lack calcified plaque (CAC = 0) generally have a very low event rate.[3] In addition, the addition of CAC to traditional risk factors results in improved risk assessment and risk reclassification.

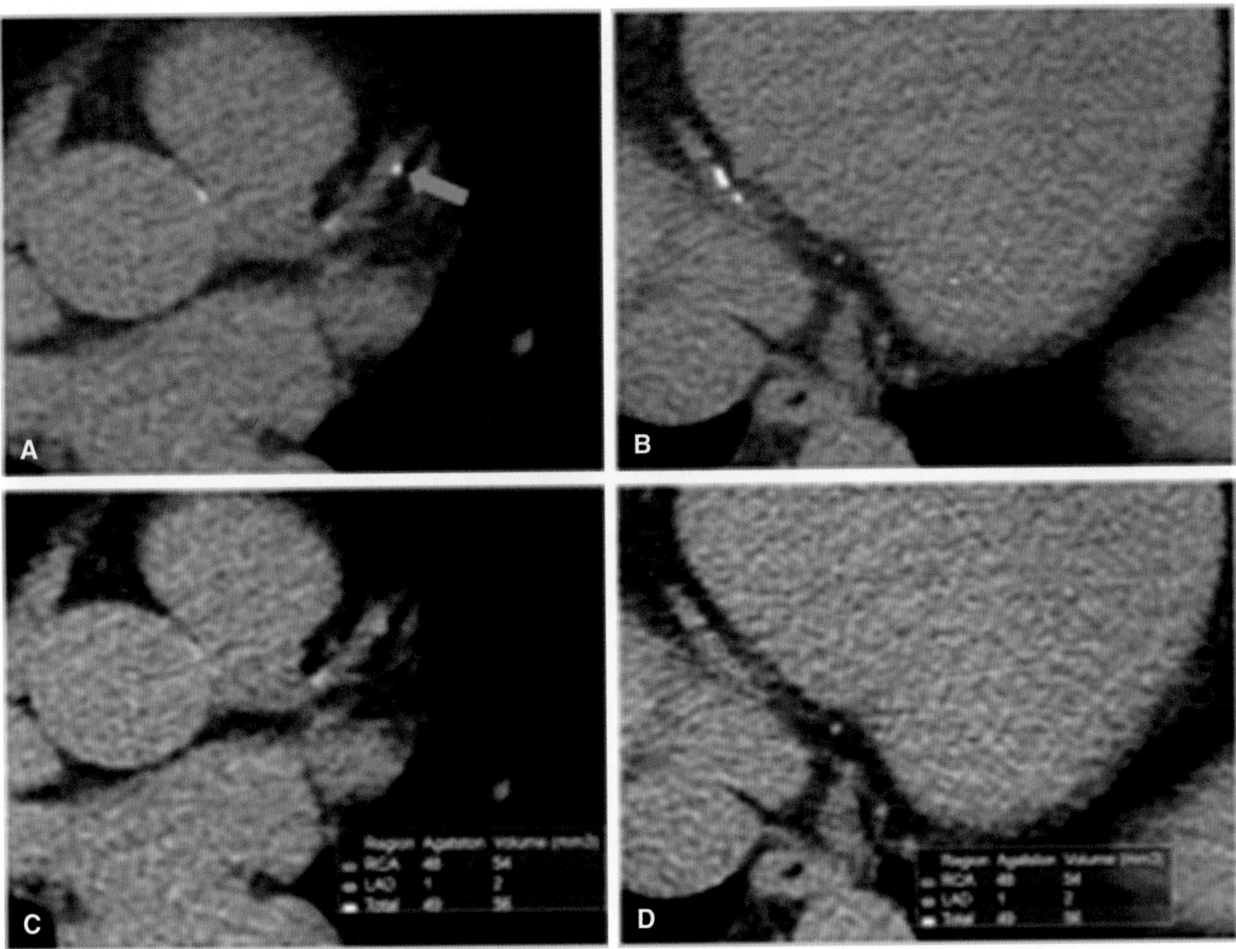

FIGURE 36.1 Example of coronary artery calcium (CAC) testing. A 54-year-old female with impaired glucose tolerance and hyperlipidemia was referred for CAC scan for cardiovascular risk assessment. A prospectively electrocardiography (ECG)-gated non-contrast computed tomography (CT) scan with field-of-view limited to the heart was obtained. Images were reconstructed at 3-mm intervals. CAC scan showing **(A)** left anterior descending artery calcifications (green arrow), **(B)** right coronary artery calcifications (red arrow), **(C,D)** overall, mild amount of coronary calcifications with an Agatston score of 49.

Indications for Coronary Artery Calcium Testing

- **Statin averse**—Improved risk assessment, in the context of shared decision-making, among individuals who meet criteria for statin therapy (ie, 10-year ASCVD risk of 5%-20%), but have a preference to defer therapy. In such patients, the presence of a CAC score of zero could be used to identify low-risk patients and defer therapy.[3-5] Notably, patients who have a high risk of ASCVD events are less likely to benefit from CAC testing because their risk may remain elevated even in the absence of CAC.
- **Statin-intolerant patients** may benefit from CAC testing to determine the likelihood that they will benefit from statin, or in some cases from additional lipid-lowering therapies that may be more costly.
- **Screening** in the lower risk cohort who have either traditional or nontraditional risk factors, when decision-making regarding risk versus benefit of statin therapy is uncertain. For example, some individuals who have a low 10-year ASCVD risk but who have a family history of premature ASCVD events may benefit from CAC testing.[4,6]
- In general, the yield of CAC testing in those who are younger than age 40 is low. However, some studies have suggested a limited role for selected use of CAC testing among men and women who are younger than age 40.[7,8] In such cases, the finding of any atherosclerosis (ie, CAC > 0) implies a higher risk of future ASCVD events; however, the absence of CAC may be less reassuring, especially when considering a longer time perspective.

Coronary Computed Tomography Angiography

CCTA is most useful for evaluating symptomatic patients with suspected CAD. In such patients, a normal CCTA, defined as having no plaque and no stenosis, is associated with excellent prognosis with a very low future rate of cardiac death or MI.[9,10]

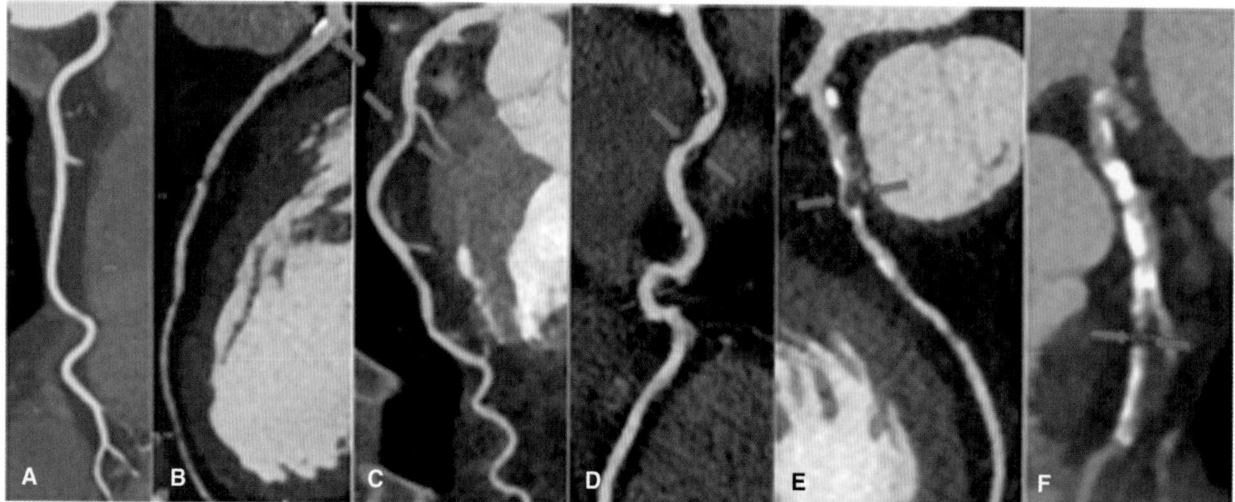

FIGURE 36.2 CAD-RADS: Coronary Artery Disease-Reporting and Data System classification. **(A)** CAD-RADS 0: coronary with no plaque or stenosis (0%). **(B)** CAD-RADS 1: There is a small amount of calcified plaque in the proximal segment of the coronary, resulting in minimal stenosis (1%-24%) (red arrows). **(C)** CAD-RADS 2: There is a small amount of noncalcified plaque in the mid segment of the coronary, resulting in mild stenosis (25%-49%) (red arrows). **(D)** CAD-RADS 3: There is a moderate amount of calcified and noncalcified plaque in the coronary, resulting in moderate stenosis (50%-69%) of the mid segment (red arrows). **(E)** CAD-RADS 4: There is a large amount of calcified and noncalcified plaque in the coronary, resulting in severe stenosis (70%-99%) of the mid segment (red arrows). **(F)** CAD-RADS 5: There is a large amount of calcified and noncalcified plaque in the coronary, resulting in total occlusion (100%) of the mid segment (red arrows).

On the other hand, patients who are found to have CAD (**Figure 36.2**) are the ones who are most likely to benefit from lifestyle and pharmacologic preventive therapies. Recently, several studies have shown that the use of CCTA results in a lower rate of subsequent myocardial infarctions or coronary heart disease death when compared with other functional approaches.[11,12] The benefits of CCTA likely reflect the fact that this test can identify the presence of atherosclerosis—and thus have an impact on patient management—in cases where functional tests (which only identify flow-limiting CAD) would otherwise be unremarkable.[13,14]

When CCTA demonstrates severe stenosis in a patient with significant symptoms (**Figure 36.3**)—or in the presence of high-risk coronary anatomy, such as left main disease or multivessel disease—coronary revascularization may be preferred to medical therapy alone. Recently, the International Study of Comparative Health Effectiveness With Medical and Invasive Approaches (ISCHEMIA) trial showed that among stable patients with symptomatic CAD, the use of coronary revascularization was not associated with a reduction in the risk of cardiovascular events, when compared to optimal medical therapy, over a median follow-up of 3.3 years.[15] This trial reinforced the importance of optimal medical therapy for treating patients with CAD, and suggested that an initial conservative management strategy of medical therapy was safe. However, among individuals with symptoms of angina, coronary revascularization was associated with a greater reduction in angina and improved quality of life. Importantly, in this trial, CCTA was used to rule out patients with underlying left main disease (~5% of included patients) and exclude individuals who did not have obstructive CAD (~14% of patients) despite an abnormal functional study.

Indications for Coronary Computed Tomography Angiography

- **Evaluation of acute chest pain** usually in the emergency department or observation unit. Use of CCTA in this setting reduces time to diagnosis and emergency department length of stay.[16] CCTA can also identify alternative explanations for a patient's symptoms (eg, aortic pathology and hiatal hernia). **Figure 36.4** presents examples of use of CCTA in the emergency department.
- **Evaluation of stable chest pain in the following patients:**
  - In patients with no prior CAD, CCTA can be used as first-line testing option. Examples of CCTA findings are shown in Figure 36.2.
  - In patients who have ischemia on functional testing, CCTA may be used to exclude high-risk anatomy, particularly if there is preference for treatment with medical therapy alone.
  - In patients with known or suspected anomalous origin of the coronary arteries, CCTA can be used to identify cases of abnormal origin of the coronary arteries, and describe high-risk features as well[17,18] (**Figure 36.5**).

Patient Management Following Coronary Computed Tomography Angiography

Patients who are found to have nonobstructive plaque (CAD RADS 1 or CAD RADS 2; Figure 36.2A,B), especially when extensive, should be prescribed preventive therapies, including lipid-lowering therapy and lifestyle changes. Studies suggest that patients who have at least a moderate amount of plaque

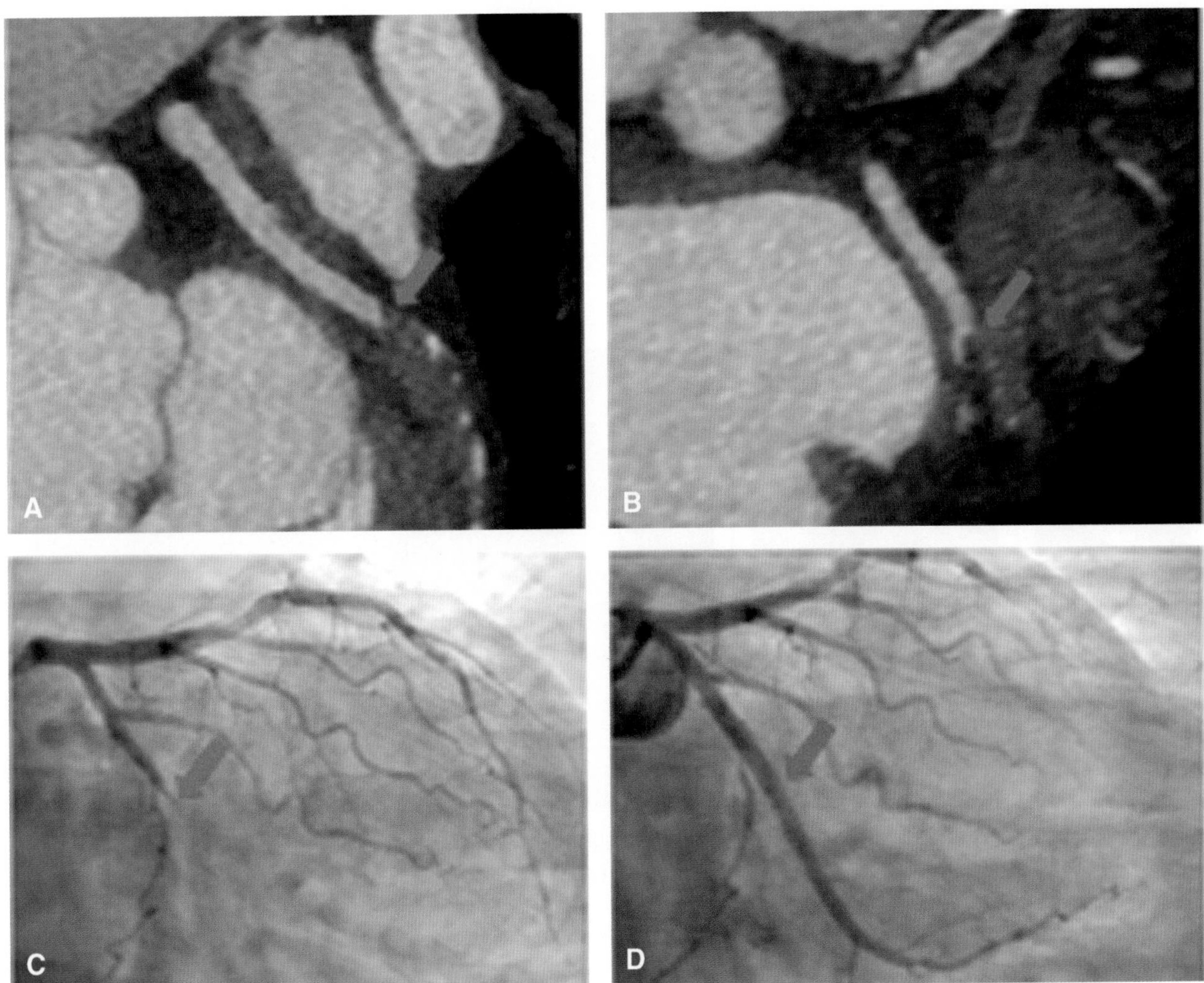

FIGURE 36.3 A 58-year-old male with hypertension and dyslipidemia presents to his outpatient cardiologist with intermittent exertional chest pain that was partially relieved with rest. Coronary computed tomography angiography (CCTA) **(A,B)** showed 100% occlusion of a large-sized second obtuse marginal (OM2) branch of the circumflex (red arrows) in orthogonal views. **(C)** Coronary angiography confirmed 100% occlusion of OM2 branch (red arrow). **(D)** The patient underwent successful percutaneous coronary intervention with three overlapping drug-eluting stents to the lesion (red arrow) with resolution of chest pain.

may also benefit from aspirin therapy,[19] if there are no contraindications or risk factors that would confer an elevated risk of bleeding. Patients who have moderate coronary stenosis (ie, 50%-69%) or severe stenosis (ie, ≥70%) also require aggressive medical therapy, but may benefit from coronary revascularization if they have frequent angina. When there is uncertainty whether a lesion is flow limiting, patients may benefit from further functional testing with exercise treadmill testing, myocardial perfusion imaging, stress echocardiography, or computed tomography estimation of fractional flow reserve (CT-FFR).

CT-FFR is a technique that applies computational fluid dynamic modeling to rest coronary CTA data to estimate invasive FFR values. The available data has shown that this is an accurate technique when compared with invasive FFR; however, it requires excellent image quality on CCTA. Registry studies found a very low rate of cardiovascular events among patients who have a CT-FFR greater than 0.8, suggesting that it is safe to defer coronary revascularization in such patients.[20,21]

Cine-Coronary Computed Tomography

In addition to evaluation of the coronary arteries, a cine-CCT can be used to obtain information on valvular function, and cardiac morphology, structure, and function.

Valvular Function

The indications for cine-CCT to evaluate valvular function (**Figure 36.6A-F**) include the following:

- **Evaluation of severity of aortic stenosis**—cine-CCT can visualize the number of leaflets on the aortic valve

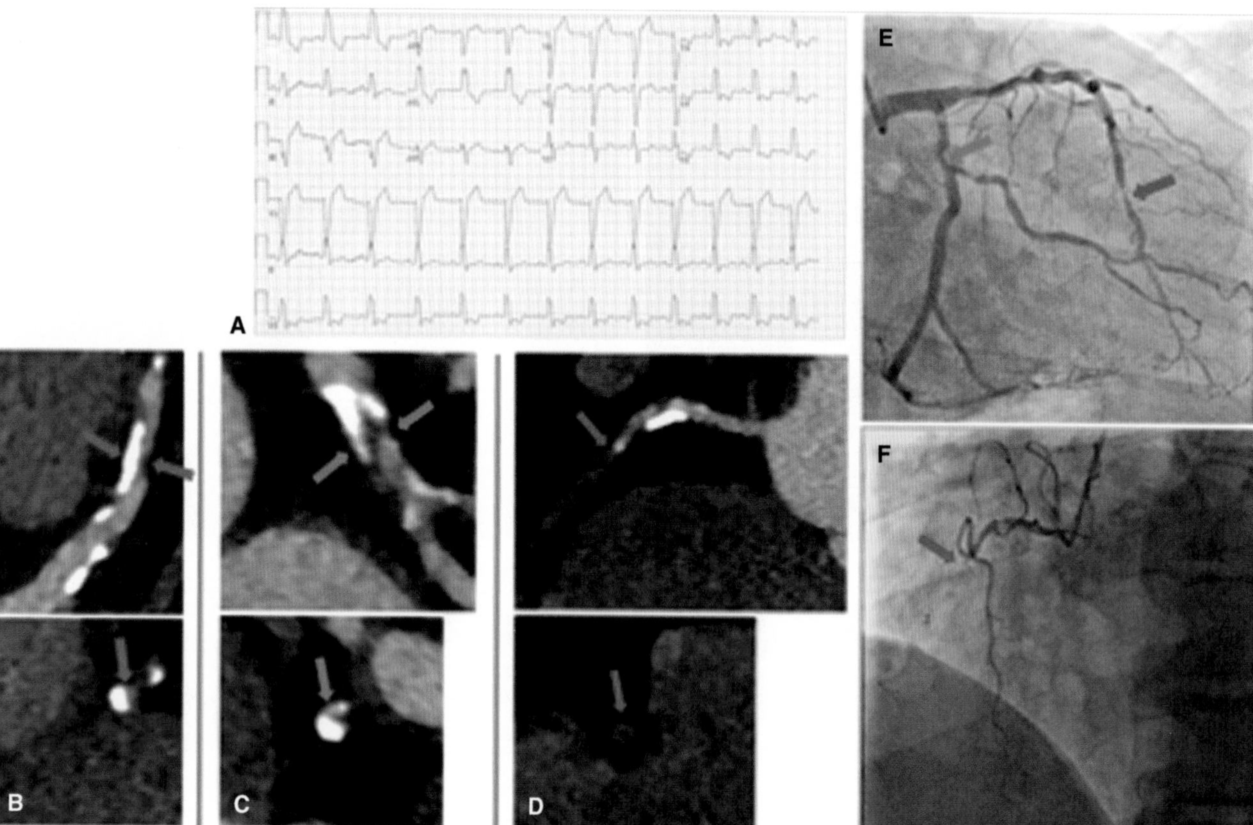

FIGURE 36.4 A 61-year-old male with obesity, dyslipidemia, and family history of premature coronary artery disease (CAD) presented to the emergency room with central chest pressure that woke him from sleep. **(A)** In the emergency room, the electrocardiography (ECG) showed normal sinus rhythm with a new left bundle branch block. High-sensitivity troponin T values procured 2 hours apart were mildly elevated at 62 and 64 ng/L (reference range: 0-14 ng/L). Coronary computed tomography angiography (CCTA) showed a large amount of calcified and noncalcified coronary plaque with severe stenoses in a multivessel distribution: **(B)** severe stenosis (70%-99%) of mid left anterior descending (red arrows), **(C)** severe stenosis (70%-99%) of proximal left circumflex (green arrows), and **(D)** total occlusion (100% stenosis) of proximal to mid right coronary arteries (blue arrows). Coronary angiography confirmed the CCTA findings. Shown here is **(E)** severe stenosis of the mid left anterior descending (red arrow) and proximal left circumflex (green arrow), and **(F)** complete occlusion of the proximal to mid right coronary arteries (blue arrow). He subsequently underwent a successful four-vessel coronary artery bypass grafting surgery.

and determine the severity of aortic stenosis. This can be performed using direct planimetry where the aortic valve opening area can be traced. In addition, aortic valve calcium score can be used to estimate the severity of aortic stenosis.[22]

- **Evaluation of aortic valve before transcatheter aortic valve replacement (TAVR)**—cine-CCT is an essential tool to select valve size and identify potential complications, such as coronary ostial occlusion.[23]
- **Evaluation of subclinical leaflet thrombosis following TAVR**[24]—see Figure 36.7D.
- **Evaluation of mitral valve before transcatheter mitral valve replacement (TMVR)**—cine-CCT can be useful in selecting valve size and for estimating the risk of LV outflow tract obstruction.[24] When there is a high risk of LV outflow tract obstruction, TMVR should be avoided.
- **Evaluation of endocarditis**—cine-CCT can be useful in evaluating patients with known or suspected endocarditis, especially when an initial evaluation using transthoracic echocardiography is inconclusive, or when transesophageal echocardiography is not feasible. Prior studies have shown that cine-CCT has a diagnostic accuracy similar to that of transesophageal echocardiography for detecting vegetations (Figure 36.6A,B). A unique advantage of cine-CCT over other imaging techniques is the ability to evaluate mechanical valves. In addition, cine-CCT is well suited for detecting perivalvular involvement, including pseudoaneurysm or fistulas. Accordingly, the current European Society of Cardiology guidelines support the modified Duke Criteria, where the identification of paravalvular involvement by CCT is considered a major criterion toward the diagnosis of infective endocarditis.[24]
- **In selected cases, cine-CCT can also evaluate the tricuspid and pulmonic valves**, although echocardiography is generally preferred for most such indications.

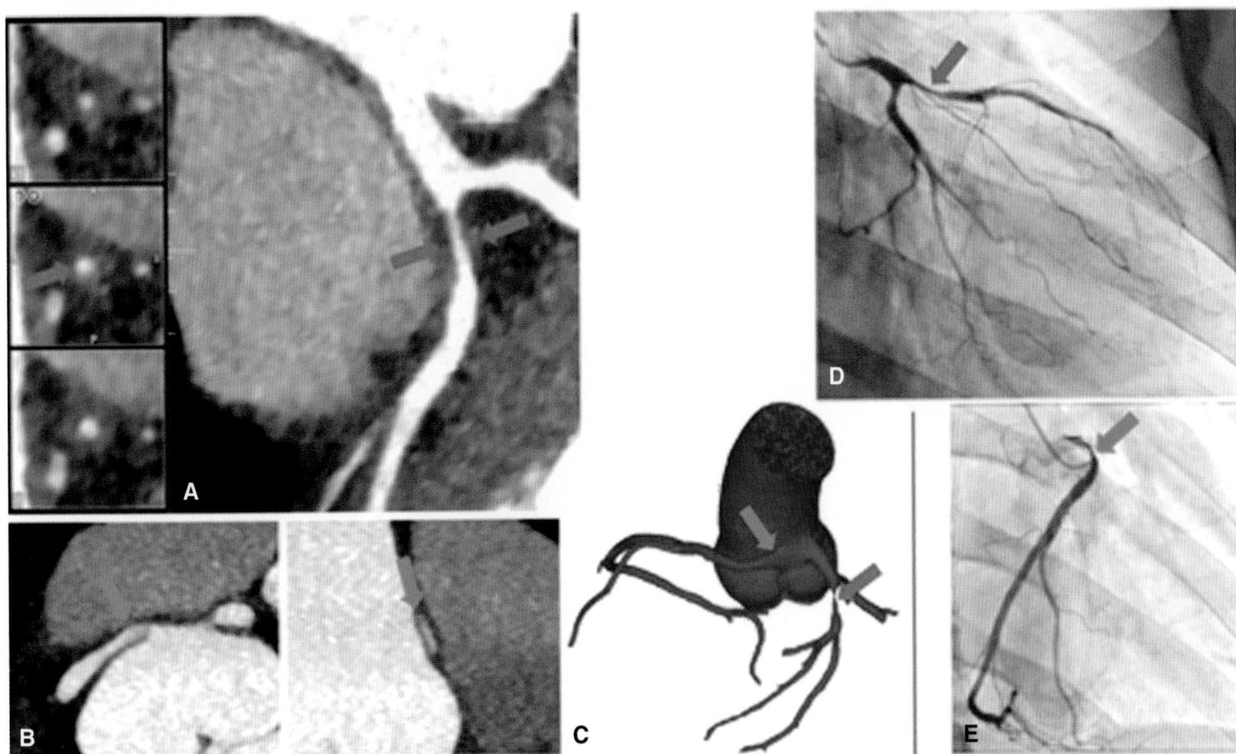

FIGURE 36.5 Example of anomalous right coronary artery (RCA) arising from the left coronary cusp. A 51-year-old male with dyslipidemia presented with exertional chest pain and decreased exercise tolerance over the past few months. Coronary computed tomography angiography (CCTA) showed **(A)** a moderate amount of noncalcified plaque causing severe stenosis of the proximal left anterior descending artery (blue arrows) and **(B)** an anomalous right coronary artery arising from the left coronary cusp via a separate ostium, via a slitlike orifice and following an interarterial course (green arrows). **(C)** Three-dimensional reconstructed images showing severe proximal left anterior descending stenosis (blue arrow) and anomalous origin of the right coronary artery (green arrow). Coronary angiogram **(D)** confirmed severe stenosis of the proximal left anterior descending (blue arrow), and **(E)** an anomalous right coronary artery arising from the left coronary cusp via a separate ostium via a slitlike orifice (green arrow). He underwent a successful single-vessel coronary artery bypass surgery and reimplantation of the right coronary artery.

Cardiac Masses

Cine-CCT can also be used to identify cardiac masses[25] (**Figure 36.7A-F**), including assessing the extent of cardiac involvement and features that may help distinguish benign from malignant masses. Cine-CCT may be particularly well suited for evaluating potential coronary involvement from cardiac masses.

Left Atrial Appendage

Cine-CCT can image the left atrial appendage and exclude the presence of a left atrial appendage thrombus.[26] Notably, a filling defect in the left atrial appendage can represent slow flow, and, therefore, postcontrast delayed imaging may be necessary in such cases to confirm the presence of a thrombus (Figure 36.7D).

Cine-CCT is also useful to procedural planning before left atrial appendage occlusion device implantation, and in selected cases to follow up to assess procedure success following such procedures.[27]

Myocardial Morphology and Cardiac Function

A multiphase cine-CCT can acquire data throughout the cardiac cycle and thus provide data on right and LV volume and function. In addition to calculating the ejection fraction, cine-CCT can also be used to identify regional wall motion abnormalities, a feature that may be helpful in detecting areas of scar from prior myocardial infarction.

With respect to evaluating myocardial morphology, cine-CCT can measure LV wall thickness in conditions ranging from hypertrophy to hypertrophic cardiomyopathy (**Figure 36.8**). In addition, cine-CCT can identify areas of prior myocardial scar. On cine-CCT, such areas can exhibit a combination of the following features: wall thinning, resting perfusion defects, abnormal wall motion, myocardial calcifications, fatty metaplasia, or late enhancement on delayed imaging (when performed).[28] Other features that can be detected on cine-CCT include myocardial crypts, aneurysms, or pseudoaneurysm.[29]

LIMITATIONS OF TECHNIQUE/PROCEDURE

CCT image quality is reduced in patients with morbid obesity (eg, body mass index [BMI] > 40 kg/m^2), those with rapid heart rate that cannot be adequately controlled with beta-blockers, or in patients who are unable to cooperate with holding their breath during the examination. In addition, image quality may be reduced in individuals who have an irregular heart rhythm, such as atrial fibrillation. In such patients,

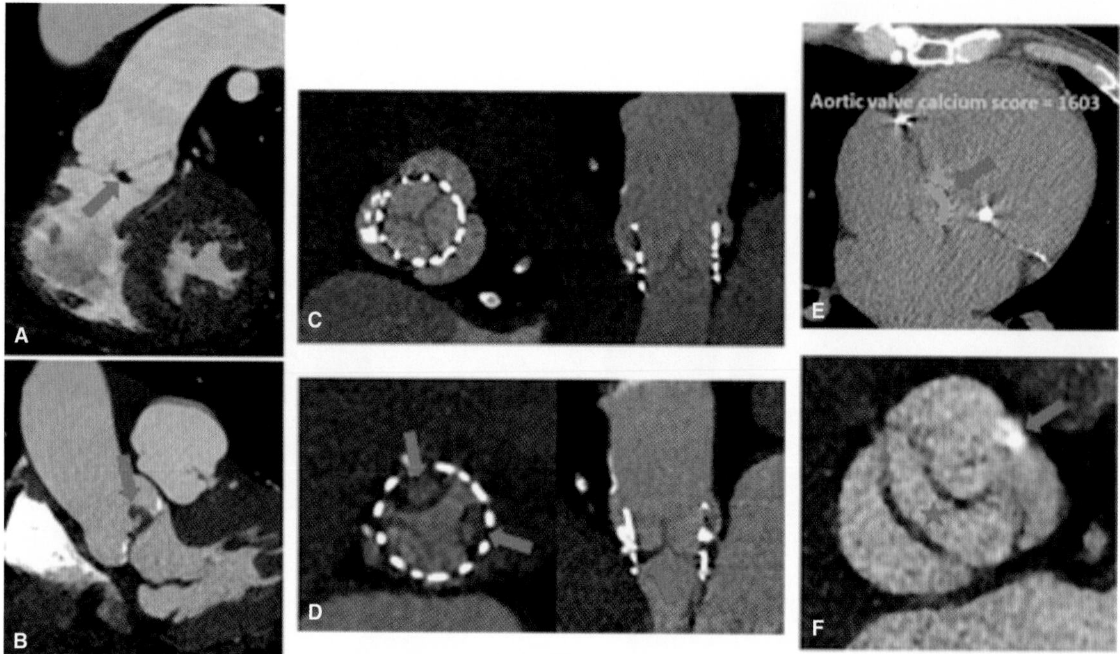

FIGURE 36.6 Examples of valvular heart disease on cine-cardiac computed tomography. **(A)** Pulmonic valve vegetation (red arrow) in a patient with intravenous drug abuse, gram-positive bacteremia, and sepsis. **(B)** Aortic valve vegetation (red arrow) in a patient with gram-positive bacteremia, epidural abscess, and sepsis. **(C)** Normal appearance of transcatheter aortic valve (TAV) leaflets in orthogonal views. **(D)** Hypoattenuating leaflet thickening (red arrows) of TAV leaflets in orthogonal views. **(E)** Severe aortic valve calcifications (red arrow) in a 72-year-old female with paradoxical low-flow, low-gradient aortic stenosis, and Agatston score of 1603 was useful in establishing the diagnosis of severe aortic stenosis. **(F)** Bicuspid aortic valve with fusion of the right and left coronary cusps. The bicuspid valve has an elliptical opening (red star) and calcification of the fusion raphe (red arrow).

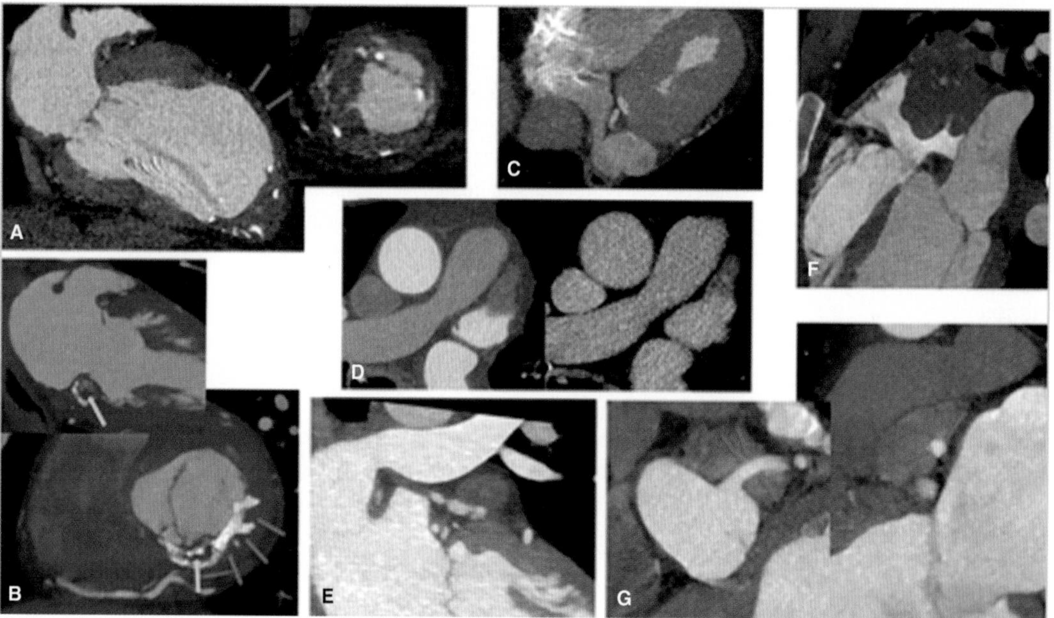

FIGURE 36.7 Examples of cardiac masses on cine-cardiac computed tomography. **(A)** Large laminated thrombus (red stars) is present within the left ventricular apex. There are calcifications within the thrombus, suggesting chronicity. The left ventricular cavity is dilated, with thinning of the mid to distal anterior wall (red arrows). The patient had chronic total occlusion of the mid left anterior descending (LAD) artery. **(B)** Large amount of severe mitral annular calcification, posteriorly (red arrows) with a large area of caseous necrosis in the center (yellow arrows). **(C)** Large enhancing soft-tissue mass (red star) in the inferior left atrioventricular groove, abutting the coronary sinus. This mass was moving with the left ventricle, and was diagnosed as a paraganglioma. Of note, on a dotatate scan, this mass also demonstrated intense uptake, consistent with a paraganglioma. **(D)** Large filling defect in the left atrial appendage on early contrast-enhanced images (red star), that persists on 60-second delayed images (blue star), consistent with a left atrial appendage thrombus. **(E)** Small, homogeneous, non–contrast-enhancing pericardial cyst (red star) adjacent to the left atrial appendage. **(F)** Large superior mediastinal mass (red star) associated with complete obliteration of the superior vena cava, and invading the superior aspect of the right atrium. Biopsy of the mass confirmed a diagnosis of lymphoma. **(G)** Large vascular pericardial mass (blue star) nearly circumferentially encasing left main coronary artery and proximal LAD (red arrows). This pericardial mass demonstrated intense dotatate uptake, most consistent with a somatostatin receptor–positive/dotatate avid tumor, such as a pericardial paraganglioma.

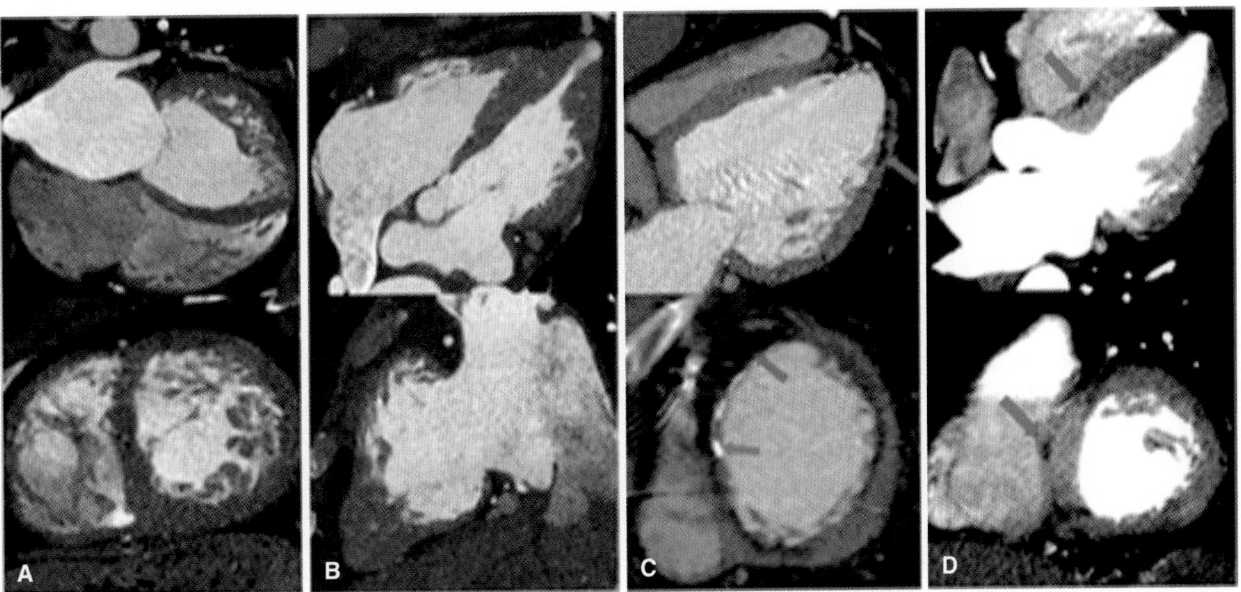

FIGURE 36.8 Examples of cardiomyopathy on cine-cardiac computed tomography. **(A)** The left ventricular (LV) cavity is severely dilated. There are prominent LV trabeculations involving the entire lateral wall and apical segments (red stars). The end-diastolic ratio of noncompacted to compacted myocardium was 4.0 (normal < 2.3), a finding that is consistent with the diagnosis of LV noncompaction. The patient had a severely reduced LV ejection fraction of 20% with global hypokinesis of the LV wall. **(B)** Increased LV apical wall thickness (red stars) in a patient with apical hypertrophic cardiomyopathy. There is an LV apical aneurysm (red arrow), without any LV cavity thrombus. In addition, there is hypertrophy of the right ventricular apex as well (blue stars). **(C)** The LV cavity is severely dilated. There is fatty metaplasia (red arrows) and calcification (blue arrow) in the LV mid to apical segments and apex consistent with a prior myocardial infarction. The patient had a severely reduced LV ejection fraction of 25% with akinesis of the mid anteroseptal and all apical segments. His left internal mammary artery graft to the left anterior descending artery was occluded. **(D)** Fat infiltration of the basal and mid interventricular septum and right ventricular wall (red arrows) in a patient with arrhythmogenic right ventricular cardiomyopathy.

misregistration artifacts may be present, although, if appropriately recognized, the scan results may still be interpretable. CCTA requires the administration of 40 to 70 cc of contrast material, and individuals who have severe renal impairment may be at risk for contrast-associated nephropathy. Thus, most centers avoid the use of CCTA when the glomerular filtration rate (GFR) is less than 30 mL/min/1.73 m^2. In addition, individuals who have severe coronary calcifications may have coronary segments that cannot be adequately visualized if the calcium obscures the lumen. Similarly, coronary stents may not be well visualized on CCTA. Despite these limitations, recent advances in CT hardware have improved image quality, and, as a result, some contemporary scanners (eg, dual-source CT) can obtain adequate images even in individuals who have elevated heart rate. In addition, the ability of CCT to image obese patients has also improved with contemporary scanners.

SPECIAL CONSIDERATIONS AND CONTRAINDICATIONS

Similar to any diagnostic imaging test, CCT should be obtained only in cases where the test results can impact patient management. Furthermore, the decision to obtain a CCT study should be made in the context of considering other available alternative testing options.

- CAC testing is only useful in patients without known CAD, and is of limited value in most individuals younger than 40 years of age.
- CCTA is most useful in symptomatic individuals who do not have known CAD. Patients who have extensive coronary plaque or prior stents may be more likely to benefit from a functional test, particularly if it is unclear whether their symptoms are related to their underlying coronary atherosclerosis.
- CCTA in asymptomatic individuals is generally not recommended, although there are current trials assessing the efficacy of such testing. A particular concern is that testing asymptomatic individuals could lead to unnecessary downstream testing and procedures such as invasive angiography and coronary revascularization.

RESEARCH AND FUTURE DIRECTIONS

Future developments will continue to expand the capabilities of CCT applications. Such developments will include technical advances that will further improve the spatial and temporal resolution of CT imaging, while also simplifying the image acquisition process so this test can be consistently performed across different settings. In addition, future research will also use CCT to help clinicians select appropriate candidates for

SECTION 2

various different cardiovascular treatments and procedures in a manner that will promote cost-effectiveness and improve safety.

Ongoing and future research will refine the predictive ability of atherosclerosis imaging—using either CAC testing or CCTA—to identify the risk of future cardiovascular events, including newer methods using machine learning to automatically quantify the amount of plaque. As importantly, future studies will need to establish how such data can inform the need for more aggressive preventive therapies. As the current armamentarium of medical therapies expands to include multiple new agents, the use of plaque imaging may allow clinicians and researchers to identify high-risk cohorts who will benefit the most from intensive treatment, and ideally before developing a cardiovascular event.

Future developments will continue to use CCT in selecting patients who are more likely to benefit from various surgical or percutaneous interventions ranging from TAVR and TMVR to left atrial appendage closure devices and ablation procedures. As more devices become available, CCT will be central in selecting between them, and also will enable advanced simulations that will be able to inform clinicians and patients about the potential benefits of various potential procedures.

KEY POINTS

- ✔ CAC testing may be useful among individuals who meet criteria for statin therapy (ie, 10-year ASCVD risk of 5%-20%) but have a preference to avoid therapy. In such patients, the presence of a CAC score of zero could be used to identify low-risk patients in whom treatment can be deferred.
- ✔ CCTA is useful for evaluating symptomatic patients with suspected CAD. In such patients, a CCTA—defined as having no plaque and no stenosis—is associated with excellent prognosis, with a very low future rate of cardiac death or myocardial infarction.
- ✔ The identification of plaque on CAC or CCTA should prompt intensification in preventive and lifestyle therapies.
- ✔ Among patients with stable CAD, the use CCTA is associated with a lower rate of subsequent myocardial infarction or coronary heart disease death when compared with other functional testing approaches.
- ✔ Patients who are found to have moderate (50%-69%) or severe (≥70%) stenosis on CCTA may benefit from functional testing if there is uncertainty regarding the potential role of coronary revascularization. One option in such cases is to use CT-FFR, whereby computational fluid dynamic modeling can estimate a measure of lesion-specific ischemia.
- ✔ Among patients presenting to the emergency department with acute chest pain, the use of CCTA is associated with a more rapid time to diagnosis and lower emergency department length of stay.
- ✔ In patients with known or suspected anomalous origin of the coronary arteries, CCTA can be used to identify cases of abnormal origin of the coronary arteries, and describe high-risk features.
- ✔ A multiphase cine-CCT is useful for evaluating valvular heart disease, and can help select candidates for TAVR and TMVR procedures.
- ✔ Cine-CCT can be useful for evaluating cardiac masses, cardiac function, and myocardial scars in patients in whom performing CMR is not feasible.

REFERENCES

1. Stocker TJ, Deseive S, Leipsic J, et al. Reduction in radiation exposure in cardiovascular computed tomography imaging: results from the PROspective multicenter registry on radiaTion dose Estimates of cardiac CT anglOgraphy iN daily practice in 2017 (PROTECTION VI). *Eur Heart J*. 2018;39:3715-3723.
2. Techasith T, Ghoshhajra BB, Truong QA, et al. The effect of heart rhythm on patient radiation dose with dual-source cardiac computed tomography. *J Cardiovasc Comput Tomogr*. 2011;5:255-263.
3. Nasir K, Bittencourt MS, Blaha MJ, et al. Implications of coronary artery calcium testing among statin candidates According to American College of Cardiology/American Heart Association Cholesterol Management Guidelines: MESA (Multi-Ethnic Study of Atherosclerosis). *J Am Coll Cardiol*. 2015;66:1657-1668.
4. Hecht H, Blaha MJ, Berman DS, et al. Clinical indications for coronary artery calcium scoring in asymptomatic patients: expert consensus statement from the Society of Cardiovascular Computed Tomography. *J Cardiovasc Comput Tomogr*. 2017;11:157-168.
5. Grundy SM, Stone NJ, Bailey AL, et al. 2018 AHA/ACC/AACVPR/AAPA/ABC/ACPM/ADA/AGS/APhA/ASPC/NLA/PCNA guideline on the management of blood cholesterol: executive summary. A Report of the American College of Cardiology/American Heart Association Task Force on Clinical Practice Guidelines. 2019;73:3168-3209.
6. Daly R, Blankstein R. Screening for atherosclerosis among low risk individuals with family history of coronary heart disease. *J Cardiovasc Comput Tomogr*. 2019;14(2):203-205.
7. Miedema MD, Dardari ZA, Nasir K, et al. Association of coronary artery calcium with long-term, cause-specific mortality among young adults. *JAMA Netw Open*. 2019;2:e197440.
8. Miedema MD, Nauffal VD, Singh A, Blankstein R. Statin therapy for young adults: a long-term investment worth considering. *Trends Cardiovasc Med*. 2020;30:48-53.
9. Hoffmann U, Ferencik M, Udelson JE, et al. Prognostic value of noninvasive cardiovascular testing in patients with stable chest pain: insights from the PROMISE Trial (Prospective Multicenter Imaging Study for Evaluation of Chest Pain). *Circulation*. 2017;135:2320-2332.
10. Knuuti J, Ballo H, Juarez-Orozco LE, et al. The performance of non-invasive tests to rule-in and rule-out significant coronary artery stenosis in patients with stable angina: a meta-analysis focused on post-test disease probability. *Eur Heart J*. 2018;39:3322-3330.
11. Bittencourt MS, Hulten EA, Murthy VL, et al. Clinical outcomes after evaluation of stable chest pain by coronary computed tomographic angiography versus usual care a meta-analysis. *Circ Cardiovasc Imaging*. 2016;9:e004419.
12. Newby DE, Adamson PD, Berry C, et al. Coronary CT angiography and 5-year risk of myocardial infarction. *N Engl J Med*. 2018;379:924-933.
13. Budoff MJ, Mayrhofer T, Ferencik M, et al. Prognostic value of coronary artery calcium in the PROMISE study (Prospective Multicenter Imaging Study for Evaluation of Chest Pain). *Circulation*. 2017;136:1993-2005.
14. Adamson PD, Williams MC, Dweck MR, et al. Guiding therapy by coronary CT angiography improves outcomes in patients with stable chest pain. *J Am Coll Cardiol*. 2019;74:2058-2070.
15. Maron DJ, Hochman JS, Reynolds HR, et al. Initial invasive or conservative strategy for stable coronary disease. *N Engl J Med*. 2020;382:1395-1407.

16. Hulten E, Pickett C, Bittencourt MS, et al. Meta-analysis of coronary CT angiography in the emergency department. *Eur Heart J Cardiovasc Imaging*. 2013;14:607.
17. Cheezum MK, Ghoshhajra B, Bittencourt MS, et al. Anomalous origin of the coronary artery arising from the opposite sinus: prevalence and outcomes in patients undergoing coronary CTA. *Eur Heart J Cardiovasc Imaging*. 2017;18:224-235.
18. Cheezum MK, Liberthson RR, Shah NR, et al. Anomalous aortic origin of a coronary artery from the inappropriate sinus of valsalva. *J Am Coll Cardiol*. 2017;69:1592-1608.
19. Miedema MD, Duprez DA, Misialek JR, et al. Use of coronary artery calcium testing to guide aspirin utilization for primary prevention: estimates from the multi-ethnic study of atherosclerosis. *Circ Cardiovasc Qual Outcomes*. 2014;7:453-460.
20. Fairbairn TA, Nieman K, Akasaka T, et al. Real-world clinical utility and impact on clinical decision-making of coronary computed tomography angiography-derived fractional flow reserve: lessons from the ADVANCE Registry. *Eur Heart J*. 2018;39(41):3701-3711.
21. Norgaard BL, Terkelsen CJ, Mathiassen ON, et al. Clinical outcomes using coronary CT angiography and FFRCT-guided management of stable chest pain patients. *J Am Coll Cardiol*. 2018;72:2123-2134.
22. Clavel MA, Pibarot P, Messika-Zeitoun D, et al. Impact of aortic valve calcification, as measured by MDCT, on survival in patients with aortic stenosis: results of an international registry study. *J Am Coll Cardiol*. 2014;64:1202-1213.
23. Blanke P, Weir-McCall JR, Achenbach S, et al. Computed tomography imaging in the context of Transcatheter Aortic Valve Implantation (TAVI)/Transcatheter Aortic Valve Replacement (TAVR): an expert consensus document of the Society of Cardiovascular Computed Tomography. *JACC Cardiovasc Imaging*. 2019;12:1-24.
24. Murphy DJ, Ge Y, Don CW, et al. Use of cardiac computerized tomography to predict neo-left ventricular outflow tract obstruction before transcatheter mitral valve replacement. *J Am Heart Assoc*. 2017;6(11):e007353.
25. Kassop D, Donovan MS, Cheezum MK, et al. Cardiac masses on cardiac CT: a review. *Curr Cardiovasc Imaging Reports*. 2014;7:9281.
26. Romero J, Husain SA, Kelesidis I, et al. Detection of left atrial appendage thrombus by cardiac computed tomography in patients with atrial fibrillation. *Circ Cardiovasc Imaging*. 2013;6:185-194.
27. Glikson M, Wolff R, Hindricks G, et al. EHRA/EAPCI expert consensus statement on catheter-based left atrial appendage occlusion—an update. *Europace*. 2019;22:184-184.
28. Blankstein R, Rogers IS, Cury RC. Practical tips and tricks in cardiovascular computed tomography: diagnosis of myocardial infarction. *J Cardiovasc Comput Tomogr*. 2009;3:104-111.
29. Hulten EA, Blankstein R. Pseudoaneurysms of the heart. *Circulation*. 2012;125:1920-1925.

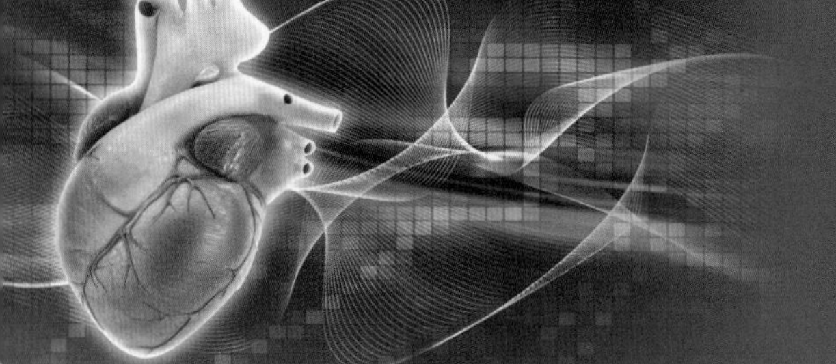

CARDIAC MAGNETIC RESONANCE IMAGING

Louis-Philippe David, Panagiotis Antiochos, and Raymond Y. Kwong

INTRODUCTION

Cardiac magnetic resonance imaging (CMR) is a noninvasive, nonionizing imaging modality, with high spatial resolution, that is considered to be the gold standard for morphologic assessment of the heart, as well as the assessment of right and left ventricular systolic and diastolic volumes, function, and mass. Using contrast agents and newer mapping techniques, CMR can, furthermore, provide unique information on tissue characterization that can improve diagnostic accuracy in the properly selected patient. The goal of this chapter is to create a comprehensive and practical reference for any general cardiologist, internist, fellow, or trainee who encounters cardiovascular magnetic resonance imaging (MRI) in their practice.

FUNDAMENTALS OF CARDIAC MAGNETIC RESONANCE

Physics for Clinicians and Instrumentation

Because of its abundance in water and lipid molecules, most clinical applications of MRI target hydrogen to generate a magnetic resonance signal. When a patient is placed inside a strong external magnetic field (B_0) such as an MRI scanner, hydrogen atoms align in the direction of B_0 resulting in a small net magnetization called M_z **(Figure 37.1)**. In order to generate an MRI signal, energy has to be transferred to the protons. Hence, a radiofrequency pulse B_1, a weaker oscillating magnetic field, is applied perpendicularly to B_o at a specific frequency called Larmor frequency. The resulting net magnetization can therefore be divided into two planes: the longitudinal plane M_z (parallel to B_0) and transverse plane M_{xy} (perpendicular to B_0). Once the regurgitant fraction (RF) pulse is turned off, hydrogen nuclei return to their equilibrium state and release energy that induces a voltage that the MRI coils can detect.[1] This relaxation process has two distinct components that happen at the same time:

- ***Longitudinal relaxation*** corresponds to the recovery of the magnetization along z direction and is defined by an exponential time constant, T1. Water molecules have long T1 values and appear dark on T1-weighted images whereas fat has a short T1 value and will appear bright.
- ***Transverse relaxation*** refers to how quickly the spins exchange energy in the xy direction. This loss of transverse magnetization follows an oscillating pattern referred to as the free-induction decay and follows a time constant: T2. Local inhomogeneities in the magnetic field further accelerate this process and lead to a faster decay called T2*. Typically, water molecules have long T2 values and appear bright on T2-weighted images that can be useful in detecting active inflammation, for example.

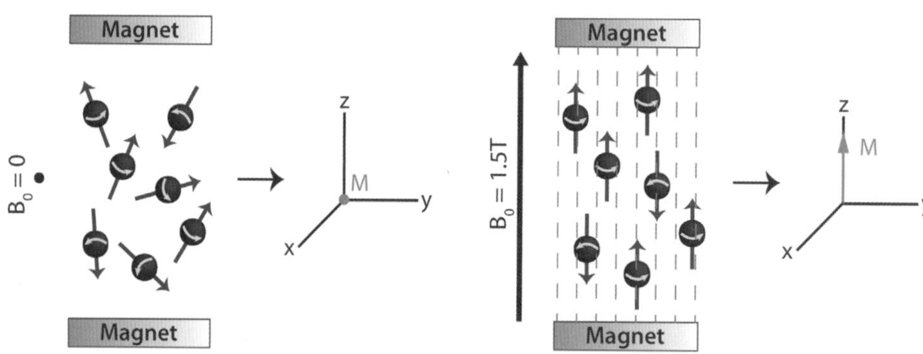

FIGURE 37.1 In the absence of a magnetic field, the hydrogen atoms in a tissue have a spin of equal magnitude but in a random direction. A vector addition of these spins results in a zero sum, that is, no net magnetization, M. If the tissue is placed within a strong magnetic field, B_0, the hydrogen atoms align with this magnetic field, resulting in a non-zero magnetization vector, M. A larger magnetic field creates greater alignment of the hydrogen protons. (Reprinted by permission from Springer: Akçakaya M, Tang M, Nezafat R. Cardiac Magnetic Resonance Imaging Physics. In: Kwong R, Jerosch-Herold M, Heydari B, eds. *Cardiovascular Magnetic Resonance Imaging. Contemporary Cardiology.* New York, NY: Springer; 2019:1-16. Copyright © 2019 Springer Science+Business Media, LLC.)

System and Signal Encoding

- The **main magnet coils** generate a strong constant, yet inhomogeneous, magnetic field (B_0). Typically, the field strength of cardiac MRI scanners ranges from 1.5 to 3 Tesla.
- When turned on, the **transmitter coils** that are built in the main structure of the magnet can emit an RF (weaker magnetic field) that will excite protons.
- Three **gradient coils** built in the main structure of the magnet along the x, y, and z directions can be turned on and off. Gradients create small variations in magnetic field along their axis and are useful for slice selection and localizing the magnetic resonance signal in space.
- **Receiving coils** are typically placed on the surface of the patient's body to maximize signal coming from the heart and are turned on during signal readout.

Cardiac Synchronization and Respiratory Gating

By synchronizing image acquisition with the cardiac cycle using ECG signal from leads attached to the patient, artifacts due to cardiac contractile motion and high velocity blood flow can be minimized. Cardiac gating depends on the quality of the ECG signal and the absence of arrhythmias. Cardiac synchronization can be prospective (R wave is detected and triggers the sequence and acquisition) or retrospective (all the data is continuously acquired over multiple R-R intervals).

Respiratory motion is another potential source of artifacts, so most sequences are performed using fast acquisition imaging techniques during breath-holding. However, some patients cannot breath-hold for 10 to 15 seconds, whereas other sequences may require longer acquisition. Respiratory gating methods such as the use of navigator sequences allow the acquisition of data in a predefined time window based on diaphragm position, at the expense of increased scan time.

Magnetic Resonance Sequences

A detailed explanation of CMR sequences is beyond the scope of this chapter. The interested reader is referred to more detailed publications on the subject.[2,3] In CMR, ***spin echo*** sequences are the cornerstone of black blood imaging and are mainly used for anatomic imaging. On the other hand, ***gradient echo*** sequences produce images where blood appears bright. Gradient recalled echo (GRE) and balanced steady-state free precession (bSSFP) are two types of gradient echo sequences frequently utilized in CMR and are typically used for cine imaging (anatomy, ventricular size, mass, and function) and phase-contrast images. ***Phase-contrast*** sequences allow quantification of blood flow and velocity and are particularly useful to assess valvular stenosis, valvular regurgitation, and intracardiac shunts.

Gadolinium-Based Contrast Agents

The use of gadolinium-based contrast agents (GBCA) in CMR provides important diagnostic and prognostic information; they are routinely used in perfusion imaging, assessment of myocardial scar, and cardiomyopathies (CMP). Based on their molecular configuration, GBCA can be classified as linear or macrocyclic agents. Macrocyclic agents are the newer generation of GBCA with a molecular structure substantially more stable in chelating the gadolinium element and thus safer than the linear agents. Allergic reactions may be seen in 0.004% to 0.7%,[4] whereas true anaphylactic reactions are rare. The most serious potential complication of exposure to GBCA was nephrogenic systemic fibrosis (NSF), observed in patients with severe kidney disease (estimated glomerular filtration rate [eGFR] $\leq$ 30 mL/min). The risk of NSF is higher during periods of rapid deterioration of renal function, acute systemic illness, or with repeated administration of GBCA within a short period of time. This irreversible process is characterized by interstitial inflammatory reaction eventually leading to skin induration, contractures, multiorgan fibrosis, and potentially death. After implementation of guidelines restricting the use of GBCA in patients with severe kidney disease and with the use of safer macrocyclic-structured GBCA, there have practically been no new reports of NSF relating to GBCA. The safety profile of GBCA has not been established in pregnant women and in general should also be avoided unless the benefits of performing the study outweighs the potential risk.

GBCA is usually injected through peripheral venous access and reaches the myocardium through coronary artery circulation within 15 to 30 seconds after injection before it diffuses into the extracellular space. Myocardial first-pass perfusion CMR and the majority of magnetic resonance angiography (MRA) are performed during this phase. At 10 to 15 minutes after injection, a wash-in/wash-out equilibrium state is reached between contrast in the blood pool and the extracellular space leading to an optimal imaging window for late gadolinium enhancement (LGE) imaging.

Late Gadolinium Enhancement

Gadolinium shortens T1 time of tissues leading to faster longitudinal recovery and a more intense magnetic resonance signal. First, an inversion time mapping sequence (TI scout) is performed to identify the optimal timing of image acquisition after an inversion recovery pulse where the normal myocardium is dark (nulled). Multiple short-axis images of the left ventricle (LV) are acquired while the inversion time (TI) is progressively increased. In patients with normal myocardium, blood pool, which contains more gadolinium, is nulled before the myocardium. In pathologies such as cardiac amyloidosis (AL) where increased extracellular volume is a hallmark of the disease, there is myocardial retention of gadolinium that may lead to nulling of the myocardium before the blood pool. Once the proper TI has been selected, images should show optimal contrast differentiation between bright LGE and the normal, nulled myocardium. Although people often associate LGE with the presence of fibrosis, it should be clear that LGE does not necessarily mean scarring. LGE reflects abnormally enlarged extracellular myocardial compartment, which can be seen in infarction, infiltration, replacement fibrosis, and also inflammation/edema.

INDICATIONS

Because of its ability to define myocardial function, volumes, and flow and provide morphologic tissue characterization, CMR is well established for a plethora of indications.[5]

With respect to ischemic heart disease (IHD), CMR is the most accurate modality for the description of myocardial infarction (MI), both in the acute and chronic phase and is important for the assessment of myocardial viability, where it is used to predict functional recovery, as well as overall risk and prognosis. In addition, the performance of stress CMR in the assessment of myocardial perfusion and ischemia in patients with suspected coronary artery disease (CAD) is at least equal to other imaging modalities.

By providing detailed myocardial scar characterization, CMR currently assumes a prominent role in the management and prognosis of patients with atrial and ventricular arrhythmias. Furthermore, for the diagnosis of CMP, CMR can separate ischemic from nonischemic CMP (NICMP) and differentiate between different etiologies of NICMP. CMR is the most important imaging modality for the diagnosis, follow-up, and prognostication of patients with myocarditis. Although echocardiography remains the initial imaging modality of choice in valvular disease, CMR is increasingly used to determine the severity of challenging valvulopathies or as an aid to evaluate the optimal timing for surgery. CMR is increasingly important in the diagnosis and follow-up of young patients with congenital heart disease, for the assessment of pericardial disease, and the characterization of cardiac masses (**Table 37.1**).

TABLE 37.1 Clinical Indications for Cardiac Magnetic Resonance (CMR)

Ischemic Heart Disease
Assessment of ventricular volumes, function, and mass
Assessment of myocardial ischemia
Assessment of myocardial infarction
Assessment of myocardial viability
Assessment of ventricular thrombus
Assessment of microvascular obstruction
Cardiomyopathies
Nonischemic cardiomyopathy
Hypertrophic cardiomyopathy: apical/nonapical
Arrhythmogenic right ventricular cardiomyopathy (dysplasia)
Restrictive cardiomyopathy
Siderotic cardiomyopathy
Left ventricular noncompaction
Cardiac involvement in Anderson-Fabry disease and amyloidosis
Cardiac sarcoidosis
Postcardiac transplantation rejection
Myocarditis
Pericardial Disease
Acute pericarditis
Pericardial effusion
Constrictive pericarditis
Arrhythmias and Prevention of Sudden Cardiac Death
Pulmonary vein anatomy for management of atrial fibrillation
Atrial function evaluation
Evaluation of patients with ventricular arrhythmias
Valvular Heart Disease
Quantification of aortic regurgitation
Quantification of mitral regurgitation
Congenital Heart Disease
Assessment of shunt size (Qp/Qs)
Anomalies of the atria and venous return
Anomalies of the valves
Anomalies of the atria, ventricles, and coronary arteries
Acquired Diseases of the Vessels
Assessment of acute aortic syndromes
Assessment and follow-up of chronic aortic syndromes
Management of aortic root dilation in patients with bicuspid aortic valve
Follow-up after aortic surgery and evaluation of CMR-compatible stent grafts
Diagnosis and follow-up of thoracic aortic aneurysm in Marfan disease
Characterization of Cardiac Masses
Future Clinical Developments
Atherosclerosis detection
Interventional CMR
Novel contrast agents
Hardware developments (high field systems)

SPECIAL CONSIDERATIONS AND CONTRAINDICATIONS

Over two million patients in the United States have implanted devices, including pacemakers and implantable cardioverter-defibrillators (ICDs), and it is estimated that more than 50% of those will require MRI after device implantation. CMR in patients with magnetic resonance-conditional devices can be performed safely as long as device restrictions are adhered to and safety precautions are taken. Although scanning of patients with non–magnetic resonance-conditional devices—especially legacy devices—is considered high risk and discouraged, it is not an absolute contraindication as long as the risk-to-benefit ratio justifies CMR.[6,7] Scanning such patients should only be considered under highly compelling circumstances and where an exit strategy in the event of device failure is firmly in place.

Apart from implanted devices, CMR is potentially problematic in patients with ferromagnetic metallic implants (**Tables 37.2** and **37.3**). Thorough screening of all patients prior to CMR is mandatory. Devices such as prosthetic heart valves, prosthetic joints, sternal wires, and intravascular stents do **not** preclude study with CMR at field strengths of 1.5 and 3.0 Tesla.

CLINICAL APPLICATIONS

Chamber Morphology and Function

Accurate quantification of LV and RV volumes can have significant diagnostic and prognostic impacts. TTE (transthoracic echocardiogram) is often the first step for clinicians to assess chamber morphology, although difficult image acquisition because of obesity, unfavorable acoustic windows, and foreshortening of the LV in apical views are potential limitations. LV evaluation by Simpson's biplane method is based on geometric assumptions and RV evaluation is often just qualitative or based on linear dimensions because of its crescentic shape. CMR can overcome these potential pitfalls, is highly reproducible, and is now considered the gold standard to assess chamber morphology.

First, a stack of short-axis SSFP cine images covering basal to apical segments of both ventricles is acquired using retrospective gating. Each slice is 6 to 8 mm thick and is acquired during breath-holding, combining information over multiple RR intervals to produce the final image. Careful planning with double-oblique orientation is crucial to avoid foreshortening of the LV. For each end-diastolic and end-systolic slices, endocardial and epicardial borders are traced. Because slice thickness is known, Simpson's method of disks can be used to accurately quantify volumes and mass. Inclusion or exclusion of papillary muscles in the LV mass is considered appropriate, as long as the given normal reference values reflect the methodology that has been used. In patients with high arrhythmia burden or respiratory motion artifacts, the use of faster free-breathing real-time cine imaging can allow evaluation of cardiac function at the expense of lower spatial resolution. Reported volumes are generally indexed to body surface area with normal reference values adapted according to the sex and age of the patient.

Estimation of atrial volumes can also be performed using four- and two-chamber long-axis views (area-length or biplane summation of disks methods). Alternatively, atrial volumes can be obtained from axial or short-axis atrial stacks.

Ischemic Heart Disease, Myocardial Infarction, and Viability

Myocardial Infarction

LGE imaging by CMR is currently the gold standard imaging modality for quantifying MI size and is able to detect small subendocardial MI (as little as 1g) with good accuracy.[8] In the acute phase of MI, CMR may detect the presence of ***microvascular obstruction***, which refers to the inability to reperfuse the coronary microcirculation in a previously ischemic region, despite opening of the epicardial vessel. On LGE sequences, microvascular obstruction appears as a dark core within the areas of hyperenhancement **(Figure 37.2 with MVO).** The extent of microvascular obstruction and infarct size increase substantially over the first 48 hours after an MI and are of prognostic value.

In patients with an acute reperfused MI, the ***area at risk*** refers to the territory supplied by the infarct-related artery that would have infarcted after MI if reperfusion had not taken place to salvage viable myocardium. The area at risk includes both the infarcted myocardium and the salvaged myocardium that surrounds it. Myocardial salvage can be calculated by subtracting the MI size from the area at risk and myocardial salvage index refers to the ratio of the myocardial salvage to the area at risk. The myocardial salvage index is considered a sensitive measure for assessing the efficacy of novel cardioprotective therapies compared with MI size alone.[9]

CMR also offers assessment of ***myocardial viability*** before coronary revascularization. The transmural extent of myocardial scar detected by LGE imaging accurately depicts a progressive stepwise decrease in functional recovery despite successful coronary revascularization. Compared to dobutamine exercise treadmill test (ETT), LGE is easy to perform and interpret and a 50% transmurality cutoff is sensitive in detecting segmental contractile recovery.[10]

Compared to other imaging modalities, CMR is the most accurate to reliably detect ***unrecognized (silent) MI***. In community-based studies that utilized CMR, MI detected by LGE imaging but unrecognized by clinical examination including ECG (thus untreated) were reported to occur in 6% to 17%, with marked increased in patient mortality consistently reported in these patients with unrecognized MI.[11]

Lastly, CMR is a valuable diagnostic tool in patients who present with acute elevation of serum biomarkers consistent

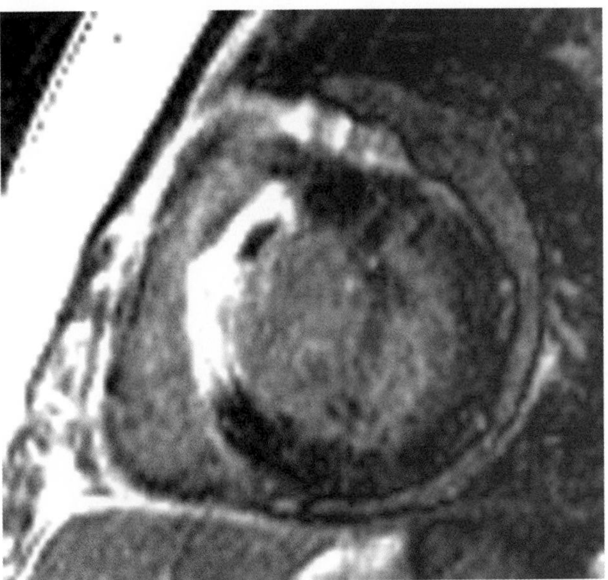

FIGURE 37.2 Short-axis phase-sensitive inversion recovery image obtained 15 min after gadolinium administration in a patient with a recent anteroseptal MI. Within the 100% transmural LGE in the anteroseptum, an area of MVO is clearly seen. LGE, late gadolinium enhancement; MI, myocardial infarction; MVO, microvascular obstruction. (Reprinted by permission from Springer: Kramer CM, Salerno M. Acute Myocardial Infarction and Postinfarction Remodeling. In: Kwong R, Jerosch-Herold M, Heydari B, eds. *Cardiovascular Magnetic Resonance Imaging. Contemporary Cardiology.* New York, NY: Springer; 2019: 161-174. Copyright © 2019 Springer Science+Business Media, LLC.)

with myocardial injury, but with nonobstructive coronary arteries (MI with no obstructive arteries [MINOCA]). By providing multicomponent assessment of myocardial structure and physiology, CMR can effectively capture various noncoronary abnormalities and guide differential diagnosis.

Stress Cardiac Magnetic Resonance Imaging for Detecting and Quantifying Myocardial Ischemia

Stress CMR has evolved to an everyday clinical tool, and is considered an effective first-line test for the evaluation, diagnosis, and risk stratification of patients with suspected IHD. Stress CMR is performed using vasodilating (eg, dipyridamole, adenosine, regadenoson) or positive inotropic pharmacologic stress agents. Following this, an intravenous bolus of GBCA is administered and three short-axis slices, each of 10 mm thickness, are acquired per cardiac cycle, at the basal, mid papillary, and apical levels of the LV, with a typical resolution of 2.5 × 2.5 mm.

In a normal scan, the wash-in (first pass) of GBCA into the myocardium can be seen as the myocardium turning from black to mid-gray uniformly throughout the whole of the LV in both the stress and rest scans. In an abnormal scan, an area of the myocardium will turn gray slower than the surrounding tissue because the blood (and hence gadolinium) enters more slowly due to a narrowing of the coronary artery supplying it. This is called a perfusion defect and usually represents myocardial ischemia. It may be seen on both the rest and stress scans in which case it is called a matched perfusion defect and is probably due to an area or scar from a previous MI. If it is only seen on the stress scan, it is called an area of inducible perfusion defect (ischemia). The positions in the LV of the perfusion defects are described using the AHA 17 segment model (**Figure 37.3**).

Multicenter studies have shown that a negative stress CMR portends to an annualized cardiac event rate of <1% in patients with an intermediate pretest likelihood of IHD.[12]

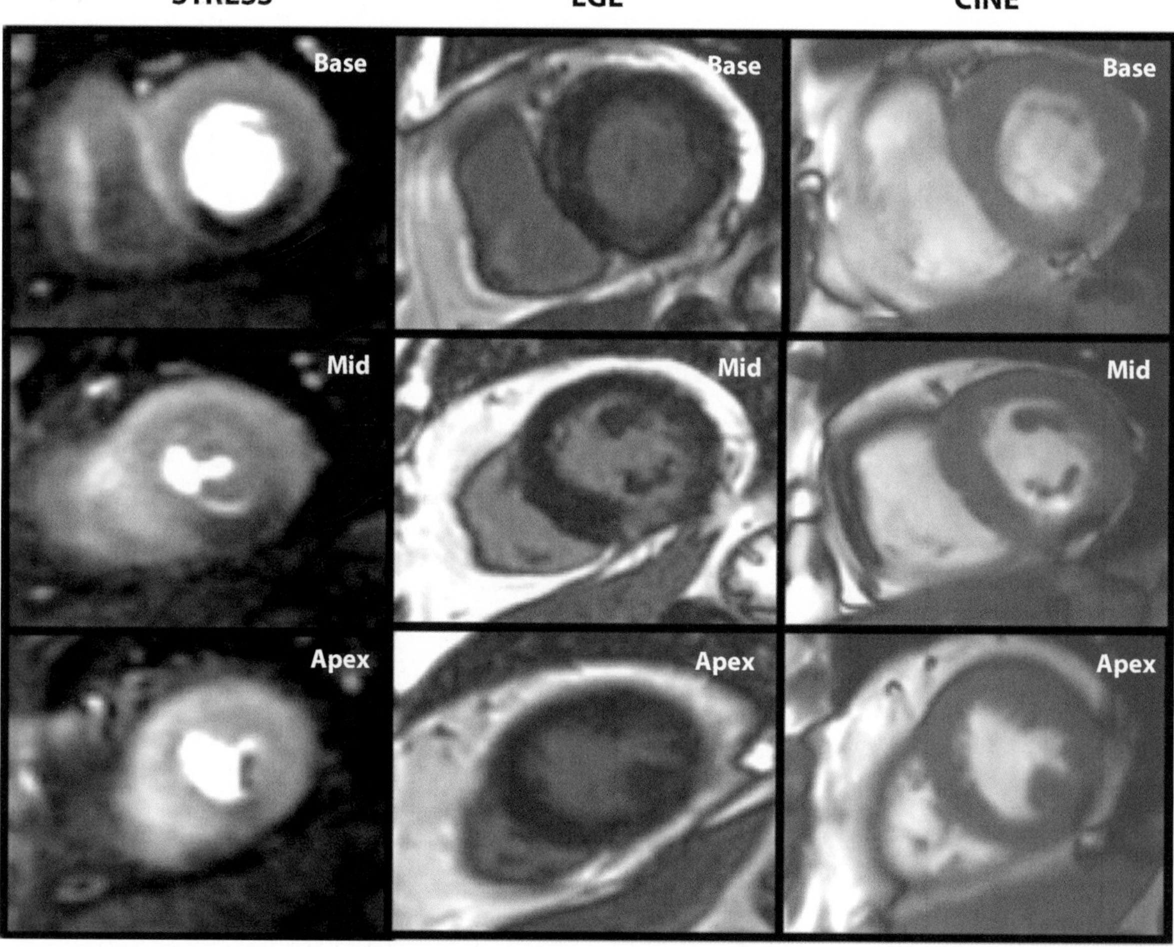

FIGURE 37.3 A 62-year-old male is referred to pharmacologic stress CMR using regadenoson to assess for coronary artery disease in the context of newly discovered hypokinesis of the inferolateral wall on echocardiogram. The study revealed a moderate size first-pass perfusion defect involving the basal inferior septum, basal inferior, mid inferior, and apical inferior segments. These areas were partially matched by subendocardial to transmural late gadolinium enhancement raising concerns for prior myocardial infarction in the distribution of the posterior descending coronary artery with significant peri-infarction ischemia. CMR, Cardiac magnetic resonance imaging; LGE, late gadolinium enhancement.

There is excellent correlation of stress CMR assessment of ischemia against invasive measurement of fractional flow reserve, showcasing its high accuracy in determining the physiologic significance of coronary stenosis, and safely guiding management in IHD.[13] Compared to cardiac single photon emission computed tomography (SPECT) imaging, stress CMR has several technical advantages: (1) it is not limited by attenuation artifacts; (2) it is free from ionizing radiation; (3) it has three- to fourfold higher spatial resolution; (4) it takes 35 to 45 minutes to complete (compared to >2 hours for dual-isotope SPECT); and (5) it performs better than SPECT in detecting single or multivessel coronary disease.[14-16]

Cardiomyopathies

Nonischemic Dilated Cardiomyopathy

Dilated cardiomyopathy is a manifestation of many disorders affecting the myocardium; this can be ischemic, but also nonischemic as in familial dilated CMP. Subendocardial or transmural LGE following a coronary artery distribution is the hallmark of ischemic CMP. Features of nonischemic forms include some degree of biventricular dilatation and biatrial enlargement, global ventricular systolic dysfunction, and functional mitral/tricuspid regurgitation. LGE is often absent, but linear mid-wall LGE involving predominantly the interventricular septum is seen in up to 30% of patients and is linked to worse prognosis[17] **(Figure 37.4)**.

Hypertrophic Cardiomyopathy

A diagnosis of hypertrophic cardiomyopathy (HCM) requires an increased LV wall thickness greater than or equal to 15 mm after other potential causes have been excluded. By virtue of its high spatial resolution, CMR allows for precise and reliable measurements of segmental LV wall thickness, including the anterolateral wall, apex, or inferior septum, areas that may not be well seen by TTE. Discrepancy in wall thickness measurements between the two techniques is often a result of underestimation of segmental areas of LV hypertrophy by ETT. Ancillary findings on CMR including aberrant LV muscle bundles, basal crypts, apical pouching, and anomalous papillary muscle insertion directly into anterior mitral leaflet may also favor a diagnosis of HCM.[18] Furthermore, in HCM patients with severe septal hypertrophy and symptomatic dynamic LV outflow tract obstruction, CMR has advantage over echocardiography in assessing the reduction of septal thickness from surgical myectomy or alcohol septal ablation.

Presence of LGE appears in approximately half of patients with HCM, is indicative of heterogeneous fibrosis and myofibril disarray, and has been associated with ventricular arrhythmias, sudden cardiac death, and progressive ventricular dilatation. LGE patterns include involvement of both RV insertion points and patchy multifocal mid-wall LGE typically in segments with increased LV wall thickness. The extent of LGE appears to be especially important for prognosis—independent of other high-risk features—when it represents greater than 15% of the total LV mass. However, even minor LGE extent provides incremental prognostic value to patient risk beyond cardiac structure and function, particularly in patients considered at low clinical risk by conventional risk stratification algorithms[19] (**e-Figure 37.1**).

A number of conditions may mimic HCM. In cases of diagnostic uncertainty, CMR plays a prominent in accurate differentiation of these entities with management implications (including participation in competitive sports, anticoagulation, and risk stratification for sudden cardiac death). First,

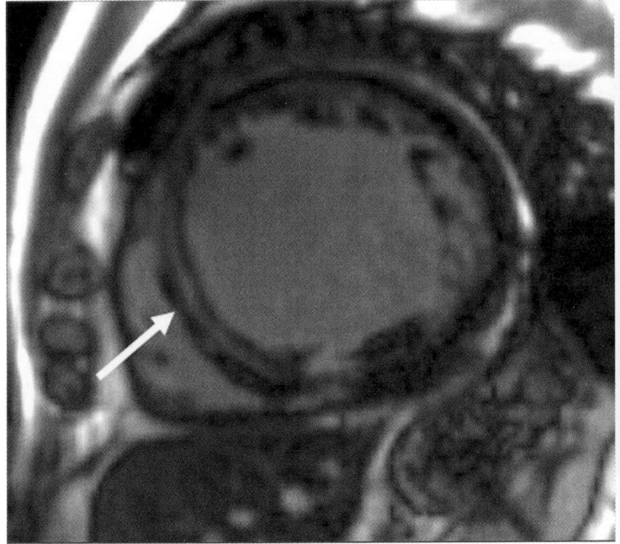
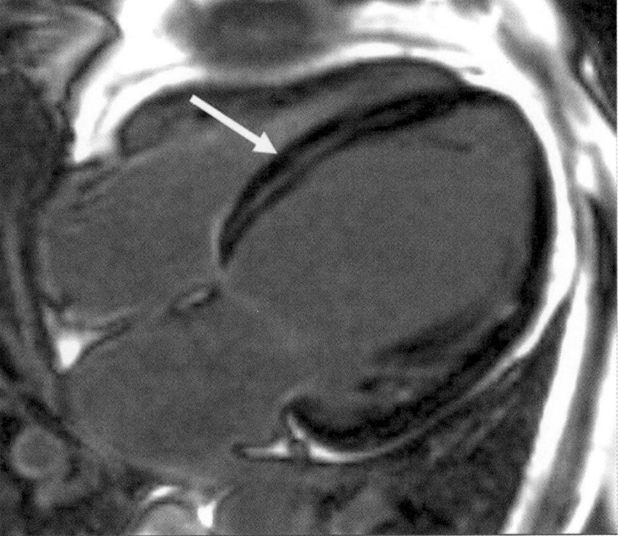

FIGURE 37.4 Short-axis (left) and four-chamber (right) views showing typical late gadolinium enhancement (LGE) distribution in a patient with severe left ventricular dilatation and markedly decreased left ventricular ejection fraction. The pattern of LGE is linear, mid-wall and involves the interventricular septum (white arrows). This is consistent with a nonischemic dilated cardiomyopathy.

when a diagnosis of HCM is suspected based on clinical profile and TTE is normal/nondiagnostic, CMR should be routinely performed to further clarify the diagnosis. LV hypertrophy associated with systemic training (ie, athlete's heart) may be difficult to differentiate from HCM. In such cases, serial CMR studies are the most reliable strategy for comparing LV wall thickness measurements before and after a period of deconditioning to distinguish pathologic from physiologic hypertrophy. A patient whose wall thickness regresses more than 2 mm supports a diagnosis of athletic heart, whereas LV hypertrophy that persists despite deconditioning supports a diagnosis of HCM.[20] LV remodeling associated with athlete's heart should not result in focal areas of myocardial scarring/fibrosis—readily identified by LGE imaging—especially in young individuals. In an athlete in whom suspicion has been raised for HCM, the presence of LGE favors a diagnosis of HCM.[20] CMR can also be helpful in the detection of changes in serial measurements of LV wall thickness after aggressive treatment with antihypertensive medication, in which a regression of hypertrophy would favor a diagnosis of hypertensive cardiomyopathy.

Cardiac Amyloidosis

Cardiac AL results from deposition of abnormally folded proteins, the amyloid fibrils, in the extracellular space of the heart. Systemic light-chain AL and transthyretin-derived (hereditary and nonhereditary TTR) AL are the two most common forms of cardiac AL. The amyloid protocol in our institution includes long-axis and short-axis cine SSFP images for LV/RV size and function, resting first-pass perfusion, TI scout, and late enhancement imaging. Classic CMR findings include concentric increase in LV wall thickness and small ventricles with biatrial enlargement suggestive of restrictive CMP. Pericardial and/or pleural effusions are also supportive findings. As amyloid proteins tend to infiltrate basal ventricular segments predominantly, careful visual assessment of LV function can reveal preserved LV apical contractility that correlates with the "cherry on top" (apical sparring) sign seen on strain imaging with ETT. Since cardiac AL is a disease of the interstitial space, gadolinium is retained in the myocardium leading to diffuse LV hyperenhancement on LGE sequences. At the equilibrium state, which is 10 to 15 minutes after contrast injection, gadolinium concentration in the myocardium can either be similar or higher than in the blood pool, which often leads to difficult nulling of the myocardium and suboptimal LGE images. On TI scout sequences, this can lead to the myocardium being nulled (appears dark) before the blood pool, a finding consistent with abnormal gadolinium kinetics. Phase-sensitive inversion recovery sequences (PSIR) can help when selection of TI is difficult. Typically, the LGE pattern is a diffuse circumferential and subendocardial involvement, although areas of transmural LGE are frequent.[21] First-pass perfusion imaging can also reveal a circumferential subendocardial perfusion deficit, which may reflect microvascular dysfunction. Newer T1 mapping techniques using precontrast (native T1), postcontrast T1, and hematocrit value allow calculation of extracellular volume (ECV)—a measure of free water in the myocardium—that is abnormally increased in case of cardiac AL **(Figure 37.5)**.

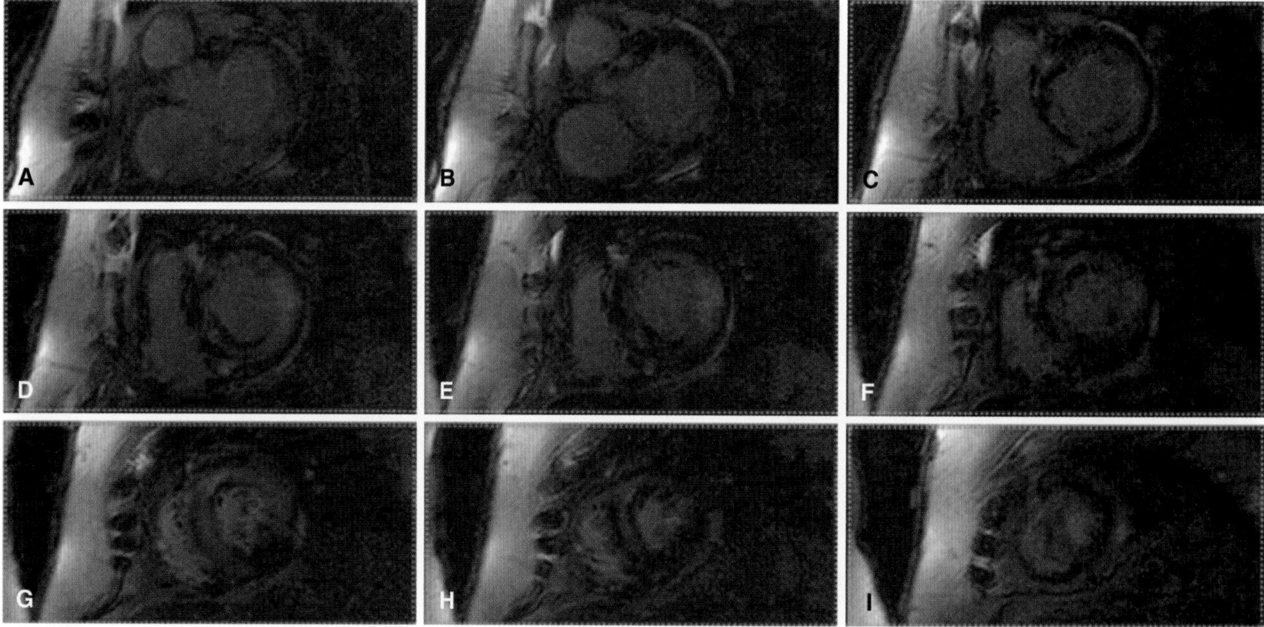

FIGURE 37.5 Cardiac amyloidosis. Late gadolinium enhancement images of the basal (**A-D**), mid (**E-G**), and apical (**H,I**) left ventricle and right ventricle reveal extensive concentric early and late gadolinium enhancement in a subendocardial pattern with relative sparing of the epicardium, in a pattern classic for cardiac amyloidosis. (Reprinted by permission from Springer: Morgan RB, Kwong RY. Assessment of Cardiomyopathies and Cardiac Transplantation. In: Kwong R, Jerosch-Herold M, Heydari B, eds. *Cardiovascular Magnetic Resonance Imaging. Contemporary Cardiology.* New York, NY: Springer; 2019:249-272. Copyright © 2019 Springer Science+Business Media, LLC.)

Cardiac Sarcoidosis

Around 5% of patients with systemic sarcoidosis have cardiac involvement. Conduction disorders as well as ventricular arrhythmias are common cardiac manifestations in these patients. The 2014 Heart Rhythm Society recommends screening with advanced imaging modality such as CMR or PET-FDG (class IIa indication) in the presence of suggestive symptoms, abnormal findings on ECG, or on echocardiogram.[22] Suggestive CMR findings include basal septal and inferolateral wall thinning or aneurysm as well as abnormal LGE. Although no LGE pattern is specific for cardiac sarcoidosis, subepicardial and mid-myocardial patchy LGE following a noncoronary distribution raises concerns for sarcoidosis, especially if basal septum is affected. However, Patel et al showed that nearly 50% of patients with cardiac sarcoidosis had at least one CAD-type of LGE lesion.[23] The presence of LGE has significant prognostic impact for all-cause mortality, cardiovascular mortality, and ventricular arrhythmias.[24] Finally, on T2-weighted images, hyperintense signal matched to abnormal LGE suggests myocardial edema and active inflammation **(Figure 37.6).**

Fabry Disease

Anderson-Fabry disease (AFD) is a rare storage disease caused by X-linked mutation in the α-galactosidase gene leading to abnormal accumulation of glycosphingolipids in lysosomes. These patients present with increased wall thickness mimicking HCM, including symmetric, asymmetric septal, and apical subtypes. In patients with concentric increase in LV wall thickness, the most frequent pattern of LGE involves the inferolateral wall, whereas more atypical scar pattern is seen in patients with nonconcentric form. Furthermore, Deva et al showed that in patients with typical inferolateral LGE pattern, around 60% of patients had at least one additional region with scar.[25] Because accumulation of lipids can shorten T1 values, the use of decreased native T1 values may support the diagnosis of AFD in certain cases.[26]

Arrhythmogenic Right Ventricular Cardiomyopathy

Arrhythmogenic right ventricular cardiomyopathy (ARVC) is a familial disease where the normal myocardium is replaced by fibrofatty tissue, increasing predisposition toward ventricular arrhythmias that precede overt morphologic abnormalities. It usually involves the right ventricle, but the LV and septum may also be affected. CMR has emerged as an important imaging modality in the diagnosis and evaluation of patients with suspected ARVC because of its superior volumetric assessment of RV function and its characterization of fibrofatty myocardial tissue. CMR does not require intravenous contrast or ionizing radiation, making it a suitable modality for follow-up in ARVC patients who are often young and require a number of repeated examinations. The main advantage of CMR is the possibility of planning any desired view so that regions such as the outflow tract, which are hard to visualize with other techniques, can be assessed with great precision.

CMR abnormalities in ARVC can broadly be divided into two groups: (1) functional abnormalities that include regional wall motion abnormalities, focal aneurysms, RV dilatation,

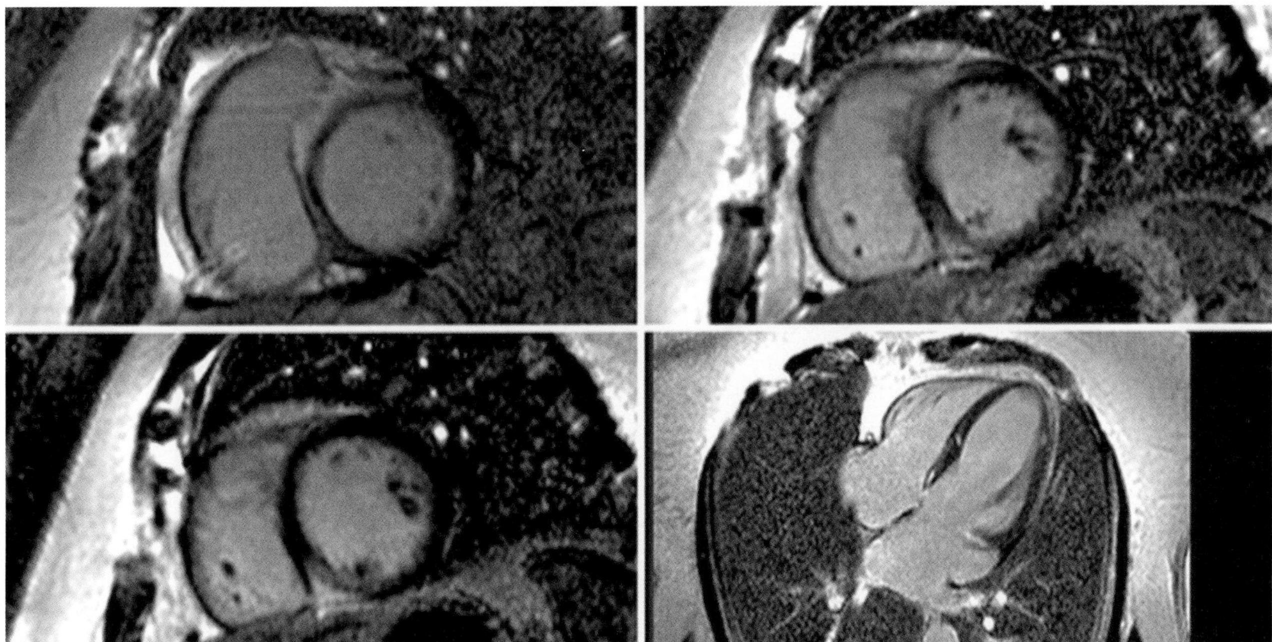

FIGURE 37.6 Cardiac sarcoidosis. Late gadolinium enhancement (LGE) images of the basal, mid, and apical left ventricle and right ventricle reveal multiple foci of epicardial LGE involving the basal and mid anteroseptum and inferoseptum at the right ventricular insertion points, in a pattern classic for cardiac sarcoidosis. (Reprinted by permission from Springer: Morgan RB, Kwong RY. Assessment of Cardiomyopathies and Cardiac Transplantation. In: Kwong R, Jerosch-Herold M, Heydari B, eds. *Cardiovascular Magnetic Resonance Imaging. Contemporary Cardiology.* New York, NY: Springer; 2019:249-272. Copyright © 2019 Springer Science+Business Media, LLC.)

and RV diastolic/systolic dysfunction; (2) morphologic abnormalities that include intramyocardial fatty infiltration, focal wall thinning, wall hypertrophy, trabecular hypertrophy and disarray, moderator band hypertrophy, and right ventricular outflow tract (RVOT) enlargement. Out of these, localized aneurysms, severe global/segmental dilatation of the RV, and global systolic dysfunction are considered major criteria whereas mild global/segmental dilatation of the RV, regional contraction abnormalities, and global diastolic dysfunction are considered minor criteria for ARVC diagnosis. Identification of fat within the myocardium is the least specific and least reproducible of any of the other parameters in the CMR evaluation of ARVC and is not a criterion for ARVC.[27] LGE imaging has the potential to identify myocardial fibrofatty changes in both RV and LV in ARVC (Figure 37.4). Overall, in patients suspected to have ARVC, CMR has a sensitivity of 96% and a specificity of 78% in detecting ARVC according to diagnostic criteria that include genotype[28] **(Figure 37.7).**

Left Ventricular Non-compaction Cardiomyopathy

Left ventricular non-compaction cardiomyopathy (LVNC) is characterized by prominent trabeculations, deep intratrabecular recesses, and compact and non-compact layers of myocardium. CMR has emerged as an imaging tool for LVNC diagnosis by offering a high contrast of myocardial tissue and accurate visualization of the LV apex, which is known to be the most commonly non-compacted area. On the basis of currently suggested CMR criteria, LVNC can be diagnosed based on linear measurements (ratio between non-compacted and compacted myocardium) at end diastole or end systole, mass ratio between total and trabeculae mass or fractal dimension—a quantitative measure of the myocardial trabeculae complexity. The most commonly used CMR criteria uses a ratio of non-compacted: compacted myocardium greater than 2.3:1 in end diastole. Other findings on CMR may include thinning of the compact LV wall—particularly in apical segments—and LV dilation with or without reduced LV function. Differentiating LVNC from normal variants remains difficult because prominent trabecular patterns, meeting diagnostic criteria for LVNC, have also been demonstrated in subjects exposed to hemodynamic loads such as pregnant women and athletes. Therefore, to avoid decreased specificity, a segmental basis for apical/mid/basal slices with reporting of the number of hypertrabeculated segments has been proposed. LVNC is more probable in subjects with three or more positive segments.[29] Finally, LGE is a common finding in LVNC, being found in up to 55% of patients. The most common pattern is septal mid-wall enhancement followed by localization at the insertion point, subendocardial, and transmural.

Iron Overload Cardiomyopathy

Chronic iron overload, for example, caused by repetitive blood transfusions for hematologic disorders, such as thalassemia major, can lead to siderotic cardiomyopathy, characterized by myocardial iron deposition. In patients with transfusion-dependent thalassemia major, cardiac death as a result of myocardial iron toxicity occurs in up to 50% of patients. Global systolic LV function is usually preserved—especially in anemic thalassemic patients—until severe cardiac toxicity has developed, and thus provides little if any guidance to chelation therapy.

CMR has a unique role in the management of iron loading disease. CMR T2* quantitation has been shown to reproducibly assess the degree of myocardial iron loading, which directly correlates with outcome. The T2* relaxation time linearly falls with increasing iron load. T2* should be assessed in the septal wall since this is the region where susceptibility artifacts are rare, in contrast to the inferolateral wall where they are common due to the proximity to the great cardiac vein. The reduction of T2* relaxation time in the presence of myocardial iron overload is only modestly associated with left ventricular ejection fraction (LVEF) and is not associated with abnormalities of diastolic function. A T2* relaxation time of less than 20 minutes has been proposed as a cutoff value for diagnosing

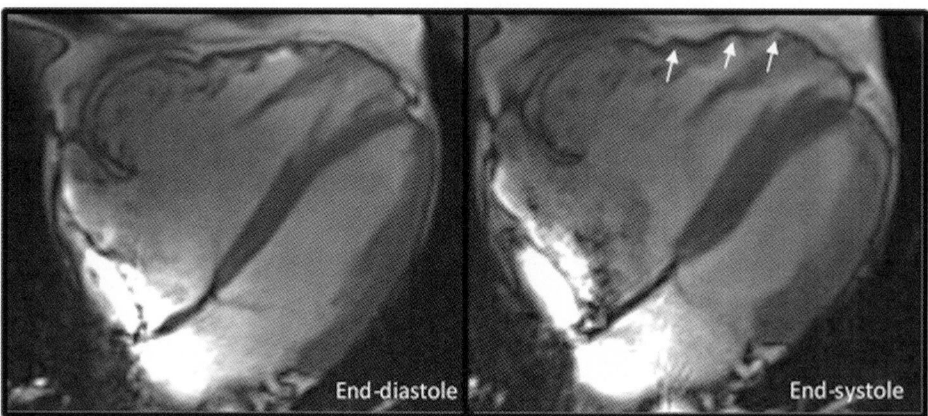

FIGURE 37.7 End-diastolic and end-systolic cine images in a 34-year-old male patient with family history of sudden cardiac death and dilated right ventricle on echocardiogram. Both images show severe right ventricular (RV) dilatation (RV end-diastolic volume: 150 mL/m^2) and RV systolic dysfunction (RV ejection fraction: 38%). There are significant wall motion abnormalities of the RV free wall (white arrows) consistent with RV microaneurysms. Imaging features fulfilled one major task force criterion for arrhythmogenic RV cardiomyopathy.

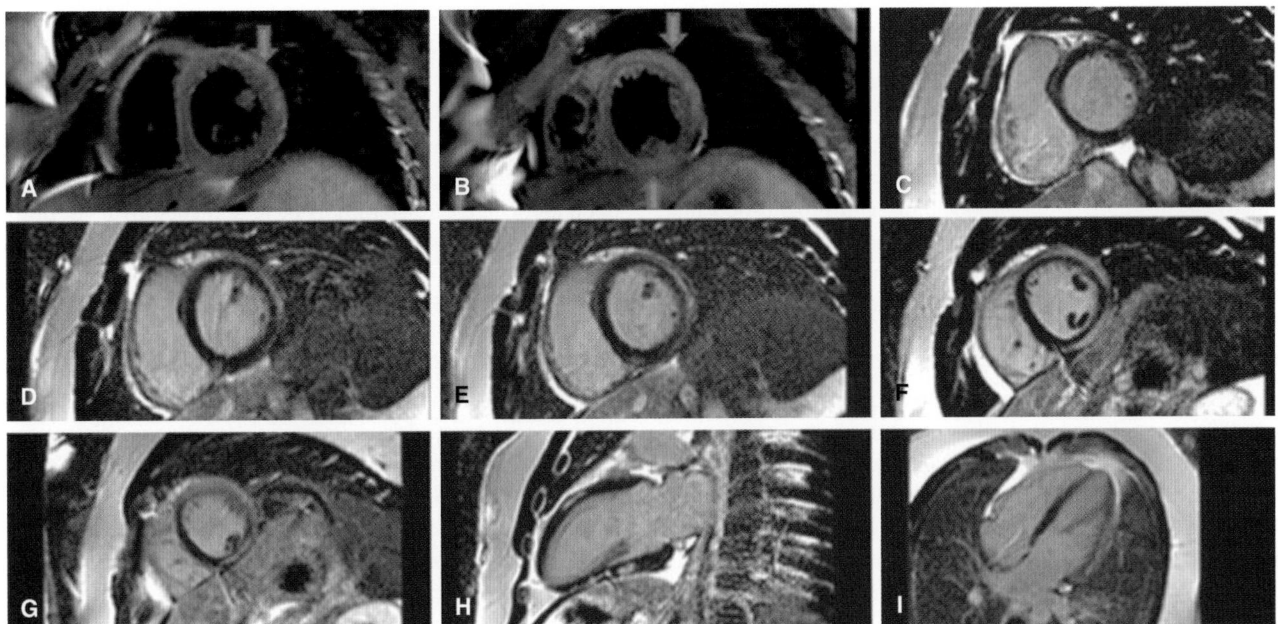

FIGURE 37.8 Myocarditis. T2 hyperintensity is seen within the basal and mid anterior, anterolateral, and inferolateral walls, as well as the mid inferior wall (**A** and **B** blue arrows indicate edema), sparing the subendocardium, suggestive of myocardial edema. On the postcontrast images (**C-I**), there is subepicardial late gadolinium enhancemtn of corresponding segments of the myocardium suggestive of inflammation/scar. In addition, there was a resting perfusion defect of the basal and mid anterolateral and inferolateral segments sparing the subendocardial layer suggestive of microvascular obstruction/myocardial necrosis. (Reprinted by permission from Springer: Morgan RB, Kwong RY. Assessment of Cardiomyopathies and Cardiac Transplantation. In: Kwong R, Jerosch-Herold M, Heydari B, eds. *Cardiovascular Magnetic Resonance Imaging. Contemporary Cardiology.* New York, NY: Springer; 2019:249-272. Copyright © 2019 Springer Science+Business Media, LLC.)

SECTION 2

cardiac siderosis, whereas a value of less than 10 minutes is associated with poor prognosis and requires initiation of iron chelation therapy.[30] T2* relaxation times can be serially monitored in patients who are receiving iron chelation therapy. Such a strategy has resulted in a significant decrease in cardiac morbidity and mortality in patients with thalassemia who require frequent blood transfusions. Similar information cannot be provided by other imaging modalities, which makes CMR an irreplaceable tool for management of siderotic cardiomyopathy and delivery of iron chelation therapy.

Myocarditis

CMR plays a key role in the diagnosis and risk stratification of patients with suspected myocarditis.[31] The updated 2018 Lake Louise Criteria now propose two main diagnostic findings for the diagnosis of myocarditis[32]: (1) ***myocardial edema*** with either regional or global increase in T2 mapping or hyperintense signal on T2 weighted images; and (2) ***nonischemic myocardial injury*** by either increased native T1 and/or ECV or the presence of LGE (**Figure 37.8**). Other supportive CMR findings also include pericardial effusion/inflammation and regional or diffuse LV systolic dysfunction. Common LGE patterns seen with nonischemic myocardial inflammation include patchy, subepicardial or mid-wall involvement, although extent can be transmural in cases of severe inflammation (Figure 37.6). Aquaro et al showed that 6 months following an acute episode of myocarditis, almost 90% of patients still had some degree of LGE on CMR.[33]

Valvular Heart Disease

Although TTE remains the first-line imaging modality for the evaluation of valvular heart disease, CMR is increasingly used in cases of inadequate echocardiographic examination and in order to provide additional information on regurgitant and cavity volumes. The CMR evaluation of valvular heart disease includes the following: (1) the quantification of lesion severity, either regurgitation or stenosis; (2) the measurement of the consequences of the valvular defect on the cardiac chambers (volume, mass, and function); and (3) the assessment of valve morphology, in selected cases. Because of its ability to accurately quantify valvular RFs, aortic regurgitation (AR) and mitral regurgitation (MR) are the most common valvulopathies referred for CMR evaluation.

The phase-contrast or velocity-encoded cine CMR pulse sequence is the imaging sequence of choice for quantifying flow and calculating velocities. For AR, phase-contrast velocity mapping just above the aortic valve enables the user to determine the volume of blood moving in anterograde and retrograde fashions within the cardiac cycle; thus, the regurgitant volume and RF can be calculated. Alternately, if the stroke volume of the pulmonary forward flow is subtracted from the stroke volume of the aortic forward flow, the regurgitant volume and RF can also be calculated. Finally, in the absence of significant mitral regurgitation and right-sided lesions, RF can be calculated by subtracting the RV stroke volume from the LV stroke volume. These internal controls help to ensure consistency of volume quantification. The reproducibility and prognostic value of CMR in quantifying the severity of valvular regurgitation using phase-contrast velocity mapping may be superior compared to TTE. In a study of patients with echocardiographic moderate or severe AR, a CMR-derived aortic RF of more than 33% was strongly associated with the development of typical symptoms and referral for aortic valve surgery.[34]

With regard to mitral regurgitation, the orientation of the regurgitant jet, such as severe obliquity, can make TTE assessment unreliable. Phase contrast for the mitral valve is more difficult because of significant movement of the mitral annulus during systole. For this reason, quantification of mitral insufficiency volume can be performed using an indirect approach. In patients with MR, the total LV stroke volume is increased and is equivalent to the aortic forward stroke volume (anterograde flow) plus the mitral regurgitant volume (retrograde flow). Since the total LV stroke volume can be calculated from planimetry of the LV end-diastolic and end-systolic contours, and the aortic forward flow can be calculated from phase-contrast CMR at the aortic root, the difference between these values will be equal to the mitral regurgitant volume.[35] Calculation of regurgitant volumes by CMR is highly reproducible, which facilitates serial assessment of MR in patients who are managed expectantly.[36]

Cardiac Thrombi and Masses

CMR is the imaging modality of choice to assess for cardiac thrombi after echocardiography has been performed. CMR allows for multiplanar reconstruction and reduces the chances of apical foreshortening, a potential limitation of echocardiography. LGE sequences with longer TI (600 msec) are particularly useful to increase differentiation between thrombus and other tissues.

CMR is also incremental to echocardiography in the assessment of cardiac masses, with the ability to assess extracardiac involvement. The main sequences used include high-resolution cine SSFP or GRE images, T1 weighted images with and without fat saturation preparation, T2 weighted images for edema/inflammation, first-pass perfusion to assess vascularity of the mass, and LGE.[37] Location, mobility, and relation with surrounding valvular and vascular structures are helpful in identifying the etiology of the mass and distinguishing between benign and malignant tumors.

Most malignant cardiac tumors are metastatic and represent either direct invasion from the mediastinum in lung or breast cancer, lymphatic spread (lymphoma or melanoma), or hematologic spread (renal cell carcinoma). Primary cardiac tumors are rare and mainly include various types of sarcomas and primary cardiac lymphoma. The presence of pericardial effusion in a patient with known metastasis should raise concern for cardiac or pericardial metastasis.

A myxoma frequently presents as a hypermobile mass located in the left atrium and attached to the interatrial septum that is isointense on T1 weighted and hyperintense on T2 weighted sequences, with some degree of heterogeneity. Other frequent benign cardiac tumors include rhabdomyomas, fibromas, and papillary fibroelastomas (**e-Figure 37.2**).

Pericardial Disease

CMR can provide superior anatomic perspective, tissue characterization, and assessment of pericardial diseases. In acute pericarditis, hyperintense signal of the pericardium on T2 weighted fast spin echo images is consistent with active pericardial inflammation. Signal intensity is inversely proportional to the chronicity of pericarditis. Typically, cine SSFP sequences are performed as part of the protocol and can accurately identify and characterize pericardial effusion and adhesions. On T1 weighted images, pericardial fat appears hyperintense and with the use of fat saturation preparation, better delineation and measurement of the pericardial thickness can be performed. A thickness up to 3 mm is considered within the normal range. In constrictive pericarditis, main CMR features include increased pericardial thickness, presence of interventricular dependence on real-time cine images, early diastolic septal bounce, small and tubular-shaped ventricles, dilated atria, inferior vena cava (IVC), and superior vena cava (SVC). Line-tagging sequences can be performed to identify pericardial adhesions. At our center, we routinely add an ECG and respiratory-gated delayed enhancement sequence (navigator) allowing detection of pericardial LGE that can represent either pericardial inflammation or scarring.

Congenital Heart Disease

Evaluation of patients with congenital heart disease (CHD) is a particular strength of CMR because of the following: (1) its ability for complete depiction of the pathologic anatomy, and (2) the lack of ionizing radiation when performing sequential studies in children and young adults. The clinical use of CMR depends on the age and the clinical condition of the patient. In neonates and infants, where sedation may be required, CMR is usually performed as an adjunct to TTE. In older children, adolescents, or adults, in more complex anatomy or at any age after surgery, CMR becomes the technique of choice because the interposition of scar tissue and lungs becomes an increasing problem for TTE.

For a complete CMR examination, the following sequences are typically performed: (1) anatomic images in the transaxial and at least one additional orthogonal plane (sagittal or coronal); (2) SSFP sequences in contiguous short-axis planes for the evaluation of biventricular function, volumes, and mass; (3) measurements of velocity and flow volume in the heart and great vessels/conduits; and (4) contrast MRA for 3D representation of the thoracic aorta, pulmonary arteries, and veins.

Atrial septal defects (ASD), coarctation of the aorta, and tetralogy of Fallot (TOF) are among the most common CHD

TABLE 37.2 Current Contraindications to Cardiac Magnetic Resonance Imaging (MRI) in Patients Without MRI-Conditional Cardiac Implanted Devices

Epicardial leads
Baseline device or lead malfunction (ie, battery at end of life, fractured lead)
Implant < 6 weeks
Pacemaker-dependent patients with implantable cardioverter defibrillator if asynchronous pacing modes are not available
Abandoned or cut endovascular leads

TABLE 37.3 Advantages and Disadvantages of Cardiac Magnetic Resonance Imaging

Advantages
Three dimensional
High spatial and temporal resolution
Intrinsic high contrast; no need for iodinated contrast
No ionizing radiation
Minimal interference from neighboring soft tissues
Multiple imaging components interrogating cardiac structures and physiology in a single study session
Disadvantages
Contraindicated with certain medical implants such as aneurysm clips, transcutaneous electrical nerve stimulation (TENS) units, and certain pacemakers
Acquisition time longer than other imaging modalities, ranging from 30 to 60 minutes
In a minority of patients, cardiac rhythm or respiratory irregularities deteriorate image quality
Claustrophobia (in about 5% of patients)
Contraindication for gadolinium contrast agents in severe chronic kidney disease

conditions referred for CMR evaluation.[38] CMR offers a less invasive alternative to diagnostic catheterization or transesophageal echocardiography for patients presenting with right-sided volume overload from a suspected left-to-right shunt. CMR can detect the presence of an ASD, assess suitability for transcatheter ASD closure, quantify right heart size and function, determine pulmonary to systemic shunt ratio (Qp/Qs) and identify any coexisting anomalous pulmonary venous return. Phase-contrast imaging positioned in a plane parallel to the atrial septum and set at a low velocity range (100 cm/sec) can visualize the ASD *en face* with good correlation with defect size measured invasively. By using the PC (phase contrast) sequence, the ratio of pulmonary blood flow (Qp) and systemic blood flow (Qs) can be accurately quantified and reflects the size of the shunt. Because most closure devices are MRI compatible, CMR can be used to assess for residual shunt and proper device deployment. Patients with a ventricular septal defect (VSD) can be assessed using similar techniques.

CMR is the first-line imaging technique for anatomic assessment of aortic arch anomalies. Coarctation of the aorta is one of the commonest forms of congenital aortic anomaly. Most patients will have had surgical repair in childhood and are followed routinely for evidence of coarctation recurrence. Gadolinium-enhanced 3D MRA is able to define the site of aortic narrowing in most cases. Cine SSFP in a long-axis "candy-cane" view can further delineate the aortic anatomy, the degree of obstruction, and any aortic valvular dysfunction. Black blood, fast spin echo sequences are useful to evaluate the entire aorta and are resistant to artifacts from implanted endovascular stents. In case of a prior coarctation repair with either a flap of the subclavian artery or a Dacron patch, focal aneurysmal dilatations of the prosthetic material may also be assessed. Phase-contrast imaging can characterize the descending to ascending aorta flow ratio and estimate pressure gradient across the coarctation and degree of collaterals formation.[39]

Finally, CMR has been firmly established as the key imaging modality for serial follow-up in surgically repaired TOF patients. Typical residual findings during follow-up include moderate to severe incompetence of the pulmonary valve, obstruction of the RVOT, and/or the branch pulmonary arteries. CMR is the only technique that allows accurate quantification of pulmonary incompetence with measurement of regurgitation volumes and fraction. Furthermore, tailored imaging planes through the RVOT, the pulmonary bifurcation, and pulmonary side branches give clear views of the anatomy. Additional functional information can be obtained by measuring the differential pulmonary perfusion and assessing the backflow separately in both pulmonary side branches. Furthermore, the presence and extent of myocardial scarring as detected by LGE has been found to be related to exercise intolerance, regional wall motion abnormalities, ventricular arrhythmias, and sudden cardiac death.[40] This information is crucial for surgical decision-making around pulmonary valve replacement.[41]

RESEARCH AND FUTURE DIRECTIONS

- A new development in CMR is the use of quantitative myocardial perfusion imaging that allows more robust and objective quantification of myocardial blood flow during rest or stress perfusion, as opposed to the standard qualitative visual approach.[42]
- 4D phase-contrast velocity mapping is a three-dimensional volumetric technique that can improve quantification of intracardiac blood flows.
- As in other imaging modalities, the use of artificial intelligence may considerably speed up image acquisition and post-processing.
- Extensive ongoing research aims to improve non–breath-hold and non–ECG-gated CMR techniques, especially in real-time cine sequences.

KEY POINTS

- ✔ CMR is a noninvasive, nonionizing imaging technique, with high spatial resolution, that is considered the gold standard for morphologic assessment of the heart, as well as the assessment of right and left ventricular systolic and diastolic function and mass.
- ✔ Owing to its ability to characterize tissue and provide morphologic definition of scar, inflammation, and necrosis (late enhancement technique), CMR is well established for the diagnosis and follow-up of CMP.
- ✔ Cardiac MRI is the most accurate modality for the description of MI, both in the acute and chronic phases. The performance of cardiac MRI in the assessment of myocardial perfusion and ischemia is more detailed than that of SPECT.
- ✔ Cardiac MRI can separate ischemic from nonischemic cardiomyopathy, and is the most important imaging modality for the diagnosis and follow-up of patients with myocarditis.
- ✔ Cardiac MRI is increasingly important in the diagnosis and follow-up of patients with CHD, usually as a complement to echocardiography.
- ✔ In valvular disease, echocardiography remains the imaging modality of choice, but cardiac MRI is increasingly used as an aid to determine the timing for surgery.
- ✔ Cardiac MRI is useful for the assessment of pericardial disease and cardiac tumors.

REFERENCES

1. Grover VPB, Tognarelli JM, Crossey MME, Cox IJ, Taylor-Robinson SD, McPhail MJW. Magnetic resonance imaging: principles and techniques: lessons for clinicians. *J Clin Exp Hepatol.* 2015;5:246-255.
2. Biglands JD, Radjenovic A, Ridgway JP. Cardiovascular magnetic resonance physics for clinicians: part II. *J Cardiovasc Magn Reson.* 2012;14:66.
3. Ridgway JP. Cardiovascular magnetic resonance physics for clinicians: part I. *J Cardiovasc Magn Reson.* 2010;12:71.
4. ACR Committee on Drugs and Contrast Media. ACR manual on contrast media. *American College of Radiology.* 2015.
5. Pennell DJ. Cardiovascular magnetic resonance. *Circulation.* 2010;121: 692-705.
6. Russo RJ, Costa HS, Silva PD, et al. Assessing the risks associated with MRI in patients with a pacemaker or defibrillator. *N Engl J Med.* 2017;376:755-764.
7. Nazarian S, Hansford R, Rahsepar AA, et al. Safety of magnetic resonance imaging in patients with cardiac devices. *N Engl J Med.* 2017;377:2555-2564.
8. Bulluck H, Dharmakumar R, Arai AE, Berry C, Hausenloy DJ. Cardiovascular magnetic resonance in acute ST-segment-elevation myocardial infarction: recent advances, controversies, and future directions. *Circulation.* 2018;137:1949-1964.
9. Ibanez B, Aletras AH, Arai AE, et al. Cardiac MRI endpoints in myocardial infarction experimental and clinical trials: JACC scientific expert panel. *J Am Coll Cardiol.* 2019;74:238-256.
10. Kim RJ, Wu E, Rafael A, et al. The use of contrast-enhanced magnetic resonance imaging to identify reversible myocardial dysfunction. *N Engl J Med.* 2000;343:1445-1453.
11. Kwong RY, Chan AK, Brown KA, et al. Impact of unrecognized myocardial scar detected by cardiac magnetic resonance imaging on event-free survival in patients presenting with signs or symptoms of coronary artery disease. *Circulation.* 2006;113:2733-2743.
12. Kwong RY, Ge Y, Steel K, et al. Cardiac magnetic resonance stress perfusion imaging for evaluation of patients with chest pain. *J Am Coll Cardiol.* 2019;74:1741-1755.
13. Nagel E, Greenwood JP, McCann GP, et al. Magnetic resonance perfusion or fractional flow reserve in coronary disease. *N Engl J Med.* 2019;380:2418-2428.
14. Schwitter J, Wacker CM, van Rossum AC, et al. MR-IMPACT: comparison of perfusion-cardiac magnetic resonance with single-photon emission computed tomography for the detection of coronary artery disease in a multicentre, multivendor, randomized trial. *Eur Heart J.* 2008;29:480-489.
15. Schwitter J, Wacker CM, Wilke N, et al. Superior diagnostic performance of perfusion-cardiovascular magnetic resonance versus SPECT to detect coronary artery disease: The secondary endpoints of the multicenter multivendor MR-IMPACT II (Magnetic Resonance Imaging for Myocardial Perfusion Assessment in Coronary Artery Disease Trial). *J Cardiovasc Magn Reson.* 2012;14:61.
16. Schwitter J, Wacker CM, Wilke N, et al. MR-IMPACT II: Magnetic Resonance Imaging for Myocardial Perfusion Assessment in Coronary artery disease Trial: perfusion-cardiac magnetic resonance vs. single-photon emission computed tomography for the detection of coronary artery disease: a comparative multicentre, multivendor trial. *Eur Heart J.* 2013;34:775-781.
17. Patel AR, Kramer CM. Role of cardiac magnetic resonance in the diagnosis and prognosis of nonischemic cardiomyopathy. *JACC Cardiovasc Imaging.* 2017;10:1180-1193.
18. Carsten R, Norbert MW, Michael J-H, et al. Utility of cardiac magnetic resonance imaging in the diagnosis of hypertrophic cardiomyopathy. *Circulation.* 2005;112:855-861.
19. Chan RH, Maron BJ, Olivotto I, et al. Prognostic value of quantitative contrast-enhanced cardiovascular magnetic resonance for the evaluation of sudden death risk in patients with hypertrophic cardiomyopathy. *Circulation.* 2014;130:484-495.
20. Gati S, Sharma S, Pennell D. The Role of cardiovascular magnetic resonance imaging in the assessment of highly trained athletes. *JACC Cardiovasc Imaging.* 2018;11:247-259.
21. Fontana M, Corovic A, Scully P, Moon JC. Myocardial amyloidosis: the exemplar interstitial disease. *JACC Cardiovasc Imaging.* 2019;12:2345-2356.
22. Birnie DH, Sauer WH, Bogun F, et al. HRS expert consensus statement on the diagnosis and management of arrhythmias associated with cardiac sarcoidosis. *Heart Rhythm.* 2014;11:1304-1323.
23. Patel MR, Cawley PJ, Heitner JF, et al. Detection of myocardial damage in patients with sarcoidosis. *Circulation.* 2009;120:1969-1977.
24. Coleman GC, Shaw PW, Balfour PC, et al. Prognostic value of myocardial scarring on CMR in patients with cardiac sarcoidosis. *JACC Cardiovasc Imaging.* 2017;10:411-420.
25. Deva DP, Hanneman K, Li Q, et al. Cardiovascular magnetic resonance demonstration of the spectrum of morphological phenotypes and patterns of myocardial scarring in Anderson-Fabry disease. *J Cardiovasc Magn Reson.* 2016;18:14.
26. Thompson RB, Chow K, Khan A, et al. T_1 mapping with cardiovascular MRI is highly sensitive for fabry disease independent of hypertrophy and sex. *Circ Cardiovasc Imaging.* 2013;6:637-645.
27. te Riele AS, Tandri H, Bluemke DA. Arrhythmogenic right ventricular cardiomyopathy (ARVC): cardiovascular magnetic resonance update. *J Cardiovasc Magn Reson.* 2014;16:50.
28. Jain A, Tandri H, Calkins H, Bluemke DA. Role of cardiovascular magnetic resonance imaging in arrhythmogenic right ventricular dysplasia. *J Cardiovasc Magn Reson.* 2008;10:32.
29. Kawel N, Nacif M, Arai AE, et al. Trabeculated (noncompacted) and compact myocardium in adults: the multi-ethnic study of atherosclerosis. *Circ Cardiovasc Imaging.* 2012;5:357-366.
30. Modell B, Khan M, Darlison M, Westwood MA, Ingram D, Pennell DJ. Improved survival of thalassaemia major in the UK and relation to T2* cardiovascular magnetic resonance. *J Cardiovasc Magn Reson.* 2008;10:42.

31. Bozkurt B, Colvin M, Cook J, et al. Current diagnostic and treatment strategies for specific dilated cardiomyopathies: a scientific statement from the American Heart Association. *Circulation.* 2016;134(23): e579-e646.
32. Ferreira VM, Schulz-Menger J, Holmvang G, et al. Cardiovascular magnetic resonance in nonischemic myocardial inflammation. *J Am Coll Cardiol.* 2018;72:3158-3176.
33. Aquaro GD, Ghebru Habtemicael Y, Camastra G, et al. Prognostic value of repeating cardiac magnetic resonance in patients with acute myocarditis. *J Am Coll Cardiol.* 2019;74:2439-2448.
34. Myerson SG, d'Arcy J, Mohiaddin R, et al. Aortic regurgitation quantification using cardiovascular magnetic resonance: association with clinical outcome. *Circulation.* 2012;126:1452-1460.
35. Uretsky S, Argulian E, Narula J, Wolff SD. Use of cardiac magnetic resonance imaging in assessing mitral regurgitation: current evidence. *J Am Coll Cardiol.* 2018;71:547-563.
36. Penicka M, Vecera J, Mirica DC, Kotrc M, Kockova R, Van Camp G. Prognostic implications of magnetic resonance-derived quantification in asymptomatic patients with organic mitral regurgitation: comparison with Doppler echocardiography-derived integrative approach. *Circulation.* 2018;137:1349-1360.
37. Mousavi N, Cheezum MK, Aghayev A, et al. Assessment of cardiac masses by cardiac magnetic resonance imaging: histological correlation and clinical outcomes. *J Am Heart Assoc.* 2019;8:e007829.
38. Babu-Narayan SV, Giannakoulas G, Valente AM, Li W, Gatzoulis MA. Imaging of congenital heart disease in adults. *Eur Heart J.* 2016;37:1182-1195.
39. Fratz S, Chung T, Greil GF, et al. Guidelines and protocols for cardiovascular magnetic resonance in children and adults with congenital heart disease: SCMR expert consensus group on congenital heart disease. *J Cardiovasc Magn Reson.* 2013;15:51.
40. Geva T, Mulder B, Gauvreau K, et al. Preoperative predictors of death and sustained ventricular tachycardia after pulmonary valve replacement in patients with repaired tetralogy of fallot enrolled in the INDICATOR Cohort. *Circulation.* 2018;138:2106-2115.
41. Bokma JP, de Wilde KC, Vliegen HW, et al. Value of cardiovascular magnetic resonance imaging in noninvasive risk stratification in tetralogy of fallot. *JAMA Cardiol.* 2017;2:678-683.
42. Salerno M, Sharif B, Arheden H, et al. Recent advances in cardiovascular magnetic resonance: techniques and applications. *Circ Cardiovasc Imaging.* 2017;10:e003951.

CHAPTER 38

HYBRID AND MULTIMODALITY IMAGING

Albert J. Sinusas

INTRODUCTION

Multimodality imaging is routinely used to facilitate the diagnosis and evaluation of cardiovascular diseases, along with risk stratification, and directing and monitoring therapy. Hybrid imaging permits the integrated assessment of structure and physiologic indices. There is now a focus on developing multimodality imaging strategies to assess the underlying cellular and molecular processes that underlie and/or participate in modulating the structural and pathophysiologic changes in the cardiovascular system. Thus, the future of multimodality imaging involves the simultaneous evaluation of structure, physiology, and molecular processes.

With the critical advancement in hybrid imaging technology, a parallel development of imaging probes for improved evaluation of these physiologic and molecular changes has occurred. The most widely used approaches for molecular imaging include radiotracers that allow for high sensitivity in vivo detection and quantification of molecular processes with single-photon emission computed tomography (SPECT) and positron emission tomography (PET).[1] Although SPECT and PET imaging provide high sensitivity for detection and quantitative assessment of molecular and physiologic processes, they suffer from limited resolution. Therefore, these radiotracer-based imaging approaches have been integrated with high-resolution anatomic imaging approaches such as x-ray computed tomography (CT) or magnetic resonance imaging (MRI) to provide anatomic co-localization and improved quantification.

Multimodality imaging can also be used to guide interventional and surgical procedures. The integration of three-dimensional (3D) imaging with cone beam tomography and real-time fluoroscopy is now part of clinical practice.

This chapter reviews the development of hybrid imaging technology for evaluation of critical physiologic and molecular processes in the cardiovascular system, including inflammation, cell death, autonomic regulation, angiogenesis, and myocardial vascular remodeling. The evolving practice of image-guided interventions is also addressed. These advancements in multimodality imaging technology should lead to improved image quantification and diagnostic accuracy, thereby promoting "precision medicine," and a more personalized approach to health care delivery.

FUNDAMENTALS OF HYBRID IMAGING

Technologic Advantage

The primary aim of multimodality hybrid imaging is to take advantage of the different physical properties of image formation from each modality to create an image set with complementary (or even synergistic) information, to produce a superior image set for research purposes, clinical applications, or a combination of both. A hybrid imaging methodology might simply improve quantification of a targeted molecular probe or imaging approach or provide anatomic localization, as would be the case for hybrid SPECT/CT, PET/CT or PET/MRI. Hybrid imaging technology may also provide new insight into a molecular pathway or pathophysiologic process or provide a link between molecular processes and associated anatomic or physiologic events. Clinical application of a hybrid imaging technology may result in improved diagnostic accuracy, improved prognostication, or monitoring a disease process or therapeutic intervention.

Therefore, the advantage of any multimodality imaging approaches is dependent on acquiring information that is more valuable than that from individual components, or even the composite sum of the components. Ideally, one should obtain unique information that can only be derived using a truly integrated hybrid technology, as opposed to acquiring images on two separate imaging systems and fusing the datasets following acquisition.

IMAGING MODALITIES AND PROCEDURES

There are many multimodality and hybrid imaging technologies currently under development for the evaluation of the cardiovascular system. This chapter cannot address all of these modalities; however, a recently published textbook that provides a very comprehensive review of hybrid imaging in cardiovascular medicine is available.[2] This chapter focuses on the most clinically relevant modalities, along with those that have translated to routine clinical application.

Single-Photon Emission Computed Tomography/ Computed Tomography

The use of hybrid SPECT/CT scanners allows the patient to be imaged on the same equipment table in the exact same position, which minimizes changes in the patient orientation between the CT and SPECT images. Thus, hybrid SPECT/CT imaging systems automatically co-register the two sets of image data, which facilitates the use of CT for SPECT attenuation correction. The CT component may be a slow-rotating nondiagnostic scanner or a fast-rotating multidetector diagnostic scanner. The slow-rotation systems generally mount the CT x-ray tube and detector on the same gantry as the SPECT detectors. Although the CT images are suboptimal for diagnostic purposes, they provide sufficient image quality for attenuation correction.[3] The hybrid SPECT/CT systems that incorporate a fast-rotating multidetector CT scanner use separate gantries for SPECT and CT imaging. Decoupling the SPECT and CT gantries allows for rapid-rotation and diagnostic CT imaging. Hybrid SPECT/CT systems have incorporated as many as 64-slice detectors. These more expensive, fast-rotation systems are capable of diagnostic CT imaging for either calcium scoring or CT angiography. However, the fast-rotation speed of the CT compared to the SPECT acquisition can result in image mismatch because of respiratory motion and introduce additional artifacts in the attenuation correction scans when performing cardiac SPECT/CT imaging. Reconstruction artifacts may also be introduced because of metal implants, or truncation of the attenuation CT scans.

Although a high-quality CT introduces some complications, these high-end hybrid systems provide valuable complementary information that improves risk stratification of patients undergoing stress perfusion imaging.[4-6] The fusion of anatomic information from CT and physiologic information from SPECT can better identify hemodynamically significant stenoses, and physiologically guided intervention may be beneficial.[7] The use of hybrid SPECT/CT imaging may be particularly helpful in the setting of complex congenital heart disease, or in the evaluation of anomalous coronary arteries. **Figure 38.1** illustrates the value of hybrid SPECT/CT imaging in evaluation of the physiologic significance of an anomalous right coronary artery that originates from the ostium of the left main coronary artery.

Other novel clinical applications of hybrid SPECT/CT include the noninvasive diagnosis of transthyretin cardiac amyloidosis (**Figure 38.2**) and the evaluation of peripheral arterial disease (**Figure 38.3**). In both clinical conditions, the registered anatomic information from CT is used to improve localization and quantification of SPECT radiotracer uptake.

Positron Emission Tomography/Computed Tomography

Hybrid imaging has become the convention for cardiac PET imaging, and hybrid PET/CT systems are generally equipped with diagnostic CT scanners. The use of CT images for attenuation correction of PET images offers the same advantages and limitations associated with hybrid SPECT/CT. Some hybrid PET/CT scanners are even capable of dual-energy CT imaging, which offers some unique advantages related to correction for beam hardening and metal artifacts, and material decomposition. Higher resolution CT scanners (64-slice and above) and hybrid imaging with PET and contrast CT imaging can provide a detailed anatomic assessment of the cardiovascular system complemented by either functional or metabolic information provided by PET, particularly if the CT images are acquired with iodinated contrast. Contrast CT images provide definition of the endocardial and epicardial surfaces of the heart, allowing for partial volume correction of the PET images and more accurate estimation of tissue activity and quantification of myocardial blood flow.

Coronary computed tomography angiography (CCTA) can characterize the epicardial coronary vessels and provide

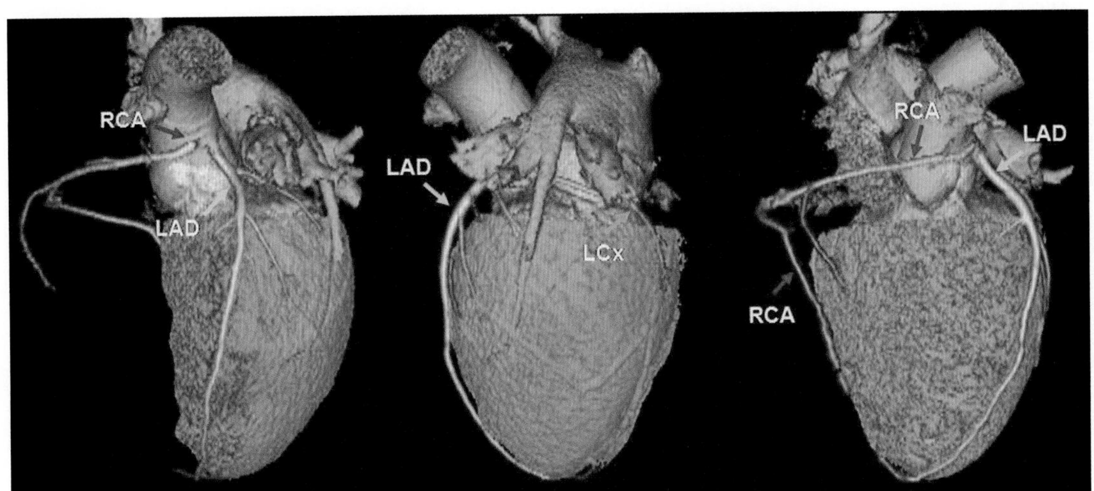

FIGURE 38.1 Hybrid exercise single-photon emission computed tomography/computed tomography (SPECT/CT) imaging. Images from a 10-year-old male who presented with chest pain and dyspnea with exertion and was found to have an anomalous RCA from left main without an intramural course. Hybrid exercise SPECT/CT imaging performed after injection of ^{99m}Tc-tetrofosmin (4.2 mCi) at peak exercise using a high-sensitivity cadmium-zinc-telluride (CZT) SPECT 64-slice CT scanner demonstrates normal myocardial perfusion. Multidetector 64-slice CT angiography did not demonstrate any significant stenosis. LAD, left anterior descending; LCx, left circumflex coronary artery; RCA, right coronary artery.

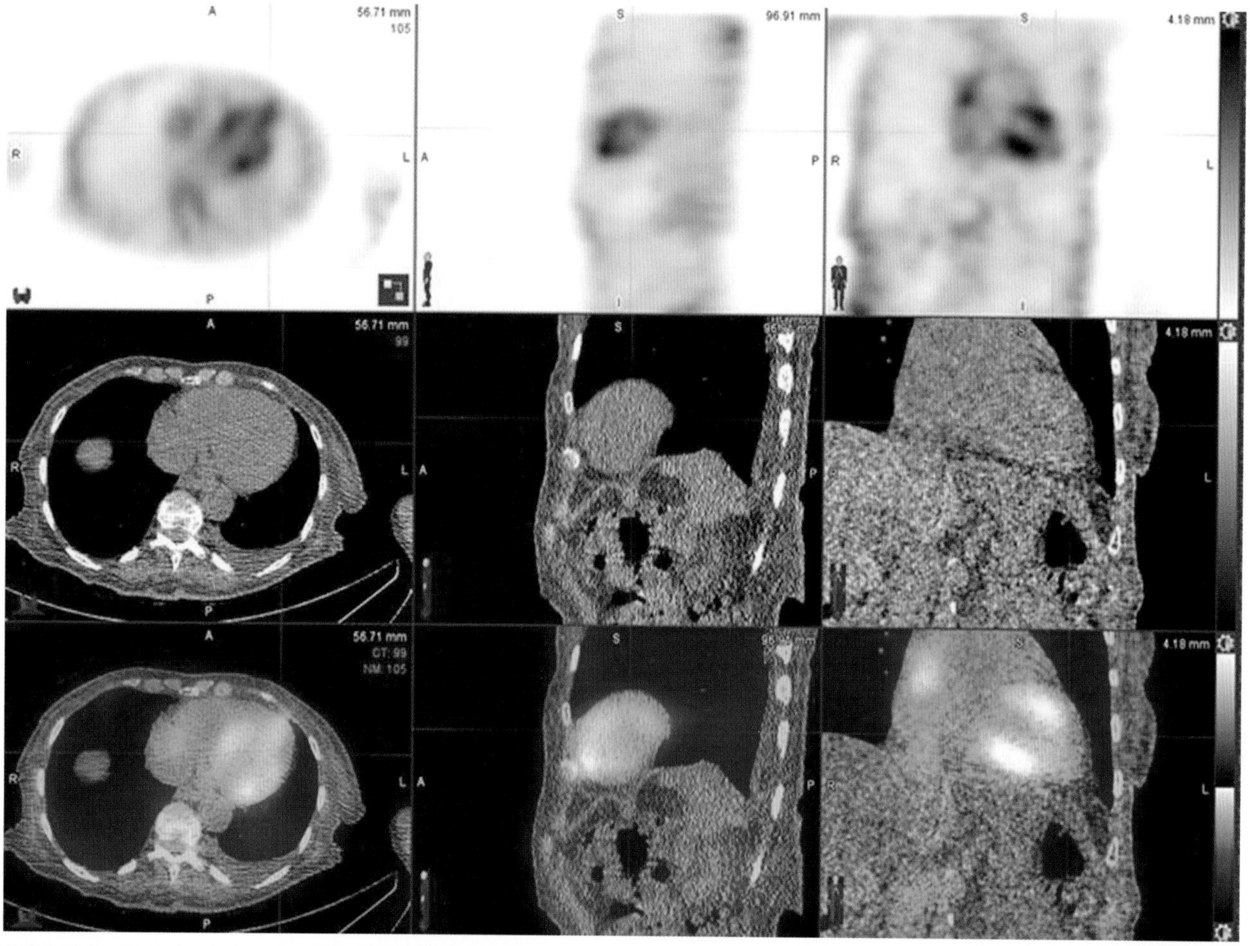

FIGURE 38.2 Digital cadmium-zinc-telluride (CZT) single-photon emission computed tomography/computed tomography (SPECT/CT) for the noninvasive diagnosis of transthyretin cardiac amyloidosis. Standard planar imaging and assessment of heart to contralateral (H/CL) uptake ratios may be confounded by blood pool activity potentially reducing the diagnostic accuracy of planar imaging. Hybrid SPECT/CT imaging with 360 degree acquisition provided better delineation of myocardial activity from the left ventricular cavity blood pool activity. (From Wojtylak P, Avril N, Kardan A. Feasibility and initial experience in the utilization of a fully digital CZT SPECT/CT system for the diagnosis of transthyretin cardiac amyloidosis (ATTR). *J Nucl Med.* 2020;61(supplement 1):3040. Reprinted with permission from Arash Kardan, MD.)

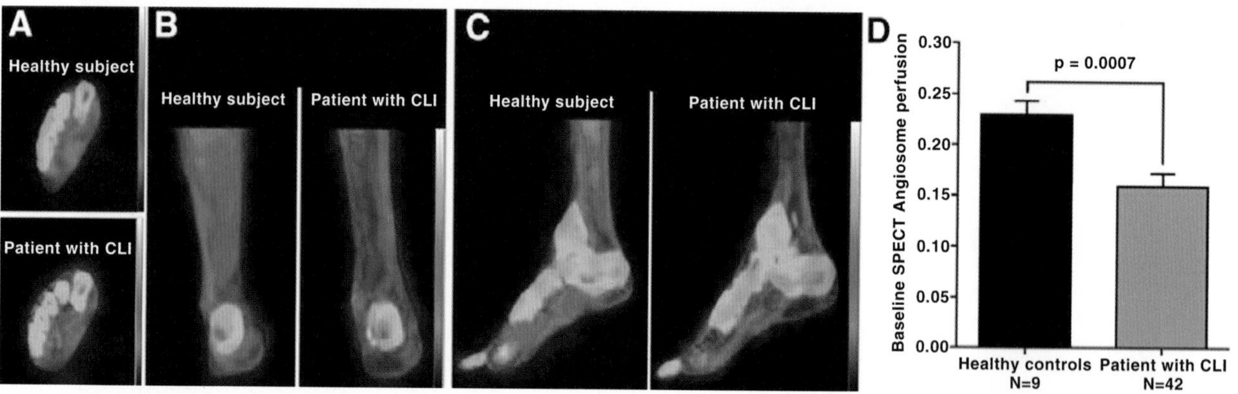

FIGURE 38.3 **(A-D):** Resting single-photon emission computed tomography/computed tomography (SPECT/CT) perfusion imaging in a healthy subject and patient with critical limb ischemia (CLI). Axial **(A)**, coronal **(B)**, and sagittal **(C)** views of ^{99m}Tc-tetrofosmin SPECT/CT images demonstrate visual differences in foot perfusion under resting conditions. **(D)** Quantitative image analysis reveals significant differences in resting foot perfusion (standardized uptake values) between healthy subjects and patients with CLI. (Reprinted with permission from Alvelo JL, Papademetris X, Mena-Hurtado C, et al. Radiotracer imaging allows for noninvasive detection and quantification of abnormalities in angiosome foot perfusion in diabetic patients with critical limb ischemia and nonhealing wounds. *Circ Cardiovasc Imaging.* 2018;11(5):e006932.)

information on the degree of stenosis within the vessel, as well as atherosclerotic plaque extent and morphology.[8] Investigators have developed algorithms that provide automated analysis of plaque features.[9,10] Although CCTA has excellent negative predictive value for ruling out obstructive disease, it tends to overestimate the severity of the stenosis.[11] Therefore, the combination of anatomic information from computed tomography angiography (CTA) and the physiologic information from PET can provide a more comprehensive assessment of coronary artery disease. Alternatively, the functional significance of a coronary stenosis detected by CCTA can be estimated with computational fluid dynamics and determination of the fractional flow reserve (FFR). The accuracy of the combined assessment with both modalities is better than with standalone PET or CCTA in several observational studies.[12-14] This improved accuracy is due to improved specificity, with either normal perfusion in the territory of a stenosis thought to be obstructive on CCTA, or normal coronary anatomy in an area thought to demonstrate abnormal perfusion. **Figure 38.4** provides an example of how hybrid PET/CT imaging can guide management in a patient with complex congenital heart disease. There is also evidence that hybrid PET-CCTA imaging can reduce referral for unnecessary downstream coronary angiography.[15] Although the evaluation of both anatomy and function with hybrid PET/CT can increase overall diagnostic accuracy, PET-CCTA is associated with both greater cost and increased radiation exposure to the patient.

Hybrid Positron Emission Tomography/Magnetic Resonance and Single-Photon Emission Computed Tomography/Magnetic Resonance Imaging

For PET/MR imaging, PET images are acquired either simultaneously or sequentially to magnetic resonance (MR) images using hybrid-scanner infrastructure. Although PET/MRI systems have been available for many years, the high cost of this hybrid technology has limited utilization to a small number of early adopters. Hybrid PET/MRI may be ideally suited for evaluation of cardiomyopathic conditions such as cardiac sarcoidosis[16] or amyloidosis,[17] or comprehensive evaluation of atherosclerosis of the coronary arteries[18] or peripheral vasculature.[19] **Figure 38.5** provides several clinical examples of hybrid PET/MR images in patients with cardiac sarcoidosis, and the relationship between MR late enhancement and PET fluorodeoxyglucose (FDG) uptake in the myocardium. The wide range of cardiovascular applications of PET/MRI was recently reviewed.[20]

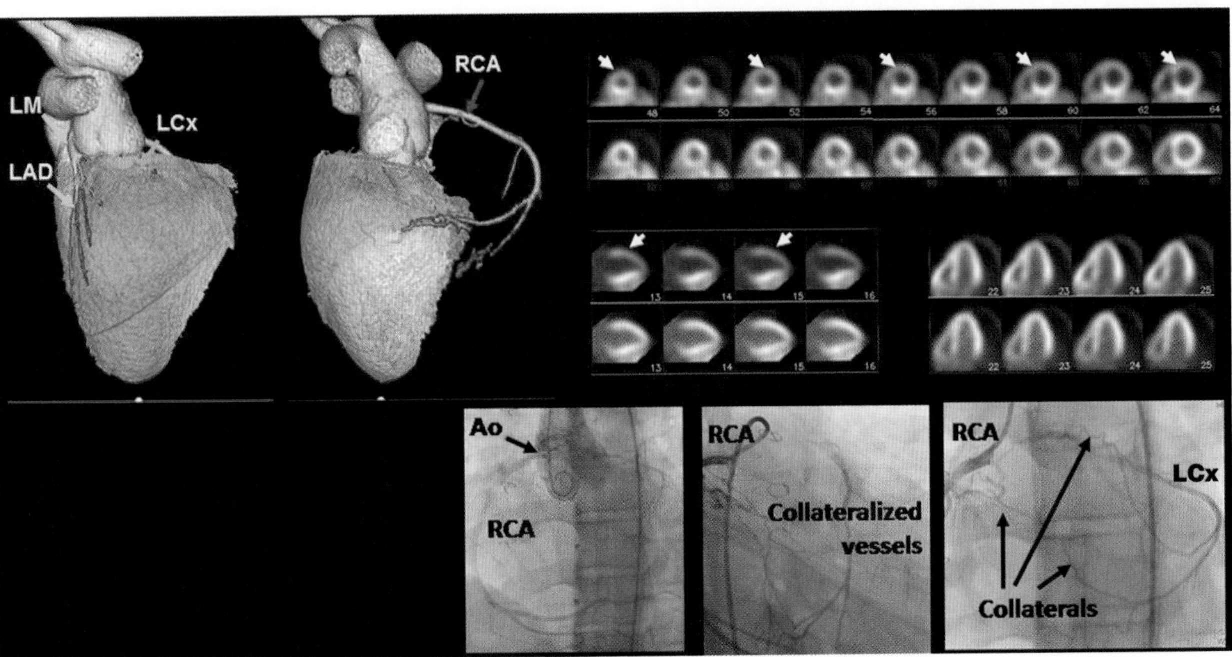

FIGURE 38.4 Hybrid ^{82}rubidium (Rb) positron emission tomography/computed tomography (PET/CT) imaging. An 18-year-old male athlete with D-transposition, s/p atrial switch operation with coronary reimplantation underwent stress testing with electrocardiographic ST depression at peak exercise without chest pain. Echocardiography demonstrated normal left ventricular (LV) function (LV ejection fraction 57%). Hybrid ^{82}Rb PET/CT imaging during regadenoson vasodilator stress demonstrated severe anteroseptal and lateral ischemia on fused images (upper left, purple area) and reconstructed PET slices (upper right, white arrows), impaired coronary flow reserve (CFR) in the left circumflex and coronary steal in the left anterior descending (LAD) territory. A coronary angiogram demonstrated near occlusion of the left main coronary ostium, with right to left collaterals (lower right). Patient underwent coronary bypass grafting with internal mammary graft to the LAD. Follow up exercise/rest ^{99m}Tc-tetrofosmin SPECT/CT imaging at workload of 17 metabolic equivalents (METs) was normal, although the patient developed 1 mm ST depression without chest pain. Ao, aorta; LCx, left circumflex coronary artery; LM, left main; RCA, right coronary artery.

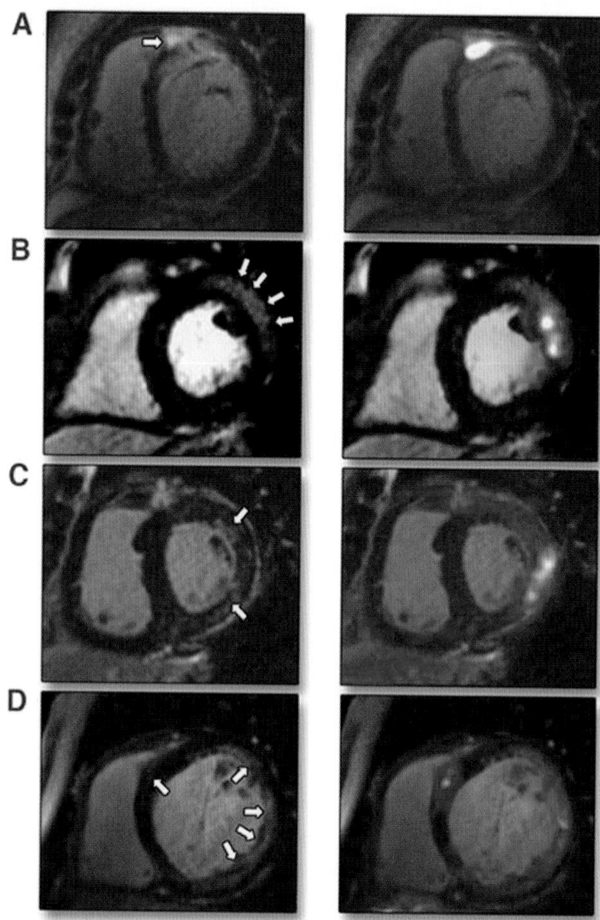

FIGURE 38.5 Hybrid positron emission tomography/magnetic resonance (PET/MR) imaging in cardiac sarcoidosis. Late gadolinium enhancement (LGE) cardiac MR images (left panels) with hybrid 18F-fluorodeoxyglucose (FDG) CMR/PET images (right panels). **(A)** Subepicardial (near transmural) LGE in the basal anteroseptum extending into the right ventricular free wall with increased FDG uptake localizing to the same region on fused CMR/PET. **(B)** Subepicardial LGE in the basal anterolateral wall with increased FDG uptake co-localizing to that region on CMR/PET. **(C)** Patchy midwall LGE in the anterolateral wall with matched increased FDG uptake on CMR/PET. **(D)** Multifocal LGE in the lateral wall with matched increased FDG uptake on CMR/PET. (Reprinted from Dweck MR, Abgral R, Trivieri MG, et al. Hybrid Magnetic Resonance Imaging and Positron Emission Tomography with fluorodeoxyglucose to diagnose active cardiac sarcoidosis. *JACC Cardiovasc Imaging.* 2018;11(1):94-107. Copyright © 2018 by the American College of Cardiology Foundation. With permission.)

The true advantage of performing PET and MRI on a hybrid imaging system versus registering PET/CT images with MR images acquired on separate, more conventional imaging systems needs to be considered, because registration and fusion of independently acquired images may be more clinically efficient and cost-effective.[21] The CT images from a hybrid PET/CT can facilitate accurate registering of separately acquired PET and MR images. In addition, the most commonly utilized PET radiotracer for myocardial perfusion imaging is rubidium-82;

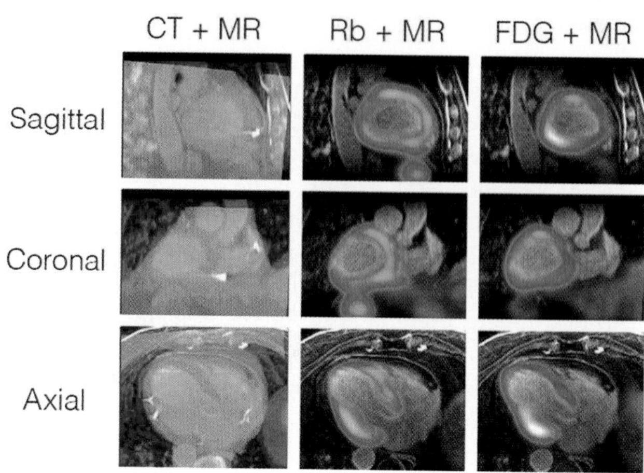

FIGURE 38.6 Positron emission tomography/computed tomography (PET/CT) and magnetic resonance (MR) image fusion. Separately acquired cardiac PET/CT and MR images were fused in a patient with cardiac sarcoidosis. CT images from a hybrid PET-CT scanner were used to fuse the PET images (color) with MR images (black and white). Shown are fused CT and CMR images (left), fused ^{82}rubidium (Rb) perfusion PET and MR (middle), and fused cardiac ^{18}fluorodeoxyglucose PET and MR (right) studies. (From Quail MA, Sinusas AJ. PET-CMR in heart failure - synergistic or redundant imaging? *Heart Fail Rev.* 2017;22(4):477-489. Image fusion and figure provided courtesy of Mary Germino. http://creativecommons.org/licenses/by/4.0/.)

and rubidium generators are not MR compatible. **Figure 38.6** provides a clinical example of the registration of separately acquired rubidium-82 and FDG PET/CT and MR images in a patient with cardiac sarcoidosis, which illustrates how one might overcome the limitation associated with bringing a rubidium generator in the magnet using image fusion.

Attenuation correction of PET images on a hybrid PET/MR scanner requires novel correction schemes, because linear attenuation corrections cannot be directly derived from MR images. The commonly used Dixon approach uses MR images to classify tissues into categories such as air, fat, and muscle to estimate attenuation coefficients of gamma emissions.[22] Other approaches use machine learning to derive attenuation correction from MR images based on libraries of paired MR and CT data sets.[23] The simultaneous acquisition of PET and MR may offer some unique advantages for partial volume correction of PET images, leading to improve absolute quantification of radiotracer uptake in the heart with incorporation of both cardiac or respiratory motion correction,[24] or improved diagnostic categorization of patients according to differential patterns of fused PET-CMR images, as in the case of evaluation of cardiac sarcoidosis or amyloidosis.[21]

Carminati et al recently reported the development of the first stationary and compact MR-compatible SPECT system for clinical application that employs thallium-activated cesium iodide (CsI(Tl)) detectors interfaced with silicon photomultipliers.[25] This hybrid SPECT/MR system facilitates simultaneous multi-isotope assessment of quantitative flow and molecular markers using readily available SPECT radiotracers.

X-ray Fluoroscopy and Computed Tomography

Current digital fluoroscopic C-arms use flat-panel x-ray detectors to generate CT-like images from rotational angiographic acquisitions. The 3D images can then be superimposed on real-time contrast fluoroscopy to help guide complex endovascular and peripheral vascular interventional procedures.[26] This 3D image–guided approach helps lower the volume of contrast and radiation exposure by reducing use of fluoroscopy and improving procedural efficiencies.[26] However, these rotational acquisitions are generally not electrocardiographic or respiratory gated; and therefore somewhat limited for cardiac applications because of the 5- to10-second acquisition times that are required to obtain the necessary 180 degree projection images. In spite of these limitations, the use of intraprocedural angiographic CT has been effectively utilized in the field of electrophysiology, especially for the guidance of atrial fibrillation ablation.[27,28]

In our laboratory, we have used commercially available software to register the segmented coronary artery tree from a prospectively acquired contrast CCTA obtained on a 64-slice CT scanner with a cone beam CT acquisition to help guide intracoronary interventions (see **Figure 38.7**) and intramyocardial delivery of theranostic iodinated hydrogels under real-time fluoroscopic guidance. Other investigators have used cone beam CT angiographic imaging to guide balloon pulmonary angioplasty and demonstrated improved safety.[29]

X-ray Fluoroscopy and Echocardiography

The 2D nature of x-ray fluoroscopy complicates the ability to reliably navigate the use and deployment of interventional devices to the optimal location under x-ray guidance alone.[30] This limitation can increase radiation exposure. To improve image guidance with fluoroscopy, other imaging modalities are often used in conjunction, including CT, MRI, and echocardiography. Echocardiography offers unique advantages in that this modality provides real-time images with both high spatial and temporal resolution. The disadvantage of echocardiography relates to the limited field of view (FOV) and variable orientation relative to the patient or organ under evaluation. There is always a trade-off between FOV and the achievable frame rate.

Cardiac ultrasound images can be acquired using transthoracic, transesophageal, or intracardiac probes. The use of transthoracic echocardiography is generally considered impractical for use in the interventional laboratory. The use of the other modalities requires registration of the echocardiographic and x-ray images. This can be accomplished by physically sensing the location and orientation of the probe or by visualizing its orientation based on the x-ray intensity profile of the probe.[30] This approach is commonly used for larger transesophageal probes. Alternatively, the probe can be tracked by fiducial markers attached to the probe, an approach more commonly used with intracardiac echocardiography.

A common application of hybrid x-ray fluoroscopy and echocardiography is guidance of placement of percutaneous aortic valves.[31] Fusion of x-ray fluoroscopy and echocardiography has also proved highly valuable for guiding electrophysiologic procedures involving atrial transeptal puncture and left atrial ablation or left atrial appendage occlusion procedures.[32] The fusion of these imaging modalities is also critical for management of acquired valvular disease and congenital heart disease,[33,34] such as placement of a mitral clip for management of mitral regurgitation and guiding closure of interatrial septal defects. Either contours of cardiac structures derived from echocardiography or real-time 3D echocardiographic images can be fused with fluoroscopic images to guide these interventional procedures (**Figure 38.8A-D**).

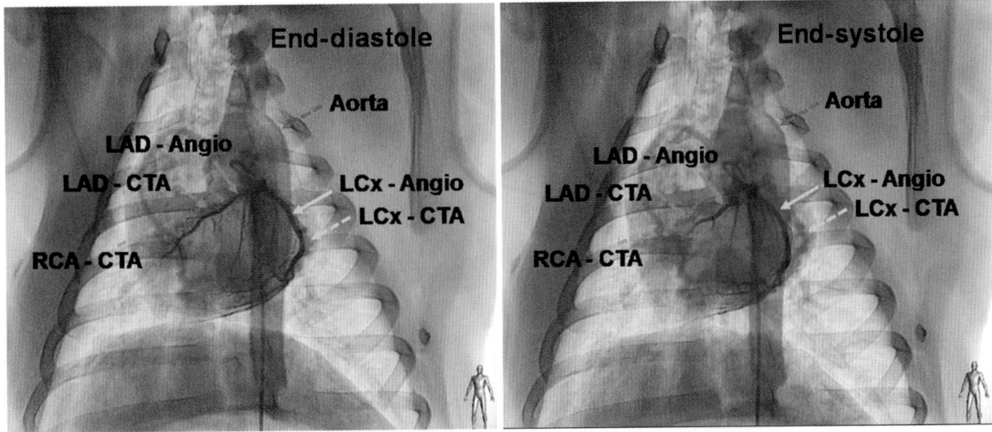

FIGURE 38.7 Fusion of contrast fluoroscopic angiography with multislice contrast coronary computed tomography angiography (CCTA). A prospective contrast CCTA was obtained using a 64-slice computed tomography (CT) scanner with the coronary anatomy frozen at end-diastole. The coronary anatomy and aorta were rendered in three-dimension (3D) and color coded (orange) and the multislice CT registered with a cone beam CT image acquired on a digital c-arm. This allowed registration of the real-time contrast angiography with the 3D CT. Images are shown at end-diastole (left) and end-systole (right). Notice that at end-diastole the coronary angiogram is superimposed on the outline of the coronary anatomy from the CT angiography. At end-systole, this registration is lost because of cardiac motion over the cardiac cycle. LAD, left anterior descending, RCA, right coronary artery, LCx, left circumflex coronary artery.

SECTION 2

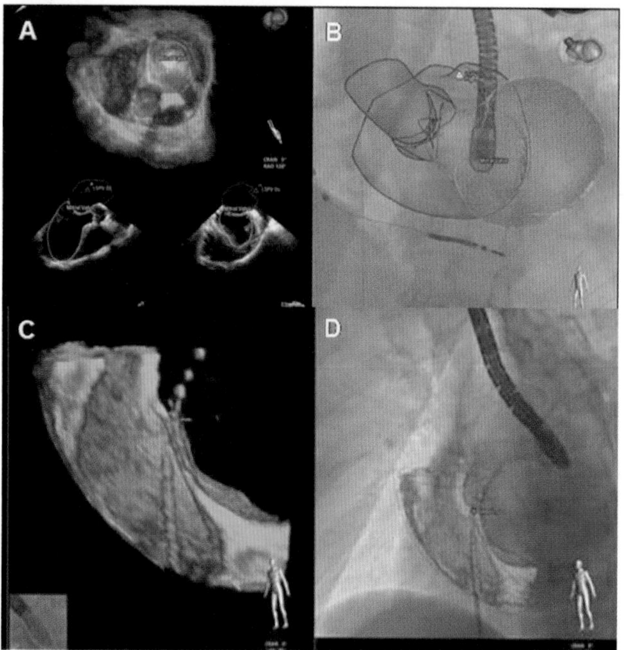

FIGURE 38.8 (A-D): Fusion of x-ray and three-dimensional (3D) transesophageal echocardiographic images using commercial software. (**A**). 3D and two-dimensional (2D) echocardiographic images are shown of aortic valve and chambers. (**B**). Contours from the 3D echocardiogram are superimposed on real-time fluoroscopic image. (**C**). 3D echocardiographic image demonstrating catheter puncturing intra-atrial septum. (**D**). Superimposition of 3D echocardiogram on fluoroscopic image.

HYBRID IMAGING PROBES

The advancement and application of hybrid imaging will require the parallel development of hybrid multimodality imaging probes.[35,36] The development of these multimodality probes offers advantages for validation of new molecularly targeted probes and hybrid imaging technologies, and may also provide complementary and unique information. The ability to track different processes in parallel offers a unique advantage, because biologic processes often are complex and involve the interaction of multiple signaling pathways and physiologic changes. Multimodality imaging probes provide a powerful mechanism to enhance the assessment of critical pathophysiologic processes and therapies by taking advantage of the individual strengths of probes for each modality. The visualization and co-localization of multiple molecular targets and the evaluation of molecular and physiologic biomarkers with structural changes, are essential to understanding complex disease processes at the molecular level and may lead to the development and evaluation of novel therapeutics. The development of these hybrid probes in combination with hybrid imaging technology has facilitated the emergence of theranostics, representing the merging of a diagnostic probe with a targeted therapeutic.

Multi-Isotope Single-Photon Emission Computed Tomography and Positron Emission Tomography Imaging

Using isotopes with gamma emissions of different energies, SPECT imaging offers (1) the unique opportunity to evaluate multiple molecularly targeted probes at the same time or (2) simultaneous imaging of targeted molecular probes and radiolabeled probes evaluating a physiologic marker. A classic example is the combined evaluation of myocardial hypoxia, angiogenesis, and tissue perfusion.[37,38] PET imaging with multiple isotopes requires use of serial imaging with radiotracer using short-lived radiotracers such as fluorine-18 (2 hours), carbon-11 (20 minutes), rubidium-82 (72 seconds), or oxygen-15 water (90 seconds).

LIMITATIONS OF HYBRID TECHNOLOGY

Combining technologies in a single hybrid device can potentially reduce the efficacy of any one technology. In the example of PET-CMR imaging, the addition of an MR magnet in the PET imaging space may limit subject eligibility for PET scanning, increase operational costs, prevent the use of generator-produced PET radioisotopes (eg, rubidium-82) within the imaging room, and complicate attenuation correction of PET scans.[21] However, recent advancements in PET and MR hardware and reconstruction software have improved efficiency of image acquisition, which may improve patient throughput. In addition, F-18–labeled PET perfusion imaging agents are on the horizon, and novel deep learning solutions have been developed for the derivation of reliable attenuation maps from MRI for application to PET images.

Introduction of new hybrid systems may lead to anxiety, confusion, and the inefficient deployment of new resources. Culture lag is considered an important aspect of social change and evolves as a result of invention, discovery, and dispersion.[39] Delays in developing the appropriate knowledge and skills needed to optimally implement a technology may impact on the efficient use of new hybrid imaging resources within the research or health care environment.

The implementation of any new hybrid technology may require the emergence of new professional identity and intercollegiate interactions. The advancement of a new hybrid technology may necessitate the establishment of new professional training pathways, and creation of professional society guidelines for training and appropriate utilization, or even creation of new professional organizations or societies. This could result in changes in certification policy and professional licensing. New technology can also require and result in changes in state or federal policy, because the shift in technology may have relevance to regulatory or licensing authorities.[40]

RESEARCH AND FUTURE DIRECTIONS

The future of hybrid imaging technology rests on the ability to achieve synergistic imaging, where nonredundant data is combined to produce information greater than the sum of the parts. Hybrid imaging will likely lead to more efficient use of imaging resources and could reduce overall health care costs by improving diagnostic accuracy and improving efficiencies in the delivery of advanced therapeutics and personalized medicine. One future goal would be to bring molecular and/or physiologic images and co-registered anatomic images generated on a hybrid imaging system into the anatomic space of a cardiovascular interventional suite or hybrid operating room to direct therapies using image guidance. Therefore, hybrid imaging will become particularly critical as the percutaneous delivery of devices and theranostics becomes more prevalent in clinical practice.

KEY POINTS

- ✔ The future of multimodality and hybrid imaging involves the simultaneous evaluation of structure, physiology, and molecular processes.
- ✔ Hybrid SPECT/CT imaging may be particularly helpful in the setting of complex congenital heart disease and in the evaluation of anomalous coronary arteries.
- ✔ The combination of anatomic information from CCTA and the physiologic information from PET can provide a more comprehensive assessment of coronary artery disease.
- ✔ Hybrid PET/MR imaging may be ideally suited for evaluation of cardiomyopathic conditions such as cardiac sarcoidosis or amyloidosis and comprehensive evaluation of atherosclerosis of the coronary arteries or peripheral vasculature.
- ✔ Hybrid x-ray fluoroscopy and echocardiography can be valuable for guidance of electrophysiologic procedures and treatment of structural heart disease.
- ✔ The advancement and application of hybrid imaging requires the parallel development of hybrid multimodality imaging probes.
- ✔ Hybrid imaging provides efficient use of imaging resources and may reduce overall health care costs by improving diagnostic accuracy and delivery of advanced therapeutics and personalized medicine.

REFERENCES

1. Boutagy NE, Feher A, Alkhalil I, Umoh N, Sinusas AJ. Molecular imaging of the heart. *Compr Physiol.* 2019;9(2):477-533.
2. Liu Y-H, Sinusas AJ. *Hybrid Imaging in Cardiovascular Medicine.* Imaging in Medical Diagnosis and Therapy (Book Series). In: Karellas A, Thomadsen B, eds. CRC Press, Taylor and Francis Group; 2018.
3. Wells R, Soueidan K, Vanderwerf K, Ruddy TD. Comparing slow-versus high-speed CT for attenuation correction of cardiac SPECT perfusion studies. *J Nucl Cardiol.* 2012;19:719-726.
4. Ghadri J, Fiechter M, Veraguth K, et al. Coronary calcium score as an adjunct to nuclear myocardial perfusion imaging for risk stratification before noncardiac surgery. *J Nucl Med.* 2012;53:1081-1086.
5. Kirisli H, Gupta V, Shahzad R, et al. Additional diagnostic value of integrated analysis of cardiac CTA and SPECT MPI using the SMARTVis system in patients with suspected coronary artery disease. *J Nucl Med.* 2014;55:50-57.
6. Mouden M, Ottervanger JP, Timmer JR, et al. The influence of coronary calcium score on the interpretation of myocardial perfusion imaging. *J Nucl Cardiol.* 2014;21:368-374.
7. De Bruyne B, Pijls HNJ, Kalesan B, et al. Fractional flow reserve-guided PCI versus medical therapy in stable coronary disease, FAME 2. *N Engl J Med.* 2012;367:991-1001.
8. Motoyama S, Ito H, Sarai M, et al. Plaque characterization by coronary computed tomography angiography and the likelihood of acute coronary events in mid-term follow-up. *J Am Coll Cardiol.* 2015;66(4):337-346.
9. Dey D, Schepis T, Marwan M, Slomka PJ, Berman DS, Achenbach S. Automated three-dimensional quantification of noncalcified coronary plaque from coronary CT angiography: comparison with intravascular US. *Radiology.* 2010;257(2):516-522.
10. Kolossvary M, Karády J, Szilveszter B, et al. Radiomic features are superior to conventional quantitative computed tomographic metrics to identify coronary plaques with napkin-ring sign. *Circ Cardiovasc Imaging.* 2017;10(12):e006843.
11. Xu R, Li C, Qian J, Ge J. Computed tomography-derived fractional flow reserve in the detection of lesion-specific ischemia: an integrated analysis of 3 pivotal trials. *Medicine.* 2015;94(46):e1963.
12. Danad I, Raijmakers PG, Appelman YE, et al. Hybrid imaging using quantitative H215O PET and CT-based coronary angiography for the detection of coronary artery disease. *J Nucl Med.* 2013;54(1):55-63.
13. Groves AM, Speechly-Dick M-E, Kayani I, et al. First experience of combined cardiac PET/64-detector CT angiography with invasive angiographic validation. *Eur J Nucl Med Mol Imaging.* 2009;36(12):2027-2033.
14. Kajander S, Joutsiniemi E, Saraste M, et al. Cardiac positron emission tomography/computed tomography imaging accurately detects anatomically and functionally significant coronary artery disease. *Circulation.* 2010;122(6):603-613.
15. Danad I, Raijmakers PG, Harms HJ, et al. Effect of cardiac hybrid (1)(5)O-water PET/CT imaging on downstream referral for invasive coronary angiography and revascularization rate. *Eur Heart J Cardiovasc Imaging.* 2014;15(2):170-179.
16. Ohira H, Tsujino I, Ishimaru S, et al. Myocardial imaging with 18F-fluoro-2-deoxyglucose positron emission tomography and magnetic resonance imaging in sarcoidosis. *Eur J Nucl Med Mol Imaging.* 2008;35(5):933-941.
17. Trivieri MG, Dweck MR, Abgral R, et al. 18F-sodium fluoride PET/MR for the assessment of cardiac amyloidosis. *J Am Coll Cardiol.* 2016;68(24):2712-2714.
18. Robson PM, Dweck MR, Trivieri MG, et al. Coronary artery PET/MR imaging: feasibility, limitations, and solutions. *JACC Cardiovasc Imaging.* 2017;10(10 Pt A):1103-1112.
19. Bini J, Eldib M, Robson PM, Calcagno C, Fayad ZA. Simultaneous carotid PET/MR: feasibility and improvement of magnetic resonance-based attenuation correction. *Int J Cardiovasc Imaging.* 2016;32(1):61-71.
20. Rischpler C, Nekolla SG, Heusch G, et al. Cardiac PET/MRI-an update. *Eur J Hybrid Imaging.* 2019;3:1-17.
21. Quail MA, Sinusas AJ. PET-CMR in heart failure—synergistic or redundant imaging? *Heart Fail Rev.* 2017;22(4):477-489.
22. Martinez-Moller A, Souvatzoglou M, Delso G, et al. Tissue classification as a potential approach for attenuation correction in whole-body PET/MRI: evaluation with PET/CT data. *J Nucl Med.* 2009;50(4):520-526.
23. Burgos N, Cardoso MJ, Thielemans K, et al. Multi-contrast attenuation map synthesis for PET/MR scanners: assessment on FDG and florbetapir PET tracers. *Eur J Nucl Med Mol Imaging.* 2015;42(9):1447-1458.
24. Petibon Y, Guehl NJ, Reese TG, et al. Impact of motion and partial volume effects correction on PET myocardial perfusion imaging using simultaneous PET-MR. *Phys Med Biol.* 2017;62(2):326-343.
25. Carminati M, D'Adda I, Morahan AJ, et al. Clinical SiPM-based MRI-compatible SPECT: preliminary characterization. *IEEE Trans Radiat Plasma Med Sci.* 2020;4:371-377.
26. Stangenberg L, Shuja F, Carelsen B, Elenbaas T, Wyers MC, Schermerhorn ML. A novel tool for three-dimensional road mapping reduces radiation exposure and contrast agent dose in complex endovascular interventions. *J Vasc Surg.* 2015;62(2):448-455.

27. Ejima K, et al. Image integration of three-dimensional cone-beam computed tomography angiogram into electroanatomical mapping system to guide catheter ablation of atrial fibrillation. *Europace.* 2010;12(1):45-51.
28. Orlov MV, Hoffmeister P, Chaudhry GM, et al. Three-dimensional rotational angiography of the left atrium and esophagus—a virtual computed tomography scan in the electrophysiology lab? *Heart Rhythm.* 2007;4(1):37-43.
29. Maschke SK, Hinrichs JB, Renne J, et al. C-Arm computed tomography (CACT)-guided balloon pulmonary angioplasty (BPA): evaluation of patient safety and peri- and post-procedural complications. *Eur Radiol.* 2019;29(3):1276-1284.
30. Housden R, Rhode K. X-ray Fluoroscopy-echocardiography. In: Liu Y-H, Sinusas AJ, eds. *Hybrid Imaging in Cardiovascular Medicine.* CRC Press, Taylor and Francis Group; 2018:137-152.
31. Lang P, Seslija P, Chu MWA, et al. US-fluoroscopy registration for transcatheter aortic valve implantation. *IEEE Trans Biomed Eng.* 2012;59(5):1444-1453.
32. Balzer J, Zeus T, Veulemans V, et al. Hybrid imaging in the catheter laboratory: real-time fusion of echocardiography and fluoroscopy during percutaneous structural heart disease interventions. *Interv Cardiol.* 2016;11(1):59-64.
33. Jone P-N, Haak A, Petri N, et al. Echocardiography-fluoroscopy fusion imaging for guidance of congenital and structural heart disease interventions. *JACC Cardiovasc Imaging.* 2019;12(7 Pt 1):1279-1282.
34. Jone P-N, Haak A, Ross M, et al. Congenital and structural heart disease interventions using echocardiography-fluoroscopy fusion imaging. *J Am Soc Echocardiogr.* 2019;32(12):1495-1504.
35. Stendahl JC, Sinusas AJ. Nanoparticles for cardiovascular imaging and therapeutic delivery, part 2: radiolabeled probes. *J Nucl Med.* 2015;56(11):1637-1641.
36. Stendahl JC, Sinusas AJ. Nanoparticles for cardiovascular imaging and therapeutic delivery, part 1: compositions and features. *J Nucl Med.* 2015;56(10):1469-1475.
37. Hedhli J, Kim M, Knox HJ, et al. Imaging the landmarks of vascular recovery. *Theranostics.* 2020;10(4):1733-1745.
38. Meoli DF, Sadeghi MM, Krassilnikova S, et al. Noninvasive imaging of myocardial angiogenesis following experimental myocardial infarction. *J Clin Invest.* 2004;113(12):1684-1691.
39. Brinkman R, Brinkman J. Cultural lag: conception and theory. *Int J Social Econ.* 1997;24(6):609-627.
40. Griffiths M. The impact of new hybrid imaging technology on the nuclear medicine workforce: Opportunities and challenges. In: International Conference on Nuclear Medicine and Radiation Therapy; July 14-15, 2016; Cologne, Germany. https://uwe-repository.worktribe.com/output/919349/the-impact-of-new-hybrid-imaging-technology-on-the-nuclear-medicine-workforce-opportunities-and-challenges

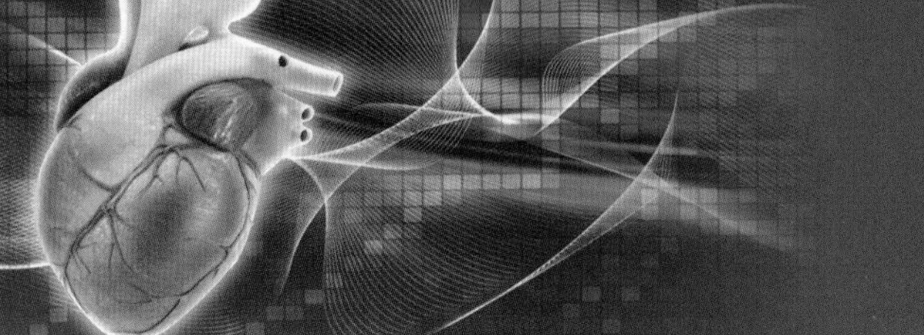

CHAPTER 39

PERIPROCEDURAL IMAGING

Federico Asch

INTRODUCTION

Historically, structural heart disease has been a field limited to surgical interventions, with periprocedural imaging providing the initial diagnosis and indication for intervention (eg, to determine the severity of mitral regurgitation). Over time, cardiac surgical procedures have become increasingly complex (ie, valve repair as an improved alternative to replacement), requiring a deeper understanding of the mechanisms involved in the disease (eg, presence of mitral prolapse, flails, perforations, clefts, annular dilatation) to guide the surgical approach and assess its success before leaving the operating room.

More recently, catheter-based procedures have been utilized in the treatment of structural heart disease because studies have shown less invasive percutaneous interventions are better tolerated, with faster recovery and favorable outcomes compared to surgery. For each intervention, multiple devices may be available, each with a specific design and with different implanting techniques. Understanding how each device is designed, how it is to be implanted, and how it is meant to work is critical for the success of these procedures.

With percutaneous interventions, the "field of view" of the operator is significantly limited when compared to open-heart surgery. Therefore, the role of cardiovascular imaging has become critical to assist in planning and guiding interventions and to evaluate immediate success or the presence of procedural complications. Accordingly, the cardiovascular imager must have a thorough understanding of multimodality imaging and the complexity of structural pathologies, devices, and procedural techniques.

INDICATIONS AND FUNDAMENTALS OF PERIPROCEDURAL IMAGING

The role and indications for imaging in patients with cardiovascular disease is dependent on the clinical characteristics, presentation, and overall patient conditions. Professional societies have developed numerous guidelines,[1-5] appropriateness use criteria, decision pathways for management,[6,7] and other standards documents that help the clinician approach patients according to their existing or suspected pathology and decide when—and which—imaging modality may be warranted.

The overall goals and roles of cardiac imaging in the patient with structural heart disease are listed in **Table 39.1**. A roadmap to the imaging needs and goals for the currently approved transcatheter procedures can be found in **Table 39.2** (transcatheter aortic valve replacement [TAVR]), **Table 39.3**, (mitral valve repair with MitraClip©) and **Table 39.4** (implantation of left atrial appendage occluder devices). Examples of images obtained during preprocedural planning and intraprocedural imaging are displayed in **Figures 39.1 through 39.4**.

Preprocedural Imaging

Transthoracic echocardiogram (TTE) is usually the initial imaging modality to evaluate patients with valvular disease or other suspected structural heart diseases, because it is widely available, noninvasive, and has almost no contraindications. A complete TTE allows for a comprehensive evaluation of cardiac chamber size and function, including visualization of valves and identification of most cardiac pathologies. The use of Doppler imaging (color and spectral) in addition to two- and three-dimensional (2D and 3D) TTE is critical to evaluate hemodynamic abnormalities such as intracardiac shunts, valvular stenosis, and valvular regurgitation. On certain occasions, TTE can be improved by using related techniques such as agitated saline injection (for detection of right-to-left shunts), ultrasound enhancing agents (for better delineation of the endocardium, intracardiac thrombus or masses, and myocardial perfusion imaging for alcohol septal ablation), or myocardial strain imaging (for left ventricular [LV] function).

Once a pathology is identified, a thorough evaluation must include quantifying severity, size, morphology, and mechanisms underlying the pathology, as well as the

TABLE 39.1 Role and Goals of Cardiac Imaging in Structural Heart Disease

Preprocedural
- Diagnose the pathology
- Determine its severity and need for intervention
- Evaluate indications and contraindications for intervention
- Determine the most appropriate procedure

Intraprocedural
- Assist in procedural planning and device selection and sizing
- Guide the procedure to maximize efficacy and safety

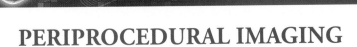

Postprocedural
- Monitor the patient post intervention, including complications
- Long-term follow-up to evaluate device function and cardiac response

consequences of the pathology to other structures within the heart (ie, ventricular or atrial remodeling, pulmonary hypertension, etc).

Although TTE frequently provides most of the information needed, the cardiac imager must understand the limitations of this modality and utilize alternative imaging modalities (ie, transesophageal echo [TEE], cardiac computed tomography [CT], cardiac magnetic resonance imaging [CMR]) when some of the needed information cannot be addressed with confidence by TTE. Although the severity of valvular disease or shunts is best assessed with TTE, detailed anatomy and morphology is best evaluated with TEE or CT. Furthermore, 3D imaging provides anatomic information that cannot be obtained from 2D imaging and allows for more accurate measurements of structures in all their dimensions, including perimeter, volume, area, and circumference, which is critical for the selection of the appropriate-sized devices. For the most part, 3D imaging for structural procedures can be obtained through TEE, multislice cardiac CT, or CMR.

TEE offers better spatial resolution than TTE (structures are better seen except those in the apex of the LV) with a similarly high temporal resolution; however, it is more invasive and requires moderate sedation. TEE's main contraindication is known or suspected obstructive disease of the upper gastrointestinal tract (ie, oropharyngeal, esophageal, or gastric).

TABLE 39.2 Role, Goals, and Types of Cardiac Imaging in Patients Undergoing TAVR

Preprocedural
- Determine aortic stenosis severity and need for intervention (TTE)
- Evaluate indications and contraindications for intervention (TTE)

Procedural planning
- Assess aortic valve anatomy (TTE, TEE, or CTA)
- Perform aortic annulus sizing (CTA or 3D TTE)
- Determine coronary artery height and aortic root dimensions (CTA or 3D TTE)
- Guide vascular access (femoral, subclavian, etc) (CTA)

Intraprocedural
- Assist in procedural planning and device selection and sizing (TEE)
- Guide the procedure to maximize efficacy and safety (TEE)

Postprocedural
- Immediate post implant, including complications (TTE, TEE)
  - Paravalvular leak
  - New or worsening LV wall motion and MR
  - Pericardial effusion or tamponade
- Long-term follow-up to evaluate device function and cardiac response (predischarge, 30 days, and yearly by TTE)
  - Paravalvular leak (TTE)
  - Valve hemodynamics: deterioration, stenosis (CTA, TEE if high gradients)
  - LV remodeling, pulmonary hypertension (TTE)

CTA, computed tomography angiography; LV, left ventricle; MR, mitral regurgitation; TAVR, transcatheter aortic valve replacement; TEE, transesophageal echocardiography; TTE, transthoracic echocardiography.

Data from Otto CM, Kumbhani DJ, Alexander KP, et al. 2017 ACC expert consensus decision pathway for transcatheter aortic valve replacement in the management of adults with aortic stenosis: a report of the American College of Cardiology Task Force on Clinical Expert Consensus Documents. *J Am Coll Cardiol.* 2017;69(10):1313–1346.

TABLE 39.3 Role and Goals of Cardiac Imaging in Patients Undergoing Mitral Valve Repair With Edge-To-Edge Leaflet Approximation

Preprocedural
- MR severity, need for intervention (TTE)
- Determine etiology (functional, degenerative, mixed; Carpentier classification) (TTE, TEE)
- Evaluate indications and contraindications for intervention (TTE)
- Determine most appropriate procedure (TEE)

Intraprocedural (TEE)
- Mitral gradients and area, MR severity
- Interatrial septal puncture and catheter guidance
- Guide clip position and number to be deployed

Postprocedural
- Monitor the patient post intervention, including complications
  - MR severity
  - Leaflet adverse events (single leaflet device attachment, laceration, etc)
  - Mitral gradients (stenosis)
  - Pericardial effusion
- Long-term follow-up to evaluate device function and cardiac response (predischarge, 30 days, every 6-12 months)
  - Valve hemodynamics (stenosis) and regurgitation (TTE)
  - Cardiac remodeling (left ventricle, atrium, pulmonary hypertension) (TTE)

MR, mitral regurgitation; TEE, transesophageal echocardiography; TTE, transthoracic echocardiography (MitraClip©).

Data from Bonow RO, O'Gara PT, Adams DH, et al. 2020 Focused Update of the 2017 ACC expert consensus decision pathway on the management of mitral regurgitation: a report of the American College of Cardiology Solution Set Oversight Committee. J Am Coll Cardiol. 2020;75(17):2236–2270.

TABLE 39.4 Role and Goals of Cardiac Imaging in Implantation of Left Atrial Appendage Occluders

Preprocedural (TEE, CTA)
- Rule out left atrial appendage thrombus
- Measure left atrial appendage dimensions
- Assess left atrial appendage anatomy (number of lobes, morphology)
- Determine the most appropriate device

Intraprocedural (TEE, ICE)
- Interatrial septal puncture
- Device positioning and expansion
- Leak peridevice

Postprocedural
- Pericardial effusion (TTE predischarge)
- Device thrombosis (TEE 30-60 days post implant)

CTA, computed tomography angiography; ICE, intracardiac echocardiography; TEE, transesophageal echocardiography; TTE, transthoracic echocardiography.

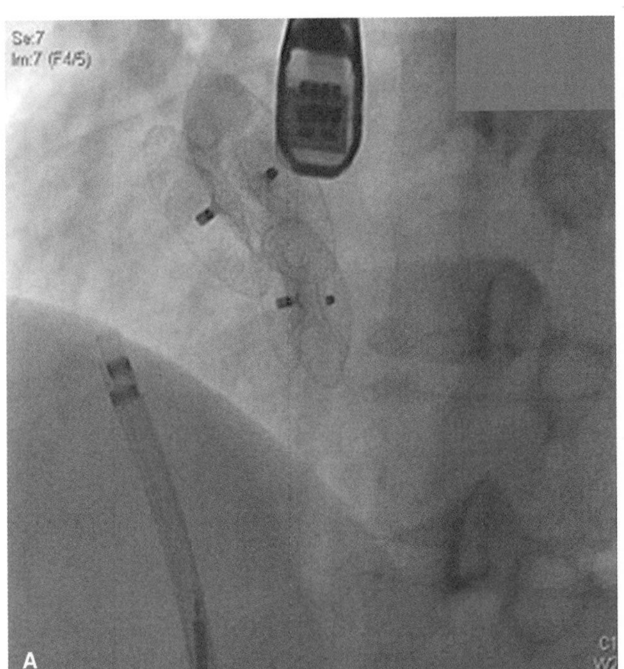

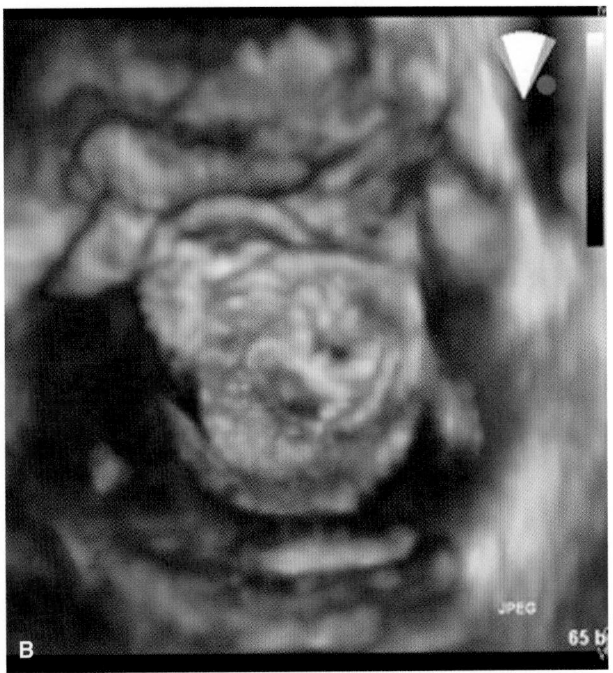

FIGURE 39.1 Intraprocedural guidance of ASD closure. **(A)** Fluoroscopic image demonstrating the presence of two side-by-side deployed Amplatzer occluder devices. At the top, the head of the TEE transducer is shown. **(B)** Real-time 3D volume rendered image of the disks deployed across the intra-atrial septum, as seen from the left atrial perspective. ASD, atrial septal defect; TEE, transthoracic echocardiography.

Cardiac CT requires, in most cases, the use of intravenous iodine contrast agents, so it may be contraindicated in patients with renal insufficiency or allergy to iodinated contrast material. Additionally, it involves exposure to radiation, which may be concerning in patients who require multiple CT studies, although this limitation has been greatly mitigated by using contemporary low-radiation protocols.

CMR is a versatile modality that has limited temporal and spatial resolutions but superior contrast resolution to allow for tissue characterization. In the event that a gadolinium-based

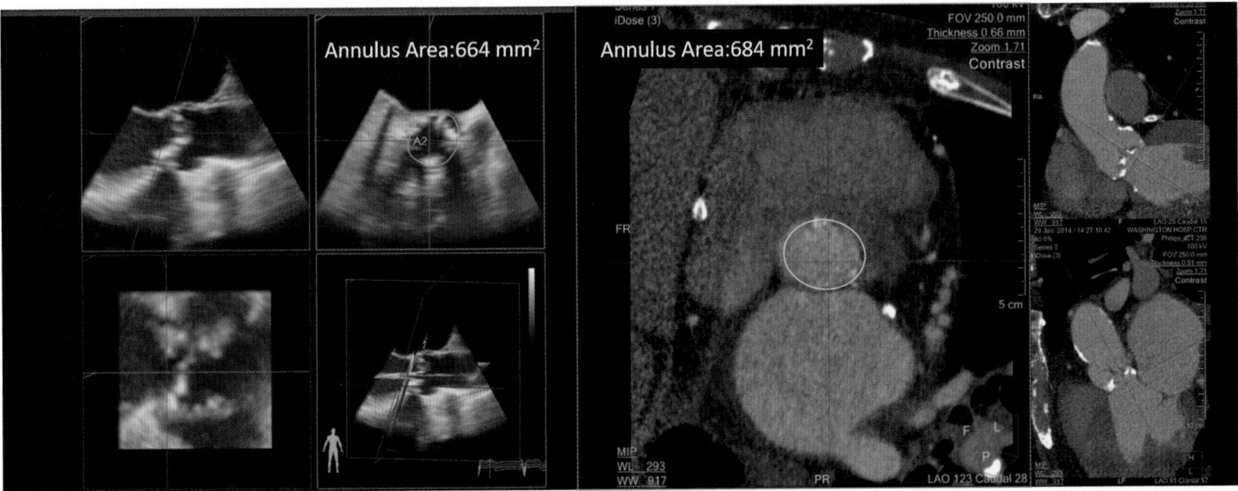

FIGURE 39.2 Aortic annular sizing for TAVR. The aortic annulus frequently has an oval shape (yellow ovals). For proper TAVR sizing, the area and perimeter are measured with 3D imaging. CT angiogram is the most commonly used modality (right panel), whereas 3D TEE could be a good alternative (left panel). In these examples, the red plane is situated at the annulus, providing a properly aligned short axis of the annulus, optimal for annulus tracing. In this case, both modalities have been used, showing a very close agreement in the measured area. CT, computed tomography; TAVR, transcatheter aortic valve replacement; TEE, transesophageal echocardiography.

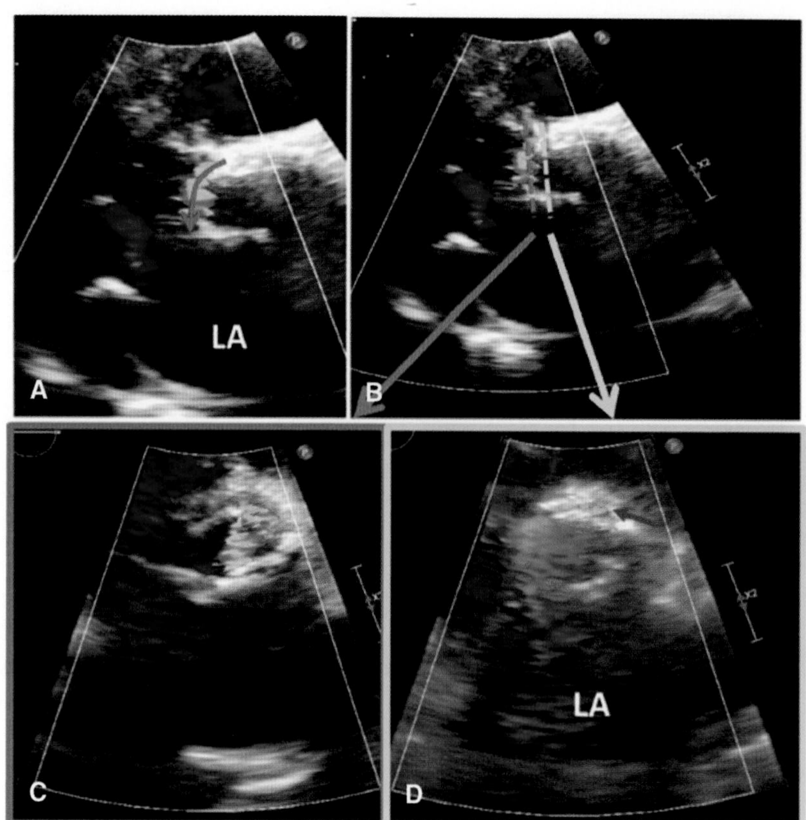

FIGURE 39.3 Paravalvular leaks in TAVR. Regurgitations around TAVR devices are common and they are usually small and multiple. These jets arise from the periphery and rapidly "spread" into the LVOT, therefore giving an impression of a large regurgitation by color Doppler (**panel A**). When scanning, it is critical to identify the jet at its origin and obtain a short axis at this plane to evaluate the percentage of the annular circumference that is leaking. When scanned too low (red plane in **B** and **panel C**), the jet will appear large and the severity of the paravalvular leak is overestimated. The proper plane (yellow in **B**, **panel D**) will reflect the real size of the regurgitant orifice. LVOT, left ventricular outflow tract. TAVR, transcatheter aortic valve replacement. (Reprinted from Zoghbi WA, Asch FM, Bruce C, et al. Guidelines for the evaluation of valvular regurgitation after percutaneous valve repair or replacement: a report from the American Society of Echocardiography developed in collaboration with the Society for Cardiovascular Angiography and Interventions, Japanese Society of Echocardiography, and Society for Cardiovascular Magnetic Resonance. *J Am Soc Echocardiogr.* 2019;32(4):431–475. Copyright © 2019 by the American Society of Echocardiography. With permission.)

contrast agent is needed, renal dysfunction may be a relative contraindication. In addition, CMR images may be limited in patients with implanted cardiac devices.

For commonly performed noninvasive imaging-guided percutaneous procedures, TAVR, edge-to-edge mitral repair, and occlusion of the left atrial appendage, the specific issues to be addressed and the most appropriate imaging modalities are listed in **Tables 39.2 to 39.4**.

Procedural Guidance

Ultrasound is the only imaging modality that displays images in real time without ionizing radiation, is portable, and can be easily integrated into the operating and catheterization suites. Hence, procedural guidance is currently limited to echocardiography, which can be done by TTE, TEE, or intracardiac echo (ICE).[8]

TEE is used to guide procedures in the operating room. In contrast, in the catheterization laboratory or hybrid operating rooms (operating room with fluoroscopy capabilities), any of the three ultrasound modalities could be used. TEE provides more detailed imaging than TTE, including Doppler and real-time 3D imaging, and can be done from the head of the procedural table without obstructing the operators. In the operating room, TEE is nowadays used by echo-trained anesthesiologists to monitor hemodynamics, even in nonstructural procedures such as coronary bypass or noncardiac surgeries.

ICE is done through special imaging catheters, which are conveniently handled by the interventional cardiologist. It provides high-quality images (similar to TEE) but with a limited depth of field. Although the interventional cardiologist typically interprets ICE images, complex procedures may still require an imager in the room. Typical procedures in which ICE is used are implantation of atrial septal defect (ASD) and patent foramen ovale (PFO) closure devices or left atrial appendage occluders in patients with atrial fibrillation (**Figure 39-5**).

Newer devices and procedures are subject to a learning curve by interventional operators; therefore, they are more dependent on guidance provided by intraprocedural imaging in

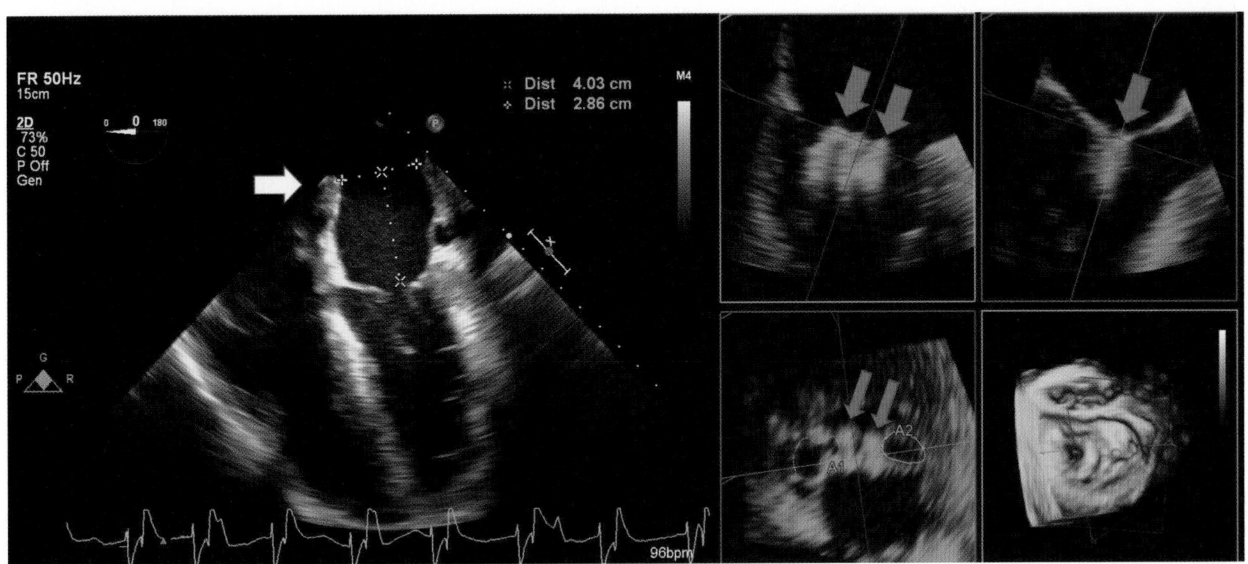

FIGURE 39.4 Critical steps in MitraClip implant. Transcatheter mitral repair with the MitraClip (edge-to-edge leaflet approximation technique) requires accessing the left atrium through an interatrial septal puncture (left panel). The exact location of the puncture is marked by the "tenting" of the septum (white arrow) and should be done at least 4 cm from the mitral annulus to allow for proper steering of the catheters and optimal positioning of the clip for deployment. Positioning of the clips usually in the central area (two clips in this case, red arrows) (A2/P2 segments) will result in a double-orifice mitral valve, which puts the patient at risk for developing mitral stenosis. For this reason, measuring the resulting area of each orifice (central lower panel) and mitral gradients is important prior to final deployment.

their early stages of procedural development. TAVR and implantation of PFO or ASD closure devices are examples of procedures that required TEE in their early days but are nowadays only assisted by fluoroscopy or ICE. Other procedures remain dependent on TEE owing to their complexity (ie, transcatheter mitral valve repair or replacement) or the need for more detailed information.

TTE is often most useful immediately after device implant, rather than to guide the intervention itself. In the case of TAVR, for example, the goal of imaging with TTE immediately after the implant is to assess efficacy and complications. The success of the implant is assessed by measuring hemodynamics (gradients), the presence and severity of regurgitation (paravalvular leak), and the position of the device. Early complications—such as device migration, embolization, pericardial effusion, and new or worsening mitral regurgitation or wall motion abnormalities—can also be detected by TTE post procedure.

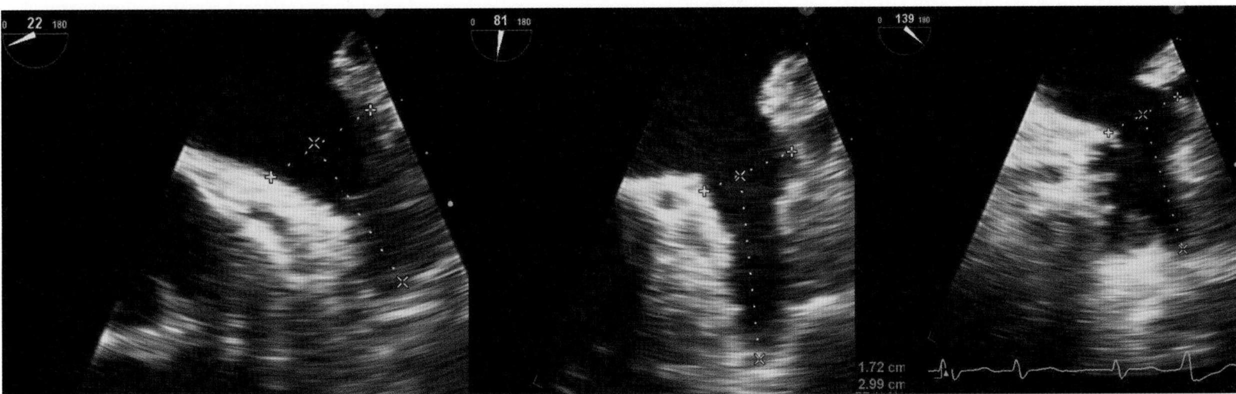

FIGURE 39.5 Left atrial appendage dimensions for occluder implant. Measurements at the ostium, landing zone, and depth are important to determine the type and size of device to be used. These measurements (which are specific to each device brand) are to be taken at multiple planes by rotating the omniplane of the TEE probe between 0 and 135 degrees. Alternatively, intracardiac echocardiography could be used during the implant, or CT angiography from preprocedural images. CT, computed tomography; TEE, transesophageal echocardiography.

TABLE 39.5 Keys to a Successful Structural Heart Imager

Preprocedural Know the pathology and the patient Be familiar with guidelines Be familiar with multiple imaging modalities Be active in the Heart Team
Intraprocedural Know the pathology Know the patient's anatomy Know your devices Understand the procedure and goals Know your operator and your team Anticipate steps and problems Take your time and ask for patience Know your tools
Postprocedural, follow-up Note the device Refer to prior images post procedure

TABLE 39.6 Strengths of Common Imaging Modalities Post TAVR

	TTE	TEE 2D+3D	4D CT
Leak severity	++	++	−
Leak location	+	++	−
Valve hemodynamics	++	+	−
Malpositioning	−	+	++
Eccentric annulus	−	++	++
Aortic root geometry	−	+	++
Frame integrity	−	+/−	++
Leaflet thrombosis	−	++	++
Leaflet degeneration	+/−	++	−
Leaflet coaptation	−	++	−

CT, computed tomography; TEE, transesophageal echocardiography; TTE, transthoracic echocardiography.

Goals and optimal imaging modalities for guidance of each procedure are listed in **Tables 39.2 to 39.4**. The success of structural heart interventions is highly dependent on the level of expertise of the implanter and the imager who assists prior to and during the procedure. Some critical aspects have to be met to become a successful "structural heart imager" (**Table 39.5**).

Postprocedural Evaluation

Immediate postprocedural imaging is accomplished with echocardiography and/or fluoroscopy and is directed at evaluating procedural success. Usually performed immediately after device deployment and prior to concluding the procedure, imaging documents proper device positioning and function, initial hemodynamic evaluation, and exclusion of complications such as pericardial effusion, thrombus, new wall motion abnormalities, or damage of other structures such as nonintervened valves, new septal defects or fistulas, cardiac wall rupture, or hematomas.

Subsequent follow-up imaging evaluation continues in a periodic manner that is specific to the type of intervention, procedural outcomes, and the patient's characteristics. After ASD or left atrial appendage closure devices, for example, close follow-up is essential over the initial 1 to 3 months to confirm device position and look for leaks and/or thrombus. For aortic and pulmonary valve implants, follow-up is recommended at 1 month and yearly thereafter,[6,9] whereas mitral and tricuspid valve interventions may require closer follow-up at 1, 6, and 12 months and yearly thereafter.[5,7] The goals are to evaluate device performance, including regurgitation, paravalvular leaks, and hemodynamics to detect early valvular degeneration or stenosis.[10-12]

Knowledge of the expected hemodynamic pattern for a given prosthetic valve is important and can be obtained from nominal values provided by the manufacturers for each valve type and size. Equally important is comparison of findings to prior studies in the same patient. In this sense, the earliest follow-up available (at discharge or 30 days) should serve as the reference or "device baseline" to be compared to in subsequent examinations. Worsening gradients, leaks, or regurgitation may warrant a more detailed evaluation with additional imaging modalities (CT, TEE, or CMR).[13] It is important to note that hemodynamic changes may occur as a result of valvular dysfunction or non–valve-related circumstances. Conditions that increase cardiac output—such as fever, hyperthyroidism, anemia, exercise, and pregnancy—can substantially increase the transvalvular gradient in the absence of valve dysfunction.

Although TTE is the main imaging modality for follow-up evaluation, it has some shortcomings. Multimodality imaging knowledge is critical for proper utilization of TEE, CT, or MRI in cases where TTE is not adequate to assess the underlying pathology. As an example, **Table 39.6** provides a framework for evaluation post TAVR, while similar concepts could be used in cases of other surgical and transcatheter interventions. A few general rules are worth mentioning:

- Evaluation of structures that lack high mobility is best achieved by gated 4D CT or by TEE. Examples include integrity and detailed position of hardware (stents or clips), immobile prosthetic disks, and thickened leaflets due to thrombosis or pannus.
- Highly mobile structures require high temporal resolution, and therefore ultrasound techniques are best suited. Examples include evaluation of the integrity of leaflets that have normal mobility, evaluation for endocarditis, etc.
- Hemodynamic interrogation is performed with ultrasound, specifically with Doppler echocardiography, because it provides high temporal resolution with good image definition in 2D or 3D imaging. Cardiac MRI can also be used to evaluate hemodynamics and regurgitation, although it is contraindicated for patients with certain metallic devices.

RESEARCH AND FUTURE DIRECTIONS

Research in the fields of structural heart disease and cardiac imaging has been occurring at a fast pace over the last decade, because imaging plays a critical role in the identification of patients in need of intervention, guiding procedures, and monitoring device performance through follow-up. As newer procedures and devices are developed, novel challenges are faced that provide new opportunities for research and developments in the fields of imaging. Areas of development include newer imaging technologies (hardware and software), application of artificial intelligence and machine learning technologies, and development of clinical applications. The success of such research and development is highly dependent on the close collaboration between industry, investigators, and professional societies.

KEY POINTS

- ✔ Rapid developments in the field of structural heart disease require a thorough understanding of cardiac anatomy and the devices in order to anticipate how they can interact and resolve or mitigate pathologic conditions.
- ✔ In percutaneous interventions, the "field of view" of the operator is significantly limited when compared to open-heart surgery. Therefore, the role of cardiovascular imaging is essential to assist in planning and conducting interventions and to evaluate the immediate success.
- ✔ The cardiovascular imager must have a thorough understanding of multimodality imaging and the complexity of structural pathologies, devices, and procedural techniques.
- ✔ Preprocedural imaging aims at identifying patients in need of an intervention and deciding which intervention is most appropriate. Once a pathology is identified, a thorough evaluation must include quantifying severity, size, morphology, and mechanisms underlying the pathology, as well as the consequences of the pathology in other structures.
- ✔ Although a TTE frequently provides most of the information needed, the cardiac imager needs to understand the limitations of this modality and alternative imaging techniques, including 3D imaging (TEE, CT, MRI) whenever appropriate.
- ✔ The success of structural heart interventions is highly dependent on the level of expertise of the implanter and the imager who assists prior to and during the procedure.
- ✔ Procedural guidance is nowadays limited to echocardiography (TEE, TTE, ICE), because ultrasound is the only modality that displays images in real time without ionizing radiation, is portable, and can be easily integrated into the operating and catheterization suites.
- ✔ Immediate postprocedural imaging is limited to echocardiography and fluoroscopy and is directed at evaluating procedural success.
- ✔ Follow-up evaluation starts at the time of patient discharge and continues in a periodic manner that is specific to the type of intervention and the patient's characteristics.
- ✔ Knowing the expected hemodynamic pattern for a given device is of utmost importance and this can be obtained from nominal values provided by the manufacturers for each device type and size.
- ✔ Worsening of gradients, leaks, or regurgitation may warrant a more detailed assessment with advanced imaging modalities (CT or TEE).

REFERENCES

1. Baumgartner H, Hung J, Bermejo J, et al. Recommendations on the echocardiographic assessment of aortic valve stenosis: a focused update from the European Association of Cardiovascular Imaging and the American Society of Echocardiography. *J Am Soc Echocardiogr.* 2017;30:372-392.
2. Nishimura RA, Otto CM, Bonow RO, et al. 2014 AHA/ACC guideline for the management of patients with valvular heart disease: a report of the American College of Cardiology/American Heart Association Task Force on Practice Guidelines. *J Am Coll Cardiol.* 2014;63:e57-e185.
3. Vahanian A, Alfieri O, Andreotti F, et al. Guidelines on the management of valvular heart disease (version 2012): the Joint Task Force on the Management of Valvular Heart Disease of the European Society of Cardiology (ESC) and the European Association for Cardio-Thoracic Surgery (EACTS). *Eur Heart J.* 2012;33:2451-2496.
4. Zoghbi WA, Enriquez-Sarano M, Foster E, et al. Recommendations for evaluation of the severity of native valvular regurgitation with two-dimensional and Doppler echocardiography. *J Am Soc Echocardiogr.* 2003;16:777-802.
5. Zoghbi WA, Asch FM, Bruce C, et al. Guidelines for the evaluation of valvular regurgitation after percutaneous valve repair or replacement: a report from the American Society of Echocardiography developed in collaboration with the Society for Cardiovascular Angiography and Interventions, Japanese Society of Echocardiography, and Society for Cardiovascular Magnetic Resonance. *J Am Soc Echocardiogr.* 2019;32:431-475.
6. Otto CM, Kumbhani DJ, Alexander KP, et al. 2017 ACC expert consensus decision pathway for transcatheter aortic valve replacement in the management of adults with aortic stenosis: a report of the American College of Cardiology Task Force on Clinical Expert Consensus Documents. *J Am Coll Cardiol.* 2017;69:1313-1346.
7. Bonow RO, O'Gara PT, Adams DH, et al. 2020 Focused update of the 2017 ACC expert consensus decision pathway on the management of mitral regurgitation: a report of the American College of Cardiology Solution Set Oversight Committee. *J Am Coll Cardiol.* 2020;75:2236-2270.
8. Zamorano JL, Badano LP, Bruce C, et al. EAE/ASE recommendations for the use of echocardiography in new transcatheter interventions for valvular heart disease. *J Am Soc Echocardiogr.* 2011;24:937-965.
9. Zoghbi WA, Chambers JB, Dumesnil JG, et al. Recommendations for evaluation of prosthetic valves with echocardiography and doppler ultrasound: a report From the American Society of Echocardiography's Guidelines and Standards Committee and the Task Force on Prosthetic Valves, developed in conjunction with the American College of Cardiology Cardiovascular Imaging Committee, Cardiac Imaging Committee of the American Heart Association, the European Association of Echocardiography, a registered branch of the European Society of Cardiology, the Japanese Society of Echocardiography and the Canadian Society of Echocardiography, endorsed by the American College of Cardiology Foundation, American Heart Association, European Association of Echocardiography, a registered branch of the European Society of Cardiology, the Japanese Society of Echocardiography, and Canadian Society of Echocardiography. *J Am Soc Echocardiogr.* 2009;22:975-1014; quiz 1082.

10. Kappetein AP, Head SJ, Généreux P, et al. Updated standardized endpoint definitions for transcatheter aortic valve implantation: the Valve Academic Research Consortium-2 consensus document. *Eur Heart J.* 2012;33:2403-2418.
11. Stone GW, Vahanian AS, Adams DH, et al. Clinical trial design principles and endpoint definitions for transcatheter mitral valve repair and replacement: part 1: clinical trial design principles: a consensus document from the mitral valve academic research consortium. *Eur Heart J.* 2015;36:1851-1877.
12. Stone GW, Adams DH, Abraham WT, et al. Clinical trial design principles and endpoint definitions for transcatheter mitral valve repair and replacement: part 2: endpoint definitions: a consensus document from the mitral valve academic research consortium. *J Am Coll Cardiol.* 2015;66:308-321.
13. Jilaihawi H, Asch FM, Manasse E, et al. Systematic CT methodology for the evaluation of subclinical leaflet thrombosis. *JACC Cardiovasc Imaging.* 2017;10:461-470.

FURTHER READINGS

Athappan G, Patvardhan E, Tuzcu EM, et al. Incidence, predictors, and outcomes of aortic regurgitation after transcatheter aortic valve replacement: meta-analysis and systematic review of literature. *J Am Coll Cardiol.* 2013;61:1585-1595.

Baumgartner H, Falk V, Bax JJ, et al. 2017 ESC/EACTS guidelines for the management of valvular heart disease. *Eur Heart* J. 2017;38:2739-2791.

Delgado V, Clavel MA, Hahn RT, et al. How do we reconcile echocardiography, computed tomography, and hybrid imaging in assessing discordant grading of aortic stenosis severity. *JACC Cardiovasc Imaging.* 2019;12:267-282.

Feldman T, Foster E, Glower DD, et al. Percutaneous repair or surgery for mitral regurgitation. *N Engl J Med.* 2011;364:1395-1406.

Hahn RT, Nicoara A, Kapadia S, Svensson L, Martin R. Echocardiographic imaging for transcatheter aortic valve replacement. *J Am Soc Echocardiogr.* 2018;31:405-433.

Jilaihawi H, Doctor N, Kashif M, et al. Aortic annular sizing for transcatheter aortic valve replacement using cross-sectional 3-dimensional transesophageal echocardiography. *J Am Coll Cardiol.* 2013;61:908-916.

Lang RM, Bierig M, Devereux RB, et al. Recommendations for chamber quantification: a report from the American Society of Echocardiography's Guidelines and Standards Committee and the Chamber Quantification Writing Group, developed in conjunction with the European Association of Echocardiography, a branch of the European Society of Cardiology. *J Am Soc Echocardiogr.* 2005;18:1440-1463.

Nishimura RA, Otto CM, Bonow RO, et al. 2017 AHA/ACC focused update of the 2014 AHA/ACC guideline for the management of patients with valvular heart disease: a report of the American College of Cardiology/American Heart Association Task Force on clinical practice guidelines. *J Am Coll Cardiol.* 2017;70:252-289.

Piazza N, de Jaegere P, Schultz C, Becker AE, Serruys PW, Anderson RH. Anatomy of the aortic valvar complex and its implications for transcatheter implantation of the aortic valve. *Circ Cardiovasc Interv.* 2008;1:74-81.

Zoghbi WA, Adams D, Bonow RO, et al. Recommendations for non-invasive evaluation of native valvular regurgitation: a report from the American Society of Echocardiography developed in collaboration with the Society for Cardiovascular Magnetic Resonance. *J Am Soc Echocardiogr.* 2017; 30:303-371.

SECTION 3

CARDIAC CATHETERIZATION AND INTERVENTION

SECTION EDITOR: Joaquin E. Cigarroa

CHAPTER 40

CARDIAC CATHETERIZATION AND HEMODYNAMIC ASSESSMENT

Punag Divanji and Joseph Yang

INTRODUCTION

Since the late 1960s, the use of the Swan-Ganz balloon-tipped catheter for the measurement of intracardiac hemodynamics has been a cornerstone in the diagnosis and management of acute myocardial infarction and cardiogenic shock.[1,2] Standard right heart catheterization involves the percutaneous placement of an introducer sheath—commonly into the internal jugular, subclavian, brachial, or femoral veins—with subsequent use of a balloon-tipped catheter for pressure waveform recording, blood co-oximetry measurement, and assessment of thermodilution cardiac output.

INDICATIONS

Right heart catheterization is indicated for the evaluation of cardiogenic shock, pulmonary hypertension, intracardiac shunting, and severe cardiomyopathy (**Table 40.1**). Invasive hemodynamics with right and left heart catheterization are also applicable in the assessment of valvular heart disease and pericardial constriction or restrictive cardiomyopathy, when echocardiography or other noninvasive imaging proves to be inconclusive or has conflicting data. Additionally, tailored therapy using a retained Swan-Ganz catheter can be useful in patients with cardiogenic shock or mixed cardiogenic/septic shock by augmenting vasopressor and inotropic medications based on filling pressures, cardiac output, and calculated resistances.[3]

ANATOMIC CONSIDERATIONS

When performed in the cardiac catheterization laboratory with fluoroscopy, right heart catheterization can be performed from a variety of venous access points, including the brachial, internal jugular, subclavian, and femoral veins. With the development of smaller caliber (5 and 6 French) catheters and hydrophilic slender sheaths, the brachial vein has become more commonly used (**Table 40.2**). An antecubital 20-gauge peripheral IV can be placed and then exchanged over a wire in the cardiac catheterization laboratory for a 5- or 6-French sheath. This access point is most comfortable for the patient and virtually eliminates the risk of pneumothorax that can be associated with internal jugular or subclavian access.[4] Bedrest is also not required for brachial venous access as compared with femoral venous access. In cases where fluoroscopic guidance is not available (such as at the bedside in the intensive care unit), the right internal jugular vein or the left subclavian vein is the preferred access point, with ultrasound-guided access and hemodynamic waveform–guided advancement.[5]

TABLE 40.1 Indications for Right Heart Catheterization

Common Indications for Right Heart Catheterization
• Heart failure • Shock • Acute myocardial infarction • Pulmonary hypertension • Valvular heart disease • Heart transplant

FUNDAMENTALS OF CARDIAC CATHETERIZATION AND HEMODYNAMIC ASSESSMENT

The basics of right heart catheterization consist of percutaneous venous access using sterile technique to place an introducer sheath into a central vein with ultrasound guidance. Pressure measurements and blood oximetry can then be obtained using a variety of catheter shapes such as the Multipurpose, Gensini, and Goodale-Lubin. However, the most commonly used catheter remains the balloon-tipped Swan-Ganz catheter, which can also be used to measure both intracardiac filling pressures and cardiac output.[2]

CLINICAL APPLICATION

Patients may present with a wide spectrum of lesions that alter normal cardiac hemodynamics, resulting in symptoms of dyspnea or heart failure. Right heart catheterization allows for the measurement of valuable clinical data to solve difficult diagnostic challenges in the patient with structural heart disease. Careful consideration of the intracardiac pressures and oxygen saturations can allow the clinician to diagnose the cause of symptoms and determine therapeutic options. There are a variety of indications for right heart catheterization, primarily in patients with heart failure, dyspnea, valvular heart disease, or suspected pulmonary hypertension (**Table 40.1**).

TABLE 40.2 Advantages and Disadvantages of Different Venous Access Sites

	Internal Jugular Vein	Femoral Vein	Brachial Vein
Advantages	• Physician familiarity • Ambulation (if retained pulmonary artery line) • Shorter fluoroscopy time	• Easily combined with other procedures.	• Less pain • Less frequent complications • Immediate ambulation
Disadvantages	• Complications: • Carotid puncture • Pneumothorax • Bradycardia (carotid sinus pressure)	• Delayed ambulation • Longer fluoroscopy time • Complications: • Infection • Femoral hematoma • Bradycardia (vagal reaction)	• Less physician familiarity • Longer fluoroscopy time • More venous tortuosity • Complications: • Brachial artery puncture

From a number of access sites, the Swan-Ganz pulmonary arterial catheter is advanced through the great veins (superior or inferior vena cava), to the right atrium (RA), the right ventricle (RV), and the pulmonary artery (PA). Importantly, these balloon-tipped, end-hole catheters can be advanced into the smaller pulmonary arterioles, ostensibly occluding inflow and allowing for measurement of the PA occlusion wedge pressure (PAWP). A plethora of data can be attained during this process, including venous and intracardiac pressures, oxygen saturation by chamber, cardiac output, and vascular resistance (by calculation). Additionally, these data can be used to calculate more advanced markers of cardiac function, including pulmonary artery pressure index (PAPi), stroke volume index (SVi), and cardiac power output (CPO) (**Table 40.3**).[6]

Hemodynamic Assessment

Right heart catheterization allows for the measurement of venous, intracardiac, and PA pressures, which can be used to determine filling pressures, resistance, and transvalvular gradients. To ensure the validity of the data prior to its clinical use, it is imperative to ensure both accuracy and precision of pressure measurements during catheterization. Thus, it is important to correctly set up the transducer system in every case. Typically, the pressure transducer is mounted on the procedure table (or patient bed, if performed outside of the catheterization laboratory) at the mid-chest level. Transducers are connected to the procedural catheter using plastic tubing filled with sterile saline. The catheter, tubing, and transducer are flushed to eliminate any bubbles, which lead to pressure waveform overdamping. After flushing, the transducer is calibrated at the mid-chest level. This process involves opening the transducer to air and allowing the system to "zero" to atmospheric pressure. Thus, measurements must be taken with a high-fidelity pressure transduction system per institutional standards, with fluid-filled tubing and optimal pressure damping to allow for appropriate interpretation of the tracings. Overdamping, often caused by air bubbles, thrombi, loose connections, or kinked catheters, can lead to underestimation of the systolic pressure, loss of the dicrotic notch, and distorted waveforms. On the other hand, underdamping, caused by excess tubing, excess components, or a defective transducer can lead to a falsely elevated systolic peak pressure, underestimated diastolic pressure, and significant waveform artifact.[7]

Accurate measurements should be taken at end expiration because the negative intrathoracic pressure produced during inspiration will lower intracardiac pressures. Of note, in intubated patients receiving mechanical ventilation with positive end-expiratory pressure, measurements are either taken at end inspiration, or an expiratory hold maneuver is performed with the ventilator to account for the impact of positive pressure. Venous and atrial pressure measurements are taken as a mean over several cardiac cycles, whereas ventricular pressure measurements are described as systolic and end-diastolic values. Arterial pressure measurements (ie, PA, aorta, peripheral arteries), are composed of systolic, diastolic, and mean values. Under fluoroscopic guidance, the flow-directed PA catheter can be advanced through the vena cava, into the RA, RV, PA, and PA wedge positions, with pressure and oxygen measurements taken in each position sequentially, either during forward advancement or during pullback. This information is then integrated with a comprehensive understanding of normal values to elucidate the clinical and hemodynamic picture.

Intracardiac Pressures

Right Atrium. The RA pressure tracing (**Figure 40.1**) consists of distinct components, with positive deflections described as "waves," and negative deflections described as "descents," with a normal mean RA pressure range of 2 to 6 mm Hg. The "a-wave" represents an increase in RA pressure caused by atrial contraction in late diastole, directly after the P-wave on the electrocardiogram (ECG). This is followed by the "c-wave," which represents the displacement of the closed tricuspid valve into the RA during the isovolumic contraction phase of early systole, typically occurring at the end of the QRS complex. As ventricular systole continues, the RA relaxes and the tricuspid annulus is pulled down toward the RV apex, resulting in a drop in atrial pressure known as the "x-descent." Corresponding to the end of the T-wave on ECG, the hemodynamic "v-wave" represents a back-pressure reflection from atrial filling against the closed tricuspid valve during ventricular systole. Finally, the "y-descent," a pressure decrease caused by the tricuspid valve opening in early diastole, occurs before the P-wave on the ECG. These components combine to form the atrial pressure tracing, and the cause of clinical various presentations can be identified via aberrations in the normal waveform (**Table 40.3**).

TABLE 40.3 Right Atrial Pressure Waveform and Common Abnormalities

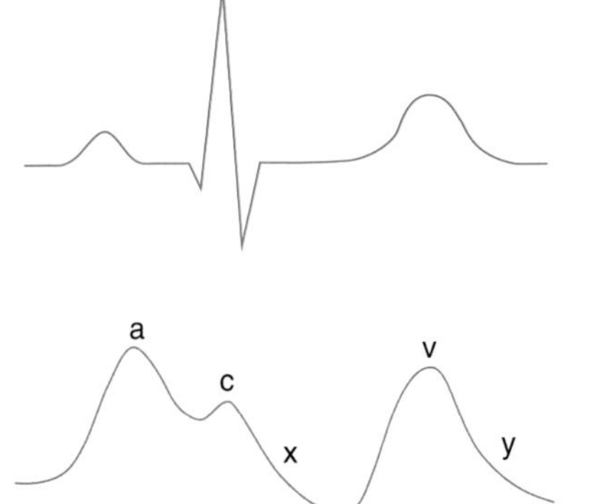

Elevated a wave • Tricuspid stenosis • Decreased RV compliance **Cannon a wave** • Third-degree AV block • Ventricular tachycardia • Ventricular pacemaker **Absent a wave** • Atrial fibrillation • Junctional rhythm **Elevated v wave** • Tricuspid regurgitation • RV failure • Reduced RA compliance • Left-to-right shunting	**Equal a and v waves** • Tamponade • Constrictive pericarditis **Prominent x descent** • Tamponade • RV ischemia **Prominent y descent** • Tricuspid regurgitation • Constrictive pericarditis • Restrictive myopathy **Blunted x descent** • Atrial fibrillation • RA ischemia **Blunted y descent** • Tricuspid stenosis • RV ischemia • Tamponade

Of note, left-to-right shunting produces a prominent v-wave in the RA if shunting occurs at the atrial level.
AV, atrioventricular; RA, right ventricle, RV, right ventricle.

Right Ventricle. Crossing the competent tricuspid valve allows measurement of the RV pressure, which is described by its peak systolic pressure (12-24 mm Hg) and end-diastolic pressure (2-6 mm Hg) (Figure 40.1). However, the pressure tracing can be subdivided into four distinct phases: systole is composed of (1) isovolumetric contraction, from tricuspid valve closure to pulmonic valve opening, and (2) ejection, from pulmonic valve opening to its closure; diastole is composed of (3) isovolumetric relaxation, from pulmonic valve closure to tricuspid valve opening, and (4) filling, from tricuspid valve opening to its closure.

Clinically, elevations in RV systolic pressure occur most commonly in the setting of pulmonary hypertension, but can also be owing to left ventricular (LV) pressure overload, pulmonic valve stenosis, RV outflow tract (RVOT) obstruction, or hemodynamically significant left-to-right shunting. Conversely, reductions in RV systolic pressure can be caused by cardiogenic shock, hypovolemia, or cardiac tamponade.

Similarly, elevations in RV end-diastolic pressure occur most commonly in the setting of volume overload of any cause, such as congestive heart failure, but can also be caused by decreased chamber compliance, ventricular hypertrophy, tricuspid regurgitation, pericardial constriction, or cardiac tamponade. Low RV end-diastolic pressure is primarily caused by hypovolemia but can also occur in the setting of tricuspid valve stenosis.

Pulmonary Artery. Beyond the pulmonic valve and into the main PA, the PA tracing is described by its peak systolic pressure (12-24 mm Hg), diastolic pressure (6-12 mm Hg), and mean pressure (10-22 mm Hg) (Figure 40.1). Similar in appearance to the aortic tracing, albeit with lower pressures, a dicrotic notch is seen in the PA, representing closure of the pulmonic valve.

An elevated PA systolic or diastolic pressure can occur in the setting of pulmonary hypertension (of any cause), mitral stenosis, mitral regurgitation, volume overload, left-to-right

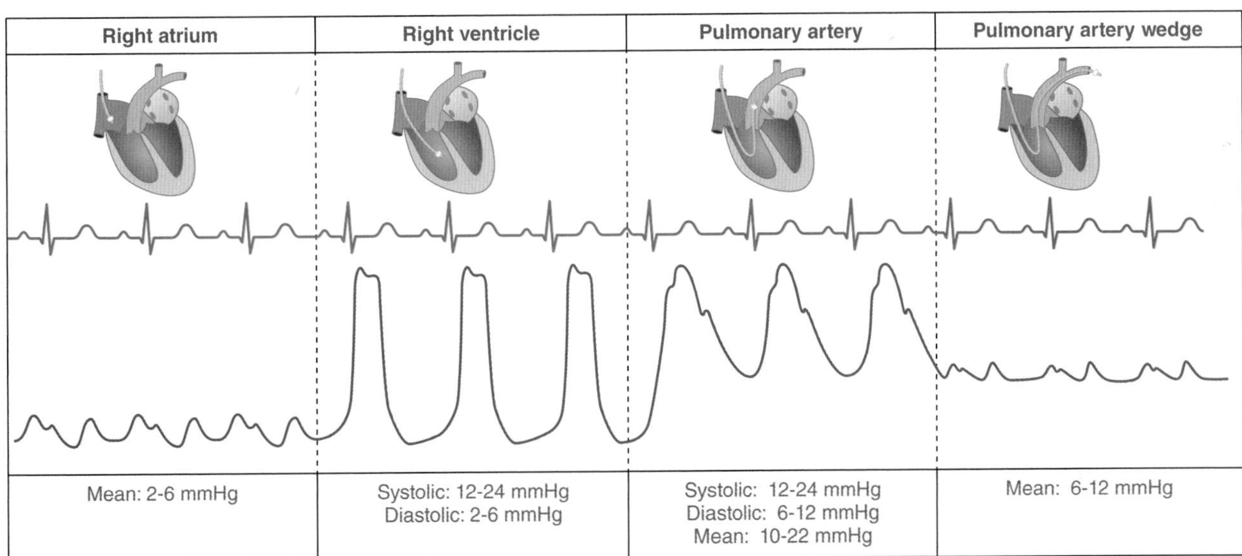

FIGURE 40.1 Right heart catheterization positions, waveforms, and normal values.

shunting, and pulmonary embolism (PE). A reduced PA systolic or diastolic pressure can occur in the setting of hypovolemia or any lesion restricting PA inflow (tricuspid valve stenosis, pulmonic valve stenosis, RVOT obstruction, tricuspid atresia, Ebstein anomaly). An isolated reduction in PA diastolic pressure (and therefore a wide PA pulse pressure) can occur because of pulmonic valve regurgitation, whereas a reduced PA pulse pressure occurs in the setting of cardiogenic shock, RV infarct, PE, or cardiac tamponade.

Pulmonary Artery Wedge Pressure. The PAWP estimates left atrial (LA) pressure and is used as a measure of left-sided intracardiac filling pressure. In the absence of mitral valve disease or cardiac disease, mean PAWP is similar to mean LV end-diastolic pressure. However, these pressures may be disparate in patients with aortic valvular disease, systemic arterial hypertension, and coronary artery disease, in whom LV end-diastolic pressure exceeds mean PAWP because of LV noncompliance and a prominent a wave. Hence, in patients with mitral valve disease or cardiac disease, mean PAWP cannot be used reliably to assess LV end-diastolic pressure.

To obtain a wedge pressure, the inflated, balloon-tipped catheter is advanced into a branch PA with the intent of blocking PA inflow. This allows the end hole of the catheter to indirectly measure the LA pressure. Therefore, the PAWP tracing is similar to the left atrial pressure tracing, consisting of the same a-c-x-v-y waveform (**Table 40.4**). Similar to the RA, the PAWP "a-wave" represents atrial systole, the "c-wave" represents the displacement of the closed mitral valve into the LA, and the "x-descent" represents LA relaxation. The "v-wave," which is intimately related to atrial compliance, represents atrial filling occurring during ventricular systole. Finally, the "y-descent" is caused by mitral valve opening in early diastole. Importantly, the PAWP tracing is often less distinct than the RA waveform and delayed compared with the ECG, as the pressure is transmitted through the pulmonary vascular system before being measured by the catheter.

With a normal mean of 6 to 12 mm Hg at end expiration, the PAWP is 0 to 6 mm Hg less than the PA diastolic pressure under normal conditions (ie, no increased pulmonary vascular resistance [PVR]). An appropriate "wedge" position should be confirmed by measuring greater than 95% oxygen saturation of blood drawn through the catheter end hole while in the wedge position. If the oxygen saturation is lower than 95%, the balloon is likely "underwedged," leading to what is essentially a damped PA measurement. Conversely, the catheter can also be "overwedged," leading to a damped PAWP waveform (nearly flat) and an estimated PAWP pressure that is higher than the PA diastolic pressure. Thus, in cases where the mean PAWP exceeds the PA diastolic pressure, "overdamping" should be considered.

There are several situations in which the PAWP does not accurately reflect mean LA pressure. Important clinical situations that disrupt the PAWP-LA pressure relationship include cor triatriatum, pulmonary veno-occlusive disease, left atrial myxoma, and anomalous pulmonary venous return.[8] In the setting of inaccurate PAWP, left heart catheterization to measure LV end-diastolic pressure can be performed to measure left-sided filling pressures. Alternatively, transseptal puncture to directly measure the LA pressure can also be considered, but this is rarely performed in contemporary practice.

TABLE 40.4 Pulmonary Artery Wedge Pressure Waveform and Common Abnormalities

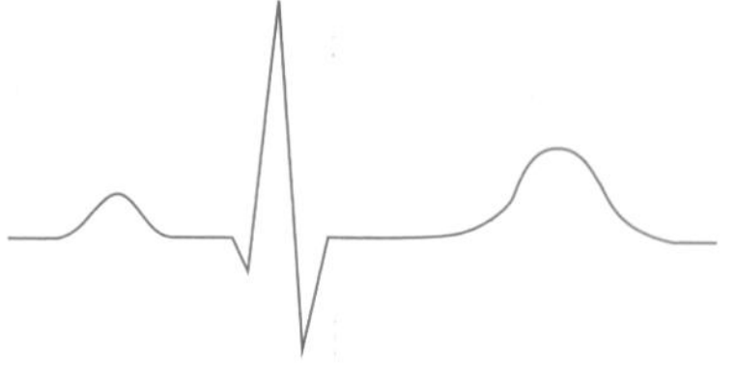

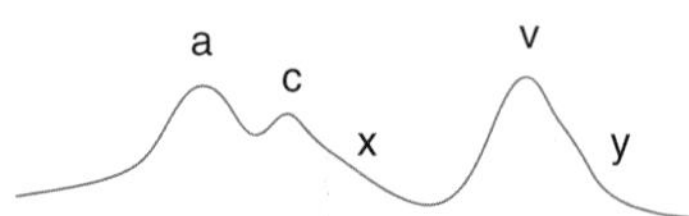

Elevated a wave	Equal a and v waves
• Mitral stenosis	• Tamponade
• Decreased LV compliance	• Constrictive pericarditis
Cannon a wave	**Prominent x descent**
• Third-degree AV block	• Tamponade
• Ventricular tachycardia	• LV ischemia
• Ventricular pacemaker	**Prominent y descent**
Absent a wave	• Mitral regurgitation
• Atrial fibrillation	• Constrictive pericarditis
• Junctional rhythm	• Restrictive myopathy
Elevated v wave	**Blunted x descent**
• Mitral regurgitation	• Atrial fibrillation
• LV failure	• LA ischemia
• Reduced LA compliance	**Blunted y descent**
• Right-to-left shunting	• Mitral stenosis
	• LV ischemia
	• Tamponade

AV, atrioventricular; LA, left atrium; LV, left ventricle.

A low PAWP is most commonly caused by hypovolemia, whereas an elevated PAWP may be caused by volume overload, valvular heart disease (mitral stenosis, mitral regurgitation, aortic stenosis, aortic regurgitation), LV failure (cardiomyopathy, ischemia), or cardiac tamponade.

Shunts

Intracardiac shunting can occur because of abnormal cardiac embryogenesis, persistent postnatal fetal communications, trauma, or mechanical complications of myocardial infarction. This includes atrial septal defects, ventricular septal defects, anomalous pulmonary venous return, and a patent ductus arteriosus. Typically, communication between the high-pressure left heart system and the low-pressure right heart system results in left-to-right shunting. This manifests as an abnormally elevated oxygen saturation, or "step-up," in right heart chambers and/or vessels, allowing for identification of the shunt (**Table 40.5**). By carefully measuring oxygen saturation in each great vessel or chamber, the location and magnitude of shunting can be determined. Meticulous measurements must be taken in multiple positions, including the vena cava, RA, RV, PA, and PAW, and systemic arterial oxygen saturation. With this information, the shunt fraction (Q_p/Q_s) of a left-to-right shunt can be calculated as follows:

$$\frac{Q_P}{Q_s} = \frac{(SaO_2 - SvO_2)}{(PvO_2 - PaO_2)}$$

Q_P = pulmonary blood flow, Q_s = systemic blood flow, SaO_2 = systemic arterial oxygen saturation,
SvO_2 = mixed venous oxygen saturation, PaO_2 = pulmonary arterial oxygen saturation
PvO_2 = pulmonary venous oxygen saturation. As it is not common to enter a pulmonary vein during right heart catheterization, systemic arterial oxygen content may be used in place of PvO_2, as long as there is no right-to-left shunting.

Under normal conditions, the ratio of pulmonary to systemic blood flow, or Q_p/Q_s, should be close to 1. At values greater than 1.5, there may be clinically significant left-to-right shunting, which, in symptomatic individuals, may warrant closure. Importantly, as noted in an elegant study by Hillis et al. evaluating intracardiac hemodynamics over a 28-year period, one-third to one-half of patients with left-to-right shunts have a significant step-up in oxygen saturation in multiple chambers, despite shunting at only one site.[8] They note, therefore, that if a patient has an intracardiac shunt in only one location by echocardiography, but has oximetric data suggesting shunting at multiple levels, further investigation may not be warranted. In contemporary practice, cardiac magnetic resonance imaging (MRI) can help to adjudicate discrepant echocardiographic and oximetric data.[9]

Cardiac Output

In addition to intracardiac pressure, the PA catheter allows for the estimation of cardiac output, which ranges from 4 to 8 L/min under normal conditions. The two primary approaches to estimate cardiac output are the Fick principle and the thermodilution method. Based on the concept of conservation of mass, Adolph Fick suggested that blood flow to an organ can be calculated by the uptake of oxygen by that organ, divided by the difference between the arterial and venous oxygen concentration. With the pulmonary circulation as a model and the assumption that pulmonary blood flow is insignificantly different from systemic blood flow, cardiac output can be estimated based on the following equation:

$$Q = \frac{VO_2}{CaO_2 - CvO_2}$$

Q = cardiac output, VO_2 = oxygen uptake, CaO_2 = arterial oxygen concentration, CvO_2 = venous oxygen concentration

TABLE 40.5 Shunt Run

Chamber	Criteria for Significant Step-up (Increase from Previous Chamber)		Potential Causes of Shunting
Inferior vena cava • Low (at L4-L5) • High (just at or below the diaphragm) **Superior vena cava** • Low (near RA junction) • High (near brachiocephalic vein)	Highest Value	Mean Value	
Right atrium • Low • Mid • High	≥11%	≥7%	ASD, PAPVR, VSD+TR
Right ventricle • Outflow tract • Mid • Tricuspid valve or apex	≥10%	≥5%	VSD, Ao-RV, PDA+PR
Pulmonary artery • Main PA • Left PA • Right PA	≥5%	≥5%	PDA, Ao-PA
Any level to PA	≥7%	≥8%	All of the above

Ao, aorta; ASD, atrial septal defect; L4-L5, 4th to 5th lumbar region; PA, pulmonary artery; PAPVR, partial anomalous pulmonary venous return; PDA, patent ductus arteriosus; PR, pulmonic regurgitation; RA, right atrium; RV, right ventricle; TR, tricuspid regurgitation; VSD, ventricular septal defect.

The direct Fick method requires measurement of oxygen consumption (VO_2), in addition to arterial and mixed venous O_2 concentrations and hemoglobin concentration. Historically, open-circuit spirometry was used to measure VO_2 by having patients breathe into a large Douglas bag, which collects all expired air over a one- to three-minute period.[10,11] The oxygen content of expired air in the Douglas bag was then compared with the known concentration of oxygen in inspired air. Given the cumbersome Douglas bag equipment, this method was used primarily in research laboratories. Thus, most clinical cardiac catheterization laboratories utilize an assumed VO_2 from published tables or predictive equations, but this method suffers from significant inaccuracy, particularly in unstable clinical settings.[10] However, routine measurement of oxygen consumption can be performed with the advent of modern metabolic carts, which utilize a portable device to measure VO_2 via facemask or mouthpiece.[12] These carts are less cumbersome than the Douglas bag method and allow for more accurate Fick cardiac output measurement than an assumed VO_2.

The second commonly used method of estimating cardiac output is thermodilution. In 1954, Fegler described the use of cold Ringer solution to determine the cardiac output of anesthetized dogs.[13] In its modern use, room temperature normal saline solution is injected through a proximal port of the catheter. A thermistor, typically located at the distal catheter tip, generates a time-temperature curve, with the area under this curve yielding a measurement of flow based on the Stewart-Hamilton equation.

$$Q = \frac{V_i\,(T_b - T_i)\,k}{\int \Delta T_b\, dt}$$

Q = cardiac output, V_i = volume of injectate, T_b = temperature of blood, T_i = temperature of injectate, k = correction factor for specific gravity and density of injectate and blood, $\int \Delta\, T_b\, dt$ = change in temperature over time (ie, time-temperature curve)

Two important conditions are assumed in order to make the required calculation: (1) constant blood flow, allowing complete mixing of the injectate and blood and (2) no loss of injectate between the injection port and thermistor. Important sources of error include variations in the volume of injectate, loss of solution, variations in temperature with the respiratory cycle. Limitations in thermodilution use include patients with very low cardiac output ($<$2 L/min) and patients with severe pulmonary or tricuspid regurgitation.[14]

Vascular Resistance

By determining intracardiac pressure and cardiac output, vascular resistance can be estimated. As described by Poiseuille in the 1800s, flow through a cylindrical vessel is determined by the pressure difference across the vessel, divided by resistance.[15] In Poiseuille equation, resistance is determined by several factors including vessel length, radius, and fluid viscosity. Thus, blood flow is determined by the pressure difference created by each cardiac cycle, divided by the dynamic resistance of the peripheral vasculature.

$$Q = \frac{\Delta P}{R} = \frac{\Delta P\, \pi\, r^4}{8\, L\, \eta}$$

Q = cardiac output, ΔP = pressure difference, R = resistance to flow
r = inside radius of the vessel, L = vessel length, η = blood viscosity

To estimate systemic vascular resistance (SVR), a measure of LV afterload, the pressure difference across the systemic circuit is calculated—by subtracting the mean right atrial pressure (mRAP) from the mean arterial pressure (MAP)—and divided by the systemic blood flow (ie, cardiac output [Q]).

$$\text{SVR} = \frac{\text{MAP} - \text{mRAP}}{\text{Q}}$$

Under normal conditions, SVR is 10 to 15 Wood units, which, when multiplied by 80, yields the metric conversion of 800 to 1200 $\text{dynes}\cdot\text{sec}\cdot\text{cm}^{-5}$. To maintain peripheral perfusion and oxygen delivery, SVR increases in response to hypovolemia, cardiogenic shock, and heart failure. Conversely, SVR decreases in response to high cardiac output and vasodilatory states, such as pregnancy, arteriovenous fistulae, cirrhosis, thyrotoxicosis, anaphylaxis, sepsis, and severe anemia.

The right heart and pulmonary system can be considered as a separate circuit. To estimate the PVR, pressure difference across the pulmonary circuit—PAWP is subtracted from mean PAP—is divided by pulmonary blood flow (which in the absence of left-to-right shunting is essentially equal to systemic blood flow [Q])

$$\text{PVR} = \frac{\text{mPAP} - \text{PAWP}}{\text{Q}}$$

Normal PVR is less than 3 Wood units, equal to 240 $\text{dynes}\cdot\text{sec}\cdot\text{cm}^{-5}$. An elevated PVR most commonly represents sequelae of left-sided heart disease, such as heart failure, or intrinsic lung disease, such as chronic obstructive pulmonary disease. Importantly, an elevated PVR is requisite in diagnosing pulmonary hypertension, either primary or owing to a variety of etiologies, such as viral infections, connective tissue disease, and pulmonary emboli. Furthermore, in patients with long-standing left-to-right shunting, the Eisenmenger syndrome can occur, with pulmonary vascular remodeling caused by chronic right-sided volume overload.

Valve Area. The degree of valvular stenosis is determined by echocardiographic estimation of two parameters: the transvalvular gradient and the valve area. However, in cases of insufficient or conflicting noninvasive data, or when additional information is needed to plan for valvular intervention, right and left heart catheterization can be used to directly measure the transvalvular gradient and calculate valve area. This relies on the Gorlin equation, which estimates valve area based on the relationship between the pressure gradient and flow.[16]

$$\text{AVA} = \frac{Q}{\text{SEP} \times \text{HR} \times 44.3 \times \sqrt{\text{MG}}}$$

Q = cardiac output, SEP = systolic ejection period, HR = heart rate, MG = mean gradient

Originally derived from patients with mitral stenosis, the Gorlin equation is most commonly used in clinical practice to assess the aortic valve, particularly in the era of transcatheter aortic valve replacement. Computer systems are able to automatically calculate valve area when provided the appropriate input data, including mean gradient and cardiac output. However, a more simplified equation can be used to quickly calculate the valve area. The Hakki equation relies on only two variables, the cardiac output and the peak-to-peak gradient, to estimate valve area.[17]

$$\text{AVA} = \frac{Q}{\sqrt{\text{PG}}}$$

Q = cardiac output, PG = peak left ventricular to peak aortic gradient

The Hakki equation may be inaccurate at extremes of heart rate (ie, <60 or >100 bpm).

In sum, right heart catheterization allows measurement of intracardiac pressures, cardiac output, and valvular gradients from which one can calculate vascular resistance and estimate valve area. Furthermore, comparative data evaluating not just the static chamber pressures, but their relation to other chambers and variation during the respiratory cycle, can allow us to differentiate other causes of shortness of breath, including pericardial constriction and restrictive cardiomyopathy (**Table 40.6**).

TABLE 40.6 Hemodynamics of Constrictive Pericarditis versus Restrictive Cardiomyopathy

	Constrictive Pericarditis	Restrictive Cardiomyopathy
Equalization of filling pressures	+	Left-sided pressures tend to be 3-5 mm Hg > right
RV/LV interdependence	Discordance	Concordance
Prominent "y" descent	+	±
"Square root" sign	+	±
PASP > 50 mm Hg	−	±
PAWP > 25 mm Hg	Less likely	Common
RVSP/RVEDP	<3	>3

LV, left ventricle; PASP, pulmonary artery systolic pressure; PAWP, pulmonary artery wedge pressure; RV, right ventricle; RVEDP, right ventricular end-diastolic pressure; RVSP, right ventricular systolic pressure; .

Mechanical Circulatory Support

Cardiogenic shock remains one of the most difficult to manage clinical conditions, with mortality approaching 50%.[18] Patients can present in extremis, often requiring advanced therapies, including inotropes, vasopressors, and mechanical circulatory support. New algorithms, including the National Cardiogenic Shock Initiative (NCSI), advocate for the use of right heart catheterization to guide the use of advanced therapies for right- and left-sided ventricular support.[19] In addition to the standard measured/calculated parameters noted above, important parameters to consider in this situation include CPO and pulmonary artery pulsatility index (PAPi) (**Table 40.7**).

$$\text{CPO} = \frac{Q \times \text{MAP}}{451}$$

Q = cardiac output, CPO = cardiac power output, MAP = mean arterial pressure

$$\text{PAPi} = \frac{\text{PASP} - \text{PADP}}{Q}$$

PAPi = pulmonary artery pulsatility index, PASP = pulmonary artery systolic pressure, PADP = pulmonary artery diastolic pressure, Q = cardiac output

CPO describes the rate of the heart's energy output and is the strongest hemodynamic correlate of outcomes in this critically ill population.[20,21] This parameter is primarily used

TABLE 40.7 Measure of Right Ventricular Function

Parameter	Calculation	Normal Value
RAP/PAWP		<0.63
Stroke volume index	CI/HR × 1000	33-47 mL/m²/beat
RV stroke work index	(MAP − RAP) × SVI	300-900 mm Hg · mL/m²
PA pulsatility index	(PASP − PADP)/RAP	>1.0
Pulmonary vascular resistance	(MPAP − PAWP)/CO	<3 Wood Units

CI, Cardiac index; CO, cardiac output; MPAP, Mean pulmonary artery pressure; PA, pulmonary artery; PAWP, pulmonary artery wedge pressure; RAP right atrial pressure; RV, right ventricle; SVI, Stroke volume index.

SECTION 3

to understand the complex state of LV performance. The current iteration of the NCSI algorithm advocates for the use of 0.6 as a threshold value for CPO, below which LV support (Impella 2.5/CP/5.0/5.5 [Abiomed, Danvers, MA, USA], TandemHeart device [Cardiac Assist Inc, Pittsburgh, PA, USA], extracorporeal membrane oxygenation) should be considered. Similarly, PAPi aids in understanding right ventricular performance, with a threshold value of 0.9, below which right ventricular support (Impella RP [Abiomed, Danvers, MA, USA], Protek Duo [TandemLife, Pittsburg, PA, USA], extracorporeal membrane oxygenation), can be considered. Conversely, when considering when/how to wean hemodynamic support (including mechanical circulatory support, inotropes, and vasopressors), CPO should be greater than 0.6, and PAPi > 0.9.[19]

Thus, right heart catheterization provides a wealth of clinical information in patients ranging from stable heart failure to cardiogenic shock in extremis. When performed appropriately, it is an invaluable clinical tool with power to guide clinical care and therapeutic implementation.

SPECIAL CONSIDERATIONS AND CONTRAINDICATIONS

As noted previously, when done at the bedside without the use of fluoroscopic guidance, the right internal jugular and left subclavian venous approaches allow for advancement of the balloon-tipped Swan-Ganz catheter to the PA based on hemodynamic tracing alone. All other access sites generally require the use of fluoroscopy to visualize the placement of the catheter to the intracardiac positions.

In patients with coagulopathy or blood dyscrasias, the brachial approach is preferred as it is a compressible site. Strict contraindications to right heart catheterization include access to vessels with known thrombus, right-sided endocarditis, and right-sided mechanical valves. Relative contraindications include the presence of recently placed pacemaker or defibrillator leads owing to risk of dislodgement. Recent PE is also a relative contraindication. Patients with known left bundle branch block on ECG may have external pacing/defibrillator pads in place, given the risk of transient complete heart block with the passage of a catheter through the RV, though this risk appears to be low (<3%).[22] In patients with retained inferior vena cava filters, the femoral approach is relatively contraindicated.

FOLLOW-UP PATIENT CARE

In general, once hemostasis is achieved, postprocedure follow-up care is dependent on the vascular access site. From the brachial approach, general wound care for the site is the only requirement. After internal jugular or subclavian access, generally chest X-ray is recommended to evaluate for pneumothorax, although this is becoming less routinely done with the generalization of ultrasound guidance for internal jugular venous access. After femoral venous access, bedrest for 2 to 4 hours is advised.

RESEARCH AND FUTURE DIRECTIONS

Over the past several years, there has been significant emphasis on the optimization of the management of cardiogenic shock. The Detroit Cardiogenic Shock Initiative assessed the feasibility of early mechanical support in patients with acute myocardial infarction and cardiogenic shock.[23] This protocol utilized a mutually agreed upon protocol with invasive hemodynamic monitoring and initiation of mechanical circulatory support. In all patients, right heart catheterization was performed to assess Fick cardiac output and filling pressures to guide Impella insertion for mechanical circulatory support prior to coronary angiography and percutaneous coronary intervention. Postintervention, CPO and PAPi were calculated based on the invasive hemodynamics to help guide weaning of vasopressors/inotropes or escalation of support. In this study, based on this shock protocol, they reported improved survival in patients who presented with acute myocardial infarction complicated by cardiogenic shock. Additionally, the NCSI, a multicenter protocol, has been initiated based on these data.[19] The Society for Cardiovascular Angiography and Interventions (SCAI) has also recently developed a clinical expert consensus statement on the classification of cardiogenic shock, with stages A-E, ranging from "at risk" to "extremis." The use of intracardiac hemodynamics via right heart catheterization to assess filling pressures, cardiac output, CPO, and PAPi can now be used to classify the stage of cardiogenic shock.[24] This will hopefully be used in the future to better define the disease state and potentially tailor therapy and use of mechanical circulatory support devices to optimize clinical outcomes.

KEY POINTS

- ✔ Use a superior vena cava (SVC) saturation rather than RA saturation for comparison to the PA saturation when confirming the absence of intracardiac shunting.
- ✔ For placement of a ballon-tipped catheter in the PA, insert a 0.014-inch coronary guidewire into the lumen if needed to navigate tortuosity from the brachial venous approach.
- ✔ For insertion from the femoral approach: once in the RA, point the balloon-tipped catheter at the lateral wall of the RA and make a loop within the RA to help direct the catheter toward the RVOT rather than the RV apex.
- ✔ Check a wedge saturation (>95%) to confirm PAWP.
- ✔ If the PAWP is not accurate, perform a left heart catheterization to assess left-sided filling pressures (ie, LV end-diastolic pressure).

REFERENCES

1. Forrester JS. A tale of serendipity, ingenuity, and chance: 50th anniversary of creation of the Swan-Ganz Catheter. *J Am Coll Cardiol.* 2019;74(1):100-103. doi:10.1016/j.jacc.2019.04.050
2. Swan HJC, Ganz W, Forrester J, Marcus H, Diamond G, Chonette D. Catheterization of the heart in man with use of a flow-directed

balloon-tipped catheter. *N Engl J Med.* 1970;283(9):447-451. doi:10.1056/NEJM197008272830902

3. Callan P, Clark AL. Invasive imaging: cardiac catheterization and angiography. Right heart catheterisation: indications and interpretation. *Heart.* 2016;102:147-157. doi:10.1136/heartjnl-2015-307786
4. Rogers T, Lederman RJ. Right heart catheterization from the arm: back to first principles. *Catheter Cardiovasc Interv.* 2014;84(1):75-76. doi:10.1002/ccd.25531
5. Mueller HS, Chatterjee K, Davis KB, et al. Present use of bedside right heart catheterization in patients with cardiac disease. *J Am Coll Cardiol.* 1998;32(3):840-864. doi:10.1016/S0735-1097(98)00327-1
6. Rab T, Ratanapo S, Kern KB, et al. Cardiac shock care centers: JACC review topic of the week. *J Am Coll Cardiol.* 2018;72(16):1972-1980. doi:10.1016/j.jacc.2018.07.074
7. Nishimura RA, Carabello BA. Hemodynamics in the cardiac catheterization laboratory of the 21st century. *Circulation.* 2012;125(17):2138-2150. doi:10.1161/CIRCULATIONAHA.111.060319
8. Ahmed S, Lange RA, Hillis LD. Inaccuracies of oximetry in identifying the location of intracardiac left-to-right shunts in adults. *Am J Cardiol.* 2008;101(2):245-247. doi:10.1016/j.amjcard.2007.07.071
9. Hundley WG, Li HF, Lange RA, et al. Assessment of left-to-right intracardiac shunting by velocity-encoded, phase-difference magnetic resonance imaging. *Circulation.* 1995;91(12):2955-2960. doi:10.1161/01.CIR.91.12.2955
10. Narang N, Thibodeau JT, Levine BD, et al. Inaccuracy of estimated resting oxygen uptake in the clinical setting. *Circulation.* 2014;129(2):203-210. doi:10.1161/CIRCULATIONAHA.113.003334
11. Dehmer GJ, Firth BG, Hillis LD. Oxygen consumption in adult patients during cardiac catheterization. *Clin Cardiol.* 1982;5(8):436-440. doi:10.1002/clc.4960050803
12. Fanari Z, Grove M, Rajamanickam A, et al. Cardiac output determination using a widely available direct continuous oxygen consumption measuring device: a practical way to get back to the gold standard. *Cardiovasc Revasc Med.* 2016;17(4):256-261. doi:10.1016/j.carrev.2016.02.013
13. Fegler G. Measurement of cardiac output in anaesthetized animals by a thermo-dilution method. *Q J Exp Physiol Cogn Med Sci.* 1954;39(3):153-164. doi:10.1113/expphysiol.1954.sp001067
14. Argueta EE, Paniagua D. Thermodilution cardiac output. *Cardiol Rev.* 2019;27(3):138-144. doi:10.1097/CRD.0000000000000223
15. Sutera SP, Skalak R. The history of Poiseuille's Law. Published 1993. Accessed October 6, 2020. https://www.annualreviews.org/doi/abs/10.1146/annurev.fl.25.010193.000245
16. Gorlin R, Gorlin SG. Hydraulic formula for calculation of the area of the stenotic mitral valve, other cardiac valves, and central circulatory shunts. I. *Am Heart J.* 1951;41(1):1-29. doi:10.1016/0002-8703(51)90002-6
17. Hakki AH, Iskandrian AS, Bemis CE, et al. A simplified valve formula for the calculation of stenotic cardiac valve areas. *Circulation.* 1981;63(5):1050-1055. doi:10.1161/01.CIR.63.5.1050
18. Helgestad OKL, Josiassen J, Hassager C, et al. Contemporary trends in use of mechanical circulatory support in patients with acute MI and cardiogenic shock. *Open Heart.* 2020;7(1):e001214. doi:10.1136/openhrt-2019-001214
19. Basir MB, Kapur NK, Patel K, et al. Improved outcomes associated with the use of shock protocols: updates from the National Cardiogenic Shock Initiative. *Catheter Cardiovasc Interv.* 2019;93(7):1173-1183. doi:10.1002/ccd.28307
20. Lim HS. Cardiac power output revisited. *Circ Heart Fail.* 2020;13(10):e007393. doi:10.1161/CIRCHEARTFAILURE.120.007393
21. Fincke R, Hochman JS, Lowe AM, et al. Cardiac power is the strongest hemodynamic correlate of mortality in cardiogenic shock: a report from the SHOCK trial registry. *J Am Coll Cardiol.* 2004;44(2):340-348. doi:10.1016/j.jacc.2004.03.060
22. Sprung CL, Elser B, Schein RMH, Marcial EH, Schrager BR. Risk of right bundle-branch block and complete heart block during pulmonary artery catheterization. *Crit Care Med.* 1989;17(1):1-3. doi:10.1097/00003246-198901000-00001
23. Basir MB, Schreiber T, Dixon S, et al. Feasibility of early mechanical circulatory support in acute myocardial infarction complicated by cardiogenic shock: The Detroit cardiogenic shock initiative. *Catheter Cardiovasc Interv.* 2018;91(3):454-461. doi:10.1002/ccd.27427
24. Baran DA, Grines CL, Bailey S, et al. SCAI clinical expert consensus statement on the classification of cardiogenic shock: this document was endorsed by the American College of Cardiology (ACC), the American Heart Association (AHA), the Society of Critical Care Medicine (SCCM), and the Society of Thoracic Surgeons (STS) in April 2019. *Catheter Cardiovasc Interv.* 2019;94(1):29-37. doi:10.1002/ccd.28329

CHAPTER 41

DIAGNOSTIC CORONARY AND PULMONARY ANGIOGRAPHY AND LEFT VENTRICULOGRAPHY

Jennifer A. Rymer, Sunil V. Rao, Richard A. Krasuski, and Rajesh V. Swaminathan

INTRODUCTION

The first selective diagnostic coronary angiogram was performed by Dr. Mason Sones in 1958 while attempting to inject contrast into the ascending aorta. He inadvertently injected the right coronary artery (RCA) selectively with 30 mL of contrast media.[1] Since that time, rapid developments have been made in the evolution of diagnostic coronary angiography and percutaneous coronary intervention (PCI), driven partly by catheter and stent development. This chapter outlines the indications and relative contraindications for performing diagnostic angiography, the various techniques for vascular access, and the potential complications of using these approaches. Also presented are the concepts surrounding radiation safety, including various measures of radiation dosage, and preventative measures to reduce exposure to both patient and operator. Finally, we present the most appropriate techniques to assess coronary, left ventriculography, and pulmonary artery (PA) angiography.

INDICATIONS

Before performing diagnostic coronary angiography, it is critical to determine whether the patient has an appropriate indication for the procedure.[2]

Suspected or Known Coronary Artery Disease

Patients with ST-segment elevation myocardial infarction (STEMI), non–ST-segment elevation myocardial infarction (NSTEMI), unstable angina, and cardiogenic shock with suspected acute coronary syndrome meet indications for diagnostic coronary angiography. In the absence of prior history of PCI, coronary artery bypass grafting (CABG), or known lesion greater than or equal to 50%, the use of diagnostic coronary angiography is considered inappropriate in asymptomatic patients with low or intermediate global coronary artery disease (CAD) risk and in symptomatic patients with low pretest probability. In symptomatic patients with high pretest probability, proceeding to coronary angiography before noninvasive testing is generally considered an appropriate strategy. In patients with a prior history of revascularization or known obstructive coronary disease on a prior angiogram, it is appropriate to perform coronary angiography if the patient has either intermediate-risk or high-risk noninvasive findings and worsening symptoms.

Arrhythmias

In patients with cardiac arrest for whom there is return of spontaneous circulation and for patients who have ventricular fibrillation or sustained ventricular tachycardia, diagnostic coronary angiography is indicated to assess for ischemic etiologies. The results of the recent COACT (COronary Angiography after Cardiac Arrest) trial demonstrated that there was no significant difference in 90-day survival for patients who had an out-of-hospital cardiac arrest with no evidence of a STEMI with regard to an immediate versus delayed strategy for coronary angiography.[3] In patients with new-onset atrial fibrillation/flutter or heart block with low- or intermediate-CAD risk, diagnostic coronary angiography is not indicated.

Valvular Heart Disease

For adult patients undergoing a preoperative assessment before valvular surgery, diagnostic coronary angiography with right heart catheterization is generally indicated. For patients with pulmonary hypertension or left ventricular (LV) dysfunction out of proportion to the severity of valvular heart disease, right heart catheterization, or diagnostic coronary angiography with right heart catheterization may be considered.

Other Indications

Right heart catheterization with or without coronary angiography/left ventriculography is often indicated in patients with newly diagnosed or suspected cardiomyopathy with or without heart failure. In situations where there has been a change in clinical status and hemodynamics are necessary, right heart catheterization is helpful. In cases of suspected constrictive or restrictive physiology, right and left heart catheterization may be necessary to assess hemodynamics.

CONTRAINDICATIONS TO CORONARY ANGIOGRAPHY

Although there are no true absolute contraindications to coronary angiography, there are multiple relative contraindications (**Table 41.1**).[4] Among those listed here, several warrant further discussion. In patients with documented prior anaphylactic reaction to contrast media, proceeding with coronary angiography is likely safe if the patient is first premedicated with a steroid and antihistamine. A common steroid preparation

TABLE 41.1 Relative Contraindications to Diagnostic Coronary Angiography

Severe or worsening anemia
Ongoing or active infection or fever
Active bleeding
Acute renal failure or advanced chronic kidney disease
Hypertensive urgency or emergency
Acute ischemic or hemorrhagic stroke
Comorbidities or concomitant illness with a shortened life expectancy
Electrolyte imbalances
Anaphylactic reaction to contrast agent
Aortic valve endocarditis or thrombosis
Acute pulmonary edema
Severe coagulopathy
Difficult or limited vascular access (ie, severe peripheral vascular disease)
Difficulty of the patient to cooperate with the procedure (because of advanced dementia, delirium, or psychological comorbidities)
Lack of patient consent

Adapted from Scanlon PJ, Faxon DP, Audet AM, et al. ACC/AHA guidelines for coronary angiography. A report of the American College of Cardiology/American Heart Association Task Force on practice guidelines (Committee on Coronary Angiography) developed in collaboration with the Society for Cardiac Angiography and Interventions. *J Am Coll Cardiol*. 1999;33(6):1756-1824. Copyright © 1999 American College of Cardiology. With permission.

includes 50 mg of oral prednisone at 13 hours, 7 hours, and 1 hour before expected contrast media injection, in addition to 50 mg intravenous (IV) diphenhydramine 1 hour before contrast media injection. Another potential regimen includes 32 mg oral methylprednisolone 12 and 2 hours before contrast media injection, in addition to an IV antihistamine.[5,6]

In patients with acute renal failure, unless there is a compelling need for urgent or emergent coronary angiography, the procedure should be deferred until dysfunction resolves. Preprocedure hydration protocols are discussed in the section "Special Considerations." For patients on oral anticoagulation, diagnostic angiography may be delayed depending on the degree of anticoagulation, or a radial artery approach may be pursued if urgently/emergently indicated. In emergent cases such as STEMI, relative contraindications may not be evident before the procedure. It is therefore always wise to utilize techniques that limit risks such as bleeding and acute kidney injury. Other relative contraindications do not preclude diagnostic coronary angiography, but may impact timing.

ANATOMIC CONSIDERATIONS

Femoral Artery Access

Femoral artery access is increasingly being replaced with radial artery access as operators change their practice because of patient preference and a decreased risk of bleeding. However, femoral access is still used, particularly for mechanical support devices and large-bore catheters, and in some patients, may be the only route of access. Therefore, appropriate technique is critical to avoid vascular complications and bleeding.

The external iliac artery becomes the common femoral artery (CFA) after passing under the inguinal ligament. Femoral arterial puncture should occur above the bifurcation of the CFA into the deep femoral artery (also known as the profunda femoris artery) and the superficial femoral artery (SFA), but below the inferior epigastric artery takeoff from the external iliac artery (**Figure 41.1**). High punctures may result in a greater risk of retroperitoneal bleed, especially if the inferior epigastric artery is punctured. Low punctures may result in pseudoaneurysms, dissection, or arteriovenous fistulae.

In most patients, the ideal puncture site lies between the superior and inferior borders of the femoral head. As such, most operators will palpate the pulse and determine where the maximal point of impulse occurs within the borders of the head of the femur using fluoroscopic guidance. Because anatomy varies between patients, ultrasound guidance can be useful to identify the CFA bifurcation, look for calcification, and assess the dimensions of the CFA (particularly helpful if large-bore access is required).

Traditionally, femoral access was obtained using the Seldinger technique, which involved a posterior wall stick and withdrawal of the access needle until pulsatile arterial flow was visualized. Because a posterior wall stick increased the risk of bleeding and access site complications, the technique has evolved such that an anterior wall stick is now the accepted manner of obtaining femoral access. After determining the ideal access site, the operator should administer local anesthetic (typically 1% lidocaine) to reduce discomfort. The anesthetic should be injected to the depth of the femoral artery. Traditionally, an 18-gauge needle is utilized to obtain access and a 0.035″ J-tip wire is then delivered through the needle into the vascular lumen. After removal of the needle, the sheath with its dilator can be delivered over the 0.035″ wire, with subsequent removal of the dilator.

Many operators now utilize a micropuncture kit (**Figure 41.2**) for femoral access.[7] With this method, a 21-gauge needle is used to obtain arterial access, and a 0.018″ wire is advanced through the needle lumen with its position confirmed fluoroscopically. The needle is then removed, and a 4-Fr sheath with introducer is inserted over the wire. The guide wire and introducer are removed, and a 0.035″ J-tip wire is passed through the 4-Fr sheath. The 4-Fr sheath may then be removed and upsized (typically 5 Fr or 6 Fr for diagnostic angiography) over the wire. A single-center, randomized trial of femoral micropuncture access versus standard 18-gauge access found no significant difference in vascular complications, including retroperitoneal bleeds, arteriovenous fistulae, pseudoaneurysms, and arterial perforations requiring intervention.[7] This study, however, was underpowered. Nevertheless, prespecified subgroups including female patients and those with final sheath sizes less than or equal to 6 Fr showed significant or near-significant reductions in complications with micropuncture access.

There is increasing evidence to suggest that obtaining femoral access via ultrasound guidance reduces the number of access attempts and potential complications. The Femoral Arterial Access with Ultrasound Trial (FAUST) is the largest randomized trial of patients undergoing CFA cannulation via ultrasound guidance compared to fluoroscopic guidance.[8] A significant improvement in first-pass success rate (83% vs. 46%, $P < .0001$), reduction in the number of access

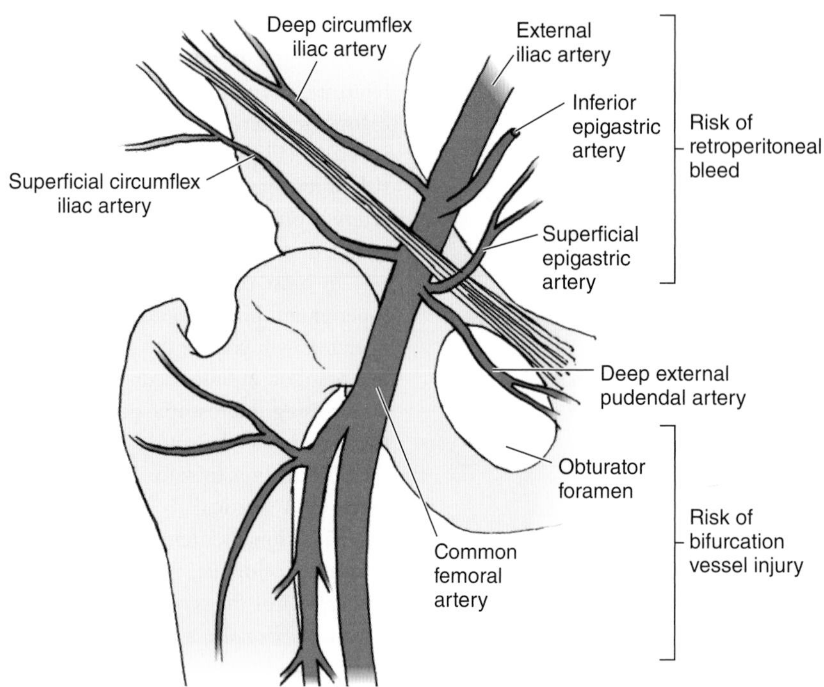

FIGURE 41.1 Femoral artery anatomy for cardiac catheterization access. Bony landmarks are useful for identifying the level of the common femoral artery. The inguinal ligament runs between the pubic tubercle and the anterior superior iliac spine, marking the top of the common femoral artery. High puncture or laceration of the inferior epigastric artery can lead to serious retroperitoneal bleeding. Puncture at or below the femoral bifurcation is also to be avoided. (Reprinted with permission from Rasmussen TE, Clouse WD, Tonnessen BH. *Handbook of Patient Care in Vascular Diseases.* 6th ed. Philadelphia, PA: Wolters Kluwer; 2018. Figure 9.1.)

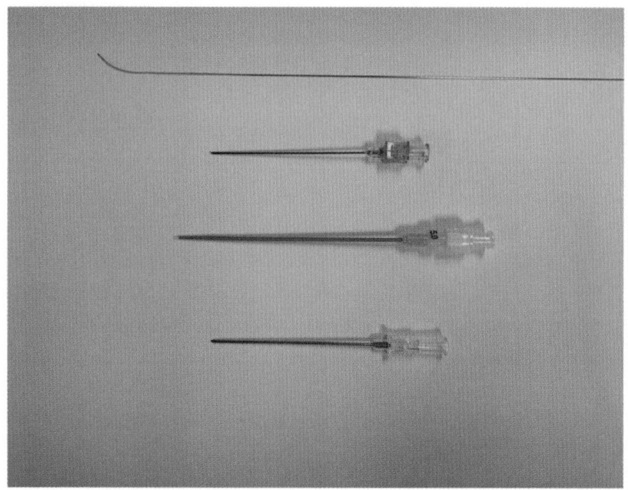

FIGURE 41.2 Illustration depicting micropuncture needle and dilator alongside an 18-gauge needle (In descending order: Micropuncture 0.018 inch guidewire, Micropuncture needle 21 gauge, Micropuncture dilatator, Standard 18-gauge arterial needle.)

attempts (1.3 vs. 3.0, $P < .0001$), and median time to access (136 seconds vs. 148 seconds, $P = .003$) was found using ultrasound. Vascular complications were also significantly reduced using ultrasound.

After obtaining successful femoral access, it is important to document a femoral angiogram. For patients with significant tortuosity, a femoral and abdominal angiogram may help decide whether a longer sheath should be utilized. A femoral angiogram can also help determine whether a vascular closure device is appropriate, because it allows for an assessment of sheath insertion site, arterial size, any access site complications, and calcification. The angiogram should be performed with the 0.035″ access wire in place to prevent the distal end of the access sheath from contacting the arterial wall and causing a retrograde dissection during angiography. A femoral angiogram can also be performed via the micropuncture sheath for the purposes of documenting an appropriate entry site before insertion of a larger sheath or inserting mechanical circulatory support.

Radial Artery Access

Although the rates of adoption of radial artery access in the United States have rapidly increased over the past decade, it still lags behind many European countries.[9,10] Although only 1.32% of PCI was performed radially from 2004 to 2007, use grew to 16% by 2011. Most recently, radial artery access has been estimated to account for up to 50% of coronary angiography[11] and it is expected to surpass femoral access over the next decade.

The brachial artery gives rise to the radial and ulnar arteries near the antecubital fossa (**Figure 41.3**). Most commonly, radial artery access is obtained with an angiocatheter or Cook needle (Cook Medical LLC, Bloomington, IN) a few

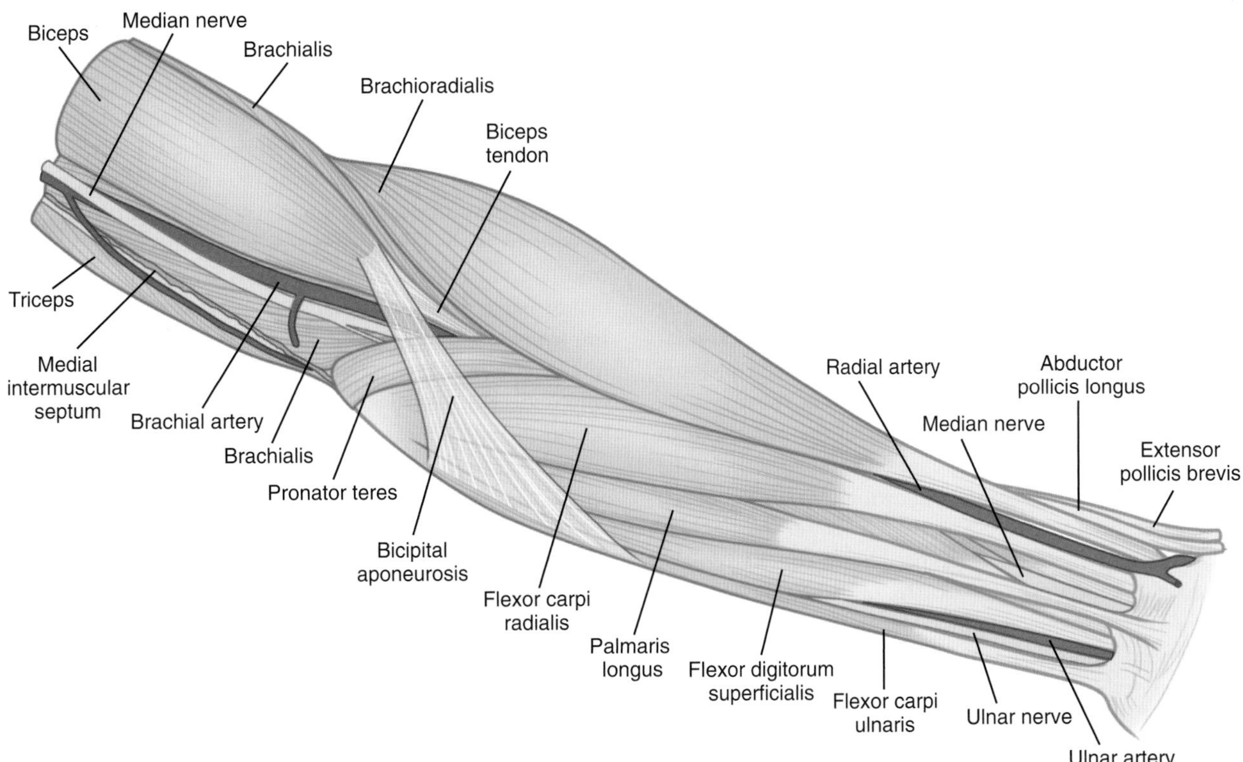

FIGURE 41.3 Anatomy of the anterior aspect of the forearm. Superficial layer of the forearm muscles. Note the position of the radial artery between the brachioradialis and flexor carpi radialis distally. (Reprinted with permission from Court-Brown CM, Heckman JD, McQueen MM, et al. *Rockwood and Green's Fractures in Adults.* 8th ed. Philadelphia, PA: Wolters Kluwer; 2015. Figure 33.16A.)

centimeters proximal to the wrist. Unlike femoral access where an anterior wall stick is the optimal approach, successful radial artery access is best obtained when the traditional Seldinger technique is used, advancing the needle "through and through" and withdrawing until the arterial flash is visualized. After passing a wire through the angiocatheter lumen, a standard 5- to 7-Fr sheath is inserted over the wire. Various radial "cocktails" including calcium channel blockers or nitrates are administered through the sheath to reduce the risk of arterial spasm. Unfractionated heparin is also administered to reduce the risk of radial occlusion.

There are several factors to consider when utilizing radial artery access for coronary angiography. If a patient has three or more of the following criteria, left radial is preferred over right radial artery access,[12,13] because it is more likely to be successful owing to lesser subclavian artery tortuosity[14]: age 70 years or older, female sex, height less than or equal to 64 inches, or hypertension. In patients with a prior history of CABG, left radial access is preferred because of ease of injection of the left internal mammary (IM) artery and vein grafts. In patients with a right IM graft, right radial artery access may be necessary. Although radial spasm can easily be managed with verapamil and increased sedation, it is best to inquire preprocedurally about previous prohibitive radial artery spasm and provide appropriate medications prophylactically.

As with femoral access, there is increasing evidence that ultrasound guidance is beneficial for radial artery access. In the Radial Artery access with Ultrasound Trial (RAUST), investigators randomized patients to undergo radial artery access via palpation compared to ultrasound guidance.[15] Use of ultrasound resulted in fewer access attempts and the first-pass success rate was significantly improved. Radial ultrasound may also help inform whether a larger sheath size (ie, 7 Fr) is possible in certain patients depending on vessel diameter. The PRIMAFACIE-TRI (Pre-procedure ultrasound IMaging of the Arm to FACIlitatE TRansradial coronary and diagnostic Interventional procedures) study examined the use of routine preprocedural ultrasound of the arm arteries to examine arm anatomy and increase procedural success,[16] and showed that procedural success using transradial or transulnar access was more likely to be successful with improved outcomes when preprocedural ultrasound was used. In some patients, examination of the arm arteries before coronary angiography will reveal a larger ulnar artery compared with the radial artery, so that transulnar access may be preferred to transradial access.

Complications of Radial Artery Access

Although bleeding complication rates are lower with radial than with femoral access, there are several potential complications of radial artery access. The primary cause of failure in transradial coronary angiography is radial artery spasm. If the sheath diameter is greater than the diameter of the patient's radial artery, radial artery stretch results in increasing vasomotor tone, leading to arterial spasm. Patients at higher risk of spasm include women, those with small wrist circumference, and younger age.[17] If significant spasm develops, device entrapment may occur. In this case, increasing force should not be used to remove equipment because this may result in avulsion of the artery. Instead, deeper sedation, local anesthetics, and additional verapamil or nitroglycerin may aid in reducing spasm. The flow-mediated vasodilation technique may also facilitate device removal.[18] In this technique, a blood pressure cuff is inflated in the upper arm to 40 mm Hg above systolic pressure for several minutes. Brisk release of the cuff results in a rapid increase in flow and vasodilation through nitric oxide release and endothelial relaxation, allowing for removal of the entrapped device.

Radial artery occlusion is another known complication of radial access, and occurs in 1% to 10% of patients undergoing transradial coronary angiography.[19] Sheath insertion can result in radial artery endothelial damage and subsequent thrombosis with arterial occlusion. Administration of 50 to 100 U/kg IV heparin once the 0.035" guidewire is successfully positioned in the ascending aorta is one strategy that significantly reduces radial artery occlusion, with evidence that high-dose heparin (100 U/kg) significantly reduces the risk compared with standard-dose heparin (50 U/kg).[20,21] The risk of radial artery occlusion is also reduced with the use of patent hemostasis,[22,23] as well as ipsilateral ulnar compression.[24] An indication of radial artery occlusion[25] may be the persistence of arm pain after the procedure, or absence of a radial pulse. However, patients may have occlusion without the loss of a radial pulse, because there may be collateral flow from the anterior interosseous artery, giving the false impression of a radial pulse. To diagnose radial artery occlusion, Doppler ultrasonography may be used, or the reverse Barbeau test, performed by occluding the ulnar artery and placing an oximeter on the ipsilateral thumb; the absence of a plethysmographic waveform indicates radial artery occlusion.

Radial artery pseudoaneurysms and arteriovenous fistulas are infrequent complications, and can usually be monitored if small and asymptomatic. Prolonged compression with a radial hemostasis device often resolves most radial artery pseudoaneurysms. If prolonged compression fails, then surgical treatment can be generally performed under local anesthesia with high success rates. A very rare complication of transradial cardiac catheterization is upper extremity compartment syndrome. In these cases, early consultation with vascular surgery is imperative.

Radial versus Femoral Artery Access

There is a large body of observational and trial data that has focused on comparing the outcomes of radial and femoral access. In patients presenting with an acute coronary syndrome, particularly in the subset presenting with STEMI, there is evidence for improved outcomes with radial access. In the RadIal Versus FemoraL RandomizED Investigation in ST-Segment Elevation Acute Coronary Syndrome (RIFLE-STEACS) study, the composite outcome of net adverse clinical events and cardiac death was reduced significantly in patients who had radial access.[26] Similarly, the RIVAL (RadIal vs. FemoraL Access for Coronary Intervention) study demonstrated a significant reduction in the primary composite outcome of death, myocardial infarction, stroke and non–CABG-related major bleeding in patients with STEMI but not in patients with NSTEMI who had radial access.[27] The MATRIX (Minimizing Adverse hemorrhagic events by TRansradial access site and systemic Implementation of angioX) trial, however, showed a reduction in all-cause mortality in patients with STEMI and NSTEMI who underwent radial access.[28] In general, radial access should be considered for most patients requiring a diagnostic coronary angiogram, particularly in patients presenting with a STEMI after operator proficiency is attained.

FUNDAMENTALS OF DIAGNOSTIC CORONARY ANGIOGRAPHY (FLUOROSCOPY AND RADIATION SAFETY)

Dosage Rates

There are several important measures of radiation exposure that are important to know. In general, *fluoroscopy time* is the most simplistic measure of radiation exposure and does not account for the fluoroscopic dose rate. Dose rates vary greatly depending on individual patient factors such as obesity. Obese patients require increased x-ray entry doses to form an image, and the obese patient is at greater risk of developing skin injury than is a thin patient who undergoes a procedure with the same *fluoroscopy time*.

KERMA, which is an acronym for "kinetic energy released per unit mass," is a radiation measure of the energy or radiation dose delivered, and represents the kinetic energy released in matter. The interventional reference point (or the dose reference point) estimates the position of the patient's skin during the procedure, and is approximately 15 cm from the isocenter. Instantaneous KERMA is a measure of beam intensity, whereas cumulative KERMA is a measure of the cumulative radiation dose to the skin. KERMA is an important measure of *deterministic risk*, where the severity of the risk is dose related. Skin injury is an example of a deterministic effect of radiation. Air KERMA (AK) is described in units of Gy.

Dose area product (DAP) is the radiation dose times the area of the irradiated field. DAP is thus a measure of the total amount of radiation exiting the tube. DAP is an important measure for *stochastic risk*, where the severity of the risk is not dose related, but the probability of an effect occurring can increase with dose. Cancer, related to DNA injury, is an example of a stochastic effect of radiation. DAP is measured in Gy*cm^2.

Radiation Complications and Strategies for Risk Reduction

Skin injury is an example of a deterministic risk of radiation exposure. Between 2 and 5 Gy, patients can experience erythema related to radiation exposure. Over 10 Gy, patients can experience permanent hair loss, and at 15 Gy, there can be skin necrosis. Although skin erythema may manifest in less than 2 weeks, hair loss and necrosis may occur anywhere from 9 to 52 weeks after the exposure.[29] Patients should be counseled whenever there is greater than 5 Gy exposure during a procedure.

Significant consideration should be given to reducing the risk of radiation-related complications. To reduce radiation exposure, the operator should minimize the use of cine, steep angles, and increased magnification, and reduce the frame rate whenever possible. Typically, 7.5 frames per second (FPS) is adequate for coronary procedures. The image receptor should be kept as close as possible to the patient, and collimation should be used as much as possible. Collimation refers to limiting the field size to the minimal required for imaging.[30] Lowering the table brings the patient closer to the x-ray tube, and can increase the risk of skin injury. The operator should monitor the radiation dose throughout the procedure, particularly if the patient is returning for a repeat procedure within 30 to 60 days. With radial procedures, particularly in inexperienced operators, there is known increase in radiation exposure compared with femoral procedures.[31,32] As radial center and operator volumes increase, radiation exposure for transradial and transfemoral procedures become similar.[33]

All personnel working in the catheterization laboratory should wear appropriate protective gear, including lead aprons for the torso and waist, a thyroid collar, and protective eyewear or glasses. Operators should consider the *inverse square law* during the procedure (where a step back during the procedure can reduce radiation exposure fourfold), and step back from the table during cine or digital subtraction imaging. Other personnel in the room should stand as far away from the table as possible, and cine and digital subtraction imaging should be stopped if staff need to approach the patient. Lead shields should be positioned to best protect the operator. Operators and other personnel should ideally wear a dose monitor on the thyroid collar and one at the waist level; but at a minimum, a dose monitor on the thyroid collar is required.

To minimize stochastic risk (and cancer risk) to the operator, the annual cumulative radiation dose should be kept below 50 mSv/year. To prevent skin injury, the annual cumulative radiation dose should be maintained below 500 mSv/year. Eye exposure should be below 150 mSv/year to prevent lens injury. All female patients of child-bearing age should undergo beta-human chorionic gonadotropin testing before undergoing fluoroscopy, and the procedure should be avoided in a pregnant patient unless absolutely necessary. For the pregnant operator, a dose monitoring badge should be worn on the thyroid collar and at the waist. The abdominal dose monitor should not exceed a reading of 1 mSv/month.[34]

CLINICAL APPLICATIONS

Performing Diagnostic Coronary Angiography

When engaging the catheter into the left main artery, a shallow left anterior oblique (LAO) projection is often used to perform angiography of the left main artery. If there is concern for a left main stenosis, a shallow right anterior oblique (RAO) or true anteroposterior (AP) view is best to examine the left main artery. Careful attention to the pressure waveform for evidence of catheter dampening should always precede an injection. In general, the left circumflex artery is best assessed using caudal views, whereas the left anterior descending (LAD) is best assessed using cranial views. For quick visualization of the left coronary system, operators may shoot the "four corners," which refers to the RAO caudal, LAO caudal, LAO cranial, and AP or RAO cranial views (**Figure 41.4A-D**).

Diagnostic Catheter Selection

Appropriate catheter selection is important when performing diagnostic angiography (**Figure 41.5**),[35] A Judkins left (JL) 3.5, 4, or 5 catheter is commonly used to engage the left coronary artery. To engage the RCA, a Judkins right (JR) 4 or 3DRC catheter may be used. For bypass angiography, the IM catheter is most frequently used to engage the left IM artery. For saphenous vein graft angiography, several catheters, including a JR 4, Amplatz left (AL) 1, or multipurpose (MP) A, are commonly used.

There are several special situations where careful catheter selection may be necessary. In cases where radial access is obtained and there may be a concern for vasospasm, the universal catheter, the Tiger (or "Tig"), may be beneficial to engage both the left and right coronary arteries to avoid an additional catheter exchange. In patients with known aortic root dilatation or thoracic aortic aneurysm, a larger curved diagnostic catheter, such as a JL 5, will likely be needed to successfully engage the left coronary artery. For LV or PA angiography, pigtail catheters (angled, straight, or Langston) are most appropriate. End-hole catheters should be avoided for LV angiography given the risk of myocardial staining, which can precipitate refractory ventricular arrhythmias, and LV perforation.

Left Coronary System

Right Anterior Oblique Caudal View. The RAO caudal view is often used to best examine the left circumflex artery with obtuse marginal (OM) branches, the ramus intermediate branch (if present), and the proximal LAD. Because the LAD overlaps with the diagonal branches, the RAO caudal view is not ideal for viewing the LAD in its entirety. Typically, this view is taken with 20 or 30° of RAO and 20 to 30° of caudal angulation.

Left Anterior Oblique Caudal View. The LAO caudal view (or the "spider" view) best projects the bifurcation of the left main coronary artery into the LAD and left circumflex. The proximal left circumflex system is well visualized in this view; however, the left main and LAD are markedly foreshortened.

Left Anterior Oblique Cranial View. The LAO cranial view is ideal for visualizing the LAD and diagonal branches. It is important to give as much LAO angulation as necessary to position the spine on the left to best separate out the course of the LAD. Typically, this view will require 40° of LAO and at least 20° of cranial angulation.

Right Anterior Oblique Cranial View. The RAO cranial view is also ideal for visualizing the proximal to mid-LAD and the diagonal

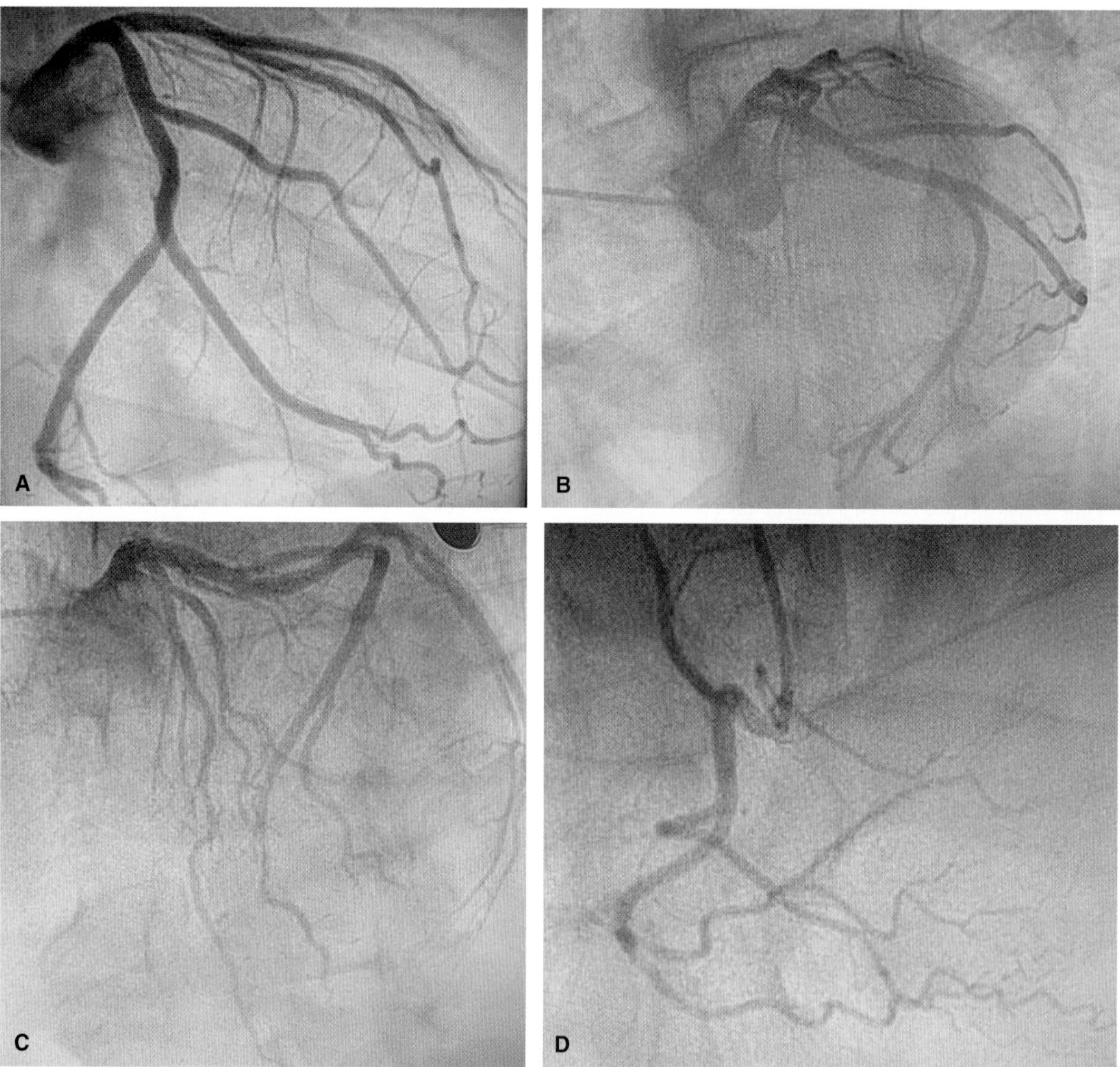

FIGURE 41.4 Standard coronary angiogram views. **(A)** Right anterior oblique caudal view. **(B)** Left anterior oblique caudal view. **(C)** Left anterior oblique cranial view. **(D)** Anterior-posterior cranial view.

branches. It is often also useful for further separating the left circumflex and LAD arteries. Typically, this is best visualized with 10 to 30° of cranial and 40° of RAO angulation.

Anteroposterior Caudal and Anteroposterior Cranial. In some patients, additional views may be necessary. The AP caudal view is best used to visualize the left main and left circumflex arteries. The AP cranial view is best used to further examine the mid-distal LAD.

Right Coronary Artery

To visualize the proximal-mid RCA, the LAO cranial (30-40° of LAO and 10-20° of cranial angulation) and RAO cranial (30-40° of RAO and 10-20° of cranial angulation) views are ideal. To display the distal RCA and bifurcation into the right posterior descending artery (PDA) and posterolateral branches, the AP cranial (20-30° cranial angulation) should be used.

Performing Diagnostic Angiography with Bypass Grafts

As a general rule, bypass grafts are best visualized in the views in which the native artery is best visualized. Views should examine the anastomosis of the graft with the aorta, the body of the graft, the anastomosis of the graft with the native artery, and any collaterals that are present. RCA grafts are best visualized using LAO cranial and RAO views. Left circumflex grafts can be examined in LAO and RAO caudal views. LAD grafts and the left IM artery are visualized using the straight AP, lateral, and cranial views.

Reading and Interpreting a Diagnostic Coronary Angiogram

The following nomenclature describes how to divide the coronary arterial tree into segments, and how to assign dominance.

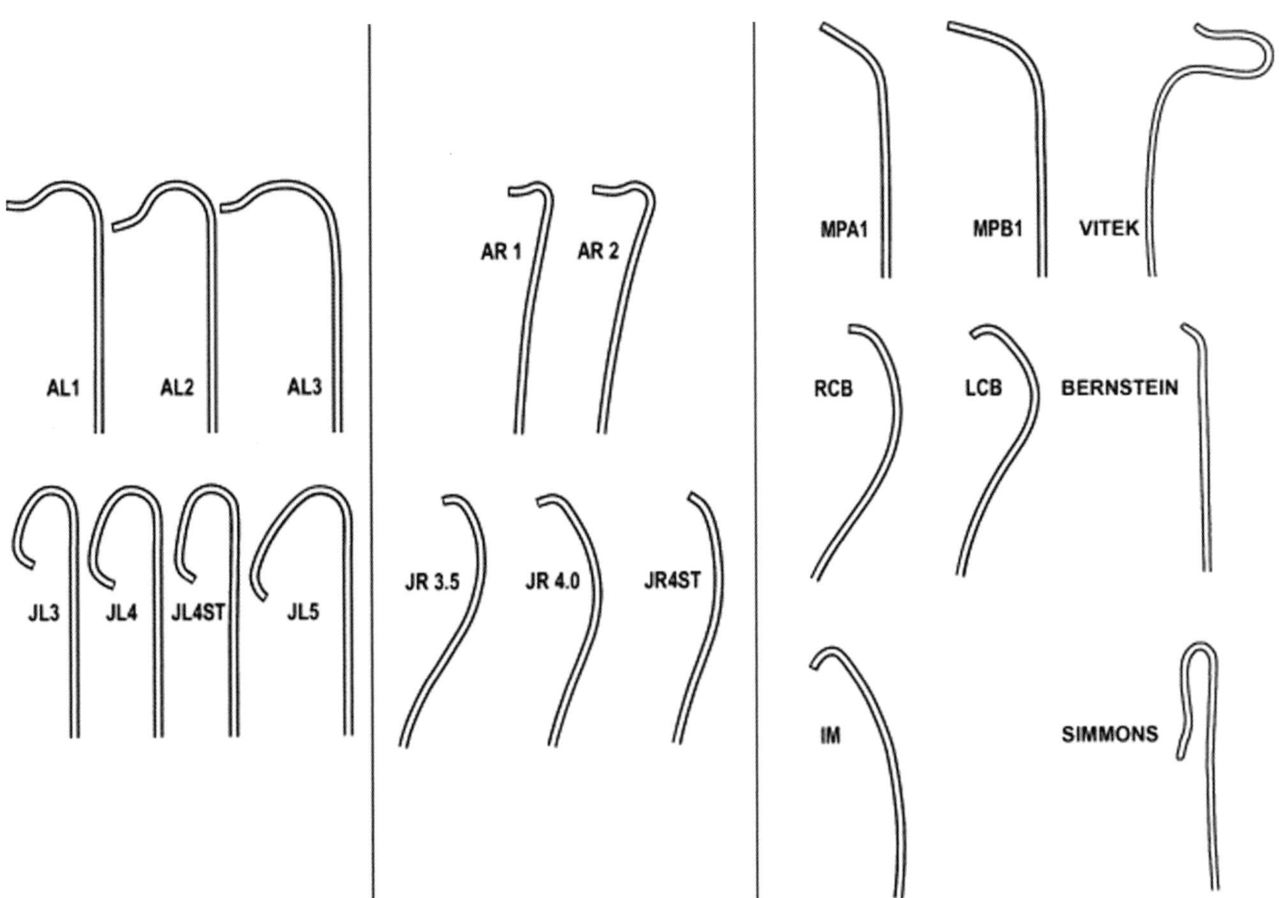

FIGURE 41.5 Diagnostic coronary angiography catheters. AL, Amplatz left; AR, Amplatz right; JL, Judkins left; JR, Judkins right; IM, internal mammary; LCB, left coronary bypass catheter; RCB, right coronary bypass catheter. (Reprinted from Casserly IP, Messenger JC. Technique and Catheters. *Cardiol Clin.* 2009;27(3):417-432. Copyright © 2009 Elsevier. With permission.)

Left Anterior Descending Artery. The proximal LAD is defined as the segment of the LAD that extends from the takeoff of the left main artery to the origin of the first septal perforator or diagonal branch. The mid-LAD runs from the end of the proximal LAD to the next diagonal branch, and the distal LAD runs from the end of the mid-LAD to the end of the artery. Diagonal arteries pass over the anterolateral surface of the left ventricle. The septal perforators originate from the LAD and extend into the interventricular septum.

Left Circumflex Artery. The proximal left circumflex arises from the left main and extends to the origin of the first OM branch. Although early classifications of the left circumflex only labeled proximal and distal segments, most operators in clinical practice characterize lesions in the "mid"-left circumflex, defined as arising from the end of the proximal left circumflex segment to where the second OM branch originates, coursing in the atrioventricular (AV) groove. The distal left circumflex also courses in the AV groove, and extends from the end of the mid-left circumflex. The OM branches arise from the left circumflex and course over the lateral surface of the LV. If an anterolateral branch arises directly off the left main artery, it is defined as a ramus intermedius rather than as an OM branch.

Right Coronary Artery. The proximal RCA extends from the right sinus of Valsalva to where the first major acute marginal branch originates. The mid-RCA originates from the end of the proximal RCA and extends to the second acute marginal artery. The distal RCA runs from the mid-RCA to the takeoff of the PDA. The right PDA originates from the distal RCA and extends to the apex, giving rise to the septal perforators, in a right-dominant system. The right posterior AV segment courses as the continuation of the distal RCA, and gives rise to the right posterolateral branches.

Dominance. The PDA supplies the posterior third of the interventricular septum and runs along the posterior interventricular sulcus to the apex of the heart. Approximately 70% to 80% of the population is right dominant, whereby the PDA will arise from the distal RCA. In a left-dominant system, the PDA arises from the left circumflex artery (5%-10% of the population), and in a codominant system, the PDA will arise from both the RCA and left circumflex arteries (10%-20% of the population).[36]

Assessing Angiographic Lesion Severity. There are several important considerations when assessing lesion severity angiographically. The percent stenosis assigned to a lesion should be estimated on

SECTION 3

the basis of the vessel diameter at the site of the lesion compared with the proximal reference vessel diameter. In addition to examining the percent stenosis, it is necessary to describe other characteristics of the lesion, including classification, calcification, eccentricity, length, and position in the vessel. The American College of Cardiology/American Heart Association (ACC/AHA) Task Force on lesion morphology established the following criteria to classify lesions[37]:

Type A lesion is typically less than 10 mm in length, is concentric, not ostial, without thrombus, calcification or any major side branch involvement.

Type B lesion is longer (10-20 mm), eccentric, may be ostial with moderate to severe calcification, and may be located at a bifurcation.

Type C lesion is commonly diffuse (at least 20 mm in length), may be a total occlusion more than 3 months old, with significant tortuosity and side branch involvement.

Type A lesions have nonangulated segments less than 45°, whereas Type C lesions may have extremely angulated segments. These lesion characteristics are important because they help predict PCI procedural success and complications. For example, PCI procedural success decreases from 92% for a Type A lesion down to 61% for a Type C lesion.

The Thrombolysis in Myocardial Infarction (TIMI) classification for coronary artery perfusion is also an important characteristic when examining a coronary angiogram[38]:

TIMI 0 flow indicates that there is no antegrade flow beyond the point of occlusion.

TIMI 1 flow indicates only faint antegrade coronary flow beyond the occlusion with incomplete filling of the distal coronary bed (ie, penetration without perfusion).

TIMI 2 flow is described by sluggish antegrade flow with complete filling of the distal coronary bed.

TIMI 3 flow is normal flow with complete filling of the distal coronary bed or opacification of the vessel within three cardiac cycles.

Performing Left Ventricular Angiography

Although LV angiography is no longer as commonly performed (given the rise of echocardiography), there are many instances in which an LV angiogram (or "v-gram") is useful during diagnostic coronary angiography. LV angiography gives valuable information regarding LV size and function, as well as quantification of mitral regurgitation or shunting through ventricular septal defects. Crossing the aortic valve retrograde *with a catheter also* provides pressure gradients to assess mid-cavitary gradients as in hypertrophic cardiomyopathies, subvalvular aortic stenosis, and valvular aortic stenosis. In cases where an acute myocardial infarction is suspected, but no culprit lesion is found, a ventriculogram can help evaluate for Takotsubo (ie, stress) cardiomyopathy (**Figure 41.6**).

Most commonly, a pigtail catheter is used to gain access into the left ventricle. The use of end-hole catheters to perform LV angiography is not recommended given the risk of

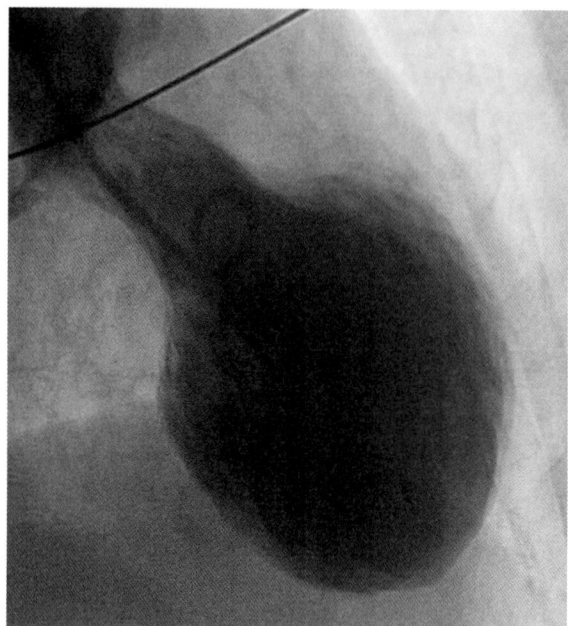

FIGURE 41.6. Left ventriculogram demonstrating findings of Takotsubo cardiomyopathy.

myocardial staining and LV perforation. If the pigtail catheter does not easily prolapse across the valve, it should be positioned in the RAO projection just above the valve and a J-wire can be advanced, straightening the pigtail and thereby advancing across the aortic valve. This may be more difficult to achieve in patients with aortic stenosis, in which case a straight 0.035" guidewire may be required. Alternatively, a hydrophilic Glidewire through an Amplatz left catheter may facilitate valve crossing. After the Amplatz left catheter is tracked into the LV, it can be exchanged for a standard pigtail catheter. Attempts to advance across the aortic valve with the guidewires should be limited to approximately 2 minutes before pausing and flushing the catheter. Ideally, the positioning of the pigtail catheter should be mid-cavitary. Common views for a ventriculogram include RAO 30° and LAO 60° (ideal for assessment of mitral valve regurgitation and LV wall motion). Performing a ventriculogram requires roughly 30 to 36 mL of contrast dye at a rate of 10 to 12 mL/sec when injected through a 5- to 6-Fr pigtail catheter.

Performing Pulmonary Angiography

Indications for performing diagnostic pulmonary angiography include assessment for suspected pulmonary embolism, determining the extent of disease in chronic thromboembolic pulmonary hypertension before planning pulmonary endarterectomy or balloon pulmonary angioplasty, and to evaluate for pulmonary arteriovenous malformations, fistulae and peripheral PA stenoses.[39] With the advent of advanced computed tomography (CT) scanning, pulmonary angiography is less commonly performed in suspected acute pulmonary embolism, given the ready availability and less invasive nature of CT.

To perform pulmonary angiography, access is obtained in the femoral, internal jugular, antecubital, or forearm vein with a 6- or 7-Fr sheath.[40,41] The operator often performs a right heart catheterization first to assess hemodynamics and cardiac output. In this case, the right heart catheter can be exchanged for the angiographic catheter with an exchange-length wire. Various diagnostic catheters can be used to perform pulmonary angiography, including the Grollman catheter (a pigtail catheter with a rightward curve and a 90° leftward curve near the tip), an Omni-flush catheter, or any angled pigtail catheter with side holes. If a Berman angiographic catheter is utilized (a dual-lumen catheter with a distal balloon and multiple holes proximal to the balloon for delivering the dye as well as recording the pressure tracing), exchange is not possible given the absence of an end hole. Because the left PA is a straight continuation of the main PA, the pigtail catheters will commonly advance easily into the left PA. The right PA takes a sharper turn off the main PA and may require wire maneuvering or a diagnostic JR catheter to access the right PA. For selective pulmonary angiography, a straight-tipped Berenstein catheter may be used. In general, we attempt to place the angiographic catheter first in the right PA, because it can then be easily pulled back and advanced into the left PA without need to disconnect from the power injector and re-prime and re-deair the circuit.

When acquiring images, the patient should be instructed to take a full breath, and then hold it for several seconds and avoid any movement. For imaging of the main PA, 30 mL of contrast should be injected over 2 seconds, and for imaging of the right or left pulmonary arteries, 25 to 30 mL of contrast should be injected over several seconds. A standard pulmonary angiogram should include both AP and lateral projections to avoid missing any lesions that could be overlapped (**Figure 41.7A-D**). In addition, some centers may use digital subtraction.

SPECIAL CONSIDERATIONS AND CONTRAINDICATIONS

Cardiac Catheterization in Patients with Renal Dysfunction

As a significant proportion of patients undergoing cardiac catheterization will either have acute renal failure or chronic kidney disease, there are several strategies that may be implemented to reduce the risk of contrast-induced nephropathy.

Biplane Imaging

Many patients undergoing coronary angiography will have chronic kidney disease or acute renal failure that necessitates limiting the amount of contrast dye. One of the best ways to accomplish this is to utilize a biplane lab where two simultaneous images can be taken from a single contrast injection. In biplane imaging, the heart is placed at the isocenter, and the lateral and AP planes are positioned in an orthogonal manner. Views should be complementary to avoid camera overlap. For example, the RAO caudal view can be combined with an LAO cranial projection. However, panning in such cases may result in loss of distal vessel imaging in one of the projections, particularly if the image is overly magnified. Setting up biplane views so that caudal views (LAO caudal and RAO caudal) and then cranial views are taken simultaneously, can prevent this from occurring as less panning (ie, movement of the patient table) is generally required.

Hydration Protocols

Many centers have instituted various pre- and post-procedural hydration protocols to reduce the risk of contrast-induced nephropathy after cardiac catheterization. In the POSEIDON (Prevention Of contraSt rEnal Injury with Different hydratiON strategies) trial, patients were randomized to a left ventricular end-diastolic pressure (LVEDP)-guided strategy compared to a standard hydration strategy.[42] Before a diagnostic catheterization or PCI, patients in the LVEDP-guided hydration arm received preprocedural hydration (0.9% NS at 3 mL/kg) and then based on LVEDP measured during the catheterization received additional postprocedural hydration (ie, 5 mL/kg/hr for <13 mm Hg; 3 mL/kg/hr for 13-18 mm Hg; and 1.5 mL/kg/hr for >18 mm Hg). Patients in the standard hydration arm received preprocedural hydration (0.9% NS at 3 mL/kg), and postprocedural hydration at 1.5 mL/kg/hr. The primary end point of contrast-induced nephropathy within 4 days of cardiac catheterization occurred in 6.7% of patients in the LVEDP-guided hydration group and in 16.3% of the standard hydration group ($P = .005$).

Anomalous Coronary Anatomy

Relevant to diagnostic coronary artery imaging is awareness of the most common anomalies and the importance of catheter selection for appropriate engagement of these arteries. The most common anomalies include separate ostia of the LAD and left circumflex arteries (incidence of 0.41%) and a left circumflex artery arising from the RCA (incidence of 0.37%).[43] Both of these are considered benign conditions. However, for other anomalous coronary artery anatomy, the course that the anomalous coronary artery takes is important in determining the risk of sudden cardiac death. For instance, an interarterial course between the aorta and the PA is associated with an increased risk of sudden cardiac death. Cardiac CT imaging should be performed to further characterize anomalous coronary artery course and can complement diagnostic cardiac catheterization for risk stratification.

FOLLOW-UP PATIENT CARE

After diagnostic cardiac catheterization, a patient should be monitored for a period, depending on the amount or type of sedation required, the access site used, and any complications experienced during the procedure. For radial access, a transradial band is placed at the end of the procedure over the access site, and is typically removed after 2 to 3 hours, with close monitoring for hemostasis. If PCI was performed or additional antithrombotic therapy was given, the transradial band may remain for a longer period. Options for femoral sheath removal include manual compression or utilization of compression or vascular closure devices. The period for monitoring

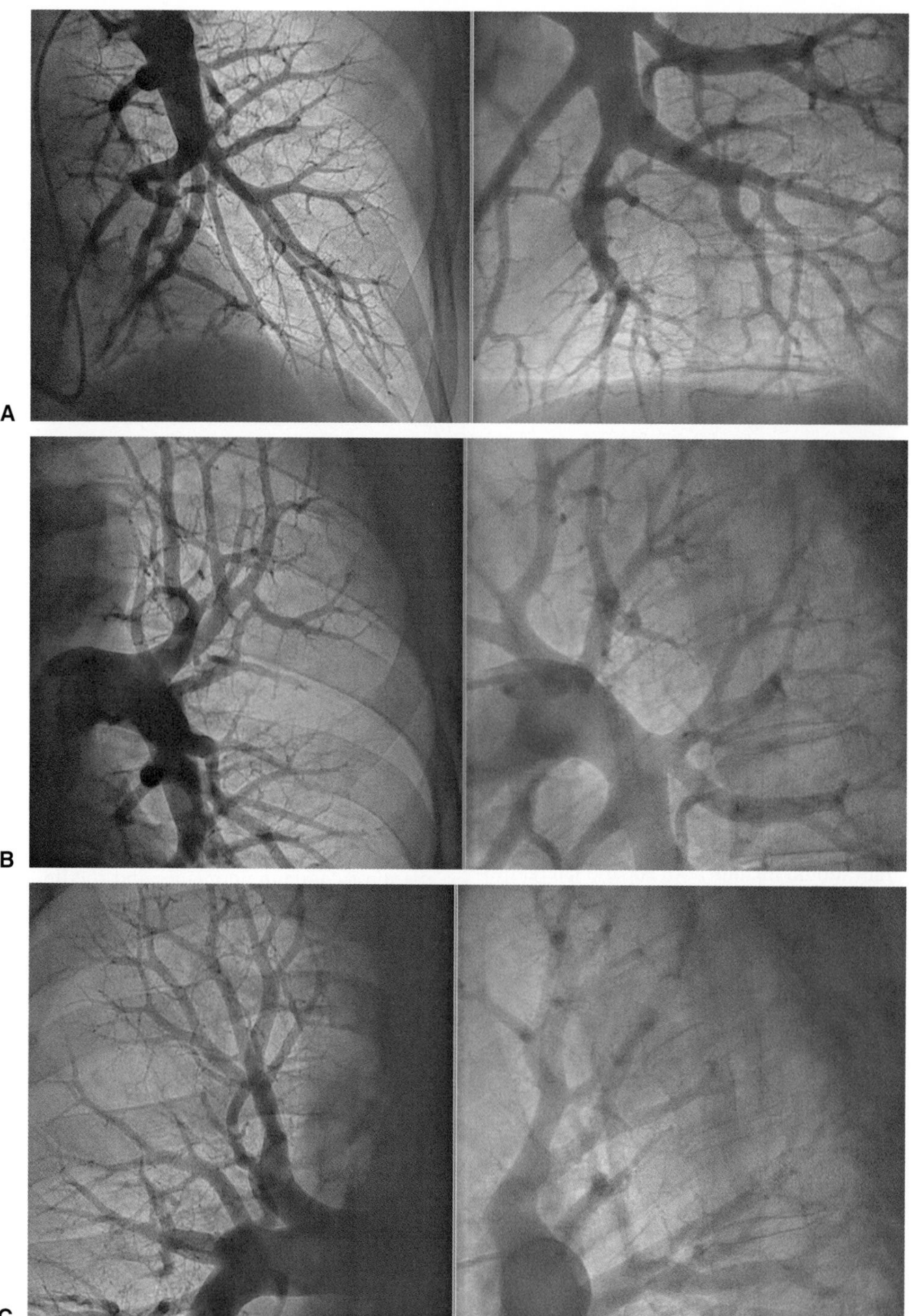

FIGURE 41.7 Pulmonary angiography standard views. **(A)** Left lower lobe anteroposterior (AP) and lateral. **(B)** Left upper lobe AP and lateral. **(C)** Right upper lobe AP and lateral.

after diagnostic angiography depends on ease of initial access, use of additional antithrombotic therapy, final sheath size, and any signs of early bleeding. Ambulation restriction can vary from 2 to 6 hours, and patients should be closely monitored for hemostasis, and potential vascular and bleeding complications. Although vascular closure devices have been shown to be noninferior to manual compression in terms of vascular complications, utilization of these devices can shorten time to hemostasis and reduce time to ambulation.[44,45]

Discharge Instructions

Before discharge, the patient should be given careful verbal and written instructions about which medications to take and who to call with concerns, complications, or questions. Patients should specifically be given information about how to monitor and initially control access site bleeding along with detailed instructions on activity restrictions. If medications were held before the procedure (ie, oral anticoagulants or metformin), instructions should be given on when to restart them.

KEY POINTS

- ✔ Perform a thorough history and physical of the patient with careful consideration of whether a diagnostic coronary angiogram is indicated, with consideration to appropriate use criteria.
- ✔ Although there are no absolute contraindications to diagnostic coronary angiography, consider patient features that may result in increased risk of complications (ie, acute renal failure, contrast dye allergy, etc).
- ✔ Consider bleeding risks, anatomic features, patient preference, and equipment needed for the procedure when choosing between femoral and radial access.
- ✔ Utilize techniques and safety equipment to reduce radiation exposure to the patient, operator, and laboratory personnel.
- ✔ When performing diagnostic coronary angiography, it is important not only to understand the standard views but also how to tailor these views to the unique anatomy of the individual patient.
- ✔ Carefully examine the coronary tree after each diagnostic catheterization to ensure that the correct nomenclature and lesion severity have been assigned.
- ✔ Utilize techniques to reduce the risk of contrast-induced nephropathy, including hydration protocols and biplane imaging.

REFERENCES

1. Bourassa MG. The history of cardiac catheterization. *Can J Cardiol.* 2005; 21:1011-1014.
2. Patel MR, Bailey SR, Bonow RO, et al. ACCF/SCAI/AATS/AHA/ASE/ASNC/HFSA/HRS/SCCM/SCCT/SCMR/STS 2012 appropriate use criteria for diagnostic catheterization. *J Am Coll Cardiol.* 2012;59(22): 1995-2027.
3. Lemkes JS, Janssens GN, van der Hoeven NW, et al. Coronary angiography after cardiac arrest without ST-segment elevation. *N Engl J Med.* 2019; 380:1397-1407.
4. Scanlon PJ, Faxon DP, Audet AM, et al. ACC/AHA guidelines for coronary angiography: a report of the ACC/AHA Task Force on Practice Guidelines (Committee on Coronary Angiography). *J Am Coll Cardiol.* 1999;33(6):1756-1824.
5. Trooboff SW, Iribarne A. Acute adverse drug reactions following cardiac catheterization: evidence-based guidance for providers and systems. *J Thorac Dis.* 2019;11:2680-2684.
6. Maddox TG. Adverse reactions to contrast material: recognition, prevention, and treatment. *Am Fam Physician.* 2002;66:1229-1234.
7. Ben-Dor I, Maluenda G, Mahmoudi M, et al. A novel, minimally invasive access technique versus standard 18-gauge needle set for femoral access. *Catheter Cardiovasc Interv.* 2012;79:1180-1185.
8. Seto AH, Abu-Fadel MS, Sparling JM, et al. Real-time ultrasound guidance facilitates femoral arterial access and reduces vascular complications: FAUST (Femoral Arterial Access with Ultrasound Trial). *JACC Cardiovasc Interv.* 2010;3:751-758.
9. Rao SV, Ou FS, Wang TY, et al. Trends in the prevalence and outcomes of radial and femoral approaches to percutaneous coronary intervention: a report from the National Cardiovascular Data Registry. *JACC Cardiovasc Interv.* 2008;1:379-386.
10. Feldman DN, Swaminathan RV, Kaltenbach LA, et al. Adoption of radial access and comparison of outcomes to femoral access in percutaneous coronary intervention: an updated report from the national cardiovascular data registry (2007-2012). *Circulation.* 2013;127:2295-2306.
11. Diagnostic and Interventional Cardiology. Radial access adoption in the United States. Published May 27, 2016. https://www.dicardiology.com/article/radial-access-adoption-united-states
12. Cha KS, Kim MH, Kim HJ. Prevalence and clinical predictors of severe tortuosity of right subclavian artery in patients undergoing transradial coronary angiography. *Am J Cardiol.* 2003;92:1220-1222.
13. Dehghani P, Mohammad A, Bajaj R, et al. Mechanism and predictors of failed transradial approach for percutaneous coronary interventions. *JACC Cardiovasc Interv.* 2009;2:1057-1064.
14. Sciahbasi A, Romagnoli E, Burzotta F, et al. Transradial approach (left vs. right) and procedural times during percutaneous coronary procedures: TALENT study. *Am Heart J.* 2011;161:172-179.
15. Seto AH, Roberts JS, Abu-Fadel MS, et al. Real-time ultrasound guidance facilitates transradial access: RAUST (Radial Artery access with Ultrasound Trial). *JACC Cardiovasc Interv.* 2015;8:283-291.
16. Chugh SK, Chugh S, Chugh Y, et al. Feasibility and utility of pre-procedure ultrasound imaging of the arm to facilitate transradial coronary diagnostic and interventional procedures (PRIMAFACIE-TRI). *Catheter Cardiovasc Interv.* 2013;82:64-73.
17. Rathore S, Stables RH, Pauriah M, et al. Impact of length and hydrophilic coating of the introducer sheath on radial artery spasm during transradial coronary intervention: a randomized study. *JACC Cardiovasc Interv.* 2010;3:475-483.
18. Pancholy SB, Karuparthi PR, Gulati R. A novel nonpharmacologic technique to remove entrapped radial sheath. *Catheter Cardiovasc Interv.* 2015;85:E35-E38.
19. Sanmartin M, Gomez M, Rumoroso JR, et al. Interruption of blood flow during compression and radial artery occlusion after transradial catheterization. *Catheter Cardiovasc Interv.* 2007;70:185-189.
20. Hahalis G, Xathopoulou I, Tsigkas G, et al. A comparison of low versus standard heparin dose for prevention of forearm artery occlusion after 5 French coronary angiography. *Int J Cardiol.* 2015;187:404-410.
21. Hahalis G, Aznaouridis K, Tsigkas G, et al. Radial artery and ulnar artery occlusions following coronary procedures and the impact of anticoagulation: ARTEMIS (Radial and Ulnar Artery Occlusion Meta-Analysis) systematic review and meta-analysis. *J Am Heart Assoc.* 2017;6:e005430.
22. Pancholy S, Coppola J, Patel T, et al. Prevention of radial artery occlusion-patent hemostasis evaluation trial (PROPHET study): a randomized comparison of traditional versus patency documented hemostasis after transradial catheterization. *Catheter Cardiovasc Interv.* 2008;72:335-340.
23. Cubero JM, Lombardo J, Pedrosa C, et al. Radial compression guided by mean artery pressure versus standard compression with a pneumatic device (RACOMAP). *Catheter Cardiovasc Interv.* 2009;73:467-472.
24. Pancholy SB, Bernatt I, Bertrand OF, Patel TM. Prevention of radial artery occlusion after transradial catheterization: the PROPHET-II randomized trial. *JACC Cardiovasc Interv.* 2016;9(19):1992-1999.
25. Avdikos G, Karatasakis A, Tsourneleas A, et al. Radial artery occlusion after transradial coronary catheterization. *Cardiovasc Diagn Ther.* 2017;7: 305-316.
26. Romagnoli E, Biondi-Zoccai G, Sciahbasi A, et al. Radial versus femoral randomized investigation in ST-segment elevation acute coronary syndrome: the RIFLE-STEACS (Radial versus femoral randomized investigation in ST-Elevation Acute Coronary Syndrome) study. *J Am Coll Cardiol.* 2012;60:2481-2489.
27. Jolly SS, Cairns J, Yusuf S, et al. Procedural volume and outcomes with radial or femoral access for coronary angiography and intervention. *J Am Coll Cardiol.* 2014;63:954-963.

28. Valgimigli M, Gagnor A, Calabro P, et al. Radial versus femoral access in patients with acute coronary syndromes undergoing invasive management: a randomized multicentre trial. *Lancet.* 2015;385:2465-2476.
29. Stecker MS, Balter S, Towbin RB, et al. Guidelines for patient radiation dose management. *J Vasc Interv Radiol.* 2009;20:S263-S273.
30. Walters TE, Kistler PM, Morton JB, et al. Impact of collimation on radiation exposure during interventional electrophysiology. *Europace.* 2012;11: 1670-1673.
31. Lange HW, von Boetticher H. Randomized comparison of operator radiation exposure during coronary angiography and intervention by radial or femoral approach. *Catheter Cardiovasc Interv.* 2006;67:12-16.
32. Shah B, Bangalore S, Feit F, et al. Radiation exposure during coronary angiography via transradial or transfemoral approaches when performed by experienced operators. *Am Heart J.* 2013;165:286-292.
33. Jolly SS, Cairns J, Niemela K, et al. Effect of radial versus femoral access on radiation dose and the importance of procedural volume: a substudy of the multicenter randomized RIVAL trial. *JACC Cardiovasc Interv.* 2013;6:258-266.
34. Duran A, Hian SK, Miller DL, et al. Recommendations for occupational radiation protection in interventional cardiology. *Catheter Cardiovasc Interv.* 2013;82:29-42.
35. Casserly IP, Messenger JC. Technique and catheters. *Cardiol Clin.* 2009; 27:417-432.
36. Shahoud JS, Ambalavanan M, Tivakaran VS. Cardiac dominance. *StatPearls.* Updated September 10, 2020. https://www.ncbi.nlm.nih.gov/books/NBK537207/
37. Ellis SG, Vandormael MG, Cowley MJ, et al. Coronary morphologic and clinical determinants of. procedural outcome with angioplasty for multi-vessel coronary disease: implications for patient selection. *Circulation.* 1990;82:1193-1202.
38. Kern MJ, Moore JA, Aguirre FV, et al. Determination of angiographic (TIMI Grade) blood flow by intracoronary Doppler flow velocity during acute myocardial infarction. *Circulation.* 1996;94:1545-1552.
39. Indications for Using Peripheral Angiography. https://radiologykey.com/angiography-and-interventions/#:~:text=%20The%20current%20indications%20for%20performing%20catheter-based%20pulmonary,congenital%20and%20acquired%20anomalies%2C%20and%20tumor...%20More%20, Accessed May 27, 2020.
40. Zuckerman DA, Sterling KM, Oser RF. Safety of pulmonary angiography in the 1990s. *J Vasc Interv Radiol.* 1996;7:199-205.
41. Grollman JH. Pulmonary arteriography, how I do it. *Cardiovasc Interv Radiol.* 1992;15:166-170.
42. Brar SS, Aharonian V, Mansukhani P, et al. Haemodynamic-guided fluid administration for the prevention of contrast-induced acute kidney injury: the POSEIDON randomized controlled trial. *Lancet.* 2014;383: 1814-1823.
43. Villa AD, Sammut E, Nair A, et al. Coronary artery anomalies overview: the normal and the abnormal. *World J Radiol.* 2016;8:537-555.
44. Lee MS, Applegate B, Rao SV, et al. Minimizing femoral artery access complications during percutaneous coronary intervention: a comprehensive review. *Catheter Cardiovasc Interv.* 2014;84:62-69.
45. Schulz-Schupke S, Helde S, Gewalt S, et al. Comparison of vascular closure devices vs manual compression after femoral artery puncture: the ISAR-CLOSURE randomized clinical trial. *JAMA.* 2014;312:1981-1987.

CHAPTER 42

INTRACORONARY IMAGING

Catalin Toma and Jeff Fowler

INTRODUCTION

Cardiac imaging technologies that involve instrumentation of the heart can provide intravascular imaging dedicated to the coronary architecture or assessment of chamber and valve function. Given the limitations of angiography, intravascular imaging was developed to better visualize the arterial lumen and the vessel wall. This technology can diagnose pathologic processes, characterize the anatomy of the coronary artery, and assist with percutaneous coronary intervention (PCI). This chapter will discuss two main clinically available technologies for coronary imaging: (1) intravascular ultrasound (IVUS) and light-based optical coherence tomography (OCT) and (2) intracardiac echocardiography (ICE).

INTRAVASCULAR ULTRASOUND

FUNDAMENTALS OF INTRAVASCULAR ULTRASOUND

IVUS relies on the reflection of ultrasonic sound waves in megahertz frequency range to reconstruct the radial architecture of a coronary vessel. IVUS imaging can be performed while maintaining normal blood flow through the vessel. The resolution of the image depends on the frequency of the ultrasound with higher resolution transducers generally having a better image quality. There are two fundamental types of IVUS catheters: fixed array and rotational. The fixed array system employs several circumferentially placed ultrasound emitter/receivers with no moving parts. These catheters (such as Eagle Eye, Phillips, Netherlands) operate at lower frequencies (20 MHz), are bulkier, and less deliverable than the rotational IVUS catheters; however, they are easy to set up and operate. Rotational IVUS catheters employ a single emitter-receiver element that is rotated via a flexible shaft connected to an external motorized drive unit, which also executes the pullback during image acquisition. These catheters (such as the Boston Scientific, Phillips, and Acist HDI) use higher frequency (ie, 40-60 MHz) resulting in higher resolution imaging. With increased frequency, however, there is more scatter of the blood cells and decreased lumen definition. They are smaller in caliber than fixed array IVUS catheters but require a slightly more elaborate preparation given the need for the external motorized drive unit.

CLINICAL APPLICATIONS

Diagnostic Utility: Intravascular Ultrasound

IVUS allows in vivo characterization of the atherosclerotic plaque morphology and the coronary lumen anatomy (**Figure 42.1A-F**). IVUS is particularly useful at detecting calcified plaque, because sound waves bounce off hardened surfaces creating distinct echoes (Figure 42.1C). IVUS has a significantly higher sensitivity for detecting vessel wall calcium than angiography.[1] Softer plaque characterization is less optimal with IVUS because of the decreased resolution (Figure 42.1A). Virtual histology (VH) IVUS, based on frequency shifts, was developed to characterize plaque composition and is currently clinically available. In a prospective natural-history study of coronary atherosclerosis, IVUS predictors of nonculprit lesion–related events had a minimal lumen area less than or equal to 4 mm^2, a plaque burden greater than or equal to 70%, and a radiofrequency thin-cap fibroatheroma. However, the clinical utility of these features in guiding therapy remains unclear.[2]

In addition to plaque characterization, IVUS data have been used to determine the hemodynamic impact of a lesion based on the lumen size. A left main artery minimal luminal cross-sectional area of less than 4.8 mm^2 by IVUS identifies a hemodynamically stenosis as determined by pressure wire measurements.[3] For non-left main disease, the anatomic assessment of functional significance is more variable; a recent meta-analysis of comparative IVUS versus fractional flow reserve (FFR) studies identified a minimal luminal cross-sectional area cutoff of 2.8 mm^2 as hemodynamically significant.[4] However, using minimal luminal area alone does not consider the length of the diseased segment, which also plays an important role in determining the pressure drop across the stenotic segment.

Procedural Guidance: Intravascular Ultrasound

The principal benefit for IVUS in the current PCI era is that of coronary procedural guidance. Historically, IVUS played a critical role in assessing stent size and placement to reduce acute stent thrombosis[5] and in preventing in-stent restenosis. In the current second-generation drug-eluting stent (DES) era (ie, with thin strut/biocompatible drug-eluting polymers), IVUS guidance retains a clinical advantage over angiographic guidance. Two randomized trials demonstrated better outcomes (ie, decrease in major adverse cardiovascular events [MACEs] and target vessel failure) when DES expansion was guided by IVUS versus angiography.[6,7] A large meta-analysis examining

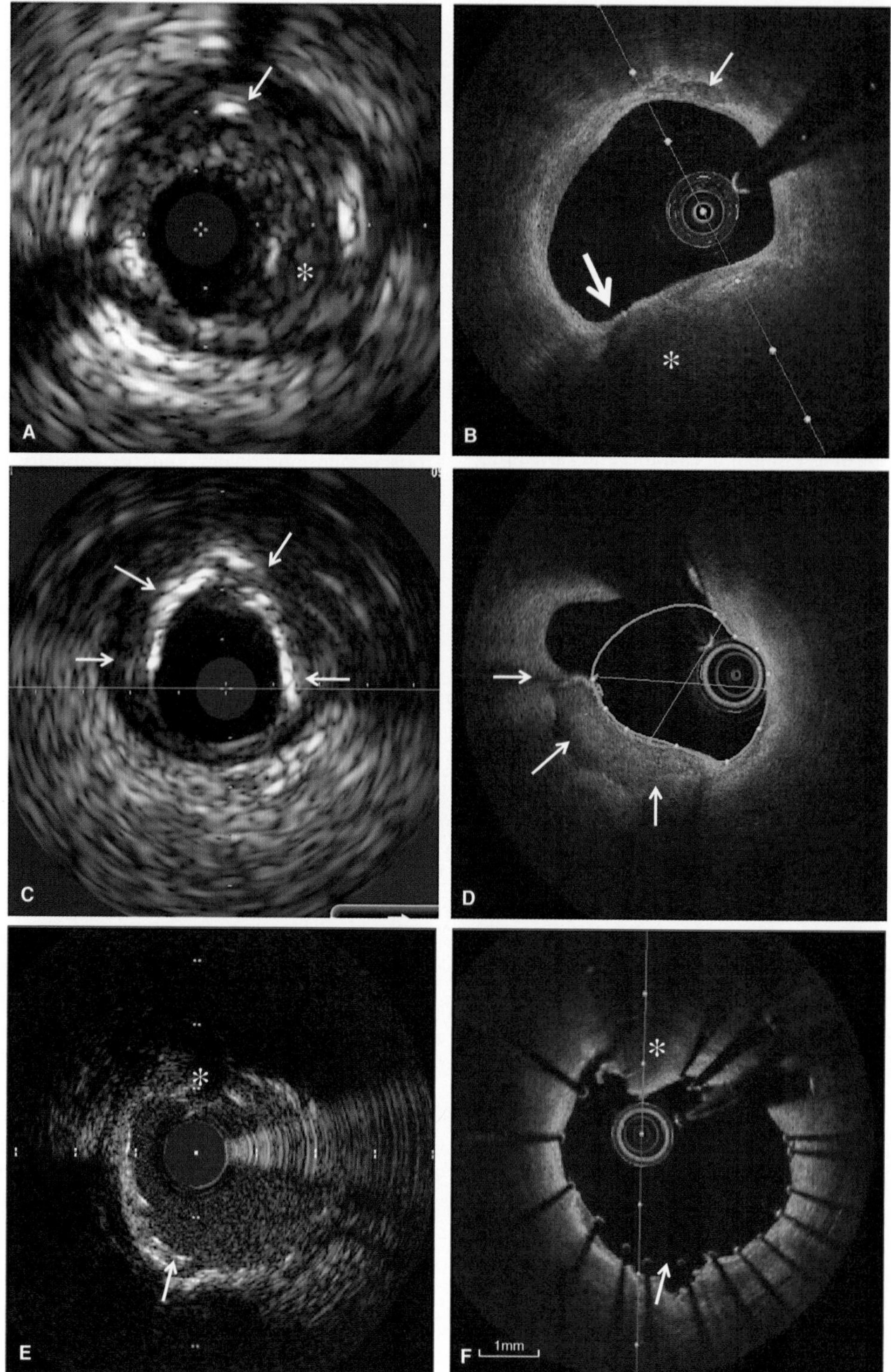

FIGURE 42.1 Lesion characterization by intravascular imaging. **(A)** Heterogenous lesion by IVUS with calcifications with characteristic signal dropout (arrow) and mixed intensity signal plaque suggestive of large necrotic core (asterisk). **(B)** OCTs higher spatial definition allows for greater detail. Calcium nodules are well-delineated (arrow), whereas lipid-rich atherosclerotic plaques have marked signal attenuation (asterisk). Thin-cap atheroma considered to be the precursor to plaque rupture can be identified by OCT at the plaque edges (arrow head). **(C)** The circumferential extent of the plaque calcification can be easily identified by IVUS (arrows, about 180 degree in this case); circumferential calcium is an important predictor of the need for atherectomy to ensure optimal stent implantation. **(D)** OCT similarly can readily detect calcified plaque (arrows), and in addition allows for an assessment of the thickness of the plaque calcium, with thicker calcium more likely to require atherectomy. **(E)** Although stent expansion can be readily assessed by IVUS, stent malapposition (arrow) and presence of thrombus (asterisk) is often challenging. **(F)** OCT is an excellent tool in detecting vascular thrombus that has a particular lobulated appearance with signal scatter (asterisk), as well as accurately assess strut malapposition (arrow). IVUS, intravascular ultrasound; OCT, optical coherence tomography.

IVUS guidance in the DES era included 31,283 patients with a 1-year follow-up demonstrating not only a significant reduction in MACE but also a favorable impact on hard endpoint, such as death and myocardial infarction.[8]

Procedural guidance involves vessel imaging before stenting for adequate sizing as well as after stenting to ensure adequate stent expansion and no significant complications such as stent edge dissection (**Figure 42.2**).

The most important element in preventing subsequent clinical events is achieving adequate stent expansion. This refers to achieving a minimal lumen area inside the stented segment as close as possible to the reference segment. The ULTIMATE (IVUS vs angiography-guided DES implantation) trial has put forward a relatively simple definition for optimal stent expansion (>90% of the distal cross-sectional area or >5 mm^2) and demonstrated the link between achieving these parameters and decreased event rates.[7] Stent expansion can be limited by the presence of heavy calcification, which can be easily identified by IVUS. An arc of calcium greater than 270 degrees (three quadrants) is considered an indication for rotational or orbital atherectomy for adequate lesion preparation prior to stenting. Lastly, stenting from "healthy to healthy vessel" or not having significant plaque burden past the stented segment is recommended. Poststenting, adequate high-pressure postdilatation based on the vessel size is essential in optimizing the PCI result. Only significant edge dissections (>3 mm) or flow limiting distal edge dissections should require additional treatment.

Patients at high risk of PCI-related complications may derive benefit from IVUS, such as those with left main, chronic total occlusions, or long lesions.[7] A number of nonrandomized studies found better outcomes for left main PCI with IVUS guidance.[9] Chronic total occlusions have a higher degree of procedural complexity when treated percutaneously, and IVUS guidance has been shown to reduce target vessel failure in a randomized controlled trial.[10]

IVUS is particularly useful in the treatment of in-stent restenosis. Although the incidence of in-stent restenosis has decreased with the newer-generation thinner struts DES, the prevalence is relatively unchanged, because more complex patients can undergo PCI. Although traditionally in-stent restenosis was associated with neointimal hyperplasia, in the era of DES other factors are commonly found; in particular, stent

Procedural Guidelines for IVUS

Pre-IVUS
- Calcification (>270°)
- Vessel sizing
  Downsize from distal media to media diameter by up to 0.5 mm
  Distal lumen average diameter (red line)
- Lesion length: co-registration and landing zones with <50% plaque burden

Treatment
- Predilate/atherectomy/intravascular lithotripsy
- Stent to nominal pressure
- Postdilate to 1:1 to measured diameters at 16 to 18 atmospheres x 30 seconds with balloon marker on stent border

Post IVUS
- Expansion: aim to achieve 90% of distal minimal lumen area or >5 mm
- Treat edge dissection only if >3 mm or flow limiting

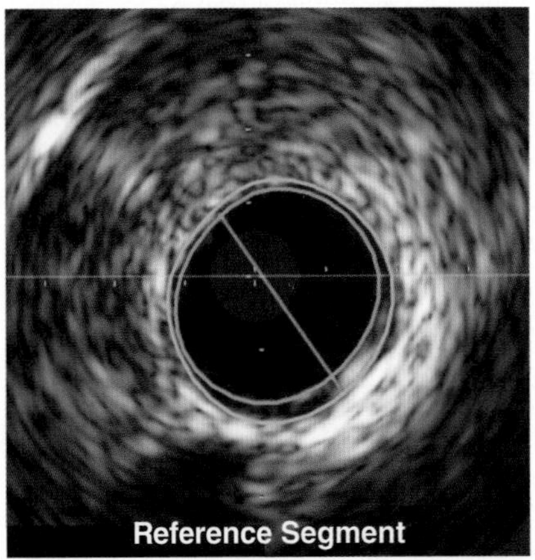

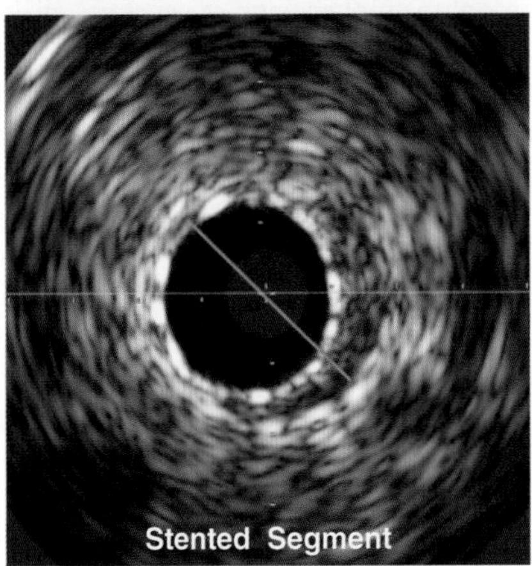

FIGURE 42.2 Coronary PCI guidance using IVUS. Assessment of the vessel before intervention allows for adequate sizing, as well as evaluating the need for atherectomy to ensure proper stent expansion. After stenting and high pressure balloon dilatation, IVUS is critical in determining adequate stent expansion relative to the reference segment, as well as the presence of any flow limiting edge dissections. IVUS, intravascular ultrasound; PCI, percutaneous coronary intervention.

underexpansion[11] and stent fracture. IVUS is particularly useful at assessing stent expansion and guiding vessel dilatation and re-stenting. The European Society of Cardiology endorses imaging for interventional guidance in cases of stent failure (Class of Recommendation IIA).[12]

Another scenario where IVUS may be particularly useful is PCI in patients with a high risk of acute kidney injury. IVUS can size vessels, determine stent length, and assess poststent outcomes without contrast injections. Ultralow contrast PCI (defined as using less contrast than the glomerular filtration rate) can thus be successfully performed, including zero contrast for PCI. In a recent series using IVUS, the average contrast volume was under 10 mL, with 0% contrast-induced kidney injury in chronic kidney disease patients undergoing PCI.[13]

LIMITATIONS AND FUTURE DIRECTIONS: INTRAVASCULAR ULTRASOUND

Despite the compelling supportive data, the penetration of IVUS for PCI guidance remains suboptimal, primarily related to limited expertise, cost, time, and lack of reimbursement. Integrated systems have been created to facilitate rapid image acquisition and coregistration with the angiographic data to support decision-making. This will likely favorably impact utilization. Newer miniaturized IVUS elements currently in development will improve catheter delivery and quality image acquisition. Automating border detection and enhancing the user interface software will speed procedural decision-making and procedure duration. The IVUS-derived lumen geometry can also be used to compute the functional pressure drop along the lesion to assess its functional significance.[14]

OPTICAL COHERENCE TOMOGRAPHY

FUNDAMENTALS OF OPTICAL COHERENCE TOMOGRAPHY

The technology behind intravascular OCT was initially developed in ophthalmology, and it generates an image based on reflected light of the vessel wall. Because the speed of light does not allow for accurate measurement of the reflected light delay to precisely assess distance from the light source (as is done with ultrasound), the interference pattern with a reference light signal is used instead. OCT uses infrared light generated by a laser source outside the body that is transmitted to the tip of the catheter via a rotating optic fiber and projected orthogonal to the inner surface of the vessel. Because OCT uses light, it has better spatial resolution (10 μm) than IVUS (200 μm), but at the cost of decreased tissue penetration. Image acquisition requires brief clearance of blood from the target vessel with a bolus of contrast or saline. The OCT imaging system currently used in the United States (Dragonfly OPTIS, Abbott Vascular) executes a rapid automatic pullback lasting a few seconds and allows for data acquisition for up to 7.5 cm of vessel length. The requirement of contrast boluses for each image runs may be an issue in patients at high risk for acute kidney injury.

CLINICAL APPLICATIONS

Diagnostic Utility: Optical Coherence Tomography

OCT creates clear images of the vessel lumen and the possibility for automatic border tracking and measurements (Figure 42.1B). The vessel size measurements obtained by OCT are closer to true values, whereas IVUS generally overestimates vessel diameters by about 10%.[15] Like IVUS, OCT can detect coronary calcification; but unlike IVUS, it can also assess the thickness of the calcified plaque, which may guide the type of atherectomy necessary for lesion optimization (Figure 42.1D). Lipid-rich and fibro-fatty areas can also be easily identified by OCT (Figure 42.1B). Similar to IVUS, there are data to show that lesions with mean lumen area less than 3.5 mm^2, thin-cap fibroatheroma, lipid arc greater than 180 degree, and OCT-identified macrophages are elements predictive of subsequent coronary events in borderline obstructive lesions.[16] One area where OCT is superior to IVUS is the detection of thrombus, which has a specific light-reflecting lobulated appearance. This is useful in identifying culprit lesions in the setting of acute coronary syndrome and in defining the mechanisms of the thrombotic event (ie, plaque rupture vs. plaque erosion).[17]

OCT is likely a better tool to characterize the pathology of stent failure, both for stent thrombosis and restenosis. For stent thrombosis, unlike IVUS, OCT can differentiate thrombus from other tissues and identify the area where the thrombus originates (Figure 42.1E,F). OCT was instrumental in identifying the most common mechanisms of late stent thrombosis, namely neoatherosclerosis, malapposition, uncovered stent struts, and underexpansion.[18,19] Knowledge of this can influence treatment decision, with repeat stenting for neoatherosclerosis and balloon dilatation for malapposition and underexpansion, although this has not been investigated prospectively.[19] For in-stent restenosis, OCT can reveal whether stent underexpansion, tissue hyperplasia, or neoatherosclerosis is the etiology, which again can tailor the interventional approach.

Another niche application for OCT is the characterization of early-stage and progression of transplant vasculopathy in donor hearts. This disease process is different from coronary atherosclerosis because it involves diffuse neointimal hyperplasia. Historically, after orthotopic heart transplant, patients get routine coronary angiograms to screen for this process. Yet angiography only detects the late stages of the disease process when significant luminal narrowing occurs. IVUS is routinely used in some centers for evaluating transplant vasculopathy; however, the resolution of OCT is far superior and can detect very early stages of the disease process, when only mild intimal thickening is present.[20]

Procedural Guidance: Optical Coherence Tomography

OCT has been utilized for procedural guidance in a similar fashion to IVUS (**Figure 42.3**). One of the early studies randomized patients with acute coronary syndrome undergoing

Procedural Guidelines for OCT

Pre-OCT
- Calcification (arc <270° and thickness >0.5 mm)
- Vessel size
  Downsize to nearest 25 mm from smallest external elastic lamina-based diameter (white line)
  Distal lumen average diameter
- Lesion length: accurate, based on pullback
- Vessel preparation is necessary to reestablish flow

Treatment
- Predilate
- Stent to nominal pressure
- Postdilate to 1:1 to measured diameters at 16 to 18 atmosopheres x 30 seconds with balloon marker on stent edge border
- Reimage

Post OCT
- Expansion: 90% of the distal reference area in the disal one-half of the stent and >90% of the proximal reference area in the proximal half of the stent
- Treat edge dissection only if >3 mm/>60° arc/flow-limiting

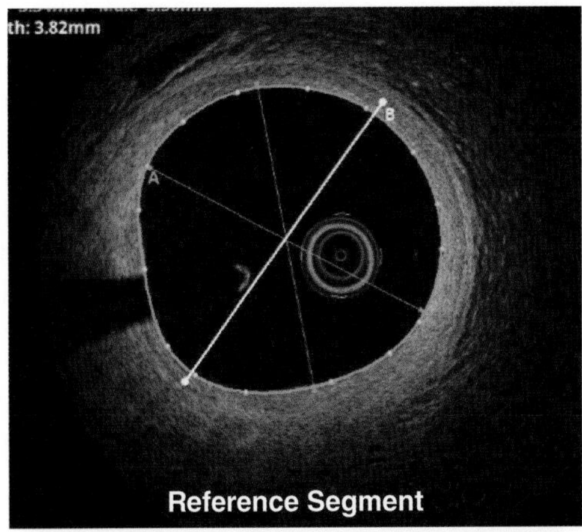

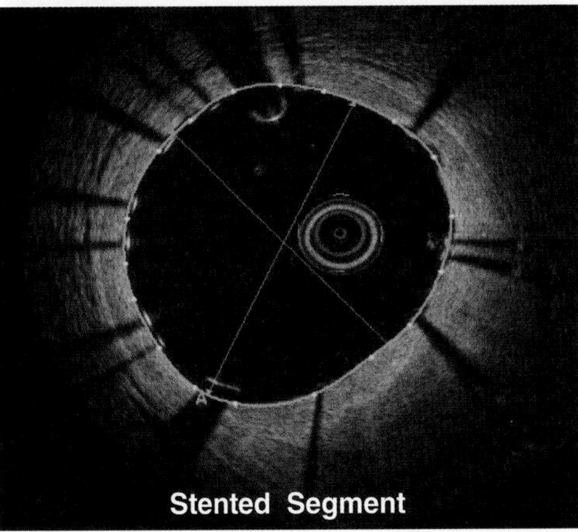

FIGURE 42.3 Coronary PCI guidance using OCT. Vessel size, lesion length, and the extent of calcium can be readily assessed with OCT pullback. Postprocedure, OCT can guide postdilatation to achieve optimal stent expansion and is more sensitive than IVUS at detecting edge dissections and plaque prolapse. IVUS, intravascular ultrasound; OCT, optical coherence tomography; PCI, percutaneous coronary intervention.

PCI to angiographic versus OCT guidance, with marginally larger expansion of the stent and improved postprocedural FFR assessment with OCT.[21] Several studies compared IVUS to OCT guidance. Cumulatively, the current data support the equivalence of OCT to IVUS in terms of procedural guidance.[22,23] A direct randomized clinical trial comparing OCT to angiographic guidance alone with clinical endpoints has completed enrolment (ILUMIEN 4).

In general, surrogate parameters such as stent cross-sectional area are slightly lower when OCT is used versus IVUS, but this could be related to the later overestimation of vessel size, although OCT may be true to size.[15] Additionally, vessel sizing for stent placement and postdilatation varies between studies and operators.

The importance of adequate stent expansion (ie, achieving a minimal stent cross-sectional area as close to the reference lumen area) has been demonstrated in multiple studies.[24] More conservative sizing is based on lumen measurements, with rounding up the stent diameter to match lumen size, whereas more aggressive approaches use the external elastic lamina rounded down to the nearest stent diameter by 0.25. Unfortunately, the external elastic lamina is not always visible by OCT. Furthermore, because of positive vessel remodeling (Glagov phenomenon), this approach can lead to marked oversizing of the stent. Given the considerable diameter range of the current stent platforms, we favor a more conservative lumen-based initial sizing approach with aggressive high-pressure postdilatation following implantation as the safer approach.

OCT is more likely than IVUS to identify subtler mechanical issues poststenting, in particular edge dissections and strut malapposition. However, most of these findings are not associated with adverse outcomes. Scoring systems have been created to define a significant edge dissection, with length (<3 mm length), arc (<60 degree arc), and depth (superficial, not extending to the media) being considered benign.[22] Additionally, proximal stent dissections are less likely to cause issues, given the tendency of blood flow to close the flap.

Strut malapposition—lack of full contact between the stent struts and the vessel wall—is also commonly observed with OCT. Malapposition can be the result of stent undersizing or a consequence of the eccentric plaque architecture, focal vessel ectasia, or side branches. It is important to underline the critical difference between stent malapposition and stent underexpansion, in which the struts may be apposed but the

SECTION 3

stented segment is not expanded sufficiently relative to the reference segment. Stent underexpansion as detected by OCT has been associated with increased target lesion failure rate.[25] Strut malapposition, on the other hand, in the absence of concomitant underexpansion, is a more benign entity. In our practice, we only attempt to correct large circumferential malapposition by using a noncompliant balloon sized 1:1 to the closest reference segment if feasible, primarily to ensure drug delivery to the vessel wall and to prevent stent deformation with subsequent instrumentation.

SPECIAL CONSIDERATIONS AND FUTURE DIRECTIONS

OCT has greater resolution than IVUS, but it requires additional contrast and can only image a relatively short segment of the vessel. The higher resolution facilitates image interpretation and quantification. Similar to IVUS, coregistration software, where the OCT data are integrated with angiography, is a positive development in procedural guidance. The pressure drop across a lesion can be calculated from the OCT-derived geometry of the vessel. The impact of OCT in procedural guidance is less established at this time in terms of hard end points, with a large-scale randomized clinical trial currently in progress.

LIMITATIONS OF INTRAVASCULAR IMAGING

Intravascular imaging requires advancing the imaging probe over an interventional wire, and as such rare procedural complications can occur (ie, vessel damage, stent deformation, thrombosis). Phased-array IVUS catheters are bulky and often cannot be advanced to the distal part of the vessel. OCT requires adequate blood displacement to obtain an image. Although intravascular imaging can provide incremental information to aid the operator, experience in obtaining and critical appraisal of these data is essential. Although intravascular imaging technology is available in most training programs, the current interventional training requirements lack specific language related to intravascular imaging in the core competencies.[26] A large number of interventionists are trained post-fellowship at various industry-sponsored events.

INTRACARDIAC ECHOCARDIOGRAPHY

FUNDAMENTALS OF INTRACARDIAC ECHOCARDIOGRAPHY

Transesophageal echocardiography (TEE) is currently the most commonly used real-time imaging modality in most structural heart disease interventions performed in the cardiac catheterization lab. The increasing trend to "simplify" these interventions using only conscious sedation in the catheterization lab has led to a renewed interest in ICE.[27] ICE is an attractive alternative because of its specific imaging benefits in some cardiac interventions, the proximity of the imaging probe to the structures being visualized, and its lack of patient discomfort and airway issues inherent to other modalities, such as TEE.[28]

The two main ICE transducer systems are mechanical/rotational and phased-array systems. Rotational ICE devices produce a cross-section image from a circular scan path perpendicular to the catheter. They are not steerable, only allow near-field imaging, and are without Doppler capabilities, which has limited their utility. Phased-array ICE systems use 64 piezoelectric elements with frequencies between 5 and 8.5 MHz to produce a single sector scan that is perpendicular to the long axis of the catheter. The probes are available between 8 and 11 French catheter, usually inserted through the femoral vein, and are steerable. Maximal tissue penetration with ICE is 10 to 20 cm, thereby allowing for near- and far-field imaging. These capabilities make phased-array ICE systems the imaging probe of choice in structural heart disease interventions. There are two phased-array ICE transducer systems commercially available in the United States: AcuNav and AcuNav V (Siemens-Acuson, Mountain View, California) and ViewFlex Xtra (Abbott Vascular, St. Paul, MN, USA). New three-dimensional capabilities are being developed and tested as well.

CLINICAL APPLICATIONS

Diagnostic Utility: Intracardiac Echocardiography

No standardized ICE imaging protocol or techniques have been developed by professional imaging societies at this time. However, several experts have recommended five standard imaging positions that are beneficial for structural heart disease interventions, including mid right atrium (RA), low RA, right ventricular (RV) inflow, RV outflow, and left atrium. The "home view" consists of neutral probe position in the mid RA where the tricuspid valve (TV) can be viewed. With progressive clockwise rotation of the probe, a general survey can first reveal the RV outflow tract and aortic valve, followed by the mitral valve and roof of the coronary sinus, followed by LA, left-sided pulmonary veins, and intra-atrial septum, followed by back-wall of the RA and finally back to the TV with a full 360 degree rotation. Anteroposterior and lateral manipulations can bring into view these structures more clearly and in orthogonal planes for three-dimensional assessment. The probe can be advanced into the superior vena cava, RV inflow, and outflow tracts, as well into the LA after a transseptal puncture, to bring structures of choice into closer proximity with the imaging probe to enhance the image clarity.

Procedural Guidance: Intracardiac Echocardiography

Currently ICE is being used to help guide a growing number of structural heart disease and electrophysiologic interventions, such as transseptal puncture for mechanical circulatory support, pulmonary vein isolation, LA appendage closures, atrial septal defect (ASD) (**Figure 42.4**), patent foramen ovale (PFO), and ventricular septal defect closure, and mitral and aortic valve intervention.

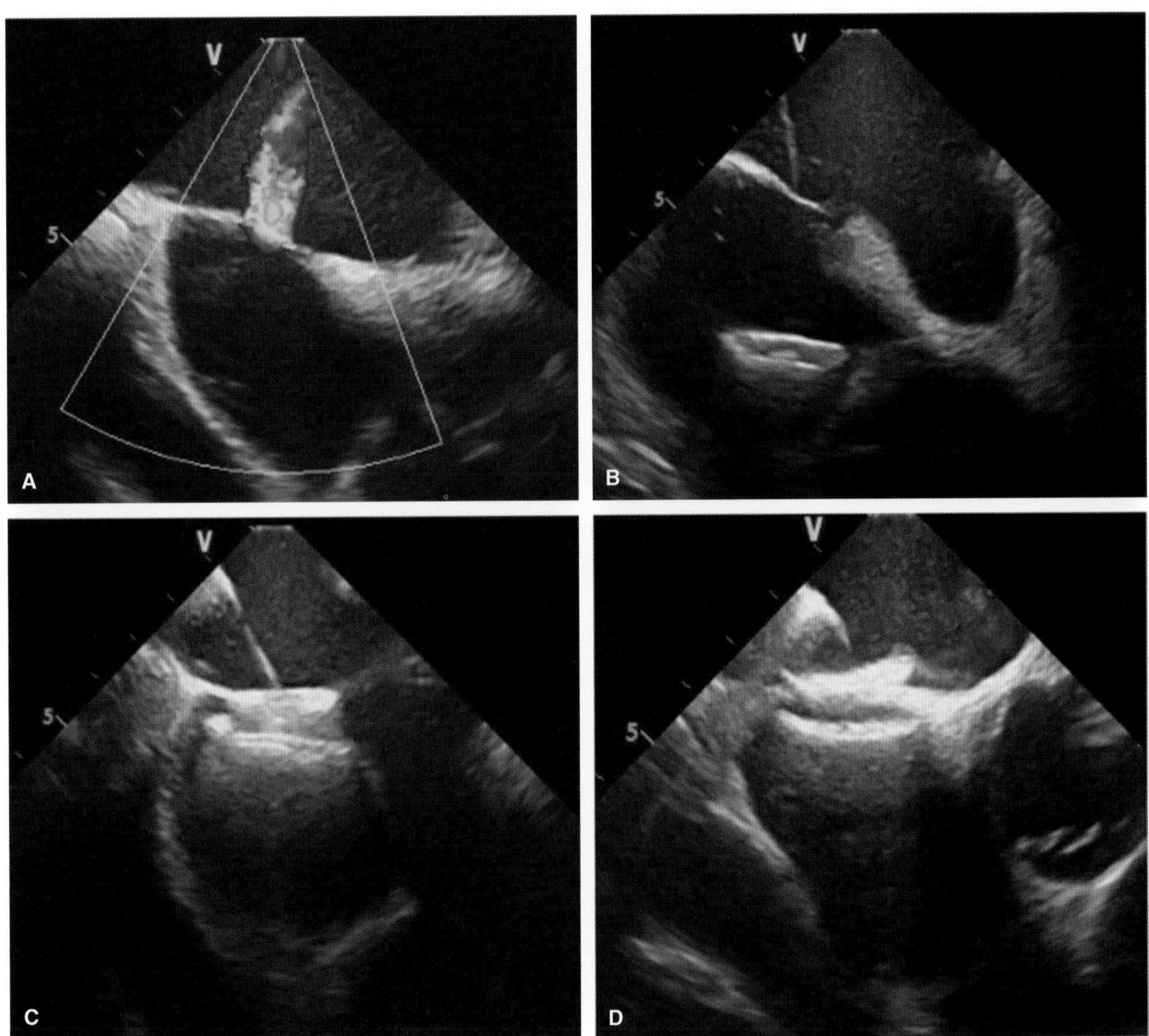

FIGURE 42.4 ICE guidance for percutaneous atrial septal occlusion **(A)** ICE septal view with color Doppler clearly identifies an ASD. **(B)** Left atrial disc of the ASD occlusion device is deployed in the left atrium. **(C)**. After pulling the disc against the intra-atrial septum, the right atrial disc is deployed. **(D)**. Aortic valve short-axis view demonstrates additional inspection of rims prior to release. ASD, atrial septal defect; ICE, intracardiac echocardiography.

ICE was first introduced to aid in transseptal punctures to guide electrophysiologic procedures[29] and provide site-specific location of transseptal puncture to access specific location in the LA for different procedures.[30,31,32] Subsequently, ICE was shown to be safe and effective in guiding PFO and ASD closures, with the ability to identify ASD rims, size the defect accurately, and identify residual leaks postprocedurally.[33] The inferior-posterior border of the intra-atrial septum is better visualized with ICE compared to TEE, which allows for complex ASD closures.[34] ICE is also utilized in arrhythmia ablations by improving tissue contact of the mapping catheters to improve successful ablations.[35] ICE can define pulmonary vein anatomy accurately to improve pulmonary vein isolation.[36] The ICE catheter can also be maneuvered into the coronary sinus, RV outflow tract, or pulmonary artery to improve visualization of the LA appendage and help guide LA appendage closure procedures.[37] ICE imaging is comparable to TEE in providing adequate imaging and hemodynamic assessment after transcatheter aortic valve replacement.[38] ICE guidance of atrioventricular valve interventions is being explored, including mitral valve edge-to-edge repair and TV edge-to-edge repair with the MitraClip (Abbott Vascular, St. Paul, MN, USA).[39,40] There are growing applications and novel indications for this imaging catheter that continue to expand and provide a safe and efficient imaging adjunct to structural heart disease interventions.

LIMITATIONS OF INTRACARDIAC ECHOCARDIOGRAPHY

There are limitations to ICE imaging including catheter oscillations because of the cardiac motion, as well as image variability because of significant anatomic variability in heart rotation and cavity size. Compared to TEE, there is limited three-dimensional capabilities and far-field and biplane imaging. ICE also is an invasive vascular modality, necessitating venous access with potential for vascular complications. ICE is an excellent complement to a growing armamentarium of multimodality imaging that can be utilized in specific and growing indications to provide superior imaging, and perhaps simplify some structural heart disease interventions.

KEY POINTS

INTRAVASCULAR IMAGING

- ✔ Expertise with intravascular imaging modalities should be a required part of interventional training and expertise.
- ✔ Integration of the intravascular imaging data with angiography can be greatly facilitated by coregistration.
- ✔ When using intravascular imaging, we favor a more conservative stent sizing with aggressive, controlled, image-based postdilatation.
- ✔ Intravascular imaging is consistently superior to angiography alone in achieving optimal stent expansion.

Intravascular imaging should be routinely employed for procedural guidance in high-risk scenarios (ie, left main disease and chronic total occlusions).

INTRACARDIAC ECHOCARDIOGRAPHY

- ✔ ICE imaging is superior to TEE in the proximity of the imaging probe to the structures being visualized and its lack of patient discomfort.
- ✔ Phased-array ICE catheters are more commonly used compared to rotational ICE catheters in structural heart interventions.
- ✔ ICE imaging is being used in an expanding number of structural heart interventions.

REFERENCES

1. Mintz GS, Popma JJ, Pichard AD, et al. Patterns of calcification in coronary artery disease. A statistical analysis of intravascular ultrasound and coronary angiography in 1155 lesions. *Circulation.* 1995;91:1959-1965.
2. Stone GW, Maehara A, Lansky AJ, et al. A prospective natural-history study of coronary atherosclerosis. *N Engl J Med.* 2011;364(3):226-235.
3. Kang SJ, Lee JY, Ahn JM, et al. Intravascular ultrasound-derived predictors for fractional flow reserve in intermediate left main disease. *JACC Cardiovasc Interv.* 2011;4(11):1168-1174.
4. Nascimento BR, de Sousa MR, Koo BK, et al. Diagnostic accuracy of intravascular ultrasound-derived minimal lumen area compared with fractional flow reserve—meta-analysis: pooled accuracy of IVUS luminal area versus FFR. *Catheter Cardiovasc Interv.* 2014;84(3):377-385.
5. Colombo A, Hall P, Nakamura S, et al. Intracoronary stenting without anticoagulation accomplished with intravascular ultrasound guidance. Circulation. 1995;91(6):1676-1688.
6. Hong SJ, Kim BK, Shin DH, et al. Effect of intravascular ultrasound-guided vs angiography-guided everolimus-eluting stent implantation: the IVUS-XPL randomized clinical trial. *JAMA.* 2015;314:2155-2163.
7. Zhang J, Gao X, Kan J, et al. Intravascular ultrasound versus angiography-guided drug-eluting stent implantation: the ULTIMATE trial. *J Am Coll Cardiol.* 2018;72(24):3126-3137.
8. Steinvil A, Chang YJ, Lee SY, et al. Intravascular ultrasound-guided drug-eluting stent implantation: an updated meta-analysis of randomized control trials and observational studies. *Int J Cardiol.* 2016;216:133-139.
9. Andell P, Karlsson S, Mohammad MA, et al. Intravascular ultrasound guidance is associated with better outcome in patients undergoing unprotected left main coronary artery stenting compared with angiography guidance alone. *Circ Cardiovasc Interv.* 2017;10:e004813.
10. Kim B-K, Shin D-H, Hong M-K, et al. Clinical impact of intravascular ultrasound-guided chronic total occlusion intervention with zotarolimus-eluting versus biolimus-eluting stent implantation: randomized study. *Circ Cardiovasc Interv.* 2015;8:e002592.
11. Goto K, Zhao Z, Matsumura M, et al. Mechanisms and patterns of intravascular ultrasound in-stent restenosis among bare metal stents and first-and second-generation drug-eluting stents. *Am J Cardiol.* 2015;116:1351-1357.
12. Windecker S, Kolh P, Alfonso F, et al. 2014 ESC/ EACTS Guidelines on myocardial revascularization: the Task Force on Myocardial Revascularization of the European Society of Cardiology (ESC) and the European Association for Cardio-Thoracic Surgery (EACTS). Developed with the special contribution of the European Association of Percutaneous Cardiovascular Interventions (EAPCI). *Eur Heart J.* 2014;35:2541-2619.
13. Azzalini L, Laricchia A, Regazzoli D, et al. Ultra-low contrast percutaneous coronary intervention to minimize the risk for contrast-induced acute kidney injury in patients with severe chronic kidney disease. *J Invasive Cardiol.* 2019;31(6):176-182.
14. Lee JG, Ko J, Hae H, et al. Intravascular ultrasound-based machine learning for predicting fractional flow reserve in intermediate coronary artery lesions. *Atherosclerosis.* 2020;292:171-177.
15. Kim IC, Nam CW, Cho YK, et al. Discrepancy between frequency domain optical coherence tomography and intravascular ultrasound in human coronary arteries and in a phantom in vitro coronary model. *Int J Cardiol.* 2016;221:860-866.
16. Prati F, Romagnoli E, Gatto L, et al. Relationship between coronary plaque morphology of the left anterior descending artery and 12 months clinical outcome: the CLIMA study. *Eur Heart J.* 2020;41(3):383-391.
17. Jia H, Abtahian F, Aguirre AD, et al. In vivo diagnosis of plaque erosion and calcified nodule in patients with acute coronary syndrome by intravascular optical coherence tomography. *J Am Coll Cardiol.* 2013; 62(19):1748-1758.
18. Souteyrand G, Amabile N, Mangin L, et al. Mechanisms of stent thrombosis analysed by optical coherence tomography: insights from the national PESTO French registry. *Eur Heart J.* 2016;37:1208-1216.
19. Jones CR, Khandhar SJ, Ramratnam M, et al. Identification of intrastent pathology associated with late stent thrombosis using optical coherence tomography. *J Interv Cardiol.* 2015;28(5):439-448.
20. Khandhar SJ, Yamamoto H, Teuteberg JJ, et al. Optical coherence tomography for characterization of cardiac allograft vasculopathy after heart transplantation (OCTCAV study). *J Heart Lung Transplant.* 2013; 32(6):596-602.
21. Meneveau N, Souteyrand G, Motreff P, et al. Optical coherence tomography to optimize results of percutaneous coronary intervention in patients with non-ST-elevation acute coronary syndrome: results of the multicenter, randomized DOCTORS study (does optical coherence tomography optimize results of stenting). *Circulation.* 2016;134(13):906-917.
22. Ali ZA, Maehara A, Genereux P, et al. Optical coherence tomography compared with intravascular ultrasound and with angiography to guide

coronary stent implantation (ILUMIEN III: oPTIMIZE PCI): a randomized controlled trial. *Lancet.* 2016;388:2618-2628.

23. Kubo T, Shinke T, Okamura T, et al. Optical frequency domain imaging vs. intravascular ultrasound in percutaneous coronary intervention (OPINION trial): one-year angiographic and clinical results. *Eur Heart J.* 2017; 38:3139-3147.
24. Song H-G, Kang S-J, Ahn J-M, et al. Intravascular ultrasound assessment of optimal stent area to prevent in-stent restenosis after zotarolimus-, everolimus-, and sirolimus-eluting stent implantation. *Catheter Cardiovasc Interv.* 2014;83:873-878.
25. Prati F, Romagnoli E, La Manna A, et al. Long-term consequences of optical coherence tomography findings during percutaneous coronary intervention: the Centro Per La Lotta Contro L'infarto—Optimization of Percutaneous Coronary Intervention (CLI-OPCI) LATE study. *EuroIntervention.* 2018;14(4):e443-e451.
26. King SB 3rd, Babb JD, Bates ER, et al. COCATS 4 Task Force 10: training in cardiac catheterization. *J Am Coll Cardiol.* 2015;65(17):1844-1853.
27. Alkhouli M. Intracardiac Echocardiography in structural heart disease interventions. *J Am Coll Cardiol Interv.* 2018;11:2133-2147.
28. Hijazi, Z. Intracardiac Echocardiography (ICE) during interventional & electrophysiological cardiac catheterization. *Circ.* 2009;119(4):587-596.
29. Epstein LM, Smith T, TenHoff H. Nonfluoroscopic transseptal catheterization: safety and efficacy of intracardiac echocardiographic guidance. *J Cardiovasc Electrophysiol.* 1998;9(6):625-630.
30. Bazaz R, Schwartzman D. Site-selective atrial septal puncture. *J Cardiovasc Electrophysiol.* 2003;14:196-199.
31. Rosu R. Intracardiac echocardiography for transseptal puncture. A guide for cardiac electrophysiologists. *Med Ultrason.* 2019;21:183-190.
32. Zamorano J. EAE/ASE recommendations for the use of echocardiography in new transcatheter interventions for valvular heart disease. *J Am Soc Echocardiogr.* 2011;24:937-965.
33. Hijazi Z, Wang Z, Cao Q, Koenig P, Waight D, Lang R. Transcatheter closure of atrial septal defects and patent foramen ovale under intracardiac echocardiographic guidance: feasibility and comparison with transesophageal echocardiography. *Catheter Cardiovasc Interv.* 2001;52(2):194-199.
34. Assaidi A, Sumian M, Mauri L, et al. Transcatheter closure of complex atrial septal defects is efficient under intracardiac echocardiographic guidance. *Arch Cardiovasc Dis.* 2014;107(12):646-653.
35. Saliba W, Thomas J. Intracardiac echocardiography during catheter ablation of atrial fibrillation. *Europace.* 2008;10(suppl 3):iii42-iii47.
36. Kanj M, Wazni O, Natale A. Pulmonary vein antrum isolation. *Heart Rhythm.* 2007;4:S73-S79.
37. Rao HB, Saksena S, Mitruka R, (ICE-CHIP) Study. Intra-cardiac echocardiography guided cardioversion to help interventional procedures (ICE-CHIP) study: study design and methods. *J Interv Card Electrophysiol.* 2005;13(suppl 1):31-36.
38. Bartel T, Bonaros N, Müller L, et al. Intracardiac echocardiography: a new guiding tool for transcatheter aortic valve replacement. *J Am Soc Echocardiogr.* 2011;24(9):966-975.
39. Patzelt J, Seizer P, Zhang YY, et al. Percutaneous Mitral Valve Edge-to-Edge Repair With Simultaneous Biatrial Intracardiac Echocardiography: First-in-Human Experience. *Circulation.* 2016 Apr 12;133(15):1517-1519.
40. Latib A, Mangieri A, Vicentini L, et al. Percutaneous tricuspid valve annuloplasty under conscious sedation (with only fluoroscopic and intracardiac echocardiography monitoring). *JACC Cardiovasc Interv.* 2017; 10:620-621.

CHAPTER 43

PERCUTANEOUS CORONARY INTERVENTION

Olabisi Akanbi and David Lee

HISTORY OF PERCUTANEOUS CORONARY INTERVENTION

Dotter performed the first angioplasty using sequential catheter dilation of a femoral arterial stenosis in 1964, and with advancement in catheter technology, Andreas Gruentzig performed the first balloon coronary angioplasty in 1977.[1] The high acute success rate and relatively low risk for percutaneous transcatheter coronary angioplasty (PTCA) allowed it to gain popularity over the next decade as a number of clinical trials confirmed its safety and utility in relieving angina. However, PTCA was limited by acute complications with abrupt closure of the vessel in 3% to 11% of procedures and restenosis, in which endothelial damage from the balloon procedure instigated a chain of events leading to a re-narrowing of the artery at the site of the injury in up to 50% of lesions weeks to months after the procedure.

Emergence of Coronary Stents

As the scientific understanding of restenosis grew, coronary stents were developed. The Cook Inc (Bloomington, Ind.) Gianturco-Roubin Flex-Stent was approved by the Food and Drug Administration (FDA) in May 1993 for the treatment of acute and threatened closure following balloon angioplasty. Designed as a balloon expandable stainless steel linear backbone with a series of coils soldered along its length, it provided mechanical scaffolding to support the vessel architecture after balloon injury and treat acute closure due to recoil and/or local vascular dissection.[2] In 1994, the Palmaz-Schatz stent (Johnson & Johnson), a mesh stent design based on a previously approved Palmaz stent for the iliac arteries, was also approved by the FDA. The impact on restenosis was quite remarkable, with the 202 subjects Stent Restenosis Study (STRESS) showing a target lesion revascularization rate of 10.2% in the stent group versus 18.4% in a balloon angioplasty-only group, a relative reduction of 45%. Despite these successes, the specter of acute and subacute stent thrombosis became a new important clinical problem. A landmark study, the Stent Anticoagulation Restenosis Study (STARS) trial,[3] established that dual antiplatelet therapy (DAPT) with aspirin and ticlopidine was the best choice for the prevention of stent thrombosis. In this trial of 1653 patients, patients treated with aspirin and ticlopidine had a stent thrombosis rate of 0.5% versus 3.6% for aspirin alone and 2.7% for aspirin and warfarin.

As the stent market grew, the number of available stents also grew. Multiple competitive stent designs became readily available with most clinically compared to previously FDA-approved stents in order to gain market approval. Despite modifications—decreasing stent bulk, improving deliverability to the target lesion, and changing cell design—the rates of restenosis and stent thrombosis remained relatively static.

Drug-Eluting Stents

The next era of coronary stenting began in April 2003 with the introduction of the Cypher stent (Cordis Corp., Santa Clara, CA, USA) in the United States. This stent incorporated the backbone of a stainless steel stent with the important additions of (1) a durable polymer coating and (2) an anti-restenosis drug (sirolimus). The coating, which consisted of a two polymer mix with sirolimus atop a base layer sprayed onto the stent surface, allowed an appreciable amount of sirolimus to be eluted into the vessel wall. The FDA pivotal Sirolimus-eluting Stents Versus Standard Stents in Patients with Stenosis in a Native Coronary Artery (SIRIUS) study[4] showed a target vessel revascularization (TVR) rate of 8.0% and target lesion revascularization (TLR) rate of 4.1% (21.0% and 16.6%, respectively, in the bare metal randomized group).

In May 2004, Boston Scientific (Natick, MA, USA) introduced its TAXUS drug-eluting stent (DES). This device used an existing bare metal stent platform with a proprietary polymer base and paclitaxel as its anti-restenosis drug. The TAXUS-IV FDA pivotal trial[5] yielded a TVR rate of 4.7% and TLR of 3.0%, with DES versus a bare metal control of 12% TVR and 11.3% TLR at 6 months.

The first major safety concern regarding DES arose in 2006 with the presentation of data from the Scandinavian national registry[6] as well as other meta-analyses, suggesting that DES was associated with worse clinical outcomes when compared with bare metal stents, especially with end points of death and late stent thrombosis after 6 months. This led to a much greater interest in stent thrombosis and concerns about premature cessation of DAPT.[7] Consequently, new guidance for duration of DAPT after DES changed to a prolonged plan of therapy, up to 1 year post-DES implantation with a bare minimum of 6 months. Subsequent data sets did not confirm the original Scandinavian findings, but concern persisted nonetheless for several years.

The next generation of DES with smaller delivery profiles, improved pharmacokinetics and greater biocompatible polymers, was delivered in 2010 and began the next wave of excitement in reducing major adverse cardiovascular events

(MACEs) related to coronary stents. As the performance of these stents improved, the interest in tackling more complex anatomies of coronary artery disease (CAD) became greater and moved the procedure forward to where we are today.

ADJUNCTIVE DEVICES

A number of adjunctive devices have been used to augment angioplasty and stenting and may be used for "vessel preparation" (ie, to allow delivery of the eventual stent). Atherectomy is used in perhaps 1% to 2% of all percutaneous coronary interventions (PCIs). This low use has been ascribed to the extra time needed for device preparation and use, cost of the devices, and general lack of data demonstrating additional clinic improvement when using atherectomy either as a primary treatment or as an adjunct to balloon angioplasty and/or coronary stenting. Atherectomy devices are the most widely used adjunctive device for vessel preparation and a variety of approaches exist. These include direct atherectomy, rotational and orbital atherectomy, excimer laser atherectomy, and, most recently, ultrasonic atherectomy.

Rotational and Orbital Atherectomy

The most widely used of atherectomy devices today are rotational and orbital atherectomy, both of which mechanistically work by plaque pulverization using a spinning diamond-tipped crown. For rotational atherectomy (Boston Scientific, Natick, MA, USA), the crown generally spins at 140 to 180,000 rpm and requires a specialized 0.009" coronary guidewire. The device is often used in calcific or densely packed lesions. As the plaque is pulverized, small 7 to 10 nm particles are created and sent downstream, increasing the risk of the no-reflow phenomenon. Several studies have shown its utility in aiding deliverability of balloons or stents but without any impact on restenosis rates or clinical outcomes.[8,9]

Orbital atherectomy has a similar mechanism of action but utilizes an eccentric diamond-tipped crown. It spins at a lower rpm while guided through the lesion and vessel, taking advantage of centrifugal force to enable differential cutting.[10] Clinical results[11] have been generally favorable but without clear improvement in TVR or clinical outcomes such as death and subsequent myocardial infarction (MI).

Excimer Laser Atherectomy

Excimer laser atherectomy involves the use of laser energy delivered to the vessel wall to vaporize plaque.[12] Traditionally, it has been used in undilatable or difficult to cross lesions as well as cases involving under-expanded stents. Its main advantage is that it can use a standard 0.014" coronary guidewire and provides a novel approach to lesion modification, which is distinctly different from rotational or orbital atherectomy.

Focused Ultrasound Energy—Intravascular Lithotripsy

Focused ultrasound energy has been developed as a tool to aid in treatment of severely calcified coronary lesions. Initial concept and success of intravascular lithotripsy has been demonstrated in the peripheral vasculature. The coronary device can be used on a standard 0.014" coronary guidewire and involves the placement of a balloon with a focused ultrasound emitter at the site of the lesion and the emitter is activated, which then destabilizes calcific plaque through microvibrations created by the sound waves. Based on reports[13-15] demonstrating safety and utility of this approach in the coronary vasculature, the FDA granted approval of the device in February 2021 for the treatment of severely calcified CAD.

INDICATIONS FOR PERCUTANEOUS CORONARY INTERVENTION

Physiologic Measurements in the Catheterization Laboratory

Pressure wire technology, most typically fractional flow reserve (FFR), has provided interventional cardiologists with a means of determining the physiologic significance of stenotic lesions during angiography. The use of coronary physiology to guide myocardial revascularization was shown to improve clinical outcomes and reduce cost in patients with CAD.[4] The majority of patients are still managed based on angiographic visual estimation of a stenosis in isolation. The main premise of coronary physiology assessment is to determine the functional significance of individual stenoses at the time of clinical decision-making, providing an objective marker to identify ischemic lesions most likely to benefit from PCI.

Fractional Flow Reserve

FFR is the most widely used pressure-derived invasive physiologic index of coronary lesion assessment and considered the gold standard for clinical physiologic assessment in the catheterization laboratory. FFR is defined as the ratio of maximum achievable coronary blood flow (CBF) in the presence of an epicardial coronary stenosis and the theoretical maximum CBF in the hypothetical absence of coronary stenosis during pharmacologic vasodilation. FFR is the ratio of the mean distal coronary pressure (P_d) to the mean proximal coronary pressure (P_a) across a stenosis during maximal hyperemia. Vasodilators are used to achieve maximal hyperemia, most commonly adenosine (**Table 43.1**). The purpose of the hyperemia is to create conditions in which pressure (P_a and P_d) and flow are linearly related.

The concept of FFR and hyperemic pressure-derived indices of coronary stenosis severity depends on the fundamental physiologic principle that coronary pressure is directly proportional to CBF when microvascular resistance is stable, achievable with hyperemic agents like adenosine. Under these conditions, the decrease in pressure across a coronary stenosis reflects the decrease in CBF to the amount of subtended myocardium. Landmark studies have shown improved patient outcomes by selecting patients for PCI with FFR (**Table 43.2**). This has led to the incorporation of FFR into coronary revascularization guidelines, which currently recommend its clinical use based on a fixed 0.8 cutoff. Of note, the current evidence on the value of FFR as a clinical decision tool is based on studies

SECTION 3

TABLE 43.1 Hyperemic Agents Used in Coronary Fractional Flow Reserve Measurements

Drug	Dose	Plateau	$T_{1/2}$	Side Effect	Pitfall
Papaverine IC	15 mg LCA 10 mg RCA	30-60 s	2 min	Transient QT prolongation and T-wave abnormalities: very rarely, ventricular tachycardia/torsade de pointes	Do not use with heparin or heparinized saline, as it forms a precipitate
Adenosine IC	40-60 μg LCA 24-36 μg RCA	5-10 s	30-60 s	Occasional transient AV block after injection in RCA	Submaximum stimulus in some patients; interruption of aortic pressure. Must repeat with escalating doses to ensure that maximal hyperemia is reached. No pullback curve possible
Adenosine IV	140 mg/kg/min	≤1-2 min	1-2 min	Decrease in blood pressure by 10%-15%. Burning or angina-like chest pain during infusion (harmless, not ischemia). Not to be used in patients with severe obstructive lung disease (potential for bronchospasm)	
Dobutamine IV	10-40 μg/kg/min	1-2 min	3-5 min	Tachycardia, mild increase in blood pressure	
Nitroprusside IC	0.3-0.9 μg/kg	20 s	1 min	20% decrease in blood pressure	

AV, atrioventricular; IC, intracoronary; IV, intravenous; min, minutes; s, seconds; $T_{1/2}$ - half life; LCA, left coronary artery; RCA, right coronary artery.

Modified from Pijls NH, Kern MJ, Yock PG, et al. Practice and potential pitfalls of coronary pressure measurement. *Catheter Cardiovasc Interv.* 2000;49(1):1-16. Copyright © 2000 Wiley-Liss, Inc. Reprinted by permission of John Wiley & Sons, Inc.

TABLE 43.2 Landmark Studies Demonstrate Improved Patient Outcomes by Selecting Patients for PCI with FFR

Trial	Study Question	Study Population	Patients (n)	Patients in the Coronary Physiology-Guided Group (n)	Study Primary Endpoint	FFR Cutoff for Treatment	Mean FFR Values	Conclusion
DEFER[6]	Safety of deferral of PCI in patients with FFR >0.75	Stable CAD	325	325	MACE[a] at 4 months	≤0.75	• Defer group: 0.87 ± 0.07 (*N* = 91) • Performance group: 0.87 ± 0.06 (*N* = 90) • Reference group: 0.56 ± 0.16 (*N* = 144)	Deferral of PCI in lesions with FFR >0.75 is safe

TABLE 43.2 Landmark Studies Demonstrate Improved Patient Outcomes by Selecting Patients for PCI with FFR (*continued*)

Trial	Study Question	Study Population	Patients (n)	Patients in the Coronary Physiology-Guided Group (n)	Study Primary Endpoint	FFR Cutoff for Treatment	Mean FFR Values	Conclusion
FAME[8]	Efficacy of FFR-guided PCI vs angiography-alone-guided PCI	Multivessel stable CAD / ACS with nonculprit stenosis	1005	509	MACE[b] at 12 months	≤0.80	• Overall cohort: 0.71 ± 0.18 • Ischemic lesions: 0.60 ± 0.14 • Nonischemic lesions: 0.88 ± 0.05	FFR-guided PCI is superior to angiography-alone-guided PCI
FAME 2[9]	FFR-guided PCI + OMT vs OMT alone in patients with FFR ≤0.80	Multivessel stable CAD	1220	1220	MACE[c] at 24 months (trial prematurely stopped at 7-month follow-up)	≤0.80	• FFR-guided PCI + OMT: 0.68 ± 0.10 • OMT alone: 0.68 ± 0.15	FFR-guided PCI + OMT reduces ischemic outcomes compared with OMT alone
Total			2550	2054				

ACS, acute coronary syndrome; CAD, coronary artery disease; FFR, fractional flow reserve; MACE, major adverse cardiac event; OMT, optimal medical treatment; PCI, percutaneous coronary intervention.

[a]Composite of all-cause mortality, myocardial infarction, coronary artery bypass graft surgery, coronary angioplasty, and any procedure-related complication necessitating major intervention or prolonged hospital stay.

[b]Composite of death, myocardial infarction, and any repeat revascularization.

[c]Composite of death from any cause, nonfatal myocardial infarction, or unplanned hospitalization leading to urgent revascularization.

that have used two different FFR criteria for defining hemodynamically significant lesions: 0.75 or 0.80. The different choice of dichotomous cutoffs has its origin in early validation studies, which demonstrated that an FFR <0.75 has 100% specificity to identify stenosis with inducible ischemia, whereas an FFR >0.80 has a sensitivity of more than 90% to exclude stenoses that cause ischemia. Recent developments spurred by wire-based FFR include other coronary functional indexes such as instantaneous wave-free ratio (iFR) and resting distal-to-aortic coronary pressure ratio (P_d/P_a), which can be performed without hyperemic agents as well as angiography-based FFR, which utilizes computational flow dynamics to estimate FFR by contrast flow[16] (**Figure 43.1A-D** and **Table 43.3**).

Irrespective of incorporation into guidelines, global adoption into clinical practice remains underutilized for a variety of reasons, including technicalities associated with FFR measurements, time consumption, inadequate reimbursement, or relative contraindications associated with hyperemia (such as severe pulmonary disease and use of adenosine).

Instantaneous Wave-Free Ratio

iFR is a pressure-based physiologic index of coronary stenosis severity that is measured under resting conditions by making use of the unique properties of baseline coronary physiology; it does not require the administration of vasodilator drugs. Consequently, it is a simpler, safe, and effective alternative to FFR to guide revascularization.

While resting P_d/P_a is the ratio of distal coronary artery pressure to aortic pressure over the entire cardiac cycle (systole and diastole), iFR is measured during a specific period of diastole known as the wave-free period, when flow is intrinsically at its highest compared with the whole cardiac cycle and there are no competing waves affecting the CBF_5. The onset of diastole is identified from the dicrotic notch, and the diastolic window is calculated beginning 25% into diastole and ending 5 ms before the end of diastole. Resting blood flow is preserved across all severities of stenosis as a result of compensatory microcirculatory vasodilation in response to the stenosis at the expense of P_d, which falls even at rest. Because pressure falls at

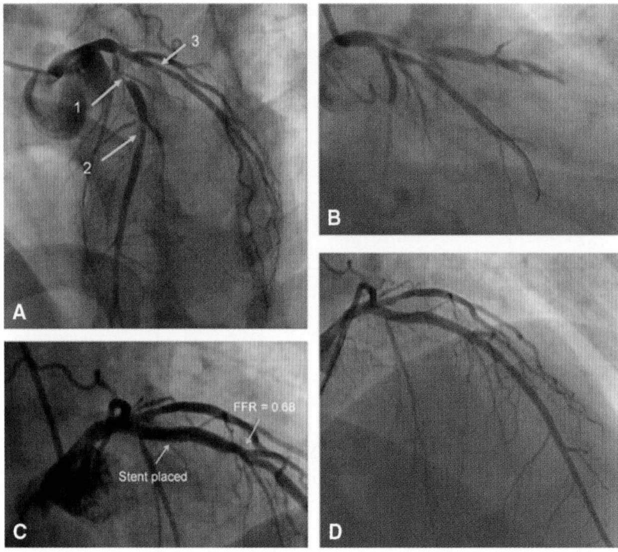

FIGURE 43.1 Angiogram and FFR of a patient with multivessel coronary artery disease (CAD). **A.** Patient with multivessel CAD undergoing PCI with an FFR-guided approach. The LAD lesion (*1*) is judged to be severe and matched with stress test result and symptoms. The mid-LAD lesion (*2*) is clearly intermediate, as is the lesion in the LCx (*3*). **B.** FFR is obtained in the LCX, with the wire positioned as shown, and is 0.88. This lesion is physiologically insignificant and is not treated with PCI. **C.** A stent is placed in the proximal LAD lesion and then FFR is performed to assess the significance of the more distal LAD lesion originally judged to be intermediate. The FFR of the LAD is 0.68, and the more distal lesion is subsequently stented as well, secondary to this significant FFR finding. **D.** Final angiogram showing the treated proximal and mid-LAD lesions with the intermediate LCX lesion left untreated. FFR, fractional flow reserve; LAD, left anterior descending; LCx, left circumflex artery; PCI, percutaneous coronary intervention.

rest with stenosis severity, a resting index should be sufficient to quantify severity, provided there is sufficient flow velocity to distinguish between stenoses. During diastole, the competing waves are quiescent, and during the wave-free period, microcirculatory resistance is at its lowest and most stable compared to the rest of the cardiac cycle. At this time, the pressure and flow velocity are linearly related, and pressure ratios can assess the flow limitation imposed by a stenosis.

Because the wave-free period exists as a proportion of diastole and changes with alterations of the R-R interval, iFR can be calculated during irregular heart rhythms like atrial fibrillation and for heart rates normally acceptable for physiologic assessment (30-130 beats/min). The ADenosine Vasodilator Independent Stenosis Evaluation (ADVISE) study[20] compared pressure-only iFR with FFR in 157 stenoses with good correlation (0.90) and receiver-operating characteristic (ROC) area under the curve (AUC) of 93%. In the VERification of Instantaneous Wave-Free Ratio and Fractional Flow Reserve for the Assessment of Coronary Artery Stenosis Severity in EverydaY Practice (VERIFY) and RESOLVE studies, FFR and iFR demonstrated no significant differences in the prediction of myocardial ischemia. The same pressure wires utilized in FFR may be used for iFR. The iFR cutoff value <0.89 is significant requiring PCI, and this has been shown to be noninferior to the FFR cutoff of 0.8. The landmark trials for iFR (DEFINE-FLAIR [Functional Lesion Assessment of Intermediate Stenosis to Guide Revascularisation] and the Instantaneous Wave-free Ratio versus Fractional Flow Reserve in Patients with Stable Angina Pectoris or Acute Coronary Syndrome [iFR-SWEDEHEART]) both compared FFR and iFR in large groups of patients and found that iFR is as reliable as FFR in predicting benefit for PCI outcomes.

TABLE 43.3 Invasive Physiologic Indices to Assess the Functional Significance of Coronary Artery Stenosis

Index	Conditions of Measurement	Interrogation Level	Advantages	Disadvantages
FFR	Hyperemia	Epicardial level	• Established cutoff	• Need for hyperemic agents • High interpatient variability in microvascular resistance during vasodilatation induced by adenosine • Affected by hemodynamic variables
iFR	Baseline	Epicardial level	• No need for hyperemic agents • Established cutoff • Assessment of tandem and/or diffuse coronary lesions	• Requires proprietary software • Longer term outcome results warranted • Outcome data in higher risk patient subgroups needed
Resting P_d/P_a	Baseline	Epicardial level	• No need for hyperemic agents	• Not validated in randomized controlled trials

TABLE 43.3 Invasive Physiologic Indices to Assess the Functional Significance of Coronary Artery Stenosis (*continued*)

Index	Conditions of Measurement	Interrogation Level	Advantages	Disadvantages
Contrast FFR	Hyperemia	Epicardial level	• Resting index correlating best with FFR	• No contrast dose established in randomized controlled trials • Contrast induces short-lived hyperemia
CFR	Hyperemia	Epicardial level and microcirculation	• Prognostic marker	• Inability to differentiate the effects of microvascular dysfunction from effects of the epicardial lesion • Need for hyperemic agents • Affected by hemodynamic variables
HSR	Hyperemia	Epicardial level	• Combination of flow and pressure measurement • Established cutoff	• Need for hyperemic agents • Largely confined to research setting owing to difficulty of measurement technique
BSR	Baseline	Epicardial level	• Combination of flow and pressure measurement • No need for hyperemic agents	• No established cutoff • Less accurate than HSR • Largely confined to research setting owing to difficulty of measurement technique

BSR, basal stenosis resistance; CFR, coronary flow reserve; FFR, fractional flow reserve; HSR, hyperemic stenosis resistance; iFR, instantaneous wave-free ratio; P_d/P_a, ratio of the mean distal coronary pressure to the mean proximal coronary pressure.

SECTION 3

INTRAVASCULAR ULTRASOUND AND OPTICAL COHERENCE TOMOGRAPHY

Angiography remains the main visual modality to determine lesion significance, but other tools are available for intracoronary imaging, including intravascular ultrasound (IVUS) and optical coherence tomography (OCT). Both are capable of high-resolute intravascular imaging and aid in improving PCI results and outcomes.

Two IVUS transducers are commercially available: a solid state and a rotating type. The solid state phased array transducer utilizes 64 transducers arranged in a circular array and emits sound at a frequency of 20 Hz. It provides good resolution on the order of 200 μm in an axial direction, with a depth penetration greater than 6 mm from its ultrasound source. The rotating transducer also provides similar resolution (150-200 μm) and slightly less penetration given its higher frequency (40-50 Hz). It utilizes a spinning transducer and mirror to capture reflected sound waves to create its image. Many studies[17-19] have demonstrated the benefit of using IVUS to improve and optimize stenting as well as to provide anatomic

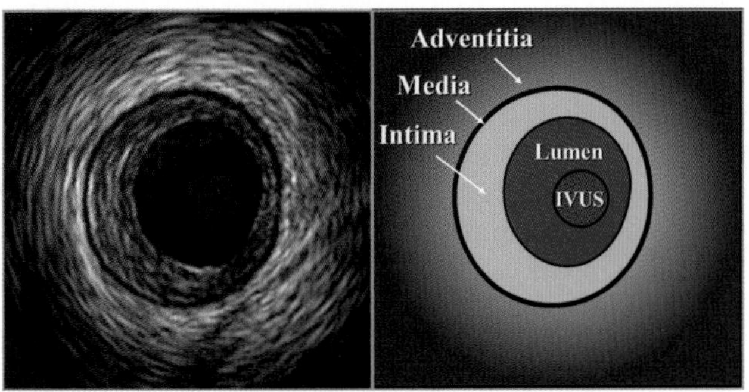

FIGURE 43.2 Intravascular ultrasound (IVUS) image showing identification of intravascular landmarks.

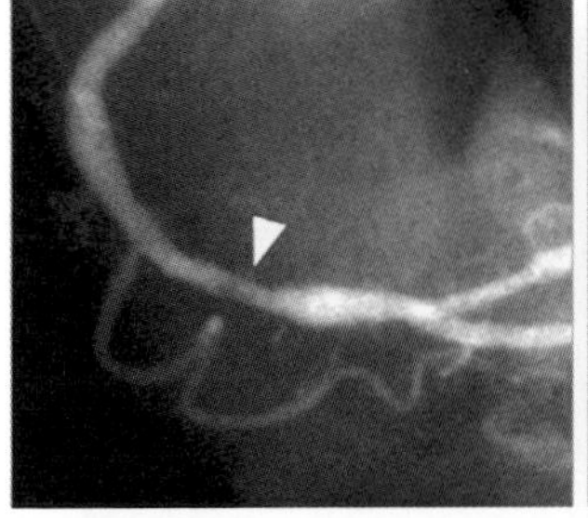
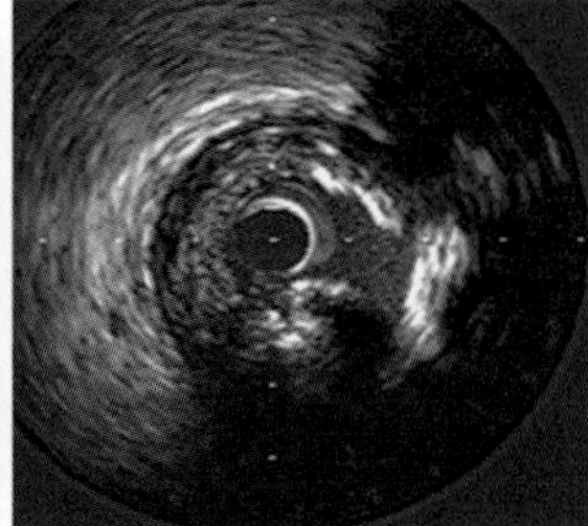

FIGURE 43.3 Intravascular ultrasound (IVUS) of an ambiguous angiographic lesion. The right coronary artery has a hazy lesion in its midsection; IVUS reveals a complex, calcified narrowing with small lumen.

data to help guide an indication for PCI, although IVUS has largely been supplanted by the functional measurements with pressure wires. IVUS has the benefit of being able to characterize soft and hard (calcific) plaque and enables appropriate measurements of vessel and lumen size to better match any intended stent usage. It can also provide longitudinal measures for estimating lesion length. It is particularly useful for ostial lesions and can help with identifying lesions that may appear ambiguous on an angiogram (**Figures 43.2** and **43.3**).

Despite its benefits, the use of IVUS has remained limited. This is due to the time required for its setup in the catheterization laboratory (although typically <5 minutes) and the need to be comfortable and well-versed with image interpretation and the use of measurement tools.

OCT uses a laser light to create an image. Its tip contains a laser emitter at a frequency of 1250 to 1350 nm with an axial resolution of 10 to 20 nm. Its depth of penetration is less than that of IVUS (typically <5 mm), and it requires a blood-free infusion during pullback through the vessel. Its superior resolution can be useful to detect small problem areas such as incomplete stent apposition or thrombus that would otherwise escape identification with IVUS imaging (**Figure 43.4**). It has been shown in studies to improve outcomes when compared to angiography alone. The main drawbacks are its cost and setup, as well as the need for flushing the vessel blood free with saline during OCT imaging. In a recent trial comparing OCT with IVUS and angiography for stenting, it was superior to angiography in terms of providing optimal stent results and similar—but not superior—to IVUS.[20]

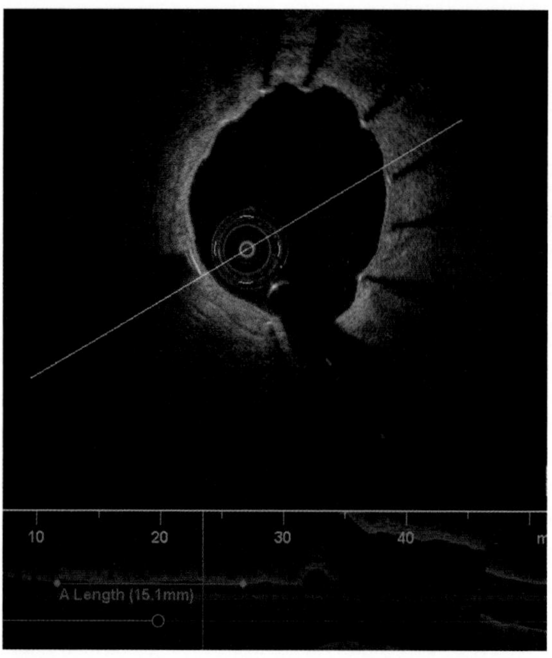

FIGURE 43.4 Optical coherence tomography image demonstrating stent struts with good apposition to the vessel wall and showing longitudinal location within the target vessel.

MULTIVESSEL DISEASE

The observation that up to one-third of patients undergoing PCI have more than one vessel with stenosis has led to great interest in performing multivessel PCI safely. To this end, multiple clinical trials compared coronary artery bypass surgery (CABG) and PCI when randomized to either strategy after review for appropriateness by a trial committee. Initial studies with bare metal stents retained an advantage for CABG in this population, largely driven by increased subsequent revascularization in patients undergoing PCI.[21,22] As a result of these trials, CABG remained the mainstay of treatment for patients with multivessel disease (MVD), especially for patients with diabetes.[23]

The introduction of DES rekindled an interest in comparing PCI and CABG, given that these stents had demonstrated a lower risk of restenosis and the need for subsequent revascularization in patients with less intensive disease. In The Synergy between Percutaneous Coronary Intervention with Taxus and Cardiac Surgery (SYNTAX) study,[24] a comparative trial of multivessel PCI with a first-generation paclitaxel-eluting stent (TAXUS) and CABG, the overall outcome favored CABG driven by the higher rate of revascularization in the PCI arm. In select anatomies (ie, less complex CAD), multivessel PCI showed similar outcomes to CABG with regard to death, MI, revascularization, and stroke (**Figure 43.5A,B**).[25] Interestingly, much of the benefit of CABG over PCI was lost by the 10-year follow-up.[26] Other studies have continued to support the notion that CABG remains superior to PCI, especially in diabetic patients, with a survival benefit with CABG extending up to 8 years.[27,28]

The ACC/AHA guidelines provide indications for multivessel PCI and appropriate revascularization strategies.[29] The interest in performing multivessel PCI remains strong in select cases when the CV surgical team is disinterested in offering CABG (**Figure 43.6**).[30]

ISOLATED LEFT MAIN CORONARY DISEASE

The SYNTAX study included an analysis of patients with isolated left main (LM) disease treated with DES that showed stenting could be done safely with a low restenosis rate. For LM lesions involving the ostium or shaft of the left main coronary artery (LMCA), patients had similar outcomes with PCI to those undergoing CABG. For lesions involving the distal LM and bifurcation, a higher acute risk and poorer outcome were noted for PCI when compared with CABG. In PRECOMBAT, a Korean study, no difference in major adverse cardiac and cerebrovascular events (MACCEs) was noted when comparing CABG to sirolimus-eluting stents for LM CAD.[31] In contrast, a German study supported the SYNTAX results, showing a higher risk of subsequent revascularization for isolated LM patients undergoing PCI[32] using sirolimus-eluting stents. A recent study using a third-generation stent—the Evaluation of XIENCE versus Coronary Artery Bypass Graft Surgery for Effectiveness of Left Main Revascularization

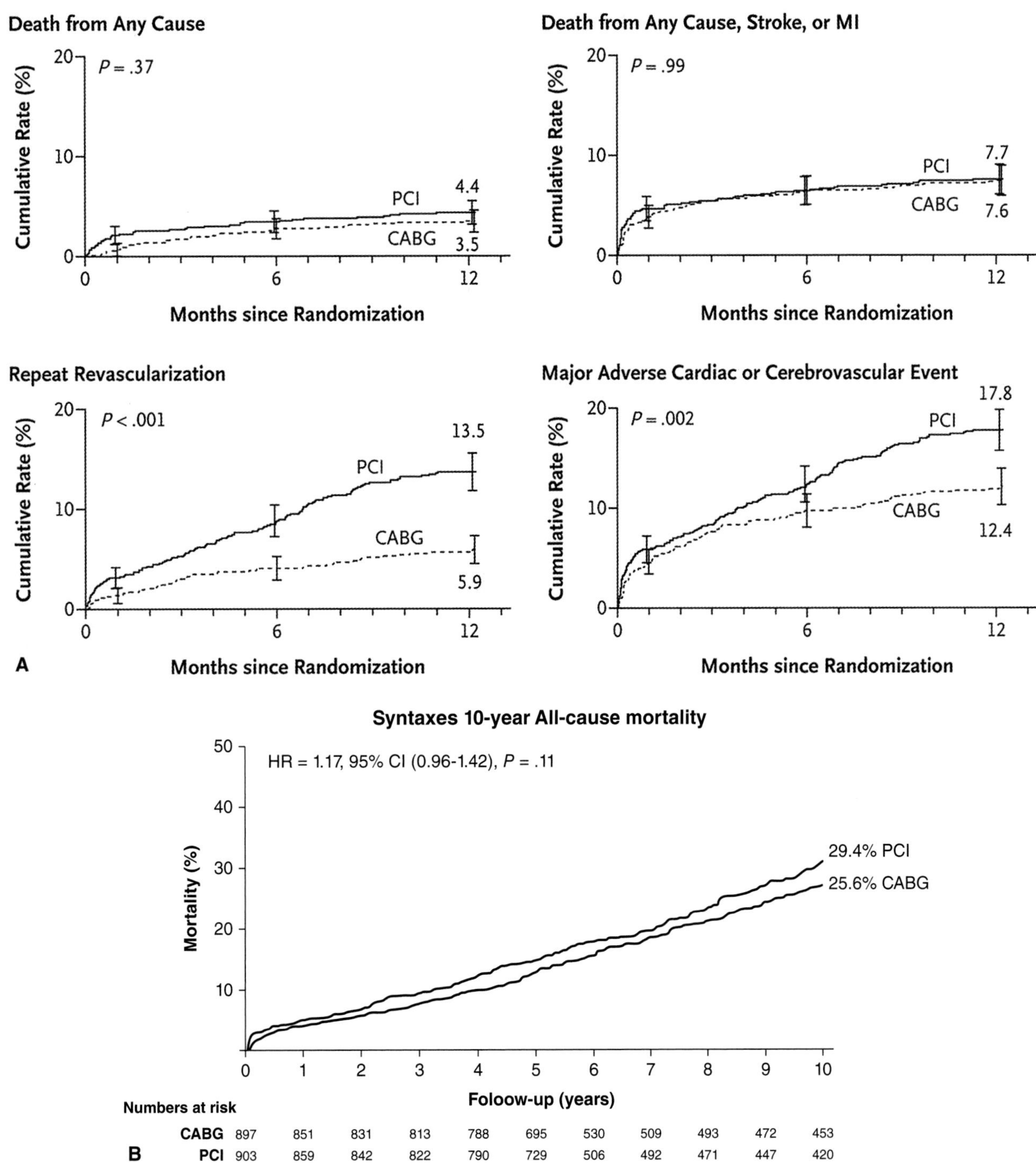

FIGURE 43.5 One-year **(A)** and 10-year outcomes **(B)** from SYNTAX. The data at 1 year demonstrate an improved outcome with CABG compared to PCI for the treatment of multivessel coronary artery disease, largely driven by repeat revascularization in the PCI arm. No significant difference in death or a composite of death, stroke, and MI was noted with CABG versus PCI. At 10 years, mortality between the two groups was similar. CABG, coronary artery bypass surgery; MI, myocardial infarction; PCI, percutaneous coronary intervention. (From Serruys PW, Morice MC, Kappetein AP, et al. Percutaneous coronary intervention versus coronary-artery bypass grafting for severe coronary artery disease. *N Engl J Med.* 2009;360(10):961-972. Copyright © 2009 Massachusetts Medical Society. Reprinted with permission from Massachusetts Medical Society.)

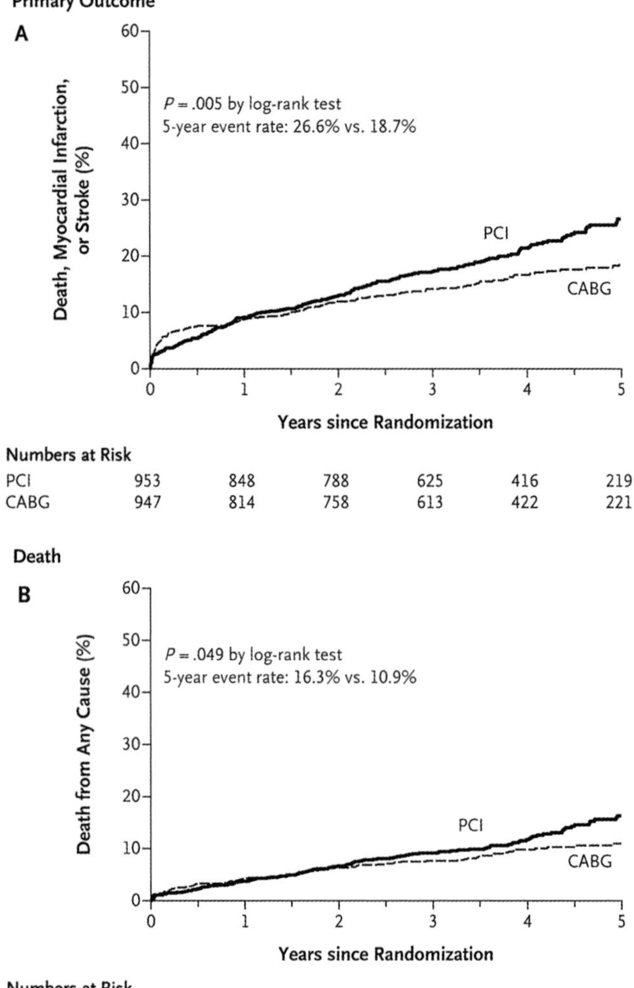

FIGURE 43.6 Five year outcomes from the Future Revascularization Evaluation in Patients with Diabetes Mellitus: Optimal Management of Multivessel Disease–FREEDOM Trial. The data demonstrate improved outcomes with CABG versus PCI in diabetic patients with multivessel disease undergoing revascularization.[28] CABG, coronary artery bypass surgery; PCI, percutaneous coronary intervention.

(EXCEL) trial[33]—studied patients with low or intermediate SYNTAX scores and isolated LM disease. In comparing an everolimus-eluting stent to CABG, no difference was noted in the composite of death, MI, stroke, and repeat revascularization at 3 years. A meta-analysis of five large trials[34] suggested that overall outcomes (death, subsequent MI, or stroke at median 5.6 years) were similar in patients treated with PCI or CABG for isolated LM disease, with a small advantage for CABG in terms of lower revascularization.

At this time, it is prudent (and per guidelines) to consult with the cardiac surgeon and interventionalist for a decision regarding the best revascularization approach in these patients. For more complex disease involving the bifurcation or with greater than one-vessel disease beyond the LM, guidelines and clinical trial data still dictate CABG over PCI.

ROLE OF PERCUTANEOUS CORONARY INTERVENTION IN STABLE ISCHEMIC HEART DISEASE

Per current guidelines, PCI should be reserved for those patients with medically refractory angina or those demonstrating large areas of ischemia on a stress test. The Clinical Outcomes Utilizing Revascularization and Aggressive Drug Evaluation (COURAGE) trial[35] demonstrated that PCI and optimal medical therapy (OMT) (including medications and lifestyle changes) were not superior to OMT alone in patients with stable symptomatic CAD: MACEs and anginal scores out to 5 years postrandomization. However, angiographic success rate for PCI was relatively low (93%), two-thirds of the patients in the initial medical therapy–alone arm eventually underwent revascularization (largely PCI) and DES use was low. In addition, most of the patients in the study were enrolled without DESs. A study comparing PCI to OMT in stable ischemic heart disease looked at the influence of ischemic burden upon short-term survival and found that PCI was superior to OMT with increasing ischemic burden.[36] These data form the basis for the guideline-directed management of stable heart disease in the United States, with a more nuanced view of PCI in Europe[37] utilizing the ischemic burden to help guide its use.

A contemporary investigation, the International Study of Comparative Health Effectiveness with Medical and Invasive Approaches (ISCHEMIA) trial,[38] examined the degree of ischemia and its relation to PCI and/or OMT outcomes. Patients with moderate or severe ischemia according to stress imaging study were randomized to PCI with OMT versus OMT alone. At a median follow-up of 3.2 years, no differences between the invasive or conservative group were noted in terms of subsequent MI or death (**Figure 43.7A-D**).

PCI remains important to help relieve angina in many patients with stable ischemic heart disease, and further investigation is warranted in higher risk groups that have been excluded from these trials, including those with heart failure or more challenging anatomy.

ROLE OF PERCUTANEOUS CORONARY INTERVENTION IN ACUTE CORONARY SYNDROMES

Unstable Angina and Non–ST-Segment Elevation Myocardial Infarction

Several trials have looked at PCI and its influence on outcomes for patients presenting with unstable angina (UA) or non–ST-segment elevation myocardial infarction (NSTEMI). In general, patients with UA/NSTEMI are medically stabilized

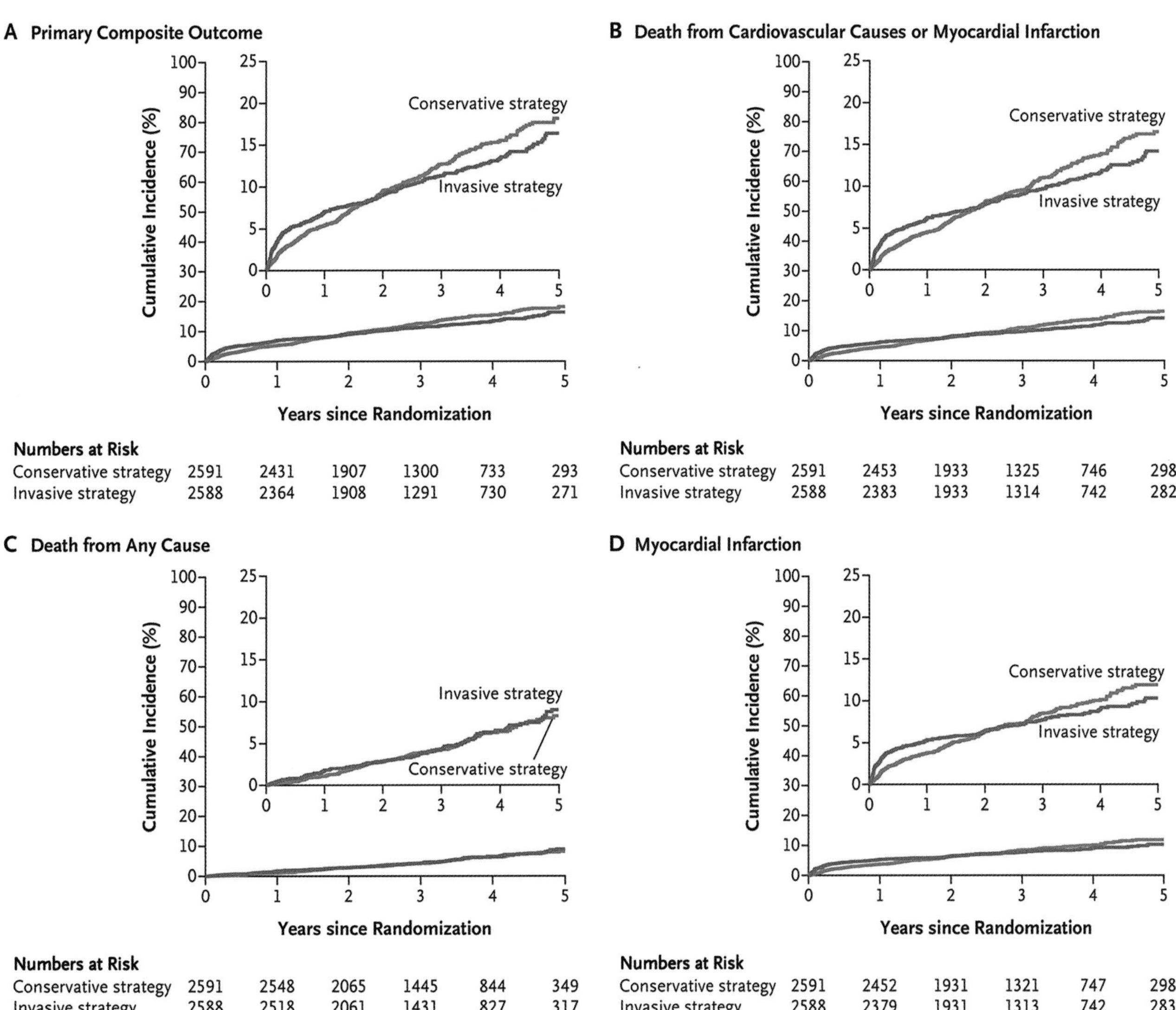

FIGURE 43.7 A-D The ISCHEMIA trial. A comparison of percutaneous coronary intervention and optimal medical therapy versus optimal medical therapy only in patients with moderate or severe ischemia showed no significant differences in outcomes. (From Maron DJ, Hochman JS, Reynolds HR, et al. Initial invasive or conservative strategy for stable coronary disease. *N Engl J Med.* 2020; 382(15):1395-1407. Copyright © 2020 Massachusetts Medical Society. Reprinted with permission from Massachusetts Medical Society.)

and consideration of angiography discussed, with angiography occurring usually within the first 24 to 48 hours. For patients refractory to medical stabilization, angiography is initiated earlier. In both groups, the goal of the angiogram is to define the coronary anatomy and identify and treat a culprit lesion. In this situation, the overwhelming evidence points to revascularization for symptom relief as well as initiation (or continuation) of aggressive medical therapy as secondary prevention.

For the past two decades, the main foci of interest have been the use of adjuvant pharmacology and the timing of PCI (or CABG when warranted). Several trials[39-41] examined the role of a routine catheterization strategy and showed its benefit over an ischemia-guided approach in lowering death, MI, and rehospitalization. The Timing of Intervention in Acute Coronary Syndromes (TIMACS) trial[42] examined the timing of angiography in patients presenting with UA/NSTEMI and found that an early invasive strategy initiated within 24 hours of hospital admission was better at preventing refractory ischemia—but not death or MI—than a delayed strategy (ie, initiated >36 hours of hospital admission), especially in those patients who were at higher risk according to the Global Registry of Acute Coronary Events (GRACE) risk score. A recent meta-analysis supported these findings and suggests that risk assessment may be important to determining who is most likely to benefit from an early invasive strategy.[43] As a result, the current guidelines from the ACCF/AHA[44] recommend the timing of the invasive strategy be based on the risk assessment of the patient.

ST-Segment Elevation Myocardial Infarction

Many trials were performed comparing the relative benefits of thrombolytic therapy and primary angioplasty, with the Primary Angioplasty in Myocardial Infarction (PAMI) study trial[45] at the forefront establishing the superiority of primary angioplasty over thrombolysis with tissue plasminogen activator (t-PA). However, in the late 1990s, only about 25% of US catheterization laboratories maintained 24-hour access for ST-segment elevation myocardial infarction (STEMI).

As delivery of quality, acute cardiac care has become a priority to patients and hospitals, most nonrural areas of the United States have access to an acute primary PCI hospital. Consequently, the DANish Acute Myocardial Infarction 2 (DANAMI-2) trial[46] showed that transfer to a PCI-capable hospital for primary PCI (with median travel time of 114 minutes) better prevented recurrent MI than administering thrombolysis in the rural hospital with subsequent transfer to a PCI-capable hospital.

Other important improvements have included assembly of multidisciplinary teams, coordinated care between the emergency department and catheterization laboratory, transmission of electrocardiograms by emergency medical systems from the field,[47] improved care at the point of first patient contact and shortening time from first patient contact to reperfusion in the catheterization laboratory ("encounter to balloon") or from the emergency department to the catheterization laboratory ("door to balloon"; D2B), and lower mortality. Survival and morbidity can be improved with timelier reperfusion with a D2B goal of less than 90 minutes.[48]

Controversy has arisen regarding the role of complete or infarct-related artery (IRA)-only revascularization in the setting of MVD during the treatment of STEMI. The Complete vs Culprit-only Revascularization to Treat Multi-vessel Disease After Early PCI for STEMI (COMPLETE) study[49] demonstrated that a strategy of complete revascularization with staged PCI of the nonculprit lesions (ie, PCI during a procedure separate from the index PCI procedure for STEMI) reduced the risk of new MI. One-third of the patients had the second procedure after hospital discharge, indicating that complete revascularization may be safely postponed until after hospital discharge in selected patients. A recent meta-analysis[50] confirmed that in patients with MVD presenting with STEMI, complete revascularization at any timing, including same sitting, staged in-hospital, and staged out-hospital, may have similar benefits. Lingering issues include (1) criteria for performing the procedure safely, (2) ideal timing of complete revascularization, and (3) the potential role of FFR or iFR in determining functional significance of borderline lesions to help guide PCI appropriateness.

Saphenous Vein Graft Interventions

Initial experience in saphenous vein graft (SVG) interventions was with balloon angioplasty and exhibited relatively poor outcomes with high restenosis rates and "no-reflow" phenomenon, in which embolic material is created by vascular injury and disruption from manipulation within the graft.[51,52] This material, typically large (>80-250 μm in diameter), plugs the native vessel microvasculature and leads to flow stasis. Predictably, poorer outcomes are associated with no-reflow.[53] Early treatments were largely pharmacologic, with use of vasodilators delivered via the guide catheter, and of very limited success. Failed approaches have included proximal protection devices with a balloon occlusion guide catheter[54] as well as covered stents to prevent atheroemboli.[55,56]

A) Balloon occlusion device

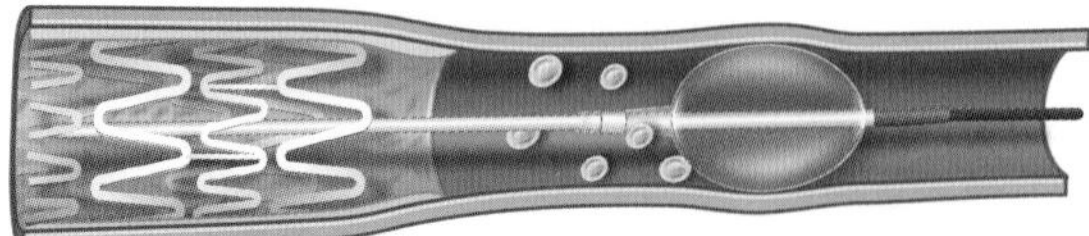

B) Filter device

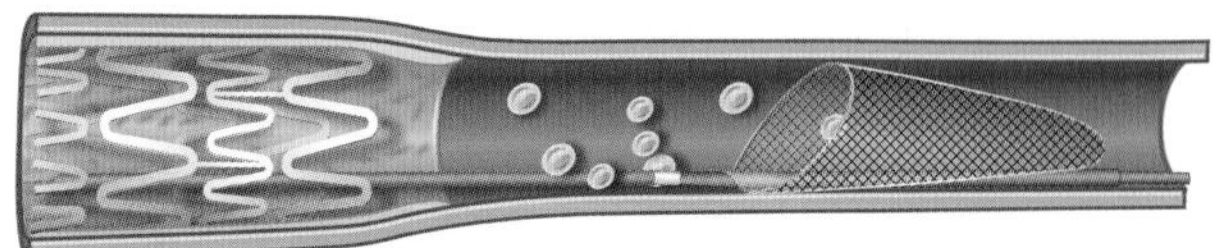

FIGURE 43.8 Embolic protection devices. **A**. Balloon occlusion device. **B**. Filter device.

Several embolic protection devices **(Figure 43.8A,B)** are currently available. With some, balloon occlusion of the SVG blood flow distal to the site of PCI allows aspiration of the debris to prevent its embolism. The Saphenous Vein Graft Free of Emboli (SAFER) trial[57] demonstrated a reduction in MACE from 16.5% in the placebo group to 9.6% in the group using a balloon occlusion and aspiration system (P <.001), and the no-reflow rate was reduced from 8% to 3.4%. Another approach to embolic protection is to combine a small filter with a guidewire. One major advantage of this system is that it allows blood flow during the intervention. In the FilterWire EX Randomized Evaluation (FIRE) trial,[57] a filter-based catheter was noninferior to a balloon occlusion and aspiration system with regard to the primary end point of MACE at 30 days.

FOLLOW-UP PATIENT CARE: DUAL ANTIPLATELET THERAPY

A number of changes have been made with respect to the use and duration of DAPT. Clopidogrel has become the standard for DAPT for many years, with continued recommendations for 1-month DAPT after bare metal stenting. For individuals who received DES, 6 to 12 months of DAPT was initially recommended.[58,59] Prospective trials such as DAPT[60] and OPTImal DUAL antiplatelet therapy (OPTIDUAL)[61] gave conflicting results regarding the ideal duration of DAPT but noted that 12 months appeared to be reasonable. However, further data showed that 6 months of DAPT poststenting with the most contemporary DESs was safe. Recent data have studied the minimum duration of DAPT in high-risk bleeding patients[62] and suggested that 1 month is reasonable and safe in these select patients.

In the 10% to 20% of patients undergoing PCI who also have a need for more intensive anticoagulation, such as with a mechanical prosthetic valve or for chronic atrial fibrillation, a number of studies have shown that a short course of DAPT with anticoagulation ("triple therapy") are at a markedly increased risk of bleeding. Subsequent studies with a single antiplatelet and anticoagulation suggest that clopidogrel (in the absence of larger data sets with prasugrel or ticagrelor) with anticoagulation ("double therapy") for at least 1 month post-PCI demonstrates an acceptable bleeding risk while preventing acute and subacute stent thrombosis.

KEY POINTS

- ✔ PCI is an important tool in managing patients with acute and chronic coronary heart disease.
- ✔ PCI has evolved from treatment of simple, focal lesions to complex multivessel, LM, and other coronary disease, include acute coronary syndrome (ACS) and STEMI.
- ✔ Improved technology and techniques have improved the safety of PCI.
- ✔ DAPT is important to prevent stent thrombosis, although the ideal duration of therapy has yet to be firmly determined.
- ✔ Adjunctive evaluation of coronary disease can aid in better decision-making and outcomes in PCI.

REFERENCES

1. Gruntzig A. Transluminal dilatation of coronary-artery stenosis. *Lancet.* 1978;1:263.
2. George BS, Voorhees WD 3rd, Roubin GS, et al. Multicenter investigation of coronary stenting to treat acute or threatened closure after percutaneous transluminal coronary angioplasty: clinical and angiographic outcomes. *J Am Coll Cardiol.* 1993;22:135-143.
3. Leon MB, Baim DS, Popma JJ, et al. A clinical trial comparing three antithrombotic-drug regimens after coronary-artery stenting. Stent Anticoagulation Restenosis Study Investigators. *N Engl J Med.* 1998;339:1665-1671.
4. Moses JW, Leon MB, Popma JJ, et al. Sirolimus-eluting stents versus standard stents in patients with stenosis in a native coronary artery. *N Engl J Med.* 2003;349:1315-1323.
5. Stone GW, Ellis SG, Cox DA, et al. A polymer-based, paclitaxel-eluting stent in patients with coronary artery disease. *N Engl J Med.* 2004;350:221-231.
6. Lagerqvist B, James SK, Stenestrand U, et al. Long-term outcomes with drug-eluting stents versus bare-metal stents in Sweden. *N Engl J Med.* 2007;356:1009-1019.
7. Airoldi F, Colombo A, Morici N, et al. Incidence and predictors of drug-eluting stent thrombosis during and after discontinuation of thienopyridine treatment. *Circulation.* 2007;116:745-754.
8. Abdel-Wahab M, Richardt G, Joachim Büttner H, et al. High-speed rotational atherectomy before paclitaxel-eluting stent implantation in complex calcified coronary lesions: the randomized ROTAXUS (Rotational Atherectomy Prior to Taxus Stent Treatment for Complex Native Coronary Artery Disease) trial. *JACC Cardiovasc Interv.* 2013;6(1):10-19.
9. Gupta T, Weinreich M, Greenberg M, Colombo A, Latib A. Rotational atherectomy: a contemporary appraisal. *Interv Cardiol.* 2019;14(3):182-189.
10. Parikh K, Chandra P, Choksi N, Khanna P, Chambers J. Safety and feasibility of orbital atherectomy for the treatment of calcified coronary lesions: the ORBIT I trial. *Catheter Cardiovasc Interv.* 2013;81:1134-1139.
11. Généreux P, Lee AC, Kim CY, et al. Orbital atherectomy for treating de novo severely calcified coronary narrowing (1-year results from the pivotal ORBIT II Trial*). Am J Cardiol.* 2015;115(12):1685-1690.
12. Tsutsui RS, Sammour Y, Kalra A, et al. Excimer Laser Atherectomy in Percutaneous Coronary Intervention: A Contemporary Review. *Cardiovasc Revasc Med.* 2021;25:75-85.
13. Brinton TJ, Ali ZA, Hill JM, et al. Feasibility of Shockwave coronary intravascular lithotripsy for the treatment of calcified coronary stenoses. *Circulation.* 2019;139:834-836.
14. Ali ZA, Nef H, Escaned J, et al. Safety and effectiveness of coronary intravascular lithotripsy for treatment of severely calcified coronary stenoses: the disrupt CAD II study. *Circ Cardiovasc Interv.* 2019;12(10):e008434.
15. Aksoy A, Salazar C, Becher MU, et al. Intravascular lithotripsy in calcified coronary lesions: a prospective, observational, multicenter registry. *Circ Cardiovasc Interv.* 2019;12(11):e008154.
16. Fearon WF, Achenbach S, Assali TEA, et al. Accuracy of fractional flow reserve derived from coronary angiography. *Circulation.* 2019;139:477-484.
17. Parise H, Maehara A, Stone GW, Leon MB, Mintz GS. Meta-analysis of randomized studies comparing intravascular ultrasound versus angiographic guidance of percutaneous coronary intervention in pre-drug-eluting stent era. *Am J Cardiol.* 2011;107:374-382.
18. Jang JS, Song YJ, Kang W, et al. Intravascular ultrasound-guided implantation of drug-eluting stents to improve outcome: a meta-analysis. *JACC Cardiovasc Interv.* 2014;7:233-243.
19. Ahn JM, Kang SJ, Yoon SH, et al. Meta-analysis of outcomes after intravascular ultrasound-guided versus angiography-guided drug-eluting stent implantation in 26,503 patients enrolled in three randomized trials and 14 observational studies. *Am J Cardiol.* 2014;113:1338-1347.
20. Ali Z, Maehara A, Genereux P, et al. Optical coherence tomography compared with intravascular ultrasound and with angiography to guide coronary stent implantation (ILUMIEN III: OPTIMIZE PCI): a randomised controlled trial. *Lancet.* 2016;388:2618-2628.
21. Booth J, Clayton T, Pepper J, et al. Randomized, controlled trial of coronary artery bypass surgery versus percutaneous coronary intervention in patients with multivessel coronary artery disease: six-year follow-up from the Stent or Surgery Trial (SoS*). Circulation.* 2008;118:381-388.
22. Daemen J, Boersma E, Flather M, et al. Long-term safety and efficacy of percutaneous coronary intervention with stenting and coronary artery bypass surgery for multivessel coronary artery disease: a meta-analysis with 5-year patient-level data from the ARTS, ERACI-II, MASS-II, and SoS trials. *Circulation.* 2008;118:1146-1154.
23. Hlatky MA, Boothroyd DB, Bravata DM, et al. Coronary artery bypass surgery compared with percutaneous coronary interventions for multivessel disease: a collaborative analysis of individual patient data from ten randomized trials. *Lancet.* 2009;373:1190-1197.
24. Serruys PW, Morice MC, Kappetein AP, et al. Percutaneous coronary intervention versus coronary-artery bypass grafting for severe coronary artery disease. *N Engl J Med.* 2009;360:961-972.
25. Kappetein AP, Feldman TE, Mack MJ, et al. Comparison of coronary bypass surgery with drug-eluting stenting for the treatment of left main and/or three-vessel disease: 3-year follow-up of the SYNTAX trial. *Eur Heart J.* 2011;32:2125-2134.
26. Thuijs DJFM, Kappetein AP, Serruys PW, et al. Percutaneous coronary intervention versus coronary artery bypass grafting in patients

with three-vessel or left main coronary artery disease: 10-year follow-up of the multicentre randomized controlled SYNTAX trial. *Lancet.* 2019;394(10206):1325-1334. Erratum in: *Lancet.* 2020;395(10227):870.
27. Farkouh ME, Domanski M, Sleeper LA, et al. Strategies for multivessel revascularization in patients with diabetes. *N Engl J Med.* 2012;367:2375-2384.
28. Farkouh ME, Domanski M, Dangas GD, et al. Long-term survival following multivessel revascularization in patients with diabetes (FREEDOM Follow-On Study*)*. *J Am Coll Cardiol.* 2019;73:629-638.
29. Patel MR, Calhoon JH, Dehmer GJ, et al. 2017 appropriate use criteria for coronary revascularization in patients with stable ischemic heart disease: a report of the American College of Cardiology Appropriate Use Criteria Task Force, American Association for Thoracic Surgery, American Heart Association, American Society of Echocardiography, American Society of Nuclear Cardiology, Society for Cardiovascular Angiography and Interventions, Society of Cardiovascular Computed Tomography, and Society of Thoracic Surgeons. *J Am Coll Cardiol.* 2017;69:2212-2241.
30. Ly HQ, Nosair M, Cartier R. Surgical turndown: "What's in a name?" for patients deemed ineligible for surgical revascularization. *Can J Cardiol.* 2019;35:959-966.
31. Ahn JM, Roh JH, Kim YH, et al. Randomized trial of stents versus bypass surgery for left main coronary artery disease: 5-year outcomes of the PRECOMBAT study. *J Am Coll Cardiol.* 2015;65:2198-2206.
32. Boudriot E, Thiele H, Walther T, et al. Randomized comparison of percutaneous coronary intervention with sirolimus-eluting stents versus coronary artery bypass grafting in unprotected left main stem stenosis. *J Am Coll Cardiol.* 2011;57:538-545.
33. Stone GW, Sabik JF, Serruys PW, et al. Everolimus-eluting stents or bypass surgery for left main coronary artery disease. *N Engl J Med.* 2016;375(23):2223-2235. Erratum in: *N Engl J Med.* 2019;381:1789.
34. Ahmad Y, Howard JP, Arnold DA, et al. Mortality after drug-eluting stents vs. coronary artery bypass grafting for left main coronary artery disease: a meta-analysis of randomized controlled trials. *Eur Heart J.* 2020;41(34):3228-3235.
35. Boden WE, O'Roarke RA, Teo KK, et al. Optimal medical therapy with or without PCI for stable coronary disease. *N Engl J Med.* 2007;356:1503-1516.
36. Gada H, Kirtane AJ, Kereiakes DJ, et al. Meta-analysis of trials on mortality after percutaneous coronary intervention compared with medical therapy in patients with stable coronary heart disease and objective evidence of myocardial ischemia. *Am J Cardiol.* 2015;115:1194-1199.
37. Neumann FJ, Sousa-Uva M, Ahlsson A, et al. 2018 ESC/EACTS Guidelines on myocardial revascularization. *Eur Heart J.* 2019;40:87-165.
38. Maron DJ, Hochman JS, Reynolds HR, et al. Initial invasive or conservative strategy for stable coronary disease. *N Engl J Med.* 2020;382:1395-1407.
39. Lagerqvist B, Husted S, Kontny F, et al. 5-year outcomes in the FRISC-II randomized trial of an invasive versus a non-invasive strategy in non-ST-elevation acute coronary syndrome: a follow-up study. *Lancet.* 2006;368:998-1004.
40. Cannon CP, Weintraub WS, Demopoulos LA, et al. Comparison of early invasive and conservative strategies in patients with unstable coronary syndromes treated with the glycoprotein IIb/IIIa inhibitor tirofiban. *N Engl J Med.* 2001;344:1879-1887.
41. Fox KA, Poole-Wilson P, Clayton TC, et al. 5-year outcome of an interventional strategy in non-ST-elevation acute coronary syndrome: the British Heart Foundation RITA 3 randomised trial. *Lancet.* 2005;366:914-920.
42. Hirsch A, Windhausen F, Tijssen JG, et al. Long-term outcome after an early invasive versus selective invasive treatment strategy in patients with non-ST-elevation acute coronary syndrome and elevated cardiac troponin T (the ICTUS trial): a follow-up study. *Lancet.* 2007;369:827-835.
43. Chahine A, Haykal T, Kanugula AK, et al. Meta-analysis of optimal timing of coronary intervention in non-ST-elevation acute coronary syndrome. *Catheter Cardiovasc Interv.* 2020;95:185-193.
44. Patel MR, Calhoon JH, Dehmer GJ, et al. ACC/AATS/AHA/ASE/ASNC/SCAI/SCCT/STS 2016 appropriate use criteria for coronary revascularization in patients with acute coronary syndromes: a report of the American College of Cardiology Appropriate Use Criteria Task Force, American Association for Thoracic Surgery, American Heart Association, American Society of Echocardiography, American Society of Nuclear Cardiology, Society for Cardiovascular Angiography and Interventions, Society of Cardiovascular Computed Tomography, and the Society of Thoracic Surgeons. *J Am Coll Cardiol.* 2017;69:570-591.
45. Grines CL, Browne KF, Marco J, et al. A comparison of immediate angioplasty with thrombolytic therapy for acute myocardial infarction. The Primary Angioplasty in Myocardial Infarction Study Group. *N Engl J Med.* 1993;328:673-679.
46. Andersen HR, Nielsen TT, Rasmussen K, et al. A comparison of coronary angioplasty with fibrinolytic therapy in acute myocardial infarction. *N Engl J Med.* 2003;349:733-742.
47. Rokos IC, French WJ, Koenig WJ, et al. Integration of pre-hospital electrocardiograms and ST-elevation myocardial infarction receiving center (SRC) networks: impact on door-to-balloon times across 10 independent regions. *JACC Cardiovasc Interv.* 2009;2:339-346.
48. Levine GN, Bates ER, Blankenship JC, et al. 2015 ACC/AHA/SCAI focused update on primary percutaneous coronary intervention for patients with ST-elevation myocardial infarction: an update of the 2011 ACCF/AHA/SCAI guideline for percutaneous coronary intervention and the 2013 ACCF/AHA guideline for the management of ST-elevation myocardial infarction. *J Am Coll Cardiol.* 2016;67(10):1235-1250.
49. Mehta SR, Wood DA., Storey RF, et al. Complete revascularization with multivessel PCI for myocardial infarction. *N Engl J Med.* 2019;381:1411-1421.
50. Ueyama H, Kuno T, Yasamura K, et al. Meta-analysis comparing same-sitting and staged percutaneous coronary intervention of non-culprit artery for ST-elevation myocardial infarction with multivessel coronary disease. *Am J Cardiol.* 2021;150:24-31.
51. Fitzgibbon GM, Kafka HP, Leach AJ, et al. Coronary bypass graft fate and patient outcome: angiographic follow-up of 5065 grafts related to survival and reoperation in 1388 patients during 25 years. *J Am Coll Cardiol.* 1996;28:616-626.
52. Kloner RA, Rude RE, Carlson N, et al. Ultrastructural evidence of microvascular damage and myocardial cell injury after coronary artery occlusion: which comes first? *Circulation.* 1980;62(5):945-952.
53. Abbo KM, Dooris M, Glazier S, et al. Features and outcome of no-reflow after percutaneous coronary intervention. *Am J Cardiol.* 1995;75(12):778-782.
54. Mauri L, Cox DA, Hermiller J, et al. The PROXIMAL trial: proximal protection during saphenous vein graft intervention using the Proxis embolic protection system: a randomized, prospective, multicenter trial. *J Am Coll Cardiol.* 2007;50(15):1142-1449.
55. Turco MA, Buchbinder M, Popma JJ, et al. Pivotal, randomized U.S. study of the Symbiot^{TM} covered stent system in patients with saphenous vein graft disease: eight-month angiographic and clinical results from the Symbiot III trial. *Catheter Cardiovasc Interv.* 2006;68(3):379-388.
56. Stone GW, Goldberg S, O'Shaughnessy C, et al. 5-year follow-up of polytetrafluoroethylene-covered stents compared with bare-metal stents in aortocoronary saphenous vein grafts the randomized BARRICADE (barrier approach to restenosis: restrict intima to curtail adverse events) trial. *JACC Cardiovasc Interv.* 2011;4(3):300-309.
57. Stone G, Rogers C, Hermiller J, et al. Randomized comparison of distal protection with a filter-based catheter and a balloon occlusion and aspiration system during percutaneous intervention of diseased saphenous vein aorto-coronary bypass grafts. *Circulation.* 2003;108(5):548-553.
58. Levine GN, Bates ER, Blankenship JC, et al. 2011 ACCF/AHA/SCAI guideline for percutaneous coronary intervention: a report of the American College of Cardiology Foundation/American Heart Association Task Force on Practice Guidelines and the Society for Cardiovascular

Angiography and Interventions. *Circulation.* 2011;124:e574-e651. Erratum in: *Circulation.* 2012;125(8):e14.

59. Windecker S, Kolh P, Alfonso F, et al. 2014 ESC/EACTS Guidelines on myocardial revascularization: The Task Force on Myocardial Revascularization of the European Society of Cardiology (ESC) and the European Association for Cardio-Thoracic Surgery (EACTS) developed with the special contribution of the European Association of Percutaneous Cardiovascular Interventions (EAPCI). *Eur Heart J.* 2014;35:2541-2619.
60. Mauri L, Keriakes DJ Yeh RW et al. Twelve or 30 Months of dual antiplatelet therapy after drug-eluting stents. *N Engl J Med.* 2014;371:2155-2166.
61. Helft G, Steg PG, Le Feuvre C, et al. Stopping or continuing clopidogrel 12 months after drug-eluting stent placement: the OPTIDUAL randomized trial. *Eur Heart J.* 2016;37:365-374.
62. Kandzari DE, Kirtane AJ, Windecker S. One-month dual antiplatelet therapy following percutaneous coronary intervention with zotarolimus-eluting stents in high-bleeding-risk patients. *Circ Cardiovasc Interv.* 2020;13(11):e009565.

CHAPTER 44

PERCUTANEOUS VALVULAR INTERVENTION

Gurion Lantz and Firas Zahr

INTRODUCTION

Over the last decade, the treatment of valvular heart disease has progressed with the introduction and maturation of transcatheter valvular interventions. Since the first transcatheter aortic valve replacement (TAVR), there has been a deluge of data supporting its role in the treatment of severe symptomatic aortic stenosis (AS) extending from extreme-risk to low-risk patients. Although much of this progress is owed to the advancement of the devices and techniques, the integration of imaging—in particular computed tomography (CT) and procedural imaging—has also greatly improved procedural success and reduced complications. Consequently, these advancements have accelerated the development of transcatheter repair and replacement of mitral and tricuspid valves.

TRANSCATHETER AORTIC-VALVE REPLACEMENT

From 2004 to 2008, surgical aortic-valve replacement (AVR) was associated with a hospital mortality of 2.8%. Furthermore, at least one-third of patients greater than 75 years of age with severe AS are deemed unsuitable for surgical AVR because of the extensive calcification of the ascending aorta (ie, so-called, porcelain aorta) or high-surgical risk. TAVR is now the standard of care for certain patients with severe aortic stenosis.

Since the first transcatheter aortic valve was placed in a human in 2002 by Alan Cribier, over 300,000 procedures have been performed worldwide.[1] This number continues to rise as indications are expanded to include low-risk patient populations. A sixfold increase in TAVR procedures occurred from 2012 to 2015, and the number of US Medicare beneficiaries receiving TAVR exceeded the number receiving surgical AVR for the first time in 2017 (30,565 vs 21,418, respectively). TAVR has become the treatment of choice for patients with severe, symptomatic AS with a prohibitive risk for surgical AVR and a viable alternative for patients with high-, intermediate-, or low-surgical risk of perioperative mortality and major morbidity depending on patient-specific risks and preferences.[2]

Landmark Clinical Trials

The PARTNER (Placement of Aortic Transcatheter Valves) trial was the first prospective, randomized controlled trial to investigate transcatheter heart valves in patients with severe, symptomatic AS. It consisted of two individually powered cohorts: PARTNER 1A and 1B. Cohort A compared TAVR to surgery among patients at high-surgical risk for operative mortality, while Cohort B compared TAVR to best medical management in patients with a prohibitive risk for surgery. PARTNER 1B showed that 1- and 5-year all-cause mortality rates were significantly lower in the TAVR arm compared with the conservative arm (31% vs 50% at 1 year and 72% vs 94% at 5 years, respectively; $P < .001$). Subsequently, PARTNER 1A demonstrated TAVR outcomes (all-cause mortality at 30 days, 1 and 5 years) to be noninferior to surgical AVR in patients at high risk for cardiac mortality.[3]

In the PARTNER 2A trial, patients considered to be at intermediate risk for surgical AVR were randomized to TAVR or surgical AVR. All-cause mortality or disabling stroke at 24 months was similar for both strategies: TAVR resulted in a significantly lower rate of death or disabling stroke in a prespecified analysis of the transfemoral access group, whereas similar outcomes to surgical AVR were seen in the transthoracic group. TAVR was associated with a lower rate of severe bleeding, acute kidney injury, and new-onset atrial fibrillation, although surgical AVR was associated with lower rates of paravalvular regurgitation and major vascular complications.[4]

Following publication of these results, the American Heart Association and American College of Cardiology (AHA/ACC) Valvular Heart Disease Focused Update recommended TAVR as an alternative to surgery for patients at intermediate surgical risk (Class of Recommendation IIA, Level of Evidence B).

The PARTNER 3 trial showed the superiority of transfemoral TAVR compared with surgical AVR for the primary composite endpoint consisting of death, stroke, or rehospitalization at 1 year in low-risk patients. Consequently, TAVR received US Food and Drug Administration (FDA) approval for low-risk patients in 2019.[5]

TYPES OF TRANSCATHETER AORTIC VALVES

There are currently two FDA–approved transcatheter heart valve systems in clinical use in the United States: the balloon-expandable SAPIEN valve series (Edwards Lifesciences Corporation, Irvine, CA, USA) (**Figure 44.1A**) and the self-expandable CoreValve series (Medtronic Inc, Minneapolis, MN, USA) (**Figure 44.1B**). The mechanically expandable LOTUS Edge valve (Boston Scientific, Marlborough, MA, USA) received FDA approval, but production was discontinued in

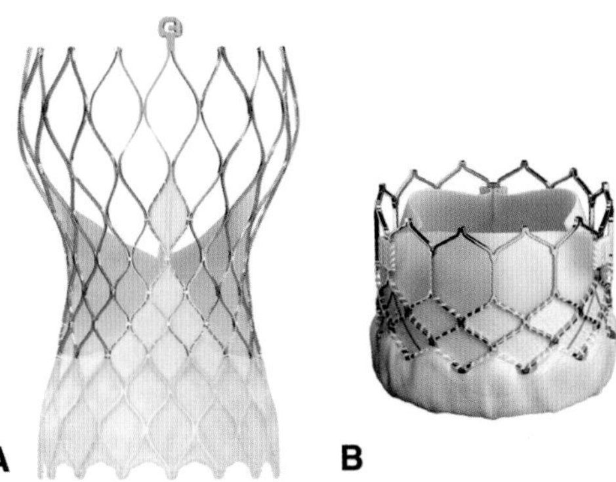

FIGURE 44.1 The latest generation of currently available FDA–approved TAVR valves in the United States include (**A**) Medtronic Evolut PRO+ and **(B)** Edwards SAPIEN 3 Ultra. FDA, US Food and Drug Administration; TAVR, transcatheter aortic valve replacement. (A, Reproduced with permission of Medtronic, Inc.; B, Courtesy of Edwards Lifesciences LLC, Irvine, CA. Edwards, Edwards Lifesciences, PASCAL, PASCAL Ace, PASCAL Precision, Edwards SAPIEN, SAPIEN, SAPIEN XT, SAPIEN 3 and SAPIEN 3 Ultra are trademarks of Edwards Lifesciences Corporation.)

January 2021 as a result of issues with the delivery system. No safety issues were noted for patients who currently have an implanted LOTUS Edge valve.

The Edwards SAPIEN valve is made from bovine pericardium mounted on a cobalt–chromium stent enveloped in an outer sealing skirt. The latest iterations of the valve, the SAPIEN 3 and SAPIEN 3 Ultra, are available in 20-, 23-, 26-, and 29-mm sizes and can be deployed through a 14 or 16-Fr sheath (for the 29- mm valve). Before delivery, the valve is tightly compressed using a crimping mechanism onto a balloon catheter that is inflated to deploy the valve in the aortic-valve annulus. Once deployed, the SAPIEN valve cannot be recaptured or repositioned (**Videos 44.1 and 44.2**).

The self-expanding Medtronic CoreValve is made from porcine pericardium mounted on a Nitinol stent, with two versions (the Evolut PRO and the Evolut PRO+) enveloped in an external pericardial wrap. The current generations of the CoreValve—the Evolut R, Evolut PRO, and Evolut PRO+—are available in 23-, 26-, and 29-mm sizes. The Evolut R and Evolut PRO+ are also available in 34 mm size. They can be delivered through either Medtronic's EnVeo R InLine sheaths (16 Fr for Evolut PRO and 14 Fr for Evolut R) or other commercially available sheaths. Because it is self-expanding, the CoreValve allows for partial deployment through the sheath, evaluation of deployment position with a functional valve, and recapturing of the valve (ie, withdrawal into the delivery sheath) if repositioning is required) (**Videos 44.3, 44.4, and 44.5**).

LIMITATIONS OF TAVR

While TAVR is now the treatment of choice for severe symptomatic AS, the potential limitations of TAVR should be considered in the treatment of younger, low-risk patients with TAVR who would otherwise be expected to have an excellent outcome following surgical AVR.

Structural Deterioration

Structural deterioration of surgically implanted bioprosthetic valves is well established. Structural valve deterioration increases with time, particularly after the first 7 to 8 years following implantation and has an incidence of less than 1%, 10% to 30%, and 20% to 50% at 1, 10, and 15 years, respectively. Structural valve deterioration of bioprosthetic valves is strongly influenced by patient age at the time of implantation, with younger patients exhibiting accelerated valvular calcification and degeneration.[6]

As the criteria for TAVR are expanded, valve durability becomes an important consideration. In a study comparing TAVR and surgical AVR using a computational approach to assess leaflet fatigue, transcatheter valve leaflets sustained higher stresses, strains, and fatigue damage. Yet, mid-term outcomes appear encouraging.[7] The 5-year follow-up of the PARTNER trial found no structural TAVR deterioration leading to hemodynamic compromise or valve replacement albeit only a minority of the study population had been followed for 5 years. The 5-year follow-up data from the Italian high-risk registry noted TAVR prosthesis failure in 1.4% and mild valve stenosis (mean gradient 20-40 mm Hg) in 2.8% although survivorship bias cannot be excluded.[8,9] Long-term follow-up is necessary to assess TAVR durability.

Paravalvular Leak

In the SURTAVI (Surgical Replacement and Transcatheter Aortic-Valve Implantation) study, the rates of moderate or severe paravalvular regurgitation at 1 year were 5.3% in the TAVR group and 0.6% in the surgical AVR group.[10] Moderate or severe paravalvular leaks were noted at 1 year in 6.8% of TAVR patients in the PARTNER A trial and only 1.5% of patients in the PARTNER S3i trial.[10,11] The decreased rate of paravalvular leaks is attributed to new device enhancements (low profile delivery system and an external skirt to prevent paravalvular regurgitation), improved case selection, increased operator experience, more precise valve positioning, and routine use of three dimensional (3D) CT reconstruction for accurate valve sizing.

The impact of paravalvular leak on mortality has yet to be fully elucidated. Assessing 2-year outcomes of the high-risk cohort in the PARTNER A trial showed even mild paravalvular leak was associated with increased mortality. On the other hand, among studies evaluating intermediate-risk groups, namely PARTNER 2A and PARTNER S3i, only moderate or severe paravalvular leak was associated with increased mortality. Patients with significant perivalvular leak should be evaluated for transcatheter occlusion device placement or surgical valve replacement.

Stroke

Mechanical manipulation of the aorta and aortic valve with transcatheter device delivery and valve placement causes embolic debris to the brain in the majority of TAVR (and surgical AVR) patients. Rates of clinical stroke and transient ischemic attack were greater after TAVR than surgical AVR in the PARTNER A trial at 30 days (5.5% vs 2.4%, respectively;

P = .04) and at 1 year (8.3% vs 4.3%, respectively; P = .04).[10] Conversely, in the CoreValve trial, the rates of stroke were similar with TAVR and surgical AVR at 30 days (4.9% vs 6.2%, respectively; P = .46) and 1 year (8.8 vs 12.6%, respectively; P = .10). In studies of intermediate-risk patients, similar rates of stroke were seen for TAVR and surgical AVR treatment.[10] Although the incidence of cerebral infarctions following TAVR is high as assessed by diffusion-weighted magnetic resonance imaging (MRI), only a fraction of these lesions manifest significant clinical neurologic findings. The role of the routine uses of neuroprotection devices to mitigate the risk of stroke remains unclear at the present time.[12]

Leaflet Dysfunction

Two registries investigated the prevalence of subclinical leaflet thrombosis, valve hemodynamics, and clinical outcomes. Subclinical leaflet thrombosis occurred frequently in bioprosthetic aortic valves (12%), more commonly in transcatheter (13%) than in surgical valves (4%).[13-15] Anticoagulation (both novel oral anticoagulants [NOACs] and warfarin), but not dual antiplatelet therapy, was effective in the prevention or treatment of subclinical leaflet thrombosis. Subclinical leaflet thrombosis was associated with increased rates of TIAs and strokes.

The true incidence of valve thrombosis, predisposing factors, clinical significance, the impact on long-term valve durability and rates of stroke, and the role of anticoagulation remain to be determined. Two ongoing pivotal trials of TAVR and surgical AVR include an FDA–mandated substudy of surveillance 4D CT in approximately one-third of the patients that will hopefully further inform the field.[13] Additionally, four trials underway are evaluating post-TAVR anticoagulation strategies.[16-19]

Conduction Abnormalities

Trials involving intermediate-risk patients show varying incidences of permanent pacemaker placement following TAVR compared with SAVR (PARTNER 2A 8.5% vs 6.7%; SURTAVI 25.9% vs 6.6%; PARTNER S3i 10.2% vs 7.3%, respectively). The self-expanding CoreValve has been associated with a higher need for permanent pacemaker placement because of the potential for deeper implantation into the left ventricular outflow tract with injury to the atrioventricular node or conduction bundles.[11] Early permanent pacemaker implantation is associated with a higher mortality and a higher composite of mortality and heart failure at 1 year. Advanced age, male gender, previous myocardial infarction, previous cardiac surgery, preexisting conduction abnormalities, and CoreValve utilization have all been identified as risk factors for new conduction defects following TAVR.

Bicuspid Valve

Bicuspid aortic-valve disease is present in 1% to 2% of the population. It presents unique anatomic challenges for TAVR in terms of valve sizing owing to a more elliptical annulus as well as higher risk for significant paravalvular regurgitation, aortic injury, and pacemaker implantation. Bicuspid aortic valves were excluded from all landmark trials until PARTNER 3, which included a bicuspid valve arm, mid- and long-term results in this patient population are not yet available. However, smaller registries and trials have shown acceptable short-term outcomes of TAVR in patients with a bicuspid aortic valve.[20]

Prosthetic Valve Endocarditis

Prosthetic valve endocarditis represents a particular challenge for patients who received TAVR because of high-operative risk associated with its treatment. An analysis of all surgical AVR and TAVR patients in the PARTNER 1 and 2 studies and found no difference in the incidence of prosthetic valve endocarditis between the two groups (5.21 vs 4.10 per 1000 person-years for TAVR and SAVR, respectively, P = .44). Independent risk factors for prosthetic valve endocarditis include younger age, male sex, prior endocarditis, end-stage renal disease, repeat TAVR procedures, lack of native valve predilation, liver and lung disease, post-TAVR acute kidney injury, and treatment in a catheterization laboratory as opposed to a hybrid operating room.[21-23]

TAVR Cost

In intermediate-risk patients in the PARTNER 2 trial, the cost of TAVR was approximately $20,000 higher than surgical AVR, owing primarily to the higher cost of the valve itself. Total hospitalization costs were $2888 higher for the second-generation SAPIEN XT valve versus surgical AVR but $4155 lower for the third-generation S3 valve, owing to a reduction in length of stay. Follow-up costs were significantly lower with both types of TAVR compared with surgical AVR. Over a lifetime horizon, TAVR was projected to lower costs by $8000 to $10,000 and increase quality-adjusted survival by 0.15 and 0.27 years compared with surgical AVR. With more minimalistic approaches to AVR increasingly favoring reduced length of stay, avoidance of general anesthesia, recovery outside of the ICU, and less alternative access, TAVR costs continue to fall; however, the largest component of the cost of TAVR remains the valve itself, which are all several times more expensive than surgical AVR valves.[24,25]

Transcatheter Aortic Valve Replacement Use in Young Patients

It is unknown how TAVR performs in young, low-risk patients. Furthermore, percutaneous coronary intervention following TAVR is more difficult because the metal valve stent can interfere with the cannulation of the coronary ostia. These factors, combined with the lower rates of paravalvular regurgitation and pacemaker placement with surgical AVR, caution against the universal adoption of TAVR, especially in young, low-risk patients.

Transcatheter Aortic Valve Replacement Use in Other Conditions

New valves and adjuncts continue to be developed for (1) additional conditions (ie, aortic insufficiency—which presents unique challenges because the aortic annulus is frequently dilated and not calcified—and failing bioprostheses); (2)

expanded indications (ie, moderate AS with depressed left ventricular function, patients with asymptomatic severe AS); and (3) prevention of procedural stroke.

TRICUSPID REGURGITATION

Surgery is currently the only Class I guideline-recommended therapy for TR, which is most often performed during left-sided heart surgery or for tricuspid valve (TV) endocarditis. Because of the paucity of evidence, American and European guideline recommendations for the management of tricuspid regurgitation (TR) are limited, and the indications and timing for surgical intervention are still debated. As the management of valvular heart disease moves toward less invasive surgical and transcatheter therapies, several techniques and devices are applied to the TV.

Currently, long-term data on the beneficial effect of isolated surgical TV therapy compared with medical therapy remains scarce. Less than 1% of cardiac patients undergo TV surgery. From 2004 to 2013, of all US patients who underwent TV surgery, only 15% had isolated TV surgery and with high in-hospital mortality (8%-10%). This is likely related to comorbidities and referral timing rather than the risk of isolated TV surgery. Residual or late significant TR after mitral-valve replacement is independently associated with poor outcomes. Since performing concomitant TV repair during left-sided heart surgery does not increase surgical risk and may result in reverse right ventricular remodeling with reduction of symptoms, a more aggressive approach to correcting TR in the presence of annular dilatation may reduce the chance of late TR progression after left-sided valve surgery.[26-28]

The TV is a complex apparatus consisting of leaflets, annulus, tendinous cords, papillary muscles, and the associated right ventricle (**Figure 44.2**). The normal tricuspid annulus is a saddle-shaped ellipsoid surrounded by several critical anatomical structures, including the atrioventricular node, right coronary artery, coronary sinus ostium, and noncoronary sinus of Valsalva. Tricuspid annulus dilation, right atrium/ventricle dilation, and TV leaflet malcoaptation are the most common changes in secondary TR. When tricuspid annulus dilation occurs, its shape becomes more circular and planar, usually in the anatomical location of the anterolateral free wall and posterior border (**Figure 44.3**). Leaflet malcoaptation may occur because of inadequate leaflet length to cover the dilated annulus or leaflet tethering from inadequate chordal redundancy. The region of malcoaptation often occurs centrally or extends from the anteroseptal commissure toward the posteroseptal commissure.[29,30]

Following the success of TAVR, there is a large interest in developing transcatheter TV devices. Multiple novel technologies are currently in the preclinical or early clinical assessment. Specific anatomical aspects should be considered according to different therapeutic targets. In addition, potential anatomical and pathophysiologic constraints of transcatheter TV interventions need to be considered.

Challenges with catheter navigation exist. The angulation between the annular plane and the superior and inferior vena cava complicate transvenous access, and the loss of anatomical landmarks under pathologic conditions (right atrial and ventricular dilation) may interfere with the proper positioning of repair/replacement devices. Preexisting device leads also interfere with device delivery and deployment. Equipment

SECTION 3

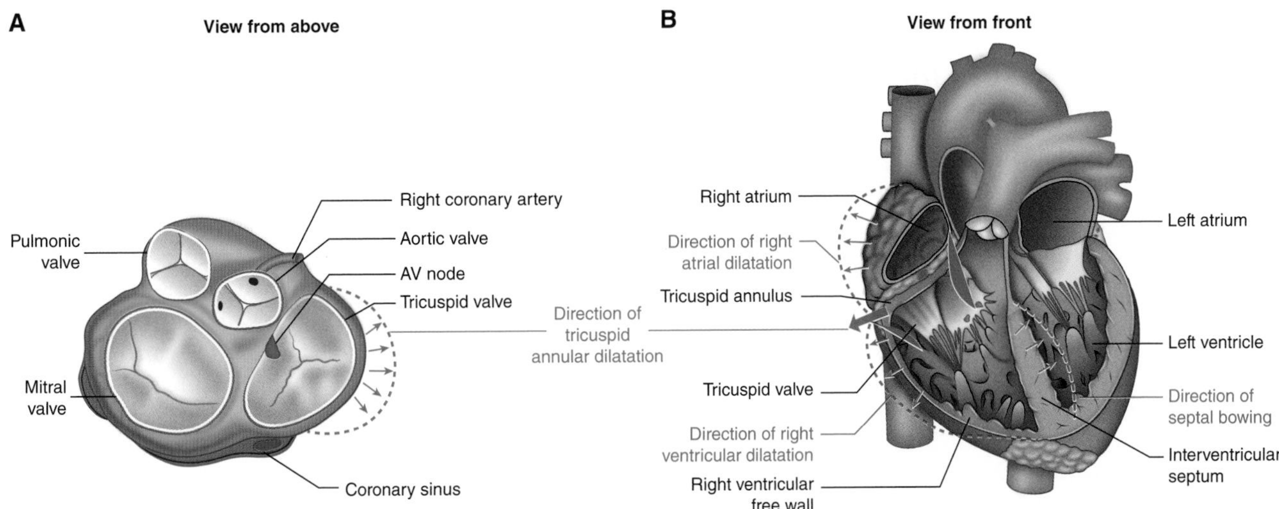

FIGURE 44.2 Complex tricuspid valve anatomy and pathophysiology of tricuspid regurgitation. **View A**: Dilation of the tricuspid annulus occurs in the portion corresponding to the right ventricular free wall, sparing the septal portion of the annulus. **View B**: Right atrial and ventricular distention and dilatation occur predominately away from the septae and drive tricuspid annular dilatation. AV, atrioventricular.

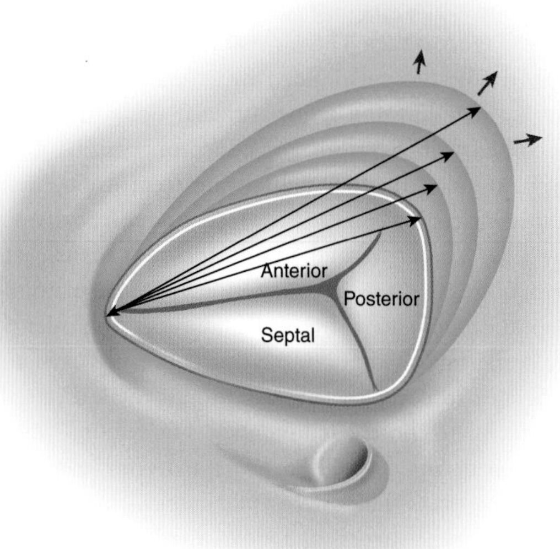

FIGURE 44.3 Tricuspid annular dilatation occurs in the area of the RV-free wall. The portion of the annulus along the septum is relatively spared.

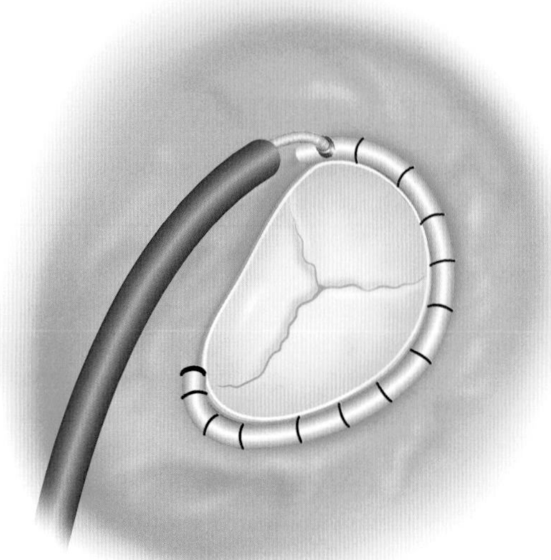

FIGURE 44.4 The Edwards tricuspid and mitral Cardioband devices are designed to mimic surgical annuloplasty.

sizing is difficult since the tricuspid annulus is significantly larger than other valves. Additionally, flexibility and fragility of the tricuspid annulus interfere with the fixation and long-term stability of transcatheter TV replacement devices. Finally, right-sided valves are at increased risk of thrombosis compared with left-sided valves because of low pressure and slow flow in the right heart chambers. This might precipitate device thrombosis, as evidenced by a rate of bioprosthetic tricuspid valve thrombosis of 12% in surgically implanted valves.

RESEARCH AND FUTURE DIRECTIONS

Devices for transcatheter TV therapy remain investigational. Currently, the most widely used technique is the edge-to-edge repair using the MitraClip device (Abbott, Santa Clara, CA, USA) in the TV position to improve leaflet coaptation.[31-33] However, clinical data are not sufficient to conclude its safety and efficacy for this use. The multicenter international TriValve (Transcatheter Tricuspid Valve Therapies) registry included 249 patients with severe TR treated with the MitraClip device in compassionate or off-label use. Procedural success (ie, patient alive with device successfully implanted with residual TR grade ≤2) was achieved in 77% of patients and was independently associated with increased survival.[34]

The tricuspid Cardioband device (Edwards Lifesciences, Irvine, CA, USA), a transcatheter direct annuloplasty device that mimics surgical annuloplasty (**Figure 44.4**), has Conformitè Europëenne (CE) mark approval and is the first commercially available transcatheter device for the treatment of significant TR. In the TRI-REPAIR study, Cardioband implantation provided favorable clinical and functional outcomes at 6 months.[35]

MANAGEMENT OF MITRAL REGURGITATION

Transcatheter mitral-valve repair (TMVr) is an alternative nonsurgical treatment option for select patients with symptomatic mitral regurgitation (MR) who are deemed by the heart team to be at high-surgical risk or inoperable.

Transcatheter Edge-to-Edge Mitral-Valve Repair MitraClip System

The initial efforts to treat MR with catheter-based methods began with the MitraClip, which was designed to mimic the surgical Alfieri stitch for patients with primary MR deemed to be at high-surgical risk for valve replacement. Most of the experience gathered so far with the MitraClip system (ie, >80,000 procedures performed worldwide) has been generated in patients with secondary MR. Prospective registry studies showed that TMVr can reduce symptoms and improve functional capacity and quality-of-life in patients with secondary MR while maintaining a low rate of complications. The current guidelines contain no strong recommendation for percutaneous correction of secondary MR; however, the recent version was released before publication of two randomized controlled clinical trials that investigated the impact of the MitraClip procedure on the outcomes of heart-failure patients (**Table 44.1**): percutaneous repair with the MitraClip device for severe functional/secondary mitral regurgitation (MITRA-FR) and cardiovascular outcomes assessment of the MitraClip percutaneous therapy for heart-failure patients with functional mitral regurgitation (COAPT).

Among patients with severe secondary mitral regurgitation in the MITRA-FR trial, the rate of death or unplanned hospitalization for heart failure at 1 year did not differ

TABLE 44.1 Notable Study Similarities and Differences Between the MITRA-FR and COAPT Trials for Evaluation of MitraClip in Patients With Severe Mitral Regurgitation and Heart Failure

	MITRA-FR	COAPT
Randomization	MitraClip and GDMT vs GDMT alone	MitraClip and GDMT vs GDMT alone
Patients enrolled	304	610
Primary endpoint	All-cause death and HF hospitalizations	HF hospitalizations
Follow-up	1 year	2 years
MR etiology	Ischemic or nonischemic functional MR	Ischemic or nonischemic functional MR
MR severity definition	Regurgitant volume >30 mL/beat or EROA > 20 mm^2	≥3+
LVEF (by echocardiography)	≥15% and ≤40%	≥20% and ≤50%
LVESD (by echocardiography)	Not specified	≤70 mm
Pulmonary hypertension	Not excluded	Excluded systolic PAP >70 mm Hg and not reversible
Right ventricular dysfunction	Not excluded	Excluded ≥ moderate-to-severe
Prior HF hospitalization	Within 12 months	Within 12 months, or corrected BNP ≥300 pg/mL, or corrected NT-proBNP ≥1500 pg/mL

BNP, brain natriuretic peptide; COAPT, Cardiovascular Outcomes Assessment of the MitraClip Percutaneous Therapy for Heart-failure Patients with Functional Mitral Regurgitation; EROA, effective regurgitant orifice area; GDMT, guideline-directed medical therapy; HF, heart failure; LVEF, left ventricular ejection fraction; LVESD, left ventricular end-systolic dimension; MITRA-FR, Multicenter Study of Percutaneous Mitral-Valve Repair MitraClip Device in Patients With Severe Secondary Mitral Regurgitation; MR, mitral regurgitation; NT-proBNP, n-terminal pro-brain natriuretic peptide; PAP, pulmonary artery pressure.

significantly between patients who underwent percutaneous mitral-valve repair in addition to receiving medical therapy and those who received medical therapy alone. Conversely, in the COAPT trial of patients with heart failure and moderate-to-severe or severe secondary mitral regurgitation who remained symptomatic despite the use of maximal doses of GDMT, transcatheter mitral-valve repair resulted in a 47% lower rate of hospitalization for heart failure and 38% lower all-cause mortality within 24 months of follow-up than medical therapy alone. Differences in patient populations, the severity of MR and left ventricular dysfunction, maximization of GDMT, and extent of postprocedure residual MR may account for the disparate results of these two studies (**Table 44.1**).[36-39] Accordingly, patients should be selected carefully to receive the MitraClip therapy.

MitraClip XTR System

A new version of the MitraClip system, the XTR system was introduced in 2018, which has an enhanced delivery system (ie, longer arms for grasping and increased maneuverability) for use in valves with large coaptation defects and high complexity. More recently, the MitraClip G4 was approved in the United States with an expanded range of clip sizes, an alternative leaflet grasping feature[40] (**Figure 44.5A,B**).

PASCAL Transcatheter Mitral-Valve Repair System

The PASCAL transcatheter mitral-valve repair system (Edwards Lifesciences Corp., Irvine, CA, USA) is another device available for edge-to-edge mitral repair (**Figure 44.5C & D**). This system allows for simpler navigation in the left atrium than currently approved systems and the potential for greater reduction of MR because of the larger size of the implant, wider paddles, and optional independent leaflet grasping for challenging anatomies. A single-arm, multicenter, prospective study to assess the safety, performance, and clinical outcomes of the PASCAL system has completed enrolment, and results are currently pending The CLASP Study Edwards PASCAL TrAnScatheter Mitral Valve RePair System Study (CLASP); NCT03170349).[41,42]

Transcatheter Direct Annuloplasty Mitral-Valve Repair

The majority of MR patients in clinical practice requiring transcatheter interventions have secondary MR. The durability of interventional functional MR repair using only the edge-to-edge technique is a matter of debate, because in mitral-valve surgery annular correction, as well as leaflet augmentation, is important to minimize the risk of recurrent MR.

Cardioband System

Among the various annuloplasty devices, percutaneous direct annuloplasty using the Cardioband system (Edwards Lifesciences Corp., Irvine, CA, USA) most closely resembles a surgical annuloplasty ring. The device is delivered via a transseptal approach, and the ring is implanted on the atrial side of the mitral annulus and cinched to reduce the annular circumference. A randomized trial comparing Cardioband implantation plus GDMT to GDMT alone in patients with functional MR was initiated but is currently on pause (ClinicalTrials.gov identifier: NCT03016975).[43]

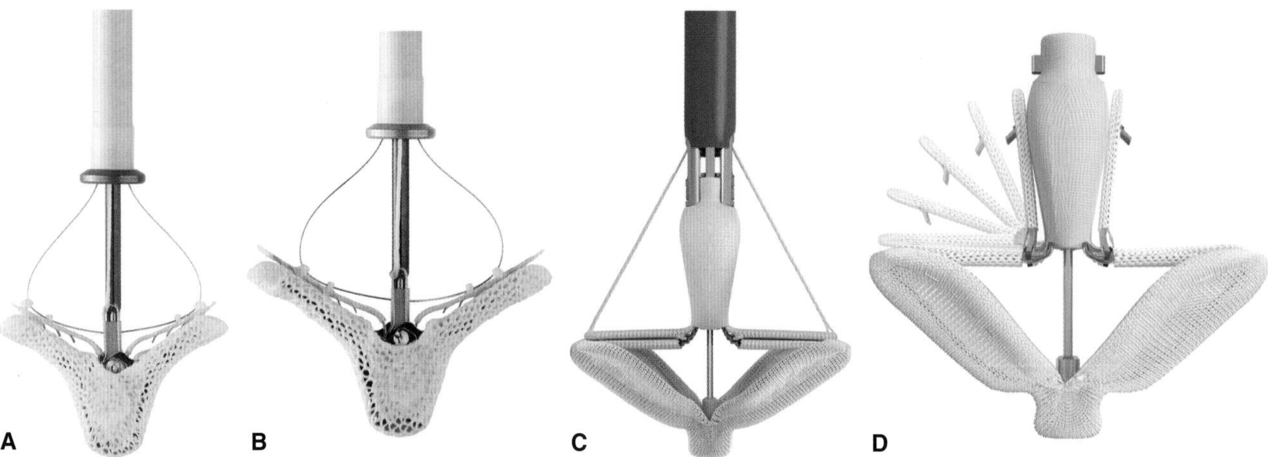

FIGURE 44.5 The latest generation of currently available devices for transcatheter edge-to-edge mitral repair include the Abbott Vascular MitraClip™G4 Clip Delivery System, NT **(A)** and XTR **(B)**, and Edwards PASCAL **(C & D)**. (MitraClip is a trademark of Abbott or its related companies. Reproduced with permission of Abbott, © 2021. All rights reserved; MitraClip is a trademark of Abbott or its related companies. Reproduced with permission of Abbott, © 2021. All rights reserved; Courtesy of Edwards Lifesciences LLC, Irvine, CA. Edwards, Edwards Lifesciences, PASCAL, PASCAL Ace, PASCAL Precision, Edwards SAPIEN, SAPIEN, SAPIEN XT, SAPIEN 3 and SAPIEN 3 Ultra are trademarks of Edwards Lifesciences Corporation.)

Research and Future Directions: Management of Secondary (Functional) Mitral Regurgitation

At present, deciding how to best treat severe functional MR in patients at high-surgical risk with minimally invasive, transcatheter-based technologies is still challenging. Surgical evidence suggests that a combination of "leaflet repair" with a concomitant ring is superior compared with single-leaflet therapy or annuloplasty alone. The principle of concomitant ring annuloplasty in mitral-valve repair can be applied to transcatheter treatment (ie, combination of MitraClip and Cardioband procedures). This strategy might become even more important if transcatheter mitral-valve repairs are expanded to younger and low-risk patients, who would require nearly perfect results and long-term durability.[44]

Percutaneous access to the mitral-valve necessitates crossing the interatrial septum. These iatrogenic ASDs are not routinely closed after edge-to-edge therapy, with as many as 50% of patients having a residual ASD following percutaneous mitral repair. This is would likely be higher following percutaneous mitral replacement since the device size is larger; however, these patients are assessed for ASD closure at the time of the index procedure.

Routine closure of iatrogenic ASDs remains controversial. In select patients with heart failure and preserved left ventricular function, creation of an ASD may reduce left atrial pressure and improve heart-failure symptoms. However, Blazek et al found that patients who presented after percutaneous mitral repair with heart-failure symptoms and iatrogenic ASD with significant left-to-right shunt showed decompression of the RV volume load, improved LV filling, increased systemic cardiac output, and an improvement in heart-failure symptoms after ASD closure.[45]

There are currently no established guidelines for closure of iatrogenic ASD after mitral intervention. Patients who present with heart-failure symptoms after percutaneous mitral intervention should be assessed for residual ASD and if found, should be considered for closure.

Transapical Off-Pump Mitral-Valve Repair With NeoChord Implantation

Transapical off-pump mitral-valve repair with artificial chorda implantation (TOP-MINI), also known as the NeoChord procedure (NeoChord Inc., St. Louis Park, MN, USA), is a relatively new option to implant neochordae via a minimally invasive approach in patients with severe MR due to leaflet prolapse or flail. Expanded polytetrafluoroethylene sutures are implanted without the need for cardiopulmonary bypass: the procedure is performed under general anesthesia using transesophageal echocardiography guidance.[46] A prospective, multicenter, randomized trial comparing the NeoChord procedure with conventional surgical mitral-valve repair is currently underway (Randomized Trial of the NeoChord DS1000 System Versus Open Surgical Repair; NCT02803957).

Transcatheter Mitral-Valve Replacement

Transcatheter mitral-valve implantation/replacement (TMVR) is an emerging treatment option for selected patients who are not suitable for surgical mitral repair or replacement. Balloon-expandable transcatheter aortic valves have been implanted in the mitral position within bioprosthetic mitral valves (valve-in-valve), mitral annuloplasty rings (valve-in-ring), and in native mitral annular calcifications (valve-in-MAC). However, left ventricular outflow tract obstruction is a major concern for patients undergoing TMVR.

An international, multicenter, observational study recently reported on the outcomes of these procedures; the technical success rates for the valve-in-valve, valve-in-ring, and valve-in-MAC procedures were 94%, 81%, and 62% ($P < .001$), respectively. All-cause mortality was higher after valve-in-MAC compared with valve-in-ring and valve-in-valve after 30 days (35% vs 19% vs 6%; $P < .001$) and 1 year (63% vs 31% vs 14%; $P < .001$).[47-50] Since identifying patients at high risk for LVOT obstruction is important, a comprehensive analysis of the mitral valve and left ventricular anatomy is essential for optimal TMVR patient selection. Recently, laceration of the mitral anterior leaflet has emerged as an option to prevent LVOT obstruction.[51]

The native mitral annulus is asymmetrical, nontubular, and frequently not calcified, and TMVR in a native mitral valve is more challenging than in the aortic position. Currently, several TMVR technologies are under development, for both the transapical and transseptal approaches. Studies of the CardiAQ (Edwards Lifesciences Corp., Irvine, CA, USA) (transapical or transseptal, self-expanding),[52] Tendyne system (Tendyne Holdings, LLC, Roseville, MN, USA) (transapical, self-expanding),[53] and the Intrepid system (Medtronic Inc., Minneapolis, MN, USA) (transapical, transseptal self-expanding)[54] to evaluate safety and effectiveness are ongoing (Tendyne, SUMMIT, NCT03433274; Intrepid, APOLLO, NCT03242642). Additional studies are being undertaken with the TIARA system (Neovasc Inc., Richmond, BC, Canada) (transapical, self-expanding) (TIARA-I, NCT02276547),[55] the Cardiovalve system (Valtech Cardio Ltd, Or Yehuda, Israel) (transseptal, self-expanding) (AHEAD, NCT03813524),[56] and the Edwards SAPIEN M3 (Edwards Lifesciences, Irvine, CA, USA). Although complications such as left ventricular outflow tract obstruction are still a concern TMVR has the potential to become a complementary option for high-risk inoperable patients.

KEY POINTS

- ✔ TAVR volume has surpassed SAVR volume in the United States.
- ✔ A decision for TAVR versus SAVR (whether with a mechanical or bioprosthetic valve) in younger patients should include a comprehensive plan for future valve interventions based on the patient's expected lifespan.
- ✔ Edge-to-edge therapy may be appropriate for primary mitral regurgitation in patients at high risk for surgery and some functional mitral regurgitation in symptomatic patients despite optimal medical therapy.
- ✔ Trials evaluating transcatheter tricuspid repair as well as mitral and tricuspid valve replacement strategies are currently undergoing.

REFERENCES

1. Cribier A, Eltchaninoff H, Bash A, et al. Percutaneous transcatheter implantation of an aortic valve prosthesis for calcific aortic stenosis: first human case description. *Circulation.* 2002;106(24):3006-3008.
2. Grover FL, Vemulapalli S, Carroll JD, et al. 2016 annual report of The Society of Thoracic Surgeons/American College of Cardiology Transcatheter Valve Therapy Registry. *J Am Coll Cardiol.* 2017;69(10):1215-1230.
3. Makkar RR, Fontana GP, Jilaihawi H, et al. Transcatheter aortic-valve replacement for inoperable severe aortic stenosis. *N Engl J Med.* 2012;366(18):1696-1704.
4. Leon MB, Smith CR, Mack MJ, et al. Transcatheter or surgical aortic-valve replacement in intermediate-risk patients. *N Engl J Med.* 2016;374(17):1609-1620.
5. Popma JJ, Deeb GM, Yakubov SJ, et al. Transcatheter aortic-valve replacement with a self-expanding valve in low-risk patients. *N Engl J Med.* 2019;380(18):1706-1715.
6. Senage T, Gillaizeau F, Tourneau TL, Marie B, Roussel J-C, Foucher Y. Structural valve deterioration of bioprosthetic aortic valves: an underestimated complication. *J Thorac Cardiovasc Surg.* 2019;157(4):1383-1390.e5.
7. Sondergaard L, Ihlemann N, Capodanno D, et al. Durability of transcatheter and surgical bioprosthetic aortic valves in patients at lower surgical risk. *J Am Coll Cardiol.* 2019;73(5):546-553.
8. Gleason TG, Reardon MJ, Popma JJ, et al. 5-year outcomes of self-expanding transcatheter versus surgical aortic valve replacement in high-risk patients. *J Am Coll Cardiol.* 2018;72(22):2687-2696.
9. Mack MJ, Leon MB, Smith CR, et al. 5-year outcomes of transcatheter aortic valve replacement or surgical aortic valve replacement for high surgical risk patients with aortic stenosis (PARTNER 1): a randomized controlled trial. *Lancet.* 2015;385(9986):2477-2484.
10. Reardon MJ, Van Mieghem NM, Popma JJ, et al. Surgical or transcatheter aortic-valve replacement in intermediate-risk patients. *N Engl J Med.* 2017;376(14):1321-1331.
11. Mack MJ, Leon MB, Thourani VH, et al. Transcatheter aortic-valve replacement with a balloon-expandable valve in low-risk patients. *N Engl J Med.* 2019;380(18):1695-1705.
12. Giustino G, Sorrentino S, Mehran R, Faggioni M, Dangas G. Cerebral embolic protection during TAVR: a clinical event meta-analysis. *J Am Coll Cardiol.* 2017;69(4):465-466.
13. Makkar RR, Blanke P, Leipsic J, et al. Subclinical leaflet thrombosis in transcatheter and surgical bioprosthetic valves: PARTNER 3 cardiac computed tomography substudy. *J Am Coll Cardiol.* 2020;75(24):3003-3015.
14. Ng ACT, Holmes DR, Mack MJ, et al. Leaflet immobility and thrombosis in transcatheter aortic valve replacement. *Eur Heart J.* 2020;41(33):3184-3197.
15. Piayda K, Zeus T, Sievert H, Kelm M, Polzin A. Subclinical leaflet thrombosis. *Lancet.* 2018;391(10124):937-938.
16. Zhu Y, Meng S, Chen M, et al. Comparing anticoagulation therapy alone versus anticoagulation plus single antiplatelet drug therapy after transcatheter aortic valve implantation in patients with an indication for anticoagulation: a systematic review and meta-analysis. *Cardiovasc Drugs Ther.* 2020 [Online ahead of print].
17. Galiuto L, Patrono C. Aspirin monotherapy vs. DAPT after TAVI: is less more? comment on the POPular TAVI trial. *Eur Heart J.* 2020;41(45):4301-4302.
18. Giustino G, Tijssen J, Windecker S, Dangas G. Rivaroxaban after transcatheter aortic valve replacement: the GALILEO trial. *Cardiovasc Res.* 2020;116(3):e39-e41.
19. Osman M, Syed M, Balla S, et al. Meta-analysis of aspirin monotherapy versus dual antiplatelet therapy after transcatheter aortic valve implantation. *Am J Cardiol.* 2020;135:187-188.
20. Forrest JK, Ramlawi B, Deeb GM, et al. Transcatheter aortic valve replacement in low-risk patients with bicuspid aortic valve stenosis. *JAMA Cardiol.* 2021;6(1):50-57.
21. Latib A, Naim C, Bonis MD, et al. TAVR-associated prosthetic valve infective endocarditis: results of a large, multicenter registry. *J Am Coll Cardiol.* 2014;64(20):2176-2178.
22. Summers MR, Leon MB, Smith CR, et al. Prosthetic valve endocarditis after TAVR and SAVR: insights from the PARTNER trials. *Circulation.* 2019;140(24):1984-1994.
23. Ullah W, Khan MS, Gowda SN, Alraies MC, Fischman DL. Prosthetic valve endocarditis in patients undergoing TAVR compared to SAVR: a systematic review and meta-analysis. *Cardiovasc Revasc Med.* 2020;21(12):1567-1572.
24. Eaton J, Mealing S, Thompson J, et al. Is transcatheter aortic valve implantation (TAVI) a cost-effective treatment in patients who are ineligible

for surgical aortic valve replacement? A systematic review of economic evaluations. *J Med Econ*. 2014;17(5):365-375.
25. McCarthy FH, Desai ND. Long-term outcomes will determine the cost-effective approach to aortic valve disease. *J Thorac Cardiovasc Surg*. 2018;155(6):2425-2426.
26. Axtell AL, Bhambhani V, Moonsamy P, et al. Surgery does not improve survival in patients with isolated severe tricuspid regurgitation. *J Am Coll Cardiol*. 2019;74(6):715-725.
27. Oh JK, Lee S, Ji H, et al. Outcomes of early surgery in patients with isolated severe tricuspid regurgitation: a prospective registry data. *JACC Cardiovasc Interv*. 2020;13(17):2086-2087.
28. Park SJ, Oh JK, Kim S-O, et al. Determinants of clinical outcomes of surgery for isolated severe tricuspid regurgitation. *Heart*. 2020;107(5).
29. Dahou A, Levin D, Reisman M, Hahn RT. Anatomy and physiology of the tricuspid valve. *JACC Cardiovasc Imaging*. 2019;12(3):458-468.
30. Dreyfus GD, Corbi PJ, John Chan KM, Bahrami T. Secondary tricuspid regurgitation or dilatation: which should be the criteria for surgical repair? *Ann Thorac Surg*. 2005;79(1):127-132.
31. Arora L, Krishnan S, Subramani S, et al. Functional tricuspid regurgitation: analysis of percutaneous transcatheter techniques and current outcomes. *J Cardiothorac Vasc Anesth*. 2021;35(3):921-931.
32. Krishnaswamy A, Navia J, Kapadia SR. Transcatheter tricuspid valve replacement. *Interv Cardiol Clin*. 2018;7(1):65-70.
33. Latib A, Ancona MB, Agricola E, et al. Percutaneous bicuspidization of the tricuspid valve. *JACC Cardiovasc Imaging*. 2017;10(4):488-489.
34. Mehr M, Taramasso M, Besler C, et al. 1-year outcomes after edge-to-edge valve repair for symptomatic tricuspid regurgitation: results from the trivalve registry. *JACC Cardiovasc Interv*. 2019;12(15):1451-1461.
35. Nickenig G, Weber M, Schüler R, et al. Two-year outcomes with the cardioband tricuspid system from the multicentre, prospective TRI-REPAIR study. *EuroIntervention*. 2021;16(15):e1264-e1271.
36. Mack MJ, Abraham WT, Lindenfeld J, et al. Cardiovascular outcomes assessment of the MitraClip in patients with heart failure and secondary mitral regurgitation: design and rationale of the COAPT trial. *Am Heart J*. 2018;205:1-11.
37. Messika-Zeitoun D, Iung B, Armoiry X, et al. Impact of mitral regurgitation severity and left ventricular remodeling on outcome after Mitraclip implantation: results from the Mitra-FR trial. *JACC Cardiovasc Imaging*. 2021;14(4):742-752.
38. Obadia JF, Armoiry X, Iung B, et al. The MITRA-FR study: design and rationale of a andomized study of percutaneous mitral valve repair compared with optimal medical management alone for severe secondary mitral regurgitation. *EuroIntervention*. 2015;10(11):1354-1360.
39. Grayburn PA, Sannino A, Packer M. Proportionate and disproportionate functional mitral regurgitation: a new conceptual framework that reconciles the results of the MITRA-FR and COAPT trials. *JACC Cardiovasc Imaging*. 2019;12(2):353-362.
40. Chakravarty T, Makar M, Patel D, et al. Transcatheter edge-to-edge mitral valve repair with the MitraClip G4 System. *JACC Cardiovasc Interv*. 2020;13(20):2402-2414.
41. Praz F, Spargias K, Chrissoheris M, et al. Compassionate use of the PASCAL transcatheter mitral valve repair system for patients with severe mitral regurgitation: a multicentre, prospective, observational, first-in-man study. *Lancet*. 2017;390(10096):773-780.
42. Praz F, Windecker S, Kapadia S. PASCAL: a new addition to the armamentarium of transcatheter repair systems for mitral leaflet approximation. *JACC Cardiovasc Interv*. 2019;12(14):1379-1381.
43. Messika-Zeitoun D, Vahanian A, Verta P, Maisano F. Perspective on the treatment of functional mitral regurgitation using the Cardioband System. *Eur Heart J*. 2019;40(38):3196-3197.
44. Latib A, Ancona MB, Ferri L, et al. Percutaneous direct annuloplasty with cardioband to treat recurrent mitral regurgitation after Mitraclip implantation. *JACC Cardiovasc Interv*. 2016;9(18):e191-e192.
45. Blazek S, Unterhuber M, Rommel K-P, et al. Biventricular physiology of iatrogenic atrial septal defects following transcatheter mitral valve edge-to-edge repair. *JACC Cardiovasc Interv*. 2021;14(1):54-66.
46. Colli A, Zucchetta F, Torregrossa G, et al. Transapical off-pump mitral valve repair with Neochord Implantation (TOP-MINI): step-by-step guide. *Ann Cardiothorac Surg*. 2015;4(3):295-297.
47. Guerrero M, Urena M, Himbert D, et al. 1-year outcomes of transcatheter mitral valve replacement in patients with severe mitral annular calcification. *J Am Coll Cardiol*. 2018;71(17):1841-1853.
48. Guerrero M, Vemulapalli S, Xiang Q, et al. Thirty-day outcomes of transcatheter mitral valve replacement for degenerated mitral bioprostheses (valve-in-valve), failed surgical rings (valve-in-ring), and native valve with severe mitral annular calcification (valve-in-mitral annular calcification) in the United States: data from the Society of Thoracic Surgeons/American College of Cardiology/Transcatheter Valve Therapy Registry. *Circ Cardiovasc Interv*. 2020;13(3):e008425.
49. Tiwana J, Aldea G, Levin DB, et al. Contemporary transcatheter mitral valve replacement for mitral annular calcification or ring. *JACC Cardiovasc Interv*. 2020;13(20):2388-2398.
50. Whisenant B, Kapadia SR, Eleid MF, et al. One-year outcomes of mitral valve-in-valve using the SAPIEN 3 transcatheter heart valve. *JAMA Cardiol*. 2020;5(11):1245-1252.
51. Khan JM, Babaliaros VC, Greenbaum AB, et al. Anterior leaflet laceration to prevent ventricular outflow tract obstruction during transcatheter mitral valve replacement. *J Am Coll Cardiol*. 2019;73(20):2521-2534.
52. Webb J, Hensey M, Fam N, et al. Transcatheter mitral valve replacement with the transseptal EVOQUE system. *JACC Cardiovasc Interv*. 2020;13(20):2418-2426.
53. Moat NE, Duncan A, Quarto C. Transcatheter mitral valve implantation: tendyne. *EuroIntervention*. 2016;12(Y):Y75-Y77.
54. Sorajja P, Bapat V. Early experience with the Intrepid system for transcatheter mitral valve replacement. *Ann Cardiothorac Surg*. 2018;7(6):792-798.
55. Verheye S, Cheung A, Leon M, Banai S. The Tiara transcatheter mitral valve implantation system. *EuroIntervention*. 2015;11(suppl W):W71-W72.
56. Maisano F, Benetis R, Rumbinaite E, et al. 2-year follow-up after transseptal transcatheter mitral valve replacement with the cardiovalve. *JACC Cardiovasc Interv*. 2020;13(17):e163-e164.

CHAPTER 45

CATHETER INTERVENTIONS IN ADULTS WITH CONGENITAL HEART DISEASE

Thomas M. Zellers, Carrie Herbert, Surendranath Veeram Reddy, and V. Vivian Dimas

TRANSCATHETER THERAPY FOR AORTIC AND PULMONARY STENOSIS

INTRODUCTION

Aortic valve stenosis (AS) and pulmonary valve stenosis (PS) are common forms of congenital heart disease, with aortic stenosis comprising 3% to 8% and PS comprising 8% to 10% of all congenital heart disease. Balloon valvuloplasty, first performed in the early 1980s, represents first-line therapy in the adolescent and young adult population, especially in AS patients who wish to avoid replacement with a mechanical valve. Following balloon valvuloplasty, AS recurrence and Aortic insufficiency (AI) progression with freedom from aortic valve replacement at 10 years is 76% and freedom from reintervention at 10 years is 46%, prompting discussions regarding surgical versus transcatheter approach as a primary intervention for AS.[1,2] In contrast, there is a low rate of reintervention for PS following balloon valvuloplasty despite a significant risk for developing at least moderate pulmonary regurgitation over time (ie, occurs in up to 60% of patients in long-term follow-up of greater than 10 years).[3]

INDICATIONS: BALLOON VALVULOPLASTY

Treatment with balloon valvuloplasty is an American Heart Association (AHA) Class I recommendation for isolated valvar AS with resting peak systolic transvalvular gradient via catheter measurement of greater than or equal to 50 mm Hg (Level of Evidence B) or greater than or equal to 40 mm Hg if there are symptoms of angina or ST-T wave changes on an electrocardiogram (EKG) at rest or with exercise (Level of Evidence C). Valvuloplasty may be considered (Class IIb recommendations) in AS patients with resting peak systolic valve gradient of greater than or equal to 40 mm Hg but without symptoms or ST-T wave changes if the patient desires to become pregnant or participate in competitive sports (Level of Evidence C) or if peak systolic valve gradient in the catheterization lab is less than 50 mm Hg in a heavily sedated or anesthetized patient if a nonsedated Doppler study finds a mean valve gradient to be greater than or equal to 50 mm Hg (Level of Evidence C)[4] (**Figure 45.1**).

Current AHA guidelines recommend pulmonary valvuloplasty for patients who have "valvar PS with peak-to-peak catheter transvalvular gradient or peak instantaneous gradient of greater than or equal to 40 mm Hg or clinically significant pulmonary valvar obstruction in the presence of right ventricular dysfunction" as Class I recommendation (Level of Evidence A).[4]

ANATOMIC CONSIDERATIONS: BALLOON VALVULOPLASTY

Aortic valve morphology is intrinsic to outcomes of balloon aortic valvuloplasty with regard to postprocedural gradient, degree of aortic insufficiency, and freedom from reintervention over time.[5,6] However, single-center and multicenter studies fail to show consensus. The presence of more than mild insufficiency, small aortic valve annulus, or presence of other cardiac lesions (such as subaortic membranes) would warrant surgical intervention rather than a transcatheter-based approach. Most pulmonary valves are amenable to valvuloplasty. Exceptions to this are severely dysplastic pulmonary valves, especially those associated with Noonan syndrome, and patients with significant subvalvular or supravalvular obstruction; patients with these conditions are better suited for surgical correction when indicated.

CLINICAL APPLICATION/METHODOLOGY: BALLOON VALVULOPLASTY

Balloon valvuloplasty is considered a nonsurgical first step to relieve significant AS or PS. The appropriate balloon(s) size(s) are important in the final result.

For AS, diagnostic catheterization, with the patient heparinized, is performed to document the gradient across the aortic valve, degree of aortic insufficiency, aortic valve annulus dimensions, and left ventricular function. Left ventricular and ascending aortic angiograms are performed to evaluate aortic valve annulus, left ventricular function, and baseline aortic insufficiency (**Figure 45.1**). A retrograde arterial or antegrade venous approach via atrial transseptal catheterization can be utilized for intervention. Single-balloon or double-balloon techniques can be utilized; double-balloon technique requires two access sites but offers smaller arterial sheath sizes than a single balloon technique. A balloon diameter is chosen that is 0.8 to 1.0 the diameter of the aortic valve annulus. Rapid right ventricular pacing can be performed to aid in the stability of the balloon during inflation (**Figure 45.2**). After each inflation, repeat pressure measurement across the valve and angiography in the ascending aorta should be performed to evaluate

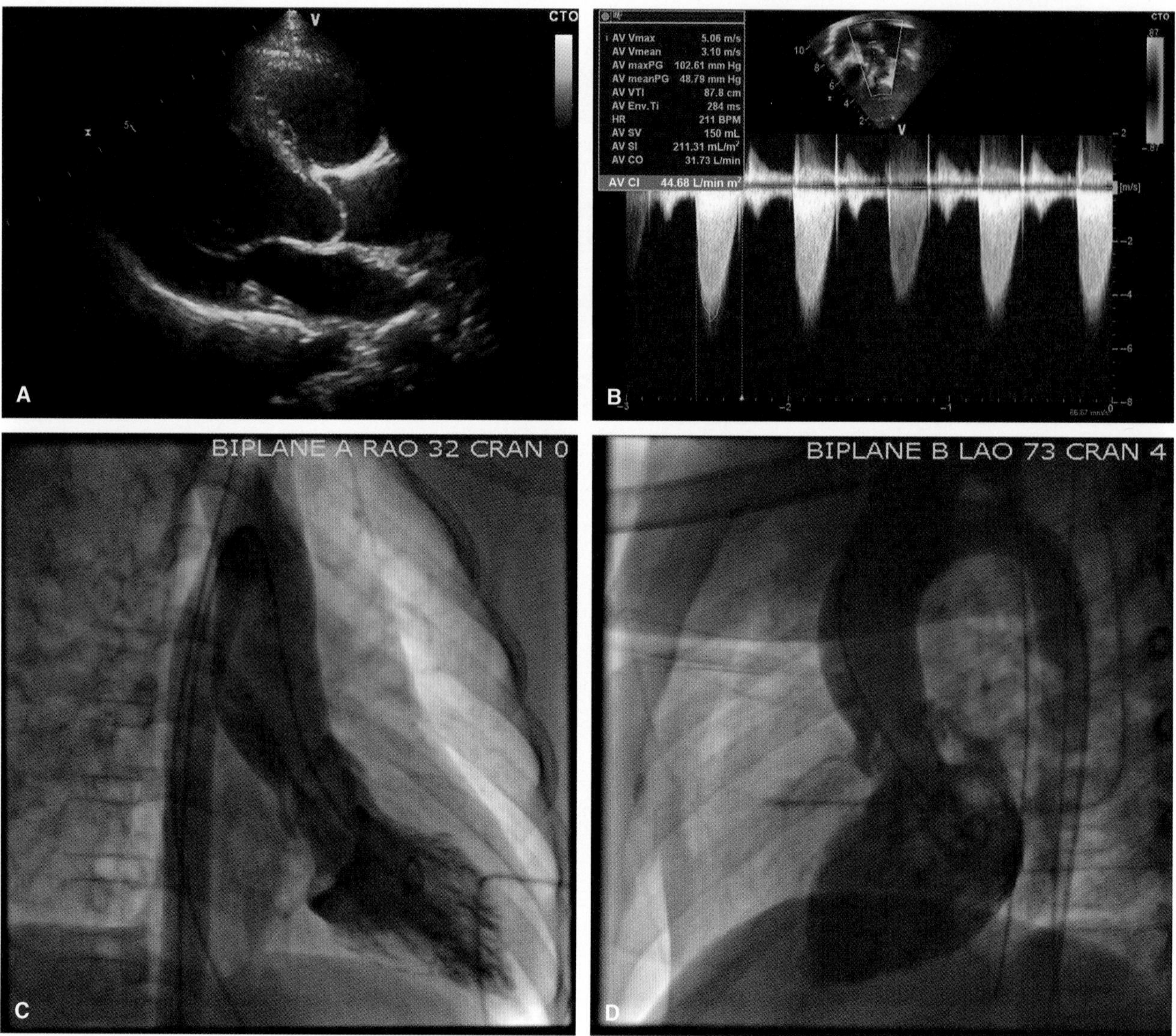

FIGURE 45.1 **(A)** Transthoracic echocardiogram parasternal long-axis imaging showing a thickened bicuspid aortic valve leaflet; **(B)** Doppler assesses peak and mean gradients; **(C)** Right anterior oblique; and **(D)** left anterior oblique projections of a patient with bicuspid aortic valve with severe aortic stenosis. The valve leaflets are thickened and doming with limited excursion.

the degree of residual stenosis and presence of aortic insufficiency (**Figure 45.2 and** **e-Figure 45.1**). Although most centers use angiography as the gold standard to assess aortic insufficiency during the procedure, echocardiography is used to assess change over time in most centers. A technically adequate dilation will often yield a residual peak-to-peak valvular systolic gradient of less than or equal to 20 to 35 mm Hg with 0 to 1 grade increase in aortic insufficiency.

For PS, a diagnostic right heart catheterization is performed to evaluate right ventricular pressure and pressure gradient across the pulmonary valve. A right ventriculogram is performed to evaluate right ventricular size and function and measure the pulmonary valve annulus, typically in cranial and straight lateral projections (**Figure 45.3**). After pulmonary valve annulus diameter is confirmed, a balloon whose diameter is 120% to 140% of the pulmonary valve annulus is chosen. A balloon size larger than 140% could lead to annulus rupture. We typically start with 120% of annulus diameter because more aggressive valvuloplasty is associated with post-valvuloplasty pulmonary regurgitation. Sufficient relief of stenosis is often achieved with one inflation of the balloon. After each inflation, repeat pressure measurements across the pulmonary valve are obtained, with a goal of postprocedure transvalvular gradient of less than 30 mm Hg (**e-Figure 45.2**). A repeat right ventriculogram is performed to evaluate for any injury to the right ventricular outflow tract. Post-valvuloplasty pulmonary insufficiency should be assessed by transthoracic echocardiography as the degree of pulmonary insufficiency is often exaggerated on angiography.

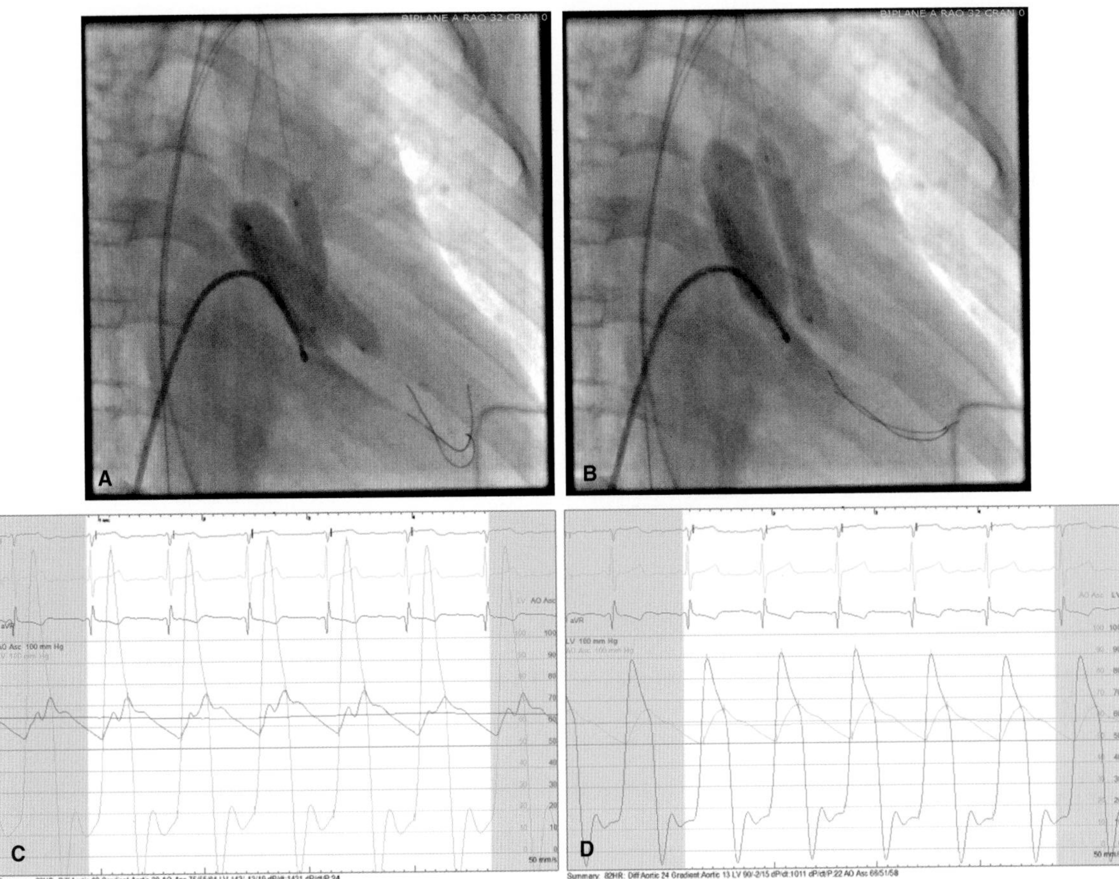

FIGURE 45.2 Fluoroscopy images of balloon aortic valvuloplasty using the double-balloon technique. A waist is seen on the smaller, more lateral balloon **(A)** that resolves with full inflation **(B)**. A pacing catheter is noted in the right ventricle, which was used for rapid pacing during valvuloplasty. Left ventricular and ascending aorta pressure waveforms before **(C)** and after **(D)** balloon aortic valvuloplasty.

LIMITATIONS: BALLOON VALVULOPLASTY

Balloon aortic valvuloplasty is considered a palliative procedure because the morphology of the valve remains abnormal and the rate of reintervention is high with both surgical valvulotomy and a transcatheter approach, with balloon aortic valvuloplasty having 10-year freedom from reintervention of 46% and surgical aortic valvuloplasty a 10-year freedom from intervention of 73%.[1,7] Technical success of the procedure is limited by valve annulus, as increasing balloon to annulus ratio increases the risk of aortic insufficiency. Balloon pulmonary valvuloplasty is limited by the size of the pulmonary valve annulus owing to the risk of annulus rupture with the use of a large balloon to annulus ratios.

FOLLOW-UP PATIENT CARE: BALLOON VALVULOPLASTY

Routine cardiology follow-up with echocardiography at 1 month, 6 months, and then yearly is typical and is imperative owing to the risk of recurrent valve stenosis and progressive valve insufficiency. Routine EKGs should be performed to evaluate for ST-T wave changes. Exercise stress testing can be considered in patients with exertional symptoms.

CLINICAL PEARLS: BALLOON VALVULOPLASTY

- Balloon aortic valvuloplasty is indicated in patients with AS with (a) peak systolic gradient greater than or equal to 50 mm Hg in asymptomatic patients or (b) greater than or equal to 40 mm Hg in patients with symptoms, EKG changes or wishing to become pregnant or play competitive sports.
- Balloon to annulus ratio of 0.8:1.0 should be used for aortic valvuloplasty to decrease the chance of creating significant aortic insufficiency.
- Balloon pulmonary valvuloplasty is indicated in patients with PS with peak-to-peak (catheter) or peak instantaneous transvalvular gradient (via echocardiogram) of greater than or equal to 40 mm Hg or in patients with clinically significant PS in the presence of right ventricular dysfunction.
- Recurrence of PS is low following balloon valvuloplasty; pulmonary insufficiency requires monitoring as these patients could require pulmonary valve replacement.

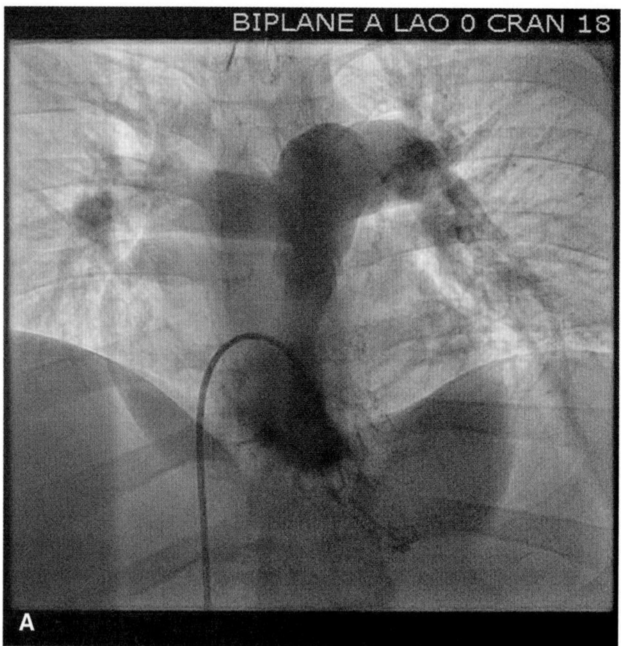

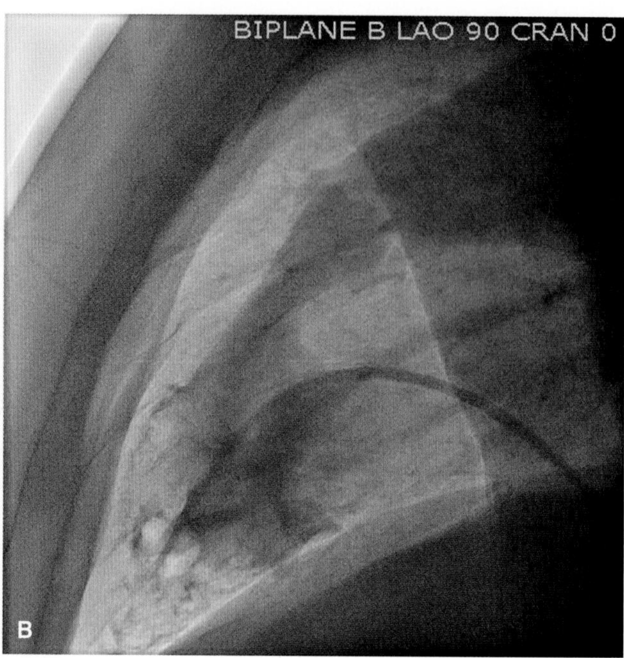

FIGURE 45.3 Right ventricular angiogram in the cranial **(A)** and lateral **(B)** projections showing a thickened and doming dysplastic pulmonary valve in a patient with severe pulmonary stenosis.

TRANSCATHETER THERAPY FOR PULMONARY ARTERY STENOSIS

INTRODUCTION

Native pulmonary artery stenosis can occur in isolation, association with genetic syndromes (ie, Alagille syndrome), or combination with other forms of congenital heart disease. In adolescents and adults, postoperative pulmonary artery stenosis is more commonly seen and is caused by scar tissue, vascular distortion, folding or extrinsic compression from surrounding structures. Long-standing branch pulmonary artery stenosis can lead to right ventricular pressure overload, pulmonary insufficiency, and eventually right ventricular failure if left untreated.

INDICATIONS: PULMONARY ANGIOPLASTY AND STENT PLACEMENT

Management of pulmonary artery stenosis is dependent upon multiple factors: the size of the patient, number of affected vessels, and concomitant lesions. In the adolescent and young adult population, most cases of pulmonary artery stenosis can be treated in the cardiac catheterization lab, either with balloon angioplasty and/or stent placement.

FUNDAMENTALS AND ANATOMIC CONSIDERATIONS: PULMONARY ANGIOPLASTY AND STENT PLACEMENT

Precatheterization planning is important, particularly in postoperative patients. Attention should be paid to the original anatomy, operative procedures including patch material used on the pulmonary arteries, and any prior cardiac catheterizations and interventions that were previously performed, including prior stents utilized. For example, patients with transposition of the great arteries who have undergone a LeCompte maneuver (draping their pulmonary arteries across the aortic root) require careful assessment of the aortic position, coronaries location, and bronchus location, particularly before pulmonary artery stent placement.

Transthoracic echocardiography should be performed prior to catheterization to evaluate right ventricular size and function, right ventricular pressure, and proximal branch pulmonary arteries. Right ventricular pressure more than half to two-third systemic pressure or a gradient greater than 20 to 30 mm Hg across the branch pulmonary artery often requires intervention.[4] Perfusion scans help evaluate the flow discrepancy between lungs in patients with unilateral branch pulmonary stenosis; flow discrepancy of 70/30% or worse is an indication of evaluation/intervention. In patients with complex disease, noninvasive imaging with computerized tomography (CT) or magnetic resonance angiograms and three-dimensional (3D) printing is particularly helpful in complex bilateral proximal stenoses (**e-Figure 45.3**).

CLINICAL APPLICATIONS: PULMONARY ANGIOPLASTY AND STENT PLACEMENT

Diagnostic right heart catheterization is performed to document hemodynamics and degree of stenosis across the branch pulmonary arteries. Main pulmonary artery angiograms are performed to delineate the areas and degree of stenosis. Choosing the appropriate camera angles is of utmost importance, as foreshortening of the vessel could lead to inappropriate measurements and stent choice. 3D rotational angiography can assist with ideal angles for intervention. When multiple lesions are present, such as in patients with repaired tetralogy of Fallot with major aortopulmonary collaterals or patients with peripheral pulmonary stenosis, interventions should be performed distal to proximal so that there are no multiple catheter and wire exchanges across freshly dilated or stented vessels. Balloon angioplasty is often performed prior to stenting, as this alone may lead to a satisfactory result and alleviate the need for stent placement. Angioplasty also gives information on the compliance of a vessel.

Although initial balloon selection for angioplasty varies by operator, a starting diameter of approximately two times the narrowest diameter of the vessel is often chosen. If there is no resolution of a waist on the balloon at full inflation, then the vessel is considered noncompliant. Cutting balloons have been shown to be effective in treating resistant lesions.[8] Despite aggressive balloon angioplasty, there remains a high rate of stenosis or restenosis. Stent placement offers better short- and long-term results.[9,10] In some patients, a prior stent that was placed when the patient was much smaller may need further dilation. If the stent cannot be enlarged to an adequate diameter, intentional fracturing of these stents has been shown to be safe and effective, allowing for the placement of a larger stent.[11,12]

Complications related to balloon pulmonary angioplasty and stent placement are not insignificant, with a serious adverse event rate of 10% noted in a multi-institutional registry. Adverse events include vascular or cardiac trauma, arrhythmia, hemodynamic compromise, pulmonary edema, and/or bleeding from reperfusion injury.[13] These procedures should be performed by operators who are well-versed in the management of these complications.

LIMITATIONS: PULMONARY ANGIOPLASTY AND STENT PLACEMENT

Vessels that are too compliant yield unsatisfactory results related to vessel recoil after balloon dilation. Noncompliant vessels can be resistant to angioplasty, even with the use of high- or ultra-high-pressure balloons and cutting balloons. Stent placement in these situations may not immediately improve the vessel stenosis, but these lesions can often be successfully re-dilated at a later date. To date, there is not a stent commercially available that will expand with somatic growth; therefore, recurrent interventions even into adulthood are often necessary to re-dilate a previously placed stent in childhood.

FOLLOW-UP PATIENT CARE: PULMONARY ANGIOPLASTY AND STENT PLACEMENT

Balloon pulmonary angioplasty has a high incidence of restenosis, and thus, these patients should be followed longitudinally. Patients with stents also require routine follow-up, as in-stent restenosis can develop, and the stent often needs to be re-dilated over time to account for patient growth.

RESEARCH AND FUTURE DIRECTIONS: PULMONARY ANGIOPLASTY AND STENT PLACEMENT

Current research includes the development of biodegradable stents, a temporary scaffold that allows for remodeling of the vessel and then disappears, thereby eliminating the need for re-dilation of a permanent stent.

CLINICAL PEARLS: PULMONARY ANGIOPLASTY AND STENT PLACEMENT

- Balloon angioplasty of pulmonary arteries may offer sufficient alleviation of stenosis; however, many patients require stent placement caused by ineffective relief of stenosis or restenosis of the vessel over time.
- Stents that can be re-dilated over time to an adult diameter should be chosen.
- Previously placed stents that cannot be expanded to an adult-sized vessel diameter may be intentionally fractured, allowing for a larger stent to be placed.
- Pulmonary angioplasty and stent placement are associated with a relatively high incidence of serious adverse events and should only be performed by experienced operators who can manage these complications.

CONDUIT ANGIOPLASTY, STENTS, AND TRANSCATHETER VALVES

INTRODUCTION

Conduits from the right ventricle to pulmonary artery are commonly used for the repair of patients with truncus arteriosus, tetralogy of Fallot with pulmonary artery atresia, pulmonary valve atresia without ventricular septal defect (VSD), Ross procedures, and various other forms of complex biventricular anatomy where there is a need to establish continuity between the right ventricle and branch pulmonary arteries. Unfortunately, bioprosthetic conduits do not grow with the patient and degenerate over time.[14] This results in conduit stenosis, insufficiency, or most commonly, both. Transcatheter intervention has become the mainstay of therapy for diseased conduits in which the conduit remains appropriately sized for the patient, and transcatheter valve technology for congenital heart disease has evolved significantly over the past decade.[15]

Valve therapy in congenital heart patients is predominantly for use in the pulmonary position. The first Food and Drug Administration (FDA)-approved transcatheter valve for use in patients in the pulmonic position was the Melody valve (Medtronic, Minneapolis, MN, USA) but was only approved for use within right ventricle to pulmonary artery conduits.[16] With the use and approval of bioprosthetic valves in adult patients with aortic valve disease, more valves have become available for use in larger diameter outflow tracts (ie, Sapien S3 and XT [Edwards Lifesciences, Irvine, CA, USA]). Although conduit therapy was a significant step in preventing congenital patients from undergoing multiple operations for conduit revisions, it did not address the large population of patients with large diameter outflow tracts whose diameter far exceeded the upper limits of the Melody valve and, in many cases, the Edwards family of valves. To meet this demand, several valves have now been developed and are undergoing trial to treat the larger outflow tracts, thus providing the interventionalist the tools to treat all dysfunctional outflow tracts whether native or conduit.

INDICATIONS: CONDUIT ANGIOPLASTY, STENTS, AND TRANSCATHETER VALVES

Conduit intervention is necessary when there is evidence of hemodynamically significant stenosis and/or insufficiency, in the presence of right ventricular dysfunction, right ventricular pressure overload, and/or progressive symptoms of exercise intolerance. The goal of conduit intervention is to relieve obstruction and, if possible, restore valve function if the conduit is of adequate size and the anatomy amenable. Transcatheter pulmonary valve implantation is indicated in patients with evidence of right ventricular volume overload; when right ventricular end-systolic volume greater than 140 mL/m^2, it does not return to normal size and volume with valve replacement. Thus, earlier intervention is warranted to optimize right ventricular remodeling.[17] Right ventricular dysfunction and even left ventricular dysfunction related to this are also indications for proceeding with transcatheter pulmonary valve replacement.

ANATOMIC CONSIDERATIONS: CONDUIT ANGIOPLASTY, STENTS, AND TRANSCATHETER VALVES

Primary anatomic considerations include conduit size, patient size, vascular access, location of the coronary arteries, and presence of any other significant lesions that may complicate the procedure such as acute angle of the branch pulmonary arteries or significant proximal branch pulmonary artery stenosis. For transcatheter valves, candidacy is related to the dimension of the outflow tract to be implanted, specifically, the size and length of the landing zone. This can be determined by 3D preprocedure imaging (CT or cardiac magnetic resonance imaging [CMRI]) but must be confirmed with balloon sizing prior to valve implantation[18] (**Figure 45.4**). The Melody valve, which is a bovine jugular vein sewn to the Cheatham-platinum stent, is suitable for conduit diameters up to 22 mm. When dilated beyond this, there is an increased risk of creating valvular insufficiency. For larger diameter outflows (ie, up to 29 mm), the Sapien family of transcatheter heart valves can be utilized. Beyond this diameter, transcatheter treatment at the time of this writing is limited to research studies. In patients who have undergone a Ross operation with dilated neoaortic roots in close proximity to the conduit, creation of aortic valve insufficiency should be assessed during compliance testing (see below) to evaluate for distortion of the neo-ascending aorta.

FUNDAMENTALS: CONDUIT ANGIOPLASTY, STENTS, AND TRANSCATHETER VALVES

Prior to catheterization, a 3D imaging study (CT or CMRI) is performed to assess the right ventricular outflow tract and conduit anatomy, the branch pulmonary artery anatomy, and the relationship of the coronary arteries to the conduit or valve landing zone, so that the operator may anticipate any potential problems[18] (**Figure 45.4**). Obstruction below the conduit should be excluded. If any concern arises regarding possible coronary artery compression, selective angiography may need to be performed during compliance testing[19] (**e-Figure 45.4**).

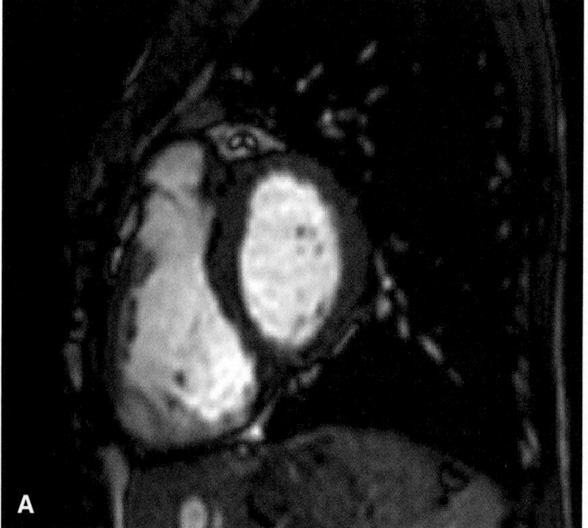

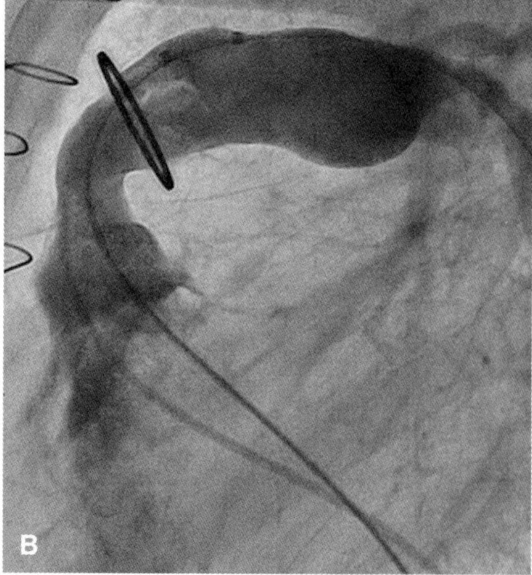

FIGURE 45.4 **(A)** The magnetic resonance image shows an enlarged right ventricle from pulmonary insufficiency. **(B)** The angiogram shows a narrowed and calcified conduit with narrowing at the valve ring and thickened valve leaflets.

CLINICAL APPLICATIONS: CONDUIT ANGIOPLASTY, STENTS, AND TRANSCATHETER VALVES

Right and left heart catheterization is performed to evaluate the right ventricular pressure, the gradient across the dysfunctional right ventricular outflow tract or conduit, the assessment of any hemodynamically significant branch pulmonary artery stenosis, and assessment of coronary artery position. Assessing ventricular compliance using diastolic pressure measurements is helpful in understanding the impact of right ventricular volume overload. Conduit interventions are limited currently by conduit size. Resolving early stenosis with a combination of angioplasty and or stent placement can help prolong the time to conduit revision.[15] However, in adolescents and adults, surgical conduit or valve replacement is indicated in patients with conduits too small for their size. In addition, transcatheter valve therapy is not indicated in conduits less than 16 mm in diameter, as the Melody valve is approved for implant conduit sizes of 16 to 22 mm. The Sapien XT is only approved for conduits greater than 20 mm in size. In patients whose conduit size is 16 mm or larger, however, restoring pulmonary valve function with a transcatheter valve is feasible. This typically requires some type of "preparation" of the conduit with bare-metal or covered stents to optimize the conduit diameter and prevent recoil and later fracture of the Melody valve stent. For heavily calcified conduits, primary covered stent placement might be indicated to prevent complications from conduit injury or rupture. Because conduit rupture may occur even in noncalcified conduits, covered stents are being considered in these conduits as well.[20] Intervention depends highly on anatomic characteristics including proximity of the coronary arteries to the conduit, other associated lesions which may or may not be amenable to transcatheter intervention, and compliance of the conduit itself. When undertaking these procedures, one must be prepared for the two most significant and potentially catastrophic complications: conduit rupture and/or coronary compression/distortion.[19-21]

Transcatheter pulmonary valve implantation can be safely performed in patients with conduit diameters greater than 16 mm and native outflow tracts up to 29 mm in diameter. Valve placement can also be successfully performed with either Melody or Sapien transcatheter valves depending on the internal diameter of the existing valve.

In native outflow tracts, balloon sizing should be performed with a compliant sizing balloon. This can be performed with or without pacing depending on the stability of the balloon during inflation. With inflation of the sizing balloon, a right ventricular angiogram determines if the balloon size completely occludes the outflow tract. Balloon sizing with a semicompliant balloon can also be used to simultaneously assess coronary artery flow with balloon occlusion of the outflow tract. If a discrete waist on the balloon with a suitable landing zone less than 29 mm in diameter is present, transcatheter valve placement can be performed based on the waist measurements. Valve placement, with or without pre-stenting of the right ventricular outflow tract, can be performed at the same procedure. For outflow tracts in which pre-stenting is needed, the decision to place the valve in a staged fashion may be warranted if there is concern about displacing the freshly placed stent with the valve delivery apparatus. Valve delivery can be performed with pacing to maintain a stable position during deployment. This is particularly helpful in patients with short landing zones. Pacing should be fast enough to reduce the blood pressure to at least the native pressure and should be tested prior to the time of valve deployment to assure that the lead captures and that pacing is well tolerated.

LIMITATIONS: CONDUIT ANGIOPLASTY, STENTS, AND TRANSCATHETER VALVES

Limitations are primarily related to the inability to relieve stenosis and reestablish valve competency (caused by valve delivery system size), conduit size or compliance, and outflow tract measuring greater than 29 mm with the available FDA-approved transcatheter valves or vascular access. An additional risk to the tricuspid valve can also occur with the use of the Edwards delivery system, as it passes uncovered through the delicate tricuspid valve apparatus and puts the tricuspid valve at significant risk of injury when multiple manipulations are required to deliver the pulmonary valve within the conduit.

SPECIAL CONSIDERATIONS AND CONTRAINDICATIONS

Smaller adolescent or adult patients represent unique challenges owing to patient size. In smaller patients with calcified conduits, consideration should be given to placing a sheath capable of accommodating a covered stent in the case of acute conduit rupture. Documented coronary artery compromise with compliance testing is a contraindication for stent or valve placement in the conduit. Recent endocarditis and inability to be anticoagulated (even with aspirin) remain contraindications for transcatheter valve placement. Limitations in patient size and vascular access have been overcome in some situations by utilizing hybrid approaches such as perventricular valve placement.

FOLLOW-UP PATIENT CARE: CONDUIT ANGIOPLASTY, STENTS, AND TRANSCATHETER VALVES

Patient follow-up is important on at least an annual basis to assess for valve performance. A follow-up 3D imaging study is helpful to assess the recovery of the right ventricle. Surveillance for valve fractures is also important, particularly with the Melody valve, requiring annual fluoroscopy for visualization. Valve stents with multiple fractures or loss of stent integrity with valve dysfunction require intervention with re-stenting and/or *re-valving*. Endocarditis prophylaxis and daily aspirin should be observed for the duration of the life of the implanted valve.

RESEARCH AND FUTURE DIRECTIONS: CONDUIT ANGIOPLASTY, STENTS, AND TRANSCATHETER VALVES

Covered delivery systems are being trialed for delivery of the Sapien family of valves, which will reduce the risk of tricuspid valve injury while using this valve. Further efforts at improving stent and valve design and profile are ongoing. In addition, the NuDel (BVM Medical Ltd, Hinckley, Leicestershire, UK) covered delivery systems are now becoming available for easier delivery of covered stents within the conduit. Two valve systems designed for larger diameter outflow tracts (ie, those >29 mm in diameter) have been studied in the United States. The Harmony valve (Medtronic, Minneapolis, MN, USA) is a covered self-expanding stent containing a bioprosthetic valve. It is available in two sizes. The Edwards Alterra adaptive pre-stent is a self-expanding partially covered nitinol stent that is hourglass-shaped to downsize the outflow tract with a central landing zone designed for a Sapien S3 transcatheter heart valve. The Alterra pre-stent will treat outflows up to 38 mm in diameter. Outside the United States, the Venus P valve (MedTech, Shanghai, China) is also a self-expanding nitinol stent with a porcine pericardial valve sewn in that is undergoing trials and treats outflows from 18 to 34 mm in diameter.

TRANSCATHETER THERAPY FOR COARCTATION IN ADULTS

INTRODUCTION

Coarctation of the aorta is a narrowing of the aorta, typically between the left subclavian artery and the origin of the patent ductus arteriosus (PDA; the juxtaductal coarctation) (**e-Figure 45.5**). It is rare to see a native coarctation in adulthood, but a recurrent coarctation (following surgical repair as an infant or child) can be seen in adolescence and adulthood. Hypertension is the primary symptom seen with a coarctation in adulthood, and occasionally this is associated with left ventricular dysfunction and congestive heart failure.

CLINICAL PEARLS: CONDUIT ANGIOPLASTY, STENTS, AND TRANSCATHETER VALVES

- Transcatheter intervention is the primary modality of therapy for dysfunctional conduits that are appropriately sized for the patient.
- For most conduits, restoration of conduit function is now possible.
- The FDA approval of covered stents and ongoing experience with conduit interventions have decreased the risk of complications related to conduit rupture.
- Careful prescreening by 3D imaging can help determine patient suitability and risks for transcatheter intervention.
- Transcatheter heart valves in congenital heart disease are almost exclusively used in the pulmonic position.
- Outflow tracts and conduits 16 to 29 mm can be treated with the currently approved transcatheter valves.
- Currently, in the United States, both Medtronic and Edwards have developed additional technology to allow for percutaneous valve placement in larger diameter outflow tracts.

INDICATIONS: TRANSCATHETER THERAPY FOR COARCTATION IN ADULTS

Persistent coarctation with a greater than 20 mm Hg upper to lower extremity blood pressure gradient, hypertension, claudication at rest or with exercise, left ventricular dysfunction, or congestive heart failure are indications for intervention. Coarctation stenting is the procedure of choice in both native and recurrent coarctations in adults.[22] Although bare-metal stenting is still the first choice, covered stents are becoming more popular, especially in patients with significant (<3 mm diameter) coarctations[23,24] (**e-Figure 45.5**).

ANATOMIC CONSIDERATIONS

MRI or CT are used to evaluate the location of the coarctation of the aorta, the diameter or the narrowed segment, size of the aorta above and below the coarctation, and location of head and neck and arm vessels, as these findings determine suitability for catheter intervention (**e-Figure 45.5**). A coarctation associated with significant transverse arch hypoplasia, however, is a much more difficult and riskier stent procedure.[23] A coarctation rarely occurs in the distal thoracic aorta or the abdominal aorta unless associated with vasculitis. Collaterals are often present and provide protective blood flow to the lower body.

FUNDAMENTALS: TRANSCATHETER THERAPY FOR COARCTATION IN ADULTS

Left heart catheterization is typically performed to measure the ascending to descending aorta pressure gradient and left ventricular pressures, including end-diastolic pressure. Angiography in the ascending aorta helps evaluate the location and severity of the coarctation. The diameters of the coarctation, the isthmus and transverse arch, the descending aorta just distal to the coarctation segment, and the aorta at the diaphragm in the anterior-posterior and lateral projections are all measured to determine the severity and the size of the balloon and length of the stent to use.

CLINICAL APPLICATIONS: TRANSCATHETER THERAPY FOR COARCTATION IN ADULTS

Left heart catheterization is typically performed from the femoral artery, but many operators prefer an additional arterial access (contralateral femoral artery, radial or brachial artery) for simultaneous pressure measurements across the coarctation, before and after angioplasty/stenting. A gradient greater than

20 mm Hg and/or a measured coarctation diameter less than 70% of the aortic diameter above the coarctation or at the diaphragm typically are indications for intervention. The severity of the coarctation influences steps taken in the procedure. For example, severe, near atresia coarctations (<3 mm in diameter) often undergo test dilation with a balloon smaller than the isthmus diameter, to enlarge the coarctation diameter before stenting and to test compliance (**Figure 45.5**). Less severe coarctations are usually tested for compliance with a balloon of 80% of the isthmus diameter (Coarctation of the Aorta Stent Trial [COAST] protocol).[25] If compliant, stenting is the next step (**Figure 45.5**). Although severe coarctations can be treated safely with bare-metal stenting, the risk of aneurysm formation (5.4%) typically prompts operators to use covered Cheatham Platinum stents (NuMed, Orlando, FL, USA) to prevent aneurysm formation (**Figure 45.6**). Covered stents also allow the use of higher-pressure balloons to maximize the expansion of the stent and resolve any residual narrowing. The stent should be expanded to the same diameter as the isthmus above the coarcted segment. Many operators choose to dilate and flare the distal stent to appose it to the descending aorta wall allowing better reendothelialization.[24-27] On occasion, bare-metal or covered stenting with incomplete dilation, followed by full dilation at a later date, has been performed. The stent is ideally mounted on a balloon the same length as the stent. Most prefer the Numed BIB (balloon-in-balloon) as deployment is predictable, and the stent position can be adjusted with only inner balloon inflation. The balloon and stent should be delivered through a long sheath at least 2 French sizes larger than recommended for the balloon alone. The balloon diameter used should be no more than 110% of the transverse arch or maximal isthmus diameter. After deployment, the balloon is carefully removed over the wire and pressures are measured across the stent, either simultaneously or as a pullback with a

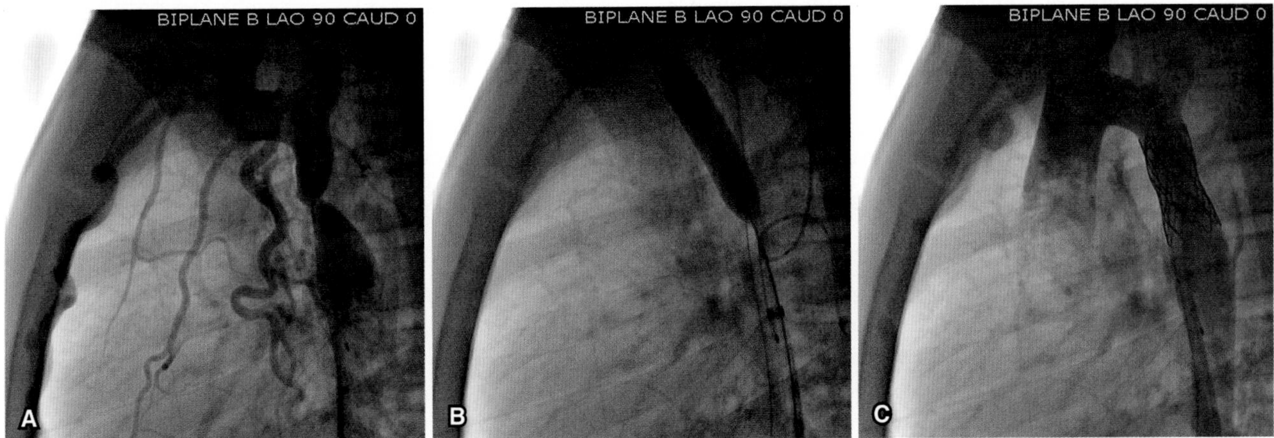

FIGURE 45.5 **(A)** Angiography in the descending aorta reveals a severe coarctation with multiple collaterals. **(B)** The coarctation is compliant by balloon testing; no waist is seen. **(C)** Post Cheatham platinum stent implantation with good apposition of the stent against the aortic wall and excellent flow through the stent and reduction of collateral flow.

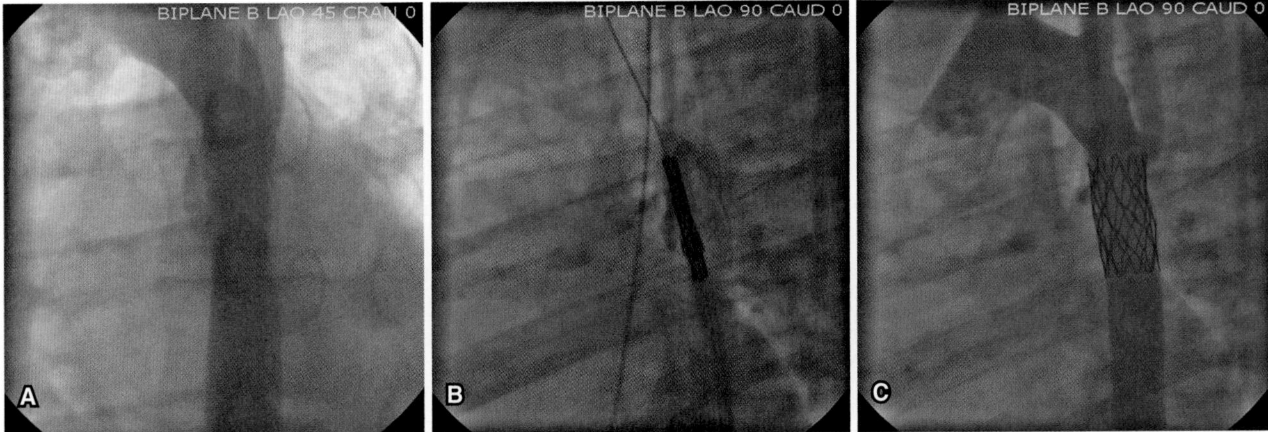

FIGURE 45.6 **View A** shows an aortic aneurysm anteriorly following stent implantation and dilation. **View B** shows the covered Cheathem Platinum stent being uncovered inside the dilated stent. Arrows show the aneurysm. **View C** shows the covered Cheathem Platinum stent in place with no residual aneurysm or wall injury.

Multitrack catheter that can be pulled back over the wire and also used for angiography. Angiography then documents the result, and aortic diameters are again measured.[24-27]

LIMITATIONS? SPECIAL CONSIDERATIONS: TRANSCATHETER THERAPY FOR COARCTATION IN ADULTS

Transverse arch hypoplasia is a special consideration. With stents in the transverse arch, there are theoretical risks for decreased carotid flow, carotid dissection, or stroke from emboli that form on the stents. In this situation, ascending to descending aortic grafting (*bucket handle* graft) may be a better long-term option. Multilevel obstructions can also be difficult to treat with a stent if the carotids or transverse arch is involved.

MRI of the brain is recommended to evaluate for intracranial aneurysms in adolescents or adults at least once. Systemic hypertension can persist despite adequate transcatheter therapy; antihypertensive therapy should be initiated or reinitiated if hypertension persists after stenting.[28] Although uncommon with stenting, mesenteric arteritis from increased blood flow to the gut after relief of coarctation can occur.

FOLLOW-UP PATIENT CARE: TRANSCATHETER THERAPY FOR COARCTATION IN ADULTS

Early follow-up for post-stent placement is typically performed at 1 month, 6 months, 1 year, and yearly thereafter with special attention to monitoring for hypertension. Echocardiography with Doppler is useful to follow residual gradients. Chest CT scans provide good imaging to detect aneurysm formation and are typically performed within 18 months and at 3 to 5 years after stent implantation. Fluoroscopy is utilized yearly to evaluate stent integrity as there is a stent fracture incidence of up to 11% with the Cheatham Platinum and covered Cheatham Platinum stents.[24-27]

RESEARCH AND FUTURE CONSIDERATIONS

The COAST and Congenital Cardiovascular Interventional Study Consortium (CCISC) studies demonstrate stent implantation as a safe, effective therapy and the treatment of choice. Thoracic endovascular aortic repair (TEVAR) self-expanding covered stents in adults with larger-sized aortas are being evaluated.

CLINICAL PEARLS: TRANSCATHETER THERAPY FOR COARCTATION IN ADULTS

- Coarctation in adulthood is usually caused by recurrent postsurgical coarctation, and hypertension is the usual presenting sign and symptom for adolescents and adults.
- Coarctation stenting is the treatment of choice for most adults.
- Bare-metal stenting is standard therapy, but covered stents are often used for severe coarctations to prevent or treat aneurysm formation.
- Hypertension can persist despite successful stent therapy, and treatment with antihypertensives is indicated.
- Brain MRI is recommended to evaluate for intracranial aneurysms at least once after adolescence in patients with coarctation of aorta.

TRANSCATHETER THERAPY FOR PATENT DUCTUS ARTERIOSUS

INTRODUCTION

Persistent PDA is uncommon in adult patients (0.05%) as it is typically discovered in childhood and treated.[29] This number may be underestimated as the incidence of inaudible PDAs in patients over 21 years of age is unknown. The risk of endocarditis in adult patients with an audible PDA is approximately 0.45% per year. Although tiny and small PDAs may be asymptomatic with minimal to no clinical findings (no heart murmur, discovered on imaging exams for other reasons), moderate to large PDAs may be associated with a continuous murmur, left heart chamber enlargement, heart failure, or pulmonary hypertension.

INDICATIONS/ANATOMIC CONSIDERATIONS: TRANSCATHETER THERAPY FOR PATENT DUCTUS ARTERIOSUS

Transcatheter PDA closure is the treatment of choice. Closure is indicated in patients (1) with congestive heart failure; (2) with volume overload and dilation of left heart structures; (3) to prevent irreversible pulmonary hypertension; and (4) to prevent endocarditis. Closure of tiny and small PDAs is controversial, as the only indication is to prevent endocarditis, and the incidence of endocarditis in inaudible PDAs is unknown. Calcified PDAs in older patients can be closed with a device or a covered graft, but the risk is higher compared to noncalcified vessels.

PDAs are classified into five different types or shapes, according to the Krichenko et al criteria.[30] Type A and E are the most common and type D is the least common type across all age groups. The type of PDA, the minimal diameter (insertion into the main pulmonary artery), and aortic ampulla diameter measurements dictate the best closure device (**Figure 45.7**).

CLINICAL APPLICATIONS: TRANSCATHETER THERAPY FOR PATENT DUCTUS ARTERIOSUS

Right and left heart catheterization is typically performed to measure pulmonary artery pressures, pulmonary (Qp) and systemic (Qs) blood flow, Qp:Qs shunt ratio, and pulmonary vascular resistance. PDA closure is contraindicated in patients with pulmonary vascular resistance greater than 8 Wood units/m^2.

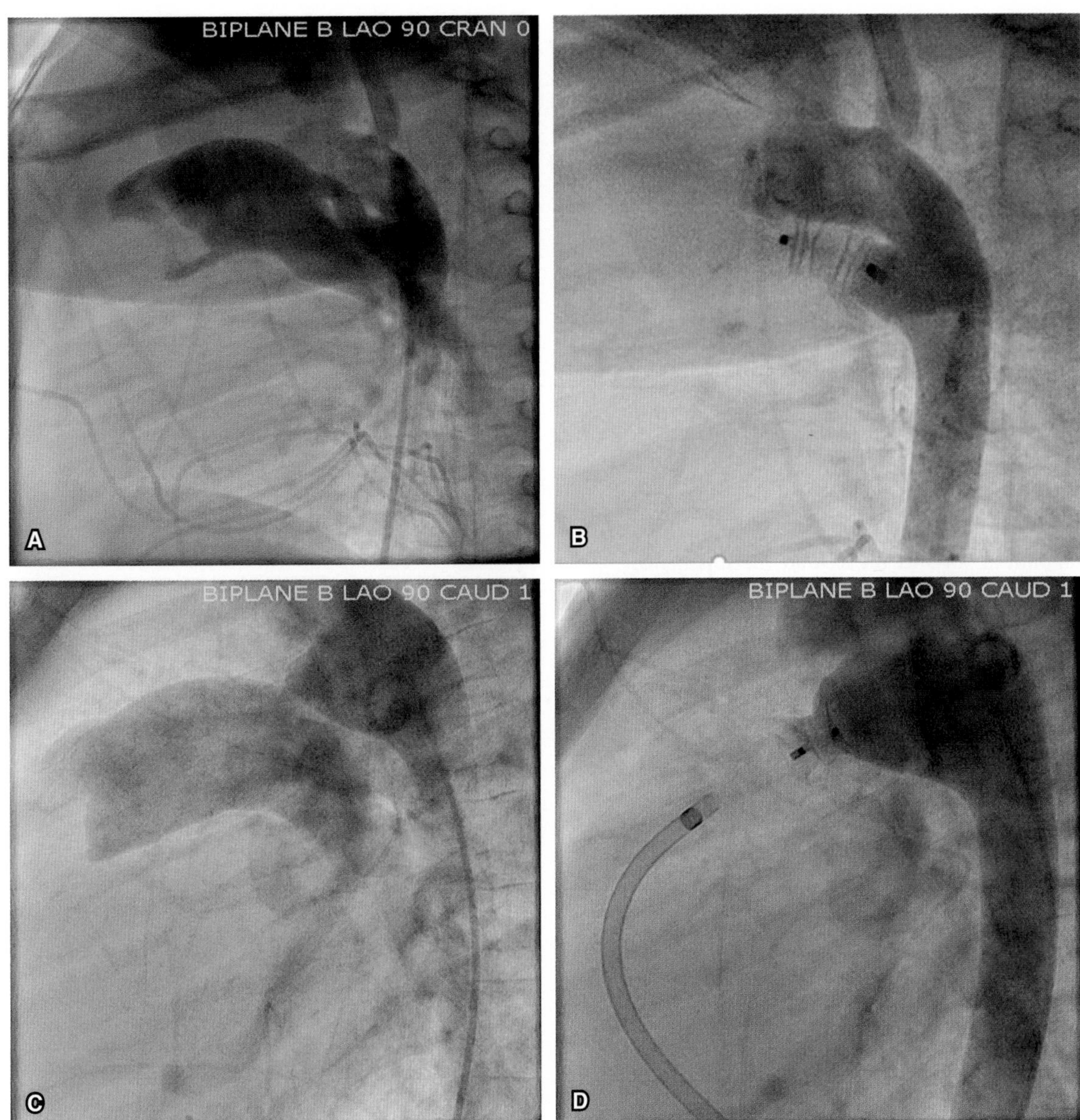

FIGURE 45.7 **(A)** Angiography reveals a Type E patent ductus arteriosus (PDA) with an elongated course. **(B)** An Amplatzer vascular plug type II has been inserted with complete closure of the PDA demonstrated by angiography in the descending aorta. **(C)** The angiogram shows a large Type A PDA with left-to-right shunting. The pulmonary end is narrowed but the aortic ampulla is quite large. **(D)** An angiogram after delivery of a large Amplatzer Duct Occluder I PDA occluder. The device is pulled far into the ampulla with the retention disc resting just distal to the insertion of the PDA into the main pulmonary artery. No residual flow is noted.

PDA closure can be accomplished using a number of embolization devices with a successful closure rate of greater than 98%. Small PDAs (minimal diameter <2 mm) can often be closed using Gianturco (Occluding Spring Emboli; Cook, Bloomington, IN, USA) or mReye (Cook Medical, Bloomington IN, USA) embolization coils. These are typically delivered free hand.[31] The NitOcclud (pfm medical ag, Cologne, Germany) coil with a controlled delivery system is made specifically for closing small to moderate PDAs. It has a high closure rate (97%) with a low rate of complications.[32] A PDA with a minimal diameter 2 mm can be closed with a variety of vascular occlusion devices, including the Amplatzer Duct Occluder (ADO) I (Abbott, Abbott Park, IL, USA),[33] the Amplatzer type II vascular plugs (Abbott, Abbott Park, IL, USA),[34] and the ADO II device (Abbott, Abbott Park, IL, USA).[35] Larger PDAs can be closed with the larger ADO I devices or the Amplatzer muscular VSD devices (typically for patients with pulmonary hypertension but pulmonary vascular resistance less than 8 Wood units/m^2; Abbott, Abbott Park, IL, USA). All of these devices are filled with Dacron to promote thrombosis of the device with closure rates greater than 98%.

Right heart catheterization is performed for hemodynamics; left heart catheterization and aortic angiography are performed to delineate the location, size, and shape of the PDA. Measurements made from this angiogram inform which devices could or should be used. Care should be taken to avoid PDA spasm with the catheter. Spasm leads to underestimating the PDA size, increasing the risk for device embolization. The decision to close from the venous or arterial side depends on the device to be used. Small PDAs are easily approached from the arterial side when using a coil or a small Amplatzer type II vascular plug. However, small PDAs can also be approached prograde when using an Amplatzer type II vascular plug or a NitOcclud coil. Moderate and large PDAs, which are typically closed with an ADO I device or VSD device, are approached from the venous side (**Figure 45.7**).

SPECIAL CONSIDERATIONS/LIMITATIONS: TRANSCATHETER THERAPY FOR PATENT DUCTUS ARTERIOSUS

Accurate measurements of the PDA by angiography are important for device selection and closure. Avoiding PDA spasm is of paramount importance for accurate measurements.

Residual shunts pose an endocarditis risk, so closure of residual shunts is important. Left pulmonary artery ostial stenosis is seen in 2% of patients following PDA closure in children. It is a very rare complication in adolescents or adults. Aortic injury or dissection can occur with device closure in older patients with calcified PDAs. In these situations, a bailout plan is required. Device embolization occurs in less than 5% of patients with current PDA devices used.

FOLLOW-UP PATIENT CARE: TRANSCATHETER THERAPY FOR PATENT DUCTUS ARTERIOSUS

Patient follow-up to document complete closure by echocardiography is important and is typically performed at 6 and 12 months postimplant. Follow-up to 5 years is typical for any noncoil device. If no complications are detected, the PDA is considered cured.

RESEARCH AND FUTURE DIRECTIONS

There is a need to evaluate which device is best in adults; but currently, there are no studies being conducted.

CLINICAL PEARLS: TRANSCATHETER THERAPY FOR PATENT DUCTUS ARTERIOSUS

- Most PDAs in adults can be closed in the cardiac catheterization lab.[36,37]
- Tiny PDAs may not need to be closed; endocarditis risk is unknown.
- Calcified PDAs in older patients are associated with higher procedural risk.
- There are many vascular occlusion devices that can be used to close PDAs successfully.
- Follow-up to at least 1 year is important to detect any residual leaks or complications.

DEVICE CLOSURE OF VENTRICULAR SEPTAL DEFECTS

INTRODUCTION

VSDs are the most common congenital heart defect, but the majority of defects seen in adulthood are small and hemodynamically insignificant. Thus, perimembranous and small muscular defects are rarely closed in adulthood. One adult-specific VSD that may require transcatheter intervention is the postinfarction VSD which historically has occurred in up to 1% to 2% of all patients with an ST-elevation myocardial infarction.[37] However, with current revascularization techniques, the incidence has decreased to less than 0.3%. One treatment option for closure of the postinfarction VSD is an Amplatzer Post Infarct VSD Occluder (Abbott, Abbott Park, IL, USA).

INDICATIONS AND ANATOMIC CONSIDERATIONS: DEVICE CLOSURE OF VENTRICULAR SEPTAL DEFECT

Postinfarction VSD closure is indicated in patients with significant left-to-right VSD shunt, left ventricular dysfunction, congestive heart failure, or cardiogenic shock who are not surgical candidates.

The majority of postinfarction VSDs are anterior or inferior/posterior septal defects. Device closure of these defects requires adequate tissue rims and defects positioned far enough away from atrioventricular valve chordal insertions that they are not entrapped by the device discs. Importantly, postinfarction VSDs are known to have friable edges early on and defects may enlarge with time with further tissue loss, making successful long-term closure difficult if addressed too early (<3-4 weeks).

FUNDAMENTALS: DEVICE CLOSURE OF VENTRICULAR SEPTAL DEFECTS

Right and left heart catheterization is indicated to evaluate hemodynamics, including left-to-right shunt and diastolic function. Left ventricular angiography (20-30 degree left anterior oblique projection with cranial angulation at 10-20 degree to profile the septum) and transesophageal echocardiography are performed to evaluate the size and location of the defect. Mechanical circulatory support may also be indicated to support the patient to improve survival before and after VSD occlusion.

CLINICAL APPLICATIONS: DEVICE CLOSURE OF VSDs

The only device FDA approved for postinfarction VSD closure is the Amplatzer Post Infarct VSD Occluder that is able to close defects 16 to 24 mm in diameter. The device chosen should be 2 to 4 mm larger than the measured VSD size to improve closure rates.[38] Transcatheter VSD closure is undertaken typically from the right internal jugular vein and retrograde from the femoral artery. An angled catheter is advanced retrograde across the aortic valve to the region of the VSD. A soft-tipped wire is advanced "left to right" across the VSD into the right ventricle (RV) and then up into the pulmonary artery. A catheter is advanced from the right internal jugular vein to the pulmonary artery, and using a snare, the soft tip of the wire is snared and brought back through the right heart and exteriorized outside the right internal jugular vein sheath. This creates a right internal jugular-VSD-femoral artery *rail*, and the right internal jugular short sheath is exchanged for a long delivery sheath, which is advanced over the wire, through the VSD to the left ventricle. An appropriately sized VSD occluder is chosen and advanced through the long sheath; the left ventricular disc is extruded, the sheath is pulled back to the septum, the waist is extruded into the defect, and the right ventricular disc is extruded against the interventricular septum. Stability is tested while residual shunt is evaluated by transesophageal echocardiography.[38]

LIMITATIONS/SPECIAL CONSIDERATIONS: DEVICE CLOSURE OF VSDs

The VSDs postinfarction can range from small to large and may have little rim anteriorly or posteriorly, which is unable to support the device. The residual significant (>moderate) shunt rate is 30%. Technical success occurs in 89% to 95% of patients, but the mortality is still 44% to 60% at 1 year despite technical successful closure.[39,40]

Infective bacterial endocarditis prophylaxis is required post-VSD closure and as long as there is any residual shunting. Device embolization can occur if septal infarction extends over time. The VSD edges should be fibrosed by 6 weeks.

FOLLOW-UP PATIENT CARE: DEVICE CLOSURE OF VENTRICULAR SEPTAL DEFECT

Follow-up depends on patient stability postclosure. Patients surviving hospital discharge should be followed at 1, 3, and 6 months and yearly thereafter. The device stability and residual shunt should be evaluated by echocardiography at each visit.

RESEARCH AND FUTURE CONSIDERATIONS

The ability to close perimembranous defects may one day be a reality if devices can be created that safely close these defects without causing aortic valve distortion or injury to the conduction system.

CLINICAL PEARLS: DEVICE CLOSURE OF VENTRICULAR SEPTAL DEFECTS

- Postinfarction VSD closure is indicated in patients with heart failure, left ventricular dysfunction, and need for mechanical circulatory support who are not surgical candidates.
- Transcatheter closure of postinfarction VSD should be delayed at least 3 to 4 weeks to allow for tissue fibrosis.
- The Amplatzer Post Infarct VSD Occluder is the only FDA-approved device for this condition.
- Technical success is greater than 90%, but 1-year mortality is high (40%-60%).

FONTAN—SINGLE VENTRICLE INTERVENTIONS

INTRODUCTION

Patients born with single ventricle anatomy undergo a three-staged palliation with the final procedure called the Fontan. The superior vena cava is anastomosed to the pulmonary artery (Glenn shunt) and the inferior vena cava, and hepatic venous blood flow is connected to the pulmonary arteries using a conduit (see Section "Anatomic considerations"). Post-Fontan palliation, patients are followed closely for development of cyanosis with or without exertion, arrhythmias, signs and symptoms of single ventricular dysfunction, and other organ system failure (ie, liver and kidney).

INDICATIONS: FONTAN—SINGLE VENTRICLE INTERVENTIONS

Cardiac catheterization is indicated for Fontan patients presenting with cyanosis, worsening heart failure symptoms, and in asymptomatic patients with noninvasive imaging evidence of Fontan pathway, branch pulmonary artery, and/or aortic arch obstruction. Routine screening cardiac catheterization is being recommended at least every 10 years to evaluate the Fontan pathway.[41,42] Other specific indications are protein-losing enteropathy and plastic bronchitis, Fontan fenestration test occlusion and closure for cyanosis, echocardiographic evidence of diastolic dysfunction, new-onset or worsening arrhythmias, presence or worsening of significant Fontan-associated liver disease (FALD), and other organ systems.

ANATOMIC CONSIDERATIONS: FONTAN—SINGLE VENTRICLE INTERVENTIONS

A patient's specific anatomy, including the surgical operative notes, should be thoroughly studied before proceeding to the catheterization laboratory. The majority of adult patients will have a fenestrated or nonfenestrated extracardiac conduit Fontan or lateral tunnel Fontan. However, older patients may have a classic Fontan (right atrium to the main pulmonary artery) or one of its variations. Other anatomical considerations include patient's femoral vessel and internal jugular vein access issues and the presence of interrupted inferior vena cava with connection to superior vena cava via azygous systems.

CLINICAL APPLICATIONS: FONTAN—SINGLE VENTRICLE INTERVENTIONS

A detailed right (Fontan pathway) and left heart cardiac catheterization should be performed to evaluate the pulmonary and systemic cardiac output (Qp and Qs, respectively). Angiograms are performed to carefully evaluate for anatomical obstructions, systemic-to-pulmonary vein collaterals, and systemic arterial to pulmonary collaterals (commonly referred to

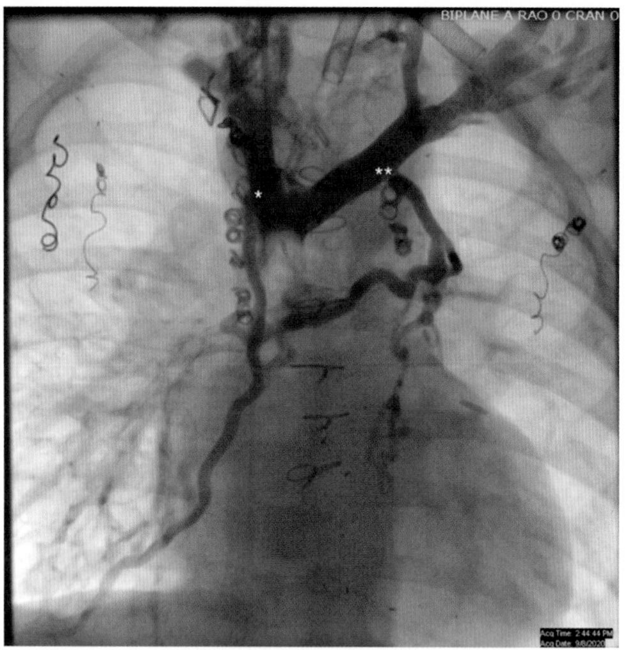

FIGURE 45.8 Balloon occlusion right superior vena cava (SVC) angiogram with a Reverse Berman angiographic catheter showing venous decompression vessels from the right SVC (*) and distal left innominate vein (**) draining caudally to the pulmonary veins acting as a right-to-left shunt.

as aortopulmonary collaterals) (**Figure 45.8, e-Figures 45.6 and 45.7**).

A comprehensive hemodynamic and angiographic evaluation should be performed to uncover areas of obstruction in the Fontan pathway, associated decompressing systemic-to-pulmonary vein channels, pulmonary arteriovenous malformations (from inadequate hepatic flow), or systemic-to-pulmonary artery collaterals. Pressure gradients greater than 1 to 2 mm Hg are hemodynamically significant in the passively flowing Fontan pathway. Measuring hepatic vein and hepatic vein wedge pressures to assess the hepatic vein-wedge gradient and liver health is customary. In patients with a patent Fontan fenestration and cyanosis or post stroke, test occlusion of and transcatheter closure of the fenestration can be considered. For stenosed systemic veins and venous connections, balloon-expandable and self-expanding stents have been used to relieve stenosis and recanalize veins.

In patients presenting with protein-losing enteropathy and plastic bronchitis, the traditional approach has been to evaluate and treat any Fontan pathway obstruction and consider creating a Fontan fenestration in patients with elevated Fontan pressures. More recently, lymphatic/thoracic duct embolization has been investigated as a treatment for failing Fontan patients with recurrent chylous effusions, plastic bronchitis, and protein-losing enteropathy.[43,44] Detailed assessment of the single ventricle systemic circulation/pathway includes evaluation of diastolic function at baseline and unmasking subclinical diastolic dysfunction with volume challenge, evaluation of recurrent aortic arch obstruction, and evaluation and closure of aortic-pulmonary artery collaterals. In some patients, especially those with heterotaxy/isomerism, careful assessment of the venous pathways should be undertaken to identify the presence of portosystemic shunts.

LIMITATIONS/SPECIAL CONSIDERATIONS: FONTAN—SINGLE VENTRICLE INTERVENTIONS

Vascular access is a concern as most of these patients have had numerous catheterizations as a child. Access from the internal jugular veins, arm vessels, or transhepatic puncture may be needed.

Bronchoscopy and 3D imaging with MRI or CT are useful in assessing Fontan anatomy, especially left pulmonary artery and/or bronchial compression by a dilated aorta. Hemoptysis presents a unique challenge and bronchoscopy may help identify the location of bleeding. In patients presenting with recurrent chylous effusions, left innominate vein patency is evaluated and if found to be stenotic, balloon and stent angioplasty should be considered to help open the egress pathway for the thoracic duct. In patients with unilateral intrapulmonary arteriovenous malformations caused by the absence of intrinsic/hepatic factor flow to that lung, surgical or transcatheter redirection of the hepatic blood flow is considered.[45]

FOLLOW-UP PATIENT CARE: FONTAN—SINGLE VENTRICLE INTERVENTIONS

Follow-up patient care for Fontan interventions is determined by the type of intervention and the type of device needed. Embolization of collaterals can be evaluated as part of the routine yearly follow-up. Device closure of fenestrations and stenting of pathways and pulmonary arteries often require closer follow-up at 1, 6, and 12 months to evaluate for any residual shunt or hemodynamically significant narrowing. Intervention for protein-losing enteropathy, effusions, or plastic bronchitis requires much closer follow-up, especially in patients with various degrees of heart failure.

RESEARCH AND FUTURE CONSIDERATIONS

Further research is needed to evaluate the optimal timing, patient candidacy, and type of lymphatic intervention. Lymphatic intervention for patients with protein-losing enteropathy is currently being investigated.

CLINICAL PEARLS: FONTAN—SINGLE VENTRICLE INTERVENTIONS

- New or worsening cyanosis, heart failure, or pathway obstruction post Fontan is important to investigate.
- Right- and left-sided Fontan obstruction can often be treated with stenting.
- T2-weighted magnetic resonance (MR) lymphangiography and dynamic contrast MR lymphangiography delineate lymphatic pathway/s prior to lymphatic intervention.
- Innominate vein patency is important for thoracic duct egress.
- Bronchoscopy can help evaluate for bronchial and left pulmonary artery compression from a dilated aorta and can help localize sites of hemoptysis.

REFERENCES

1. Hill GD, Ginde S, Rios R, et al. Surgical valvotomy versus balloon valvuloplasty for congenital aortic valve stenosis: a systematic review and meta-analysis. *J Am Heart Assoc.* 2016;5:e003931.
2. Atik SU, Eroglu AG, Cinar B, et al. Comparison of balloon dilatation and surgical valvuloplasty in non-critical congenital aortic valve stenosis at long-term follow-up. *Pediatr Cardiol.* 2018;39:1554-1560.
3. Devanagondi R, Peck D, Sagi J, et al. Long-term outcomes of balloon valvuloplasty for isolated pulmonary valve stenosis. *Pediatr Cardiol.* 2017;38:247-254.
4. Feltes TF, Bacha E, Beekman RH, et al. Indications for cardiac catheterization and intervention in pediatric cardiac disease: a scientific statement from the american heart association. *Circulation.* 2011;123:2607-2652.
5. Masakatia SA, Justino H, Ing FF, et al. Aortic valve morphology is associated with outcomes following balloon valvuloplasty for congenital aortic stenosis. *Catheter Cadiovasc Interv.* 2013;81:90-95.
6. Petit CJ, Gao K, Goldstein BH, et al. Relation of aortic valve morphologic characteristics to aortic valve insufficiency and residual stenosis in children with congenital aortic stenosis undergoing balloon valvuloplasty. *Am J Cardiol.* 2016;117:972-979.
7. Torres A, Vincent JA, Everett A, et al. Balloon valvuloplasty for congenital aortic stenosis: multi-center safety and efficacy outcome assessment. *Catheter Cardiovasc Interv.* 2015;86:808-820.
8. Bergersen L, Gauvreau K, Justino H, et al. Randomized trial of cutting balloon compared with high-pressure angioplasty for the treatment of resistant pulmonary artery stenosis. *Circulation.* 2011;124:2388-2396.
9. Ing FF, Khan A, Kobayashi D, et al. Pulmonary artery stents in the recent era: immediate and intermediate follow-up. *Catheter Cardiovasc Interv.* 2014;84:1123-1130.
10. Law MA, Shamszad P, Nugent AW, et al. Pulmonary artery stents: long-term Follow-up. *Catheter Cardiovasc Interv.* 2010;75(5):757-764.
11. Morray BH, McElhinney DB, Marshall AC, et al. Intentional fracture of maximally dilated balloon-expandable pulmonary artery stents using ultra-high-pressure balloon angioplasty: a preliminary analysis. *Circ Cardiovasc Interv.* 2016;9:e003281.
12. Agrawal H, Qureshi AH, Justino H. Intentional longitudinal and side-cell stent fractures: intermediate term follow up. *Catheter Cardiovasc Interv.* 2018;91(6):1110-1118.
13. Holzer RJ, Gauvreau K, Kreutzer J, et al. Balloon angioplasty and stenting of branch pulmonary arteries—adverse events and procedural characteristics: results of a mulit-institutional registry. *Circ Cardiovasc Interv.* 2011;4:287-296.
14. Shinkawa T, Chipman C, Bozzay T, et al. Outcome of right ventricle to pulmonary artery conduit for biventricular repair. *Ann Thorac Surg.* 2015;99(4):1357-1366.
15. Aggarwal S, Garekar S, Forbes TJ, et al. Is stent placement effective for palliation of right ventricle to pulmonary artery conduit stenosis? *J Am Coll Cardiol.* 2007;49:480-484.
16. McElhinney DB, Hellenbrand WE, Zahn EM, et al. Short-and medium-term outcomes after transcatheter pulmonary valve placement in the expanded multicenter US melody valve trial. *Circulation.* 2010;122(5):507-516.
17. Ran L, Wang W, Secchi F, et al. Percutaneous pulmonary valve implantation in patients with right ventricular outflow tract dysfunction: a systematic review and meta-analysis. Ther Adv Chronic Dis. 2019;10:2040622319857635.
18. Chung R, Taylor AM. Imaging for preintervention planning: transcatheter pulmonary valve therapy. *Circ Cardiovasc Imaging.* 2014;7:182-189.
19. Morray BH, McElhinney DB, Cheatham JP, et al. Risk of coronary artery compression among patients referred for transcatheter pulmonary valve implantation: a multicenter experience. Circ Cardiovasc Interv. 2013;6(5):535-542.
20. Delaney JW, Goldstein BH, Bishnoi RN, et al. Covered CP stent for treatment of right ventricular conduit injury during Melody transcatheter pulmonary valve replacement. *Circ Cardiovasc Interv.* 2018;11(10):e006598.
21. Gewillig M, Brown S. Coronary compression caused by stenting a right pulmonary artery conduit. *Catheter Cardiovasc Interv.* 2009;74(1);144-147.
22. Alkashkari W, Albugami S, Hijazi ZM. Management of coarctation of the aorta in adult patients. *Korean Circ J.* 2019;49(4):298-313.
23. Batlivala SP, Goldstein BH. Current transcatheter approaches for the treatment of aortic coarctation in children and adults. *Interv Cardiol Clin.* 2019;8(1):47-58.
24. Taggart NW, Minahan M, Cabalka AK, et al. Immediate outcomes of covered stent placement for treatment or prevention of aortic wall injury associated with coarctation of the aorta (COAST II). *JACC Cardiovasc Interv.* 2016;9(5):484-493.
25. Meadows J, Minahan M, McElhinney DB, et al. Intermediate outcomes in the prospective, multicenter Coarctation of the Aorta Stent Trial (COAST). *Circulation.* 2015;131(19):1656-1664.
26. Forbes TJ, Kim DW, Du W, et al. Comparison of surgical, stent, and balloon angioplasty treatment of native coarctation of the aorta: an observational study by the CCISC (Congenital Cardiovascular Interventional Study Consortium). *J Am Coll Cardiol.* 2011;58(25):2664-2674.
27. Holzer R, Qureshi S, Ghasemi A, et al. Stenting of aortic coarctation: acute, intermediate, and long-term results of a prospective multi-institutional registry—Congenital Cardiovascular Interventional Study Consortium (CCISC). *Catheter Cardiovasc Interv.* 2010;76(4):553-563.
28. van der Burg JJ, Warmerdam EG, Krings GJ, et al. Effect of stent implantation on blood pressure control in adults with coarctation of the aorta. *Cardiovasc Revasc Med.* 2018;19(8):944-950.
29. Warnes CA, Liberthson R, Danielson GK, et al. Task force 1: the changing profile of congenital heart disease in adult life. *J Am Coll Cardiol.* 2001;37:1170-1175.
30. Krichenko A, Benson LN, Burrows P, et al. Angiographic classification of the isolated, persistently patent ductus arteriosus and implications for percutaneous catheter occlusion. *Am J Cardiol.* 1989;63(12):877-880.
31. Cambier PA, Kirby WC, Wortham DC, et al. Percutaneous closure of the small (less than 2.5 mm) patent ductus arteriosus using coil embolization. *Am J Cardiol.* 1992;69:815-816.
32. Moore JW, Greene J, Palomares S, et al. Results of the combined US Multicenter pivotal study and the continuing access study of the NitOccluld PDA device for percutaneous closure of patent ductus arteriosus. *JACC Cardiovasc Interv.* 2014;7:1430-1436.
33. Pass RH, Hijazi ZM, Hsu DT, et al. Multicenter USA Amplatzer patent ductus arteriosus occlusion device trial. Initial and one-year results. *J Am Coll Cardiol.* 2004;44:513-519.
34. VanLoozen D, Sandoval JP, Delaney JW, et al. Use of the Amplatzer vascular plugs and Amplatzer duct occluder II additional sizes for occlusion of patent ductus arteriosus: a multiinstitutional study. *Catheter Cardiovasc Interv.* 2018;92:1323-1328.

35. Gruenstein DH, Ebeid M, Radtke W, et al. Transcatheter closure of patent ductus arteriosus using the AMPLATZER duct occlude II (ADO II). *Catheter Cardiovasc Interv.* 2017;89:1118-1128.
36. Alkashkari W, Albugami S, Alrahimi J, et al. Percutaneous device closure of patent ductus arteriosus in adult patients with 10-year follow up. *Heart Views.* 2019;20(4):139-145.
37. Behjati-Ardakani M, Rafiel M, Behjati-Ardakani MA, et al. Long-term results of transcatheter closure of patent ductus arteriosus in adolescents and adults with Amplatzer duct occluder. *N Am J Med Sci.* 2015;7(5):208-211.
38. Schlotter F, de Waha S, Eitel I, et al. Interventional post-myocardial infarction ventricular septal defect closure: a systematic review of current evidence. *EuroIntervention.* 2016;12:94-102.
39. Sathananthan J, Ruygrok P. Evolution in the management of postinfarct ventricular septal defects from surgical to percutaneous approach: a single-center experience. *J Invasive Cardiol.* 2013;25(7):339-343.
40. Holzer R, Balzer D, Amin Z, et al. Transcatheter closure of postinfarction ventricular septal defects using the new Amplatzer muscular VSD occluder: results of a U.S. Registry. *Catheter Cardiovasc Interv.* 2004;61:196-201.
41. Rychik J, Atz AM, Celermajer DS, et al. Evaluation and management of the child and adult with Fontan circulation: a scientific statement from the American Heart Association. *Circulation.* 2019;140:e234-e284.
42. Stout KK, Daniels CJ, Aboulhosn JA, et al. 2018 AHA/ACC Guideline for the management of adults with congenital heart disease: a report of the American College of Cardiology/American Heart Association Task Force on Clinical Practice Guidelines. *J Am Coll Cardiol.* 2019;73(12):1494-1563.
43. Savla JJ, Itkin M, Rossano JW, et al. Post-operative chylothorax in patients with congenital heart disease. *J Am Coll Cardiol.* 2017;69:2410-2422.
44. Dori Y, Keller MS, Rome JJ, et al. Percutaneous lymphatic embolization of abnormal pulmonary lymphatic flow as treatment of plastic bronchitis in patients with congenital heart disease. *Circulation.* 2016;133(12):1160-1170.
45. Dori Y, Sathanandam S, Glatz AC, et al. Catheter approach to redirect hepatic venous return for treatment of unilateral pulmonary arteriovenous malformations after Fontan. *Catheter Cardiovasc Interv.* 2014;84(1):86-93.

CHAPTER 46

PERCUTANEOUS CLOSURE OF PATENT FORAMEN OVALE AND ATRIAL SEPTAL DEFECT

Ricardo Cigarroa and Ignacio Inglessis

PATENT FORAMEN OVALE CLOSURE

INTRODUCTION

Patent foramen ovale (PFO) is the most common intracardiac shunt encountered in clinical practice. The foramen ovale is an essential component of the fetal circulation, allowing highly oxygenated placental blood to flow directly from the right to left atrium, bypassing the fetal lungs and directly supplying the coronary arteries and fetal brain. A communication between septum secundum and septum primum, the foramen ovale typically closes in most individuals in the first year of life following hemodynamic changes that increase left atrial (LA) pressure and decrease right atrial (RA) pressure. The LA pressure rise is the result of an increase in systemic vascular resistance after interruption of the umbilical cord and rising pulmonary venous return to the LA after lung expansion. In addition, RA pressure falls as a result of reducing blood return to the RA after ductus venosus closure and decreasing pulmonary vascular resistance after lung expansion. The competent valve of the foramen ovale is then pressed to the interatrial limbus, and functional closure of the foramen ovale, without left-to-right interatrial shunt, occurs as a result of LA pressure in excess of RA pressure.

The foramen ovale remains patent in about one-third of the population for unknown reasons, although there is evidence to suggest a genetic predisposition.[1] The prevalence of PFO appears to decrease with age, whereas older age is associated with larger PFOs.[2] The majority of individuals with a PFO will remain asymptomatic, but a small percentage develop clinically significant pathology from this communication and benefit from percutaneous closure.

DIAGNOSIS

Echocardiography

Echocardiography is the primary modality for diagnosing PFO. Although doppler assessment of the interatrial septum may reveal flow across a PFO (**Figure 46.1A**), bubble studies are often needed to document communication between the two atria and obtain preliminary data on PFO size based on the timing and number of bubbles that appear in the left atrium (**Figure 46.1B**). A bubble study is performed by injecting agitated saline through a peripheral IV while visualizing both atria, often in the apical four chamber view on transesophageal echocardiography (TTE). Images should be captured at both rest and with provocative maneuvers, such as Valsalva or cough,

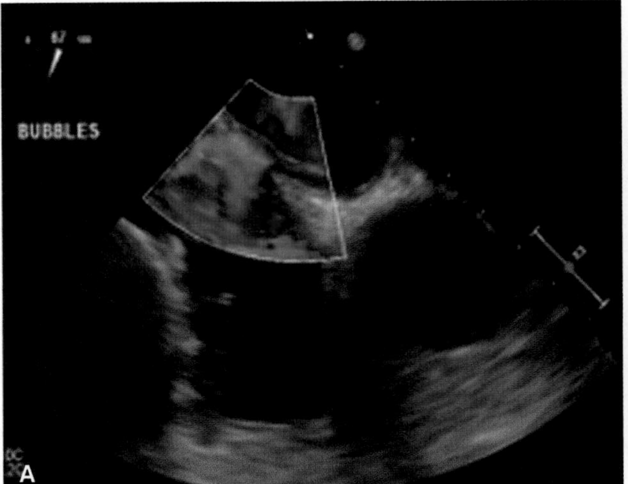

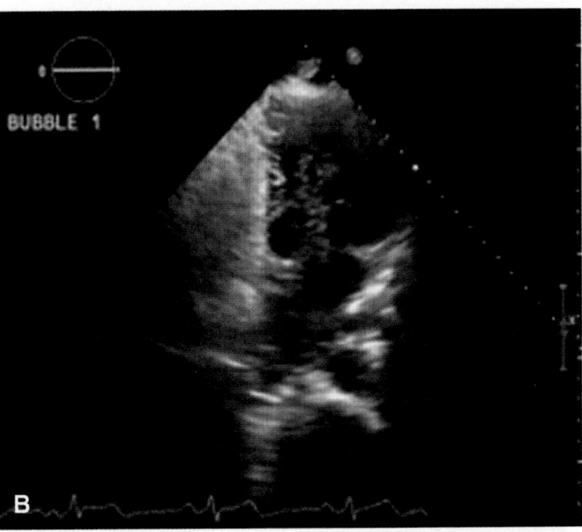

FIGURE 46.1 **(A)** Transesophageal echocardiographic imaging of patent foramen ovale. **(B)** Transthoracic echocardiography with positive agitated saline/bubble study.

which increase the pressure in the right atrium and more forcefully eject bubbles through a shunt if present. Indicators of a high-quality bubble study include complete opacification of the right atrium and atrial septal shift to the left after release of Valsalva maneuver.[3]

The most inclusive criteria for a "positive" bubble study include bubbles appearing in the LA within 5 to 7 cardiac cycles following Valsalva release, with earlier appearance (<3 beats) more strongly favoring PFO and later appearance (after 5-7 beats) suggesting extracardiac shunt, such as pulmonary arterial-venous malformation.[3-5] TEE can diagnose PFO by both doppler ultrasound and bubble study, but is often unnecessary with a well-performed TTE.[4] Although TTE shows the presence of bubbles in the LA, TEE (**Figure 46.2**) and intracardiac echo (ICE) can also directly visualize the atrial septal flap, and thus may be more sensitive than TTE for the detection of PFO.[4,6] However, if the PFO is not easily visualized, TEE diagnosis may be hindered by requiring sedation, which both decreases RA pressure and impairs the ability to perform provocative testing.

Transcranial doppler (TCD) is another noninvasive method useful in the initial screening for PFO. TCD measures cerebral blood flow and can identify microbubbles passing through intracranial arteries for the detection of right to left shunt. A recent study by Maffe et al.,[7] using TEE as the gold standard, found that both TTE and TCD showed high sensitivity for PFO detection, whereas TTE showed improved specificity when using the appearance of bubbles in the left atrium within 3 cardiac cycles as cutoff for PFO detection (**Table 46.1**).

Anatomic Characteristics as Prognostic Indicator and Device Selection

Information about the size and anatomic characteristics of PFO determined by echocardiography are important both prognostically—as risk factors for stroke—and for proper device selection and sizing. The number of bubbles that cross into the left atrium can be used as a rough estimate for PFO size, which is an important variable in determining the benefit of PFO closure. Subanalysis of the REDUCE and RESPECT trials did not find a benefit in preventing recurrent stroke with closure versus medical therapy in patients with small shunts (defined as <6 bubbles in the LA within 3 cardiac cycles) or trace to moderate shunts (<20 bubbles in the LA within 3 cardiac cycles), respectively.[8,9] Additionally, the CLOSE trial excluded patients altogether who had small to moderate shunts, defined as less than 30 bubbles in the left atrium within 3 cardiac cycles.[10] Being able to accurately quantify shunt size on TTE requires high-quality imaging, including well-performed provocative maneuvers.

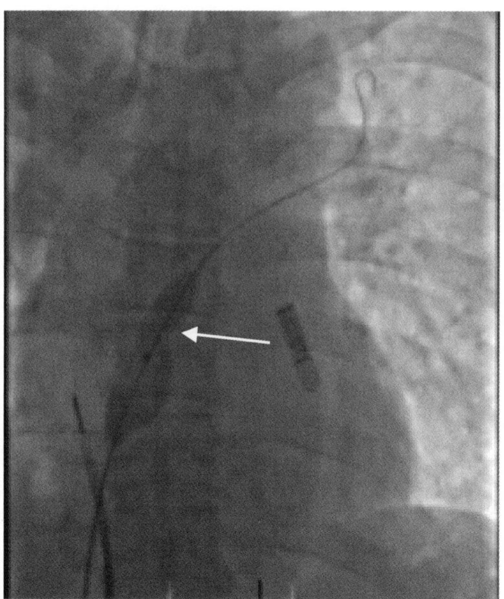

FIGURE 46.2 Balloon sizing of patent foramen ovale.

TABLE 46.1 Sensitivity and Specificity of TTE and TCD When Compared to the Gold Standard of TEE

Modality	Sensitivity (%)	Specificity (%)
TTE	89	100
TCD	85	90

TEE, transesophageal echocardiography; TCD, transcranial doppler; TTE, transesophageal echocardiography.
Adapted from Maffè S, Dellavesa P, Zenone F, et al. Transthoracic second harmonic two- and three-dimensional echocardiography for detection of patent foramen ovale. *Eur J Echocardiogr*. 2010;11(1):57-63. Reproduced by permission of Oxford University Press.

Another prognostically significant anatomic feature is the presence of an atrial septal aneurysm (ASA), which is an excursion of the septum primum of 10 mm or greater beyond the plane of the atrial septum.[1] ASAs are present in 2% to 3% of the general population, are associated with intracardiac shunts,[11-13] and have increased prevalence in patients with ischemic stroke, possibly by acting as a nidus for thrombus formation and thus a source of embolus in the setting of shunt. Furthermore, PFO with septal aneurysms are thought to be larger than those without an associated ASA, further increasing the risk for paradoxical emboli.[13-15] In the RESPECT trial, PFO closure in the setting of ASA was found to be significantly protective against recurrent stroke when compared to medical therapy (1.7% vs. 7.6%, hazard ratio [HR] 0.20, P = .005).[9] Finally, the presence of an ASA led to subject inclusion in the studies, regardless of PFO size in the CLOSE trial.[10]

INDICATIONS FOR PATENT FORAMEN OVALE CLOSURE

Cryptogenic Stroke

PFOs are implicated in the pathophysiology of cryptogenic strokes by allowing clot formed in the venous system to cross into the arterial circulation.[16,17] However, multiple early investigations failed to show definitive benefit of routine PFO closure for this indication.[18-20] A diagnosis of cryptogenic stroke may be made when there is clinical and radiologic evidence of an ischemic stroke and no cause is readily identifiable.[21,22] Important etiologies to investigate prior to making the diagnosis of cryptogenic stroke include atrial fibrillation, peripheral artery disease, endocarditis, and hypercoagulable state. Cryptogenic strokes are more common in younger patients who lack risk factors for stroke that accrue with age.[23,24]

Recently, three large randomized control trials found a significant reduction in recurrent stroke in patients who underwent transcatheter PFO closure when compared with patients who were treated with antiplatelet therapy alone after experiencing cryptogenic stroke[8-10] (**Table 46.2**). These trials enrolled patients who were unlikely to have a stroke from reasons other than paradoxical embolus by ruling out atrial fibrillation, hypercoagulable states, and carotid disease prior to closure. Furthermore, older patients and patients with uncontrolled risk factors for stroke were excluded from the studies. Important eligibility criteria included an age limit of 60 years, moderate or large PFO size, and the presence of an interatrial septal aneurysm, which has been associated with recurrent cryptogenic stroke.[11]

Decompression Sickness

Decompression sickness is a severe illness that affects individuals exposed to increased atmospheric pressures. It is most commonly encountered in scuba divers, although it also can occur during high-altitude or unpressurized air travel.[25] This condition occurs when nitrogen dissolved in the blood and tissues by high pressure forms bubbles as pressure decreases. These bubbles may cross into the arterial system through a PFO and lead to stroke. Other symptoms include musculoskeletal pain, rash, confusion, paresthesias, paralysis, and respiratory distress. Severe decompression syndrome requires expedient treatment with hyperbaric chamber therapy. Although there are no large studies to recommend routine closure in divers, one small randomized study found that subjects who underwent PFO closure had less arterial bubbles when compared to those who did not in patients exposed to similar conditions.[26] After PFO closure, patients should be counseled that they are at similar risk for decompression sickness (DCS) as those who do not have PFOs and should continue to take routine precautions.

Hypoxia

Under the proper conditions, PFO may allow for significant right to left shunting leading to clinically significant hypoxia. Platypnea-orthodeoxia syndrome is one manifestation of this and is associated with hypoxia and breathlessness in the upright position that improves when the patient is recumbent.[27] The upright position changes or stretches the conformation of the interatrial communication, increasing the proportion of blood flow from the inferior vena cava through the defect and into the LA. Other clinical scenarios in which the RA pressure is higher than the LA (ie, pulmonary hypertension, Ebstein anomaly, tricuspid stenosis) may also lead to clinically significant hypoxia when an interatrial communication is present.

FUNDAMENTALS OF PERCUTANEOUS PFO CLOSURE

Successful PFO closure requires adequate intraprocedural imaging of the PFO. Although this may be done with TEE, intracardiac echo (ICE) provides excellent views of interatrial septal anatomy and allows for the procedure to be done under conscious sedation. Accordingly, ICE is the imaging method of choice for PFO closure.

Vascular Access

Bilateral femoral venous access is obtained with 7-French venous sheaths. Through the right sheath, a multipurpose guide is used to place a 0.035-inch J-tipped wire at the inferior vena cava–RA junction. The left sheath is then upsized to a 10-French long sheath through which the ICE catheter (9-French) is advanced into the RA and positioned to visualize the PFO: this is often achieved with posterior tilt and clockwise rotation of the ICE catheter. In patients with severe obstruction of the left venous system because of May-Thurner anatomy, "double sticking" the right femoral vein provides access for both the imaging catheter and the delivery system.

Sizing the PFO

PFO sizing can be done with direct echocardiographic measurement, balloon sizing (**Figure 46.2**), or visual estimation based on echo images by an experienced operator. In determining the

TABLE 46.2 Key Findings from Recent Trials of Patent Foramen Ovale Closure Versus Medical Therapy After Stroke

	Recurrent Stroke	Procedural Complications	Atrial Fibrillation	No Residual Shunt 1 year
CLOSE[10]	0% vs. 6% (HR 0.03-0.26, $P < .001$)	5.9%	4.6% vs. 0.9%, $P = .02$	93%
REDUCE[8]	1.4% vs. 5.4% (HR 0.23, 0.09-0.62, $P = .002$)	2.5%	6.6% vs. 0.4%, $P < .001$	76%
RESPECT[9]	3.8% vs. 5.4% (HR 0.55, 0.31-0.999, $P = .046$)	5.0%	Not significantly different, $P = .36$[a]	Not available

[a]Seven episodes of atrial fibrillation were reported periprocedurally, all resolved prior to discharge. No significant difference in atrial fibrillation between groups beyond the periprocedural period.

Adapted from Saver JL, Carroll JD, Thaler DE, et al. Long-term outcomes of patent foramen ovale closure or medical therapy after stroke. *N Engl J Med.* 2017;377(11):1022-1032.

size of device to be used, important considerations are length of the PFO "tunnel" and size of interatrial septum.

Crossing the PFO

Over the 0.035 inches J-tipped wire, a 5-French multipurpose catheter is introduced into the RA. Under fluoroscopic and ICE guidance, the wire is advanced through the patent foramen ovale and positioned into the left upper pulmonary vein. If there is difficulty passing the wire through the PFO, the multipurpose catheter may be advanced ahead of the wire and with a counterclockwise rotation may pass through the PFO (**Figure 46.3**). Once the catheter is advanced over the wire into the left upper pulmonary vein, a double-exchange stiff wire, such as the Amplatz extra stiff wire, is carefully inserted into the left upper pulmonary vein. At that point, the catheter and sheath are withdrawn while leaving the wire in place. The support wire is needed to exchange the venous sheath for a long 11-French sheath in the right femoral vein if using the GORE® Cardioform device, whereas the Amplatzer™ PFO Occluder delivery system is introduced directly through the venotomy.

Device Insertion

There are currently two Food and Drug Administration (FDA)–approved devices for PFO closure: the GORE® Cardioform Septal Occluder and the Amplatzer™ PFO Occluder.

GORE® Cardioform Septal Occluder

The GORE® Cardioform Septal Occluder's design includes two self-expanding discs formed over an expanded polytetrafluoroethylene (ePTFE)-covered nitinol frame, covered with woven fabric (**Figure 46.4**). The device sizes include 20, 25, and 30 mm, which are the disc diameters.

The GORE® Cardioform Septal Occluder device is prepackaged connected to its delivery system, fully expanded. Prior to insertion in the patient, the device is submerged under water, and a large (30 mL) saline-filled syringe is connected to the proximal side-port of the delivery catheter to flush it to remove air from the system. The operator then loads the occluder into the delivery catheter, and the system is flushed through again until no bubbles are seen exiting from the distal tip of the catheter.

The device is advanced over the wire, under fluoroscopic and echocardiographic guidance, until the tip of the sheath is in the LA. After removing the wire, the occluder device is extruded through the delivery catheter until the left disc is deployed, while carefully keeping the device from advancing further into the LA. Once the left disc is fully deployed, the delivery system is retracted until the left disc makes contact with the interatrial septum. At that point, the right disc is deployed. Once both discs are fully deployed and the position appears satisfactory on imaging, the occluder device is detached from the delivery device.

Amplatzer™ PFO Occluder

The Amplatzer™ PFO Occluder is designed with two discs made of an external nitinol wire frame encasing a polyester fabric thread (**Figure 46.5**). The device sizes include 18, 25, and 35 mm. The larger devices are designed with asymmetric discs, with the smaller disc residing in the left atrium and the larger disc in the right atrium, while the 18-mm device has two discs of equal size.

The Amplatzer™ PFO Occluder is delivered through an 8-French (18- and 25-mm device) or 9-French (35-mm device) TorqVue sheath. The PFO Occluder is attached to its delivery cable via clockwise rotating motion. Once securely attached, the occluder device is withdrawn into the delivery sheath while submerged in water, and the system is flushed with saline to remove air.

The delivery sheath is then advanced over a supportive wire and dilator until it crosses the PFO. The wire and dilator

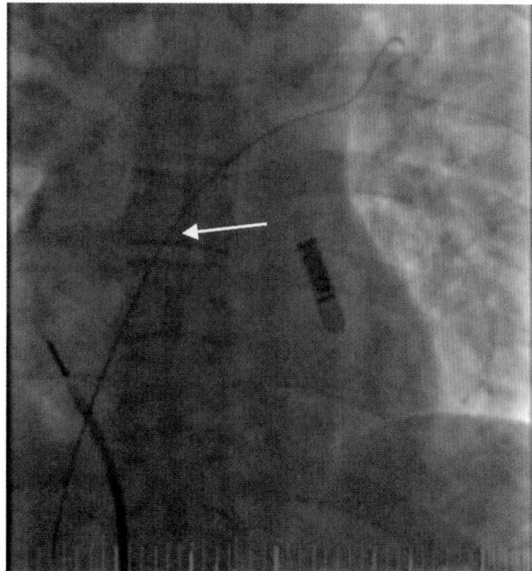

FIGURE 46.3 Patent foramen ovale (PFO) crossed with wire. Arrow shows guidewire across the PFO.

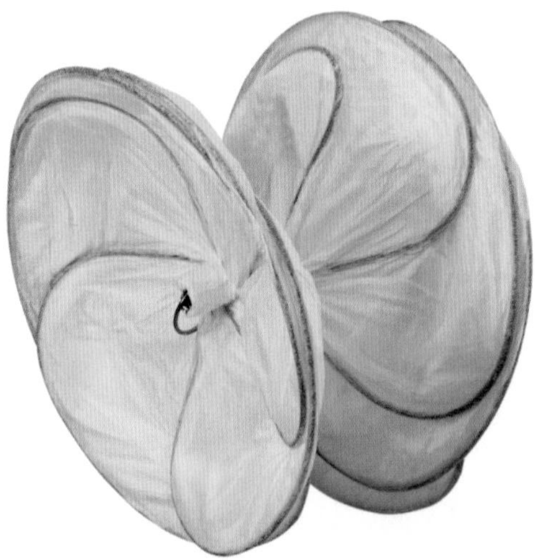

FIGURE 46.4 GORE® Cardioform Septal Occluder. The GORE® Cardioform Septal Occluder's design includes two self-expanding discs formed over an expanded polytetrafluoroethylene (ePTFE)-covered nitinol frame, covered with woven fabric. The device sizes include 20, 25, and 30 mm. (Courtesy of W. L. Gore & Associates, Inc.)

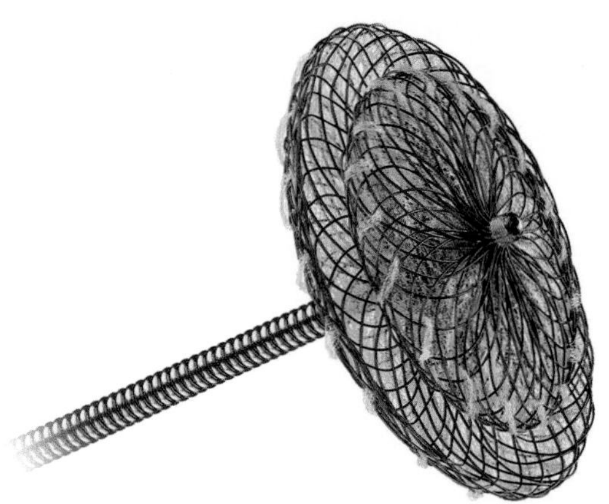

FIGURE 46.5 The Amplatzer™ PFO Occluder is designed with two discs made of an external nitinol wire frame encasing a polyester fabric thread. The device sizes include 18, 25, and 35 mm. (Amplatzer is a trademark of Abbott or its related companies. Reproduced with permission of Abbott, © 2021. All rights reserved.)

are removed, and the LA disc is unsheathed from the catheter and positioned adjacent to the atrial septum. Once adjacent to the septum, the RA disc is then unsheathed. Device position and function is evaluated on fluoroscopy and echocardiography. If the position is satisfactory, the occluder is released by a counterclockwise rotation of the delivery cable.

LIMITATIONS AND ANATOMICAL CHALLENGES

In patients who have very long tunnels (defined as ≥12 mm), tunnel length and angle of passage can interfere with proper functioning of the PFO closure device because of deformity of the device, leading to incomplete closure. One strategy proposed to overcome this issue is performing transseptal puncture through the septal flap of the PFO, allowing an improved closure profile of the defect.[28,29] In experienced centers, transseptal puncture is associated with low morbidity and mortality, and the safety is further improved under TEE or ICE guidance.[30,31]

ATRIAL SEPTAL DEFECT CLOSURE

INTRODUCTION

Atrial septal defects (ASDs) are among the most common adult congenital cardiac defects, occurring in an estimated 1.6 per 1000 live births worldwide.[32] Unlike PFOs, where a normal interatrial communication in the fetus persists into adulthood, ASDs are congenital defects of the atrial septum. However, the techniques for percutaneous intervention are similar. This section will highlight the differences in workup, indication for closure, and percutaneous approach to closure for ASD when compared to PFO.

Diagnostic Modalities to Evaluate ASD

ASDs are often detected on TTE; however, TEE offers more detailed information about ASD size, tissue rim characteristics, and proximity to surrounding structures.[33,34] Magnetic resonance imaging (MRI) has emerged as a noninvasive option of evaluating ASD anatomy providing high-quality imaging of ASD anatomy and associated pathology, as well as the ability to calculate shunt fraction.[35,36] Routine diagnostic catheterization prior to ASD closure is no longer necessary, but if noninvasive modalities are inconclusive, directly measuring pulmonary artery pressure, cardiac output, shunt magnitude, as well as hemodynamic response to temporary balloon occlusion is helpful in guiding treatment. Invasive testing is even more important when ASD exists in the presence of pulmonary hypertension to rule out the pathology of Eisenmenger, as closure in this setting is associated with adverse outcomes.[37]

ANATOMIC CONSIDERATIONS: ASD

Percutaneous closure of ASD is currently only offered as an alternative to surgery for secundum ASD, the second most common cause of an atrial level shunt after PFO. Other lesions such as primum ASD, sinus venosus defects, and coronary sinus defects should be closed surgically because of the absence of suitable rim tissue for device placement and potential device interference with the conduction system and mitral/tricuspid valves.[37] A secundum ASD is a defect within the fossa ovalis, often because of defective development of the septum primum. These lesions are often well-formed and avoid neighboring structures such as superior and inferior vena cava, pulmonary veins, and coronary sinus.[34]

Percutaneous closure of isolated secundum ASDs has largely replaced surgical closure in patients with appropriate anatomy because of observational and randomized-controlled studies showing lower complication rate, shorter length of stay, and lower cost in favor of percutaneous closure versus surgical closure with similar closure success rates for both.[38-40] Large ASD size and deficient rim tissue around the defect are factors that may influence the decision to treat surgically, because ASD closure devices require adequate tissue (ie, 5 mm of tissue from ASD to the vena cavae, pulmonary veins, coronary sinus, AV valves, and aorta) to support the device while avoiding neighboring structures.[33] Hence, high-quality imaging is necessary to evaluate suitability for percutaneous closure. One study evaluating the feasibility of transcatheter closure of isolated, large ASDs (balloon stretched diameter ≥34 mm in adults) found that transcatheter closure was safe and effective in this population; however, superior and posterior rim deficiencies predicted procedural failure.[41] The risk of device erosion is rare but serious, and patients can present with pericardial effusion and tamponade years after device placement.

INDICATIONS FOR PERCUTANEOUS ASD CLOSURE

The indications for ASD closure expand on those for PFO closure by also addressing the increased hemodynamic burden that may culminate in right ventricular dysfunction. Indeed, left ventricular compliance decreases with age, leading to increased left-to-right flow.[34,42] Furthermore, patients with ASD are at risk of developing exercise intolerance, atrial arrhythmias, and paradoxical emboli.[43,44] The 2018 AHA/ACC guidelines for the management of adults with congenital heart disease recommend considering closure of ASD when (1) left-to-right shunting is large enough to cause physiologic effects, corresponding to a shunt magnitude (ratio of pulmonary to systemic blood flow) of 1.5:1 or higher; (2) if RA or right ventricular enlargement is noted on imaging; or (3) if the ASD is thought to be the cause of impaired exercise capacity. The presence of pulmonary hypertension is also an indication for ASD, as long as the systolic pulmonary artery pressure is less than 50% of systemic pressure and pulmonary vascular resistance is less than one-third of the systemic vascular resistance. The guidelines recommend against closing the ASD when pulmonary artery systolic pressure is greater than two-thirds systemic pressure or pulmonary vascular resistance is greater than two-thirds systemic resistance.[37]

CLINICAL APPLICATIONS: PERCUTANEOUS ASD CLOSURE

The technique and devices for ASD closure are similar to those for PFO closure discussed earlier. Although ICE and TTE have been found to be effective in periprocedural guidance,[37,41] the majority of cases use TEE to guide the procedures because of superior imaging of atrial anatomy and familiarity of use. TEE guidance, however, requires general sedation. Balloon sizing is more commonly used in ASD closure than PFO closure, and data suggest avoiding device oversize greater than 2 mm beyond stretched atrial defect size to decrease the risk of device erosion.[45]

The GORE® Cardioform Septal Occluder is approved for closure of ASDs up to 17 mm in diameter, whereas the GORE® Cardioform ASD Occluder (**Figure 46.6A**) was recently approved for closure of ASDs up to 35 mm in diameter. The Amplatzer™ ASD device (**Figure 46.6B**) has been FDA-approved since the early 2000s for ASDs up to 38 mm in diameter, whereas the Amplatzer™ Cribriform Multifenestrated Septal Occluder (**Figure 46.6C**), which has a narrower waist, is FDA-approved for the closure of fenestrated ASDs.

FOLLOW-UP PATIENT CARE FOR PFO/ASD CLOSURE

After PFO/ASD closure, follow-up TTE is performed at 1 day, 1 month, 6 months, and 1 year postprocedure, and then yearly to evaluate device position and function. Dual-antiplatelet therapy is prescribed for 3 to 6 months, then aspirin 81 mg daily indefinitely. Antibiotic prophylaxis for dental procedures is recommended only for the first 6 months postprocedure. Careful observation and clinical suspicion are warranted to detect the development of atrial fibrillation, which occurs in 4% to 6% of patients in clinical trials within 6 weeks of the procedure, and usually resolves around 6 months postprocedure.[8,10]

LIMITATIONS AND CONTRAINDICATIONS: PFO/ASD CLOSURE

Although both PFO and ASD closure are low-risk outpatient procedures, there are short- and long-term risks that patients should be counseled about. Atrial arrhythmias, such as atrial fibrillation, have been observed in 4% to 6% of patients shortly after PFO and ASD closure. Device erosion years after placement is a rare but serious complication of ASD closure. It occurs most commonly in patients with a deficient aortic and/or superior rim or otherwise oversized device. Accordingly, closure devices should not be oversized, greater than 2 mm, beyond the stretched atrial defect diameter obtained by balloon sizing.[45,46] Device embolization, aortic erosion, pericardial effusion with tamponade, device thrombus, stroke, and endocarditis are rare complications.

Contraindications for PFO/ASD closure include (1) intracardiac masses such as vegetations, thrombus, or tumor near the PFO/ASD; (2) access site issues, including inadequate vessels to accommodate large diameter sheaths; and (3) documented thrombus along the venous pathway to the RA.

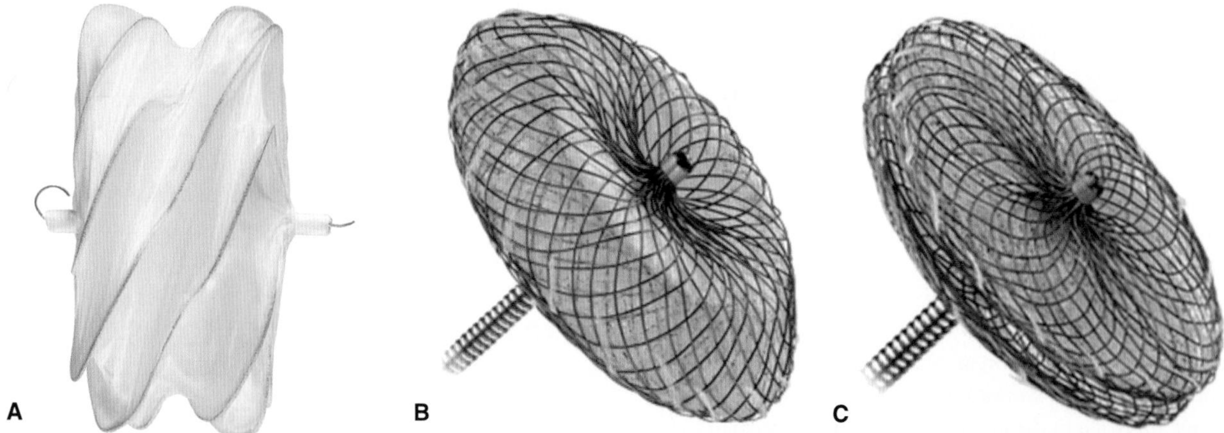

FIGURE 46.6 **(A)** GORE® Cardioform ASD Occluder. **(B)** Amplatzer™ ASD device. **(C)** Amplatzer™ Cribriform Multifenestrated Septal Occluder. (Courtesy of W. L. Gore & Associates, Inc.; Amplatzer is a trademark of Abbott or its related companies. Reproduced with permission of Abbott, © 2021. All rights reserved.)

RESEARCH AND FUTURE DIRECTIONS

In addition to cryptogenic stroke, migraines have been associated with the presence of PFO.[47,48] Observational studies have suggested that PFO closure may have an effect on migraine burden.[49,50] However, no study has shown that PFO closure significantly reduces migraine burden.[51] The GORE® Cardioform Septal Occluder Migraine Clinical Study (ClinicalTrials.gov NCT04100135) will randomize patients with at least one migraine headache a week to PFO closure versus a sham procedure, and both arms will be treated with either clopidogrel or prasugrel for at least 6 months postprocedure, and will provide further information on the benefit of this procedure for treatment of migraines.

KEY POINTS

- ✔ Cryptogenic stroke is the most common indication for PFO closure.
- ✔ Thorough investigation for identifiable causes of stroke prior to PFO closure includes history, physical exam, electrocardiogram, 30-day event monitoring for atrial fibrillation, imaging of carotid arteries, and a hypercoagulable workup. Ideally, both neurology and cardiology should be involved in the evaluation and decision-making process.
- ✔ Patients with large PFOs or associated atrial septal aneurysms appear to benefit more from PFO closure after cryptogenic stroke than those with smaller shunt burden and no aneurysm.
- ✔ Although TEE can be used for intraprocedural guidance of PFO closure, ICE avoids the need for general sedation.
- ✔ Echocardiographic imaging after PFO device positioning is necessary to ensure good contact and stable positioning.
- ✔ Suitable tissue rim is necessary to support percutaneous ASD closure devices, thus high-quality TEE imaging is necessary in preprocedural assessment and for intraprocedural guidance.

REFERENCES

1. Arquizan C, Coste JL, Touboul P-J, Mas J-L. Is patent foramen ovale a family trait? *Stroke.* 2001;32(7):1563-1566.
2. Hagen PT, Scholz DG, Edwards WD. Incidence and size of patent foramen ovale during the first 10 decades of life: an autopsy study of 965 normal hearts. *Mayo Clinic Proc.* 1984;59(1):17-20.
3. Attaran RR, Ata I, Kudithipudi V, Foster L, Sorrell VL. Protocol for optimal detection and exclusion of a patent foramen ovale using transthoracic echocardiography with agitated saline microbubbles. *Echocardiography.* 2006;23(7):616-622.
4. Thanigaraj S, Valika A, Zajarias A, Lasala JM, Perez JE. Comparison of transthoracic versus transesophageal echocardiography for detection of right-to-left atrial shunting using agitated saline contrast. *Am J Cardiol.* 2005;96(7):1007-1010.
5. Rahmouni HW, Keane MG, Silvestry FE, et al. Failure of digital echocardiography to accurately diagnose intracardiac shunts. *Am Heart J.* 2008;155(1):161-165.
6. Di Tullio M, Sacco RL, Venketasubramanian N, Sherman D, Mohr JP, Homma S. Comparison of diagnostic techniques for the detection of a patent foramen ovale in stroke patients. *Stroke.* 1993;24(7):1020-1024.
7. Maffe S, Dellavesa P, Zenone F, et al. Transthoracic second harmonic two-and three-dimensional echocardiography for detection of patent foramen ovale. *Eur J Echocardiogr.* 2010;11:57-63. doi:10.1093/ejechocard/jep165
8. Sondergaard L, Kasner SE, Rhodes JF, et al. Patent foramen ovale closure or antiplatelet therapy for cryptogenic stroke. *N Engl J Med.* 2017;377(11):1033-1042.
9. Saver JL, Carroll JD, Thaler DE, et al. Long-term outcomes of patent foramen ovale closure or medical therapy after stroke. *N Engl J Med.* 2017;377(11):1022-1032.
10. Mas JL, Derumeaux G, Guillon B, et al. Patent foramen ovale closure or anticoagulation vs. antiplatelets after stroke. *N Engl J Med.* 2017;377(11):1011-1021.
11. Mas J-L, Arquizan C, Lamy C, et al. Recurrent cerebrovascular events associated with patent foramen ovale, atrial septal aneurysm, or both. *N Engl J Med.* 2001;345(24):1740-1746.
12. Olivares-Reyes A, Chan S, Lazar EJ, Bandlamudi K, Narla V, Ong K. Atrial septal aneurysm: a new classification in two hundred five adults. *J Am Soc Echocardiogr.* 1997;10(6):644-656.
13. Mattioli A. Atrial septal aneurysm as a cardioembolic source in adult patients with stroke and normal carotid arteries. A multicentre study. *Eur Heart J.* 2001;22(3):261-268.
14. Mugge A, Daniel WG, Angermann C, et al. Atrial septal aneurysm in adult patients. A multicenter study using transthoracic and transesophageal echocardiography. *Circulation.* 1995;91(11):2785-2792.
15. Cabanes L, Mas JL, Cohen A, et al. Atrial septal aneurysm and patent foramen ovale as risk factors for cryptogenic stroke in patients less than 55 years of age. A study using transesophageal echocardiography. *Stroke.* 1993;24(12):1865-1873.
16. Windecker S, Stortecky S, Meier B. Paradoxical embolism. *J Am Coll Cardiol.* 2014;64(4):403-415.
17. Lechat P, Mas JL, Lascault G, et al. Prevalence of patent foramen ovale in patients with stroke. *N Engl J Med.* 1988;318(18):1148-1152.
18. Carroll JD, Saver JL, Thaler DE, et al. Closure of patent foramen ovale versus medical therapy after cryptogenic stroke. *N Engl J Med.* 2013;368(12):1092-1100.
19. Meier B, Kalesan B, Mattle HP, et al. Percutaneous closure of patent foramen ovale in cryptogenic embolism. *N Engl J Med.* 2013;368(12):1083-1091.
20. Furlan AJ, Reisman M, Massaro J, et al. Closure or medical therapy for cryptogenic stroke with patent foramen ovale. *N Engl J Med.* 2012;366(11):991-999.
21. Adams HP, Bendixen BH, Kappelle LJ, et al. Classification of subtype of acute ischemic stroke. Definitions for use in a multicenter clinical trial. TOAST. Trial of Org 10172 in Acute Stroke Treatment. *Stroke.* 1993;24(1):35-41.
22. Arsava EM, Ballabio E, Benner T, et al. The Causative Classification of Stroke system: an international reliability and optimization study. *Neurology.* 2010;75(14):1277-1284.
23. Jacobs BS, Boden-Albala B, Lin IF, Sacco RL. Stroke in the young in the Northern Manhattan stroke study. *Stroke.* 2002;33(12):2789-2793.
24. White H, Boden-Albala B, Wang C, et al. Ischemic stroke subtype incidence among whites, blacks, and hispanics. *Circulation.* 2005;111(10):1327-1331.
25. Moon RE, Camporesi EM, Kisslo JA. Patent foramen ovale and decompression sickness in divers. *Lancet.* 1989;1(8637):513-514.
26. Honěk J, Šrámek M, Šefc L, et al. Effect of catheter-based patent foramen ovale closure on the occurrence of arterial bubbles in scuba divers. *JACC: Cardiovasc Interv.* 2014;7(4):403-408.
27. Cheng TO. Platypnea-orthodeoxia syndrome: etiology, differential diagnosis, and management. *Catheter Cardiovasc Interv.* 1999;47(1):64-66.
28. McMahon CJ. Use of the transseptal puncture in transcatheter closure of long tunnel-type patent foramen ovale. *Heart.* 2002;88(2):e3.
29. Thompson AJ, Hagler DJ, Taggart NW. Transseptal puncture to facilitate device closure of "long-tunnel" patent foramen ovale. *Catheter Cardiovasc Interv.* 2015;85(6):1053-1057.

30. Fagundes RL, Mantica M, De Luca L, et al. Safety of single transseptal puncture for ablation of atrial fibrillation: retrospective study from a large cohort of patients. *J Cardiovasc Electrophysiol.* 2007;18(12):1277-1281.
31. Roelke M, Smith AJ, Palacios IF. The technique and safety of transseptal left heart catheterization: the Massachusetts General Hospital experience with 1,279 procedures. *Cathet Cardiovasc Diagn.* 1994;32(4):332-339.
32. Van Der Linde D, Konings EEM, Slager MA, et al. Birth prevalence of congenital heart disease worldwide. *J Am Coll Cardiol.* 2011;58(21):2241-2247.
33. Tobis J, Shenoda M. Percutaneous treatment of patent foramen ovale and atrial septal defects. *J Am Coll Cardiol.* 2012;60(18):1722-1732.
34. Wyman W. Lai LLM, Meryl S. Cohen, Tal Geva. *Echocardiography in Pediatric and Congenital Heart Disease.* 2nd ed. John Wiley & Sons; 2015.
35. Valente AM, Sena L, Powell AJ, Del Nido PJ, Geva T. Cardiac magnetic resonance imaging evaluation of sinus venosus defects: comparison to surgical findings. *Pediatr Cardiol.* 2007;28(1):51-56.
36. Durongpisitkul K, Tang NL, Soongswang J, Laohaprasitiporn D, Nana A, Kangkagate C. Cardiac magnetic resonance imaging of atrial septal defect for transcatheter closure. *J Med Assoc Thai.* 2002;85 Suppl 2:S658-S666.
37. Stout KK, Daniels CJ, Aboulhosn JA, et al. 2018 AHA/ACC Guideline for the management of adults with congenital heart disease: executive summary: a report of the American College of Cardiology/American Heart Association Task Force on Clinical Practice Guidelines. *Circulation.* 2019;139(14):e637-e697.
38. Du Z-D, Hijazi ZM, Kleinman CS, Silverman NH, Larntz K. Comparison between transcatheter and surgical closure of secundum atrial septal defect in children and adults. *J Am Coll Cardiol.* 2002;39(11):1836-1844.
39. Jones TK, Latson LA, Zahn E, et al. Results of the U.S. multicenter pivotal study of the HELEX septal occluder for percutaneous closure of secundum atrial septal defects. *J Am Coll Cardiol.* 2007;49(22):2215-2221.
40. Losay J, Petit J, Lambert V, et al. Percutaneous closure with Amplatzer device is a safe and efficient alternative to surgery in adults with large atrial septal defects. *Am Heart J.* 2001;142(3):544-548.
41. Baruteau A-E, Petit J, Lambert V, et al. Transcatheter closure of large atrial septal defects. *Circ: Cardiovasc Interv.* 2014;7(6):837-843.
42. Engelfriet P, Meijboom F, Boersma E, Tijssen J, Mulder B. Repaired and open atrial septal defects type II in adulthood: an epidemiological study of a large European cohort. *Int J Cardiol.* 2008;126(3):379-385.
43. Saxena A, Divekar A, Soni NR. Natural history of secundum atrial septal defect revisited in the era of transcatheter closure. *Indian Heart J.* 2005;57(1):35-38.
44. Shah D, Azhar M, Oakley CM, Cleland JGF, Nihoyannopoulos P. Natural history of secundum atrial septal defect in adults after medical or surgical treatment: a historical prospective study. *Br Heart J.* 1994;71(3):224-228.
45. Amin Z, Hijazi ZM, Bass JL, Cheatham JP, Hellenbrand WE, Kleinman CS. Erosion of Amplatzer septal occluder device after closure of secundum atrial septal defects: review of registry of complications and recommendations to minimize future risk. *Catheter Cardiovasc Interv.* 2004;63(4):496-502.
46. McElhinney DB, Quartermain MD, Kenny D, Alboliras E, Amin Z. Relative risk factors for cardiac erosion following transcatheter closure of atrial septal defects. *Circulation.* 2016;133(18):1738-1746.
47. Lip PZ, Lip GY. Patent foramen ovale and migraine attacks: a systematic review. *Am J Med.* 2014;127(5):411-420.
48. Takagi H, Umemoto T. A meta-analysis of case-control studies of the association of migraine and patent foramen ovale. *J Cardiol.* 2016;67(6):493-503.
49. Wilmshurst PT, Nightingale S, Walsh KP, Morrison WL. Effect on migraine of closure of cardiac right-to-left shunts to prevent recurrence of decompression illness or stroke or for haemodynamic reasons. *Lancet.* 2000;356(9242):1648-1651.
50. Ben-Assa E, Rengifo-Moreno P, Al-Bawardy R, et al. Effect of residual interatrial shunt on migraine burden after transcatheter closure of patent foramen ovale. *JACC Cardiovasc Interv.* 2020;13(3):293-302.
51. Tobis JM, Charles A, Silberstein SD, et al. Percutaneous closure of patent foramen ovale in patients with migraine. *J Am Coll Cardiol.* 2017;70(22):2766-2774.

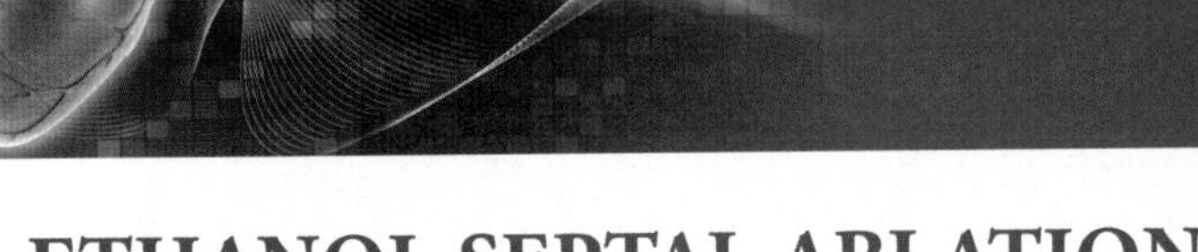

CHAPTER 47

ETHANOL SEPTAL ABLATION

Srikanth Yandrapalli, Risheek Kaul, and Srihari S. Naidu

INTRODUCTION

Hypertrophic cardiomyopathy (HCM) is the most commonly inherited cardiac disease, with estimates suggesting a prevalence approximating 1 in 500.[1,2] More recently, increased awareness and genotyping has revealed a genotypic prevalence as high as 1 in 300.[1] It has been linked to more than 1500 mutations in genes encoding sarcomeric proteins and is transmitted in an autosomal dominant pattern.[1,3] However the penetrance, phenotypic expression, and clinical manifestations are extremely diverse even in patients with the same genotypic background.[3] HCM is defined as the presence of an increase in left ventricular (LV) wall thickness (usually > 15 mm in adults or two standard deviations from normal in children) in the absence of abnormal loading conditions that could elicit a similar magnitude response.[4,5] Most patients with a positive phenotype are asymptomatic or minimally symptomatic.[2,6] Approximately 75% of patients have an obstructive cardiomyopathy that is characterized by dynamic LV outflow tract (LVOT) obstruction at rest or on provocation most typically because of apposition of a hypertrophied basal septum with the anterior leaflet of the mitral valve. The presence of this LVOT obstruction is an independent predictor of progressive heart failure and subsequent mortality.[7] Roughly 10% of patients with HCM progress to medically refractory heart failure and are candidates for septal reduction therapy with surgical myectomy or ethanol septal ablation.[4–6] In contemporary practice, the threshold for septal reduction has reduced to include lesser degrees of heart failure, those with recurrent obstruction-related lightheadedness, those who cannot tolerate optimal doses of pharmacotherapy, and those who continue to have severe systemic hypertension.[8] Favorable outcome, including a significant improvement of survival in observational experience, has further fueled interest in and performance of these procedures.

Since first performed by Cleland in 1958, surgical myectomy has been the preferred septal reduction therapy for more than 50 years, with mortality <1% in high-volume tertiary care centers.[4,5,9,10] Alcohol (ethanol) septal ablation is an alternate percutaneous catheter-based procedure that has gained increasing popularity in the last two decades owing to its less invasive nature, shorter recovery period, and similar long-term clinical outcomes. Currently, patient databases suggest that in the United States alcohol septal ablation (ASA) and surgical myectomy are roughly evenly split in terms of cumulative performance volumes, whereas those in Europe and Asia strongly favor ASA over surgical myectomy.[5,11]

ASA was first reported in 1994 by Professor Ulrich Sigwart in a case series involving 3 patients who had failed medical therapy and pacemaker insertion and were poor surgical candidates.[12] He had previously observed that balloon occlusion of the first major septal branch of the left anterior descending (LAD) coronary artery led to a temporary—yet striking—reduction in LVOT gradients in all 3 patients. Based on this evidence, he developed a protocol for permanent ablation of septal myocardial tissue using pure alcohol to create a *therapeutic myocardial infarction* with hopes of yielding a more sustained result.[12] ASA generally involves the injection of 1 to 2 mL of 98% ethanol into a proximal septal perforator branch of the LAD coronary artery to produce a myocardial infarction of the basal septum with a decrease in septal contractility (initially) and thinning (chronically). An overview of the procedure is presented in **Figure 47.1**. The combination eliminates turbulence in the outflow tract, resolves related mitral regurgitation, and over time widens the outflow tract to mirror the surgical myectomy result. More specifically, ASA causes necrosis of the hypertrophied part of the basal interventricular septum at the point of contact of the anterior mitral valve leaflet, causing an immediate reduction in septal contractility in 90% of patients and a subsequent fall in LVOT gradients.[13] Over the next 6 to 12 months, there is LV remodeling, scar retraction and regression of the hypertrophy, leading to widening of the outflow tract, reduction in mitral regurgitation and improvement in diastolic function globally.[14–16] Multiple studies have now shown that long-term survival of patients with HCM after successful ASA is comparable to the general disease-free population.[17,18] This latter point is intriguing because it would imply improvement in both heart failure and sudden cardiac arrest-related mortality, and indeed this appears to be the case for both ASA and surgical myectomy.[8]

INDICATIONS AND ANATOMIC CONSIDERATIONS

The 2011 American College of Cardiology/American Heart Association (ACC/AHA) guidelines recommend that septal reduction therapy be offered to HCM patients with severe symptoms (generally New York Heart Association [NYHA] Functional Class III or IV) that persist despite optimal medical treatment utilizing negative inotropic drugs. A Class IIa recommendation is given for surgical myectomy as the treatment of choice, with ASA recommended when surgery

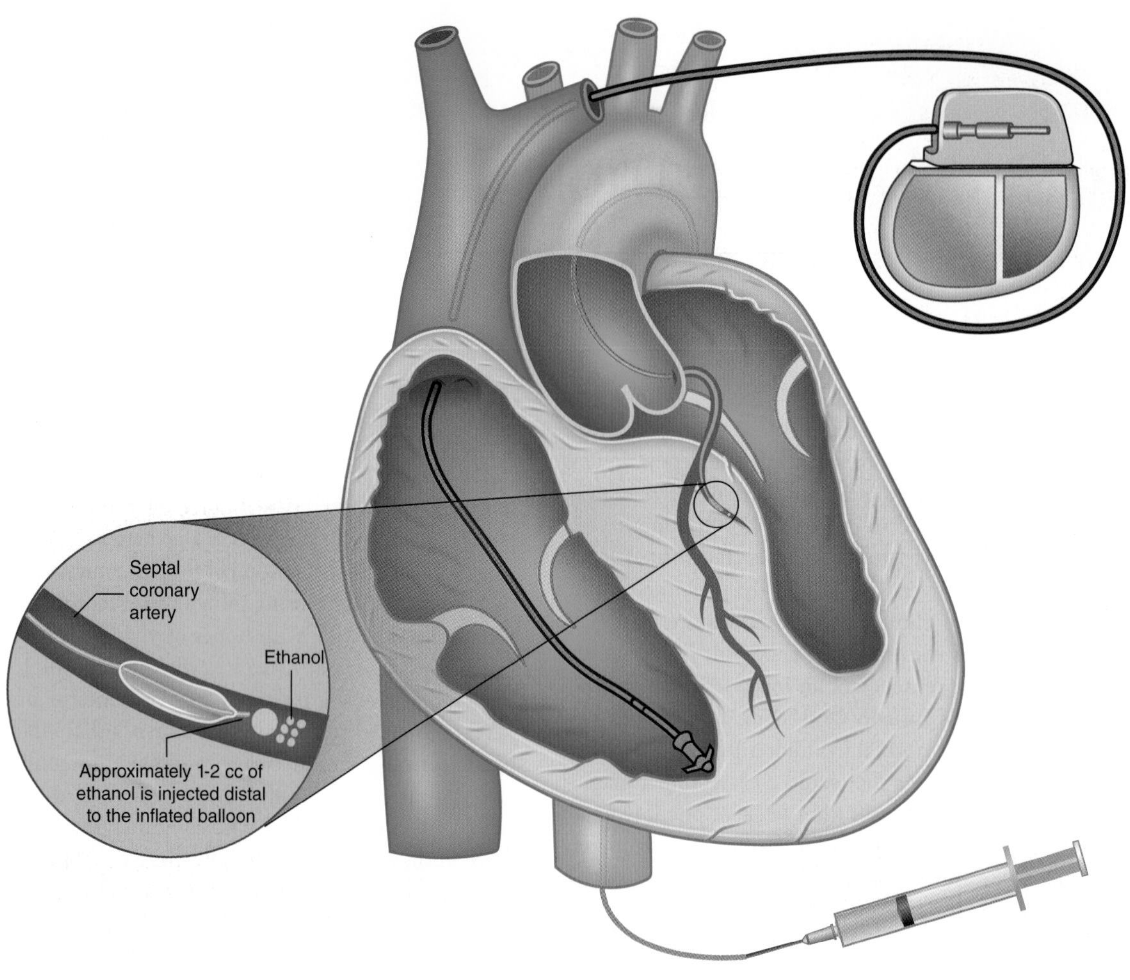
Septal
coronary
artery
Ethanol
Approximately 1-2 cc of
ethanol is injected distal
to the inflated balloon

FIGURE 47.1 Alcohol septal ablation procedure

is contraindicated (Class IIa) or considered high risk.[4] ASA is a Class IIb in patients who are candidates for both procedures. The more recent European Society of Cardiology (ESC) guidelines published in 2014, however, give septal reduction therapy a Class I indication and list both techniques as being comparable with the choice of therapy based on anatomy, clinical profile, patient and physician preference, and institutional experience.[5,19,20] These more recent guidelines are based on intervening data suggesting equipoise between the two procedures in the absence of other surgical disease. Invasive treatments should also be considered in patients with resting or provoked gradients ≥50 mm Hg and patients that experience recurrent exertional syncope despite maximally tolerated drug therapy.[4,5] As opposed to the ACC/AHA guidelines, the ESC guidelines also reduce the allowable symptoms to NYHA Class II. Septal reduction therapy should not be performed on patients who are asymptomatic with normal exercise tolerance or whose symptoms are controlled on optimal medical therapy (Class III)[4]; **Table 47.1** illustrates indications and contraindications for ASA.

Surgical myectomy is considered the gold standard therapy for LVOT obstruction reduction based on tradition and the fact that it was developed and fine-tuned decades earlier than ASA. However, no randomized controlled trial has compared the two modalities. Several observational data and single center studies have demonstrated comparable clinical efficacy in terms of functional status improvement and mortality of ASA and surgical myectomy in the long term despite an increased need for reintervention and permanent pacemaker (PPM) implantation with ASA therapy; **Tables 47.2 and 47.3**. At high-volume tertiary care centers and in large databases, mortality for surgical myectomy and ASA are both <1%, despite ASA patients typically having more comorbidities and being roughly 10 to 15 years older at the time of procedure.[19,21]

In observational experience, while surgical myectomy resulted in greater improvements in LVOT gradients than ASA,

TABLE 47.1 Indications and Contraindications for Alcohol Septal Ablation

Indications for Alcohol Septal Ablation

- Symptoms that interfere substantially with lifestyle despite optimal medical therapy (New York Heart Association [NYHA] class II, III, or IV; CCS (Canadian Cardiovascular) class 2, 3, or 4 angina or recurrent gradient-related lightheadedness or syncope).
- Resting or provoked left ventricular outflow tract gradient of >50 mm Hg.
- Adequately sized and accessible septal branches supplying the target myocardial segment.
- Absence of important intrinsic abnormality of mitral valve and of other conditions for which cardiac surgery is independently indicated.

Contraindications to Alcohol Septal Ablation

- Asymptomatic disease or minimal symptoms.
- Septal thickness <15 mm at point of systolic anterior motion (SAM) contact.
- Patients with well-controlled symptoms on optimal medical therapy.
- Children and adults aged <21 years.
- Apical and mind-cavitary phenotypes are absolute and contra-indications, respectively

clinical efficacy was similar between strategies in terms of reduction in NYHA class, syncope, and angina.[20] The difference in outcomes lies primarily in the development of conduction system abnormalities with a 2% to 3% PPM implantation rate after surgical myectomy and a 10% to 15% rate after ASA. Importantly, much of this difference is related to the age difference in the two populations, given more subclinical conduction disease in older patients and those with more comorbidities slated for ASA.[4,21] More recent data from specialized and experienced centers have confirmed the procedural safety of ASA and the rarity of previously well-documented complications with ASA like heart block, ventricular arrhythmias, and need for PPM. With the refinement of the ASA technique, including the use of myocardial contrast echocardiography guidance and decreased alcohol infusion dosages, now as low as 0.5 cc, the PPM implantation rate has improved in the current era to 7% to 10%.[4,19]

Several clinical and anatomic criteria guide the selection of either ASA or surgical myectomy for LVOT reduction and clinical improvement in HCM; **Table 47.4**. ASA is preferred in older patients (>60 years of age) with significant noncardiac comorbidities, adult patients of any age with particularly favorable coronary and septal anatomy, patients with gradients localized to the proximal basal septum, those with preexisting right bundle branch block (RBBB) or PPM/defibrillator, those who have

SECTION 3

TABLE 47.2 Study Comparison of Efficacy and Safety of Septal Ablation and Septal Myectomy

Number of Patients	Efficacy	Safety (Ablation vs Myectomy)
ASA: 41 Myectomy: 41	No difference in NYHA functional class, exercise capacity, or gradient.	Mortality: 2% vs 0% PPM implantation: 22% vs 2%
ASA: 25 Myectomy: 26	No difference in NYHA functional class.	Mortality: no difference PPM implantation: 24% vs 8%
ASA: 20 Myectomy: 24	More improvements in exercise capacity after myectomy, no difference in gradient, NYHA functional class.	Mortality: 5 vs 4% PPM implantation: 15% vs 4%
ASA: 54 Myectomy: 48	Greater improvement in symptoms in myectomy.	Mortality: 11% vs 0% PPM implantation: N/A
ASA: 123 Myectomy: 123	No difference in survival of severe symptoms.	Mortality: no difference PPM implantation: 23% vs 2%
ASA: 91 Myectomy: 40	Not reported	Higher rate of cardiac death after ablation
ASA: 161 Myectomy: 102	No difference in survival, symptoms, hospitalizations.	Mortality: no difference PPM implantation: no difference More tamponade in myectomy group.
ASA: 316 Myectomy: 250	No difference in gradient reduction but higher failure rate in ablation group.	Mortality: no difference PPM implantation: N/A More ICD discharges after ablation.
ASA: 167 Myectomy: 334	Better reductions in gradient in patients with myectomy, fewer reinterventions in myectomy group.	Mortality: no difference PPM implantation: not reported.

ASA, alcohol septal ablation; ICD, Implantable Cardioverter Defibrillator; NYHA, New York Heart Association; PPM, permanent pacemaker.

TABLE 47.3 Meta-Analyses Comparing Efficacy and Safety of Septal Ablation and Septal Myectomy

Studies	Efficacy	Safety (Ablation vs Myectomy)
12 comparative studies	No difference in NYHA functional class or gradient.	Mortality: No significant difference. PPM implantation: OR 2.57 favor myectomy.
19 ablation and 8 myectomy studies	No difference in NYHA functional class, greater improvement in gradient after myectomy.	Mortality: 2.1% vs 1.8% SCD: 0.3% vs 0.4% PPM Implantation:1 1% vs 5%
24 studies	Lower rate of re-intervention after myectomy.	Mortality: No difference PPM implantation: 10% vs 4%
40 studies	Lower rates of reintervention after myectomy.	Periprocedural Mortality: 1.2% vs 2& Long term mortality: no difference PPM implantation: 10% vs 5%

NYHA, New York Heart Association; OR, odds ratio; PPM, permanent pacemaker; SCD, sudden cardiac death.

TABLE 47.4 Factors Favoring Alcohol Septal Ablation and Septal Myomectomy in Hypertrophic Obstructive Cardiomyopathy

	Factors Favoring Septal Ablation	Factors Favoring Septal Myectomy
Patient & Clinical Factors	• Patients> 60 years of age • Adults of any age with particularly favorable anatomy • Patients at high or prohibitive cardiac risk • Patients with preexisting RBBB • Patients with preexisting PPM/ICD • Prior failed myectomy	• Younger patients, especially those <21 years of age • Patients with surgically correctable cardiac comorbidities • Preexisting Left Bundle Branch Block • Prior failed alcohol septal ablation
Anatomic & Hemodynamic Factors	• Septal thickness >15 mm • Resting or provoked gradient >50 mm Hg • Accessible septal branches supplying the target myocardium • Presence of a focal septal bulge • Obstructive LVOT gradients localized to the proximal basal ventricular septum	• Septal thickness <15 mm • Lack of accessible septal branches • Massive diffuse LVH with septal thickness >25-30 mm • Presence of midventricular obstruction • Presence of subvalvular membranes • Presence of anomalous papillary muscles • Severe LVOT gradients of >100 mm Hg resting and > 200 mm Hg provoked

LVH, left ventricular hypertrophy; LVOT, left ventricular outflow tract; PPM, permanent pacemaker; RBBB, right bundle branch block.

recurrent obstruction after myectomy, and individuals with a strong desire to avoid open heart surgery after a thorough physician-patient discussion (Class IIb in the ACC/AHA guidelines). Surgical myectomy, on the other hand, is preferred in patients that are younger (<40 years of age), have surgically correctable cardiac comorbidities, especially intrinsic mitral valvular abnormalities, preexisting left bundle branch block (LBBB), unfavorable anatomy for ASA, or a history of failed ASA unamenable to repeat ablation.[4,5,20,22] In patients under 21 years of age, ASA is contraindicated (Class III recommendation).[4]

The younger versus older preference is driven largely by comorbidities, but also by the septal hypertrophy anatomy. Younger patients typically have massive, diffuse hypertrophy extending beyond the basal septum, with significant cavity size reduction and higher gradients. Such patients are well suited for surgical myectomy and poorly suited for ASA. On the other hand, older patients tend to have basal septum focal thickening amenable to a small aliquot of alcohol directed to one location. Therefore, in clinical practice, the number of patients who truly could have either procedure remains a small fraction of the overall population. In our practice, where both surgical myectomy and ASA are available at high volume, ASA is performed roughly 60% of the time and surgical myectomy 40% of the time; the percentage of patients going for one or the other procedure in the de novo population appears to be roughly 50%.

ASA relies heavily on the presence of adequately sized and accessible septal branches supplying the target hypertrophied myocardium of at least 15 mm in thickness. It is strongly discouraged in patients with septal thickness <15 mm owing to an increased risk of iatrogenic ventricular septal defect formation.[17] The presence of a focal septal bulge is also an anatomically favorable scenario for ASA. Patients that do not have accessible septal branches have massive or diffuse LV hypertrophy with septal thickness > 25 to 30 mm, midventricular obstruction, subvalvular membranes, anomalous papillary muscles, intrinsic mitral valve abnormalities or severe LVOT gradients of >100 mm Hg resting and >200 mm Hg with provocation are not favorable for ASA, although it can be performed with some reduction in predicted efficacy. These patients will have better outcomes with surgical myectomy because the experienced surgeon can tailor the operation under direct visualization to address any specific anatomic abnormalities producing the LVOT gradient. It is important to note that experience matters in both techniques, because there are notable failures of both ASA and surgical myectomy, requiring one or the other repeat procedure. Thus, volume requirements for both techniques currently require 10 procedures per year for maintenance of proficiency.[9,20,23]

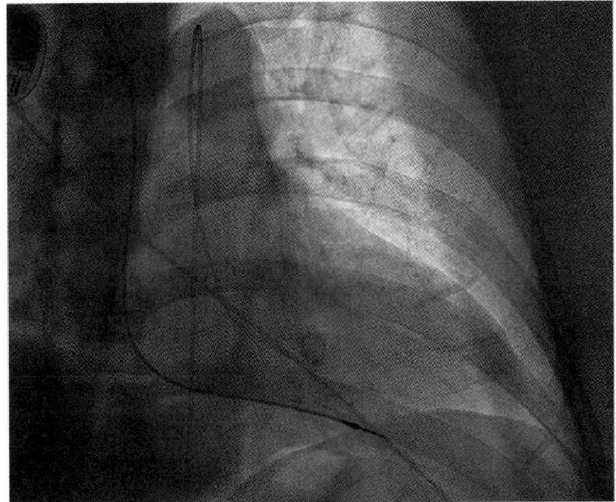

FIGURE 47.2 Screw-in transvenous semipermanent pacemaker lead placed in the right ventricular apex via the right internal jugular venous approach. This lead is connected to an externalized generator.

FUNDAMENTALS OF ALCOHOL SEPTAL ABLATION

After appropriate patient selection for ASA, the procedure should be performed at an HCM center of excellence by an experienced operator. An experienced center is one that has performed more than 50 procedures cumulatively, whereas an experienced operator performs more than 10 per year.[20,24] Coronary anatomy and hemodynamic data should be available prior to planning the procedure, ideally in a separate cardiac catheterization. This is because the ASA procedure is coordinated between interventional cardiology, electrophysiology and echocardiography and not well suited to ad hoc performance.

The original ASA technique has undergone several modifications to improve both the identification of the target septal branch and hemodynamic efficacy and to decrease the risk of major acute complications (heart block, arrhythmias, alcohol spillage and PPM requirement), and any long-term impact of resultant myocardial scar. In this section, we discuss the procedural detail from our institution's experience.

Transvenous Pacing

In patients without an implanted cardiac electronic device with ventricular sensing and pacing feature, a temporary transvenous pacemaker (TVP) is placed from the internal jugular vein with a screw-in pacing lead (active fixation) positioned in the right ventricular apex, attached to an externalized generator; **Figure 47.2**. This is in anticipation of any conduction system damage and atrioventricular (AV) block from the ablation procedure, which is most often transient. The pacing wire tip should be directed away from the basal septum and toward the right ventricular apex because septal ablation can cause fluctuations of the pacing threshold given ablation of the right ventricular side of the basal septum. Further, pacing at the right ventricular apex reverses the activation sequence of the LV and promotes an apical to basal activation of the LV, which may be beneficial in some patients. Balloon-tip pacemaker wires may also be used, but the use of a flexible screw-in pacemaker electrode may lower the incidence of pericardial tamponade resulting from cardiac perforation, improve lead stability and threshold, and promote earlier ambulation and more prolonged monitoring. Indeed, given that heart block often improves over time, it is possible that prolonged monitoring will reduce the need for PPMs in this population, although data for this remain in development. Once the lead position is confirmed in position and with optimal threshold, we then proceed to the ablation procedure. To ensure appropriate functioning of the transvenous pacing lead after the ablation, lead parameters and pacing threshold are also tested after the ASA procedure prior to transfer of the patient from the catheterization laboratory to the intensive care unit. Although this is most important for balloon-tipped, nonactive fixation leads, it is also recommended for active-fixation leads to confirm thresholds have not changed at the conclusion of the case.

Vascular Access

The right internal jugular vein is accessed for temporary transvenous pacer insertion, as discussed previously. Femoral venous access can be utilized as well, if a temporary balloon-tipped TVP is used, although, as previously seen, this is less favored in contemporary practice. For arterial access, we prefer the right femoral artery to allow for ease of catheter handling and more secure and predictable guide backup, by avoiding mechanical transmission of respiratory variation, which can be encountered with transradial arterial access. Radial access was also successfully used for ASA and is the standard in some hospitals. Ultimately, vascular access depends on accessibility and operator experience.

Procedural Hemodynamic Assessment

Historically, the procedure required hemodynamic guidance of LVOT gradients to determine the completeness of myocardial ablation, and therefore β-blocker therapy was discontinued and intravenous fluid boluses were avoided in order to allow for maximal provocation of the LVOT gradient. In our practice, however, we generally continue these medications, including disopyramide, because we had already determined that gradients persisted on these medications at the time of initial diagnostic cardiac catheterization, and because continuing all medications makes the assessment of postprocedure conduction abnormalities more easily attributable to the ablation itself rather than medication changes. Accordingly, we utilize myocardial contrast echo, basal hypokinesis, improvement of systolic anterior motion (SAM), and reduction in turbulence to document a successful result rather than measuring pre- and posthemodynamics. In addition, because these medications (β-blockers and calcium channel blockers) will need to be continued at least for the next 6 months until remodeling occurs, and for ongoing blood pressure control in some patients, we find it better to continue them preoperatively and throughout the hospitalization.

Methods of procedural hemodynamic assessment of LVOT gradients differ between centers. Most operators prefer intraprocedural hemodynamic measurements with either retrograde (transaortic) or anterograde (transseptal) catheterization into the LV. A retrograde approach is commonly preferred by many operators to avoid risks of transseptal puncture. Simultaneous pressure recordings from the LV and ascending aorta with a pigtail catheter positioned in the LV and another in the ascending aorta can help in accurate measurement of obstructive gradients (**Figure 47.3A-D**). In patients with no aortoiliac disease, one pigtail catheter in the LV apex that can be compared to the femoral arterial sheath is often sufficient to record

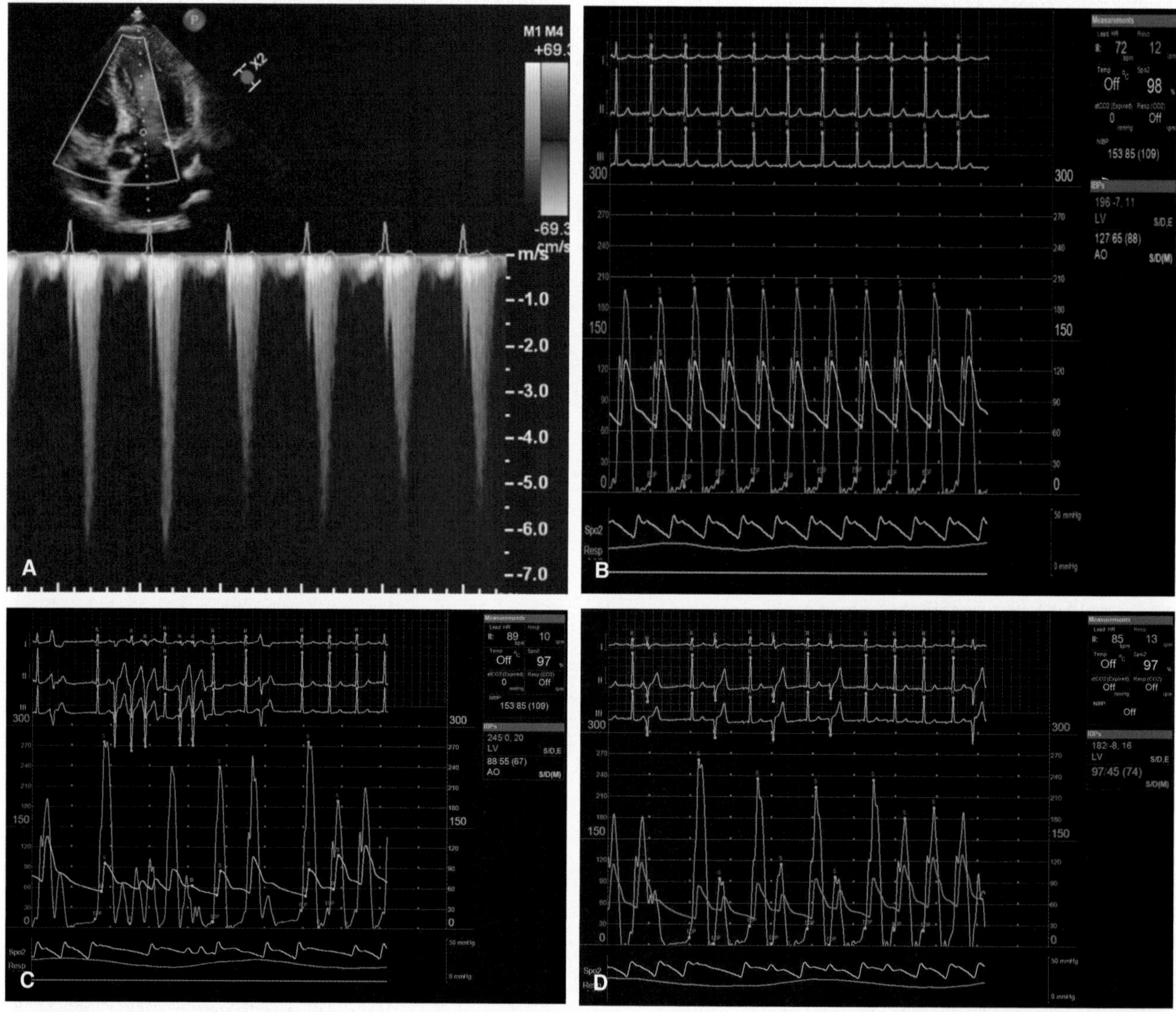

FIGURE 47.3 Echocardiographic and hemodynamic assessment of preprocedural left ventricular outflow tract (LVOT) gradients. **Panel A**: Preprocedural echocardiogram showing a provocable LVOT gradient (Valsalva) of 140 mm Hg. **Panel B**: Preprocedural hemodynamic assessment with pigtail catheter in the LV apex (orange) and the aorta (blue) showing a resting LVOT gradient of 80 mm Hg, which increased to 160 mm Hg (**Panel C)** during the induction of extrasystoles (Brockenbrough-Braunwald-Morrow sign). **Panel D**: In patients with no aortoiliac disease, one pigtail catheter in the LV apex (orange) that can be compared with the femoral arterial sheath (pink) is often sufficient to record gradients.

gradients and is the standard at our center (**View D**). This approach requires only 1 arterial access site, thereby minimizing the risk of access site complications. Catheter entrapment is avoided by use of a multiholed pigtail catheter, with the catheter positioned in the midventricle. Intraprocedural provoked LVOT gradients can be measured after the administration of a positive inotropic drug such as isoproterenol or dobutamine or a vasodilator such as nitroglycerin or amyl nitrite, by induction of extrasystoles with programmed stimulation utilizing the temporary pacemaker, or by the Valsalva maneuver. Most centers, including our own, do not use inotropes or nitroglycerin, however, and prefer physiologic provocation with Valsalva and Brockenbrough-Braunwald-Morrow sign in the awake patient; importantly, if sedation is utilized, other more aggressive maneuvers may be required as aforementioned (**View C**). The LVOT gradients may be masked or attenuated in the presence of increased afterload (arterial hypertension), and in such cases, the use of intraprocedural arterial vasodilators (nitroglycerin) may be helpful to accurately assess the gradients.

At our center, we also rely on LVOT gradient assessments obtained from intraprocedural echocardiography. We obtain immediate preprocedural transthoracic myocardial contrast enhanced echocardiography while on the table to visualize and quantify the myocardial septum to be ablated and to accurately determine the resting and provoked (Valsalva) LVOT gradients (**View A**). Notably, the echocardiogram can be performed while the operator has the pigtail in the LV. In this manner, simultaneous gradients may invasively and noninvasively be obtained, and the operator can assist the echocardiography technician in recording the maximal provoked gradients via stimulation of extrasystoles during a continuous wave Doppler recording. Echocardiography is obtained during alcohol injection to visualize the extent of basal septal opacification, lack of alcohol in other sites, and to measure LVOT obstructive gradient improvement and SAM in real time. The septal thickness on echocardiography also helps determine the total amount of alcohol, as 1 mL is generally used for every 1 cm septal thickness at the point of septal contact of mitral valve SAM.

ASA Procedure

Standard guiding catheters and long coronary wires are used for the procedure. The left coronary ostium is cannulated using an appropriately sized guide catheter (6F JL4, if femoral approach) and angiography performed to visualize the septal perforator artery arising from the most proximal region of the LAD. A steep right anterior oblique cranial projection is typically utilized. Bolus and continuous infusion of bivalirudin is started to prevent thrombus formation associated with catheter and wire manipulation. Heparin can also be used alternatively, with periodic activated clotting time checks to confirm adequate anticoagulation throughout the procedure. Although there are no data comparing either anticoagulant in ASA, we prefer bivalirudin because, unlike heparin, it is shorter acting and does not require frequent activated clotting time checks to monitor for anticoagulant activity. Given the longer potential length of these procedures, we have preferred bivalirudin infusion. A 0.014-inch-long coronary angioplasty guidewire is then positioned in the target septal artery and an over-the-wire balloon catheter is advanced into the target proximal septal artery and inflated. The size of the balloon approximates the diameter of the chosen septal and can range from 1.25 to 2.5 mm. The length is usually 6 mm. We generally use the noncompliant Sprinter balloon (Medtronic Inc., Mounds View, MN) or a Flextome cutting balloon (Boston Scientific, Maple Grove, MN). The Flextome cutting balloon with its atherotomes offers enhanced balloon stability owing to increased friction between the balloon and the arterial wall, although it does not come in a size of less than 2.0-mm diameter.[25] Precise balloon position and stability are essential to prevent watermelon-seeding and remote myocardial infarction down the LAD. After the septal is wired, the balloon is brought past the ostium of the septal perforator and inflated to completely occlude the vessel. Aggressive inflation is avoided because distal dissection can occur in the septal perforator, eliminating the possibility of alcohol infusion. Complete occlusion of anterograde septal flow is confirmed with angiography through the guide catheter, and the coronary guidewire is removed. A small amount of contrast medium (undiluted omnipaque) is injected through the central balloon lumen to opacify the septal and its branches, delineate the area supplied by the septal branch on simultaneous echo, and to ensure no reflux of contrast (later alcohol) into the LAD after balloon inflation. Abnormal collateral connections from the septal artery to other coronary arteries is also ruled out during this part of the procedure, because this would contribute to distant, unintended myocardial infarction.

As visualized on transthoracic myocardial contrast echocardiography, the contrast injection (undiluted omnipaque) delineates the area to be infarcted and excludes contrast (and subsequently alcohol) deposition in remote myocardial regions such as the LV anterior or posterior walls, papillary muscles, and right ventricular free wall or moderator band. The optimal septal branch supplies the area in the basal septum, which is adjacent to the zone of maximal acceleration of the outflow jet and includes the point of coaptation between septum and anterior mitral leaflet. The target septal branch usually originates from the proximal segment of the LAD artery, but is not always the first septal. It may be the second or third septal, or it may originate from diagonal or ramus intermediate branches of the left coronary artery (**Figure 47.4A,B**). Selective septal artery branch occlusion (of diagonal branches, or LV branch of a first septal perforator, for example) and ablation (if anatomically feasible) can also be performed to produce favorable improvements in hemodynamics with an anticipated lower rate of complete AV block in our experience.

Once the appropriate septal branch is identified, approximately 1 to 2 mL of 98% alcohol is injected slowly into the septal artery through the lumen of the inflated balloon catheter over 2 to 3 minutes and left in place for 5 minutes. The amount of alcohol required is usually guided by the septal thickness (1 mL per 1 cm thickness) adjacent to the location of maximal flow acceleration and includes the point of coaptation between septum and anterior mitral leaflet. Echocardiography is done

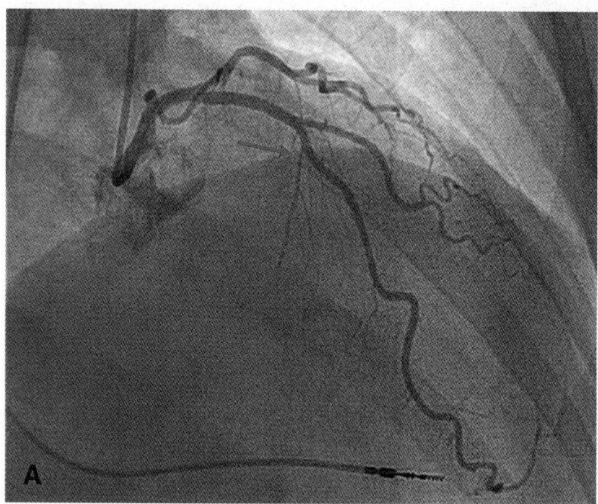

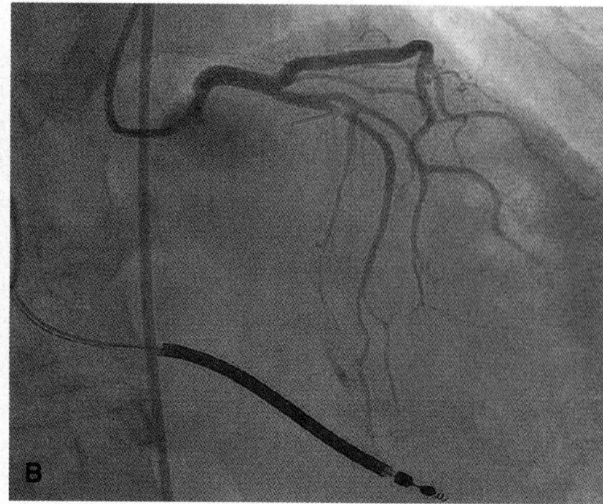

FIGURE 47.4 Coronary angiograms showing origins of the target septal perforator arteries (arrows). Left: Target septal perforator arising as the first branch of the left anterior descending artery (LAD). Right: Target septal perforator arising as a branch of the first diagonal branch of the LAD.

to localize the area of myocardial infarction during alcohol injection and determine improvements in LVOT gradient and SAM in real time. Echocardiography is also rotated between multiple views to confirm no opacification/ablation of distant sites. Continuous echocardiographic assessment of septal wall motion abnormality and other regions of the heart is important during alcohol injection and for a 5-minute period following the infusion to make sure that there is no spillage of ethanol into LAD distribution beyond the septal artery being injected. Immediate improvement in LVOT gradient is observed and a > 50% reduction in provoked gradient and to less than 30 mm Hg is historically required to ensure procedural success. Echocardiogram may also show improvement in SAM in real time. Provoked gradients can be measured by inducing extrasystoles with the pigtail catheter in the LV. Complete AV block may occur during this time. In addition, nonsustained ventricular tachycardia may be seen. Both can be minimized by slowing the rate of infusion when seen. After the 5-minute period, the balloon catheter is deflated and withdrawn from the septal artery while maintaining negative pressure through the indeflator. Coronary angiography is then performed, after flushing the guide, to confirm the patency of the LAD artery and occlusion of the target septal branch. Hemodynamic measurements are repeated again using echocardiography to obtain a postprocedure baseline, or repeat invasive hemodynamics may be performed.

FOLLOW-UP PATIENT CARE

In-Hospital Postprocedure Care

Because the mechanism behind the ASA is the creation of a myocardial infarction in the septal artery territory, patients are at risk for complications that can result from ischemia in the jeopardized myocardial territory. Important among these are anginal chest pain, which usually resolves within an hour of procedure completion, the development of ventricular arrhythmias or AV conduction system disease. Post procedure, patients are continued on their outpatient medications and admitted to the coronary care unit (CCU) with the TVP in place. Patients may develop significant ventricular ectopy during the first 24 to 48 hours, although cases of ventricular tachycardia are rare. Creatinine phosphokinase and troponin levels are obtained at 6-hour intervals. Peak myocardial enzyme levels (creatinine phosphokinase elevation to 500-2000 units) correlate well with the infarct size[26] and also procedural success and longer term efficacy.[27] Six-hour intervals allow more accurate assessment of the peak. Peak serum creatinine phosphokinase values should be in the 800 to 1200 units range, in general. Lower amounts indicate potentially too small a septal myocardial ablation, whereas higher amounts indicate potential spillage of ethanol to other regions of the myocardium.

Damage to the AV conduction system is a frequent complication of ASA, and AV conduction recovery may require several days of in-hospital monitoring. We prefer a 3-day monitoring period at our center with the TVP in place, because patients do not go home until 4 days after the procedure, and the screw-in TVP allows for safer longer monitoring in these patients while the patient can ambulate freely. Patients with preexisting PPM or ICD may be safely discharged at 2 to 3 days post procedure depending on infarct size. Patients are placed on continuous telemetric monitoring for the duration of their hospitalization to monitor for any tachy- or bradyarrhythmias. In addition to postprocedural 12-lead EKG, daily EKGs are obtained to monitor for the development or progression of conduction system abnormalities, including PR interval prolongation, AV block, bundle branch block, or complete heart block. Although a new RBBB is the most common EKG development after ASA, baseline LBBB and first-degree AV block appear to be associated with the highest risk of the development of compete AV block.

Clinically stable patients are downgraded to the step-down telemetry unit for an additional 2 to 3 days of monitoring prior to discharge. They are monitored for any signs of clinical decompensation, including access site complications, cardiac tamponade, progressive heart failure, and, most importantly, conduction or rhythm abnormalities. Approximately 40% to

60% of patients will develop a RBBB, and 20% of them will have an associated left anterior fascicular block.[28-31] Around 10% to 15% develop a new LBBB, and first degree AV block complicates 7% to 17% of procedures.[31,32] Around 25% to 55% of individuals will develop transient complete AV block during the ASA procedure. In most cases, the conduction system recovers by day 3 to 4 post ASA (can take as long as 13 days), and 10% to 20% of patients will have persistent AV block.[28] Certain electrocardiographic and electrophysiologic variables predict the development of delayed or subacute complete AV block necessitating permanent pacing. Patients with acute complete heart block during the ASA, preexisting or new bundle branch conduction disturbances, and post-ASA prolonged PR duration/first-degree AV block, and absence of retrograde AV nodal conduction after ASA are associated with delayed development of complete AV block.[31,32] Patients who develop these electrocardiographic changes definitely require a longer monitoring period with the TVP in place (3 days).[33] Patients without any of the aforementioned predictors could be considered for a shorter TVP duration (24 hours), although in our practice we prefer the 72-hour monitoring period more routinely.

The decision to explant the TVP or implant a permanent device is made on day 3 or 4 of the hospitalization on a case-by-case basis.[4] Permanent devices are implanted in patients with persistent complete or high-grade AV block and in those with delayed onset complete AV block (>36 hours post procedure) or recurrence of complete AV block after initial recovery (1%-25%). In patients with no evidence of conduction abnormalities, recovered AV block, and in those who have remained clinically stable, we explant the temporary pacemaker on post-procedure day 3. In some cases of fluctuating EKG intervals, patients can be watched longer, up to one week, prior to the determination of need for PPM. In our center, however, we have found that most patients with PPM implanted in this manner do not end up in heart block weeks later. Therefore, there may be a role for longer term monitoring prior to the decision to implant a PPM. However, as previously discussed, 7% to 15% of patients require a PPM prior to discharge. Importantly, patients should not receive a defibrillator (ICD) in lieu of a PPM, unless they meet independent criteria for ICD placement. The ASA procedure itself does not modify this decision, unless late> 48 hours ventricular tachycardia or fibrillation develops.

Discharge PostProcedure Care

After discharge, patients are followed for clinical improvement in symptoms and NYHA functional class, and with serial echocardiograms (1, 3, 6 months) to monitor resting and provoked (by exercise or valsalva maneuver) LVOT gradients, widening of the outflow tract, resolution of SAM and mitral regurgitation, and overall remodeling. The obstructive gradients continue to decline over the first few months and may take 3 to 12 months to attain stable levels.[13,15] Diastolic function improvement and regression of LV hypertrophy may continue up to 2 years later.[14,15] Improvement in NYHA functional class by at least 1 class and a >50% reduction in the peak resting or provoked LVOT gradient and a final resting gradient of <20 mm Hg is required for procedural success and occurs in roughly 80% to 90% of the procedures.[28,34] Although there are no specific criteria to guide the management of β-blocker or calcium channel blocker therapy after ASA, we prefer to continue them immediately after the procedure. Medical therapy should be carefully optimized during the follow-up period, with most patients coming off disopyramide immediately and other medications gradually withdrawn as symptoms and blood pressure allow.[2] There are no data that indicate an increase in incidence of ventricular arrhythmias or sudden death after ASA. As such, β-blocker use post ASA should be guided by obstructive symptoms but not to reduce the risk of arrhythmias or sudden cardiac death.[35] Diuretic therapy, however, is usually continued in the postoperative period because the diastolic changes in the hypertrophied myocardium require time to improve. Over half of the patients who get a PPM will have resumption in normal conduction within 6 months from the procedure.

For roughly 10% of patients, repeat septal reduction therapy is required for procedural failure or recurrent symptoms with dynamic obstruction despite optimization of medical therapy.[17,18,28,34] At that juncture, either ASA or surgical myectomy can be pursued based on anatomy, clinical profile, and patient and physician preference, although in most cases ASA of a second septal perforator chosen based on the echocardiographic location of the area of ablation (either more proximal or more distal) can be easily performed if additional perforators are available. In our experience of over 200 patients, all such patients with recurrent obstruction have been managed successfully with a combination of medication optimization and repeat ASA.

CLINICAL CASE

A 64-year-old man with recently diagnosed HCM presented to our HCM Center of Excellence for evaluation of heart failure symptoms and frequent lightheadedness. Echocardiogram revealed normal LV ejection fraction, a 20-mm basal septum, and a resting LVOT gradient of 70 mm Hg provocable to 140 mm Hg with Valsalva (**Figure 47.3A**). SAM of the anterior mitral valve leaflet was seen with septal contact. Left heart catheterization with coronary angiography performed as part of the initial evaluation revealed mild coronary artery disease in the proximal LAD artery, and a large first septal perforator to the basal septum likely at the region of SAM was noted (**Figure 47.5A**). The patient was on maximally tolerable doses of metoprolol and verapamil at the time of this examination. The patient met indications for septal reduction based on symptoms, anatomy, and severe gradients. After a thorough physician-patient discussion in the ambulatory setting regarding the risks and benefits of either septal reduction strategy, we decided to proceed with ASA.

The patient was electively admitted to the hospital and brought to the catheterization lab and a screw-in TVP was placed via the right internal jugular venous approach (**Figure 47.2**).

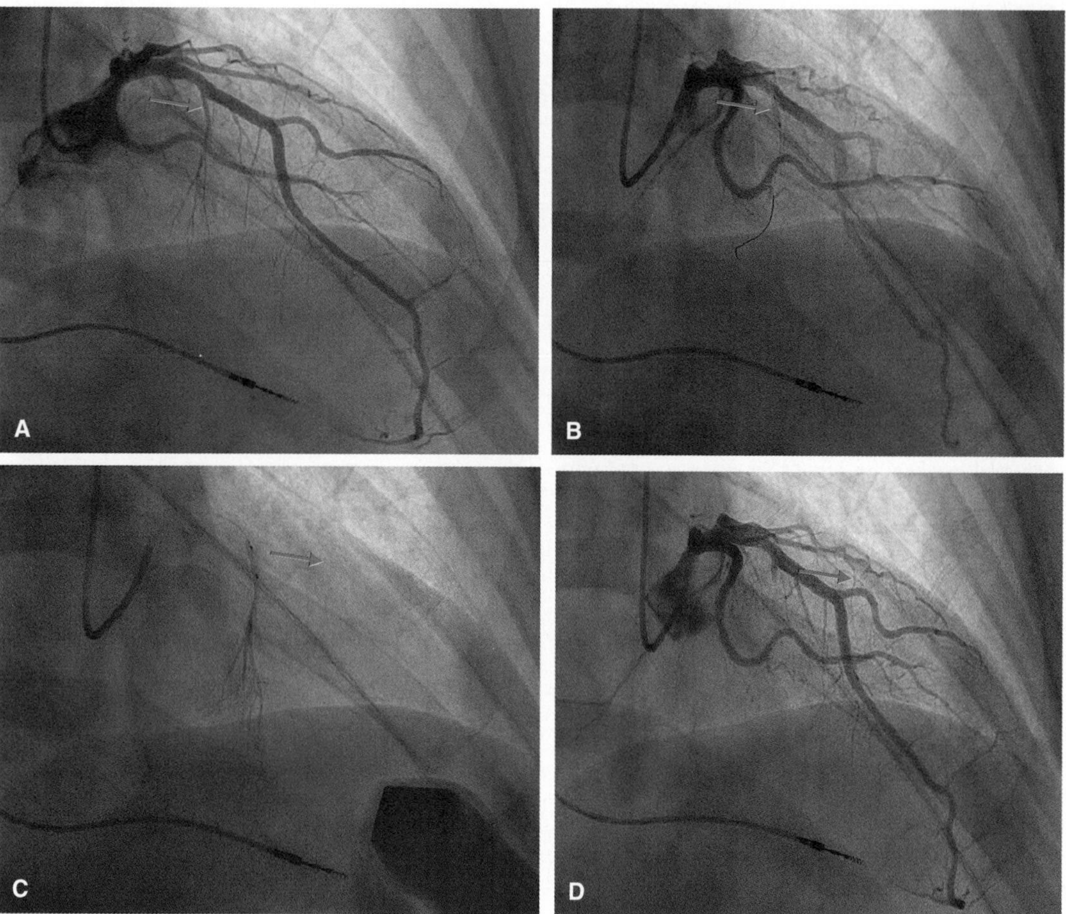

FIGURE 47.5 **A-D:** Alcohol septal ablation procedure. **Panel A:** Left heart catheterization with coronary angiography revealed mild coronary artery disease in the proximal left anterior descending artery, and a large first septal perforator to the main basal septum likely at the region systolic anterior motion was noted. **Panel B:** A 2.0 × 6 mm Flextome over-the-wire cutting balloon was passed over a 0.014″-long coronary wire and positioned at the proximal part of the target artery and inflated to 6 atm. **Panel C:** A myocardial contrast echocardiogram was performed after injecting omnipaque contrast into the septal perforator distal to the inflated balloon. **Panel D:** Angiogram of the left coronary artery after alcohol ablation now demonstrated an occluded target septal perforator.

Aspirin 325 mg was administered orally before the procedure. Utilizing the right femoral arterial approach and a 6F JL4 guiding catheter, the target septal perforator was identified (**Figure 47.5A**). Bivaluridin bolus followed by an infusion was initiated when the left coronary artery was engaged. A 2.0 × 6 mm Flextome over-the-wire cutting balloon was passed over a 0.014″ coronary wire and positioned at the proximal part of the target artery and inflated to 6 atm (**Figure 47.5B**). A myocardial contrast echocardiogram was performed after injecting omnipaque contrast into the septal perforator distal to the inflated balloon (**Figure 47.5C**). Identification of the hyperechogenic area of the basal septum after contrast injection confirmed the appropriateness of the septal artery chosen for ablation. After the administration of 2-mg intravenous morphine for pain control, 2.5 mL of 98% ethyl alcohol was injected intracoronary into the septal perforator distal to the inflated balloon. The balloon was deflated after 10 minutes of continuous inflation. Immediate intraprocedural transthoracic echocardiogram done at this time revealed significant improvement in the resting LVOT gradient to 8 mm Hg (**Figure 47.6A**). Angiogram of the left coronary artery now demonstrated an occluded target septal perforator (**Figure 47.5D**). The right femoral artery was appropriately closed with an Angioseal device, and bivalirudin infusion was discontinued.

An immediate EKG was performed to document postprocedure conduction changes. The patient was then admitted to the CCU, and his outpatient medications were continued. Enzyme testing and telemetry monitoring were done as described previously. Preprocedural ECG demonstrated sinus rhythm without any conduction abnormalities (**Figure 47.7A**). Immediate post-ASA ECG demonstrated sinus rhythm with a normal PR interval and new RBBB (**Figure 47.7B**). ECG findings were stable at 3 days post ASA without the need for pacing (**Figure 47.7C**), at which time the TVP was removed. At 3-month follow-up, the patient experienced significant improvement in symptoms, and echocardiography showed minimal resting LVOT gradient (**Figure 47.6B**) and a provoked LVOT gradient of 32 mm Hg (**Figure 47.6C**).

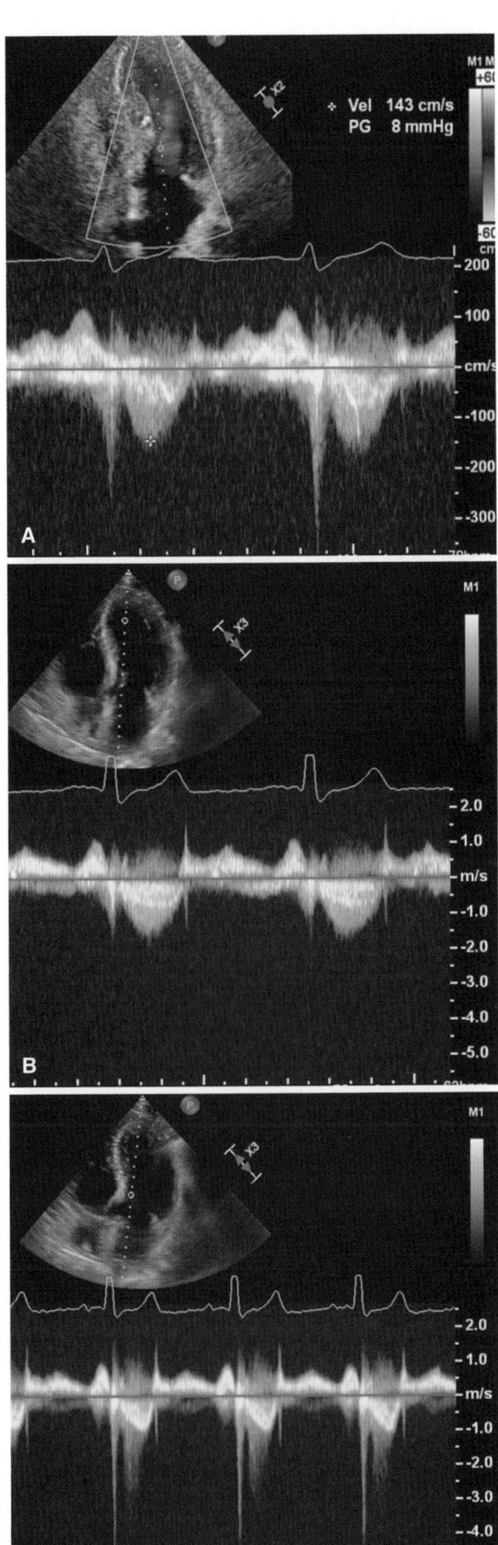

FIGURE 47.6 Left ventricular outflow tract (LVOT) gradients during the procedure and at follow-up. **Panel A:** Immediate intraprocedural transthoracic echocardiogram done after intracoronary alcohol injection into the target septal perforator artery revealed significant improvement in the resting LVOT gradient to 8 mm Hg from a baseline of 70 mm Hg. **Panel B:** At 3-month follow-up, patient had significant improvement in resting (minimal) and provoked (**Panel C**; 32 mm Hg) LVOT gradients.

SPECIAL CONSIDERATIONS

ASA has been utilized in some cases of midventricular obstruction rather than LVOT obstruction. This approach will depend on the identification of a septal artery that supplies the target midventricular myocardium and usually requires more than one septal to be ablated, and higher doses of alcohol. ASA has been successfully performed in patients who had a prior myectomy and residual LVOT obstruction.[36] Careful anatomic evaluation can guide successful ablation in such cases. Another important consideration is the presence of obstructive or significant coronary artery disease in the LAD around the origin of the target septal perforator artery. In such a clinical scenario, it is preferred to proceed with the ASA prior to necessary indicated percutaneous coronary intervention of the diseased LAD segment to avoid difficulties in accessing the septal artery for the ASA. Finally, there is a growing need for ASA prior to transcatheter aortic valve replacement (pre-TAVR) in older patients with both aortic stenosis and LVOT obstruction.[37] Recent studies support preemptive ASA to increase the predicted neo-LVOT area prior to transcatheter mitral valve replacement. Such a strategy may enable safe transcatheter mitral valve replacement in patients usually excluded secondary to prohibitive risk of LVOT obstruction.[38]

RESEARCH/FUTURE DIRECTIONS

The greatest challenge for septal reduction therapy choice in HCM is the absence of randomized data comparing the reduction strategies. Such a trial is unlikely given the low prevalence of the disease and the requirement of almost 35,000 HCM patients to be screened to randomize 1200 patients with medically refractory obstruction to either strategy. In the absence of randomized data, available observation data and center experiences guide procedural strategies. Studies comparing medical therapy with septal reduction for mortality benefit are currently lacking in the HCM population, but it is widely assumed that medications do not offer a survival advantage, whereas septal reduction appears to normalize survival curves.

Percutaneous intramyocardial septal radiofrequency ablation from a transapical approach is a novel technique that could be useful in minimizing complications, namely conduction injury, from the currently available and guideline-supported techniques. However, efficacy and long-term followup data for this technique are limited.[38] Cryoablation techniques are also under investigation. Enhanced imaging guidance with intracardiac echocardiography for continuous intraprocedural imaging of the treated segment of the septum can be utilized. Studies evaluating the benefit of utilizing CT/MRI guidance for the ablation procedure are needed. The use of polyvinyl alcohol foam particles, microspheres, absorbable gelatin sponges, or septal coils as alternatives to alcohol may further reduce the incidence of complete heart block associated with ASA, although data to date have not been favorable.[35] Finally, in some patients, particularly those with a thinner septum of <1.5 cm, mitraclip may help pull the anterior mitral leaflet more posterior and out of the outflow tract, eliminating SAM and obstruction.

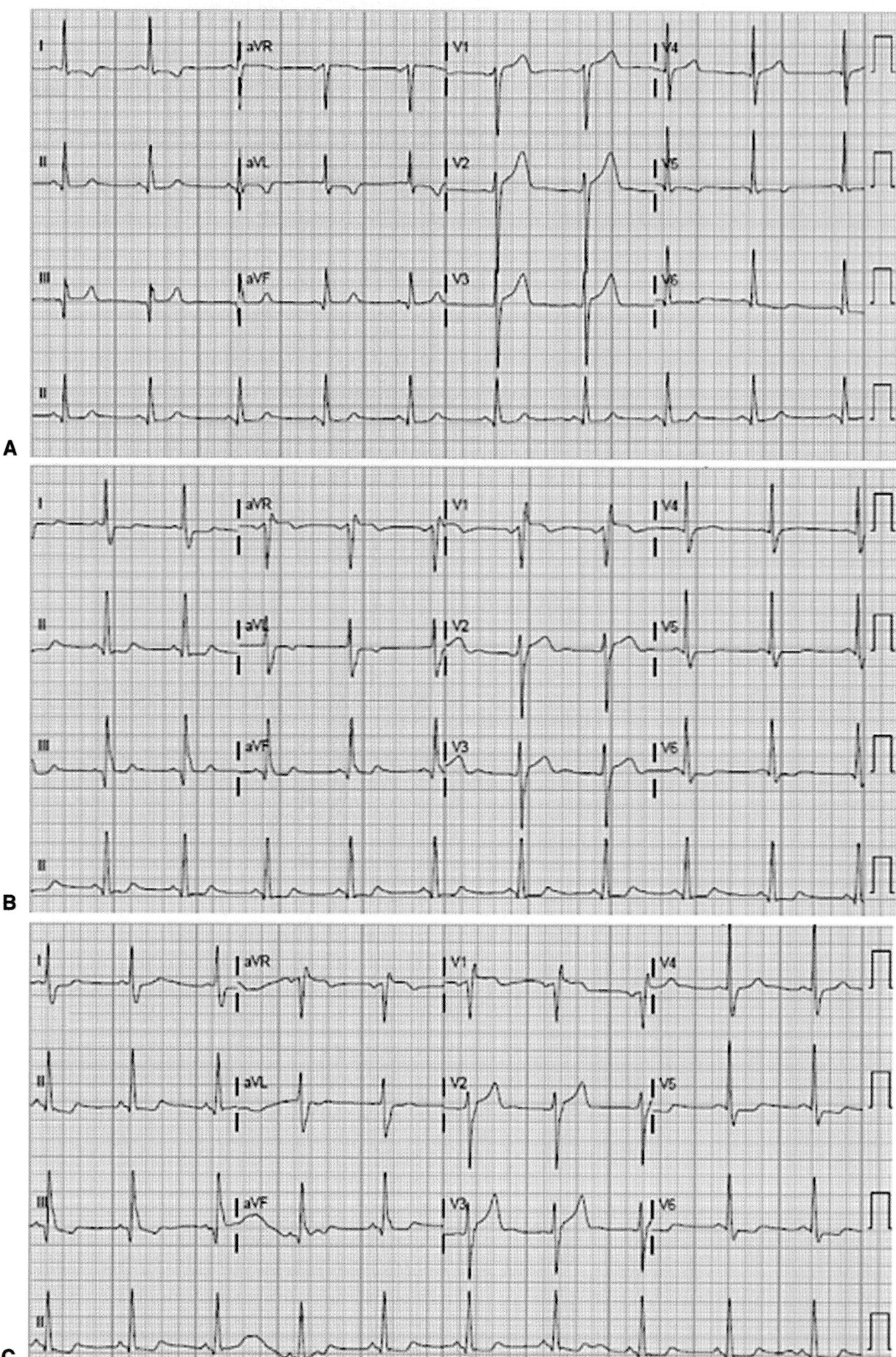

FIGURE 47.7 Electrocardiogram (ECG) monitoring in the peri-ablation period. **Panel A:** Pre-alcohol septal ablation ECG with normal sinus rhythm and left ventricular hypertrophy. **Panel B:** Immediate post-alcohol septal ablation ECG with new right bundle branch block (RBBB). **Panel C:** ECG 3 days post ECG with sinus rhythm and stable RBBB.

KEY POINTS

- ✔ A screw-in TVP with externalized generator can allow for reduced complication rates, earlier mobilization and ambulation, and prolonged monitoring. As the true incidence of long-term complete heart block is very low, prolonged monitoring up to a week may obviate the need for permanent pacing in some patients.
- ✔ Avoid too rapid infusion of alcohol, and too high a dose of alcohol, in order to avoid complications, including ventricular tachycardia or fibrillation during the procedure (acutely) or ventricular septal defect after the procedure. In general, no more than 1 mL for every 1-cm maximal wall thickness at the point of SAM contact or at the point of maximal flow acceleration should be used, with average alcohol doses of approximately 1 to 2 cc.
- ✔ Do not assume the first septal is always the correct septal; sometimes, it is the second or even third septal, or a septal off a non-LAD vessel such as the ramus or diagonal. Look for these septal perforator arteries in multiple angiographic projections.
- ✔ Peak serum creatinine phosphokinase values should be in the 800 to 1200 range, in general. Lower amounts indicate potentially too small an ablation, whereas higher amounts indicate potential spillage to other regions of the heart.
- ✔ Continue medications in the postprocedure period, especially in patients with severely elevated provocable gradients over 100 mm Hg and hypertension. Edema of the septum within the first 2 to 3 days may increase LVOT gradients during this period and need to be managed carefully to avoid recurrent in-hospital heart failure.
- ✔ In the adequately hydrated patient, a small amount of intracoronary nitroglycerin (100 mcg) can dilate the septal arteries and help choose the appropriate size of the balloon needed for the ablation procedure.
- ✔ Myocardial contrast echocardiography guidance is pivotal during the procedure, and institutions should train echocardiography technicians for the procedure and have one or two technicians who routinely assist in these cases.

REFERENCES

1. Semsarian C, Ingles J, Maron MS, Maron BJ. New perspectives on the prevalence of hypertrophic cardiomyopathy. *J Am Coll Cardiol.* 2015;65(12):1249-1254. doi:10.1016/j.jacc.2015.01.019
2. Andries G, Yandrapalli S, Naidu SS, Panza JA. Novel pharmacotherapy in hypertrophic cardiomyopathy. *Cardiol Rev.* 2018;26(5):239-244. doi:10.1097/CRD.0000000000000211
3. Panza JA, Naidu SS. Historical perspectives in the evolution of hypertrophic cardiomyopathy. *Cardiol Clin.* 2019;37(1):1-10. doi:10.1016/j.ccl.2018.08.001
4. Gersh BJ, Maron BJ, Bonow RO, et al. ACCF/AHA guideline for the diagnosis and treatment of hypertrophic cardiomyopathy: executive summary: a report of the American College of cardiology foundation/American heart association task force on practice guidelines. *Circulation.* 2011;124(24):2761-2796. doi:10.1161/CIR.0b013e318223e230
5. Elliott PM, Anastasakis A, Borger MA, et al. ESC guidelines on diagnosis and management of hypertrophic cardiomyopathy. *Eur Heart J.* 2014;35(39):2733-2779. doi:10.1093/eurheartj/ehu284
6. McKay J, Nagueh SF. Alcohol septal ablation to reduce heart failure. *Interv Cardiol Clin.* 2017;6(3):445-452. doi:10.1016/j.iccl.2017.03.012
7. Maron MS, Olivotto I, Betocchi S, et al. Effect of left ventricular outflow tract obstruction on clinical outcome in hypertrophic cardiomyopathy. *N Engl J Med.* 2003;348(4):295-303. doi:10.1056/NEJMoa021332
8. Naidu SS, Panza JA, Spielvogel D, Malekan R, Goldberg J, Aronow WS. Does relief of outflow tract obstruction in patients with hypertrophic cardiomyopathy improve long-term survival? Implications for lowering the threshold for surgical myectomy and alcohol septal ablation. *Ann Transl Med.* 2016;4(24):485. doi:10.21037/atm.2016.12.47
9. Kim LK, Swaminathan R V., Looser P, et al. Hospital volume outcomes after septal myectomy and alcohol septal ablation for treatment of obstructive hypertrophic cardiomyopathy: US nationwide inpatient database, 2003-2011. *JAMA Cardiol.* 2016;1(3):324-332. doi:10.1001/jamacardio.2016.0252
10. Liebregts M, Vriesendorp PA, Ten Berg JM. Alcohol septal ablation for obstructive hypertrophic cardiomyopathy: a word of endorsement. *J Am Coll Cardiol.* 2017;70(4):481-488. doi:10.1016/j.jacc.2017.02.080
11. Maron BJ, Yacoub M, Dearani JA. Controversies in cardiovascular medicine. Benefits of surgery in obstructive hypertrophic cardiomyopathy: bring septal myectomy back for European patients. *Eur Heart J.* 2011;32(9):1055-1058. doi:10.1093/eurheartj/ehr006
12. Sigwart U. Non-surgical myocardial reduction for hypertrophic obstructive cardiomyopathy. *Lancet.* 1995;346(8969):211-214. doi:10.1016/S0140-6736(95)91267-3
13. Yoerger DM, Picard MH, Palacios IF, Vlahakes GJ, Lowry PA, Fifer MA. Time course of pressure gradient response after first alcohol septal ablation for obstructive hypertrophic cardiomyopathy. *Am J Cardiol.* 2006;97(10):1511-1514. doi:10.1016/j.amjcard.2005.12.040
14. Jassal DS, Neilan TG, Fifer MA, et al. Sustained improvement in left ventricular diastolic function after alcohol septal ablation for hypertrophic obstructive cardiomyopathy. *Eur Heart J.* 2006;27(15):1805-1810. doi:10.1093/eurheartj/ehl106
15. Mazur W, Nagueh SF, Lakkis NM, et al. Regression of left ventricular hypertrophy after nonsurgical septal reduction therapy for hypertrophic obstructive cardiomyopathy. *Circulation.* 2001;103(11):1492-1496. doi:10.1161/01.cir.103.11.1492
16. van Dockum WG, Beek AM, ten Cate FJ, et al. Early onset and progression of left ventricular remodeling after alcohol septal ablation in hypertrophic obstructive cardiomyopathy. *Circulation.* 2005;111(19):2503-2508. doi:10.1161/01.CIR.0000165084.28065.01
17. Nagueh SF, Groves BM, Schwartz L, et al. Alcohol septal ablation for the treatment of hypertrophic obstructive cardiomyopathy: a multicenter north american registry. *J Am Coll Cardiol.* 2011;58(22):2322-2328. doi:10.1016/j.jacc.2011.06.073
18. Sorajja P, Ommen SR, Holmes DR, et al. Survival after alcohol septal ablation for obstructive hypertrophic cardiomyopathy. *Circulation.* 2012;126(20):2374-2380. doi:10.1161/CIRCULATIONAHA.111.076257
19. Naidu SS. Survival and pacemaker risk after alcohol septal ablation: informing the choice of invasive therapy for hypertrophic cardiomyopathy. *Can J Cardiol.* 2013;29(11):1369-1370. doi:10.1016/j.cjca.2013.05.003
20. Naidu SS. Performance volume thresholds for alcohol septal ablation in treating hypertrophic cardiomyopathy: guidelines, competency statements, and now data. *Can J Cardiol.* 2018;34(1):13-15. doi:10.1016/j.cjca.2017.11.017
21. Heldman AW, Wu KC, Abraham TP, Cameron DE. Myectomy or alcohol septal ablation surgery and percutaneous intervention go another round. *J Am Coll Cardiol.* 2007;49(3):358-360. doi:10.1016/j.jacc.2006.10.029
22. Fifer MA. Choice of septal reduction therapies and alcohol septal ablation. *Cardiol Clin.* 2019;37(1):83-93. doi:10.1016/j.ccl.2018.08.009
23. Gersh BJ, Maron BJ, Bonow RO, et al. 2011 ACCF/AHA guideline for the diagnosis and treatment of hypertrophic cardiomyopathy: executive summary: a report of the American College of Cardiology Foundation/American Heart Association Task Force on Practice Guidelines. *J Am Coll Cardiol.* 2011;58(25):2703-2738. doi:10.1016/j.jacc.2011.10.825

24. Veselka J, Faber L, Jensen MK, et al. Effect of institutional experience on outcomes of alcohol septal ablation for hypertrophic obstructive cardiomyopathy. *Can J Cardiol.* 2018;34(1):16-22. doi:10.1016/j.cjca.2017.10.020
25. Polin N, Feldman D, Naidu SS. Alcohol septal ablation for hypertrophic obstructive cardiomyopathy: novel application of the cutting balloon. *J Invasive Cardiol.* 2006;18(9):436-437.
26. Hage FG, Aqel R, Aljaroudi W, et al. Correlation between serum cardiac markers and myocardial infarct size quantified by myocardial perfusion imaging in patients with hypertrophic cardiomyopathy after alcohol septal ablation. *Am J Cardiol.* 2010;105(2):261-266. doi:10.1016/j.amjcard.2009.08.680
27. Chang SM, Lakkis NM, Franklin J, Spencer WH, Nagueh SF. Predictors of outcome after alcohol septal ablation therapy in patients with hypertrophic obstructive cardiomyopathy. *Circulation.* 2004;109(7):824-827. doi:10.1161/01.CIR.0000117089.99918.5A
28. Reinhard W, Ten Cate FJ, Scholten M, de Laat LE, Vos J. Permanent pacing for complete atrioventricular block after nonsurgical (alcohol) septal reduction in patients with obstructive hypertrophic cardiomyopathy. *Am J Cardiol.* 2004;93(8):1064-1066. doi:10.1016/j.amjcard.2003.12.065
29. Talreja DR, Nishimura RA, Edwards WD, et al. Alcohol septal ablation versus surgical septal myectomy: comparison of effects on atrioventricular conduction tissue. *J Am Coll Cardiol.* 2004;44(12):2329-2332. doi:10.1016/j.jacc.2004.09.036
30. Liebregts M, Steggerda RC, Vriesendorp PA, et al. Long-term outcome of alcohol septal ablation for obstructive hypertrophic cardiomyopathy in the young and the elderly. *JACC Cardiovasc Interv.* 2016;9(5):463-469. doi:10.1016/j.jcin.2015.11.036
31. Lawrenz T, Lieder F, Bartelsmeier M, et al. Predictors of complete heart block after transcoronary ablation of septal hypertrophy: results of a prospective electrophysiological investigation in 172 patients with hypertrophic obstructive cardiomyopathy. *J Am Coll Cardiol.* 2007;49(24):2356-2363. doi:10.1016/j.jacc.2007.02.056
32. Chen AA, Palacios IF, Mela T, et al. Acute predictors of subacute complete heart block after alcohol septal ablation for obstructive hypertrophic cardiomyopathy. *Am J Cardiol.* 2006;97(2):264-269. doi:10.1016/j.amjcard.2005.08.032
33. El-Sabawi B, Nishimura RA, Barsness GW, Cha Y-M, Geske JB, Eleid MF. Temporal occurrence of arrhythmic complications after alcohol septal ablation. *Circ Cardiovasc Interv.* 2020;13(2):e008540. doi:10.1161/CIRCINTERVENTIONS.119.008540
34. Fernandes VL, Nielsen C, Nagueh SF, et al. Follow-up of alcohol septal ablation for symptomatic hypertrophic obstructive cardiomyopathy the Baylor and Medical University of South Carolina experience 1996 to 2007. *JACC Cardiovasc Interv.* 2008;1(5):561-570. doi:10.1016/j.jcin.2008.07.005
35. Fifer MA, Sigwart U. Hypertrophic obstructive cardiomyopathy: alcohol septal ablation. *Eur Heart J.* 2011;32(9):1059-1064. doi:10.1093/eurheartj/ehr013
36. Cherif E, Ghazal S. Alcohol septal ablation after suboptimal surgical septal myomectomy. *CASE (Phila).* 2018;2(5):210-217. doi:10.1016/j.case.2018.02.004
37. Shenouda J, Silber D, Subramaniam M, et al. Evaluation and management of concomitant hypertrophic obstructive cardiomyopathy and valvular aortic stenosis. *Curr Treat Options Cardiovasc Med.* 2016;18(3):17. doi:10.1007/s11936-016-0440-3
38. Wang DD, Guerrero M, Eng MH, et al. Alcohol septal ablation to prevent left ventricular outflow tract obstruction during transcatheter mitral valve replacement: First-in-Man Study. *JACC Cardiovasc Interv.* 2019;12(13):1268-1279. doi:10.1016/j.jcin.2019.02.034

CHAPTER 48

LEFT ATRIAL APPENDAGE CLOSURE

Thomas A. Dewland and Randall J. Lee

INTRODUCTION

For decades, clinicians have recognized the association between atrial fibrillation (AF) and thromboembolic stroke.[1] This risk has traditionally been mitigated through oral anticoagulant therapy.[2-4] A sizeable proportion of patients, however, are poor candidates for long-term anticoagulation because of an elevated bleeding risk. While data from contemporary clinical trials suggest that the yearly risk of major bleeding on anticoagulation is approximately 2% to 4% per year,[3,5,6] this risk is likely higher in certain patient populations with more severe comorbidities compared with carefully selected trial participants. Concern for bleeding complications has prompted the development of alternative therapies to mitigate AF–associated stroke risk.

The left atrial appendage (LAA) plays a central role in the pathogenesis of AF–associated stroke.[7,8] The reduction in mechanical atrial function and LAA contractility that accompanies AF frequently results in a substantial decrease in appendage blood flow velocity. In addition to other factors including inflammation and endothelial dysfunction,[9] this stasis increases the propensity for thrombus formation; approximately, 90% of the thrombi that develop secondary to AF originate in the LAA.[7] This finding, coupled with the clinical need for nonpharmacologic stroke prevention strategies, has led to the development of invasive techniques to anatomically eliminate this vulnerable LAA substrate through mechanical closure.

Several techniques currently exist for LAA closure. Broadly, these techniques can be classified as percutaneous versus surgical. Percutaneous closure is typically performed via a transseptal puncture using femoral venous access, with some techniques also requiring percutaneous subxiphoid epicardial access. Surgical LAA closure typically utilizes either a lateral thoracotomy, lateral thoracoscopic, or median sternotomy approach. Various terms are indiscriminately used in the literature to describe mechanical LAA interventions, including appendage closure, occlusion, exclusion, ligation, and removal. Closure is a general term for the methods described in this chapter. Occlusion specifically refers to the use of an endocardial device to seal the appendage, although exclusion/ligation describes closure via an external ligature. Only open surgical techniques can effectively remove or excise LAA tissue.

Currently, the Watchman device (Boston Scientific, Natick, MA, USA) is the only LAA closure system approved by the US Food and Drug Administration (FDA) for AF–associated stroke prevention. Two randomized trials have compared this therapy to warfarin.[10,11] Collectively, these trials suggest that Watchman implantation is noninferior to warfarin for AF stroke prevention.

Additional devices that utilize a conceptually similar approach and implant technique have been developed, including the Amplatzer Cardiac Plug (Abbott Laboratories, Chicago, IL, USA), and WaveCrest LAA Occlusion System (Coherex Medical, Salt Lake City, UT, USA), but none have received FDA approval as of early 2021. The LARIAT device (SentreHEART, Redwood City, CA, USA) is an alternative approach that uses a suture-based epicardial ligation system that is delivered with simultaneous left atrial endocardial and percutaneous subxiphoid epicardial access. This technology has notably not been evaluated with regard to AF stroke prevention in a prospective, randomized clinical trial. Several open surgical techniques have also been developed for LAA closure, including oversewing the appendage or placement of a mechanical clip on the epicardial surface near the appendage ostium (AtriClip [AtriCure, Mason, OH, USA]).

INDICATIONS

In general, LAA closure is indicated for individuals with an elevated risk of AF–associated thromboembolic stroke and a compelling reason to discontinue or avoid long-term anticoagulant therapy. The threshold used to define an appropriate "elevated risk" will continue to evolve as the long-term efficacy of the LAA closure is better defined and advances in implant technology, technique, and experience influence procedural safety. The CHA_2DS_2-VASc score is the guideline-recommended clinical scoring system used to estimate annual stroke risk among nonanticoagulated patients with AF,[12] and this scoring system plays a central role in defining LAA closure candidacy. While the initial clinical trials evaluating the efficacy of Watchman therapy relative to warfarin enrolled individuals with different minimum stroke risk profiles (including a $CHADS_2$ score ≥ 1 for PROTECT AF [PROTECTion in Patients With Atrial Fibrillation]),[10,11] current US Medicare and private insurer reimbursement protocols only cover Watchman implantation for individuals with a $CHADS_2$ score greater than or equal to 2 or a CHA_2DS_2-VASc score greater than or equal to 3. The stroke risk threshold to justify alternative, non-FDA–approved LAA closure techniques is not defined, although an absolute stroke risk similar to or higher than that used for the Watchman device is likely appropriate. Because surgical LAA closure can be accomplished with minimal additional risk or procedural length during open cardiac surgery performed for other indications, current surgical guidelines indicate that it is reasonable to surgically close the LAA in all patients with a history of AF at the time of their concomitant open surgical procedure, regardless of thromboembolic risk.[13]

In addition to having an elevated AF stroke risk, current candidates for LAA closure should also be identified by their treating clinicians as poor long-term candidates for anticoagulation. Explicit criteria to establish poor anticoagulation candidacy have not been rigorously defined. A prior history of clinically significant bleeding is the main justification for LAA closure, although closure can be considered among individuals who have occupations or hobbies that confer an elevated risk of traumatic bleeding or are at high risk of bleeding due to medical comorbidities (eg, thrombocytopenia or frequent mechanical falls with resultant head trauma).

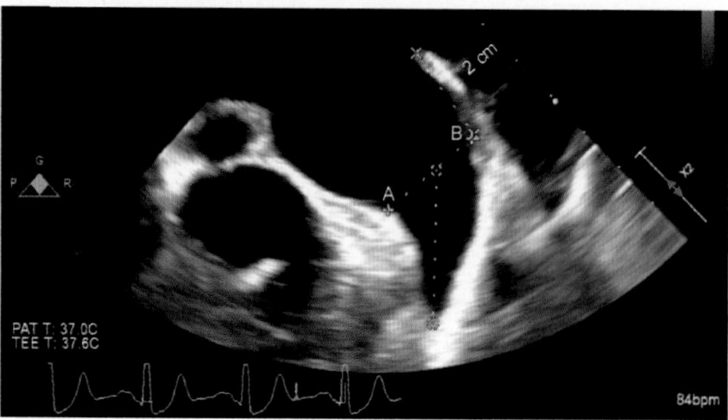

FIGURE 48.1 Measurement of left atrial appendage ostial width by transesophageal echocardiogram. Ostial appendage width should be measured using a transesophageal echocardiogram; the distance between the left circumflex coronary artery/mitral valve annulus **(A)** and a point 2 cm from the tip of the left upper pulmonary vein/LAA ridge **(B)** should be assessed. LAA, left atrial appendage.

ANATOMIC CONSIDERATIONS

The growth and clinical adoption of LAA closure have resulted in renewed interest in appendage anatomy. The internal orifice of the LAA is typically ovoid, although a minority of patients will demonstrate more complex, alternative morphologies.[14] A defined neck usually extends from this orifice, beyond which the body/dominant lobe of the appendage extends and gives rise to a variable number of secondary lobes. Several terms have been used to describe the anatomy of the main appendage body. In general, most appendages demonstrate one of the following four patterns, listed in order of decreasing prevalence: (1) chicken wing, characterized by a sharp bend in the dominant lobe in its proximal or middle portion; (2) cactus, with multiple branches arising from the dominant lobe; (3) windsock, with a relatively straight dominant lobe; or (4) cauliflower, distinguished by complex branching of multiple lobes without a dominant central lobe.[15]

The Watchman device currently comes in five sizes (21, 24, 27, 30, and 33 mm), and individuals with an appendage ostium that is less than 17 mm or greater than 31 mm are not currently candidates for closure with this device. As the Watchman device is circular, it may prove difficult or impossible to circumferentially occlude appendages with severely eccentric ostial shapes. Ostial width should be measured using transesophageal echocardiography (TEE); the distance between the left circumflex coronary artery/mitral valve annulus and a point 2 cm from the tip of the left upper pulmonary vein/LAA ridge should be assessed at 0, 45, 90, and 135° transducer angles (**Figure 48.1**). The device is considered "square" in its dimensions, as the length of the device is identical to the maximal ostial diameter. For this reason, appendages with ostial diameters that substantially exceed the depth of the dominant lobe, as is more commonly seen in a chicken wing and cauliflower morphologies, can be particularly challenging to safely and successfully close. Device size selection must therefore incorporate maximal ostial width, appendage depth, and overall appendage anatomy. The device should be compressed between 8% and 20% once successfully implanted to mitigate the risk of embolization. To achieve adequate compression, a device diameter of 5 to 7 mm larger than the maximally measured ostial diameter is typically chosen, provided the appendage depth is also adequate.

The next-generation Watchman FLX device, approved, and currently available overcomes some of the limitations of the previous generation Watchman device. The Watchman FLX comes in five sizes (20, 24, 27, 31, and 35 mm) for ostia measuring 15 to 32 mm, allowing closure of both smaller and larger LAA ostia compared with the current Watchman device. Additionally, because of the redesign of the profile and fixation struts of the Watchman FLX, only 10 mm of LAA depth is required, making the device more amenable to LAA morphologies where the ostium width is greater than the depth of the dominant lobe.

The LARIAT snare is 50 mm in diameter, and attempted closure is not safe when the maximal appendage diameter exceeds this dimension. Some individuals with ostial diameters too large to be closed with a Watchman device (>31 mm) may be candidates for this technique. Because of technical aspects of LARIAT implant, the LAA cannot be closed when the distal tip of the appendage is posteriorly directed or when it lies behind the pulmonary artery.

FUNDAMENTALS OF LEFT ATRIAL APPENDAGE CLOSURE

Preprocedure

It should be emphasized that Watchman LAA closure is best considered as a treatment *strategy* rather than a single invasive procedure for stroke reduction. Patients who receive this device require postimplant TEE imaging and months of anticoagulation or antiplatelet therapy to prevent thrombus formation during implant endothelialization. Before proceeding with device implantation, it is crucial that patients understand this postprocedure regimen. Detailed counseling and thoughtful patient selection are especially important with respect to the postprocedure anticoagulation regimen, as the very nature of Watchman candidacy implies a heightened risk of bleeding complication. If a patient is determined to have an absolute contraindication to anticoagulant or antiplatelet therapy, remaining closure options include percutaneous LAA ligation or open surgical closure.

Intraprocedure

Transseptal puncture location is critically important for the success of the procedure. Because of the anterior and superior orientation of the dominant lobe in most appendages, puncture of the fossa ovalis in an inferior and posterior location is necessary to allow for catheter manipulation and coaxial orientation of the delivery sheath and appendage (**Figure 48.2**). In cases where it is difficult to place the delivery sheath into an appropriate lobe, repeat transseptal access should be considered, especially if review of the initial attempt suggests a lower or more posterior puncture can be safely obtained.

The operator should have a complete understanding of the appendage anatomy before selecting and deploying the device. This will require the integration of both the TEE and fluoroscopic images. These imaging modalities are complementary and, when used together, will ensure adequate device sizing. As echocardiographic measurements can underestimate the ostial diameter and depth of the appendage, careful attention to fluoroscopic assessment of these dimensions is important. In addition to using the depth measurement markers on the access sheath, fluoroscopic estimation of LAA ostial diameter can be quickly performed by remembering that the access sheath is approximately 5 mm in width. Many patients presenting for this procedure will have had a prior contrast-enhanced chest computed tomographic (CT) scan for unrelated clinical care; these studies should also be reviewed. In some cases, three dimensional (3D) reconstruction of appendage anatomy may be possible, which gives the operator further insight into the often-complex structure of the appendage.

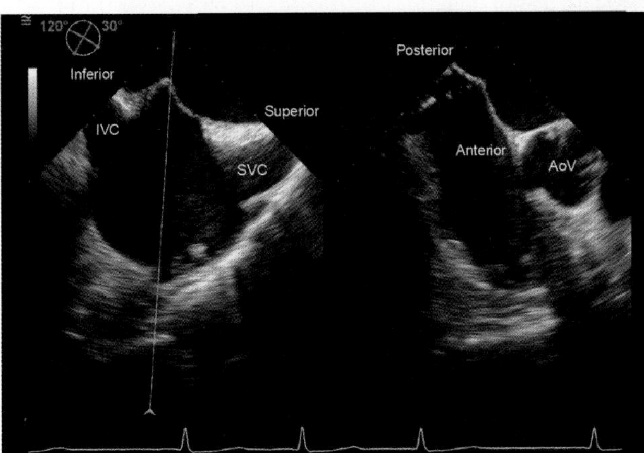

FIGURE 48.2 Transesophageal echocardiogram–guided transseptal puncture. Because of the anterior and superior orientation of the dominant lobe in most appendages, puncture of the fossa ovalis in an inferior and posterior location is necessary to allow for catheter manipulation and coaxial orientation of the delivery sheath and appendage. Bicaval (left) and short-axis (right) transesophageal echocardiographic views are helpful for guiding the puncture. AoV, aortic valve; IVC, inferior vena cava; SVC, superior vena cava.

CLINICAL APPLICATIONS

Watchman Methodology

Most patients undergo a preprocedure screening TEE in the weeks before implant to confirm that appendage anatomy is appropriate for closure. The necessity of this preprocedure imaging is debatable, as a TEE is also performed at the time of device implantation. Omitting this preprocedure TEE may improve patient convenience, reduce overall healthcare costs, and slightly diminish patient risk. On the other hand, obtaining a screening TEE allows for the early identification of patients with anatomy that is either difficult or not feasible to close. This allows for more tailored preprocedure patient counseling, discussion of alternative closure techniques if necessary, more efficient patient flow in the procedure laboratory, and avoidance of preprocedure anticoagulation in high-risk patients who cannot be treated with a Watchman device.

We typically perform Watchman implantation with the patient taking uninterrupted anticoagulation to minimize the risk of LAA thrombus.[16] For individuals not already on anticoagulation, this therapy is usually started 1 week before implant. It should be noted that the randomized trials establishing the clinical efficacy of Watchman were performed with periprocedure warfarin, although observational data suggests direct oral anticoagulation (DOAC) therapy is also reasonable from a safety and efficacy standpoint.[16] Warfarin is continued with a target international normalized ratio (INR) of less than 3.0 on the morning of the procedure, although DOAC dosing is held the morning of the implant (last dose the evening before the procedure). Aspirin 81 mg daily is started the day before implant. Watchman implantation is performed under general anesthesia to facilitate paralysis and apnea during device deployment. Before femoral access, a TEE is performed to exclude LAA thrombus and to measure ostial LAA diameter (Figure 48.1). As above, ostial diameter measurements are made in the 0, 45, 90, and 135° transducer planes and the maximum diameter is used for sizing.

Ultrasound-guided right femoral vein access is obtained, and a short 11 Fr sheath is inserted. The use of the 11 Fr short sheath results in predilation at the femoral venotomy site and allows for easy insertion of the 14 Fr access sheath. We then administer a bolus of heparin before transseptal puncture, targeting an activated clotting time (ACT) of 300 seconds. Transseptal puncture is performed with an SL0 sheath that has been inserted through the 11 Fr short sheath. As noted above, we target an inferior and posterior transseptal puncture location within the fossa ovalis. Bicaval and short-axis TEE views are helpful for guiding the puncture (Figure 48.2). After transseptal puncture, left atrial pressure is measured through the SL0 sheath. If required, intravenous fluid is administered to obtain a left atrial pressure greater than or equal to 10 mm Hg; this will ensure that the LAA is adequately distended and helps to avoid undersizing the device. A 0.035" exchange length, extra stiff J wire is then positioned within the left upper pulmonary vein (LUPV). The SL0 sheath and 11 Fr short sheaths are then removed over this wire and replaced with the Watchman access sheath. The J wire in the LUPV can be visualized on TEE, allowing for most of the sheath exchange to occur with real-time confirmation of wire stability but without fluoroscopic exposure. In most cases, a double-curved access sheath shape is used.

A 5 Fr angled pigtail catheter is then inserted into the access sheath and is positioned within the LAA using a combination of fluoroscopic and echocardiographic guidance. The angulation of the pigtail is necessary to manipulate the catheter into the appendage. Appendage anatomy is then defined using hand injection of intravenous contrast in an RAO 30° caudal 15 to 20° projection. This fluoroscopic information is complementary to the echocardiographic data, and it is very helpful for sizing determination. This RAO caudal view roughly corresponds to the 135° view on TEE. The tip of the access catheter is then advanced, using the pigtail catheter as a rail, to the distal aspect of the most anterior and superior lobe of the appendage. To prevent traumatic injury of the appendage, the access sheath should never be advanced beyond the distal curvature of the pigtail catheter. Continuous application of counterclockwise torque is often needed to maintain the tip of the access sheath in the superior/anterior appendage.

An appropriately sized Watchman device is then prepped using serial saline flushes to eliminate all trapped air. Slight retraction/advancement of the delivery knob should be performed to ensure the device is engaged with the core wire. Before insertion of the delivery sheath into the access sheath, the distal aspect of the constrained device should align with the distal marker band on the delivery sheath. Under apnea, the pigtail catheter is removed, the Watchman delivery sheath is inserted into the access sheath until the distal markers align, and the device is then deployed by slowly unsheathing the delivery sheath via retraction of the access sheath. As the device exits the access sheath, its architecture results in immediate self-expansion. Apnea is used to minimize movement within the thorax while manipulating the sheaths and device in the appendage without the protection afforded by the pigtail catheter, reducing the risk of cardiac perforation/tamponade (**Figure 48.3**).

After device delivery, assessment for compression, appropriate positioning, and adequate seal is performed using TEE (both 2D and color Doppler imaging) in the 0, 45, 90, and 135° views (**Figure 48.4**). To ensure accurate assessment of maximal compression, measurements should be taken in a plane that also images the central threaded insert. Hand injection of contrast through the access sheath against the face of the device is recommended to further exclude leak and to ensure closure of proximal lobes that may be missed by TEE (Figure 48.3). If the device is too distal in the appendage, a partial recapture may be performed under apnea. This is accomplished by using the access sheath to

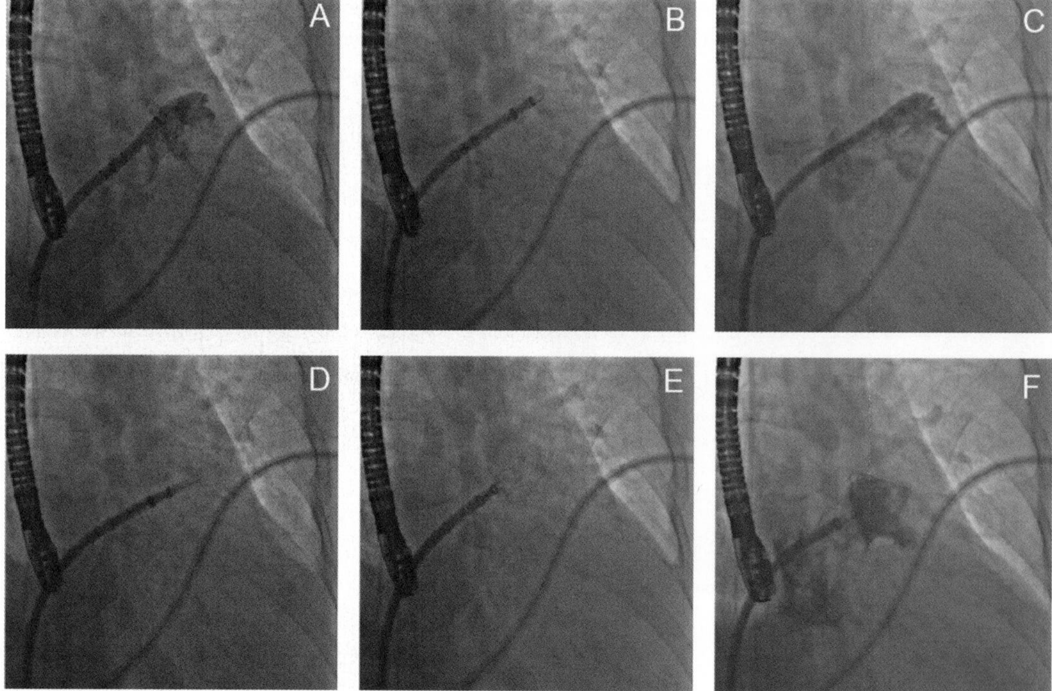

FIGURE 48.3 Watchman deployment under fluoroscopic guidance. **A.** Hand injection of contrast material through the pigtail catheter delineates appendage anatomy. After injection, the access sheath is further advanced over the pigtail catheter into the most superior/interbranch of the appendage. **B-E.** The device is deployed by withdrawing the access sheath. During deployment, contrast material can be injected **(C)** to understand the relationship between the Watchman device and the appendage borders. After deploying the device **(F)**, contrast agent injection demonstrates an ostial position with coverage of all lobes. All views are in a right anterior oblique projection with 15° of caudal angulation.

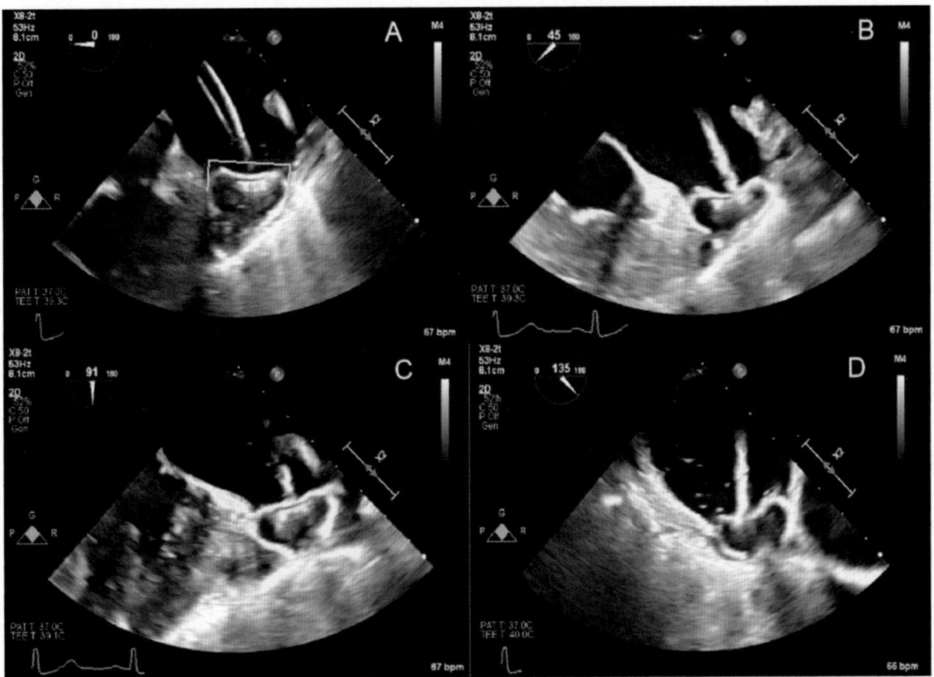

FIGURE 48.4 Post-deployment Watchman transesophageal echocardiographic evaluation. After device delivery, assessment for compression, appropriate positioning, and adequate seal is performed using transesophageal echocardiography in the 0° **(A)**, 45° **(B)**, 90° **(C)**, and 135° **(D)** views. To ensure accurate assessment of maximal compression, diameter measurements (**A**, yellow line) should be obtained in a plane that also images the central threaded insert.

collapse the shoulders of the device, slightly retracting the entire assembly, then redeploying the device. If the device is positioned too proximally, a full recapture should be performed under apnea and a new device should be used. Depending on patient anatomy and implant depth, the device may exhibit a "shoulder" at the appendage ostium. While a slight shoulder is acceptable if the device is otherwise well seated, it is important to remember that the fabric cap only covers the proximal half of the device and a large shoulder may result in a residual leak around the cap (**Figure 48.5**).

After confirming appropriate positioning, a tug test is performed. With the hemostasis valve completely loosened and the access sheath withdrawn from the face of the device, gentle traction should then be applied to the deployment knob. This "tug" should result in slight movement of the device on fluoroscopy or TEE with a spontaneous return to its initial position. In some instances, this test will slightly improve the position of a device that was initially implanted too deeply. If the device moves too proximally on TEE, repositioning or device upsizing is necessary.

Fulfillment of the PASS criteria (position, anchor, size, and seal) should be confirmed before the final deployment of the device. For **position**, the proximal aspect of the device should sit at the appendage ostium and cover all lobes. **Anchor** criteria are fulfilled by documenting the stability of the device after the tug test. The **size** of the device should be between 80% and 92% of the nominal diameter (8%-20% compressed), and this should be confirmed in all four TEE views (0, 45, 90, 135°). Finally, the adequate **seal** is defined as the absence or minimal flow (<5 mm) around the device using TEE color Doppler and fluoroscopic contrast injection.

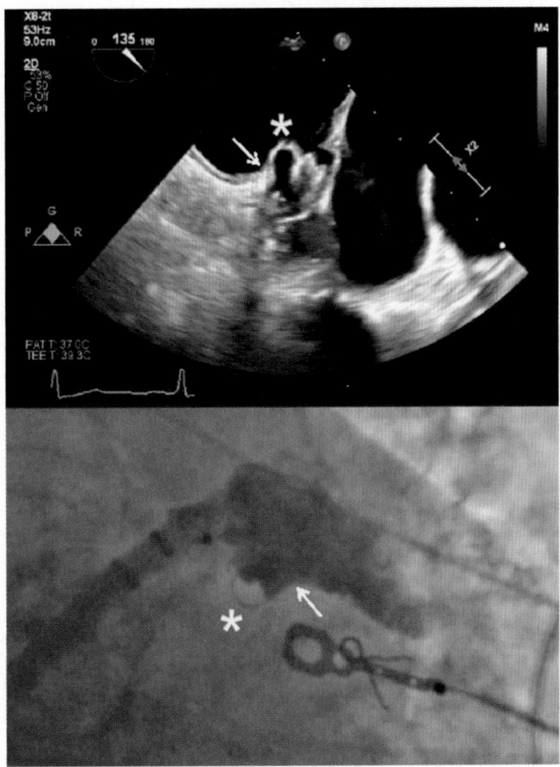

FIGURE 48.5 Unacceptable Watchman device shoulder. An example of a Watchman device placed too proximally, resulting in a large inferior shoulder (*) that extends far beyond the appendage ostium (arrow). This particular device was recaptured and repositioned.

SECTION 3

After all PASS criteria are confirmed, the device is released by rotating the deployment knob approximately five revolutions in a counterclockwise direction. The delivery sheath and core wire are then completely withdrawn into the access sheath, which is pulled back across the septum and into the inferior vena cava. We use the combination of a 0-silk, figure-of-eight suture, and manual compression to achieve hemostasis without heparin reversal.

Postprocedure, patients maintain a supine position for 4 to 6 hours to ensure hemostasis. The figure-of-eight suture is typically removed the following morning. Anticoagulation and aspirin 81 mg PO are restarted the evening of the procedure. Patients are typically observed overnight and discharged to home the following morning.

LARIAT Methodology

A preprocedure CT scan is necessary to assess LAA anatomy, to exclude patients with an appendage apex that is directed either posteriorly or superiorly behind the pulmonary artery, and to ensure that the maximal appendage diameter is less than 50 mm. The implant procedure is performed under general anesthesia with TEE guidance. Subxiphoid epicardial access is obtained using an anterior approach with anterior–posterior (AP) and cross-table lateral fluoroscopic views. The optimal epicardial needle access angle in an AP view can be estimated from the CT scan; the needle and subsequent sheath should be directed just lateral to the apex of the LAA (toward the left shoulder). The epicardium should be entered approximately 2 cm above the left ventricular apex. The use of a 21-gauge micropuncture needle for epicardial puncture has been shown to reduce procedural complications.[17] After serial dilation, a 14 Fr epicardial sheath is inserted into the pericardial space. Systemic anticoagulation is then administered using heparin targeting an ACT of 300 seconds. Transseptal puncture is then performed with insertion of an SL1 sheath. After left atrial access is obtained, contrast is injected through the sheath to visualize the appendage. An EndoCATH balloon occlusion catheter (AtriCure, Mason, OH, USA) containing a 0.025" magnet-tipped wire is placed through the SL1 sheath, and the magnet is maneuvered into the most superior and anterior aspect of the LAA. Placing a slight bend at the distal centimeter of the magnet wire can help with magnet maneuverability. A magnet-tipped 0.035" wire is then placed through the epicardial sheath. The epicardial magnet is advanced until the two magnets connect. The rail provided by the two magnet wires is used to guide the LARIAT suture device over the appendage (**Figure 48.6**). The EndoCATH balloon is then inflated to mark the LAA ostium. The snare is closed near the ostium of the appendage and endocardial closure of the appendage is confirmed using TEE and contrast injection under fluoroscopic imaging. The balloon is then deflated, and the endocardial magnet/catheter assembly is withdrawn into the left atrium. The suture is then fully deployed with two applications of the TenSURE tensioning system performed 5 minutes apart. The LARIAT handle must be held in a stable position while tensioning the suture to avoid tearing the appendage. Finally, the suture is cut in the pericardial space near the appendage using a suture cutter that is advanced over the

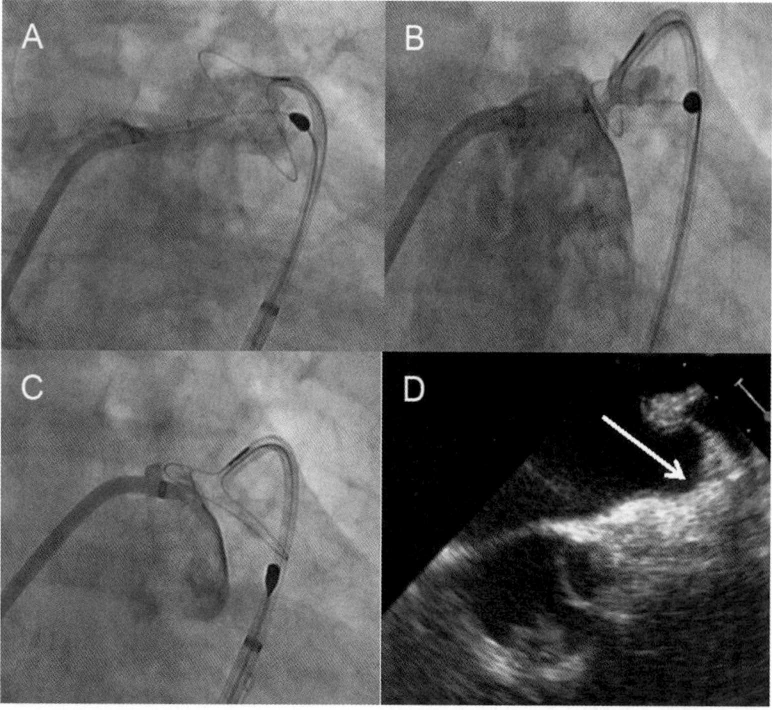

FIGURE 48.6 LARIAT delivery. **A.** Injection of contrast through the endocardial sheath. The endocardial and epicardial wires are connected, and the LARIAT suture device is advanced over the appendage. **B.** The snare is tightened around the appendage ostium. **C.** After suture delivery, endocardial contrast injection demonstrates that the appendage is completely closed. **D.** Transesophageal echocardiographic imaging confirms complete closure of the appendage (white arrow).

suture tail. A pigtail catheter is usually left in the pericardial space overnight. It is removed the following morning if drainage is less than 50 mL during a 12-hour period and after a TTE document the absence of a pericardial effusion.

Case Presentation

A 61-year-old woman was admitted to the hospital after suffering a stroke. Ambulatory monitoring after hospital discharge demonstrated paroxysmal AF. Additional stroke risk factors included hypertension and diabetes. She was not immediately started on anticoagulation because of a history of gastric arteriovenous malformations that had resulted in prior gastrointestinal bleeding. She was referred for Watchman implant in light of her CHA_2DS_2-VASc score of 5 (hypertension, diabetes, prior stroke, female gender) and poor candidacy for long-term anticoagulation. A preimplant TEE demonstrated appropriate appendage anatomy (Figure 48.2), including an appendage depth greater than ostial width. Warfarin was started 1 week before the procedure, and aspirin was started the day before the procedure. A 24-mm Watchman device was implanted (Figures 48.3 and 48.4). Her postprocedure course was uneventful, and she was discharged home the following day on warfarin and aspirin.

LIMITATIONS

Not all thromboembolic strokes related to AF arise from the LAA. As it is well recognized that anticoagulation does not completely eliminate the risk of thromboembolism, it also must be acknowledged that closure of the LAA will not prevent embolism of an intracardiac thrombus that forms at a site remote from the appendage (eg, nonappendage left atrium due to "atrial myopathy" or the left ventricle in the setting of systolic dysfunction). LAA closure will similarly not impact strokes due to noncardioembolic etiologies, including aortic and cerebral atherosclerotic disease.

The optimal duration of anticoagulant and antiplatelet therapy following Watchman LAA occlusion remains to be defined. Until the endothelialization of the Watchman device is complete, the exposed titanium threaded insert and the polyethylene terephthalate fabric cap may serve as the nidus for thrombus formation if anticoagulant/antiplatelet therapy is prematurely discontinued. Notably, there is observational data to suggest that patients treated with dual antiplatelet therapy alone after Watchman implantation have a similar risk of postprocedure stroke compared with patients treated with the usual anticoagulation/antiplatelet regimen.[18] Further investigation is ongoing.

While successful LAA closure allows patients to stop anticoagulation and therefore minimizes/eliminates the heightened risk of bleeding with long-term anticoagulation, this benefit is offset by the acute risk of procedural complication and periprocedural bleeding. Notably, in a meta-analysis that combined 5 years of patient-level data from the PROTECT AF and PREVAIL (Prospective Randomized EVAluatIon of the Watchman Left atrial appendage closure device in patients with atrial fibrillation versus long-term warfarin therapy) randomized trials, the overall risk of major bleeding was 3.1% with Watchman compared with 3.5% with warfarin (P = .60).[19] It was only after the exclusion of periprocedural bleeding events that the difference in the rate of major bleeding was statistically significant between treatment groups (**Table 48.1**). This highlights the importance of procedural safety and is a reminder that the overall benefit of LAA closure can be eliminated in the setting of procedural complication rates that exceed those observed in the Watchman clinical trials. The PINNACLE FLX study evaluated the safety and effectiveness of the next-generation Watchman FLX LAA closure device in patients with nonvalvular AF in whom anticoagulation is indicated, but who have an appropriate rationale to seek a nonpharmaceutical alternative. This study reported that LAA closure with this next-generation LAA closure device was associated with a low incidence of adverse events and a high incidence of anatomic closure.[20]

Residual leak between the LAA and the left atrium is observed in up to one-third of patients after Watchman implantation.[21] The optimal management of these leaks are not completely defined. Continued anticoagulation is recommended when the residual leak is more than 5 mm in diameter (**Figure 48.7**), although a retrospective analysis notably did not demonstrate a conclusive association between

TABLE 48.1 Combined Event Rates from the PREVAIL and PROTECT AF Trials

	Rate (per 100 patient-years)		
	Watchman	Warfarin	
Outcome	n = 732	n = 382	P
Stroke or systemic embolism	1.7%	1.8%	0.87
Major bleeding, all	3.1%	3.5%	0.60
Major bleeding, periprocedural excluded	1.7%	3.6%	0.0003
All cause death	3.6%	4.9%	0.035

Adapted from Reddy VY, Doshi SK, Kar S, et al. 5-Year Outcomes After Left Atrial Appendage Closure: From the PREVAIL and PROTECT AF Trials. *J Am Coll Cardiol.* 2017;70(24):2964-2975. Copyright © 2017 Elsevier. With permission.

SECTION 3

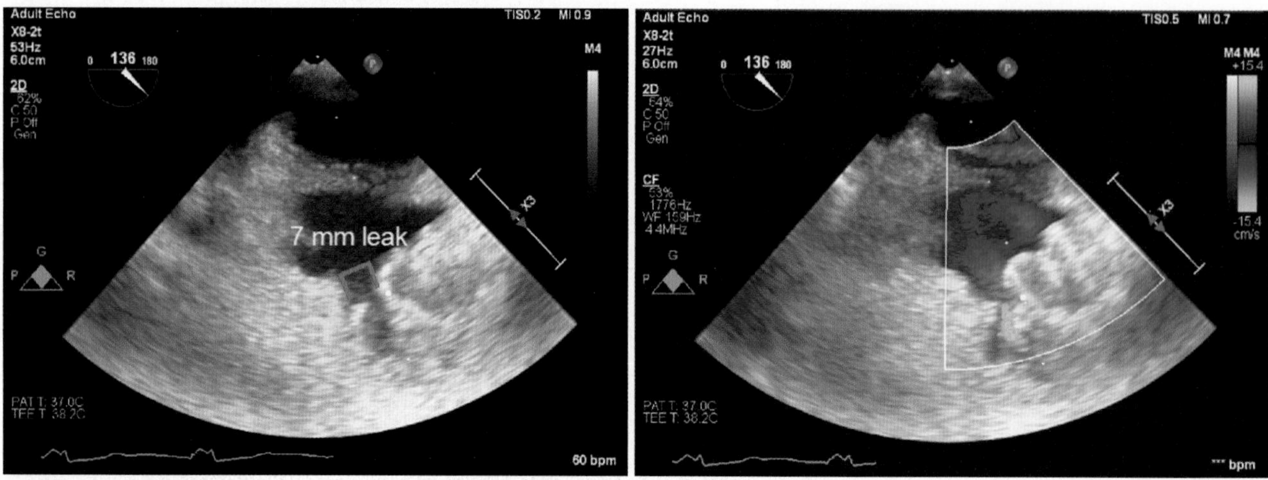

FIGURE 48.7 Residual left atrial appendage leak after Watchman implantation. Transesophageal echocardiography images demonstrate a residual left atrial appendage leak (>5 mm) seen at 6 weeks of follow-up.

stroke outcomes and either the presence or size of the residual leak.[21] Closure of the residual leak can be considered in individuals who are at high-thromboembolic risk and cannot be continued on anticoagulation, although the size of leak prompting intervention and the optimal closure device (eg, endovascular coil, vascular plug, septal occluder) has yet to be determined.[22]

Percutaneous left atrial closure using a snare device requires epicardial access for delivery of the suture over the appendage. Individuals who have previously undergone cardiac surgery are poor candidates for this procedure because of the resultant dense pericardial adhesions. For similar reasons, percutaneous epicardial access may not be possible in patients with prior pericarditis or left-sided chest/breast radiation therapy. Severe obesity and pectus excavatum may also limit the ability to obtain epicardial access.

SPECIAL CONSIDERATIONS AND CONTRAINDICATIONS

The presence of an LAA thrombus, as identified using either the pre- or intraprocedural TEE, is an absolute contraindication to percutaneous closure. As percutaneous closure devices require transseptal puncture for left atrial access, prior closure of an atrial septal defect, especially when this was accomplished using a large occluder device that completely covers the fossa ovalis, may limit the ability to safely and successfully perform transseptal puncture.

When measuring the LAA ostial diameter and selecting the appropriate Watchman device, there is a tendency to choose the largest feasible device size to ensure adequate compression and maximize stability. Compression of the device more than 30%, however, should be avoided. Potential risks of device oversizing include excessive or potentially harmful radial pressure on the surrounding atrial/ostial appendage tissue and wrinkling of the fabric cap, which may result in an inadequate seal.

For patients who have undergone LAA closure and require cardioversion for AF management, the optimal anticoagulation and imaging protocol remain unclear. Initial data using a precardioversion TEE to exclude thrombus followed by cardioversion without further anticoagulation has been shown to have a reasonable safety profile, although confirmatory studies are necessary.[23]

It should be recognized that individuals at very high risk of bleeding complication, including those who are likely to derive the greatest benefit from mechanical LAA closure, may not be able to tolerate the recommended Watchman postimplant anticoagulant and antiplatelet regimen. Because neither percutaneous nor open surgical LAA ligation techniques leave foreign material in contact with the blood pool, these strategies do not require postprocedure anticoagulation. Despite the current absence of evidence supporting their efficacy, percutaneous, or stand-alone open surgical LAA ligation procedures are, therefore, still considered and performed among certain high-risk patients who cannot tolerate the Watchman postimplant anticoagulation/antiplatelet protocol.

FOLLOW-UP PATIENT CARE

All Watchman patients have discharged on daily oral anticoagulation and aspirin 81 mg. A repeat TEE is performed after 45 days. After documenting the absence of left atrial thrombus and adequate LAA seal (defined as no peridevice leak >5 mm), anticoagulation can be stopped. Aspirin is increased to 325 mg by mouth daily, and clopidogrel 75 mg by mouth daily is administered for a total of 6 months postimplant. Continued aspirin is currently recommended by the manufacturer.

All LARIAT patients should be discharged on colchicine 0.6 mg twice daily. This should be continued for approximately 4 weeks to minimize pericardial pain and to reduce the risk of Dressler syndrome/pericardial effusion.

RESEARCH AND FUTURE DIRECTIONS

As additional LAA closure devices gain FDA approval for AF–associated stroke prevention, comparative trials will be necessary to determine, which techniques provide the optimal risk/benefit profile. It is also important to remember that the PROTECT AF[11] and PREVAIL[10] trials were conducted in an era when warfarin was the dominant AF anticoagulation strategy. Because DOAC therapy has been shown to be both more effective and safer than warfarin,[24] further research is necessary to determine if Watchman LAA closure is noninferior to this class of anticoagulants. In addition, the LAA has been shown to play an important role in AF pathogenesis.[25] Percutaneous LAA ligation, in contrast to percutaneous endocardial occlusion techniques, results in necrosis and electrical quiescence of the LAA tissue.[26] An ongoing randomized clinical trial with the LARIAT device (aMAZE trial, ClinicalTrials.gov, Registration No. NCT02513797) is currently underway to evaluate whether this treatment improves AF outcomes when combined with pulmonary vein isolation.[27]

KEY POINTS

- ✔ It is important for patients to understand that Watchman LAA closure, in its current form, is a longitudinal treatment strategy that requires multiple procedures (at a minimum, the implant procedure, and a 45-day post-procedure TEE) and 6 months of postimplant anticoagulation/antiplatelet therapy.
- ✔ Understanding appendage anatomy is important for screening patients and for intraprocedural decision making.
- ✔ Echocardiography and fluoroscopy provide complementary intraprocedural data; familiarity with both modalities is critical for optimal and efficient device delivery.
- ✔ A posterior and inferior transseptal locations are usually necessary to facilitate efficient device delivery.
- ✔ For patients in whom percutaneous LAA closure is not possible or is unsuccessful, surgical closure options exist, although these techniques are more invasive, and there is currently sparse data supporting their efficacy for stroke prevention.

REFERENCES

1. Wolf PA, Dawber TR, Thomas HE, Kannel WB. Epidemiologic assessment of chronic atrial fibrillation and risk of stroke: the Framingham study. *Neurology.* 1978;28(10):973-977.
2. Warfarin versus aspirin for prevention of thromboembolism in atrial fibrillation: stroke prevention in atrial fibrillation II study. *Lancet.* 1994;343(8899):687-691.
3. Granger CB, Alexander JH, McMurray JJ, et al. Apixaban versus warfarin in patients with atrial fibrillation. *N Engl J Med.* 2011;365(11):981-992.
4. Hart RG, Pearce LA, Aguilar MI. Meta-analysis: antithrombotic therapy to prevent stroke in patients who have nonvalvular atrial fibrillation. *Ann Intern Med.* 2007;146(12):857-867.
5. Connolly SJ, Ezekowitz MD, Yusuf S, et al. Dabigatran versus warfarin in patients with atrial fibrillation. *N Engl J Med.* 2009;361(12):1139-1151.
6. Patel MR, Mahaffey KW, Garg J, et al. Rivaroxaban versus warfarin in nonvalvular atrial fibrillation. *N Engl J Med.* 2011;365(10):883-891.
7. Blackshear JL, Odell JA. Appendage obliteration to reduce stroke in cardiac surgical patients with atrial fibrillation. *Ann Thorac Surg.* 1996;61(2):755-759.
8. Stoddard MF, Dawkins PR, Prince CR, Ammash NM. Left atrial appendage thrombus is not uncommon in patients with acute atrial fibrillation and a recent embolic event: a transesophageal echocardiographic study. *J Am Coll Cardiol.* 1995;25(2):452-459.
9. Guazzi M, Arena R. Endothelial dysfunction and pathophysiological correlates in atrial fibrillation. *Heart.* 2009;95(2):102-106.
10. Holmes DR, Kar S, Price MJ, et al. Prospective randomized evaluation of the Watchman Left Atrial Appendage Closure device in patients with atrial fibrillation versus long-term warfarin therapy: the PREVAIL trial. *J Am Coll Cardiol.* 2014;64(1):1-12.
11. Holmes DR, Reddy VY, Turi ZG, et al. Percutaneous closure of the left atrial appendage versus warfarin therapy for prevention of stroke in patients with atrial fibrillation: a randomized non-inferiority trial. *Lancet.* 2009;374(9689):534-542.
12. January CT, Wann LS, Calkins H, et al. 2019 AHA/ACC/HRS focused update of the 2014 AHA/ACC/HRS guideline for the management of patients with atrial fibrillation: a report of the American College of Cardiology/American Heart Association Task Force on Clinical Practice Guidelines and the Heart Rhythm Society. *J Am Coll Cardiol.* 2019;74(1):104-132.
13. Badhwar V, Rankin JS, Damiano RJ, et al. The Society of Thoracic Surgeons 2017 clinical practice guidelines for the surgical treatment of atrial fibrillation. *Ann Thorac Surg.* 2017;103(1):329-341.
14. Wang Y, Di Biase L, Horton RP, Nguyen T, Morhanty P, Natale A. Left atrial appendage studied by computed tomography to help planning for appendage closure device placement. *J Cardiovasc Electrophysiol.* 2010;21(9):973-982.
15. Di Biase L, Santangeli P, Anselmino M, et al. Does the left atrial appendage morphology correlate with the risk of stroke in patients with atrial fibrillation? Results from a multicenter study. *J Am Coll Cardiol.* 2012;60(6):531-538.
16. Enomoto Y, Gadiyaram VK, Gianni C, et al. Use of non-warfarin oral anticoagulants instead of warfarin during left atrial appendage closure with the Watchman device. *Heart Rhythm.* 2017;14(1):19-24.
17. Gunda S, Reddy M, Pillarisetti J, et al. Differences in complication rates between large-bore needle and a long micropuncture needle during epicardial access: time to change clinical practice? *Circ Arrhythm Electrophysiol.* 2015;8(4):890-895.
18. Reddy VY, Mobius-Winkler S, Miller MA, et al. Left atrial appendage closure with the Watchman device in patients with a contraindication for oral anticoagulation: the ASAP study (ASA Plavix Feasibility Study With Watchman Left Atrial Appendage Closure Technology). *J Am Coll Cardiol.* 2013;61(25):2551-2556.
19. Reddy VY, Doshi SK, Kar S, et al. 5-year outcomes after left atrial appendage closure: from the PREVAIL and PROTECT AF trials. *J Am Coll Cardiol.* 2017;70(24):2964-2975.
20. Kar S, Doshi SK, Sadhu A, et al. Primary outcome evaluation of a next generation left atrial appendage closure device: results from the PINNACLE FLX trial. *Circulation.* 2021;143(18):1754-1762. doi:10.1161/CIRCULATIONAHA.120.050117
21. Viles-Gonzalez JF, Kar S, Douglas P, et al. The clinical impact of incomplete left atrial appendage closure with the Watchman Device in patients with atrial fibrillation: a PROTECT AF (Percutaneous Closure of the Left Atrial Appendage Versus Warfarin Therapy for Prevention of Stroke in Patients With Atrial Fibrillation) substudy. *J Am Coll Cardiol.* 2012;59(10):923-929.

SECTION 3

22. Della Rocca DG, Horton RP, Di Biase L, et al. First experience of transcatheter leak occlusion with detachable coils following left atrial appendage closure. *JACC Cardiovasc Interv.* 2020;13(3):306-319.
23. Sharma SP, Turagam MK, Gopinathannair R, et al. Direct current cardioversion of atrial fibrillation in patients with left atrial appendage occlusion devices. *J Am Coll Cardiol.* 2019;74(18):2267-2274.
24. Lopez-Lopez JA, Sterne JAC, Thom HHZ, et al. Oral anticoagulants for prevention of stroke in atrial fibrillation: systematic review, network meta-analysis, and cost effectiveness analysis. *BMJ.* 2017;359:j5058.
25. Di Biase L, Burkhardt JD, Mohanty P, et al. Left atrial appendage: an underrecognized trigger site of atrial fibrillation. *Circulation.* 2010;122(2):109-118.
26. Han FT, Bartus K, Lakkireddy D, et al. The effects of LAA ligation on LAA electrical activity. *Heart Rhythm.* 2014;11(5):864-870.
27. Lee RJ, Lakkireddy D, Mittal S, et al. Percutaneous alternative to the Maze procedure for the treatment of persistent or long-standing persistent atrial fibrillation (aMAZE trial): rationale and design. *Am Heart J.* 2015;170(6):1184-1194.

SECTION 4

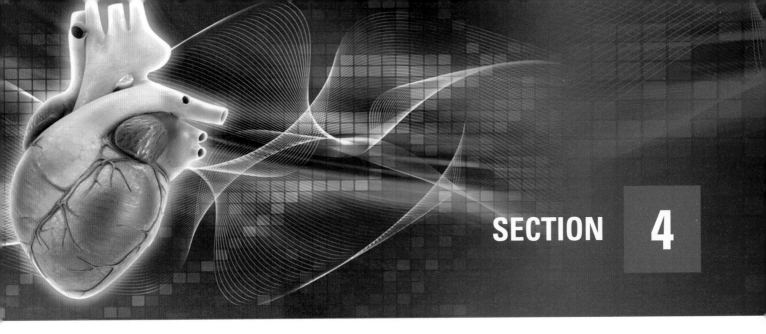

ELECTROPHYSIOLOGY

SECTION EDITOR: Kalyanam Shivkumar

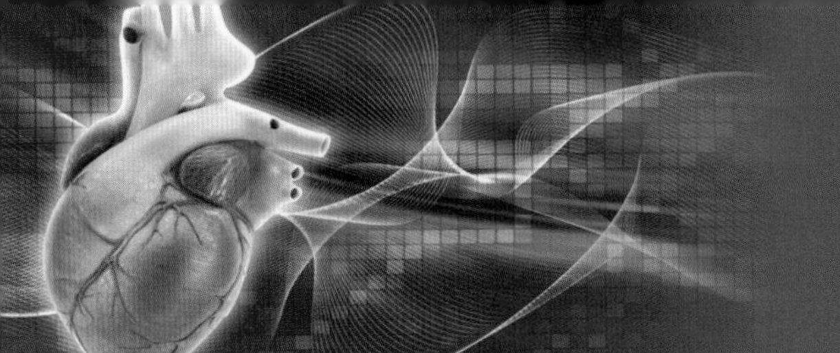

CHAPTER 49

THE ELECTROCARDIOGRAM

Duc H. Do and Noel G. Boyle

INTRODUCTION

The electrocardiogram (ECG) is one of the main diagnostic tools of the clinician, whether in the clinic, emergency department, or hospital. The first ECG machine was developed by William Einthoven in 1901 in Leiden, the Netherlands, for which he received the 1924 Nobel Prize in Medicine. Since then the ECG has undergone many improvements, including an increase in the number of leads recorded, electrical noise filtering, automated algorithms for ECG interpretation, and miniaturization of the necessary equipment. But it fundamentally performs the same task: recording the electrical activity of the heart.[1]

INDICATIONS

The ECG has many applications. A standard 12-lead ECG records a 10-second snapshot of the heart's electrical activity. This is useful in diagnosing causes of chest pain, including myocardial infarction, causes of palpitation, including supraventricular and ventricular arrhythmias, causes of syncope, including tachyarrhythmias and bradyarrhythmias and other conduction abnormalities. Continuous ECG recording can be used to monitor a patient's cardiac electrical activity in the hospital, a procedural suite (operating room, catheterization lab, etc.), or in the outpatient setting and to alert for the presence of ischemia, arrhythmias, and QT interval prolongation following the administration of certain medications.[2] Stress ECGs utilize continuous ECG monitoring during treadmill exercise or simulated pharmacologic stress to detect signs of ischemia. Continuous ambulatory ECG monitoring can be used to record cardiac rhythm on a patient at home for periods between 24 hours and 1 month to diagnose causes of palpitations and/or syncope. ECG recording is also combined with other types of testing to correlate cardiac electrical activity and other organ functions, such as in sleep studies and electroencephalography. A new application of a body vest of 224 electrodes, called ECG imaging (ECGI), has also been in use in recent years predominantly in the evaluation and research of arrhythmias.

Use of the ECG can be broadly defined as for both diagnostic and screening purposes. Specific populations where screening ECGs have been advocated include elderly patients at risk of atrial fibrillation who may benefit from anticoagulation for stroke prevention, competitive athletes to evaluate for genetic abnormalities (ie, long QT syndrome, Brugada syndrome, hypertrophic cardiomyopathy, arrhythmogenic right ventricular cardiomyopathy), which may increase the risk of sudden cardiac death during exercise, and individuals in high-risk occupations such as military service and pilots to evaluate for the preceding conditions and other abnormalities such as Wolff-Parkinson-White (WPW) pattern. The positive predictive value of a test for various abnormalities of interest should be considered when recommending general screening requirements; a high false positive rate can lead to a significant amount of unnecessary medical testing. For example, normal variants and physiologic mimics of pathologic states (eg, physiologic ventricular hypertrophy from intense athletic training) can result in a high rate of false positive reading by inexperienced readers or if the clinical setting is unknown.[3]

ANATOMIC CONSIDERATIONS

The heart in young adults is generally more vertically oriented and gradually shifts leftward throughout life. Hence, a vertical axis of 90 to 100° is normal in young individuals (axis discussed in detail further on). Particularly in females with pendulous breasts, placement of the precordial leads in the standard locations may be difficult; it is generally recommended to place the electrodes immediately under the left breast line. Placement of the precordial leads outside of the standard locations or in patients with a deformed chest, orthotopic heart transplant, prior cardiac surgery, and prior pneumonectomy may result in changes in R wave progression (discussed further later) owing to changes in the heart position within the chest cavity.

FUNDAMENTALS OF ELECTROCARDIOGRAPHY

An ECG is recorded by attaching electrodes (flat paper stickers with adhesive) to the patient's skin. Each electrode records electrical potentials from the heart's depolarization and repolarization. In a standard 12-lead ECG, electrodes are placed on the patient's right arm (RA), left arm (LA), and left leg (LL), and a ground electrode is generally placed on the right leg to reduce interference. Six precordial leads are placed across the patient's chest. Three types of lead exist in modern-day ECG: (1) bipolar leads; (2) augmented leads; and (3) unipolar leads. Bipolar leads measure the difference in potential between two electrodes, whereas unipolar leads measure the electrical activity directly beneath the electrode only. Augmented leads are calculated from bipolar leads.

The standard bipolar leads are leads I, II, III. These are calculated by subtracting the potentials between the (LA-RA), (LL-RA), and (LL-LA), respectively (**Figure 49.1**). Based on the "Einthoven triangle," the third bipolar lead can always be calculated if the other two leads are recorded through the formula Lead I + Lead III = Lead II.

The augmented leads are then calculated from a combination of the bipolar leads using the following formulas:

$$aVR = RA - \frac{1}{2}(LA + LL)$$

$$aVL = LA - \frac{1}{2}(RA + LL)$$

$$aVF = LL - \frac{1}{2}(RA + LA)$$

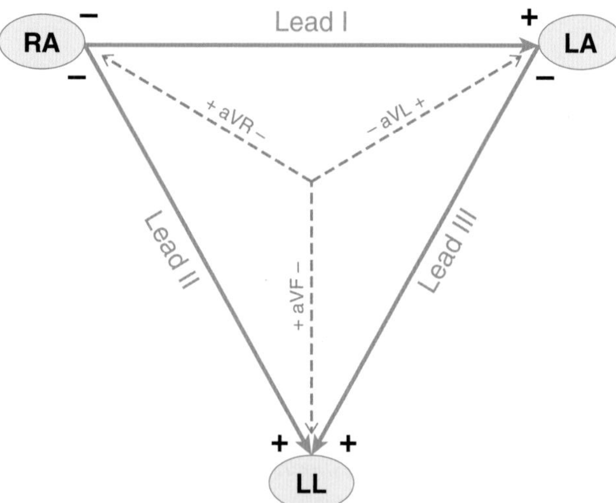

FIGURE 49.1 Einthoven triangle. Einthoven triangle is created by the three bipolar limb leads I, II, III, which are formed by three electrodes placed on the right arm (RA), left arm (LA), and left leg (LL). The augmented leads (aVR, aVL, and aVF) are calculated from leads I, II, and III.

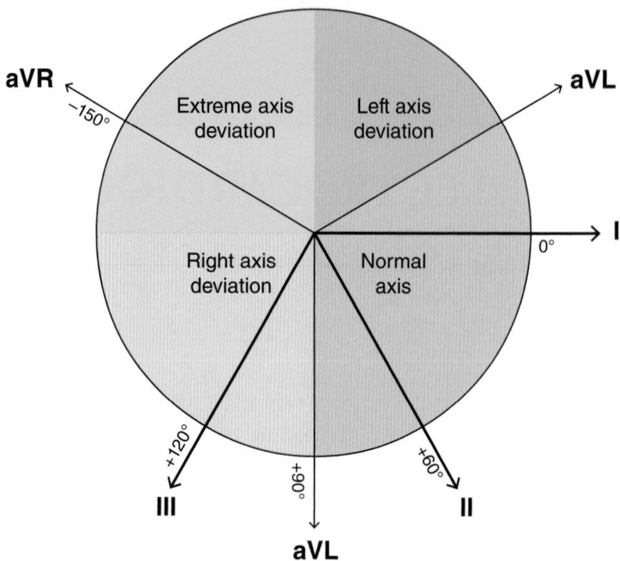

FIGURE 49.2 The frontal plane of the electrocardiogram (ECG) formed by the standard bipolar limb leads (bold arrows) and the augmented leads. Using the vector in these ECG leads, the net QRS vector can be determined. Normal QRS axis is –30° to +90°.

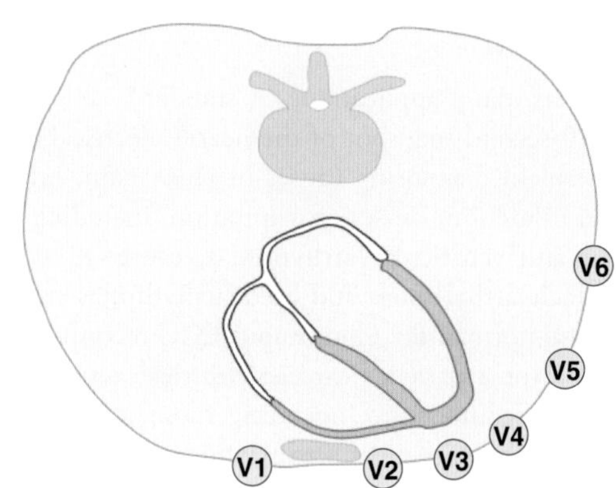

FIGURE 49.3 The precordial leads (V1-V6) record the horizontal plane of the heart.

The bipolar limb leads and augmented leads together can be described as the "frontal plane" of the heart (**Figure 49.2**). The precordial leads are unipolar leads and are placed across the chest to record the horizontal plane of the heart (**Figure 49.3**). The most common configuration in a 12-lead ECG system is V1 to V6. In specific situations for diagnosing myocardial infarction, discussed in more detail further on, right-sided (V3R-V6R) or posterior precordial leads (V7-V9) can be placed (**Table 49.1**).

The 12 standard ECG leads can be further categorized by which part of the left ventricle it records potentials from, this being most useful for the purposes of diagnosing myocardial infarction (**Table 49.2**).

In some specific uses of ECG, such as continuous telemetry ECG monitoring in the hospital or ambulatory Holter monitoring, a more limited set of leads are typically used. A standard 5-electrode continuous ECG system in the hospital generally provides all 6 frontal leads and 1 precordial lead, generally in the V1 or V2 position. A standard 4-lead Holter monitoring system generally provides 3 limb bipolar leads.

In general, when electrical depolarization of the heart occurs in the direction of a particular lead, the deflection is positive (above the isoelectric baseline). If depolarization is away from the lead, the deflection is negative below the isoelectric baseline.

Standard ECG paper consists of large boxes and small boxes. Each large box is comprised of 5 × 5 small boxes, which are in turn 1 × 1 mm. Standard ECGs are printed at a speed of 25 mm/s (ie, 25 horizontal small boxes [5 large boxes] make up

TABLE 49.1 Precordial Leads

Standard 12-Lead Electrocardiogram	Right-Sided Leads	Posterior Leads
V1	V1R	V1
V2	V2R	V2
V3	V3R	V3
V4	V4R	V7
V5	V5R	V8
V6	V6R	V9

Precordial Lead Position	
V1	Fourth intercostal space, right parasternal
V2	Fourth intercostal space, left parasternal
V3	Halfway between V2 and V4
V4	Fifth intercostal space, left midclavicular line
V5	Horizontal from V4, left anterior-axillary line
V6	Horizontal from V4 and V5, left midaxillary line
V7	Horizontal from V6, left posterior axillary line
V8	Horizontal from V6, tip of left scapula
V9	Horizontal from V6, left paraspinal
V1R	Fourth intercostal space, left parasternal
V2R	Fourth intercostal space, right parasternal
V3R	Halfway between V2R and V4R
V4R	Fifth intercostal space, right midclavicular line
V5R	Horizontal from V4R, right anterior-axillary line
V6R	Horizontal from V4R and V5R, right midaxillary line

TABLE 49.2 Lead Position Categorization (in Relation to Left Ventricle)

Lateral	Leads I, aVL, V5, V6
Inferior	Leads II, III, aVF
Septal	Leads V1, V2
Anterior	Leads V3, V4
Posterior	Leads V7, V8, V9

1 second). Hence, each horizontal small box is equal to 40 ms, and each large box represents 200 ms. The vertical calibration (amplitude) is most commonly 10 mm/1 mV. Hence, each small vertical box equals 0.1 mV (**Figure 49.4**). In rare cases, such as in ECGs with very large QRS complexes, the calibration may be different (eg, 5 mm/mV, **Figure 49.5**). Amplitude interpretations need to be performed carefully with this different scale. Typically, a calibration box is recorded at the beginning of the ECG tracing to inform the reader of the paper speed (ie, mm/s) and amplitude (ie, mm/mv) calibration.

CLINICAL APPLICATIONS

P-QRS-T Waves

The heart normally depolarizes electrically first in the atria and then in the ventricle. This is reflected on the ECG by a lower amplitude P wave, reflecting atrial depolarization, followed by an isoelectric segment (PR segment) when electrical activity traverses the atrioventricular (AV) node and the His-Purkinje system within the heart, which does not generate sufficient depolarization to show up on the surface ECG. A taller amplitude QRS complex reflects ventricular depolarization. The Q wave component is the initial negative deflection, the R wave the first positive deflection, the S wave a negative deflection that occurs after an R wave. In cases where there is another positive deflection after the S wave, that deflection is termed R' (read R-prime). The ST segment is the segment between the QRS and T wave that reflects ventricular repolarization (**Figure 49.6**). Occasionally, another low-amplitude wave is seen after the T wave, which is called the U wave. The origin of the U wave is widely debated and may represent repolarization of the Purkinje fibers.

A systematic approach should always be utilized to interpret an ECG. Although each clinician may choose a different approach, one should maintain a consistent approach so as not to miss important diagnoses. We generally approach ECG by assessing the following: rate; rhythm; axis; intervals; hypertrophy; ischemia; infarction; and other findings (eg, electrolyte or drug effects, clinical diagnosis patterns, lead misplacements, etc.)

Structured Approach to ECG Analysis Includes:

- Rate
- Rhythm
- Axis
- Intervals
- Hypertrophy
- Ischemia & infarction
- Other findings: electrolyte or drug effects; clinical diagnosis patterns; lead misplacements

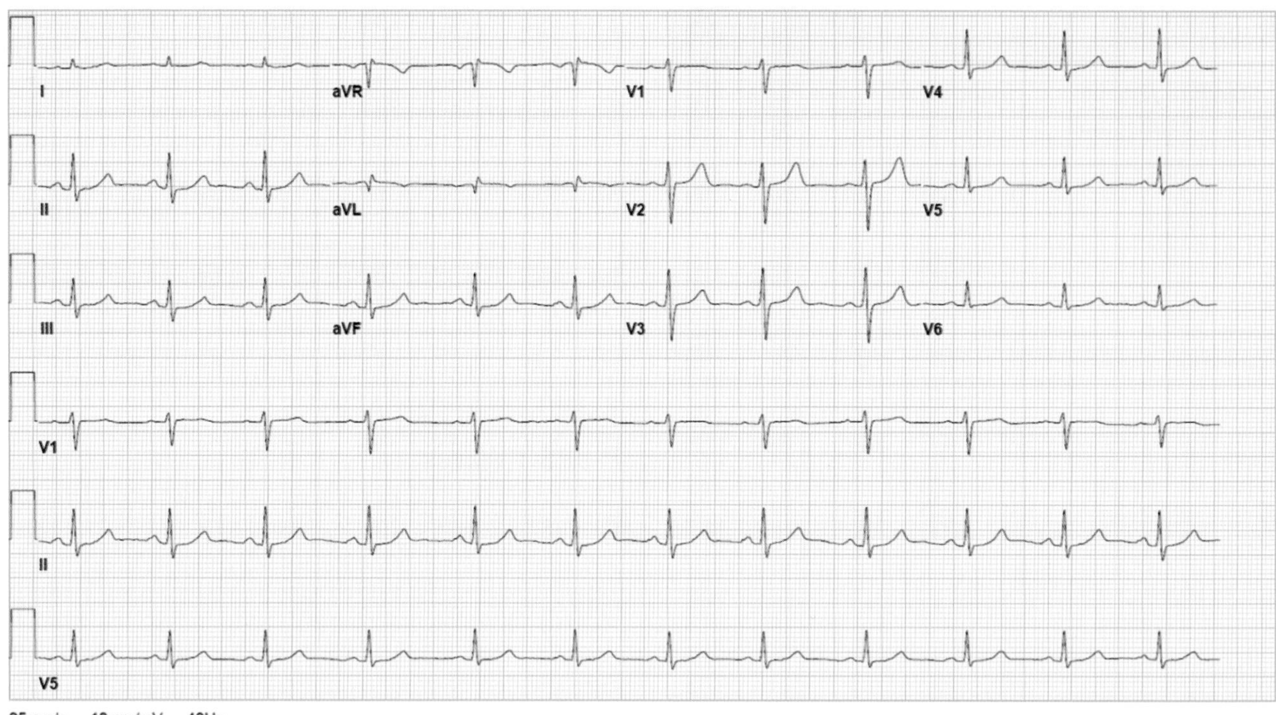

FIGURE 49.4 A normal electrocardiogram showing normal sinus rhythm at approximately 75 beats per minute. Note the standard scales. Each small box on the paper is 1 × 1 mm. The standard paper speed is 25 mm/s (5 large horizontal boxes = 1 second; hence, each large horizontal box = 200 ms, each small horizontal box = 40 ms). The standard amplitude scale is 10 mm/mV (10 small boxes = 1 mV, each small box = 0.1 mV). The calibration for amplitude is seen by the rectangular wave at the far left.

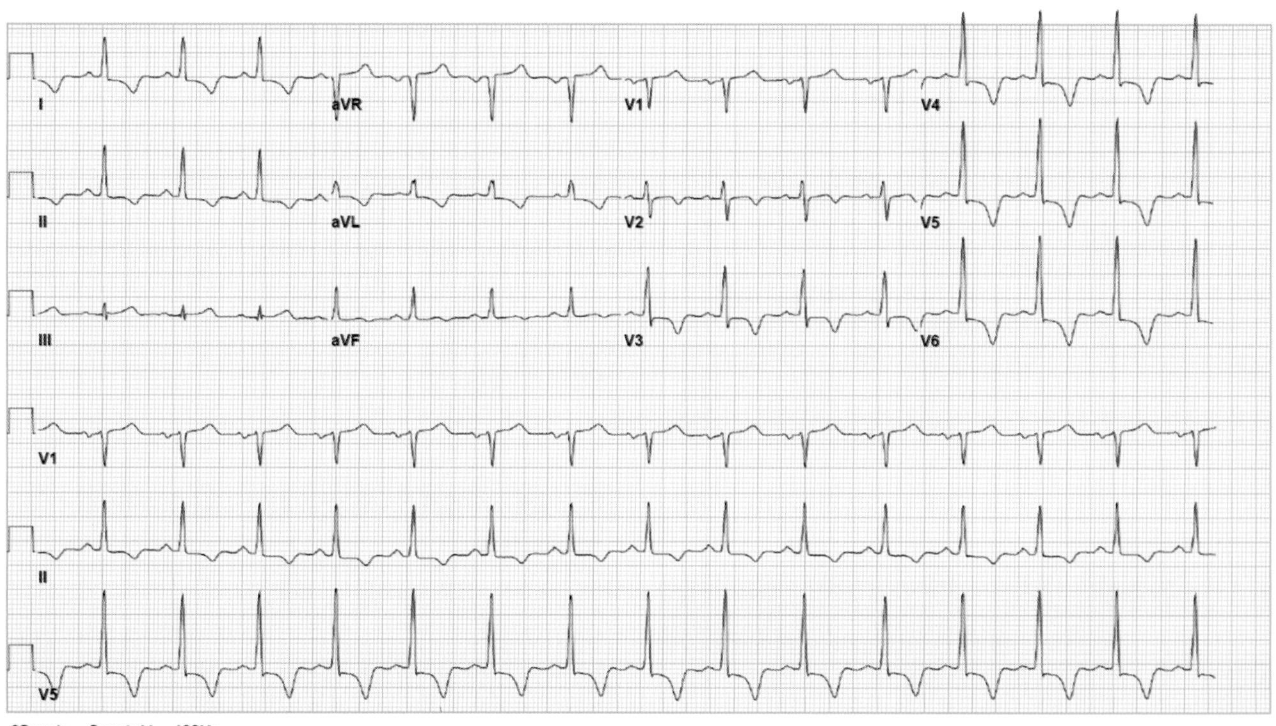

FIGURE 49.5 Left ventricular hypertrophy. Note the amplitude scaling on this electrocardiogram (ECG) is 5 mm/mV, as seen by the calibration marker on the far left. This ECG shows sinus rhythm at a rate of approximately 90 bpm with left ventricular hypertrophy. Note the asymmetrically inverted T waves in the inferolateral leads, representing repolarization abnormalities attributable to left ventricular hypertrophy.

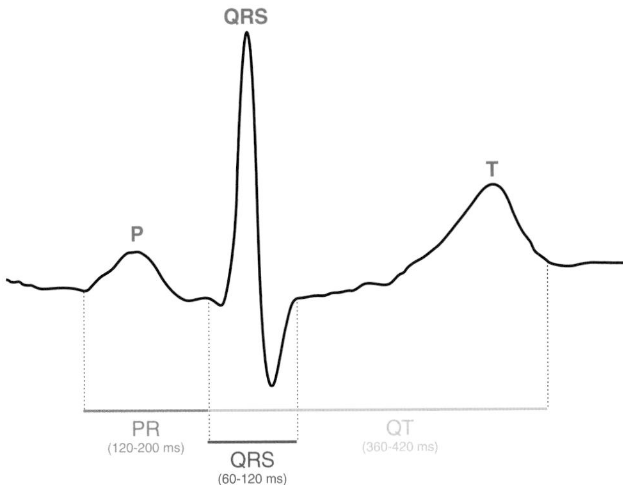

FIGURE 49.6 P-QRS-T complex. The P, QRS, T waves are marked in red. The PR interval is measured from the beginning of the P wave to the beginning of the QRS. The QRS interval (duration) is measured from the beginning to the end of the QRS complex. The QT interval is measured from the beginning of the QRS to the end of the T wave (where the line tangent to the downslope of the T wave crosses the isoelectric line). Normal ranges for each interval are displayed within parentheses. The ST segment is the normally isoelectric segment between the orange arrows.

Rate

When the rhythm is regular, the ventricular rate can initially be roughly estimated by counting the number of large boxes between one QRS complex and the next (eg, if there is 1 large box between two QRS complexes, the rate is 300 beats per minute [bpm]; 2 large boxes: 150 bpm; 3 large boxes: 100 bpm; 4 large boxes: 75 bpm; 5 large boxes: 60 bpm; etc.) (Figure 49.5). When there is an irregular rhythm, the number of QRS complexes can be counted within the standard 10-second recording and multiplied by 6 (eg, if there are 10 QRS complexes across the 10-second recording strip, the heart rate is approximately 60 bpm). Rates <60 bpm are considered bradycardic, 60 to 100 bpm are normal, and >100 bpm are tachycardic. However, many normal healthy individuals have resting heart rates in the 45 to 60 range, or even lower.

While the atrial and ventricular rate is generally the same, this may not be the case in various arrhythmias. An atrial rate can be calculated separately from a ventricular rate using a similar manner, but using the P waves instead of the QRS deflections.

Rhythm

Correct diagnosis of the rhythm requires identification of P waves and their morphology when they exist. In normal cardiac electrical activity, the atrium depolarizes starting at the sinus node, the main pacemaker of the heart, which lies in the high right atrium near the superior vena cava. Sinus rhythm (ie, an atrial rhythm that originates from the sinus node) can be identified by a P wave that is upright in leads I, II, and III and usually inverted in lead aVR. The P wave is also generally biphasic (±) in lead V1. Normal sinus rhythm refers to a sinus rate that is 60 to 100 bpm, sinus bradycardia <60 bpm, and sinus tachycardia >100 bpm.

If P waves are present but not of a sinus morphology, this represents an ectopic atrial rhythm (ie, atrial depolarization originating from a different area of the atrium). Other common atrial rhythms include atrial fibrillation, where there is no organized atrial activity and therefore no organized P waves are present and the intervals between the QRS complexes are variable (the pulse is generally described as "irregularly irregular" in atrial fibrillation) (**Figure 49.7**), or atrial flutter, where there is a macroreentrant circuit around the atrium and is characterized by "sawtooth" pattern flutter waves, best seen in leads II, III, aVF, and V1.

The AV node conducts electrical activity from the atrium to the ventricle and also slows down the impulses that reach the ventricle. Under normal circumstances, each P wave should be followed by a QRS on the ECG. If there are P waves without following QRS complexes, there is heart block (ie, AV node block). A "normal ECG," hence, generally has a rhythm with a sinus rate of 60 to 100 bpm with a sinus P wave before each QRS.

AV nodal AV block is divided into first degree, second degree, and third degree. In first-degree AV block, there is prolonged conduction time between the atrium and the ventricle, reflected as a prolonged PR interval >200 ms (discussed more in detail further on). In second-degree AV block, every few P waves are blocked in the AV node. In second-degree Type I block (also called Mobitz I block or Wenckebach), the PR interval increases until a QRS is dropped (**Figure 49.8**). In second-degree Type II block (also called Mobitz II block), the PR interval does not change when a QRS is dropped. In third-degree heart block (also called complete heart block, **Figure 49.9**), there is no electrical communication between the atrium and the ventricles. When the conduction ratio is 2:1, 3:1, or higher, this pattern is referred to as "high degree AV block" because it does not fit into the first-, second-, or third-degree block classification.

Many other arrhythmias, both originating from the atrium or AV node (ie, supraventricular tachycardia, **Figure 49.10**) and the ventricles (ie, ventricular tachycardia, **Figure 49.11**), can be identified on ECG. Premature ventricular complexes (PVCs, Figure 49.10), or premature atrial complexes (PACs), are common findings and are generally benign (**Figure 49.12**). However, patients with a very high burden of PVCs (ie, >25% of all beats) may be at risk for PVC-mediated cardiomyopathy.

Axis

The axis of ventricular depolarization represents the net vector of all electrical depolarization vectors in the heart. Since the left ventricular myocardial mass is generally larger than the right ventricular myocardial mass, the net vector of depolarization points toward the left ventricle. Hence, normal axis is considered between –30° and +90°. Left axis deviation is diagnosed with the axis between–30° and –90°, right axis deviation between +90° and +180°, and extreme right axis deviation between –90° and –180° (Figure 49.2).

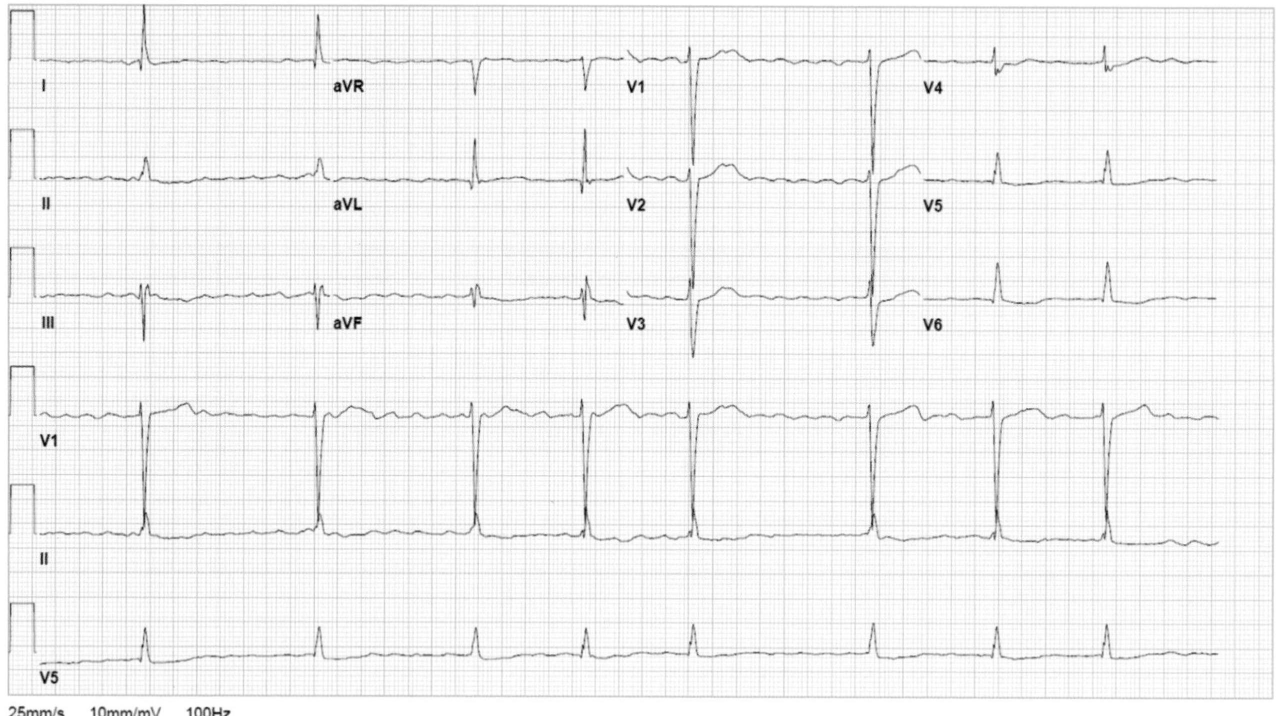

FIGURE 49.7 Atrial fibrillation. Electrocardiogram shows an irregularly irregular rhythm with no organized atrial activity (ie, no discrete P waves). Instead, fibrillatory waves are seen.

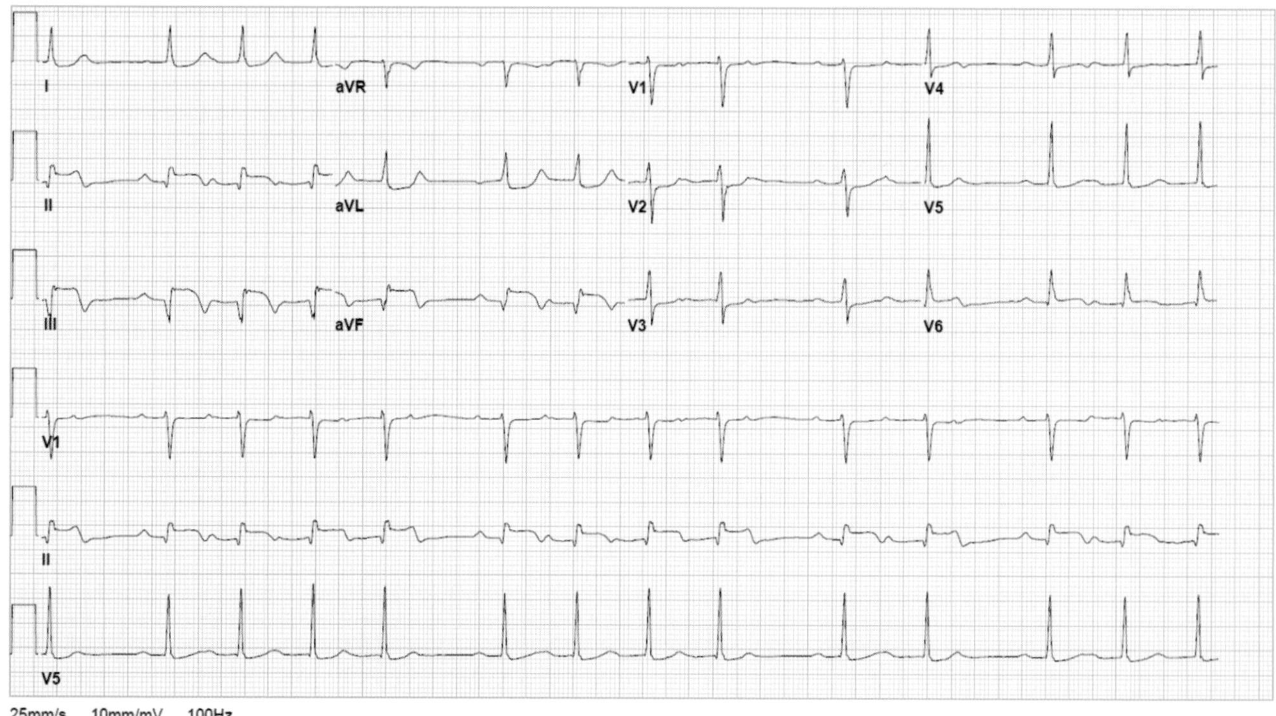

FIGURE 49.8 Second degree type I block. Note the "grouped beating" pattern of QRS complexes in this electrocardiogram. The PR interval increases with each beat up to the dropped beat, diagnostic of second degree type I block (also referred to as Mobitz I block or Wenckebach). There are also Q waves, ST elevations, and T wave inversions in the inferolateral leads, indicating an acute ST-elevation MI.

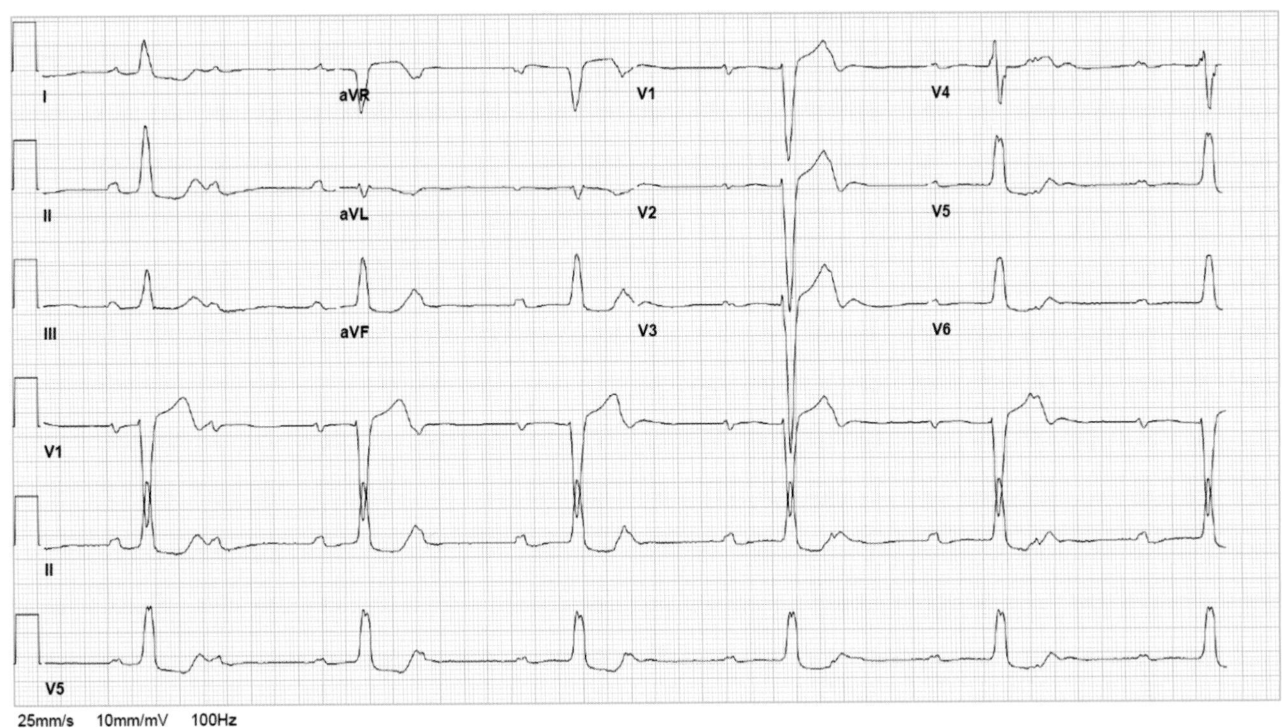

FIGURE 49.9 Complete heart block. Electrocardiogram shows sinus rhythm at a rate of approximately 65 bpm with a QRS rate of approximately 35 bpm. There is no relationship between the P waves and QRS complexes, diagnostic of complete heart block. Note that the QRS complexes demonstrate a left bundle branch block pattern.

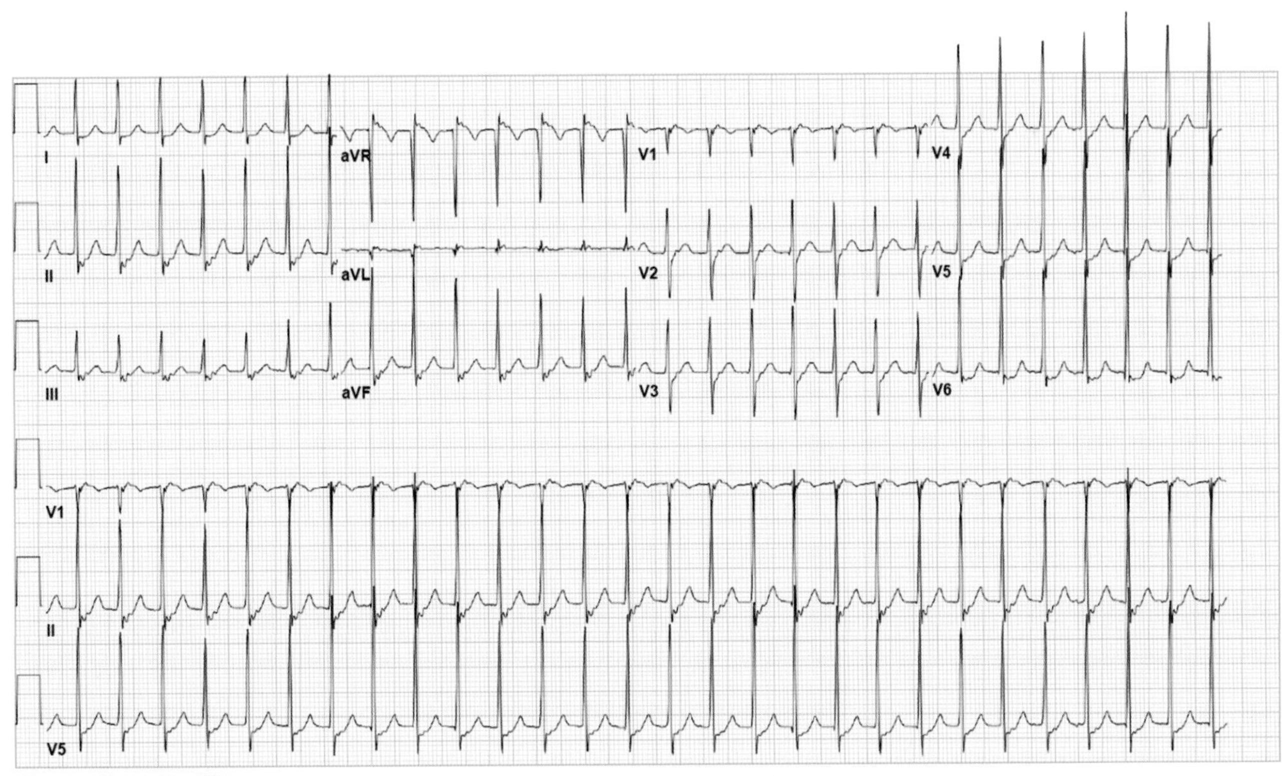

FIGURE 49.10 Supraventricular tachycardia. Electrocardiogram shows a regular narrow complex tachycardia (generally referred to as a supraventricular tachycardia) at a rate of 170 bpm. This likely represents an atrioventricular nodal reentrant tachycardia, as noted by the retrograde P wave immediately after the QRS complex (best seen in lead V1).

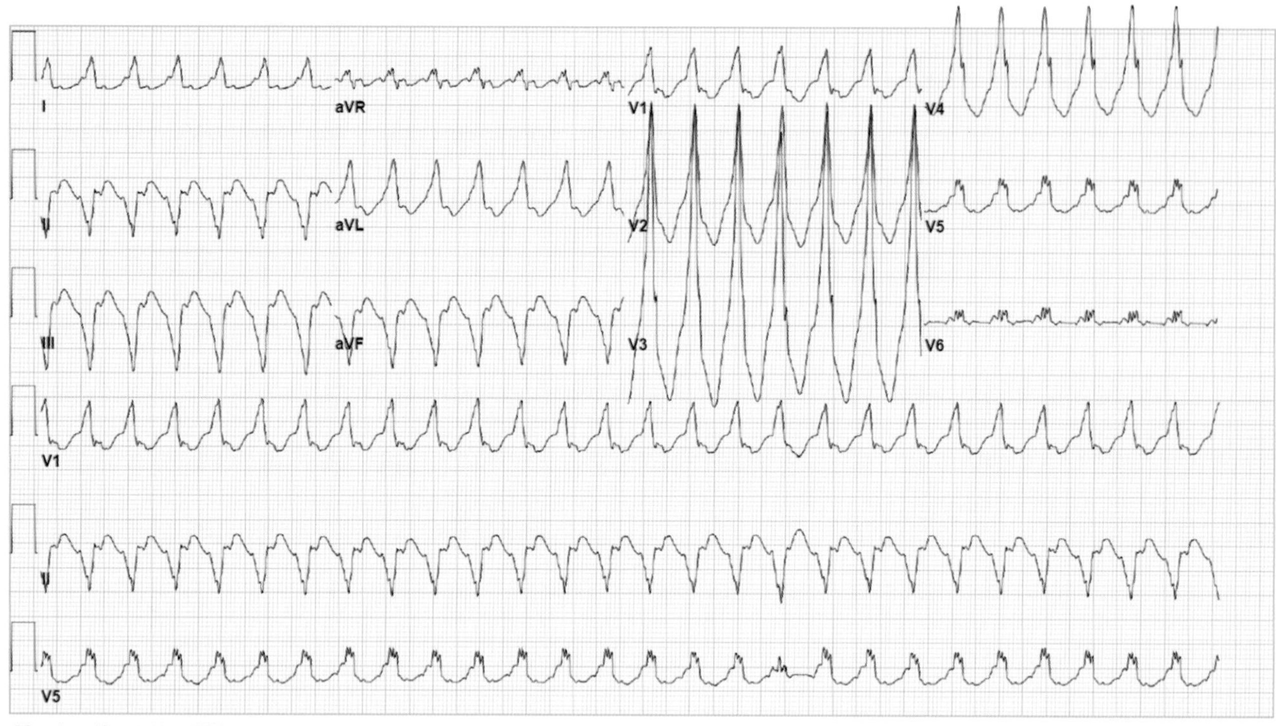

FIGURE 49.11 Ventricular tachycardia. Electrocardiogram shows a regular wide complex tachycardia at a rate of approximately 150 bpm. Given the precordial concordance (R waves in all precordial leads), this is most consistent with a ventricular tachycardia.

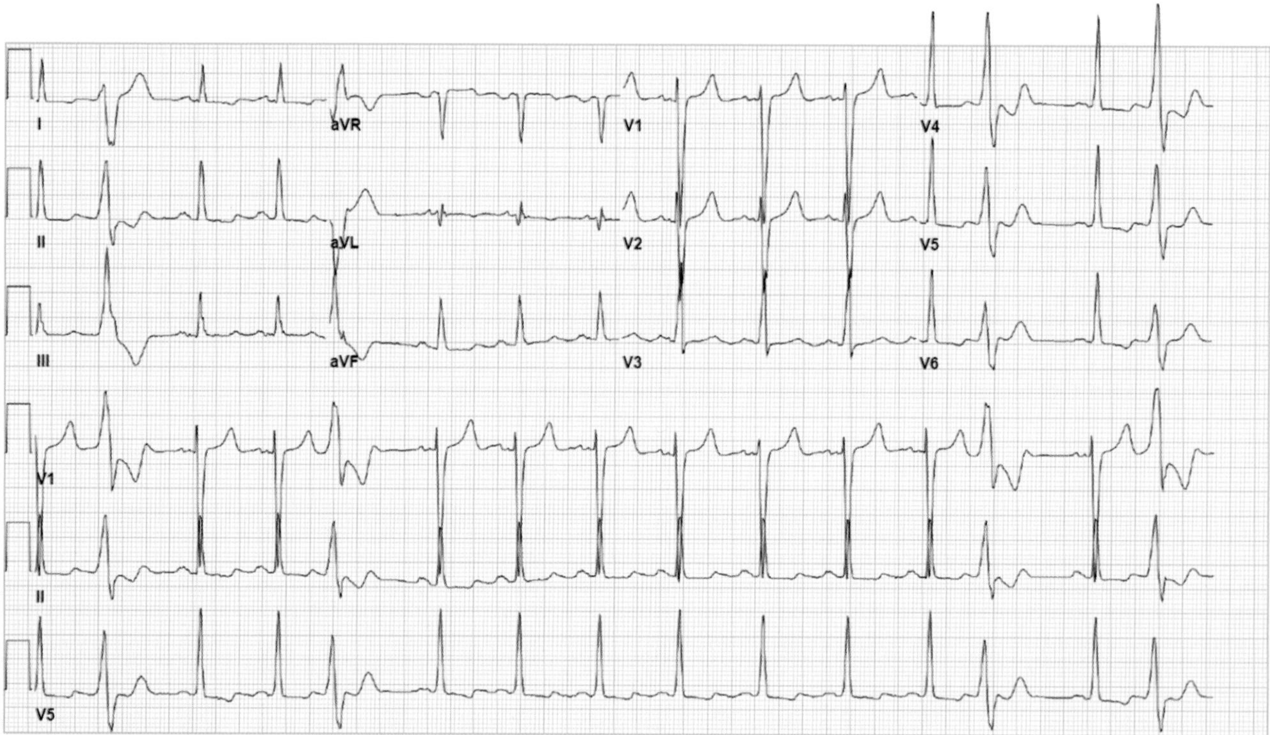

FIGURE 49.12 Premature ventricular complex. Electrocardiogram shows sinus rhythm with occasional premature complexes with a wider QRS duration, suggestive of a ventricular origin (hence, premature ventricular complex).

Axis can be quickly determined by using the quadrant method. Depending on whether the QRS is positive or negative in leads I and aVL, the quadrant of the axis can be determined (Figure 49.2). Hence, if lead I and aVL are both positive, the axis is normal. If lead I is positive, but aVL is negative, lead II is evaluated: If positive, the axis is still normal; if negative, there is left axis deviation. If lead I is negative, there is right axis or extreme right axis deviation.

Different pathologies (or normal variants) can lead to various axis deviations (**Table 49.3**).

Intervals

Different intervals can be measured from the ECG, which reflect the time required for depolarization or repolarization in the heart; normal ranges exist for each of these intervals (Figure 49.6).

The PR interval includes the amount of time required from the initiation of atrial depolarization to the beginning of ventricular depolarization. Prolongation of the PR interval is most commonly attributable to conduction delay in the AV node but also potentially to slow atrial depolarization or conduction delay in the His-Purkinje system. Short PR intervals may be attributable to normal variant (ie, rapid conduction through the AV node) or to the presence of an abnormal electrical connection between the atrium and the ventricle (ie, accessory pathway, also referred to as a bypass tract or Bundle of Kent). This is evidenced by the presence of a slurred upstroke of the QRS (delta wave, **Figure 49.13**). The presence of a delta wave on ECG with associated symptoms such as palpitations makes for a diagnosis of WPW syndrome, which may

TABLE 49.3 Causes of Axis Deviation

Left Axis Deviation	Right Axis Deviation
Left ventricular hypertrophy	Right ventricular hypertrophy
Left anterior fascicular block	Left posterior fascicular block
Left bundle branch block	Lateral myocardial infarction
Inferior myocardial infarction	Ostium secundum atrial septal defect
Ostium primum atrial septal defect	Wolff-Parkinson-White syndrome
Wolff-Parkinson-White syndrome	Normal variant (young individuals)

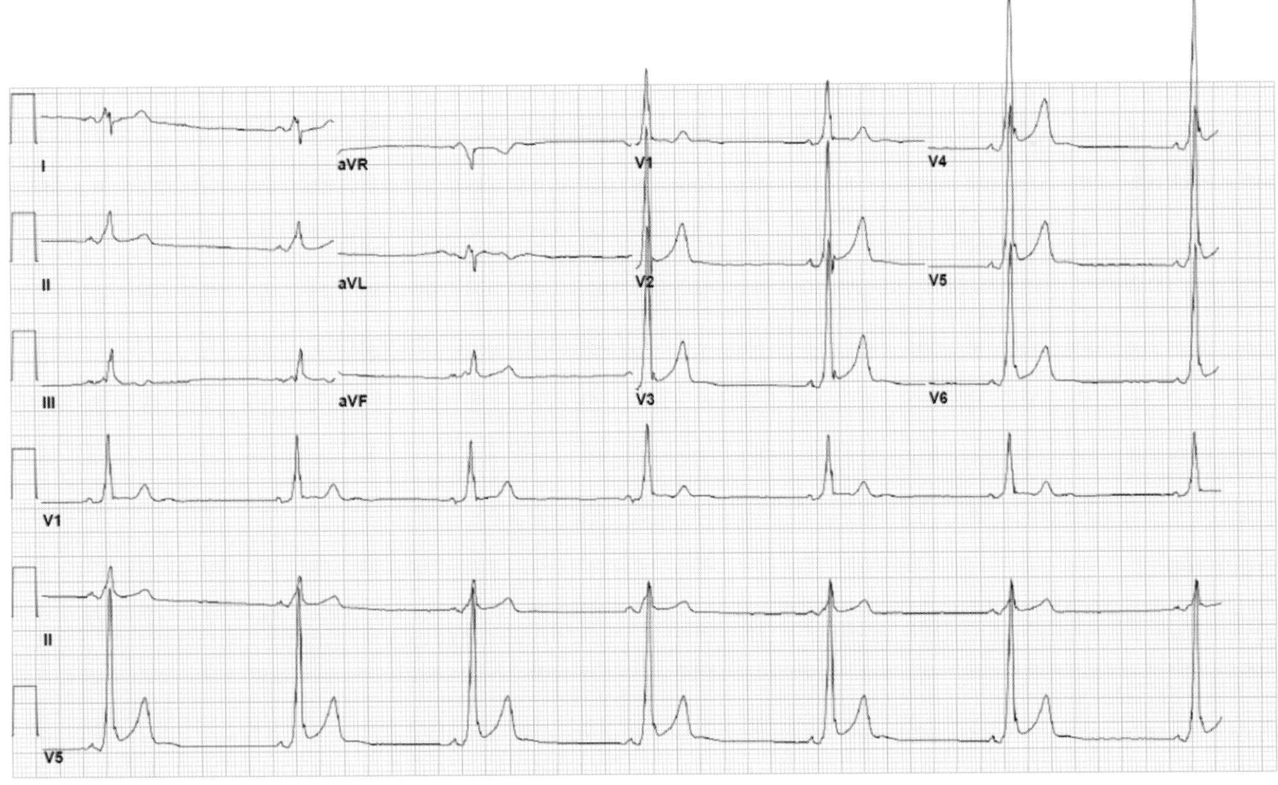

FIGURE 49.13 Wolff-Parkinson-White. Electrocardiogram shows sinus bradycardia with a short PR and a delta wave, representing conduction via an accessory pathway. Many patients with such accessory pathways are symptomatic from arrhythmias. This pathway was successfully ablated along the anterior mitral isthmus (left anterior).

be a cause of supraventricular tachycardias, or in severe cases syncope or sudden cardiac death.

The QRS duration represents the time required for the ventricle to depolarize. In normal physiology, the majority of the ventricles are depolarized after the electrical impulse has traveled quickly through the His-Purkinje system, and hence the QRS complex has sharp deflections and is short. If there is delay or block in the His-Purkinje system, the QRS duration prolongs owing to some myocardium being depolarized through myocardial cell-to-cell electrical propagation, which is much slower. If the QRS duration is greater than 120 ms, the conduction delay can be categorized as a right bundle branch block (characterized by an RR' or rSR' pattern in lead V1 and slurred S wave in leads V5, V6, I), left bundle branch block (QS in lead V1 with wide R waves in V5 and V6), or nonspecific intraventricular conduction delay when the morphology does not fit either pattern. Other reasons for a wide QRS include ventricular paced rhythm, ventricular rhythm, hyperkalemia, or artifact.

The QT interval is measured from the beginning of the QRS complex to the end of the T wave (using a tangent line along the steepest downslope of the T wave, the end of the T wave is marked where this crosses the isoelectric line). The QT interval should be measured in the lead with the longest such interval. This represents ventricular repolarization. The QT is dependent on the ventricular rate and is therefore generally reported as the corrected QT (QTc). The most common formula for correction is the Bazett formula ($QTc = \frac{QT}{\sqrt{RR}}$). However, this formula results in an overcorrection of the QT interval at fast heart rates and undercorrection at slow heart rates. Normal QTc differ between men (<440 ms) and women (<460 ms). By rule of thumb, a QT interval that is less than half the RR interval is generally normal. Patients with prolonged QT, whether because of genetic abnormalities in ion channels or because of the effect of medication that acts on the cardiac potassium channels, are at increased risk for a form of polymorphic ventricular tachycardia known as "torsades de pointes." Electrolyte abnormalities can also affect the QT interval: hypocalcemia, hypomagnesemia, and hypokalemia prolong the QT; hyperkalemia and hypercalcemia shorten the QT interval. Short QT can also be attributable to a genetically inherited channelopathy, which can also predispose individuals to ventricular arrhythmias.

Hypertrophy

The presence of concentric or eccentric ventricular hypertrophy increases the corresponding QRS amplitudes. The presence of atrial enlargement increases the corresponding P wave amplitude or prolongs conduction time (**Table 49.4**).

The presence of conduction delay can make the ECG diagnosis of ventricular hypertrophy more difficult. With left bundle branch block, it is generally recommended not to attempt an ECG diagnosis of left ventricular hypertrophy. With left anterior fascicular block, the R wave in aVL criteria is increased to >1.3 mV (compared with >1.1 mV normally).

TABLE 49.4 Atrial and Ventricular Enlargement/Hypertrophy Criteria

Right atrial enlargement	P wave amplitude >0.25 mV in lead II P wave positive deflection in lead V1 >0.15 mV in amplitude
Left atrial enlargement	P wave duration >100 ms in lead II Duration between two peaks in Lead II P wave >40 ms P wave in lead V1 negative deflection >1 × 1 small box
Left ventricular hypertrophy	S wave in lead V1 + R wave in lead V5/V6 >0.35 mV R wave in lead aVL >1.1 mV R wave in lead aVL + S wave in lead V3 >0.28 mV in males, >0.20 mV in females
Right ventricular hypertrophy	R wave in lead V1 >7 mm or R/S ratio >1 with supporting findings: right atrial enlargement, right axis deviation R wave amplitude in right bundle branch block > 1.1 mV

Ventricular hypertrophy is generally accompanied by repolarization abnormalities.[4]

Decreases in QRS voltage can be seen if there is either a significant amount of fluid (pericardial effusion), fat (obesity), or air (chronic obstructive pulmonary disease [COPD]) between the heart and the chest wall. Infiltrative cardiomyopathies, classically cardiac amyloidosis, may also present with low QRS voltages and pseudo-infarction patterns. Low voltage criteria can either be fulfilled with limb lead (QRS amplitude [ie, R peak to Q/S trough] <0.5 mV in all leads) or precordial lead criteria (QRS amplitude <1.0 mV in all leads).

Ischemia and Infarction

Evaluation of chest pain is one of the most common uses of the ECG. Evidence of ischemia by ECG should always be interpreted in the context of the patient's clinical presentation.[5]

The most important thing to rule out in every ECG is evidence of an ST-elevation myocardial infarction (STEMI), which requires emergent revascularization in most situations. A STEMI presents in the earliest phases (<30 minutes) as hyperacute T waves (ie, large peaked T waves) often with no ST segment elevations. After approximately 30 minutes, ST segment elevations become apparent. ST segment elevation is diagnosed based on the presence of ≥0.1 mV elevation of the ST segment (in leads V2 and V3 ≥0.15 mV in females, ≥0.2 mV in males ≥40 years old, ≥0.25 mV in males <40 years old) in two contiguous leads compared with the PR or TP segment.[6] In the posterior (V7-V9) and right-sided (V3R and V4R) leads, ≥0.05 mV ST elevation is considered abnormal.[6] After several hours, as tissue is infarcted, Q waves begin developing with persistence

TABLE 49.5 Differential for ST Segment Elevations

Diagnosis	Electrocardiogram Findings	Clinical Presentation
Pericarditis	Diffuse ST elevations, PR segment depression in all leads except aVR, where PR elevation is present; Downsloping TP segment	Pleuritic chest pain, worse with supine position.
Brugada syndrome	Coved ST segment elevation in leads V1 and V2 with T wave inversions	May be asymptomatic or present with signs and symptoms of ventricular arrhythmias. Findings of Brugada syndrome may be induced by fever or drugs.
Early repolarization (normal variant)	J waves with ST segment elevation	Asymptomatic patient or noncardiac chest pain presentation. Generally young males, particularly of African descent.
Hyperkalemia	Peaked T waves may also be present	ST segment elevation is an early finding in hyperkalemia and can sometimes be seen in conjunction with peaked T waves ([K+] 5.5-6.5 mmol/L).

of ST segment elevations. When the entire myocardium in the arterial territory is infarcted (by 12 hours), there is a QS wave in the affected territories with residual ST segment elevations. Over the next 24 hours, the ST segments resolve, and T waves invert, which may remain inverted for weeks to years, or indefinitely.

The territories where ST segment elevations are present localize the area of infarction (Table 49.2). The differential for ST segment elevations includes many other pathologic and benign diagnoses, which need to be considered in the context of the clinical presentation (**Table 49.5**).

Diagnosing a STEMI in a patient with a left bundle branch block presents many difficulties. A new left bundle branch block may be a STEMI equivalent, although many studies have shown that the prevalence in such patients is low, generally owing to lack of knowledge of preexisting left bundle branch block. The Sgarbossa criteria were developed to assist with the diagnosis of a STEMI in patients with a left bundle branch block.[7]

The presence of pathologic Q waves (classically defined as a Q wave duration ≥40 ms, or depth ≥25% of the R wave in the same lead, or presence of Q wave equivalent) in two contiguous leads represents evidence of an infarct. In the presence of ST segment elevations, the infarct is "acute/recent"; in their absence, it is "age indeterminate" or "old." Q waves can appear normally in leads III and aVR, although they should not also be present in contiguous leads if normal (ie, leads III and aVF). Delta waves can sometimes masquerade as a Q wave. A Q wave equivalent in the anterior precordial leads is "poor R wave progression," defined as the lack of a transition to R > S by lead V4 and R wave amplitude in lead V3 <3 mm. A large R wave in lead V1 may be a Q wave equivalent in the posterior leads. Both of these findings have other differentials that should be evaluated in the context of other ECG findings and clinical presentation (**Table 49.6**).

Subendocardial ischemia may be evidenced by either T wave inversions or, in more severe cases, ST segment depression (≥0.05 mV ST depression). Inverted T waves in leads III, aVR, and V1 may be a normal variant. ST segment depressions and T wave inversions attributable to ischemia should be differentiated from repolarization abnormalities attributable to ventricular hypertrophy (the former generally presents with symmetric T wave inversions, the latter with asymmetric T wave inversions like a reverse check mark; Figure 49.5). Diffuse deep T wave inversions with QT prolongation can represent an acute neurologic event, particularly subarachnoid hemorrhage, which must be clinically differentiated from myocardial ischemia (**Figure 49.14**).

Specific Diagnoses

There are several ECG patterns that are pathognomonic of a disease state and that require pattern recognition in relation to clinical presentation. These include the following: the peaked T wave in hyperkalemia (**Figure 49.15**), sine wave pattern of severe hyperkalemia (**Figure 49.16**), electrical alternans in large pericardial effusion, short QT in hypercalcemia, neurologic T waves (Figure 49.14), diffuse ST segment elevation in acute pericarditis (**Figure 49.17**), prominent Osborn waves (J waves) in hypothermia, and "scooped" ST segments in digoxin effect (**Figure 49.18**). Abnormalities in axis or R wave progression should also raise suspicion for lead reversal (**Figure 49.19**), and rarely dextrocardia (**Figure 49.20**).

LIMITATIONS

The ECG should always be interpreted within the clinical context. This is particularly imperative in the setting of a potential myocardial infarction accompanied by equivocal ECG findings. When the patient's symptoms are suggestive of a myocardial infarction, but the ECG does not meet diagnostic criteria for a STEMI, rapid reevaluation every few minutes with serial ECGs should be performed. Right-sided and posterior ECGs should also be ordered. Strong clinical suspicion should trump ECG and/or troponin findings in the setting of an acute

TABLE 49.6 Differential for Q Wave Equivalents

Diagnosis	Other Potential Electrocardiogram Findings
Poor R Wave Progression[a]	
Left ventricular hypertrophy	Voltage criteria for left ventricular hypertrophy, repolarization abnormalities
Left anterior fascicular block	Left axis deviation, qR in leads I and aVL, rS in leads II and III and aVF
Anterior myocardial infarction	T wave inversions may be present
Poor lead placement	Normal T waves
Normal variant	
Large R Wave in Lead V1[b]	
Right ventricular hypertrophy	Right axis deviation, right atrial enlargement, repolarization abnormalities
Right bundle branch block	QRS duration > 120 ms
Wolff-Parkinson-White	Delta wave, short PR
Posterior myocardial infarction	Upright T waves in V1, inferior myocardial infarction, Q waves in leads V7-V9
Duchenne muscular dystrophy	Similar to posterior myocardial infarction
Lead misplacement	V1 and V3 are the most commonly mixed up lead pair
Hypertrophic cardiomyopathy	Voltage criteria for left ventricular hypertrophy, repolarization abnormalities
Normal variant	

[a]R/S transition later than V4, R wave in lead V3 less than 3 mm.
[b]R/S > 1 in lead V1.

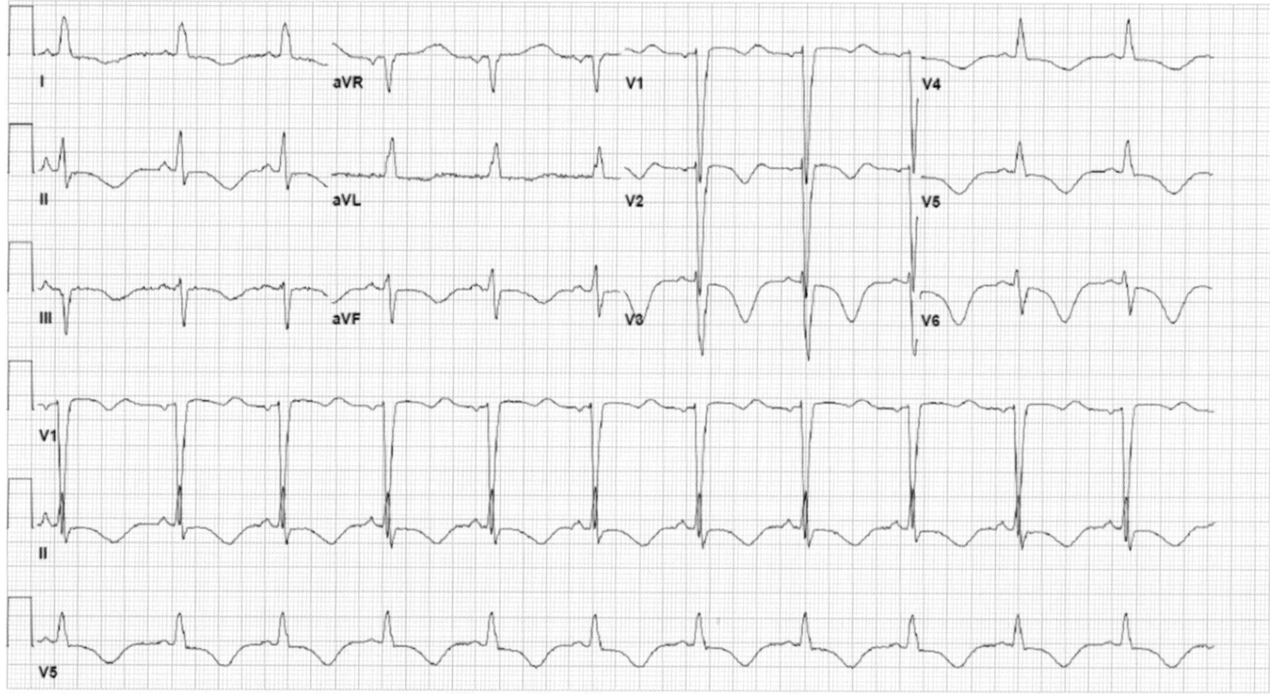

FIGURE 49.14 Neurologic T waves. Electrocardiogram (ECG) shows diffuse deeply inverted T waves with QT prolongation. This ECG is highly concerning for an acute neurologic event, including subarachnoid hemorrhage.

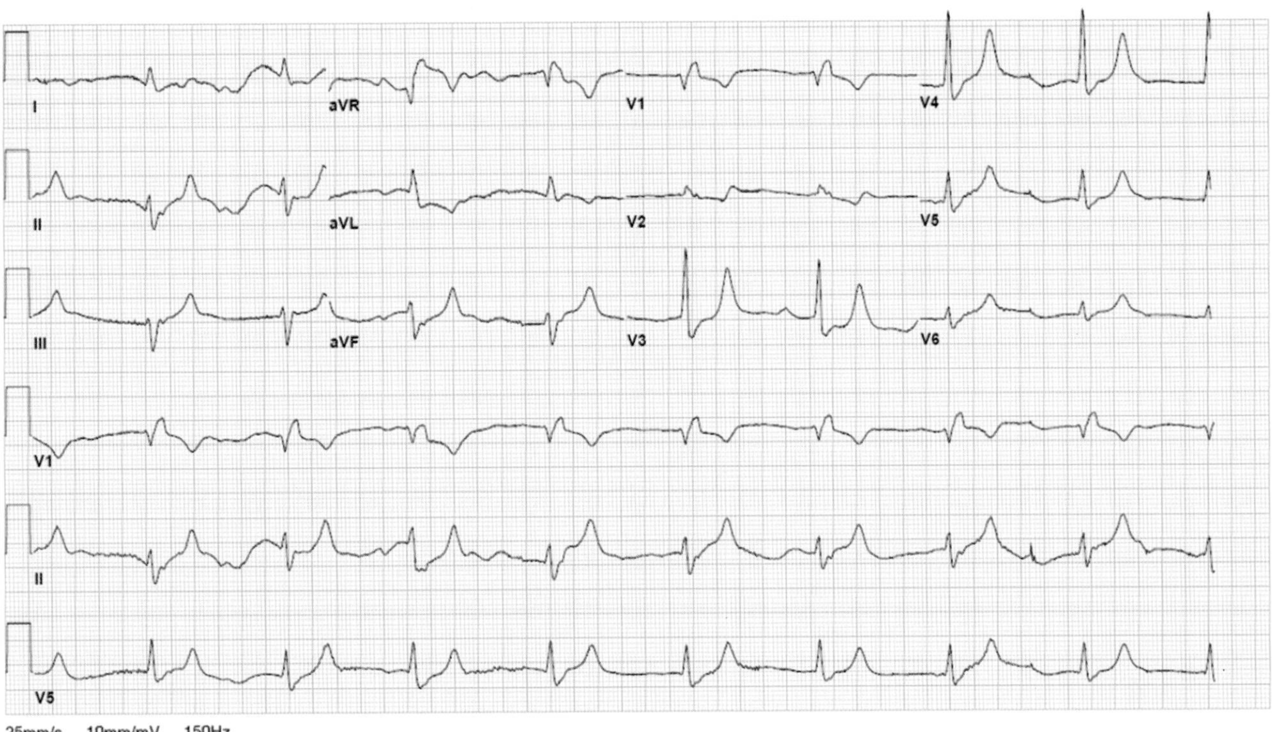

FIGURE 49.15 Moderate hyperkalemia. Electrocardiogram (ECG) shows many signs of moderate hyperkalemia, including peaked T waves, low amplitude P wave (in this ECG, indiscernible), and widened QRS. This patient had a potassium level of 7.8.

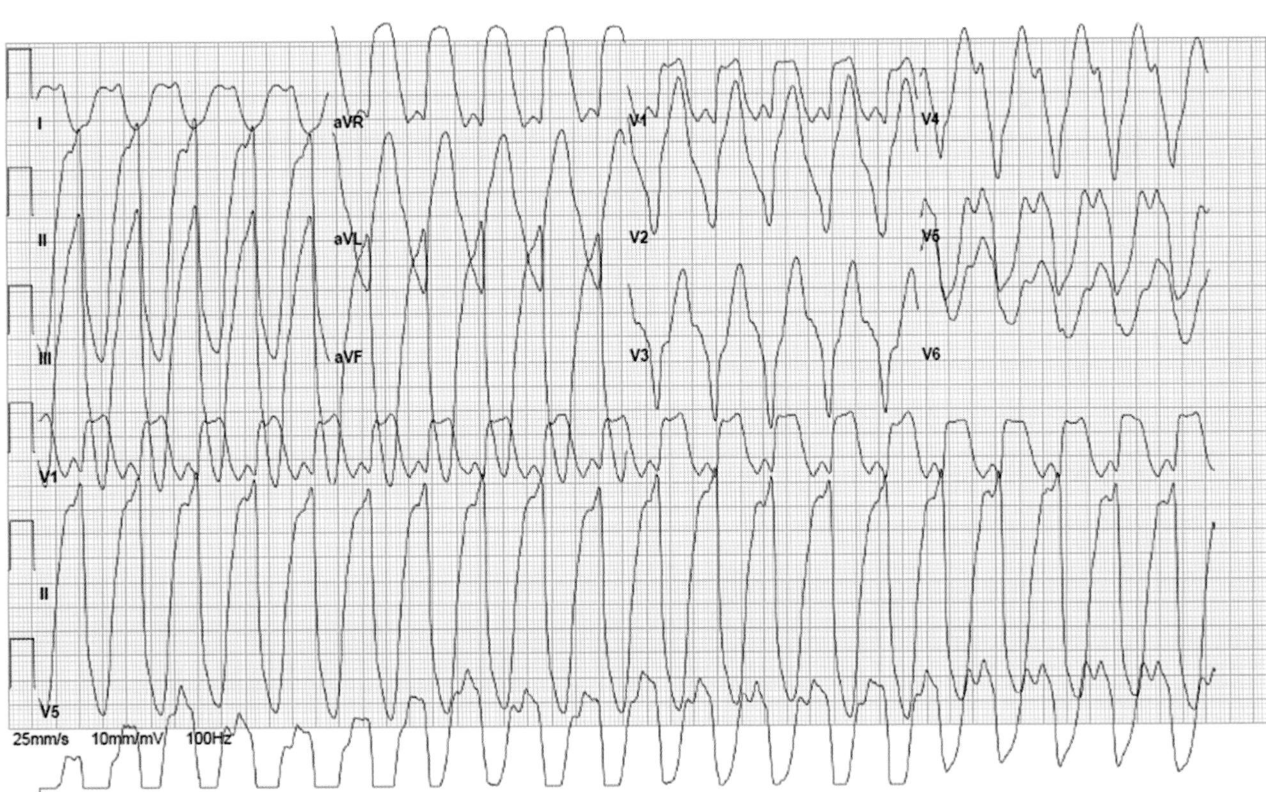

FIGURE 49.16 Severe hyperkalemia. Electrocardiogram (ECG) shows a nearly sinusoidal QRS-T wave. This pattern should raise concern for severe hyperkalemia, warranting emergent treatment, including dialysis. This patient had a potassium level of 8.5 mEq/L.

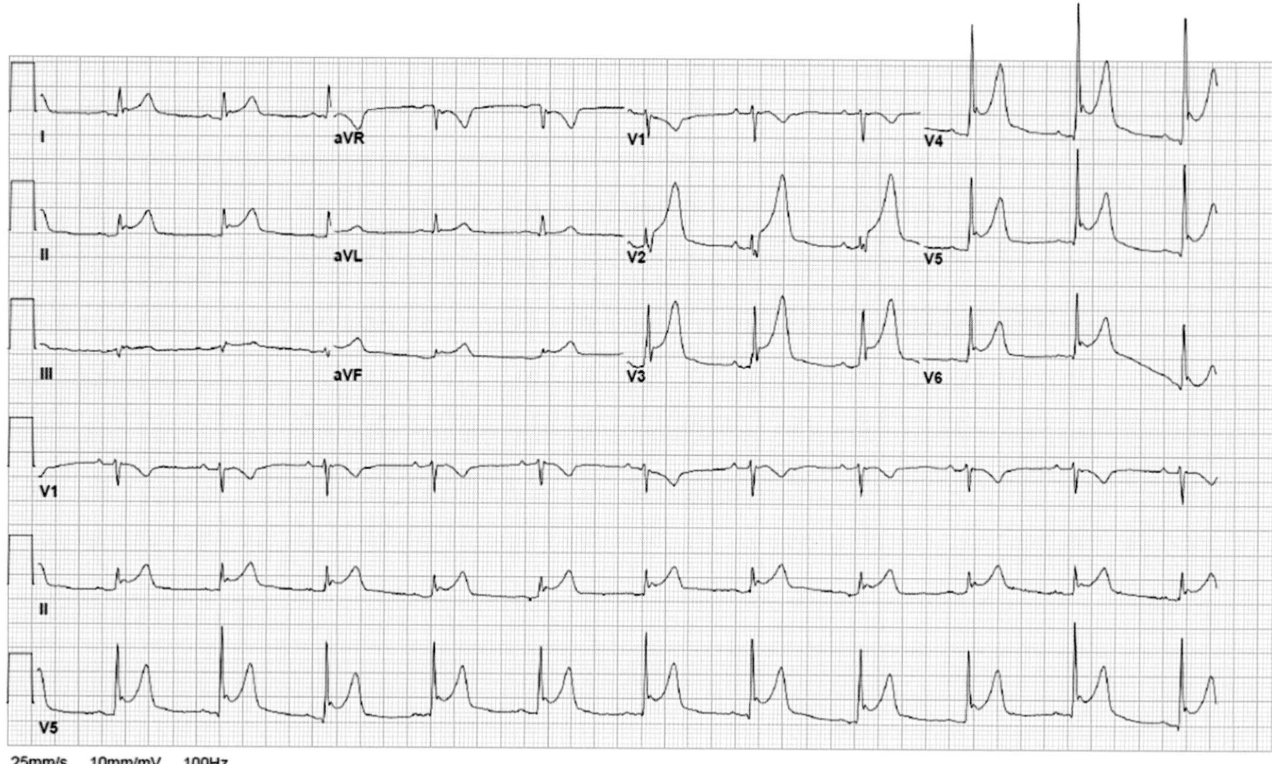

FIGURE 49.17 Acute pericarditis. Electrocardiogram shows diffuse ST segment elevation and PR segment depression, diagnostic of acute pericarditis.

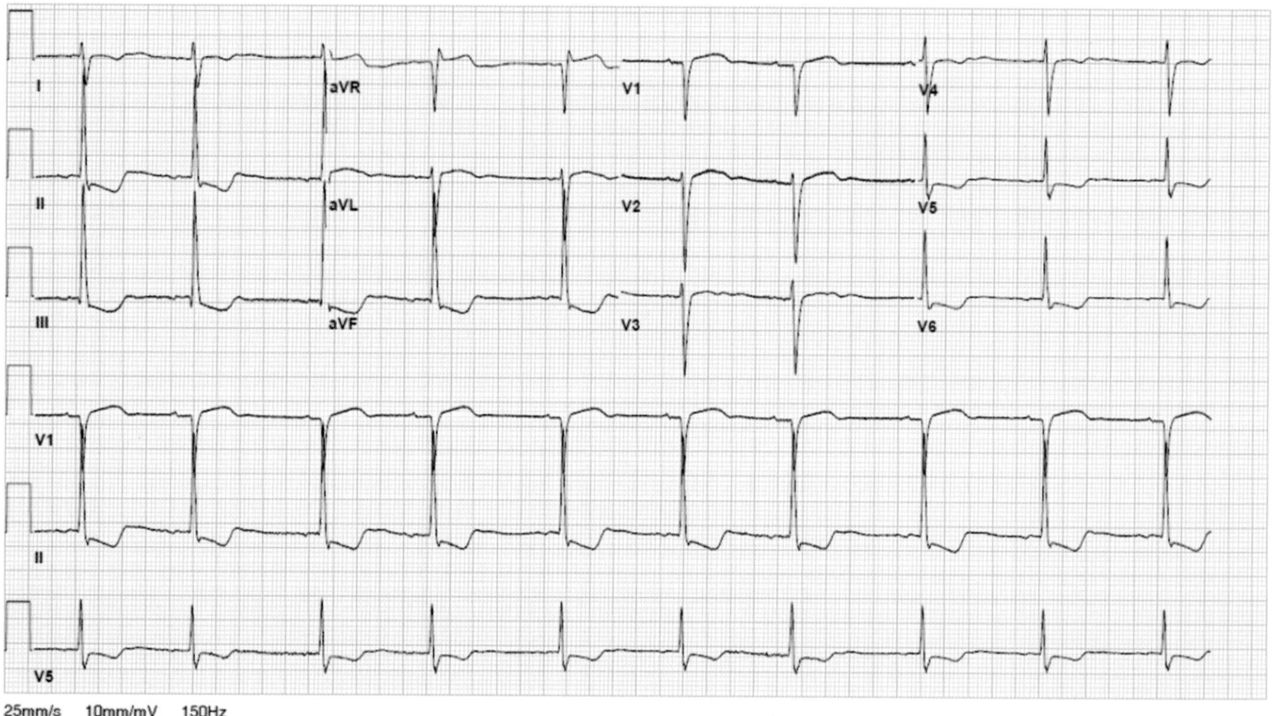

FIGURE 49.18 Digoxin effect. Electrocardiogram shows the "scooped" ST segment and T wave inversions that are an effect of digoxin. This sign alone is insufficient to diagnose digoxin toxicity. Note that the rhythm here is an ectopic atrial rhythm, likely attributable to sinus node suppression caused by digoxin. Sinus rhythm returned following cessation of digoxin.

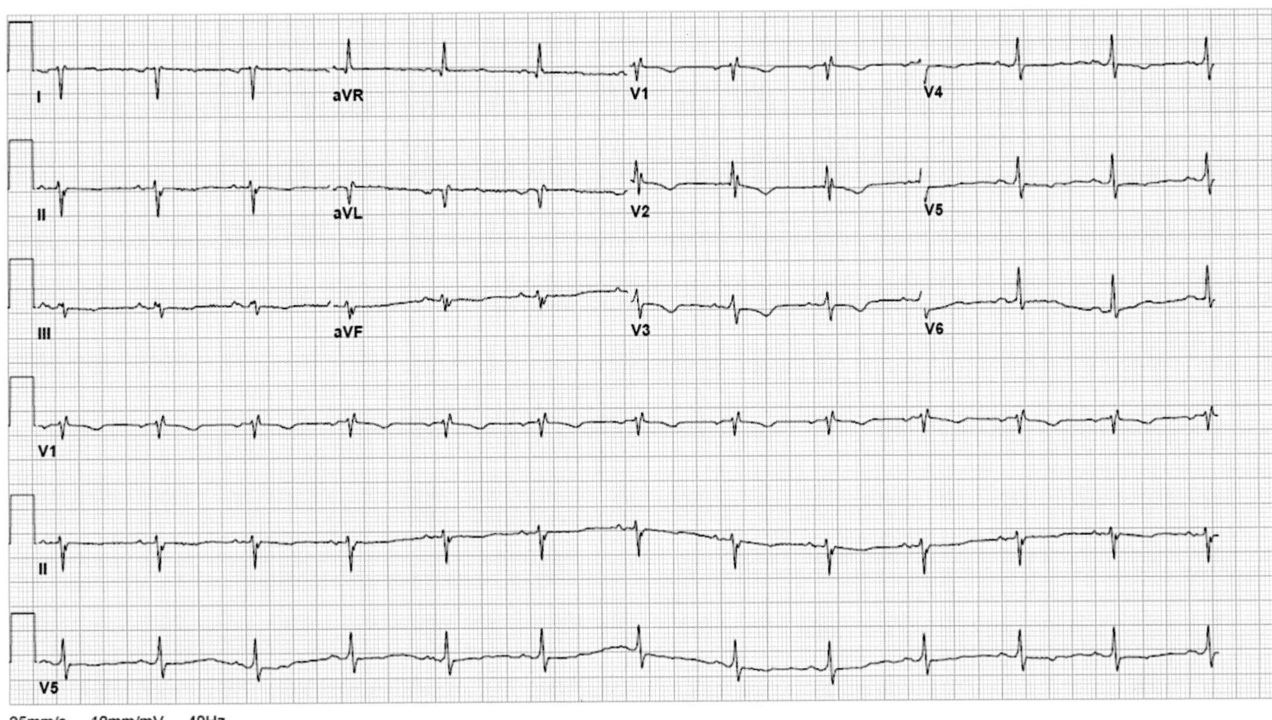

FIGURE 49.19 Lead reversal. Electrocardiogram shows an example of right arm-left arm lead reversal in a patient with normal sinus rhythm. This results in inversion of lead I, switching of lead II and III, and switching of lead aVR and aVL. Note that there is normal precordial R wave progression and normal sinus P wave morphology in lead V1, excluding dextrocardia as the diagnosis.

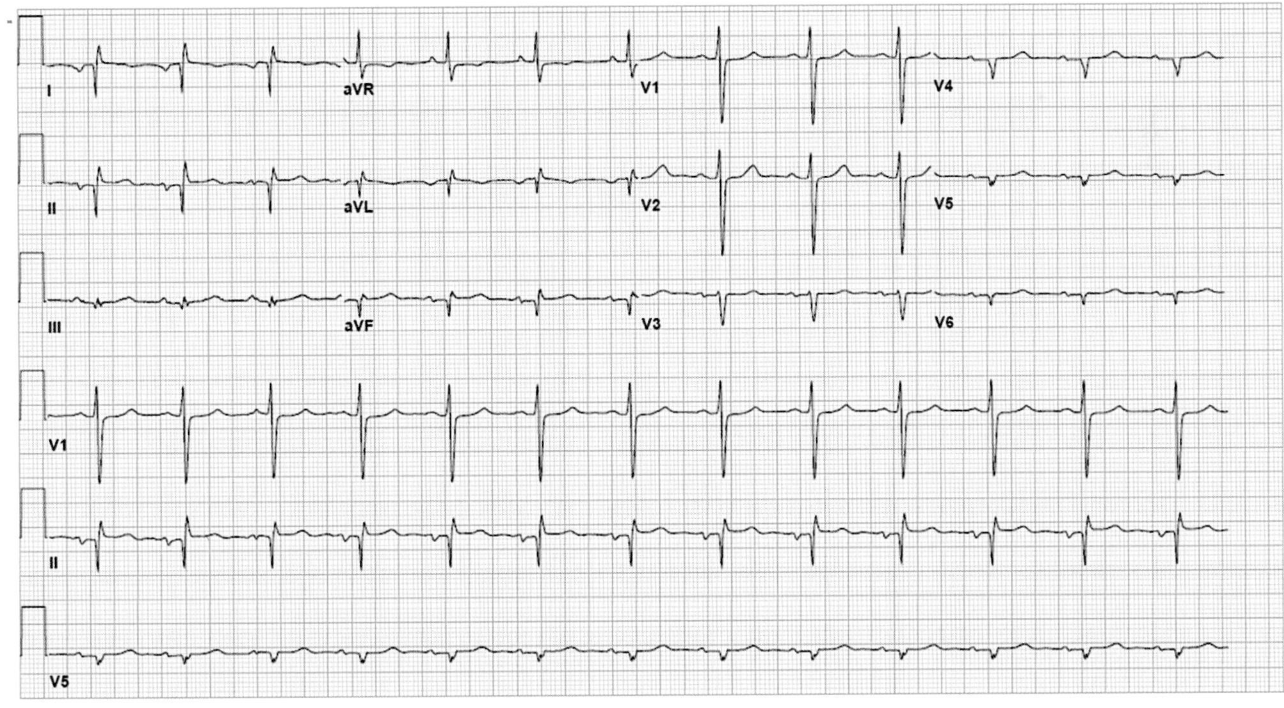

FIGURE 49.20 Dextrocardia. Electrocardiogram (ECG) for a patient with dextrocardia using ECG leads in the standard position. Diagnostic features include a negative R wave progression from V1 to V6, positive P wave in lead V1, inverted P wave in lead I, and positive QRS in lead aVR. Contrast this with right arm-left arm lead reversal in Figure 49.19, where precordial R wave progression is normal and the P wave in lead V1 is negative, as expected with sinus rhythm.

STEMI. Automated ECG reads should also always be overread by an experienced clinician.[8]

A standard 12-lead ECG may not always capture the pathology that the patient presents with (particularly syncope and palpitations), particularly if the symptoms are paroxysmal (ie, intermittent). Continuous monitoring, including continuous ambulatory monitoring, has a higher chance of identifying such arrhythmic etiologies. In cases where symptoms are infrequent, an implantable loop recorder (which is implanted subcutaneously in the chest and can record for 3 or more years) may be appropriate.

Arrhythmias may also not be correctly diagnosed with an ECG, or a broad differential may remain. The differentiation between supraventricular and ventricular tachycardia or etiology of syncope (bradyarrhythmia vs ventricular tachyarrhythmia) is particularly important in the management of patients. In cases where the distinction is not clear, an invasive electrophysiology study may be indicated to clarify the diagnosis.

Normal measurement for intervals, particularly the QT interval, are based on population studies. There is significant overlap in QT interval between patients with long-QT syndrome and those without long-QT syndrome, which makes diagnosis difficult. Patients with long-QT syndrome also manifest varying degrees of QT prolongation throughout the ECG, further complicating diagnosis. Provocative testing such as an epinephrine challenge, ambulatory monitoring, and genetic testing can help confirm or exclude this diagnosis.[9]

Other applications of the ECG also have many limitations; stress ECG, for example, has approximately 70% sensitivity and specificity for diagnosing ischemia. In patients where a strong clinical suspicion exists, additional imaging modalities such as stress echocardiogram or myocardial perfusion scan should be considered, or proceeding with anatomic evaluation by computed tomography angiography or coronary angiography.

Currently, telemetry monitoring also has many inherent limitations, including false alarms that are either incorrect diagnoses, caused by artifact or misinterpretation of the ECG signal, or removal of electrodes. Most alarms in current clinical practice are not actionable and can lead to alarm fatigue.[10]

SPECIAL ISSUES OR CONTRAINDICATIONS

The ECG is a safe and noninvasive procedure and does not pose risks to the patient besides potential skin reactions to the electrodes. Patients with hairy skin should have the areas where electrodes will be placed shaved and abraded for optimal contact. Stress testing, including stress ECG, should not be performed in patients with acute infarcts or symptomatic severe aortic stenosis attributable to the risk of sudden cardiac death.

RESEARCH AND FUTURE DIRECTIONS

Over the past several years, several consumer-level ECG devices have been developed that can record single-lead or multiple-limb-lead ECG rhythm strips. Automated algorithms are then utilized to classify the rhythm strips as normal or abnormal, which patients can then send to their physicians for review. These are particularly helpful for documenting rare arrhythmia symptoms. Although these devices may be an excellent modality to screen high-risk patients for atrial fibrillation and need for anticoagulation to reduce the risk of stroke, technical issues caused by signal noise and difficulties with high-quality recording of the P wave still limit the accurate diagnosis of atrial fibrillation. More research will need to be done in this area as the technology evolves and improves.

KEY POINTS

- ✔ The ECG records the electrical activity of the heart. This can be performed in single 10-second snapshots, or continuously.
- ✔ The standard 12-lead ECG includes 6 limb leads and 6 precordial leads. Fewer leads are generally used for continuous monitoring.
- ✔ The normal electrical activity of the heart is manifested by the P wave, QRS complex, and T wave. The P wave represents atrial depolarization, QRS ventricular depolarization, and T wave ventricular repolarization.
- ✔ A systematic approach should always be used when interpreting ECGs.
- ✔ Abnormalities in the ECG can be used to diagnose a variety of cardiac and noncardiac conditions, including myocardial infarction, pulmonary embolism, cardiac arrhythmias, drug toxicity, and electrolyte disorders.
- ✔ Interpretation of the ECG should always be made in the context of the patient presentation.

REFERENCES

1. Fye WB. A history of the origin, evolution, and impact of electrocardiography. *Am J Cardiol.* 1994;73(13):937-949.
2. Sandau KE, Funk M, Auerbach A, et al. Update to practice standards for electrocardiographic monitoring in hospital settings: a scientific statement from the American Heart Association. *Circulation.* 2017;136(19):e273-e344. doi:10.1161/CIR.0000000000000527
3. Brosnan M, Gerche AL, Kumar S, et al. Modest agreement in ECG interpretation limits the application of ECG screening in young athletes. *Heart Rhythm.* 2015;12(1):130-136. doi:10.1016/j.hrthm.2014.09.060
4. Hancock EW, Deal BJ, Mirvis DM, et al. AHA/ACCF/HRS recommendations for the standardization and interpretation of the electrocardiogram: part V: electrocardiogram changes associated with cardiac chamber hypertrophy a scientific statement from the American Heart Association Electrocardiography and Arrhythmias Committee, Council on Clinical Cardiology; the American College of Cardiology Foundation; and the Heart Rhythm Society Endorsed by the International Society for Computerized Electrocardiology. *J Am Coll Cardiol.* 2009;53(11):992-1002. doi: 10.1016/j.jacc.2008.12.015
5. Wagner GS, Macfarlane P, Wellens H, et al. AHA/ACCF/HRS recommendations for the standardization and interpretation of the electrocardiogram: part VI: acute ischemia/infarction: a scientific statement from the American Heart Association Electrocardiography and Arrhythmias Committee, Council on Clinical Cardiology; the American College of Cardiology Foundation; and the Heart Rhythm Society. Endorsed by the

International Society for Computerized Electrocardiology. *J Am Coll Cardiol.* 2009;53(11):1003-1011. doi:10.1016/j.jacc.2008.12.016

6. Thygesen K, Alpert JS, Jaffe AS, et al. Fourth universal definition of myocardial infarction (2018). *J Am Coll Cardiol.* 2018;72(18):2231-2264. doi:10.1016/j.jacc.2018.08.1038
7. Sgarbossa EB, Pinski SL, Barbagelata A, et al. Electrocardiographic diagnosis of evolving acute myocardial infarction in the presence of left bundle-branch block. *N Engl J Med.* 1996;334(8):481-487.
8. Salerno SM, Alguire PC, Waxman HS. Training and competency evaluation for interpretation of 12-lead electrocardiograms: recommendations from the American College of Physicians. *Ann Intern Med.* 2003;138(9):747-750. doi:10.7326/0003-4819-138-9-200305060-00012
9. Al-Khatib SM, Stevenson WG, Ackerman MJ, et al. AHA/ACC/HRS guideline for management of patients with ventricular arrhythmias and the prevention of sudden cardiac death: a report of the American College of Cardiology/American Heart Association Task Force on Clinical Practice Guidelines and the Heart Rhythm Society. *Circulation.* 2017;72(14):e91-e220. doi:10.1161/cir.0000000000000549
10. Drew BJ, Harris P, Zègre-Hemsey JK, et al. Insights into the problem of alarm fatigue with physiologic monitor devices: a comprehensive observational study of consecutive intensive care unit patients. *PLoS One.* 2014; 9(10):e110274.

CHAPTER 50

MECHANISMS OF CARDIAC ARRHYTHMIAS

Peter Hanna, Kalyanam Shivkumar, and James N. Weiss

INTRODUCTION

For several billion heartbeats in a lifetime, electromechanical coupling ensures normal electrical activity, and activates working myocardium to contract and perform its mechanical function to maintain the circulation. Normal electrical activity necessitates impulse formation and conduction, and electrophysiologic disturbances in impulse formation or conduction result in cardiac arrhythmias that can significantly compromise cardiac contraction (**Algorithm 50.1**). Mechanisms of such aberrations are discussed in this chapter.

IMPULSE FORMATION

Spontaneous Automaticity

Specialized conducting cells in the heart are found in the sinoatrial (SA) node, atrioventricular (AV) node, and the His-Purkinje system and exhibit automaticity to self-generate spontaneous, rhythmic action potentials. A cardinal attribute of these pacemaking cells is the spontaneous diastolic depolarization during phase 4 that follows an action potential, originally attributed to the "funny" current (I_f) identified in the late 1970s.[1] This current is now known to be mediated by sarcolemmal potassium (K^+)/sodium (Na^+) hyperpolarization–activated cyclic nucleotide-gated channels (HCN4 in the heart), distinct among voltage-sensitive ion channels in their activation upon hyperpolarization rather than depolarization (**Figure 50.1**).[2,3] Permeable to both Na^+ and K^+ ions, I_f is an inward current that depolarizes the diastolic resting potential. Assisted by a host of other sarcolemmal ion channels constituting the membrane clock, I_f brings the cell to the threshold for voltage-gated L-type calcium Ca^{2+} channels to generate the action potential upstroke. In the early 2000s, improved confocal microscopic imaging demonstrated that the membrane clock is integrally coupled to a Ca^{2+} clock that plays an essential shared role in automaticity.[4] The Ca^{2+} clock, driven by progressive Ca^{2+} release from the sarcoplasmic reticulum (SR) into the cytoplasm during diastole, activates inward current via electrogenic Na^+-Ca^{2+} exchange (ie, three Na^+ in, one Ca^{2+} out) to assist in depolarizing diastolic membrane potential sufficiently to activate voltage-gated L-type Ca^{2+} channels and generate the upstroke of the action potential.[5] Overall, the heart rate is regulated by phosphorylation of key proteins in both clocks in response to changes in autonomic tone and other factors.

In tissues with pacemaking ability, the SA node normally has the fastest intrinsic rate and serves as the primary pacemaker. Impairment of SA nodal function results in latent or subsidiary pacemakers in atria or ventricles taking over, albeit at slower rates, with atrial and AV junctional subsidiary pacemakers also responsive to autonomic tone. Normally, quiescent cardiac tissue can also develop automaticity or triggered activity under pathophysiologic conditions or due to a host of genetic abnormalities, as discussed in a later chapter.

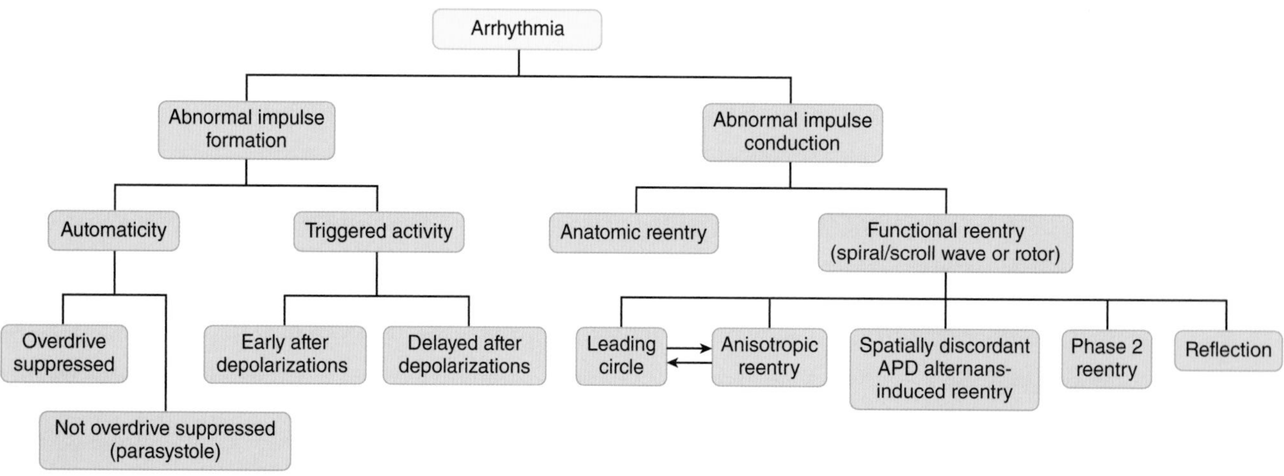

ALGORITHM 50.1 Classification of cardiac arrhythmias. APD, action potential duration.

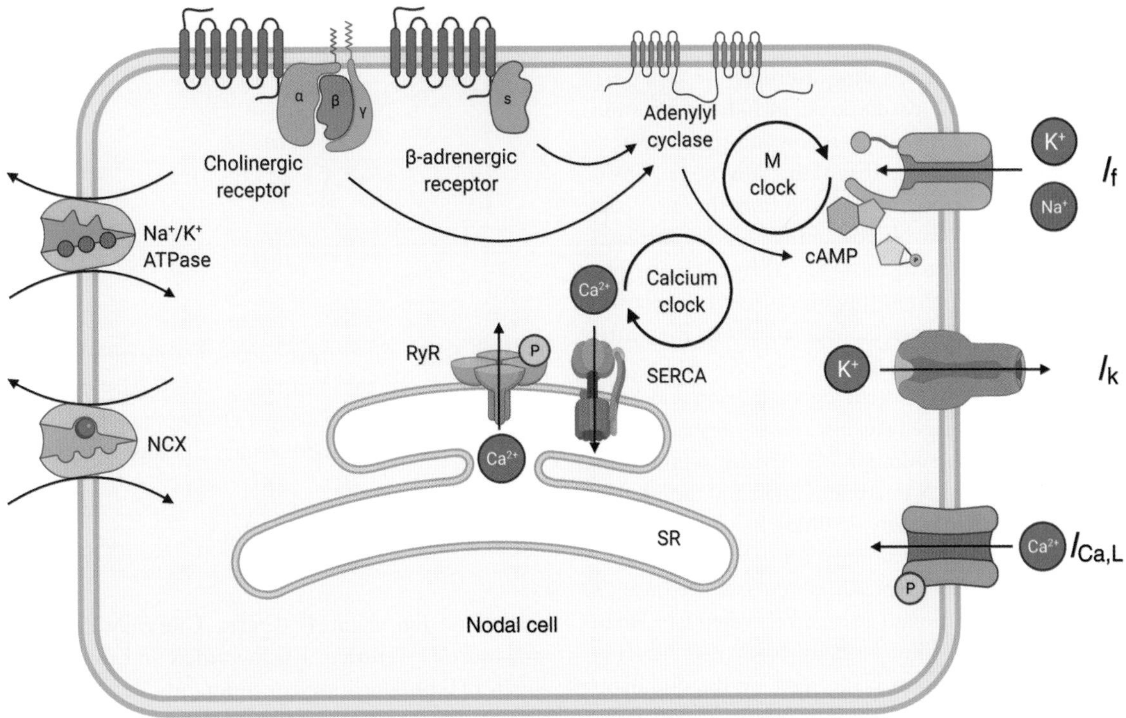

FIGURE 50.1 Schematic of regulation of automaticity in pacemaker cells. The membrane and calcium (Ca^{2+}) clocks are coupled to regulate spontaneous, rhythmic action potentials. The membrane clocks involve the HCN4 channels at the sarcolemmal membrane. The calcium clock regulates (1) intracellular Ca^{2+} cycling between the SR and myoplasm and (2) Ca^{2+} balance via Ca^{2+} channels at the sarcolemmal membrane. ATPase, adenosine triphosphatase; cAMP, cyclic adenosine monophosphate; Ca^{2+}, calcium; K^+, potassium; M clock, membrane clock; NCX, Na^+/Ca^{2+} exchanger; RyR, ryanodine receptor; SERCA, sarco/endoplasmic reticulum calcium-ATPase; SR, sarcoplasmic reticulum. Created with BioRender.com.

Changes in Spontaneous Automaticity

The SA node is densely innervated and under neural control that regulates the heart rate. The enhanced automaticity mediates physiologic responses to stress such as exercise, anxiety, or hypovolemia. Autonomic modulation of heart rate occurs through affecting both the Ca^{2+} and membrane clocks (Figure 50.1). The sympathetic nervous system provides adrenergic input to increase the heart rate through multiple ionic currents, including I_f, to increase the rate of diastolic depolarization and shorten diastole.[4] For example, β-adrenergic stimulation increases intracellular cyclic adenosine monophosphate (cAMP), which then directly binds HCN4 channels to augment I_f.[6] The Ca^{2+} clock is also modulated by phosphorylation of Ca^{2+} cycling proteins (eg, phospholamban, L-type Ca^{2+} channels, and ryanodine receptors) that regulate $[Ca^{2+}]_i$ balance and spontaneous SR Ca^{2+} cycling.[7] The resultant changes in rate may be accompanied by shifts in the dominant pacemaking site within the SA node or to a subsidiary pacemaker site. Enhanced automaticity in other foci may cause ectopic beats or rhythms to emerge. For example, insults to the AV node such as acute myocardial infarction, digitalis toxicity, isoproterenol, or cardiac surgery may result in enhanced automaticity. In such instances, the firing rate of the AV junction may supersede that of the SA node and result in an accelerated junctional rhythm.

Conversely, the parasympathetic nervous system activates muscarinic K^+ channels and decreases I_f to decrease the rate of diastolic depolarization and reduce heart rate. Acetylcholine (ACh) binds muscarinic receptors to inhibit adenylate cyclase and reduce cAMP levels at low-moderate vagal stimulation.[4] Decreased automaticity of the SA node may further result in escape rhythms to become the dominant rhythm. In short, in each SA nodal pacemaking cycle, the membrane and calcium clocks are continuously coupled and are modulated by the autonomic nervous system to maintain spontaneous, rhythmic action potentials across a wide physiologic range.

Enhanced Automaticity

Abnormal automaticity may also develop in normally non-pacemaking cells. A high resting K^+ conductance together with a high intracellular-to-extracellular ratio of K^+ maintained by Na^+-K^+ adenosine triphosphatase (ATPase) generate a negative resting membrane potential that approaches the K^+ equilibrium potential (~−95 mV by the Nernst equation), rendering working atrial and ventricular cardiomyocytes quiescent during diastole. However, multiple different mechanisms can cause abnormal automaticity in such normally quiescent cells, such as membrane depolarization.[8] Some factors, such as hypokalemia, can also induce automaticity in association with membrane hyperpolarization. At normally polarized resting membrane potentials, Na^+ channels are activated and contribute to a rapid upstroke. At depolarized resting membrane potentials, Ca^{2+} currents mediate a slow upstroke.

Automaticity of most pacemakers, including the sinus node, is inhibited by overdrive suppression and remains latent unless their intrinsic rate exceeds that of the sinus node.[9] Overdrive suppression of automaticity can result from the faster pacing rate, causing intracellular Na^+ accumulation that increases outward current via electrogenic Na^+-K^+ ATPase activity. The resulting hyperpolarizing current opposes phase 4 depolarization to slow spontaneous diastolic depolarization. Even after overdrive pacing terminates, continued Na^+-K^+ ATPase activity suppresses the rate of diastolic depolarization and heart rate until the elevated intracellular Na^+ levels normalize. The faster the rate or longer the duration of overdrive suppression, the greater the intracellular Na^+ accumulation and duration of increased Na^+-K^+ ATPase activity, resulting in a longer period of quiescence after cessation of stimulation.

Latent pacemakers are typically suppressed because of resetting by the faster dominant pacemaker, whereas a latent pacemaker site can also exhibit entrance block that insulates it either fully or partially from being reset by the dominant pacemaker. The result is a parasystole or modulated parasystole, an ectopic rhythm that marches independently or quasi-independently through the dominant rhythm. This situation can arise when the dominant pacemaker is surrounded by ischemic, infarcted, or otherwise electrically compromised tissues that inhibit resetting of the latent pacemaker. This activity is typically characterized by premature ventricular contractions that march through the sinus rate and rarely result in a life-threatening ventricular arrhythmia.

Triggered Activity

Afterdepolarizations are abnormal impulses that are classified as early afterdepolarization (EAD) or delayed afterdepolarization (DAD) depending on whether they arise during or following an action potential, respectively. Unlike automaticity, they require an antecedent action potential, whether spontaneous, triggered, or artificially paced. If an EAD or DAD depolarizes the membrane potential to threshold, an action potential results, and is referred to as triggered activity (**Figure 50.2**). In cardiac tissue, such triggered beats can propagate from regions with EADs into regions without EADs, generating tachycardias and initiating reentry when dispersion of refractoriness is sufficient.[10] Unfortunately, EADs and DADs cannot be directly detected clinically from an electrocardiogram.

Early Afterdepolarizations

EADs occur during phase 2 or phase 3 of the cardiac action potential before repolarization is complete. They typically occur in the setting of a prolonged action potential such as in long QT syndromes. Multiple conditions may result in QT prolongation including myocardial injury, electrolyte disturbances (hypokalemia, hypomagnesemia), acidosis, hypoxia, catecholamines, QT prolonging drugs (antiarrhythmic and noncardiac drugs), left ventricular hypertrophy, heart failure, and congenital ion channels defects. Clinically, EADs can cause polymorphic ventricular tachycardias and torsades de pointes when QT prolongation concomitantly increases dispersion of refractoriness and makes tissue vulnerable to reentry.

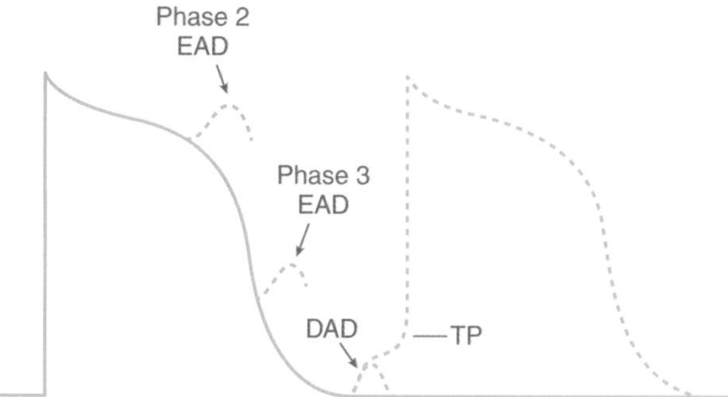

FIGURE 50.2 Afterdepolarizations are classified on the basis of occurrence during cardiac action potential. Early afterdepolarizations (EADs; dashed line) and delayed afterdepolarizations (DADs; dashed line) that reach threshold potential (TP) trigger an action potential (dashed line).

Action potential duration (APD) prolongation occurs when net outward current during the action potential plateau is reduced so that repolarization reserve becomes impaired. The imbalance can be caused by uncompensated increases in inward currents such as the late sodium (I_{Na}) or Ca^{2+} currents (I_{Ca} or I_{NCX}) or decreases in outward repolarizing potassium currents (I_{Kr}, I_{KS}, I_{K1}). If sufficiently severe, reactivation of the L-type Ca^{2+} channels during phase 2 or 3 can reverse repolarization altogether and cause the upstroke of EAD[11] to trigger a new action potential that propagates into surrounding tissue that has already repolarized.

EADs occurring late in phase 3 have also been associated with APD shortening when intracellular Ca^{2+} continues to rise during the rapid repolarization phase of the action potential.[12] In this case, activation of inward I_{NCX} can reverse repolarization and cause triggered activity. These late EADs are clinically relevant, because they can occur after cessation of other types of tachycardia such as atrial fibrillation, atrial tachycardia, ventricular tachycardia, and ventricular fibrillation.[13,14]

EADs that induce triggered activity are sensitive to heart rate. Class III antiarrhythmic agents tend to induce EADs at slow heart rates because of their reverse use-dependence property, whereas β-agonists may induce EADs at faster heart rates by augmenting the L-type Ca^{2+} current to further reduce repolarization reserves.[15]

Delayed Afterdepolarizations

DADs occur in phase 4 of the cardiac action potential after repolarization is complete. DADs are caused by spontaneous SR Ca^{2+} release during diastole, typically occurring in the setting of intracellular Ca^{2+} overload. Normally, Ca^{2+} influx during the action potential upstroke and early phases of the plateau triggers Ca^{2+} release from the SR, followed by Ca^{2+}

reuptake into the SR during repolarization and early diastole. SR Ca^{2+} uptake is potentiated by high intracellular Ca^{2+}, cAMP, and catecholamines. Elevation of SR Ca^{2+} during repolarization may result in subsequent spontaneous calcium release from the SR, leading to activation of a transient inward current I_{TI}, due to I_{NCX}, the Ca^{2+}-activated nonselective cationic current $I_{NS(Ca)}$, and/or the Ca^{2+}-activated chloride current $I_{Cl(Ca)}$,[16-18] which underlies the DAD. DADs are more likely to be induced, persist, and reach the threshold for triggered activity at faster rates, whether spontaneous or pacing induced, in contrast to the slower rates often associated with EADs. DADs are thought to be the mechanism underlying catecholaminergic polymorphic ventricular tachycardia, which is caused by mutations of the type 2 ryanodine receptor or calsequestrin that result in "leaky" ryanodine receptors promoting spontaneous SR Ca^{2+} release.[19] The leakiness of ryanodine receptor is further enhanced during catecholamine stimulation.

DADs are more likely to reach threshold and result in action potential firing in the setting of digitalis toxicity, catecholamines, and electrolyte abnormalities (hypokalemia, hypomagnesemia, and hypercalcemia), as well as structural heart disease such as hypertrophy, heart failure, and post-myocardial infarction.[15,20] Digitalis toxicity causes DAD-dependent triggered arrhythmias by inhibiting the Na^+-K^+ ATPase, resulting in accumulation of intracellular Na^+.[21] This reduces the driving force for Na^+ influx, thereby inhibiting the ability of NCX (Na^+/Ca^{2+} exchanger) to remove calcium from the cytoplasm, resulting in Ca^{2+} overload.

Catecholamines increase intracellular Ca^{2+} loading by multiple mechanisms, including increasing Ca^{2+} influx through L-type Ca^{2+} current and stimulating Ca^{2+} uptake into the SR, thereby increasing Ca^{2+} stores for subsequent release. These effects are mediated largely by increased cAMP in response to β-adrenergic stimulation.

ABNORMAL IMPULSE CONDUCTION

Reentry

Reentry occurs when a wavefront corresponding to a propagating action potential upstroke circulates continuously through the tissue by reactivating repolarized tissue that has recovered its excitability. It is the most common mechanism of clinical arrhythmias including AV reentrant tachycardia using a bypass tract, AV nodal reentrant tachycardia, atrial flutter, atrial fibrillation, and ventricular tachycardia and fibrillation. Reentry can circulate around a fixed anatomic obstacle or a region of functionally refractory tissue (**Figure 50.3**). In the latter case, the functional reentry circuit can be stationary (producing a monomorphic tachycardia) or can meander throughout the tissue (producing polymorphic tachycardia) or break up into multiple wavefronts (fibrillation).

Reentry Around a Fixed Anatomic Obstacle

Circus-type reentry was initially hypothesized by McWilliam in 1887 and experimentally demonstrated in jelly fish rings by Mayor in 1906.[22,23] Mines was the first to demonstrate reentry in the heart, using rings of tissue cut from tortoise hearts.[24] He determined that the maintenance of reentry required the length of the anatomic circuit or pathway to exceed the wavelength (distance between the wavefront and the waveback), which is calculated as

$$\lambda = CV \times RP$$

where λ is the wavelength; CV, the conduction velocity; and RP, the refractory period that usually can be approximated by the APD. In other words, there has to be an excitable gap between the waveback and wavefront of the returning wave. From this simple relationship, a reduction in conduction velocity (CV) or APD reduces the wavelength and, hence, the path length required for the initiation or maintenance of reentry.

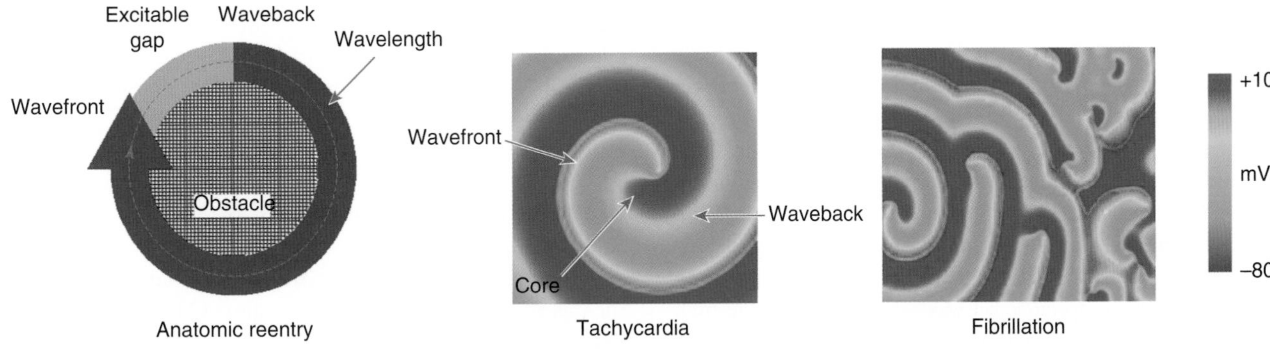

FIGURE 50.3 Models of anatomic and functional reentry. In anatomic reentry, the circuit around an obstacle (cross-hatched region) requires that a segment of the loop has fully recovered (excitable gap; gray). The anatomic path around the obstacle must exceed the length of the wavelength (distance between wavefront and waveback; dashed line). In functional reentry, the core of the rotor is functionally refractory and may be either stationary (tachycardia) or mobile (fibrillation). (Reprinted from Weiss JN, Qu Z, Shivkumar K. Ablating atrial fibrillation: A translational science perspective for clinicians. *Heart Rhythm.* 2016;13(9):1868-1877. Copyright © 2016 Heart Rhythm Society. With permission.)

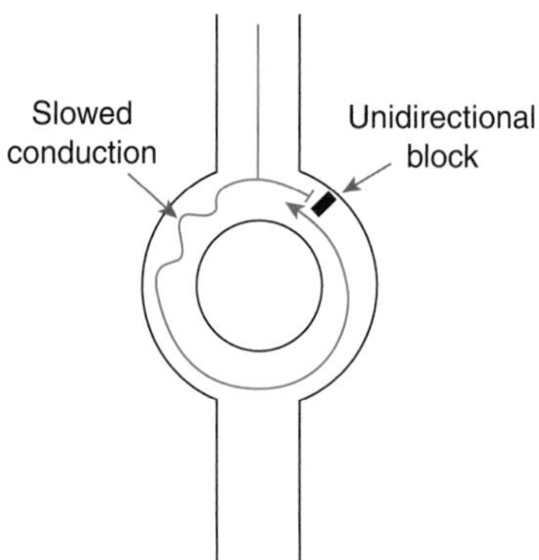

FIGURE 50.4 Schematic of anatomic circus movement reentry. As a wavefront approaches an obstacle such as a branch in conduction pathway, the impulse propagates down both limbs. If unidirectional block is present, antegrade conduction is blocked. If conduction down the other pathway is sufficiently slow, the area of block may recover from refractoriness to allow retrograde conduction. If this occurs, a reentrant circuit is formed.

Initiation of reentry also requires unidirectional conduction block to start the process (**Figure 50.4**). Unidirectional block, whether transient or permanent, is usually a product of heterogeneous electrophysiologic properties in the myocardium. A premature stimulus is most likely to initiate reentry when it both induces unidirectional block and slows conduction so that the area of conduction block has time to recover before the propagating wavefront returns to that site. Of note, this premature stimulus may be caused by a distinct arrhythmic mechanism such as automaticity or triggered activity. A clinical example of this type of reentry is typical atrial flutter, whose anatomic pathway circulates around the tricuspid valve and its isthmus with the inferior vena cava.

Functional Reentry

Garrey postulated that reentry could occur in the absence of an anatomic obstacle in 1914,[25] but it was not until the 1970s that Allessie et al convincingly demonstrated functional reentry experimentally in isolated rabbit atrial preparations.[26] Early mechanistic explanations included the leading circle hypothesis and anisotropic reentry, which are now known to be variants of spiral wave reentry (called *scroll wave reentry* in three dimensions), a generic property of excitable media including chemical systems such as the Belousov-Zhabotinsky reaction and Ca^{2+}-induced Ca^{2+} release in addition to cardiac electrical propagation.[27] In this type of reentry, the functionally refractory core of the spiral/scroll wave rotor is due to the high curvature of the wavefront in this region such that the source of depolarizing current from the curved wavefront is inadequate to bring the repolarized tissue in the core to the threshold of excitation due to the source-sink mismatch. Depending on the electrophysical properties of the tissue, the core of a spiral/scroll wave rotor can be stationary, meandering, or hypermeandering, corresponding to monomorphic or polymorphic tachycardia, respectively. In some cases, the arm of the rotor can also be unstable, such that the rotor breaks up into multiple fibrillatory waves, producing electrocardiographic fibrillation (Figure 50.3). The breakup of the arm of the rotor can be caused either by fibrillatory conduction block, if the tissue distant from the core cannot maintain 1:1 conduction (called *mother rotor fibrillation*), or by intrinsic unstable dynamic oscillations of the rotor's arm (called *multiple wavelet fibrillation*).[10] Dispersion of excitability or refractoriness sets the conditions for functional reentry. Clinically, these mechanisms are relevant to both atrial and ventricular tachycardias and fibrillation.

Spatially Discordant Action Potential Duration Alternans

As noted earlier, the initiation of reentry can be caused by properly timed premature stimuli in electrophysiologically heterogeneous tissue with preexisting dispersion of refractoriness and/or excitability. However, rapid pacing can also dynamically create electrophysiologic dispersion, leading to unidirectional conduction block and reentry due to spatially discordant action potential alternans,[28] in which regions of long APD alternate with regions of short APD in the same tissue (**Figure 50.5**). This occurs because both APD and CV vary with the previous diastolic interval, causing both to oscillate at rapid heart rates in which the diastolic interval is short. Both the incomplete recovery of ionic currents and Ca^{2+} cycling elements at short diastolic intervals (known as APD and Ca^{2+} cycling restitution properties) contribute to the action potential oscillations, whereas incomplete recovery of the Na^+ current I_{Na} (or the L-type Ca^{2+} current in depolarized tissue) underlie the oscillations in CV. In the setting of spatially discordant APD alternans, a premature extrasystole arising in a region where the APD is short can block as it propagates into an adjacent region with long APD (asterisk in Figure 50.5). The resulting unidirectional conduction block may then initiate reentry. This is the major mechanism by which very rapid pacing (>250 bpm) induces fibrillation in even normal hearts. In heart failure, electrical and Ca^{2+} cycling remodeling result in spatially discordant alternans at much slower heart rates, often in the physiologic range, predisposing to sudden cardiac death. Electrocardiographic detection of QT alternans at modestly increased heart rates is used clinically to assess the risk of sudden cardiac death in patients with heart failure.

Other Variations of Functional Reentry

Another important type of functional reentry known as *phase 2 reentry* occurs in the setting of excessive repolarization reserve such as acute myocardial ischemia, short QT syndromes, and Brugada syndrome.[10,29,30] Under these conditions, regions of the heart with excessive repolarization reserve become predisposed to all-or-none early repolarization of the action potential, creating regions with very short plateau-less action potentials juxtaposed next to regions with action potentials exhibiting a prominent dome in the plateau (phase 2) caused by reactivation of the L-type Ca^{2+} current. Regions of the heart with a high density of the transient outward K^+ current (I_{to}),

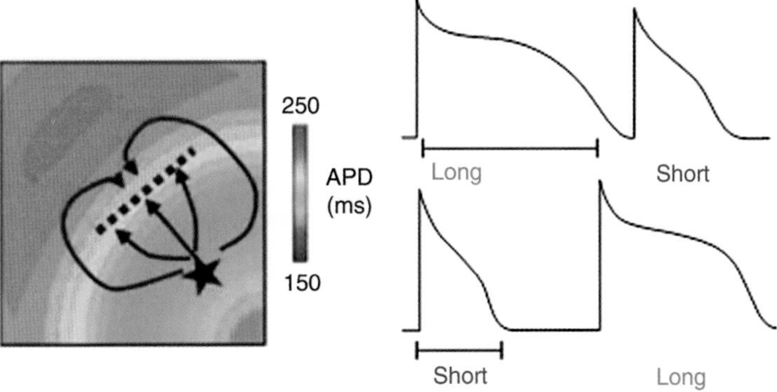

FIGURE 50.5 Mechanism of initiation of reentry by a premature ectopic beat during spatially discordant alternans. A premature ectopic beat (asterisk) occurring in the region of short action potential duration (APD; blue) blocks (dashed line) as it propagates across the nodal line (yellow), where APD does not alternate, into the region with long APD (red). Meanwhile, the ectopic beat successfully propagates laterally, waiting for the long APD region to repolarize and then reenters the blocked region to initiate figure-of-eight reentry. (Adapted with permission from Weiss JN, Garfinkel A, Karagueuzian HS, et al. Perspective: a dynamics-based classification of ventricular arrhythmias. *J Mol Cell Cardiol.* 2015;82:136-152. Copyright © 2015 Elsevier and Weiss JN, Karma A, Shiferaw Y, et al. From pulsus to pulseless: the saga of cardiac alternans. *Circ Res.* 2006;98(10):1244-1253.)

such as the right ventricular epicardium, are particularly susceptible to phase 2 reentry. The marked dispersion of refractoriness can allow electrical currents from the action potential dome regions to flow into and re-excite adjacent short-action potential regions that have already repolarized, creating a premature extrasystole. Under the right conditions, the premature extrasystole can induce functional reentry that rapidly degenerates into fibrillation, especially when slow conduction due to acute ischemia or chronic fibrosis is also present. Clinically, this mechanism is thought to be an important cause of sudden cardiac death following acute coronary artery occlusion and congenital short QT and Brugada syndromes.

Finally, in addition to dispersion of refractoriness inducing phase 2 reentry, dispersion of excitability can also induce a variant of reentry known as *reflection*.[31-33] Reflection has been demonstrated in excised canine Purkinje fibers with a central gap region made inexcitable by high extracellular potassium concentrations or pure sucrose. Although reflection by itself only produces a single extrasystole, the extrasystole can potentially serve as a trigger to induce reentry in adjacent tissue. Whether reflection is clinically important is uncertain.

KEY POINTS

- ✔ Cardiac arrhythmias result from disruption of both normal impulse formation and impulse conduction. These etiologies are implicated in both congenital and acquired cardiac arrhythmias.
- ✔ Clinically, more than one mechanism may be involved in the same patient.
- ✔ A firm understanding of the mechanistic basis of these arrhythmias is required to distinguish which are most critical in a given patient.
- ✔ Understanding the molecular, cellular, and tissue-level mechanisms of cardiac arrhythmias are critical for developing and implementing appropriate pharmacologic and/or ablative therapies for these heart rhythm disorders.

REFERENCES

1. Carmeliet E. Pacemaking in cardiac tissue. From IK2 to a coupled-clock system. *Physiol Rep.* 2019;7(1):e13862.
2. DiFrancesco D. Characterization of single pacemaker channels in cardiac sino-atrial node cells. *Nature.* 1986;324(6096):470-473.
3. Ludwig A, Zong X, Jeglitsch M, Hofmann F, Biel M. A family of hyperpolarization-activated mammalian cation channels. *Nature.* 1998; 393(6685):587-591.
4. Lakatta EG, Maltsev VA, Vinogradova TM. A coupled SYSTEM of intracellular Ca^{2+} clocks and surface membrane voltage clocks controls the timekeeping mechanism of the heart's pacemaker. *Circ Res.* 2010;106(4): 659-673.
5. Bogdanov KY, Maltsev VA, Vinogradova TM, et al. Membrane potential fluctuations resulting from submembrane Ca^{2+} releases in rabbit sinoatrial nodal cells impart an exponential phase to the late diastolic depolarization that controls their chronotropic state. *Circ Res.* 2006;99(9): 979-987.
6. Bucchi A, Baruscotti M, Robinson RB, DiFrancesco D. Modulation of rate by autonomic agonists in SAN cells involves changes in diastolic depolarization and the pacemaker current. *J Mol Cell Cardiol.* 2007; 43(1):39-48.
7. Vinogradova TM, Bogdanov KY, Lakatta EG. β-Adrenergic stimulation modulates ryanodine receptor Ca^{2+} release during diastolic depolarization to accelerate pacemaker activity in rabbit sinoatrial nodal cells. *Circ Res.* 2002;90(1):73-79.
8. Katzung B. Electrically induced automatically in ventricular myocardium. *Life Sci.* 1974;14(6):1133-1140.
9. Vassalle M. The relationship among cardiac pacemakers. Overdrive suppression. *Circ Res.* 1977;41(3):269-277.
10. Weiss JN, Garfinkel A, Karagueuzian HS, et al. Perspective: a dynamics-based classification of ventricular arrhythmias. *J Mol Cell Cardiol.* 2015;82: 136-152.
11. January CT, Riddle JM. Early afterdepolarizations: mechanism of induction and block. A role for L-type Ca^{2+} current. *Circ Res.* 1989; 64(5):977-990.

12. Szabo B, Sweidan R, Rajagopalan CV, Lazzara R. Role of Na^+: Ca^{2+} exchange current in Cs^+-induced early afterdepolarizations in Purkinje fibers. *J Cardiovasc Electrophysiol.* 1994;5(11):933-944.
13. Burashnikov A, Antzelevitch C. Reinduction of atrial fibrillation immediately after termination of the arrhythmia is mediated by late phase 3 early afterdepolarization–induced triggered activity. *Circulation.* 2003; 107(18):2355-2360.
14. Patterson E, Lazzara R, Szabo B, et al. Sodium-calcium exchange initiated by the Ca^{2+} transient: an arrhythmia trigger within pulmonary veins. *J Am Coll Cardiol.* 2006;47(6):1196-1206.
15. Priori SG, Corr PB. Mechanisms underlying early and delayed afterdepolarizations induced by catecholamines. *Am J Physiol.* 1990;258(6):H1 796-H1805.
16. Karagueuzian HS, Katzung BG. Voltage-clamp studies of transient inward current and mechanical oscillations induced by ouabain in ferret papillary muscle. *J Physiol.* 1982;327(1):255-271.
17. Hill J Jr, Coronado R, Strauss H. Reconstitution and characterization of a calcium-activated channel from heart. *Circ Res.* 1988;62(2):411-415.
18. Zygmunt AC. Intracellular calcium activates a chloride current in canine ventricular myocytes. *Am J Physiol.* 1994;267(5):H1984-H1995.
19. Priori SG, Napolitano C, Tiso N, et al. Mutations in the cardiac ryanodine receptor gene (hRyR2) underlie catecholaminergic polymorphic ventricular tachycardia. *Circulation.* 2001;103(2):196-200.
20. Rosen MR, Gelband H, Merker C, Hoffman BF. Mechanisms of digitalis toxicity: effects of ouabain on phase four of canine Purkinje fiber transmembrane potentials. *Circulation.* 1973;47(4):681-689.
21. Kass R, Tsien R, Weingart R. Ionic basis of transient inward current induced by strophanthidin in cardiac Purkinje fibres. *J Physiol.* 1978; 281(1):209-226.
22. Mayor AG. *Rhythmical Pulsation in Scyphomedusae, I.* Carnegie Institution of Washington; 1906.
23. McWilliam JA. Fibrillar contraction of the heart. *J Physiol.* 1887;8(5): 296-310.
24. Mines GR. On dynamic equilibrium in the heart. *J Physiol.* 1913;46(4-5): 349-383.
25. Garrey WE. The nature of fibrillary contraction of the heart—Its relation to tissue mass and form. *Am J Physiol.* 1914;33(3):397-414.
26. Allessie MA, Bonke FI, Schopman FJ. Circus movement in rabbit atrial muscle as a mechanism of tachycardia. *Circ Res.* 1973;33(1):54-62.
27. Winfree AT, Tyson JJ. When time breaks down: the three-dimensional dynamics of electrochemical waves and cardiac arrhythmias. *PhT.* 1988; 41(12):107.
28. Qu Z, Garfinkel A, Chen P-S, Weiss JN. Mechanisms of discordant alternans and induction of reentry in simulated cardiac tissue. *Circulation.* 2000;102(14):1664-1670.
29. Antzelevitch C, Burashnikov A. Overview of basic mechanisms of cardiac arrhythmia. *Card Electrophysiol Clin.* 2011;3(1):23-45.
30. Lukas A, Antzelevitch C. Phase 2 reentry as a mechanism of initiation of circus movement reentry in canine epicardium exposed to simulated ischemia. *Cardiovasc Res.* 1996;32(3):593-603.
31. Schmitt FO, Erlanger J. Directional differences in the conduction of the impulse through heart muscle and their possible relation to extrasystolic and fibrillary contractions. *Am J Physiol.* 1928;87(2):326-347.
32. Wit AL, Hoffman BF, Cranefield PF. Slow conduction and reentry in the ventricular conducting system: I. Return extrasystole in canine Purkinje fibers. *Circ Res.* 1972;30(1):1-10.
33. Antzelevitch C, Jalife J, Moe GK. Characteristics of reflection as a mechanism of reentrant arrhythmias and its relationship to parasystole. *Circulation.* 1980;61(1):182-191.

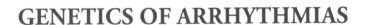

GENETICS OF ARRHYTHMIAS

Aadhavi Sridharan, Jason S. Bradfield, and James N. Weiss

INTRODUCTION

Cardiac arrhythmias comprise a wide spectrum of abnormalities of the heart rhythm; these can be benign, can increase the risk of stroke or embolism, or can even be life-threatening, resulting in sudden cardiac death (SCD). Because of the significant advances in the area of cardiovascular genetics over the past three decades, several arrhythmia syndromes previously considered idiopathic are now known to be caused by mutations in genes primarily encoding ion channels.[1] This has facilitated an improved understanding of the pathophysiology of these disorders and recognition of important genotype-phenotype associations, which has in turn resulted in significant diagnostic, prognostic, and therapeutic implications. This chapter includes a brief discussion of the cardiac action potential and associated ion channels, followed by the genetic basis and genotype-phenotype correlations of common hereditary arrhythmia syndromes.

CARDIAC ACTION POTENTIAL AND ION CHANNELS

A fundamental knowledge of the cardiac action potential is necessary to understand the genetics of cardiac arrhythmias. The cardiac action potential is a brief change in voltage across the cell membrane of myocytes, achieved through a complex, orchestrated change in permeability of sodium (Na^+), potassium (K^+), calcium (Ca^{2+}), and chloride (Cl^-) ions through different types of ion channels.

The action potential in a typical ventricular myocyte is divided into five phases, named phase 0 through phase 4 (**Figure 51.1**). During phase 4, also termed the resting phase, there is a higher concentration of Na^+ and Ca^{2+} outside the cell and a higher concentration of K^+ inside the cells. During this phase, an abundance of open K^+ channels allowing slow leakage of K^+ out of the cell maintain the membrane potential at approximately −90 mV, near the equilibrium potential of K^+. When these resting myocytes reach a threshold voltage of approximately −70 mV, they enter phase 0. During phase 0, also known as rapid depolarization, a transient increase in Na^+ conductance and decrease in inward rectifier K^+ current results in a positive membrane potential closer to the equilibrium potential of Na^+. Phase 1 represents an initial, rapid repolarization phase that is caused by a transient outward K^+ current. During phase 2, also termed the plateau phase, there is inward Ca^{2+} current through the L-type calcium channels that are activated when the membrane potential depolarizes to −40 mV. Inward Ca^{2+} currents and outward K^+ currents are relatively balanced during this plateau phase. Phase 3 is the repolarization phase during which there is inactivation of Ca^{2+} current and an increase in outward K^+ current caused by activation of several different time-dependent potassium channels.[2,3]

Maintenance of normal sinus rhythm is thus dependent on the coordinated movement of ions mediating the cardiac action potential. Ion channel dysfunction can have significant consequences that present as arrhythmias, some potentially lethal.

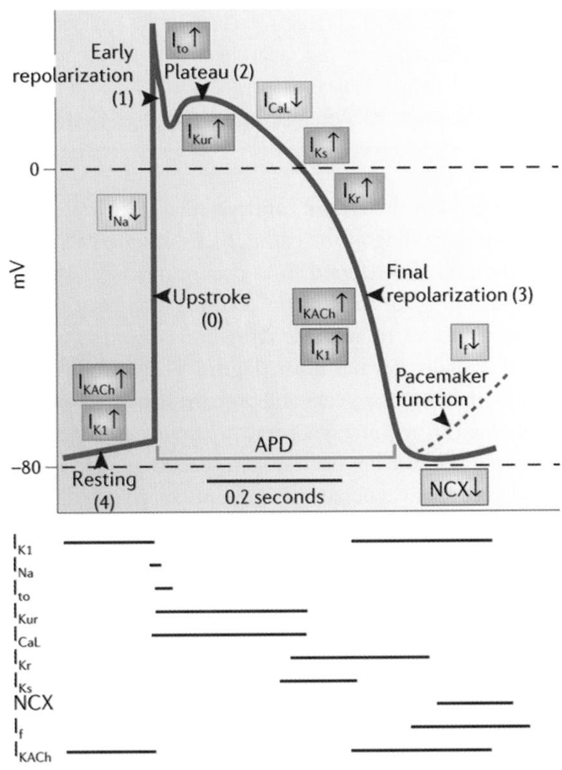

FIGURE 51.1 Cardiac action potential and respective ion currents during various phases. IK1, inward rectifier K current; INa, Na current; Ito, transient outward K current; IKur, ultrarapid component of the delayed rectifier K current; IKr, rapid component of the delayed rectifier K current; IKs, slow component of the delayed rectifier K current; NCX, Na-Ca exchanger; If, hyperpolarization-activated nonselective pacemaker "funny" current; IKACh, Acetylcholine-activated K current. (Reprinted by permission from Nature: Nattel S, Carlsson L. Innovative approaches to anti-arrhythmic drug therapy. *Nat Rev Drug Discov.* 2006;5(12):1034-1049. Copyright © 2006 Springer Nature.)

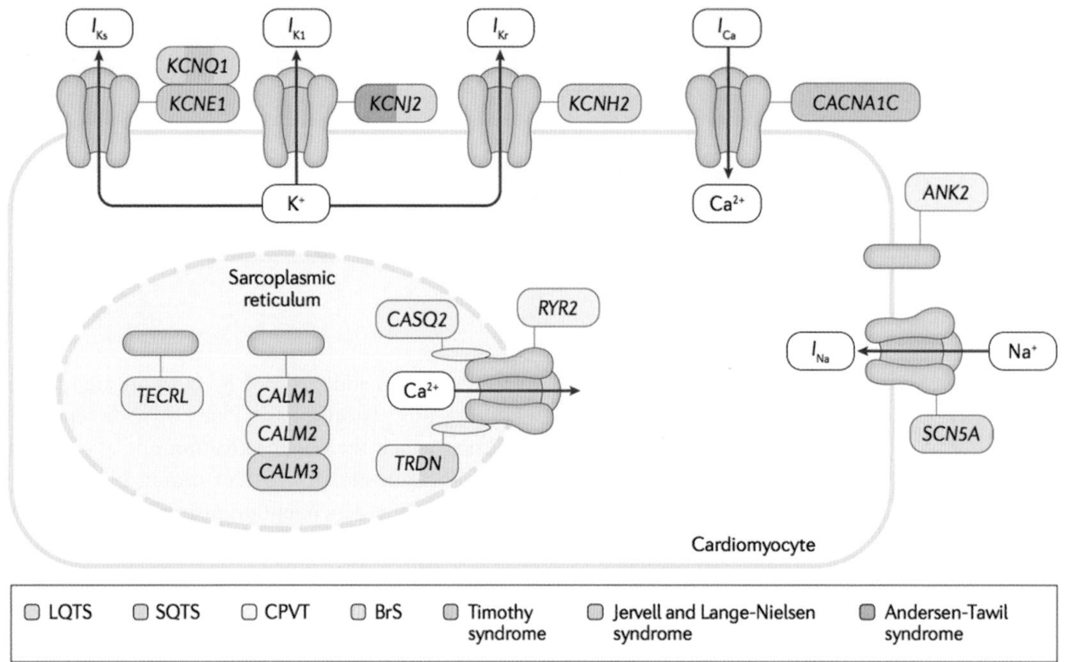

FIGURE 51.2 Genes and proteins involved in the pathogenesis of hereditary cardiac arrhythmias. The genes that encode ion channels and proteins in the sarcoplasmic reticulum are color-coded according to the inherited arrhythmia disorder in which they are implicated. BrS, Brugada syndrome; CPVT, catecholaminergic polymorphic ventricular tachycardia; LQTS, long QT syndrome; SQTS, short QT syndrome. Reprinted with permission from Schwartz PJ, Ackerman MJ, Antzelevitch C, et al. Inherited cardiac arrhythmias. *Nat Rev Dis Primers.* 2020;6:58.

Recent progress in the area of cardiovascular genetics has led to a better understanding of the pathogenesis of inherited arrhythmia syndromes, also referred to as channelopathies. Mutations in genes encoding for specific ion channels have been shown to cause specific forms of heritable arrhythmia disorders occurring in the structurally normal heart. **Figure 51.2** and **Table 51.1** summarize the common genes and proteins associated with common inherited arrhythmia syndromes. Current guidelines recommend genetic counseling or mutation-specific genetic screening of first-degree relatives of patients with inherited arrhythmia syndromes to identify affected family members, caused by increased risk of adverse cardiac events in genotype-positive patients.[4]

COMMON HEREDITARY ARRHYTHMIA SYNDROMES

Long QT Syndrome

Congenital long QT syndrome (LQTS), the most prevalent of the inherited arrhythmias occurring in about 1 in 2000 people,[5] is characterized by delayed myocardial repolarization and prolongation of the QT interval (corrected QT [QTc] >470 msec), resulting in an increased risk of syncope owing to torsades de pointes, seizures, and SCD in otherwise healthy children and adolescents with structurally normal hearts.[1,6] It is most commonly inherited in an autosomal dominant manner (and was previously known as Romano-Ward syndrome), and rarely as a recessive disorder (known as Jervell and Lange-Nielsen syndrome,[7] characterized by a severe cardiac phenotype and sensorineural hearing loss). At the genetic and molecular levels, LQTS is a heterogeneous disorder consisting of several distinct cardiac channelopathies. Approximately 90% of patients with a clinical diagnosis of LQTS have mutations in one of the three major LQTS-susceptibility genes that encode ion channels essential in coordinating the duration of the cardiac action potential: *KCNQ1*-encoded I_{Ks} (K_v7.1) potassium channel, *KCNH2*-encoded I_{Kr} (K_v11.1) potassium channel, or *SCN5A*-encoded I_{Na} (Na_v1.5) sodium channel. Loss-of-function mutations in *KCNQ1* underlie about 30% to 35% of LQTS type 1 (LQT1). Loss-of-function *KCNH2* mutations cause approximately 25% to 40% of LQTS type 2 (LQT2). These loss-of-function mutations can directly impair channel function or indirectly reduce their trafficking to the cell membrane, resulting in prolongation of the action potential at the cellular level and hence QT prolongation. Gain-of-function *SCN5A* mutations account for roughly 5% to 10% of LQTS type 3 (LQT3). Gain-of-function mutations in the Na^+ channel prolong the action potential duration by impairing channel inactivation and increasing late Na^+ currents, which results in increased vulnerability to early afterdepolarizations and triggered activity initiating torsades de pointes, polymorphic ventricular tachycardia, and ventricular fibrillation. About 15% to 20% of patients with a definite clinical diagnosis of LQTS remain genotype-negative even after extensive genetic testing.[1,6]

Mutations in genes encoding ion channel subunits (*KCNE1, KCNE2, KCNJ5,* and *SCN4B*) or proteins that regulate ion channel function (*CALM1, CALM2, CALM3, AKAP9, CAV3, ANK2, SNTA1,* and *TRDN*) have also been implicated in LQTS pathogenesis and account for about 5% of cases.[1,6]

TABLE 51.1 Genes Implicated in Inherited Cardiac Arrhythmia Syndromes

Gene	Protein	Function	Associated Disorder	Inheritance
KCNQ1	Potassium voltage-gated channel $K_v7.1$	Subunit of the voltage-gated potassium channel responsible for the I_{Ks} current	LQTS (LQT1)	AD
			Jervell and Lange-Nielsen syndrome	AR
			SQTS (SQT2)	AD
KCNH2	Potassium voltage-gated channel subfamily H member 2 (also known as K_V 11.1)	Pore-forming subunit of the voltage-gated potassium channel responsible for the I_{Kr} current	LQTS (LQT2) and SQTS (SQT1)	AD
KCNE1	Potassium voltage-gated channel subfamily E member 1	Subunit of the potassium channel responsible for the I_{Ks} current	Jervell and Lange-Nielsen syndrome	AR
KCNJ2	Inward rectifier potassium channel 2 (Kir2.1)	Potassium channel responsible for the I_{K1} current	Andersen-Tawil syndrome and SQTS (SQT3)	AD
SCN5A	Sodium channel protein type 5 subunit-a (also known as Na_v 1.5)	Subunit of the voltage-gated sodium channel responsible for the I_{Na} current	LQTS (LQT3)	AD
			BrS	Complex inheritance
CALM1	Calmodulin 1	Calcium-binding protein	LQTS and CPVT	AD
CALM2	Calmodulin 2	Calcium-binding protein	LQTS and CPVT	AD
CALM3	Calmodulin 3	Calcium-binding protein	LQTS	AD
ANK2	Ankyrin B	Protein involved in the localization and membrane stabilization of ion transporters and ion channels	CPVT	AD
TRDN	Triadin	Sarcoplasmic reticulum component of the calcium release unit	LQTS and CPVT	AR
CACNA1C	Voltage-dependent L-type calcium channel subunit a1C (also known as Ca_v 1.2)	Pore-forming subunit of the calcium channel responsible for the L-type calcium currents	Timothy syndrome	AD
RYR2	Ryanodine receptor 2	Sarcoplasmic reticulum calcium channel	CPVT	AD
CASQ2	Calsequestrin 2	Component of the sarcoplasmic reticulum calcium release unit	CPVT	AR
TECRL	Trans-2,3-enoyl-CoA reductase -like	Endoplasmic reticulum protein	CPVT	AR

AD, autosomal dominant; AR, autosomal recessive; BrS, Brugada syndrome; CPVT, catecholaminergic polymorphic ventricular tachycardia; If, hyperpolarization-activated nonselective pacemaker «funny» current; IK1, inward rectifier K current; IKACh, Acetylcholine-activated K current; IKr, rapid component of the delayed rectifier K current; IKs, slow component of the delayed rectifier K current; IKur, ultrarapid component of the delayed rectifier K current; INa, Na current; Ito, transient outward K current; LQT1, LQT2, LQT3, types 1-3 long QT syndrome; long QT syndrome; LQTS, long QT syndrome; LQTS3, Long QT Syndrome type 3; NCX, Na-Ca exchanger; SQTS, short QT syndrome; SQT1, SQT2, SQT3, types 1-3 short QT syndrome; SQTS2, Short QT Syndrome type 2; SQTS3, Short QT Syndrome type 3.
(Reprinted with permission from Schwartz PJ, Ackerman MJ, Antzelevitch C, et al. Inherited cardiac arrhythmias. *Nat Rev Dis Primers.* 2020;6:58)

Genotype-Phenotype Correlations

Relatively specific genotype-phenotype correlations have been described in LQTS. Swimming- and exertion-induced cardiac events are strongly associated with LQT1, auditory-triggered events and those occurring in the postpartum period are associated with LQT2, and events occurring during periods of sleep or rest are associated with LQT3. On electrocardiogram (ECG), LQT1 is typically characterized by a broad-based T wave (**Figure 51.3A**), LQT2 by a low-amplitude notched or biphasic T wave (**Figure 51.3B**), and LQT3 by a long isoelectric segment followed by a narrow-based T wave (**Figure 51.3C**). Efficacy of β-blocker therapy is greater among LQT1 patients compared to LQT2 and LQT3 patients.[6,8] Although a vast majority of mutations are single nucleotide substitutions or small insertion/deletions, approximately 5% to 10% of LQTS patients have multiple mutations in these genes. These patients typically present at a younger age with a more severe phenotype than patients with a single mutation.

Diagnosis and Treatment

Although the diagnosis of LQTS is clear in a young patient presenting with an episode of syncope in the setting of physical or emotional stress and prolonged QTc interval on ECG, it may be more challenging in asymptomatic individuals with

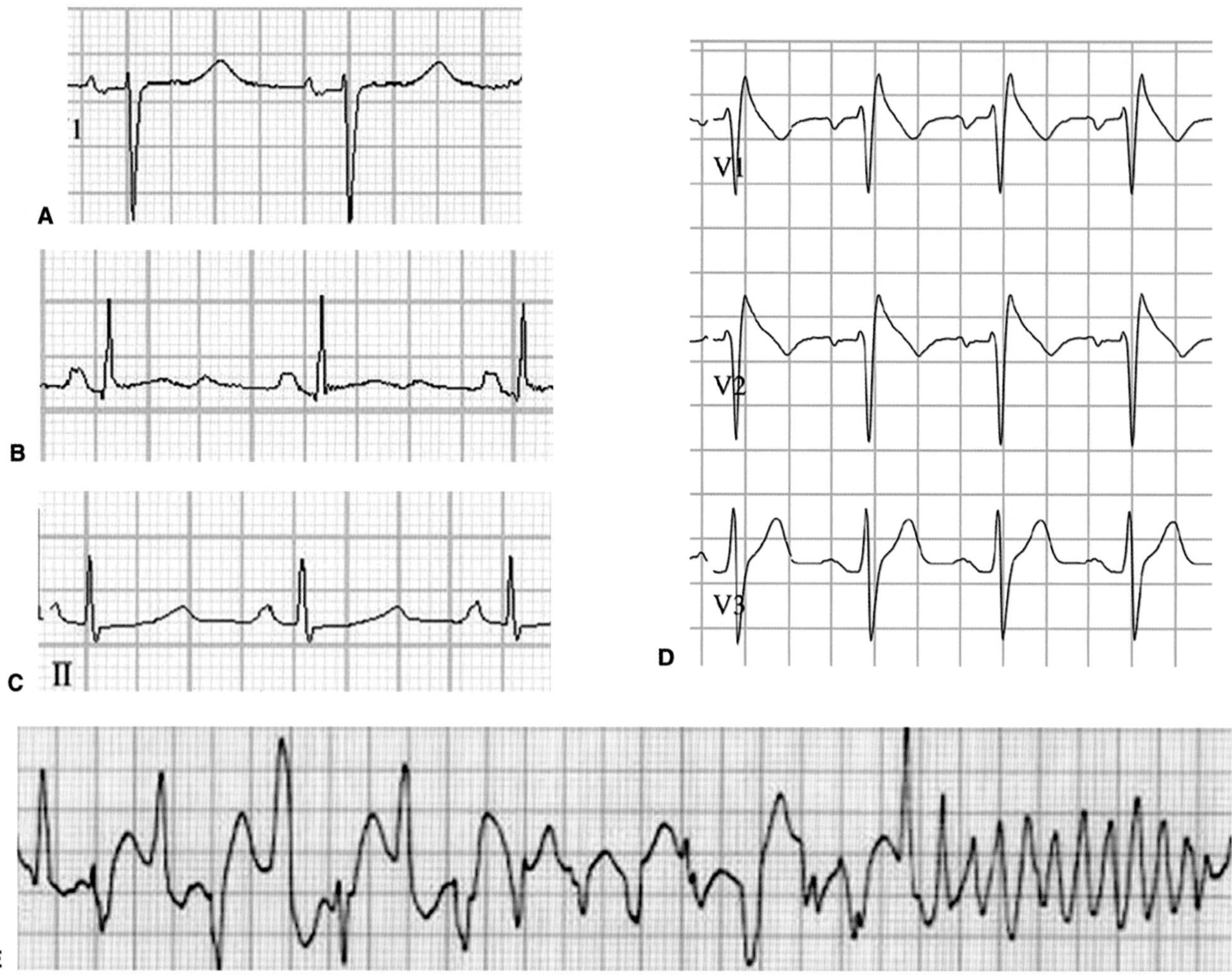

FIGURE 51.3 Representative electrocardiogram tracings from patients with genetic arrhythmia syndromes. **(A)** In long QT syndrome type 1, the typical electrocardiographic (ECG) pattern consists of a broad-based T wave. **(B)** In long QT syndrome type 2, there is a prolonged QT interval with a clear and characteristic notch on the T wave. **(C)** In long QT syndrome type 3, there is a long isoelectric segment following the QRS complex, followed by a late-onset T wave. **(D)** In Brugada type I pattern ECG, there is a coved-type ST segment in the right precordial leads followed by a terminal negative T wave. (A-D: Reprinted with permission from Al-Khatib SM, Stevenson WG, Ackerman MJ, et al. 2017 AHA/ACC/HRS guideline for management of patients with ventricular arrhythmias and the prevention of sudden cardiac death: a report of the ACC/AHA Task Force on Clinical Practice Guidelines and the Heart Rhythm Society. *Heart Rhythm.* 2018;15:e190-e252). **(E)** Bidirectional ventricular tachycardia followed by polymorphic ventricular tachycardia then ventricular fibrillation is shown in a patient with catecholaminergic polymorphic ventricular tachycardia. (E: Reprinted with permission from Roses-Noguer F, Jarman JW, Clague JR, Till J. Outcomes of defibrillator therapy in catecholaminergic polymorphic ventricular tachycardia. *Heart Rhythm.* 2014;11:58-66.) ACC, American College of Cardiology; AHA, American Heart Association; HRS, Heart Rhythm Society.

only modestly prolonged QTc intervals, with such cases being detected during mandatory screening prior to participation in sports. Secondary causes of QT prolongation (such as medications, disease states, or electrolyte disturbances) must be excluded. Exercise testing should be performed to assess for exercise-induced arrhythmias (although rare in LQTS), changes in T wave morphology, and presence of a maladaptive QT response during the recovery phase. Ambulatory rhythm monitoring can provide supportive information, including intermittent QT prolongation and underlying dynamic T wave changes, especially at night. The LQTS diagnostic score, also known as the *Schwartz Score*,[9] first developed in 1985 and most recently updated in 2011, should be calculated (**Table 51.2**). A high probability Schwartz score (≥3.5 points) carries ~80% likelihood of a positive LQTS genetic test. Genetic testing should not be pursued in patients with a low Schwartz score (<1 point). The likelihood of LQTS is ~5% to 20% for an intermediate probability Schwartz score, and negative genetic testing in this situation would not warrant a diagnosis of LQTS. Genetic testing not only aids in the diagnosis of LQTS in the presenting patient but also helps identify asymptomatic but at-risk family members who may not have been otherwise diagnosed and received life-saving therapy.[1]

All patients with LQTS should receive β-blocker therapy unless contraindicated; nadolol and propranolol are the most effective. Mexiletine confers a protective effect in patients with LQT3 because of its QT-attenuating effect by blocking late sodium current. Left cardiac sympathetic denervation can be effective for LQTS patients with persistent arrhythmias despite β-blocker therapy and also for those who cannot tolerate β-blockers. Secondary prevention implantable cardioverter-defibrillator (ICD) is indicated for LQTS patients who present with resuscitated SCD or those who have recurrent events despite β-blockers. Primary prevention ICD may be considered for symptomatic LQTS patients despite β-blockers, and for asymptomatic patients with high-risk features (such as QTc > 500 msec, genotypes LQT2 and LQT3, females with genotype LQT2, <40 years of age, onset of symptoms at <10 years of age, and recurrent syncopal episodes) after β-blocker therapy has been initiated. Avoidance of QT-prolonging drugs, hypokalemia, and hypomagnesemia are also recommended.[4]

TABLE 51.2 Diagnostic Criteria for Long QT Syndrome (LQTS)

	Points
Electrocardiographic findings[a]	
(A) QTc[b]	
≥480 ms	3
460-479 ms	2
450-459 ms (in males)	1
(B) QTc[b] ≥480 ms in 4th minute of recovery from exercise stress test	1
(C) Torsade de pointes[c]	2
(D) T wave alternans	1
(E) Notched T wave in three leads	1
(F) Low heart rate for age[d]	0.5
Clinical history	
(A) Syncope[c]	
With stress	2
Without stress	1
(B) Congenital deafness	0.5
Family history	
(A) Family members with definite LQTS[e]	1
(B) Unexplained sudden cardiac death below age 30 years among immediate members[e]	0.5

Note: SCORE: ≤1 point: low probability of LQTS. 1.5-3 points: intermediate probability of LQTS. ≥3.5: points high probability.

[a]In the absence of medications or disorders known to affect these electrocardiographic features.

[b]QTc calculated by Bazett formula where $QTc = QT/\sqrt{RR}$.

[c]Mutually exclusive.

[d]Resting heart rate below the second percentile for age.

[e]The same family member cannot be counted in A and B.

(Reprinted with permission from Schwartz PJ, Crotti L. QTc behavior during exercise and genetic testing for the long-QT syndrome. *Circulation.* 2011;124:2181-2184)

Andersen-Tawil Syndrome

First described by Andersen in a case report in 1971[10] and later described by Tawil in 1994,[11] Andersen-Tawil syndrome (ATS) is a rare, multisystem disorder characterized by periodic paralysis, dysmorphic features, and ventricular arrhythmias (VA). It is a heterogeneous disorder that occurs sporadically or is inherited in an autosomal dominant fashion. ECG abnormalities manifested in ATS include marked QTU prolongation, prominent U waves, and ventricular ectopy, including polymorphic ventricular tachycardia, ventricular bigeminy, and bidirectional ventricular tachycardia.[1,12] Although ATS was initially proposed as LQTS type 7 (LQT7) given extreme prolongation of the QT interval, it has been argued that these QT measurements erroneously included the prominent U wave and should therefore be considered as its own clinical entity.[1,13] Loss-of-function mutations in *KCNJ2* encoding the inward rectifier potassium channel Kir2.1 responsible for the I_{K1} current accounts for approximately two-thirds of cases of ATS[14]; the genetic cause of the remaining one-third remains to be elucidated.

Timothy Syndrome

An extremely rare disorder, Timothy syndrome is characterized by fetal bradycardia, extreme prolongation of the QT interval (QTc >500 msec), macroscopic T wave alternans, and a 2:1 atrioventricular (AV) block at birth. The extracardiac manifestations of Timothy syndrome include webbing of the toes and fingers, dysmorphic facial features, abnormal dentition, immune deficiency, severe hypoglycemia, cognitive abnormalities, and autism. Most cases of Timothy syndrome have been attributed to recurrent sporadic *de novo* occurrences of G406R missense mutation in the *CACNA1C*-encoded cardiac L-type calcium channel (Cav1.2) that cause defective inactivation of the Ca^{2+} current, thus prolonging the action potential duration and QT interval.[1,15]

Short QT Syndrome

Short QT syndrome (SQTS), first described only in 2000,[16] is characterized by a short QT interval (typically 340 msec or less, although the exact cutoff value remains a matter of debate) on ECG with underlying structurally normal hearts, and is associated with paroxysmal atrial fibrillation (AF), syncope, and increased risk for SCD caused by VA. Although SQTS is most commonly inherited in an autosomal dominant manner, some *de novo* sporadic cases have also been reported. Eight subtypes of SQTS caused by mutations in eight different genes have been described to date. These include gain-of-function mutations in the potassium channel-encoding genes *KCNH2* (SQT1), *KCNQ1* (SQT2), and *KCNJ2* (SQT3) and loss-of-function mutations in *CACNA1C* (SQT4), *CACNB2b* (SQT5), and *CACNA2D1* (SQT6), which encode for the alpha, beta, and delta subunits of the L-type Ca^{2+} channel, respectively, as well as a carnitine transporter *SLC22A5* (SQT7) and chloride-bicarbonate anion exchanger *SLC4A3* (SQT8).[1,17] An increase in net outward current caused by either augmentation of outward repolarizing K^+ currents or a reduction in inward depolarizing currents from Ca^{2+} channels, or a combination thereof, results in early repolarization and shortening of the action potential, refractoriness, and QT interval, predisposing the heart to phase 2 reentry initiating ventricular tachycardia and fibrillation, similar to other early repolarization syndromes.[18]

Genotype-Phenotype Correlations

In addition to a short QT interval, the typical ECG of SQTS demonstrates tall, peaked T waves in the precordial leads with either a short or no ST segment, with symmetric T waves in SQT1 but asymmetric in SQT2 to SQT4. SQTS patients with *KCNH2* mutations have a shorter QT interval and show a greater response to hydroquinidine therapy compared to patients with non-*KCNH2* mutations.[17]

Diagnosis and Treatment

The presence of a shorter than normal QT interval, in the absence of other clinical history, family history, or genetic findings, may represent a normal variant. Diagnostic criteria,[19] based on ECG characteristics, clinical presentation, family history, and genetic findings, have been proposed to aid in the evaluation of patients suspected to have SQTS (**Table 51.3**). Other potential causes of QT shortening such as electrolyte imbalances and medication effects should be ruled out.

For patients with a low probability of SQTS, no pharmacologic or device therapy is recommended. For patients with SQTS who have a cardiac arrest or sustained VA, ICD is recommended. For SQTS patients with recurrent sustained VA in whom ICD therapy is declined or contraindicated, or in those with recurrent ICD therapies, treatment with QT-prolonging drugs may be useful, especially quinidine in the setting of SQT1.[4]

TABLE 51.3 Proposed Diagnostic Criteria for Short QT Syndrome

	Points
QT_C	
<370 ms	1
<350 ms	2
<330 ms	3
J point-Tpeak interval <120 ms	1
Clinical history[a]	
History of sudden cardiac arrest	2
Documented polymorphic VT or VF	2
Unexplained syncope	1
Atrial fibrillation	1
Family history[a]	
First- or second-degree relative with high-probability SQTS	2
First- or second-degree relative with autopsy-negative sudden cardiac death	1
Sudden infant death syndrome	1
Genotype[a]	
Genotype positive	2
Mutation of undetermined in a culprit gene	1

Note: High-probability SQTS: ≥4 points; intermediate-probability SQTS: 3 points; low-probability SQTS: ≤2 points; Electrocardiogram: must be recorded in the absence of modifiers to shorten the QT, and Jpoint-Tpeak interval must be measured in the precordial lead with the greatest amplitude T wave. Clinical history: events must occur in the absence of an identifiable etiology, including structural heart disease. Points can only be received for one of cardiac arrest, documented polymorphic VT, or unexplained syncope. Family history: points can only be received once in this section.

QTc, corrected QT; SQTS, short QT syndrome; VF, ventricular fibrillation; VT, ventricular tachycardia.

[a]A minimum of 1 point must be obtained in the electrocardiographic section in order to obtain additional points.

(Reprinted with permission from Gollob MH, Redpath CJ, Roberts JD. The short QT syndrome: proposed diagnostic criteria. *J Am Coll Cardiol.* 2011;57:802-812)

Brugada Syndrome

First described in 1992,[20] Brugada syndrome (BrS) is an inherited arrhythmia characterized by coved-type greater than or equal to 2 mm ST-segment elevation followed by a negative T wave in the right precordial leads (V1-V2) on ECG (type 1 pattern, **Figure 51.3D**), and an increased risk for SCD caused by polymorphic VA, especially during sleep, in the absence of underlying structural heart disease.[21,22] (Type 2 Brugada ECG pattern consists of a *saddleback* ST-segment configuration, in which the elevated ST segment descends toward the baseline, then rises again to form an upright or biphasic T wave.) Although it can be inherited as an autosomal dominant disorder, most cases of BrS may be sporadic. The only gene that has strong evidence supporting a causal link in BrS is loss-of-function mutations in the *SCN5A*-encoded cardiac sodium channel, but *SCN5A* mutations account for only about 15% to 30% of families with BrS. Loss of function of the Na^+ channel predisposes to early repolarization and slowing of conduction in regions of the heart with high I_{to} density, such as the right ventricular epicardium. Both phase 2 reentry and fibrosis contribute to the increased risk of VA. At least 20 other genes have been associated with BrS through genetic studies in single individuals or small families, highlighting the largely sporadic presentation of the disorder.[1]

Genotype-Phenotype Correlations

Because of the sporadic nature of the disorder, genotype-phenotype correlations are not as well elucidated in BrS patients. *SCN5A* mutations are associated with a higher incidence of conduction abnormalities in BrS patients.[1]

Diagnosis and Treatment

BrS is most commonly diagnosed following a clinically significant event such as syncope or SCD, and the patient is found to have the classic Brugada pattern findings on ECG. Some patients are diagnosed based on the presence of typical ECG findings and positive family history of SCD or Brugada ECG patterns. Diagnosis of BrS is established when a type 1 ST-segment elevation is observed either spontaneously or after intravenous administration of a Na^+ channel blocker in at least one right precordial lead (V1 or V2) placed in a standard or superior position. Patients with suspected BrS and asymptomatic patients with Brugada pattern on ECG should undergo comprehensive evaluation including cardiac imaging with echocardiography, magnetic resonance imaging, and stress testing. Alternative causes of ST-segment elevation including acute right ventricular ischemia, atypical right bundle branch block, and arrhythmogenic right ventricular cardiomyopathy need to be ruled out.[23]

In patients with BrS with spontaneous type 1 ECG pattern and history of SCD or syncope, ICD is recommended. In patients with BrS experiencing recurrent ICD shocks for sustained VA, or those who decline or are not candidates for ICD therapy, pharmacologic therapy with quinidine or catheter ablation is recommended. In patients with suspected BrS without a spontaneous type 1 ECG pattern, a pharmacologic challenge with Na^+ channel blockers can be useful to aid in the diagnosis, but a positive test alone in the absence of symptoms is not an indication for ICD. In asymptomatic patients with BrS and spontaneous type 1 ECG pattern, an electrophysiology study may be considered for further risk stratification, though the value of this remains controversial.[24] Timely treatment of fever and avoidance of aggravating drugs are also recommended in all patients with BrS.[4]

Catecholaminergic Polymorphic Ventricular Tachycardia

Catecholaminergic polymorphic ventricular tachycardia (CPVT) is a hereditary arrhythmia that classically presents as exercise-induced syncope or SCD in young and otherwise healthy patients with completely normal resting ECG and structurally normal hearts. The hallmark of this disorder is bidirectional ventricular tachycardia that is similar to that described in digitalis toxicity **(Figure 51.3E)**. Accounting for 60% of cases of CPVT and with an autosomal dominant inheritance pattern, mutations in the *RyR2*-encoded cardiac ryanodine receptor/Ca^{2+} release channel represent the most common genetic subtype of CPVT (CPVT1). *RyR2* mediates the release of Ca^{2+} from the sarcoplasmic reticulum, which is required for myocardial contraction. The mutations in *RyR2* interfere with the stabilization of *RyR2* by associated binding proteins, leading to spontaneous Ca^{2+} release from the sarcoplasmic reticulum, especially in the setting of increased adrenergic stress, such as with exercise. This spontaneous Ca^{2+} release from the sarcoplasmic reticulum by *leaky RyR2* activates inward Na-Ca exchange current, which can trigger life-threatening arrhythmias caused by delayed afterdepolarizations. CPVT type 2 (CPVT2), a much less common autosomal recessive form, is caused by mutations in *CASQ2*, which encodes the Ca^{2+}-binding sarcoplasmic reticulum protein calsequestrin 2 and also regulates *RyR2 leakiness*. Mutations in other genes involved in Ca^{2+} homeostasis, including *CALM1* and *TRDN*, have also been implicated in the pathogenesis of CPVT.[1,25]

Genotype-Phenotype Correlations

Patients with *CASQ2* mutations exhibit a more severe phenotype with earlier onset, higher penetrance, and younger age at death than those with mutations in *RyR2*. Among patients with mutations in *RyR2*, those with mutations in the C-terminal channel-forming domain have an increased frequency of nonsustained ventricular tachycardia when compared to those with mutations in the N-terminal domain.[1,26]

Diagnosis and Treatment

Exercise stress test is the primary diagnostic test necessary for the diagnosis of CPVT; drug testing with epinephrine may be used for adult patients who are unable to exercise, or annual ambulatory rhythm monitoring may be used in children and those unable to exercise.[25]

For patients with CPVT, β-blocker therapy is recommended. In CPVT patients with recurrent, sustained VA or syncope already receiving maximally tolerated β-blocker therapy, intensification of pharmacologic therapy with flecainide, left cardiac sympathetic denervation, and/or ICD is recommended.[4]

Progressive Cardiac Conduction Disease

Also known as Lev-Lenegre disease, progressive cardiac conduction disease (PCCD) is characterized by an age-related, progressive alteration in impulse propagation through the His-Purkinje system, with right or left bundle branch block and QRS widening leading to complete AV and intraventricular block, syncope, and sometimes SCD, in the absence of structural heart disease. Mutations in several genes, including *SCN5A*, *SCN1B*, and *TRPM4*, have been causally linked to PCCD. It is most frequently inherited in an autosomal dominant pattern, although autosomal recessive inheritance and sporadic cases have rarely been reported as well.[1,27]

Atrial Fibrillation

AF is the most common arrhythmia and is associated with increased morbidity (such as heart failure and stroke) and mortality. Although most cases of AF are associated with well-defined risk factors such as older age, hypertension, obesity, myocardial infarction, heart failure, valvular heart disease, and alcohol consumption, up to 30% of AF patients have no underlying known risk factors. Recent epidemiologic and genetic studies have highlighted the heritability of AF. Mutations in potassium and sodium channels as well as non-ion channel variants (such as connexin 40, atrial natriuretic peptide, and the renin-angiotensin system) have been reported. These ultimately result in changes in conduction, inflammation, and fibrosis that predispose to the development of AF.[28]

KEY POINTS

- ✔ Inherited cardiac arrhythmias can lead to sudden death in young and otherwise healthy individuals with structurally normal hearts.

SECTION 4

- ✔ An understanding of the cardiac action potential and ion channels is critical in understanding the genetic basis of inherited arrhythmia syndromes.
- ✔ Because of advances in cardiovascular genetics, an improved understanding of the pathophysiology of these hereditary arrhythmia disorders has resulted in significant diagnostic, prognostic, and therapeutic impact.

REFERENCES

1. Schwartz PJ, Ackerman MJ, Antzelevitch C, et al. Inherited cardiac arrhythmias. *Nat Rev Dis Primers.* 2020;6:58.
2. Shah M, Akar FG, Tomaselli GF. Molecular basis of arrhythmias. *Circulation.* 2005;112:2517-2529.
3. Grant AO. Cardiac ion channels. *Circ Arrhythm Electrophysiol.* 2009;2:185-194.
4. Al-Khatib SM, Stevenson WG, Ackerman MJ, et al. 2017 AHA/ACC/HRS guideline for management of patients with ventricular arrhythmias and the prevention of sudden cardiac death: executive summary: a report of the American College of Cardiology/American Heart Association Task Force on Clinical Practice Guidelines and the Heart Rhythm Society. *Heart Rhythm.* 2018;15:e190-e252.
5. Schwartz PJ, Stramba-Badiale M, Crotti L, et al. Prevalence of the congenital long-QT syndrome. *Circulation.* 2009;120:1761-1767.
6. Tester DJ, Ackerman MJ. Genetics of long QT syndrome. *Methodist Debakey Cardiovasc J.* 2014;10:29-33.
7. Schwartz PJ, Spazzolini C, Crotti L, et al. The Jervell and Lange-Nielsen syndrome: natural history, molecular basis, and clinical outcome. *Circulation.* 2006;113:783-790.
8. Priori SG, Napolitano C, Schwartz PJ, et al. Association of long QT syndrome loci and cardiac events among patients treated with beta-blockers. *JAMA.* 2004;292:1341-1344.
9. Schwartz PJ, Crotti L. QTc behavior during exercise and genetic testing for the long-QT syndrome. *Circulation.* 2011;124:2181-2184.
10. Andersen ED, Krasilnikoff PA, Overvad H. Intermittent muscular weakness, extrasystoles, and multiple developmental anomalies. A new syndrome? *Acta Paediatr Scand.* 1971;60:559-564.
11. Tawil R, Ptacek LJ, Pavlakis SG, et al. Andersen's syndrome: potassium-sensitive periodic paralysis, ventricular ectopy, and dysmorphic features. *Ann Neurol.* 1994;35:326-330.
12. Peters S, Schulze-Bahr E, Etheridge SP, Tristani-Firouzi M. Sudden cardiac death in Andersen-Tawil syndrome. *Europace.* 2007;9:162-166.
13. Zhang L, Benson DW, Tristani-Firouzi M, et al. Electrocardiographic features in Andersen-Tawil syndrome patients with KCNJ2 mutations: characteristic T-U-wave patterns predict the KCNJ2 genotype. *Circulation.* 2005;111:2720-2726.
14. Plaster NM, Tawil R, Tristani-Firouzi M, et al. Mutations in Kir2.1 cause the developmental and episodic electrical phenotypes of Andersen's syndrome. *Cell.* 2001;105:511-519.
15. Sepp R, Hategan L, Bacsi A, et al. Timothy syndrome 1 genotype without syndactyly and major extracardiac manifestations. *Am J Med Genet A.* 2017;173:784-789.
16. Gussak I, Brugada P, Brugada J, et al. Idiopathic short QT interval: a new clinical syndrome? *Cardiology.* 2000;94:99-102.
17. Dewi IP, Dharmadjati BB. Short QT syndrome: the current evidences of diagnosis and management. *J Arrhythm.* 2020;36:962-966.
18. Antzelevitch C, Yan GX. J-wave syndromes: Brugada and early repolarization syndromes. *Heart Rhythm.* 2015;12:1852-1866.
19. Gollob MH, Redpath CJ, Roberts JD. The short QT syndrome: proposed diagnostic criteria. *J Am Coll Cardiol.* 2011;57:802-812.
20. Brugada P, Brugada J. Right bundle branch block, persistent ST segment elevation and sudden cardiac death: a distinct clinical and electrocardiographic syndrome. A multicenter report. *J Am Coll Cardiol.* 1992;20:1391-1396.
21. Polovina MM, Vukicevic M, Banko B, Lip GYH, Potpara TS. Brugada syndrome: a general cardiologist's perspective. *Eur J Intern Med.* 2017;44:19-27.
22. Chen PS, Priori SG. The Brugada syndrome. *J Am Coll Cardiol.* 2008;51:1176-1180.
23. Sieira J, Dendramis G, Brugada P. Pathogenesis and management of Brugada syndrome. *Nat Rev Cardiol.* 2016;13:744-756.
24. Adler A, Rosso R, Chorin E, Havakuk O, Antzelevitch C, Viskin S. Risk stratification in Brugada syndrome: clinical characteristics, electrocardiographic parameters, and auxiliary testing. *Heart Rhythm.* 2016;13:299-310.
25. Baltogiannis GG, Lysitsas DN, di Giovanni G, et al. CPVT: arrhythmogenesis, therapeutic management, and future perspectives. A brief review of the literature. *Front Cardiovasc Med.* 2019;6:92.
26. van der Werf C, Nederend I, Hofman N, et al. Familial evaluation in catecholaminergic polymorphic ventricular tachycardia: disease penetrance and expression in cardiac ryanodine receptor mutation-carrying relatives. *Circ Arrhythm Electrophysiol.* 2012;5:748-756.
27. Asatryan A, Boussiba S, Zarka A. Stimulation and isolation of *Paraphysoderma sedebokerense* (Blastocladiomycota) propagules and their infection capacity toward their host under different physiological and environmental conditions. *Front Cell Infect Microbiol.* 2019;9:72.
28. Ragab AAY, Sitorus GDS, Brundel B, de Groot NMS. The genetic puzzle of familial atrial fibrillation. *Front Cardiovasc Med.* 2020;7:14.

CHAPTER 52

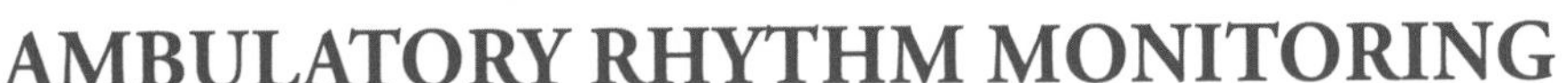

AMBULATORY RHYTHM MONITORING

Kevin Sung, Justin Hayase, and Jason S. Bradfield

INTRODUCTION

Ambulatory monitoring is a diagnostic tool performed in the outpatient setting to evaluate symptomatic patients for cardiac arrhythmias, risk stratify patients with underlying conditions, or guide therapeutic arrhythmia management.[1] With new advances in technology, the various modalities to perform ambulatory monitoring have also become more portable and provide more accurate data. This chapter seeks to discuss clinical indications for ambulatory monitoring, different modalities of monitoring, and the current state of the field (**Table 52.1**).

INDICATIONS

Syncope

Syncope is a common condition with an estimated lifetime prevalence of 35%.[2] Finding the underlying cause of syncope can be challenging and requires a detailed history and physical examination. The most useful information, however, may be difficult to obtain during patient encounters unless the patient has active symptomatic episodes.[3]

Ambulatory monitoring plays a key role in diagnosing underlying cardiac arrhythmias that may occur during symptomatic episodes. The selection of an ambulatory monitoring device depends primarily on the predicted duration of the monitoring period needed to capture a symptomatic event. Patients may be placed on a Holter monitor, an extended Holter monitor (EHM), or an event monitor. Inconclusive studies with recurrent episodes may warrant more long-term monitoring such as an implantable loop recorder. The advantages and disadvantages of the different monitoring methods are discussed later in the chapter.

Identifying underlying cardiac arrhythmias can have significant implications for patient outcomes. In elderly patients with unexplained falls, as many as 20% of patients with an implantable loop recorder can be found to have an arrhythmia as the etiology of their falls.[4]

Palpitations

Palpitations can be due to various arrhythmias that cause noticeable change, acceleration, or irregularity in heart rhythm noticed by patients. A common cause of palpitations is atrial fibrillation (AF) with a rapid ventricular rate. Ambulatory monitoring is often recommended, with the choice of modality dependent on the frequency of the symptomatic episodes when AF is suspected. Automated algorithms have improved detection of AF with a high degree of sensitivity and specificity.[5]

Initiation of antiarrhythmic drugs for patients may warrant a period of ambulatory monitoring to evaluate the efficacy of therapy. For example, in a patient with symptomatic premature ventricular complexes (PVCs), ambulatory monitoring can help quantify burden before and after initiation of antiarrhythmic medications to determine treatment effect. According to the American Heart Association/American College of Cardiology (AHA/ACC) guidelines, for a patient with an

TABLE 52.1 Summary of Ambulatory Monitoring Modalities

Modality	Time Frame	Advantages	Disadvantages
Holter monitor	24-48 hours	Noninvasive Low cost Continuous monitoring	Cumbersome device with wires Short time frame Cannot shower
Extended Holter monitor	7-30 days	Noninvasive Continuous monitoring Small wearable device	May or may not shower depending on device
Event monitor	Up to 30 days	Noninvasive Real-time provider notification of prespecified arrhythmia criteria	Patient must activate during symptomatic events
Implantable loop recorders	Up to 3 years	Continuous monitoring Length of monitoring	Invasive procedure required

underlying arrhythmia with confirmed reproducibility, initiating an antiarrhythmic medication would warrant ambulatory monitoring.[6]

Risk Stratification

Several congenital conditions, such as Brugada syndrome and congenital long-QT syndrome, may predispose an individual to developing ventricular arrhythmias (VAs). Ambulatory monitoring can help guide risk stratification and associated medical/interventional therapy for management of VAs.

In patients with Wolff-Parkinson-White syndrome, ambulatory monitoring may also play a role in risk stratification.[7] Electrocardiographic (ECG) monitoring can identify the heart rate at which preexcitation is lost, generally correlating with the risk of developing life-threatening VA.[8] Because the demographic of preexcitation pathways commonly affect younger patients, ambulatory monitoring may guide risk-benefit discussions regarding subsequent participation in sports and the need for further evaluation with an electrophysiology study and catheter ablation.

Preablation Assessment

Patients with arrhythmias refractory to medical treatment may be candidates for ablation procedures. These include the spectrum of arrhythmias from supraventricular tachycardias (SVTs) to VAs. For these patients, ambulatory monitoring can provide an assessment of the characteristics of the specific arrhythmia, the arrhythmia burden, and elucidating morphology (P wave or QRS complex) suggestive of anatomic origin.

PVCs occur sporadically in most healthy individuals; however, with increased frequency, they may be associated with PVC-induced cardiomyopathy and poorer cardiovascular outcomes.[9] Ambulatory monitoring helps assess the burden of PVCs in patients, and guides further management regarding medical therapy or potential ablative management. Furthermore, the morphologies of the PVCs help localize the site of origin for the ablation procedure.[10]

AF is the most common arrhythmia in the United States and Europe. Patient symptom profiles can vary, and may not accurately represent the amount of time a patient spends in AF. Ambulatory monitoring may help in distinguishing persistent (ie, occurs for longer than 7 days) versus paroxysmal (lasts <1 week) AF, and aid in discussions regarding risk, prognosis, and procedural outcomes.[11] Catheter ablation success rates for paroxysmal AF are estimated at 70% to 80%, whereas for persistent AF, ablation provides 30% to 60% success.[12,13] Because AF has been shown to progress from paroxysmal to persistent to permanent in a subset of patients, ambulatory monitoring may also help monitor the AF burden in patients over time.

Cardiomyopathy

Inherited cardiomyopathies such as hypertrophic cardiomyopathy (HCM) or arrhythmogenic right ventricular cardiomyopathy (ARVC) place patients at high risk for sudden cardiac death (SCD). HCM is one of the most common inherited cardiac disorders worldwide, and is associated with increased risk of SCD in young adulthood. Approximately 20% of adults with HCM have non–sustained ventricular tachycardia (NSVT), which is associated with increased risk of SCD. Ambulatory monitoring is thus recommended as part of the initial evaluation of patients with HCM.[14] Similarly, in patients with suspected ARVC, the presence of VA forms part of the diagnostic criteria, so ambulatory monitoring should be obtained in patients undergoing evaluation for ARVC.[15] Furthermore, any symptoms such as palpitations, presyncope, or syncope would warrant additional monitoring of patients with high-risk cardiomyopathies. This data may then be used to risk stratify patients and assess the need for implantable cardioverter-defibrillator (ICD) placement.[14,16,17]

FUNDAMENTALS OF AMBULATORY RHYTHM MONITORING

Holter Monitoring

The Holter monitor is a tool that allows continuous monitoring of patient heart rhythm for 24 to 48 hours. It is one of the oldest technologies of ambulatory monitoring, and has a diagnostic yield of 15% to 39%.[18] The major benefit of a Holter monitor is continuous monitoring. Traditional Holter monitors use either a two- or three-lead setup, and the wearer carries a recording device (**Figure 52.1**). A more expansive 12-lead Holter monitor setup may provide a greater degree of diagnostic utility.[19] Certain Holter monitors also have a feature where patients are able to press a button to mark any symptomatic periods during the recording timeframe.

A disadvantage of Holter monitoring is the relatively poor diagnostic sensitivity, largely owing to short recording time frame relative to other modalities. Another downside is the requirement for patients to wear leads and an external device

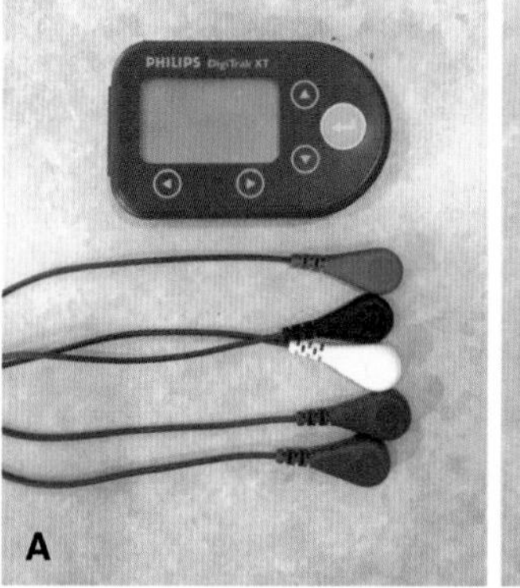

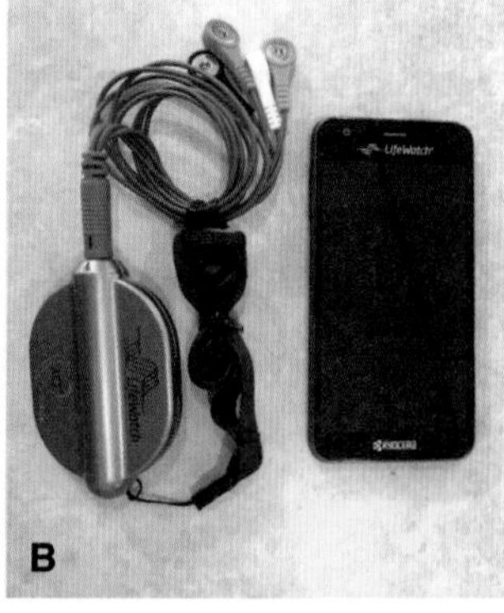

FIGURE 52.1 Holter and event monitors offered by BioTelemetry Inc. (Malvern, PA). **(A)** Philips DigiTrak XT® Holter monitor provides 24 to 48 hours of three-lead ECG continuous data. **(B)** BioTel LifeWatch® Mobile Cardiac Telemetry three-lead monitor can be worn for up to 30 days and allows patients to wirelessly transmit data in real time. There is also a patient reporting system for symptoms to be time stamped to ECG rhythm tracings. ECG, electrocardiographic. (A & B, Used with permission of Koninklijke Philips N.V.)

for the duration of the monitoring, which can be cumbersome as well as prone to frequent detachments. A large percentage of patients report that they prefer the patch-based extended monitors over the traditional 24- to 48-hour Holter monitors based on comfort.[18]

Extended Holter Monitor

The EHM is an alternative recording device that allows for continuous monitoring for a more prolonged time compared to traditional Holter monitors. The patient typically wears a patch or other small device containing a single lead over the upper left anterior chest. An EHM may continue monitoring for up to 14 days. There are numerous companies that offer various EHM devices, each with their own advantages. The iRhythm Ziopatch and Biotel ePatch devices provide a single lead over the left upper chest, which is more convenient for patients than is the traditional Holter monitor requiring multiple leads (**Figure 52.2**). Preventice Solutions also offers a patch, which has the added benefit of being waterproof, allowing patients to swim while wearing the device. DMS-Service manufactures the myPatch, which comes in different sizes, including pediatric and neonatal. MediLynx provides an additional product that allows the wearer to interface with their own device, indicate specific symptoms, and transmit data in real time. This is somewhat of a hybrid device because this feature is more typical of event monitors (discussed in the section "Event Monitoring").

Because a major advantage of the EHM is a less conspicuous, compact device, patients experience less interference with everyday life compared to traditional Holter monitors and have a higher monitoring completion rate.[20] The downside is that the device can only record a limited number of leads, sometimes limiting interpretation of results. However, in conditions such as AF, significant bradyarrhythmias, and VT, the EHM can be very accurate in recording these events.

Event Monitoring

The event monitor is an ECG monitoring tool with usually two or three leads. Patients are connected to an external device for up to a 30-day period. When patients become symptomatic, they will activate the device, and the event monitor will record for a short period of time. An important benefit of the event monitor is real-time notification of any potentially life-threatening or critical events such as complete heart block, VT, and so on.

The device allows for an extended period of monitoring; however, it is limited by the presence of symptoms in the patient. Although event monitors have automated notification triggers for certain high-risk arrhythmias (eg, complete heart block, VT), they may potentially miss asymptomatic episodes of arrhythmia if the programmed criteria are not met. Furthermore, the event monitor introduces the possibility of user error, because it is up to the patient to activate the device during the episode of arrhythmia for the effective recording. As a result, event monitoring has largely given way to Holter monitoring and EHMs, particularly because the technology for EHMs has improved, allowing for patients to indicate when they have symptoms as well as transmit data in real time with some products. However, given the event monitor's ability to alert providers of any potentially life-threatening events, it may still be a favorable option for higher risk patients.

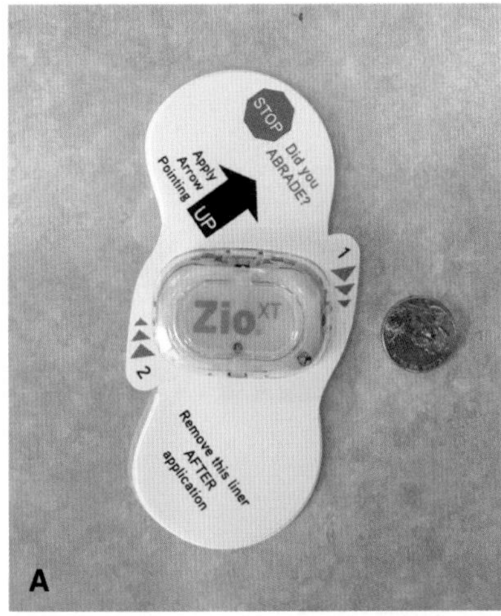

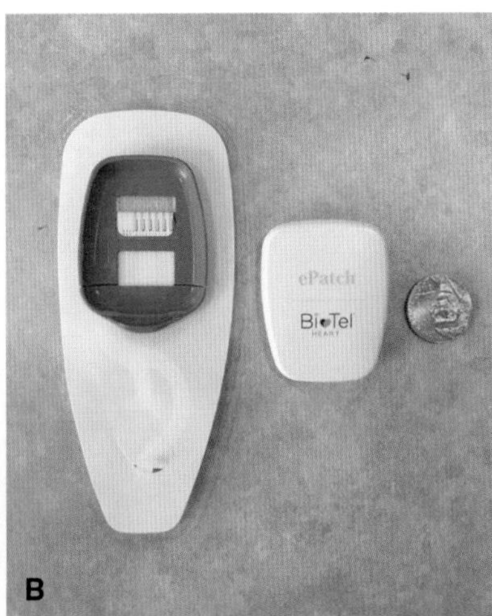

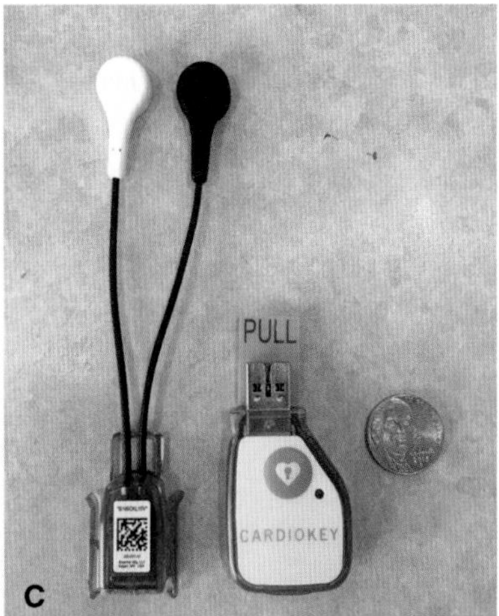

FIGURE 52.2 Examples of extended Holter monitors. For all the devices shown, patients can press a button to indicate when they experience symptoms. A nickel is included in all the photographs for size reference. **(A)** ZioPatch® offered by iRhythm (San Francisco, CA) provides single-lead continuous data for up to 14 days with a water-resistant patch device. Patients can shower while wearing the device. **(B)** ePatch® provided through Biotel Heart (Malvern, PA) provides single-lead continuous data for up to 14 days in the form of a water-resistant patch monitor. Patients can shower while wearing the device. **(C)** CardioKey® offered through Biotel Heart (Malvern, PA) provides single-lead continuous data for up to 14 days in the form of a miniature device connected to two electrodes. Patients cannot shower with the device. (A, Courtesy of iRhythm Technologies, Inc.; B & C, Used with permission of Koninklijke Philips N.V.)

Implantable Loop Recorder

The loop recorder is an implantable device smaller than the size of a universal serial bus (USB) memory stick (**Figure 52.3**) that can be inserted into the subcutaneous tissue of a patient through a minimally invasive, outpatient procedure. The loop recorder may record information for up to 3 years. Once the recording time has lapsed or its diagnostic value has been fulfilled, the device may be removed. Advantages of the loop recorder include the prolonged recording length and the convenience for the patient during the monitoring session. Disadvantages include risks typical of any minor procedure including bleeding, infection, and hematoma formation at the implant site. Furthermore, owing to the compact nature of the device, it contains only two electrodes measuring a single lead.

Multiple studies have shown the effectiveness of the loop recorder in diagnosing conditions, such as AF, compared to the Holter monitor.[21,22] However, given the invasiveness and long-term commitment of the loop recorder, it is usually reserved for patients who have failed a traditional Holter or EHM.

SPECIAL CONSIDERATIONS AND CONTRAINDICATIONS

The previously described noninvasive ambulatory monitors such as Holters, EHMs, and event monitors are safe and have no absolute contraindications. The main risk to patients is the potential for skin irritation from the adhesives required to wear the monitors. Certain occupational or lifestyle limitations are considerations as well (eg, competitive swimmers, divers). Loop recorders require a small procedure to implant them subcutaneously. Relative contraindications to their use include ongoing infection or history of bleeding disorder.[23]

Direct-to-Consumer Products and Research

With the advent of portable smart devices, direct-to-consumer ambulatory ECG monitoring has become a rapidly expanding field. Currently, there are more than 10 options of consumer ambulatory monitoring.[24] A few of the more widely used devices are the AliveCor© (Mountain View, CA) Kardia system, and the Apple Watch® by Apple© (Cupertino, CA) (**Figure 52.4**).

The AliveCor© KardiaMobile® product is a pocket-sized device that connects wirelessly to the consumer's handheld smartphone. The KardiaMobile® provides the capability of obtaining a single-lead or a six-lead ECG conveniently within 30 seconds. Early studies in head-to-head comparisons between the AliveCor© Kardia system and the standard 12-lead ECG showed very similar interpretations.[25]

Furthermore, preliminary data have suggested that direct-to-consumer ambulatory monitoring may add value for specific measurements such as the QT interval. This can be particularly useful when monitoring patients on medications such as dofetilide or sotalol. In a small pilot study of five patients, the AliveCor© QTC measurement correlated well with standard ECG QTC measurements.[26] This study was hypothesis generating and requires further confirmation before clinical application. Recently, the REHEARSE-AF trial demonstrated the efficacy of detecting asymptomatic AF in patients with elevated CHADS2-VASc score using aggressive AliveCor© monitoring.[27] However, owing to device costs and biweekly AliveCor© ECG commercial analysis with cardiologist overreads over the course of a year, the cost per diagnosis in this study was over \$10,000, raising significant cost-benefit concerns.

Apple also introduced a photoplethysmograph (PPG)-based algorithm within its third generation of the Apple Watch® to

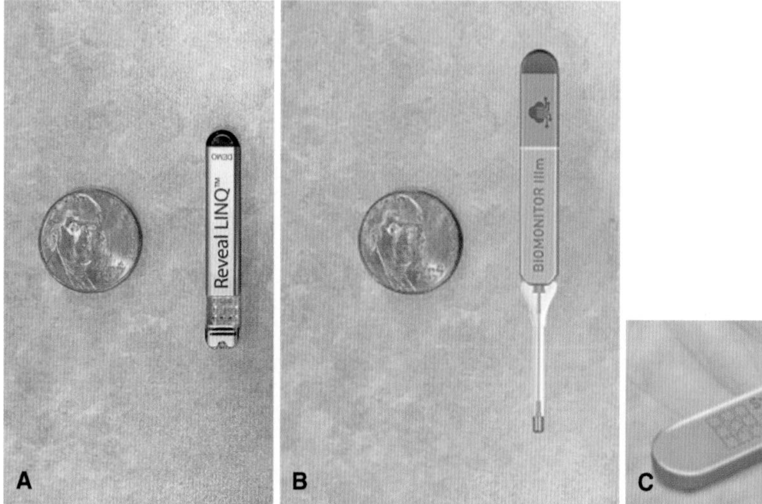

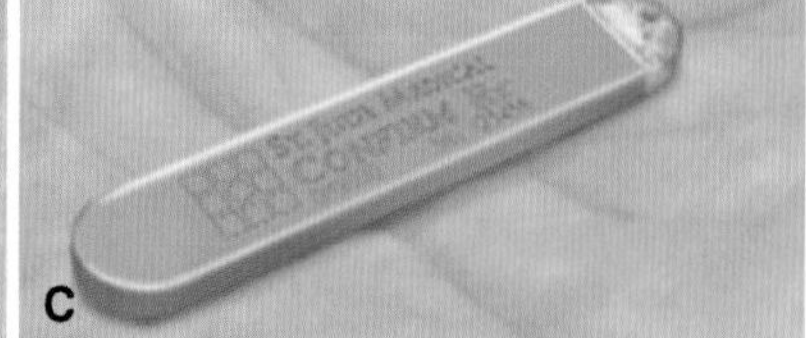

FIGURE 52.3 Examples of implantable loop recorders. All loop recorders shown are placed in the subcutaneous tissue during a minimally invasive procedure under local anesthesia. A nickel is shown in each photograph for size reference. **(A)** Reveal LINQ offered by Medtronic (Minneapolis, MN). **(B)** BioMonitor 2 offered by Biotronik (Berlin, Germany). **(C)** ConfirmRx offered by Abbott/St. Jude Medical (Chicago, IL). (A, Reproduced with permission of Medtronic, Inc.; B, Reproduced with permission of Biotronik SE & Co. KG.; C, ConfirmRx is a trademark of Abbott or its related companies. Reproduced with permission of Abbott, © 2021. All rights reserved.)

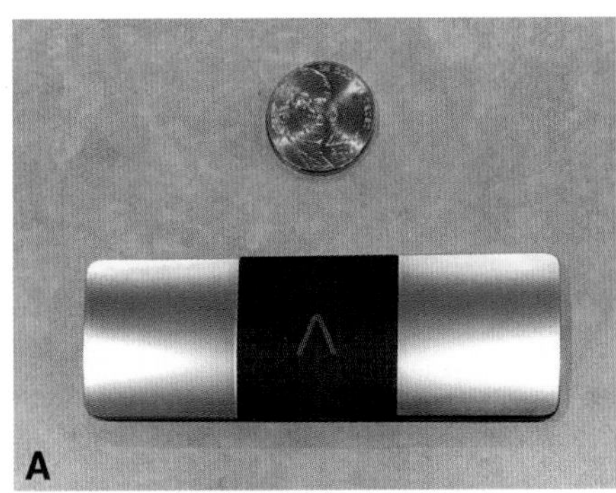

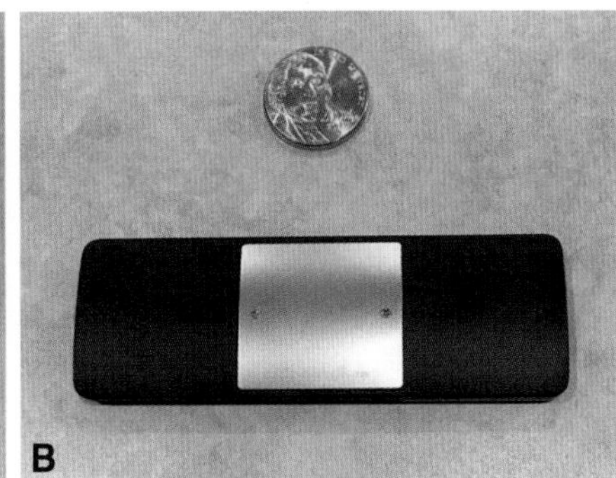

FIGURE 52.4 Direct-to-consumer products. The front **(A)** and back **(B)** of the six-lead KardiaMobile device offered by AliveCor (Mountain View, CA) with a nickel shown for size reference. (A & B, Courtesy of AliveCor, Inc.)

detect AF, with a clinical study in 2019, demonstrating feasibility of enrollment via digital recruitment methods of over 400,000 participants.[28] The clinical implications of such data (ie, the detection of subclinical AF in patients who are otherwise asymptomatic) is a topic of considerable debate. In addition, the newer version of the Apple Watch® utilizes ECG technology that essentially makes the PPG technology of the prior version obsolete. Methods of obtaining a full 12-lead ECG with use of the Apple Watch® have been proposed, which, if shown to be reliable, could greatly increase patient access to an important cardiovascular diagnostic tool.[29]

Although additional studies are needed to further validate these devices, it is a highly proliferative field that may improve accessibility and cost of monitoring for patients in the future. Importantly, in the United States, current procedural terminology (CPT) billing codes now allow providers to obtain reimbursement for reviewing rhythm tracings of these direct-to-consumer products. Because these products generate significant public interest, they are likely to become more popular with increasing usage among technologically capable patients.

FUTURE DIRECTIONS

With the increasing number of modalities of ECG monitoring and growing access of direct-to-consumer devices, there will be an escalating burden of digital ECG data interpretation. Key developments in machine learning will improve the accuracy and access of ambulatory monitoring data analysis. Recent machine learning algorithms reading single-lead recordings have outperformed general cardiologists for 12 core rhythm categories including AF, atrial bigeminy, SVT, and Wenckebach heart block.[30] The application of these neural networks to cloud-based user monitoring systems can distinguish clinical arrhythmias with increasing speed and with over 91% accuracy for numerous arrhythmias.[31] The reliability of these machine learning algorithms and their application, especially in direct-to-consumer products, for clinical decision-making will require further study.

KEY POINTS

- ✔ Technologic advancements have allowed ambulatory rhythm monitors to become increasingly more compact, comfortable, and convenient for patient use.
- ✔ A number of ambulatory rhythm monitoring devices can help providers diagnose arrhythmias when symptoms are present, risk stratify patients with underlying cardiac diseases, or quantify burden of arrhythmias.
- ✔ The selection of an ambulatory rhythm monitor should be guided by the frequency of patient symptoms, patient preferences, and the strengths and limitations of each modality.
- ✔ Providers should be aware of a number of direct-to-consumer products that are available on the market as they increase in popularity and patient use.
- ✔ CPT billing codes now provide a means of reimbursement for reviewing direct-to-consumer product rhythm tracings.

REFERENCES

1. Steinberg JS, Varma N, Cygankiewicz I, et al. 2017 ISHNE-HRS expert consensus statement on ambulatory ECG and external cardiac monitoring/telemetry. *Heart Rhythm*. 2017;14:e55-e96.
2. Subbiah R, Chia PL, Gula LJ, et al. Cardiac monitoring in patients with syncope: making that elusive diagnosis. *Curr Cardiol Rev*. 2013;9:299-307.
3. Shen WK, Sheldon RS, Benditt DG, et al. 2017 ACC/AHA/HRS Guideline for the evaluation and management of patients with syncope: a report of the American College of Cardiology/American Heart Association Task Force on Clinical Practice Guidelines and the Heart Rhythm Society. *Circulation*. 2017;136:e60-e122.
4. Bhangu J, McMahon CG, Hall P, et al. Long-term cardiac monitoring in older adults with unexplained falls and syncope. *Heart*. 2016;102:681-686.
5. Logan B, Healey J. Robust detection of atrial fibrillation for a long term telemonitoring system. *Comput Cardiol*. 2005;32:619-622.
6. Kusumoto FM, Schoenfeld MH, Barrett C, et al. 2018 ACC/AHA/HRS Guideline on the evaluation and management of patients with bradycardia and cardiac conduction delay: a report of the American College of Cardiology/American Heart Association Task Force on Clinical Practice Guidelines and the Heart Rhythm Society. *J Am Coll Cardiol*. 2019;140:e382-e482.

7. Rao AL, Salerno JC, Asif IM, Drezner JA. Evaluation and management of wolff-Parkinson-white in athletes. *Sports Health.* 2014;6:326-332.
8. Pediatric and Congenital Electrophysiology Society, Heart Rhythm Society, American College of Cardiology Foundation, et al. PACES/HRS expert consensus statement on the management of the asymptomatic young patient with a Wolff-Parkinson-White (WPW, ventricular preexcitation) electrocardiographic pattern: developed in partnership between the Pediatric and Congenital Electrophysiology Society (PACES) and the Heart Rhythm Society (HRS). Endorsed by the governing bodies of PACES, HRS, the American College of Cardiology Foundation (ACCF), the American Heart Association (AHA), the American Academy of Pediatrics (AAP), and the Canadian Heart Rhythm Society (CHRS). *Heart Rhythm.* 2012;9:1006-1024.
9. Panizo JG, Barra S, Mellor G, Heck P, Agarwal S. Premature ventricular complex-induced cardiomyopathy. *Arrhythm Electrophysiol Rev.* 2018;7:128-134.
10. Al-Khatib SM, Stevenson WG, Ackerman MJ, et al. 2017 AHA/ACC/HRS Guideline for management of patients with ventricular arrhythmias and the prevention of sudden cardiac death: executive summary: a report of the American College of Cardiology/American Heart Association Task Force on Clinical Practice Guidelines and the Heart Rhythm Society. *J Am Coll Cardiol.* 2018;138:e210-e271.
11. Pillarisetti J, Patel A, Boc K, et al. Evolution of paroxysmal atrial fibrillation to persistent or permanent atrial fibrillation: predictors of progression. *J Atr Fibrillation.* 2009;2:191.
12. Ouyang F, Tilz R, Chun J, et al. Long-term results of catheter ablation in paroxysmal atrial fibrillation: lessons from a 5-year follow-up. *Circulation.* 2010;122:2368-2377.
13. Brooks AG, Stiles MK, Laborderie J, et al. Outcomes of long-standing persistent atrial fibrillation ablation: a systematic review. *Heart Rhythm.* 2010;7:835-846.
14. Gersh BJ, Maron BJ, Bonow RO, et al. 2011 ACCF/AHA Guideline for the Diagnosis and Treatment of Hypertrophic Cardiomyopathy: a report of the American College of Cardiology Foundation/American Heart Association Task Force on Practice Guidelines. Developed in collaboration with the American Association for Thoracic Surgery, American Society of Echocardiography, American Society of Nuclear Cardiology, Heart Failure Society of America, Heart Rhythm Society, Society for Cardiovascular Angiography and Interventions, and Society of Thoracic Surgeons. *J Am Coll Cardiol.* 2011;58:e212-e260.
15. Towbin JA, McKenna WJ, Abrams DJ, et al. 2019 HRS expert consensus statement on evaluation, risk stratification, and management of arrhythmogenic cardiomyopathy. *Heart Rhythm.* 2019;16:e301-e372.
16. Kawasaki T, Sakai C, Harimoto K, et al. Holter monitoring and long-term prognosis in hypertrophic cardiomyopathy. *Cardiology.* 2012;122:44-54.
17. Wang W, James CA, Calkins H. Diagnostic and therapeutic strategies for arrhythmogenic right ventricular dysplasia/cardiomyopathy patient. *Europace.* 2019;21:9-21.
18. Barrett PM, Komatireddy R, Haaser S, et al. Comparison of 24-hour Holter monitoring with 14-day novel adhesive patch electrocardiographic monitoring. *Am J Med.* 2014;127:95.e11-e17.
19. Su L, Borov S, Zrenner B. 12-lead Holter electrocardiography. Review of the literature and clinical application update. *Herzschrittmacherther Elektrophysiol.* 2013;24:92-96.
20. Fung E, Jarvelin MR, Doshi RN, et al. Electrocardiographic patch devices and contemporary wireless cardiac monitoring. *Front Physiol.* 2015;6:149.
21. Galli A, Ambrosini F, Lombardi F. Holter monitoring and loop recorders: from research to clinical practice. *Arrhythm Electrophysiol Rev.* 2016;5:136-143.
22. Bisignani A, De Bonis S, Mancuso L, Ceravolo G, Bisignani G. Implantable loop recorder in clinical practice. *J Arrhythm.* 2019;35:25-32.
23. Vilcant V, Kousa O, Hai O. Implantable loop recorder. StatPearls [Internet]. Updated July 31, 2020. https://www.ncbi.nlm.nih.gov/books/NBK470398/
24. Bansal A, Joshi R. Portable out-of-hospital electrocardiography: a review of current technologies. *J Arrhythm.* 2018;34:129-138.
25. Baquero GA, Banchs JE, Ahmed S, Naccarelli GV, Luck JC. Surface 12 lead electrocardiogram recordings using smart phone technology. *J Electrocardiol.* 2015;48:1-7.
26. Chung EH, Guise KD. QTC intervals can be assessed with the AliveCor heart monitor in patients on dofetilide for atrial fibrillation. *J Electrocardiol.* 2015;48:8-9.
27. Halcox JPJ, Wareham K, Cardew A, et al. Assessment of remote heart rhythm sampling using the alivecor heart monitor to screen for atrial fibrillation: the REHEARSE-AF Study. *Circulation.* 2017;136:1784-1794.
28. Perez MV, Mahaffey KW, Hedlin H, et al. Large-scale assessment of a smartwatch to identify atrial fibrillation. *N Engl J Med.* 2019;381:1909-1917.
29. Cobos Gil MA. Standard and precordial leads obtained with an Apple Watch. *Ann Intern Med.* 2019;172(6):436-437.
30. Hannun AY, Rajpurkar P, Haghpanahi M, et al. Cardiologist-level arrhythmia detection and classification in ambulatory electrocardiograms using a deep neural network. *Nat Med.* 2019;25:65-69.
31. Yildirim O, Plawiak P, Tan RS, Acharya UR. Arrhythmia detection using deep convolutional neural network with long duration ECG signals. *Comput Biol Med.* 2018;102:411-420.

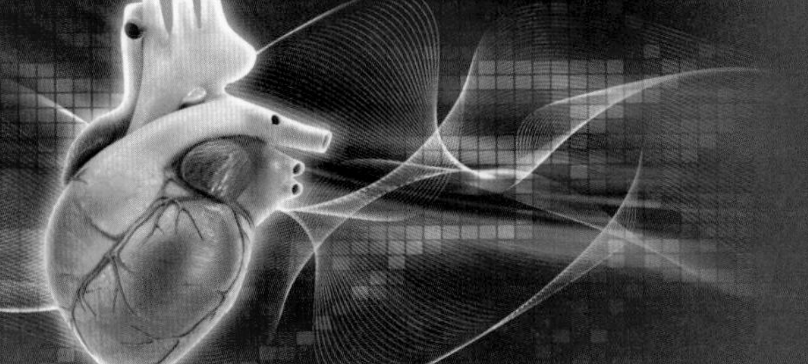

CHAPTER 53

ELECTROPHYSIOLOGY TESTING

Duc H. Do and Noel G. Boyle

INTRODUCTION

An electrophysiology (EP) test (study) is a minimally invasive procedure where electrode-tipped catheters are placed into the heart to record electrical activity in various areas. The EP study may be used as an isolated diagnostic procedure or in combination with an ablation procedure. As a diagnostic procedure, the EP study may clarify a diagnosis that is not clear from surface electrocardiograms (ECGs), allowing for informed decision-making regarding further treatment options. In combination with ablation procedures, the EP study clarifies the mechanism of an arrhythmia to guide an ablation treatment strategy.[1]

INDICATIONS

As a diagnostic procedure, the EP study is indicated whenever an arrhythmia diagnosis is unknown or unclear based on the available information (including ambulatory or inpatient telemetry monitoring, implantable loop recorder–stored electrograms (EGMs), and surface ECG). Common clinical indications for EP study include palpitations and syncope of unclear etiology. Wide complex tachycardias where the diagnosis of supraventricular tachycardia (SVT) versus ventricular tachycardia (VT) is not clear can also be an indication for EP study. Current indications for EP study are shown in **Table 53.1**. An EP study an also be used to risk stratify patients such as those with ischemic cardiomyopathy with a borderline left ventricular ejection fraction that may not meet standard criteria for primary prevention implantable cardioverter-defibrillator (ICD) (**Table 53.2**). As a combined procedure with ablation, the EP study is used to clarify the mechanism of an arrhythmia such that an ablation treatment strategy can be planned. The EP study is generally tailored to the indication because not all maneuvers are important in all clinical scenarios.

ANATOMIC CONSIDERATIONS

Venous access from the femoral veins and/or the internal jugular veins is required to perform an EP study. The presence of deep venous thrombosis or venous occlusion is a contraindication to performing an EP study.

Two main fluoroscopic views are utilized to localize which structures a catheter is in during an EP study: right anterior oblique (RAO), which shows anterior and posterior positions in the heart, and left anterior oblique (LAO), which delineates

TABLE 53.1 Indications for Electrophysiology Study

Clinical Diagnosis	Potential Causative Arrhythmias	Helpful EP Study Maneuvers
Syncope	• Sinus node dysfunction • Atrioventricular block (particularly infrahisian) • Ventricular tachycardia • Accessory pathway	• Sinus node recovery time (SNRT) • Baseline intervals (particularly HV) • Atrial pacing to block cycle length • Atrial programmed electrical stimulation • Drug administration (eg, flecainide, procainamide) • Ventricular programmed electrical stimulation • Ventricular pacing, evaluating for VA conduction • Atrial pacing to block cycle length, evaluating for preexcitation
Palpitations	• Supraventricular tachycardia • Ventricular tachycardia	• Atrial programmed electrical stimulation • Atrial burst pacing • Ventricular programmed electrical stimulation • Isoproterenol administration • Ventricular programmed electrical stimulation • Isoproterenol administration

EP, electrophysiology; HV, His-ventricular; VA, ventriculoatrial.

TABLE 53.2 Risk Stratification With Electrophysiology Study

Clinical Indication	Diagnostic Maneuvers
ischemic cardiomyopathy	Ventricular programmed electrical stimulation for inducible VT/VF
cardiac sarcoidosis	Ventricular programmed electrical stimulation for inducible VT/VF.
Wolff-Parkinson-White	Accessory pathway effective refractory period Shortest preexcited RR in atrial fibrillation
second degree AV block	Baseline HV, determine level of AV block (AV nodal vs infrahisian)

AV, atrioventricular; HV, His-ventricular; ICD, implantable cardioverter-defibrillator; LVEF, left ventricular ejection fraction; VF, ventricular fibrillation; VT, ventricular tachycardia

right and left orientation in the heart (**Figure 53.1**). Using a combination of these two views, recordings from the catheter, and an understanding of cardiac anatomy, the location of catheters can be determined.

Because most catheters are placed into the central veins, they will first enter the right atrium. The sinus node is the primary pacemaker site in the heart and lies in the high lateral right atrium near the junction with the superior vena cava. A catheter placed in this area should record the earliest atrial depolarization during sinus rhythm.

A catheter can be placed into the coronary sinus by advancing it to the inferior tricuspid annulus and then rotating it posteriorly. The coronary sinus lies anterior to the fossa ovalis (ie, interatrial septum), which is itself anterior to the plane of the superior and inferior vena cava junction with the right atrium. The coronary sinus courses within the left atrioventricular (AV) groove between the left atrium and left ventricle, and is closer to the atrium than to the left circumflex artery. Hence, recordings from catheters within the coronary sinus generally have near-field atrial signals and far-field ventricular signals (discussed in more detail subsequently). Catheters in the coronary sinus can sometimes be advanced further toward the great cardiac vein (along the anterolateral AV groove) and the anterior interventricular vein (which lies along the interventricular septum, and generally rightward of the left anterior descending artery). Ventricular branches of the coronary sinus course anteriorly from the body of the coronary sinus. It is common for the tip of a catheter within the coronary sinus to be wedged into a ventricular branch, leading to a more near-field ventricular signal.

The bundle of His is the only normal AV connection across the central fibrous body of the heart. It connects the compact AV node with the His-Purkinje system (the right and left bundles). It can be located along the superior aspect of the membranous septum. A catheter wedged between the septal and anterior leaflet of the tricuspid valve can record electrical activity in the His bundle. The His-bundle EGM can also be recorded from the left side of the membranous septum (left ventricular aspect). The aortic valve, specifically the junction

RAO

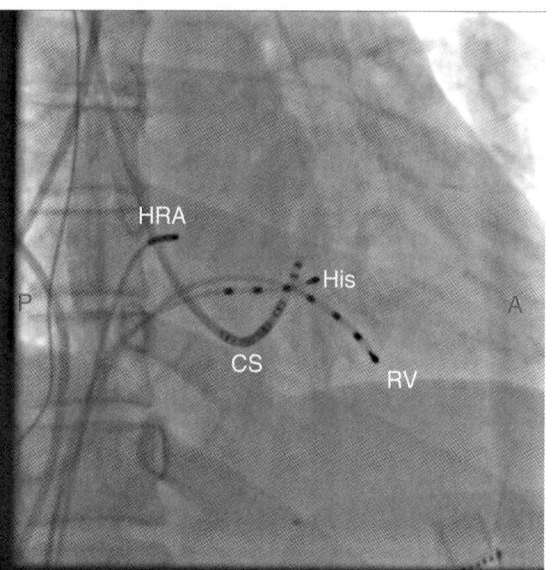

LAO

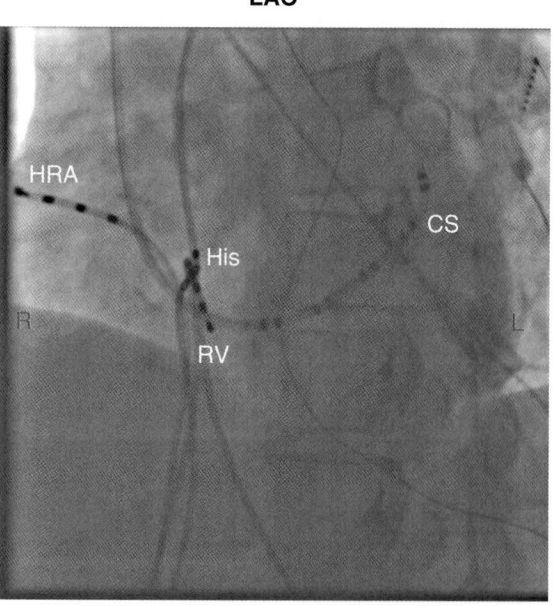

FIGURE 53.1 Fluoroscopic image of standard catheter positions in electrophysiology study. The standard fluoroscopic views for electrophysiology studies are RAO (right anterior oblique) which shows A (anterior) and P (posterior) positions in the heart and LAO (left anterior oblique) which shows R (right) and L (left) orientation in the heart. The standard catheters in an electrophysiology study are placed in the HRA (high right atrium), HIS (His bundle), RV (right ventricle), and CS (coronary sinus).

of the noncoronary cusp and right coronary cusp, lies just superior and leftward of the His bundle.

The right bundle extends down the right side of the interventricular septum and then across to the free wall of the right ventricle via the moderator band. There are many exits for the right bundle into the right ventricular myocardium near the apex of the right ventricle and from branches off the moderator band to the free wall. For an electrical impulse from the right ventricle to propagate retrograde via the AV node to the atrium in the absence of an accessory pathway (ie, in the majority of patients), the impulse must enter the right bundle near the apex (near the standard position of a right ventricular catheter) or moderator band branches.

In cases where catheters need to be placed in the left atrium, access can be obtained through a patent foramen ovale, atrial septal defect, or by performing transseptal puncture through the interatrial septum at the fossa ovalis. The fossa ovalis lies posterior to the coronary sinus and aortic root. Crossing the interatrial septum requires significant caution and guidance with fluoroscopy and/or intracardiac echocardiography to avoid crossing anteriorly into the aorta or posteriorly into the pericardial space. Access to the left ventricle can be performed via transseptal (by crossing the mitral valve) or retrograde aortic (by crossing the aortic valve) approaches. Anticoagulation with heparin should be performed before placing catheters and sheaths in the left atrium or ventricle to prevent formation of blood clots and potential stroke or systemic embolism. Significant care should also be taken to prevent air within sheaths and catheters in the left side of the heart or arterial system to avoid air embolisms.

FUNDAMENTALS OF ELECTROPHYSIOLOGIC TESTING

The EP study is performed by inserting electrode-tipped catheters into the body through central venous sheaths (generally from the right/left femoral veins and/or right internal jugular vein) and positioning them within the heart (Figure 53.1). Catheters are placed within the specific chambers/vessels using fluoroscopy and/or three-dimensional electroanatomic mapping (EAM). There are many shapes and sizes of electrode-tipped catheters, based on the purpose of the catheter. The most standard catheters are quadripolar (four recording electrodes) and have a preformed curve, and are manipulated only by torqueing and advancing/retracting the catheter. Many catheters designed for placement in structures such as the coronary sinus, or for mapping cardiac structures have more electrodes (10+) and are deflectable. Most catheters are between 4 and 8 French in diameter. The specific catheters used are tailored toward the purpose of the EP study. At the end of the EP study procedure, all catheters and sheaths are removed and hemostasis is obtained by manual compression and/or vascular closure device.

Intracardiac EGMs are recordings from these electrodes. In contrast to surface ECG that records the summation of cardiac electrical activity, EGMs record localized cardiac activity only between two electrodes on the catheter, called a *bipolar electrode*. Hence, this provides electrical information only within the vicinity of the recording electrodes. EGMs contain several rapid deflections, representing depolarization of myocardial tissue between the two recording electrodes. Remote (far-field) cardiac electrical activity can also be seen, characterized by less rapid deflections (**Figure 53.2**). Less commonly used are unipolar lead configurations that measure cardiac electrical activity directly beneath the electrode. High-pass and low-pass filters are applied to EGMs for display to reduce noise and interference. The usual filter range for bipolar EGMs is 30 to 500 Hz. A notch filter is also generally applied to remove electrical noise (50 or 60 Hz).

EGMs are displayed on the recording screen by the position of the catheter (eg, HRA for high right atrium, HIS for His bundle, CS for coronary sinus, RV for right ventricle) or by the name of the catheter (eg, DD for duodecapolar or Abl for ablation catheter) and the pair of electrodes from which the recording is originating. Basic catheters inserted in the HRA, HIS, and RV are quadripolar, with two or three EGMs displayed for each catheter. Other catheters are multipolar catheters with multiple pairs of recording electrodes. Pairs of electrodes can be distinguished by a subscript *p* for proximal, *m* for middle, and *d* for distal (eg, HIS_p, HIS_m, HIS_d) or by number pair, where by convention, electrode 1 is the most distal (eg, CS 1,2 representing the most distal bipolar recording pair of electrodes, CS 3,4 representing the second most distal pair) (Figure 53.2).

The amplitude of EGMs depends on multiple factors: electrode contact to the myocardial tissue, the proximity of an electrode to the tissue from where the EGM originates, and the health of the myocardial tissue. Contact against a myocardial surface can be determined by tactile sensation, visualization of catheter bend by fluoroscopy or EAM, presence of sharp near-field EGMs, or springs within the catheter shaft that can measure contact force (generally available with ablation catheters only). Catheters placed on the annulus will record both atrial and ventricular EGMs with approximately the same amplitude. As the catheter moves away from the annulus and toward the atrium, the atrial EGM will progressively become higher amplitude than does the ventricular EGM, and vice versa for a catheter moving away from the annulus from the ventricular side. Areas of myocardium with a significant amount of fibrosis will have relatively lower amplitudes than will the normal myocardial tissue. On the display screen, the gain can be adjusted to improve visualization of low-amplitude signals. The standard sweep speed for visualization during an EP study is also much faster than that of surface ECG to enable better resolution of temporal relationships (100-200 mm/second during EP study vs 25 mm/second on surface ECG).

Baseline Intervals

Intervals measured by EP study are reported in milliseconds (ms). The interval between two consecutive instances of the same recurring EGM is called the cycle length. To convert cycle length to beats per minute (bpm), which is used more routinely

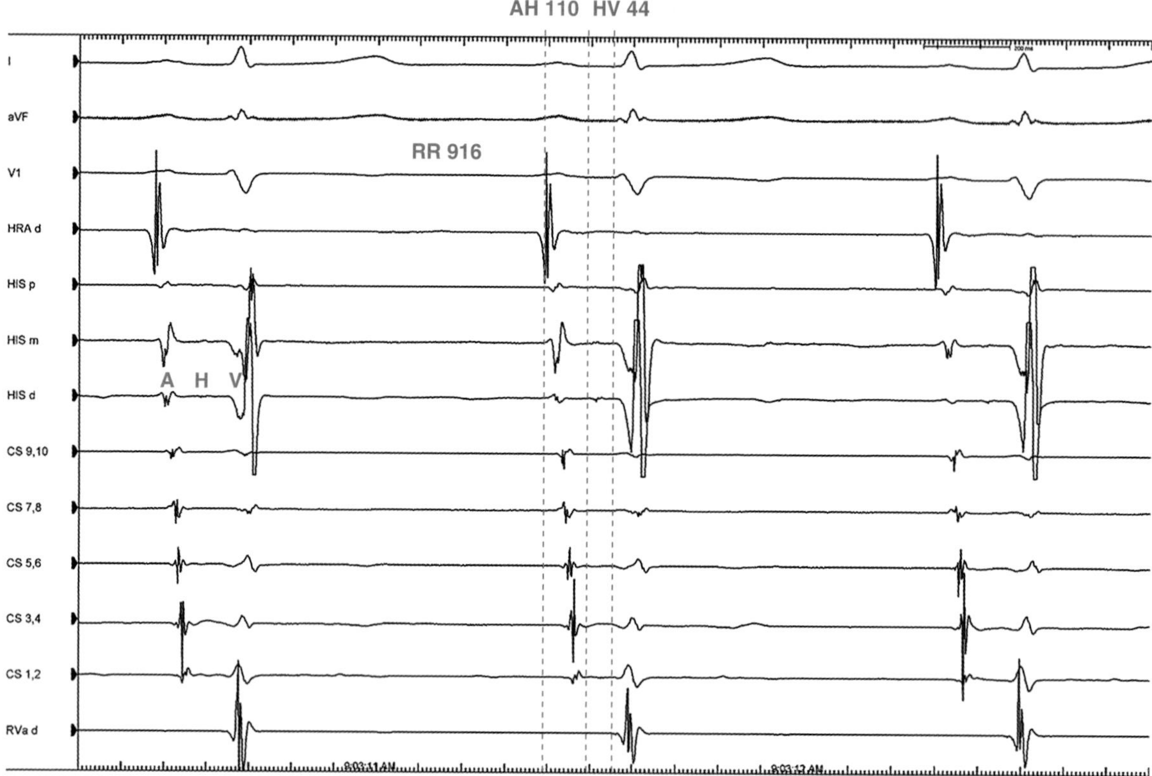

FIGURE 53.2 Basic intervals. All measurements are in milliseconds (ms). In the standard arrangement for a diagnostic EP study, three surface electrocardiographic (ECG) leads are shown along with high right atrium (HRA), His bundle (His), coronary sinus (CS), and right ventricle (RV) electrogram (EGM) recordings. Subscripts denote recording pair of electrodes on each quadripolar catheter: p: proximal, m: middle, d: distal. The CS catheter is a decapolar catheter with five recording bipoles: CS 1,2 of the most distal bipole, and CS 9,10 is the most proximal bipole positioned at the CS ostium. The RR interval (916 ms) is measured between two R waves and can be measured on any lead from surface ECG or from ventricular EGMs on intracardiac recordings. The AH and HV intervals are measured on the distal His-bundle catheter in this case, where the onset of the His-bundle EGM, denoted by H is most clearly seen as a small sharp deflection. The AH interval (110 ms, normal 50-120 ms) is measured from the beginning of the atrial EGM (A) to the His-bundle EGM (H) on the HISd channel. The HV interval (44 ms, normal 35-55 ms) is measured from the His-bundle EGM (H) to the first ventricular activation (V) on any surface ECG lead or intracardiac lead.

in surface ECG terminology, one simply applies a conversion formula: heart rate (HR; bpm) = 60,000/cycle length (ms).

Precise measurements of AV conduction can be performed with intracardiac recording. In addition to the basic surface ECG measurements of the PR, QRS, QT, PP, and RR intervals, in an EP study, AV conduction can be further broken down into the AH and HV intervals. These are measured at the His-bundle catheter, which, because of its location on the superior tricuspid annulus between atrial and ventricular tissue, can simultaneously record atrial, His bundle, and ventricular depolarization (Figure 53.2). If a recording in this general area does not show an atrial EGM, the sharp deflection is likely from the right bundle, not the His bundle.

The AH interval is the time measured between the initial atrial depolarization and the His-bundle depolarization as measured by the His-bundle catheter. Normal values are 50 to 120 ms. This measures conduction across the AV node, and is highly dependent on vagal, sympathetic tone, as well as medications such as beta-blockers or calcium channel blockers that slow conduction (negative dromotropy), or isoproterenol that speeds up conduction (positive dromotropy). Significantly prolonged AH intervals in the lack of reversible factors may represent high vagal tone, intrinsic AV nodal disease, or conduction down the slow pathway of the AV node.

The HV interval is the time measured between His-bundle depolarization and the earliest ventricular depolarization either on surface ECG or on EGM. Normal values are 35 to 55 ms. Shorter values generally represent preexcitation via bypass tracts that depolarize ventricular tissue independent of the AV node and the His-Purkinje system (**Figure 53.3**). Longer values usually represent Purkinje system disease, although in rare cases, this may be the manifestation of conduction delay within the His bundle itself.

Distinguishing the site of conduction delay or block by recording the AH and HV intervals during EP study can assist with determining whether a pacemaker should be implanted in cases where the etiology of AV block is uncertain. AV block that occurs below the level of the His bundle (ie, infrahisian)

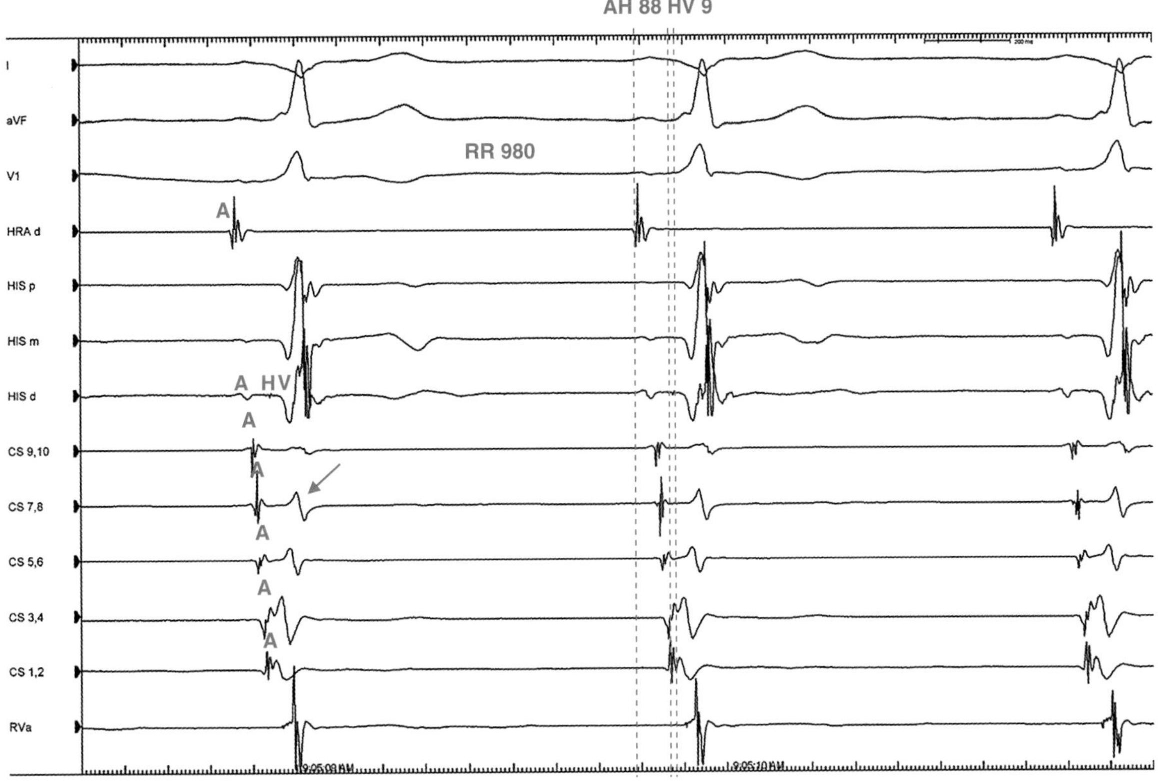

FIGURE 53.3 Intracardiac recording in sinus rhythm in a patient with a left-sided anterior bypass tract. This shows three surface electrocardiographic leads with a standard array of electrogram (EGM) recordings obtained from four catheters: HRA, high right atrium; HIS, His bundle; CS, coronary sinus; RVa, right ventricular apex. Subscripts denote recording pair of electrodes on each quadripolar catheter: p: proximal, m: middle, d: distal. Number pairs denote recording pair of electrodes on a multipolar catheter where 9,10 is the most proximal pair and 1,2 is the most distal pair. The atrial EGM is labeled "A" in the figure, and activation moves from HRA to His to CS (proximal to distal). The dotted vertical lines show the time of first ventricular activation (V) and intracardiac His (H) EGM, resulting in a short HV interval of 9 ms (normal 35-55 ms), indicative of a bypass tract. A far-field ventricular EGM, denoted by the arrow, is seen in the CS bipoles.

generally represents a poorer prognosis in regard to progression to complete heart block with slow or no escape rhythm, and, therefore, is an indication for a permanent pacemaker.

Retrograde conduction, measured by the ventriculoatrial (VA) interval, the time measured between ventricular depolarization to the earliest atrial depolarization, is also helpful in the study of SVT. The manner by which the atrium is depolarized in the retrograde direction can also give clues as to whether a bypass tract is present. Retrograde conduction through the AV node depolarizes the atrium in a midline (or concentric) manner where atrial EGMs propagate from CS 9,10, which is the most midline electrode pair in the CS catheter, toward CS 1,2, which is the most lateral electrode pair. Other patterns of depolarization are consistent with bypass tracts, although midline depolarization does not rule out the presence of a septal bypass tract that can insert into the atrium at a location very similar to that of the AV node (**Figure 53.4 A,B**). Adenosine, which generally blocks AV nodal conduction but not accessory pathway conduction, can be administered by rapid intravenous push to distinguish AV nodal versus accessory pathway conduction.

Pacing Maneuvers

Various pacing maneuvers can be performed to gain further insights into the conduction system or to induce arrhythmias.

The sinus node recovery time (SNRT) is a marker of how quickly it recovers following a rapid atrial rhythm such as atrial tachycardia or atrial fibrillation, and serves as a surrogate for sinus node dysfunction and propensity for conversion pauses if prolonged. This measurement is performed after an atrial pacing train of 30 to 60 seconds. This can be repeated at multiple atrial pacing cycle lengths (eg, 600, 500, 400 ms). The SNRT is measured as the time to first EGM in the HRA catheter following cessation of atrial pacing. A normal SNRT is less than 1500 ms. The SNRT can also be corrected (cSNRT) for the baseline sinus cycle length (AA) using the formula cSNRT = SNRT – AA. A normal cSNRT is less than 500 ms. A prolonged SNRT or cSNRT may be an indication for pacemaker for sinus node dysfunction.

The AV Wenckebach cycle length is the atrial pacing cycle length at which there is a block in the AV node. At progressively faster pacing rates, there will always be a point at which the

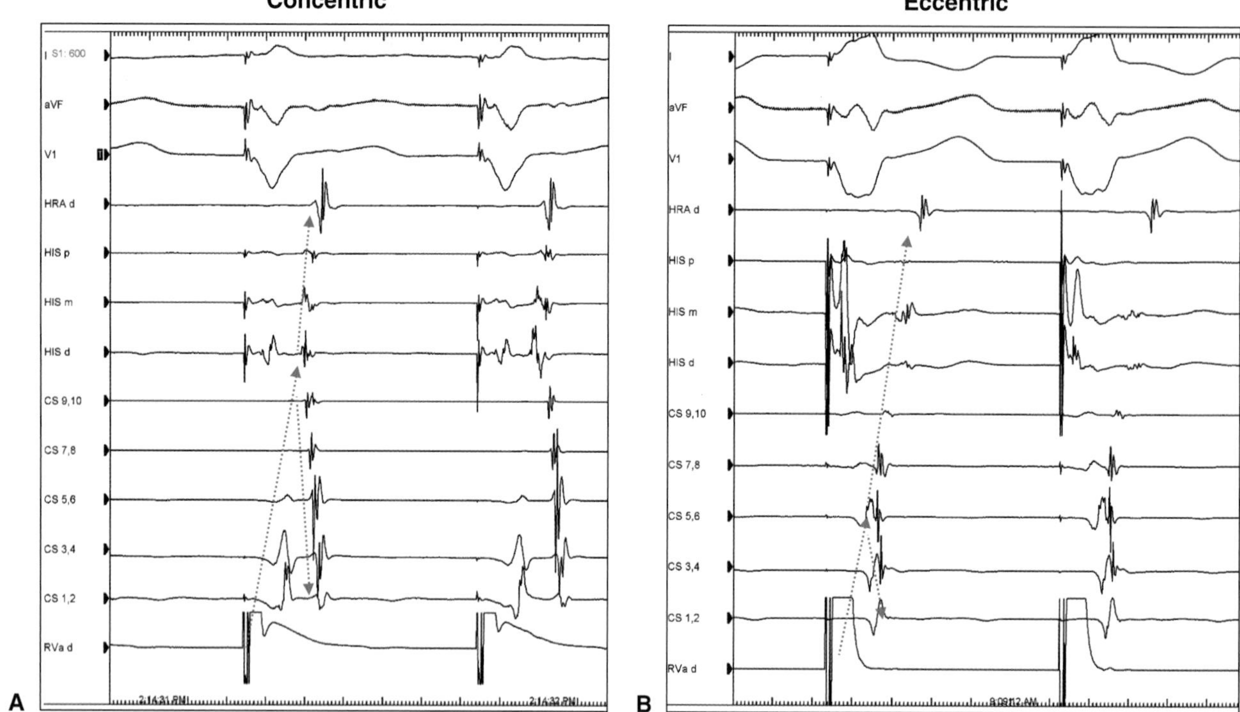

FIGURE 53.4 (A,B) Retrograde ventriculoatrial activation patterns. **Panel A** shows a concentric (midline) pattern of activation where the earliest atrial activation is along the His-bundle catheter. This pattern is consistent with retrograde conduction up the atrioventricular node or a septal pathway. **Panel B** shows an eccentric pattern of activation where the earliest atrial activation is along the mid-coronary sinus indicative of the presence of a left-sided accessory pathway.

AV node blocks conduction down to the ventricle. In young healthy individuals, the AV Wenckebach cycle length is generally short (<400 ms, corresponding with HR >150 bpm). However, this cycle length may be longer even in young healthy individuals who are deeply sedated given the influence of vagal tone on AV node function. In general, patients with diseased AV nodes will have a much longer AV Wenckebach cycle length (>600 ms, corresponding to HR <100 bpm). The AV Wenckebach cycle length alone should not inform decision-making regarding pacemaker need because this represents physiologic AV nodal function. The clinical presentation needs to be considered.

Arrhythmias that are reentrant in mechanism can often be induced using programmed electrical stimulation: delivering extrastimuli (ie, progressively earlier pacing stimuli). These are delivered after a pacing train of 8 to 10 beats at a fixed cycle length (eg, 600 ms). All myocardial tissues have an effective refractory period (ERP), the shortest interval at which an electrical input to the tissue can be conducted. Up to three extrastimuli may be given when attempting induction of arrhythmias, with the shortest coupling interval of each being at the ERP or 200 ms (with coupling intervals <200 ms, atrial/ventricular fibrillation (VF) can often be induced, which is of limited or no value in most EP studies). S1 refers to the pacing train cycle length, S2 the coupling interval for the first extrastimulus, S3 the second extrastimulus, and S4 the third extrastimulus.

The addition of medications such as isoproterenol can increase the chance of inducing arrhythmias, particularly SVT. Atrial arrhythmias are generally induced using atrial extrastimuli (**Figure 53.5**), although some atrioventricular nodal reentrant tachycardia (AVNRT) and many atrioventricular reentrant tachycardias (AVRTs) can be induced using ventricular extrastimuli. Likewise, ventricular arrhythmias are generally induced using ventricular extrastimuli (**Figure 53.6**), although some rare forms of VT such as fascicular VT or bundle branch reentrant VT can be induced using atrial extrastimuli. Arrhythmias caused by triggered activity may also be initiated by burst pacing by building up intracellular calcium levels. Arrhythmias due to enhanced automaticity generally are best induced with isoproterenol. Once an arrhythmia is induced, various pacing maneuvers such as overdrive pacing can be performed to distinguish the mechanism. Discussion of these maneuvers and their interpretation are beyond the scope of this chapter.[2,3] Differentiating SVT from VT can be easily done with an EP study by proving the presence of AV dissociation (**Figure 53.7**).

Electroanatomic Mapping

In more advanced applications of EP studies, particularly in combination with catheter ablation of arrhythmias, three-dimensional EAM can also be performed. This allows for three-dimensional localization of catheters and representation of cardiac anatomy based on catheter movement. Three main commercially available EAM systems exist today: Navx Ensite

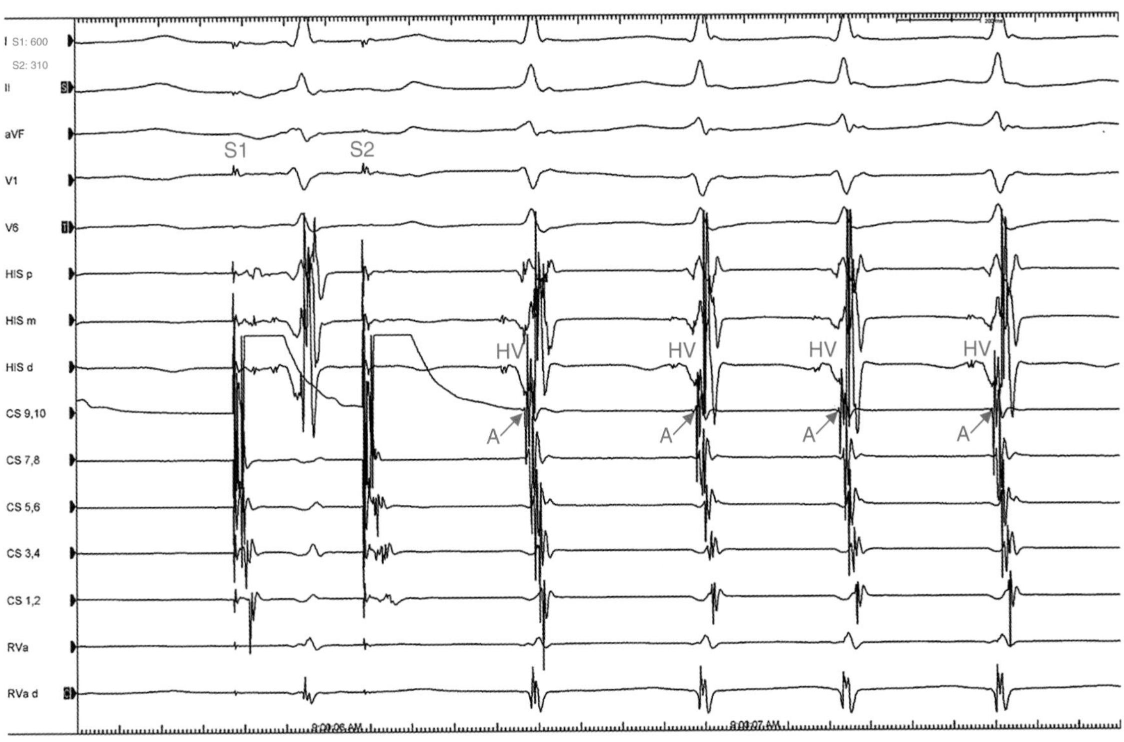

FIGURE 53.5 Initiation of atrioventricular nodal reentrant tachycardia (AVNRT) with atrial programmed electrical stimulation. An atrial drive train (S1) at 600 ms is followed by a single extrastimulus (S2) at 310 ms, resulting in a change in antegrade conduction from the fast pathway (after S1) to the slow pathway (after S2)—as evidenced by a sudden increase in the A2H2 interval. This is followed by retrograde conduction over the fast pathway, leading to initiation of AVNRT. Note that retrograde atrial activation (A) and ventricular activation (V) are near simultaneous during tachycardia, which is characteristic of AVNRT. In this example, the pacing stimuli are delivered from the proximal coronary sinus (CS) electrode (9,10).

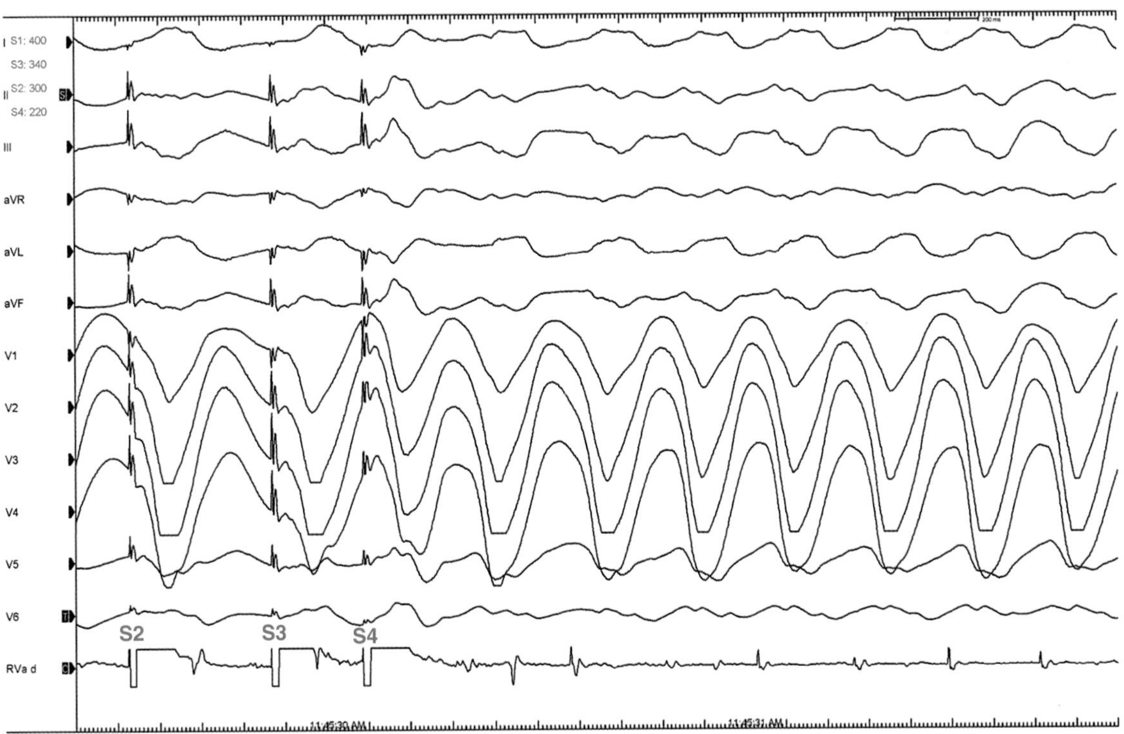

FIGURE 53.6 Initiation of ventricular tachycardia from ventricular programmed electrical stimulation. Triple extrastimuli from the right ventricular apex (RVa) are delivered inducing ventricular tachycardia. The first (S2), second (S3), and third (S4) extrastimuli at 340/300/220 ms are seen here following a drive train (S1) of 400 ms (not shown).

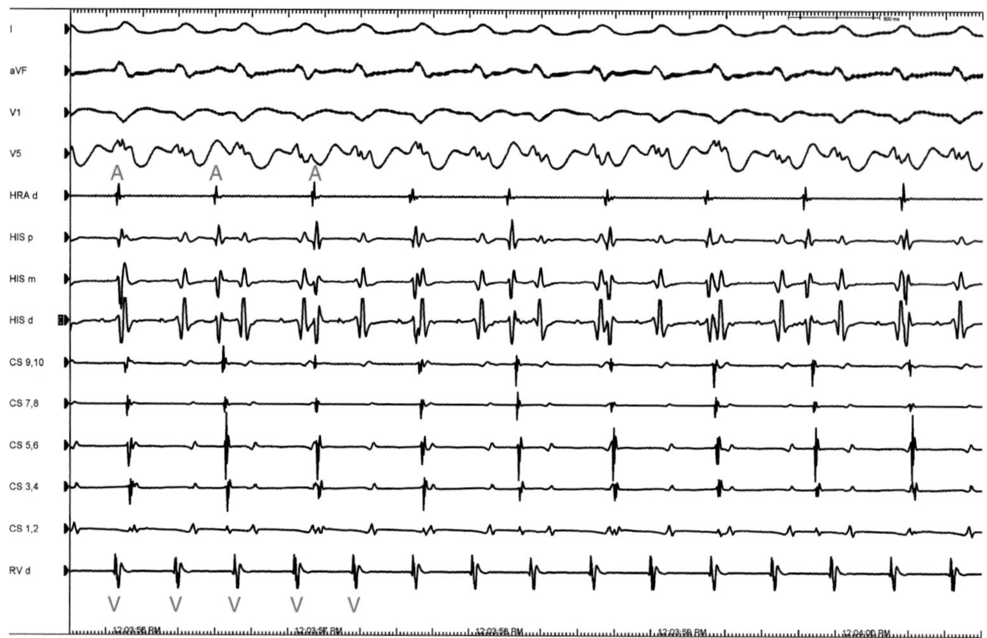

FIGURE 53.7 Ventricular tachycardia with atrioventricular (AV) dissociation. AV dissociation can be easily determined during EP study by separate catheters in the atrium (A) and ventricle (V) showing AV dissociation, or a single catheter in the coronary sinus where both A and V can be recorded as in this tracing. In this tracing, catheters in the high right atrium (HRA), His-bundle position, coronary sinus (CS), and right ventricle (RV) clearly show fewer A than V, and clear AV dissociation. Note that a far-field V signal can be seen in the CS catheter.

(Abbott, St Paul, MN), Carto (Biosense Webster, Irvine, CA), and Rhythmia (Boston Scientific, MA). Navx Ensite allows for localization of any electrode-tipped catheter by measuring the impedance of the various electrodes on the catheter in relationship to patches on the chest and back. Carto and Rhythmia localize proprietary catheters with built-in magnets by measuring the magnetic field, generated by a magnet located under the cath lab table, at the catheter tip. Navx Ensite is also able to secondarily detect catheter position using a magnetic field, and Carto/Rhythmia can detect other catheters using impedance measurements. All three systems are able to create a shell of the cardiac chambers through the creation of a three-dimensional model based on where the catheters have been previously moved. Use of EAM allows for significantly reduced fluoroscopy use, and for some experienced operators, no fluoroscopy.

Information regarding timing and voltage of EGMs can be incorporated with spatial data to create voltage maps or activation maps, among many other possibilities. Voltage maps can show areas of scar within a cardiac chamber. Because many reentrant arrhythmias, such as VT in patients with structural heart disease or atypical atrial flutters, are dependent on areas of slow conduction generally located in partially scarred myocardium, voltage maps can help localize such areas for ablation (**Figure 53.8 A,B**). Activation maps show timing of electrical activity at different areas in the heart. This can help establish the anatomic mechanism of arrhythmias (ie, macroreentrant or focal) or localize the site of an accessory pathway, and help guide an ablation strategy (**Figure 53.9 A,B**). Details about ablation are presented elsewhere.

Advanced applications of EAM include EAM-guided endomyocardial biopsy, which can help increase biopsy yield, and EAM-guided pacemaker implantation, which is particularly helpful in pregnant patients to reduce or eliminate the need for fluoroscopy.

Complications

The EP study is generally a low-risk procedure with a less than 1% risk of major complication including myocardial infarction, stroke, or death. Most complications are due to vascular access including hematomas, pseudoaneurysm, and arteriovenous fistulas. These can potentially be avoided by performing ultrasound-guided vascular access. Although rare when ablation is not performed, cardiac perforation can occur if excessive force is applied to areas with thin walls such as the atria, right ventricle, or aneurysms. This is a potentially life-threatening complication resulting in cardiac tamponade that must be treated with emergent pericardiocentesis and may even require open heart surgery to repair.

CLINICAL APPLICATIONS OF ELECTROPHYSIOLOGY TESTING

Patients with syncope whose history is concerning for a cardiogenic cause of syncope (ie, no or very short prodrome before syncope and facial or head injury) and without any revealing findings on 12-lead ECG or monitoring, may be considered for an EP study to help guide the decision on whether to implant a permanent pacemaker, ICD, or implantable loop recorder.

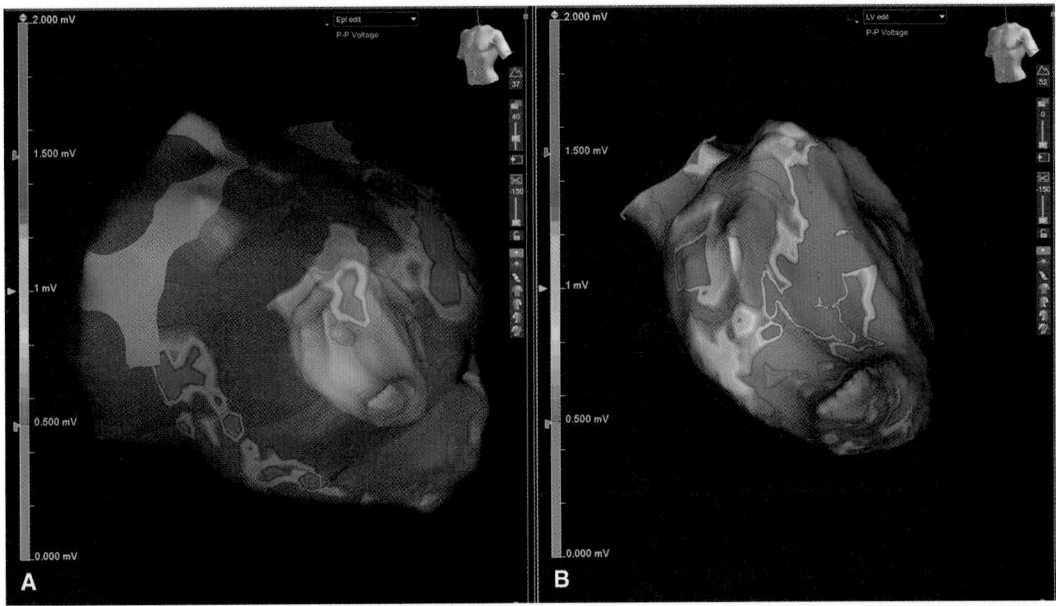

FIGURE 53.8 **(A,B)** Voltage electroanatomic maps. Voltage maps incorporate three-dimensional anatomic information based on where catheters have moved, along with electrogram (EGM) voltages at those locations. Voltage maps in this case of ventricular tachycardia ablation were created using the Navx Ensite system (Abbott, St Paul, MN). Normal myocardium (voltage >1.5 mV) is displayed in purple. Dense scar (voltage <0.5 mV) is displayed in gray, and border zone tissue (voltage 0.5-1.5 mV) is displayed with other colors of the rainbow. **Panel A** shows a voltage map of the epicardium overlying the left ventricular endocardium, shown in **panel B**. A large septal scar is noted in **panel B**. **Panel B** shows scar along the entire septal epicardium, anterior wall of the right ventricle, and apex. These are consistent with scar in the territory of the left anterior descending artery. This information can be used to guide ablation in areas likely to contribute to ventricular tachycardia.

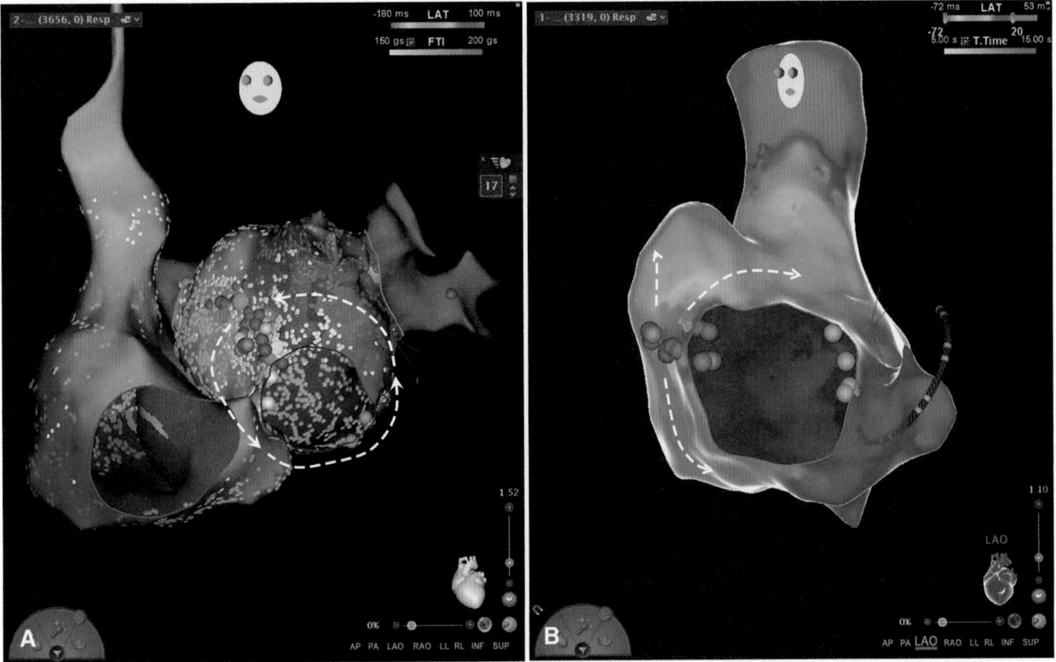

FIGURE 53.9 **(A,B)** Activation electroanatomic maps. Activation maps incorporate three-dimensional anatomic information with activation timing, and allows for determination of arrhythmia mechanism to help guide ablation. Relative timing of local electrograms (EGMs) are labeled with red (earliest) and purple (latest). **Panel A** shows a reentrant arrhythmia (counterclockwise mitral-isthmus atrial flutter) where the colors of the rainbow are spread across the left atrium around the mitral annulus. Ablation (red dots) along the anterior mitral-isthmus line (from mitral annulus to right superior pulmonary vein) resulted in termination (at the green dot) and noninducibility of the arrhythmia. **Panel B** shows a focal arrhythmia (atrial tachycardia originating from tricuspid annulus anterior to the right atrial appendage). Ablation performed around the atrial tachycardia focus led to noninducibility of the arrhythmia. Electroanatomic maps were created using the Carto system (Biosense Webster, Irvine, CA).

Potential indications for implantation of a pacemaker include findings of significant infrahisian disease (HV > 100 ms), infrahisian AV block, or significantly prolonged SNRT. Class I agents such as procainamide or flecainide may also be sometimes administered to unmask infrahisian disease.[4] Inducible VT, particularly in patients with coronary artery disease or nonischemic cardiomyopathy with reduced left ventricular systolic function generally would be an indication for implantation of an ICD. Because the negative predictive value of a normal EP study is not 100%, patients with presumed cardiogenic syncope may benefit from implantation of a loop recorder for continuous monitoring in case they have another syncopal episode.

Patients with ischemic cardiomyopathy and left ventricular ejection fraction of 35% to 40% (which does not meet indications for primary prevention with an ICD) may still be at risk for VT and hence benefit from an EP study to assess for inducibility of VT. Those with readily inducible VT or VF may benefit from an ICD for primary prevention. Similarly, patients with cardiac sarcoidosis with left ventricular ejection fraction less than 35% but no prior ventricular arrhythmias may also be candidates for an EP study for risk stratification to determine whether they may benefit from an ICD.[5]

An EP study can also be helpful in risk stratification for patients with asymptomatic preexcitation (Wolff-Parkinson-White pattern on ECG), particularly individuals in high-risk professions (eg, pilot, firefighter). An exercise stress test is generally a first step in risk stratification; demonstration of an abrupt cessation in preexcitation during exercise suggests that the pathway is low risk for rapidly conducting atrial fibrillation that may degenerate into VF. The negative predictive value of an exercise stress test is only 30%, and hence EP study is generally recommended for further risk stratification. Induction of atrial fibrillation during EP study by rapid atrial pacing and observation of a shortest preexcited RR interval of greater than 240 ms suggests that a pathway is low risk. Attempts at inducing SVT can also be performed during the EP study. If a pathway is low risk by EP study and does not sustain SVT, catheter ablation can be safely deferred.[6]

LIMITATIONS OF ELECTROPHYSIOLOGY TESTING

An EP study may not always induce patients' clinical arrhythmia. Because this procedure is often done under at least light sedation, some arrhythmias that are sympathetically driven may fail to be induced even with administration of medications such as isoproterenol. Not all arrhythmias induced during an EP study may be relevant clinically. This is true for both atrial and ventricular arrhythmias induced with extrastimulus testing. The clinical significance of polymorphic VT or VF induced during EP study with multiple closely coupled pacing extrastimuli is particularly difficult to determine.

SPECIAL CONSIDERATIONS—PREGNANCY

Fluoroscopy is generally required to perform an EP study and hence should not be performed in pregnant patients. There are methods to perform this study without fluoroscopy using three-dimensional EAM if there is an absolute need to perform this procedure during pregnancy.

KEY POINTS

- ✔ The EP study is a minimally invasive study using electrode-tipped catheters placed in the heart. It can be performed as a stand-alone procedure or in combination with ablation for treatment of arrhythmias.
- ✔ One major indication for EP study is the evaluation of bradyarrhythmias. In cases of heart block, the precise level of block (ie, AV node, intrahisian, or infrahisian) can be determined with a catheter placed in the His-bundle position.
- ✔ EP studies can be used to risk stratify patients at high risk for ventricular arrhythmias.
- ✔ Arrhythmias, both supraventricular and ventricular, can be induced during an EP study using programmed extrastimulation. The addition of medications such as isoproterenol may be necessary to induce some arrhythmias.
- ✔ EAM can be performed in conjunction with EP studies to provide spatial information. This is particularly helpful when the EP study is performed in conjunction with an ablation.

REFERENCES

1. Josephson ME. *Josephson's Clinical Cardiac Electrophysiology*. Lippincott Williams & Wilkins; 2015.
2. Knight BP, Ebinger M, Oral H, et al. Diagnostic value of tachycardia features and pacing maneuvers during paroxysmal supraventricular tachycardia. *J Am Coll Cardiol.* 2000;36:574-582.
3. Stevenson WG, Friedman PL, Sager PT, et al. Exploring postinfarction reentrant ventricular tachycardia with entrainment mapping. *J Am Coll Cardiol.* 1997;29:1180-1189.
4. Roca-Luque I, Francisco-Pasqual J, Oristrell G, et al. Flecainide versus procainamide in electrophysiological study in patients with syncope and wide QRS duration. *JACC Clin Electrophysiol.* 2019;5:212-219.
5. Al-Khatib SM, Stevenson WG, Ackerman MJ, et al. 2017 AHA/ACC/HRS Guideline for management of patients with ventricular arrhythmias and the prevention of sudden cardiac death: a report of the American College of Cardiology/American Heart Association Task Force on Clinical Practice Guidelines and the Heart Rhythm Society. *Circulation.* 2017;72:e91-e220.
6. Page RL, Joglar JA, Caldwell MA, et al. 2015 ACC/AHA/HRS guideline for the management of adult patients with supraventricular tachycardia: a report of the American College of Cardiology/American Heart Association Task Force on Clinical Practice Guidelines and the Heart Rhythm Society. *Circulation.* 2016;67:e27-e115.

CHAPTER 54

BRADYCARDIAS: SINUS NODE DYSFUNCTION AND ATRIOVENTRICULAR CONDUCTION DISTURBANCES

Osamu Fujimura† and Houman Khakpour

INTRODUCTION

Bradycardia is generally defined as a heart rate less than 60 beats per minute (bpm) and is caused by sinus node dysfunction, disturbances of the atrioventricular (AV) conduction system, or both. Causes can be reversible or irreversible. In the absence of reversible causes, permanent pacing is the only reliable treatment for patients with symptomatic bradycardia and asymptomatic type II second-degree and third-degree AV block.

SINUS NODE DYSFUNCTION

Epidemiology and Etiology

The precise prevalence of sinus node dysfunction is difficult to study because of its wide range of presentations including asymptomatic patients. Studies on sick sinus syndrome have shown an incidence rate of 0.5 to 3.5 per 1000 person-years.[1]

Analysis of two large epidemiologic studies comprised of more than 20,000 patients showed a sick sinus syndrome incidence of 0.8 cases per 1000 person-years during a mean follow-up of 17 years.[2-4] Advanced age was the most significant risk factor among several identified variables, with most patients presenting in their 70s and 80s.[2]

Sinus node dysfunction is classified as intrinsic or extrinsic (**Table 54.1**). The differentiation is crucial because the extrinsic causes of sinus node dysfunction are often reversible, and permanent pacing can largely be avoided.

Intrinsic Bradycardia

Sinus node dysfunction is most often seen in the elderly population as a result of age-related progressive fibrosis in the sinus node and its adjacent atrial tissue. This may result in abnormalities of impulse formation, conduction, or both and manifest as a variety of clinical abnormalities (**Figure 54.1A**).[5] Patients with sinus node dysfunction often have underlying cardiac conditions, including ischemic heart disease, infiltrative disorders (amyloidosis, hemochromatosis, and sarcoidosis), collagen vascular disease, musculoskeletal disorders,[6] and prior cardiac surgeries including orthotopic heart transplantation and congenital heart surgery.[7] Familial forms of sinus node dysfunction related to autosomal dominance and recessive inheritance have been reported.[8]

Extrinsic (Functional) Bradycardia

Extrinsic factors include medications and perturbances in the autonomic nervous system leading to an increase in the parasympathetic tone. Medications that directly suppress sinoatrial nodal tissue or indirectly affect it via the autonomic nervous system include digoxin, beta-blockers, non-dihydropyridine calcium channel blockers (verapamil and diltiazem), clonidine, and antiarrhythmic drugs (type IA, IC, and III).[9,10] Increase in parasympathetic tone is seen in carotid sinus hypersensitivity (**Figure 54.1B**), neurally mediated syncope (vasovagal syncope), and situational syncope.[11] Sleep apnea can cause a variety of arrhythmias including significant sinus bradycardia and AV block, primarily because of an increase in vagal tone.[12] Significant bradycardia is well documented in patients with grand mal seizure and anorexia nervosa.[13] Well-trained athletes can have a resting heart rate of less than 40 bpm and a type I AV block.[14] Hypothyroidism may also lead to sinus bradycardia.

Clinical Presentation of Sinus Node Dysfunction

Common Signs and Symptoms

Abnormalities in sinus node can be persistent or intermittent. Bradycardia produces a wide variety of symptoms such as fatigue, shortness of breath, light-headedness, and syncope, whereas some patients experience little to no symptoms. It is often difficult to determine if vague symptoms, such as lack of energy, are in fact caused by bradycardia. Thus, it is crucial to correlate the presenting symptoms with electrocardiographic (ECG) findings. Sinus node dysfunction is generally considered significant when sinus pause is greater than 3 seconds while awake and sinus rate less than 40 bpm, although significant overlap exists between asymptomatic and symptomatic individuals.

Diagnosis of Sinus Node Dysfunction

History and Physical Examination

Comprehensive history taking is crucial and should focus on duration, frequency, and severity of symptoms. Evaluation for extrinsic causes should include symptoms provoked or preceded by cough, defecation, urination, food swallowing, shaving, prolonged standing, dehydration, and unpleasant experiences. Medications, family and surgical history should be carefully reviewed.

Physical examination includes vital signs (ie, heart rate and blood pressure) and orthostatic changes in vital signs. Carotid sinus massage can be performed at the bedside by

†Deceased author.

TABLE 54.1 Intrinsic and Extrinsic Causes of Sinus Node Dysfunction

Extrinsic Causes	
Medication	Beta-blockers, digoxin, CCB, clonidine, class I and III AAD, lithium, methyldopa, risperidone, cisplatin, interferon
Increased vagal tone	Pain, increased intra-abdominal pressure
Hypoxemia/Hypercapnia	Sleep apnea, respiratory insufficiency (suffocation, drowning, stroke, drug overdose)
Metabolic	Acidosis, hyperkalemia, hypokalemia, hypoglycemia, anorexia nervosa, seizure
Infection	Lyme disease, legionella, psittacosis, typhoid fever, typhus, Listeria, malaria, leptospirosis, Dengue fever, viral hemorrhagic fevers
Hypothermia	
Hypothyroidism	
Carotid sinus hypersensitivity	
Neurologic	Elevated intracranial pressure, traumatic spinal cord injury above sixth thoracic spine
Acute myocardial ischemia or infarction	
Intrinsic Causes	
Degenerative	Progressive fibrotic process usually related to aging
Neurologic diseases	Mutations in lamin A/C gene including limb-girdle and Emery-Dreifuss muscular dystrophies, tuberous sclerosis
Infiltrative disorders	Amyloidosis, hemochromatosis, lymphoma
Immune disease	SLE
Cardiac surgery	Maze procedure, valve replacement
Familial	

AAD, antiarrhythmic drug; CCB, non-dihydropyridine calcium channel blocker; SLE, systemic lupus erythematosus.

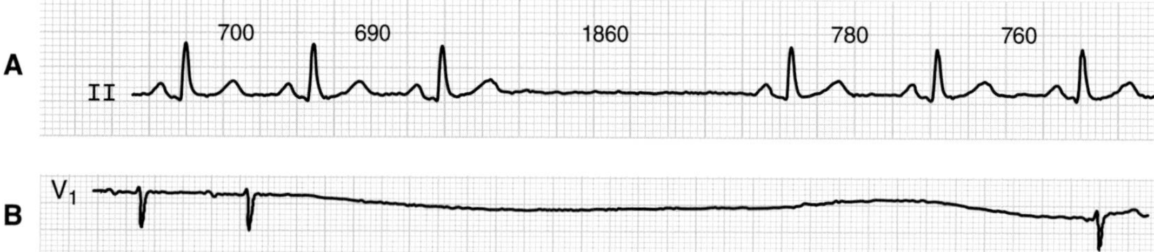

FIGURE 54.1 **(A)** Sinus pause. Note modest sinus arrhythmia as measured by slight variation in PP intervals. **(B)** Carotid sinus hypersensitivity: during carotid massage, PR interval prolongs followed by cessation of atrial and ventricular activity for about 6 seconds.

applying gentle pressure over the carotid sinus with the patient in the supine position. It is contraindicated if there is an ipsilateral carotid bruit.

Noninvasive Testing

A 12-lead ECG is important to evaluate the overall electrical activation of the heart but is often insufficient unless the symptomatic episode is present during the ECG recording. A variety of extended ambulatory ECG monitors are available and can continuously record the cardiac rhythm up to 30 days. US Food and Drug Administration (FDA)-cleared portable ECG devices with one- or six-lead capability also are commercially available. An echocardiogram may be performed to evaluate for any underlying cardiac pathology. Exercise testing is used not only to evaluate stress-induced ischemia but importantly for its effects on sinus rate. For example, a normal chronotropic response is present in well-trained athletes with resting sinus bradycardia.[14] Patients with chronotropic incompetence show a variety of abnormalities in response to exercise.[9,10] Screening for sleep apnea can be performed with a sleep study.[12] Genetic testing and counseling may be required in select cases.[15]

Electrocardiographic Features

Sinus node dysfunction manifests as sinus bradycardia, sinus pause—caused by sinus arrest, sinoatrial conduction block, or overdrive suppression (tachycardia-bradycardia)—and chronotropic incompetence.

Patients with chronotropic incompetence are not able to adequately increase their heart rate during exercise to meet metabolic demands. There is no uniformly acceptable definition, as a variety of heart rate responses to exercise have been reported.[9,10] Inability to achieve a sinus rate to 100 to 120 bpm or 70% to 75% of the predicted maximum heart rate for age (220–age) is a commonly used target.[10]

Sick sinus syndrome is defined by symptoms directly caused by bradycardia. A pause greater than 3 seconds and heart rate less than 40 bpm while awake are generally considered to be diagnostic once extrinsic bradycardia is excluded. Upon gentle carotid sinus massage, a pause greater than 3 seconds during carotid massage is diagnostic for carotid sinus hypersensitivity when associated with symptoms, but this can be seen in asymptomatic elderly individuals.[9,10]

Electrophysiologic Features

An electrophysiologic study (EPS) is beneficial in select patients suspected of sick sinus syndrome.[16] The test involves placement of a pacing catheter in the high right atrium. Atrial pacing is performed at multiple constant rates (usually from 100 to 200 bpm) for at least 30 seconds. Sinus node recovery time (SNRT) is measured from the last atrial pacing beat to the first spontaneous sinus beat. The SNRT is abnormal when greater than 1500 ms and diagnostic of sick sinus syndrome if it is greater than 3000 ms especially if associated with symptoms. SNRTs have about 80% sensitivity and 90% specificity for the diagnosis of sick sinus syndrome. The sinoatrial conduction time (ie, the time in milliseconds that it takes for a high-rate atrial paced beat to enter and reset the sinus node) may be prolonged in patients with sick sinus syndrome. It can be measured directly or indirectly, with normal being 45 to 125 ms. It is, however, a less sensitive method than SNRTs for detecting sick sinus syndrome.[10,16]

Management of Sinus Node Dysfunction

- *Immediate management:* No immediate therapy is generally required with the exception of the patient with frequent and profound symptomatic sinus pauses or bradycardia in whom medication (such as atropine, or beta-agonists such as isoproterenol or dopamine) or temporary pacing may be required. A search for reversible causes should simultaneously be undertaken (see management for AV conduction disturbances for detail).
- *Long-term management:* Because sinus node dysfunction is not a life-threatening condition, the search for a reversible cause can generally be performed in the outpatient setting and, if present, stopped. Occasionally, medications identified to be the culprit cannot be stopped because of the lack of alternative therapy. In the absence of a reversible cause, the only effective therapy for sick sinus syndrome is permanent pacing (**Table 54.2**).[9]

ATRIOVENTRICULAR CONDUCTION DISTURBANCES

Epidemiology

Although AV conduction abnormalities are common, advanced degree of AV block is relatively infrequent. Analysis of a cohort of greater than 6000 individuals with a follow-up of 25 years revealed an incidence of hospitalization because of second- or third-degree AV block of 0.9%.[17] Older age, male gender, a history of myocardial infarction, a history of heart failure, elevated blood pressure, and elevated glucose levels were individually linked to AV block.[17] Patients with sick sinus syndrome also have a higher incidence of development of AV block. Analysis of the collected data from 28 studies on atrial pacing used for sick sinus syndrome disclosed a median annual incidence of complete AV block of 0.6% (0%-4.5%).[18] The DANPACE trial comprised of 1384 patients with a mean follow-up of 8.9 years showed the annual rate of mode change from atrial pacing to dual-chamber pacing was 4.5%.[19]

Pathogenesis

Disturbances in the AV conduction system can be defined as a delayed or interrupted electric signal transmission from the atrium to the ventricle. They can be caused by a variety of factors and can be transient or permanent.

TABLE 54.2 Indications for Permanent Pacemaker in SND

Indications for Permanent Pacemaker in SND	COR
In patients with symptoms that are directly attributable to SND, permanent pacing is indicated to increase heart rate and improve symptoms.	Class I
In patients who develop symptomatic sinus bradycardia as a consequence of guideline-directed therapy for which there is no alternative treatment and continued treatment is clinically necessary, permanent pacing is recommended to increase heart rate and improve symptoms.	Class I
For patients with tachy-brady syndrome and symptoms attributable to bradycardia, permanent pacing is reasonable to increase heart rate and reduce symptoms.	Class IIa
In patients with symptomatic chronotropic incompetence, permanent pacing with rate-responsive programming is reasonable to increase exertional heart rates and improve symptoms.	Class IIa

COR, class of recommendation; SND, sinus node dysfunction.

Adapted from Kusumoto FM, Schoenfeld MH, Barrett C, et al. 2018 ACC/AHA/HRS guideline on the evaluation and management of patients with bradycardia and cardiac conduction delay: a report of the American College of Cardiology/American Heart Association Task Force on Clinical Practice Guidelines and the Heart Rhythm Society. *Circulation.* 2019;140(8):e382-e482.

Congenital Atrioventricular Block

Congenital complete heart block (CHB) is considered to be a result of embryonic maldevelopment of the AV node and less frequently the His-Purkinje system.[20] The incidence is reported to be about 1 in 22,000 live births. Neonatal lupus is associated with 60% to 90% of these cases, and 50% of diagnosed patients have other cardiac malformations, such as congenitally corrected transposition of the great vessels, ventricular septal defects, AV canal defects, and Ebstein anomaly.[20]

Acquired Atrioventricular Block

The following causes are associated with development of acquired AV block (**Table 54.3**).[21]

- **Degenerative diseases of the conduction system.** This is the most common cause of acquired AV block accounting for approximately 50% of cases and is attributed to fibrosis and sclerosis of the conduction system.
- **Medications.** Beta-blockers and digoxin impair or block the AV node indirectly via the autonomic nervous system. Calcium channel blockers and amiodarone directly slow or block the AV node. Class I and III antiarrhythmic medications can affect conduction in the His-Purkinje system, which leads to block within or below the His bundle, especially in the presence of preexisting disease of the conduction system.[22]
- **Acute myocardial infarction.** Before reperfusion interventions became widely available, the incidence of AV block was 12% to 25% in patients with acute myocardial infarction. First-degree AV block occurred in 2% to 12%, second-degree AV block in 3% to 10%, and third-degree AV block in 3% to 7%.[21] It is unclear whether reperfusion therapy has altered the incidence of AV block. First- and second-degree type I AV block occurs more commonly with inferior myocardial infarction than anterior or lateral infarctions. In patients with CHB as a complication of acute inferior myocardial infarction, the site of the AV block is usually the AV node with a junctional escape beat of 40 to 60 bpm. It generally responds to atropine and resolves spontaneously within several days. Some patients with AV block occurring during the early phase of acute inferior wall myocardial infarction are resistant to atropine. Small series showed reversal of atropine-resistant AV block with aminophylline, a competitive adenosine antagonist. The release of adenosine during myocardial infarction may be responsible in such cases.[23] In the setting of acute anterior wall myocardial infarction, CHB is associated with a large amount of myocardial damage that involves the His-Purkinje system. The escape beat stems from the His-Purkinje system with a rate of 30 to 40 bpm. The AV block is less likely transient and should be treated with permanent pacing. Conversely, current guidelines recommend against permanent pacing in patients with acute myocardial infarction and transient second- or third-degree AV block that subsequently resolves.[10]
- **Cardiac infections.** Infective endocarditis involving the aortic valve (ie, with perivalvular abscess) and myocarditis with viral, bacterial, or parasitic etiologies—including Lyme disease, rheumatic fever, Chagas disease (caused by *Trypanosoma cruzi*), tuberculosis, measles, and mumps—can all cause a variety of AV block. With Lyme disease (caused by *Borrelia burgdorferi* and transmitted by the *Ixodes* deer

TABLE 54.3 Causes of Acquired Atrioventricular Block

Degenerative diseases	Approximately 50% of cases. Because of sclerosis of the conduction system
Medication	Beta-blockers, digoxin, CCB, amiodarone, class I and III AAD, acute MI
Infection	Infective endocarditis involving the aortic valve, myocarditis, Lyme disease, rheumatic fever, Chagas disease, tuberculosis, measles, mumps
Rheumatic disease	SLE, reactive arthritis, rheumatoid arthritis, sclerodermn, ankylosing spondylitis, polymyositis
Infiltrative diseases	Sarcoidosis, amyloidosis, hemochromatosis, cardiac tumors
Neuromyopathies	Kearns-Sayre syndrome, myotonic muscular dystrophy
Iatrogenic	Aortic and mitral valve surgery, CABG, TAVR, congenital heart surgery near conduction system, catheter ablation
Vagally mediated	Micturition, swallowing, cough, OSA
Paroxysmal AV block	Initiation and termination by PAC or PVC
Metabolic	Hyperkalemia, hypermagnesemia, hypothyroidism, adrenal insufficiency

AAD, antiarrhythmic drug; AV, atrioventricular; CABG, coronary artery bypass grafting; CCB, non-dihydropyridine calcium channel blocker; MI, myocardial infarction; OSA, obstructive sleep apnea; PAC, premature atrial contraction; PVC, premature ventricular contraction; SLE, systemic lupus erythematosus; TAVR, transcatheter aortic valve replacement.

tick) CHB is usually at the level of the AV node. Temporary pacing is often needed for CHB because of Lyme disease, but permanent pacing is required only rarely after treatment with antibiotics.[24]

- **Rheumatic disease.** Systemic lupus erythematosus, reactive arthritis, rheumatoid arthritis, ankylosing spondylitis, polymyositis, and scleroderma result in varying degrees of AV block.
- **Infiltrative cardiac disease.** AV block occurs in association with sarcoidosis, amyloidosis, hemochromatosis, and cardiac tumors (benign and malignant).
- **Neuromyopathies.** Kearns-Sayre syndrome and neuromuscular disorders such as myotonic muscular dystrophy and Becker muscular dystrophy can cause AV block.
- **Iatrogenic.** Trauma in the proximity of the conduction system can cause AV block. Most commonly this is in association with aortic valve surgery *and* less commonly with coronary bypass or mitral valve surgery. Congenital heart surgery for endocardial cushion defect and ventricular septal defect can result in AV block (transient or permanent). Transcatheter aortic valve replacement (TAVR) is associated with AV block. AV block (temporary or permanent) is a well-recognized complication of catheter ablation performed near the conduction system.
- **Vagally mediated AV block.** AV block can occur in vagally enhanced conditions, such as micturition, swallowing, and cough. The episode is usually preceded by gradual slowing of the sinus rate and prolongation of the PR interval. Slowing of sinus rate (ie, increasing PP interval) is noted during ventricular asystole and acceleration of the sinus rate ensues upon resumption of AV conduction. The block occurs in the AV node and is usually benign.[11]
- **Paroxysmal AV block.** This condition is characterized by sudden loss of AV conduction and ventricular asystole. Clear distinction between vagally mediated AV block and paroxysmal AV block may not always be straightforward, but the following observations are characteristic of paroxysmal AV block. First, CHB is usually preceded by a premature atrial or ventricular contraction (PAC or PVC) and is terminated by another PAC or PVC. Second, AV block can be initiated upon tachycardia termination because of overdrive suppression of AV conduction. Third, acceleration of the sinus rate (ie, decreased PP interval) is usually observed during ventricular asystole. The exact mechanism is not clear but is thought to be due to local phase 4 block in the His bundle.[25]
- **Obstructive sleep apnea.** A variety of arrhythmias (atrial, ventricular, and AV block) occur in association with this condition. Severity of hypoxia seems to be related to atrial fibrillation, ventricular arrhythmias, and sudden death. Bradycardia and AV block appear to be caused by vagal stimulation during apnea and hypoxia.
- **Genetics.** Familial heart block has been linked to mutations in the cardiac sodium channel gene (*SCN5A*) and chromosomes 1 and 19.[8,15]
- **Metabolic.** Bradycardia including AV block can occur in association with hyperkalemia, hypermagnesemia, hypothyroidism, and adrenal insufficiency.
- **Long QT syndrome.** Extremely prolonged QT intervals are seen in some patients with long QT syndrome such as LQT2, LQT3, LQT8, and LQT9. A prolonged ventricular refractory period can cause 2:1 AV block because of functional block below the His bundle.[15]
- **Congenital heart disease.** In addition to congenital CHB, congenitally corrected transposition of the great vessels is associated with acquired CHB that develops at a rate of 2% per year.

Clinical Presentation of Atrioventricular Conduction Disturbances

Symptoms are generally related to the severity of bradycardia and include fatigue, presyncope, syncope, worsening heart failure, or even sudden death. First-degree AV block usually does not cause any symptoms but marked PR prolongation (>300 ms) can result in atrial systole occurring shortly after the preceding ventricular systole. As a result, some patients especially with left ventricular dysfunction can develop worsening heart failure symptoms. Second-degree AV block may produce no symptoms or "skipped beats." Persistent 2:1 AV block may produce symptoms associated with chronic bradycardia. CHB can often cause presyncope, syncope, and rarely sudden death.

Diagnosis of Atrioventricular Conduction Disturbances

As in sinus node dysfunction, a thorough history and physical examination are imperative and should include a search for any underlying etiologies.

A 12-lead ECG is crucial in the diagnosis of AV block as well as associated cardiac conditions. Extended ambulatory ECG monitoring may be required in some cases. Echocardiography is useful in assessing the underlying cardiac pathology. Exercise testing is valuable in the assessment of site of AV block as well as the presence of myocardial ischemia. Exercise results in withdrawal of vagal tone and enhancement in sympathetic drive, leading to an increase in the sinus rate and improved AV node conduction with minimal effect on the His-Purkinje system.

In first-degree AV block because of a delay in the AV node, exercise shortens PR intervals. In second-degree type I AV block with the site of block in the AV node, exercise improves AV conduction, leading to higher AV conduction ratios (eg, from 3:2 to 4:3) or restoration of 1:1 AV conduction. In second-degree type II AV block with the site of block in or below the His bundle, exercise can worsen the AV block by increasing the sinus rate and improving the AV node conduction, which in turn renders the His-Purkinje system refractory. Exercise testing is beneficial in determining the site of block in patients with 2:1 AV block by assessing the effect of exercise on the AV conduction ratio (improvement vs deterioration). Development of AV block during exercise suggests the location of the AV block to be within or below the His bundle. Rare cases of exercise-induced AV node block provoked by ischemia to the AV node artery have been reported. Bradycardia after completion of stress testing usually is caused by a vagally mediated response.[10]

Atropine increases the sinus rate and improves AV node conduction in second-degree AV block with the block in the AV node but can worsen conduction if the block is within or below the His bundle. **Table 54.4** summarizes clues and maneuvers that can aid in identifying the site of conduction block.

EPS is rarely needed for diagnosis and treatment of AV block because the aforementioned noninvasive tests are sufficient. Electrophysiologic testing is useful in symptomatic patients in whom an arrhythmic etiology including AV block is suspected but cannot be documented on the standard tests. In such instances, EPS is indicated and involves assessment of sinus node, AV node, and His-Purkinje system as well as attempt at induction of supraventricular and ventricular tachycardia. Medications such as atropine, isoproterenol, and procainamide are often used to facilitate arrhythmia induction.[16]

Electrocardiographic and Electrophysiologic Features

First-Degree AV Block. First-degree AV block is defined as prolonged PR interval of greater than 200 ms on a surface ECG. It is typically caused by delayed conduction in the AV node. Occasionally, it can result from conduction delay in the right atrium or in the His-Purkinje system (HV interval), especially in the presence of structural heart disease with right atrial enlargement or bundle branch block. His bundle recording is essential to correctly localize the site of the conduction delay. First-degree AV block has a good prognosis. This entity does not cause bradycardia by itself.

Second-Degree AV Block. The prognosis of second-degree AV block is dependent on the site of conduction block. Disease in the His-Purkinje system is associated with a less favorable prognosis, whereas the prognosis of AV node block is generally favorable. Second-degree AV block is divided into two types: Type I AV block (Wenckebach, Mobitz I) and type II AV block (Mobitz II). Type I AV block is characterized by progressive PR prolongation leading to a nonconducted P wave (**Figure 54.2A**), whereas the RR interval progressively shortens. The QRS interval is usually normal, and the site of AV block is usually in the AV node. If type I AV block occurs in the setting of bundle branch block, the site of the block occasionally occurs within the His bundle or below the His. His bundle recording is required to reach the correct diagnosis. Type II AV block exhibits a constant PR interval before a blocked P wave (**Figure 54.2B**). The QRS morphology is usually wide with the site of the block below the His bundle. When the QRS interval is normal, the site of the block is within the His bundle. On occasion, junctional extrasystole with bidirectional block (concealed His extrasystole) can produce the same ECG feature.

2:1 AV Block and High-Grade AV Block. When the sinus rate (PP interval) is regular, the PR interval is constant for conducted beats in patients with 2:1 AV block. High-degree AV block refers to failure of AV conduction of two or more consecutive P waves (**Figure 54.3A**). The site of conduction block can be in the AV node, within, or below the His bundle. The general principle in diagnosis of site of conduction is the same as for second-degree AV block.

Third-Degree (Complete) AV Block. With third-degree AV block, the atrial rhythm is totally blocked in the AV node, within, or below the His bundle. Escape rhythm occurs in the AV junction or ventricle. In junctional escape beat, the QRS rhythm is the same as the normally conducted beat with an escape rate of 40 to 60 bpm, whereas ventricular escape beat shows a wide QRS different than that of conducted beat with an escape rate of 30 to 40 bpm. The hallmark ECG feature is called AV dissociation where both atrial and ventricular rhythms are occurring independently at different rates (**Figure 54.3B**).[26]

TABLE 54.4 Clues and Maneuvers for Determining Level of AV Block

Site of Block	AV Node	His-Purkinje System
Type of block	Wenckebach more common than 2:1	Mobitz II/2:1 more common than Wenckebach
QRS complex	Usually narrow	BBB common
PR of conducted beats	Long	Normal
Carotid sinus pressure	Worsens block	Improves block
Exercise	Improves block	Worsens block
Atropine	Improves block	Worsens block
Isoproterenol	Improves block	Variable effect
Escape rhythm	Narrow QRS, reliable	Wide QRS, unreliable

AV, atrioventricular; BBB, bundle branch block.

Differential Diagnosis

Nonconducted premature atrial contractions: A PAC with a short coupling interval can occur during the effective refractory period of the AV conduction system—usually the AV node—and fails to conduct to the ventricle. This can be misdiagnosed as type I or type II AV block. Nonconducted PACs can be distinguished from second-degree AV block because they occur prematurely and usually have a different P-wave morphology than that of sinus rhythm, whereas second-degree AV block shows fairly constant PP intervals and the P-wave morphologies are the same.

AV dissociation: AV dissociation is defined as the presence of independent atrial and ventricular rhythms each at a different rate. There are four types of AV dissociation. AV dissociation associated with CHB shows a sinus rate that is faster than the ventricular rate with no evidence of AV conduction. This is an important distinguishing factor for accurate diagnosis of CHB. When sinus rate is slower than the ventricular rate, as in the case of sinus bradycardia with a junctional escape rhythm, diagnosis of AV block/CHB cannot be made. Another example is ventricular tachycardia in which the ventricular rate is usually greater than sinus rate with evidence of AV dissociation. Meticulous analysis of relation between atrial and ventricular rates is a key to reaching the correct diagnosis.[27]

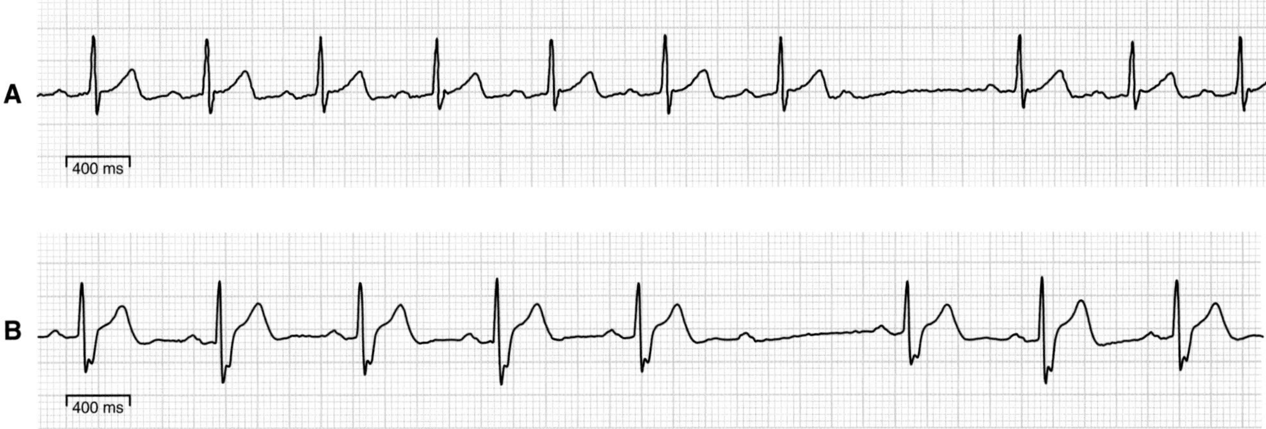

FIGURE 54.2 **(A)** Second-degree Mobitz type I (Wenckebach) atrioventricular (AV) block. Note PR prolongation prior to nonconducted P wave. **(B)** Second-degree type II AV block. The PR interval remains constant. (American Heart Association, Inc.)

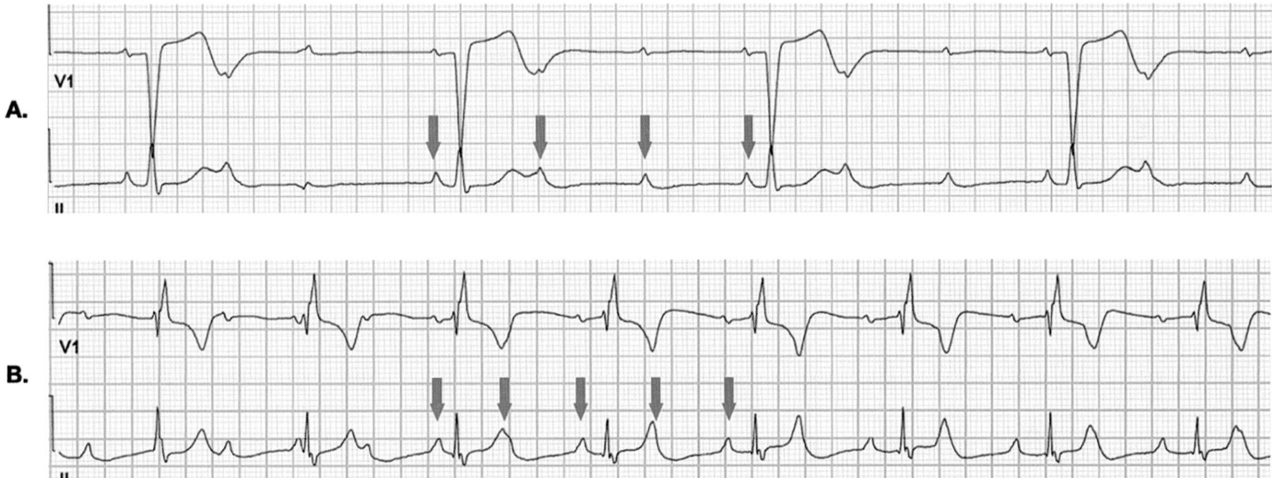

FIGURE 54.3 **(A)** High-grade AV block. Tracing shows sinus rhythm with 3:1 AV conduction and wide QRS with LBBB. **(B)** Complete AV block. There is sinus rhythm at a rate of 110 bpm. There is no AV conduction. A junctional escape rhythm with RBBB morphology at a rate of ~50 bpm is present. Red arrows are marking P waves. AV, atrioventricular; LBBB, left bundle branch block; RBBB, right bundle branch block.

Concealed His extrasystole: A junctional premature beat that blocks in both directions reveals an ECG finding of type II second-degree AV block. Sudden and unexpected PR prolongation without change in PP interval during ECG tracing implicates this mechanism. His bundle recording during AV block is essential for the correct diagnosis.[28]

Management of Atrioventricular Conduction Disturbances

Immediate Management

Urgent therapy may be required in patients with symptomatic bradycardia caused by second-degree AV block (type I and type II) and third-degree (complete) heart block. In hemodynamically stable patients, close observation with backup transcutaneous pacing and continuous ECG monitoring is acceptable until a final decision regarding long-term therapy (permanent pacing) is made. Reversible causes should be investigated including acute ischemia or myocardial infarction, medications, Lyme disease, and metabolic abnormalities.

Pharmacologic Therapy. Atropine (0.5-2 mg) blocks the muscarinic acetylcholine receptor and improves sinus rate and AV node conduction but does not have any effect on the His-Purkinje system. In rare cases, atropine can paradoxically worsen AV block when the block is occurring in the His-Purkinje system. Of note, lower doses of atropine (<0.5 mg) can result in slowing of heart rate.

Beta-adrenergic agonists such as isoproterenol, dopamine, and epinephrine increase sinus rate and improve AV node conduction (and to a lesser degree that of His-Purkinje system). In patients with acute myocardial infarction or unstable angina, these drugs may induce ventricular tachyarrhythmias and myocardial ischemia.

Aminophylline is a nonselective adenosine receptor antagonist and phosphodiesterase inhibitor. Small studies have shown immediate reversal of atropine-nonresponsive CHB complicated by acute inferior wall myocardial infarction.[23]

Digoxin-specific antibody (Fab) is a monovalent immunoglobulin that binds to intravascular digoxin. Review of studies comprising of greater than 2000 patients revealed a rapid response with improvements of symptoms in 50% to 90% of patients with AV block because of digoxin overdose.[29]

Calcium infusion can provide modest improvement in AV block in patients with calcium channel blocker overdose. Glucagon has also been used in patients with calcium channel blocker and beta-blocker overdose.

Temporary Pacing. Pacing is indicated for patients with significant symptoms such as persistent bradycardia with hemodynamic instability, prolonged pauses, and bradycardia-dependent ventricular tachycardia (*Torsade de pointes*). Temporary pacing can be performed in such patients if reversible causes are suspected or if permanent pacing is contraindicated (in case of systemic infection for example). Pacing should ideally be performed transvenously. Transcutaneous pacing can be used in an urgent situation, but it is painful for awake patients and myocardial capture is often difficult to confirm. When a permanent pacing lead is placed, externalized, and connected to a reusable pacemaker generator (outside the body), the procedure is referred to as a *tempo-perm* pacing. This type of pacemaker has minimal risk of lead dislodgement and stable pacing threshold for a much longer period than traditional temporary pacemakers (for up to 2-4 weeks). This is particularly useful in pacemaker-dependent patients who have contraindication(s) for a permanent pacemaker placement because of acute conditions such as systemic infection.[10]

Long-Term Management

First-degree AV block is associated with a benign course and it usually requires no therapy. Second-degree AV block within or below the His bundle is associated with progression to CHB that may lead to presyncope, syncope, polymorphic ventricular tachycardia, or even sudden death. Conversely, second-degree AV block within the AV node generally has a benign course and does not require therapy unless the patient becomes symptomatic related to bradycardia.

It is generally agreed that permanent pacing is indicated for nonreversible acquired type II second- and third-degree AV block (CHB) regardless of symptoms. For congenital CHB, permanent pacing is indicated for symptomatic patients including those with syncope, heart failure, or chronotropic incompetence. Pacing is also indicated for asymptomatic patients considered at risk of syncope or sudden death, heralded by a wide QRS escape rhythm, complex ventricular ectopy, ventricular dysfunction, average escape rate less than 50 bpm, or abrupt pauses of 2 or 3 times the basic cycle length. If symptoms, such as syncope, are suggestive of but not proven to be caused by bradycardia after extensive evaluation, careful follow-up with placement of an implantable loop monitor is a reasonable option.[30] **Table 54.5** summarizes management of bradycardia in patients with adult congenital heart disease.

Permanent Pacing. Indications for permanent pacing in patients with acquired AV block are listed in **Table 54.6.** Scenarios in which permanent pacing is not recommended and potentially harmful are summarized in **Table 54.7**. Ideal pacing modes for specific conditions are not fully established. Patients with bradycardia who have chronic left ventricular

TABLE 54.5 Recommendations for Management of Bradycardia in Adult Congenital Heart Disease

Management of Bradycardia in Adult Congenital Heart Disease (ACHD)	COR
Atrial-based permanent pacing is recommended in ACHD patients with SND or chronotropic incompetence.	Class I
Permanent pacing is recommended in ACHD patients with symptomatic AV block.	Class I
In patients with congenital complete AV block and any of the following, permanent pacing is recommended: 1. Symptomatic bradycardia 2. Wide QRS escape rhythm 3. Mean daytime heart rate below 50 bpm 4. Complex ventricular ectopy 5. Ventricular dysfunction.	Class I
Permanent pacing is recommended in ACHD patients with postoperative second-degree type II, high-grade or third-degree AV block that is not expected to resolve.	Class I
In asymptomatic patients with congenital complete AV block, permanent pacing is reasonable.	Class IIa
In patients with repaired ACHD who require a pacemaker, a pacing device with atrial antitachycardia pacing capability is reasonable.	Class IIa
In ACHD patients with SND or AV conduction disease undergoing cardiac surgery, intraoperative placement of permanent epicardial pacing system is reasonable.	Class IIa
In ACHD patients with venous to systemic intracardiac shunts, placement of endocardial pacing leads may be harmful.	Class III: Harm

ACHD, adult congenital heart disease; AV, atrioventricular; COR, class of recommendation; SND, sinus node dysfunction.
American Heart Association, Inc.

TABLE 54.6 Indications for Permanent Pacemaker in Acquired AV Block

Indications for Permanent Pacemaker in Acquired AV Block	COR
Second-degree Mobitz type II, high-grade, or third-degree AV block not attributable to reversible or physiologic causes, regardless of symptoms	Class I
Neuromuscular diseases associated with conduction disorders, including muscular dystrophy with evidence of second- or third-degree AV block regardless of symptoms. Consider defibrillator capability if needed and meaningful survival of >1 year is expected	Class I
Permanent AF with symptomatic bradycardia	Class I
Symptomatic AV block as a consequence of guideline-directed therapy for which there is no alternative treatment and continued treatment is clinically necessary	Class I
Infiltrative cardiomyopathy, such as cardiac sarcoidosis or amyloidosis, and second-degree Mobitz type II, high-grade or third-degree AV block. Consider defibrillator capability if needed and meaningful survival of >1 year is expected	Class IIa
Lamin A/C gene mutations, including limb-girdle and Emery-Dreifuss muscular dystrophies, with a PR interval >240 ms and LBBB. Consider defibrillator capability if needed and meaningful survival of >1 year is expected	Class IIa
Marked first-degree or second-degree Mobitz type I (Wenckebach) AV block with symptoms that are clearly attributable to the AV block	Class IIa
Neuromuscular diseases, such as myotonic dystrophy type 1, with a PR interval >240 ms, a QRS duration >120 ms, or fascicular block. Consider defibrillator capability if needed and meaningful survival of >1 year is expected	Class IIb

AF, atrial fibrillation; AV, atrioventricular; COR, class of recommendation; LBBB, left bundle branch block.
American Heart Association, Inc.

TABLE 54.7 Recommendations Against Permanent Pacemaker Implantation

Recommendations Against Permanent Pacemaker Implantation	COR
In asymptomatic individuals with sinus bradycardia or sinus pauses that are secondary to physiologically elevated parasympathetic tone, permanent pacing should not be performed.	Class III: Harm
In patients with asymptomatic SND, or sleep-related sinus bradycardia or transient sinus pauses occurring during sleep or in those in whom the symptoms have been documented to occur in the absence of bradycardia or chronotropic incompetence, permanent pacing should not be performed.	Class III: Harm
In patients with first- or second-degree Mobitz type I (Wenckebach) or 2:1 AV block believed to be at the level of the AV node, with symptoms that do not temporally correspond to the AV block, permanent pacing should not be performed.	Class III: Harm
In asymptomatic patients with first- or second-degree Mobitz type I (Wenckebach) or 2:1 AV block believed to be at the level of the AV node, permanent pacing should not be performed.	Class III: Harm
In patients who had acute AV block attributable to a known reversible and nonrecurrent cause, and have had complete resolution of the AV block with treatment of the underlying cause, permanent pacing should not be performed.	Class III: Harm
In patients with asymptomatic vagally mediated AV block, permanent pacing should not be performed.	Class III: Harm
In patients with an acute MI and transient AV block that resolves, permanent pacing should not be performed.	Class III: Harm
In patients with an acute MI and a new BBB or isolated fascicular block in the absence of second- or third-degree AV block, permanent pacing should not be performed.	Class III: Harm

AV, atrioventricular; BBB, bundle branch block; COR, class of recommendation; MI, myocardial infarction; SND, sinus node dysfunction.
American Heart Association, Inc.

dysfunction should be evaluated for a cardiac defibrillator with pacing capabilities. Cardiac resynchronization therapy should be considered for patients with left ventricular dysfunction and marked QRS prolongation or patients with second- or third-degree AV block that requires predominant right ventricular pacing.[10]

SPECIAL CONSIDERATIONS AND FUTURE DIRECTIONS

An increasing number of cases of inflammatory disease that affect the heart, such as sarcoidosis, have been reported. CHB can be the first manifestation of cardiac sarcoidosis without classic findings such as hilar lymphadenopathy on chest radiograph. Ventricular tachycardia often occurs as well. Cardiac magnetic resonance imaging (MRI) or positron emission tomography with computed tomography is recommended to detect inflammation.[31] Chagas disease—caused by *T. cruzi* infection and leading to conduction disease, ventricular tachycardia, and cardiomyopathy—has been increasingly recognized in the United States.[32]

New devices are now available for clinical use. His bundle pacing has been increasingly used in lieu of left ventricular pacing via coronary sinus pacing.[33] Leadless pacemakers are now available for selected patients.[34] Most current devices are MRI conditional. For nonconditional devices, MRI can be offered at selected facilities.[35]

FOLLOW-UP PATIENT CARE

Patients not undergoing device therapy require careful clinical observation.

Patients who undergo device therapy need to have the device checked regularly. Home monitoring devices can be used to monitor the device from home.

KEY POINTS

- ✔ Sinus node dysfunction is classified as intrinsic or extrinsic. The extrinsic causes of sinus node dysfunction are often reversible, and permanent pacing can largely be avoided in these cases.
- ✔ In the absence of a reversible cause, the only effective therapy for sick sinus syndrome is permanent pacing.
- ✔ Degenerative conduction system disease accounts for half of cases of acquired AV block and is attributed to fibrosis and sclerosis of the conduction system.
- ✔ In patients with acquired AV block, permanent pacing is indicated for symptomatic second-degree AV block (type I or II) and third-degree AV block. In addition, it is generally agreed that pacing is indicated for asymptomatic second-degree (type II) and third-degree AV block.
- ✔ Current guidelines recommend against permanent pacing in patients with acute myocardial infarction and transient second- or third-degree AV block that subsequently resolves.
- ✔ The most common cardiac arrhythmia manifestation of Lyme disease is CHB. Temporary pacing is often required, but permanent pacing is rarely needed after treatment with antibiotics.
- ✔ Paroxysmal AV block is a condition characterized by sudden loss of AV conduction and ventricular asystole. Clear distinction between vagally mediated AV block and paroxysmal AV block may not always be straightforward.
- ✔ An increasing number of cases of sarcoidosis have been reported. CHB can be the first manifestation of cardiac sarcoidosis without classic findings. Ventricular tachycardia often occurs as well. Chagas disease leading to conduction disease, ventricular tachycardia, and cardiomyopathy has been increasingly recognized in the United States.

REFERENCES

1. Baine WB, Yu W, Weis KA. Trends and outcomes in the hospitalization of older Americans for cardiac conduction disorders or arrhythmias, 1991-1998. *J Am Geriatr Soc.* 2001;49(6):763-770. doi:10.1046/j.1532-5415.2001.49153.x
2. Jensen PN, Gronroos NN, Chen LY, et al. Incidence of and risk factors for sick sinus syndrome in the general population. *J Am Coll Cardiol.* 2014;64(6):531-538. doi:10.1016/j.jacc.2014.03.056
3. Investigators TA. The Atherosclerosis Risk in Communities (ARIC) Study: design and objectives. The ARIC investigators. *Am J Epidemiol.* 1989; 129(4):687-702. http://www.ncbi.nlm.nih.gov/pubmed/2646917
4. Fried LP, Borhani NO, Enright P, et al. The cardiovascular health study: design and rationale. *Ann Epidemiol.* 1991;1(3):263-276. doi:10.1016/1047-2797(91)90005-W
5. Evans R, Shaw DB. Pathological studies in sinoatrial disorder (sick sinus syndrome). *Heart.* 1977;39(7):778-786. doi:10.1136/hrt.39.7.778
6. Sanders P, Kistler PM, Morton JB, Spence SJ, Kalman JM. Remodeling of sinus node function in patients with congestive heart failure: reduction in sinus node reserve. *Circulation.* 2004;110(8):897-903. doi:10.1161/01.CIR.0000139336.69955.AB
7. Sherwin ED, Triedman JK, Walsh EP. Update on interventional electrophysiology in congenital heart disease evolving solutions for complex hearts. *Circ Arrhythm Electrophysiol.* 2013;6(5):1032-1040. doi:10.1161/CIRCEP.113.000313
8. Ruan Y, Liu N, Priori SG. Sodium channel mutations and arrhythmias. *Nat Rev Cardiol.* 2009;6(5):337-348. doi:10.1038/nrcardio.2009.44
9. Benditt DG, Sakaguchi S, Goldstein MA, Lurie KG, Gornick CC, Adler SW. Sinus node dysfunction: pathophysiology, clinical features, evaluation and treatment. In: Zipes JJ, ed. *Cardiac Electrophysiology: From Cell to Bedside.* Vol 2. 1st ed. WB Sanders; 1995:1215-1247.
10. Kusumoto FM, Schoenfeld MH, Barrett C, et al. 2018 ACC/AHA/HRS Guideline on the evaluation and management of patients with bradycardia and cardiac conduction delay: a report of the American College of Cardiology/American Heart Association Task Force on Clinical Practice Guidelines and the Heart Rhyth. *Circulation.* 2019;140(8):e382-e482. doi:10.1161/CIR.0000000000000628
11. Calkins H, Zipes DP. Hypotension and syncope. In: Zipes DP, Libby P, Bonow RO, Mann DL, eds. *Braunwald's Heart Disease: A Textbook of Cardiovascular Medicine.* 11th ed. Elsevier; 2012:885-895. doi:10.1016/b978-1-4377-0398-6.00042-1
12. Miller WP. Cardiac arrhythmias and conduction disturbances in the sleep apnea syndrome. Prevalence and significance. *Am J Med.* 1982;73(3):317. doi:10.1016/0002-9343(82)90706-9
13. Bestawros M, Darbar D, Arain A, et al. Ictal asystole and ictal syncope: insights into clinical management. *Circ Arrhythm Electrophysiol.* 2015;8(1):159-164. doi:10.1161/CIRCEP.114.001667
14. Stein R, Medeiros CM, Rosito GA, Zimerman LI, Ribeiro JP. Intrinsic sinus and atrioventricular node electrophysiologic adaptations in endurance athletes. *J Am Coll Cardiol.* 2002;39(6):1033-1038. doi:10.1016/S0735-1097(02)01722-9
15. Ackerman MJ, Priori SG, Willems S, et al. HRS/EHRA expert consensus statement on the state of genetic testing for the channelopathies and cardiomyopathies. *Europace.* 2011;13(8):1077-1109. doi:10.1093/europace/eur245
16. Fujimura O, Yee R, Klein GJ, Sharma AD, Boahene KA. The diagnostic sensitivity of electrophysiologic testing in patients with syncope caused by transient bradycardia. *N Engl J Med.* 1989;321(25):1703-1707. doi:10.1056/nejm198912213212503
17. Kerola T, Eranti A, Aro AL, et al. Risk factors associated with atrioventricular block. *JAMA Netw Open.* 2019;2(5):e194176. doi:10.1001/jamanetworkopen.2019.4176
18. Rosenqvist M, Obel IWP. Atrial pacing and the risk for AV block: is there a time for change in attitude? *Pacing Clin Electrophysiol.* 1989; 12(1 I):97-101. doi:10.1111/pace.1989.12.p1.97
19. Brandt NH, Kirkfeldt RE, Nielsen JC, et al. Single lead atrial vs. dual chamber pacing in sick sinus syndrome: Extended register-based follow-up in the DANPACE trial. *Europace.* 2017;19(12):1981-1987. doi:10.1093/europace/euw364

20. Friedman D, Duncanson L, Glickstein J, Buyon J. A review of congenital heart block. *Images Paediatr Cardiol.* 2003;5(3):36-48. http://www.ncbi.nlm.nih.gov/pubmed/22368629%0Ahttp://www.pubmedcentral.nih.gov/articlerender.fcgi?artid=PMC3232542
21. Stambler BS, Rahimtoola SH, Ellenbogen KA. Pacing for atrioventricular conduction system disease. In: Ellenbogen KA, ed. *Clinical Cardiac Pacing, Defibrillation, and Resynchronization Therapy.* 3rd ed. Elsevier; 2007:429-472. doi:10.1016/B978-1-4160-2536-8.50019-4
22. Zeltser D, Justo D, Halkin A, et al. Drug-induced atrioventricular block: prognosis after discontinuation of the culprit drug. *J Am Coll Cardiol.* 2004;44(1):105-108. doi:10.1016/j.jacc.2004.03.057
23. Altun A, Kirdar C, Özbay G. Effect of aminophylline in patients with atropine-resistant late advanced atrioventricular block during acute inferior myocardial infarction. *Clin Cardiol.* 1998;21(10):759-762. doi:10.1002/clc.4960211012
24. Steere AC. Lyme disease. *N Engl J Med.* 1989;321(9):586-596. doi:10.1056/NEJM198908313210906
25. Lee S, Wellens HJJ, Josephson ME. Paroxysmal atrioventricular block. *Heart Rhythm.* 2009;6(8):1229-1234. doi:10.1016/j.hrthm.2009.04.001
26. McConachie I, Wilkinson K. Atrioventricular block. In: *Anaesthesia.* 1985;40:923-924. doi:10.1111/j.1365-2044.1985.tb11081.x
27. Olgin JE. AV dissociation. In: Libby P, Bonow RO, Mann DL, eds. *Braunwald's Heart Disease: A Textbook of Cardiovascular Medicine.* 8th ed. Elsevier; 2008:919-920.
28. Fisch C, Zipes DP, McHenry PL. Electrocardiographic manifestations of concealed junctional ectopic impulses. *Circulation.* 1976;53(2):217-223. doi:10.1161/01.CIR.53.2.217
29. Antman EM, Wenger TL, Butler VP, Haber E, Smith TW. Treatment of 150 cases of life-threatening digitalis intoxication with digoxin-specific Fab antibody fragments. Final report of a multicenter study. *Circulation.* 1990;81(6):1744-1752. doi:10.1161/01.CIR.81.6.1744
30. Krahn AD, Klein GJ, Yee R, Skanes AC. Randomized assessment of syncope trial: conventional diagnostic testing versus a prolonged monitoring strategy. *Circulation.* 2001;104(1):46-51. doi:10.1161/01.CIR.104.1.46
31. Tung R, Bauer B, Schelbert H, et al. Incidence of abnormal positron emission tomography in patients with unexplained cardiomyopathy and ventricular arrhythmias: the potential role of occult inflammation in arrhythmogenesis. *Heart Rhythm.* 2015;12(12):2488-2498. doi:10.1016/j.hrthm.2015.08.014
32. Nunes MCP, Beaton A, Acquatella H, et al. Chagas cardiomyopathy: an update of current clinical knowledge and management: a scientific statement from the American Heart Association. *Circulation.* 2018;138(12):e169-e209. doi:10.1161/CIR.0000000000000599
33. Ajijola OA, Upadhyay GA, Macias C, Shivkumar K, Tung R. Permanent His-bundle pacing for cardiac resynchronization therapy: initial feasibility study in lieu of left ventricular lead. *Heart Rhythm.* 2017;14(9):1353-1361. doi:10.1016/j.hrthm.2017.04.003
34. El-Chami MF, Bonner M, Holbrook R, et al. Leadless pacemakers reduce risk of device-related infection: Review of the potential mechanisms. *Heart Rhythm.* 2020;17(8):1393-1397. doi:10.1016/j.hrthm.2020.03.019
35. Nazarian S, Hansford R, Rahsepar AA, et al. Safety of magnetic resonance imaging in patients with cardiac devices. *N Engl J Med.* 2017;377(26):2555-2564. doi:10.1056/nejmoa1604267

CHAPTER 55

SUPRAVENTRICULAR TACHYCARDIAS

Roberto G. Gallotti, Kevin M. Shannon, and Jeremy P. Moore

INTRODUCTION

Epidemiology and Risk Factors

Supraventricular tachycardia (SVT) is a general term that is used to describe any arrhythmia with a ventricular rate greater than 100 bpm that originates at or above the level of the His bundle. This term encompasses atrioventricular nodal reentrant tachycardia (AVNRT), atrioventricular reentrant tachycardia (AVRT), ectopic atrial tachycardia (EAT), atrial flutter, focal atrial tachycardia (AT), junctional tachycardia, and inappropriate sinus tachycardia. The epidemiology of SVT is difficult to define given the wide range of rhythms that fall in this category; however, it is estimated that the prevalence of SVT in the general population is 2.29 per 1000 persons with approximately 89,000 new cases diagnosed per year.[1] Gender and age are independent risk factors, with women having twice the risk of men, and those older than 65 years of age being at fivefold risk for developing paroxysmal SVT when compared to those younger than 65 years of age.[1,2] The frequency of the different types of SVT changes over the course of a person's life. AVRT is the most common form of SVT in childhood and adolescence; however, in those middle-aged and older, AVNRT and AT are more common.[1,2]

PATHOGENESIS

To define the pathogenesis of SVT, one must first identify the basic tachycardia mechanism. These can be divided into two principal forms: (1) disorders of reentry and (2) those of impulse formation. A reentrant tachycardia occurs when there is continuous wavefront propagation over an anatomic or functional pathway. For this to occur, three distinct criteria must be met. First, there must be two distinct pathways present forming a closed loop, thus allowing continuous circular movement of the tachycardia wavefront. Second, unidirectional conduction block must be possible in one of the two pathways. Third, an area of this loop must have slow conduction or the loop must be adequately large enough to allow recovery of conduction before the next electrical wavefront returns.

The second major mechanism of SVT occurs when there is an abnormal impulse formation from either enhanced automaticity or triggered activity. Enhanced automaticity can be simplified as a rapidly firing focus that competes with or suppresses the sinus node. Triggered activity occurs when there is spontaneous cell membrane depolarization occurring either during or after repolarization.[3,4]

Atrioventricular Nodal Reentrant Tachycardia

As implied by the name, this rhythm is a reentrant tachycardia that utilizes two functional limbs of the atrioventricular (AV) node, in the setting of a phenomenon known as dual AV node physiology. Dual AV node physiology can be recognized when invasive testing shows that the conduction pattern into the AV node is discontinuous, reflecting separate slowly and rapidly conducting pathways with distinct refractory periods. The typical form of AVNRT is most often initiated when a premature atrial contraction (PAC) blocks in one of these functional pathways (the fast pathway) and instead enters the AV node through the alternate pathway (the slow pathway). By the time the electrical impulse has traveled through the alternate pathway, the first pathway has recovered. This permits retrograde conduction back to the atrium where it can perpetually reenter the circuit. This is the most common form of AVNRT; however, atypical forms exist, where impulse propagation occurs through "fast-slow" or "slow-slow" AV nodal pathways.

Accessory Pathway-Mediated Reentrant Tachycardia

This is a second form of reentry, and is the most common form of SVT in children. Accessory pathways (APs) are extranodal AV muscular connections that are classified by their conduction properties (decremental vs. nondecremental) and by the direction over which the electrical wavefront travels (antegrade, retrograde, or both). APs with antegrade conduction will display a classic delta-wave on the surface electrocardiogram (ECG; **Figure 55.1**). This is the result of early ventricular depolarization at the insertion of the AP. If this finding is present and there are symptoms compatible with SVT, this is termed Wolff-Parkinson-White (WPW) syndrome. Reentry occurs when a PAC blocks in the AP but conducts down the AV node and the His-Purkinje system; by the time the electrical impulse reaches the AP, it has recovered and allows the electrical impulse to travel in a retrograde direction from the ventricle to the atria, thus completing the loop needed for reentrant tachycardia. Reentry can also initiate when a premature ventricular complex (PVC) occurs and blocks in the His-Purkinje system but conducts to the atrium by the AP.

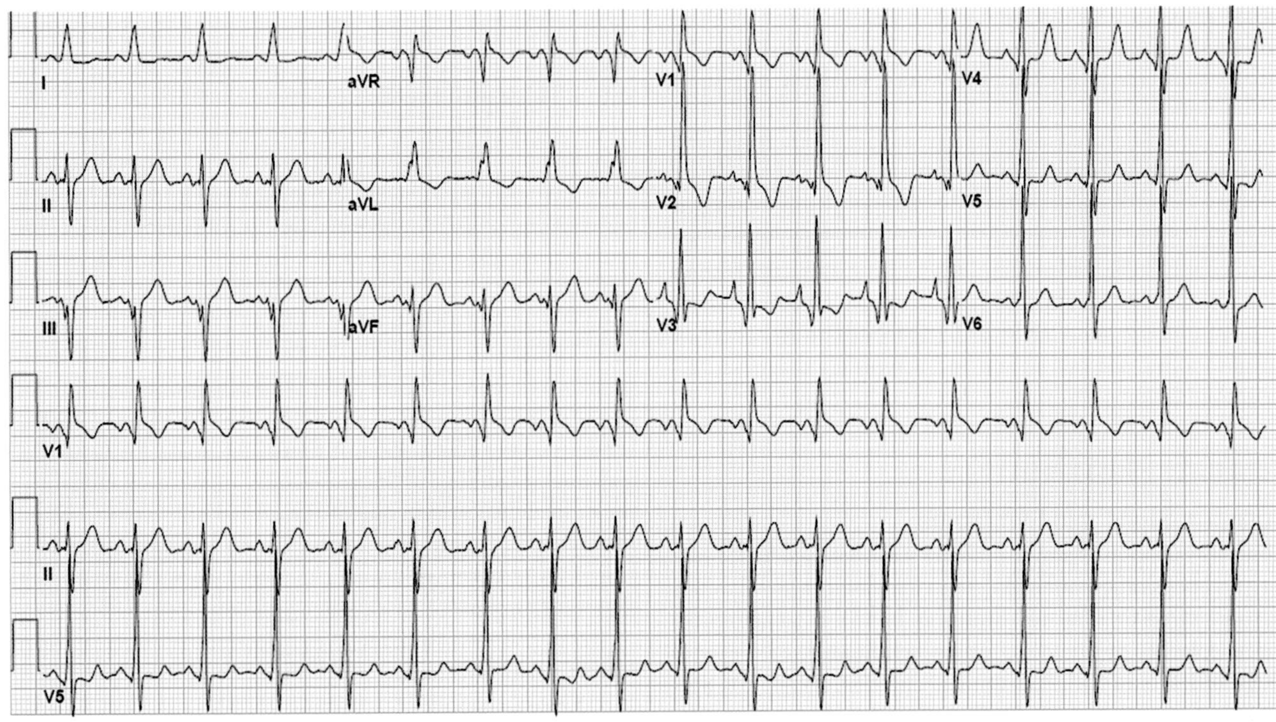

FIGURE 55.1 A 12-lead electrocardiogram of Wolff-Parkinson-White. Note the delta wave at the onset of the QRS.

Concealed APs are those that only allow retrograde conduction (from the ventricle to the atria). The mechanism of SVT is identical to that of WPW; however, there will be no evidence of preexcitation during sinus rhythm. Paroxysmal junctional reciprocating tachycardia is a unique type of concealed AP where the pathway has decremental properties with repetitive or incessant behavior, sometimes associated with tachycardia-induced cardiomyopathy. Mahaim fibers are another rare type of APs. These are AV node–like structures that are located in the right parietal AV annulus with insertions into the distal right bundle branch or surrounding myocardium. They have antegrade decremental conduction, but unlike the AV node, have not been shown to exhibit retrograde conduction.

Atrial Flutter

Atrial flutter is another broad term that is used to describe any tachycardia with a macroreentrant circuit in the atria. The most common of these is cavotricuspid isthmus–dependent flutter, also referred to as counterclockwise atrial flutter or typical atrial flutter. This rhythm is characterized by an electrical wavefront that propagates around the tricuspid annulus (up the atrial septum and down the right atrial free wall) with obligate conduction through the isthmus between the inferior vena cava and tricuspid valve.[5] In cases where the electrical wavefront propagates in the reverse direction, the tachycardia is referred to as reverse typical flutter or clockwise atrial flutter.

Atypical flutters are macroreentrant circuits that do not involve the cavotricuspid isthmus. These reentrant circuits are particularly prevalent in patients with congenital heart disease or patients with prior cardiac surgery, and will often use incisional or scar-related substrates as isthmuses for reentry.

Atrial Ectopic Tachycardia

Atrial ectopic tachycardia (AET) is a form of enhanced automaticity where single or multiple foci in either the right or left atrium fire rapidly. In the largest study to date, 63% of these foci were in the right atrium, predominantly along the crista terminalis.[6] Left-sided foci commonly localize to the pulmonary veins. AETs can be paroxysmal or incessant, the latter potentially resulting in tachycardia-induced cardiomyopathy.[7] Multifocal atrial tachycardia (MAT) is a form of AT where greater than or equal to three distinct P-wave morphologies can be identified; this is an irregular rhythm.

Focal Atrial Tachycardia

Focal ATs historically referred to ATs from enhanced automaticity; however, in more recent decades, the term has been expanded to include ATs of focal origin from automatic, triggered, and microreentrant etiologies. The pathogenesis of focal ATs cannot be distinguished by the surface ECG. Focal ATs account for 5% to 15% of arrhythmias in adult patients undergoing invasive electrophysiology studies.[8]

Junctional Tachycardia

This form of SVT occurs when there is abnormal impulse formation originating from the AV junction including the His node. This form of SVT more commonly occurs in the pediatric population and can occur as congenital or in the postcardiac surgery period. Congenital junctional tachycardia classically presents shortly after birth, and is associated with high morbidity and mortality resulting from an increased incidence of systolic dysfunction.[9]

Inappropriate Sinus Tachycardia

A relatively rare form of tachycardia defined as sinus in origin (normal P-wave axis, normal PR interval), inappropriate sinus tachycardia has an average 24-hour heart rate greater than 90 bpm in adults without identifiable cause. The mechanism of inappropriate sinus tachycardia is related to disorders of the autonomic nervous system and is typically diagnosed after secondary causes of sinus tachycardia have been excluded.

CLINICAL PRESENTATION

Common Signs and Symptoms

Clinical evaluation of any arrhythmia starts with a detailed history and physical examination. The chief complaint will often be palpitations or a "racing" heartbeat, but SVT can also present as episodes of dizziness, feeling lightheaded, or syncope. Questions should focus on timing, duration, frequency, and quality of symptoms because these clues can direct the medical provider toward the specific form of SVT. How symptoms start and stop are critical; SVT will typically have a sudden onset and abrupt termination, contrary to sinus tachycardia that is characterized by a gradual increase at the onset followed by a gradual slowing of the heart rate as it returns to normal. Frequency of symptoms is important and can be a clue to the magnitude of the problem, and can direct the provider on the best diagnostic modality to confirm the diagnosis. Beyond palpitations, there are a number of associated symptoms; these can include chest discomfort, shortness of breath, lightheadedness, or even syncope.

Special attention should be paid to syncope, defined as a transient loss of consciousness due to impaired cerebral blood flow, because this could be a "red flag" of a more serious problem. Syncope during tachycardia may represent a hemodynamic compromise. SVT does not commonly present with syncope; thus, syncope could suggest a different arrhythmia such as ventricular tachycardia (VT) or ventricular fibrillation. Patients with preexcitation on their ECG may present with ventricular fibrillation secondary to rapid conduction of atrial fibrillation over their AP. In this setting, this would be a life-threatening event, and urgent evaluation and treatment is warranted. A second exception involves elderly patients with AVNRT; this population is more vulnerable to syncope with the onset of SVT.[10]

Physical Examination Findings

The physical examination is rarely useful for patients with SVT. The sensation of rapid regular pounding in the neck during tachycardia has been shown to be a positive predictor of AVNRT.[11] Nonspecific findings such as a systolic or diastolic murmur could indicate a congenital cardiac anomaly, some of which are associated with specific forms of SVT.

DIAGNOSIS

Diagnostic evaluation should begin with a resting 12-lead ECG. This is used to evaluate for preexcitation (seen in WPW), classically described as a delta wave preceding the QRS and a resultant short PR interval (Figure 55.1). The resting ECG also serves as a nonspecific screening tool for congenital heart disease, myocardial abnormalities (cardiomyopathies), and conduction abnormalities (first-, second-, or third-degree AV block). Any of these diagnoses can be associated with SVT, but would warrant a different diagnostic and therapeutic approach.

The key to diagnosing SVT is capturing the arrhythmic event on an ECG (**Figure 55.2**). This can be challenging, especially in patients with paroxysmal SVT where episodes are sporadic and brief in duration. A thorough clinical history is thus essential in guiding which ambulatory monitoring modality is most likely to capture one of the arrhythmic events. Historically, Holter monitoring has been used for 24-hour ambulatory ECG recording; however, in recent years, this technology has vastly expanded, with patch monitors now lasting up to 4 weeks and wearable single-lead electrode monitoring being commercially available.

Once an episode of tachycardia has been recorded, the onset and offset of tachycardia should be carefully evaluated because this often provides the most diagnostic clues to the subtype of SVT. For a narrow complex tachycardia (QRS <120 ms), a stepwise approach is recommended (**Algorithm 55.1**). If the documented arrhythmia is a wide complex tachycardia (QRS >120 ms) the differential includes either a VT or an SVT with aberrancy with delayed conduction through any portion of the conduction system. Identifying VA dissociation with V>A, or fusion complexes (the resultant QRS from two sources of ventricular activation) can help readily identify VT. Differentiating between these two rhythms, however, can be challenging at times, and a number of criteria and ECG algorithms have been described, such as the Brugada criteria[12] or Vereckei algorithm.[13] VT can be a life-threatening arrhythmia; therefore, differentiating it from SVT is crucial.

Risk Stratification in Wolff-Parkinson-White Syndrome

Patients with WPW pattern on their ECG warrant a prompt evaluation because of the risk of sudden cardiac death (SCD) with an incidence of 4.5 episodes per 1000 patient-years.[14,15] Even in the so-called asymptomatic patient, one without SVT, the risk of sudden cardiac arrest has been well defined, and in 50% to 65% of these cases, sudden cardiac arrest was the sentinel symptom.[16,17] Stratifying patients with WPW and identifying those at highest risk is vital, but unfortunately remains an imperfect science reliant on ambulatory monitoring and exercise treadmill tests. Intermittent preexcitation, also termed nonpersistent preexcitation, has been used as a marker to indicate low risk of life-threatening events. Recent large studies have shown that although nonpersistent preexcitation is associated with fewer high-risk APs, it does not exclude the risk of SCD.[18] Other markers have thus been developed to stratify

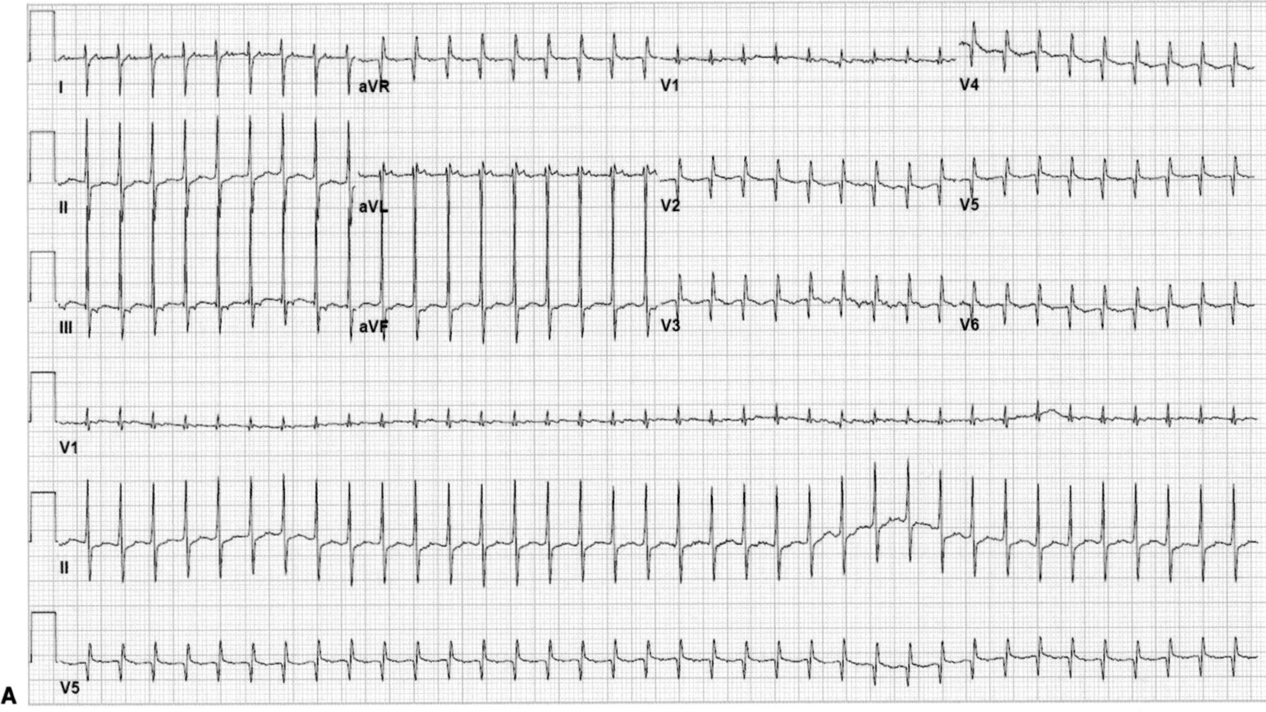

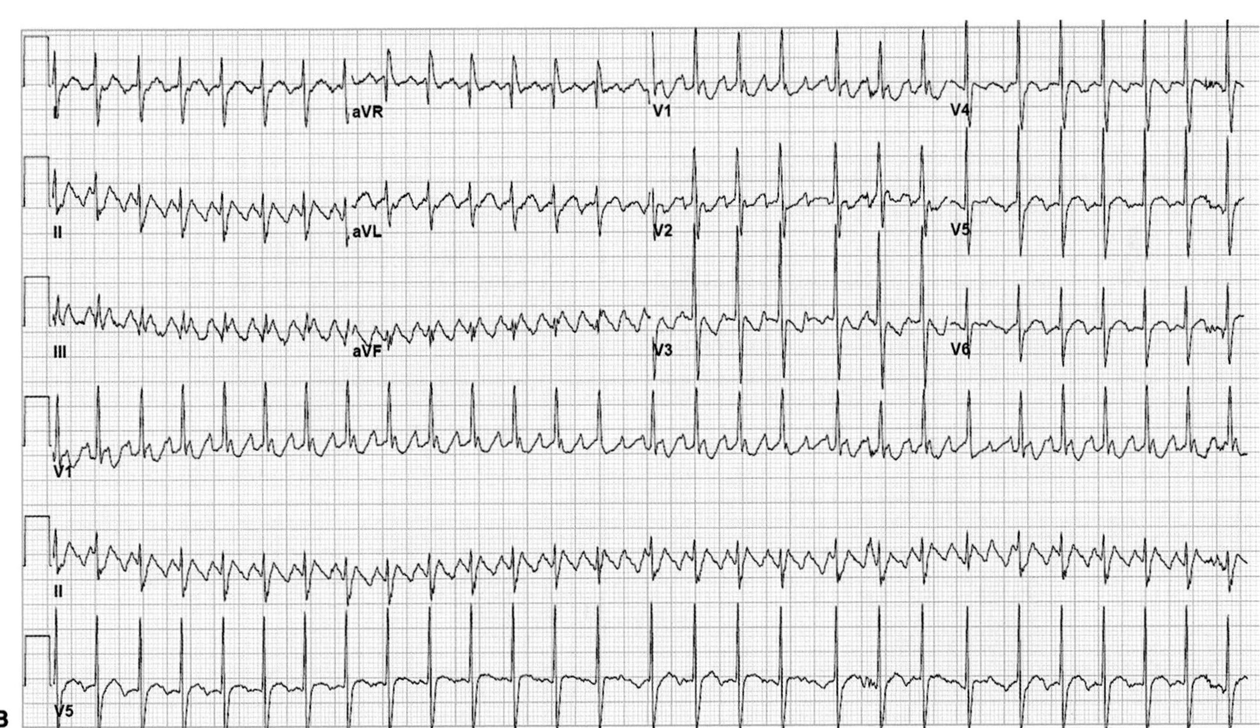

FIGURE 55.2 Twelve-lead electrocardiogram examples of supraventricular tachycardia (SVT). **(A)** Narrow complex tachycardia with visible retrograde P-waves and a 1:1 atrioventricular (AV) relationship. **(B)** Narrow complex tachycardia with atrial flutter waves with a 2:1 AV relationship.

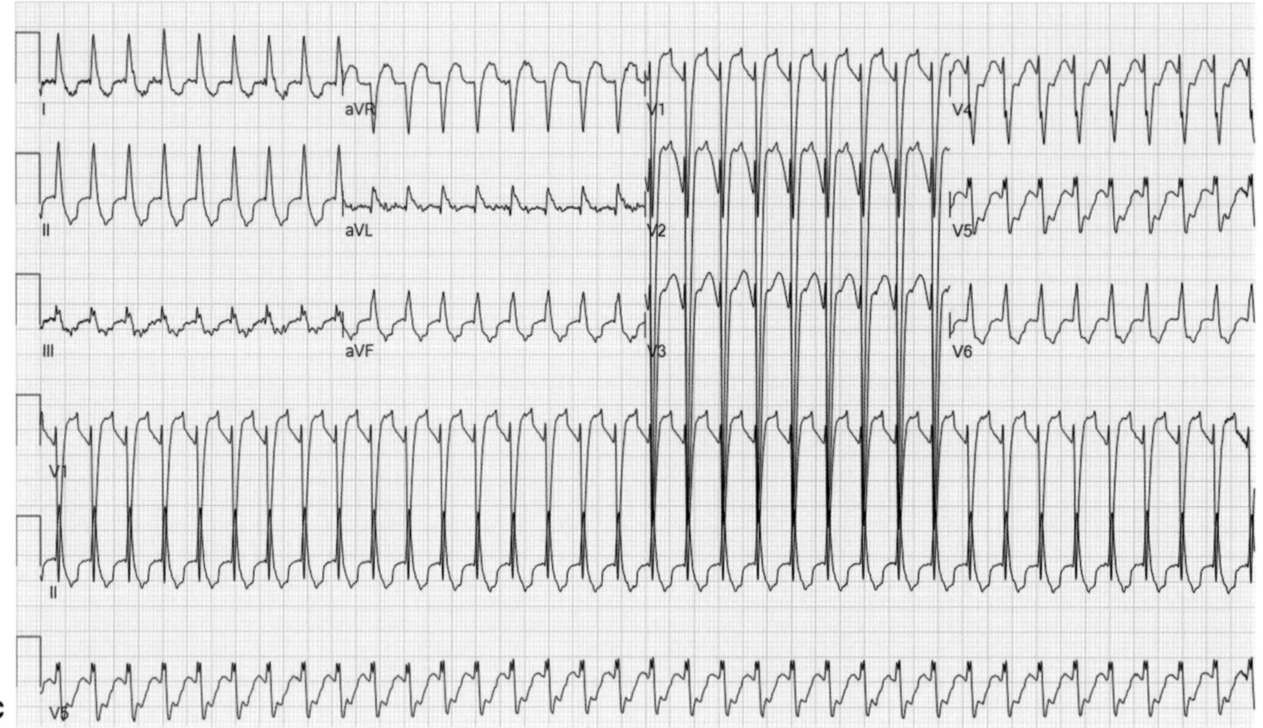

FIGURE 55.2 (*Continued*) **(C)** Wide complex tachycardia demonstrating SVT with aberrant conduction.

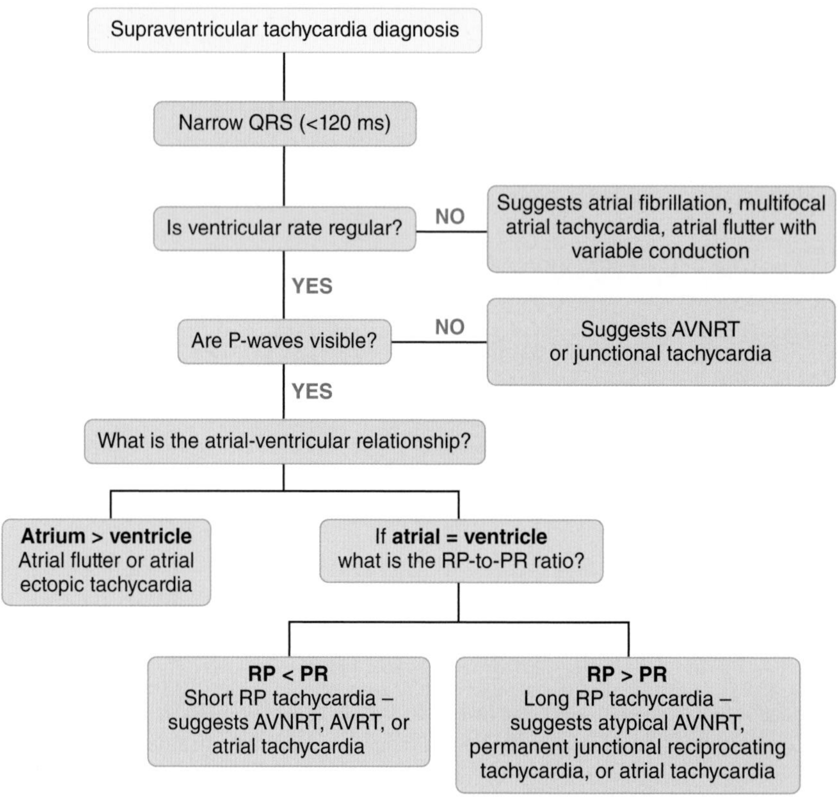

ALGORITHM 55.1 Diagnostic algorithm for supraventricular tachycardia. A, atrial; AVNRT, atrioventricular nodal reentrant tachycardia; AVRT, atrioventricular reentrant tachycardia; MAT, multifocal atrial tachycardia; V, ventricular. (Reprinted with permission from Blomström-Lundqvist C, Scheinman MM, Aliot EM, et al. ACC/AHA/ESC guidelines for the management of patients with supraventricular arrhythmias—executive summary: a report of the American College of Cardiology/American Heart Association Task Force on Practice Guidelines and the European Society of Cardiology Committee for Practice Guidelines (Writing Committee to Develop Guidelines for the Management of Patients With Supraventricular Arrhythmias). *Circulation.* 2003;108(15):1871-1909.)

the risk of SCD among patients with WPW. The shortest preexcited R-R interval (SPERRI) is one of these markers. Historically, a SPERRI less than 250 ms was associated with patients with WPW who had experienced a sudden cardiac arrest event[19,20]; however, these values are derived from invasive electrophysiology studies in patients without general anesthesia. Recent studies have shown that a SPERRI less than 250 ms was only 64% sensitive in identifying pediatric patients with WPW who had experienced a life-threatening event.[16] In the modern era of catheter ablation, a low threshold for ablation of WPW APs has been advocated, especially when the pathway location suggests that collateral damage is not a major concern.

MANAGEMENT

Guidelines for the management of SVT were set forth per the 2015 American College of Cardiology/American Heart Association/Heart Rhythm Society (ACC/AHA/HRS) task force.[21] Management can be grossly divided into management of an acute episode of SVT versus ongoing management.

Acute Management

For the patient who presents with SVT, diagnostic evaluation as described earlier should be commenced, paying attention to distinguish SVT from aberrancy versus VT, because management of these will be significantly different. Once the diagnosis of SVT is confirmed, the mainstay of initial treatment involves slowing or temporarily blocking AV conduction. This will work to terminate any reentrant tachycardia in which the AV node participates in the circuit, such as AVRT or AVNRT. Vagal maneuvers are first line, and can be quickly performed or taught to patients; for adults, these maneuvers include Valsalva and carotid massage,[22] whereas in pediatrics, particularly in infants, an ice bag applied to the face or rectal stimulation may work better.[23] If vagal maneuvers do not work, adenosine is recommended for the patient with regular SVT. Even if adenosine does not work to terminate tachycardia, it can be a useful diagnostic tool to unmask P waves in AT or atrial flutter. For this reason, it is important to have continuous ECG recording while adenosine is administered. Other acute therapies include intravenous metoprolol or verapamil.

Synchronized cardioversion holds a Class I recommendation for patients who present with either hemodynamically unstable SVT in whom vagal maneuvers or adenosine are ineffective or not feasible, and for patients with hemodynamically stable SVT that is refractory to pharmacologic therapy or in whom such treatment is contraindicated.[21] As defined by the advanced cardiovascular life support (ACLS) guidelines, hemodynamic instability for persistent SVT is defined by hypotension, acutely altered mental status, signs of shock, ischemic chest discomfort, or acute heart failure symptoms.[24]

Ongoing Management

Long-term treatment options for SVT include observation, drug therapy, and catheter ablation. The option to consider is dependent on the frequency and duration of SVT and a shared decision between the patient and electrophysiologist. Medical management can be the optimal choice for patients who are deemed too high risk for an ablation because of comorbidities, or those who do not wish to undergo a procedure (**Table 55.1**).

Catheter Ablation

The goal of the invasive electrophysiology study is to establish the mechanism of SVT and elimination of the tachycardia substrate when performed with a catheter ablation. Standards for equipment and training of operators were set forth by the HRS 2014 consensus.[25] The general principle of an electrophysiology study involves placement of one or more catheters in the high right atrium, His bundle, ventricle, and coronary sinus. From these locations, electrograms are recorded and programmed stimulation is performed. Catheter positions may have to be modified in patients with congenital heart disease, particularly in univentricular patients palliated with a Fontan operation. Complications from an electrophysiology study are rare, but can be life threatening.[26] These procedures can be done with conscious sedation or general anesthesia; however, special care should be taken with the choice of anesthetic because many of these agents can have an electrophysiologic effect in suppressing arrhythmias.[27,28]

Once catheters are in place, baseline intervals from the surface ECG (PR, QRS, QT, RR intervals) and intracardiac measurements of the atrial-His (AH) and His-ventricular (HV) intervals are documented. There are two basic pacing maneuvers that are performed in both the atria and ventricle: incremental pacing and timed extrastimuli. With incremental pacing at specific cycle lengths, the electrophysiologist

TABLE 55.1 Drug Therapy for Supraventricular Tachycardia

Classification	Drug	Adverse Effect
Beta-blockade	Atenolol Metoprolol Nadolol Propranolol	Hypotension, bronchospasm, bradycardia
Calcium channel antagonist	Diltiazem Verapamil	Hypotension, bradycardia, hepatic injury
Cardiac glycoside	Digoxin	Bradycardia, heart block, nausea, vomiting
Sodium channel antagonist	Flecainide Propafenone	QT prolongation, torsades de pointes
Class III	Sotalol Dofetilide Amiodarone	QT prolongation, torsades de pointes QT prolongation, torsades de pointes, hypo/hyperthyroidism, pulmonary fibrosis, hepatic toxicity, optic neuritis, peripheral neuropathy, photosensitivity

can determine the AV and ventriculoatrial (VA) block cycle lengths. Programmed electrical stimulation can also consist of a drive train followed by a premature extra stimulus that is delivered progressively earlier until the stimulus fails to capture the myocardium or functionally blocks in the electrical connection being studied. This maneuver determines the effective refractory period (ERP) of the tested site (atria, antegrade, and retrograde AV node, AP, ventricle). During the diagnostic testing, the electrophysiologist pays close attention to the pattern of atrial activation during ventricular pacing, and presence of dual AV node physiology.

In patients in whom VA conduction occurs through the AV node, the pattern of atrial activation is concentric (earliest in the His catheter) and decremental. If the pattern of activation is eccentric, this is suggestive of an AP. Dual AV node physiology is defined by a marked increase in the AH interval of 50 ms in response to a 10 ms decrease in the atrial premature stimuli that follows the drive train.[29] When this phenomenon occurs, the AV has properties of both fast and slow pathways and has the substrate necessary for AVNRT. Sustained slow pathway conduction occurs when there is 1:1 AV conduction where the PR interval exceeds the R-R interval during atrial pacing. This reflects the AV node's ability to sustain antegrade conduction over the slow pathway necessary for typical AVNRT.[30]

Once SVT is induced, the electrophysiologist works to determine the mechanism of tachycardia before performing an ablation. A few important observations from the intracardiac electrograms while SVT is ongoing include the following:

- If A is greater than V, this excludes AVRT.
- The pattern of atrial activation (eccentric suggests presence of AP).
- If septal VA time is less than 70 ms, this makes AVRT less likely.
- A bundle branch block that prolongs VA time is diagnostic of AVRT.

Specific pacing maneuvers can also be used to prove the mechanism of SVT. Pacing in the ventricle at a cycle length 10 to 40 ms shorter than the tachycardia cycle length is referred to as ventricular overdrive pacing; this maneuver distinguishes AVRT and AET from AVNRT (**Figure 55.3**).

PVCs are also routinely used during the electrophysiology study, and are timed to occur when the His is in its refractory period; these are called His-refractory PVCs. How these beats affect the conduction to the atrium can be telling of the SVT mechanism. A His-refractory PVC that terminates tachycardia without conduction to the atria is diagnostic of AVRT (Figure 55.3). One that advances the atrial signal excludes AVNRT, but does not separate AVRT from a focal AT.

Entrainment is yet another diagnostic maneuver that can be used during an electrophysiology study to help define the anatomic substrates involved in SVT. The maneuver involves pacing at a cycle length faster than the tachycardia cycle length without interrupting the arrhythmia.[31] The response to pacing allows the electrophysiologist to determine whether the area in question is involved in the tachycardia circuit. This technique is commonly employed in atypical flutters that do not use the cavotricuspid isthmus.

Electroanatomic Mapping

The introduction of electroanatomic mapping revolutionized the field of invasive electrophysiology over the past two decades. Electroanatomic mapping is a computer-based technology that creates a three-dimensional visual of the anatomy and electrical information (**Figure 55.4A**). It allows the user to map the propagation of electrical signals to determine the optimal site for radiofrequency ablation while minimizing the use of fluoroscopy. Modern iterations of this technology now involve catheters that enable rapid and simultaneous acquisition of points for more accurate delineation of complex arrhythmias.[32] This is particularly useful in patients with congenital heart disease who have a high burden of scar-related arrhythmias,[33] often postsurgical, and inconsistent anatomic landmarks because of their underlying congenital disease (**Figure 55.4B**).

Ablation Outcomes

Ablation outcomes have continued to improve in recent decades with the increased availability of electroanatomic mapping, multipolar catheters, and contact force catheters. Single-procedure ablation success across all SVT subtypes is reported to be 90% to 98%, with a 3% to 6% recurrence rate.[34,35] Efficacy and safety in pediatric patients is excellent, with success rates comparable to that of adults.[36,37] Complication rates are higher in those weighing less than 15 kg.[37,38]

FOLLOW-UP PATIENT CARE

Follow-up care for patients receiving treatment for SVT is driven by their mechanism of SVT, burden of arrhythmia, and the chosen treatment approach. Patients who chose medications will be followed up in ambulatory clinics to assess the efficacy of the medication and screen for medication side effects. Patients choosing to undergo catheter ablation will be routinely seen in the ambulatory setting within 1 to 2 weeks of their procedure to check the venipuncture sites. They will then have periodic assessments in the first 12 months following ablation to assess for recurrence. Adult patients with congenital heart disease are often followed up for longer periods given their increased burden of arrhythmia.[39]

RESEARCH AND FUTURE DIRECTIONS

- Medications: Clinical trials on choice of antiarrhythmic remain limited; further randomized data is needed.
- Sudden cardiac arrest: Noninvasive risk stratification of patients with WPW pattern on the surface ECG remains imperfect, and better predictive models are needed. Empiric ablation of WPW in asymptomatic children is being explored.
- Technology: Optimal parameters for contact force catheters are needed for different populations (pediatric and congenital patients). Linear ablation catheters are being developed to optimize success and efficiency during atrial flutter ablations.

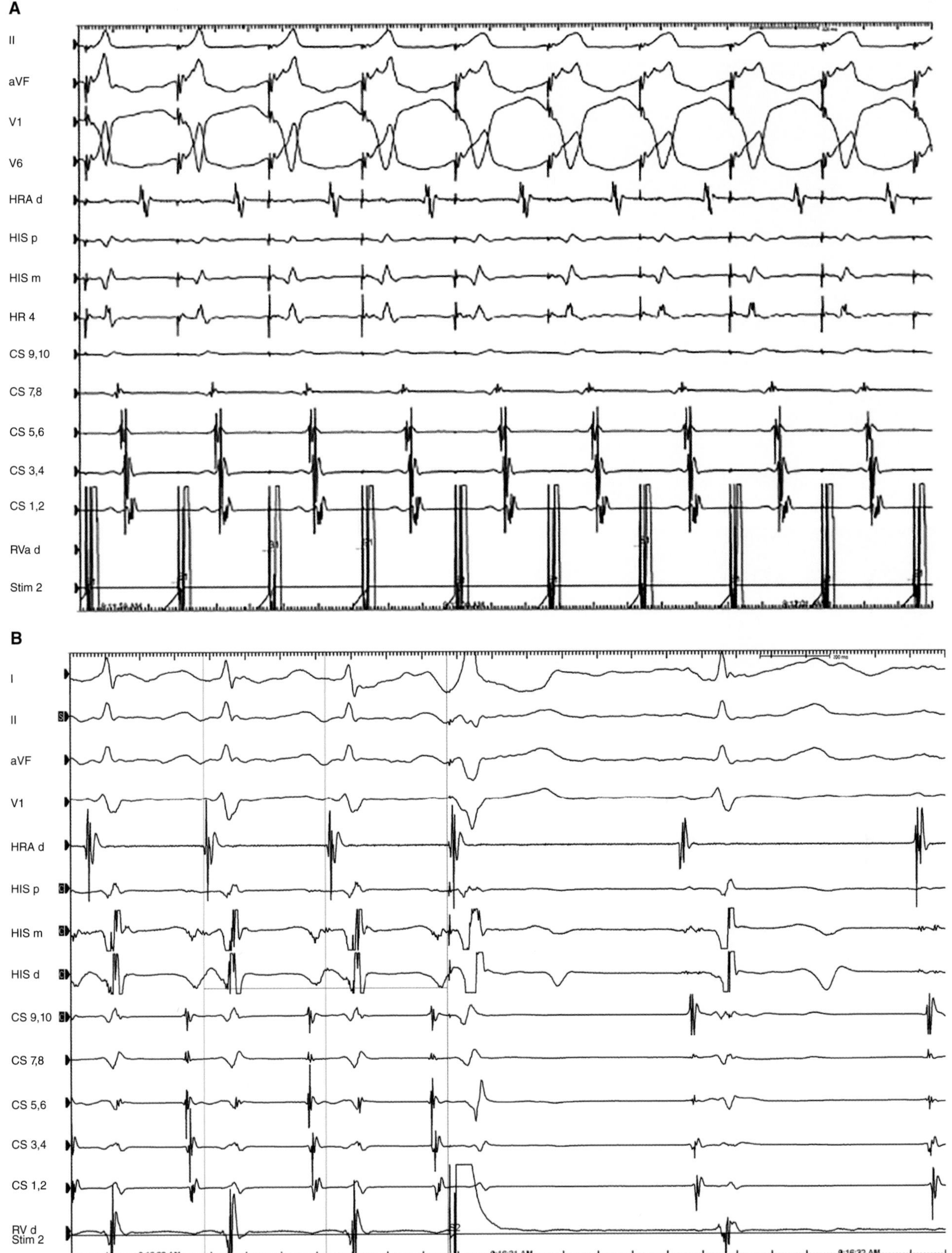

FIGURE 55.3 Pacing maneuvers during an electrophysiology study. Diagnostic catheters show atrial and/or ventricular signals at distinct sites—high right atrium (HRA), His, coronary sinus (CS), right ventricle (RV). **(A)** Ventricular overdrive pacing (VOP)—diagnostic maneuver in which the ventricle is paced during SVT. This maneuver is used to differentiate between different forms of SVT. **(B)** His-refractory premature ventricular contraction that terminates supraventricular tachycardia (SVT) without conduction to the atrium is diagnostic of pathway-mediated reentrant tachycardia. Note the absence of an atrial signal on the HRA catheter following the ventricular paced beat.

SECTION 4

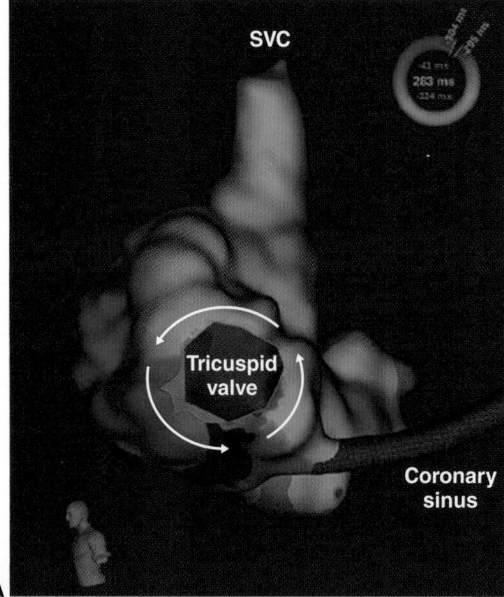

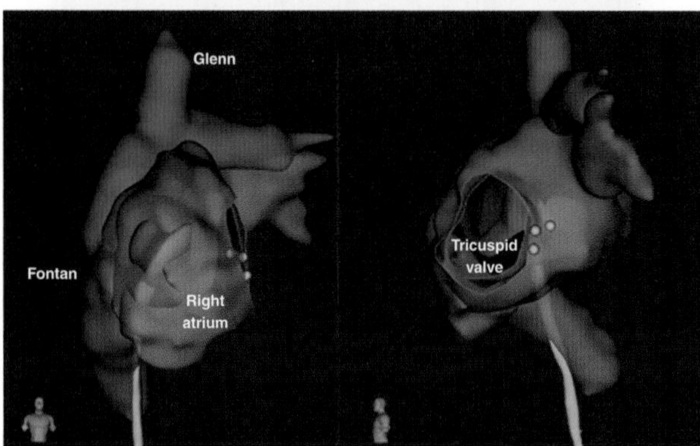

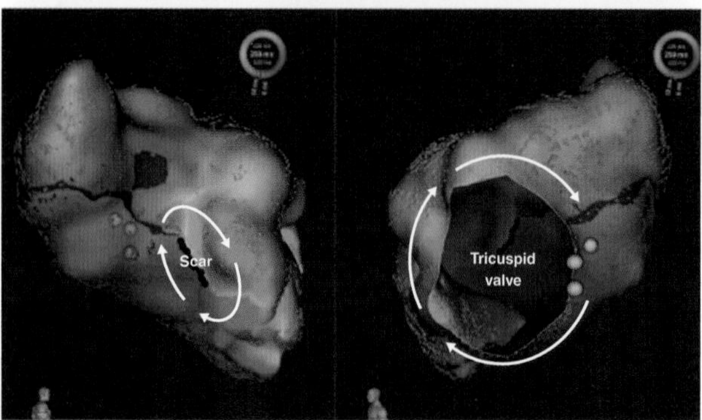

FIGURE 55.4 Electroanatomic mapping (Rhythmia HDx™, Boston Scientific, Marlborough, MA). **(A)** Example of cavotricuspid atrial flutter. Colors on the map represent different timing intervals of the circuit, with the composite image showing a wave front traveling counterclockwise around the tricuspid valve annulus. **(B)** Example of a patient with complex single-ventricle anatomy. The upper inset shows a three-dimensional (3D) rendition of the anatomy created at the time of the electrophysiology study. The lower inset shows a complex "dual loop," where the patient has two competing atrial flutter circuits.

KEY POINTS

- ✔ SVT is a broad all-encompassing term that describes tachycardias with atrial rates greater than 100 bpm originating from the His bundle or above.
- ✔ Diagnosing what form of SVT a patient has will allow for shared decision-making with the patient on what therapeutic modality to choose.
- ✔ Percutaneous ablations offer a high success rate for elimination of the arrhythmia substrate.
- ✔ Patients with congenital heart disease have higher burdens of SVT and anatomic barriers to traditional ablation approaches.

REFERENCES

1. Orejarena LA, Vidaillet H Jr, DeStefano F, et al. Paroxysmal supraventricular tachycardia in the general population. *J Am Coll Cardiol.* 1998; 31(1):150-157.
2. Porter MJ, Morton JB, Denman R, et al. Influence of age and gender on the mechanism of supraventricular tachycardia. *Heart Rhythm.* 2004; 1(4):393-396.
3. Zimetbaum PJ, Josephson ME. *Practical Clinical Electrophysiology.* Wolters Kluwer Health/Lippincott Williams & Wilkins; 2009:xiv, 304pp.
4. Gillette PC, Garson A Jr. Electrophysiologic and pharmacologic characteristics of automatic ectopic atrial tachycardia. *Circulation.* 1977;56(4 Pt 1): 571-575.
5. Shah DC, Jais P, Haissaguerre M, et al. Three-dimensional mapping of the common atrial flutter circuit in the right atrium. *Circulation.* 1997; 96(11):3904-3912.
6. Kistler PM, Roberts-Thomson KC, Haqqani HM, et al. P-wave morphology in focal atrial tachycardia: development of an algorithm to predict the anatomic site of origin. *J Am Coll Cardiol.* 2006;48(5):1010-1017.
7. Salerno JC, Kertesz NJ, Friedman RA, Fenrich AL, Jr. Clinical course of atrial ectopic tachycardia is age-dependent: results and treatment in children <3 or ≥3 years of age. *J Am Coll Cardiol.* 2004;43(3):438-444.
8. Chen SA, Chiang CE, Yang CJ, et al. Sustained atrial tachycardia in adult patients. Electrophysiological characteristics, pharmacological response, possible mechanisms, and effects of radiofrequency ablation. *Circulation.* 1994;90(3):1262-1278.
9. Alasti M, Mirzaee S, Machado C, et al. Junctional ectopic tachycardia (JET). *J Arrhythm.* 2020;36(5):837-844.
10. Haghjoo M, Arya A, Heidari A, Fazelifar AF, Sadr-Ameli MA. Electrophysiologic characteristics and results of radiofrequency catheter ablation in elderly patients with atrioventricular nodal reentrant tachycardia. *J Electrocardiol.* 2007;40(2):208-213.
11. Gonzalez-Torrecilla E, Almendral J, Arenal A, et al. Combined evaluation of bedside clinical variables and the electrocardiogram for the differential diagnosis of paroxysmal atrioventricular reciprocating tachycardias in patients without pre-excitation. *J Am Coll Cardiol.* 2009;53(25):2353-2358.
12. Brugada P, Brugada J, Mont L, Smeets J, Andries EW. A new approach to the differential diagnosis of a regular tachycardia with a wide QRS complex. *Circulation.* 1991;83(5):1649-1659.
13. Vereckei A, Duray G, Szenasi G, Altemose GT, Miller JM. New algorithm using only lead aVR for differential diagnosis of wide QRS complex tachycardia. *Heart Rhythm.* 2008;5(1):89-98.
14. Pappone C, Santinelli V, Manguso F, et al. A randomized study of prophylactic catheter ablation in asymptomatic patients with the Wolff-Parkinson-White syndrome. *N Engl J Med.* 2003;349(19):1803-1811.

15. Munger TM, Packer DL, Hammill SC, et al. A population study of the natural history of Wolff-Parkinson-White syndrome in Olmsted County, Minnesota, 1953-1989. *Circulation.* 1993;87(3):866-873.
16. Etheridge SP, Escudero CA, Blaufox AD, et al. Life-threatening event risk in children with Wolff-Parkinson-White syndrome: a multicenter international study. *JACC Clin Electrophysiol.* 2018;4(4):433-444.
17. Montoya PT, Brugada P, Smeets J, et al. Ventricular fibrillation in the Wolff-Parkinson-White syndrome. *Eur Heart J.* 1991;12(2):144-150.
18. Escudero CA, Ceresnak SR, Collins KK, et al. Loss of ventricular preexcitation during noninvasive testing does not exclude high-risk accessory pathways: a multicenter study of WPW in children. *Heart Rhythm.* 2020;17(10):1729-1737.
19. Bromberg BI, Lindsay BD, Cain ME, Cox JL. Impact of clinical history and electrophysiologic characterization of accessory pathways on management strategies to reduce sudden death among children with Wolff-Parkinson-White syndrome. *J Am Coll Cardiol.* 1996;27(3):690-695.
20. Santinelli V, Radinovic A, Manguso F, et al. The natural history of asymptomatic ventricular pre-excitation a long-term prospective follow-up study of 184 asymptomatic children. *J Am Coll Cardiol.* 2009;53(3):275-280.
21. Page RL, Joglar JA, Caldwell MA, et al. 2015 ACC/AHA/HRS Guideline for the management of adult patients with supraventricular tachycardia: executive summary: a report of the American College of Cardiology/American Heart Association Task Force on Clinical Practice Guidelines and the Heart Rhythm Society. *Circulation.* 2016;133(14):e471-e505.
22. Waxman MB, Wald RW, Sharma AD, Huerta F, Cameron DA. Vagal techniques for termination of paroxysmal supraventricular tachycardia. *Am J Cardiol.* 1980;46(4):655-664.
23. Wayne MA. Conversion of paroxysmal atrial tachycardia by facial immersion in ice water. *JACEP.* 1976;5(6):434-435.
24. Neumar RW, Otto CW, Link MS, et al. Part 8: adult advanced cardiovascular life support: 2010 American Heart Association Guidelines for Cardiopulmonary Resuscitation and Emergency Cardiovascular Care. *Circulation.* 2010;122(18 suppl 3):S729-S767.
25. Haines DE, Beheiry S, Akar JG, et al. Heart Rythm Society expert consensus statement on electrophysiology laboratory standards: process, protocols, equipment, personnel, and safety. *Heart Rhythm.* 2014;11(8):e9-e51.
26. Horowitz LN, Kay HR, Kutalek SP, et al. Risks and complications of clinical cardiac electrophysiologic studies: a prospective analysis of 1,000 consecutive patients. *J Am Coll Cardiol.* 1987;9(6):1261-1268.
27. Wutzler A, Huemer M, Boldt LH, et al. Effects of deep sedation on cardiac electrophysiology in patients undergoing radiofrequency ablation of supraventricular tachycardia: impact of propofol and ketamine. *Europace.* 2013;15(7):1019-1024.
28. Guerra F, Stronati G, Capucci A. Sedation in cardiac arrhythmias management. *Expert Rev Cardiovasc Ther.* 2018;16(3):163-173.
29. Denes P, Wu D, Dhingra RC, Chuquimia R, Rosen KM. Demonstration of dual A-V nodal pathways in patients with paroxysmal supraventricular tachycardia. *Circulation.* 1973;48(3):549-555.
30. Kannankeril PJ, Fish FA. Sustained slow pathway conduction: superior to dual atrioventricular node physiology in young patients with atrioventricular nodal reentry tachycardia? *Pacing Clin Electrophysiol.* 2006;29(2):159-163.
31. Waldo AL. Atrial flutter: entrainment characteristics. *J Cardiovasc Electrophysiol.* 1997;8(3):337-352.
32. Nakagawa H, Ikeda A, Sharma T, Lazzara R, Jackman WM. Rapid high resolution electroanatomical mapping: evaluation of a new system in a canine atrial linear lesion model. *Circ Arrhythm Electrophysiol.* 2012;5(2):417-424.
33. Moore JP, Buch E, Gallotti RG, Shannon KM. Ultrahigh-density mapping supplemented with global chamber activation identifies noncavotricuspid-dependent intra-atrial re-entry conduction isthmuses in adult congenital heart disease. *J Cardiovasc Electrophysiol.* 2019;30(12):2797-2805.
34. Spector P, Reynolds MR, Calkins H, et al. Meta-analysis of ablation of atrial flutter and supraventricular tachycardia. *Am J Cardiol.* 2009;104(5):671-677.
35. Okishige K, Okumura K, Tsurugi T, et al. Japan ablation registry: cryoablation in atrioventricular nodal reentrant tachycardia ("JARCANRET study"): results from large multicenter retrospective investigation. *J Interv Card Electrophysiol.* 2020;58(3):289-297.
36. Krause U, Paul T, Bella PD, et al. Pediatric catheter ablation at the beginning of the 21st century: results from the European Multicenter Pediatric Catheter Ablation Registry 'EUROPA'. *Europace.* 2021;23(3):431-440.
37. Kugler JD, Danford DA, Houston K, Felix G. Radiofrequency catheter ablation for paroxysmal supraventricular tachycardia in children and adolescents without structural heart disease. Pediatric EP Society, Radiofrequency Catheter Ablation Registry. *Am J Cardiol.* 1997;80(11):1438-1443.
38. Lee PC, Hwang B, Chen SA, et al. The results of radiofrequency catheter ablation of supraventricular tachycardia in children. *Pacing Clin Electrophysiol.* 2007;30(5):655-661.
39. Bouchardy J, Therrien J, Pilote L, et al. Atrial arrhythmias in adults with congenital heart disease. *Circulation.* 2009;120(17):1679-1686.

CHAPTER 56

ATRIAL FIBRILLATION AND ATRIAL FLUTTER

Aron Bender, Joseph Hadaya, Peyman Benharash, Eric Buch, and Richard J. Shemin

INTRODUCTION

Epidemiology

Atrial fibrillation is the most common arrhythmia encountered clinically, and is a major driver of health care utilization. Data from the 2010 Global Burden of Disease Study estimate the prevalence of atrial fibrillation at approximately 33 million affected individuals worldwide, with higher prevalence in males.[1] The incidence of atrial fibrillation continues to increase, with approximately 70 new cases per 100,000 person-years as of 2010.[1] A recent database analysis reported a 10% to 20% cumulative risk of developing atrial fibrillation by the age of 80 years.[2] Although assessing the cost burden associated with atrial fibrillation presents a challenge given the presence of comorbid conditions, there are at least 450,000 admissions for atrial fibrillation per year, and the annual incremental cost in the United States from atrial fibrillation alone is at least $6 billion.[3]

Atrial flutter often coexists with atrial fibrillation. As a result, atrial flutter is seen in more than one-third of patients with atrial fibrillation, and the majority of patients presenting with atrial flutter will also have atrial fibrillation.

Risk Factors

The risk factors for both atrial fibrillation and atrial flutter include age, male sex, genetic predisposition, hypertension, heart failure, valvular or ischemic heart disease, obesity, thyroid dysfunction, obstructive sleep apnea, lung disease, and excessive alcohol consumption. For atypical atrial flutter, prior atrial surgery or ablation is nearly a prerequisite.

PATHOGENESIS

Atrial fibrillation is a consequence of a variety of pathologic conditions that result in structural and electrophysiologic remodeling in the atria. The proposed mechanisms for the initiation and maintenance of atrial fibrillation are based on the concepts of triggers and substrate. Focal atrial tachycardia (most commonly originating in the pulmonary veins, less commonly in the right atrium, superior vena cava, left atrial appendage, or coronary sinus) can initiate fibrillation in the susceptible atria.[4] As the duration and burden of atrial fibrillation increases, changes occur in the electrophysiologic characteristics of atrial myocytes, including shortening of the atrial effective refractory period and slowing of conduction velocity, which promote reentry and lead to longer episodes of atrial fibrillation.[5] As the burden and duration of atrial fibrillation increases, there is also an increase in triggers beyond the pulmonary veins.[6] The autonomic nervous system and a dense network of atrial innervation are also implicated in the initiation and maintenance of atrial fibrillation; procedural modification of ganglionic plexuses is one mechanistic explanation for the efficacy of ablation.[7]

As opposed to the disorganized electrical activity seen in atrial fibrillation, atrial flutter is an organized macroreentrant rhythm. The most common form of atrial flutter, cavotricuspid isthmus (CTI)–dependent atrial flutter, involves a circuit around the right atrium including a narrow corridor between the tricuspid valve and the inferior vena cava that is usually targeted in catheter ablation. Atypical atrial flutters can occur in either atrium, often as a result of prior surgery or ablation, where electrically inert atrial scar tissue forms an obstacle around which the flutter circuit can propagate (**Figure 56.1 A-C**).

CLINICAL PRESENTATION

Common Signs and Symptoms

Symptoms of atrial fibrillation and atrial flutter are variable across patients and even between episodes in the same patient. Common symptoms include palpitations, fatigue, dizziness, dyspnea, chest pressure, and exercise intolerance. Some patients are asymptomatic and diagnosed incidentally. The ventricular rate, duration, and stage of atrial fibrillation, as well as the presence of concurrent conditions, all play a role in the development of symptoms. The hemodynamic consequences of an irregular heart rhythm and loss of atrial contraction can be amplified in patients with underlying structural heart disease.[8,9] As a result, the development of atrial fibrillation or flutter can lead to decompensated heart failure or angina. Chronically uncontrolled (ie, rapid) ventricular rates and irregularity can lead to cardiomyopathy and heart failure, even in patients without prior evidence of ventricular dysfunction. Syncope occurring in patients with atrial fibrillation or atrial flutter is uncommon, and is most often a result of sinus node dysfunction and resulting post-conversion pauses following termination of episodes.

Thromboembolism is a serious complication of atrial fibrillation and flutter, and may account for up to 15% of ischemic strokes in the United States. Stroke may be the first presentation of atrial fibrillation or flutter in a previously asymptomatic patient.[10]

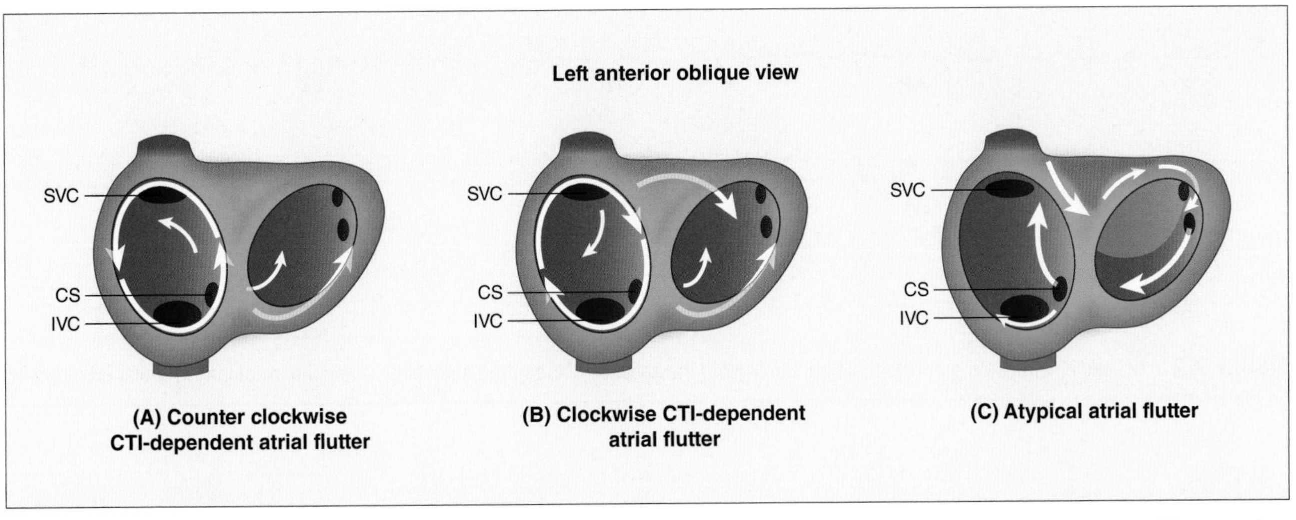

FIGURE 56.1 **(A,B,C)** Representative images of counterclockwise cavotricuspid isthmus (CTI)–dependent atrial flutter, clockwise CTI–dependent atrial flutter, and atypical atrial flutter, in this case utilizing the mitral annulus. CS, coronary sinus; CTI, cavotricuspid isthmus; IVC, inferior vena cava; SVC, superior vena cava.

Physical Examination Findings

The physical examination in atrial fibrillation is characterized by irregularity or variability in the pulse rate and intensity, loss of the atrial wave in the jugular venous waveform, and variability in the intensity of S1. In very rapidly conducted atrial fibrillation, the auscultated heart rate will be greater than is the heart rate measured by radial artery palpation, resulting in a "pulse deficit."

DIAGNOSIS

The diagnosis of atrial fibrillation or flutter is confirmed electrocardiographically. Although the 12-lead electrocardiogram (ECG) is the gold standard for diagnosis of both atrial fibrillation and atrial flutter, these rhythms are often diagnosed on outpatient rhythm monitors ordered to evaluate for suggestive signs and symptoms or as part of the workup after a thromboembolic event. Atrial arrhythmias are also diagnosed via interrogation of pacemakers and defibrillators.

Atrial fibrillation is characterized on 12-lead ECG by rapid, irregular atrial activity without clear P waves and irregularity in the timing of QRS complexes (**Figure 56.2**).

The classification of atrial fibrillation is based on duration of episodes and is an important consideration in the planned treatment approach:

- *Paroxysmal atrial fibrillation:* Episodes last less than 7 days, either terminating spontaneously or with intervention.
- *Persistent atrial fibrillation:* Episodes last 7 days or longer.
- *Longstanding persistent atrial fibrillation:* Continuous atrial fibrillation lasting at least 1 year in duration.
- *Permanent atrial fibrillation:* This designation marks persistent atrial fibrillation with acknowledgment by both physician and patient that rhythm control will not be pursued.

The identification of CTI-dependent atrial flutter has important implications for developing a treatment plan. "Typical" counterclockwise atrial flutter is characterized by constant, repetitive, undulating atrial activity at 240 to 340 beats per minute (**Figure 56.3**). These flutter waves are negative in the inferior leads (II, III, aVF) with a gradual downsloping segment, followed by a sharper negative deflection, and then a sharp positive deflection returning above the baseline before the next cycle. Flutter waves tend to be positive in V1, with transition to negative across the precordium by V6. The ventricular rate is most commonly half the atrial rate because of the 2:1 conduction through the atrioventricular (AV) node, although depending on medications and balance in adrenergic input to the AV node, conduction can be a lower integer (3:1 or 4:1 conduction) or at times variable. Clockwise CTI–dependent atrial flutter has a variable ECG appearance, although it can be thought of as the opposite of the counterclockwise version with positive, notched flutter waves in the inferior leads and negative, notched deflections in V1 transitioning to positive deflections by V6.

Atypical atrial flutter is identified by rapid, organized atrial activity that does not fit the patterns consistent with CTI-dependent mechanisms and should be suspected in patients with prior atrial surgery or ablation (**Figure 56.4**).

MANAGEMENT OF ATRIAL FIBRILLATION

Medical Approach

The goals of treatment in atrial fibrillation and atrial flutter are to reduce the risk of thromboembolism, alleviate symptoms, and prevent the deleterious effects of rapid ventricular rates. The mainstays of therapy are therefore anticoagulation as directed by risk of thromboembolic events, risk factor modification, rate control strategies, and rhythm control strategies, both medical and procedural. The results of the 2002 AFFIRM trial, where a rhythm control approach did not demonstrate

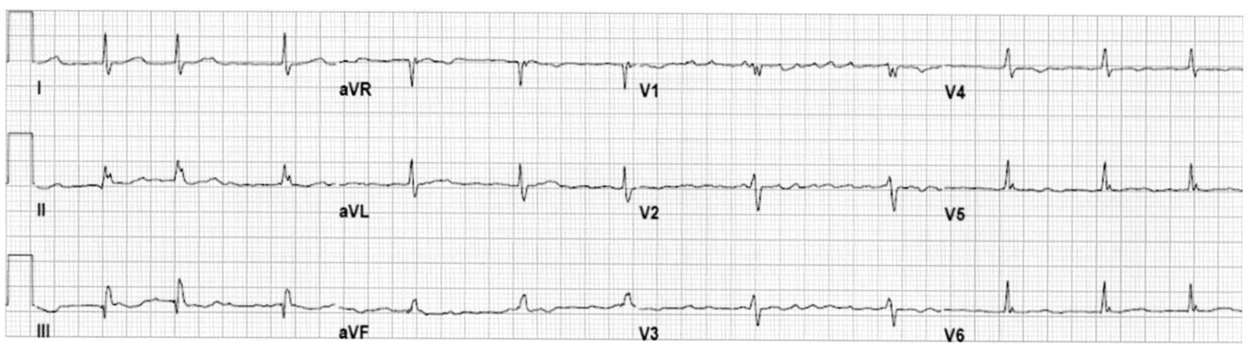

FIGURE 56.2 12 Lead electrocardiogram of atrial fibrillation. Note the absence of organized atrial activity and the irregularly irregular RR intervals.

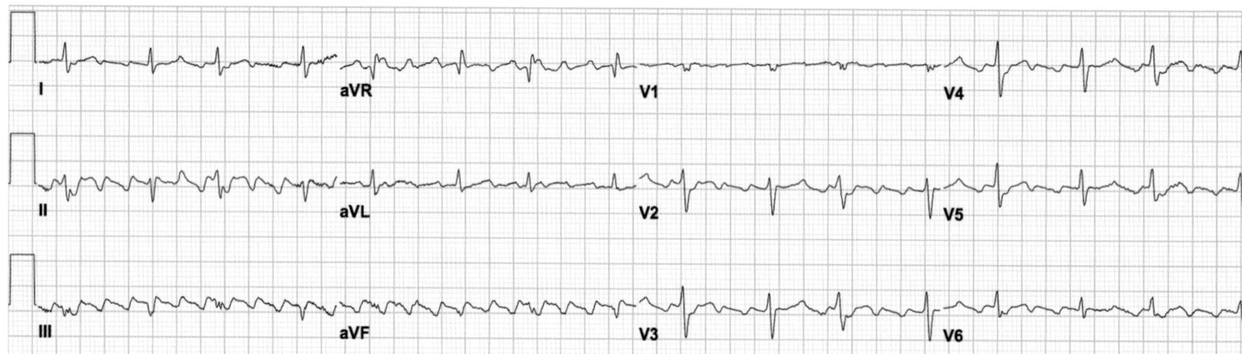

FIGURE 56.3 12 Lead electrocardiogram of "typical" counterclockwise cavotricuspid isthmus–dependent atrial flutter with variable ventricular conduction (3:1 and 4:1). Note negative flutter waves in the inferior leads and positive flutter waves in V1 transitioning to negative by V6.

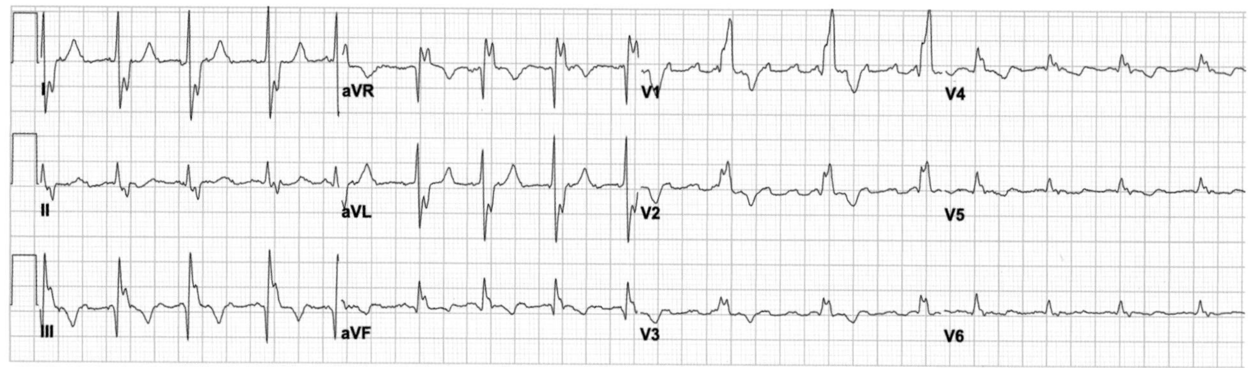

FIGURE 56.4 12 Lead electrocardiogram of "atypical" atrial flutter with variable ventricular conduction. Note flutter waves seen best in lead V1. This flutter circuit encircled the left-sided pulmonary veins utilizing scar surgical implantation of left-sided pulmonary veins after left lung transplant.

a mortality benefit over a rate control approach, have guided treatment of atrial fibrillation.[11] In most patients, a rhythm control approach is indicated for symptom relief, not to prevent stroke or increase life expectancy (**Algorithm 56.1**). An exception is patients with tachycardia-induced cardiomyopathy despite optimal achievable rate control, in whom rhythm control is the preferred strategy. There is also emerging evidence that patients with left ventricular systolic dysfunction of any etiology might especially benefit from maintenance of sinus rhythm.

Prevention of Thromboembolic Events

Thromboembolic events, particularly stroke, present the greatest risk of morbidity and mortality in atrial fibrillation and flutter. The decision to pursue anticoagulation therapy should be based on an assessment of the individualized risk for both stroke and bleeding events, regardless of whether a rate control or a rhythm control approach is planned (**Table 56.1**). The most prominent risk stratification scheme is the CHA_2DS_2-VASc scoring system, where one point each is assigned for a history of congestive heart failure, female sex, hypertension, age

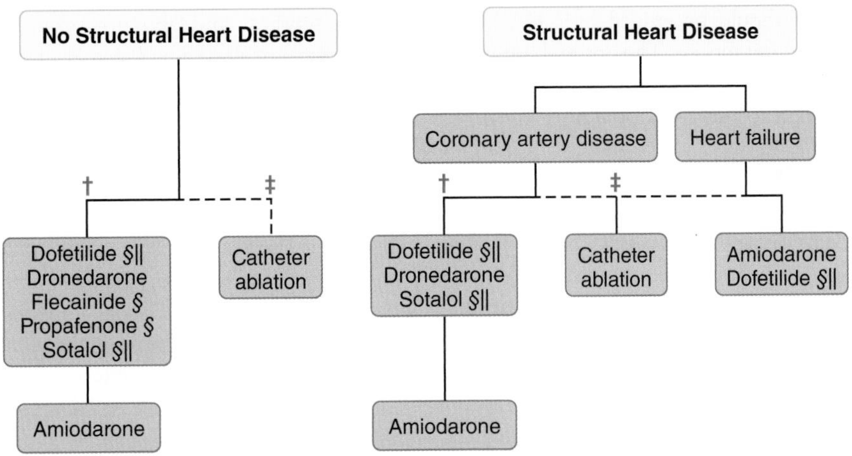

ALGORITHM 56.1 Approach to rhythm control strategy in patients with paroxysmal or persistent atrial fibrillation. (Adapted from January CT, Wann LS, Alpert JS, et al.; American College of Cardiology/American Heart Association Task Force on Practice Guidelines. 2014 AHA/ACC/HRS guideline for the management of patients with atrial fibrillation: a report of the American College of Cardiology/American Heart Association Task Force on Practice Guidelines and the Heart Rhythm Society. *J Am Coll Cardiol*. 2014;64(21):e1-e76. Copyright © 2014 American Heart Association, Inc., the American College of Cardiology Foundation, and the Heart Rhythm Society. With permission.)

*Catheter ablation is only recommended as first-line therapy for patients with paroxysmal atrial fibrillation (Class IIa recommendation).

TABLE 56.1 Anticoagulation Medications, Mechanism, and Dosage

Drug	Mechanism	Dose
Apixaban	Factor Xa inhibitor	5 mg twice daily, or 2.5 mg daily in patients with at least two of following: weight < 60 kg, Cr > 1.5, age older than 80 years
Dabigatran	Direct thrombin inhibitor	150 mg twice daily, or 75 mg twice daily with creatinine clearance 15-30 mL/min
Edoxaban	Factor Xa inhibitor	60 mg daily, or 30 mg daily with creatinine clearance 15-50 mL/min. Do not use if >95 mL/min
Rivaroxaban	Factor Xa inhibitor	20 mg daily, or 15 mg daily with creatinine clearance 15-50 mL/min
Warfarin	Vitamin K antagonist	Variable

between 65 and 75 years, diabetes mellitus, or vascular disease, and two points are assigned for either age 75 years or older, or prior transient ischemic attack/stroke. Patients with a CHA_2DS_2-VASc score of zero are considered at greater risk of bleeding from anticoagulation relative to the benefit derived from anticoagulation; therefore, chronic anticoagulation is not recommended. Therapeutic anticoagulation is recommended for patients with a CHA_2DS_2-VASc score of 2 or greater unless bleeding risk is felt to be prohibitive. In intermediate-risk patients (CHA_2DS_2-VASc = 1), either aspirin or anticoagulation is a reasonable approach. Female sex alone without an additional risk factor does not increase stroke risk and should, therefore, be treated as low risk.

It is worth noting that the CHA_2DS_2-VASc score does not apply in patients with mechanical valves, hypertrophic cardiomyopathy, or moderate to severe rheumatic mitral stenosis. These populations are at high risk for thromboembolism, warranting anticoagulation regardless of the CHA_2DS_2-VASc score.

In patients with ischemic stroke not known to have atrial fibrillation, cardiac monitoring is recommended for at least 24 hours after presentation to detect this rhythm. In patients with cryptogenic stroke, it is reasonable to pursue additional ambulatory cardiac monitoring. Although several trials have demonstrated increased detection of atrial fibrillation following cryptogenic stroke with either wearable or implantable monitors, the optimal modality and duration of monitoring have not been established.

Periprocedural Considerations

The most common source of thromboembolism in patients with atrial fibrillation or flutter is thrombus in the left atrial appendage. Transesophageal echocardiogram (TEE) is the most sensitive and specific imaging modality for the detection of left atrial appendage thrombus. Although 3 to 4 weeks of uninterrupted anticoagulation before cardioversion or ablation has been shown to lead to the resolution of 85% of thrombi, some centers use TEE to rule out intracardiac thrombus in all patients undergoing cardioversion or ablation for atrial fibrillation, regardless of anticoagulation status. Anticoagulation should be continued for at least 30 days following cardioversion and at least 2 months following atrial fibrillation ablation, although subsequent anticoagulation should be guided by CHA_2DS_2-VASc risk rather than procedural success. The optimal duration of anticoagulation is uncertain for patients following successful flutter ablation without prior documented atrial fibrillation.

Anticoagulation Agents

In the 2019 American Heart Association/American College of Cardiology/Heart Rhythm Society (AHA/ACC/HRS) guidelines, the direct oral anticoagulants are recommended over warfarin in eligible patients, except for those with mechanical prosthetic valves or moderate to severe rheumatic mitral stenosis.[12] Although more expensive, these drugs are easier to manage than is warfarin (ie, they do not require regular laboratory monitoring) and show equal or better safety and efficacy in randomized controlled trials.

Left Atrial Appendage Closure

The majority of cardiac thrombi in patients with atrial fibrillation or flutter originate in the left atrial appendage.[13] In patients with elevated stroke risk and either an increased risk of bleeding or poor adherence to medical therapy, left atrial appendage occlusion via a percutaneous procedure or minimally invasive surgical thoracoscopic approach is an alternative to oral anticoagulation to reduce the risk of stroke.[12] In patients with atrial fibrillation undergoing cardiac surgery, a concomitant maze procedure and closure of the left atrial appendage should be considered; this is a class I recommendation in patients undergoing mitral valve repair or replacement.

Risk Factor Modification

All patients with atrial fibrillation and atrial flutter should undergo an evaluation for treatable risk factors. This includes a history, physical, and laboratory examination to screen for hyperthyroidism, sleep apnea, hypertension, heart failure, diabetes, structural heart disease, and excessive alcohol consumption (**Algorithm 56.2**). In the LEGACY trial, optimal risk factor management resulted in freedom from arrhythmias without antiarrhythmic medications in nearly 40% of patients with at least 10% sustained weight loss.[14] Increased cardiorespiratory fitness has also shown a correlation with reduction in arrhythmic burden.[15] In addition, because even moderate alcohol intake increases the risk of atrial fibrillation, patients should be counseled on reducing or eliminating alcohol consumption.[16] Although the association between sleep-disordered breathing and atrial fibrillation is well established, there is currently a lack of randomized data demonstrating an arrhythmic benefit to sleep apnea therapy. Current guidelines recommend intensive risk factor modification as an important adjunct to any other treatment strategy.[17]

Rate Control

Pharmacologic Rate Control Agents

Control of the ventricular rate is an important mainstay in the management of atrial fibrillation and flutter, both to prevent symptoms and the deleterious effects of rapid ventricular rates. The target for average ventricular rate in atrial fibrillation was studied in the RACE II trial, and a lenient strategy targeting an average rate less than 110 bpm was found to be noninferior and more readily achieved than was a strict rate control strategy (resting heart rate < 80 bpm and heart rate during moderate exercise < 110 bpm), although it should be noted that the average heart rate in the lenient strategy was closer to 90 bpm.[18] The average rate can be assessed with ambulatory Holter monitors or from interrogation of pacemakers and defibrillators.

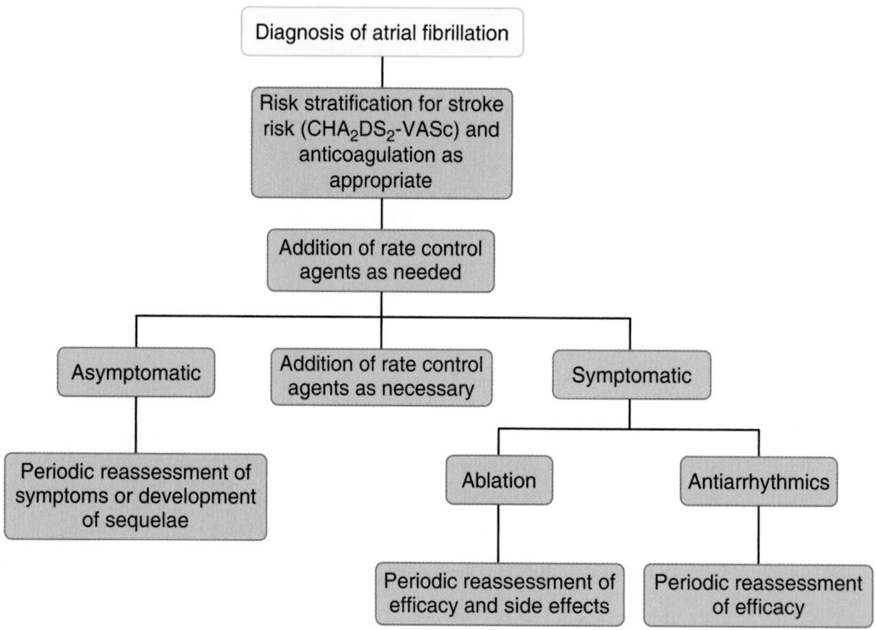

ALGORITHM 56.2 Approach to management of atrial fibrillation.

AV nodal blocking agents including β-blockers, nondihydropyridine calcium channel blockers (CCBs), and digoxin are all used in the control of ventricular rates. Many patients with atrial fibrillation have another indication for β-blocker therapy (ie, heart failure, coronary artery disease, etc), so this is a logical first option as a rate control agent in these patients. Although both β-blockers and CCBs are effective, CCBs may be preferred in patients with reactive airway disease and should be avoided in patients with heart failure and ventricular dysfunction. Digoxin is less effective as a rate control agent and its use is associated with greater mortality risk in patients with atrial fibrillation, so it is often reserved for short-term therapy in patients with decompensated heart failure or hypotension that limits the use of β-blockers or CCBs.

Atrioventricular Junction Ablation

In patients who have otherwise failed medical approaches to achieve rate control, a combined pace and ablate strategy may be employed, with implantation of a permanent pacemaker followed by AV junction ablation. This strategy offers regularization of the RR interval and control of the ventricular rate; however, it is a considered a last resort because it renders the patient pacemaker dependent and fails to restore AV synchrony.

Rhythm Control

Options for achieving and maintaining sinus rhythm include electrical cardioversion, antiarrhythmic medications, and percutaneous and surgical procedures. Because there has not been demonstration of a mortality benefit for a rhythm control strategy, the goals of restoration of sinus rhythm include reducing symptom burden, improving quality of life, and prevention of tachycardia and its long-term consequences. Because atrial fibrillation tends to be a progressive disease, patients should be advised that treatment focuses on a reduction in the frequency and duration of episodes, as opposed to the expectation of a permanent cure.

Cardioversion

Cardioversion is often the first approach in newly diagnosed persistent atrial fibrillation and an important tool for acute management of patients with hemodynamic instability or ventricular preexcitation. Cardioversion is also a useful tool for patients with infrequent persistent episodes of atrial fibrillation or atrial flutter.

Synchronized direct current cardioversion is the most commonly utilized form of cardioversion because of its high rate of acute success and low risk. In cases where sedation is contraindicated, acute pharmacologic cardioversion with intravenous ibutilide can restore sinus rhythm in up to 50% of patients. Ibutilide is associated with a small (1.2%-2.4%) risk of torsades de pointes, and caution should be employed in patients with prolonged QT intervals, hypokalemia, or severe left ventricular dysfunction. Dofetilide is also up to 60% effective in pharmacologic cardioversion, although it requires initiation over several in-hospital days with telemetry and QT monitoring. Amiodarone has a low rate of acute success in terminating atrial fibrillation, although it is typically well tolerated and provides a concurrent intermediate-term strategy for management of atrial fibrillation, either in preparation for cardioversion or as a pharmacologic bridge strategy. It is particularly useful in the treatment of postoperative atrial fibrillation, which is commonly seen after cardiothoracic surgery.

Antiarrhythmic Medications

Antiarrhythmic agents are a pharmacologic option for long-term maintenance of sinus rhythm in patients with symptomatic atrial fibrillation. The choice of antiarrhythmic agent should be guided by the features specific to each patient (see Figure 56.2).

Class IC Antiarrhythmics. Flecainide and propafenone are good first-line options for patients with atrial fibrillation and no structural heart disease. Owing to positive use dependence, these agents are most effective with rapid rates, and can be used for a pill-in-pocket strategy for paroxysmal atrial fibrillation. Owing to the risk of organizing atrial fibrillation into slow atrial flutter with 1:1 ventricular conduction, class IC agents should be used in conjunction with an AV nodal blocker.

Class III Antiarrhythmics. Dofetilide provides up to a 65% rate of sinus rhythm maintenance at 1 year. Sotalol is a less effective agent, with a 30% to 50% rate of sinus rhythm maintenance at 1 year. Owing to QT prolongation and risk of ventricular arrhythmias, these class III antiarrhythmics should be initiated in the hospital with continuous telemetry and ECG monitoring of QTc.

Amiodarone. Amiodarone is the most effective and most commonly prescribed option for pharmacologic management of atrial fibrillation, with a 65% rate of sinus rhythm maintenance at 1 year. Amiodarone is generally well tolerated in the short term and can be used in most patients. Owing to its iodine moiety and lipophilic nature, amiodarone has a large volume of distribution and carries the potential for adverse effects including pulmonary, thyroid, hepatic, ophthalmic, and neurologic toxicity. Owing to its cytochrome P450 induction, amiodarone can also increase the concentrations of other common medications including warfarin, digoxin, and statins. Long-term amiodarone use requires surveillance for thyroid, liver, and lung dysfunction.

Dronedarone. Dronedarone is an amiodarone analog without the iodine moiety. Although it is associated with fewer side effects than is amiodarone, it is also less effective. Dronedarone has been demonstrated to increase mortality in patients with NYHA class III or IV heart failure or recent heart failure decompensation, and those with permanent atrial fibrillation.

Percutaneous Catheter Ablation for Atrial Fibrillation

Catheter ablation offers higher efficacy rates than do antiarrhythmic medications and can be considered as a first-line therapy for patients with symptomatic paroxysmal or persistent atrial fibrillation.[19] Published success rates vary for paroxysmal atrial fibrillation across various studies, with single-procedure success rates between 59% and 89%.[20]

In persistent atrial fibrillation, a recent meta-analysis demonstrated a 67% single-procedure success rate from pulmonary vein isolation alone.[21] Allowing for multiple procedures, long-term success rates approach 80%.

For paroxysmal atrial fibrillation, the goal of ablation is primarily to eliminate triggers from the most common site of origin, the pulmonary veins.[4] The standard ablation strategy for atrial fibrillation is therefore antral electrical isolation of the pulmonary veins with either radiofrequency (RF) ablation or balloon-based cryoablation (**Figure 56.5**). These two modalities were compared head-to-head in the Fire and Ice trial, in which no difference was found between the two techniques in terms of either efficacy or safety.[22] In persistent atrial fibrillation, there is no consensus regarding the best approach beyond pulmonary vein isolation, although options include substrate modification with electrical isolation of the posterior wall or targeting of triggers beyond the pulmonary veins including additional spontaneous or induced ectopic foci, Ligament of Marshall ablation, or left atrial appendage ablation.

The risks of catheter ablation include vascular complications, pericarditis, damage to the phrenic nerve, and esophageal complications including atrioesophageal fistula, with the overall risk of a major complication around 3%.

Percutaneous Catheter Ablation for Atrial Flutter

Catheter ablation for typical atrial flutter offers success rates of over 85%. For CTI-dependent flutter, the goal of ablation is to achieve a line of block along the floor of the right atrium from the tricuspid annulus to the inferior vena cava. It should be noted that catheter ablation for atrial flutter does not impact the risk of development of atrial fibrillation. The ablation of atypical flutter involves mapping of the flutter circuit and ablation of a critical isthmus of the circuit, often at the left atrial roof or mitral isthmus, although other circuits are also seen.

Surgical Procedures for Atrial Fibrillation

Surgical approaches for atrial fibrillation have experienced major advances over the past three decades, with the first systematically studied surgical lesion set introduced by Dr. James Cox and his colleagues. The initial lesion sets were designed to isolate the pulmonary veins and disrupt common macroreentrant circuits in both atria, while allowing for propagation of the sinoatrial node impulse to both atria and the AV node.[2] Since the introduction of this operation, multiple iterations and modifications have been made. The lesions of the Cox maze procedure have been created using a "cut-and-sew" technique and provided excellent efficacy despite technical complexity, because this technique ensured contiguous and transmural ablation lines. With advances in energy sources adapted to surgical application, incisions have been replaced with ablation lines using primary bipolar RF and cryogenic ablation energy sources.

Biatrial versus left atrial lesion sets remain debated. Pulmonary vein isolation alone or as part of a complete left atrial maze lesion set is sufficient for paroxysmal atrial fibrillation. Current evidence suggests biatrial ablation is more efficacious than are left atrial lesion sets alone in persistent atrial fibrillation.[24] In addition, the traditional operation is performed on cardiopulmonary bypass through a median sternotomy, whereas less invasive approaches have been developed to avoid sternotomy and cardiopulmonary bypass. For example, the thoracoscopic maze procedure can be performed using ports in both chest cavities, and allows for creation of a nearly complete lesion set as well as epicardial occlusion of the left atrial appendage with a clip. This procedure in selected patients shows high success rates.[25,26]

The efficacy of surgical ablation is in part due to the ability to generate contiguous transmural lesions, as well as the ability to deliver both epicardial and endocardial energy under direct visualization with reduced risk of damage to the esophagus

A

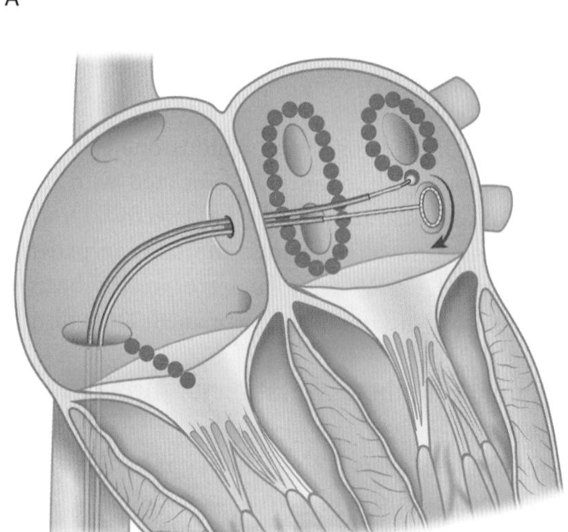

B

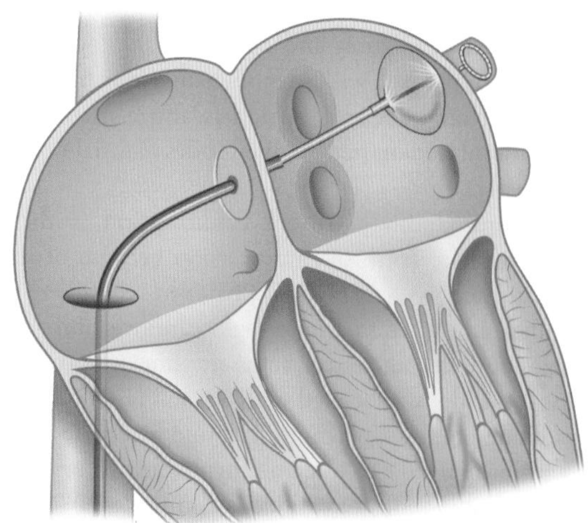

FIGURE 56.5 (**A,B**) Schematic of radiofrequency (left panel) and cryoballoon (right panel) pulmonary vein isolation.

and surrounding structures.[27] Moreover, testing of conduction block and modulation of ganglionic plexi is readily performed using surgical methods. Needless to say, the efficacy of the surgical maze procedure appears to depend on the type of atrial fibrillation and its duration with patients in new-onset paroxysmal atrial fibrillation having the greatest likelihood of success.

Although there is variation in the use of surgical ablation during cardiac surgery, partly due to surgeon practice and experience, national use of surgical ablation has increased.[28] The Society for Thoracic Surgery 2017 Clinical Practice Guidelines recommend concomitant surgical ablation for atrial fibrillation at the time of mitral valve surgery as a class I indication. Likewise, guidelines advise that ablation can be safely performed at the time of isolated aortic valve surgery or coronary artery bypass grafting. In conjunction with surgical ablation, left atrial appendage exclusion or ligation is recommended for reduction of thromboembolic risk.[28] Complete exclusion of the left atrial appendage is perhaps the most important contributor to the improved survival of patients following the Cox maze operation (**Figure 56.6**).

Although most surgical ablation is performed concomitantly with other cardiac procedures, a subset of patients can be considered for isolated surgery for atrial fibrillation with the goal of restoring sinus rhythm. In the modern era, these patients typically experience symptoms refractory to medical management and often have failed at least one attempt at catheter ablation.

Outcomes for surgical management of atrial fibrillation have generally been excellent. Institutional series and meta-analyses of modern renditions of the operation have reported freedom from atrial fibrillation of 78% to 85% at 1 to 5 years postoperatively.[29,30] The original "cut-and-sew" biatrial Cox maze III procedure performed for atrial fibrillation was found to have a sustained freedom from atrial fibrillation of 95% at 10 years without any strokes at follow-up. The added risk to a concomitant surgical procedure is minimal.[31]

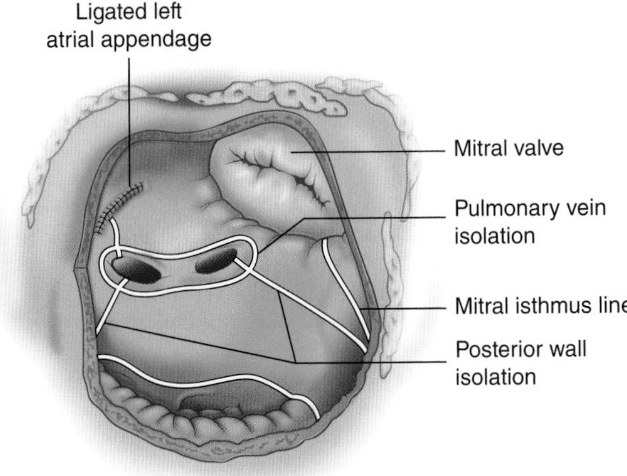

FIGURE 56.6 A demonstration of the left atrial lesion sets of the modern rendition of the Maze procedure (Cox Maze IV), whereby lesions are made with a combination of bipolar radiofrequency ablation and cryogenic energy to isolate the pulmonary veins, posterior wall, and include a mitral isthmus ablation line. Right atrial lesions are also performed (not shown).

Surgical patients undergoing a maze procedure are best evaluated and followed by a heart team including cardiothoracic surgeons and cardiac electrophysiologists. This approach ensures evidence-based recommendations and follow-up care. Ambulatory monitoring at 3, 6, and 12 months after surgery guides management of antiarrhythmic drugs, need for cardioversion or "touch-up" catheter ablation, and anticoagulation management.

Management of Postoperative Atrial Fibrillation

Atrial fibrillation is common in the perioperative setting, particularly following cardiac or thoracic surgery. With respect to prevention, it is a class I recommendation to continue outpatient β-blockers in the perioperative setting, and prevention of hypomagnesemia has been demonstrated to be effective in a thoracic surgery population. Amiodarone is effective and may be used for prevention of perioperative atrial fibrillation in high-risk patients. Management of incident perioperative atrial fibrillation can be approached either with a primary rate control or rhythm control strategy. Anticoagulation is recommended for episodes lasting longer than 48 hours in patients with elevated stroke risk as determined by CHA_2DS_2-VASc score, while taking into account risk of bleeding in general and as guided by the surgery performed. Although there is a clear association between development of perioperative atrial fibrillation and increased risk of stroke, the optimal duration of anticoagulation has not been studied definitively. The 2014 American Association of Thoracic Surgery guidelines recommend considering discontinuation of anticoagulation 4 weeks after documented return to sinus rhythm.

FOLLOW-UP PATIENT CARE

Subsequent care for patients undergoing treatment for atrial fibrillation and atrial flutter is guided by the treatment approach chosen. For all patients, clinic visits provide the opportunity for periodic assessment of the efficacy of the current treatment approach, monitoring for side effects from medications, and a discussion regarding the risks and benefits of an alternative approach.

For patients on antiarrhythmic therapy, follow-up should include evaluation of efficacy, development of side effects, abnormal conduction, or prolongation of the QT interval.

Following catheter ablation for atrial fibrillation, it is recommended to perform periodic assessments for recurrence of atrial fibrillation with ambulatory rhythm monitoring at 3, 6, and 12 months after ablation.

For patients undergoing a rate control approach, ambulatory monitoring can show average heart rate, burden of tachycardia, and the coexistence of significant bradyarrhythmias. Patients should also be evaluated for bleeding complications from anticoagulation.

RESEARCH AND FUTURE DIRECTIONS

- Alternatives to anticoagulation: Ongoing trials are evaluating the efficacy of percutaneous left atrial appendage closure for stroke reduction, even in patients eligible for long-term anticoagulation.
- Risk factor modification: Further randomized data are required for evaluating the optimal strategy and benefit of management of treatment of obstructive sleep apnea, weight loss, exercise, and metabolic risk factors.
- Technology: The next wave of developments in the treatment of atrial fibrillation include alternative ablation energy sources, such as pulsed field ablation, and alternative delivery mechanisms of current energy sources, including lattice-tip RF catheters, as well as laser and RF balloon catheters.
- Approaches: Further randomized studies are needed to determine the optimal strategy for catheter ablation and surgical maze.

KEY POINTS

✔ Atrial fibrillation is the most common arrhythmia and is a major driver of morbidity and health care utilization.

✔ Symptoms of atrial fibrillation and atrial flutter are variable, and the approach to patient care should be guided by patient symptoms and the presence of concurrent conditions.

✔ Anticoagulation for the prevention of thromboembolic events should be guided by estimated stroke risk and bleeding risk, regardless of the subtype of atrial fibrillation or the treatment approach selected.

✔ Both percutaneous and surgical ablation offer higher success rates than do antiarrhythmic medications in atrial fibrillation.

✔ Patients with atrial fibrillation underdoing cardiac surgery should have concurrent surgical ablation (concomitant maze) especially if undergoing mitral valve repair or replacement. Surgical patients with atrial fibrillation should have left atrial appendage exclusion. Selected patients can benefit from stand-alone surgical ablation.

✔ Risk factor modification is an important component of the management of atrial fibrillation and flutter. Patients should be assessed and treated for areas of potential reversible risk factors.

REFERENCES

1. Chugh SS, Havmoeller R, Narayanan K, et al. Worldwide epidemiology of atrial fibrillation: a Global Burden of Disease 2010 Study. *Circulation.* 2014;129(8):837-847.
2. Alonso A, Agarwal SK, Soliman EZ, et al. Incidence of atrial fibrillation in whites and African-Americans: the Atherosclerosis Risk in Communities (ARIC) study. *Am Heart J.* 2009;158(1):111-117.
3. Kim MH, Johnston SS, Chu B-C, Dalal MR, Schulman KL. Estimation of total incremental health care costs in patients with atrial fibrillation in the United States. *Circ Cardiovasc Qual Outcomes.* 2011;4(3):313-320.
4. Haissaguerre M, Jaïs P, Shah DC, et al. Spontaneous initiation of atrial fibrillation by ectopic beats originating in the pulmonary veins. *N Engl J Med.* 1998;339(10):659-666.
5. Wijffels MC, Kirchhof CJ, Dorland R, Allessie MA. Atrial fibrillation begets atrial fibrillation. A study in awake chronically instrumented goats. *Circulation.* 1995;92(7):1954-1968.
6. Lim HS, Hocini M, Dubois R, et al. Complexity and distribution of drivers in relation to duration of persistent atrial fibrillation. *J Am Coll Cardiol.* 2017;69(10):1257-1269.
7. Chen PS, Chen LS, Fishbein MC, Lin S-F, Nattel S. Role of the autonomic nervous system in atrial fibrillation: pathophysiology and therapy. *Circ Res.* 2014;114(9):1500-1515.
8. Garimella RS, Chung EH, Mounsey JP, Schwartz JD, Pursell I, Gehi AK. Accuracy of patient perception of their prevailing rhythm: a comparative analysis of monitor data and questionnaire responses in patients with atrial fibrillation. *Heart Rhythm.* 2015;12(4):658-665.
9. Xiong Q, Proietti M, Senoo K, Lip GYH. Asymptomatic versus symptomatic atrial fibrillation: a systematic review of age/gender differences and cardiovascular outcomes. *Int J Cardiol.* 2015;191:172-177.
10. Pistoia F, Sacco S, Tiseo C, Degan D, Ornello R, Carolei A. The epidemiology of atrial fibrillation and stroke. *Cardiol Clin.* 2016;34(2):255-268.
11. Wyse DG, Waldo AL, DiMarco JP, et al. A comparison of rate control and rhythm control in patients with atrial fibrillation. *N Engl J Med.* 2002;347(23):1825-1833.
12. January CT, Wann LS, Calkins H, et al. 2019 AHA/ACC/HRS focused update of the 2014 AHA/ACC/HRS Guideline for the management of patients with atrial fibrillation: a report of the American College of Cardiology/American Heart Association Task Force on Clinical Practice Guidelines and the Heart Rhythm Society. *J Am Coll Cardiol.* 2019;74(1):104-132.
13. Yaghi S, Song C, Gray WA, Furie KL, Elkind MSV, Kamel H. Left atrial appendage function and stroke risk. *Stroke.* 2015;46(12):3554-3559.
14. Pathak RK, Middeldorp ME, Meredith M, et al. Long-Term Effect of Goal directed weight management on Atrial Fibrillation Cohort: A 5 Year follow-up study (LEGACY). *J Am Coll Cardiol.* 2015;65(20):2159-2169.
15. Pathak RK, Elliott A, Middeldorp ME, et al. Impact of CARDIOrespiratory FITness on arrhythmia recurrence in obese individuals with atrial fibrillation: the CARDIO-FIT Study. *J Am Coll Cardiol.* 2015;66(9):985-996.
16. Larsson SC, Drca N, Wolk A. Alcohol consumption and risk of atrial fibrillation: a prospective study and dose-response meta-analysis. *J Am Coll Cardiol.* 2014;64(3):281-289.
17. Chung MK, Eckhardt LL, Chen LY, et al. Lifestyle and risk factor modification for reduction of atrial fibrillation: a scientific statement from the American Heart Association. *Circulation.* 2020;141(16):e750-e772. doi:10.1161/CIR0000000000000748
18. Van Gelder IC, Groenveld HF, Crijns HJGM, et al. Lenient versus strict rate control in patients with atrial fibrillation. *N Engl J Med.* 2010;362(15):1363-1373.
19. Calkins H, Hindricks G, Cappato R, et al. 2017 HRS/EHRA/ECAS/APHRS/SOLAECE expert consensus statement on catheter and surgical ablation of atrial fibrillation. *Heart Rhythm.* 2017;14(10):e275-e444.
20. Ganesan AN, Shipp NJ, Brooks AG, et al. Long-term outcomes of catheter ablation of atrial fibrillation: a systematic review and meta-analysis. *J Am Heart Assoc.* 2013;2(2):e004549.
21. Voskoboinik A, Moskovitch JT, Harel N, Sanders P, Kistler PM, Kalman JM. Revisiting pulmonary vein isolation alone for persistent atrial fibrillation: a systematic review and meta-analysis. *Heart Rhythm.* 2017;14(5):661-667.
22. Kuck KH, Brugada J, Fürnkranz A, et al. Cryoballoon or radiofrequency ablation for paroxysmal atrial fibrillation. *N Engl J Med.* 2016;374(23):2235-2245.

23. Cox JL, Schuessler RB, D'Agostino HJ, Jr, et al. The surgical treatment of atrial fibrillation. III. Development of a definitive surgical procedure. *J Thorac Cardiovasc Surg*. 1991;101(4):569-583.
24. Blackstone EH, Chang HL, Rajeswaran J, et al. Biatrial maze procedure versus pulmonary vein isolation for atrial fibrillation during mitral valve surgery: new analytical approaches and end points. *J Thorac Cardiovasc Surg*. 2019;157(1):234-243.e9.
25. Sirak J, Jones D, Sun B, Sai-Sudhakar C, Crestanello J, Firstenberg M. Toward a definitive, totally thoracoscopic procedure for atrial fibrillation. *Ann Thorac Surg*. 2008;86(6):1960-1964.
26. Krul SP, Driessen AHG, van Boven WJ, et al. Thoracoscopic video-assisted pulmonary vein antrum isolation, ganglionated plexus ablation, and periprocedural confirmation of ablation lesions: first results of a hybrid surgical-electrophysiological approach for atrial fibrillation. *Circ Arrhythm Electrophysiol*. 2011;4(3):262-270.
27. Prasad SM, Maniar HS, Diodato MD, Schuessler RB, Damiano RJ Jr. Physiological consequences of bipolar radiofrequency energy on the atria and pulmonary veins: a chronic animal study. *Ann Thorac Surg*. 2003;76(3):836-841; discussion 841-842.
28. Badhwar V, Rankin JS, Damiano RJ Jr, et al. The Society of Thoracic Surgeons 2017 Clinical Practice Guidelines for the surgical treatment of atrial fibrillation. *Ann Thorac Surg*. 2017;103(1):329-341.
29. Barnett SD, Ad N. Surgical ablation as treatment for the elimination of atrial fibrillation: a meta-analysis. *J Thorac Cardiovasc Surg*. 2006;131(5):1029-1035.
30. Henn MC, Lancaster TS, Miller JR, et al. Late outcomes after the Cox maze IV procedure for atrial fibrillation. *J Thorac Cardiovasc Surg*. 2015;150(5):1168-1176, 1178.e1-2.
31. Musharbash FN, Schill MR, Sinn LA, et al. Performance of the Cox-maze IV procedure is associated with improved long-term survival in patients with atrial fibrillation undergoing cardiac surgery. *J Thorac Cardiovasc Surg*. 2018;155(1):159-170.

SECTION 4

CHAPTER 57

VENTRICULAR TACHYCARDIA

Justin Hayase and Jason S. Bradfield

INTRODUCTION

Ventricular tachycardia (VT) is an important cause of sudden cardiac death that is estimated to affect between 230,000 and 350,000 people in the United States annually.[1] VT is defined as greater than or equal to 3 beats originating from the ventricles at a rate greater than 100 beats per minute. Sustained VT is defined as lasting longer than 30 seconds or VT requiring intervention for termination because of hemodynamic compromise. Nonsustained VT is defined as lasting less than 30 seconds and self-terminating. VT can be either monomorphic (having the same beat-to-beat electrocardiographic [ECG] morphology) or polymorphic (changing QRS morphology beat to beat). Ventricular fibrillation is defined as rapid and disorganized, irregular electrical activity, typically at a rate greater than 300 bpm (**Figure 57.1**).

PATHOGENESIS

Monomorphic VT and polymorphic VT typically have different underlying mechanisms/pathophysiology. Polymorphic VT may often be driven by ischemia, whereas monomorphic VT is rarely due to an ischemic insult. A form of polymorphic VT, known as *torsades de pointes*, can be precipitated by a long QT interval. There are many causes of a long QT interval including electrolyte abnormalities, drug effects, or inherited channelopathies. Monomorphic VT is most commonly due to either focal mechanisms (either triggered activity or automaticity) or scar-based reentry (most often in the setting of structural heart disease).[2] Focal mechanisms are often implicated in idiopathic VT entities, such as outflow tract VTs or Purkinje fiber–associated VTs, which can occur in the absence of structural heart disease; however, their occurrence does not exclude structural heart disease. In contrast to focal VT, the presence of scar promotes a macro-reentrant mechanism for myocardial VT. The heterogeneous conduction properties of scarred myocardium create the critical isthmuses that promote wave break and create excitable gaps, which can sustain a macro-reentrant circuit for monomorphic VT[3] (**Figure 57.2**).

CLINICAL PRESENTATION

Patients can present with a variety of symptoms depending on the VT characteristics, comorbidities, and underlying etiology. Symptoms can include chest pain, shortness of breath,

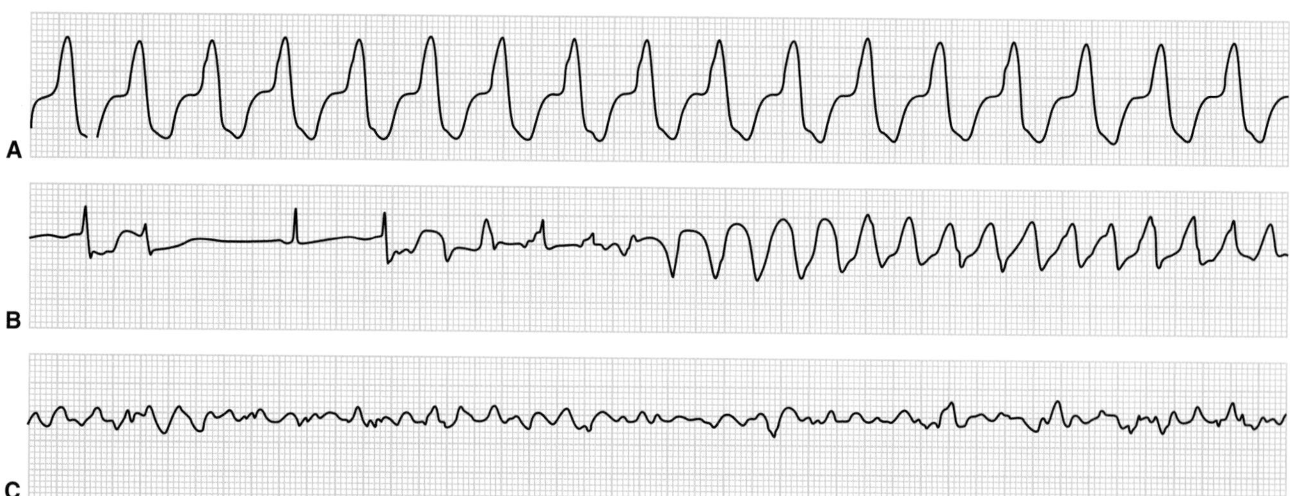

FIGURE 57.1 Different types of ventricular tachyarrhythmias. **(A)** Monomorphic ventricular tachycardia characterized by a wide QRS complex rhythm, rate greater than 100 bpm, with the same beat-to-beat electrocardiographic (ECG) morphology. **(B)** Polymorphic ventricular tachycardia with beat-to-beat variability in QRS morphology. Prolonged QT interval can be appreciated at the beginning of the rhythm strip, which predisposes to torsades de pointes. **(C)** Ventricular fibrillation with disorganized, irregular electrical activity at a rate greater than 300 bpm.

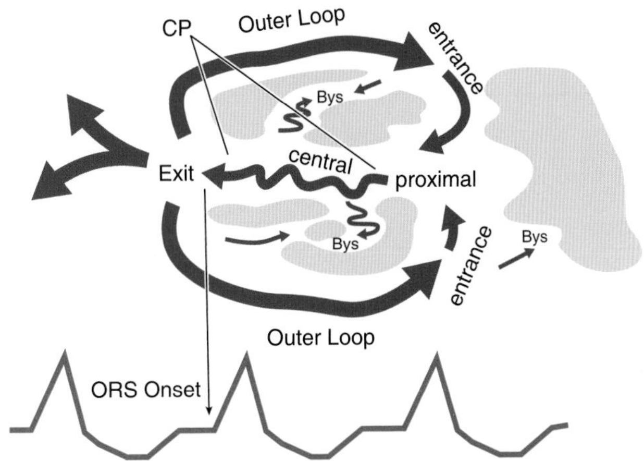

FIGURE 57.2 Mechanisms of scar-mediated ventricular tachycardia. Scar tissue is indicated by gray stippled areas. A circuit that contains two loops and a common pathway (CP), through which conduction is slowed, is illustrated with a "figure-of-eight" configuration. The common pathway has an exit and central and proximal regions. The onset of the QRS complex occurs as the excitation wavefront exits the common pathway and begins propagating around the two outer loops. The wavefront then enters the infarct zone via the proximal entrance then processes to the central region, thus completing the circuit. Several regions that are in the chronic infarct but do not participate in the circuit are labeled as bystanders (Bys). (Adapted from Stevenson WG, Friedman PL, Sager PT, et al. Exploring postinfarction reentrant ventricular tachycardia with entrainment mapping. *J Am Coll Cardiol.* 1997;29(6):1180-1189. Copyright © 1997 Elsevier. With permission.)

palpitations, dizziness, diaphoresis, weakness, and/or syncope. Symptoms are typically abrupt in onset, and if the VT rate is fast, then hemodynamic compromise can be sudden.[4] Less commonly, if the VT rate is much slower, symptoms can be more subacute if the VT has been ongoing for some time.

DIAGNOSIS

As always, a history and physical examination must initiate every patient evaluation. Attention to the patient's general appearance and vital signs is critical because hemodynamic collapse can occur rapidly in a patient with VT. Tachycardia, weak and thready pulse, pallor, diaphoresis, and marginal blood pressure are important signs to note. A basic assessment according to advanced cardiac and life support algorithms is imperative, with prompt intervention to maintain support of the patient's airway, breathing, and circulation (**Algorithm 57.1**).

The most important tool for establishing a diagnosis of VT, however, is the 12-lead ECG. The presence of a wide complex tachycardia on ECG should immediately raise the clinician's concern for VT, although there are other possibilities that should also be considered. Multiple criteria have been developed to differentiate VT from other causes of wide complex tachycardia with a high degree of sensitivity and specificity. Brugada and colleagues developed an algorithm in which an absence of an RS complex in all precordial leads, an R to S interval of greater than 100 ms, the presence of atrioventricular (AV) dissociation, or morphology criteria in leads V1 and V6 can identify VT with a sensitivity of 98.7% and specificity of 96.5%.[5] Another algorithm utilizing only lead aVR can also distinguish VT from supraventricular tachycardia with aberrancy with sensitivity of 96.5% and specificity of 95.7%[6] (**Algorithm 57.2**). The presence of structural heart disease also greatly increases the probability that the wide complex tachycardia is VT.[1]

MANAGEMENT OF VENTRICULAR TACHYCARDIA

As previously mentioned, management of VT initially should follow the algorithm provided by advanced cardiac life support recommendations, with an emphasis on circulatory support and airway protection. Electrical cardioversion is often recommended if VT does not self-terminate. If VT remains refractory to supportive measures, medications should be administered, typically via intravenous formulation. Guideline recommendations suggest the use of amiodarone, sotalol, or procainamide.[1] In the guidelines, procainamide received a stronger recommendation than did amiodarone or sotalol[1]; however, this is based on limited data,[7] and procainamide use is associated with toxicities that require close monitoring. For this reason, in our practice, we prefer the use of amiodarone as an initial agent in cases of refractory VT in the acute setting. Lidocaine has fallen out of favor as a primary agent for management of VT; however, it may still have a role where ischemia is suspected, or when used in combination with other antiarrhythmic agents such as amiodarone.[8] Lidocaine can also be useful in suppressing arrhythmias in the short term, owing to its short half-life, when subsequent electrophysiology procedures are planned, whereas other agents with longer half-lives could affect arrhythmia inducibility and thus decrease procedural efficacy.

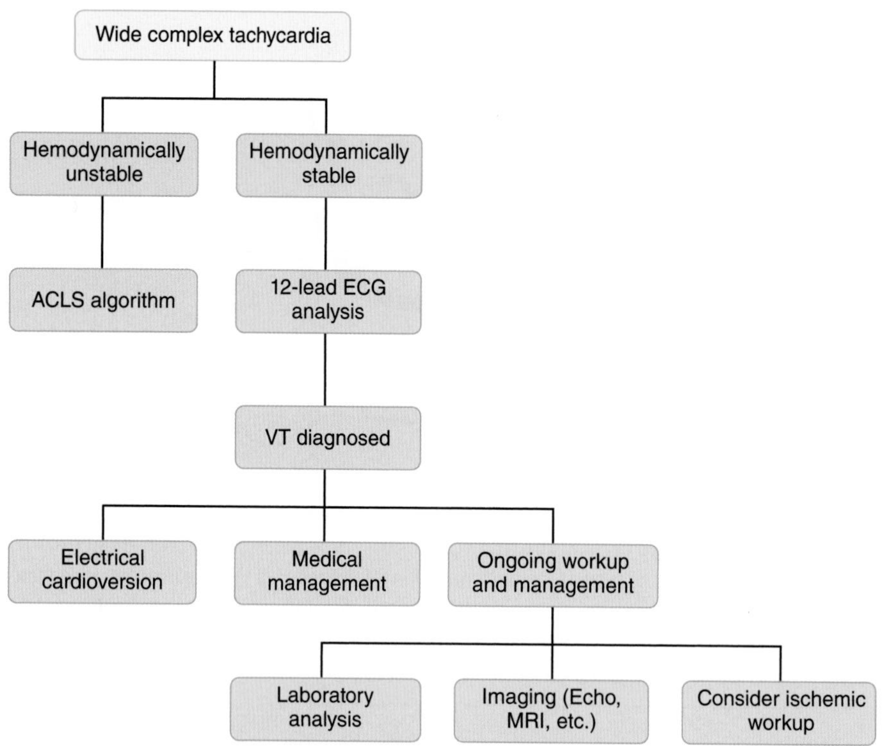

ALGORITHM 57.1 Diagnostic approach to wide complex tachycardia. ACLS, advanced cardiac life support; ECG, electrocardiogram; echo, echocardiogram; MRI, magnetic resonance imaging; VT, ventricular tachycardia.

Once stabilized, an evaluation for underlying causes of VT should be performed, such as electrolyte imbalances, drug toxicities, endocrine disorders, inherited channelopathies, or acute coronary syndromes (**Algorithm 57.3**). If patients continue to have ongoing ventricular arrhythmias in spite of addressing any underlying causes and initiation of antiarrhythmic medications, consideration for intubation and sedation should be made. Advanced imaging such as a cardiac magnetic resonance imaging (MRI) can be performed to assess for myocardial scar, and a positron emission tomography-computed tomography (PET-CT) scan may also be useful in identifying inflammatory conditions such as myocarditis that could be contributing to the arrhythmias.[9]

The management of VT also varies greatly depending on whether it is an idiopathic versus a scar-mediated mechanism. The surface ECG morphology of VT is critical in guiding management because certain 12-lead ECG features can suggest an idiopathic etiology.[10] In cases of scar-mediated VT, the 12-lead ECG can also localize exit sites and direct future invasive procedural management.[11]

Medical Approach

Management approaches vary depending on whether the VT is idiopathic and occurs in a structurally normal heart, or whether it is a scar-mediated one in the case of a structurally abnormal heart. Idiopathic VT or premature ventricular complexes (PVCs) commonly originate from the outflow tract, AV annular regions, papillary muscles/moderator band, or the fascicular conduction system.[1] Medication management commonly includes beta-blockers or non-dihydropyridine calcium channel blockers. Antiarrhythmic medications may also be considered. If patients remain refractory to medical therapy or do not tolerate medications, then catheter ablation should be offered, which is discussed further in the section "Percutaneous Interventions."

Patients with sustained monomorphic VT and structural heart disease should receive an implantable cardioverter defibrillator (ICD) as a class I recommendation.[1] Particularly in patients with a reduced left ventricular ejection fraction, the ICD has demonstrated mortality benefit in multiple clinical trials.[12,13] However, although the ICDs can abort potential life-threatening ventricular arrhythmias, they do not prevent VT from occurring, and ICD shocks have been associated with poorer outcomes as well as reduced quality of life.[14] Certain cardiac device programming parameters, such as the use of anti-tachycardia pacing (ATP), can decrease the likelihood of ICD shocks and improve quality of life.[15] Nonetheless, the management options for patients who continue to experience VT include (1) medications, (2) catheter-based interventions, or (3) surgical therapies.

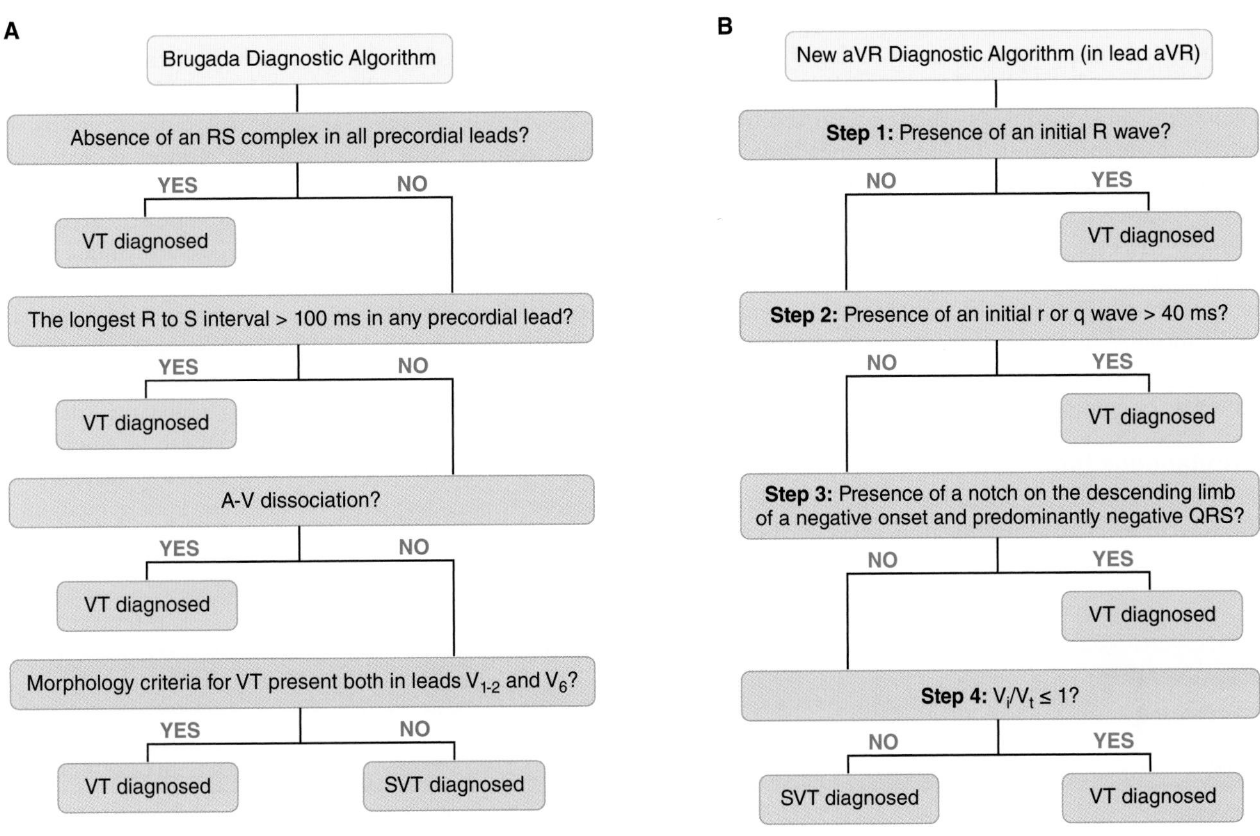

ALGORITHM 57.2 Electrocardiographic (ECG) diagnostic algorithms for ventricular tachycardia. SVT, supraventricular tachycardia. **(A)** Stepwise Brugada algorithm for diagnosis of ventricular tachycardia (VT). Any one of the four criteria can establish the diagnosis of VT. **(B)** Stepwise approach for diagnosis of VT using only lead AVR. V_i/V_t represents the ventricular activation velocity ratio, with V_i being the vertical excursion in millivolts during the initial 40 ms of the QRS complex and V_t being the vertical excursion in millivolts during the terminal 40 ms of the QRS complex. (Adapted from Vereckei A, Duray G, Szénási G, et al. New algorithm using only lead aVR for differential diagnosis of wide QRS complex tachycardia. *Heart Rhythm*. 2008;5(1):89-98. Copyright © 2008 Heart Rhythm Society. With permission.)

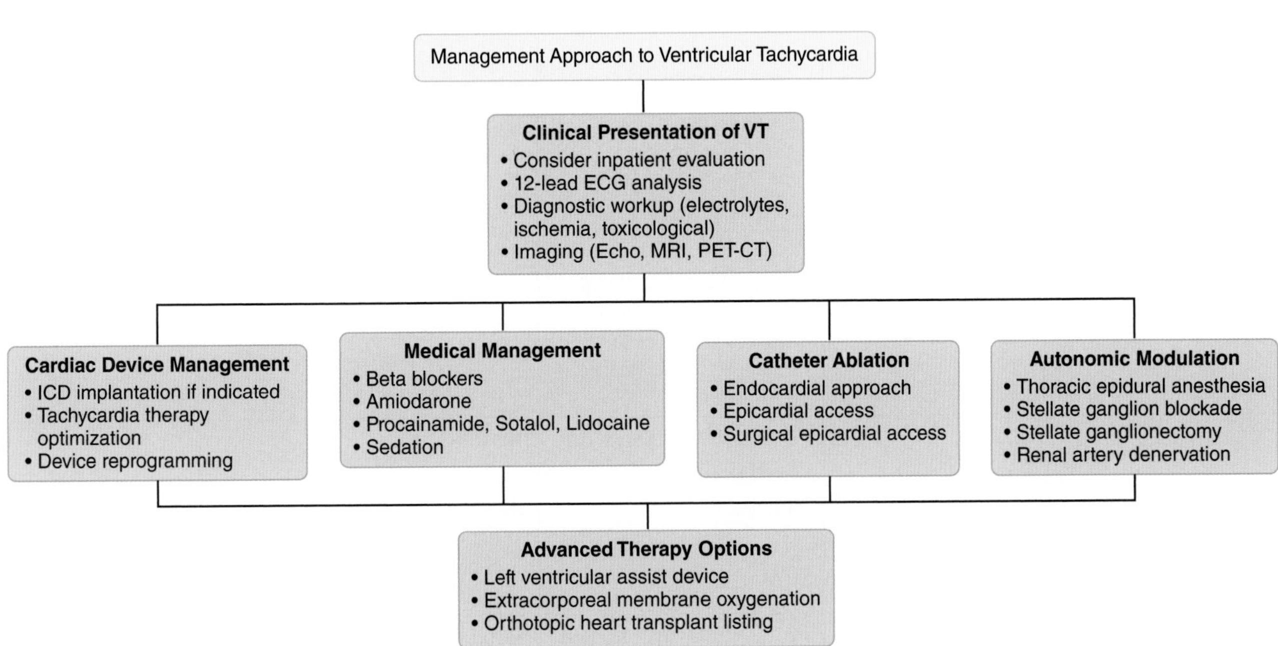

ALGORITHM 57.3 Management approach to ventricular tachycardia. ECG, electrocardiogram; echo, echocardiogram; ICD implantable cardioverter defibrillator MRI, magnetic resonance imaging; PET-CT, positron emission tomography-computed tomography; VT, ventricular tachycardia.

Beta-blockers are a mainstay in the management of ventricular arrhythmias, particularly in the setting of left ventricular dysfunction, owing to their demonstrated mortality benefit. A number of antiarrhythmic medications can also be considered, which are included in **Table 57.1**. Amiodarone is often the primary agent of choice because of its comparatively higher efficacy[16]; however, in the long term, because of the multitude of adverse effects of amiodarone, many practitioners prefer to stop this agent or minimize its use. Long-term antiarrhythmic medication options for VT include amiodarone (if necessary),[17] sotalol,[18] mexiletine,[19] ranolazine,[20] or dofetilide.[21] In the absence of structural heart or coronary artery disease, other agents may be considered such as flecainide or propafenone.[22]

Percutaneous Interventions

In cases of symptomatic, idiopathic VT or PVCs that remain refractory to medical management or where medications are not tolerated or preferred, catheter ablation is a recommended management option.[1] Catheter ablation is most effective when there is one predominant morphology of the VT or PVCs (**Figure 57.3A**). In addition, an elevated PVC burden (typically >15%) can cause an associated cardiomyopathy, for which catheter ablation can result in recovery of ventricular function.[23]

For patients with structural heart disease, catheter ablation for VT has been shown to reduce arrhythmic events, particularly in those with ICDs, as a means of reducing ICD shocks.[24] Catheter ablation is also recommended in patients with VT refractory to medical management.[1] In particular, the VANISH trial showed the greatest benefit for catheter ablation in patients already taking amiodarone therapy.[25] Various mapping and ablation strategies can be employed to achieve procedural success including activation mapping, entrainment, pace mapping, or substrate homogenization[26,27] (**Figure 57.3B**).

TABLE 57.1 Medications for Treatment of Ventricular Tachycardia

Drug	Vaughn Williams Class	Dose	Side Effects	Special Consideration
Amiodarone	III	IV: 300-mg bolus for VF/pulseless VT arrest; 150-mg bolus for stable VT; 1 mg/min × 6 h, then 0.5 mg/min × 18 h PO: 400 mg every 8-12 h while loading (total 10 gm), maintenance dose 200-400 mg daily	Hypotension, bradycardia, QT prolongation, corneal deposits, thyrotoxicity, neurotoxicity, hepatotoxicity, pulmonary toxicity, dermatologic abnormalities	Increases defibrillation threshold in long term
Sotalol	III	IV: 75 mg every 12 h PO: 80-120 mg every 12 h, may increase dose every 3 d; max 320 mg/d	QT prolongation, hypotension, bradycardia	Decreases defibrillation threshold
Procainamide	IA	IV: loading dose 10-17 mg/kg at 20-50 mg/min Maintenance dose: 1-4 mg/min	QT prolongation, AV block, lupus-like symptoms, hypotension,	Must monitor metabolite (NAPA) levels
Lidocaine	IB	IV: 1-1.5 mg/kg bolus, Repeat 0.5-0.75 mg/kg bolus every 5-10 min (max cumulative dose 3 mg/kg). Maintenance 1-4 mg/min	Bradycardia, hypotension, neurotoxicity	Monitor levels, goal <5 μg/mL
Mexiletine	IB	PO: 150-300 mg every 8 h or every 12 h	Neurotoxicity	
Beta-blockers: metoprolol, carvedilol, propranolol, nadolol	II	Variable	Heart failure exacerbation, bradycardia, hypotension	Mortality benefit in systolic dysfunction with metoprolol succinate and carvedilol
Ranolazine	N/A	PO: 500-1000 mg every 12 h	QT prolongation, hypotension	Antianginal effects

AV, atrioventricular; d, day; h, hour; IV, intravenous; NAPA; *N*-acetyl procainamide; PO, orally; VF, ventricular fibrillation; VT, ventricular tachycardia.

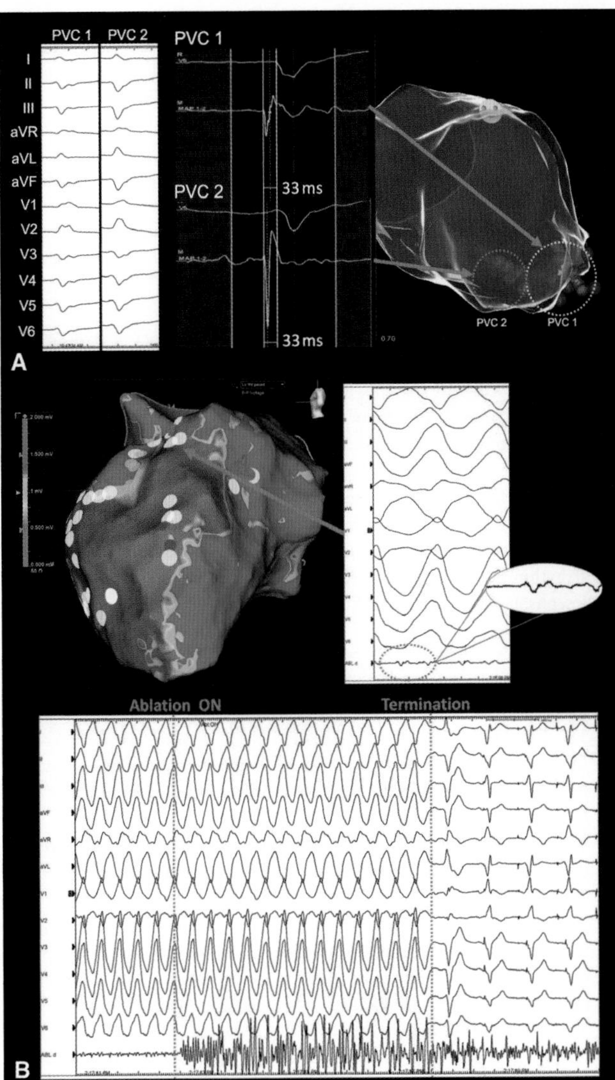

FIGURE 57.3 Catheter ablation for ventricular arrhythmias. **(A)** Catheter ablation of symptomatic idiopathic premature ventricular complexes (PVCs) originated from the inferomedial papillary muscle. Left: 12-lead surface electrocardiographic (ECG) of two different PVC morphologies with similar, but slightly different, exit sites. Middle: Local bipolar electrogram signals obtained at the lateral and medial base of the papillary muscle, each approximately 33 ms before the onset of the QRS complex. Right: electroanatomic map (Carto, Biosense Webster, Irvine, CA) with no significant areas of scar and corresponding sites of origin targeting areas of earliest activation for each PVC. Ablation lesions indicated by red dots. **(B)** Catheter ablation of monomorphic ventricular tachycardia (VT) in a patient with ischemic cardiomyopathy with prior total occlusion of the left anterior descending artery and extensive anterior and anteroseptal scar. Top: Electroanatomic map (NavX, Abbott Medical, Chicago, IL) with corresponding 12-lead ECG of monomorphic VT with local electrogram signal demonstrating nearly continuous, fractionated, diastolic activity indicative of a region of slow conduction. Bottom: ablation in this region resulted in termination of VT.

Depending on a number of patient and VT factors, catheter ablation either with an endocardial, epicardial, or a combined endocardial and epicardial approach can be considered.[28] It is important to establish a strategy upfront because the need for epicardial access can significantly impact procedural planning. Once catheters are placed within the left ventricle, either via transseptal or retrograde aortic approach, heparinization is required, which complicates the potential need for percutaneous epicardial access.

Some 12-lead ECG features can suggest the presence of an epicardial exit site, depending on myocardial substrate. For ischemic cardiomyopathy, these include a pseudodelta wave interval of greater than 34 ms, intrinsicoid deflection time in V2 of greater than 85 ms, and RS complex of >121 ms.[29] In nonischemic cardiomyopathy, the absence of inferior Q waves, a pseudodelta of greater than or equal to 75 ms, a maximum deflection index of greater than 0.59, or the presence of an inferior Q wave in lead I can indicate the presence of an epicardial circuit.[30]

Cardiac imaging with contrast-enhanced MRI can also help guide the ablation strategy based on scar characteristics. Subepicardial or mid-myocardial scar can favor an epicardial or combined epicardial/endocardial approach. Patient factors such as prior unsuccessful endocardial ablation or the presence of nonischemic cardiomyopathy or arrhythmogenic right ventricular cardiomyopathy also may suggest the need for an epicardial approach to achieve success.[28]

Aside from catheter ablation, a number of other percutaneous options for autonomic modulation are also effective in treating VT. Thoracic epidural anesthesia, stellate ganglion blockade, and renal artery denervation are minimally invasive approaches that modulate the sympathetic input to the cardiac neuraxis, for which there is demonstrated efficacy in the treatment of ventricular arrhythmias.[31]

Surgical Approach

In patients with a history of cardiac surgery, pericardial adhesions can be a significant limitation to obtaining epicardial access for catheter ablation procedures. In these cases, surgical epicardial access is a feasible strategy with outcomes similar to standard VT catheter ablation procedures.[32] Importantly, owing to technical and anatomic factors, in patients with previous cardiac surgery, the area of exposure via surgical access can be more limited compared to patients with no prior pericardial interventions. For this reason, it is important to consider surface ECG and imaging features of the VT to determine the best surgical approach, either via subxiphoid (for inferior and inferolateral access) or lateral thoracotomy (for anterior and anterolateral access) to facilitate the best chance for ablation success.

Surgical cardiac sympathetic denervation is a procedure in which the lower one-half of the stellate ganglia and the T2 to T4 ganglia of the thoracic sympathetic chain are resected via a video-assisted thoracoscopic approach. This therapy has been utilized for congenital arrhythmogenic conditions such as long QT syndrome[33] or catecholaminergic polymorphic VT.[34] This has also demonstrated efficacy in management of refractory ventricular arrhythmias, with significant reductions in arrhythmia burden and ICD therapies.[35] Observational data for refractory VT suggest that bilateral stellate ganglia resection may be more effective than is unilateral.[36] In patients with VT refractory to medications or catheter ablation, sympathetic denervation carries a class IIb recommendation.[1]

Finally, advanced heart failure treatment options may also be considered for those with refractory ventricular arrhythmias, such as left ventricular assist devices or orthotopic heart transplant. Temporary support with extracorporeal membrane oxygenation may also be used as a bridge to more definitive therapy such as durable mechanical support device or cardiac transplantation.

EMERGING THERAPIES AND FUTURE DIRECTIONS

An emerging therapy for VT employs the use of radiation therapy to perform substrate modification in a noninvasive manner for the reduction of ventricular arrhythmias. This treatment modality has demonstrated promise in a small number of patients.[37] Whether this or other noninvasive therapies can be applied in a broader selection of patients will require further study.

KEY POINTS

- ✔ Wide complex tachycardia is most often due to VT, especially in patients with structural heart disease.
- ✔ Management of VT should focus on airway and circulatory support, with prompt cardioversion indicated as per advanced cardiac life support guidelines.
- ✔ Long-term treatment options for VT include antiarrhythmic medications, catheter ablation, and surgical intervention.
- ✔ Autonomic modulation can provide marked reduction in VT episodes in patients with otherwise refractory ventricular arrhythmias.

REFERENCES

1. Al-Khatib SM, Stevenson WG, Ackerman MJ, et al. 2017 AHA/ACC/HRS Guideline for management of patients with ventricular arrhythmias and the prevention of sudden cardiac death: executive summary: a report of the American College of Cardiology/American Heart Association Task Force on Clinical Practice Guidelines and the Heart Rhythm Society. *J Am Coll Cardiol.* 2017. 2018 Oct 2;72(14):e91-220.
2. Cronin EM, Bogun FM, Maury P, et al. 2019 HRS/EHRA/APHRS/LAHRS expert consensus statement on catheter ablation of ventricular arrhythmias. *Heart Rhythm.* 2019;1(8):1143-1144.
3. Stevenson WG, Friedman PL, Sager PT, et al. Exploring postinfarction reentrant ventricular tachycardia with entrainment mapping. *J Am Coll Cardiol.* 1997;29:1180-1189.
4. Hamer AW, Rubin SA, Peter T, Mandel WJ. Factors that predict syncope during ventricular tachycardia in patients. *Am Heart J.* 1984;107:997-1005.
5. Brugada P, Brugada J, Mont L, Smeets J, Andries EW. A new approach to the differential diagnosis of a regular tachycardia with a wide QRS complex. *Circulation.* 1991;83:1649-1659.
6. Vereckei A, Duray G, Szenasi G, Altemose GT, Miller JM. New algorithm using only lead aVR for differential diagnosis of wide QRS complex tachycardia. *Heart Rhythm.* 2008;5:89-98.
7. Ortiz M, Martin A, Arribas F, et al. Randomized comparison of intravenous procainamide vs. intravenous amiodarone for the acute treatment of tolerated wide QRS tachycardia: the PROCAMIO study. *Eur Heart J.* 2017;38:1329-1335.
8. Yoshie K, Tomita T, Takeuchi T, et al. Renewed impact of lidocaine on refractory ventricular arrhythmias in the amiodarone era. *Int J Cardiol.* 2014;176:936-940.
9. Tung R, Bauer B, Schelbert H, et al. Incidence of abnormal positron emission tomography in patients with unexplained cardiomyopathy and ventricular arrhythmias: The potential role of occult inflammation in arrhythmogenesis. *Heart Rhythm.* 2015;12:2488-2498.
10. Enriquez A, Baranchuk A, Briceno D, Saenz L, Garcia F. How to use the 12-lead ECG to predict the site of origin of idiopathic ventricular arrhythmias. *Heart Rhythm.* 2019;16:1538-1544.
11. Josephson ME, Callans DJ. Using the twelve-lead electrocardiogram to localize the site of origin of ventricular tachycardia. *Heart Rhythm.* 2005;2:443-446.
12. Bardy GH, Lee KL, Mark DB, et al. Amiodarone or an implantable cardioverter-defibrillator for congestive heart failure. *N Engl J Med.* 2005; 352:225-237.
13. Moss AJ, Zareba W, Hall WJ, et al. Prophylactic implantation of a defibrillator in patients with myocardial infarction and reduced ejection fraction. *N Engl J Med.* 2002;346:877-883.
14. Poole JE, Johnson GW, Hellkamp AS, et al. Prognostic importance of defibrillator shocks in patients with heart failure. *N Engl J Med.* 2008;359:1009-1017.
15. Wathen MS, DeGroot PJ, Sweeney MO, et al. Prospective randomized multicenter trial of empirical antitachycardia pacing versus shocks for spontaneous rapid ventricular tachycardia in patients with implantable cardioverter-defibrillators: Pacing Fast Ventricular Tachycardia Reduces Shock Therapies (PainFREE Rx II) trial results. *Circulation.* 2004;110:2591-2596.
16. Effect of prophylactic amiodarone on mortality after acute myocardial infarction and in congestive heart failure: meta-analysis of individual data from 6500 patients in randomised trials. Amiodarone Trials Meta-Analysis Investigators. *Lancet.* 1997;350:1417-1424.
17. Connolly SJ, Dorian P, Roberts RS, et al. Comparison of beta-blockers, amiodarone plus beta-blockers, or sotalol for prevention of shocks from implantable cardioverter defibrillators: the OPTIC Study: a randomized trial. *JAMA.* 2006;295:165-171.
18. Pacifico A, Hohnloser SH, Williams JH, et al. Prevention of implantable-defibrillator shocks by treatment with sotalol. d,l-Sotalol Implantable Cardioverter-Defibrillator Study Group. *N Engl J Med.* 1999;340: 1855-1862.
19. Podrid PJ, Lown B. Mexiletine for ventricular arrhythmias. *Am J Cardiol.* 1981;47:895-902.
20. Bunch TJ, Mahapatra S, Murdock D, et al. Ranolazine reduces ventricular tachycardia burden and ICD shocks in patients with drug-refractory ICD shocks. *Pacing Clin Electrophysiol.* 2011;34:1600-1606.
21. Baquero GA, Banchs JE, Depalma S, et al. Dofetilide reduces the frequency of ventricular arrhythmias and implantable cardioverter defibrillator therapies. *J Cardiovasc Electrophysiol.* 2012;23:296-301.
22. Echt DS, Liebson PR, Mitchell LB, et al. Mortality and morbidity in patients receiving encainide, flecainide, or placebo. The Cardiac Arrhythmia Suppression Trial. *N Engl J Med.* 1991;324:781-788.
23. Lee GK, Klarich KW, Grogan M, Cha YM. Premature ventricular contraction-induced cardiomyopathy: a treatable condition. *Circ Arrhythm Electrophysiol.* 2012;5:229-236.

24. Delacretaz E, Brenner R, Schaumann A, et al. Catheter ablation of stable ventricular tachycardia before defibrillator implantation in patients with coronary heart disease (VTACH): an on-treatment analysis. *J Cardiovasc Electrophysiol.* 2013;24:525-529.
25. Sapp JL, Wells GA, Parkash R, et al. Ventricular tachycardia ablation versus escalation of antiarrhythmic drugs. *N Engl J Med.* 2016;375:111-121.
26. Di Biase L, Burkhardt JD, Lakkireddy D, et al. Ablation of stable VTs versus substrate ablation in ischemic cardiomyopathy: the VISTA randomized multicenter trial. *J Am Coll Cardiol.* 2015;66:2872-2882.
27. Marchlinski F, Garcia F, Siadatan A, et al. Ventricular tachycardia/ventricular fibrillation ablation in the setting of ischemic heart disease. *J Cardiovasc Electrophysiol.* 2005;16(suppl 1):S59-S70.
28. Boyle NG, Shivkumar K. Epicardial interventions in electrophysiology. *Circulation.* 2012;126:1752-1769.
29. Berruezo A, Mont L, Nava S, Chueca E, Bartholomay E, Brugada J. Electrocardiographic recognition of the epicardial origin of ventricular tachycardias. *Circulation.* 2004;109:1842-1847.
30. Valles E, Bazan V, Marchlinski FE. ECG criteria to identify epicardial ventricular tachycardia in nonischemic cardiomyopathy. *Circ Arrhythm Electrophysiol.* 2010;3:63-71.
31. Zhu C, Hanna P, Rajendran PS, Shivkumar K. Neuromodulation for ventricular tachycardia and atrial fibrillation: a clinical scenario-based review. *JACC Clin Electrophysiol.* 2019;5:881-896.
32. Li A, Hayase J, Do D, et al. Hybrid surgical versus percutaneous access epicardial ventricular tachycardia ablation. *Heart Rhythm.* 2018;15(4):512-519.
33. Moss AJ, McDonald J. Unilateral cervicothoracic sympathetic ganglionectomy for the treatment of long QT interval syndrome. *N Engl J Med.* 1971;285:903-904.
34. Wilde AA, Bhuiyan ZA, Crotti L, et al. Left cardiac sympathetic denervation for catecholaminergic polymorphic ventricular tachycardia. *N Engl J Med.* 2008;358:2024-2029.
35. Ajijola OA, Lellouche N, Bourke T, et al. Bilateral cardiac sympathetic denervation for the management of electrical storm. *J Am Coll Cardiol.* 2012;59:91-92.
36. Vaseghi M, Barwad P, Malavassi Corrales FJ, et al. Cardiac sympathetic denervation for refractory ventricular arrhythmias. *J Am Coll Cardiol.* 2017;69:3070-3080.
37. Cuculich PS, Schill MR, Kashani R, et al. Noninvasive cardiac radiation for ablation of ventricular tachycardia. *N Engl J Med.* 2017;377:2325-2336.

CHAPTER 58

ANTIARRHYTHMIC DRUGS

Aadhavi Sridharan and Noel G. Boyle

INTRODUCTION

Antiarrhythmic drugs are pharmacologic agents that primarily affect specific ion channel activity, thereby altering membrane conductance and ultimately the cardiac action potential. The goal of antiarrhythmic drug therapy is to restore and maintain sinus rhythm and to prevent recurrence of arrhythmias.[1] Antiarrhythmic agents were the mainstay of treatment for arrhythmias until the advent of implantable cardioverter defibrillators (ICDs) and catheter ablation in the 1980s. Despite these advances, antiarrhythmic drug therapy still plays a central role in the management of patients with arrhythmias, often in combination with other treatment modalities. A detailed understanding of the underlying mechanism of action, side-effect profile, and potential proarrhythmic effects of these drugs is therefore critical for their safe and appropriate use in clinical practice.[2] This chapter first reviews the anatomy of the cardiac electrical conduction system and the cardiac action potential, and then describes the mechanisms of action, side-effect profiles, and proarrhythmic potential of various antiarrhythmic agents.

ANATOMY OF THE CARDIAC ELECTRICAL CONDUCTION SYSTEM

The electrical impulse of each heartbeat originates in the sinoatrial (SA) node, located in the superior aspect of the right atrium (**Figure 58.1**). SA nodal cells are specialized pacemaker cells that are able to spontaneously generate rhythmic impulses and typically comprise the natural pacemaker of the heart. This impulse then travels radially to the left atrium as well as inferiorly to reach the atrioventricular (AV) node located in the posteroinferior region of the interatrial septum, near the opening of the coronary sinus. The AV node consists of highly specialized conducting cells that conduct the electrical impulse from the atria to the ventricles and can significantly slow the conduction of rapid electrical impulses as in atrial flutter (AFL) or atrial fibrillation (AF), a property known as decremental conduction. The impulse then reaches the bundle of His at the base of the ventricles and travels rapidly down the right and left bundle branches in the interventricular septum. The left bundle branch further separates into the left anterior and left posterior fascicles. The bundle branches ultimately terminate into numerous Purkinje fibers, which then stimulate small areas of the myocardium to contract. The AV node and His-Purkinje systems are latent pacemakers and may exhibit automaticity if the SA node is suppressed.[3,4]

This organization of the cardiac electrical conduction system allows for the sequential contraction of the atria followed by the ventricles with each heartbeat. Decremental conduction through the AV node ensures atrial contraction with complete emptying of the atria and occurs before the electrical impulse reaches the ventricles. Rapid conduction of the electrical impulse through the His-Purkinje fibers then allows for brisk and synchronous contraction of the ventricles beginning at the apex of the heart.

CARDIAC ACTION POTENTIAL

Understanding the mechanism of action of antiarrhythmic drugs requires a fundamental knowledge of the cardiac action potential. The cardiac action potential is a brief change in voltage across the cell membrane of myocytes; this is achieved through a complex, coordinated change in permeability of sodium (Na^+), potassium (K^+), and calcium (Ca^{2+}) ions through different types of ion channels.

The action potential in a typical ventricular myocyte is divided into five phases, named phase 0 through phase 4 (**Figures** 58.1 and **58.2**). During phase 4, also termed the resting phase, there is a higher concentration of Na^+ and Ca^{2+} outside the cell than inside and a higher concentration of K^+ inside the cells than outside. During this phase, the membrane is impermeable to Na^+ and Ca^{2+}, but there is an abundance of open K^+ channels allowing slow leakage of K^+ out of the cell, thus maintaining the membrane potential at approximately −90 mV, near the equilibrium potential of K^+. When these resting myocytes reach a threshold voltage of approximately −70 mV, they enter phase 0.

The most common stimulus that raises the resting transmembrane potential to the threshold voltage is the depolarization of a nearby myocyte, thus spreading the wave of depolarization across the myocardium one cell at a time. During phase 0, also known as rapid depolarization, there is a transient increase in Na^+ conductance through voltage-dependent fast sodium channels and cessation of K^+ current. This results in a positive membrane potential closer to the equilibrium potential of Na^+. Phase 1 represents an initial, rapid repolarization phase that is caused by a transient outward K^+ current through rapidly activating K^+ channels. During phase 2, also termed the plateau phase, there is inward Ca^{2+} current through the

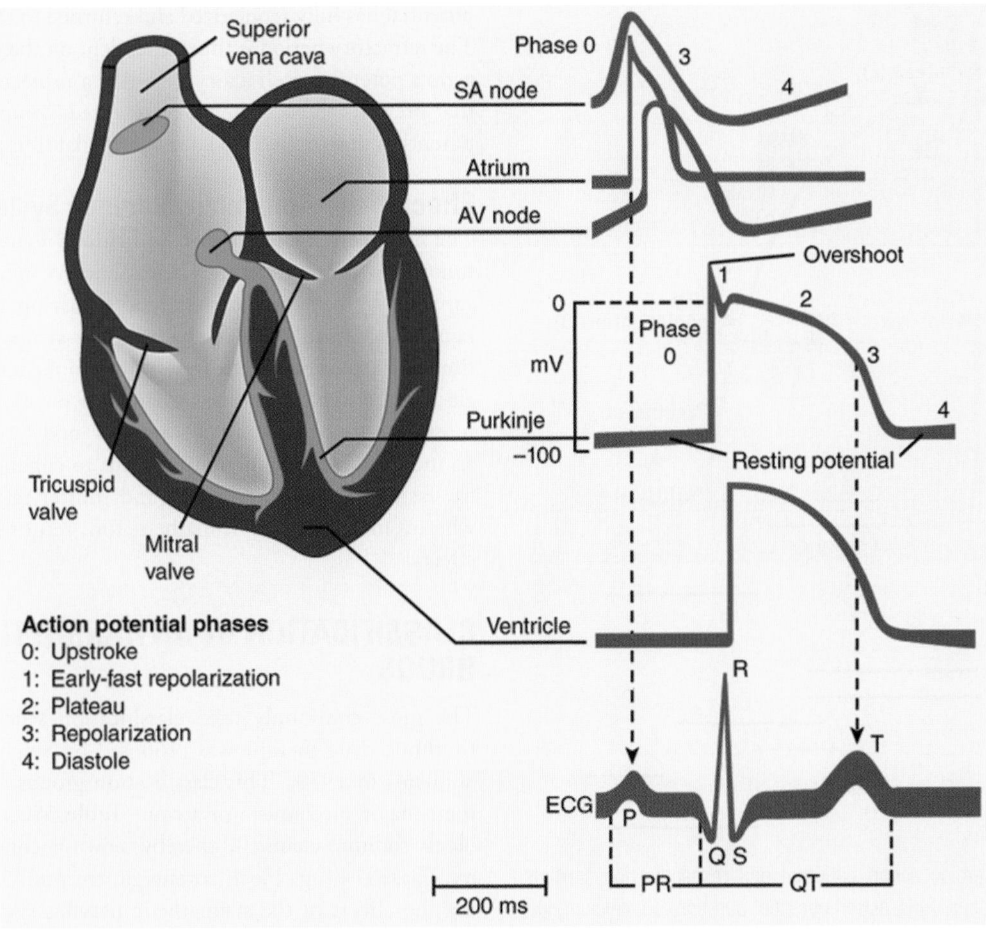

FIGURE 58.1 Schematic representation of the heart, electrical conduction system, and representative cardiac action potentials of various myocardial cells. AV, atrioventricular; SA, sinoatrial. (Republished with permission of McGraw Hill LLC from Antiarrhythmic Drugs. In: Katzung BG, Kruidering-Hall M, Trevor AJ, eds. *Katzung & Trevor's Pharmacology: Examination & Board Review.* 12th ed. New York, NY: McGraw-Hill, 2019:122-133; permission conveyed through Copyright Clearance Center, Inc.)

L-type calcium channels that are activated when the membrane potential depolarizes to −40 mV. Inward Ca^{2+} currents and outward K^+ currents are relatively balanced during this plateau phase. Phase 3 is the repolarization phase during which there is cessation of Ca^{2+} movement and increase in outward K^+ current through several (at least six) different potassium channels.[3-6]

In pacemaker cells such as in the SA node, the action potential typically consists of three phases (Figure 58.1). During phase 4, there is no true resting membrane potential. Rather there is spontaneous depolarization because of slow, inward Na^+ current through "funny" channels and inward Ca^{2+} current through T-type calcium channels. This is followed by depolarization in phase 0 once the membrane potential reaches approximately −40 to −30 mV; depolarization is primarily because of inward Ca^{2+} current through L-type calcium channels. Repolarization in phase 3 occurs mainly because of outward, hyperpolarizing K^+ currents, which brings the membrane potential back to −60 mV.[7] Thus, unlike in non-pacemaker cardiac action potentials, there is no contribution from fast sodium channel in SA nodal cells, resulting in a slower rate of depolarization (ie, slope of phase 0). The cardiac action potential in various other myocardial cells is depicted in Figure 58.1.

Conduction Velocity

The speed of depolarization of a myocyte determines the rate at which its neighboring myocyte is stimulated to depolarize, thereby determining the speed of propagation of the electrical impulse through myocardial tissue. Therefore, the slope of phase 0 determines the conduction velocity of the action potential through the myocardium. Conduction velocity is fastest in the Purkinje system and slowest in the AV node to allow for ventricular filling.[4]

Refractory Period

Once an action potential is initiated in a myocyte, during the time of phases 0, 1, 2, and most of phase 3, the cell is unable to initiate another action potential; this period of time is termed the refractory period. In other words, the refractory period of an excitable cell refers to the period of time during which it is unable to respond to or propagate a second stimulus. This is due to ion channels that remain inactive until the membrane

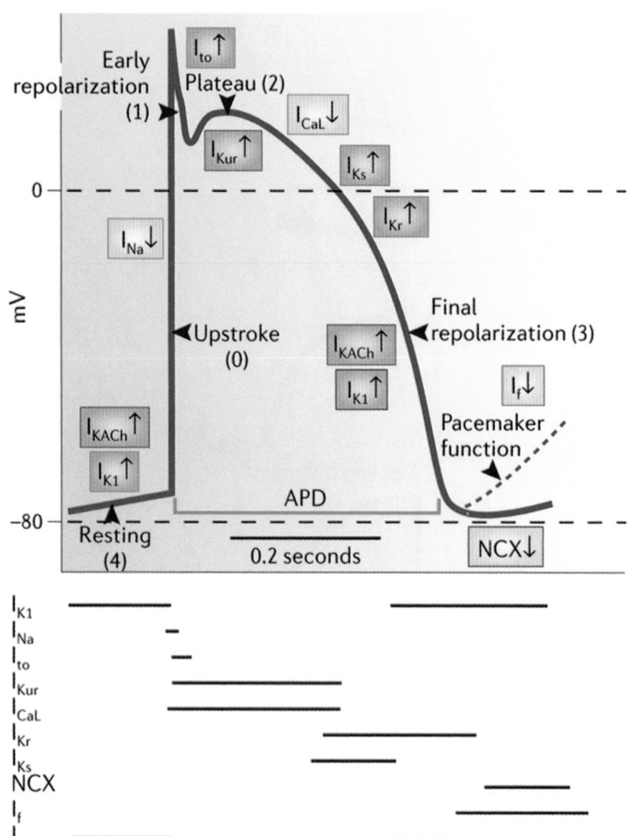

FIGURE 58.2 Cardiac action potential and respective ion currents during various phases. APD, action potential duration; Ca, calcium; I(K-ACh), acetylcholine-regulated K current; I(CaL), L-type Ca-channel current; I(f) = "funny" pacemaker current; I(Kr), rapid delayed-rectified current, I(Ks), slow delayed rectifier current; I(Kur), ultra-rapid delayed-rectifier current, I(to), transient outward current; K, potassium; Na, sodium; NCX, Na/Ca-exchanger. (Reprinted by permission from Nature: Nattel S, Carlsson L. Innovative approaches to anti-arrhythmic drug therapy. *Nat Rev Drug Discov.* 2006;5(12):1034-1049. Copyright © 2006 Springer Nature.)

potential has fully repolarized and returned to the resting state. The refractory period is thus dependent on the duration of the action potential. Refractory period is a protective mechanism that prevents the occurrence of repeated, compounded action potentials that can lead to poor ventricular filling and ejection.[4]

Effect of the Autonomic Nervous System

The heart is richly innervated and closely regulated by the autonomic nervous system.[8] The SA and AV nodes are directly supplied by both sympathetic and parasympathetic nerve fibers. In contrast, there is much greater sympathetic innervation than parasympathetic innervation in the rest of the cardiac electrical system. Therefore, change in parasympathetic tone most directly affects the SA and AV nodal tissues. Overall, an increase in sympathetic tone leads to enhanced automaticity, faster conduction velocity, and shorter refractory period, whereas increased parasympathetic tone results in the opposite effects.

CLASSIFICATION OF ANTIARRHYTHMIC DRUGS

The most commonly used classification scheme for antiarrhythmic drug therapy was proposed by Singh and Vaughan Williams in 1970.[9] This classification groups drugs based on their major mechanism of action (**Table 58.1**). Class I drugs block sodium channels, thereby slowing conduction velocity; Class II drugs block adrenergic receptors, thereby blunting the effects of the sympathetic nervous system on cardiac electrophysiology; Class III drugs block potassium channels, thereby increasing the refractory period; and Class IV drugs block calcium channels, thereby affecting nodal cells that are depolarized mainly via calcium currents. **Figure 58.3** is a schematic that demonstrates the effect of these agents on the cardiac action potential. Critics of this classification system argue that some drugs can affect multiple ion channels, thus having

TABLE 58.1 Singh-Vaughan Williams Classification of Antiarrhythmic Drugs

Class	Drug(s)	Clinical Use	Major Adverse Effects
Ia (sodium channel blocker, intermediate kinetics; potassium channel blocker)	Quinidine, Procainamide, Disopyramide	AF and ventricular arrhythmias	QT prolongation, torsades de pointes Procainamide: Lupus-like syndrome
Ib (sodium channel blocker, fast kinetics)	Lidocaine, Mexiletine	Ventricular arrhythmias (especially ischemic)	Neurologic (tremor, drowsiness, seizures, coma) and gastrointestinal (nausea) effects
Ic (sodium channel blocker, slow kinetics)	Flecainide, Propafenone	PSVT, AF, ventricular arrhythmias in the absence of structural heart disease	Proarrhythmic potential in causing reentrant VT
II (beta-adrenoceptor blockers)	Propranolol, Nadolol, Metoprolol, Esmolol, and many others	Ventricular rate control in SVT, AF, AFL, and ventricular arrhythmia in CPVT and LQTS	Beta-adrenergic blocking effects (bronchospasm, bradycardia, fatigue)

(*Continued*)

TABLE 58.1 Singh-Vaughan Williams Classification of Antiarrhythmic Drugs (*Continued*)

III (potassium channel blockers)	Amiodarone (also has Class I, II, and IV properties)	Atrial and ventricular arrhythmias	Thyroid, pulmonary, hepatic, cutaneous, and neurologic side effects
	Dronedarone	AF	Increases mortality in heart failure and permanent AF
	Sotalol (also has Class II properties)	AF, ventricular arrhythmias	QT prolongation, torsades de pointes
	Dofetilide	AF	QT prolongation, torsades de pointes
	Ibutilide	Acute treatment of AF conversion	QT prolongation, torsades de pointes
IV (calcium channel blockers)	Verapamil, Diltiazem	Ventricular rate control in SVT, AF, AFL	Hypotension, negative inotropic effect, bradycardia
Others	Adenosine	Acute treatment of AV node-dependent arrhythmias	Risk of transient asystole
	Digoxin	Ventricular rate control in AF	Common gastrointestinal and neurologic side effects

AF, atrial fibrillation; AFL, atrial flutter; AV, atrioventricular; CPVT, catecholaminergic polymorphic ventricular tachycardia; LQTS, long QT syndrome; PSVT, paroxysmal supraventricular tachycardia; SVT, supraventricular tachycardia; VT, ventricular tachycardia.

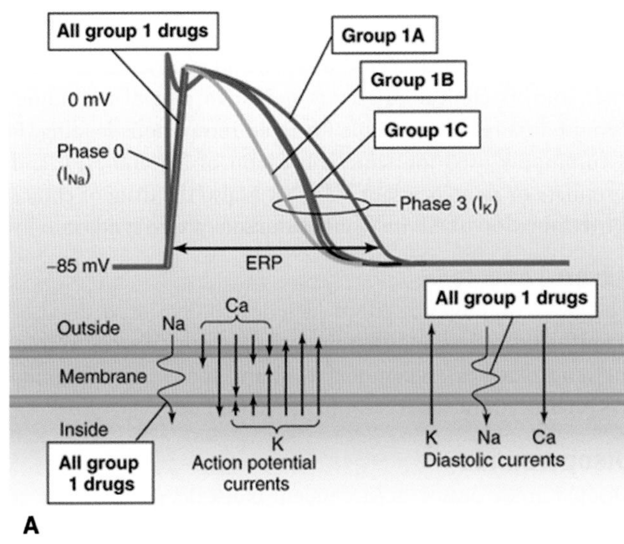

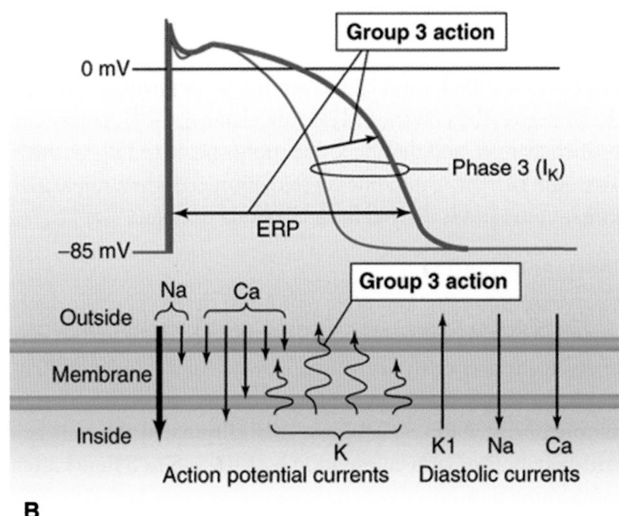

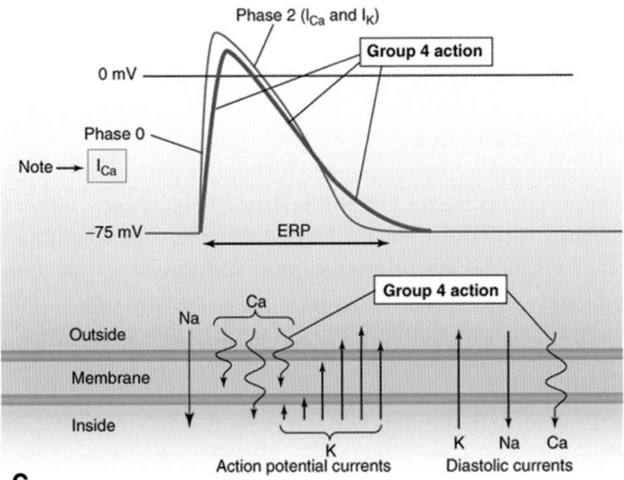

FIGURE 58.3 Schematic diagram depicting the effects of Class **(A)** I, **(B)** III, and **(C)** IV antiarrhythmic drugs. Ca, calcium; ERP, effective refractory period; K, potassium; and Na, sodium. (Republished with permission of McGraw Hill LLC from Antiarrhythmic Drugs. In: Katzung BG, Kruidering-Hall M, Trevor AJ, eds. *Katzung & Trevor's Pharmacology: Examination & Board Review.* 12th ed. New York, NY: McGraw-Hill, 2019:122-133; permission conveyed through Copyright Clearance Center, Inc.)

mixed effects on the action potential, and drugs within the same class can have clinically distinct effects from one another.

CLASS IA DRUGS

Class IA drugs block the rapid sodium channel at high concentrations, resulting in slowing of the conduction velocity, and moderately block potassium channels at lower concentrations, resulting in longer action potential duration and increase in refractory period. Class IA drugs have intermediate kinetics of onset and offset of action; they bind and unbind from sodium channels more slowly than Class IB agents, but more rapidly than Class IC agents. Because they affect both atrial and ventricular tissue, they have the potential to treat both atrial and ventricular arrhythmias. Because of their effect on potassium channels resulting in prolongation of action potential duration and thus refractory period, these drugs have proarrhythmic potential because of QT prolongation, leading to the potential for early afterdepolarizations and risk of developing a polymorphic ventricular tachycardia (VT) known as torsades de pointes. All Class I drugs also exhibit use dependence such that their sodium channel blocking effects are more pronounced at faster heart rates.[1,2]

Quinidine

Quinidine blocks several channels including the rapid inward sodium channel, the I_{Kr} and I_{to} potassium rectifier channels, and, to a lesser degree, the slow inward calcium channel, the I_{Ks} potassium rectifier channel, and the adenosine triphosphate (ATP)-sensitive potassium current. Quinidine is a stereoisomer of the antimalarial drug quinine and is derived from cinchona tree bark.[10]

Pharmacokinetics

After oral administration, 80% to 90% of the drug is absorbed, reaching peak plasma concentration within 3 to 4 hours. It can be given intravenously if infused slowly. Approximately 80% of quinidine in circulation is protein bound, and it has a large volume of distribution. It is primarily eliminated through hepatic metabolism, and elimination half-life is 5 to 8 hours after oral administration.[1,2,11]

Clinical Use

Quinidine was historically the first medication used to treat both atrial and ventricular arrhythmias and in recent years has found an application in the treatment of Brugada syndrome and short QT syndrome because of its I_{to} (transient outward potassium channel) blockade properties.[11,12] Starting in the 1920s, it was the drug of choice to treat AF, often in conjunction with digoxin, until its proarrhythmic potential was recognized in the 1990s.[13] Quinidine may result in torsades de pointes leading to syncope (quinidine syncope) or sudden cardiac death, and because of its significant side-effect profile and drug-drug interactions, its use in clinical practice has markedly declined in recent years.

Adverse Effects of Quinidine

The most common side effects are gastrointestinal, including diarrhea, nausea, vomiting, abdominal pain, and anorexia. Central nervous system (CNS) toxicity (tinnitus, visual disturbances, confusion, delirium, psychosis) and allergic reactions (rash, fever, hemolytic anemia, and rarely anaphylaxis) are not uncommon. Because quinidine is an inhibitor of the cytochrome P450 enzyme system, it can increase blood levels and potentiate the effect of other drugs including warfarin and flecainide.

Procainamide

Procainamide primarily blocks the inactivated state of I_{Na} and to a lesser extent also blocks I_{Kr} and $I_{K.ATP}$. The electrophysiologic effects and therapeutic uses of procainamide are similar to those of quinidine.[14]

Pharmacokinetics

Procainamide's onset of action is immediate with intravenous infusion and approximately 1 hour after oral administration. Approximately 80% of the oral drug is bioavailable. Elimination half-life of procainamide is 3 to 5 hours, with 50% to 60% of the drug excreted in the urine and 10% to 30% undergoing hepatic metabolism. In the liver, procainamide is acetylated to *N*-acetylprocainamide, an active metabolite with Class III antiarrhythmic properties, which is primarily eliminated by the kidneys with an elimination half-life of 7 to 8 hours (although it can exceed 10 hours if high doses of procainamide are used).[14]

Clinical Use

It can be used to treat reentrant atrial and ventricular arrhythmias, and its clinical efficacy is similar to that of quinidine. Because it is readily available for rapid intravenous loading, it is commonly used for acute conversion of AF and AFL and terminate or slow incessant VTs.[15] It is also the drug of choice for termination of AF in Wolff-Parkinson-White syndrome.[16]

Adverse Effects

The most common side effects include hypotension with intravenous administration, gastrointestinal effects (nausea, vomiting, and diarrhea), agranulocytosis, and lupus. Procainamide has proarrhythmic effects similar to quinidine.

Disopyramide

Disopyramide causes use-dependent block (ie, greater effect at faster rates) of I_{Na}, and also blocks of I_{Kr} and $I_{K.ATP}$, with similar electrophysiologic effects to quinidine. Because of its anticholinergic effects, it can increase SA node discharge rate and shorten AV nodal conduction time and refractoriness when the nodes are under cholinergic (vagal) influence.[1,2,14]

Pharmacokinetics

Oral absorption of disopyramide is high (80%-90%), and peak concentrations are reached within 1 to 2 hours. About 60% of the drug is eliminated by the kidneys, and the remainder is metabolized in the liver; therefore, renal and hepatic dysfunction prolongs its elimination time and requires dose adjustment. The mean elimination half-life is 8 to 9 hours in healthy individuals.[14]

Clinical Use

Similar to quinidine and procainamide, it can be used to treat atrial and ventricular arrhythmias. However, its clinical use has been limited because of its negative inotropic and anticholinergic effects. It is effective in treating premature ventricular contractions (PVCs) and preventing recurrent VT. Although it can also be used to treat AF or AFL, the ventricular rate must be controlled prior to its use to prevent 1:1 AV conduction.[15] It may improve symptoms and reduce left ventricular outflow gradient in hypertrophic cardiomyopathy.[17]

Adverse Effects

Because of its anticholinergic effects, the most common side effects are urinary hesitancy or retention, constipation, dry mouth, and blurred vision. In addition to the proarrhythmic potential similar to quinidine and procainamide, disopyramide can rarely cause cardiovascular collapse in patients with reduced left ventricular systolic function because of its negative inotropic effects.[14]

CLASS IB DRUGS

This class of drugs leads to a decrease in the duration of the action potential and therefore a decrease in the refractory period; they have no effect on the conduction velocity. These drugs have rapid onset and offset kinetics compared to Class IA and Class IC drugs. Because of their limited effect on atrial tissue, they are primarily used to treat ventricular arrhythmias. Class IB agents do not have significant proarrhythmic potential.[1,2]

Lidocaine

Lidocaine blocks I_{Na} in the open and inactivated states. First introduced as a local anesthetic agent in 1948, lidocaine came to be used as an antiarrhythmic drug for the treatment of ventricular arrhythmias during the 1950s.

Pharmacokinetics

Because of extensive first-pass metabolism in the liver leading to unpredictably low plasma levels, lidocaine is administered intravenously. Most (50%-80%) of the drug is protein bound. Hepatic metabolism of the drug depends on hepatic blood flow; severe hepatic dysfunction or poor hepatic blood flow such as in shock states can therefore result in decreased lidocaine metabolism. Its elimination half-life averages 1 to 2 hours in healthy individuals, more than 4 hours in the setting of uncomplicated myocardial infarction, more than 10 hours in the setting of myocardial infarction with heart failure, and even longer in the setting of cardiogenic shock.[18]

Clinical Use

Lidocaine is especially effective against ischemia-related ventricular arrhythmias. Because lidocaine primarily binds to the sodium channel in the inactivated state, it exhibits greater efficacy in ischemic myocardium with reduced membrane potential, which results in delayed recovery of voltage-dependent sodium channel inactivation. Because of its rapid onset of action, it is commonly used in the acute treatment of ventricular arrhythmias.[15] It is generally ineffective for treatment of supraventricular arrhythmias.

Adverse Effects

Dose-related adverse effects are due to CNS toxicity such as dizziness, confusion, delirium, coma, seizures, and rarely malignant hyperthermia. Lidocaine does not have any significant proarrhythmic effects.[18]

Mexiletine

An oral analog of lidocaine, mexiletine has similar electrophysiologic properties and side-effect profile to that of lidocaine.[2]

Pharmacokinetics

Mexiletine is almost completely absorbed after oral administration and has minimal first-pass hepatic metabolism. Peak plasma levels are reached in 2 to 4 hours, and elimination half-life is 10 hours in healthy individuals and 17 hours in patients after myocardial infarction. It is primarily metabolized in the liver and is 70% protein bound.[18]

Clinical Use

Similar to lidocaine, mexiletine is used in the treatment of ventricular arrhythmias.[15]

Adverse Effects

The most common side effects include CNS (tremor, blurred vision, ataxia) and gastrointestinal (nausea, vomiting, dyspepsia) symptoms. Mexiletine, like lidocaine, does not have significant proarrhythmic effects.

CLASS IC DRUGS

Class IC drugs primarily slow conduction velocity by blocking the rapid sodium channels, and only minimally prolong refractory period. They exhibit slow onset and offset kinetics compared to Class IA and Class IB drugs. Because they have similar effects on atrial and ventricular tissue, they can be used to treat both atrial and ventricular arrhythmias. Because of their effect of slowing conduction velocity with no effect on refractoriness, these drugs have the proarrhythmic potential of causing reentrant ventricular tachyarrhythmias.[1,2]

Flecainide

Flecainide blocks the rapid sodium channel in a use-dependent manner and has significant depressant effect on cardiac systolic performance. As a Class IC agent, flecainide causes a significant slowing in conduction velocity.

Pharmacokinetics

Flecainide is well absorbed after oral administration, and peak plasma concentrations are reached after 2 to 4 hours. It is mostly (70%) metabolized by the liver, and elimination half-life is 12 to 24 hours. Approximately 40% of the drug is protein bound.[19]

Clinical Use

It is effective in terminating and preventing AF and AFL and in suppressing PVCs.[15,19-22]

Adverse Effects

The most important adverse effect of flecainide is related to its proarrhythmic potential causing reentrant VT in patients with underlying structural heart disease. The Cardiac Arrhythmia Suppression Trial (CAST) showed increased mortality with the use of flecainide in patients with recent myocardial infarction.[23] It has a significant negative inotropic effect similar to that of disopyramide; therefore, it should not be used in patients with left ventricular systolic dysfunction. CNS (blurred

SECTION 4

vision, confusion) and gastrointestinal effects have been occasionally reported.[19,20]

Propafenone

Similar to flecainide, propafenone is a potent blocker of the sodium channels, resulting in slower conduction velocity. Additionally, it also has mild beta-blocking properties unlike flecainide, and its negative inotropic effect is less than that of flecainide and disopyramide.[1,2]

Pharmacokinetics

Propafenone is well absorbed from the gastrointestinal tract and reaches peak plasma levels 2 to 3 hours following oral dose. It undergoes extensive first-pass hepatic metabolism, resulting in nonlinear kinetics. As the dose is increased and hepatic metabolism is saturated, a relatively small dosage increase can result in significant increases in plasma drug concentrations. The drug is mostly (>90%) protein bound, with an elimination half-life of 5 to 8 hours.[24]

Clinical Use

It is indicated for the treatment of paroxysmal supraventricular tachycardia (SVT) and AF, and in suppressing spontaneous PVCs as well as nonsustained and sustained VT.[21,22]

Adverse Effects

Side effects are uncommon and include CNS (taste disturbances and blurred vision) and gastrointestinal effects; exacerbation of bronchospastic lung disease may occur because of its mild beta-blocking effects. The proarrhythmic effect of propafenone is less than that of flecainide and occurs more often in patients with a history of sustained VT and depressed left ventricular ejection fraction.[24]

CLASS II DRUGS

This class of drugs includes beta-adrenoceptor blockers that exert their antiarrhythmic effect by competitively blocking adrenergic receptors. Their major electrophysiologic effects are manifested in SA and AV nodal cells (where there is greatest sympathetic innervation). They lead to decrease in automaticity in the SA node and slowing in conduction and prolonged refractoriness in the AV node.[1,2] Cardioselective agents (such as atenolol, esmolol, and metoprolol) primarily block beta-1 receptors in the heart, whereas nonselective agents (such as propranolol and carvedilol) have more systemic effects.

Beta-adrenoceptor Blockers

Pharmacokinetics

Although different beta-blockers have similar pharmacologic effects, their pharmacokinetics vary widely. For instance, propranolol is available in short- and long-acting oral as well as intravenous formulations. Following oral administration, it is almost 100% absorbed but first-pass hepatic clearance reduces its bioavailability to 30%. Esmolol, given intravenously, has a rapid and very short duration of action, is metabolized by erythrocyte esterase, and has an elimination half-life of 9 minutes. It is therefore most useful in clinical settings where immediate beta-blockade effect is required.

Clinical Use

Beta-adrenoceptor blockers are particularly efficacious in treating tachyarrhythmias that include the SA or AV nodes within the reentrant pathway such as AV nodal reentrant tachycardia and AV reciprocating tachycardia. In atrial tachycardia, AF, and AFL, they can be effective in controlling the ventricular rate by allowing fewer impulses to be conducted to the ventricles by increasing AV nodal conduction time and refractoriness. Beta-blockers are also useful in the treatment of catecholamine-dependent or ischemia-related ventricular arrhythmias.[15,21,22]

Adverse Effects

Adverse effects are directly related to adrenergic blockade and include bradycardia, bronchospasm, Raynaud phenomenon, fatigue, sexual dysfunction, and mental depression.[1,2]

CLASS III DRUGS

Class III drugs predominantly exert their effect by blocking potassium channels and thus prolong repolarization, action potential duration, and refractory period. These agents exhibit varying degrees of reverse use dependence such that their effect is more pronounced at slower heart rates. Because of this effect, these drugs have the proarrhythmic effect of causing pause-dependent torsades de pointes.[1,2]

Amiodarone

Although amiodarone has predominant potassium channel–blocking effects (by decreasing the transient outward delayed rectifier and inward delayed rectifier currents), it also has inhibitory effects on sodium channels (in the inactivated state), adrenergic receptors, as well as calcium channels.[25,26] Amiodarone is a structural analog of thyroid hormone.

Pharmacokinetics

Amiodarone is variably and unpredictably absorbed, with an oral bioavailability of 30% to 50%. Gastrointestinal absorption is improved if taken with a diet rich in fat, and plasma concentrations peak 3 to 7 hours after a single oral dose. Onset of action is within 1 to 2 hours after intravenous administration and may take 2 to 3 days (or even longer) after oral administration. There is minimal first-pass effect, and it undergoes CYP3A4-mediated hepatic metabolism to desethylamiodarone, which is an active metabolite. It is highly (96%) protein bound and has a large but variable volume of distribution. As it is highly lipophilic and is concentrated in multiple tissues, the elimination half-life is long, typically 50 to 60 days.[25]

Clinical Use

Amiodarone is most commonly used to treat AF, AFL, and ventricular tachyarrhythmias[15,21,22] and rarely used to treat SVT. Amiodarone is the first-line agent in the treatment of ventricular fibrillation (refractory to shock therapy or otherwise), hemodynamically stable VT, and prevention of recurrent VT in patients receiving appropriate defibrillator therapy for ventricular arrhythmias.[27] It is the only antiarrhythmic drug recommended by the American Heart Association in the Advanced Cardiovascular Life Support algorithm. Amiodarone is also commonly used for rhythm control in patients with AF after electrical cardioversion and less commonly to slow rapid ventricular response in patients with AF.

Adverse Effects

Its use is limited because of significant organ toxicity, some of which is due to the iodine contained within the drug. Amiodarone most commonly leads to gastrointestinal (nausea, vomiting, anorexia) and pulmonary adverse effects, but hepatic, thyroid, ocular, cutaneous, and neurologic effects also occur frequently.[28] Although gastrointestinal and pulmonary toxicities were previously reported in up to 15% to 30% of patients receiving high-dose amiodarone therapy, recent findings suggest the incidence is much less (<5%), with lower maintenance doses used in contemporary practice. Adverse effects are more common with long-term therapy, especially at higher dose activity. Most adverse effects are reversible with dose reduction or discontinuation of treatment, although resolution of adverse effects may be slow because of the drug's long half-life. Although amiodarone can result in prolongation of the QT interval, the risk of proarrhythmia with amiodarone is lower compared to other Class III agents. It can cause sinus bradycardia and AV nodal blockade because of its calcium channel blocking activity. Drug interactions are common (with medications such as warfarin, statins, antiretrovirals), and amiodarone can lead to increased serum levels of Class I drugs with concurrent therapy.

Dronedarone

Dronedarone is a noniodinated derivative of amiodarone. Dronedarone blocks the rapid and slow components of the delayed rectifier potassium current, more potently blocks the rapid sodium current than amiodarone, and exhibits similar effects on the L-type calcium current as amiodarone.[29]

Pharmacokinetics

Dronedarone is 70% to 90% absorbed after oral administration, especially if taken with food, reaching peak plasma concentrations within 3 to 4 hours. Unlike the long elimination half-life of amiodarone, dronedarone has an elimination half-life of 13 to 19 hours. Dronedarone is metabolized by and moderately inhibits the activity of the hepatic CYP3A4 system; therefore, it should not be used in combination with medications with similar inhibitory effects on these enzyme complexes.[26,29]

Clinical Use

Dronedarone is used to facilitate cardioversion of AF/AFL or in the maintenance of sinus rhythm after restoration of sinus rhythm.[21]

Adverse Effects

Because of increased risk of mortality, dronedarone should not be used in patients with heart failure[30] or permanent AF as a rate control agent.[31] Side effects include rash, photosensitivity, nausea, diarrhea, and headache; lung and thyroid abnormalities are less common compared to amiodarone, likely because of the absence of the iodine moiety.

Sotalol

Sotalol is a noncardioselective beta-blocker and produces a prolongation of the cardiac action potential in both atrial and ventricular cells. Sotalol blocks the I_{Kr} channel and has beta-blocking properties, which results in a negative inotropic effect.[32]

Pharmacokinetics

Sotalol is well absorbed following oral administration, achieving peak plasma concentrations within 2 to 3 hours. The drug is not metabolized; it is excreted unchanged by the kidneys; therefore, the dosage should be reduced in patients with renal dysfunction. The elimination half-life is 7 to 8 hours.[1,2,33]

Clinical Use

It is indicated in the treatment of AF and significant ventricular arrhythmias. It is used for maintenance of sinus rhythm after cardioversion mainly in patients with AF and underlying coronary artery disease. It can prevent recurrence of sustained VT or ventricular fibrillation, and is second-line therapy to empiric amiodarone. It is typically used as adjunctive therapy to an ICD to reduce the frequency of appropriate shocks or of inappropriate shocks because of supraventricular arrhythmias.[15,21]

Adverse Effects

It leads to a dose-related prolongation of the QT interval and has the proarrhythmic potential of causing torsades de pointes. It displays reverse use dependence; therefore, its effect is more evident at lower heart rates. It has a significant negative inotropic effect because of its beta-blocker properties; therefore, it should not be used in patients with left ventricular systolic dysfunction.[34] Other side effects seen with beta-blockers may also apply to sotalol.

Ibutilide

Ibutilide is a methanesulfonamide derivative with structural similarities to sotalol. It blocks the I_{Kr} channel and also activates a slow inward sodium current.[35]

Pharmacokinetics

Ibutilide is administered intravenously and is extensively metabolized. It is renally cleared, with an average elimination half-life of 6 hours.[35]

Clinical Use

Ibutilide is used for the acute cardioversion of AF and AFL.[21]

Adverse Effects

Like sotalol, it leads to a dose-related prolongation of the QT interval, displays reverse use dependence, and its most serious adverse effect is related to its proarrhythmic potential.[1,2]

Dofetilide

Unlike other Class III drugs, dofetilide is a "pure" Class III agent as its sole electrophysiologic effect is to block the rapid component of I_{Kr}.[36]

Pharmacokinetics

Dofetilide is fully absorbed after oral administration. Although it undergoes both renal and hepatic metabolism, dose adjustment is required in patients with renal dysfunction. The elimination half-life is 8 to 10 hours in healthy individuals.[36]

Clinical Use

It is used for the acute cardioversion of AF and chronic suppression of recurrent AF.[21] It has minimal hemodynamic effects and therefore can be used in patients with heart failure.[37]

Adverse Effects

Like other Class III agents, dofetilide exhibits reverse use dependence and proarrhythmic potential (torsades de pointes); therefore, it should not be used in conjunction with other Class I and Class III antiarrhythmic agents. Its use is also contraindicated with other drugs that increase the plasma concentration of dofetilide (such as verapamil, ketoconazole, and trimethoprim). Noncardiac effects such as headache, gastrointestinal disturbances, sleep disorders, and flu-like symptoms have been reported.[36]

CLASS IV DRUGS

The nondihydropyridine calcium channel blockers (verapamil and diltiazem) exert their effect on the slow calcium channels responsible for the depolarization phase in SA and AV nodal tissues, thus decreasing automaticity and prolonging conduction and refractoriness in these tissues.

Calcium Channel Blockers

Pharmacokinetics

With oral administration, both verapamil and diltiazem are well absorbed but undergo extensive first-pass hepatic metabolism. Both drugs are highly protein bound. The elimination half-life of verapamil is 5 to 12 hours, whereas that of diltiazem is 3.5 hours.

Clinical Use

Calcium channel blockers are most effective in treating arrhythmias that use the SA or AV node within the reentrant circuit. Like Class I agents, these drugs also exhibit use dependence. These drugs are used in the treatment of AV nodal reentrant and reciprocating tachycardias, as well as to control ventricular rates in AF and AFL.

Adverse Effects

Adverse effects include negative inotropic effects, hypotension, and bradycardia, especially when used in conjunction with beta-blockers.[1,2]

UNCLASSIFIED ANTIARRHYTHMIC DRUGS

Adenosine

A naturally occurring purine nucleoside, adenosine interacts with the A1 receptors, which in turn activates potassium channels leading to hyperpolarization of cells.[38] It has a significant, transient effect on SA and AV nodes, manifested as slowing of the SA node and/or high-degree AV block.

Pharmacokinetics

Adenosine is rapidly eliminated from circulation because of uptake into cells and inactivation by adenosine deaminase. Its elimination half-life is less than 10 seconds.

Clinical Use

Adenosine is quite useful in the termination of reentrant tachyarrhythmias involving the AV node. Because of its transient effect, it is useful for the diagnosis, but not treatment, of AF and AFL.

Adverse Effects

Side effects of the drug are also transient and include flushing, dyspnea, chest pressure, and sinus bradycardia or arrest.[39]

Digoxin

A member of the cardiac glycoside family, digoxin exerts its antiarrhythmic effects mainly by increasing central and peripheral vagal tone, as well as by increasing intracellular calcium concentration (by inhibiting the sodium-potassium adenosine triphosphatase, which in turn leads to decreased activity of the sodium-calcium exchanger) leading to increased inotropy.

Pharmacokinetics

Digoxin is well absorbed after oral administration, although absorption varies slightly depending on preparation. When used intravenously, peak effect occurs after 1.5 to 3 hours. It is eliminated unchanged primarily by the kidneys, with an elimination half-life of 36 hours in healthy individuals.

Clinical Use

It is most useful in the treatment of AV nodal reentrant arrhythmias and in controlling the ventricular response in AF and AFL.[21] Because of its narrow therapeutic window, its clinical use has decreased in recent years.[40]

Adverse Effects

Digoxin toxicity results in gastrointestinal (nausea, vomiting, diarrhea, cramps, anorexia), neurologic (visual changes, delirium), and arrhythmic (SA nodal dysfunction, AV block, VT) effects. Hypokalemia worsens the effects of digoxin toxicity. Significant life-threatening arrhythmias related to digoxin toxicity are treated with digoxin-specific antibody.

Ranolazine

Although initially used for the treatment of chronic angina, ranolazine has significant electrophysiologic properties. It inhibits the late sodium current as well as the delayed rectifier current, prolonging the QT interval.[41]

Pharmacokinetics

Peak plasma concentration is obtained 2 to 6 hours after administration, and half-life is about 7 hours. Ranolazine undergoes extensive metabolism in the liver through the cytochrome P450 enzyme system and is mainly excreted through the kidneys.[41]

Clinical Use

Although not approved for use as an antiarrhythmic agent, ranolazine has been shown to be effective in the prevention of AF in patients with acute coronary syndromes, prevention as well as conversion of postoperative AF after cardiac surgery, conversion of recent-onset AF, and maintenance of sinus rhythm in recurrent AF. It has also been shown to reduce VT and drug-refractory ICD shocks.[41]

Adverse Effects

The most common side effects of ranolazine are dizziness, nausea, constipation, and headache. Despite its effect of QT prolongation, ranolazine rarely causes torsades de pointes.[41]

OTHER CLASSIFICATION SCHEMES

Although the Singh-Vaughan Williams classification scheme remains the most commonly used because of its simplicity, it has significant limitations such as oversimplification, grouping drugs with dissimilar effects into the same class, and inability to account for multiple effects of the same drug, some of which were discovered long after the classification system was introduced. Thus, other antiarrhythmic drug classification schemes have since been proposed attempting to overcome the limitations of the Singh-Vaughan Williams classification.

One such classification scheme is the Sicilian Gambit,[42] which takes into account a host of additional factors such as a drug's effect on various channels, receptors, and pumps; effect on second messenger cascades; and other hemodynamic effects (**Figure 58.4**). The Sicilian Gambit is more of a tabular listing of a drug's multitude pharmacologic effects than a true classification system. This scheme thus describes the precise mechanism(s) of action of each drug more thoroughly, allowing for better prediction of the overall pharmacologic effect of any given antiarrhythmic agent. However, because of its inherent complexity and lack of generalizations about antiarrhythmic agents, this scheme is not useful for everyday clinical practice.[43]

A more recent report[44] proposed a modernized, more expanded version of the Singh-Vaughan Williams classification and groups currently available as well as investigational new drugs through their known molecular, ion channel, transporter,

Table 24. The Effects of Antiarrhythmic Drugs on Cardiac Function: Classification of Drugs Proposed by the Members of Sicilian Gambit

Drug	Ion channels						Receptors				Pumps	Clinical efficacy			ECG findings		
	Na			Ca	K	If	α	β	M_2	A_1	Na-K ATPase	LV function	Sinus rhythm	Extra-cardiac	PR	QRS	JT
	Fast	Med	Slow														
Lidocaine	○											→	→	◐			↓
Mexiletine	○											→	→	◐			↓
Procainamide		Ⓐ			◐							↓	→	●	↑	↑	↑
Disopyramide			Ⓐ		◐				○			↓	→	◐	↑↓	↑	↑
Quinidine		Ⓐ			◐		○		○			→	↑	◐	↑↓	↑	↑
Propafenone		Ⓐ						◐				↓	↓	○	↑	↑	
Aprindine		Ⓘ		○	○	○						→	→	◐	↑	↑	→
Cibenzoline			Ⓐ	○	◐				○			↓	→	○	↑	↑	→
Pirmenol			Ⓐ		◐				○			↓	↑	○	↑	↑	↑→
Flecainide			Ⓐ		○							↓	→	○	↑	↑	
Pilsicainide			Ⓐ									↓	→	○	↑	↑	
Bepridil	○			●	◐							?	→	○			↑
Verapamil	○			●			◐					↓	↓	○	↑		
Diltiazem				◐								↓	↓	○	↑		
Sotalol					●			●				↓	↓	○	↑		↑
Amiodarone	○			○	●		◐	◐				→	↓	●	↑		↑
Nifekalant					●							→	→	○			↑
Nadolol								●				↓	↓	○	↑		
Propranolol	○							●				↓	↓	○	↑		
Atropine									●			→	↑	◐	↓		
ATP										■		?	↓	○	↑		
Digoxin									■		●	↑	↓	●	↑		↓

Relative intensity of blockage: ○=low; ◐=moderate; and ●=strong.
A=activated channel blocker, I=inactivated channel blocker, ■=agonist.
ATP, adenosine triphosphate.
Modified from Members of the Sicilian Gambit, Antiarrhythmic therapy: a pathophysiologic approach. New York: Futura Publishing Company, Inc; 1994.

FIGURE 58.4 Sicilian Gambit Classification. (Reprinted by permission from Springer: Lau W, Newman D, Dorian P. Can antiarrhythmic agents be selected based on mechanism of action? *Drugs*. 2000;60(6):1315-1328. Copyright © 2000 Springer Nature.)

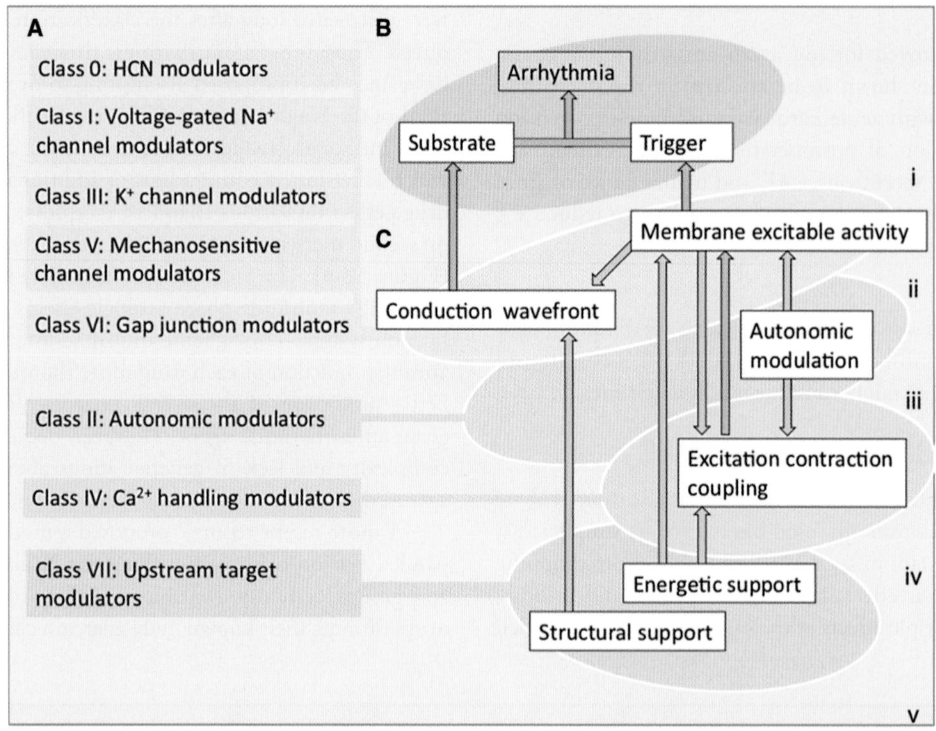

FIGURE 58.5 Modern Oxford Classification of antiarrhythmic drugs, showing correlation between the classes **(A)** and arrhythmia substrate or trigger **(B)**, or the underlying cellular or physiologic cascade **(C)**. Ca^{2+}, calcium; HCN, hyperpolarization-activated cyclic nucleotide gated; K^+, potassium; Na^+, sodium. (From Huang CL, Wu L, Jeevaratnam K, et al. Update on antiarrhythmic drug pharmacology. *J Cardiovasc Electrophysiol.* 2020;31(2):579-592. Reprinted by permission of John Wiley & Sons, Inc.)

receptor, or intracellular cell signaling targets (**Figure 58.5**).[45] While preserving the basic simplicity of the widely accepted classic Vaughan Williams framework, this system also incorporates advances in antiarrhythmic drug therapy over the past half-century and facilitates the addition of novel antiarrhythmic drugs currently under investigation.

CONCLUSIONS

Antiarrhythmic agents still play a critical role in the treatment of arrhythmias, both as lone and hybrid therapy in combination with device and catheter ablation strategies. The decision of when to initiate antiarrhythmic drug therapy depends on the specific arrhythmia and requires careful consideration of patient characteristics, drug interactions, and comorbid conditions. Patients on antiarrhythmic drugs should be closely monitored for evidence of symptom alleviation and side effects.

KEY POINTS

- ✔ Antiarrhythmic drugs play an integral role in the management of arrhythmias, either alone or in combination with device and catheter ablation therapies.
- ✔ An understanding of the cardiac conduction system and cardiac action potential is critical in understanding the effect of antiarrhythmic drugs.
- ✔ The Singh-Vaughan Williams classification of antiarrhythmic drugs groups drugs based on their primary mechanism of action.
- ✔ Antiarrhythmic drugs also have proarrhythmic effects and can potentially result in the development of life-threatening ventricular tachyarrhythmias.
- ✔ Initiation of antiarrhythmic drug therapy therefore necessitates careful consideration of specific patient characteristics, drug and disease interactions, and requires close follow-up for evidence of symptom alleviation and development of adverse effects.

REFERENCES

1. Dan GA, Martinez-Rubio A, Agewall S, et al. Antiarrhythmic drugs-clinical use and clinical decision making: a consensus document from the European Heart Rhythm Association (EHRA) and European Society of Cardiology (ESC) Working Group on Cardiovascular Pharmacology, endorsed by the Heart Rhythm Society (HRS), Asia-Pacific Heart Rhythm Society (APHRS) and International Society of Cardiovascular Pharmacotherapy (ISCP). *Europace.* 2018;20:731an-732an.
2. Mankad P, Kalahasty G. Antiarrhythmic drugs: risks and benefits. *Med Clin North Am.* 2019;103:821-834.
3. Anderson RH, Yanni J, Boyett MR, Chandler NJ, Dobrzynski H. The anatomy of the cardiac conduction system. *Clin Anat.* 2009;22:99-113.
4. Nattel S, Carlsson L. Innovative approaches to anti-arrhythmic drug therapy. *Nat Rev Drug Discov.* 2006;5:1034-1049.

5. Grant AO. Cardiac ion channels. *Circ Arrhythm Electrophysiol.* 2009;2: 185-194.
6. Shah M, Akar FG, Tomaselli GF. Molecular basis of arrhythmias. *Circulation.* 2005;112:2517-2529.
7. Murphy C, Lazzara R. Current concepts of anatomy and electrophysiology of the sinus node. *J Interv Card Electrophysiol.* 2016;46:9-18.
8. Goldberger JJ, Arora R, Buckley U, Shivkumar K. Autonomic nervous system dysfunction: JACC focus seminar. *J Am Coll Cardiol.* 2019;73: 1189-1206.
9. Singh BN, Vaughan Williams EM. A third class of anti-arrhythmic action. Effects on atrial and ventricular intracellular potentials, and other pharmacological actions on cardiac muscle, of MJ 1999 and AH 3474. *Br J Pharmacol.* 1970;39:675-687.
10. Grace AA, Camm AJ. Quinidine. *N Engl J Med.* 1998;338:35-45.
11. Vitali Serdoz L, Rittger H, Furlanello F, Bastian D. Quinidine-A legacy within the modern era of antiarrhythmic therapy. *Pharmacol Res.* 2019;144: 257-263.
12. Sieira J, Dendramis G, Brugada P. Pathogenesis and management of Brugada syndrome. *Nat Rev Cardiol.* 2016;13:744-756.
13. Coplen SE, Antman EM, Berlin JA, Hewitt P, Chalmers TC. Efficacy and safety of quinidine therapy for maintenance of sinus rhythm after cardioversion. A meta-analysis of randomized control trials. *Circulation.* 1990;82: 1106-1116.
14. Ribeiro C, Longo A. Procainamide and disopyramide. *Eur Heart J.* 1987; 8(suppl A):11-19.
15. Al-Khatib SM, Stevenson WG, Ackerman MJ, et al. 2017 AHA/ACC/HRS guideline for management of patients with ventricular arrhythmias and the prevention of sudden cardiac death: executive summary: a report of the American College of Cardiology/American Heart Association Task Force on Clinical Practice Guidelines and the Heart Rhythm Society. *Heart Rhythm.* 2018;15:e190-e252.
16. Boahene KA, Klein GJ, Sharma AD, Yee R, Fujimura O. Value of a revised procainamide test in the Wolff-Parkinson-White syndrome. *Am J Cardiol.* 1990;65:195-200.
17. Sherrid MV, Barac I, McKenna WJ, et al. Multicenter study of the efficacy and safety of disopyramide in obstructive hypertrophic cardiomyopathy. *J Am Coll Cardiol.* 2005;45:1251-1258.
18. Rizzon P, Di Biase M, Favale S, Visani L. Class 1B agents lidocaine, mexiletine, tocainide, phenytoin. *Eur Heart J.* 1987;8(suppl A):21-25.
19. Paolini E, Stronati G, Guerra F, Capucci A. Flecainide: electrophysiological properties, clinical indications, and practical aspects. *Pharmacol Res.* 2019;148:104443.
20. Salvage SC, Chandrasekharan KH, Jeevaratnam K, et al. Multiple targets for flecainide action: implications for cardiac arrhythmogenesis. *Br J Pharmacol.* 2018;175:1260-1278.
21. January CT, Wann LS, Alpert JS, et al. 2014 AHA/ACC/HRS guideline for the management of patients with atrial fibrillation: a report of the American College of Cardiology/American Heart Association Task Force on Practice Guidelines and the Heart Rhythm Society. *J Am Coll Cardiol.* 2014;64:e1-e76.
22. Page RL, Joglar JA, Caldwell MA, et al. 2015 ACC/AHA/HRS Guideline for the management of adult patients with supraventricular tachycardia: a report of the American College of Cardiology/American Heart Association Task Force on Clinical Practice Guidelines and the Heart Rhythm Society. *J Am Coll Cardiol.* 2016;67:e27-e115.
23. Echt DS, Liebson PR, Mitchell LB, et al. Mortality and morbidity in patients receiving encainide, flecainide, or placebo. The cardiac arrhythmia suppression trial. *N Engl J Med.* 1991;324:781-788.
24. Funck-Brentano C, Kroemer HK, Lee JT, Roden DM. Propafenone. *N Engl J Med.* 1990;322:518-525.
25. Hamilton D Sr, Nandkeolyar S, Lan H, et al. Amiodarone: a comprehensive guide for clinicians. *Am J Cardiovasc Drugs.* 2020;20(6):549-558.
26. Vamos M, Hohnloser SH. Amiodarone and dronedarone: an update. *Trends Cardiovasc Med.* 2016;26:597-602.
27. Dorian P, Cass D, Schwartz B, Cooper R, Gelaznikas R, Barr A. Amiodarone as compared with lidocaine for shock-resistant ventricular fibrillation. *N Engl J Med.* 2002;346:884-890.
28. Epstein AE, Olshansky B, Naccarelli GV, Kennedy JI Jr, Murphy EJ, Goldschlager N. Practical management guide for clinicians who treat patients with amiodarone. *Am J Med.* 2016;129:468-475.
29. Patel C, Yan GX, Kowey PR. Dronedarone. *Circulation.* 2009;120: 636-644.
30. Kober L, Torp-Pedersen C, McMurray JJ, et al. Increased mortality after dronedarone therapy for severe heart failure. *N Engl J Med.* 2008; 358:2678-2687.
31. Connolly SJ, Camm AJ, Halperin JL, et al. Dronedarone in high-risk permanent atrial fibrillation. *N Engl J Med.* 2011;365:2268-2276.
32. Hohnloser SH, Woosley RL. Sotalol. *N Engl J Med.* 1994;331:31-38.
33. Kpaeyeh JA Jr, Wharton JM. Sotalol. *Card Electrophysiol Clin.* 2016;8: 437-452.
34. Waldo AL, Camm AJ, deRuyter H, et al. Survival with oral d-sotalol in patients with left ventricular dysfunction after myocardial infarction: rationale, design, and methods (the SWORD trial). *Am J Cardiol.* 1995;75: 1023-1027.
35. Naccarelli GV, Lee KS, Gibson JK, VanderLugt J. Electrophysiology and pharmacology of ibutilide. *Am J Cardiol.* 1996;78:12-16.
36. Shenasa F, Shenasa M. Dofetilide: electrophysiologic effect, efficacy, and safety in patients with cardiac arrhythmias. *Card Electrophysiol Clin.* 2016;8: 423-436.
37. Torp-Pedersen C, Moller M, Bloch-Thomsen PE, et al. Dofetilide in patients with congestive heart failure and left ventricular dysfunction. Danish Investigations of Arrhythmia and Mortality on Dofetilide Study Group. *N Engl J Med.* 1999;341:857-865.
38. Layland J, Carrick D, Lee M, Oldroyd K, Berry C. Adenosine: physiology, pharmacology, and clinical applications. *JACC Cardiovasc Interv.* 2014; 7:581-591.
39. Wilbur SL, Marchlinski FE. Adenosine as an antiarrhythmic agent. *Am J Cardiol.* 1997;79:30-37.
40. Turakhia MP. Digoxin in atrial fibrillation?: leave it out of the medicine cabinet. *J Am Coll Cardiol.* 2018;71:1075-1077.
41. Saad M, Mahmoud A, Elgendy IY, Richard Conti C. Ranolazine in cardiac arrhythmia. *Clin Cardiol.* 2016;39:170-178.
42. The 'Sicilian Gambit'. A new approach to the classification of antiarrhythmic drugs based on their actions on arrhythmogenic mechanisms. The Task Force of the Working Group on Arrhythmias of the European Society of Cardiology. *Eur Heart J.* 1991;12:1112-1131.
43. Garratt CJ, Griffith MJ. The Sicilian gambit: an opening move that loses the game? *Eur Heart J.* 1996;17:341-343.
44. Lei M, Wu L, Terrar DA, Huang CL. Modernized classification of cardiac antiarrhythmic drugs. *Circulation.* 2018;138:1879-1896.
45. Huang CL, Wu L, Jeevaratnam K, Lei M. Update on antiarrhythmic drug pharmacology. *J Cardiovasc Electrophysiol.* 2020;31:579-592.

CHAPTER 59

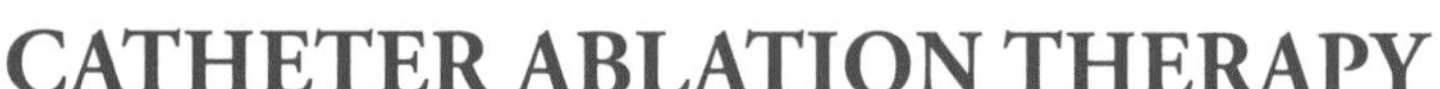

CATHETER ABLATION THERAPY

Darshan Krishnappa and Kalyanam Shivkumar

INTRODUCTION

Cardiac rhythm disorders are a frequent cause of morbidity and mortality occurring in 2% to 3% of the general population, with the prevalence increasing with advanced age and comorbidities such as hypertension, diabetes mellitus, chronic kidney disease, heart failure, and other structural heart diseases.[1] Although pharmacotherapy has long been the mainstay in the management of cardiac arrhythmias, its use is restricted by limited efficacy and side effects leading to an increasing interest in surgical and interventional therapies. Although the era of invasive arrhythmia management was heralded by open surgical approaches, the high rates of morbidity and mortality associated with these procedures led to the development and widespread adoption of percutaneous catheter-based strategies. The safety and efficacy of catheter-based ablation therapies for cardiac arrhythmias has been established in numerous observational, registry-based and randomized controlled studies involving patients of diverse racial and ethnic groups conducted at multiple centers across the world and has become the first-line therapy for several arrhythmias.[2,3]

In this chapter, we will first discuss catheter-based mapping for the diagnosis and localization of arrhythmias followed by a discussion on the energy sources used for catheter ablation of arrhythmias. We will then discuss the current literature on the efficacy and safety of catheter ablation in various cardiac arrhythmias before highlighting the complications associated with these procedures.

FUNDAMENTALS OF CATHETER-BASED MAPPING OF CARDIAC ARRHYTHMIAS

Catheter ablation of cardiac arrhythmias begins with the induction and precise localization of the arrhythmia under investigation so as to maximize procedural success while limiting the amount of cardiac tissue that is ablated/damaged.

Catheters used for electrophysiology (EP) studies and mapping of arrhythmias have electrodes (ranging from four to multiple) at their distal end, which are capable of recording intracardiac electrical signals when placed in contact with excitable cardiac tissue. These diagnostic catheters are capable not only of sensing and recording signals from the heart but also stimulating or pacing the heart. An EP study begins with the placement of these diagnostic catheters (usually quadripolar and decapolar) at strategic locations within the heart—most commonly the high right atrium close to the superior vena cava—right atrial junction, at the atrioventricular (AV) junction where the bundle of His is located, at the right ventricular apex/base or right ventricular outflow tract and within the coronary sinus from where coronary sinus musculature and left atrial signals can be recorded. The electrogram characteristics (timing and morphology) at each of these sites along with a knowledge of fluoroscopic cardiac anatomy aid in the precise placement of these diagnostic catheters (**Figure 59.1**). Signals recorded from these catheters also aid in assessing the conduction properties of the AV conduction axis of the heart.

Pacing maneuvers from these intracardiac catheters are used to induce clinical arrhythmia, and interpretation of information recorded from these catheters placed at several vantage points within the heart (based on the timing of signals recorded by these catheters) during the induced arrhythmia—along with additional diagnostic pacing maneuvers performed during the arrhythmia—aid in its precise diagnosis. Although information from these catheters approximates the likely location of origin of cardiac arrhythmias (focus of origin or location of accessory pathway [AP] or reentrant circuit), a roving diagnostic or ablation catheter is then used for more precise localization.

Three-Dimensional Electroanatomic Mapping Systems

More recently, advances in technology have led to the development of three-dimensional (3D) electroanatomic mapping (EAM) systems—CARTO® (Biosense, Diamond Bar, CA), EnSite NavX® (Abbott, Abbott Park, IL), Rhythmia® (Boston Scientific, Cambridge, MA)—which enable in situ catheter visualization and reconstruction of cardiac chambers (atrial, ventricular, and vascular structures) with the ability to mark or tag the location of various cardiac structures (including the AV, aortic and pulmonary valves; papillary muscles; and the location of the AV conduction axis). The use of 3D EAM systems helps minimize fluoroscopic use and radiation exposure both for the patient and the interventional EP team. These 3D EAM systems are impedance- and/or magnetic-based and utilize electrical fields and magnetic fields, respectively, to precisely localize the position of the diagnostic and ablation catheters. Simultaneously, electrical signals are recorded using these catheters from the different cardiac chambers during sinus rhythm (voltage and activation mapping), during pacing (pace mapping and voltage mapping), and/or during the arrhythmia

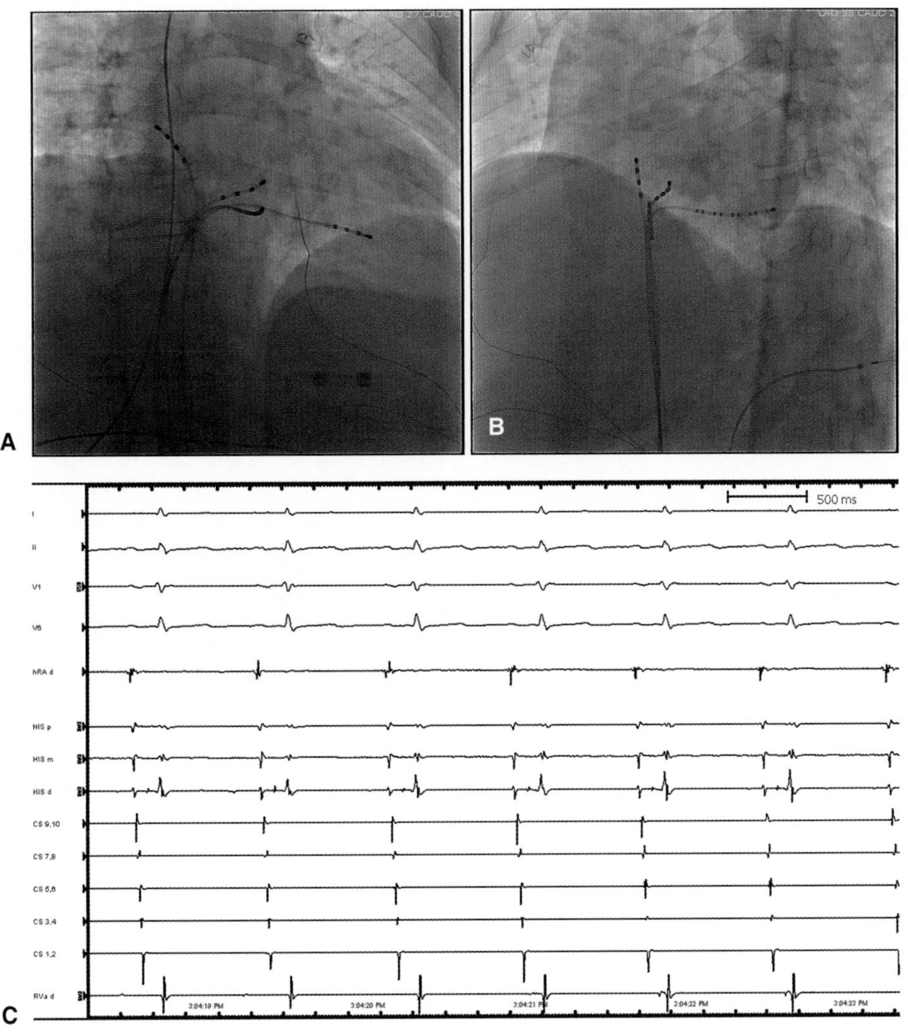

FIGURE 59.1 Right anterior oblique **(A)** and left anterior oblique **(B)** views of catheters placed during a standard EP study. Intracardiac signals **(C)** recorded by these catheters. CS, coronary sinus; EP, electrophysiology; Discovered in 1893 by Swiss-born cardiologist and anatomist Wilhelm His, not an abbreviation hRA, high right atrium; RVa, right ventricular apex.

(activation, voltage, and entrainment mapping). In addition, multielectrode catheters (with electrodes ranging from 20 to 64 per catheter) that are capable of rapidly recording electrical signals simultaneously from multiple areas of the heart permitting the construction of high-density EAMs are now available, thus improving the precision of arrhythmia mapping. The use of preprocedural computerized tomography (CT) or magnetic resonance imaging (MRI) and intraprocedural intracardiac echocardiography and image integration into 3D EAM systems further helps improve the precision of anatomical mapping particularly in patients undergoing ablation of complex arrhythmias including atrial fibrillation (AF) and ventricular arrhythmias (VAs).

Voltage Mapping

Voltage mapping consists of measuring the amplitude of electrical signals recorded from different sites within the chamber of interest to help identify areas of scarring which are often the site of location of critical isthmus of reentrant arrhythmias. Thresholds for normal voltage in the atria and ventricles have been suggested by prior studies, which serve as a guide to identify scarred tissue, though variations are often observed based on differences in myocardial thickness and activation wavefront directionality[4-6] (**Figure 59.2**). Identification of such abnormal tissue helps focus further mapping efforts on specific areas of the heart in an attempt to identify critical sites responsible for cardiac arrhythmia.

Activation Mapping

During activation mapping, signals are recorded from the chamber of interest—the atrium during atrial arrhythmias, atrioventricular nodal reentrant tachycardia (AVNRT) or orthodromic AV reentrant tachycardia (AVRT), and the ventricle during VAs or antidromic AVRT—to determine the pattern of chamber activation during the arrhythmia to identify the site of earliest chamber activation and/or the reentrant circuit responsible for

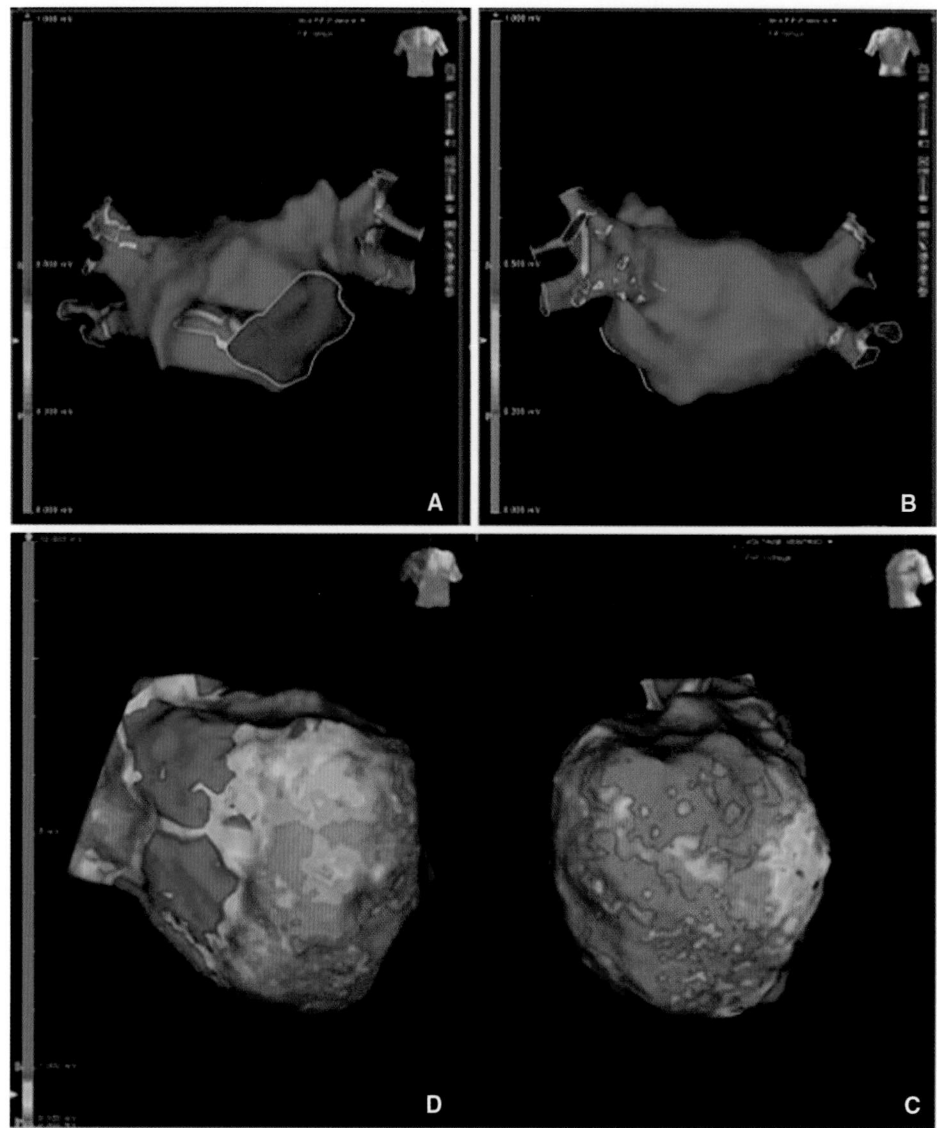

FIGURE 59.2 Voltage mapping during sinus rhythm. Voltage map of the left atrium (LA) during sinus rhythm showing the anterior **(A)** and posterior aspect **(B)** of the LA, respectively. This color-coded map depicts the voltage of the different regions of the LA. The color scale is shown on the left of each image with purple representing areas of normal voltage and gray representing areas of dense scar. Voltage map of the left ventricle (LV) in a patient with ischemic cardiomyopathy and scar-mediated ventricular tachycardia in right anterior oblique **(C)** and left anterior oblique **(D)** views, respectively. The gray areas represent dense scar with a transition (scar border zone) to healthy tissue (purple areas) being represented by other colors in the spectrum of the color scale used.

the arrhythmia. Activation mapping during focal arrhythmias helps identify the site of origin of tachycardia whereas in orthodromic AVRT and antidromic AVRT, the site of earliest chamber activation helps localize the site of attachment of APs which are then targeted for ablation. Activation at successful ablation sites usually precedes the P-wave or QRS complexes (during atrial arrhythmias and VAs) by 30 milliseconds or more. In reentrant tachycardias (atrial flutter and scar-based reentrant ventricular tachycardia [VT]) activation mapping helps identify reentrant circuits, with localization of areas critical for the tachycardia (critical isthmus—typically areas of low-voltage fractionated signals with slow conduction) that are then targeted for ablation (**Figure 59.3**). Although activation mapping helps achieve precise localization of the site of origin of tachycardia, it is not always feasible because several tachycardias (especially VT) are hemodynamically unstable. In such scenarios, other mapping techniques such as pace mapping and voltage mapping are useful.

Pace Mapping

Another useful mapping technique in VAs is pace mapping. During pace mapping, pacing is performed from different sites within the heart, and the QRS morphology during pacing is then compared to that during the arrhythmia to help localize the site of origin (focal arrhythmias) or site of exit (reentrant arrhythmias) of arrhythmias. A pace match greater

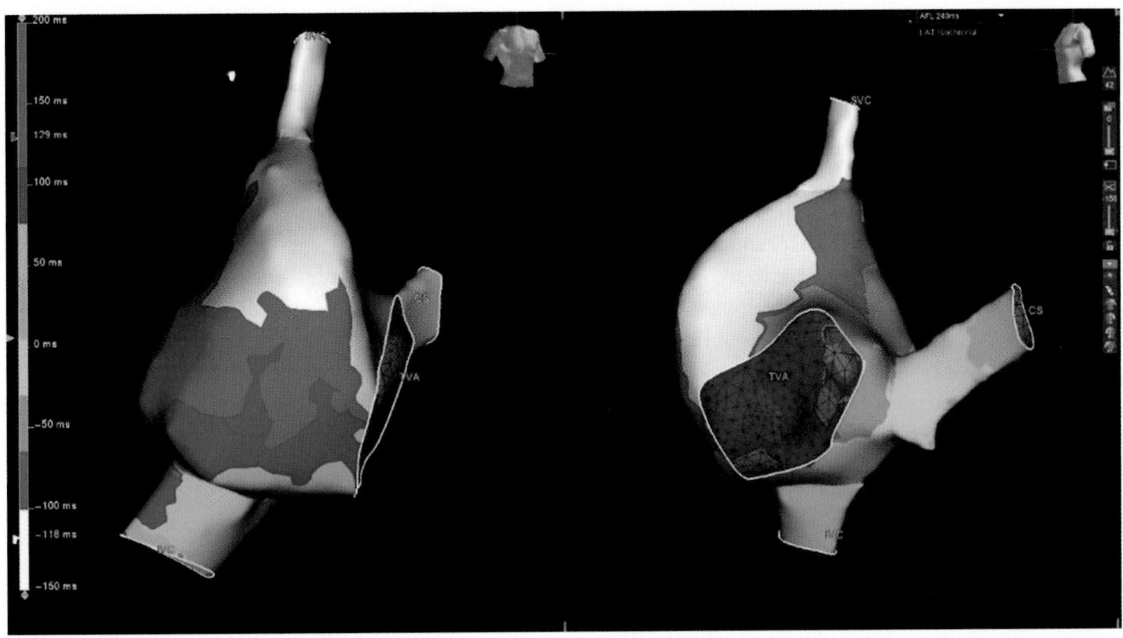

FIGURE 59.3 Activation mapping of the right atrium during cavotricuspid isthmus-dependent typical flutter. CS, coronary sinus; IVC, inferior vena cava; SVC, superior vena cava; TVA, tricuspid valve annulus.

than or equal to 11/12 ECG leads or greater than or equal to 95% using clinically available pace match software (CARTO® PASO™, Biosense Webster, Diamond Bar, CA; Score Map, Abbott, Abbott Park, IL) is usually seen at sites of successful ablation. Although pace mapping is useful, it has several limitations including the inability to capture (1) local myocardium within areas of scarring at lower outputs and (2) neighboring tissue at higher outputs, thus reducing its accuracy. Further, pace mapping is not useful for atrial arrhythmias because surface P-waves are often not clearly discernible during atrial tachycardia, which limits any comparisons.

Entrainment mapping of arrhythmias is performed during mapping of hemodynamically stable reentrant arrhythmias to aid in confirming areas that have been identified as potential isthmuses during activation mapping. This is particularly useful in patients with large areas of scar with abnormal fractionated low-voltage signals seen at multiple sites which may represent either areas critical to the reentrant arrhythmia or passive bystander areas. During entrainment, pacing is performed from suspected areas during the tachycardia at a cycle length 20 to 30 milliseconds shorter than the tachycardia cycle length (ie, at a rate slightly faster than the tachycardia rate) and the response of the tachycardia to such a pacing maneuver is analyzed to determine if the site of pacing is a part of the reentrant circuit.[7,8]

ENERGY SOURCES FOR CATHETER ABLATION OF ARRHYTHMIAS

Catheter ablation of cardiac arrhythmias was first achieved by delivering direct current energy, via an intracardiac electrode catheter, to the His bundle region so as to disrupt AV conduction in patients with supraventricular arrhythmias refractory to medical therapy. Although successful, the degree of control over tissue ablated with this form of catheter ablation was limited and resulted in damage to a large mass of cardiac tissue and was associated with a high rate of complications.[9] Several other energy sources, with a higher efficacy and more favorable safety profile, have been developed and adopted into clinical use.

Radiofrequency Ablation

Radiofrequency ablation (RF) was first used in 1987 for the treatment of cardiac arrhythmias and has since become the most common form of energy used for the ablation of arrhythmias. RF energy achieves tissue injury via resistive and conductive heating of tissue, with irreversible injury resulting from heating of tissues to a temperature greater than 50 °C. RF ablation uses energy in the 500 to 1000 kHz spectrum. RF energy from an RF generator is delivered between a platinum-iridium electrode at the tip of the ablation catheter (that serves as the cathode) and a dispersive grounding patch (that serves as the anode) usually applied on the abdomen, thigh, or calf. The small surface area of the distal end of the ablation catheter results in a high current density leading to resistive heating of tissue in contact with the catheter tip. With current density being inversely proportional to the square of the distance from the energy source, the degree of resistive tissue heating decreases exponentially as one moves away from the energy source. Thus, only tissue that is in immediate contact with the catheter tip undergoes resistive heating, thereby limiting and controlling tissue injury. Heat then radiates away from this area of resistive heating to neighboring tissue, resulting in conductive heating and damage to a small area of adjacent tissue in 3D space.

The current then flows through the body and returns via the grounding patch to the RF generator completing the circuit. The larger surface area of the dispersive electrode prevents heating and injury to the skin in contact with the grounding patch. Since its inception, the RF ablation catheter has undergone several iterations including changes in size, electrode type (platinum-iridium vs gold), and use of tip irrigation (closed-loop vs open-loop irrigation) in an attempt to achieve relatively larger and deeper lesions as compared to the initial nonirrigated catheters. Monitoring of the electrode tip-tissue interface temperature via thermocouples at the electrode tip is useful to titrate power in nonirrigated 4-mm tip catheters. However, they are not useful with larger tip (8 mm) and irrigated catheters owing to the greater passive and active cooling of the catheter tip, respectively, thus lowering the tip temperature although the temperature of tissue just beneath the surface is much greater.

Cryoablation

Cryoablation consists of inflicting tissue injury by cooling tissues to subzero temperatures. Cooling of tissue is achieved using a steerable catheter with a hollow shaft through which a hollow tube delivers a compressed cryorefrigerant such as nitrous oxide to the distal electrode tip. Expansion of the compressed nitrous oxide as it is released to the catheter tip leads to a liquid to gaseous phase transition with resulting cooling of the electrode tip via the Joule-Thompson effect. This cooled catheter tip subsequently extracts heat from the surrounding tissue resulting in tissue cooling. Whereas cooling tissue to 0 to −5 °C (probe temperature of 0 to −30 °C) results in reversible loss of function, freezing to lower temperatures of −20 to −30 °C (probe temperature of −70 to −80 °C) for longer durations of 2 to 3 minutes will result in permanent damage and loss of function. Cryoablation produces tissue injury via two mechanisms: direct cellular injury through intra- and extracellular ice crystal formation, which results in mechanical and osmotic cellular damage during both the freezing and thawing phase; and ischemic cell death caused by microcirculatory damage during the thawing phase. Cryoablation has certain advantages over RF ablation. The efficacy and safety of ablation at a site can be assessed by cooling to temperatures between 0 and −5 °C, which results in reversible loss of function. If the desired effect is not seen or significant collateral damage is seen, ablation at this site can be stopped, thereby preventing irreversible damage. Further, with freezing, the catheter tip adheres to the adjacent myocardium, resulting in assured catheter stability during ablation as opposed to the respirophasic and cardiophasic catheter motion during RF ablation. However, cryoablation is associated with a higher recurrence rate as compared to RF ablation in patients with AVNRT and AVRT, and hence in such patients is preferred only when ablation is required close to the conduction axis such as during ablation of superoparaseptal and midseptal APs which lie close to the bundle of His and AV node, respectively.[10,11] Although cryoablation was first used to ablate AVNRT using steerable electrode tip catheters, more recently steerable cryoballoon catheters have been developed to aid in catheter ablation of AF. Several observational and randomized studies have shown the noninferiority (and even superiority in some studies) of cryoballoon ablation to RF ablation in patients with paroxysmal AF, while being associated with lower rates of pulmonary vein reconnection and shorter procedural times. These advantages have led to the increased use of cryoballoon ablation in preference to RF ablation in patients with paroxysmal AF.[12-15]

Laser Ablation

Laser ablation has only been studied for the management of paroxysmal AF. Endoscopic laser ablation uses a 980-nm diode laser to cause tissue heating and injury. Similar to cryoballoon ablation, multilumen balloon tip catheters have been developed for use in laser catheter ablation of AF. Initial studies with newer generation ablation catheters have shown noninferiority of laser ablation to RF ablation in patients with paroxysmal AF.[16,17]

Other Sources of Energy

Despite the considerable progress made in the field of catheter ablation of arrhythmias, the relatively high recurrence rate seen with some arrhythmias, such as AF and VT, and the potential for injury to neighboring structures during ablation has led to continued interest in identifying newer safer sources of energy to further improve efficacy rates and minimize complications. Electroporation is a newer form of ablation that uses pulsed electrical fields (created with high-voltage direct current) delivered locally to cardiac tissue via steerable sheaths. Electroporation works by creating pores in the cell membrane, thus increasing membrane permeability and causing irreversible cell injury. The tissue selectivity of different current pulses has led to considerable interest in this modality of ablation. Initial preclinical and clinical studies are promising with short procedural times and minimal collateral injury.[18-20]

INDICATIONS FOR CATHETER ABLATION

Supraventricular Arrhythmias Focal Atrial Tachycardia

Focal atrial tachycardia (FAT) is an organized tachycardia arising from a discrete region within the atria with atrial rates ranging from 100 to 250 bpm with variable ventricular rates. Although FAT may arise from any site within the atria, they most commonly arise from the crista terminalis, pulmonary veins, coronary sinus, superior vena cava, atrial appendages, perimitral/tricuspid annulus, and the parahisian location. Although pharmacotherapy has long been the mainstay of management of these patients, the high efficacy rates and low rates of complications of catheter ablation have led to it becoming a Class I indication for FAT especially if incessant or causing tachycardia-induced cardiomyopathy.[2,3] Activation mapping during the tachycardia helps localize the focus of origin which can then be targeted for ablation. Several studies have demonstrated an acute success rate of 80% to 95%, with a recurrence rate of 4% to 20% and a low complication rate of 1% to 2%.[21-23] The site of origin of the tachycardia considerably influences outcomes, with FAT arising from the parahisian location, superior vena cava, and pulmonary veins being associated with higher recurrence rates. The development of pulmonary vein isolation procedures for FAT arising from the pulmonary veins and AF has further helped refine the ablation of these arrhythmias with improvements in outcomes (**Table 59.1**).

Atrioventricular Nodal Reentrant Tachycardia

AVNRT refers to reentry occurring at the AV junction and involving the different extensions of the AV node (fast pathway located posterosuperiorly and/or one or more of the slow pathways—right inferior extension, left inferior extension, or the inferolateral extension). The most common form of AVNRT—the so-called typical AVNRT—involves the right inferior slow pathway as the antegrade limb of the circuit whereas the fast pathway serves as the retrograde limb of the circuit. Other atypical forms of AVNRT involve different permutations of the different AV nodal extensions as parts of the circuit. Although beta-blockers and calcium channel blockers are useful in preventing and terminating episodes of AVNRT, their low efficacy, need for long-term medication, and the high success rates with catheter ablation have made catheter ablation a Class I indication in the management of patients with AVNRT. Although initial strategies of catheter ablation of AVNRT targeted the fast pathway, current approaches to catheter ablation involve ablating the slow pathway—most frequently the right inferior extension located anterior to the coronary sinus ostium—which is associated with a lower risk of complete AV block. Catheter ablation is highly successful with a reported success rate of 97% and a recurrence rate of 2% to 5% with a less than 1% risk of complete AV block (Table 59.1).[2,3,24-26] Cryoablation carries a lower risk of AV block but a higher risk of recurrence.[11]

Accessory Pathways

APs are additional conduction channels, apart from the normal AV conduction axis (AV node and His-Purkinje system), between the atria and ventricles that bypass the normal AV conduction axis. The most common forms of these pathways extend between atrial and ventricular myocardium whereas rarer forms exist that connect directly to the AV node or other components of the His-Purkinje conduction system. Anatomically, the majority of APs are located in the left lateral location around the mitral annulus, followed by the paraseptal locations with APs around the tricuspid annulus being less common. The vast majority of these APs have similar electrophysiologic characteristics as working atrial and ventricular myocardium, with sodium-dependent action potentials and fast conduction as compared to the AV node which exhibits calcium-dependent slow conduction. These APs can conduct antegrade, retrograde, or in both directions. These APs in concert with the normal AV conduction axis (or rarely with another AP) create a substrate for AV reentry, giving rise to orthodromic AP-mediated tachycardia/ AVRT with retrograde conduction in the AP or antidromic AVRT with antegrade conduction in the AP. APs are also associated with a higher risk of AF with the added risk of sudden cardiac death resulting from rapid conduction down the AP leading to ventricular fibrillation (VF). A number of pharmacological agents targeting different components of the reentrant circuit are available and have been used in the management of patients with AVRT. However, given the high

TABLE 59.1 Catheter Ablation of Supraventricular Arrhythmias

		Acute Success Rate (%)	Recurrence Rate (%)	Complication Rate (%)
Atrial tachycardia	Crista terminalis[70,71]	98.5	9	<1
	Tricuspid annulus[72]	100	11	<1
	Coronary sinus[73]	88	<1	<1
	Superior vena cava[74]	100	0	20
	Parahisian[75,76]	95-100	0-7	1-6
	Mitral annulus[77,78]	100	0	0-8
	Atrial appendages[79,80]	75-95	0-20	0-5
AVNRT[2,24]		95-97	2-5	1
Accessory pathway–mediated tachycardia	Left free wall[27,81,82]	95-98	2-3	<1
	Right free wall[83,84]	95	5-20	1
	Superior paraseptal[85-87]	95	15	1
	Inferior paraseptal[88-91]	95-98	5-6	1-2
CTI-dependent atrial flutter[50,51]		90-95	6-9	1
Non-CTI-dependent atrial flutter[92-95]		75-90	10-45	1-2

AVNRT, atrioventricular nodal reentrant tachycardia; CTI, cavotricuspid isthmus.

success rates associated with catheter ablation, it has now become the treatment of choice (Class I recommendation) for the management of symptomatic patients and certain groups of asymptomatic patients at a high risk of sudden cardiac death.[2,3] APs can be mapped and localized during tachycardia, mapping the site of earliest atrial activation during orthodromic AVRT or the earliest ventricular activation during antidromic AVRT; during sinus rhythm or atrial pacing for antegrade-conducting pathways to map the site of earliest ventricular activation; and/or during ventricular pacing for retrogradely conducting pathways to localize the site of earliest atrial activation. Often, conduction through the AP as represented by an AP potential can also be identified.[27] Once localized, these APs can be targeted using either nonirrigated or irrigated catheters or cryoablation. RF ablation is associated with a lower risk of recurrence and is preferred to cryoablation. However, cryoablation may be particularly useful for APs located close to the conduction system such as superior paraseptal APs to lower the risk of AV block. Although most centers continue to use a fluoroscopic guided approach, there has been an increasing use of 3D EAM systems to increase the accuracy of mapping and ablation while reducing radiation exposure. Current data from several multicenter studies suggest a success rate of 92% with a recurrence rate of around 8%. However, the recurrence rate is influenced by the site of AP, with a much higher recurrence seen with superior paraseptal (anteroseptal) APs.[2,3,27-29]

Atrial Fibrillation

AF is the most common cardiac arrhythmia and is associated with considerable morbidity and mortality. The history, epidemiology, clinical manifestations, complications, and pharmacological management of AF are discussed in Chapter 56. Initial attempts at catheter ablation of AF were designed to mimic the surgical Cox-Maze procedure that was designed to interrupt macroreentrant circuits within the atria and reduce the mass of electrically active atrial tissue, thereby preventing the initiation and maintenance of AF. The seminal observation by Haïssaguerre et al of pulmonary vein ectopics initiating AF ushered in a new era of invasive AF management with an increasing focus on identifying and eliminating "triggers" of AF.[30] The pulmonary veins, including their antral regions, are the most frequent source of AF triggers, whereas nonpulmonary vein triggers are seen in 15% to 30% of patients, including from the posterior wall of the left atrium, left atrial appendage, vein of Marshall, and the interatrial septum. Right atrial sites of triggers include the crista terminalis, the coronary sinus, and the superior vena cava.[31-33] Additionally, areas of scar/fibrosis are frequently seen in patients with persistent AF, which create areas of electrophysiological heterogeneity predisposing to wave breaks and reentry contributing to AF initiation and maintenance. Accordingly, current strategies of AF ablation involve targeting the triggers of AF either alone or in combination with additional substrate-based ablation. The low efficacy of pharmacological agents in maintaining sinus rhythm has led to a Class I indication for catheter ablation of AF in patients not responding to or intolerant of antiarrhythmic agents. Additionally, catheter ablation has a Class IIa indication as a first-line therapy for AF.

The current practice of catheter ablation of paroxysmal AF varies among centers with most performing electrical isolation of the pulmonary veins and antrum alone. 3D EAM systems are used to construct the left atrial and pulmonary vein geometry, with preoperative CT or MRI being used in most centers to clearly delineate left atrial and pulmonary venous anatomy. RF, cryoballoon, or laser balloon is used to ablate left atrial tissue around the ostium of the pulmonary veins including the pulmonary vein antrum with the goal of electrically isolating the pulmonary veins and antra from the left atrium. Isolation of the pulmonary veins is confirmed using pacing maneuvers from within the veins and the atria. Additional triggers are targeted in patients with recurrences following ablation. Alternatively, some centers attempt to identify and target additional triggers during the index procedure using provocative agents such as isoproterenol. Pulmonary vein isolation has a 1-year success rate of 60% to 80% in patients with paroxysmal AF.[34-36] Although additional nonpulmonary vein triggers play a role in some patients with recurrences, the majority of patients are found to have a reconnection of the pulmonary veins. Thus, durable isolation of the pulmonary veins remains a challenge in AF ablation, with close proximity to neighboring structures such as the esophagus and the phrenic nerve limiting energy delivery and transmural lesion formation. Accordingly, a number of strategies have been adopted to improve the durability of the lesion set including the use of irrigated catheters that are associated with wider and deeper lesions, contact force sensing catheters that enable monitoring of catheter tissue contact, high-power short-duration ablation, mechanical esophageal deviation during ablation of the posterior wall of the left atrium, and balloon ablation to create large confluent lesions.[12,37,38] The shorter procedural time, large overlapping confluent lesions created, and similar efficacy to RF ablation have led to the increasing use of cryoballoon ablation, with some studies showing lower rates of pulmonary vein reconnection at follow-up.[12,15] The high tissue selectivity of electroporation makes it an attractive option in the future to enable the use of higher energy to achieve irreversible transmural lesions particularly in the posterior wall of the left atrium in close proximity to the esophagus.

The outcomes of pulmonary vein isolation are less encouraging in patients with persistent and long-standing persistent AF, with recurrence rates ranging from 30% to 60% being described in multiple studies.[39-42] Ablation of additional triggers in the form of superior vena caval isolation, left atrial appendage isolation, or coronary sinus ablation have not significantly improved outcomes. Isolation of the left atrial appendage is associated with a higher risk of stroke, and while some centers have shown added value in isolation of the left atrial appendage in patients with persistent AF, the small number of patients having triggers arising from the left atrial appendage likely confer an unfavorable risk-benefit ratio.[42-44] Additional strategies that have been tried include linear lesions in the left and right atria to interrupt reentrant circuits and reduce the excitable left atrial mass, ablation of areas showing complex fractionated electrograms, isolation of the posterior wall of the left atrium (given its embryologic relationship with the pulmonary veins), and rotor mapping.[45-47] However, none of these ablation strategies have consistently been shown to have additive value to pulmonary vein isolation alone.[41] Currently, catheter ablation for persistent AF is a Class IIa indication in symptomatic patients with persistent AF. Catheter ablation appears to be especially useful in patients with AF and heart failure, with improvements in quality of life, ejection fraction, and mortality rates being demonstrated in a number of studies.[35,48,49] Although all patients with persistent AF undergoing catheter ablation should undergo pulmonary vein isolation, the benefits of additional ablation strategies are still unclear.[35]

Macroreentrant Atrial Tachycardia (MRAT)/Atrial Flutter

The term atrial flutter was initially used to describe atrial tachycardia with a rate greater than 240 bpm, in the absence of an isoelectric interval between P-waves on the surface electrocardiogram (ECG); signifying a reentrant arrhythmia utilizing a macroreentrant circuit. The presence of scar tissue within the atria however confounds this definition with low-voltage and slow-conduction areas in scarred atria resulting in absence of isoelectric intervals in patients with atrial tachycardia and presence of apparent isoelectric intervals in patients with atrial flutter. MRAT includes cavotricuspid isthmus (CTI)-dependent atrial tachycardias/flutter—described as typical atrial flutter—and non-CTI-dependent atrial flutters constituting the atypical atrial flutters.

CTI-dependent atrial flutter involves a large reentrant circuit around the tricuspid annulus with the activation wavefront traveling in clockwise direction (down the interatrial septum and up the lateral wall) or counterclockwise direction. Both activation and entrainment mapping with pacing from the CTI (the isthmus between the tricuspid annulus and the inferior vena cava) are useful in confirming the diagnosis of CTI-dependent atrial flutter. CTI-dependent atrial flutter is highly amenable to catheter ablation and involves the creation of a linear lesion set extending from the tricuspid annulus to the inferior vena cava to achieve a line of block across the CTI, thus interrupting the reentrant circuit. Catheter ablation of CTI-dependent flutter has a success rate of greater than 90% with a recurrence rate ranging from 6% to 9% and a complication rate of 1%.[2,3,50,51]

Non-CTI-dependent atrial flutter typically occurs in individuals with structural heart disease usually following surgical or catheter ablation of AF or following open-heart surgery involving creation of atriotomies or lung transplant. Atrial fibrosis resulting from prior ablation or atriotomy-related scars create conditions for slow conduction, thereby predisposing to macro reentry. Perimitral flutter and roof-dependent flutter are the most common atypical forms of atrial flutter and along with CTI-dependent flutter account for 90% of all atrial flutters. Atypical atrial flutters may also be seen de novo (in the absence of prior ablations or surgeries) in a small number of individuals with atrial scarring secondary to structural heart disease and increased left atrial pressures. Activation mapping during the tachycardia helps identify the reentrant circuit with entrainment mapping helping confirm the diagnosis. The approach to ablation of these macroreentrant flutters involves the creation of a linear lesion between two anatomical obstacles transecting the reentrant circuit. Accordingly, a perimitral flutter is treated with a mitral isthmus line (between the left inferior pulmonary vein and mitral annulus) or an anterior septal line (between the right superior pulmonary vein and the mitral annulus) whereas a roof-dependent flutter is treated with a linear roofline (between the right and left superior pulmonary veins). Owing to a poor response to pharmacological agents and a high rate of recurrence, catheter ablation is the treatment of choice for atypical atrial flutter. Outcomes of catheter ablation are less promising for non-CTI-dependent than for typical CTI-dependent atrial flutter with 1-year recurrence rates ranging from 15% to 50% depending on the etiology, underlying atrial substrate, and degree of fibrosis, though the reentrant circuit responsible for the recurrent arrhythmia may be different from that of the initial tachycardia.[2]

Ventricular Arrhythmias

Premature Ventricular Contractions and Idiopathic Ventricular Arrhythmias

The mechanisms and site of origin of premature ventricular contractions (PVC) and idiopathic ventricular arrhythmias (IVA) have been described in a previous chapter. Briefly, the right ventricular outflow tract is the most common site of origin of PVCs and IVA accounting for nearly 50% of all cases with less frequent sites being the aortic sinuses of Valsalva, left ventricular outflow tract, left ventricular summit, endocavitary structures such as the papillary muscles and moderator band, peritricuspid and perimitral annular locations, inferoseptal recess of the left ventricle, and the parahisian location. Although these VAs are caused by abnormal automaticity or triggered activity, idiopathic fascicular VT is one of the most common left-sided VTs occurring in individuals with structurally normal hearts that is caused by reentry involving the fascicular system. Pharmacologic therapy in the form of beta-blockers, calcium channel blockers, and occasionally amiodarone represent the first-line therapy in symptomatic patients with frequent PVCs and idiopathic VAs and those with PVC-induced cardiomyopathy. Catheter ablation is increasingly being used and is indicated in symptomatic patients or patients with PVC-induced cardiomyopathy who are not responding to antiarrhythmic agents or when antiarrhythmic agents are not tolerated. Considerable experience has accrued with catheter ablation of idiopathic VAs with the establishment of relatively high success rates, particularly for VAs arising from the ventricular outflow tracts and idiopathic fascicular VT and may even be preferred over antiarrhythmic agents in these patients.[52] The 12-lead EKG is useful for localizing the site of origin of idiopathic VAs, and several algorithms have been published. During catheter mapping, both activation and pace mapping are useful in the localization of idiopathic VAs. Activation at successful sites usually precedes the QRS complex by 30 milliseconds or more, while pace mapping is useful in patients with infrequent PVCs or VTs that cannot be mapped during the EP study. Mapping of idiopathic fascicular VT involves activation mapping during VT with identification of fascicular potentials that precede the onset of the QRS (the so-called P1 and P2 signals) and entrainment mapping to confirm the circuit components.[53-57]

Owing to the proximity of the different cardiac chambers to each other, particularly the outflow tracts of the ventricles, it is essential to carefully map all neighboring structures to precisely identify sites with the earliest activation prior to ablation. Use of intracardiac echocardiography to visualize endocavitary structures and the location of the aortic sinuses and to guide catheter movement and stability is particularly useful in these patients. The outcomes of catheter ablation vary depending on the site of origin, with long-term success rates ranging from 65% to 100% (**Table 59.2**). Ablation of right ventricular outflow tract VAs has a high success rate with a rate of recurrence of around 5%. Similarly, a high success rate is seen in patients with left ventricular outflow tract VAs and idiopathic fascicular VT. Success rates are lower with ablation of papillary muscle VAs owing to the greater anatomical challenges involved, including the thickness of the papillary muscles, intramural location of the focus of origin in a majority of patients, and the difficulties in achieving catheter stability at these sites owing to the vigorous contractions of the papillary muscles. The use of cryoablation may be useful in patients in whom RF ablation is not successful. The combined use of these ablation modalities in combination with intracardiac echocardiographic imaging results in a success rate of 80% to 90% in most described series.[54] Similarly, ablation of parahisian VAs is challenging owing to the proximity to the conduction system and the risk for complete heart block and bundle branch blocks. However, careful and high-density mapping helps precisely localize the focus of origin, thus minimizing the number of ablation lesions required to eliminate these arrhythmias and limiting damage to the conduction system.

Scar-Mediated Ventricular Tachycardia

Scar-mediated reentrant VT is the leading mechanism of VT in patients with structural heart disease. Electrical heterogeneity, both in conduction/propagation and in repolarization, gives rise to areas of slow conduction and conduction block predisposing to reentry. Ischemic heart disease is the leading cause for scar-mediated VT followed by nonischemic causes such as sarcoidosis, hypertrophic cardiomyopathy, arrhythmogenic cardiomyopathy, myocarditis, and Chagas disease. The location of scar varies based on etiology with the majority of patients with ischemic cardiomyopathy having a subendocardial scar whereas a substantial proportion of patients with nonischemic cardiomyopathy have scar epicardially and intramurally requiring epicardial cardiac mapping and ablation. Epicardial mapping is achieved via a percutaneous sub-xiphoid access to the pericardial cavity. Catheter ablation of VT is recommended in patients refractory to antiarrhythmic agents or not tolerant of or unwilling to take medications (Class I indication).

Preprocedural risk stratification involves assessment of severity of left ventricular dysfunction and heart failure, and comorbidities including chronic kidney disease, chronic lung disease, and atrial arrhythmias. The use of preoperative cardiac MRI is useful in characterizing the scar substrate whereas a positron emission tomography scan is useful in patients with nonischemic cardiomyopathy to look for evidence of active myocarditis. Hemodynamic support measures such as extracorporeal membrane oxygenation, mechanical circulatory support devices, or intra-aortic balloon pump may be used in patients with severe left ventricular systolic dysfunction. Mapping of scar-mediated VT involves a combination of voltage, pace, activation, and entrainment mapping in an attempt to decipher the various components of the reentrant circuit. A limitation to activation and entrainment mapping is the hemodynamic instability of more than 70% of all VTs induced in the EP laboratory, thereby increasing the reliance on other mapping techniques. Once mapped, ablation strategies consist of targeting the clinical VT induced and mapped and additionally

TABLE 59.2 Catheter Ablation of Idiopathic Ventricular Arrhythmias

	Acute Success Rate (%)	Recurrence Rate (%)	Complication Rate (%)
Right ventricular/left ventricular outflow tract[96,97]	95-98	5	<1
Parahisian[98]	88-90	14	<1
Tricuspid annular[99,100]	60-90	0	<20
Moderator band[101]	80	60	<1
Papillary muscles[102,103]	88-94	0-30	7
Mitral annular[104,105]	80-100	0-30	<1
Inferoseptal recess[56,106]	100	0	<1

modifying the scar substrate by ablating areas of abnormal signals within the scar.[58,59]

The benefits of catheter ablation of VT have been demonstrated in several randomized, observational, and registry-based studies with reductions in recurrence of VT and implantable cardiodefibrillator interventions, though a mortality benefit has not been consistently demonstrated. The benefits remain even in patients with VT storm—defined as three or more episodes of sustained VT or implantable cardiodefibrillator interventions in a 24-hour period.[60-63] Success rates of scar-mediated VT ablation range from 40% to 80% depending on the underlying etiology, degree of left ventricular dysfunction, and comorbidities.[52] In the majority of patients with a recurrence, a reduction in the frequency of episodes and implantable cardiodefibrillator interventions is seen following VT ablation.

COMPLICATIONS OF CATHETER ABLATION

The rate of complications during catheter ablation of cardiac arrhythmias ranges from less than 1% to 5% depending on the procedure performed, anticoagulation use, and underlying comorbidities.[29,64] The most frequent complication encountered is related to vascular access, occurring in 1% to 2% of patients, with the most frequent occurrences being bleeding and hematoma formation. Femoral pseudoaneurysm and arteriovenous fistula are less common being seen in less than 0.5% of patients.[64] Radiation exposure—both to the patient and the interventional electrophysiologist—is a cause for concern particularly for complex cases with long procedural durations, though the advent of 3D EAM has led to significant reductions in the use of fluoroscopy.

Complete heart block occurs in less than 1% in patients undergoing catheter ablation with a higher risk of up to 10% in patients with superior paraseptal (anteroseptal) and midseptal APs.[65,66] Cryoablation is associated with a lower risk of complete heart block than RF ablation but a higher risk of recurrence. Phrenic nerve injury is reported to have an incidence of 0.2% to 0.5% during AF ablation. High output pacing to localize the phrenic nerve and pacing to capture the phrenic nerve during ablation helps recognize and avoid this complication.[67]

Cardiac perforation and tamponade are rare but are more common during catheter ablation of AF owing to the thin wall of the left atrium, occurring in up to 2% of patients as compared to 0.2% during supraventricular tachycardia (SVT) ablation.[29,68] Stroke during left-sided catheter ablation is reported in less than 1% of patients, although silent cerebral infarcts have been reported in several studies. The use of irrigated catheters, continued preprocedural anticoagulation, and optimal intraprocedural anticoagulation—coupled with safety strategies to avoid air embolization—have led to significant reductions in silent cerebral infarcts. Coronary artery injury during catheter ablation is rare, with the incidence being reported in less than 0.2% of cases. A precise understanding of anatomy and obtaining coronary angiograms when ablating close to arterial structures helps avoid this potentially fatal complication. Atrio-esophageal fistula is a rare complication that can occur during AF ablation with a reported incidence of less than 0.1%.[67] Monitoring the esophageal temperature during AF ablation helps identify esophageal heating and has considerably reduced the incidence of this devastating complication.

Mortality during catheter ablation of supraventricular arrhythmias is extremely rare, occurring in less than 0.1% of cases while a mortality rate of 0.1% to 3% has been described during VT ablation. Risk factors for mortality include older age, female sex, diabetes mellitus, hypertension, severity of left ventricular dysfunction and heart failure, chronic kidney disease, chronic lung disease, and VT storm.[69]

PATIENT FOLLOW-UP CARE

Follow-up of patients following catheter ablation of cardiac arrhythmias is influenced by numerous factors including type of cardiac arrhythmia, procedural characteristics and outcomes, and cardiac function and comorbidities.

Following successful ablation of SVTs, patients return to follow-up after 2 weeks. Assessment includes a general physical examination with particular emphasis on ensuring no vascular access site complications and an ECG to document the rhythm and to assess for any recurrence of preexcitation (in case of APs). Subsequently, patients continue regular follow-up with their primary care physicians or cardiologists (in the presence of underlying cardiac dysfunction). The follow-up of patients undergoing AF or atrial flutter ablation is further individualized depending on the need for antiarrhythmic agents to maintain sinus rhythm.

Following VT ablation, follow-up is usually scheduled after 2 weeks, with an earlier patient visit scheduled in patients with severe left ventricular (LV) dysfunction or patients undergoing complex procedures including epicardial ablation. Antiarrhythmic drugs are usually continued for 6 to 12 months after which a decision to discontinue them is taken based on underlying cardiac function, success of the procedure, and occurrence of other VTs.

KEY POINTS

- ✔ The advent of percutaneous therapies has revolutionized the management of cardiac arrhythmias by achieving effective outcomes while avoiding the undesirable side effects seen with antiarrhythmic medications.
- ✔ Ablation of supraventricular arrhythmias such as AVNRT and AVRT is associated with a high success rate of greater than 90% and is curative in the vast majority of patients.
- ✔ Catheter ablation is highly effective in the management of AF and atrial flutter, with continued technological advances leading to increasing success rates with lower rates of recurrence.
- ✔ Ablation therapy is an important tool in the management of VAs with high success rates in patients with idiopathic and ischemic scar-related VT. Although success

rates currently are lower in patients with nonischemic cardiomyopathy, the increasing use of advanced cardiac imaging is contributing to continued advances in this challenging cohort of patients.

- ✔ With more advanced mapping tools and newer forms of ablation such as electroporation on the horizon, further improvements in success rates of ablation are anticipated while minimizing the risk of complications.

REFERENCES

1. Shaan K, Choi SH, Weng LC, et al. Frequency of cardiac rhythm abnormalities in a half million adults. *Circ Arrhythm Electrophysiol.* 2018;11:e006273.
2. Brugada J, Katritsis DG, Arbelo E, et al. 2019 ESC Guidelines for the management of patients with supraventricular tachycardia. The Task Force for the management of patients with supraventricular tachycardia of the European Society of Cardiology (ESC) Developed in collaboration with the Association for European Paediatric and Congenital Cardiology (AEPC). *Eur Heart J.* 2020;41:655-720.
3. Page RL, Joglar JA, Caldwell MA, et al. 2015 ACC/AHA/HRS Guideline for the management of adult patients with supraventricular tachycardia. *Circulation.* 2016;133:e506-e574.
4. Marchlinski FE, Callans DJ, Gottlieb CD, Zado E. Linear ablation lesions for control of unmappable ventricular tachycardia in patients with ischemic and nonischemic cardiomyopathy. *Circulation.* 2000;101:1288-1296.
5. Hutchinson MD, Gerstenfeld EP, Desjardins B, et al. Endocardial unipolar voltage mapping to detect epicardial ventricular tachycardia substrate in patients with nonischemic left ventricular cardiomyopathy. *Circ Arrhythm Electrophysiol.* 2011;4:49-55.
6. Tung R, Kim S, Yagishita D, et al. Scar voltage threshold determination using ex vivo magnetic resonance imaging integration in a porcine infarct model: Influence of interelectrode distances and three-dimensional spatial effects of scar. *Heart Rhythm.* 2016;13:1993-2002.
7. Waldo AL. From bedside to bench: entrainment and other stories. *Heart Rhythm.* 2004;1:94-106.
8. Stevenson WG, Friedman PL, Sager PT, et al. Exploring postinfarction reentrant ventricular tachycardia with entrainment mapping. *J Am Coll Cardiol.* 1997;29:1180-1189.
9. Gallagher JJ, Svenson RH, Kasell JH, et al. Catheter technique for closed-chest ablation of the atrioventricular conduction system. *N Engl J Med.* 1982;306:194-200.
10. Opel A, Murray S, Kamath N, et al. Cryoablation versus radiofrequency ablation for treatment of atrioventricular nodal reentrant tachycardia: cryoablation with 6-mm-tip catheters is still less effective than radiofrequency ablation. *Heart Rhythm.* 2010;7:340-343.
11. Hanninen M, Yeung-Lai-Wah N, Massel D, et al. Cryoablation versus RF ablation for AVNRT: a meta-analysis and systematic review. *J Cardiovasc Electrophysiol.* 2013;24:1354-1360.
12. Kuck K-H, Brugada J, Fürnkranz A, et al. Cryoballoon or radiofrequency ablation for paroxysmal atrial fibrillation. *N Engl J Med.* 2016;374:2235-2245.
13. Andrade JG, Champagne J, Dubuc M, et al. Cryoballoon or radiofrequency ablation for atrial fibrillation assessed by continuous monitoring: a randomized clinical trial. *Circulation.* 2019;140:1779-1788.
14. Mörtsell D, Arbelo E, Dagres N, et al. Cryoballoon vs. radiofrequency ablation for atrial fibrillation: a study of outcome and safety based on the ESC-EHRA atrial fibrillation ablation long-term registry and the Swedish catheter ablation registry. *Europace.* 2019;21:581-589.
15. Kuck K-H, Albenque J-P, Chun KRJ, et al. Repeat ablation for atrial fibrillation recurrence post cryoballoon or radiofrequency ablation in the FIRE AND ICE trial. *Circ Arrhythm Electrophysiol.* 2019;12:e007247.
16. Dukkipati Srinivas R, Kuck KH, Neuzil P, et al. Pulmonary vein isolation using a visually guided laser balloon catheter. *Circ Arrhythm Electrophysiol.* 2013;6:467-472.
17. Šedivá L, Petrů J, Škoda J, et al. Visually guided laser ablation: a single-centre long-term experience. *Europace.* 2014;16:1746-1751.
18. Reddy VY, Neuzil P, Koruth JS, et al. Pulsed field ablation for pulmonary vein isolation in atrial fibrillation. *J Am Coll Cardiol.* 2019;74:315-326.
19. Reddy VY, Koruth J, Jais P, et al. Ablation of atrial fibrillation with pulsed electric fields: an ultra-rapid, tissue-selective modality for cardiac ablation. *JACC Clin Electrophysiol.* 2018;4:987-995.
20. Koruth J, Kuroki K, Iwasawa J, et al. Preclinical evaluation of pulsed field ablation: electrophysiological and histological assessment of thoracic vein isolation. *Circ Arrhythm Electrophysiol.* 2019;12:e007781.
21. Kistler PM, Sanders P, Fynn SP, et al. Electrophysiological and electrocardiographic characteristics of focal atrial tachycardia originating from the pulmonary veins: acute and long-term outcomes of radiofrequency ablation. *Circulation.* 2003;108:1968-1975.
22. Anguera I, Brugada J, Roba M, et al. Outcomes after radiofrequency catheter ablation of atrial tachycardia. *Am J Cardiol.* 2001;87:886-890.
23. Biviano AB, Bain W, Whang W, et al. Focal left atrial tachycardias not associated with prior catheter ablation for atrial fibrillation: clinical and electrophysiological characteristics. *Pacing Clin Electrophysiol.* 2012;35:17-27.
24. Katritsis DG, Josephson ME. Classification, electrophysiological features and therapy of atrioventricular nodal reentrant tachycardia. *Arrhythm Electrophysiol Rev.* 2016;5:130-135.
25. Jazayeri MR, Hempe SL, Sra JS, et al. Selective transcatheter ablation of the fast and slow pathways using radiofrequency energy in patients with atrioventricular nodal reentrant tachycardia. *Circulation.* 1992;85:1318-1328.
26. Katritsis DG, Zografos T, Siontis KC, et al. Endpoints for successful slow pathway catheter ablation in typical and atypical atrioventricular nodal re-entrant tachycardia: a contemporary, multicenter study. *JACC Clin Electrophysiol.* 2019;5:113-119.
27. Haïssaguerre M, Gaïta F, Marcus FI, Clémenty J. Radiofrequency catheter ablation of accessory pathways. *J Cardiovasc Electrophysiol.* 1994;5:532-552.
28. Keegan R, Aguinaga L, Fenelon G, et al. The first Latin American Catheter Ablation Registry. *Europace.* 2015;17:794-800.
29. Bohnen M, Stevenson WG, Tedrow UB, et al. Incidence and predictors of major complications from contemporary catheter ablation to treat cardiac arrhythmias. *Heart Rhythm.* 2011;8:1661-1666.
30. Haïssaguerre M, Jaïs P, Shah DC, et al. Spontaneous initiation of atrial fibrillation by ectopic beats originating in the pulmonary veins. *N Engl J Med.* 1998;339:659-666.
31. Valles E, Fan R, Roux JF, et al. Localization of atrial fibrillation triggers in patients undergoing pulmonary vein isolation: importance of the carina region. *J Am Coll Cardiol.* 2008;52:1413-1420.
32. Yamaguchi T, Tsuchiya T, Miyamoto K, Nagamoto Y, Takahashi N. Characterization of non-pulmonary vein foci with an EnSite array in patients with paroxysmal atrial fibrillation. *Europace.* 2010;12:1698-1706.
33. Chang H-Y, Lo L-W, Lin Y-J, et al. Long-term outcome of catheter ablation in patients with atrial fibrillation originating from nonpulmonary vein ectopy. *J Cardiovasc Electrophysiol.* 2013;24:250-258.
34. Hakan O, Knight BP, Hiroshi T, et al. Pulmonary vein isolation for paroxysmal and persistent atrial fibrillation. *Circulation.* 2002;105:1077-1081.
35. Calkins H, Hindricks G, Cappato R, et al. 2017 HRS/EHRA/ECAS/APHRS/SOLAECE expert consensus statement on catheter and surgical ablation of atrial fibrillation. *Europace.* 2018;20:e1-e160.
36. Di Biase L, Conti S, Mohanty P, et al. General anesthesia reduces the prevalence of pulmonary vein reconnection during repeat ablation when compared with conscious sedation: results from a randomized study. *Heart Rhythm.* 2011;8:368-372.
37. Reddy VY, Shah D, Kautzner J, et al. The relationship between contact force and clinical outcome during radiofrequency catheter ablation of atrial fibrillation in the TOCCATA study. *Heart Rhythm.* 2012;9:1789-1795.
38. Winkle RA, Mohanty S, Patrawala RA, et al. Low complication rates using high power (45-50 W) for short duration for atrial fibrillation ablations. *Heart Rhythm.* 2019;16:165-169.

39. Tscholl V, Lsharaf AK-A, Lin T, et al. Two years outcome in patients with persistent atrial fibrillation after pulmonary vein isolation using the second-generation 28-mm cryoballoon. *Heart Rhythm.* 2016;13:1817-1822.
40. Voskoboinik A, Moskovitch JT, Harel N, Sanders P, Kistler PM, Kalman JM. Revisiting pulmonary vein isolation alone for persistent atrial fibrillation: A systematic review and meta-analysis. *Heart Rhythm.* 2017;14:661-667.
41. Verma A, Jiang C, Betts TR, et al. Approaches to catheter ablation for persistent atrial fibrillation. *N Engl J Med.* 2015;372:1812-1822.
42. Romero J, Michaud GF, Avendano R, et al. Benefit of left atrial appendage electrical isolation for persistent and long-standing persistent atrial fibrillation: a systematic review and meta-analysis. *Europace.* 2018;20:1268-1278.
43. Al Rawahi M, Liang JJ, Kapa S, et al. Incidence of left atrial appendage triggers in patients with atrial fibrillation undergoing catheter ablation. *JACC Clin Electrophysiol.* 2020;6:21-30.
44. Kim YG, Shim J, Oh S-K, Lee K-N, Choi J-I, Kim Y-H. Electrical isolation of the left atrial appendage increases the risk of ischemic stroke and transient ischemic attack regardless of postisolation flow velocity. *Heart Rhythm.* 2018;15:1746-1753.
45. Narayan SM, Krummen DE, Shivkumar K, Clopton P, Rappel W-J, Miller JM. Treatment of atrial fibrillation by the ablation of localized sources: CONFIRM (Conventional Ablation for Atrial Fibrillation With or Without Focal Impulse and Rotor Modulation) trial. *J Am Coll Cardiol.* 2012;60:628-636.
46. O'Neill MD, Jaïs P, Takahashi Y, et al. The stepwise ablation approach for chronic atrial fibrillation—evidence for a cumulative effect. *J Interv Card Electrophysiol.* 2006;16:153-167.
47. Nademanee K, McKenzie J, Kosar E, et al. A new approach for catheter ablation of atrial fibrillation: mapping of the electrophysiologic substrate. *J Am Coll Cardiol.* 2004;43:2044-2053.
48. Marrouche NF, Brachmann J, Andresen D, et al. Catheter ablation for atrial fibrillation with heart failure. *N Engl J Med.* 2018;378:417-427.
49. Di Biase L, Mohanty P, Mohanty S, et al. ablation versus amiodarone for treatment of persistent atrial fibrillation in patients with congestive heart failure and an implanted device: results from the AATAC multicenter randomized trial. *Circulation.* 2016;133:1637-1644.
50. Pérez FJ, Schubert CM, Parvez B, Pathak V, Ellenbogen KA, Wood MA. Long-term outcomes after catheter ablation of cavo-tricuspid isthmus dependent atrial flutter. *Circ Arrhythm Electrophysiol.* 2009;2:393-401.
51. Da Costa A, Thévenin J, Roche F, et al. Results from the Loire-Ardèche-Drôme-Isère-Puy-de-Dôme (LADIP) trial on atrial flutter, a multicentric prospective randomized study comparing amiodarone and radiofrequency ablation after the first episode of symptomatic atrial flutter. *Circulation.* 2006;114:1676-1681.
52. Cronin EM, Bogun FM, Maury P, et al. 2019 HRS/EHRA/APHRS/LAHRS expert consensus statement on catheter ablation of ventricular arrhythmias. *Heart Rhythm.* 2020;17:e2-e154.
53. Enriquez A, Malavassi F, Saenz LC, et al. How to map and ablate left ventricular summit arrhythmias. *Heart Rhythm.* 2017;14:141-148.
54. Enriquez A, Supple GE, Marchlinski FE, Garcia FC. How to map and ablate papillary muscle ventricular arrhythmias. *Heart Rhythm.* 2017;14:1721-1728.
55. Enriquez A, Tapias C, Rodriguez D, et al. How to map and ablate parahisian ventricular arrhythmias. *Heart Rhythm.* 2018;15:1268-1274.
56. Li A, Zuberi Z, Bradfield JS, et al. Endocardial ablation of ventricular ectopic beats arising from the basal inferoseptal process of the left ventricle. *Heart Rhythm.* 2018;15:1356-1362.
57. Kapa S, Gaba P, DeSimone CV, Asirvatham SJ. Fascicular ventricular arrhythmias: pathophysiologic mechanisms, anatomical constructs, and advances in approaches to management. *Circ Arrhythm Electrophysiol.* 2017;10(1):e002476.
58. Briceño DF, Romero J, Gianni C, et al. Substrate ablation of ventricular tachycardia: late potentials, scar dechanneling, local abnormal ventricular activities, core isolation, and homogenization. *Card Electrophysiol Clin.* 2017;9:81-91.
59. Jaïs P, Maury P, Khairy P, et al. Elimination of local abnormal ventricular activities: a new end point for substrate modification in patients with scar-related ventricular tachycardia. *Circulation.* 2012;125:2184-2196.
60. Sapp JL, Wells GA, Parkash R, et al. Ventricular tachycardia ablation versus escalation of antiarrhythmic drugs. *N Engl J Med.* 2016;375:111-121.
61. Martinez BK, Baker WL, Konopka A, et al. Systematic review and meta-analysis of catheter ablation of ventricular tachycardia in ischemic heart disease. *Heart Rhythm.* 2020;17:e206-e219.
62. Santangeli P, Frankel DS, Tung R, et al. Early mortality after catheter ablation of ventricular tachycardia in patients with structural heart disease. *J Am Coll Cardiol.* 2017;69:2105-2115.
63. Tzou WS, Tung R, Frankel DS, et al. Outcomes after repeat ablation of ventricular tachycardia in structural heart disease: an analysis from the International VT Ablation Center Collaborative Group. *Heart Rhythm.* 2017;14:991-997.
64. Cappato R, Calkins H, Chen S-A, et al. Worldwide survey on the methods, efficacy, and safety of catheter ablation for human atrial fibrillation. *Circulation.* 2005;111:1100-1105.
65. Mandapati R, Berul CI, Triedman JK, Alexander ME, Walsh EP. Radiofrequency catheter ablation of septal accessory pathways in the pediatric age group. *Am J Cardiol.* 2003;92:947-950.
66. Feldman A, Voskoboinik A, Kumar S, et al. Predictors of acute and long-term success of slow pathway ablation for atrioventricular nodal reentrant tachycardia: a single center series of 1,419 consecutive patients. *Pacing Clin Electrophysiol.* 2011;34:927-933.
67. Bhaskaran A, Chik W, Thomas S, Kovoor P, Thiagalingam A. A review of the safety aspects of radio frequency ablation. *Int J Cardiol Heart Vasc.* 2015;8:147-153.
68. Bhaskaran A, Tung R, Stevenson WG, Kumar S. Catheter ablation of VT in non-ischaemic cardiomyopathies: endocardial, epicardial and intramural approaches. *Heart Lung Circ.* 2019;28:84-101.
69. Vergara P, Tzou WS, Tung R, et al. Predictive score for identifying survival and recurrence risk profiles in patients undergoing ventricular tachycardia ablation. *Circ Arrhythm Electrophysiol.* 2018;11:e006730.
70. Kalman JM, Olgin JE, Karch MR, Hamdan M, Lee RJ, Lesh MD "Cristal tachycardias": origin of right atrial tachycardias from the crista terminalis identified by intracardiac echocardiography. *J Am Coll Cardiol.* 1998;31:451-459.
71. Morris GM, Segan L, Wong G, et al. Atrial tachycardia arising from the crista terminalis, detailed electrophysiological features and long-term ablation outcomes. *JACC Clin Electrophysiol.* 2019;5:448-458.
72. Morton JB, Sanders P, Das A, Vohra JK, Sparks PB, Kalman JM. Focal atrial tachycardia arising from the tricuspid annulus: electrophysiologic and electrocardiographic characteristics. *J Cardiovasc Electrophysiol.* 2001;12:653-659.
73. Kistler PM, Fynn SP, Haqqani H, et al. Focal atrial tachycardia from the ostium of the coronary sinus: electrocardiographic and electrophysiological characterization and radiofrequency ablation. *J Am Coll Cardiol.* 2005;45:1488-1493.
74. Zhao Z, Li X, Guo J. Electrophysiologic characteristics of atrial tachycardia originating from the superior vena cava. *J Interv Card Electrophysiol.* 2009;24:89-94.
75. Wang Z, Ouyang J, Liang Y, et al. Focal atrial tachycardia surrounding the anterior septum. *Circ Arrhythm Electrophysiol.* 2015;8:575-582.
76. Pap R, Makai A, Szilágyi J, et al. Should the aortic root be the preferred route for ablation of focal atrial tachycardia around the AV node?: support from intracardiac echocardiography. *JACC Clin Electrophysiol.* 2016;2:193-199.
77. Gonzalez MD, Contreras LJ, Jongbloed MRM, et al. Left atrial tachycardia originating from the mitral annulus–aorta junction. *Circulation.* 2004;110:3187-3192.
78. Wang Y, Li D, Zhang J, et al. Focal atrial tachycardia originating from the septal mitral annulus: electrocardiographic and electrophysiological characteristics and radiofrequency ablation. *Europace.* 2016;18:1061-1068.
79. Guo X, Zhang J, Ma J, et al. Management of focal atrial tachycardias originating from the atrial appendage with the combination of radiofrequency

catheter ablation and minimally invasive atrial appendectomy. *Heart Rhythm.* 2014;11:17-25.

80. Yang Q, Ma J, Zhang S, Hu J, Liao Z. Focal atrial tachycardia originating from the distal portion of the left atrial appendage: characteristics and long-term outcomes of radiofrequency ablation. *Europace.* 2012;14:254-260.
81. Brugada J, Garcia-Bolao I, Figueiredo M, Puigfel M, Matas M, Navarro-López F. Radiofrequency ablation of concealed left free-wall accessory pathways without coronary sinus catheterization. *J Cardiovasc Electrophysiol.* 1997;8:249-253.
82. Yamane T, Jaïs P, Shah DC, et al. Efficacy and safety of an irrigated-tip catheter for the ablation of accessory pathways resistant to conventional radiofrequency ablation. *Circulation.* 2000;102:2565-2568.
83. Calkins H, Yong P, Miller JM, et al. Catheter ablation of accessory pathways, atrioventricular nodal reentrant tachycardia, and the atrioventricular junction: final results of a prospective, multicenter clinical trial. The Atakr Multicenter Investigators Group. *Circulation.* 1999;99:262-270.
84. Telishevska M, Faelchle J, Buiatti A, et al. Irrigated-tip catheters for radiofrequency ablation of right-sided accessory pathways in adolescents. *Pacing Clin Electrophysiol.* 2017;40:1167-1172.
85. Haissaguerre M, Marcus F, Poquet F, Gencel L, Le Métayer P, Clémenty J. Electrocardiographic characteristics and catheter ablation of parahissian accessory pathways. *Circulation.* 1994;90:1124-1128.
86. Brugada J, Puigfel M, Mont L, et al. Radiofrequency ablation of anteroseptal, para-Hisian, and mid-septal accessory pathways using a simplified femoral approach. *Pacing Clin Electrophysiol.* 1998;21:735-741.
87. Gaita F, Haissaguerre M, Giustetto C, et al. Safety and efficacy of cryoablation of accessory pathways adjacent to the normal conduction system. *J Cardiovasc Electrophysiol.* 2003;14:825-829.
88. Wen MS, Yeh SJ, Wang CC, King A, Lin FC, Wu D. Radiofrequency ablation therapy of the posteroseptal accessory pathway. *Am Heart J.* 1996;132:612-620.
89. Takahashi A, Shah DC, Jaïs P, Hocini M, Clementy J, Haïssaguerre M. Specific electrocardiographic features of manifest coronary vein posteroseptal accessory pathways. *J Cardiovasc Electrophysiol.* 1998;9:1015-1025.
90. Gatzoulis KA, Apostolopoulos T, Costeas X, et al. Radiofrequency catheter ablation of posteroseptal accessory pathways–results of a step-by-step ablation approach. *J Interv Card Electrophysiol.* 2001;5:193-201.
91. Sun Y, Arruda M, Otomo K, et al. Coronary sinus-ventricular accessory connections producing posteroseptal and left posterior accessory pathways: incidence and electrophysiological identification. *Circulation.* 2002;106:1362-1367.
92. Coffey JO, d'Avila A, Dukkipati S, et al. Catheter ablation of scar-related atypical atrial flutter. *Europace.* 2013;15:414-419.
93. Yokokawa M, Latchamsetty R, Ghanbari H, et al. Characteristics of atrial tachycardia due to small vs large reentrant circuits after ablation of persistent atrial fibrillation. *Heart Rhythm.* 2013;10:469-476.
94. Markowitz SM, Brodman RF, Stein KM, et al. Lesional tachycardias related to mitral valve surgery. *J Am Coll Cardiol.* 2002;39:1973-1983.
95. Jaïs P, Shah DC, Haïssaguerre M, et al. Mapping and ablation of left atrial flutters. *Circ Am Heart Assoc.* 2000;101:2928-2934.
96. Yamada T, McElderry HT, Doppalapudi H, et al. Idiopathic ventricular arrhythmias originating from the aortic root: prevalence, electrocardiographic and electrophysiologic characteristics, and results of radiofrequency catheter ablation. *J Am Coll Cardiol.* 2008;52:139-147.
97. Konstantinidou M, Koektuerk B, Wissner E, et al. Catheter ablation of right ventricular outflow tract tachycardia: a simplified remote-controlled approach. *Europace.* 2011;13:696-700.
98. Ban J-E, Chen Y-L, Park H-C, et al. Idiopathic ventricular arrhythmia originating from the para-Hisian area: Prevalence, electrocardiographic and electrophysiological characteristics. *J Arrhythmia.* 2014;30:48-54.
99. Tada H, Tadokoro K, Ito S, et al. Idiopathic ventricular arrhythmias originating from the tricuspid annulus: prevalence, electrocardiographic characteristics, and results of radiofrequency catheter ablation. *Heart Rhythm.* 2007;4:7-16.
100. Yamada T, Yoshida N, Itoh T, et al. Idiopathic ventricular arrhythmias originating from the parietal band. *Circ Arrhythm Electrophysiol.* 2017;10:e005099.
101. Sadek MM, Benhayon D, Sureddi R, et al. Idiopathic ventricular arrhythmias originating from the moderator band: Electrocardiographic characteristics and treatment by catheter ablation. *Heart Rhythm.* 2015;12:67-75.
102. Peichl P, Baran J, Wichterle D, et al. The tip of the muscle is a dominant location of ventricular ectopy originating from papillary muscles in the left ventricle. *J Cardiovasc Electrophysiol.* 2018;29:64-70.
103. Gordon JP, Liang JJ, Pathak RK, et al. Percutaneous cryoablation for papillary muscle ventricular arrhythmias after failed radiofrequency catheter ablation. *J Cardiovasc Electrophysiol.* 2018;29:1654-1663.
104. Tada H, Ito S, Naito S, et al. Idiopathic ventricular arrhythmia arising from the mitral annulus: a distinct subgroup of idiopathic ventricular arrhythmias. *J Am Coll Cardiol.* 2005;45:877-886.
105. Wasmer K, Köbe J, Dechering DG, et al. Ventricular arrhythmias from the mitral annulus: patient characteristics, electrophysiological findings, ablation, and prognosis. *Heart Rhythm.* 2013;10:783-788.
106. Santangeli P, Hutchinson MD, Supple GE, Callans DJ, Marchlinski FE, Garcia FC. Right atrial approach for ablation of ventricular arrhythmias arising from the left posterior–superior process of the left ventricle. *Circ Arrhythm Electrophysiol.* 2016;9:e004048.

CHAPTER 60

IMPLANTABLE CARDIOVERTER-DEFIBRILLATORS

Jonathan Lerner and Noel G. Boyle

INTRODUCTION

Since the first implant in 1980, and Food and Drug Administration (FDA) approval in 1985, implantable cardioverter-defibrillators (ICDs) have become the mainstay for treatment of ventricular arrhythmias and the prevention of sudden cardiac death (SCD).[1] ICD implantation is increasing exponentially worldwide. During the last world survey in 2009, it was estimated that there were 328,027 ICDs implanted, with 222,407 new implants and 105,620 replacements.[2] In the 40 years since their introduction, ICDs have become much smaller, longer-lasting, and multifeatured. As a result, the implantation of a dual-chamber ICD system is very similar to the implantation of a permanent pacemaker. Beyond defibrillation, modern ICDs are able to apply antitachycardia pacing to terminate up to 83% of ventricular arrhythmias, characterize and record arrhythmias, assess activity levels and monitor heart failure parameters, and provide cardiac resynchronization therapy (CRT).[3] As the indications for ICDs and CRT have expanded, so too has the number of these devices implanted. In the last decade, the development of a subcutaneous ICD (S-ICD) has provided yet another option in the prevention of SCD.[4]

INDICATIONS

The indications for implantation of an ICD can broadly be divided into primary and secondary prevention of SCD. Secondary prevention describes those patients who have already experienced a life-threatening arrhythmia (eg, ventricular tachycardia [VT] or ventricular fibrillation [VF]) whereas primary prevention describes those at elevated risk for SCD who have not yet experienced an event. A summary of the most recent American Heart Association/American College of Cardiology/Heart Rhythm Society (AHA/ACC/HRS) consensus guidelines of common ICD indications is provided in **Table 60.1**.[5]

TABLE 60.1 Major Indications for Implantable Cardioverter-Defibrillator Therapy

Class of Recommendation	Patient Population
Secondary Prevention	
I	Patients with NICM who survive sudden cardiac arrest caused by VT/VF or experience hemodynamically unstable VT or stable sustained VT not owing to reversible causes
I	Unexplained syncope in a patient with ischemic cardiomyopathy with inducible sustained monomorphic VT on EP study
IIa	Syncope presumed to be caused by ventricular arrhythmias in a NICM patient who does not meet LVEF criteria for a primary prevention ICD
Primary Prevention	
I	LVEF ≤35% with NYHA Class II or III heart failure despite GDMT
I	Ischemic cardiomyopathy with LVEF ≤30% and NYHA Class I heart failure
I	Ischemic cardiomyopathy with (a) NSVT and (b) LVEF ≤40% with inducible sustained VT or VF at EP study
IIa	Nonhospitalized patients with NYHA Class IV who are also candidates for cardiac transplantation or a LVAD
IIb	NICM with (a) LVEF ≤35% despite GDMT and (b) NYHA Class I heart failure

EP, electrophysiology; GDMT, guideline-directed medical therapy; ICD, implantable cardioverter-defibrillator; LVAD, left ventricular assist device; LVED, LVEF, left ventricular ejection fraction; NICM, nonischemic cardiomyopathy; NSVT, nonsustained ventricular tachycardia; NYHA, New York Heart Association; VF, ventricular fibrillation; VT, ventricular tachycardia.

Adapted from Al-Khatib SM, Stevenson WG, Ackerman MJ, et al. 2017 AHA/ACC/HRS guideline for management of patients with ventricular arrhythmias and the prevention of sudden cardiac death: A Report of the American College of Cardiology/American Heart Association Task Force on Clinical Practice Guidelines and the Heart Rhythm Society. *Heart Rhythm.* 2018;15(10):e73-e189. © 2018 by the American College of Cardiology Foundation, the American Heart Association, Inc., and the Heart Rhythm Society. With permission.

Secondary Prevention

Implantation of an ICD is indicated in all patients who have survived sudden cardiac arrest caused by VT or VF, those with an episode of hemodynamically unstable VT or stable sustained VT not owing to a reversible cause.[5] Three major multicenter randomized trials have studied the use of ICD in this patient population: Antiarrhythmics Versus Implantable Defibrillators (AVID) (1997), Canadian implantable defibrillator study (CIDS) (2000), and Cardiac Arrest Study Hamburg (CASH) (2000) which are summarized in **Table 60.2.** Each of the three trials randomized patients who had suffered sudden cardiac arrest or a sustained, life-threatening ventricular arrhythmia to antiarrhythmic medications versus ICD and antiarrhythmic medications.[6-8] Although all three trials showed a reduction in all-cause mortality in the ICD groups, this only reached statistical significance in the AVID trial.[6] A subsequent meta-analysis of all three trials showed a reduction of death by 28% in ICD groups. This was almost entirely attributable to a 50% reduction in arrhythmic death.[9] Because of the results of these studies, ICDs have become the first-line treatment for secondary prevention of SCD. Antiarrhythmic medications have been relegated to adjunctive treatments to reduce arrhythmia recurrence and appropriate ICD therapy.

Primary Prevention

Ischemic Cardiomyopathy

Multiple studies have confirmed that ICDs reduce all-cause mortality in selected patients with ischemic cardiomyopathy (**Table 60.3**). The Multicenter Automatic Defibrillator Implantation Trial (MADIT, 1996) and Multicenter Unsustained Tachycardia Trial (MUSTT, 1999) were the first large, multicenter trials of ICDs used for primary prevention. In spite of differences in study design, common inclusion criteria were coronary artery disease, reduced ejection fraction (EF), nonsustained VT, and inducible sustained monomorphic VT. In the MADIT trial, patients were randomized to receive medical therapy (typically amiodarone) or an ICD.[10] In the MUSTT study, patients were randomized to electrophysiologic study-guided drug therapy (ie, those with inducible VT) and received medications versus no antiarrhythmic therapy.[11] Although MUSTT was not a specific ICD trial for primary prevention of SCD, the results of the trial revealed that only with ICD backup was a significant reduction of arrhythmic death or cardiac arrest achieved. In 46% of the treatment group, ICDs were implanted owing to failure of medical therapy to suppress inducible VT. Both trials ultimately showed a decrease of greater than 50% in all-cause mortality in the ICD groups. The broader applicability of these trials has been questioned owing to the strict inclusion criteria of documented nonsustained VT and requirement for electrophysiologic studies.[12,13]

In response to these criticisms, the next generation of trials attempted to simplify and broaden inclusion criteria. The MADIT II trial (2002) randomized 1232 subjects with previous myocardial infarction (MI) and left ventricular ejection fraction (LVEF) less than or equal to 30% to conventional medical therapy versus ICD implantation.[14] Notably, neither documentation of nonsustained VT nor electrophysiologic study was required for randomization. Patients in the study had an average LVEF of 23%, and two-thirds of the patients had congestive heart failure with New York Heart Association (NYHA) Class II to IV symptoms. In the 20 months of follow-up analyzed in the initial report, the risk of death from any cause in the ICD group was 31% lower than in the conventional medical therapy arm. This benefit persisted up to

TABLE 60.2 Major Trials of ICD in Secondary Prevention of Sudden Cardiac Death

Trial	Number of Patients	Major Inclusion Criteria	Comparison Therapy	HR Mortality (ICD)	*P* Value
AVID	1013	Resuscitated VF, sustained VT+ syncope, sustained VT+LVEF ≤ 40% + hemodynamic compromise	Class III antiarrhythmics	0.62	<0.02
CIDS	659	Resuscitated VF, out of hospital cardiac arrest requiring defibrillation, sustained VT+ syncope, VT ≥ 150 bpm + symptoms +LVEF ≤ 35%, EPS-inducible monomorphic VT+ documented spontaneous VT	Amiodarone	0.8	0.142
CASH	288+58 (propafenone group stopped early)	Resuscitated cardiac arrest secondary to VT/VF	Amiodarone, propafenone, metoprolol	0.76	0.081

AVID, Antiarrhythmics Versus Implantable Defibrillators; bpm, beats per minute; CASH, Cardiac Arrest Study Hamburg; CIDS, Canadian Implantable Defibrillator Study; EPS, electrophysiology study; HR, heart rate; ICD, implantable cardioverter-defibrillator; LVEF, left ventricular ejection fraction SCD, sudden cardiac death; VF, ventricular fibrillation; VT, ventricular tachycardia.

Data from Antiarrhythmics Versus Implantable Defibrillators (AVID) Investigators. A comparison of antiarrhythmic drug therapy with implantable defibrillators in patients resuscitated from near-fatal ventricular arrhythmias. *N Engl J Med.* 1997;337(22):1576-1583. doi:10.1056/NEJM199711273372202; Connolly SJ, Gent M, Roberts RS, et al. Canadian implantable defibrillator study (CIDS): a randomized trial of the implantable cardioverter defibrillator against amiodarone. *Circulation.* 2000;101(11):1297-1302. doi:10.1161/01.cir.101.11.1297; Kuck KH, Cappato R, Siebels J, Rüppel R. Randomized comparison of antiarrhythmic drug therapy with implantable defibrillators in patients resuscitated from cardiac arrest: the Cardiac Arrest Study Hamburg (CASH). *Circulation.* 2000;102(7):748-754. doi:10.1161/01.cir.102.7.748

TABLE 60.3 Major Trials of ICD Benefit in Primary Prevention of Sudden Cardiac Death

Trial	Number of Patients	Etiology	Major Inclusion Criteria	HR Mortality (ICD)	*P* Value
MADIT	196	ICM	LVEF ≤ 35%, NSVT, inducible VT	0.46	.009
MUSTT	704	ICM	LVEF ≤ 40%, NSVT, inducible VT	0.45	<.001
MADIT II	1232	ICM	LVEF ≤ 30%, prior MI	0.69	.016
SCD-HeFT	2521	ICM and NICM	LVEF ≤ 35%, CHF NYHA Class II or III	0.77	.007
DEFINITE	458	NICM	LVEF ≤ 35%, VPCs or NSVT	0.65	.05
COMPANION	1520	ICM and NICM	LVEF ≤ 35%, CHF NYHA Class II or III, QRS ≥ 120 ms	0.64	.003
DINAMIT	676	ICM	LVEF ≤ 35%, HRV, recent MI (<40 days)	1.08	.66
CABG Patch	900	ICM	LVEF ≤ 35%, CABG, abnormal SAECG	1.07	.64
DANISH	556	NICM	NYHA Class II, III or IV (if CRT), LVEF ≤ 35%, increased NT-proBNP	0.87	.28

B-type natriuretic peptide; CABG, coronary artery bypass graft surgery; CHF, congestive heart failure; CRT, cardiac resynchronization therapy; HR, heart rate; HRV, heart rate variability; ICM, ischemic cardiomyopathy; LVEF, left ventricular ejection fraction; MI, myocardial infarction; NICM, nonischemic cardiomyopathy; NSVT, nonsustained ventricular tachycardia; NT-proBNP, N terminal-pro-hormone brain natriuretic protein; NYHA, New York Heart Association; NICM, nonischemic cardiomyopathy; SAECG, signal averaged electrocardiogram; SCD, sudden cardiac death; VPC, ventricular premature complexes.

Adapted from Sroubek J, Buxton AE. Primary Prevention Implantable Cardiac Defibrillator Trials: What Have We Learned? *Card Electrophysiol Clin.* 2017;9(4):761-773.

8 years, as was shown in a follow-up study. The number of ICDs needed to prevent one death was six over that time period.[15]

The Sudden Cardiac Death in Heart Failure Trial (SCD-HeFT), reported in 2005, is the largest primary prevention study with 2521 patients enrolled. It was the first major trial to include both ischemic and nonischemic cardiomyopathy; the inclusion criteria were NYHA Class II or III congestive heart failure and an LVEF less than or equal to 35%. Patients were randomized to medical therapy plus placebo, medical therapy plus amiodarone, or medical therapy plus ICD. The trial showed a 23% reduction in all-cause mortality in the ICD group and no improvement in all-cause mortality in the amiodarone group.[16] It should be noted that the ICD arm received single-lead, shock-only ICDs, which may affect the generalizability of the results to a more typical population seen in current clinical practice with dual-chamber ICD and CRT devices.

Nonischemic Cardiomyopathy

Although patients with nonischemic cardiomyopathy have an increased risk of SCD, unlike patients with ischemic cardiomyopathy, the evidence supporting the use of ICDs for primary prevention is notably weaker. As noted above, the SCD-HeFT trial was the first to include patients with nonischemic cardiomyopathy. The results of subgroup analyses of the trial showed similar beneficial effects in both ischemic and nonischemic cardiomyopathy.[16]

Beyond SCD-HeFT, two subsequent randomized trials of ICD use in nonischemic cardiomyopathy, the Defibrillators in Non-Ischemic Cardiomyopathy Treatment Evaluation (DEFINITE) trial and the Danish Study to Assess the Efficacy of ICDs in Patients with Nonischemic Systolic Heart Failure on Mortality (DANISH) trial, did not show an overall survival benefit. DEFINITE (2004) enrolled 229 patients with nonischemic cardiomyopathy, an LVEF less than 36% and ventricular premature complexes or nonsustained VT. Patients were randomized to medical therapy versus medical therapy plus ICD and followed for a mean of 29 months. All-cause mortality was lower in the ICD group; however, this was not statistically significant. ICDs did significantly reduce the rate of SCD in the treatment group.[17]

The most recent trial of ICD use in nonischemic cardiomyopathy, DANISH, was reported in 2016. The trial enrolled 560 patients with nonischemic cardiomyopathy, (NYHA Classes II or III) with LVEF less than or equal to 35% and an elevated serum N-terminal pro-B-type natriuretic peptide to usual care versus usual care plus ICD.[18] Greater than 50% of enrolled patients in both groups received CRT, a notable difference from prior trials. DANISH did not show a significant difference in overall survival between the two groups. The ICD group had a 50% lower risk of SCD compared with the control group. The DANISH trial is unique among prior trials of ICDs in nonischemic cardiomyopathy for a number of reasons. The observed mortality rate in the control arm and ICD group was 3% to 4% at 8 years, which was significantly lower than in prior trials. There was high utilization of CRT in both groups; CRT has been independently shown to reduce all-cause mortality and SCD.[19] Finally, medical therapy has significantly improved in the decade since prior studies were done, further reducing mortality in the control group. The high utilization of CRT and changes in medical therapy likely reduced the statistical power to detect a difference in mortality between the two groups. Subsequent meta-analyses support current guidelines that recommend placement of an ICD for primary prevention in patients with nonischemic cardiomyopathy and EF less than or equal to 35% after optimization on medical therapy for 3 months.[20]

TABLE 60.4 Implantable Cardioverter-Defibrillator (ICD) Indications for Rare Cardiomyopathies and Channelopathies

Condition	Inclusion Criteria	Class of Recommendation for ICD Placement
Arrhythmogenic right ventricular cardiomyopathy	ARVC with an additional marker of increased risk for SCD (resuscitated SCA, sustained VT, LVEF or RVEF ≤35%)	**I**
	ARVC with syncope presumed to be caused by ventricular arrhythmias	**IIa**
Hypertrophic cardiomyopathy	HCM with SCA or spontaneous sustained VT causing syncope or hemodynamic compromise	**I**
	HCM with either: a. maximum LV wall thickness ≥30 mm b. SCD in one or more first-degree relatives presumably caused by HCM c. One or more episodes of unexplained syncope within the preceding 6 months	**IIa**
	HCM with spontaneous NSVT or an abnormal blood pressure response with exercise who also have additional SCD risk modifiers or high-risk features	**IIa**
Catecholaminergic polymorphic ventricular tachycardia	CPVT and recurrent sustained VT or syncope, while receiving adequate or maximally tolerated β-blocker	**I**
Brugada syndrome	Brugada syndrome with spontaneous type 1 Brugada pattern on ECG and SCA, sustained ventricular arrhythmia, or recent history of syncope presumed to be caused by ventricular arrhythmia	**I**
Cardiac sarcoidosis	Cardiac sarcoidosis with sustained VT or SCA or LVEF ≤35%	**I**
	Cardiac sarcoidosis and LVEF >35% who have syncope and/or evidence of myocardial scar by cardiac MRI or PET scan, and/or have an indication for permanent pacing	**IIa**
Long-QT syndrome	High-risk symptomatic long-QT syndrome patients in whom a β-blocker is ineffective or not tolerated	**I**
	Asymptomatic patients with long-QT syndrome and a resting QTc >500 ms while receiving β-blocker	**IIb**
Emery-Dreifuss or limb-girdle type 1B muscular dystrophies	Emery-Dreifuss or limb-girdle type 1B muscular dystrophies with progressive cardiac involvement	**IIa**
Lamin A/C mutation	Nonischemic cardiomyopathy caused by lamin A/C mutation who have two or more risk factors (NSVT, LVEF <45%, non-missense mutation, and male sex)	**IIa**
Myotonic dystrophy type 1	Myotonic dystrophy type 1 with an indication for a permanent pacemaker	**IIb**

ARVC, arrhythmogenic right ventricular cardiomyopathy; CPVT, catecholaminergic polymorphic ventricular tachycardia; ECG, electrocardiogram; HCM, hypertrophic cardiomyopathy; NSVT, nonsustained ventricular tachycardia; LV, left ventricle; LVEF, left ventricular ejection fraction; MRI, magnetic resonance imaging; PET, positron emission tomography; RVEF, right ventricular ejection fraction; SCA, sudden cardiac arrest; SCD, sudden cardiac death; VT, ventricular tachycardia.

Adapted from Al-Khatib SM, Stevenson WG, Ackerman MJ, et al. 2017 AHA/ACC/HRS guideline for management of patients with ventricular arrhythmias and the prevention of sudden cardiac death: A Report of the American College of Cardiology/American Heart Association Task Force on Clinical Practice Guidelines and the Heart Rhythm Society. *Heart Rhythm.* 2018;15(10):e73-e189.

Genetic and Acquired Disorders

Numerous genetic and acquired disorders confer an increased risk of SCD. These include Brugada syndrome, arrhythmogenic right ventricular cardiomyopathy, hypertrophic cardiomyopathy, long-QT and short-QT syndromes, as well as infiltrative diseases like amyloidosis and cardiac sarcoidosis. Evidence for the use of ICDs in these patient populations in primary prevention is limited to case series and expert opinions. The consequences of ICD placement in these patients should not be minimized. ICD implantation in these often-young patients exposes them to lifetime risks of device infection, lead malfunction, and the need for repeated generator changes. Guidelines for ICD placement in some of these conditions are summarized in **Table 60.4**.

"High-Risk" Syncope

Patients with unexplained syncope and structural heart disease comprise a small portion of the total number of ICD implants. Very little data are available in this patient population that can be used to guide therapy. Trials of secondary prevention did not include these patients, and syncope was often part of the exclusion criteria for primary prevention studies. Among patients with ischemic cardiomyopathy and unexplained syncope, electrophysiologic study can be used for risk stratification; inducible monomorphic VT is a Class I indication for ICD implantation. In those patients with nonischemic cardiomyopathy, the role of electrophysiologic testing remains unclear; the presence of syncope presumed to be secondary to ventricular arrhythmia is a Class IIa indication for ICD implantation by current guidelines.[5,21]

CONTRAINDICATIONS: IMPLANTABLE CARDIOVERTER-DEFIBRILLATORS

Even among those appropriately selected for ICD placement, only one-third will receive an appropriate shock for VT/VF in the first 5 years after placement. Many high-risk patients will not benefit from their ICD because of the elevated incidence of nonarrhythmic death caused by other comorbidities, in spite of their risk of VT/VF.

Important exclusions to primary prevention ICD implantation are coronary artery bypass graft (CABG) or percutaneous coronary intervention (PCI) within the prior 90 days, MI within the prior 40 days, and treatment of heart failure for less than 3 months. In addition, ICD implantation is not indicated in patients with NYHA Class IV heart failure who are not candidates for CRT or advanced therapies such as left ventricular assist device or cardiac transplantation.[5] This is owing to their high rate of nonarrhythmic death.

Two important studies underlie the waiting period requirements following revascularization or MI. The Defibrillator in Acute Myocardial Infarction Trial (DINAMIT), reported in 2004, randomized patients with acute MI, LVEF less than or equal to 35%, and reduced heart rate variability to ICD plus medical therapy versus medical therapy alone. Patients were enrolled 6 to 40 days after an MI. No difference in overall mortality was observed between the two groups.[22] Similarly, the CABG Patch trial (1997) randomized patients with ischemic cardiomyopathy and abnormal electrocardiograms to receive an ICD or no antiarrhythmic treatment at the time of CABG. After follow-up, no difference in mortality was observed between the two cohorts.[23]

DEVICE SELECTION

Transvenous ICDs

There are two major variables to consider when selecting an ICD system: single- versus dual-chamber device and single- versus dual-coil shocking lead. For patients with a pacing indication and who are in sinus rhythm, dual-chamber devices are preferred. For patients whose only indication is for prevention of arrhythmic events or are in permanent atrial fibrillation, single-chamber devices are appropriate. Single-chamber devices have a reduced rate of complications related to lead placement (eg, dislodgement or perforation).[24] Dual-chamber devices were thought to provide a theoretical advantage of better discrimination between atrial and ventricular arrhythmias to avoid inappropriate shocks; however, data from the Primary Prevention ICD French Registry (DAI-PP) and National Cardiovascular Data Registry (NCDR) showed no significant difference in inappropriate therapies between the two types of devices.[24,25] No prospective studies have been conducted on this topic and, in the current era of improved discrimination algorithms, the data suggest that single-chamber devices are adequate to prevent inappropriate shocks.

Early transvenous ICD systems developed in the 1990s required two separate shocking leads, for defibrillation (one in the right ventricle and one in the innominate/superior vena cava (SVC)), as the defibrillator "can" was inactive ("cold") (**Figure 60.1 upper row**). In more modern systems, with active participation of the "can" in defibrillation, the second lead is no longer necessary (Figure 60.1 **lower row**). The advantage of dual-coil leads was a reportedly improved defibrillation efficacy caused by decreased shock impedance and a greater number of shock vectors. However, a recent meta-analysis found a statistically significant decrease in defibrillation thresholds with dual-coil leads of 0.81 J, which was clinically insignificant.[26] Dual-coil leads are more complex, have higher failure rates, and are more difficult to extract. Because of the disadvantages of dual-coil leads, coupled with their limited advantages, single-coil leads are now generally preferred.[27]

Subcutaneous ICDs

Transvenous leads have long been the Achilles heel of implantable cardiac devices. Because of perioperative risks (eg, pneumothorax, perforation) and late complications (eg, infection, lead fracture, or malfunction), an entirely subcutaneous device was developed.[4] S-ICDs offer both advantages and disadvantages compared with transvenous systems. S-ICDs are only capable of defibrillation and brief postshock transcutaneous

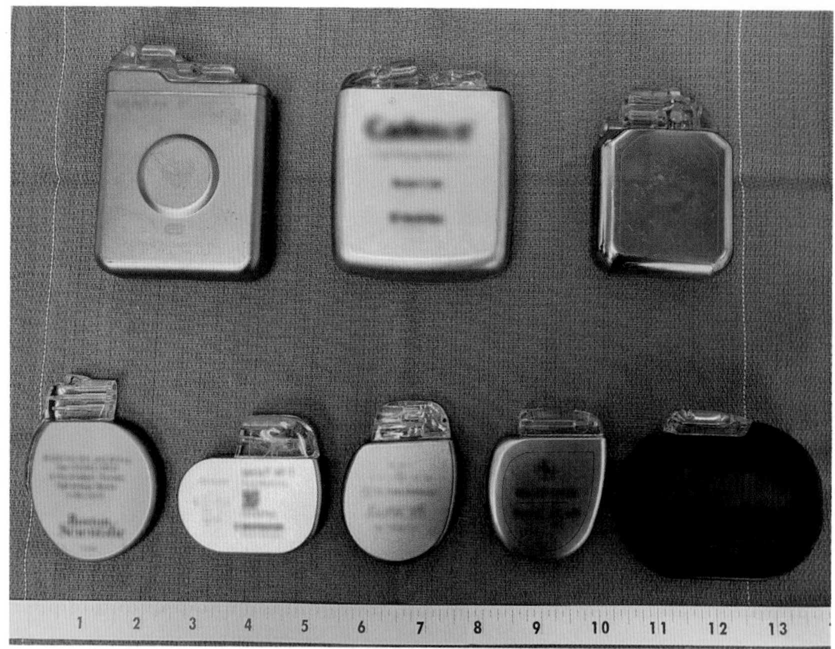

FIGURE 60.1 Examples of early and current implantable cardioverter-defibrillator devices. Upper row: Early model devices (upper left and center) from 1990s which were abdominal implants with epicardial patches and initial pectoral implanted device with transvenous leads (upper right). Lower row: Current pectoral ICD devices and modern SQ ICD device (right). [scale is in inches]

pacing. They cannot be used in patients with a pacing indication nor can they be used in patients who might benefit from antitachycardia pacing. S-ICDs are preferred in patients with a history of device infection or endocarditis, those with poor venous access, and are often the patient choice for younger patients.[5]

ANATOMIC CONSIDERATIONS

Site Selection

The process of selection of an implant site is similar to that of permanent pacemakers with the caveat that ICD generators are somewhat larger and more prominent. Most devices are implanted adjacent to the site of venous access, the vast majority of which are in the left upper chest, near the subclavian, axillary, or cephalic vein. Similarly, most ICD devices are placed on the left side to optimize defibrillation vector with an "active" can and right ventricular shocking coil. The left-sided venous system also has the advantage of a "shallower" angle between the left subclavian and innominate veins, making lead advancement easier. Important reasons to choose the alternative side include a history of breast cancer or the presence of an arteriovenous dialysis fistula. Both issues typically require implantation on the contralateral side.[28]

Venography

A venogram performed prior to the implantation procedure will define the venous anatomy and the feasibility of each approach to implantation. The procedure is done with an injection of 10 to 15 mL of contrast through an IV in the ipsilateral arm. Storing fluoroscopic images for later use in the procedure helps to guide attempts at venous access. The venogram may also reveal an absent or atretic cephalic vein, as well as more central stenosis (**Figure 60.2**). The risk/benefit of venography should be carefully considered in patients with renal insufficiency who are at risk for contrast-induced nephropathy; in such cases, ultrasound imaging can be used to assess the patency of the venous system.

Implant Techniques

There are a variety of approaches to implanting transvenous ICDs which are identical to the implantation of permanent pacemakers. The two most common sites of access for the leads are the cephalic and axillary veins. The cephalic implantation technique requires a surgical cutdown to the vein prior to lead advancement. Although this approach is somewhat more technically challenging, it virtually eliminates the risk of pneumothorax and also decreases the risk of later lead fractures from subclavian crush syndrome. Access to the axillary or subclavian veins is obtained through a modified Seldinger technique with leads advanced through peel-away sheaths. Other, less common sites of venous access are the external jugular and iliofemoral veins.[29]

Implantation of an S-ICD is significantly different from the placement of a transvenous device. The generator is placed in the subcutaneous tissues of the fifth or sixth left intercostal space near the mid-axillary line. The shocking coil is typically placed in the left parasternal region and connected to the generator with a specialized tunneling tool. The placement of the shocking coil requires one or two additional small incisions on the chest wall.

After placement of an ICD, patients were typically monitored overnight for observation, although many hospitals now

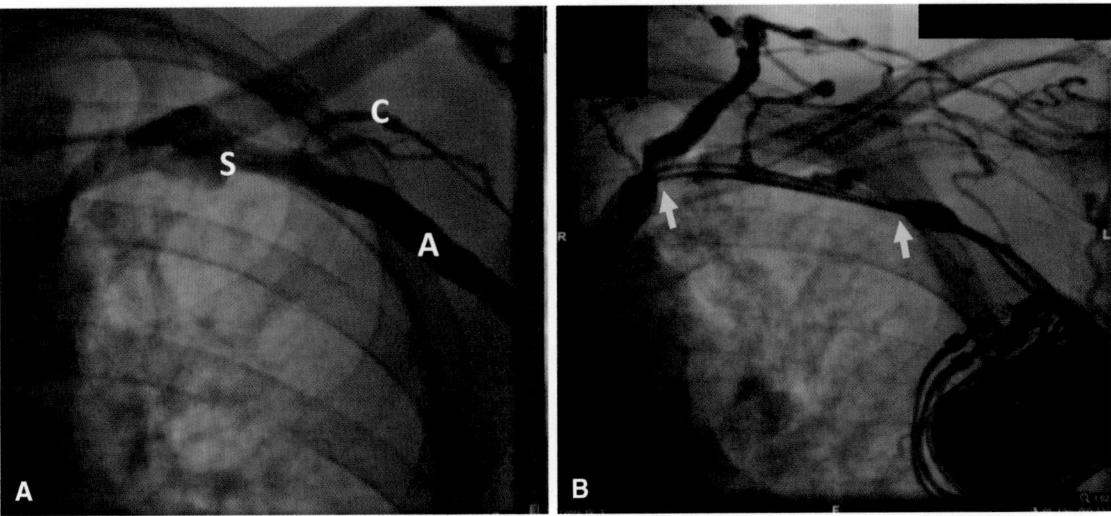

FIGURE 60.2 **(A)** Venogram showing patent left axillary (A), subclavian (S), and cephalic (C) veins. **(B)** Venogram showing occlusion extending from axillary to subclavian veins (between arrows) with extensive collateral veins in a patient with an implanted dual-chamber pacemaker.

discharge these patients on the same day. A chest x-ray is obtained to exclude pneumothorax and confirm lead position, and a 12-lead electrocardiogram is obtained. The device is interrogated to ensure it is functioning properly, prior to discharge.

CLINICAL ASPECTS OF ICD MANAGEMENT

Device Programming

Optimal ICD programming is important to ensure appropriate shocks will be delivered when indicated and that inappropriate shocks are avoided. A number of studies have investigated ICD programming strategies and their effects on appropriate and inappropriate shocks, as well as on all-cause mortality. The Primary Prevention Parameters Evaluation (PREPARE) Study, (MADIT-RIT), and ALTITUDE REDUCES studies generally showed that multiple detection zones, longer detection intervals, and the use of antitachycardia pacing reduced the number of total, appropriate, and inappropriate shocks without any effect on mortality.[30-32] ICD programming guidelines released by the Heart Rhythm Society in 2015 and updated in 2019 are summarized in **Table 60.5**.[33]

PATIENT AND DEVICE FOLLOW-UP

After implantation, an initial follow-up visit should be scheduled within 2 weeks to ensure the implant incision site is healed and without infection. Initial interrogation should take place within 3 months of implantation and should continue every 3 to 6 months thereafter. Modern devices allow for remote interrogation so that lead parameters, battery status, and events may be reviewed remotely.

SPECIAL CONSIDERATIONS—WEARABLE DEFIBRILLATORS

Patients who are post-MI and with new heart failure with reduced EF must wait 40 days and 3 months, respectively, before implantation of an ICD for primary prevention. As discussed above, the trials involving these populations, DINAMIT and CABG Patch did not show a mortality benefit of ICD placement in these populations as each population is not sufficiently selected to have a high risk of arrhythmic death. Nevertheless, there may be patients who are at high short-term risk for SCD (eg, myocarditis) who fall into the current exclusion criteria for ICD placement. In these cases, a wearable defibrillator is an option until the patient becomes eligible for ICD or their clinical condition improves.

The Vest Prevention of Early Sudden Death Trial (VEST) is the only randomized trial to evaluate wearable defibrillators. The trial tested whether a wearable defibrillator reduced SCD in the early period after acute MI with an LVEF less than or equal to 35%. No benefit was observed in the reduction of arrhythmic death.[34,35] Current guidelines give a Class IIa recommendation to the use of wearable defibrillators in the setting of temporary ICD removal (eg, infection) for patients with a history of SCD or sustained VT. There is a Class IIb recommendation for wearable defibrillator use for patients with an increased risk of SCD who fall into two categories: those with active cardiac inflammation and those who fall into the 40-day or 3-month ICD exclusion windows.[5]

RESEARCH AND FUTURE DIRECTIONS

ICD technology has advanced remarkably since initial developments in the 1980s. Implantation techniques approach the simplicity of permanent pacemaker insertion. The addition of features like event recording, antitachycardia pacing, and recording of physiologic parameters have expanded ICD's functionality and usefulness in the treatment of a variety of cardiac patients. Subcutaneous systems have afforded some key advantages to selected patients. Reliability of transvenous leads remains a major limitation, and continued innovation both in lead design and in subcutaneous devices will likely contribute to improved performance in these devices.

TABLE 60.5 General Implantable Cardioverter-Defibrillator (ICD) Programming Guidelines

Detection parameters	Program tachyarrhythmia detection duration to require the tachycardia to continue for at least 6-12 seconds or for 30 intervals
	Slowest tachycardia therapy zone between 185 and 200 bpm in primary prevention patients
	Enable SVT discriminators
	Program SVT discriminators to include rates >200 bpm
	For secondary prevention patients in whom clinical VT rate is known, program the slowest tachycardia therapy zone at least 10 bpm below the tachycardia rate but not faster than 200 bpm
	Program more than one tachycardia detection zone to allow effective use of tiered therapy and/or SVT-VT discriminators
	For subcutaneous ICDs, program two tachycardia detection zones: a. Zone with tachycardia discriminators at rate ≤200 bpm b. Zone without discriminators at rate ≥230 bpm
	Program tachycardia monitoring zone to record untreated arrhythmias
	Activate all lead failure alerts
	Disable SVT discriminator timeout
	Activate lead "noise" algorithms
	Active T-wave oversensing algorithms
Therapy parameters	Program ATP therapy "on" for all VT detection zones up to 230 bpm in patients with structural heart disease
	Program ATP to deliver at least one ATP attempt with a minimum of eight stimuli at a cycle length of 84%-88% arrhythmia cycle length
	Use burst ATP therapy in preference to ramp ATP therapy
	Program the initial shock energy to the maximum available energy in the highest detection rate zone (unless specific DFT testing demonstrates efficacy at lower energies)

ATP, antitachycardia pacing; bpm, beats per minute; DFT, defibrillation threshold; ICD, implantable cardioverter-defibrillator; SVT, supraventricular tachycardia; TCL, tachycardia cycle; VT, ventricular tachycardia.

Adapted from Stiles MK, Fauchier L, Morillo CA, et al. 2019 HRS/EHRA/APHRS/LAHRS focused update to 2015 expert consensus statement on optimal implantable cardioverter-defibrillator programming and testing. *Heart Rhythm.* 2020;17(1):e220-e228. https://creativecommons.org/licenses/by/4.0/.

KEY POINTS

- ✔ Since their development in the 1980s, ICDs remain an effective treatment for the prevention of SCD.
- ✔ The survival benefit seen from ICD implantation is driven by the reduction in arrhythmic death. Appropriate patient selection is key: patients with a high risk of nonarrhythmic death or low risk of arrhythmic death are unlikely to benefit from an ICD.
- ✔ Modern ICD systems have become small enough that the implantation technique is identical to permanent pacemakers.
- ✔ Selection of an ICD system and implant site should be based on patient and clinical factors. An S-ICD may be optimal for patients with high infection risk or with poor venous access and no pacing indication.
- ✔ Dual-chamber ICDs do not seem to provide a benefit in the discrimination of VF versus supraventricular tachycardia and should be reserved for patients with sinus node dysfunction or conduction abnormalities.
- ✔ Device programming should be based on guideline recommendations in order to minimize the number of inappropriate shocks.
- ✔ Routine ICD interrogation is now an integral part of device follow-up and allows for earlier detection of device malfunction and greater patient convenience.
- ✔ Wearable defibrillators may be considered in patients who have a high short-term risk of SCD but are not candidates for an implanted device because of extrinsic limitations; however, no trials have shown a reduction in mortality with their use.

REFERENCES

1. Mirowski M, Reid PR, Mower MM, et al. Termination of malignant ventricular arrhythmias with an implanted automatic defibrillator in human beings. *N Engl J Med.* 1980;303(6):322-324. doi:10.1056/NEJM198008073030607
2. Mond HG, Proclemer A. The 11th world survey of cardiac pacing and implantable cardioverter-defibrillators: calendar year 2009—a World Society of Arrhythmia's project. *Pacing Clin Electrophysiol.* 2011;34(8):1013-1027. doi:10.1111/j.1540-8159.2011.03150.x
3. Cantillon DJ, Wilkoff BL. Antitachycardia pacing for reduction of implantable cardioverter-defibrillator shocks. *Heart Rhythm.* 2015;12(6):1370-1375. doi:10.1016/j.hrthm.2015.02.024
4. Bardy GH, Smith WM, Hood MA, et al. An entirely subcutaneous implantable cardioverter-defibrillator. *N Engl J Med.* 2010;363(1):36-44. doi:10.1056/NEJMoa0909545

5. Al-Khatib SM, Stevenson WG, Ackerman MJ, et al. 2017 AHA/ACC/HRS Guideline for management of patients with ventricular arrhythmias and the prevention of sudden cardiac death: a report of the American College of Cardiology/American Heart Association Task Force on Clinical Practice Guidelines and the Heart Rhythm Society. *Heart Rhythm.* 2018;15(10):e73-e189. doi:10.1016/j.hrthm.2017.10.036
6. Antiarrhythmics versus Implantable Defibrillators (AVID) Investigators. A comparison of antiarrhythmic-drug therapy with implantable defibrillators in patients resuscitated from near-fatal ventricular arrhythmias. *N Engl J Med.* 1997;337(22):1576-1583. doi:10.1056/NEJM199711273372202
7. Connolly SJ, Gent M, Roberts RS, et al. Canadian implantable defibrillator study (CIDS): a randomized trial of the implantable cardioverter defibrillator against amiodarone. *Circulation.* 2000;101(11):1297-1302. doi:10.1161/01.cir.101.11.1297
8. Kuck KH, Cappato R, Siebels J, Rüppel R. Randomized comparison of antiarrhythmic drug therapy with implantable defibrillators in patients resuscitated from cardiac arrest: the Cardiac Arrest Study Hamburg (CASH). *Circulation.* 2000;102(7):748-754. doi:10.1161/01.cir.102.7.748
9. Connolly SJ, Hallstrom AP, Cappato R, et al. Meta-analysis of the implantable cardioverter defibrillator secondary prevention trials. AVID, CASH and CIDS studies. Antiarrhythmics vs Implantable Defibrillator study. Cardiac Arrest Study Hamburg. Canadian Implantable Defibrillator Study. *Eur Heart J.* 2000;21(24):2071-2078. doi:10.1053/euhj.2000.2476
10. Moss AJ, Hall WJ, Cannom DS, et al. Improved survival with an implanted defibrillator in patients with coronary disease at high risk for ventricular arrhythmia. Multicenter Automatic Defibrillator Implantation Trial Investigators. *N Engl J Med.* 1996;335(26):1933-1940. doi:10.1056/NEJM199612263352601
11. Buxton AE, Lee KL, Fisher JD, Josephson ME, Prystowsky EN, Hafley G. A randomized study of the prevention of sudden death in patients with coronary artery disease. Multicenter Unsustained Tachycardia Trial Investigators. *N Engl J Med.* 1999;341(25):1882-1890. doi:10.1056/NEJM199912163412503
12. Buxton AE, Lee KL, DiCarlo L, et al. Electrophysiologic testing to identify patients with coronary artery disease who are at risk for sudden death. Multicenter Unsustained Tachycardia Trial Investigators. *N Engl J Med.* 2000;342(26):1937-1945. doi:10.1056/NEJM200006293422602
13. Meissner MD, Lieberman RA. Electrophysiologic testing to identify patients at risk for sudden death. *N Engl J Med.* 2000;343(24):1813-1814. doi:10.1056/NEJM200012143432414
14. Moss AJ, Zareba W, Hall WJ, et al. Prophylactic implantation of a defibrillator in patients with myocardial infarction and reduced ejection fraction. *N Engl J Med.* 2002;346(12):877-883. doi:10.1056/NEJMoa013474
15. Goldenberg I, Gillespie J, Moss AJ, et al. Long-term benefit of primary prevention with an implantable cardioverter-defibrillator: an extended 8-year follow-up study of the Multicenter Automatic Defibrillator Implantation Trial II. *Circulation.* 2010;122(13):1265-1271. doi:10.1161/CIRCULATIONAHA.110.940148
16. Bardy GH, Lee KL, Mark DB, et al. Amiodarone or an implantable cardioverter-defibrillator for congestive heart failure. *N Engl J Med.* 2005;352(3):225-237. doi:10.1056/NEJMoa043399
17. Kadish A, Dyer A, Daubert JP, et al. Prophylactic defibrillator implantation in patients with nonischemic dilated cardiomyopathy. *N Engl J Med.* 2004;350(21):2151-2158. doi:10.1056/NEJMoa033088
18. Køber L, Thune JJ, Nielsen JC, et al. Defibrillator implantation in patients with nonischemic systolic heart failure. *N Engl J Med.* 2016;375(13):1221-1230. doi:10.1056/NEJMoa1608029
19. Cleland JG, Daubert JC, Erdmann E, et al. The effect of cardiac resynchronization on morbidity and mortality in heart failure. *N Engl J Med.* 2005;352(15):1539-1549. doi:10.1056/NEJMoa050496
20. Al-Khatib SM, Fonarow GC, Joglar JA, et al. Primary prevention implantable cardioverter defibrillators in patients with nonischemic cardiomyopathy: a meta-analysis. *JAMA Cardiol.* 2017;2(6):685-688. doi:10.1001/jamacardio.2017.0630
21. Gatzoulis KA, Vouliotis AI, Tsiachris D, et al. Primary prevention of sudden cardiac death in a nonischemic dilated cardiomyopathy population: reappraisal of the role of programmed ventricular stimulation. *Circ Arrhythm Electrophysiol.* 2013;6(3):504-512. doi:10.1161/CIRCEP.113.000216
22. Hohnloser SH, Kuck KH, Dorian P, et al. Prophylactic use of an implantable cardioverter-defibrillator after acute myocardial infarction. *N Engl J Med.* 2004;351(24):2481-2488. doi:10.1056/NEJMoa041489
23. Bigger JT. Prophylactic use of implanted cardiac defibrillators in patients at high risk for ventricular arrhythmias after coronary-artery bypass graft surgery. Coronary Artery Bypass Graft (CABG) Patch Trial Investigators. *N Engl J Med.* 1997;337(22):1569-1575. doi:10.1056/NEJM199711273372201
24. Defaye P, Boveda S, Klug D, et al. Dual-vs. single-chamber defibrillators for primary prevention of sudden cardiac death: long-term follow-up of the Défibrillateur Automatique Implantable-Prévention Primaire registry. *Europace.* 2017;19(9):1478-1484. doi:10.1093/europace/euw230
25. Dewland TA, Pellegrini CN, Wang Y, Marcus GM, Keung E, Varosy PD. Dual-chamber implantable cardioverter-defibrillator selection is associated with increased complication rates and mortality among patients enrolled in the NCDR implantable cardioverter-defibrillator registry. *J Am Coll Cardiol.* 2011;58(10):1007-1013. doi:10.1016/j.jacc.2011.04.039
26. Kumar P, Baker M, Gehi AK. Comparison of single-coil and dual-coil implantable defibrillators: a meta-analysis. *JACC Clin Electrophysiol.* 2017;3(1):12-19. doi:10.1016/j.jacep.2016.06.007
27. Pokorney SD, Parzynski CS, Daubert JP, et al. Temporal trends in and factors associated with use of single-versus dual-coil implantable cardioverter-defibrillator leads: data from the NCDR ICD registry. *JACC Clin Electrophysiol.* 2017;3(6):612-619. doi:10.1016/j.jacep.2016.11.014
28. Ellenbogen KA, Kaszala K. *Cardiac Pacing and ICDs.* 7th ed. John Wiley & Sons; 2020:1. (online resource).
29. Lau EW. Upper body venous access for transvenous lead placement—review of existent techniques. *Pacing Clin Electrophysiol.* 2007;30(7):901-909. doi:10.1111/j.1540-8159.2007.00779.x
30. Wilkoff BL, Williamson BD, Stern RS, et al. Strategic programming of detection and therapy parameters in implantable cardioverter-defibrillators reduces shocks in primary prevention patients: results from the PREPARE (Primary Prevention Parameters Evaluation) study. *J Am Coll Cardiol.* 2008;52(7):541-550. doi:10.1016/j.jacc.2008.05.011
31. Moss AJ, Schuger C, Beck CA, et al. Reduction in inappropriate therapy and mortality through ICD programming. *N Engl J Med.* 2012;367(24):2275-2283. doi:10.1056/NEJMoa1211107
32. Gilliam FR, Hayes DL, Boehmer JP, et al. Real world evaluation of dual-zone ICD and CRT-D programming compared to single-zone programming: the ALTITUDE REDUCES study. *J Cardiovasc Electrophysiol.* 2011;22(9):1023-1029. doi:10.1111/j.1540-8167.2011.02086.x
33. Stiles MK, Fauchier L, Morillo CA, Wilkoff BL. 2019 HRS/EHRA/APHRS/LAHRS focused update to 2015 expert consensus statement on optimal implantable cardioverter-defibrillator programming and testing. *Heart Rhythm.* 2020;17(1):e220-e228. doi:10.1016/j.hrthm.2019.02.034
34. Olgin JE, Pletcher MJ, Vittinghoff E, et al. Wearable cardioverter-defibrillator after myocardial infarction. *N Engl J Med.* 2018;379(13):1205-1215. doi:10.1056/NEJMoa1800781
35. Sroubek J, Buxton AE. Primary prevention implantable cardiac defibrillator trials: what have we learned? *Card Electrophysiol Clin.* 2017;9(4):761-773. doi:10.1016/j.ccep.2017.08.006

CHAPTER 61

SYNCOPE

Humberto Butzke da Motta and Olujimi A. Ajijola

INTRODUCTION

Syncope is defined as a transient loss of consciousness (TLOC) and loss of postural tone because of cerebral hypoperfusion. It is characterized by rapid onset, short duration (minutes or less), and spontaneous recovery; is not associated with prior head trauma, use of alcohol or other substances or metabolic abnormalities; and must be differentiated from seizure.[1,2] It can cause secondary traumatic injury and be the only warning sign of severe cardiac disease before sudden cardiac death.

Syncope is a common clinical problem, accounting for up to 3% of all emergency department (ED) visits[3] for an estimate of over 156,000 hospital admissions in the United States in 2013, with increasing costs in the last decade.[4] Among the 7814 participants in the Framingham Heart Study, in an average follow-up of 17 years, 822 patients (11%) reported having syncope, with an incidence of a first episode of 6.2 per 1000 patient-years.[5] In the general population, up to 50% of people report having had at least one episode of syncope, most of whom never come to medical attention, with peaks at around 20, 60, and 80 years of age.[6]

PATHOGENESIS, CAUSES, AND CLASSIFICATION

Syncope is the result of a fall in systemic blood pressure (BP), leading to a global decrease in cerebral perfusion. BP is the result of the interaction between cardiac output and systemic vascular resistance—with these two mechanisms acting together in different degrees depending on the underlying cause—leading to hypotension.

The causes of syncope can be divided into three major groups: reflex syncope, orthostatic hypotension, and cardiac syncope. These are summarized in **Table 61.1** and **Figure 61.1**.

Reflex Syncope

Reflex syncopes, also called neurally mediated syncopes or vasovagal syncopes (VVSs), are caused by a loss of sympathetic tone or increase in vagal tone. The mechanisms involved determine two hemodynamic patterns: either a vasodepressive state, with decreased systemic vascular resistance, or a cardioinhibitory state, with bradycardia and low cardiac output. These mechanisms are not associated with specific triggers and can predominate or occur simultaneously. Reflex syncopes can be subdivided into: *situational*—that is, associated with specific actions, such as micturition, stimulation of the gastrointestinal tract (swallowing, defecation), cough, post–strenuous exercise, laughter; *vasovagal*—occurring either with prolonged standing or emotional and physical stimulation (eg, pain, blood phobia, other forms of emotional stress); and associated with *carotid sinus hypersensitivity*. There are also cases in which no specific trigger can be identified or the patient presents with nontypical symptoms. These cases are denominated *reflex syncope of unknown cause*, and the diagnosis is probable if cardiac causes are excluded and/or the symptoms are reproduced in a tilt-table test. Reflex syncope is considered to have a more benign course than that of cardiac syncope or orthostatic hypotension.[7]

TABLE 61.1 Causes of Syncope

Reflex syncope or neurally-mediated syncope • Vasovagal syncope • Situational syncope • Syncope triggered by carotid sinus hypersensitivity • Syncope induced by mechanical factors (self-induced syncope, straining, micturition, cough, playing wind instruments, etc)
Orthostatic hypotension • Primary autonomic failure • Secondary autonomic failure • Drugs (vasodilators, diuretics, phenothiazines, antidepressants, etc) • Volume depletion
Cardiac syncope • Bradyarrhythmias • Sinus node dysfunction • Atrioventricular conduction system disease • Tachyarrhythmias • Supraventricular tachycardia • Ventricular tachycardia • Structural heart disease (aortic stenosis, ischemic heart disease, hypertrophic cardiomyopathy, cardiac masses, pericardial disease/tamponade, prosthetic valve dysfunction) • Great vessels disease (pulmonary embolism, aortic dissection, pulmonary hypertension)

With data from Brignole M, Moya A, de Lange FJ, et al. 2018 ESC Guidelines for the diagnosis and management of syncope. *Eur Heart J.* 2018;39(21):1883-1948. doi:10.1093/eurheartj/ehy037; Saal DP, van Dijk JG. Classifying syncope. *Auton Neurosci.* 2014;184:3-9. doi:10.1016/j.autneu.2014.05.007

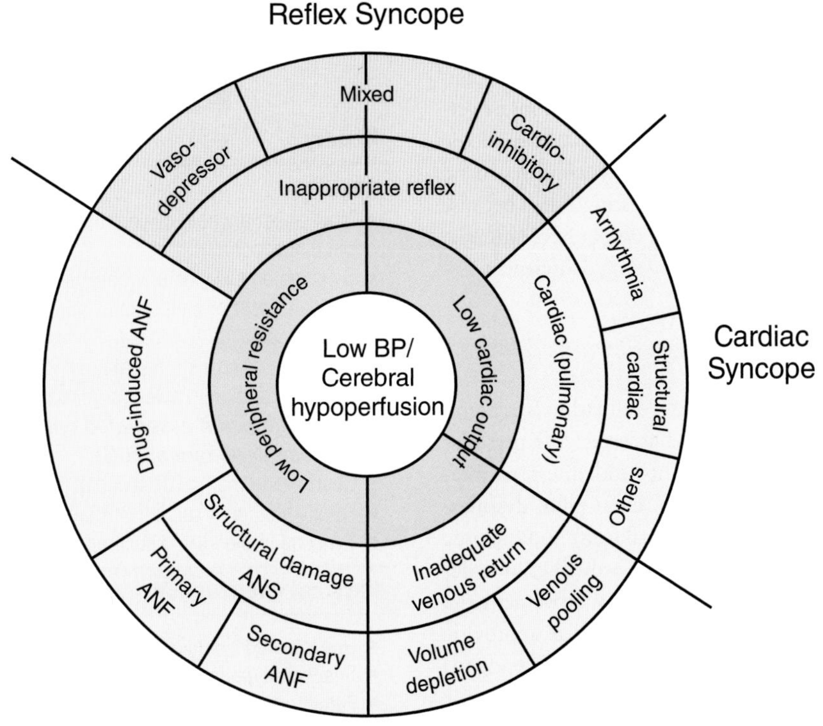

FIGURE 61.1 Pathophysiologic basis of the classification of syncope. ANF, autonomic failure; ANS, autonomic nervous system; BP, blood pressure. (From Brignole M, Moya A, de Lange FJ, et al.; ESC Scientific Document Group. 2018 ESC Guidelines for the diagnosis and management of syncope. *Eur Heart J.* 2018;39(21):1883-1948. Reproduced by permission of The European Society of Cardiology.)

Orthostatic Syncope

Moving to an upright position is associated with a significant shift of blood to the lower segments of the body, leading to a decrease in preload. In physiologic states, this activates the sympathetic nervous system, which counteracts by increasing the systemic vascular tone, thereby restoring blood flow toward the heart and maintaining cardiac output. In pathologies that cause autonomic failure, this compensation mechanism may be impaired. In these patients, changing from a recumbent or sitting position to the upright posture may trigger syncope or presyncope. This is denominated *orthostatic hypotension* and is defined as a 20 mm Hg or more drop in systolic BP or a 10 mm Hg or more drop in diastolic BP after 3 minutes of standing.[8] Autonomic failure may occur as a primary phenomenon in neurodegenerative diseases such as Parkinson disease, multiple system atrophy, or pure autonomic failure, as well as a secondary effect of other systemic illnesses, such as diabetes mellitus or amyloidosis. It can also be an adverse effect of drugs (eg, alpha- or beta-adrenergic antagonists, diuretics) and occur in volume-depleted states.

The *postural orthostatic tachycardia syndrome* (POTS), a condition related to orthostatic hypotension, is defined as an increment of 30 bpm in heart rate within 10 minutes of standing or after being tilted head-up, in the absence of hypotension. Patients may complain of symptoms of cerebral hypoperfusion or autonomic reactivity. It is associated with recent viral illness, deconditioning, chronic fatigue, or restricted autonomic neuropathy. Symptoms tend to be relieved by returning to the recumbent position.

Cardiac Syncope

Cardiac or *cardiopulmonary syncopes*, which occur when the cardiac output is dramatically decreased, can be subdivided into two categories: *arrhythmic syncope* and *structural cardiac disease*. The most frequent form of arrhythmic syncope is that caused by bradyarrhythmias, usually happening when the ventricular rate is lower than 30 bpm for 15 to 30 seconds.[9] Tachyarrhythmias, notably ventricular tachycardia but also supraventricular tachycardia, can also present with syncope. Particular heart diseases that lead to syncope are covered in depth in specific chapters in this book.

Some conditions may be confused with syncope. *Generalized epileptic seizures*, with concomitant disorganized electrical activity of both cerebral hemispheres, cause TLOC, but generally last longer and present with one-sided limb movements, tongue bites, and more prolonged postictal mental confusion and somnolence. *Psychogenic pseudosyncope* does not have the characteristic changes in BP and heart rate that accompany syncope; it usually has increased frequency, longer duration, and patients tend to maintain their eyes closed, which is unusual in syncope.

Cerebrovascular disease, notably *subclavian steal syndrome*, which was previously described as a cause of syncope, does not fit the more modern definition. This syndrome, as well as transient ischemic attacks (TIAs) arising from carotid obstructions or vertebrobasilar ischemia, does not present without focal neurologic signs, being relatively easy to distinguish from syncope in general practice. *Cataplexy*, a rare diagnosis, can be distinguished because of the fact that patients with this condition do not have amnesia, being able to describe the event after recovering conscience.

DIAGNOSIS

The most important part of the diagnostic evaluation is a careful and thorough patient history. It should ascertain the presence of any prodromal symptoms such as light-headedness, palpitations, sweating, tunnel and faded vision, chest pain, dyspnea, and neurologic symptoms (eg, focal weakness, tonic-clonic movements). An eyewitness account is also valuable, in order to establish the duration of the attack and any movement the patient may have done while unconscious, as well as to provide a description of the recovery period. The presence of previous episodes of syncope should also be evaluated, as well as possible triggers. The physical examination should focus on measuring the BP while the patient is in a supine position, after sitting, immediately after standing, and after being upright for 3 minutes. Also, the physician should pay attention to heart rate and rhythm and any signs of possible structural heart disease, such as gallops, murmurs, rubs, or bruits. A summary neurologic examination looking for focal signs is also warranted.

All patients presenting with syncope should have a 12-lead electrocardiogram (ECG) performed. An abnormal ECG in the context of syncope is associated with increased all-cause mortality.[10]

According to the most recent guidelines on the diagnosis and management of syncope,[1,2] the initial evaluation should answer four questions, which will guide the subsequent management:

1. Was the event a TLOC?
2. Was it syncopal or nonsyncopal in origin?
3. In the case of syncope, is there a clear etiology?
4. Is there evidence to suggest a high risk of cardiovascular events or death?

Clinical and ECG features associated with higher risk are summarized in **Table 61.2**. Patients who do not have structural heart disease, ECG abnormalities, family history of sudden cardiac death, and no evidence of supine or exertional syncope or palpitations at the time of syncope are considered to be at low risk for cardiac syncope and should be managed in the outpatient setting.[11]

Routine comprehensive laboratory testing is not recommended. Selected tests should be ordered according to clinical suspicion. The usefulness of high-sensitivity troponin and B-type natriuretic peptide is uncertain when not guided by a specific clinical hypothesis, such as a clinical suspicion of ischemia or heart failure.

TABLE 61.2 High-Risk Clinical and Electrocardiographic Features in Patients With Syncope

History

Major
- New onset of chest discomfort, breathlessness, abdominal pain, headache
- Syncope on exertion or when supine
- Sudden onset of palpitations immediately followed by syncope
- History of severe structural heart disease (heart failure, low ejection fraction, previous myocardial infarction)

Minor (high risk if associated with structural heart disease or abnormal ECG)
- Short prodrome (<10 seconds)
- Family history of sudden cardiac death at young age
- Syncope in the sitting position

Physical examination

- Unexplained systolic BP in the ED <90 mm Hg
- Suspected gastrointestinal bleed
- Persistent bradycardia (<40 bpm) when awake
- Undiagnosed systolic murmur

Electrocardiogram

Major
- Acute ischemia
- Mobitz II second- or third-degree AV block
- Atrial fibrillation with slow ventricular response (<40 bpm) or repetitive sinoatrial block or sinus pauses >3 seconds
- Bundle branch block, intraventricular conduction disturbance, ventricular hypertrophy, Q-waves consistent with ischemic heart disease or cardiomyopathy
- Sustained or nonsustained VT
- Brugada pattern
- QTc >460 ms in repeated 12-lead ECGs
- Pacemaker malfunction

Minor (high risk if history consistent with arrhythmic syncope)
- Mobitz I second-degree AV block or first-degree AV block with markedly prolonged PR interval
- Asymptomatic mild sinus bradycardia (40-50 bpm) or slow atrial fibrillation (ventricular rate 40-50 bpm)
- Paroxysmal SVT or atrial fibrillation
- Preexcited QRS complex
- Short QTc (<340 ms)
- Atypical Brugada pattern
- Features suggestive of ARVC

ARVC, arrhythmogenic right ventricular cardiomyopathy; AV, atrioventricular; BP, blood pressure; bpm, beats per minute; ECG, electrocardiogram; ED, emergency department; ms, milliseconds; QTc, corrected QT interval; SVT, supraventricular tachycardia; VT, ventricular tachycardia.

With data from Brignole M, Moya A, de Lange FJ, et al. 2018 ESC Guidelines for the diagnosis and management of syncope. *Eur Heart J.* 2018;39(21):1883-1948. doi:10.1093/eurheartj/ehy037; Mereu R, Sau A, Lim PB. Diagnostic algorithm for syncope. *Auton Neurosci.* 2014;184:10-16. doi:10.1016/j.autneu.2014.05.008

Continuous ECG monitoring with telemetry is warranted for high-risk hospitalized patients and should be initiated as soon as possible, despite its low diagnostic yield. Other modalities of monitors should be indicated according to the frequency of symptoms. External loop recorders have a better diagnostic performance when compared to Holter monitoring, but also have a low diagnostic yield. Implantable loop recorders (ILRs) have shown to be more cost-effective than a combined strategy with external loop recorder, tilt-table test, and electrophysiologic study,[12] with the most common association with syncope being asystole and bradycardia.[13] The ILR is indicated in the investigation of recurrent unexplained syncope without high-risk criteria, as well as to evaluate the indication for cardiac pacing in patients with reflex syncope.[14]

Transthoracic echocardiography (TTE) should be performed in patients in whom structural heart disease is suspected. It can be useful to demonstrate left ventricular systolic dysfunction and, in some cases, identify the cause of syncope and eliminate the need for further testing (eg, severe aortic stenosis, atrial myxoma).

An exercise stress test should be performed in those who have syncope during or after exertion. Syncope during exercise is considered to be a rare event and is usually associated with structural or arrhythmic causes, whereas syncope during recovery mostly reflects an increased vagal tone.

An electrophysiologic study has a low diagnostic yield when performed in patients with normal ECG and TTE. Also, its role has decreased in the last few years because of the advancement of noninvasive monitors as well as the expansion of indication of implantable cardioverter-defibrillators (ICDs) for primary prevention in all patients with heart failure and left ventricular ejection fraction less than or equal to 35%. However, it still can be useful to measure the His bundle-ventricular interval in patients with bundle branch block and syncope, as well as to diagnose and treat supraventricular tachycardias.

Tilt-table test has been used to investigate syncope since the 1980s. The patient is placed in the supine position for at least 20 minutes, with assessment of baseline heart rate and BP. The table is then rapidly tilted up to 60 to 80 degrees to the horizontal to place the patient in a head-up position. This provides a gravitational stimulus without the counteraction of muscular contraction. Sensitizing agents, such as sublingual nitroglycerin or isoproterenol, can be used, with the caveat of decreasing the specificity of the test.[15,16] The end point is to reproduce symptoms alongside a typical hemodynamic pattern (cardioinhibitory, vasodepressive, or mixed). The most appropriate setting to perform a tilt-table test is in patients with suspected VVS, orthostatic hypotension, or POTS. It can also be useful to diagnose psychogenic pseudosyncope. It cannot be used to evaluate response to pharmacologic treatment.[17] Unfortunately, in the situation in which it could be most useful, that is, to evaluate unexplained syncope, the test has not performed well, with positivity rates around 30%.[18]

Some clinical maneuvers may help identify patients with syncope because of orthostatic hypotension or reflex.

- Abnormal *heart rate variability with deep breathing* may signal a dysfunctional autonomic system. This test is performed by having the patient take deep breaths with continuous heart rate monitoring.[19]
- The *Valsalva maneuver* consists of a forced expiration against a closed glottis or closed loop system while BP and heart rate are continuously monitored. The hemodynamic changes induced can be divided into four phases: phase 1—increased intrathoracic pressure with mechanical compression of the aorta and transient increase in BP; early phase 2—compression of the vena cava with decreased venous return and decreased cardiac output, with consequent fall in BP; late phase 2—detection of drop in BP by baroreceptors, leading to sympathetic discharge and vasoconstriction, increasing systemic resistance and BP; phase 3—patient stops exhaling, which decreases intrathoracic pressure, leading to an interruption in BP rise; phase 4—arteriolar vasoconstriction with "overshoot" of BP. These phases can be better visualized in **Figure 61.2**. Failure to increase heart rate when BP drops or absence of BP increase in phases 2 and 4 may indicate autonomic dysfunction.
- *A carotid sinus massage* is recommended to investigate patients with syncope compatible with reflex mechanism. It is deemed positive when there is a ventricular pause longer than 3 seconds and/or a drop in systolic BP greater than 50 mm Hg, with reproduction of symptoms. This maneuver should be avoided or undertaken with caution in patients with previous stroke, TIAs, or known carotid stenosis greater than 70%.
- During the *active standing test* the patient is asked to stand after being in supine position for at least 5 minutes. It provides a different assessment from the tilt-table test, as it simulates the physiologic changes associated with moving to the upright position in daily life. It is positive when systolic BP decreases 20 mm Hg or more or diastolic BP decreases 10 mm Hg or more from baseline, or systolic BP falls under 90 mm Hg, with reproduction of symptoms.

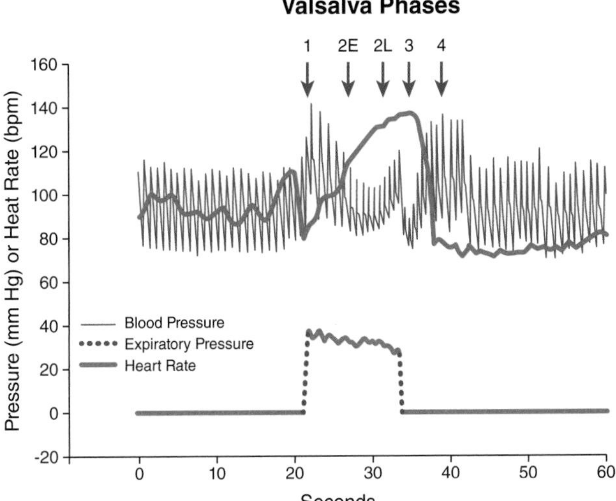

FIGURE 61.2 The Valsalva maneuver. (Reprinted from Jones PK, Gibbons CH. The role of autonomic testing in syncope. *Auton Neurosci.* 2014;184:40-45. Copyright © 2014 Elsevier. With permission.)

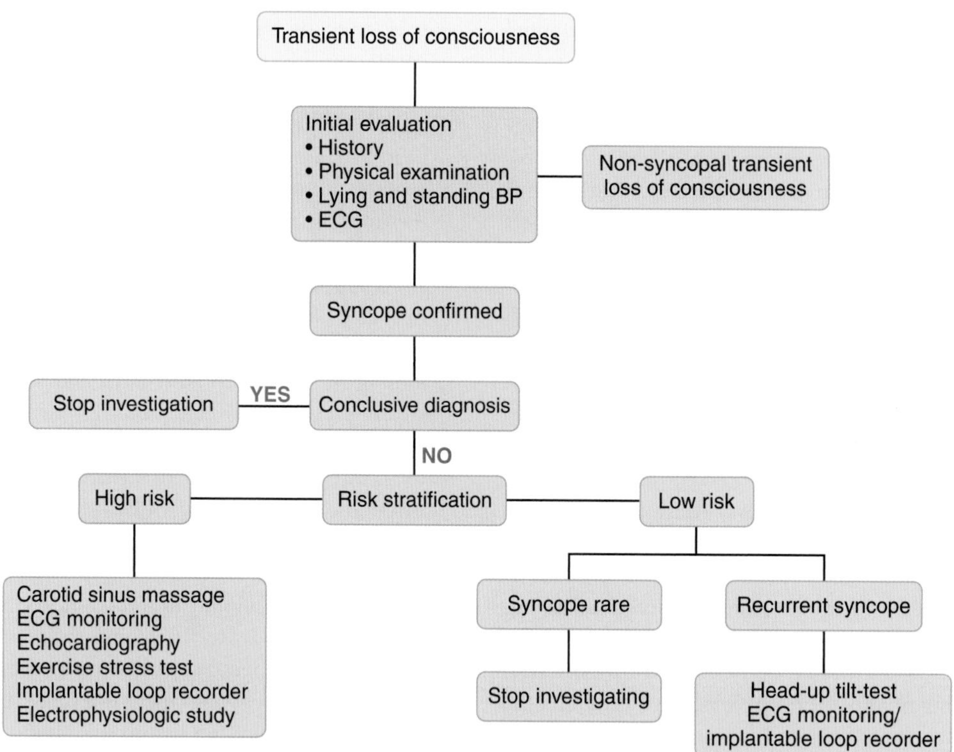

ALGORITHM 61.1 Diagnostic management of syncope. BP, blood pressure; ECG, electrocardiogram. (Adapted from Mereu R, Sau A, Lim PB. Diagnostic algorithm for syncope. *Auton Neurosci.* 2014;184:10-16. Copyright © 2014 Elsevier. With permission.)

- Ambulatory BP monitoring may be used to identify patients who are "non-dippers" or even have increased BP during sleep, which is associated with orthostatic hypotension.[20]

The diagnostic management of syncope is summarized in **Algorithm 61.1**.

MANAGEMENT

As stated earlier, the initial evaluation should aim to identify patients who are at high risk for cardiac syncope and sudden cardiac death, as well as those who are symptomatic because of another severe acute illness. These patients should be admitted and treated accordingly. Those who do not have high-risk features should be subdivided into intermediate or low risk. Patients who do not fit into high- or low-risk categories should be observed in the ED, preferably in a syncope unit, but not admitted to the hospital. They are likely to need expert consultation, which in most cases can be done safely in the outpatient setting. Low-risk features are described in **Table 61.3**.

Scoring systems have been developed in the past two decades to assist with the management of syncope in the emergency room, focusing on trying to identify patients with worse short-term prognosis. The most well-known criteria are the San Francisco Syncope Rule,[21] the Rose rule,[22] the Boston rule,[23] the Osservatorio Epidemiologico della Sincope nel Lazio (OESIL) risk score,[24] and the EGSYS) score.[25] Not all of them have been externally validated, and they are generally not considered to be superior to clinical judgment, so they should not be used alone.[26]

The management of reflex syncope and orthostatic hypotension will be presented. Syncope because of structural cardiac disease and because of arrhythmogenic disorders is thoroughly covered in other chapters.

The current European Society of Cardiology (ESC) and American Heart Association/American College of Cardiology/Heart Rhythm Society (AHA/ACC/HRS) guidelines regarding the treatment of orthostatic hypotension recommend that all patients should be educated about their condition. They also

TABLE 61.3 Low-Risk Clinical and Electrocardiographic Features in Patients With Syncope

- Normal physical examination
- Normal electrocardiogram
- Associated with typical prodrome of reflex syncope
- After unpleasant sensation
- After prolonged standing
- During meal or postprandial
- Associated with specific triggers as cough, defecation, micturition
- Triggered by head rotation or pressure on carotid sinus
- Standing from supine/sitting position
- Long history of recurrent syncope with same characteristics of current episode
- Absence of structural cardiac disease

With data from Brignole M, Moya A, de Lange FJ, et al. 2018 ESC Guidelines for the diagnosis and management of syncope. *Eur Heart J.* 2018;39(21):1883-1948. doi:10.1093/eurheartj/ehy037 should maintain a daily water intake of 2 to 3 L and adequate salt consumption. Rapid ingestion of water, as well as counterpressure maneuvers, such as squatting, leg crossing, handgrip, and lower body muscle tension, can also relieve symptoms temporarily. Other measures such as compressive stockings and sleeping with the bed tilted greater than 10 degrees may also be beneficial. Intensive treatment for hypertension may exacerbate symptoms, especially when diuretics or beta-blockers are used. Some pharmacologic treatments have also been studied. Midodrine (2.5-10 mg three times daily), an alpha-agonist, may be effective for some patients, but the evidence is of low quality[27]. Fludrocortisone (0.1-0.3 mg/day), a mineralocorticoid, may also be beneficial, but its use may be limited by supine hypertension and excessive fluid retention. More recently, the US Food and Drug Administration (FDA) has approved droxidopa, a precursor of norepinephrine, for the treatment of orthostatic hypotension, after symptomatic improvement was shown without increasing the risk for supine hypertension.[28] Other agents, such as pyridostigmine and octreotide, have an uncertain benefit.

The management of reflex syncope may include nonpharmacologic treatment, medications, and implanted devices. Patients should be educated about the benign course of their condition, considering the absence of structural heart disease and the young age with which many patients present. They should be taught to identify triggers and avoid them as much as possible, keep hydrated, as well as to lie down and activate counterpressure measures as soon as prodromal symptoms ensue. Careful avoidance or reduction in doses of antihypertensive drugs, nitrates, diuretics, neuroleptic antidepressants, or dopaminergic drugs is recommended. In the SPRINT trial, patients assigned to a systolic BP goal of 120 mm Hg had an increased risk of syncope compared to those assigned to a 140 mm Hg goal.[29] In motivated, symptomatic subjects, tilt-training (progressive periods in upright posture) has been proposed, with conflicting results.

Educational measures tend to control symptoms and reduce the recurrence in the majority of patients with VVS. For those in whom these interventions fail or experience syncope in high-risk activities (eg, driving, machine operation, flying, athletes), have a short prodrome that puts them at risk for traumatic lesions, or have very frequent episodes, more intensive treatment is warranted.

Many drugs have been tested for VVS, most with disappointing results. Fludrocortisone (0.05-0.2 mg/day) may be an option for patients without contraindications (ie, heart failure or hypertension). Treatment with alpha-agonists (etilefrine, midodrine) is probably of little use as a result of reduced compliance because of frequent dosing and side effects (ie, hypertension, urinary obstruction). The use of beta-blockers to treat reflex syncope is controversial, particularly in patients younger than 42 years. Other drugs such as paroxetine, theophylline, and sibutramine are under evaluation.

Patients with a documented cardioinhibitory mechanism may benefit from cardiac pacing. Based on the ISSUE-3 trial, the most recent ESC and AHA/ACC/HRS guidelines give a class IIa recommendation for cardiac pacing in patients 40 years or older with cardioinhibitory VVS and a documented correlation between symptoms and ECG recording. This includes patients with asystole of 3 seconds or more and syncope

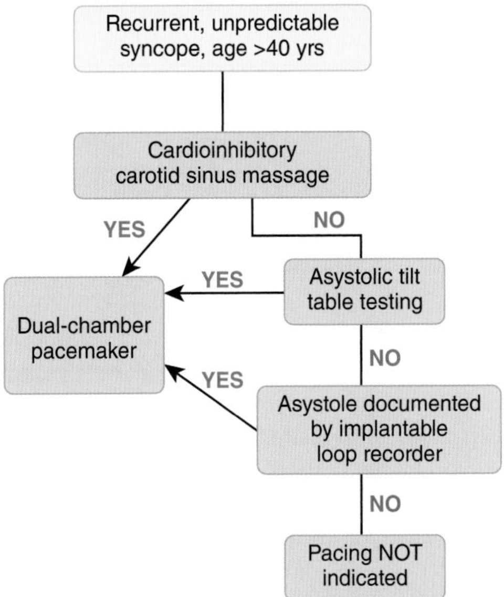

ALGORITHM 61.2 Cardiac pacing for patients with reflex syncope. (From Brignole M, Moya A, de Lange FJ, et al.; ESC Scientific Document Group. 2018 ESC Guidelines for the diagnosis and management of syncope. *Eur Heart J.* 2018;39(21):1883-1948. Reproduced by permission of The European Society of Cardiology.)

or asystole of 6 seconds or more irrespective of syncope, recorded on ILR.[30] Consideration for pacemaker implantation is also warranted for patients with carotid sinus syndrome–associated syncope with predominant cardioinhibitory response. There is diverging opinion regarding pacing in cases of tilt-table test–induced cardioinhibitory syncope. For those with mixed or vasodepressive mechanisms, pacing is not warranted. The proposed algorithm for cardiac pacing in VVS, adapted from the ESC guidelines, is shown in **Algorithm 61.2**. The decision to implant a device should always be shared with the patient, taking into consideration the quality of life, burden of syncope, and risks associated with the pacemaker.

SPECIAL CONSIDERATIONS AND FUTURE RESEARCH

TLOC because of cerebral hypoperfusion is a very common problem, leading to around 3% of ED evaluations. In many cases, it leads to unnecessary testing, procedures, and cost. The main focus of the initial evaluation should be to ascertain that the patient indeed had syncope by excluding other causes of TLOC and to evaluate the likelihood of an underlying structural heart disease or severe illness. Patients considered to be at high risk for structural heart disease or severe illness should be admitted for further evaluation and treatment. Those without these features most likely can be safely managed as outpatients. If a diagnosis of neurally mediated syncope or orthostatic hypotension is made, nonpharmacologic treatment is successful in most cases. However, some patients may eventually need medications as described earlier or even cardiac pacing. More research is needed to further the understanding of autonomic dysfunction as a cause of reflex syncope, leading the way to more targeted therapies.

KEY POINTS

- ✔ Syncope—TLOC caused by global cerebral hypoperfusion—is a common medical problem very frequently associated with expensive and unnecessary investigation.
- ✔ Causal mechanisms can be subdivided into three groups: reflex syncope, orthostatic hypotension, and cardiac syncope.
- ✔ Only patients with high-risk features need to be hospitalized for investigation and treatment of syncope. Most patients may be observed for a short period and be discharged and reevaluated in the outpatient setting.
- ✔ Investigation must include a detailed history, focused physical examination, and ECG. These tests should guide the necessity for further evaluation.
- ✔ The treatment of orthostatic hypotension involves educational measures and avoiding excessive vasodilators and diuretics. Pharmacologic treatment with fludrocortisone, midodrine, or droxidopa may also be needed.
- ✔ The treatment of reflex syncope is most often successful with education, but pharmacologic treatment and even implanted pacemakers may be necessary in carefully selected cases.

REFERENCES

1. Shen W-K, Sheldon RS, Benditt DG, et al. 2017 ACC/AHA/HRS Guideline for the evaluation and management of patients with syncope: a report of the American College of Cardiology/American Heart Association Task Force on Clinical Practice Guidelines and the Heart Rhythm Society. *Circulation.* 2017;136(5):e25-e59. doi:10.1161/CIR.0000000000000499
2. Brignole M, Moya A, de Lange FJ, et al. 2018 ESC Guidelines for the diagnosis and management of syncope. *Eur Heart J.* 2018;39(21): 1883-1948. doi:10.1093/eurheartj/ehy037
3. Day SC, Cook EF, Funkenstein H, Goldman L. Evaluation and outcome of emergency room patients with transient loss of consciousness. *Am J Med.* 1982;73(1):15-23. doi:10.1016/0002-9343(82)90913-5
4. Anand V, Benditt DG, Adkisson WO, Garg S, George SA, Adabag S. Trends of hospitalizations for syncope/collapse in the United States from 2004 to 2013—an analysis of national inpatient sample. *J Cardiovasc Electrophysiol.* 2018;29(6):916-922. doi:10.1111/jce.13479
5. Soteriades ES, Evans JC, Larson MG, et al. Incidence and prognosis of syncope. *N Engl J Med.* 2002;347(12):878-885. doi:10.1056/NEJMoa012407
6. Ruwald MH, Hansen ML, Lamberts M, et al. The relation between age, sex, comorbidity, and pharmacotherapy and the risk of syncope: a Danish nationwide study. *Europace.* 2012;14(10):1506-1514. doi:10.1093/europace/eus154
7. Toarta C, Mukarram M, Arcot K, et al. Syncope prognosis based on emergency department diagnosis: a prospective cohort study. *Acad Emerg Med.* 2018;25(4):388-396. doi:10.1111/acem.13346
8. Freeman R, Wieling W, Axelrod FB, et al. Consensus statement on the definition of orthostatic hypotension, neurally mediated syncope and the postural tachycardia syndrome. *Clin Auton Res.* 2011;21(2):69-72. doi:10.1007/s10286-011-0119-5
9. Saal DP, van Dijk JG. Classifying syncope. *Auton Neurosci.* 2014;184:3-9. doi:10.1016/j.autneu.2014.05.007
10. Pérez-Rodon J, Martínez-Alday J, Barón-Esquivias G, et al. Prognostic value of the electrocardiogram in patients with syncope: data from the Group for Syncope Study in the Emergency Room (GESINUR). *Heart Rhythm.* 2014;11(11):2035-2044. doi:10.1016/j.hrthm.2014.06.037
11. Mereu R, Sau A, Lim PB. Diagnostic algorithm for syncope. *Auton Neurosci.* 2014;184:10-16. doi:10.1016/j.autneu.2014.05.008
12. Edvardsson N, Wolff C, Tsintzos S, Rieger G, Linker NJ. Costs of unstructured investigation of unexplained syncope: insights from a micro-costing analysis of the observational PICTURE registry. *Europace.* 2015;17(7):1141-1148. doi:10.1093/europace/euu412
13. Brignole M, Vardas P, Hoffmann E, et al. Indications for the use of diagnostic implantable and external ECG loop recorders. *Europace.* 2009;11(5):671-687. doi:10.1093/europace/eup097
14. Solbiati M, Sheldon RS. Implantable rhythm devices in the management of vasovagal syncope. *Auton Neurosci.* 2014;184:33-39. doi:10.1016/j.autneu.2014.05.012
15. Raviele A, Menozzi C, Brignole M, et al. Value of head-up tilt testing potentiated with sublingual nitroglycerin to assess the origin of unexplained syncope. *Am J Cardiol.* 1995;76(4):267-272. doi:10.1016/S0002-9149(99)80079-4
16. Morillo CA, Klein GJ, Zandri S, Yee R. Diagnostic accuracy of a low-dose isoproterenol head-up tilt protocol. *Am Heart J.* 1995;129(5):901-906. doi:10.1016/0002-8703(95)90110-8
17. Moya A, Permanyer-Miralda G, Sagrista-Sauleda J, et al. Limitations of head-up tilt test for evaluating the efficacy of therapeutic interventions in patients with vasovagal syncope: Results of a controlled study of etilefrine versus placebo. *J Am Coll Cardiol.* 1995;25(1):65-69. doi:10.1016/0735-1097(94)00336-O
18. Furukawa T, Maggi R, Solano A, Croci F, Brignole M. Effect of clinical triggers on positive responses to tilt-table testing potentiated with nitroglycerin or clomipramine. *Am J Cardiol.* 2011;107(11):1693-1697. doi:10.1016/j.amjcard.2011.01.057
19. Jones PK, Gibbons CH. The role of autonomic testing in syncope. *Auton Neurosci.* 2014;184:40-45. doi:10.1016/j.autneu.2014.05.011
20. Voichanski S, Grossman C, Leibowitz A, et al. Orthostatic hypotension is associated with nocturnal change in systolic blood pressure. *Am J Hypertens.* 2012;25(2):159-164. doi:10.1038/ajh.2011.191
21. Quinn JV, Stiell IG, McDermott DA, Sellers KL, Kohn MA, Wells GA. Derivation of the San Francisco Syncope Rule to predict patients with short-term serious outcomes. *Ann Emerg Med.* 2004;43(2):224-232. doi:10.1016/S0196-0644(03)00823-0
22. Reed MJ, Newby DE, Coull AJ, Prescott RJ, Jacques KG, Gray AJ. The ROSE (Risk Stratification of Syncope in the Emergency Department) Study. *J Am Coll Cardiol.* 2010;55(8):713-721. doi:10.1016/j.jacc.2009.09.049
23. Grossman SA, Fischer C, Lipsitz LA, et al. Predicting adverse outcomes in syncope. *J Emerg Med.* 2007;33(3):233-239. doi:10.1016/j.jemermed.2007.04.001
24. Ammirati F. Diagnosing syncope in clinical practice. Implementation of a simplified diagnostic algorithm in a multicentre prospective trial—the OESIL 2 Study (Osservatorio Epidemiologico della Sincope nel Lazio). *Eur Heart J.* 2000;21(11):935-940. doi:10.1053/euhj.1999.1910
25. Del Rosso A, Ungar A, Maggi R, et al. Clinical predictors of cardiac syncope at initial evaluation in patients referred urgently to a general hospital: the EGSYS score. *Heart.* 2008;94(12):1620-1626. doi:10.1136/hrt.2008.143123
26. Matthews R, Young A. Did this patient have cardiac syncope? the rational clinical examination systematic review. *J Emerg Med.* 2019;57(5): 751-752. doi:10.1016/j.jemermed.2019.11.005
27. Parsaik AK, Singh B, Altayar O, et al. Midodrine for orthostatic hypotension: a systematic review and meta-analysis of clinical trials. *J Gen Intern Med.* 2013;28(11):1496-1503. doi:10.1007/s11606-013-2520-3
28. Strassheim V, Newton JL, Tan MP, Frith J. Droxidopa for orthostatic hypotension: a systematic review and meta-analysis. *J Hypertens.* 2016;34(10):1933-1941. https://journals.lww.com/jhypertension/Fulltext/2016/10000/Droxidopa_for_orthostatic_hypotension__a.4.aspx
29. Wright JT Jr, Williamson JD, Whelton PK, et al. A randomized trial of intensive versus standard blood-pressure control. *N Engl J Med.* 2015;373(22):2103-2116. doi:10.1056/NEJMoa1511939
30. Brignole M, Menozzi C, Moya A, et al. Pacemaker therapy in patients with neurally mediated syncope and documented asystole. *Circulation.* 2012;125(21):2566-2571. doi:10.1161/CIRCULATIONAHA.111.082313

CHAPTER 62

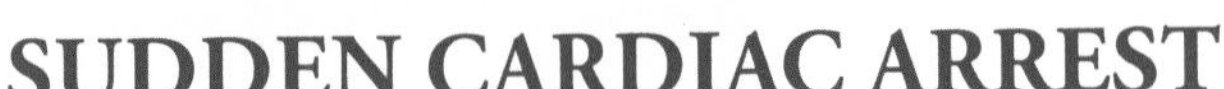

SUDDEN CARDIAC ARREST

Yuliya Krokhaleva and Marmar Vaseghi

INTRODUCTION

Sudden cardiac arrest (SCA) is defined as the cessation of all mechanical activity of the heart resulting in the absence of circulation with the onset of symptoms within 1 hour preceding the otherwise unexpected event. When resuscitation is not attempted or not successful, SCA leads to sudden cardiac death (SCD). Overall survival from SCA remains poor, and out-of-hospital cardiac arrest portends a worse prognosis compared to in-hospital cardiac arrest. However, recent progress in prevention and treatment of cardiovascular diseases has been linked to improved outcomes over the years, with an increase in survival to hospital discharge after out-of-hospital cardiac arrest from 10.2% in 2006 to 12.4% in 2015 and from 28.5% in 2000 to 48.7% in 2018 after in-hospital cardiac arrest.[1] Cardiovascular mortality is the leading cause of death in the United States, with SCD accounting for over half of all cases.[2] Owing to its significant fatality toll, SCA has a profound impact on global public health and utilization of medical resources with far-reaching socioeconomic consequences.

Epidemiology of SCD

Over the course of the last 20 to 30 years, approximately 230,000 to 450,000 deaths per year in the United States have been attributed to SCD.[2] In 2017, mortality from SCD was reported to be 379,133. The incidence of SCA tends to increase with age in both sexes. However, at any age, SCA is more common in men, who are two to three times more likely to fall victim, than women.[1] The projected rate of SCA in younger subjects (less than or equal to 34 years of age) is 1 per 100,000 a year. As the population ages, the annual rate of SCA surges from the age of 35 to 75 years (1 per 1,000) and decreases after that.[2]

Age also affects the etiology of SCD. Autopsy studies demonstrate that younger victims (median age of 29 years) may have structurally normal hearts in up to 42% of cases, whereas older individuals (mean age 54.7 years) are found to have no structural cardiac abnormalities in only 4% of postmortem evaluations.[3] In young victims, predominant causes of SCD are congenital channelopathies; inherited dilated, hypertrophic, and arrhythmogenic cardiomyopathies; and coronary artery anomalies. Other common autopsy findings include idiopathic fibrotic cardiomyopathy, obesity-associated cardiomyopathy, and hypertensive cardiomyopathy.[4] Structural heart disease (SHD) is identified in the majority of older individuals with SCA, with coronary artery disease (CAD) accounting for 70% of cases.[2] Other types of SHD found in 10% to 15% of instances include nonischemic cardiomyopathy (NICM), left ventricular hypertrophy (LVH), hypertrophic cardiomyopathy (HCM), arrhythmogenic right ventricular cardiomyopathy (ARVC), myocarditis, congenital coronary anomalies, and mitral valve prolapse.[2] Primary arrhythmic causes include channelopathies, such as congenital long QT syndrome, Brugada syndrome, catecholaminergic polymorphic ventricular tachycardia (VT), Wolff-Parkinson-White (WPW) syndrome, as well as early repolarization syndrome, idiopathic VT, or ventricular fibrillation (VF). They are implicated in 1% to 2% of cases.[5-7] Noncardiac and other unidentified etiologies account for the remaining 5% to 25% of SCA and encompass trauma, bleeding, drug overdose, pulmonary embolism, central airway obstruction, hypoxia, intracranial hemorrhage, and near-drowning. Etiologies of SCA in adults in the United States are summarized in **Figure 62.1**.[1,2,6,7]

Risk Factors Associated With SCA

Many of the risk factors for CAD and SCA are the same: hypertension, hyperlipidemia, type 2 diabetes mellitus, smoking, obesity, and a sedentary lifestyle. Most of these risk factors are treatable and/or preventable. General preventative measures tend to work on a population level but seem to have limited effects on an individual's risk of SCA. Congestive heart failure (CHF), previous stroke or transient ischemic attack, atrial fibrillation, hypertension, diabetes mellitus, peripheral arterial disease, chronic kidney disease, obstructive sleep apnea, and chronic obstructive pulmonary disease (COPD) are independently associated with increased risk of ventricular tachyarrhythmias and SCD, particularly in patients over the age of 75 years.[8] The risk of SCD in individuals with adult congenital heart disease is higher than in the general population and increases depending on the complexity of the heart defect. Eisenmenger syndrome has the highest incidence of SCA, whereas transposition of the great arteries—either after atrial switch surgery or congenitally corrected—and Fontan physiology carry moderate risk.[9]

Genetics

SCA in a first-degree relative is a well-known risk factor for SCD. The presence of a genetic predisposition was suggested by studies that reported SCA as the first presentation of cardiac disease in several generations of families independent of other

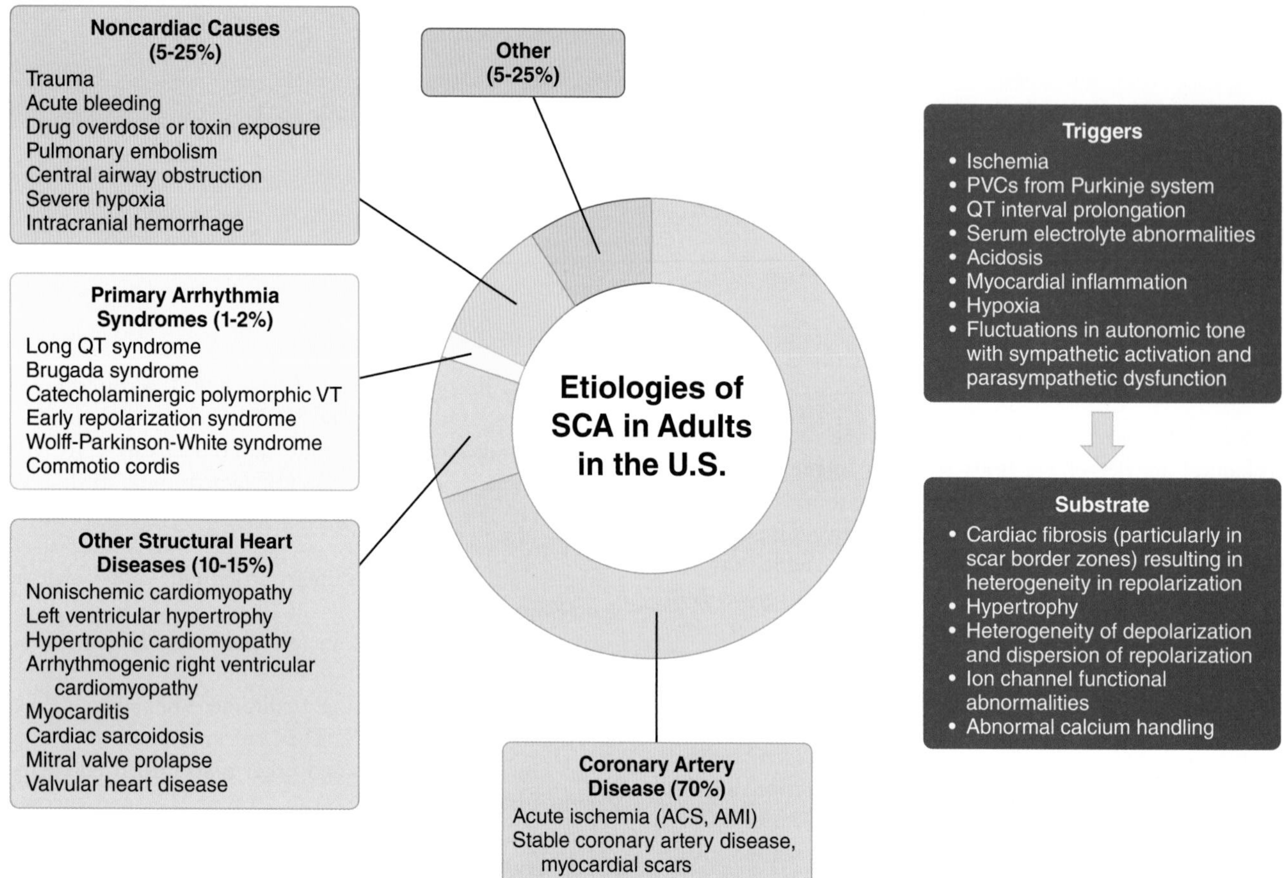

FIGURE 62.1 Etiologies of sudden cardiac arrest in adults in the United States.ACS, acute coronary syndrome; AMI, acute myocardial infarction; PVC, premature ventricular complex; SCA, sudden cardiac arrest; VT, ventricular tachycardia.

cardiovascular risk factors. The rate of SCA or acute myocardial infarction (AMI) was reported to be 1.5- to 2-fold higher in first-degree relatives of SCD victims who had no previous history of heart disease as compared to those without a family history.[10,11] Moreover, the risk of SCA in individuals with no prior history of cardiac disease was approximately 10-fold higher when there was a family history of SCD in more than one first-degree relative when compared to just one relative.[11] Mutation-specific genetic testing is recommended for screening of family members of survivors of unexplained SCA to identify those with the subclinical disease who are at risk.[12]

Between 3% and 45% of autopsies in previously healthy children, adolescents, and adults less than 35 years of age find no anatomical or histologic pathology, and therefore, fail to determine the cause of sudden death.[3,13] Common cardiac channelopathies, such as long QT syndrome, catecholaminergic polymorphic VT, and Brugada syndrome are not associated with any morphologic abnormalities on postmortem examination and can be categorized as unexplained SCD. Molecular autopsy may identify a pathologic mechanism and clarify the cause of death in in up to 27% of such cases.[5] A combination of histologic and molecular autopsy examination coupled with family screening may increase the likelihood of determining the cause of SCD and help prevent it in surviving relatives.

Risk Prediction

The difference between population and individual risk is at the core of suboptimal prediction of the probability of SCA. The highest risk group is comprised of adults with underlying SHD and traditional cardiovascular risk factors, yet patients with SHD constitute a small proportion of all sudden deaths. At the same time, the overwhelming majority of SCDs occur in the general population without traditional CAD risk factors. This presents a challenging quandary of how to identify susceptible subjects at higher risk within a general population that is overall at low risk, particularly because in up to 50% of patients SCA may be the initial manifestation of cardiac disease.[2] It is this group of patients who are concealed within the general population that contemporary state-of-the-art research is targeting to identify reliable predictors of SCA.

Left ventricular ejection fraction (LVEF) remains the key parameter currently used for risk stratification of SCD. Implantation of internal cardioverter defibrillators (ICDs) in patients with SHD and LVEF less than or equal to 35% provides a survival benefit.[14,15] Accordingly, the presence of severe left ventricular dysfunction is the chief determinant of whether or not ICD for primary prevention of SCA is implanted. However, LVEF has limited effectiveness in providing a reliable assessment of risk, leading to both underuse and overuse of

ICDs. A small proportion of subjects with ICDs receive appropriate anti-tachycardia pacing and defibrillation therapies. Only 1% to 5% of patients with an ICD require device therapy each year, and up to 65% of patients implanted with ICDs will not receive an appropriate therapy over the 3-year period after device implantation.[16] Similarly, 15% to 18% of biventricular defibrillator recipients do not require appropriate ICD therapies over a 2.4-year follow-up.[17] In addition, up to 70% of all SCDs occur in individuals with LVEF greater than 35%, with half of these individuals having a normal LVEF.[18] None of these subjects qualify for an ICD based on current implantation criteria. Perhaps the risk of SCD associated with LVEF less than or equal to 35% should not be viewed as a binary parameter but rather as a continuous variable over a range of values.

A number of parameters outside of LVEF have been suggested for risk stratification of SCD, but none is superior to LVEF as a predictor. Part of the challenge is that most of these parameters—both individually and in combination—predict overall cardiovascular mortality and are not specific for SCD. Moreover, the low magnitude of the predictive value (1.5- to 3-fold) of proposed non-LVEF risk factors substantially limits their clinical utility.[19]

The electrocardiogram (ECG) is an inexpensive and widely available test that can help detect signs of CAD and assess QRS morphology as well as QT interval. In a Spanish study of those over the age of 40 years, between 0.6% and 1.2% of individuals had ECG features that portended an increased risk of SCD, including long or short QT interval or spontaneous Brugada type 1 pattern. Moreover, when borderline ECGs were added (QT interval between normal and overtly abnormal as well as Brugada type 2 pattern), the prevalence increased to 8.3%.[20] The ECG parameters associated with a higher risk of SCD are summarized in **Table 62.1**.[19]

Various imaging modalities, such as echocardiography, cardiac magnetic resonance imaging (CMR), positron emission tomography (PET), and others, allow detailed characterization of the pathologic myocardial substrate to aid in the assessment of the individual risk of SCA (see **Table 62.2**). The primary CMR finding associated with increased risk of SCA is the presence and extent of a left ventricular scar.[21] Several echocardiographic parameters have also been linked to increased risk of SCD, ventricular tachyarrhythmias, and ICD therapies. These include the presence of LVH and abnormal longitudinal strain.[21,22] The PET evidence of sympathetic denervation has

TABLE 62.1 Electrocardiographic and Autonomic Variables Associated with Increased Risk of Sudden Cardiac Arrest Beyond Left Ventricular Ejection Fraction

Parameter	Variable
Heart rate	Resting heart rate >75 bpm
	Heart rate profile (resting heart rate >75 bpm and increase in heart rate to <89 bpm during exercise)
	Reduced heart rate variability
	Abnormal heart rate turbulence
Baroreceptor sensitivity	Decreased baroreflex sensitivity
Abnormal depolarization	Longer QRS duration
	Fragmentation of the QRS
	Left ventricular hypertrophy by ECG criteria
	Delayed intrinsicoid deflection of the QRS
	Delayed QRS transition zone (R wave transition in V5-V6)
Abnormal repolarization	Idiopathic QT prolongation
	Tpe prolongation
	T wave morphology restitution and T wave amplitude
	Early repolarization pattern
	Microvolt T wave alternans
	Late potentials on signal-averaged ECG
	Prolonged P wave duration
	ECG imaging of regions of delayed activation after exercise
Depolarization and repolarization combined index	QRS-T angle
Electrical risk score	Combination of resting heart rate, left ventricular hypertrophy, QRS transition zone, QRS-T angle, QTc, Tpe

bpm, beats per minute; ECG, electrocardiogram; QTc, corrected QT interval; Tpe, T peak to T end interval.

TABLE 62.2 Imaging Parameters Associated with Increased Risk of Sudden Cardiac Arrest Independent of Left Ventricular Ejection Fraction

Imaging Modality	Parameter	Associated Risk
Cardiac magnetic resonance imaging	LGE scar mass >10 g and border zone mass >5.3 g	SCD, ICD therapies
	LGE scar 26%-75% of wall thickness	Inducible VT
	Mid-wall LGE	SCD in nonischemic cardiomyopathy
	LGE % peri-infarct zone	All-cause mortality and arrhythmic death, ICD therapy in patients with ischemic cardiomyopathy and left ventricular dysfunction
	LGE scar	VA or SCD in nonischemic cardiomyopathy
	LGE scar >17% and circumferential strain >−7.2%	Late adverse remodeling as a marker of SCD after myocardial infarction
	LGE and global extracellular volume	SCD in hypertrophic cardiomyopathy
	High signal intensity with T2-weighted CMR	SCD in hypertrophic cardiomyopathy
Echocardiography	• Left ventricular hypertrophy by imaging • Left ventricular mass >143 g/m^2 in men and >102 g/m^2 in women • Each 50 g/m^2 increment in left ventricular mass is associated with 45% increase in risk of SCD	SCD
	• Strain and speckle tracking echocardiography • Mechanical dispersion • Longitudinal systolic strain • Global longitudinal strain[212]	SCD, VA, and ICD therapies in ischemic cardiomyopathy
	• Right ventricular strain[214]	Composite of SCD, admission for VA, or ICD therapy in ischemic cardiomyopathy
^{123}I-MIBG SPECT	Decreased heart/mediastinum ratio <1.6	SCD and ICD therapy in heart failure patients
	Increased regional and global washout rate	SCD and ICD therapy in heart failure patients
	Increased regional washout rate	VA in hypertrophic and arrhythmogenic right ventricular cardiomyopathy
	Reduced ^{123}I-MIBG uptake	SCD in Brugada syndrome
Positron emission tomography	Sympathetic denervation by ^{11}C-HED PET	SCD in ischemic cardiomyopathy
	Perfusion defects (^{82}Rb or $^{13}NH_3$) and inflammation (increased uptake of 18-FDG)	VA in cardiac sarcoidosis

^{11}C-HED PET, carbon-11-metahydroxyephedrine positron emission tomography; CMR, cardiac magnetic resonance imaging; ^{18}FDG, ^{18}F-2-fluorodeoxyglucose; g, gram; ICD, implantable cardioverter defibrillator; ^{123}I-MIBG, iodine-123-labeled norepinephrine analog meta-iodobenzylguanidine; LGE, late gadolinium enhancement; m^2, square meter; ^{13}NH3, ^{13}N-ammonia; ^{82}Rb, ^{82}-rubidium; SCD, sudden cardiac death; SPECT, single-photon emission computed tomography; VA, ventricular tachyarrhythmia; VT, ventricular tachycardia.

predictive value for SCA in ischemic cardiomyopathy ischemic cardiomyopathy (ICM), whereas perfusion defects and the presence of inflammation have been associated with ventricular tachyarrhythmias in cardiac sarcoidosis.[23]

A number of biomarkers, including C-reactive protein, B-natriuretic peptide, and nonesterified fatty acids (n-3 fatty acids), as well as decreased serum calcium level, have been linked to an increased risk of SCD in both men and women.[24,25]

Finally, as illustrated in Table 62.1, impaired cardiac autonomic activity, including decreased heart rate variability and heart rate turbulence as well as diminished baroreflex sensitivity, has been shown to predict not only cardiovascular mortality but also increased risk of SCA and ventricular tachyarrhythmias specifically, as reported in patients after myocardial infarction (MI) and in the setting of congenital heart disease.[26] Overall, using a combination of these clinical, genetic, autonomic, imaging, and ECG parameters may provide increasingly incremental value in risk stratification for SCA compared to LVEF alone.

PATHOGENESIS

Historically, VT and VF were implicated in the majority of SCA events. Bradyarrhythmias, such as high-grade atrioventricular block without sufficient escape rhythm leading to asystole, are responsible for approximately 10% of cardiac arrests.[2]

Catecholamine surge occurring during SCA worsens ventricular tachyarrhythmias but tends to be beneficial in the setting of bradycardia, increasing the rate of the escape rhythm. Pulseless electrical activity (PEA) was the third most common mechanism of SCA. However, temporal trends show a decrease in the incidence of ventricular tachyarrhythmias and an increase in PEA and asystole as a cause of SCD.[2] Reduction in arrhythmic death can be attributed to efforts targeting cardiovascular risk factors, advances in the medical treatment of CAD, and timely coronary reperfusion, as well as widespread use of ICDs. On the contrary, the rise in the incidence of PEA mirrors an increase in population aging and higher prevalence of patients with advanced heart failure.[27]

Ventricular tachyarrhythmias can manifest as monomorphic VT, polymorphic VT, or VF. Monomorphic VT usually occurs in the presence of a myocardial scar that has formed after a previous ischemic injury. Cardiac fibrosis, interspersed with channels of surviving myocardium within scar and border zone regions, is a typical example of the pathologic substrate. Slow electrical conduction in the border zone predisposes to the formation of reentry circuits and subsequent VT. Border zones can also serve as sites of premature ventricular complexes (PVCs) that trigger VT initiation. A rare form of monomorphic VT that utilizes right and left bundle branches or left fascicles of the electrical conduction system as a reentry circuit is called bundle branch reentry VT. It accounts for 5% to 8% of all monomorphic VTs in SHD. It is usually very rapid and tends to occur in patients with severely diseased hearts, such as those with dilated cardiomyopathy.

Polymorphic VT usually occurs in the setting of acute ischemia, inflammation, serum electrolyte abnormalities, QT interval prolongation, or autonomic nervous system imbalance. Catecholaminergic polymorphic VT is a rare disease caused by mutations in the ryanodine receptor or calsequestrin genes. It manifests as exercise- or stress-induced polymorphic VT without underlying QT prolongation.

Both monomorphic VT and polymorphic VT may accelerate and degenerate into VF. VF can also occur as the primary ventricular tachyarrhythmia. VF is characterized by chaotic multiple areas of microreentry and rotating spiral waves. Heterogeneity of depolarization and dispersion of repolarization serve as underlying conditions for VF.

Most ventricular tachyarrhythmias are initiated by a PVC trigger. In one-third of cases, it is an early PVC, falling on the T wave of the preceding QRS complex (R on T phenomenon). In two-thirds of instances, a late PVC triggers ventricular tachyarrhythmias.

CLINICAL PRESENTATION

As the definition of SCA suggests, patients present pulseless in a state of complete hemodynamic collapse. Patients with shockable rhythms are found to have ventricular tachyarrhythmias, whereas those with nonshockable rhythms have either asystole or PEA. Although survival after SCA is generally poor, shockable rhythms have better outcomes compared to nonshockable rhythms (25%-40% vs <5%, respectively).[1] Analysis of SCA data from 648 patients from the Oregon Sudden Unexpected Death Study showed that the type of heart failure was associated with the presenting rhythm at the time of the arrest. Patients with heart failure with reduced ejection fraction with LVEF less than or equal to 40% and borderline heart failure with preserved ejection fraction with LVEF 41% to 49% were more likely (2 and 2.5 times, respectively) to present with shockable rhythms compared to those with heart failure with preserved ejection fraction with LVEF ≥50%. Only 27% of individuals with heart failure with preserved ejection fraction and cardiac arrest presented with a shockable rhythm. Individuals with heart failure with preserved ejection fraction also had the lowest rates of survival to hospital discharge of 9.9%.[28]

Clinical triggers often lead to SCA in patients with an underlying substrate. Common triggers of SCA owing to ventricular tachyarrhythmias are outlined in **Figure 62.1** and **Table 62.3**. Sympathetic activation is considered to be one of the primary triggers of SCA. Despite this, the occurrence of SCD during competitive sports or sexual activity is rare. Interestingly, there exists a so-called sports paradox as described by Chugh and Weiss.[29] Sedentary older adults (>35 years of age) have a substantially increased risk of SCD during periods of vigorous physical activity. The relative risk of SCA during 30 minutes of vigorous physical exertion and 30 minutes immediately following exertion was 16.9 times higher than at other times. Of note, the risk of SCA during and 30 minutes after exertion was particularly high in individuals who exercised less than once per week (relative risk, 74.1). In contrast, subjects who exercised greater than or equal to five times a week had a markedly lower risk (relative risk, 10.9) of SCA during exercise, though it was still greater than the risk at rest.[30] However, the increased risk of SCD is counteracted by well-known benefits of fitness, highlighting the importance of the gradual introduction of exercise in sedentary individuals as well as an emphasis on the frequency of physical activity as opposed to intensity, especially at the beginning of training. In addition, physical exertion and particularly strenuous exercise are often implicated in the initiation of ventricular tachyarrhythmias in patients with long QT syndrome type 1, catecholaminergic polymorphic VT, and ARVC.

The majority of SCAs are not witnessed to ascertain symptoms preceding the event. Moreover, patients surviving SCA tend to have retrograde amnesia precluding recollection of symptoms. However, literature shows that half of SCA victims may have nonspecific complaints preceding SCA by 24 hours and up to 4 weeks. The most common precursor symptoms are chest pain and dyspnea. Data show that seeking medical attention as opposed to not doing so at the onset of new unstable symptoms is associated with better survival (32.1% vs 6%).[31]

Differential Diagnosis

The only difference between the presentation of syncope and SCA is that the subject spontaneously wakes up after a few

TABLE 62.3 Triggers for Sudden Cardiac Arrest

Trigger	Clinical Significance
Ischemia	• Acute ischemia should be suspected in all SCA victims • May range from ACS to transient ischemia in an otherwise stable CAD patient to coronary spasm • Acute ischemia is associated with polymorphic VT, VF, or rapid monomorphic VT (ventricular flutter) • Chronic CAD with myocardial scar usually leads to slower monomorphic VT
Serum electrolyte abnormalities	• Particularly hypokalemia, hypomagnesemia, and hyperkalemia • Unlikely to cause VA but usually potentiates effects of other conditions (eg, ischemia, prolonged QT interval)
Acidosis	• Either metabolic or respiratory acidosis • Unlikely to cause VA, usually potentiates effects of other conditions
QT interval prolongation	• Congenital or acquired • Often precipitated by QT-prolonging medications (azithromycin, levofloxacin, ketoconazole, metoclopramide, sertraline, lithium, methadone, etc) • Many internet sites list QT prolonging medications (www.crediblemeds.org) • Bradycardia potentiates QT prolongation • Usually associated with polymorphic VT, VF, and TdP
Anti-arrhythmic medications	• All anti-arrhythmics may cause proarrhythmia, especially in patients with SHD • May be challenging to differentiate if SCA is caused by underlying condition that anti-arrhythmic is prescribed for or because of proarrhythmia
Myocardial inflammation	• Myocarditis, active inflammatory phase of cardiac sarcoidosis, inflammatory cardiomyopathy
Heart failure	• Risk of SCA is elevated in all patients with CHF, but particularly during CHF exacerbation
Severe hypoxemia	• More commonly associated with PEA arrest but may lead to VA caused by exacerbating underlying ischemia
Fluctuations in the autonomic tone	• Sympathetic activation, parasympathetic withdrawal • Often implicated in SCA occurring during exercise, physical or emotional stress • Associated with LQT1, catecholaminergic polymorphic VT, ARVC, polymorphic VT, VF, and monomorphic VT with faster tachycardia rates

ACS, acute coronary syndrome; ARVC, arrhythmogenic right ventricular cardiomyopathy; CAD, coronary artery disease; CHF, congestive heart failure; LQT1, long QT 1 syndrome; PEA, pulseless electrical activity; SCA, sudden cardiac arrest; SHD, structural heart disease; TdP, torsades de pointes; VA, ventricular tachyarrhythmia; VF, ventricular fibrillation; VT, ventricular tachycardia.

seconds of unconsciousness in the event of syncope but remains in a state of cardiocirculatory arrest in the setting of SCA.

A more important differential diagnosis concerns the underlying etiology, triggers, and acute conditions leading to SCA. Between 15% and 25% of SCAs are of noncardiac etiology (see **Figure 62.1**). Identification of the precipitating conditions that result in SCA is of paramount importance because it has significant implications for patient management.

DIAGNOSIS

Evaluation Upon Initial Presentation

Evaluation for conditions that have resulted in SCA begins at the time of ongoing resuscitation efforts. Identification of acute reversible causes of SCA may lead to lifesaving interventions. Such examples include cardiac tamponade and tension pneumothorax that could be alleviated by emergent pericardiocentesis or large-bore needle decompression of the pleural space, respectively. Targeted history from relatives, medical personnel, or chart review obtained before SCA or after the return of spontaneous circulation (ROSC), as well as laboratory analysis of the blood work obtained from the patient during resuscitation, is invaluable in trying to ascertain the etiology of SCA.

Given that CAD is the predominant underlying etiology in most adult patients, an ECG should be obtained as soon as possible upon ROSC. The ECG is useful in the assessment of ST segment changes consistent with ischemia, any rate or rhythm abnormalities, as well as QT interval and patterns consistent with specific diseases. Recent history of invasive cardiac procedures or surgery, malignancy, or radiation in the past should alert for the possibility of cardiac tamponade. The diagnosis is confirmed with a quick bedside echocardiogram.

Electrolyte abnormalities and acidosis are evident in venous and arterial blood samples. They rarely lead to SCA on their own, but rather potentiate another condition that may be the primary cause, such as myocardial ischemia or QT prolongation. Moreover, electrolyte disturbances could both precipitate SCA and occur as a result of one. Attempts at correction of metabolic derangements should be undertaken immediately, using intravenous (IV) potassium and magnesium infusion for hypokalemia and hypomagnesemia, respectively, or calcium, bicarbonate, and insulin with glucose for hyperkalemia.

Continuous bicarbonate infusion and initiation of hemodialysis may be required for the correction of severe hyperkalemia and metabolic acidosis. Institution of mechanical ventilation could be needed for marked respiratory acidosis. Anemia and hypovolemia are diagnosed based on laboratory work and physical examination. They are corrected by administration of IV fluids as well as blood products in cases of severe anemia while a simultaneous search for the source of acute bleeding is undertaken.

Tension pneumothorax should be suspected in patients who had a recent internal jugular or subclavian central venous line placement, pacemaker implantation, thoracentesis, chest trauma, or those with severe COPD and emphysema. History of recent long-distance travel, prolonged immobilization, such as after surgery, particularly orthopedic surgery, central venous access with indwelling lines, or recent cardiac catheter ablation procedure as well as a history of hypercoagulable state should alert the physician to the increased likelihood of pulmonary embolism. Exposure to a toxin or drug overdose needs to be considered as potential reversible causes of SCA. The diagnosis can be confirmed by a toxicologic screening.

Evaluation After Return of Spontaneous Circulation

After ruling out noncardiac causes of SCA, the focus shifts to evaluation for SHD. In addition to history, physical examination, ECG and laboratory studies, cardiac catheterization, and echocardiography are performed. Coronary angiography is usually performed emergently as soon as ROSC is achieved in nearly all adult patients as CAD is the cause of SCA in approximately 2/3 of adults.[2]

Echocardiography is another diagnostic modality that is commonly used as a part of the emergent evaluation of SCA victims. It is easily available at the bedside and may detect many structural heart abnormalities by assessing left and right ventricular chamber size and function, wall thickness and motion abnormalities, valvular pathology, and whether or not a pericardial effusion is present. CMR with delayed gadolinium enhancement provides superior spatial resolution and tissue characterization as compared to the echocardiogram and is capable of diagnosing underlying SHD in almost 50% of SCA patients.[32]

Despite standard diagnostic evaluations outlined earlier, the etiology of SCA remains unknown in up to two-thirds of patients without SHD.[33,34] Data from Cardiac Arrest Survivors with Preserved Ejection Fraction Registry (CASPER) indicate that further testing may lead to a diagnosis of the underlying cause of SCA in up to 56% of patients with no SHD by echocardiography and preserved LVEF. Additional diagnostic studies in all patients comprised signal-averaged ECG, exercise stress test, CMR, and IV epinephrine, and procainamide challenge tests. Select patients also had electrophysiologic study, electroanatomic voltage mapping, and right ventricular endomyocardial biopsy.[33,35]

Genetic testing is often beneficial not only for confirmation of diagnosis but also for identification of familial mutations and subsequent screening of asymptomatic relatives who may be at risk. Targeted genetic testing, rather than whole-genome testing, is recommended based on the clinical evaluation and diagnostic data.[12]

MANAGEMENT

Management of Sudden Cardiac Arrest Upon Initial Presentation

Management of patients presenting with SCA, both before and after ROSC, is outlined in **Algorithm 62.1**.[36] Once it is recognized that the patient is in cardiac arrest, American Heart Association (AHA) cardiac arrest advanced cardiac life support (ACLS) algorithm should be implemented without delay.[37] After help is requested and cardiopulmonary resuscitation (CPR) is initiated, either an automatic external defibrillator (AED) or regular defibrillator should be connected to the patient. The rhythm is then classified as either shockable or nonshockable. If the rhythm is shockable (VT, VF), then defibrillation with 200 J biphasic shock should be delivered as soon as possible immediately followed by CPR for 2 minutes. If the patient remains in a shockable rhythm, another defibrillation is performed followed by CPR and administration of 1 mg of epinephrine IV or via intraosseous approach, which can be repeated every 3 to 5 minutes. After another 2-minute round of CPR, the rhythm should be reassessed and if the patient is still in a shockable rhythm, then another defibrillation is performed followed by

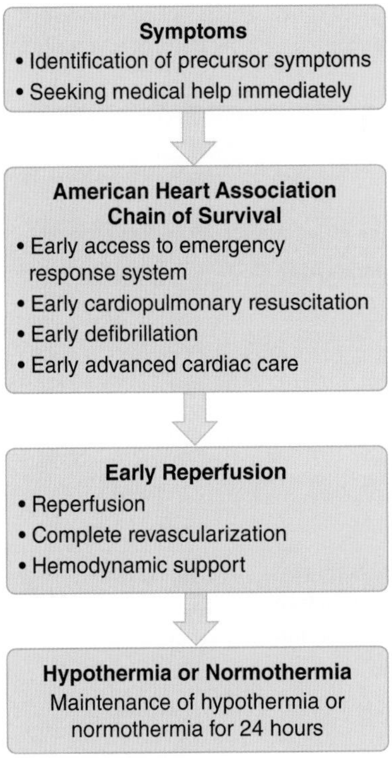

Symptoms
• Identification of precursor symptoms
• Seeking medical help immediately
American Heart Association Chain of Survival
• Early access to emergency response system
• Early cardiopulmonary resuscitation
• Early defibrillation
• Early advanced cardiac care
Early Reperfusion
• Reperfusion
• Complete revascularization
• Hemodynamic support
Hypothermia or Normothermia
Maintenance of hypothermia or normothermia for 24 hours

ALGORITHM 62.1 Treatment of sudden cardiac arrest upon initial presentation. (Reprinted from Krokhaleva Y, Vaseghi M. Update on prevention and treatment of sudden cardiac arrest. *Trends Cardiovasc Med* 2019;29(7):394-400. Copyright © 2018 Elsevier. With permission.)

SECTION 4

2 minutes of CPR and administration of either 300 mg of amiodarone or 1 to 1.5 mg/kg of lidocaine IV. A second dose of amiodarone (150 mg) or lidocaine (0.5-0.75 mg/kg) IV can be given after 3 to 5 minutes from the time of the first-dose administration. The cycle of CPR, rhythm assessment, and defibrillation, as well as epinephrine, amiodarone, or lidocaine IV administration, is to be repeated until ROSC or the decision is made to terminate resuscitation efforts. If the patient is found to be in a nonshockable rhythm during the next rhythm check, ACLS algorithm must be switched to cardiac arrest with nonshockable rhythm.

If the rhythm is classified as nonshockable (PEA, asystole), then CPR for 2 minutes should be initiated, and 1 mg epinephrine IV given as soon as possible. The cycles of CPR for 2 minutes, rhythm reassessment, and epinephrine administration every 3 to 5 minutes, must be repeated until ROSC or the decision is made to stop resuscitation. If the rhythm changes to shockable, then the shockable rhythm cardiac arrest ACLS protocol is applied.

It is very important to continuously monitor the quality of CPR. When CPR, rhythm assessment, and drug administration are being performed, rescue breathing followed by advanced airway and waveform capnography should be implemented. Search and treatment of any reversible causes is usually performed during ongoing resuscitation efforts.

Management After Return of Spontaneous Circulation

Once ROSC is achieved, most patients are taken for emergent coronary angiography, unless an obvious noncardiac cause of SCA is identified. Early coronary reperfusion is of vital importance, given the preponderance of CAD as a cause of SCA in the majority of victims. Coronary angiography not only allows for the diagnosis of acute coronary events but also provides treatment in the same setting. Percutaneous revascularization is usually achieved by coronary stent deployment. Hemodynamic support may be needed in patients with severe circulatory instability, which may include insertion of an intra-aortic balloon pump, percutaneous left ventricular assist device, or the initiation of external extracorporeal oxygenation.

Targeted temperature management, also known as therapeutic hypothermia, was introduced for the management of SCA victims after ROSC based on observations of better neurologic recovery in avalanche victims. Body temperature is lowered to 32 °C to 34 °C and maintained for 24 hours followed by rewarming. Targeted temperature management has been shown to improve survival after ROSC and should be initiated as soon as possible.[38]

Many patients will require advanced airway, sedation, and hemodynamic support with an infusion of inotropic (dobutamine, milrinone, low-dose dopamine less than or equal to 5 μg/kg/min) and/or vasopressor (dopamine 5-20 μg/kg/min, norepinephrine, phenylephrine, epinephrine, vasopressin) medications.

Once ROSC is achieved and the patient is stabilized, a search for the culprit substrate, triggers, and acute conditions that resulted in SCA should be started promptly if not done already. Subsequent management depends on the underlying etiology. Medical, percutaneous, and surgical management options of various conditions that may lead to SCA are outlined in **Table 62.4**.[2,39]

TABLE 62.4 Management and Prevention of Sudden Cardiac Arrest After Return of Spontaneous Circulation in the Acute and Chronic Setting by Etiology

Condition	Medical Therapy	Percutaneous Intervention	Surgery
Acute ischemia (AMI, ACS); chronic CAD	Beta-blocker	Revascularization with percutaneous coronary intervention	Coronary artery bypass grafting
	ACEI		
	Dual antiplatelet therapy		
	Lipid lowering medications (statins, PCSK9 inhibitors—evolocumab [repatha])		
	Nitrate if needed		
Heart failure with reduced ejection fraction, acute or acute on chronic	Beta-blocker	IABP, Impella in the acute setting	Orthotopic heart transplantation
	ACEI	CRT	LVAD, BIVAD as a destination therapy or bridge to transplantation
	ARB		
	Sacubitril/Valsartan		
	Diuretics		
	Nitrate and hydralazine combination		
	Inotropes in the acute setting (dobutamine, milrinone)		

TABLE 62.4 Management and Prevention of Sudden Cardiac Arrest After Return of Spontaneous Circulation in the Acute and Chronic Setting by Etiology (*continued*)

Condition	Medical Therapy	Percutaneous Intervention	Surgery
Monomorphic ventricular tachycardia	Beta-blocker	Catheter ablation of VT	Hybrid surgical epicardial and percutaneous endocardial ablation of VT in select patients with epicardial or transmural scar
	Anti-arrhythmic medication (class III)		
Polymorphic ventricular tachycardia	Beta-blocker	CSD	
		Catheter ablation of PVC triggers	
Torsades de pointes	Avoid QT-prolonging medications	Temporary pacemaker	
	Replenish serum potassium and magnesium	Permanent pacemaker implantation for bradycardia-dependent TdP	
Arrhythmogenic right ventricular cardiomyopathy	Guideline-directed heart failure therapies (see heart failure with reduced ejection fraction)	ICD implantation	Orthotopic heart transplantation
	Anti-arrhythmic medications	Combined epicardial and endocardial VT ablation	VAD
Long QT syndrome	Avoid QT-prolonging medications	ICD implantation	
	Beta-blocker (nadolol preferred for LQT2)	CSD	
	Sodium channel blockers (flecainide, mexiletine, ranolazine) for LQT3		
Brugada syndrome	Quinidine for patients with history of ES, SVT, or contraindications for ICD	ICD implantation	
	Isoproterenol infusion for ES	Catheter ablation of PVC triggers in right ventricular outflow tract	
Catecholaminergic polymorphic VT	Quinidine	ICD implantation	
	Beta-blocker	CSD	
	Flecainide		
Short QT syndrome	Quinidine	ICD implantation	
	Sotalol		
Early repolarization	Isoproterenol infusion for ES	ICD implantation	
	Quinidine		
Idiopathic VF	Beta-blocker	ICD implantation	
	Quinidine	Catheter ablation of PVC triggers in Purkinje system	
		CSD	
Severe bradycardia	Avoid negative chronotropic medications (beta-blockers, non-dihydropyridine calcium channel blockers, digoxin, class III anti-arrhythmic medications)	Permanent pacemaker implantation	Epicardial pacemaker (rare)
	Isoproterenol, dobutamine, dopamine infusion		
	Temporary pacemaker (intravenous)		
	Transcutaneous pacing		

ACEI, angiotensin converting enzyme inhibitor; ACS, acute coronary syndrome; AMI, acute myocardial infarction; ARB, angiotensin II receptor blocker; ARVC, arrhythmogenic right ventricular cardiomyopathy; BIVAD, biventricular assist device; CAD, coronary artery disease; CHF, congestive heart failure; CRT, cardiac resynchronization therapy; CSD, cardiac sympathetic denervation; ES, electrical storm; IABP, intra-aortic balloon pump; ICD, implantable cardioverter defibrillator; LQT2, long QT syndrome type 2; LQT3, long QT syndrome type 3; LQTS, long QT syndrome; LVAD, left ventricular assist device; PVC, premature ventricular complex; SVT, supraventricular tachycardia; TdP, torsades de pointes; VT, ventricular tachycardia.

Preventing Sudden Cardiac Arrest and Reducing Burden of Ventricular Tachycardia/Ventricular Fibrillation Episodes

ICDs have been firmly established as an effective intervention to prevent SCD from ventricular tachyarrhythmias. Accordingly, they are implanted for either primary or secondary prevention of SCA. Unfortunately, ICD-unresponsive SCD from VT/VF has been reported to be 5% to 17%. Moreover, appropriate ICD shocks are associated with a sixfold higher all-cause mortality compared to no shocks, as well as substantial patient discomfort that may lead to the development of post-traumatic stress disorder.[40] Catheter ablation of VT is a percutaneous procedure that has been shown to reduce the frequency of VT episodes and ICD therapies, both shocks and anti-tachycardia pacing. Depending on the substrate, mapping and catheter ablation can be performed via the endocardium, epicardium, or as a combined epicardial and endocardial ablation. In cases of previous open cardiac surgery or known adhesions in the pericardial space (eg, history of pericardial tamponade), a hybrid epicardial/endocardial ablation is usually done. In this circumstance, endocardial ablation is performed via percutaneous approach, whereas epicardial ablation is done through a small thoracotomy. Epicardial substrate is frequently present or even predominant in patients with NICM and ARVC, which is why in such cases, a combined epicardial and endocardial VT ablation is typically performed as the first approach for ablation. Ventricular tachycardia ablation and outcome for different etiologies of ventricular tachyarrhythmias are depicted in **Algorithm 62.2**.[36]

In secondary prevention ICD patients, two randomized controlled trials (SMASH-VT and VTACH) demonstrated a 35% to 39% reduction in ICD shocks for VT at 2 years of follow-up in subjects with ICM who had undergone VT ablation as compared to medical therapy only. Neither trial showed a reduction in mortality.[41,42] However, observational or retrospective data of patients with implanted ICDs both for primary and secondary prevention of SCD who received appropriate ICD shocks reported not only a decrease in the frequency of ICD shocks but also a mortality benefit after successful catheter ablation of VT.[43-45] Procedural success of VT ablation is dependent on the etiology, extent of scar, and the number of VT morphologies observed. In the Thermocool Ventricular Tachycardia Ablation trial of patients with VT and advanced SHD caused by ICM or NICM, 53% of patients were VT free or had a reduction in treated VT episodes 6 months after ablation, whereas 20% had an increase in the number of VT occurrences.[46]

VT ablation outcomes are better for some etiologies than for others. Data from the International Ventricular Tachycardia Ablation Center Collaborative Study and other single-center reports indicate that after VT ablation, combined endpoint of survival free from VT, death, or heart transplantation as well as a reduction in the frequency of VT episodes are superior in patients with dilated cardiomyopathy, myocarditis, and ARVC compared to individuals with HCM, valvular heart disease, and sarcoidosis.[47]

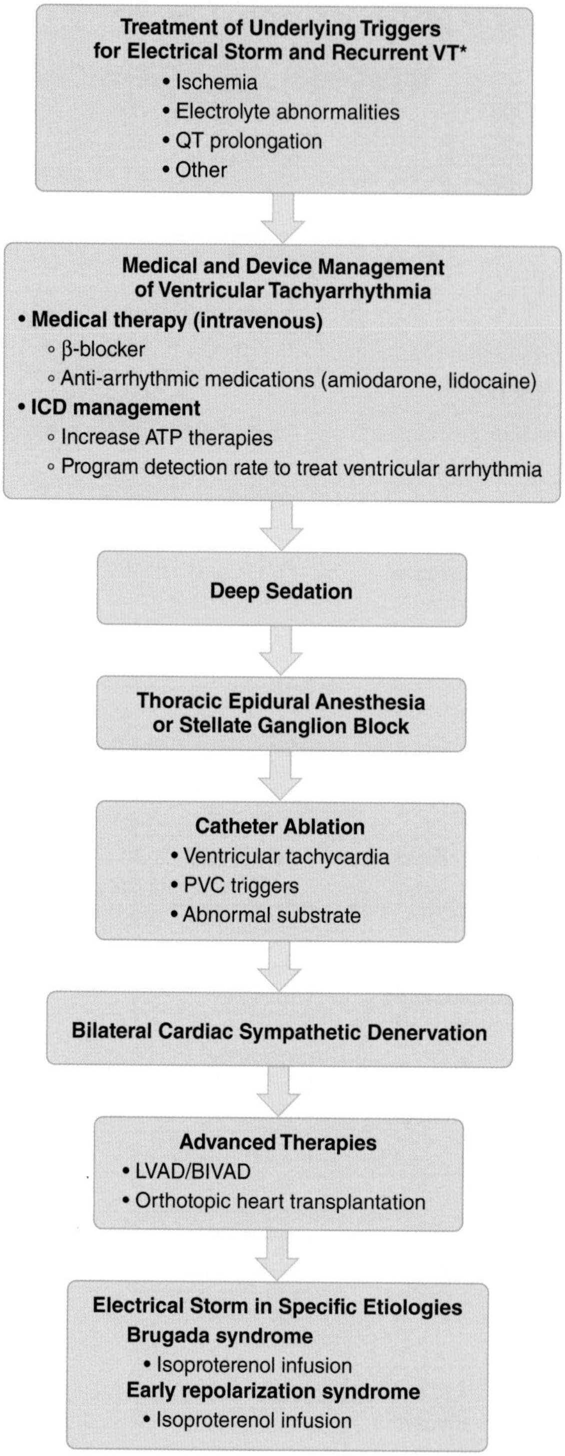

Treatment of Underlying Triggers for Electrical Storm and Recurrent VT*
- Ischemia
- Electrolyte abnormalities
- QT prolongation
- Other

↓

Medical and Device Management of Ventricular Tachyarrhythmia
- **Medical therapy (intravenous)**
  - β-blocker
  - Anti-arrhythmic medications (amiodarone, lidocaine)
- **ICD management**
  - Increase ATP therapies
  - Program detection rate to treat ventricular arrhythmia

↓

Deep Sedation

↓

Thoracic Epidural Anesthesia or Stellate Ganglion Block

↓

Catheter Ablation
- Ventricular tachycardia
- PVC triggers
- Abnormal substrate

↓

Bilateral Cardiac Sympathetic Denervation

↓

Advanced Therapies
- LVAD/BIVAD
- Orthotopic heart transplantation

↓

Electrical Storm in Specific Etiologies

Brugada syndrome
- Isoproterenol infusion

Early repolarization syndrome
- Isoproterenol infusion

ALGORITHM 62.2 Ventricular tachycardia ablation and outcomes for different etiologies of ventricular tachyarrhythmias. ATP, anti-tachycardia pacing; BIVAD, biventricular assist device; ICD, implantable cardioverter defibrillator; LVAD, left ventricular assist device; PVC, premature ventricular complex; VT, ventricular tachycardia. (Modified from Krokhaleva Y, Vaseghi M. Update on prevention and treatment of sudden cardiac arrest. *Trends Cardiovasc Med.* 2019;29(7):394-400. Copyright © 2018 Elsevier. With permission.)

VT ablation in patients with heart failure can be a long complex procedure that is usually performed in ill patients with advanced SHD, low LVEF, and comorbidities. The reported rate of procedural complications is 3% to 8% depending on medical center volume, operator experience, ablation techniques, availability of advanced hemodynamic support intraoperatively, as well as the patient's clinical status and duration of ablation.[41,42,46]

Bundle branch reentry VT is an infrequent reentrant monomorphic VT in patients with conduction system disease and a circuit that involves the bundle branches. The first-line therapy for bundle branch reentry VT is endocardial ablation, which is reported to have a nearly 100% success rate.[2] Because this form of VT tends to occur in diseased hearts with marked dilated cardiomyopathy where other forms of VT may also occur, ICD implantation is recommended for all patients with bundle branch reentry VT.

Because Purkinje fibers appear to be more resistant to ischemia than does the rest of the myocardium, PVCs originating from the Purkinje system—often the left posterior fascicle and peri-infarct border zones—are frequently implicated as triggers of polymorphic VT and VF during acute ischemia as well as in the setting of idiopathic VF. The reported success rate of catheter ablation of PVC triggers is 80% to 100%, which may effectively prevent recurrent VF episodes, including electrical storm.[48,49] There are preliminary data suggesting that PVC triggers of VF storm in Brugada syndrome are located in the region of the right ventricular outflow tract and that combined epicardial and endocardial ablation of those PVCs may treat electrical storm in this population.[50]

Management of Electrical Storm

Electrical storm is defined as three or more episodes of sustained ventricular tachyarrhythmia in 24 hours or incessant VT for 12 hours or longer. Electrical storm is a life-threatening emergency and a harbinger of increased mortality rate. Electrical storm is estimated to occur in 4% to 7% of primary prevention ICD recipients and 10% to 58% of secondary prevention ICD recipients.[51] Most triggers that are implicated in arrhythmic SCA may also initiate electrical storm. Identification and correction of acute reversible causes of electrical storm is of utmost importance. Then stepwise approach to patient management in electrical storm is outlined in **Algorithm 62.3**.

The main medication used in electrical storm is an IV beta-blocker. There are data indicating that a nonselective beta-blocker propranolol may be superior to a selective beta1-blocker metoprolol in patients with electrical storm, when it is concomitantly used with IV amiodarone.[52]

Sympathetic activation plays a crucial role in the pathogenesis of electrical storm because it leads to ventricular tachyarrhythmias and it is also potentiated by the patient's anxiety, fear, and pain from ICD shocks. Therefore, a number of medications and procedures used during electrical storm aim to block sympathetic activation on multiple levels, which has

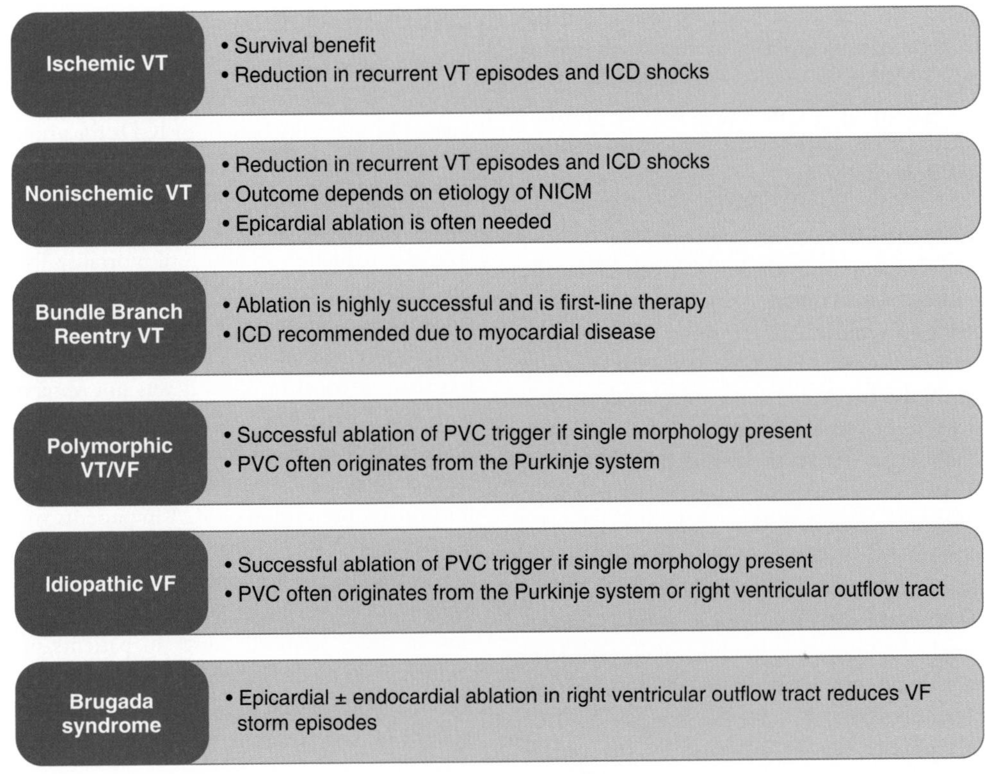

Ischemic VT
• Survival benefit
• Reduction in recurrent VT episodes and ICD shocks
Nonischemic VT
• Reduction in recurrent VT episodes and ICD shocks
• Outcome depends on etiology of NICM
• Epicardial ablation is often needed
Bundle Branch Reentry VT
• Ablation is highly successful and is first-line therapy
• ICD recommended due to myocardial disease
Polymorphic VT/VF
• Successful ablation of PVC trigger if single morphology present
• PVC often originates from the Purkinje system
Idiopathic VF
• Successful ablation of PVC trigger if single morphology present
• PVC often originates from the Purkinje system or right ventricular outflow tract
Brugada syndrome
• Epicardial ± endocardial ablation in right ventricular outflow tract reduces VF storm episodes

ALGORITHM 62.3 Management of electrical storm: an algorithm for the management of electrical storm is described. ICD, implantable cardioverter defibrillator; NICM, nonischemic cardiomyopathy; PVC, premature ventricular complex; VF, ventricular fibrillation; VT, ventricular tachycardia.

been shown to improve survival in patients with SCA compared to standard ACLS protocol.[53] These approaches encompass administration of beta-blocker, deep sedation, thoracic epidural anesthesia, and stellate ganglion block.

Medical therapy consists of IV beta-blocker and anti-arrhythmic medications (usually lidocaine or amiodarone IV bolus followed by continuous infusion). Patients' ICDs may require reprogramming to reduce shocks and treat the majority of ventricular tachyarrhythmias with anti-tachycardia pacing. It is important to emphasize that if an individual does not have an ICD in place at the time of electrical storm, the electrical storm should be terminated first before ICD implantation is performed.

If medical therapy proves insufficient to suppress ventricular tachyarrhythmias, deep sedation may be effective. This usually requires endotracheal intubation and mechanical ventilation. The next steps include thoracic epidural anesthesia or stellate ganglion block, which by targeting the sympathetic nervous system, can reduce the burden of ventricular tachyarrhythmias. These can be performed at bedside by an anesthesiologist or pain specialist. Thoracic epidural anesthesia includes placement of an epidural catheter at the T2 vertebral level in the epidural space to provide cardiac sympathetic blockade. Thoracic epidural anesthesia has been shown to be beneficial in the suppression of medication-refractory electrical storm.[54] Stellate ganglion block is achieved by injection of an anesthetic in the region of stellate ganglia.

Catheter ablation of ventricular tachyarrhythmias is usually performed once the patient is stabilized and electrical storm is suppressed. However, in recalcitrant cases, ablation may be performed in the setting of electrical storm and has been reported to terminate ventricular tachyarrhythmias in 90% of subjects.[55] Ablation targets include mappable VTs, PVC triggers of polymorphic VT or VF, as well as substrate modification targeting areas of abnormal myocardial voltage, late activation, and slow conduction.

Autonomic Modulation

Autonomic nervous system is intrinsically involved in the pathogenesis of cardiac arrhythmias. Fluctuations in autonomic tone resulting in sympathetic activation and parasympathetic dysfunction are known to be associated with SCA and ventricular tachyarrhythmias. At the same time, vagal stimulation has been shown to be protective against ventricular tachyarrhythmias.[56] Pathologic neural remodeling following heart injury involves (1) local denervation of sympathetic fibers with subsequent heterogeneous reinnervation at localized border zone sites, (2) abnormal denervation of the normal myocardium distal to the injured site, and (3) extracardiac remodeling involving the intrathoracic and extrathoracic ganglia, including the stellate ganglia.[57] Autonomic modulation at each level of the cardiac neuraxis can provide additional tools for malignant arrhythmia management.

Sympathetic blockade can be achieved by the use of beta-blockers, angiotensin converting enzyme inhibitors, angiotensin II receptor blockers, aldosterone antagonists, thoracic epidural anesthesia, stellate ganglion block, cardiac sympathetic denervation, spinal cord stimulation, and renal denervation. Cardiac sympathetic denervation is performed by surgical resection of 1/3 to 1/2 of the stellate and T1-T4 thoracic ganglia. Although initially introduced for the treatment of long QT syndrome and catecholaminergic polymorphic VT, cardiac sympathetic denervation was subsequently demonstrated to be beneficial in patients with SHD owing to reduction in ventricular tachyarrhythmia episode frequency and ICD shocks.[58,59] Renal denervation involves catheter ablation of renal nerve fibers surrounding the renal arteries. A number of small studies have illustrated the benefit of renal denervation as an adjunctive therapy in patients with refractory VT in addition to catheter ablation and cardiac sympathetic denervation. Renal denervation is associated with a reduction in ventricular tachyarrhythmia burden and number of ICD shocks.[60-62]

The purpose of increasing parasympathetic tone is to counteract the adverse effects of sympathetic stimulation. Methods to achieve this include vagal nerve stimulation, spinal cord stimulation, transcutaneous vagal nerve stimulation, and carotid body stimulation. Vagal nerve stimulation is performed through bipolar electrodes implanted around the cervical vagal trunk. Spinal cord stimulation involves stimulation at the T1 to T4 levels via a catheter placed in the epidural space. Vagal nerve stimulation and spinal cord stimulation reduce the frequency of ventricular tachyarrhythmias in animal studies both during ischemia and after chronic MI, but data in humans are relatively sparse and stimulation parameters, such as dose, duration, and frequency, still need to be tested and verified.[63-69]

PREVENTION OF SUDDEN CARDIAC ARREST

Primary prevention of arrhythmic SCA involves implantation of ICDs in patients at high risk of ventricular tachyarrhythmias. The mortality benefit of ICDs for primary prevention of SCA in patients with LVEF less than or equal to 35% and ICM or NICM was firmly established in two seminal randomized controlled trials, MADIT-II and SCD-HeFT. They demonstrated a reduction in all-cause mortality by 23% to 28% in the ICD group compared to the medical therapy group.[14,15] A subsequent randomized clinical trial suggested that although mortality reduction was consistently seen in ICM with LVEF less than or equal to 35%, it was not observed in all patients with NICM and low LVEF. Only younger, but not older, patients (age ≤68 years) with NICM had a 36% all-cause mortality reduction.[70] Nevertheless, ICD implantation is indicated for primary prevention of SCA in patients with both ICM and NICM and LVEF less than or equal to 35%.[2]

A number of randomized controlled trials for secondary prevention of SCA with ICDs showed a 20% to 23% reduction in death from all causes in patients in the ICD group compared to medical therapy group.[71] ICD implantation for secondary prevention of SCA, not owing to reversible causes, is a class I indication in the ACC/AHA guidelines.[2]

RESEARCH AND FUTURE DIRECTIONS

Because SCD remains the leading cause of mortality that occurs with little warning, better risk assessment in the general population with normal left ventricular function is needed. An additional direction of future research involves the development of new pharmacologic agents to treat conditions that lead to SCA as well as avenues to increase the percentage of patients achieving ROSC and survival with full neurologic recovery. Innovations in catheter ablation tools and techniques to improve outcomes and shorten VT ablation procedure time represent an additional area for research. Finally, neurocardiology is an exciting and rapidly evolving field with an immense potential to improve the management of ventricular tachyarrhythmias. Further studies are necessary to better understand mechanisms of autonomic modulation and its effect as well as identify the best modalities and stimulation protocols.

KEY POINTS

- ✔ The presenting rhythm during SCA has a major impact on outcomes. Shockable rhythms (VT/VF) are associated with better survival compared to nonshockable rhythms (PEA, asystole).
- ✔ Given the short time from the onset of symptoms to SCA, identification of patients at elevated risk on an individual and population level is the key toward prevention of SCA in subjects without traditional risk factors, specifically in those with preserved LVEF, who comprise the majority of patients suffering SCA.
- ✔ Targeted genetic testing and screening of family members of survivors of SCA to identify those with subclinical disease who are at risk are warranted.
- ✔ Most subjects with ROSC after SCA should have emergent coronary angiography to evaluate the status of coronary arteries and provide prompt revascularization if needed because CAD accounts for approximately 70% of SCA cases.
- ✔ Targeted temperature management improves survival in victims of SCA and should be started as soon as possible after ROSC.
- ✔ Treatment of ventricular tachyarrhythmia episodes in patients with and without SHD usually involves a combination of medical therapy and catheter ablation. Catheter ablation of VT and PVC triggers for VF is an effective strategy to decrease the frequency of recurrent ventricular tachyarrhythmias and should be used early on in patients with documented sustained VT or ICD shocks.
- ✔ ICDs are the cornerstone strategy to prevent arrhythmic death in patients with SHD and left ventricular dysfunction (primary prevention) as well as improve mortality in survivors of SCA (secondary prevention).
- ✔ Management of electrical storm requires a multimodal and multidisciplinary approach, including medications, ICD management, sedation, autonomic modulation, and catheter ablation.
- ✔ Autonomic modulation may have the potential to provide an incremental benefit in the management of SCA.

REFERENCES

1. Virani SS, Alonso A, Benjamin EJ, et al. Heart disease and stroke statistics-2020 update: a report from the American Heart Association. *Circulation.* 2020;141:e139-e596.
2. Al-Khatib SM, Stevenson WG, Ackerman MJ, et al. 2017 AHA/ACC/HRS Guideline for management of patients with ventricular arrhythmias and the prevention of sudden cardiac death: executive summary: a report of the American College of Cardiology/American Heart Association Task Force on Clinical Practice Guidelines and the Heart Rhythm Society. *Heart Rhythm.* 2018;15:e190-e252.
3. Landry CH, Allan KS, Connelly KA, et al. Sudden cardiac arrest during participation in competitive sports. *N Engl J Med.* 2017;377:1943-1953.
4. Bagnall RD, Weintraub RG, Ingles J, et al. A prospective study of sudden cardiac death among children and young adults. *N Engl J Med.* 2016;374:2441-2452.
5. Extramiana F, Stordeur B, Furioli V, et al. Spectrum and outcome of patients who have undergone implantation of an implantable cardioverter defibrillator after aborted-sudden cardiac arrest. *Am J Cardiol.* 2018;121:149-155.
6. Chugh SS, Reinier K, Teodorescu C, et al. Epidemiology of sudden cardiac death: clinical and research implications. *Prog Cardiovasc Dis.* 2008;51:213-228.
7. Hayashi M, Shimizu W, Albert CM. The spectrum of epidemiology underlying sudden cardiac death. *Circ Res.* 2015;116:1887-1906.
8. Koene RJ, Norby FL, Maheshwari A, et al. Predictors of sudden cardiac death in atrial fibrillation: the Atherosclerosis Risk in Communities (ARIC) study. *PLoS One.* 2017;12:e0187659.
9. Moore B, Yu C, Kotchetkova I, Cordina R, Celermajer DS. Incidence and clinical characteristics of sudden cardiac death in adult congenital heart disease. *Int J Cardiol.* 2018;254:101-106.
10. Friedlander Y, Siscovick DS, Weinmann S, et al. Family history as a risk factor for primary cardiac arrest. *Circulation.* 1998;97:155-160.
11. Jouven X, Desnos M, Guerot C, Ducimetière P. Predicting sudden death in the population: the Paris Prospective Study I. *Circulation.* 1999;99:1978-1983.
12. Ackerman MJ, Priori SG, Willems S, et al. HRS/EHRA expert consensus statement on the state of genetic testing for the channelopathies and cardiomyopathies this document was developed as a partnership between the Heart Rhythm Society (HRS) and the European Heart Rhythm Association (EHRA). *Heart Rhythm.* 2011;8:1308-1339.
13. Winkel BG, Holst AG, Theilade J, et al. Nationwide study of sudden cardiac death in persons aged 1-35 years. *Eur Heart J.* 2011;32:983-990.
14. Moss AJ, Zareba W, Hall WJ, et al. Prophylactic implantation of a defibrillator in patients with myocardial infarction and reduced ejection fraction. *N Engl J Med.* 2002;346:877-883.
15. Bardy GH, Lee KL, Mark DB, et al. Amiodarone or an implantable cardioverter–defibrillator for congestive heart failure. *N Engl J Med.* 2005;352:225-237.
16. Moss AJ, Greenberg H, Case RB, et al. Long-term clinical course of patients after termination of ventricular tachyarrhythmia by an implanted defibrillator. *Circulation.* 2004;110:3760-3765.
17. Moss AJ, Hall WJ, Cannom DS, et al. Cardiac-resynchronization therapy for the prevention of heart-failure events. *N Engl J Med.* 2009;361:1329-1338.
18. Stecker EC, Vickers C, Waltz J, et al. Population-based analysis of sudden cardiac death with and without left ventricular systolic dysfunction: two-year findings from the Oregon Sudden Unexpected Death Study. *J Am Coll Cardiol.* 2006;47:1161-1166.
19. Chugh SS. Einthoven and electrical risk: value of the electrocardiogram to predict sudden cardiac death. *J Cardiovasc Electrophysiol.* 2018;29:61-63.
20. García PA, Martín JJA, Abad CG, et al. Prevalence of electrocardiographic patterns associated with sudden cardiac death in the Spanish population aged 40 years or older. Results of the OFRECE study. *Rev Esp Cardiol (Engl Ed).* 2017;70:801-807.

21. Suzuki T, Nazarian S, Jerosch-Herold M, Chugh SS. Imaging for assessment of sudden death risk: current role and future prospects. *Europace.* 2016;18:1491-1500.
22. Ersboll M, Valeur N, Andersen MJ, et al. Early echocardiographic deformation analysis for the prediction of sudden cardiac death and life-threatening arrhythmias after myocardial infarction. *JACC Cardiovasc Imaging.* 2013;6:851-860.
23. van der Bijl P, Delgado V, Bax JJ. Sudden cardiac death: the role of imaging. *Int J Cardiol.* 2017;237:15-18.
24. Albert CM, Ma J, Rifai N, Stampfer MJ, Ridker PM. Prospective study of C-reactive protein, homocysteine, and plasma lipid levels as predictors of sudden cardiac death. *Circulation.* 2002;105:2595-2599.
25. Yarmohammadi H, Uy-Evanado A, Reinier K, et al. Serum calcium and risk of sudden cardiac arrest in the general population. *Mayo Clin Proc.* 2017;92:1479-1485.
26. De Ferrari GM, Sanzo A, Bertoletti A, Specchia G, Vanoli E, Schwartz PJ. Baroreflex sensitivity predicts long-term cardiovascular mortality after myocardial infarction even in patients with preserved left ventricular function. *J Am Coll Cardiol.* 2007;50:2285-2290.
27. Keller SP, Halperin HR. Cardiac arrest: the changing incidence of ventricular fibrillation. *Curr Treat Options Cardiovasc Med.* 2015;17:392.
28. Woolcott OO, Reinier K, Uy-Evanado A, et al. Sudden cardiac arrest with shockable rhythm in patients with heart failure. *Heart Rhythm.* 2020;17(10):1672-1678.
29. Chugh SS, Weiss JB. Sudden cardiac death in the older athlete. *J Am Coll Cardiol.* 2015;65:493-502.
30. Albert CM, Mittleman MA, Chae CU, Lee IM Hennekens CH, Manson JE. Triggering of sudden death from cardiac causes by vigorous exertion. *N Engl J Med.* 2000;343:1355-1361.
31. Marijon E, Uy-Evanado A, Dumas F, et al. Warning symptoms are associated with survival from sudden cardiac arrest. *Ann Intern Med.* 2016;164:23-29.
32. Muser D, Santangeli P, Selvanayagam JB, Nucifora G. Role of cardiac magnetic resonance imaging in patients with idiopathic ventricular arrhythmias. *Curr Cardiol Rev.* 2019;15:12-23.
33. Krahn AD, Healey JS, Chauhan V, et al. Systematic assessment of patients with unexplained cardiac arrest: Cardiac Arrest Survivors With Preserved Ejection Fraction Registry (CASPER). *Circulation.* 2009;120:278-285.
34. Herman ARM, Cheung C, Gerull B, et al. Outcome of apparently unexplained cardiac arrest. *Circ Arrhythm Electrophysiol.* 2016;9(1):e003619.
35. Krahn AD, Gollob M, Yee R, et al. Diagnosis of unexplained cardiac arrest: role of adrenaline and procainamide infusion. *Circulation.* 2005;112:2228-2234.
36. Krokhaleva Y, Vaseghi M. Update on prevention and treatment of sudden cardiac arrest. *Trends Cardiovasc Med.* 2019;29:394-400.
37. Panchal AR, Bartos JA, Cabañas JG, et al. Part 3: adult basic and advanced life support: 2020 American Heart Association Guidelines for cardiopulmonary resuscitation and emergency cardiovascular care. *Circulation.* 2020;142:S366-S468.
38. Bernard SA, Gray TW, Buist MD, et al. Treatment of comatose survivors of out-of-hospital cardiac arrest with induced hypothermia. *N Engl J Med.* 2002;346:557-563.
39. Priori SG, Wilde AA, Horie M, et al. HRS/EHRA/APHRS expert consensus statement on the diagnosis and management of patients with inherited primary arrhythmia syndromes: document endorsed by HRS, EHRA, and APHRS in May 2013 and by ACCF, AHA, PACES, and AEPC in June 2013. *Heart Rhythm.* 2013;10:1932-1963.
40. Poole JE, Johnson GW, Hellkamp AS, et al. Prognostic importance of defibrillator shocks in patients with heart failure. *N Engl J Med.* 2008;359:1009-1017.
41. Reddy VY, Reynolds MR, Neuzil P, et al. Prophylactic catheter ablation for the prevention of defibrillator therapy. *N Engl J Med.* 2007;357:2657-2665.
42. Kuck KH, Schaumann A, Eckardt L, et al. Catheter ablation of stable ventricular tachycardia before defibrillator implantation in patients with coronary heart disease (VTACH): a multicentre randomised controlled trial. *Lancet.* 2010;375:31-40.
43. Tung R, Vaseghi M, Frankel DS, et al. Freedom from recurrent ventricular tachycardia after catheter ablation is associated with improved survival in patients with structural heart disease: an International VT Ablation Center Collaborative Group study. *Heart Rhythm.* 2015;12:1997-2007.
44. Bella PD, Baratto F, Tsiachris D, et al. Management of ventricular tachycardia in the setting of a dedicated unit for the treatment of complex ventricular arrhythmias. *Circulation.* 2013;127:1359-1368.
45. Bunch TJ, Weiss JP, Crandall BG, et al. Patients treated with catheter ablation for ventricular tachycardia after an ICD shock have lower long-term rates of death and heart failure hospitalization than do patients treated with medical management only. *Heart Rhythm.* 2014;11:533-540.
46. Stevenson WG, Wilber DJ, Natale A, et al. Irrigated radiofrequency catheter ablation guided by electroanatomic mapping for recurrent ventricular tachycardia after myocardial infarction: the multicenter thermocool ventricular tachycardia ablation trial. *Circulation.* 2008;118:2773-2782.
47. Vaseghi M, Hu TY, Tung R, et al. Outcomes of catheter ablation of ventricular tachycardia based on etiology in nonischemic heart disease: an international ventricular tachycardia ablation center collaborative study. *JACC Clin Electrophysiol.* 2018;4:1141-1150.
48. Haissaguerre M, Shoda M, Jais P, et al. Mapping and ablation of idiopathic ventricular fibrillation. *Circulation.* 2002;106:962-967.
49. Bansch D, Oyang F, Antz M, et al. Successful catheter ablation of electrical storm after myocardial infarction. *Circulation.* 2003;108:3011-3016.
50. Nademanee K, Veerakul G, Chandanamattha P, et al. Prevention of ventricular fibrillation episodes in Brugada syndrome by catheter ablation over the anterior right ventricular outflow tract epicardium. *Circulation.* 2011;123:1270-1279.
51. Guerra F, Palmisano P, Dell'Era G, et al. Cardiac resynchronization therapy and electrical storm: results of the OBSERVational registry on long-term outcome of ICD patients (OBSERVO-ICD). *Europace.* 2018;20:979-985.
52. Chatzidou S, Kontogiannis C, Tsilimigras DI, et al. Propranolol versus metoprolol for treatment of electrical storm in patients with implantable cardioverter-defibrillator. *J Am Coll Cardiol.* 2018;71:1897-1906.
53. Nademanee K, Taylor R, Bailey WE, Rieders DE, Kosar EM. Treating electrical storm: sympathetic blockade versus advanced cardiac life support-guided therapy. *Circulation.* 2000;102:742-747.
54. Do DH, Bradfield J, Ajijola OA, et al. Thoracic epidural anesthesia can be effective for the short-term management of ventricular tachycardia storm. *J Am Heart Assoc.* 2017;6(11):e007080.
55. Geraghty L, Santangeli P, Tedrow UB, Shivkumar K, Kumar S. Contemporary management of electrical storm. *Heart Lung Circ.* 2019;28:123-133.
56. Huang WA, Boyle NG, Vaseghi M. Cardiac innervation and the autonomic nervous system in sudden cardiac death. *Card Electrophysiol Clin.* 2017;9:665-679.
57. Ajijola OA, Hoover DB, Simerly TM, et al. Inflammation, oxidative stress, and glial cell activation characterize stellate ganglia from humans with electrical storm. *JCI Insight.* 2017;2(18):e94715.
58. Vaseghi M, Barwad P, Corrales FJM, et al. Cardiac sympathetic denervation for refractory ventricular arrhythmias. *J Am Coll Cardiol.* 2017;69:3070-3080.
59. Dusi V, Gornbein J, Do DH, et al. Arrhythmic risk profile and outcomes of patients undergoing cardiac sympathetic denervation for recurrent monomorphic ventricular tachycardia after ablation. *J Am Heart Assoc.* 2021;10:e018371.
60. Bradfield JS, Hayase J, Liu K, et al. Renal denervation as adjunctive therapy to cardiac sympathetic denervation for ablation refractory ventricular tachycardia. *Heart Rhythm.* 2020;17:220-227.
61. Evranos B, Canpolat U, Kocyigit D, Coteli C, Yorgun H, Aytemir K. Role of adjuvant renal sympathetic denervation in the treatment of ventricular arrhythmias. *Am J Cardiol.* 2016;118:1207-1210.
62. Armaganijan LV, Staico R, Moreira DA, et al. 6-month outcomes in patients with implantable cardioverter-defibrillators undergoing renal sympathetic denervation for the treatment of refractory ventricular arrhythmias. *JACC Cardiovasc Interv.* 2015;8:984-990.
63. Yamaguchi N, Yamakawa K, Rajendran PS, Takamiya T, Vaseghi M. Antiarrhythmic effects of vagal nerve stimulation after cardiac sympathetic denervation in the setting of chronic myocardial infarction. *Heart Rhythm.* 2018;15:1214-1222.

64. Vaseghi M, Salavatian S, Rajendran PS, et al. Parasympathetic dysfunction and antiarrhythmic effect of vagal nerve stimulation following myocardial infarction. *JCI Insight.* 2017;2:e86715.
65. Vanoli E, De Ferrari GM, Stramba-Badiale M, Hull SS Jr, Foreman RD, Schwartz PJ. Vagal stimulation and prevention of sudden death in conscious dogs with a healed myocardial infarction. *Circ Res.* 1991;68:1471-1481.
66. Kent KM, Smith ER, Redwood DR, Epstein SE. Electrical stability of acutely ischemic myocardium. Influences of heart rate and vagal stimulation. *Circulation.* 1973;47:291-298.
67. Yoon MS, Han J, Tse WW, Rogers R. Effects of vagal stimulation, atropine, and propranolol on fibrillation threshold of normal and ischemic ventricles. *Am Heart J.* 1977;93:60-65.
68. Issa ZF, Zhou X, Ujhelyi MR, et al. Thoracic spinal cord stimulation reduces the risk of ischemic ventricular arrhythmias in a postinfarction heart failure canine model. *Circulation.* 2005;111:3217-3220.
69. Waxman MB, Wald RW. Termination of ventricular tachycardia by an increase in cardiac vagal drive. *Circulation.* 1977;56:385-391.
70. Kober L, Thune JJ, Nielsen JC, et al. Defibrillator implantation in patients with nonischemic systolic heart failure. *N Engl J Med.* 2016;375:1221-1230.
71. Connolly SJ, Hallstrom AP, Cappato R, et al. Meta-analysis of the implantable cardioverter defibrillator secondary prevention trials. AVID, CASH and CIDS studies. Antiarrhythmics vs Implantable Defibrillator study. Cardiac Arrest Study Hamburg. Canadian Implantable Defibrillator Study. *Eur Heart J.* 2000;21:2071-2078.

CHAPTER 63

PERMANENT CARDIAC PACEMAKERS

Carlos Macias

INTRODUCTION

The history of cardiac implantable electrical devices (CIEDs), and specifically cardiac pacemakers indicated for the management of bradyarrhythmias, dates back 60 years to the development of a postoperative external pacing system at the University of Minnesota by Dr Walton Lillehei in collaboration with Earl Bakken, a hospital engineer who later founded Medtronics. The first fully implantable human permanent pacemaker was employed in 1958 when Dr Ake Senning, a thoracic surgeon at Karolinska Hospital in Stockholm, implanted myocardial electrodes and a pulse generator with a rechargeable nickel-cadmium battery in a 40-year-old patient with complete heart block. The first generator lasted 8 hours, and the patient went on to have more than two dozen pulse generator replacements but lived until age 86 years.[1,2]

It is difficult to imaging modern medicine without these remarkable devices which now number over 1 million implants yearly worldwide with 200,000 in the United States. Implants are projected to continue to increase owing to an aging population, with an estimated 7 million people globally living with CIEDs. Knowledge of the clinical indications, basic function, troubleshooting, reprogramming, perioperative management, risks and complications, new techniques and technologies (physiologic pacing, leadless pacemakers), and future direction of these devices is invaluable for practitioners caring for patients with heart disease.[3]

CLINICAL INDICATIONS

The executive summary from the American College of Cardiology and the American Heart Association guideline for implantation of cardiac pacemakers and anti-arrhythmia devices provides guidance for CIED appropriateness use. Among the most frequently encountered Class I indications in clinical practice are sinus node dysfunction, acquired high-degree atrioventricular (AV) block and tachybrady syndrome. The two most frequent clinical indications remain sinus node dysfunction and acquired high-degree AV block (see **Tables 63.1** and **63.2** for guideline recommendations for permanent pacemaker implant).[3,4]

Cardiac Native Conduction

Intrinsic automaticity is responsible for sinus node cellular depolarization with a subsequent electrical wavefront propagation to the AV node, the bundle of His, and the His-Purkinje system and distally to the right bundle branch and anterior and posterior fascicles of the left bundle branch. Failure at any level interrupts native electrical propagation necessary for normal cardiac contractility and function. A permanent pacemaker system delivers a timed electrical impulse that results

TABLE 63.1 Permanent Pacemaker in Sinus Node Dysfunction
Class I Indications for Permanent Pacemaker *Symptomatic* sinus bradycardia and sinus pauses or sinus arrest *Symptomatic* chronotropic incompetence *Symptomatic* sinus bradycardia from required medical therapy
Class IIa Indications for Permanent Pacemaker Sinus node dysfunction with heart rate <40 bpm without clear association with symptoms Unexplained syncope when significant abnormalities with sinus node are noted during electrophysiology study
Class IIb Indications for Permanent Pacemaker Minimally *Symptomatic* patients with chronic heart rate <40 bpm
Class III Contraindications for Permanent Pacemaker Asymptomatic patients Symptomatic sinus bradycardia from nonessential medical therapy

TABLE 63.2 Permanent Pacemaker in Acquired Atrioventricular (AV) Conduction Disease

Class I Indications for Permanent Pacemaker
Third- or second-degree type 2 AV block Recurrent syncope, reproduced by carotid sinus massage with >3-second asystole
Class IIa Indications for Permanent Pacemaker
Persistent third-degree AV block in asymptomatic patients Asymptomatic second-degree AV block with His-ventricular interval >100 ms Symptomatic first- or second-degree AV block Symptomatic neurocardiogenic syncope with documented bradycardia during tilt table testing
Class IIb Indications for Permanent Pacemaker
Neuromuscular disease (muscular dystrophy, Erb dystrophy) with any degree AV block with or without symptoms AV block secondary to necessary drug therapy
Class III Contraindications for Permanent Pacemaker
Asymptomatic first-degree or fascicular AV block Type 1 second-degree AV block Asymptomatic cardioinhibitory response to carotid sinus massage Situational vasovagal syncope when possible to avoid triggers

in downstream depolarization, thereby bypassing the region(s) with significant conduction disease.

PACEMAKER SYSTEM AND BASICS OF PACING

A transvenous pacemaker system is comprised of the pulse generator and the lead(s). The number of the leads gives the device functionality as a single-chamber, dual-chamber (ie, atrium and ventricle), or biventricular pacemaker. The pulse generator is comprised of the battery/energy source, the device circuitry, and the header, which will serve to secure the connection of the lead to the generator. The leads are used for the dual purpose of sensing for intrinsic atrial and ventricular signals and pacing when required. The lead is comprised of the electrode (conductor) with its tip fixation mode (active or passive), the insulation, connection pin, and tie-down sleeves used to secure the lead to the pectoral muscle.

Pacemakers must be able to reliably sense local or near field impulses in a given cardiac chamber (atrium or ventricle). This is known as sensing, which is measured and reported in amplitude as millivolts (mV). For a lead placed in the atrium, the usual atrial sensing amplitude ranges between 1.0 and 5.0 mV, with the majority falling between 2 and 3 mV, which allows for appropriate discrimination of atrial fibrillatory waves and associated device mode switch, will be discussed later. For leads placed in or adjacent to the ventricle, ventricular sensing amplitude ranges between 5 and 15 mV.

Current leads have a bipolar configuration and design but can be programmed to sense and pace in a bipolar or unipolar setting. Bipolar programming is preferred as it decreases the possibility of sensing noncardiac electrical signals causing inappropriate pacing inhibition. A lead programmed in the unipolar setting has the cathode (−) at the tip of the lead and the pulse generator serving as the anode (+), which creates a wider antenna and more susceptible for sensing noncardiac signals. The bipolar lead will have both the cathode (−) and anode (+) located just proximal to the distal end of the lead in the intracardiac chamber which results in a smaller antenna, which is less likely to pick up external electrical potentials. Bipolar leads are the standard of care for newly implanted systems, though some unipolar leads still exist from previously implanted devices. Once a lead is deployed, the stability of the cardiac tissue and lead interface is critical for appropriate and stable sensing and pacing parameters and so, active fixation (deployed helix) is the primary mode of lead delivery to the myocardial tissue for right atrial and right ventricular leads. The use of passive (ie, not active) fixation mechanisms with fixating tines or wings is used in select cases primarily to reduce the risk of cardiac chamber perforation; however, passive leads represent less than 5% of implanted leads in use because of limitations with stability. The exception is the almost exclusive use of passive fixation mechanisms for stability in coronary sinus leads owing to the risk of venous perforation with active mechanisms.[1-3]

FOLLOW-UP PATIENT CARE

The most inquired parameter when discussing pacemaker follow-up care relates to pacing mode and the lower/upper programmed rates.

Programmed Modes and Application

The mode is identified by chamber paced, chamber sensed, response to sensing, rate modulation, and multisite pacing and represented by a combination of three to five capitalized letters (O = none, A = atrium, V = ventricle, D = dual A+V, T = triggered, and I = inhibited). For example, a device programmed DDD will pace both the atrium and the ventricle, sense both atria and ventricle, and based on the sensing will respond with either a triggered (paced event) or inhibited response to reset the timing for the next pacemaker timing cycle. In comparison, a VVIR programmed pacemaker will pace and sense the ventricle, will be inhibited by a sensed event, and has rate modulation (also referred commonly as rate response) enabled to increase the pacing rate to approximate the appropriate heart rate relative to the activity of the person (**Table 63.3**).

The VVI mode with or without R (rate response) is reserved for single-chamber ventricular pacemakers in the setting of permanent atrial fibrillation or a dual-chamber system in a person who now has permanent atrial fibrillation without expectation of restoration of sinus rhythm in which case the device can be programmed to a single-chamber mode. AAI mode with a single-chamber device and lead in the right atrium is not frequently implanted in the United States for patients with sinus node dysfunction without AV nodal conduction disease; however, in other parts of the world, it is the preferred mode for isolated sinus node dysfunction (**Figure 63.1**). However, AAI-DDD programming is frequently employed as a means to primarily pace the right atrium and allow intrinsic conduction to the ventricle to reduce ventricular pacing, which is the ideal programmed mode for those with sinus node dysfunction but intact AV node conduction. All current manufacturers have this programmable feature with a different nomenclature. Although the device is programmed to AAI mode, it surveils for ventricular sensed events following atrial sensing or pacing. If no ventricular sensing is recorded, the device will switch to a DDD mode and scan for native ventricular sensing which, when present, will revert the pacemaker to an AAI mode and scanning for native ventricular sensing starts again. AOO, VOO, or DOO modes are asynchronous pacing for the atrium, ventricular, or both respectably and are rarely used other than for temporary periods such as during electrocautery to prevent oversensing and pacing inhibition and during magnetic resonance imaging.

Rate-Response Programming

Rate-response programming aims at achieving an appropriate rate increase with physical activity and is most beneficial in those with sinus node dysfunction and chronotropic incompetence. This mode is also employed with single-chamber devices with slow ventricular response as a result of atrial fibrillation or complete heart block. Accelerometers embedded in the pulse generator are the most common sensors employed for this purpose, but changes in minute ventilation, thoracic impedance, and cardiac contractility are also employed to assess rate response needs with programmable features on the slope increase and recovery. As noted above, rate response corresponds to the fourth letter of the programmed settings (ie, DDDR).

Atrial Mode Switch

Atrial mode switch (AMS) is the change from a dual-chamber atrial sensing mode to a nontracking mode and occurs if the atrial rate is usually above 170 bpm. The goal is to prevent continued pacing at the upper tracking rate, leading to symptoms from pacing at high rates and paced-induced cardiomyopathy if the arrhythmia is sustained. Once the atrial arrhythmia stops, the device will resume the tracking at the programmed settings. Additionally, during routine device interrogation, the number and duration of arrhythmia events and the percentage of time spent in AMS will be available to guide strategies for rhythm and rate control. It should be noted that a single-chamber device cannot assess for AMS because of lack of atrial sensing, and the atrial detection rate is also a programmable feature.

Pacemaker-Mediated Tachycardia

Pacemaker-mediated tachycardia (PMT) is characteristically an atrial sensed rhythm followed by a ventricular paced rate at the upper programmed rate which commonly is 130 bpm for most patients. Initiation of PMT occurs during ventricular sensing or pacing with retrograde AV node conduction and P waves sensed and tracked with subsequent ventricular pacing. Although most current device platforms have algorithms for PMT detection and termination, this can be avoided by extending the postventricular atrial refractory period (PVARP) or switching to a nontracking mode if frequent episodes occur. The hallmark is the presence of a ventricular paced rate at the programmed upper rate which is not associated with physical activity.[1-3] PMT can be terminated by placing a 90-gauss round magnet over the device, which will achieve DOO mode for the duration of the time the magnet is placed over the pulse generator, thereby preventing the atrial lead from sensing P waves that arise from retrograde AV node conduction.

TABLE 63.3 Permanent Pacemaker Mode Nomenclature

Position	I	II	III	IV	V
Category	Chamber(s) Paced	Chamber(s) Sensed	Response to Sensing	Rate Modulation	Multisite Pacing
	0 = none	0 = none	0 = none	0 = none	0 = none
	A = atrium	A = atrium	T = triggered	R = rate response	A = atrium
	V = ventricle	V = ventricle	I = inhibited	–	V = ventricle
	D = dual (A+V)	D = dual (A+V)	D = dual (T+I)	–	D = dual (A+V)

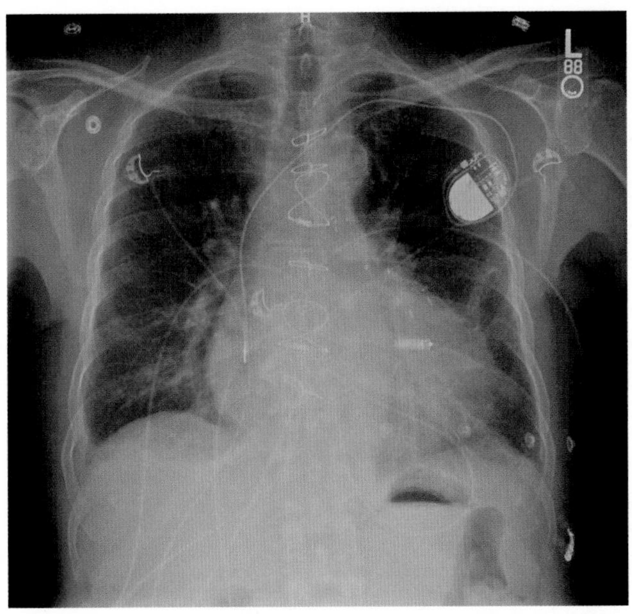

FIGURE 63.1 AAI Pacemaker with single transvenous lead to the right atrium.

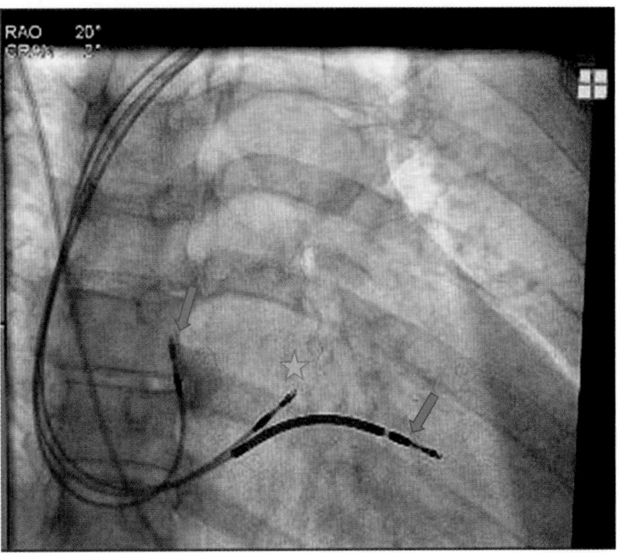

FIGURE 63.2 His bundle lead system (biventricular implantable cardio-defibrillator with His bundle lead). Blue arrows correspond to right atrial lead and right ventricular leads. Yellow star corresponds to His bundle lead.

Physiologic Pacing

The association between dyssynchrony from right ventricular pacing and paced-induced cardiomyopathy is well known especially in those individuals with an expected right ventricular paced burden greater than 40% and those with a left ventricular ejection fraction of less than 50%. Physiologic pacing targets right ventricular lead delivery to the conduction system—either the His bundle or distally to the left bundle branch—resulting in a narrow QRS duration and activation that directly engages the native conduction system with less potential dyssynchrony compared with the traditional right ventricular apical pacing. The current lead for conduction system pacing is a 4.1 French actively deployed helix lead (Select Secure Model 3830, Medtronic, Inc) delivered using a fixed curve or deflectable sheath designed for His lead implantation, although additional leads from other manufacturers are coming to market. There is much enthusiasm within the electrophysiology community that physiologic ventricular pacing will become the standard to preserve near-native conduction during ventricular pacing (**Figure 63.2**).[5-12]

Leadless Permanent Pacemaker

For patients with an indication for a single-chamber device, an alternative to the traditional transvenous pacemaker system is available. The MICRA (Medtronic, Inc) is a transfemoral delivery system to the right ventricle with components (generator and pacing and sensing electrode) that are integrated into a device that is ~3 cm long. This device can only pace the ventricle; however, two programmed modes are available, VVI mode and VDI. The initial leadless device to market only had ventricular sensing with programmable rate response to (ie, a VVI or VVIR device) and thus, not suitable for patients in which atrial sensing (sinus rhythm) needed to be tracked to preserve AV synchrony. A second-generation device (MICRA AV, Medtronic, Inc) allows atrial sensing and hence AV synchrony in patients with high-degree AV block: this device paces the ventricle but can sense both atria and ventricle. However, because of lack of right atrial pacing, it is not indicated for patients with sinus node dysfunction. Among the benefits of leadless devices, the risk of acute pocket infection is eliminated compared with a transvenous device; however, there is a slightly higher risk of bleeding and vascular complications with its use[13] (**Figure 63.3**).

PERMANENT PACEMAKER COMPLICATIONS

Acute (Procedure-Related) Complications

Complications from permanent pacemakers are divided into acute (procedure related) and chronic (device related). Among the more frequent acute complications are pneumothorax (<1%) during attempts at vascular access: this is reduced by the use of fluoroscopic guidance with contrast venography, ultrasound-guided venous access, and cephalic vein cut down that avoids direct venous puncture. Cardiac perforation and tamponade (<1%), perioperative hematoma, infection 1% (subacute), lead dislodgement, and venous thrombosis (1%-3%) are other acute complications.

Infection is reported around 1% and secondary to common perioperative skin and nosocomial pathogens like *Staphylococcus*

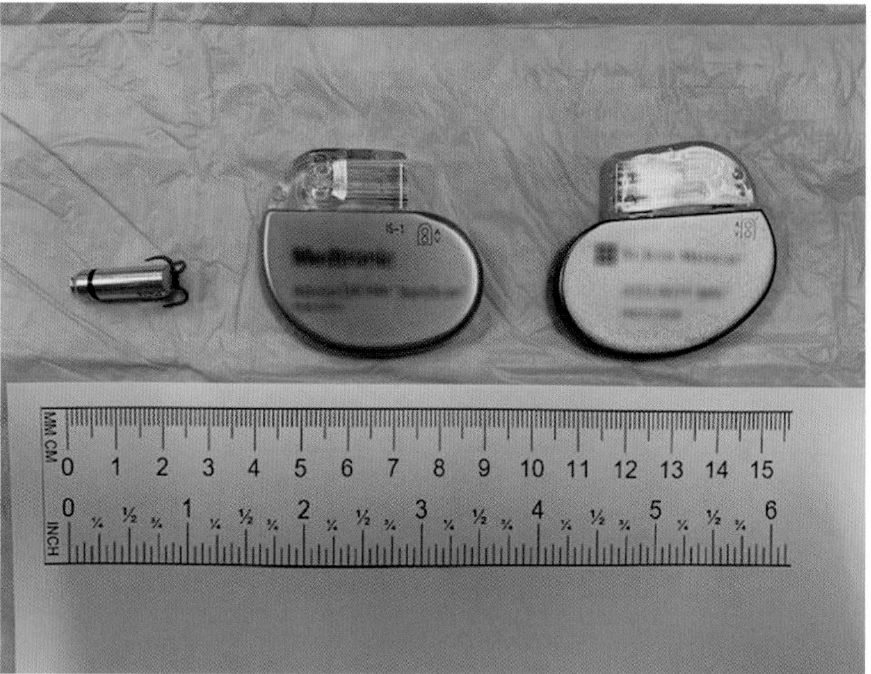

FIGURE 63.3 Comparison of leadless pacemaker (left) and transvenous pacemaker middle and (right).

aureus and *Staphylococcus epidermidis*, primarily related to pocket infection which can result in bacteremia. Extraction of the entire system is usually required in these cases, and the infection must be cleared prior to implantation of a second device on the contralateral side. Although the risk of infection is low when standard sterile procedure protocols are followed, some factors such as diabetes mellitus, hemodialysis, and recent infection leading to bacteremia are known to result in higher infection rates. Minor and localized infections along the superficial incision site can occur; however, these rarely progress to removal of CIEDs and are commonly managed with oral antibiotic therapy.

Chronic (Device-Related) Complications

Chronic or late complications are related primarily to device malfunction such as premature battery depletion or lead failure caused by lead fracture or insulation breach and those related to chronic device implant such as venous occlusion or stenosis such as seen in superior vena cava (SVC) syndrome. These are usually discovered during routine office follow-up and remote monitoring evaluation and when changes in lead impedance, sensing, and/or pacing threshold are noted. Lead failure is concerning when found in pacemaker-dependent patients. Although programming changes can be considered in select cases, replacement of the nonfunctional component is usually required.[14-16]

Although risk infection of an implanted cardiac device remains a concern, when presenting late after implant (>2 years) it is usually associated with an infection source not related to the implant but rather leading to bacteremia seeding of the device leads, which is an important consideration when distinguishing from primary implant infections.

Management of infected pacemaker leads or generator is done with the removal of the pacemaker system (explant or extraction); however, in very limited and specific scenarios in which the morbidity and mortality risk of procedural extraction is unacceptably high and the goals of care support a conservative approach to management, suppressive antibiotic management can be considered.

Device Malfunction: Undersensing/Oversensing

Device "undersensing" is a failure of the system to recognize a true cardiac electrical signal resulting in pacing output when there should be none. In the case of ventricular pacing, this can have the potential of inducing ventricular fibrillation should the paced event fall during the relative refractory period during repolarization—also known as "R on T phenomenon"—when the myocardial is ischemic. The factors leading to undersensing can be patient-related such as electrolyte or acid–base disorders and myocardial ischemia. However, more frequently, it is related to a device component (ie, lead failure from fracture or dislodgement) or programmed sensitivity above or near the intrinsic sensing.

"Oversensing" is the detection of electrical signals that the device erroneously considers cardiac in origin, resulting in inappropriate inhibition of pacing. This is especially concerning for those who are device-dependent. Common causes include myopotentials (ie, oversensing of extrinsic electric potential from skeletal muscle activity) and electromagnetic interference. Lead fracture and insulation breach are other common causes of oversensing and also result in lead impedance being out of the normal range (**Figure 63.4**).

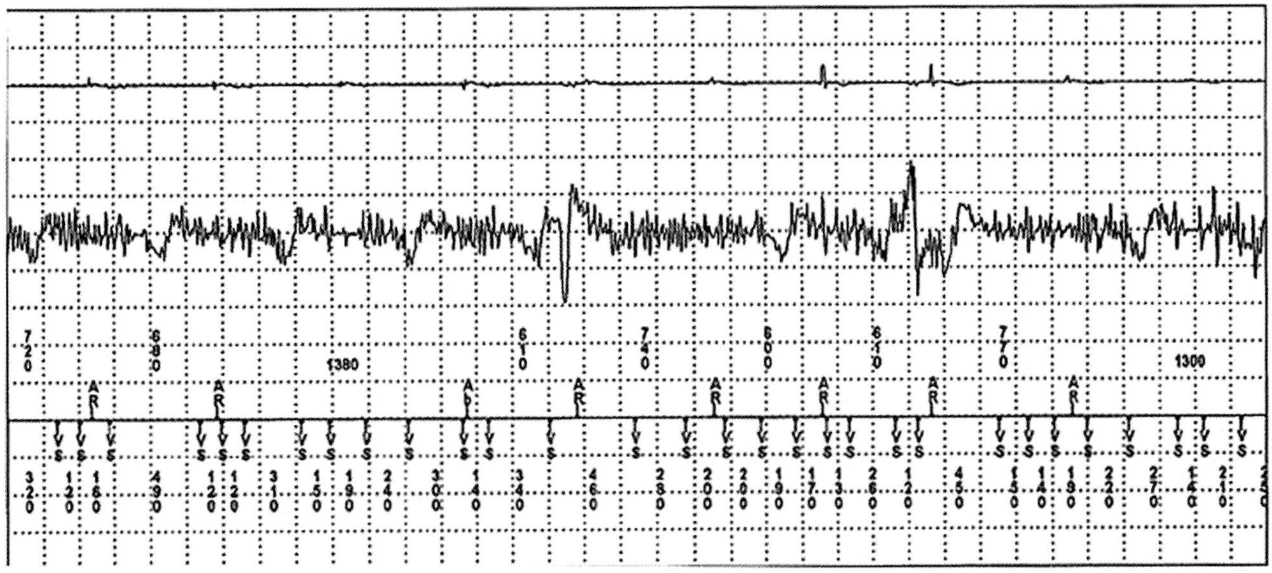

FIGURE 63.4 Right ventricle lead noise with short V-V intervals 120 to 140 milliseconds secondary to lead fracture resulting in "oversensing." AR, atrial refractory (the atrial electrogram recording is within the programmed ventriculoatrial refractory period, ie, is seen by the device but not taken into account in the atrial-ventricular pacing timing). VS, ventricular sensed event, an electrogram recorded by the ventricular lead.

SPECIAL CONSIDERATIONS (PERIOPERATIVE MANAGEMENT AND MAGNETIC RESONANCE IMAGING)

Perioperative pacemaker management is a frequent cardiac consultation request, with the primary focus on determining if the patient is device-dependent and assessing the risk of device inhibition from oversensing related to surgical tools used for hemostasis (ie, cautery) and those commonly used in orthopedic procedures. Electrocautery application, when performed in bipolar mode, is much less likely to result in a wide pulse field and cause pacemaker inhibition. So whenever possible, electrocautery should be performed in bipolar mode and away from the pacemaker site. However, if monopolar mode is used or the surgery site is above the diaphragm in a patient who is device-dependent, the perioperative programming recommendation is an asynchronous pacing mode (DOO or VOO). The use of a 90 Gauss round magnet over the device will achieve DOO mode for the duration of the time the magnet is placed over the pulse generator.

Pacemaker systems implanted as of 2017 obtained from the four major CIED manufacturers in the United States are magnetic resonance imaging (MRI) conditional and considered safe, including the leadless Micra device. Devices with an MRI conditional pulse generator but with older non-MRI conditional leads should be evaluated on an individual case-by-case basis if MR imaging can be done safely.[17]

KEY POINTS

- ✔ Permanent pacemaker implant is the standard of care of nonreversible symptomatic bradyarrhythmias with low periprocedural risk.
- ✔ An understanding of basic pacemaker function, pacing mode, and programmable features are necessary in the practice of medicine owing to the prevalence of these devices, which will continue to increase with an aging population.
- ✔ Ventricular pacing produces dysynchrony that has opened the field of physiologic pacing (coronary sinus pacing, conduction system pacing) with new implant techniques and lead development.
- ✔ The development of leadless devices along with physiologic pacing are two areas of development which will likely have the most influence in the near term.
- ✔ MRI conditional devices are the standard for new implants and require minimal device programing for those patients having MRI scans.

SECTION 4

REFERENCES

1. Mulpuru SK, Madhavan M, McLeod CJ, Cha YM, Friedman PA. Cardiac pacemakers: function, troubleshooting, and management: part 1 of a 2-part series. *J Am Coll Cardiol.* 2017;69(2):189-210. doi:10.1016/j.jacc.2016.10.061
2. Madhavan M, Mulpuru SK, McLeod CJ, Cha YM, Friedman PA. Advances and future directions in cardiac pacemakers: part 2 of a 2-part series. *J Am Coll Cardiol.* 2017;69(2):211-235. doi:10.1016/j.jacc.2016.10.064

3. Jeffrey K, Parsonnet V. Cardiac pacing, 1960-1985: a quarter century of medical and industrial innovation. *Circulation.* 1998;97(19):1978-1991. doi:10.1161/01.cir.97.19.1978
4. Epstein AE, DiMarco JP, Ellenbogen KA, et al. 2012 ACCF/AHA/HRS focused update incorporated into the ACCF/AHA/HRS 2008 guidelines for device-based therapy of cardiac rhythm abnormalities: a report of the American College of Cardiology Foundation/American Heart Association Task Force on Practice Guidelines and the Heart Rhythm Society. *Circulation.* 2013;127:e283-e352.
5. Healey JS, Crystal E, Connolly SJ. Physiologic pacing: where pacing mode selection reflects the indication. *Heart.* 2004;90(6):593-594. doi:10.1136/hrt.2003.022111
6. Lewis AJM, Foley P, Whinnett Z, Keene D, Chandrasekaran B. His bundle pacing: a new strategy for physiological ventricular activation. *J Am Heart Assoc.* 2019;8(6):e010972. doi:10.1161/JAHA.118.010972. Erratum in: *J Am Heart Assoc.* 2019;8(11):e002310.
7. Sharma AD, Rizo-Patron C, Hallstrom AP, et al. Percent right ventricular pacing predicts outcomes in the DAVID trial. *Heart Rhythm.* 2005;2(8):830-834. doi:10.1016/j.hrthm.2005.05.015
8. Curtis AB, Worley SJ, Adamson PB, et al. Biventricular pacing for atrioventricular block and systolic dysfunction. *N Engl J Med.* 2013;368(17):1585-1593. doi:10.1056/NEJMoa1210356
9. Upadhyay GA, Tung R. His bundle pacing for cardiac resynchronization. *Card Electrophysiol Clin.* 2018;10(3):511-517. doi:10.1016/j.ccep.2018.05.010
10. Zhang S, Zhou X, Gold MR. Left bundle branch pacing: JACC review topic of the week. *J Am Coll Cardiol.* 2019;74(24):3039-3049. doi:10.1016/j.jacc.2019.10.039
11. Vijayaraman P, Dandamudi G, Zanon F, et al. Permanent His bundle pacing: recommendations from a Multicenter His Bundle Pacing Collaborative Working Group for standardization of definitions, implant measurements, and follow-up. *Heart Rhythm.* 2018;15(3):460-468. doi:10.1016/j.hrthm.2017.10.039
12. Ajijola OA, Upadhyay GA, Macias C, Shivkumar K, Tung R. Permanent His-bundle pacing for cardiac resynchronization therapy: initial feasibility study in lieu of left ventricular lead. *Heart Rhythm.* 2017;14(9):1353-1361. doi:10.1016/j.hrthm.2017.04.003
13. Bhatia N, El-Chami M. Leadless pacemakers: a contemporary review. *J Geriatr Cardiol.* 2018;15(4):249-253. doi:10.11909/j.issn.1671-5411.2018.04.002
14. Clémenty N, Fernandes J, Carion PL, et al. Pacemaker complications and costs: a nationwide economic study. *J Med Econ.* 2019;22(11):1171-1178. doi:10.1080/13696998.2019.1652186
15. Polyzos KA, Konstantelias AA, Falagas ME. Risk factors for cardiac implantable electronic device infection: a systematic review and meta-analysis. *Europace.* 2015;17(5):767-777. doi:10.1093/europace/euv053
16. Al-Hadithi AB, Do DH, Boyle NG. Vein management for cardiac device implantation. *Card Electrophysiol Clin.* 2018;10(4):561-571. doi:10.1016/j.ccep.2018.05.003
17. Russo RJ, Costa HS, Silva PD, et al. Assessing the risks associated with MRI in patients with a pacemaker or defibrillator. *N Engl J Med.* 2017;376(8):755-764. doi:10.1056/NEJMoa1603265

CHAPTER 64

LEAD EXTRACTION

Munish Kannabhiran and Noel G. Boyle

INTRODUCTION AND HISTORY

The use of cardiovascular implantable electronic devices (CIEDs) has increased dramatically over the last few decades, with almost 1.2 to 1.4 million CIEDs implanted annually worldwide.[1] In parallel with this, device- or lead-related complications and extractions have also risen significantly—especially in the aging population who tend to have more medical comorbidities. Although newer technological advancements allow the implantation of leadless pacemakers and subcutaneous implantable cardioverter-defibrillators (ICDs) in select populations, the majority of implanted devices are still transvenous.

Lead extraction via heart surgery, primarily used until the 1980s, is now reserved for certain scenarios such as failed percutaneous lead extraction, leads with very large vegetations in endocarditis, and when other cardiac surgery is needed, such as valve replacement. Early nonsurgical techniques introduced in the 1960s included simple mechanical traction and the use of weight and pulley systems to provide sustained traction.[2] Telescoping mechanical sheaths made of stainless steel, polypropylene, or Teflon were introduced in the 1980s, resulting in superior transvenous extraction rates approaching 80%. The availability of locking stylets in the 1990s allowed for lead reinforcement, and powered sheaths using excimer laser system became available in the mid-1990s.

Transvenous lead extraction (TLE), as a part of overall lead management, has grown markedly since the 1990s, not only as a consequence of growth in CIED implants and increasing rates of infection and lead failure but also because of increased awareness of indications for lead management and the development of more advanced and safer extraction tools.[3]

Removing the pulse generator is generally uncomplicated, as is transvenous removal of recently implanted leads (<12 months). However, extraction of chronic leads is often challenging with inherent life-threatening complications owing to scar or fibrous adhesions as well as calcifications.[4] The degree of endothelial fibrosis is related to the length of time the lead has been implanted and the patient's vascular inflammatory reactivity. Fibrotic attachments are found not only at the lead tip, but can occur anywhere along the entire length of the lead—between the lead and the innominate vein, superior vena cava (SVC), tricuspid valve, or myocardium[5] as depicted in **Figure 64.1**. Common sites are the innominate-SVC junction, the SVC-right atrial junction, the tricuspid valve, and the lead tip site. The earlier techniques of TLE relied on simple manual traction, frequently proved ineffective for chronically implanted leads, and carried a significant risk of myocardial avulsion, tamponade, and death. This limited the initial indications for TLE to life-threatening situations such as sepsis and uncontrolled infection. However, with the advancement in technology and availability of new extraction tools, TLE has become safer and more effective, with expanded indications.

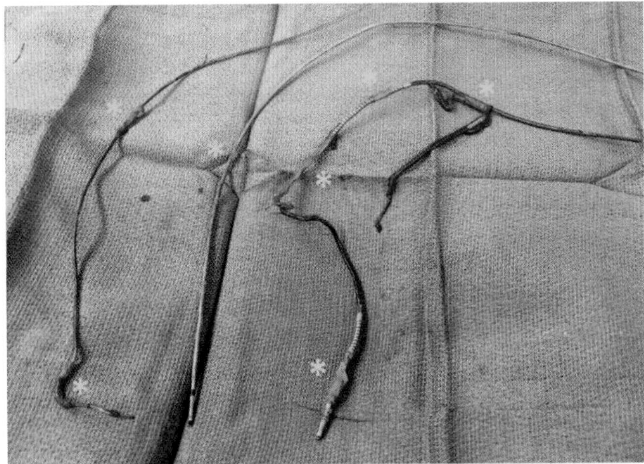

FIGURE 64.1 Explanted leads to coronary sinus (left), right atrium (middle), and right ventricle (right) which demonstrate scar/fibrous tissue (yellow asterisks) attached to the lead tips and mid-portion of the leads.

Lead extraction is defined as a procedure where the removal of at least one pacing or defibrillator lead requiring the assistance of equipment not typically employed during lead implantation or at least one lead was implanted for greater than 1 year according to the Heart Rhythm Society (HRS) expert consensus statement on CIED lead management and extraction.[1] The term "lead explant" is used when all leads are removed without tools or with implantation stylets and all the removed leads were implanted for less than 1 year. "Lead removal" indicates the removal of a lead using any technique, regardless of time since implantation.

INDICATIONS FOR LEAD EXTRACTION

Infection remains the most common indication for lead extraction, constituting almost half of all cases.[6,7] There has been a slight downtrend in infectious indications in the last 10 years not because of a lower incidence of infections, but rather because of increasing indications for lead removal owing to other conditions such as lead dysfunction. The Lead Extraction in the CONtemporary setting (LExICon) study[8] from 2010 reported 57% cases had infectious indications, decreasing to 53% in the European Lead Extraction ConTRolled registry (ELECTRa) study from 2017,[7] and to 48% in the most recent Patient-Related Outcomes of Mechanical lead Extraction Techniques (PROMET) study[9] published in early 2020. Lead dysfunction, abandoned functional leads, thrombosis/vascular access issues, and severe tricuspid regurgitation (TR) are the next most common indications for lead extraction. Chronic pain, recalled leads, malignant arrhythmias from abandoned leads, and the need for radiation therapy are other rare indications for lead extraction.

The current indications for lead removal are based on the updated HRS expert consensus statement from 2017,[1] and the complete list is provided in **Tables 64.1** and **64.2**. The infectious indication for removal is based on mortality benefit and reduced morbidity associated with infected CIED removal as well as the inability to medically treat the contaminated devices. However, the decision-making process regarding lead extraction for noninfectious indications needs to be individualized. There are no randomized clinical trials to guide treatment in these situations. Hence, a careful assessment of the risks of extraction versus the potential clinical benefits related to that particular indication needs to be weighed on a case-by-case basis.

FACILITY CONSIDERATIONS

Lead extractions should optimally be performed in high-volume centers with experienced operators, given the risks associated with the procedure, especially for older leads and multiple leads in high-risk patient populations. The key requirement is that the facility provides the necessary equipment and personnel to perform lead extractions and manage complications safely.[10] These extraction procedures are usually undertaken in operating rooms or hybrid laboratories, whereas removal of younger leads can often be safely performed in electrophysiology laboratories. A subanalysis of ELECTRa registry showed that TLEs are performed in the operating room in 53% of patients, hybrid rooms in 20% of patients, and catheterization laboratories in 27% of the patients.[11] The ability to provide immediate surgical intervention in cases of major complications—such as an SVC tear or cardiac avulsion with tamponade—makes the operating room and the hybrid laboratory the best options to perform lead extractions in high-risk cases. The cardiac surgeon and a full support team—including cardiopulmonary perfusionist and equipment—must be available to provide emergent open-chest surgical repair within 5 to 10 minutes.[12] Although studies have shown increased complication rates (including SVC tear and death) when both the cardiologist and cardiothoracic surgeon are performing the case compared to cardiologists alone, this actually reflects the high-risk profile and complexity of these cases which warranted the procedure being done in the operating room in the first place.[11] Hence, in our institution, we adopt an integrative approach between the cardiac electrophysiologist and the cardiac surgeon, where both are scrubbed in for the cases, which are predominantly performed in the operating room or hybrid laboratory with cardiopulmonary bypass standby.[12]

Risk Stratification

Preprocedural risk stratification of patients helps to identify and carefully select which procedures need to be undertaken

TABLE 64.1 Recommendations for Lead Extraction (Infectious)

Class	Recommendations
I	If antibiotics are going to be prescribed, drawing at least two sets of blood cultures before starting antibiotic therapy is recommended for all patients with suspected cardiovascular implantable electronic device (CIED) infection to improve the precision and minimize the duration of antibiotic therapy.
I	Gram stain and culture of generator pocket tissue and the explanted lead(s) are recommended at the time of CIED removal to improve the precision and minimize the duration of antibiotic therapy.
I	Preprocedural transesophageal echocardiography (TEE) is recommended for patients with suspected systemic CIED infection to evaluate the absence or size, character, and potential embolic risk of identified vegetations.
I	Evaluation by physicians with specific expertise in CIED infection and lead extraction is recommended for patients with *documented* CIED infection.
IIa	TEE can be useful for patients with CIED pocket infection with and without positive blood cultures to evaluate the absence or size, character, and potential embolic risk of identified vegetations.
IIa	Evaluation by physicians with specific expertise in CIED infection and lead extraction can be useful for patients with *suspected* CIED infections.
IIb	Additional imaging may be considered to facilitate the diagnosis of CIED pocket or lead infection when it cannot be confirmed by other methods.

Reprinted from Kusumoto FM, Schoenfeld MH, Wilkoff BL, et al. 2017 HRS expert consensus statement on cardiovascular implantable electronic device lead management and extraction. *Heart Rhythm.* 2017;14(12):e503-e551.

TABLE 64.2 Recommendations for Lead Extraction (Noninfectious)

Class	Recommendations
Thrombosis/Vascular Issues	
I	Lead removal is recommended for patients with clinically significant thromboembolic events attributable to thrombus on a lead or a lead fragment that cannot be treated by other means.
I	Lead removal is recommended for patients with superior vena cava (SVC) stenosis or occlusion that prevents implantation of a necessary lead.
I	Lead removal is recommended for patients with planned stent deployment in a vein already containing a transvenous lead, to avoid entrapment of the lead.
I	Lead removal as part of a comprehensive plan for maintaining patency is recommended for patients with SVC stenosis or occlusion with limiting symptoms.
IIa	Lead removal can be useful for patients with ipsilateral venous occlusion preventing access to the venous circulation for required placement of an additional lead.
Chronic Pain	
IIa	Device and/or lead removal can be useful for patients with severe chronic pain at the device or lead insertion site or believed to be secondary to the device, which causes significant patient discomfort, is not manageable by medical or surgical techniques, and for which there is no acceptable alternative.
Other	
I	Lead removal is recommended for patients with life-threatening arrhythmias secondary to retained leads.
IIa	Lead removal can be useful for patients with a cardiovascular implantable electronic device (CIED) location that interferes with the treatment of malignancy.
IIa	Lead removal can be useful for patients if a CIED implantation would require more than four leads on one side or more than five leads through the SVC.
IIa	Lead removal can be useful for patients with an abandoned lead that interferes with the operation of a CIED system.
IIb	Lead removal may be considered for patients with leads that, because of their design or their failure, pose a potential future threat to the patient if left in place.
IIb	Lead removal may be considered for patients to facilitate access to magnetic resonance imaging (MRI).
IIb	Lead removal may be considered in the setting of normally functioning nonrecalled pacing or defibrillation leads for selected patients after a shared decision-making process.

Reprinted from Kusumoto FM, Schoenfeld MH, Wilkoff BL, et al. 2017 HRS expert consensus statement on cardiovascular implantable electronic device lead management and extraction. *Heart Rhythm.* 2017;14(12):e503-e551. Copyright © 2017 Heart Rhythm Society. With permission.

in the operating or hybrid room with appropriate expertise to manage potential lethal complications. Several studies have identified high-risk features that are more commonly associated with periprocedural complications including death. They include age (>68 years), female gender, lower body mass index (<25 kg/m^2), anemia (hemoglobin <11.5 g/dL), number of prior CIED procedures, low-volume centers, New York Heart Association (NYHA) Class III to IV symptoms, chronic kidney disease, long lead dwell time (>10 years), and systemic infectious indication.[7,11,13,14] Among these, advanced patient age, low-volume centers, NYHA Class III to IV symptoms, and systemic infection were directly related to increased all-cause mortality.[7,11] A chest radiography showing multiple device leads (three active and two abandoned) is shown in **Figure 64.2**, which is one of the high-risk features associated with increased risk of periprocedural complications. Recently, Jachec et al[14] developed a calculator to risk stratify the patients undergoing TLE to predict the probability of major complications **(Table 64.3)**.

IMAGING CONSIDERATIONS

Fluoroscopy remains the primary imaging modality used periprocedurally during lead extractions along with transesophageal echocardiography (TEE). Other imaging tools such as cardiac computerized tomography (CT) and tagged white blood cell scan may be helpful preprocedurally for assessing venous stenosis and confirming infection in questionable cases, respectively. A chest radiograph will identify undocumented old leads, show whether the implanted leads were actively or passively fixed, and may show areas of calcification. Actively fixated leads can be identified with a corkscrew helix attached to the myocardium, whereas passively fixated leads have conical tips or tines at the lead tip.[15] TEE has a primary role preprocedurally to establish the diagnosis of endocarditis, evaluate the size of vegetations, and document any preexisting pericardial effusion. It is also used periprocedurally to monitor cardiac function and integrity.

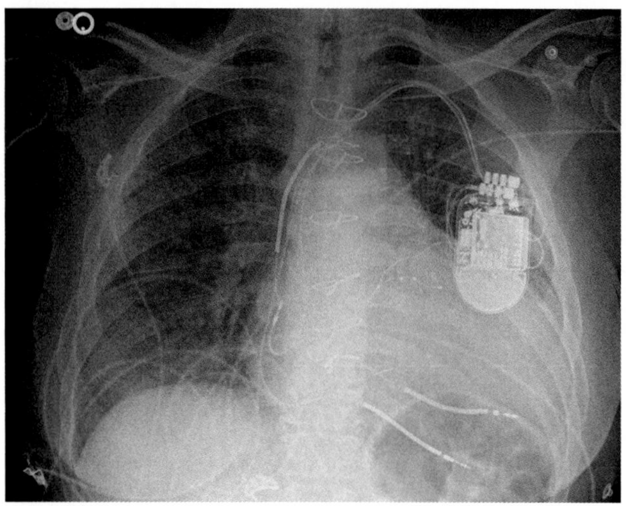

FIGURE 64.2 Chest x-ray showing a cardiac resynchronization therapy defibrillator (CRT-D) device with five leads (current and abandoned)—one right atrial, two right ventricular, and two coronary sinus leads.

TABLE 64.3 Calculator of Probability of Major Complications of Transvenous Lead Extractions

No.	Predictors of the Risk of Major Complications	Score
1	Sum of dwell times of leads planned for extraction (>16.5 years)	6.0
2	Young patient (first implantation under the age of 30 years)	2.2
3	Hemoglobin concentration <11.5 g/dL	2.3
4	Female gender	2.7
5	Number of previous CIED procedures per patient	1.4
	Total Score	-

Total Score	0-4.0	4.1-10	10.1-16	>16
Complications	0.2%-0.5%	0.5%-2.5%	2.5%-11.8%	>11.8%
Risk	Low Risk	Intermediate Risk	High Risk	Very High Risk

CIED, cardiovascular implantable electronic device.
From Jacheć W, Polewczyk A, Polewczyk M, et al. Transvenous Lead Extraction SAFeTY Score for Risk Stratification and Proper Patient Selection for Removal Procedures Using Mechanical Tools. *J Clin Med.* 2020;9(2):361. https://creativecommons.org/licenses/by/4.0/.

ANATOMIC CONSIDERATIONS

Most CIEDs are implanted subcutaneously in the left chest wall, and hence a left subclavian/axillary/cephalic venous approach is the most common approach for lead removal. This may allow the operator to perform the entire procedure using a single incision on the ipsilateral side. Also, for selected procedures, an SVC balloon[16] can be "parked" in the inferior vena cava via the right femoral vein on standby for acute management of an SVC tear. Additionally, femoral arterial and venous sheaths may be placed for potential perfusion pump access if emergent sternotomy is needed. In other complicated scenarios, femoral vein, internal jugular vein, contralateral subclavian vein approaches, or a combination thereof can be used, especially if there is a need to retrieve broken lead fragments.

FUNDAMENTALS OF LEAD EXTRACTION

The patient is prepped and draped in the same manner as for any open-heart surgery. After general anesthesia is administered, a TEE probe is inserted. Usually, an incision is made through the original CIED implantation site to gain access to the device pocket. In cases where there is a localized pocket infection, the pocket is debrided, and microbial cultures of the pocket tissue are obtained. If no infection is present, only minimal debridement needs to be performed while freeing the leads from the fibrotic constraints in the pocket.[17] The leads are then disconnected from the generator and are dissected away from the fibrous tissue to proximal to the protective "sleeves." If the leads have active fixation, they should be unscrewed at this stage, although this is not likely to be effective in chronic leads. Next, to minimize lead disintegration, a lead locking stylet is deployed inside the lead's central lumen to fixate it inside the lead's distal conductor coil (as far distal as possible). This helps to prevent the lead from unraveling as well as allowing application of traction along the entire length of the lead. Additionally, ties are applied to stabilize the outer insulation and provide further traction support. If the lead locking device cannot be inserted, a lead extender cable can be used.[18] It is essential that careful attention is given to lead preparation, and many experienced operators emphasize the importance of this step.

Lead explantation for relatively recent leads can be performed by simple traction on the leads accessed via the implant vein with mild to moderate force, after the fixation screws have been unscrewed (often with a standard nonlocking stylet in place). This is the simplest and most basic technique for lead removal being performed for decades and was found to be effective in the removal of 27% of the leads in the ELECTRa registry.[7] This approach is successful in removing leads that move freely in the vein but remain attached at the tip to the myocardium.[1]

For lead extractions involving older leads with dense scar tissue or calcifications, specialized sheaths or tools are almost always required. There are three main specialized sheaths/tools used in lead extraction: telescoping sheaths, laser sheaths, and rotational mechanical cutting sheaths. Optimal tool selection depends upon the characteristics and severity of adhesions at the lead-tissue interface as well as operator experience and training. Often, no single tool is sufficient for all types of fibrous or calcified adhesions encountered during lead extractions, and switching extraction tools and approaches is frequently necessary.[1]

Telescoping Sheaths

Brodell et al[19] described this early transvenous technique of lead extraction in 1990 using flexible, telescoping sheaths advanced over the lead to dilate scar tissue while applying traction on the lead. In this method, the telescoping sheath (made of Teflon or polypropylene) is advanced coaxially over the implanted lead until it reaches the distal tip of the lead at the myocardial interface. Once the sheath reaches the myocardial interface, the sheath is fixed with countertraction applied to the myocardium as traction is applied to the lead, resulting in "traction-countertraction" forces to release the lead tip from the myocardium.[17] Countertraction is the direct force to the myocardium at the lead tip by the extraction sheath. A representation of traction and countertraction forces applied during lead extraction using a telescoping sheath is shown in **Figure 64.3**. Telescoping sheaths can effectively disrupt fibrous adhesions, but stainless-steel sheaths are needed for dense fibrotic or heavily calcified lesions.

Laser Sheaths

The excimer laser (Spectranetics Inc, Philips, Eindhoven, Holland) is a xenon chloride "cool" cutting laser with a wavelength of 308 nm and an absorption depth of 0.06 mm, cutting tissue only in contact with its tip. This is commercially available in 12F, 14F, and 16F sizes (external diameter). As only proteins and fats absorb the laser energy, it can cut through fibrous adhesions surrounding the pacemaker lead without damaging the lead insulation.[20] The laser sheath replaces the inner sheath of the Teflon telescoping sheath with optic fibers forming a single circumferential ring of light sandwiched between the inner and outer walls of the tip as shown in **Figure 64.4**. The flexible laser sheath is advanced over the implanted lead with mild pressure while lasing, and moderate traction pressure is supplied through the locking stylet to provide a stable "rail" for the laser sheath to advance. The technique is similar to that used with dilator sheaths, except that the laser takes the place of the inner sheath with less force required and the emphasis placed on cutting, not pushing, with the laser. The outer Teflon sheath provides additional support and can be used to disrupt more dense fibrotic adhesions. The laser sheath often has to be completely advanced to the myocardial insertion point to free all adhesions. Laser application should stop 0.5 cm from the distal end of the lead tip to prevent damage to the myocardium. The Pacing Lead Extraction with The Excimer Sheath (PLEXES) trial reported in 1999 demonstrated superiority of excimer laser over standard telescopic extraction sheaths with complete extraction success rate of 94% compared to 64% for 465 leads.[21] Laser sheaths can sever fibrous lesions efficiently but are ineffective with heavily calcified lesions.

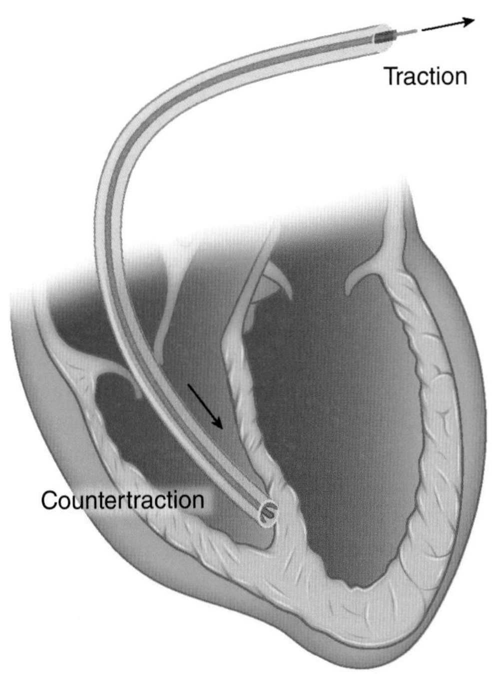

FIGURE 64.3 Diagrammatic representation of traction (with locking stylet) and countertraction (by sheath) forces applied during lead extraction.

Rotational Mechanical Cutting Sheaths

The Evolution® (Cook Medical, Bloomington, IN) mechanical dilator sheath was introduced in early 2010 as an additional tool to facilitate lead extractions. Its inner sheath has a rotational stainless-steel bladed tip to overcome dense fibrosis and calcified adhesions as shown in **Figure 64.4**. The rotational mechanism allows the sheath to advance along the lead body while cutting fibrotic attachments. The outer sheath covers the cutting edge when cutting activity is not desired, so that venous walls are protected from damage.[22] Subsequently, the TightRail® (Spectranetics Inc, Philips, NV) rotating mechanical sheath was introduced in 2014. The first-generation mechanical dilators had a unidirectional rotational mechanism that sometimes resulted in "wrapping or winding" of nontarget leads, whereas current-generation rotational sheaths are bidirectional, avoiding this problem. As with the telescoping and laser sheaths, the lead is first prepared using a locking stylet with additional silk ties to secure the insulation. The mechanical dilator sheath is then passed over the lead until it reaches a fibrous obstacle. Light traction is applied to maintain the lead as a rail while the mechanical sheath cuts through the fibrous adhesions in a rotational manner. There is a trigger activation handle at the end of the sheath, which activates the rotational cutting mechanism. Once the sheath cuts past the adhesion, one can resume gliding the sheath gently over the lead again without mechanical rotation until it hits another adhesion, and the process is repeated. A shorter mechanical dilator sheath known as the Evolution® Shortie Mechanical Dilator Sheaths (Cook Medical, Bloomington, IN) has been designed to overcome the difficulties of initial venous access in cases of extensive scarred

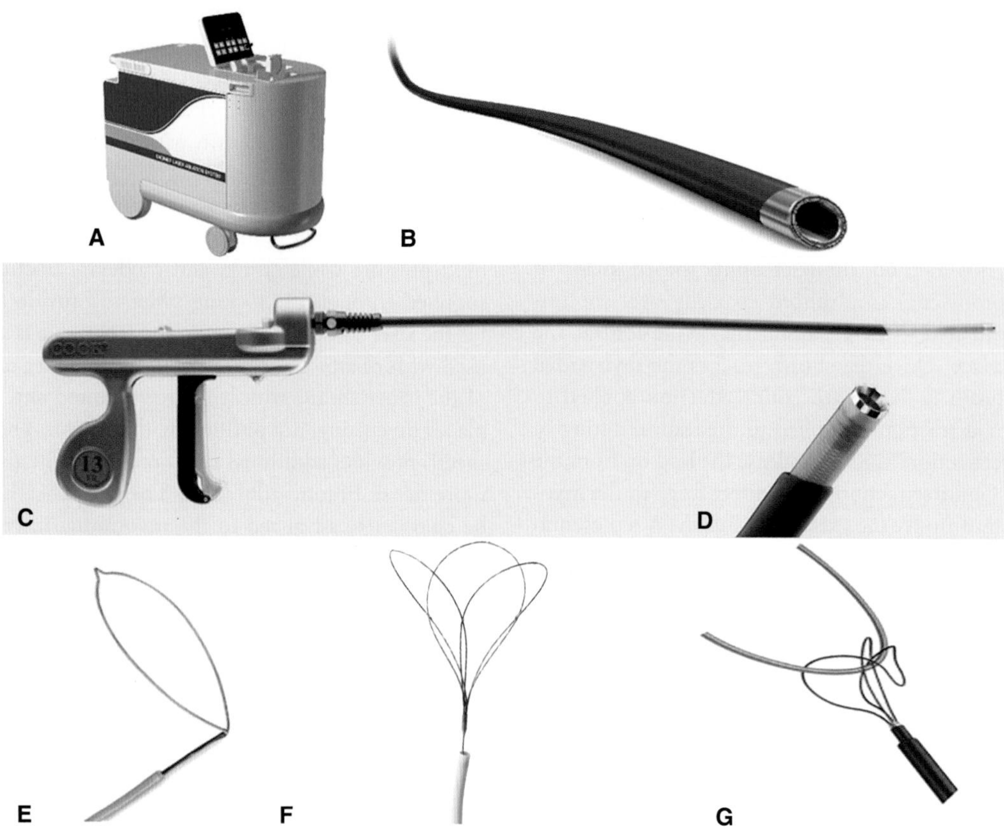

FIGURE 64.4 Lead extraction tools. **(A)** CVX 300, the generator that emits an excimer laser utilizing xenon chloride; **(B)** Spectranetics Laser sheath constructed using 82 optical fibers; **(C)** Evolution RL hand-powered flexible sheath with a specialized dissection tip; **(D)** Close-up view of mechanical dilator sheath showing stainless-steel tip; **(E)** Amplatz Goose Neck snare; **(F)** Merit Medical EN snare, and **(G)** Cook Needle's Eye Snare. (A & B, Used with permission of Koninklijke Philips N.V.; C, D, & G, Courtesy of Cook Medical; E, Reproduced with permission of Medtronic, Inc.; © Merit Medical. Reprinted by permission.)

or calcified tissue around the target vein lead access.[23] Among the three specialized tools, mechanical cutting tools are most efficient at traversing densely calcified fibrotic lesions.[1]

LIMITATIONS OF TRANSVENOUS LEAD EXTRACTION

The major limitation of TLE is when lead fracture or unraveling prevents its removal via the implant vein. Additional tools such as femoral snaring may help in retrieving the broken lead fragments in those cases. Sometimes, it may be impossible to retrieve all the fragments and the patient may end up with retained lead remnants. Occasionally, these lead remnants cause mechanical complications such as embolization into the pulmonary vasculature[24] or recurrent infection.[25] TLE is not suitable for large lead masses (ie, vegetation or thrombus >2.5 cm)[1]: cardiac surgery is indicated for lead extraction in these cases.

SPECIAL CONSIDERATIONS

Femoral Snaring

Femoral snaring is now generally considered a secondary approach for lead removal most often used only after a failure of the primary approach via the implant vein. It is very helpful for the retrieval of severed leads, retained lead segments or lead fragments with free ends floating in the venous system, heart, or pulmonary arteries. These femoral snares can also help in maintaining traction of the distal end of leads with severe adhesions, whereas the extraction sheath advances through the occluded veins. The Byrd Workstation™ (Cook Medical, Bloomington, IN), initially described in 1991,[26] consists of a 16F outer sheath with a one-way valve that is advanced over a wire into the femoral vein, and a 12F inner sheath through which a number of retrieval snares can be advanced such as Needle's Eye Snare® (Cook Medical, Bloomington, IN), EN snare® (©Merit Medical, UT), or the Amplatz GooseNeck® Snare (Covidien, Dublin, Ireland). Some of the various snares used in current clinical practice are shown in **Figure 64.4A-G**.

For leads or lead fragments that are fixed at both ends, a multicomponent snare such as the Needle's Eye™ Snare (Cook Medical, Bloomington, IN) can be used for the initial attempt. A closed loop is created by catching the lead with the hook-shaped portion (hood) of the snare (placed behind the lead) and then advancing a needle (in front of the lead) through the hood.[27] Once the lead is grasped, a telescoping sheath is then advanced over the system to tighten the loop around the lead and downward traction can be applied to pull the lead toward the inferior vena cava. Compared to the multicomponent snare approach, a single or multiloop snares are helpful in retrieving retained leads or lead fragments with loose ends. A deflectable sheath can be used to manipulate the snare into close proximity of the free end of the retained lead. The free end of the lead is then captured with one or more of the loops of the snaring tool (Goose-Neck snare or Ensnare) loaded on a bioptome forceps for additional support.

Coronary Sinus Leads

TLE of coronary sinus (CS) leads can be achieved with a high procedural success rate, similar to other atrial or ventricular leads (98%).[28] The major complication rate is similar to that seen with non-CS lead extraction (2.1% vs 1.8%). CS lead tip location (CS ostium/mid-CS/CS tributaries) influences the procedural and radiological success rates and procedural complexity but not complications.[28] Although most CS leads can be removed with simple manual traction, long-standing chronic leads may still require specialized extraction tools. Fibrous adhesions are not commonly seen in the CS as in other venous structures, likely because of smaller lead diameter. Hence, the detachment of CS leads from connective tissue scars in the venous and atrial areas to the CS ostium is generally sufficient for further removal of the lead using simple traction.

Ghosts

Small fibrinous sheaths or strands and even possibly vegetations may be noted in the right atrium and SVC following lead extraction, which appear as tubular as intracardiac masses on echocardiography or CT scans. These are termed as "ghosts," which have an incidence ranging from 8% to 14% and are most commonly observed in patients with infectious indications for extraction.[29] A recent study actually showed that patients who have residual "ghosts" after TLE had a higher mortality than those without "ghosts" (28% vs 5%; $P < .001$).[29] A possible reason for the higher mortality in patients with a "ghost" is suspected secondary to uncontrolled severe systemic infection, residual endocarditis/vegetation, or pulmonary embolism after TLE. Hence, it is prudent to assess and measure all the details of any "ghosts" via imaging modalities such as echocardiography and CT scan at the end of a procedure, and they should be documented for future reference. There are currently no guidelines on the management of these "ghosts."

COMPLICATIONS

Complications are classified by their severity into major and minor, with major complications being those that pose an immediate threat to life or result in death. Major complications usually arise from perforation or tear to the venous vasculature or myocardium. These include death, cardiac avulsion, vascular laceration, pericardial tamponade, hemothorax, and thromboembolic events. Overall, the incidence of mortality from several studies has been reported in the range of 0.19% to 1.20%.[1] The potential for life-threatening complications necessitates the importance of having a cardiac surgeon on standby along with the necessary equipment needed for emergent thoracotomy. Intraoperative TEE monitoring allows for prompt recognition of some of these life-threatening complications such as pericardial tamponade, hemorrhagic pleural effusion, and tricuspid valve injury. It also helps in visualizing inversion of the cardiac walls during lead traction, obliterating the right ventricular lumen as a cause of hypotension during the procedure.

Minor complications are adverse events that require medical intervention, including minor procedural interventions, but do not significantly affect the patient's function.[1] Minor complications include bleeding, pneumothorax necessitating chest tube placement, venous thrombosis, and migrated lead fragment. A complete list of complications with the reported incidence is provided in **Table 64.4**.[1] To minimize complications and perform lead extractions in a safe environment, it is important to utilize a joint approach between cardiac electrophysiologists and cardiothoracic surgeons performing the case together either in the operating room or hybrid laboratory with cardiopulmonary bypass standby.[12]

Rescue Device

Rescue devices, such as an SVC balloon that can occlude the SVC from the innominate veins to the right atrium, can be deployed quickly in SVC tears. The Bridge™ Occlusion Balloon

TABLE 64.4 Periprocedural Complications of Lead Extraction

Complications	Incidence (%)
Major Complications	**0.19-1.80**
Death	0.19-1.20
Cardiac avulsion	0.19-0.96
Vascular laceration	0.19-0.96
Respiratory arrest	0.20
Pericardial effusion requiring intervention	0.23-0.59
Hemothorax requiring intervention	0.07-0.20
Massive pulmonary embolism	0.08
Minor Complications	**0.60-6.20**
Hematoma requiring evacuation	0.90-1.60
Pneumothorax requiring chest tube	1.10
Bleeding requiring blood transfusion	0.08-1.00
Worsening tricuspid valve function	0.32-0.59
Pulmonary embolism	0.24-0.59
Venous thrombosis requiring medical intervention	0.10-0.21
Migrated lead fragment without sequelae	0.20
Pericardial effusion without intervention	0.07-0.16

Reprinted from Kusumoto FM, Schoenfeld MH, Wilkoff BL, et al. 2017 HRS expert consensus statement on cardiovascular implantable electronic device lead management and extraction. *Heart Rhythm.* 2017;14(12):e503-e551.

(Spectranetics) is a low-pressure, compliant balloon measuring 8 cm in length that is designed to conform to the SVC in the majority of individuals. In high-risk extractions, these balloons can be prophylactically placed in the inferior vena cava and then quickly advanced into the SVC with inflation time less than 15 seconds in case of SVC tear.[30] This acts as a temporary measure to tamponade the torn SVC and stabilizes the patient's hemodynamics until the cardiac surgeon can perform emergent thoracotomy and repair the tear surgically. High-risk patients include females, low body mass index ($<$25 kg/m^2), low left ventricular ejection fraction, dual-coil ICD leads, multiple indwelling leads ($\geq$4), combined age of leads over 10 years (sum of implant duration for each implanted lead), and requirement for use of multiple extraction tools.[16]

PATIENT FOLLOW-UP

Postprocedure management emphasizes monitoring for complications, wound care, adequate duration of antibiotic treatment, and determining the appropriate timing for CIED reimplantation, if indicated. A chest radiograph is routinely obtained postprocedure to rule out pneumothorax or hemothorax and check for retained lead fragments. Transthoracic echocardiography can be repeated as needed to assess for delayed pericardial effusion, "ghost" fragments, and tricuspid valve function/damage. The need for CIED replacement should be carefully reevaluated as the patient may have recovered sinus node function (for pacemaker) or left ventricular ejection fraction (for defibrillators) in the interim. The risks versus benefits of CIED reimplantation should be evaluated on a case-by-case basis in these scenarios. However, for patients who definitely need a CIED reimplant (such as complete heart block, pacemaker dependent patients), a temporary pacemaker—using a permanent transvenous lead connected to an external device—may be placed until a definite decision is made on the timing of the reimplantation.[31]

The optimal timing of device reimplantation is unknown because there are no prospective trials comparing the timing of new device reimplantation with the risk of recurrent infection. Current HRS expert consensus statement from 2017[1] suggests that new device implantation should be postponed until blood cultures are negative for at least 72 hours, although implantation should be delayed longer if the patient has other undrained sources of infection. Replacement device implantation should be performed in an alternative location such as the contralateral side or using an epicardial or subcutaneous approach. Same day device reimplantation may be considered for select cases that have only localized pocket infection.[1]

RESEARCH AND FUTURE DIRECTIONS

Newer and more effective tools to disrupt adhesions safely will likely be developed. These may employ a completely different technology than the current mechanical cutting or laser energy methods. The ultimate goal in lead management is avoiding infections, lead dysfunction, and complications with the devices. The newer leadless devices may provide an alternative in selected patients, as they completely eliminate the transvenous leads and their associated problems.

Currently, only single-chamber leadless pacemakers are available, but dual-chamber leadless pacemakers may soon be available. Retrieval of leadless pacemaker devices is a major area of concern; however, deflectable sheaths introduced via the femoral vein along with snares can be used with an approach similar to retrieving retained lead fragments. However, in cases with longer dwell time, open-heart surgery may be needed, given the risk of ventricular septal perforation.

For people requiring defibrillators, subcutaneous ICDs are a promising alternative to traditional defibrillators with transvenous leads. This is especially true for people undergoing lead extractions for recurrent infectious indications. In patients who require pacing along with defibrillation, there have been case reports of leadless pacemaker insertion (single chamber in the right ventricle) in combination with subcutaneous ICDs to provide the same benefit.[32] Although the two systems do not communicate with each other, device-device communication is likely to be developed in the near future.[33]

Leadless cardiac resynchronization therapy may also become a reality in the future. Currently, resynchronization is achieved using transvenous left ventricular epicardial leads placed in the coronary venous tributaries. Endovascular left ventricular pacing for cardiac resynchronization has shown promising results in a recent study,[34] and this combined with leadless technology in the future may help us circumvent the issues with current transvenous cardiac resynchronization therapy devices.

KEY POINTS

- ✔ Device or lead-related complications and the need for lead extractions have risen in parallel with the overall increase in implantation of CIEDs.
- ✔ Infection is the most common indication for lead extraction, constituting almost half of all the cases, followed by lead dysfunction.
- ✔ Lead extractions should be performed in high-volume centers with experienced operators.
- ✔ The overall mortality in recent years with TLE is lower than 2%.
- ✔ Explantation for relatively recent leads can be performed by simple traction of the lead after it has been unscrewed (with a standard nonlocking stylet in place). This is the oldest and simplest technique for lead removal.
- ✔ For lead extractions involving older leads with dense scar tissue or calcifications, specialized sheaths or tools are often required. The three main specialized sheaths/tools currently used in lead extraction are telescoping sheaths, laser sheaths, and rotational mechanical cutting sheaths.
- ✔ No one tool is adept at negotiating all types of fibrous adhesions encountered during lead extractions, and switching between extraction tools and approaches is frequently necessary.

- ✔ Femoral snares may be used to retrieve broken lead fragments as well as in maintaining traction in the distal end of the leads with severe adhesions.
- ✔ Leadless cardiac devices including cardiac resynchronization therapy and defibrillators represent the future of CIEDs, which may avoid many of the current issues with transvenous leads.

REFERENCES

1. Kusumoto FM, Schoenfeld MH, Wilkoff BL, et al. 2017 HRS expert consensus statement on cardiovascular implantable electronic device lead management and extraction. *Heart Rhythm*. 2017;14(12):e503-e551.
2. Bilgutay AM, Jensen NK, Schmidt WR, Garamella JJ, Lynch MF. Incarceration of transvenous pacemaker electrode. Removal by traction. *Am Heart J*. 1969;77(3):377-379.
3. Bongiorni MG, Burri H, Deharo JC, et al. 2018 EHRA expert consensus statement on lead extraction: recommendations on definitions, endpoints, research trial design, and data collection requirements for clinical scientific studies and registries: endorsed by APHRS/HRS/LAHRS. *Europace*. 2018;20(7):1217.
4. Becker AE, Becker MJ, Claudon DG, Edwards JE. Surface thrombosis and fibrous encapsulation of intravenous pacemaker catheter electrode. *Circulation*. 1972;46(2):409-412.
5. Robboy SJ, Harthorne JW, Leinbach RC, Sanders CA, Austen WG. Autopsy findings with permanent pervenous pacemakers. *Circulation*. 1969;39(4):495-501.
6. Deshmukh A, Patel N, Noseworthy PA, et al. Trends in use and adverse outcomes associated with transvenous lead removal in the United States. *Circulation*. 2015;132(25):2363-2371.
7. Bongiorni MG, Kennergren C, Butter C, et al. The European Lead Extraction ConTRolled (ELECTRa) study: a European Heart Rhythm Association (EHRA) registry of transvenous lead extraction outcomes. *Eur Heart J*. 2017;38(40):2995-3005.
8. Wazni O, Epstein LM, Carrillo RG, et al. Lead extraction in the contemporary setting: the LExICon study: an observational retrospective study of consecutive laser lead extractions. *J Am Coll Cardiol*. 2010;55(6):579-586.
9. Starck CT, Gonzalez E, Al-Razzo O, et al. Results of the Patient-Related Outcomes of Mechanical lead Extraction Techniques (PROMET) study: a multicentre retrospective study on advanced mechanical lead extraction techniques. *Europace*. 2020;22(7):1103-1010.
10. Franceschi F, Dubuc M, Deharo JC, et al. Extraction of transvenous leads in the operating room versus electrophysiology laboratory: a comparative study. *Heart Rhythm*. 2011;8(7):1001-1005.
11. Sidhu BS, Gould J, Bunce C, et al. The effect of centre volume and procedure location on major complications and mortality from transvenous lead extraction: an ESC EHRA EORP European Lead Extraction ConTRolled ELECTRa registry subanalysis. *Europace*. 2020;22(11):1718-1728.
12. Bernardes de Souza B, Benharash P, Esmailian F, Bradfield J, Boyle NG. Value of a joint cardiac surgery-cardiac electrophysiology approach to lead extraction. *J Card Surg*. 2015;30(11):874-876.
13. Fu HX, Huang XM, Zhong LI, et al. Outcomes and complications of lead removal: can we establish a risk stratification schema for a collaborative and effective approach? *Pacing Clin Electrophysiol*. 2015;38(12):1439-1447.
14. Jachec W, Polewczyk A, Polewczyk M, Tomasik A, Kutarski A. Transvenous lead extraction SAFeTY score for risk stratification and proper patient selection for removal procedures using mechanical tools. *J Clin Med*. 2020;9(2):361.
15. Aguilera AL, Volokhina YV, Fisher KL. Radiography of cardiac conduction devices: a comprehensive review. *Radiographics*. 2011;31(6):1669-1682.
16. Wilkoff BL, Kennergren C, Love CJ, Kutalek SP, Epstein LM, Carrillo R. Bridge to surgery: best practice protocol derived from early clinical experience with the Bridge Occlusion Balloon. Federated Agreement from the Eleventh Annual Lead Management Symposium. *Heart Rhythm*. 2017;14(10):1574-1578.
17. Perez AA, Woo FW, Tsang DC, Carrillo RG. Transvenous lead extractions: current approaches and future trends. *Arrhythm Electrophysiol Rev*. 2018;7(3):210-217.
18. Love CJ. Lead management and lead extraction. *Card Electrophysiol Clin*. 2018;10(1):127-136.
19. Brodell GK, Castle LW, Maloney JD, Wilkoff BL. Chronic transvenous pacemaker lead removal using a unique, sequential transvenous system. *Am J Cardiol*. 1990;66(12):964-966.
20. Levy T, Walker S, Paul V. Initial experience in the extraction of chronically implanted pacemaker leads using the Excimer laser sheath. *Heart*. 1999;82(1):101-104.
21. Wilkoff BL, Byrd CL, Love CJ, et al. Pacemaker lead extraction with the laser sheath: results of the pacing lead extraction with the excimer sheath (PLEXES) trial. *J Am Coll Cardiol*. 1999;33(6):1671-1676.
22. Hussein AA, Wilkoff BL, Martin DO, et al. Initial experience with the Evolution mechanical dilator sheath for lead extraction: safety and efficacy. *Heart Rhythm*. 2010;7(7):870-873.
23. Mazzone P, Migliore F, Bertaglia E, et al. Safety and efficacy of the new bidirectional rotational Evolution(R) mechanical lead extraction sheath: results from a multicentre Italian registry. *Europace*. 2018;20(5):829-834.
24. Robinson T, Oliver J, Sheridan P, Sahu J, Bowes R. Fragmentation and embolization of pacemaker leads as a complication of lead extraction. *Europace*. 2010;12(5):754-755.
25. Kim D, Baek YS, Lee M, et al. Remnant pacemaker lead tips after lead extractions in pacemaker infections. *Korean Circ J*. 2016;46(4):569-573.
26. Byrd CL, Schwartz SJ, Hedin N. Intravascular techniques for extraction of permanent pacemaker leads. *J Thorac Cardiovasc Surg*. 1991;101(6):989-997.
27. Mulpuru SK, Hayes DL, Osborn MJ, Asirvatham SJ. Femoral approach to lead extraction. *J Cardiovasc Electrophysiol*. 2015;26(3):357-361.
28. Kutarski AW, Jachec W, Tulecki L, et al. Safety and effectiveness of coronary sinus leads extraction—single high-volume centre experience. *Adv Interv Cardiol*. 2019;15(3):345-356.
29. Narducci ML, Di Monaco A, Pelargonio G, et al. Presence of 'ghosts' and mortality after transvenous lead extraction. *Europace*. 2017;19(3):432-440.
30. Tsang DC, Azarrafiy R, Pecha S, Reichenspurner H, Carrillo RG, Hakmi S. Long-term outcomes of prophylactic placement of an endovascular balloon in the vena cava for high-risk transvenous lead extractions. *Heart Rhythm*. 2017;14(12):1833-1838.
31. Braun MU, Rauwolf T, Bock M, et al. Percutaneous lead implantation connected to an external device in stimulation-dependent patients with systemic infection—a prospective and controlled study. *Pacing Clin Electrophysiol*. 2006;29(8):875-879.
32. Ito R, Kondo Y, Winter J, et al. Combination of a leadless pacemaker and subcutaneous implantable cardioverter defibrillator therapy for a Japanese patient with prosthetic valve endocarditis. *J Arrhythm*. 2019;35(2):311-313.
33. Tjong FVY, Brouwer TF, Koop B, et al. Acute and 3-month performance of a communicating leadless antitachycardia pacemaker and subcutaneous implantable defibrillator. *JACC Clin Electrophysiol*. 2017;3(13):1487-1498.
34. Morgan JM, Biffi M, Geller L, et al. ALternate Site Cardiac ResYNChronization (ALSYNC): a prospective and multicentre study of left ventricular endocardial pacing for cardiac resynchronization therapy. *Eur Heart J*. 2016;37(27):2118-2127.

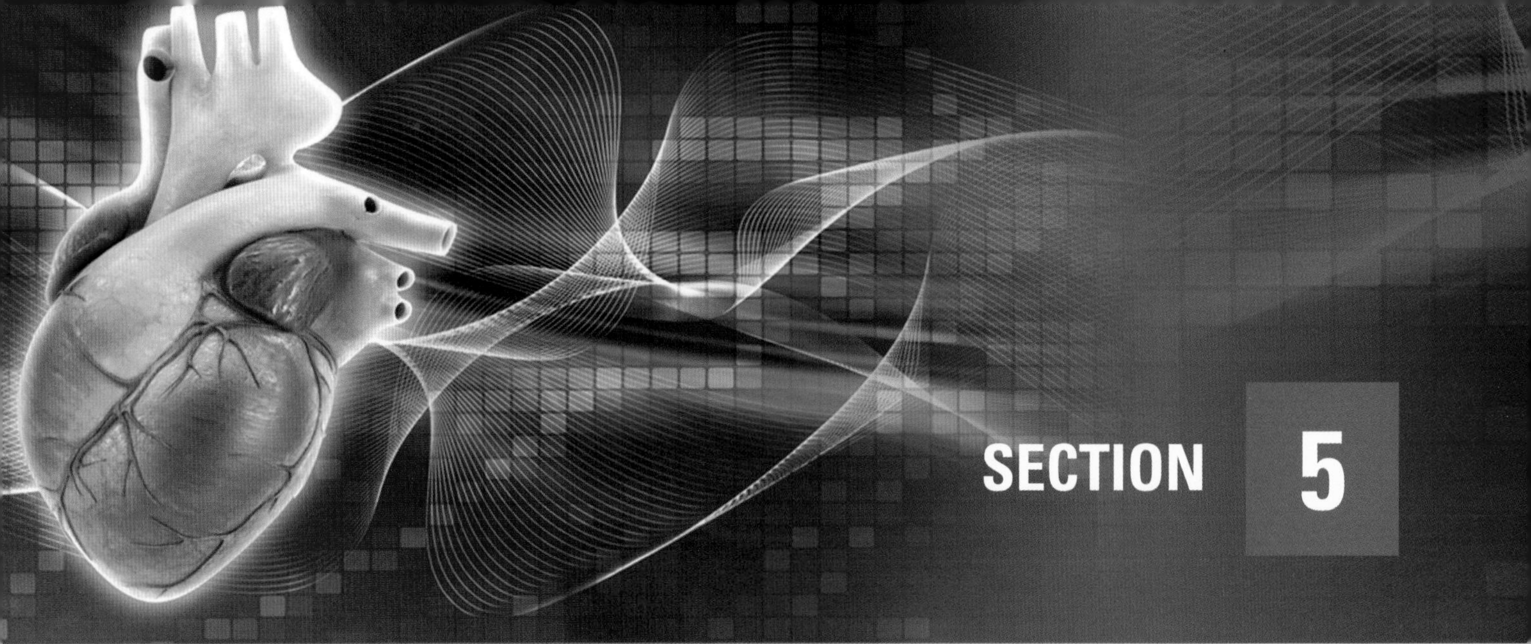

HEART FAILURE

SECTION EDITOR: Biykem Bozkurt

CHAPTER 65

HEART FAILURE: EPIDEMIOLOGY, CHARACTERISTICS, AND PROGNOSIS

Justin Ezekowitz

INTRODUCTION

Heart failure (HF) is a major public health problem affecting up to 2% of the population and ~10% of elderly individuals in the Western world[1,2] and over 37.7 million globally.[3]

The definitions and taxonomies have evolved significantly from the first description of the disease by the German pathologist, Rudolf Virchow in 1858, and it is expected to evolve further as we make progress in understanding the pathophysiology of the disease.[4] This change of definitions may have contributed partly to the change of the epidemiological statistics over time.

The statistics reported in different studies relied heavily on the diagnostic criteria, the method of ascertaining diagnosis, and the population under study (elderly vs all, hospitalized patients vs all, trial-based vs population-based, etc). Several criteria—including the Framingham,[5] Boston (aka Carlson),[6] Gothenburg,[7] Duke,[8] and European Society of Cardiology (ESC) criteria[9]—have been developed over several decades to help us with the task of diagnosing HF, with variable performances in the validation studies (**Table 65.1**).

CLASSIFICATIONS OF HEART FAILURE

Midrange Ejection Fraction, Preserved Ejection Fraction, and Reduced Ejection Fraction

One of the classifications widely used over the last few decades in randomized clinical trials (RCTs) and in practice guidelines is classifying symptomatic patients with HF based on their left ventricular ejection fraction (LVEF) status into those with preserved (HFpEF), midrange (HFmrEF), or reduced (HFrEF) ejection fraction, which are defined as LVEF ≥50%, 40% to 49%, and less than 40%, respectively (**Table 65.2**). It is important to note that although HFrEF generally refers to systolic HF and contractile dysfunction, the patients with HFrEF may have both systolic and diastolic dysfunctions. On the other hand, HFpEF does not necessarily imply diastolic HF.[10] Diastolic function, which is about ventricular relaxation and filling during diastole, might be impaired in HFpEF, and they may have overlapping clinical features, but the two terms are not equivalent to each other. On the other hand, abnormalities of systolic function such as impaired global longitudinal strain have been reported in patients with HFpEF.[11] Although the above-mentioned groups have similarities in terms of clinical symptoms and presentation, they differ in terms of demographics, underlying factors, structural heart abnormalities, and response to therapies.[12]

Stages of Heart Failure

One of the widely used functional classifications of HF is the New York Heart Association (NYHA) functional classification, which classifies patients predominantly based on HF symptoms and functional limitations. Hence, it helps in assessing the severity of patient symptoms, indicating the need for escalation of HF treatments, and evaluating the response to treatment (**Table 65.3**). Of note, patients can move back and forth between the different NYHA classes.

Subsequently, the American College of Cardiology (ACC)/American Heart Association (AHA) guideline suggested a classification based on disease progression, which classifies patients with HF into four stages from A to D (Table 65.3).[13]

Risk Factors

Many risk factors have been evaluated and identified through different cohort studies. To name a few, hypertension (present in 44%-91% of patients at incident HF diagnosis), diabetes mellitus (DM; 18%-23%), coronary artery disease (CAD; 29%-63%), obesity (25%), smoking (51%), arrhythmias, congenital heart diseases and cardiomyopathies.[12,14] The above-mentioned traditional risk factors have been responsible for over half of incident HF cases in the Olmsted County, MN cohort.[15] Hypertension, older age, female sex, and DM are the greatest risk factors for HFpEF. Although the HFpEF population is shown to be more obese than HFrEF population, body mass index was a risk factor for both, and there was no difference in its prognostic effect on the incidence of HFpEF and HFrEF.[16] Dyslipidemia, inflammation, hyperglycemia, exposure to cardiotoxic agents (such as alcohol, amphetamines, chemotherapy, and radiation therapy), micronutrient deficiency, family history of HF or other cardiovascular diseases, and poorer socioeconomic status are other risk factors for HF.[14]

One-third of the U.S.population has at least one risk factor for HF.[17] The number of risk factors per person increased by 30% from 1979 to 2002 in patients with incident HF.[18] Prevention and controlling these risk factors can lead to a reduction in the incidence of HF, although the reduction of these might be a herculean endeavor itself. According to the National

TABLE 65.1 Different Diagnostic Criteria for the Diagnosis of Patients With Heart Failure

Diagnostic Model	Components	Diagnosis of HF
Framingham criteria	**Major criteria:** acute pulmonary edema, jugular vein distension, hepatojugular reflux, paroxysmal nocturnal dyspnea or orthopnea, pulmonary rales, S3 heart sound, weight loss >4.5 kg in 5 days in response to treatment, cardiomegaly on chest x-ray **Minor criteria**: ankle edema, dyspnea on exertion, hepatomegaly, nocturnal cough, pleural effusion, tachycardia, weight loss >4.5 kg in 5 days with diuretics	≥2 major or 1 major and ≥2 minor criteria
Boston criteria	**History** (dyspnea at rest, orthopnea, paroxysmal nocturnal dyspnea, dyspnea while walking, dyspnea on climbing, leg fatigue while walking), **physical examination** (tachycardia, jugular vein distension, lung crackles, wheezing, S3), and **chest radiography** (alveolar pulmonary edema, interstitial pulmonary edema, bilateral pleural effusion, cardiothoracic ratio ≥0.5, upper zone flow redistribution) criteria	Definite HF: 8-12 points; Possible HF: 5-7 points; Unlikely HF: ≤4 points
Gothenburg criteria	**Cardiac score:** coronary heart disease in past, within past year, angina in past, within past year, leg edema, pulmonary rales, atrial fibrillation, **Pulmonary disease score:** history of bronchitis in past, chronic bronchitis in past year, asthma, asthma in past year, coughing, phlegm, or wheezing, rhonchi at physical examination, **Therapy score:** history of digoxin or diuretic use	Graded 0 if all scores zero, Grade 1 (latent) if cardiac score >0 but other two zero, Grade 2 (manifest) if cardiac score >0 and either pulmonary or therapy score >0, Grade 3 if all scores >0, and Grade 4 if death owing to heart failure
Duke criteria	**Cardiomegaly** by radiography, S3 gallop, other congestive heart symptoms including dyspnea, orthopnea, paroxysmal nocturnal dyspnea, edema in history or by examination, history of inotrope therapy, rales, tachycardia, jugular vein distension, hepatojugular reflux	
ESC criteria	Clinical history (orthopnea, paroxysmal nocturnal dyspnea, history of CAD, history of arterial hypertension, exposure to cardiotoxic drugs/radiation, use of diuretics), physical examination (rales, bilateral ankle edema, heart murmurs, jugular vein distension, laterally displaced and broadened apical beat), any abnormality on ECG, elevated natriuretic peptides (BNP ≥ 35 pg/mL and NT-proBNP ≥ 125 pg/mL), echocardiography	HF unlikely if all criteria absent or if at least one clinical/physical examination/ECG criterion was present but with no elevated serum natriuretic peptide level or with elevated serum natriuretic peptide level but no findings in favor of HF on echocardiography

BNP, brain-type natriuretic peptide; CAD, coronary artery disease; ECG, electrocardiogram; ESC, European Society of Cardiology; HF, heart failure; NT-proBNP, N-terminal pro-brain-type natriuretic peptide.

TABLE 65.2 The Classification of HF Based on Left Ventricular Ejection Fraction Status

	LVEF	Other Criteria	Proportion	Clinical Features
HFrEF	<40%	-	40%-50%	Systolic HF, but diastolic dysfunction may also present
HFmrEF	40%-49%	Elevated natriuretic peptide levels, and structural cardiac disease or diastolic dysfunction	10%-20%	Either borderline HFpEF in transition to HFrEF or patients with recovered HFrEF; Hence, sharing features of both HFrEF and HFpEF
HFpEF	≥50%	Elevated natriuretic peptide levels, and structural cardiac disease or diastolic dysfunction	40%-50%	Predominantly older, more often female with more comorbidities such as hypertension, diabetes, atrial fibrillation, or obesity, but less ischemic heart diseases compared to patients with HFrEF

HF, heart failure; HFmrEF, heart failure with midrange ejection fraction; HFpEF, heart failure with preserved ejection fraction; HFrEF, heart failure with reduced ejection fraction; LVEF, left ventricular ejection fraction.

TABLE 65.3 New York Heart Association and American College of Cardiology/American Heart Association Functional Classifications of Patients With Heart Failure

	Class	Definition
NYHA	Class I	Cardiac disease without limitations of physical activity. Ordinary physical activity does not cause undue fatigue, palpitation, shortness of breath, or chest pain.
	Class II	Cardiac disease resulting in a slight limitation of physical activity. Comfortable at rest, but ordinary physical activity results in fatigue, palpitation, shortness of breath, or chest pain.
	Class III	Cardiac disease resulting in marked limitation of physical activity. Comfortable at rest, but less than ordinary activity causes fatigue, palpitation, shortness of breath, or chest pain.
	Class IV	Cardiac disease with inability to conduct physical activity without discomfort. Symptoms may be present even at rest.
ACC/AHA	Stage A	Patients at risk of heart failure (ie, those with hypertension, diabetes, or atherosclerotic coronary disease) who have not yet developed structural heart changes
	Stage B	Patients have structural heart disease (ie, reduced ejection fraction, left ventricular hypertrophy, chamber enlargement) but have not yet developed signs or symptoms of heart failure.
	Stage C	Patients with clinical heart failure
	Stage D	Patients with advanced heart failure requiring advanced interventions such as cardiac resynchronization therapy, left ventricular assist device, or heart transplantation

ACC, American College of Cardiology; AHA, American Heart Association; NYHA, New York Heart Association.

Health and Nutrition Examination Survey (NHANES) study, the prevalence of hypertension, myocardial infarction, and smoking has declined, but the prevalence of obesity and DM has increased over the past few decades.[19,20]

HF could result from a wide range of etiologies, from hereditary and structural conditions to infective and inflammatory causes. Causes may originate from the cardiovascular system or other organ systems. The Global Burden of Disease (GBD) study has identified up to 17 etiologies for HF.[21] The underlying etiologies and risk factors may vary from one age, sex, or racial group to another. Ischemic heart disease and chronic obstructive pulmonary disease (COPD) are the leading etiologies for HF in high-income countries, whereas major underlying etiologies in the low-income countries have been hypertensive heart disease, rheumatic heart disease, cardiomyopathy, and myocarditis.[22]

Ischemic Heart Disease

HF has a prevalence of ~20% in patients with ischemic heart disease, whereas the prevalence is significantly lower (1%-2%) in those without ischemic heart disease.[23] This etiology is responsible for two-thirds of HFrEF cases and a third of HFpEF cases.[24,25] According to the GBD study, the prevalence of ischemic HF increased from 240 per 100,000 person-years in 1990 to 270 per 100,000 person-years in 2010 among men, but was relatively stable among women (190 per 100,000 person-years).[26]

Hypertensive Heart Disease

Hypertension is a risk factor but is also one of the most frequent comorbidities in HF.[27,28] Besides community-based cohort studies, having subsequent HF among the end points of RCTs on hypertension has provided the opportunity to know more about the effects of these conditions on the development or worsening of HF. A majority of patients with HF (73.6% in HFrEF and 89.3% in HFpEF according to Olmsted County study)[25] have hypertension. Although patients with blood pressure greater than 160/90 mm Hg had double the risk of HF compared to those with blood pressure less than 140/90 mm Hg,[29] medical treatment is shown to reduce the risk in both patients with moderate and severe hypertension by 87%.[30] However, the management has been suboptimal in many cases, for example, in the Prospective Urban Rural Epidemiology (PURE) study, only 46.7% and 31.7% of patients with hypertension were receiving treatment and only 19% and 12.7% were at the target blood pressure range, respectively, in high- and low-income countries.[31]

Valvular Heart Disease

Moderate to severe valve disease is estimated to be present in 2.5% of the U.S. population.[32] In a prospective study of adult patients with moderate to severe native or acquired valvular heart disease, congestive HF was present in 21.3% of patients at the time of valvular intervention.[33] Among community patients with suspected HF in the United Kingdom (UK), 37.5%, 11.3%, and 2.7% were shown to have mild, moderate, and severe valvular disease, respectively.[34] The highest population-attributable risk related to the valvular disease is rheumatic heart disease, which is reduced substantially in the developed world, owing to improved living conditions and increased antibiotic therapy. The incidence rate of rheumatic fever varies from 1 case per 100,000 person-years in the developed countries to greater than 100 cases per 100,000 person-years in sub-Saharan Africa.[35]

Cardiomyopathies

Cardiomyopathy generally refers to the structural and functional abnormalities of the heart muscle in the absence of CAD, hypertension, valvular heart disease, and congenital heart disease that may progress to HF, and is categorized based on morphology and function into five phenotypes of hypertrophic, dilated, restrictive, arrhythmogenic right ventricular, and unclassified cardiomyopathies.[4,36] Cardiomyopathies are major causes of HF in the Western world.[13] Although the number of deaths secondary to cardiomyopathy has increased by 40.8% from 1990 to 2010, the age-standardized death rates were decreased by 9.8% from 6.7 to 6.1 per 100,000 in the same time period.[37]

OTHER IMPORTANT COMORBIDITIES

Coexisting comorbidities such as CAD, COPD, DM, renal failure, and pneumonia or a combination of those are prevalent in patients with HF (**Figure 65.1**)[85]. They may contribute to the development of disease as mentioned above, make the diagnosis more complex, worsen the severity of HF symptoms, interact with the treatment effects, and are sometimes, but not always, harbingers of poorer outcomes.

Based on the data from the NHANES cohort, the proportion of patients with HF with greater than five comorbid conditions increased from 42.1% in 1988 to 1994 to 58.0% in 2003 to 2008,[38] with increase in hypercholesterolemia (41%-54%), DM (25%-38%), obesity (33%-47%), kidney disease (35%-46%), thyroid disease (10%-23%), and osteoporosis (5%-16%) being the main drivers of this increase.[14] Patients with HFpEF are shown to have more comorbidities compared to HFrEF with an average of one more comorbidities.[39]

Diabetes Mellitus

In the Framingham Heart Study (FHS), 14% of men and 26% of women with HF had DM as a comorbidity. Male

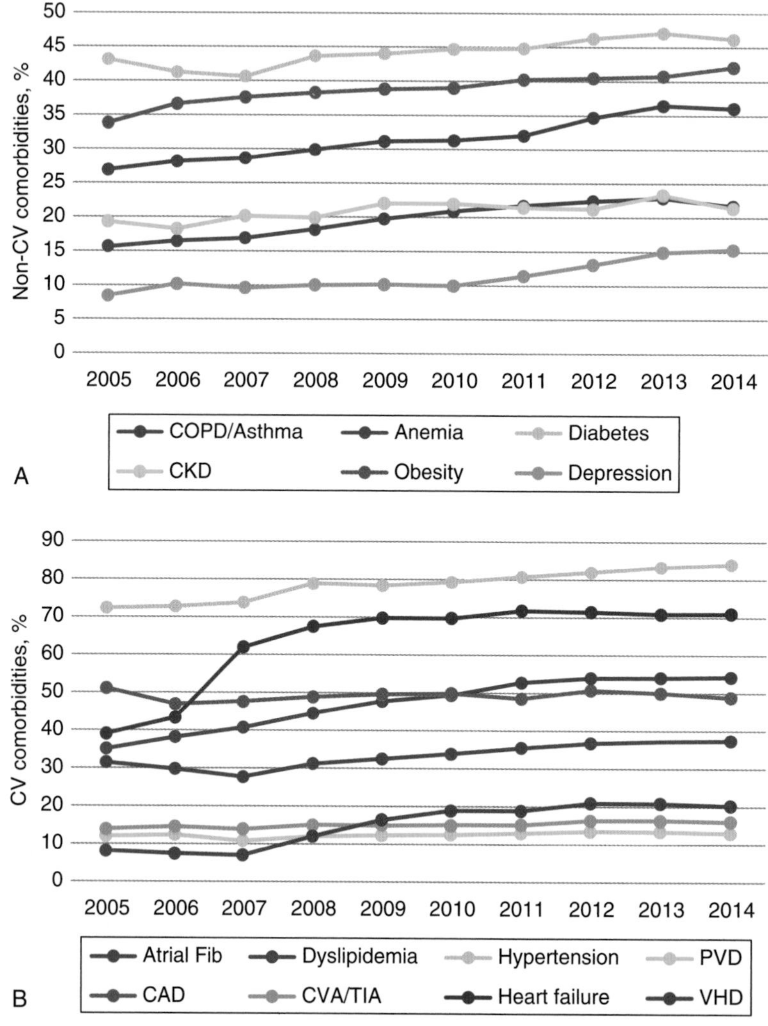

FIGURE 65.1 Temporal trends in the prevalence of **(A)** noncardiovascular and **(B)** cardiovascular comorbidities in patients with heart failure. CAD, coronary artery disease; CKD, chronic kidney disease; COPD, chronic obstructive pulmonary disease; CV, cardiovascular; CVA, cerebrovascular accident; PVD, peripheral vascular disease; TIA, transient ischemic attack; VHD, valvular heart disease. (Data from Sharma A, Zhao X, Hammill BG, et al. Trends in Noncardiovascular Comorbidities Among Patients Hospitalized for Heart Failure. *Circ Heart Fail.* 2018;11(6):e004646.)

and female patients with DM had, respectively, twofold and fivefold increased risk of developing HF[27,40] compared to their counterparts without DM. In a study pooling the data from FHS, the Cardiovascular Health Study (CHS), and the Prevention of Renal and Vascular End-Stage Disease (PREVEND) cohort, DM was not an independent predictor of developing HFpEF but an independent risk factor for HFrEF, when adjusted for other covariates.[16] Although the age-, sex-, and ethnicity-adjusted incidence rates of hypertension and CAD have stabilized over the recent decades, the incidence rates are still increasing and projected to increase for DM and obesity in the coming decades. Whether DM can directly cause clinical HF, independent of other causes, is to be determined.

Chronic Kidney Disease

Chronic kidney disease (CKD) is a common comorbidity (40%-60%) among patients with HF and an independent predictor of adverse outcomes in patients with HF.[41] Various mechanisms such as inflammatory, immunologic, neurohormonal, and stress-related pathways and metabolic, hemodynamic, and volume changes are involved in the deleterious effects of CKD on heart function or the effect of HF on renal function, all known as cardiorenal syndrome. Studies have shown an increase in the rate of CKD comorbidity among patients with HF from 34% in the 1980s to 46% in the early 2000s.[38]

Chronic Obstructive Pulmonary Disease

COPD occurs as a comorbidity in a third of patients with HF. The proportion of patients with HF and concurrent COPD remained stable (26%-30%) over a time period between 1988 and 2008.[38] The overlapping symptoms can be a cause of misdiagnosis for patients presenting with acute decompensated HF. COPD is shown to be more prevalent and more associated with adverse outcomes, such as mortality, in HFpEF than in HFrEF.[39,42]

Arrhythmias

Atrial fibrillation is the most common cardiac rhythm abnormality in patients with HF. Roughly, one-third of patients with HF enrolled in community-based studies or trials have atrial fibrillation as a comorbidity,[43] and inadequate control of the ventricular response is a major cause of decompensation in HF.

Anemia

Anemia is relatively prevalent (>30%) among patients with HF and anemic patients with HF are demonstrated to have poorer clinical outcomes.[44] The probability of anemia is correlated with the severity of HF.[45] Besides anemia, iron deficiency is another comorbidity in HF that can coexist with anemia (43%-68% of patients with anemia and 15%-35% of those without anemia).[46]

Frailty

Given the high prevalence of HF among elderly individuals, many patients with HF suffer from frailty (40%-55%), and frailty is considered a prognostic factor in HF, conferring a twofold increase in the risk of death.[47]

Depression

The frequency of depression among patients with HF is reported to be around 30% to 50%, with poorer quality of life reported in those with depression.[46]

Cognitive Disorder

Several studies have reported the presence of cognitive disorders and dementia in patients with chronic HF, which is mainly attributed to vascular disease and reduced cardiac output and subsequent cerebral hypoperfusion.[43]

EPIDEMIOLOGY

Incidence

Each year, up to 1 million new cases are being diagnosed with HF in the United States.[48] The incidence of HF increases by age from 0.3 patients per 1000 person-year in those with age less than 55 years to 18 cases per 1000 person-year among those with age over 85 years.[12] In the FHS, the incidence rate is close to 10 per 1000 population after 65 years of age,[29] but the rate is estimated to be much higher and approaching 21 per 1000 population above the age of 65 years in a pooled cohort of three studies sponsored by the National Heart, Lung and Blood Institute (NHLBI).[49]

In the CHS, the annual rates per 1000 population of new HF events doubled per each decade increase in age after 45 years in White men (15.2 for 65-74 years of age, 31.7 for 75-84 years of age, and 65.2 for ≥85 years). For White women, the rates were 8.2, 19.8, and 45.6, respectively, for the same age groups. The respective rates were 16.9, 25.5, and 50.6 for African American men, and 14.2, 25.5, and 44.0, for African American women.[50] A similar increase in incidence rates by age is reported by other studies.[14,48]

Secular Trends

According to the literature, the incidence of HF increased until the mid-1990s[51] and has declined afterward.[25,52-59] Although the incidence declined for both HFpEF and HFrEF, the slope was steeper for HFrEF.[25] This stabilization of the incidence of HF in the developed countries is most likely owing to improvement in the primary prevention of cardiovascular diseases and proper treatment of ischemic heart disease.[4]

In the FHS, the incidence of HF among women decreased from 420 per 100,000 person-year in 1950 to 327 per 100,000 person-year in 1999, without a similar reduction among men (564 cases per 100,000 person-year).[57] In the Olmsted County, MN cohort study, age- and sex-adjusted incidence rates decreased significantly from 315.8 per 100,000 in 2000 to 219.3 per 100,000 in 2010, with a more pronounced reduction in the HFrEF subgroup than in those with HFpEF.[25] Hence, the proportion of patients with HFpEF among new cases increased over time (from 38% in 1986 to 57% in 2010), reflecting an incremental interest and awareness about HF and HFpEF and proper prevention and treatment of ischemic heart disease as the major risk for HFrEF.

Prevalence

Based on data from 2013 to 2016, over 6.2 million adult Americans are estimated to have HF.[48] By 2030, the prevalence of HF (not adjusted for age) in the United States is projected to increase by 46% when compared to that of 2012 to over 8 million people (2.97% of U.S. population).[60] Similar prevalence rates of 2% to 3% were reported from Europe.[61]

The prevalence of HF ranges from 1% to 14% in Western countries.[12,60] Besides a growing and aging population, improved survival after HF diagnosis has led to an increase in the prevalence of this condition.[12] The prevalence of HF approximately doubles per decade of life,[4] and the lifetime risk of HF is estimated to be around 20% to 33%.[12]

The prevalence of HFpEF has increased over two decades, and roughly half of the patients with HF are diagnosed with HFpEF.[10,39] As mentioned above, in the Olmsted County cohort, the proportion of patients with HFpEF has increased from 38% in 1986 to 48% in 2000 and eventually to 57% in 2010, with a lower decline in incidence rates compared to patients with HFrEF in the same study period.[25]

Gender and Racial Differences

The incidence and prevalence of HF vary by demographic variables including gender and race.

Gender: Gender differences exist in terms of the HF incidence, disease phenotypes, and outcome, with males having more HFrEF and ischemic etiology, whereas HFpEF and nonischemic causes are more prominent among women.[46]

Female patients with HF are generally older than men with HF, with higher LVEF, less structural cardiac diseases, more HF symptoms, and worse NYHA class at presentation. They tend to have more comorbidities including hypertension, DM, renal disease, atrial fibrillation, arthritis, iron deficiency, anemia, frailty, depression, and thyroid abnormalities, but better outcomes in terms of mortality or hospital admissions.[46] The above-mentioned decline in the incidence rate of HF from 2000 to 2010 was shown to be higher in women compared to men (43% vs 29%). In spite of the higher incidence of HF in males across all ages, the lifetime risk of HF is equal between the two sexes, owing to a longer life span among women. Given the differences in the clinical features of HF in males and females, it is important to have a balanced representation of both sexes in the studies and trials of therapeutic interventions.

Ethnicity: Many studies have reported a higher incidence of HF in Blacks as compared to Caucasians.[12] In the Multi-Ethnic Study of Atherosclerosis (MESA), the incidence rate was highest for Blacks, followed by Hispanics, Whites, and Chinese individuals (4.6, 3.5, 2.4, and 1.0 per 1000 person-years, respectively).[62] The lower lifetime risk reported for Black men (20%-29%) and women (24%-46%) in three NHLBI-sponsored cohort studies compared to White men (30%-42%) and women (32%-39%) can be attributed to competing risk of premature death.[49] Similarly, in the NHANES cohort (2007-2010), non-Hispanic Blacks had the highest prevalence of HF, followed by non-Hispanic Whites and Mexican Americans.[14] Black women and men present at an earlier age with incident HF (approximately 10 years earlier),[62] and they have the highest proportion of nonischemic HF.[14] The heterogeneity in risk of developing HF across different ethnicities is attributed to differential comorbidity burden and socioeconomic factors in different racial groups. As an example of differential comorbidity burden, African Americans have a different response to antihypertensive treatments such as angiotensin-converting enzyme inhibitors or angiotensin receptor blockers compared to Caucasians, mainly because of low renin levels.[43] After adjustment for known cardiovascular risk factors, low socioeconomic status is shown to be associated with higher rates of HF.[4]

In a population-based study from Canada, status Aboriginal patients with HF were shown to have increased mortality at 1 and 5 years compared with their White counterparts, after adjustment for demographic and clinical confounders.[63] Other studies from Australia showed higher age- and sex-specific HF incidence rates among Aboriginals as compared to White patients,[64] and reported an increase in the risk-adjusted mortality of Aboriginal patients with HF from 2000 to 2008, whereas the rate was decreased in the same period in their non-Aboriginal counterparts.[65]

Geographical Variability and Global Burden

Geographical and regional variabilities in the prevalence and outcome of the disease have been reported. The majority of the evidence at our disposal regarding the epidemiology and management of HF is from the developed and high-income countries, whereas there is a paucity of data from low- and middle-income countries (LMICs).[66] Fifteen million people are estimated to have HF in 51 European countries represented by the ESC, representing 2% to 3% of the population.[61] In 2014, China had 4.5 million patients with HF.[67] The prevalence was estimated to range between 1.3 and 4.6 million in India in 2010[68] and around 1 million in Japan in 2003.[69]

Also, there is significant geographical variability in terms of patient characteristics, with the mean age in the patients with HF in the Sub-Saharan region being roughly 20 years lower than the mean in the Western world, but with worse clinical outcomes.[70] Similar lower ages at disease onset (~10 years younger than developed countries) were reported from the countries in the Middle East.[71] A cohort study using the data from the Tanzania HF study and Swedish HF registry reported a younger HF population, with more female patients, different comorbidity profiles, and a more severe disease stage in the Tanzanian cohort.[72] Regarding the geographical variability of HF subtypes, the data from a multinational randomized controlled trial showed the prevalence of HFpEF to be highest in Northern America, intermediate in Western Europe, and lowest in Eastern Europe and Russia.[73]

PROGNOSIS

Overall, the prognosis is poor among patients with HF, with high rates of death and rehospitalization reported following an HF diagnosis.

Mortality

Many studies have shown an improvement in survival over time in patients with HF.[4,12] In the United States, the absolute 5-year survival has improved by 9% from 1979 to 2000.[58] This decline in mortality is attributed to the improved delivery of care and implementation of HF therapies such as medical therapy, coronary revascularization, and device therapies, and it mirrors the reduced mortality from cardiovascular disease observed in the GBD study.[74] However, the survival curve plateaued afterward,[25] and the outcome is still poor with high mortality and rehospitalization rates across the HF spectrum. The 1-year and 5-year survival after acute HF diagnosis is estimated to be 72% to 78%,[12,48] and 35% to 60%,[12,14,39,48] respectively; similar to that in cancer patients.[75] The survival decreases with an increase in the comorbidity burden.

In-hospital and 1-year mortality is shown to be higher in LMICs. The International Congestive Heart Failure (INTER-CHF) study reported a geographical variability in the 1-year mortality from HF, ranging from 7% in China, and 9% in South America or the Middle East to 23% in India and 34% in Africa.[70] Other studies from LMICs have reported similarly high mortality rates. For example, in-hospital and 1-year mortality rates were 19% and 35%, respectively, in a study from the Democratic Republic of Congo.[76] In India, approximately half (44.8%) of patients with HF die within 3 years.[77] After adjustment for demographics such as age and sex, the case fatality rate was 3.72 times higher in low-income countries, and 2.61 times higher in middle-income countries when compared to high-income countries.[4] That being said, according to some studies, the observed differences in the crude mortality rates disappear after adjustment for demographic and clinical variables.[72]

In the United States, the any-mention HF mortality rates per 100,000 population for the year of 2015 varied across subgroups from 112.6 for Black men to 107.4 for White men, 93.9 for Black women, and 79.6 per 100,000 population for White women.[48] Similarly, in the NHLBI-sponsored Atherosclerosis Risk in Communities (ARIC) study, 5-year case fatality rates were higher for Blacks compared to Whites.[78] Some studies have shown higher mortality in men compared to women (59% vs 45% at 5 years).[57]

Cardiovascular death is the major cause of demise in patients with HF in almost every region except for Africa.[70] In the Olmsted County cohort study, 43% of deaths at 5-year follow-up were noncardiovascular, the proportion increased over time (from 26% in 1979-1984 to 49% in 1997-2002), and it was higher for HFpEF, although the difference attenuated after adjustment for comorbidities.[12] The Meta-Analysis Global Group in Chronic Heart Failure (MAGGIC) study pooled the data from 17 observational studies and clinical trials consisting of 24,501 patients in total and showed a 32% lower risk of death in patients with HFpEF compared to HFrEF subgroup.[79] Patients with HFpEF have lower rates of cardiovascular death but relatively similar rates of noncardiovascular death compared to patients with HFrEF.[25]

Hospitalization and Health Care Burden

HF is the leading cause of hospitalization among the elderly.[12] HF hospitalizations are responsible for a major portion of health care burden attributed to HF[60] with a risk-adjusted 30-day rehospitalization rate of greater than 20% after index hospitalization[4] and an average of 1.34 hospitalizations per person-year in patients with established HF diagnosis.[25] In the United States, there are more than 1 million hospitalizations with a primary diagnosis of HF each year.[48] The number of hospitalizations that listed HF as primary or secondary diagnosis increased from 1.27 million in the year 1979 to 3.86 million in the year 2004, and is projected to continue to increase by 50% up to the year 2035, owing to the aging population and increase in HF prevalence.[4]

Three-quarter of the total annual direct cost associated with HF is attributed to HF hospitalizations.[80] Although the rate of hospitalization for other major cardiovascular diseases (eg, CAD or stroke) decreased from the 1980s to 2000s, the rate of HF hospitalization increased in both women and men in the same period.[81]

A quarter and a half of the patients who are hospitalized for HF are readmitted to the hospital within 30-days and 1-year, respectively.[12] The risk of hospitalization is comparable between HFpEF and HFrEF subgroups,[12,25,48] and the majority of rehospitalizations are noncardiovascular (50%-62%),[4,12,25] demonstrating the high comorbidity burden in this patient population.

Cost and Financial Burden

HF has a considerable burden on health care systems. A study in 2012 pooled the known national expenditures and estimated the global cost of HF care to be around 108 billion USD annually, with 86% of expenditure occurring in high-income countries that have only 18% of the world population, and the remaining 15 billion dollars being spent in the developing world.[82] Each HF hospitalization was estimated to cost 10,775 USD on average in the United States, which is significantly higher than the annual cost of care per HF patient in the developing world (eg, ~2000 USD per year in Nigeria).[4] The total direct and indirect cost associated with HF in the United States is expected to increase from about 30.7 billion USD in the year 2012 to 69.8 billion USD by 2030.[12,60]

Challenges in Underresourced Regions: Health Care Access and Quality of Care

With an increase in the prevalence of HF, providing long-term, evidence-based care for these patients is a necessity and becomes incrementally challenging and complex. Disposition from hospital to skilled nursing facilities, assisted living, or hospice centers have increased over the past few decades.[83] Roughly, a quarter of the Medicare beneficiaries with HF hospitalization in the Get With the Guideline program were discharged to a skilled nursing home.[84] Based on the data from Medicare beneficiaries and Olmsted County cohorts, nearly 40% of HF patients enroll to hospice months prior to death.[12]

A few procedures and therapies, such as mechanical circulatory support devices, with proven efficacy for improving survival and quality of life in selected advanced patients with HF are not universally available to all eligible patients throughout the world, as they are capital-intensive and not feasible to be covered by the health care systems of the LMICs.

Studies have indicated that traditional demographic, clinical, and socioeconomic variables altogether only explain less than 50% of the regional variability observed for the mortality from HF,[66,70] hence, other issues such as health care access, health care infrastructure, and the quality of care are some potential factors that may play a role.

KEY POINTS

- ✔ HF is a global public health problem.
- ✔ The incidence peaked in the mid-1990s and subsequently stabilized or decreased.
- ✔ The prevalence has increased over the past decades, mainly owing to the aging population and the improvement in survival after HF diagnosis.
- ✔ The prevalence and incidence increase with age and multicomorbidities.
- ✔ Risk factors are evolving with a trend for a decrease in hypertension but an increase in DM and obesity. Prevention and controlling these risk factors can lead to a reduction in the incidence of HF.
- ✔ HF is associated with higher morbidity and mortality and impaired quality of life.
- ✔ The epidemiology of HF may evolve over the next few decades owing to the change in the prevalence and control of known risk factors, the aging population, and improved survival from ischemic and valvular heart disease.

REFERENCES

1. Lund LH, Rich MW, Hauptman PJ. Complexities of the global heart failure epidemic. *J Card Fail.* 2018;24(12):813-814.
2. Metra M, Teerlink JR. Heart failure. *Lancet.* 2017;390(10106):1981-1995.
3. Mozaffarian D, Benjamin EJ, Go AS, et al. Heart disease and stroke statistics-2016 update: a report from the American Heart Association. *Circulation.* 2016;133(4):e38-e360.
4. Ziaeian B, Fonarow GC. Epidemiology and aetiology of heart failure. *Nat Rev Cardiol.* 2016;13(6):368-378.
5. McKee PA, Castelli WP, McNamara PM, Kannel WB. The natural history of congestive heart failure: the Framingham study. *N Engl J Med.* 1971;285(26):1441-1446.
6. Carlson KJ, Lee DC, Goroll AH, Leahy M, Johnson RA. An analysis of physicians' reasons for prescribing long-term digitalis therapy in outpatients. *J Chronic Dis.* 1985;38(9):733-739.
7. Eriksson H, Caidahl K, Larsson B, et al. Cardiac and pulmonary causes of dyspnoea—validation of a scoring test for clinical-epidemiological use: the Study of Men Born in 1913. *Eur Heart J.* 1987;8(9):1007-1014.
8. Harlan WR, oberman A, Grimm R, Rosati RA. Chronic congestive heart failure in coronary artery disease: clinical criteria. *Ann Intern Med.* 1977;86(2):133-138.
9. Ponikowski P, Voors AA, Anker SD, et al. 2016 ESC Guidelines for the diagnosis and treatment of acute and chronic heart failure: the Task Force for the diagnosis and treatment of acute and chronic heart failure of the European Society of Cardiology (ESC)Developed with the special contribution of the Heart Failure Association (HFA) of the ESC. *Eur Heart J.* 2016;37(27):2129-2200.
10. Yoon S, Eom GH. Heart failure with preserved ejection fraction: present status and future directions. *Exp Mol Med.* 2019;51(12):1-9.
11. Shah AM, Claggett B, Sweitzer NK, et al. Prognostic importance of impaired systolic function in heart failure with preserved ejection fraction and the impact of spironolactone. *Circulation.* 2015;132(5):402-414.
12. Dunlay SM, Roger VL. Understanding the epidemic of heart failure: past, present, and future. *Curr Heart Fail Rep.* 2014;11(4):404-415.
13. Hunt SA, Abraham WT, Chin MH, et al. 2009 focused update incorporated into the ACC/AHA 2005 guidelines for the diagnosis and management of heart failure in adults: a report of the American College of Cardiology Foundation/American Heart Association Task Force on Practice Guidelines: developed in collaboration with the International Society for Heart and Lung Transplantation. *Circulation.* 2009;119(14):e391-479.
14. Liu L, Eisen HJ. Epidemiology of heart failure and scope of the problem. *Cardiol Clin.* 2014;32(1):1-8, vii.
15. Dunlay SM, Weston SA, Jacobsen SJ, Roger VL. Risk factors for heart failure: a population-based case-control study. *Am J Med.* 2009;122(11):1023-1028.
16. Ho JE, Enserro D, Brouwers FP, et al. Predicting heart failure with preserved and reduced ejection fraction: the international collaboration on heart failure subtypes. *Circ Heart Fail.* 2016;9(6).
17. Kovell LC, Juraschek SP, Russell SD. Stage A heart failure is not adequately recognized in US adults: analysis of the National Health and Nutrition Examination Surveys, 2007-2010. *PloS One.* 2015;10(7):e0132228.
18. Dunlay SM, Redfield MM, Weston SA, et al. Hospitalizations after heart failure diagnosis a community perspective. *J Am Coll Cardiol.* 2009;54(18):1695-1702.
19. Flegal KM, Carroll MD, Ogden CL, Johnson CL. Prevalence and trends in obesity among US adults, 1999-2000. *JAMA.* 2002;288(14):1723-1727.
20. Gregg EW, Cheng YJ, Cadwell BL, et al. Secular trends in cardiovascular disease risk factors according to body mass index in US adults. *JAMA.* 2005;293(15):1868-1874.
21. Hawkins NM, Petrie MC, Jhund PS, Chalmers GW, Dunn FG, McMurray JJ. Heart failure and chronic obstructive pulmonary disease: diagnostic pitfalls and epidemiology. *Eur J Heart Fail.* 2009;11(2):130-139.
22. Vos T, Flaxman AD, Naghavi M, et al. Years lived with disability (YLDs) for 1160 sequelae of 289 diseases and injuries 1990-2010: a systematic analysis for the Global Burden of Disease Study 2010. *Lancet.* 2012;380(9859):2163-2196.
23. Public Health Agency of Canada. *Report from the Canadian Chronic Disease Surveillance System: Heart Disease in Canada, 2018.* Public Health Agency of Canada; 2018:49-50.
24. McMurray JJ, Adamopoulos S, Anker SD, et al. ESC Guidelines for the diagnosis and treatment of acute and chronic heart failure 2012: the Task Force for the Diagnosis and Treatment of Acute and Chronic Heart Failure 2012 of the European Society of Cardiology. Developed in collaboration with the Heart Failure Association (HFA) of the ESC. *Eur Heart J.* 2012;33(14):1787-1847.
25. Gerber Y, Weston SA, Redfield MM, et al. A contemporary appraisal of the heart failure epidemic in Olmsted County, Minnesota, 2000 to 2010. *JAMA Intern Med.* 2015;175(6):996-1004.
26. Moran AE, Forouzanfar MH, Roth GA, et al. The global burden of ischemic heart disease in 1990 and 2010: the Global Burden of Disease 2010 study. *Circulation.* 2014;129(14):1493-1501.

27. Kenchaiah S, Vasan RS. Heart failure in women—insights from the Framingham Heart Study. *Cardiovasc Drugs Ther.* 2015;29(4):377-390.
28. Levy D, Larson MG, Vasan RS, Kannel WB, Ho KK. The progression from hypertension to congestive heart failure. *JAMA.* 1996;275(20):1557-1562.
29. Lloyd-Jones DM, Larson MG, Leip EP, et al. Lifetime risk for developing congestive heart failure: the Framingham Heart Study. *Circulation.* 2002;106(24):3068-3072.
30. Yusuf S, Thom T, Abbott RD. Changes in hypertension treatment and in congestive heart failure mortality in the United States. *Hypertension.* 1989;13(suppl 5):I74-79.
31. Chow CK, Teo KK, Rangarajan S, et al. Prevalence, awareness, treatment, and control of hypertension in rural and urban communities in high-, middle-, and low-income countries. *JAMA.* 2013;310(9):959-968.
32. Nkomo VT, Gardin JM, Skelton TN, Gottdiener JS, Scott CG, Enriquez-Sarano M. Burden of valvular heart diseases: a population-based study. *Lancet.* 2006;368(9540):1005-1011.
33. Iung B, Baron G, Butchart EG, et al. A prospective survey of patients with valvular heart disease in Europe: the Euro Heart Survey on Valvular Heart Disease. *Eur Heart J.* 2003;24(13):1231-1243.
34. Marciniak A, Glover K, Sharma R. Cohort profile: prevalence of valvular heart disease in community patients with suspected heart failure in UK. *BMJ Open.* 2017;7(1):e012240.
35. Essop MR, Nkomo VT. Rheumatic and nonrheumatic valvular heart disease: epidemiology, management, and prevention in Africa. *Circulation.* 2005;112(23):3584-3591.
36. Elliott P, Andersson B, Arbustini E, et al. Classification of the cardiomyopathies: a position statement from the European Society of Cardiology Working Group on myocardial and pericardial diseases. *Eur Heart J.* 2007;29(2):270-276.
37. Lozano R, Naghavi M, Foreman K, et al. Global and regional mortality from 235 causes of death for 20 age groups in 1990 and 2010: a systematic analysis for the Global Burden of Disease Study 2010. *Lancet.* 2012;380(9859):2095-2128.
38. Wong CY, Chaudhry SI, Desai MM, Krumholz HM. Trends in comorbidity, disability, and polypharmacy in heart failure. *Am J Med.* 2011;124(2):136-143.
39. Dunlay SM, Roger VL, Redfield MM. Epidemiology of heart failure with preserved ejection fraction. *Nat Rev Cardiol.* 2017;14(10):591-602.
40. Kannel WB, Hjortland M, Castelli WP. Role of diabetes in congestive heart failure: the Framingham study. *Am J Cardiol.* 1974;34(1):29-34.
41. Silverberg D, Wexler D, Blum M, Schwartz D, Iaina A. The association between congestive heart failure and chronic renal disease. *Curr Opin Nephrol Hypertens.* 2004;13(2):163-170.
42. Richards M, Di Somma S, Mueller C, et al. Atrial fibrillation impairs the diagnostic performance of cardiac natriuretic peptides in dyspneic patients: results from the BACH Study (Biomarkers in ACute Heart Failure). *JACC Heart Fail.* 2013;1(3):192-199.
43. Krum H, Gilbert RE. Demographics and concomitant disorders in heart failure. *Lancet.* 2003;362(9378):147-158.
44. Kosiborod M, Curtis JP, Wang Y, et al. Anemia and outcomes in patients with heart failure: a study from the National Heart Care Project. *Arch Intern Med.* 2005;165(19):2237-2244.
45. Silverberg DS, Wexler D, Blum M, et al. The use of subcutaneous erythropoietin and intravenous iron for the treatment of the anemia of severe, resistant congestive heart failure improves cardiac and renal function and functional cardiac class, and markedly reduces hospitalizations. *J Am Coll Cardiol.* 2000;35(7):1737-1744.
46. Savarese G, D'Amario D. Sex differences in heart failure. *Adv Exp Med Biol.* 2018;1065:529-544.
47. McNallan SM, Chamberlain AM, Gerber Y, et al. Measuring frailty in heart failure: a community perspective. *Am Heart J.* 2013;166(4):768-774.
48. Benjamin EJ, Muntner P, Alonso A, et al. Heart disease and stroke statistics-2019 update: a report from the American Heart Association. *Circulation.* 2019;139(10):e56-e528.
49. Huffman MD, Berry JD, Ning H, et al. Lifetime risk for heart failure among white and black Americans: cardiovascular lifetime risk pooling project. *J Am Coll Cardiol.* 2013;61(14):1510-1517.
50. Roger VL, Go AS, Lloyd-Jones DM, et al. Heart disease and stroke statistics—2012 update: a report from the American Heart Association. *Circulation.* 2012;125(1):e2-e220.
51. Croft JB, Giles WH, Pollard RA, Casper ML, Anda RF, Livengood JR. National trends in the initial hospitalization for heart failure. *J Am Geriatr Soc.* 1997;45(3):270-275.
52. Curtis LH, Whellan DJ, Hammill BG, et al. Incidence and prevalence of heart failure in elderly persons, 1994-2003. *Arch Intern Med.* 2008;168(4):418-424.
53. Barasa A, Schaufelberger M, Lappas G, Swedberg K, Dellborg M, Rosengren A. Heart failure in young adults: 20-year trends in hospitalization, aetiology, and case fatality in Sweden. *Eur Heart J.* 2014;35(1):25-32.
54. Teng TH, Finn J, Hobbs M, Hung J. Heart failure: incidence, case fatality, and hospitalization rates in Western Australia between 1990 and 2005. *Circ Heart Fail* 2010;3(2):236-243.
55. Yeung DF, Boom NK, Guo H, Lee DS, Schultz SE, Tu JV. Trends in the incidence and outcomes of heart failure in Ontario, Canada: 1997 to 2007. *CMAJ* 2012;184(14):E765-773.
56. Stewart S, MacIntyre K, MacLeod MM, Bailey AE, Capewell S, McMurray JJ. Trends in hospitalization for heart failure in Scotland, 1990-1996. An epidemic that has reached its peak? *Eur Heart J.* 2001;22(3):209-217.
57. Levy D, Kenchaiah S, Larson MG, et al. Long-term trends in the incidence of and survival with heart failure. *N Engl J Med.* 2002;347(18):1397-1402.
58. Roger VL, Weston SA, Redfield MM, et al. Trends in heart failure incidence and survival in a community-based population. *JAMA.* 2004;292(3):344-350.
59. Barker WH, Mullooly JP, Getchell W. Changing incidence and survival for heart failure in a well-defined older population, 1970-1974 and 1990-1994. *Circulation.* 2006;113(6):799-805.
60. Heidenreich PA, Albert NM, Allen LA, et al. Forecasting the impact of heart failure in the United States: a policy statement from the American Heart Association. *Circ Heart Fail.* 2013;6(3):606-619.
61. Dickstein K, Cohen-Solal A, Filippatos G, et al. ESC Guidelines for the diagnosis and treatment of acute and chronic heart failure 2008: the Task Force for the Diagnosis and Treatment of Acute and Chronic Heart Failure 2008 of the European Society of Cardiology. Developed in collaboration with the Heart Failure Association of the ESC (HFA) and endorsed by the European Society of Intensive Care Medicine (ESICM). *Eur Heart J.* 2008;29(19):2388-2442.
62. Bahrami H, Kronmal R, Bluemke DA, et al. Differences in the incidence of congestive heart failure by ethnicity: the multi-ethnic study of atherosclerosis. *Arch Intern Med.* 2008;168(19):2138-2145.
63. Kaul P, McAlister FA, Ezekowitz JA, Grover VK, Quan H. Ethnic differences in 1-year mortality among patients hospitalised with heart failure. *Heart.* 2011;97(13):1048-1053.
64. Teng TH, Katzenellenbogen JM, Thompson SC, et al. Incidence of first heart failure hospitalisation and mortality in Aboriginal and non-Aboriginal patients in Western Australia, 2000-2009. *Int J Cardiol.* 2014;173(1):110-117.
65. Teng TH, Katzenellenbogen JM, Hung J, et al. A cohort study: temporal trends in prevalence of antecedents, comorbidities and mortality in Aboriginal and non-Aboriginal Australians with first heart failure hospitalization, 2000-2009. *Int J Equity Health.* 2015;14:66.
66. Mensah GA. Heart failure in low-income and middle-income countries: rising burden, diverse etiology, and high mortality. *J Card Fail.* 2018;24(12):833-834.
67. Weiwei C, Runlin G, Lisheng L, et al. Outline of the report on cardiovascular diseases in China, 2014. *Eur Heart J.* 2016;18(suppl F):F2-F11.
68. Huffman MD, Prabhakaran D. Heart failure: epidemiology and prevention in India. *The Natl Med J India.* 2010;23(5):283-288.
69. Shiba N, Nochioka K, Miura M, Kohno H, Shimokawa H. Trend of westernization of etiology and clinical characteristics of heart failure patients in Japan—first report from the CHART-2 study. *Circ J.* 2011;75(4):823-833.
70. Dokainish H, Teo K, Zhu J, et al. Global mortality variations in patients with heart failure: results from the International Congestive Heart Failure (INTER-CHF) prospective cohort study. *Lancet Glob Health.* 2017;5(7):e665-e672.
71. Al-Shamiri MQ. Heart failure in the Middle East. *Curr Cardiol Rev.* 2013;9(2):174-178.

72. Makubi A, Hage C, Sartipy U, et al. Heart failure in Tanzania and Sweden: Comparative characterization and prognosis in the Tanzania Heart Failure (TaHeF) study and the Swedish Heart Failure Registry (SwedeHF). *Int J Cardiol.* 2016;220:750-758.
73. Kristensen SL, Kober L, Jhund PS, et al. International geographic variation in event rates in trials of heart failure with preserved and reduced ejection fraction. *Circulation.* 2015;131(1):43-53.
74. GBD 2017 Causes of Death Collaborators. Global, regional, and national age-sex-specific mortality for 282 causes of death in 195 countries and territories, 1980-2017: a systematic analysis for the Global Burden of Disease Study 2017. *Lancet.* 2018;392(10159):1736-1788.
75. Askoxylakis V, Thieke C, Pleger ST, et al. Long-term survival of cancer patients compared to heart failure and stroke: a systematic review. *BMC Cancer.* 2010;10:105.
76. Malamba-Lez D, Ngoy-Nkulu D, Steels P, Tshala-Katumbay D, Mullens W. Heart failure etiologies and challenges to care in the developing world: an observational study in the Democratic Republic of Congo. *J Card Fail.* 2018;24(12):854-859.
77. Sanjay G, Jeemon P, Agarwal A, et al. In-hospital and three-year outcomes of heart failure patients in South India: the Trivandrum Heart Failure Registry. *J Card Fail.* 2018;24(12):842-848.
78. Loehr LR, Rosamond WD, Chang PP, Folsom AR, Chambless LE. Heart failure incidence and survival (from the Atherosclerosis Risk in Communities study). *Am J Cardiol.* 2008;101(7):1016-1022.
79. Meta-analysis Global Group in Chronic Heart Failure (MAGGIC). The survival of patients with heart failure with preserved or reduced left ventricular ejection fraction: an individual patient data meta-analysis. *Eur Heart J.* 2012;33(14):1750-1757.
80. Dunlay SM, Shah ND, Shi Q, et al. Lifetime costs of medical care after heart failure diagnosis. *Circ Cardiovasc Qual Outcomes.* 2011;4(1):68-75.
81. Liu L. Changes in cardiovascular hospitalization and comorbidity of heart failure in the United States: findings from the National Hospital Discharge Surveys 1980-2006. *Int J Cardiol.* 2011;149(1):39-45.
82. Cook C, Cole G, Asaria P, Jabbour R, Francis DP. The annual global economic burden of heart failure. *Int J Cardiol.* 2014;171(3):368-376.
83. Fang J, Mensah GA, Croft JB, Keenan NL. Heart failure-related hospitalization in the U.S., 1979 to 2004. *J Am Coll Cardiol.* 2008;52(6):428-434.
84. Allen LA, Hernandez AF, Peterson ED, et al. Discharge to a skilled nursing facility and subsequent clinical outcomes among older patients hospitalized for heart failure. *Circ Heart Fail* 2011;4(3):293-300.
85. Sharma A, Zhao X, Hammill Bradley G, et al. Trends in noncardiovascular comorbidities among patients hospitalized for heart failure: insights from the Get With The Guidelines-Heart Failure Registry. *Circ Heart Fail.* 2018;11(6):e004646.

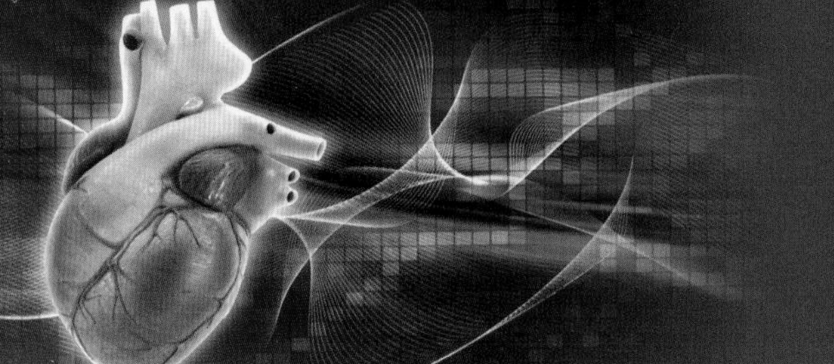

CHAPTER 66

HEART FAILURE PATHOPHYSIOLOGY

Luise Holzhauser and Paul J. Mather

INTRODUCTION AND CLASSIFICATIONS

Regardless of the etiology, heart failure (HF) is a complex clinical syndrome that results from any structural or functional impairment of ventricular filling or ejection of blood. The cardinal manifestations of HF are dyspnea and fatigue, which may limit exercise tolerance and cause or lead to fluid retention, which may lead to pulmonary and/or splanchnic congestion and/or peripheral edema. Some patients have exercise intolerance but with little evidence of fluid retention, whereas others complain primarily of edema, dyspnea, or fatigue. The left ventricular ejection fraction (LVEF) is a crude measure of actual cardiac function but is the clinically most widely accepted method of HF characterization and prognostication.

The categories of HF have recently been updated as follows: (1) HF with reduced EF (HFrEF), which includes patients with symptomatic HF and LVEF less than or equal to 40%; (2) HF with mid-range EF (HFmrEF), which includes patients with symptomatic HF and LVEF 41% to 49%; (3) HF with preserved EF (HFpEF), which includes patients with symptomatic HF and LVEF more than 50%; and (4) HF with improved EF (HFimpEF), which identifies patients with symptomatic HF with a baseline LVEF less than or equal to 40%, a greater than or equal to 10-point increase from baseline LVEF, and a second measurement of LVEF more than 40%.[1]

The causative pathophysiology is considered to be distinctly different between HFrEF and HFpEF despite a certain degree of overlap in risk factors. HFrEF is caused by either an inciting event or an inherited mechanism eventually leading to loss of cardiomyocytes, dysfunction, and dilation of the left ventricle (LV), resulting in pump failure setting off a vicious cycle of neurohormonal activation triggering further disease progression. HFpEF, on the other hand, is less a primary cardiac phenomenon but rather the cardiac manifestation of a systemic pathology. It is hypothesized that comorbidities defined by pro-inflammatory states—such as hypertension, diabetes, chronic obstructive pulmonary disease, obesity, and chronic kidney disease—eventually lead to cardiomyocyte hypertrophy and resultant stiffening of the heart muscle leading to increased filling pressures.[2] Thus, although inflammation is implied among all spectrums of HF, inflammatory biomarkers are more strongly associated with HFpEF, and endothelial dysfunction and reduced bioavailability of nitric oxide are hallmarks of HFpEF pathophysiology.[3]

This chapter focuses on classic concepts of HFrEF pathophysiology.

VICIOUS CYCLE OF NEUROHORMONAL ADAPTIVE AND MALADAPTIVE MECHANISMS IN HEART FAILURE WITH REDUCED EJECTION FRACTION

Independent of the inciting event of HFrEF, the ultimate consequence is a reduced cardiac output (CO) detected by baroreceptors in the peripheral circulation as a low volume state leading to activation of both the renin-angiotensin-aldosterone system (RAAS) and the sympathetic nervous system (SNS). CO is maintained via increase in both contractility and heart rate (HR) accompanied by increased circulatory volume via salt and water retention and peripheral vasoconstriction. This initial adaptive response, triggered by neurohormonal activation to maintain cardiac hemostasis, ultimately leads to adverse remodeling in conditions of persistent stress. The degree of neurohormonal activation correlates with disease severity and prognosis in HF.[4] Notably in chronic HFrEF, there is decrease in baroreceptor activity, increase in chemosensitivity to hypoxia and hypercarbia leading to further enhanced neurohormonal activation, and imbalance between SNS and parasympathetic nervous system with decreased parasympathetic tone manifest as enhanced HR, myocardial contractility, and peripheral vasoconstriction.[5]

SNS activation triggers release of renin via vasoconstriction of the renal artery and renal hypoperfusion as well as direct effects via β1-receptors on the juxtaglomerular apparatus.[6] An additional trigger for renin release is decreasing chloride in the macula densa of the loop of Henle, which may be worsened by loop diuretics. Renin converts circulating angiotensinogen secreted by the liver to angiotensin I, which is then cleaved by angiotensin-converting enzyme (ACE) to angiotensin II. Angiotensin II is a potent vasoconstrictor and the most potent stimulator of aldosterone release from the adrenal glands. Both angiotensin II at the proximal tubule and aldosterone at the distal tubule increase salt and water retention. In chronic HF non-osmotic and angiotensin II triggered release of arginine-vasopressin from the thirst center in the brain further decrease free water clearance in the kidney and thus contribute to hyponatremia.[4,7]

RAAS activation is a pivotal player in the pathophysiology of HF, and chronic RAAS activation is a hallmark of adverse cardiac remodeling, fluid retention, and clinical manifestation of HF **(Algorithm 66.1)**.[4] Several short chain peptides including angiotensin 1-7 are derived from angiotensin II and counteract its effects on adverse LV remodeling.[8]

With the recent development of angiotensin receptor-neprilysin inhibition (ARNI), the important role of the natriuretic peptide systems has been recognized, including natriuretic peptide and B-type natriuretic peptide that are released following myocardial and atrial stretch and counteract adverse downstream effects of RAAS activity extraction via cGMP production, but peripheral resistance to natriuretic peptides in HF is common.[4,9]

The unique benefit of the ARNI compound lies in antagonizing downstream effects of angiotensin II and at the same time augmenting natriuretic peptide function by inhibiting neprilysin-mediated cleavage of these peptides. Thus, it augments vasodilation and natriuresis inhibited by natriuretic peptide resistance.[4]

Peripheral vascular vasoconstriction in HF is mediated via β1-receptors, and it augments blood pressure at the cost of reduced renal blood flow and increased myocardial afterload. In addition, neurohormonal activation enhances vascular tone, resulting in increased filling of the failing LV, thereby contributing to adverse remodeling, pump failure, and enhanced neurohormonal activation.[4]

MOLECULAR AND CELLULAR CHANGES

LV remodeling is driven by chronic neurohormonal activation, resulting in myocardial molecular structural and cellular changes, including alterations in myocyte biology and gene expression.

Myocardial Structural Changes and Extracellular Matrix

Initially, cardiomyocyte hypertrophy is compensatory and occurs in either a concentric pattern in cases of pressure overload with addition of sarcomeres in parallel or an eccentric pattern with elongated myocytes and sarcomeres added in sequence as a response to volume overload. With ongoing myocardial stress, remodeling transitions from adaptive to maladaptive, characterized by myocyte elongation, sarcomere disarray, decrease in α-myosin heavy chain (*MYH6*) gene expression, and increase in β-myosin heavy chain (*MYH7*) gene.[10] α-Myosin heavy chain (MHC) has a higher adenosine triphosphate (ATP)ase activity and shortening velocity; thus, hearts expressing *MYH6* have higher contractile velocity than hearts expressing β-MHC. This shift in relative gene expression is reminiscent of expression levels of the fetal gene program of these contractile proteins in the embryonic heart.[11]

Neurohormonal activation with elevated norepinephrine and angiotensin II levels triggers necrotic cardiomyocyte death.[12,13] The human heart has minimal regenerative capacity, and cardiomyocyte necrosis, apoptosis, and autophagy are commonly observed in the failing myocardium.[4,14] Aside from cardiomyocytes loss, molecular and structural alterations within the extracellular matrix (ECM) also play a pivotal role in the adverse remodeling process. The ECM not only preserves tissue integrity and facilitates force transmission, but it also serves as

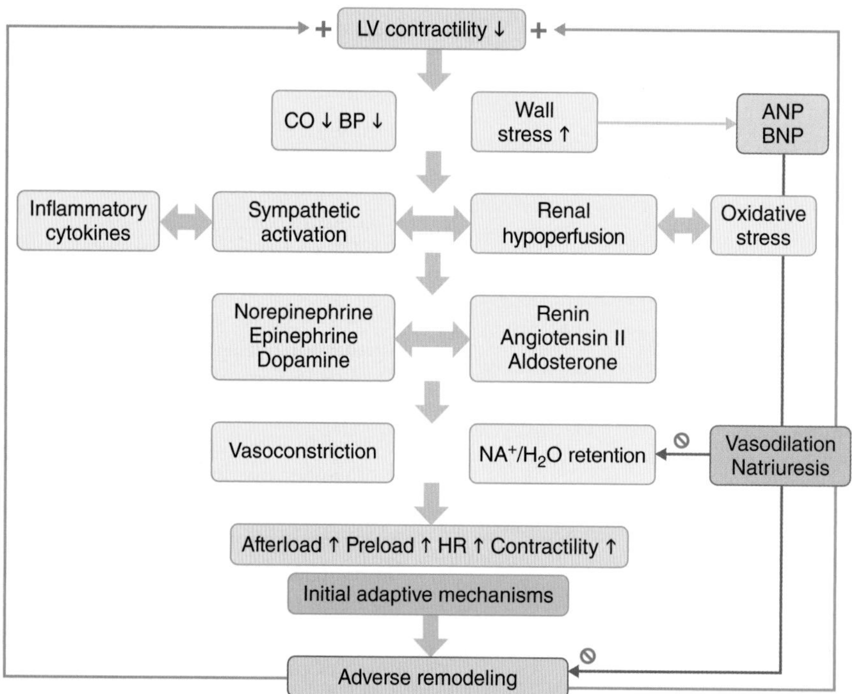

ALGORITHM 66.1 The vicious cycle of neurohormonal activation in HFrEF. A decrease in cardiac output and blood pressure leads to activation of the sympathetic nervous system and the renin-angiotensin-aldosterone system. The resulting increase in preload and afterload as well as heart rate and contractility maintain cardiac output and perfusion. However, this initially adaptive process leads to adverse remodeling and sets off the vicious cycle of neurohormonal activation in chronic HF. ANP, atrial natriuretic peptide; BNP, B-type natriuretic peptide; HFrEF, heart failure with reduced ejection fraction. BP, blood pressure; CO, cardiac output; HR, heart rate; H20, water; LV, left ventricular; Na, sodium

a signaling hub for cardiomyocytes and as a reservoir of growth factors allowing for a fast response to injury with activation of a repair program.[15] RAAS activation stimulates myocardial fibrosis via fibroblast proliferation and collagen production.[16]

As with cardiomyocytes, different injury patterns lead to different structural changes in the ECM, including activation of a matrix-synthetic program in cardiac fibroblasts with conversion to myofibroblasts and synthesis of ECM proteins. The resulting expansion in ECM can increase myocardial stiffness, thereby aggravating diastolic dysfunction of the failing LV. Further, conditions of pressure overload lead to dilative remodeling and systolic failure, possibly mediated by changes in the interstitial metalloproteinase-protease/antiprotease balance. In ischemic injury patterns, however, more dynamic changes in the cardiac ECM contribute to regulation of inflammation and repair and can mediate adverse cardiac remodeling.[17]

Any cardiac injury, however, leads to initiation of tissue repair mechanisms, which are closely linked to innate immunity. Tumor necrosis factor α (TNF-α), transforming growth factor β (TGF-β), and interleukins (IL) including IL-1, IL-12, IL-8, and IL-18 are major mediators of this pro-inflammatory response. TNF-α and IL-1 have negative inotropic effects mediated via β-receptor uncoupling and impaired calcium (Ca^{2+}) signaling, which negatively affects diastolic function.[18,19] In addition to adversely affecting excitation-contraction coupling, TNF-α triggers hypertrophy of cardiomyocytes and ECM remodeling via regulation of tissue inhibitors of metalloproteinases.[20,21] Although preclinical data showed beneficial effects of inhibiting TNF-α signaling, clinical trials using anti-TNF therapy showed an increased risk of all-cause death and/or HF hospitalization. This could in part be explained by inhibiting nuclear factor-κB (NF-κB), a transcription regulator and key effector of TNF-α. Aside from mediating inflammation, apoptosis, and ECM remodeling, NF-κB also has cardioprotective effects, including antioxidant activity, improving mitochondrial function, and inhibiting cell death.[3] This example describes the delicate balance between a necessary inflammatory response to initiate tissue repair, especially in acute ischemic injury, and the deleterious effects of persistent inflammation aggravating the adverse remodeling process.

In advanced HF injury, neurohormonal activation and inflammation eventually lead to changes in cellular composition of the failing myocardium and alterations in LV ECM, with chamber dilation, wall thinning, and change in shape toward a spherical appearance further aggravating LV dysfunction.[4]

Molecular Changes in the Failing Heart

β-Receptor Signaling

Persistent SNS activation with high levels of catecholamines further aggravates pathologic changes in the heart, and sustained β-receptor stimulation has been shown to correlate with worsening LV dysfunction and mortality.[22] Chronic Ca^{2+} overload mediated by β-receptor signaling may contribute to cardiomyocyte death.[23] β1-Receptors mediate cardiac function via the stimulatory G-protein (guanyl nucleotide binding protein [Gs]) pathway, adenylyl cyclase, and subsequent cAMP generation. Downstream activation of protein kinase A (PKA) then leads to phosphorylation of several targets, including phospholamban (PLB) and the sarcoplasmic/endoplasmic reticulum calcium ATPase (SERCA), thereby maintaining intracellular Ca^{2+} dynamics, lusitropy (rate of myocardial relaxation), and positive inotropy. The β1-receptor is the main receptor subtype expressed by cardiomyocytes with a ratio of 4:1 to β2-receptors. In the failing heart, however, chronic adrenergic stimulation leads to downregulation of β1-receptors with a 1:1 ratio of β1 and β2 as well as decreased sensitivity of cardiomyocytes to endogenous and exogenous catecholamines with decoupling from downstream G-protein activation.[24,25] The process of β-receptor downregulation and decoupling is initialed by phosphorylation via G protein–coupled receptor kinase (GRK), thus facilitating internalization of the receptors mediated via β-arrestin (**Algorithm 66.2**).

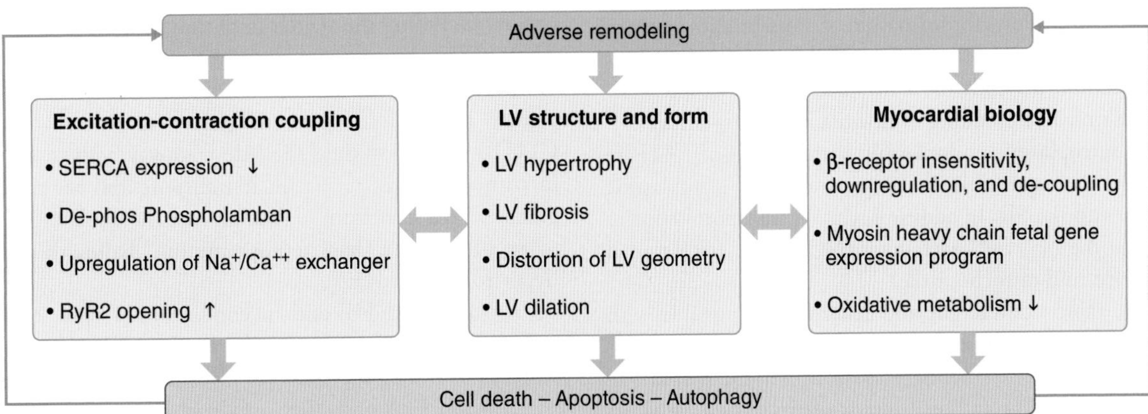

ALGORITHM 66.2 Myocardial structural and molecular changes of adverse remodeling. Adverse remodeling is characterized by myocardial molecular structural and cellular changes, including alterations in myocyte biology, excitation-contraction coupling, and gene expression. De-phos, de-phosphorylation; LV, left ventricular; Na/Ca, sodium-calcium; RyR2, ryanodine receptor; SERCA, sarcoplasmic-endoplasmic reticulum Ca^{2+} ATPase.

Along with β-arrestin, other mediators are recruited, including mitogen-activated protein kinase (MAPK). These signaling pathways are crucial components of adverse remodeling and apoptosis. The main kinase involved in the phosphorylation process is elevated in HF and inhibited by β-blocker therapy.[4,26,27]

There is now growing evidence for cross talk between β-receptors and other signaling pathways. For example, β1-receptors can mediate proapoptotic signaling via several pathways, including calcium and MAPK signaling. On the other hand, persistent β2-receptor activation can lead to coupling of the receptor to the Gα.I (inhibitory) pathway linked to activation of a cell survival pathway and attenuation of the positive inotropic effects of β-receptor stimulation. However, β-receptor subtypes cannot simply be labeled as "cardiotoxic" or "cardioprotective." These β-receptor functions seem mostly dependent on the type and duration of cardiac stress. It is, however, important to note that the role of β-receptor signaling in HF far exceeds downstream effects of PKA phosphorylation.[28]

Calcium Signaling

Ca^{2+} shifts play a crucial role in excitation-contraction coupling. Contraction is initiated by a transient increase in cytosolic Ca^{2+} concentration to activate cross-bridge formation between the actin and myosin myofilament proteins. Myofibrils are interwoven with the Ca^{2+}-storing sarcoplasmic reticulum (SR) and mitochondria. Voltage-gated ion channels, exchangers, and the Na^+/K^+ ATPase pump are located on the transverse tubular membranes (L-type channels) and in close proximity to the intracellular ryanodine receptor (RyR2) Ca^{2+} release channels on the SR membrane.[29] Voltage-dependent opening of L-type Ca^{2+} channels permits Ca^{2+}influx, which triggers opening of RyR2 channels and resulting in release of Ca^{2+} from the SR. The Ca^{2+} released from the SR contributes the major portion of myofilament activating Ca^{2+}. Ca^{2+} then binds to troponin C on the troponin-tropomyosin complex on the actin filaments, which moves tropomyosin away from the binding sites and allows for formation of cross-bridges between actin and myosin to initiate myocardial contraction. Subsequent relaxation depends on a decrease in cytoplasmic Ca^{2+} concentration and unbinding of myofilament cross-bridges.

The sarcoplasmic-endoplasmic reticulum Ca^{2+} ATPase (SERCA2a) is responsible for sequestration of cytoplasmic Ca^{2+} back into the SR. In addition, Ca^{2+} is transported out of the cell via the Na^+/Ca^{2+} exchanger (NCX), the sarcolemmal Ca^{2+} ATPase, and mitochondria.

Thus, rapid contraction and relaxation is possible with Ca^{2+} cycling between the extracellular space, cytosol, and SR.[29]

Changes in Ca^{2+} signaling play an important role in HF and arrhythmias. The failing heart is characterized by alterations of key Ca^{2+} signaling proteins, resulting in decreased SR Ca^{2+} release, enhanced diastolic SR Ca^{2+} "leak," and reduced SR Ca^{2+} sequestration. The consequence is further impaired contractility with decreased Ca^{2+} release to myofilaments and aggravated diastolic dysfunction (**Algorithm 66.2**).[29]

The reduced SR Ca^{2+} is attributable to several mechanism, including reduced SERCA expression and activity as well as dephosphorylation of phospholamban, which further inhibits SERCA activity.[30] PKA mediated hyperphosphorylation of RyR2 resulting in increased diastolic SR Ca2+ likely plays a key role in further promoting $Ca2^+$-dependent remodeling.[29,31]

HF is characterized by abnormal energy metabolism, with decreased energy production and utilization. Maintaining cardiomyocyte Ca^{2+} homeostasis with SERCA2a and the Na^+-K^+ ATPase function are major sources of ATP consumption. Thus, ATP deficiency in Ca^{2+} signaling may further contribute to myocardial dysfunction in HF.[29] β-Blockers decrease energy consumption and have been shown to normalize Ca^{2+} handling in failing human hearts.[31] Mechanical unloading with left ventricular assist devices (LVADs) also improves Ca^{2+} homeostasis in the failing heart, highlighting the relationship between Ca^{2+} homeostasis and metabolism improved with HF therapies.[29]

CARDIAC AND SYSTEMIC METABOLISM WITH DEVELOPMENT OF INSULIN RESISTANCE

The myocardium is a high energy-dependent tissue. The source of ATP generation differs in physiologic and pathologic conditions. Under physiologic conditions, 60% to 90% of myocardial ATP is derived from fatty acid oxygenation, and the residual 10% to 40% is generated equally from glycolysis and lactate oxidation. However, free fatty acid (FFA) oxidation requires high oxygen consumption but results in three times more ATP generation than aerobic glycolysis.[33]

Thus, in an oxygen-rich state, FFAs appear as a superior fuel. However, both acute and chronic myocardial failures alter the availability of oxygen, and fuel metabolism must adapt accordingly to avoid organ failure. In early stages of HF, FFA utilization is only slightly decreased. But with disease progression, mitochondrial oxidative metabolism further declines, and the myocardium becomes more reliant on glycolysis for energy production. A complex array of metabolic adaptations occurs, including the switch to glycolysis away from FFA utilization. This is promoted by activation of glucose metabolism pathways, such as adenosine monophosphate (AMP)-activated protein kinase, leading to stimulation of glucose uptake via GLUT4 as well as the PI3K/Akt pathway activation, which, in turn, promotes intracellular transport and metabolism of glucose. This shift from FFA to glucose metabolism is thought to be part of the "fetal reprogramming" hallmark of cardiac hypertrophy and HF.[34,35]

In advanced HF and in conditions of type 2 diabetes, the myocardium develops insulin resistance. Insulin resistance worsens with the progression of HF, further compromising the switch from FFA utilization to glycolysis and resulting in increased dependence on FFA metabolism (**Algorithm 66.3**).

Increased FFA serum levels in HF further aggravate impaired insulin signaling and mitochondrial dysfunction with decreased ATP production from β-oxidation and increased oxygen requirements. Loss of mitochondria and mitochondrial

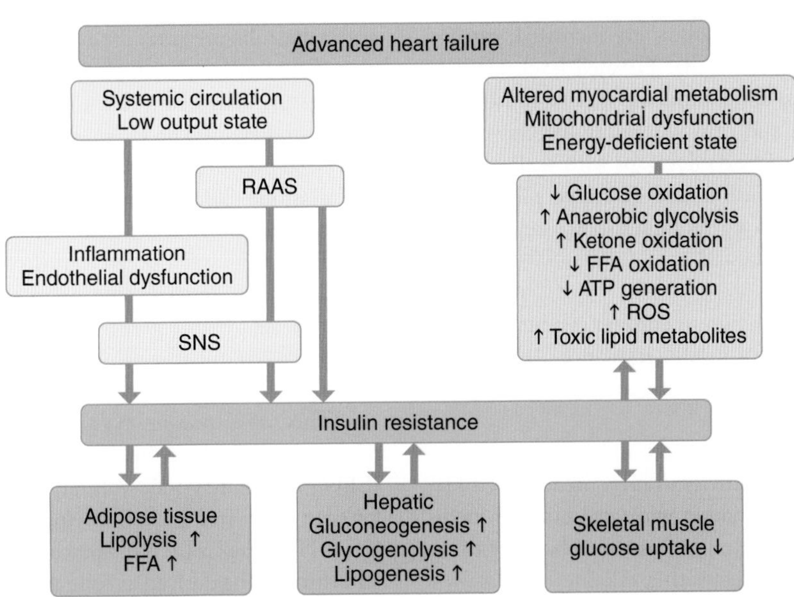

ALGORITHM 66.3 Metabolism in heart failure: An energy-deficient state and the role of insulin resistance. In chronic heart failure, a shift away from free fatty acid (FFA) to glucose metabolism occurs. Mitochondrial dysfunction and uncoupling between glycolysis and glucose oxidation further aggravate the decline in cardiac efficiency. In advanced heart failure, insulin resistance develops, which compromises the transition from FFA utilization to glycolysis and increases dependence on FFA metabolism. In the systemic circulation, neurohormonal activation with elevated FFA, increased hepatic gluconeogenesis and glycolysis as well as cardiac cachexia are the drivers of insulin resistance. ATP, adenosine triphosphate; FFA, free fatty acid; RAAS, renin-angiotensin-aldosterone system; ROS, reactive oxygen species; SNS, sympathetic nervous system.

dysfunction further contributes to the reduced glucose oxidation and energy production in advanced HF. This uncoupling between glycolysis and glucose oxidation aggravates the decline in cardiac efficiency.[36]

Moreover, insulin resistance is associated with diminished transport of FFAs into the mitochondria primarily via reduced activity of the transport protein carnitine palmitoyltransferase 1. The loss of mitochondrial hemostasis results in FFA accumulation, which further impairs mitochondrial integrity and structure triggering mitochondrial-mediated cell death. Toxic storage molecules, including triglycerides, diacylglycerol, and ceramide, inhibit insulin signaling and further contribute to adverse myocardial remodeling. Mitochondrial hemostasis is regulated by multiple factors, including ceramides, the level of mitochondrial redox stress, and expression of metabolic genes. These may serve as potential therapeutic targets in HF in the future.[37] Mechanical unloading with LVADs has already been shown to correct both systemic and local metabolic dysfunction, reducing myocardial levels of toxic lipid intermediates and improving cardiac insulin signaling.[38,39]

Ketone production increases proportionally to HF severity and neurohormonal activation. Ketone bodies can be used as fuel in the myocardium instead of FFA, especially in advanced HF with downregulated *FFA* gene expression. Myocardial ketone utilization becomes especially relevant in conditions of insulin resistance and cardiac.[40] Notably, sodium glucose co-transporter-2 (SGLT2) inhibitors increase levels of circulating ketones and cardiac ketone oxidation, thus providing fuel for the "energy-starved heart" and improving cardiac performance. Importantly, this increase in ketone oxidation is not associated with a decrease in glucose or FFA oxidation, which results in increased ATP production.[41] The major source for the energy deprivation in advanced HF is mitochondrial dysfunction, and SGLT2 inhibitors have been shown to improve mitochondrial respiratory function, which also may contribute to improving energy production in the heart.[42] Thus, SGLT2 inhibitors may not increase cardiac efficiency but supply an extra source of fuel to the energy-compromised failing heart (**Algorithm 66.3**).[43]

There is now mounting evidence for a potentially protective role of purinergic signaling in HF metabolism. Preclinical studies suggest that partial adenosine-1 receptor agonists can enhance expression of the GLUT-1 and GLUT-4 glucose transporters to near-normal levels and improve mitochondrial function with enhanced FFA oxidation and reduction FFA plasma levels.[44,45]

Among established HF therapies, β-blocker therapy reduces myocardial oxygen consumption and improves myocardial energy efficiency, possibly via a switch in myocardial substrate utilization from FFA to glucose oxidation. Carvedilol specifically has been shown to induce a "metabolic shift," with a decreased ratio of myocardial FFA and glucose utilization.[46]

SNS activation, a hallmark compensatory mechanism in acute and chronic HF, leads to increased serum levels of FFAs, glucocorticoids, and epinephrine. Subsequently, elevated FFA levels further increase SNS activation. This compensatory hyperadrenergic state has been described as the core of metabolic derangements in HF.[47,48] Under these conditions, hepatic gluconeogenesis and glycolysis are increased, causing hyperglycemia and hyperinsulinemia. Elevated levels of FFAs adversely affect insulin signaling, inducing skeletal muscle and hepatic insulin resistance and thus worsening hyperglycemia. In advanced HF, cardiac cachexia develops with skeletal muscle hypoperfusion, muscle wasting and decreased physical activity associated with growth hormone resistance, and further worsening of insulin resistance and accumulation of toxic lipid storage molecules.[39,49,50]

In addition, RAAS activation in chronic HF further contributes to the development of insulin resistance. Angiotensin II directly inhibits pancreatic insulin secretion and glucose uptake by the skeletal muscle system.[51,52]

ACE inhibitors increase FFA uptake and improve myocardial energetics and insulin sensitivity in HF.[53] In advanced HF, LVAD implantation in combination with goal-directed medical therapy has been shown to improve the metabolic dysfunction complicating and likely aggravating HF.[54]

HEMODYNAMICS IN HEART FAILURE

LV pressure-volume loops are derived from plotting LV pressure against LV volumes throughout the cardiac cycle **(Figure 66.1A)**. The cardiac cycle is typically divided into four basic phases: diastole, isovolumetric contraction, systole, and isovolumetric relaxation.

During diastole, there is a constant increase in LV pressure and volume as LV filling occurs. At the end of diastole, the ventricle contracts, whereupon the LV pressure exceeds left atrial pressure resulting in closure of the mitral valve and beginning of isovolumetric contraction. When LV pressure exceeds aortic diastolic pressure, the aortic valve opens and ejection begins. Ejection ends with closure of the aortic valve when the LV pressure falls below the aortic pressure and isovolumetric relaxation begins. The LV pressure continues to fall, and once left, atrial pressure exceeds LV pressure, the mitral valve opens, and diastolic filling begins. It is important to note that the height of the pressure volume loop (PVLP) equals the systolic blood pressure and the left ventricular end-diastolic pressure (LVEDP) also reflects pulmonary capillary wedge pressure (PCWP).[55] The time points representing end diastole and end systole are typically used to assess diastolic and systolic properties of the LV, respectively.

The *stroke volume* (SV) is defined by the width of the pressure-volume loop (ie, the difference end-diastolic volume [EDV] and end-systolic volume [ESV]) **(Figure 66.1B)**. The CO can be derived by multiplying the SV with the HR: CO = SV × HR. The LVEF is the percentage volume ejected per beat and thus can be derived as follows: LVEF = SV/EDV.

The lower end of the pressure-volume loop is defined by the end-diastolic pressure-volume relationship (EDPVR), the passive filling curve for the ventricle. THE EDPVR describes the amount of volume required to create a certain pressure in the LV and consequently the diastolic volume for a defined pressure. This relationship is reflected by LV chamber geometry, wall thickness, and myocardial structure. Thus, the EDPVR is nonlinear, and the slope defines diastolic stiffness, whereas ventricular compliance can be expressed as the reciprocal 1/EDPVR **(Figure 66.1C)**. EDPVR is altered in HF, reflecting the fact that diastolic stiffness increases with loading.[56]

The upper boundary of the pressure-volume loop is formed by the end-systolic pressure-volume relationship (ESPVR).

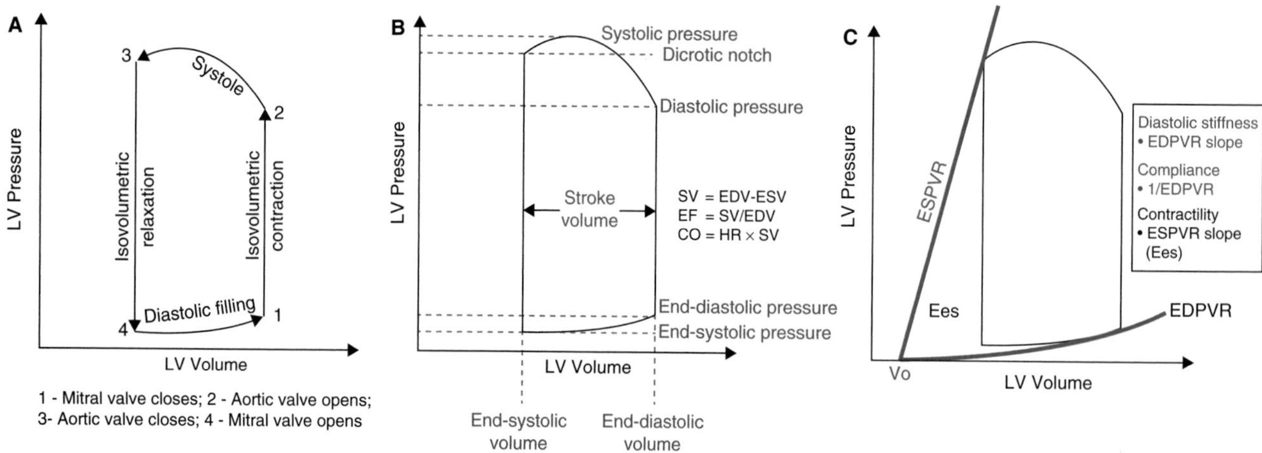

FIGURE 66.1 Pressure-volume loops. The four phases of the cardiac cycle are depicted in the pressure-volume loop by plotting left ventricular (LV) pressure against LV volumes **(A)**. These time points correlate with distinct pressures and volumes **(B)**. The end-diastolic pressure-volume relationship (EDPVR) is nonlinear and is descriptive of the diastolic properties of the LV (C). The end-systolic pressure-volume relationship (ESPVR) is linear and load independent, and its slope (Ees) describes the LV contractility **(C)**. CO, cardiac output; EDV, end-diastolic volume; Ees, end-systolic elastance; EF, ejection fraction; ESV, end-systolic volume; HR, heart rate; SV, stroke volume V_0, volume at end-systolic pressure of 0 mmHg. (Adapted from Burkhoff D, Wang J. Mechanical properties of the heart and its interaction with the vascular system. 2002.)

The ESPVR is linear and defined by the slope end-systolic elastance (Ees) and volume-axis intercept (Vo). ESPVR shifts occur with changes in ventricular contractility; in HFrEF, both ESPVR and EDPVR shift toward larger volumes but decreased SV (**Figure 66.2A, B**).

Importantly, Ees is independent of preload and afterload and is thus a load-independent marker of contractility. Ees increases with inotropic therapy, whereas an acute or chronic decrease in contractility will reduce the slope (**Figure 66.2C**). Ventricular preload and afterload define the shape and location of the loop. Preload is reflected by EDP or EDV (**Figure 66.2B**). Afterload is defined by the total peripheral resistance (TPR = mean arterial pressure/cardiac output) depicted as "effective arterial elastance" (Ea).[55] The failing LV in HFrEF is afterload sensitive, and small shifts in Ea can have drastic effects on the SV: this is in contrast to HFpEF. Thus, LVEF varies not only with contractility but also with afterload changes, whereas preload only has a minor effect (**Figure 66.2A**). When progressing from acute (**Figure 66.3A**) to chronic heart failure, EDPVR will shift up and to the right when pictured on the pressure-volume loop (**Figure 66.3B**). Diastolic capacity is reflective of chamber size and describes LV volume at a given pressure; it differs between conditions of hypertrophy (inappropriately reduced) versus LV dilation (increased).[55,56]

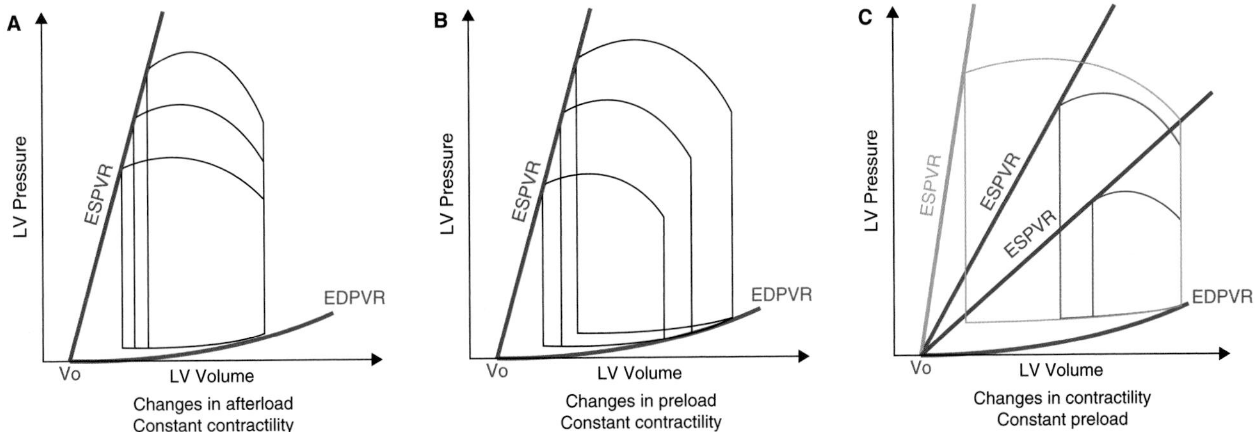

FIGURE 66.2 Changes in afterload, preload, and contractility. An increase in left ventricular (LV) afterload reduces stroke volume (SV) **(A)**. The failing LV in heart failure with reduced ejection fraction is very sensitive to afterload increase, and even a small change can reduce SV substantially. Under normal conditions, an increase in preload or contractility will increase the SV **(B, C)**. EDPVR, end-diastolic pressure-volume relationship; ESPVR, end-systolic pressure-volume relationship; LV, left ventricular V_0, volume at end-systolic pressure of 0 mmHg. (Adapted from Burkhoff D, Wang J. Mechanical properties of the heart and its interaction with the vascular system. 2002.)

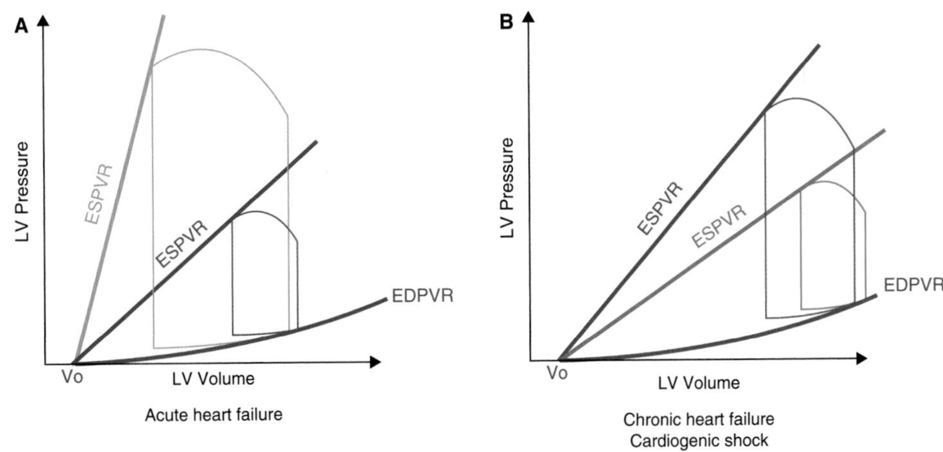

FIGURE 66.3 Acute and chronic heart failure. An acute decrease in contractility lowers blood pressure and stroke volume but will only have a minor effect on the end-diastolic pressure-volume relationship (EDPVR) **(A)**. In contrast, in chronic heart failure, the EDPVR moves up and to the right reflective of gradual increase in diastolic stiffness of the failing heart **(B)**. EDPVR, end-diastolic pressure-volume relationship; ESPVR, end-systolic pressure-volume relationship; LV, left ventricular V_0, volume at end-systolic pressure of 0 mmHg. (Adapted from Burkhoff D, Wang J. Mechanical properties of the heart and its interaction with the vascular system. 2002.)

KEY POINTS

- ✔ The definitions of symptomatic HF categories have recently been updated:
  - HF with reduced EF (HFrEF): symptomatic HF, LVEF ≤ 40%
  - HF with mid-range EF (HFmrEF): LVEF 41-49%
  - HF with preserved EF (HFpEF): LVEF 50%
  - HF with improved EF (HFimpEF): baseline LVEF ≤ 40%, a ≥ 10 point increase from baseline LVEF, and a second measurement of LVEF > 40%.
- ✔ The causative pathophysiology of HFrEF and HFpEF differs greatly despite a certain degree of overlap in risk factors with a greater link to inflammation in HFpEF.
- ✔ HFrEF is characterized by a vicious cycle of neuro-hormonal adaptive and maladaptive mechanisms triggered by decreased cardiac output and low blood pressure.
- ✔ Myocardial molecular structural and cellular changes including alterations in myocyte biology and gene expression such as switch to fetal gene program and changes in Beta-receptor and key Ca2+ signaling proteins are hallmarks of the adverse remodeling progress which further decreases contractility.
- ✔ Resulting advanced heart failure is an energy deficient state with loss of mitochondria and development of myocardial and systemic insulin resistance as well as cardiac cachexia.
- ✔ Pressure volume loops plot LV pressure against LV volumes throughout the cardiac cycle and can describe the interplay of loading conditions, afterload, and contractility in HF.
- ✔ In HFrEF in contrast to HFpEF even small changes in afterload can drastically reduce stroke volume. Consequently, LVEF not only varies with contractility but also with afterload whereas pre-load has a much smaller impact.

REFERENCES

1. Bozkurt B, Coats A, Tsutsui H, et al. A report of the Heart Failure Society of America, Heart Failure Association of the European Society of Cardiology, Japanese Heart Failure Society and Writing Committee of the Universal Definition of Heart Failure Consensus Conference. *Eur J Heart Fail.* 2021;23(3):352-380.
2. Borlaug BA. The pathophysiology of heart failure with preserved ejection fraction. *Nat Rev Cardiol.* 2014;11(9):507-515.
3. Murphy SP, Kakkar R, McCarthy CP, Januzzi JL Jr. Inflammation in Heart Failure: JACC State-of-the-Art Review. *J Am Coll Cardiol.* 2020;75(11):1324-1340.
4. Hartupee J, Mann DL. Neurohormonal activation in heart failure with reduced ejection fraction. *Nat Rev Cardiol.* 2017;14(1):30-38.
5. Giannoni A, Emdin M, Bramanti F, et al. Combined increased chemosensitivity to hypoxia and hypercapnia as a prognosticator in heart failure. *J Am Coll Cardiol.* 2009;53(21):1975-1980.
6. Weinberger MH, Aoi W, Henry DP. Direct effect of beta-adrenergic stimulation on renin release by the rat kidney slice in vitro. *Circ Res.* 1975;37(3):318-324.
7. Bekheirnia MR, Schrier RW. Pathophysiology of water and sodium retention: edematous states with normal kidney function. *Curr Opin Pharmacol.* 2006;6(2):202-207.
8. McCollum LT, Gallagher PE, Ann Tallant E. Angiotensin-(1-7) attenuates angiotensin II-induced cardiac remodeling associated with upregulation of dual-specificity phosphatase 1. *Am J Physiol Heart Circ Physiol.* 2012;302(3):H801-H810.
9. McMurray JJ, Packer M, Desai AS, et al. Angiotensin-neprilysin inhibition versus enalapril in heart failure. *N Engl J Med.* 2014;371(11):993-1004.
10. Lowes BD, Minobe W, Abraham WT, et al. Changes in gene expression in the intact human heart. Downregulation of alpha-myosin heavy chain in hypertrophied, failing ventricular myocardium. *J Clin Invest.* 1997;100(9):2315-2324.
11. Miyata S, Minobe W, Bristow MR, Leinwand LA. Myosin heavy chain isoform expression in the failing and nonfailing human heart. *Circ Res.* 2000;86(4):386-390.
12. Tan LB, Jalil JE, Pick R, Janicki JS, Weber KT. Cardiac myocyte necrosis induced by angiotensin II. *Circ Res.* 1991;69(5):1185-1195.
13. Todd GL, Baroldi G, Pieper GM, Clayton FC, Eliot RS. Experimental catecholamine-induced myocardial necrosis. I. Morphology, quantification and regional distribution of acute contraction band lesions. *J Mol Cell Cardiol.* 1985;17(4):317-338.
14. Kostin S, Pool L, Elsasser A, et al. Myocytes die by multiple mechanisms in failing human hearts. *Circ Res.* 2003;92(7):715-724.
15. Hynes RO. The extracellular matrix: not just pretty fibrils. *Science.* 2009;326(5957):1216-1219.
16. Sadoshima J, Izumo S. Molecular characterization of angiotensin II—induced hypertrophy of cardiac myocytes and hyperplasia of cardiac fibroblasts. Critical role of the AT1 receptor subtype. *Circ Res.* 1993;73(3):413-423.
17. Frangogiannis NG. The extracellular matrix in ischemic and nonischemic heart failure. *Circ Res.* 2019;125(1):117-146.
18. Yokoyama T, Vaca L, Rossen RD, Durante W, Hazarika P, Mann DL. Cellular basis for the negative inotropic effects of tumor necrosis factor-alpha in the adult mammalian heart. *J Clin Invest.* 1993;92(5):2303-2312.
19. McTiernan CF, Lemster BH, Frye C, Brooks S, Combes A, Feldman AM. Interleukin-1 beta inhibits phospholamban gene expression in cultured cardiomyocytes. *Circ Res.* 1997;81(4):493-503.
20. Yokoyama T, Nakano M, Bednarczyk JL, McIntyre BW, Entman M, Mann DL. Tumor necrosis factor-alpha provokes a hypertrophic growth response in adult cardiac myocytes. *Circulation.* 1997;95(5):1247-1252.
21. Li YY, McTiernan CF, Feldman AM. Proinflammatory cytokines regulate tissue inhibitors of metalloproteinases and disintegrin metalloproteinase in cardiac cells. *Cardiovasc Res.* 1999;42(1):162-172.
22. Thomas JA, Marks BH. Plasma norepinephrine in congestive heart failure. *Am J Cardiol.* 1978;41(2):233-243.
23. Communal C, Singh K, Pimentel DR, Colucci WS. Norepinephrine stimulates apoptosis in adult rat ventricular myocytes by activation of the beta-adrenergic pathway. *Circulation.* 1998;98(13):1329-1334.
24. Fowler MB, Laser JA, Hopkins GL, Minobe W, Bristow MR. Assessment of the beta-adrenergic receptor pathway in the intact failing human heart: progressive receptor down-regulation and subsensitivity to agonist response. *Circulation.* 1986;74(6):1290-1302.
25. Port JD, Bristow MR. Altered beta-adrenergic receptor gene regulation and signaling in chronic heart failure. *J Mol Cell Cardiol.* 2001;33(5):887-905.
26. Iaccarino G, Tomhave ED, Lefkowitz RJ, Koch WJ. Reciprocal in vivo regulation of myocardial G protein-coupled receptor kinase expression by beta-adrenergic receptor stimulation and blockade. *Circulation.* 1998;98(17):1783-1789.
27. Najafi A, Sequeira V, Kuster DW, van der Velden J. beta-adrenergic receptor signalling and its functional consequences in the diseased heart. *Eur J Clin Invest.* 2016;46(4):362-374.
28. Bernstein D, Fajardo G, Zhao M. The role of beta-adrenergic receptors in heart failure: differential regulation of cardiotoxicity and cardioprotection. *Prog Pediatr Cardiol.* 2011;31(1):35-38.
29. Luo M, Anderson ME. Mechanisms of altered Ca(2)(+) handling in heart failure. *Circ Res.* 2013;113(6):690-708.
30. Schwinger RH, Munch G, Bolck B, Karczewski P, Krause EG, Erdmann E. Reduced Ca(2+)-sensitivity of SERCA 2a in failing human myocardium due to reduced serin-16 phospholamban phosphorylation. *J Mol Cell Cardiol.* 1999;31(3):479-491.

31. Kushnir A, Wajsberg B, Marks AR. Ryanodine receptor dysfunction in human disorders. *Biochim Biophys Acta Mol Cell Res.* 2018;1865(11 Pt B):1687-1697.
32. Kubo H, Margulies KB, Piacentino V 3rd, Gaughan JP, Houser SR. Patients with end-stage congestive heart failure treated with beta-adrenergic receptor antagonists have improved ventricular myocyte calcium regulatory protein abundance. *Circulation.* 2001;104(9):1012-1018.
33. Glatz JFC, Nabben M, Young ME, Schulze PC, Taegtmeyer H, Luiken J. Re-balancing cellular energy substrate metabolism to mend the failing heart. *Biochim Biophys Acta Mol Basis Dis.* 2020;1866(5):165579.
34. Razeghi P, Young ME, Alcorn JL, Moravec CS, Frazier OH, Taegtmeyer H. Metabolic gene expression in fetal and failing human heart. *Circulation.* 2001;104(24):2923-2931.
35. Stanley WC, Recchia FA, Lopaschuk GD. Myocardial substrate metabolism in the normal and failing heart. *Physiol Rev.* 2005;85(3):1093-1129.
36. Zhang L, Jaswal JS, Ussher JR, et al. Cardiac insulin-resistance and decreased mitochondrial energy production precede the development of systolic heart failure after pressure-overload hypertrophy. *Circ Heart Fail.* 2013;6(5):1039-1048.
37. Kretzschmar T, Wu JMF, Schulze PC. Mitochondrial homeostasis mediates lipotoxicity in the failing myocardium. *Int J Mol Sci.* 2021;22(3):1498.
38. Chokshi A, Drosatos K, Cheema FH, et al. Ventricular assist device implantation corrects myocardial lipotoxicity, reverses insulin resistance, and normalizes cardiac metabolism in patients with advanced heart failure. *Circulation.* 2012;125(23):2844-2853.
39. Khan RS, Kato TS, Chokshi A, et al. Adipose tissue inflammation and adiponectin resistance in patients with advanced heart failure: correction after ventricular assist device implantation. *Circ Heart Fail.* 2012;5(3):340-348.
40. Lommi J, Kupari M, Koskinen P, et al. Blood ketone bodies in congestive heart failure. *J Am Coll Cardiol.* 1996;28(3):665-672.
41. Verma S, Rawat S, Ho KL, et al. Empagliflozin increases cardiac energy production in diabetes: novel translational insights into the heart failure benefits of SGLT2 inhibitors. *JACC Basic Transl Sci.* 2018;3(5):575-587.
42. Shao Q, Meng L, Lee S, et al. Empagliflozin, a sodium glucose co-transporter-2 inhibitor, alleviates atrial remodeling and improves mitochondrial function in high-fat diet/streptozotocin-induced diabetic rats. *Cardiovasc Diabetol.* 2019;18(1):165.
43. Lopaschuk GD, Verma S. *Mechanisms of cardiovascular benefits of sodium glucose co-transporter* 2 (SGLT2) inhibitors: A State-of-the-Art Review. *JACC Basic Transl Sci.* 2020;5(6):632-644.
44. Sabbah HN, Gupta RC, Kohli S, et al. Chronic therapy with a partial adenosine A1-receptor agonist improves left ventricular function and remodeling in dogs with advanced heart failure. *Circ Heart Fail.* 2013;6(3):563-571.
45. Staehr PM, Dhalla AK, Zack J, et al. Reduction of free fatty acids, safety, and pharmacokinetics of oral GS-9667, an A(1) adenosine receptor partial agonist. *J Clin Pharmacol.* 2013;53(4):385-392.
46. Bayeva M, Sawicki KT, Ardehali H. Taking diabetes to heart–deregulation of myocardial lipid metabolism in diabetic cardiomyopathy. *J Am Heart Assoc.* 2013;2(6):e000433.
47. Opie LH, Knuuti J. The adrenergic-fatty acid load in heart failure. *J Am Coll Cardiol.* 2009;54(18):1637-1646.
48. Paolisso G, Manzella D, Rizzo MR, et al. Elevated plasma fatty acid concentrations stimulate the cardiac autonomic nervous system in healthy subjects. *Am J Clin Nutr.* 2000;72(3):723-730.
49. Doehner W, von Haehling S, Anker SD. Insulin resistance in chronic heart failure. *J Am Coll Cardiol.* 2008;52(3):239; author reply 239-240.
50. Riehle C, Abel ED. Insulin signaling and heart failure. *Circ Res.* 2016;118(7):1151-1169.
51. Underwood PC, Adler GK. The renin angiotensin aldosterone system and insulin resistance in humans. *Curr Hypertens Rep.* 2013;15(1):59-70.
52. Sauder MA, Liu J, Jahn LA, Fowler DE, Chai W, Liu Z. Candesartan acutely recruits skeletal and cardiac muscle microvasculature in healthy humans. *J Clin Endocrinol Metab.* 2012;97(7):E1208-E1212.
53. Yamauchi S, Takeishi Y, Minamihaba O, et al. Angiotensin-converting enzyme inhibition improves cardiac fatty acid metabolism in patients with congestive heart failure. *Nucl Med Commun.* 2003;24(8):901-906.
54. Nguyen AB, Imamura T, Besser S, et al. Metabolic dysfunction in continuous-flow left ventricular assist devices patients and outcomes. *J Am Heart Assoc.* 2019;8(22):e013278.
55. Burkhoff D, Wang J. Mechanical properties of the heart and its interaction with the vascular system. 2002:1-23.
56. Ten Brinke EA, Burkhoff D, Klautz RJ, et al. Single-beat estimation of the left ventricular end-diastolic pressure-volume relationship in patients with heart failure. *Heart.* 2010;96(3):213-219.

CHAPTER 67

GENETICS OF CARDIOMYOPATHIES

Gary S. Beasley, Hugo Martinez, and Jeffrey A. Towbin

INTRODUCTION

Primary cardiomyopathies, which include dilated cardiomyopathy (DCM), hypertrophic cardiomyopathy (HCM), restrictive cardiomyopathy (RCM), arrhythmogenic cardiomyopathy (ACM), and left ventricular noncompaction cardiomyopathy (LVNC), remain major causes of morbidity and mortality in the world.[1-4] These classified forms of cardiomyopathy have diverse clinical, structural, morphological, and functional presentations. Among the various types of cardiomyopathies, DCM represents the most common form in adults and children, accounting for approximately 40% of all cases in children. This is followed by HCM, LVNC, and, least commonly, ACM and RCM.[1-4]

After over three decades of genetic and molecular research, many causative genes have been identified, and overlap in the genetic causes of the various forms of cardiomyopathies have also been identified in which defects in the same gene could lead to allelic disorders.[1-8] Generally, there are mechanistic "final common pathways" that predominate for each of the forms of cardiomyopathy (**Figure 67.1**).[9,10] For instance, DCM is typically caused by variants in genes encoding structural proteins such as cytoskeletal and sarcomeric proteins and, in this case, usually presents with features of heart failure.[10] HCM is considered a disease of the sarcomere and usually presents with syncope or sudden death and may develop features of heart failure with preserved ejection fraction (HFpEF).[11-13] Arrhythmias, which are most commonly caused by pathogenic variants in genes encoding ion channels when isolated, may also be a late manifestation in DCM or other forms of cardiomyopathy.[14] This chapter will present the different forms of cardiomyopathy and what is currently known about the genetic basis and the pathophysiological mechanisms responsible for the disorders.

DILATED CARDIOMYOPATHY

Dilated cardiomyopathy (DCM) is characterized by an enlarged left ventricular chamber, left ventricular wall thinning, and systolic dysfunction in the absence of abnormal loading conditions (ie, hypertension and valvular disease) or coronary artery disease sufficient to cause global systolic impairment (**Figure 67.2A**).[1-5,15] Individuals with DCM commonly present with symptomatic heart failure, arrhythmias, or conduction disturbance.[1-4] DCM in children has an estimated incidence of approximately 0.57 per 100,000 cases compared with the report of 1/2500 incidence in adult subjects.[16] However, the actual incidences could be far higher because of the reduced

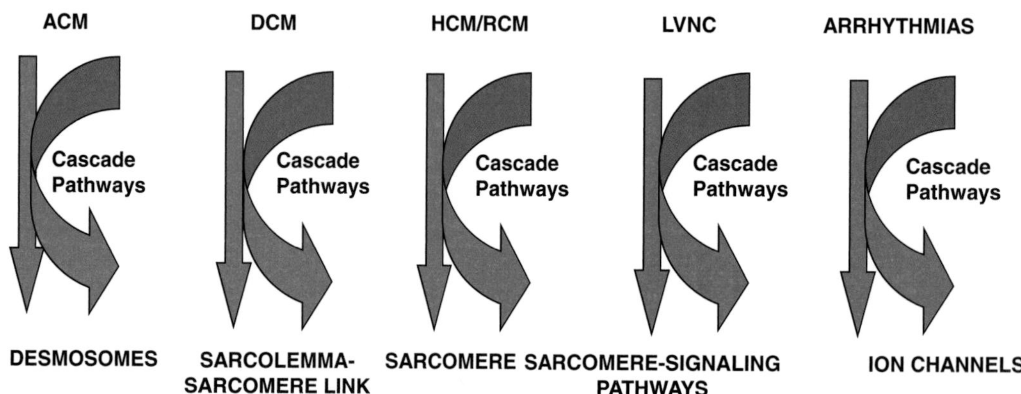

FIGURE 67.1 Primary pathways responsible for the different cardiomyopathy and arrhythmia phenotypes. The cascade pathways include interacting proteins, medications, mitochondrial disturbance, or other modifying factors. ACM, arrhythmogenic cardiomyopathy; DCM, dilated cardiomyopathy; HCM, hypertrophic cardiomyopathy; LVNC, left ventricular noncompaction; RCM, restrictive cardiomyopathy.

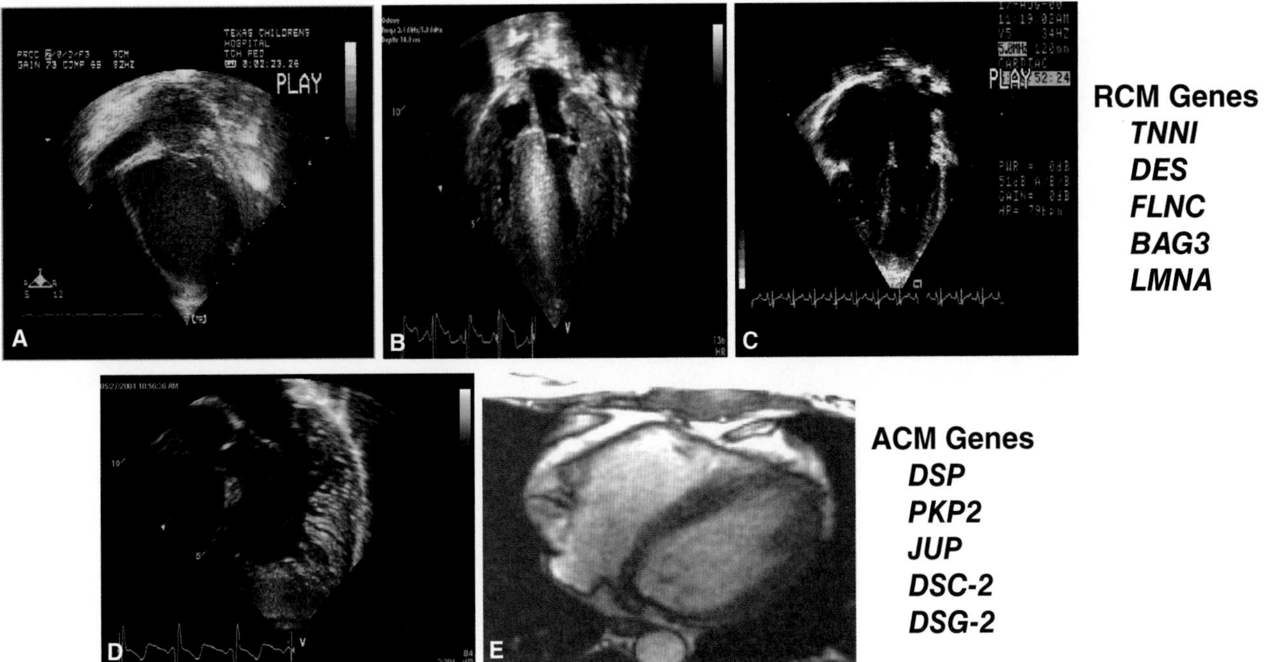

FIGURE 67.2 The different forms of classified cardiomyopathies. Causative genes for restrictive cardiomyopathy (RCM) and arrhythmogenic cardiomyopathy (ACM). **A.** Dilated cardiomyopathy with dilated left ventricle and depressed systolic function. **B.** Hypertrophic cardiomyopathy with severe hypertrophy, small ventricular chambers, and mildly dilated left atrium. Systolic function is hypercontractile, and there is diastolic dysfunction. **C.** Restrictive cardiomyopathy with dilated atria, normal ventricular size and systolic function, and diastolic dysfunction. **D.** Left ventricular noncompaction cardiomyopathy. Note the heavy trabeculations in the left ventricular apex and posterior wall. **E.** Cardiac magnetic resonance imaging of arrhythmogenic right ventricular cardiomyopathy. Note the markedly dilated right ventricle.

detection rate caused by incomplete penetrance and variable expressivity observed in DCM, which can lead to a prolonged asymptomatic period preceding the development of overt heart failure.[1-4,16] A disease prevalence of 1:250 to 500 for DCM has been reported in adults.[17]

Although a proportion of DCM could be attributed to infections causing myocarditis, with reports estimating 16% to 34% of DCM cases in childhood and 12% to 17% in adults in North America,[1,2,8,16,18-20] a large fraction of DCM is genetic in origin. These may be either sporadic, if there is no previous family history and screening of first-degree relatives is negative, or familial, if it occurs in two or more close relatives.[1-4,16] Although familial DCM is reported in approximately 20% to 35% of adult cases,[15,21,22] it is estimated to occur in up to 67% of cases after accurate screening of the relatives of idiopathic DCM subjects.[8] Most cases are inherited as autosomal dominant, X-linked, or autosomal recessive traits, and, less frequently, as mitochondrial inheritance.[23-26] In approximately 30% of familial cases, a genetic cause can be identified.

DCM is caused by disturbances in "final common pathways" that result in disturbance of force transmission and can include sarcomere, Z-disk, and cytoskeleton proteins that are affected by relevant gene mutations.[6,8-10] Genes encoding proteins of the ion channels, the nuclear envelope, mitochondrial proteins, transcription factors, and heat shock chaperones are alternative sites of gene mutation[27] (**Table 67.1**). Although more than 100 genes are implicated as mutation targets in familial DCM, very few of them have been shown to account for greater than or equal 5% of this disease.[28] Most of the genes with pathogenic mutations are missense mutations (different amino acids in a protein sequence), but nonsense, frameshift, deletion, and other forms of mutations may occur. "Private" or unique to a family and very rare mutations are the standard finding in DCM.[29,30]

In DCM, pathogenic gene variants that affect critical pathways of contractile function, ion distribution, or cellular function have the potential to result in a DCM phenotype. This was initially demonstrated by the identification of the dystrophin (*DMD*) gene, the gene responsible for Duchenne and Becker muscular dystrophy and causative of the associated skeletal myopathy and DCM. The *DMD* gene was subsequently identified as the gene responsible for the X-linked form of DCM as well.[31,32] However, defects in the *DMD* gene could explain only a fraction of all DCM cases; later, other genes responsible for DCM were identified, defining DCM as a genetically heterogeneous entity. Based on these findings, we formulated the "final common pathway" hypothesis (1998) in which it was suggested that abnormalities in other genes encoding for dystrophin-associated proteins and proteins involved in the structural formation and maintenance of cardiomyocyte structure and contractile function could also potentially lead to the development of DCM.[9,10] It is now known that

TABLE 67.1 Genes Associated With Cardiomyopathies and Their Allelic Disorders

Gene	OMIM[a]	Locus	Gene Name[b]	Associated Phenotypes[b]
ABCC9	601439	12p12.1	ATP-binding cassette, sub-family C (CFTR/MRP), member 9	DCM
ACTC1	102540	15q14	Actin, α, cardiac muscle 1	DCM HCM RCM
ACTN2	102573	1q42-q43	Actinin, α 2	DCM HCM
BAG3	603883	10q25.2-q26.2	BCL2-associated athanogene 3	MFM DCM
CSRP3	600824	11p15.1	Cysteine and glycine-rich protein 3 (cardiac LIM protein)	DCM LVNC HCM
DES	125660	2q35	Desmin	MFM DCM RCM
DMD	300377	Xp21.2	Dystrophin	DMD BMD DCM
DSC2	125645	18q12.1	Desmocollin 2	ARVC
DSG2	125671	18q12.1	Desmoglein 2	ARVC ALVC DCM
DSP	125647	6p24	Desmoplakin	ARVC ALVC DCM
DTNA	601239	18q12.1	Dystrobrevin, α	LVNC
EMD	300384	Xq28	Emerin	EDMD DCM
EYA4	603550	6q23-q24	Eyes absent homolog 4 (Drosophila)	DFNA DCM
FKTN	607440	9q31	Fukutin	FCMD DCM
HCN4	605206	15q24.1	Hyperpolarization activated cyclic nucleotide-gated potassium channel 4	LVNC CD MVP
HSPB7	610692	1p36.13	Heat shock 27kDa protein family, member 7	DCM
JUP	173325	17q21	Junctional plakoglobin	ARVC ND
LAMP2	309060	Xq24	Lysosomal-associated membrane protein 2	DD HCM DCM
LDB3	605906	10q22-q23	LIM-domain binding 3	DCM ± LVNC MFM
LMNA	150330	1q21.2	Lamin A/C	DCM ± CD CMT2B1 EDMD HGPS LGMD MADA FPLD2

TABLE 67.1 Genes Associated With Cardiomyopathies and Their Allelic Disorders *(Continued)*

Gene	OMIM[a]	Locus	Gene Name[b]	Associated Phenotypes[b]
MYBPC3	600958	11p11.2	Myosin-binding protein C, cardiac	DCM HCM
MYH6	160710	14q12	Myosin, heavy chain 6, cardiac muscle, α	DCM HCM
MYH7	160760	14q12	Myosin, heavy chain 7, cardiac muscle, β	DCM HCM RCM LVNC
MYL2	160781	12q23-q24	Myosin, light chain 2, regulatory, cardiac, slow	HCM
MYL3	160790	3p21.3-21.2	Myosin, light chain 3, alkali light chain; ventricular isoform, skeletal isoform, slow	HCM
MYPN	608517	10q21.1	Myopalladin	DCM RCM HCM
NEBL	605491	10p13-p12	Nebulette	DCM
NEXN	613121	1p31.1	Nexilin (F actin binding protein)	DCM HCM
PKP2	602861	12p11	Plakophilin 2	ARVC
PKP4	604276	2q23-q31	Plakophilin 4	ARVC
PLN	172405	6q22.1	Phospholamban	DCM
PRKAG2	602743	7q36.1	Protein kinase, AMP-activated, γ2 noncatalytic subunit	HCM ± WPW FCNCG
PSEN1	104311	14q24.3	Presenilin 1	AD DCM FAI
PSEN2	600759	1q31-q42	Presenilin 2 (Alzheimer disease 4)	AD-4 DCM
RBM20	613171	10q25.2	RNA binding motif protein 20	DCM
RYR2	180902	1q43	Ryanodine receptor 2 (cardiac)	ARVC CPVT1
SCN5A	600163	3p21	Sodium channel, voltage-gated, type V, α subunit	BRS LQTS DCM ± CD
SGCB	600900	13q12	Sarcoglycan, β	LGMD2E DCM
SGCD	601411	5q33-q34	Sarcoglycan, delta	LGMD2F DCM
TAZ	300394	Xq28	Tafazzin	BTS LVNC DCM
TCAP	604488	17q12	Titin-cap (telethonin)	LGMD2G HCM DCM
TGFB3	190230	14q24	Transforming growth factor, β 3	ARVC
TMEM43	612048	3p25.1	Transmembrane protein 43	ARVC
TMPO	188380	12q22	Thymopoietin	DCM
TNNC1	191040	3p21.1	Troponin C type 1 (slow)	DCM HCM

(continued)

TABLE 67.1 Genes Associated With Cardiomyopathies and Their Allelic Disorders *(Continued)*

Gene	OMIM[a]	Locus	Gene Name[b]	Associated Phenotypes[b]
TNNI3	191044	19q13.4	Troponin I type 3 (cardiac)	DCM HCM RCM
TNNT2	191045	1q32	Troponin T type 2 (cardiac)	DCM HCM RCM
TPM1	191010	15q22.1	Tropomyosin 1 (α)	DCM HCM
TTN	188840	2q31	Titin	TMD LGMD2J EOMFC DCM HCM HMERF
VCL	193065	10q22.1-q23	Vinculin	DCM HCM

[a]OMIM, online Mendelian inheritance in man (http://www.ncbi.nlm.nih.gov/omim)
[b]Genetic Home References (http://ghr.nlm.nih.gov/)
AD, Alzheimer disease; ARVC, arrhythmogenic right ventricular cardiomyopathy; ATP, adenosine triphosphate; BCL-2, B-cell lymphoma 2; BMD, Becker muscular dystrophy; BRS, Brugada syndrome; CD, conduction defects; CFTR, cystic fibrosis transmembrane conductance regulator; CMT2B1, Charcot-Marie-Tooth disease type 2B1; CPVT, catecholaminergic polymorphic ventricular tachycardia; DCM, dilated cardiomyopathy; DD, Danon disease; DFNA, autosomal dominant late-onset progressive nonsyndromic deafness; DMD, Duchenne muscular dystrophy; EDMD, Emery-Dreifuss muscular dystrophy; EOMFC, early-onset myopathy with fatal cardiomyopathy; FAI, familial acne inverse; FCMD, Fukuyama congenital muscular dystrophy; FCNCG, fatal congenital nonlysosomal cardiac glycogenosis; FPLD2, familial partial lipodystrophy of the Dunnigan type; HCM, hypertrophic cardiomyopathy; HGPS, Hutchinson-Gilford progeria syndrome; HMERF, myopathy with early respiratory muscle involvement; LGMD, limb-girdle muscular dystrophy; LQTS, long-QT syndrome; LVNC, left ventricular noncompaction; MADA, mandibuloacral dysplasia type A with partial lipodystrophy; MFM, myofibrillar myopathy; MRP, multidrug resistance-associated protein; MVP, mitral valve prolapse; ND, Naxos disease; nNOS, neuronal nitric oxide synthase; RCM, restrictive cardiomyopathy; TMD, tibial muscular dystrophy, tardive; VCFS, velocardiofacial syndrome; WPW, Wolff-Parkinson-White syndrome.

perturbation of cardiomyocyte proteins involved in contractile force generation and transmission (eg, cytoskeletal, sarcomeric, and ion channel proteins) are involved in the pathogenesis of DCM.[6-8,11-14,17,27,33] *In vitro* models and animal models recapitulating the human disease suggest that alteration of the protein continuum connecting the cardiomyocyte plasma membrane (sarcolemma) to the sarcomere, and through the intermediate filaments, to the perinuclear membrane, can lead to a transient hypertrophic phase, followed by decompensated systolic performance, left ventricular wall thinning, and left ventricular chamber dilation.[34-36]

Additionally, more than 30 genes identified to cause DCM in isolation, genes have also been identified that are associated with syndromic forms of DCM, such as genes involved in metabolism and mitochondrial function, besides loci allelic to other cardiomyopathic phenotypes.[37] In particular, primary diseases of the skeletal muscle, such as various forms of muscular dystrophy and other skeletal myopathies, frequently present with a DCM phenotype.[38-41]

Despite the large number of genes associated with DCM, they account for only approximately 40% of all cases. Horvat et al performed genetic screening in 532 DCM patients and 527 healthy control subjects.[42] Variants that were protein-altering (truncating, missense) and rare (defined here by minor allele frequency less than 0.1% in the European subgroup in the Exome Sequencing Project database) in a set of 41 cardiomyopathy-associated genes were evaluated. Variants that met these criteria were found in 407 (77%) DCM cases and in 348 (66%) control subjects ($P = .0002$), with the number of rare variants per person ranging from 0 to 13 (mean 1.63) in DCM cases and from 0 to 8 (mean 1.24) in controls ($P < .0001$). With notable exceptions—such as titin (*TTN*), lamin A/C (*LMNA*), β-myosin heavy chain 7 (*MYH7*), and RNA binding motif protein 20 (*RBM20*)—relatively few genes carried a statistically significant excess burden of rare variants in DCM versus control cases.[42] Indeed, from a comprehensive search of publications that included family studies, in vitro data, and animal models, we found that only 14 of 41 genes (34%) represented on two genetic testing panels had robust genetic and functional evidence for roles in DCM causation.[42] Interestingly, this refined set of 14 genes encoded a range of cardiomyocyte components and did not alter the prevailing hypothesis that familial DCM has heterogeneous molecular origins.[42]

In addition, genes encoding for ion channels, such as the cardiac sodium channel (*SCN5A*), which causes long-QT syndrome (LQTS) and Brugada syndrome, is also implicated in the pathogenesis of DCM and, in particular, mutations in *SCN5A* that affect the S4-voltage sensor are seen in subjects with DCM and arrhythmias.[14,43-46] This suggests that ion channels not only influence the electrocardiographic (ECG) findings and potentiate arrhythmias in DCM[14] but may also weaken the cardiomyocytes structure leading to DCM and vice versa, as demonstrated in a mouse model harboring the *LDB3*-encoded ZASP (Z-band alternatively spliced PDZ-motif) mutation causing DCM in humans.[47] Another potential mechanism, particularly in the case of SCN5A, is its relationship with dystrophin. SCN5A binds to dystrophin and could potentially disrupt the function of dystrophin and lead to a dystrophin-related cardiomyopathy, as would be predicted by the "final common pathway" hypothesis.[9,10]

Clinically, the presentation of idiopathic, acquired, and genetic forms of DCM is indistinguishable. This suggests that clinical evaluation of relatives of children with DCM should always be considered when a diagnosis of DCM is reached. Unfortunately, a significant proportion of DCM remains idiopathic, where a firm etiologic diagnosis cannot be reached. This suggests that more genes are yet to be discovered and that modifiers likely play a significant role in disease development.

HYPERTROPHIC CARDIOMYOPATHY

Hypertrophic cardiomyopathy (HCM) is one of the most common genetic disorders with a prevalence of 1/500, representing one of the most frequent causes of sudden cardiac death in young athletes in the United States.[48,49] HCM is characterized by excessive thickening generally limited to the left ventricular myocardium and interventricular septum, in the absence of conditions that increase afterload such as aortic stenosis or systemic hypertension, and morphologically is typically characterized by myocyte disarray (**Figure 67.2B**).[3,4,8,49] The interventricular septal thickening most commonly demonstrates asymmetric hypertrophy but focal areas of septal hypertrophy or concentric hypertrophy may occur. Left ventricular outflow tract obstruction may also occur. Individuals with HCM may be asymptomatic or present with or develop signs of heart failure or sudden death.[48,49] Clinical presentations therefore include syncope or nonresuscitated sudden death, dyspnea, diaphoresis, chest pain, palpitations, or arrhythmias. The age of onset of HCM-related symptoms varies from infancy to adulthood. However, most appear in adolescence.[49]

As previously described for DCM, primary HCM has a genetic basis in most cases. Many genes, with many encoding for sarcomeric proteins[11] that are mainly involved in force generation, have been identified to cause HCM, and many of them are allelic to DCM and other cardiomyopathies (**Table 67.1**).[50]

Similar to DCM, HCM is characterized by significant genetic and allelic heterogeneity and variable expressivity.[11-13] However, contrary to DCM, genetic testing in HCM using the current technology has a high-detection rate because mutations in four sarcomeric genes, β-myosin heavy chain (*MYH7)*, myosin-binding protein C (*MYBPC3)*, cardiac troponin T (*TNNT2)*, and cardiac troponin I (*TNNI3*), appear to cause approximately 80% of all familial HCM cases. Mutations can also be identified in about 40% of sporadic and idiopathic cases of HCM.[11] Although genotype-phenotype correlation is imperfect, it has been reported that mutations in *MYH7* are associated with early-onset disease, and in some cases, a more severe phenotype, while *MYBPC3* mutations have been identified in subjects with later onset presentation, and *TNNT2* mutations are associated with a high incidence of sudden cardiac death.[11,51] That said, both *MYH7* and *MYBPC3* mutations have been identified in children as young as less than 1 year of age.[52-54]

HCM is a monogenic disorder in most cases, although double heterozygote mutations have been described and may be associated with earlier-onset and a more dramatic phenotype.[11,55]

Despite the high-detection rate of clinical genetic testing in HCM, the lack of good genotype-phenotype correlation has lessened the clinical utility of genetic screening in affected patients, although this is improving. Lopes et al demonstrated that the presence of any sarcomere variant is associated with an asymmetric septal hypertrophy pattern, younger age at presentation, family history of HCM and sudden cardiac death, and female gender.[56] This study also showed that patients with pathogenic variants in sarcomeric genes and proteins had higher cardiovascular and sudden death-related mortality during follow-up. Patients with more than one pathogenic sarcomere variant had more sudden cardiac death risk markers, consistent with previously published suggestions of a gene dose effect.[13,26-28,57,58] A low number of outcome events occurred during follow-up, and this may have biased the survival analysis and precluded an analysis of other associations, including the effect of carrying multiple compared with single variants. More recently, Robyns and colleagues, using the stringent American College of Medical Genetics and Genomics (ACMG)/Association for Molecular Pathology (AMP) criteria, identified a mutation in 37% of patients studied with the majority of them in MYBPC3, MYH7, and the troponin complex.[59] The genetic yield was very similar to what was previously published in a large cohort of almost 3000 unselected index patients.[59] Patients with a mutation were younger at diagnosis and had more severe disease including more pronounced hypertrophy and more frequent syncope. However, the sudden cardiac death rate was very similar. *MYBPC3* mutation carriers had a worse outcome compared with troponin complex mutations and a trend toward worse outcome compared to *MYH7* mutation carriers and mutation-negative patients. This contrasts with earlier reports claiming worse survival in *MYH7* mutation carriers compared with *MYBPC3*.[60,61] In addition, the presence of negative T waves in the lateral ECG leads was a negative predictor of carrying a mutation.

In addition, clinical genetic testing is quite useful for the screening of clinically affected and unaffected family members because of the lack of symptoms in most people with HCM and the relatively high risk of sudden death compared to the general population. Genetic counseling by trained professionals is highly recommended for accurate familial risk assessment and to reduce the potential psychological impact of the genetic testing.

ARRHYTHMOGENIC CARDIOMYOPATHY

Arrhythmogenic cardiomyopathy (ACM) is defined as an arrhythmogenic heart muscle disorder, which is not explained by ischemic, hypertensive, or valvular heart disease. ACM is relatively uncommon, with an estimated prevalence of between 1/1000 and 1/5000.[62] It is characterized by frequent sustained ventricular arrhythmias (average 10.6% per year)[63] progressive ventricular dysfunction (deterioration in right ventricular fractional area change averaging 0.7% per year)[64] and a high risk of sudden cardiac death. Patients typically present between 12 and 50 years of age with symptoms associated with arrhythmias but pediatric and elderly cases have been described.[65] Clinical presentation may be with symptoms or documentation of atrial fibrillation, conduction disease, and right or left ventricular arrhythmia.[66] In addition to the distinguishing feature of ACM being the clinical presentation with documented or symptomatic arrhythmia, the ACM phenotype may overlap with other cardiomyopathies, particularly DCM, where the arrhythmia presentation may be associated with moderate to severe ventricular dilatation and impaired systolic function (eg, arrhythmogenic right ventricular cardiomyopathy [ARVC], arrhythmogenic left ventricular cardiomyopathy [ALVC], or arrhythmogenic DCM [aDCM] caused by *desmoplakin, filamin C, lamin A/C, SCN5A,* or *phospholamban* variants).[63-65] Like all forms of genetically based cardiovascular disease, the mechanisms responsible for the phenotype that develops also rely on the dysfunction of final common protein pathways.[66,67] This distinction between an arrhythmic versus a heart failure presentation in patients who fulfill current DCM diagnostic criteria is important, as the genetic basis, sudden death risk, prognosis, and focus of management are different in these two scenarios.[66-74]

ARRHYTHMOGENIC RIGHT VENTRICULAR CARDIOMYOPATHY

ARVC is a myocardial disease, morphologically characterized by fibrosis with or without fatty infiltration and dilation of the right ventricle, along with thinning of the right ventricular wall, arrhythmias, and sudden cardiac death.[66] Left ventricular involvement may also be identified.[66] This patient group will be more fully described later.

ARVC is often diagnosed secondary to arrhythmias, palpitations, syncope, and aborted sudden death.[62,63,66,69] ARVC can manifest in the early teenage years with the majority of patients being in their late teenage years or young adulthood, especially in athletes.[75,76] ARVC is predominantly genetically determined and often inherited within families, mostly as an autosomal dominant trait with reduced penetrance and variable expression.[66] However, autosomal recessive inheritance has been observed in individuals affected by Naxos disease presenting with ARVC, diffuse nonepidermolytic palmoplantar keratoderma, and woolly hair, as well as in Carvajal syndrome, characterized by striate palmoplantar keratoderma, woolly hair, and left ventricular cardiomyopathy.[73,77-79]

The histopathology of ARVC demonstrates replacement of myocytes by fibrous or fibroadipose tissue in the right ventricular free wall. Lesions extend from the epicardium to the endocardium and predominantly involve the area between the anterior part of the pulmonary infundibulum, the apex, and the infero-posterior wall (the so-called "triangle of dysplasia"). Myocyte loss and fibrous replacement are most often segmental and usually do not involve the interventricular septum. Left ventricular histological involvement in the infero-lateral wall is frequently reported in autopsy cases or explanted hearts, even in the absence of macroscopic left ventricular involvement.[66,80-83] This left ventricular involvement has led to the term "quadrangle of ARVC." Lymphocytic or histiocytic inflammatory infiltrates, focal necrosis, and signs of apoptosis are frequent.[83] Diagnostic assessment for ARVC includes cardiac magnetic resonance imaging (CMRI), echocardiography, and ECG.[66,73] The CMRI classically demonstrates a dilated right ventricle with wall thinning and fatty replacement of the myocardium, systolic dysfunction, and the right ventricular outflow tract may be aneurysmal.[66,84,85] Late gadolinium enhancement (LGE) on CMRI typically identifies areas of fibrosis. The left ventricle may also be affected with a DCM appearance. The echocardiogram may demonstrate a dilated right or left ventricle with systolic dysfunction, and the ECG demonstrates T-wave inversion in leads V_1 through V_3, QRS duration 110 ms in V_1 through V_3, an epsilon wave (electric potentials after the end of the QRS complex), an ST-elevation pattern similar to that seen in Brugada syndrome may be noted, and a prolonged S-wave upstroke in V_1 through V_3 measuring 55 ms.[66,73] Right ventricular endomyocardial biopsy may be definitive when typical fibrofatty replacement of the myocardium and inflammation is visible; this is more obvious in advanced disease.[66,73] Commonly, only fibrosis and inflammatory infiltrates are seen, particularly in earlier disease presentations. Since the primary area of fibrofatty replacement is in the "triangle of dysplasia" in the apical and infundibular regions of the right ventricle, this makes a biopsy diagnosis more challenging. Autopsy or explant after transplantation will commonly demonstrate classic histopathologic diagnostic criteria.[73]

ACM is currently considered a genetically determined, autosomal dominant inherited disease with reduced penetrance and variable clinical expression.[66,73] It is considered a disease of the desmosomes since causative variants in genes coding for desmosomal components are found in about 50% of ACM patients.[86] Variants in nondesmosomal genes have been reported in a minority (1%-3%) of ACM patients (**Table 67.1**).[66] Most of the genes causing ARVC encode proteins of the cardiac desmosome such as plakoglobin (PG), desmoplakin (DSP), plakophilin-2 (PKP2), plakophilin-4 (PKP4), desmocollin-2 (DSC2), and desmoglein-2 (DSG2), resulting in defective cell-to-cell adhesion and altered nuclear signaling, leading to diminished desmosomal protein localization (**Figure 67.3**), and dramatic reduction in immunoreactive

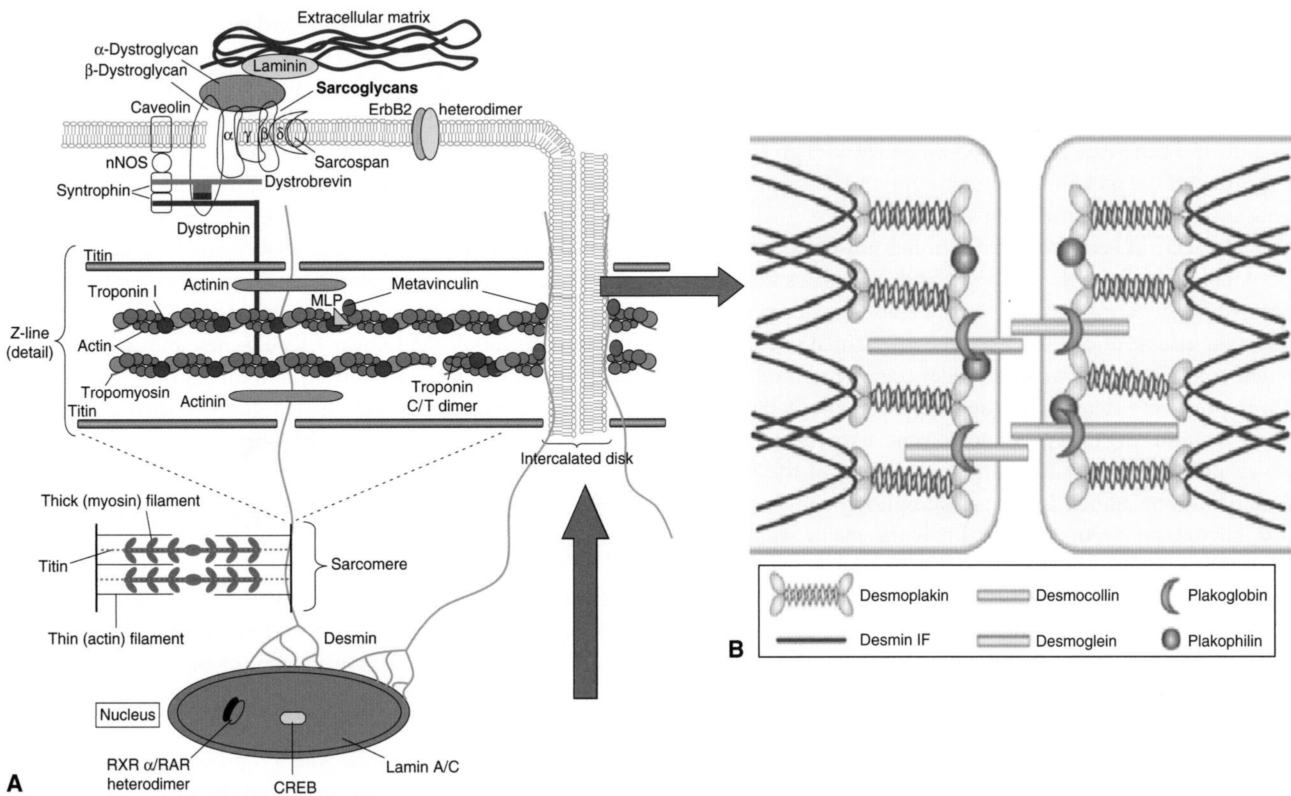

FIGURE 67.3 Cardiomyocyte. **A.** Cardiomyocyte demonstrating extracellular matrix, sarcolemma, intercalated disk, sarcomere, and nucleus and key proteins. **B.** Desmosome with key proteins. CREB, cAMP-response element binding protein; ErbB2, erb-b2 receptor tyrosine kinase 2; MLP, muscle LIM protein; RAR, retinoic acid receptor; RXR, retinoid X receptor

signal for the *GJA1*-encoded gap junction protein connexin-43 (Cx43) at the intercalated disks.[66,87-91]

Connexin-43 is a highly phosphorylated protein, whose phosphorylation pattern plays important roles in the regulation of protein turnover, trafficking, intercalated disk assembly, internalization, degradation, and channel gating properties.[91] In the failing right ventricle, altered phosphorylation of Cx43 leads to a nonphosphorylated protein, causing a weaker immunoreactive signal to be observed in the right ventricular myocardium of patients and animal models with ARVC.[89,90] Gehmlich and colleagues suggested that the cytoplasmic portion of a highly phosphorylated Cx43 protein binds the DSC2a isoform, connecting the gap junction to the desmosome.[89] They identified a novel variant in DSC2 as well as a DSG2 variant in an individual with a family history of sudden death, mild ECG abnormalities in the proband and her daughter, and immunohistochemistry demonstrated severe depression of the PG signal at the intercalated disk, whereas Western blot showed minimal reduction of DSG2 and DSC2 expression levels and mild reduction of Cx43. Electrophoretic mobility of Cx43 was abnormal and consistent with differential phosphorylation, suggesting a lower proportion of the highly phosphorylated protein. All other desmosomal proteins were normal. Therefore, the authors suggested that the DSC2a isoform provides a critical link between the desmosome and gap junction and that disruption leads to the clinical features of disease upon physiologic trigger. They also suggested that the combination of PG loss and Cx43 disturbance is an early indicator of developing clinical disease, with the risk of arrhythmias (and therefore sudden death) lurking for future clinical presentation. An extension of this suggestion leads to the possibility that mutations in desmosomal proteins could possibly alter Cx43 phosphorylation and weaken the linkage between the gap junction and desmosome, causing loss of electrical coupling between cardiac myocytes, and leading to myocyte cell death, fibrofatty replacement and arrhythmias.[87-91] These findings were felt to be potentially useful for early genotype-phenotype biomarker disease diagnosis, risk stratification, and outcome prediction, and possibly preventive therapy, but that significant caution should be used before assuming this to be correct.

In addition to abnormalities in desmosomal genes, mutations in the nondesmosomal genes have been also associated with ARVC and are thought to cause ARVC via secondary disruption of the desmosome.[62,66,87,92] These genes include transmembrane protein 43 (*TMEM43*), transforming growth factor β-3 *(TGF3)*, ryanodine receptor 2 *(RYR2)*, phospholamban (*PLN*), sodium voltage-gated channel α subunit 5 *(SCN5A)*, ankyrin-B (*ANK2*), desmin (*DES*), filamin C (*FLNC*), lamin A/C (*LMNA*), titin (*TTN*), αT catenin (*CTNNA3*), and cadherin-2 (*CDH2*).[62,66,92] More recently, variants in *TJP1* which encodes tight junction protein 1 were identified via exome sequencing of an ACM family.[93] Additional *TJP1* variants were subsequently detected in several patients in a multinational cohort. *ANK2* was proposed as an ACM gene based on identification of a rare variant segregating in a large family, confirmation of rare *ANK2* variants in numerous ACM cohorts, and recapitulation of the phenotype in a mouse model.[94] Finally, Poloni et al identified a nonsense variant segregating in a family in a candidate gene, *TP63* which encodes p63 protein, a member of the p53 family of transcription factors previously associated with ectodermal dysplasias.[95]

The *TGF β3*-encoded transforming growth factor 3 is a cytokine, which stimulates fibrosis and modulates cell adhesion, while the *RYR2*-encoded human ryanodine receptor 2 induces the release of calcium from the myocardial sarcoplasmic reticulum. *TMEM43*, which encodes transmembrane protein 43, is a response element for the peroxisome proliferator-activated receptor γ (PPARγ), an adipogenic transcription factor, which may explain the fibrofatty replacement of the myocardium. Phospholamban is a small phosphoprotein in the cardiac sarcoplasmic reticulum, and it is the major regulator of SERCA2a activity and calcium-cycling.[96,97] It normally inhibits the sarcoplasmic reticulum calcium transport ATPase, which is the pump that transports calcium ions to regulate cardiac contractions. Ankyrins are a family of proteins implicated in the membrane targeting of ion channels and transporters in both excitable and nonexcitable cells. Ankyrin-B (AnkB, encoded by *ANK2*) targets the Na^+/Ca^{++} exchanger and Na^+/K^+ ATPase to the cardiac transverse tubule network.[98] It has been suggested that disturbance of AnkB results in loss of protein phosphatase 2A activity, increased phosphorylation of the ryanodine receptor, exaggerated delayed afterdepolarization-mediated trigger activity, and arrhythmogenesis. *SCN5A* encodes the α-subunit of the cardiac sodium channel NaV1.5, which is responsible for the rapid depolarization of cardiac cells, thus allowing for their contraction.[99] At adherens junctions, classical cadherins such as cadherin 2—also known as N-cadherin, a calcium-dependent cell surface adhesion molecule—join neighboring cardiomyocytes through interactions with the actin cytoskeleton via catenin-α3 (*CTNNA3)* and a paralogue, catenin-α1, encoded by *CTNNA1.*[100] The *TJP1* gene encodes the multifunctional protein zonula occludens-1 (ZO-1), which interacts with proteins of the intercalated disk. In cardiomyocytes, ZO-1 is essential for a normal organization of both gap junctions and area composita (made up of desmosomal and adherens junction proteins), interacting with Cx43 and cadherin 2, respectively.[101,102] It has been reported that ZO-1 regulates the number, size, and distribution of gap junctions, binding Cx43 molecules in an area adjacent to the functional gap junctions.[103,104]

Although most ARVC cases follow an autosomal dominant pattern, autosomal recessive pattern was recognized with homozygous mutations in the plakoglobin-encoding gene causing Naxos disease, and homozygous mutations in *DSP* in Carvajal syndrome.[78,79,105,106] However, because of the reduced penetrance and variable expressivity, which characterizes ARVC, single mutations in individual genes may not be sufficient to cause the development of the disease.[107,108] Compound heterozygous mutations or double heterozygous, digenic mutations in desmosomal genes may be required for disease development and clinical manifestation.[107,108] In fact, although frameshift mutations are regarded as deleterious changes according to the current recommendations, many *PKP2* (plakophilin 2) mutations demonstrate low penetrance and an additional mutation in another ARVC gene is necessary to develop the disease. Therefore, despite much literature suggesting that *PKP2* mutations cause approximately 25% to 30% of ARVC cases, this is not the primary cause of the disease in a percentage of subjects. This complex genetic behavior makes clinical genetic testing challenging to interpret.[107,108] Therefore, despite the apparent autosomal dominant mode of inheritance, clinical genetic testing should be comprehensive and multimodal for all the known ARVC genes, and genetic-based diagnosis should be conservatively and thoughtfully considered. In addition, most gene elusive patients have isolated disease suggesting oligogenic or multifactorial inheritance.[81]

ARRHYTHMOGENIC LEFT VENTRICULAR CARDIOMYOPATHY

Left ventricular involvement in ARVC is now known to be common, occurring in 65% to 85% of cases of ACM.[109] In left ventricular ACM, the electrocardiogram typically demonstrates T-wave inversion in the anterior and inferolateral leads along with low-QRS voltages in limb leads and monomorphic sustained ventricular tachycardia with a right bundle branch block morphology of the QRS, and structural changes predominantly affecting the left ventricle.[82,110] The extent of arrhythmia, which typically originates in the left ventricle, can be incongruent with the degree of ventricular dysfunction and dilatation. Left ventricular involvement in ARVC is common and characterized phenotypically by clinical and CMRI features, which allow differential diagnosis with DCM. The most distinctive feature of ARVC-left ventricular phenotype is the large amount of left ventricular myocardial fibrosis/LGE, which is directly related to the left ventricular systolic dysfunction. The remodeling pattern of "hypokinetic, nondilated, and fibrotic" left ventricle fits better with an ARVC-left ventricular phenotype than with a phenotypically less expressed DCM. The fibro-fatty myocardial replacement of a significant proportion of left ventricular musculature accounts for the low-QRS voltages on the ECG and acts as a substrate for life-threatening ventricular arrhythmias.

Similar to right ventricular disease, myocardial thinning, local aneurysm, and wall motion abnormalities can be present. Cardiac MRI can be used to identify extensive LGE in an epicardial and midmyocardial distribution, which can precede clinical features in children and young adults. This pattern of enhancement can mimic acute infective myocarditis during inflammatory phases of the disease.

Biventricular ACM is defined by active and equal involvement of both ventricles, and patients can have features of both classical and left-dominant disease. Severe biventricular dysfunction can ensue or be evident at presentation. These patients can be diagnosed as having DCM with right ventricular involvement, although ventricular ectopy and arrhythmias originating from either ventricle are a cardinal feature. Left ventricular LGE is more frequently seen affecting the subepicardial layers of the left ventricle.

LEFT VENTRICULAR NONCOMPACTION

Left ventricular noncompaction (LVNC) is a genetic disease characterized by cardiomyopathy with excessive and unusual trabeculations within the mature left ventricle.[111,112] LVNC has been considered to be a developmental failure of the heart to form fully the compact myocardium during the later stages of cardiac development. Clinically and pathologically, LVNC is characterized by a spongy morphological appearance of the myocardium occurring primarily in the left ventricle with the abnormal trabeculations typically being most evident in the apical and mid-lateral-inferior portions of the left ventricle.[111,112] The right ventricle may also be affected alone or in conjunction with the left ventricle. In LVNC, in addition to the regional presence of prominent trabeculae and intertrabecular recesses in the left ventricle, thickening of the myocardium in two distinct layers composed of compacted and noncompacted myocardium is also classically noted.[111,112]

At least eight different LVNC phenotypes appear to exist, all having different outcomes (**Figure 67.4**). A brief description of the subtypes that we developed[10] is described here:

- **"Benign" Form of LVNC:** This subtype is characterized by normal left ventricular size and wall thickness with preserved systolic and diastolic function (**Figure 67.4A**). This subtype accounts for up to ~35% of LVNC patients and is a predictor of good outcome in the absence of significant arrhythmias.[52]
- **LVNC with Arrhythmias:** This subtype is defined by preserved systolic function with normal left ventricular size and wall thickness but has evidence of underlying arrhythmias, usually identified at the time of diagnosis. This subtype appears to have a worse outcome compared with the normal population or those with similar forms of rhythm disturbance.
- **Dilated Cardiomyopathy Form of LVNC:** This subtype is characterized by concomitant left ventricular dilation and systolic dysfunction (**Figure 67.4B**).[3,10,14,42,43,48,52]
- **Hypertrophic Cardiomyopathy Form of LVNC:** This subtype is characterized by left ventricular thickening, usually with asymmetric septal hypertrophy, in addition to diastolic dysfunction and hypercontractile systolic function (**Figure 67.4C**).[10,52]
- **Hypertrophic and Dilated Cardiomyopathy Form of LVNC:** This subtype, also known as a mixed phenotype, is characterized by left ventricular thickening, dilation, and depressed systolic function at presentation.
- **Restrictive Cardiomyopathy Form of LVNC:** This rare form of LVNC is characterized by left atrial or biatrial dilation and diastolic dysfunction (**Figure 67.4D**). This phenotype mimics the clinical behavior of restrictive cardiomyopathy.
- **Right Ventricular or Biventricular Cardiomyopathy Form of LVNC:** This subtype is characterized by hypertrabeculation of both the right ventricle and left ventricle (**Figure 67.4E**).
- **LVNC with Congenital Heart Disease:** LVNC has been reported in association with most all congenital heart lesions and may contribute to myocardial dysfunction or arrhythmias. Right-sided lesions, especially Ebstein anomaly, pulmonic stenosis, pulmonary atresia, tricuspid atresia, and double outlet right ventricle are most common, with septal defects and left heart defects less commonly seen (**Figure 67.5**).

Affected individuals are at risk of left or right ventricular failure or both. Heart failure symptoms can be exercise-induced or persistent at rest, but many patients are asymptomatic. Chronically treated patients sometimes present acutely with decompensated heart failure. Other life-threatening risks are ventricular arrhythmias and atrioventricular block, presenting clinically as syncope, and sudden death. Genetic inheritance arises in at least 30% and 50% of patients. LVNC is thought to occur in approximately 1 per 7000 live births.[111,112] It occurs in newborns, young children, and adults, with the worst reported outcomes seen in infants, particularly those with associated systemic disease and metabolic derangement. In some families, a consistent phenotype of LVNC is seen in affected relatives, but quite commonly individuals with features of LVNC are found in families where other affected relatives have typical HCM, DCM, or RCM. Mutations in ~80 genes have been implicated and include cytoskeletal, sarcomeric, ion channel, and mitochondrial genes, with sarcomere-encoding genes being most common.[111-113] In the case of LVNC with congenital heart disease, disturbance of the Notch, TGF-β superfamily, or Wnt signaling pathways appear to be part of a "final common pathway" for this form of the disease.[114,115] In addition, disrupted mitochondrial function and metabolic abnormalities have a causal role as well.[111-115] Treatments focus on improvement of cardiac efficiency and reduction of mechanical stress in those with systolic dysfunction. Further, arrhythmia therapy and implantation of an automatic implantable cardioverter-defibrillator (ICD) for prevention of sudden death are mainstays of treatment when deemed necessary and appropriate. Patients with LVNC associated with congenital heart disease commonly require surgical- or catheter-based interventions.

The genetic cause of LVNC, like the clinical phenotype itself, is heterogeneous. However, like the genetic causes of other forms of cardiomyopathy, LVNC genetics also follows a "final common pathway."[100,111-116] The specific "final common pathway," however, depends on the clinical phenotype and mirrors the genetic causes of the clinical subtype in cardiomyopathies devoid of LVNC. For instance, HCM is a disease of sarcomere dysfunction while ARVC is a disease of desmosome dysfunction. However, in LVNC, there appears to be a disturbance of more than a single "final common pathway" and, in most cases, probably disturbs a primary pathway (such as the sarcomere) and a developmental pathway (such as the NOTCH pathway) via a disturbance of protein-protein binding caused by the primary genetic mutation.

The first genetic cause of LVNC without evidence of congenital heart disease was initially described by Bleyl et al, who

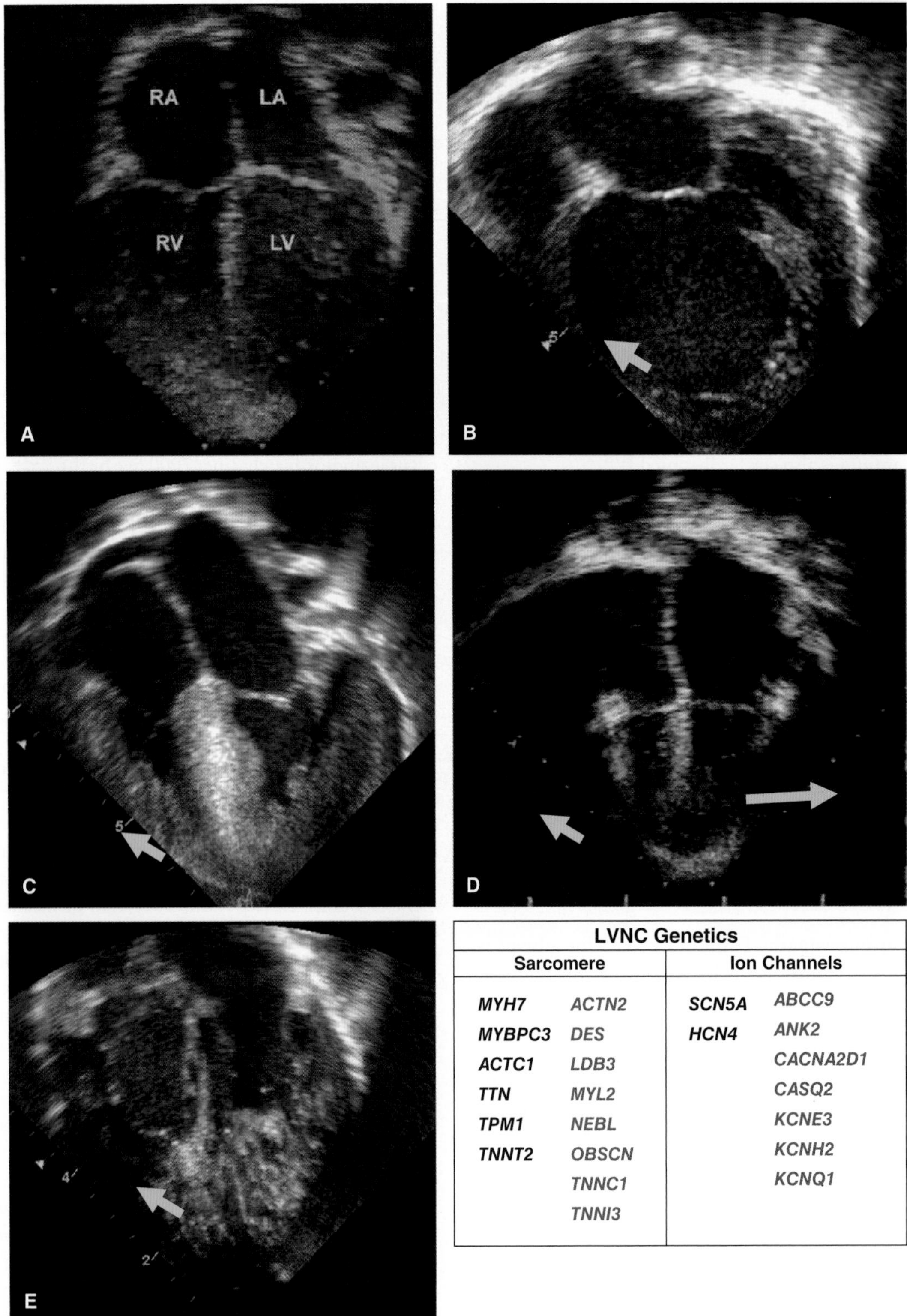

LVNC Genetics			
Sarcomere		Ion Channels	
MYH7	*ACTN2*	***SCN5A***	*ABCC9*
MYBPC3	*DES*	***HCN4***	*ANK2*
ACTC1	*LDB3*		*CACNA2D1*
TTN	*MYL2*		*CASQ2*
TPM1	*NEBL*		*KCNE3*
TNNT2	*OBSCN*		*KCNH2*
	TNNC1		*KCNQ1*
	TNNI3		

FIGURE 67.4 Phenotypic heterogeneity of left ventricular noncompaction (LVNC) and genetic causes. Sarcomere- and ion channel-encoding genes are involved in the pathogenesis of LVNC. Arrows demonstrate areas of hypertrabeculation. **A.** Hypertrabeculation of left ventricle with normal left ventricular size, thickness, systolic and diastolic function and normal atria. This is a benign form. **B.** Dilated cardiomyopathy form of LVNC. **C.** Hypertrophic cardiomyopathy form of LVNC. **D.** Restrictive cardiomyopathy form of LVNC. **E.** Biventricular cardiomyopathy form of LVNC.

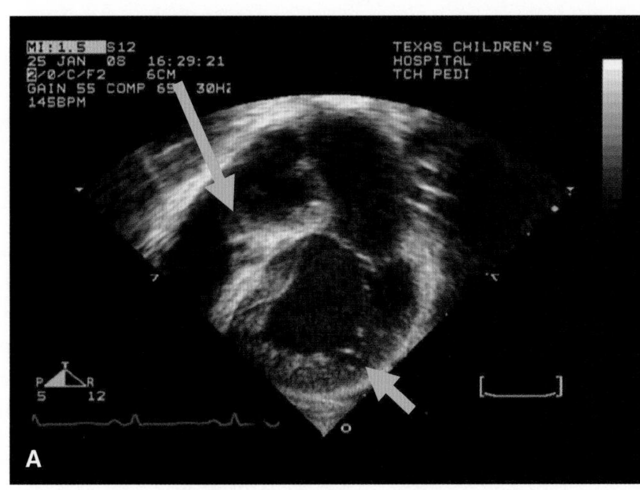

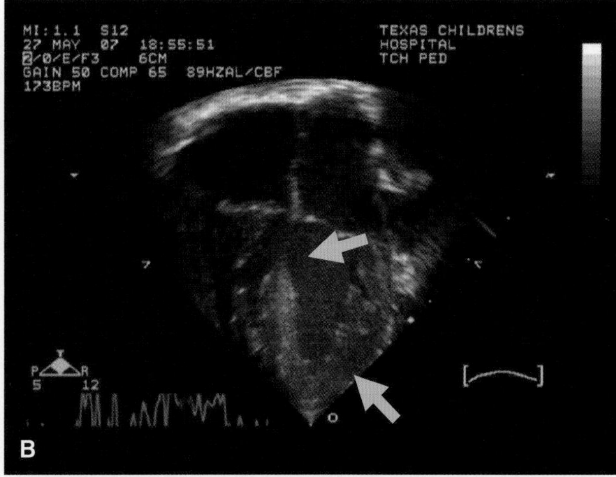

LVNC + CHD GENETICS

MYH7
NKX2.5
DTNA
KLHL26
MIB1

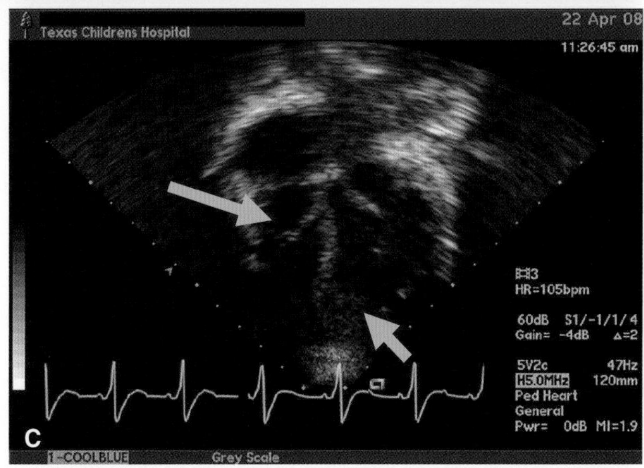

FIGURE 67.5 Left ventricular noncompaction cardiomyopathy (LVNC) is associated with congenital heart disease (CHD). **A.** LVNC with tricuspid atresia. The top arrow demonstrates the tricuspid valve abnormality and the bottom arrow points to the apical hypertrabeculation. **B.** LVNC with a large ventricular septal defect. The top arrow demonstrates the ventricular septal defect and the bottom arrow points to the apical hypertrabeculation. **C.** LVNC with Ebstein anomaly. The top arrow demonstrates the Ebstein tricuspid valve abnormality and the bottom arrow points to the apical hypertrabeculation. Genes associated with the development of LVNC with congenital heart disease (CHD).

identified mutations in the X-linked TAZ gene in patients and carrier females. TAZ encodes the tafazzin protein, a phospholipid transacylase that is important for membrane function and, when mutated typically causes the multisystem human disorder called Barth syndrome, which is characterized by cardiomyopathy (commonly LVNC), skeletal myopathy, cyclic neutropenia, 3-methylglutaconic aciduria (a marker of mitochondrial dysfunction), and deficiency of a key membrane phospholipid of cardiomyocytes and mitochondria called cardiolipin.[117] It is believed that this defect disturbs mitochondrial function, leading to a combination of an energy production-energy utilization abnormality and, because the sarcomere requires energy in the form of adenosine triphosphate (ATP), sarcomere dysfunction occurs.

Multiple genes causing autosomal dominant LVNC have since been identified, including mutations in genes causing congenital heart disease with LVNC. Mutations in ~20 genes have been implicated and mostly include cytoskeletal, sarcomeric, and ion channel genes, with sarcomere-encoding genes being most common. In addition, disorders such as Barth syndrome and muscular dystrophies are known to be associated with LVNC as well. In patients with hypoplastic left heart syndrome and LVNC, α-dystrobrevin mutations were identified as causative, while mutations in Nkx-2.5 were identified in children with LVNC and atrial septal defect. Further, both β-myosin heavy chain (MYH7) mutations and α-tropomyosin (TPM1) mutations have been reported in patients with LVNC and Ebstein anomaly.[118-120]

The most common genes identified include the sarcomere-encoding genes β-myosin heavy chain (*MYH7*), α-cardiac actin (*ACTC1*), cardiac troponin T (*TNNT2*), myosin-binding protein C (MYBPC3), and ZASP (also called LIM-domain binding protein 3, LBD3).[118-121] In addition, mutations in α-tropomyosin (TPM1) and cardiac troponin I (TNNI3) also have been identified. Hoedemaekers et al[121] additionally demonstrated an association of LVNC with genetic variants in two calcium handling genes, as well as TAZ and lamin A/C (LMNA).[121] Probst et al[122] further showed that sarcomere gene mutations are important in LVNC, showing a prevalence of 29%, with MYH7 and MYBPC3 most frequently mutated (13% and 8%, respectively). Dellefave et al also identified sarcomere mutations in LVNC, including those presenting with heart failure in infancy.[123] Further, Hastings et al performed whole genome sequencing, linkage analysis, and functional studies on two families with LVNC and identified missense mutations in titin (TTN), which encodes the giant titin protein found in the Z-disk and sarcomere.[124] Bagnall and colleagues showed an association of LVNC, idiopathic ventricular fibrillation, and sudden death with a mutation in the ACTN2 gene in a family.[125] van Waning et al reported 104 genetic cases with mutations, and 82% involved a sarcomere gene. In most of these cases (71%), a mutation was identified in *MYH7*, *MYBPC3*, or *TTN*, and 11% had a mutation in *ACTC1*, *ACTN2*, *MYL2*, *TNNC1*, *TNNT2*, or *TPM1*.[126] In children, no TTN mutations were noted. These authors also identified mutations in the non-sarcomere encoding genes DES, DSP, FKTN (fukutin), HCN4 (hyperpolarization activated cyclic nucleotide gated potassium channel 4), KCNQ1, LAMP2 (lysosomal-associated membrane protein 2), *LMNA*, MIB1 (mindbomb E3 ubiquitin protein ligase 1), NOTCH1, PLN, RYR2, SCN5A, and *TAZ*.[126]

Along with sarcomere-encoding and cytoskeleton-encoding genes, pathogenic variants in the sodium channel gene (SCN5A) have been associated with LVNC and rhythm disturbance.[127,128] Another cytoskeletal protein associated with LVNC is dystrophin, the defective protein causing Duchenne and Becker muscular dystrophy in boys.[129]

In addition, homozygous deletions in desmoplakin and plakophilin 2—desmosomal protein-encoding genes known to cause arrhythmogenic cardiomyopathy and dilated cardiomyopathy—have also been identified in LVNC patients.[1,65,66,130,131] Mitochondrial genome mutations have also been identified to be associated with LVNC[132,133] and chromosomal abnormalities and syndromic patients also have been identified with LVNC including 1p36 deletion, 7p14.3p14.1 deletion, 18p subtelomeric deletion, 22q11.2 deletion, distal 22q11.2, trisomies 18 and 13, 8p23.1 deletion, tetrasomy 5q35.2-5q35, Coffin-Lowry syndrome (RPS6KA3 mutation), Sotos syndrome (NSD1 mutation), and Charcot-Marie-Tooth disease type 1A (PMP22 duplication).[134-144]

Diagnostic testing in patients with LVNC appear to have a detection rate of clinically significant variants in 35% to 40% of individuals, with sarcomere-encoding genes most commonly found to be mutated.[145]

RESTRICTIVE CARDIOMYOPATHY

Restrictive cardiomyopathy (RCM) is uncommon, accounting for up to 5% of cardiomyopathies in children and adults.[146-149] In the 2006 classification consensus statement by the American Heart Association, primary restrictive cardiomyopathy was defined as a rare form of heart disease characterized by "normal or decreased volume of both ventricles associated with biatrial enlargement, normal left ventricular wall thickness and atrioventricular valves, impaired ventricular filling with restrictive physiology, and normal (or near normal) systolic function."[3]

The most common presenting signs and symptoms in children with RCM include dyspnea that is frequently exacerbated by an intercurrent respiratory illness or "asthma," fatigue, exercise intolerance, syncope, and sudden death.[146-149] The ECG is typically abnormal, with the most common abnormalities being right or left atrial enlargement; however, ST segment depression and ST-T-wave abnormalities are frequently present. Right or left ventricular hypertrophy can also be seen, as well as conduction abnormalities.[3,4,8] The Holter and event monitors are useful to evaluate for rhythm disturbances, conduction abnormalities, and evidence of ischemia based on ST segment analysis.[3,4,8,146-149] Arrhythmias have been reported in approximately 15% of pediatric patients and include atrial flutter, high-grade second- and third-degree atrioventricular block, atrial fibrillation, atrial tachycardias, Wolff-Parkinson-White syndrome with supraventricular tachycardia and ventricular tachycardia and torsades de pointes.[3,4,8,146,150-152] Symptomatic sinus bradycardia requiring pacing has also been reported. The most striking finding on echocardiography is massive atrial dilatation in the absence of atrioventricular valve regurgitation.[153] In children, findings consistent with restrictive filling and increased left ventricular end-diastolic pressure are noted.[153] Systolic function is typically preserved although some degree of systolic dysfunction has been seen in some patients at presentation and deterioration of systolic dysfunction over time has also been reported in children.[146,147,152,153] Ventricular hypertrophy is not prominent, but some degree of concentric increase in septal and left ventricular posterior wall thickness is seen in a significant proportion of cases otherwise fulfilling all the other criteria for RCM. Cardiac catheterization may demonstrate elevated left or right ventricular end-diastolic pressures. Pulmonary hypertension is frequently present at the time of initial catheterization, and markedly elevated pulmonary vascular resistance can occur within 1 to 4 years of diagnosis.[146,153] EMB reveals myofiber hypertrophy and mild-to-moderate interstitial fibrosis.

In children in the United States and Australia, RCM accounts for 2.5% to 5% of the diagnosed cardiomyopathies, with the majority having no specific cause identified.[2,3,154] In Australia, RCM accounted for 2.5% of the cardiomyopathies diagnosed in children less than 10 years of age,[154] while the US report from the Pediatric Cardiomyopathy Registry investigators reported that RCM accounted for 3% of the cardiomyopathies in children less than 18 years of age.[3] The estimated annual incidence in the United States and Australia is 0.04/100,000 and 0.03/100,000 children, respectively.[2,154] Multiple causes of RCM have been described in adults and children.

Some cases are inherited and these most commonly cardiac, α-actin (ACTC1).[36,49] *Pathogenic variants* in filamin C (FLNC), BCL2 associated athanogene 3 (BAG3), myopalladin (MYPN), and desmin (DES) have also been reported.[155-162] Another complex subgroup of patients has been identified with

RCM associated with atrioventricular block and skeletal myopathy, and these are usually caused by mutations in desmin or lamin A/C.[155-157]

The prognosis in children with RCM is poor.[146-151] Half of the children die or undergo transplant within 3 years of diagnosis. Sudden cardiac death has been reported to be a common mode of death in children with RCM.[146-151] Patients who appear to be at greater risk for sudden death include those who present with signs and symptoms of ischemia, such as syncope and chest pain. However, heart failure related deaths are the most common.

MITOCHONDRIAL GENOME AND NUCLEAR GENES WITH MITOCHONDRIAL FUNCTION AND CARDIOMYOPATHIES

Mitochondria provide the major energy source for the myocardium, and abnormalities of the mitochondrial genome (mtDNA) and nuclear genes encoding proteins involved in mitochondrial respiratory chain function are seen in cardiomyopathies.[132,133,163-165] The mitochondrial respiratory chain consists of five enzyme complexes (I-V) in the inner membrane of the mitochondria, and the energy that is generated is used to produce ATP via oxidative phosphorylation.[133,165] Defects in oxidative phosphorylation could originate from alterations in any of the five complexes of the respiratory chain, although the most frequently affected include complexes I (NADH-CoQ reductase) and IV (cytochrome-*c* oxidase).[132,133,163-165] Mitochondrial diseases usually manifest in early childhood, although different levels of heteroplasmy in various tissues may be associated with pleiotropic effects clinically and age-dependent expressivity. Children affected by mitochondrial diseases commonly present with cardiomyopathy (17%) and cardiac involvement is generally associated with worse prognosis and increased mortality.[133,163]

Mitochondria occupy a significant portion (20%-30%) of cardiac cell volume, and their dynamic nature allow them to respond to the level of energy requirement by altering their unit number. In cardiomyocytes, mitochondria are not only functionally related to cardiac contraction and energy homeostasis, but they are also physically linked to the sarcoplasmic reticulum through the intermediate filament protein desmin, which provides the necessary ratio of mitochondria to intermediate filament for the optimal exchange of ions, lipids, and other metabolites.[163,165]

Thus, it should not be surprising that altered integrity of the mitochondria could lead to functional and structural impairment of cardiac cells. In fact, the absence of desmin in mouse hearts leads to an abnormal accumulation of subsarcolemmal clusters of mitochondria, degeneration of the mitochondrial matrix, and proliferation associated with the development of DCM and heart failure.[132,133,163-164]

The mtDNA is approximately 16 kb in length and encodes 13 of the 69 proteins required for oxidative metabolism performed by Complex I-V, 22 transfer RNA (tRNAs), and two ribosomal RNA (rRNA). Mitochondria are inherited from the mother, and they can vary in number within the cells from various tissues (heteroplasmy), accounting for the pleiotropic effect. Mutations leading to mitochondrial defects have been identified in subjects with isolated LVNC, as well as DCM and HCM,[132,133,163-165] thus supporting the importance of mitochondrial genome screening in primary cardiomyopathies. In addition, complex mitochondrial diseases such as Kearns-Sayre syndrome, myoclonic epilepsy with ragged red muscle fibers (MERRF) syndrome, and mitochondrial encephalopathy with lactic acidosis and stroke-like episodes (MELAS) have also been associated with cardiomyopathies, suggesting that a multimodal approach including novel technologies for the screening of the nuclear DNA (nDNA) and the mtDNA should be employed in both research and clinical testing in individuals with cardiomyopathies, particularly babies.[132,133,163-165] The currently available technologies such as whole genome or exome sequencing, multiplex ligation-dependent probe amplification, array-based comparative genomic hybridization for nDNA and mtDNA, and high-density array combining single nucleotide polymorphism and copy number variation probes using the currently available platforms allow for rapid results with increasingly lower cost, improvements in turn-around times, and comprehensive investigation of the underlying genetic etiologies involved in cardiomyopathies.

MUSCLE IS MUSCLE: CARDIOMYOPATHY AND SKELETAL MYOPATHY GENES OVERLAP

Many of the genes identified for inherited cardiomyopathy, especially DCM, are also known to cause skeletal myopathy in humans or mouse models. Well-described examples include the genes encoding dystrophin, δ-sarcoglycan, and lamin A/C. Mutations in the genes encoding desmin, tafazzin, α-dystrobrevin, ZASP/LBD3, MLP/CSRP3, α-actinin 2, and titin also resulted in an associated skeletal myopathy. This suggests that cardiac and skeletal muscle function are interrelated and that the skeletal muscle fatigue seen in patients with DCM may be because of primary skeletal muscle disease and not simply the cardiac dysfunction. This concept has recently been supported by Song et al who evaluated skeletal muscle structure and function in wild-type (WT) mice and compared that with cardiac myosin-binding protein C null mice (t/t), which develop DCM-induced heart failure. The t/t mice indeed developed DCM-induced heart failure in association with profound exercise intolerance. Compared with WT, t/t mouse hearts demonstrated significant hypertrophy of the atria and ventricles and systolic and diastolic dysfunction. In parallel, the skeletal muscles of t/t mice were shown to exhibit weakness and myopathy. Compared with WT, plantar flexor muscles of t/t null mice produced less peak isometric plantar torque (Po), developed torque more slowly (+dF/dt), and relaxed more slowly (−dF/dt, longer half-relaxation times, 1/2RT). Gastrocnemius muscles of t/t mice had a greater number of fibers with smaller diameters and central nuclei. Oxidative fibers, both type I and type IIa, showed significantly smaller cross-sectional areas and more central nuclei. These fiber phenotypes suggested ongoing repair and regeneration under homeostatic conditions. In addition, the ability of muscles to recover and regenerate after acute injury was impaired in the t/t mice. They concluded that DCM-induced heart failure induces a unique skeletal myopathy characterized by decreased muscle strength, atrophy of oxidative fiber types, ongoing inflammation and damage under homeostasis, and impaired regeneration after acute muscle injury and likely exacerbates exercise intolerance.

KEY POINTS

- ✔ Dilated Cardiomyopathy is typically caused by variants in genes encoding structural proteins such as cytoskeletal and sarcomeric proteins.
- ✔ Arrhythmogenic cardiomyopathy is currently considered a genetically determined, autosomal dominant inherited disease with reduced penetrance and variable clinical expression.
- ✔ Left ventricular noncompaction is a genetic disease characterized by cardiomyopathy with excessive and unusual trabeculations within the mature left ventricle.
- ✔ Complex mitochondrial diseases such as Kearns-Sayre syndrome, myoclonic epilepsy with ragged red muscle fibers
- ✔ (MERRF) syndrome, and mitochondrial encephalopathy with lactic acidosis and stroke-like episodes (MELAS) have also been associated with cardiomyopathies

REFERENCES

1. Heron, M, Sutton PD, Xu J, et al. Annual summary of vital statistics: 2007. *Pediatrics.* 2010;125:4-15.
2. Lipshultz SE, Sleeper LA, Towbin JA, et al. The incidence of pediatric cardiomyopathy in two regions of the United States. *N Engl J Med.* 2003;348:1647-1655.
3. Maron BJ, Towbin JA, Thiene G, et al. Contemporary definitions and classification of the cardiomyopathies: an American Heart Association Scientific Statement from the Council on Clinical Cardiology, Heart Failure and Transplantation Committee; Quality of Care and Outcomes Research and Functional Genomics and Translational Biology Interdisciplinary Working Groups; and Council on Epidemiology and Prevention. *Circulation.* 2006;113(14):1807-1816.
4. Elliott P, Andersson B, Arbustini E, et al. Classification of the cardiomyopathies: a position statement from the European Society of Cardiology Working Group on Myocardial and Pericardial Diseases. *Eur Heart J.* 2008;29(2):270-276.
5. Ramchand J, Wallis M, Macciocca I, et al. Prospective evaluation of the utility of whole exome sequencing in dilated cardiomyopathy. *J Am Heart Assoc.* 2020;9(2):e013346. doi:10.1161/JAHA.119.013346
6. Burke MA, Cook SA, Seidman JG, Seidman CE. Clinical and mechanistic insights into the genetics of cardiomyopathy. *J Am Coll Cardiol.* 2016;68(25):2871-2886. doi:10.1016/j.jacc.2016.08.079
7. Hershberger RE, Givertz MM, Ho CY, et al. ACMG Professional Practice and Guidelines Committee. Genetic evaluation of cardiomyopathy: a clinical practice resource of the American College of Medical Genetics and Genomics (ACMG). *Genet Med.* 2018;20(9):899-909.
8. Lipshultz SE, Law YM, Asante-Korang A, et al. Cardiomyopathy in children: classification and diagnosis: a scientific statement from the American Heart Association. *Circulation.* 2019;140(1):e9-e68.
9. Bowles NE, Bowles KR, Towbin, JA. The "Final Common Pathway" hypothesis and inherited cardiovascular disease: the role of cytoskeletal proteins in dilated cardiomyopathy. *Herz.* 2000;25:168-175.
10. Towbin, JA. The role of cytoskeletal proteins in cardiomyopathies. *Curr Opin Cell Biol.* 1998;10(1):131-139.
11. Marian AJ, Braunwald E. Hypertrophic cardiomyopathy: genetics, pathogenesis, clinical manifestations, diagnosis, and therapy. *Circ Res.* 2017;121(7):749-770.
12. Teekakirikul P, Zhu W, Huang HC, Fung E. Hypertrophic cardiomyopathy: an overview of genetics and management. *Biomolecules.* 2019;9(12):878. doi:10.3390/biom9120878
13. Maron BJ, Maron MS, Maron BA, Loscalzo J. Moving beyond the sarcomere to explain heterogeneity in hypertrophic cardiomyopathy: JACC Review Topic of the Week. *J Am Coll Cardiol.* 2019;73(15):1978-1986.
14. Wilde AAM, Amin AS. Clinical spectrum of SCN5A mutations: long QT syndrome, Brugada syndrome, and cardiomyopathy. *JACC Clin Electrophysiol.* 2018;4(5):569-579.
15. Pinto YM, Elliott PM, Arbustini E, et al. Proposal for a revised definition of dilated cardiomyopathy, hypokinetic non-dilated cardiomyopathy, and its implications for clinical practice: a position statement of the ESC working group on myocardial and pericardial diseases. *Eur Heart J.* 2016;37(23):1850-1858.
16. Towbin JA, Lowe AM, Colan SD, et al. Incidence, causes, and outcomes of dilated cardiomyopathy in children. *JAMA.* 2006;296(15):1867-1876.
17. Hershberger RE, Hedges DJ, Morales A. Dilated cardiomyopathy: the complexity of a diverse genetic architecture. *Nat Rev Cairdiol.* 2013;10:531-547.
18. Hsu DT, Canter CE. Dilated cardiomyopathy and heart failure in children. *Heart Fail Clin.* 2010;6(4):415-432.
19. Herskowitz A, Campbell S, Deckers J, et al. Demographic features and prevalence of idiopathic myocarditis in patients undergoing endomyocardial biopsy. *Am J Cardiol.* 1993;71:982-986.
20. Kasper EK, Agema WR, Hutchins GM, Deckers JW, Hare JM, Baughman KL. The causes of dilated cardiomyopathy: a clinicopathologic review of 673 consecutive patients. *J Am Coll Cardiol.* 1994;23(3):586-590.
21. Grünig E, Tasman JA, Kücherer H, Franz W, Kübler W, Katus HA. Frequency and phenotypes of familial dilated cardiomyopathy. *J Am Coll Cardiol.* 1998;31(1):186-194.
22. Petretta M, Pirozzzi F, Sasso L, Paglia A, Bonaduce D. Review and meta-analysis of the frequency of familial dilated cardiomyopathy. *Am J Cardiol.* 2011;108:1171-1176.
23. Burkett EL, Hershberger RE. Clinical and genetic issues in familial dilated cardiomyopathy *J Am Coll Cardiol.* 2005;45(7):969-981.
24. Mahon NG, Murphy RT, Macrae CA, Caforio AL, Elliott PM, Mckenna WJ. Echocardiographic evaluation in asymptomatic relatives of patients with dilated cardiomyopathy reveals preclinical disease *Ann Intern Med.* 2005;143(2):108-115.
25. Anastasakis A, Sevdalis E, Papatheodorou E, Stefanadis C. Anderson-Fabry disease: a cardiomyopathy that can be cured. *Hellenic J Cardiol.* 2011;52(4):316-326.
26. Hershberger RE, Cowan J, Morales A, Siegfried JD. Progress with genetic cardiomyopathies: screening, counseling, and testing in dilated, hypertrophic, and arrhythmogenic right ventricular dysplasia/cardiomyopathy. *Circ Heart Fail.* 2009;2(3):253-261.
27. Hershberger RE, Siegfried JD. Update 2011: clinical and genetic issues in familial dilated cardiomyopathy. *J Am Coll Cardiol.* 2011;57(16):1641-1649.
28. Sturm AC, Hershberger RE. Genetic testing in cardiovascular medicine: current landscape and future horizons. *Curr Opin Cardiol.* 2013;28(3):317-325.
29. Norton N, Robertson PD, Rieder MJ, et al. Evaluating pathogenicity of rare variants from dilated cardiomyopathy in the exome era. *Circ Cardiovasc Genet.* 2012;5(2):167-174.
30. Pan S, Caleshu CA, Dunn KE, et al. Cardiac structural and sarcomere genes associated with cardiomyopathy exhibit marked intolerance of genetic variation. *Circ Cardiovasc Genet.* 2012;5(6):602-610.
31. Towbin JA, Hejtmancik JF, Brink P, et al. X-linked dilated cardiomyopathy. Molecular genetic evidence of linkage to the Duchenne

muscular dystrophy (dystrophin) gene at the Xp21 locus. *Circulation.* 1993;87(6):1854-1865.

32. Muntoni F, Cau M, Ganau A, et al. Brief report: deletion of the dystrophin muscle-promoter region associated with X-linked dilated cardiomyopathy. *N Engl J Med.* 1993;329(13):921-925.
33. Koenig X, Ebner J, Hilber K. Voltage-dependent sarcolemmal ion channel abnormalities in the dystrophin-deficient heart. *Int J Mol Sci.* 2018;19:3296. doi:10.3390/ijms19113296
34. Petrof, BJ, Shragert, JB, Stedmant, HH, Kellyt, AM, Sweeney HL. Dystrophin protects the sarcolemma from stresses developed during muscle contraction (Muscular Dystrophy/Muscle Injury/Mdx Mouse). *Med Sci.* 1993;90:3710-3714.
35. Markham LW, Michelfelder EC, Border WL, et al. Abnormalities of diastolic function precede dilated cardiomyopathy associated with Duchenne muscular dystrophy. *J Am Soc Echocardiogr.* 2006;19:865-871.
36. Dadson K, Hauck L, Billia F. Molecular mechanisms in cardiomyopathy. *Clin Sci (Lond).* 2017;131(13):1375-1392.
37. Vasilescu C, Ojala TH, Brilhante V, et al. A genetic basis of severe childhood-onset cardiomyopathies. *J Am Coll Cardiol.* 2018;72(19):2324-2338.
38. D'Ambrosio P, Petillo R, Torella A, et al. Cardiac diseases as a predictor warning of hereditary muscle diseases. The case of laminopathies. *Acta Myol.* 2019;38(2):33-36.
39. Feingold B, Mahle WT, Auerbach S, et al. Management of cardiac involvement associated with neuromuscular diseases: a scientific statement from the American Heart Association. *Circulation.* 2017;136(13):e200-e231.
40. Sommerville RB, Vincenti MG, Winborn K, et al. Diagnosis and management of adult hereditary cardio-neuromuscular disorders: a model for the multidisciplinary care of complex genetic disorders. *Trends Cardiovasc Med.* 2017;27(1):51-58.
41. Arbustini E, Di Toro A, Giuliani L, Favalli V, Narula N, Grasso M. Cardiac phenotypes in hereditary muscle disorders: JACC State-of-the-Art Review. *J Am Coll Cardiol.* 2018;72(20):2485-2506.
42. Horvat C, Johnson R, Lam L, et al. A gene-centric strategy for identifying disease-causing rare variants in dilated cardiomyopathy. *Genet Med.* 2019;21:133-143.
43. Peters S, Kumar S, Elliott P, Kalman JM, Fatkin D. Arrhythmic genotypes in familial dilated cardiomyopathy: implications for genetic testing and clinical management. *Heart Lung Circ.* 2019;28(1):31-38.
44. McNair WP, Sinagra G, Taylor MR, et al. SCN5A mutations associate with arrhythmic dilated cardiomyopathy and commonly localize to the voltage-sensing mechanism. *J Am Coll Cardiol.* 2011;57:2160-2168.
45. Moreau A, Chahine M. A new cardiac channelopathy: from clinical phenotypes to molecular mechanisms associated with $Na_v1.5$ gating pores. *Front Cardiovasc Med.* 2018;5:139. doi:10.3389/fcvm.2018.00139
46. Cheng J, Morales A, Siegfried JD, et al. SCN5A rare variants in familial dilated cardiomyopathy decrease peak sodium current depending on the common polymorphism H558R and common splice variant Q1077del. *Clin Transl Sci.* 2010;3(6):287-294.
47. Li Z, Ai T, Samani K, Xi Y, et al. A ZASP missense mutation, S196L, leads to cytoskeletal and electrical abnormalities in a mouse model of cardiomyopathy. *Circ Arrhythm Electrophysiol.* 2010;3(6):646-656.
48. Udelson JE. Evaluating and reducing the risk of sudden death in hypertrophic cardiomyopathy. *Circulation.* 2019;139(6):727-729.
49. Maron BJ. Clinical course and management of hypertrophic cardiomyopathy. *N Engl J Med* 2018;379(7):655-668.
50. Fatkin D, Graham RM. Molecular mechanisms of inherited cardiomyopathies. *Physiol Rev.* 2002;82(4):945-980.
51. Ho CY, Day SM, Ashley EA, et al. Genotype and lifetime burden of disease in hypertrophic cardiomyopathy: insights from the Sarcomeric Human Cardiomyopathy Registry (SHaRe). *Circulation.* 2018;138(14):1387-1398.
52. Kaski JP, Syrris P, Esteban MT, et al. Prevalence of sarcomere protein gene mutations in preadolescent children with hypertrophic cardiomyopathy. *Circ Cardiovasc Genet.* 2009;2(5):436-441.
53. Rupp S, Felimban M, Schänzer A, et al. Genetic basis of hypertrophic cardiomyopathy in children. *Clin Res Cardiol.* 2019;108(3):282-289.
54. Morita H, Rehm HL, Menesses A, et al. Shared genetic causes of cardiac hypertrophy in children and adults. *N Engl J Med.* 2008;358:1899-1908.
55. Bales ND, Johnson NM, Judge DP, Murphy AM. Comprehensive versus targeted genetic testing in children with hypertrophic cardiomyopathy. *Pediatr Cardiol.* 2016;37(5):845-851.
56. Lopes LR, Syrris P, Guttmann OP, et al. Novel genotype-phenotype associations demonstrated by high-throughput sequencing in patients with hypertrophic cardiomyopathy. *Heart.* 2015;101(4):294-301.
57. Keren A, Syrris P, McKenna WJ. Hypertrophic cardiomyopathy: the genetic determinants of clinical disease expression. *Nat Clin Pract Cardiovasc Med.* 2008;5:158-168.
58. Girolami F, Ho CY, Semsarian C, et al. Clinical features and outcome of hypertrophic cardiomyopathy associated with triple sarcomere protein gene mutations. *J Am Coll Cardiol.* 2010;55:1444-1453.
59. Robyns T, Breckpot J, Nuyens D, et al. Clinical and ECG variables to predict the outcome of genetic testing in hypertrophic cardiomyopathy. *Eur J Med Genet.* 2020;63(3):103754. doi:10.1016/j.ejmg.2019.103754
60. Charron P, Dubourg O, Desnos M, et al. Clinical features and prognostic implications of familial hypertrophic cardiomyopathy related to the cardiac myosin-binding protein C gene. *Circulation.* 1998;97:2230-2236.
61. Corrado D, Basso C, Judge DP. Arrhythmogenic cardiomyopathy. *Circ Res.* 2017;121:784-802.
62. Bosman LP, Sammani A, James CA, et al. Predicting arrhythmic risk in arrhythmogenic right ventricular cardiomyopathy: a systematic review and meta-analysis. *Heart Rhythm.* 2018;15:1097-1107.
63. Chivulescu M, Lie OH, Popescu BA, et al. High penetrance and similar disease progression in probands and in family members with arrhythmogenic cardiomyopathy. *Eur Heart J.* 2020;41(14):1401-1410. doi:10.1093/eurheartj/ehz570
64. James CA, Calkins H. Arrhythmogenic right ventricular cardiomyopathy: progress toward personalized management. *Annu Rev Med.* 2019;70:1-18.
65. Towbin JA, McKenna WJ, Abrams DJ, et al. 2019 HRS Expert consensus statement on evaluation, risk stratification, and management of arrhythmogenic cardiomyopathy: executive summary. *Heart Rhythm.* 2019;16(11):e373-e407.
66. Vatta M, Marcus FI, Towbin JA. Arryhthmogenic right ventricular cardiomyopathy: a "final common pathway" that defines clinical phenotype. *Eur Heart J.* 2007;28:529-530.
67. Corrado D, Thiene GC. Arrhythmogenic right ventricular cardiomyopathy/dysplasia: clinical impact of molecular genetic studies. *Circulation.* 2006;113(13):1634-1647.
68. Goff ZD, Calkins H. Sudden death related cardiomyopathies: arrhythmogenic right ventricular cardiomyopathy, arrhythmogenic cardiomyopathy, and exercise-induced cardiomyopathy. *Prog Cardiovasc Dis.* 2019;62(3):217-226.
69. Towbin JA. Genetic arrhythmias complicating patients with dilated cardiomyopathy: how it happens. *Heart Rhythm.* 2020;17(2):313-314.
70. Hoorntje ET, Te Rijdt WP, James CA, et al. Arrhythmogenic cardiomyopathy: pathology, genetics, and concepts in pathogenesis. *Cardiovasc Res.* 2017;113(12):1521-1531.
71. Gandjbakhch E, Redheuil A, Pousset F, Charron P, Frank R. Clinical diagnosis, imaging, and genetics of arrhythmogenic right ventricular cardiomyopathy/dysplasia: JACC State-of-the-Art Review. *J Am Coll Cardiol.* 2018;72(7):784-804.
72. Marcus FI, McKenna WJ, Sherrill D, et al. Diagnosis of arrhythmogenic right ventricular cardiomyopathy/dysplasia: proposed modification of the Task Force Criteria. *Eur Heart J.* 2010;31(7):806-814.
73. Karmouch J, Zhou QQ, Miyake CY, et al. Distinct cellular basis for early cardiac arrhythmias, the cardinal manifestation of arrhythmogenic cardiomyopathy, and the skin phenotype of cardiocutaneous syndromes. *Circ Res.* 2017;121(12):1346-1359.
74. James CA, Bhonsale A, Tichnell C, et al. Exercise increases age-related penetrance and arrhythmic risk in arrhythmogenic right ventricular dysplasia/cardiomyopathy-associated desmosomal mutation carriers. *J Am Coll Cardiol.* 2013;62(14):1290-1297.
75. Te Riele ASJM, James CA, Sawant AC, et al. Arrhythmogenic right ventricular dysplasia/cardiomyopathy in the pediatric population: clinical

characterization and comparison with adult-onset disease. *JACC Clin Electrophysiol.* 2015;1(6):551-560.
76. Nitoiu D, Etheridge SL, Kelsell DP. Insights into desmosome biology from inherited human skin disease and cardiocutaneous syndromes. *Cell Commun Adhes.* 2014;21(3):129-140.
77. Protonotarios N, Tsatsopoulou A, Patsourakos P, et al. Cardiac abnormalities in familial palmoplantar keratosis. *Br Heart J.* 1986;56:321-326.
78. Carvajal-Huerta L Epidermolytic palmoplantar keratoderma with woolly hair and dilated cardiomyopathy. *J Am Acad Dermatol.* 1998;39:418-421.
79. Peters S, Trümmel M, Meyners W. Prevalence of right ventricular dysplasia-cardiomyopathy in a non-referral hospital. *Int J Cardiol.* 2004;97:499-501.
80. Groeneweg JA, Bhonsale A, James CA, et al. Clinical presentation, long-term follow-up, and outcomes of 1001 arrhythmogenic right ventricular dysplasia/cardiomyopathy patients and family members. *Circ Cardiovasc Genet.* 2015;8:437-446.
81. Corrado D, Basso C, Thiene G, et al. Spectrum of clinicopathologic manifestations of arrhythmogenic right ventricular cardiomyopathy/dysplasia: a multicenter study. *J Am Coll Cardiol.* 1997;30:1512-1520.
82. Asimaki A, Saffitz JE. The role of endomyocardial biopsy in ARVC: looking beyond histology in search of new diagnostic markers. *J Cardiovasc Electrophysiol.* 2011;22:111-117.
83. Femia G, Semsarian C, McGuire M, Sy RW, Puranik R. Long term CMR follow up of patients with right ventricular abnormality and clinically suspected arrhythmogenic right ventricular cardiomyopathy (ARVC). *J Cardiovasc Magn Reson.* 2019;21:76.
84. Haugaa KH, Basso C, Badano, LP, et al. Comprehensive multi-modality imaging approach in arrhythmogenic cardiomyopathy—an expert consensus document of the European Association of Cardiovascular Imaging. *Eur Heart J Cardiovac Imaging.* 2017;18(3):237-253.
85. van Lint FHM, Murray B, Tichnell C, et al. Arrhythmogenic right ventricular cardiomyopathy-associated desmosomal variants are rarely de novo. *Circ Genom Precis Med.* 2019;12:e002467.
86. Austin KM, Trembley MA, Chandler SF, et al. Molecular mechanisms of arrhythmogenic cardiomyopathy. *Nat Rev Cardiol.* 2019;16(9):519-537.
87. Noorman M, Hakim S, Kessler E, et al. Remodeling of the cardiac sodium channel, connexin43, and plakoglobin at the intercalated disk in patients with arrhythmogenic cardiomyopathy. *Heart Rhythm.* 2013;10(3):412-419.
88. Gehmlich K, Lambiase PD, Asimaki A, et al. A novel desmocollin-2 mutation reveals insights into the molecular link between desmosomes and gap junctions. *Heart Rhythm.* 2011;8(5):711-718.
89. Asimaki A, Kleber AG, Saffitz JE. Pathogenesis of arrhythmogenic cardiomyopathy. *Can J Cardiol.* 2015;31:1313-1324.
90. Xue J, Yan X, Yang Y, et al. Connexin 43 dephosphorylation contributes to arrhythmias and cardiomyocyte apoptosis in ischemia/reperfusion hearts. *Basic Res Cardiol.* 2019;114(5):40. doi:10.1007/s00395-019-0748-8
91. James CA, Syrris P, van Tintelen JP, Calkins H. The role of genetics in cardiovascular disease: arrhythmogenic cardiomyopathy. *Eur Heart J.* 2020;41(14):1393-1400.
92. De Bortoli M, Postma AV, Poloni G, et al. Whole-exome sequencing identifies pathogenic variants in TJP1 gene associated with arrhythmogenic cardiomyopathy. *Circ Genom Precis Med.* 2018;11:e002123. doi:10.1161/CIRCGEN.118.002123
93. Roberts JD, Murphy NP, Hamilton RM, et al. Ankyrin-B dysfunction predisposes to arrhythmogenic cardiomyopathy and is amenable to therapy. *J Clin Invest.* 2019;129:3171-3184.
94. Poloni G, Calore M, Rigato I, et al. A targeted next-generation gene panel reveals a novel heterozygous nonsense variant in the TP63 gene in patients with arrhythmogenic cardiomyopathy. *Heart Rhythm.* 2019;16:773-780.
95. MacLennan DH, Kranias EG. Phospholamban: a crucial regulator of cardiac contractility. *Nat Rev Mol Cell Biol.* 2003;4(7):566-577.
96. Kranias EG, Hajjar RJ. The phospholamban journey 4 decades after setting out for ithaka. *Circ Res.* 2017;120:781-783.
97. Sucharski HC, Dudley EK, Keith CBR, El Refaey M, Koenig SN, Mohler PJ. Mechanisms and alterations of cardiac ion channels leading to disease: role of ankyrin-B in cardiac function. *Biomolecules.* 2020;10(2):211. doi:10.3390/biom10020211
98. Li W, Yin L, Shen C, Hu K, Ge J, Sun A. *SCN5A* Variants: association with cardiac disorders. *Front Physiol.* 2018;9:1372. doi:10.3389/fphys.2018.01372
99. Li Y, Merkel CD, Zeng X, et al. The N-cadherin interactome in primary cardiomyocytes as defined using quantitative proximity proteomics. *J Cell Sci.* 2019;132(3):jcs221606. doi:10.1242/jcs.221606
100. Bruce AF, Rothery S, Dupont E, Severs NJ. Gap junction remodelling in human heart failure is associated with increased interaction of connexin43 with ZO-1. *Cardiovasc Res.* 2008;77:757-765.
101. Palatinus JA, O'Quinn MP, Barker RJ, Harris BS, Jourdan J, Gourdie RG. ZO-1 determines adherens and gap junction localization at intercalated disks. *Am J Physiol Heart Circ Physiol.* 2011;300:H583-H594.
102. Rhett JM, Gourdie RG. The perinexus: a new feature of Cx43 gap junction organization. *Heart Rhythm.* 2012;9:619-623.
103. Rhett JM, Jourdan J, Gourdie RG. Connexin 43 connexon to gap junction transition is regulated by zonula occludens-1. *Mol Biol Cell.* 2011;22:1516-1528.
104. McKoy G, Protonotarios N, Crosby A, et al. Identification of a deletion in plakoglobin in arrhythmogenic right ventricular cardiomyopathy with palmoplantar keratoderma and woolly hair (Naxos disease) *Lancet.* 2000;355:2119-2124.
105. Norgett EE, Hatsell SJ, Carvajal-Huerta L, et al. Recessive mutation in desmoplakin disrupts desmoplakin-intermediate filament interactions and causes dilated cardiomyopathy, woolly hair and keratoderma. *Hum Mol Genet.* 2000;9:2761-2766.
106. Xu T, Yang Z, Vatta M, et al. Multidisciplinary study of right ventricular dysplasia investigators. Compound and digenic heterozygosity contributes to arrhythmogenic right ventricular cardiomyopathy. *J Am Coll Cardiol.* 2010;55(6):587-597.
107. Rowe MK, Roberts JD. The evolution of gene-guided management of inherited arrhythmia syndromes: peering beyond monogenic paradigms towards comprehensive genomic risk scores. *J Cardiovasc Electrophysiol.* 2020;31(11):2998-3008. doi:10.1111/jce.14415
108. Miles C, Finocchiaro G, Papadakis M, et al. Sudden death and left ventricular involvement in arrhythmogenic cardiomyopathy. *Circulation.* 2019;139:1786-1797.
109. Cipriani A, Zorzi A, Sarto P, et al. Predictive value of exercise testing in athletes with ventricular ectopy evaluated by cardiac magnetic resonance. *Heart Rhythm.* 2019;16:239-248.
110. Towbin JA. Left ventricular noncompaction: a new form of heart failure. *Heart Fail Clin.* 2010;6(4):453-469.
111. Towbin JA, Lorts A, Jefferies JL. Left ventricular non-compaction cardiomyopathy. *Lancet.* 2015;386(9995):813-825.
112. van Waning JI, Moesker J, Heijsman D, Boersma E, Majoor-Krakauer D. Systematic review of genotype-phenotype correlations in noncompaction cardiomyopathy. *J Am Heart Assoc.* 2019;8(23):e012993. doi:10.1161/JAHA.119.012993
113. Ajima R, Bisson JA, Helt JC, et al. Cohen ED DAAM1 and DAAM2 are co-required for myocardial maturation and sarcomere assembly. *Dev Biol.* 2015;408(1):126-139.
114. D'Amato G, Luxán G, de la Pompa JL. Notch signalling in ventricular chamber development and cardiomyopathy. *FEBS J.* 2016;283(23):4223-4237.
115. Towbin JA, Jefferies JL. Cardiomyopathies due to left ventricular noncompaction, mitochondrial and storage diseases, and inborn errors of metabolism. *Circ Res.* 2017;121:838-885.
116. Bleyl SB, Mumford BR, Brown-Harrison MC, et al. Xq28-linked noncompaction of the left ventricular myocardium: prenatal diagnosis and pathologic analysis of affected individuals. *Am J Med Genet.* 1997;72(3):257-265.
117. Ouyang P, Saarel E, Bai Y, et al. A de novo mutation in NKX2.5 associated with atrial septal defects, ventricular noncompaction, syncope and sudden death. *Clin Chim Acta.* 2011;412:170-175.
118. Postma AV, van Engelen K, van de Meerakker J, et al. Mutations in the sarcomere gene MYH7 in Ebstein anomaly. *Circ Cardiovasc Genet.* 2011;4:43-50.
119. Kelle AM, Bentley SJ, Rohena LO, Cabalka AK, Olson TM. Ebstein anomaly, left ventricular non-compaction, and early onset heart failure associated with a de novo α-tropomyosin gene mutation. *Am J Med Genet A.* 2016;170(8):2186-2190.

120. Hoedemaekers YM, Caliskan K, Michels M, et al. The importance of genetic counseling, DNA diagnostics, and cardiologic family screening in left ventricular noncompaction cardiomyopathy. *Circ Cardiovasc Genet.* 2010;3:232-239.
121. Probst S, Oechslin E, Schuler P, et al. Sarcomere gene mutations in isolated left ventricular noncompaction cardiomyopathy do not predict clinical phenotype. *Circulation Cardiovasc Genet.* 2011;4:367-374.
122. Dellefave LM, Pytel P, Mewborn S, et al. Sarcomere mutations in cardiomyopathy with left ventricular hypertrabeculation. *Circ Cardiovasc Genet.* 2009;2:442-449.
123. Hastings R, de Villiers CP, Hooper C, et al. Combination of whole genome sequencing, linkage, and functional studies implicates a missense mutation in titin as a cause of autosomal dominant cardiomyopathy with features of left ventricular noncompaction. *Circ Cardiovasc Genet.* 2016;9:426-435.
124. Bagnall RD, Molloy LK, Kalman JM, Semsarian C. Exome sequencing identifies a mutation in the ACTN2 gene in a family with idiopathic ventricular fibrillation, left ventricular noncompaction, and sudden death. *BMC Med Genet.* 2014;15:99.
125. van Waning JI, Caliskan K, Hoedemaekers YM, et al. Genetics, clinical features, and long-term outcome of noncompaction cardiomyopathy. *J Am Coll Cardiol.* 2018;71(7):711-722.
126. Shan L, Makita N, Xing Y, et al. SCN5A variants in Japanese patients with left ventricular noncompaction and arrhythmia. *Mol Genet Metab.* 2008;93:468-474.
127. Finsterer J, Stollberger C. Primary myopathies and the heart. *Scand Cardiovasc J.* 2008;42:9-24.
128. Ramond F, Janin A, Di Filippo S, et al. Homozygous PKP2 deletion associated with neonatal left ventricle noncompaction. *Clin Genet.* 2017;91:126-130.
129. Williams T, Machann W, Kuhler L, et al. Novel desmoplakin mutation: juvenile biventricular cardiomyopathy with left ventricular non-compaction and acantholytic palmoplantar keratoderma. *Clin Res Cardiol.* 2011;100:1087-1093.
130. Tang S, Batra A, Zhang Y, Ebenroth ES, Huang T. Left ventricular noncompaction is associated with mutations in the mitochondrial genome. *Mitochondrion.* 2010;10:350-357.
131. El-Hattab AW, Scaglia F, Mitochondrial cardiomyopathies. *Front Cardiovasc Med.* 2016;3:25. doi:10.3389/fcvm.2016.00025
132. Digilio M, Bernardini L, Gagliardi M, et al. Syndromic non-compaction of the left ventricle: associated chromosomal anomalies. *Clin Genet.* 2013;84(4):362-367.
133. Eldomery MK, Akdemir ZC, Vögtle FN, et al. MIPEP recessive variants cause a syndrome of left ventricular non-compaction, hypotonia, and infantile death. *Genome Med.* 2016;8(1):106.
134. Beken S, Cevik A, Turan O, et al. A neonatal case of left ventricular noncompaction associated with trisomy 18. *Genet Counsel.* 2011;22(2):161-164.
135. Yukifumi M, Hirohiko S, Fukiko I, Mariko M. Trisomy 13 in a 9-year-old girl with left ventricular noncompaction. *Pediatr Cardiol.* 2011;32(2):206-207.
136. Blinder JJ, Martinez HR, Craigen WJ, Belmont J, Pignatelli RH, Jefferies JL. Noncompaction of the left ventricular myocardium in a boy with a novel chromosome 8p23.1 deletion. *Am J Med Genet Part A.* 2011;155A(9):2215-2220.
137. Martinez HR, Niu MC, Sutton VR, et al. Coffin-Lowry syndrome and left ventricular noncompaction cardiomyopathy with a restrictive pattern. *Am J Med Genet Part A.* 2011;155A(12):3030-3034.
138. Martinez HR, Belmont JW, Craigen WJ, Taylor MD, Jefferies JL. Left ventricular noncompaction in Sotos syndrome. *Am J Med Genet Part A.* 2011;155A(5):1115-1118.
139. Zechner U, Kohlschmidt N, Kempf O, et al. Familial Sotos syndrome caused by a novel missense mutation, C2175S, in NSD1 and associated with normal intelligence, insulin dependent diabetes, bronchial asthma, and lipedema. *Eur J Med Genet.* 2009;52(5):306-310.
140. Sellars EA, Zimmerman SL, Smolarek T, Hopkin RJ. Ventricular noncompaction and absent thumbs in a newborn with tetrasomy 5q35.2-5q35.3: an association with Hunter-McAlpine syndrome? *Am J Med Genet Part A.* 2011;155A(6):1409-1413.
141. Corrado G, Checcarelli N, Santarone M, Stollberger C, Finsterer J. Left ventricular hypertrabeculation/noncompaction with PMP22 duplication-based Charcot-Marie-Tooth disease type 1A. *Cardiol.* 2006;105(3):142-145.
142. Arndt AK, Schafer S, Drenckhahn JD, et al. Fine mapping of the 1p36 deletion syndrome identifies mutation of PRDM16 as a cause of cardiomyopathy. *Am J Hum Genet.* 2013;93:67-77.
143. Pearce FB, Litovsky SH, Dabal RJ, et al. Pathologic features of dilated cardiomyopathy with localized noncompaction in a child with deletion 1p36 syndrome. *Congenit Heart Dis.* 2012;7:59-61.
144. Anderson HN, Cetta F, Driscoll DJ, Olson TM, Ackerman MJ, Johnson JN, Idiopathic restrictive cardiomyopathy in children and young adults. *J Am Coll Cardiol.* 2018;121(10):1266-1270.
145. Denfield SW, Webber SA. Restrictive cardiomyopathy in childhood. *Heart Fail Clin.* 2010;6:445-452.
146. Wittekind SG, Ryan TD, Gao Z, et al. Contemporary outcomes of pediatric restrictive cardiomyopathy: a single-enter experience. *Pediatr Cardiol.* 2019;40(4):694-704.
147. Webber SA, Lipshultz SE, Sleeper LA, et al. Outcomes of restrictive cardiomyopathy in childhood and the influence of phenotype: a report from the Pediatric Cardiomyopathy Registry. Pediatric Cardiomyopathy Registry Investigators. *Circulation.* 2012;126(10):1237-1244.
148. Walsh MA, Grenier MA, Jefferies JL, Towbin JA, Lorts A, Czosek RJ. Conduction abnormalities in pediatric patients with restrictive cardiomyopathy. *Circ Heart Fail.* 2012;5(2):267-273.
149. Rivenes SM, Kearney DL, Smith EO, et al. Sudden death and cardiovascular collapse in children with restrictive cardiomyopathy. *Circulation.* 2000;102:876-882.
150. Pereira NL, Grogan M, Dec GW. Spectrum of restrictive and infiltrative cardiomyopathies: part 1 of a 2-part series. *J Am Coll Cardiol.* 2018;71:1130-1148.
151. Ryan TD, Madueme PC, Jefferies JL, et al. Utility of echocardiography in the assessment of left ventricular diastolic function and restrictive physiology in children and young adults with restrictive cardiomyopathy: a comparative echocardiography-catheterization study. *Pediatr Cardiol.* 2017;38:381-389.
152. Nugent AW, Daubeney P, Chondros P, et al. The epidemiology of childhood cardiomyopathy in Australia, *N Engl J Med.* 2003 348:1639-1646.
153. Fitzpatrick AP, Shapiro LM, Rickards AF, et al. Familial restrictive cardiomyopathy with atrioventricular block and skeletal myopathy. *Br Heart J.* 1990;63:114-118.
154. Goldfarb LG, Dalakas MC. Tragedy in a heartbeat: malfunctioning desmin causes skeletal and cardiac muscle disease. *J Clin Invest.* 2009;119(7):1806-1813.
155. Muchtar E, Blauwet LA, Gertz MA. Restrictive cardiomyopathy: genetics, pathogenesis, clinical manifestations, diagnosis, and therapy. *Circ Res.* 2017;121(7):819-837.
156. Kiselev A, Vaz R, Knyazeva A, et al. De novo mutations in FLNC leading to early-onset restrictive cardiomyopathy and congenital myopathy. *Hum Mutat.* 2018;39(9):1161-1172.
157. Schänzer A, Rupp S, Gräf S, et al. Dysregulated autophagy in restrictive cardiomyopathy due to Pro209Leu mutation in BAG3. *Mol Genet Metab.* 2018;123(3):388-399.
158. Finsterer J, Stöllberger C, Höftberger R. Restrictive cardiomyopathy as a cardiac manifestation of myofibrillar myopathy. *Heart Lung.* 2011;40:e123-e127.
159. Gu Q, Mendsaikhan U, Khuchua Z, et al. Dissection of Z-disc myopalladin gene network involved in the development of restrictive cardiomyopathy using system genetics approach. *World J Cardiol.* 2017;9(4):320-331.
160. Huby AC, Mendsaikhan U, Takagi K, et al. Disturbance in Z-disk mechanosensitive proteins induced by a persistent mutant myopalladin causes familial restrictive cardiomyopathy. *J Am Coll Cardiol.* 2014;64(25):2765-2776.
161. Lee S, Kim N, Noh Y, et al. Mitochondrial DNA, mitochondrial dysfunction, and cardiac manifestations. *Front Biosci (Landmark Ed).* 2016;21:1410-1426.
162. Finsterer J, Kothari S. Cardiac manifestations of primary mitochondrial disorders. *Int J Cardiol.* 2014;177:754-763.
163. Kanungo S, Morton J, Neelakantan M, Ching K, Saeedian J, Goldstein A. Mitochondrial disorders. *Ann Transl Med.* 2018;6(24):475.
164. Song T, Manoharan P, Millay DP, et al. Dilated cardiomyopathy-mediated heart failure induces a unique skeletal muscle myopathy with inflammation. *Skelet Muscle.* 2019;9(1):4. doi:10.1186/s13395-019-0189-y

CHAPTER 68

HEART FAILURE WITH PRESERVED EJECTION FRACTION

Tyler Moran, Anita Deswal, and Arunima Misra

INTRODUCTION

Cardiovascular (CV) disease is the number one cause of death worldwide.[1] Although there have been major advances in the management of many CV disease states, including heart failure with reduced ejection fraction (HFrEF) which has robust evidence for a multitude of therapies, heart failure with preserved ejection fraction (HFpEF) remains a notable exception. Consequently, HFpEF remains a challenging clinical syndrome to diagnose and treat. HFpEF has almost similar morbidity and mortality compared to HFrEF[2]; however, there exists limited evidence for the treatment of HFpEF to improve clinical outcomes. This chapter presents the epidemiology, diagnosis, and management of HFpEF based on currently available data.

Definition and Guidelines

The definition of heart failure (HF) is complex, but the fundamental basis for HF is the inability of the ventricle to pump or fill effectively with normal filling pressure. These failures result in the common symptoms and signs of HF including dyspnea and fatigue, as well as edema or fluid retention. Historically, pump failure was reported as systolic HF and filling failure as diastolic HF. As our understanding of physiology and pathophysiology advanced, the mechanisms for HF were shown to overlap as most patients with HF have pump or systolic dysfunction, albeit sometimes subtle, as well as filling or diastolic dysfunction. Therefore, the initial terminology of systolic HF or diastolic HF was changed to include the terms reduced or preserved ejection fraction.[3]

The American College of Cardiology (ACC)/American Heart Association (AHA)/Heart Failure Society of America (HFSA) HF guidelines define HFpEF as HF with left ventricular ejection fraction (LVEF) ≥50%. Nonetheless, trials studying treatment for HFpEF have used varying definitions and have often included patients with LVEF ≥45%. The borderline or midrange group (HFmEF) with LVEF between 40% and 49% appears to have similarities to both HFrEF and HFpEF, and is a group that includes HFrEF patients in whom LVEF has improved, those with HFpEF where the LVEF appears to progressively decline over time, and patients with an acute injury such as myocardial infarction that causes a reduction in LVEF to this range.[4] The LVEF remains important in the classification of patients with HF because of some differences in patient demographics, comorbid conditions, etiology and pathophysiology, prognosis, response to therapies, as well as the ease of a phenotypic differentiation by LVEF. Also, most clinical trials in HF selected and continue to select patients based on LVEF. However, LVEF values are dependent not only on the disease condition but also on loading conditions, the imaging technique used, the method of analysis, and the interoperator variability, making it even more challenging to accurately classify all patients into nonoverlapping groups of preserved LVEF, reduced LVEF, and midrange LVEF. Currently, most definitions of HFpEF include (1) clinical symptoms and/or signs of HF; (2) normal or near-normal LVEF; and (3) evidence of structural and/or functional cardiac abnormalities or of elevated left ventricular (LV) filling pressures.

Epidemiology

In the United States, about 6.2 million adults (2.2% of the population) have HF. It is the number one reason for hospitalizations in patients aged greater than or equal to 65 years. Of the patients hospitalized for HF, almost half have HFpEF. The prevalence of HF continues to rise as the population ages. Specifically, the prevalence of HFpEF, compared with the prevalence of HFrEF, appears to be increasing over time along with the aging of the population.[5] HFpEF is associated with substantial morbidity and mortality, and the frequency of clinical events markedly increases once a patient is hospitalized for HF.[6] Because patients with HFpEF have a normal or near-normal LVEF, the diagnosis is more difficult and the management less defined than HFrEF. This is in part owing to fewer clinical trials as compared to HFrEF, but also because several completed clinical trials demonstrated no benefit on mortality and morbidity in HFpEF patients. Understanding the pathophysiology and comorbidities that define HFpEF is germane to developing better treatments and to changing the trajectory of associated significant morbidity and possibly mortality.

Risk Factors

Both HFrEF and HFpEF share a number of risk factors, including coronary artery disease (CAD), hypertension, diabetes mellitus, obesity, and smoking.[7] However, there are some differences in the HF subtypes. As a group, patients with HFpEF are older; are more likely to be female; and have a greater prevalence of hypertension, obesity, renal dysfunction, sleep disorders, chronic obstructive pulmonary disease, atrial fibrillation, and anemia, than those with HFrEF.[8] In addition to being a comorbidity, renal disease is a significant contributor to hypertension, cardiac dysfunction, LV stiffening, delayed LV relaxation, and sodium and water retention resulting in the syndrome of HFpEF.[9] Furthermore, when right HF progresses with venous congestion, worsening renal function may be noted, underlining the importance of cardiorenal interactions in HF.[10]

PATHOGENESIS

To fully understand the heterogeneity within HFpEF, one should appreciate the varying mechanisms that may underlie the clinical syndrome. Etiologies of HFpEF are multiple (**Table 68.1**). Hypertension is the most common underlying cause associated with HFpEF. It is present in a majority of patients with HFpEF regardless of age, gender, or racial group, and may result in LV hypertrophy. In addition, CAD has been noted in 35% to 60% of patients with HFpEF[11] and is associated with a greater risk of developing HFrEF and higher mortality.[12] Other contributors or precipitants for the development of HFpEF include atrial fibrillation, diabetes mellitus (in 20%-30%), and obesity (in at least 50%). In fact, obesity may be even more prevalent, with HFpEF being underdiagnosed because of the difficult physical examination and lower natriuretic peptide levels in obese patients.[11] Valvular heart disease leading to HF in the presence of normal LVEF also presents as HFpEF. Other etiologies include toxic, inflammatory, and metabolic causes, which may be mediated through comorbidities such as diabetes mellitus and chronic kidney disease, as well as restrictive cardiomyopathies, including infiltrative disorders and transplant rejection, and hypertrophic cardiomyopathy.[13] Given the importance of cardiac amyloidosis, it is discussed in detail in Chapter 30.

TABLE 68.1 Potential Etiologies of HFpEF

Abnormalities of the Myocardium	
Ischemic	Coronary artery disease with a scar or active ischemia Microvascular disease and endothelial dysfunction
Toxic	Drugs: alcohol, cocaine, anabolic steroids Metals: iron, lead Medications: chemotherapy, immunomodulators
Immune and inflammatory	Radiation: high cardiac radiation doses Infectious: HIV, Chagas Noninfectious: lymphocytic myocarditis, autoimmune diseases, eosinophilic myocarditis, immune checkpoint inhibitor therapy
Infiltrative	Malignant: direct involvement or metastases Nonmalignant: amyloidosis, sarcoidosis, hemochromatosis, storage diseases including Fabry disease
Metabolic	Thyroid, growth hormone diseases, adrenal hormone diseases, pregnancy, diabetic cardiomyopathy
Genetic	Hypertrophic cardiomyopathy, muscular dystrophy
Endomyocardial	Endocardial fibroelastosis, hypereosinophilic syndrome, carcinoid
Abnormalities of Loading Conditions	
Hypertension	Primary and secondary forms of hypertension
Valvular/structural disease	Heart valve disease Septal defects
Pericardial disease	Constrictive pericarditis
High output states	Severe anemia, sepsis, thyrotoxicosis, AV fistula, pregnancy
Volume overload	Renal failure
Obesity-related HFpEF	Metabolic/inflammatory with microvascular dysfunction/volume expansion/pericardial and chest wall, abdominal restraint
Abnormalities of Cardiac Rhythm	
Rhythm disorders	Atrial or ventricular arrhythmias, eg, atrial fibrillation, pacing, conduction disorders

AV, arteriovenous; HFpEF, heart failure preserved ejection fraction.

Modified from How to diagnose heart failure with preserved ejection fraction: the HFA–PEFF diagnostic algorithm: a consensus recommendation from the Heart Failure Association (HFA) of the European Society of Cardiology. *Eur Heart J.* 2019; 40(40):3297-3317. Reproduced by permission of Oxford University Press.

Underlying Mechanisms and Multisystem Involvement

Although initially thought to be caused only by diastolic dysfunction, HFpEF is now recognized to have complex pathophysiology, and in a majority of patients is related to multisystem involvement. The clinical syndrome of HFpEF may result from cardiac, pulmonary, vascular, peripheral reserve, or renal abnormalities, all finally resulting in increased LV diastolic pressure and the common clinical manifestations of HF. Various cardiac abnormalities leading to the phenotype of HFpEF can include myocyte hypertrophy, diastolic and early systolic ventricular dysfunction, atrial dysfunction, energy metabolism abnormalities, interstitial fibrosis, inflammation, increased oxidative stress, endothelial dysfunction, and impaired density and autoregulation of the microcirculation. Also contributing to HFpEF are volume overload secondary to renal disease, neurohormonal (specifically renin-angiotensin-aldosterone system) activation, reduced vasodilator reserve, chronotropic incompetence during exercise, and impaired right ventricular-pulmonary artery coupling.[14,15] Cardiometabolic diseases common in HFpEF—including obesity, hypertension, and diabetes—induce a systemic pro-inflammatory state, which in turn triggers systemic and coronary microvascular inflammation. This results in a reduction of nitric oxide bioavailability downstream, which promotes myocyte and myocardial hypertrophy, cardiomyocyte stiffness, and interstitial fibrosis.[16]

Cardiac Abnormalities

In HFpEF, the rise in end-diastolic pressure is caused by a complex interaction between diastolic dysfunction, underlying although not overt systolic dysfunction, atrial and LV stiffness, and reduced arterial compliance.[17] There is an elevation of LV filling pressures either only with exercise or also at rest with worsening during exercise.[18] In a significant proportion of patients, elevation in LV filling pressure is contributed by diastolic dysfunction with impaired active relaxation and increased LV passive chamber stiffness leading to the LV diastolic pressure-volume relationship shifted up and to the left.[19] In these patients, during exercise or with other increases in heart rate, the baseline abnormalities may be accentuated leading to increases in LV diastolic pressure.[18] Although there has been significant progress in noninvasive measurement of diastolic function, it is not possible to accurately assess a significant proportion of patients, especially in light of differing methods and uncertain abnormal thresholds in aging populations using echocardiography. For example, in an older Olmsted County epidemiologic study of HF patients, 78% of those with HFpEF had diastolic dysfunction, 10% had normal diastolic function, and the remainder were indeterminate.[20] More recently, in the Treatment of Preserved Cardiac Function Heart Failure With an Aldosterone Antagonist (TOPCAT) trial, diastolic function was measured using the ratio between transmitral E wave velocity and tissue Doppler e' velocities, and graded based on the ratio of E/e', transmitral E/A, and deceleration time of transmitral E velocity. Owing to the presence of atrial fibrillation, missing tissue Doppler, or transmitral E velocity, only 52% of patients with HFpEF could have diastology assessed. In these patients, diastolic dysfunction was present in only 66%; 44% had moderate to severe dysfunction. Nonetheless, regardless of the method of noninvasive diastolic assessment, studies have shown that worse diastolic function is associated with adverse outcomes in patients with HFpEF, including mortality and HF hospitalization.[21]

Other cardiac mechanisms are likely to contribute to HFpEF but are less easily assessed and not well studied in epidemiologic studies or clinical trials. These include extrinsic LV restraint by the pericardium and the right heart causing an elevation of LV filling pressures, especially during exercise. For example, HFpEF patients with severe obesity may have increased pericardial restraint owing to increased mediastinal, chest wall, and abdominal fat.[22] LV systolic dysfunction may also be present as measured by strain and without necessarily impacting LVEF.[23] In the TOPCAT trial, longitudinal strain was abnormal in over half the patients and was associated with a higher risk of CV death or HF hospitalization. Thus, in the setting of HFpEF, impaired longitudinal strain predicts a worse prognosis.[24]

Furthermore, elevated filling pressure in HFpEF results in left atrial remodeling and dysfunction, which may lead to pulmonary hypertension (PH) and eventually right ventricular failure. When atrial fibrillation is present, as it is in many patients with HFpEF, PH and subsequent right HF can ensue more quickly, sometimes irreversibly. In fact, left atrial dysfunction has been associated with worse exercise capacity, more advanced pulmonary vascular disease, and higher mortality.[25]

Pulmonary Hypertension

Left heart-related or Group 2 PH is defined as an increase in mean pulmonary artery pressure (PAP) greater than 20 to 25 mm Hg with a pulmonary capillary wedge pressure (PCWP) $\geq$15 mm Hg.[26] Some epidemiologic studies suggest that HFpEF may be a more common cause of PH than other forms of PH[27] and may occur in up to 36% to 53% of patients with HFpEF.[21] This group of patients are often older, have more CV comorbidities, worse exercise capacity, and more impaired renal function compared to patients with idiopathic PH.[28] With long-standing PH, the right ventricle (RV) can hypertrophy, dilate, and eventually fail especially if significant tricuspid regurgitation develops and there is concomitant renal failure.[28] Importantly, the development of RV dysfunction predicts a worse prognosis and a marked increased risk of death in patients with HFpEF.[29]

Role of Peripheral Abnormalities

In addition to cardiac abnormalities, systemic vasculature, endothelium, adipocytes, and skeletal muscle play a role in HFpEF.[18,22,30] Clinically, these abnormalities may be latent at rest and only reveal themselves during stress; thus, symptoms may only occur during exercise or other stress.[18] A major contributor to HFpEF is the systemic circulation whereby the aortic and conduit stiffness result in excessive blood pressure variability and greater arterial afterload mismatch, especially during exercise. Endothelial dysfunction and abnormal nitric oxide–mediated vasodilation are found in almost half of patients with HFpEF[18] and are associated with a worse prognosis compared to those with normal vasodilator response.[31] Skeletal muscle alterations have also been observed in HFpEF, with increased fatty infiltration and reduced sarcomeres, along with an impaired ability to extract oxygen, contributing to exercise intolerance.[30] Similar underlying mechanisms contribute to both chronic kidney disease and HFpEF, and subsequent sodium and volume overload further contribute to both kidney and heart dysfunction in a vicious cycle. In chronic kidney disease, CV events are more likely in those with modest degrees of volume overload with or without concomitant hypertension.[32]

The comorbidity-inflammation paradigm proposed by Paulus and Tschöpe suggests that HFpEF may be the result of a comorbidity-induced systemic pro-inflammatory state, which leads to endothelial dysfunction, coronary microvascular dysfunction, and abnormal cardiac structure and function.[16] Comorbidities including diabetes, obesity, and hypertension may induce a systemic pro-inflammatory state, which causes coronary microvascular endothelial inflammation. The endothelial inflammation reduces nitric oxide bioavailability, cyclic guanosine monophosphate content, and protein kinase G (PKG) activity in adjacent cardiomyocytes, which in turn induces hypertrophy and increases resting tension from hypophosphorylation of titin. Both the stiff cardiomyocytes and interstitial fibrosis then contribute to high diastolic LV stiffness and HF. A recent study undertook a comprehensive proteomic evaluation of this inflammatory paradigm.[33] The investigators found that the comorbidity burden was associated with heightened systemic inflammation, which in turn was associated with worse cardiac function and hemodynamic stress. Thus, anti-inflammatory strategies may hold promise in the treatment of this HFpEF phenotype.

Inflammation from visceral and epicardial fat is a contributor to the higher incidence of HFpEF with obesity. However, other mechanisms such as abnormal sodium retention leading to increased plasma volume and LV and RV dilation, alterations in energy substrate metabolism, PH leading to RV failure, and mechanical epi/pericardial, chest wall or abdominal restraint leading to diastolic ventricular interactions may all play a role.[22,34]

CLINICAL PRESENTATION

Clinical Symptoms and Associated Comorbidities

With regard to history, important clinical risk factors for HFpEF include elderly age, female sex, hypertension, atrial fibrillation, diabetes, and obesity. Symptoms of HFpEF are similar to HFrEF and include dyspnea, fatigue, and swelling. Dyspnea is the hallmark symptom notably occurring with exertion. Clinical awareness of the risk factors is important; when a patient presents with these symptoms, one should consider HFpEF in the differential diagnosis.

Physical Examination

The physical examination may show signs of volume overload, including rales, elevated jugular venous pressure, and lower extremity edema. An S4, and less commonly an S3, gallop may be present. In a significant proportion, the physical examination is without obvious signs of volume overload.

DIAGNOSIS

The diagnosis of HFpEF is challenging, given the symptoms of dyspnea, fatigue and edema in the presence of a normal LVEF can often be attributed to advanced age as well as comorbidities that are present in many of the patients. Various definitions have been proposed but when evaluated against a gold standard of rest and stress invasive hemodynamic testing, the correlations have been inconsistent.[35]

The 2019 recommendations for diagnosis by the Heart Failure Association of the European Society of Cardiology (ESC/HFA) along with an algorithm H_2FPEF, based on an evidence-based approach, may facilitate the diagnosis of HFpEF[39,43] **(Algorithm 68.1)**. This algorithm is based on clinical suspicion from a thorough history and physical examination followed by diagnostic tests to include electrocardiography, chest x-ray, echocardiography, and assessment of natriuretic peptides. The algorithm scores the patient based on clinical and diagnostic assessment. Further testing is recommended using echocardiography stress testing or invasive hemodynamic monitoring if the diagnosis remains unclear.

With the algorithm provided by the consensus statement from ESC/HFA or the use of the H_2FPEF score, diagnosis of HFpEF may be more accurate. Clinical suspicion based on risk factors and symptoms of dyspnea warrants a thorough workup including biomarkers, echocardiography, and even invasive evaluation if needed, so that a definitive diagnosis can be made. It is important to rule out other causes of dyspnea as well including mimickers of HFpEF including constrictive pericarditis, severe valvular disease, hypertrophic cardiomyopathy, congenital heart disease, and amyloid heart disease or cor pulmonale owing to pulmonary pathology or primary PH.

Diagnostic Testing

Serum Natriuretic Peptides

Diagnostic testing including serum natriuretic peptides should be performed. They are more sensitive in nonobese patients (obesity is associated with lower values) and less specific in more elderly patients (elderly patients can have elevated serum natriuretic peptides without HF). Serum levels of N-terminal pro-brain natriuretic peptide (NT-proBNP) less than 125 pg/mL or B-type natriuretic peptide (BNP) less than 35 pg/mL have high negative predictive value to exclude HF.[36] Importantly, because

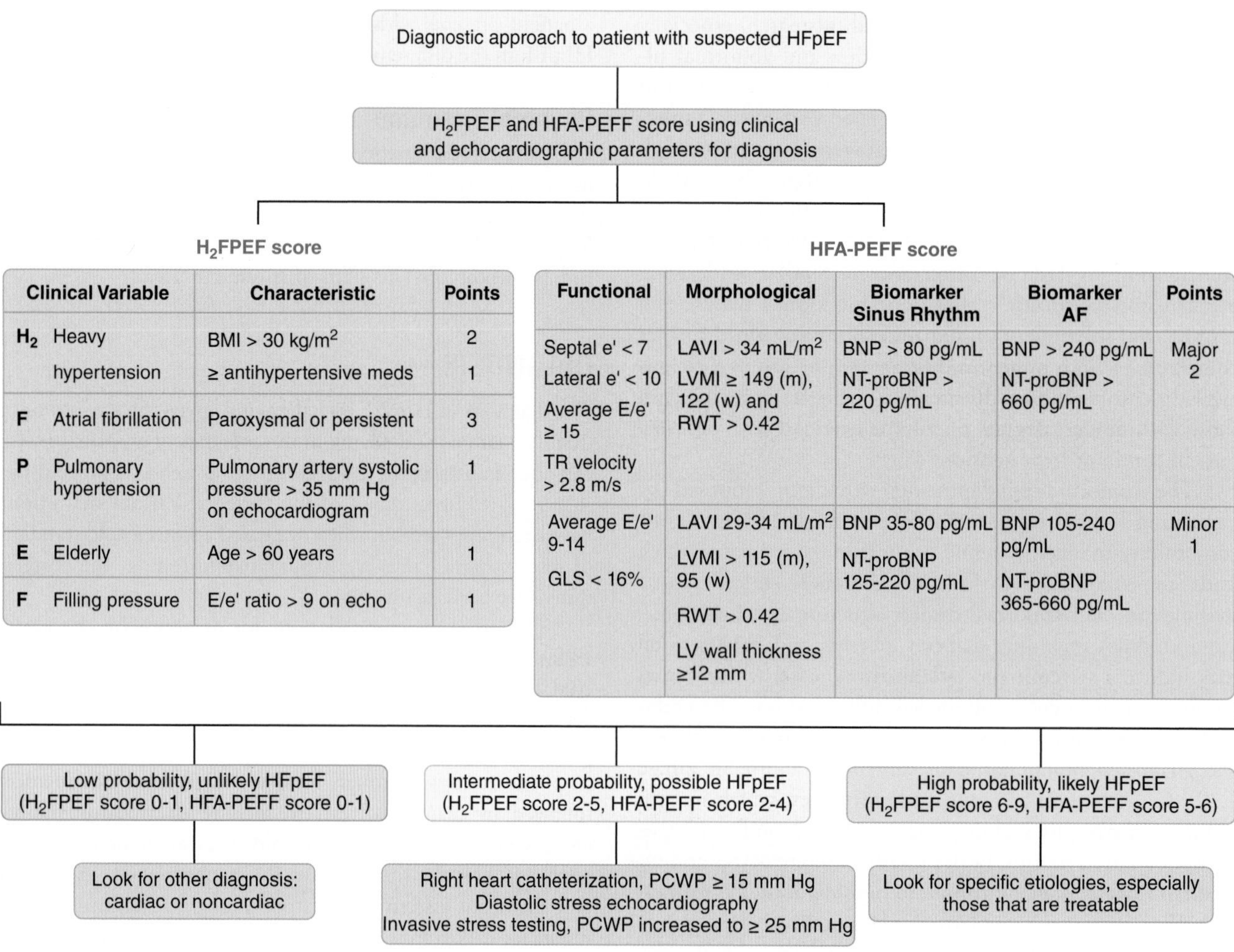

H_2FPEF score

Clinical Variable		Characteristic	Points
H_2	Heavy	BMI > 30 kg/m²	2
	hypertension	≥ antihypertensive meds	1
F	Atrial fibrillation	Paroxysmal or persistent	3
P	Pulmonary hypertension	Pulmonary artery systolic pressure > 35 mm Hg on echocardiogram	1
E	Elderly	Age > 60 years	1
F	Filling pressure	E/e' ratio > 9 on echo	1

HFA-PEFF score

Functional	Morphological	Biomarker Sinus Rhythm	Biomarker AF	Points
Septal e' < 7 Lateral e' < 10 Average E/e' ≥ 15 TR velocity > 2.8 m/s	LAVI > 34 mL/m² LVMI ≥ 149 (m), 122 (w) and RWT > 0.42	BNP > 80 pg/mL NT-proBNP > 220 pg/mL	BNP > 240 pg/mL NT-proBNP > 660 pg/mL	Major 2
Average E/e' 9-14 GLS < 16%	LAVI 29-34 mL/m² LVMI > 115 (m), 95 (w) RWT > 0.42 LV wall thickness ≥12 mm	BNP 35-80 pg/mL NT-proBNP 125-220 pg/mL	BNP 105-240 pg/mL NT-proBNP 365-660 pg/mL	Minor 1

ALGORITHM 68.1 Diagnostic approach to patient with suspected HFpEF. BNP, brain natriuretic peptide; GLS, global longitudinal strain; HFA-PEFF, Heart Failure Association-Pretest assessment, Echocardiogram and natriuretic peptide, Functional testing and Final etiology workup; HFpEF, heart failure preserved ejection fraction; H_2FPEF, heavy, hypertension, (atrial) fibrillation, pulmonary hypertension, elderly, filling pressure; LAVI, left atrial volume index; LVMI, left ventricular mass index; NT-proBNP, N-terminal pro-brain natriuretic peptide; PCWP, pulmonary capillary wedge pressure; RWT, relative wall thickness; TR, tricuspid regurgitation.

NPs are released owing to increased wall stress, they are more predictive of HF in HFrEF than in HFpEF where wall stress can be normalized in the setting of LV hypertrophy. In fact, 18% of patients with invasively proven HFpEF have serum natriuretic peptide levels below diagnostic thresholds.[37] On the other hand, elevated serum natriuretic peptide levels may be present in the absence of HF in patients with renal dysfunction or atrial fibrillation, and higher thresholds may be needed for diagnosis in these situations. Thus, serum natriuretic peptide testing cannot be used as a stand-alone test to rule out HFpEF, and instead must be taken into consideration with other diagnostic tests.

Metabolic Panel

In addition, a complete metabolic panel including electrolytes, blood urea nitrogen, creatinine as well as liver function tests, hemoglobin A1c, thyroid-stimulating hormone, complete blood count should be assessed. Abnormalities can suggest comorbid conditions (ie, kidney disease, diabetes, anemia, thyroid dysfunction) that can contribute to HFpEF or exacerbate associated symptoms, especially anemia.[38]

Electrocardiogram and Chest X-Ray

Electrocardiography is nonspecific, but may suggest LV hypertrophy or left atrial enlargement. Importantly, if atrial fibrillation is present, HFpEF should be considered because it is highly predictive of coexisting HFpEF.[39] The chest x-ray may or may not be helpful, but if it shows pulmonary congestion, then the diagnosis of HFpEF is much more likely.

Echocardiography

Echocardiography should be performed in patients with dyspnea. Even if clinical suspicion for HFpEF is low, echocardiography should be done to evaluate for HFrEF, valvular disease, PH, and pericardial effusion.[40] Standard echocardiography should include measurement of ejection fraction by quantitative means with preserved LVEF ≥50%. A diagnosis of HFpEF is suggested if the LV is not dilated and there is concentric remodeling or LV hypertrophy and left atrial enlargement. Other findings suggestive of HFpEF include abnormal diastology and longitudinal strain.[41] The American Society of Echocardiography guidelines recommend measurement of early diastolic tissue velocity (septal and lateral e'), the average transmitral E wave velocity to tissue Doppler e' ratio (E/e'), left atrial volume indexed to body surface area (LAVI), and tricuspid regurgitation velocity (TRV) to assess pulmonary artery systolic pressure. Taken together, these echocardiographic features may suggest the diagnosis of HFpEF but are not definitive.[42]

A 2019 consensus statement from the ESC/HFA suggests a step-by-step approach toward diagnosing HFpEF and uses similar criteria for echocardiographic measurements as described in the American Society of Echocardiography guidelines with some variations for age and presence of atrial fibrillation. It also includes other echocardiographic parameters (LV longitudinal strain) and incorporates functional (diastolic echocardiographic measures and global longitudinal strain), morphologic (left atrial volume, LV mass, and thickness), and biomarker (serum natriuretic peptide) measurements into a scoring system (detailed in **Algorithm 68.1**).[43]

If the score based on the above criteria is nondiagnostic, further testing for HFpEF using invasive assessment or diastolic echocardiographic stress testing can be performed. If right heart catheterization shows PCWP ≥15 mm Hg, then HFpEF is present. However, because both symptoms and hemodynamic changes may only occur with exertion, invasive hemodynamic testing during exercise (PCWP increased to ≥ 25 mm Hg is diagnostic) or with echocardiographic measurements of diastology are indicated when the diagnosis of HFpEF under resting conditions is in doubt.[42]

The H_2FPEF score (0-9 points) has also been proposed for the discrimination of HF with preserved ejection fraction from noncardiac causes of dyspnea.[39] The six clinical and echocardiographic variables that constitute the H_2FPEF score include the following: (1) obesity with body mass index greater than 30 kg/m^2 (H); (2) the use of greater than or equal to 2 antihypertensive drugs (H); (3) atrial fibrillation (F); (4) PH with pulmonary artery systolic pressure greater than 35 mm Hg (P); (5) age greater than 60 years (E); and (6) elevated filling pressures with E/e' greater than 9 (F) **(Algorithm 68.1)**.[39]

Identify Etiology and Rule Out HFpEF Mimickers

Once the diagnosis of HFpEF is confirmed, it is essential to try to identify the etiology, if possible, in order to guide specific therapy for reversible or modifiable conditions **(Table 68.1)**.[43] These include common conditions such as hypertension, CAD, valvular disease, infiltrative diseases including hemochromatosis and cardiac amyloidosis, autoimmune diseases, glycogen storage diseases, drug or radiation toxicity, metabolic and hormonal causes. Even more important are to rule out HFpEF mimickers such as severe valvular disease, constrictive pericarditis, hypertrophic cardiomyopathy, and congenital heart disease, as well as cor pulmonale owing to lung disease or primary PH.

MANAGEMENT OF PATIENT WITH HFPEF

Once the diagnosis of HFpEF is made, however, the evidence for treatment to impact its morbidity and mortality remains scant as demonstrated by the guidelines from both ACC/AHA/HFSA and ESC/HFA in **Table 68.2.**

The overall treatment rests on the management of volume and congestion and treatment of any underlying cause, in particular hypertension and CAD. Consensus of experts recommends revascularization of CAD for ischemia, treatment of atrial fibrillation, and optimal treatment of uncontrolled hypertension. Although specific classes of drugs do not show strong evidence for improved morbidity or

TABLE 68.2 Treatment of HFpEF From ACC/AHA/HFSA and ESC/HFA Guidelines

COR	LOE	Recommendation ACC/AHA/HFSA[4]	Recommendation ESC/HFA[40]
I	B	Systolic and diastolic blood pressure should be controlled in accordance with clinical practice guidelines to prevent morbidity.	Diuretics are recommended in congested patients to alleviate symptoms and signs of HF.*
I	C	Diuretics should be used for relief of symptoms owing to volume overload.	Treatment of all cardiac and noncardiac comorbidities is recommended to improve symptoms, well-being, and/or prognosis.*
IIa	C	Coronary revascularization is reasonable in patients with CAD in whom angina or demonstrable ischemia is adversely affecting HFpEF symptoms.	*in ESC/HFA Guidelines, above applies for HFpEF and HFmEF.
IIa	C	Management of AF according to published clinical practice guidelines in patients to improve symptoms of HF	
IIa	C	Use of BBs, ACEIs, and ARBs in patients with hypertension is reasonable to control blood pressure.	

TABLE 68.2 Treatment of HFpEF From ACC/AHA/HFSA and ESC/HFA Guidelines (*continued*)

COR	LOE	Recommendation ACC/AHA/HFSA[4]	Recommendation ESC/HFA[40]
IIb	B-R	In select patients with HFpEF (LVEF ≥45%), elevated BNP levels or HF admission within 1 year, eGFR >30 mL/min, creatinine <2.5 mg/dL, potassium <5.0 mEq/L, MRAs may be considered to reduce hospitalizations.	
IIb	B	Use of ARBs may be considered to decrease hospitalizations for patients with HFpEF.	
III	B-R	Routine use of nitrates or phosphodiesterase-5 inhibitors to increase the activity of QoL in patients with HFpEF is ineffective.	

ACC, American College of Cardiology; ACEI, angiotensin-converting enzyme inhibitor; AF, atrial fibrillation; AHA, American Heart Association; ARB, angiotensin receptor blocker; BB, beta-blocker; BNP, brain natriuretic peptide; CAD, coronary artery disease; COR, class of recommendation; eGFR, estimated glomerular filtration rate; ESC, European Society of Cardiology; HF, heart failure; HFA, Heart Failure Association; HSFA, Heart Failure Society of America; HFpEF, heart failure preserved ejection fraction; LOE, level of evidence; LVEF, left ventricular ejection fraction; MRA, mineralocorticoid receptor antagonist; QoL, quality of life.

ACC/AHA/HFSA guidelines reprinted from Yancy CW, Jessup M, Bozkurt B, et al. 2017 ACC/AHA/HFSA Focused Update of the 2013 ACCF/AHA Guideline for the Management of Heart Failure: A Report of the American College of Cardiology/American Heart Association Task Force on Clinical Practice Guidelines and the Heart Failure Society of America. *J Card Fail.* 2017;23(8):628-651. Copyright © 2017 Elsevier. With permission. ESC/HFA guidelines adapted from Baumgartner H, Falk V, Bax JJ, et al. 2017 ESC/EACTS Guidelines for the management of valvular heart disease. *Eur Heart J.* 2017;38(36):2739-2791.

mortality, there is some evidence for the use of beta-blockers, angiotensin-converting enzyme inhibitors (ACEIs), and angiotensin receptor blockers (ARBs) for the management of hypertension and in specific high-risk populations of HFpEF, mineralocorticoid receptor antagonists (MRA) and perhaps angiotensin receptor-neprilysin inhibitors (ARNIs) **(see Algorithm 68.2).**

A summary of risk factors, gender differences, and effective therapies by class is shown in **Figure 68.1** for HFrEF, HFpEF including overlap syndrome HF with "midrange EF" (HFmEF). Specific etiologies or contributing factors will require specific treatment (eg, treatment with amyloid fibril stabilizers for transthyretin amyloidosis, aortic valve replacement for severe aortic stenosis, or treatment for LV outflow tract obstruction in hypertrophic cardiomyopathy). Subsequently, the goal becomes the treatment of HF itself including management of congestion and comorbidities.

Treat congestion
- Loop diuretics +/– MRA
- Modest sodium restriction

Treat underlying causes
- Hypertension with goal < 130/80 mmHg
- Coronary artery disease
- Valvular disease
- Infiltrative diseases
- Hypertrophic cardiomyopathy
- Others

Treat precipitating factors and comorbidities
- Atrial fibrillation: rate vs rhythm control
- Ongoing ischemia
- Anemia
- Sleep apnea
- Diabetes
- Obesity plus sedentary lifestyle: Consider exercise plus weight loss

Patients with recurrent HF hospitalization & elevated NPs
- MRAs, ARBs, ARNI might be helpful to decrease HF hospitalization, especially if LVEF at lower end of normal range
- Consider remote hemodynamic monitoring

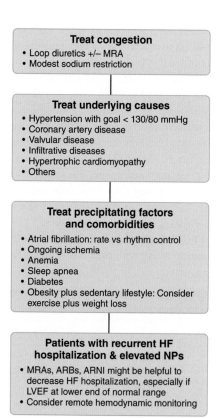

ALGORITHM 68.2 Treatment approach to HFpEF. ARB, angiotensin receptor blockers; ARNI, angiotensin receptor-neprilysin inhibitors; HF, heart failure; HFpEF, heart failure preserved ejection fraction; LVEF, left ventricular ejection fraction; MRA, mineralocorticoid receptor antagonists; NP, natriuretic peptides.

Nonpharmacologic Measures

Sodium and Fluid Restriction

HFpEF is accompanied by volume overload in most instances. Owing to a lack of data, considerable debate has ensued about whether sodium restriction is beneficial and, if so, what target is needed in patients with HF. Guidelines have given a weaker level of recommendation for sodium restriction or avoidance of excessive salt intake to reduce congestive symptoms. Similarly, the efficacy of fluid restriction in patients with HF has even less of an evidence base, but may be considered with severe HF, especially with hyponatremia.[9,44]

Exercise and Weight Loss

Studies have shown that exercise is safe, and exercise training may be beneficial in patients with HFpEF to improve exercise capacity and quality of life. Types of exercise studied include walking and cycling.[45] Additionally, obesity is a risk factor for HFpEF, and therapeutic weight loss has been associated with an

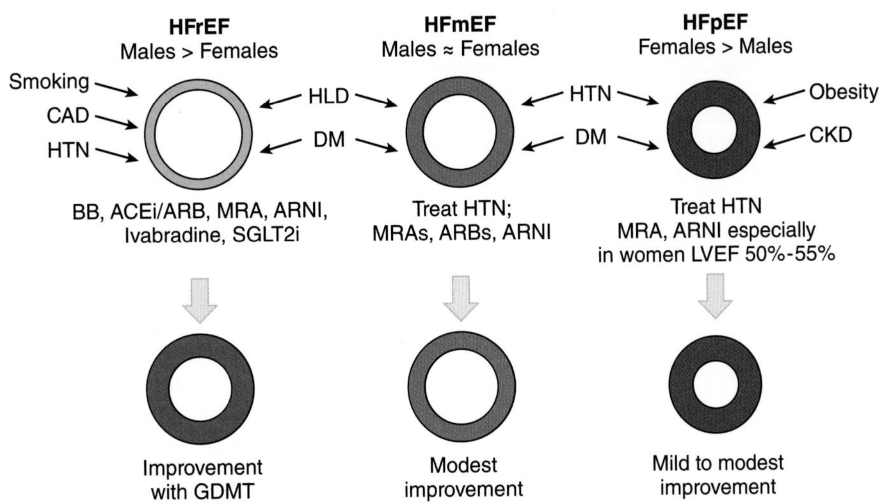

FIGURE 68.1 Comparison of risk factors, gender, and recommended therapies for HFrEF. ACEI, angiotensin-converting enzyme inhibitor; ARB, angiotensin receptor blocker; ARNI: angiotensin receptor-neprilysin inhibitor; BB, beta-blocker; CAD, coronary artery disease; CKD, chronic kidney disease; DM, diabetes mellitus; GDMT, guideline-directed medical therapy; HFmEF, heart failure with midrange ejection fraction; HFpEF, heart failure preserved ejection fraction; HFrEF, heart failure reduced ejection fraction; HLD, hyperlipidemia; HTN, hypertension; LVEF, left ventricular ejection fraction; MRA, mineralocorticoid receptor antagonist; SGLT2i, sodium-glucose linked transporter type-2 inhibitor.

improvement in hemodynamic measures: lower heart rate, mean arterial pressure, oxygen consumption, PCWP, and right-sided pressures including mean PAP and right atrial pressure.[46] In older patients with HFpEF, either exercise or weight loss can improve maximum oxygen consumption and their effects may be additive.[47] Therefore, in patients with excess body mass, weight loss in addition to exercise should be an important component of the treatment plan. Severely obese individuals may benefit from bariatric surgery, based on observational data.[48] However, prospective clinical trial data are not currently available.

Medical and Pharmacologic Approaches

Table 68.3 outlines the classes of drugs studied, the potential mechanisms underlying use, the clinical trials studying efficacy, and current recommendations for use in the treatment of HFpEF.

TABLE 68.3 Drug Classes, Study Results, and Recommended Treatment of HFpEF

Drug Class	Mechanism	Clinical Trials	Results	Recommendations
Nitrates and nitrites	Preload lowering agents, nitric oxide donors, venodilators	**NEAT-HFpEF:** isosorbide mononitrate vs placebo[82] **INDIE-HFpEF:** inhaled inorganic nitrite vs control[83]	No difference, in activity, quality of life or NT-proBNP in either trial	Data do not support the routine use of nitrates or nitrites
RAAS antagonists	Improve systemic blood pressure, myocardial relaxation, myocardial fibrosis	**CHARM-Preserved:** candesartan vs placebo[84] **PEP-CHF:** perindopril in elderly vs placebo[85] **I-PRESERVE:** irbesartan vs placebo[86]	No significant difference in CV death or HF hospitalization Borderline significant benefit on reduction in HF hospitalization No difference in all-cause mortality or HF hospitalization No difference in all-cause mortality or CV hospitalization	In CHARM-Preserved: Data do not support routine use of ACEI or ARBs specifically for HFpEF; can be used to control underlying hypertension or if indicated in select patients with diabetes

(continued)

TABLE 68.3 Drug Classes, Study Results, and Recommended Treatment of HFpEF (*continued*)

Drug Class	Mechanism	Clinical Trials	Results	Recommendations
Mineralocorticoid receptor antagonists	Less sodium and more potassium retention, attenuating endothelial dysfunction, reducing vascular inflammation and fibrosis	**Aldo-DHF:** spironolactone vs placebo[65] **RAAM-PEF:** eplerenone vs placebo[87] **TOPCAT:** spironolactone vs placebo[66]	Improved echo diastolic parameters E/e′, LV mass index, and NT pro-BNP; no change in QoL or functional capacity Improved E/e′, reduced collagen turnover, but no change in functional capacity No difference in CV death/HF hospitalization/aborted cardiac arrest; HF hospitalization was lower but not total hospitalizations, more hyperkalemia, and renal failure; post hoc analysis showed reduced HF hospitalizations/CV death/aborted cardiac arrest in the Americas	Based on **TOPCAT** showing improved outcomes in North America, updated ACC/AHA HF Guideline 2017 Focused update: MRA may be considered to reduce HF hospitalizations in patients with: LVEF ≥ 45% Elevated BNP levels HF admission within 1 year eGFR >30 mL/min, creatinine <2.5 mg/dL and potassium <5 mEq/L
Angiotensin receptor-neprilysin inhibitors	Elevate circulating natriuretic peptides to improve sodium excretion, vasodilation, and inhibit RAAS	**PARAMOUNT:** sacubitril/valsartan vs valsartan alone[88] **PARAGON-HF:** sacubitril/valsartan vs valsartan[68]	Reduced NT pro-BNP levels No significant difference in HF hospitalizations or CV death	No recommendations for use of ARNIs yet although some suggest that select populations including women, those with recent HF hospitalizations, and mildly reduced EF may benefit; more studies are needed
Beta-blockers and Ivabradine (I_f channel blocker)	Increase diastolic filling time with reduced heart rate	**J-DHF:** carvedilol vs placebo[89] **ELANDD:** nebivolol vs placebo[90] **EDIFY:** ivabradine vs placebo[91]	Underpowered study but no differences in HF hospitalization or CV death No difference in 6-min walk test or oxygen consumption No difference in E/e′, 6-min walk test, or NT pro-BNP	No recommendations for beta-blockers in HFpEF; concern for worsening chronotropic incompetence in some patients; may be used for coexisting indications of angina, post-myocardial infarction, rate control in atrial fibrillation, and in some for hypertension No recommendations for ivabradine

TABLE 68.3 Drug Classes, Study Results, and Recommended Treatment of HFpEF (*continued*)

Drug Class	Mechanism	Clinical Trials	Results	Recommendations
Selective phosphodiesterase type 5 inhibition (PDE-5 inhibition)	Enhance nitric oxide–mediated vasodilation as well as effects on pulmonary artery pressure and right ventricular hypertrophy	**RELAX:** sildenafil vs placebo[92]	No change in peak oxygen consumption, exercise tolerance, diastolic parameters, or pulmonary artery pressure	Not recommended routinely for HFpEF
Endothelin antagonists	To reduce pulmonary hypertension in HFpEF	**BADDHY**: bosentan[93] and sitaxsentan[94]	No benefit	Not recommended for pulmonary hypertension owing to HFpEF
Lusitropic agents	Improve relaxation	**RALI-DHF**: ranolazine[95]	No change in echo parameters or NT-proBNP	
Soluble guanylate cyclase stimulator	Generate cyclic guanosine monophosphate and restore sensitivity of soluble guanylate cyclase to endogenous nitric oxide	**VITALITY-HFpEF:** vericiguat[96]	No improvement in QoL	
Partial adenosine A1 receptor agonist	Improve mitochondrial function, enhance sarcoplasmic reticulum 2a activity, optimize energy substrate metabolism, reverse cardiac remodeling	**PANACHE**: neladenoson[97]	No initial benefit noted on 6-minute walk distance, QoL, NT-proBNP levels	Early clinical phase IIb trial data not encouraging

ACC, American College of Cardiology; ACEI, angiotensin-converting enzyme inhibitor; AHA, American Heart Association; ARB, angiotensin receptor blocker; BNP, brain natriuretic peptide; CV, cardiovascular; eGFR, estimated glomerular filtration rate; HF, heart failure; HFpEF, heart failure preserved ejection fraction; HSFA, Heart Failure Society of America; LV, left ventricular; LVEF, left ventricular ejection fraction; MRA, mineralocorticoid receptor antagonist; NT-proBNP, N-terminal pro-brain natriuretic peptide; QoL, quality of life; RAAS, renin-angiotensin-aldosterone system.

Treatment of Volume Overload and Congestion—Diuretics

The clinical presentation of patients with HFpEF is often mediated by increased right- and left-sided filling pressures and is associated with peripheral edema, abdominal congestion, and pulmonary vascular congestion. Therefore, diuretic use to facilitate excess volume removal is a mainstay for symptom management for many patients. This group has a high prevalence of renal dysfunction with inappropriate sodium and water retention. This also leads to salt-sensitive hypertension and further worsening of diastolic function. Some HFpEF patients with significant hypertension may have larger LV end-diastolic volumes contributed to by other underlying conditions (ie, renal dysfunction and anemia) resulting in more volume overload. Although there are no clinical trials definitively evaluating the use of diuretics on clinical outcomes specifically in patients with HFpEF, diuretics are used for the treatment of hypertension and HF. Diuretics are indicated in all HFpEF patients with evidence of volume overload and in most patients with a prior history of volume overload to maintain a decongested state. Small, clinical trials of diuretics demonstrated their effects on increasing urinary sodium excretion, decreasing physical signs of fluid retention, and improving symptoms and exercise tolerance.[49,50] A recent observational, propensity-matched study demonstrated a reduction in short-term HF hospitalization and mortality in patients with HF (irrespective of LVEF) who were discharged with diuretics when compared to those discharged without diuretics.[51] It is important to note that while diuretic use can frequently offer symptom relief with improvement in blood pressure, a subgroup of patients with significant LVH and small LV cavities may have reduced cardiac output with rapid diuresis. This could result in hypotension and prerenal azotemia, so caution should be exercised. Also, judicious diuretic use is important for patients with right ventricular dysfunction because this group has also been associated with worsening renal function during acute HF.[52]

Treatment of Hypertension

Hypertension is nearly universally present in patients with HFpEF. The effects of hypertension on the development of HFpEF are due at least in part to LV hypertrophy with impaired relaxation and diastolic dysfunction. Appropriately managing hypertension remains one of the most important treatment options for these patients. Elevated arterial pressures increase afterload, which further impairs LV relaxation and filling.[53] Also, poor compliance of aortic and LV walls can enhance arterial and left atrial coupling, resulting in higher left atrial pressures caused by elevated arterial systolic pressures.[54] Further, impaired LV relaxation and elevated filling pressures can reduce coronary vascular reserve, resulting in myocardial ischemia without epicardial coronary disease. Trials evaluating the reduction of blood pressure using ACEIs or ARBs compared with other agents have suggested that blood pressure control—rather than the specific class of antihypertensive agents used—may be the major determinant of regression of hypertrophy and improvement in diastolic function.[55,56] Although some classes of antihypertensive medications may offer incremental benefit over others, emphasis on adequate blood pressure control is paramount. Those adequately treated for hypertension have ~50% reduction in the incidence of HF.[57]

The most recent update of the AHA/ACC guidelines for the management of hypertension recommends that those at a higher risk of cardiac events should have a goal blood pressure less than 130/80 mm Hg.[58] Although clinical trials demonstrate a substantial decrease in the incidence of HF with the treatment of hypertension and with more intensive blood pressure control in higher-risk patients, clinical trials have not specifically examined ideal blood pressure targets in patients with HFpEF. Therefore, at present, patients with HFpEF can be treated to a target of less than 130/80 mm Hg, as recommended for higher-risk hypertensive patients.[4] Finally, if pharmacotherapy for hypertension fails to achieve adequate blood pressure control, more invasive strategies may be needed for resistant hypertension including renal denervation and baroreceptor manipulation with chronic electrical stimulation of the carotid sinus to prevent or treat HFpEF.

Treatment of Atrial Fibrillation and Other Underlying Comorbidities

Atrial fibrillation is common in HFpEF patients and associated with worse outcomes, but as HFpEF progresses and atrial dysfunction worsens, the risk of developing paroxysmal atrial fibrillation also increases.[59,60] Once paroxysmal atrial fibrillation progresses to permanent atrial fibrillation, patients display severe atrial dysfunction with abnormal RV-pulmonary vascular coupling compared with patients with HFpEF in sinus rhythm.[25,61] Whether treating underlying atrial fibrillation for rhythm control improves outcomes in HFpEF is unclear.[60] Although select patients who are very symptomatic with atrial fibrillation may do better with rhythm control, prospective selection of this patient group as well as mode for rhythm control (medications vs ablation) is not clear at present.

No randomized studies for rate versus rhythm control in HFpEF with atrial fibrillation are available. In patients with HFrEF, a large, randomized control trial of rate control versus rhythm control (with antiarrhythmic medications) did not demonstrate a benefit on clinical outcomes, quality of life, or functional strategy with either strategy.[62] Some small trials of atrial fibrillation ablation have demonstrated benefit of rhythm control over rate control in symptoms, functional capacity, and quality of life.[63,64] Similar trials are not yet available in HFpEF.

Significant underlying CAD can be a contributor to symptoms and should be treated as per current guidelines. Observational studies have shown that CAD is common in patients with HFpEF and is associated with worse outcomes which may be improved with treatment and revascularization.[12]

Other comorbidities are even less well studied and it is unclear if treating anemia or obstructive sleep apnea has any effect on HF outcomes in HFpEF. As we increasingly study HFpEF, new data may emerge to underscore the benefit of treating these and other comorbid conditions.

Research and Future Directions

Clinical trials in the general HFpEF population have not demonstrated significant efficacy for several drug classes that have proven benefit in HFrEF such as renin-angiotensin system blockers (ACEIs, ARBs) or beta-blockers. However, ACEIs, ARBs, and beta-blockers may be used to treat hypertension or comorbidities such as CAD.

Two drug classes, MRAs and ARNIs, however, have been shown to have some efficacy in certain subgroups of HFpEF and deserve additional discussion. The basis of MRA use in HFpEF is their ability to improve measures of diastolic function, such as E/e' ratios on echocardiography in patients with HFpEF and induced reverse remodeling as demonstrated by a decline in LV mass index as well as improved strain and reduced left atrial area.[65]

Treatment of Preserved Cardiac Function Heart Failure With an Aldosterone Antagonist or TOPCAT Trial

The TOPCAT trial investigated the effects of spironolactone on the combined primary end point of death, aborted cardiac death, and HF hospitalization in 3445 patients with HFpEF having LVEF ≥45%. Although the overall trial did not show statistically significant efficacy (hazard ratio (HR) = 0.89: 95% confidence interval [CI], 0.77-1.04; $P = .14$), post hoc subgroup analysis demonstrated benefit in some groups in the Americas (HR = 0.82, 95% CI, 0.69-0.98) but not in Russia/Georgia (HR = 1.10, 95% CI, 0.79-1.51). The premise of this analysis was that patients enrolled from the Americas had significantly higher rates of clinical events in the placebo arm compared to those enrolled in Russia/Georgia, and that adherence to study medication was questionable in a sample of patients treated in Russia/Georgia. These analyses suggest that in appropriately selected patients with symptomatic HFpEF having EF ≥45%, elevated BNP level or recent HF hospitalization, and appropriate renal function and potassium levels, MRAs might be considered with close monitoring of potassium and renal function.[66,67]

Prospective Comparison of ARNI With ARB Global Outcomes in HFpEF PARAGON-HF Clinical Trial

After the success of ARNIs for the treatment of HFrEF, attention shifted to investigating their efficacy in HFpEF. In the PARAGON-HF (Prospective Comparison of ARNI with ARB Global Outcomes in HFpEF) trial, the ARNI sacubitril/valsartan was compared to the ARB valsartan in 4822 patients with LVEF ≥45% with mostly New York Heart Association (NYHA) Class II and III HF, elevated serum natriuretic peptide levels, and structural heart disease. The primary end point was a composite of total hospitalizations for HF or death from CV causes. The primary end point fell short of statistical significance in favor of the ARNI (HR = 0.87, 95% CI, 0.75-1.01; $P = .06$).[68] In a post hoc analysis, sacubitril-valsartan showed a relative risk reduction in the primary outcomes in patients hospitalized within 30 days (HR = 0.73) compared to those never hospitalized (HR = 1.00).[69] The suggestion of trend toward improvement in the PARAGON-HF trial led to the PARALLAX trial, A Randomized, Double-blind Controlled Study Comparing LCZ696 to Medical Therapy for Comorbidities in HFpEF Patients. In this study, sacubitril/valsartan was compared to individualized renin-angiotensin-aldosterone system (RAAS) blockade. At 12 weeks, there was a significant (16.4%) reduction of NT-proBNP in the sacubitril-valsartan group compared to the group with individualized medical therapy ($P < .0001$) with no change in functional status. In addition, a post hoc analysis showed that sacubitril-valsartan reduced the risk for HF hospitalization by 50% ($P = .005$) (abstract from ESC presented on August 30, 2020, study design as published).[70] FDA has approved an expanded indication for sacubitril/valsartan "to reduce the risk of cardiovascular death and hospitalization for heart failure in adult patients with chronic heart failure," and that, "Benefits are most clearly evident in patients with LVEF below normal."

Ongoing Trial: PARAGLIDE-HF (Changes in NT-proBNP and Outcomes, Safety, and Tolerability in HFpEF Patients With Acute Decompensated Heart Failure [ADHF] Who Have Been Stabilized During Hospitalization and Initiated In-hospital or Within 30 Days Post-discharge)

The improved outcomes in hospitalized patients in PARAGON-HF are the basis for the ongoing PARAGLIDE-HF trial (Changes in NT-proBNP and Outcomes, Safety, and Tolerability in HFpEF Patients with Acute Decompensated Heart Failure (ADHF) Who Have Been Stabilized During Hospitalization and Initiated In-hospital or Within 30 Days Post-discharge). The estimated study completion is March 2022.

In summary, two separate trials investigating ARNIs in HFpEF show signals, but not definitive benefit, for the use of ARNIs in patients with HFpEF, possibly those at higher risk of HF hospitalization, such as those with recent HF hospitalization. However, the role of ARNI in HFpEF still needs clarification.

Because HFpEF is a heterogeneous syndrome, grouping patients into pathophysiologic and phenotypical groups may be more beneficial in identifying specific therapies for the subgroups. Targeting inflammation, fibrosis, microvascular, and metabolic abnormalities among others may prove helpful.

Emerging Pharmacotherapy

Selective Inhibitors of the Sodium-Glucose Cotransporter 2 (SGLT-2) Inhibitors—Promising Results

Perhaps the most promising medications in many years are the newer hypoglycemic agents, the selective inhibitors of the sodium-glucose cotransporter 2 (SGLT-2) inhibitors. This diabetic treatment convincingly impacts CV events, especially with the reduction in incident HF, in addition to modest improvements in glycemic control, blood pressure, and weight loss.[71,72] Consistent results with ~30% reduction in HF hospitalizations were also noted with other SGLT2 inhibitors, dapagliflozin, and ertugliflozin.[73,74]

The investigational SGLT1/2 inhibitor sotagliflozin is the first agent clearly shown in a prespecified analysis of randomized trials to improve clinical outcomes in patients with HFpEF. The Effect of Sotagliflozin on Cardiovascular and Renal Events in Patients With Type 2 Diabetes and Moderate Renal Impairment Who Are at Cardiovascular Risk (SCORED) study randomized patients with type 2 diabetes and chronic kidney disease to treatment with sotagliflozin or placebo on top of guideline-directed medical therapy (GDMT) (https://clinicaltrials.gov/ct2/show/NCT03315143). The Effect of Sotagliflozin on Cardiovascular Events in Patients With Type 2 Diabetes Post Worsening Heart Failure (SOLOIST-WHF) trial randomized patients with type 2 diabetes who were recently hospitalized for worsening HF (https://clinicaltrials.gov/ct2/show/NCT03521934). A meta-analysis of these two trials included 4500 patients with type 2 diabetes and diagnosed with HF at entry (https://www.abstractsonline.com/pp8/#!/9228/presentation/24035).

The primary end point, which was the same in both trials, was the combined incidence of CV death and the total number of either hospitalization for HF or urgent outpatient visits for HF. Compared with placebo, treatment with sotagliflozin for a median of about 15 months reduced this composite end point by a relative 33% among the 1931 with HFpEF (LVEF ≥50%) and by 43% among the 811 patients with an LVEF of 40% to 49% (HFmEF).

With this evidence, one can consider using these agents in diabetic patients with HF or those at risk for HF. Mechanisms unrelated to glycemic control are likely to be responsible for the laudable CV benefits. Proposed mechanisms are natriuresis, systemic blood pressure lowering, reduction in arterial stiffness and preservation of renal function along with renal sodium and glucose handling, and possibly positive effects on cardiac metabolism with a shift from fatty acids to ketone bodies.[75]

Emerging data for the SGLT-2 inhibitors class show promise in reducing CV death and HF hospitalizations irrespective of the presence or absence of diabetes mellitus, but specific data for HFpEF are still not yet available. Multiple clinical trials in patients irrespective of diabetes status are ongoing to test the effects of SGLT2 inhibitors on HFpEF outcomes.

Potential Device-Based Therapies

Left Atrial Pressure Reduction

Elevated left atrial pressure with concomitant pulmonary congestion plays a central role in dyspnea for patients with HFpEF, both at rest and particularly during activity. Dyspnea on exertion with poor exercise tolerance is highly correlated with poor outcomes in patients with HF. For this reason, nonmedical (mechanical) therapies have been pursued to reduce left atrial pressures for patients with HFpEF. The REDUCe Elevated Left Atrial Pressure in Patients with Heart Failure (REDUCE-LAP-HF) trial was a single-arm phase 1 study to evaluate the safety and efficacy of an 8-mm interatrial shunt device (IASD, Corvia Medical, Tewksbury, MA) in patients with symptomatic HFpEF (LVEF >40%) despite medical therapy, who had PCWP >15 mm Hg at rest or >25 mm Hg during exercise.[76] The device was placed percutaneously and allowed for left-to-right shunting across the interatrial septum to decompress the left atrial pressure. At 6 months of follow-up, of the 64 patients who had the device implanted, there were no periprocedural or major adverse cardiac or cerebrovascular events and 52% had improvement in PCWP at rest, and 58% had PCWP reduction with exertion. Additionally, 1 year after implantation, patients had improvement in NYHA scores, quality of life scores, and 6-minute walk distances.[77]

In phase II of REDUCE-LAP-HF I trial, 44 patients with HFpEF with NYHA class III or ambulatory class IV, LVEF ≥40%, exercise PCWP ≥25 mm Hg, and PCWP-right atrial pressure gradient greater than or equal to 5 mm Hg were randomized (22 in each group) to IASD implant or sham procedure where subjects had femoral access and intracardiac echo but no IASD placement. At 1-month follow-up, PCWP decreased by 3.5 ± 6.4 mm Hg in the treatment group versus 0.5 ± 5.0 mm Hg in the control group ($P = .14$).[78] Based on data from these small trials, it seems IASD can reduce PCWP and improve functional measures in HFpEF patients up to 1 year. However, long-term safety and effectiveness are yet to be determined. A larger phase III trial is ongoing (REDUCE LAP-HF Trial II).

Pressure Monitoring Devices

Annually, there are over 1 million admissions in the United States for primary diagnosis of HF.[79] Of those admitted with HF, it is estimated that ~50% have HFpEF. Because these admissions typically occur from symptoms of edema and dyspnea related to pulmonary congestion, considerable research has evaluated methods of monitoring the volume status of patients outside the hospital in hopes of reducing the frequency of hospitalizations. The CardioMEMS Heart Sensor Allows Monitoring of Pressure of Improve Outcomes in NYHA Class III Heart Failure Patients (CHAMPION) trial randomly assigned patients with HF (regardless of LVEF)—with only patients being blinded to assignment group—to either wireless implantable pulmonary artery hemodynamic monitoring system or control group that included weight monitoring, for at least 6 months. Medical management, predominantly through diuretic dose adjustments, was based on pulmonary artery diastolic pressure values. After a mean 15-month follow-up, the treatment group was associated with a 37% reduction in HF admissions ($P < .0001$).[80] Of the subgroup ($N = 119$ subjects) with LVEF ≥40%, those with the pulmonary artery hemodynamic monitoring system ($N = 62$) had a 50% lower incidence of HF compared with control after an average follow-up of 17.6 months ($P < .0001$), suggesting benefit in patients with HFpEF.[81]

Although there are some uncertainties regarding long-term cost-effectiveness, risk, and data management issues related to permanent pulmonary artery hemodynamic monitoring systems, the data are promising. A large trial, Hemodynamic-GUIDEd management of Heart Failure (GUIDE-HF) is ongoing and will include ~3600 patients to confirm the benefit of PAP monitoring compared to standard of care on HF hospitalization/urgent visits for HF or CV mortality.

KEY POINTS

- ✔ Consider the diagnosis of HFpEF in patients with unexplained dyspnea and normal LVEF, especially in the presence of risk factors including older age, obesity, hypertension, diabetes, and coexisting atrial fibrillation.
- ✔ Given the difficulty in the diagnosis of HFpEF, consider the use of the H_2FPEF or the HFA-PEFF scores to exclude or confirm the diagnosis of HFpEF.
- ✔ If the diagnosis of HFpEF is uncertain following application of the scoring systems, consider invasive hemodynamic testing.
- ✔ Once HFpEF is diagnosed, evaluate the etiology of HFpEF.
- ✔ Treat symptoms and signs of congestion with diuretics.
- ✔ Treat comorbid conditions including hypertension, CAD, atrial fibrillation, and obesity with a focus on symptom relief and prevention of hospitalizations.
- ✔ Consider the use of spironolactone or ARNI in patients with LVEF toward the lower end of normal and those at high risk for HF hospitalization.

REFERENCES

1. World Health Organization. The top 10 causes of death. Published 2018. Accessed November 11, 2020. https://www.who.int/news-room/fact-sheets/detail/the-top-10-causes-of-death
2. Lam CSP, Gamble GD, Ling LH, et al. Mortality associated with heart failure with preserved vs. reduced ejection fraction in a prospective international multi-ethnic cohort study. *Eur Heart J.* 2018;39:1770-1780.
3. Yancy CW, Jessup M, Bozkurt B, et al. 2013 ACCF/AHA guideline for the management of heart failure: a report of the American College of

Cardiology Foundation/American Heart Association Task Force on Practice Guidelines. *J Am Coll Cardiol.* 2013;62:e147-e239.

4. Yancy CW, Jessup M, Bozkurt B, et al. 2017 ACC/AHA/HFSA focused update of the 2013 ACCF/AHA guideline for the management of heart failure. *J Cardiac Fail.* 2017;23:628-651.
5. Benjamin EJ, Muntner P, Alonso A, et al. Heart disease and stroke statistics-2019 update: a report from the American Heart Association. *Circulation.* 2019;139:e56-e528.
6. Ather S, Chan W, Bozkurt B, et al. Impact of noncardiac comorbidities on morbidity and mortality in a predominantly male population with heart failure and preserved versus reduced ejection fraction. *J Am Coll Cardiol.* 2012;59:998-1005.
7. Dunlay SM, Weston SA, Jacobsen SJ, Roger VL Risk factors for heart failure: a population-based case-control study. *Am J Med.* 2009;122:1023-1028.
8. Steinberg BA, Zhao X, Heidenreich PA, et al. Trends in patients hospitalized with heart failure and preserved left ventricular ejection fraction: prevalence, therapies, and outcomes. *Circulation.* 2012;126:65-75.
9. van de Wouw J, Broekhuizen M, Sorop O, et al. Chronic kidney disease as a risk factor for heart failure with preserved ejection fraction: a focus on microcirculatory factors and therapeutic targets. *Front Physiol.* 2019;10:1108.
10. Tabucanon T, Tang WHW. Right heart failure and cardiorenal syndrome. *Cardiol Clin.* 2020;38:185-202.
11. Lam CSP, Donal E, Kraigher-Krainer E, Vasan RS. Epidemiology and clinical course of heart failure with preserved ejection fraction. *Eur J Heart Fail.* 2011;13:18-28.
12. Hwang S-J, Melenovsky V, Borlaug BA. Implications of coronary artery disease in heart failure with preserved ejection fraction. *J Am Coll Cardiol.* 2014;63:2817-2827.
13. Little WC, Brucks S. Therapy for diastolic heart failure. *Prog Cardiovasc Dis.* 2005;47:380-388.
14. Franssen C, Chen S, Hamdani N, Paulus WJ From comorbidities to heart failure with preserved ejection fraction: a story of oxidative stress. *Heart.* 2016;102:320-330.
15. Mohammed SF, Hussain S, Mirzoyev SA, Edwards WD, Maleszewski JJ, Redfield MM. Coronary microvascular rarefaction and myocardial fibrosis in heart failure with preserved ejection fraction. *Circulation.* 2015;131:550-559.
16. Paulus WJ, Tschöpe C. A novel paradigm for heart failure with preserved ejection fraction. *J Am Coll Cardiol.* 2013;62:263-271.
17. Borlaug BA. The pathophysiology of heart failure with preserved ejection fraction. *Nat Rev Cardiol.* 2014;11:507-515.
18. Borlaug BA, Olson TP, Lam CSP, et al. Global cardiovascular reserve dysfunction in heart failure with preserved ejection fraction. *J Am Coll Cardiol.* 2010;56:845-854.
19. Westermann D, Kasner M, Steendijk P, et al. Role of left ventricular stiffness in heart failure with normal ejection fraction. *Circulation.* 2008;117:2051-2060.
20. Bursi F, Weston SA, Redfield MM, et al. Systolic and diastolic heart failure in the community. *JAMA.* 2006;296:2209-2216.
21. Shah AM, Shah SJ, Anand IS, et al. Cardiac structure and function in heart failure with preserved ejection fraction: baseline findings from the echocardiographic study of the Treatment of Preserved Cardiac Function Heart Failure with an Aldosterone Antagonist trial. *Circ Heart Fail.* 2014;7:104-115.
22. Obokata M, Reddy YNV, Pislaru SV, Melenovsky V, Borlaug BA. Evidence supporting the existence of a distinct obese phenotype of heart failure with preserved ejection fraction. *Circulation.* 2017;136:6-19.
23. Tan YT, Wenzelburger F, Lee E, et al. The pathophysiology of heart failure with normal ejection fraction: exercise echocardiography reveals complex abnormalities of both systolic and diastolic ventricular function involving torsion, untwist, and longitudinal motion. *J Am Coll Cardiol.* 2009;54:36-46.
24. Shah AM, Claggett B, Sweitzer NK, et al. Prognostic importance of impaired systolic function in heart failure with preserved ejection fraction and the impact of spironolactone. *Circulation.* 2015;132:402-414.
25. Melenovsky V, Hwang S-J, Redfield MM, Zakeri R, Lin G, Borlaug BA. Left atrial remodeling and function in advanced heart failure with preserved or reduced ejection fraction. *Circ Heart Fail.* 2015;8:295-303.
26. Simonneau G, Montani D, Celermajer DS, et al. Haemodynamic definitions and updated clinical classification of pulmonary hypertension. *Eur Respir J.* 2019;53(1):1801913. doi:10.1183/13993003.01913-2018
27. Hurdman J, Condliffe R, Elliot CA, et al. ASPIRE registry: assessing the Spectrum of Pulmonary hypertension identified at a REferral centre. *Eur Respir J.* 2012;39:945-955.
28. Thenappan T, Shah SJ, Gomberg-Maitland M, et al. Clinical characteristics of pulmonary hypertension in patients with heart failure and preserved ejection fraction. *Circ Heart Fail.* 2011;4:257-265.
29. Mohammed SF, Hussain I, AbouEzzeddine OF, et al. Right ventricular function in heart failure with preserved ejection fraction: a community-based study. *Circulation.* 2014;130:2310-2320.
30. Houstis NE, Eisman AS, Pappagianopoulos PP, et al. Exercise intolerance in heart failure with preserved ejection fraction: diagnosing and ranking its causes using personalized O_2 pathway analysis. *Circulation.* 2018;137:148-161.
31. Akiyama E, Sugiyama S, Matsuzawa Y, et al. Incremental prognostic significance of peripheral endothelial dysfunction in patients with heart failure with normal left ventricular ejection fraction. *J Am Coll Cardiol.* 2012;60:1778-1786.
32. Hung S, Lai Y, Kuo K, Tarng D. Volume overload and adverse outcomes in chronic kidney disease: clinical observational and animal studies. *J Am Heart Assoc.* 2015;4(5):e001918. doi:10.1161/JAHA.115.001918
33. Sanders-van Wijk S, Tromp J, Beussink-Nelson L, et al. Proteomic evaluation of the comorbidity-inflammation paradigm in heart failure with preserved ejection fraction: results from the PROMIS-HFpEF study. *Circulation.* 2020;142:2029-2044.
34. Packer M, Kitzman DW. Obesity-related heart failure with a preserved ejection fraction. *JACC Heart Fail.* 2018;6:633-639.
35. Ho JE, Zern EK, Wooster L, et al. Differential clinical profiles, exercise responses, and outcomes associated with existing HFpEF definitions. *Circulation.* 2019;140:353-365.
36. Chow SL, Maisel AS, Anand I, et al. Role of biomarkers for the prevention, assessment, and management of heart failure: a scientific statement from the American Heart Association. *Circulation.* 2017;135:e1054-e1091.
37. Obokata M, Kane GC, Reddy YNV, Olson TP, Melenovsky V, Borlaug BA. Role of diastolic stress testing in the evaluation for heart failure with preserved ejection fraction: a simultaneous invasive-echocardiographic study. *Circulation.* 2017;135:825-838.
38. Kasner M, Aleksandrov AS, Westermann D, et al. Functional iron deficiency and diastolic function in heart failure with preserved ejection fraction. *Int J Cardiol.* 2013;168:4652-4657.
39. Reddy YNV, Carter RE, Obokata M, Redfield MM, Borlaug BA. A simple, evidence-based approach to help guide diagnosis of heart failure with preserved ejection fraction. *Circulation.* 2018;138:861-870.
40. Baumgartner H, Falk V, Bax JJ, et al. 2017 ESC/EACTS guidelines for the management of valvular heart disease. *Eur Heart J.* 2017;38:2739-2791.
41. Wan S-H, Vogel MW, Chen HH. Pre-clinical diastolic dysfunction. *J Am Coll Cardiol.* 2014;63:407-416.
42. Nagueh SF, Smiseth OA, Appleton CP, et al. Recommendations for the evaluation of left ventricular diastolic function by echocardiography: an update from the American Society of Echocardiography and the European Association of Cardiovascular Imaging. *J Am Soc Echocardiogr.* 2016;29:277-314.
43. Pieske B, Tschöpe C, de Boer RA, et al. How to diagnose heart failure with preserved ejection fraction: the HFA-PEFF diagnostic algorithm: a consensus recommendation from the Heart Failure Association (HFA) of the European Society of Cardiology (ESC). *Eur Heart J.* 2019;40:3297-3317.
44. Ponikowski P, Voors AA, Anker SD, et al. 2016 ESC Guidelines for the diagnosis and treatment of acute and chronic heart failure: The Task Force

for the diagnosis and treatment of acute and chronic heart failure of the European Society of Cardiology (ESC)Developed with the special contribution of the Heart Failure Association (HFA) of the ESC. *Eur Heart J.* 2016;37:2129-2200.

45. Fukuta H, Goto T, Wakami K, Kamiya T, Ohte N. Effects of exercise training on cardiac function, exercise capacity, and quality of life in heart failure with preserved ejection fraction: a meta-analysis of randomized controlled trials. *Heart Fail Rev.* 2019;24:535-547.
46. Reddy YNV, Anantha-Narayanan M, Obokata M, et al. Hemodynamic effects of weight loss in obesity: a systematic review and meta-analysis. *JACC Heart Fail.* 2019;7:678-687.
47. Kitzman DW, Brubaker P, Morgan T, et al. Effect of caloric restriction or aerobic exercise training on peak oxygen consumption and quality of life in obese older patients with heart failure with preserved ejection fraction: a randomized clinical trial. *JAMA.* 2016;315:36-46.
48. Sundström J, Bruze G, Ottosson J, Marcus C, Näslund I, Neovius M. Weight loss and heart failure: a nationwide study of gastric bypass surgery versus intensive lifestyle treatment. *Circulation.* 2017;135:1577-1585.
49. Felker GM, Stevenson LW, Rouleau JL, McNulty SE, Givertz MM, Braunwald E. Diuretic strategies in patients with acute decompensated heart failure. *N Engl J Med.* 2011;364:797-805.
50. Goebel KM. Six-week study of torsemide in patients with congestive heart failure. *Clin Ther.* 1993;15:1051-1059.
51. Faselis C, Arundel C, Patel S, et al. Loop diuretic prescription and 30-day outcomes in older patients with heart failure. *J Am Coll Cardiol.* 2020;76:669-679.
52. Mukherjee M, Sharma K, Madrazo JA, Tedford RJ, Russell SD, Hays AG. Right-sided cardiac dysfunction in heart failure with preserved ejection fraction and worsening renal function. *Am J Cardiol.* 2017;120:274-278.
53. Leite-Moreira AF, Correia-Pinto J. Load as an acute determinant of end-diastolic pressure-volume relation. *Am J Physiol Heart Circ Physiol.* 2001;280:H51-H59.
54. Kawaguchi M, Hay I, Fetics B, Kass DA. Combined ventricular systolic and arterial stiffening in patients with heart failure and preserved ejection fraction: implications for systolic and diastolic reserve limitations. *Circulation.* 2003;107:714-720.
55. Solomon SD, Janardhanan R, Verma A, et al. Effect of angiotensin receptor blockade and antihypertensive drugs on diastolic function in patients with hypertension and diastolic dysfunction: a randomised trial. *Lancet.* 2007;369:2079-2087.
56. Devereux RB, Palmieri V, Sharpe N, et al. Effects of once-daily angiotensin-converting enzyme inhibition and calcium channel blockade-based antihypertensive treatment regimens on left ventricular hypertrophy and diastolic filling in hypertension: the prospective randomized enalapril study evaluating regression of ventricular enlargement (preserve) trial. *Circulation.* 2001;104:1248-1254.
57. Moser M, Hebert PR. Prevention of disease progression, left ventricular hypertrophy and congestive heart failure in hypertension treatment trials. *J Am Coll Cardiol.* 1996;27:1214-1218.
58. Whelton PK, Carey RM, Aronow WS, et al. 2017 ACC/AHA/AAPA/ABC/ACPM/AGS/APhA/ASH/ASPC/NMA/PCNA guideline for the prevention, detection, evaluation, and management of high blood pressure in adults: a report of the American College of Cardiology/American Heart Association Task Force on Clinical Practice Guidelines. *Hypertension.* 2018;71:e13-e115.
59. Zakeri R, Borlaug BA, McNulty SE, et al. Impact of atrial fibrillation on exercise capacity in heart failure with preserved ejection fraction: a RELAX trial ancillary study. *Circ Heart Fail.* 2014;7:123-130.
60. Zafrir B, Lund LH, Laroche C, et al. Prognostic implications of atrial fibrillation in heart failure with reduced, mid-range, and preserved ejection fraction: a report from 14 964 patients in the European Society of Cardiology Heart Failure Long-Term Registry. *Eur Heart J.* 2018;39:4277-4284.
61. Obokata M, Reddy YNV, Melenovsky V, Pislaru S, Borlaug BA. Deterioration in right ventricular structure and function over time in patients with heart failure and preserved ejection fraction. *Eur Heart J.* 2019;40: 689-697.
62. Roy D, Talajic M, Nattel S, et al. Rhythm control versus rate control for atrial fibrillation and heart failure. *N Engl J Med.* 2008;358:2667-2677.
63. Prabhu S, Taylor AJ, Costello BT, et al. Catheter ablation versus medical rate control in atrial fibrillation and systolic dysfunction: the CAMERA-MRI study. *J Am Coll Cardiol.* 2017;70:1949-1961.
64. Khan MN, Jaïs P, Cummings J, et al. Pulmonary-vein isolation for atrial fibrillation in patients with heart failure. *N Engl J Med.* 2008;359:1778-1785.
65. Edelmann F, Wachter R, Schmidt AG, et al. Effect of spironolactone on diastolic function and exercise capacity in patients with heart failure with preserved ejection fraction: the Aldo-DHF randomized controlled trial. *JAMA.* 2013;309:781-791.
66. Pitt B, Pfeffer MA, Assmann SF, et al. Spironolactone for heart failure with preserved ejection fraction. *N Engl J Med.* 2014;370:1383-1392.
67. Pfeffer MA, Claggett B, Assmann SF, et al. Regional variation in patients and outcomes in the Treatment of Preserved Cardiac Function Heart Failure With an Aldosterone Antagonist (TOPCAT) trial. *Circulation.* 2015;131:34-42.
68. Solomon SD, McMurray JJV, Anand IS, et al. Angiotensin–Neprilysin inhibition in heart failure with preserved ejection fraction. *N Engl J Med.* 2019;381:1609-1620.
69. Vaduganathan M, Claggett BL, Desai AS, et al. Prior heart failure hospitalization, clinical outcomes, and response to Sacubitril/Valsartan compared with Valsartan in HFpEF. *J Am Coll Cardiol.* 2020;75: 245-254.
70. Wachter R, Shah SJ, Cowie MR, et al. Angiotensin receptor neprilysin inhibition versus individualized RAAS blockade: design and rationale of the PARALLAX trial. *ESC Heart Fail.* 2020;7:856-864.
71. Fitchett D, Zinman B, Wanner C, et al. Heart failure outcomes with empagliflozin in patients with type 2 diabetes at high cardiovascular risk: results of the EMPA-REG OUTCOME* trial. *Eur Heart J.* 2016;37:1526-1534.
72. Rådholm K, Figtree G, Perkovic V, et al. Canagliflozin and heart failure in type 2 Diabetes mellitus: results from the CANVAS program. *Circulation.* 2018;138:458-468.
73. Wiviott SD, Raz I, Bonaca MP, et al. Dapagliflozin and cardiovascular outcomes in type 2 diabetes. *N Engl J Med.* 2019;380:347-357.
74. Cosentino F, Cannon CP, Cherney DZI, et al. Efficacy of ertugliflozin on heart failure-related events in patients with type 2 diabetes mellitus and established atherosclerotic cardiovascular disease: results of the VERTIS CV trial. *Circulation.* 2020;142:2205-2215.
75. Butler J, Handelsman Y, Bakris G, Verma S. Use of sodium-glucose co-transporter-2 inhibitors in patients with and without type 2 diabetes: implications for incident and prevalent heart failure. *Eur J Heart Fail.* 2020;22:604-617.
76. Hasenfuß G, Hayward C, Burkhoff D, et al. A transcatheter intracardiac shunt device for heart failure with preserved ejection fraction (REDUCE LAP-HF): a multicentre, open-label, single-arm, phase 1 trial. *Lancet* .2016;387:1298-1304.
77. Kaye DM, Hasenfuß G, Neuzil P, et al. One-year outcomes after transcatheter insertion of an interatrial shunt device for the management of heart failure with preserved ejection fraction. *Circ Heart Fail.* 2016;9:e003662.
78. Feldman T, Mauri L, Kahwash R, et al. Transcatheter interatrial shunt device for the treatment of heart failure with preserved ejection fraction (REDUCE LAP-HF I [Reduce Elevated Left Atrial Pressure in Patients With Heart Failure]): a phase 2, randomized, sham-controlled trial. *Circulation.* 2018;137:364-375.
79. Jackson SL, Tong X, King RJ, Loustalot F, Hong Y, Ritchey MD. National burden of heart failure events in the United States, 2006 to 2014. *Circ Heart Fail.* 2018;11(12):e004873. doi:10.1161/CIRCHEARTFAILURE.117.004873

80. Abraham WT, Adamson PB, Bourge RC, et al. Wireless pulmonary artery haemodynamic monitoring in chronic heart failure: a randomised controlled trial. *Lancet.* 2011;377:658-666.
81. Adamson PB, Abraham WT, Bourge RC, et al. Wireless pulmonary artery pressure monitoring guides management to reduce decompensation in heart failure with preserved ejection fraction. *Circ Heart Fail.* 2014;7:935-944.
82. Redfield MM, Anstrom KJ, Levine JA, et al. Isosorbide mononitrate in heart failure with preserved ejection fraction. *N Engl J Med.* 2015;373:2314-2324.
83. Reddy YNV, Lewis GD, Shah SJ, et al. INDIE-HFpEF (Inorganic Nitrite Delivery to Improve Exercise Capacity in Heart Failure With Preserved Ejection Fraction): rationale and design. *Circ Heart Fail.* 2017;10(5):e003862. doi:10.1161/CIRCHEARTFAILURE.117.003862
84. Yusuf S, Pfeffer MA, Swedberg K, et al. Effects of candesartan in patients with chronic heart failure and preserved left-ventricular ejection fraction: the CHARM-preserved trial. *Lancet.* 2003;362:777-781.
85. Cleland JGF, Tendera M, Adamus J, et al. The perindopril in elderly people with chronic heart failure (PEP-CHF) study. *Eur Heart J.* 2006;27:2338-2345.
86. Massie BM, Carson PE, McMurray JJ, et al. Irbesartan in patients with heart failure and preserved ejection fraction. *N Engl J Med.* 2008;359:2456-2467.
87. Deswal A, Richardson P, Bozkurt B, Mann DL. Results of the Randomized Aldosterone Antagonism in Heart Failure With Preserved Ejection Fraction Trial (RAAM-PEF). *J Card Fail.* 2011;17:634-642.
88. Solomon SD, Zile M, Pieske B, et al. The angiotensin receptor neprilysin inhibitor LCZ696 in heart failure with preserved ejection fraction: a phase 2 double-blind randomised controlled trial. *Lancet.* 2012;380:1387-1395.
89. Yamamoto K, Origasa H, Hori M, J-DHF Investigators. Effects of carvedilol on heart failure with preserved ejection fraction: the Japanese Diastolic Heart Failure Study (J-DHF). *Eur J Heart Fail.* 2013;15:110-118.
90. Conraads VM, Metra M, Kamp O, et al. Effects of the long-term administration of nebivolol on the clinical symptoms, exercise capacity, and left ventricular function of patients with diastolic dysfunction: results of the ELANDD study. *Eur J Heart Fail.* 2012;14:219-225.
91. Komajda M, Isnard R, Cohen-Solal A, et al. Effect of ivabradine in patients with heart failure with preserved ejection fraction: the EDIFY randomized placebo-controlled trial. *Eur J Heart Fail.* 2017;19:1495-1503.
92. Redfield MM, Chen HH, Borlaug BA, et al. Effect of phosphodiesterase-5 inhibition on exercise capacity and clinical status in heart failure with preserved ejection fraction: a randomized clinical trial. *JAMA.* 2013;309:1268-1277.
93. Koller B, Steringer-Mascherbauer R, Ebner CH, et al. Pilot study of endothelin receptor Blockade in Heart Failure with Diastolic Dysfunction and Pulmonary Hypertension (BADDHY-Trial). *Heart Lung Circ.* 2017;26:433-441.
94. Zile MR, Bourge RC, Redfield MM, Zhou D, Baicu CF, Little WC. Randomized, double-blind, placebo-controlled study of sitaxsentan to improve impaired exercise tolerance in patients with heart failure and a preserved ejection fraction. *JACC Heart Fail.* 2014;2:123-130.
95. Maier LS, Layug B, Karwatowska-Prokopczuk E, et al. RAnoLazIne for the treatment of diastolic heart failure in patients with preserved ejection fraction: the RALI-DHF proof-of-concept study. *JACC Heart Fail.* 2013;1:115-122.
96. Armstrong PW, Lam CSP, Anstrom KJ, et al. Effect of vericiguat vs placebo on quality of life in patients with heart failure and preserved ejection fraction: the VITALITY-HFpEF randomized clinical trial. *JAMA.* 2020;324:1512-1521.
97. Shah SJ, Voors AA, McMurray JJV, et al. Effect of Neladenoson Bialanate on exercise capacity among patients with heart failure with preserved ejection fraction: a randomized clinical trial. *JAMA.* 2019;321:2101-2112.

CHAPTER 69

HEART FAILURE WITH REDUCED EJECTION FRACTION

John M. Suffredini and Savitri E. Fedson

INTRODUCTION

A variety of structural or functional cardiac abnormalities can result in the clinical condition of heart failure (HF), although the majority result from left ventricular (LV) dysfunction with filling or ejection of blood. Although imaging modalities are critical in the diagnosis and management of HF, the condition itself remains a clinical diagnosis, with classic presenting features including dyspnea on exertion, orthopnea, weight gain, and peripheral edema. Previously, patients with reduced left ventricular ejection fraction (LVEF) were defined as having systolic HF, whereas patients with normal LVEF were defined as having diastolic HF. However, increased recognition of the significant overlap of both systolic and diastolic dysfunction in clinical HF has led to a change in nomenclature. The condition now is subcategorized into heart failure with reduced ejection fraction (HFrEF) and heart failure with preserved ejection fraction (HFpEF). HFrEF has been defined by the American College of Cardiology (ACC)/American Heart Association (AHA) 2013 Heart Failure Guidelines as clinical HF with an LVEF less than or equal to 40%, whereas HFpEF is defined as clinical HF with an LVEF greater than or equal to 50%.[1,2] HF patients with LVEF between 41% and 49% are defined as HFpEF with borderline ejection fraction or as heart failure with mid-range ejection fraction (HFmrEF). Patients with reduced LVEF but remain without clinical evidence or manifestations of HF are best defined as asymptomatic LV dysfunction.[1]

Epidemiology

There are currently estimated to be 6.2 million individuals over 20 years of age in the United States with HF and 23 million individuals worldwide.[3,4] The prevalence and incidence of HF is on the rise in the United States and other developed countries, and it is estimated that more than 750,000 new cases of HF will be diagnosed each year in the United States by 2040.[5] A major factor contributing to this rise is the aging population. The incidence of HF doubles for each decade of life, with the lifetime likelihood of developing HF approximately 20%.[6]

HFrEF specifically is estimated to account for approximately 50% of all HF diagnoses, although, as a proportion of all HF, it is decreasing over time.[1,3] Male gender has been associated with new diagnosis of HFrEF, whereas female gender is associated with HFpEF, likely related to higher incidences of ischemic cardiomyopathy in male patients. The lifetime risk for the development of HFrEF is 10.6% in males in comparison to 5.8% for females.[7] New diagnosis of HFrEF has also been associated with active tobacco abuse, elevated high-sensitivity troponin, and prior myocardial infarction (MI).[8]

Approximately 6% of the population have asymptomatic LV dysfunction without clinical symptoms consistent with HF. These patients have an annual risk of 10% for developing clinical HF.[1]

Racial Disparities

Racial differences between the incidence and prevalence rates of HF have been observed. Black males are the highest risk group for the development of HFrEF and have a significantly higher 5-year mortality rate in comparison to non-hispanic white patients with HFrEF. Overall, the prevalence in Black males is 4.5% in comparison to 2.7% in non-hispanic white males, and similar differences have been demonstrated between Black and non-hispanic white females.[9] Other studies have observed no significant difference in HFrEF prevalence rates when the populations are adjusted for prior MI, suggesting that atherosclerotic disease burden and implementation of guideline-based therapy likely is an important factor in racial disparities in HFrEF.

Hospitalizations

HF exacerbations are one of the most frequent causes for hospitalization in the United States. Every year, there are more than 1 million hospitalizations related to HF, accounting for more than 20% of hospitalizations in patients over the age of 65 years.[1] Approximately 50% of these hospitalizations involve patients with HFrEF specifically. After discharge, this patient population is at increased risk for rehospitalization, with more than 25% of patients requiring repeat hospitalization within 1 month. Despite a growing prevalence of the disease, hospitalizations with the primary diagnosis of HF exacerbation have trended downward over the past two decades, which has been attributed to more effective therapies and increased programs focused on reduction in re-admission rates for these patients.[10]

Prognosis and Mortality

HF is associated with a 5-year mortality of approximately 50% and accounts for 7% of cardiovascular (CV) deaths in the United States. The mortality rates in patients with HFrEF and HFpEF are thought to be similar, although some analyses have suggested a lower mortality rate in patients with HFpEF. In a recent meta-analysis, the annual mortality for HFrEF was

14.2% compared to 12.1% for HFpEF, irrespective of age, gender, and a number of CV risks.[11] However, increasingly trends point to improvements in HFrEF mortality over time, whereas mortality rates in HFpEF patients have remained stable, which is likely related to a growing number of effective therapy options for HFrEF patients. From 1993 to 2005, 30-day posthospitalization mortality improved from 12.6% to 10.8% in one study, and other studies have demonstrated similar improvements in mortality rates since 1980s.[1,12] HF hospitalizations are one of the strongest predictors for mortality, and average median survival falls to approximately 2 years after first hospitalization for HF exacerbation.[13] Other strong predictors for mortality include renal function, serum sodium concentration, age, and systolic blood pressure.

Health Care Cost Burden

The economic burden of HF is significant, and total costs associated with the health care services and lost worker productivity are estimated to be more than $30 billion a year in the United States and more than $100 billion worldwide.[1] HF accounts for 2% of total health care spending in the United States. A strong contributor to these costs is HF exacerbations requiring hospitalization, with a HF hospitalization costing more than a mean of $20,000 and a high number of patients requiring multiple hospitalizations per year.[14] Among patients with HFrEF, new pharmacologic agents as well as device therapy—such as internal cardiac defibrillators and cardiac resynchronization therapy—have improved outcomes while also contributing significantly to the rising cost of care. By 2030, it is expected that the direct health care costs associated with HF will exceed $50 billion in the United States.[15]

Etiologies of Heart Failure with Reduced Ejection Fraction

There is a wide variety of underlying etiologies associated with HFrEF. The most common etiology is ischemic cardiomyopathy, in which a combination of acute coronary events and chronic supply-demand ischemia results in declining LV systolic function. Overall, coronary artery disease accounts for approximately 40% of patients with HFrEF.[16] Owing to the high prevalence of ischemic-induced HFrEF, all patients with HFrEF must undergo an ischemic evaluation and then are generally characterized as either ischemic cardiomyopathy or nonischemic cardiomyopathy.

Among patients with nonischemic cardiomyopathy, the most common identified etiologies are hypertension and valvular heart disease. However, a significant portion of patients with nonischemic cardiomyopathy are without a clearly identifiable etiology and are labeled as idiopathic or dilated cardiomyopathy. Important etiologies of nonischemic cardiomyopathy to consider include those related to increased and abnormal cardiac energetics, such as tachycardia- or stress-induced cardiomyopathy; toxin related, such as substance abuse associated or chemotherapy-related cardiomyopathy; and inflammation related, such as peripartum cardiomyopathy and myocarditis.[17,18] In addition, dilated cardiomyopathy can be attributed to genetic causes in approximately 30% to 40% of cases, and in these, there may be an identifiable genetic variant in 40%.[19] Other etiologies include infiltrative processes such as amyloidosis, sarcoidosis, and hemochromatosis. Congenital heart disease accounts for approximately 0.4% (**Table 69.1**).[20]

PATHOGENESIS

The primary mechanism of the clinical syndrome of HFrEF is reduction in the pumping efficiency of the myocardium with (1) failure to deliver sufficient oxygen to meet the metabolic needs of the body and/or (2) elevated filling pressures. However, owing to the numerous diverse etiologies of HF, there is no single unified mechanism to explain the underlying pathophysiology of the syndrome. HFrEF begins with an initial insult, which can have a rapid onset such as an acute MI, or it can result from a gradual process, such as infiltrative cardiomyopathies. These events are followed by progressive LV remodeling driven by changes in neurohormonal axes and the increased pressures and volumes experienced by the myocardial tissue. This process is characterized by changes in the gross structure of the ventricle, with concentric hypertrophy and/or spherical dilation, and by changes in the underlying cellular structure of the myocardium as cardiac myocytes are replaced by fibrosis. It is now understood that in most patients with HFrEF, this process of LV remodeling begins before clinical manifestation of the disease. Many modern pharmacologic and device therapies for HFrEF are focused on preventing or reversing LV remodeling.

Neurohormonal Axes

As cardiac output falls and/or filling pressures rise in a patient with HFrEF, various hormonal compensatory mechanisms are activated. Initially, a fall in cardiac output and blood pressure will be detected by baroreceptors in the carotid sinus and aortic arch. In order to maintain blood pressure and end-organ perfusion, the sympathetic nerves system (SNS) is activated, resulting in the release of catecholamines primarily by the adrenal medulla but also from the myocardium itself. This is accompanied by a simultaneous reduction in parasympathetic activation. Increased levels of circulating norepinephrine effect a number of organ systems. In the myocardium, activation of β-1 receptors increases contractility and heart rate, resulting in an initial increase in cardiac output while also increasing myocardial oxygen demand. Eventually, there is downregulation of the cardiac β-adrenergic receptors. In the peripheral vasculature, stimulation of α-1 receptors results in peripheral vasoconstriction, increasing system blood pressure, and increasing LV afterload.

In the kidneys, sympathetic activation induces the production of renin via two mechanisms. Peripheral vasoconstriction results in decreased blood flow to the glomerular juxtaglomerular apparatus, which induces renin production; renin production is also triggered directly by the activation of β-1 receptors on the juxtaglomerular apparatus. Renin begins the hormonal activation of the renin-angiotensin-aldosterone

TABLE 69.1 Etiologies of Heart Failure with Reduced Ejection Fraction
Ischemic Cardiomyopathy
Hypertension
Valvular Heart Disease
Familial (Genetic)
Tachycardia-Mediated Cardiomyopathy
Toxin-Induced Cardiomyopathies: • Chemotherapy (anthracyclines, trastuzumab, thymidine kinase inhibitors) • Alcohol • Amphetamine, cocaine • Heavy metals • Hemochromatosis
Metabolic • Thyroid dysfunction • Acromegaly • Pheochromocytoma • Diabetes
Myocarditis • Coxsackievirus • COVID-19 (Sars-Covid 19) • Parvovirus B19 • Cytomegalovirus • Epstein-Barr virus • Human immunodeficiency virus • Influenza • Hepatitis • Chagas disease (*Trypanosoma cruzi*) • Lyme disease (*Borrelia burgdorferi*) • Autoimmune
Pregnancy-Associated Cardiomyopathies • Eclampsia-induced cardiomyopathy • Peripartum cardiomyopathy
Nutritional Deficiencies • Thiamine deficiency • Selenium deficiency • Vitamin C deficiency
Infiltrative Processes • Amyloidosis • Sarcoidosis
Inflammatory Processes • Systemic lupus erythematosus • Eosinophilic myocarditis
Congenital/Genetic Heart Disease • Muscular dystrophies (Becker, Duchenne) • Lysosomal storage diseases (Fabry, Gaucher, etc) • Congenital heart defects
Stress-Induced Cardiomyopathy

system (RAAS). Renin converts angiotensinogen, produced by the liver, to angiotensin I. Angiotensin I is converted to the active form angiotensin II by angiotensin-converting enzyme (ACE) in vascular endothelial cells, primarily in the pulmonary vascular beds. Angiotensin II results in the retention of both sodium and water via both direct and indirect mechanisms. Angiotensin II directly stimulates sodium channels and sodium pumps in the proximal tubule, the ascending loop of Henle, and in the collecting ducts. The protein also induces the release of the mineralocorticoid hormone aldosterone from the zona glomerulosa in the adrenal cortex and antidiuretic hormone (ADH) from the posterior pituitary gland. Aldosterone upregulates the expression of Na^+/K^+ pumps in the cells of distal tubule and collecting ducts, allowing for the increased reabsorption of sodium. Aldosterone also promotes collagen synthesis and fibrosis within the myocardium. ADH induces its effect by increasing the insertion of aquaporin-2 water channels in the collecting duct, allowing reabsorption of water.

Ultimately, the activation of the RAAS results in significant retention of sodium and water through several mechanisms, increasing blood volume and pressure. Initially, activation of these neurohormonal axes allows for short-term compensation for declining cardiac output by increasing blood volume, inducing peripheral vasoconstriction, and increasing cardiac contractility and heart rate. However, these processes increasingly become maladaptive as the disease progresses.[21,22]

Ventricular Remodeling

In response to increased pressures and volumes, the myocardium begins to undergo a remodeling process with changes to the LV structure and underlying histopathology. Myocyte hypertrophy develops in response to increased LV wall strain and loading. In patients with HFrEF, LV wall stress is primarily driven by volume overload, resulting in progressive dilation of the ventricle. At the cellular level, sarcomeres within the myocytes are deposited in series, allowing the individual cells to elongate in response to rising diastolic wall stress. This process is known as "eccentric hypertrophy" in contrast to concentric hypertrophy, which traditionally develops because of elevated pressures in systole. In concentric hypertrophy, additional sarcomeres are deposited in a parallel manner within the cardiac myocytes. As the LV continues to dilate and progresses from the normal ellipsoid shape of the ventricle to a spherical one in HFrEF, the geometric changes to the ventricle worsen the mechanical pumping efficiency of the heart, which correlates with a worsening prognosis. Dilatation of the ventricle and sarcomere stretch leads to increased ventricular preload.

As chamber dilation and wall thinning progress, cardiac myocytes are progressively lost via several mechanisms of cellular death, including apoptosis, autophagy, and necrosis. At this stage, neurohormonal axis activation induces a direct impact on LV remodeling by triggering cardiac myocyte death via necrosis and apoptosis. Both norepinephrine and angiotensin II at sufficient serum concentrations are capable of inducing myocyte cell death. Increased rates of cell death and the resulting inflammation within the cardiac tissue signal an inappropriate proliferation of fibroblasts and increase deposition of extracellular matrix collagen proteins, in part due to aldosterone signaling. This slow, chronic loss of cardiac myocytes followed by myocardial fibrosis formation contributes to the continued decline in cardiac reserve and the progressive nature of the disease course.[23,24]

Protective Counterregulatory Mechanisms

In response to increased wall strain on the atrium and ventricle, several counterregulatory mechanisms exist to induce excretion of water and sodium, lower systemic blood pressure, and slow the progression of LV remodeling. The most important hormones involved in this protective mechanism are the natriuretic peptides: the brain (or b-type) natriuretic peptide (BNP) and atrial natriuretic peptide (ANP). Although both hormones are produced and released primarily by cardiac cells, BNP derived its name from its originally isolation from brain tissue in 1988 and is the most relevant in clinical practice. ANP is released rapidly in response to acute changes in atrial pressure and has a short in vivo half-life of approximately 3 minutes. BNP is released more slowly in response to chronic changes in myocardial pressures and has a slightly longer half-life of 20 minutes in vivo. Both peptides bind to natriuretic peptide receptors, NPR-A and NPR-B, found in several tissues, including the kidneys, vascular smooth muscle, adrenal glands, and myocardium itself. Once ANP or BNP binds to the receptor, it induces the production of guanosine cyclic monophosphate (cGMP). In the kidneys, cGMP reduces sodium and water reabsorption by inhibition of Na^+-Cl^- co-transporters in the distal convoluted tubule and inhibits activation of the RAAS by reducing renin secretion from the juxtaglomerular apparatus. RAAS activation is further inhibited by cGMP action in the adrenal cortex, thereby reducing the secretion of aldosterone. Vasodilation is induced in the vascular smooth muscle. In the myocardium itself, cGMP has a cardioprotective effect against LV remodeling by inhibition of cardiac myocyte apoptosis and inhibition of cardiac fibroblast proliferation. The natriuretic peptides are relatively quickly degraded enzymatically by neutral endopeptidase (NEP), also known as *neprilysin.* As HF progresses, expression of natriuretic peptides increases and assists in counterbalancing the maladaptive SNS and RAAS activations. Over time, however, the tissues develop increased resistance to natriuretic peptides by downgrading of NPR-A and NPR-B receptors, counteracting its efficiency, and accelerating disease progression.[25,26]

TABLE 69.2 New York Heart Association Functional Class

Class I	No significant limitation in physical activity. Patient is asymptomatic.
Class II	Slight limitation in physical activity. Patient becomes symptomatic with marked activity, such as climbing flights of stairs or ambulating multiple blocks.
Class III	Significant limitation in physical activity. Patient becomes symptomatic with minimal exertion, such as ambulating short distances.
Class IV	Severe limitation in physical activity. Patient experiences symptoms such as dyspnea even at rest.

History and Common Signs and Symptoms

Most patients with HFrEF initially present with signs and symptoms of volume overload. The most common presenting symptoms are dyspnea and fatigue, which patients often report have been progressively worsening for weeks or months (**Table 69.2**). As the LV fails and cardiac output decreases, pulmonary pressures rise, resulting in extravasation of fluid into the interstitial spaces. The etiology of the sensation of dyspnea is multifactorial and results from the resulting decreased pulmonary compliance, elevated pulmonary pressures, and hypoxia. Dyspnea in HF is often exacerbated by lying flat (orthopnea), which results in an increase in venous return and pulmonary pressures. Other possible pulmonary symptoms can include decreased exercise tolerance, nonproductive cough, or wheezing. Increased venous capillary bed pressures results in fluid extravasation into third spaces throughout the body. Lower extremity swelling results from accumulation of peripheral edema. Abdominal distention, increased girth, and discomfort may result from cardiac ascites and abdominal wall edema. This can be accompanied by early satiety and poor appetite. The development of third space edema in multiple systems results in progressive weight gain. Patients can report palpitations from HFrEF-associated arrhythmias. Increasingly, there is growing understanding of the psychological symptoms of HFrEF, including depression, insomnia, and anxiety. Late presenting patients with near cardiogenic shock may report cool extremities, confusion, lightheadedness, and severe fatigue.

Beyond physical symptoms, the interviewer should obtain a complete assessment of the patient's medical, social, and family histories with a particular focus on CV risk factors.[27]

Physical Examination

Despite the number of and availability of modern imaging modalities to assess a suspected HFrEF patient, HF remains a clinical diagnosis, with the physical examination playing a central role in initial evaluation. Even in resource-unlimited health care systems, the physical examination is particularly important because it will often guide initial management before confirmatory imaging studies can be obtained. The majority of physical examination findings in the new-onset HFrEF patient will be related to clinical manifestation of congestion (**Table 69.3**).

Pulmonary congestion can manifest as pulmonary edema or pleural effusions. On physical examination, pulmonary edema can manifest as fine crackles. The finding of bilateral basilar crackles has low sensitivity but strong specificity for HF exacerbation. The presence of bilateral or unilateral (usually favoring the right side) pleural effusion(s) can be detected by diminished breath sounds on the affected size. Cardiac wheezing can also occasionally be heard due to secondary bronchospasm in the setting of pulmonary congestion.

TABLE 69.3 Physical Examination Signs in Heart Failure

Physical Examination Signs	Underlying Pathology
Cardiac Examination	
S3 gallop	Increased intravascular volume
S4 gallop	Ventricular hypertrophy
Displaced PMI	Ventricular hypertrophy or dilation
Elevated jugular venous pulse	Increased intravascular volume
Positive hepatojugular reflex	Increased intravascular volume
Tachycardia	Low cardiac output
Pulmonary Examination	
Rales	Pulmonary edema
Cardiac wheeze	Pulmonary edema
Diminished breath sounds	Pleural effusion
Abdominal Examination	
Distended abdomen	Cardiac ascites or intestinal wall edema
Abdominal fluid wave	Cardiac ascites
Organomegaly	Organ interstitial edema
Extremities	
Peripheral pitting edema	Extremity edema
Diminished pulses	Poor extremity perfusion
Pulsus alternans	Low cardiac output
Cool distal extremities	Poor extremity perfusion

PMI, point of maximal impulse.

Central venous pressure can be assessed by evaluating the level of the jugular venous pulse (JVP). When the patient's upper body is elevated at a 45-degree angle, a JVP with a height of greater than 4 to 5 cm above the sternal angle is suggestive of elevated central venous pressures. The hepatojugular reflex can also be used to assess central venous pressure by applying firm compression to the right upper quadrant of abdomen for at least 10 seconds while monitoring for elevation of the JVP. An increase in JVP of greater than 3 cm is considered a positive test consistent with elevated central venous pressures. Both tests can be limited by body habitus.

A cardiac examination should include careful auscultation for third (S3) and fourth (S4) heart sounds. Detection of a S3 gallop is highly specific for HF and occurs in early diastole due to an increased volume of blood entering the ventricle during passive filling. The S4 heart sound occurs in late diastole and is produced by blood propelled by atrial contraction striking the hypertrophied LV. The point of maximal impulse (PMI) can also be evaluated; in patients with a hypertrophied LV and resulting cardiomegaly, the PMI will move downward and laterally.

An abdominal examination may detect distention, fluid wave secondary to ascites, or organomegaly.

The lower extremities should be evaluated for peripheral pitting edema, which is a common sign of volume overload, although not specific to HF. Long-standing edema will result in stasis dermatitis changes in the skin with hyperpigmentation, skin thickening, pruritus, and ulcer formation. Cool or pale distal extremities can be signs of low-output HF and cardiogenic shock.[27]

DIAGNOSIS

Metabolic Laboratory Data

Although HF cannot be diagnosed based on laboratory data, metabolic abnormalities are commonly seen in patients with HF. Patients with significant volume overload may present with significant hyponatremia and renal insufficiency. These can also be a marker of poor systemic perfusion and a reduced cardiac output state. Patients receiving aggressive diuresis must be monitored for electrolyte abnormalities, such as hypokalemia or hypomagnesemia. Renal and liver dysfunction can be suggestive of a decompensated low-output state or worsening venous congestion of those organ systems.

Serum Biomarkers

In modern clinical practice, natriuretic peptides are the most commonly used serum biomarkers in the diagnosis and management of HFrEF. BNP, with a half-life of approximately 20 minutes, and N-terminal pro b-type natriuretic peptide (NT-proBNP), with a half-life of approximately 80 minutes, are the most commonly used assays. Both BNP and NT-proBNP are released from the ventricle during periods of increased wall strain and, therefore, clinically often used to distinguish patients with possible HF exacerbation from other etiologies of dyspnea.[28] A cutoff of 100 pg/mL for BNP or 900 pg/mL for NT-proBNP is typically suggested, but both assays can be significantly impacted by other conditions. It is well established that serum natriuretic peptide levels rise with age, regardless of LV function. Renal dysfunction results in impaired clearance of BNP and NT-proBNP and can elevate the circulating levels of both peptides. Serum natriuretic peptide levels can be artificially depressed in overweight and obese patients, with up to 20% reduction in overweight and 60% reduction in obese patients. In addition, there are known racial differences, with African Americans typically having lower levels of circulating BNP. As such, both BNP and NT-proBNP assays must be interpreted in the setting of each patient's individual clinical situation **(Table 69.4)**. Beyond the initial diagnosis, natriuretic peptide assays can also be used to track response to diuresis in admitted patients with acute HF exacerbations when other indicators are limited or present conflicting information. Multiple studies have also demonstrated that both BNP and NT-proBNP have a correlation with prognosis and can be used to predict mortality.[25,26,29,30] ANP and midregional pro-ANP have been examined as biomarkers for HF but as yet have not shown to be equivalent to BNP.

Troponin elevation can occur in HFrEF patient even in the absence of an acute coronary syndrome or overt myocardial injury. Increased LV wall strain during periods of acute HF exacerbation will produce supply-demand ischemia that can

TABLE 69.4 Noncardiac Influence on Natriuretic Peptides

Diagnosis of Heart failure	
BNP > 100 pg/mL NT-PROBNP > 900 pg/mL	90% Sensitivity
Noncardiac factors that decrease BNP/NT-proBNP	**Obesity African American race**
Noncardiac factors that increase BNP/ NT-proBNP	Significant pulmonary disease Pulmonary embolism Older age Renal disease Sepsis

BNP, brain (or b-type) natriuretic peptide; ml, milliliters NT-proBNP, N-terminal pro b-type natriuretic peptide pg, picograms.

result with high-sensitivity cardiac troponin T elevation, which does correlate with increased in-hospital mortality.[31,32]

A number of other biomarkers have been investigated for clinical usefulness. Specifically, soluble suppression of tumorigenicity 2 (sST2) is a member of the interleukin (IL)-1 receptor family and is a receptor protein for IL-33. It is upregulated in cardiac myocytes and cardiac fibroblasts in response to cardiac strain or injury. The soluble form of the receptor likely acts as a decoy receptor and inhibitor to the cardioprotective protein IL-33. ST2 used in conjunction with NT-proBNP significantly improves diagnostic and prognostic accuracy in both acute and chronic HF patients. Although the ST2 assay is Food and Drug Administration (FDA) approved and currently commercially available, the assay has not found widespread clinical use at this time.[33,34]

Galectin (GAL)-3 is a β-galactoside-binding lectin that is upregulated in HF. It is secreted by activated macrophages, myofibroblasts, and monocytes as a mediator of fibrosis and associated with incident HF, CV mortality, and all-cause death. However, there are no clear data at present about how to manage those with elevated levels, or the response of GAL-3 to guideline therapies.[28,35,36] Renal biomarkers, such as cystatin C and neutrophil gelatinase-associated lipocalin (NGAL), have been used in the context of cardiorenal syndromes.

In addition, recent analyses of biomarker banks have shown that in addition to NT-proBNP, HFrEF is associated with increased levels of growth differentiation factor 15 (GDF-15), IL-1, and, in general, DNA-binding transcription factors and proteins associated with nitric oxide synthetic processes and cellular protein metabolic processes. In the future, recognition of these pathways in the clinical spectrum of HF will probably lead to identification of other biomarkers with clinical utility.[37]

Electrocardiogram

An electrocardiogram (ECG) should be obtained in all patients with suspected or new diagnosis of HFrEF. Although sinus tachycardia is the most common ECG abnormality seen in acute HF, rhythm disturbances such as atrial fibrillation, atrial flutter, or ventricular arrhythmias are commonly seen in patients with structurally abnormal hearts. Patients may demonstrate increased voltages consistent with chamber enlargement. Ischemic changes in the form of Q waves, ST segment, or T wave changes could suggest an underlying ischemic etiology. QRS duration should be assessed because this can be an indication for cardiac resynchronization therapy.[38]

Imaging

All patients with suspected HF should be evaluated with a transthoracic echocardiogram (TTE). Echocardiography allows for a relatively low-cost, noninvasive, comprehensive assessment of cardiac structure, ventricular function, and valvular function (**Table 69.5**). LV systolic function can be assessed by LVEF, LV outflow track velocity-time integral, or strain imaging. Doppler assessment of the mitral valve inflow pattern and the mitral annulus allows for evaluation of diastolic dysfunction and LV filling pressures. The individual valves can be assessed for function. The central venous pressure can be assessed by evaluating the inferior vena cava diameter and respiratory variation.[39]

Nuclear medicine studies are widely used in cardiology to assess myocardial perfusion. They can also be used to evaluate LV systolic function in patients with poor acoustic TTE windows, with a technique known as radionuclide ventriculography or multigated acquisition (MUGA). These imaging techniques can also provide useful information about the diastolic properties of the ventricle. Nuclear medicine studies can also be used to evaluate for specific etiologies of HFrEF; F-18 fluorodeoxyglucose (FDG) positron emission tomography (PET) can be used both to diagnosis cardiac sarcoidosis and to monitor disease activity. Bone-avid tracers such as technetium-99m pyrophosphate (Tc-99m PYP) can be used in the diagnosis of familial or transthyretin amyloidosis. ^{123}I-meta-iodobenzylguanidine (mIBG), an established tracer for imaging myocardial denervation, has been utilized to image myocardial denervation in familial transthyretin cardiac amyloidosis and may have a role in prognostic determination for patients with HFrEF.[40-42]

Cardiac magnetic resonance (CMR) imaging is a growing area of cardiac imaging. In HF patients, it allows for a detailed assessment of cardiac structure and function similar to TTE while also allowing for assessment of infiltrative processes and fibrosis. CMR fibrosis data can add to prognostic determination beyond ejection fraction. In addition, in early dilated cardiomyopathy, the degree of myocardial edema, fibrosis, and injury can help identify patients who are likely to have myocardial recovery.[43-45]

The use of gadolinium allows for the evaluation of myocardial viability, scar, and myocarditis, and the pattern of late gadolinium enhancement and tissue characterization can help discriminate between certain etiologies, such as amyloidosis and hemochromatosis. When combined with chemical stress testing techniques, CMR imaging can also be used to evaluate myocardial perfusion.[46]

Invasive Testing

When noninvasive assessments of cardiac function, volume status, or hemodynamics are inadequate or limited, a right heart catheterization can be used to directly measure intracardiac

TABLE 69.5 Imaging Modalities for Heart Failure

	Function	Anatomy	Pros	Cons
Echocardiography	Biventricular systolic and diastolic function, estimates of right atrial and pulmonary artery pressures	Chamber size, valvular disease, pericardial effusion	Portable, no radiation, common; hemodynamic and functional assessment	Limited by acoustic windows, subjective interpretation of function
Cardiac MR	Biventricular function; can be used to assess for ischemia, viability	Able to assess chamber size, pericardial pathology; can help with anatomy (congenital)	Can aid in diagnosis of dilated cardiomyopathy, myocarditis or suggest etiologies (such as noncompaction, hemochromatosis, myocarditis, amyloidosis, sarcoidosis)	Limited compatibility with ferrous metals; can be limited by tachycardia
Cardiac CT	Biventricular function	Define anatomy (congenital, great vessels), coronary artery assessment, ventricular volumes	High negative predictive value for coronary artery disease	Radiation and iodinated contrast; limited by tachycardia
Nuclear Imaging				
MUGA	LV systolic function and can assess diastolic parameters	LV volume	Quantitative EF, reproducible	Radiation exposure
SPECT	LV function, ischemia		Diagnosis of transthyretin amyloidosis with bone-avid tracers	Radiation exposure, may miss balanced three-vessel coronary artery disease
PET	LV function, myocardial perfusion and viability, diagnose sarcoid, evaluate hibernating myocardium		Diagnosis and follow cardiac sarcoidosis	Radiation exposure, may miss three-vessel coronary artery disease

CT, computed tomography; EF, ejection fraction; LV, left ventricular; MR, magnetic resonance; MUGA, multigated acquisition scan; SPECT, single photon emission computed tomography; PET, positron emission tomography.

pressures and assess cardiac output. In undifferentiated patients with new diagnosis of HFrEF, selective coronary angiography is often performed at the same time to evaluate for coronary artery disease as the underlying etiology. Although routine use of right heart catheterization is not supported by clinical guidelines, it is essential in the evaluation of patients for advanced surgical therapies, such as cardiac transplantation or mechanical circulatory support, and is indicated for those patients if the clinical assessment of volume status or cardiac output is unclear.[1]

In patients in whom the etiology of their HFrEF remains unclear despite noninvasive evaluations, a myocardial biopsy can be performed during right heart catheterization. Although, owing to the related procedural risks, noninvasive diagnostic techniques are preferred for the majority of patients, there remains a role for myocardial biopsy in certain patient populations. Patients with new-onset HFrEF with rapid decompensation in which there is a suspicion for giant cell myocarditis are one population in which early myocardial biopsy is recommended. Myocardial biopsy is also frequently used to monitor for signs of allograft rejection in cardiac transplant patients.[1]

Although continuous pulmonary artery pressure monitoring was previously limited to patients in intensive care units, in 2014, the first FDA-approved wireless pulmonary artery pressure monitor became available, which allows for long-term monitoring of pulmonary artery pressures in the ambulatory setting, allowing for the outpatient practice of hemodynamically tailored therapy. This has been demonstrated to reduce HF-related hospitalizations in patients with New York Heart Association (NYHA) class III HF.[47]

MANAGEMENT OF THE PATIENT WITH HEART FAILURE WITH REDUCED EJECTION FRACTION

Therapeutic Targets in Modern Heart Failure Therapy

A firm understanding of the underlying pathophysiology of HFrEF is crucial in understanding modern guideline-directed medical and device therapy. The principal goal of the long-term management of HFrEF is directed at preventing or reversing ventricular remodeling. Current therapeutic targets for mortality-reducing therapies include inhibition of maladaptive neurohormonal axes, reduction of ventricular wall stress, and, more recently, promotion of intrinsic cardioprotective counterregulatory axes.

Neprilysin inhibitors are a more recent therapeutic target that have emerged for HFrEF. By inhibition of the neprilysin enzyme that is responsible for the rapid breakdown of ANP and BNP, neprilysin inhibitors increase the circulating levels of the natriuretic peptides that act as a counterregulatory mechanism to RAAS and SNS overactivation. Currently, there is one medication available in this class, sacubitril, which is sold as a combination pill with the ARB valsartan. Given the medication's combination with an ARB, the side-effect profile is similar, with hypotension and hyperkalemia being common. Based on the results of the Prospective Comparison of ARNI with ACE-I to Determine Impact on Global Mortality and Morbidity in Heart Failure (PARADIGM-HF) trial demonstrating improvements in outcomes including hospitalizations and mortality compared to an ACE-I alone, the sacubitril/valsartan combination was given a Class I indication for the management of HFrEF by the ACCF/AHA 2016 Focused Update on New Pharmacological Therapy for Heart Failure Guideline.[48]

ACE inhibitors (ACE-Is) were one of the first classes of medications to demonstrate mortality benefit in patients with HFrEF. ACE-Is inhibit the conversion of angiotensin I to the active form angiotensin II. By doing so, they block activation of the RAAS and induce vasodilation, promote sodium and water wasting, and inhibit ventricle remodeling. The peripheral vasodilation reduces LV wall strain. Vasodilation in the glomerular afferent and efferent arterioles often results with a mild decrease in glomerular filtration rate, and inhibition of aldosterone release can result in hyperkalemia. ACE-Is also increase bradykinin levels by inhibition of their degradation, which contribute to their antihypertensive effects but also can induce a nonproductive cough in approximately 10% of patients who take the medication. In rare cases, ACE-Is can cause bradykinin-induced angioedema. The ACC/AHA 2013 Guideline for Management of Heart Failure recommends ACE-Is as a class I indication in all patients with HFrEF unless the patient has a contraindication.

In patients who cannot tolerate ACE-Is, angiotensin II receptor blockers (ARBs) are used as an alternative therapy. ARBs inhibit the RAAS by antagonism of the angiotensin II receptor in several tissues. The result is similar pharmacologic effects as observed with ACE-Is without any significant increase in bradykinin levels. Similar to ACE-Is, several randomized controlled trials have demonstrated a mortality benefit when ARBs are used in patients with HFrEF. However, no benefit has been demonstrated from the combination of an ACE-I and an ARB, and there is a significantly elevated risk of side effects. Consequently, only one class of these medications is recommended for use at a time. The ACCF/AHA 2013 Guideline recommends the use of ARBs in any HFrEF patient unable to tolerate an ACE-I, unless otherwise contraindicated, as a Class I indication.

Further inhibition of the RAAS is achieved via mineralocorticoid receptor antagonists (MRAs), such as spironolactone or eplerenone, which block the binding of aldosterone to its receptors. While ACE-Is and ARBs reduce production of aldosterone, it has been demonstrated that over time aldosterone production returns to normal despite the inhibition. This has been described as "aldosterone breakthrough." MRAs are thought to counter this long-term return of normal aldosterone production. Similar to ACE-I/ARBs, MRAs have demonstrated a mortality benefit in patients with HFrEF in randomized controlled trials. ACCF/AHA 2013 Guideline for Management of Heart Failure gives a Class I indication for the use of MRAs in HFrEF patients with LVEF 35% or less and NYHA Class II to IV symptoms.

Renin inhibitors have also been investigated as a novel approach to RAAS inhibition in HFrEF. Aliskiren is a direct renin inhibitor that has been investigated in HFrEF. However, two randomized controlled trials failed to demonstrate any significant improvement in HF outcomes, and the medication is not currently recommended for the management of HF.

β-Adrenergic blockers are a major component of chronic HF management. They function as competitive antagonist to β-adrenergic and, in some cases, α-adrenergic receptors. By doing so, they mitigate the sustained sympathetic activation that becomes maladaptive in patients with HFrEF. Long-term, β-adrenergic blockade with carvedilol, metoprolol succinate, or bisoprolol has been demonstrated to reverse LV remodeling and significantly improve outcomes with reductions in hospitalizations and mortality. Despite the benefits, initialization of β-blocker therapy must be done cautiously, as the negative chronotropic and inotropic effects can result in decompensation if started too aggressively in a clinically borderline patient. The ACCF/AHA 2013 Guideline recommends the use of carvedilol, metoprolol succinate, or bisoprolol in all HFrEF patients who do not have a contraindication.[1]

Finally, new therapeutic targets continue to be investigated. Most recently, the diabetes medication dapagliflozin, an inhibitor of sodium-glucose co-transporter 2 (SGLT2), has demonstrated an improvement in CV mortality and hospitalizations in patients with HFrEF in the randomized controlled Dapagliflozin and Prevention of Adverse Outcomes in Heart Failure (DAPA-HF) trial. This effect was seen in both patients with and without diabetes. The exact mechanism is not fully understood, but may be related to the class' diuretic effect.[49]

For a more complete discussion of the management of acute and chronic HFrEF, see Chapters 68 and 75.

RECOVERY

With modern pharmacologic and device therapies, the overall prognosis of HFrEF has improved over the past two decades. There remains debate over whether the LV can recover, or whether reverse remodeling only represents partial normalization of myocardial maladaptation. Variably defined LV recovery has been accepted to mean normalization of LVEF to more than 50%, with additional normalization of the molecular, cellular, and gross structural changes of the heart; this is in distinction to a reversely remodeled LV where there is a shift in the LV end-diastolic pressure-volume relationship to normal, an absolute increase in LVEF of 10% to over 35%, and a decrease in LV end-diastolic dimension (LVEDD) of 10%. Guideline-directed medical therapies' inhibition of the RAAS and SNS allows for reversal of the maladaptive LV remodeling over time. Among patient receiving guideline-directed medical therapy, approximately 40% will demonstrate an improvement in LVEF and reduction in chamber dilation.[50] The likelihood of LVEF recovery and reversal of LV remodeling correlates closely with medical therapy dosages. Reverse remodeling has been seen in dilated cardiomyopathy in particular and is associated with a shorter duration of cardiac dysfunction, less fibrosis, and less total cardiac injury. CMR imaging may help identify those patients who are most likely to have recovery of some function **(Table 69.6)**. Patients who have any degree of LV recovery have a 49% reduction in mortality and improvements in quality-of-life metrics. Recent data suggest that even patients with a LVEF recovery to more than 50% have improved outcomes if they remain on guideline-directed medical therapy indefinitely.[51]

RESEARCH AND FUTURE DIRECTIONS

Despite modern therapies, recovery of scarred, nonviable myocardium remains an elusive goal and major area of cardiac research. After a cardiac injury occurs, resulting in the replacement of a large region of myocytes with fibrosis, the myocardium lacks the ability to restore a significant number of newly generated myocytes and, therefore, contractile function to the region. An ongoing focus of research is inducing the production of new myocytes in this patient population. The randomized controlled Myoblast Autologous Grafting in Ischemic Cardiomyopathy (MAGIC) trial evaluated an early approach to this by implanting autologous skeletal muscle myoblasts surgically into postinfarction scars. Unfortunately, this approach failed to demonstrate any clinical benefit, and patients had an increased risk of arrhythmic complications.[52] Many strategies have evaluated converting cardiac fibroblasts into induced cardiomyocyte cells, and although a number of techniques have been demonstrated to be effective in vitro, there remains significant challenges to achieving fully functioning induced cardiomyocytes in vivo.[53] The first clinical trial to evaluate implanting sheets of induced cardiomyocytes into myocardial scar is currently underway in Japan, led by Osaka University. Despite the challenges, cardiac myocyte regeneration in HF remains an active area of research.

TABLE 69.6 Predictors for Left Ventricular Recovery

Etiologies	Clinical Factors
Stress induced	Hypertension
Hyperthyroidism	Non-African American race
Tachycardia-induced	Less fibrosis
Chemotherapy related	Lower NYHA class
Alcohol	
Viral myocarditis	
Peripartum	
Recent-onset DCM	

DCM, dilated cardiomyopathy; NYHA, New York Heart Association.

KEY POINTS

- ✔ HFrEF has been defined by the American College of Cardiology (ACC)/American Heart Association (AHA) 2013 Heart Failure Guidelines as clinical HF with an LVEF less than or equal to 40%.
- ✔ The primary mechanism of the clinical syndrome of HFrEF is reduction in the pumping efficiency of the myocardium with failure to deliver sufficient oxygen to meet the metabolic needs of the body and/or elevated filling pressures.
- ✔ All patients with suspected HF should be evaluated with a transthoracic echocardiogram (TTE).
- ✔ When noninvasive assessments of cardiac function, volume status, or hemodynamics are inadequate or limited, a right heart catheterization can be used to directly measure intracardiac pressures and cardiac output.
- ✔ Current therapeutic targets for mortality-reducing therapies for HFrEF include inhibition of maladaptive neurohormonal axes, reduction of ventricular wall stress, and, more recently, promotion of intrinsic cardioprotective counterregulatory axes.

REFERENCES

1. Yancy CW, Jessup M, Bozkurt B, et al. 2013 ACCF/AHA guideline for the management of heart failure: a report of the American College of Cardiology Foundation/American Heart Association Task Force on practice guidelines. *Circulation.* 2013;128(16):e240-e327. doi:10.1161/CIR.0b013e31829e8776
2. Vasan RS, Benjamin EJ, Levy D. Prevalence, clinical features and prognosis of diastolic heart failure: an epidemiologic perspective. *J Am Coll Cardiol.* 1995;26(7):1565-1574. doi:10.1016/0735-1097(95)00381-9
3. Benjamin EJ, Muntner P, Alonso A, et al. Heart disease and stroke statistics-2019 update: a report from the American Heart Association. *Circulation.* 2019;139:e56-e528. doi:10.1161/CIR.0000000000000659

4. McMurray JJ, Petrie MC, Murdoch DR, Davie AP. Clinical epidemiology of heart failure: public and private health burden. *Eur. Heart J.* 1998;19(suppl P):P9-P16.
5. Owan TE, Redfield MM. Epidemiology of diastolic heart failure. *Prog Cardiovasc Dis.* 2005;47(5):320-332. doi:10.1016/j.pcad.2005.02.010
6. Lloyd-Jones DM, Larson MG, Leip EP, et al. Lifetime risk for developing congestive heart failure: the Framingham Heart Study. *Circulation.* 2002;106(24):3068-3072. doi:10.1161/01.CIR.0000039105.49749.6F
7. Pandey A, Omar W, Ayers C, et al. Sex and race differences in lifetime risk of heart failure with preserved ejection fraction and heart failure with reduced ejection fraction. *Circulation.* 2018;137(17):1814-1823. doi:10.1161/CIRCULATIONAHA.117.031622
8. Brouwers FP, de Boer RA, van der Harst P, et al. Incidence and epidemiology of new onset heart failure with preserved vs. reduced ejection fraction in a community-based cohort: 11-year follow-up of PREVEND. *Eur Heart J.* 2013;34(19):1424-1431. doi:10.1093/eurheartj/eht066
9. Go AS, Mozaffarian D, Roger VL, et al. Heart disease and stroke statistics-2013 update: a report from the American Heart Association. *Circulation.* 2013;127(1):e6-e245. doi:10.1161/CIR.0b013e31828124ad
10. Blecker S, Paul M, Taksler G, Ogedegbe G, Katz S. Heart failure-associated hospitalizations in the United States. *J Am Coll Cardiol.* 2013;61(12):1259-1267. doi:10.1016/j.jacc.2012.12.038
11. Berry C, Doughty RN, Granger C, et al. The survival of patients with heart failure with preserved or reduced left ventricular ejection fraction: an individual patient data meta-analysis: Meta-analysis Global Group in Chronic Heart Failure (MAGGIC*). Eur Heart J.* 2012;33(14):1750-1757. doi:10.1093/eurheartj/ehr254
12. Levy D, Kenchaiah S, Larson MG, et al. Long-term trends in the incidence of and survival with heart failure. *N Engl J Med.* 2002;347(18):1397-1402. doi:10.1056/NEJMoa020265
13. Jhund PS, Macintyre K, Simpson CR, et al. Long-term trends in first hospitalization for heart failure and subsequent survival between 1986 and 2003. A population study of 5.1 million people. *Circulation.* 2009;119(4):515-523. doi:10.1161/CIRCULATIONAHA.108.812172
14. Lesyuk W, Kriza C, Kolominsky-Rabas P. Cost-of-illness studies in heart failure: a systematic review 2004-2016. *BMC Cardiovasc Disord.* 2018;18(1):74. doi:10.1186/s12872-018-0815-3
15. Heidenreich PA, Albert NM, Allen LA, et al. Forecasting the impact of heart failure in the United States a policy statement from the American Heart Association. *Circ Heart Fail.* 2013;6(3):606-619. doi:10.1161/HHF.0b013e318291329a
16. Baldasseroni S, Opasich C, Gorini M, et al. Left bundle-branch block is associated with increased 1-year sudden and total mortality rate in 5517 outpatients with congestive heart failure: a report from the Italian Network on Congestive Heart Failure. *Am Heart J.* 2002;143(3):398-405. doi:10.1067/mhj.2002.121264
17. Givertz MM, Mann DL. Epidemiology and natural history of recovery of left ventricular function in recent onset dilated cardiomyopathies. *Curr Heart Fail Rep.* 2013;10(4):321-330. doi:10.1007/s11897-013-0157-5
18. Japp AG, Gulati A, Cook SA, Cowie MR, Prasad SK. The diagnosis and evaluation of dilated cardiomyopathy. *J Am Coll Cardiol.* 2016;67(25):2996-3010. doi:10.1016/j.jacc.2016.03.590
19. McNally EM, Mestroni L. Dilated cardiomyopathy: genetic determinants and mechanisms. *Circ Res.* 2017;121:731-748. doi:10.1161/CIRCRESAHA.116.309396
20. Ziaeian B, Fonarow GC. Epidemiology and aetiology of heart failure. *Nat Rev Cardiol.* 2016;13(6):368-378. doi:10.1038/nrcardio.2016.25
21. Francis GS, Goldsmith SR, Levine TB, Olivari MT, Cohn JN. The neurohumoral axis in congestive heart failure. *Ann Intern Med.* 1984;101(3):370-377. doi:10.7326/0003-4819-101-3-370
22. Hartupee J, Mann DL. Neurohormonal activation in heart failure with reduced ejection fraction. *Nat Rev Cardiol.* 2017;14(1):30-38. doi:10.1038/nrcardio.2016.163
23. St. John Sutton MG, Sharpe N. Left ventricular remodeling after myocardial infarction: pathophysiology and therapy. *Circulation.* 2000;101:2981-2988. doi:10.1161/01.cir.101.25.2981
24. Konstam MA, Kramer DG, Patel AR, Maron MS, Udelson JE. Left ventricular remodeling in heart failure: current concepts in clinical significance and assessment. *JACC Cardiovasc Imaging.* 2011;4(1):98-108. doi:10.1016/j.jcmg.2010.10.008
25. Chow SL, Maisel AS, Anand I, et al. Role of biomarkers for the prevention, assessment, and management of heart failure: a scientific statement from the American Heart Association. *Circulation.* 2017;135(22):e1054-e1091. doi:10.1161/CIR.0000000000000490
26. Nishikimi T, Maeda N, Matsuoka H. The role of natriuretic peptides in cardioprotection. *Cardiovasc Res.* 2005;69(2):318-328. doi:10.1016/j.cardiores.2005.10.001
27. Yancy CW, Jessup M, Bozkurt B, et al. 2016 ACC/AHA/HFSA focused update on new pharmacological therapy for heart failure: an update of the 2013 ACCF/AHA guideline for the management of heart failure. *J Am Coll Cardiol* 2016; doi:10.1016/j.jacc.2016.05.011
28. McMurray JJV, Solomon SD, Inzucchi SE, et al. Dapagliflozin in patients with heart failure and reduced ejection fraction. *N Engl J Med.* 2019;381(21):1995-2008. doi:10.1056/NEJMoa1911303
29. Bloom MW, Greenberg B, Jaarsma T, et al. Heart failure with reduced ejection fraction. *Nat Rev Dis Primers.* 2017;3:17058. doi:10.1038/nrdp.2017.58
30. Yancy CW, Jessup M, Bozkurt B, et al. 2017 ACC/AHA/HFSA focused update of the 2013 ACCF/AHA guideline for the management of heart failure. *J Am Coll Cardiol.* 2017;70(6):776-803. doi:10.1016/j.jacc.2017.04.025
31. De Lemos JA, McGuire DK, Drazner MH. B-type natriuretic peptide in cardiovascular disease. *Lancet.* 2003;362(9380):316-322. doi:10.1016/S0140-6736(03)13976-1
32. Zile MR, Claggett BL, Prescott MF, et al. Prognostic implications of changes in N-terminal pro-B-type natriuretic peptide in patients with heart failure. *J Am Coll Cardiol.* 2016;68(22):2425-2436. doi:10.1016/j.jacc.2016.09.931
33. Kociol RD, Pang PS, Gheorghiade M, et al. Troponin elevation in heart failure. *J Am Coll Cardiol* 2010;56(14):1071-1078. doi:10.1016/j.jacc.2010.06.016
34. Peacock 4th WF, Marco TD, Fonarow GC, et al. Cardiac troponin and outcome in acute heart failure. *N Engl J Med.* 2008;358(20):2117-2126. doi:10.1056/NEJMoa0706824
35. Ciccone MM, Cortese F, Gesualdo M, et al. A novel cardiac bio-marker: ST2: a review. *Molecules.* 2013;18(12):15314-15328. doi:10.3390/molecules181215314
36. Wettersten N, Maisel AS. Biomarker developments in heart failure: 2016 and beyond. *Curr Opin Cardiol.* 2019;34(2):218-224. doi:10.1097/HCO.0000000000000596
37. Aimo A, Gaggin HK, Barison A, Emdin M, Januzzi JL. Imaging, biomarker, and clinical predictors of cardiac remodeling in heart failure with reduced ejection fraction. *JACC Heart Fail.* 2019;7(9):782-794. doi:10.1016/j.jchf.2019.06.004
38. Ebong I, Mazimba S, Breathett K. Cardiac biomarkers in advanced heart failure: how can they impact our pre-transplant or pre-LVAD decision-making. *Curr Heart Fail Rep.* 2019;16(6):274-284. doi:10.1007/s11897-019-00447-w
39. Tromp J, Westenbrink BD, Ouwerkerk W, et al. Identifying pathophysiological mechanisms in heart failure with reduced versus preserved ejection fraction. *J Am Coll Cardiol.* 2018;72(10):1081-1090. doi:10.1016/j.jacc.2018.06.050
40. Fonseca, C. Diagnosis of heart failure in primary care. *Heart Fail Rev.* 2006;11(2):95-107. doi:10.1007/s10741-006-9481-0
41. Lang RM, Badano LP, Mor-Avi V, et al. Recommendations for cardiac chamber quantification by echocardiography in adults: an update from the American Society of Echocardiography and the European Association of Cardiovascular Imaging. *J Am Soc Echocardiogr* 2015;28(1):1-39.e14. doi:10.1016/j.echo.2014.10.003
42. Dorbala S, Ando Y, Bokhari S, et al. ASNC/AHA/ASE/EANM/HFSA/ISA/SCMR/SNMMI expert consensus recommendations for multimodality imaging in cardiac amyloidosis: part 1 of 2—evidence base and standardized methods of imaging. *J Card Fail* 2019;25(11):e1-e39. doi:10.1016/j.cardfail.2019.08.001
43. Fontana M, Pica S, Reant P, et al. Prognostic value of late gadolinium enhancement cardiovascular magnetic resonance in cardiac amyloidosis. *Circulation.* 2015;132(16):1570-1579. doi:10.1161/CIRCULATIONAHA.115.016567

44. Divakaran S, Stewart GC, Lakdawala NK, et al. Diagnostic accuracy of advanced imaging in cardiac sarcoidosis. *Circ Cardiovasc Imaging.* 2019;12(6):e008975. doi:10.1161/CIRCIMAGING.118.008975
45. Kubanek M, Sramko M, Maluskova J, et al. Novel predictors of left ventricular reverse remodeling in individuals with recent-onset dilated cardiomyopathy. *J Am Coll Cardiol* 2013;61(1):54-63. doi:10.1016/j.jacc.2012.07.072
46. Arnold JR, McCann GP. Cardiovascular magnetic resonance: applications and practical considerations for the general cardiologist. *Heart.* 2020; 106(3):174-181. doi:10.1136/heartjnl-2019-314856
47. Patel AR, Kramer CM. Role of cardiac magnetic resonance in the diagnosis and prognosis of nonischemic cardiomyopathy. *JACC Cardiovasc Imaging.* 2017;10(10 Pt A):1180-1193. doi:10.1016/j.jcmg.2017.08.005
48. Saeed M, Van TA, Krug R, Hetts SW, Wilson MW. Cardiac MR imaging: current status and future direction. *Cardiovasc Diagn Ther.* 2015; 5(4):290-310. doi:10.3978/j.issn.2223-3652.2015.06.07
49. Givertz MM, Stevenson LW, Costanzo MR, et al. Pulmonary artery pressure-guided management of patients with heart failure and reduced ejection fraction. *J Am Coll Cardiol.* 2017;70(15):1875-1886. doi:10.1016/j.jacc.2017.08.010
50. Yancy CW, Jessup M, Bozkurt B, et al. 2016 ACC/AHA/HFSA focused update on new pharmacological therapy for heart failure: an update of the 2013 ACCF/AHA guideline for the management of heart failure. *J Am Coll Cardiol* 2016; doi:10.1016/j.jacc.2016.05.011
51. McMurray JJV, Solomon SD, Inzucchi SE, et al. Dapagliflozin in patients with heart failure and reduced ejection fraction. *N Engl J Med.* 2019;381(21):1995-2008. doi:10.1056/NEJMoa1911303
52. Merlo M, Pyxaras SA, Pinamonti B, Barbati G, Lenarda AD, Sinagra G. Prevalence and prognostic significance of left ventricular reverse remodeling in dilated cardiomyopathy receiving tailored medical treatment. *J Am Coll Cardiol.* 2011;57(13):1468-1476. doi:10.1016/j.jacc.2010.11.030
53. Halliday BP, Wassall R, Lota AS, et al. Withdrawal of pharmacological treatment for heart failure in patients with recovered dilated cardiomyopathy (TRED-HF): an open-label, pilot, randomised trial. *Lancet.* 2019;393(10166):61-73. doi:10.1016/S0140-6736(18)32484-X
54. Menasché P, Alfieri O, Janssens S, et al. The myoblast autologous grafting in ischemic cardiomyopathy (MAGIC) trial: first randomized placebo-controlled study of myoblast transplantation. *Circulation.* 2008;117(9): 1189-1200. doi:10.1161/CIRCULATIONAHA.107.734103
55. Talman V, Ruskoaho H. Cardiac fibrosis in myocardial infarction—from repair and remodeling to regeneration. *Cell Tissue Res.* 2016;365(3):563-581. doi:10.1007/s00441-016-2431-9

CHAPTER 70

DILATED CARDIOMYOPATHY

Reema Hasan, Taylor Alexander Lebeis, Supriya Shore, and Monica Mechele Colvin

INTRODUCTION

Cardiomyopathy is a disease of the heart muscle, which can include dilatation and impaired contraction of one or both ventricles as well as infiltrative diseases of the myocardium. Due to the dilatation and hypertrophy that develops after myocardial injury, patients may develop impaired systolic function, resulting in dilated cardiomyopathy (DCM).[1] DCM has many causes and all of them affect ventricular function to a varying degree. While most patients with DCM have symptoms, some may be asymptomatic because of compensatory mechanisms. Continued enlargement of the ventricles leads to a decline in ventricular function followed by conduction system abnormalities, ventricular arrhythmias, thromboembolism, and heart failure.

The earlier patients are identified and treated, the better the prognosis.

Without medical therapy, DCM is progressive, leading to heart failure and death. Once end-stage heart failure develops, survival rates are poor without heart transplants. In this chapter, we discuss the various etiologies of DCM, its pathogenesis, diagnosis, and management.

Definition and Classifications

The classification of DCM has evolved over time with advances in genetics and disease recognition. Currently, DCM refers to a spectrum of heterogeneous myocardial disorders that are characterized by ventricular dilation and depressed myocardial performance in the absence of hypertension, valvular, congenital, or ischemic heart disease. In clinical practice, the etiology of heart failure (HF) has been categorized as ischemic or nonischemic cardiomyopathy, with the latter interchangeably used with DCM. However, this fails to recognize that nonischemic cardiomyopathy can include cardiomyopathies caused by volume or pressure overload (such as hypertension or valvular heart disease) that are not conventionally accepted under the definition of DCM.

Classification schemes, such as the one proposed by the American Heart Association (AHA), divide cardiomyopathies into two major groups based on predominant organ involvement: primary cardiomyopathies (ie, genetic, nongenetic, and acquired) are those solely or predominantly confined to heart muscle, whereas secondary cardiomyopathies have myocardial involvement as part of a generalized systemic (multiorgan) disorder (ie, amyloidosis, hemochromatosis, sarcoidosis, autoimmune/collagen vascular diseases, toxins, cancer therapy, and endocrine disorders such as diabetes mellitus).

The European Society of Cardiology (ESC) Working Group on Myocardial and Pericardial Diseases takes a different approach based on a clinically oriented classification in which heart muscle disorders are grouped into specific morphologic and functional phenotypes, including hypertrophic cardiomyopathies, DCM, arrhythmogenic right ventricular dysplasia, restrictive cardiomyopathies, and unclassified cardiomyopathies. Each phenotype is then subclassified into familial and nonfamilial forms.

Most recently, the MOGE(S) nosology system was developed, which incorporates the morphofunctional phenotype (M), organ(s) involvement (O), genetic inheritance pattern (G), etiologic annotation (E) including genetic defect or underlying disease/substrate, and the functional status (S) of the disease using both the American College of Cardiology (ACC)/AHA HF stages and New York Heart Association (NYHA) functional class. This nomenclature is endorsed by the World Heart Federation and is supported by an internet-assisted application. It also assists in the description of cardiomyopathy in symptomatic and asymptomatic patients, as well as family members in the context of genetic testing.

Epidemiology

The reported incidence and prevalence of dilated cardiomyopathies worldwide are affected by geographic differences, evolving diagnostic criteria, and socioeconomic factors. In the United States, the age-adjusted prevalence of DCM is reported to be approximately equal to 36 cases per 100,000 population or 1:2500 individuals.[2] Approximately, 30% to 40% of patients diagnosed with DCM have a nonischemic origin.[3] DCM is more commonly seen in men than women. While DCM typically occurs in the third or fourth decade of life, it can be seen in children and the elderly. Age is an independent risk factor for mortality in DCM.

PATHOGENESIS

Enlargement of the left ventricle (LV) or both the right and left ventricles occurs in DCM due to LV failure or a secondary myopathic process that is causing biventricular failure. Reduced systolic function is thought to be due to myocardial remodeling that causes an increase in both end-systolic and end-diastolic volumes (**Figure 70.1**). Dilatation of the ventricles can lead to

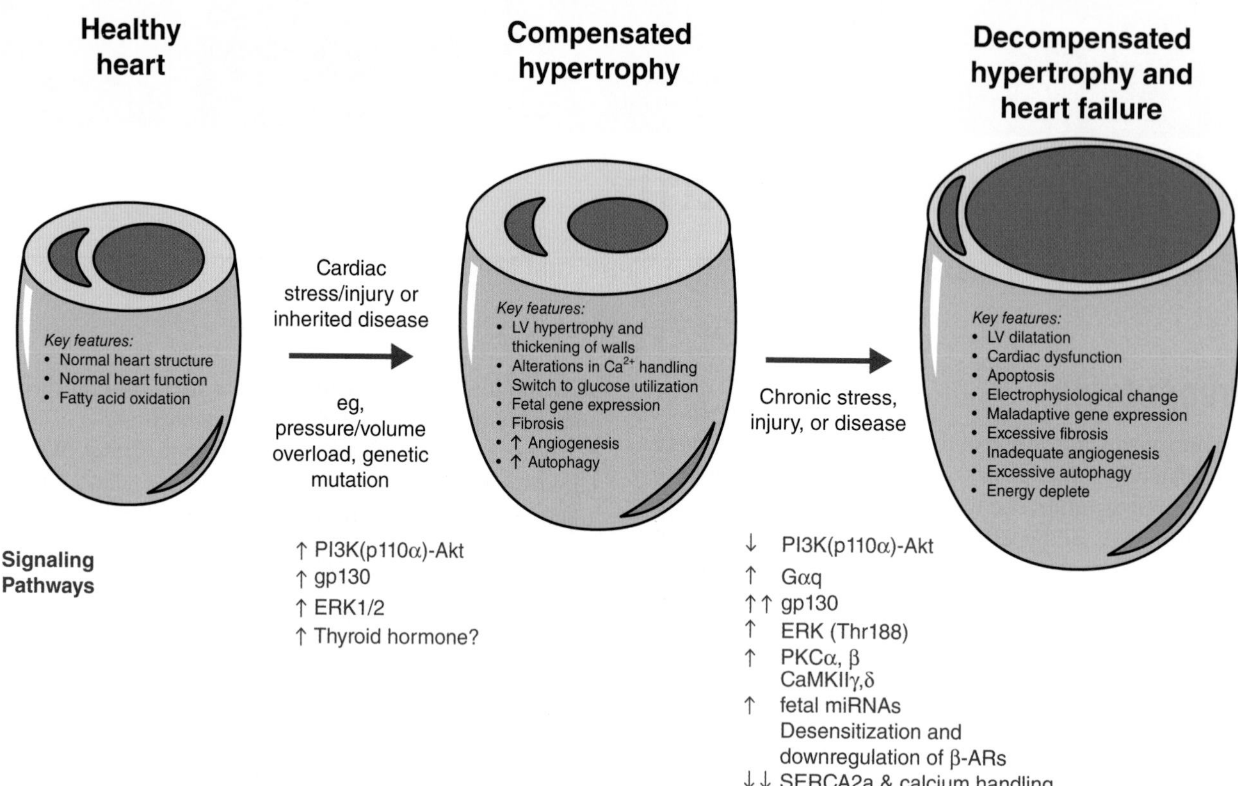

FIGURE 70.1 Pathogenesis of cardiomyopathy. (Reprinted by permission from Springer: Tham YK, Bernardo BC, Ooi JY, et al. Pathophysiology of cardiac hypertrophy and heart failure: signaling pathways and novel therapeutic targets. *Arch Toxicol.* 2015;89(9):1401-1438. Copyright © 2015 Springer Nature.)

tricuspid or mitral insufficiency. Over time, this will lead to a reduced ejection fraction and increased ventricular wall stress. To compensate, heart rate and peripheral vascular tone increase, resulting in additional myocardial injury. Neurohormonal activation of the renin–angiotensin–aldosterone system and an increase in catecholamines are compensatory mechanisms that occur. Natriuretic peptides levels also increase. Ultimately, the compensatory mechanisms become injurious creating myocardial ischemia. Eventually, the heart becomes overwhelmed and fails. Histologic examination of the myocardium typically shows nonspecific changes of fibrosis and hypertrophy, although myocardial injury with an infiltrate of inflammatory cells is also seen.

CLINICAL PRESENTATION AND EVALUATION

History and Physical

DCM can be asymptomatic for many years. If untreated, most patients will develop the syndrome of HF. Symptoms of HF include paroxysmal nocturnal dyspnea, orthopnea, leg swelling, and shortness of breath with exertion or at rest. Nonspecific symptoms include fatigue, malaise, and weakness. More advanced cases can include thromboembolic complications, conduction disturbances, arrhythmias, or sudden cardiac death. Since symptoms can be nonspecific, it is not uncommon for the diagnosis to be missed or confused with asthma.

Physical exam findings include crackles in the lungs, elevated jugular venous pressures, peripheral edema, and a S3 gallop. The point of maximum impulse, or PMI, may be displaced laterally. Tricuspid or mitral regurgitation murmurs can be present because of ventricular enlargement and annular dilation. Neck examination can reveal jugular venous distention, large V-waves, brisk Y descent, and a positive hepatojugular reflux. The murmur of mitral regurgitation may not be holosystolic, and the usual inspiratory increase in the murmur of tricuspid regurgitation (Carvallo's sign) is frequently absent.

The initial diagnostic approach should exclude all potentially reversible causes of LV dysfunction (**Algorithm 70.1**). Laboratory testing should include thyroid function tests, HIV serology, electrolytes, hemoglobin A1c, hematocrit, and iron studies. Urine toxicology screen and alcohol level can be checked when substance abuse is suspected. Excess alcohol consumption has been reported in up to 40% of patients with idiopathic DCM. A history of alcohol consumption is important since abstinence may result in a dramatic increase in ejection fraction. A recent viral illness, particularly one accompanied by myalgias or pericarditis, may suggest a role for myocarditis. Ischemic heart disease should be considered whenever coronary risk factors or chest pain on exertion is present. If a complete family history suggests a familial cardiomyopathy, echocardiography may need to be performed in close relatives to rule out asymptomatic abnormalities.

Hypothyroidism, hyperthyroidism, and anemia should be excluded before diagnosing DCM. A chest x-ray may show cardiomegaly and evidence of pulmonary effusions and venous

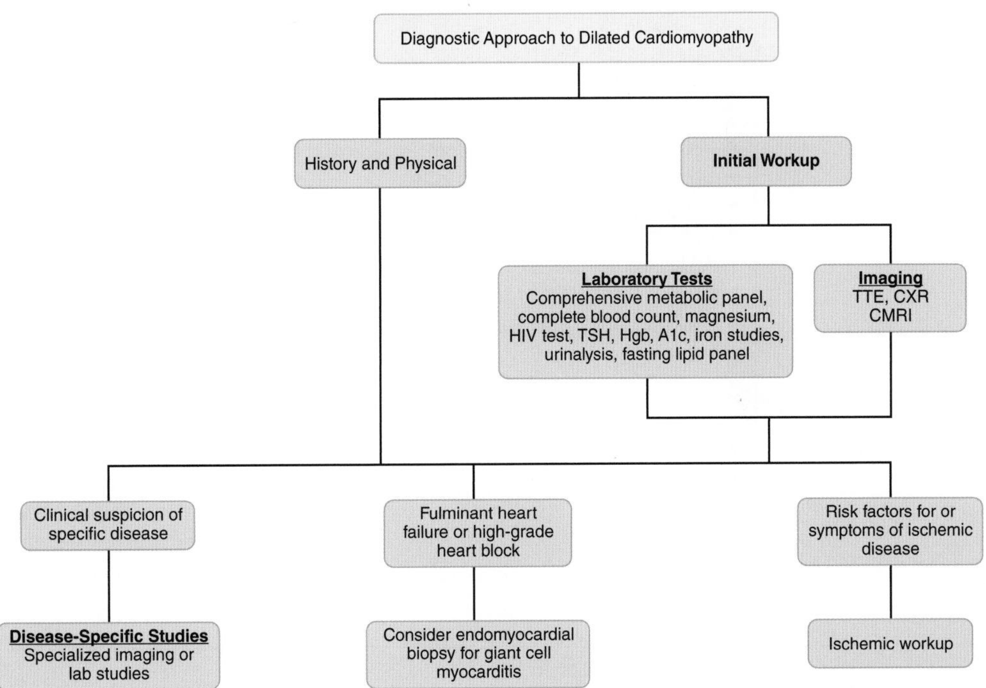

ALGORITHM 70.1 Diagnostic approach to dilated cardiomyopathy. CMRI, cardiac magnetic resonance imaging; CXR, chest radiograph; Hgb, hemoglobin; HIV, human immunodeficiency virus; TSH, thyroid-stimulating hormone; TTE, transthoracic echocardiogram. (Data from Yancy CW, Jessup M, Bozkurt B, et al. 2017 ACC/AHA/HFSA focused update of the 2013 ACCF/AHA Guideline for the management of heart failure: A Report of the American College of Cardiology/American Heart Association Task Force on Clinical Practice Guidelines and the Heart Failure Society of America. *J Am Coll Cardiol.* 2017;70(6):776-803.)

congestion. Electrocardiogram (ECG) may show nonspecific ST-segment and T-wave abnormalities or even atrial fibrillation. Oxygen consumption of less than 14 mL/kg/min on a metabolic stress test indicates a poor prognosis.

DIAGNOSIS

Dilated cardiomyopathy describes a heterogeneous collection of disorders causing myocardial dysfunction without significant valvular, ischemic, congenital, or hypertensive disease.[1] The general diagnostic workup for dilated cardiomyopathy is described in this section; refer to **Algorithm 70.1** regarding the approach. The initial evaluation of dilated cardiomyopathy begins with a thorough clinical history and physical examination. Special attention needs to be made for clinical risk factors and comorbid conditions that predispose the patient for HF and warrant additional investigation. Additionally, a detailed family history of HF, heart disease, sudden cardiac death, exercise intolerance, or other unexplained dyspnea needs to be obtained.

After completing the general clinical examination, an ischemic evaluation should be performed to determine whether coronary artery disease is the cause of the reduced ejection fraction. Not all patients require an ischemic evaluation. Generally, those under the age of 35 years do not require an ischemic evaluation unless risk factors for such exist or there is a high clinical suspicion.[9] For those who warrant an investigation, the type of ischemic evaluation is dependent upon the patient characteristics and risk factors. Common methods of evaluating for ischemia include left heart catheterization, coronary computed tomography angiography, or stress testing (nuclear medicine, cardiac magnetic resonance imaging [CMRI], or echocardiography). After establishing that the origin of the patient's cardiomyopathy is nonischemic, it is important to determine whether there is a reversible etiology.

The 2016 AHA Scientific Statement on Current Diagnostic and Treatment Strategies for Specific Dilated Cardiomyopathies describes the general approach to the workup of DCM.[1] The path of evaluation is determined by clinical suspicion of disease states based on the presentation of the specific patient and whether there is high-enough pretest probability to indicate specific testing. A list of disease states and specific testing is found in **Table 70.1**.

Diagnostic Testing

Echocardiography

Transthoracic echocardiography (TTE) is the backbone of the imaging evaluation of cardiomyopathy. It is able to provide information about the structure and function of the heart at a low cost in real time. TTE allows for evaluation of wall motion and has the ability to survey for structural changes that may be the cause of the cardiomyopathy including congenital abnormalities and valvular dysfunction. Contrast echocardiography can help enhance images for estimation of the ejection fraction and identification of LV thrombi. If there is a question about the presence of thrombus, CMRI can be used to more accurately assess.

TABLE 70.1 Imaging Findings and Specialized Testing for Specific Cardiomyopathies

Disease	Specialized Testing	Imaging Findings
Amyloidosis	• SPEP, UPEP, Bence Jones protein • Decreased QRS amplitude on ECG • NM pyrophosphate scan • Definitive diagnosis from biopsy • Abdominal fat pad, gingiva, rectum, bone marrow, heart, liver, or kidney • DNA mutational analysis of biopsied tissue	**TTE** • Thickened ventricular walls, biatrial dilatation, valvular thickening, and pericardial effusion • Restrictive filling pattern • Apical sparing on longitudinal strain bull's eye plot **CMRI** • Global subendocardium LGE **NM Pyrophosphate Scan** • Tracer uptake
Hypertrophic cardiomyopathy	• Genetic Testing • Holter monitor	**TTE** • Dynamic LVOT obstruction secondary to LVH • Systolic anterior motion of the mitral valve • Apical aneurysms can be seen • Reduced strain in the hypertrophied areas **CMRI** • Fibrosis
Infectious (viral, bacterial, fungal, spirochetal, protozoal, rickettsial)	• Targeted serologic testing • Screen for HIV in appropriate clinical setting • *Trypanosoma cruzi* (travel or residence in South and/or Central America)	**TTE** • Dilated LV with depressed LV function
Peripartum cardiomyopathy	• Serial measurement of LVEF • Stress echocardiography to risk stratify • Genetic testing and counseling can be helpful	**TTE** • Dilated LV • LV thrombus commonly present
Cardiac sarcoidosis	• ECG with bundle branch block, new AV block, frequent PVCs, VT, pathologic Q waves, and ST-T changes • Holter monitor to evaluate for heart block and ventricular arrhythmias • EMB can be performed through limited sensitivity	**TTE** • Wall motion abnormalities, abnormal septal thickness, and abnormal LV systolic and diastolic function **CMRI** • Early enhancement of granulomas suggests inflammation and edema on T2-weighted gadolinium images • Late enhancement in T2-weighted gadolinium images suggest fibrosis and scar • Lesions typically present in mid-myocardial basal segments of septal and lateral walls
		Nuclear Medicine • PET imaging with FDG detects active inflammation
Myocarditis	• Troponin level, ESR, CRP, eosinophil count • ECG with widened QRS, PR depression or diffuse ST-segment elevation, low voltage, or new heart block • EMB can be considered in appropriate clinical setting	**TTE** • Dilated LV with abnormal LV systolic function **CMRI** • Increased epicardial or midwall signal intensity on T1-weighted, post-gadolinium contrast sequences in a non-coronary distribution
Tachycardia-mediated cardiomyopathy	• Holter monitor, Zio patch, or implantable cardiac monitor	
Endocrine (Hyperthyroidism/hypothyroidism, acromegaly, Cushing, pheochromocytoma)	• Thyroid function studies, urine metanephrines • Testing for acromegaly or GH deficiency in the appropriate setting	**TTE** • Pericardial effusion in hypothyroidism

Disease	Specialized Testing	Imaging Findings
Autoimmune (PAN, SLE, Scl, RA, dermatomyositis, diabetic cardiotoxins)	• Autoimmune panel • EMB can be performed when hydroxychloroquine-mediated HF is suspected • Cardiac biomarkers	**TTE** • Pericardial effusions with RA **CMRI** • Early after injection enhancement LGE present in a minority of patients with SLE • Patchy fibrosis in Scl
Cardiotoxins (alcohol, amphetamines, cocaine, anthracyclines, trastuzumab, clozapine, chloroquine, carbon monoxide, cobalt, lead, mercury)	• Urine or serum drug screening • Thorough toxin exposure history • History of radiotherapy to the mediastinum • EMB can be considered but is not routinely performed	**TTE** • Globally depressed EF **CMRI** • Significant fibrosis can be seen
Nutritional (Carnitine, thiamine, selenium)	• Trace element nutritional screening	

CMRI, cardiac magnetic resonance imaging; CRP, C-reactive protein; ECG, electrocardiogram; EMB, endomyocardial biopsy; ESR, erythrocyte sedimentation rate; FDG, fluorodeoxyglucose; GH, growth hormone; LGE, late gadolinium enhancement; LV, left ventricular; LVH, left ventricular hypertrophy; LVOT, Left ventricular outflow tract; NM, Nuclear medicine; PAN, polyarteritis nodosa; PET, positron emission tomography; RA, rheumatoid arthritis; Scl, scleroderma; SLE, systemic lupus erythematosus; SPEP, serum protein electrophoresis; TTE, Transthoracic echocardiogram; UPEP, urine protein electrophoresis.

Three-dimensional (3D) echocardiography has been used with increasing frequency due to improved accuracy and reproducibility. As opposed to TTE, 3D echocardiography allows for better spatial resolution between structures, and estimation of both RV and LV ejection fractions is not affected by geometric assumptions, although it is limited by lower temporal resolution, image quality, and less published data.[4]

Speckle tracking echocardiography is another echocardiographic feature that involves tracking the displacement of speckles in the myocardium and represents myocardial deformation (ie, strain). It can be used to detect cardiomyopathy and is independent of the beam angle, which can be limiting in other echocardiographic measurements. Speckle tracking can be used to identify specific patterns consistent with specific disease states. Global longitudinal strain is an independent predictor of all-cause mortality in patients with heart failure due to reduced ejection fraction (HFrEF). The overall assessment of cardiomyopathy by TTE involves the incorporation of all available data to have a complete evaluation.

Cardiac Magnetic Resonance Imaging

CMRI is a useful tool in the evaluation of DCM. CMRI is often more accurate than echocardiography in determining the left and right ventricular volumes and function, especially in those with suboptimal imaging windows. CMRI can further characterize the severity of valvular disease and its contribution to cardiomyopathy. Additionally, CMRI has the ability to evaluate for myocardial inflammation, edema, fibrosis, and ischemia. In T2-weighted images, myocardial edema can be identified in active myocarditis.[3] In ischemic disease, there is often regional subendocardial late gadolinium enhancement (LGE)—which represents expansion of the extracellular space and delayed contrast washout, most commonly due to fibrosis—whereas there are multiple patterns of LGE in patients with DCM (ie, midwall striae or patches, subepicardial, or subendocardial enhancement). Nevertheless, the presence of LGE portends a poor prognosis.[3]

CMRI is particularly helpful in certain cardiomyopathies. In cardiac hemochromatosis, CMRI is able to quantitatively assess iron load in the myocardium with changes in signal time and shorter relaxation time. Global subendocardial LGE is typically seen in cardiac amyloidosis. Lesions in cardiac sarcoidosis typically present in the mid-myocardial basal segments of the septal and lateral walls, and early enhancement of granulomas is suggestive of inflammation and edema. CMRI is limited by the cost, availability, and incompatibility with some implanted cardiac devices.

Cardiac Computed Tomography

Typically used as part of the ischemic evaluation and for congenital disease, cardiac computed tomography (CT) can be used when CMRI cannot be safely performed such as with a ventricular assist device or when the images are otherwise disrupted by the body habitus or cardiac implants. Cardiac CT is noninvasive and has a high sensitivity for coronary artery disease. It is able to accurately measure LV wall thickness, mass, and volume, and can also provide a functional assessment of the heart, but some assessments require administration of a contrast agent and a stable rhythm for ECG gating. Cardiac CT is a reasonable option when there are limitations to echocardiography and CMRI.

Nuclear Medicine Imaging

Nuclear medicine imaging is able to assess the left and right ventricular function and provide additional information about the diagnosis. Multigated radionuclide angiography (MUGA) is a reproducible method of measuring ejection fraction. However, MUGA is limited in its ability to evaluate for structural abnormalities and requires administration of a radioactive agent that over time amounts to a significant radiation dose to the patient.

The diagnosis of some cardiomyopathies can be performed with nuclear medicine studies. Technetium pyrophosphate (^{99m}Tc-PYP) uptake is seen with amyloid infiltration of the myocardium. Further, ^{99m}Tc-3,3-diphosphono-1,2-propanodicarboxylic acid (^{99m}Tc-DPD) has been demonstrated as being useful for differentiating between transthyretin and light-chain amyloidosis.[5] Positron emission tomography imaging with fluorodeoxyglucose (PET-FDG) is considered a standard imaging modality for the diagnosis of cardiac sarcoidosis and helps identify active inflammation around the granulomas. The ability to recognize inflammation helps identify those patients who would derive benefit from immunosuppressive therapy. The monitoring of improvement in the sarcoid inflammation is commonly performed and is helpful in reducing steroid use while maintaining disease control.[6]

Endomyocardial Biopsy

Endomyocardial biopsy (EMB) is the process by which a transvenous bioptome collects cardiac tissue from the right ventricular septum. The LV can also undergo biopsy in situations where it is the primarily affected site, although this carries the additional risk of stroke. Generally, EMB is considered safe. Significant risks include myocardial perforation causing pericardial tamponade, cardiac arrhythmia, bundle branch block, heart block, tricuspid valve injury, arterial injury, and pneumothorax. The complication rate is reported as being between 1% and 6%.[7] Given the risk, EMB should not be performed in the routine workup of HF. EMB should be considered in certain situations where the predicted prognostic and diagnostic value outweighs the risk of the procedure and the anticipated yield of the procedure is reasonable, as some cardiomyopathies are patchy or located in areas not amenable to biopsy. Consideration should also be given to whether EMB results would impact therapy.

The AHA/ACC/ESC guidelines on HF management recommend EMB in unexplained, new-onset fulminant HF that is less than 2 weeks in duration and new-onset HF of 2 weeks to 3 months associated with a dilated LV and new ventricular arrhythmias, second- or third-degree heart block or failure to respond to typical care within a few weeks. EMB should also be considered in the setting of rapidly progressing HF when the cause can only be confirmed by biopsy and there is effective available therapy.[1] There is less support for EMB in HF of a duration greater than 3 months with a new arrhythmia, HF associated with allergic reaction or eosinophilia, anthracycline cardiomyopathy, unexplained restrictive cardiomyopathy, new-onset HF without ventricular arrhythmia or heart block, HF with unexplained hypertrophic cardiomyopathy, and arrhythmogenic right ventricular dysplasia.

Genetic Testing

Familial occurrence comprises 30% to 50% of patients with dilated cardiomyopathy.[8] Often, the genes involved in DCM are those that affect the functional link between the cytoskeleton and sarcomere.[8] Autosomal dominant inheritance is the most common pattern in familial DCM although X-linked, autosomal recessive, and mitochondrial inheritance patterns have also been seen.[8] To identify those who would benefit from genetic screening, it is important to conduct a thorough three-generation family history. First-degree relatives should be screened periodically. If a DCM-causative mutation is detected, then appropriate family members should be screened. Genetic counseling is often helpful when genetic testing is completed.

MANAGEMENT OF DILATED CARDIOMYOPATHY

Medical Management

Guideline-directed medical therapy (GDMT) consisting of neurohormonal blockade forms the cornerstone of managing DCM, and treatment is stratified based on the presence or absence of HF symptoms. In general, neurohormonal blocking agents (angiotensin-converting enzyme inhibitors [ACEIs], angiotensin II receptor blockers [ARBs], angiotensin receptor neprilysin inhibitor [ARNI]), β-blockers (metoprolol succinate, carvedilol, bisoprolol), and mineralocorticoid receptor antagonists (MRA) (eplerenone and spironolactone) are considered standard therapy, depending on the presence and severity of HF symptoms (**Algorithm 70.2**). This section provides a broad overview of the general principles involved in management of dilated cardiomyopathy with specific considerations based on HF etiology detailed later.

Asymptomatic Left Ventricular Systolic Dysfunction

For asymptomatic patients with a LV ejection fraction of less than 40%, guidelines recommend treatment with an ACEI or ARB in cases of intolerance to ACEI, in addition to β-blockers.[9] Randomized trials have consistently demonstrated a mortality benefit and lower rates of hospitalization with ACEI.[10] Data supporting ARBs are weaker, and, hence, ARBs are recommended only in cases with ACEI intolerance. Both ACEIs and ARBs prevent reverse remodeling and cardiac fibrosis mediated by activation of the renin–angiotensin cascade and are potent vasodilators that reduce afterload leading to improved hemodynamics.[10]

Beta-blockers, specifically carvedilol, metoprolol succinate, and bisoprolol, have a morbidity and mortality benefit independent of ACEI/ARB in patients with chronic HF.[10] Similar to angiotensin antagonists, β-blockers also prevent cardiac reverse remodeling by blocking compensatory adrenergic activation. Agents with α-blocking properties like carvedilol reduce afterload as well.

Symptomatic Left Ventricular Systolic Dysfunction

Primary Therapy: For patients with symptomatic DCM, first-line therapy consists of angiotensin antagonists, β-blockers, aldosterone antagonists in selected patients, usually accompanied by diuretics for symptom relief.[9] In patients tolerating ACEI or ARB, replacement with an ARNI is recommended to further lower morbidity and mortality (COR I, LOE B-R).[9]

MRAs (spironolactone or eplerenone) are recommended for patients with NYHA Class II symptoms or worse, serum potassium less than 5 mmol/L, and creatinine clearance greater than 30 mL/min.[9] Furthermore, among African American patients with NYHA Class III to IV symptoms or in patients

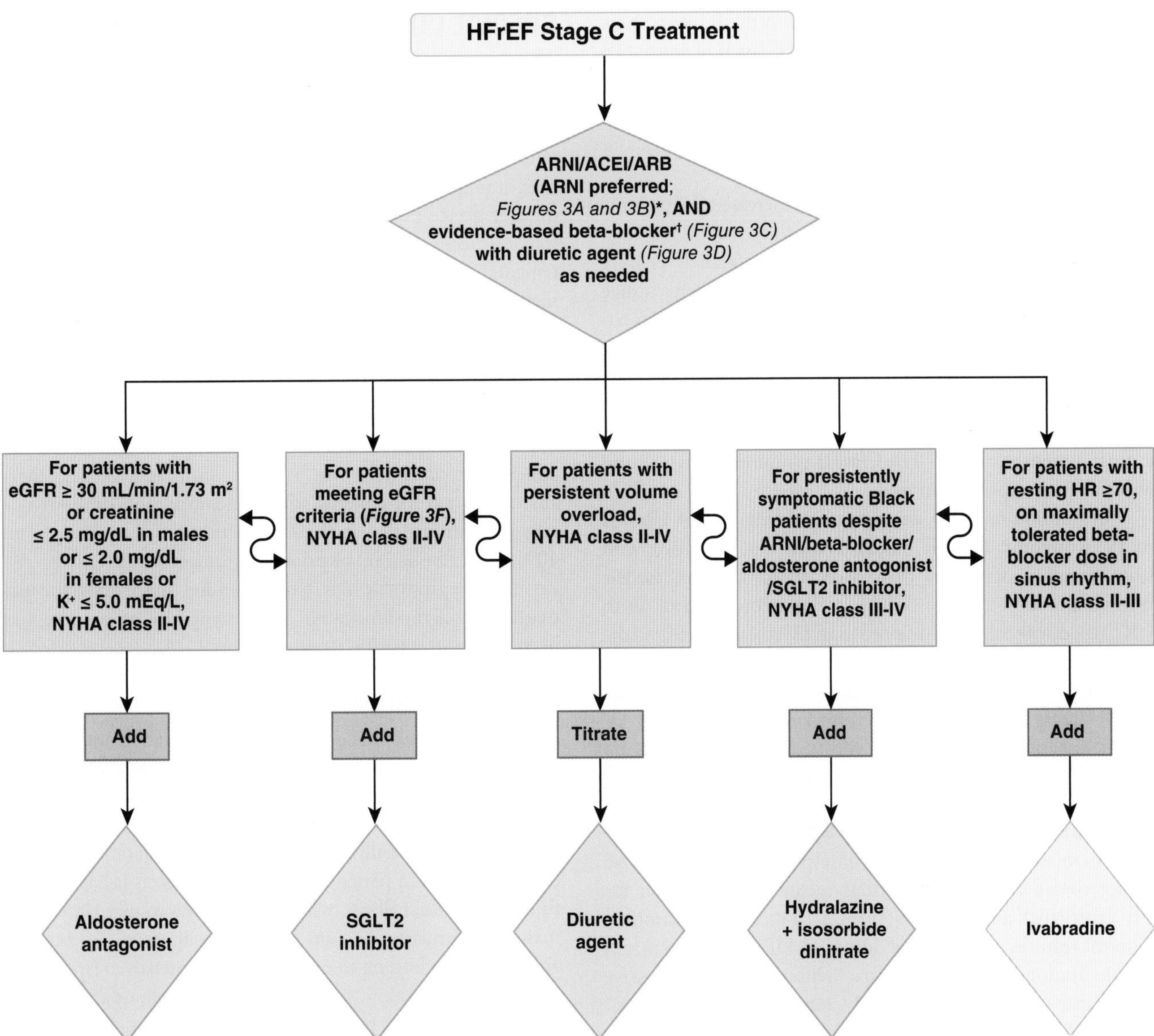

ALGORITHM 70.2 Guideline-Directed Management of Symptomatic Heart Failure. (Reprinted from Maddox TM, Januzzi JL Jr, Allen LA, et al. 2021 Update to the 2017 ACC Expert Consensus Decision Pathway for Optimization of Heart Failure Treatment: Answers to 10 Pivotal Issues About Heart Failure With Reduced Ejection Fraction: A Report of the American College of Cardiology Solution Set Oversight Committee. *J Am Coll Cardiol.* 2021;77(6):772-810. Copyright © 2021 by the American College of Cardiology Foundation. With permission.)

intolerant of angiotensin antagonists, hydralazine, and nitrate in combination is recommended. The benefit of aldosterone antagonists and hydralazine-nitrate is additive to angiotensin antagonists and β-blockers.[10]

Secondary Therapy: Ivabradine is a selective inhibitor of the sinoatrial pacemaker and provides heart rate reduction. It may be considered in patients with NYHA Class II to III symptoms who have a resting heart rate over 70 beats per minute in sinus rhythm, despite being on maximally tolerated dose of β-blockers to reduce HF hospitalizations. Ivabradine did not have a mortality benefit in randomized trials.[11]

Digoxin, a Na^+-K^+ ATPase inhibitor that increases cardiac contractility by increasing intracellular calcium and reduces heart rate by parasympathetic stimulation, may be added in patients with persistent NYHA Class III to IV symptoms despite maximally tolerated GDMT. While randomized trials show that it reduces HF hospitalizations without a mortality benefit, contemporary data from registries suggests a potential harm with digoxin withdrawal.[12] Adverse events from digoxin correlate with serum levels and, hence, the target level to maximize efficacy and minimize adverse events is between 0.5 and 0.8 ng/mL.[13]

Sodium-glucose cotransporter 2 (SGLT-2) inhibitors reduce preload by causing osmotic diuresis and natriuresis in patients with or without diabetes. They may also promote vasodilatation and reduce afterload while improving myocardial energy metabolism. Randomized trials with these agents show improved survival in patients with NYHA Class II or worse HF, with or without diabetes mellitus, and thus may be considered as adjunct therapy.[14]

Device Therapy

The risk of ventricular arrhythmias is increased in patients with nonischemic DCM with an LV ejection fraction less than or equal to 35%. Randomized trials and meta-analyses have consistently showed a reduced incidence of sudden cardiac death with implantable cardioverter defibrillators (ICD) in patients with symptomatic DCM and LVEF less than or equal to 35%.[15] Accordingly, guidelines recommend ICD in all patients with LV ejection fraction less than or equal to 35% secondary to nonischemic DCM despite maximally tolerated GDMT for at least 3 months with NYHA Class II symptoms or worse and at least 1 year expected survival.

In addition to ICDs, among patients with NYHA Class II to IV symptoms and left bundle branch block (LBBB) with QRS duration of greater than or equal to 150 ms, cardiac resynchronization therapy (CRT) is also recommended. With CRT, a pacemaker lead is advanced to an LV epicardial vein via the coronary sinus to facilitate simultaneous pacing of the right and LV, thereby leading to improved cardiac contractile synchronization.[9] Among responders, CRT is associated with improved LV systolic function and remodeling with reduced mitral regurgitation, all leading to improved symptoms and prolonged survival.[16]

Advanced Heart Failure Therapies

For patients with refractory HF, unresponsive to GDMT and device therapy, additional options include consideration for left ventricular assist devices (LVADs) or cardiac transplant. Clinical features suggestive of advanced HF include recurrent hospitalizations, cardiac cachexia, hyponatremia, progressive intolerance to GDMT and NYHA Class IIIb to IV symptoms.[9]

LVADs provide long-term mechanical circulatory support as either a bridge to transplant strategy or as permanent therapy for advanced HF. Survival has improved progressively with newer generation devices. Important factors to consider before device implantation include right ventricular function and renal function. Common complications for these patients receiving these devices include infections, gastrointestinal bleeding, thromboembolic complications including stroke, and right ventricular dysfunction.[17]

Cardiac transplantation improves the quality of life and survival for a well-selected group of patients with refractory end-stage HF. Posttransplant management is comprised of life-long immunosuppression typically with calcineurin inhibitors, cell proliferation inhibitors, mammalian target of rapamycin inhibitors, and steroids. Associated complications include infections and acute rejection (cellular and antibody mediated) in the initial few years. Over the long term, complications include malignancies and chronic allograft vasculopathy associated with progressive narrowing of coronary arteries due to concentric proliferation of endothelial cells.[18] Presently, 1-year survival postcardiac transplant is 90%, and median 10-year survival is 50%.[19]

SPECIAL CONSIDERATIONS

Genetic/Familial Cardiomyopathy

Current guidelines recommend treatment of cardiomyopathy based on phenotype as described earlier. Specific genetic mutations currently do not modify medical therapy for HF. However, among patients with significant arrhythmia or conduction disease, device therapy may be considered before LV ejection fraction declines below 35%. This is particularly true among patients whose risk of ventricular arrhythmias is considerably higher, such as those with arrhythmogenic cardiomyopathy (previously known as arrhythmogenic right ventricular dysplasia), lamin A/C mutations, hypertrophic cardiomyopathy, or SCN5A mutations.[20] Management of thromboembolic complications in patients with noncompaction cardiomyopathy is an important component of therapy. Although the role of routine anticoagulation is unknown, systemic anticoagulation is generally considered for patients with noncompaction cardiomyopathy and left ventricular ejection fraction less than or equal to 40%, atrial fibrillation, or prior thromboembolic events.[21]

Activity restriction is recommended specifically for patients with arrhythmogenic cardiomyopathy as exercise has been shown to expedite its progression.[20]

Cardiac Amyloidosis

The use of standard GDMT is challenging in amyloidosis due to accompanying hypotension. Diuretics and vasodilators should be used carefully due to restrictive cardiac physiology. Similarly, β-blockers should be used cautiously since cardiac output is substantially dependent on heart rate. Digoxin is contraindicated in patients with amyloidosis, as it has high affinity for amyloid fibrils, which predisposes to digoxin cardiotoxicity.[22] Similarly, calcium channel antagonists also bind to amyloid fibrils leading to exaggerated hypotensive response.[23]

Conduction abnormalities frequently accompany amyloidosis, and the need for pacemakers is common. Prognosis of patients with amyloidosis should be carefully considered before offering device therapy. Treatment of the underlying amyloidosis based on subtype should also be considered.

AL Amyloidosis

Two types of amyloid commonly involve the heart: immunoglobulin light chain (AL) and transthyretin (ATTR). AL cardiac disease, when untreated, is associated with poor prognosis and median survival less than 1 year after diagnosis. High-dose chemotherapy with hematopoietic cell transplantation is used to eliminate blood cell dyscrasia. The intensity of chemotherapy depends on the extent of organ involvement. The most common regimen used comprises bortezomib, cyclophosphamide, and dexamethasone.[1] Stem-cell transplantation is contraindicated in the presence of NYHA Class III to IV symptoms.

ATTR Amyloidosis

ATTR may be familial or sporadic, also known as senile. ATTR cardiomyopathy is caused by the deposition of transthyretin amyloid fibrils in the myocardium.[7] Both diflunisal and tafamidis stabilize the transthyretin tetramer and reduce the formation of transthyretin amyloid. In a randomized trial, tafamidis reduced mortality and symptom burden in patients with ATTR cardiomyopathy.[24] Tafamidis is now recommended, and U.S. Food and Drug Administration (FDA) approved for patients with ATTR cardiac disease and NYHA Class I to III symptoms, although the cost may be prohibitive for some patients.

While there are no randomized clinical trials of diflunisal in ATTR cardiac disease, single-center and retrospective studies suggest tolerability. Newer agents such as patisiran, which is an anti-TTR small interfering ribonucleic acid, lower serum natriuretic protein levels and improve LV remodeling.[24] Inotersen is an antisense oligonucleotide, which inhibits the production of hepatic TTR.[24]

Epigallocatechin-3-gallate (EGCG), the main polyphenol in green tea, disrupts ATTR fibrils in mice. Observational studies of EGCG in humans have been provocative, but currently, there are no randomized controlled trials.[25] Doxycycline is currently being investigated.

In individuals with familial ATTR, liver transplantation is curative and should be considered if diagnosed early before the onset of cardiomyopathy.[1] Since cardiac disease may progress after liver transplantation, combined liver, and heart transplant may be indicated for those with cardiac involvement.[26]

Myocarditis

Recommended treatment for myocarditis presenting as DCM is per current guidelines for HF with neurohormonal blockade. Immunosuppression with steroids is recommended in specific scenarios such as sarcoidosis, eosinophilic myocarditis, and giant cell myocarditis. Sustained aerobic exercise during acute viral myocarditis is associated with increased mortality in animal models. Hence, competitive sports should be avoided for 3 to 6 months after diagnosis. Nonsteroidal anti-inflammatory agents should be avoided due to the increased risk for mortality. Management of acute arrhythmias and conduction abnormalities is largely supportive since these resolve with improvement of underlying inflammation.[1]

HIV/Chagas Disease

Treatment for dilated cardiomyopathy secondary to HIV and Chagas is the same as for HF with reduced ejection fraction with the exception of added treatment for HIV and *Trypanosoma cruzi*, respectively. An additional consideration in Chagas cardiomyopathy is antithrombotic therapy for the prevention of systemic and pulmonary thromboembolism. Current Latin American guidelines recommend antithrombotic therapy based on a cardioembolic risk score (1 point each for age > 48 years, primary ST-T wave changes, apical aneurysm, and 2 points for LV systolic dysfunction). For patients with a score of 3 or over, systemic anticoagulation is recommended.[27]

Toxic Cardiomyopathy

Toxic cardiomyopathies arise most commonly from alcohol or cocaine abuse and the use of stimulants. Complete abstinence from the offending agent is recommended. There is limited evidence evaluating the use of GDMT in patients with toxic cardiomyopathy. For cocaine abusers, preferentially combined α- and β-blockers should be considered to oppose α-stimulation from cocaine use. Since alcohol abuse is associated with thiamine and folate deficiency, these should be supplemented.[1]

Chemotherapy-Induced Cardiomyopathy

If a new decline in LV systolic function is noted in patients with preexisting LV systolic dysfunction, the risk of continued therapy should be weighed against benefits, especially in the case of anthracyclines. Standard guideline–directed neurohormonal therapy is recommended for the treatment of HF with reduced ejection fraction in these patients.

Since the cardiotoxic effect of anthracyclines is dose dependent, total cumulative dose of doxorubicin should be restricted to under 450 mg/m^2. For patients needing higher doses, liposomal formulations should be considered. Additionally, infusional regimens have been shown to reduce the risk of cardiotoxicity as opposed to bolus regimens. Dexrazoxane is currently the only FDA-approved drug available for the prevention of anthracycline-mediated cardiomyopathy and is currently approved for use in individuals with metastatic breast cancer receiving over 300 mg/m^2 of doxorubicin.[28]

Most recently, immune checkpoint inhibitors have been noted to cause immune-mediated myocarditis. For patients presenting with signs of HF while on therapy, these agents should be immediately stopped and the use of high-dose corticosteroids be considered. For those with an immediate response to corticosteroids, immunosuppression with mycophenolate mofetil or thymoglobulin should be considered.[29]

Peripartum Cardiomyopathy

Peripartum cardiomyopathy is defined as cardiomyopathy with LV ejection fraction less than 45% presenting during the last month of pregnancy or within the first 5 months postpartum in the absence of other causes of HF and cardiomyopathy. Although the cause is unknown, genetic and inflammatory mechanisms are suspected. Risk factors include age greater than 30 years, African descent, multiparity, and preeclampsia or hypertension. Similar to HF of other etiologies, management is based on neurohormonal blockade and volume management.

Peripartum cardiomyopathy is associated with higher rates of thromboembolism, and the postpartum period is a hypercoagulable state; therefore, anticoagulation is recommended during pregnancy and the first 2 months after delivery. Heparin and unfractionated heparin are recommended during pregnancy.

ACE-inhibitors and ARBs are contraindicated during pregnancy, and hydralazine combined with nitrates is favored. Beta-blockers are considered to be safe during pregnancy, and β-1 selective agents may be preferable during pregnancy as nonselective β-blockers may promote uterine contractions.

Both β-blockers and ACEI/ARBs may be used during breastfeeding. Digoxin may also be safely used during pregnancy, but its role is unclear. In a small, randomized clinical trial, bromocriptine, in addition to standard therapy for HF, was associated with a higher rate of full recovery[30]; however, safety concerns remain, and currently, there is not enough evidence to suggest its use.

The majority of women will experience recovery within 6 months[31]; however, the recurrence rate with subsequent pregnancies is high, especially in those with persistent LV dysfunction before a subsequent pregnancy.[32] In addition, of those who do not have recovery before subsequent pregnancy, 16% died.

Autoimmune Cardiomyopathy

Autoimmune diseases can cause cardiomyopathy via several mechanisms: atherosclerotic disease and ischemic cardiomyopathy, immune-mediated myocarditis, apoptosis, and toxicity related to the treatment of an autoimmune disorder (**Table 70.2**). The most common autoimmune disorder associated with cardiac disease is systemic lupus erythematosus. Twenty-five percent of patients with SLE have cardiac manifestations, and cardiac disease is the third leading cause of death for patients with SLE.[33] Myocarditis is a rare but potentially fatal manifestation of SLE, which may be subclinical in presentation.[34] African American ethnicity is significantly associated with the development of SLE myocarditis.[35] SLE myocarditis is typically treated with high-dose methylprednisolone, followed by oral corticosteroids in combination with immunosuppressive drugs, such as azathioprine, cyclophosphamide, or intravenous immunoglobulin (IVIg).[36] EMB may be useful in excluding infectious myocarditis before administering high-dose immunosuppressants.[37] In addition, EMB may be useful in excluding chloroquine/hydroxychloroquine cardiomyopathy.[38]

Other autoimmune and inflammatory disorders with cardiac manifestations are shown in Table 70.2. Treatment of autoimmune/inflammatory cardiac disease should be targeted at the underlying mechanism. HF and LV dysfunction should be treated according to ACC/AHA guidelines.

Arrhythmia-Associated Cardiomyopathy

Tachycardia-Induced Cardiomyopathy

Tachycardia-induced cardiomyopathy is a potentially reversible cause of cardiomyopathy and is defined as cardiac dysfunction caused by a high or irregular ventricular rate that is completely or partially reversible after the normalization of heart rate. Pure tachycardia-induced cardiomyopathy occurs in a healthy heart, where tachycardia is the only identifiable abnormality whereas impure tachycardia-induced cardiomyopathy causes deterioration of cardiac function in the setting of structural heart.[39]

Management is directed at maintaining sinus rhythm or controlling ventricular rate while using GDMT for HF to prevent adverse remodeling. Involvement of electrophysiology for the management of specific arrhythmias is essential. Secondary causes for tachyarrhythmias should be investigated.

TABLE 70.2 Autoimmune and Inflammatory Causes of and Contributors to Cardiomyopathy

Autoimmune/Inflammatory Disorders Associated With Cardiomyopathy and Heart Failure	Mechanism
Rheumatoid arthritis	Cardiomyopathy, myocardial fibrosis, pulmonary hypertension, valvular disease, myocarditis, arrhythmias, coronary artery disease
Polyarteritis nodosa	Coronary involvement from vasculitis and myocardial infarction
Systemic sclerosis	LV systolic and diastolic dysfunction, myocarditis
Dermatomyositis	LV enlargement, LV diastolic dysfunction, LVH, pulmonary hypertension, valvular disease
Systemic lupus erythematosus	Atherosclerosis, myocarditis
Sarcoid	LV systolic and diastolic dysfunction, arrhythmias
Eosinophilic granulomatosis with polyangiitis (EGPA) (formerly Churg-Strauss)	Endomyocarditis, dilated cardiomyopathy, restrictive cardiomyopathy
Granulomatosis with polyangiitis (GPA) (formerly Wegener granulomatosis)	Cardiomyopathy, pericarditis, valvular lesions, coronary arteritis, arrhythmias
Spondyloarthritis	Valvular disease, myocarditis
Myasthenia gravis (MG)	Myocarditis in thymoma-related MG, giant cell myocarditis, stress-induced cardiomyopathy
Primary Sjögren syndrome	Myocarditis (rare), endocardial fibroelastosis (in children with complete heart block)

LV, left ventricular; LVH, left ventricular hypertrophy.

Left Bundle Branch Block-Associated Cardiomyopathy

While the presence of LBBB is often an indicator of underlying cardiac disease, LBBB has also been associated with the development of cardiomyopathy.[40] The diagnosis of LBBB-associated is established ideally by the presence of LBBB before the development of cardiomyopathy in the absence of other identifiable causes. Documentation of LBBB before the development of LV dysfunction can be challenging.

CRT is associated with improvement in symptoms in patients with HF and LBBB. While GDMT is recommended for 3 months in patients with HF before initiating CRT, patients with LBBB-associated cardiomyopathy appear to have less improvement in ejection fraction with GDMT at 3 months than those with narrow QRS.[41] Greater than one-third of those with HF and LBBB receiving CRT have an improvement in ejection fraction, with most having substantial improvement.[41] A retrospective analysis suggests greater likelihood of improvement in ejection fraction with earlier CRT (≤9 months vs >9 months).[42] Prospective clinical trials of early CRT have not been performed; therefore, the decision to initiate CRT early should be made in conjunction with electrophysiology consultation and on an individual basis. Patients with LV dysfunction and LBBB should also receive GDMT.

Premature Ventricular Contractions

Isolated premature ventricular contractions (PVCs) have been implicated as a cause of DCM and resolution of cardiomyopathy has been reported after elimination of PVCs with ablation therapy.[43,44] Proposed mechanisms include ventricular dyssynchrony and increased myocardial oxygen demand. Similar to LBBB-induced cardiomyopathy, establishing PVCs as causative rather than a result of cardiomyopathy can be challenging. Risk factors for the development of PVC-induced cardiomyopathy include PVC QRS duration greater than or equal to 156 ms, PVC burden greater than or equal to 26%, male sex, and LV site of origin.[45] Twenty-four hour Holter may be inadequate in assessing the frequency of PVCs. PVC burden greater than 24% had a sensitivity and specificity of 79% and 78%.[46] Since RFA may be curative in these patients,[47] frequent PVCs should be evaluated as a cause for cardiomyopathy in consultation with electrophysiology.[48]

Metabolic/Endocrine Causes

Diabetes is independently associated with the risk of HF and can result in both a restrictive and a dilated phenotype, although the mechanisms vary (Figure 70.2). Diagnosis of the restrictive phenotype is based on an LV ejection fraction greater than or equal to 50%, LV end-diastolic volume index (LVEDVI) less than or equal to 97 mL/m^2, diastolic dysfunction in the setting of diabetes, usually Type II, and absence of another identifiable cause. The dilated phenotype is characterized by LV ejection fraction less than 50%, LVEDVI greater than 97 mL/m^2 in the setting of diabetes, typically Type I, and no other identifiable cause. The mainstay of treatment of diabetic restrictive cardiomyopathy phenotype is volume management and diuretics, as well as management of comorbid conditions which can worsen heart symptoms, such as hypertension, sleep apnea, and obesity. Patients with the dilated phenotype should be managed according to HF guidelines.[49]

Obesity is associated with hypertension, diabetes, inactivity, and atherosclerosis, which increase the risk for HF and cardiovascular disease. In addition, obesity is independently associated with cardiomyopathy.[50] Obesity, particularly severe obesity, can predispose to morphologic cardiac changes, right ventricular systolic dysfunction, LV systolic and diastolic dysfunction, and left ventricular hypertrophy.[51] Given the associated risk factors, in the setting of obesity other causes of cardiomyopathy should be investigated. GDMT is recommended, however, efforts should also target weight loss and increasing activity level. Bariatric surgery appears to be associated with improvement in cardiac remodeling.[52] Aggressive weight loss efforts should be considered with input from surgical and medical specialists.

Both hyper- and hypothyroidism can result in structural cardiac changes, and thyroid disease should be excluded as a cause of DCM. Endocrinology consult may help differentiate hypothyroidism as a cause of DCM as opposed to sick euthyroid syndrome.

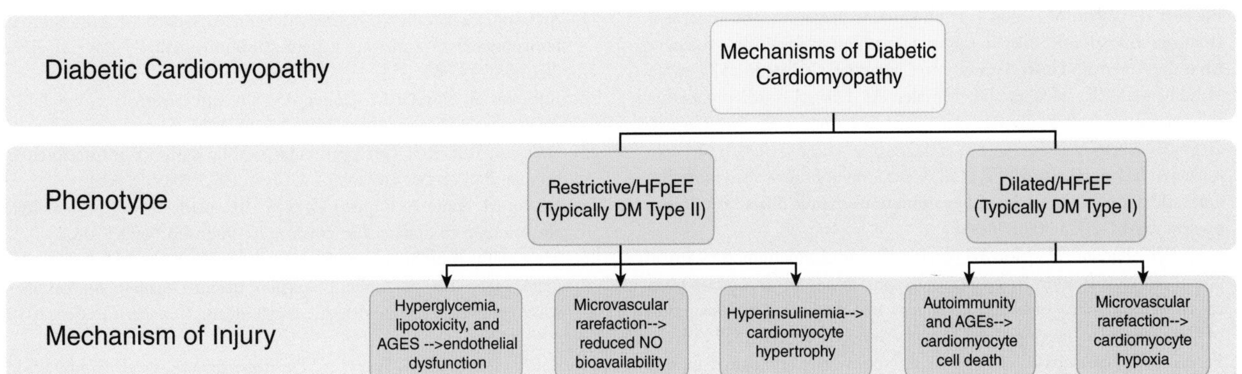

FIGURE 70.2 Diabetes-associated cardiomyopathy and mechanisms of injury. AGEs, advanced glycation end products; DM, diabetes mellitus; NO, nitric oxide.

FOLLOW-UP PATIENT CARE

Patients with DCM require close follow-up to ensure medication compliance, symptom surveillance, medication titration, and laboratory monitoring. For patients with clinical changes, echocardiography should be considered to evaluate for progression of disease. Appropriate preventative measures including immunization against influenza, severe acute respiratory coronavirus 2 (SARS-CoV-2), and pneumococcal disease should be strongly encouraged.

Among patients who recover cardiac function with medical and device therapy, neurohormonal blockade should be continued in the absence of side effects. This is primarily due to risk for recurrence of LV systolic dysfunction even with complete LV recovery if neurohormonal blockade is withdrawn.[9]

KEY POINTS

- ✔ DCM is a common cause of HF with many etiologies. Reversible causes of cardiomyopathy should be excluded.
- ✔ Transthoracic echocardiography is the backbone of imaging in cardiomyopathy; CMRI is useful in determining etiology of HF and may be beneficial in evaluating new cardiomyopathy of unknown etiology.
- ✔ Inherited cardiomyopathy may occur in up to 50% of DCM, and genetic counseling is useful when inherited cardiomyopathy is suspected.
- ✔ The transthyretin mutation is prevalent in African Americans and is associated with ATTR amyloid cardiomyopathy. Tafamidis is recommended for patients with NYHA I-III HF due to ATTR amyloid.
- ✔ Although specific cardiomyopathies may warrant variations in treatment, in general, patients benefit from GDMT; management of heart failure due to DCM should proceed in accordance with the AHA/ACC HF guidelines.

REFERENCES

1. Bozkurt B, Colvin M, Cook J, et al. Current diagnostic and treatment strategies for specific dilated cardiomyopathies: a scientific statement from the American Heart Association. *Circulation.* 2016;134:e579-e646.
2. Hershberger RE, Hedges DJ Morales A. Dilated cardiomyopathy: the complexity of a diverse genetic architecture. *Nat Rev Cardiol.* 2013;10:531-547.
3. Gulati A, Jabbour A, Ismail TF, et al. Association of fibrosis with mortality and sudden cardiac death in patients with nonischemic dilated cardiomyopathy. *JAMA.* 2013;309:896-908.
4. Lang RM, Badano LP, Mor-Avi V, et al. Recommendations for cardiac chamber quantification by echocardiography in adults: an update from the American Society of Echocardiography and the European Association of Cardiovascular Imaging. *J Am Soc Echocardiogr.* 2015;28:1-39.e14.
5. Perugini E, Guidalotti PL, Salvi F, et al. Noninvasive etiologic diagnosis of cardiac amyloidosis using 99mTc-3,3-diphosphono-1,2-propanodicarboxylic acid scintigraphy. *J Am Coll Cardiol.* 2005;46:1076-1084.
6. Ning N, Guo HH, Iagaru A, et al. Serial cardiac FDG-PET for the diagnosis and therapeutic guidance of patients with cardiac sarcoidosis. *J Card Fail.* 2019;25:307-311.
7. Yilmaz A, Kindermann I, Kindermann M, et al. Comparative evaluation of left and right ventricular endomyocardial biopsy: differences in complication rate and diagnostic performance. *Circulation.* 2010;122:900-909.
8. Hershberger RE, Siegfried JD. "Update 2011: clinical and genetic issues in familial dilated cardiomyopathy." *J Am Coll Cardiol.* 2011;57(16):1641-1649.
9. Yancy CW, Jessup M, Bozkurt B, et al. 2017 ACC/AHA/HFSA focused update of the 2013 ACCF/AHA guideline for the management of heart failure: a report of the American College of Cardiology/American Heart Association Task Force on Clinical Practice Guidelines and the Heart Failure Society of America. *Circulation.* 2017;136:e137-e161.
10. Yancy CW, Jessup M, Bozkurt B, et al. 2013 ACCF/AHA guideline for the management of heart failure: executive summary: a report of the American College of Cardiology Foundation/American Heart Association Task Force on practice guidelines. *Circulation.* 2013;128:1810-1852.
11. Swedberg K, Komajda M, Bohm M, et al. Ivabradine and outcomes in chronic heart failure (SHIFT): a randomised placebo-controlled study. *Lancet.* 2010;376:875-885.
12. Malik A, Masson R, Singh S, et al. Digoxin discontinuation and outcomes in patients with heart failure with reduced ejection fraction. *J Am Coll Cardiol.* 2019;74:617-627.
13. Rathore SS, Curtis JP, Wang Y, Bristow MR, Krumholz HM. Association of serum digoxin concentration and outcomes in patients with heart failure. *JAMA.* 2003;289:871-878.
14. McMurray JJV, Solomon SD, Inzucchi SE, et al. Dapagliflozin in patients with heart failure and reduced ejection fraction. *N Engl J Med.* 2019;381:1995-2008.
15. Desai AS, Fang JC, Maisel WH, Baughman KL. Implantable defibrillators for the prevention of mortality in patients with nonischemic cardiomyopathy: a meta-analysis of randomized controlled trials. *JAMA.* 2004;292:2874-2879.
16. McAlister FA, Ezekowitz J, Hooton N, et al. Cardiac resynchronization therapy for patients with left ventricular systolic dysfunction: a systematic review. *JAMA.* 2007;297:2502-2514.
17. Feldman D, Pamboukian SV, Teuteberg JJ, et al. The 2013 International Society for Heart and Lung Transplantation Guidelines for mechanical circulatory support: executive summary. *J Heart Lung Transplant.* 2013;32:157-187.
18. Kittleson MM, Kobashigawa JA. Cardiac transplantation: current outcomes and contemporary controversies. *JACC Heart Fail.* 2017;5:857-868.
19. Khush KK, Cherikh WS, Chambers DC, et al. The International Thoracic Organ Transplant Registry of the International Society for Heart and Lung Transplantation: thirty-fifth adult heart transplantation report-2018; focus theme: multiorgan transplantation. *J Heart Lung Transplant.* 2018;37:1155-1168.
20. Ackerman MJ, Priori SG, Willems S, et al. HRS/EHRA expert consensus statement on the state of genetic testing for the channelopathies and cardiomyopathies this document was developed as a partnership between the Heart Rhythm Society (HRS) and the European Heart Rhythm Association (EHRA). *Heart Rhythm.* 2011;8:1308-1339.
21. Arbustini E, Favalli V, Narula N, Serio A, Grasso M. Left ventricular noncompaction: a distinct genetic cardiomyopathy? *J Am Coll Cardiol.* 2016;68:949-966.
22. Rubinow A, Skinner M, Cohen AS. Digoxin sensitivity in amyloid cardiomyopathy. *Circulation.* 1981;63:1285-1288.
23. Pollak A, Falk RH. Left ventricular systolic dysfunction precipitated by verapamil in cardiac amyloidosis. *Chest.* 1993;104:618-620.
24. Emdin M, Aimo A, Rapezzi C, et al. Treatment of cardiac transthyretin amyloidosis: an update. *Eur Heart J.* 2019;40(45):3699-3706.
25. Mereles D, Buss SJ, Hardt SE, Hunstein W, Katus HA. Effects of the main green tea polyphenol epigallocatechin-3-gallate on cardiac involvement in patients with AL amyloidosis. *Clin Res Cardiol.* 2010;99:483-490.
26. Reich HJ, Awad M, Ruzza A, De Robertis MA, et al. combined heart and liver transplantation: the Cedars-Sinai experience. *Transplant Proc.* 2015;47:2722-2726.
27. Andrade JP, Marin Neto JA, Paola AA, et al. I Latin American guidelines for the diagnosis and treatment of Chagas' heart disease: executive summary. *Arq Bras Cardiol.* 2011;96:434-442.

28. Henriksen PA. Anthracycline cardiotoxicity: an update on mechanisms, monitoring and prevention. *Heart.* 2018;104:971-977.
29. Brahmer JR, Lacchetti C, Thompson JA. Management of immune-related adverse events in patients treated with immune checkpoint inhibitor therapy: American Society of Clinical Oncology clinical practice guideline summary. *J Oncol Pract.* 2018;14:247-249.
30. Hilfiker-Kleiner D, Haghikia A, Berliner D, et al. Bromocriptine for the treatment of peripartum cardiomyopathy: a multicentre randomized study. *Eur Heart J.* 2017;38:2671-2679.
31. McNamara DM, Elkayam U, Alharethi R, et al. Clinical outcomes for peripartum cardiomyopathy in North America: results of the IPAC Study (Investigations of Pregnancy-Associated Cardiomyopathy). *J Am Coll Cardiol.* 2015;66:905-914.
32. Elkayam U. Risk of subsequent pregnancy in women with a history of peripartum cardiomyopathy. *J Am Coll Cardiol.* 2014;64:1629-1636.
33. Szekanecz Z, Shoenfeld Y. Lupus and cardiovascular disease: the facts. *Lupus.* 2006;15:3-10.
34. Jacobsen S, Petersen J, Ullman S, et al. A multicentre study of 513 Danish patients with systemic lupus erythematosus. I. Disease manifestations and analyses of clinical subsets. *Clin Rheumatol.* 1998;17:468-477.
35. Apte M, McGwin Jr G, Vilá L, et al. Associated factors and impact of myocarditis in patients with SLE from LUMINA, a multiethnic US cohort. *Rheumatology.* 2008;47:362-367.
36. Tincani A, Rebaioli C, Taglietti M, Shoenfeld Y. Heart involvement in systemic lupus erythematosus, anti-phospholipid syndrome and neonatal lupus. *Rheumatology.* 2006;45:iv8-iv13.
37. Caforio AL, Pankuweit S, Arbustini E, et al. Current state of knowledge on aetiology, diagnosis, management, and therapy of myocarditis: a position statement of the European Society of Cardiology Working Group on Myocardial and Pericardial Diseases. *Eur Heart J.* 2013;34:2636-2648.
38. Jain D, Halushka MK. Cardiac pathology of systemic lupus erythematosus. *J Clin Pathol.* 2009;62:584-592.
39. Fenelon G, Wijns W, Andries E, Brugada P. Tachycardiomyopathy: mechanisms and clinical implications. *Pacing Clin Electrophysiol.* 1996 ;19:95-106.
40. Barot HV, Sharma S, Schwartzman A, Patten R. Incidence of left bundle branch block—associated cardiomyopathy. *J Card Fail.* 2017;23:S55.
41. Wang NC, Singh M, Adelstein EC, et al. New-onset left bundle branch block-associated idiopathic nonischemic cardiomyopathy and left ventricular ejection fraction response to guideline-directed therapies: the NEOLITH study. *Heart Rhythm.* 2016;13:933-942.
42. Wang NC, Li JZ, Adelstein EC, et al. New-onset left bundle branch block-associated idiopathic nonischemic cardiomyopathy and time from diagnosis to cardiac resynchronization therapy: the NEOLITH II study. *Pacing Clin Electrophysiol.* 2018;41:143-154.
43. Chugh SS, Shen WK, Luria DM, Smith HC. First evidence of premature ventricular complex-induced cardiomyopathy: a potentially reversible cause of heart failure. *J Cardiovasc Electrophysiol.* 2000;11:328-329.
44. Huizar JF, Ellenbogen KA, Tan AY, Kaszala K. Arrhythmia-induced cardiomyopathy: JACC state-of-the-art review. *J Am Coll Cardiol.* 2019;73 :2328-2344.
45. Park K-M, Im SI, Park S-J, Kim JS, On YK. Risk factor algorithm used to predict frequent premature ventricular contraction-induced cardiomyopathy. *Int J Cardiol.* 2017;233:37-42.
46. Baman TS, Lange DC, Ilg KJ, et al. Relationship between burden of premature ventricular complexes and left ventricular function. *Heart Rhythm.* 2010;7:865-869.
47. El Kadri M, Yokokawa M, Labounty T, et al. Effect of ablation of frequent premature ventricular complexes on left ventricular function in patients with nonischemic cardiomyopathy. *Heart Rhythm.* 2015;12:706-713.
48. Cha Y-M, Lee GK, Klarich KW, Grogan M. Premature ventricular contraction-induced cardiomyopathy: a treatable condition. *Circ Arrhythm Electrophysiol.* 2012;5:229-236.
49. Seferović PM, Paulus WJ. Clinical diabetic cardiomyopathy: a two-faced disease with restrictive and dilated phenotypes. *Eur Heart J.* 2015;36:1718-1727.
50. Kenchaiah S, Sesso HD, Gaziano JM. Body-mass index and vigorous physical activity and the risk of heart failure among men. *Circulation.* 2009;119:44-52.
51. Alpert MA, Agrawal H, Aggarwal K, Kumar SA, Kumar A. Heart failure and obesity in adults: pathophysiology, clinical manifestations and management. *Curr Heart Fail Rep.* 2014;11:156-165.
52. Owan T, Avelar E, Morley K, et al. Favorable changes in cardiac geometry and function following gastric bypass surgery: 2-year follow-up in the Utah obesity study. *J Am Coll Cardiol.* 2011;57:732-739.

CHAPTER 71

HYPERTROPHIC CARDIOMYOPATHY

Ali J. Marian

INTRODUCTION

Hypertrophic cardiomyopathy (HCM) is a genetic disorder of cardiac myocytes that is diagnosed by the presence of cardiac hypertrophy, not explained by secondary causes; a nondilated left ventricle; and typically an increased left ventricular ejection fraction (LVEF). Cardiac hypertrophy is often asymmetric with a predominant involvement of the interventricular septum, which is referred to as asymmetric septal hypertrophy (ASH). However, hypertrophy may involve the apex of the left ventricle only, which is denoted as apical HCM. Rarely, hypertrophy is restricted to other regions of the left ventricle, including the lateral or posterior wall. The expression of cardiac hypertrophy is age-dependent. It is infrequent in childhood, typically develops during adolescence, and seldom initially manifests after the fifth decade of life.[1]

A unique phenotypic feature of HCM is the presence of left ventricular outflow tract obstruction (LVOTO), which is present at rest in about one-third of the patients and inducible by exercise or inotropic stimulation in another third. Myocyte disarray is the pathologic hallmark of HCM. Other pathologic features include myocyte hypertrophy and interstitial fibrosis.

Epidemiology

HCM is among the most common genetic cardiovascular disorders. The estimated prevalence of HCM varies between 1:300 and 1:600 individuals in the general adult population without a particular geographic, ethnic, or sex predilection.[2] Estimates of the HCM prevalence are based on detection of a left ventricular wall thickness of greater than or equal to 13 mm (or ≥15 mm in some centers) on an echocardiogram. Estimating the prevalence of HCM based on the expression of cardiac hypertrophy is confounded by age-dependent expression of cardiac hypertrophy. Accordingly, about half of the family members of patients with known HCM mutations express cardiac hypertrophy by the third decade of life and approximately three quarter by the sixth decade.[1,3] Conversely, using cardiac hypertrophy alone to estimate the prevalence of HCM has the risk of including phenocopy conditions, such as storage diseases. At the genetic level, approximately 1:167 individuals (0.6%) carry pathogenic variants in the known HCM genes and hence might develop HCM.[4]

Genetic Basis of Hypertrophic Cardiomyopathy

HCM is a familial disease with an autosomal dominant pattern of inheritance in about 60% of the patients. It is sporadic in the remainder. Whether sporadic or familial, HCM is a genetic disease, commonly caused by mutations in genes encoding sarcomere proteins.[5] Accordingly, a single mutation is responsible and sufficient to cause familial HCM, albeit with variable penetrance. Moreover, phenotypic expression of the disease, including age of onset and severity of the disease, is influenced by a number of factors other than the causal mutation.

Christine and Jonathan Seidman identified the first causal mutation for HCM as a missense mutation in the *MYH7* gene, encoding the sarcomere protein myosin heavy chain 7 (or βMYH).[6] The discovery led to partial elucidation of the molecular genetic basis of HCM upon identification of additional genes. The well-established causal genes for HCM primarily code for proteins involved in sarcomere structure and function. Therefore, HCM to a large degree is considered a disease of the sarcomere.

Mutations in the *MYH7* and *MYBPC3* genes, the latter coding for myosin binding protein C3, are the most common causes for HCM, being responsible for 40% to 50% of HCM.[5] Mutations in the *TNNT2* (cardiac troponin T), *TNNI3* (cardiac troponin I), *TPM1* (a-tropomyosin), *ACTC1* (cardiac a-actin), *MYL2* (myosin light chain), *MYL3* (myosin light chain 3), and *CSRP3* (muscle LIM protein) genes are responsible for less than 10% of the HCM cases. Genes implicated as causes of HCM are listed in **Table 71.1**.

Despite these remarkable discoveries, the causal genes in approximately 40% of HCM have been difficult to identify. The so-called missing causal genes primarily pertain to HCM in sporadic cases and small families, as the causal genes in large families have been identified through genetic linkage, co-segregation analysis, and candidate gene sequencing. This is in contrast to sporadic cases or small families, wherein unambiguous ascertainment of pathogenicity of the genetic variants is difficult to establish. The challenge is further compounded by the incomplete and often low penetrance of the pathogenic variants in the sporadic cases and small families, which is reflective of their modest- to moderate-effect sizes. Finally, two or more pathogenic variants have been reported in ~5% of patients with sporadic cases or small families with HCM, suggesting that a small subset of HCM is oligogenic.[7-10]

Cardiac Histopathology

Gross cardiac pathology is notable for increased heart weight and left ventricular wall thickness, but a small ventricular

TABLE 71.1 Potential Pathogenicity of Variants in Genes Associated with Hypertrophic Cardiomyopathy (HCM)

		Pathogenicity (95% Confidence Interval of the Ratio of Observed to Expected Variants in the GnomAD Population)	
Gene	**Protein**	**Missense**	**Nonsense and Splice Acceptor or Donor Variants**
ACTC1	Cardiac α-actin	0.13-0.22	0.06-0.48
TNNC1	Cardiac troponin C	0.39-0.63	0.04-0.59
MYH7	β-Myosin heavy chain	0.63-0.71	0.35-0.57
VCL	Vinculin	0.64-0.76	0.17-0.4
JPH2	Junctophilin 2	0.68-0.81	0.30-0.78
TNNT2	Cardiac troponin T	0.64-0.86	0.22-0.64
TPM1	α-tropomyosin	0.28-0.44	0.25-0.78
ACTN2	Actinin, α 2	0.78-0.91	0.07-0.24
MYBPC3	Myosin binding protein-C	0.80-0.91	0.32-0.59
CAV3	Caveolin 3	0.62-0.92	0.32-1.47
MYL3	Essential myosin light chain	0.68-0.95	0.16-0.9
FHL1	Four-and-a-half LIM domains 1	0.67-0.92	0.0-0.28
PLN	Phospholamban	0.47-0.98	0-1.56
MYH6	Myosin heavy chain α	0.88-0.98	0.57-0.86
TNNI3	Cardiac troponin I	0.57-0.81	0.15-0.69
MYOZ2	Myozenin 2 (calsarcin 1)	0.75-1.01	0.30-1.07
TTN	Titin	1.01-1.04	0.3-0.35
LDB3	Lim domain binding 3	0.89-1.04	0.28-0.68
MYL2	Regulatory myosin light chain	0.74-1.06	0.69-1.75
FLNC	Filamin C	0.77-0.85	0.12-0.25
MYLK2	Myosin light chain kinase 2	0.88-1.06	0.13-0.48
ANKRD1	Ankyrin repeat domain 1	0.84-1.09	0.59-1.34
NEXN	Nexilin	0.94-1.13	0.40-0.78
TCAP	TCAP (Telethonin)	0.83-1.15	0.12-0.95
FHOD3	Formin homology 2 domain containing 3	0.86-0.97	0.17-0.37
TRIM63	Muscle ring finger protein 1	0.92-1.16	0.70-1.47
CASQ2	Calsequestrin 2	0.93-1.16	0.65-1.38

Note: Table lists genes and the encoded protein associated with HCM. It includes data on tolerance of gene to missense and loss of function variants; the latter defined as nonsense and splice acceptor or donor variants. The lower the ratio of observed to the expected number of variants indicates stronger selection against predicted loss-of-function (ie, the gene is less tolerant to loss of function variants). Although these indices might serve as guides, the pathogenicity of each variant should be assessed based on exquisite phenotyping of the individual.

cavity. Hypertrophy might also involve the right ventricle but seldom in isolation. Cardiac hypertrophy is typically asymmetric with predominant involvement of the basal interventricular septum. HCM may be restricted to the cardiac apex as in apical HCM. It occasionally involves the posterior or lateral wall only. Other morphologic features include elongation of the mitral valve leaflets or abnormal insertion of the papillary muscles.

Myocyte hypertrophy, disarray, is defined as disorganized orientation of myocytes; and interstitial fibrosis comprise histologic features of HCM (**Figure 71.1**). Although myocyte hypertrophy and interstitial fibrosis are common to various myocardial diseases, disarray, typically involving greater than 10% of the myocardium, is the pathologic hallmark of HCM. Interstitial fibrosis, clinically assessed by detection of late gadolinium enhancement (LGE) on cardiac magnetic resonance (CMR) imaging, is common in patients with HCM.[11]

Cardiac Physiology

HCM is characterized by a hyperdynamic left ventricle and therefore an increased or a high-normal LVEF. Left ventricular end-diastolic volume is either normal or reduced because of concentric hypertrophy, and end-systolic volume is small because of the hyperdynamic contraction. Despite an increased LVEF, regional systolic myocardial dysfunction, detected by various imaging modalities, is common in HCM and often precedes expression of cardiac hypertrophy.[12] Left ventricular relaxation is commonly impaired because of the increased bound state of the actomyosin complex, elevated diastolic intracellular calcium (Ca^{2+}) concentration, and increased myocardial fibrosis. Diastolic dysfunction leads to elevated left atrial pressure and symptoms of heart failure. It is also associated with the development of atrial fibrillation in HCM. Diastolic dysfunction is worse during physical exertion and is the main reason for exercise-induced dyspnea.

A unique characteristic of HCM is the presence of LVOTO, which occurs because of encroachment of the hypertrophic septum on the left ventricular outflow tract (LVOT) and systolic anterior motion of the mitral valve anterior leaflet owing to Venturi effect induced by the hyperdynamic contraction. LVOTO is typically detected by Doppler echocardiography or cardiac catheterization upon documentation of a systolic pressure gradient between the left ventricular cavity and the subaortic valve region (**Figure 71.2**). LVOTO varies with changes in contractility, preload, and afterload. Increased contractility or reduced left ventricular volume increases LVOTO. Conversely, negative inotropic agents and increased left ventricular volume reduce LVOTO. The Valsalva maneuver provokes or increases LVOTO during the straining phase.

Approximately one-third of patients with HCM have LVOTO at rest, whereas it could be provoked upon Valsalva or other interventions in another third. Patients with severe obstruction usually have elevated left ventricular diastolic pressure and experience exertional dyspnea. A small subfraction of patients with HCM—particularly the elderly with long-standing LVOTO, severe myocardial fibrosis, and concomitant coronary artery disease—develop heart failure with reduced LVEF.

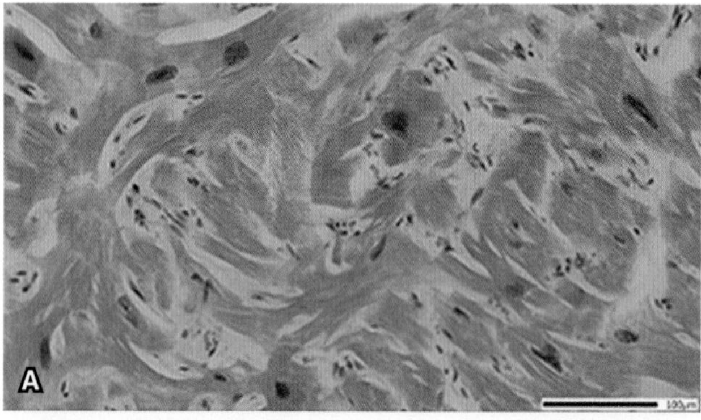

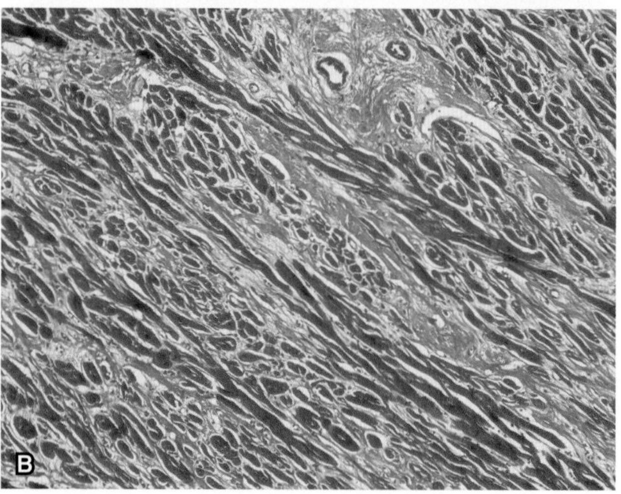

FIGURE 71.1 Histologic phenotypes of hypertrophic cardiomyopathy. **(A)** H&E stained thin myocardial section showing severe myocyte disarray. **(B)** A thin myocardial section stained with Masson trichrome showing severe myocardial fibrosis. H&E, hematoxylin and eosin.

PATHOGENESIS

For simplicity, pathogenesis of HCM could be classified into sequential sets of events, comprised of the primary effect, functional defects, secondary molecular changes, histologic and physiologic phenotype, and clinical features.

Primary Effect

The primary defect in HCM, a genetic disease, is the causal mutation (aka, pathogenic variant). Therefore, the initial stimulus in the pathogenesis of the phenotype has to originate from the causal pathogenic variant(s). In view of the genetic diversity of HCM, the initial impetus is diverse according to the type of the genetic variant and the function(s) of the gene involved.

HCM is commonly caused by a heterozygous mutation; therefore, only one copy of the gene is affected. A gene carrying the missense mutation is typically expressed into messenger ribonucleic acid (mRNA) and protein, albeit somewhat at a lower efficiency. Nevertheless, both normal and mutant proteins are expressed in the heart and to a large extent equally.

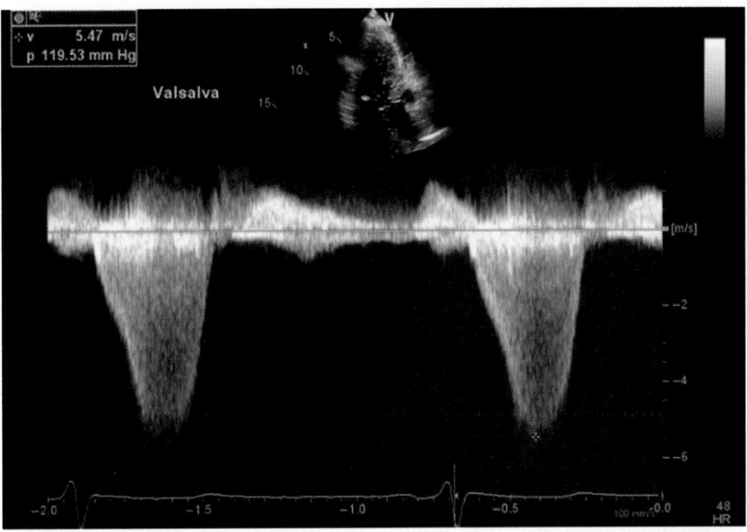

FIGURE 71.2 Echocardiographic detection of left ventricular outflow tract obstruction. Doppler velocities at the left ventricular outflow tract record about 5.5 m/s flow, corresponding to a gradient of 120 mm Hg.

The mutant protein carrying the missense mutation is typically incorporated into the sarcomere, although the efficiency of incorporation might be reduced. The phenotypic effect results from a dominant-negative effect of the mutant protein.

Alternatively, the mutation could lead to premature truncation of the protein because of a gain or loss of a stop codon or insertion/deletion mutation shifting the codon frame. Intracellular mechanisms target such mutant mRNAs for decay. Whenever the mutant mRNA escapes the surveillance mechanisms, the encode truncated protein is expressed but is quickly targeted by unfolded protein response and the ubiquitin-proteasome pathways for degradation. The net effect is haploinsufficiency because the protein is expressed from the healthy but not the mutant copy of the gene. Haploinsufficiency is relatively an uncommon mechanism in HCM because most mutations are missense mutations except those in the *MYBPC3* gene.

Functional Defects

Sarcomeres containing the mutant proteins exhibit a diverse array of functional effects, such as impaired Ca^{2+} sensitivity, altered actin-myosin cross-bridge cycling, and inefficient force generation. Functional effects of the mutations vary among different mutations and the involved genes. Mutations in the *MYH7* and *MYBPC3* proteins typically affect adenosine diphosphate/adenosine triphosphate (ADP/ATP)-dependent association and dissociation of actin and myosin molecules during a cardiac cycle, and consequently, inefficient force generation. Likewise, increased Ca^{2+} sensitivity of the myofilaments is the main effect of mutations involving the thin filament proteins. The net effect of this functional phenotype at the molecular level is an increased number of myosin molecules bound to actin at any given moment during a cardiac cycle.

Secondary Molecular Changes

The initial functional defects in the sarcomeres provoke expression and activation of stress-responsive and Ca^{2+}-activated transcriptional regulators, which then induce the expression of genes involved in cardiac hypertrophy and fibrosis, among others. A large set of transcriptional regulators and biologic pathways are activated in HCM, including calcineurin, mitogen-activated protein kinases, and transforming growth factor β pathways.[13,14] Overall, these secondary molecular changes are largely similar to those involved in various forms of secondary cardiac hypertrophy and fibrosis, with some variability pertaining to the biologic functions of the causal HCM genes.

Histologic and Morphologic Phenotypes

Histologic phenotype of HCM such as myocyte hypertrophy and myocardial fibrosis are tertiary phenotypes, resulting from activation of the molecular pathways consequent of function defects in sarcomeres.

Clinical Phenotype

Histologic and molecular changes induce gross morphologic and functional changes in HCM, which are responsible for the clinical manifestations of HCM, including heart failure with preserved ejection fraction (HFpEF), LVOTO, and cardiac arrhythmias.

CLINICAL PRESENTATION

Symptoms and Signs

The majority of patients with HCM are asymptomatic or have minimal symptoms that do not interfere with their lifestyle. Symptoms are typically reflective of cardiac arrhythmias, diastolic dysfunction, and LVOTO. Reduced exercise capacity and exertional dyspnea are the early symptoms that occur because of worsening of diastolic dysfunction during exercise. Chest pain is also a relatively common symptom and occurs because of increased oxygen demand of a hypertrophic myocardium often in the presence of reduced blood flow as a result of microvascular abnormalities.

Palpitations, often caused by supraventricular tachycardia (SVT) or nonsustained ventricular tachycardia (NSVT), is a common symptom in patients with HCM. NSVT is present in 20% to 30% of the patients and is a risk factor for sudden cardiac death (SCD), particularly in the symptomatic young patients.[15] Syncope is relatively uncommon but a serious manifestation of HCM, as it is usually caused by cardiac arrhythmias and less commonly by severe LVOTO or autonomic dysfunction.

The annual incidence of atrial fibrillation in patients with HCM is ~2% to 3%.[16] A quarter of patients with HCM experience atrial fibrillation, which is poorly tolerated by most patients because of (1) shortening of the left ventricular filling period resulting from the rapid ventricular rate and (2) loss of the atrial contribution to ventricular filling.[16] Atrial fibrillation is particularly common in patients with LVOTO, HFpEF, and left atrial enlargement.[16] It is also a major risk factor for thromboembolic stroke, and when detected, an oral anticoagulant should be administered to prevent stroke.

Physical examination of patients with HCM is notable for the finding of a forceful, leftward displaced, sometimes bifid, and occasionally triplet apical impulse. The carotid pulse is brisk and bifid, the latter in those with LVOTO, reflective of tidal and percussion waves. The jugular venous pulse might show a prominent A wave. Cardiac auscultation is remarkable for a prominent fourth heart sound, and in those with LVOTO, a harsh, mid-systolic murmur, which is the loudest between the apex and the left sternal border. The intensity and duration of the murmur vary with changes in ventricular loading conditions and myocardial contractility, as discussed earlier. Patients with LVOTO also typically have mitral regurgitation, which is characterized by a pansystolic blowing murmur at the apex.

DIAGNOSIS

Detailed history taking and physical examination supplemented with a 12-lead electrocardiogram (ECG) and thorough transthoracic echocardiographic study are commonly used in the evaluation of patients with HCM. In addition, cardiac rhythm monitoring, preferably for 30 days, is indicated in those with palpitations, presyncope, or syncope. Cardiopulmonary exercise testing provides useful information in assessing the functional capacity of the patients. CMR is often used to verify the diagnosis in difficult cases and to assess myocardial fibrosis. Genetic testing is routinely applied for the accurate diagnosis of HCM as well as preclinical identification of those at risk.

Electrocardiogram

The ECG, the most commonly used test, often provides the first clue to the diagnosis of HCM by showing evidence of cardiac hypertrophy. ECG abnormalities, found in most patients with HCM, often precedes expression of cardiac hypertrophy on the echocardiogram.[1] The ECG findings are notable for the presence of increased QRS voltage, secondary ST and T changes, left atrial enlargement, and deep Q waves in the inferior and/or lateral leads that mimic myocardial infarction. Apical HCM has characteristic electrocardiographic manifestations with deep T wave inversions in the precordial leads (**Figure 71.3A**). In addition, pre-excitation and delta wave, resembling Wolff-Parkinson-White, is detected in 2% to 3% of patients with HCM. The presence of pre-excitation findings on ECG suggests a phenocopy condition.

Echocardiography

Unexplained cardiac hypertrophy, typically detected on an echocardiogram, is the clinical diagnostic hallmark of HCM (**Figure 71.3B**). The diagnosis is commonly based on detection of a left ventricular wall thickness of 13 mm or greater, unexplained by the loading conditions, and a preserved or increased LVEF, as discussed earlier. Using a cutoff point of 15 mm of greater increases specificity of the diagnosis but reduces sensitivity of the echocardiographic diagnosis. A Z score representing a deviation from the expected values in a matched group is used to detect cardiac hypertrophy in children. LVOTO is a characteristic finding in HCM, as discussed earlier.

Cardiac Magnetic Resonance

CMR is a valuable tool whenever the diagnosis of HCM is suspected but unconfirmed by ECG and echocardiography. LGE on CMR is commonly used to detect and quantify LGE as a surrogate marker for myocardial fibrosis. Presence and extent of LGE is associated with adverse clinical outcomes, including heart failure, cardiac arrhythmias, and SCD.[11,17,18]

Biomarkers

Blood level of N-terminal pro-brain natriuretic protein (NT-proBNP), the most commonly used circulating biomarker in HCM, is typically elevated in patients with HCM, in particular in those with LVOTO and HFpEF. It is a valuable marker for assessing a patient's response to interventions as well as in prognostication. Circulating cardiac troponins and cytokines are also often elevated in HCM patients with LVOTO, atrial fibrillation, or heart failure, reflective of myocyte stress and injury.[19] Elevated circulating levels of cleaved products of collagen synthesis and degradation, matrix metalloproteinase 2, apelin, and galectin 3 are considered biomarkers for detection of interstitial fibrosis.[20,21] Finally, circulating microRNAs and circular RNAs have been detected in patients with HCM.

Genetic Testing

Genetic testing, which is routinely used in patients with HCM, leads to the identification of the causal variants in about a third to half of the probands with HCM.[10,22] The commonly used approach is whole-exome sequencing followed by an analysis of the pathogenic variants in genes known to cause HCM. The main challenge in genetic testing is in discerning the pathogenicity of the genetic variants, particularly in sporadic cases and in small families. The difficulty is in part because of the

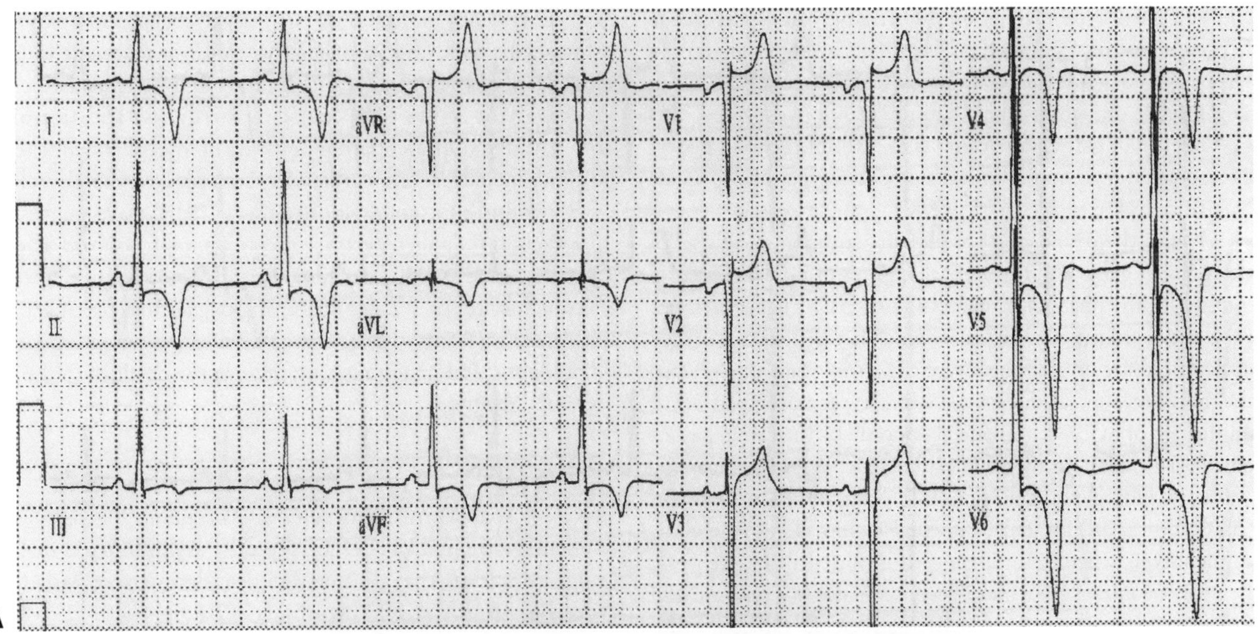

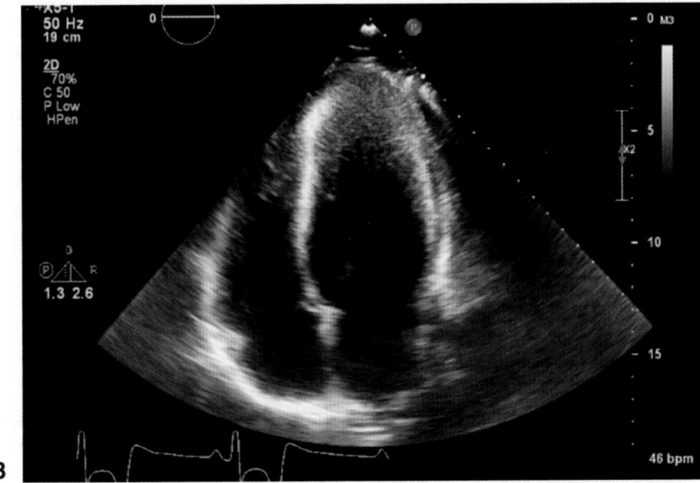

FIGURE 71.3 Electrocardiogram and echocardiogram in apical HCM. **(A)** 12-lead electrocardiographic recording in apical HCM, showing the characteristic findings, which are notable for deep T wave inversion in the precordial leads. **(B)** The corresponding four-chamber echocardiographic view showing extensive apical hypertrophy. HCM, hypertrophic cardiomyopathy.

presence of a very large number of genetic variants in each genome, shortcomings of the algorithms to predict pathogenicity, and genetic heterogeneity of HCM, among others. Identification of a pathogenic variant in a well-established causal gene might be reassuring but does not totally eliminate the challenge in ascertaining pathogenicity.

Clinical utilities of genetic testing include accurate diagnosis of HCM from the phenocopy conditions and the preclinical diagnosis and stratification of the family members at risk.[10] Family members who carry the pathogenic variant are at increased risk and require periodic phenotypic evaluation to detect HCM early and intervene to prevent major events such as SCD.[12,23] This is clinically impactful because SCD is often the first manifestation of HCM.[24-26] Conversely, family members who have not inherited the pathogenic variants are not at an increased risk of HCM and do not require frequent clinical evaluation. Moreover, identification of the causal gene/mutation might enable gene/mutation-specific therapies, as they become available. Finally, genetic testing could lead to the identification of the phenocopy conditions that mimic HCM, which encompasses about 3% to 5% of the adult HCM patients.[10] The distinction is clinically valuable as the natural history and treatment of the phenocopy conditions differ and specific therapies might be available, such as enzyme replacement therapy for Anderson-Fabry disease, a lysosomal storage disorder.

Genotype-Phenotype Correlation in Hypertrophic Cardiomyopathy

Patients with HCM exhibit considerable variability in the phenotypic expression, including clinical manifestations, rendering genotype-phenotype correlation challenging. Variability in the phenotypic expression of HCM is evident even among family members who share the same pathogenic variant, indicating the influence of factors other than the causal pathogenic variant. Presence of pathogenic variants in multiple genes is generally associated with more pronounced phenotype such as severe ventricular hypertrophy and LVOTO.[7-9]

Overall, there is no clear correlation between a specific set of mutations or genes and the clinical features of HCM. The prerequisite for the phenotypic expression of HCM is the presence of the causal pathogenic variant(s), which is expected to exert the largest effect size on the phenotype. The severity of the phenotype, however, such as the age of onset, severity of hypertrophy, and the risk of SCD, is influenced not only by the causal pathogenic variant but also by other pathogenic variants; epigenetic factors, including noncoding RNAs; posttranslational protein modifications; and the environmental factors. Thus, the clinical phenotype, whether in single-gene disorders or in polygenic disease, is a complex trait, and the consequence of stochastic and nonlinear interactions between the pathogenic variants, other genetic factors (modifier genes), and the environmental factors.

Genes known to cause HCM could also cause other hereditary cardiomyopathies, such as dilated cardiomyopathy, restrictive cardiomyopathy, and left ventricular noncompaction syndrome.[27,28] The basis for such extreme phenotypic pleiotropy resulting from mutations in a single gene is unknown. Differential effects of the mutations on Ca^{2+} sensitivity of the thin filaments and differential protein-protein interactions are plausible mechanisms.[29,30]

Differential Diagnosis

HCM is a great masquerader. It is not uncommon for a patient with HCM to present to the emergency department with chest pain and undergo investigation for acute coronary syndromes because of the presence of ECG abnormalities and on occasion elevated plasma levels of cardiac troponin T or I. In such cases, HCM is often diagnosed during a left ventricular angiography.

Cardiac hypertrophy, the clinical diagnostic hallmark of HCM, per se is a nonspecific finding, as it is present in various loading conditions and in athlete's hearts. The classic definition of HCM requires exclusion of such conditions; nevertheless, concomitant presence of hypertension and valvular heart disease could make the clinical diagnosis of HCM challenging. Likewise, athlete's heart, particularly those who routinely perform isometric exercises, could exhibit a significant degree of left ventricular hypertrophy with a wall thickness of up to 18 mm.[31] The distinction between HCM and athlete's heart is important as HCM is among the most common causes of SCD in young athletes.[25] Presence of ASH, LVOTO, and a small left ventricular cavity size would indicate HCM as opposed to athlete's hearts and other forms of secondary hypertrophy.[31] In addition, the presence of abnormal Q waves, prominent repolarization abnormalities, left atrial enlargement, and evidence of diastolic dysfunction would support the diagnosis of HCM. Genetic testing by defining the pathogenic variants might solidify the diagnosis of HCM.

Phenocopy conditions, such as glycogen and lysosomal storage diseases, mitochondrial diseases, and several musculoskeletal disorders may also mimic HCM. The distinction is important as the time course of the disease and treatment often differ. Differentiating features of the phenocopy conditions include severe cardiac hypertrophy, very high-voltage QRS complexes, conduction defects, delta wave suggesting pre-excitation, and detection of concomitant noncardiac phenotypes, such as skin, renal, or skeletal abnormalities. Specific biochemical tests, such as measuring α-galactosidase A activity in Anderson-Fabry disease, myocyte disarray on endomyocardial biopsy, and genetic testing might provide clues to the differential diagnosis.

PROGNOSIS

HCM has an annual mortality rate of about 1% per year.[32] Patients without LVOTO are typically asymptomatic or have mild symptoms that do not significantly interfere with their lifestyle. Approximately two-thirds of patients with HCM live a normal life span without significant limitations.[33] Nevertheless, HCM is among the common causes of SCD in adolescents and young adults, particularly among competitive athletes.[24-26] Patients with long-standing LVOTO are at an increased risk of HFpEF as well as atrial fibrillation. Effective therapies for LVOTO, such as alcohol septal ablation and surgical myectomy, are available, which lead to significant improvement in the overall prognosis of this subset of patients with HCM.

MANAGEMENT

Phenotypic expression as well as the evolution of the phenotype in HCM is age-dependent. Therefore, periodic evaluation of those at risk and their family members, as well as those who have expressed the disease, is required. Evaluation of HCM patients includes detailed history taking, with special emphasis on symptoms of palpitations, pre-syncope, and syncope, as well as symptoms of heart failure. Family history is an essential part of evaluation of patients with HCM, as it provides valuable information about the course of the disease, including the risk of SCD. Cardiac rhythm monitoring for an extended period of time could provide valuable data on assessment of cardiac arrhythmias, and hence, the risk of SCD and stroke. Echocardiography and CMR are invaluable in detecting and quantifying hypertrophy and fibrosis, LVOTO, and concomitant mitral regurgitation. Treadmill exercise or cardiopulmonary exercise testing enables assessment of the patient's functional capacity and risk of exercise-induced arrhythmias.

Pharmacologic Therapy

The majority of patients, particularly those without LVOTO, are asymptomatic and do not require pharmacologic treatment. For those with symptoms, the first and likely cornerstone of therapy is a β-adrenergic receptor blocker (β-blocker), specifically, one without intrinsic sympathetic activity. β-blockers are useful for relieving or attenuating symptoms of palpitations, chest pain, and dyspnea as well as exercise-induced LVOTO.

The benefits of β-blockers in reducing the risk of SCD are unclear. Their typical side effects, such as excessive fatigue, exercise intolerance, and central nervous system symptoms, are the main hindrance in the use of β-blockers in patients with HCM. The second line of therapy—and the first line in those who do not tolerate βblockers—are the L-type calcium channel blockers, such as verapamil or diltiazem. The potential beneficial effects of the L-type calcium channel blockers are in accord with our understanding of the role of altered Ca^{2+} currents in diastolic dysfunction in HCM. Calcium channel blockers are also helpful in the management of SVT and possibly in slowing the development of HCM in those who carry pathogenic variants in the *MYBPC3* gene.[34]

Disopyramide, a negative inotropic agent, in conjunction with a β-blocker—the latter to reduce parasympatholytic effects of disopyramide—is used to reduce LVOTO.[35] Diuretics are useful in a subset of patients who have symptoms of heart failure, elevated left ventricular filling pressure, and elevated serum NT-proBNP levels. The risk associated with the use of diuretics includes hypovolemia and consequently hypotension and syncope. Anti-arrhythmic drugs are used judiciously in the treatment of SVT or NSVT because of the risk of pro-arrhythmias in the background of a pathologic ventricular substrate.

An implantable cardioverter-defibrillator (ICD) is the first choice in symptomatic patients with recurrent NSVT or SVT. The intervention is often complemented with radiofrequency ablation and the use of anti-arrhythmic drugs to prevent or reduce the frequency of arrhythmias. New-onset atrial fibrillation is best managed with direct cardioversion after exclusion of an intracardiac clot by transesophageal echocardiography. Persistent and recurrent atrial fibrillation requires rate or rhythm control and long-term oral anticoagulation to reduce the risk of thromboembolism.[16]

Management of Patients at Risk of Sudden Cardiac Death

HCM is among the common causes of SCD in the young, particularly in young athletes.[24-26] The risk of SCD in an adult patient with HCM ranges from 0.5% to 2% per year. The main challenge in the management of patients with HCM is to identify those who are at an increased risk and hence, intervene to prevent SCD. Overall, ICD is safe and effective in reducing the risk of SCD in patients with HCM, albeit not without complications.[36] The complication rate of an ICD implantation is less than 5% per year, whereas its effective appropriate shock rate, indicative of serious arrhythmias, ranges from 3% to 15% per year and higher in those with a prior arrhythmic event and in children.[37-39]

Although none of the known risk factors reliably predict the risk of SCD, several algorithms have been developed to stratify and identify the high-risk individuals. Implantation of an ICD is indicated in those with a prior episode of cardiac arrest or SVT. A history of recurrent syncope, suggestive of arrhythmias as the cause, as well as the presence of symptomatic NSVT, identifies high-risk individuals. Indication for an ICD indication is less clear in asymptomatic patients with recurrent NSVT. A history of SCD in more than one family member also denotes a genetic background that is susceptible to cardiac arrhythmias and hence, increased risk of SCD. The increased susceptibility might reflect the presence of multiple pathogenic variants and/or presence of pathogenic variants in genes coding for ion channels. Patients with severe left ventricular hypertrophy are generally considered at an increased risk of cardiac arrhythmias, although those with extreme hypertrophy might not be at an increased risk. The extent of LGE on CMR has been associated with an increased risk of SCD, albeit there is variability in the quantification of LGE, requiring center-specific data interpretation. Whereas severe LVOTO is a risk factor for heart failure and atrial fibrillation, its role in increasing the risk of SCD is unclear.

Management of Left Ventricular Outflow Tract Obstruction

LVOTO is a major risk factor for heart failure and atrial fibrillation in patients with HCM. Pharmacologic therapy with a β-blocker and disopyramide is often beneficial in attenuating symptoms but not fully effective or well tolerated. Catheter-based or surgical interventions are indicated in those who remain symptomatic, despite pharmacologic therapy, and have a significant LVOTO, defined arbitrarily as a systolic pressure gradient greater than or equal to 50 mm Hg at rest or with exercise.[40] Surgical septal myectomy, known as Morrow procedure, and alcohol septal ablation are highly effective in reducing LVOTO and improving symptoms.[41] The clinical outcomes are largely equal and therefore the choice of alcohol septal ablation or surgical myectomy is mainly dictated by secondary factors. For example, the presence of concomitant cardiac diseases, such as coronary artery disease, or the absence of a suitable septal perforator, would necessitate surgical myectomy. In contrast, alcohol septal ablation is preferred in the presence of comorbid conditions that increase the risk of general anesthesia and surgery. Alcohol septal ablation is associated with 10% to 20% risk of advanced conduction defect, requiring implantation of a permanent pacemaker. Because of concern about possible induction of an arrhythmogenic substrate after alcohol septal ablation, implantation of an ICD might be justified in those who are judged to be at high risk for serious cardiac arrhythmias. In contrast, surgical myectomy is typically associated with a lower risk of cardiac arrhythmias postsurgery, albeit, it does not eliminate the risk.

Several professional organizations have published clinical practice guidelines for the diagnosis and management of patients with HCM, including a very recent report by the American College of Cardiology and American Heart Association, which might be informative to the practicing physicians.[42]

RESEARCH AND FUTURE DIRECTIONS

Delineation of the genetic basis of HCM has led to partial elucidation of its molecular pathogenesis and hence, subsequent development of small molecules that target myosin ATPase activity. Mavacamten (MYK-461) is an orally administered small-molecule inhibitor of myosin ATPase activity that has been tested in preclinical and phase I-II clinical studies. Preclinical studies suggest beneficial effects of this mechanistically designed drug in reducing cardiac hypertrophy, myocyte disarray, and fibrosis in experimental models.[43] Phase II clinical trials with Mavacamten point to a promising safety profile along with beneficial effects in reducing LVOTO, partly through reducing LVEF, increasing peak oxygen consumption, and improving symptoms.[44] The main risk associated with its use is a dose-dependent reduction in LVEF.[44] Clinical studies are ongoing to assess the beneficial effects of this drug on obstructive and nonobstructive HCM.

Experimental data in models organisms suggest beneficial effects of treatment with angiotensin II receptor blockers, 3-hydroxy-3-methyglutaryl-coenzyme A reductase inhibitors (statins), mineralocorticoid receptor blockers, and antioxidant N-acetylcysteine in preventing, attenuating, or reversing the HCM-like phenotypes.[45] The results of the pilot studies in human patients with HCM have not been promising, albeit the studies by design were not efficacy studies.[46-48]

Various gene therapy approaches have been used in experimental models to attenuate the HCM-like phenotype, including adeno-associated virus serotype 9 (AAV9)-mediated gene expression, short hairpin RNA (shRNA)-based targeting of the mutant mRNA, and clustered regularly interspaced short palindromic repeats (CRISPR)-Cas9 editing of the mutation.[49-51] Clinical applications of these experimental approaches remain to be explored.

KEY POINTS

- ✔ HCM is a relatively common disease characterized by unexplained cardiac hypertrophy and a preserved or increased LVEF.
- ✔ HCM, whether familial or sporadic, is a genetic disease caused mainly by mutations in genes coding for sarcomeric or sarcomere-associated proteins.
- ✔ The causal genes in about 40% of the HCM cases are unknown. Genetic testing identifies the causal genes in less than half of the cases.
- ✔ HCM is an important cause of SCD in the young.
- ✔ An ICD is highly effective in terminating VT and converting ventricular fibrillation. An ICD should be implanted in those with a previous history of cardiac arrest, VT, and symptomatic NSVT.
- ✔ LVOTO is a major cause of symptoms of heart failure and risk of atrial fibrillation.
- ✔ Surgical septal ablation and surgical myectomy are highly effective in reducing LVOTO and improving patients' symptoms. The choice should be tailored according to patient-specific conditions.
- ✔ A new small-molecule inhibitor of myosin ATPase activity, designed based on the underpinning pathogenesis of HCM, is being tested for safety and efficacy in patients with HCM.

REFERENCES

1. Charron P, Dubourg O, Desnos M, et al. Diagnostic value of electrocardiography and echocardiography for familial hypertrophic cardiomyopathy in a genotyped adult population. *Circulation.* 1997;96:214-219.
2. Maron BJ, Gardin JM, Flack JM, Gidding SS, Kurosaki TT, Bild DE. Prevalence of hypertrophic cardiomyopathy in a general population of young adults. Echocardiographic analysis of 4111 subjects in the CARDIA Study. Coronary Artery Risk Development in (Young) Adults. *Circulation.* 1995;92:785-789.
3. Niimura H, Bachinski LL, Sangwatanaroj S, et al. Mutations in the gene for cardiac myosin-binding protein C and late-onset familial hypertrophic cardiomyopathy. *N Engl J Med.* 1998;338:1248-1257.
4. Semsarian C, Ingles J, Maron MS, Maron BJ. New perspectives on the prevalence of hypertrophic cardiomyopathy. *J Am Coll Cardiol.* 2015;65:1249-1254.
5. Marian AJ, Braunwald E. Hypertrophic cardiomyopathy: genetics, pathogenesis, clinical manifestations, diagnosis, and therapy. *Circ Res.* 2017;121:749-770.
6. Geisterfer-Lowrance AA, Kass S, Tanigawa G, et al. A molecular basis for familial hypertrophic cardiomyopathy: a beta cardiac myosin heavy chain gene missense mutation. *Cell.* 1990;62:999-1006.
7. Blair E, Price SJ, Baty CJ, Ostman-Smith I, Watkins H. Mutations in cis can confound genotype-phenotype correlations in hypertrophic cardiomyopathy. *J Med Genet.* 2001;38:385-388.
8. Girolami F, Ho CY, Semsarian C, et al. Clinical features and outcome of hypertrophic cardiomyopathy associated with triple sarcomere protein gene mutations. *J Am Coll Cardiol.* 2010;55:1444-1453.
9. Li L, Bainbridge MN, Tan Y, Willerson JT, Marian AJ. A potential oligogenic etiology of hypertrophic cardiomyopathy: a classic single-gene disorder. *Circ Res.* 2017;120:1084-1090.
10. Alfares AA, Kelly MA, McDermott G, et al. Results of clinical genetic testing of 2,912 probands with hypertrophic cardiomyopathy: expanded panels offer limited additional sensitivity. *Genet Med.* 2015;17:880-888.
11. Mc LA, Ellims AH, Prabhu S, et al. Diffuse ventricular fibrosis on cardiac magnetic resonance imaging associates with ventricular tachycardia in patients with hypertrophic cardiomyopathy. *J Cardiovasc Electrophysiol.* 2016;27:571-580.
12. Nagueh SF, McFalls J, Meyer D, et al. Tissue Doppler imaging predicts the development of hypertrophic cardiomyopathy in subjects with subclinical disease. *Circulation.* 2003;108:395-398.
13. Lim DS, Roberts R, Marian AJ. Expression profiling of cardiac genes in human hypertrophic cardiomyopathy: insight into the pathogenesis of phenotypes. *J Am Coll Cardiol.* 2001;38:1175-1180.
14. Helms AS, Alvarado FJ, Yob J, et al. Genotype-dependent and -independent calcium signaling dysregulation in human hypertrophic cardiomyopathy. *Circulation.* 2016;134:1738-1748.
15. Monserrat L, Elliott PM, Gimeno JR, Sharma S, Penas-Lado M, McKenna WJ. Non-sustained ventricular tachycardia in hypertrophic cardiomyopathy: an independent marker of sudden death risk in young patients. *J Am Coll Cardiol.* 2003;42:873-879.
16. Guttmann OP, Rahman MS, O'Mahony C, Anastasakis A, Elliott PM. Atrial fibrillation and thromboembolism in patients with hypertrophic cardiomyopathy: systematic review. *Heart.* 2014;100:465-472.
17. O'Hanlon R, Grasso A, Roughton M, et al. Prognostic significance of myocardial fibrosis in hypertrophic cardiomyopathy. *J Am Coll Cardiol.* 2010;56:867-874.
18. Schelbert EB, Piehler KM, Zareba KM, et al. Myocardial fibrosis quantified by extracellular volume is associated with subsequent hospitalization for heart failure, death, or both across the spectrum of ejection fraction and heart failure stage. *J Am Heart Assoc.* 2015;4(12):e002613.
19. Moreno V, Hernandez-Romero D, Vilchez JA, et al. Serum levels of high-sensitivity troponin T: a novel marker for cardiac remodeling in hypertrophic cardiomyopathy. *J Card Fail.* 2010;16:950-956.
20. Lombardi R, Betocchi S, Losi MA, et al. Myocardial collagen turnover in hypertrophic cardiomyopathy. *Circulation.* 2003;108:1455-1460.

21. Ho CY, Lopez B, Coelho-Filho OR, et al. Myocardial fibrosis as an early manifestation of hypertrophic cardiomyopathy. *N Engl J Med.* 2010;363:552-563.
22. Gruner C, Ivanov J, Care M, et al. Toronto hypertrophic cardiomyopathy genotype score for prediction of a positive genotype in hypertrophic cardiomyopathy. *Circ Cardiovasc Genet.* 2013;6:19-26.
23. Nagueh SF, Bachinski LL, Meyer D, et al. Tissue Doppler imaging consistently detects myocardial abnormalities in patients with hypertrophic cardiomyopathy and provides a novel means for an early diagnosis before and independently of hypertrophy. *Circulation.* 2001;104:128-130.
24. Bagnall RD, Weintraub RG, Ingles J, et al. A prospective study of sudden cardiac death among children and young adults. *N Engl J Med.* 2016;374:2441-2452.
25. Maron BJ, Doerer JJ, Haas TS, Tierney DM, Mueller FO. Sudden deaths in young competitive athletes: analysis of 1866 deaths in the United States, 1980-2006. *Circulation.* 2009;119:1085-1092.
26. O'Mahony C, Jichi F, Pavlou M, et al. A novel clinical risk prediction model for sudden cardiac death in hypertrophic cardiomyopathy (HCM risk-SCD). *Eur Heart J.* 2014;35:2010-2020.
27. Mogensen J, Kubo T, Duque M, et al. Idiopathic restrictive cardiomyopathy is part of the clinical expression of cardiac troponin I mutations. *J Clin Invest.* 2003;111:209-216.
28. Hoedemaekers YM, Caliskan K, Majoor-Krakauer D, et al. Cardiac beta-myosin heavy chain defects in two families with non-compaction cardiomyopathy: linking non-compaction to hypertrophic, restrictive, and dilated cardiomyopathies. *Eur Heart J.* 2007;28:2732-2737.
29. Lombardi R, Bell A, Senthil V, et al. Differential interactions of thin filament proteins in two cardiac troponin T mouse models of hypertrophic and dilated cardiomyopathies. *Cardiovasc Res.* 2008;79:109-117.
30. Debold EP, Schmitt JP, Patlak JB, et al. Hypertrophic and dilated cardiomyopathy mutations differentially affect the molecular force generation of mouse alpha-cardiac myosin in the laser trap assay. *Am J Physiol Heart Circ Physiol.* 2007;293:H284-H291.
31. Grazioli G, Usin D, Trucco E, et al. Differentiating hypertrophic cardiomyopathy from athlete's heart: an electrocardiographic and echocardiographic approach. *J Electrocardiol.* 2016;49:539-544.
32. Pelliccia F, Pasceri V, Limongelli G, et al. Long-term outcome of nonobstructive versus obstructive hypertrophic cardiomyopathy: a systematic review and meta-analysis. *Int J Cardiol.* 2017;243:379-384.
33. Maron BJ, Rowin EJ, Casey SA, et al. Hypertrophic cardiomyopathy in adulthood associated with low cardiovascular mortality with contemporary management strategies. *J Am Coll Cardiol.* 2015;65:1915-1928.
34. Ho CY, Lakdawala NK, Cirino AL, et al. Diltiazem treatment for pre-clinical hypertrophic cardiomyopathy sarcomere mutation carriers: a pilot randomized trial to modify disease expression. *JACC Heart Fail.* 2015;3:180-188.
35. Sherrid MV, Barac I, McKenna WJ, et al. Multicenter study of the efficacy and safety of disopyramide in obstructive hypertrophic cardiomyopathy. *J Am Coll Cardiol.* 2005;45:1251-1258.
36. Maron BJ, Shen WK, Link MS, et al. Efficacy of implantable cardioverter-defibrillators for the prevention of sudden death in patients with hypertrophic cardiomyopathy. *N Engl J Med.* 2000;342:365-373.
37. Maron BJ, Spirito P, Ackerman MJ, et al. Prevention of sudden cardiac death with implantable cardioverter-defibrillators in children and adolescents with hypertrophic cardiomyopathy. *J Am Coll Cardiol.* 2013;61:1527-1535.
38. Maron BJ, Spirito P, Shen WK, et al. Implantable cardioverter-defibrillators and prevention of sudden cardiac death in hypertrophic cardiomyopathy. *JAMA.* 2007;298:405-412.
39. Vriesendorp PA, Schinkel AF, Van Cleemput J, et al. Implantable cardioverter-defibrillators in hypertrophic cardiomyopathy: patient outcomes, rate of appropriate and inappropriate interventions, and complications. *Am Heart J.* 2013;166:496-502.
40. Nishimura RA, Seggewiss H, Schaff, HV. Hypertrophic obstructive cardiomyopathy: surgical myectomy vs septal ablation. *Circ Res.* 2017;121(7):771-783.
41. Batzner A, Pfeiffer B, Neugebauer A, Aicha D, Blank C, Seggewiss H. Survival after alcohol septal ablation in patients with hypertrophic obstructive cardiomyopathy. *J Am Coll Cardiol.* 2018;72:3087-3094.
42. Ommen SR, Mital S, Burke MA, et al. 2020 AHA/ACC Guideline for the diagnosis and treatment of patients with hypertrophic cardiomyopathy: a report of the American College of Cardiology/American Heart Association Joint Committee on Clinical Practice Guidelines. *Circulation.* 2020;142:e558-e631.
43. Green EM, Wakimoto H, Anderson RL, et al. A small-molecule inhibitor of sarcomere contractility suppresses hypertrophic cardiomyopathy in mice. *Science.* 2016;351:617-621.
44. Heitner SB, Jacoby D, Lester SJ, et al. Mavacamten treatment for obstructive hypertrophic cardiomyopathy: a clinical trial. *Ann Intern Med.* 2019;170:741-748.
45. Marian AJ. Experimental therapies in hypertrophic cardiomyopathy. *J Cardiovasc Transl Res.* 2009;2:483-492.
46. Marian AJ, Tan Y, Li L, et al. Hypertrophy regression with N-acetylcysteine in hypertrophic cardiomyopathy (HALT-HCM): a randomized, placebo-controlled, double-blind pilot study. *Circ Res.* 2018;122:1109-1118.
47. Shimada YJ, Passeri JJ, Baggish AL, et al. Effects of losartan on left ventricular hypertrophy and fibrosis in patients with nonobstructive hypertrophic cardiomyopathy. *JACC Heart Fail.* 2013;1:480-487.
48. Nagueh SF, Lombardi R, Tan Y, Wang J, Willerson JT, Marian AJ. Atorvastatin and cardiac hypertrophy and function in hypertrophic cardiomyopathy: a pilot study. *Eur J Clin Invest.* 2010;40:976-983.
49. Mosqueira D, Mannhardt I, Bhagwan JR, et al. CRISPR/Cas9 editing in human pluripotent stem cell-cardiomyocytes highlights arrhythmias, hypocontractility, and energy depletion as potential therapeutic targets for hypertrophic cardiomyopathy. *Eur Heart J.* 2018;39:3879-3892.
50. Mearini G, Stimpel D, Geertz B, et al. Mybpc3 gene therapy for neonatal cardiomyopathy enables long-term disease prevention in mice. *Nat Commun.* 2014;5:5515.
51. Jiang J, Wakimoto H, Seidman JG, Seidman CE. Allele-specific silencing of mutant Myh6 transcripts in mice suppresses hypertrophic cardiomyopathy. *Science.* 2013;342:111-114.

CHAPTER 72

RESTRICTIVE CARDIOMYOPATHIES

Gurusher Panjrath and Joseph M. Krepp

INTRODUCTION

Restrictive cardiomyopathies are a cluster of distinct myocardial diseases with a similar pathophysiology of myocardial muscle stiffening and impaired ventricular filling. The phenotypic expression of this group of cardiomyopathies may be quite different, ranging from hereditary, infiltrative, dilated, or hypertrophic cardiomyopathy (**Table 72.1**). However, the characteristic pathophysiology of restrictive cardiomyopathy is similar and represented by a rapid rise in intraventricular pressure with a small increase in volume.[1] The diastolic volumes may be preserved or reduced. Usually, it may be associated with preserved biventricular systolic function; however, it may change late in the course of disease. Anatomically, the hallmarks of this group of disorders include substantial atrial dilatation and normal or reduced left ventricular size in the absence of pericardial disease. Depending on the stage of presentation and severity of disease, the anatomic features may vary widely. In its classic form, the restrictive pattern of ventricular filling may be apparent in the form of a diastolic "dip and plateau" on the hemodynamic tracing. Advanced stages of diastolic dysfunction with restrictive filling patterns may be apparent on echocardiography. The etiology of restrictive cardiomyopathy can be genetic, inherited, or acquired. Compared to other forms of cardiomyopathy, restrictive cardiomyopathies are less common and more likely to be underdiagnosed. As a heterogeneous group of disorders (**Table 72.1**) with varying degrees of restrictive physiology, the diagnosis can be challenging and requires a high degree of suspicion. An important differential diagnosis of restrictive cardiomyopathy is constrictive pericarditis, which has significant overlap in presentation and clinical features. A thickened pericardium may be seen in constrictive pericarditis on imaging, but 18% of patients with constrictive pericarditis may not have a thickened pericardium. Advanced echocardiographic techniques can sometimes help differentiate between the two, but endomyocardial biopsy may be needed in specific cases. Similarly, often, several diagnostic modalities need to be employed to specifically identify the cause of restrictive cardiomyopathy (**Algorithm 72.1**), as discussed in later subsections.

Epidemiology, pathogenesis, diagnostic, and management approaches are discussed in more detail under each subsection of some of the common forms of restrictive cardiomyopathies.

CARDIAC SARCOIDOSIS

Sarcoidosis is a systemic, multiorgan disease of uncertain etiology involving noncaseating granulomas, most commonly involving the lungs. Other organs involved include eyes, the nervous system, skin, and myocardium. While cardiac involvement was historically thought to occur in only 5% of pulmonary sarcoid cases, the prevalence is much higher, ranging up to 25% in recently reported autopsy studies.[2] Cardiac sarcoid is frequently underdiagnosed and requires a high degree of suspicion. While the most common presentation leading to a diagnosis may be sudden cardiac death, cardiac sarcoid may present as heart block, ventricular arrhythmias, ventricular aneurysms, and restrictive or dilated cardiomyopathy.

Cardiac sarcoidosis is more prevalent among African Americans and women in the United States; the annual incidence is 10.9 per 100,000 among whites and 35.5 per 100,000 among African Americans.[3] Outside the United States, the highest prevalence is reported among Scandinavians and Japanese. It is uncommon to observe sarcoidosis in patients who are young (<15 years of age) or older (>70 years of age).

Multiple environmental and genetic factors have been postulated as contributing factors to the development of sarcoidosis. Geographic, seasonal, and occupational clustering suggests possible infectious, environmental, or occupational etiologies. Recent evidence suggests an immunologic response to an unidentified antigen, which is triggered in genetically susceptible individuals. Association with human leukocyte antigen (HLA)—specifically HLA DQB1*0601 and HLADRB1*—has been reported.[4,5]

Most often, granulomatous involvement of the myocardium is patchy, rendering the utility of endomyocardial biopsy limited in detecting granulomas. The granulomas are composed of macrophages, histiocytes, and lymphocytes and result in myocardial edema, granulomatous infiltration, and fibrosis. The most common cardiac sites for granulomas are the basal septum, atrioventricular (AV) node, bundle of His, ventricular free walls, and papillary muscles. In cases of severe disease, especially presenting as dilated cardiomyopathy, granulomas maybe absent, and extensive fibrosis may be present instead. Although left ventricular dysfunction is common, it not uncommon to have right ventricular dysfunction, especially in patients with sarcoid-related pulmonary hypertension. Cardiac sarcoid can masquerade as arrhythmogenic right ventricular

TABLE 72.1 Etiologies of Restrictive Cardiomyopathy

Myocardial Causes
Infiltrative
Amyloidosis
Sarcoidosis
Noninfiltrative
Idiopathic
Myofibrillar myopathies
Scleroderma
Storage Disorders
Fabry disease
Gaucher disease
Hereditary hemochromatosis
Mucopolysaccharidoses
Niemann-Pick disease
Endomyocardial Causes
Carcinoid
Chemotherapeutic toxicity (eg, anthracyclines)
Drugs (busulfan, ergotamine, serotonin)
Endomyocardial fibrosis
Hypereosinophilic syndrome
Metastatic malignancy
Radiation toxicity

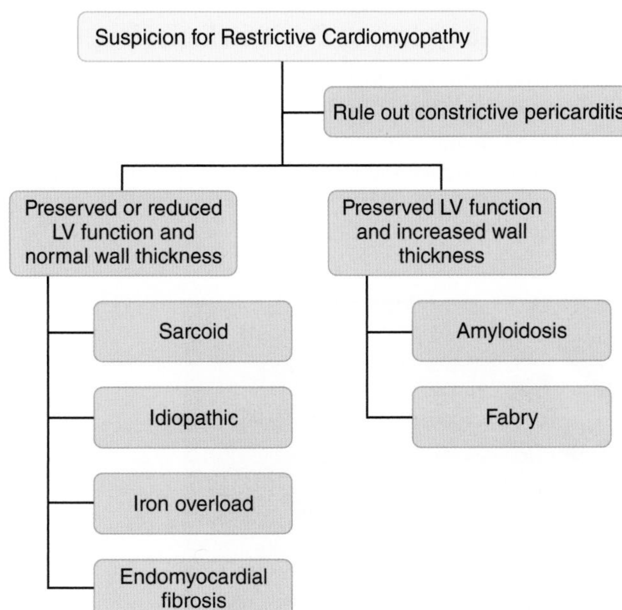

ALGORITHM 72.1 Differential diagnosis for common types of restrictive cardiomyopathy. LV, left ventricular.

dysplasia, including aneurysm formation and predominant right ventricular involvement.

Clinical Presentation: Cardiac Sarcoidosis

The most common presentation of sarcoidosis results from pulmonary involvement. More than half of patients with sarcoidosis have parenchymal tissue involvement, and a quarter of the patients have hilar lymphadenopathy. Isolated cardiac involvement occurs in about 35% to 65% of all initial cardiac presentations, including brady and tachyarrhythmias. The clinical presentation is variable based on the extent, location, and activity of the granulomatous lesions. The most common presentations among cardiac sarcoidosis patients is cardiomyopathy with or without clinical heart failure, ventricular or atrial arrhythmias, heart block, and AV valvular regurgitation, which may be due to papillary muscle infiltration or direct involvement of the myocardium.[6]

Heart failure symptoms may be due to direct myocardial involvement, or secondary from valvular regurgitation or right ventricular dysfunction as a result of pulmonary involvement. Atrial arrhythmias are common and likely result from ventricular diastolic dysfunction, elevated filling pressure, and subsequent atrial dilation and scarring.[7] Supraventricular arrhythmias can occur in one-third of the patients with cardiac sarcoidosis. Ventricular arrhythmias are also common as a result of myocardial fibrosis and arise from late-onset scar formation and re-entrant circuit in areas of slow conduction. Most cases of recurrent ventricular arrhythmia arise from the right ventricular or left ventricular septal endocardial wall. In late-stage cardiac sarcoidosis, these arrhythmias can be hard to manage despite medications or ablations. Sudden death is a common presentation for ventricular arrhythmias and can occur in 25% of cases.[8] Conduction abnormalities are common, with complete heart block the most common conduction abnormality (25%-30%) and may present as syncope or sudden cardiac death.[9]

DIAGNOSIS: CARDIAC SARCOIDOSIS

Initial workup (**Algorithm 72.2**) involves the electrocardiogram (ECG), which may be abnormal in patients with clinically manifest cardiac disease.[10] Findings may include fragmentation of the QRS complex, right bundle branch block, left bundle branch block, or varying degrees of heart block. Rarely, pathologic Q waves or epsilon waves may occur.

Echocardiography may be helpful in those with symptomatic disease but can be normal in clinically silent cardiac sarcoidosis or even in cases of sudden cardiac death. Echocardiographic abnormalities can be seen in 14% to 56% of patients with cardiac sarcoidosis.[11] Unfortunately, these findings can be variable and not specific to cardiac sarcoidosis. They commonly include ventricular diastolic and/or systolic dysfunction, regional wall motion abnormalities in a noncoronary pattern, basal septal thinning, and discrete aneurysms.

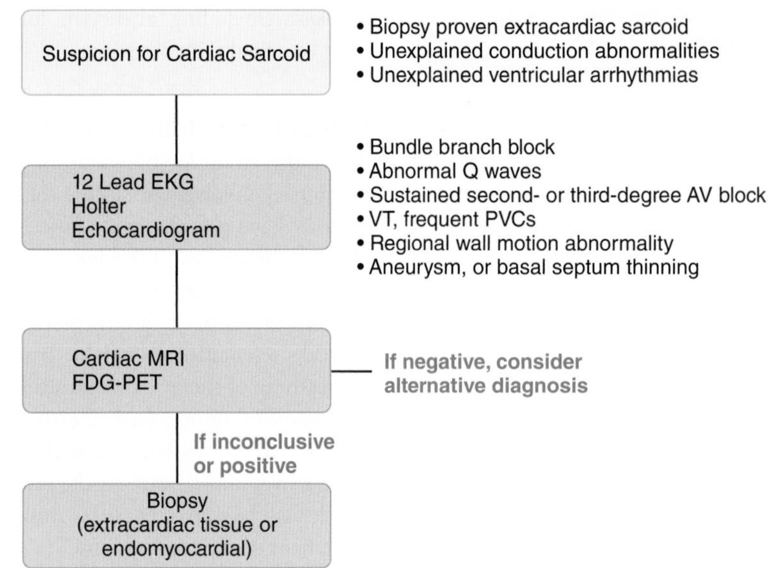

ALGORITHM 72.2 Simplified algorithm for diagnosis of cardiac sarcoidosis. AV, atrioventricular; EKG, electrocardiography; FDG-PET, ^{18}F-fluorodeoxyglucose positron emission tomography; MRI, magnetic resonance imaging; PVCs, premature ventricular contractions; VT, ventricular tachycardia.

Cardiac Magnetic Resonance Imaging: Cardiac Sarcoidosis

CMRI has emerged as an important diagnostic tool for cardiac sarcoidosis with good sensitivity and specificity. CMRI findings may vary based on the phase of sarcoid involvement. An acute myocarditis-like inflammatory picture including myocardial edema on T2 imaging during the acute phase may be observed[2] **(Figure 72.1A,B)**. Later in the disease, late gadolinium enhancement (LGE) can identify areas of fibrosis. Although there is no definitive diagnostic pattern of LGE—it can show a coronary or noncoronary pattern—it usually spares the endocardium and is patchy and multifocal. LGE is more commonly present in the basal septum and lateral walls in the mid-myocardium and epicardium.[12] Right ventricular free wall and transmural involvement may also be seen in selected cases. The extent of LGE burden is associated with the risk of adverse events including ventricular arrhythmias[13] and is useful in predicting response to treatment, with a higher LGE burden predictive of lack of corticosteroid responsiveness and less likelihood of improvement in left ventricular systolic function.

^{18}F-Fluorodeoxyglucose Positron Emission Tomography Imaging: Cardiac Sarcoidosis

^{18}F-fluorodeoxyglucose positron emission tomography (FDG-PET) imaging is complementary to CMRI for diagnosing cardiac sarcoid and in monitoring response to therapy.

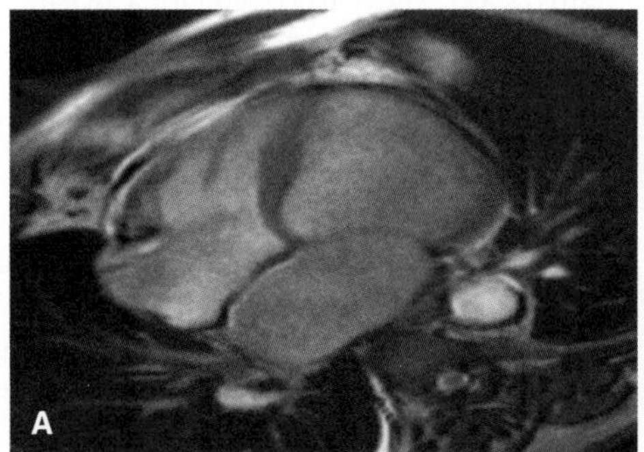

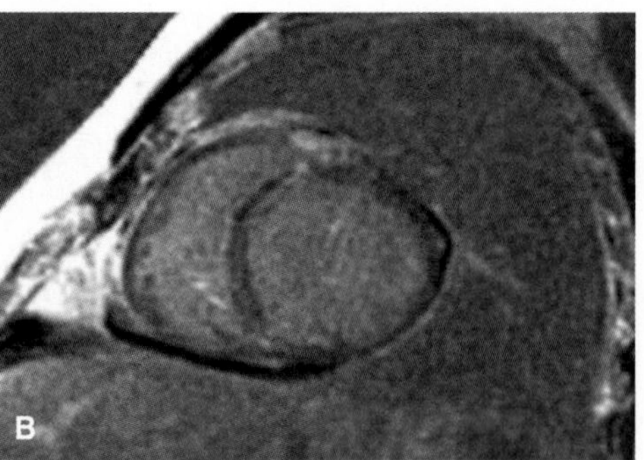

FIGURE 72.1 Cardiac sarcoid. A four-chamber FIESTA (steady-state) view showing the enlarged left ventricle and left atrium (**panel A**) and T1-weighted post-gadolinium contrast magnetic resonance imaging showing late gadolinium enhancement diffusely in the mid-wall of the septum and a couple foci in the lateral wall (**panel B**).

FDG-PET can identify active inflammation due to affinity of activated macrophages to have higher metabolic rate and thus greater uptake of FDG. Essentially, FDG uptake signifies active disease and, when combined with a perfusion tracer, can provide information on fibrotic activity **(Figure 72.2A,B)**. It also allows longitudinal monitoring of response to treatment.

Endomyocardial biopsy allows histologic confirmation of noncaseating granulomas. The yield is, however, low; a sensitivity of less than 25%, which may go up to 50% in cases where biopsy is guided by intracardiac echo, PET, or magnetic resonance imaging (MRI). Endomyocardial biopsy is useful in select cases to distinguish cardiac sarcoidosis from other forms of restrictive or inflammatory cardiomyopathies. Targeted biopsy of an extracardiac organ—such as lymph nodes or lungs—may be preferable initially, with endomyocardial biopsy reserved for select cases where extracardiac tissue may not be easily available or is nondiagnostic.

MANAGEMENT: CARDIAC SARCOIDOSIS

Management of cardiac sarcoid revolves around pharmacotherapy for heart failure, immunosuppressants, arrhythmia management, and decision on implantable cardioverter device (ICD) placement. Although there is a paucity of randomized clinical trials in the management of cardiac sarcoid, it is common practice to initiate and optimize guideline-driven medical therapy in those with ventricular systolic dysfunction. Immunosuppressive therapy remains the cornerstone in management strategy.[14] Multiple nonrandomized trials have demonstrated the utility of immunosuppressants in patients with cardiac sarcoid, with steroids being the main agent.[15] Steroids have been beneficial for treating atrial and ventricular tachyarrhythmias and ventricular systolic dysfunction, particularly in early disease before fibrosis is evident on CMRI. Prednisone is the agent of choice and is usually started at 1 mg/kg daily up to 40 mg/day, which is gradually tapered off to a maintenance dose. The level of scar burden and ventricular arrhythmias may predict response to steroids. Methotrexate is the second-line agent that is commonly used concomitantly with steroids in nonresponders or in a steroid-sparing strategy.[16] Other agents that have been reported to be useful include mycophenolate mofetil, anti–tumor necrosis factor α antibodies, azathioprine, cyclophosphamide, infliximab, adalimumab, and rituximab.

Arrhythmia management includes steroids to reduce the risk of ventricular arrhythmia and reverse heart block. The consensus is that ICD implantation is reasonable in patients with ventricular dysfunction (left ventricular ejection fraction <50%) and sustained ventricular arrhythmias, syncope, or sustained ventricular tachycardia on electrophysiologic study.[17] Similarly, pacemaker implantation is considered appropriate among those with second -or third-degree conduction block. A pacemaker/ICD may be considered in those patients requiring a pacemaker for heart block but with concomitant left ventricular dysfunction. The role of ICD in those with preserved ejection fraction is not clear. A strategy for ablation for sustained or recurrent ventricular tachycardia due to cardiac sarcoid has shown to be successful.

For patients with severe left ventricular dysfunction, advanced therapies such as left ventricular assist devices (VADs) and cardiac transplantation should be considered. While the total number of patients undergoing cardiac transplantation because of underlying cardiac sarcoidosis is low, it may be underestimated due to under diagnosis. More importantly, post-transplant outcomes in patients with sarcoidosis are similar to those with other underlying etiologies.[18]

CARDIAC AMYLOIDOSIS

Cardiac amyloidosis is a disorder of protein misfolding due to unstable tertiary structures leading to insoluble fibrils that can accumulate in various organs, most notably the myocardium, ultimately leading to clinical heart failure. It is subcategorized according to the type of misfolded protein, and, although there are more than 30 identified proteins that can result in amyloidosis, there are only 5 that typically result in cardiac involvement: immunoglobulin light chain, immunoglobulin heavy chain, serum amyloid A, apolipoprotein A1, and transthyretin.

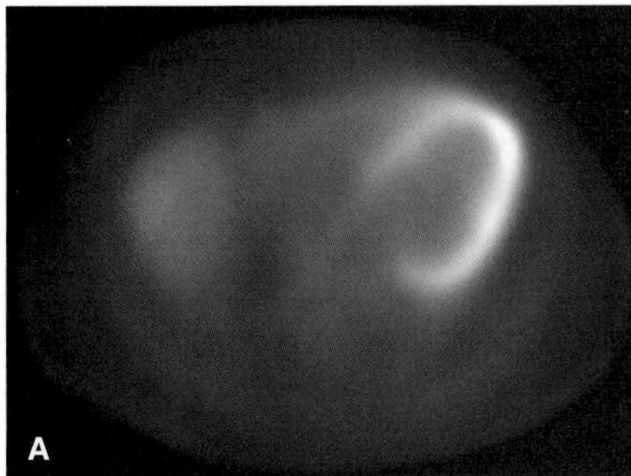

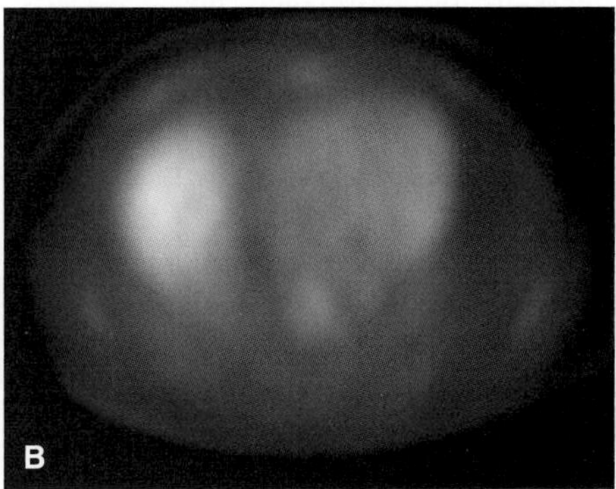

FIGURE 72.2 Utility of FDG-PET in cardiac sarcoid. The pre-steroid image **(A)** shows diffuse FDG uptake consistent with inflammation. The post-steroid image **(B)** shows significant improvement with mild residual uptake only in the basilar lateral wall. FDG-PET, ^{18}F-fluorodeoxyglucose positron emission tomography.

The vast majority of cases of cardiac amyloidosis can be categorized into either primary light-chain (AL) amyloidosis or transthyretin amyloidosis (ATTR).

The amyloid fibrils found in AL amyloidosis are the result of immunoglobulins that are produced by a clonal plasma cell dyscrasia, such as multiple myeloma. These light chains can be characterized as having either a κ or λ predominant pattern, which can be detected on a serum free light-chain assay. Estimates suggest that there are approximately 3000 new cases of AL amyloidosis every year, and half of patients with AL amyloidosis have evidence of cardiac involvement, highlighting the importance of recognizing the presence of AL amyloidosis.[19] The degree of cardiac involvement is strongly associated with poor survival, with median survival of 6 months for untreated AL cardiac amyloidosis after onset of heart failure.

Conversely, the fibrils formed in ATTR are the result of destabilization of the quaternary protein structure of transthyretin. Transthyretin, previously known as *prealbumin*, is a protein that is produced by the liver, which circulates in a tetrameric form and transports thyroid hormone and retinol (vitamin A). Through varying mechanisms, the tetramers dissociate into oligomers and monomers, which ultimately deposit in various organ systems, most notably the heart. According to autopsy data, 17% of subjects older than 80 years with heart failure with preserved ejection fraction (HFpEF) demonstrated deposition of transthyretin within cardiac tissue.[20] Hereditary ATTR (ATTRh) is secondary to an autosomal dominant condition, which results in an amino acid substitution of transthyretin, subsequently causing tetramer destabilization and formation of amyloid fibrils. ATTRh can result in a primarily familial amyloid polyneuropathy, a predominant familial amyloid cardiomyopathy, or an overlap of the two syndromes. The three principal genetic polymorphisms that result in familial amyloid cardiomyopathy include Val122Ile, Leu111Met, and Ile68Leu. ATTRh is considered to be rare owing to variable penetrance, though an estimated 3% to 4% of persons of African or Caribbean descent are carriers of the Val122Ile mutation.[21]

Clinical Presentation: Cardiac Amyloidosis

Cardiac amyloidosis may manifest with signs and symptoms of heart failure as a result of diastolic heart failure; however, a later disease stage may present with ventricular systolic dysfunction. Patients may exhibit symptoms consistent with a low cardiac output state (ie, early fatigue), chest pain, and exertional dyspnea. Owing to a rise in atrial pressures and resultant atrial dilatation, concomitant atrial arrhythmias are also common.[22] Orthostasis and intolerance to standard heart failure therapies including angiotensin-converting enzyme inhibitors, angiotensin receptor blockers, and β-blockers is fairly common.

Patients with AL amyloid typically present between the ages of 40 and 70 years with a relatively equal male-to-female ratio and exhibit periorbital ecchymoses and macroglossia.[23] Isolated cardiac infiltration is rare, and patients tend to present with multiorgan involvement because of amyloid fibril deposition in the kidneys, liver, lungs, gastrointestinal tract, soft tissues, and nervous system (**Table 72.2**).[24] Renal deposition with resultant proteinuria is a common manifestation of AL amyloidosis, whereas ATTR uncommonly has renal involvement. A triad of heart failure, hepatomegaly, and proteinuria should prompt consideration for the presence of AL amyloidosis.

There are various clinical features of ATTRh and wild-type ATTR (ATTRwt) that are unique from those of AL amyloidosis, as well as between each other (**Table 72.2**). As previously discussed, patients with ATTRh may present with primary cardiac infiltration, primary neurologic involvement, or an overlap syndrome.[25] The age of onset varies depending on the genetic polymorphism; however, the cardiomyopathy tends to occur after the sixth decade of life, whereas the polyneuropathy tends to present two decades earlier. Patients with the Val30Met mutation can present with an earlier onset aggressive polyneuropathy versus a later onset mixed disease process.[21] Val122Ile results in a primary cardiomyopathy phenotype among persons of African and Caribbean descent, and more than 50% of patients present with concurrent sensory neuropathies. Alternatively, Ile18Leu and Leu111Met are endemic to Italy and Denmark, resulting in an early-onset severe restrictive cardiomyopathy.[23] In general, the kidneys are not involved in

TABLE 72.2 Extracardiac Manifestations of Amyloidosis

Organ System	Clinical Features
Light-Chain Amyloidosis	
Hematologic	Periorbital purpura, easy bruising
Nervous system	Polyneuropathy, autonomic dysfunction, gastroparesis
Kidney	Proteinuria, renal failure
Liver	Hepatomegaly
Gastrointestinal	Early satiety, constipation, diarrhea
Pulmonary	Pleural effusions, diffuse alveolar infiltrates
Soft tissue/musculoskeletal	Bilateral carpal tunnel syndrome, rash, macroglossia
Transthyretin Amyloidosis	
Nervous system	Polyneuropathy, autonomic dysfunction, gastroparesis
Kidney	Renal impairment (rarely ATTRh)
Gastrointestinal	Early satiety, constipation, diarrhea
Soft tissue/musculoskeletal	Carpal tunnel syndrome, lumbar spinal stenosis, spontaneous biceps tendon rupture
Ocular	Vitreous opacification (ATTRh)
Urologic	Hematuria

ATTRh, hereditary transthyretin amyloidosis.

transthyretin amyloid cardiomyopathy (ATTR-CM); however, renal failure can accompany Val30Met mutation. In contrast to AL amyloidosis, the gastrointestinal symptoms of diarrhea, constipation, and early satiety that accompany individuals with ATTRh are the result of a neuropathy rather than direct amyloid fibril infiltration of the gastrointestinal tract.

The average age of presentation for ATTRwt is the seventh decade, with a male predominance. There is an overlap in the demographics among patients with ATTRwt and aortic stenosis. Among patients undergoing transcatheter aortic valve replacement, 16% had evidence of ATTRwt on nuclear scintigraphy.[26] Furthermore, a diagnosis of low-flow, low-gradient severe aortic stenosis in an elderly patient with heart failure should prompt consideration for underlying ATTR-CM.

DIAGNOSIS: CARDIAC AMYLOIDOSIS

Central to the diagnostic algorithm for cardiac amyloidosis is heart failure in the presence of left ventricular hypertrophy on echocardiography without an identifiable underlying etiology. The phenotype of cardiac amyloidosis can appear similar to hypertensive cardiomyopathy and hypertrophic cardiomyopathy, with more than one-third of patients with ATTRwt being misdiagnosed as hypertensive heart disease.[27]

Owing to multisystemic involvement, an accurate diagnosis requires a high degree of clinical suspicion. A diagnostic overview is highlighted in **Algorithm 72.3**. In patients with a history of diastolic heart failure and/or echocardiographic left ventricular hypertrophy, it is important to recognize diagnostic "red flags" whose presence should raise suspicion for cardiac amyloidosis, particularly ATTR-CM[28] **(Table 72.3)**.

Amyloid fibril deposition in the tenosynovial tissue of the carpal tunnel results in nerve entrapment, causing carpal tunnel syndrome. The presence of bilateral carpal tunnel syndrome often predates the cardiomyopathy, and a history of biceps tendon muscle rupture or lumbar spinal stenosis should heighten clinical suspicion. Other highlights include the presence of polyneuropathies and/or dysautonomia, particularly due to orthostatic hypotension as well as intolerance to standard heart failure therapies (ie, angiotensin-converting enzyme inhibitors, angiotensin receptor blockers, and β-blockers).

Classically, patients with cardiac amyloidosis exhibit concentric left ventricular hypertrophy with septal and posterior wall thicknesses greater than or equal to 12 m. Additional findings include atrial enlargement, right ventricular free wall hypertrophy, thickened AV valves, and pericardial effusion. Although a "speckled" appearance on nonharmonic echocardiographic imaging was touted to be diagnostic of cardiac amyloidosis (ie, due to the echogenic nature of amyloid within the myocardium), recent studies have shown that it is neither specific nor sensitive for cardiac amyloidosis **(Figure 72.3A-D)**. Abnormal diastolic function is present with restrictive physiology seen in

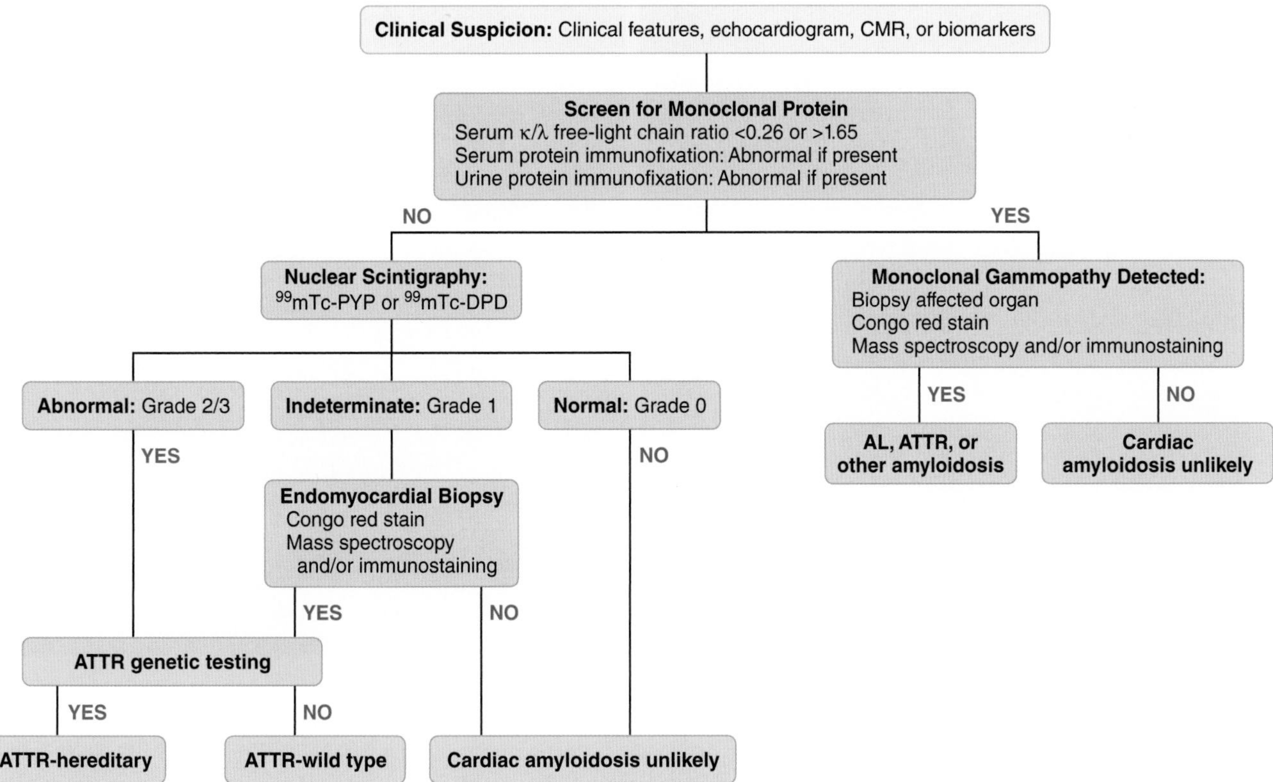

ALGORITHM 72.3 Diagnostic overview for cardiac amyloidosis. AL, primary light-chain amyloidosis; ATTR, transthyretin amyloidosis; CMR, cardiac magnetic resonance imaging; ^{99}mTc-PYP, 99m-technetium pyrophosphate; ^{99}mTc-DPD, 99m technetium-3,3-diphosphono-1,2-propanodicarboxylic.

TABLE 72.3 "Red Flags" Features in Suspected Cardiac Amyloidosis

Clinical Features
Orthopedic manifestations: carpal tunnel syndrome, lumbar spinal stenosis, biceps tendon rupture
Symptoms of polyneuropathy or dysautonomia
Intolerance to standard heart failure therapies and/or antihypertensive medications
Family history of cardiomyopathy and/or polyneuropathy
Diagnostic Features
Discordance between QRS voltage on electrocardiogram and echocardiographic left ventricular hypertrophy
Unexplained left ventricular hypertrophy, right ventricular hypertrophy, and/or atrial wall thickening
Reduced global longitudinal strain with apical-sparing pattern
Unexplained atrioventricular block
Persistent mildly elevated troponin levels

late stages. Global longitudinal strain typically demonstrates an "apical-sparing" pattern with a base-to-apex strain gradient (**Figure 72.4**).

Diagnostic Testing

The most sensitive ECG feature of cardiac amyloidosis is the discrepancy between the presence of ventricular hypertrophy and a low QRS voltage on the ECG, termed an *abnormal voltage/mass ratio*, which is present in 73% to 80% of patients with cardiac amyloidosis.[29] The presence of AV block, atrial arrhythmias, and pseudo-infarction patterns in the precordial leads is common.

Classically, amyloidosis exhibits a pattern of global subendocardial LGE on CMRI; however, this pattern can be varied, leading to significant challenges with obtaining an accurate diagnosis. False-negative results can occur if myocardial tissue is not correctly "nulled," and attention must be paid when choosing an appropriate inversion time for accurate nulling of

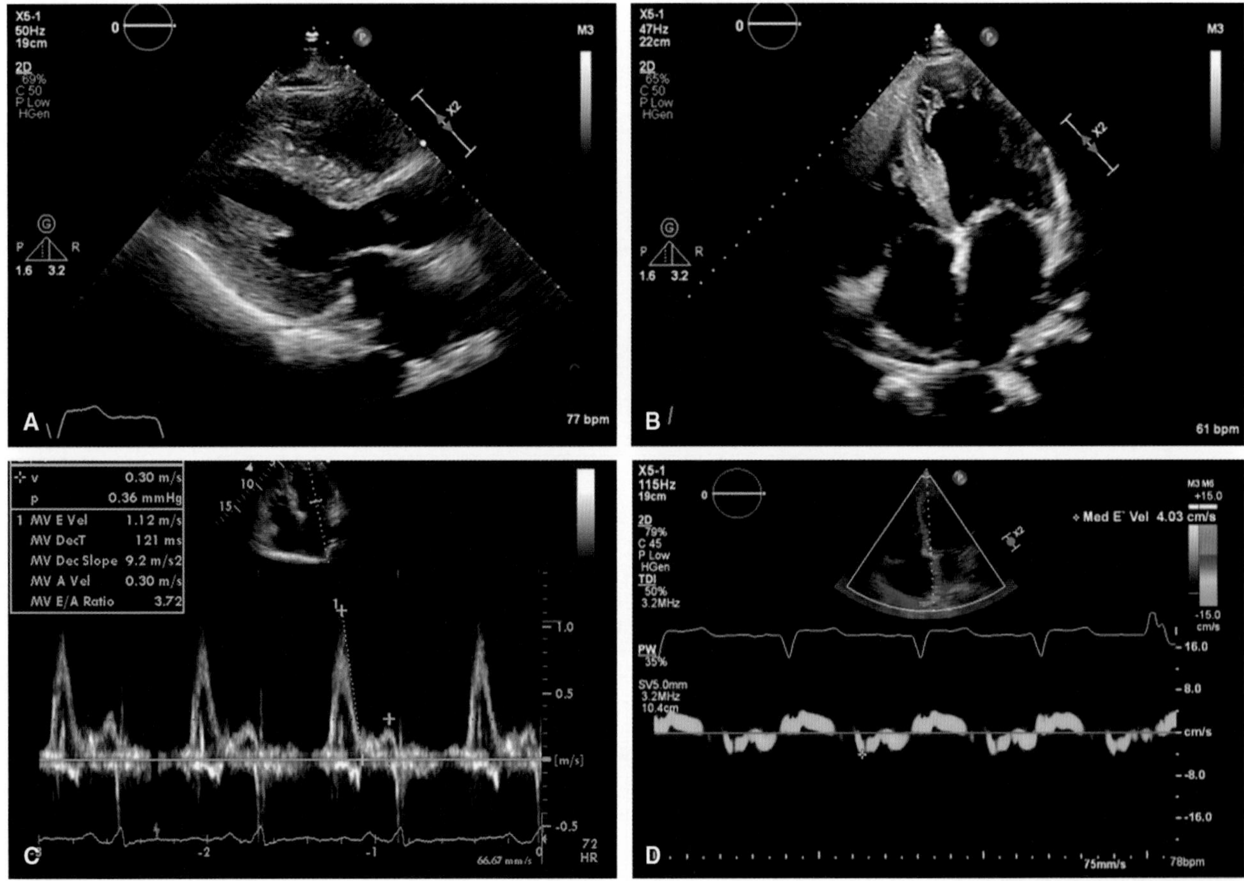

FIGURE 72.3 Echocardiographic features of cardiac amyloidosis. Images demonstrating typical features of cardiac amyloidosis. **A.** Two-dimensional parasternal long-axis view demonstrating concentric left ventricular hypertrophy and myocardial speckling. **B.** Two-dimensional apical four chamber demonstrating concentric left ventricular hypertrophy, biatrial enlargement, mitral leaflet thickening, and a small pericardial effusion. **C.** Pulse-wave Doppler of mitral inflow showing a marked increase in *E*/*A* ratio with a prominent *E* wave, rapid *E* wave deceleration time, and with a marked reduction in transmitral *A* velocity. **D.** Tissue Doppler of the medial mitral annulus demonstrating a significant reduction in *e*′ diastolic velocities.

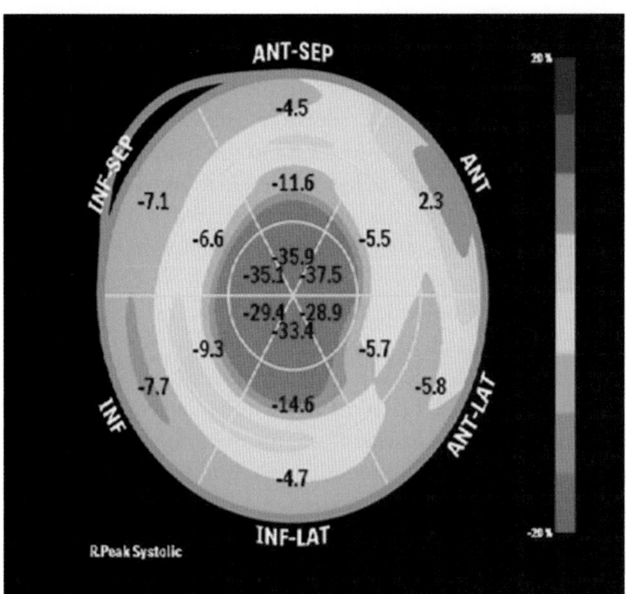

FIGURE 72.4 Myocardial strain in cardiac amyloidosis. Bull's-eye color-coded strain image depicting preserved apical strain and significantly reduced basal strain ("apical-sparing" pattern).

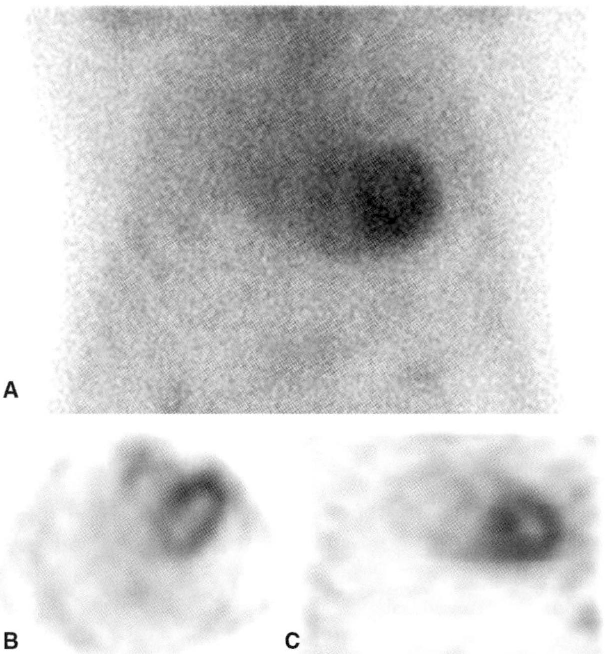

FIGURE 72.5 99m-Technetium pyrophosphate (99^{m}Tc-PYP) scintigraphy. **A.** A 3-hour planar Technetium-99m Pyrophosphate (PYP) showing marked myocardial uptake with nearly absent rib uptake: Perugini grade 3. **B and C.** Lower panels: Corresponding SPECT images in transverse and coronal planes depicting intense myocardial uptake with absence of radiotracer in the blood pool.

the myocardium. T1 mapping along with myocardial extracellular volume fraction both enhance the diagnostic utility of CMRI.[30]

Definitive diagnosis must be obtained and subtyped according to the amyloid fibrils as either AL or ATTR. First, a diagnosis of AL cardiac amyloidosis must be excluded via evaluation for a monoclonal gammopathy. The presence of a band on either serum or urine immunofixation electrophoresis, or an abnormal serum free light-chain ratio (<0.26 or >1.65) signifies the presence of a monoclonal protein.[31] Once a monoclonal gammopathy has been excluded, diagnosis of ATTR-CM can be pursued with myocardial scintigraphy, using 99m-technetium phosphate derivatives **(Figure 72.5A-C)**. 99m-technetium pyrophosphate (^{99}mTc-PYP) or 99m technetium-3,3-diphosphono-1,2-propanodicarboxylic (^{99}mTc-DPD) in Europe is particularly avid for ATTR-CM (both ATTRwt and ATTRh), although they demonstrate minimal to no uptake in AL cardiac amyloidosis. When a circular region of interest is made around the heart (to represent myocardial ^{99}mTc-PYP uptake) and this is compared to a "mirror image" over the contralateral chest, a heart/contralateral lung (H/CL) ratio of greater than 1.5 is highly sensitive and specific in the identification of ATTR-CM.[32] A semiquantitative visual scoring system is an additional means of identification of ATTR-CM, with an excellent sensitivity (>99%) for the detection of ATTR-CM, as subjects with myocardial uptake equal to or more than the contralateral ribs representing a "positive" study.[33] Importantly, AL cardiac amyloidosis can occasionally result in a mildly "positive" test; therefore, laboratory testing to exclude a monoclonal protein is mandatory.[34]

Endomyocardial Biopsy

Endomyocardial biopsy remains the gold standard for the diagnosis of cardiac amyloidosis with high sensitivity and specificity. Although biopsy should not be used as a first-line diagnostic strategy, it is particular useful in clarifying the diagnosis when ^{99}mTc-PYP is indeterminate and laboratory testing has excluded AL amyloidosis.[35] Apple-green birefringence is visualized under polarized light following Congo red staining of the myocardial sample. Proteomic and mass spectrometry technology is used to determine particular amyloid proteins. The diagnostic yield of extracardiac tissue depends on the underlying etiology of the amyloidosis. Generally, a fat pad biopsy is not a recommended strategy for the diagnosis of cardiac amyloidosis owing to its low sensitivity, particularly in patients with ATTR-CM.

Genetic Testing

Upon establishment of a diagnosis of ATTR-CM, *TTR* gene sequencing is recommended as this is the only method of differentiating ATTRh from ATTRwt. Depending on the mutation, there can be varying degrees of neuropathies, cardiac involvement, and ages of presentation; some patients may present with a more prominent polyneuropathy, whereas others, including African Americans with the Val122Ile mutation, may present with a predominant cardiomyopathy.[36,37]

MANAGEMENT: AMYLOIDOSIS

Treatment of AL amyloidosis involves the use of chemotherapeutic agents, including steroids, alkylating agents such as melphalan, proteasome inhibitors, and immunomodulatory agents, which largely have been used in the treatment of multiple myeloma, with the goal of therapy to target the plasma cells involved in the clonal expansion of the free light chains.[38] Autologous stem cell transplantation (SCT) can provide lasting hematologic and cardiac responses; however, patients with advanced cardiac involvement and heart failure are the poor candidates for high-dose chemotherapy with SCT, making patient selection critical in this process.[23,39] Subjects with elevation in cardiac biomarkers, significant renal impairment, symptomatic heart failure, and those with depressed left ventricular ejection fractions are at high risk of morbidity and mortality with SCT.

Patients who are the poor candidates for SCT may be the candidates for bortezomib-based regimens, including cyclophosphamide, bortezomib, and dexamethasone (CyBorD) or bortezomib, melphalan, and dexamethasone. Immunomodulatory agents, including lenalidomide, thalidomide, and pomalidomide, are beneficial to patients with relapsed AL amyloidosis, with resistance to alkylating agents and bortezomib-based therapies.[40] Monoclonal antibodies, including daratumumab, an anti-CD38 monoclonal antibody, have demonstrated promise in the treatment of multiple myeloma, with evidence of good efficacy in early clinical trials of patients with refractory AL amyloidosis. Lastly, concurrent off-label use of doxycycline, which is an inhibitor of matrix metalloproteinases, along with chemotherapy has shown promise in patients with AL amyloidosis, with improved survival based on retrospective analyses.

Therapies for ATTR-CM can be divided into TTR stabilization, TTR silencing, and the emerging area of TTR disruption (**Table 72.4**). Transthyretin tetramer stabilizers prevent further breakdown of TTR and, thus, prevent continued deposition of the amyloid fibrils. Tafamidis binds selectively to the thyroxine-binding site of TTR and slows dissociation of TTR tetramers into monomers. In the ATTR-ACT trial, tafamidis was associated with a reduction in all-cause mortality and cardiovascular-related hospitalizations in both patients with ATTRwt or ATTRh.[41] The nonsteroidal anti-inflammatory medication, diflunisal, has been demonstrated to stabilize TTR in vitro. Although limited data exist, diflunisal has been associated with survival benefit in patients with ATTR-CM. The synthetic small molecule ligand, AG10, binds to TTR with great affinity to stabilize the tetramer and has demonstrated a favorable safety profile. It is currently under investigation.

In contrast, TTR protein silencers target the hepatic synthesis of TTR. Patisiran, an intravenously administered double-stranded small interfering RNA, and inotersen, a subcutaneously administered antisense oligonucleotide, reduce circulating TTR and progression of ATTRh-related polyneuropathy.[42,43] Although not prespecified end points, both therapies were associated with favorable cardiovascular outcomes in patients with cardiac involvement. Ongoing trials are evaluating the safety and efficacy of various TTR protein silencers in ATTR-CM.

Lastly, therapies targeting the clearance of amyloid deposits, including doxycycline plus tauroursodeoxycholic acid (TUDCA), green tea, and turmeric, have demonstrated limited efficacy, with significant side effects in the case of doxycycline administered concomitantly with TUDCA.

Orthotopic Heart Transplant

Mechanical circulatory support with a VAD as a bridge for orthotopic heart transplant (OHT) is generally an ineffective treatment strategy with poor outcomes, owing to the relatively small left ventricular chamber size, concentric left ventricular hypertrophy, and restrictive physiology, resulting in suction events and right heart failure. OHT in cardiac amyloidosis has

TABLE 72.4 Disease-Modifying Therapies for Transthyretin Amyloidosis

Drug	Indication	Mechanism of Action	Dose/Delivery	Side Effects
Tafamidis	ATTRwt-CM ATTRh-CM	TTR stabilizer	20 mg, 80 mg, 61 mg once daily (oral)	Gastrointestinal upset
Diflunisal	Off-label use ATTRwt-CM/N ATTRh-CM/N	TTR stabilizer	250 mg once daily (oral)	Fluid retention Renal dysfunction Bleeding
Patisiran	ATTRh-N	TTR silencer	0.3 mg/kg IV every 3 weeks	Vitamin A deficiency Infusion reaction
Inotersen	ATTRh-N	TTR silencer	284 mg/wk SQ	Vitamin A deficiency Infusion reaction Thrombocytopenia Glomerulonephritis

ATTRwt-CM, wild-type transthyretin cardiac amyloidosis; ATTRh-CM, hereditary transthyretin cardiac amyloidosis; ATTRh-N, neuropathy due to hereditary transthyretin amyloidosis; IV, intravenous; kg, kilogram; mg, milligram; SQ, subcutaneous; TTR, transthyretin.

proven to be an effective strategy in patients with end-stage cardiomyopathy with appropriate patient identification and selection.[44] In individuals with AL cardiac amyloidosis, it is important to ascertain the number of involved organ systems as those with extensive extracardiac involvement and advanced heart failure have poor clinical outcomes, and selection for OHT must be carefully scrutinized. Furthermore, it is paramount to target the plasma cell dyscrasia to prevent disease recurrence and amyloid deposition into the transplanted heart. In ATTR-CM, heart-liver transplantation may be performed in patients with ATTRh at risk of progression of neuropathy with OHT alone; however, TTR silencer therapy may result in an evolution of this treatment paradigm.

FABRY CARDIOMYOPATHY

Fabry disease is an X-linked, lysosomal storage disorder resulting from mutations in the gene that codes for the enzyme α-galactosidase. Deficiency in this enzyme results in progressive lysosomal accumulation of neutral glycosphingolipids, specifically sphingolipid (GL3).

CLINICAL PRESENTATION

Classically, the disease affects males early in life, with clinical onset in childhood. Progressive accumulation of globotriaosylceramide results in multiorgan involvement and progressive organ dysfunction and failure. The most commonly affected organs include the kidneys, nervous system, skin, eyes, vascular endothelium, and the heart. Although it typically occurs in men with transmission from women carriers (ie, X-linked), it can also affect women, though, usually later in life. In the absence of identified affected family members, the disease can progress unidentified and result in a missed diagnosis. Clinical manifestation may be subtle and may be misdiagnosed as malingering or are mistakenly attributed to other disorders, such as rheumatic fever, erythromelalgia, neurosis, Raynaud syndrome, multiple sclerosis, chronic intermittent demyelinating polyneuropathy, lupus, acute appendicitis, and growing pains.

Progressive glycosphingolipid accumulation occurs in the vascular endothelium and leads to cardiac, renal, brain involvement and results in early death. Among patients with Fabry disease, more than 50% have cardiac involvement, which presents as hypertrophic cardiomyopathy. Most patients have concentric left ventricular hypertrophy, without outflow tract obstruction, preserved ventricular ejection fraction, and diastolic dysfunction. Regional longitudinal function is abnormal, usually involving the basal posterolateral wall. Fibrosis starts from mid-myocardium and progresses to transmural involvement. The plasma α-galactosidase activity is undetectable or low, with the latter usually having mild disease.

Two types of clinical presentation may occur, including classic disease or a milder, late-onset, renal or cardiac apical variant.[45] Fabry disease usually presents in childhood and may manifest as intermittent episodes of acute pain in extremities (acroparesthesias) characterized by burning pain in the distal end of extremities, resulting in ischemic injury of peripheral nerves; red and purple punctate skin lesions (angiokeratomas) involving the lower midsection, buttocks, thighs, and upper parts of the legs; a corneal opacity that does not affect vision; hypohidrosis; extreme temperature and exercise intolerance; mild proteinuria; and gastrointestinal problems. Cardiac manifestations include left ventricular hypertrophy, valvular insufficiency (especially mitral insufficiency), ascending aortic dilatation, small-vessel coronary artery disease, and conduction abnormalities, such as nonspecific conduction delays and bradycardia. Some patients may have palpitations or arrhythmia and require pacemakers. Some may have angina due to small-vessel disease and left ventricular hypertrophy rather than epicardial coronary artery disease. Cerebrovascular manifestations include early stroke, transient ischemic attacks, white matter lesions, hemiparesis, and vertigo. The underlying pathophysiology is small-vessel vascular disease from the deposition of glycosphingolipid and resultant vascular insufficiency. Age at onset and phenotypic variability correlate with the degree of α-galactosidase enzyme activity-level deficiency. Low enzyme activity is associated with early onset and severity of disease, whereas carriers may remain asymptomatic, few may develop renal or cardiac involvement in childhood and adulthood, including left ventricular hypertrophy and cardiomyopathy.[46] Late-onset phenotype may be present in atypical male variants who have a milder disease without any early manifestations of classic Fabry disease. This is partly due to low residual α-galactosidase levels. However, they may present with late-onset cardiomegaly and mild proteinuria—usually after 40 years of age—and this may be an under-recognized etiology of idiopathic left ventricular hypertrophy or late-onset hypertrophic cardiomyopathy.

DIAGNOSIS: FABRY CARDIOMYOPATHY

Diagnosis is made by determining α-galactosidase levels in plasma or peripheral leukocytes. Female carriers can have normal to very low α-galactosidase A activity, and molecular genetic testing may demonstrate their specific gene mutation. A comprehensive genetic panel will also evaluate for sarcomeric mutations typical for hypertrophic cardiomyopathy. ECG may show a short PR interval, left ventricular hypertrophy, heart block, or nonspecific intraventricular conduction delays. Echocardiography may demonstrate mild-to-severe left ventricular hypertrophy and diastolic abnormalities; systolic function is usually preserved. An endomyocardial biopsy may show inclusions in vascular endothelial cytoplasm on light or electron microscopy.

MANAGEMENT: FABRY CARDIOMYOPATHY

Management of Fabry cardiomyopathy involves accurate diagnosis, specifically in those patients with unexplained hypertrophic cardiomyopathy or late-onset cardiac variants with low residual enzyme activity, including evaluation of the severity of fibrosis.[47] Treatment involves enzyme replacement therapy with recombinant α-galactosidase A intravenously every 2 weeks, which has been shown to arrest progression and, possibly, reverse early cardiomyopathy. Owing to multisystem organ involvement, a multidisciplinary approach in staging and management of various organ systems is recommended.

ENDOMYOCARDIAL FIBROSIS

Endomyocardial fibrosis (EMF) or tropical EMF is the most common form of restrictive cardiomyopathy in developing countries.[48] The pathogenesis is not understood but may be due to genetic and environmental factors and is more prevalent in certain countries, such as Nigeria, Uganda, Brazil, Asia, and Equatorial Africa. There is a predominance among youth from lower socioeconomic status.

The natural history of EMF includes an active phase characterized by recurrent flares of inflammation, which subsequently leads to a chronic phase resulting in restrictive cardiomyopathy. During the active phase, EMF usually presents with a febrile illness associated with pancarditis and eosinophilia, dyspnea, itching, and periorbital swelling. Myocardial injury involves edema, eosinophilic infiltration, subendocardial myofibril necrosis, and vasculitis. Pericardial effusion and mural thrombi are frequent. Recurrent active episodes progress to the chronic phase, where biventricular failure or isolated right-sided heart failure is common, and isolated left-sided disease is rare.

CLINICAL PRESENTATION AND DIAGNOSTIC TESTING: ENDOMYOCARDIAL FIBROSIS

The clinical presentation includes facial edema, exophthalmos, jugular venous distension, hepatomegaly, splenomegaly, and abdominal swelling. Ascites can be profound. More specific features of EMF include hypertrophy of the parotid gland, periorbital edema, and proptosis.

Atrial fibrillation is common. Patients may have severe pulmonary hypertension from recurrent pulmonary emboli.

ECG may show conduction abnormalities, such as first-degree AV block, right bundle branch block, right ventricular hypertrophy, or right-axis deviation. Radiography may show pronounced cardiomegaly, biatrial dilatation, pulmonary infundibular dilatation, and pleural and pericardial effusions.

In the chronic form of EMF, the echocardiogram is consistent with restrictive cardiomyopathy with shrunken ventricles, severe biatrial dilation, and AV valvular abnormalities. The cardiac apex may be severely retracted, and the trabecular chamber almost virtually obliterated in right-sided EMF, leading to dilatation of the outflow tract. Obliterative fibrosis of the posterior tricuspid pocket results in severe tricuspid regurgitation. Other features include a restrictive inflow pattern, dilated inferior vena cava, and pericardial effusion.

CMRI may be valuable in the diagnosis of early EMF disease because it outlines the degree of chamber distortion and extent of thrombosis and fibrosis and may be useful before surgery to detail anatomic involvement and guide planning.

MANAGEMENT: ENDOMYOCARDIAL FIBROSIS

Medical management involves treatment of symptomatic heart failure using diuretics and angiotensin-converting enzyme inhibitors combined with anticoagulation for intracardiac thrombi. Although paracentesis offers short-term relief of ascites, its utility is limited because ascites often reaccumulates rapidly. Open heart surgery—surgical endocardectomy and valve repair—increases survival compared to medical treatment, but its availability is limited in many poor areas.[49]

IRON OVERLOAD CARDIOMYOPATHY

Iron overload cardiomyopathy occurs as a result of changes in iron hemostasis and is characterized by early restrictive cardiomyopathy, which may proceed to dilated cardiomyopathy. Excess iron deposition may result from increased absorption or excessive parenteral iron administration or blood transfusion. In elderly patients, increased use of parenteral iron for myelodysplastic syndrome or end-stage renal disease leads to higher risk of iron overload cardiomyopathy. Hereditary conditions such as hemochromatosis, thalassemia major, and sickle cell disease along with myelodysplasia or aplastic anemia may result in excessive iron or blood transfusion. In iron overload, the amount of iron is in excess of serum transferrin iron-binding capacity, leading to non-transferrin-bound iron and an increase in iron pool formation.

Hereditary hemochromatosis is an autosomal recessive disease typically resulting from the homozygous mutation Cys282Tyr in the "high iron" (*HFE*) gene. *HFE* gene impairs iron metabolism and increases gastrointestinal iron absorption. A minority (<10%) of cases are due to heterozygous mutations in Cys282Tyr and His63Asp. There is variable penetrance of disease, even with Cys282Tyr homozygotes. Iron is deposited in organs, including the heart, liver, thyroid, gonads, skin, and pancreatic islet cells, resulting in cirrhosis, cardiomyopathy, and diabetes, among other conditions. The presentation of hereditary hemochromatosis may vary widely with different genetic types. For example, type 2 usually presents by the second decade, whereas types 1 and 4 usually manifest in adulthood.

In type 1 hemochromatosis, mutations in the *HFE* gene involve either a single base pair change (C282Y) or a substitution (H63D). Type 2 is associated with mutations of the *HFE2* gene that encodes for hemojuvelin or in the hepcidin antimicrobial peptide (*HAMP*) gene that encodes for hepcidin. Type 3 hereditary hemochromatosis involves mutations in the *TfR2* gene that encodes for transferrin receptor 2. Type 4 is caused by mutations in the *SLC40A1* gene that encodes for ferroportin.

CLINICAL PRESENTATION: IRON OVERLOAD CARDIOMYOPATHY

Early stages in iron overload tend to present with nonspecific findings. Patients may have exertional dyspnea, supraventricular arrhythmias, first-degree AV block, and infrequently sudden death.

Screening tests for iron load include serum ferritin and percent transferrin saturation. A serum iron level of less than 200 ng/mL in women and 300 ng/mL in men or transferrin saturation of less than 45% in women and 50% in men exclude iron overload. Genetic testing for C282Y and H63D is recommended when elevated transferrin saturation is identified.

DIAGNOSIS: IRON OVERLOAD CARDIOMYOPATHY

Echocardiography is the primary screening tool to screen patients with suspected iron overload. Usually, left ventricular wall thickness is not increased, but impaired left ventricular diastolic function, restrictive filling pattern with or without atrial dilation, and biventricular dysfunction and dilation are present. Restrictive left ventricular filling with right ventricular dilation may be present. Longitudinal and circumferential strain rates may be reduced. CMRI is useful in quantification of myocardial iron burden. Shortened T2-weighted relaxation time is a measure of myocardial iron load and is useful in longitudinal monitoring and assessing response to therapy.

MANAGEMENT: IRON OVERLOAD CARDIOMYOPATHY

The primary management of iron overload—especially in hemochromatosis—involves phlebotomy. Each session of phlebotomy removes 200 to 250 mg of iron and may need to be performed one to two times per week to bring the transferrin saturation less than 30% and serum ferritin less than 50 ng/mL.[50] Subsequently, maintenance phlebotomy is performed to maintain serum ferritin levels less than 100 mg/mL or transferrin saturation less than 50%. Chelation therapy is an alternative when phlebotomy is not feasible. It is also instituted in transfusion-dependent patients to prevent myocardial iron deposition. Currently used chelators include parenteral deferoxamine, oral deferiprone, and deferasirox. CMR-based T2* imaging–guided early chelation can prevent iron overload cardiomyopathy and related complications. In those with iron overload cardiomyopathy, chelation therapy can lead to improvement in ventricular function and prevent arrhythmias and mortality.

FOLLOW-UP PATIENT CARE

Patients with restrictive cardiomyopathy require regular follow-up to evaluate clinical status, monitor adherence and proper use of medications, evaluate response to therapy, and assess potential need for changes in management. Each visit should assess ability to perform activities of daily living, volume status and body weight as well as diet and sodium intake. In addition, pneumococcal vaccination and annual influenza vaccination are indicated in these high-risk individuals.

RESEARCH AND FUTURE DIRECTIONS

Future developments focused on etiology of poorly understood restrictive cardiomyopathies such as sarcoidosis and EMF are needed. This will allow early diagnosis and tailored management. Disease awareness and a multidisciplinary approach to the management of some of the diseases involving multiple organ system need better adoption. As newer therapies become available for specific etiologies such as cardiac amyloid, awareness and appropriate implementation of algorithms will be required to tailor options to individual patients and their specific dominant phenotype. Lastly, better measures are needed to define prognosis and to identify patients who may benefit from existing and emergent therapies and consideration for palliation with poor prognosis.

KEY POINTS

- ✔ Unexplained hypertrophic cardiomyopathy needs further evaluation to exclude causes of restrictive cardiomyopathies.
- ✔ Constrictive pericarditis and restrictive cardiomyopathy present with similar symptoms and hemodynamic findings.
- ✔ Multimodality imaging approach needs to be utilized when a definitive diagnosis is absent.
- ✔ Immunosuppressants should be considered when appropriate in confirmed cases of cardiac sarcoid.
- ✔ Monitoring for atrial arrhythmias in restrictive cardiomyopathies is important to evaluate the need for anticoagulation.
- ✔ Evaluation of light-chain amyloidosis should be performed early in the workup for cardiac amyloidosis.
- ✔ ATTR-CM should be treated with recently approved drugs.
- ✔ If clinical suspicion persists despite noninvasive testing, endomyocardial biopsy should be considered.
- ✔ Female Fabry carriers can have normal to very low residual enzyme activity. Thus, molecular genetic testing for specific mutations in the α-galactosidase gene must be performed.
- ✔ Cardiac transplantation may be considered in select cases with advanced restrictive cardiomyopathy of varying etiology that is refractory to tailored management.

REFERENCES

1. Ammash NM, Seward JB, Bailey KR, Edwards WD, Tajik AJ. Clinical profile and outcome of idiopathic restrictive cardiomyopathy. *Circulation.* 2000;101(21):2490-2496.
2. Patel MR, Cawley PJ, Heitner JF, et al. Detection of myocardial damage in patients with sarcoidosis. *Circulation.* 2009;120(20):1969-1977.
3. Rybicki BA, Major M, Popovich J Jr, Maliarik MJ, Iannuzzi MC. Racial differences in sarcoidosis incidence: a 5-year study in a health maintenance organization. *Am J Epidemiol.* 1997;145(3):234-241.
4. Rossman MD, Thompson B, Frederick M, et al. HLA-DRB1*1101: a significant risk factor for sarcoidosis in blacks and whites. *Am J Hum Genet.* 2003;73(4):720-735.
5. Naruse TK, Matsuzawa Y, Ota M, et al. HLA-DQB1*0601 is primarily associated with the susceptibility to cardiac sarcoidosis. *Tissue Antigens.* 2000;56(1):52-57.

6. Pereira NL, Grogan M, Dec GW. Spectrum of restrictive and infiltrative cardiomyopathies: part 2 of a 2-part series. *J Am Coll Cardiol.* 2018;71(10):1149-1166.
7. Cain MA, Metzl MD, Patel AR, et al. Cardiac sarcoidosis detected by late gadolinium enhancement and prevalence of atrial arrhythmias. *Am J Cardiol.* 2014;113(9):1556-1560.
8. Hamzeh N, Steckman DA, Sauer WH, Judson MA. Pathophysiology and clinical management of cardiac sarcoidosis. *Nat Rev Cardiol.* 2015;12(5):278-288.
9. Nery PB, Beanlands RS, Nair GM, et al. Atrioventricular block as the initial manifestation of cardiac sarcoidosis in middle-aged adults. *J Cardiovasc Electrophysiol.* 2014;25(8):875-881.
10. Birnie DH, Nery PB, Ha AC, Beanlands RS. Cardiac sarcoidosis. *J Am Coll Cardiol.* 2016;68(4):411-421.
11. Hyodo E, Hozumi T, Takemoto Y, et al. Early detection of cardiac involvement in patients with sarcoidosis by a non-invasive method with ultrasonic tissue characterisation. *Heart.* 2004;90(11):1275-1280.
12. Ichinose A, Otani H, Oikawa M, et al. MRI of cardiac sarcoidosis: basal and subepicardial localization of myocardial lesions and their effect on left ventricular function. *AJR Am J Roentgenol.* 2008;191(3):862-869.
13. Greulich S, Deluigi CC, Gloekler S, et al. CMR imaging predicts death and other adverse events in suspected cardiac sarcoidosis. *JACC Cardiovasc Imaging.* 2013;6(4):501-511.
14. Hamzeh NY, Wamboldt FS, Weinberger HD. Management of cardiac sarcoidosis in the United States: a Delphi study. *Chest.* 2012;141(1):154-162.
15. Sadek MM, Yung D, Birnie DH, Beanlands RS, Nery PB. Corticosteroid therapy for cardiac sarcoidosis: a systematic review. *Can J Cardiol.* 2013;29(9):1034-1041.
16. Nagai S, Yokomatsu T, Tanizawa K, et al. Treatment with methotrexate and low-dose corticosteroids in sarcoidosis patients with cardiac lesions. *Intern Med.* 2014;53(23):2761.
17. Birnie DH, Sauer WH, Bogun F, et al. HRS expert consensus statement on the diagnosis and management of arrhythmias associated with cardiac sarcoidosis. *Heart Rhythm.* 2014;11(7):1305-1323.
18. Perkel D, Czer LS, Morrissey RP, et al. Heart transplantation for end-stage heart failure due to cardiac sarcoidosis. *Transplant Proc.* 2013;45(6):2384-2386.
19. Muchtar E, Buadi FK, Dispenzieri A, Gertz MA. Immunoglobulin light-chain amyloidosis: from basics to new developments in diagnosis, prognosis and therapy. *Acta Haematol.* 2016;135(3):172-190.
20. Mohammed SF, Mirzoyev SA, Edwards WD, et al. Left ventricular amyloid deposition in patients with heart failure and preserved ejection fraction. *JACC Heart Fail.* 2014;2(2):113-122.
21. Quarta CC, Falk RH, Solomon SD. V122I transthyretin variant in elderly black Americans. *N Engl J Med.* 2015;372(18):1769.
22. Longhi S, Quarta CC, Milandri A, et al. Atrial fibrillation in amyloidotic cardiomyopathy: prevalence, incidence, risk factors and prognostic role. *Amyloid.* 2015;22(3):147-155.
23. Maurer MS, Elliott P, Comenzo R, Semigran M, Rapezzi C. Addressing common questions encountered in the diagnosis and management of cardiac amyloidosis. *Circulation.* 2017;135(14):1357-1377.
24. Grogan M, Scott CG, Kyle RA, et al. Natural history of wild-type transthyretin cardiac amyloidosis and risk stratification using a novel staging system. *J Am Coll Cardiol.* 2016;68(10):1014-1020.
25. Rapezzi C, Merlini G, Quarta CC, et al. Systemic cardiac amyloidoses: disease profiles and clinical courses of the 3 main types. *Circulation.* 2009;120(13):1203-1212.
26. Castaño A, Narotsky DL, Hamid N, et al. Unveiling transthyretin cardiac amyloidosis and its predictors among elderly patients with severe aortic stenosis undergoing transcatheter aortic valve replacement. *Eur Heart J.* 2017;38(38):2879-2887.
27. Gonzβlez-López E, Gagliardi C, Dominguez F, et al. Clinical characteristics of wild-type transthyretin cardiac amyloidosis: disproving myths. *Eur Heart J.* 2017;38(24):1895-1904.
28. Witteles RM, Bokhari S, Damy T, et al. Screening for transthyretin amyloid cardiomyopathy in everyday practice. *JACC Heart Fail.* 2019;7(8):709-716.
29. Cyrille NB, Goldsmith J, Alvarez J, Maurer MS. Prevalence and prognostic significance of low QRS voltage among the three main types of cardiac amyloidosis. *Am J Cardiol.* 2014;114(7):1089-1093.
30. Banypersad SM, Sado DM, Flett AS, et al. Quantification of myocardial extracellular volume fraction in systemic AL amyloidosis: an equilibrium contrast cardiovascular magnetic resonance study. *Circ Cardiovasc Imaging.* 2013;6(1):34-39.
31. Drayson M, Tang LX, Drew R, Mead GP, Carr-Smith H, Bradwell AR. Serum free light-chain measurements for identifying and monitoring patients with nonsecretory multiple myeloma. *Blood.* 2001;97(9):2900-2902.
32. Bokhari S, Castaño A, Pozniakoff T, Deslisle S, Latif F, Maurer MS. (99m)Tc-pyrophosphate scintigraphy for differentiating light-chain cardiac amyloidosis from the transthyretin-related familial and senile cardiac amyloidoses. *Circ Cardiovasc Imaging.* 2013;6(2):195-201.
33. Perugini E, Guidalotti PL, Salvi F, et al. Noninvasive etiologic diagnosis of cardiac amyloidosis using 99mTc-3,3-diphosphono-1,2-propanodicarboxylic acid scintigraphy. *J Am Coll Cardiol.* 2005;46(6):1076-1084.
34. Gillmore JD, Maurer MS, Falk RH, et al. Nonbiopsy diagnosis of cardiac transthyretin amyloidosis. *Circulation.* 2016;133(24):2404-2412.
35. Ardehali H, Qasim A, Cappola T, et al. Endomyocardial biopsy plays a role in diagnosing patients with unexplained cardiomyopathy. *Am Heart J.* 2004;147(5):919-923.
36. Rapezzi C, Quarta CC, Obici L, et al. Disease profile and differential diagnosis of hereditary transthyretin-related amyloidosis with exclusively cardiac phenotype: an Italian perspective. *Eur Heart J.* 2013;34(7):520-528.
37. Dungu JN. Cardiac amyloid—an update. *Eur Cardiol.* 2015;10(2):113-117.
38. Merlini G, Seldin DC, Gertz MA. Amyloidosis: pathogenesis and new therapeutic options. *J Clin Oncol.* 2011;29(14):1924-1933.
39. Cibeira MT, Sanchorawala V, Seldin DC, et al. Outcome of AL amyloidosis after high-dose melphalan and autologous stem cell transplantation: long-term results in a series of 421 patients. *Blood.* 2011;118(16):4346-4352.
40. Palladini G, Russo P, Foli A, et al. Salvage therapy with lenalidomide and dexamethasone in patients with advanced AL amyloidosis refractory to melphalan, bortezomib, and thalidomide. *Ann Hematol.* 2012;91(1):89-92.
41. Maurer MS, Schwartz JH, Gundapaneni B, et al. Tafamidis treatment for patients with transthyretin amyloid cardiomyopathy. *N Engl J Med.* 2018;379(11):1007-1016.
42. Adams D, Gonzalez-Duarte A, O'Riordan WD, et al. Patisiran, an RNAi therapeutic, for hereditary transthyretin amyloidosis. *N Engl J Med.* 2018;379(1):11-21.
43. Benson MD, Waddington-Cruz M, Berk JL, et al. Inotersen treatment for patients with hereditary transthyretin amyloidosis. *N Engl J Med.* 2018;379(1):22-31.
44. Barrett CD, Alexander KM, Zhao H, et al. Outcomes in patients with cardiac amyloidosis undergoing heart transplantation. *JACC Heart Fail.* 2020;8(6):461-468.
45. Eng CM, Fletcher J, Wilcox WR, et al. Fabry disease: baseline medical characteristics of a cohort of 1765 males and females in the Fabry Registry. *J Inherit Metab Dis.* 2007;30(2):184-192.
46. Drechsler C, Schmiedeke B, Niemann M, et al. Potential role of vitamin D deficiency on Fabry cardiomyopathy. *J Inherit Metab Dis.* 2014;37(2):289-295.
47. Weidemann F, Niemann M, Breunig F, et al. Long-term effects of enzyme replacement therapy on Fabry cardiomyopathy: evidence for a better outcome with early treatment. *Circulation.* 2009;119(4):524-529.
48. Grimaldi A, Mocumbi AO, Freers J, et al. Tropical endomyocardial fibrosis: natural history, challenges, and perspectives. *Circulation.* 2016;133(24):2503-2515.
49. Schneider U, Jenni R, Turina J, Turina M, Hess OM. Long-term follow up of patients with endomyocardial fibrosis: effects of surgery. *Heart.* 1998;79(4):362-367.
50. Kremastinos DT, Farmakis D. Iron overload cardiomyopathy in clinical practice. *Circulation.* 2011;124(20):2253-2263.

CHAPTER 73

MYOCARDITIS

Melissa A. Lyle, Lori A. Blauwet, and Leslie T. Cooper

INTRODUCTION

Myocarditis refers to inflammation of the myocardium and incorporates a broad spectrum of clinical and histopathologic presentations.[1] Acute myocarditis results from either an external event or an endogenous trigger. External causes include viruses, bacteria, parasites, drugs, and direct toxins, while internal triggers are associated with host autoantigen-mediated myocarditis. The initial cardiac injury precipitates an immunologic response, which results in cardiac inflammation. This chapter focuses on the diagnosis and management of common causes of acute and chronic myocarditis. The diagnosis and management of cardiac sarcoidosis are covered elsewhere.

The clinical presentation can range from subclinical disease to fulminant myocarditis that requires inotropic or mechanical circulatory support.[2] The host immune response can downregulate after clearance of damage with little scar or result in more persistent or extensive inflammation that permanently damages heart tissue. Usually the process is self-limited, but if the immune response persists, then cardiac remodeling can lead to chronic dilated cardiomyopathy (DCM). Up to 20% of patients with myocarditis develop chronic DCM.[1,3]

The Dallas criteria, proposed in 1986, defined acute myocarditis as an inflammatory cellular infiltrate with associated myocyte necrosis or degeneration of adjacent myocytes, noted on conventionally stained myocardial tissue sections.[4] However, these criteria have been criticized because of interreader variability and low sensitivity. Immunohistologic criteria, which rely on cell-specific immunoperoxidase stains for surface antigens including anti-CD3 (T lymphocytes), anti-CD68, and class I and II human leukocyte antigens, are thought to have greater sensitivity and better prognostic value.[5] Myocarditis accounts for 10% of initially unexplained DCM when the Dallas criteria are used. The rate of myocarditis increases from 20% to 30% when immunohistology establishes the diagnosis.[6]

Epidemiology

The true incidence of myocarditis is difficult to quantify given the wide range of clinical presentations; however, in 2019, an estimated 820,000 incident cases of myocarditis occurred in men and 608,000 cases in women. The overall global incidence of myocarditis during 2019 was estimated at 1.4 million or 19 per 100,000 population.[7] As a percentage of heart failure prevalence, the myocarditis burden varies from 0.5% to 4.0%. From 1990 to 2015, the death rate from myocarditis and cardiomyopathy together was approximately 5 per 100,000.[8] Based on autopsy and clinical case series, myocarditis is thought to be one of the leading causes of sudden cardiac death.[9] There is a bimodal distribution by age. Notably, the prevalence of myocarditis as a cause of cardiomyopathy is high in the first year of life. The increased rate and more fulminant presentation in infants can be attributed to an immature immune system. Myocarditis is responsible for approximately 2% of infant sudden cardiovascular deaths.[2] The prevalence of myocarditis relative to all heart failure declines between ages 1 and 12 years, then the risk again increases after puberty. The mean age of adults with most forms of myocarditis ranges between 20 and 51 years,[10] while the mean age of patients with giant cell myocarditis (GCM) is 42 years.[11]

Most case studies of myocarditis illustrate a male predominance, which is strongly influenced by sex hormones. In mice, estrogenic hormones protect against viral infection of cardiomyocytes and decrease the myocardial inflammatory response. Testosterone exerts a deleterious effect through inhibition of regulatory components and promotion of inflammasome-mediated, profibrotic pathways.[12] The severity of disease as assessed by the degree of delayed gadolinium enhancement on magnetic resonance imaging (MRI) is greater in men with myocarditis than women. In patients with severe myocarditis requiring mechanical circulatory support, female sex predicts a higher likelihood of bridge to recovery.[13]

PATHOGENESIS

Current understanding of cellular and molecular pathogenesis of acute myocarditis as being caused by an inciting event, such as a viral infection or a primary immunologic abnormality, is based mostly on animal models. Viral infection is one of the most common causes of myocarditis, and most of our understanding regarding the pathophysiology of viral myocarditis is specifically derived from mouse models with heightened autoimmunity with or without enteroviral infection. The pathogenesis of viral myocarditis may be conceptualized into overlapping phases of viral infection and replication, an immunologic response including innate and adaptive immune responses, and chronic cardiac remodeling. Viruses can enter the host via the gastrointestinal or respiratory systems and subsequently undergo replication in host organs such as the liver, spleen, and pancreas. Enteroviruses eventually reach the heart by hematogenous or lymphatic spread. At the cellular level, viruses are internalized after binding to a cell surface receptor leading to viral genome and proteome interaction with host cellular machinery. The mechanism varies by virus with coxsackieviruses and adenoviruses using a transmembrane molecule known as the coxsackievirus-adenovirus receptor (CAR), which triggers receptor-associated kinases such as p56lck, Fyn, and Abl to facilitate viral entry.[14] In immature cardiomyocytes, CAR is found on the entire surface of cardiac myocytes, which could partly explain the apparent susceptibility of infants to coxsackievirus B3-mediated myocarditis.[15] A recent study involving inducible CAR knockout mice illustrated that elimination of CAR prevented virus entry into myocytes and subsequent signs of inflammatory cardiomyopathy.[16] After entry of the enterovirus into the cell, the positive, single-strand RNA is released from the icosahedral capsid and translated using host translational mechanisms. Enteroviruses such as coxsackievirus B produce protease 2A, which can then cleave dystrophin and damage cytoskeletal components such as the dystrophin-sarcoglycan complex with disruption of the sarcolemmal membrane. Thus, viral proteases can cause cardiomyopathy in the absence of enteroviral replication.

Innate and antigen-specific immunity both play an important role in the pathogenesis of viral and autoimmune myocarditis. An antigen-independent tissue repair mechanism is initiated within days of enteroviral infection and serves to contain viral replication. During the innate immunity phase, multiple inflammatory markers—including cytokines, histamine, inducible nitric oxide, and complement components—are rapidly upregulated or released. Damage receptors, such as the toll-like receptor (TLR), signaling through the NLRP3 inflammasome are one of the earliest innate immune pathways. Damage receptors recognize pathogen motifs, such as double-stranded RNA, and activate cytosolic and nuclear signaling mechanisms, thereby increasing master proinflammatory cytokines such as interferon-1β. The downstream molecules activated by TLR signaling, specifically myeloid differentiation factor-88 (MyD88), which binds to toll-like receptor 4, play an important role in myocarditis, particularly viral infections. Mice with global knockout of MyD88 are noted to have decreased susceptibility to viral infections, indicating that the absence of MyD88 offers a degree of host protection from myocarditis.[17] Some viruses continue to replicate at a low level, causing ongoing direct myocardial injury. Viral proteases can inhibit host cell protein synthesis, induce apoptosis, and cleave dystrophin, resulting in cardiomyocyte injury and cardiomyopathy.

Antigen-specific, cell-mediated immunity begins 4 to 5 days after viral infection. Acquired immunity is an antigen-specific response directed to a single antigen, mediated by T and B cells. T cells are targeted to danger signals and attempt to limit infection by destroying the host cell and secreting cytokines. T-cell mediated immunity is important for limiting viral replication but can have detrimental effects on the host organ. Helper T cell types 1 and 2 (Th1 and Th2) secrete tumor necrosis factor (TNF) and interleukins, which are associated with resultant autoimmune cardiomyopathy. Helper T cells that produce interleukin 17 (TH17) can result in a higher rate of chronic DCM.

Cardiac injury associated with myocarditis may be caused by the virus directly entering the endothelial cells (as in parvovirus B19) and myocytes (enterovirus). In the majority of patients with viral myocarditis, the specific pathogen is cleared and removed, with the immune system being subsequently downregulated. However, in a minority of patients, the virus is not cleared and there is persistent myocyte infection. Cytokines such as TNF α can also cause cellular dysfunction without acute or persistent infection. As noted previously, up to 20% of myocarditis patients develop chronic DCM, with some due to persistent viral infection.[3] Treatments that regulate steps in pathogenesis, including the mechanism of viral entry and replication, components of innate and acquired immunity, and integrity of the sarcolemmal membrane are under investigation as detailed here.

Host factors can affect susceptibility to myocarditis. Genetic susceptibilities, including HLA-DQB1* polymorphisms, can increase the risk of progressive inflammatory cardiomyopathy. There has been speculation that microbial components contribute to this process as well. A recent study using a mouse model of spontaneous autoimmune myocarditis illustrated that progression of myocarditis depended on cardiac myosin-specific T helper cells imprinted in the intestine by a *Bacteroides* species peptide mimic. This study found that distinct bacterial communities, particularly *Bacteroides*, provide mimic peptides that can activate MYH6-specific $CD4^+$ T cells. Modification of the microbiome by antibiotic treatment reduced cardiac inflammation and prevented lethal cardiomyopathy.[18] Other environmental factors can modify the cardiac immune response to injury in murine models. For example, the endocrine disrupter bisphenol A (BPA), commonly found in plastic water bottles and plastic food storage containers, increases myocardial inflammation. Bruno et al found that exposure to BPA dissolved in water at a high-human relevant dose (5 μg BPA/kg body weight) administered to adult female BALB/c mice increased the severity of coxsackievirus B3 (CVB3) myocarditis and pericarditis. The BPA exposure increased the estrogen receptor β (ERβ) expression in the heart, which has been previously found to promote other cardiovascular diseases.[19,20] BPA also increased the number of T cells, mast cells, proinflammatory cytokines such as IFNγ, IL-1β, and IL-17A, and the TLR/caspase-1 signaling pathway. Additionally, BPA that leaked from the plastic bottles, with no additional BPA added to the water, activated cardiac mast cells, and increased cardiac fibrosis.[19] Other environmental factors, including low levels of selenium and high levels of mercury, can also increase myocardial damage in viral myocarditis.[21,22] Finally, in a clinical study of checkpoint inhibitor myocarditis, chronic use of prednisone at doses greater than 20 mg per day increases the severity of disease.

Infectious Etiologies

Enterovirus

From the 1950s to 1990s, enterovirus species, specifically coxsackievirus, were the most frequently identified viruses in patients with myocarditis. Enteroviruses are nonenveloped, lytic viruses with a single, positive-strand RNA genome of approximately 7.4 kb. Molecular studies during the late 1980s and 1990s utilizing polymerase chain reaction (PCR) identified an enterovirus genome in heart biopsies of 15% to 30% of patients with acute myocarditis.

Adenovirus

Adenoviruses are nonenveloped, double-stranded DNA viruses that cause myocarditis in a common rat model. The incidence of adenovirus in myocarditis patients varies between a high of 23% and a low of 2%. In the past decade, the prevalence of enteroviruses and adenoviruses detected in the myocardium of patients with myocarditis has decreased to the single digits. The most commonly detected viral genomes on endomyocardial biopsy samples are now parvovirus B19 (B19V) and human herpesvirus 6.

B19V of the Genus Erythrovirus

B19V of the genus Erythrovirus is a nonenveloped, nonlytic virus with a single-strand, positive-strand DNA genome, and parvoviruses do not cross species. Its primary receptor is globoside, known as group P antigen. Group P antigen is found primarily on erythroid progenitors, erythroblasts, megakaryocytes, and endothelial cells. This tropism translates to a reported association with the relatively common clinical syndrome of chest pain because of microvascular dysfunction. The B19V genome has been identified by PCR studies in 11% to 56% of patients with myocarditis and in 10% to 51% of patients with DCM. Because of a high prevalence of B19V in heart tissue from subjects without apparent heart conditions, B19V may often have a bystander role, particularly in subjects with low copy numbers detected on endomyocardial biopsy (EMB) samples.[23] Studies that demonstrated a correlation of much higher viral loads with more acute myocarditis support this conclusion.

Human Immunodeficiency Virus (HIV)

HIV is associated with myocarditis and DCM, either through direct toxicity of the gp120 protein or through secondary viral infections. Myocarditis is the most common cardiac pathologic finding at autopsy in patients with severe HIV.[1] The incidence of myocarditis, in addition to cardiomyopathy and pericardial disease, correlates with the severity of HIV infection as measured by a low $CD4^+$ count or high-viral titers. Since the introduction of highly active antiretroviral therapy (HAART), the incidence of myocarditis in HIV-infected patients has dramatically decreased in developed countries. In regions with limited availability to HAART, HIV-associated myocarditis remains clinically important.[24]

Influenza A and B

Influenza A and B viruses are known causes of myocarditis, with H1N1 having a particularly severe clinical syndrome. The incidence of myocarditis in severe influenza A infections may be as high as 5% with reports of electrocardiographic changes suggestive of subclinical cardiac involvement as high as 11%. Some cases of influenza A resulted in fulminant myocarditis with a high rate of recovery after supportive medical care. If myocardial tissue is obtained in the course of ventricular assist device (VAD) placement, histopathologic examination illustrates a cellular inflammatory infiltrate.[25]

COVID-19

In the setting of the COVID-19 pandemic, it has been demonstrated that patients admitted to the hospital with COVID-19 infection had a 13% to 41% incidence of myocardial injury, but classic lymphocytic myocarditis was relatively uncommon. Further research will be needed to clearly define the mechanism of cardiac injury and risk of myocarditis following infection with SARS-CoV2.

Nonviral Pathogens (Bacteria and Parasites)

Nonviral pathogens, including bacteria and parasites, can also affect the heart and incite an immune reaction resulting in myocarditis. Globally, bacterial- and protozoal-related myocarditis is much less common than viral myocarditis. Important bacterial infections associated with myocarditis include *Corynebacterium diphtheriae* that causes heart block and group A streptococcus species that cause poststreptococcal valvulitis and myocarditis. The tick-borne spirochete *Borrelia burgdorferi* causes Lyme disease, which usually begins with the characteristic rash of erythema chronicum migrans, followed by neurologic, joint, and cardiac involvement. Lyme carditis, frequently characterized by a heart block, is an uncommon manifestation, complicating only 1.1% of patients with Lyme disease.[26] In central and northern South America, infections involving the protozoa *Trypanosoma cruzi* (ie, Chagas disease) is a common cause of cardiomyopathy. Occasionally helminths, including *Echinococcus granulosus* and *Trichinella spiralis*, can result in clinical myocarditis, sometimes with profound eosinophilia.

Noninfectious Etiologies

A variety of noninfectious causes, including toxic and autoimmune reactions, can damage the heart with an inflammatory infiltrate and myocyte necrosis. Causes with specific treatments include adverse drug hypersensitivity reactions, systemic disorders such as eosinophilic granulomatosis with polyangiitis, cancer, and hypereosinophilic syndrome. These are associated with specific forms of eosinophilic myocarditis. Checkpoint inhibitor chemotherapeutic drugs are a recently described cause for severe and frequently fatal myocarditis.

Drug Toxicity

Adverse drug reactions manifest as a direct toxic effect on the heart or hypersensitivity myocarditis. Drug-induced hypersensitivity typically occurs within 8 weeks of initiation of the drug. Common offenders include antiepileptics, antimicrobials, and sulfa-based drugs. The inotrope dobutamine, often used for additional hemodynamic support in patients with cardiogenic shock or end-stage heart failure, is associated with eosinophilic myocarditis. Because of adverse outcomes associated with dobutamine-associated hypersensitivity myocarditis, this agent should be discontinued when significant eosinophilia occurs in association with an otherwise unexplained decline in ventricular function. The antipsychotic drug clozapine has also been associated with myocarditis, with reported rates as high as 1% to 10% of patients. Myocarditis can occur anytime during treatment but usually is diagnosed within the first 2 months after initiation of clozapine.

Chemotherapeutic Agents

Chemotherapeutic agents, including anthracyclines, can cause cardiac toxicity and sometimes myocardial inflammation. Immune checkpoint inhibitors are newer chemotherapeutic agents that have substantially improved the outcome of several cancers by releasing restrained antitumor immune responses; however, they can be associated with myocarditis in up to 1% of patients. Ipilimumab, an anticytotoxic T-lymphocyte-associated antigen 4 (CTLA-4) antibody, and nivolumab, an antiprogrammed death-1 (PD-1) antibody, improve survival in patients with melanoma and can be used in combination to augment antitumor activity. The prevalence of myocarditis associated with immune checkpoint inhibitors is 1.14%, with a median onset time of 34 days after initiation of therapy. Myocarditis after immune checkpoint inhibitor therapy can result in a fulminant process, which may respond to corticosteroids as initial treatment.[27] Fulminant myocarditis may be more common in patients who receive more than one checkpoint inhibitor, as it occurs in 0.27% of patients treated with a combination of ipilimumab and nivolumab.[28]

Giant Cell Myocarditis and Arrhythmogenic Right Ventricular Cardiomyopathy/Dysplasia

Idiopathic GCM is a rare, autoimmune form of myocarditis histologically defined by the presence of multinucleated giant cells, lymphocytic inflammatory infiltrate, and myocyte necrosis.[1] GCM is thought to be autoimmune given the association with other autoimmune disorders. Usually occurring in young adults, GCM carries a high risk of death without cardiac transplantation. Plakoglobin remodeling at cardiac myocyte junctions is known to occur in arrhythmogenic right ventricular cardiomyopathy/dysplasia (ARVD) but is also seen in GCM with ventricular arrhythmias.[29] Occasionally, myocarditis and ARVD can coexist or myocarditis can mimic ARVD or acute left ventricular dysplasia (ALVD). Greater than 50% of ARVD patients have associated desmosomal gene mutations. Nondesmosomal gene mutations have also been identified in association with ARVD. Lopez-Ayala et al identified seven patients with acute myocarditis, four with ALVD, and two with classic ARVD. All patients had defined gene mutations, and microsatellite analysis identified that they were all relatives or had a common ancestor, providing evidence for familial distribution of myocarditis. In this study, there appeared to be a higher incidence of myocarditis in desmoplakin mutation carriers, illustrating that signs of acute myocarditis should raise the possibility of ARVD, particularly if the pattern occurs in patient's relatives.[29]

CLINICAL PRESENTATION

Myocarditis presents with a wide array of clinical presentations, which can contribute to delayed diagnosis. A viral prodrome including fever, myalgias, fatigue, and rash may precede the myocarditis presentation by several days to weeks. The initial presentation can range from an asymptomatic patient with abnormal electrocardiographic or echocardiographic abnormalities to a patient presenting with heart failure and hemodynamic collapse. A recent series of 245 patients with clinical suspicion of myocarditis illustrated the most common initial symptoms are nonspecific: fatigue (82%), dyspnea on exertion (81%), arrhythmias (55%), palpitations (49%), and chest pain at rest (26%).[30]

Chest pain from myocarditis can mimic typical angina and myocardial infarction, but the pattern of chest pain is more frequent pericarditis with elevated troponin levels and mildly reduced left ventricular systolic function (termed myopericarditis). Isolated epicardial inflammation with adjacent pericardial involvement generally has a less than 1% risk of death or transplantation. Even with preserved left ventricular ejection fraction (LVEF), the risk of ventricular arrhythmia, death or transplant varies with the pattern of late gadolinium enhancement (LGE) on MRI.[31]

Cardiac rhythm disturbances, such as premature ventricular contractions (PVC), are very common as the initial presentation. The prevalence of ventricular arrhythmias varies by the histologic type of myocarditis, with sustained or symptomatic arrhythmias more common in GCM and hypersensitivity myocarditis compared with lymphocytic myocarditis.[32]

DIAGNOSIS

Electrocardiography

Myocarditis is likely underdiagnosed because of the low availability of cardiac MRI and EMB. A high level of clinical suspicion is necessary to make the appropriate clinical diagnosis. Electrocardiography is recommended in the American Heart Association (AHA) scientific statement and European Society of Cardiology (ESC) position statement for all patients with suspected myocarditis.[33,34] There are no pathognomonic electrocardiographic findings but nonspecific T wave abnormalities and sinus tachycardia frequently occur. Low voltage can suggest diffuse edema seen in fulminant myocarditis.[32] PR segment depression may signal associated pericarditis. High-degree heart block or ventricular arrhythmias suggest a higher risk of a specific disorder such as GCM.

Chest Radiography and Biomarkers

Chest radiography may reveal cardiomegaly secondary to chamber dilatation or pericardial effusion. Cardiac biomarkers of myocardial injury, if elevated, can help confirm the diagnosis of myocarditis. Higher levels of troponin T are associated with lower LVEF and are known to be a prognostic indicator for poor outcome in adult patients with acute myocarditis.[35]

Echocardiography and Magnetic Resonance Imaging

Imaging studies to exclude coronary artery disease, valvular heart disease, and congenital heart disease include echocardiography and coronary angiography in patients with possible acute myocarditis. Echocardiography is also helpful in regard to assessment of left and right ventricular systolic function. The presence of right ventricular dysfunction was a significant predictor of death or need for cardiac transplantation in a series of 23 patients with biopsy-confirmed myocarditis.[36] There are no specific echocardiographic features of myocarditis but patients with fulminant myocarditis may present with a normal end-diastolic dimension and thickened walls. In patients with suspected myocarditis and a low clinical risk of death or transplant, cardiac MRI can predict the risk of subsequent arrhythmias and provide a probable diagnosis.

The evaluation for specific forms of cardiomyopathy in the setting of acute DCM (**Algorithm 73.1**) depends on the severity of disease. The American College of Cardiology (ACC)/AHA and the Heart Failure Society of America (HFSA) 2016 scientific statement on the management of specific cardiomyopathies recommends an endomyocardial biopsy (EMB) if an acute dilated or nondilated cardiomyopathy is complicated by sustained or symptomatic ventricular arrhythmias, high-grade heart block, failure to respond to guideline-directed medical therapy, or the need for inotropes or mechanical circulatory support.[37]

If none of those clinical features are present, then cardiac MRI should be considered. Cardiac MRI can distinguish between ischemic and nonischemic cardiomyopathy, and can evaluate intracellular and interstitial edema, hyperemia and capillary leakage, and necrosis and fibrosis. The International Consensus Group on Cardiovascular Magnetic Resonance in Myocarditis suggests that a cardiac MRI should be performed in patients with clinical suspicion of myocarditis if the MRI results will affect management.[38] MRI is most accurate for the diagnosis of acute myocarditis within the first several weeks of symptom onset. Accuracy is increased when T1 and T2 parametric mapping techniques are used in addition to standard LGE and T2 weight imaging.[39] Recent data suggest that the persistence or increase of LGE at 6 months is associated with a worse prognosis following acute myocarditis and that risk increases as the extent of LGE increases.[31] In the same study, resolution of LGE was associated with a better prognosis. Positron emission tomographic imaging, used primarily to detect active inflammation in suspected cardiac sarcoidosis, does not currently have an established role in the diagnosis of acute myocarditis.

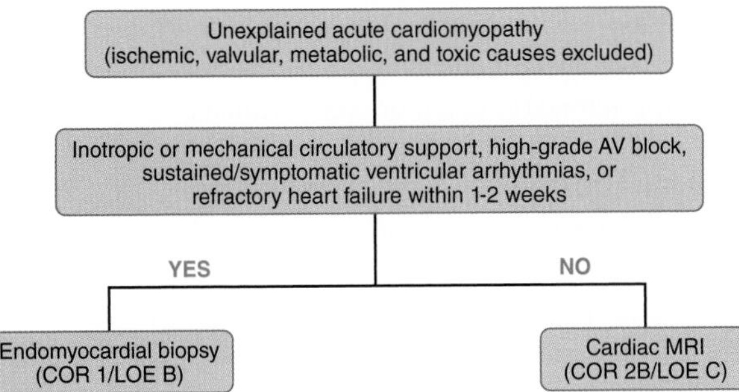

ALGORITHM 73.1 Approach to diagnosis in unexplained acute cardiomyopathy. AV, atrioventricular; COR, class of recommendation; LOE, level of evidence; MRI, magnetic resonance imaging

Endomyocardial Biopsy

Endomyocardial biopsy remains essential in more severe cases of acute myocarditis. Two scenarios exist in which both the ACC and ESC give EMB a class I or equivalent recommendation ("should be performed"): (1) unexplained new-onset heart failure symptoms less than 2 weeks in duration with hemodynamic compromise, concerning for fulminant myocarditis and (2) unexplained new-onset heart failure with symptoms of 2 weeks to 3 months duration associated with ventricular arrhythmias or high-grade atrioventricular (AV) block (Mobitz type II second degree or third-degree AV block), concerning for GCM. In addition, an EMB is reasonable in the setting of suspected eosinophilic myocarditis or myocarditis associated with systemic conditions such as rheumatoid arthritis, lupus, or scleroderma.

The role of persistent inflammation in the pathogenesis of chronic DCM is an area of active research. In this setting, an EMB demonstrating the presence of a high number of T lymphocytes or macrophages has unique value in predicting an increased risk of mortality or transplantation over the next decade.[40] The ESC position statement and a number of more recent review articles recommend using the presence of viral genomes or inflammation on EMB to guide immunosuppressive and antiviral therapy in this setting.

MANAGEMENT OF THE PATIENT WITH MYOCARDITIS

Acute Myocarditis Presenting With Dilated Cardiomyopathy

Patients with acute myocarditis who present with DCM should be treated according to current heart failure guidelines from the ACC, AHA, HFSA, and ESC.[41] Guideline-directed medical therapy—including β blockers, angiotensin-converting-enzyme inhibitors/angiotensin-receptor blockers/angiotensin receptor-neprilysin inhibitors, mineralocorticoid receptor antagonists, and diuretics if needed—are relevant to myocarditis as well as other causes of heart failure. Candesartan improved survival in a murine model of viral myocarditis (60% vs 18% with no candesartan treatment)[42] and nonselective β-blockers have been shown to improve histopathological results in coxsackievirus B myocarditis. Digoxin should generally be avoided in acute myocarditis because digoxin increased mortality in mice with viral myocarditis (**Algorithm 73.2**).[43]

Tachyarrhythmias and Conduction Abnormalities

Tachyarrhythmias and conduction abnormalities frequently seen with acute myocarditis can be treated with supportive therapy. Arrhythmias and heart block may resolve within several weeks.

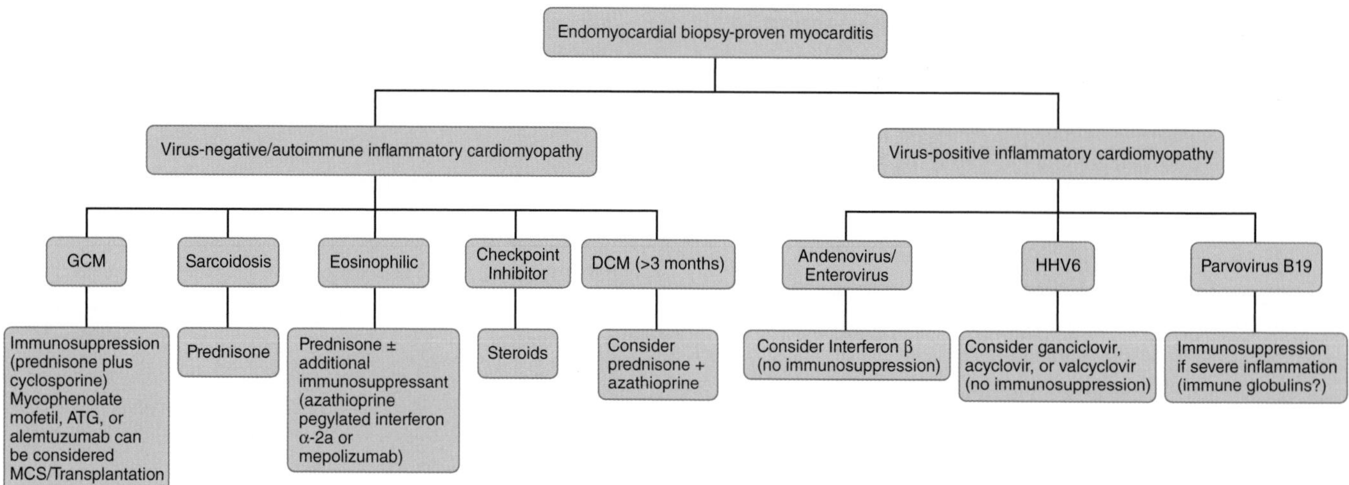

ALGORITHM 73.2 Management of myocarditis or inflammatory cardiomyopathy. ATG, anti-thymocyte globulin; DCM, dilated cardiomyopathy; GCM, giant cell myocarditis; HHV6, human herpesvirus 6; MCS, mechanical circulatory support.

A temporary pacemaker may be utilized for patients with symptomatic bradycardia or complete heart block. Individuals with symptomatic or sustained ventricular arrhythmias may require an implantable cardioverter-defibrillator (ICD) or further advanced heart failure therapies if the arrhythmias continue after the acute inflammatory phase. The ACC/AHA/ESC guidelines for the management of arrhythmias recommend that acute arrhythmia emergencies be conventionally managed in the setting of myocarditis and patients transferred to a center where hemodynamic support (mechanical circulatory support or transplantation) can be provided.[44] The same guideline recommends an ICD be placed in all patients with GCM who have ventricular arrhythmias and who are thought to have a 1 year or more life expectancy.

Fulminant Myocarditis and Altered Hemodynamics

In fulminant myocarditis, altered hemodynamics may require additional support such as inotropes or mechanical circulatory support, such as VADs, or extracorporeal membrane oxygenation (ECMO). Mechanical circulatory support may serve as a bridge to recovery or a bridge to cardiac transplantation. The recovery time can vary from weeks to months, and cardiac transplantation is an alternative for patients with myocarditis who have refractory heart failure despite optimal medical therapy and mechanical circulatory support. Despite higher rates of early rejection, survival rates after transplantation for GCM have similar survival rates compared with other causes of cardiac transplantation.[45]

Immunosuppressive Therapy

In patients with acute lymphocytic myocarditis and DCM, immunosuppression with prednisone combined with either azathioprine or cyclosporine did not improve LVEF at 28 weeks or transplant-free survival at 5 years in a randomized controlled trial.[1]

In contrast to acute myocarditis, chronic virus-negative DCM diagnosed by immunohistology and that is unresponsive to standard guideline therapy may respond to a 6-month course of prednisone and azathioprine. Three studies have shown that azathioprine and prednisone in virus-negative DCM of more than 6 months duration may increase LVEF and lower New York Heart Association (NYHA) functional class.[1] Alternate treatment regimens, including corticosteroid-based therapy combined with cyclosporine or mycophenolate mofetil, have been suggested.[3] Rituximab, a monoclonal antibody against the B-cell surface molecule CD20, has also been described as a treatment option for chronic myocarditis.[3]

In patients with GCM, immunosuppressive therapy including cyclosporine and corticosteroids increases transplant-free survival in patients with less than 3 months of symptoms. In subjects who do not respond or are intolerant of the initial regimen, mycophenolate mofetil, antithymocyte globulin (ATG), or alemtuzumab (Campath) may be considered. Abrupt cessation of immunosuppression in GCM after 1 year of treatment has been associated with GCM recurrence in two cases.[46]

Eosinophilic necrotizing myocarditis is also responsive to immunosuppression, with the most common regimen including corticosteroids sometimes combined with azathioprine, pegylated interferon (IF) α-2a, or mepolizumab.[47]

Antiviral Therapy

Viral infection may be a therapeutic target in acute and chronic myocarditis (the latter termed inflammatory cardiomyopathy). Viral myocarditis is defined by the presence of viral genomes on EMB. The presence of viral genomes has been associated with worsening heart failure and increased mortality. In murine viral myocarditis, antiviral therapy with ribavirin and interferon-α decreased severity of the myocardial lesions and reduced mortality.[1]

Interferon β has been used in patients with chronic DCM and evidence of viral persistence. The Betaferon in Chronic Viral Cardiomyopathy Trial (BICC trial) included patients with chronic DCM and viral genomes detected by PCR assay on heart biopsy tissue. In the 15 subjects with enteroviral or adenoviral infection, 6 million international units (MIU) of interferon β (IFN-β) subcutaneously three times per week eliminated the genomes and improved NYHA class.[48] Viral clearance was also associated with improvement in left ventricular function. In the BICC trial, IFN-β was not associated with B19V clearance. Given B19V and HHV-6 are now more common than adenovirus and enterovirus, antiviral therapy would need to be directed against these specific viruses. For HHV-6, there may be a role for the use of immunosuppressive drugs in combination with antiviral medications including ganciclovir, acyclovir, or valacyclovir.

B19V-Related Myocarditis: Intravenous Immunoglobulins, Telbivudine, and Prednisone Plus Azathioprine

There are ongoing studies evaluating anti-B19V treatment in subjects with more chronic syndromes. Currently, three different treatment options are being investigated for B19V-related myocarditis: intravenous immunoglobulins, telbivudine, and prednisone plus azathioprine.[3] Antiviral and immunomodulatory effects in experimental models previously suggested a role for intravenous immune globulin (IVIG) in acute myocarditis; however, in the Intervention in Myocarditis and Acute Cardiomyopathy trial, patients with acute DCM who were treated with IVIG did not have improved outcomes compared with those given placebo.[49] Therefore, IVIG is not routinely used for acute myocarditis therapy, but ongoing trials are investigating whether high doses of IVIG in addition to traditional heart failure therapy in patients with chronic DCM and B19V persistence improve cardiac function with virus elimination. Telbivudine is an antiviral synthetic nucleoside, which preferentially inhibits the DNA-dependent single-stranded DNA synthesis and may interfere with the replication of B19V. However, additional studies are currently lacking. Finally, recent preliminary findings from the CAPACITY (Cortisone in Parvovirus Inflammatory Cardiomyopathy) single-center observational investigation illustrated that the combination of prednisone and azathioprine in addition to standard heart failure treatment in patients with B19V positive DCM was associated with an improved LVEF, but these results need further validation in a randomized controlled trial.[3,50]

FOLLOW-UP PATIENT CARE

All patients with acute myocarditis, including those who have normal LVEF or recover quickly, should refrain from aerobic activity, with the timing of reintroduction of exercise based on the decrease of left ventricular dysfunction and extent of recovery. A minimum of 3 to 6 months abstinence from competitive sports is recommended with an echocardiogram, symptom-limited treadmill test, and arrhythmia monitor performed before the clearance. This recommendation is based on epidemiological studies and mouse models of myocarditis that illustrated an increased rate of death with sustained exercise.[1]

RESEARCH AND FUTURE DIRECTIONS

Clinical and translational research is focused on refining diagnosis and improving management strategies for acute myocarditis and chronic inflammatory cardiomyopathy. Recent translational studies have illustrated a causal link between microribonucleic acids (miRNAs), small RNA molecules that posttranscriptionally regulate gene expression, and myocarditis. Certain miRNAs regulate the virulence of cardiotropic viruses and inflammatory pathways, and novel miRNA therapeutic targets are currently being investigated as emerging therapies for myocarditis.[8] Other emerging therapies for the treatment of myocarditis (**Table 73.1**) include a number of new antiinflammatory treatments. Briefly, interleukin (IL)-1 is a

TABLE 73.1 Emerging/Experimental Therapies in Myocarditis

	Mechanism of Action	Evidence
IL-1β Inhibitors		
Anakinra	IL-1 receptor antagonist	Beneficial in recurrent pericarditis. Clinical trial phase IIB evaluation of Anakinra versus placebo in the treatment of acute myocarditis (ARAMIS)[a]
Canakinumab	Anti-IL1β monoclonal antibody	Found to reduce IL-1β levels in stable coronary artery disease with further investigation needed for myocarditis
Colchicine	Inhibits the NLRP3 inflammasome assembly	First-line treatment for pericarditis and may be beneficial for myocarditis through reduction of NLRP3 activity
Rilonacept	Blocks IL-1α and IL-1β signaling	Phase 2 clinical trials illustrated improved outcomes in recurrent pericarditis; Phase 3 trial RHAPSODY[b] ongoing

(continued)

TABLE 73.1 Emerging/Experimental Therapies in Myocarditis (*continued*)

	Mechanism of Action	Evidence
HMGB1 Inhibitors	Inhibition of high-mobility group box-1 (HMGB1), a nuclear protein involved in transcription regulation and DNA replication, released by necrotic tissue	Levels of HMB1 are elevated on endomyocardial biopsy in patients with acute myocarditis, making HMBG1 a potential target of therapy for acute autoimmune myocarditis
S100A9 Inhibitors	Inhibition of alarmins	S100A8/A9 are associated with CVB3 myocarditis and are thought to be involved in activation of the NLRP3 inflammasome, making S100 A8/A9 a potential therapeutic target for acute CVB3 myocarditis
Modulation of T Cells		
Treg cells transfer	Restoration of the Treg/Th17 balance via direct Treg cell application and expansion	CD4+CD25+FoxP3+regulatory T (Treg) cells are thought to play a pivotal role in myocarditis, with impaired Treg cells in myocarditis and a lower proportion of Treg cells with enhanced Th17 response
IL-2 agonists	Promotes Treg cell production and mature Treg cell survival	
Mesenchymal Cells	Immunomodulatory properties	Mesenchymal stromal cells have been shown to have cardioprotective and immunomodulatory properties helpful in models of CVB3-induced myocarditis
Nanocarriers	Nanomaterials used to transport biological or pharmacological agents	In the setting of myocarditis, nanocarriers have been evaluated to reduce monocyte maturation, target fibroblasts to reduce fibrosis, and target myocytes to reduce apoptosis

[a]Anakinra versus placebo for the treatment of acute myocarditis (ARAMIS) http://www.clinicaltrials.gov. Unique identifier: NCT03018834).
[b]Phase 3 Study to Assess the Efficacy and Safety of Rilonacept Treatment in Subjects with Recurrent Pericarditis (RHAPSODY) http://www.clinicaltrials.gov. Unique identifier: NCT03737110).
CVB3, coxsackie B3; DNA, deoxyribonucleic acid; IL, interluekin; NLRP3, NLR family pyrin domain containing 3; S100A8/A9, S100 calcium-binding protein A8/A9; Treg, T regulatory cells

proinflammatory cytokine that increases the innate immune response. Upstream of IL-1 is the inflammasome, a cytosolic aggregate structure composed of an adaptor protein, procaspase-1, and a sensor molecule. The best-described inflammasome has a sensor molecule known as NLRP3 (nucleotide-binding domain and leucine-rich repeat pyrin domain containing-3), which can be activated by infectious pathogens such as coxsackievirus or endogenous triggers.[3] Treatments that block the IL-1 pathway, including IL-1 receptor antagonist anakinra, the anti-IL-1β monoclonal antibody canakinumab, and colchicine, which inhibits the NLRP3 assembly, may have a role in the treatment of myocarditis. As more evidence regarding the pathophysiology of myocarditis is uncovered, advancements regarding therapeutic options will increasingly enter clinical trials.

KEY POINTS

- ✔ Myocarditis refers to inflammation of the myocardium.
- ✔ Classic myocarditis typically results from exposure to an external antigen, such as virus, bacteria, parasite, or toxin, or an internal trigger.
- ✔ Viral infections are the most common infectious cause of myocarditis.
- ✔ Parvovirus B19 and human herpesvirus 6 are now most frequently associated with myocarditis.
- ✔ Prevalence of myocarditis is high during the first year of life, declines during childhood, and rises again after puberty until the fifth decade.
- ✔ Pathogenesis of viral myocarditis includes viral infection and replication, the immunologic response, which can include an innate and adaptive immune response, and chronic cardiac remodeling.
- ✔ Myocarditis is likely underdiagnosed because of the low availability of cardiac MRI and endomyocardial biopsy. A high level of clinical suspicion is necessary to make the appropriate clinical diagnosis.
- ✔ The clinical picture of myocarditis can range from an asymptomatic patient with only electrocardiographic or echocardiographic abnormalities to someone with mild chest pain, dysrhythmias, or heart failure symptoms, to someone who presents with fulminant myocarditis with hemodynamic collapse requiring mechanical circulatory support.
- ✔ First-line therapy for myocarditis is supportive care.
- ✔ Routine treatment of mild to moderately severe myocarditis with immunosuppression is not recommended.

- ✔ Immunosuppression is the treatment of choice for GCM, cardiac sarcoidosis, eosinophilic myocarditis, and some types of autoimmune myocarditis.
- ✔ There may be a role for a short course of immunosuppression in patients with chronic dilated cardiomyopathy that is not responsive to guideline-directed medical therapy.

REFERENCES

1. Cooper LT Jr. Myocarditis. *N Engl J Med.* 2009;360:1526-1538.
2. Blauwet LA, Cooper LT. Myocarditis. *Prog Cardiovasc Dis.* 2010;52:274-288.
3. Tschope C, Cooper LT, Torre-Amione G, Van Linthout S. Management of myocarditis-related cardiomyopathy in adults. *Circ Res.* 2019;124:1568-1583.
4. Leone O, Veinot JP, Angelini A, et al. 2011 consensus statement on endomyocardial biopsy from the Association for European Cardiovascular Pathology and the Society for Cardiovascular Pathology. *Cardiovasc Pathol.* 2012;21:245-274.
5. She RC, Hammond EH. Utility of immunofluorescence and electron microscopy in endomyocardial biopsies from patients with unexplained heart failure. *Cardiovasc Pathol.* 2010;19:e99-e105.
6. Rigopoulos AG, Klutt B, Matiakis M, Apostolou A, Mavrogeni S, Noutsias M. Systematic review of PCR proof of parvovirus B19 genomes in endomyocardial biopsies of patients presenting with myocarditis or dilated cardiomyopathy. *Viruses.* 2019;11(6):566.
7. GBD 2019 Viewpoint Collaborators. Five insights from the Global Burden of Disease Study 2019. Lancet. 2020;396:1135-1159.
8. Heymans S, Eriksson U, Lehtonen J, Cooper LT Jr. The quest for new approaches in myocarditis and inflammatory cardiomyopathy. *J Am Coll Cardiol.* 2016;68:2348-2364.
9. Harmon KG, Asif IM, Maleszewski JJ, et al. Incidence and etiology of sudden cardiac arrest and death in high school athletes in the United States. *Mayo Clin Proc.* 2016;91:1493-1502.
10. Fenoglio JJ Jr, Ursell PC, Kellogg CF, Drusin RE, Weiss MB. Diagnosis and classification of myocarditis by endomyocardial biopsy. *N Engl J Med.* 1983;308:12-18.
11. Cooper LT Jr, Berry GJ, Shabetai R. Idiopathic giant-cell myocarditis—natural history and treatment. Multicenter Giant Cell Myocarditis Study Group Investigators. *N Engl J Med.* 1997;336:1860-1866.
12. Lyden DC, Olszewski J, Feran M, Job LP, Huber SA. Coxsackievirus B-3-induced myocarditis. Effect of sex steroids on viremia and infectivity of cardiocytes. *Am J Pathol.* 1987;126:432-438.
13. Atluri P, Ullery BW, MacArthur JW, et al. Rapid onset of fulminant myocarditis portends a favourable prognosis and the ability to bridge mechanical circulatory support to recovery. *Eur J Cardiothorac Surg.* 2013;43:379-382.
14. Coyne CB, Bergelson JM. Virus-induced Abl and Fyn kinase signals permit coxsackievirus entry through epithelial tight junctions. *Cell.* 2006;124:119-131.
15. Kashimura T, Kodama M, Hotta Y, et al. Spatiotemporal changes of coxsackievirus and adenovirus receptor in rat hearts during postnatal development and in cultured cardiomyocytes of neonatal rat. *Virchows Arch.* 2004;444:283-292.
16. Shi Y, Chen C, Lisewski U, et al. Cardiac deletion of the Coxsackievirus-adenovirus receptor abolishes Coxsackievirus B3 infection and prevents myocarditis in vivo. *J Am Coll Cardiol.* 2009;53:1219-1226.
17. Marty RR, Dirnhofer S, Mauermann N, et al. MyD88 signaling controls autoimmune myocarditis induction. *Circulation.* 2006;113:258-265.
18. Gil-Cruz C, Perez-Shibayama C, De Martin A, et al. Microbiota-derived peptide mimics drive lethal inflammatory cardiomyopathy. *Science.* 2019;366:881-886.
19. Bruno KA, Mathews JE, Yang AL, et al. BPA alters estrogen receptor expression in the heart after viral infection activating cardiac mast cells and T cells leading to perimyocarditis and fibrosis. *Front Endocrinol (Lausanne).* 2019;10:598.
20. Xiong Q, Liu X, Shen Y, et al. Elevated serum Bisphenol A level in patients with dilated cardiomyopathy. *Int J Environ Res Public Health.* 2015;12:5329-5337.
21. Beck MA, Levander OA, Handy J. Selenium deficiency and viral infection. *J Nutr.* 2003;133:1463S-1467S.
22. Cooper LT, Rader V, Ralston NV. The roles of selenium and mercury in the pathogenesis of viral cardiomyopathy. *Congest Heart Fail.* 2007;13:193-199.
23. Koepsell SA, Anderson DR, Radio SJ. Parvovirus B19 is a bystander in adult myocarditis. *Cardiovasc Pathol.* 2012;21:476-481.
24. Pugliese A, Isnardi D, Saini A, Scarabelli T, Raddino R, Torre D. Impact of highly active antiretroviral therapy in HIV-positive patients with cardiac involvement. *J Infect.* 2000;40:282-284.
25. Rezkalla SH, Kloner RA. Influenza-related viral myocarditis. *WMJ.* 2010;109:209-213.
26. Forrester JD, Meiman J, Mullins J, et al. Notes from the field: update on Lyme carditis, groups at high risk, and frequency of associated sudden cardiac death—United States. *MMWR Morb Mortal Wkly Rep.* 2014;63:982-983.
27. Mahmood SS, Fradley MG, Cohen JV, et al. Myocarditis in patients treated with immune checkpoint inhibitors. *J Am Coll Cardiol.* 2018;71:1755-1764.
28. Johnson DB, Balko JM, Compton ML, et al. Fulminant myocarditis with combination immune checkpoint blockade. *N Engl J Med.* 2016;375:1749-1755.
29. Lopez-Ayala JM, Pastor-Quirante F, Gonzalez-Carrillo J, et al. Genetics of myocarditis in arrhythmogenic right ventricular dysplasia. *Heart Rhythm.* 2015;12:766-773.
30. Kuhl U, Pauschinger M, Noutsias M, et al. High prevalence of viral genomes and multiple viral infections in the myocardium of adults with "idiopathic" left ventricular dysfunction. *Circulation.* 2005;111:887-893.
31. Aquaro GD, Ghebru Habtemicael Y, Camastra G, et al. Prognostic value of repeating cardiac magnetic resonance in patients with acute myocarditis. *J Am Coll Cardiol.* 2019;74:2439-2448.
32. Kociol RD, Cooper LT, Fang JC, et al. Recognition and initial management of fulminant myocarditis: a scientific statement from the American Heart Association. *Circulation.* 2020;141(6):e69-e92.
33. Bozkurt B, Colvin M, Cook J, et al. Current diagnostic and treatment strategies for specific dilated cardiomyopathies: a scientific statement from the American Heart Association. *Circulation.* 2016;134:e579-e646.
34. Caforio AL, Pankuweit S, Arbustini E, et al. Current state of knowledge on aetiology, diagnosis, management, and therapy of myocarditis: a position statement of the European Society of Cardiology Working Group on Myocardial and Pericardial Diseases. *Eur Heart J.* 2013;34:2636-2648, 2648a-2648d.
35. Al-Biltagi M, Issa M, Hagar HA, Abdel-Hafez M, Aziz NA. Circulating cardiac troponins levels and cardiac dysfunction in children with acute and fulminant viral myocarditis. *Acta Paediatr.* 2010;99:1510-1516.
36. Mendes LA, Dec GW, Picard MH, Palacios IF, Newell J, Davidoff R. Right ventricular dysfunction: an independent predictor of adverse outcome in patients with myocarditis. *Am Heart J.* 1994;128:301-307.
37. Yancy CW, Jessup M, Bozkurt B, et al. 2016 ACC/AHA/HFSA focused update on new pharmacological therapy for heart failure: an update of the 2013 ACCF/AHA guideline for the management of heart failure: a report of the American College of Cardiology/American Heart Association Task Force on Clinical Practice Guidelines and the Heart Failure Society of America. *J Am Coll Cardiol.* 2016;68:1476-1488.

38. Friedrich MG, Sechtem U, Schulz-Menger J, et al. Cardiovascular magnetic resonance in myocarditis: a JACC white paper. *J Am Coll Cardiol.* 2009;53:1475-1487.
39. Ferreira VM, Schulz-Menger J, Holmvang G, et al. Cardiovascular magnetic resonance in nonischemic myocardial inflammation: expert recommendations. *J Am Coll Cardiol.* 2018;72:3158-3176.
40. Nakayama T, Sugano Y, Yokokawa T, et al. Clinical impact of the presence of macrophages in endomyocardial biopsies of patients with dilated cardiomyopathy. *Eur J Heart Fail.* 2017;19:490-498.
41. Dickstein K, Cohen-Solal A, Filippatos G, et al. ESC guidelines for the diagnosis and treatment of acute and chronic heart failure 2008: the Task Force for the Diagnosis and Treatment of Acute and Chronic Heart Failure 2008 of the European Society of Cardiology. Developed in collaboration with the Heart Failure Association of the ESC (HFA) and endorsed by the European Society of Intensive Care Medicine (ESICM). *Eur Heart J.* 2008;29:2388-2442.
42. Saegusa S, Fei Y, Takahashi T, et al. Oral administration of candesartan improves the survival of mice with viral myocarditis through modification of cardiac adiponectin expression. *Cardiovasc Drugs Ther.* 2007;21:155-160.
43. Matsumori A, Igata H, Ono K, et al. High doses of digitalis increase the myocardial production of proinflammatory cytokines and worsen myocardial injury in viral myocarditis: a possible mechanism of digitalis toxicity. *Jpn Circ J.* 1999;63:934-940.
44. Al-Khatib SM, Stevenson WG, Ackerman MJ, et al. 2017 AHA/ACC/HRS guideline for management of patients with ventricular arrhythmias and the prevention of sudden cardiac death: executive summary: a report of the American College of Cardiology/American Heart Association Task Force on Clinical Practice Guidelines and the Heart Rhythm Society. *Heart Rhythm.* 2018;15:e190-e252.
45. Elamm CA, Al-Kindi SG, Bianco CM, Dhakal BP, Oliveira GH. Heart transplantation in giant cell myocarditis: analysis of the united network for organ sharing registry. *J Card Fail.* 2017;23:566-569.
46. Maleszewski JJ, Orellana VM, Hodge DO, Kuhl U, Schultheiss HP, Cooper LT. Long-term risk of recurrence, morbidity and mortality in giant cell myocarditis. *Am J Cardiol.* 2015;115:1733-1738.
47. Bleeker JS, Syed FF, Cooper LT, Weiler CR, Tefferi A, Pardanani A. Treatment-refractory idiopathic hypereosinophilic syndrome: pitfalls and progress with use of novel drugs. *Am J Hematol.* 2012;87:703-706.
48. Schultheiss HP, Piper C, Sowade O, et al. Betaferon in chronic viral cardiomyopathy (BICC) trial: effects of interferon-beta treatment in patients with chronic viral cardiomyopathy. *Clin Res Cardiol.* 2016;105:763-773.
49. McNamara DM, Holubkov R, Starling RC, et al. Controlled trial of intravenous immune globulin in recent-onset dilated cardiomyopathy. *Circulation.* 2001;103:2254-2259.
50. Tschope C, Elsanhoury A, Schlieker S, Van Linthout S, Kuhl U. Immunosuppression in inflammatory cardiomyopathy and parvovirus B19 persistence. *Eur J Heart Fail.* 2019;21:1468-1469.

CHAPTER 74

TOXIN-INDUCED CARDIOMYOPATHIES

Omar Jawaid, Suparna C. Clasen, Abhishek Khemka, and Maya Guglin

INTRODUCTION

Various substances have been associated with cardiomyopathies. This includes legally available substances, illicit substances of abuse, and prescribed medications. The epidemiology, pathophysiology, and outcomes of substance-induced cardiomyopathy are varied. In addition to guideline-directed medical therapy, identification of the offending substances and prompt cessation are key features in the management of substance abuse cardiomyopathy.

ALCOHOLIC CARDIOMYOPATHY

Although widely consumed, only a small subset of patients with long-standing abuse of ethanol develop a dilated cardiomyopathy. Those with consumption of greater than 90 g/day of ethanol for greater than 5 years are at the highest risk for developing cardiomyopathy, although individual genetic predisposition also plays a role. As ethanol exposure increases, so does the risk of cardiomyopathy, with those ingesting greater than 200 g/day of ethanol having the highest risk of developing cardiomyopathy.

The pathogenesis of alcoholic cardiomyopathy includes various mechanisms, such as direct toxic effects on cardiomyocytes, mitochondrial dysfunction, disruption of calcium homeostasis, increased β-adrenergic tone, increased arrhythmogenic potential, and inappropriate activation of the renin-angiotensin-aldosterone (RAAS) axis. Ethanol's effects on cardiomyocyte mitochondria have been well-documented, leading to free radical generation. Ethanol also disrupts the sarcoplasmic reticulum causing inappropriate calcium release and derangement of calcium metabolism.[1] This in turn leads to aberrant cardiac remodeling and increased arrhythmogenic tendencies including reentry dependent tachycardias, atrial fibrillation, ventricular tachycardia and ventricular fibrillation.[2] Finally, RAAS and sympathetic tone is increased by various mechanisms including fluid shifts, poor nutrition, inappropriate systemic vasodilation, and aberrant hormonal signaling. Abstinence of ethanol can often reverse these changes; however, when dose exposure increases, left ventricular dysfunction often becomes irreversible.[3]

Clinical manifestations of alcoholic cardiomyopathy, as well as treatment, are similar to idiopathic dilated cardiomyopathy, but long-term outcomes are more favorable, especially if the patient maintains abstinence.[3] Observational data demonstrate that at 140 months of follow-up, between 35% and 85% of patients with alcoholic cardiomyopathy will be alive as compared to 40% to 70% with idiopathic dilated cardiomyopathy. However, several characteristics portend a poor outcome including continued ethanol use, atrial fibrillation, and electrocardiographic QRS duration greater than 120 ms. Patients with these risk factors have poor outcomes ranging from 0% to 65% survival at 12 years, with accumulating risk factors associated with the worst outcomes. Identifying and modifying these risk factors are key components in the management of alcoholic cardiomyopathy, with ethanol cessation forming the basis of treatment.

COCAINE-INDUCED CARDIOMYOPATHY

Cocaine is a semisynthetic alkaloid derived from the leaves of the *Erythroxylum coca* plant. It can be consumed in a variety of manners including inhalation, intravenous injection, insufflation, and ingestion. Cocaine acts on dopaminergic and sympathetic receptors in the brain as well as in the periphery and exerts a variety of effects including euphoria. After ethanol, cocaine is the second most commonly used drug and the most commonly encountered drug in patients presenting with chest pain. Postmortem data suggest that up to 28% of regular cocaine users have significant coronary artery disease even among those of young age at the time of death (ie, median age 34 years).[4]

Cocaine exerts its effects by excessively stimulating the dopaminergic and sympathetic nervous systems. This in turn has multiple effects on the heart through hypertension, tachyarrhythmias, cardiomyocyte toxicity, coronary vasospasm, and dissection. In addition, cocaine causes accelerated atherosclerosis as well as microvascular ischemia through inappropriate platelet activation, which contributes to myocardial dysfunction. Hypertension is a well-documented effect of sympathetic activation. In one series, up to 47% of documented cocaine users developed severe, chronic hypertension.[4] The resultant increased afterload on the heart causes multiple downstream effects including left ventricular hypertrophy, microvascular disease, and maladaptive remodeling through neurohormonal pathways. In addition, cocaine users are at higher risk of developing tachyarrhythmias, most notably atrial fibrillation but also ventricular tachyarrhythmias. This is in part caused by increased sympathetic activation brought on by cocaine use, as well as myocardial remodeling. Cocaine is also directly toxic to cardiomyocytes, causing oxidative damage, free radical generation, disruption of calcium stores, and eventually myonecrosis.

Finally, cocaine exerts direct toxic effects on the vasculature by causing endothelial disruption. This in turn leads to vascular inflammation, plaque formation and erosion, and intra-arterial thrombosis through direct platelet aggregation induced by cocaine and its metabolites.

The outcomes of cocaine-induced cardiomyopathy are directly linked to continued cocaine abuse. Cocaine cessation often results in reversal of cardiomyopathy, although up to 30% of patients will not recover cardiac function.[5]

METHAMPHETAMINE-INDUCED CARDIOMYOPATHY

Amphetamines are a class of semisynthetic chemicals with profound dopaminergic and sympathetic activity. In controlled settings, amphetamines and their derivatives provide relief from multiple conditions including attention deficit disorder, but when consumed in excess, methamphetamine exhibits short- and long-term consequences to the cardiovascular system. Methamphetamine ingestion provides a long-lasting high that has proven resistant to substance abuse counseling and treatment, leading to a significant dependency on the substance. Data from hospital diagnosis codes reveal that up to 5% of admissions for heart failure (HF) exacerbations are caused by methamphetamine use. Patients with methamphetamine-associated cardiomyopathy are typically younger (ie, average age at diagnosis is 49.7 years) than individuals with idiopathic dilated cardiomyopathy and with significant left ventricular dysfunction, with up to 30% of patients having left ventricular ejection fractions (LVEF) less than 40% at the time of diagnosis. Those with the highest amounts of methamphetamine consumption have more severely depressed LVEF.[6]

Methamphetamine exerts numerous effects on the cardiovascular system, which in turn promote aberrant remodeling, myocardial loss, and ultimately cardiomyopathy. Methamphetamine abuse results in catecholamine excess, increased reactive oxygen species, direct myocardial toxic effects, mitochondrial dysfunction with aberrant coupling of the electron transport chain, and coronary vasospasm and ischemia. In addition, catecholamine excess causes increased left ventricular afterload, aberrant cardiac remodeling, and myocyte necrosis. Endomyocardial biopsy of methamphetamine users demonstrates extensive fibrosis, with higher levels of fibrosis corresponding to more severe left ventricular dysfunction. In addition to left ventricular dysfunction, methamphetamine use is emerging as a significant cause of pulmonary arterial hypertension (PAH). Long-standing PAH can lead to right ventricular failure. Direct endothelial injury by methamphetamine results in aberrant pulmonary vascular remodeling. Methamphetamine also causes dysfunction of key modulators of vascular function including endothelin, carboxylesterase 1, and bone morphogenetic protein receptor type 2. Although pulmonary vasodilators can provide some relief, early intervention and methamphetamine cessation are key in preventing the progression of PAH. However, even with cessation, return of normal pulmonary vascular function may not occur.

In a case series in Germany, 57% of patients presenting with decompensated HF attributed to methamphetamine with continued abuse had high mortality; median time to death was approximately 6 months. Furthermore, survivors demonstrated persistent left ventricular dysfunction and repeated admissions for HF exacerbations. However, in those who were able to cease methamphetamine abuse, 80% were alive at 26 months. Moreover, these patients saw drastic increases in their left ventricular function: mean LVEF increased from 23% on initial discharge to 47% at follow-up. In comparison, those with continued methamphetamine use had a decline in LVEF from 19% to 17%, despite similar prescription rates of guideline-directed medical therapy.[7]

OTHER DRUG-INDUCED CARDIOMYOPATHIES

Several prescription medications have been associated with cardiomyopathy. A limited list of drugs associated with cardiomyopathy is provided in **Table 74.1**.

Chloroquine and its derivatives are immunomodulators used in the treatment of a variety of rheumatologic conditions including rheumatoid arthritis. Chloroquine and derivatives are increasingly recognized as cardiomyocyte toxic agents leading to drug-induced cardiomyopathy. Frequently a restrictive cardiomyopathy occurs, although dilated and hypertrophic variants have been described as well. In addition to direct cardiomyocyte toxicity, chloroquine can exert toxic effects on the cardiac conduction system including the sinoatrial and atrioventricular nodes. Cardiomyopathy may become evident within weeks of the beginning of therapy or manifest after years of treatment. Cessation of chloroquine can reverse cardiomyopathy; however, persistent myocardial dysfunction requiring advanced therapies including transplantation has been reported.[8] Although endomyocardial biopsy is the gold standard for diagnosis, a careful history and review of the medication list can often provide clues. Endomyocardial biopsy reveals vacuolization of cardiomyocytes, confirming the diagnosis.

Clozapine is a dopamine antagonist most commonly used in schizophrenic spectrum psychiatry disorders. Although agranulocytosis is the most commonly associated adverse effect of clozapine, IgE-mediated myocarditis resulting in cardiomyopathy is a recognized complication. Although most often encountered in the first few weeks of treatment, clozapine-induced myocarditis can also present later, even years after clozapine treatment. In addition to a careful review of the medication list, laboratory assessments of C-reactive protein and troponin I or T levels may provide clues to a developing cardiomyopathy. Prompt cessation of clozapine often results in reversal of the cardiomyopathy.

MANAGEMENT OF THE PATIENT WITH DRUG-INDUCED CARDIOMYOPATHY

Drug-induced cardiomyopathies are an important cause of non-ischemic cardiomyopathy. Prompt detection and cessation of offending drugs is key in reversing myocardial dysfunction.

TABLE 74.1 Drug-induced Cardiomyopathy

Drug	Mechanism	Onset	Reversibility
Ethanol	Cardiotoxicity, neurohormonal and electrical derangement	Years	Often reversible, can be permanent
Cocaine	Cardiotoxicity, coronary vasospasm, accelerated atherosclerosis, neurohormonal derangement	Years	Often reversible, can be permanent
Methamphetamine and derivatives	Cardiotoxicity, accelerated atherosclerosis, neurohormonal derangement, pulmonary arterial hypertension	Months to years	Cardiomyopathy may be reversible, pulmonary arterial hypertension may persist
Chloroquine/hydroxychloroquine	Lysosomal inhibition, myocardial vacuolization	Weeks to years	Usually reversible
Clozapine	IgE hypersensitivity reaction, myocarditis	Weeks to years	Usually reversible
Anagrelide	Derangement of phosphodiesterase activity	Weeks	Reversible
Itraconazole	Negative inotropy	Immediate to days	Reversible
Amphotericin B	Unknown, possibly mitochondrial dysfunction	Immediate	Reversible
Bromocriptine	Adrenergic surge	Immediate to weeks	Reversible
Etanercept, adalimumab, infliximab	Unknown, likely cytokine derangement	Immediate to weeks	Often reversible, can be permanent

The fundamentals of cardiomyopathy treatment remain similar, namely neurohormonal blockade and fluid management to treat congestive symptoms. It is unclear whether treatment must be continued after cessation of the offending agent and myocardial recovery is observed. More research is needed to help guide specific therapies as well as identify potential causes of cardiomyopathy as the list of pharmacologic agents ever expands.

CHEMOTHERAPY-INDUCED CARDIOMYOPATHY

Advances in chemotherapy, novel immune- and targeted therapies have been lifesaving for patients with cancer. These treatments are not thought of as "toxins" *per se,* but they do have the potential for adverse cardiac side effects. For example, treatment of breast cancer involves chemotherapy with anthracycline-containing regimens, targeted therapy with antihuman epidermal growth factor receptor 2 (HER2) agents, and radiation therapy. The use of these agents may result in treatment-associated cardiotoxicity. Furthermore, the presence of concomitant cardiovascular risk factors and comorbidities can affect the timing, severity, and potentially the reversibility of cancer therapy–related cardiotoxicities. Cardiotoxic effects of chemotherapeutics can occur immediately upon exposure or years later depending on the anticancer therapy.

Cancer therapy–related cardiomyopathy may present as asymptomatic left ventricular systolic dysfunction, subclinical diastolic dysfunction, symptomatic HF, and even cardiogenic shock. Chemotherapy-induced cardiomyopathy is estimated to affect up to 10% of cancer survivors and has among the poorest prognosis compared to other causes of cardiomyopathy.

ANTHRACYCLINES

Anthracyclines have been used for a variety of cancers including solid (eg, breast cancer, sarcoma, lung cancer) and hematologic (eg, leukemia, lymphomas) malignancies. Anthracyclines (doxorubicin, epirubicin, daunorubicin, idarubicin, and mitoxantrone) were first implicated as potential culprits for cardiomyopathy in 1967 when daunomycin was being used for leukemias.

In the Childhood Cancer Survivor Study, administration of less than or equal to 250 mg/m^2 anthracycline therapy was associated with 2.4× increased risk for developing HF, but that rose to a 5.2× risk if greater than 250 mg/m^2 doxorubicin was administered. In contrast, some patients have received doses as high as 1000 mg/m^2 without significant cardiac events, whereas others developed cardiac dysfunction after doses as low as 100 mg/m^2.[9] Overall, the risk of cardiotoxicity increases with cumulative doses of anthracycline; for instance, with doxorubicin, there is an approximately 5% risk at a cumulative dose of 400 mg/m^2, a 26% risk at a dose of 550 mg/m^2, and up to a 48% risk at a cumulative dose of 700 mg/m^2.[10] Factors associated with an increased incidence of anthracycline-induced cardiomyopathy include total dose, dose fractions, concomitant therapies (ie, other chemotherapy or radiotherapy), female sex, cardiovascular risk factors (including tobacco use, hypertension, dyslipidemia, obesity, diabetes mellitus, underlying left ventricular dysfunction), and age (>65 years or <4 years).[11,12] Genetic factors may also play a role. Decreased expression of topoisomerase 2b has been associated with a variant of the retinoic receptor g gene, which predicts predisposition to cardiotoxicity in childhood cancer patients receiving anthracycline therapy.[13]

Pathogenesis

Anthracyclines are thought to cause cardiac dysfunction by damaging topoisomerase-IIβ in cardiomyocytes and decreasing expression of genes promoting antioxidative and electron transport expression. Consequently, this leads to deoxyribonucleic acid double strand breaks, defects in mitochondrial biogenesis, formation of reactive oxygen species, and subsequent cardiomyocyte death.[14] Endomyocardial biopsies show myocyte damage with vacuolar swelling, myofibrillar disarray, and cell death. Anthracyclines may also affect pathways regulating the growth of heart muscle during maturation.

On a macroscopic scale, anthracycline-induced cardiomyopathy is typically described as new-onset HF or evidence of left ventricular dysfunction, usually based on assessment of LVEF. In a longitudinal study of childhood acute lymphoblastic leukemia survivors over 15 years after anthracycline treatment, decreased left ventricular mass and restrictive cardiomyopathy were noted. Myocardial mass declined by 5% as early as 6 months after receiving anthracyclines along with increased afterload and associated HF symptomology. Cardiotoxicity occurs during anthracycline treatment with progressive injury that can extend for years after treatment is completed. Hence, acute (sometimes noted with only symptoms or troponin elevation without LVEF decline) and/or late manifestations may occur following anthracycline therapy.

Clinical Presentation: Anthracycline Toxicity

Three time courses of anthracycline toxicity have been described. An acute episode of symptomatic HF may occur after a single dose or course of anthracyclines with clinical manifestations seen within 2 weeks of treatment. Subacute episodes—occurring within 1 year of anthracycline treatment—manifest as a dilated cardiomyopathy with symptoms of HF, and this is the most common presentation. The final form is a chronic or late-onset cardiomyopathy, presenting years to decades after the chemotherapy course.

A more recent prospective study suggests that anthracycline cardiotoxicity may not be discrete in presentation. Rather, it exists in a spectrum, and myocardial damage can be seen histologically after the first dose. The median time from the last dose of anthracycline to the development of cardiotoxicity was 3.5 months, with 98% of cases occurring within the first year of follow-up and most having asymptomatic LVEF depression. Accordingly, later diagnosis of symptomatic HF in the original retrospective studies may have been preceded by undiagnosed asymptomatic left ventricular dysfunction in an era when LVEF monitoring was less ubiquitous. There is also a consideration for the multiple-hit hypothesis where the myocardium is made susceptible by anthracyclines and then subsequently has further deterioration with the introduction of additional cardiovascular risk factors.[15]

In the era of modern chemotherapy treatment, about 9% of anthracycline-treated patients develop cardiotoxicity, with 81% having New York Heart Association (NYHA) class I-II symptoms and another 19% having NYHA Class III-IV symptoms. The majority (82%) of patients have some degree of recovery (mean time 8 ± 5 months, 11% full recovery, 71% partial recovery) following completion of their anthracycline regimen. Of those who do not develop frank cardiotoxicity, there is still a slight decline in LVEF from baseline (ie, from 64% to 61%). Earlier detection of cardiomyopathy with guideline-directed HF therapy was associated with recovery of LVEF.

Management of Patient with Anthracycline Toxicity

A preventative strategy for cancer therapy-related cardiotoxicity involves a multidisciplinary approach including oncologists, cardiologists, pharmacists, and nursing. All patients receiving anthracycline therapy should have a baseline history and physical, optimization of cardiovascular risk factors and pretherapy assessment of cardiac function by echocardiogram or other imaging modalities (**Algorithms 74.1**). All modifiable cardiovascular risk factors such as smoking, diabetes, and hypertension should be addressed. If a patient has symptomatic HF or LVEF less than 40%, anthracycline therapy should be avoided if possible. In patients with asymptomatic left ventricular dysfunction with LVEF greater than 40%, clinicians should optimize goal-directed HF therapy and risk factors. Patients should also have regular imaging during therapy and after completion to assess for LVEF decline. In cancer patients who develop cardiomyopathy, the ideal scenario would utilize non-anthracycline-containing regimens while maintaining chemotherapeutic efficacy.

Anthracycline-induced cardiomyopathy is treated according to guideline-directed management of HF, with no specific interventions for this etiology. However, the focus should be on prevention. Because anthracycline-induced cardiotoxicity is dose-dependent, dose limitation plays a major role. The generally accepted safe cumulative dose is less than 400 mg/m^2 as there is an estimated 5% risk of HF at a cumulative dose of 400 mg/m^2. However, cardiac safety needs to be balanced with optimal cancer therapy efficacy for the greatest chance of patient longevity, which may mean higher doses of anthracyclines.[12]

Based on the 2017 guidelines, patients who receive high-dose anthracycline therapy (eg, doxorubicin ≥250 mg/m^2, epirubicin ≥600 mg/m^2) or lower dose therapy in combination with radiotherapy where the heart is in the treatment field are at increased risk for developing cardiac dysfunction.[16] Patients who receive lower dose anthracyclines that are older (≥60 years), have two or more risk factors (ie, diabetes

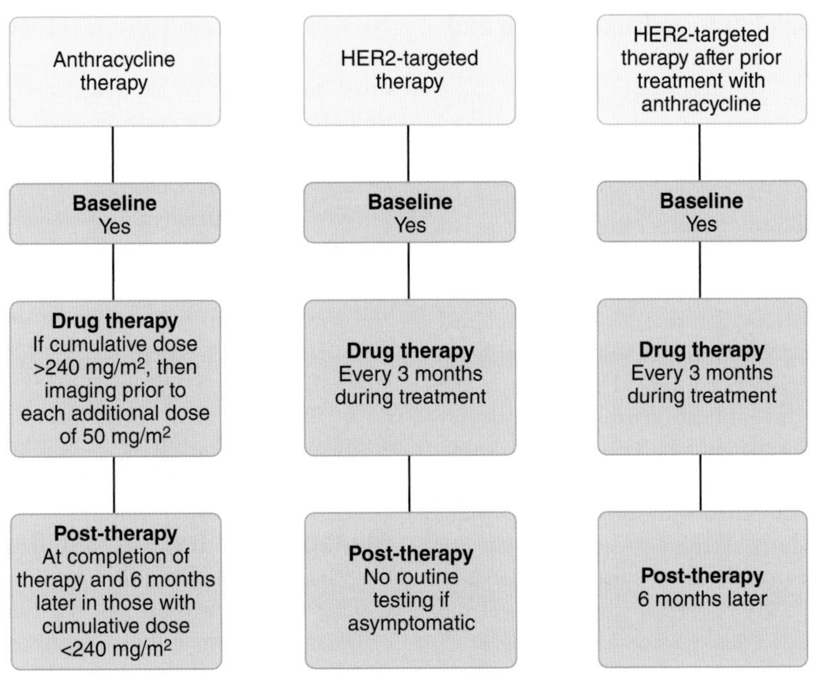

ALGORITHM 74.1 Echocardiographic surveillance during and after treatment with anthracycline therapy or HER2-targeted therapy.

mellitus, dyslipidemia, hypertension, obesity, smoking), or receive subsequent trastuzumab therapy are also at increased risk of cardiomyopathy. These patients should be monitored and have modifiable risk factors actively managed. For those receiving high-dose anthracyclines, there is also consideration to use a liposomal formulation of doxorubicin to prevent cardiotoxicity or include the cardioprotectant dexrazoxane, continuous infusion. Liposomal formulations of anthracyclines selectively enter cancer cells (thought to be secondary to damaged microvasculature and lymphatic systems) and have limited effect on cardiomyocytes.[17] Dexrazoxane chelates intracellular iron, thereby blocking free radical formations and inhibiting the topoisomerase II-β isoenzyme.[18] Although there is some controversy concerning whether dexrazoxane inhibits the anticancer benefits of anthracyclines, a large Cochrane meta-analysis suggested use of dexrazoxane did not diminish response rates.[19]

Research and Future Directions

Additional efforts are underway to study β-blockers (ie, metoprolol, carvedilol, nebivolol), angiotensin-converting enzyme inhibitors (ACEi) (ie, enalapril), angiotensin receptor blockers (ARBs) (ie, candesartan), statins, and other agents for prevention of cardiotoxicity. Cardinale et al[20] reported nearly complete prevention of anthracycline-induced cardiomyopathy with enalapril, and Kalay et al[21] achieved similar effects with carvedilol. The outcomes of later studies were more heterogeneous. In patients treated for early breast cancer with adjuvant anthracyclines with or without trastuzumab, concomitant treatment with candesartan, but not metoprolol, prevented early decline in LVEF.[22] Conversely, Kaya et al showed beneficial effects of nebivolol.[23] In the OVERCOME (preventiOn of LV dysfunction with Enalapril and caRvedilol in patients submitted to intensive ChemOtherapy for the treatment of Malignant hEmopathies) trial, where patients were mostly treated with anthracyclines, a combination of an ACEi and a β-blocking agent was shown to be cardioprotective.[24] Recently, a prospective, randomized, double-blind, placebo-controlled study on prevention of anthracycline cardiotoxicity (The Carvedilol Effect in Preventing Chemotherapy Induced Cardiotoxicity trial) failed to find any difference in LVEF between carvedilol- and placebo-treated patients.[25]

In patients who develop left ventricular dysfunction or clinical HF, a shared decision-making approach should be pursued, evaluating the risk/benefit of holding further anthracycline treatment and using alternative cancer therapies if possible. Patients should be treated according to goal-directed HF therapy and have contributing factors, such as hypertension, optimized.

HER2-TARGETED AGENTS: TRASTUZAMAB AND PERTUZUMAB

Trastuzumab (Herceptin)[26] is indicated for adjuvant treatment of HER2-overexpressing breast cancer. It is typically used (1) as a treatment regimen containing doxorubicin, cyclophosphamide, and either paclitaxel or docetaxel; (2) with docetaxel and carboplatin; or (3) as a single agent following multimodality anthracycline-based therapy. Trastuzumab is also used in the treatment of gastric cancers. Pertuzumab (Perjetz) is approved for use in combination with trastuzumab and docetaxel in people who have metastatic HER2-positive breast cancer.

Epidemiology and Risk Factors: Trastuzumab and Pertuzumab Therapy

Left ventricular dysfunction associated with targeted therapies has been most extensively evaluated with trastuzumab. The incidence of trastuzumab cardiac toxicity is dependent on a number of risk factors including anthracycline chemotherapy exposure, patient age, and cardiovascular comorbidities. In patients with advanced breast cancer disease, the incidence of left ventricular dysfunction ranges from 2% to 7% when trastuzumab is used as monotherapy, 2% to 13% when combined with paclitaxel, and up to 27% when in combination with anthracyclines.[27] In the Herceptin Adjuvant (HERA) study, the incidence of trastuzumab discontinuation owing to cardiac disorders was low (4.3%). Most patients with cardiac dysfunction recovered in less than 6 months after cessation of therapy.[28]

Clinical risk factors associated with increased risk of developing trastuzumab-induced cardiomyopathy include age greater than 50 years, decreased LVEF, obesity, and previous or concurrent anthracycline use,[29-36] particularly those receiving concurrent anthracyclines at a dose greater than 300 mg/m^2.[29] For this reason, trastuzumab is typically given in sequential therapy after anthracycline-containing regimens. Trastuzumab in combination with taxanes has low rates of cardiotoxicity.

In one small study of elderly women (age >70 years) treated with trastuzumab, those with diabetes had a greater than fivefold increased risk of cardiotoxicity compared to those without diabetes. For patients with nonmetastatic HER2 positive breast cancer, radiotherapy is commonly administered concurrently with adjuvant trastuzumab.[37] Fortunately, concurrent treatment with trastuzumab and adjuvant radiation therapy does not increase the risk of cardiovascular toxicity.

Pathogenesis: Trastuzumab and Pertuzumab Toxicity

Trastuzumab binds to the extracellular domain of the HER2 receptor that prevents activation of intracellular tyrosine kinase and subsequently leads to reduced HER2 signaling via several mechanisms.[38] Pertuzumab binds farther from the extracellular membrane and imposes a similar downstream cascade on the HER2 receptor pathway. Cardiac dysfunction associated with trastuzumab appears to be a direct consequence of HER2 inhibition in cardiomyocytes: trastuzumab dysregulates HER2 signaling and suppresses autophagy in cardiomyocytes to trigger the accumulation of toxic reactive oxygen species. There are no distinct biopsy findings typical or pathognomonic for trastuzumab-induced cardiomyopathy.

Diagnosis and Cardiac Monitoring: Trastuzumab and Other HER2-Targeted Agents

Trastuzumab-induced cardiotoxicity is diagnosed by a decrease in LVEF with or without symptoms of HF. In case of asymptomatic left ventricular dysfunction, most clinical trials use an absolute decrease in LVEF of greater than 10% to below the lower limit of normal or greater than 15% from the baseline value.[39] In order to ensure timely diagnosis of asymptomatic left ventricular dysfunction, The National Comprehensive Cancer Network recommends that LVEF be monitored at baseline and every 3 months during trastuzumab therapy.[10] Recently, other assessments of left ventricular function have emerged as more sensitive for early diagnosis of HER2 therapy-related cardiotoxicity. Baseline global longitudinal strain (GLS) and changes in GLS have emerged as powerful adjunctive tools,[40] as they are independently prognostic for developing cancer therapy-related cardiotoxicity. Further, GLS has additive predictive value in addition to the traditional clinical parameters and baseline LVEF in predicting the development of cardiotoxicity. Using serum cardiac biomarkers—such as troponin and natriuretic peptides—in screening for trastuzumab cardiotoxicity has poor discriminative ability as a stand-alone tool. Nevertheless, elevated serum troponin levels during cancer therapy portend a poor cardiovascular prognosis.

Management: Trastuzumab Cardiotoxicity

Several algorithms for cardiac monitoring during trastuzumab therapy have been proposed, but there is limited consensus on when trastuzumab should be discontinued. The European Society for Medical Oncology's (ESMO) guidelines has proposed a *stopping/starting* rule based on trastuzumab trial data (**Algorithm 74.2**). If the LVEF absolute decline is greater than 15% from baseline to below the lower limit of normal (50%), trastuzumab is withheld for 4 weeks, and LVEF is reassessed.[41] In clinical practice, the use of cardioprotective strategies with ACEi, ARB, and β-blocker therapy may be deployed in this setting. If the LVEF remains below these levels after treatment interruption, then typically trastuzumab is discontinued. Additionally, those who develop symptomatic HF on therapy should stop further trastuzumab cycles.

A number of clinical trials have assessed cardioprotective strategies with ACEis, ARBs, and β-blockers in breast cancer patients undergoing trastuzumab therapy. The Multidisciplinary Approach to Novel Therapies in Cardiology Oncology Research trial (MANTICORE) assessed 94 patients with early HER2-positive breast cancer receiving trastuzumab with or without anthracyclines treated with perindopril or bisoprolol, as compared to placebo.[42] The study authors did not find statistically significant changes in LVEF with perindopril or bisoprolol, but there were modest improvements in left ventricular (LV) end-diastolic volumes and asymptomatic LVEF reduction.

In the largest study to date of 468 patients with HER2-positive breast cancer, Guglin et al assessed the effect of lisinopril versus carvedilol versus placebo in preventing trastuzumab cardiotoxicity.[43] Neither lisinopril nor carvedilol was effective at preventing cardiomyopathy compared with placebo. However, among those treated with an anthracycline prior to trastuzumab therapy, lisinopril and carvedilol appeared to be effective at preventing cardiomyopathy and minimizing treatment interruptions.

The SAFE-HEaRt study (A pilot study assessing the cardiac SAFEty of HER2-targeted therapy in patients with HER2 positive breast cancer and reduced left ventricular function; ClinicalTrials.gov, Identifier: NCT01904903) of 30 patients

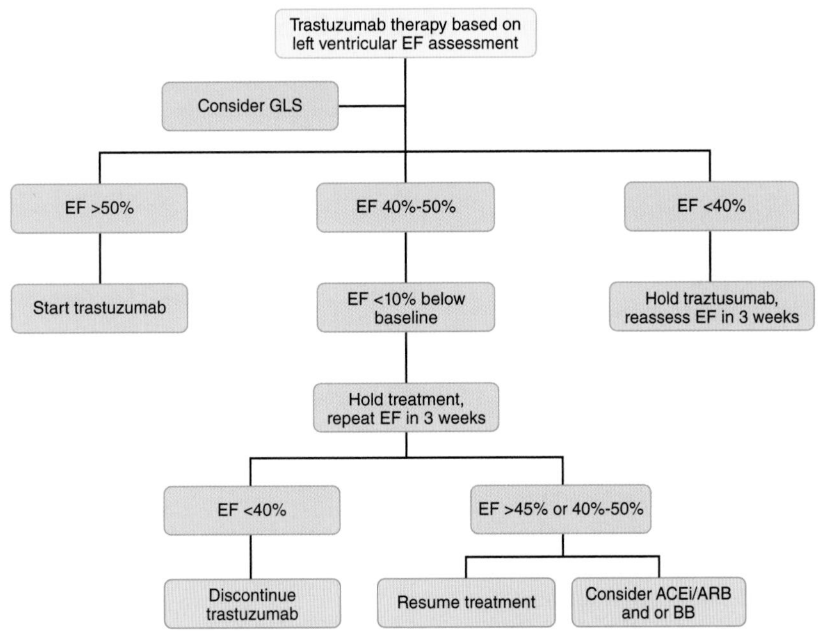

ALGORITHM 74.2 Algorithm for trastuzumab continuation or discontinuation based on left ventricular ejection fractions (LVEF) assessment. ACEi, angiotensin-converting enzyme inhibitor; ARB, angiotensin receptor blocker; BB, β-blocker; EF, ejection fraction; GLS, global longitudinal strain. (Reprinted from Curigliano G, Cardinale D, Suter T, et al. Cardiovascular toxicity induced by chemotherapy, targeted agents and radiotherapy: ESMO Clinical Practice Guidelines. *Ann Oncol.* 2012;23(Suppl 7):vii155-vii166. Copyright © 2012 European Society for Medical Oncology. With permission.)

sought to prospectively assess if trastuzumab can safely be used in patients with mildly reduced left ventricular systolic function (defined as LVEF between 40% and 49%). Despite small numbers, these data suggest that HER2-targeted therapy can be safely administered to women with reduced LVEF in the setting of ongoing treatment with β-blocker and ACEi or an ARB.[44] Future research is needed to translate these studies into clinical practice.

As new evidence emerges, there are limited harmonizing guidelines on what the optimal strategies are for mitigating trastuzumab cardiotoxicity. There is consensus that overt changes in LVEF (ie, decline to less than 40%) or symptomatic HF warrant trastuzumab interruption and treatment with an ACEi or ARB and β-blocker per standard of care. In practice, the threshold LVEF for initiation of cardioprotective treatment may be less than 50% (ie, patients with LVEF 40% to 50%, may be started on an ACEi or ARB and β-blocker). Several risk scores have been developed to predict the cardiac risk of HF or cardiomyopathy with or without anthracycline exposures, but these tools need additional validation and are not used in general clinical practice.

Research and Long-term Implications of Trastuzumab Cardiotoxicity

Most patients tolerate trastuzumab-associated changes in left ventricular function. Moreover, these changes may be reversible. A recent pooled analysis of[41,45-47] trastuzumab-treated patients—most of whom also received anthracycline chemotherapy—showed 11.3% experienced a cardiac event, with most (8.7%) being mildly symptomatic or asymptomatic LVEF decrease. In long-term follow-up,[36] severe HF was more common in trastuzumab-treated patients (2.3%) than in those who did not receive trastuzumab as part of their chemotherapeutic regiment (0.8%). However, a large majority of patients completed trastuzumab treatment (76.2%).

OTHER CHEMOTHERAPY

Besides anthracyclines and targeted therapies, other cancer therapies may potentially increase the risk for patients developing cardiomyopathies. This includes antimetabolites, microtubule-targeting agents, and alkylating agents. Newer cancer therapies can also cause cardiomyopathy including vascular endothelial growth factor signaling pathway inhibitors and proteasome inhibitors.

A unique class of cancer treatment medications includes immunotherapy. Checkpoint inhibitors enhance the body's natural immune system, via antibodies, to attack cancer cells for a variety of tumors including Hodgkin lymphoma, non-small cell lung cancer, melanoma, renal cell carcinoma, head and neck cancers, and others. The primary targets for these agents include programmed cell death receptor 1 (nivolumab, pembrolizumab), programmed cell death ligand 1 (atezolizumab, avelumab, and durvalumab), and cytotoxic T-lymphocyte associated antigen 4 (ipilimumab). Although they provide significant benefits, significant immune-related adverse effects may occur with the antibodies attacking healthy tissue thereby causing dermatologic (vitiligo), gastrointestinal (diarrhea and colitis), endocrine (hypothyroidism, hyperthyroidism, adrenal insufficiency, diabetes mellitus), and pulmonary (pneumonitis) manifestations in the setting of an intensified immune system. Although rare, cardiotoxicity may also occur, with a higher incidence with multiple versus single-agent therapy (0.27% vs 0.06%, respectively).[48]

Signs and symptoms of HF typically develop after only one to two doses of checkpoint inhibitors. In one study, death occurred in 46% of patients with checkpoint inhibitor–associated myocarditis.[49] If patients on immunotherapy develop chest pain, palpitations, edema, dyspnea, fatigue, or clinical signs of HF, an electrocardiogram and cardiac biomarkers should be obtained. If abnormal, immune checkpoint inhibitor therapy should be discontinued until cardiology consultation and further diagnostic workup (ie, echocardiogram, cardiac magnetic resonance imaging) are obtained. Initial treatment should focus on managing symptoms based on the American College of Cardiology (ACC)/American Heart Association (AHA) HF guidelines with additional consideration given for high-dose corticosteroids (1-2 mg/kg of prednisone). If patients do not respond to oral steroids, intravenous methylprednisolone (1 g q daily) can be considered along with immunosuppressants (eg, mycophenolate or antithymocyte globulin).

KEY POINTS

- ✔ Many addictive drugs—such as alcohol, cocaine, and methamphetamine—may cause cardiomyopathy, which is frequently reversible on cessation of use of the offensive drug.
- ✔ In a small proportion of cases, cardiomyopathies caused by addictive drugs, cause long-lasting or irreversible damage to the cardiac muscle.
- ✔ Some prescription drugs also can cause cardiomyopathy.
- ✔ Anthracyclines cause dose-dependent cardiomyopathy.
- ✔ Anthracycline cardiac toxicity can be alleviated by using dexrazosan or liposomal formulation of doxorubicin.
- ✔ Anthracycline-induced cardiomyopathy may be partially reversible if treated according to HF guidelines.
- ✔ β-blockers, ACEis, and ARBs, used prophylactically, may be able to minimize or prevent anthracycline-induced cardiotoxicity.
- ✔ Trastuzumab causes mild and mostly reversible cardiomyopathy.
- ✔ Cardiotoxic effects from HER2-targeted therapy remain a challenging and important clinical entity.
- ✔ Despite the cardiac risks associated with HER2-targeted agents, the benefits favor their use.
- ✔ Patients receiving HER2-targeted agents must undergo vigilant cardiovascular monitoring, management of baseline cardiovascular risk factors, and early initiation of cardioprotective strategies.

REFERENCES

1. Varga ZV, Ferdinandy P, Liaudet L, Pacher P. Drug-induced mitochondrial dysfunction and cardiotoxicity. *Am J Physiol Heart Circ Physiol.* 2015;309(9):H1453-H1467.
2. Voskoboinik A, Prabhu S, Ling LH, Kalman JM, Kistler PM. Alcohol and atrial fibrillation: a sobering review. *J Am Coll Cardiol.* 2016;68(23):2567-2576.
3. Maisch B. Alcoholic cardiomyopathy: the result of dosage and individual predisposition. *Herz.* 2016;41(6):484-493.
4. Havakuk O, Rezkalla SH, Kloner RA. The cardiovascular effects of cocaine. *J Am Coll Cardiol.* 2017;70(1):101-113.
5. Zaca V, Lunghetti S, Ballo P, Focardi M, Favilli R, Mondillo S. Recovery from cardiomyopathy after abstinence from cocaine. *Lancet.* 2007;369(9572):1574.
6. Diercks DB, Fonarow GC, Kirk JD, et al. Illicit stimulant use in a United States heart failure population presenting to the emergency department (from the Acute Decompensated Heart Failure National Registry Emergency Module). *Am J Cardiol.* 2008;102(9):1216-1219.
7. Voskoboinik A, Ihle JF, Bloom JE, Kaye DM. Methamphetamine-associated cardiomyopathy: patterns and predictors of recovery. *Intern Med J.* 2016;46(6):723-727.
8. Yogasundaram H, Hung W, Paterson ID, Sergi C, Oudit GY. Chloroquine-induced cardiomyopathy: a reversible cause of heart failure. *ESC Heart Fail.* 2018;5(3):372-375.
9. Nysom K, Holm K, Lipsitz SR, et al. Relationship between cumulative anthracycline dose and late cardiotoxicity in childhood acute lymphoblastic leukemia. *J Clin Oncol.* 1998;16(2):545-550.
10. Mehta LS, Watson KE, Barac A, et al. Cardiovascular disease and breast cancer: where these entities intersect: a scientific statement from the American Heart Association. *Circulation.* 2018;137(8):e30-e66.
11. Plana JC, Galderisi M, Barac A, et al. Expert consensus for multimodality imaging evaluation of adult patients during and after cancer therapy: a report from the American Society of Echocardiography and the European Association of Cardiovascular Imaging. *J Am Soc Echocardiogr.* 2014;27(9):911-939.
12. Swain SM, Whaley FS, Ewer MS. Congestive heart failure in patients treated with doxorubicin: a retrospective analysis of three trials. *Cancer.* 2003;97(11):2869-2879.
13. Aminkeng F, Bhavsar AP, Visscher H, et al. A coding variant in RARG confers susceptibility to anthracycline-induced cardiotoxicity in childhood cancer. *Nat Genet.* 2015;47(9):1079-1084.
14. Zhang S, Liu X, Bawa-Khalfe T, et al. Identification of the molecular basis of doxorubicin-induced cardiotoxicity. *Nat Med.* 2012;18(11):1639-1642.
15. Cardinale D, Colombo A, Bacchiani G, et al. Early detection of anthracycline cardiotoxicity and improvement with heart failure therapy. *Circulation.* 2015;131(22):1981-1988.
16. Armenian SH, Lacchetti C, Barac A, et al. Prevention and monitoring of cardiac dysfunction in survivors of adult cancers: American Society of Clinical Oncology Clinical Practice Guideline. *J Clin Oncol.* 2017;35(8):893-911.
17. Batist G. Cardiac safety of liposomal anthracyclines. *Cardiovasc Toxicol.* 2007;7(2):72-74.
18. Hasinoff BB, Herman EH. Dexrazoxane: how it works in cardiac and tumor cells. Is it a prodrug or is it a drug? *Cardiovasc Toxicol.* 2007;7(2):140-144.
19. van Dalen EC, Caron HN, Dickinson HO, Kremer LC. Cardioprotective interventions for cancer patients receiving anthracyclines. *Cochrane Database Syst Rev.* 2011;(6):CD003917.
20. Cardinale D, Colombo A, Sandri MT, et al. Prevention of high-dose chemotherapy-induced cardiotoxicity in high-risk patients by angiotensin-converting enzyme inhibition. *Circulation.* 2006;114(23):2474-2481.

21. Kalay N, Basar E, Ozdogru I, et al. Protective effects of carvedilol against anthracycline-induced cardiomyopathy. *J Am Coll Cardiol.* 2006;48(11):2258-2262.
22. Gulati G, Heck SL, Ree AH, et al. Prevention of cardiac dysfunction during adjuvant breast cancer therapy (PRADA): a 2 × 2 factorial, randomized, placebo-controlled, double-blind clinical trial of candesartan and metoprolol. *Eur Heart J.* 2016;37(21):1671-1680.
23. Kaya MG, Ozkan M, Gunebakmaz O, et al. Protective effects of nebivolol against anthracycline-induced cardiomyopathy: a randomized control study. *Int J Cardiol.* 2013;167(5):2306-2310.
24. Bosch X, Rovira M, Sitges M, et al. Enalapril and carvedilol for preventing chemotherapy-induced left ventricular systolic dysfunction in patients with malignant hemopathies: the OVERCOME trial (preventiOn of left Ventricular dysfunction with Enalapril and caRvedilol in patients submitted to intensive ChemOtherapy for the treatment of Malignant hEmopathies). *J Am Coll Cardiol.* 2013;61(23):2355-2362.
25. Avila MS, Ayub-Ferreira SM, de Barros Wanderley MR Jr, et al. Carvedilol for prevention of chemotherapy related cardiotoxicity. *J Am Coll Cardiol.* 2018;71(20):2281-2290.
26. Genentech. HERCEPTIN® (trastuzumab). https://www.accessdata.fda.gov/drugsatfda_docs/label/2010/103792s5250lbl.pdf
27. Oncology. Chemotherapy-related heart failure. Chapter 1—Cardiac Complications of Cancer and Anti-Cancer Treatment. https://oncologypro.esmo.org/Education-Library/Handbooks/Oncological-Emergencies/Chemotherapy-related-Heart-Failure
28. Suter TM, Procter M, van Veldhuisen DJ, et al. Trastuzumab-associated cardiac adverse effects in the herceptin adjuvant trial. *J Clin Oncol.* 2007;25(25):3859-3865.
29. Seidman A, Hudis C, Pierri MK, et al. Cardiac dysfunction in the trastuzumab clinical trials experience. *J Clin Oncol.* 2002;20(5):1215-1221.
30. Slamon D, Eiermann W, Robert N, et al. Adjuvant trastuzumab in HER2-positive breast cancer. *N Engl J Med.* 2011;365(14):1273-1283.
31. Valero V, Forbes J, Pegram MD, et al. Multicenter phase III randomized trial comparing docetaxel and trastuzumab with docetaxel, carboplatin, and trastuzumab as first-line chemotherapy for patients with HER2-gene-amplified metastatic breast cancer (BCIRG 007 study): two highly active therapeutic regimens. *J Clin Oncol.* 2011;29(2):149-156.
32. Bergman I, Barmada MA, Griffin JA, Slamon DJ. Treatment of meningeal breast cancer xenografts in the rat using an anti-p185/HER2 antibody. *Clin Cancer Res.* 2001;7(7):2050-2056.
33. Slamon DJ, Leyland-Jones B, Shak S, et al. Use of chemotherapy plus a monoclonal antibody against HER2 for metastatic breast cancer that overexpresses HER2. *N Engl J Med.* 2001;344(11):783-792.
34. Harbeck N, Ewer MS, De Laurentiis M, Suter TM, Ewer SM. Cardiovascular complications of conventional and targeted adjuvant breast cancer therapy. *Ann Oncol.* 2011;22(6):1250-1258.
35. Curigliano G, Cardinale D, Suter T, et al. Cardiovascular toxicity induced by chemotherapy, targeted agents and radiotherapy: ESMO Clinical Practice Guidelines. *Ann Oncol.* 2012;23(suppl 7):vii155-vii166.
36. de Azambuja E, Ponde N, Procter M, et al. A pooled analysis of the cardiac events in the trastuzumab adjuvant trials. *Breast Cancer Res Treat.* 2020;179(1):161-171.
37. Sayan M, Abou Yehia Z, Gupta A, Toppmeyer D, Ohri N, Haffty BG. Acute cardiotoxicity with concurrent trastuzumab and hypofractionated radiation therapy in breast cancer patients. *Front Oncol.* 2019;9:970.
38. Hudis CA. Trastuzumab—mechanism of action and use in clinical practice. *N Engl J Med.* 2007;357(1):39-51.
39. Dang CT, Yu AF, Jones LW, et al. Cardiac surveillance guidelines for trastuzumab-containing therapy in early-stage breast cancer: getting to the heart of the matter. *J Clin Oncol.* 2016;34(10):1030-1033.
40. Clasen SC, Scherrer-Crosbie M. Applications of left ventricular strain measurements to patients undergoing chemotherapy. *Curr Opin Cardiol.* 2018;33(5):493-497.
41. Romond EH, Jeong JH, Rastogi P, et al. Seven-year follow-up assessment of cardiac function in NSABP B-31, a randomized trial comparing doxorubicin and cyclophosphamide followed by paclitaxel (ACP) with ACP plus trastuzumab as adjuvant therapy for patients with node-positive, human epidermal growth factor receptor 2-positive breast cancer. *J Clin Oncol.* 2012;30(31):3792-3799.
42. Pituskin E, Mackey JR, Koshman S, et al. Multidisciplinary Approach to Novel Therapies in Cardio-Oncology Research (MANTICORE 101-Breast): a randomized trial for the prevention of trastuzumab-associated cardiotoxicity. *J Clin Oncol.* 2017;35(8):870-877.
43. Guglin M, Krischer J, Tamura R, et al. Randomized trial of lisinopril versus carvedilol to prevent trastuzumab cardiotoxicity in patients with breast cancer. *J Am Coll Cardiol.* 2019;73(22):2859-2868.
44. Lynce F, Barac A, Geng X, et al. Prospective evaluation of the cardiac safety of HER2-targeted therapies in patients with HER2-positive breast cancer and compromised heart function: the SAFE-HEaRt study. *Breast Cancer Res Treat.* 2019;175(3):595-603.
45. Piccart-Gebhart MJ, Procter M, Leyland-Jones B, et al. Trastuzumab after adjuvant chemotherapy in HER2-positive breast cancer. *N Engl J Med.* 2005;353(16):1659-1672.
46. Romond EH, Perez EA, Bryant J, et al. Trastuzumab plus adjuvant chemotherapy for operable HER2-positive breast cancer. *N Engl J Med.* 2005;353(16):1673-1684.
47. Perez EA, Romond EH, Suman VJ, et al. Trastuzumab plus adjuvant chemotherapy for human epidermal growth factor receptor 2-positive breast cancer: planned joint analysis of overall survival from NSABP B-31 and NCCTG N9831. *J Clin Oncol.* 2014;32(33):3744-3752.
48. Johnson DB, Balko JM, Compton ML, et al. Fulminant myocarditis with combination immune checkpoint blockade. *N Engl J Med.* 2016;375(18):1749-1755.
49. Moslehi JJ, Salem JE, Sosman JA, Lebrun-Vignes B, Johnson DB. Increased reporting of fatal immune checkpoint inhibitor-associated myocarditis. *Lancet.* 2018;391(10124):933.

CHAPTER 75

ACUTE HEART FAILURE

Nicholas S. Hendren, Justin L. Grodin, and Mark H. Drazner

INTRODUCTION

Acute decompensated heart failure (ADHF) is defined as new or recurrent symptoms and signs of heart failure (HF) requiring unscheduled care for impromptu therapies. Clinically, this is manifest by typical symptoms (eg, orthopnea) that may also be accompanied by signs of increased intracardiac pressure (eg, rales). HF is a clinical diagnosis based on a combination of symptoms, physical exam findings, radiographic, and/or laboratory abnormalities. Left ventricular ejection fraction (LVEF) is a key descriptor of HF. Heart failure with reduced ejection fraction (HFrEF) is typically defined as an LVEF less than or equal to 40%, and heart failure with preserved ejection fraction (HFpEF) as an LVEF greater than or equal to 50%. Heart failure with mildly reduced ejection fraction (HFmrEF) represents an LVEF of 41% to 49%. Differentiation based on LVEF is important owing to different underlying etiologies, demographics, comorbidities, and responses to therapy.

Epidemiology

ADHF remains a common reason for hospitalization. In the United States, the total estimated annual cost of HF is projected to increase to nearly $70 billion by 2030.[1] An aging population, increasing rates of obesity, lower myocardial infarction mortality, and improved survival with chronic left ventricular (LV) systolic dysfunction have all resulted in a larger population with chronic HF at risk for acute decompensation.[12,13]

Disease Burden, Incidence, and Trends

Based on data from the U.S. National Inpatient Sample, between 2001 and 2014 more than 57 million admissions occurred for ADHF as the primary or secondary diagnosis.[2] Approximately 25% of these admissions were caused by a primary HF diagnosis.[2] From 2001 to 2014, the rate of hospitalization for the primary diagnosis of HF declined 3% annually from 563/100,000 U.S. adults in 2001 to 398/100,000 U.S. adults in 2014.[2] This is in contrast to the rates of hospitalization for a secondary diagnosis of HF, which remained stable between 2010 and 2014 at approximately 1388/100,000 U.S. adults.[2] From 2013 to 2017, on the other hand, an increase in primary HF admissions was observed, including increases in crude rates of overall and unique patient hospitalizations (JAMA Cardiol. 2021 Feb 10;e207472. doi:10.1001/jamacardio.2020.7472, PMID: 33566058).). Owing to an expanding population, the absolute number of hospitalizations for ADHF is anticipated to increase.

Hospitalization and Outcomes

Large HF registries such as the Acute Decompensated Heart Failure National Registry (ADHERE), Organized Program to Initiate Lifesaving Treatment in Hospitalized Patients with Heart Failure (OPTIMIZE-HF) and EuroHeart Failure Survey II (EHFS II) have helped to inform our understanding of ADHF. Registries have observed that new onset HF represents 12% to 37% of admissions while patients with a known HF history represent 63% to 88% of admissions.[3-5] These registries have demonstrated that despite declining primary HF admissions, the proportion of admissions for HFpEF is increasing. Data from Olmstead County, Minnesota, observed that admissions for HFpEF relative to HFrEF increased at a rate of 1% per year from 1987 to 2001.[6] Similarly, the Get With The Guidelines–Heart Failure (GWTG-HF) registry demonstrated that the proportion of patients hospitalized with ADHF and HFpEF increased from 33% in 2005 to 39%, and those with HFrEF decreased from 52% to 47% in 2010.[7] Presently, the proportions of hospitalizations for ADHF with HFrEF versus HFpEF are roughly equivalent.[8,9]

Demographics and Risk Factors

ADHF is the most common cause of hospitalization for patients greater than or equal to 65 years, and about 75% of HF admissions occur in patients greater than or equal to 65 years old (**Figure 75.1A**).[2] Although the lifetime risk for HF is equal for men[10] and women,[2] women hospitalized for ADHF are more likely to present with HFpEF and are typically older than men.[14-16] Women with HF are less likely to have coronary artery disease (CAD) and are more likely to have hypertension and diabetes.[14-16] In the absence of CAD, the lifetime risk of HF is 11.4% for men and 15.4% for women, suggesting differences partly attributable to hypertension.[11]

Disparities for HF among different races have also been observed. The U.S. National Inpatient Sample from 2001 to 2014 observed that White patients comprised the majority of primary HF hospitalizations (~65%), followed by Black (~20%), Hispanic (~10%), Asian (~2%) patients and other races (~3%).[2] In the Multi-Ethnic Study of Atherosclerosis (MESA), incident HF was highest in Black Americans, followed by Hispanic, White, and Chinese Americans (4.6, 3.5, 2.4, and 1.0 per 1000 person-years, respectively) (**Figure 75.1B**).[17] Black Americans have a higher rate of hospitalization and HF death, at least partially attributed to increased comorbid conditions and lower socioeconomic status.[17,18] Payer status and

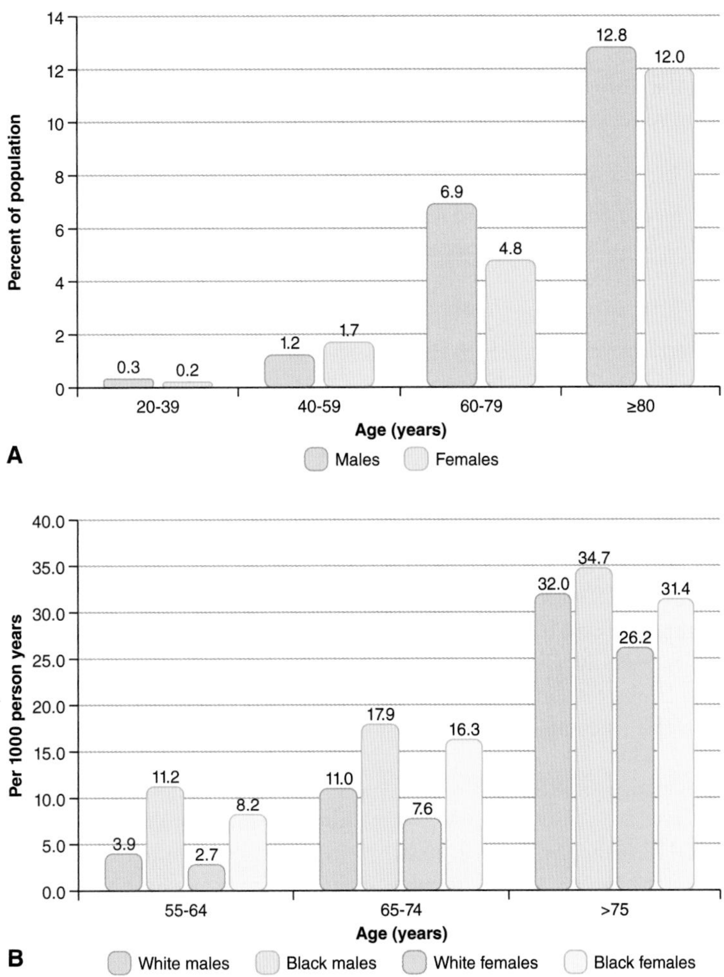

FIGURE 75.1 **A.** Prevalence of heart failure for adults greater than or equal to 20 years by sex and age (statistics from National Health and Nutrition Examination Survey, 2013-2016). **B.** First acute decompensated heart failure annual event rates per 1000 from Atherosclerosis Risk in Communities Study (2005-2014). (Reprinted with permission from Benjamin EJ, Muntner P, Alonso A, et al. Heart Disease and Stroke Statistics—2019 Update: A report from the American Heart Association. *Circulation.* 2019;139(10):e56-e528. Copyright © 2019 American Heart Association, Inc.)

socioeconomic status are strongly associated with clinical outcomes in ADHF.[19] HF patients without insurance are typically younger with fewer comorbidities; however, the absence of insurance is associated with longer hospitalization for ADHF, lower rate of implantable cardioverter defibrillator (ICD) implantation, lower rate of beta-blockade, decreased quality of care, and a trend toward increased in-hospital mortality compared with private payer status.[19] Medicaid insurance is associated with increased risk of rehospitalization or death and repeated hospitalization compared with private payer status.[20] Decreased quality of care and modest increases in adjusted length of stay for HF have also been observed for Medicare groups compared with private payer status.[19] Limited data also suggest that HF may disproportionately affect lower socioeconomic classes. Approximately one-third of the admissions have been reported to occur among patients within the lowest quartile of household income.[2] Lower socioeconomic status has been associated with increased mortality and higher risk of readmission for ADHF.[20-22]

Finally, patients admitted for ADHF are increasingly complex with comorbidies including CAD (50%-60%), chronic obstructive pulmonary disease (20%-30%), chronic renal disease (20%-30%), atrial arrhythmias (30%-35%), and other medical problems.[2,6,15] Frailty is increasingly identified as a comorbidity (18%-54% in the elderly)[23] and has been associated with a higher rate of hospitalization for ADHF, worse prognosis, and higher mortality compared with nonfrail elderly patients with HF.[23]

PATHOPHYSIOLOGY

ADHF is caused principally by a deterioration of cardiac function in combination with simultaneous central and peripheral processes, leading to congestion through sodium and fluid retention.

Myocardial Injury

During ADHF, cardiac injury can be caused both by a decrease in the myocardial oxygen supply and by an increase in the myocardial oxygen demand. Acute ischemia from acute coronary syndrome (ACS) can dramatically reduce myocardial function. Subacute oxygen supply mismatch in the absence of ACS may be related to a combination of low coronary diastolic blood pressure and high LV diastolic pressure, resulting in decreased coronary artery perfusion; tachycardia, reducing coronary artery perfusion time; and reduced oxygen delivery.[8,24] Increased myocardial oxygen demand can be caused by tachycardia, increased LV wall stress, activation of inflammatory cascades, and/or inotrope therapy, which may all exacerbate oxygen demand mismatch.[8]

Evidence of myocardial injury during ADHF is often demonstrated by elevation in plasma troponin levels. The ADHERE registry demonstrated that 6.2% of patients hospitalized with ADHF had an abnormally elevated plasma cardiac troponin T (>0.1 µg/L) or I (>1 µg/L) concentration, which was associated with a lower systolic blood pressure and higher-in-hospital mortality (8.0% vs 2.7%) compared with a normal troponin.[25] More recently, in the RELAX-AHF 9 (RELAXi in Acute Heart Failure) trial, 93% of patients had an abnormal high-sensitivity troponin (>0.013 µg/L), and a higher troponin level was independently associated with a higher, 180-day, mortality.[26] Both observations demonstrate that myocardial injury during ADHF is common and associated with a worse prognosis.

Cardiorenal Mechanisms

An important component of ADHF pathophysiology is renal function. Worsening renal function during ADHF, termed "cardiorenal syndrome," is common (25%-35%) during hospitalization and is associated with worse outcomes and a longer hospital stay.[27] A general definition is a rise in creatinine of at least 0.3 mg/dL. [27] However, it is important to distinguish between transient fluctuations in renal function versus frank renal injury. During treatment for ADH, transient changes in creatinine are common and are not associated with adverse outcomes if effective decongestion is achieved.[28]

Classically, worsening renal function is attributed to the cardiac output due to a failing heart resulting in pre-renal hypoperfusion. More recent investigations suggest this may be a minor contributor.[28] The relationship between intracardiac hemodynamics and renal function is complex. For instance, elevated central venous pressure is a strong predictor of worsening renal function rather than reduced cardiac output.[29] Elevated right atrial pressures lead to elevated central venous pressures, resulting in renal venous hypertension and increased renal vascular resistance, and impaired intrarenal blood flow increases the pressure within Bowman capsule, leading to "backward congestion."[28,30] On the other hand, inadequate cardiac output can activate the renin-angiotensin-aldosterone system (RAAS) and the sympathetic nervous system (SNS), leading to fluid retention, increased preload, increased catecholamines, and worsening cardiac pump failure.[28,31]

Therapies to decrease congestion may reduce intravascular volume, leading to decreased glomerular perfusion pressure, increased neurohormonal activation, and vasoconstriction, paradoxically leading to temporarily worse renal function.[28] Activation of the neurohormonal mediators results in increased proximal tubular sodium and water reabsorption, often resulting in oliguria and worsening congestion.[28] Finally, the low resistance of the renal vasculature and the low oxygen tension in the outer medulla make the kidneys sensitive to hypotension-induced injury.[28]

Vascular Mechanisms

There is increasing recognition that the vascular system has an important role in the pathophysiology of ADHF. Peripheral arterial vasoconstriction increases LV afterload and LV filling pressures and redistributes blood flow centrally, leading to increased vascular congestion. Several studies suggest that increases in body weight can precede clinical symptoms of congestion; however, studies using implantable hemodynamic monitors have also demonstrated that increases in LV diastolic filling pressures can occur without changes in body weight.[32] This suggests that intravascular redistribution, rather than frank overload, is one of the mechanisms leading to adverse hemodynamics. The venous system stores about 70% of the total blood volume, and the splanchnic system approximately 25% in healthy individuals.[33,34] The splanchnic system is more compliant than arterial vessels and has a large capacitance to act as a reservoir for excess blood volume.[33]

SNS activation can result in active blood transfer into the systemic circulation, whereas passive splanchnic recruitment can contribute to congestion.[33,35] Splanchnic blood volume shifts may contribute to the rapid improvement of HF symptoms within a few hours of treatment despite minimal changes in body weight.[33,36] Mechanisms of HF pathology may include a reduced storage capacity and inability to tolerate extra volume; visceral congestion; contributing to cardiorenal syndrome; and increased sympathetic tone, contributing to increased venous pressures and peripheral edema.[33] Contributions of the splanchnic vasculature to HF pathology remains an area of active research.

CLINICAL PRESENTATION AND DIAGNOSTIC EVALUATION

The initial evaluation of the patient with suspected ADHF should focus on an efficient and expeditious diagnosis of HF, defining the clinical profile of the patient, triaging to an appropriate level of care, and providing urgent therapies for potentially life-threatening conditions.

Symptoms

Most patients presenting with ADHF have gradual progression of symptoms over days or weeks before seeking care. However, symptoms occasionally develop suddenly in the setting of ACS, acute valvular dysfunction, or a hypertensive crisis. Symptoms from HF are characterized by a diverse composite of physiologic, psychological, and social factors, leading to a high degree of heterogeneity between patients.[37] Dyspnea is the predominant left HF symptom, occurring in greater than 90% of patients, and can occur at rest, with exertion, or in specific positions (eg, orthopnea or bendopnea). Peripheral and abdominal edema are additional hallmark right-sided HF symptoms in addition to nausea, anorexia, early satiety, and right upper quadrant pain. A list of symptoms is provided in **Table 75.1.**

Physical Examination

Despite advancements in biomarkers, imaging and labs, the clinical exam remains fundamental to identifying the hemodynamic status of the patient (**Table 75.2**). Heart rate and blood pressure are important assessments in patients with ADHF. Tachycardia is often present either owing to arrhythmias or as a compensatory mechanism to maintain cardiac output with a reduced stroke volume. Most patients presenting with ADHF are normotensive or hypertensive. Based on the ADHERE registry, about 50% of patients presenting with ADHF have a systolic blood pressure greater than 140 mm Hg, and about 15% of patients have a systolic blood pressure greater than 175 mm Hg.[38] Hypotension with a systolic blood pressure less than 90 mm Hg occurs in a minority of patients admitted with ADHF but is strongly associated with worse outcomes.[3] Pulse pressure (difference between systolic and diastolic blood pressure) and proportional pulse pressure (pulse pressure/systolic blood pressure) are useful indirect crude assessments of LV stroke volume and, thus, cardiac index. For acute and chronic systolic HF, a proportional pulse pressure less than 25% is associated with a cardiac index (CI) less than 2.2 L/min/m^2.[39-41] Increased pulse pressure may indicate underlying anemia, aortic insufficiency, thyroid abnormalities, and/or poor vascular compliance.

Jugular venous distention (JVD) is a useful estimate of right atrial pressure, but accurate assessment is highly dependent on the skills of the examiner. For most patients, higher right atrial pressure is related to a higher pulmonary capillary wedge pressure (PCWP).[42] However, this association may not be true in the setting of significant tricuspid regurgitation, isolated right ventricular failure, pericardial constriction, restrictive cardiomyopathy, or a large pulmonary embolism.

Careful auscultation can reveal clinical clues about underlying cardiac function and valvular abnormalities. Despite poor interobserver agreement,[43] extra heart sounds (S3 or S4) are present in at least 30% of patients admitted for ADHF.[44] The presence of a third heart sound and elevated jugular venous pressure (JVP) were independently associated with all-cause death, HF death, and increased HF hospitalization.[44] A right ventricular heave, pulsatile liver, or enlarged point of maximal impulse may also provide ancillary information about cardiac function.

The hepatojugular or abdominojugular reflux is an assessment of venous congestion. A positive test is defined as greater than 3 cm H_2O sustained increase in JVP after ten continuous seconds of pressure on the abdomen. In the absence of isolated right ventricular failure, a positive result reliably predicts a PCWP greater than 15 mm Hg.[45] Bendopnea is a recently described symptom of HF that may be present in at least 50% of patients with ADHF, reliably predicts a PCWP greater than 15 mm Hg, and may be associated with adverse long-term clinical outcomes.[42,46] Bendopnea can be tested by having a patient bend at the waist while sitting to touch their feet for up to 30 seconds to assess for dyspnea.[42]

Rales and peripheral edema are a common physical exam finding present in half to two-thirds of patients presenting with ADHF.[36] Lower extremity edema is typically symmetric, pitting and predominates in gravity dependent areas, including the legs, ankles, thighs, sacrum, abdomen, or back. Redness and erythema are often present in patients with ADHF, and bilateral erythema rarely represents cellulitis.[47] Visceral congestion is common, and patients frequently report abdominal distention independent of lower extremity edema. Right-sided congestion can also result in hepatomegaly and splenomegaly, leading to right upper quadrant pain, hemorrhoids, and ascites. However, the absence of rales and peripheral edema is also frequent in patients with chronic HF caused by hypertrophy of the lymphatic system to accommodate increased venous drainage. Thus, the absence of rales and edema does not

TABLE 75.1 Symptoms and Physical Exam Findings of Heart Failure

Signs and Symptoms of Heart Failure	Physical Exam Findings of Heart Failure
General	Anasarca
Altered mental status	Ascites
Cachexia	Cool extremities
Edema (abdominal, lower extremities, or scrotal)	Displaced or enlarged point of maximal impulse
Fatigue	Elevated jugular venous pressure
Malaise	Lower extremity edema
Weight Gain	Hepatojugular reflux
Gastrointestinal	Hepatomegaly or pain to liver palpation
Abdominal Pain	Kussmaul sign
Anorexia	Narrow pulse pressure
	Parasternal lift
Bloating	Pleural effusion
Early satiety	Pulsus alternans
Respiratory	Rales
Bendopnea	S3 and/or S4 gallop
Cough, possibly productive	Slow capillary refill
Dyspnea	Systolic or diastolic murmur
Orthopnea	Tachycardia
Paroxysmal nocturnal dyspnea	Tachypnea
Shortness of breath at rest or with exertion	Weight gain

TABLE 75.2 Utility of Clinical Exam Findings in ADHF

	Exam Finding	Sensitivity	Specificity	PPV	NPV	(+)LR	(−)LR
Perfusion[a]	S3 Gallop	62	32	61	33	0.92	0.85
	SBP < 100 mm Hg	42	66	77	29	1.24	1.14
	PPP < 25%	10	96	88	28	2.54	1.07
	Cool Extremities	20	88	82	28	1.68	1.10
	"Cold" Profile	33	86	87	32	2.33	1.28
Congestion[b]	Ascites	21	92	81	40	2.44	1.15
	Rales > 1/3	15	89	69	38	1.32	1.04
	Edema > 2+	41	66	67	40	1.20	1.11
	Orthopnea > 2 pillows	86	25	66	51	1.15	1.80
	JVP > 12 mm Hg	65	64	75	52	1.79	1.82
	HJR	83	27	65	49	1.13	1.54

ADHF, acute decompensated heart failure; HJR, hepatojugular reflux; JVP, jugular venous pressure; LR, likelihood ratio; NPV, negative predictive value; PPP; proportional pulse pressure; PPV, positive predictive value; SBP, systolic blood pressure.

[a]Cardiac index < 2.2 L/min/m^2.

[b]Pulmonary capillary wedge pressure > 22 mm Hg.

Adapted with permission from Drazner MH, Hellkamp AS, Leier CV, et al. Value of clinician assessment of hemodynamics in advanced heart failure: the ESCAPE trial. *Circ Heart Fail.* 2008;1(3):170-177.

exclude ADHF. Cool extremities with sluggish capillary refill are frequently invoked as a sign of decreased perfusion and low cardiac output. However, assessment is highly subjective and is neither a sensitive nor a specific sign of cardiac output and is thus not a reliable clinical exam finding.[41] For example, in the Evaluation Study of Congestive Heart Failure and Pulmonary Artery Catheterization Effectiveness (ESCAPE), trial cool extremities only had a sensitivity of 20% to detect a CI less than 2.3 L/min/m^2.[41] We summarize these observations to our trainees by saying, "If patients are cold, they are cold; but if they are warm, they may still be cold."

Biomarkers

In the context of ADHF, B-type natriuretic peptide (BNP) and N-terminal pro-B-type natriuretic peptide (NT-proBNP) are useful for the diagnosis of ADHF when clinical symptoms and exam findings are equivocal. In the Breathing Not Properly study, a sensitivity and specificity cutoff of 100 pg/mL maximized the discriminatory characteristics of BNP. A value less than 100 pg/mL had an 89% negative predictive value to rule out HF, whereas the positive predictive value was more modest, at only 79%.[48] NT-proBNP has similar operating characteristics, albeit with different values for sex and age. Like any test, clinical and exam findings must be integrated to most accurately interpret the value. False positives can result from increased age, anemia, arrhythmias, infection, LV hypertrophy, pulmonary embolism, malignancy, renal failure, chemotherapy, illicit drugs, and/or myocardial infarction, among other etiologies[8]. False negative test results can be related to obesity or HFpEF.[8] Importantly, for patients recently started on angiotensin receptor-neprilysin inhibition (ARNI) therapy, BNP may be elevated owing to inhibition of BNP degradation.[49] Higher absolute levels of NT-proBNP are associated with increased risk for adverse outcomes, including HF hospitalization or cardiac death.[50]

With effective decongestion, NT-proBNP or BNP typically declines by >50%, and a decrease of at least 30% by discharge may be associated with better clinical outcomes.[51] Studies with natriuretic peptide-guided therapies with serial measurements of natriuretic peptides have not shown clear and consistent evidence for improvement in mortality and cardiovascular outcomes and are therefore not recommended for reducing hospitalization or death in the guidelines. [8]

Radiography, Electrocardiogram, and Echocardiography

A chest x-ray is commonly performed in patients with suspected ADHF. In patients with chronic HF and appropriate symptoms, radiographic changes are often subtle, and most patients do not have evidence of pulmonary edema. In EuroHeart Failure Survey II (EHFS II), only 16% of patients presenting with ADHF had evidence of pulmonary edema.[4] The chest x-ray may also identify causes of dyspnea other than ADHF. The electrocardiogram (ECG) is an appropriate test to assess for signs of coronary ischemia, cardiac strain, and arrhythmias. Echocardiography is fundamental to the management and risk assessment of patients with HF to assess systolic function, diastolic function, valvular function, wall motion, chamber sizes, pericardial disease, other structural abnormalities and provide hemodynamic estimates.

MANAGEMENT OF PATIENT WITH ACUTE HEART FAILURE

Triage of Patients With Acute Heart Failure

Most unscheduled treatment for ADHF occurs in the emergency department.[51] Risk stratification is important to identify patients both with high- and low-risk features to triage for appropriate levels of care. However, the accuracy of these risk prediction tools is limited. Low-risk patients may be discharged home; however, about 80% of patients who present to the emergency department with ADHF are admitted to the hospital. Generally, admission is warranted for patients with resting hypoxia, significant weight gain, hypotension, poor perfusion, acute renal injury, new diagnosis of ADHF, and ICD discharges. Beyond diuretics, treatment strategies for ADHF are limited with few evidence-based therapies for acute management. Currently, hospitalization focuses on relieving congestion, limiting end-organ damage, addressing comorbid conditions, and optimizing long-term evidence-based therapies.

ADHF often has an inciting clinical trigger, and multiple precipitants are often identified in patients presenting for ADHF (**Table 75.3**). Precipitating events were identified in 61% of patients presenting with ADHF, and more than one factor was observed in 19.2% in the OPTIMIZE-HF registry.[52] Common precipitants of decompensation include a respiratory infection (15%), ACS (15%), arrhythmia (14%), uncontrolled hypertension (11%), and medication nonadherence (9%).[52] Of note, the contribution of dietary and medication nonadherence may be overstated, and care should be taken to investigate alternative reversible causes of decompensation. Hospitalization is also an opportunity to provide additional education about HF and its management, including dietary sodium restriction.

Clinical Classifications and Profiles

A useful framework for clinical assessment is the Stevenson profiles (**Figure 75.2**). These profiles focus on simple clinical markers of perfusion (cold vs warm) and congestion (wet vs dry). Profiles are also useful to help guide clinical therapy. An etiology other than HF should be sought to explain the patient's symptoms in profile A (warm and dry). Patients in profile B (wet and warm) typically respond to escalation of diuretic therapy. However, the sensitivity of the clinical exam for a reduced CI is low, and some patients thought to be profile B will actually be profile C. This concept is important to consider in presumed profile B patients who have a suboptimal response to diuretics. Patients in profile C require a therapy in addition to diuretics; typically, the choice is between adding intravenous vasodilators or inotropic therapy and, in severe cases, mechanical circulatory support. Options for patients with profile L and persistent symptoms include digoxin, cardiac resynchronization (where appropriate), advanced therapies and/or palliative care. For patients in profile L, sometimes an attempt is made to allow the ventricular filling pressures to rise by holding diuretics or providing intravenous fluids, in the hope that the CI will rise and the patient will transition to profile A. However, our experience suggests that you often convert a profile L patient to a profile C patient.

TABLE 75.3 Precipitating Causes of Acute Decompensated Heart Failure

Precipitants of ADHF
Factors Related to Acute Events
Acute atrial fibrillation or other tachyarrhythmias
Bradyarrhythmias
Electrolyte disturbances
Fever
Myocardial ischemia
Poorly controlled hypertension
Pulmonary thromboembolism
Systemic infection and/or sepsis
Factors Related to Physicians
Insufficient or inappropriate prescription doses
Intravenous fluid overload during hospitalization
Lack of patient education for heart failure management (eg, diet)
Undetected volume overload
Factors Related to Medical Comorbidities
Anemia
Arterovenous fistulas
Decompensated diabetes
Depression
Hyperthyroidism and hypothyroidism
Pregnancy
Renal failure
Factors Related to Patients
Excessive alcohol consumption
Use of illicit drugs (cocaine, methamphetamine, etc)
Excessive water and salt intake
Nonadherence to treatment and/or lack of access to medication
Nutritional deficiencies
Self-medication or alternative therapies
Factors Related to Medications
Beta-blockers (negative inotropy)
Calcium channel antagonists (negative inotropy)
Digitalis intoxication
Drugs toxic to the myocardium (eg, adriamycin)
Estrogens
Group I antiarrhythmic drugs (negative inotropy)
Nonsteroidal anti-inflammatory drugs
Tricyclic antidepressants (negative inotropy)
Steroids

The Stevenson profile conveys prognostic information. Admission Stevenson profile B or C compared with profile A is associated with increased risk of death and increased risk of urgent cardiac transplantation at 1 year.[53] At discharge, profile B, C, or L is independently associated with 50% increased risk for rehospitalization or death compared with profile A.[41]

Another classification is based on the relative degrees of right- and/or left-sided HF. Approximately 75% of patients with elevated JVP have an elevated PCWP. However, the remaining 25% of patients have discordant right- and left-sided pressures that can occur regardless of LVEF.[42] Disproportionate elevations of right compared with LV pressures is evident with an elevated right atrial pressure (RAP)/PCWP ratio greater than 0.66.[42] Patients with right to left equalizer patterns have disproportionately more right- than left-sided elevation of ventricular filling pressures, and this profile is associated with impaired renal function and an increased risk of subsequent HF hospitalization and death.[54,55] These patients are anecdotally more challenging to decongest compared with patients with an RAP/PCWP ratio less than 0.66. In sum, the characterization as right, left, or biventricular HF may help guide therapy and provide prognostic information.

Medical Approach

Respiratory Management for Acute Decompensated Heart Failure

Dyspnea is the most common symptom during presentation, and therapies are typically aimed at addressing this complaint. Supplemental oxygen therapy should be provided for patients with sustained hypoxia (pulse oximetry < 90%). In patients with hypoxemia attributed to pulmonary edema, noninvasive continuous positive airway pulmonary pressure (CPAP) or bilevel positive airway pressure (BiPap) helps alleviate symptoms.[56] In a multicenter prospective randomized trial, 1069 patients with acute cardiogenic pulmonary edema were assigned to standard oxygen therapy, CPAP (5-15 cm H_2O), or BiPap (inspiratory pressure, 8-20 cm H_2O; expiratory pressure, 4-10 cm H_2O). Compared with standard therapy, noninvasive positive pressure more rapidly improved respiratory distress and metabolic derangements but did not affect 7-day all-cause mortality or the rate of intubation.[57] Noninvasive positive pressure plus nitrates are particularly effective therapy for hypertensive or acute "flash" pulmonary edema and may avert the need for invasive ventilation. Contraindications for use include the indication for invasive ventilation, unconsciousness, altered mental status, vomiting, or patient inability to tolerate the mask.

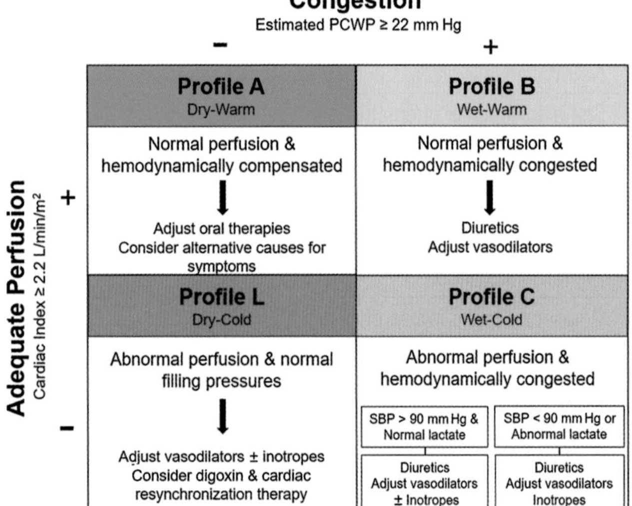

FIGURE 75.2 Stevenson clinical profiles and suggested clinical therapies. PCWP, pulmonary capillary wedge pressure.

Blood Pressure

Most patients with ADHF present with normal or increased blood pressure.[3] Hypotension is associated with a worse prognosis for patients admitted with ADHF. The OPTIMIZE-HF registry observed that lower systolic blood pressure at admission was associated with increased in-hospital mortality: 7.2% (<120 mm Hg), 3.6% (120-139 mm Hg), 2.5% (140-161 mm Hg), and 1.7% (>161 mm Hg)[3]. Systolic blood pressure greater than 160 mm Hg was not associated with increased in-hospital mortality.[3] Admission systolic blood pressure was also independently associated with risk of post-discharge mortality with an 18% increase in hazard ratio for each 10-mm Hg decrease in systolic blood pressure less than 140 mm Hg.[3] These findings may be partially attributable to differences in tolerance of evidence-based medical therapy.

Treating disorders that may contribute to hypotension, for example, ACS, pulmonary embolism, or hypovolemia, is essential. Asymptomatic hypotension in the absence of congestion and poor perfusion does not necessitate emergent therapies; however, inotropic therapy may be considered for persisting symptomatic hypotension or hypoperfusion.

Invasive Hemodynamic Monitoring

Invasive hemodynamic monitoring with a pulmonary artery (PA) catheter may be a useful strategy for the management of some patients with ADHF. These catheters provide real-time data on cardiac output, pulmonary arterial pressures, and right- and left-sided filling pressures. Routine use was evaluated in the ESCAPE trial, which randomized 433 patients with ADHF to management with a PA catheter or routine care. There was no difference in the duration of hospitalization (8.7 vs 8.3 days), 6-month mortality, or total nonhospitalized days at 6 months.[58] However, one limitation of ESCAPE is that the sickest subset of patients may not have been enrolled as the clinician may not have had clinical equipoise about the need for invasive monitoring.

Despite the absence of randomized evidence of benefit, PA catheters continue to have a role in patients with severe hemodynamic derangement, refractory shock, clinical deterioration despite clinical assessment guided therapy, or uncertainty about the hemodynamic status. In patients with advanced HF, targeting a right atrial pressure less than 8 mm Hg, PCWP of less than 18 mm Hg, and systemic vascular resistance of ~1000 to 1200 dynes-sec/cm² may be useful targets.[58]

Volume Status and Decongestion

Patients with clinical congestion typically have at least 4 to 5 L of excess fluid, and more than 10 L is not uncommon.[59] Loop diuretics are the primary pharmacologic therapy for ADHF and are commonly initiated in the emergency department. Despite long-standing and widespread use, the impact of diuretics on clinical outcomes has not been extensively tested in adequately powered clinical trials except for the Diuretic Optimization Strategies Evaluation (DOSE) trial.[59] For patients who are diuretic naive, 20 to 40 mg of IV furosemide is a reasonable starting dose. For patients on outpatient diuretics, the initial dose should be approximately 2.5 times the oral outpatient loop diuretic equivalent and can be administered via either intermittent boluses or a continuous infusion, given that either strategy achieved similar decongestion[59] (**Table 75.4**).

Although no specific guidelines exist, 3 to 5 L of urine output daily until the achievement of adequate decongestion is a reasonable target.[60] If a desired response is not achieved, owing to the steep dose-response curve, titration of the diuretic dose should be rapid (within a few hours), the dose being doubled until adequate response is achieved or the maximal dose is achieved. Diuretic resistance is a common problem with HF, and high doses of diuretics are markers of a poorer prognosis associated with increased mortality and sudden death[61] (**Table 75.5**).

During ADHF, sodium retention is more avid, and increased gut edema slows oral diuretic absorption, thus reducing peak plasma levels and promoting less natriuresis.[62] Intravenous administration avoids variations in bioavailability and allows for rapid onset within 30 to 60 minutes. A typical dose of a loop diuretic increases urinary excretion of sodium chloride for several hours, but this is then followed by a period of low sodium excretion and sodium retention because the half-life of the drug is shorter than the typical dosing interval (**Figure 75.3A-C**). To induce a negative sodium chloride balance, sodium excretion must exceed sodium intake. This is the rationale for the 2-g sodium diet restriction during hospitalization for ADHF. As effective diuresis is achieved, less extracellular fluid leads to a decreased response to each subsequent dose of diuretic, termed the "braking response."[62] This response leads to increased SNS activation and RAAS activation and promotes diuretic resistance, contributing to the increasing dose of diuretics required for diuresis during subsequent hospitalizations.

In the setting of diuretic resistance, adjunctive therapies to loop diuretics are often required. Administration of a thiazide-like diuretic that blocks the distal tubule can significantly augment diuresis. Intravenous chlorothiazide (500-1000 mg) or oral metolazone (2.5-10 mg) are effective, but volume status, electrolytes, and renal function must be monitored more frequently. If hypokalemia is a persisting problem, administration of a potassium sparing diuretic such as spironolactone or eplerenone can be considered. The Aldosterone Targeted Neurohormonal Combined With Natriuresis Therapy in Heart Failure (ATHENA-HF) trial evaluated the addition of daily spironolactone versus placebo to usual care as an adjunct diuretic for patients with ADHF. Despite being well tolerated without increased adverse events, there was no significant difference in decongestion or improvement in NT-proBNP between treatment groups at 96 hours.[63] Finally, carbonic anhydrase inhibition (eg, acetazolamide 250-500 mg) may also augment natriuresis and may result in less

TABLE 75.4 Diuretic Approach to Acute Decompensated Heart Failure

Equivalent Oral Furosemide Dose	Intravenous Bolus Dose	Infusion Rate	Metolazone[a]
<80 mg	40 mg BID-TID	5 mg/hr	NA
80-160 mg	80 mg BID-TID	10 mg/hr	NA
161-240 mg	80 mg BID-TID	20 mg/hr	NA
>240 mg	80 mg TID-QID	30 mg/hr	2.5-5 mg daily

Initial starting diuretics dose should be approximately 2.5 times the oral baseline regimen in divided doses based on DOSE trial. Diuretics should be increased until goal of daily urine output of 3-5 L daily is achieved. A dose of 40 mg of oral furosemide is equivalent to 20 mg of torsemide and 1 mg of bumetanide.
[a]Hydrochlorothiazide (50 mg BID), chlorthalidone (25 mg daily), acetazolamide (250-500 mg), or chlorothiazide (500 mg) can be administered 30 minutes prior to furosemide to augment diuresis. BID, twice daily; NA, not applicable; QID, four times daily; TID, three times daily.
Data derived from Ellison DH, Felker GM. Diuretic Treatment in Heart Failure. *N Engl J Med*. 2018;378(7):684-685.

TABLE 75.5 Factors Contributing to Diuretic Resistance

Reasons for Diuretic Resistance
Inaccurate diagnosis or hemodynamic status
Increased sodium intake
Insufficient dose of diuretic
Nonadherence to medications
Hypotension
Poor absorption of diuretic due to gut edema
Increased age
Low renal blood flow
Reduced glomerular filtration (chronic kidney disease)
Nephron remodeling
Neurohormonal activation (renin-angiotensin-aldosterone system activation)
Impairment by uremic toxins
Use of nonsteroidal anti-inflammatory drugs
Reduced intravascular volume despite increased total extracellular fluid volume

Data derived from Ellison DH, Felker GM. Diuretic Treatment in Heart Failure. *N Engl J Med*. 2018;378(7):684-685.

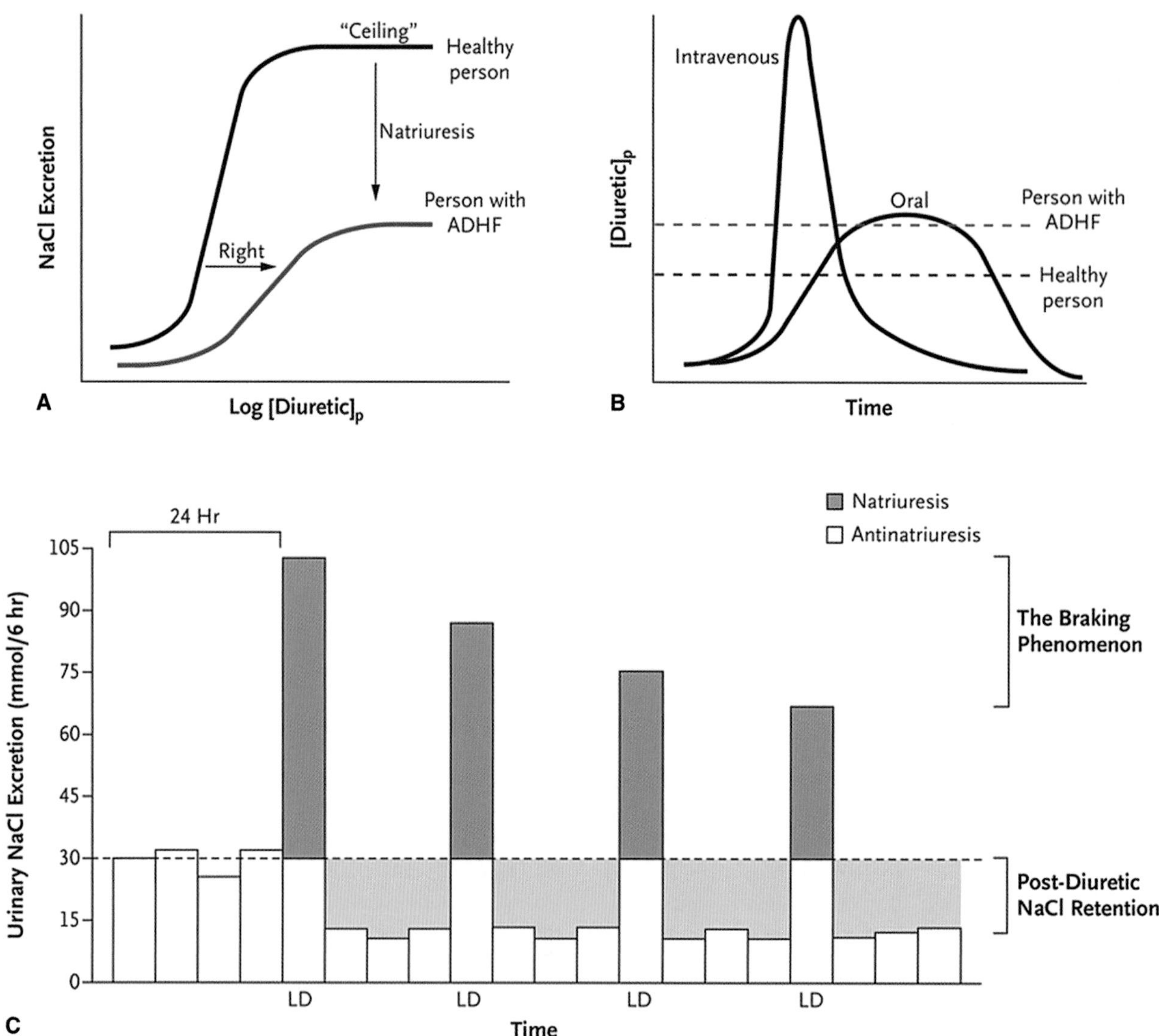

FIGURE 75.3 Properties of loop diuretics. **A**. Relationship between the log of the plasma diuretic concentration ($[\text{Diuretic}]_p$) and sodium chloride excretion. Acute decompensated heart failure (ADHF) shifts the curve to the right and reduces the "ceiling" natriuresis. **B**. Relationship of the plasma concentration of loop diuretic $[\text{Diuretic}]_p$ as a function of time after an intravenous or oral dose. The natriuretic threshold (dashed lines) is higher in patients with ADHF than in healthy persons. Natriuresis is a function of the time above the natriuretic threshold. **C**. The effects of repeated daily doses of a loop diuretic (LD) on NaCl excretion, viewed in 6-hour blocks. Postdiuretic NaCl retention and the braking phenomenon are shown. To be effective, natriuresis must exceed antinatriuresis. (From Ellison DH, Felker GM. Diuretic Treatment in Heart Failure. *N Engl J Med*. 2018;378(7):684-685. Copyright © 2018 Massachusetts Medical Society. Reprinted with permission from Massachusetts Medical Society.)

neurohormonal activation compared with thiazide-like diuretics.[64] Diuretic strategies with acetazolamide are under active clinical investigation.

Electrolyte Management

Electrolyte abnormalities of potassium and magnesium are common in patients with HF. Low serum magnesium occurs in over 1/3 of patients on chronic diuretic therapy.[65] Serum magnesium is typically measured; however, less than 1% of magnesium exists extracellularly, and serum levels are not representative of total body magnesium stores.[66] Maintenance of serum levels greater than 1.9 mg/dL is recommended; however, there is minimal high-quality evidence to support this recommendation in the absence of torsades de pointes. Recommendations stem from retrospective studies associating lower levels of magnesium with hypokalemia, increased risk of cardiac arrhythmias, and increased risk for cardiac death.[66] In a small double-blind placebo-controlled study, oral magnesium repletion versus placebo in patients ($N = 70$) with an ICD was not associated with reduced ICD shocks.[67] As such, daily serum assessment of magnesium during hospitalization for ADHF may not be beneficial, and oral replacement is likely sufficient.

In patients with HF, the goal serum potassium is generally greater than 3.9 mEq/L and less than 5 mEq/L to reduce the risk of sudden cardiac death attributable to arrhythmias. Moderate quality evidence has observed increased risk of all-cause death, HF death, and HF hospitalization even with modest hypokalemia 3.5 to 3.9 mEq/L.[68] During administration of parenteral diuretics, serum potassium should be monitored at least daily, followed by either oral or intravenous repletion, as necessary.

Both hypochloremia and hyponatremia are associated with adverse clinical outcomes in patients with ADHF.[69,70] Lower admission and discharge serum chloride levels were independently associated with increased mortality.[69] Although these findings may relate to a dilutional effect attributable to increased vasopressin, they may also represent relative electrolyte depletion attributable to chronic diuretic use.[69] Likewise, hyponatremia in patients with ADHF is associated with a longer length of admission, increased in-hospital mortality and increased postdischarge mortality.[70] The presence of both metabolic derangements identifies patients at increased risk for adverse outcomes.

Pharmacologic Therapy for Acute Decompensated Heart Failure

General Principles

Guideline-directed medical therapy (GDMT) has dramatically improved outcomes for HFrEF. In general, most cardiac medications should be continued in patients admitted with profile B ADHF, and discharge on maximally tolerated GDMT should be strongly considered. An exception would include temporarily holding angiotensin-converting enzyme inhibitors (ACEI), angiotensin receptor blockers (ARB), or ARNI for significant hypotension, oliguric acute renal failure, or hyperkalemia. However, these conditions might also identify individuals with more advanced HF at increased long-term risk of death.[71] Digoxin improves hemodynamics without increasing heart rate or decreasing blood pressure in patients with a low cardiac output. However, digoxin should not be continued in patients with advanced atrioventricular block, active ischemia, or severe renal impairment.

Beta-Blockers

For patients in profile C HF, shock and evidence of inadequate perfusion of end-organs, beta-blockers may be held or have their dose reduced until hemodynamic stabilization. Once patients are adequately compensated, resumption of low-dose metoprolol succinate, carvedilol, or bisoprolol should be considered prior to discharge. For patients who required inotropic therapy or who were discontinued from beta-blockers, the optimal timing of reinitiation needs to be individualized depending on hemodynamic stability.

Renin-Angiotensin-Aldosterone System Inhibitor Therapy

For patients with profile C ADHF and HFrEF, in the absence of hypotension, vasodilators can be used with diuretics to improve symptoms of congestion and improve hemodynamics. For patients with profile B HFrEF and stable blood pressure, maximizing ACEi, ARB, or ARNI therapy should be considered, given the association of these therapies with improved outcomes post discharge.[51] For patients with tenuous hemodynamics, captopril can be initiated and rapidly up-titrated. Owing to the short half-life of the medication, captopril is an excellent choice for patients with borderline blood pressures or during weaning of parenteral therapies. A small randomized trial demonstrated that captopril, compared with enalapril, was better tolerated and associated with fewer adverse events in patients with advanced HF.[72] If the patient cannot tolerate ACEI owing to progressively worsening renal function, angioedema, persistent cough, or allergies, then hydralazine can also be considered. Like captopril, the shorter half-life of the drug allows for a rapid up-titration of the medication to reduce afterload and stabilize the hemodynamic status. Additionally, organic nitrates (nitroglycerin, isosorbide dinitrate) and sodium nitroprusside all promote vasodilation, reduce preload, and reduce PCWP.

Angiotensin Receptor-Neprilysin Inhibitors

Most well-designed clinical trials evaluating medications or medical strategies for management of ADHF have demonstrated no or minimal clinical benefit beyond standard care (Table 75.8). A recent notable exception is the PIONEER-HF trial. PIONEER-HF randomized 881 patients with ADHF and an LVEF less than 40% to either sacubitril-valsartan or enalapril after a period of inpatient clinical stability.[73] Initiation of sacubitril-valsartan versus enalapril during the index hospitalization was associated with a larger decline in NT-proBNP after 4 and 8 weeks of follow-up, and there was no increased risk of adverse safety outcomes.[73] A subsequent prespecified exploratory post hoc analysis of blinded adjudicated events observed that the cumulative incidence of cardiovascular death or rehospitalization was 8.5% versus 13.6%, favoring sacubitril-valsartan at 8 weeks.[74] Thus, if the patient can afford the medication and is hemodynamically stable, initiation of sacubitril-valsartan for patients with ADHF and resolving congestion during the hospital stay appears safe and is associated with a greater reduction of NT-proBNP and possibly a lower rate of rehospitalization. However, further prospective data are needed to confirm the benefit of sacubitril-valsartan in ADHF.

Nitrates

Organic nitrates are potent venodilators with rapid decreases in pulmonary venous and LV filling pressures, leading to improvement in pulmonary congestion, dyspnea, and myocardial oxygen demand.[75] At higher doses, they also act as arterial vasodilators, effectively reducing afterload and potentially increasing cardiac output. Nitrates are more selective for epicardial rather than intramyocardial coronary arteries and useful in patients with concomitant CAD. Nitrates can be rapidly up-titrated every few minutes to achieve a target blood pressure. Unfortunately, tachyphylaxis to continuous nitrate infusions typically begins after 24 hours. Additionally, there are no robust randomized data showing benefit of nitrates on hard clinical outcomes e.g., risk of subsequent hospitalization or mortality, in patients with ADHF.

Sodium Nitroprusside

Sodium nitroprusside is a powerful afterload reducing agent that is titratable with a half-life of seconds to minutes (**Table 75.6**). It is particularly useful in the setting of low output ADHF with elevated afterload (ie, high systemic vascular resistance) and/or significant mitral regurgitation in the setting of normal to mild renal dysfunction. Sodium nitroprusside should not be routinely used in patients with restrictive cardiomyopathy (relatively fixed stroke volume), aortic stenosis (fixed afterload), and known obstructive CAD, including myocardial infarction owing to potential coronary steal syndrome. Typically, sodium nitroprusside is administered in an intensive care setting and rapidly titrated to a mean arterial blood pressure of 60 to 65 mm Hg (Table 75.6). Nitroprusside is metabolized to nitric oxide and cyanide, which can produce toxic side effects because of thiocyanate production. Accumulation of cyanide is rare, but impaired hepatic function and doses greater than 200 μg/min for 48 hours increase the risk.[76] Nausea, headache, or altered sensorium are clinical manifestations of cyanide toxicity. Despite the benefits of potent afterload reduction leading to improved cardiac output without increased myocardial work, nitroprusside is administered to less than 1% of patients with ADHF.[77] Nonrandomized studies have demonstrated a profound reduction of PCWP, reduced afterload, and improved cardiac output.[77] In a cohort of 175 patients with severe ADHF, intravenous sodium nitroprusside was also associated with greater hemodynamic improvement and lower rates of inotropic support or worsening renal function during hospitalization compared with usual care.[77]

Inotropes and Inodilators

The inotropic drugs (dobutamine, milrinone) and inodilators (levosimendan) increase cardiac output through cyclic adenosine monophosphate (cAMP)-mediated inotropy and calcium sensitization[78] (**Table 75.7**). Retrospective registry data suggest that even short-term use (hours to days) of intravenous inotropes is associated with significant side effects, including hypotension, atrial or ventricular arrhythmias, increased in-hospital and increased long-term mortality.[79] As such, these agents are typically reserved for patients with refractory shock when

TABLE 75.6 Protocol for Initiation and Weaning of Sodium Nitroprusside in ADHF

Protocol for Initiation and Weaning of Sodium Nitroprusside
Sodium Nitroprusside
Initiation: 10-40 μg/min or 0.1-0.4 μg/kg/min infusion
Titration: Titrate to mean arterial pressure (MAP) 60-65 mm Hg or systolic blood pressure 90-100 mm Hg. Do not exceed 400 μg/min or 4 μg/kg/min.
Weaning: Decrease infusion while maintaining MAP goals after stabilization of hemodynamics for >12 hours while initiating/increasing oral vasodilators.
Captopril
Incremental dosing: 6.25 mg → 12.5 mg → 25 mg → 50 mg → 75 mg
Initiation: 6.25-12.5 mg
If tolerated, after 2 hours increase to next dose.
If tolerated, after 2 additional hours, increase to next dose.
If tolerated, after 6 additional hours, then start 50-75 mg three times daily.
If tolerated for 24 hours at stable dose, consider transition to losartan or valsartan.
If losartan is well tolerated for 48 hours, consider transition to sacubitril-valsartan.
Hydralazine
Initiation: 25 mg
If tolerated, after 2 hours increase to 50 mg.
If tolerated, after additional 6 hours increase dose to 75 mg.
If tolerated, after additional 8 hours increase to 100 mg three times daily.
Isosorbide
Initiation: 10 mg
If tolerated, after 2 hours increase dose to 20 mg.
If tolerated, after 6 additional hours increase to 40 mg three times daily.

Data derived from Mullens W, Abrahams Z, Francis GS, et al. Sodium nitroprusside for advanced low-output heart failure. *J Am Coll Cardiol.* 2008;52(3):200-207.

TABLE 75.7 Intravenous Vasoactive Medications for Acute Decompensated Heart Failure

Drug	Dose	Side Effects	Hemodynamic Effects
Dobutamine	1-10 μg/kg/min	Tachycardia, arrhythmias, myocardial ischemia, and possibly cardiomyocyte necrosis due to direct cytotoxic effects	Stimulation of β_1 and β_2 receptors with variable effects on the α-adrenergic receptors. Increased inotropy, chronotropy, and mild vasodilation. Tachyphylaxis may occur with infusions >48 hours due to β-receptor desensitization.
Dopamine	2-20 μg/kg/min	Atrial and ventricular tachyarrhythmias	Preferential stimulation of dopamine receptor stimulation at low doses (<5 μg/kg/min) with increasing β_1 and α_1 receptor stimulation at higher doses (>5 μg/kg/min), causing chronotropy and vasoconstriction
Epinephrine	0.01-1.0 μg/kg/min	Tachycardia, nausea, anxiety, and skin necrosis	Stimulates β_1, β_2, and α_1 receptors, resulting in increased inotropy with balanced vasodilator and vasoconstrictor effects
Milrinone	0.10-0.25 μg/kg/min and titrated max dose 0.75 μg/kg/min	Hypotension and atrial or ventricular arrhythmias	Cyclic AMP is a signaling molecule that increases inotropy, chronotropy, and lusitropy in cardiomyocytes and vasorelaxation in vascular smooth muscle.
Nitroglycerin	5-200 μg/min	Headache, hypotension	Activation of guanylate cyclase and relaxation of vascular smooth muscle. Tachyphylaxis may occur with continuous infusions >48 hours.
Norepinephrine	0.01-3.0 μg/kg/min	Tachycardia, nausea, anxiety, and skin necrosis	β_1 and α_1 receptor stimulation with weaker agonism of the $beta_2$ receptors, causing vasoconstriction
Sodium nitroprusside	Initiated at 10 μg/min or 0.1 μg/kg/min and titrated to a max dose of 400 μg/min or 4.0 μg/kg/min	Nausea and abdominal discomfort. Rare side effects include seizures, metabolic acidosis, and methemoglobinemia.	Increased production of nitric oxide, leading to activation of guanylate cyclase and relaxation of vascular smooth muscle. Results in a marked reduction of afterload

alternative interventions have failed to prevent hemodynamic collapse and as a palliative measure for patients with end-stage HF. Inotropes should be discontinued once adequate hemodynamics have been restored. If adequate hemodynamics cannot be restored or these therapies are unable to be weaned, consultation with an advanced HF team and/or palliative care should be considered.

Dobutamine

Dobutamine is a commonly used inotropic agent, resulting in increased inotropy and chronotropy through increases in cAMP and calcium sensitization.[80] In general, dobutamine is preferred (as compared with milrinone) in patients with cardiogenic shock with hypotension and moderate to severe renal insufficiency. Beta-blocker therapy will result in competitive antagonism of dobutamine, such that higher doses are needed or, preferentially, alternative therapy with milrinone. Dobutamine should be weaned off with adjustments of afterload reducing agents to mitigate hemodynamic rebound. The Calcium Sensitizer or Inotrope or None in Low-Output Heart Failure (CASINO) trial demonstrated significantly increased mortality with dobutamine versus placebo similar to the results of prior studies with this class of agents.[81]

Phosphodiesterase Inhibitors

Phosphodiesterase IIIa (PDE IIIa) inhibitors such as milrinone and enoximone (available in Europe) augment cardiac hemodynamics via stimulation of the cAMP pathway. This mechanism is independent of adrenergic cell receptors and bypasses receptor downregulation or antagonism by beta-blockers.[80] This mechanism allows for synergy with patients on dobutamine and hemodynamic inotropic effect in those on beta-blockers. PDE IIIa inhibitors cause peripheral and pulmonary vasodilation, reducing afterload and preload while increasing inotropy.[80] Owing to the prolonged effect of milrinone, patients should be observed for at least 48 hours after cessation to ensure clinical stability. Milrinone is renally excreted, necessitating a dose adjustment or avoidance for renal dysfunction.

In the Outcomes of a Prospective Trial of Intravenous Milrinone for Exacerbations of Chronic Heart Failure (OPTIME-CHF) trial,[82] 951 patients hospitalized with ADHF were randomized to milrinone versus placebo. There was no difference in the primary end point of days hospitalized for HF within 30 days, but increased hypotension, arrhythmias, and mortality in patients with ischemic heart disease was observed with milrinone.[79]

Vasopressors

Vasopressors should be reserved for patients with profound hypotension and evidence of end-organ injury because these agents will preferentially redirect blood flow centrally at the expense of peripheral tissue and increased afterload. Phenylephrine is a selective α_1 receptor agonist with potent arterial vasoconstrictor effects useful for hypotension related to vasodilation rather than reduced cardiac output.[80] Epinephrine is a full β receptor agonist and potent inotropic agent with balanced vasodilator and vasoconstrictor effects. The direct effect of increasing inotropy independent of myocardial catecholamine stores makes it a useful agent in the treatment of posttransplant patients with denervated hearts.[80] Dopamine is often used as a vasoconstrictor and for theoretical effects on renal perfusion. However, the Renal Optimization Strategies Evaluation (ROSE) trial showed no benefit of low-dose dopamine versus placebo for decongestion or improvement of renal function.[83] A meta-analysis suggested that low-dose dopamine may increase urine output on the first day with no association with renal function and a trend toward increased adverse events.[84]

Arginine Vasopressin (AVP) Antagonists

Vasopressin is a major regulator of serum osmolality and inappropriately high levels appear to play a major role in hyponatremia for patients with HF. In the Efficacy of Vasopressin Antagonism in Heart Failure Outcome Study with Tolvaptan (EVEREST) trial, tolvaptan modestly improved the rate of diuresis in ADHF without further impairing renal function or blood pressure; however, clinical outcomes, including survival and readmission rates, were not affected. AVP antagonists (eg, tolvaptan) have been approved for patients with severe hypervolemic and euvolemic hyponatremia, but they are not routinely indicated because they have not demonstrated improved clinical outcomes in patients with HF.

Vasodilators

Numerous vasodilators have been tested in ADHF and are summarized in **Table 75.8**. Trials testing recombinant human brain-type natriuretic peptide (nesiritide), recombinant form of human relaxin-2 (relaxin), endothelin receptor A/B antagonist (tezosentan), adenosine A_1-receptor antagonist (rolofylline), and urodilatin (ularitide) in ADHF have been largely disappointing without significant improvements in clinical outcomes or symptomatic improvement beyond standard care.

Nonpharmacologic Therapies

Extracorporeal isotonic fluid removal with ultrafiltration can be used to remove sodium and water in patients with ADHF. The theoretical advantage is to remove isotonic fluid, resulting in a predictable volume without the neurohormonal or

TABLE 75.8 Major Clinical Trials for Patients with Acute Decompensated Heart Failure

Trial for ADHF	Treatment	Cohort	Results
VMAC (2002, *N* = 489)	Double-blind IV nitroglycerin vs IV nesiritide (recombinant human B-type natriuretic peptide) vs placebo	Hospitalized with ADHF and SBP >90 mm Hg	Greater reduction of PCWP with IV nesiritide vs nitroglycerin at 24 hours (−8.2 mm Hg, −6.3 mm Hg, −2 mm Hg; *P* = .04). No difference in patient-reported dyspnea at 24 hours (*P* = .13)
OPTIME-CHF (2003, *N* = 949)	Double-blind, IV milrinone (0.5 μg/kg/min) vs placebo for 48-72 hours	Hospitalized ADHF without cardiogenic shock	No difference in number of days hospitalized within 60 days (*P* = .20)
ESCAPE (2005, *N* = 433)	Unblinded pulmonary artery catheter vs standard care	Hospitalized ADHF with LVEF <30% and SBP <125 mm Hg	No difference in mortality (*P* = .35) or number of hospitalized days (*P* = .67) at 180 days
REVIVE-2 (2005, N = 600)	Double-blind, IV levosimendan or placebo	Hospitalized with ADHF, LVEF <35% and dyspnea at rest despite IV diuretics	Mild improvement of clinical course at 5 days with levosimendan; however, numerically more deaths
EVEREST (2007, *N* = 4133)	Double-blind, tolvaptan (vasopressin V_2 receptor blocker) vs placebo	Hospitalized ADHF and LVEF <40% without cardiogenic shock	No difference in mortality (*P* = .68) or composite of CV death and HF hospitalization (*P* = .55) during 9.9-month median follow-up
SURVIVE (2007, *N* = 1327)	Double-blind, IV dobutamine vs IV levosimendan (calcium sensitizing inodilator)	Hospitalized ADHF, LVEF <30% and required inotropic support	No difference in all-cause mortality at 31 (*P* = .29) or 180 days (*P* = .40)
UNLOAD (2007, *N* = 200)	Unblinded ultrafiltration vs usual care for 48 hours	Hospitalized with ADHF and serum creatinine <3.0 mg/dL	At 48 hours greater weight loss in ultrafiltration arm (*P* = .001), but no difference in dyspnea improvement

(*continued*)

TABLE 75.8 Major Clinical Trials for Patients with Acute Decompensated Heart Failure (*continued*)

Trial for ADHF	Treatment	Cohort	Results
VERITAS (2007, *N* = 1435)	Double-blind, IV tezosentan (endothelin receptor A/B antagonist) vs placebo	Hospitalized with ADHF and LVEF <40%	No difference in patient-reported symptoms at 24 hours (*P* > .50) or the incidence of death or worsening HF at 7 days (*P* = .95)
PROTECT (2010, *N* = 2033)	Double-blind, Rolofylline (adenosine A_1 receptor antagonist) vs placebo	Hospitalized with ADHF and eGFR 20-80 mL/min/1.73 m^2	No difference in clinical improvement (*P* = .35) or renal function (*P* = .44) at 60 days
ASCEND-HF (2011, *N* = 7141)	Double-blind, IV nesiritide (recombinant human B-type natriuretic peptide) vs placebo	Hospitalized with ADHF and SBP <100 mm Hg	No difference in composite end point of HF and all-cause death at 30 days (*P* = .31) or 24-hour improvement in dyspnea
DOSE (2011, *N* = 308)	Double-blind, 1:1:1:1 low-dose (intermittent vs continuous IV) or high-dose (intermittent vs continuous IV) furosemide	Hospitalized with ADHF and SBP <90 mm Hg	No difference in symptoms at 70 hours between treatment arms. Mild increase in weight loss in high-dose arm at 72 hours (*P* = .01)
SMAC-HF (2011, *N* = 1771)	Single-blind, hypertonic saline solution (150 mL 1.4%-4.6% NaCl) twice daily and 120 mmol vs 80 mmol Na restriction	Single center, hospitalized for ADHF, LVEF <40% and NYHA class III	Primary outcome of all-cause death (*P* < .001) or HF rehospitalization (*P* < .001) at mean 57-month follow-up favoring hypertonic saline arm
CARRESS-HF (2012, *N* = 188)	Ultrafiltration (200 mL/h) vs usual care with diuretics to resolution of congestion	Hospitalized with ADHF and increase in serum creatinine of at least 0.3 mg/dL within 12 weeks	Increase of composite end point of change in weight and increase of creatinine at 96 hours for ultrafiltration arm (*P* = .003)
ROSE (2013, *N* = 360)	Double-blind, IV dopamine (2 μg/kg/min) vs nesiritide (recombinant human B-type natriuretic peptide) vs placebo	Hospitalized with ADHF and eGFR 15-60 mL/min/1.73 m^2	No difference in 72-hour urine output for low-dose dopamine (*P* = .59) or nesiritide (*P* = .49) vs placebo
ATHENA (2017, *N* = 360)	Double-blind, daily spironolactone 100 mg vs spironolactone 25 mg vs placebo	Hospitalized with ADHF and eGFR >30 mL/min/1.73 m^2	No difference in the change in NT-proBNP at 96 hours (*P* = .57) or secondary 30-day mortality or HF rehospitalization rate
TRUE-AHF (2017, *N* = 2157)	Double-blind, IV Ularitide (urodilatin) vs placebo for 48 hours	Hospitalized ADHF with SBP >115 mm Hg	No difference in CV death at 2 years (*P* = .75) or median length of stay at 30 days (*P* = .16)
PIONEER-HF (2019, *N* = 881)	Double-blind, sacubitril-valsartan vs enalapril	Hospitalized with ADHF with an LVEF <40%	Greater reduction of NT-proBNP (*P* < .001) and death or HF hospitalization (*P* = .007) at 16-week follow-up in sacubitril-valsartan arm
RELAX-AHF-2 (2019, *N* = 6545)	Double-blind, IV serelaxin (recombinant human relaxin-2) vs placebo for 48 hours	Hospitalized with ADHF and SBP >125 mm Hg	No difference in CV death at 180 days (*P* = .77) or worsening HF at 5 days (*P* = .19)

cardiorenal activation seen with diuretics. Cardiorenal Rescue Study in Acute Decompensated Heart Failure (CARRESS-HF) randomized 188 patients with ADHF, worsening renal function and persisting congestion to ultrafiltration (200 mL/hour) versus aggressive diuresis (target 3-5 L of urine output daily). Ultrafiltration resulted in similar weight loss (~12 lbs), but more fluid removal, and worse renal function without a difference in 60-day clinical outcomes.[60,85] Given that randomized trials have largely not shown clinical benefit, the role of ultrafiltration remains limited in ADHF.

Hypertonic Saline

Administration of hypertonic (3%) saline concomitant with high-dose diuretics and fluid restriction may facilitate diuresis and improve clinical outcomes. The Self-Management and Care of Heart Failure (SMAC-HF) trial randomly assigned 1771 patients hospitalized with ADHF to a single blind strategy of 150 mL of 3% saline, furosemide, and a sodium restriction versus furosemide and sodium restriction.[86] The hypertonic saline arm had a shorter length of stay, increased creatinine clearance, reduced readmission rate, and improved survival.[86] Although these results are intriguing, they should be interpreted with caution given the unblinded nature of the study, and further studies are warranted.

Clinical Trajectories During Hospitalization for ADHF

After admission, most patients rapidly improve with standard treatment; however, monitoring of a patient's clinical trajectory is important to identify nonresponders (**Figure 75.4**). Three main clinical trajectories are improving toward target, stalled after initial response, and no improvement and/or worsening[51] (**Figure 75.5**). Patients that demonstrate clinical improvement with standard therapy should be optimized on GDMT. Patients with clinical deterioration or unresponsiveness should have therapy escalated and consideration of advanced or palliative therapies in case of further hemodynamic decline. Patients with initial improvement but stalled clinical response often have persisting congestion and require consideration for escalation of therapies to complete decongestion or compromise with incomplete decongestion.[51] Patients with a stalled clinical response often have more advanced disease, higher baseline diuretic doses, and worse baseline renal function.[51] For some of these patients, additional decongestion will result in worsening renal function or hypotension, and discharge with residual decongestion is necessary ("compromise with congestion").

Decongestion

The primary goal of hospitalization is complete decongestion because the rate of rehospitalization or death is lowest in patients with complete clinical decongestion.[51] Average weight loss during admission is 4 to 8 kg.[51,59] Clinical symptoms often resolve before physical exam findings resolve, and 30% to 50% of patients are discharged prior to complete decongestion.[51] Once admitted for ADHF, the median length of stay is approximately 4 to 5 days in the United States, 7 days in Canada, 8 days in Europe, and 5 days in South America without significant differences in case mix.[87,88] Inpatient mortality for ADHF is about 5% to 7% and has declined approximately by 2% to 3% since 2001.[2] Yet patients admitted with cardiogenic shock continue to have a 25% to 50% risk of mortality.[89] Each hospitalization for ADHF is associated with an increased risk of recurrent hospitalizations and worse prognosis.[90] Any HF hospitalization is associated with an estimated 25% risk of death within the next year.[51]

DISCHARGE AND FOLLOW-UP PATIENT CARE

Predischarge Planning

Discharge should mark a time to review optimal GDMT, review the overall clinical trajectory, and ensure adequate follow-up for continuity of care. The discharge phase marks a transition toward assessing clinical readiness, safety and care transitions to outpatient care. This includes optimization of oral regimens,

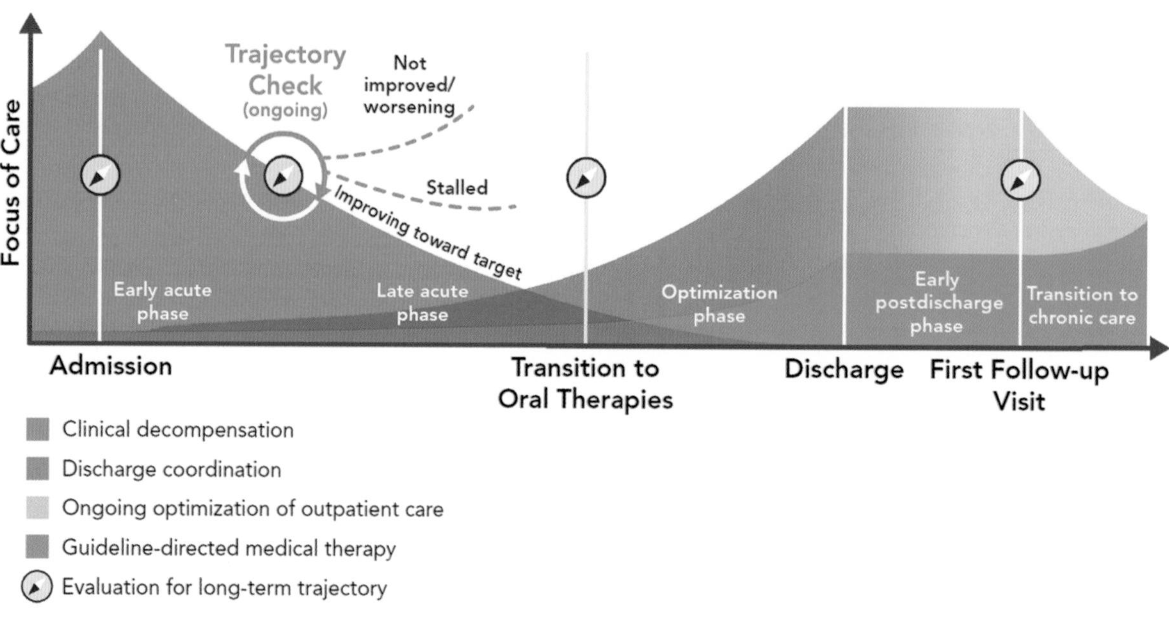

FIGURE 75.4 Graphic depiction of the clinical course of hospitalized acute decompensated heart failure, showing the degree of focus on clinical decompensation (red), discharge coordination (blue), ongoing coordination of outpatient care (light blue), and optimization of guideline-directed medical therapy (green), with ongoing assessment of the clinical course (circle with arrows), and key time points for review and revision of the long-term disease trajectory for the heart failure journey (compass signs). (Reprinted from Hollenberg SM, Warner Stevenson L, Ahmad T, et al. 2019 ACC Expert Consensus Decision Pathway on Risk Assessment, Management, and Clinical Trajectory of Patients Hospitalized With Heart Failure: A Report of the American College of Cardiology Solution Set Oversight Committee. *J Am Coll Cardiol.* 2019;74(15):1966-2011. Copyright © 2019 by the American College of Cardiology Foundation. With permission.)

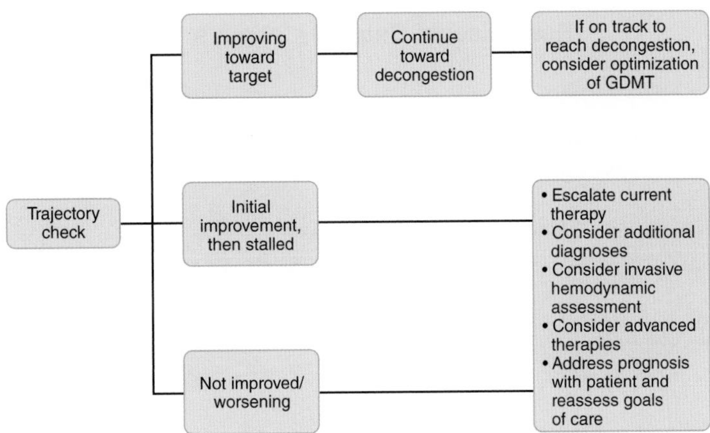

FIGURE 75.5 Clinical trajectories and therapeutic implications during hospitalization for acute decompensated heart failure. GDMT, guideline-directed medical therapy. (Reprinted from Hollenberg SM, Warner Stevenson L, Ahmad T, et al. 2019 ACC Expert Consensus Decision Pathway on Risk Assessment, Management, and Clinical Trajectory of Patients Hospitalized With Heart Failure: A Report of the American College of Cardiology Solution Set Oversight Committee. *J Am Coll Cardiol.* 2019;74(15):1966-2011. Copyright © 2019 by the American College of Cardiology Foundation. With permission.)

establishment of postdischarge appointments, and discussing mechanisms to prevent readmission. Maintenance doses of diuretics are typically lower than required for diuresis, and the need for potassium supplementation should be considered.

Rehospitalization Problem

The high rate of rehospitalization has become a significant focus of therapeutic efforts in the United States. Approximately 25% of elderly patients admitted for ADHF are rehospitalized within 30 days.[91] Adjudication of these events reveal that about 50% are attributable to HF, 25% to additional cardiac causes, and 25% to noncardiac factors[92] **(Figure 75.6)**. It is estimated that up to 75% of these readmissions may be preventable.[93] In HFpEF, the rehospitalization rate within 60 to 90 days of discharge is about 30% and is equal to that of HFrEF. [94] Early reoccurrence of congestion is common in the days to weeks following hospital discharge, and discharge prior to resolution of hemodynamic congestion appears to be a common risk for rehospitalization.[95] Social factors, including income, employment, insurance status, lack of social support and location, are associated with the risk of HF readmission.[51] A Medicare rehospitalization reduction program was implemented in an attempt to reduce cost and the rate of rehospitalizations, but concerns have risen that it may paradoxically have led to increased postdischarge mortality rates[96] If true, some theorize that appropriate readmissions are prevented owing to financial incentives, leading to increased patient mortality.[96] However, this remains a highly debated topic of active research. Early postdischarge follow-up within 7 to 10 days is associated with a lower risk of rehospitalization.[93] Improved use of GDMT is also associated with reduced rates of rehospitalization.[92]

RESEARCH AND FUTURE DIRECTIONS

ADHF remains a challenging condition manifest in a clinically heterogeneous population with a high risk of readmission at 30 days or death at 1 year. Despite marked advances in the management of chronic systolic HF, most pharmacotherapies or management strategies have largely failed to significantly improve the outcomes of patients with ADHF (Table 75.8). Early data suggest that ARNI may have a role in this setting, but confirmatory evidence is warranted. For now, patients with ADHF should be completely decongested via diuresis, have GDMT administered as tolerated, be educated about their condition, and have early follow-up after transition back to the outpatient setting. Clinicians should also consider their patient's clinical trajectory and be alert to the possibility that consultation by an advanced HF or palliative care specialist is warranted. Studies examining safety and efficacy of initiation of sodium-glucose cotransporter-2 (SGLT2) inhibitors, ARNI, and other evolving HF therapies are ongoing and will provide further information for treatment of patients with ADHF.

KEY POINTS

- ✔ ADHF is a complex process with highly heterogeneous symptoms and variable overlapping pathogenic processes.
- ✔ ADHF represents a downward inflection point in the natural history of a patient with chronic HF, associated with a high risk of readmission at 30 days and death at 1 year.
- ✔ Resolution of symptoms may not indicate a resolution of hemodynamic congestion, illustrating that clinical and hemodynamic congestion are not synonymous.
- ✔ The physical exam is fundamental to identifying the clinical hemodynamic status of the patient to guide acute therapies, risk stratification, and prognosis.
- ✔ Most cardiac medications should be continued for patients admitted with ADHF, and discharge on maximally tolerated GDMT for HF is strongly recommended.

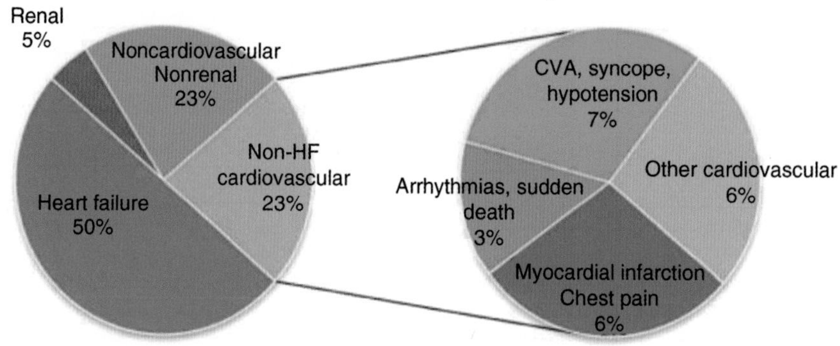

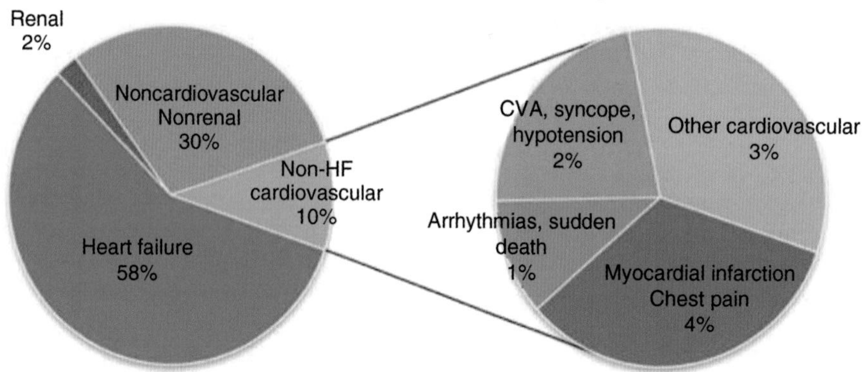

FIGURE 75.6 Etiology of readmissions within 30 and 31 to 60 days after discharge attributable to a hospitalization for acute decompensated heart failure. CVA, cerebrovascular; HF, heart failure. (Reprinted from Vader JM, LaRue SJ, Stevens SR, et al. Timing and Causes of Readmission After Acute Heart Failure Hospitalization-Insights From the Heart Failure Network Trials. *J Card Fail.* 2016;22(11):875-883. Copyright © 2016 Elsevier. With permission.)

- ✔ The use of inotropes should be avoided except for refractory shock or low-output HF attributable to the increased mortality associated with even short-term use.
- ✔ Three main clinical trajectories during hospitalization for ADHF have been described: improving toward target, stalled after initial response, and not improved and/or worsening.
- ✔ The objective of diuretics is to induce a net negative sodium and water balance of at least 3 to 5 L of urine output daily until resolution of congestion or a compromise on decongestion is achieved.
- ✔ Hospital discharge prior to complete decongestion is associated with a higher risk of long-term rehospitalization and death.

REFERENCES

1. Benjamin EJ, Muntner P, Alonso A, et al. Heart disease and stroke statistics-2019 update: a report from the American Heart Association. *Circulation.* 2019;139(10):e56-e528.
2. Akintoye E, Briasoulis A, Egbe A, et al. National trends in admission and in-hospital mortality of patients with heart failure in the United States (2001-2014). *J Am Heart Assoc.* 2017;6(12):e006955.
3. Gheorghiade M, Abraham WT, Albert NM, et al. Systolic blood pressure at admission, clinical characteristics, and outcomes in patients hospitalized with acute heart failure. *JAMA.* 2006;296(18):2217-2226.
4. Nieminen MS, Brutsaert D, Dickstein K, et al. EuroHeart Failure Survey II (EHFS II): a survey on hospitalized acute heart failure patients: description of population. *Eur Heart J.* 2006;27(22):2725-2736.
5. Yancy CW, Lopatin M, Stevenson LW, et al. Clinical presentation, management, and in-hospital outcomes of patients admitted with acute decompensated heart failure with preserved systolic function: a report from the Acute Decompensated Heart Failure National Registry (ADHERE) Database. *J Am Coll Cardiol.* 2006;47(1):76-84.
6. Owan TE, Hodge DO, Herges RM, Jacobsen SJ, Roger VL, Redfield MM. Trends in prevalence and outcome of heart failure with preserved ejection fraction. *N Engl J Med.* 2006;355(3):251-259.
7. Steinberg BA, Zhao X, Heidenreich PA, et al. Trends in patients hospitalized with heart failure and preserved left ventricular ejection fraction: prevalence, therapies, and outcomes. *Circulation.* 2012;126(1):65-75.
8. Yancy CW, Jessup M, Bozkurt B, et al. 2013 ACCF/AHA guideline for the management of heart failure: executive summary: a report of the American College of Cardiology Foundation/American Heart Association Task Force on practice guidelines. *Circulation.* 2013;128(16):1810-1852.
9. Mozaffarian D, Benjamin EJ, Go AS, et al. Executive summary: heart disease and stroke statistics—2016 update: a report from the American Heart Association. *Circulation.* 2016;133(4):447-454.
10. Djousse L, Driver JA, Gaziano JM. Relation between modifiable lifestyle factors and lifetime risk of heart failure. *JAMA.* 2009;302(4):394-400.

11. Lloyd-Jones DM, Larson MG, Leip EP, et al. Lifetime risk for developing congestive heart failure: the Framingham Heart Study. *Circulation.* 2002;106(24):3068-3072.
12. Mosterd A, Hoes AW, de Bruyne MC, et al. Prevalence of heart failure and left ventricular dysfunction in the general population; The Rotterdam Study. *Eur Heart J.* 1999;20(6):447-455.
13. Redfield MM, Jacobsen SJ, Burnett JC Jr, Mahoney DW, Bailey KR, Rodeheffer RJ. Burden of systolic and diastolic ventricular dysfunction in the community: appreciating the scope of the heart failure epidemic. *JAMA.* 2003;289(2):194-202.
14. Fonarow GC, Abraham WT, Albert NM, et al. Age-and gender-related differences in quality of care and outcomes of patients hospitalized with heart failure (from OPTIMIZE-HF). *Am J Cardiol.* 2009;104(1):107-115.
15. Hsich EM, Grau-Sepulveda MV, Hernandez AF, et al. Sex differences in in-hospital mortality in acute decompensated heart failure with reduced and preserved ejection fraction. *Am Heart J.* 2012;163(3):430-437, 437.e1-3.
16. Lee DS, Gona P, Vasan RS, et al. Relation of disease pathogenesis and risk factors to heart failure with preserved or reduced ejection fraction: insights from the Framingham heart study of the national heart, lung, and blood institute. *Circulation.* 2009;119(24):3070-3077.
17. Bahrami H, Kronmal R, Bluemke DA, et al. Differences in the incidence of congestive heart failure by ethnicity: the multi-ethnic study of atherosclerosis. *Arch Intern Med.* 2008;168(19):2138-2145.
18. Loehr LR, Rosamond WD, Chang PP, Folsom AR, Chambless LE. Heart failure incidence and survival (from the Atherosclerosis Risk in Communities study). *Am J Cardiol.* 2008;101(7):1016-1022.
19. Kapoor JR, Kapoor R, Hellkamp AS, Hernandez AF, Heidenreich PA, Fonarow GC. Payment source, quality of care, and outcomes in patients hospitalized with heart failure. *J Am Coll Cardiol.* 2011;58(14):1465-1471.
20. Foraker RE, Rose KM, Suchindran CM, Chang PP, McNeill AM, Rosamond WD. Socioeconomic status, Medicaid coverage, clinical comorbidity, and rehospitalization or death after an incident heart failure hospitalization: Atherosclerosis Risk in Communities cohort (1987 to 2004). *Circ Heart Fail.* 2011;4(3):308-316.
21. Rathore SS, Masoudi FA, Wang Y, et al. Socioeconomic status, treatment, and outcomes among elderly patients hospitalized with heart failure: findings from the National Heart Failure Project. *Am Heart J.* 2006;152(2):371-378.
22. Philbin EF, Dec GW, Jenkins PL, DiSalvo TG. Socioeconomic status as an independent risk factor for hospital readmission for heart failure. *Am J Cardiol.* 2001;87(12):1367-1371.
23. Jha SR, Ha HS, Hickman LD, et al. Frailty in advanced heart failure: a systematic review. *Heart Fail Rev.* 2015;20(5):553-560.
24. Olsen CO, Attarian DE, Jones RN, et al. The coronary pressure-flow determinants left ventricular compliance in dogs. *Circ Res.* 1981;49(4):856-865.
25. Peacock WF 4th, De Marco T, Fonarow GC, et al. Cardiac troponin and outcome in acute heart failure. *N Engl J Med.* 2008;358(20):2117-2126.
26. Metra M, Cotter G, Davison BA, et al. Effect of serelaxin on cardiac, renal, and hepatic biomarkers in the Relaxin in Acute Heart Failure (RELAX-AHF) development program: correlation with outcomes. *J Am Coll Cardiol.* 2013;61(2):196-206.
27. Forman DE, Butler J, Wang Y, et al. Incidence, predictors at admission, and impact of worsening renal function among patients hospitalized with heart failure. *J Am Coll Cardiol.* 2004;43(1):61-67.
28. Rangaswami J, Bhalla V, Blair JEA, et al. Cardiorenal syndrome: classification, pathophysiology, diagnosis, and treatment strategies: a scientific statement from the American Heart Association. *Circulation.* 2019;139(16):e840-e878.
29. Mullens W, Abrahams Z, Francis GS, et al. Importance of venous congestion for worsening of renal function in advanced decompensated heart failure. *J Am Coll Cardiol.* 2009;53(7):589-596.
30. Grodin JL. Hemodynamically, the kidney is at the heart of cardiorenal syndrome. *Cleve Clin J Med.* 2018;85(3):240-242.
31. Zhang DY, Anderson AS. The sympathetic nervous system and heart failure. *Cardiol Clin.* 2014;32(1):33-45, vii.
32. Zile MR, Bennett TD, St John Sutton M, et al. Transition from chronic compensated to acute decompensated heart failure: pathophysiological insights obtained from continuous monitoring of intracardiac pressures. *Circulation.* 2008;118(14):1433-1441.
33. Fudim M, Hernandez AF, Felker GM. Role of volume redistribution in the congestion of heart failure. *J Am Heart Assoc.* 2017;6(8):e006817.
34. Rapaport E, Weisbart MH, Levine M. The splanchnic blood volume in congestive heart failure. *Circulation.* 1958;18(4 Part 1):581-587.
35. Gelman S, Mushlin PS. Catecholamine-induced changes in the splanchnic circulation affecting systemic hemodynamics. *Anesthesiology.* 2004;100(2):434-439.
36. Hendren NS, Drazner MH, Pandey A, Tang WHW, Grodin JL. Implications of perceived dyspnea and global well-being measured by visual assessment scales during treatment for acute decompensated heart failure. *Am J Cardiol.* 2019;124(3):402-408.
37. Pang PS, Cleland JG, Teerlink JR, et al. A proposal to standardize dyspnoea measurement in clinical trials of acute heart failure syndromes: the need for a uniform approach. *Eur Heart J.* 2008;29(6):816-824.
38. Adams KF, Jr., Fonarow GC, Emerman CL, et al. Characteristics and outcomes of patients hospitalized for heart failure in the United States: rationale, design, and preliminary observations from the first 100,000 cases in the Acute Decompensated Heart Failure National Registry (ADHERE). *Am Heart J.* 2005;149(2):209-216.
39. Petrie CJ, Ponikowski P, Metra M, et al. Proportional pulse pressure relates to cardiac index in stabilized acute heart failure patients. *Clin Exp Hypertens.* 2018;40(7):637-643.
40. Stevenson LW, Perloff JK. The limited reliability of physical signs for estimating hemodynamics in chronic heart failure. *JAMA.* 1989;261(6):884-888.
41. Drazner MH, Hellkamp AS, Leier CV, et al. Value of clinician assessment of hemodynamics in advanced heart failure: the ESCAPE trial. *Circ Heart Fail.* 2008;1(3):170-177.
42. Thibodeau JT, Drazner MH. The role of the clinical examination in patients with heart failure. *JACC Heart Fail.* 2018;6(7):543-551.
43. Joshi N. The third heart sound. *South Med J.* 1999;92(8):756-761.
44. Drazner MH, Rame JE, Stevenson LW, Dries DL. Prognostic importance of elevated jugular venous pressure and a third heart sound in patients with heart failure. *N Engl J Med.* 2001;345(8):574-581.
45. Ewy GA. The abdominojugular test: technique and hemodynamic correlates. *Ann Intern Med.* 1988;109(6):456-460.
46. Baeza-Trinidad R, Mosquera-Lozano JD, El Bikri L. Assessment of bendopnea impact on decompensated heart failure. *Eur J Heart Fail.* 2017;19(1):111-115.
47. Yek C, Hendren NS, Dominguez AR. Edema and ulceration of the lower extremities-all that's red is not infection: a teachable moment. *JAMA Intern Med.* 2018;178(2):277-278.
48. Maisel AS, Krishnaswamy P, Nowak RM, et al. Rapid measurement of B-type natriuretic peptide in the emergency diagnosis of heart failure. *N Engl J Med.* 2002;347(3):161-167.
49. McMurray JJ, Packer M, Desai AS, et al. Angiotensin-neprilysin inhibition versus enalapril in heart failure. *N Engl J Med.* 2014;371(11):993-1004.
50. Kristensen SL, Jhund PS, Mogensen UM, et al. Prognostic value of N-terminal pro-B-type natriuretic peptide levels in heart failure patients with and without atrial fibrillation. *Circ Heart Fail.* 2017;10(10):e004409.
51. Hollenberg SM, Stevenson LW, Ahmad T, et al. 2019 ACC expert consensus decision pathway on risk assessment, management, and clinical trajectory of patients hospitalized with heart failure: a report of the American College of Cardiology Solution Set Oversight Committee. *J Am Coll Cardiol.* 2019;74(15):1966-2011.
52. Fonarow GC, Abraham WT, Albert NM, et al. Factors identified as precipitating hospital admissions for heart failure and clinical outcomes: findings from OPTIMIZE-HF. *Arch Intern Med.* 2008;168(8):847-854.
53. Nohria A, Tsang SW, Fang JC, et al. Clinical assessment identifies hemodynamic profiles that predict outcomes in patients admitted with heart failure. *J Am Coll Cardiol.* 2003;41(10):1797-1804.
54. Drazner MH, Velez-Martinez M, Ayers CR, et al. Relationship of right-to left-sided ventricular filling pressures in advanced heart failure: insights from the ESCAPE trial. *Circ Heart Fail.* 2013;6(2):264-270.

55. Grodin JL, Drazner MH, Dupont M, et al. A disproportionate elevation in right ventricular filling pressure, in relation to left ventricular filling pressure, is associated with renal impairment and increased mortality in advanced decompensated heart failure. *Am Heart J.* 2015;169(6):806-812.
56. Vital FM, Saconato H, Ladeira MT, et al. Non-invasive positive pressure ventilation (CPAP or bilevel NPPV) for cardiogenic pulmonary edema. *Cochrane Database Syst Rev.* 2008(3):CD005351.
57. Gray A, Goodacre S, Newby DE, et al. Noninvasive ventilation in acute cardiogenic pulmonary edema. *N Engl J Med.* 2008;359(2):142-151.
58. Binanay C, Califf RM, Hasselblad V, et al. Evaluation study of congestive heart failure and pulmonary artery catheterization effectiveness: the ESCAPE trial. *JAMA.* 2005;294(13):1625-1633.
59. Felker GM, Lee KL, Bull DA, et al. Diuretic strategies in patients with acute decompensated heart failure. *N Engl J Med.* 2011;364(9):797-805.
60. Bart BA, Goldsmith SR, Lee KL, et al. Ultrafiltration in decompensated heart failure with cardiorenal syndrome. *N Engl J Med.* 2012;367(24):2296-2304.
61. Neuberg GW, Miller AB, O'Connor CM, et al. Diuretic resistance predicts mortality in patients with advanced heart failure. *Am Heart J.* 2002;144(1):31-38.
62. Ellison DH, Felker GM. Diuretic treatment in heart failure. *N Engl J Med.* 2018;378(7):684-685.
63. Butler J, Anstrom KJ, Felker GM, et al. Efficacy and safety of spironolactone in acute heart failure: the ATHENA-HF randomized clinical trial. *JAMA Cardiol.* 2017;2(9):950-958.
64. Mullens W, Verbrugge FH, Nijst P, et al. Rationale and design of the ADVOR (Acetazolamide in Decompensated Heart Failure with Volume Overload) trial. *Eur J Heart Fail.* 2018;20(11):1591-1600.
65. Gottlieb SS. Importance of magnesium in congestive heart failure. *Am J Cardiol.* 1989;63(14):39G-42G.
66. DiNicolantonio JJ, Liu J, O'Keefe JH. Magnesium for the prevention and treatment of cardiovascular disease. *Open Heart.* 2018;5(2):e000775.
67. Baker WL, Kluger J, Coleman CI, White CM. Impact of Magnesium L-Lactate on occurrence of ventricular arrhythmias in patients with implantable cardioverter defibrillators: a randomized, placebo-controlled trial. *Open Cardiovasc Med J.* 2015;9:83-88.
68. Bowling CB, Pitt B, Ahmed MI, et al. Hypokalemia and outcomes in patients with chronic heart failure and chronic kidney disease: findings from propensity-matched studies. *Circ Heart Fail.* 2010;3(2):253-260.
69. Grodin JL, Simon J, Hachamovitch R, et al. Prognostic role of serum chloride levels in acute decompensated heart failure. *J Am Coll Cardiol.* 2015;66(6):659-666.
70. Gheorghiade M, Abraham WT, Albert NM, et al. Relationship between admission serum sodium concentration and clinical outcomes in patients hospitalized for heart failure: an analysis from the OPTIMIZE-HF registry. *Eur Heart J.* 2007;28(8):980-988.
71. Gilstrap LG, Fonarow GC, Desai AS, et al. Initiation, continuation, or withdrawal of angiotensin-converting enzyme inhibitors/angiotensin receptor blockers and outcomes in patients hospitalized with heart failure with reduced ejection fraction. *J Am Heart Assoc.* 2017;6(2):e004675.
72. Packer M, Lee WH, Yushak M, Medina N. Comparison of captopril and enalapril in patients with severe chronic heart failure. *N Engl J Med.* 1986;315(14):847-853.
73. Velazquez EJ, Morrow DA, DeVore AD, et al. Angiotensin-neprilysin inhibition in acute decompensated heart failure. *N Engl J Med.* 2019;380(6):539-548.
74. Morrow DA, Velazquez EJ, DeVore AD, et al. Clinical outcomes in patients with acute decompensated heart failure randomly assigned to sacubitril/valsartan or enalapril in the PIONEER-HF trial. *Circulation.* 2019;139(19):2285-2288.
75. Publication Committee for the VMAC Investigators. Intravenous nesiritide vs nitroglycerin for treatment of decompensated congestive heart failure: a randomized controlled trial. *JAMA.* 2002;287(12):1531-1540.
76. Hottinger DG, Beebe DS, Kozhimannil T, Prielipp RC, Belani KG. Sodium nitroprusside in 2014: a clinical concepts review. *J Anaesthesiol Clin Pharmacol.* 2014;30(4):462-71.
77. Mullens W, Abrahams Z, Francis GS, et al. Sodium nitroprusside for advanced low-output heart failure. *J Am Coll Cardiol.* 2008;52(3):200-207.
78. Nagy L, Pollesello P, Papp Z. Inotropes and inodilators for acute heart failure: sarcomere active drugs in focus. *J Cardiovasc Pharmacol.* 2014;64(3):199-208.
79. Felker GM, Benza RL, Chandler AB, et al. Heart failure etiology and response to milrinone in decompensated heart failure: results from the OPTIME-CHF study. *J Am Coll Cardiol.* 2003;41(6):997-1003.
80. Overgaard CB, Dzavik V. Inotropes and vasopressors: review of physiology and clinical use in cardiovascular disease. *Circulation.* 2008;118(10):1047-1056.
81. Coletta AP, Cleland JG, Freemantle N, Clark AL. Clinical trials update from the European Society of Cardiology Heart Failure meeting: SHAPE, BRING-UP 2 VAS, COLA II, FOSIDIAL, BETACAR, CASINO and meta-analysis of cardiac resynchronisation therapy. *Eur J Heart Fail.* 2004;6(5):673-676.
82. Cuffe MS, Califf RM, Adams KF Jr, et al. Short-term intravenous milrinone for acute exacerbation of chronic heart failure: a randomized controlled trial. *JAMA.* 2002;287(12):1541-1547.
83. Chen HH, Anstrom KJ, Givertz MM, et al. Low-dose dopamine or low-dose nesiritide in acute heart failure with renal dysfunction: the ROSE acute heart failure randomized trial. *JAMA.* 2013;310(23):2533-2543.
84. Friedrich JO, Adhikari N, Herridge MS, Beyene J. Meta-analysis: low-dose dopamine increases urine output but does not prevent renal dysfunction or death. *Ann Intern Med.* 2005;142(7):510-524.
85. Grodin JL, Carter S, Bart BA, Goldsmith SR, Drazner MH, Tang WHW. Direct comparison of ultrafiltration to pharmacological decongestion in heart failure: a per-protocol analysis of CARRESS-HF. *Eur J Heart Fail.* 2018;20(7):1148-1156.
86. Paterna S, Fasullo S, Parrinello G, et al. Short-term effects of hypertonic saline solution in acute heart failure and long-term effects of a moderate sodium restriction in patients with compensated heart failure with New York Heart Association class III (Class C) (SMAC-HF Study). *Am J Med Sci.* 2011;342(1):27-37.
87. Samsky MD, Ambrosy AP, Youngson E, et al. Trends in readmissions and length of stay for patients hospitalized with heart failure in Canada and the United States. *JAMA Cardiol.* 2019;4(5):444-453.
88. Khan H, Greene SJ, Fonarow GC, et al. Length of hospital stay and 30-day readmission following heart failure hospitalization: insights from the EVEREST trial. *Eur J Heart Fail.* 2015;17(10):1022-1031.
89. van Diepen S, Katz JN, Albert NM, et al. Contemporary management of cardiogenic shock: a scientific statement from the American Heart Association. *Circulation.* 2017;136(16):e232-e268.
90. Solomon SD, Dobson J, Pocock S, et al. Influence of nonfatal hospitalization for heart failure on subsequent mortality in patients with chronic heart failure. *Circulation.* 2007;116(13):1482-1487.
91. Khera R, Wang Y, Nasir K, Lin Z, Krumholz HM. Evaluation of 30-day hospital readmission and mortality rates using regression-discontinuity framework. *J Am Coll Cardiol.* 2019;74(2):219-234.
92. Vader JM, LaRue SJ, Stevens SR, et al. Timing and causes of readmission after acute heart failure hospitalization-insights from the heart failure network trials. *J Card Fail.* 2016;22(11):875-883.
93. Desai AS, Stevenson LW. Rehospitalization for heart failure: predict or prevent? *Circulation.* 2012;126(4):501-506.
94. Fonarow GC, Stough WG, Abraham WT, et al. Characteristics, treatments, and outcomes of patients with preserved systolic function hospitalized for heart failure: a report from the OPTIMIZE-HF Registry. *J Am Coll Cardiol.* 2007;50(8):768-777.
95. Blair JE, Khan S, Konstam MA, et al. Weight changes after hospitalization for worsening heart failure and subsequent re-hospitalization and mortality in the EVEREST trial. *Eur Heart J.* 2009;30(13):1666-1673.
96. Wadhera RK, Joynt Maddox KE, Wasfy JH, Haneuse S, Shen C, Yeh RW. Association of the hospital readmissions reduction program with mortality among medicare beneficiaries hospitalized for heart failure, acute myocardial infarction, and pneumonia. *JAMA.* 2018;320(24):2542-2552.

CHAPTER 76

CHRONIC HEART FAILURE MANAGEMENT

Ray Hu, Edo Y. Birati, and Lee R. Goldberg

INTRODUCTION

Heart failure is estimated to affect over 26 million adults worldwide[1] and is one of the leading causes of inpatient admissions and mortality in Western countries.[2] In the United States, it is estimated that 30 billion dollars per year is spent on the treatment of at least 5 million heart failure patients, and both numbers are expected to grow significantly in the next decade.[3] The past several decades have seen significant progress in the standardization of optimal medical therapy and the use of device therapy including implantable cardiac defibrillators, chronic resynchronization therapy, and left ventricular (LV) assist devices for select populations. This chapter will focus on the medical management of heart failure, and device-specific therapies will be discussed separately. Medical treatment is the cornerstone of heart failure therapy and is essential prior to and in concert with device therapy. Furthermore, while this chapter focuses on symptomatic and disease-modifying therapies of heart failure, identifying and treating potentially reversible causes (coronary disease, thyroid disease, high output states, hemochromatosis, etc) is paramount.

GOALS OF CHRONIC HEART FAILURE TREATMENT

Broadly speaking, the goals of heart failure treatment are to improve patient symptoms and quality of life, slow disease progression, and prolong survival.[4] These goals are achieved through combining classes of medications with device therapies and lifestyle changes. Heart failure symptoms generally arise from excessive fluid retention and from inability of the heart to generate adequate cardiac output with subsequent circulatory congestion and inadequate organ perfusion. As such therapies aimed at relieving symptoms are generally targeted to improve volume status and to decrease cardiac afterload in an effort to improve forward flow. Conversely, therapies aimed at slowing and reversing disease progression work to dampen the maladaptive overactivation of the various neurohormonal pathways. This can lead not only to improved cardiac performance but also to positive cardiac structural changes known as reverse remodeling.

PHARMACOLOGIC THERAPY

Diuretics

Clinical manifestations of heart failure may result from inappropriate intravascular and extravascular volume expansion caused by excessive sodium and fluid retention. As such, diuretics are fundamental in achieving and maintaining proper fluid balance to alleviate symptoms of heart failure. They are used both acutely and chronically to manage volume status. Although anecdotal studies have shown that diuretics can improve cardiac function, symptoms, and exercise tolerance,[5] diuretics activate the sympathetic system and over time are thought to be detrimental in heart failure. Therefore, the use of diuretics alone, without neurohormonal blockade, is not recommended, as adrenergic activation has been associated with worse outcomes in heart failure.

Loop diuretics such as furosemide, bumetanide, and torsemide are the most commonly prescribed diuretics for heart failure. These compounds act to reversibly inhibit the Na^+-K^+-2Cl symporter in the ascending loop of Henle to enhance urinary sodium and water excretion. Loop diuretics also have venodilatory effects and have been shown to decrease right atrial and pulmonary venous wedge pressure within minutes of intravenous (IV) infusion.[6] Oral bioavailability varies significantly and can be as low as 40% for furosemide and greater than 80% for bumetanide and torsemide. Thus, bumetanide and torsemide may be more effective in patients with significant volume overload or right-sided heart failure and subsequent intestinal edema.

Observational studies have suggested an association between higher dose diuretics and worse clinical outcomes,[7] which may be mediated through increased renal injury, electrolyte abnormalities, and neurohormonal activation.[8] The Diuretic Optimization Strategies Evaluation (DOSE) study, a randomized double-blind study, compared diuretic strategies in acute heart failure with IV furosemide using either twice daily bolus dosing or a continuous infusion at two doses (equivalent to outpatient dose vs. 2.5 times the outpatient dose). There was no difference in the co-primary endpoints of global assessment of symptoms or a change in creatinine at 72 hours in either the low- versus high-dose groups or the bolus versus continuous infusion groups.[9] Of note, there was a trend toward greater relief of dyspnea and net fluid loss at 72 hours in the high-dose group.

Of note, loop diuretics initiate a renal homeostatic mechanism that increases distal solute and water resorption and in turn decreases diuretic effectiveness. This phenomenon can be overcome with a coadministration of a thiazide-like diuretic (eg, metolazone or chlorothiazide) that acts on the distal tubule to block sodium reabsorption. Adding a thiazide-like diuretic can often precipitate a brisk diuresis and close monitoring is required to prevent excessive fluid and electrolyte loss (particularly hypokalemia and hyponatremia).

Angiotensin Converting Enzyme Inhibitors

There is tremendous evidence supporting the use of angiotensin converting enzyme (ACE) inhibitors in patients with reduced (<40%) left ventricular ejection fraction (LVEF), and the use of these agents is indicated in all patients with LV systolic dysfunction. ACE inhibitors block ACE that is responsible for the conversion of angiotensin I to angiotensin II. In addition, they enhance kinin activity through the inhibition of kininase II. ACE inhibitors have been shown in several clinical trials to stabilize LV remodeling, improve symptoms, prevent hospitalizations, and prolong life in patients with reduced LVEF.[10-13] These large, randomized trials included varied patients, such as asymptomatic and symptomatic patients, elderly patients, women, and a wide range of etiologies of LV systolic dysfunction. The Studies on Left Ventricular Dysfunction (SOLVD) Prevention Study[11] and the Survival and Ventricular Enlargement (SAVE) Study[13] have shown that enalapril and captopril, respectively, can reduce the development of symptoms, decrease hospitalizations, and prolong life, in asymptomatic patients with LV dysfunction. Furthermore, the Cooperative North Scandinavian Enalapril Survival Study (CONSENSUS I)[10] demonstrated that the absolute benefit is greatest in patients with more severe disease (New York Heart Association [NYHA] Class IV heart failure), as the study showed a much larger effect size of enalapril than the SOLVD treatment and prevention trials. The impact of ACE inhibitors on heart failure outcomes appears to be a class effect. The beneficial effects of ACE inhibitors are dose dependent,[14] and thus doses should be titrated as tolerated until they reach those used in clinical trials (**Table 76.1**).

Side effects of ACE inhibitors, such as azotemia and hypotension, are related to the suppression of renin-angiotensin system activity. These effects are generally well tolerated and do not require dose adjustment unless the patient is symptomatic, or the magnitude of hypotension or azotemia is significant. Hyperkalemia may also occur, especially with potassium supplementation or treatment with potassium-sparing diuretics such as spironolactone. The kinin effects of ACE inhibitors can lead to side effects including dry cough (up to 10% of patients) and angioedema. Replacement of the ACE inhibitor with an angiotensin receptor antagonist may alleviate the kinin-mediated side effects but not hyperkalemia or renal insufficiency. Patients with bilateral renal artery stenosis may experience acute renal failure upon the initiation of ACE inhibitors. In all patients, laboratories including electrolytes and renal function should be monitored on initiation and titration of ACE inhibitors.

Angiotensin Receptor Blockers

Angiotensin receptor blockers (ARBs) antagonize the angiotensin type 1 receptor to inhibit the adverse biologic effects of angiotensin II on cardiac remodeling. This mechanism has no effect on bradykinin activity and thus avoids some of the adverse effects of ACE inhibitors. In systolic heart failure patients intolerant of ACE inhibitors, aggregate data suggest that ARBs are as effective as ACE inhibitors in reducing symptoms, hospitalizations, and mortality. In the Candesartan in Heart Failure: Assessment of Reduction in Mortality and Morbidity (CHARM-Alternative)[15] trial, candesartan reduced mortality and hospital admissions irrespective of background β-blocker therapy. Similar findings were seen in a study on valsartan (Valsartan Heart Failure Trial).[16] There is also evidence to suggest that ARBs may be beneficial when added to ACE inhibitors. In the CHARM-Added trial, the addition of candesartan resulted in a 4% to 5% reduction in cardiovascular death and hospitalizations in patients taking a β-blocker and ACE inhibitor.[12] Of note, significantly higher rates of renal injury and hyperkalemia occurred in the candesartan group, and there was overall a low usage of spironolactone. As such, the general consensus has been that ACE inhibitors are first-line agents for renin-angiotensin-aldosterone system (RAAS) blockade, and ARBs should be used in patients intolerant to ACE inhibitors, though this may be shifting with the advent of angiotensin receptor neprilysin inhibitor (ARNI) therapy. Per current practice guidelines, there is a Class IIb recommendation[4] for combination therapy with ACE inhibitors and ARBs in patients intolerant to spironolactone, though the utility of this strategy in the context of modern therapies is uncertain.

The side effects of ARBs are similar to the non-kinin-mediated effects of ACE and include hypotension, azotemia, and hyperkalemia. An ARB can be used for patients who have an ACE cough and patients who have experienced angioedema with an ACE inhibitor can receive an ARB with enhanced monitoring. Initial and target doses of ARBs are listed in **Table 76.2**.

Angiotensin Receptor Neprilysin Inhibitors

ARNIs are a newer class of RAAS antagonists for the treatment of heart failure, which combines an ARB and a neprilysin inhibitor. The first and currently only approved agent combines sacubitril with valsartan. Neprilysin is a zinc-dependent membrane endopeptidase and cleaves a variety of peptides including natriuretic peptides, bradykinin, and adrenomedullin. Inhibition of neprilysin increases levels of atrial natriuretic peptide, B-type natriuretic peptide, C-type natriuretic peptide and adrenomedullin which results in increased vasodilatation, natriuresis, and decreased left ventricular fibrosis and hypertrophy.[17] Of note, neprilysin also breaks down angiotensin II, and its inhibition can lead to vasoconstriction and increased afterload. Thus, neprilysin inhibitors are combined with RAAS inhibitors to prevent deleterious potentiation of angiotensin II.

In the PARADIGM-HF (Prospective Comparison of ARNI with ACEI to Determine Impact on Global Mortality and Morbidity in Heart Failure) trial, the use of sacubitril/valsartan resulted in a 20% relative risk reduction as compared to enalapril in the combined endpoint of cardiovascular mortality and heart failure hospitalizations[18] in stable NYHA Class II to IV patients with LVEF less than 35%. A significant decrease in all-cause mortality was also noted. It is important to note

TABLE 76.1 Angiotensin Converting Enzyme Inhibitors and Associated Initial, Maximum (Max), and Randomized Controlled Trial (RCT) Dose

Mechanism of Action	Drug	Initial Daily Dose(s)	Max Dose(s)	Mean RCT Dose
Inhibits the conversion of angiotensin I to angiotensin II and upregulates bradykinin, thereby counteracting the overactivation of the renin-angiotensin system and the effects of adverse cardiac remodeling	Captopril	6.25 mg tid	50 mg tid	122.7 mg daily
	Enalapril	2.5 mg bid	10-20 mg bid	16.6 mg daily
	Fosinopril	5-10 mg qd	40 mg qd	NA
	Lisinopril	2.5-5 mg qd	20-40 mg qd	32.5-35.0 mg daily
	Perindopril	2 mg qd	8-16 mg qd	NA
	Quinapril	5 mg bid	20 mg bid	NA
	Ramipril	1.25-2.5 mg qd	10 mg qd	NA
	Trandolapril	1 mg qd	4 mg qd	NA

bid, twice a day; NA, not available; qd, every day; tid, three times a day.

TABLE 76.2 Commonly Used Angiotensin Receptor Blockers and Associated Initial, Maximum (Max), and Randomized Controlled Trial (RCT) Dose

Mechanism of Action	Drug	Initial Daily Dose(s)	Max Dose(s)	Mean RCT Dose
Inhibits angiotensin II receptors, thereby counteracting the overactivation of the renin-angiotensin-aldosterone system and counteracting the effects of adverse cardiac remodeling	Candesartan	4-8 mg qd	32 mg qd	24 mg daily
	Losartan	25-50 mg qd	50-150 mg qd	129 mg daily
	Valsartan	20-40 mg bid	160 mg bid	254 mg daily

bid, twice a day; qd, every day.

that there was no placebo arm in the PARADIGM-HF trial, and sacubitril/valsartan was being compared to the standard of care enalapril revealing an incremental benefit. PIONEER-HF (Comparison of Sacubitril–Valsartan versus Enalapril on Effect on NT-proBNP in Patients Stabilized from an Acute Heart Failure Episode), a study on in-hospital initiation of sacubitril/valsartan in acute heart failure patients, showed no difference in adverse events when compared to enalapril.[19] Current guidelines recommend replacement with ARNI in Class II to III patients tolerating ACE inhibitor or ARB therapy.[20] The starting dose of sacubitril/valsartan is dependent on the dose of ACE inhibitor or ARB that the patient tolerates with a target dose of sacubitril/valsartan being 93 mg/107 mg. Recent guidelines suggest that ARNI can be initial therapy for systolic heart failure avoiding the need to transition from an ACE or ARB.

The most common side effect of ARNI is hypotension which can occur in up to 18% of patients. Hyperkalemia is also common; cough and angioedema are rarely observed. The combination of an ACE inhibitor and neprilysin inhibitor significantly increases the risk of angioedema thought to be secondary to high levels of bradykinin. Therefore, administration of an ARNI with an ACE inhibitor is contraindicated. When transitioning from an ACE inhibitor to ARNI, a 36-hour washout period following discontinuation of the ACE inhibitor is required prior to the first dose of ARNI.

β-Blockers

β-Blockers alleviate the harmful effects of sustained cardiac adrenergic stimulation by blocking one or more α- and β-adrenergic receptors. Most of the harmful effects of β-adrenergic stimulation in the heart are thought to be mediated through the β1 receptor. Three β-blockers have been shown to improve outcomes in patients with heart failure: carvedilol (The Carvedilol Prospective Randomized Cumulative Survival [COPERNICUS] trial[21]), bisoprolol (Cardiac Insufficiency Bisoprolol Study II [CIBIS-II] trial[22]), and sustained-release metoprolol succinate (Metoprolol CR/XL Randomized Intervention Trial in Congestive Heart Failure [MERIT-HF] trial[23]). Carvedilol blocks α1, β1, and β2 receptors whereas bisoprolol and metoprolol are β1 selective. When given in combination with a RAAS blocker (ACE inhibitor or ARB) to patients with an LVEF less than 40%, these β-blockers decrease symptoms and hospitalizations, prolong survival, and promote reverse LV remodeling. Not all β-blockers improve clinical outcomes in heart failure[24-26]; unlike with ACE inhibitors and ARBs, the benefits of β-blockers in heart failure do not represent a class effect.

β-Blockers should be initiated in low doses and titrated to target doses as tolerated. Titration of β-blockers should occur slowly (increase dose no more often than every 2 weeks) and should not occur in the setting of volume overload or borderline-low cardiac output, as inhibition of the adrenergic system in these settings can exacerbate acute heart failure. Patients do not need to be on maximum tolerated dose of a RAAS blocker prior to the initiation of a β-blocker; the majority of patients enrolled in β-blocker trials were not on high-dose ACE inhibitors. A clinical trial of low- versus high-dose ACE inhibitor found that most of the mortality benefit of ACE inhibitors occurred at low- to moderate dose.[14] This suggests that the mortality benefit of adding moderate- to high-dose β-blocker to lower dose ACE inhibitor exceeds that of increasing the dose of ACE inhibitor and only being able to introduce low-dose β-blocker. Therefore, the current guidance is that patients should be on low- to moderate-dose ACE inhibitor combined with maximally tolerated β-blocker.[14]

In addition to fluid overload, β-blockers can cause hypotension, bradycardia, and a general feeling of fatigue. Dose reduction should be considered if the patient experiences symptomatic hypotension or if the heart rate is less than 50 bpm without the presence of a pacemaker. Traditionally, β-blockers were held or reduced in the setting of acute decompensated heart failure; however, there is evidence that acute withdrawal of β-blockers can lead to increased complications including arrhythmias, and studies have suggested continuation during acute heart failure is safe.[27] β-Blockers should be held in the setting of acute decompensation requiring the use of inotropes. Initial and target doses of β-blockers are listed in **Table 76.3**.

Mineralocorticoid Receptor Antagonists

Mineralocorticoid receptor antagonists (MRAs) are potassium-sparing diuretics that competitively bind to the aldosterone receptor and increase the secretion of sodium and water in the distal tubule at the expense of potassium retention. The beneficial effects of MRAs are independent of its effect on sodium balance as the doses given for heart failure are much lower than doses required to achieve diuresis. Administration of an MRA reduces symptoms, hospitalizations, and mortality in patients with systolic dysfunction (LVEF $< 35\%$) after an acute myocardial infarction in the Eplerenone Post-AMI Heart Failure Efficacy and Survival Study (EPHESUS) trial,[28] or in chronic systolic heart failure patients who are receiving ACE inhibitor alone in the Randomized Aldactone Evaluation Study (RALES) trial[29] or ACE inhibitor with a β-blocker in the Eplerenone in Patients with Systolic Heart Failure and Mild Symptoms (EMPHASIS-HF) trial.[30] The administration of an MRA is recommended in patients with NYHA Class II to IV heart failure with an LVEF less than 35% and who are receiving an ACE inhibitor or ARB and a β-blocker. MRA should be initiated in the setting of baseline serum potassium less than 5 mEq/L and an estimated glomerular filtration rate (eGFR) greater than 30 mL/min/1.73 m^2. Initial and target doses of MRAs are listed in **Table 76.4**.

The most significant side effect of MRA is hyperkalemia, which can be life-threatening. Potassium supplementation should be stopped upon initiation of an MRA, and patients should be counseled on avoiding potassium-rich foods. Patients with renal dysfunction are at increased risk, and MRAs are generally avoided in patients with a serum creatinine clearance less than 30 mL/min/1.73 m^2 or potassium greater than 5.0 mEq/L.[31] Renal function and potassium levels should be checked within 1 week of MRA initiation to monitor for stability. In the RALES trial, 10% of men who used spironolactone developed gynecomastia. This is due to off-target sex hormone effects that can also cause menstrual irregularities in women. A second-generation MRA, such as eplerenone, is more mineralocorticoid receptor-selective and is recommended when spironolactone is not tolerated due to endocrine side effects. Finerenone, a nonsteroidal, selective MRA designed to bypass endocrine side effects, has been shown to have a similar efficacy profile as steroidal MRAs and to reduce CKD chronic kidney disease progression and cardiovascular events in patients with chronic kidney disease and type 2 diabetes mellitus[32,33] and is currently awaiting Food and Drug Administration (FDA) approval.

Isosorbide Dinitrate and Hydralazine

The combination of hydralazine, a peripheral vasodilator, and isosorbide dinitrate, a nitrate that is converted to nitric oxide, has been shown to reduce symptoms and mortality in African American NYHA Class III and IV patients with LVEF less than 40% who are already receiving RAAS and β-blockade. The efficacy of this combination in other racial groups is not known. One possible explanation is that African Americans may have less RAAS activity and a higher incidence of angioedema,[34] which decreases their net benefit from RAAS inhibition when compared to the general population. Hydralazine and isordil can also be used in patients who cannot tolerate RAAS due to renal insufficiency or hyperkalemia. The Vasodilator Heart Failure Trial (V-HeFT) study showed improved mortality in those randomized to hydralazine and nitrates as compared to placebo in the pre-ACE inhibitor and β-blocker era.[35] Of note, the V-HeFT trial showed that ACE inhibitors were superior to hydralazine and nitrates; therefore, hydralazine and nitrates should be used alone only when ACE inhibitors are not tolerated.

Both isosorbide dinitrate and hydralazine are well tolerated, and the biggest barrier to medication adherence is the onerous dosing schedule for the patient (both given three times a day). Hypotension can occur with both medications, and headaches are sometimes seen with nitrates which generally subside over time. Because hydralazine is a peripherally selective vasodilator, a reflex tachycardia can occur. Importantly, hydralazine may cause drug-induced lupus, with various clinical presentations, including rash, vasculitis, and pericarditis.[36]

Ivabradine

Ivabradine selectively reduces heart rate but, unlike β-blockers, does not impact cardiac contractility. Ivabradine selectively blocks the I_f (funny) channel current, a mixed sodium-potassium channel that activates with hyperpolarization and supplies an inward current which starts the phase 4 diastolic depolarization; thus, it controls the rate of spontaneous activity of the sinoatrial (SA) node and the cardiac cycle. The degree of I_f inhibition is directly related to the frequency of channel

TABLE 76.3 Beta-blockers With Heart Failure Clinical Benefit and Associated Initial, Maximum (Max), and Randomized Controlled Trial (RCT) Dose

Mechanism of Action	Drug	Initial Daily Dose(s)	Max Dose(s)	Mean RCT Dose
Blocks various adrenergic receptors	Bisoprolol	1.25 mg qd	10 mg qd	8.6 mg daily
	Carvedilol	3.125 mg bid	50 mg bid	37 mg daily
	Carvedilol CR	10 mg qd	80 mg qd	NA
	Metoprolol CR/XL	12.5-25 mg qd	200 mg qd	159 mg daily

bid, twice a day; NA, not applicable; qd, every day.

TABLE 76.4 Commonly Used Mineralocorticoid Receptor Antagonists With Associated Initial, Maximum (Max), and Randomized Controlled Trial (RCT) Dose

Mechanism of Action	Drug	Initial Daily Dose(s)	Max Dose(s)	Mean RCT Dose
Competitively binds to the aldosterone receptor, which increases the secretion of water and sodium in the distal tubule and decreases the secretion of potassium	Spironolactone	4-8 mg qd	32 mg qd	24 mg daily
	Eplerenone	25-50 mg qd	50-150 mg qd	129 mg daily

qd, every day.

opening. Hence, ivabradine is expected to be most effective at high heart rates and tends to not cause severe bradycardia. The Systolic Heart Failure Treatment with the I_f Inhibitor Ivabradine Trial (SHIFT) showed that compared to placebo ivabradine reduced the combined endpoint of heart failure hospitalizations and mortality in patients with an LVEF less than 35% and a heart rate greater than 70 bpm on standard guideline-directed medical therapy, including a β-blocker.[37] This effect was driven mainly by reductions in hospitalizations as secondary analyses did not show an improvement in cardiovascular or all-cause mortality. Of note, only 25% of the studied population was on guideline-recommended doses of β-blockers and up to half of the patients were on 50% or lower of the recommended doses. It is possible that titrating β-blockers to recommended doses may have reduced hospitalizations to a similar degree. Furthermore, ivabradine has not been shown to improve clinical outcomes in studies in patients with ischemic heart disease.[38,39] Currently, there is a Class IIa recommendation by both the European Society of Cardiology ESC and American Heart Association (AHA)/American College of Cardiology (ACC) guidelines to consider the addition of ivabradine in those with LVEF ≤35%, NYHA Class II to III symptoms, who are on maximum tolerated β-blocker dose and whose heart rate remains above 70 bpm. In clinical practice, ivabradine is most useful in patients who are unable to tolerate maximal β-blockers due to side effects or bronchospastic pulmonary disease.

Ivabradine is generally well tolerated, but it should not be used in patients who are pacemaker dependent or with persistent atrial fibrillation since the mechanism of action involves the SA node. Interestingly, the aggregate clinical data on ivabradine use suggest that it increases the frequency of atrial fibrillation; hence, its use should be avoided in patients with paroxysmal atrial fibrillation. The mechanism for this effect is not well understood.

Sodium Glucose Cotransporter 2 Inhibitors

Sodium glucose cotransporter 2 (SGLT2) inhibitors are a class of antidiabetic medications that block filtered glucose resorption in the kidneys to promote glucosuria and decrease serum glucose concentration. As part of the regulatory review of this class of drugs, cardiovascular outcomes were evaluated because other classes of antidiabetic agents had been associated with increased cardiovascular risk. Initial trials of SGLT2 inhibitors for diabetes demonstrated reductions in heart failure hospitalizations in patients who largely did not have heart failure at enrollment, suggesting prevention of heart failure development.[40-42] Furthermore, the risk reduction was observed early after randomization, suggesting a mechanism that was independent of the benefits of optimal glucose control. These observations led to the Dapagliflozin and Prevention of Adverse Outcomes in Heart Failure (DAPA-HF) trial, which showed a striking reduction in heart failure hospitalizations and mortality in NYHA Class II to III patients with LVEF less than 40% treated with 10 mg daily of dapagliflozin independent of the presence of diabetes.[43]

The mechanism of the clinical impact of SGLT2 inhibitors in heart failure is not well understood. Because cardiomyocytes lack SGLT2 receptors, indirect mechanisms are likely. SGLT2 inhibitors have been shown to produce favorable changes in blood pressure, weight loss, uricosuria, intravascular volume, and ketosis which may all contribute to the observed clinical benefit.[44] The US Food and Drug Administration approved dapagliflozin for adults with heart failure and reduced ejection fraction with or without diabetes to reduce the risk of cardiovascular death or hospitalization. These developments are not yet reflected in the ACC/AHA or ESC guidelines and are widely expected to be incorporated in the next iteration. Of note, while dapagliflozin is the only SGLT2 inhibitor currently approved and formally started as a primary treatment for heart failure, the benefits are believed to be a class effect. Recently, the EMPagliflozin outcomE tRial in Patients With chrOnic heaRt Failure With Reduced Ejection Fraction (EMPEROR-Reduced) trial showed similar clinical and mortality improvements with empagliflozin.[45]

Mycotic urinary tract infections are more common in patients taking SGLT2 inhibitors due to enhanced glucosuria and are generally well tolerated and easily treated. Rarely, euglycemic ketoacidosis can occur, and thus SGLT2 inhibitors are avoided in type 1 diabetics. In addition, patients on SGLT2 inhibitors can experience euglycemic ketoacidosis in the setting of surgery, infection, trauma, major illness, or decreased oral intake. For this reason, SGLT2 inhibitors may need to be held prior to surgery, periods of fasting, or during major illnesses. Heart failure patients should be monitored for excessive diuresis and resultant electrolyte abnormalities, especially when concurrently treated with a loop diuretic and ARNI. The increase in urine output can be profound in these patients who may require reduction or cessation of loop diuretics.

Intravenous Iron

Although the cause of morbidity in heart failure is multifactorial, impaired oxygen delivery is believed to be a major contributor. Iron deficiency has been shown to impair aerobic performance, and the incidence of iron deficiency is increased in heart failure. Despite these observations, oral iron supplementation has not demonstrated clinical benefit.[46] Oral iron formulation is less effective at replenishing iron stores than parental formulations, and first-generation IV formulations had an unacceptable side effect profile, most notably anaphylactic shock. Newer generation IV formulations with carbohydrate shells that slow the release of iron are much safer. Trials of IV iron therapy in symptomatic NYHA Class II to III heart failure patients with LVEF less than or equal to 40% and evidence of iron deficiency (ferritin < 300 ng/mL, transferrin saturation $\leq 20\%$) demonstrated improvements in NYHA functional class, 6-minute walk test, and quality of life.[47,48] IV iron, such as iron sucrose and ferric carboxymaltose, is well tolerated and safe. There is a theoretical risk of exacerbating existing bloodstream infections, and although this has not been demonstrated in clinical trials, its use should be avoided with systemic infection. In addition, these solutions may cause hypophosphatemia.

Digoxin

Digoxin is a cardiac glycoside that inhibits the Na^+/K^+-ATPase in cell membranes, which ultimately increases intercellular calcium and myocardial contractility. It has been used in the treatment of heart failure for over 100 years. Despite its long history, considerable debate exists about its clinical utility. Studies have demonstrated that discontinuation of digoxin may result in worse outcomes. The Digitalis Investigation Group (DIG) trial addressed the prospective utility of digoxin in heart failure and showed decreased hospitalizations but no reduction in mortality compared to placebo.[49] Subgroup analyses suggested a strong trend toward decreased death due to pump failure which was offset by increased nonpump failure cardiac deaths including ventricular arrhythmias. Recent studies demonstrated that digoxin may increase mortality in patients with atrial fibrillation.

The main side effects of digoxin are heart block, arrhythmias, neurologic symptoms, and gastrointestinal symptoms. These side effects are generally minimized by maintaining trough plasma digoxin levels between 0.5 and 0.8 ng/mL for men and 0.5 and 0.7 ng/mL for women. Women, the elderly, and those with renal dysfunction are at higher risk of digoxin toxicity, and hypokalemia and hypomagnesemia can lower the threshold for digoxin toxicity. For the majority of patients, the oral dose should be 0.125 mg daily, and doses greater than 0.25 mg daily are generally not recommended. Digoxin toxicity can be reversed by the administration of digoxin-specific antibodies.

Pharmacotherapeutic Approach to Heart Failure

Despite compelling evidence that ACE inhibitors/ARBs/ARNIs, β-blockers, and MRAs reduce hospitalization and mortality in patients with heart failure, these therapies continue to be underutilized. Furthermore, because many heart failure therapies have effects on hemodynamics, renal function, and electrolyte levels, initiation or titration of one therapy may come at the expense of the patient's ability to tolerate another. Given that some therapies offer greater benefits than others and that these effects are often dose dependent, it is important to establish a "core therapy" of treatments with most clinical benefit and titrating these therapies to guideline-directed doses prior to the addition of other therapies.

ACE inhibitors/ARBs/ARNIs and β-blockers have been shown to confer the greatest clinical benefit in heart failure and should be titrated to the maximum tolerated doses prior to initiation of a third agent. Of note, ARNIs have superior clinical benefit compared to ACE inhibitors and ARBs, and emerging evidence demonstrates that its use as initial therapy is likely safe. Thus, it is likely to become the first-line RAAS blockade agent as clinicians become more comfortable with its use. Once the core therapy of a RAS blocking agent or ARNI in conjunction with a β-blocker has been established at target doses, additional therapies should be considered. Generally, an MRA is added as the third agent and titrated to the target dose, though striking clinical benefits seen in recent trials of SGLT2 inhibitors in both diabetic and nondiabetic heart failure patients may increase its priority in future guidelines. Additional therapies such as hydralazine, nitrates, ivabradine, and digoxin should be considered in patient populations in which they have demonstrated clinical benefit.

NONPHARMACOLOGIC THERAPIES

Several nonpharmacologic interventions have been shown to be potentially beneficial in heart failure patients. The most established of these is the use of implantable biventricular pacemakers and defibrillators for cardiac resynchronization in patients with conduction abnormalities and prevention of sudden cardiac death. Several trials consisting of over 9000 patients with NYHA Class I to IV heart failure with LVEF less than or equal to 35% have demonstrated that biventricular pacing can reduce morbidity, mortality, and improve left ventricular remodeling in combination with comprehensive neurohormonal blockade. The Multicenter InSync Randomized Clinical Evaluation (MIRACLE) trial[50] included ambulatory NYHA Class III to IV heart failure patients with LVEF less than or equal to 35% and QRS duration greater than or equal to 130 ms and showed that compared to placebo, cardiac resynchronization therapy (CRT) improved symptoms, functional capacity, and reduced hospitalizations for heart failure. Furthermore, the trial showed evidence of reverse remodeling with improvements in LV size and function by echocardiography in the CRT arm. Subsequently, the CArdiac REsynchronization in Heart Failure (CARE-HF) trial[51] demonstrated a mortality benefit of CRT in a similar patient population. The Multicenter Automatic Defibrillator Implantation Trial with Cardiac Resynchronization therapy (MADIT-CRT)[52] and Resynchronization/defibrillation for Ambulatory heart Failure Trial (RAFT)[53] both showed morbidity and mortality benefit of CRT in NYHA Class II and ischemic NYHA Class I patients with LVEF less than 30%. Of note, prespecified subgroup analysis demonstrated greater benefit with CRT in women, in patient with a QRS duration of 150 ms or longer, and in patients with left bundle branch block. Importantly, CRT does not benefit patients with normal QRS duration. The Echocardiography-guided Cardiac Resynchronization Therapy (EchoCRT) trial demonstrated that CRT provided no benefit and higher mortality in patients with QRS duration less than 130 ms and echocardiographic evidence of desynchrony.[54] Current guideline recommendations define dyssynchrony by electrocardiogram (ECG) alone, and CRT is most strongly recommended in NYHA Class II, III, or ambulatory Class IV patients with LVEF less than or equal to 35% and in sinus rhythm with a left bundle branch block and a QRS duration greater than or equal to 150 ms.[4] Weaker recommendations are provided for ischemic Class I patients, patients without a left bundle branch block, and patients with a QRS duration between 130 and 150 ms. Consideration is also made for patients who do not meet the prior criteria but require significant right ventricular pacing which has been associated with worsening left ventricular function.[55]

Sudden cardiac death is a leading cause of mortality in patients with heart failure and occurs several times more frequently than in the general population.[3] This observation has led to numerous studies investigating the utility of implantable cardioverter defibrillators (ICDs) to reduce mortality in patients with heart failure. The landmark Sudden Cardiac Death-Heart Failure Trial (SCD-HeFT)[56] enrolled over 2500 patients with NYHA Class II or III symptoms and LVEF less than 35% of either ischemic or nonischemic etiology. Participants were randomized to ICD, amiodarone, or placebo in a background of guideline-directed medical therapy (85% ACE inhibitor or ARB, 69% β-blocker, and 19% aldosterone antagonists). The study found that ICD treatment was associated with a statistically significant 23% reduction in all-cause mortality compared to placebo and that there was no mortality difference in the amiodarone group compared to placebo. Based largely on the findings of this study, the current guidelines provide strong level I recommendation for ICD therapy for primary prevention of sudden cardiac death in ischemic (at least 40 days after myocardial infarction) and nonischemic NYHA Class II and III heart failure patients with LVEF less than 35%. These patients should also have been chronically treated with appropriate guideline-directed medical therapy and have an expected life expectancy of greater than 1 year. ICD therapy is also recommended in Class I patients with ischemic heart failure at least 40 days after myocardial infarction who have an LVEF less than 35%.

Patient-level educational programs covering a wide variety of topics including disease knowledge, medication management, fluid management, diet, and physical activity have been studied for the treatment of heart failure. A systematic review of 35 programs suggests modest aggregate benefit of these programs, though rigorous evaluation is limited by a wide range of interventions used and measured outcomes.[57]

Sleep-disordered breathing is prevalent in patients with reduced LVEF with the majority experiencing central sleep apnea and another 10% with obstructive sleep apnea. The main clinical significance of central sleep apnea in heart failure is its association with adverse clinical outcomes, although whether this association is a reflection of advanced cardiac disease or the presence of a separate risk factor is not clear. The presence of central sleep apnea generally reflects a need to escalate heart failure therapy rather than initiate noninvasive ventilation. In obstructive sleep apnea, initial studies suggested reduced cardiac events in heart patients treated with continuous positive airway pressure. However, a more recent randomized clinical trial of over 2700 patients demonstrated no cardiovascular benefit.[58]

Although most patients with reduced LVEF respond well to guideline-directed medical therapy and enjoy a good quality of life, some patients do not improve or will experience a rapid recurrence and progression of symptoms despite optimal therapies. These patients should be considered for advanced treatment strategies including continuous parental inotropic therapy, mechanical circulatory support, and referral for cardiac transplantation. These therapies are discussed in detail in other chapters. In patients who are not candidates for advanced treatment strategies, palliative and hospice care is a critical aspect of their care and have been shown to improve clinical outcomes.[59]

RESEARCH AND FUTURE DIRECTIONS

Heart Failure with Preserved Ejection Fraction

Unlike heart failure with reduced ejection fraction, evidence from prospective randomized controlled trials is lacking for patients with heart failure with preserved ejection fraction (HFpEF). No treatment has been convincingly shown to reduce morbidity or mortality in patients with HFpEF. β-Blockers, ACE inhibitors, ARBs, digoxin, MRAs, sildenafil, nitrates, and ARNIs have all been studied and have not shown convincing clinical benefit. As such, the general approach for these patients is to aggressively treat hypertension to prevent or reverse left ventricular hypertrophy, maintain euvolemia to reduce symptoms and congestion, minimize ischemia, and to maximize diastolic filling by maintaining sinus rhythm. The only Class I treatments for HFpEF are blood pressure control and diuretics for symptom management.[31]

Although no randomized clinical trial in HFpEF met its primary clinical endpoint, there are a few trials that should be highlighted for suggestions of clinical benefit which has translated into guideline recommendations.

The CHARM-Preserved trial[60] studied the effects of candesartan in patients with an LVEF greater than 40% and found that, if adjusted for differences in baseline characteristics, fewer patients in the candesartan arm reached the primary endpoint of cardiovascular death or heart failure–related hospitalization. There was no effect on mortality. This finding led to a Class IIb recommendation for the use of ARB to decrease hospitalizations in HFpEF.[4]

The Treatment of Preserved Cardiac Function Heart Failure with an Aldosterone Antagonist (TOPCAT) trial studied spironolactone in HFpEF and found no difference in the primary composite outcome of cardiovascular death, cardiac arrest, or HF hospitalization for spironolactone compared to placebo. However, further analysis found that there were regional variations in clinical benefits, and patients enrolled from Russia and Georgia had no clinical benefit or significant changes in creatinine, blood pressure, or potassium, raising questions about treatment adherence in this population. A nonprespecified post hoc analysis that excluded patients from Russia and Georgia showed a significant reduction in the primary endpoint with spironolactone compared to placebo.[61] This finding led to a Class IIb recommendation in the 2017 ACC/AHA/HFSA Heart Failure Society of America-focused guideline update[62] for the use of MRAs to decrease hospitalizations in appropriately selected patients with HFpEF (with EF ≥45%, elevated brain natriuretic peptide [BNP] levels or heart failure admission within 1 year, eGFR >30 mL/min, creatinine <2.5 mg/dL, potassium <5.0 mEq/L).

FOLLOW-UP PATIENT CARE

As discussed earlier, the goals of heart failure management are to improve patient symptoms and quality of life, slow disease progression, and prolong survival. Management of heart failure requires adherence to a complex medical regimen, daily self-monitoring, and maintaining specific lifestyle modifications. Frequent follow-up allows for reinforcement of adherence to medical and lifestyle changes as well as evaluation for side effects, disease progression, and development of comorbidities. Patients should be followed serially with assessment for dyspnea, orthopnea, and paroxysmal nocturnal dyspnea as well as weight, jugular venous pressure, presence of peripheral edema. At each visit, patients should be assessed for the ability to increase to target doses of guideline-directed medical therapies. Surveillance laboratories and serum drug levels should be obtained regularly. Current guidelines recommend against the routine assessment of left ventricular size and function with a transthoracic echocardiogram in the absence of clinical or therapeutic change.

Dietary indiscretion is a major cause of acute decompensated heart failure in previously stable patients and as such patients should be advised to restrict dietary sodium to 2 to 3 g daily. Patients should also be advised to limit alcohol consumption and certain drugs known to exacerbate heart failure including nonsteroidal anti-inflammatory drugs (NSAIDs). Patients should be advised to weigh themselves regularly and notify providers of acute weight gain so diuretics can be adjusted to avoid further decompensation.

The recognition that guideline-directed therapies for heart failure remain underutilized has led to the investigation of various models to optimize care for chronic heart failure patients. A Cochrane review of over 20 studies investigating various disease management programs including case management interventions and utilization of multimodality care team found that these programs improved morbidity and mortality in heart failure patients.[63] Although these studies are limited by heterogeneity of intervention and outcomes measured, it is widely believed that optimal heart failure care requires a specialized integrated heart failure clinic with a multimodality team including heart failure cardiologists, nurses, case managers, pharmacists, dietitians, and psychologists.

KEY POINTS

- ✔ Heart failure is a leading cause of morbidity and mortality worldwide.
- ✔ The main goals of heart failure treatment are to improve patient symptoms and quality of life, slow disease progression, and prolong survival.
- ✔ Loop diuretics are effective in relieving congestion and symptoms of heart failure but do not alter mortality or disease progression.
- ✔ ACE inhibitors/ARBs/ARNIs and β-blockers have been shown to confer the greatest clinical benefit in heart failure and should be titrated to the maximum tolerated doses to constitute a core heart failure therapy. MRAs and SGLT2 inhibitors should be considered in most patients after established core therapy. Additional therapies such as hydralazine, nitrates, ivabradine, and digoxin should be considered in selected patient populations in which they have demonstrated clinical benefit.
- ✔ Nonpharmacologic therapies with the most clinical benefit for chronic heart failure include ICDs for the prevention of sudden cardiac death and biventricular pacing for cardiac resynchronization.

REFERENCES

1. Savarese G, Lund LH. Global public health burden of heart failure. *Card Fail Rev.* 2017;3(1):7-11. doi:10.15420/cfr.2016
2. Neumann T, Biermann J, Neumann A, et al. Heart failure: the commonest reason for hospital admission in Germany. *Dtsch Arztebl.* 2009;106(16):269-275. doi:10.3238/arztebl.2009.0269
3. Benjamin EJ, Blaha MJ, Chiuve SE, et al. Heart disease and stroke statistics' 2017 update: a report from the American Heart Association. *Circulation.* 2017;135(10):e146-e603. doi:10.1161/CIR.0000000000000485
4. Yancy CW, Jessup M, Bozkurt B, et al. 2013 ACCF/AHA guideline for the management of heart failure: executive summary: a report of the American College of Cardiology Foundation/American Heart Association task force on practice guidelines. *Circulation.* 2013;128(16):1810-1852. doi:10.1161/CIR.0b013e31829e8807
5. Faris RF, Flather M, Purcell H, Poole-Wilson PA, Coats AJ. Diuretics for heart failure. *Cochrane Database Syst Rev.* 2016;4(4):CD003838. doi:10.1002/14651858.CD003838.pub4
6. Jhund PS, McMurray JJV, Davie AP. The acute vascular effects of frusemide in heart failure. *Br J Clin Pharmacol.* 2000;50(1):9-13. doi:10.1046/j.1365-2125.2000.00219.x
7. Hasselblad V, Stough WG, Shah MR, et al. Relation between dose of loop diuretics and outcomes in a heart failure population: results of the ESCAPE trial. *Eur J Heart Fail.* 2007;9(10):1064-1069. doi:10.1016/j.ejheart.2007.07.011
8. Francis GS, Siegel RM, Goldsmith SR, Olivari MT, Levine TB, Cohn JN. Acute vasoconstrictor response to intravenous furosemide in patients with chronic congestive heart failure. Activation of the neurohumoral axis. *Ann Intern Med.* 1985;103(1):1-6. doi:10.7326/0003-4819-103-1-1
9. Felker GM, Lee KL, Bull DA, et al. Diuretic strategies in patients with acute decompensated heart failure. *N Engl J Med.* 2011;364(9):7907-7805. doi:10.1056/NEJMoa1005419
10. Swedberg K, Kjekshus J. Effects of enalapril on mortality in severe congestive heart failure: results of the Cooperative North Scandinavian Enalapril Survival Study (CONSENSUS). *Am J Cardiol.* 1988;60(2):60-66. doi:10.1016/S0002-9149(88)80087-0
11. SOLVD Investigators; Yusuf S, Pitt B, Davis CE, Hood WB Jr, Cohn JN. Effect of enalapril on mortality and the development of heart failure in asymptomatic patients with reduced left ventricular ejection fractions. *N Engl J Med.* 1992;327(10):685-691. doi:10.1056/NEJM199209033271003
12. McMurray JJV, Östergren J, Swedberg K, et al. Effects of candesartan in patients with chronic heart failure and reduced left-ventricular systolic function taking angiotensin-converting-enzyme inhibitors: the CHARM-Added trial. *Lancet.* 2003;362(9386):767-771. doi:10.1016/S0140-6736(03)14284-5
13. Pfeffer MA, Braunwald E, Moyé LA, et al. Effect of captopril on mortality and morbidity in patients with left ventricular dysfunction after myocardial infarction: results of the survival and ventricular enlargement trial. *N Engl J Med.* 1992;327(10):669-677. doi:10.1056/NEJM199209033271001
14. Packer M, Poole-Wilson PA, Armstrong PW, et al. Comparative effects of low and high doses of the angiotensin-converting enzyme inhibitor, lisinopril, on morbidity and mortality in chronic heart failure. *Circulation.* 1999;100(23):12-18. doi:10.1161/01.CIR.100.23.2312
15. Granger CB, McMurray JJV, Yusuf S, et al. Effects of candesartan in patients with chronic heart failure and reduced left-ventricular systolic function intolerant to angiotensin-converting-enzyme inhibitors: the CHARM-alternative trial. *Lancet.* 2003;362(9386):772-776. doi:10.1016/S0140-6736(03)14284-5
16. Cohn JN, Tognoni G; Valsartan Heart Failure Trial Investigators. A randomized trial of the angiotensin-receptor blocker valsartan in chronic heart failure. *N Engl J Med.* 2001;345(23):1667-1675. doi:10.1056/NEJMoa010713
17. Corti R, Burnett JC, Rouleau JL, Ruschitzka F, Lüscher TF. Vasopeptidase inhibitors: a new therapeutic concept in cardiovascular disease? *Circulation.* 2001;104(15):1856-1862. doi:10.1161/hc4001.097191
18. McMurray JJV, Packer M, Desai AS, et al. Angiotensin-neprilysin inhibition versus enalapril in heart failure. *N Engl J Med.* 2014;371(11):993-1004. doi:10.1056/NEJMoa1409077
19. Velazquez EJ, Morrow DA, DeVore AD, et al. Angiotensin-neprilysin inhibition in acute decompensated heart failure. *N Engl J Med.* 2019;380:539-548. doi:10.1056/NEJMoa1812851
20. Hunt SA, Abraham WT, Chin MH, et al. 2009 focused update incorporated into the ACC/AHA 2005 guidelines for the diagnosis and management of heart failure in adults: a report of the American College of Cardiology Foundation/American Heart Association Task Force on practice guidelines: develop. *Circulation.* 2009;119(14):e391-e479. doi:10.1161/CIRCULATIONAHA.109.192065
21. Packer M, Fowler MB, Roecker EB, et al. Effect of carvedilol on the morbidity of patients with severe chronic heart failure: results of the carvedilol prospective randomized cumulative survival (COPERNICUS) study. *Circulation.* 2002;106(17):2194-2199. doi:10.1161/01.CIR.0000035653.72855.BF
22. The Cardiac Insufficiency Bisoprolol Study II (CIBIS-II): a randomised trial. *Lancet.* 1999;353(9146):9-13. doi:10.1161/HYPERTENSIONAHA.117.10280
23. MERIT-HF Study Group. Effect of metoprolol CR/XL in chronic heart failure: Metoprolol CR/XL Randomised Intervention Trial in Congestive Heart Failure (MERIT-HF). *Lancet.* 1999;353(9169):2001-2007. doi:10.1016/S0140-6736(99)04440-2
24. The Beta-Blocker Evaluation of Survival Trial Investigators; Eichhorn EJ, Domanski MJ, Krause-Steinrauf H, Bristow MR, Lavori PW. A trial of the beta-blocker bucindolol in patients with advanced chronic heart failure. *N Engl J Med.* 2001;344(22):1659-1667. doi:10.1056/NEJM200105313442202
25. Group TX in SHFS. Xamoterol in severe heart failure. *Lancet.* 1990;336(8706):1-6. doi:10.1016/0140-6736(90)91517-E
26. Poole-Wilson PA, Swedberg K, Cleland JGF, et al. Comparison of carvedilol and metoprolol on clinical outcomes in patients with chronic heart failure in the Carvedilol Or Metoprolol European Trial (COMET): randomised controlled trial. *Lancet.* 2003;362(9377):7-13. doi:10.1016/S0140-6736(03)13800-7
27. Jondeau G, Neuder Y, Eicher JC, et al. B-CONVINCED: Beta-blocker CONtinuation Vs. INterruption in patients with Congestive heart failure hospitalizED for a decompensation episode. *Eur Heart J.* 2009;30(18):2186-2192. doi:10.1093/eurheartj/ehp323
28. Pitt B, Remme W, Zannad F, et al. Eplerenone, a selective aldosterone blocker, in patients with left ventricular dysfunction after myocardial infarction. *N Engl J Med.* 2003;348(14):9-21. doi:10.1056/NEJMoa030207
29. Pitt B, Zannad F, Remme WJ, et al. The effect of spironolactone on morbidity and mortality in patients with severe heart failure. *N Engl J Med.* 1999;341(10):709-717. doi:10.1056/NEJM199909023411001
30. Zannad F, McMurray JJV, Krum H, et al. Eplerenone in patients with systolic heart failure and mild symptoms. *N Engl J Med.* 2011;364(1):11-21. doi:10.1056/NEJMoa1505949
31. Hunt SA, Abraham WT, Chin MH, et al. ACC/AHA 2005 Guideline update for the diagnosis and management of chronic heart failure in the adult: a report of the American College of Cardiology/American Heart Association Task Force on practice guidelines (writing committee to update the 2001 Guidelines for the evaluation and management of heart failure). *J Am Coll Cardiol.* 2005;46(6):e1-e82. doi:10.1016/j.jacc.2005.08.022
32. Bakris GL, Agarwal R, Anker SD, et al. Effect of finerenone on chronic kidney disease outcomes in type 2 diabetes. *N Engl J Med.* 2020;383(23):2219-2229. doi:0.1056/NEJMoa2025845
33. Filippatos G, Anker SD, Böhm M, et al. A randomized controlled study of finerenone vs. eplerenone in patients with worsening chronic heart failure and diabetes mellitus and/or chronic kidney disease. *Eur Heart J.* 2016;37(27):2105-2114. doi:10.1093/eurheartj/ehw132
34. Bloche MG. Race-based therapeutics. *N Engl J Med.* 2004;351(20):35-37.
35. Cohn JN, Archibald DG, Ziesche S, et al. Effect of vasodilator therapy on mortality in chronic congestive heart failure. *N Engl J Med.* 1986;314(24):1547-1552. doi:10.1056/NEJM198606123142404
36. Iyer P, Dirweesh A, Zijoo R. Hydralazine induced lupus syndrome presenting with recurrent pericardial effusion and a negative antinuclear antibody. *Case Rep Rheumatol.* 2017;2017:5245904. doi:10.1155/2017/5245904
37. Swedberg K, Komajda M, Böhm M, et al. Ivabradine and outcomes in chronic heart failure (SHIFT): a randomised placebo-controlled study. *Lancet.* 2010;376(9744):875-885. doi:10.1016/S0140-6736(10)61198-1

38. Fox K, Ford I, Steg PG, et al. Ivabradine for patients with stable coronary artery disease and left-ventricular systolic dysfunction (BEAUTIFUL): a randomised, double-blind, placebo-controlled trial. *Lancet.* 2008; 372(9641):807-816. doi:10.1016/S0140-6736(08)61170-8
39. Fox K, Ford I, Steg PG, Tardif JC, Tendera M, Ferrari R. Ivabradine in stable coronary artery disease without clinical heart failure. *N Engl J Med.* 2014;371:1091-1099. doi:10.1056/NEJMoa1406430
40. Neal B, Perkovic V, Mahaffey KW, et al. Canagliflozin and cardiovascular and renal events in type 2 diabetes. *N Engl J Med.* 2017;377(7):644-657. doi:10.1056/NEJMoa1611925
41. Zinman B, Wanner C, Lachin JM, et al. Empagliflozin, cardiovascular outcomes, and mortality in type 2 diabetes. *N Engl J Med.* 2015;373(22):2117-2128. doi:10.1056/NEJMoa1504720
42. Wiviott SD, Raz I, Bonaca MP, et al. Dapagliflozin and cardiovascular outcomes in type 2 diabetes. *N Engl J Med.* 2019;380(4):347-357. doi:10.1056/NEJMoa1812389
43. McMurray JJV, Solomon SD, Inzucchi SE, et al. Dapagliflozin in patients with heart failure and reduced ejection fraction. *N Engl J Med.* 2019;381(21):1995-2008. doi:10.1056/NEJMoa1911303
44. Selvaraj S, Kelly DP, Margulies KB. Implications of altered ketone metabolism and therapeutic ketosis in heart failure. *Circulation.* 2020;141:1800-1812. doi:10.1161/CIRCULATIONAHA.119.045033
45. Packer M, Anker SD, Butler J, et al. Cardiovascular and renal outcomes with empagliflozin in heart failure. *N Engl J Med.* 2020;383(15):1413-1424. doi:10.1056/nejmoa2022190
46. Lewis GD, Malhotra R, Hernandez AF, et al. Effect of oral iron repletion on exercise capacity in patients with heart failure with reduced ejection fraction and iron deficiency the IRONOUT HF randomized clinical trial. *JAMA - J Am Med Assoc.* 2017;317(19):1958-1966. doi:10.1001/jama.2017.5427
47. Anker SD, Colet JC, Filippatos G, et al. Ferric carboxymaltose in patients with heart failure and iron deficiency. *N Engl J Med.* 2009;361(25):36-48. doi:10.1056/NEJMoa0908355
48. Ponikowski P, Van Veldhuisen DJ, Comin-Colet J, et al. Beneficial effects of long-term intravenous iron therapy with ferric carboxymaltose in patients with symptomatic heart failure and iron deficiency. *Eur Heart J.* 2015;36(11):657-668. doi:10.1093/eurheartj/ehu385
49. Garg R, Gorlin R, Smith T, Yusuf S. The effect of digoxin on mortality and morbidity in patients with heart failure. *N Engl J Med.* 1997;336(8):525-533. doi:10.1056/NEJM199702203360801
50. Abraham WT, Fisher WG, Smith AL, et al. Cardiac resynchronization in chronic heart failure. *N Engl J Med.* 2002;346(24):1846-1853.
51. Cleland JGF, Daubert JC, Erdmann E, et al. The effect of cardiac resynchronization on morbidity and mortality in heart failure. *N Engl J Med.* 2005;352(15):1539-1549. doi:10.1056/NEJMoa050496
52. Moss AJ, Zareba W, Hall WJ, et al. Prophylactic implantation of a defibrillator in patients with myocardial infarction and reduced ejection fraction. *N Engl J Med.* 2002;346(12):877-883. doi:10.1097/00132586-200304000-00009
53. Tang ASL, Wells GA, Talajic M, et al. Cardiac-resynchronization therapy for mild-to-moderate heart failure. *N Engl J Med.* 2010;363(25):2385-2395.
54. Ruschitzka F, Abraham WT, Singh JP, et al. Cardiac-resynchronization therapy in heart failure with a narrow QRS complex. *N Engl J Med.* 2013;369(15):1395-1405. doi:10.1056/nejmoa1306687
55. Curtis AB, Worley SJ, Adamson PB, et al. Biventricular pacing for atrioventricular block and systolic dysfunction. *N Engl J Med.* 2013;368:1585-1593. doi:10.1056/NEJMoa1210356
56. Bardy GH, Lee KL, Mark DB, et al. Amiodarone or an implantable cardioverter–defibrillator for congestive heart failure. *N Engl J Med.* 2005;352(3):225-237.
57. Allen D, Gillen E, Rixson L. Systematic review of the effectiveness of integrated care pathways: what works, for whom, in which circumstances? *Int J Evid Based Healthc.* 2009;7(2):61-74. doi:10.1111/j.1744-1609.2009.00127.x
58. McEvoy RD, Antic NA, Heeley E, et al. CPAP for prevention of cardiovascular events in obstructive sleep apnea. *N Engl J Med.* 2016;375(10):919-931. doi:10.1056/NEJMoa1606599
59. Diop MS, Rudolph JL, Zimmerman KM, Richter MA, Skarf LM. Palliative care interventions for patients with heart failure: a systematic review and meta-analysis. *J Palliat Med.* 2017;20(1):84-92. doi:10.1089/jpm.2016.0330
60. Yusuf S, Pfeffer MA, Swedberg K, et al. Effects of candesartan in patients with chronic heart failure and preserved left-ventricular ejection fraction: the CHARM-preserved trial. *Lancet.* 2003;362(9386):777-781. doi:10.1016/S0140-6736(03)14285-7
61. Pfeffer MA, Claggett B, Assmann SF, et al. Regional variation in patients and outcomes in the treatment of preserved cardiac function heart failure with an aldosterone antagonist (TOPCAT) trial. *Circulation.* 2015;131(1):34-42. doi:10.1161/CIRCULATIONAHA.114.013255
62. Shen W-K, Sheldon RS, Benditt DG, et al. 2017 ACC/AHA/HRS Guideline for the evaluation and management of patients with syncope: a report of the American College of Cardiology/American Heart Association Task Force on Clinical Practice Guidelines and the Heart Rhythm Society. *J Am Coll Cardiol.* 2017;70(16):2101-2102. doi:10.1016/j.jacc.2017.08.024
63. Takeda A, Martin N, Taylor RS, Taylor SJC. Disease management interventions for heart failure. *Cochrane Database Syst Rev.* 2019;1(1):CD002752. doi:10.1002/14651858.CD002752.pub4

CHAPTER 77

CARDIAC ELECTRONIC IMPLANTABLE DEVICE THERAPY

Yang Yang, Irakli Giorgberidze, and Lorraine Cornwell

INTRODUCTION

The first case of successful defibrillation in a human was performed in 1947 by Dr Claude Beck, a cardiothoracic surgeon, on a 14-year-old boy whose rhythm had degenerated into ventricular fibrillation (VF) during surgery for pectus excavatum.[1] Based on the contemporary studies of Carl Wiggers, who showed that timely defibrillation restored sinus rhythm in animals with VF,[2] Beck applied a direct shock to the heart cardioverting it back to sinus rhythm.

With time, both open- and closed-chest defibrillation became the mainstay of resuscitation from cardiac arrest. Michel Mirowski and Morton Mower invented and built the first implantable cardioverter-defibrillator (ICD)[3] that was implanted in February 1980.[4] The first ICD weighed over 200 g and used large epicardial patches for defibrillation while requiring a thoracotomy for implantation.

Over time the ICD attained indications for sudden death prevention in patients who survived ventricular tachycardia (VT) or cardiac arrest (secondary prevention) and those with left ventricular (LV) systolic dysfunction at risk of sudden death (primary prevention).[5] Subsequently, studies demonstrated that simultaneously pacing both right and left ventricle (ie, biventricular pacing) in electrically dyssynchronous ventricles could improve mechanical synchrony, LV systolic function, and the functional status of patients[6] and decrease mortality.[7] With those findings, biventricular pacing or cardiac resynchronization therapy (CRT) has become the standard of care for heart failure patients with a wide QRS complex on the electrocardiogram. Thus, the benefits of ICD therapy in sudden death prevention and the benefits of CRT in the improvement of heart failure led to the combination of biventricular pacing with defibrillation (ie, implantable CRT-defibrillators [CRT-D] device).

Due to the initial limitations of both generator size and need for epicardial patches, the earliest ICDs required cardiothoracic and abdominal wall surgery. With advances in technology, the device (ie, generator) is now a fifth its original size and implanted via minimally invasive surgery via the creation of small subcutaneous pocket in a pectoral region. Epicardial patches have been replaced by intracardiac leads (wire electrodes) that use sheath-based introducer techniques for transvenous implantation under fluoroscopic guidance.

ICDs consist of a pulse generator and up to three intracardiac leads for CRT-D systems. The pulse generator—also known as "the can"—contains the high-voltage capacitor, battery, and sensing circuitry for the device. Contemporary ICDs function as a defibrillator and also incorporate all functions of a pacemaker. The defibrillator lead, which consists of a pace/sensing electrode and one or two coils for defibrillation, is usually implanted into the right ventricle. In dual-chamber ICDs, a regular pacing lead is also implanted into the right atrium. With CRT devices, LV pacing is accomplished by a lead that is advanced into one of the epicardial LV veins via the coronary sinus (CS).

Contemporary techniques for ICD and CRT-D implantation are minimally invasive procedures that use local anesthesia and conscious sedation, percutaneous venous access through the Seldinger technique and only one incision for the creation of the generator pocket. The right ventricular and right atrial leads are then guided into the appropriate location under fluoroscopic guidance. Specially designed guiding sheaths are used for delivery of the LV lead to the selected branch of the CS. The generator is secured in either a subcutaneous or submuscular pocket. The whole procedure can be done on a same-day basis requiring minimal hospitalization.

INDICATIONS

Table 77.1 lists the current indications for ICD implantation for both primary and secondary prevention.

Secondary Prevention

Early observations showed both VF and VT are leading causes of sudden cardiac death (SCD), and patients who survived the initial event remained at high risk of recurrent life-threatening arrhythmias. Accordingly, patients with documented VT or VF were among the first to be enrolled in clinical trials demonstrating the effectiveness of ICDs in reducing mortality.

The first trial to enroll sudden death survivors was the Cardiac Arrest Study Hamburg (CASH), which evaluated 346 patients with prior cardiac arrest. Patients were randomized to either ICD, metoprolol, amiodarone, or propafenone. Propafenone therapy was discontinued early due to excess mortality secondary to the presumed increased proarrhythmic effect of the drug. At a mean follow-up of 57 months, the trial demonstrated a trend toward a decrease in total mortality when comparing ICD to antiarrhythmic drugs (36.4% vs 44.4%, $P = .08$).[8]

TABLE 77.1 Class I and IIa Indications for Implantable Cardioverter-Defibrillator Therapy

Class I Indications for ICD Therapy
Survivors of cardiac arrest due to VF or hemodynamically unstable sustained VT after evaluation to determine the cause and to exclude any completely reversible causes (LOE: A)
Structural heart disease and spontaneous sustained VT, whether hemodynamically stable or unstable (LOE: B)
Syncope of undetermined origin with clinically relevant, hemodynamically significant sustained VT/VF induced at EPS (LOE: B)
LVEF ≤ 35% due to prior MI who are at least 40 days post-MI and are in NYHA class II or III heart failure (LOE: A)
Left ventricular dysfunction due to prior MI who are at least 40 days post-MI, have an LVEF ≤30%, and are in NYHA functional class I heart failure (LOE: A)
Nonsustained VT due to prior MI, LVEF ≤40%, and inducible VF or sustained VT at EPS
Class IIa Indications
Sustained VT and normal or near-normal ventricular function (LOE: C)
Catecholaminergic polymorphic VT who have syncope and documented sustained VT while receiving β-blockers (LOE: C)
Brugada syndrome who have had syncope or documented VT that has not resulted in cardiac arrest (LOE: C)
Unexplained syncope, significant LV dysfunction, and nonischemic dilated cardiomyopathy (LOE: C)
Hypertrophic cardiomyopathy that has one or more major risk factors for SCD (LOE: C)
Cardiac sarcoidosis, giant cell myocarditis, or Chagas disease (LOE: C)

EPS, electrophysiology study; ICD, implantable cardioverter-defibrillator; LOE, level of evidence; LVEF, left ventricular ejection fraction; MI, myocardial infarction; NYHA, New York Heart Association; SCD, sudden cardiac death; VF, ventricular fibrillation; VT, ventricular tachycardia.

Adapted from Epstein AE, DiMarco JP, Ellenbogen KA, et al. ACC/AHA/HRS 2008 Guidelines for Device-Based Therapy of Cardiac Rhythm Abnormalities: a report of the American College of Cardiology/American Heart Association Task Force on Practice Guidelines (Writing Committee to Revise the ACC/AHA/NASPE 2002 Guideline Update for Implantation of Cardiac Pacemakers and Antiarrhythmia Devices) developed in collaboration with the American Association for Thoracic Surgery and Society of Thoracic Surgeons. *J Am Coll Cardiol.* 2008;51(21):e1-e62.

Similarly, the Canadian Implantable Defibrillator Study (CIDS) randomized patients with prior cardiac arrest, hemodynamically significant or sustained VT, and LV ejection fraction (LVEF) < 35% to either ICD (*N*=328) or amiodarone (*N* = 331). At 5 years, a trend toward decreased mortality with ICD therapy (8.3% per year in ICD group vs 10.2% per year in amiodarone group, *P* = .14) was observed.[9]

The Antiarrhythmics Versus Implantable Defibrillators (AVID) trial provided the crucial evidence which prior trials were hinting toward. It compared ICD therapy with antiarrhythmic drug therapy (amiodarone or sotalol) in 1016 patients with LVEF < 40% and life-threatening arrhythmias (ie, either prior VF or sustained VT with syncope or signs of hemodynamic compromise). The study was stopped early at 18 months when it showed a significant mortality benefit for ICD therapy (15.8% vs 24.0%).[10]

These studies provide the backbone for current guidelines, which make ICD implantation a class I recommendation (ie, therapy should be performed) for patients with prior SCD not due to a reversible cause such as ischemia.

Primary Prevention

Patients with LV dysfunction, prior myocardial infarction, and frequent ventricular ectopy are known to be at increased risk of life-threatening arrhythmias.[11,12] Based on these observations, studies were designed to evaluate the efficacy of ICD in reducing mortality in "high-risk" patients who had not yet suffered cardiac arrest (ie, primary prevention).

The first such patients studied were those with spontaneous nonsustained VT who had inducible sustained VT in the electrophysiology laboratory. The Multicenter Automatic Defibrillator Implantation Trial (MADIT) enrolled 196 patients with LVEF ≤ 35%, nonsustained VT, and inducible and nonsuppressible (with procainamide) sustained VT induced during electrophysiologic study and randomized them to ICD versus optimal medical therapy (including antiarrhythmics). After a mean follow-up period of 27 months, there was a significant reduction in all-cause mortality with ICD (38.6% vs 15.8%, *P* = .009).[13]

The Multicenter Unsustained Tachycardia Trial (MUSTT) randomized patients with recent myocardial infarction (ranging from 4 days to 3 years before randomization), LVEF ≤ 40%, spontaneous nonsustained VT, and inducible VT to either conservative treatment (angiotensin-converting enzyme inhibitors/β-blockers) or antiarrhythmic therapy (intervention arm). Patients randomized to the intervention group received antiarrhythmic drug therapy (Class I agent, amiodarone, or sotalol) and underwent repeat testing for inducible sustained VT. Those who failed multiple drugs received an ICD. Overall, 46% of patients received ICDs. At a mean follow-up of 39 months, there was a significant difference in mortality between non-ICD and ICD patients regardless of antiarrhythmic therapy (24% vs 55%, *P* < .001).[14]

Moving beyond risk stratification by electrophysiology testing, the MADIT II trial enrolled 1232 postmyocardial infarction patients with LVEF ≤ 30%—regardless of prior ventricular ectopy—to receive prophylactic ICD or conventional medical therapy. The trial was terminated early at 20 months due to significant reduction in overall mortality in the ICD group (14.2% vs 19.8%, *P* = .016), driven almost entirely by reduction in SCD (3.8% vs 10.0%, *P* < .01).[15]

The Defibrillators in Non-Ischemic Cardiomyopathy Treatment Evaluation (DEFINITE) trial of 458 patients with nonischemic cardiomyopathy, LVEF ≤35%, and PVCs or nonsustained VT showed that implantation of an ICD significantly reduced the risk of SCD from arrhythmia (1% vs 6%, *P* = .006) and was associated with a nonsignificant reduction in the risk of death from any cause (9.4% vs 17.5%, *P* = .08) at 29 months.[16]

The large-scale trial that showed ICD benefit in patients with LV systolic dysfunction irrespective of ischemic versus nonischemic etiology was Sudden Cardiac Death in Heart Failure Trial (SCD-HeFT). The study enrolled patients with both ischemic and nonischemic cardiomyopathy, New York Heart

Association (NYHA) Class II or III heart failure symptoms and LVEF ≤ 35%, and randomized them to ICD, amiodarone, or conventional therapy. The study demonstrated significant reduction in mortality with ICD at 45 months (ICD 22% vs amiodarone 28% vs placebo 29%, $P < .01$).[17]

Cardiac Resynchronization Therapy

A common issue for patients with heart failure, particularly for those with a wide QRS complex on the electrocardiogram, is dyssynchronous mechanical contraction of the dilated LV. Consequently, pacing the lateral wall of the LV was hypothesized to restore mechanical synchrony of the LV, improve systolic function, and prevent pump failure.

Cardiac resynchronization therapy was evaluated in the Comparison of Medical Therapy, Pacing, and Defibrillation in Heart Failure (COMPANION) trial. Patients ($N = 1624$) with NYHA Class III or IV heart failure, QRS interval of >120 ms and LVEF ≤ 35% were randomized to optimal medical therapy, biventricular pacing (CRT-P), or CRT-D. A significant reduction in the combined endpoint of heart failure and mortality was noted for both CRT therapies (HR = 0.81 for CRT-P, $P = .014$; HR = 0.80 for CRT-D, $P = .01$). This was powered by reduction in heart failure hospitalizations (HR = 0.66 for CRT-P, $P < .002$; HR = 0.60 for CRT-D, $P < .001$). A significant decrease in mortality was observed in CRT-D patients (HR = 0.64, $P = .003$) and a trend for such in CRT-P patients (HR = 0.74, $P = .059$).[18]

The first trial to show definitive mortality benefit for CRT was the Cardiac Resynchronization-Heart Failure (CARE-HF) study, which randomized 813 patients with NYHA Class III/IV heart failure, LVEF ≤ 35% and QRS ≥ 120 ms to either CRT-P or medical therapy. CRT-P was associated with a significant (36%) reduction in mortality ($P < .002$).[19]

Incremental mortality benefit of CRT compared with ICD therapy only was demonstrated in MADIT-CRT trial, which randomized 1820 patients (NYHA Class I or II heart failure, LVEF ≤ 30% and QRS ≥ 130 ms) to CRT-D or ICD-only therapy. During long-term follow-up of 854 patients, CRT-D therapy showed a significant reduction in mortality when compared with ICD-only therapy (HR = 0.59, $P < .001$).[20]

Additional trials have further identified the specific populations of patients most likely to benefit from CRT therapy. Current American Heart Association (AHA)/American College of Cardiology (ACC)/Heart Rhythm Society (HRS) guidelines for CRT therapy are summarized in **Table 77.2**.

ANATOMIC CONSIDERATIONS

The left pectoral region is the preferred site for implantation for most ICD systems. This allows for lower defibrillation threshold when compared with right-sided implant and is less onerous for most right-handed patients. Other considerations for site selection include prior surgery sites (ie, mastectomy), presence of other cardiac devices, and viable vascular access. An ICD device should not be implanted on the same side as indwelling venous catheters or arteriovenous fistulas.

For vascular access, the cephalic, subclavian, or axillary veins are used for implantation of intracardiac leads. The selection is operator dependent although there are some innate advantages and disadvantages of each of these methods. The cephalic vein is usually accessed by the cutdown technique while subclavian and axillary veins are accessed percutaneously. A cephalic cutdown precludes the risk of pneumothorax and allows for easier exposure of the lateral deltopectoral muscle, which carries an advantage in patients with little subcutaneous fat who may need a submuscular pocket creation. Conversely, the size of the cephalic vein greatly varies and at times, it may be challenging to accommodate more than one lead. The axillary vein has the advantage of being distal enough to minimize the risk of pneumothorax and also allows visualization of the vein with ultrasound. Subclavian vein access is associated with the highest risk of pneumothorax and lead fracture due to passage of the lead between the clavicle and the first rib before entering the vein ("subclavian crush").

TABLE 77.2 Indications for Cardiac Resynchronization Therapy

NYHA Functional Class			
	Left Bundle Branch Block		
	QRS 120-129 ms	QRS 130-149 ms	QRS > 150 ms
II	COR IIa (LOE B)	COR IIa (LOE B)	COR I (LOE B)
III and IV	COR IIa (LOE B)	COR IIa (LOE B)	COR I (LOE A)
	Non-Left Bundle Branch Block		
	QRS 120-129 ms	QRS 130-149	QRS > 150 ms
II	COR III (LOE B)	COR III (LOE B)	COR IIb (LOE B)
III and IV	COR IIb (LOE B)	COR IIb (LOE B)	COR IIa (LOE B)

COR, classification of recommendation; LOE, level of evidence; ms, milliseconds; NYHA, New York Heart Association.

Data from Yancy CW, Jessup M, Bozkurt B, et al. 2013 ACCF/AHA Guideline for Management of Heart Failure. A report of the American College of Cardiology Foundation/American Heart Association Task Force on Practice Guidelines. *Circulation*. 2013;128:e240–e327.

Contrast venography is helpful in patients with potentially difficult venous access and for some operators is routinely done for every device implant. Venous anatomy and patency can be visualized through the injection of 10 to 20 mL of contrast into a distal vein in the ipsilateral arm and then observing the pectoral region under fluoroscopy.

FUNDAMENTALS OF IMPLANTABLE CARDIOVERTER-DEFIBRILLATOR AND CRT IMPLANTATION

Preoperative Preparation

Prophylactic antibiotics are routinely used for the prevention of device-related infections. Cephalosporins such as cefazolin are often given immediately preprocedural to reduce the risk of device infection due to their effectiveness against skin flora. Once anatomic considerations above have been considered and a site has been selected, the operator will obtain vascular access through a plethora of options.

Vascular Access

Subclavian and axillary vein approaches are the most common transvenous routes used and will be described in detail. Knowledge of the underlying anatomy is crucial for successful access, as it is often done without the benefit of direct visualization or ultrasound guidance. The subclavian vein courses underneath the clavicle and exits the thoracic cavity at the junction of the first rib and the clavicle to become the axillary vein (which some refer to as the extrathoracic portion of the subclavian vein). In normal anatomic position, the apex of the lung lies lateral to the juncture.

After local infiltration of lidocaine, the needle is placed 1 to 2 cm inferolateral to the junction of the first rib and the clavicle and advanced with a medial and cephalad angulation. A more lateral approach risks puncture of the apical lung and pneumothorax, while a more medial approach may result in compression of the ICD lead between the first rib and clavicle risking subclavian crush phenomenon.

For accessing the axillary vein more laterally, a lower approach is used. Under fluoroscopy, the needle is inserted lateral to the second rib with a 45-degree angle to the body surface and a cephalad angulation. The intended target is the most proximal portion of the axillary vein, as it courses over the first rib. The medial border for this approach is the first rib, which will prevent inadvertent puncture of the underlying structures including the lung. Sometimes, it may be necessary to adjust the angle to the body surface steeper up to 60 degrees, especially in patients with significant subcutaneous fat. Venography of the axillary-subclavian vein often is performed before accessing the vein (**Figure 77.1**).

An ultrasound may be used to guide access by placing the vascular probe on the sagittal plane over the middle third of the clavicle and tracing the axillary vein laterally until it no longer overlaps with the axillary artery. The vein then can be entered under ultrasound guidance to avoid accidental arterial puncture.

Alternatively, the cephalic approach utilizes a venous cutdown to visualize the entry site located at the deltopectoral groove, which can be localized by palpating for the coracoid process of the scapula. After infiltration with local anesthetic, a 2 to 4 cm vertical incision is made at the level of the coracoid process to accommodate for the lead placement. Once exposed, careful dissection is made to the pectoral fascial plane. The deltopectoral groove is formed by the borders of the pectoral and deltoid muscles, which are separated carefully to expose the cephalic vein. In cases where the cephalic vein is too small for lead placement, the dissection can be extended proximally until the axillary vein is visualized.

Regardless of the route of access, if multiple leads are to be implanted (eg, for CRT-D), it is preferred to obtain separate access sites for each lead to minimize the potential for inadvertent lead dislodgment.

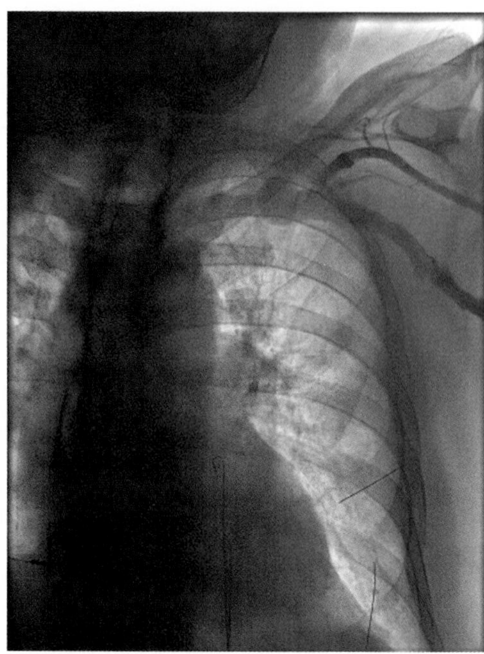

FIGURE 77.1 Left-sided venogram showing the axillary vein coursing between the first rib and clavicle.

Pocket Creation

Before skin incision, it is imperative to ensure the patency of the vein by either first obtaining access or advancing guidewires all the way to the right atrium or performing a venogram and demonstrating patency of the access vein (**Figure 77.1**).

For most patients with sufficient subcutaneous tissue, an incision between 5 and 7 cm is made and carried to the prepectoral fascia while using electrocautery to achieve hemostasis. The prepectoral fascial plane is then opened with blunt dissection to an adequate size to accommodate the generator. However, in emaciated patients, it may be necessary to create a subpectoral pocket instead due to the lack of overlying subcutaneous tissue. In that case, an incision must be made to expose the deltopectoral groove. Once identified, the lateral edge of the deltopectoral muscle is separated gently from the pectoralis minor using blunt dissection to create a space for the generator underneath.

Placement of the Leads

The technique for intracardiac lead placement is largely independent of access site selection. Up to three intracardiac leads can be implanted depending on the need of the patient.

For ICD implantation, in patients with no indication for pacing, recent trends have leaned toward implanting only the RV lead for primary prevention as the addition of atrial lead does not significantly improve discrimination algorithms for VT.[21] A dual-chamber device is implanted in patients with pacing indications (bradycardia, conduction system disease), dual-chamber system also is preferred in patients with paroxysmal atrial fibrillation with rapid ventricular response, or slow VT. There has also been a trend toward simpler, single-coil RV leads, which avoid superior vena cava (SVC) stenosis that can arise with SVC defibrillation coils and are associated with significantly less risk of superior vena cava damage during the lead extraction.

All intracardiac leads are soft tipped and have very little intrinsic support. An inner stylet must be used at most times to steer and position the lead. The stylets are usually straight or curve-tipped to allow for different lead positioning. Care must be taken while advancing the lead with a stylet as considerable forces are transmitted and can lead to inadvertent intracardiac damage and even cardiac perforation.

For RV lead implantation, a curved stylet should be used to facilitate crossing the tricuspid valve. After crossing the tricuspid valve, the lead tip is directed into the RV outflow tract to confirm its position in the RV. This is an important step to ensure the lead did not inadvertently advance into the CS or cross to the LV through an atrial septal defect, patent foramen ovale, or ventricular septal defect. During RV lead placement, premature ventricular complexes localized to the RV may also help in identifying the correct position. Careful fluoroscopic verification of the lead positioning in right anterior oblique (RAO) and left anterior oblique (LAO) views is essential to ensure that the RV lead is not placed in the CS or one of its branches or in the LV by crossing the above-mentioned anatomical defects. Once the lead position is confirmed to be in the RV, the curved stylet is then changed for a soft-tipped straight stylet. The lead is slowly withdrawn from the RV outflow tract, and counterclockwise torque is applied to allow the lead tip to softly drop toward the RV apex. Ideally, the RV lead should be fixed to the apical septum rather than the RV apex proper. Septal position can be confirmed on an LAO view with the lead pointing toward the right of the screen. Once the lead position is confirmed, the extendable-retractable active fixation mechanism is deployed to fix the lead in place, and the stylet is withdrawn by one-third of its length under fluoroscopic guidance to ensure the lead position remains stable. If the lead needs to be repositioned, the fixation mechanism is retracted and the lead is repositioned to a different site via gentle maneuvering of the stylet.

Once a satisfactory position is obtained and the lead is fixed in place, pacing and sensing thresholds of the lead can be assessed using a pacing system analyzer. The intracardiac signal should be scrutinized for a "current of injury," which is seen as "ST elevation" on the local bipolar electrogram. The current injury size that is roughly one-third of the local electrogram amplitude indicates sufficient contact and fixation of the lead tip with the myocardium. For the RV lead, generally accepted electrical parameters are as follows: R wave amplitude at least 5 mV, capture threshold <2.5 V at 0.5 ms pulse width, and an impedance between 350 and 1000 Ω. In addition, signals should be examined for the far-field detection of P waves and T waves oversensing. High-voltage pacing testing (1 ms at 10 V) should be done to ensure there is no phrenic nerve (ie, diaphragmatic) stimulation. After ensuring a proper amount of slack in the RV lead, the proximal portion of the lead is secured by anchoring it down in the pocket with nonabsorbable sutures around the suture sleeve. Multiple sutures should be used to secure the lead snugly, and acute angles of the lead should be avoided to avoid future lead injury.

The right atrial lead, if required, is then implanted. A straight stylet is first used to advance the lead into the lower right atrium and then exchanged for a curved, J-tipped stylet. At this point, the tip of the intracardiac lead should sit in the middle of the right atrium and be pointed upward. The lead and stylet can be withdrawn until the tip of the lead snaps into the right atrial appendage or anterolateral right atrial wall. Some clockwise or counterclockwise motion will help locate the stable implant site. Once the appropriate location is found, the same process of fixation and signal analysis is conducted to ensure adequate lead positioning before securing the lead.

Left Ventricular Lead

In the case of CRT device implantation, a third lead must be guided into the CS and advanced to a cardiac vein on the epicardial surface of the LV lateral wall. The CS lies in the posterior coronary groove between the left ventricle and the left atrium, with the ostium located at the posteroseptal region of the right atrium near the tricuspid valve. The opening is approximately 1 cm in diameter and sometimes inadvertently cannulated during routine implantation of the RV lead. Cannulation of the CS requires the use of specially curved guiding sheaths to direct the guidewire posteroseptal toward the CS ostium. Usually, an inner sheath is used for cannulation of the CS and an outer sheath is then advanced for lead delivery. Under fluoroscopic guidance, advancing the inner sheath distal to the eustachian ridge—which lies in the anterior aspect of the CS ostium—in the RAO view and then gently moving it posteriorly and rotating toward the septum in the LAO view helps direct the guidewire figure into the CS. The position of the guidewire in the CS must be verified in RAO and LAO projections before advancing inner and outer sheaths over the guidewire into the CS. Once in the CS, the guidewire and inner sheath are removed, and a small amount of the contrast is injected into the outer sheath to confirm proper location of the sheath in the CS and rule out inadvertent CS dissection during the cannulation. After this, balloon occlusive venography of the CS and its ventricular branches is performed with injection of contrast while occluding the CS ostium with a balloon

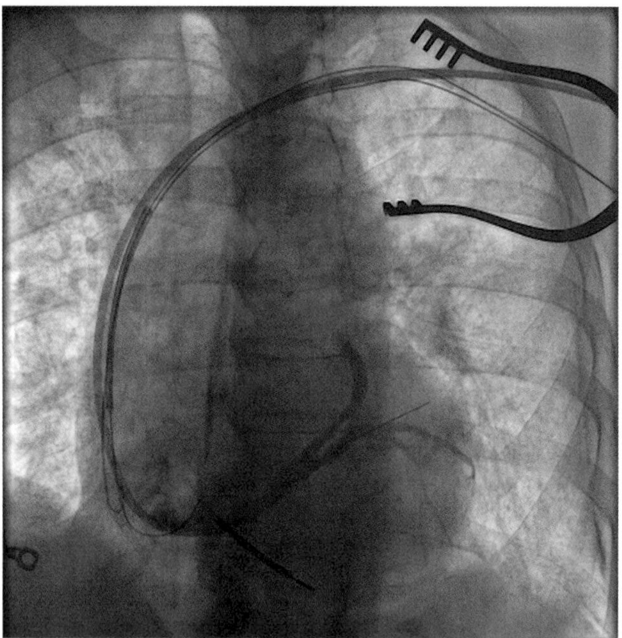

FIGURE 77.2 Venogram of the coronary sinus. The posterolateral branch of the middle cardiac vein is identified as a target vein for implantation of the left ventricular lead.

catheter (**Figure 77.2**). This visualizes appropriate candidate branches for LV lead implantation, with the referred location a lateral or posterolateral branch that would ensure the pacing of the LV regions most remote from the septum and displaying the most delay of activation in the setting of the left-bundle branch block. Absence of phrenic nerve stimulation also must be ensured before accepting final lead position, after which the delivery system is gently withdrawn from the CS and slit away with the use of a special tool, that ensures lead stability during delivery system removal. The main electrical criteria for accepting LV lead placement are pacing threshold and absence of the phrenic nerve stimulation. Once the final lead position is accepted and a proper amount of slack ensured in the right atrium, the lead is secured to the pocket as described above. If no appropriate branch exists, thoracoscopic LV epicardial lead placement may be considered. **Figure 77.3** shows the final lead positioning in LAO and RAO views. **Figure 77.4** shows the chest radiograph of CRT-D system.

Generator Placement

Once all leads are secured in the pocket, the proximal connector pins are cleaned with gauze and then inserted into the appropriate ports on the header of the generator. For high-voltage defibrillation leads such as the IS-1 connectors, the torque wrench must be inserted into the device before connecting the lead. After ensuring full insertion of the pins inside the generator header, the pins are permanently secured in the device with a torque wrench.

After all, leads are securely connected, the pocket is irrigated with an antibiotic solution. While no large, randomized controlled trials exist validating the use of antibiotic irrigation solution, it is routinely used in clinical care. After irrigation, the leads are gently coiled into the pocket, and the generator is inserted and placed on top of the leads. Some operators use an additional nonabsorbable suture to secure the device inside the pocket. A variety of different closure methods can be used to close the pocket sterilely and securely.

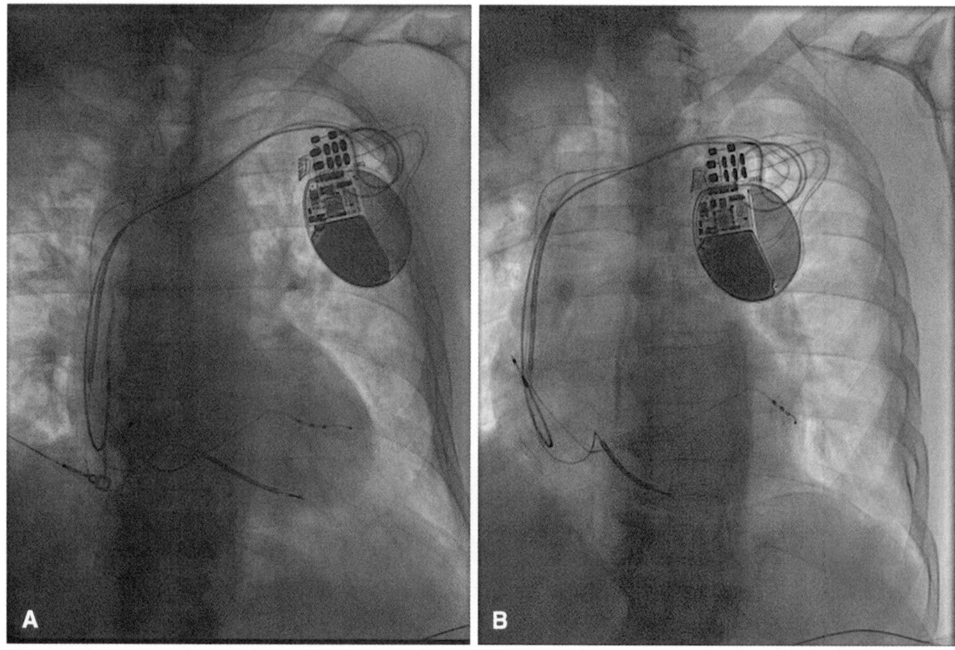

FIGURE 77.3 Final position of right atrial, right ventricular, and left ventricular leads in right anterior oblique **(A)** and left anterior oblique **(B)** radiographic views.

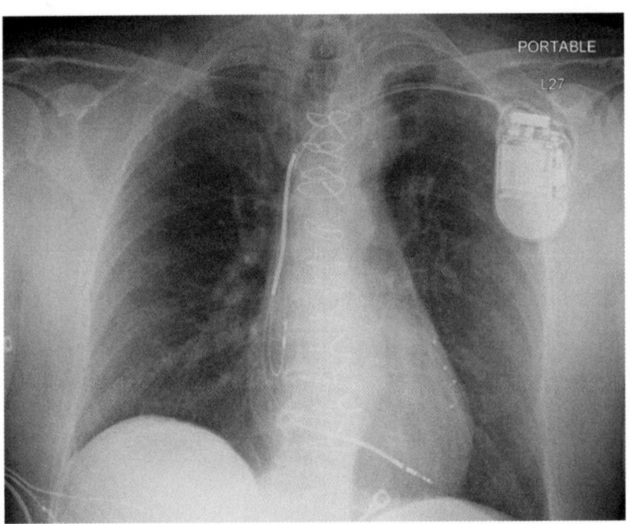

FIGURE 77.4 Postoperative chest x-ray showing three intracardiac leads in the right atrium, right ventricle, and lateral branch of the middle cardiac vein. There is no evidence of pneumothorax or enlarged cardiac silhouette.

Postprocedural Care

A chest radiogram is obtained routinely postprocedure to rule out pneumothorax. The ipsilateral arm is immobilized with a sling. After a new device implantation, patients are usually admitted for overnight observation. Although little evidence exists to support postprocedural oral antibiotics, oral regimens covering skin flora are almost always prescribed for patients for 3 to 5 days postimplantation.

SPECIAL CONSIDERATIONS AND CONTRAINDICATIONS

Contraindications

Although ICDs have been shown to be effective in preventing mortality by reducing the incidence of SCD, they cannot stop progression of heart failure or mitigate other causes of mortality. ICD implantation is contraindicated in four groups of patients:

- Estimated life expectancy of less than 1 year or poor functional capacity.
- Incessant ventricular tachyarrhythmias.
- NYHA Class IV patients who fail to respond to the guideline-directed medical therapy and are not deemed suitable for cardiac transplantation or CRT.

Ventricular tachycardia in the absence of structural heart disease that is amenable to catheter ablation or ventricular tachyarrhythmias secondary to reversible causes.

Noninfectious Complications of Implantation

Properly obtained venous access is the first and most crucial step to the prevention of both acute and chronic complications. Inadvertent arterial puncture can lead to hemothorax, and accidental puncture of the underlying lung can cause pneumothorax. If the access site is located too medial, the lead can be compressed by the narrow angle of the clavicle and the first rib, leading to lead malfunction and fragmentation ("subclavian crush").

Although the use of active fixation leads has led to a significant decrease in the incidence of lead dislodgement, it still remains a fairly common issue in device implantation, with the majority of dislodgements being associated with atrial leads.[22] It is most commonly due to poor attachment of the lead to the myocardium. Close attention must be paid to the current of injury at the time of implantation to ensure there is sufficient contact. Additionally, one must ensure the appropriate amount of slack in the intracardiac lead during implantation to prevent tension on the lead once the patient assumes an upright position.

Pocket hematomas can form if insufficient attention is paid to achieve careful hemostasis during pocket creation. Bleeding from the venous access site can also lead to a hematoma in the device pocket, especially in patients with elevated venous pressure.

Venous stenosis and thrombosis are common problems in the chronic setting due to the long-term presence of intravenous leads. Although peripheral venous thrombosis or stenosis is rarely a clinically significant issue, it propagates to the central venous system systemic anticoagulation or intervention may be required.

Risks of cardiac perforation are minimal with contemporary active fixation leads, with most estimates ranging from 0.1% to 0.4%.[23] They are mostly self-limited and require only close monitoring. In rare cases when tamponade occurs, emergent pericardiocentesis is crucial and life-saving. In the chronic setting, the decision to extract the lead must be made with care and is often a collaborative effort between electrophysiologists and surgeons.

Infectious Complications

The rate of periprocedure infections related to cardiac implantable devices remained steady until 2005 when the indication of ICDs for primary prevention led to a significant increase in the number of patients with multiple comorbidities being implanted with a device. The rate of periprocedure infections is now ~2.5% per year.[24]

Sterile technique is crucial to prevention of infection in any invasive procedure and even more so with device implantation. Most operators double-glove when preparing for implantation. Periprocedural antibiotics reduce the incidence of periprocedural infections by up to 80%. While little evidence exists for continuing them postprocedure, most operators routinely give oral antibiotics for 3 to 5 days—and up to 10 days—postimplant. Infections can range from cellulitis over the device pocket to lead endocarditis. The presence of intravascular infection with persistent bacteremia almost ensures the need for removal of the generator and all leads.

FOLLOW-UP PATIENT CARE

After device implantation, a routine in-person postprocedural clinic visit is made for all patients to ensure proper wound healing and appropriate device function. In addition to analyzing intracardiac signals, modern devices have become increasingly sophisticated and are capable of recording, identifying, and analyzing a plethora of diagnostic data regarding their own performance and the patient's clinical status. To ensure proper functioning of the device, periodic in-person evaluations are recommended postimplant. However, only a minority of patients adhere to such a rigorous schedule of in-office visits. This prompted the development of remote or home monitoring of cardiac implantable electrical devices, which now has become standard of care.[25]

Almost all modern cardiac implantable electrical devices now have a mechanism of communication that can relay clinical information from the patient's home to the appropriate medical personnel. Patients are given a small external device capable of receiving transmitted data from their ICD. This monitoring device, if close enough to the ICD, is capable of remotely downloading all relevant clinical information, which can then be sent digitally to the appropriate health care professionals. Scheduled remote interrogations that involve full transmission of device function and all relevant clinical data on an established scheduled and unscheduled remote monitoring that involves automatic transmission when specified alert events such as abnormal lead impedance or tachycardia episodes occur are advised. Home monitoring has been shown to be safe and effective across all devices and has been responsible for reducing the burden of in-office visits while also providing a safety net for daily surveillance.[26]

RESEARCH AND FUTURE DEVELOPMENTS IN CRT

Although many years of accumulated experience and the introduction of better delivery tools have increased the rate of successful LV lead implantation, the venous anatomy of some patients, as well as anatomical interactions with the phrenic nerve, do not allow for pacing of the LV lateral wall in some patients. This population can comprise up to 25% of all attempted CRT devices.[27] Accordingly, efforts toward alternative methods for pacing the left ventricle are ongoing.

His-bundle[28] or the left-bundle branch area pacing[29] has been introduced as a potential alternative to traditional CRT. Pilot studies show that His-bundle or the left-bundle pacing has beneficial effects on heart failure patients.

Finally, wireless pacing devices are being developed that can be directly implanted to stimulate the LV myocardium.[30]

KEY POINTS

- ✔ ICDs are a key component of primary and secondary prevention of SCD. In patients with reduced LVEF (<35%), primary prevention ICDs reduce mortality and arrhythmic death.
- ✔ Patients with limited life expectancy (<1 year), incessant VT, and class IV heart failure who are not candidates for transplant or Ventricular Assist Device (VAD) do not benefit from ICD implantation.
- ✔ CRT utilizes two pacing leads in the RV apex and LV-free wall to regain electrical and mechanical synchrony in chronic heart failure.
- ✔ Appropriate utilization of CRT can improve mortality, reduce hospitalizations, and reverse LV dilatation.
- ✔ Patients with NYHA Class III/IV, wide QRS > 150 ms, and LBBB are more likely to benefit from CRT.
- ✔ Patients with narrow QRS < 120 ms do not benefit from CRT.

REFERENCES

1. Meyer JA. Claude Beck and cardiac resuscitation. *Ann Thorac Surg.* 1988;45:103-105.
2. Wiggers CJ. The physiologic basis for cardiac resuscitation from ventricular fibrillation—Method for serial defibrillation. *Am Heart J.* 1940;20:413-422.
3. Mirowski M, Mower MM, Reid PR. The automatic implantable defibrillator. *Am Heart J.* 1980;100:1089-1092.
4. Mirowski M, Reid PR, Mower MM, et al. Termination of malignant ventricular arrhythmias with an implanted automatic defibrillator in human beings. *N Engl J Med.* 1980;303:322-324.
5. Al-Khatib SM, Stevenson WG, Ackerman MJ, et al. 2017 AHA/ACC/HRS Guideline for management of patients with ventricular arrhythmias and the prevention of sudden cardiac death. *Circulation.* 2018;138:e272-e391.
6. Kosmala W, Marwick TH. Meta-analysis of effects of optimization of cardiac resynchronization therapy on left ventricular function, exercise capacity, and quality of life in patients with heart failure. *Am J Cardiol.* 2014;113:988-994.
7. Shah RM, Patel D, Molnar J, Ellenbogen KA, Koneru JN. Cardiac-resynchronization therapy in patients with systolic heart failure and QRS interval ≤130 ms: insights from a meta-analysis. *Europace.* 2015;17:267-273.
8. Kuck KH, Cappato R, Siebels J, Rüppel R. Randomized comparison of antiarrhythmic drug therapy with implantable defibrillators in patients resuscitated from cardiac arrest: the Cardiac Arrest Study Hamburg (CASH). *Circulation.* 2000;102:748-754.
9. Connolly SJ, Gent M, Roberts RS, et al. Canadian implantable defibrillator study (CIDS): a randomized trial of the implantable cardioverter defibrillator against amiodarone. *Circulation.* 2000;101:1297-1302.
10. Antiarrhythmics versus Implantable Defibrillators (AVID) Investigators. A comparison of antiarrhythmic-drug therapy with implantable defibrillators in patients resuscitated from near-fatal ventricular arrhythmias. *N Engl J Med.* 1997;337:1576-1583.
11. Multicenter Postinfarction Research Group. Risk stratification and survival after myocardial infarction. *N Engl J Med.* 1983;309:331-336.
12. Curtis JP, Sokol SI, Wang Y, et al. The association of left ventricular ejection fraction, mortality, and cause of death in stable outpatients with heart failure. *J Am Coll Cardiol.* 2003;42:736-742.
13. Moss AJ, Hall WJ, Cannom DS, et al. Improved survival with an implanted defibrillator in patients with coronary disease at high risk for ventricular arrhythmia. *N Engl J Med.* 1996;335:1933-1940.
14. Buxton AE, Lee KL, Fisher JD, Josephson ME, Prystowsky EN, Hafley G. A randomized study of the prevention of sudden death in patients with coronary artery disease. Multicenter Unsustained Tachycardia Trial Investigators. *N Engl J Med.* 1999;341:1882-1890.
15. Moss AJ, Zareba W, Hall WJ, et al. Prophylactic implantation of a defibrillator in patients with myocardial infarction and reduced ejection fraction. *N Engl J Med.* 2002;346:877-883.
16. Kadish A, Dyer A, Daubert JP, et al. Prophylactic defibrillator implantation in patients with nonischemic dilated cardiomyopathy. *N Engl J Med.* 2004;350:2151-2158.

17. Bardy GH, Lee KL, Mark DB, et al. Amiodarone or an implantable cardioverter–defibrillator for congestive heart failure. *N Engl J Med.* 2005;352:225-237.
18. Bristow MR, Saxon LA, Boehmer J, et al. Cardiac-resynchronization therapy with or without an implantable defibrillator in advanced chronic heart failure. *N Engl J Med.* 2004;350:2140-2150.
19. Cleland JGF, Daubert J-C, Erdmann E, et al. The effect of cardiac resynchronization on morbidity and mortality in heart failure. *N Engl J Med.* 2005;352:1539-1549.
20. Moss AJ, Hall WJ, Cannom DS, et al. Cardiac-resynchronization therapy for the prevention of heart-failure events. *N Engl J Med.* 2009;361:1329-1338.
21. Corbisiero R, Lee MA, Nabert DR, et al. Performance of a new single-chamber ICD algorithm: discrimination of supraventricular and ventricular tachycardia based on vector timing and correlation. *Europace.* 2006;8:1057-1061.
22. Ghani A, Delnoy PPHM, Ramdat Misier AR, et al. Incidence of lead dislodgement, malfunction and perforation during the first year following device implantation. *Neth Heart J.* 2014;22:286-291.
23. Ellenbogen KA, Hellkamp AS, Wilkoff BL, et al. Complications arising after implantation of DDD pacemakers: the MOST experience. *Am J Cardiol.* 2003;92:740-741.
24. Kirkfeldt RE, Johansen JB, Nohr EA, Jørgensen OD, Nielsen JC. Complications after cardiac implantable electronic device implantations: an analysis of a complete, nationwide cohort in Denmark. *Eur Heart J.* 2014;35:1186-1194.
25. Burri H, Senouf D. Remote monitoring and follow-up of pacemakers and implantable cardioverter defibrillators. *Europace.* 2009;11:701-709.
26. Varma N, Epstein AE, Irimpen A, Schweikert R, Love C. TRUST Investigators: Efficacy and safety of automatic remote monitoring for implantable cardioverter-defibrillator follow-up: the Lumos-T Safely Reduces Routine Office Device Follow-up (TRUST) trial. *Circulation.* 2010;122:325-332.
27. Khan FZ, Virdee MS, Gopalan D, et al. Characterization of the suitability of coronary venous anatomy for targeting left ventricular lead placement in patients undergoing cardiac resynchronization therapy. *Europace.* 2009;11:1491-1495.
28. Deshmukh P, Casavant DA, Romanyshyn M, Anderson K. Permanent, direct His-bundle pacing: a novel approach to cardiac pacing in patients with normal His-Purkinje activation. *Circulation.* 2000;101:869-877.
29. Huang W, Su L, Wu S, et al. A novel pacing strategy with low and stable output: pacing the left bundle branch immediately beyond the conduction block. *Can J Cardiol.* 2017;33:1736.e1-1736.e3.
30. Reddy VY, Miller MA, Neuzil P, et al. Cardiac resynchronization therapy with wireless left ventricular endocardial pacing: the SELECT-LV study. *J Am Coll Cardiol.* 2017;69:2119-2129.

CHAPTER 78

MECHANICAL CIRCULATORY SUPPORT

Anju Bhardwaj, Alexis Shafii, Andrew Civitello, and Ajith Nair

INTRODUCTION

Heart failure (HF) is a syndrome that affects over 6.5 million individuals in the United States. Despite significant advances in medical therapy, it remains a leading cause of death with a 5-year mortality of greater than 50%.[1] Patients with HF refractory to medical therapy may qualify for advanced therapies including heart transplantation or implantation of mechanical circulatory support devices. Although heart transplantation is considered a definitive therapy for patients with advanced HF, its use is limited by a paucity of organs, prolonged wait times, and stringent selection criteria. With improvements in technology and the advent of smaller, durable continuous flow pumps, the use of implantable left ventricular assist devices (LVADs) has emerged as an effective and viable option.

Over the last decade, most patients treated with an implantable LVAD received continuous flow devices that have smaller profiles and a single moving impeller/rotor. Three pumps have been approved by the US Food and Drug Administration (FDA): the HeartMate II axial flow pump (Abbott Laboratories, Abbott Park, IL, USA); the HeartWare centrifugal pump ventricular assist device system (Medtronic, St. Paul, MN, USA); and the HeartMate III magnetically levitated centrifugal pumps (St. Jude Medical, Pleasanton, CA, USA). See **Figure 78.1A-C.**

These pumps are driven electrically by a percutaneous driveline that is connected to a small controller and an external energy source with either replaceable batteries or a direct alternating current power source. The LVAD unloads the heart and pumps blood from the left ventricle to the ascending aorta.

INDICATIONS

Candidate Selection

Four major indications for LVAD implantation are discussed here. These pumps were initially used for shorter periods of time as a "bridge to transplantation" to ensure survival of patients until a donor organ became available.[2] The landmark REMATCH (Randomized Evaluation of Mechanical Assistance for the Treatment of Congestive Heart Failure) trial demonstrated that pulsatile LVADs were associated with a survival benefit and could be used as "destination therapy" with improved quality of life in patients on guideline-directed medical therapy who were not deemed candidates for transplant.[3] Continuous flow LVADs subsequently demonstrated improved survival and freedom from device complications compared to pulsatile LVADs.[4]

Patients with acute hemodynamic instability in whom candidacy of transplant cannot be evaluated until after LVAD

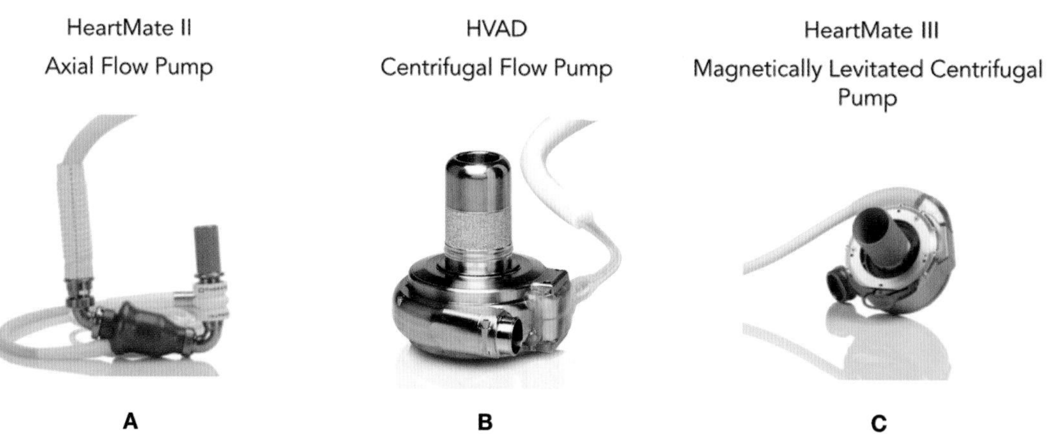

FIGURE 78.1 HeartMate II, HeartWare ventricular assist device (HVAD), and HeartMate III. **(A)** HeartMate II axial flow pump. **(B)** HVAD centrifugal flow pump and ventricular assist device system. **(C)** HeartMate III: magnetically levitated centrifugal pump. (A, HeartMate II is a trademark of Abbott or its related companies. Reproduced with permission of Abbott, © 2021. All rights reserved.; B, Reproduced with permission of Medtronic, Inc.; C, HeartMate 3 is a trademark of Abbott or its related companies. Reproduced with permission of Abbott, © 2021. All rights reserved.)

implantation are deemed as "bridge to decision." These patients may have relative contraindications or comorbidities—like renal dysfunction, pulmonary hypertension, or obesity—that may be reversible after prolonged hemodynamic support.[5] Finally, "bride to recovery" is used in patients with potentially reversible myocardial dysfunction, such as fulminant myocarditis or peripartum cardiomyopathy, where LVAD support may function as a bridge to myocardial recovery.[6]

Criteria for LVAD implantation are based on inclusion and exclusion criteria from clinical LVAD trials and are listed in **Table 78.1**. LVAD implantation is considered reasonable in patients with stage D HF who are advanced to medical and device-based therapies.

The Interagency Registry for Mechanically Assisted Circulatory Support (INTERMACS) profiles for advanced HF are listed in **Table 78.2** and may aid in identification of patients likely to benefit from mechanical support devices.[7] LVAD implantation can be considered in selected INTERMACS profile 1 to 2 patients, in all INTERMACS profile 3 patients, and in severely symptomatic INTERMACS profile 4 to 7 patients after a frank, well-informed discussion with the patient regarding risk of adverse events versus benefits of better functional status and survival.[7-9]

Rigorous evaluation is required to assess candidacy for LVAD therapy. Major considerations include clinical necessity (assessed by patient's clinical and functional status and hemodynamic studies), presence of absolute and relative contraindications as mentioned in **Table 78.3**, and psychosocial factors and patient goals of care. LVAD is still an evolving therapy fraught with complications, which makes ideal candidate selection imperative to maximize its benefit.

TABLE 78.1 Indications For Mechanical Circulatory Support

- Left ventricular ejection fraction ≤35%
- New York Heart Association Class IIIB/IV or persistently elevated natriuretic peptides
- End-organ dysfunction
- Patient requiring inotropes
- Recurrent hospitalizations
- Edema despite escalating diuretics
- Hemodynamic instability (hypotension/tachycardia)
- Inability to tolerate guideline-directed medical therapy because of hypotension or renal failure
- High filling pressures with low cardiac output
- Cardiac cachexia
- Limited functional status (usually assessed by inability to exercise, peak oxygen consumption <14 mL/kg/min or a 6-minute walk test <300 m)

TABLE 78.2 INTERMACS Ventricular Assist Device Placement According to INTERMACS Profiles

INTERMACS Profile	Description	% VAD implants
7	Advanced NYHA Class III symptoms	0.5%
6	Exertion limited	0.9%
5	Exertion intolerant	2.3%
4	Resting symptoms (home on oral therapy)	13.0%
3	Stable but inotrope dependent	31.7%
2	Progressive decline on inotropic support	36.5%
1	Critical cardiogenic shock	15.1%

INTERMACS, Interagency Registry for Mechanically Assisted Circulatory Support; NYHA, New York Heart Association; VAD, ventricular assist device

PREIMPLANTATION CONSIDERATIONS: VALVE DISEASE AND PULMONARY HYPERTENSION

Aortic Valve Disease

Significant aortic regurgitation requires concomitant aortic valve repair or replacement with LVAD placement as regurgitant flows can diminish the hemodynamic support.[10] Another strategy to address aortic regurgitation involves oversewing the aortic valve. Patients with oversewn valves are completely LVAD dependent, and pump dysfunction can be fatal. Mechanical aortic valves are associated with high risk of thrombosis and may necessitate valve replacement with a bioprosthetic valve or placement of a patch on top of the mechanical valve to mitigate the risk of valvular thrombosis and thromboembolism.[11,12] Aortic stenosis does not warrant any intervention as systemic flow occurs through the device and bypasses the aortic valve.

Mitral Valve Disease

Functional mitral regurgitation does not routinely require intervention, as unloading of the ventricle by the LVAD leads to a reduction in regurgitation.[13,14] Transcatheter edge-to-edge mitral valve repair has been performed for persistent mitral regurgitation despite LVAD support.[15] Moderate-to-severe mitral stenosis may compromise left ventricular filling, reduce LVAD flows, and require prosthetic valve replacement. Both mechanical and bioprosthetic mitral valves are not associated with increased risk of thrombosis following LVAD insertion.[16]

Tricuspid Valve Regurgitation

Right ventricular failure is a major cause of morbidity and mortality after LVAD implantation. Tricuspid regurgitation may exacerbate right ventricular failure, and valve repair may

TABLE 78.3 Absolute and Relative Contraindications to Left Ventricular Assist Devices

Absolute	Relative
Sepsis or current active infection	Morbid obesity
Right heart failure	Chronic renal dysfunction, not on dialysis
Untreated and severe carotid artery disease	Malnutrition
Severe pulmonary disease	Severe or untreated mitral stenosis
Severe irreversible cerebral injury	
Dialysis-dependent renal failure	
Elevated INR from liver failure	
Disseminated intravascular coagulation	
Severe end-organ failure	
Noncardiac illness with survival <2 years	

INR, international normalized ratio.

decrease the risk of postoperative right ventricular failure.[17] As LVADs generally lead to an improvement in tricuspid regurgitation via reductions in pulmonary pressures and right ventricular dimension,[18] valve repair may be considered for isolated cases of severe tricuspid regurgitation during LVAD implant.[19]

Pulmonary Hypertension

In patients with advanced HF, pulmonary hypertension is primarily the consequence of left heart disease. In this setting, the mean pulmonary arterial (PA) pressure is greater than or equal to 20 mm Hg and mean pulmonary capillary wedge pressure (PCWP) is greater than or equal to 15 mm Hg.[20] Combined precapillary and postcapillary pulmonary hypertension is characterized by a pulmonary vascular resistance (PVR) greater than or equal to 3 Wood units, and the transpulmonary gradient (mean PA pressure—PCWP) is greater than 12 mm Hg. Patients with fixed and elevated PVR are not candidates for heart transplant because of the high risk of posttransplantation right ventricular failure.[21] Patients bridged with an LVAD may show improvement in PVR after LVAD over 3 to 6 months, thus altering their transplant eligibility.[22-24]

OTHER PREIMPLANTATION CONSIDERATIONS: PATIENT COMORBIDITIES

Renal Dysfunction

Renal dysfunction in advanced HF may be multifactorial. Cardiorenal syndrome related to low cardiac output and increased venous congestion generally improves after LVAD support, whereas intrinsic kidney disease related to chronic poor perfusion, hypertension, or diabetes mellitus may result in persistent and progressive renal failure.[25]

Renal dysfunction is associated with poor outcomes post-LVAD, and end-stage renal disease requiring dialysis is an absolute contraindication for LVAD because of high short-term mortality.[26,27] However, there is no clear consensus on a glomerular filtration rate below which an LVAD would not be considered. Postoperative renal dysfunction may result from massive fluid shifts, acute blood loss, arrhythmias, and use of vasoactive medications, and transient renal replacement therapy may be required.[28]

Hepatic Dysfunction

Hepatic dysfunction is associated with increased mortality and morbidity in HF; it is usually attributed to ischemic hepatitis because of decreased hepatic blood flow, congestive hepatopathy related to increased hepatic venous pressures, and cardiac cirrhosis because of chronic right ventricular dysfunction.[29] Elevated liver enzymes and bilirubin are associated with worse post-LVAD outcomes, and a liver biopsy may be required to exclude noncardiac causes of liver dysfunction prior to LVAD implantation. Hepatic dysfunction associated with HF has been shown to improve after LVAD implantation.[25]

Obesity

Morbid obesity is associated with worse outcomes post-LVAD implantation because of increased risk of device-related infections and thromboembolism.[30] A body mass index greater than or equal to 35 kg/m^2 is considered a contraindication for heart transplantation, but weight loss may reverse this eligibility. Bariatric surgery is an efficacious weight loss modality, and concomitant gastric sleeve during LVAD implantation has been performed with success.[31]

Age, Malnutrition, and Debilitation

Advanced age is associated with mortality and prolonged hospitalizations post-LVAD implant, but it should not be used as a criterion to exclude LVAD therapy.[32] Carefully selected elderly patients can have excellent outcomes. Rather than age alone, frailty may be a better surrogate to assess candidacy.[33]

Cachexia and malnutrition are associated with poor postoperative outcomes; therefore, patients with poor nutritional status should undergo a nutritional assessment to develop a strategy based on their individual needs before LVAD implantation.[34]

Psychosocial Considerations

Given the complexity of care associated with LVAD therapy, each patient should have a thorough psychosocial and behavioral evaluation before implantation. Compliance, self-care, and psychosocial and behavioral assessment are critical to ascertain appropriate management and support strategies for the patient. Factors evaluated for heart transplant can be followed for LVAD implantation as well.[35]

SURGICAL IMPLANTATION TECHNIQUE

LVAD implantation is performed by insertion of an inflow cannula into the left ventricular apex and attaching an outflow graft to the ascending aorta. A sewing ring that is sutured to the myocardial surface secures the inflow cannula in place and the myocardial tissue inside the sewing ring is removed with a coring knife. The typical location of the inflow cannula is slightly anterior to the left ventricular apex and 1 to 2 cm lateral to the left anterior descending coronary artery. Intraoperative transesophageal echocardiography (TEE) can facilitate pinpointing the proper insertion location of the inflow cannula, which is aligned with the long axis of the mitral valve inlet and is parallel to the intraventricular septum. The HeartMate II pump requires the creation of a preperitoneal pocket in the abdominal wall, but this device is no longer utilized as newer generation centrifugal pumps are entirely intrapericardial. Once the inflow cannula of the LVAD has been secured to the sewing ring, the outflow graft can then be directed to the ascending aorta. The outflow graft is attached to the mid-ascending aorta in an end-to-side fashion with a beveled angle directing blood toward the aortic arch. The outflow graft length must be carefully approximated as excessive length can lead to kinking and a short graft may be at risk for occlusion and bleeding.[32] The device driveline is then tunneled with a lance through the rectus abdominis muscle and subcutaneous tissue to an exit site on the upper abdominal wall, where it is connected to the device controller module.

The median sternotomy incision is the most common surgical approach for device implantation. More recently, the lateral thoracotomy approach has been utilized with the smaller intrapericardial devices. Attributed advantages of this minimally invasive approach are reduction in blood loss and hospital stay as well as a reduction in right ventricular dysfunction.[36] Concomitant valve procedures may be performed as stated earlier but are not feasible through the thoracotomy approach. Following device implantation, intraoperative coagulopathy is commonly encountered and is managed with blood product repletion. Rapidly acquired von Willebrand deficiency can also complicate postoperative surgical bleeding. Anticoagulation with heparin is initiated 6 to 24 hours after surgery and Partial thromboplastin time (PTT) goals are adjusted based on the degree of hemostasis.

Right Ventricular Assessment

Right ventricular failure after LVAD implantation is a cause of significant morbidity and mortality and decreased survival to transplantation,[37] and it is identified as the most significant risk factor of death after implantation.[38] Predicting patients who are at risk improves patient selection and allows clinicians to implement strategies to avoid right ventricular failure. There are multiple predictors of post-LVAD right ventricular failure that have been identified,[39,40] but all these studies lack consensus, and no absolute measures of right ventricular function have been identified that would preclude an LVAD implant.

Clinical predictors of right ventricular failure include the presence of pulmonary hypertension, coagulopathy, previous cardiac surgery, hypotension, vasopressor requirement, and elevated aspartate aminotransferase, bilirubin, or creatinine. Echocardiographic parameters for right ventricular failure have not been uniformly validated, but include dilation and reduced contractility, low tricuspid annular plane systolic excursion (TAPSE <7.5 mm), reduced right ventricular fractional change area ($<35\%$), short- to long-axis ratio greater than 0.6, and severe tricuspid regurgitation.[41] Right heart catheterization is required prior to LVAD implantation. Parameters associated with right ventricular dysfunction include central venous pressure/PCWP ratio greater than 0.6, decreased right ventricular stroke work index (<300 mm Hg · mL/m^2), and a PA pulsatility index (systolic PA pressure—diastolic PA pressure/central venous pressure) less than 2.[42,43] Patients at high risk of right ventricular failure need close hemodynamic PA catheter–guided monitoring and volume optimization with aggressive diuresis, and ultrafiltration if needed. Rarely, percutaneous temporary mechanical circulatory support has been utilized for optimizing hemodynamics and end-organ function prior to LVAD implant. Planned biventricular support has been demonstrated to yield superior survival benefits to late right ventricular support.[44]

FUNDAMENTALS OF MANAGEMENT

Clinical Assessment

The history for patients with LVAD implementation must include assessment of HF symptoms, implantable cardioverter defibrillator (ICD) shocks, clinical evidence of bleeding, recent device parameters and alarms, driveline site condition and discharge, and signs of hemolysis including hematuria. Physical examination includes assessment of pulse, blood pressure, auscultation of the LVAD, and examination of the driveline and device connections. Blood pressure is best assessed manually using a Doppler ultrasound probe and sphygmomanometer.[45] If the aortic valve opens and the patient has a consistent pulse, the opening pressure likely represents the systolic pressure. However, if a patient has minimal or inconsistent pulsatility, the opening pressure is more likely an estimate of the mean arterial pressure. The centrifugal pumps are afterload-sensitive pumps, and typical mean arterial pressure targets are between 75 and 90 mm Hg.[46] Mean arterial pressures greater than or equal to 90 mm Hg may lead to diminished forward flow and increased risk of stroke.[47,48]

Device Interrogation

Monitoring of device parameters provides significant insight into the hemodynamic status of the patient. Device parameters include speed (in revolutions per minute), power (in watts), estimated flow (L/min), and, in the HeartMate devices, pulsatility index: waveforms should be analyzed for HeartWare LVAD devices.[49] Device parameters should be reviewed each visit to assess for trends or acute changes (see **Table 78.4**).[50] Pump flows in centrifugal devices are calculated as a function of the set speed, power consumption, and blood viscosity (hematocrit). The flow is proportional to the speed and power consumption and inversely correlated to the blood viscosity. The pulsatility index corresponds to magnitude of flow through the LVAD averaged over 15-second intervals and is a specific parameter for HeartMate devices (**Figure 78.2**).

Diagnostic Laboratory Tests

Laboratory testing particularly relevant to LVAD patients includes evaluation for anemia, international normalized ratio (INR) with predefined anticoagulation goals, and hemolysis. Screening for hemolysis is done by plasma-free hemoglobin (>40 mg/dL specific for hemolysis) and lactate dehydrogenase (2.5× the upper limit of normal, >600 IU) and should be performed routinely during follow-up evaluation.[47]

Imaging

Echocardiography is essential for assessment of LVAD function. Key parameters include right and left ventricular function, inflow cannula position and orientation, inflow and outflow velocities, left ventricular dimensions, aortic valve excursion, valvular pathology, and vena cava size. Speed adjustments during echocardiography allow for optimization of LVAD speed and can assist in diagnosing LVAD dysfunction.[51]

Comprehensive guidelines for echocardiographic imaging of LVAD patients have been published.[52] Recommended surveillance intervals include postoperative week 2, and at 1, 3, 6, and 12 months for stable patients and then every 6 to 12 months thereafter.

Cardiac computed tomography (CT) angiography is used to diagnose cannula malposition, outflow graft kinking, narrowing, or thrombosis.[53] In cases of suspected infection when CT scan is unrevealing, nuclear imaging with radioisotope-tagged white blood cells can help identify the presence and extent of infection.[54]

CHRONIC MANAGEMENT

Neurohormonal Antagonists

Neurohormonal antagonists should be continued after LVAD implantation to treat blood pressure, regulate intravascular volume, and abrogate progressive myocardial remodeling.[55] Diuretics are used to treat volume overload. Angiotensin-converting enzyme inhibitors or angiotensin II receptor blockers treat hypertension and additionally have been shown to reduce the incidence of gastrointestinal (GI) bleeding in LVAD patients.[56] Additional antihypertensive medications can be used to achieve optimal blood pressure goals, and pulmonary vasodilators have been used to treat persistent elevations in PVR after LVAD.

Antithrombotic Therapy

Warfarin is used to prevent pump thrombosis, and INR goals are typically 2 to 3. These goals can be increased in patients with a history of pump thrombosis despite therapeutic INR or decreased in the setting of recurrent bleeding. The device manufacturer recommends daily aspirin dose 81 mg in HeartMate devices and 325 mg for the HeartWare LVAD.[47]

TABLE 78.4 Characteristics of HeartMate II, HeartWare, and HeartMate III

Device	Speed (rpm)	Average Speed (rpm)	Flow	Intrinsic Pulse	Pulsatility Index	Speed Adjustments and Testing
HeartMate II	6000-15,000	9400	Axial	No	4-6	400 rpm increments (8000 to 12,000 rpm)
HeartWare	1800-6000	2800	Centrifugal	Optional Lavare Cycle 200 rpm ramp down for 2 sec and increase 400 rpm for 1 sec. This 3-sec cycle repeated every minute	2-4 L/min difference between peak and trough	100 rpm increments 2400 to 3200 rpm
HeartMate III	4800-6500	5400	Centrifugal	Yes every 2 sec, 2000 rpm decrease from set speed for 0.15 s and then increase by 4000 rpm for 0.2 s	1-4	100 rpm increments (4600 to 6200 rpm)

L, liters; min,. minutes; rpm, revolutions per minute; sec, seconds

Reprinted by permission from Springer: Albert CL, Estep JD. How to optimize patient sSelection and device performance of the newest generation left ventricular assist devices. *Curr Treat Options Cardiovasc Med.* 2019;21(9):48. Copyright © 2019 Springer Nature.

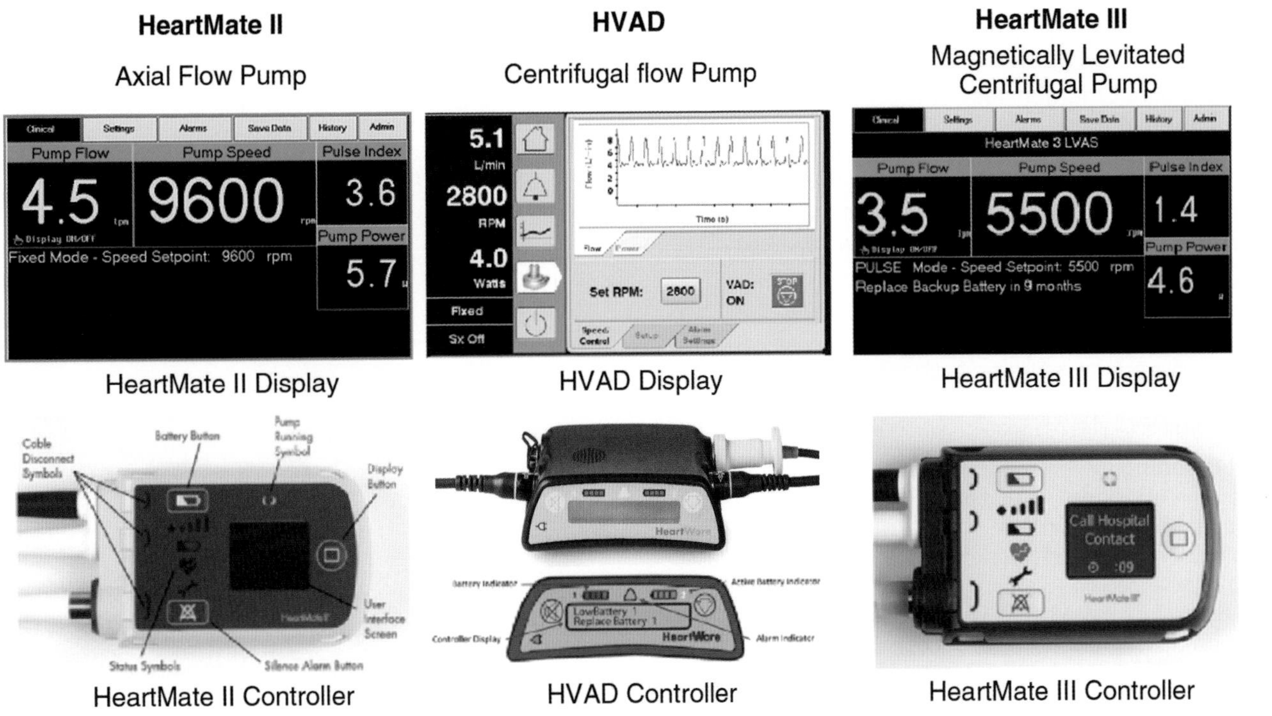

FIGURE 78.2 Left ventricular assist devices (LVADs) display screens and controllers. The HeartMate devices display pump flow, pump speed, pump power, and pulsatility index (top panel). The HeartWare ventricular assist device (HVAD) provides pump flow, pump speed, and pump power in addition to flow waveforms. The HeartMate devices have similar controllers. The LVAD drivelines connect to the controllers, which can be connected to batteries or an electrical outlet. HeartMate II and HeartMate 3 are trademarks of Abbott or its related companies. Reproduced with permission of Abbott, © 2021. All rights reserved. HeartWare HVAD Controller images reproduced with permission of Medtronic.

Device Therapy

The majority of LVAD patients have a preexisting ICD. Patients without an existing ICD typically do not require de novo ICD unless there is a significant history of ventricular arrhythmias. For patients with biventricular pacing, there is no clear benefit of continuing cardiac resynchronization therapy.[57]

COMPLICATIONS OF LEFT VENTRICULAR ASSIST DEVICES

See **Table 78.5** for a summary of assessment and treatment of LVAD complications.

Neurologic Emergencies

Ischemic and hemorrhagic stroke remain a substantial cause of mortality and morbidity in LVAD patients. The annual incidence is roughly 9%, accounting for 19% of deaths and shows a bimodal distribution with the highest risk being in the perioperative period and then 1 year after implant. Most of the neurologic events in LVADs are cardioembolic in nature.[58,59] In the ENDURANCE trial, the HeartWare LVAD was associated with higher incidence of stroke compared to the HeartMate II device, although stricter blood pressure control was associated with improvement in the incidence of stroke.[48] The HeartMate III has been associated with lesser incidence of strokes compared to HeartMate II, but no head-to-head comparisons have been available with the HeartWare device.[60] Other predisposing factors to neurologic events include inadequate anticoagulation, driveline infection, uncontrolled hypertension, and stasis because of pump inflow or outflow obstruction. Early diagnosis and immediate assessment are crucial, and if applicable, the stroke team should be activated with immediate assessment of INR and emergent CT brain evaluation. In case of hemorrhagic stroke, INR reversal (with vitamin K, fresh frozen plasma, and/or prothrombin protein complex in rare cases) and neurosurgical consultation remain the mainstay of therapy. Hemorrhagic strokes may also be associated with mycotic aneurysms associated with LVAD infections.[61] Ischemic strokes may be treated with mechanical thrombectomy.

Left Ventricular Assist Device Infection

Most LVAD infections originate from the driveline exit site and may range from local cellulitis to systemic pump infections. Infections occur in 15% to 30% of LVAD recipients and are most commonly caused by *Pseudomonas* or *Staphylococcus*. LVAD infections are associated with trauma to the driveline site, younger age, obesity, and exposed driveline velour.[62] Evaluation includes driveline drainage cultures, blood cultures, and imaging with CT or positron emission tomography scan to assess for drainable collections. Treatment strategies include intravenous antibiotics in tandem with surgical debridement (with or without antibiotic bead placement). This is followed by oral suppressive therapy. Pump exchange is invariably associated with recurrent infections, and cardiac transplantation is the only definitive treatment of LVAD infections.

TABLE 78.5 Assessment and Treatment of Left Ventricular Assist Device Complications

Neurologic Emergencies
Activate stroke team
Hold anticoagulation until imaging and INR obtained
Obtain head CT
Ischemic stroke—order CT angiogram head and neck, MAP optimization to ensure perfusion, endovascular thrombectomy if indicated
Hemorrhagic stroke—INR reversal, neurosurgery evaluation

LVAD Infection
Obtain driveline drainage cultures and blood cultures
CT or PET scan imaging
Intravenous antibiotics followed by chronic suppressive antibiotics
Surgical debridement with or without antibiotic beads placement
Transplant in eligible candidates if advanced local infection but no evidence of active bacteremia

GI Bleeding
Assessment of hemodynamic status
Hold aspirin and warfarin
Consider reversal of anticoagulation if hemodynamically unstable
Transfuse as needed
GI consult for colonoscopy for lower GI bleeding and EGD/enteroscopy for upper GI bleeding
If rapid bleeding, tagged RBC scan recommended
If source identified and massive bleeding present may consider IR embolization
Lowering goal INR and/or decreasing/discontinuing antiplatelet therapy for recurrent bleeding
Long-term agents like octreotide (somatostatin analogue), thalidomide (antiangiogenic agent), and danazol may be considered

Ventricular Arrhythmias
Assessment of hemodynamic status
Defibrillation if hemodynamically unstable
If stable, obtain echocardiogram and/or speed optimization for a reversible cause
Antiarrhythmic drugs
Catheter ablation for select cases of scar VT

Heart Failure
Assess left-sided vs right-sided or biventricular HF
For left-sided or biventricular HF
- Systemic vasodilators for hypertension
- If aortic insufficiency present, diuresis, increasing LVAD support, inotropic support, TAVR in select cases
- Pump speed optimization for inadequate unloading

For right-sided HF
- Diuretics
- Inotropic agents
- Pulmonary vasodilators
- Right ventricular assist device, if indicated

LVAD Malfunction
Assessment of hemodynamic status and check if VAD dependent
Evaluate device connections
Evaluate driveline for tear/fracture
Review LVAD flows and alarms
Check batteries and controller
Consult LVAD engineer

Pump Thrombosis
Assessment of hemodynamic status
Laboratory evaluation for markers of hemolysis
Echocardiography with ramp study (LVEDD is recorded at increasing LVAD speeds)
CT angiogram if concern for outflow graft thrombus
Intravenous heparin or direct thrombin inhibitors depending on INR
Pump exchange is definitive therapy and should be done promptly to avoid renal failure/end-organ damage
Increase goal INR and intensify antiplatelet therapy if preceding INRs are therapeutic.

CT, computed tomography; EGD, esophagogastroduodenoscopy; GI, gastrointestinal; HF, heart failure; INR, international normalized ratio; IR, interventional radiology; LVAD, left ventricular assist device; LVEDD, left ventricular end-diastolic diameter; MAP, mean arterial pressure; PET, positron emission tomography; RBC, red blood cells; TAVR, transcatheter aortic valve replacement; VT, ventricular tachycardia.

Gastrointestinal Bleeding

GI bleeding is one of the most frequent complications associated with high readmission rates. Patient presentations range from an asymptomatic decline in hemoglobin to fatigue/dyspnea because of chronic anemia or frank bleeding with hemodynamic instability. The bleeding is multifactorial and attributed to use of antithrombotic and antiplatelet therapy, acquired coagulopathy (because of shear stress by the pump), and formation of arteriovenous malformations in the gastric mucosa because of continuous flow.[63] Initial treatment includes assessment of hemodynamic status, discontinuing anticoagulation, transfusion as needed, and GI consultation. Active reversal of INR is not pursued unless the patient is hemodynamically unstable. Endoscopy, including capsule endoscopy, is usually warranted to locate arteriovenous malformations, and small bowel enteroscopy may be required if located in the jejunum.

For active bleeding, angiography, tagged red blood scans, or CT angiography may be used to locate the culprit site, and embolization by interventional radiology may be required in refractory cases. In addition to adjusting anticoagulation and antiplatelet therapies, long-term agents for recurrent events include octreotide (somatostatin analogue), omega-3 fatty acids, thalidomide (antiangiogenic agent), and danazol.[64]

Ventricular Arrhythmias

The reported prevalence of ventricular arrhythmias following LVAD implant varies from 22% to 59%.[65,66] Mechanisms of the ventricular arrhythmias include suction events (high speeds, hypovolemia, cannula malposition), scar related, and withdrawal of beta-blockers.[67] Although ventricular arrhythmias may be initially tolerated, progressive right ventricular failure can result in diminished LVAD flows and hemodynamic instability. Initial evaluation involves assessment of hemodynamic stability, echocardiogram to rule out any treatable etiology like hypovolemia or suction because of high speed, and need for antiarrhythmic therapy or defibrillation. Catheter ablation of ventricular tachycardia (VT) may be considered in selected cases.

Heart Failure

HF in LVAD patients can result from late right ventricular failure, persistent left HF, and biventricular failure. Left heart and biventricular HF could be attributed to hypertension, LVAD dysfunction (because of pump thrombosis or technical fault), aortic insufficiency, and inadequate left ventricular unloading. Treating the underlying etiology is essential. Hypertension responds to adjusting or adding systemic vasodilators. Management of aortic insufficiency is challenging and treatment involves diuresis, increasing LVAD speed, and possible inotropic support.[68] If the patient is not a candidate for transplant, surgical aortic valve replacement may be required. In case of inadequate left ventricular unloading, speed optimization via echocardiography and catheterization should be performed to achieve optimal hemodynamics. Right ventricular failure may be acute or chronic. Chronic right ventricular failure may present months to years after implant, with signs of venous congestion, increased diuretic requirements, and decreased LVAD flows and pulsatility.[69] The etiology is complex and has not been fully elucidated but may be attributed to distortion of right ventricular geometry or progressive myocardial dysfunction. Severe right ventricular failure in LVAD patients necessitates consideration for transplantation.

Left Ventricular Assist Device Malfunction

LVAD malfunction or failure may result from a variety of causes, including electrical malfunction and pannus formation or thrombosis. Mechanical pump failure is extremely rare with current devices. Electrical malfunction typically presents with LVAD alarms or pump stoppage. Initial evaluation involves hemodynamic assessment followed by examining device connections and the driveline, reviewing LVAD alarms and flows, and ensuring the controller is connected to the power source and the batteries are charged. Controller exchange should be performed by well-trained personnel because of the potential for hemodynamic collapse during temporary pump stoppage.[70]

Pump Thrombosis

LVAD thrombosis can occur on the inflow cannula, pump, or outflow graft.[71] Predisposing factors are inadequate antithrombotic or antiplatelet therapy, low pump speed, driveline infection, outflow graft stenosis or obstruction, interruption of anticoagulation, and cannula malposition (**Figure 78.3**). The clinical presentation varies from asymptomatic hemolysis, high-power or low-flow alarms, multiorgan failure, or even cardiogenic shock. Laboratory markers of hemolysis and echocardiographic evaluation with speed adjustments aid in diagnosis. CT angiography may help identify an outflow graft thrombus. Administration of intravenous heparin or direct thrombin inhibitors is recommended if thrombus is detected. Definitive therapy is pump exchange. Thrombolytics like recombinant tissue-type plasminogen activator (rt-PA) or glycoprotein IIb/IIIa inhibitors have also been used in stable patients. After initial therapy, the INR goal is intensified, and antiplatelet therapy is intensified with the addition of clopidogrel or dipyridamole.

SPECIAL CONSIDERATIONS

Recovery

Sufficient myocardial recovery with the subsequent explanation of an LVAD has been reported in about 1% to 2% of the cases, but limited data are available on long-term outcomes. A European registry demonstrated excellent survival after LVAD explanation, with only a minority of the patients relapsing.[72] However, there are potential concerns regarding LVAD explanation. Moreover, if hardware remains inside the heart, anticoagulation has to be continued because of the risk of thrombosis. A recent study demonstrated that LVAD therapy combined with the standardized guideline-directed medical therapy improvement in left ventricular ejection fraction reached explantation criteria over 18 months follow-up and maintained their left ventricular ejection fraction the following year after explantation.[73]

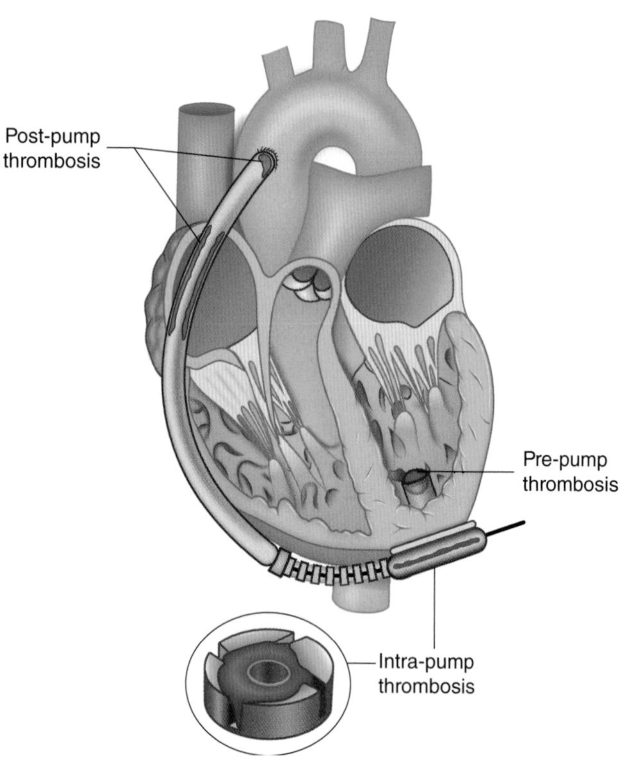

FIGURE 78.3 Left ventricular assist devices thrombosis sites.

Transplantation

LVADs are known to improve survival for patients on the cardiac transplant wait-list, but their effects on morbidity and survival after a heart transplantation remain unclear. Device-related complications may adversely affect the posttransplant outcomes. Right HF while on LVAD support may result in posttransplant vasoplegia and primary graft dysfunction. Alloimmunization may also limit donor selection and increase rejection risk after transplantation.[74]

Palliative Care and Shared Decision Making

End-of-life care in LVAD patients requires preimplantation discussions and assessments of goals of care including circumstances for LVAD deactivation.[75] Shared decision making between the patient, caregivers, and health care team can help prevent ethical dilemmas related to end-of-life issues for LVAD patients. A multidisciplinary team approach is required prior to LVAD implantation to provide education on benefits and complications associated with LVADs, as well as outlining advanced directives in LVAD patients.[76]

FUTURE DIRECTIONS

LVADs have evolved over the last five decades. Further refinement of the technology will likely result in decreased complications and improved long-term survival. Future developments include completely implantable micro-pumps with subcutaneously charging battery unit to avoid driveline infections and improve quality of life. Smaller pumps, though they may provide less support, can be implanted earlier and percutaneously and may aid in myocardial recovery or used in conjunction with guideline-directed medical therapy for extended support. The potentially can obviate the need for transplant or surgically implanted pumps.[77] Finally, a contemporary total artificial heart that provides full biventricular support, either as a bridge to transplant or as destination therapy, will be key for patients with right ventricular failure, biventricular failure, and restrictive cardiomyopathies.[78]

KEY POINTS

- ✔ LVAD therapy is indicated for patients with severe left ventricular systolic dysfunction and Stage D (end-stage) HF.
- ✔ Appropriate selection of candidates with attention to comorbid conditions such as renal, hepatic, and pulmonary disease is important to ensure optimal outcomes.
- ✔ Surgical implantation of the LVADs is best performed at high-volume centers. Right ventricular assessment before, during, and after surgery is essential.
- ✔ Patients are managed with neurohormonal antagonists and anticoagulation after LVAD implantation. Combined imaging and catheterization can be utilized to optimize LVAD settings.
- ✔ Complications of LVADs include cerebrovascular accidents (hemorrhagic and thrombotic), driveline and device infections, mucosal bleeding, and right ventricular failure.
- ✔ Pump thrombosis and malfunction can occur after LVAD implantation. Laboratory testing, imaging including echocardiography and CT scan, and catheterization can be utilized to diagnose and identify the location of pump thrombosis.

REFERENCES

1. Benjamin EJ, Blaha MJ, Chiuve SE, et al. Heart disease and stroke statistics-2017 update: a report from the American Heart Association. *Circulation.* 2017;135:e146-e603.
2. Miller LW, Pagani FD, Russell SD, et al. Use of a continuous-flow device in patients awaiting heart transplantation. *N Engl J Med.* 2007;357:885-896.
3. Rose EA, Gelijns AC, Moskowitz AJ, et al. Long-term use of a left ventricular assist device for end-stage heart failure. *N Engl J Med.* 2001;345:1435-1443.
4. Slaughter MS, Rogers JG, Milano CA, et al. Advanced heart failure treated with continuous-flow left ventricular assist device. *N Engl J Med.* 2009;361:2241-2251.
5. Elhenawy AM, Algarni KD, Rodger M, et al. Mechanical circulatory support as a bridge to transplant candidacy. *J Card Surg.* 2011;26:542-547.
6. Farrar DJ, Holman WR, McBride LR, et al. Long-term follow-up of Thoratec ventricular assist device bridge-to-recovery patients successfully

removed from support after recovery of ventricular function. *J Heart Lung Transplant.* 2002;21:516-521.
7. Stevenson LW, Couper G. On the fledgling field of mechanical circulatory support. *J Am Coll Cardiol.* 2007;50:748-751.
8. Estep JD, Starling RC, Horstmanshof DA, et al. Risk assessment and comparative effectiveness of left ventricular assist device and medical management in ambulatory heart failure patients: results from the ROADMAP study. *J Am Coll Cardiol.* 2015;66:1747-1761.
9. Jorde UP, Kushwaha SS, Tatooles AJ, et al. Results of the destination therapy post-food and drug administration approval study with a continuous flow left ventricular assist device: a prospective study using the INTERMACS registry (Interagency Registry for Mechanically Assisted Circulatory Support). *J Am Coll Cardiol.* 2014;63:1751-1757.
10. Park SJ, Liao KK, Segurola R, Madhu KP, Miller LW. Management of aortic insufficiency in patients with left ventricular assist devices: a simple coaptation stitch method (Park's stitch). *J Thorac Cardiovasc Surg.* 2004;127:264-266.
11. Feldman CM, Silver MA, Sobieski MA, Slaughter MS. Management of aortic insufficiency with continuous flow left ventricular assist devices: bioprosthetic valve replacement. *J Heart Lung Transplant.* 2006;25:1410-1412.
12. Rao V, Slater JP, Edwards NM, Naka Y, Oz MC. Surgical management of valvular disease in patients requiring left ventricular assist device support. *Ann Thorac Surg.* 2001;71:1448-1453.
13. Slaughter MS, Pagani FD, Rogers JG, et al. Clinical management of continuous-flow left ventricular assist devices in advanced heart failure. *J Heart Lung Transplant.* 2010;29:S1-S39.
14. Kanwar MK, Rajagopal K, Itoh A, et al. Impact of left ventricular assist device implantation on mitral regurgitation: an analysis from the MOMENTUM 3 trial. *J Heart Lung Transplant.* 2020;39:529-537.
15. Cork DP, Adamson R, Gollapudi R, Dembitsky W, Jaski B. Percutaneous repair of postoperative mitral regurgitation after left ventricular assist device implant. *Ann Thorac Surg.* 2018;105:e45-e46.
16. Wang TS, Hernandez AF, Felker GM, Milano CA, Rogers JG, Patel CB. Valvular heart disease in patients supported with left ventricular assist devices. *Circ Heart Fail.* 2014;7:215-222.
17. Krishan K, Nair A, Pinney S, Adams DH, Anyanwu AC. Liberal use of tricuspid-valve annuloplasty during left-ventricular assist device implantation. *Eur J Cardiothorac Surg.* 2012;41:213-217.
18. Atluri P, Fairman AS, MacArthur JW, et al. Continuous flow left ventricular assist device implant significantly improves pulmonary hypertension, right ventricular contractility, and tricuspid valve competence. *J Card Surg.* 2013;28:770-775.
19. Saeed D, Kidambi T, Shalli S, et al. Tricuspid valve repair with left ventricular assist device implantation: is it warranted? *J Heart Lung Transplant.* 2011;30:530-535.
20. Simonneau G, Montani D, Celermajer DS, et al. Haemodynamic definitions and updated clinical classification of pulmonary hypertension. *Eur Respir J.* 2019;53(1):1801913.
21. Mehra MR, Kobashigawa J, Starling R, et al. Listing criteria for heart transplantation: International Society for Heart and Lung Transplantation guidelines for the care of cardiac transplant candidates—2006. *J Heart Lung Transplant.* 2006;25:1024-1042.
22. Selim AM, Wadhwani L, Burdorf A, Raichlin E, Lowes B, Zolty R. Left ventricular assist devices in pulmonary hypertension group 2 with significantly elevated pulmonary vascular resistance: a bridge to cure. *Heart Lung Circ.* 2019;28:946-952.
23. Tsukashita M, Takayama H, Takeda K, et al. Effect of pulmonary vascular resistance before left ventricular assist device implantation on short- and long-term post-transplant survival. *J Thorac Cardiovasc Surg.* 2015;150:1352-1360, 1361.e1-e2.
24. Gulati G, Ruthazer R, DeNofrio D, Vest AR, Kent D, Kiernan MS. Understanding longitudinal changes in pulmonary vascular resistance after left ventricular assist device implantation. *J Card Fail.* 2021;27(5):552-559.
25. Russell SD, Rogers JG, Milano CA, et al. Renal and hepatic function improve in advanced heart failure patients during continuous-flow support with the HeartMate II left ventricular assist device. *Circulation.* 2009;120:2352-2357.
26. Bansal N, Hailpern SM, Katz R, et al. Outcomes associated with left ventricular assist devices among recipients with and without end-stage renal disease. *JAMA Intern Med.* 2018;178:204-209.
27. Walther CP, Niu J, Winkelmayer WC, et al. Implantable ventricular assist device use and outcomes in people with end-stage renal disease. *J Am Heart Assoc.* 2018;7(14):e008664.
28. Demirozu ZT, Etheridge WB, Radovancevic R, Frazier OH. Results of HeartMate II left ventricular assist device implantation on renal function in patients requiring post-implant renal replacement therapy. *J Heart Lung Transplant.* 2011;30:182-187.
29. Gelow JM, Desai AS, Hochberg CP, Glickman JN, Givertz MM, Fang JC. Clinical predictors of hepatic fibrosis in chronic advanced heart failure. *Circ Heart Fail.* 2010;3:59-64.
30. Clerkin KJ, Naka Y, Mancini DM, Colombo PC, Topkara VK. The impact of obesity on patients bridged to transplantation with continuous-flow left ventricular assist devices. *JACC Heart Fail.* 2016;4:761-768.
31. Jeng EI, Miller AH, Friedman J, et al. Ventricular assist device implantation and bariatric surgery: a route to transplantation in morbidly obese patients with end-stage heart failure. *ASAIO J.* 2021;67:163-168.
32. Kirklin JK, Naftel DC, Pagani FD, et al. Seventh INTERMACS annual report: 15,000 patients and counting. *J Heart Lung Transplant.* 2015;34:1495-1504.
33. Adamson RM, Stahovich M, Chillcott S, et al. Clinical strategies and outcomes in advanced heart failure patients older than 70 years of age receiving the HeartMate II left ventricular assist device: a community hospital experience. *J Am Coll Cardiol.* 2011;57:2487-2495.
34. Holdy K, Dembitsky W, Eaton LL, et al. Nutrition assessment and management of left ventricular assist device patients. *J Heart Lung Transplant.* 2005;24:1690-1696.
35. Eshelman AK, Mason S, Nemeh H, Williams C. LVAD destination therapy: applying what we know about psychiatric evaluation and management from cardiac failure and transplant. *Heart Fail Rev.* 2009;14:21-28.
36. McGee E Jr, Danter M, Strueber M, et al. Evaluation of a lateral thoracotomy implant approach for a centrifugal-flow left ventricular assist device: The LATERAL clinical trial. *J Heart Lung Transplant.* 2019;38:344-351.
37. Dang NC, Topkara VK, Mercando M, et al. Right heart failure after left ventricular assist device implantation in patients with chronic congestive heart failure. *J Heart Lung Transplant.* 2006;25:1-6.
38. Deng MC, Loebe M, El-Banayosy A, et al. Mechanical circulatory support for advanced heart failure: effect of patient selection on outcome. *Circulation.* 2001;103:231-237.
39. Atluri P, Goldstone AB, Fairman AS, et al. Predicting right ventricular failure in the modern, continuous flow left ventricular assist device era. *Ann Thorac Surg.* 2013;96:857-863; discussion 863-864.
40. Cordtz J, Nilsson JC, Hansen PB, et al. Right ventricular failure after implantation of a continuous-flow left ventricular assist device: early haemodynamic predictors. *Eur J Cardiothorac Surg.* 2014;45:847-853.
41. Raina A, Seetha Rammohan HR, Gertz ZM, Rame JE, Woo YJ, Kirkpatrick JN. Postoperative right ventricular failure after left ventricular assist device placement is predicted by preoperative echocardiographic structural, hemodynamic, and functional parameters. *J Card Fail.* 2013;19:16-24.
42. Bellavia D, Iacovoni A, Scardulla C, et al. Prediction of right ventricular failure after ventricular assist device implant: systematic review and meta-analysis of observational studies. *Eur J Heart Fail.* 2017;19:926-946.
43. Kang G, Ha R, Banerjee D. Pulmonary artery pulsatility index predicts right ventricular failure after left ventricular assist device implantation. *J Heart Lung Transplant.* 2016;35:67-73.
44. Takeda K, Naka Y, Yang JA, et al. Outcome of unplanned right ventricular assist device support for severe right heart failure after implantable left ventricular assist device insertion. *J Heart Lung Transplant.* 2014;33:141-148.
45. Lanier GM, Orlanes K, Hayashi Y, et al. Validity and reliability of a novel slow cuff-deflation system for noninvasive blood pressure monitoring in

patients with continuous-flow left ventricular assist device. *Circ Heart Fail.* 2013;6:1005-1012.
46. Cowger JA, Shah P, Pagani FD, et al. Outcomes based on blood pressure in patients on continuous flow left ventricular assist device support: an Interagency Registry for Mechanically Assisted Circulatory Support analysis. *J Heart Lung Transplant.* 2020;39:441-453.
47. Feldman D, Pamboukian SV, Teuteberg JJ, et al. The 2013 International Society for Heart and Lung Transplantation Guidelines for mechanical circulatory support: executive summary. *J Heart Lung Transplant.* 2013;32:157-187.
48. Milano CA, Rogers JG, Tatooles AJ, et al. HVAD: the ENDURANCE supplemental trial. *JACC Heart Fail.* 2018;6:792-802.
49. Rich JD, Burkhoff D. HVAD flow waveform morphologies: theoretical foundation and implications for clinical practice. *ASAIO J.* 2017;63:526-535.
50. Albert CL, Estep JD. How to optimize patient selection and device performance of the newest generation left ventricular assist devices. *Curr Treat Options Cardiovasc Med.* 2019;21:48.
51. Uriel N, Morrison KA, Garan AR, et al. Development of a novel echocardiography ramp test for speed optimization and diagnosis of device thrombosis in continuous-flow left ventricular assist devices: the Columbia ramp study. *J Am Coll Cardiol.* 2012;60:1764-1775.
52. Stainback RF, Estep JD, Agler DA, et al. Echocardiography in the management of patients with left ventricular assist devices: recommendations from the American Society of Echocardiography. *J Am Soc Echocardiogr.* 2015;28:853-909.
53. Vivo RP, Kassi M, Estep JD, et al. MDCT assessment of mechanical circulatory support device complications. *JACC Cardiovasc Imaging.* 2015;8:100-102.
54. Kim J, Feller ED, Chen W, Liang Y, Dilsizian V. FDG PET/CT for early detection and localization of left ventricular assist device infection: impact on patient management and outcome. *JACC Cardiovasc Imaging.* 2019;12:722-729.
55. McCullough M, Caraballo C, Ravindra NG, et al. Neurohormonal blockade and clinical outcomes in patients with heart failure supported by left ventricular assist devices. *JAMA Cardiol.* 2020;5:175-182.
56. Converse MP, Sobhanian M, Taber DJ, Houston BA, Meadows HB, Uber WE. Effect of angiotensin II inhibitors on gastrointestinal bleeding in patients with left ventricular assist devices. *J Am Coll Cardiol.* 2019;73:1769-1778.
57. Gopinathannair R, Roukoz H, Bhan A, et al. Cardiac resynchronization therapy and clinical outcomes in continuous flow left ventricular assist device recipients. *J Am Heart Assoc.* 2018;7(12):e009091.
58. DeVore AD, Patel PA, Patel CB. Medical management of patients with a left ventricular assist device for the non-left ventricular assist device specialist. *JACC Heart Fail.* 2017;5:621-631.
59. Kormos RL, Cowger J, Pagani FD, et al. The Society of Thoracic Surgeons Intermacs database annual report: Evolving indications, outcomes, and scientific partnerships. *J Heart Lung Transplant.* 2019;38:114-126.
60. O'Horo JC, Abu Saleh OM, Stulak JM, Wilhelm MP, Baddour LM, Rizwan Sohail M. Left ventricular assist device infections: a systematic review. *ASAIO J.* 2018;64:287-294.
61. Trachtenberg BH, Cordero-Reyes AM, Aldeiri M, et al. Persistent blood stream infection in patients supported with a continuous-flow left ventricular assist device is associated with an increased risk of cerebrovascular accidents. *J Card Fail.* 2015;21:119-125.
62. Mehra MR, Uriel N, Naka Y, et al. A fully magnetically levitated left ventricular assist device—final report. *N Engl J Med.* 2019;380:1618-1627.
63. Suarez J, Patel CB, Felker GM, Becker R, Hernandez AF, Rogers JG. Mechanisms of bleeding and approach to patients with axial-flow left ventricular assist devices. *Circ Heart Fail.* 2011;4:779-784.
64. Tabit CE, Chen P, Kim GH, et al. Elevated angiopoietin-2 level in patients with continuous-flow left ventricular assist devices leads to altered angiogenesis and is associated with higher nonsurgical bleeding. *Circulation.* 2016;134:141-152.
65. Nakahara S, Chien C, Gelow J, et al. Ventricular arrhythmias after left ventricular assist device. *Circ Arrhythm Electrophysiol.* 2013;6:648-654.
66. Greet BD, Pujara D, Burkland D, et al. Incidence, predictors, and significance of ventricular arrhythmias in patients with continuous-flow left ventricular assist devices: a 15-year institutional experience. *JACC Clin Electrophysiol.* 2018;4:257-264.
67. Vollkron M, Voitl P, Ta J, Wieselthaler G, Schima H. Suction events during left ventricular support and ventricular arrhythmias. *J Heart Lung Transplant.* 2007;26:819-825.
68. Grant AD, Smedira NG, Starling RC, Marwick TH. Independent and incremental role of quantitative right ventricular evaluation for the prediction of right ventricular failure after left ventricular assist device implantation. *J Am Coll Cardiol.* 2012;60:521-528.
69. Rich JD, Gosev I, Patel CB, et al. The incidence, risk factors, and outcomes associated with late right-sided heart failure in patients supported with an axial-flow left ventricular assist device. *J Heart Lung Transplant.* 2017;36:50-58.
70. Singhvi A, Trachtenberg B. Left ventricular assist devices 101: shared care for general cardiologists and primary care. *J Clin Med.* 2019;8(10):1720.
71. Scandroglio AM, Kaufmann F, Pieri M, et al. Diagnosis and treatment algorithm for blood flow obstructions in patients with left ventricular assist device. *J Am Coll Cardiol.* 2016;67:2758-2768.
72. Antonides CFJ, Schoenrath F, de By T, et al. Outcomes of patients after successful left ventricular assist device explantation: a EUROMACS study. *ESC Heart Fail.* 2020;7:1085-1094.
73. Birks EJ, Drakos SG, Patel SR, et al. Prospective multicenter study of myocardial recovery using left ventricular assist devices (RESTAGE-HF [Remission from Stage D Heart Failure]): medium-term and primary end point results. *Circulation.* 2020;142:2016-2028.
74. Pal N, Gay SH, Boland CG, Lim AC. Heart transplantation after ventricular assist device therapy: benefits, risks, and outcomes. *Semin Cardiothorac Vasc Anesth.* 2020;24:9-23.
75. Pak ES, Jones CA, Mather PJ. Ethical challenges in care of patients on mechanical circulatory support at end-of-life. *Curr Heart Fail Rep.* 2020;17:153-160.
76. Allen LA, McIlvennan CK, Thompson JS, et al. Effectiveness of an intervention supporting shared decision making for destination therapy left ventricular assist device: the DECIDE-LVAD randomized clinical trial. *JAMA Intern Med.* 2018;178:520-529.
77. Annamalai SK, Esposito ML, Reyelt LA, et al. Abdominal positioning of the next-generation intra-aortic fluid entrainment pump (Aortix) improves cardiac output in a swine model of heart failure. *Circ Heart Fail.* 2018;11:e005115.
78. Kleinheyer M, Timms DL, Greatrex NA, Masuzawa T, Frazier OH, Cohn WE. Pulsatile operation of the BiVACOR TAH—motor design, control and hemodynamics. *Annu Int Conf IEEE Eng Med Biol Soc.* 2014;2014:5659-5662.

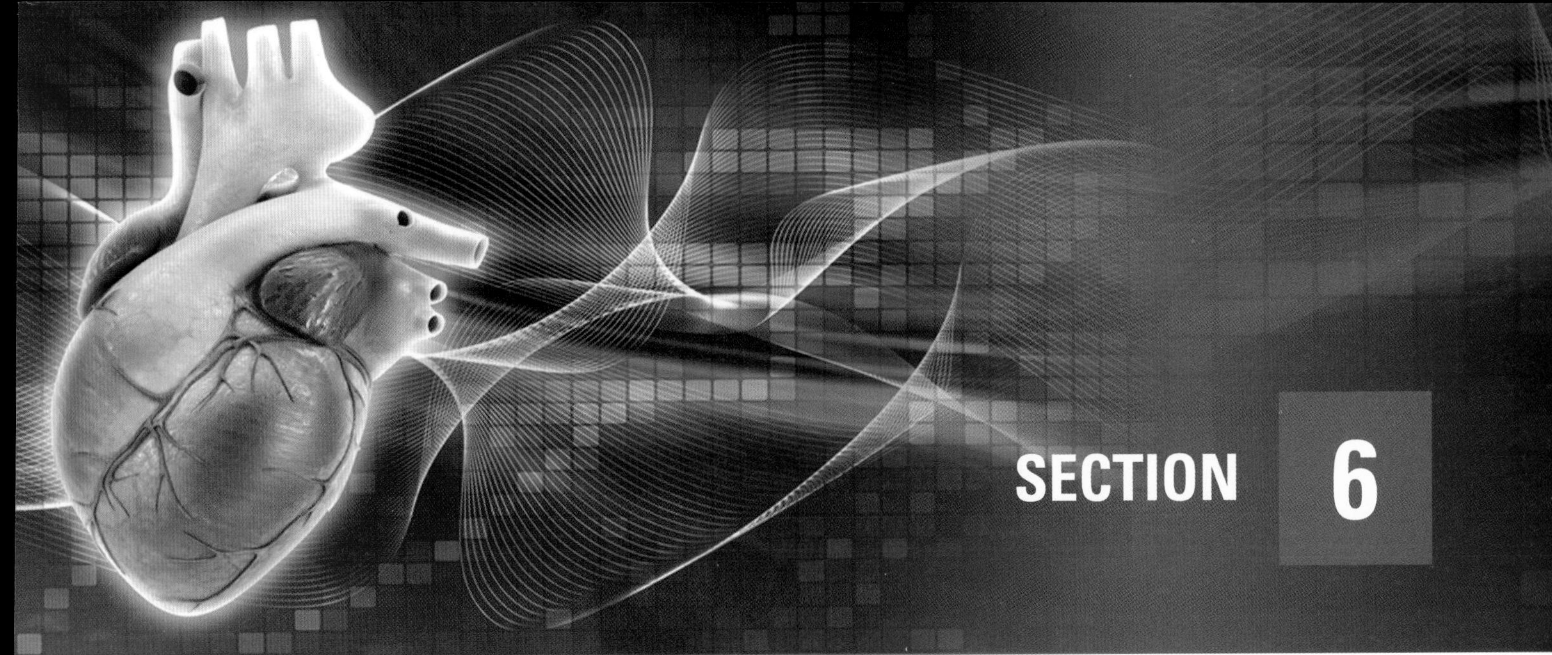

VASCULAR MEDICINE

SECTION EDITOR: Steve Bailey

CHAPTER 79

AORTIC DISEASES

Dawn S. Hui, Lalithapriya Jayakumar, and Andrea J. Carpenter

GENERAL INTRODUCTION

AORTIC DISSECTION

An aortic dissection is a tear in the aortic intima, with the separation of the intima and media and the creation of a false lumen. Clinical manifestations are related to structural changes in the aortic wall and the subsequent rheologic alterations, both in the aorta itself and in the branch vessels. Because all end-organ perfusion originates from the aorta, aortic dissection is one of the most fatal vascular diseases.

Epidemiology

In the United States, the estimated incidence of thoracic aortic dissection is 2.9 to 4.3 cases per 100,000 persons annually.[1] The increasing incidence over time is likely due to the growing use and improved quality of diagnostic imaging; however, the true incidence may remain underestimated due to the exclusion of prehospital deaths from studies. There is a gender and age differential, with the age-adjusted incidence of men being 5.2 compared with 2.2 per 100,000 in women.[2] The average age of onset is 65 years, although specific risk factors are associated with aortic dissection at a younger age, including connective tissue disorders, bicuspid aortic valve, inflammatory or infectious conditions leading to arteritis, a family history of aortic dissection, cocaine use, and pregnancy. Other risk factors associated with aortic dissection include male gender, hypertension, smoking, and atherosclerosis. A well-known risk factor is an aortic aneurysm, with dissection risk related to aneurysm diameter.

Pathogenesis

The sine qua non of an aortic dissection is an intimal tear. However, the inciting event leading to intimal disruption remains under investigation, with classical theory holding that the intimal tear is the inciting event. Newer evidence suggests an alternate theory highlighting the role of the tunica media.[3-5] This layer, rich in lamellar units with elastic laminae, smooth muscle cells, collagen fibers, and elastic fibers, provides the strength of the aortic wall, tolerating pressures up to 600 mm Hg.[3] Changes in medial architecture occur with processes such as cystic medial necrosis or ischemia from longstanding hypertension causing rupture of the vasa vasorum.[4] Medial weakness then leads to the intimal tear.

Regardless of the preceding events, the intimal tear occurs most commonly as a spontaneous event, while trauma and iatrogenic etiologies (such as coronary angiography) account for a minority of events. Pressurized blood flows through this tear, leading to progressive separation of the intima from the media and adventitia. This channel is known as the false lumen, with the intimo-medial septum ("intimal flap") separating it from the true lumen. As flowing blood propagates longitudinally, either antegrade or retrograde, more and more aortic segments become involved. Shear forces may produce additional tears along the aorta, leading to additional communication sites between the two lumens. Thrombus may develop, limiting propagation of the dissection.

Complications of dissection include malperfusion, aneurysm, and rupture. Malperfusion occurs when localized thrombus, or the intimal flap, obstructs the ostium of a branch vessel. The intimal flap location is dynamic and sensitive to relative true and false lumen pressurization. The compromised integrity of the media and adventitia can lead to aneurysmal dilation. If an aortic rupture occurs, the cardiac output is displaced into the extravascular space. Localized thrombi may limit egress of blood into the extravascular space (ie, "contained rupture"), but aortic rupture is a near-universally fatal event. Immediate treatment priorities in prehospital and emergency room settings are aimed at preventing or mitigating these complications until definitive treatment can be rendered.

CLINICAL PRESENTATION

The most common presenting symptom of an acute aortic dissection is pain in the chest (79%), back (47%), or abdomen (22%). Common descriptors of the pain include abrupt (85%), severe or "the worst ever" (90%), sharp (62%), and a tearing or ripping sensation (49%).[6] When malperfusion exists, symptoms related to the end-organ ischemia predominate, such as syncope or focal weakness with cerebrovascular malperfusion and extremity pain or numbness with extremity malperfusion. Visceral malperfusion may present as abdominal pain, nausea, vomiting, or renal failure.

The differential diagnosis is variable, depending on the presenting symptoms. Since many thoracic aortic dissection patients have risk factors for coronary artery atherosclerosis, the differential diagnosis includes myocardial ischemia or infarction (MI). Other chest pain- related differential diagnoses include pulmonary embolism or pneumonia. Because these diagnoses are generally more common or more often suspected than thoracic aortic dissection, workup including electrocardiogram (ECG), cardiac enzymes, or pulmonary embolism-protocol computed tomography (CT) can lead to a delay in the true diagnosis. Malperfusion syndromes may direct suspicion toward more localized processes, such as intra-abdominal processes in the case of visceral malperfusion, classical ischemic or hemorrhagic stroke in the case of cerebral malperfusion, and peripheral vascular disease in the case of extremity malperfusion. When malperfusion is advanced, particularly with visceral ischemia, mentation may be altered, limiting the reliability of the history or physical examination.

Propagation of the dissection into the aortic root can lead to a special subset of clinical sequelae. If the flap involves the coronary ostia leading to coronary malperfusion, the patient may present with a concomitant acute MI, clouding the picture or masking the true diagnosis. Aortic valve commissures may shear from their aortic wall attachments, leading to acute aortic insufficiency and acute heart failure.

Patients may not present for evaluation at the time of the initial dissection event. In etiologies such as catheter-induced dissection or trauma, the patient may not recall a history of symptoms. Rarely, the dissection may be undetected for years and discovered on chest imaging incidentally or due to symptoms from aneurysm degeneration of a longstanding dissection. The classification by time course is acute (≤2 weeks since the onset of symptoms), subacute (15-90 days from symptoms), and chronic (91 days or more).

DIAGNOSIS

History should focus on the characteristics and location of pain in addition to risk factors, particularly hypertension, known connective tissue disorders, bicuspid aortic valve, or a family history of dissection. Physical examination should include a focused heart and lung exam, a gross neurologic assessment, vascular exam, abdominal exam, and bilateral arm blood pressure measurement. ECG and chest radiography are routinely obtained in the acute evaluation of chest pain; chest radiograph may show a widened mediastinum or otherwise unexplained pleural effusion, raising the suspicion for thoracic aortic dissection.

The diagnostic test of choice is CT angiography (CTA). While magnetic resonance angiography has a sensitivity and specificity of ~100%, the long acquisition time and lack of emergent availability make it less desirable. In the contemporary era, multidetector helical CT (MDCT) is an excellent rapid, minimally invasive, and safe imaging modality. It allows assessment of both the thoracic and abdominal aorta. False-positive MDCT examinations can be minimized with attention to optimal contrast bolus timing, ECG gating to reduce motion artifact, and narrow collimation to improve resolution. False negatives can be minimized with "thin cuts" of images (ie, ≤3 mm). Recent studies have shown MDCT to have 100% sensitivity and specificity. Other modalities include angiography and transesophageal echocardiography which are invasive and require sedation. Transthoracic echocardiography, while noninvasive and not requiring sedation, has a sensitivity of only 59% to 85% and specificity of 93% to 96%, but it may be the initial test of choice for hemodynamically unstable patients.[7]

Because the differential for chest pain includes MI, pulmonary embolism, and thoracic aortic dissection, CT protocols to evaluate all three diagnoses in a single examination have been investigated. However, these protocols use higher contrast and radiation doses, often exclude the abdominal aorta, and lack data on sensitivity and specificity. If the clinical judgment can differentiate among the likelihood of these three diagnoses, the most appropriate test for that diagnosis should be chosen. Regardless, ECG and cardiac enzymes are recommended as part of the initial workup. D-dimer testing may be useful in differentiating pulmonary embolism and thoracic aortic dissection, with a serum D-dimer level less than 500 ng/dL less likely to be associated with aortic dissection.[8]

An important part of the evaluation includes the identification of the dissection location. The Stanford classification system is practical and widely used due to its simplicity in stratifying patients for treatment (**Figure 79.1**). Stanford type A thoracic aortic dissection is one involving the ascending aorta, regardless of whether the descending aorta is involved. Stanford type B thoracic aortic dissection involves only the descending aorta. This classification system becomes unclear when the dissection originates or propagates retrograde to the aortic arch, leading to the contemporary term "acute non-A non-B aortic dissection."[9] Which aortic segments need to be treated varies according to the extent of dissection, long-term rupture risk, and the surgeon's clinical judgment balancing operative complexity and benefit. The details of surgical repair exceed the scope of this chapter, but some references may be of interest to the reader.[9,10]

MANAGEMENT OF PATIENT

When a thoracic aortic dissection is suspected, immediate management priorities include (1) performing a prompt history and physical examination; (2) confirmation of diagnosis with testing; (3) minimizing the rupture risk and optimizing perfusion of the true lumen; and (4) excluding other cardiovascular diagnoses. The differential of MI, pulmonary embolism, and thoracic aortic dissection have important implications for treatment, due to the impact of immediate management decisions. Antiplatelet and anticoagulation therapy are indicated for acute coronary syndrome and pulmonary embolism respectively, but in the 39% of thoracic aortic dissections initially misdiagnosed, these therapies lead to worse outcomes.[11]

Immediate medical management of thoracic aortic dissection is blood pressure and heart rate control using medications that decrease pulsatile pressure in the aorta, including treating pain to mitigate the catecholamine surge. Goal systolic pressure is 100 to 120 mm Hg and heart rate is 60 to

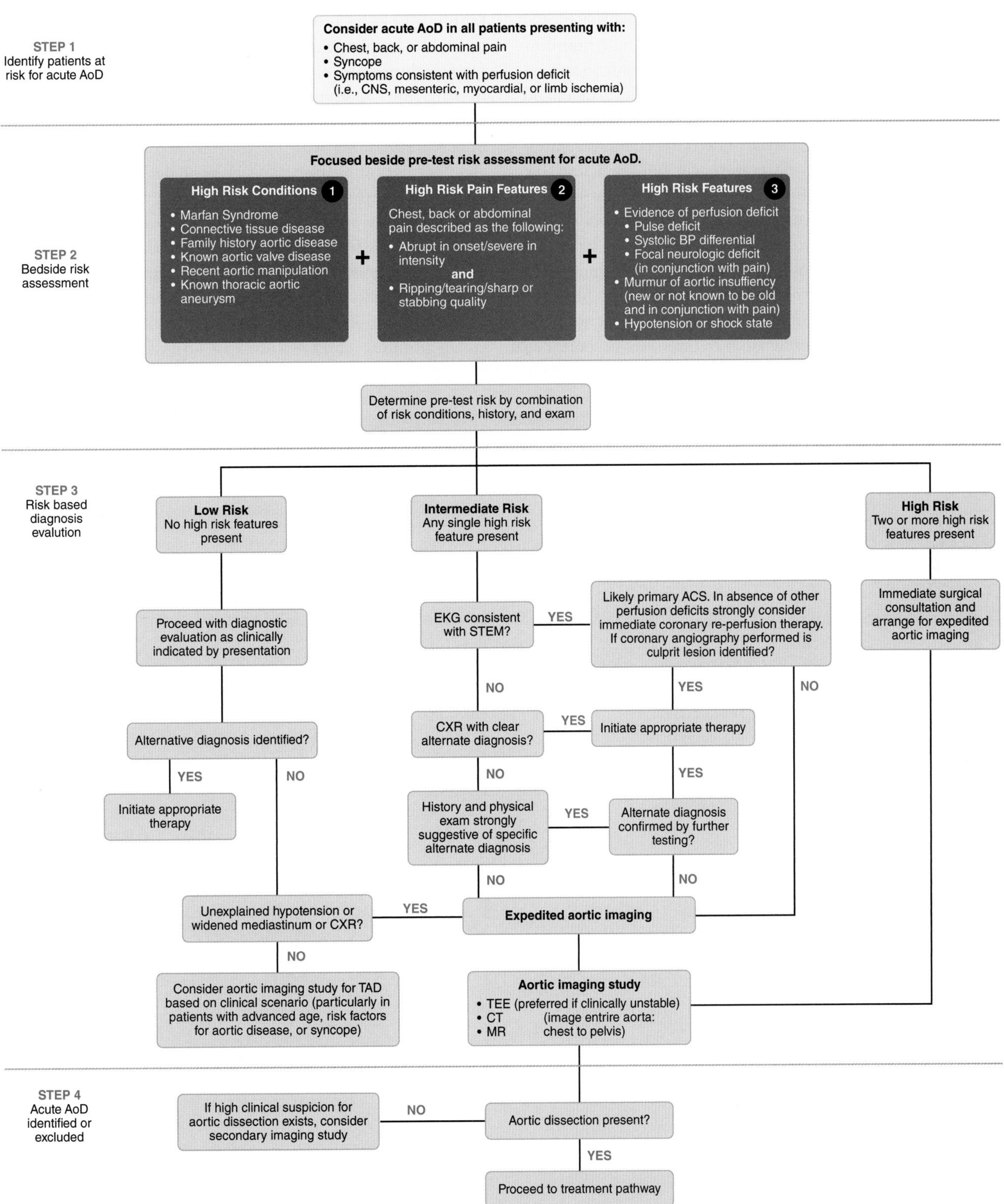

FIGURE 79.1 Flowchart for evaluation of suspected thoracic aortic dissection. AoD, aortic; dissection; BP, blood pressure; CNS, central nervous system; CT, computed tomography; CXR, chest radiograph; MR, magnetic resonance imaging; TAD, thoracic aortic dissection; TEE, transesophageal echocardiography. (Reprinted with permission from Hiratzka LF, Bakris GL, Beckman JA, et al. 2010 ACCF/AHA/AATS/ACR/ASA/SCA/SCAI/SIR/STS/SVM Guidelines for the Diagnosis and Management of Patients With Thoracic Aortic Disease: Executive Summary: A report of the American College of Cardiology Foundation/American Heart Association Task Force on Practice Guidelines, American Association for Thoracic Surgery, American College of Radiology, American Stroke Association, Society of Cardiovascular Anesthesiologists, Society for Cardiovascular Angiography and Interventions, Society of Interventional Radiology, Society of Thoracic Surgeons, and Society for Vascular Medicine. *Circulation.* 2010;121(13):1544–1579.)

80 beats per minute. A large-bore intravenous catheter should be placed for rapid resuscitation, and hemodynamic monitoring should be established. Short-acting intravenous agents are used due to the potential for rapid hemodynamic changes and instability. Beta-blockers are first-line agents given their effect on both blood pressure and heart rate (Class I, LOE C).[12] If vasodilators are initiated before heart rate control (Class III), reflex tachycardia may ensue, thereby increasing aortic shear stress. For patients with suspected or confirmed cocaine use, selection of a β-blocker with α and β dual receptor blockade, such as carvedilol or labetalol, is preferred to avoid unopposed α-stimulation. For patients who cannot tolerate β-blockade due to bradycardia, calcium channel blockers may be administered. Vasodilators are considered once heart rate is controlled (**Table 79.1**). Infusion concentrations should be maximized to avoid administering large volumes of crystalloid and subsequent volume overload. Intravenous opioids for pain may aid in managing hypertension. Finally, a blood sample for type and crossmatch should be submitted in anticipation of emergent intervention, along with electrolytes, complete blood count, and coagulation parameters. Metabolic derangements, as a sequela of malperfusion, should be promptly treated.

If patients present with or develop sudden hypotension, concern for acute rupture or hemopericardium with tamponade must be considered immediately. Permissive relative hypotension to a systolic blood pressure of 80 mm Hg and judicious administration of fluids may mitigate sequela of rupture, but emergent intervention is critical for survival.

TABLE 79.1 Antihypertensive Agents for Aortic Dissection

	Drug	Initial IV Dose	Infusion Dose	Onset/Duration of Action	Side Effects	Considerations
Beta-adrenergic receptor blockers	Esmolol	250-500 µg/kg over 1 minute	25-50 µg/kg/min, titrate up to max 300 µg/kg/min	1-2 minutes; 10-30 minutes	Nausea, flushing, bronchospasm, bradycardia, first-degree heart block	Nonhepatic, nonrenal clearance Avoid in acutely decompensated heart failure
	Labetalol	20 mg followed by 20-50 mg bolus every 10 minutes up to 300 mg	0.5-2 mg/min, titrate to max 10 mg/min	2-5 minutes; 2-6 hours	Nausea, vomiting, paresthesias, bronchospasm, dizziness, bradycardia, first-degree heart block	Avoid in acutely decompensated heart failure; use with caution in obstructive airway disease
Nondihydropyridine calcium channel blockers	Diltiazem	0.25-0.35 mg/kg	5-20 mg/hr	1-3 minutes, 0.5-10 hours	Nausea, bradycardia, first-degree heart block, dizziness	Avoid in acutely decompensated heart failure
	Verapamil	5-10 mg, may repeat in 5-10 minutes		3-5 minutes; 0.5-6 hours	Nausea, bradycardia, first-degree heart block, dizziness	Avoid in acutely decompensated heart failure
Vasodilators	Nitroprusside		0.25-0.5 µg/kg/min, titrate to max 10 µg/kg/min	Immediate; 1-10 minutes	Elevated intracranial pressure, decreased cerebral blood flow, reduced coronary flow in coronary artery disease, cyanide and thiocyanate toxicity, nausea, vomiting, muscle spasm, flushing, sweating	To minimize cyanide toxicity, infusion duration should be as short as possible and ≤2 µg/kg/min. For patients with higher doses (ie, >500 µg/kg and >2 µg/kg/min) administer sodium thiosulfate infusion to avoid cyanide toxicity.
	Nicardipine		2.5-5 mg/hr, titrate to max 15-30 mg/hr	5-15 minutes; 0.5-8 minutes	Tachycardia, headache, dizziness, nausea, flushing, local phlebitis, edema	

(continued)

TABLE 79.1 Antihypertensive Agents for Aortic Dissection (*continued*)

	Drug	Initial IV Dose	Infusion Dose	Onset/Duration of Action	Side Effects	Considerations
Second-line agents	Clevidipine		1-2 mg/hr, titrate up to 16 mg/hr	2-4 minutes; 5-15 minutes	Atrial fibrillation, nausea, lipid allergy	Nonrenal, nonhepatic clearance
	Nitroglycerin		5-200 µg/min	2-5 minutes; 5-10 minutes	Hypoxemia, reflex sympathetic activation with tachycardia, headache, vomiting, flushing, methemoglobinemia, tolerance	Useful in patients with coronary ischemia or acute pulmonary edema
	Enalaprilat	1.25-5 mg IV every 6 hr		15-30 minutes; 6 hours	Precipitous fall in pressure with high-renin states; variable response, headache, dizziness	Slow onset, variable response, long duration of effect; avoid in acute myocardial infarction, renal impairment, or pregnancy

IV, intravenous; hr, hour; kg, kilogram; mg, milligram; min, minutes; µg, microgramshr, hour.
Adapted from Black JH III, Manning WJ. Management of acute aortic dissection. In K.A. Collins (Ed.). UpToDate; 2019. Retrieved December 18, 2019 from https://www.uptodate.com/contents/management-of-acute-aortic-dissection; Hiratzka LF, Bakris GL, Beckman JA, et al. 2010 ACCF/AHA/AATS/ACR/ASA/SCA/SCAI/SIR/STS/SVM Guidelines for the Diagnosis and Management of Patients With Thoracic Aortic Disease: A report of the American College of Cardiology Foundation/American Heart Association Task Force on Practice Guidelines, American Association for Thoracic Surgery, American College of Radiology, American Stroke Association, Society of Cardiovascular Anesthesiologists, Society for Cardiovascular Angiography and Interventions, Society of Interventional Radiology, Society of Thoracic Surgeons, and Society for Vascular Medicine. *Circulation.* 2010;121:e266; Tsai TT, Nienaber CA, Eagle KA. Acute aortic syndromes. *Circulation.* 2005;112:3802; Marik PE, Rivera R. Hypertensive emergencies: an update. *Curr Opin Crit Care.* 2011;17:569.

MEDICAL VERSUS SURGICAL APPROACH

The management for thoracic aortic dissection is the emergent open surgical repair for Stanford type A dissection with a 30-day mortality of 26%, as opposed to a 58% survival for medical management. Conversely, medical management results in better outcomes for uncomplicated Stanford type B dissection (30-day mortality 10.7% vs 31.4% with open surgical management). Complicated Stanford type B thoracic aortic dissections (ie, with malperfusion, leak, or impending rupture) are best treated with immediate medical therapy followed promptly by surgical or endovascular repair (Class I, LOE B).[12,13] Advancements in thoracic endovascular aortic repair (TEVAR) have resulted in markedly improved long-term outcomes for type B thoracic aortic dissection compared to open surgical repair. Long-term benefits of medical therapy plus TEVAR versus medical therapy alone,[14] favor medical therapy plus early TEVAR in select patients even without evidence of malperfusion.

Percutaneous Intervention

In acute thoracic aortic dissection, the goals of TEVAR are to occlude the primary entry tear, re-establish flow to malperfused beds, and maintain existing perfusion to branch vessels. When the primary entry tear is successfully occluded, increased pressure in the true lumen relative to the false lumen leads to shifting of the dynamic intimal flap, increasing flow to the previously malperfused bed. The dissected layers may not completely reappose but with time the false lumen may thrombose, leading to long-term aortic remodeling and reduced risk of dilation and rupture. Additional tears along the aorta may contribute to continued false lumen perfusion. Whether to treat these additional tears at the index operation is a matter of clinical judgment involving assessment of organs that are primarily or exclusively supplied by false lumen flow, and the likelihood of false lumen thrombosis with time. Two other percutaneous techniques for branch vessel malperfusion include fenestration, in which additional communications between the true and false lumen are created to support flow to vessels arising from the false lumen and stenting of branch vessels.

Surgical Approaches

The standard of care for acute type A thoracic aortic dissection is emergent open surgical operation, with resection and replacement of the aortic portion containing the primary tear. Type A thoracic aortic dissection is associated with a high mortality and morbidity, due to involvement of the coronary arteries, aortic valve, and great vessels, or rupture leading to cardiac tamponade. Historic data suggests that acute type A thoracic aortic dissection carries a mortality rate of 1% per hour until definitively treated by surgical intervention. With improvements in imaging, early management of blood pressure and heart rate, and hospital transport, contemporary mortality rates are 0.15% per hour for surgically managed cases and 0.77% per hour for medically managed cases.[15]

PATIENT FOLLOW-UP CARE

Even after repair, thoracic aortic dissection carries a lifetime risk of future aortic events. Percutaneous and surgical intervention reduce the immediate risk of rupture but do not always result in complete reapposition of the layers, which is at risk of aneurysmal degeneration. This is best mitigated by risk factor modification. Patients are counseled on hypertension management, with optimal ambulatory systolic blood pressure 90 to 120 mm Hg (90-130 mm Hg patients with diabetes or renal disease). Ambulatory blood pressure monitoring and lifestyle changes—such as smoking cessation, physical activity, and reduction in dietary sodium—are part of this counseling. Other lifestyle modifications include avoiding increased intrathoracic pressures associated with chronic constipation, obstructive sleep apnea, Valsalva maneuvers, or isometric exercises such as weight- lifting. Dynamic, aerobic exercise is associated with only a moderate increase in blood pressure and should not be discouraged by clinicians. Guidelines do not specify a weight-lifting limit[11]; rather, patients who wish to maintain a weight-lifting program are counseled to lift to the point that they do not "bear down." Degeneration and dilation of chronic aortic aneurysms are typically asymptomatic. Serial imaging is recommended to chart the growth rate of the aneurysm and identify patients who may require intervention to prevent rupture. Following acute thoracic aortic dissection repair, imaging is recommended before hospital discharge and at 1, 6, and 12 months to identify early aneurysmal degeneration. If stable, annual imaging suffices thereafter. Subsequent intervention is recommended according to size criteria for aortic aneurysms.

Finally, family counseling is important given the familial patterns of aortopathy. First-degree relatives of patients who have experienced an aortic dissection should undergo imaging to assess for aneurysms. First-degree relatives of patients with bicuspid aortic valves should undergo an echocardiogram to evaluate for a bicuspid valve and proximal aortic dilation. Patients of a young age, a strong family history of aortopathy, or clinical features suggestive of genetic disorder may benefit from genetic testing for mutations; if positive, then first-degree relatives should also undergo genetic testing.

RESEARCH AND FUTURE DIRECTIONS

Areas of ongoing research in aortic dissection include prevention, workup, and management. There is no good screening test for future development of thoracic aortic dissection. Only a minority of patients with acute thoracic aortic dissection have known preoperative risk factors of connective tissue disorders, familial history, or bicuspid aortic valve. The remainder often has a history of hypertension or smoking, but most patients with these risk factors will not develop thoracic aortic dissection. While aortic aneurysm diameter size is a predisposing condition to thoracic aortic dissection, many occur at a diameter below the 5.5 cm recommended for prophylactic replacement.[16]

As discussed above, the differential for a patient with chest pain includes MI and pulmonary embolism. Identification of sensitive and specific biomarkers would expedite the care of these patients and potentially improve outcomes, especially given the dilemma of whether to administer antiplatelet or anticoagulant therapy in unstable patients.

For type A thoracic aortic dissection, surgical therapy is standard of care, but subgroups have demonstrated extreme mortality. Patients with malperfusion and severe acidosis (base deficit ≥ 10) have a 92% surgical mortality rate; those with abdominal malperfusion have a 100% mortality.[17] New algorithms propose correction of malperfusion using percutaneous techniques initially, followed by open surgical replacement.[18] Another surgical modification is the addition of concomitant antegrade stenting of the descending thoracic aorta at the time of surgical acute type A repair, with the goal of stabilizing the descending aorta and promoting aortic remodeling.[19,20]

Plaque Rupture/Penetrating Atherosclerotic Ulcer

Penetrating aortic ulcer (PAU) describes an entity in which ulceration of an atherosclerotic lesion penetrates the internal elastic lamina into the media. Of note, PAU is a disease of the intima (i.e. atherosclerosis), whereas aortic dissection and intramural hematoma are diseases of the media. Asymptomatic PAU without complications may be treated conservatively while PAU with persistent pain, with an intramural or periaortic haemorrhage should be treated surgically or with endovascular stenting.

Intramural Hematoma

In aortic intramural haematoma (IMH), hemorrhage occurs in the media of the aortic wall in the absence of a demonstrable two-lumen flow and primary intimal tear. Acute IMH accounts for ~6% of nontraumatic acute aortic syndromes. Involvement of the ascending aorta carries substantial mortality, and urgent or emergent operative or endovascular intervention is typically indicated, whereas arch and descending IMH are less likely to be associated with an adverse outcome and a nonsurgical initial approach may be appropriate[21]. Invasive treatment of type B IMH is indicated if maximum aortic diameter is >55 mm or mean growth rate is ≥5 mm/year.

AORTIC ANEURYSM

An aortic aneurysm is a localized dilation of all three layers of the aorta, defined as a 50% increase in diameter compared with a normal adjacent segment of aorta. Absolute size criteria are typically greater than or equal to 3 cm for an abdominal aortic aneurysm (AAA) and greater than or equal to 3.5 cm for a thoracic aortic aneurysm (TAA). Clinical manifestations are related to rupture (impending, acute, or chronic), rapid expansion, compression of nearby structures, thrombosis, distal embolic phenomena, or dissection.

EPIDEMIOLOGY

In the United States, the number of new cases of TAA and AAA has steadily increased since 1970.[22] This is attributed to improved diagnostic modalities, patient and physician awareness, and increased life expectancy. Risk factors include hypertension, smoking, and atherosclerotic arterial disease. Aortic aneurysmal disease tends to affect white men over age 65 with a history of tobacco use. While AAAs tend to arise as a result of atherosclerotic degeneration, 20% of TAAs are attributed to aneurysmal degeneration of chronic aortic dissection.[23]

In screening studies, the incidence of AAA is 3% to 5% across all age groups. The incidence increases steadily with age greater than 55 years; the male to female ratio is 4:1 until age 60 to 70 years, nearing 1:1 in those greater than or equal to 80 years of age. The incidence is increased in selected patient populations, such as those with coronary or peripheral atherosclerotic disease (5%-10%) and femoral or popliteal aneurysms (50%).[22] The incidence of TAA is 10.4 cases per 100,000, with a male to female ratio of 1.7:1.[24] Multiple aneurysms are present in 3.4% of TAAs and 13% of AAAs. There is a familial component in 15% to 25%.[25,26]

PATHOGENESIS OF AORTIC ANEURYSMS

The etiology of aortic aneurysm varies by location, with atherosclerotic degeneration causing 90% of AAA and medial degeneration causing 80% of TAA. The second-most common etiology for both is aneurysmal degeneration of a chronic aortic dissection. Uncommon causes include collagen vascular disorders (eg, vascular Ehler's Danlos syndrome-type IV, Marfan syndrome, Loeys-Dietz), aortitis, and autoimmune pathologies (eg, Takayasu's arteritis), and infectious etiologies (eg, tuberculous, mycotic, syphilitic, and HIV).[22,23]

The aortic wall is made up of mainly types I and III collagen, elastin, and vascular smooth muscle cells. Lamellar elastin units are more abundant in the thoracic aorta than the abdominal aorta, with a further abrupt decrease in the infrarenal abdominal aorta.[22] This finding, in addition to chronic inflammatory components and the mechanical differences between the thoracic and abdominal aorta (ie, more pulsatile motion in the abdominal portion), contributes to the elastin fragmentation found in histopathologic analysis of aortic aneurysms. The disruption and remodeling of the extracellular matrix in aortic aneurysms, specifically of collagen and elastin, led to the identification of matrix metalloproteinases (MMP-9) as important components in aneurysm formation. Systemic MMP levels are elevated in 50% of patients with aortic aneurysm, but not in those with aorto-occlusive disease. Interestingly, these levels decrease to normal after aortic aneurysm repair.[23]

Aneurysm enlargement is a gradual process. Rapid enlargement is an indication of instability or impending rupture and the need for urgent repair. Growth rates for both TAA and AAA are nonlinear, rendering individual growth rates unpredictable. But patterns have been established. The median growth rate is 0.5 cm per year for both TAA and AAA. However, growth rates increase as aneurysm size increases.[24] Aneurysm morphology analysis has shown that rupture occurs not at the greatest diameter but rather the area of maximum wall stress, which is influenced by the shape, curvature, thickness, calcification, shear stress, and mural thrombus.[27,28]

Multiple trials have evaluated rupture risk. The annual risk of rupture in AAA is 1% for aneurysms 4.0 to 5.4 cm in diameter. Each subsequent centimeter increase carries an annual 10% relative increase.[22] The steep increase in rupture risk beyond 5.0 cm is the basis for recommending elective aneurysm repair for AAA more than 5.0 cm in diameter (**Figure 79.2A,B**). TAA rupture risk rises even more dramatically, at 1% annually at less than or equal to 5.0 cm, 37.5% annually at 5.1 to 6.0 cm and 62.5% annually at more than 6 cm diameter.[29] Rapid growth (>1 cm/year), saccular morphology, systolic hypertension, female gender, and chronic obstructive pulmonary disease are other risk factors for rupture of both AAA and TAA.

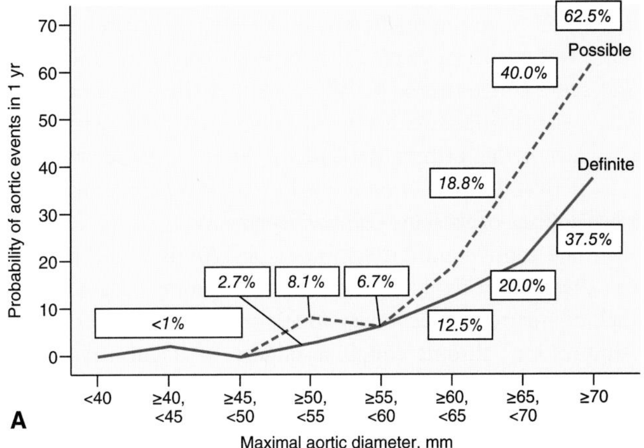

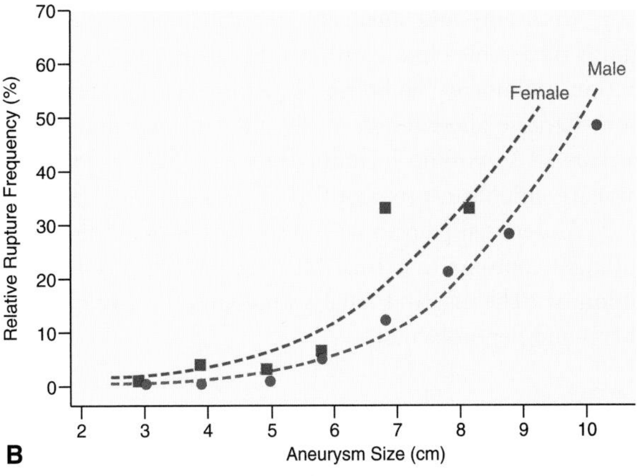

FIGURE 79.2 Rupture risk of descending thoracic aortic aneurysm according to aneurysm diameter **(A)** (Reprinted with permission from Kim JB, Kim K, Lindsay ME, et al. Risk of rupture or dissection in descending thoracic aortic aneurysm. *Circulation*. 2015;132(17):1620-1629. Copyright ©2015 American Heart Association, Inc.) and abdominal aortic aneurysm according to aneurysm diameter and modified by gender **(B)**. (Reprinted from Skibba AA, Evans JR, Hopkins SP, et al. Reconsidering gender relative to risk of rupture in the contemporary management of abdominal aortic aneurysms. *J Vasc Surg*. 2015;62(6):1429-1436. Copyright © 2015 Elsevier. With permission.)

CLINICAL FEATURES OF THORACIC AND ABDOMINAL AORTIC ANEURYSMS

Most (70%-75%) TAAs and AAAs are asymptomatic when first detected, although up to 60% develop symptoms before rupture.[30] The diagnosis most commonly results from imaging for unrelated symptoms.

AAA symptoms result from compression of nearby structures, typically duodenum or ureters resulting in nausea/vomiting or hydronephrosis, respectively. Abdominal, flank, or back pain occurs from aneurysmal pressure on overlying peritoneum or somatosensory nerves. Chronic abdominal or back pain is the most common symptom presenting in 30% of patients. Tenderness to palpation on the exam has been shown to correlate with the impending risk of rupture.[22] The classic presentation of a ruptured AAA is a tender, pulsatile abdominal mass and shock. Pain associated with rupture tends to be steady and severe, ranging from minutes to days in duration. Abdominal distension is common. Rarely an AAA can rupture into the iliac vein or inferior vena cava resulting in an aortocaval fistula and acute congestive heart failure, or into the gastrointestinal tract with life-threatening hematochezia. Patients with such may have reflex tachycardia and angina from blood loss anemia. If an abdominal exam is overlooked, this may result in the misdiagnosis of an acute coronary syndrome.

The most common symptom of TAA is vague pain in the chest, back, flank, or abdomen. Symptoms of large TAAs include hoarseness secondary to left recurrent laryngeal nerve compression, chronic cough secondary to tracheal compression, dysphagia secondary to esophageal compression, and life-threatening hemoptysis or hematemesis from erosion into pulmonary structures or the esophagus, respectively.[25]

The differential diagnosis is variable, depending on presenting symptoms and aneurysm location. The differential diagnosis of chronic chest pain includes myocardial ischemia/infarction, pulmonary embolism, pneumonia, and aortic dissection. Because alternate diagnoses are generally more common than TAA, workup including ECG, cardiac enzymes, or pulmonary embolism-protocol CT can lead to a delay in diagnosis. Abdominal pain in AAA also has a broad differential including symptomatic hernia, biliary conditions, bowel obstruction or ischemia, and renal pathologies including pyelonephritis and nephrolithiasis.

DIAGNOSIS OF THORACIC AND ABDOMINAL AORTIC ANEURYSMS

The history should focus on the characteristics and location of pain and risk factors for aortic aneurysms including hypertension, connective tissue disorders, family history of aneurysm, and smoking. Physical examination should include (1) a focused heart and lung exam; (2) careful search for arterial perfusion differences in upper and lower extremities; (3) evidence of chest or abdominal bruits; (4) assessment of organ malperfusion (ie, visceral ischemia or focal neurologic deficits); and (5) a comprehensive peripheral pulse assessment noting any pulsatile masses, particularly in the popliteal fossa. An ECG and chest or abdominal radiography are routinely obtained in the acute evaluation of chest pain and/or abdominal pain. The chest radiograph may show a widened enlarged aortic knob, tracheal deviation, left mainstem bronchus displacement, or calcifications outlining the aortic silhouette.

The gold standard for evaluation of TAA is MDCT with three-dimensional (3D) reconstruction, with sensitivity and specificity for detecting aortic aneurysms more than 95%.[25] MDCT also allows for the detection of other pathologies that may affect patient management including malignancy or infectious processes. In patients with renal insufficiency, noncontrast MDCT may be useful to estimate aneurysm size, but it does not permit assessment of the extent of atherosclerotic disease, associated dissection, branch vessel patency, and the presence of intercostal arteries contributing to spinal cord perfusion. 3D reconstruction is important for operative planning including stent-graft positioning. Magnetic resonance imaging and angiography can be considered for diagnostic purposes of thoracoabdominal aortic aneurysm, but limitations include increased cost and study time, poorer spatial resolution, limited visualization of thrombus and calcium, and interference from metallic implants.[25] There are no currently accepted biomarkers for the diagnosis of aneurysm. Erythrocyte sedimentation rate and C-reactive protein are useful but nonspecific biomarkers in narrowing a differential for inflammatory or mycotic aneurysm etiology, which can have implications in treatment approaches.

The imaging modality of choice for AAA diagnosis and surveillance is B-mode ultrasound. It involves no ionizing radiation and provides accurate aneurysm size measurement, with sensitivity and specificity approaching 100%. While it can identify structural details such as thrombus burden and calcifications, it is less helpful in measuring the distance from the renal arteries, which is critical piece for endovascular operative planning. The visceral segment, where celiac, superior mesenteric, and renal arteries arise, may be poorly visualized. Other factors that affect ultrasound imaging include body habitus and overlying bowel gas.[21] MDCT provides major structural information including calcification, involvement of the visceral segment, distance from the renal arteries, congenital anomalies affecting surgical planning (eg, horseshoe kidney), and periaortic stranding or fibrosis indicating inflammatory or infected aneurysm. MDCT is the most essential imaging modality when determining endograft suitability for operative treatment.

Important aspects of aortic aneurysm assessment include identification of its location and morphology. The Crawford classification is widely used for thoracoabdominal aneurysms, as it has important therapeutic and outcome implications (**Figure 79.3**). The most common type, accounting for 30% of thoracoabdominal aneurysms, is the Crawford type II aneurysm (ie, from above the sixth intercostal extending distal to the infrarenal aortic segment). Involvement of the aortic arch, visceral segment, relationship to the renal vessels, and morphology (fusiform vs saccular) are the features in treatment planning.

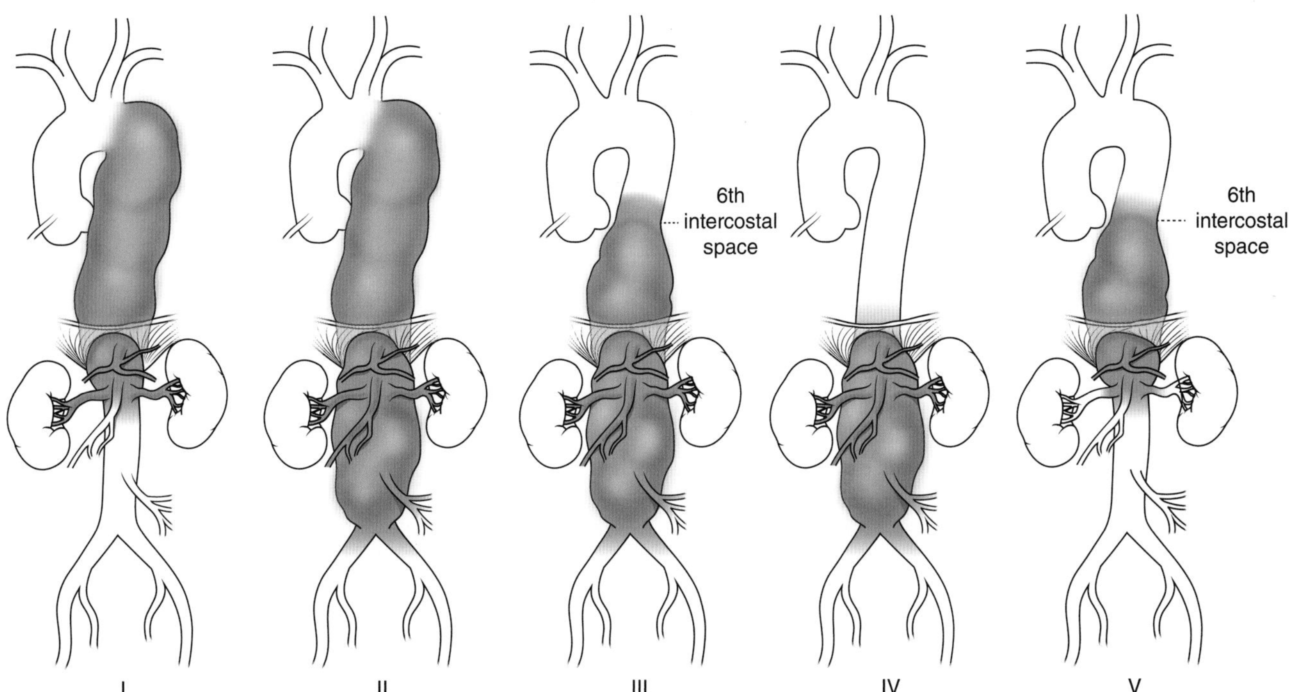

FIGURE 79.3 Crawford's classification of thoracoabdominal aortic aneurysms defines the aneurysmal extent. Extent I, distal to the left subclavian artery and extends to include the origins of the celiac axis and superior mesenteric arteries. The renal arteries can also be involved, but the aneurysm does not extend into the infrarenal segment. Extent II, distal to the left subclavian artery to below the renal arteries. Extent III, from the sixth intercostal space into the abdominal aorta. Extent IV, the entire abdominal aorta. Extent V, below the sixth intercostal space to just above the renal arteries. (Reprinted with permission from Grover FL, Mack MJ. *Cardiac Surgery.* Philadelphia, PA: Wolters Kluwer; 2016. Figure 15.1.)

MANAGEMENT OF AORTIC ANEURYSMS

In an elective setting when an AAA is suspected, management priorities are to obtain a history and physical examination to aid in the clinician's judgment, confirm the diagnosis using the appropriate imaging modality, optimize medical management of comorbidities and rule out other cardiovascular diagnoses. Screening for AAA with abdominal duplex ultrasound is recommended in men ages 65 to 75 years who have ever smoked.[31,32] Ultrasound screening is also recommended for men and women over 75 years in good health and for 65 to 75 years old first-degree relatives of a patient with a known AAA. Referral to a vascular or cardiothoracic surgeon is recommended once an AAA or TAA is discovered.[32]

The Society for Vascular Surgery recommends repair—open or endovascular—for all patients of acceptable perioperative risk with an ascending or descending TAA or thoracoabdominal aneurysm greater than or equal to 5.5 cm in diameter as well as all patients with saccular and symptomatic aneurysms. However, treatment decisions must also consider patient characteristics. Patients with Marfan syndrome or other genetically mediated disorders (vascular Ehlers-Danlos syndrome, Turner syndrome, bicuspid aortic valve, or familial TAA and dissection) should undergo an elective operation at smaller diameters (4.0-5.0 cm depending on the condition) to avoid acute dissection or rupture.[12]

In patients with rupture, management priorities include stabilizing the patient and preparing them for definitive operative treatment, which may include facilitation of emergent transfer to a higher level of care. Mortality rate after rupture is greater than 90% in the first 24 hours; most patients die before arriving in an emergency room.[33] Resuscitation is ideally performed in the operating room, as proximal vascular control of the aorta is required for these efforts to be effective. Resuscitation may include the use of permissive hypotension while maintaining perfusion to end organs (ie, systolic arterial pressures of 70-80 mm Hg are tolerated for short periods to limit the ongoing loss of blood), administration of platelets, and associated coagulation factors.[34] If the rupture is suspected, massive blood transfusion protocols should be immediately initiated. The patient should be prepped and draped in the operating room, with the surgical team scrubbed before the induction of general anesthesia, which can result in severe hypotension when the tamponade effect of the chest and abdominal wall musculature is relieved during the administration of anesthetic agents. Preinduction aortic control can also be obtained rapidly by trans-femoral or trans-brachial balloon occlusion of the aorta proximal to the rupture site.

Approaches to Aortic Aneurysm Repair

Repair techniques include an open replacement, endovascular stent placement, or a combination (hybrid repair). Choice of technique depends on the aneurysm anatomy including involvement of branch vessels and the ability to completely exclude (endovascular) or excise and replace (surgical) the abnormal aorta. Other factors affecting the suitability of the endovascular approach include large aortic diameter, tortuosity, excessive calcifications of access vessels, or inadequate proximal or distal landing zones for the endograft.[35] If multiple nonconsecutive broad segments are concurrently involved, a staged approach may be required, with the largest or symptomatic segment treated first.

At the time of this writing, there are no US Food and Drug Administration-approved endovascular options for repair of ascending aortic aneurysms. Aortic arch aneurysms require open surgery with hybrid approaches increasingly chosen to limit morbidity. Aneurysms involving the descending thoracic aorta are preferentially treated with endovascular stenting, given the high morbidity rate of open repair, particularly pulmonary complications which occur in up to 27% of affected patients.[36] Both open and endovascular repair of this region carry the risk of spinal cord ischemia. With open repair, this risk can be mitigated by surgical reimplantation of the intercostal arteries. During endovascular treatment, spinal cord ischemia risk factors include aortic coverage greater than or equal to 20 cm, aortic coverage between T9 and T12 (ie, at the origin of artery of Adamkiewicz), coverage of the left subclavian artery, occluded or covered internal iliac arteries, perioperative hypotension, female gender, prolonged procedure, and prior aortic surgery of any type. The risk of spinal ischemia is mitigated by prophylactic cerebrospinal fluid drainage and maintaining elevated systemic pressures to maximize spinal artery perfusion pressure.[36]

FOLLOW-UP OF PATIENTS WITH AORTIC ANEURYSMS

Surveillance after repair of TAA and AAA is indicated to prevent late rupture and aneurysm-related death. After endovascular repair, surveillance is intended to identify changes in aneurysmal sac size, endovascular device leak, device migration, or failure. MDCT angiography imaging of the repaired segment should be done 1 month postendovascular repair. In the absence of aneurysmal sac enlargement or endovascular device leak, ultrasound imaging can be performed at 6 and 12 months for AAA, and then annually.[37] Given the location of the thoracic aorta, MDCT is the best imaging modality for surveillance of a thoracic endograft 1, 6, and 12 months, and then annually for 5 years, after which CT is performed every 5 years if there are no concerning changes.[38]

KEY POINTS

- ✔ An aortic dissection is a tear in the aortic intima, with the separation of the intima and media and the creation of a false lumen.
- ✔ Penetrating aortic ulcer (PAU) describes an entity in which ulceration of an atherosclerotic lesion penetrates the internal elastic lamina into the media.
- ✔ In aortic intramural haematoma (IMH), hemorrhage occurs in the media of the aortic wall in the absence of a demonstrable two-lumen flow and primary intimal tear.
- ✔ Involvement of the ascending aorta in IMH carries substantial mortality, and urgent or emergent operative or endovascular intervention is typically indicated, whereas arch and descending IMH are less likely to be associated with an adverse outcome and a nonsurgical initial approach may be appropriate.
- ✔ The management for thoracic aortic dissection is emergent open surgical repair for Stanford type A dissection with a 30-day mortality of 26%, as opposed to a 58% survival for medical management.
- ✔ Conversely, medical management results in better outcomes for uncomplicated Stanford type B dissection (30-day mortality 10.7% vs 31.4% with open surgical management).
- ✔ Even after repair, thoracic aortic dissection carries a lifetime risk of complications which is best mitigated by risk factor modification.

REFERENCES

1. LeMaire SA, Russell L. Epidemiology of thoracic aortic dissection. *Nat Rev Card.* 2011;8:103-113.
2. Clouse WD, Hallett JW Jr, Schaff HV, et al. Acute aortic dissection: population-based incidence compared with degenerative aortic aneurysm rupture. *Mayo Clin Proc.* 2004;79:176-180.
3. Nakashima Y. Pathogenesis of aortic dissection: elastic fiber abnormalities and aortic medial weakness. *Ann Vasc Dis.* 2010;3:28-36.
4. Akutsu K. Etiology of aortic dissection. *Gen Thorac Cardiovasc Surg.* 2019;67:271-276.
5. Osada H, Kyogoku M, Ishidou M, Morishima M, Nakajima H. Aortic dissection in the outer third of the media: what is the role of the vasa vasorum in the triggering process? *Eur J Cardiothorac Surg.* 2013;43:e82-e88.
6. Hagan PG, Nienaber CA, Isselbacher EM, et al. The International Registry of Acute Aortic Dissection (IRAD): new insights into an old disease. *JAMA.* 2000;283(7):897-903.
7. American College of Radiology ACR Appropriateness Criteria® Suspected Acute Aortic Syndrome. https://acsearch.acr.org/docs/69402/Narrative/
8. Shimony A, Filion KB, Mottillo S, Dourian T, Eisenberg MJ. Meta-analysis of usefulness of d-dimer to diagnose acute aortic dissection. *Am J Cardiol.* 2011;107:1227-1234.
9. Rylski B, Perez M, Beyersdorf F, et al. Acute non-A non-B aortic dissection: incidence, treatment, and outcome. *Eur J Cardiothorac Surg.* 2017;52:1111-1117.
10. Sultan I, McGarvey J, Vallabhajosyula P, Desai ND, Bavaria JE, Szeto WY. Routine use of hemiarch during acute type A aortic dissection repair. *Ann Cardiothorac Surg.* 2016;5:245-247.
11. Hansen MS, Nogardea GJ, Hutchins SJ. Frequency of and inappropriate treatment of misdiagnosis of acute aortic dissection. *Am J Cardiol.* 2007;99(6):852-856.
12. Hiratzka LF, Bakris GL, Beckman JA. 2010 ACCF/AHA/AATS/ACR/ASA/SCA/SCAI/SIR/STS/SVM Guidelines for the diagnosis and management of patients with thoracic aortic disease: executive summary. *Circulation.* 2010;121:1544-1579.
13. Fattori R, Piergiorgio C, De Rango P, et al. Interdisciplilnary expert consensus document on management of type B aortic dissection. *J Am Coll Card.* 2013;61:1661-1678.
14. Nienaber CA, Kische S, Rousseau H, et al. Endovascular repair of type B aortic dissection: long-term results of the randomized investigation of stent grafts in aortic dissection trial. *Circ Cardiovasc Interv.* 2013;6:407-416.

15. Strauss C, Harris K, Hutchison S, et al. "Time is Life": early mortality in type A acute aortic dissection: insights from the IRAD registry. *J Am Coll Cardiol.* 2013;61:E1516.
16. Pape LA, Tsai TT, Isselbacher EM, et al. Aortic diameter >5.5 cm is not a good predictor of type A aortic dissection: observations from the International Registry of Acute Aortic Dissection (IRAD). *Circulation.* 2007;116:1120-1127.
17. Lawton JS, Moon MR, Liu J, et al. The profound impact of combined severe acidosis and malperfusion on operative mortality in the surgical treatment of type A aortic dissection. *J Thorac Cardiovasc Surg.* 2018;155:897-904.
18. Leshnower B, Keeling WB, Duwayri Y, Jordan WD, Chen EP. The "thoracic endovascular aortic repair-first" strategy for acute type A dissection with mesenteric malperfusion: initial results compared to conventional algorithms. *J Thorac Cardiovasc Surg.* 2019;158:1516-1524.
19. Preventza O, Olive JK, Liao JL, et al. Acute type I aortic dissection with or without antegrade stent delivery: mid-term outcomes. *J Thorac Cardiovasc Surg.* 2019;158:1273-1281.
20. Vallabhajosyula P, Szeto WY, Pulsipher A, et al. Antegrade thoracic stent grafting during repair of acute Debakey type I dissection promotes distal aortic remodeling and reduces late open distal reoperation rate. *J Thorac Cardiovasc Surg.* 2014;147:942-948.
21. Evangelista A, Mukherjee D, Mehta RH, et al. Acute intramural hematoma of the aorta: a mystery in evolution. *Circulation.* 2005;111(8):1063-1070. doi:10.1161/01.CIR.0000156444.26393.80
22. Goldstone, J. Aneurysms of the aorta and iliac arteries. *In*: Moore WS, Lawrence PF, Oderich GS, eds. *Vascular and Endovascular Surgery: A Comprehensive Review.* Elsevier/Saunders; 2019:633-658.
23. White JV, Mazzacco SL. Formation and growth of aortic aneurysms induced by adventitial elastolysis. *Ann N Y Acad Sci.* 1996;800:97-120. doi:10.1111/j.1749-6632.1996.tb33302.x
24. Elefteriades JA. Thoracic aortic aneurysm: reading the enemy's playbook. *Curr Prob Cardiol.* 2008;33(5):203-277. doi:10.1016/j.cpcardiol.2008.01.004
25. Upchurch GR, Perry RJT. Thoracic and thoracoabdominal aortic aneurysms: etiology, epidemiology, natural history, medical management, and decision making. In: Sidawy AN, Perler BA, Rutherford RB, eds. *Rutherford's Vascular Surgery and Endovascular Therapy Volume 1.* Elsevier; 2019:970-985.
26. Clouse WD, Hallett JW Jr, Schaff HV, Gayari MM, Ilstrup DM, Melton III LJ. Improved prognosis of thoracic aortic aneurysms. *JAMA.* 1998;280(22):1926-1929. doi:10.1001/jama.280.22.1926
27. Crawford ES. Aortic aneurysm: a multifocal disease. *Arch Surg.* 1982;117(11):1393. doi:10.1001/archsurg.1982.01380350001001
28. Gloviczki P, Pairolero P, Welch T, et al. Multiple aortic aneurysms: the results of surgical management. *J Vasc Surg.* 1990;11(1):19-28. doi:10.1067/mva.1990.16620
29. Kim JB, Kim K, Lindsay ME, et al. Risk of rupture or dissection in descending thoracic aortic aneurysm. *Circulation.* 2015;132(17):1620-1629. doi:10.1161/circulationaha.114.015177
30. Panneton JM, Hollier LH. Nondissecting thoracoabdominal aortic aneurysms: part I. *Ann Vasc Surg.* 1995;9(5):503-514. doi:10.1007/bf02143869
31. Clinical Summary: Abdominal aortic aneurysm: screening. United States Preventive Services Taskforce. Published December 2019. Accessed January 14, 2021. https://uspreventiveservicestaskforce.org/uspstf/document/ClinicalSummaryFinal/abdominal-aortic-aneurysm-screening
32. Chaikof EL, Dalman RL, Eskandari MK, et al. The Society for Vascular Surgery practice guidelines on the care of patients with an abdominal aortic aneurysm. *J Vasc Surg.* 2018;67:2.e2-77.e2. doi: 10.1016/j.jvs.2017.10.044
33. Charlton-Ouw, KM, Pratt WB, Miller CC, Azizzadeh A, Estrera AL, Safi HJ. Descending thoracic and thoracoabdominal aortic aneurysms: general principles and open surgical repair. *In*: Moore WS, Lawrence PF, Oderich GS, eds. *Vascular and Endovascular Surgery: A Comprehensive Review.* Elsevier/Saunders; 2019:540-553.
34. Lindsay, TF. Ruptured aortoiliac aneurysms and their management. In: Sidawy AN, Perler BA, Rutherford RB, eds. *Rutherford's Vascular Surgery and Endovascular Therapy Volume 1.* Elsevier; 2019:944-960.
35. Nation D, Wang G. TEVAR: Endovascular repair of the thoracic aorta. *Semin Interv Radiol.* 2015;32(03):265-271. doi:10.1055/s-0035-1558824
36. Wortmann M, Böckler D, Geisbüsch P. Perioperative cerebrospinal fluid drainage for the prevention of spinal ischemia after endovascular aortic repair. *Gefässchirurgie.* 2017;22(S2):35-40. doi:10.1007/s00772-017-0261-z
37. Malik R, Kölbel T, Kelly P, Mckinsey J. What is your protocol for following patients after TEVAR? Ask the experts. *Endovascular Today.* 2017;16(11). Accessed January 14, 2021. https://evtoday.com/pdfs/et1117_F8_ATE2.pdf
38. Meena RA, Benarroch-Gampel J, Leshnower BG, et al. Surveillance recommendations after thoracic endovascular aortic repair should be based on initial indication for repair. *Ann Vasc Surg.* 2019;57:51-59. doi:10.1016/j.avsg.2018.11.001

CHAPTER 80

PERIPHERAL ARTERIAL DISEASE

Joseph J. Ingrassia, Matt Finn, and Sahil Parikh

INTRODUCTION

Epidemiology

The Centers for Disease Control and Prevention (CDC) estimates that around 8.5 million Americans suffer from peripheral arterial disease (PAD).[1] Some estimate that the true prevalence of PAD in the United States is closer to 20 million and is expected to increase in the coming years as the population ages.[2] Up to one-third of patients above the age of 50 years with either diabetes or smoking history or above the age of 70 years are afflicted with PAD.[3] The disparate estimates regarding the prevalence of PAD likely represent a combination of a lack of awareness in the medical community and asymptomatic or atypical presentation of the disease in patients.[4]

Risk Factors

Common atherosclerotic risk factors such as age, hypertension, hyperlipidemia, diabetes mellitus (DM), and smoking contribute to the risk of developing lower extremity PAD.[5]

Smoking, particularly, is a powerful risk factor for PAD development.[6] Depending on the measurements used, smoking contributes to 1.9 to 3.4 times increased risk for the odds of the development of PAD.[7] Among U.S. male professionals, smoking is the most contributable risk factor for the occurrence of PAD.[8] Chronic kidney disease[9] is associated with incident PAD and worse clinical outcomes. African American race[10] even after adjustment for multiple risk factors, including inflammatory markers, had an odds ratio of 1.7 to 2.9 for PAD compared to non-Hispanic whites.[11]

DM that is poorly controlled and/or longstanding is associated with the development of PAD, whereas new-onset diabetes is not as strongly associated.[12] Patients with PAD who have DM are more likely to have an amputation and are at an increased risk of mortality compared to patients who are non-DM with PAD.[13]

Hyperlipidemia is closely linked with PAD; however, compared with healthy controls patients with PAD have been found to have lower levels of high-density lipoprotein (HDL) with higher concentrations of very low-density lipoprotein (vLDL) and triglycerides. Interestingly, the levels of LDL were lower in patients with established PAD compared with healthy controls.[14] Reasons for these findings are not fully elucidated, but the complex interplay between both biologic and mechanical forces acting on the lower extremity vasculature may partially explain why the protective effect of HDL seems to be more important than is low-density lipoprotein (LDL) elevation in the development of PAD.

Different risk factors may predispose patients to different anatomic presentations of PAD, with male gender and cigarette smoking associated with higher incidence of iliac disease, whereas older age and diabetes are associated more with the development of tibial level disease.[15]

PATHOGENESIS

PAD is a spectrum of disease that is the result of progressive arterial insufficiency most commonly because of atherosclerosis. In addition to the traditional mechanisms of progression of atherosclerosis, the lower extremity arteries, specifically the superficial femoral artery, are subject to mechanical forces that promote the progression of atherosclerosis[16] (**Table 80.1**).

In patients with chronic limb-threatening ischemia (CLTI), progressive luminal narrowing may not be the only or most important factor in the development of ischemia. Postmortem study indicates that thrombotic occlusion with insignificant atherosclerotic changes of the affected vessels is seen in a significant portion of limbs with CLTI.[17] This supports a mechanism of chronic subclinical atheroembolism leading to progressive arterial insufficiency. Traditionally, large thromboembolic causes of acute arterial occlusion and/or insufficiency from causes such as atrial fibrillation, paradoxical embolism, endocarditis, and/or thromboembolism from aneurysms more proximally typically present acutely as acute limb ischemia and represent medical emergencies.

CLINICAL PRESENTATION

Acute Limb Ischemia

Acute limb ischemia is most often due to arterial thromboembolism. In patients without preexisting PAD, there is an abrupt onset of symptoms. Pain in the affected leg distal to the occlusion, paresthesias, and/or paralysis or diminished motor function are common complaints in patients with acute limb ischemia.

Patients with preexisting PAD may have developed sufficient arterial collateralization that acute limb ischemia may present as a sudden worsening of preexisting symptoms.

Clinical presentation and physical examination of patients with acute limb ischemia are often remembered by the "Six P's": **p**ainful and **p**ale limb distal to the level of occlusion,

TABLE 80.1 Nonatherosclerotic Causes of Lower Extremity Peripheral Arterial Disease

Condition	Pathology	Diagnostics	Treatment	Additional Recommendations
Fibromuscular Dysplasia	Fibroplasia of the medial arterial layer (most common), the intimal or adventitial layers and may affect the iliac, femoral, or popliteal arteries	Anatomic evaluation of the renal and cerebrovascular arteries. Imaging of other vascular beds (mesenteric, upper and lower extremities) is reasonable depending on symptoms. Duplex ultrasound is a reasonable initial screening test in experienced centers. CTA MRA	Conventional ASCVD risk factor management. PTA if symptoms develop though symptomatic involvement of the lower extremities is not as common as renal and/or carotid arteries.	SCAD is associated with FMD. It is reasonable to screen for FMD in patients with a history of SCAD.[18]
Large and Medium Vessel Vasculitides (Takayasu, Giant Cell, Polyarteritis Nodosa)	Inflammation of the arterial wall	Laboratory: Complete blood count, inflammatory markers, complement levels, ANCA Vascular Imaging: CTA, MRA, Ultrasound PET imaging may detect vessel wall inflammation.	Disease-specific medical treatment	Disease-specific immunosuppression in order to induce disease remission and periodic monitoring to detect subclinical disease flares
Popliteal Artery Entrapment Syndrome	Anatomic abnormalities in the course of the popliteal artery combined with some degree of hypertrophy of the surrounding gastrocnemius muscles produce arterial Insufficiency.	CTA MRA DSA	Surgical popliteal artery release and/or bypass	These patients are at elevated risk of acute limb ischemia.[19]
External Iliac Artery Endofibrosis[20]	Fibrosis due to repetitive trauma seen in cyclists and runners.	Duplex ultrasound CTA MRA DSA Intravascular imaging	Patch angioplasty, interposition grafts	Diagnostic criteria and treatment are not standardized.
Cystic Adventitial Disease of the Lower Extremity Arteries	Arterial luminal compression due to cystic collection of mucinous material within the adventitia. Resolution of claudication takes longer than typical intermittent claudication.	Duplex ultrasound CTA MRA	Optimal treatment strategies have not yet been identified. PTA has not demonstrated benefit.	MRA allows for characterization of the vessel wall.

ANCA, antineutrophil cytoplasmic antibodies; ASCVD, atherosclerotic cardiovascular disease; CTA, computed tomography angiography; DSA, digital subtraction angiography; FMD, fibromuscular dysplasia; MRA, magnetic resonance angiography; PET, positron emission tomography; PTA, percutaneous transluminal angioplasty; SCAD, spontaneous coronary artery dissection.

(Adapted from Hayes SN, Kim ESH, Saw J. et al. Spontaneous coronary artery dissection: current state of the science: a scientific statement from the American Heart Association. Circulation. 2018;137:e523-e557)

SECTION 6

TABLE 80.2 Rutherford Classification for Acute Limb Ischemia

Category	Sensory Impairment	Motor Impairment	Arterial Doppler Signal	Venous Doppler Signal
Class I Viable—No immediate threat	No	No	Audible	Audible
Class IIa Marginally threatened	Minimal or none	No	±	Audible
Class IIb Immediately threatened	Involves forefoot ± rest pain	Mild to moderate	Usually inaudible	Audible
Class III Irreversible	Anesthetic	Paralytic/Rigor	Inaudible	Inaudible

Data from Rutherford RB, Baker JD, Ernst C, et al. Recommended standards for reports dealing with lower extremity ischemia: revised version. J Vasc Surg. 1997;26:517-538.

with diminished or absent **p**ulses that can eventually progress to **p**oikilothermia, **p**aresthesias, and **p**aralysis if left untreated. Therapy for this condition includes prompt revascularization if the limb is deemed viable and amputation for nonviable limbs. The Rutherford Classification of acute limb ischemia is presented in **Table 80.2.**[21] Consultation with a vascular specialist is recommended in all cases of suspected acute limb ischemia.

Chronic Limb Ischemia: Intermittent Claudication to Chronic Limb-Threatening Ischemia

Patients with arterial insufficiency of the lower extremities present with claudication symptoms distal to the hemodynamically significant lesion. Aortoiliac disease may present with exertional cramping of the buttocks and thighs as well as impotence and atrophy of the musculature in the lower limbs (Leriche syndrome). Disease in the common and superficial femoral arteries presents with claudication in the calves (typical intermittent claudication). Isolated tibial level disease typically does not produce symptoms of claudication.

Most patients with PAD, however, do not present with typical claudication symptoms.[3] Patients with established vascular disease in one territory (coronary, cerebrovascular) or those who are at high risk for atherosclerotic vascular disease should be questioned closely regarding atypical manifestations of lower extremity PAD. These symptoms may include muscle groups that are easily fatigued out of proportion to the level of activity, aching and/or tingling that are exacerbated by exertion and relieved with rest, fatigue with periods of prolonged standing, etc.

Physical examination of the patient with chronic ischemia of the lower extremities may reveal loss of hair over the lower legs and feet; pale, shiny, and/or atrophic skin; disturbances in nail growth; elevation pallor; dependent rubor progressing to minor tissue loss; and/or frank gangrene.

Patients that are classified within Rutherford Classes 4 to 6 for more than 2 weeks with an additional abnormal hemodynamic parameter (ankle-brachial index [ABI] < 0.4, absolute highest ankle systolic pressure <50 mm Hg, absolute toe pressure <30 mm Hg, transcutaneous oximetry [$TcPO_2$] < 30 mm Hg, and/or flat or minimally pulsatile pulse volume recording) are deemed to have critical limb ischemia (CLI) or CLTI.[22] **Table 80.3** outlines commonly used classification systems for patients with chronic limb ischemia.[21,23]

TABLE 80.3 Fontaine and Rutherford Classification for Chronic Limb Ischemia

Classification	Stage	Description
Fontaine	1	Asymptomatic
	IIa	Mild claudication
	IIb	Moderate–severe claudication
	III	**Rest pain**
	IV	**Ulceration or gangrene**
Rutherford	0	Asymptomatic
	1	Mild claudication
	2	Moderate claudication
	3	Severe claudication
	4	**Rest pain**
	5	**Minor tissue loss**
	6	**Severe tissue loss or gangrene**

Note: Bold denotes critical limb ischemia.

Patients with claudication are at an increased risk of cardiovascular-related morbidity and mortality. Some datasets show PAD is associated with hazard ratios above six for related cardiovascular disease morbidity and mortality.[7]

Specifically, regarding the risk of future limb events, 21% of patients with intermittent claudication progress to CLTI within 5 years,[24] making the identification and early medical management of these patients of paramount importance.

Aneurysmal Disease

Aneurysmal disease is defined as a focal dilation that is increased greater than 50% of the vessel's normal reference diameter involving all components of the vessel wall (intima, media, and adventitia).

Iliac Artery Aneurysms

Isolated iliac artery aneurysms are rare. More commonly, iliac artery aneurysms are associated with abdominal aortic aneurysms (AAAs), and the management of iliac artery aneurysms is dependent on the management of the AAA. In cases where the common iliac artery aneurysm is larger than 1.6 cm in diameter, the iliac aneurysm should be followed independently from the AAA. Repair is indicated for symptomatic iliac aneurysms, aneurysms greater than 3 cm in diameter, those that expand greater than or equal to 7 mm in 6 months or greater than 1 cm in 1 year.[25] For patients with concomitant AAA, any common iliac artery aneurysm is treated in order to assure a proper seal. In isolated iliac artery aneurysm, consideration of the location of internal iliac artery with respect to the aneurysm must be given as this may impact the endovascular treatment options.

Popliteal Artery Aneurysms

Popliteal aneurysms are the most common type of aneurysm in the lower extremity. There is a strong male prevalence, and it occurs most commonly in the fifth and sixth decades. Typically, popliteal aneurysms are detected incidentally on imaging testing and are strongly associated with atherosclerotic disease. Symptoms range from an asymptomatic pulsatile mass to limb ischemia from thromboembolism. Thromboembolism is more common in larger aneurysms (>2 cm). Patients with popliteal artery aneurysms are at high risk for aneurysm formation in the contralateral limb, femoral arteries, and abdominal aorta. These areas should be screened with vascular imaging when a popliteal artery aneurysm is detected. Repair is indicated for symptomatic aneurysms of any size, especially patent aneurysms greater than 2 cm in diameter[26] given the increased risk of limb ischemia or those that have expanded >0.5 cm per year. Thrombus within the aneurysm sac may be a relative indication for repair. Open surgical or endovascular repair with a covered stent may be undertaken. Given the anatomic location behind the knee and relatively straightforward open surgical approach, surgical excision is preferred in patients who are candidates for both approaches.

DIAGNOSTIC TESTING IN PERIPHERAL ARTERIAL DISEASE

The diagnostic evaluation of PAD utilizes several different testing modalities that can be used to detect, quantify, and provide descriptive information about the disease state.

When deciding which testing modalities to employ, familiarity with the strengths and weakness of each test can help to minimize the amount of unnecessary testing and increase the clinical return per test performed. **Algorithm 80.1** outlines the suggested imaging modalities to employ depending on the arterial segment(s) as detected on arterial duplex ultrasound.

Ankle-Brachial Index

The ABI is a bilevel screening test that is considered the cornerstone and first test in patients with confirmed or suspected PAD. Patients are placed in a supine position ideally after 5 to 10 minutes of rest. A blood pressure cuff is wrapped around the ankle and Doppler probes are used to insonate the anterior tibial and posterior tibial arteries distal to the cuff. The highest arm systolic pressure is divided by the highest of the two pedal artery systolic pressure.

Normal ABI values range from 1 to 1.39. Values less than 0.9 or greater than 1.4 are considered abnormal. Values between 0.9 and 0.99 are considered to be borderline and may prompt further investigation. Any drop in blood pressure greater than 20 mm Hg between two adjacent segments is concerning for significant interval stenosis. The ABI has a sensitivity 68% to 84% and a specificity of 84% to 99% for lower extremity arterial disease.[27] In patients with diabetes and/or end-stage renal disease, medial calcification may dampen or falsely normalize

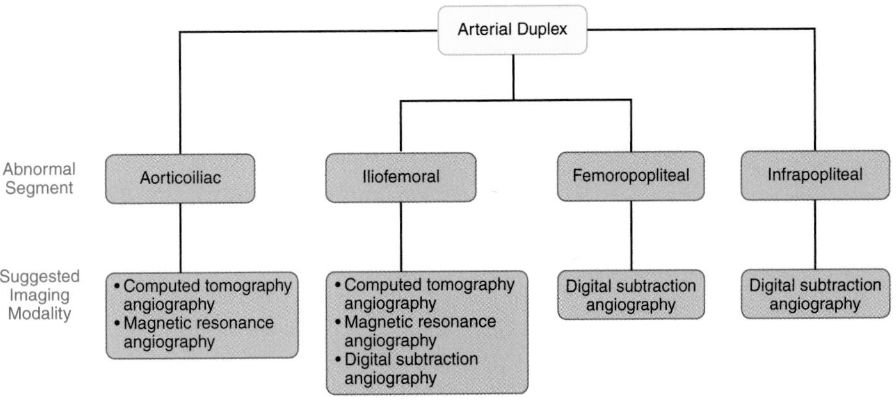

ALGORITHM 80.1 Diagnostic imaging approach to the patient with claudication prior to revascularization.

SECTION 6

ABI values. In these patients, a toe brachial index (TBI) might be a better indicator of disease.

Pulse Volume Recording

Pulse volume recording (PVR) is commonly combined with the ABI to provide diagnostic information about the degree of arterial insufficiency along the lower extremity. The PVR measures the volumetric change with each pulse at the site of interest. Typically, PVR measurements are made at several levels (high thigh, low thigh, calf, ankle, metatarsal, and toes). The normal contour of a PVR recording consists of a sharp systolic upstroke, a dicrotic notch in the downstroke, and a gradual descent to baseline. As the severity of stenosis proximal to the site of measurement increases, the waveform will (1) lose the dicrotic notch, (2) show a slower systolic upstroke and (3) demonstrate a loss of amplitude with a more rounded appearance. In instances when blood pressures cannot be accurately obtained, the PVR can give important information about the health of the vasculature (**Figure 80.1**).

Exercise Ankle-Brachial Index

In patients with a borderline abnormal ABI, or a normal ABI with signs and symptoms suggestive of aortoiliac disease

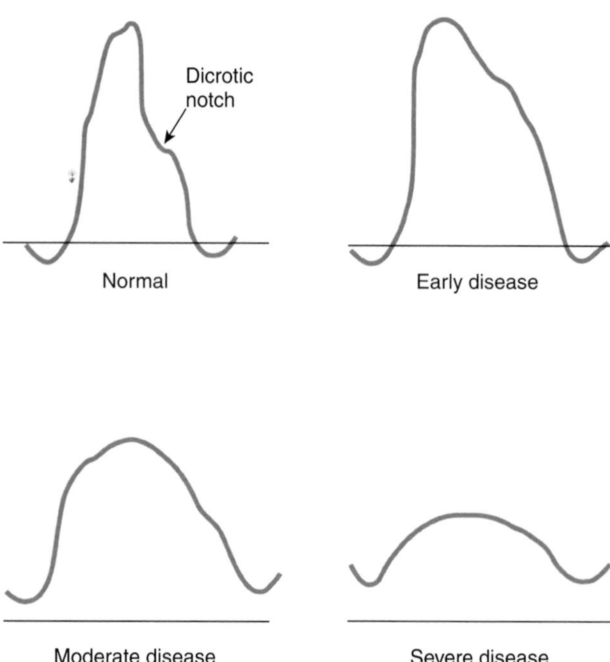

FIGURE 80.1 Segmental volume plethysmography in peripheral vascular disease. Variations in the contours of the pulse volume recording with segmental volume plethysmography reflect the severity of peripheral vascular disease. Mild disease is characterized by the absence of a dicrotic notch. With progressive obstruction, the upstroke and downstroke become equal, and with severe disease, the amplitude of the waveform is blunted. (Adapted with permission from Rajagopalan S, Dean SM, Mohler ER, et al. *Manual of Vascular Diseases.* 2nd ed. Philadelphia, PA: Wolters Kluwer Health/Lippincott Williams & Wilkins; 2011. Figure 16.4.)

(weak femoral pulse, typical thigh, and/or buttock claudication), the exercise ABI can help to unmask aortoiliac disease and/or determine the functional severity of moderate stenoses. Additionally, the exercise ABI provides the ability to get an objective assessment of a patient's walking tolerance as well as claudication distance. To perform the test, patients have an ABI/PVR performed at rest. Next, patients are disconnected from the ABI/PVR machine with blood pressure cuffs left in place. Patients then walk on a treadmill according to a protocol that increases the speed and incline with time. The speed and incline vary depending on patient factors. At the point that the patient's claudication symptoms are so severe that the patient requests to stop walking, the treadmill is stopped and the patient is transitioned off of the treadmill and has new ABI/PVR recording completed in a supine position. Postexercise, a systolic blood pressure (SBP) decrease greater than 30 mm Hg or post-ABI decrease greater than 20% is considered a positive test for PAD.

Arterial Duplex Ultrasound

Arterial duplex ultrasound consists of two tests, the first is an ultrasound anatomic evaluation of the artery and surrounding structures that can identify calcifications, aneurysms, pseudoaneurysms, and vessel size/diameter. The duplex portion of the examination consists of a Doppler evaluation of blood flow that utilizes the conservation of mass principle to quantify the degree of stenosis along a blood vessel. Arterial duplex ultrasound has high sensitivity and specificity to detect a 50% stenosis within a vessel (aortoiliac sensitivity 86%, specificity 97%, femoropopliteal sensitivity 86%, specificity 97%, infrapopliteal sensitivity 83%, specificity 84%).[28] This is frequently the first test to evaluate the arterial anatomy in patients being considered for revascularization after an abnormal ABI or exercise ABI. The advantages to arterial duplex that include the noninvasive nature of the examination, the ability to obtain physiologic as well as some anatomic data and contrast-free nature of the examination allow for indiscriminate use in patients with renal dysfunction. Because of the ability to repeat the test without consequence to the renal function and its noninvasive nature, the arterial duplex is the test of choice for follow-up after revascularization for the evaluation of bypass grafts as well as native vessels that have undergone endovascular intervention. The quality of the examination, however, is highly dependent upon the technician performing the examination, and therefore, a quality improvement and assurance program are recommended to maintain high-quality, reproducible examinations.

Computed Tomography Angiogram

Computed tomography angiogram (CTA) provides excellent anatomic information about the lower extremity vasculature. With a sensitivity and specificity of 99% to detect mild stenosis,[29] CTA is a useful diagnostic tool for an anatomic evaluation of the lower extremity vasculature. Particularly in patients with occlusive aortoiliac disease, a CTA can be helpful in balloon and stent sizing. CTA is not without its limitations. The need for intravenous contrast may limit the use of this testing modality in patients with chronic kidney disease. Vessel wall calcifications can also preclude accurate luminal assessments and for this reason a CTA is generally of limited utility in the evaluation of infrapopliteal vessels that are often plagued with medial calcifications.

Magnetic Resonance Angiogram

Magnetic resonance angiogram (MRA) has similar strengths with respect to vessel sizing as CTA. Because of a relatively long imaging time, motion artifacts are more frequent with MRA compared to CTA. This may explain a sensitivity (93%) and specificity (89%)[30] that are slightly worse than CTA. Whereas calcifications may preclude accurate vessel sizing in CTA, in MRA, the degree of vascular calcifications may be underestimated. MRA therefore is useful in evaluating infrapopliteal runoff vessels. MRA is also not reliable for the evaluation of endovascular scaffolds.

Transcutaneous Oxygen Pressure

$TcPO_2$ is a test for the local microcirculation that may be helpful to monitor the efficacy of revascularization and to predict wound healing. $TcPO_2$ is not widely available and is time intensive to perform, with tests taking around 45 to 60 minutes. Local edema limits the accuracy of the test. Further studies are required to provide validation before its widespread use can be recommended.

Skin Perfusion Pressure

Skin perfusion pressure (SPP) similar to $TcPO_2$ is most useful to assess the microcirculation in patients with CLTI to monitor the efficacy and revascularization and predict wound healing. Compared with $TcPO_2$ there is a shorter testing time (~10 minutes); however, SPP is subject to anatomic and technical factors (such as probe size and shape relative to the area of interest) that may affect measurements. As with $TcPO_2$ further validation studies are needed before its widespread use can be recommended.

Invasive Angiography/Digital Subtraction Angiography

Digital subtraction angiography (DSA) is considered the gold standard for anatomic evaluation. Given the invasive nature of this test, its use is best reserved for instances of planned endovascular revascularization and/or for evaluation of below-the-knee disease.

MANAGEMENT OF PERIPHERAL ARTERIAL DISEASE

Medical Approach

Patients with PAD are at an increased risk of cardiovascular events that are associated with a high risk of morbidity and mortality. Patients with PAD and vascular disease in another territory are among the highest risk patients in cardiovascular medicine. The early application of guideline-directed medical therapy and risk factor control has been shown to have large clinical benefits. Thus, early identification of these patients in clinical practice is of paramount importance in preventing future morbidity and mortality. The European Society of Cardiology Guidelines on the Diagnosis and Treatment of Peripheral Arterial Diseases makes the point of differentiating asymptomatic PAD from "masked" PAD. Patients with PAD typically have multiple comorbidities (heart failure, chronic obstructive pulmonary disease [COPD], diabetes, neuropathy) and/or sedentary lifestyles that can prevent the appreciation of the severity of the disease burden. Patients at high risk for PAD should be screened with ABI/TBI and if positive an objective assessment of their walking tolerance should be undertaken. Patients that have "masked" PAD rather than truly asymptomatic PAD should be treated with more aggressive medical therapy.

Patients with PAD broadly fall into two categories, claudicants and CLTI. In claudicants, revascularization should only be considered in patients who remain intolerably symptomatic despite application of optimal medical therapy and an exercise walking program. **Algorithms 80.2 and 80.3** outline the

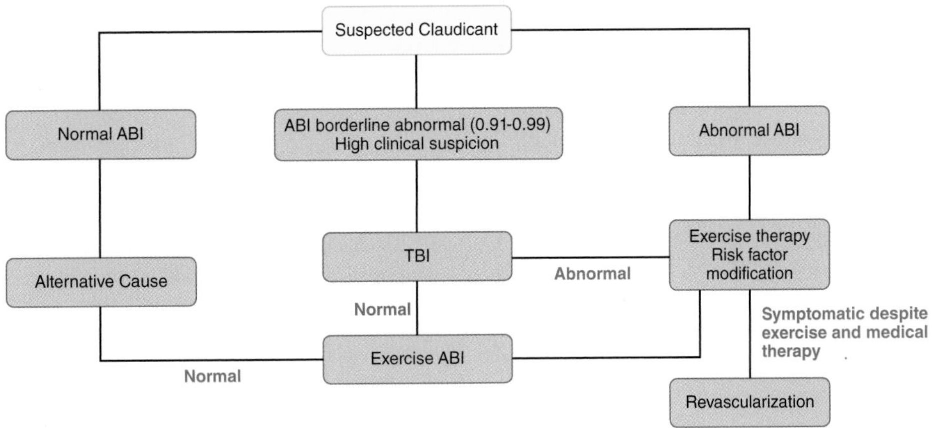

ALGORITHM 80.2 Diagnostic and therapeutic approach to the patient with claudication. ABI, ankle-brachial index; TBI, toe brachial index.

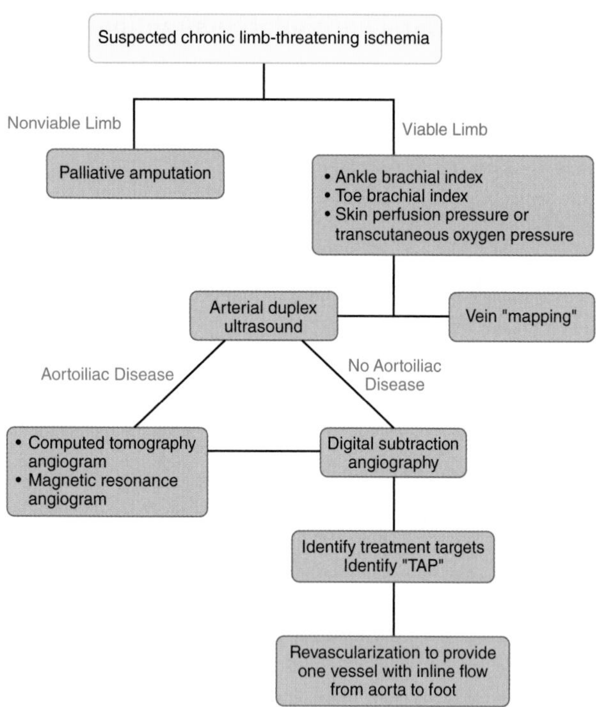

ALGORITHM 80.3 Diagnostic and therapeutic approach to the patient with chronic limb threatening ischemia. TAP, target arterial path;

approach to patients with suspected claudication. **Table 80.4** identifies important comorbid conditions and evidence-based medications that should be used in their management in patients with PAD.

Lifestyle, Diet, and Exercise Program

After diagnosis of PAD, patients should be advised on a healthy lifestyle including diet and a cardiovascular exercise program specifically aimed at walking if the patient is symptomatic. Blood pressure should be tightly controlled with the preferential use of angiotensin-converting enzyme inhibitor (ACEI) or angiotensin receptor blocker (ARB). Antithrombotic therapy should be applied as outlined in **Table 80.5**. High-dose statin therapy should be started to prevent future cardiovascular events and improve walking distance. In patients with diabetes, tight glucose control should be pursued with metformin and a sodium-glucose cotransporter 2 (SGLT2) inhibitor agent. Efforts at tobacco cessation should be undertaken. In patients with concomitant coronary artery disease, PCSK9 inhibitors should be considered.[31]

If the patient has claudication, a supervised exercise therapy (SET) should be prescribed to improve walking distance. Formal supervised exercise programs in the United States should consist of 12 weeks of sessions at least three times per week of 30 to 60 minutes per session. Baseline measurements of peak walking distance, walking distance and time to claudication onset, 6-minute walk test, heart rate and blood pressure before, during, and after exercise, as well as timed "get up and go" are all variables that should be collected in a formal SET program. Quality-of-life questionnaires and the Walking Impairment Questionnaire are available to track patients' responses to SET. Patients are monitored on a treadmill at a speed that will bring about claudication in 2 to 5 minutes. Patients walk to a moderate amount of claudication before resting until the pain completely resolves. The patients then walk again until experiencing a moderate amount of claudication. This process is repeated for the duration of the session.

The use of the phosphodiesterase inhibitor cilostazol has been shown to improve walking distance in claudicants[32]; however, the rates of discontinuation are high because of high incidence of side effects including headache and gastrointestinal (GI) upset, and the medication is contraindicated in patients with any degree of symptomatic heart failure. The additional benefits of cilostazol beyond statin therapy, ACE, and a walking program are not clearly defined. The European Society of Cardiology Guidelines on the management of PAD do not recommend the routine use of this agent, whereas the American College of Cardiology guidelines give the use of cilostazol a 1A recommendation in order to improve symptoms and walking distance.[27]

Chronic Limb-Threatening Ischemia

Patients with CLTI (Rutherford Class 4-6) should be approached differently from those with claudication. Algorithm 80.3

Comorbid Conditions

Comorbid Condition	Goal	Medication
Hypertension	<130/80 mmHg	ACEI/ARB
Diabetes mellitus	HbA1c: 7-8% (< 7% if CLTI present)	Metformin SGLT2i
Blood cholesterol	LDL <70 mg/dL LDL <50 mg/dL if concomitant CAD	High-intensity statin Ezetimibe,[a,34] PCSK9i,[a,31] Icosapent ethyl[b,35]
Tobacco dependence	Tobacco abstinence	Varenicline Nicotine replacement short term Cognitive behavioral therapy

ACEI, angiotensin-converting enzyme inhibitor; ARB, angiotensin II receptor blocker; CAD, coronary artery disease; CLTI, chronic limb-threatening ischemia; HbA1c, hemoglobin A1c; LDL, low-density lipoprotein; PCSK9i, proprotein convertase subtilisin/kexin type 9 inhibitor; SGLT2i, sodium-glucose cotransporter-2 inhibitor.

[a]In select populations such as those with coronary artery disease and history of myocardial infarction

[b]In select populations with elevated triglycerides

TABLE 80.5 Antithrombotic Medical Regimens

PAD Category	Antithrombotic Treatment Strategy	Notes
PAD without prior revascularization	SAPT	Clopidogrel preferred over ASA[36] Ticagrelor[37] or ASA if contraindication to clopidogrel exists
PAD periprocedural revascularization	DAPT 1 month; followed by ASA + rivaroxaban 2.5 mg orally twice daily[38]	± PPI based on bleeding risk
PAD with remote prior revascularization	ASA Clopidogrel 75 mg daily ASA + rivaroxaban 2.5 mg orally twice daily	
PAD with stable CAD	ASA + rivaroxaban 2.5 mg orally twice daily[39]	Independent of history of revascularization
PAD with CAD and recent ACS or PCI	DAPT for length of CAD indication followed by ASA + ticagrelor 60 mg orally twice daily OR ASA + rivaroxaban 2.5 mg orally twice daily	Factors favoring ticagrelor over rivaroxaban: complex coronary artery disease, bifurcation stents, multivessel PCI
PAD with indication for anticoagulation without prior revascularization	OAC + clopidogrel 75 mg daily OR OAC monotherapy	Addition of clopidogrel based upon bleeding risk
PAD with indication for anticoagulation with prior revascularization	OAC + clopidogrel 75 mg daily 1 month post-revascularization followed by OAC +/- clopidogrel	Maintenance of clopidogrel based upon bleeding risk
PAD, asymptomatic without history of revascularization or additional vascular disease	No antithrombotic treatment	

ACS, acute coronary syndrome ASA, acetylsalicylic acid; CAD, coronary artery disease; DAPT, dual antiplatelet therapy; OAC, oral anticoagulation; PAD, peripheral arterial disease; PCI, percutaneous coronary intervention; PPI, proton pump inhibitor; SAPT, single antiplatelet therapy.

outlines the approach to patients with CLTI. These patients should also be evaluated by a multidisciplinary team whose efforts within their respective disciplines should coalesce around the healing of the patient's wound or to limit the level of amputation.

In patients with CLTI, the initial presentation of PAD may be a nonhealing lower extremity wound. In these patients, the clinical evaluation and application of medical therapy should be done as expeditiously as possible. Revascularization is the cornerstone of therapy in CLTI and should be performed as soon as feasibly possible in eligible candidates.

WiFi (Wound, ischemia, foot infection) score[33] should be calculated for all patients with CLTI to determine the viability of the limb and expected benefit from revascularization. For those patients with viable limbs that would benefit from revascularization, an anatomic evaluation of the arterial and venous system (in case of the need for bypass the conduit status will be known) should be promptly undertaken. For patients with concern for aortoiliac disease, further anatomic assessment with CTA/MRA should be completed prior to invasive DSA in order to obtain accurate vessel sizing of the aortoiliac segments in the event that endovascular revascularization is required. At the time of invasive evaluation, angiography down to the level of the foot should be completed. Particular attention should be paid to the degree of inflow disease, degree and extent of calcification, length of occlusion, the runoff in the infrapopliteal segment, the presence of inframalleolar disease, and completeness of the pedal arch. CLTI is an anatomically heterogeneous disease; however, in patients with CLTI, involvement of more than one arterial segment (aortoiliac, femoropopliteal, infrapopliteal) is the rule rather than the exception.

Percutaneous Interventions in Peripheral Arterial Disease

Endovascular approaches to the treatment of lower extremity disease are possible from a variety of different access sites including femoral retrograde, femoral antegrade, radial, brachial, and pedal/infrapopliteal.

Endovascular treatment of PAD includes a strategy of percutaneous transluminal angioplasty (PTA) with some combination of plaque modification, anti-restenotic drug application, and scaffolding as needed. There are many devices on the market that accomplish these tasks.

Revascularization Strategy

In patients who have claudication despite the initiation of guideline-directed medical therapy including an antiplatelet agent, high-intensity statin and blood pressure control with an ACE/ARB should be initiated. A walking program preferably with a supervised exercise component should be initiated to improve claudication symptoms and exercise tolerance. In patients with claudication that is lifestyle-limiting in spite of the above-mentioned measures, revascularization to improve symptoms is a reasonable approach. Revascularization should not be performed proactively to prevent the progression to CLTI.

After diagnostic angiography, a plan for revascularization should be established that may include endovascular, open surgical, or a hybrid approach depending on the segments involved, and technical, anatomic, and patient factors.

For patients with claudication with aortoiliac involvement, an endovascular first approach is preferred. In femoropopliteal segments with stenotic but not occluded vessels, an endovascular is preferred over an open surgical approach. In femoropopliteal occlusions, there is felt to be equipoise between endovascular and open surgical approach. Below-the-knee endovascular interventions may be appropriate for claudicants but are rarely appropriate for open surgical bypass.[40]

In CLTI the optimal strategy for revascularization is not known. Ideally inline blood flow from the distal aorta to the foot should be established via endovascular and/or surgical techniques.[27]

Robust data comparing bypass grafting to endovascular therapy are lacking. The BASIL trial, published in 2010, randomized 452 patients with CLI to bypass or endovascular intervention without a significant difference in overall survival or amputation-free survival. Patients who survived past 2 years may have better outcomes with surgery.[41] Endovascular therapies have improved significantly since the time of the BASIL trial and the forthcoming BASIL-2 (ISRCTN27728689) and BEST-CLI (NCT02060630) trials will randomize patients with CLI to bypass versus "best endovascular therapy"; these trials should help inform revascularization strategies in the future.

Surgical Approach—Special Considerations

For patients being evaluated for surgical endarterectomy or bypass surgery, several additional factors must be taken into account prior to proceeding to the operating room.

Operative Risk

Surgical patients referred for infrainguinal bypass have high rates of coronary artery disease. In patients with stable coronary artery disease, a strategy of revascularization prior to vascular surgery was not found to be beneficial.[42] In patients with CLTI, coronary revascularization should precede infrainguinal bypass only in situations of cardiac instability, or a high ratio of benefit to risk favors coronary revascularization (ie, recent ST-elevation myocardial infarction with residual proximal vessel obstructive coronary artery disease, severe proximal left anterior descending artery disease). All patients should be managed with blood pressure control in the perioperative period. Antiplatelet medications should be resumed as soon as feasible postoperatively. β-blockers especially should be continued throughout the perioperative period.

Define Bypass Vessels

DSA down to the level of the foot should be performed to identify suitable vessels for bypass. In certain scenarios, noninvasive imaging techniques are acceptable; however, these are rare. Particular attention should be paid to both inflow and outflow from the intended grafting sites as adequate inflow and outflow are important factors to maintain graft patency.

Conduit Status

Greater saphenous vein (GSV) and autologous grafts are preferred to prosthetic grafts because of superior patency rates. Small saphenous and upper extremity veins can be potentially used as bypass conduits. Ideally, vein diameter should be above 3 mm and without calcifications or sclerosis. Smaller veins can be utilized in certain instances if needed.

Often the length of vein needed to complete a bypass is a limiting factor. Prosthetic grafts include: polytetrafluoroethylene (PTFE), expanded PTFE, Dacron, heparin-bonded PTFE. These grafts can be used in patients when suitable autologous vein grafts are not available for bypass, but in patients with CLTI the use of these grafts is highly discouraged.[22]

RESEARCH AND FUTURE DIRECTIONS

In the endovascular space, the use of intravascular imaging to help guide plaque modification strategies and device sizing may be of particular value in increasing primary patency rates of endovascular intervention. Studies currently underway specifically for below-the-knee therapies in the form of sirolimus-based drug delivery technologies and bioresorbable scaffolds may offer improved options for endovascular treatment in the below-the-knee space, which is of critical importance for patients with CLTI. Further, slim sheaths and devices have been developed that allow for the treatment of all lower extremity lesions from the radial access site. Presently, the technology is limited by the availability of devices with the appropriate length; however, this limitation will likely not persist far into the future. Infrapopliteal access has been shown to be safe and effective and offers additional access options outside of the common femoral artery.[43,44]

Ongoing clinical trials—BEST-CLI (NCT02060630), BASIL-2 (ISRCTN27728689), BASIL-3 (ISRCTN14469736), and SWEDEPAD 1 and 2 (NCT02051088)—should be completed and reported in the coming years and will provide more robust data regarding optimal revascularization strategies in patients with both claudication and CLTI.

FOLLOW-UP PATIENT CARE

Aneurysms

In patients with iliac artery aneurysms and concomitant AAA, the follow-up and imaging schedule should be based on the state of the AAA. In patients with isolated iliac artery aneurysms, it is reasonable to perform an imaging evaluation at 0, 6, and 12 months to ascertain the rates of expansion. The choice of imaging modality may depend on local expertise as well as patient factors. For popliteal artery aneurysms, a similar imaging protocol should be followed; however, duplex ultrasound is the optimal test. In patients with popliteal artery aneurysms, clinicians should pay careful attention to distal vascular beds to detect any thromboembolic events that would prompt repair regardless of size.

TABLE 80.6 Follow-up Of Patients With Peripheral Arterial Disease After Revascularization

Category	4-12 Weeks	6 Months	12 Months and Annually
Intermittent claudication	ABI Arterial duplex Serum lipids	ABI Arterial duplex	ABI Arterial duplex Serum lipids
Chronic limb-threatening ischemia	ABI $TcPO_2$ WiFi classification Arterial duplex Serum lipids	ABI $TcPO_2$ WiFi classification Arterial Dupplex Serum lipids	ABI $TcPO_2$ WiFi classification Arterial duplex Serum lipids

ABI, ankle-brachial index; $TcPO_2$, transcutaneous oximetry; WiFi, wound, ischemia, and foot infection.

Chronic Limb Ischemia

Routine follow-up to ensure adequate control of risk factors is advised for all patients. At follow-up visits patients should have, at a minimum, an assessment of blood pressure, pulses, and visual inspection of the feet. Serum lipids and hemoglobin A1c (HbA1c) should be checked every 6 months with intensification of lifestyle and medication treatment to ensure adequate control. In patients who have undergone revascularization, outpatient follow-up within 1 month post-revascularization with an assessment of ABI/TBI, arterial duplex, and wound healing is applicable. **Table 80.6** shows a schedule of recommended tests that should be completed at various points of follow-up.[45] Careful attention should be paid to any changes in symptoms and/or noninvasive testing (even in the absence of definitive worsening or change in symptoms) in patients post-revascularization as these changes could indicate an impending threat to the patency of the revascularization intervention.

KEY POINTS

- ✔ ABI/PVR in high-risk patients to establish early diagnosis and prompt medical therapy to aggressively address atherosclerotic cardiovascular disease (ASCVD) risk factors.
- ✔ Walking exercise therapy is indicated for all claudicants, especially after revascularization.
- ✔ Refrain from anatomic evaluation of patients unless revascularization is being considered.
- ✔ In patients with CLTI, a multidisciplinary approach including wound care experts and careful management of comorbid conditions, specifically diabetes mellitus, are important factors in promoting wound healing and/or limiting the level of amputation.

REFERENCES

1. Centers for Disease Control and Prevention. Peripheral arterial disease fact sheet. 2017. https://www.cdc.gov/dhdsp/data_statistics/fact_sheets/fs_pad.htm
2. Beaufort SC. THE SAGE GROUP releases new estimates for the United States Prevalence and Incidence of Peripheral Artery Disease (PAD) and Critical Limb Ischemia (CLI). Published October 25, 2016. https://www.businesswire.com/news/home/20161025006420/en/SAGE-GROUP-Releases-New-Estimates-United-States
3. Hirsch AT, Criqui MH, Treat-Jacobson D. Peripheral arterial disease detection, awareness, and treatment in primary care. *JAMA.* 2001;286:1317-1324.
4. Dhaliwal G, Mukherjee D. Peripheral arterial disease: epidemiology, natural history, diagnosis and treatment. *Int J Angiol.* 2007;16:36-44.
5. Mukherjee D, Yadav JS. Update on peripheral vascular diseases: from smoking cessation to stenting. *Cleve Clin J Med.* 2001;68:723-733.
6. Planas A, Clarβ A, Marrugat J, et al. Age at onset of smoking is an independent risk factor in peripheral artery disease development. *J Vasc Surg.* 2002;35:506-509.
7. Criqui MH, Aboyans V. Epidemiology of peripheral artery disease. *Circ Res.* 2015; 116:1509-1526.
8. Joosten MM, Pai JK, Bertoia ML, et al. Associations between conventional cardiovascular risk factors and risk of peripheral artery disease in men. *JAMA.* 2012;308:1660-1667.
9. Wattanakit K, Folsom AR, Selvin E, et al. Kidney function and risk of peripheral arterial disease: results from the Atherosclerosis Risk in Communities (ARIC) Study. *J Am Soc Nephrol.* 2007;18:629-636.
10. Criqui MH, Vargas V, Denenberg JO, et al. Ethnicity and peripheral arterial disease. *Circulation.* 2005;112:2703-2707.
11. Ix JH, Allison MA, Denenberg JO, Cushman M, Criqui MH. Novel cardiovascular risk factors do not completely explain the higher prevalence of peripheral arterial disease among African Americans. *J Am Coll Cardiol.* 2008;51:2347-2354.
12. Beks PJ, Mackaay AJ, de Neeling JN, de Vries H, Bouter LM, Heine RJ. Peripheral arterial disease in relation to glycaemic level in an elderly Caucasian population: the Hoorn Study. *Diabetologia.* 1995;38:86-96.
13. Jude EB, Oyibo SO, Chalmers N, Boulton AJM. Peripheral arterial disease in diabetic and nondiabetic patients: a comparison of severity and outcome. *Diabetes Care.* 2001;24:1433-1437.
14. Mowat BF, Skinner ER, Wilson HM, Leng GC, Fowkes FG, Horrobin D. Alterations in plasma lipids, lipoproteins and high density lipoprotein subfractions in peripheral arterial disease. *Atherosclerosis.* 1997;131:161-166.
15. Diehm N, Shang A, Silvestro A, et al. Association of cardiovascular risk factors with pattern of lower limb atherosclerosis in 2659 patients undergoing angioplasty. *Eur J Vasc Endovasc Surg.* 2006;31:59-63.
16. Banerjee S. Superficial femoral artery is not left anterior descending artery. *Circulation.* 2016;134:901-903.
17. Narula N, Dannenberg AJ, Olin JW, et al. Pathology of peripheral artery disease in patients with critical limb ischemia. *J Am Coll Cardiol.* 2018;72:2152-2163.
18. Hayes SN, Kim ESH, Saw J, et al. Spontaneous coronary artery dissection: current state of the science: a scientific statement from the American Heart Association. *Circulation.* 2018;137:e523-e557.
19. Igari K, Sugano N, Kudo T, et al. Surgical treatment for popliteal artery entrapment syndrome. *Ann Vasc Dis.* 2014;7:28-33.

20. Chevalier J-M, Enon B, Walder J, et al. Endofibrosis of the external iliac artery in bicycle racers: an unrecognized pathological state. *Ann Vasc Surg.* 1986;1:297-303.
21. Rutherford RB, Baker JD, Ernst C, et al. Recommended standards for reports dealing with lower extremity ischemia: revised version. *J Vasc Surg.* 1997;26:517-538.
22. Conte MS, Bradbury AW, Kolh P, et al. Global vascular guidelines on the management of chronic limb-threatening ischemia. *Eur J Vasc Endovasc Surg.* 2019;58:S1-S109.e33.
23. Fontaine R, Kim M, Kieny R. [Surgical treatment of peripheral circulation disorders]. *Helv Chir Acta.* 1954:21:499-533.
24. Sigvant B, Lundin F, Wahlberg E. The risk of disease progression in peripheral arterial disease is higher than expected: a meta-analysis of mortality and disease progression in peripheral arterial disease. *Eur J Vasc Endovasc Surg.* 2016;51:395-403.
25. Kasirajan V, Hertzer NR, Beven EG, O'Hara PJ, Krajewski LP, Sullivan TM. Management of isolated common iliac artery aneurysms. *Cardiovasc. Surg.* 1998;6:171-177.
26. Hirsch AT, Haskal ZJ, Hertzer NR, et al. ACC/AHA 2005 Practice Guidelines for the management of patients with peripheral arterial disease (lower extremity, renal, mesenteric, and abdominal aortic): a collaborative report from the American Association for Vascular Surgery/Society for Vascular Surgery, Society for Cardiovascular Angiography and Interventions, Society for Vascular Medicine and Biology, Society of Interventional Radiology, and the ACC/AHA Task Force on Practice Guidelines (Writing Committee to Develop Guidelines for the Management of Patients With Peripheral Arterial Disease): endorsed by the American Association of Cardiovascular and Pulmonary Rehabilitation; National Heart, Lung, and Blood Institute; Society for Vascular Nursing; TransAtlantic Inter-Society Consensus; and Vascular Disease Foundation. *Circulation.* 2006;113:e463-e654.
27. Gerhard-Herman MD, Gornik HL, Barrett C, et al. 2016 AHA/ACC Guideline on the management of patients with lower extremity peripheral artery disease: a report of the American College of Cardiology/American Heart Association Task Force on Clinical Practice Guidelines. *J Am Coll Cardiol.* 2017;69:e726-e779.
28. Koelemay MJ, den Hartog D, Prins MH, Kromhout JG, Legemate DA, Jacobs MJ. Diagnosis of arterial disease of the lower extremities with duplex ultrasonography. *Br J Surg.* 1996;83:404-409.
29. Ota H, Takase K, Igarashi K, et al. MDCT compared with digital subtraction angiography for assessment of lower extremity arterial occlusive disease: importance of reviewing cross-sectional images. *AJR Am J Roentgenol.* 2004;182:201-209.
30. Burbelko M, Augsten M. Kalinowski MO, Heverhagen, JT. Comparison of contrast-enhanced multi-station MR angiography and digital subtraction angiography of the lower extremity arterial disease. *J Magn Reson Imaging.* 2013;37:1427-1435.
31. Bonaca MP, Nault P, Giugliano RP, et al. Low-density lipoprotein cholesterol lowering with evolocumab and outcomes in patients with peripheral artery disease: insights from the FOURIER Trial (Further Cardiovascular Outcomes Research With PCSK9 Inhibition in Subjects With Elevated Risk). *Circulation.* 2018;137:338-350.
32. Cleanthis M, Robless P, Mikhailidis DP, Stansby G. Cilostazol for peripheral arterial disease. doi:10.1002/14651858.CD003748.pub4
33. Mills JL Sr, Conte MS, Armstrong DG, et al. The Society for Vascular Surgery Lower Extremity Threatened Limb Classification System: risk stratification based on wound, ischemia, and foot infection (WIfI). *J Vasc Surg.* 2014;59:220-234.e1-e2.
34. Cannon CP, Blazing MA, Giugliano RP, et al. Ezetimibe added to statin therapy after acute coronary syndromes. *N Engl J Med.* 2015;372: 2387-2397.
35. Bhatt DL, Steg PG, Miller M, et al. Cardiovascular risk reduction with icosapent ethyl for hypertriglyceridemia. *N Engl J Med.* 2019;380:11-22.
36. CAPRIE Steering Committee. A randomised, blinded, trial of clopidogrel versus aspirin in patients at risk of ischaemic events (CAPRIE). CAPRIE Steering Committee. *Lancet.* 1996;348:1329-1339.
37. Hiatt WR, Fowkes FGR, Heizer G, et al. Ticagrelor versus clopidogrel in symptomatic peripheral artery disease. *N Engl J Med.* 2017;376:32-40.
38. Bonaca MP, Bauersachs RM, Anand SS, et al. Rivaroxaban in peripheral artery disease after revascularization. *N Engl J Med.* 2020;382:1994-2004.
39. Eikelboom JW, Connolly SJ, Bosch J, et al. Rivaroxaban with or without aspirin in stable cardiovascular disease. *N Engl J Med.* 2017:377:1319-1330.
40. Bailey SR, Beckman JA, Dao TD, et al. ACC/AHA/SCAI/S:IR/SVM 2018 appropriate use criteria for peripheral artery intervention. *J Am Coll Cardiol.* 2019:73:214-237.
41. Bradbury AW, Adam DJ, Bell J, et al. Bypass versus Angioplasty in Severe Ischaemia of the Leg (BASIL) trial: an intention-to-treat analysis of amputation-free and overall survival in patients randomized to a bypass surgery-first or a balloon angioplasty-first revascularization strategy. *J Vasc Surg.* 2010;51:5S-17S.
42. McFalls EO, Ward HB, Moritz TE, et al. Coronary-artery revascularization before elective major vascular surgery. *N Engl J Med.* 2004;351: 2795-2804
43. Mustapha JA, Saab F, McGoff T, et al. Tibio-pedal arterial minimally invasive retrograde revascularization in patients with advanced peripheral vascular disease: the TAMI technique, original case series. *Catheter Cardiovasc Interv.* 2014;83:987-994.
44. Schmidt A, Bausback Y, Piorkowski M, et al. Retrograde tibioperoneal access for complex infrainguinal occlusions: short-and long-term outcomes of 554 endovascular interventions. *JACC Cardiovasc Interv.* 2019;12:1714-1726.
45. Venermo M, Sprynger M, Desormais I, et al. Follow-up of patients after revascularisation for peripheral arterial diseases: a consensus document from the European Society of Cardiology Working Group on Aorta and Peripheral Vascular Diseases and the European Society for Vascular Surgery. *Eur J Prev Cardiol.* 2019;6(18):1971-1984. doi:10.1177/2047487319846999

CHAPTER 81

CEREBROVASCULAR DISEASE

Steven R. Bailey

INTRODUCTION

Disease of the cerebrovascular system reflects intrinsic alterations of blood flow that occur because of ischemia, hemorrhage, or mass effect. This chapter provides an overview of the clinically important aspects regarding ischemic and hemorrhagic stroke.

Cerebrovascular disease and stroke remain the fifth leading cause of death and the most frequent causes of disability in the United States and the world. In the United States, there are an estimated 795,000 new or recurrent strokes each year, with 147,810 stroke-related deaths reported in 2018.[1]

PATHOGENESIS

Stroke is due to the interruption of blood flow to the brain tissue because of blockage of an artery or hemorrhage from an artery resulting in vascular spasm and compression. Ischemic stroke accounts for over 70% of all strokes,[2] and can be secondary to multiple etiologies including intracerebral atherosclerosis, embolization of plaque/thrombus from an extracerebral vessel, or cardioembolic events. Rare events that are not discussed in greater detail include arteriovenous malformations, vasculitis, and venous sinus thromboses.

One of the most common arterial causes of ischemic stroke is an embolus of an atherosclerotic plaque, with or without thrombus, that originates from arteries within the neck, aortic arch, or intracranial vessels. Inflammation and ulceration of these large vessels occurs as part of the systemic atherosclerotic process involving the heart, peripheral aorta, and cerebral vessels. Occasionally, the carotid artery may progress to complete occlusion; however, in the setting of an intact circle of Willis, this rarely causes a stroke as the primary lesion. More commonly, ulceration and exposure of the lipid-rich core of the atherosclerotic lesion initiates a thrombus that most commonly embolizes to the internal carotid arteries, distal to the bifurcation of the common carotid artery.

Intracranial atherosclerosis, as an etiology of ischemic stroke, shows marked geographic and racial disparities. It is the etiology of ischemic stroke in only 10% to 15% of White patients, typically in diabetic patients who are heavy smokers. This rate increases in Black individuals and is as high as 30% to 50% of Asian patients.[3] Not only is the likelihood of stroke higher in Black as compared to White individuals but they also have a larger burden of intracerebral atherosclerosis.[4] As discussed later, therapy for intracranial occlusion is far more challenging than are large vessel embolic events.

CLINICAL PRESENTATION

Patients suffering a stroke most often present with facial asymmetry, alteration of speech, or arm weakness. This has given rise to the pneumonic "FAST," which stands for *f*acial asymmetry, *a*rm weakness, *s*peech changes, and *t*ime to call 911, as promoted by the American Stroke Association. This was modified to include changes in *b*alance, especially gait-related and *e*ye changes with diplopia or visual changes. This has given rise to the BEFAST mnemonic because it is estimated to identify more than 95% of patients who present with an acute stroke syndrome.

Middle Cerebral Artery Stroke

The middle cerebral artery (MCA) is the most commonly affected vascular distribution. It is divided into four anatomic segments, M1, M2, M3, and M4. M1 supplies the horizontal segment of the MCA that is responsible for blood flow to the basal ganglia.[5] The basal ganglia control emotions, executive function, motor control, and motor learning. The M2 or Sylvian segment supplies blood to the parietal lobe, the insula, inferolateral temporal lobe, and the superior temporal lobe. Branches from this segment supply areas of the brain that process sound and integrate experience and emotion. The M3 (opercular) segment nourishes the surface of the frontoparietal and temporal operculum and extends to the sylvian fissure. The M4 (cortical) segment supplies the surface of the sylvian fissure extending over the cortex.

An MCA infarction typically results in contralateral hemiparesis, facial paralysis, and sensory loss of the face and upper extremity. Gaze preferences toward the side of the lesion may be seen. The lower extremity is less commonly involved. Other findings of an MCA stroke include dysarthria, aphasia, and hemispheric neglect.

The Anterior Cerebral Artery Stroke

The anterior cerebral arteries (ACAs) supply the medial segments of the sylvian fissure forward. It often divides into two branches, A1 and A2. The central artery supplies the caudate nucleus, corpus callosum, and anterior putamen. The cortical branches supply the frontal and olfactory lobes via the orbital branches, parietal lobe from the parietal branches, and cingulate, superior, central, and paracentral gyri. The ACA runs above the optic chiasm and pituitary glands.

An ACA infarct is a rare event, seen in only 3% of all strokes. Typical symptoms include contralateral hemiplegia that is worse in the leg than in the arm (crural hemiparesis). The eye fields may deviate away from the side of hemiplegia. Sensory loss is minimal. Reduced verbal expression or mutism can resemble aphasia.

Posterior Cerebral Artery Stroke

Posterior cerebral artery (PCA) blood flow is related to multiple interconnected vessels. PCA is divided into four segments, P1, P2, P3, and P4. The posterior circulation is supplied by the vertebral, basilar, posterior inferior cerebellar, anterior inferior cerebellar, and superior cerebellar arteries. The PCA supplies the lower part of the optic tract radiations.

Stroke in the posterior circulation is associated with symptoms of diplopia vertigo, visual field defects, dysphagia, memory impairment, and altered consciousness. Unilateral PCA infarction may result in contralateral homonymous hemianopia with sparing of macular vision. Less severe involvement may result in quadrantanopia. Aggressive behavior, hypersomnolence hallucinations, and aggressive behavior or pure sensory stroke may be presenting symptoms as well.

Differential Diagnosis of Acute Stroke

Patients with systemic infections, brain tumors, seizure disorders, metabolic disorders (ie, hypoglycemia or hyponatremia), positional vertigo, or conversion disorders may manifest neurologic symptoms that simulate stroke. Features that suggest non-stroke etiologies include younger age, mild symptoms, no history of vascular risk factors, and arrival to the emergency room by personal transportation rather than by emergency medical services.

The clinical diagnosis of an individual suffering a stroke can be difficult, and in more than 30% of cases, the neurologic symptoms are not due to an acute cerebrovascular event but are due to other etiologies.[6] Neurologic symptoms that can resemble a stroke may be due to systemic infection, seizure, brain tumor, toxic or metabolic disorders (hyponatremia or hypoglycemia), positional vertigo, or psychiatric problems such as a conversion disorder.

Hemorrhagic Stroke

Intracerebral hemorrhage (ICH) is most often the result of hypertension or vascular abnormalities resulting in the rupture of smaller penetrating arteries in contrast to ischemic stroke due to large vessel occlusion. ICH accounts for 10% to 20% of strokes worldwide, but varies widely across social and ethnic strata. In low-income countries, the rates of ICH are nearly double compared to that in high-income countries (22 vs 10 per 100,000 person-years[7]). Non-modifiable risk factors include, age, sex, ethnicity, chronic kidney disease, and cerebral amyloid angiopathy. Rates vary widely across races, with Asian and Black individuals having rates much higher than do Whites and Hispanics. The rates are higher in men than in women. The greatest disparity is seen with age. The rate of ICH increases from 37.2 per 100,000 person-years in men aged 55 to 74 years to 176.3 per 100,000 person-years in men aged 75 to 94 years.[8] Cerebral microbleeds increase with age and are more common in men. These are associated with an increased risk of warfarin-associated ICH as well as spontaneous ICH.

Modifiable risk factors for ICH are hypertension, cigarette smoking, excessive alcohol consumption, and pharmacotherapy with anticoagulant, antithrombotic, or sympathomimetic drugs. These risk factors account for nearly 90% of attributable risk.[9]

Cardioembolic Stroke

Cardioembolic stroke is increasing in frequency, because treatments for hypertension and hyperlipidemia decrease other causes of ischemic stroke. Importantly, cardioembolic strokes are associated with larger strokes than are other etiologies of ischemic stroke.[10] A number of risk factors are associated with cardioembolic stroke including atrial fibrillation, patent foramen ovale, recent myocardial infarction, systolic heart failure, infective endocarditis, prosthetic heart valve, and aortic arch atheroma. Rare causes include atrial myxoma, papillary fibroelastoma, and mitral calcification.

Types of Stroke

Hemorrhagic stroke often presents differently than does ischemic stroke.[11] As the putamen is the most common location for ICH, the most common symptoms are the development over many minutes or a few hours of headache, nausea, and vomiting. Although vomiting may occur in 50% of hemispheric ICH, almost all of cerebellar ICHs have this symptom. Seizures that occur in 10% of patients with ICH are seen in up to 50% of patients with lobar hemorrhage. Decreased level of consciousness may occur because of increased intracranial pressure. Stupor or coma in the setting of ICH defines a subset with involvement of the brainstem reticular activation system.

Cardioembolic strokes typically present with neurologic defects that are maximal at onset and are more likely to affect the cerebral cortex in contrast to small vessel or lacunar strokes with slower progression of symptoms. The involvement of the cerebral cortex is more likely to result in aphasia or visual field defects. Approximately 50% of cardioembolic strokes involve multiple vascular segments.[12]

DIAGNOSTIC APPROACH

Referral to Stroke Center

It is recommended by the American Heart Association (AHA)/ American Stroke Association (ASA) 2019 guidelines that the early management of patients for potential stroke occurs within a regional system of care.[6] Patients at high clinical suspicion should be referred to a certified stroke center capable of administering thrombolytic therapy (ie, intravenous tissue plasminogen activator [IV t-PA]). The benefit, in the setting of multiple thrombolytic-capable facilities, of referring to a center that has mechanical thrombectomy capability is uncertain at this time.

The treatment of stroke should begin with a determination of symptom onset, because this is critical for decisions regarding therapy and prognosis. If the time of symptom onset is unknown, the time the patient was last known to be normal without new neurologic symptoms should be used as the time of onset.

An expeditious neurologic assessment should be performed for all patients with suspected stroke. The most common tool is the National Institutes of Health Stroke Scale (NIHSS), which reviews 11 categories including level of consciousness, gaze, visual, facial palsy, motor function of arms and legs, ataxia, language, dysarthria, extinction, and inattention. Vertigo is associated with vertebrobasilar artery system occlusion, and may be either central or peripheral. A focused physical examination is also important as part of the initial evaluation. Vital signs, breathing, circulation, and airway need to be assessed. Patients with respiratory compromise due to elevated intracranial pressure are at increased risk for aspiration and asphyxiation, and they should be evaluated for the need for endotracheal intubation.

Reversible causes of neurologic defects should be excluded. Blood glucose using a finger stick should be determined immediately. Other laboratory testing including complete blood count and platelets, troponin, prothrombin time, international normalized ratio, and activated partial thromboplastin time may be indicated, but should not delay the start of thrombolytic therapy. Additional laboratory testing can be deferred until the acute stroke management has occurred.

Diagnostic Modalities

The clinical diagnosis of stroke is based on clinical presentation, but confirmed with imaging. The imaging tools available include computed tomography (CT) without contrast, computed tomography angiography (CTA), CT perfusion, CT venography, magnetic resonance imaging (MRI), magnetic resonance angiography (MRA), magnetic resonance perfusion, ultrasonography, nuclear medicine, and invasive angiography. CT imaging is readily available and non-contrast CT imaging studies do not increase the risk of renal dysfunction. Conversely, imaging using contrast—iodinated and gadolinium—can result in renal injury.

The initial imaging performed for patients with suspected stroke is CT without contrast, which is excellent at excluding hemorrhage. The identification of ischemic stroke by non-contrast CT varies with the age of infarction. In the hyperacute phase (<12 hours) non-contrast CT is most valuable for excluding hemorrhage. Occasionally a thrombus can be detected because of high attenuation in the images. In the acute phase (12-24 hours), the findings are subtle: loss of gray/white matter interface due to increased water content secondary to cell edema. The subacute phase (24 hours to 5 days) demonstrates edema due to altered blood vessels with well-defined margins and mass effect. Old strokes are visualized by non-contrast CT as volume loss of parenchyma and hypoattenuation due to encephalomacia.[13] The non-contrast CT image can be used in risk assessment and decisions regarding thrombolytic therapy. The ASPECTS (Alberta Stroke Program Early CT Score) scale is a 10-point quantitative score used to assess early ischemic changes on non-contrast head CT. A score of less than 7 is associated with worse outcomes.[14]

CTA is performed by injection of IV contrast, typically into an antecubital vein, to better identify vessel thrombosis or occlusion, aneurysm, and dissection. Reconstructions of three-dimensional (3D) images and maximal intensity projections can assist with determination of clot length and distal stenosis.

MRI with or without gadolinium plays an important role in stroke imaging. MRI has higher soft-tissue contrast imaging ratios than does CT, particularly in the hyperacute and acute phases of stroke, with changes seen as early as 3 hours. Multiple protocols may be used, including fluid-attenuated inversion recovery (FLAIR), T2-weighted imaging (T2WI), T1-weighted imaging (T1WI), and diffusion-weighted imaging (DWI). DWI utilizes the impairment of mitochondrial function resulting in a shift of water into the cell, causing restricted water motion, and is considered the best sequence to detect brain infarctions as early as minutes after onset. It has a sensitivity ranging from 88% to 100% and a specificity of 95% to 100%, with an accuracy of 95%.[15] MRA is similar to CTA, but is more time consuming to obtain, is not available in every center, and is typically used for patients allergic to iodinated contrast material.

MANAGEMENT

Medical Approach

In the setting of an acute stroke, medical management consists of a focused history to determine timing of onset of stroke and assessment of indications and contraindications to thrombolytic therapy or mechanical thrombectomy (**Algorithm 81.1**). The current goal for door-to-needle time is 60 minutes or less. Within this goal is a door-to-initial physician contact (<2.5 minutes), door-to-stroke team (within 5 minutes), door-to-CT/MRI acquisition (within 25 minutes), door-to-CT/MRI interpretation (within 45 minutes), and door-to-needle time of less than 60 minutes. If there is a decision to perform mechanical thrombectomy, the door-to-device time should be less than 90 minutes. Innovative protocols such as direct door-to-CT can yield even shorter times to definitive therapy.

While treating the patient, blood pressure should be maintained in the less than 185/110 mm Hg range and blood sugar greater than the 50 mg/dL level.

Within the initial brief clinical evaluation, the indication for thrombolytic therapy should be determined on the basis of time of presentation from symptom onset as well as other risk factors. Currently, patients 18 years or older who present within 3 hours of symptom onset having mild but disabling stroke or severe stroke without contraindications have a Class I indication for IV t-PA administration (**Table 81.1**). Patients presenting at 3 to 4.5 hours between the ages of 18 and 80 years without prior stroke or diabetes with an NIHSS score less than or equal to 25, not taking oral anticoagulants, and without imaging evidence of involvement of greater than one-third of the MCA territory are also considered Class I for IV t-PA administration. **Table 81.2** provides information regarding risk assessment and contraindications to IV t-PA administration.

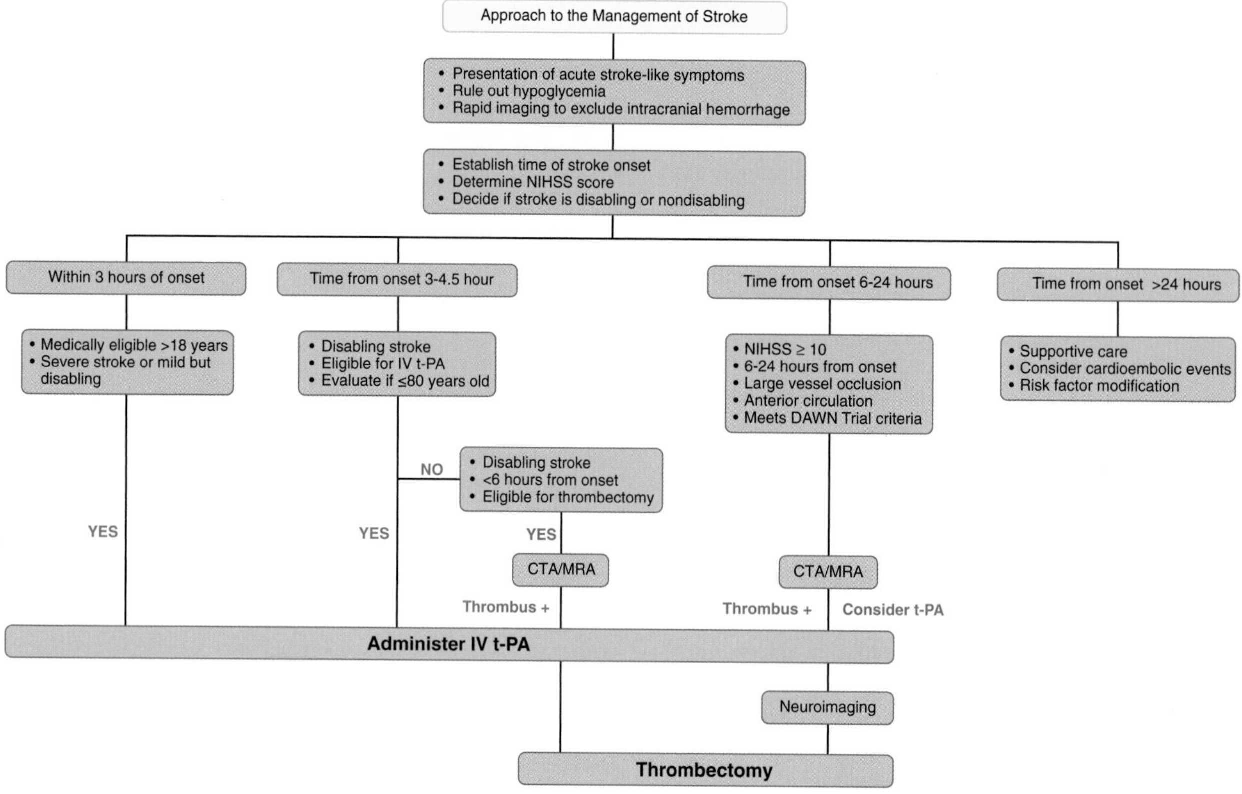

ALGORITHM 81.1 Approach to the management of acute stroke. CTA, computed tomography angiogram; DAWN, Diffusion weighted imaging or computerized tomography perfusion Assessment with clinical mismatch in the triage of Wake up and late presenting strokes undergoing Neurointervention; IV t-PA, intravenous tissue plasminogen activator; MRA, magnetic resonance angiogram; NIHSS, National Institutes of Health Stroke Scale. (Adapted from Powers WJ, Rabinstein AA, Ackerson T, et al. Guidelines for the early management of patients with acute ischemic stroke: 2019 update to the 2018 guidelines for the early management of acute ischemic stroke: a guideline for healthcare professionals American Heart Association/American Stroke Association. *Stroke.* 2019;50(12):e344-e418. doi:10.1161/STR.0000000000000211; Nogueira RG, Jadhav AP, Haussen DC, et al. Thrombectomy 6 to 24 hours after stroke with a mismatch between deficit and infarct. *N Engl J Med.* 2018;378:11-21. doi:10.1056/NEJMoa1706442)

TABLE 81.1 Indications for Intravenous Tissue Plasminogen Activator Therapy

Current indications: Class I recommendations

Stroke symptom(s) onset within 3 hours and the following are present:

- 18 years of age or older
- Severe stroke[a]
- Mild but disabling stroke[b]

Stroke symptom(s) onset 3-4.5 hours ago and the following are present:

- 18-79 years of age
- Without a history of both diabetes mellitus and prior stroke
- NIHSS score ≤25
- Not taking oral anticoagulants
- Without imaging evidence of ischemic injury involving more than one-third of the middle cerebral artery territory
- Blood pressure can be lowered safely and maintained <185/110 mm Hg
- Blood glucose >50 mg/dL
- Mild to moderate early ischemic changes on non-contrast CT scan
- With antiplatelet drug monotherapy or combination therapy
- With end-stage renal disease with normal aPTT

aPTT, activated partial thromboplastin time; CT, computed tomography; t-PA, tissue plasminogen activator.

[a]Severe stroke is defined as National Institutes of Health Stroke Scale (NIHSS) score of 21 or greater.

[b]Mild but disabling is a NIHSS score of 20 or less but with significant mental or physical disability.

Data from Powers WJ, Rabinstein AA, Ackerson T, et al. Guidelines for the early management of patients with acute ischemic stroke: 2019 update to the 2018 guidelines for the early management of acute ischemic stroke: a guideline for healthcare professionals from the American Heart Association/American Stroke Association. *Stroke.* 2019;50(12):e344-e418.

TABLE 81.2 Contraindications to Intravenous Tissue Plasminogen Activator (t-PA) Therapy

Patients presenting 3-4.5 hours from stroke symptom onset
- 80 years of age or older (COR IIa)
- Both prior stroke and diabetes mellitus (COR IIb)
- Mild but disabling stroke (COR IIb)
- NIHSS score >25 (COR IIb)

Relative contraindications
- Preexisting dementia (COR IIb)
- Moderate to severe ischemic stroke with early improvement, but remains moderately impaired and potentially disabled (COR IIa)
- Seizure at the time of onset, if evidence suggests that residual impairments are secondary to stroke (COR IIa)
- Preexisting disability (mRS ≥ 2 COR IIb)
- Initial blood glucose levels <50 or >400 mg/dL that are subsequently normalized (COR IIb)
- Clinical history of potential bleeding diathesis or coagulopathy (COR IIb)
- History of warfarin use and an INR ≤ 1.7 or a PT < 15 s (COR IIb)
- Lumbar dural puncture in the preceding 7 days (COR IIb)
- Arterial puncture of a noncompressible blood vessel in the preceding 7 days (COR IIb)
- Recent major trauma (within 14 days) not involving the head (COR IIb)
- Major surgery in the preceding 14 days (COR IIb)
- History of gastrointestinal or genitourinary bleeding (>21 days) (COR IIb)
- Women who are menstruating and do not have a history of menorrhagia (COR IIa)
- Women with recent or active history of menorrhagia without clinically significant anemia or hypotension (COR IIb)
- Recent or active vaginal bleeding causing clinically significant anemia (after emergency consultation with a gynecologist) (COR IIa)
- Extracranial cervical arterial dissection (COR IIa)
- Intracranial arterial dissection (COR IIb)
- Small or moderately sized unruptured and unsecured intracranial aneurysm (COR IIa)
- Giant unruptured and unsecured intracranial aneurysm (COR IIb)
- Unruptured and untreated intracranial vascular malformation, if high likelihood of morbidity and mortality outweigh the anticipated risk of ICH (COR IIb)
- Small number of cerebral microbleeds demonstrated on MRI (COR IIa)
- Previously high burden of cerebral microbleeds (>10) demonstrated on MRI if there is potential for substantial benefit (COR IIb)
- Extra-axial intracranial neoplasm (COR IIb)
- Concurrent acute MI, followed by percutaneous coronary angioplasty and stenting, if indicated (COR IIa)
- MI in the past 3 months: non-STEMI or STEMI involving the right or inferior myocardium (COR IIa)
- MI in the past 3 months: STEMI involving the left anterior myocardium (COR IIb)
- Major AIS likely to produce severe disability and acute pericarditis (COR IIb), after urgent consultation with cardiologist
- Moderate AIS likely to produce mild disability and acute pericarditis (COR IIb)
- Major or moderate AIS likely to produce severe or mild disability and known left atrial or ventricular thrombus (COR IIb)
- Major AIS likely to produce severe disability and cardiac myxoma or papillary fibroelastoma (COR IIb)
- AIS due to complications of cardiac or cerebral angiographic procedures (COR IIa)
- Systemic malignancy and >6-month life expectancy in the absence of other contraindications (COR IIb)
- Pregnancy, when anticipated benefits of treating severe or moderate stroke outweigh increased risk of uterine bleeding (COR IIb)
- Early postpartum period (<14 days after delivery) (COR IIb)
- History of diabetic hemorrhagic retinopathy or other hemorrhagic ophthalmic conditions, but potential increased risk of visual loss should be weighed against anticipated benefits (COR IIa)
- Sickle cell disease in adults (COR IIa)
- Hyperdense middle cerebral artery sign (COR IIa)
- Illicit drug use (COR IIa)
- Stroke mimics (COR IIa)

Contraindications (Class III—Harm)
- CT reveals an acute intracranial hemorrhage
- CT brain imaging exhibits extensive regions of clear hypoattenuation
- Prior ischemic stroke within 3 months
- Recent severe head trauma within 3 months
- Acute head trauma (posttraumatic infarction that occurs during the acute in-hospital phase)
- Intracranial/spinal surgery within the prior 3 months
- History of intracranial hemorrhage
- Symptoms and signs most consistent with a subarachnoid hemorrhage
- Structural gastrointestinal malignancy
- Gastrointestinal bleeding event within 21 days

Continued

TABLE 81.2 Contraindications to Intravenous Tissue Plasminogen Activator (t-PA) Therapy (*Continued*)

- Platelets < 100,000/mm^3
- INR > 1.7
- aPTT > 40 s
- PT > 15 s
- Treatment dose of LMWH within the previous 24 hours
- Taking direct thrombin inhibitors or direct factor Xa inhibitors unless laboratory tests are normal or the patient has not received a dose of these agents for >48 hours (assuming normal renal metabolic function)
- Symptoms consistent with infective endocarditis
- Known or suspected to be associated with aortic arch dissection
- Intra-axial intracranial neoplasm

Contraindications (Class III—No benefit)

- Otherwise eligible patients with mild but nondisabling stroke

AIS, acute ischemic stroke; aPTT, activated partial thromboplastin time; COR, Class of Recommendation; CT, computed tomography; ICH, intracerebral hemorrhage; INR, international normalized ratio; LMWH, low-molecular-weight heparin; MI, myocardial infarction; MRI, magnetic resonance imaging; mRS, modified Rankin Score; NIHSS, National Institutes of Health Stroke Scale; PT, partial thromboplastin time; STEMI, ST-elevation myocardial infarction.

Data from Powers WJ, Rabinstein AA, Ackerson T, et al. Guidelines for the early management of patients with acute ischemic stroke: 2019 update to the 2018 guidelines for the early management of acute ischemic stroke: a guideline for healthcare professionals from the American Heart Association/American Stroke Association. *Stroke.* 2019;50(12):e344-e418.

Percutaneous Approaches

Mechanical thrombectomy with stent thrombus retrievers (Class I C-EO) is increasingly utilized for those patients presenting less than 6 hours after the onset of an acute stroke.[16] Mechanical thrombectomy is recommended over intra-arterial fibrinolysis as first-line therapy.[16] Mechanical thrombectomy has a Class I indication for individuals older than 18 years who have a prestroke modified Rankin Score (mRS) less than 1, occlusion of the internal carotid artery or proximal MCA, NIHSS score greater than or equal to 6, and ASPECTS score greater than or equal to 6. Patients who present greater than 6 hours and less than 24 hours after the onset of symptoms with an occlusion of the internal carotid artery or M1 segment of the MCA and a disproportionately severe clinical deficit relative to infarct volume on imaging can be considered for mechanical thrombectomy as well.[17,18] One series estimates that the current procedure rate of mechanical thrombectomy (3 per 100,000 patients) could rise to as many 24 per 100,000 patients if it was applied more often in patients presenting between 6 and 24 hours after symptom onset.[19]

Surgical Management of Stroke

Surgical or percutaneous stent management of stroke, except in the setting of an acute complication of an endarterectomy or stent procedure, has limited utility in the setting of the patient with an acute stroke.

Acute Medical Management Post a Stroke

Acute management includes maintenance of airway and attention to oxygenation. Supplemental oxygen is indicted if the oxygen saturation falls below 94%. Regulation of blood pressure post a stroke is often dynamic. Although permissive hypertension to 220/120 mm Hg during the first 24 to 48 hours may be acceptable if no acute intervention is performed, a blood pressure target of 180/105 mm Hg is recommended if IV t-PA or mechanical thrombectomy is administered[20] to decrease hypertensive encephalopathy, hemorrhagic transformation, and cardiac, pulmonary, and renal complications. The optimal blood pressure post interventional therapy is currently uncertain.

Severe hyperglycemia is associated with worse outcomes. Aggressive glucose lowering (target 80-130 mg/dL) does not improve outcomes, and results in more hypoglycemic events than permissive hyperglycemia. The current guidelines recommend maintaining glucose levels between 140 and 180 mg/dL.[21] Hyperosmolar therapy does not improve outcomes. Decompressive hemicraniectomy[22] may decrease mortality and improve functional outcomes, but timing for this procedure remains to be answered. Targeted temperature control has not been shown to improve outcomes.

Enteral feedings beginning in the first 48 hours improves outcomes. Investigation of speech and swallowing functions assists in determining the need for long-term enteral alimentation using a percutaneous enteral gastrostomy. Early mobilization after the acute stroke and initiation of rehabilitation beginning in the intensive care unit is associated with improved outcomes and functional recovery.[23]

Evaluation of Unknown Etiology of Acute Stroke

As discussed earlier, acute ischemic stroke is classified as (1) large artery atherosclerosis; (2) cardioembolic; (3) small vessel occlusion; (4) stroke of other determined etiology; or (5) stroke of undetermined etiology. In patients with an unknown etiology, evaluation for a vascular, cardiac, or hypercoagulable etiology should be undertaken. This can include vascular imaging, MRI, echocardiography with agitated saline contrast imaging, hemoglobin A_{1C}, lipid panel, and hypercoagulability workup, among others.

Secondary Prevention

Administration of aspirin within 48 hours of ischemic stroke decreases the risk of a second stroke. A meta-analysis of 16 trials demonstrated a 22% reduction in recurrent ischemic stroke in the first several weeks post ischemic stroke.[24] The Platelet-Oriented Inhibition in New TIA and minor ischemic stroke (POINT) trial of aspirin and clopidogrel demonstrated a reduction in recurrent ischemic strokes with their use at 90 days.

In patients with dyslipidemia, early initiation of high-intensity statin therapy decreases both fatal and nonfatal strokes[25] in a diverse patient population with small vessel occlusion, large vessel atherosclerosis, and unknown causes (excluding cardioembolic events). Although still the subject of investigation, the recommended target low-density lipoprotein cholesterol level is 70 mg/dL. This seems to encompass not only the cholesterol-lowering effects but also the pleotropic effects of endothelial protection, decreased thrombosis, and inflammation.

INTRACRANIAL ANEURYSM

Demographics

Intracranial aneurysms represent an abnormal dilatation of the arterial wall. The anterior segment of the circle of Willis is the site of 85% of aneurysms.[26] Approximately 2.8% of the U.S. population (>6 million individuals) have one or more unruptured intracranial aneurysms. They are most prevalent in patients between the ages of 35 and 60 years, with women being 1.5 times more likely to have an intracranial aneurysm than do men. Although only 0.25% of aneurysms rupture, they still represent 3% to 5% of all new strokes, primarily related to secondary subarachnoid hemorrhage. The incidence of intracranial aneurysm rupture peaks in the fifth decade. A number of risk factors are associated with aneurysm growth and rupture, including genetic conditions, family history, female sex, hormonal therapy, uncontrolled hypertension, older age, alcohol abuse, and cigarette smoking. Aortic aneurysm, bicuspid aortic valve, coarctation of the aorta, and Marfan syndrome are also associated with intracranial aneurysms.

Clinical Presentation

The common presenting symptoms are headache (25%), transient cerebral ischemia (10%), and "spells," otherwise undefined (7%). Other symptoms can include seizures, cranial neuropathy, or visual disturbances. A sentinel headache days to weeks before intracranial aneurysm hemorrhage has been reported in 10% to 43% of cases, and appears to represent patients at high risk of death.[27]

Aneurysm rupture is often lethal with death in 4% to 14% of cases within the first 24 hours, with most within 6 hours of presentation, and 50% of patients will die by 6 months without treatment. Intracranial aneurysm recurrent hemorrhage carries a 50% to 85% mortality.[28]

Diagnosis

Most intracranial aneurysms are discovered during evaluation for intracranial hemorrhage or incidental evaluation for other symptoms. A non-contrast CT is positive in approximately 98% of cases within the first 12 hours of intracranial aneurysm hemorrhage and over 90% at 24 hours. The finding of intracranial hemorrhage decreases over time. If the CT finding is negative but clinical suspicion is high, an MRI with FLAIR imaging or a lumbar puncture is indicated to establish the diagnosis. Angiography (CTA, MRA, or invasive) is useful to identify location and size of intracranial aneurysms.

Currently, guidelines do not recommend CTA/MRA screening for intracranial aneurysms in the general population.[29] Patients should be screened if they have two or more family members with an intracranial aneurysm, polycystic kidney disease, fibromuscular dysplasia, aortic aneurysms, or osteodysplastic dwarfism.[29]

Medical Therapy

Medical therapy to include control of blood pressure and smoking cessation have been demonstrated in small studies to decrease the risk of intracranial aneurysm rupture, although the small sample size leaves uncertainty. Use of aspirin does not seem to increase the size of intracranial aneurysm hemorrhage and, in one randomized trial, decreased the risk of hemorrhage from unruptured intracranial aneurysms. Anticoagulants are poorly studied, but seem to increase the risk and severity of intracranial aneurysm hemorrhage.

Vasospasm post aneurysm rupture is seen in 40% to 70% of patients, peaking at 7 to 10 days post the rupture. Although vasospasm may be symptomatic or asymptomatic, it can lead to recurrent stroke and should be managed with calcium channel blocker administration.[30]

Percutaneous and Surgical Approaches

In patients with aneurysmal subarachnoid hemorrhage, the decision on treatment depends on the surgical and endovascular expertise of the group, admission subarachnoid hemorrhage grade, aneurysm location, presence or potential of vasospasm, and occurrence of a space-occupying hematoma. Early studies demonstrated higher rates of closure using surgical clipping with lower procedural morbidity and mortality than in those treated endovascularly. Flow diverters, or stents, have been introduced to treat intracranial aneurysms without rupture. Use of flow diverters in subarachnoid hemorrhage has demonstrated acceptable acute sealing of the aneurysm, but shows an increased risk of thrombosis in the posterior circulation and with multiple devices. There is also concern about the need for dual antiplatelet therapy in patients with subarachnoid hemorrhage treated with these therapies.

SPECIAL CONSIDERATIONS

The optimal device for intracranial aneurysm treatment remains to be defined. Outcomes reflect institutional expertise, operator experience, patient selection, and patient choices. The choice of therapy is complex, should occur in a multidisciplinary setting, and optimally involve the patient and family members.

There are no guidelines that specify surveillance intervals. The typical initial evaluations are at 6 to 12 months, with follow-up at 2 to 3 years after the initial evaluation. Poststroke and hemorrhage protocols that examine imaging and potential proteomic markers will assist in risk stratifying patients.

RESEARCH AND FUTURE DIRECTIONS

Stroke identification and access to timely care remains a critical need. Unfortunately, unlike acute myocardial infarction that is diagnosed by an electrocardiogram and serum biomarkers, stroke has no single, quick, and simple test. Development of reliable scales that can predict stroke severity on presentation is needed. Field-deployed CT scanners are not feasible in most geographic settings, thus leaving clinicians with the need for easy, quick, and reliable clinical scales, because the current ones are cumbersome and have limited predictive value. New deep learning and artificial intelligence programs are being developed—such as CVaid (Tel Aviv, Israel) and Pulsara (Bozeman, MT)—to assist in patient assessment, establish testing and triage plans, and decrease dependency on access to stroke centers. Finally, once diagnostic imaging is obtained, new protocols for automated assessment using the ASPECTS score are being developed to assist sites with improved diagnostic accuracy and optimal therapeutic plans.

An additional opportunity is to extend the time window for definitive therapy using adjunctive pharmacology. Recent trials using NA-1 have promising early results, but larger, longer term trials in patients who do not receive IV t-PA are required to understand the potential of such agents.[31]

KEY POINTS

- ✔ Stroke mortality is decreasing in the United States but remains the leading cause of disability worldwide.
- ✔ The BEFAST criteria should be used to screen patients for potential stroke, because it can identify more than 95% of patients who present with an acute stroke.
- ✔ Stroke multidisciplinary teams improve patient outcomes and functional recovery.
- ✔ Intracranial aneurysms and subarachnoid hemorrhage require a multidisciplinary team to decide on optimal device and procedures.
- ✔ Deep learning and artificial intelligence offer opportunities to improve stroke diagnosis.
- ✔ Adjunctive pharmacology to extending the treatment time window is being evaluated in prospective trials.

REFERENCES

1. Virani SS, Alonso A, Aparicio HJ, et al. Heart disease and stroke statistics—2021 update: a report from the American Heart Association. *Circulation.* 2021;143:e254-e743.
2. Feigin VL, Nguyen G, Cercy K, et al. Global, regional, and country-specific lifetime risks of stroke, 1990 and 2016. *N Engl J Med.* 2018;379:2429-2437.
3. Kim JS, Kim YJ, Ahn SH, Kim BJ. Location of cerebral atherosclerosis: why is there a difference between East and West? *Int J Stroke.* 2018;13(1):35-46.
4. Qiao Y, Suri FK, Zhang Y, et al. Racial differences in prevalence and risk for intracranial atherosclerosis in a US community-based population. *JAMA Cardiol.* 2017;2(12):1341-1348. doi:10.1001/jamacardio.2017.4041
5. Cho L, Mukherjee D. Basic cerebral anatomy for the carotid interventionalist: the intracranial and extracranial vessels. *Catheter Cardiovasc Interv.* 2006;68(1):104-111.
6. Powers WJ, Rabinstein AA, Ackerson T, et al. Guidelines for the early management of patients with acute ischemic stroke: 2019 update to the 2018 guidelines for the early management of acute ischemic stroke: a guideline for healthcare professionals from the American Heart Association/American Stroke Association. *Stroke.* 2019;50(12):e344-e418. doi:10.1161/STR.0000000000000211
7. Feigin VL, Lawes CM, Bennett DA, Barker-Collo SL, Parag V. Worldwide stroke incidence and early case fatality reported in 56 population-based studies: a systematic review. *Lancet Neurol.* 2009;8:355-369.
8. Jolink WM, Klijn CJ, Brouwers PJ, Kappelle LJ, Vaartjes I. Time trends in incidence, case fatality, and mortality of intracerebral hemorrhage. *Neurology.* 2015;85:1318-1324.
9. Charidimou A, Kakar P, Fox Z, Werring DJ. Cerebral microbleeds and recurrent stroke risk: systematic review and meta-analysis of prospective ischemic stroke and transient ischemic attack cohorts. *Stroke.* 2013;44:995-1001.
10. O'Donnell MJ, Xavier D, Liu L, et al. Risk factors for ischaemic and intracerebral haemorrhagic stroke in 22 countries (the INTERSTROKE study): a case-control study. *Lancet.* 2010;376(9735):112-123.
11. Runchey S, McGee S. Does this patient have a hemorrhagic stroke?: clinical findings distinguishing hemorrhagic stroke from ischemic stroke. *JAMA.* 2010;303(22):2280-2286.
12. Adams HP, Bendixen BH, Kappelle LJ, et al. Classification of subtype of acute ischemic stroke. Definitions for use in a multicenter clinical trial. TOAST. Trial of Org 10172 in Acute Stroke Treatment. *Stroke.* 1993;24:35-41.
13. Birenbaum D, Bancroft LW, Felsberg GJ. Imaging in acute stroke. *West J Emerg Med.* 2011;12(1):67-76.
14. Puetz V, Dzialowski I, Hill MD, Demchuk AM. The Alberta Stroke Program Early CT Score in clinical practice: what have we learned? *Int J Stroke.* 2009;4(5):354-364.
15. Kamalian S, Lev MH. Stroke imaging. *Radiol Clin North Am.* 2019;57(4):717-732.
16. Goyal M, Menon BK, van Zwam WH, et al. Endovascular thrombectomy after large-vessel ischaemic stroke: a meta-analysis of individual patient data from five randomised trials. *Lancet.* 2016;387(10029):1723-1731.
17. Albers GW, Marks MP, Kemp S, et al. Thrombectomy for stroke at 6 to 16 hours with selection by perfusion imaging. *N Engl J Med.* 2018;378(8):708-718.
18. Nogueira RG, Jadhav AP, Haussen DC, et al. Thrombectomy 6 to 24 hours after stroke with a mismatch between deficit and infarct. *N Engl J Med.* 2018;378(1):11-21. doi:10.1056/NEJMoa1706442
19. Rai AT, Seldon AE, Boo S, et al. A population-based incidence of acute large vessel occlusions and thrombectomy eligible patients indicates significant potential for growth of endovascular stroke therapy in the USA. *J Neurointerv Surg.* 2017;9:722-726.
20. Rasmussen M, Schönenberger S, Hendèn PL, et al. Blood pressure thresholds and neurologic outcomes after endovascular therapy for acute ischemic stroke: an analysis of individual patient data from 3 randomized clinical trials. *JAMA Neurol.* 2020;77:622-631.
21. Johnston KC, Bruno A, Pauls Q, et al. Intensive vs standard treatment of hyperglycemia and functional outcome in patients with acute ischemic stroke: the SHINE randomized clinical trial. *JAMA.* 2019;322:326-335.
22. Vahedi K, Hofmeijer J, Juettler E, et al. Early decompressive surgery in malignant infarction of the middle cerebral artery: a pooled

analysis of three randomised controlled trials. *Lancet Neurol.* 2007;6: 215-222.
23. Hu MH, Hsu SS, Yip PK, et al. Early and intensive rehabilitation predicts good functional outcomes in patients admitted to the stroke intensive care unit. *Disabil Rehabil.* 2010;32:1251-1259.
24. Rothwell PM, Algra A, Chen Z, et al. Effects of aspirin on risk and severity of early recurrent stroke after transient ischaemic attack and ischaemic stroke: time-course analysis of randomised trials. *Lancet.* 2016;388:365-375.
25. Amarenco P, Bogousslavsky J, Callahan A III, et al. High-dose atorvastatin after stroke or transient ischemic attack. *N Engl J Med.* 2006;355:549-559.
26. Schievink WI. Intracranial aneurysms. *N Engl J Med.* 1997;336:28-40.
27. Beck J, Raabe A, Szelenyi A, et al. Sentinel headache and the risk of rebleeding after aneurysmal subarachnoid hemorrhage. *Stroke.* 2006;37: 2733-2737.
28. Naidech AM, Janjua N, Kreiter KT, et al. Predictors and impact of aneurysm rebleeding after subarachnoid hemorrhage. *Arch Neurol.* 2005;62:410-416.
29. Thompson BG, Brown RD Jr, Amin-Hanjani S, et al. Guidelines for the management of patients with unruptured intracranial aneurysms: a guideline for healthcare professionals from the American Heart Association/ American Stroke Association. *Stroke.* 2015;46:2368-2400.
30. Connolly ES Jr, Rabinstein AA, Carhuapoma JR, et al. Guidelines for the management of aneurysmal subarachnoid hemorrhage: a guideline for healthcare professionals from the American Heart Association/American Stroke Association. *Stroke.* 2012;43:1711-1737.
31. Hill MD, Goyal M, Menon BK, et al. Efficacy and safety of nerinetide for the treatment of acute ischaemic stroke (ESCAPE-NA1): a multicentre, double-blind, randomised controlled trial. *Lancet.* 2020;395:878-887. doi:10.1016/S0140-6736(20)30258-0

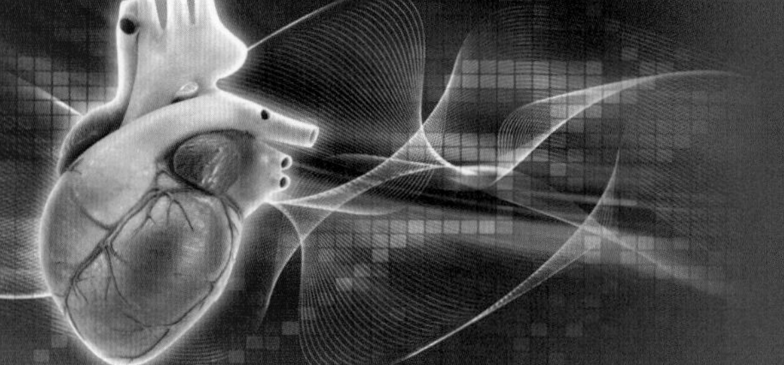

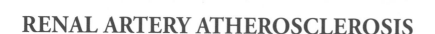

CHAPTER 82

RENAL ARTERY ATHEROSCLEROSIS

Jose D. Tafur and Christopher J. White

INTRODUCTION

Atherosclerotic renal artery stenosis (ARAS) is an important cause of secondary hypertension. It also threatens renal function and increases the risk of cardiovascular decompensation syndromes such as acute coronary syndromes and flash pulmonary edema.[1,2] Understanding the pathophysiology and clinical manifestation of ARAS is crucial in optimizing care for patients with the condition. In each individual with ARAS, it is important to determine whether it is hemodynamically significant and causing a clinical problem such as uncontrolled hypertension, fluid retention, or renal insufficiency.

Epidemiology

It is estimated that about 7% of individuals older than age 65 years have ARAS.[3] An autopsy series showed ARAS with greater than or equal to 50% luminal diameter narrowing (ie, stenosis) in 27% of patients older than 50 years and 53% of patients with prior history of diastolic hypertension.[4] Another autopsy series found that 8% of patients with diabetes and 10% of patients with both diabetes and hypertension had evidence of ARAS.[5] Coronary artery disease, hypertension, diabetes, smoking, and age are associated with an increased prevalence of ARAS. The strongest predictor of ARAS is the presence of atherosclerotic peripheral vascular disease (PAD).[2]

Risk Factors

The patient with ARAS frequently has atherosclerotic vascular disease involving other vascular beds such as the coronaries, lower extremities, and carotids. A study to determine the prevalence of ARAS in patients with atherosclerosis elsewhere found ARAS—defined as greater than 50% renal artery diameter stenosis—in 38% of subjects with an abdominal aortic aneurysm and 39% of those with PAD. Another multicenter cohort study evaluated the association of ARAS with age, gender, and other potential risk factors among participants in the cardiovascular health study (CHS). ARAS (≥60% stenosis) was found in 6.8% of study participants, including 5.5% women and 9.1% of men ($P = 0.053$). ARAS was found in 6.9% of white and 6.7% of African American participants ($P = 0.993$).[3]

ARAS represents more than 90% of all causes of renal artery stenosis (RAS). It predominantly affects patients of advanced age and those with other risk factors for atherosclerotic disease (diabetes, dyslipidemia, and tobacco use).[6] ARAS may be unilateral or bilateral, usually involving the ostium and more proximal segments of the renal arteries.

PATHOGENESIS

Neurohormonal activation from unilateral or bilateral renal hypoperfusion will result in renin release, an early stimulator in the renin-angiotensin-aldosterone system (RAAS).[7,8] When hypoperfusion occurs, the ischemic kidney releases renin from juxtaglomerular cells. Renin stimulates the release of angiotensin I, which is converted to angiotensin II by angiotensin-converting enzyme (ACE) in the pulmonary endothelium. In unilateral ARAS, this neurohormonal activation will lead to vasoconstriction and pressure diuresis of the unaffected kidney known as *pressure natriuresis*; this prevents systemic volume overload causing hypertension and hyponatremia. Angiotensin II also stimulates the release of antidiuretic hormone from the posterior pituitary gland, stimulating the release of aldosterone from the adrenal cortex. Aldosterone exerts effects on the renal tubules, causing more sodium and water retention. With bilateral (or solitary ARAS with a single functioning kidney), the lack of natriuresis leads to fluid and sodium retention, resulting in congestive heart failure (CHF).[9]

Ischemic nephropathy occurs in severe ARAS when there is a significant decrease in renal cortical oxygenation that leads to excretory dysfunction. There are several mechanisms explaining how a hemodynamically significant lesion ultimately results in interstitial fibrosis.[10] By one pathway, recurrent local ischemia causes tubulointerstitial injury and microvascular damage, which contributes to oxidative injury, increased production of fibrogenic cytokines, and inflammation that eventually leads to atrophy and fibrosis. In moderate ARAS, renal cortical and medullary oxygenation are preserved by a compensatory decrease in oxygen consumption.[11]

CLINICAL PRESENTATION

Common Signs and Symptoms

The main clinical syndromes associated with hemodynamically significant ARAS include renovascular hypertension, ischemic nephropathy, and/or cardiac destabilization syndromes.

Renovascular Hypertension

Resistant (refractory) hypertension is defined as blood pressure (BP) above goal on three different classes of antihypertensive medications, ideally including a diuretic drug.[12,13] Patients with resistant hypertension should be evaluated for secondary causes of hypertension. Studies of resistant hypertension commonly reveal a high prevalence of previously unrecognized renovascular disease, particularly in older patients. In patients older than 50 years of age who were referred to a hypertension center, 13% had a secondary cause of hypertension, the most common of which was ARAS.[6]

ARAS is a common finding in patients with hypertension undergoing cardiac catheterization to assess coronary artery disease. In a population of veterans with hypertension referred for coronary angiography, more than 20% were found to have hemodynamically significant ARAS (stenosis >70%).[14]

Ischemic Nephropathy

ARAS is a potentially reversible form of renal insufficiency. However, if unrecognized, it can lead to end-stage renal disease (ESRD). Some studies suggest that 11% to 14% of ESRD is attributable to chronic ischemic nephropathy from ARAS.[15] Favorable predictors of improvement with renal revascularization include a rapid recent increase in serum creatinine concentration, decrease in glomerular filtration rate (GFR) during angiotensin-converting enzyme inhibitor (ACEI) or angiotensin receptor blocker (ARB) treatment, absence of glomerular or interstitial fibrosis on kidney biopsy, and kidney pole-to-pole length greater than 8.0 cm.[16] In 73 patients with chronic renal failure (creatinine clearance <50 mL/min) and clinical evidence of renal vascular disease and a mean follow-up of 2 years, renal function improved in 34 of 59 patients (58%). The most important predictor of improvement was the slope of the reciprocal serum creatinine plot before revascularization, suggesting that rapidly progressive renal failure is associated with a more favorable response after revascularization in patients with vascular nephropathy and ARAS.[17]

Cardiac Destabilization Syndromes

Exacerbations of coronary ischemia and CHF caused by increased systemic vasoconstriction and/or volume overload can be attributed to ARAS. The most widely recognized example of a cardiac destabilization syndrome is "flash" pulmonary or Pickering syndrome.[1,18] Renovascular disease may also complicate the treatment of patients with heart failure by preventing the administration of angiotensin antagonist therapy (ie, ACEI or ARB worsening kidney function because of a decrease in renal perfusion pressure).

The importance of renal artery revascularization in the treatment of cardiac disturbance syndromes has been described in a series of patients presenting with either CHF or an acute coronary syndrome.[19] Successful renal stent placement resulted in a significant decrease in BP and symptom improvement in 88% (42 of 48) of patients. For those patients who presented with unstable angina, renal artery stenting improved the Canadian Class Society (CCS) symptoms at least by one class, independent of concomitant coronary intervention. In patients presenting with CHF, the New York Heart Association (NYHA) Class of symptoms improved by at least one, also independent of coronary revascularization. Among 207 patients with decompensated CHF, 19% had severe ARAS and underwent renal artery stenting with a decreased frequency of CHF admissions, flash pulmonary edema, reduced NYHA Class symptoms, and tolerance to ACEI.[20]

Differential Diagnosis

Understanding the pathophysiology and clinical manifestations of ARAS is crucial when developing an appropriate differential diagnosis for resistant hypertension. Essential hypertension, other causes of secondary hypertension, and other causes of worsening renal function can coexist. When ARAS is detected, it is very important to determine whether it is hemodynamically significant and causing a clinical problem such as resistant hypertension, CHF, or renal insufficiency, because nonobstructive ARAS may be an innocent bystander. Importantly, not all patients with ARAS will develop a clinical syndrome, and, certainly, only a minority of patients with hypertension and/or CHF have ARAS.

Besides atherosclerosis, other conditions may result in RAS. Fibromuscular dysplasia is the cause in 10% to 30% of patients with RAS, most commonly affecting women younger than 50 years of age and typically involving the middle and distal main renal artery or the intrarenal branches. Other less common causes (<10%) of RAS include thromboembolic disease, arterial dissection, infrarenal aortic aneurysm, vasculitis (ie, Takayasu arteritis, Buerger disease, polyarteritis nodosa, and post radiation), neurofibromatosis type 1, and retroperitoneal fibrosis.

DIAGNOSIS

There are multiple diagnostic modalities available for the diagnosis of ARAS. According to the American College of Cardiology/American Heart Association (ACC/AHA) clinical practice guidelines, magnetic resonance angiography (MRA), computed tomographic angiography (CTA), and duplex ultrasonography (DUS) all receive a class I indication (level of evidence B) as a screening test to establish ARAS.[13] When the clinical suspicion is high for ARAS and the result of the noninvasive test is inconclusive, catheter angiography is then recommended for screening. Each diagnostic test has its own advantages and disadvantages, allowing physicians to have different approaches to different patients (**Figure 82.1**).

Doppler Ultrasound Evaluation

Renal artery Doppler ultrasound, or DUS, is useful for screening for ARAS. It carries a sensitivity of 84%, specificity of 97%, and positive predictive value of 94% for the detection of significant ARAS.[21] The accuracy of this test is highly dependent on the technicians' skill in performing the examination.

A peak systolic velocity (PSV) greater than180 cm/sec has a 95% sensitivity and 90% specificity for identifying significant ARAS. When the ratio of the PSV of the stenosed renal artery to the aortic PSV (ie, renal to aortic ratio [RAR]) is greater than 3.5, DUS predicts greater than 60% RAS with a 92% sensitivity.[22,23] DUS also allows follow-up of stent patency in patients who have undergone renal artery stenting; however, the criteria for native RAS overestimates the degree of

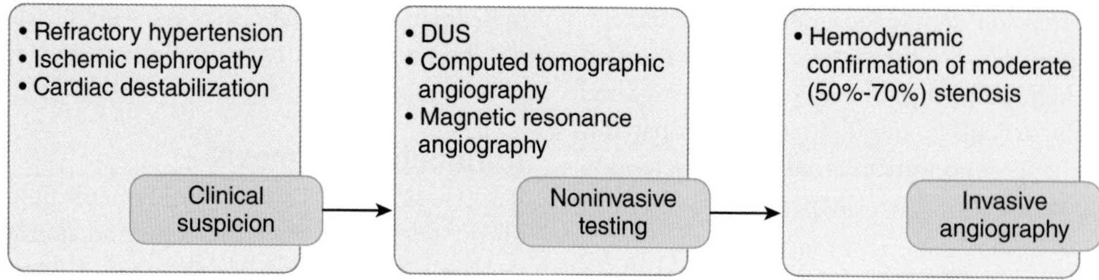

FIGURE 82.1 Diagnostic approach to the patient with renal artery stenosis.

angiographic in-stent restenosis (ISR). Surveillance monitoring for renal stent patency should take into account that PSV and RAR obtained by DUS are higher for any given degree of arterial narrowing within the stent. PSV greater than 395 cm/sec or RAR greater than 5.1 were the most predictive of angiographically significant ISR.[24]

DUS can be performed without risk to the patient, because there is no iodinated contrast or ionizing radiation required. The main limitations for DUS include unsatisfactory examinations because of bowel gas or large body habitus. There is a requirement for a capable sonographer who is allowed enough time to perform the examination.

The intrarenal resistive index (RI) is the ratio of the peak-systolic to end-diastolic velocity within the renal parenchyma at the level of the cortical blood vessels.[25] The RI is a representation of small vessel glomerulosclerosis or nephrosclerosis. There have been conflicting reports regarding the usefulness of RI to predict individual patient response to revascularization, and as such is of uncertain or doubtful clinical value.

Computed Tomographic Angiography

CTA can provide high-resolution cross-sectional imaging of ARAS while supplying three-dimensional (3D) angiographic images of the aorta, renal, and visceral arteries, allowing localization and enumeration of the renal arteries, including accessory branches.[26] Sensitivity (59%-96%) and specificity (82%-99%) of CTA for detecting significant ARAS compare well with invasive angiography.[27] CTA requires the administration of 100 to 150 mL of iodinated contrast and, therefore, carries the potential risk of contrast-induced nephropathy (CIN), especially in patients with estimated GFR of less than 60 mL/1.73 m^2, diabetes mellitus, or anemia.[28,29] In addition, CTA requires the use of ionizing radiation. However, as CTA scanner technology advances, spatial resolution will improve, scanning time will decrease, the administered contrast load may be reduced, and the amount of radiation will be decreased.[30,31] In addition, iso-osmolar contrast media are now available, with decreased potential for nephrotoxicity.[32] CTA allows the clinician to follow up patients with prior stents to detect ISR, an advantage over MRA in which metallic stents generate artifact.

Magnetic Resonance Angiography

This imaging modality, with contrast enhancement using gadolinium, allows localization and enumeration of the renal arteries and characterization of the stenosis. When compared to invasive angiography, it has sensitivity of 92% to 97% and specificity of 73% to 93% for detection of ARAS.[33,34] MRA does not require the use of ionizing radiation. Limitations of MRA include the association of gadolinium with nephrogenic systemic fibrosis when administered to patients with estimated GFR less than 30 mL/1.73 m^2 and metal-causing artifacts; therefore, it is not useful in patients with prior renal stents. Other patients who are not good candidates for MRA include those with claustrophobia or those with implanted ferromagnetic medical devices (eg, artificial joints and permanent pacemakers).[35]

Invasive Renal Angiography

Invasive angiography remains the "gold standard" for the diagnosis of renal artery disease. However, the visual estimate of the severity of stenosis can be inaccurate. When a single operator performed visual estimation of angiographic diameter stenosis in patients with moderate or severe RAS (ie, 50%-90% diameter stenosis), the correlation was poor between the visually estimated angiographic diameter stenosis and resting mean translesional pressure gradient ($r = 0.43$; $P = 0.12$); hyperemic mean translesional pressure gradient ($r = 0.22$; $P = 0.44$); and renal fractional flow reserve (RFFR) ($r = 0.18$; $P = 0.54$).[36] Tortuous anatomy of the renal arteries and the inability to obtain extreme craniocaudal angulation during invasive angiography limits the accuracy of the angiographic determination of the severity of ARAS. Therefore, a physiologic assessment should always be performed with invasive angiography in the patient with moderate (50%-70%) stenoses. Functional measurements include translesional resting or hyperemic systolic (>20 mm Hg) and mean (>10 mm Hg) gradients, and RFFR.[36-38]

MANAGEMENT OF THE PATIENT WITH RENAL ARTERY STENOSIS

Medical Approach

Medical treatment is the first-line treatment of ARAS. Controlling risk factors—smoking, dyslipidemia, and hyperglycemia—is important. No randomized study has analyzed the effects of different antihypertensive regimens in patients with ARAS, because they often have refractory hypertension and require multiple antihypertensive medications. According to ACC/AHA guidelines, ARBs, calcium channel blockers, ACEIs, and beta-blockers are a class I recommendation in treating secondary hypertension due to ARAS. The Cardiovascular Outcomes in Renal Atherosclerotic Lesion (CORAL) trial showed no difference in outcomes between medical treatment versus medical treatment plus renal artery stenting in patients with moderate ARAS and hypertension, highlighting the importance of medical therapy.[39]

Traditionally, the use of RAAS antagonists (ACEI or ARBs) has been cautioned because of the theoretical risk of worsening kidney function due to a decrease in perfusion pressure to the kidney. However, many studies have shown better outcomes after using these medications. An observational study found that 53% of patients included with renovascular disease were taking a RAAS antagonist, and these patients had a lower risk of the primary outcome (myocardial infarction, stroke, and death) (hazard ratio 0.70 and confidence interval 0.53-0.90) than those not taking a RAAS antagonist. Using a RAAS antagonist in ARAS patients should be accompanied by close monitoring of renal function. RAAS antagonists were tolerated in 357 out of 378 patients (94%) when used prospectively and in 54 of 69 patients (78%) with bilateral RAS (stenosis >60%).[40]

The benefit from statins and antiplatelet therapy in populations of patients with atherosclerosis supports their use in patients with ARAS. An association between statin use and improved survival in patients with ARAS was reported in a large case series of patients who underwent renal artery stenting.[41]

Percutaneous Interventions

Renal artery stenting (**Figure 82.2**) for ARAS has been evaluated in three randomized controlled trials (RCTs). Stent Placement in Patients with Atherosclerotic Renal Artery Stenosis and Impaired Renal Function: A Randomized Trial (STAR) enrolled patients with ARAS with stenoses greater than 50% and a creatinine clearance less than 80 mL/min/1.73m^2. Medical therapy alone was compared with medical therapy and renal artery stenting. Renal artery stenting had no effect on progression of chronic kidney disease, and BP improved in both groups. However, a major limitation of this study was that 30% of the patients randomized to the revascularization arm had ARAS less than 50% and were not candidates for revascularization.[42]

Revascularization was not superior than was medical therapy in the Angioplasty and Stenting for Renal Artery Lesions (ASTRAL) trial. Several criticisms of this trial have been voiced, including employing only ultrasound as the modality used to measure the severity of RAS, so that many of the patients in the trial did not have significant stenoses (ie, only 60% of the patients had stenosis >70%) and were unlikely to benefit from revascularization. In addition, the revascularization group was on less antihypertensive medications than was the medical group (2.77 vs 2.97, respectively; P = 0.03) making comparison of the groups difficult. There was also a 9% complication rate in the revascularization group, which is much higher than has been reported in other studies, suggesting that many of these operators were inexperienced.[43,44]

In the most recent RCT—the Cardiovascular Outcomes in Renal Atherosclerotic Lesions (CORAL) trial—medical therapy outperformed renal revascularization. However, the study enrolled patients without resistant hypertension by including patients with a systolic BP greater than or equal to 155 mm Hg despite taking greater than or equal to two antihypertensive medications. In fact, many patients in the medical group had significant improvement in their BP once started on the trial medications, corroborating that they did not have resistant hypertension at enrollment. In addition, the severity of moderate (50%-70% diameter stenosis) lesions was not hemodynamically confirmed. Hence, patients with nonobstructive ARAS may have been enrolled in the trial.[39]

Despite the negative results of the trials, a 2016 comparative effectiveness analysis concluded that there was low strength of evidence for the relative benefits of percutaneous transluminal renal artery balloon angioplasty and renal artery stenting versus medical therapy alone in patients with ARAS.[45] The ASTRAL and the CORAL trials demonstrated that in hypertensive patients with moderate ARAS (50%-70%

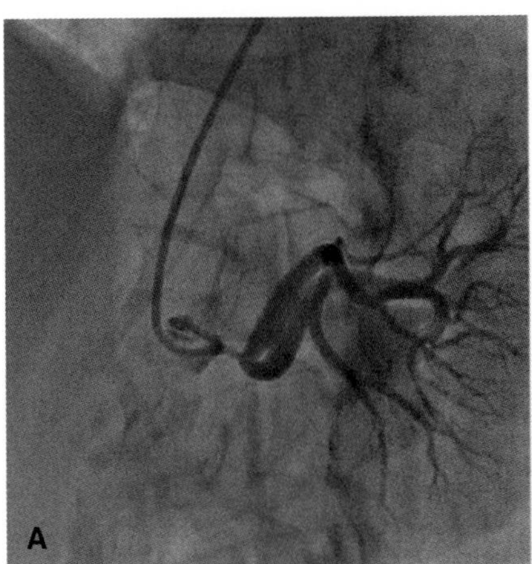

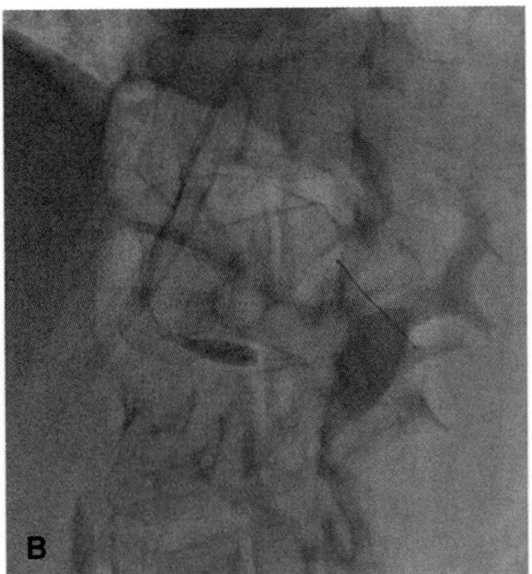

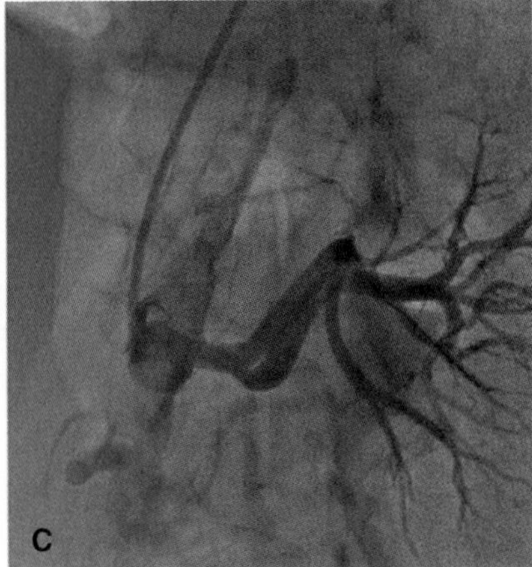

FIGURE 82.2 Renal intervention via right radial access. **A.** Diagnostic angiogram. **B.** A 6-mm balloon-expandable stent deployment. **C.** Final result.

diameter stenosis) and unconfirmed hemodynamic severity of RAS, there was no benefit of revascularization over medical therapy alone. As noted by the Agency for Healthcare Research Quality (AHRQ) report on Comparative Effectiveness Statement on Renal Artery Stenting, selection bias may have prevented enrollment of patients who would have likely benefited from revascularization (ie, those with very severe stenoses and resistant hypertension, sudden onset, "flash" pulmonary edema, or ischemic nephropathy).[39,44,45] There was equipoise for ARAS patients with borderline or unclear indications for stenting allowing their randomization in the trials, but those with the most severe ARAS may not have been randomized in the trials. In many RCTs, this remains a common limitation, which may be addressed with a parallel registry.[39] The current ACC/AHA appropriate use criteria for renal revascularization guidelines are summarized in **Table 82.1**. The approach to management of the patient with ARAS is summarized in **Figure 82.3**.

TABLE 82.1 Current Appropriate Use Criteria from the Society for Cardiovascular Angiography and Interventions and American Heart Association/American College of Cardiology Guideline Recommendations

Hemodynamically Significant RAS[a] Scenario	SCAI Appropriate Use Criteria	AHA/ACC Recommendations	
		Class	Level of Evidence
Cardiac disturbance syndrome with hypertension • Flash pulmonary edema, NSTEMI • Unstable angina	Appropriate	I IIa	B
CKD stage IV with kidney size >7 cm • Bilateral ARAS	Appropriate	IIa	B
CKD stage IV without another explanation • Bilateral or unilateral with solitary kidney ARAS	Appropriate	IIb	B
Resistant hypertension (failing maximally tolerated doses of at least three agents including a diuretic) • Bilateral or unilateral with solitary kidney ARAS • Unilateral ARAS	Appropriate May be appropriate	IIa	B
Recurrent CHF with unilateral ARAS	May be appropriate	I	B
Asymptomatic	Rarely appropriate	IIb	C

ACC, American College of Cardiology; ACS, acute coronary syndrome; AHA, American Heart Association; ARAS, atherosclerotic renal artery stenosis; CHF, congestive heart failure; CKD, chronic kidney disease; NSTEMI, non–ST-elevation myocardial infarction; SCAI, Society for Cardiovascular Angiography and Interventions.
[a]Hemodynamically significant renal artery stenosis (RAS) = (a) 50%-70% (moderate) stenosis with resting/hyperemic translesional mean gradient greater than 10 mm Hg, and/or systolic gradient greater than 20 mm Hg; or renal fractional flow reserve (RFFR) less than or equal to 0.8 or (b) greater than 70%-99% (severe) stenosis.

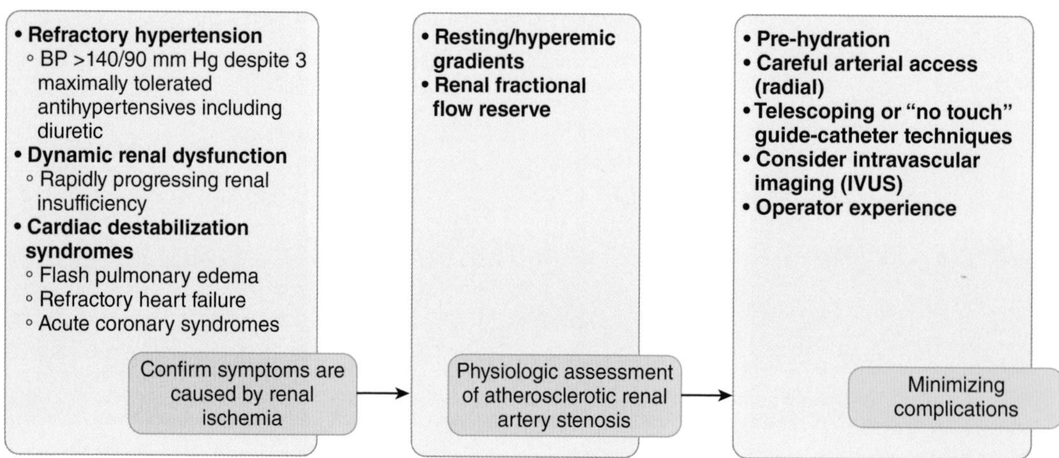

FIGURE 82.3 Approach to treatment of patient with renal artery stenosis. BP, blood pressure.

Surgical Approach

Initial attempts to revascularize severe ARAS were limited to open renal artery surgery. In a 500-patient cohort with ARAS and hypertension who underwent surgical revascularization, 12% were cured of hypertension and 73% improved. However, the surgical complication rate was 5% to 7%, which included bleeding and infections.[29] A small (N = 58) RCT compared open renal artery surgery to balloon angioplasty in patients with unilateral severe ARAS and uncontrolled hypertension. There were no differences between the surgical group and the balloon angioplasty group with regard to BP improvement, renal function improvement, or renal artery patency at 24 months, so the less invasive endovascular procedures have largely replaced open surgery.[46]

SPECIAL CONSIDERATIONS

Renal artery stenting is the preferred technique to treat severe ARAS unresponsive to medical therapy. When performed by experienced operators, the complication rate approaches 2%, with the most common complications related to femoral access (hematoma, pseudoaneurysm, and arteriovenous fistula); however, atheroembolism, retroperitoneal hematoma, renal artery rupture, aortic and renal artery dissection, contrast nephropathy, renal infarction, and death have also been reported.[47,48] To reduce complications, some procedural considerations to consider include radial artery vascular access, embolic protection devices, the catheter-in-catheter technique, the no-touch technique, stent sizing with intravascular ultrasound, and vigorous hydration before and after contrast exposure.

FOLLOW-UP PATIENT CARE

Once a renal artery stent has been placed, patients should be assessed at 1, 6, and 12 months with renal artery DUS.[24] The DUS criteria for patency in a stented artery are different than that in a native vessel, because decreased compliance within the stent will cause higher velocities. ISR greater than 70% can be confirmed with a PSV greater than 395 cm/sec.[49] If DUS suggests restenosis, one should confirm the recurrence of clinical symptoms before reintervention is performed.[24] If DUS is inconclusive, then CTA would be the next best test for determining stent patency. MRA is affected by metal artifact with previous renal stenting, so it should not be used in patients with suspected renal stent ISR.[27] If ultrasound and CTA are still inconclusive and the patient has recurrent clinical symptoms, then angiography with hemodynamic confirmation of the severity of the stenosis is indicated.

KEY POINTS

- ✔ RAS is a frequent cause of secondary hypertension, renal insufficiency, and cardiac destabilization syndromes.
- ✔ Noninvasive screening for RAS can be done with Doppler ultrasonography (DUS), CTA, and MRA.
- ✔ Patients with medically controlled renovascular hypertension should not undergo renal stenting because there is no added benefit of revascularization.
- ✔ Patients with (1) uncontrolled renovascular hypertension having failed three maximally tolerated antihypertensive medications (one of which is a diuretic), (2) ischemic nephropathy, and (3) cardiac destabilization syndromes with hemodynamically significant RAS are those most likely to benefit from renal artery stenting.
- ✔ Moderate (50%-90% diameter narrowing) RAS should undergo hemodynamic evaluation. A hemodynamically significant lesion has a translesional resting or hyperemic systolic gradient (>20 mm Hg) or mean gradient (>10 mm Hg); an RFFR ≤0.8) may also be used to establish a significant gradient.
- ✔ Following renal artery stent placement, patients should have routine 1-, 3-, 6-, 12-month, and annual clinical, laboratory, and imaging follow-up for surveillance of ISR.

SECTION 6

REFERENCES

1. Messerli FH, Bangalore S, Makani H, et al. Flash pulmonary oedema and bilateral renal artery stenosis: the Pickering syndrome. *Eur Heart J.* 2011;32(18):2231-2235.
2. Benjamin MM, Fazel P, Filardo G, Choi JW, Stoler RC. Prevalence of and risk factors of renal artery stenosis in patients with resistant hypertension. *Am J Cardiol.* 2014;113(4):687-690.
3. Hansen KJ, Edwards MS, Craven TE, et al. Prevalence of renovascular disease in the elderly: a population-based study. *J Vasc Surg.* 2002;36(3):443-451.
4. Holley KE, Hunt JC, Brown AL Jr, Kincaid OW, Sheps SG. Renal artery stenosis. A clinical-pathologic study in normotensive and hypertensive patients. *Am J Med.* 1964;37:14-22.
5. Sawicki PT, Kaiser S, Heinemann L, Frenzel H, Berger M. Prevalence of renal artery stenosis in diabetes mellitus—an autopsy study. *J Intern Med.* 1991;229(6):489-492.
6. Anderson GH Jr, Blakeman N, Streeten DH. The effect of age on prevalence of secondary forms of hypertension in 4429 consecutively referred patients. *J Hypertens.* 1994;12(5):609-615.
7. Agarwal M, Lynn KL, Richards AM, Nicholls MG. Hyponatremic-hypertensive syndrome with renal ischemia: an underrecognized disorder. *Hypertension.* 1999;33(4):1020-1024.
8. Eirin A, Lerman LO. Darkness at the end of the tunnel: poststenotic kidney injury. *Physiology.* 2013;28(4):245-253.
9. Textor SC, Lerman L. Renovascular hypertension and ischemic nephropathy. *Am J Hypertens.* 2010;23(11):1159-1169.
10. Textor SC, Lerman LO. Paradigm shifts in atherosclerotic renovascular disease: where are we now? *J Am Soc Nephrol.* 2015;26(9):2074-2080.
11. Gloviczki ML, Glockner JF, Lerman LO, et al. Preserved oxygenation despite reduced blood flow in poststenotic kidneys in human atherosclerotic renal artery stenosis. *Hypertension.* 2010;55(4):961-966.
12. Pimenta E, Calhoun DA. Resistant hypertension: incidence, prevalence, and prognosis. *Circulation.* 2012;125(13):1594-1596.
13. Calhoun DA, Jones D, Textor S, et al. Resistant hypertension: diagnosis, evaluation, and treatment: a scientific statement from the American Heart Association Professional Education Committee of the Council for High Blood Pressure Research. *Circulation.* 2008;117(25):e510-e526.
14. Aqel RA, Zoghbi GJ, Baldwin SA, et al. Prevalence of renal artery stenosis in high-risk veterans referred to cardiac catheterization. *J Hypertens.* 2003;21(6):1157-1162.

15. Preston RA, Epstein M. Ischemic renal disease: an emerging cause of chronic renal failure and end-stage renal disease. *J Hypertens.* 1997; 15(12 Pt 1):1365-1377.
16. Garovic VD, Textor SC. Renovascular hypertension and ischemic nephropathy. *Circulation.* 2005;112(9):1362-1374.
17. Muray S, Martin M, Amoedo ML, et al. Rapid decline in renal function reflects reversibility and predicts the outcome after angioplasty in renal artery stenosis. *Am J Kidney Dis.* 2002;39(1):60-66.
18. Messerli FH, Bangalore S. The Pickering Syndrome—a pebble in the mosaic of the cardiorenal syndrome. *Blood Press.* 2011;20(1):1-2.
19. Khosla S, White CJ, Collins TJ, Jenkins JS, Shaw D, Ramee SR. Effects of renal artery stent implantation in patients with renovascular hypertension presenting with unstable angina or congestive heart failure. *Am J Cardiol.* 1997;80(3):363-366.
20. Gray BH, Olin JW, Childs MB, Sullivan TM, Bacharach JM. Clinical benefit of renal artery angioplasty with stenting for the control of recurrent and refractory congestive heart failure. *Vasc Med.* 2002;7(4):275-279.
21. Taylor DC, Kettler MD, Moneta GL, et al. Duplex ultrasound scanning in the diagnosis of renal artery stenosis: a prospective evaluation. *J Vasc Surg.* 1988;7(2):363-369.
22. Strandness DE Jr. Duplex imaging for the detection of renal artery stenosis. *Am J Kidney Dis.* 1994;24(4):674-678.
23. Olin JW, Piedmonte MR, Young JR, DeAnna S, Grubb M, Childs MB. The utility of duplex ultrasound scanning of the renal arteries for diagnosing significant renal artery stenosis. *Ann Intern Med.* 1995; 122(11):833-838.
24. Chi YW, White CJ, Thornton S, Milani RV. Ultrasound velocity criteria for renal in-stent restenosis. *J Vasc Surg.* 2009;50(1):119-123.
25. Radermacher J. [Ultrasonography of the kidney and renal vessels. I. Normal findings, inherited and parenchymal diseases]. *UrologeA.* 2005;44(11): 1351-1363; quiz 1364.
26. Kawashima A, Sandler CM, Ernst RD, Tamm EP, Goldman SM, Fishman EK. CT evaluation of renovascular disease. *Radiographics.* 2000; 20(5):1321-1340.
27. Kim TS, Chung JW, Park JH, Kim SH, Yeon KM, Han MC. Renal artery evaluation: comparison of spiral CT angiography to intra-arterial DSA. *J Vasc Interv Radiol.* 1998;9(4):553-559.
28. McCullough PA, Adam A, Becker CR, et al. Risk prediction of contrast-induced nephropathy. *Am J Cardiol.* 2006;98(6A):27K-36K.
29. McCullough PA, Adam A, Becker CR, et al. Epidemiology and prognostic implications of contrast-induced nephropathy. *Am J Cardiol.* 2006;98(6A):5K-13K.
30. Cho ES, Yu JS, Ahn JH, et al. CT angiography of the renal arteries: comparison of lower-tube-voltage CTA with moderate-concentration iodinated contrast material and conventional CTA. *AJR Am J Roentgenol.* 2012;199(1):96-102.
31. Lufft V, Hoogestraat-Lufft L, Fels LM, et al. Contrast media nephropathy: intravenous CT angiography versus intraarterial digital subtraction angiography in renal artery stenosis: a prospective randomized trial. *Am J Kidney Dis.* 2002;40(2):236-242.
32. Davenport MS, Khalatbari S, Cohan RH, Dillman JR, Myles JD, Ellis JH. Contrast material-induced nephrotoxicity and intravenous low-osmolality iodinated contrast material: risk stratification by using estimated glomerular filtration rate. *Radiology.* 2013;268(3):719-728.
33. Turgutalp K, Kiykim A, Ozhan O, Helvaci I, Ozcan T, Yildiz A. Comparison of diagnostic accuracy of Doppler USG and contrast-enhanced magnetic resonance angiography and selective renal arteriography in patients with atherosclerotic renal artery stenosis. *Med Sci Monit.* 2013;19:475-482.
34. Tan KT, van Beek EJ, Brown PW, van Delden OM, Tijssen J, Ramsay LE. Magnetic resonance angiography for the diagnosis of renal artery stenosis: a meta-analysis. *Clin Radiol.* 2002;57(7):617-624.
35. Dellegrottaglie S, Sanz J, Rajagopalan S. Technology insight: clinical role of magnetic resonance angiography in the diagnosis and management of renal artery stenosis. *Nat Clin Pract Cardiovasc Med.* 2006;3(6):329-338.
36. Subramanian R, White CJ, Rosenfield K, et al. Renal fractional flow reserve: a hemodynamic evaluation of moderate renal artery stenoses. *Catheter Cardiovasc Interv.* 2005;64(4):480-486.
37. Mitchell JA, Subramanian R, White CJ, et al. Predicting blood pressure improvement in hypertensive patients after renal artery stent placement: renal fractional flow reserve. *Catheter Cardiovasc Interv.* 2007;69(5):685-689.
38. Mulumudi MS, White CJ. Renal frame count: a quantitative angiographic assessment of renal perfusion. *Catheter Cardiovasc Interv.* 2005;65(2): 183-186.
39. Cooper CJ, Murphy TP, Cutlip DE, et al. Stenting and medical therapy for atherosclerotic renal-artery stenosis. *N Engl J Med.* 2014;370(1):13-22.
40. Hackam DG, Duong-Hua ML, Mamdani M, et al. Angiotensin inhibition in renovascular disease: a population-based cohort study. *Am Heart J.* 2008;156(3):549-555.
41. Bates MC, Campbell JE, Stone PA, Jaff MR, Broce M, Lavigne PS. Factors affecting long-term survival following renal artery stenting. *Catheter Cardiovasc Interv.* 2007;69(7):1037-1043.
42. Bax L, Woittiez AJ, Kouwenberg HJ, et al. Stent placement in patients with atherosclerotic renal artery stenosis and impaired renal function: a randomized trial. *Ann Intern Med.* 2009;150(12):840-848, W150-W151.
43. Wheatley K, Ives N, Gray R, et al. Revascularization versus medical therapy for renal-artery stenosis. *N Engl J Med.* 2009;361(20):1953-1962.
44. Rump LC, Nitschmann S. [Medical vs. interventional therapy of renal artery stenosis: ASTRAL study (Angioplasty and STenting for Renal Artery Lesions)]. *Internist (Berl).* 2011;52(2):218-220.
45. Raman G, Adam GP, Halladay CW, Langberg VN, Azodo IA, Balk EM. Comparative effectiveness of management strategies for renal artery stenosis: an updated systematic review. *Ann Intern Med.* 2016;165(9):635-649.
46. Weibull H, Bergqvist D, Bergentz SE, Jonsson K, Hulthen L, Manhem P. Percutaneous transluminal renal angioplasty versus surgical reconstruction of atherosclerotic renal artery stenosis: a prospective randomized study. *J Vasc Surg.* 1993;18(5):841-850; discussion 850-852.
47. Klein AJ, Jaff MR, Gray BH, et al. SCAI appropriate use criteria for peripheral arterial interventions: an update. *Catheter Cardiovasc Interv.* 2017;90(4):E90-E110.
48. Rocha-Singh K, Jaff MR, Rosenfield K, ASPIRE 2 Trial Investigators. Evaluation of the safety and effectiveness of renal artery stenting after unsuccessful balloon angioplasty: the ASPIRE-2 study. *J Am Coll Cardiol.* 2005;46(5):776-783.
49. Granata A, Fiorini F, Andrulli S, et al. Doppler ultrasound and renal artery stenosis: an overview. *J Ultrasound.* 2009;12(4):133-143.

CHAPTER 83

MESENTERIC ARTERIAL DISEASE

Stefanos Giannopoulos and Ehrin J. Armstrong*

INTRODUCTION

Epidemiology

Mesenteric ischemia constitutes overall a rare entity that commonly presents among the elderly, and is attributed to reduced blood flow in the intestinal circulation that does not meet the metabolic demands of the corresponding viscera.[1] Depending on the clinical scenario, mesenteric ischemia is divided into two types: acute and chronic mesenteric ischemia. The pathophysiologic mechanisms resulting in reduced blood flow include (1) mesenteric venous thrombosis; (2) arterial thrombosis; (3) nonocclusive mesenteric ischemia; and (4) arterial embolism.[1,2] Independent of the underlying cause, both types (ie, acute mesenteric ischemia and acute on chronic mesenteric ischemia) of mesenteric ischemia eventually lead to intestinal wall necrosis, perforation, peritonitis, and death.[2] The prevalence of acute mesenteric ischemia is estimated to be around 0.1% of all hospital admissions; however, the mortality associated with the disease rises to 80% in certain cases. Hence, early diagnosis and treatment are crucial to alter the disease's course.[3]

Risk Factors

Atherosclerosis is one of the main causes of chronic mesenteric ischemia (almost 90% of cases), and therefore populations with a higher prevalence of comorbidities or conditions that are predisposed to advanced atherosclerosis (eg, smoking, hypertension, dyslipidemia, diabetes mellitus, metabolic syndrome, sedentary lifestyle) are at higher risk for chronic mesenteric ischemia. On the other hand, acute mesenteric ischemia has been attributed to embolic occlusion in 40% to 50% of cases, to arterial thrombosis of a stenosed mesenteric vessel in 20% to 35% of the cases, and to arteritis in almost 5% of the cases.[1] Thus, several other factors that predispose to thrombus formation or embolization have been correlated with mesenteric ischemia as well, including but not limited to cardiac diseases (ie, arrhythmias, congestive heart failure, recent myocardial infarction, valvular disease), hypovolemia, and intra-abdominal tumor.[1,2,4] Additionally, there has been observed an association between acute mesenteric ischemia incidence and increased age and female sex.[5]

PATHOGENESIS

Mesenteric ischemia is caused by an imbalance between intestinal blood supply and oxygen demand, which occurs either acutely or is a chronic process. Insufficient perfusion of the large and small intestines can be caused either from embolic/thrombotic arterial occlusion, venous thrombosis, or from nonocclusive entities, such as arterial vasospasm, hypovolemia, reduced effective blood flow (eg, congestive heart failure, states of low cardiac output), and reduced oxygen-carrying capacity from red blood cells (eg, anemia, methemoglobinemia, carboxyhemoglobinemia).[1,2] Less frequently, dissection of the superior mesenteric artery is the trigger of acute mesenteric ischemia.[6,7] The result of reduced arterial or venous blood flow is a hemorrhagic infarction and the severity of the disease depends on (1) the vessels affected; (2) the duration of occlusion/ischemia; (3) the overall hemodynamic status (ie, systemic blood pressure, volume status, blood flow); and (4) the collateral blood supply. Thus, damage to the intestinal vessel wall varies from reversible ischemia to permanent injury owing to transmural infarction, eventually causing bowel wall necrosis, perforation, and peritonitis.

CLINICAL PRESENTATION

Common Signs and Symptoms

Patients diagnosed with chronic mesenteric ischemia usually have a long-standing history of progressive, worsening epigastric postprandial pain (ie, 10-180 min after a meal), which leads to avoidance of eating and subsequent significant weight loss.[8] Additionally, patients with chronic mesenteric ischemia often have history of vascular disease, including cerebrovascular accidents, coronary artery disease, and symptomatic peripheral artery disease.[8] Nonspecific symptoms are gastrointestinal discomfort, experienced as nausea with/without vomiting and changes in bowel habits, such as diarrhea/constipation and flatulence.[8-10]

Patients with acute mesenteric ischemia present differently from those with chronic mesenteric ischemia, with the most important observation being the disproportionate pain that the patient experiences compared to physical examination findings. Traditionally, the pain associated with acute

* Ehrin Armstrong, MD, is a consultant to Abbott Vascular, Boston Scientific, Cardiovascular Systems Incorporated (CSI), Medtronic, Philips, and PQ Bypass. All other authors have no relationship to disclose.

mesenteric ischemia is described as diffuse, constant, difficult to localize, and moderate to severe in intensity. Related gastrointestinal symptoms that commonly present synchronously with the pain include nausea with/without vomiting in almost three quarters of acute mesenteric ischemia cases and abdominal discomfort/distension with/without diarrhea. As the bowel ischemia persists, intestinal bleeding, obstipation, and signs of sepsis may become more apparent. Among the different pathogenic mechanisms of acute mesenteric ischemia, acute arterial embolization is the most rapidly evolving and is associated with the most painful and robust presentation.

Patients presenting with acute mesenteric ischemia owing to intestinal arterial thrombosis usually have a history of chronic mesenteric ischemia with postprandial pain, whereas coronary artery disease and peripheral vascular disease are also commonly observed in this population. Thus, those patients usually develop acute mesenteric ischemia on a background of chronic mesenteric ischemia. However, due to the chronic course of the disease, collateral blood flow is better developed and, as such, the signs/symptoms at presentation are less severe than cases of arterial embolization. Similarly, patients with acute mesenteric ischemia attributed to nonocclusive arterial or venous disease (often elderly) usually develop symptoms of intestinal ischemia (eg, postprandial pain, acute abdominal pain, obstipation, intestinal bleeding) over several days and often these are preceded by a prodrome of intestinal irritation, discomfort, and/or malaise. The fourth type of acute mesenteric ischemia, caused by mesenteric venous thrombosis, usually affects the small intestine and is observed among younger patients with hypercoagulable states (eg, coagulopathies, malignancy, immobility, drug-induced hypercoagulability). It is characterized by insidious onset (over several days) and less severe abdominal pain compared to the other types of acute mesenteric ischemia.

Physical Examination Findings

The examination findings are relevant to the type of mesenteric ischemia, the different pathogenic mechanisms, and the progress of the disease at the time of presentation.[1,2] Thus, the main findings of chronic mesenteric ischemia are signs of malnutrition, owing to the postprandial pain and fear of eating, whereas in some cases signs of peripheral vascular disease are apparent (eg, intermittent claudication, stable angina, decreased distal pulses).[8,11] However, patients with chronic mesenteric ischemia may also present with acute on chronic mesenteric ischemia. The pathognomonic finding of acute mesenteric ischemia is that the patient complains of severe abdominal pain, although the abdominal examination is inconclusive. Nonetheless, if the disease has progressed (ie, intestinal wall infarction with necrosis and perforation), signs of peritonitis may be present. Moreover, in severe cases the patient may present with signs of sepsis and hemodynamic instability.[1,2,11]

Differential Diagnosis

Owing to the indolent course and nonspecific symptoms at onset, a high degree of clinical suspicion is required. Because most patients present with abdominal pain, all conditions that can cause abdominal pain should be considered in the differential diagnosis. See **Table 83.1** for a list of differential diagnoses for abdominal pain. In addition, because of presenting signs of malnutrition, chronic mesenteric ischemia should be differentiated from malignancies and malabsorption syndromes.

TABLE 83.1 Differential Diagnosis of Abdominal Pain

Diagnosis	Characteristics of Abdominal Pain	Typical Physical Findings, if Present
Cardiovascular		
Stable ischemic heart disease	Chronic typical or atypical angina	Postprandial epigastric pain, abdominal angina
Acute coronary syndrome	Unstable angina (progressive, new onset, or new occurrence of rest angina)	Severe constant epigastric pain
Aortic dissection	Sharp or *tearing*, sudden onset radiating from substernal to intrascapular, might involve epigastric area	Loss of carotid or upper extremity pulses, stroke
Abdominal aortic aneurysm	Back, flank, abdominal pain (when the aneurysm ruptures)	Symptoms from local compression, hemodynamic instability, embolic phenomena affecting the lower limbs, pulsatile abdominal mass
Pulmonary		
Bacterial pneumonia	Pleuritic pain with dyspnea	Pleural friction rub
Gastrointestinal		
Abdominal abscess	Abdominal pain, focal tenderness, signs of peritonitis may be present	Fever, ileus, tenderness to palpation, reduced bowel sounds
Acute cholecystitis	Biliary colic, right hypochondriac pain, pain radiating to back or scapula	Murphy sign (+), tenderness to deep palpation, mass at the right hypochondriac region

Diagnosis	Characteristics of Abdominal Pain	Typical Physical Findings, if Present
Cholangitis	Acute or chronic RUQ pain	Fever, chills, jaundice, RUQ tenderness, +/- septic shock, +/-confusion
Acute pancreatitis	Epigastric pain, may be *boring* radiating to back	Epigastric tenderness
Acute pyelonephritis	Flank pain that may radiate to the groin	Costovertebral angle tenderness, chills, fever
Appendicitis	Periumbilical or epigastric pain that migrates to the RLQ	Rebound tenderness, rigidity, guarding, Rovsing sign, obturator sign, psoas sign, Dunphy sign
Diverticulitis	Sharp pain in LLQ	Rebound tenderness, rigidity, guarding
Intussusception	Pain is colicky, severe, and intermittent	RUQ sausage-shaped mass and RLQ emptiness (Dance sign), abdominal distension if obstruction is complete, currant jelly stools
Intestinal volvulus	Severe colicky abdominal pain	Abdominal distension, abdomen very tympanic to percussion, obstipation, rebound tenderness if peritoneal irritation
Intestinal perforation	Sharp, severe, sudden-onset epigastric pain	Rebound tenderness, rigidity, bowel sounds are usually absent in generalized peritonitis
Intestinal obstruction (eg, malignancy)	Crampy abdominal pain	Increased bowel sounds, tenderness, rigidity, guarding, fullness
Esophageal disease (eg, rupture, tear)	Substernal pain or pressure, sharp or dull	Nonspecific
Gastroesophageal reflux	Substernal and/or epigastric burning	Bad odor with breathing
Other Causes of Abdominal Pain That Should be Considered		
Septic shock	Abdominal pain to deep palpation, signs of perforation and peritonitis	Fever, hypotension, tachycardia, altered mental status, petechiae, or purpura in disseminated intravascular coagulation
Testicular torsion	Sudden onset of severe testicular, inguinal, abdominal pain	Scrotal pain that does not resolve with elevation of the testicle, tender and high-riding testicle, horizontal lie of the testicle, absent cremasteric reflex
Ectopic pregnancy	Lower abdominal pain	Vaginal bleeding, pelvic pain, acute onset severe pain with tubal rupture followed by hemodynamic instability
Metabolic (eg, acute intermittent porphyria)	Severe, colicky, poorly localized abdominal pain	Signs and symptoms specific for the metabolic pathology (eg, skin lesions, urine discoloration, neurologic symptoms)
Lactic acidosis	Diffuse abdominal pain that cannot be easily localized	Nausea, vomiting, Kussmaul breathing, hypotension, oliguria, altered mental status

LLQ, left lower quadrant; RLQ, right lower quadrant; RUQ, right upper quadrant.

DIAGNOSIS

Acute Mesenteric Ischemia

Although medical advancements have improved several diagnostic modalities over the last decades, the early recognition and diagnosis of acute mesenteric ischemia remains challenging and a high level of clinical suspicion is warranted for timely diagnosis and treatment[12,13]. Owing to the often inconclusive findings of physical examination and the nonspecific history, additional tests may be needed to establish the diagnosis. Although the diagnosis cannot be established with laboratory studies, they are helpful in assessing the following: (1) fluid and electrolytes; (2) acid-base status (eg, lactic acidosis); (3) potential infectious causes; (4) blood volume status; and (5) the degree of malnutrition in cases of acute mesenteric ischemia on chronic mesenteric ischemia (eg, tests for albumin, transferrin, C-reactive protein, transthyretin).[1] When a hypercoagulable status is suspected, laboratory tests for protein C/S and anti-thrombin III levels are recommended, and further testing for autoimmune diseases is warranted (eg, tests for systemic lupus erythematosus, antiphospholipid syndrome). Although several biomarkers have been investigated for the diagnosis of intestinal ischemia, currently no clinically helpful biomarkers have been validated for the diagnosis of acute or chronic mesenteric ischemia.[1,14,15]

SECTION 6

Valuable imaging studies that help in the diagnosis of acute mesenteric ischemia include plain abdominal radiographs, duplex ultrasonography (DUS), computed tomographic angiography (CTA), magnetic resonance angiography (MRA), and catheter angiography. Plain abdominal radiographs are useful in detecting/excluding other causes of abdominal pain (see Table 83.1) (eg, intestinal perforation, intestinal volvulus, free intraperitoneal air). However, at the onset of acute mesenteric ischemia, the abdominal radiograph is usually normal and should not be used to exclude acute mesenteric ischemia.[16] Furthermore, radiographic signs of acute mesenteric ischemia are mostly non-disease specific—including paralytic ileus, thickened intestinal wall, intestinal obstruction—whereas more specific signs, such as pneumatosis intestinalis and thumbprinting, present later during the course of the disease.[1,16]

DUS constitutes an alternative useful tool in identifying absent or reduced blood flow in the involved vessels, while excluding other causes of abdominal pain such as biliary disease. Additionally, risk factors for acute mesenteric ischemia such as cardiac valvular disease can be detected by DUS. However, several limitations apply to ultrasound use. Its sensitivity decreases in the presence of intestinal dilation, obesity, and calcified vessels, and only proximal arterial occlusions can be detected.[1] Moreover, this test depends on the skills of the ultrasonographer and physician, which can significantly affect the test's reliability and reproducibility.[1]

CTA has been shown to have a sensitivity of 96% to 100% and a specificity up to 94% for mesenteric ischemia, and, as such, it has been increasingly used for the diagnosis of acute mesenteric ischemia.[17] CTA can identify the cause of mesenteric ischemia (ie, provides clues for the source of embolization and identifies other pathologic processes such as malignancies) while determining the severity of ischemia (ie, free intra-abdominal air, pneumatosis intestinalis, lack of intestinal wall contrast enhancement, evidence of gas in the portal vein).[18,19] However, the accuracy of CTA is limited for venous thrombosis compared to arterial occlusion, although two-phase imaging, enhancing intestinal venous blood flow imaging, has been shown to be sufficient to diagnosis acute mesenteric ischemia because of venous thrombosis.[20,21]

MRA constitutes a reasonable alternative to CTA for assessing mesenteric ischemia, avoiding ionizing radiation exposure and being particularly effective for detecting venous occlusions, although it may overestimate the severity of occlusion in some cases.[22] MRA has excellent sensitivity (100%) and specificity rates (91%) for detecting mesenteric ischemia. However, because of the time required to perform MRA and its higher cost, CTA remains the more practical option for acute mesenteric ischemia diagnosis.[23]

Conventional arterial angiography, previously used for diagnosis of mesenteric ischemia, is now usually utilized for preoperative planning after the diagnosis of acute mesenteric ischemia has been established.[1] Furthermore, selective angiography can be combined with several endovascular treatment modalities, including thrombolysis, vasodilator infusion, stenting, or balloon angioplasty of the affected vessels.[24,25] Although conventional angiography has the benefit of offering contemporary revascularization options, it should be performed with caution in critically ill patients who might eventually require surgical therapy, so that actual treatment is not delayed. Thus, it is at the discretion of the operator whether to perform arterial angiography in an emergency or to proceed with exploratory laparotomy.

Chronic Mesenteric Ischemia

The diagnostic approach of mesenteric ischemia is generally similar for both acute and chronic mesenteric ischemia despite differences in symptom onset and disease course, because most patients with chronic mesenteric ischemia present with an acute/subacute exacerbation of previous symptoms (ie, acute mesenteric ischemia on chronic mesenteric ischemia). Laboratory tests play an important role in evaluating the nutritional status of the patient with chronic mesenteric ischemia (not complicated by acute mesenteric ischemia). A complete blood cell count with differential may be useful to detect any blood dyscrasias attributed to poor nutrition. Blood chemistries, coagulation studies, liver function, and stool testing may evaluate the severity of the disease and provide additional information, helping identify potential pathogenic mechanisms. However, the diagnosis for chronic mesenteric ischemia is mainly based on (1) medical history indicating inadequate intestinal blood flow (eg, postprandial abdominal pain, abdominal discomfort, frequent changes in bowel habits); (2) stenosis greater than 70% of a mesenteric artery; and (3) evidence of actual ischemia.[26,27]

DUS of the mesenteric vessels can visualize the superior mesenteric and celiac arteries in up to 90% and 80% of cases, respectively.[16] Therefore, it has been considered a good screening option for detection of proximal vessel disease.[28] However, several technical considerations limit its applicability (eg, skill of the operator, obesity, dilated bowel loops).[29,30] Although DUS can be a useful tool for the diagnosis of chronic mesenteric ischemia, it has largely been replaced by CTA,[13] given its high sensitivity (96%) and specificity (94%) for detecting chronic mesenteric ischemia.[18] Thus, patients with known atherosclerotic disease and clinical symptoms that indicate chronic intestinal ischemia should undergo CTA, in order to confirm mesenteric atherosclerosis.[13,31,32] CTA can confirm or exclude mesenteric atherosclerotic disease, while identifying other abdominal pathologies as the source of the presenting symptoms.[16,33] Additionally, MRA constitutes a reasonable screening test with high sensitivity, and it can also be performed without contrast in patients who have a contraindication to intravenous contrast infusion.[34] However, when the results of noninvasive imaging studies are inconclusive, conventional arterial angiography is recommended.

Several functional studies for the diagnosis of chronic mesenteric ischemia have been investigated, including but not limited to measurement of postprandial intestinal (ie, jejunal) pH, assessment of mucosal oxygen saturation, and determination of mesenteric vein blood flow after a meal. Unfortunately, none of these studies has provided sufficient beneficial evidence.

Accordingly, no functional test is performed routinely in clinical practice, and larger prospective studies are warranted to evaluate those diagnostic modalities.[35,36]

MANAGEMENT OF ACUTE MESENTERIC ARTERIAL DISEASE

Medical Approach

Once acute mesenteric ischemia (either acute mesenteric ischemia or acute mesenteric ischemia on chronic mesenteric ischemia) is diagnosed, resuscitation with aggressive intravenous fluid infusion (ie, normal saline, blood products as needed), supplemental oxygen, and broad-spectrum antibiotics is required, because patients with acute mesenteric ischemia are often in a highly toxic state.[37] Vasopressors for improvement of hemodynamic status should be avoided if possible because they can exacerbate the intestinal ischemia. Additionally, adequate pain management (eg, opioid analgesics) and proton pump inhibitors should be provided.[38] After stabilization of the patient, several treatment modalities (ie, medical, surgical, or endovascular therapy) are available, with the most optimal therapeutic approach depending on the clinical status of the patient, the cause of acute mesenteric ischemia, and the affected vessel.

In selected patients, pharmacologic therapy can alleviate symptoms (eg, vasodilators in nonocclusive acute mesenteric ischemia) or limit thrombus propagation (eg, heparin administration in cases of mesenteric venous thrombosis).[39] Thrombolytics may be lifesaving in emergency cases of arterial occlusion.[39] However, it is generally recommended that patients with hemodynamic instability, signs of peritonitis, and advanced intestinal ischemia who are not high risk for surgery should undergo immediate exploratory laparotomy. Stable patients with less severe clinical and radiologic findings can safely undergo endovascular therapy. Previous studies demonstrate noninferiority of endovascular therapy compared to traditional surgical management of acute mesenteric ischemia.[40,41] Further research is warranted to determine the late-term outcomes of endovascular interventions.[42,43]

Percutaneous Interventional Approaches

Endovascular interventions when compared to surgery are considered safer in terms of periprocedural outcomes owing to shorter procedural time, less blood loss, and minimal invasive nature of the procedures. However, only hemodynamically stable patients without advanced intestinal ischemia are suitable candidates. Endovascular approaches for the treatment of acute mesenteric ischemia mainly include mechanical thrombectomy, thrombolysis, and percutaneous transluminal angioplasty (ie, balloon angioplasty with/without stenting). Several endovascular treatment options are presented in **Table 83.2**.

Surgical Approaches

Surgical evaluation is warranted when clinical and/or radiologic signs of advanced intestinal ischemia are apparent or the patient is hemodynamically unstable. Arterial revascularization techniques are preferred. However, in cases of intestinal perforation or nonviable intestinal segments, resection of the ischemic intestine with end-to-end anastomosis is inevitable. When the viability of the affected intestinal segment is questionable, bowel rescue with revascularization should be attempted, and the viability of the affected segment should be reassessed intraoperatively. Surgical revascularization techniques include embolectomy/thromboendarterectomy and mesenteric bypass with autologous or synthetic conduits.[44,45] Details regarding surgical revascularization techniques are presented in Table 83.2.

MANAGEMENT OF CHRONIC MESENTERIC ISCHEMIA

Medical Approach

In patients diagnosed with chronic mesenteric ischemia (~90% of the cases attributed to atherosclerotic plaques in the mesenteric arteries), elimination of modifiable risk factors for atherosclerosis is crucial in order to delay the disease course. Thus, smoking cessation, lipid control, blood pressure regulation, adequate diabetes control, and exercise are recommended for secondary atherosclerosis prevention, while the need for antiplatelet therapy should be evaluated. Moreover, as chronic mesenteric ischemia is correlated with postprandial pain and fear of eating, many patients experience significant weight loss, so assessment of the patient's nutritional status is necessary.[45] In cases of severe malnutrition (eg, low body mass index, hypoalbuminemia, endocrine disorders), parenteral nutrition can be given as rescue therapy.[46]

Percutaneous Interventional Approaches

When patients have overt clinical symptoms despite conservative care, a revascularization approach should be evaluated, with the optimal goal being the prevention of intestinal infarction.[47] Similar to acute mesenteric ischemia management, revascularization for the treatment of chronic mesenteric ischemia includes surgical and endovascular interventions. Although open surgical repair has been traditionally considered to have more durable results, endovascular interventions are increasingly utilized as first-line therapy. However, it is at the operator's discretion whether the patient will undergo surgery or percutaneous transluminal angioplasty, taking into account life expectancy, potential cardiovascular comorbidities, the severity of the disease (eg, number of vessels affected, degree of stenosis), and the overall clinical status.

In general, endovascular therapy consists of either balloon angioplasty or angioplasty with stenting. Bare metal stent deployment or covered graft utilization has been associated with better patency rates and lower revascularization rates during follow-up compared to balloon angioplasty alone.[48-50] Complications associated with an endovascular procedure mainly include (1) distal embolization; (2) acute vessel thrombosis; (3) iatrogenic perforation; (4) arterial dissection; and (5) access site complications (eg, local hematoma, compartment syndrome if branchial access). Details regarding angioplasty techniques are presented in Table 83.2.

Surgical Approaches

The type of open surgical repair for the treatment of chronic mesenteric ischemia mainly depends on the anatomy/diseased vessels.[51] In most diffuse mesenteric arterial disease, an aortomesenteric or aortoceliac bypass is performed with either synthetic or autologous vein conduits.[47] Endarterectomy constitutes a reasonable alternative to bypass surgery, offering superior rates of freedom from symptom recurrence compared to mesenteric bypass.[52] However, complex anatomy and multivessel disease limit its application. Several revascularization approaches are presented in Table 83.2.

TABLE 83.2 Treatment Modalities for Acute and Chronic Mesenteric Ischemia

A. Contemporary Endovascular Treatment Options for Mesenteric Ischemia

Endovascular Approach	Indications	Technique	Considerations	Recommended Surveillance Imaging
Thrombolysis	Acute arterial occlusion, distal lesions	Anticoagulation with heparin	• Within 8-10 hours from symptoms onset • No signs of advanced ischemia Consider vasodilation; • Risk for bleeding	• CTA • Duplex ultrasound measuring hemodynamic variables; • Adjust follow-up imaging according to patients risk factors for disease recurrence • Timely reintervention
Mechanical thrombectomy	Acute arterial occlusion	Aspiration, stent retriever, atherectomy, combined approach	• Within 8-10 hours from symptom onset • No signs of advanced ischemia, if unsuccessful consider open conversion	
Percutaneous transluminal angioplasty +/- stenting	• Usually for acute on chronic mesenteric ischemia; • Chronic mesenteric ischemia	Balloon angioplasty with bailout stenting, primary stenting with bare metal stents or covered grafts	• Risk for dissection • Plain balloon angioplasty has higher restenosis rates than stenting • Consider antithrombotic therapy, especially when stents or covered grafts are deployed	

B. Contemporary Surgical Treatment Options for Mesenteric Ischemia

Endovascular Approach	Indications	Technique	Considerations	Recommended Surveillance Imaging
Exploratory laparotomy	• Severe intestinal ischemia • Advanced disease with signs of peritonitis	Abdominal exploration to identify: Ischemic intestinal segments and perforations, bleeding sites	• Nonviable intestinal segments should be resected • If intestinal viability is questionable, consider revascularization and reassessment	• Consider second exploratory laparotomy • CTA • Imaging studies at 3, 6, 12 months, and every year thereafter
Revascularization	• Hemodynamically unstable patients • Advanced intestinal ischemia • Radiologic findings of necrotic intestines	• Embolectomy and full intestinal inspection • Mesenteric bypass • Endarterectomy • Translocation of superior mesenteric artery	• Endarterectomy and translocation of the superior mesenteric artery should be avoided in acute arterial occlusion; • Autologous grafts should be preferred for mesenteric bypass, especially when perforation and peritonitis have occurred • Reevaluate intestinal blood flow after revascularization • Leave abdominal wall open if a second laparotomy is planned	

CTA, computed tomography angiography.

SPECIAL CONSIDERATIONS REGARDING MORTALITY

Acute Mesenteric Ischemia

Despite medical advancements in the urgent/emergent treatment of acute mesenteric ischemia, the overall mortality remains high. A previous study investigating the outcomes of both endovascular and surgical revascularization for the treatment of acute mesenteric ischemia reported an all-cause mortality of 22% and a periprocedural complication in almost 70% of the cases.[41] Generally, most periprocedural deaths are attributed to progression of intestinal ischemia, which leads eventually to peritonitis, septic shock, and multiorgan failure. Therefore, a multidisciplinary approach and intensive postoperative/postintervention surveillance are crucial for improved outcomes and better survival rates. Additionally, future research determining the risk factors for poor prognosis after endovascular or open repair is warranted.

Chronic Mesenteric Ischemia

Selective interventional treatment of chronic mesenteric ischemia is associated with a perioperative all-cause incidence ranging from 0% to 16%. However, emergent treatment of acute mesenteric ischemia on chronic mesenteric ischemia is complicated with death in up to 50% of the cases.[53,54] Generally, open surgical repair has been associated with higher morbidity rates, whereas percutaneous transluminal angioplasty has been associated with higher target repeat revascularization rates during follow-up.[47] Moreover, it is important to note that in contrast to acute mesenteric ischemia, most all-cause death events during follow-up are attributed to causes other than worsening intestinal ischemia, with cardiovascular disease and malignancy being the most common.[47] Therefore, secondary prevention of atherosclerosis progression is crucial to the management of chronic mesenteric ischemia in order to avoid/delay restenosis of mesenteric arteries.

FOLLOW-UP PATIENT CARE

Follow-up for Acute Mesenteric Ischemia

Patients presenting with acute mesenteric ischemia are critically ill and usually require prolonged hospitalization. A previous systematic review suggested that after a surgical revascularization procedure, an additional laparotomy 24 to 48 hours after the index procedure is needed in order to reevaluate the intestinal blood flow.[41] This study showed that almost 30% of patients undergoing second-look laparotomy had necrotic intestinal segments requiring resection.[41] After the patient is discharged, long-term management is focused on preventing future ischemic events. Therefore, appropriate antithrombotic therapy with anticoagulants should be prescribed in cases of mesenteric embolism and antiplatelet agents and statin therapy are recommended for patients with acute thrombotic arterial occlusion of an atherosclerotic mesenteric lesion.

In addition to optimized medical therapy, surveillance imaging with DUS or CTA is recommended for patients who undergo percutaneous transluminal angioplasty for the treatment of acute mesenteric ischemia, although the data regarding the most optimal follow-up imaging intervals after stenting are sparse. However, imaging studies at 3, 6, 12 months, and every year thereafter may be reasonable. In cases of restenosis, evaluation by a vascular specialist is warranted, as reintervention may be needed.

Follow-up for Chronic Mesenteric Ischemia

After revascularization for chronic mesenteric ischemia, a diet should be started. However because patients with chronic mesenteric ischemia are often malnourished, adjunctive parental nutrition should be considered if enteral nutrition does not meet their metabolic demands. Additionally, as chronic mesenteric ischemia is a sequela of atherosclerosis in almost 90% of cases, secondary prevention of atherosclerosis progression is crucial to the management of patients presenting with chronic mesenteric ischemia to delay disease propagation and avoid future ischemic events. Therefore, modification of modifiable risk factors for arterial disease plays an important role in the follow-up care of this high-risk population.

Regarding imaging surveillance, because there are not any specific guidelines, the type of imaging evaluation depends on the preference of the physician and the institutional resources/protocols.[55] Available options for assessment of mesenteric blood flow include DUS, CTA, and MRI with/without contrast infusion. In the patient who has undergone mesenteric revascularization, a baseline imaging study should be performed as soon as the patient is stable and has recovered from the intervention. Surveillance imaging at 3, 6, 12 months, and every year thereafter is reasonable, because most restenosis events will occur in the first six months.[56] The incidence of restenosis is higher among patients receiving endovascular therapy versus surgical repair, ranging from 5% to 15%.[56] Restenosis usually presents with symptom recurrence, and reevaluation of the need for a second revascularization procedure is crucial. Data regarding the most optimal treatment approach (repeat stenting/balloon angioplasty, surgery, etc) for the treatment of restenosis after endovascular therapy or surgical repair are sparse, and, as such, the choice of the therapeutic modality is at the discretion of the operator.

RESEARCH AND FUTURE DIRECTIONS

Although the main pathogenic mechanisms of acute mesenteric ischemia and chronic mesenteric ischemia are well defined, future research is warranted in this field. Several open surgical modalities and endovascular interventions with favorable short- and long-term outcomes have been proposed. However, specific indications for one type of intervention over another are lacking because there are no direct comparative studies. Moreover, additional data are required in order to optimize surveillance imaging for patients undergoing procedures for acute mesenteric ischemia or chronic mesenteric ischemia, because no guidelines indicate the most appropriate imaging study. Furthermore, future prospective studies should determine the most optimal time intervals for surveillance imaging, because early detection of disease recurrence and timely

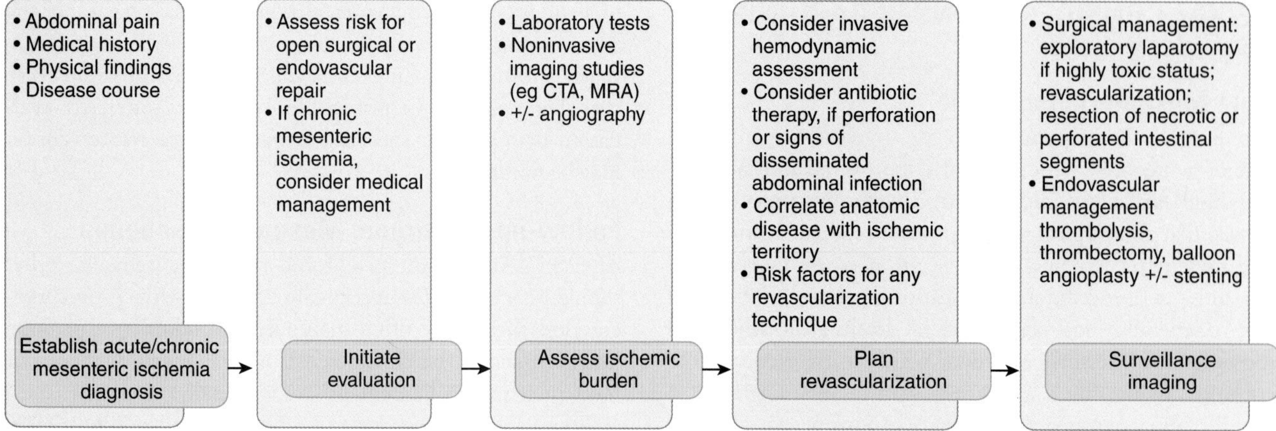

FIGURE 83.1 Treatment algorithm for mesenteric arterial disease.

reintervention may prevent subsequent devastating complications (eg, necrotic intestinal ischemia requiring bowel resection, long hospitalizations, advanced disease with peritonitis, or sepsis). Lastly, studies should guide decision-making for the treatment of recurrent disease (ie, repeat endovascular repair or surgery).

KEY POINTS

- ✔ Diagnosis of mesenteric ischemia requires a high index of clinical suspicion, because in most cases the clinical findings are nonspecific.
- ✔ Patients presenting with acute mesenteric ischemia are usually at a highly toxic status and intervention should not be delayed. A multidisciplinary approach with evaluation of all available therapeutic modalities is of high importance for optimal decision-making. See **Figure 83.1**.
- ✔ In most chronic mesenteric ischemia cases, advanced atherosclerotic disease is apparent, and, as such, this population is at high risk for cardiovascular mortality. Therefore, patients diagnosed with chronic mesenteric ischemia should be evaluated for coronary artery disease before undergoing any type of procedure.
- ✔ Patients with symptomatic chronic mesenteric ischemia usually present with malnutrition. Because the severity of malnutrition potentially affects the outcomes of the index procedure, the nutritional status should be assessed in all patients. When abnormal, parenteral nutrition should be considered.
- ✔ Surveillance imaging after mesenteric revascularization is recommended at 3-, 6-, 12-month intervals and every year thereafter. However, patients at high risk for disease recurrence should be screened more frequently.
- ✔ In patients treated with endovascular therapy, symptom recurrence is correlated with disease recurrence (ie, restenosis). Accordingly, prompt evaluation for reintervention should be made.

REFERENCES

1. Clair DG, Beach JM. Mesenteric Ischemia. *N Engl J Med.* 2016;374(10):959-968.
2. Tilsed JV, Casamassima A, Kurihara H, et al. ESTES guidelines: acute mesenteric ischaemia. *Eur J Trauma Emerg Surg.* 2016;42(2):253-270.
3. Leone M, Bechis C, Baumstarck K, et al. Outcome of acute mesenteric ischemia in the intensive care unit: a retrospective, multicenter study of 780 cases. *Intensive Care Med.* 2015;41(4):667-676.
4. Lawson RM. Mesenteric Ischemia. *Crit Care Nurs Clin North Am.* 2018;30(1):29-39.
5. Cardin F, Fratta S, Perissinotto E, et al. Clinical correlation of mesenteric vascular disease in older patients. *Aging Clin Exp Res.* 2012;24(Suppl 3):43-46.
6. Acosta S. Mesenteric ischemia. *Curr Opin Crit Care.* 2015;21(2):171-178.
7. Zhao Y, Yin H, Yao C, et al. Management of acute mesenteric ischemia: a critical review and treatment algorithm. *Vasc Endovascular Surg.* 2016;50(3):183-192.
8. Bakhtiar A, Yousphi AS, Ghani AR, Ali Z, Ullah W. Weight loss: a significant cue to the diagnosis of chronic mesenteric ischemia. *Cureus.* 2019;11(8):e5335.
9. Van Damme H, Boesmans E, Creemers E, Defraigne JO. How to manage chronic mesenteric ischemia? A deliberated strategy. *Acta Chir Belg.* 2020;120(1):1-5.
10. Blauw JTM, Pastoors HAM, Brusse-Keizer M, et al. The Impact of Revascularisation on Quality of Life in Chronic Mesenteric Ischemia. *Can J Gastroenterol Hepatol.* 2019;2019:7346013.
11. Cleveland Clinic. Intestinal ischemic syndrome. Accessed December, 2019. https://my.clevelandclinic.org/health/diseases/17136-intestinal-ischemic-syndrome
12. Ambe PC, Kang K, Papadakis M, Zirngibl H. Can the preoperative serum lactate level predict the extent of bowel ischemia in patients presenting to the emergency department with acute mesenteric ischemia? *Biomed Res Int.* 2017;2017:8038796.
13. Barret M, Martineau C, Rahmi G, et al. Chronic mesenteric ischemia: a rare cause of chronic abdominal pain. *Am J Med.* 2015;128(12):1363.e1361-1368.
14. Acosta S, Nilsson T. Current status on plasma biomarkers for acute mesenteric ischemia. *J Thromb Thrombolysis.* 2012;33(4):355-361.
15. Evennett NJ, Petrov MS, Mittal A, Windsor JA. Systematic review and pooled estimates for the diagnostic accuracy of serological markers for intestinal ischemia. *World J Surg.* 2009;33(7):1374-1383.
16. Oliva IB, Davarpanah AH, Rybicki FJ, et al. ACR Appropriateness Criteria® imaging of mesenteric ischemia. *Abdom Imaging.* 2013;38(4):714-719.
17. Hagspiel KD, Flors L, Hanley M, Norton PT. Computed tomography angiography and magnetic resonance angiography imaging of the mesenteric vasculature. *Tech Vasc Interv Radiol.* 2015;18(1):2-13.

18. Kirkpatrick ID, Kroeker MA, Greenberg HM. Biphasic CT with mesenteric CT angiography in the evaluation of acute mesenteric ischemia: initial experience. *Radiology.* 2003;229(1):91-98.
19. Aschoff AJ, Stuber G, Becker BW, et al. Evaluation of acute mesenteric ischemia: accuracy of biphasic mesenteric multi-detector CT angiography. *Abdom Imaging.* 2009;34(3):345-357.
20. Alvi AR, Khan S, Niazi SK, Ghulam M, Bibi S. Acute mesenteric venous thrombosis: improved outcome with early diagnosis and prompt anticoagulation therapy. *Int J Surg.* 2009;7(3):210-213.
21. Barmase M, Kang M, Wig J, Kochhar R, Gupta R, Khandelwal N. Role of multidetector CT angiography in the evaluation of suspected mesenteric ischemia. *Eur J Radiol.* 2011;80(3):e582-587.
22. Wyers MC. Acute mesenteric ischemia: diagnostic approach and surgical treatment. *Semin Vasc Surg.* 2010;23(1):9-20.
23. Acosta S, Bjornsson S, Ekberg O, Resch T. CT angiography followed by endovascular intervention for acute superior mesenteric artery occlusion does not increase risk of contrast-induced renal failure. *Eur J Vasc Endovasc Surg.* 2010;39(6):726-730.
24. Di Minno MN, Milone F, Milone M, et al. Endovascular thrombolysis in acute mesenteric vein thrombosis: a 3-year follow-up with the rate of short and long-term sequaelae in 32 patients. *Thromb Res.* 2010;126(4):295-298.
25. Arthurs ZM, Titus J, Bannazadeh M, et al. A comparison of endovascular revascularization with traditional therapy for the treatment of acute mesenteric ischemia. *J Vasc Surg.* 2011;53(3):698-704; discussion 704-695.
26. Kolkman JJ, Geelkerken RH. Diagnosis and treatment of chronic mesenteric ischemia: an update. *Best Pract Res Clin Gastroenterol.* 2017;31(1):49-57.
27. Foley TR, Rogers RK. Endovascular therapy for chronic mesenteric ischemia. *Curr Treat Options Cardiovasc Med.* 2016;18(6):39.
28. Nicoloff AD, Williamson WK, Moneta GL, Taylor LM, Porter JM. Duplex ultrasonography in evaluation of splanchnic artery stenosis. *Surg Clin North Am.* 1997;77(2):339-355.
29. van Petersen AS, Meerwaldt R, Kolkman JJ, et al. The influence of respiration on criteria for transabdominal duplex examination of the splanchnic arteries in patients with suspected chronic splanchnic ischemia. *J Vasc Surg.* 2013;57(6):1603-1611.e1601-1610.
30. Seidl H, Tuerck J, Schepp W, Schneider AR. Splanchnic arterial blood flow is significantly influenced by breathing-assessment by duplex-Doppler ultrasound. *Ultrasound Med Biol.* 2010;36(10):1677-1681.
31. Bjornsson S, Resch T, Acosta S. Symptomatic mesenteric atherosclerotic disease-lessons learned from the diagnostic workup. *J Gastrointest Surg.* 2013;17(5):973-980.
32. Schaefer PJ, Pfarr J, Trentmann J, et al. Comparison of noninvasive imaging modalities for stenosis grading in mesenteric arteries. *Rofo.* 2013;185(7):628-634.
33. Cademartiri F, Palumbo A, Maffei E, et al. Noninvasive evaluation of the celiac trunk and superior mesenteric artery with multislice CT in patients with chronic mesenteric ischaemia. *Radiol Med.* 2008;113(8):1135-1142.
34. Cardia PP, Penachim TJ, Prando A, Torres US, D'Ippolito G. Non-contrast MR angiography using three-dimensional balanced steady-state free-precession imaging for evaluation of stenosis in the celiac trunk and superior mesenteric artery: a preliminary comparative study with computed tomography angiography. *Br J Radiol.* 2017;90(1075):20170011.
35. Mensink PB, Geelkerken RH, Huisman AB, Kuipers EJ, Kolkman JJ. Twenty-four hour tonometry in patients suspected of chronic gastrointestinal ischemia. *Dig Dis Sci.* 2008;53(1):133-139.
36. Friedland S, Benaron D, Coogan S, Sze DY, Soetikno R. Diagnosis of chronic mesenteric ischemia by visible light spectroscopy during endoscopy. *Gastrointest Endosc.* 2007;65(2):294-300.
37. Kozuch PL, Brandt LJ. Review article: diagnosis and management of mesenteric ischaemia with an emphasis on pharmacotherapy. *Aliment Pharmacol Ther.* 2005;21(3):201-215.
38. Corcos O, Castier Y, Sibert A, et al. Effects of a multimodal management strategy for acute mesenteric ischemia on survival and intestinal failure. *Clin Gastroenterol Hepatol.* 2013;11(2):158-165.e152.
39. Alhan E, Usta A, Cekic A, Saglam K, Turkyilmaz S, Cinel A. A study on 107 patients with acute mesenteric ischemia over 30 years. *Int J Surg.* 2012;10(9):510-513.
40. Bjorck M, Orr N, Endean ED. Debate: whether an endovascular-first strategy is the optimal approach for treating acute mesenteric ischemia. *J Vasc Surg.* 2015;62(3):767-772.
41. Ryer EJ, Kalra M, Oderich GS, et al. Revascularization for acute mesenteric ischemia. *J Vasc Surg.* 2012;55(6):1682-1689.
42. Jia Z, Jiang G, Tian F, et al. Early endovascular treatment of superior mesenteric occlusion secondary to thromboemboli. *Eur J Vasc Endovasc Surg.* 2014;47(2):196-203.
43. Becquemin JP. Management of the diseases of mesenteric arteries and veins: clinical practice guidelines of the European Society for Vascular Surgery (ESVS). *Eur J Vasc Endovasc Surg.* 2017;53(4):455-457.
44. Roussel A, Castier Y, Nuzzo A, et al. Revascularization of acute mesenteric ischemia after creation of a dedicated multidisciplinary center. *J Vasc Surg.* 2015;62(5):1251-1256.
45. Yamamoto M, Orihashi K, Nishimori H, et al. Indocyanine green angiography for intra-operative assessment in vascular surgery. *Eur J Vasc Endovasc Surg.* 2012;43(4):426-432.
46. Mansukhani NA, Hekman KE, Yoon DY, et al. Impact of body mass index on outcomes after mesenteric revascularization for chronic mesenteric ischemia. *Ann Vasc Surg.* 2018;48:159-165.
47. Oderich GS. Current concepts in the management of chronic mesenteric ischemia. *Curr Treat Options Cardiovasc Med.* 2010;12(2):117-130.
48. Tallarita T, Oderich GS, Macedo TA, et al. Reinterventions for stent restenosis in patients treated for atherosclerotic mesenteric artery disease. *J Vasc Surg.* 2011;54(5):1422-1429.e1421.
49. Aburahma AF, Campbell JE, Stone PA, et al. Perioperative and late clinical outcomes of percutaneous transluminal stentings of the celiac and superior mesenteric arteries over the past decade. *J Vasc Surg.* 2013;57(4):1052-1061.
50. Oderich GS, Erdoes LS, Lesar C, et al. Comparison of covered stents versus bare metal stents for treatment of chronic atherosclerotic mesenteric arterial disease. *J Vasc Surg.* 2013;58(5):1316-1323.
51. Keese M, Schmitz-Rixen T, Schmandra T. Chronic mesenteric ischemia: time to remember open revascularization. *World J Gastroenterol.* 2013;19(9):1333-1337.
52. Mell MW, Acher CW, Hoch JR, Tefera G, Turnipseed WD. Outcomes after endarterectomy for chronic mesenteric ischemia. *J Vasc Surg.* 2008; 48(5):1132-1138.
53. Oderich GS, Bower TC, Sullivan TM, Bjarnason H, Cha S, Gloviczki P. Open versus endovascular revascularization for chronic mesenteric ischemia: risk-stratified outcomes. *J Vasc Surg.* 2009;49(6):1472-1479.e1473.
54. Schermerhorn ML, Giles KA, Hamdan AD, Wyers MC, Pomposelli FB. Mesenteric revascularization: management and outcomes in the United States, 1988-2006. *J Vasc Surg.* 2009;50(2):341-348.e341.
55. Tallarita T, Oderich GS, Gloviczki P, et al. Patient survival after open and endovascular mesenteric revascularization for chronic mesenteric ischemia. *J Vasc Surg.* 2013;57(3):747-755; discussion 754-745.
56. Sharafuddin MJ, Olson CH, Sun S, Kresowik TF, Corson JD. Endovascular treatment of celiac and mesenteric arteries stenoses: applications and results. *J Vasc Surg.* 2003;38(4):692-698.

CHAPTER 84

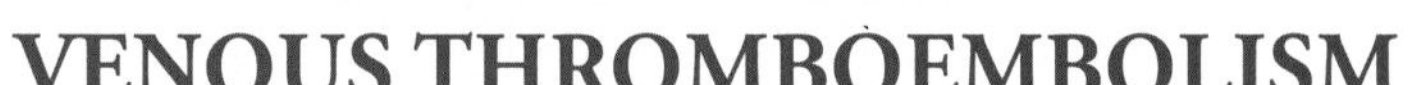

VENOUS THROMBOEMBOLISM

Stephanie M. Madonis and J. Stephen Jenkins

INTRODUCTION

Venous thromboembolic (VTE) disease is a condition in which a thrombus forms in the venous circulation and includes both deep vein thrombosis (DVT) and pulmonary embolism (PE). Although the true incidence of VTE is unknown, according to the U.S. Centers for Disease Control and Prevention, it is estimated at 900,000 individuals in the United States each year.[1] This disease burden accrues substantial health care costs and leads to significant morbidity and mortality. The purpose of this chapter is to describe the various clinical features and presentations of VTE with a particular focus on DVT. An overview regarding the different treatment options in addition to the evaluation and management of long-term sequelae from DVT is also provided.

PATHOPHYSIOLOGY

In the simplest sense, DVT is the development of thrombus in a deep vein that may either partially or completely obstruct blood flow through the affected blood vessel.

Thrombus consists of a network of fibrin products that forms a mesh around platelets, white blood cells, and red blood cells via the coagulation cascade. The pathogenesis of thrombus formation can be condensed into three well-described factors, otherwise known as *Virchow triad*. This triad consists of (1) endothelial cell injury that leads to activation and secretion of procoagulant tissue factors, (2) venous stasis, and (3) hypercoagulability. Different disease processes and/or conditions may result in the activation of one or more of these three factors, and ultimately predispose an individual to the development of DVT.

Once a thrombus has formed, it has a few different fates or outcomes. This includes propagation of thrombus along the blood vessel wall because of additional platelet and fibrin deposition, organization and recanalization of the thrombus within the blood vessel and, lastly, embolization or dislodgment from the blood vessel wall, allowing it to travel to other vasculature sites via the systemic circulation.[2] DVT itself is not a life-threatening condition unless the thrombus detaches and embolizes to the vasculature of the lungs, resulting in a PE.

NOMENCLATURE

Oftentimes, DVT is categorized as having been (1) provoked by an identifiable patient-related or environmental risk factor or (2) unprovoked with no identifiable provoking event evident. This distinction is made because of important prognostic and management implications. Current guidelines advocate for at least 3 months of anticoagulation for provoked DVTs, whereas long-term anticoagulation is recommended for patients with unprovoked events because of a high risk of recurrence.

Provoking risk factors can be further subdivided into transient or persistent. Transient risk factors are those that resolve after they have "provoked" a DVT, and include events such as recent surgery, trauma, confinement to bed or prolonged immobilization, use of oral contraceptives or hormone replacement therapy, and pregnancy. Potential permanent or persistent risk factors include malignancy, hereditary thrombophilia, inflammatory bowel disease, collagen vascular disease, chronic renal disease, congestive heart failure, obesity, and tobacco use disorder.

It is approximated that 25% to 50% of DVT cases have no identifiable predisposing risk factor or trigger, and are therefore, classified as being unprovoked.[3]

ANATOMIC CONSIDERATIONS

Most DVTs arise in the deep venous system of the lower extremities or pelvis, but they can also affect other venous parts of the body, including the upper extremities, brain, liver, intestines, or kidney(s). Although upper extremity DVTs are far less common than are lower extremity DVTs, they still account for approximately 4% to 10% of all DVT cases.[4] Upper extremity DVTs may arise in the internal jugular, subclavian, axillary, or brachial veins, and are often associated with, or related to, indwelling central venous catheters, pacemaker or defibrillator leads, and thoracic outlet syndrome.

Lower extremity DVTs have traditionally been categorized by the anatomic location of thrombus as either proximal or distal (**Figure 84.1**). Proximal DVT is routinely used to describe thrombus that is located in the inferior vena cava (IVC) and iliac, femoral, or popliteal veins. Distal DVT is used to describe thrombus confined to the calf veins, which includes the peroneal, posterior, and anterior tibial veins, and muscular calf veins (ie, the soleal or gastrocnemius). Compared to proximal DVTs, distal DVTs are not as common and oftentimes do not require treatment or intervention.[5]

Although this anatomic subdivision is appropriate for clinical purposes, a new anatomic division at the level of the iliofemoral veins is being widely adopted, and is particularly useful when it comes to risk stratification of patients

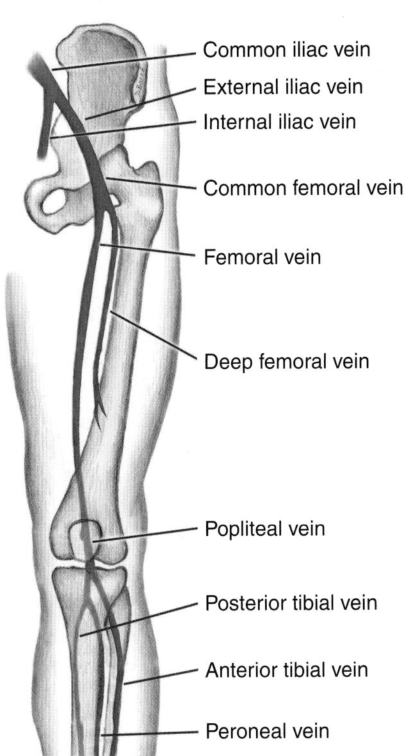

FIGURE 84.1 Anatomy of the deep venous system. (Image created by James Jenkins and Darren Barre, John Ochsner Heart and Vascular Institute, New Orleans, Louisiana)

with lower extremity DVTs that may benefit from early invasive catheter-based treatment. Studies have demonstrated that proximal DVTs involving the common femoral vein and/or iliac veins portend worse prognosis and carry higher risk for adverse outcomes when compared to proximal DVTs that do not involve the common femoral vein or iliac veins.[6,7] Consequently, these patients with iliofemoral thrombosis are likely to benefit from invasive strategies such as catheter-directed thrombolysis (CDT) and/or mechanical or aspiration thrombectomy.[8,9]

The 2012 guidelines of the Society for Vascular Surgery and the American Venous Forum recognize the need for this important distinction in the diagnosis of lower extremity DVTs, with guideline 1.1 stating: "We recommend use of precise terminology to characterize the most proximal extent of venous thrombosis as involving the iliofemoral veins, with or without extension into the IVC; the femoropopliteal veins; or isolated to the calf veins in preference to simple characterization of a thrombus as proximal or distal."[10]

DIAGNOSIS

Clinical Presentation and Laboratory Testing

Clinical signs and symptoms of acute DVT are highly variable. Some individuals with DVT may be asymptomatic, whereas others may experience pain and swelling in the affected limb, erythema, skin discoloration, superficial venous dilatation, unexplained fever, and even cyanosis in cases with severe venous obstruction.

Clinical suspicion and pretest probability is the first step in the diagnostic algorithm of DVT.

The likelihood that DVT is present can be assessed using prediction tools such as the widely validated Wells Scoring System for DVT (**Table 84.1**). Although this structured scoring system is helpful, the value of clinical judgment or gestalt is also well recognized.

D-dimer testing, in combination with structured clinical risk assessment, can also be utilized to rule out DVT. When the clinical pretest probability for DVT is low or intermediate, a negative quantitative D-dimer assay has a high negative predictive value, and therefore is adequate to safely exclude DVT. It is imperative to recognize, however, that because of its low specificity, an elevated D-dimer does not confirm the diagnosis of DVT. In this situation, or in a patient with a high pretest probability for DVT, D-dimer testing alone is not sufficient, and further assessment is warranted.

TABLE 84.1 Pretest Probability of Deep Vein Thrombosis (Wells Score)

Clinical Finding	Points
• Paralysis, paresis, or recent orthopedic casting of lower extremity	1
• Recently bedridden for more than 3 days or major surgery within 4 weeks	1
• Localized tenderness along distribution of deep venous system	1
• Swelling of entire leg	1
• Calf swelling by more than 3 cm when compared to the asymptomatic leg (measured 10 cm below tibial tuberosity)	1
• Pitting edema (greater in the symptomatic leg)	1
• Collateral superficial veins (non-varicose vein)	1
• Active cancer or cancer treated within previous 6 months	1
• Alternative diagnosis more likely than that of DVT (eg, Baker's cyst, cellulitis, superficial vein thrombosis, post-phlebitic syndrome, inguinal lymphadenopathy)	−2
Risk Score Interpretation	**Points**
High probability of DVT	3-8
Moderate probability	1-2
Low probability	−2 to 0

Wells scoring system for DVT: −2 to 0 points: low probability; 1-2 points: moderate probability; 3-8 points: high probability.

Modified from Wells PS, Anderson DR, Bormanis J, et al. Value of assessment of pretest probability of deep-vein thrombosis in clinical management. *Lancet.* 1997;350(9094):1795-1798. Copyright © 1997 Elsevier. With permission.

Noninvasive Imaging

Venous ultrasonography (VUS) is considered the first-line imaging modality for assessment and diagnosis of DVT given its safety, availability, accuracy, and cost-effectiveness. VUS provides an overall sensitivity of 94.2% for proximal and 63.5% for isolated distal DVT, with an overall specificity of 93.8%.[11] Combination with color Doppler ultrasound (CDUS) increases sensitivity; however, it lowers specificity.[11]

A comprehensive evaluation of the lower extremities with VUS includes examination from the common femoral confluence to the calf veins. The upper extremities should be evaluated from the subclavian vein, including the internal jugular through the brachial veins. CDUS findings that support the presence of DVT include the following:

- Direct visualization of thrombus with vein enlargement
- Inability to compress the walls of the vein(s)
- Blunted augmentation or absence of blood flow in response to distal (calf) compression
- Abnormal spectral Doppler (ie, lack of respiratory variation in the venous spectral Doppler flow pattern)
- Abnormal color Doppler (ie, lack of flow or partial recanalization on color flow ultrasound)

If VUS finding is negative and clinical suspicion for DVT remains high, or when DVT is suspected in the pelvis or IVC, alternative imaging with computed tomographic venography or magnetic resonance venography should be considered.

Venography

Contrast venography was considered to be the gold standard test for the diagnosis of DVT in the past. However, owing to its invasive nature and need for potentially harmful contrast agents, it has largely been replaced by noninvasive tests such as VUS.

MANAGEMENT

Algorithm 84.1 provides basic treatment for the management of patients with a new diagnosis of DVT.

Medical Approach

Systemic anticoagulation is the mainstay of therapy for patients with acute DVT. If clinical suspicion for DVT is intermediate or high, anticoagulation should be initiated while further testing is performed to confirm the diagnosis, particularly if no contraindication(s) to anticoagulation exist.

Several anticoagulation options are available (**Table 84.2**), and agent selection largely depends on patient characteristics as well as on patient and physician preference.

Warfarin, which disrupts vitamin K metabolism, thereby inhibiting clotting factors II, VII, IX, and X, was the most

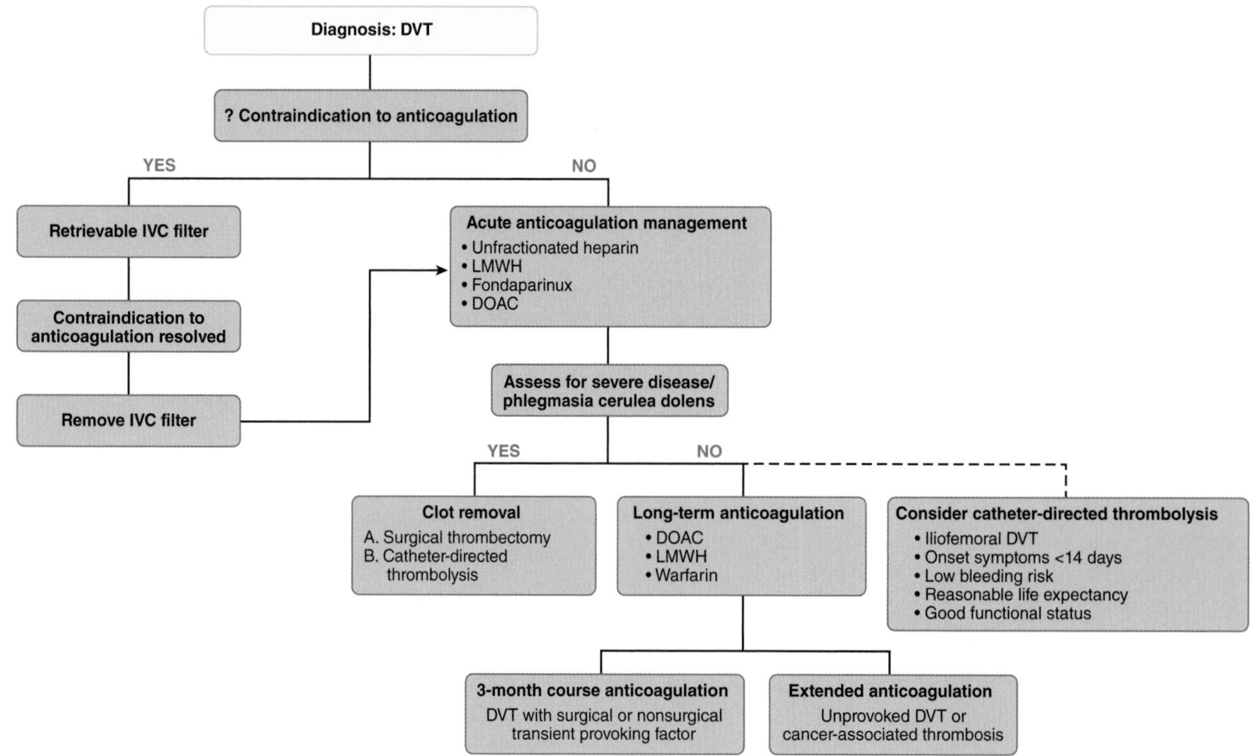

ALGORITHM 84.1 Approach to the management of acute deep vein thromboembolism. DOAC, direct oral anticoagulant; DVT, deep vein thrombosis; IVC, inferior vena cava; LMWH, low-molecular-weight heparin. (Adapted with permission from Liu D, Peterson E, Dooner J, et al. Diagnosis and management of iliofemoral deep vein thrombosis: clinical practice guideline. *CMAJ*. 2015;187(17):1288-1296.)

TABLE 84.2 Anticoagulation Reference for Treatment of Deep Vein Thrombosis

Drug Class/Drugs	Initial Dose	Maintenance Dose	Side Effects
		Low-Molecular-Weight Heparins	
Enoxaparin	1.0 mg/kg SC twice daily *or* 1.5 mg/kg SC once daily	1.0 mg/kg SC twice daily *or* 1.5 mg/kg SC once daily	• Bleeding • Heparin-induced thrombocytopenia (HIT) • Osteoporosis • Hypersensitivity/anaphylaxis • Limited use in renal insufficiency
Tinzaparin	175 IU/kg SC once daily	175 IU/kg SC once daily	
Dalteparin	100 IU/kg SC twice daily *or* 200 IU/kg SC once daily	100 IU/kg SC twice daily *or* 200 IU/kg SC once daily	
		Unfractionated Heparin	
Heparin	Bolus: 80 IU/kg IV (max 10,000 IU)	Continuous: 18 IU/kg/h IV with aPTT monitoring (goal is to achieve aPTT of 1.5-2× baseline)	• Bleeding • HIT (more likely than with LMWH) • Osteoporosis • Hypersensitivity/anaphylaxis
		Pentasaccharide	
Fondaparinux	<50 kg: 5 mg SC once daily 50-100 kg: 7.5 mg SC once daily >100 kg: 10 mg SC once daily	<50 kg: 5 mg SC once daily 50-100 kg: 7.5 mg SC once daily >100 kg: 10 mg SC once daily	• Bleeding • Limited use in renal insufficiency and patients with low body weight
		Vitamin K Antagonist	
Warfarin[a]	–	Adjust to target INR 2-3	• Bleeding • Warfarin-induced skin necrosis (increased in protein C or S deficiency) • Teratogen • Osteoporosis • Agranulocytosis
		Direct Oral Anticoagulants	
Apixaban	10 mg PO twice daily for 7 days	5 mg PO twice daily	• Bleeding
Dabigatran[b]	–	150 mg PO twice daily	
Edoxaban[b]	–	60 mg PO once daily	
Rivaroxaban	15 mg PO twice daily for 21 days	20 mg PO once daily	

aPTT, activated partial thromboplastin time; INR, international normalized ratio; LMWH, low-weight-molecular heparin; IU, international units; IV, intravenous; PO, oral; SC, subcutaneous.

[a]Parenteral overlap with unfractionated heparin (UFH), low-weight-molecular heparin (LMWH), or fondaparinux must be administered for a minimum of 5 days and until the international normalized ratio (INR) is within target range of 2 to 3 for 2 consecutive days.

[b]Parenteral overlap with unfractionated heparin (UFH), low-weight-molecular heparin (LMWH), or fondaparinux must be administered for a minimum of 5 days before maintenance dosing is initiated with the designated agent.

widely used oral anticoagulant of choice for well over 50 years. The international normalized ratio (INR) is used to monitor warfarin concentrations. An INR value between 2.0 and 3.0 is considered to be "therapeutic range" for most clinical situations, including treatment of acute DVT. When warfarin is chosen as the oral agent, treatment must be initiated and overlapped with a parenteral drug until the INR is therapeutic (ie, >2) for two consecutive INR values.

Approved parenteral agents include indirect anticoagulants (unfractionated heparin [UFH], low-molecular-weight heparin [LMWH], or fondaparinux) and the direct anticoagulants that target thrombin (lepirudin, desirudin, bivalirudin, and argatroban). In patients with a creatinine clearance (CrCl) greater than 30 mL/min, the preferred overlapping parenteral agent is LMWH or fondaparinux. In patients with CrCl less than 30 mL/min, UFH is preferred.

Recently, direct oral anticoagulants (DOACs), including apixaban, rivaroxaban, edoxaban, and dabigatran, have emerged as valid treatment options for DVT. Per current guideline recommendations, DOACs are actually preferred to warfarin as first-line oral agents, particularly for patients with low-risk DVT.[12] DOACs are at least as effective and probably safer than is treatment with vitamin K antagonists (ie, warfarin) or parenteral drugs. This statement is supported by a meta-analysis of 27,023 patients that showed similar VTE recurrence rates in patients receiving DOACs versus conventional therapy (2.0% vs 2.2%, respectively; relative risk [RR] 0.90). The same study showed that treatment with a DOAC significantly reduced the risk of major bleeding events (RR 0.61) and lowered the risk of intracranial bleeding, fatal bleeding, and clinically relevant non-major bleeding.[13]

Another advantage of DOACs over warfarin therapy is that they are given as fixed once- or twice-daily regimens, contingent on the patient's renal function, and do not require regular monitoring of clotting parameters (ie, INR) to guide dosage adjustment. Because apixaban and rivaroxaban provide their effects immediately, they do not require bridging with UFH, LMWH, or fondaparinux when starting treatment. This is in contrast to the other DOACs—edoxaban and dabigatran—that do require pretreatment with a parenteral agent for a minimum of 5 days.

The decision regarding drug choice should be influenced by bleeding risk, patient comorbidities, cost, and convenience. Factors associated with an increased tendency for bleeding, which must be taken into consideration, include advanced age, previous bleeding, renal failure, liver failure, anemia, thrombocytopenia, malignancy, previous stroke, diabetes mellitus, poor functional status, concomitant antiplatelet therapy, and/or erratic anticoagulation control. Unique or specialized patient subsets that require more distinctive approaches to tailoring anticoagulation therapy have been identified. Among the ones mentioned here briefly are patients with malignancy and pregnant women.

Absolute contraindications to anticoagulation include intracranial bleeding; severe active bleeding; recent brain, eye, or spinal cord surgery; and malignant hypertension. Relative contraindications include recent cerebrovascular accident, recent major surgery, and severe thrombocytopenia.

Malignancy

For patients with active malignancy and cancer-associated thrombosis, LMWH is preferred as the initial and long-term anticoagulant, although there is emerging data now to support the use of DOACs.[14] All four DOACs have demonstrated comparable safety and efficacy in conventional treatment in this setting.[15] Conversely, it should be recognized that warfarin, and other vitamin K antagonists, are not recommended as preferred treatment in the cancer subpopulation, and are considered "third choice." Warfarin should only be administered when neither a DOAC nor an LMWH is feasible in these patients.

Pregnancy

The incidence of DVT in pregnant women is about six times the incidence in nonpregnant women.[16] Warfarin should be avoided in the treatment of acute DVT in this patient population because of its adverse effects on the fetus. Vitamin K antagonists cross the placenta readily and are associated with adverse pregnancy outcomes including miscarriage, prematurity, low birthweight, neurodevelopment problems, and characteristic embryopathy (ie, fetal warfarin syndrome) following fetal exposure in the first trimester. DOACs have not been adequately tested, and are therefore currently contraindicated. The preferred anticoagulants are LMWH or UFH because they do not cross the placenta.

Duration of Medical Therapy

Optimal duration of anticoagulation therapy must take into account (1) the presence or absence of provoking risk factors, (2) the risk of DVT recurrence compared to the risk of bleeding, and (3) the individual patient's preferences and values.

There is general agreement that 3 months is the minimum length of time for treatment of acute DVT with anticoagulation. Cessation of anticoagulant therapy after 3 months of treatment is typically recommended in those with (1) surgery-associated DVT, (2) DVT provoked by a nonsurgical transient risk factor, and (3) a first unprovoked DVT in a patient with a high risk of bleeding complications.[12]

Indefinite therapy is recommended for patients with recurrent episodes of DVT or VTE regardless of the cause. In one study, the risk of recurrent VTE during a 4-year follow-up period was reduced from 21% to 3% with continued anticoagulation; however, the incidence of major bleeding increased from 3% to 9%.[17]

Patients with malignancy have a particularly higher rate of DVT recurrence than do non-cancer patients. Therefore, after a recommended 6 months of therapy in this patient population, the decision to continue anticoagulation should be based on the individual evaluation of cancer activity, patient tolerability, and the overall benefit-to-risk ratio.

Endovascular Interventions

Percutaneous Approach

The primary objectives of treatment of acute DVT are to prevent PE, reduce morbidity and mortality, and prevent or minimize the risk of developing post-thrombotic syndrome. When this cannot be achieved with systemic anticoagulation alone, endovascular therapy may be considered. Percutaneous transcatheter treatment in patients with DVT consists of thrombus removal with CDT, percutaneous mechanical thrombectomy, angioplasty, and/or stenting of venous obstructions.

CDT may be performed in association with percutaneous mechanical thrombectomy, which includes fragmentation, maceration, and aspiration of thrombus. Although routine use of thrombolysis is not warranted, depending on current guidelines, patients who are most likely to benefit from aggressive management with CDT are those with proximal iliofemoral DVT, symptom duration less than 14 days, low bleeding risk, life expectancy greater than 1 year, and good functional status.[18]

Several randomized controlled trials comparing CDT to conventional anticoagulation, including CaVenT (catheter-directed venous thrombolysis) and ATTRACT (Acute Venous Thrombosis: Thrombus Removal with Adjunctive Catheter-Directed Thrombolysis), demonstrated a lower incidence of post-thrombotic syndrome and improved iliofemoral patency in patients with a high proximal DVT who were treated with CDT compared to those treated with anticoagulation alone. However, this benefit came at the expense of excess major bleeding.[8,9]

Important contraindications to thrombolysis are summarized in **Table 84.3**. Furthermore, it should be acknowledged that patients with DVT who receive CDT (with or without percutaneous mechanical thrombectomy) must also be placed on appropriate anticoagulation therapy.

Surgical Approach

Surgical venous thrombectomy is an alternative option for the management of extensive acute DVT; however, it has traditionally been reserved for patients presenting with phlegmasia cerulea dolens in which thrombus completely occludes venous outflow, causing massive limb swelling, and eventually ischemia and necrosis. It is performed by surgically exposing the common femoral vein and saphenofemoral junction through a longitudinal incision in the skin. The patient must be heparinized before the procedure.

TABLE 84.3 Contraindications to Catheter-Directed Thrombolysis

Absolute Contraindications
• Active internal bleeding
• Cerebrovascular event (including transient ischemic attacks), neurosurgical procedure (including spinal and paraspinal surgery), or cerebral trauma in the past 3 months
• Severe coagulopathy, such as disseminated intravascular coagulation
• Absolute contraindication to anticoagulation
Relative Contraindications
• Age older than 75 years
• Internal bleeding in the past 3 months
• Intracranial tumor or lesion, or seizure disorder
• Recent cardiopulmonary resuscitation, major surgery, obstetric delivery, organ biopsy, or major trauma in the past 10 days
• Severe allergy to thrombolytic agent, anticoagulant, or contrast media (not controlled by steroid/antihistamine pretreatment)
• Severe thrombocytopenia
• Uncontrolled hypertension (systolic >180 mm Hg, diastolic >110 mm Hg)
• Right-to-left cardiac or pulmonary shunt
• Suspicion for infected venous thrombus
• Bacterial endocarditis
• Left ventricular thrombus
• Current use of anticoagulation
• Renal failure
• Severe hepatic dysfunction
• Diabetic hemorrhagic retinopathy
• Pregnancy or lactation
• Dementia

Venous Thromboembolism Recurrence

Recurrence of VTE is common. The most important factors determining recurrence risk are whether the event was unprovoked or provoked by a transient or persistent risk factor. Other determinants include (1) DVT location (ie, distal versus proximal DVT), (2) ongoing nonmodifiable risk factors, and (3) whether the episode was a first event versus a recurrent event. The lowest annual recurrence rates after stopping anticoagulation is observed in DVT after surgery (1% at 1 year; 3% at 5 years). The rate rises to 3% at 1 year and 15% at 5 years for patients with provoked DVT in which the trigger was not surgery. The highest recurrence rates are for unprovoked DVT (5%-10% at 1 year and 30% at 5 years).[19] The 2019 European Society of Cardiology guidelines recommend an extended duration of anticoagulation in patients with the highest risk of DVT recurrence.[20] In fact, all patients with an unprovoked DVT should be considered for indefinite therapy if overall bleeding risk is low. In patients with an intermediate risk of recurrence, further discussion regarding treatment duration should be based on risk of bleeding and patient preference, as mentioned previously.

Inferior Vena Cava Filters

An IVC filter is a retrievable device that is designed to mechanically trap or capture venous emboli larger than 4 mm, thereby preventing thrombus migration from the lower extremities to the pulmonary arteries, in turn causing a PE. The device is typically placed in the infrarenal portion of the IVC. Although they are made to be deployed and later retrieved (typically within 60-90 days), all devices can theoretically remain in the body permanently; however, long-term durability data are lacking.

In general, IVC filters are not recommended, and offer little benefit for patients with DVT who are tolerating treatment with systemic anticoagulation. They are strictly reserved for those with acute DVT who have an absolute contraindication to anticoagulation or for patients who experience anticoagulation failure (ie, documented recurrence of DVT, progression of DVT, or complication requiring discontinuation of anticoagulation therapy).

In the randomized controlled PREPIC (Prevention du Risque d'Embolie Pulmonaire par Interruption Cave) trial, the addition of an IVC filter to anticoagulation for DVT increased the risk of DVT recurrence (11.6%-20.8%) and did not improve the 2-year survival rate. However, those who received a filter had significantly fewer PEs than did those treated with anticoagulation alone (1.1% vs 4.8%).[21] Therefore, if a patient is felt to be at increased risk for bleeding complications, the risks and benefits may favor use of a filter. As soon as bleeding risk is acceptable, however, resumption of anticoagulation followed by filter removal is recommended. PREPIC 2 demonstrated that the risk of recurrent PE was not reduced by the presence of an IVC filter when used in combination with anticoagulation when compared to anticoagulation alone.[22]

IVC filter insertion is not without potential short- and long-term complications, which include access site–related ones (eg, hematoma, access site DVT) and device- and deployment-related issues (eg, filter migration, strut fracture, strut perforation, or erosion through the IVC wall and adjacent structures). Thrombotic complications of IVC filters are an important and complex issue that can be avoided by prompt retrieval of the filter. Unfortunately, in clinical practice, the majority of filters inserted are never removed (retrieval rates ranging from 12% to 45%).[23] This is mainly due to lack of organized patient follow-up.

Retained IVC filters are not a straightforward indication for chronic anticoagulation despite the associated risk of increased filter-related thrombosis. Although many authors recommend extended anticoagulation in this setting to minimize the potential for such complications, the evidence supporting this is still open to debate.[23-26]

Long-Term Sequelae

Post-thrombotic Syndrome

Important sequelae of DVT include PE, post-thrombotic syndrome, VTE recurrence, varicose veins, chronic venous insufficiency, and secondary lymphedema. Post-thrombotic syndrome is the most common long-term complication of DVT and can affect between 20% and 50% of patients within 2 years of the diagnosis. Post-thrombotic syndrome is thought to develop from venous hypertension that is the result of persistent venous obstruction and valvular reflux due to venous valve damage. Venous hypertension ultimately leads to reduced calf muscle perfusion, increased tissue permeability, and promotion of the associated clinical manifestations of post-thrombotic syndrome.[27] Signs and symptoms of post-thrombotic syndrome may include pain, heaviness, itching or tingling, swelling, varicose veins, skin discoloration, and/or ulceration. Symptoms typically occur within 3 to 6 months of the initial DVT episode, but occasionally can occur up to 2 years or even longer.

There is no gold standard test to establish the diagnosis of post-thrombotic syndrome; it is primarily a clinical diagnosis based on the presence of typical symptoms in a patient with a previous DVT. The Villalta scale (**Table 84.4**) has been adopted to both diagnose and grade the severity of post-thrombotic syndrome as well as to guide further management. A score of 5 to 9 signifies mild disease, 10 to 14 moderate disease, and a score greater than or equal to 15 and/or if a venous ulcer is present, is consistent with severe disease.

A conservative treatment strategy with elastic compression stockings is favored for patients with mild to moderate post-thrombotic syndrome based on the Villalta scale. In those with moderate to severe disease that is uncontrolled by elastic compression stockings alone, intermittent compression devices or pneumatic compression sleeve units may be used preferentially. In severe post-thrombotic syndrome that is lifestyle limiting and/or refractory to conservative measures, endovascular treatment with CDT (with or without percutaneous mechanical thrombectomy), or even surgical repair, may be considered.

TABLE 84.4 Villalta Post-Thrombotic Syndrome Scale

	None	Mild	Moderate	Severe
Symptoms				
Pain	0	1	2	3
Heaviness	0	1	2	3
Cramps	0	1	2	3
Pruritus	0	1	2	3
Paresthesia	0	1	2	3
Clinical Signs				
Pretibial edema	0	1	2	3
Redness	0	1	2	3
Skin induration	0	1	2	3
Hyperpigmentation	0	1	2	3
Venous ectasia	0	1	2	3
Pain on calf compression	0	1	2	3
Venous ulcer	Absent	–	–	Present
Risk Score Interpretation			*Points*	
Mild disease			5-9	
Moderate disease			10-14	
Severe disease			≥15 and/or venous ulcer	

Modified with permission from Villalta S, Bagatella P, Piccioli A, et al. Assessment of validity and reproducibility of a clinical scale for the post-thrombotic syndrome. *Haemostasis.* 1994;24:158a. Copyright © 1994 Karger Publishers, Basel, Switzerland.

SPECIAL CONSIDERATIONS

Superficial Vein Thrombosis

In contrast to DVT, superficial vein thrombosis is characterized by thrombosis and inflammation in a superficial vein. In the upper extremity, superficial vein thrombosis occurs in the basilic and/or cephalic vein(s), whereas in the lower extremity, it occurs in the greater and/or lesser saphenous vein(s). The majority of cases (60%-80%) involve the greater saphenous vein, followed by the lesser saphenous vein. Many of the predisposing risk factors that are associated with superficial vein thrombosis are also associated with other thrombotic conditions, including, but not limited to, obesity, trauma, prolonged immobilization, and hypercoagulable states. Uniquely, however, the most commonly associated predisposing condition in superficial vein thrombosis of the lower extremities is varicose veins, which are identified in up to 62% of patients.[28]

Superficial vein thrombosis was previously thought to have a benign prognosis and be of limited clinical significance; however, studies have shown that superficial vein thrombosis may be associated with a considerable risk of concomitant DVT (24.9%-26.3%) or PE (3.9%-6.8%).[29-31] These observations highlight the importance that superficial vein thrombosis should no longer be considered as a separate entity, but rather be included under the umbrella term of VTE.

Superficial vein thrombosis is recognized by the presence of warmth, erythema, and tenderness over a superficial vein, and may also manifest as a hard "cordlike" structure upon palpation.

It is recommended that all patients with clinically suspected superficial vein thrombosis should undergo VUS to (1) confirm the diagnosis of superficial vein thrombosis, (2) determine the precise location and extent of superficial vein thrombosis, and (3) potentially diagnose or rule out the presence of concomitant DVT. Treatment of superficial vein thrombosis largely depends on these aforementioned features.

The vast majority of patients with superficial vein thrombosis are managed conservatively with local compression, heat application, and use of nonsteroidal anti-inflammatory agents aimed at reducing pain and inflammation. Patients diagnosed with an associated DVT should be started on appropriate anticoagulation therapy. Individuals who are diagnosed with a lower extremity superficial vein thrombosis within 3 to 5 cm of the saphenofemoral or saphenopopliteal junctions are considered to be equivalent in risk for developing DVT, and are therefore treated with anticoagulation as well. Surgery (ie, ligation and stripping and/or local thrombectomy) is also an option in this setting depending on patient characteristics; however, this treatment approach remains controversial.

It should be mentioned that patients with lower extremity superficial vein thrombosis that is not associated with varicose veins are more likely to have an associated genetic hypercoagulable disorder; therefore, appropriate investigation is advised in this patient subset.

May-Thurner Syndrome

May-Thurner syndrome or Cockett syndrome is a well-described anatomic anomaly where the left common iliac vein is compressed between the right common iliac artery and lower lumbar spine. This clinical entity is simultaneously associated with increased risk of DVT in the left lower limb. Patients often present with significant left lower extremity pain and swelling that is out of proportion with the extent of venous thrombosis. Failure or poor response to initial anticoagulation therapy is also commonly encountered. The majority of cases follow the classic left-sided description, although other variants such as right-sided May-Thurner syndrome have been reported.[32,33]

If May-Thurner syndrome is suspected, the diagnosis can be confirmed by noninvasive imaging with computed tomographic venography or magnetic resonance venography, although false-positive results are common. Contrast venography and intravascular ultrasound with transvenous pressure measurements is the definitive diagnostic test of choice.

The treatment for iliofemoral venous thrombosis secondary to May-Thurner syndrome combines use of initial anticoagulation followed by CDT and placement of a stent in the compressed iliac vein. Antiplatelet agents are also often prescribed in conjunction with anticoagulation after venous stent deployment; however, their efficacy in preventing reocclusion has not been adequately assessed.

Paget-Schroetter Disease

Paget-Schroetter disease is a rare form of upper extremity DVT. It refers to axillosubclavian vein thrombosis that is associated with strenuous and repetitive activity of the upper extremities and tends to occur in younger, active adults. The pathogenesis is "effort related" and therefore distinct from other VTE disorders. Treatment involves initial venous thrombolysis and endovascular venoplasty, followed by prompt surgical alleviation of compression because recurrence after thrombolysis is high. Patients who are left untreated, or who are treated with anticoagulation alone, may develop long-term complications such as post-thrombotic syndrome that leads to significant residual disability.[34]

FOLLOW-UP PATIENT CARE

Once the diagnosis of acute DVT is established, it is important to arrange close follow-up to monitor not only for potential complications related to the DVT but also to monitor both patient compliance and tolerance to anticoagulation therapy. Anticoagulation treatment should be reviewed and tailored to the patient at each follow-up visit, addressing optimal treatment duration by taking the patient's bleeding risk and risk of DVT recurrence into consideration. Furthermore, individuals who had an unprovoked DVT event should be screened for the possibility of undiagnosed cancer and/or should be offered thrombophilia testing with referral to a hematologist, as deemed appropriate, to help guide management.

It should be noted that surveillance VUS testing is not warranted in patients on adequate anticoagulation, unless a change in the VUS scan results will lead to a change in patient management. Repeat ultrasound testing should only be performed at or near the end of anticoagulation treatment to establish a new baseline and determine whether fibrosis and/or scarring are present.[35] Following acute DVT, the affected vein may heal completely or scar, leading to partial venous obstruction. This scarring process was formerly referred to as chronic thrombus or residual thrombus; however, these terms have lost favor because they are frequently misinterpreted by providers, leading to inappropriate overtreatment with anticoagulation for presumed persistent or acute thrombus. Chronic post-thrombotic change is now the preferred term for the residual material that persists on ultrasound after acute DVT.

RESEARCH AND FUTURE DIRECTIONS

Venous disease encompasses a full spectrum of clinical signs and symptoms, ranging from potentially devastating acute DVT to post-thrombotic syndrome, which can markedly impact a patient's quality of life. Comprehensive evaluation is needed to determine optimal management strategies. Anticoagulation is the mainstay of treatment for acute DVT. Although parenteral heparins and oral vitamin K antagonists have been available on the market for several decades, DOACs have now emerged as preferred agents for treatment in most clinical situations. Endovascular interventional tools, including catheter-based treatment and surgery, are also available for the management of DVT in specific unique circumstances. Ongoing clinical trials will help improve patient selection for these advanced therapies in this rapidly evolving field.

KEY POINTS

- ✔ Algorithms for the diagnosis of DVT offer the greatest accuracy when incorporating an assessment of pretest clinical probability (ie, Wells Score) with appropriate use of D-dimer testing and imaging.
- ✔ The mainstay treatment of DVT is systemic anticoagulation. DOACs are safe and effective agents, and are recommended as first-line anticoagulants for most patients with DVT.
- ✔ Determination of optimal duration of anticoagulation for DVT is determined by balancing (1) the patient's long-term risk for DVT recurrence after treatment of initial episode and (2) the patient's bleeding risk.
- ✔ With the exception of May-Thurner syndrome, interventional treatment for lower extremity DVT is still being investigated. Emerging data and clinical experience favor use of percutaneous transcatheter strategies for select cases of proximal iliofemoral DVT.
- ✔ There is no role for prophylactic IVC filter insertion. The indications for IVC filter insertion is the inability to anticoagulate in the presence of acute DVT.
- ✔ May-Thurner syndrome should be recognized clinically in a young adult with unilateral left leg swelling and DVT from extrinsic compression of the left common iliac vein by the right common iliac artery.
- ✔ Post-thrombotic syndrome is an important sequela of DVT. Management is typically conservative and based on scoring from the Villalta scale.

REFERENCES

1. Centers for Disease Control and Prevention. Venous thromboembolism (blood clots): data and statistics. Retrieved March 2, 2020. https://www.cdc.gov/ncbddd/dvt/data.html
2. Zagaria ME. Venous thrombosis: pathogenesis and potential for embolism. *US Pharm.* 2009;34(2):22-24.
3. Beckman MG, Hooper WC, Critchley SE, et al. Venous thromboembolism: a public health concern. *Am J Prev Med.* 2010;38:S495-S501.
4. Heil J, Miesbach W, Vogl T, et al. Deep vein thrombosis of the upper extremity: a systematic review. *Dtsch Arztebl Int.* 2017;114(14):244-249.
5. Sule AA, Chin TJ, Handa P, et al. Should symptomatic, isolated distal deep vein thrombosis be treated with anticoagulation? *Int J Angiol.* 2009; 18(2):83-87.
6. Jenkins JS, Michael P. Deep venous thrombosis: an interventionalist's approach. *Ochsner J.* 2014;14(4):633-640.
7. De Maeseneer MGR, Bochanen N, van Rooijen G, et al. Analysis of 1,338 patients with acute lower limb deep venous thrombosis (DVT) supports inadequacy of the term "proximal DVT." *Eur J Vasc Endovasc Surg.* 2016;51:415-420.
8. Enden T, Haig Y, Klow NE, et al. Long-term outcome after additional catheter-directed thrombolysis versus standard treatment for acute iliofemoral deep vein thrombosis (the CaVenT study): a randomized controlled trial. *Lancet.* 2012;379(9810):31-38.
9. Vedantham S, Goldhaber SZ, Julian JA, et al. Acute venous thrombosis: thrombus removal with adjunctive catheter-directed thrombolysis (ATTRACT Trial). *N Engl J Med.* 2017;377(23):2240-2252.
10. Meissner MH, Gloviczki P, Comerota AJ, et al. Early thrombus removal strategies for acute deep venous thrombosis: clinical practice guidelines of the Society for Vascular Surgery and the American Venous Forum. *J Vasc Surg.* 2012;55:1449-1462.
11. Goodacre S, Sampson F, Thomas S, et al. Systematic review and meta-analysis of the diagnostic accuracy of ultrasonography for deep vein thrombosis. *BMC Med Imaging.* 2005;5:6.
12. Kearon C, Akl EA, Ornelas J, Blaivas A, et al. Antithrombotic therapy for VTE disease: CHEST guideline and expert panel report. *Chest.* 2016;149(2):315-352.
13. van Es N, Coppens M, Schulman S, et al. Direct oral anticoagulants compared with vitamin K antagonists for acute venous thromboembolism: evidence from phase 3 trials. *Blood.* 2014;124(12):1968-1975.
14. Wang TF, Li A, Garcia, D. Managing thrombosis in cancer patients. *Res Pract Thromb Haemost.* 2018;2(3):429-438.
15. Vedovati MC, Germini F, Agnelli G, et al. Direct oral anticoagulants in patients with VTE and cancer. *Chest.* 2015;147(2):475-483.
16. Michota F, Merli G. Anticoagulation in special patient populations: are special dosing considerations required? *Cleve Clin J Med.* 2005; 72:S37-S42.
17. Schulman S, Granqvist S, Holmstrom M, et al. The duration of oral anticoagulant therapy after a second episode of venous thromboembolism. The Duration of Anticoagulation Trial Study Group. *N Engl J Med.* 1997;336(6):393-398.
18. Charalel RA, Vedantham S. Deep vein thrombosis interventions in cancer patients. *Semin Intervent Radiol.* 2017;34(1):50-53.
19. Khan F, Rahman A, Carrier M, et al. Long-term risk of recurrence after discontinuing anticoagulants for a first unprovoked venous thromboembolism: protocol for a systematic review and meta-analysis. *BMJ Open.* 2017;7:1-7.
20. Konstantinides SV, Meyer G, Becattini C, et al. 2019 ESC Guidelines for the diagnosis and management of acute pulmonary embolism deployed in collaboration with the European Respiratory Society (ERS): The Task Force for the diagnosis and management of acute pulmonary embolism of the European Society of Cardiology (ESC). *Eur Heart J.* 2020;41(4):543-600.
21. Decousus H, Leizorovicz A, Parent F, et al. A clinical trial of vena caval filters in the prevention of pulmonary embolism in patients with proximal deep-vein thrombosis. *N Engl J Med.* 1998;338:409-416.
22. Mismetti P, Laporte S, Pellerin O, et al. Effect of a retrievable inferior vena cava filter plus anticoagulation vs anticoagulation alone on risk of recurrent pulmonary embolism. *JAMA.* 2015;313(16):1627-1635.
23. Duffett L, Carrier M. Inferior vena cava filters. *J Thromb Haemost.* 2016;15(1):3-12.
24. Weinberg I, Jaff MR. Inferior vena cava filters: truth or dare? *Circ Cardiovasc Interv.* 2013;6:498-500.
25. Ray CE Jr, Prochazka A. The need for anticoagulation following inferior vena cava filter placement: systematic review. *Cardiovasc Intervent Radiol.* 2008;31(2):316-324.
26. Yale SH, Mazza JJ, Glurich I, et al. Recurrent venous thromboembolism in patients with and without anticoagulation after inferior vena caval filter placement. *Int Angiol.* 2006;25(1):60-66.
27. Kahn SR. The post-thrombotic syndrome. *Hemato Am Soc Hematol Educ Program.* 2016;1:413-418.
28. Litzendorf ME, Satiani B. Superficial venous thrombosis: disease progression and evolving treatment approaches. *Vasc Health Risk Manag.* 2011;7:569-575.
29. Decousus H, Quéré I, Presles E, et al. Superficial venous thrombosis and venous thromboembolism: a large, prospective epidemiologic study. *Ann Intern Med.* 2010;152(4):218-224.

30. Sevestre MA, Labarere J, Brin S, et al. Optimizing history taking for evaluating the risk of venous thromboembolism: the OPTIMEV study. *J Mal Vasc*. 2005;30(4):217-227.
31. Frappé P, Buchmuller-Cordier A, Bertoletti L, et al. Annual diagnosis rate of superficial vein thrombosis of the lower limbs: the STEPH community-based study. *J Thromb Haemost*. 2014;12(6):831-838.
32. Abboud G, Midulla M, Lions C, et al. Right-sided May-Thurner syndrome. *Cardiovasc Intervent Radiol*. 2010;33(5):1056-1059.
33. Burke RM, Rayan SS, Kasirajan K, et al. Unusual case of right-sided May-Thurner syndrome and review of its management. *Vascular*. 2006;14(1):47-50.
34. Alla VM, Natarajan N, Kaishik M, et al. Paget-Schroetter Syndrome: review of pathogenesis and treatment of effort thrombosis. *West J Emerg Med*. 2010;11(4):358-362.
35. Needleman L, Cronan JJ, Lilly MP, et al. Ultrasound for lower extremity deep venous thrombosis. *Circulation*. 2018;137:1505-1515.

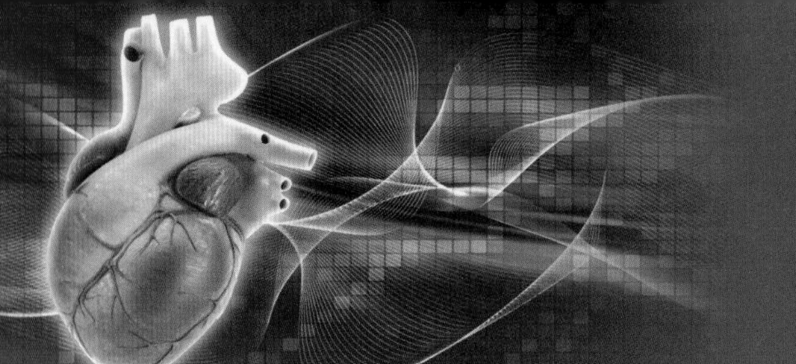

CHAPTER 85

PULMONARY EMBOLISM

Debabrata Mukherjee and Richard A. Lange

INTRODUCTION

Pulmonary embolism (PE), which refers to obstruction of the pulmonary artery or its branches, is an important cause of morbidity and mortality with 150,000 to 250,000 hospitalizations and 100,000 deaths annually, making it the third most common cause of cardiovascular death in the United States and with a quarter of these patients presenting with sudden death.[1,2] Although tumor, air, amniotic fluid, or fat can cause PE, the most common cause is thrombotic obstruction, which will be the focus of this chapter.

PATHOGENESIS

The pathogenesis of PE is related to the formation of thrombus and involves venous stasis, endothelial injury, and a hypercoagulable state. Most PE arise from thrombus in the lower extremity proximal (ie, iliac or femoral) and popliteal veins with thrombi developing at sites of decreased flow, such as valve cusps or bifurcations.

Predisposing factors for venous thromboembolism and PE have been categorized into strong, moderate, or weak risk factors. Strong risk factors include lower-limb fractures; hospitalization for heart failure or atrial fibrillation/flutter (within previous 3 months); hip or knee replacement; major trauma; myocardial infarction (within previous 3 months); any previous venous thromboembolism or PE; and spinal cord injury.[3-5] Moderate risk factors include arthroscopic knee surgery, autoimmune diseases, blood transfusions, central venous lines, intravenous catheters and leads, oral contraceptive therapy, postpartum period, infection (specifically pneumonia, urinary tract infection, and human immunodeficiency virus), inflammatory bowel disease, malignancy, paralytic stroke, and thrombophilia. Relatively weak risk factors include bed rest more than 3 days, diabetes mellitus, systemic hypertension, immobility owing to sitting (ie, prolonged car or air travel), increasing age, laparoscopic surgery, obesity, pregnancy, and presence of varicose veins.[3-5] Estrogen-containing oral contraceptive agents are associated with an elevated thromboembolism risk, and their use is the most frequent risk factor for thromboembolism and PE in women of reproductive age.[6]

PE interferes with both circulation and gas exchange in the lungs, but acute right ventricular (RV) failure owing to acute pressure overload is the primary cause of death in severe PE.[4] Acute RV failure, with impaired RV filling and/or reduced RV flow output, is a critical determinant of clinical severity and outcome in acute PE.[7] Clinical symptoms and signs of overt RV failure and hemodynamic instability indicate a high risk of early (in-hospital or 30-day) mortality in individuals with PE and are important prognostic signs.

CLINICAL PRESENTATION

PE may present at one end of the spectrum with no symptoms to the other extreme with shock or sudden death. However, the most common presentation is dyspnea followed by pleuritic chest pain and cough. Hemoptysis may be present occasionally in those who have developed pulmonary infarction. Individuals with a large PE may also present with shock, arrhythmia, or syncope. Signs on physical examination may include tachycardia, tachypnea, jugular venous distension, parasternal heave, a loud pulmonary component of the second heart sound and pulsatile liver. Given the heterogeneity of symptoms and signs and lack of symptoms in some patients, it is important to have a high index of suspicion to avoid a missed diagnosis.

DIAGNOSIS

The diagnosis of PE should incorporate clinical and pretest probability assessment, D-dimer testing, and imaging. Because most common symptoms include dyspnea, chest pain, and cough, other conditions such as pericarditis, acute myocardial infarction, acute aortic syndrome, and pleuritis should be considered in the differential diagnosis. Of note, the three most prevalent diagnoses associated with high risk of adverse outcomes in patients presenting with nontraumatic chest pain include acute coronary syndrome, thoracic aortic dissection, and PE. Accordingly, these three need to be considered in any individual presenting with chest pain and dyspnea.[8] When imaging is indicated (ie, the patient is suspected of having a moderate or high probability of PE), computed tomographic pulmonary angiography (CTPA) is the imaging modality of choice with ventilation perfusion (V/Q) scanning used less often. For hemodynamically unstable patients, bedside echocardiography or venous ultrasound may be used for presumptive diagnosis of PE.

The combination of clinical symptoms, signs, and predisposing factors for thromboembolism helps categorize patients with suspected PE into low-, intermediate-, and high-risk categories for the likelihood of PE. The most frequently used prediction rules are the revised Geneva rule (**Table 85.1**) and the Wells rule to assess the probability of PE.

Using the Geneva score, the proportion of patients with confirmed PE can be expected to be ~10% in the low-probability category, 30% in the moderate-probability category, and 65% in the high-probability category.[11]

For the Wells score, 3 points are assigned to clinical symptoms of deep vein thrombosis (DVT), 3 points if PE is the most likely diagnosis, 1.5 points for heart rate > 100 beats/min, 1.5 points for immobilization or surgery within 4 weeks, 1.5 points for previous DVT or PE, 1 point for hemoptysis, and 1 point for malignancy. Note that all the criteria can be obtained from the history and physical examination: heart rate is the only parameter that is measured. Everything else comes from history. The modified Wells criteria for PE categorizes

TABLE 85.1 The Revised Geneva Clinical Prediction Rule for Pulmonary Embolism

Items	Clinical Decision Rule Points	
	Original Version[9]	Simplified Version[10]
Previous PE or DVT	3	1
Heart rate		
75-94 bpm	3	1
≥95 bpm	5	2
Surgery or fracture within the past month	2	1
Hemoptysis	2	1
Active cancer	2	1
Unilateral lower-limb pain	3	1
Pain on lower-limb deep venous palpation and unilateral edema	4	1
Age >65 years	1	1
Clinical probability		
Three-level score		
Low	0-3	0-1
Intermediate	4-10	2-4
High	≥11	≥5
Two-level score		
PE unlikely	0-5	0-2
PE likely	≥6	≥3

bpm, beats per minute; DVT, deep vein thrombosis; PE, pulmonary embolism.
(From Konstantinides SV, Meyer G, Becattini C, et al.; ESC Scientific Document Group. 2019 ESC Guidelines for the diagnosis and management of acute pulmonary embolism developed in collaboration with the European Respiratory Society (ERS): The Task Force for the diagnosis and management of acute pulmonary embolism of the European Society of Cardiology (ESC). *Eur Heart J.* 2020;41(4):543-603. Reproduced by permission of The European Society of Cardiology.)

suspected patients with PE to less than 2 as low risk, 2-6 as intermediate risk, and greater than 6 as high risk.[12] The simplified Wells criteria define PE as unlikely if the patient has a score of less than or equal to 4 whereas PE is likely for those with a score greater than 4. A further simplified Wells rule assigns one weight for the presence of all individual variables in the model with a score between 0 and 7. One study suggested that this simplification of the Wells rule by assigning only one point to each of the seven variables had similar diagnostic accuracy and clinical utility as the original Wells criteria.[13]

The Wells score has a slightly lower sensitivity (81% vs 84%) and a higher specificity (82% vs 77%) compared with the revised Geneva score. In the high-probability group, the positive predictive value for the Wells score is reported to be superior to that of the revised Geneva score (80% vs 58%).[14]

Electrocardiography is fairly nonspecific, and findings may include sinus tachycardia, anterior precordial T wave inversion, an S1Q3T3 pattern (ie, a deep S wave in lead I with Q wave and T wave inversion in lead III), and precordial ST-segment elevation.

The chest radiography is neither sensitive nor specific for PE. It is more useful in assessing for differential diagnostic possibilities such as pneumonia and pneumothorax rather than establishing the diagnosis of PE. Nevertheless, described chest radiographic signs include enlarged pulmonary artery; Hampton hump (ie, peripheral wedge of airspace opacity owing to lung infarction); Westermark sign (ie, regional oligemia); pleural effusion (35%); enlarged right descending pulmonary artery with sudden cutoff; and elevated diaphragm.

Performing definitive diagnostic imaging in every patient with dyspnea or pleuritic chest pain will lead to unnecessary testing with inherent risks and costs so a targeted approach is indicated. The pulmonary embolism rule-out criteria (PERC) were developed for patients presenting to the emergency department for selecting patients whose likelihood of having PE is so low that diagnostic imaging should not be considered.[15] The criteria include eight clinical variables significantly associated with an absence of PE: age less than 50 years; pulse less than 100 beats/min; arterial oxygen saturation greater than 94%; no unilateral leg swelling; no hemoptysis; no recent trauma or surgery; no history of thromboembolism; and no oral hormone use.[15] A prospective validation study and a randomized management study demonstrated that PE can be safely excluded in patients with low clinical probability who met all criteria of the PERC rule.[16,17]

Serum D-dimer levels are elevated in acute thrombosis because of activation of coagulation and fibrinolysis. The negative predictive value of D-dimer testing is high, with a normal serum D-dimer level making the diagnosis of PE quite unlikely. On the other hand, the positive predictive value of elevated serum D-dimer levels is low; hence, an elevated D-dimer is not useful for confirmation of PE. Of note, the specificity of D-dimer in establishing the diagnosis PE decreases with age to ~10% in patients greater than 80 years of age, and the use of age-adjusted cutoff levels is recommended to improve the performance of D-dimer testing in the elderly.[18] A prospective study evaluated an age-adjusted cutoff for serum D-dimer levels (age × 10 µg/L, for patients aged >50 years) in 3346 patients and reported that its use increased the number of patients in whom PE could be excluded from 6.4% to 30%, without additional false-negative findings, thus avoiding many unnecessary imaging tests.[19] The 2020 European Society of Cardiology (ESC) Guidelines for the diagnosis and management of acute PE specifically recommends that serum D-dimer cutoff values adjusted for age or adapted to clinical probability can be used as an alternative to fixed D-dimer cutoff values[4] to better avoid unnecessary imaging.

CTPA is the diagnostic modality of choice for patients with suspected PE, as it allows excellent visualization of the pulmonary arteries down to the subsegmental level with a sensitivity of 83% and a specificity of 96% for PE diagnosis using older four-detector scans.[20] V/Q lung scintigraphy is an older established diagnostic test for suspected PE and is less often used these days. Compared to CTPA, V/Q scans use lower radiation and no iodinated contrast. Thus, it may be preferred in outpatients with a low clinical probability and a normal chest radiography, in young (especially female) patients, in pregnant individuals, in patients with a history of contrast-induced anaphylaxis, and patients with severe kidney disease.[21] Finally, invasive pulmonary angiography—once the gold standard for the diagnosis of PE—is now rarely used because less-invasive CTPA offers similar diagnostic accuracy and information and is associated with significantly lower procedural risk.[22]

Acute PE may lead to RV pressure overload and dysfunction, which can be detected by echocardiography and may be considered in patients with suspected PE and hemodynamic instability. Echocardiography has a reported negative predictive value of 40% to 50%; hence, a negative result does not exclude PE.[23] The combination of a pulmonary ejection acceleration time less than 60 ms with a peak systolic tricuspid valve gradient less than 60 mm Hg (the "60/60" sign), or depressed contractility of the RV free wall compared to the RV apex—known as the McConnell sign—is suggestive of PE but is present in only 12% to 20% of patients with PE.[24]

PE typically originates from lower-limb thrombosis, and venous ultrasound showing proximal DVT in patients suspected of having PE should be adequate grounds for anticoagulation therapy. In patients with suspected PE and hemodynamic instability who are unable to undergo CTPA or a V/Q scan, venous ultrasound and/or echocardiography may help guide diagnostic and therapeutic choices.

MANAGEMENT OF THE PATIENT

The initial focus on therapy for PE should be on adequate oxygenation and resuscitation in unstable patients. Supplemental oxygen is indicated in patients with PE and arterial oxygen saturation less than 90%. The cornerstone of therapy for PE is immediate anticoagulation, but some patients with massive or life-threatening PE may require treatment beyond anticoagulation, including thrombolysis, and percutaneous or surgical embolectomy. It is important to risk stratify individuals with PE using clinical, imaging, and laboratory findings in order to target aggressive therapies for those at the highest risk of having a poor outcome. The pulmonary embolism severity index (PESI) **(Table 85.2)** reliably identifies patients at low or high risk for 30-day mortality.[25,26] A simplified version of the PESI (sPESI) has been validated, given the complexity of the original PESI,[27] and provides robust risk stratification.

A helpful classification of PE severity and the risk of early (in-hospital or 30-day) death is depicted in **Table 85.3**. It is critical to identify patients with (suspected) high-risk PE early because these individuals require aggressive therapeutic strategies in addition to anticoagulation.[29]

In general, for patients with high or intermediate clinical probability of PE, anticoagulation is indicated while awaiting the results of diagnostic tests. Choices for anticoagulation are subcutaneous, weight-adjusted low-molecular-weight heparin (LMWH) or fondaparinux, or intravenous unfractionated heparin (UFH). Among parenteral anticoagulants for PE, LMWH and fondaparinux are preferred over UFH for initial anticoagulation, as they carry a lower risk of inducing major bleeding and heparin-induced thrombocytopenia. UFH is preferred in those with hemodynamic instability in whom catheter-based reperfusion treatment will be needed.

Oral alternatives to LMWH and fondaparinux that provide rapid anticoagulant effects are the non-vitamin K antagonist oral anticoagulants (NOACs), such as dabigatran, apixaban, edoxaban, and rivaroxaban. Table 85.4 presents dosing recommendations for various anticoagulants. LMWH is the treatment of choice for PE during pregnancy as it does not cross the placenta—in contrast to vitamin K antagonists and NOACs—and consequently does not confer a risk of fetal hemorrhage or teratogenicity.[30]

Primary treatment refers to the minimal length of time a patient must be on therapeutic anticoagulation to treat the initial PE before consideration is given to discontinuing anticoagulation or switching to a long-term anticoagulation regimen aimed at preventing thromboembolic recurrence (secondary prevention). For primary treatment of patients with PE—whether provoked by a transient risk factor or by a chronic risk factor or unprovoked—the American Society of Hematology (ASH) guideline panel suggests using a shorter course of anticoagulation (3-6 months) over a longer course of anticoagulation (6-12 months).[31] After completion of primary treatment in patients with PE provoked by a chronic risk factor or for unprovoked PE, the ASH guideline panel suggests indefinite antithrombotic therapy with a vitamin K antagonist or NOAC over stopping anticoagulation.[31] Furthermore, for patients with breakthrough PE during therapeutic vitamin K antagonist treatment, the guideline recommends using LMWH over NOAC therapy.

Thrombolytic therapy may be indicated for certain intermediate- to high-risk PE patients as it leads to rapid improvements in pulmonary obstruction, pulmonary artery pressure, and pulmonary vascular resistance, compared with UFH alone accompanied by a reduction in RV dilation on echocardiography. A meta-analysis of 16 thrombolysis trials

TABLE 85.2 Original and Simplified Pulmonary Embolism Severity Index

Parameter	Original Version[28]	Simplified Version[27]
Age	Age in years	1 point (if age > 80 years)
Male sex	+10 points	–
Cancer	+30 points	1 point
Chronic heart failure	+10 points	1 point
Chronic pulmonary disease	+10 points	
Pulse rate ≥ 110 bpm	+20 points	1 point
Systolic BP < 100 mmHg	+30 points	1 point
Respiratory rate > 30 breaths/minute	+20 points	–
Temperature < 36°C	+20 points	–
Altered mental status	+60 points	–
Arterial oxyhemoglobin saturation < 90%	+20 points	1 point
	Risk strata[a]	
	Class I: ≤65 points: very low 30-day mortality risk (0%-1.6%) **Class II: 66-85 points**: low mortality risk (1.7%-3.5%)	**0 points =** 30-day mortality risk 1.0%, (95% CI 0.0%-2.1%)
	Class III: 86-105 points: moderate mortality risk (3.2%-7.1%) **Class IV: 106-125 points**: high mortality risk (4.0%-11.4%) **Class V: >125 points**: very high mortality risk (10.0%-24.5%)	**≥1 point(s) =** 30-day mortality risk 10.9% (95% CI 8.5%-13.2%)

BP, blood pressure; bpm, beats per minute; CI, confidence interval.
[a]Based on the sum of points.
From Konstantinides SV, Meyer G, Becattini C, et al.; ESC Scientific Document Group. 2019 ESC Guidelines for the diagnosis and management of acute pulmonary embolism developed in collaboration with the European Respiratory Society (ERS): The Task Force for the diagnosis and management of acute pulmonary embolism of the European Society of Cardiology (ESC). *Eur Heart J.* 2020;41(4):543-603. Reproduced by permission of The European Society of Cardiology.

with 2115 individuals with PE and RV dysfunction reported that thrombolysis was associated with lower rates of all-cause mortality but increased risks of major bleeding and intracranial hemorrhage.[1]

Catheter-based therapy entails the insertion of a catheter into the pulmonary arteries for mechanical fragmentation of the thrombus, thrombus aspiration, or more commonly a pharmacomechanical approach combining mechanical or ultrasound fragmentation of the thrombus with locally administered reduced-dose thrombolysis. Specific catheters for PE management include the EKOS EkoSonic (BTG PLC; London, UK) catheter for ultrasound-assisted catheter-directed thrombolysis; and the Penumbra Indigo (Penumbra, Inc.; Alameda, CA, USA) and FlowTriever (Inari Medical, Inc.; Irvine, CA, USA) catheters for mechanical thrombectomy. A scientific statement from the American Heart Association on interventional therapies for acute PE suggests that systemic thrombolysis, surgical embolectomy, catheter-directed PE therapy, and mechanical circulatory support should be strongly considered in patients with PE and hemodynamic instability, as they lead to improved outcomes in these selected patients.[32] Conversely, the use of either catheter-based lysis or embolectomy in patients with intermediate-risk PE has, thus far, been correlated only with more rapid improvement of RV dysfunction than anticoagulation alone, but not improved short- or long-term clinical or functional outcomes.[32]

The ASH 2020 guidelines for the management of venous thromboembolism recommend the use of thrombolytic therapy with anticoagulation for patients with PE and hemodynamic instability as opposed to anticoagulation alone.[31] These recommendations for thrombolytic therapy for patients with PE and hemodynamic instability are consistent with the American College of Chest Physicians (ACP) Evidence-Based Clinical Practice Guidelines.[33] However, the 2016 ACP Guidelines recommend systemic thrombolytic therapy over catheter-directed thrombolysis,[33] whereas the 2020 ASH guidelines recommend catheter-directed thrombolysis over systemic thrombolysis.[31] This likely reflects additional data acquired between 2016 and 2020 on the efficacy of catheter-directed thrombolysis and the known bleeding risks associated with systemic

TABLE 85.3 Classification of Pulmonary Embolism Severity and the Risk of Early (In-Hospital or 30-Day) Death

Early Mortality Risk		Indicators of Risk			
		Hemodynamic Instability[a]	Clinical Parameters of PE Severity and/or Comorbidity PESI Class III-V or sPESI ≥I	RV Dysfunction on TTE or CTPA[b]	Elevated Cardiac Troponin Levels[c]
High		+	(+)[d]	+	(+)
Intermediate	Intermediate-high	–	+[e]	+	+
	Intermediate-low	–	+[e]	One (or none) positive	
Low		–	–	–	Assessment optional: if assessed, negative

CTPA, computed tomography pulmonary angiography; PE, pulmonary embolism; PESI, Pulmonary Embolism Severity Index; RV, right ventricular; sPESI, simplified Pulmonary Embolism Severity Index; TTE, transthoracic echocardiogram.
[a]One of the following clinical presentations: cardiac arrest, obstructive shock (systolic blood pressure [BP] < 90 mm Hg or vasopressors required to achieve a BP ≥90 mm Hg despite an adequate filling status, in combination with end-organ hypoperfusion), or persistent hypotension (systolic BP < 90 mm Hg or a systolic BP drop ≥40 mm Hg for >15 minutes, not caused by new-onset arrhythmia, hypovolemia, or sepsis).
[b]Prognostically relevant imaging (echocardiography or CTPA) findings in patients with acute PE.
[c]Elevation of further laboratory biomarkers, such as plasma N-terminal pro-B-type natriuretic peptide ≥600 ng/L, plasma heart-type fatty acid-binding protein ≥6 ng/mL, or copeptin ≥24 pmol/L, may provide additional prognostic information.
[d]Hemodynamic instability, combined with PE confirmation on CTPA and/or evidence of RV dysfunction on TTE, is sufficient to classify a patient into the high-risk PE category. In these cases, neither calculation of the PESI nor measurement of troponins or other cardiac biomarkers is necessary.
[e]Signs of RV dysfunction on TTE (or CTPA) or elevated cardiac biomarker levels may be present despite a calculated PESI of I-II or an sPESI of 0. Until the implications of such discrepancies for the management of PE are fully understood, these patients should be classified into the intermediate-risk category.
From Konstantinides SV, Meyer G, Becattini C, et al.; ESC Scientific Document Group. 2019 ESC Guidelines for the diagnosis and management of acute pulmonary embolism developed in collaboration with the European Respiratory Society (ERS): The Task Force for the diagnosis and management of acute pulmonary embolism of the European Society of Cardiology (ESC). *Eur Heart J.* 2020;41(4):543-603. Reproduced by permission of The European Society of Cardiology.

thrombolysis.[34,35] For patients with PE with echocardiography and/or biomarkers compatible with RV dysfunction but without hemodynamic compromise (submassive PE), the ASH guideline panel suggests anticoagulation alone over the routine use of thrombolysis in addition to anticoagulation.[31] The ASH guidelines also prefer home treatment over hospital-based treatment for uncomplicated PE at low risk for complications and recommend NOACs over vitamin K antagonists for primary treatment of thromboembolism.[31]

Algorithm 85.1 depicts the management of patients with hemodynamic instability suspected to be at high risk for PE, and **Algorithm 85.2** for patients with suspected PE without hemodynamic instability or high-risk features. In general, primary reperfusion therapy with systemic thrombolysis is the treatment of choice for patients with high-risk PE. Surgical pulmonary embolectomy and percutaneous catheter-directed treatment are typically alternative reperfusion options in patients with contraindications to systemic thrombolysis. In patients with PE at very high risk of death with cardiogenic shock, cardiac arrest, or impending hemodynamic collapse, mechanical support may be considered. Venoarterial extracorporeal membrane oxygenation (VA ECMO) has shown benefit when used in combination with thrombolysis, with improved survival rates and reasonable safety.[36,37] For patients with acute PE and no evidence of hemodynamic compromise, parenteral or oral anticoagulation without reperfusion techniques is adequate initial treatment as depicted in Algorithm 85.2. Early discharge of low-risk patients with acute PE and continuation of anticoagulant treatment at home is reasonable if proper outpatient care and anticoagulant treatment can be provided.

SPECIAL CONSIDERATIONS

Pulmonary Embolism Response Teams

The concept of multidisciplinary rapid-response teams for the management of PE has recently emerged with increasing acceptance from clinicians. Such pulmonary embolism response teams (PERTs) include specialists from cardiovascular medicine, pulmonary/critical care, hematology, vascular medicine, anesthesiology, cardiothoracic surgery, and either interventional cardiology or interventional radiology.[38,39] The guidelines from the PERT consortium recommend using a multidisciplinary PERT in patients with high- or intermediate-risk PE, as well as for PE patients in whom there is uncertainty regarding treatment.[2]

TABLE 85.4 Anticoagulation Reference for Treatment of Deep Vein Thrombosis

Drug Class	Initial Dose	Maintenance Dose	Side Effects
Low-molecular-weight heparins			
Enoxaparin	1.0 mg/kg SC twice daily *or* 1.5 mg/kg SC once daily	1.0 mg/kg SC twice daily *or* 1.5 mg/kg SC once daily	• Bleeding • Heparin-induced thrombocytopenia (HIT) • Osteoporosis • Hypersensitivity/anaphylaxis • Limited use in renal insufficiency
Tinzaparin	175 IU/kg SC once daily	175 IU/kg SC once daily	
Dalteparin	100 IU/kg SC twice daily *or* 200 IU/kg SC once daily	100 IU/kg SC twice daily *or* 200 IU/kg SC once daily	
Unfractionated heparins			
Heparin	Bolus: 80 IU/kg IV (max 10,000 IU)	Continuous: 18 IU/kg/h IV with aPTT monitoring (goal is to achieve aPTT of 1.5-2× baseline)	• Bleeding • HIT (more likely than with LMWH) • Osteoporosis • Hypersensitivity/anaphylaxis
Pentasaccharide			
Fondaparinux	<50 kg: 5 mg SC once daily 50-100 kg: 7.5 mg SC once daily >100 kg: 10 mg SC once daily	<50 kg: 5 mg SC once daily 50-100 kg: 7.5 mg SC once daily >100 kg: 10 mg SC once daily	• Bleeding • Limited use in renal insufficiency and patients with low body weight
Vitamin K antagonist			
Warfarin[a]	–	Adjust to target INR 2-3	• Bleeding • Warfarin-induced skin necrosis (increased in protein C or S deficiency) • Teratogen • Osteoporosis • Agranulocytosis
Direct oral coagulants			
Apixaban	10 mg PO twice daily for 7 days	5 mg PO twice daily	• Bleeding
Dabigatran[b]	–	150 mg PO twice daily	
Edoxaban[b]	–	60 mg PO once daily	
Rivaroxaban	15 mg PO twice daily for 21 days	20 mg PO once daily	

aPTT, activated partial thromboplastin time INR, international normalized ratio; IU, international units; IV, intravenous; PO, oral; SC, subcutaneous.
[a]Parenteral overlap with unfractionated heparin (UFH), low-molecular-weight heparin (LMWH), or fondaparinux must be administered for a minimum of 5 days and until the INR is within the target range of 2-3 for two consecutive days.
[b]Parenteral overlap with UFH, LMWH, or fondaparinux must be administered for a minimum of 5 days before maintenance dosing is initiated with the designated agent.
Table created by Stephanie M. Madonis, MD & James S. Jenkins, MD authors of Chapter 84 Venous Thromboembolism and reprinted with permission.

Coronavirus Disease 2019 and Pulmonary Embolisms

An increased risk of thromboembolism and PE has been reported with coronavirus disease 2019 (COVID-19) pandemic. A systematic review and meta-analysis[40] reported increased rates of venous and arterial thromboembolism in patients infected with COVID-19, with the overall PE rate in patients with COVID-19 being 13% (95% CI: 11%-16%); in those in the intensive care unit 19% (95% CI: 14%-25%); and postmortem PE rates 22% (95% CI: 16%-28%). Furthermore, patients with COVID-19 who developed thromboembolism were at a significantly higher odds of mortality compared to those who did not.[40] One study reported that anticoagulant therapy, mainly with LMWH, was associated with a better prognosis in COVID-19 patients with sepsis-induced coagulopathy or with markedly elevated D-dimer.[41] The diagnosis and management of PE associated with COVID-19 represent a challenging clinical scenario. PERT can facilitate fast, appropriate, multidisciplinary, team-based approach in these complex patients with a goal to tailor the best therapeutic decision-making, prioritizing optimal patient care, especially given the lack of evidence-based clinical practice guidelines in the setting of COVID-19.[42]

FOLLOW-UP PATIENT CARE

Close follow-up of patients with PE is indicated to monitor for early complications of PE, which is predominantly recurrent

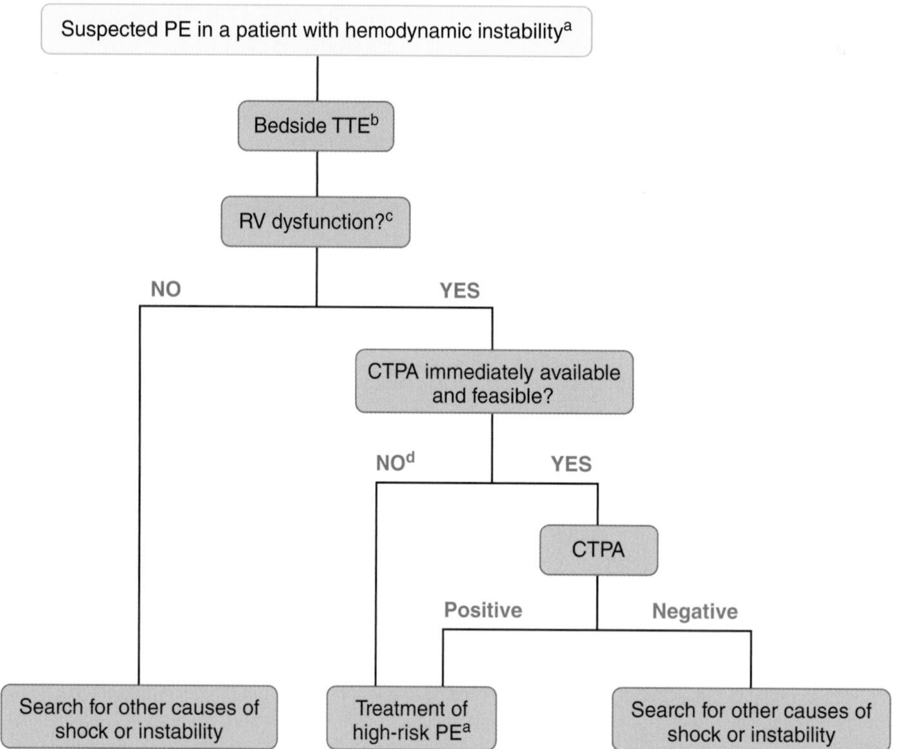

ALGORITHM 85.1 Diagnostic algorithm for patients with hemodynamic instability suspected to be at high risk for pulmonary embolism. CTPA, computed tomography pulmonary angiography; PE, pulmonary embolism; RV, right ventricular; TTE, transthoracic echocardiogram. [a]Need for cardiopulmonary resuscitation; systolic blood pressure (BP) < 90 mm Hg or vasopressors required to achieve a BP ≥ 90 mm Hg despite adequate filling status or systolic BP < 90 mm Hg or systolic BP drop ≥ 40 mm Hg, lasting longer than 15 minutes and not caused by new-onset arrhythmia, hypovolemia, or sepsis; and end-organ hypoperfusion (altered mental status; cold, clammy skin; oliguria/anuria; increased serum lactate). [b]Ancillary bedside imaging tests may include transesophageal echocardiography, which may detect emboli in the pulmonary artery and its main branches; and bilateral venous compression ultrasonography, which may confirm deep vein thrombosis and thus venous thromboembolism. [c]In the emergency situation of suspected high-risk PE, this refers mainly to a right/left ventricular diameter ratio > 1.0; and the echocardiographic findings of RV dysfunction. [d]Includes the cases in which the patient's condition is so critical that it only allows bedside diagnostic tests. In such cases, echocardiographic findings of right ventricular dysfunction confirm high-risk PE and emergency reperfusion therapy is recommended. (From Konstantinides SV, Meyer G, Becattini C, et al.; ESC Scientific Document Group. 2019 ESC Guidelines for the diagnosis and management of acute pulmonary embolism developed in collaboration with the European Respiratory Society (ERS): The Task Force for the diagnosis and management of acute pulmonary embolism of the European Society of Cardiology (ESC). *Eur Heart J.* 2020;41(4):543-603. Reproduced by permission of The European Society of Cardiology.)

thromboembolism, and for late complications of PE (ie, chronic thromboembolic pulmonary hypertension [CTEPH]). The goal of anticoagulation after acute PE is to complete the treatment of the acute episode and prevent recurrence of PE over the long term. Patients with PE who are on anticoagulants should be monitored for bleeding and adverse effects of medications.

RESEARCH AND FUTURE DIRECTIONS

PE is a common clinical condition with varied manifestations and with significant morbidity and mortality. Given the complexities of diagnostic and therapeutic modalities, a collaborative multidisciplinary approach with PERT is helpful and may improve clinical outcomes, especially in high-risk PE. Further development of novel therapeutic options and randomized clinical trials are needed to delineate optimal approaches for these patients.

KEY POINTS

- ✔ Anticoagulation therapy should be started in patients with suspected acute PE as soon as possible, while diagnostic workup is ongoing, unless the patient is bleeding or has contraindications to anticoagulation.
- ✔ Validated diagnostic algorithms for PE, including standardized assessment of clinical probability and plasma D-dimer testing, should be incorporated into the patient's evaluation. They may help avoid unnecessary and potentially harmful imaging tests and exposure to ionizing radiation in patients unlikely to have a PE.
- ✔ In patients presenting with PE and hemodynamic instability, bedside echocardiography is useful to differentiate suspected PE from other acute life-threatening situations.

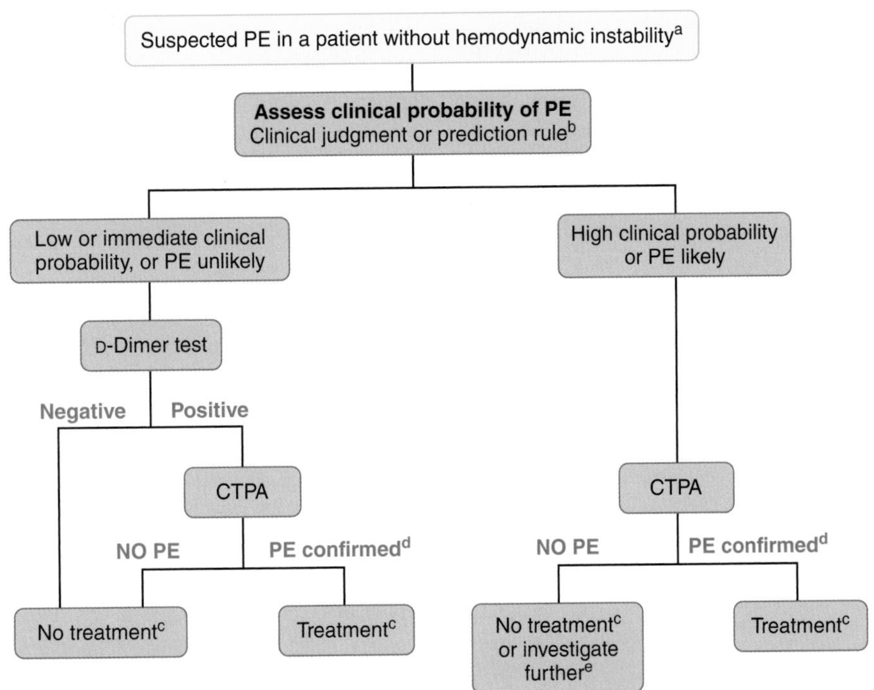

ALGORITHM 85.2 Suspected PE in a patient without hemodynamic instability. Diagnostic algorithm for patients with suspected pulmonary embolism without hemodynamic instability. CTPA, computed tomography pulmonary angiography/angiogram; PE, pulmonary embolism. [a]No need for resuscitation and no evidence of shock. [b]Two alternative classification schemes may be used for clinical probability assessment, that is, a three-level scheme (clinical probability defined as low, intermediate, or high) or a two-level scheme (PE unlikely or PE likely). [c]Treatment refers to anticoagulation treatment for PE. [d]CTPA is considered diagnostic of PE if it shows PE at the segmental or more proximal level. [e]In case of a negative CTPA in patients with high clinical probability, investigation by further imaging tests may be considered before withholding PE-specific treatment. (From Konstantinides SV, Meyer G, Becattini C, et al.; ESC Scientific Document Group. 2019 ESC Guidelines for the diagnosis and management of acute pulmonary embolism developed in collaboration with the European Respiratory Society (ERS): The Task Force for the diagnosis and management of acute pulmonary embolism of the European Society of Cardiology (ESC). *Eur Heart J.* 2020;41(4):543-603. Reproduced by permission of The European Society of Cardiology.)

- ✔ Thrombolytic therapy with anticoagulation is recommended for patients with PE and hemodynamic instability rather than anticoagulation alone.
- ✔ For patients with PE without hemodynamic instability, anticoagulation alone (ie, without thrombolysis) is the treatment of choice, even in those with echocardiographic and/or biomarkers compatible with RV dysfunction (ie, submassive PE).
- ✔ In patients with PE at very high risk of death (ie, with cardiogenic shock, cardiac arrest, or impending hemodynamic collapse), mechanical support may be considered.
- ✔ Anticoagulation with an NOAC is preferred over LMWH or vitamin K antagonist regimen in PE patients without hemodynamic instability.
- ✔ After completion of primary anticoagulation treatment, patients should be reexamined after the first 3 to 6 months of anticoagulation, weighing the benefits versus risks of continuing treatment to decide on the extension and dose of anticoagulant therapy.
- ✔ For PE in a pregnant patient, diagnostic pathways and algorithms including CTPA or V/Q lung scan should be considered, which can be used safely during pregnancy.

REFERENCES

1. Chatterjee S, Chakraborty A, Weinberg I, et al. Thrombolysis for pulmonary embolism and risk of all-cause mortality, major bleeding, and intracranial hemorrhage: a meta-analysis. *JAMA.* 2014;311:2414-2421.
2. Rivera-Lebron B, McDaniel M, Ahrar K, et al. Diagnosis, treatment and follow up of acute pulmonary embolism: Consensus Practice from the PERT Consortium. *Clin Appl Thromb Hemost.* 2019;25:1076029619853037.
3. Anderson FA Jr, Spencer FA. Risk factors for venous thromboembolism. *Circulation.* 2003;107.
4. Konstantinides SV, Meyer G, Becattini C, et al. 2019 ESC Guidelines for the diagnosis and management of acute pulmonary embolism developed in collaboration with the European Respiratory Society (ERS). *Eur Heart J.* 2020;41:543-603.
5. Rogers MA, Levine DA, Blumberg N, Flanders SA, Chopra V, Langa KM. Triggers of hospitalization for venous thromboembolism. *Circulation.* 2012;125:2092-2099.

6. Blanco-Molina A, Rota LL, Di Micco P, et al. Venous thromboembolism during pregnancy, postpartum or during contraceptive use. *Thromb Haemost.* 2010;103:306-311.
7. Harjola VP, Mebazaa A, Celutkiene J, et al. Contemporary management of acute right ventricular failure: a statement from the Heart Failure Association and the Working Group on Pulmonary Circulation and Right Ventricular Function of the European Society of Cardiology. *Eur J Heart Fail.* 2016;18:226-241.
8. Bautz B, Schneider JI. High-risk chief complaints i: chest pain-the big three (an update). *Emerg Med Clin North Am.* 2020;38:453-498.
9. Le Gal G, Righini M, Roy PM, et al. Prediction of pulmonary embolism in the emergency department: the revised Geneva score. *Ann Intern Med.* 2006;144:165-171.
10. Klok FA, Mos IC, Nijkeuter M, et al. Simplification of the revised Geneva score for assessing clinical probability of pulmonary embolism. *Arch Intern Med.* 2008;168:2131-2136.
11. Ceriani E, Combescure C, Le Gal G, et al. Clinical prediction rules for pulmonary embolism: a systematic review and meta-analysis. *J Thromb Haemost.* 2010;8:957-970.
12. Wells PS, Anderson DR, Rodger M, et al. Derivation of a simple clinical model to categorize patients probability of pulmonary embolism: increasing the models utility with the SimpliRED D-dimer. *Thromb Haemost.* 2000;83:416-420.
13. Gibson NS, Sohne M, Kruip MJ, et al. Further validation and simplification of the Wells clinical decision rule in pulmonary embolism. *Thromb Haemost.* 2008;99:229-234.
14. Ma Y, Huang J, Wang Y, et al. Comparison of the Wells score with the revised Geneva score for assessing pretest probability of pulmonary embolism in hospitalized elderly patients. *Eur J Intern Med.* 2016;36:e18-e19.
15. Kline JA, Mitchell AM, Kabrhel C, Richman PB, Courtney DM. Clinical criteria to prevent unnecessary diagnostic testing in emergency department patients with suspected pulmonary embolism. *J Thromb Haemost.* 2004;2:1247-1255.
16. Penaloza A, Soulie C, Moumneh T, et al. Pulmonary embolism rule-out criteria (PERC) rule in European patients with low implicit clinical probability (PERCEPIC): a multicentre, prospective, observational study. *Lancet Haematol.* 2017;4:e615-e621.
17. Freund Y, Cachanado M, Aubry A, et al. Effect of the pulmonary embolism rule-out criteria on subsequent thromboembolic events among low-risk emergency department patients: the PROPER randomized clinical trial. *JAMA.* 2018;319:559-566.
18. Righini M, Goehring C, Bounameaux H, Perrier A. Effects of age on the performance of common diagnostic tests for pulmonary embolism. *Am J Med.* 2000;109:357-361.
19. Righini M, Van Es J, Den Exter PL, et al. Age-adjusted D-dimer cutoff levels to rule out pulmonary embolism: the ADJUST-PE study. *JAMA.* 2014;311:1117-1124.
20. Stein PD, Fowler SE, Goodman LR, et al. Multidetector computed tomography for acute pulmonary embolism. *N Engl J Med.* 2006;354:2317-2327.
21. Reid JH, Coche EE, Inoue T, et al. Is the lung scan alive and well? Facts and controversies in defining the role of lung scintigraphy for the diagnosis of pulmonary embolism in the era of MDCT. *Eur J Nucl Med Mol Imaging.* 2009;36:505-521.
22. Qanadli SD, Hajjam ME, Mesurolle B, et al. Pulmonary embolism detection: prospective evaluation of dual-section helical CT versus selective pulmonary arteriography in 157 patients. *Radiology.* 2000;217:447-455.
23. Roy PM, Colombet I, Durieux P, Chatellier G, Sors H, Meyer G. Systematic review and meta-analysis of strategies for the diagnosis of suspected pulmonary embolism. *BMJ.* 2005;331:259.
24. Kurnicka K, Lichodziejewska B, Goliszek S, et al. Echocardiographic pattern of acute pulmonary embolism: analysis of 511 consecutive patients. *J Am Soc Echocardiogr.* 2016;29:907-913.
25. Elias A, Mallett S, Daoud-Elias M, Poggi JN, Clarke M. Prognostic models in acute pulmonary embolism: a systematic review and meta-analysis. *BMJ Open.* 2016;6:e010324.
26. Kohn CG, Mearns ES, Parker MW, Hernandez AV, Coleman CI. Prognostic accuracy of clinical prediction rules for early post-pulmonary embolism all-cause mortality: a bivariate meta-analysis. *Chest.* 2015;147:1043-1062.
27. Jimenez D, Aujesky D, Moores L, et al. Simplification of the pulmonary embolism severity index for prognostication in patients with acute symptomatic pulmonary embolism. *Arch Intern Med.* 2010;170:1383-1389.
28. Aujesky D, Obrosky DS, Stone RA, et al. Derivation and validation of a prognostic model for pulmonary embolism. *Am J Respir Crit Care Med.* 2005;172:1041-1046.
29. Erythropoulou-Kaltsidou A, Alkagiet S, Tziomalos K. New guidelines for the diagnosis and management of pulmonary embolism: key changes. *World J Cardiol.* 2020;12:161-166.
30. Regitz-Zagrosek V, Roos-Hesselink JW, Bauersachs J, et al. 2018 ESC Guidelines for the management of cardiovascular diseases during pregnancy. *Eur Heart J.* 2018;39:3165-3241.
31. Ortel TL, Neumann I, Ageno W, et al. American Society of Hematology 2020 guidelines for management of venous thromboembolism: treatment of deep vein thrombosis and pulmonary embolism. *Blood Adv.* 2020;4:4693-4738.
32. Giri J, Sista AK, Weinberg I, et al. Interventional therapies for acute pulmonary embolism: current status and principles for the development of novel evidence: a scientific statement from the American Heart Association. *Circulation.* 2019;140:e774-e801.
33. Kearon C, Akl EA, Ornelas J, et al. Antithrombotic therapy for VTE disease: CHEST Guideline and Expert Panel Report. *Chest.* 2016;149:315-352.
34. Robertson L, McBride O, Burdess A. Pharmacomechanical thrombectomy for iliofemoral deep vein thrombosis. *Cochrane Database Syst Rev.* 2016;11:CD011536.
35. Zheng JJ, Zhang ZH, Shan Z, et al. Catheter-directed thrombolysis in the treatment of acute deep venous thrombosis: a meta-analysis. *Genet Mol Res.* 2014;13:5241-5249.
36. George B, Parazino M, Omar HR, et al. A retrospective comparison of survivors and non-survivors of massive pulmonary embolism receiving veno-arterial extracorporeal membrane oxygenation support. *Resuscitation.* 2018;122:1-5.
37. Yusuff HO, Zochios V, Vuylsteke A. Extracorporeal membrane oxygenation in acute massive pulmonary embolism: a systematic review. *Perfusion.* 2015;30:611-616.
38. Porres-Aguilar M, Rivera-Lebron BN, Anaya-Ayala JE, Leon MCG, Mukherjee D. Perioperative acute pulmonary embolism: a concise review with emphasis on multidisciplinary approach. *Int J Angiol.* 2020;29:183-188.
39. Porres-Aguilar M, Anaya-Ayala JE, Jimenez D, Mukherjee D. Pulmonary embolism response teams: pursuing excellence in the care for venous thromboembolism. *Arch Med Res.* 2019;50:257-258.
40. Malas MB, Naazie IN, Elsayed N, et al. Thromboembolism risk of COVID-19 is high and associated with a higher risk of mortality: a systematic review and meta-analysis. *EClinicalMedicine.* 2020;29:100639.
41. Tang N, Bai H, Chen X, Gong J, Li D, Sun Z. Anticoagulant treatment is associated with decreased mortality in severe coronavirus disease 2019 patients with coagulopathy. *J Thromb Haemost.* 2020;18:1094-1099.
42. Porres-Aguilar M, Tapson VF, Rivera-Lebron BN, et al. Impact and role of pulmonary embolism response teams in venous thromboembolism associated with COVID-19. *J Investig Med.* 2021; jim-2021-001856.

SECTION 7

CARDIOVASCULAR SURGERY

SECTION EDITOR: Michael E. Jessen

CHAPTER 86

CORONARY ARTERY BYPASS GRAFTING

Michael E. Jessen

HISTORY/BACKGROUND

Coronary arterial bypass grafting (CABG) is a surgical technique used to improve myocardial blood supply by creating vascular conduits that allow blood flow past obstructive lesions in the coronary arteries. The technique appeared after the introduction of selective coronary arteriography by Sones in 1958 and has seen considerable evolution over six decades. Although the first conventional coronary bypass operations were performed using a saphenous-vein graft by Sabiston in 1962 and using a left internal thoracic artery graft by Kolesov in 1964, it was the pioneering work of Rene Favaloro that led to the broad acceptance of the operation for treatment of ischemic heart disease.[1] The operation has since undergone modifications to include other bypass conduits to avoid the use of cardiopulmonary bypass and to utilize less invasive techniques (**Figure 86.1**). Today it remains the most commonly performed cardiovascular operation in the world and is one of the most rigorously studied operations in history. By current guidelines, CABG represents the most highly recommended procedure for the treatment of ischemic heart disease in patients with complex coronary artery disease, left main coronary artery stenosis, depressed left ventricular (LV) systolic function, and some associated conditions such as diabetes mellitus.[2,3]

INDICATIONS FOR CORONARY ARTERIAL BYPASS GRAFTING

Clinical Indications and Coronary Anatomy Considerations

In broad terms, CABG is used today for treating patients with significant coronary artery disease to achieve control of angina or to prolong survival, or both.[4] CABG remains one of the most effective means for control of angina, and disabling angina is a Class I indication for CABG. In patients with multivessel coronary disease, CABG offers better relief of angina than guideline-directed medical therapy (GDMT), and when compared with both medical therapy and percutaneous coronary intervention (PCI), CABG reduces the incidence of subsequent myocardial infarction and the need for additional revascularization.[5]

Many contemporary indications for CABG focus on the survival benefit that has been observed with CABG compared with GDMT. CABG prolongs survival in patients with several defined coronary anatomic conditions. CABG is indicated in patients with >50% stenosis of the left main coronary artery with or without symptoms of angina. PCI is occasionally used in these patients, although results may be less favorable (see discussion below). CABG also appears to improve survival in patients with >70% stenosis in three major coronary arteries or with >70% stenosis in two major coronary arteries when one is the proximal left anterior descending (LAD). These benefits may be seen in asymptomatic patients, those with mild or stable angina, and those found to have high-risk criteria on stress testing, abnormal intracoronary hemodynamic evaluation, or sizeable (>20%) perfusion defects on myocardial perfusion stress imaging.[4] CABG has been extensively compared to revascularization by PCI. A discussion of trials comparing these treatment options is provided later in the chapter.

Survival benefits of CABG are more apparent in patients with impaired LV function. A meta-analysis of 20 studies, including 54,173 patients, comparing CABG and PCI in patients with decreased left ventricular ejection fraction (LVEF) found significantly lower hazard ratios for mortality (HR 0.763; 95% confidence interval [CI] 0.678-0.859; $P < .001$), myocardial infarction (HR 0.481; 95% CI 0.365-0.633; $P < .001$), and repeat revascularization (HR 0.321; 95% CI 0.241-0.428; $P < .001$) in the CABG group than in the PCI group.[6] These data support the selection of CABG over PCI to improve survival in this higher risk subset. The mechanism behind this benefit may be a reduction in new myocardial infarction.[7]

Patients diagnosed with acute ST-segment elevation myocardial infarctions (STEMI) typically undergo urgent coronary arteriography and PCI. A small portion of these patients have coronary anatomy that is unsuitable for PCI or coronary occlusions that cannot be opened. Patients with these conditions and evidence of ongoing myocardial ischemia can benefit from emergency CABG, although the peri-procedural risk is higher than when CABG is performed electively. Similarly, patients who develop an acute coronary occlusion with ongoing ischemia while undergoing an elective PCI procedure should be considered for emergency CABG to preserve LV function providing their risk profile is not prohibitive.

Patients who present with non-ST segment elevation myocardial infarctions (NSTEMI) are typically treated medically initially. However, those who experience ongoing ischemia that is unresponsive to medical therapy can be treated with urgent revascularization. This is most commonly accomplished by PCI, but CABG has an important role in this

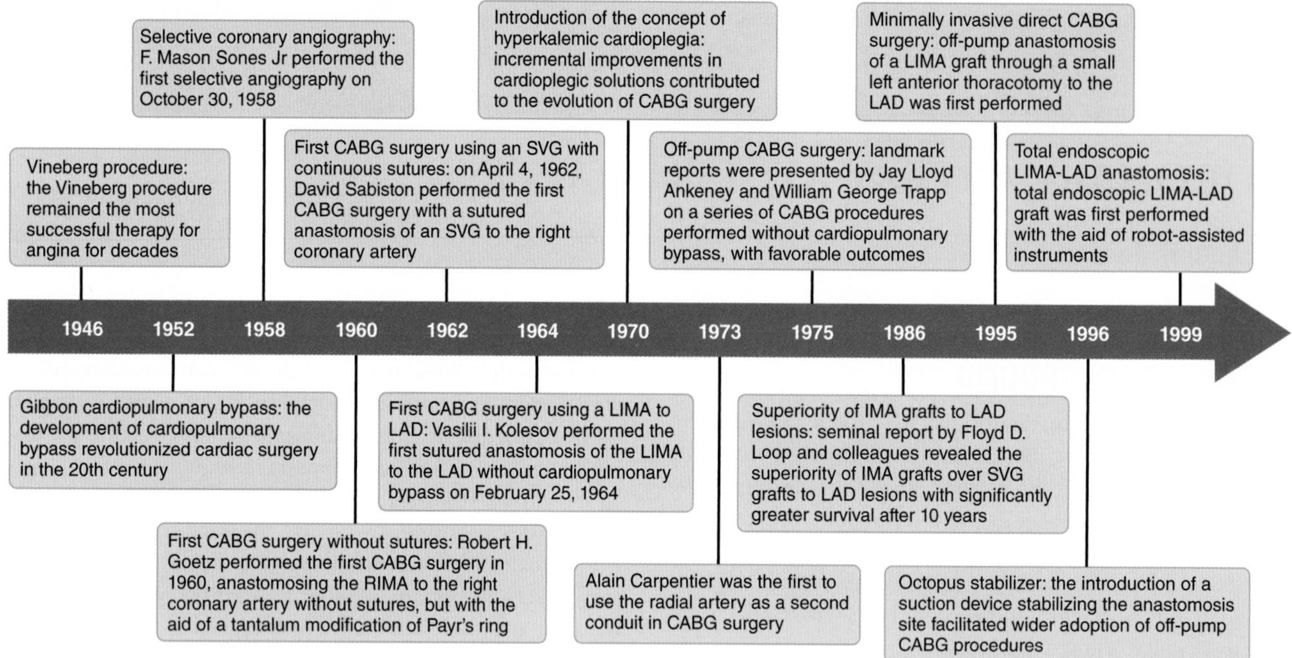

FIGURE 86.1 Milestones in the evolution of CABG surgery—the history of CABG can be traced to the 1940s, when the Vineberg procedure was introduced as an effective strategy to treat symptomatic angina. Since then, great strides have been made optimizing CABG surgery techniques, including off-pump surgery and less invasive surgical revascularization techniques. CABG, coronary arterial bypass grafting; IMA, internal mammary artery; LAD, left anterior descending coronary artery; LIMA, left internal mammary artery; RIMA, right internal mammary artery; SVG, saphenous vein graft. (Reprinted by permission from Nature: Caliskan E, de Souza DR, Böning A, et al. Saphenous vein grafts in contemporary coronary artery bypass graft surgery. *Nat Rev Cardiol.* 2020;17(3):155-169. Copyright © 2019 Springer Nature.)

group of patients. In an observational study that included 5112 patients presenting with STEMI or unstable angina between 2000 and 2016, propensity score-matching analysis was used to compare early outcomes and all-cause mortality in groups treated with PCI or CABG.[8] Multivariable analysis showed that CABG was independently associated with a significant 65% reduction in 10-year mortality ($P < .001$). Interestingly, this long-term advantage was seen among male patients and not female patients. Thus, CABG has an important role in the treatment of a wide range of patients with disabling angina, high-risk coronary anatomy, STEMI and NSTEMI, and impaired LV systolic function.

Current ACC/AHA guidelines[2,3] recommend CABG as Class I for the following patient groups:

Special Subgroups

Important survival benefits from CABG may accrue in other subgroups of patients. One group that has received much

Revascularization to Improve Survival: Recommendations: Class I

1. CABG to improve survival is recommended for patients with significant (≥50% diameter stenosis) left main coronary artery stenosis (*Level of Evidence: B*).
2. CABG to improve survival is beneficial in patients with significant (≥70% diameter) stenoses in three major coronary arteries (with or without involvement of the proximal LAD artery) or in the proximal LAD plus 1 other major coronary artery (*Level of Evidence: B*).
3. CABG or PCI to improve survival is beneficial in survivors of sudden cardiac death with presumed ischemia-mediated ventricular tachycardia caused by significant (≥70% diameter) stenosis in a major coronary artery (*CABG Level of Evidence: B; PCI Level of Evidence: C*[3,4,5]).

Revascularization to Improve Symptoms: Recommendations Class I

1. CABG to improve symptoms is beneficial in patients with one or more significant (≥70% diameter) coronary artery stenoses amenable to revascularization and unacceptable angina despite GDMT (*Level of Evidence: A*).

CABG in Patients With Acute Myocardial Infarction: Recommendations Class I

1. Emergency CABG is recommended in patients with acute MI in whom (1) primary PCI has failed or cannot be performed, (2) coronary anatomy is suitable for CABG, and (3) persistent ischemia of a significant area of myocardium at rest and/or hemodynamic instability refractory to nonsurgical therapy is present *(Level of Evidence: B)*.
2. Emergency CABG is recommended in patients undergoing surgical repair of a postinfarction mechanical complication of MI, such as ventricular septal rupture, mitral valve insufficiency because of papillary muscle infarction and/or rupture, or free wall rupture *(Level of Evidence: B)*.
3. Emergency CABG is recommended in patients with cardiogenic shock and who are suitable for CABG irrespective of the time interval from MI to onset of shock and time from MI to CABG *(Level of Evidence: B)*.
4. Emergency CABG is recommended in patients with life-threatening ventricular arrhythmias (believed to be ischemic in origin) in the presence of left main stenosis greater than or equal to 50% and/or three-vessel CAD *(Level of Evidence: C)*.

CABG, coronary arterial bypass grafting; CAD, coronary artery disease; GDMT, guideline-directed medical therapy; LAD, left anterior descending; MI, myocardial infarction; PCI, percutaneous coronary intervention

scrutiny is patients with diabetes mellitus. The Future Revascularization Evaluation in Patients with Diabetes Mellitus: Optimal Management of Multivessel Disease (FREEDOM) trial randomized 1900 diabetic patients with multivessel coronary artery disease to PCI or CABG (**Table 86.1**).[9] The primary composite outcome of death, myocardial infarction, and stroke at 5 years was significantly higher with PCI as compared with CABG (26.6% vs 18.7%, $P = .005$). Notably, a significant reduction in all-cause mortality (16.3% vs 10.9%, $P = .049$) and myocardial infarction (13.9% vs 6.0%, $P < .001$) was observed with CABG, although the incidence of stroke was higher (2.4% vs 5.2%, $P = .03$). At 1 year, repeat revascularization was significantly higher in the PCI group (13% vs 5%, $P < .0001$). All events were higher in patients with insulin-dependent diabetes as compared with non-insulin-dependent diabetes, including the primary end point (29% vs 19% at 5 years, $P < .001$). In a study of 943 FREEDOM patients with extended follow-up, all-cause mortality rate was higher in the PCI group compared with CABG (23.7% vs 18.7%, $P = .076$).[10] CABG is considered the preferred revascularization option in patients with diabetes.

Some retrospective studies have suggested a survival benefit with CABG in patients with mild-to-moderate chronic kidney disease (CKD) and end-stage renal disease (ESRD). A recent study examined mortality in 971 veterans with incident ESRD, who underwent CABG ($N = 582$) or PCI ($N = 389$) up to 5 years prior to dialysis initiation. Compared to PCI, patients who underwent CABG had a 34% lower risk of death ($P = .002$) after initiation of dialysis.[11] Although randomized trials are needed, CABG appears to be the preferred revascularization option in patients with advanced kidney disease.

SURGICAL TECHNIQUES

The majority of coronary bypass operations are performed through a median sternotomy incision, with the patient cannulated for cardiopulmonary bypass via the ascending aorta and

TABLE 86.1 Kaplan-Meier Estimates of Key Outcomes at 2 Years and 5 Years After Randomization

Outcome	2 Years After Randomization		5 Years After Randomization		Patients With Event		*P* Value[a]
	PCI (N=953)	CABG (N=947)	PCI (N=953)	CABG (N=947)	PCI (N=953)	CABG (N=947)	
	number (percent)				*number*		
Primary composite[b]	121 (13.0)	108 (11.9)	200 (26.6)	146 (18.7)	205	147	0.005[c]
Death from any cause	62 (6.7)	57 (6.3)	114 (16.3)	83 (10.9)	118	86	0.049
Myocardial infarction	62 (6.7)	42 (4.7)	98 (13.9)	48 (6.0)	99	48	<0.001
Stroke	14 (1.5)	24 (2.7)	20 (2.4)	37 (5.2)	22	37	0.03[d]
Cardiovascular death	9 (0.9)	12 (1.3)	73 (10.9)	52 (6.8)	75	55	0.12

CABG, coronary arterial bypass grafting; PCI, percutaneous coronary intervention.
[a] *P* values were calculated with the use of the log-rank test on the basis of all available follow-up data (ie, more than 5 years).
[b] The primary composite outcome was the rate of death from any cause, myocardial infarction, or stroke.
[c] $P = .006$ in the as-treated (non-intention-to-treat) analysis.
[d] $P = .16$ by the Wald test of the Cox regression estimate for study-group assignment in 1712 patients after adjustment for the average glucose level after the procedure.
From Farkouh ME, Domanski M, Sleeper LA, et al. Strategies for multivessel revascularization in patients with diabetes. *N Engl J Med.* 2012;367(25):2375-2384. Copyright © 2012 Massachusetts Medical Society. Reprinted with permission from Massachusetts Medical Society.

right atrium. Bypass conduits, most commonly the left internal thoracic artery and greater saphenous vein, are harvested, the aorta is cross clamped, and the heart is arrested with a potassium-containing cardioplegia solution to achieve a diastolic arrest, reduce myocardial oxygen demand and provide a bloodless operating field. Bypass grafts are constructed to allow blood flow beyond coronary obstructions, the cross clamp is removed, cardiac activity is reestablished, and the patient is weaned from cardiopulmonary bypass. Surgical drains are placed, the sternum is reapproximated with wires, and the incisions are closed. While this framework comprises the commonest form of the operation, several noteworthy variations are applied.

Conduits for Coronary Bypass Grafts

The most common conduit used for bypass grafting is the greater saphenous vein. However, vein grafts become diseased or occluded over time at significant rates. Vein graft failure occurs in three distinct phases: (1) early (<1 month) graft occlusion results from graft thrombosis owing to technical imperfections in the construction of the graft, poor runoff in the target vessel, or vein graft endothelial injury during harvest; (2) intermediate (1-12 months) graft stenosis attributable to development of intimal hyperplasia near anastomotic sites; and (3) late graft disease (>12 months) from the development of atherosclerosis in the vein graft itself **(Figure 86.2)**. Up to 15% of saphenous-vein grafts occlude by 1 year, and angiographic studies have shown a 40% to 50% occlusion rate at 10 years. Clinical outcomes are worse when graft occlusion occurs, with higher rates of recurrent angina, myocardial infarction, and need for repeat revascularization. Vein graft patency is improved with the use of antiplatelet therapy.

Vein grafts can be harvested through open incisions or through endoscopic approaches.

Randomized trials have shown no difference in cardiovascular outcomes between these methods, although wound complications are reduced with endoscopic vein harvesting.[12]

The left internal mammary artery (LIMA) is unquestionably the preferred conduit for use in CABG, and grafting of the LAD with this conduit is firmly entrenched as the standard of care. This construct results in the highest 10-year patency rate (>90%), survival, and freedom from cardiac events compared with any other conduit. The LIMA can be harvested as a pedicle graft or as a "skeletonized" graft that may offer greater length and lower sternal complication rates. The vast majority of LIMA grafts are placed as in situ grafts, although the LIMA can be used as a free graft or Y-graft in select situations.

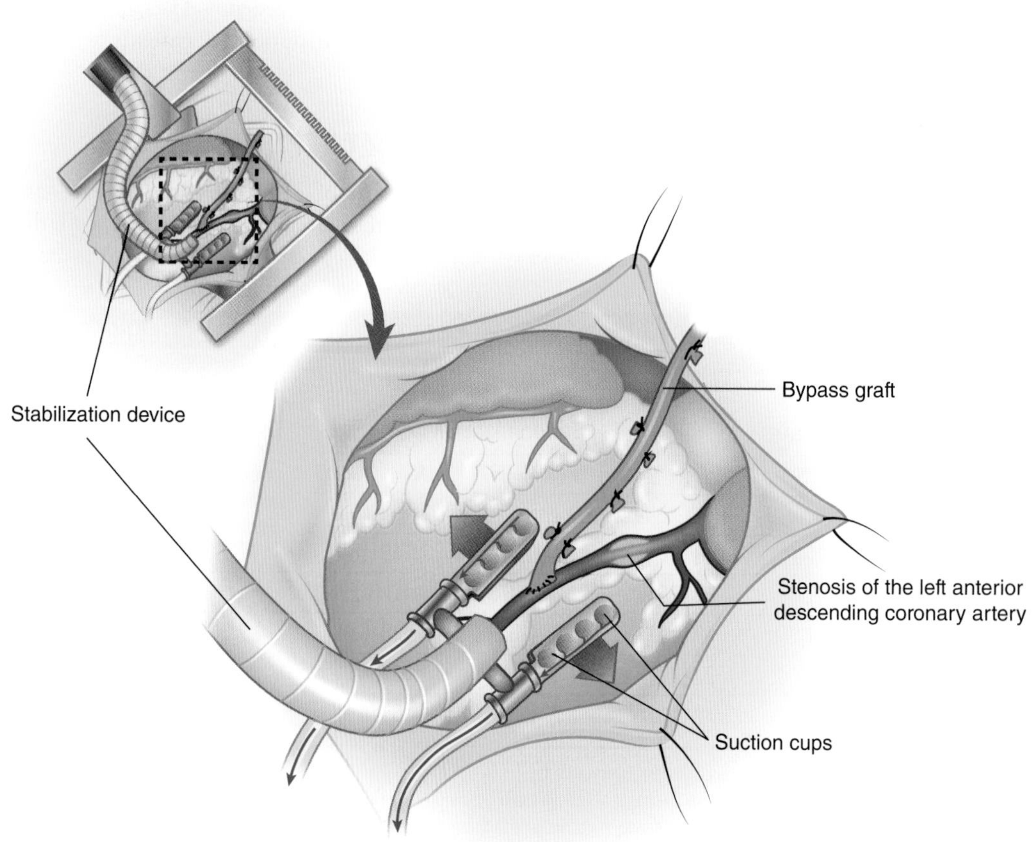

FIGURE 86.2 Deployed stabilization device for off-pump coronary artery bypass surgery.

Owing to superior results observed with the LIMA graft, surgeons have considered the use of bilateral internal mammary artery (IMA) grafting as a mechanism to further improve CABG outcomes. A number of observational studies and meta-analyses have suggested high graft patency rates, superior survival rates, and lower rates of recurrent angina, late myocardial infarction, and hospitalization for cardiac events in patients undergoing CABG with multiple arterial grafts compared with single arterial grafts. However, the multicenter, prospective randomized Arterial Revascularization Trial (ART trial), in which patients were randomly assigned to undergo single or bilateral IMA grafting did not identify significant differences in mortality or rates of adverse cardiovascular events between groups at 10 years of follow-up.[13] In this trial, patients with bilateral IMA grafting sustained a significantly higher rate of sternal wound complications. Interpretation of the study has been complicated by a high crossover rate (14% of patients allocated to bilateral IMA actually received a single IMA) and by the fact that 22% of patients allocated to single IMA receiving an additional radial artery.

The other conduit that has received considerable attention is the radial artery. This artery has morphologic differences from IMAs and is more prone to spasm after grafting. Multiple randomized, controlled trials comparing radial-artery grafts and saphenous-vein grafts (all patients in both groups also received one IMA graft) suggested benefits but were underpowered to detect differences in clinical outcomes. A patient-level combined analysis of six randomized, controlled trials comparing radial-artery grafts and saphenous-vein grafts was reported in 2018.[14] At a mean follow-up of 5 years, the incidence of adverse cardiac events was significantly lower with radial-artery grafts than with saphenous-vein grafts (hazard ratio, 0.67), as was the rate of graft occlusion (hazard ratio, 0.44), the incidence of myocardial infarction (hazard ratio, 0.72), and the need for repeat revascularization (hazard ratio, 0.50). The incidence of death from any cause was not different between groups. These data suggest an advantage associated with the use of the radial artery as a second conduit in CABG operations. Despite these studies, the use of bilateral IMA grafting remains low worldwide, and only 10% to 20% of patients in Europe and 5% in the United States undergo CABG with multiple arterial grafting.

Use of Cardiopulmonary Bypass

For many years, CABG was performed almost exclusively with the use of cardiopulmonary bypass to support the circulation and allow a bloodless, motionless field for the conduct of the operation. Cardiopulmonary bypass requires a period of intense anticoagulation, creates a systemic inflammatory response, and involves significant aortic manipulation. Surgeons questioned whether eliminating cardiopulmonary bypass could reduce some of the adverse effects of CABG, particularly bleeding complications, stroke, and neurocognitive changes. Techniques and surgical equipment evolved to allow positioning of the heart to gain access to all regions of the myocardium and to allow effective stabilization of coronary vessels to perform the anastomoses (**Figure 86.3**).

Enthusiasm for these procedures—off-pump coronary artery bypass surgery (OPCAB)—increased in the early 2000s, and multiple randomized trials comparing OPCAB and conventional on-pump CABG emerged. Some of the large early trials showed no beneficial effects on early or long-term outcomes and suggested that OPCAB may result in less complete revascularization and possibly inferior graft patency. A systematic review of 86 trials reported in 2012 did not demonstrate any significant benefit of OPCAB compared with on-pump CABG regarding mortality, stroke, or myocardial infarction.[15] The analysis identified better long-term survival in patients undergoing on-pump CABG, suggesting that it should remain the standard surgical treatment. A subsequent meta-analysis of 100 studies involving over 19,000 patients found no difference between the two techniques with respect to all-cause mortality and myocardial infarction. OPCAB was associated with a significant 28% reduction in the odds of stroke. This study also suggested that the technique may prove effective in reducing mortality and morbidity in patients at higher risk for adverse events.[16] The use of OPCAB has waned in the United States in recent years, although its use remains robust in developing countries, where the availability of cardiopulmonary bypass is limited by high procedural costs.

Minimally Invasive Approaches

Some CABG procedures are performed through small anterolateral mini-thoracotomy incisions. This approach usually limits the operation to anastomosis of the LIMA to the LAD and a few other vessels. In some centers, a hybrid revascularization approach has emerged for treatment of multivessel coronary artery disease with minimally invasive surgery revascularization of the LAD followed by PCI for revascularization of the other vessels. Finally, a robot-assisted total endoscopic approach that may allow complete revascularization has been pioneered. Data on short and intermediate outcomes are limited, and acceptance of these methods awaits the results of further studies.

PATIENT RISK ASSESSMENT

In order to accurately inform patients of their risk of mortality or of the development of important complications following CABG, several robust predictive models have been developed based on large prospective databases in which data are collected by trained personnel. Almost all cardiac surgery programs participate in a database, and current guidelines consider participation in a state, regional, or national clinical data registry that provides periodic reports of risk-adjusted outcomes an important component of any program.[4] The most widely used risk models are the Society of Thoracic Surgeons (STS), Adult Cardiac Surgery Database Predictive Risk of Mortality (PROM), and the European System for Cardiac Operative Risk Evaluation (EuroSCORE II). Both models use multiple preoperative patient variables to calculate a perioperative mortality estimate. A recent systematic review comparing these two established risk models for prediction of perioperative mortality suggested similar performance.[17] Preoperative calculation of mortality risk is valuable in counseling patients before CABG, and

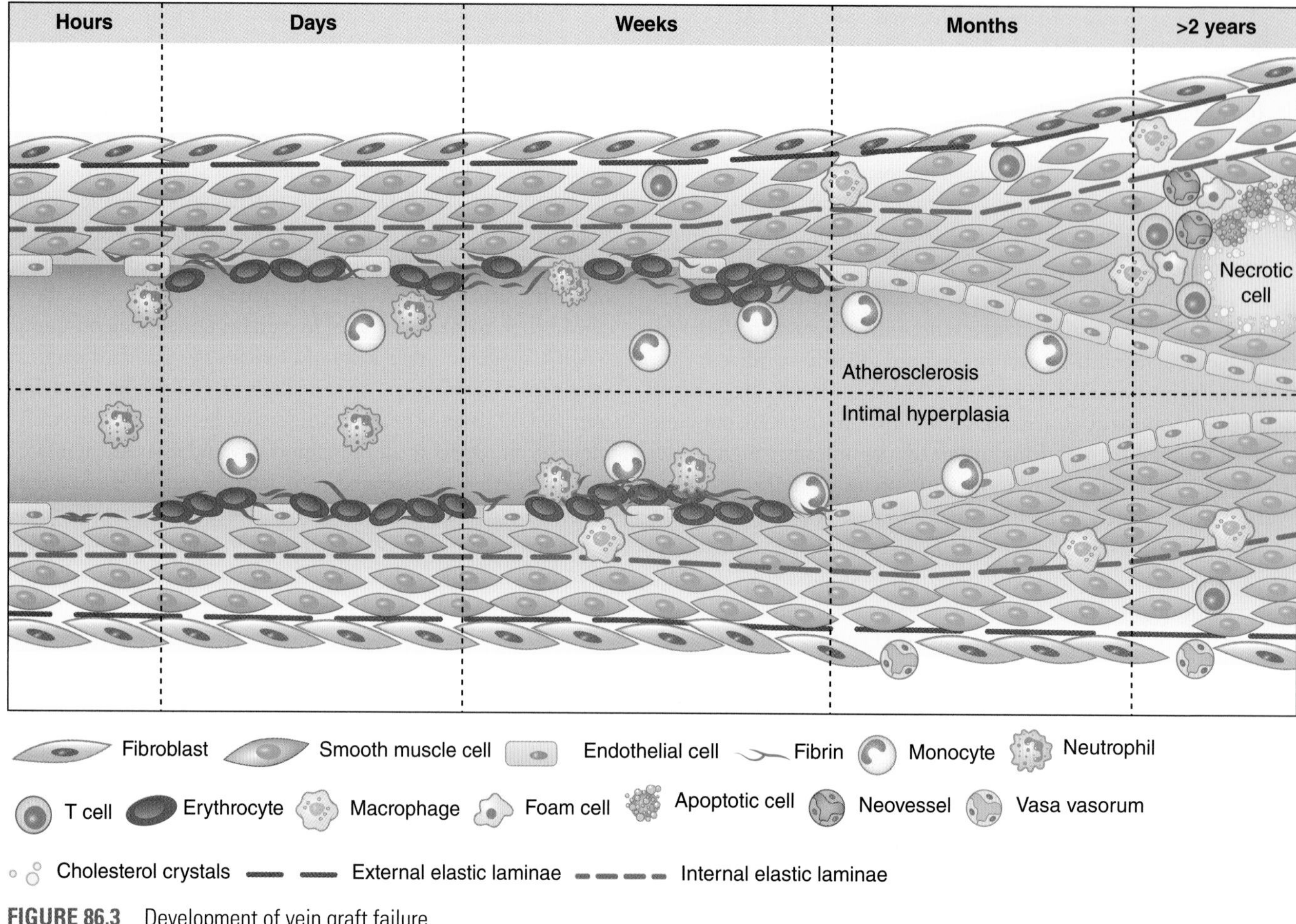

FIGURE 86.3 Development of vein graft failure.

the STS now considers this process a component of defining high-performing programs.

Recently, machine learning algorithms for estimating operative mortality risk in cardiac surgery have been developed and show promise in further refining our ability to estimate mortality and adverse outcomes following CABG.[18] Further research in this dynamic area is ongoing.

LIMITATIONS AND COMPLICATIONS

Limitations of CABG

Coronary bypass surgery offers important relief from angina and survival benefits for many patients but has significant limitations that can be grouped into three general areas. First, there are limitations based on coronary anatomy. Some patients have very diffuse coronary disease or disease that extends very distally in the coronary artery. These patients may be at risk for an incomplete revascularization, which diminishes the benefit of the operation, or may not be eligible for CABG at all. The decision of suitability for bypass grafting is usually within the purview of the surgical team. In some instances, coronary endarterectomy can be an adjunctive procedure that improves coronary artery outflow and allows grafting of vessels that otherwise may be unsuitable. However, outcomes in patients who require endarterectomy are, in general, inferior to those who do not.[19] Some patients may have had such previous extensive stent placement throughout the coronary arteries that inadequate target vessels remain. Another limitation relates to the degree of LV systolic dysfunction in the patient. CABG offers a survival benefit to many patients with complex coronary disease, and the magnitude of the benefit tends to be greater in patients who have worse degrees of ventricular dysfunction. However, extreme LV dysfunction, particularly when accompanied by profound degrees of LV remodeling may tip the risk-benefit ratio away from CABG. In a propensity matched study comparing patients with poor LV function (EF $<$ 20%) with those with good LV function (EF $>$ 60%) undergoing CABG, patients with depressed LV function were found to have higher mortality and major morbidity rates compared to patients with good LV function. Of note, the subgroup of patients with both LVEF less than 20% and ventricular enlargement had the worst outcomes, with perioperative mortality rates over 12%. Thus, the combination of LV size and LVEF may aid in the decision-making process to determine whether CABG is the most appropriate revascularization strategy.[20] An evaluation of myocardial viability may also be useful in patients with severely depressed LV function, particularly in those without angina. Finally, associated noncardiac conditions may limit the benefit of CABG. Patients with ESRD, underlying malignancies, or severe pulmonary or hepatic dysfunction are examples in which the decision for CABG is more complex because the additional conditions increase the surgical risk and limit the survival benefit. In these cases, a "heart team" approach—with input from the primary physician, cardiothoracic surgeon, cardiologist, and patient—is beneficial in selecting the optimal treatment pathway.[4]

Complications of Coronary Arterial Bypass Grafting

Any consideration of CABG also needs to consider the potential complications that may result from the operation. Complications can occur in any organ system after CABG, but the most serious adverse sequelae include stroke, perioperative myocardial infarction, low-output state, renal failure, respiratory failure, prolonged ventilation, postoperative bleeding, reoperation, and infection or septicemia. Overall, approximately 14% of patients undergoing CABG will experience at least one serious complication.[21] Rates of transfusion of blood products vary widely among institutions: at U.S. hospitals performing at least 100 on-pump CABG operations in 2008 (82,446 cases at 408 sites), the rates of red blood cell blood transfusion ranged from 7.8% to 92.8%.[22] Approximately 10% of allogeneic blood transfusions in the United States are given to subjects undergoing cardiac surgery. Wound infections may occur from conduit harvest sites or from the sternotomy incision. A detailed review of sternal wound infections is provided in Chapter 95. The commonest complication after cardiac surgery is perioperative atrial fibrillation, although this complication is typically effectively treated in hospital without a significant impact on early mortality rates.

Not surprisingly, operative mortality rates increase with the occurrence of major complications. Despite quality initiatives, the sequelae of these complications vary greatly among institutions. Recent data have suggested that a significant factor related to mortality is the failure to rescue the patient when one or more complications arise. CABG mortality rates correlate more strongly with failure to rescue than with absolute complication rates.[23] Complications have a major impact on duration of hospitalization, long-term outcomes, and hospital resource utilization and costs.[21]

LONG-TERM OUTCOMES

Although early mortality in patients undergoing CABG is now approaching 2% overall, the long-term mortality rates are less well studied. A Dutch cohort study reported survival estimates of 92% at 5 years, 77% at 10 years, 57% at 15 years, and 40% at 20 years.[24] A Danish population-based cohort study examining more than 50,000 CABG patients and more than 500,000 individuals from the general population matched by age, sex, and calendar year of surgery found a higher mortality rate in the isolated CABG cohort than in the general population, especially within the first 10 years of surgery.[25] Long-term survival is affected by multiple coexisting clinical variables. Using data on nearly 350,000 CABG patients from the STS Adult Cardiac Surgery Database and Centers for Medicare and Medicaid Services, Shahian and colleagues developed a long-term survival prediction model for isolated CABG.[26] LV systolic dysfunction, diabetes mellitus, female sex, renal insufficiency, and chronic lung disease all had a negative impact on late survival (**e-Figure 86.1**). Nevertheless, both early and late survival rates are improving for patients undergoing CABG, and aggressive treatment of underlying comorbid conditions is likely to continue this trend.

REOPERATIONS

Over time many CABG patients develop progression of disease in the native coronary system or disease in the bypass grafts. When this occurs, symptomatic patients may be considered for revascularization, either by PCI or repeat CABG. Using data from the STS Adult Cardiac Surgery Database, Fosbol and colleagues reported on 723,134 patients greater than or equal to 65 years of age who underwent CABG between 2001 and 2007.[27] The cumulative incidence of repeat revascularization at 1, 5, 10, and 18 years was 2%, 7%, 13%, and 16% respectively, but the vast majority of repeat revascularization was accomplished with PCI. The prevalence of repeat CABG was 0.1%, 0.6%, 1.3%, and 1.7%, respectively at these time-points, and the rate appears to be declining.[28] Repeat CABG now comprises only about 2% of all CABG operations in the United States,[29] likely because of greater use of arterial grafts in initial operations, better treatment of risk factors, and expanded use of PCI. Repeat CABG presents a number of technical challenges, including the potential for inadequate bypass conduits, cardiac injury during sternal reentry, difficulties in identifying target coronary vessels and controlling patent IMA grafts, and avoiding embolization of atherosclerotic debris from diseased vein grafts.[30] The in-hospital mortality risk of repeat CABG is increased compared to primary CABG but is still relatively low (~3%) despite more operations being performed on patients with higher risk profiles.[29] Cardiac, vascular, and respiratory complications are more frequent in repeat, compared to primary, CABG, and length of hospitalization is longer. A heart team approach, with careful consideration of all treatment options is important in this patient group.

COMPARISONS WITH MEDICAL THERAPY AND PERCUTANEOUS CORONARY INTERVENTION

Coronary Arterial Bypass Grafting Versus Medical Therapy in Ischemic Cardiomyopathy (the STITCH Trial)

Many studies have suggested that CABG may offer a survival benefit to patients with severe coronary artery disease and depressed LV systolic function, but most were conducted in an era when medical therapy was not well defined, and very few patients enrolled had severe LV dysfunction or symptomatic heart failure.[31] One of the largest trials that sought to examine the survival benefit of a strategy of CABG added to GDMT as compared with GDMT alone was conducted between July 2002 and May 2007: the Surgical Treatment for Ischemic Heart Failure (STICH) study.[32] In this prospective randomized trial, 1212 patients with a LVEF less than or equal to 35% and coronary artery disease amenable to CABG were randomly assigned to undergo CABG plus GDMT (610 patients) or GDMT therapy alone (602 patients). The primary outcome was death from any cause, and major secondary outcomes included death from cardiovascular causes and death from any cause or hospitalization for cardiovascular causes. At a median follow-up of 56 months, there was no significant difference between the CABG group and the medical therapy group in the rate of death from any cause, although the rates of death from cardiovascular causes and of death from any cause or hospitalization for cardiovascular causes were lower among patients in the CABG group. Close observation continued out to a median duration of follow-up of 9.8 years in an extended follow-up study STICH Extension Study (STICHES)[33] (**e-Figure 86.2**). The primary outcome occurred in 58.9% of the CABG group and in 66.1% of the medical therapy group ($P = .02$). A total of 40.5% of the CABG group and 49.3% of the medical therapy group died from cardiovascular causes ($P = .006$). Death from any cause or hospitalization for cardiovascular causes occurred in 76.6% of the CABG group and 87% of the medical therapy group ($P < .001$). Thus, CABG with medical therapy was found to confer a significant survival benefit at 10 years compared with medical therapy alone, and median survival was extended by nearly 18 months. CABG should be considered as an addition to medical therapy in patients with ischemic cardiomyopathy.

CABG Versus PCI in Patients With Complex Coronary Artery Disease (SYNTAX Trial)

Multiple clinical trials comparing CABG and PCI have been published. A large meta-analysis of the most pertinent randomized trials demonstrated a survival advantage of CABG over PCI in patients with multivessel disease.[34] One trial that quantified the complexity of coronary disease as well was the Synergy Between PCI with TAXUS and Cardiac Surgery (SYNTAX) trial. The trial was first reported in 2009 when only 1-year results were available[35] but showed that CABG, as compared with PCI, resulted in lower rates of the combined end point of major adverse cardiac or cerebrovascular events (MACCE) in patients with three-vessel or left main coronary artery disease. Importantly, this trial used a predefined scoring system to quantify the severity of coronary disease, in which lower scores indicated less severe or complex disease. Patients with low (0-22) or intermediate (22-32) scores had similar rates of MACCE with CABG or PCI, whereas among patients with high scores (>32), the event rate was significantly higher in the PCI group than in the CABG group. Results after 5 years of follow-up were reported in 2013.[36] In this analysis, outcomes with CABG were superior to those with PCI in patients with both intermediate or high SYNTAX scores. Rates of major adverse coronary and cerebral events (MACCE) were significantly increased with PCI in intermediate score patients (25.8% of the CABG group vs 36.0% of the PCI group; $P = .008$) and in high-score patients (26.8% vs 44.0%; $P < .0001$). (**see e-Figure 86.3**). An investigator-driven follow-up extension of this trial up to 10 years has also been reported: The SYNTAX Extended Survival (SYNTAXES) study.[37] The only end point that was monitored was all-cause mortality. At 10 years, no significant difference was observed in all-cause death between PCI and CABG. However, CABG provided a significant survival benefit in patients with three-vessel disease but not in patients with left main coronary artery disease. Taken together, the SYNTAX trial supports the concept that CABG offers a survival benefit compared to PCI, the largest impact being in patients with complex, multivessel coronary disease.

CABG Versus PCI in Patients With Left Main Disease (The EXCEL and NOBLE Trials)

Two major trials have randomized patients with left main coronary artery disease to treatment with CABG or PCI and have reported follow-up out to 5 years. The Evaluation of XIENCE versus Coronary Artery Bypass Surgery for Effectiveness of Left Main Revascularization (EXCEL) trial of 1905 patients in 17 countries compared CABG with PCI in patients with left main disease and a SYNTAX score less than 32. No significant difference in the primary outcome (the combination of death, myocardial infarction, and stroke) was reported. At 5 years, a primary outcome event had occurred in 22% of the patients in the PCI group and in 19.2% of the patients in the CABG group ($P = .13$). Of note, death from any cause occurred more frequently in the PCI group than in the CABG group (13.0% vs 9.9%), and ischemia-driven revascularization was more frequent after PCI than after CABG (16.9% vs 10.0%). The trial has been criticized in part for the definition of peri-procedural myocardial infarction used. The Nordic-Baltic-British Left Main Revascularization (NOBLE) trial randomized 1201 patients from nine European countries with left main coronary artery disease requiring revascularization to CABG or PCI.[38,40] The primary end point was MACCE, a composite of all-cause mortality, nonprocedural myocardial infarction, repeat revascularization, and stroke. CABG was found to be superior to PCI for the primary composite end point ($P = .0002$). In subanalyses, all-cause mortality was similar (9% after PCI vs 9% after CABG, $P = .68$), but nonprocedural myocardial infarction was greater after PCI (8% vs 3%, $P = .0002$), and repeat revascularization was greater after PCI (17% vs 10%, $P = .0009$) (**Figure 86.4**). Differences in outcomes between the trials may relate to definitions of myocardial infarction, types of stents used in the PCI arm, and the components of the primary outcome. CABG remains strongly recommended for patients with left main disease, whereas further studies are warranted to assess the value of PCI in this group.

FOLLOW-UP PATIENT CARE

Antiplatelet Therapy

Paramount to the success of CABG is long-term patency of the bypass grafts. Early studies found that the combination of aspirin (ASA) and dipyridamole led to improved vein graft patency

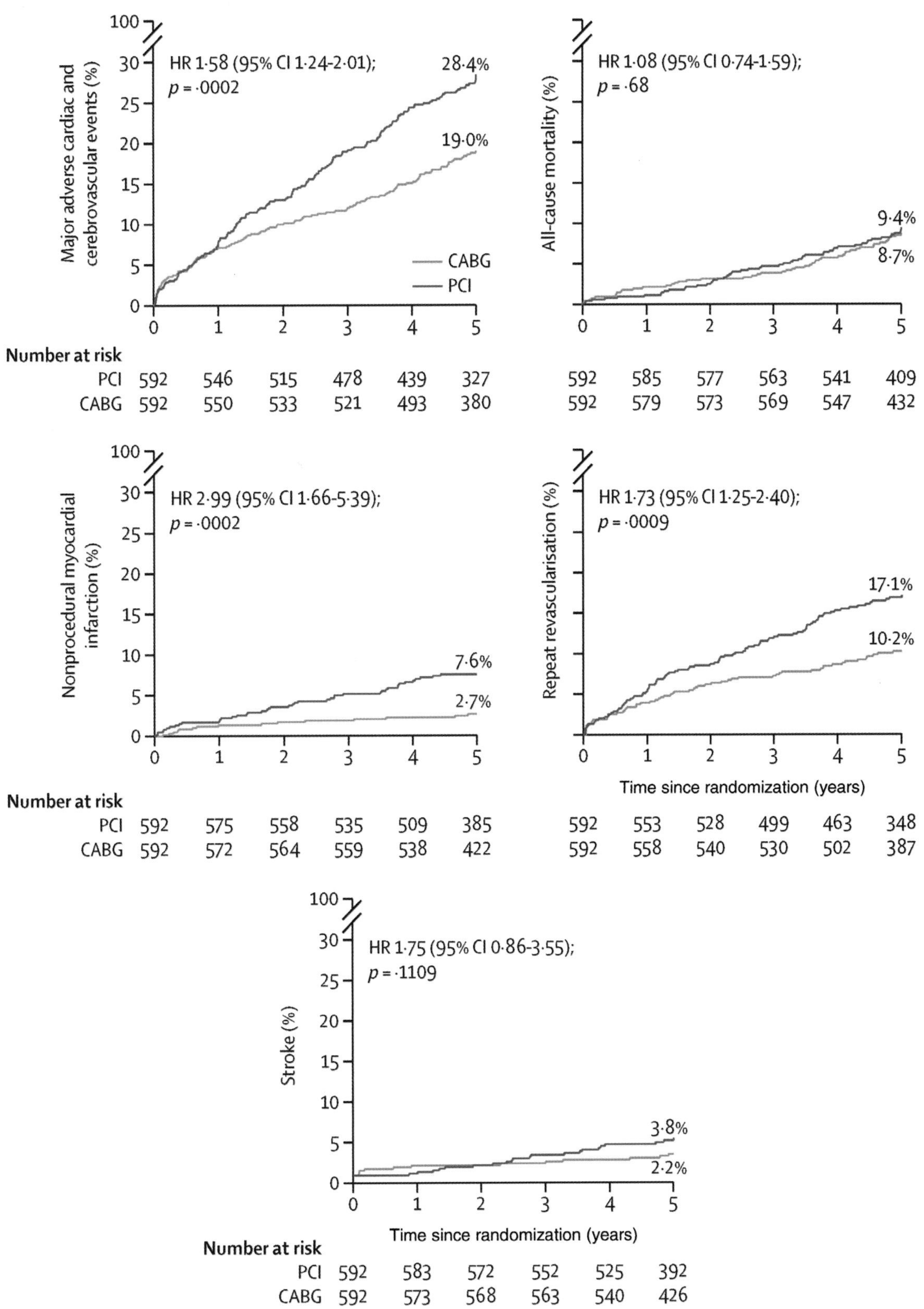

FIGURE 86.4 The Nordic-Baltic-British Left Main Revascularization (NOBLE) trial randomized 1201 patients from nine European countries with left main coronary artery disease requiring revascularization to CABG or PCI. The primary end point was a composite of all-cause mortality, nonprocedural myocardial infarction, repeat revascularization, and stroke. CABG was found to be superior to PCI for the primary composite end point. In subanalyses, all-cause mortality was similar, but nonprocedural myocardial infarction, and repeat revascularization was greater after PCI. CABG, Coronary arterial bypass grafting; PCI, percutaneous coronary intervention. (Reprinted from Holm NR, Mäkikallio T, Lindsay MM, et al.; NOBLE investigators. Percutaneous coronary angioplasty versus coronary artery bypass grafting in the treatment of unprotected left main stenosis: updated 5-year outcomes from the randomised, non-inferiority NOBLE trial. *Lancet.* 2020;395(10219):191-199. Copyright © 2019 Elsevier. With permission.)

after CABG. Later, the incremental benefit of dipyridamole was deemed to be minimal, and guidelines recommended postoperative ASA only. The 2011 AHA/ACC CABG Guidelines advocated lifelong ASA monotherapy at a dose ≥ 100 mg.[4] However, these guidelines have been further refined as additional information on clinical outcomes and graft patency has appeared. ASA in a dose of 100 to 325 mg daily is safe and effective and, ideally, should be administered within 6 hours after surgery.[39] In addition, multiple studies have evaluated dual antiplatelet therapy after CABG. A meta-analysis of five randomized studies comparing the combination of ASA and clopidogrel with ASA monotherapy showed a significantly lower incidence of vein graft occlusion at 1 year with dual antiplatelet therapy: no difference in arterial graft patency was observed.[40]

A 2015 American Heart Association scientific statement recommends the combination of aspirin and clopidogrel after OPCAB.[41] A systematic review and network meta-analysis examining 20 randomized trials concluded that dual antiplatelet therapy with ASA plus ticagrelor or ASA plus clopidogrel is effective in reducing saphenous-vein graft failure when compared with aspirin monotherapy. This analysis did not identify a significant difference in major bleeding, myocardial infarction, or death.[42] As a result, many surgical teams now initiate a P2Y12 inhibitor (usually clopidogrel) in the early postoperative period and continue it for up to 12 months. This is now a Class IIB recommendation of the American College of Cardiology/American Heart Association Task Force on Clinical Practice Guidelines.[40] Data are limited in assessing the effect of other strategies such as oral anticoagulants, but saphenous-vein graft failure was not reduced by the combination of ASA and rivaroxaban in one large trial.[43] Risks of bleeding should be considered when tailoring long-term therapy.

Secondary Prevention Measures—Guideline-Directed Strategies

A large amount of data has accumulated on postoperative management of patients following CABG. Many of the current recommendations follow guideline-directed strategies for managing patients with coronary artery disease, modified for patients who have undergone CABG.[41] Patients should undergo intensive lipid management after surgery, with a goal low-density lipoprotein cholesterol (LDL) of less than 100 mg/dL because evidence supports a reduction in progression of atherosclerosis in bypass grafts and the native coronary circulation as well as reduction in overall cardiovascular events when this is accomplished.[44] Current guidelines recommend high-intensity statin therapy (atorvastatin 40-80 mg or rosuvastatin 20-40 mg) as the preferred pharmacologic approach. Beta blocker drugs are also recommended in almost all patients following CABG. These agents are effective in preventing postoperative atrial fibrillation and have been shown to improve survival following myocardial infarction. Patients with preexisting LV systolic dysfunction may also gain a survival benefit with beta blocker therapy.

CABG patients frequently have associated cardiovascular risk factors, and appropriate treatment of these conditions improves long-term outcomes. This includes treatment of hypertension (with a focus on the use of beta blockers and angiotensin-converting enzyme inhibitors), diabetes (to achieve an HbA1c level <7%), and aggressive efforts at smoking cessation. Weight loss should be recommended for obese patients, even with consideration for bariatric surgery if lifestyle interventions are not effective. The subset of CABG patients who have LV dysfunction (LVEF < 40%) and a prior myocardial infarction deserve special consideration. Evidence suggests that these patients will realize benefits from beta blocker therapy, treatment with angiotensin-converting enzyme inhibitors or angiotensin receptor blocker, and, possibly, aldosterone antagonists. Patients with severely depressed LV function (EF < 35%) should have their LV function reassessed 3 months following CABG. If LV dysfunction of this magnitude persists, they should be considered for insertion of an implantable cardioverter-defibrillator. Finally, patients should be screened for depression after CABG, because depression is common and is associated with adverse outcomes,[45] and treatment can be effective. Enrollment in formal outpatient cardiac rehabilitation programs has also been found to be beneficial and should be recommended for all post-CABG patients.

RESEARCH AND FUTURE DIRECTIONS

Despite more than five decades of experience with CABG worldwide, the operation continues to be studied and to evolve. This evolution is progressing in multiple domains and includes refinement of indications to evaluate specific subgroups that may experience the greatest benefit from surgical revascularization, particularly in patients with reduced LV systolic function. The optimal method of assessing myocardial viability has not been established, and accurate prediction of myocardial viability may expand the use of CABG in patients with advanced heart failure. More work to expand our understanding of the benefits or limitations of multiple arterial grafts, particularly bilateral IMA grafts, is needed to guide surgical revascularization strategies. Additionally, future trials specifically assessing perioperative and postoperative antiplatelet and anticoagulant therapies are needed to optimize long-term graft patency and long-term patient outcomes. CABG has not seen as much progress in the area of minimally invasive approaches as valvular heart surgery, and novel approaches that offer smaller incisions with faster recovery are likely to appear. Studies examining methods to promote early recovery after surgery hold promise in reducing morbidity after CABG. Hybrid approaches, in which CABG and PCI are performed in combination to achieve myocardial revascularization deserve further clinical evaluation. As both CABG and PCI are dynamic fields, further comparisons between the two methods will continue. Furthermore, studies assessing the economic impact of CABG on health care costs and on overall cost-effectiveness in patients with advanced ischemic heart disease are needed.

KEY POINTS

- ✔ CABG has evolved over nearly six decades and remains the commonest cardiovascular operation performed in the world today.
- ✔ Indications for CABG fall into two broad categories: to control angina or prolong survival (or both). CABG is the preferred revascularization strategy in patients with more complex coronary artery disease (higher SYNTAX scores), left main coronary artery disease, depressed LV systolic function, and certain comorbidities such as diabetes mellitus.
- ✔ The commonest conduit used in bypass operations is the saphenous vein. Vein grafts are at risk for occlusion at rates that increase over time after CABG. ASA therapy reduces this risk, and recent data suggest that dual antiplatelet therapy may offer additional benefits on vein graft patency.
- ✔ The LIMA graft is the preferred conduit, particularly when used to graft the LAD, and has been shown to have superior patency rates and superior patient survival rates. The added value of bilateral IMA grafts is controversial. Radial-artery conduits have been shown to be superior to vein grafts up to 5 years after CABG.
- ✔ CABG can be performed without cardiopulmonary bypass (OPCAB procedure), but studies have not shown consistent advantages of OPCAB, and several studies suggest inferior bypass graft patency and less complete revascularization.
- ✔ Robust risk models have been developed that predict risk of early mortality following CABG. These have value in assessing treatment options and informing patients.
- ✔ The value of CABG is decreased in patients with diffuse coronary artery disease, severely depressed LV function with significant remodeling, and serious comorbidities. In these patients, a "heart team" approach—with input from the primary physician, cardiothoracic surgeon, cardiologist, and patient—is beneficial in selecting the optimal treatment pathway.
- ✔ The most serious complications after CABG include stroke, perioperative myocardial infarction, low-output state, renal failure, respiratory failure, prolonged ventilation, postoperative bleeding, reoperation, and infection or septicemia. A significant factor related to mortality is the failure to rescue the patient when one or more complications arise. CABG mortality rates correlate more strongly with failure to rescue than with absolute complication rates.
- ✔ Patients should receive GDMT after CABG to improve outcomes. This includes antiplatelet therapy, intensive lipid lowering therapy, treatment of hypertension, treatment of diabetes (if present), weight loss therapy, and aggressive efforts at smoking cessation.

REFERENCES

1. Favaloro RG. Critical analysis of coronary artery bypass graft surgery: a 30-year journey. *J. Am. Coll. Cardiol.* 1998;31:1b-63b.
2. Neumann FJ, Sousa-Uva M, Ahlsson A, et al. 2018 ESC/EACTS Guidelines on myocardial revascularization. *Eur. Heart J.* 2019;40 :87-165.
3. Fihn SD, Blankenship JC, Alexander KP, et al. 2014 ACC/AHA/AATS/PCNA/SCAI/STS focused update of the guideline for the diagnosis and management of patients with stable ischemic heart disease: a report of the American College of Cardiology/American Heart Association Task Force on Practice Guidelines, and the American Association for Thoracic Surgery, Preventive Cardiovascular Nurses Association, Society for Cardiovascular Angiography and Interventions, and Society of Thoracic Surgeons. *J. Am. Coll. Cardiol.* 2014;64:1929-1949.
4. Hillis LD, Smith PK, Anderson JL, et al. 2011 ACCF/AHA guideline for coronary artery bypass graft surgery: a report of the American College of Cardiology Foundation/American Heart Association Task Force on Practice Guidelines. *Circulation.* 2011;124:e652-e735. doi:10.1161/CIR.0b013e31823c074
5. Hueb W, Lopes N, Gersh BJ, et al. Ten-year follow-up survival of the Medicine, Angioplasty, or Surgery Study (MASS II): a randomized controlled clinical trial of 3 therapeutic strategies for multivessel coronary artery disease. *Circulation.* 2010;122(10):949-957. doi:10.1161/CIRCULATIONAHA.109.911669
6. Sá MPBO, Perazzo ÁM, Saragiotto FAS, et al. Coronary artery bypass graft surgery improves survival without increasing the risk of stroke in patients with ischemic heart failure in comparison to percutaneous coronary intervention: a meta-analysis with 54,173 patients. *Braz J Cardiovasc Surg.* 2019;34(4):396-405. doi:10.21470/1678-9741-2019-0170
7. Lee PH, Park H, Lee JS, Lee SW, Lee CW. Meta-analysis comparing the risk of myocardial infarction following coronary artery bypass grafting versus percutaneous coronary intervention in patients with multivessel or left main coronary artery disease. *Am J Cardiol.* 2019;124(6):842-850. doi:10.1016/j.amjcard.2019.06.009
8. Ram E, Sternik L, Klempfner R, et al. Outcomes of different revascularization strategies among patients presenting with acute coronary syndromes without ST elevation. *J Thorac Cardiovasc Surg.* 2020;160(4):926-935.e6. doi:10.1016/j.jtcvs.2019.08.130
9. Farkouh ME, Domanski M, Sleeper LA, et al. Strategies for multivessel revascularization in patients with diabetes *N Engl J Med.* 2012;367:2375-2384.
10. Farkouh ME, Domanski M, Dangas GD, et al. Long-term survival following multivessel revascularization in patients with diabetes: the FREEDOM follow-on study. *J Am Coll Cardiol.* 2019;73(6):629-638. doi:10.1016/j.jacc.2018.11.001
11. Gaipov A, Molnar MZ, Potukuchi PK, et al. Predialysis coronary revascularization and postdialysis mortality. *J Thorac Cardiovasc Surg.* 2019;157(3):976-983.e7. doi:10.1016/j.jtcvs.2018.08.107
12. Zenati MA, Bhatt DL, Bakaeen FG, et al. Randomized trial of endoscopic or open vein-graft harvesting for coronary-artery bypass. N Engl J Med. 2019;380:132-141.
13. Taggart DP, Benedetto U, Gerry S, et al. Bilateral versus single internal-thoracic-artery grafts at 10 years. *N Engl J Med.* 2019;380:437-446 doi:10.1056/NEJMoa1808783
14. Gaudino M, Benedetto U, Fremes S, et al. Radial-artery or saphenous-vein grafts in coronary-artery bypass surgery *N Engl J Med.* 2018;378:2069-2077. doi:10.1056/NEJMoa1716026
15. Møller CH, Penninga L, Wetterslev J, Steinbrüchel DA, Gluud C. Off-pump versus on-pump coronary artery bypass grafting for ischaemic heart disease. *Cochrane Database Syst Rev.* 2012 Mar 14;(3):CD007224. doi:10.1002/14651858.CD007224.pub2
16. Kowalewski M, Pawliszak W, Malvindi PG, et al. Off-pump coronary artery bypass grafting improves short-term outcomes in high-risk patients compared with on-pump coronary artery bypass grafting: Meta-analysis.

J Thorac Cardiovasc Surg. 2016;151(1):60-77.e58 doi:10.1016/j.jtcvs.2015.08.042

17. Sullivan PG, Wallach JD, Ioannidis JP. Meta-analysis comparing established risk prediction models (EuroSCORE II, STS Score, and ACEF Score) for perioperative mortality during cardiac surgery. *Am J Cardiol.* 2016;118(10):1574-1582. doi:10.1016/j.amjcard.2016.08.024
18. Kilic A, Goyal A, Miller JK, et al. Predictive utility of a machine learning algorithm in estimating mortality risk in cardiac surgery. *Ann Thorac Surg.* 2020;109(6):1811-1819. doi:10.1016/j.athoracsur.2019.09.049
19. Wang J, Gu C, Yu W, Gao M, Yu Y. Short-and long-term patient outcomes from combined coronary endarterectomy and coronary artery bypass grafting: a meta-analysis of 63,730 patients (PRISMA). *Medicine (Baltimore).* 2015;94(41):e1781. doi:10.1097/MD.0000000000001781
20. Fukunaga N, Ribeiro RVP, Lafreniere-Roula M, Manlhiot C, Badiwala MV, Rao V. Left ventricular size and outcomes in patients with left ventricular ejection fraction less than 20. *Ann Thorac Surg.* 2020 110(3):863-869. doi:10.1016/j.athoracsur.2020.01.005
21. Brown PP, Kugelmass AD, Cohen DJ, et al. The frequency and cost of complications associated with coronary artery bypass grafting surgery: results from the United States Medicare program. *Ann Thorac Surg.* 2008;85(6):1980-1986. doi:10.1016/j.athoracsur.2008.01.053
22. Bennett-Guerrero E, Zhao Y, O'Brien SM, et al. Variation in use of blood transfusion in coronary artery bypass graft surgery. *JAMA.* 2010;304(14):1568-1575. doi:10.1001/jama.2010.1406
23. Edwards FH, Ferraris VA, Kurlansky PA, et al. Failure to rescue rates after coronary artery bypass grafting: an analysis from the society of thoracic surgeons adult cardiac surgery database. *Ann Thorac Surg.* 2016;102(2):458-464. doi:10.1016/j.athoracsur.2016.04.051
24. Veldkamp RF, Valk SD, van Domburg RT, van Herwerden LA, Meeter K. Mortality and repeat interventions up until 20 years after aorto-coronary bypass surgery with saphenous vein grafts. A follow-up study of 1041 patients. *Eur Heart J.* 2000;21:747-753. doi:10.1053/euhj.1999.1867
25. Adelborg K, Horváth-Puhó E, Schmidt M, et al. Thirty-year mortality after coronary artery bypass graft surgery. *Circ Cardiovasc Qual Outcomes.* 2017;10:e002708. doi:10.1161/CIRCOUTCOMES.116.002708
26. Shahian DM, O'Brien SM, Sheng S, et al. Predictors of long-term survival after coronary artery bypass grafting surgery. *Circulation.* 2012;125:1491-1500 doi:10.1161/CIRCULATIONAHA.111.066902
27. Fosbol EL, Zhao Y, Shahian DM, Grover FL, Edwards FH, Peterson ED. Repeat coronary revascularization after coronary artery bypass surgery in older adults: the Society of Thoracic Surgeons' national experience, 1991-2007. *Circulation.* 2013;127:1656-1663.
28. Mori M, Wang Y, Murugiah K, et al. Trends in reoperative coronary artery bypass graft surgery for older adults in the United States, 1998 to 2017. *J Am Heart Assoc.* 2020;9(20):e016980. doi:10.1161/JAHA.120.016980
29. Elbadawi A, Hamed M, Elgendy IY, et al. Outcomes of reoperative coronary artery bypass graft surgery in the United States. *J Am Heart Assoc.* 2020;9(15):e016282. doi:10.1161/JAHA.120.016282
30. Bakaeen FG, Akras Z, Svensson LG. Redo coronary artery bypass grafting. Indian *J Thorac Cardiovasc Surg.* 2018;34(suppl 3):272-278. doi:10.1007/s12055-018-0651-1
31. Yusuf S, Zucker D, Peduzzi P, et al. Effect of coronary artery bypass graft surgery on survival: overview of 10-year results from randomised trials by the Coronary Artery Bypass Graft Surgery Trialists Collaboration. *Lancet.* 1994;344:563-570.
32. Velazquez EJ, Lee KL, Deja MA, et al. Coronary-artery bypass surgery in patients with left ventricular dysfunction. *N Engl J Med.* 2011;364:1607-1616.
33. Velazquez EJ, Lee KL, Jones RH, et al. Coronary-artery bypass surgery in patients with ischemic cardiomyopathy. *N Engl J Med.* 2016;374:1511-1520.
34. Head SJ, Milojevic M, Daemen J, et al. Mortality after coronary artery bypass grafting versus percutaneous coronary intervention with stenting for coronary artery disease: a pooled analysis of individual patient data. *Lancet.* 2018;391(10124):939-948. doi:10.1016/S0140-6736(18)30423-9. Erratum in: *Lancet.* 2018;392(10146):476.
35. Serruys PW, Morice MC, Kappetein AP, et al. Percutaneous coronary intervention versus coronary-artery bypass grafting for severe coronary artery disease. *N Engl J Med.* 2009;360(10):961-972. doi:10.1056/NEJMoa0804626. Erratum in: *N Engl J Med.* 2013;368(6):584.
36. Mohr FW, Morice MC, Kappetein AP, et al. Coronary artery bypass graft surgery versus percutaneous coronary intervention in patients with three-vessel disease and left main coronary disease: 5-year follow-up of the randomised, clinical SYNTAX trial. *Lancet.* 2013;381(9867):629-638. doi: 10.1016/S0140-6736(13)60141-5
37. Thuijs DJFM, Kappetein AP, Serruys PW, et al. Percutaneous coronary intervention versus coronary artery bypass grafting in patients with three-vessel or left main coronary artery disease: 10-year follow-up of the multicentre randomised controlled SYNTAX trial. *Lancet.* 2019;394(10206):1325-1334. doi:10.1016/S0140-6736(19)31997-X. Erratum in: *Lancet.* 2020;395(10227):870.
38. Holm NR, Mäkikallio T, Lindsay MM, et al. Percutaneous coronary angioplasty versus coronary artery bypass grafting in the treatment of unprotected left main stenosis: updated 5-year outcomes from the randomised, non-inferiority NOBLE trial. *Lancet.* 2020;395(10219):191-199. doi:10.1016/S0140-6736(19)32972-1
39. Fremes SE, Levinton C, Naylor CD, Chen E, Christakis GT, Goldman BS. Optimal antithrombotic therapy following aortocoronary bypass: a metaanalysis. *Eur J Cardiothorac Surg.* 1993;7:169-180.
40. Nocerino AG, Achenbach S, Taylor AJ. Meta-analysis of effect of single versus dual antiplatelet therapy on early patency of bypass conduits after coronary artery bypass grafting. *Am J Cardiol.* 2013;112:1576-1579.
41. Kulik A, Ruel M, Jneid H, et al. Secondary prevention after coronary artery bypass graft surgery: a scientific statement from the American Heart Association. *Circulation.* 2015;131:927-964. doi:10.1161/CIR.0000000000000182
42. Solo K, Lavi S, Kabali C, et al. Antithrombotic treatment after coronary artery bypass graft surgery: systematic review and network meta-analysis. *BMJ.* 2019;367:l5476 doi:10.1136/bmj.l5476
43. Lamy A, Eikelboom J, Sheth T, et al. Rivaroxaban, aspirin, or both to prevent early coronary bypass graft occlusion: the COMPASSCABG study. *J Am Coll Cardiol.* 2019;73:121-130. doi:10.1016/j.jacc.2018.10.048
44. Knatterud GL, Rosenberg Y, Campeau L, et al Long-term effects on clinical outcomes of aggressive lowering of low-density lipoprotein cholesterol levels and low-dose anticoagulation in the Post Coronary Artery Bypass Graft Trial: Post CABG Investigators. *Circulation.* 2000;102:157-165.
45. Blumenthal JA, Lett HS, Babyak MA, et al. Depression as a risk factor for mortality after coronary artery bypass surgery. *Lancet.* 2003;362:604-609. doi:10.1016/S0140-6736(03)14190-6

CHAPTER 87

AORTIC VALVE SURGERY

Andres Samayoa Mendez and Amy E. Hackmann

INTRODUCTION

Aortic valve surgery has evolved from aortic valvotomy in the 1940s to the technologically advanced percutaneous techniques of today. Much improvement has been made through the years in surgical approach, valve design, and patient management. Surgical replacement of the aortic valve remains the gold standard for treating aortic valve disease.

INDICATIONS

The most common indications for aortic valve surgery are valve stenosis and regurgitation, with aortic stenosis (AS) being the most prevalent heart valve disease. Indications for aortic valve surgery are based on the 2014 American Heart Association (AHA)/American College of Cardiology (ACC) Valvular Heart Disease Guidelines and the focused 2017 update.[1,2] Diagnosis is most commonly made after physical examination findings demonstrate a murmur, leading to a transthoracic echocardiogram or a patient presents with typical symptoms. Adjunctive diagnostic studies may include angiography for measurement of pressure gradients across the aortic valve or to identify regurgitant flow. Cardiac-gated computed tomography (CT) scan and cardiac magnetic resonance imaging may also be used to assess aortic valve pathology.

Aortic Stenosis

The primary indication for intervention is symptomatic (stage D) severe AS, which is typically characterized by echocardiographic peak flow velocity (V_{max}) ≥4 m/s, mean gradient (MG) of ≥40 mm Hg, or an aortic valve area (AVA) ≤1.0 cm^2. However, there are actually three defined stages of symptomatic, severe AS by echocardiographic criteria. Stage D1 is high-gradient AS with V_{max} of ≥4m/s, MG of ≥40 mm Hg, and AVA ≤1.0 cm^2. D2 is commonly referred to as low-flow, low-gradient AS and is characterized by V_{max} ≤4 m/s, MG of ≤40 mm Hg, and AVA of ≤1.0 cm^2 with reduced left ventricular ejection fraction (LVEF < 50%). Stage D3 is low-gradient with normal LVEF or paradoxical low flow with AVA of ≤1.0 cm^2, V_{max} ≤4 m/s or MG of ≤40 mm Hg, indexed AVA ≤0.6 cm^2/m^2, or stroke volume index <35 mL/m^2.

Typical symptoms of severe stenosis are syncope or presyncope by history or on exercise testing, exertional dyspnea, reduced exercise tolerance, angina, and heart failure. Indications for aortic valve surgery are summarized in **Table 87.1**.

Surgical Aortic Valve Replacement Versus Transcatheter Aortic Valve Replacement for Aortic Stenosis

When deciding upon surgical aortic valve replacement (SAVR) versus transcatheter aortic valve replacement (TAVR), a comprehensive Heart Valve Team should aid in the candidacy for either approach. The Heart Team is usually integrated by cardiac surgery, cardiology, interventional cardiology, and cardiac anesthesia.[3] The decisions are made based on the Society of Thoracic Surgeons (STS) predicted risk of mortality, with intermediate risk being 4% to 8% and high risk ≥8%, patient frailty, comorbid conditions, and patient preference. The indications for TAVR are rapidly changing with evolving technologies and mounting TAVR long-term data.[4,5] Primary recommendations are (1) surgical SAVR for patients who meet aortic valve replacement (AVR) indications with low or intermediate surgical risk; (2) TAVR or high-risk SAVR in high surgical risk patients based on Heart Team assessment; and (3) TAVR is recommended in patients with prohibitive surgical risk and/or a predictive postprocedure survival of more than 12 months. TAVR is a reasonable alternative (Class IIa) in patients with severe AS and intermediate surgical risk based on the Heart Team assessment. Percutaneous aortic balloon dilation may be considered (Class IIb) as a bridge to SAVR or TAVR in patients with severe AS who are severely symptomatic or need a delay in definitive therapy for other reasons.

Aortic Regurgitation

Indications for intervention depend on the acuity of aortic regurgitation (AR). Acute AR secondary to aortic dissection or infective endocarditis is a surgical emergency, and early AVR results in better outcomes.[1,6] Patients may present with hypotension, systemic hypoperfusion, and/or pulmonary edema. Chronic AR can present with symptoms of angina, exertional dyspnea, or heart failure symptoms. Severe AR characteristics include jet width more than 65% of left ventricular outflow tract, vena contracta greater than 0.60 cm, holo-diastolic flow reversal in the proximal abdominal aorta, regurgitant volume greater than or equal to 60 mL/beat, regurgitant fraction greater than or equal to 50%, effective regurgitant orifice area (EROA) ≥0.30 cm^2, angiography grade 3+ to 4+, and left ventricular dilation. Recommendations for aortic valve surgery are summarized in Table 87.1. Surgical AVR is the treatment for AR; however, a growing number of reports in the literature demonstrate TAVR as a potential therapy in highly selected cases.

TABLE 87.1 Indications for Aortic Valve Replacement

	Class of Recommendation	Recommendations
Aortic stenosis	Class I (should)	Stage D1 AS
		Asymptomatic severe AS and LVEF < 50%
		Severe AS undergoing other cardiac surgery
	Class IIa (reasonable)	Asymptomatic critical AS (MG ≥ 60 mm Hg and V_{max} ≥ 5 m/s) and low surgical risk
		Asymptomatic severe AS with decreased exercise tolerance or decreased blood pressure during exercise
		Stage D2 with V_{max} ≥ 4m/s or MG ≥ 40 mm Hg on low-dose dobutamine stress test
		Stage D3, normotensive, LVEF > 50% with AS as the most likely cause of symptoms
		Moderate AS undergoing other cardiac surgery
	Class IIb (may be considered)	Asymptomatic severe AS, rapid disease progression, and low surgical risk
Aortic regurgitation (chronic)	Class I (should)	Symptomatic severe AR
		Asymptomatic severe AR and LVEF < 50%
		Severe AR undergoing other cardiac surgery
	Class IIa (reasonable)	Asymptomatic severe AR, LVEF ≥ 50%, and severe LV dilation (LVESD > 50 mm)
		Moderate AR undergoing other cardiac surgeries
	Class IIb (may be considered)	Asymptomatic severe AR, LVEF < 50%, and progressive severe LV dilation (LVEDD > 65 mm)

AR, aortic regurgitation; AS, aortic stenosis; LV, left ventricle; LVEDD, left ventricular end-diastolic dimension; LVEF, left ventricular ejection fraction; LVESD, left ventricular end-systolic ejection fraction; MG, mean gradient; V_{max}, maximum aortic velocity.

Choice of Valve Type

The choice of valve type for each patient includes a number of factors, many of which are nonmedical. For patients younger than 50 years and able to take chronic anticoagulation, mechanical valves are generally preferred.[7,8] For those older than 70 years, bioprosthetic valves are recommended. For those with occupations or hobbies that prohibit anticoagulants, or patients unable to take anticoagulation routinely, bioprosthetic valves should be considered. For women of childbearing age, the risk of fetal complications associated with chronic anticoagulation for a mechanical valve needs to be weighed against the rapid deterioration that may occur with a bioprosthesis. With the approval of TAVR for valve-in-valve replacement, the age at which more bioprosthetic valves than mechanical valves are used is decreasing rapidly.[9]

ANATOMIC CONSIDERATIONS

The aortic root components include the sinuses of Valsalva, interleaflet triangles, and the cusps of the leaflets. It extends from the aortic annulus to the sinotubular junction and typically measures 2 to 3 cm in length. The aortic annulus has multiple definitions. The surgical annulus is where the cusps attach to the aortic wall and is the anatomic division between the left ventricle and the sinus of Valsalva (**Figure 87.1**). Radiographically, the annulus is the virtual basal ring that is formed by an imaginary line connecting the base of each cusp.[10,11]

The aortic valve opens and closes 2 to 3 billion times during an average lifetime and is normally formed by three semilunar valves that prevent retrograde flow to the left ventricle during diastole. The valve cusps attach to the aortic wall in a crescentic fashion. Adjacent cusps come together forming the commissures. The sinuses of Valsalva are the dilated pockets in the aortic root behind the cusps.[12] The sinuses are named based on the position of the coronary ostia: left, right, and noncoronary sinuses. The left coronary ostium diameter measures 3 to 5 mm. The right coronary ostium diameter is usually smaller, 2 to 3 mm.[13]

Important structural relationships need to be taken into consideration while operating in this space. The right noncoronary commissure is related to the membranous septum. The noncoronary sinus and the left noncoronary commissure are in continuity with the aortomitral curtain. The left bundle of His lies beneath the right noncoronary commissure, which is also in close relationship to the right atrium, and the right-left commissure is in close relationship with the right ventricular outflow tract. The left noncoronary commissure and the left coronary sinus are in close relation to the dome of the left atrium.[11]

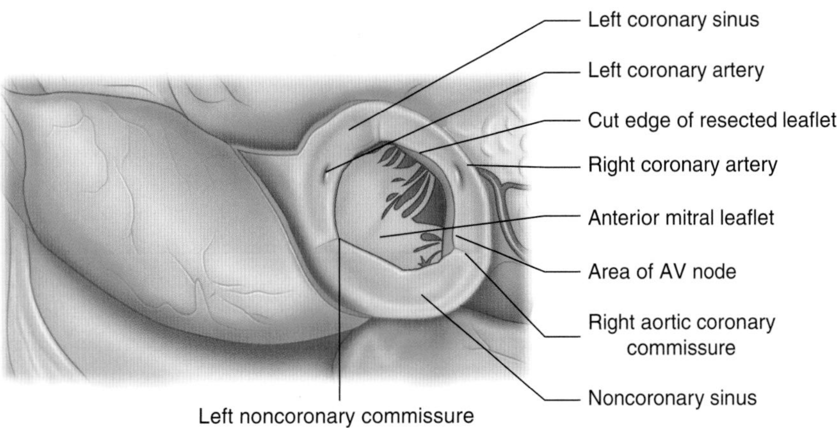

FIGURE 87.1 Relevant surgical anatomy and the aortic valve as seen from the surgeon's view. The valve leaflets have been excised to demonstrate the aortic annulus and relevant structures.

FUNDAMENTALS OF AORTIC VALVE REPLACEMENT

The typical surgical approach is via median sternotomy. Alternative approaches are partial sternotomy and right thoracotomy with good results.[14,15] After dividing the pericardium and exposing the ascending aorta, the patient is placed on cardiopulmonary bypass via cannulas in the ascending aorta and right atrium. A left ventricular vent can be placed through the right superior pulmonary vein or directly through the aortic valve into the ventricle to avoid fibrillation or left ventricular dilation. The patient is cooled depending on local practices, commonly to 32 °C. Cardioplegia can be administered antegrade, retrograde, directly in the coronary ostia, or by some combination of these approaches. Cardioplegia should be re-dosed as needed, being mindful that most patients with AS have some degree of left ventricular hypertrophy.

To allow for aortic cross-clamping as well as the aortotomy closure, the aortopulmonary window is dissected with electrocautery. Carbon dioxide can be instilled in the chest cavity to help displace room air. Once the heart is arrested, an aortotomy is made at least 1 cm above the right coronary artery. The right and left coronary ostia are identified. The aortotomy is extended with a transverse or oblique incision using scissors. The aorta can be transected if needed, but usually a transverse or oblique incision will give sufficient exposure for AVR (**Figure 87.2A,B**).

The valve is excised sharply. Any annular calcium is debrided sharply and with blunt crushing using heavy graspers or a pituitary rongeur. Sufficient calcium needs to be removed to allow placement of the annular stitches and permit the sewing cuff of the valve to contact the annular tissue circumferentially. Attention must be paid to avoid denuding the endocardium or injure neighboring structures. After completing the annular debridement, the area is irrigated with abundant cold saline to remove any calcium or other small debris.

The annulus is sized using valve sizers specific to the type of valve chosen and is not interchangeable. Annular stitches are placed 1 mm apart using braided, nonabsorbable sutures, commonly 2-0 or 3-0 Ethibond (ie, polyester). The valve is implanted in a supra-annular technique, with horizontal mattress, pledgeted sutures going from ventricle to aorta, thus the pledgets stay in the subannular position (**e-Figure 87.1 A,B**).

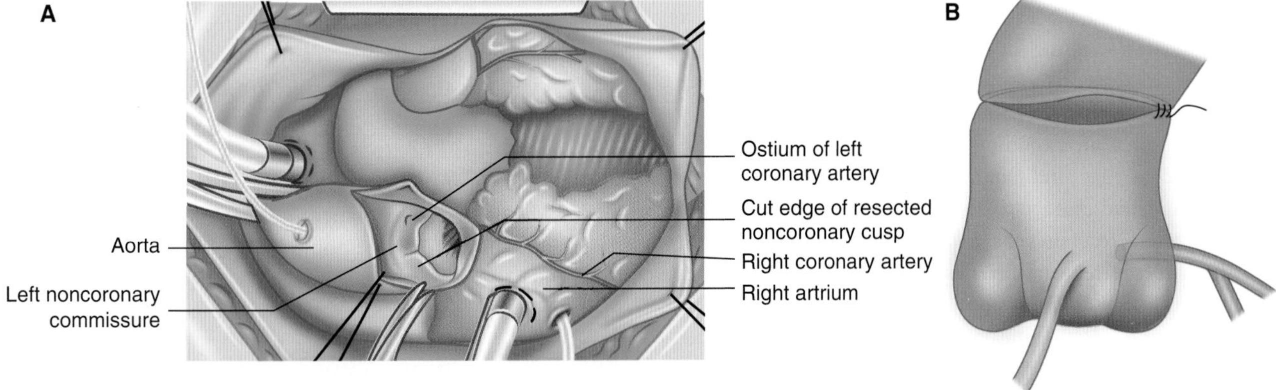

FIGURE 87.2 **A,B:** After the aorta is cross-clamped and the heart is arrested, an anterior transverse aortotomy is made. The valve is visualized through the initial aortotomy, and the incision is extended toward the noncoronary sinus. The aortic valve leaflets are resected and annular calcium debrided. The valve is sized using standard valve sizers. **B:** The initial aortic incision is made a minimum of 1 cm above the right coronary artery and extended toward the noncoronary cusp. This incision can be transverse as depicted or curvilinear toward the nadir of the noncoronary sinus. Stay sutures can be placed as needed to aid visualization.

The supra-annular valve positioning has shown superior transvalvular hemodynamics compared with the intra-annular position.[16] If using nonpledgeted sutures, studies have shown a low perivalvular leak rate and decreased cross-clamp and cardiopulmonary bypass times.[17,18] For the smaller annulus, simple interrupted sutures or a continuous running suture might increase the effective orifice area (EOA), hence reducing the risk of patient-prosthesis mismatch.[19]

After suture placement, the annulus is assessed for the final valve size. It is best to place a valve of appropriate size, as either over- or undersizing can negatively impact valve function and long-term durability. The sutures are passed through the sewing ring and then tied or secured with an automated fastener. The valve is examined to ensure there is no valve damage during implant and proper opening and closing of the leaflets (mechanical valves). Both left and right coronary arteries are examined for obstruction by the sewing ring. A dental mirror can also be used to examine the position of the valve and the pledgets.

The aortotomy is closed in two layers, using polypropylene sutures with or without pledgets. The patient is rewarmed and then the cross-clamp is removed after Valsalva maneuvers to evacuate air from the pulmonary veins and the left ventricle. Transesophageal echocardiography is used to examine the adequacy of de-airing of the heart before removing the left ventricular vent and separating from cardiopulmonary bypass. The valve is evaluated with echocardiography for heart function, perivalvular leak, prosthetic valve function, and mitral valve function. Temporary pacing wires are placed.

FUNDAMENTALS OF TRANSCATHETER AORTIC VALVE REPLACEMENT

Transcatheter AVR is a rapidly changing field, with newer devices often developed before the previous generation completes clinical trials. The main types of transcatheter valves currently available are balloon-expandable and self-expanding devices. The type and size of the device is selected using preoperative studies, usually a contrast-enhanced, electrocardiogram-gated CT scan of the aorta, iliac, and femoral arteries. Multiple factors are considered in selecting the correct valve size, type, and access site. Preoperative aortic root evaluation is necessary for assessing the left ventricular outflow tract, annulus, sinuses of Valsalva, sinotubular junction, ascending aorta, and coronary ostia. The ascending aorta, iliac, and femoral arteries need to be evaluated for size, shape, and characteristics of calcium deposits.[20]

Multiple access sites have been described. The preferable sites are the femoral arteries, and with smaller devices, this access is suitable in approximately 95% of patients (**e-Figure 87.2**).[21] Other access sites are transcarotid, axillary or subclavian, transaortic, transapical, brachiocephalic, and transcaval.[22]

In the hybrid operating room or the cardiac catheterization laboratory, the patient is placed in the supine position. Commonly, a cardiac surgeon and an interventional cardiologist perform the procedure together. General anesthesia or deep sedation can be used based on local experience and patient comorbidities. The patient is prepared with monitoring lines, and a temporary transvenous pacemaker is placed in the right ventricle. The common femoral arteries are accessed with small sheaths, and preclosure sutures can be placed on the valve access site. A pigtail catheter is placed in the coronary cusp that will be used as a marker of the annulus. The base of the leaflets is identified with angiography, and all leaflets are placed at a coplanar level to determine the best fluoroscopic deployment view. The aortic valve is crossed with a flexible wire and subsequently exchanged to a stiff wire. Predeployment balloon dilatation can then be performed under rapid ventricular pacing if indicated. The valve delivery device is passed over the wire, positioned, and deployed. The deployment position and mechanism vary depending on the type of valve. After the valve is placed, an echocardiogram is performed to further assess the valve function and position, coronary flow, and paravalvular leak and to rule out a new pericardial effusion. A postdeployment balloon dilatation can be performed if a significant paravalvular leak is identified. At the end of the procedure, the femoral access points are closed with percutaneous techniques, or with open femoral repair if the percutaneous route fails or in heavily diseased vessels.

SPECIAL CONSIDERATIONS AND CONTRAINDICATIONS

Small Annulus and Patient-Prosthesis Mismatch

Patients with a small aortic annulus have an increased risk of receiving an aortic valve with a small EOA. If the EOA is small in relation to the patient's body surface area (BSA), the patient may suffer from patient-prosthesis mismatch. This can affect cardiac function, prosthetic thrombosis, cardiac events, rehospitalizations, sudden death, and overall mortality.[23-27] To identify patient-prosthesis mismatch, the indexed EOA (ie, EOA divided by BSA) needs to be calculated. An indexed EOA $\leq 0.85\ cm^2/m^2$ is considered the threshold for patient-prosthesis mismatch. Furthermore, an indexed EOA of 0.65 to $0.85\ cm^2/m^2$ is classified as moderate and less than $0.65\ cm^2/m^2$ as severe.[26] The impact on outcome correlates with the severity of patient-prosthesis mismatch and the age of the patient, with patients younger than 60 years old the most affected.[26,28]

To prevent patient-prosthesis mismatch, the minimal valve size for the patient needs to be calculated to obtain an indexed EOA $> 0.85\ cm^2/m^2$. This can affect the type and brand of valve that will be offered to the patient because the EOA for each differs. If, after measuring the annulus, the minimal valve size is too small and patient-prosthesis mismatch is expected, a root enlargement should be considered, especially in younger, active patients.

Aortic Root Enlargement

Aortic root enlargement is a safe addition to the AVR operation. In a meta-analysis of nine observational studies, no difference in early and late mortality was observed with aortic root enlargement followed by AVR compared to AVR alone. Furthermore, there was no difference in permanent pacemaker implantation, reoperation for bleeding, or stroke. Longer cardiopulmonary bypass and cross-clamp times were observed with aortic root involvement, with a mean difference of 20 and 14 minutes, respectively.[29]

Two main techniques are used to enlarge the aortic root in adults: Nicks and Manouguian (e-Figure 87.3 A-C). Several modifications exist to these procedures, but the main principles to achieve aortic root enlargement persist.

Nicks Technique, first described in 1970 by Nicks et al, the aorta is incised, the leaflets and calcium are removed, and the aortic incision is extended across the noncoronary sinus and through the annulus, finishing at the origin of the mitral valve.[30] A bovine pericardial patch is sewn with continuous sutures starting at the mitral valve origin and continuing to cover the entire aortotomy. The valve is implanted in the usual fashion at the level of the annulus. This often allows an increase in aortic root diameter of 2 mm or one valve size.

Manouguian Technique described in 1979 by Manouguian et al, the aorta is incised, the leaflets and calcium are removed, then the aortotomy is extended into the left and noncoronary commissure.[31] The incision is extended through the fibrous trigone and about 1 cm into the anterior mitral leaflet. This results in an opening in the left atrium which needs to be patched. A separate ovoid or diamond-shaped patch is sutured in a running fashion, starting at the mitral valve defect. The valve is implanted in the standard fashion and the remaining patch is integrated into the aortotomy closure.

Porcelain Aorta

The prevalence of porcelain aorta (ie, severe circumferential calcification of the aorta) was 7.5% in a study of consecutive patients undergoing AS evaluation.[32] The risk is increased in patients with chronic kidney disease, radiation-induced heart disease, and systemic inflammatory diseases.[33] The presence of extensive calcifications during cardiac surgery is associated with an increased risk of stroke and death. A porcelain aorta can be identified preoperatively with a chest x-ray or with CT scan. Intraoperatively, the best tool for identification is epiaortic ultrasonography, as it assists with choosing cannulation and cross-clamp sites in cases with patchy aortic calcifications.[34] If unsafe to cannulate or clamp the aorta, an alternative cannulation site can be chosen, and the valve replacement can be done in deep hypothermic circulatory arrest. Alternatively, an area of the ascending aorta can be endarterectomized under circulatory arrest, then the cross-clamp is applied and the valve replaced while rewarming the patient. For heavily calcified ascending aortas, a tube graft is rarely used to replace the ascending aorta. TAVR is a viable option for the porcelain aorta and is used with increasing frequency; currently, it is the preferred method for AVR for heavily calcified aortas.

FOLLOW-UP PATIENT CARE

Patients after AVR require follow-up for heart and valve function over time. Most commonly, an echocardiogram is performed annually and with any symptoms that might indicate valve dysfunction such as shortness of breath or heart failure. Endocarditis prophylaxis for procedures is recommended lifelong. Antiplatelet and anticoagulant management varies based on local protocols and valve choice.

RESEARCH AND FUTURE DIRECTIONS

The most rapidly changing valve technologies are the transcatheter valves and delivery systems. Lessons learned have been applied to surgical valve technology, as well, such as "suture-less" aortic valves or valves stored dry, rather than in glutaraldehyde. One type of bioprosthetic valve is designed to expand when a TAVR is deployed valve-in-valve. Selected centers perform AVR for AR, using an annuloplasty ring and leaflet repair.[35] Long-term data on this technique are minimal. Studies are ongoing of lower anticoagulation targets for selected mechanical valves and could include the use of direct oral anticoagulants in place of warfarin in the future.

KEY POINTS

- ✔ Aortic stenosis is often detected by physical examination.
- ✔ Acute AR is a surgical emergency, and early AVR results in better outcomes.
- ✔ Mechanical valves are recommended for patients younger than 50 years and bioprosthetic valves for those 70 years of age and older.
- ✔ Patient-prosthesis mismatch is related to worse outcomes, especially in patients younger than 60 years.
- ✔ The Heart Team approach to decision-making for AVR benefits patients chosen for both surgical and transcatheter approaches.
- ✔ Aortic root enlargement techniques can allow larger valve sizes, thus reducing the risk of patient-prosthesis mismatch.
- ✔ Especially with more advanced transcatheter technologies, younger patients are choosing bioprosthetic valves.

REFERENCES

1. Nishimura RA, Otto CM, Bonow RO, et al. 2014 AHA/ACC guideline for the management of patients with valvular heart disease: a report of the American College of Cardiology/American Heart Association Task Force on Practice Guidelines [published correction appears in *J Thorac Cardiovasc Surg.* 2014;64(16):1763. Dosage error in article text]. *J Thorac Cardiovasc Surg.* 2014;148(1):e1-e132. doi:10.1016/j.jtcvs.2014.05.014
2. Nishimura RA, Otto CM, Bonow RO, et al. 2017 AHA/ACC focused update of the 2014 AHA/ACC guideline for the management of patients with valvular heart disease: a report of the American College of Cardiology/American Heart Association Task Force on Clinical Practice Guidelines. *Circulation.* 2017;135(25):e1159-e1195. doi:10.1161/CIR.0000000000000503
3. Sintek M, Zajarias A. Patient evaluation and selection for transcatheter aortic valve replacement: the heart team approach. *Prog Cardiovasc Dis.* 2014;56(6):572-582. doi:10.1016/j.pcad.2014.02.003

4. Blackman DJ, Saraf S, MacCarthy PA, et al. Long-term durability of transcatheter aortic valve prostheses. *J Am Coll Cardiol.* 2019;73(5):537-545. doi:10.1016/j.jacc.2018.10.078
5. Daubert MA, Weissman NJ, Hahn RT, et al. Long-term valve performance of TAVR and SAVR: a report from the PARTNER I Trial. *JACC Cardiovasc Imaging.* 2016;S1936-878X(16)30895-6. doi:10.1016/j.jcmg.2016.11.004
6. Akinseye OA, Pathak A, Ibebuogu UN. Aortic valve regurgitation: a comprehensive review. *Curr Probl Cardiol.* 2018;43(8):315-334. doi:10.1016/j.cpcardiol.2017.10.004
7. Goldstone AB, Chiu P, Baiocchi M, et al. Mechanical or biologic prostheses for aortic-valve and mitral-valve replacement. *N Engl J Med.* 2017;377(19):1847-1857. doi:10.1056/NEJMoa1613792
8. Briffa NP. Results of mechanical versus tissue AVR: caution in young patients with tissue AVR. Heart 2019;105(suppl 2):s34-s37. doi: 10.1136/heartjnl-2018-313516
9. Hirji SA, Kolkailah AA, Ramirez-Del Val, F, et al. Mechanical versus bioprosthetic aortic valve replacement in patients aged 50 years and younger. *Ann Thorac Surg.* 2018;106(4):1113-1121. https://doi.org/10.1016/j.athoracsur.2018.05.073
10. Kunihara T. Anatomy of the aortic root: implications for aortic root reconstruction. *Gen Thorac Cardiovasc Surg.* 2017;65(9):488-499. doi:10.1007/s11748-017-0792-y
11. De Paulis R, Salica A. Surgical anatomy of the aortic valve and root-implications for valve repair. *Ann Cardiothorac Surg.* 2019;8(3):313-321. doi:10.21037/acs.2019.04.16
12. Schoen FJ. Evolving concepts of cardiac valve dynamics: the continuum of development, functional structure, pathobiology, and tissue engineering. *Circulation.* 2008;118(18):1864-1880. doi:10.1161/CIRCULATIONAHA.108.805911
13. James TN. Anatomy of the coronary arteries in health and disease. *Circulation.* 1965;32(6):1020-1033. doi:10.1161/01.cir.32.6.1020
14. Ghanta RK, Lapar DJ, Kern JA, et al. Minimally invasive aortic valve replacement provides equivalent outcomes at reduced cost compared with conventional aortic valve replacement: a real-world multi-institutional analysis. *J Thorac Cardiovasc Surg.* 2015;149(4):1060-1065. doi:10.1016/j.jtcvs.2015.01.014
15. Tabata M, Umakanthan R, Cohn LH, et al. Early and late outcomes of 1000 minimally invasive aortic valve operations. *Eur J Cardiothorac Surg.* 2008;33(4):537-541. doi:10.1016/j.ejcts.2007.12.037
16. Kim SH, Kim HJ, Kim JB, et al. Supra-annular versus intra-annular prostheses in aortic valve replacement: impact on haemodynamics and clinical outcomes. *Interact Cardiovasc Thorac Surg.* 2019;28(1):58-64. doi:10.1093/icvts/ivy190
17. Chan PG, Chan EG, Seese L, et al. Safety and feasibility of a nonpledgeted suture technique for heart valve replacement. *JAMA Surg.* 2019;154(3):260-261. doi:10.1001/jamasurg.2018.4243
18. LaPar DJ, Ailawadi G, Bhamidipati CM, et al. Use of a nonpledgeted suture technique is safe and efficient for aortic valve replacement. *J Thorac Cardiovasc Surg.* 2011;141(2):388-393. doi:10.1016/j.jtcvs.2010.04.011
19. Tabata M, Shibayama K, Watanabe H, et al. Simple interrupted suturing increases valve performance after aortic valve replacement with a small supra-annular bioprosthesis. *J Thorac Cardiovasc Surg.* 2014;147(1):321-325. doi:10.1016/j.jtcvs.2012.11.020
20. Francone M, Budde RPJ, Bremerich J, et al. CT and MR imaging prior to transcatheter aortic valve implantation: standardisation of scanning protocols, measurements and reporting-a consensus document by the European Society of Cardiovascular Radiology (ESCR) [published correction appears in *Eur Radiol.* 2020 Mar 2]. *Eur Radiol.* 2020;30(5):2627-2650. doi:10.1007/s00330-019-06357-8
21. Dahle TG, Kaneko T, McCabe JM. Outcomes following subclavian and axillary artery access for transcatheter aortic valve replacement. *J Am Coll Cardiol Interv.* 2019;12(7):662-669. doi:10.1016/j.jcin2019.01.219
22. Madigan M, Atoui R. Non-transfemoral access sites for transcatheter aortic valve replacement. *J Thorac Dis.* 2018;10(7):4505-4515. doi:10.21037/jtd.2018.06.150
23. Tasca G, Mhagna Z, Perotti S, et al. Impact of prosthesis-patient mismatch on cardiac events and midterm mortality after aortic valve replacement in patients with pure aortic stenosis [published correction appears in *Circulation.* 2006;113(7):e288. Quiani, Eugenio [corrected to Quaini, Eugenio]]. *Circulation.* 2006;113(4):570-576. doi:10.1161/CIRCULATIONAHA.105.587022
24. Walther T, Rastan A, Falk V, et al. Patient prosthesis mismatch affects short- and long-term outcomes after aortic valve replacement. *Eur J Cardiothorac Surg.* 2006;30(1):15-19. doi:10.1016/j.ejcts.2006.04.007
25. Daneshvar SA, Rahimtoola SH. Valve prosthesis-patient mismatch (VP-PM): a long-term perspective. *J Am Coll Cardiol.* 2012;60(13):1123-1135. doi:10.1016/j.jacc.2012.05.035
26. Honda K, Okamura Y. Prosthesis-patient mismatch in aortic stenosis. *Gen Thorac Cardiovasc Surg.* 2014;62(2):78-86. doi:10.1007/s11748-013-0331-4
27. Herrmann HC, Daneshvar SA, Fonarow GC, et al. Prosthesis-patient mismatch in patients undergoing transcatheter aortic valve replacement: from the STS/ACC TVT Registry. *J Am Coll Cardiol.* 2018;72(22):2701-2711. doi:10.1016/j.jacc.2018.09.001
28. Weber A, Noureddine H, Englberger L, et al. Ten-year comparison of pericardial tissue valves versus mechanical prostheses for aortic valve replacement in patients younger than 60 years of age. *J Thorac Cardiovasc Surg.* 2012;144(5):1075-1083. doi:10.1016/j.jtcvs.2012.01.024
29. Yu W, Tam DY, Rocha RV, Makhdoum A, Ouzounian M, Fremes SE. Aortic root enlargement is safe and reduces the incidence of patient-prosthesis mismatch: a meta-analysis of early and late outcomes. *Can J Cardiol.* 2019;35(6):782-790. doi:10.1016/j.cjca.2019.02.004
30. Nicks R, Cartmill T, Bernstein L. Hypoplasia of the aortic root. The problem of aortic valve replacement. *Thorax.* 1970;25(3):339-346. doi:10.1136/thx.25.3.339
31. Manouguian S, Seybold-Epting W. Patch enlargement of the aortic valve ring by extending the aortic incision into the anterior mitral leaflet. New operative technique. *J Thorac Cardiovasc Surg.* 1979;78(3):402-412.
32. Faggiano P, Frattini S, Zilioli V, et al. Prevalence of comorbidities and associated cardiac diseases in patients with valve aortic stenosis. Potential implications for the decision-making process. *Int J Cardiol.* 2012;159(2):94-99. doi:10.1016/j.ijcard.2011.02.026
33. Abramowitz Y, Jilaihawi H, Chakravarty T, Mack MJ, Makkar RR. Porcelain aorta: a comprehensive review [published correction appears in *Circulation.* 2015;131(12):e386]. *Circulation.* 2015;131(9):827-836. doi:10.1161/CIRCULATIONAHA.114.011867
34. Whitley WS, Glas KE. An argument for routine ultrasound screening of the thoracic aorta in the cardiac surgery population. *Semin Cardiothorac Vasc Anesth.* 2008;12(4):290-297. doi:10.1177/1089253208328583
35. Lansac E, de Kerchove L. Aortic valve repair techniques: state of the art. *Eur J Cardiothorac Surg.* 2018;53(6):1101-1107. doi:10.1093/ejcts/ezy176

CHAPTER 88

MITRAL VALVE SURGERY: A PATHOANATOMIC APPROACH

Vinay Badhwar, Jahnavi Kakuturu, and Chris C. Cook

INTRODUCTION

The most prevalent adult valvular heart disease is mitral valve (MV) disease, and its most common presentation is regurgitation.[1] Mitral stenosis (MS) is associated with fusion or calcification of the leaflets preventing their adequate opening or closing throughout the cardiac cycle. Mitral regurgitation (MR) may be primary, secondary, or mixed.[2] Primary MR is an abnormality of the leaflets or subvalvular chordal apparatus. Secondary MR occurs because of the restriction of leaflet motion, with or without mitral annular dilatation, secondary to ventricular, and papillary muscle pathology. Mixed MR occurs when pathoanatomic features of primary and secondary MR coexist in the same patient. Strategies and techniques of surgical correction of MV disease are tailored to treat the precise pathoanatomy.

Untreated severe primary MR is associated with significant longitudinal morbidity including a 30% incidence of atrial fibrillation and 63% incidence of heart failure.[3] Similar sequela accompany severe MS. Once the presence of severe MR has been established, MV surgery is indicated to prevent further left ventricular dilatation and symptoms of heart failure, even in asymptomatic patients. For patients with severe MS who are not candidates for percutaneous mitral balloon commissurotomy (PMBC), mitral valve replacement (MVR) is necessary to treat pulmonary hypertension, symptoms of dyspnea and fatigue, and prevention of secondary right ventricular dysfunction. Whenever anatomically possible and appropriate, MV repair should be performed as it may confer a survival advantage over MVR of 12% to 21% at 15 years.[4,5] This chapter will review the indications and pathoanatomic approach to current MV surgery.

INDICATIONS

For patients with severe primary MR without symptoms or with symptoms but without ventricular compromise, early surgical intervention compared with watchful waiting confers superior 10-year survival (86% vs 69%, respectively), with repair rates in high-volume centers exceeding 95% and a mortality of less than 1%.[6] Techniques of MV surgery have shifted from prosthetic MVR as the principle therapy for all pathology, to one based on the primary strategy of MV repair whenever possible, which has been applied with increasing consistency for the last 25 years. A recent analysis of the Society of Thoracic Surgeons (STS) Adult Cardiac Surgery Database revealed that 17,907 isolated nonredo MV surgeries were performed across the United States, a 24% increase over 5 years previously, the majority of which were MV repair with an overall repair rate for primary MR of 82.5%.[7] Durability of MV repair is generally excellent with a freedom from reoperation rate of 94% at 10 years.[8] The surgical approach to isolated MV operations has also changed, with 23% of patients in the STS study having received minimally invasive thoracotomy or robotic techniques.[7] Current indications for MV surgery are based largely on these principles, as well as similar findings in the literature that have been summarized by the 2020 American College of Cardiology (ACC)/American Heart Association (AHA) Clinical Practice Guidelines released in December 2020 and highlighted later.[9]

For severe MS, defined by an MV area of less than or equal 1.5 cm^2, diastolic pressure half time of greater than or equal to 150 ms, and pulmonary artery systolic pressures greater than 50 mm Hg, MVR is the principle therapy for nonrheumatic calcific pathology and symptoms.[9] For patients with symptomatic severe rheumatic MS who have failed PMBC or deemed not a candidate for it, MV surgery is a Class 1 recommendation.

For primary MR, MV surgery is a Class 1 recommendation for symptomatic severe MR regardless of left ventricular (LV) function or asymptomatic patients with an LV ejection fraction (LVEF) less than or equal 60% or LV end-systolic dimension (ESD) greater than or equal to 40 mm by echocardiography. It is further a Class 1 recommendation that MV repair is performed whenever possible for primary MR. For patients with preserved LVEF and focal degenerative MV disease involving less than half of the posterior leaflet only, MVR is considered Class 3, or harmful. For asymptomatic patients with normal LVEF greater than 60%, MV repair is a Class 2a indication provided a durable repair can be provided greater than 95% of the time at a mortality rate of less than 1%. For asymptomatic patients with preserved LVEF but LV dilatation or recent decline in LVEF, MV surgery is a Class 2b recommendation. Finally, for patients of high or prohibitive risk for MV surgery, transcatheter edge-to-edge repair (TEER) is considered a Class 2a recommendation (**Algorithm 88.1**).[9]

For rheumatic MR (primary or mixed), associated with symptoms, MV repair is a Class 2b recommendation provided it is performed in an experienced comprehensive valve center.

For secondary MR, ongoing controversy remains as to the optimal treatment at the optimal time given its dynamic nature and the impact on the degree of LV dysfunction on both short-term and long-term outcomes.[10-13] Consistent across all

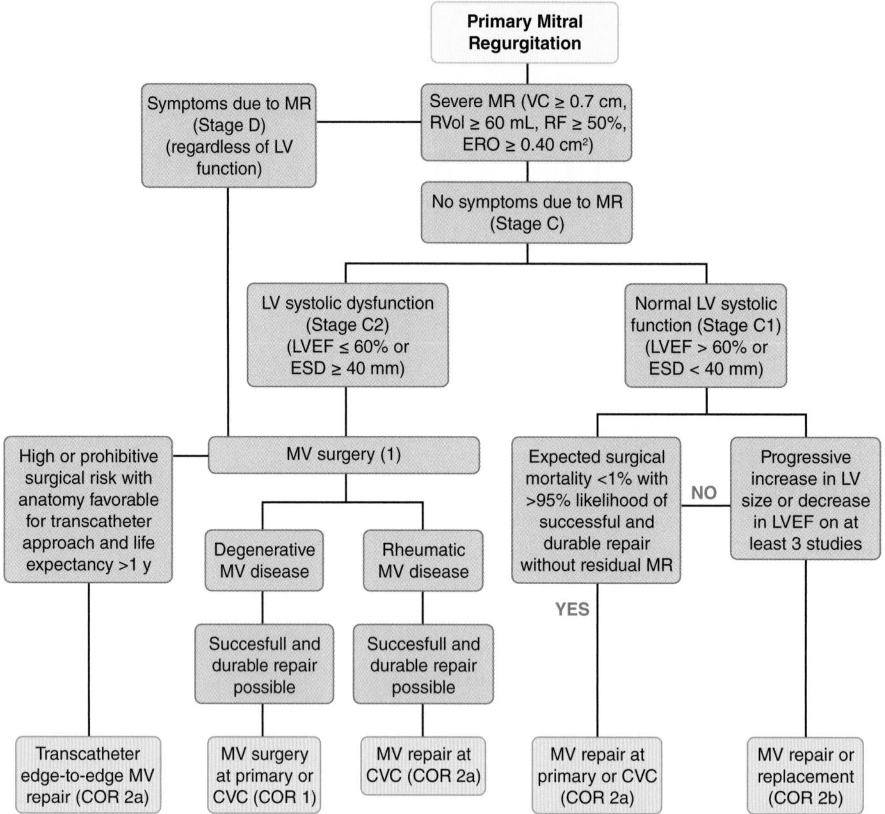

ALGORITHM 88.1 Guidelines for the management of primary mitral regurgitation. COR, class of recommendation CVC, cardiovascular center; ERO, effective regurgitant orifice area; ESD, end-systolic volume; LV, left ventricular; LVEF, left ventricular ejection fraction; MR, mitral regurgitation; MV, mitral valve; RF, regurgitant fraction RVol, regurgitant volume; VC, vena contracta; y, year. (Reprinted from Otto CM, Nishimura RA, Bonow RO, et al. 2020 ACC/AHA Guideline for the Management of Patients With Valvular Heart Disease: A Report of the American College of Cardiology/American Heart Association Joint Committee on Clinical Practice Guidelines. *J Am Coll Cardiol*. 2021;77(4):e25-e197. Copyright © 2021 by the American College of Cardiology Foundation and the American Heart Association, Inc. With permission.)

planned MV interventions is the role of guideline-directed medical therapy (GDMT) on optimizing loading conditions before MV surgery or TEER.[9-13] As such, all patients presenting with secondary MR should have initial attempts at GDMT optimization, preferably with a heart failure specialist.[9] For patients with symptomatic severe secondary MR, MV surgery is a Class 2a recommendation when coronary artery bypass grafting (CABG) is performed for myocardial ischemia. MV surgery also holds a Class 2b recommendation for MR secondary to annular dilatation and atrial fibrillation (or atrial MR), and symptomatic severe MR due to LVEF less than 50%. Although some patients may benefit from MV repair techniques, chord-sparing MVR for secondary MR may be reasonable in certain individuals, and it carries a Class 2b recommendation (**Algorithm 88.2**).[9]

ANATOMIC CONSIDERATIONS

For the MV surgeon, it is essential to have a working mastery of echocardiographic structural interpretation, for it is the prediction of pathoanatomic mechanisms and the identification of potential anatomic pitfalls that provides the guidance for surgical strategy.[14] Quantitative parameters consistent with severe MR should be identified before anesthetic induction and include a vena contracta width greater than 7 mm, effective regurgitant orifice area greater than 40 mm^2, regurgitant volume greater than 60 mL, regurgitant fraction greater than 50%, or the presence of a flail leaflet or ruptured chorda.[2] Important for surgical planning is the two-dimensional (2D) or three-dimensional (3D) identification of surgically relevant items such as clefts, annular/leaflet calcification, perforations, or possible coexistent chordal tethering that may impact the tailoring of the precise steps to achieve a successful surgical outcome.

Pathoanatomy at every level of the mitral apparatus may coexist in the same patient, and the preoperative or intraoperative imaging must be carefully reviewed so that the MV surgeon may make an effort to develop the surgical plan before making incision. This is of particular importance when the mechanism is anything more than focal single scallop disease. The MV apparatus is subdivided into the annulus, anterior and posterior leaflets, and the subvalvular chordae tendineae

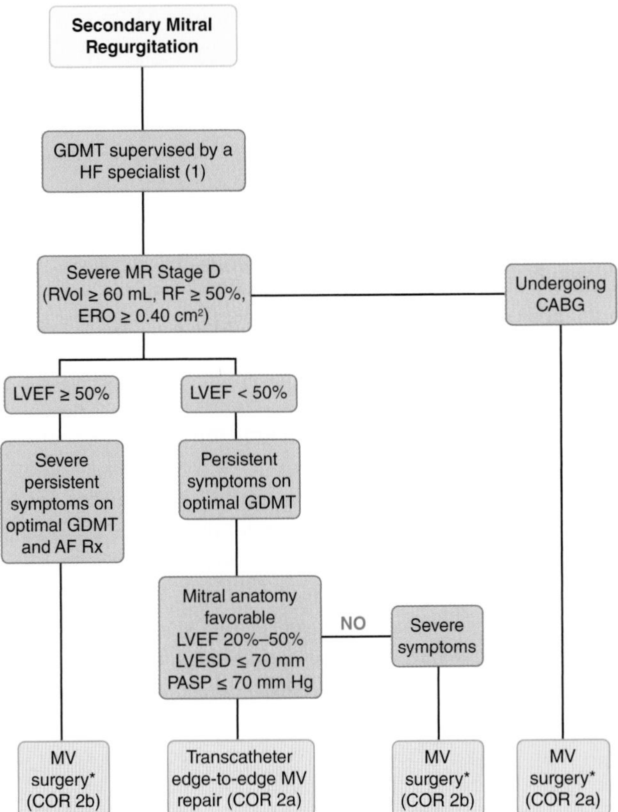

ALGORITHM 88.2 Guidelines for the management of secondary mitral regurgitation. *Chordal-sparing MV replacement may be reasonable to choose over downsized annuloplasty repair. AF, atrial fibrillation; CABG, coronary artery bypass grafting; COR, class of recommendation; ERO, effective regurgitant orifice area; GDMT, guideline-directed medical therapy; HF, heart failure; LVEF, left ventricular ejection fraction; LVESD, left ventricular end-systolic volume; MR, mitral regurgitation; MV, mitral valve; PASP, pulmonary artery systolic pressure; RF, regurgitant fraction; RVol, regurgitant volume Rx, treatment. (Reprinted from Otto CM, Nishimura RA, Bonow RO, et al. 2020 ACC/AHA Guideline for the Management of Patients With Valvular Heart Disease: A Report of the American College of Cardiology/American Heart Association Joint Committee on Clinical Practice Guidelines. *J Am Coll Cardiol.* 2021;77(4):e25-e197. Copyright © 2021 by the American College of Cardiology Foundation and the American Heart Association, Inc. With permission.)

and papillary muscles. The posterior leaflet is subdivided from lateral to medial into P1, P2, and P3 segments, with corresponding A1, A2, and A3 segments of the anterior leaflet. The anterior leaflet constitutes two-thirds of the valve orifice area and one-third of the annular circumference, while the posterior leaflet constitutes one-third of the valve area and two-thirds of the circumference. The subvalvular apparatus is composed of the anterolateral and posteromedial papillary muscles that give rise to primary chords attached to the free edge of the leaflet, secondary chords attached to the mid-leaflet ventricular surface, and tertiary chords attached to base of the leaflet.

The Carpentier classification is most commonly used to define leaflet motion to describe the possible etiology of MR.[2,15] Type 1 is normal leaflet motion, and the MR may be due to congenital clefts, endocarditis/perforation, or annular dilation. Type 2 is excessive leaflet motion, and it is associated with primary degenerative leaflet prolapse or flail leaflet accompanied with chordal rupture. Type 3 is restricted leaflet motion. Type 3A occurs when leaflet motion is restricted in systole and diastole such as with rheumatic disease or radiation, and Type 3B occurs when leaflet motion is restricted in systole only such as with ischemic or nonischemic ventricular secondary MR. Type 3B secondary MR may further be subclassified into grades of severity (1-4) based on the amount of annular dilation, amount of leaflet tethering, and LVEF (**Table 88.1**).[12,13]

As valve complexity increases, so does the coexistence of different pathoanatomic mechanisms. The MV surgeon must incorporate the echocardiographic structural imaging (eg, clefts and leaflet height) and the pathologic mechanism (eg, excess or restricted motion) to formulate the reconstructive strategy.

FUNDAMENTALS OF MITRAL VALVE SURGERY

Important steps in the delivery of high-quality MV surgery include optimal surgical approach and exposure, careful valve analysis to confirm pathoanatomy, and meticulous technique for MV repair or replacement.

The approach to MV surgery is conventionally performed via a median sternotomy, facilitated by central arterial and bicaval venous cannulation for cardiopulmonary bypass, and hypothermic cardioplegic arrest. The roof of the left atrium is entered and retracted anterolaterally to provide exposure for all types of MV operations. Exposure is often facilitated by marsupialization of the ride-sided pericardium and dissection of the bicaval pericardial reflection. The successful performance of all MV surgery is based not only on meticulous valvular technique but maintenance of excellent venous drainage and myocardial protection. These fundamental principles provide reproducibly excellent results and mortality rates from isolated MVR of less than 4% and isolated MV repair of less than 1%.[16]

In recent years, minimally invasive approaches to MV surgery have been performed with durability results equivalent to traditional sternotomy but with slightly faster recovery and potentially less morbidity. Rib-sparing right mini-thoracotomy with either direct-vision or video assistance and peripheral arterial and venous cannulation has become a standard platform used successfully in multiple experienced MV centers across the world for 20 years.[17] Robotic-assisted MV surgery was developed in parallel with other minimally invasive techniques[18]. However, initial adoption was slow until the last decade when the advancement of robotic telemanipulation technology and instrumentation markedly improved the reproducibility of results. This has facilitated a recent rapid increase in robotic application with excellent quality outcomes, such that nearly 15% of all isolated MV operations in the United States are now performed robotically.[16] Robotic MV repair, replacement, and concomitant procedures such as surgical ablation and tricuspid

TABLE 88.1 Pathoanatomic Grading of Type IIIB Secondary Mitral Regurgitation

Grade	Annular Dilatation	Leaflet Tethering	Left Ventricular Ejection Fraction (%)
1	Mild to moderate (<4 cm)	Mild (<5 mm)	>45
2	Moderate to severe (4-5 cm)	Moderate (5-10 mm)	35-45
3	Severe (>5 cm)	Severe (>10 mm)	25-35
4	Severe (>5 cm)	Severe (>10 mm)	<25 or presence of inferobasal dysfunction

Reprinted from Badhwar V, Alkhouli M, Mack MJ, et al. A pathoanatomic approach to secondary functional mitral regurgitation: Evaluating the evidence. *J Thorac Cardiovasc Surg*. 2019;158(1):76-81. Copyright © 2019 by The American Association for Thoracic Surgery. With permission.

valve repair are now performed with increasing regularity in many centers. For several centers, this has become the standard routine approach to perform MV surgery with longitudinal durability outcomes and cost equivalency to sternotomy.[17]

Following MV exposure with excellent visualization, the next fundamental step is a careful examination of the mitral leaflets, annulus, and subvalvular apparatus to confirm or modify the preoperative echocardiographically derived pathoanatomically based surgical plan. Given the general "repair-first" strategy for all MV surgery, this step is important to confirm safety and efficacy of MV repair. Should preoperative imaging or intraoperative anatomic confirmation steps identify pathoanatomy unfavorable for a durable repair within the surgeon's experience, then chord-sparing MVR may be the safest and more optimal solution. Predictors of potential failure of MV repair include leaflet calcium or restriction, prior MV repair, mitral annular calcification (MAC) involving the base of the leaflet, and tissue destruction such as from endocarditis.[2,12,14,19] This noted, some of these cases may be successfully and durably repaired in experienced high-volume comprehensive valve centers.[2,9,19] Chord-sparing MVR is often the best solution for calcific mitral stenosis or severe Type 3 disease.[9,13] Determinants of durably successful MV repair include achieving a coaptation depth of greater than 5 mm, stabilizing the mitral valve annulus, and restoring normal motion of the leaflets with no more than trace to mild MR on an immediate postrepair transesophageal echocardiogram.[2,14,19]

The technique for MVR is well established. This involves the excision of the offending pathology while preserving the annular-ventricular continuity through chordal preservation. The degree of resection must be sufficient to safely place the largest prosthesis possible without injury or compression to surrounding anatomic structures. Chordal preservation is performed by either maintaining the posterior leaflet chordal attachments only, preserving both posterior and anterior attachments by dividing the anterior leaflet and incorporating its chords in the posterior annular suture line, or using artificial chords of polytetrafluoroethylene (PTFE) when the native subvalvular apparatus is heavily diseased and in need of resection. Suture placement is most commonly performed from the ventricular side of the annulus to facilitate larger prostheses, but this may also be performed from the atrial side in an everting manner. The use of supportive Teflon pledgets with each suture is optional. Following circumferential annular suture placement with appropriate depth and precision to avoid adjacent structures such as the circumflex coronary artery, aortic valve leaflet, and atrioventricular node, the sutures are placed through the sewing ring of the prosthesis and tied to securely seat the valve without paravalvular defects.

The two foundations of successful MV repair are the preoperative and intraoperative clear identification of pathoanatomy, followed by targeted lesion-based methods to restore durable leaflet coaptation. Pathoanatomy-directed MV repair techniques may include a nonresection strategy using PTFE artificial chords, limited triangular resection, or, when significant posterior leaflet height reduction is required, a more extensive resection and sliding valvuloplasty.[19-22] While some surgeons may prefer one technique over another, there is little to no difference in long-term outcome as long as the fundamental principles of coaptation depth restoration, annular stability, and preservation of leaflet motion are adhered to. Most MV surgeons use all techniques, and often in combination, to successfully repair pathologies with increasing complexity. This becomes particularly important in the patient with excess leaflet tissue or posterior leaflet height and a small LV size where other predictors of systolic anterior motion may exist.[23] The gradation of primary MR pathology starts with focal single leaflet prolapse or flail (eg, P2) that involves less than half of the posterior leaflet (**Figure 88.1**), followed by diffuse posterior leaflet disease involving multiple scallops if not all of the leaflets (**Figure 88.2**), bileaflet disease with dominant posterior flail (**Figure 88.3**), anterior leaflet flail (**Figure 88.4**), and diffuse bileaflet myxomatous degeneration or Barlow disease (**Figure 88.5**). Each gradation of complexity is often accompanied by a need to augment techniques to durably restore leaflet coaptation.

CLINICAL ASPECTS OF APPLICATION

As mitral disease states advance in complexity, often more than one mechanism or pathology is involved. Surgeons and cardiologists often use multiple sources of information to guide referral timing and reparability. Surgical teams advancing in their management of case complexity must be prepared to apply lesion-directed techniques. To assimilate the fundamental principles and techniques for MV surgery, a pathoanatomic

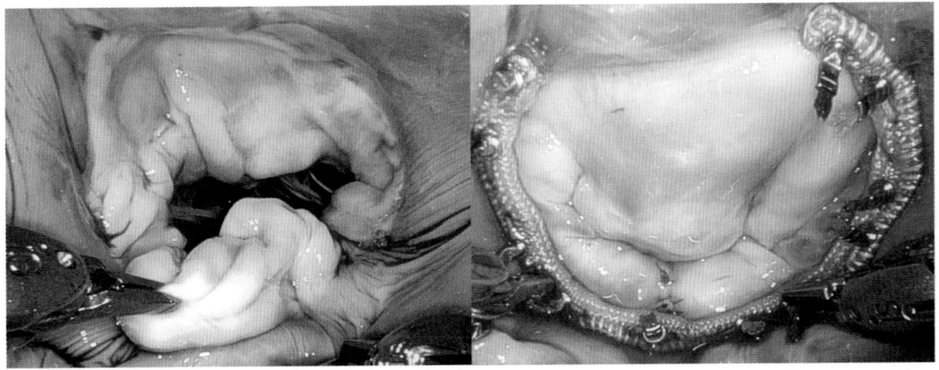

FIGURE 88.1 Repair of focal P2 prolapse with or without flail. Focal P2 disease (left) may be repaired by either a nonresection technique using artificial chords to support the primary leaflet edge or by limited focal resection as was used in this case (right). All valve repairs should include an annuloplasty ring or band to support the repair and prevent longitudinal annular dilatation. These lesions should be reparable greater than 95% of the time with a mortality rate less than 1%.

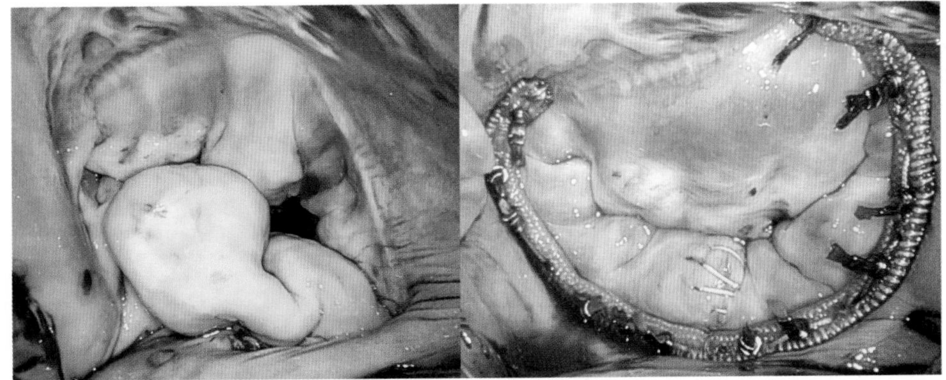

FIGURE 88.2 Repair of diffuse posterior leaflet prolapse or flail. Diffuse multiscallop involvement of the posterior leaflet (left) often requires efforts to reduce posterior leaflet height while preserving leaflet motion. This may be accomplished by resection or nonresection supportive techniques. In this case, both were applied by a central focal resection and a single polytetrafluoroethylene (PTFE) suture that both repaired the resected leaflet and supported the repair to the papillary muscle at the same time (right). (From Roberts HG, Rankin JS, Wei LM, et al. Respectful resection to enhance the armamentarium of mitral valve repair: is less really more? *J Thorac Cardiovasc Surg.* 2018;156:1854-1855.)

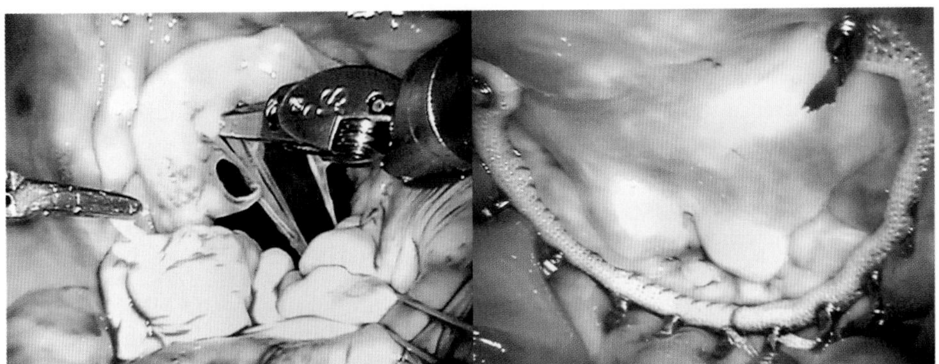

FIGURE 88.3 Repair of bileaflet prolapse. When prolapse or flail involves both leaflets (left), repair may involve both leaflets or, in some cases, a strategy to reduce posterior leaflet height alone that permits normalization of the anterior and posterior coaptation relationship. This case involved a posterior leaflet resection and sliding valvuloplasty (right).

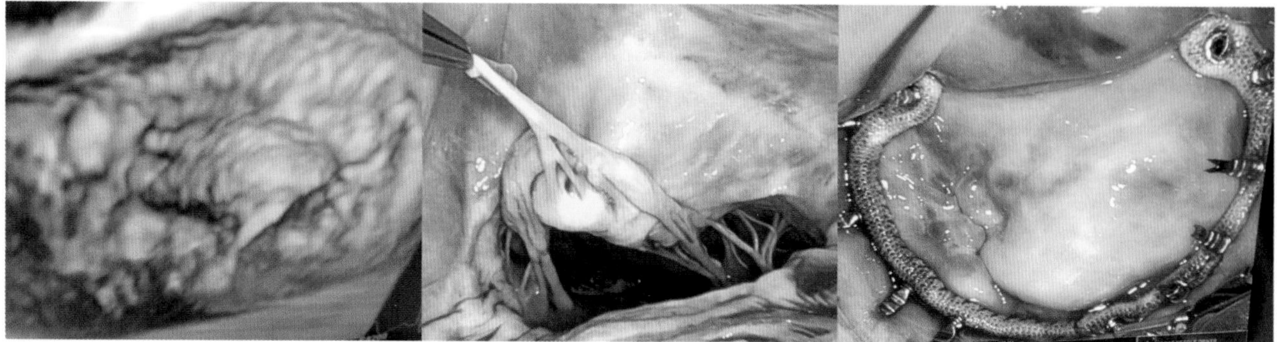

FIGURE 88.4 Repair of anterior leaflet flail. With severe anterior leaflet prolapse or flail due to elongated or ruptured primary chords (left), there is often normal or tethered secondary or tertiary anterior chorda (center). This complex lesion may be repaired by the addition of primary polytetrafluoroethylene (PTFE) chords to support the flail segment, or, as in this case, perform ipsilateral chordal transfer of robust secondary chords by detaching them from the mid-portion of the leaflet and reimplanting them in the primary position (right).

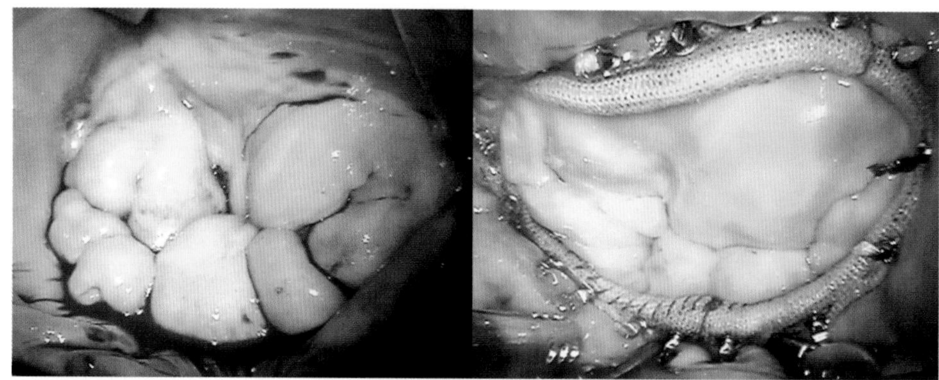

FIGURE 88.5 Repair of diffuse bileaflet myxomatous degeneration (Barlow Disease). When there is a diffuse myxomatous disease manifested by excess tissue of both leaflets, there are often multiple pathoanatomic issues such as multiscallop prolapse, chordal elongation/rupture, focal chordal restriction, leaflet clefts, and possible annular calcification (left). Durable repair must address the specific pathology in a targeted lesion-specific approach. This case involved closure of clefts in the posterior leaflet, focal resection, and partial sliding valvuloplasty, and division of restricted secondary chorda to A1 and A3 (right).

complexity score from Grade 1 to 4 has been introduced to guide applicable technical advances (**Figure 88.6**).[19] Grade 1 complexity involves focal leaflet or annular pathology that can be treated by straightforward focal repair that may involve limited resection, chordal support, and annuloplasty. The successful repair rate for this category should approach 100%. Grade 2 lesions involve more diffuse posterior leaflet disease that often involves multiscallop reconstructive techniques and should be repairable greater than 90% of the time. Grade 3 complexity involves multisegment bileaflet pathology with/without concomitant MAC and may require a combination of several techniques as illustrated in Figure 88.5. Grade 4 complexity is one that may confer the highest level of difficulty due to pathologies such as perforations or annular abscess associated with infective endocarditis, or severe mixed restrictive disease due to leaflet, annular, or ventricular reasons requiring additional techniques such as autologous pericardial patch augmentation. Grade 3 and 4 patients have a higher likelihood of MVR and may require teams in a comprehensive valve center with extensive experience to deliver a durable and successful repair using several advanced techniques.

LIMITATIONS OF TECHNIQUE OR PROCEDURE

Successful MV surgery and MV repair, in particular, require experience of the surgeon and the operative team to achieve the best possible outcomes.[24] This involves cardiac anesthesia, perfusion, and the surgical team to work as an effective unit to facilitate all of the principles outlined: effective imaging, effective perfusion, and effective technique. If the team functions suboptimally, inferior outcomes may follow.

Grade	Pathoanatomic Features	Echocardiography	Operative Findings	Repair Options
1	• Annular dilatation • Isolated posterior leaflet prolapse or single segment flail	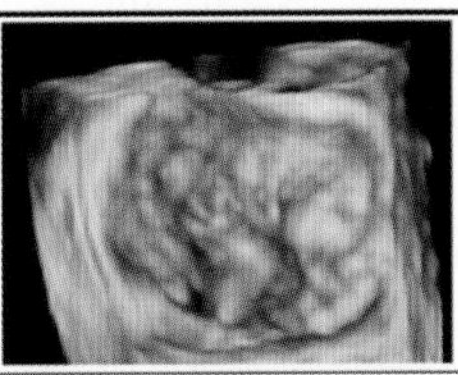	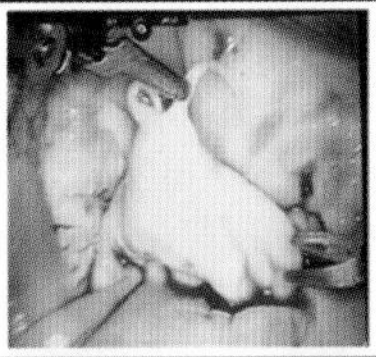	• Focal resection and valvuloplasty with ring annuloplasty • PTFE neochord support • Ring/band annuloplasty
2	• Diffuse myxomatous disease predominantly of posterior leaflet (forme fruste)	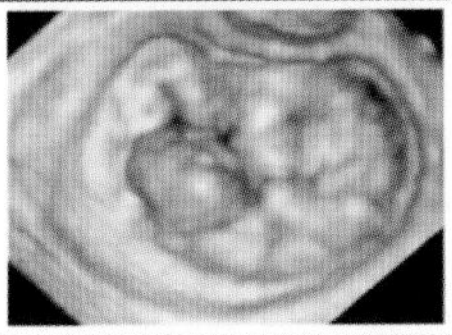	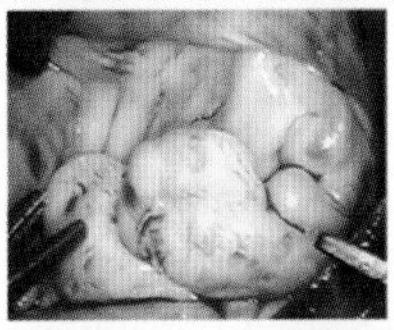	• Partial resection and sliding leaflet valvuloplasty • Multi-segment PTFE neochord support • Ring/band annuloplasty
3	• Diffuse bi-leaflet myxomatous disease (Barlow) • Anterior leaflet flail • Multi-segment flail • Focal posterior mitral annular calcification	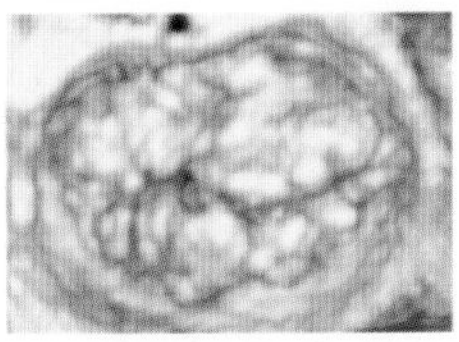	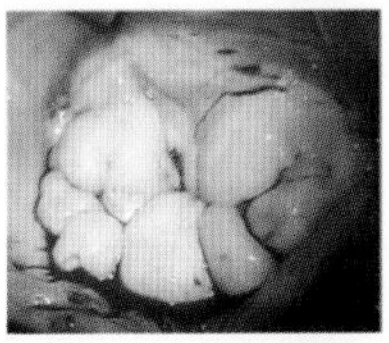	• Partial resection and sliding leaflet valvuloplasty • Multi-segment PTFE neochord support • Secondary chordal transfer • Focal calcium resection • Ring/band annuloplasty
4	• Endocarditis ± leaflet perforation or annular abscess • Rheumatic Type IIIA disease • Secondary Type IIIB disease with severe tethering • Severe mitral annular calcification	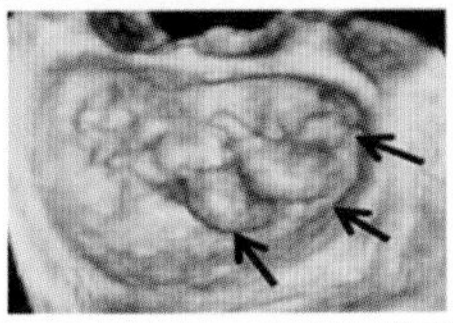	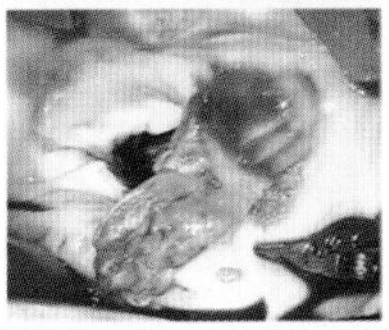	• Reconstruction with patch augmentation • Subvalvular mobilization • Radical annular reconstruction • Ring/band annuloplasty

FIGURE 88.6 Pathoanatomic grading system to guide mitral valve repair. To assimilate the principles of pathoanatomic guided mitral valve surgery, this pathoanatomic complexity score from Grade 1 to 4, helps guide the augmentation of techniques that may facilitate successful outcome. PTFE, polytetrafluoroethylene (From Alreshidan M, Herron RD, Wei LM, et al. Surgical techniques for mitral valve repair: A pathoanatomic grading system. *Semin Cardiothorac Vasc Anesth.* 2019;23(1):20-25. Copyright © 2019 SAGE Publications. Reprinted by permission of SAGE Publications, Inc.)

The majority of open-heart programs and surgeons are able to effectively perform MVR and focal MV repair operations (Grade 1 complexity) with excellent outcomes.[5,16] As complexity increases, maintaining successful repair rates for primary MR may be influenced by experience. A volume-outcome association has been found for repair rate of primary MR.[25] The inflection point of this relationship is estimated to occur at 35 annual MV surgery cases at the surgeon level and 75 annual cases at the institutional level. Interestingly, access to these higher volume centers in the United States may be far more ubiquitous than once recognized. Nearly 80% of the population lives within a hospital referral region with at least one such center.[25]

SPECIAL CONSIDERATIONS

Several special considerations associated with optimal short-term and long-term outcomes in the management of MV disease warrant brief review. These include the management of concomitant atrial fibrillation, identification, and avoidance of systolic anterior motion, navigating severe MAC, and the treatment of high- or prohibitive-risk patients with MV disease.

Patients commonly present with atrial fibrillation at the time of MV surgery. In fact, the development of valvular atrial fibrillation serves as one of the markers of MV disease severity. Surgical ablation at the time of MV surgery confers short-term and long-term reduction in morbidity and mortality. Thus, the performance of concomitant surgical ablation at the time of MV surgery has received multisocietal Class 1 guideline recommendation.[26,27] The most accepted method of ablation procedure at the time of MV surgery is the full biatrial Cox-Maze IV lesion set.[28]

Before MV surgery, and particularly MV repair, identification of risk factors for systolic anterior motion is of particular importance. Risk factors for the development of systolic anterior motion include a small hyperkinetic left ventricle with reduced end-diastolic volume, lower ratio of anterior to posterior leaflets (<1.3), presence of bilateral leaflet prolapse or excessive leaflet tissue, an acute aortomitral angle (<120°), a thick basal interventricular septum (>15 mm), decreased distance between the coaptation point and interventricular septum (<25 mm), and anterior papillary muscle displacement.[14,19,23] When these are identified, MV repair technique navigation should include avoiding undersized annuloplasty rings and strategies that reduce posterior leaflet height to ensure that postrepair coaptation occurs as far posterior as possible while maintaining good coaptation depth to avoid proximate crowding of the LV outflow tract.

SECTION 7

The existence of moderate to severe MAC may significantly complicate MV repair or replacement. All efforts to identify and quantify the extent of MAC preoperatively are most helpful for clinical decision-making. Echocardiography is the principle manner in which to determine the impact of MAC on leaflet motion, but computed tomography is often of added assistance to identify the depth and breadth of ventricular involvement in severe cases. Operative techniques used to address MAC can range from avoidance to radical resection.[29] When MAC exists with less than 25% involvement of the annular circumference and it does not involve the primary MV lesion, it is often left alone as part of lesion-directed MV repair since annular sutures and ring placement are often possible without MAC disruption. When MAC involves greater than 25% of the annular circumference or it is immediately involved in the MV lesion, it is often required to focally or more radically resect the MAC as part of the MV repair or replacement. Depending on the depth of MAC, this resection may or may not require autologous pericardial annular reinforcement or reconstruction. When the MAC is mostly circumferential and not predicted to readily hold sutures for conventional MVR, two alternatives have emerged. One is the open valve-in-MAC technique that involves excision of the anterior mitral leaflet and the off-label deployment of an inverted balloon-expandable Sapien transcatheter aortic valve prosthesis (Edwards Lifesciences, Irvine, CA, USA) supported by 3 to 4 anchoring sutures. The other is to pursue primary transcatheter mitral valve replacement (TMVR) strategies within existing U.S. Food and Drug Administration (FDA)-sponsored clinical trials.[30]

Many patients with MR may be of high to prohibitive predicted STS risk of operative mortality (≥8%) associated with elevated comorbidities and frailty. For these patients with primary MR with an acceptable anatomy and predicted minimum 1-year survival, TEER with the FDA-approved MitraClip device (Abbott, Santa Clara, CA, USA) has been shown to improve symptoms and quality of life and meets a Class 2a indication.[9] For patients with severe secondary MR of high to prohibitive risk, the management decision is more nuanced.[12,13] While TEER has been shown to improve outcomes in some patients with limited ventricular distortion, some patients have shown no benefit.[12,13] Patients with larger ventricles, more MV leaflet tethering, and lower LVEF, who are not candidates for advanced heart failure therapies such as transplant, have shown promising early results with TMVR performed within existing clinical trials.[12,13]

RESEARCH AND FUTURE DEVELOPMENTS

The search for innovative therapies to treat MV disease has recently spawned no less than 50 start-up companies and over $1 billion in investment.[31] There are over 20 devices currently in various stages of clinical trials. These include novel ways to perform TEER, percutaneously augment MV coaptation by endovascular or extra-anatomic means, replace chorda via a transapical approach, and perform TMVR via a transapical or transseptal approach. Of these devices, the two most promising to reach U.S. approval are the Medtronic Intrepid TMVR (Medtronic, Minneapolis, MN, USA) and the Abbott Tendyne TMVR (Abbott, Santa Clara, CA, USA). Both have achieved large enrollment in their clinical trials with respectable early outcomes, or as is the case with Tendyne, commercial approval in Europe. However, all of these devices will need to prove superior to the high bar of established benchmarks of safety and outcome of MV surgery.

KEY POINTS

- ✔ Surgical MV replacement has a significant survival advantage over MVR and should be attempted whenever feasible.
- ✔ Indications for MV surgery include symptomatic patients with severe MR, and asymptomatic patients with LVEF less than 60% or an LVEDD (left ventricular end-diastolic diameter) greater than 40 mm in whom successful MV repair can be reasonably assured.
- ✔ Echocardiographic assessment is essential in identifying the mechanism of MV disease and planning repair technique strategy based on detailed pathoanatomy.
- ✔ Risk factors for systolic anterior motion should be identified preoperatively and preventive surgical strategies should be utilized.
- ✔ If MVR is performed for nondegenerative disease, chordal sparing techniques must be utilized whenever possible.

REFERENCES

1. Wu S, Chai A, Arimie S, et al. Incidence and treatment of severe primary mitral regurgitation in contemporary clinical practice. *Cardiovasc Revasc Med.* 2018;19:960-963.
2. O'Gara PT, Grayburn PA, Badhwar V, et al. 2017 ACC expert consensus decision pathway on the management of mitral regurgitation: a report of the American College of Cardiology Task Force on Expert Consensus Decision Pathways. *J Am Coll Cardiol.* 2017;70:2421-2449.
3. El Sabbagh A, Reddy YNV, Nishimura RA. Mitral valve regurgitation in the contemporary era: insights into diagnosis, management, and future directions. *JACC Cardiovasc Imaging.* 2018;11:628-643.
4. Suri RM, Schaff HV, Dearani JA, et al. Survival advantage and improved durability of mitral repair for leaflet prolapse subsets in the current era. *Ann Thorac Surg.* 2006;82:819-826.
5. Daneshmand MA, Milano CA, Rankin JS, et al. Mitral valve repair for degenerative disease: a 20-year experience. *Ann Thorac Surg.* 2009;88:1828-1837.
6. Suri RM, Vanoverschelde JL, Grigioni F, et al. Association between early surgical intervention vs watchful waiting and outcomes for mitral regurgitation due to flail mitral valve leaflets. *JAMA.* 2013;310:609-616.
7. Gammie JS, Chikwe J, Badhwar V, et al. Isolated mitral valve surgery: The Society of Thoracic Surgeons adult cardiac surgery database analysis. *Ann Thorac Surg.* 2018;106:716-727.
8. Gillinov AM, Blackstone EH, Nowicki ER, et al. Valve repair versus valve replacement for degenerative mitral valve disease. *J Thorac Cardiovasc Surg.* 2008;135:885-893.
9. Otto CM, Nishimura RA, Bonow RO, et al. 2020 ACC/AHA guideline for the management of patients with valvular heart disease: a report of the American College of Cardiology/American Heart Association

Joint Committee on Clinical Practice Guidelines. *J Am Coll Cardiol.* 2021:77(4):e25-e197. doi:10.1016/j.jacc.2020.11.018

10. Goldstein D, Moskowitz AJ, Gelijns AC, et al. Two-year outcomes of surgical treatment of severe ischemic mitral regurgitation. *N Engl J Med.* 2016;374:344-353.
11. Michler RE, Smith PK, Parides MK, et al. Two-year outcomes of surgical treatment of moderate ischemic mitral regurgitation. *N Engl J Med.* 2016;374:1932-1941.
12. Badhwar V, Alkhouli M, Mack MJ, Thourani VH, Ailawadi G. A pathoanatomic approach to secondary functional mitral regurgitation: evaluating the evidence. *J Thorac Cardiovasc Surg.* 2019;158:76-81.
13. Badhwar V. Transcatheter mitral valve intervention: consensus, quality, and equipoise. *J Thorac Cardiovasc Surg.* 2020;160:93-98.
14. Badhwar V, Smith AJ, Cavalcante JL. A pathoanatomic approach to the management of mitral regurgitation. *Trends Cardiovasc Med.* 2016;26:126-134.
15. Carpentier A. Cardiac valve surgery—the "French correction". *J Thorac Cardiovasc Surg.* 1983;86:323-337.
16. Badhwar V, Rankin JS, He X, et al. The Society of Thoracic Surgeons mitral repair/replacement composite score: a report of The Society of Thoracic Surgeons Quality Measurement Task Force. *Ann Thorac Surg.* 2016;101:2265-2271.
17. Holzhey DM, Seeburger J, Misfeld M, Borger MA, Mohr FW. Learning minimally invasive mitral valve surgery: a cumulative sum sequential probability analysis of 3895 operations from a single high-volume center. *Circulation.* 2013;128:483-491.
18. Coyan G, Wei LM, Althouse A, et al. Robotic mitral valve operations by experienced surgeons are cost-neutral and durable at 1 year. *J Thorac Cardiovasc Surg.* 2018;156:1040-1047.
19. Alreshidan M, Herron RD, Wei LM, et al. Surgical techniques for mitral valve repair: a pathoanatomic grading system. *Semin Cardiothorac Vasc Anesth.* 2019;23:20-25.
20. Bonow RO, O'Gara PT, Adams DH, et al. 2020 focused update of the 2017 ACC expert consensus decision pathway on the management of mitral regurgitation. *J Am Coll Cardiol.* 2020;75:2236-2270.
21. Seeburger J, Falk V, Borger MA, et al. Chordae replacement versus resection for repair of isolated posterior mitral leaflet prolapse: à ègalité. *Ann Thorac Surg.* 2009;87:1715-1720.
22. Roberts HG, Rankin JS, Wei LM, et al. Respectful resection to enhance the armamentarium of mitral valve repair: is less really more? *J Thorac Cardiovasc Surg.* 2018;156:1854-1855.
23. Ashikhmina E, Schaff HV, Daly RC, et al. Risk factors and progression of systolic anterior motion after mitral valve repair. *J Thorac Cardiovasc Surg.* 2020. doi:10.1016/j.jtcvs.2019.12.106 [Online ahead of print].
24. El-Eshmawi A, Castillo JG, Tang GHL, Adams DH. Developing a mitral valve center of excellence. *Curr Opin Cardiol.* 2018;33:155-161.
25. Badhwar V, Vemulapalli S, Mack MA, et al. Volume-outcome association of mitral valve surgery in the United States. *JAMA Cardiol.* 2020;5:1-10.
26. Badhwar V, Rankin JS, Damiano RJ Jr, et al. The Society of Thoracic Surgeons 2017 clinical practice guidelines for the surgical treatment of atrial fibrillation. *Ann Thorac Surg.* 2017;103:329-341.
27. Calkins H, Hindricks G, Cappato R, et al. 2017 HRS/EHRA/ECAS/APHRS/SOLAECE expert consensus statement on catheter and surgical ablation of atrial fibrillation. *Heart Rhythm.* 2017;14:e275-e444.
28. Alreshidan M, Roberts HG, Rankin JS, Wei LM, Badhwar V. Current approach to surgical ablation for atrial fibrillation. *Semin Thorac Cardiovasc Surg.* 2019;31:141-145.
29. Edelman JJ, Badhwar V, Larbalestier R, Yadav P, Thourani VH. Contemporary surgical and transcatheter management of mitral annular calcification. *Ann Thorac Surg.* 2021;111(2):390-397. doi:10.1016/j.athoracsur.2020.04.148
30. Clinicaltrials.gov. Clinical trial to evaluate the safety and effectiveness of using the tendyne mitral valve system for the treatment of symptomatic mitral regurgitation (SUMMIT). Accessed December 1, 2020. https://clinicaltrials.gov/ct2/show/NCT03433274
31. Badhwar V, Thourani VH, Ailawadi G, Mack MJ. Transcatheter mitral therapy: the event horizon. *J Thorac Cardiovasc Surg.* 2016;152:330-336.

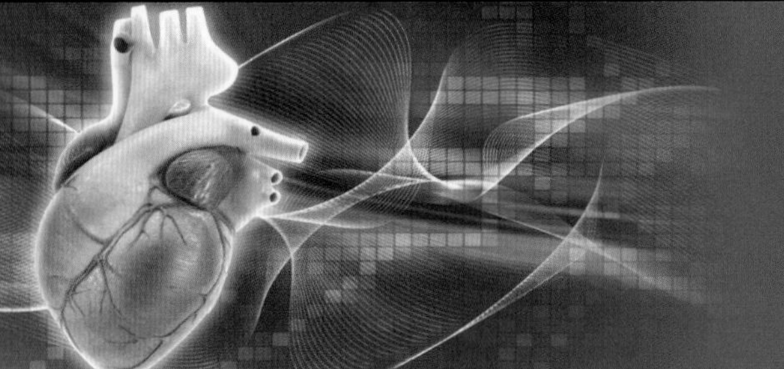

CHAPTER 89

THORACIC AORTIC SURGERY

Yuki Ikeno, Akiko Tanaka, and Anthony L. Estrera

INTRODUCTION

The aorta is the conduit that carries almost 200 million L of blood to the body in a lifetime. Yet despite its critical role, it is subject to a variety of disease processes that can have serious health consequences. This chapter describes the anatomy of the aorta, the classification and pathogenesis of aortic diseases, and the epidemiology and risk factors associated with specific aortic conditions. As the principal treatment of serious aortic disease is surgery, surgical strategies, including organ protection during aortic repair, will also be reviewed.

ANATOMY OF THE AORTA

The aorta is anatomically divided into the aortic root, ascending aorta, transverse aortic arch, descending thoracic aorta, and abdominal aorta (**Figure 89.1**). The aortic wall is composed of three layers: intima, media, and adventitia. The intima is the innermost layer and made of a single layer of endothelium.

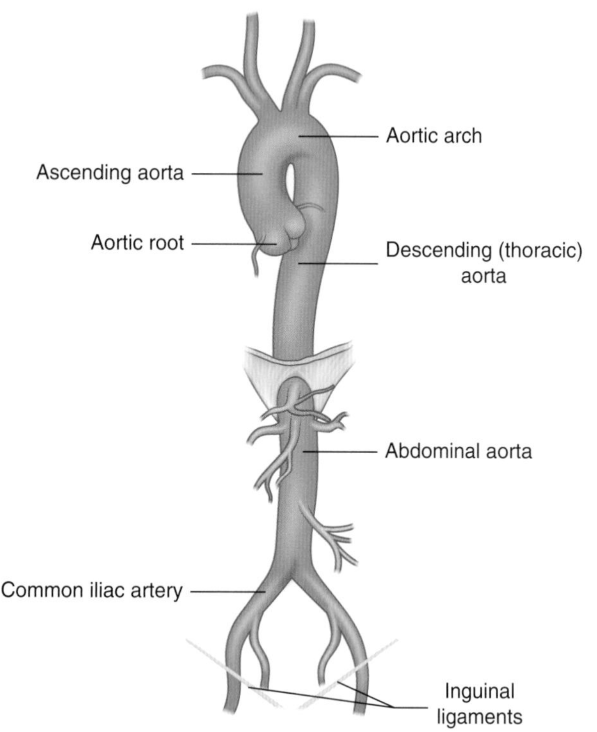

FIGURE 89.1 Anatomy of the aorta.

The media lies between intima and adventitia and is made of smooth muscle cells, elastic tissue, and collagen. The adventitia is the outmost layer, mainly composed of collagen, lymphatics, and a network of small blood vessels (vasa vasorum). The intima and inner one-third of media are directly nourished by blood from the aortic lumen, whereas the vasa vasorum feeds the outer two-thirds of media and adventitia.

DEFINITION AND CLASSIFICATIONS OF THORACIC AORTIC DISEASE

Aortic diseases can be classified into the following categories: true aneurysm, false aneurysm (pseudoaneurysm), aortic dissection, and penetrating aortic ulcer.[1] A true aortic aneurysm is a dilatation of the aorta, involving all three layers of the aortic wall. An aneurysm is defined by a diameter of 50% or greater than the normal. The aneurysm location is described using the anatomy mentioned earlier, and the descending thoracic aortic aneurysm is further divided into three extents (ie, A, B, and C) and the thoracoabdominal aneurysm is subdivided into five extents (ie, I-V)[2,3] (**Figure 89.2**). In a false aneurysm, the aneurysmal wall consists of adventitia or periaortic tissue.

Aortic dissection occurs when blood enters through an intimal tear and rapidly separates the media, forming a false lumen. Two classifications of aortic dissection based on the extent of the dissection are widely used: the DeBakey and Stanford classifications.[4] In DeBakey type I or Stanford type A dissection, the dissection involves the ascending aorta. In DeBakey type II, only the ascending aorta is involved. In DeBakey type III, or Stanford type B, spares the ascending aorta and involves the descending/thoracoabdominal aorta (**Figure 89.3A,B**). However, these classifications are confusing when the dissection flap extends from the transverse arch without the ascending aorta involved, the so-called non-A and non-B. Thus, recently, the Society of Vascular Surgery and Society of Thoracic Surgeons described a new classification system, focusing on the location of the entry tear: Any dissection with the entry tear in the ascending aorta is named type A; tear in the arch or dissection is type B, regardless of the proximal extension; and type I is defined as unidentified tear but dissection involving the ascending aorta.[5] This classification is useful when evaluating the indication for thoracic endovascular aortic repair (TEVAR).

Aortic dissection is also classified based on the time elapsed since initial clinical presentation (hyperacute: <24 hours,

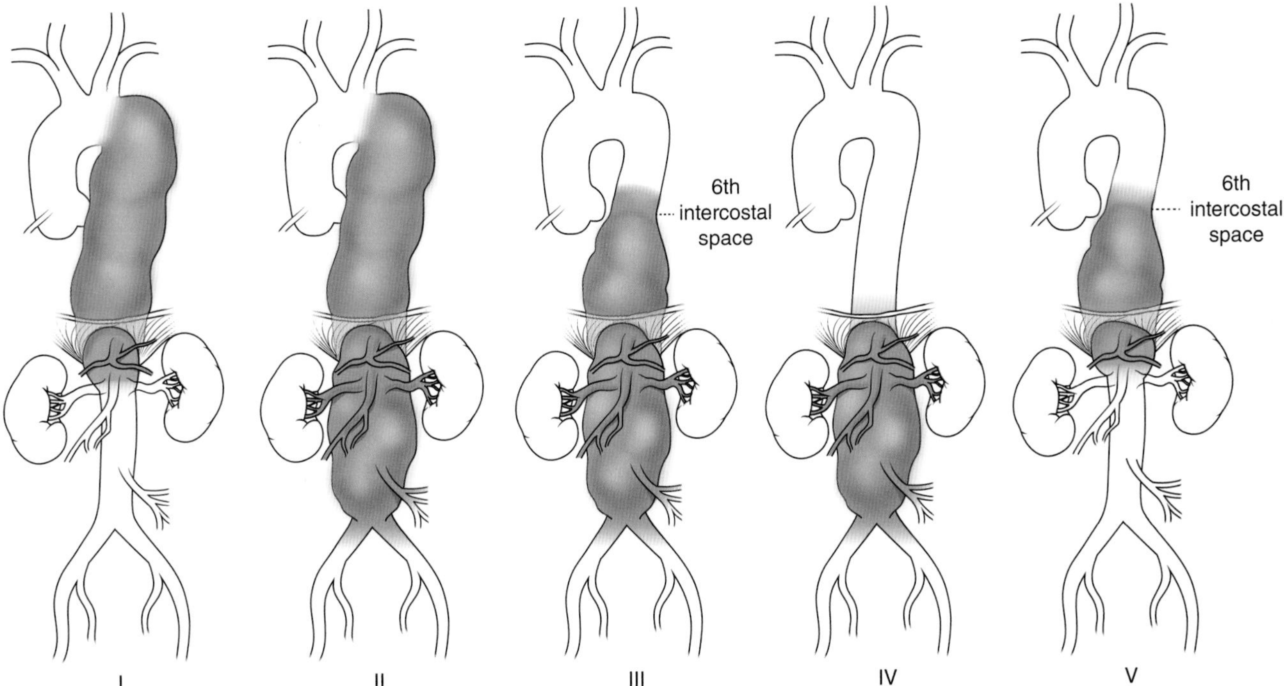

FIGURE 89.2 Crawford's classification of thoracoabdominal aortic aneurysms defines the aneurysmal extent. Extent I, distal to the left subclavian artery to above the renal arteries. Extent II, distal to the left subclavian artery to below the renal arteries. Extent III, from the sixth intercostal space to below the renal arteries. Extent IV, entire abdominal aorta. Extent V, below the sixth intercostal space to just above the renal arteries. (Reprinted with permission from Grover FL, Mack MJ. *Cardiac Surgery*. Philadelphia, PA: Wolters Kluwer; 2016. Figure 15.1.)

acute: 2-7 days, subacute: >7-30 days, chronic: >30 days).[6] Chronic aortic dissection may develop aneurysmal dilatation of the aortic wall.

Penetrating arteriosclerotic ulcer is an aortic disorder, which penetrates and ulcerates the internal elastic lamina of the aortic wall. It is a form of diffuse arteriosclerotic disease with sessile, mobile, or pedunculated atheroma composed of lipid deposition in the intimal layer of the aorta.

PATHOGENESIS

Thoracic Aortic Aneurysms

A variety of conditions involve the development of aortic disease: congenital, degenerative, traumatic, inflammatory, infectious, and anastomotic. Genetic/congenital conditions—such as Marfan syndrome, Loeys-Dietz syndrome, Ehlers-Danlos syndrome, Turner syndrome, Noonan syndrome, and autosomal dominant polycystic kidney disease—carry higher risks for aortic dissection and rupture.[7,8] Aneurysmal changes can also occur in the aorta distal to stenotic aortic valves or coarctation. Patients with a bicuspid aortic valve are at risk for developing ascending aortic dilatation from structural aortic wall abnormalities and turbulent flow.[9] Cystic medial degeneration and atherosclerosis are the common causes of a degenerative aneurysm. Cystic medial degeneration, the loss of elastic tissue and smooth muscle cells because of the inflammation and apoptosis, is most frequently observed in the ascending aorta,[10] while atherosclerosis mainly affects the descending thoracic and abdominal aortic segments. Blunt aortic trauma can also cause aortic disease, most frequently occurring at the isthmus.[11] Inflammatory diseases are rare but can also cause aortic disease. These include Takayasu arteritis, Behçet disease, and giant cell arteritis.[12] Infection from bacteria and fungus can cause aneurysmal degeneration.

Incidence and Survival

The incidence of thoracic aortic aneurysms is 5.9 new aneurysms per 100,000 person-years in the United States.[13] The major causes of deaths in people with these aneurysms are aortic rupture and dissection. Joyce and colleagues[14] reported a survival rate of 50% at 5 years and 30% at 10 years in 107 patients with a thoracic aortic aneurysm. Of those, 32% died of rupture. Aneurysm diameter correlates with the survival: patients whose aortic diameter was more than 6 cm showed significantly lower survival than patients with an aortic diameter of less than 6 cm (36.6% vs 61.1%, at 5 years, respectively).

Aortic Growth Rate and Aortic Events

Elefteriades and colleagues reported in a retrospective study that the mean growth rate of the ascending aorta was 0.14 cm per year, and that of the descending/thoracoabdominal aortic aneurysm was 0.19 cm per year, with an incremental increase in growth rate as the diameter continues to enlarge. In addition,

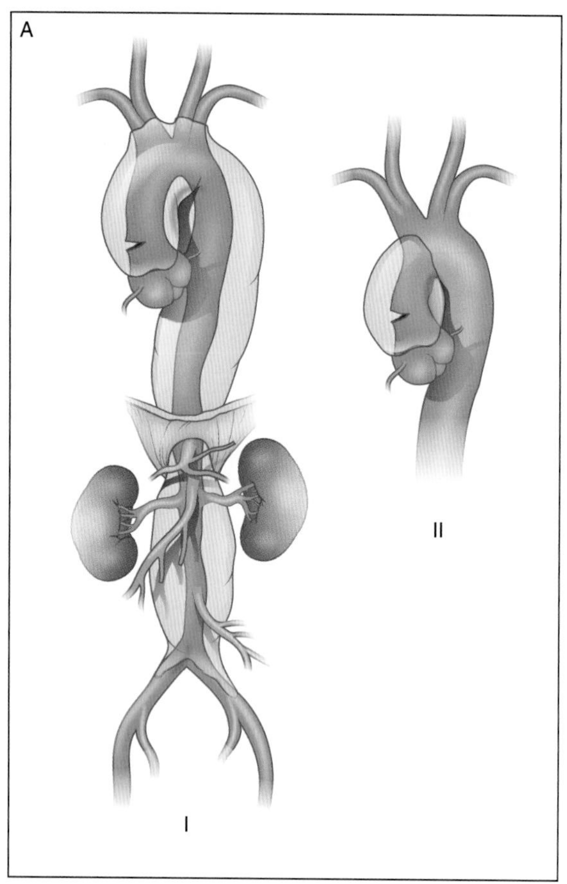

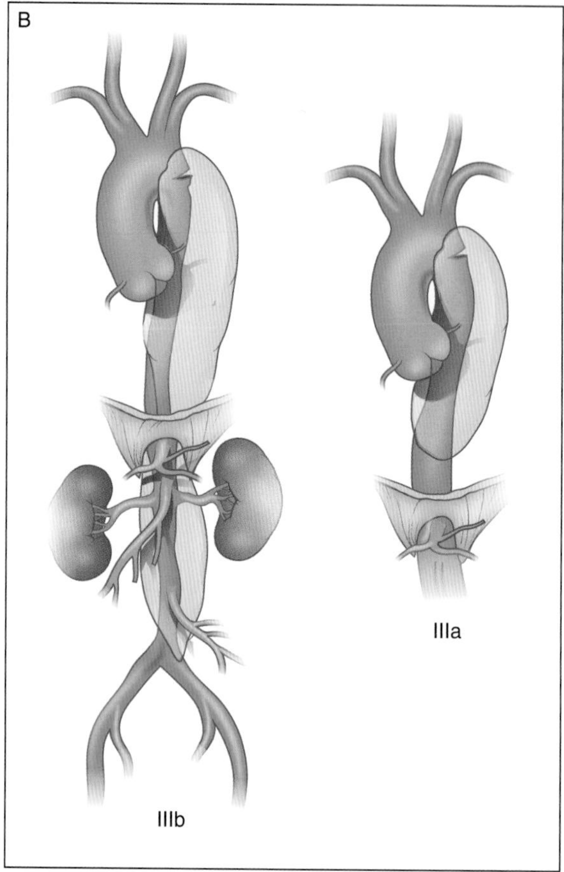

FIGURE 89.3 Classification of aortic dissection. DeBakey type I (Stanford type A) involves the ascending aorta. In DeBakey type II, only the ascending aorta is involved. DeBakey type III (Stanford type B) spares the ascending aorta and involves the descending/thoracoabdominal aorta.

the aortic diameter following aortic dissection grew at a faster rate of 0.37 cm per year.[15,16] In the ascending aorta, the yearly incidence of adverse aortic events (ie, a composite of rupture, dissection, and death) was significantly associated with aortic size (3.5-3.9 cm, 2.2%; 4.0-4.4 cm, 4.3%; 4.5-4.9 cm, 4.0%; 5.0-5.4 cm, 5.8%; 5.5-5.9 cm, 6.8%; >6.0 cm, 15.0%). The rate of adverse events increased sharply at the size of 5.25 and 5.5 cm and then again between 5.75 and 6 cm. Likewise, the yearly rate of adverse aortic events in the descending/thoracoabdominal aorta increased markedly at a size of 6 cm and 6.5 cm (3.0-3.4 cm, 0.6%; 3.5-4.0 cm, 4.1%; 4.0-4.4 cm, 7.3%; 4.5-4.9 cm, 10.2%; 5.0-5.4 cm, 3.0%; 5.5-5.9 cm, 7.8%; 6.0-6.4 cm, 18.7%; 6.5-6.9 cm, 21.0%; >7 cm, 18.9%). Connective tissue disease is also known as an independent risk factor for aortic events.

Aortic Dissection

Epidemiology and Risk Factors

In population-based studies, the incidence of acute aortic dissection is estimated at 2 to 6 per 100,000 person-years.[17,18] The incidence is higher in men than in women and increases with age. In the International Registry of Acute Aortic Dissection (IRAD), the mean age was 63 years, 65% of which were men. Other risk factors for aortic dissection include preexisting aortic disease, aortic valve disease, a family history of aortic diseases, a history of cardiac surgery, cigarette smoking, blunt chest trauma, and use of drugs, such as cocaine and amphetamines.[19]

Clinical Presentation: Acute Aortic Dissection

Abrupt onset of chest/back pain is the most frequent symptom of acute aortic dissection. Other symptoms and presentations are aortic rupture, aortic valve regurgitation, cardiac tamponade, myocardial ischemia, congestive heart failure, and end-organ malperfusion (ie, neurological deficit, spinal cord injury, mesenteric ischemia, renal failure, and limb ischemia). P pulse deficits may be observed in as many as 30%. Because of these lethal complications, the prognosis of the disease without prompt treatment is devastating. Hirst and colleagues reported that 3% of patients with acute type A dissection died immediately after the onset, 21% within 24 hours, 74% within 2 weeks, 80% within a month, and 93% within a year.[20] Thus, the acute phase (2 weeks within onset) is considered a critical time with high mortality.[21]

However, the prognosis of acute aortic dissection highly depends on its extension. In the autopsy study of acute aortic dissection, patients with Stanford type A dissection emerged as a cause of sudden cardiovascular death more frequently than Stanford type B (65.0% vs 6.5%),[22] and most deaths occurred in the acute phase. The mortality rate for Stanford type B dissection in the acute phase is approximately 50% in patients with end-organ ischemia or rupture and 10% in patients without complications.[23]

HISTORY OF AORTIC SURGERY

The history of aortic surgery has been a series of challenges against the lethal natural history of aortic disease and complexity of the procedures. A vital contribution to the modern aortic surgery was made by Rudolph Matas in 1902, when he first performed the endoaneurysmorrhaphy with controlling proximal and distal artery.[1] Throughout the first half of the 20th century, sporadic attempts were made to treat aortic aneurysms, almost all in the abdominal aorta. In 1944, Alexander and Byron successfully resected a thoracic aortic aneurysm secondary to coarctation without reconstruction of aortic continuity.[24] In 1948, Gross and colleagues replaced the coarctation with an aortic allograft, although the result was unsatisfactory. In 1950, Swan and colleagues reported a successful series for treating coarctations and aneurysms using an allograft replacement. In 1953, DeBakey and Cooley reported the first successful application of resection and grafting to a descending thoracic aortic aneurysm.[25] Three years later, they reported the first successful modern operation for ascending aortic aneurysm by graft replacement under cardiopulmonary bypass (CPB). In 1964, Wheat and colleagues reported a simultaneous but separate replacement of the ascending aorta and aortic valve, with reimplantation of the coronary ostia into the graft. Bentall and De Bono, in 1968, accomplished a root replacement with a composite of a valve and polyester tube graft.

Transverse arch repair, a more complicated surgical challenge, saw technical advances, and improved outcomes with the development of strategies for brain protection. In 1957, DeBakey and colleagues reported the first successful aortic arch aneurysm with allograft replacement under CPB and antegrade cerebral perfusion. Morris and colleagues reported the first acute type A dissection repair in 1963. In 1975, Griepp and colleagues established the hypothermic circulatory arrest for aortic arch repair,[26] which pioneered subsequent brain protection strategies.

The thoracoabdominal aneurysm also remained a challenge, not only because of the magnitude of the operation but also due to the potential for multiorgan dysfunction after repair, including in the intestinal, renal, and spinal cord ischemic complications. In 1955, Ellis and colleagues reported a repair of an aneurysm involving a renal artery by graft replacement. In the same year, Etheredge and colleagues reported a successful repair of the thoracoabdominal aneurysm, including the celiac and superior mesenteric arteries. Finally, in 1956, DeBakey and colleagues reported a successful repair of thoracoabdominal aneurysm involving all the visceral arteries.

The development of devices also has contributed to the improvement of surgical outcomes. Instead of an allograft, the first satisfactory synthetic aortic substitute was a fabric tube made of polyvinyl chloride cloth in 1954. Since Deterling and colleagues reported the utility of polyester, it has been widely used. Impregnating the polyester graft with collagen, gelatin, or albumin has demonstrated a considerable reduction in blood loss through the grafts. Guilmet and colleagues described the use of gelatin-resorcinol-formaldehyde glue to reinforce the dissected aortic wall before anastomoses in 1979.[27] An albumin and glutaraldehyde-based adhesive, the BioGlue (CryoLife Inc, Kennesaw, GA, USA), has been approved for use in the United States.

Endovascular stent grafting—thoracic endovascular aortic repair (TEVAR)—was introduced by Dake and colleagues in the early 1990s, using a custom-designed graft.[28] Currently, a variety of off-the-shelf grafts have become available for clinical use.

SURGICAL INDICATIONS AND RISK EVALUATION

The surgical indications of chronic thoracic aortic disease are determined by the balance of surgical risks and the expected adverse events due to the aortic disease. Guidelines suggest optimal treatment options for each condition.[18,19,29] Patients who have an acute aortic syndrome (ie, ruptured aneurysm, acute aortic dissection, intimal hematoma, and symptomatic aortic ulcer) are indicated for emergent/urgent surgical repair, due to their highly lethal nature. In patients with acute type B dissection, interventions should be recommended when patients have organ malperfusion syndrome, progression of dissection, aneurysm expansion, or uncontrolled hypertension (complicated type B dissection). Medical management had been preferred when patients do not have these features (uncomplicated type B dissection), but endovascular options may be considered to prevent late complications.[30] The Investigation of Stent Grafts in Aortic Dissection (INSTEAD) trial compared TEVAR and optimal medical therapy (OMT) for patients with subacute and chronic uncomplicated type B dissection (2-52 weeks after initial diagnosis). At early follow-up, patients treated with TEVAR were found to have improved aortic remodeling but no difference in mortality. However, after 5 years, TEVAR significantly reduced the incidence of aneurysm formation, and aortic-related mortality compared with OMT.[30] As a result, some surgical teams recommend a more aggressive approach, advocating TEVAR for treatment of patients with uncomplicated type B dissection.

In patients with chronic thoracic aortic disease, computed tomography, or magnetic resonance imaging is used to evaluate the aorta. Small aortic aneurysm (3.5-4.4 cm) can be monitored by annual imaging, while those with an aneurysm (4.5-5.4 cm) require semiannual imaging follow-up until they reach the criteria for surgical treatment.[18] Stringent control of hypertension, lipid profile optimization, smoking cessation, and other atherosclerosis risk-reduction measures should be instituted for these patients. However, no medical treatment has been established to reverse aortic dilatation.

Surgical interventions are recommended for asymptomatic patients with aortic root or ascending aortic aneurysm when (1) the aortic diameter is 5.5 cm or greater; (2) growth rate is more than 0.5 cm per year; and (3) aortic size is greater than 4.5 cm, and the patient is undergoing aortic valve repair/replacement. Patients with Marfan syndrome and hereditary aortic disease, bicuspid aortic disease, small body size, or planned pregnancy are indicated for aortic repair at lower thresholds.[19,29]

Few data exist on the natural history of isolated aortic arch aneurysms since they are frequently associated with adjacent aortic aneurysms. Currently, interventions to the asymptomatic aortic arch are considered in patients with an arch diameter exceeding 5.5 cm and those who are already planned for the adjacent aneurysm repair.

The surgical/endovascular repairs of descending thoracic or thoracoabdominal aortic aneurysm have been reoriented with the development of stent grafts. However, there are no randomized trials that compare the outcomes of endovascular repair with a conventional open operation and nonoperative management. Currently, TEVAR is the first line for descending thoracic aortic aneurysm and indicated with aneurysm size of more than 5.5 cm. Open surgery is reserved for patients whose anatomy is not suitable for TEVAR. Surgical intervention is considered in thoracoabdominal aneurysms exceeding 5.5 to 6.0 cm. In patients with connective tissue disorders, open repair is generally preferred to endovascular treatment and may be recommended at a smaller diameter.

Perioperative Risk Evaluation

Preoperative evaluation includes imaging studies to determine the extent of disease, limits of the planned procedure, and risks of the procedure. Myocardial infarction, low-cardiac output state, respiratory failure, renal failure, and stroke are the principal causes of mortality and morbidity after aortic repairs—and preoperative assessment of these organ systems is essential.[31] Intraoperative transesophageal echocardiography is recommended in all open surgical repairs of the thoracic aorta.

AORTIC ANEURYSM REPAIR

Surgical techniques of aortic aneurysm repair are described by the location of the aneurysm.

Aortic Root Replacement

In patients with aortic root dilation with aortic valve disease, composite valve graft replacement with either biological or mechanical valves (modified Bentall operation) is indicated. The aorta and the heart are exposed via median sternotomy. After the CPB is established with dual-stage venous drainage, proximal arch cannulation, and left ventricular venting through the right upper pulmonary vein the ascending aorta is clamped and antegrade cardioplegia is administered. Subsequent myocardial protection is achieved with continuous retrograde and selective antegrade cardioplegia. If severe aortic insufficiency is present, retrograde cardioplegia alone may be given initially. The ascending aorta is opened, and the aortic valve resected. The Valsalva sinus is trimmed, leaving coronary artery cuffs and an aortic sinus rim to be used for a hemostatic second row (described later). When bioprosthetic valves are used, a composite of the valve is created using a branched Sienna™ Collared Graft (Terumo Cardiovascular Group, Ann Arbor, MI, USA) with a single sidearm using the following steps. The size of the Dacron graft is determined by adding 3 mm to the size of the annulus. For example, a 30-mm graft is used when the annulus is sized to 27 mm. Once the valve is washed and ready, the collar of the Dacron graft is trimmed, leaving 1-cm remnant at the base. Three to four crimps of the proximal end of the Dacron graft are left, to suture the bioprosthetic valve cuff with a running 4-0 polypropylene suture (**Figure 89.4A**). If the right coronary is distant from the graft, the sidearm may be utilized for a bypass. If the right coronary artery button is to be directly reimplanted to the main Dacron graft, 2-0 polyester pledgeted mattress sutures are placed through the annulus then through the composite graft. The sutures are tied, and the composite graft is seated in a supra-annular position. Continuous 3-0 polypropylene sutures are used for the second row, holding the collar to the remnant of the sinus rim to secure the hemostasis (**Figure 89.4B**). On-X Ascending Aortic Prosthesis (CryoLife, Inc., Kennesaw, GA, USA) is used for mechanical composite graft, whose generous valve cuff is also suitable for the second row. After completing implantation in the annulus, the distal end of the composite graft is trimmed to the length appropriate for the distal anastomosis. The coronary buttons are reattached to the graft using a running 5-0 polypropylene sutures with bovine pericardial strip reinforcement. If the coronary artery ostia are displaced far laterally by a large aortic root aneurysm, the modified Cabrol technique (interposition using a second graft between the coronary button and aortic graft) is used (**Figure 89.4 C,D**).[32] The distal anastomosis is constructed using a 4-0 continuous polypropylene suture.

In the 1990s, valve-sparing root techniques were reported to preserve the intact native valve, especially in the young population, to avoid anticoagulation. David proposed the reimplantation technique,[33] and Yacoub reported the remodeling technique.[34] The critical difference between these two procedures is annular stabilization. In the reimplantation technique, the entire native aortic valve and the sinus rim is sutured inside the root graft, with the first row sewed to the level of atrioventricular junction, and the rim of the native aortic valve is sutured to the inside of the graft (second row). The reimplantation procedure is preferred in patients with connective tissue disease to prevent late aortic annulus dilation with the annular stabilization. On the other hand, the remodeling procedure tailors the graft by making three incisions and trimming the flaps for sinus reconstruction and is sutured to the small rims of aortic sinus wall. Thus, the remodeling procedure theoretically provides more physiologic dynamics than the reimplantation.

The expected result for the risk of death for composite valve graft is 5.6% in the current meta-analysis.[32] Additional comorbidities and emergency operations are associated with increased risk. The surgical mortality for valve-sparing aortic

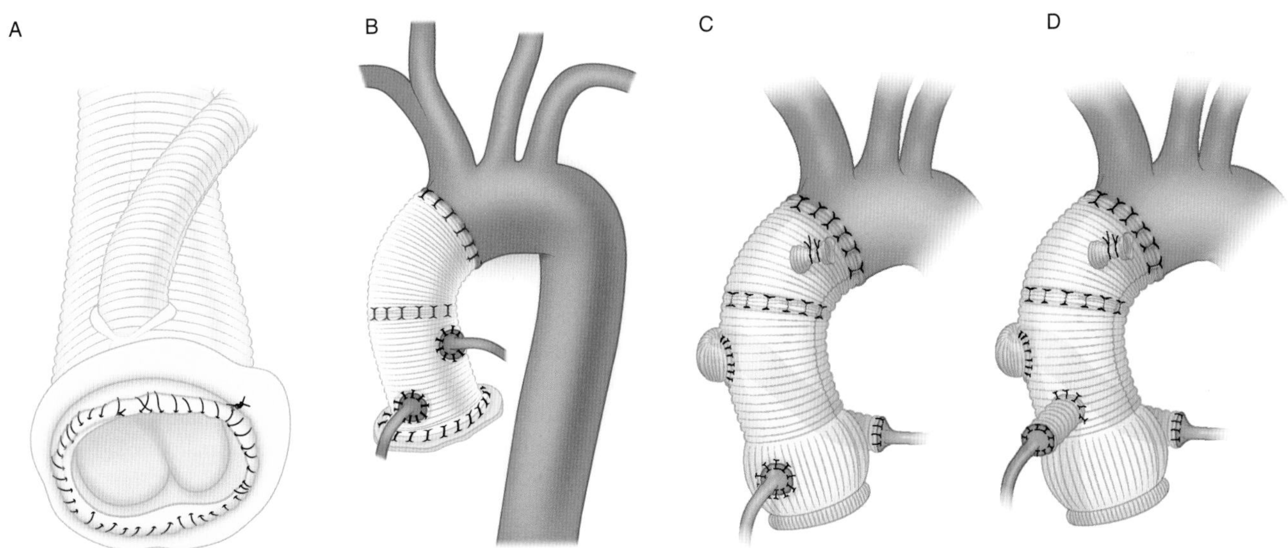

FIGURE 89.4 Aortic root replacement: **A**. Composite bioprosthetic graft. **B**. Completion of aortic root procedure after second-row hemostatic suture line. **C**. Modified Cabrol procedures; and **D**. Reimplantation procedure.

root reconstruction is less than 1.5%, since these patients are mostly young and otherwise healthy.[35]

Ascending and Proximal Arch Replacement

To eliminate all the diseased wall, ascending and proximal arch replacement is recommended for proximal aortic disease rather than simple ascending aortic replacement. Steps proceed as follows. The chest is entered through a full median sternotomy. After establishing CPB with bicaval drainage, ascending aortic cannulation, and left ventricular sump, the patient is cooled to deep hypothermia. The ascending aorta is clamped, and antegrade cardioplegic solution is administered to induce cardiac arrest, followed by continuous retrograde cardioplegia. CPB is stopped after reaching the target temperature and retrograde cerebral perfusion is initiated, via a superior vena cava cannula. The aorta is transected just proximal to the brachiocephalic artery and at the sinotubular junction. A Dacron graft with a single sidearm is typically used (commonly size 28 or 30 mm). The distal anastomosis is completed first, the graft is clamped, and systemic circulation is reestablished through the sidearm. If an aortic valve procedure is required, this is performed before the proximal anastomosis during systemic warming. In patients with aortic dissection, the dissected aorta may be reinforced with circumferential 4-0 polypropylene-pledgeted sutures or the dissected aortic wall may be approximated using surgical glue and Teflon felt strips. Some reports have described development of late wall necrosis when glue is used.[36] Once all the anastomoses are completed, the patient is weaned from CPB.

The reported mortality after the proximal aortic repair is 1% to 5%.[37] Comorbid conditions, such as advanced age, impaired renal function, concomitant coronary bypass graft surgery, and emergency operation, are associated with increased mortalities.[38] Endovascular stent grafts for the treatment of aneurysms or other conditions of the ascending aorta or aortic root have not been approved by the US Food and Drug Administration (FDA), but a clinical trial evaluating endovascular ascending aortic repair for acute type A aortic dissection is currently underway.

Transverse Arch Replacement

Total arch replacement with the distal suture line distal to the left subclavian artery (zone 3) has been the conventional approach for treating diseases of the aortic arch (**Figure 89.5**). However, to minimize surgical risks, zone 2 arch replacement with suture line proximal to the left subclavian artery has become popular. The elephant trunk procedure is a useful technique to prepare for a two-stage surgery when the disease extends to the descending thoracic aorta.[39] In this variation, a distal extension of the graft is left free floating within the lumen of the remaining descending thoracic aorta. A subsequent open or endovascular operation is performed to replace the descending thoracic aorta using the extension as the proximal site of the repair. With the advent of TEVAR, open arch vessel debranching (hybrid aortic arch repair) with zone 1 TEVAR is now an option.[40] These procedures may be considered as an alternative to conventional surgery in selected patients. However, there is no device approved by the FDA for the aortic arch disease.

Our technique for transverse arch replacement with elephant trunk is as follows. A multibranched Dacron graft with a surrounding collar (Sienna™ Collared Graft [Terumo Cardiovascular Group, Ann Arbor, MI, USA]) is selected, as it allows easy size adjustment of the distal anastomosis by trimming the collar. After establishment of hypothermic circulatory arrest, retrograde cerebral perfusion is initiated through the superior vena cava cannula. Antegrade cerebral perfusion can also be used. The distal anastomosis is performed proximal to the left subclavian with a continuous 4-0 polypropylene suture

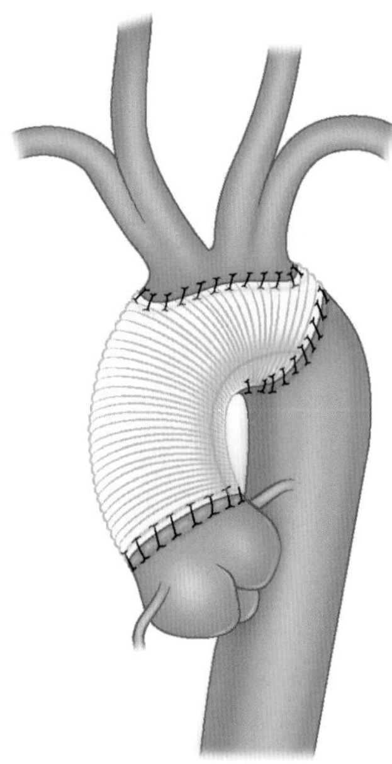

FIGURE 89.5 Total arch replacement with the distal suture line distal to the left subclavian artery (zone 3).

(zone 2). The elephant trunk is truncated to approximately 7 cm, short enough to avoid spinal cord injury but long enough to facilitate the future procedure. The innominate artery and left common carotid artery are commonly reconstructed as a single cuff, but these are individually reconstructed in case of connective tissue disorders. The systemic circulation is then restored through the sidearm of the graft, and the proximal anastomosis performed at the level of sinotubular junction during the warming.

Some groups prefer to perform proximal anastomosis before the arch vessel reconstruction while using antegrade cerebral perfusion[41] to minimize the cardiac ischemic time. Others perform the arch vessel reconstruction first (arch first technique) to minimize the cerebral perfusion time. Near-infrared spectroscopy or electroencephalography is a commonly utilized intraoperative neuromonitor by experienced team, and changes seen on the monitors during surgery may prompt alterations in cerebral protective strategies.[42] There is a 1% to 7% risk of stroke, even in elective surgery.[43] The optimal strategies for arterial cannulation technique and cerebral protection are still controversial. The ascending aorta, right axially artery, innominate artery, and femoral artery are possible options for cannulation site, and no option has emerged as clearly superior. Depending on the brain protection methods, aortic anatomy, or atherosclerotic plaques, the approach should be tailored on a case-by-case basis. As an adjunct to deep hypothermic circulatory arrest (14-20 °C) or moderate hypothermia (20-28 °C), contemporary brain protection strategies apply antegrade or retrograde cerebral perfusion. Retrograde cerebral perfusion was first introduced by Ueda and colleagues in 1988,[44] perfusing cold-oxygenated blood into the superior vena cava. This procedure also allows the washout of particulate emboli from the brain. Antegrade cerebral perfusion techniques have undergone several modifications over the past six decades. In a nonrandomized comparison from cases reported in the Society of Thoracic Surgeons database, patients receiving hypothermic circulatory arrest without cerebral perfusion showed higher mortality and morbidity than groups treated with adjunctive retrograde or antegrade perfusion. However, there were no significant differences observed between the two cerebral perfusion techniques.[45]

The mortality after a total arch replacement is 2% to 6% in elective procedures but increases to 15% in emergent cases.[43] Meticulous brain and myocardial protection, correction of coagulopathies, and improved operative techniques have led to improved outcomes compared to the mortality of 17% in the late 1990s.[46]

Descending/Thoracoabdominal Aortic Replacement

Multiorgan protection, especially of the spinal cord, is crucial to the success of aortic repair involving the descending thoracic aorta and thoracoabdominal aorta. We routinely use adjuncts of cerebral spinal fluid drainage, distal aortic perfusion with left heart bypass, and neuromonitoring-guided intercostal artery reattachment to prevent spinal cord ischemia.[47]

The technique is briefly described. Under general anesthesia with double-lumen endotracheal intubation to isolate separate the lung, the patient is placed in the right lateral decubitus position with the hip rotated to the left at 60 degrees. A thoracoabdominal incision is used to enter the sixth intercostal space and the retroperitoneal space. The peritoneal sac and the left kidney are rotated anteriorly and to the right. A table-fixed self-retractor (THeOmni® [Integra Lifesciences, NJ, USA]) is used to assist the exposure. The left pulmonary vein is cannulated for venous drainage and left femoral artery for arterial return to establish a left heart bypass. The proximal anastomosis is performed under segmental clamping to minimize the duration of organ ischemia. Hypothermic circulatory arrest after cooling using full CPB is used in cases in which when there is no space to apply a proximal clamp. The distal anastomosis is performed before the reattachment of the visceral and renal arteries to increase spinal cord perfusion by restoring pulsatile flow to the pelvic circulation (**Figure 89.6**). In most cases, the T8 to T12 segmental (intercostal) arteries are attached to the aortic graft, as they are important to the spinal perfusion.[48]

Mortality following descending aortic repair is 2% to 5%. The incidence of spinal cord ischemia ranges from 3% to 16%,[49] but can be less than 3% for elective surgical repairs.[50] The risk of mortality after the thoracoabdominal aortic repair is strongly influenced by the urgency of surgery, comorbid disease, and extent of repair. The reported mortality is 5% for extent I repair and 10% for extent II.[51]

Endovascular Thoracic Aortic Repair

TEVAR is now the preferred option for the treatment of descending thoracic aortic lesions when anatomically feasible. Primary requisites for TEVAR are suitable landing zones

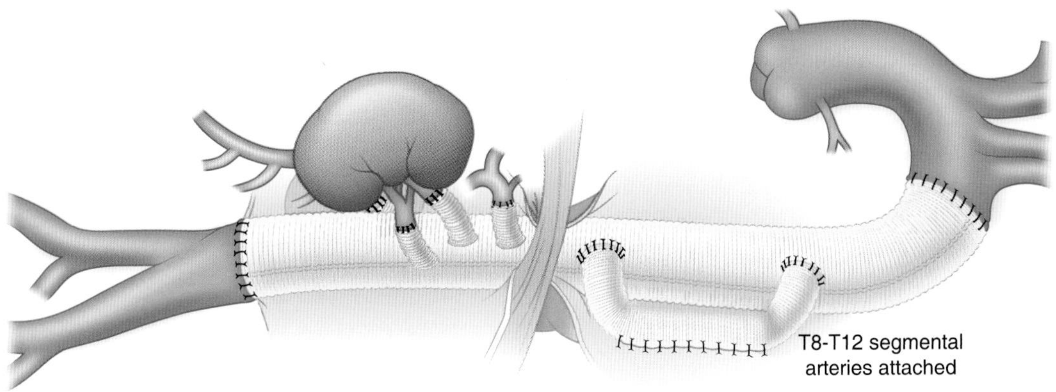

FIGURE 89.6 Thoracoabdominal aortic repair.

proximal and distal to the diseased segment (approximately 2 cm in length), and diameters of these landing segments need to be more than 16 mm and less than 45 mm. If coverage of the left subclavian artery is required, a left carotid artery bypass to left subclavian artery bypass or transposition may need to be performed before stent grafting. There are no available off-the-shelf devices for thoracoabdominal aortic disease in the US market. Thus, hybrid surgery with debranching of the visceral and renal artery segments or physician-modified fenestrated devices are used. Currently, clinical trials are ongoing for branched and fenestrated endograft in the United States and outcomes are awaited.

PATIENT FOLLOW-UP CARE

Medical management of patients with known aortic aneurysms or chronic aortic dissection is mainly focused on blood pressure control and surveillance imaging. In general blood pressure targets below 130/80 mm Hg are appropriate, and beta-blockers are the commonest antihypertensive agents prescribed. Some data suggest that beta-blockers may reduce aortic expansion and improve survival with aortic dissection. Calcium channel blockers and renin-angiotensin inhibitors are also frequently used. Angiotensin-1 antagonists (particularly losartan) have been shown to decrease the rate of aortic enlargement in patients with Marfan syndrome and Lowes-Dietz syndrome. As such, angiotensin-1 blockers are frequently selected as a second agent in patients with aortic aneurysm or dissection if beta-blockers alone do not achieve the blood pressure target. Most centers recommend that patients with aortic aneurysm or dissection avoid isometric heavy weightlifting and body contact sports. Leisure activities including sports with lower static and dynamic stress levels are typically allowed.[19]

For patients primarily receiving medical therapy, surveillance should be performed 6 months after initial diagnosis, then at yearly intervals unless the aortic diameter is approaching the criteria for further treatment. For patients who have undergone aortic surgery or TEVAR, follow-up imaging should be performed at 1 month after surgery to exclude the presence of early complications. Surveillance imaging should be repeated after 6 months, 12 months, and then yearly. Imaging will evaluate disease progression in other untreated parts of the aorta. If no progression of the disease has been observed for several years, a 2-year surveillance interval may be appropriate.[19]

RESEARCH AND FUTURE DIRECTIONS

Aortic surgery has made much progress over the decades, with significant advances in perioperative care, surgical techniques, and organ protection strategies. Stent grafting has replaced the first-line treatment for descending thoracic aortic disease. However, open surgical repair remains the mainstay in the remaining lesions at this time. Further studies are needed to establish preferred options for cerebral protection, with a particular focus on comparing antegrade and retrograde cerebral perfusion techniques. The best option for early management of uncomplicated acute type B aortic dissection has not been established and well-powered randomized trials with long-term follow-up comparing TEVAR with OMT would be welcome. Use of endovascular devices for treatment of aortic diseases involving the ascending aorta and transverse arch is another frontier that is now beginning to be explored, and device manufacturers are initiating trials of custom-built endografts, tailored in size to the individual patient. Other options for aortic repair, including novel personalized external support devices manufactured with three dimensional printing have been developed and early clinical use has begun.[52] Clinical trials exploring all of these techniques are anxiously awaited.

KEY POINTS

- ✔ Aortic disease is an important contributor to cardiovascular mortality and morbidity.
- ✔ The two main forms of aortic disease are aneurysm formation and aortic dissection. These have different etiologies and treatment strategies.

- ✔ Aortic diseases have a number of etiologies: congenital, degenerative, traumatic, inflammatory, infectious, and anastomotic. Genetic conditions, particularly Marfan syndrome, Loeys-Dietz syndrome, Ehlers-Danlos syndrome, and Turner syndrome carry higher risks for aortic dissection and rupture. Aneurysmal changes can also occur in the aorta distal to stenotic aortic valves or coarctation and are more common in patients with a bicuspid aortic valve.
- ✔ The natural history of aortic aneurysms is one of slow growth over time. Surveillance imaging is critical to assessing aortic dimensions. Size criteria for elective surgical intervention depend on the location (ascending aorta, transverse arch, descending, or thoracoabdominal aorta) and the presence or absence of a genetic syndrome.
- ✔ Acute aortic dissection involving the ascending aorta (Stanford type A) is treated with emergency surgical repair. Acute aortic dissection involving the descending thoracic aorta (Stanford type B), when uncomplicated, can be treated medically with pain control, blood pressure control, and close monitoring. Early use of TEVAR in this setting is being used by some centers with encouraging early results.
- ✔ Open surgery for thoracic aortic aneurysms has evolved and techniques used are tailored to the portion of the aorta that is replaced. Important strategies to protect the brain (often using hypothermia and selective cerebral perfusion) and the spinal cord (using cerebrospinal fluid drainage, distal aortic perfusion with left heart bypass, and neuromonitoring-guided intercostal artery reattachment) have been developed and reduce the risk of neurologic complications.
- ✔ Follow-up in patients with known aneurysms below size criteria, and in patients who have undergone prior aortic interventions, focuses on blood pressure control and ongoing surveillance imaging of all portions of the aorta.

REFERENCES

1. Kouchoukos NT, Blackstone EH, Hanley FL, Kirklin JK. *Kirklin/Barratt-Boyes Cardiac Surgery E-book*. Elsevier Health Sciences; 2012.
2. Crawford ES, Crawford JL, Safi HJ, et al. Thoracoabdominal aortic aneurysms: Preoperative and intraoperative factors determining immediate and long-term results of operations in 605 patients. *J Vasc Surg.* 1986;3(3):389-404.
3. Safi HJ, Miller CC 3rd. Spinal cord protection in descending thoracic and thoracoabdominal aortic repair. *Ann Thorac Surg.* 1999;67(6):1937-1939; discussion 1953-1938.
4. Kouchoukos NT, Dougenis D. Surgery of the thoracic aorta. *N Engl J Med.* 1997;336(26):1876-1889.
5. Lombardi JV, Hughes GC, Appoo JJ, et al. Society for Vascular Surgery (SVS) and Society of Thoracic Surgeons (STS) reporting standards for type B aortic dissections. *Ann Thorac Surg.* 2020;109(3):959-981.
6. Booher AM, Isselbacher EM, Nienaber CA, et al. The IRAD classification system for characterizing survival after aortic dissection. *Am J Med.* 2013;126:730.e19-730.e24. doi:10.1016/j.amjmed.2013.01.020
7. Francke U, Furthmayr H. Genes and gene products involved in Marfan syndrome. *Semin Thorac Cardiovasc Surg.* 1993;5(1):3-10.
8. Loeys BL, Schwarze U, Holm T, et al. Aneurysm syndromes caused by mutations in the tgf-β receptor. *N Engl J Med.* 2006;355(8):788-798.
9. Lindsay J. Coarctation of the aorta, bicuspid aortic valve and abnormal ascending aortic wall. *Am J Cardiol.* 1988;61(1):182-184.
10. Olson LJ, Subramanian R, Edwards WD. Surgical pathology of pure aortic insufficiency: a study of 225 cases. *Mayo Clin Proc.* 1984;59(12):835-841.
11. Azizzadeh A, Keyhani K, Miller CC III, Coogan SM, Safi HJ, Estrera AL. Blunt traumatic aortic injury: Initial experience with endovascular repair. *J Vasc Surg.* 2009;49(6):1403-1408.
12. Yajima M, Numano F, Park YB, Sagar S. Comparative studies of patients with Takayasu arteritis in Japan, Korea and India: comparison of clinical manifestations, angiography and HLA-B antigen. *Japanese Circ J.* 1993;58(1):9-14.
13. Bickerstaff LK, Pairolero PC, Hollier LH, et al. Thoracic aortic aneurysms: a population-based study. *Surgery.* 1982;92(6):1103-1108.
14. Joyce JW, Fairbairn JF 2nd, Kincaid OW, Juergen JL. Aneurysms of the thoracic aorta. A clinical study with special reference to prognosis. *Circulation.* 1964;29:176-181.
15. Zafar MA, Chen JF, Wu J, et al. Natural history of descending thoracic and thoracoabdominal aortic aneurysms. *J Thorac Cardiovasc Surg.* 2021;161(2):498-511.e1.
16. Elefteriades JA, Farkas EA. Thoracic aortic aneurysm clinically pertinent controversies and uncertainties. *J Am Coll Cardiol.* 2010;55(9):841-857.
17. Howard DP, Banerjee A, Fairhead JF, Perkins J, Silver LE, Rothwell PM. Population-based study of incidence and outcome of acute aortic dissection and premorbid risk factor control: 10-year results from the oxford vascular study. *Circulation.* 2013;127(20):2031-2037.
18. Hiratzka LF, Bakris GL, Beckman JA, et al. 2010 ACCF/AHA/AATS/ACR/ASA/SCA/SCAI/SIR/STS/SVM guidelines for the diagnosis and management of patients with thoracic aortic disease. A report of the American College Of Cardiology Foundation/American Heart Association task force on practice guidelines, an American Association for Thoracic Surgery, American College of Radiology, American Stroke Association, Society of Cardiovascular Anesthesiologists, Society for Cardiovascular Angiography and Interventions, Society of Interventional Radiology, Society of Thoracic Surgeons, and Society for Vascular Medicine. *J Am Coll Cardiol.* 2010;55(14):e27-e129.
19. Erbel R, Aboyans V, Boileau C, et al. 2014 ESC guidelines on the diagnosis and treatment of aortic diseases. *Eur Heart J.* 2014;35(41):2873-2926.
20. Hirst AE Jr, Johns Jr VJ, Kime SW Jr. Dissecting aneurysm of the aorta: A review of 505 cases. *Medicine (Baltimore).* 1958;37(3):217-279.
21. Miller DC, Stinson EB, Oyer PE, et al. Operative treatment of aortic dissections: experience with 125 patients over a sixteen-year period. *J Thorac Cardiovasc Surg.* 1979;78(3):365-382.
22. Murai T, Baba M, Ro A, et al. Sudden death due to cardiovascular disorders: a review of the studies on the medico-legal cases in Tokyo. *Keio J Med.* 2001;50(3):175-181.
23. Nauta FJ, Trimarchi S, Kamman AV, et al. Update in the management of type B aortic dissection. *Vasc Med.* 2016;21(3):251-263.
24. Alexander J, Byron FX. Aortectomy for thoracic aneurysm. *JAMA.* 1944;126(18):1139-1145.
25. DeBakey ME, Cooley DA. Successful resection of aneurysm of thoracic aorta and replacement by graft. *JAMA.* 1953;152(8):673-676.
26. Griepp RB, Stinson EB, Hollingsworth JF, Buehler D. Prosthetic replacement of the aortic arch. *J Thorac Cardiovasc Surg.* 1975;70(6):1051-1063.
27. Guilmet D, Bachet J, Goudot B, et al. Use of biological glue in acute aortic dissection: preliminary clinical results with a new surgical technique. *J Thorac Cardiovasc Surg.* 1979;77(4):516-521.
28. Dake MD, Miller DC, Semba CP, Mitchell RS, Walker PJ, Liddell RP. Transluminal placement of endovascular stent-grafts for the treatment of descending thoracic aortic aneurysms. *N Engl J Med.* 1994; 331(26):1729-1734.
29. JCS Joint Working Group. Guidelines for diagnosis and treatment of aortic aneurysm and aortic dissection (JCS 2011): digest version. *Circulation.* 2013;77(3):789-828.
30. Nienaber CA, Kische S, Rousseau H, et al. Endovascular repair of type B aortic dissection: long-term results of the randomized investigation of stent grafts in aortic dissection trial. *Circ Cardiovasc Interv.* 2013;6(4):407-416.

31. Kouchoukos NT. Composite graft replacement of the ascending aorta and aortic valve with the inclusion-wrap and open techniques. *Semin Thorac Cardiovasc Surg.* 1991;3(3):171-176.
32. Tanaka A, Al-Rstum Z, Zhou N, et al. Feasibility and durability of the modified cabrol coronary artery reattachment technique. *Ann Thorac Surg.* 2020;110(6):1847-1853. doi:10.1016/j.athoracsur.2020.04.125
33. David TE, Feindel CM. An aortic valve-sparing operation for patients with aortic incompetence and aneurysm of the ascending aorta. *J Thorac Cardiovasc Surg.* 1992;103(4):617-621; discussion 622.
34. Sarsam MA, Yacoub M. Remodeling of the aortic valve annulus. *J Thorac Cardiovasc Surg.* 1993;105(3):435-438.
35. David TE, David CM, Feindel CM, Manlhiot C. Reimplantation of the aortic valve at 20 years. *J Thorac Cardiovasc Surg.* 2017;153(2):232-238.
36. Ikeno Y, Yokawa K, Yamanaka K, et al. The fate of aortic root and aortic regurgitation after supracoronary ascending aortic replacement for acute type A aortic dissection. *J Thorac Cardiovasc Surg.* 2021;161(2):483-493.
37. Svensson LG, Longoria J, Kimmel WA, Nadolny E. Management of aortic valve disease during aortic surgery. *Ann Thorac Surg.* 2000;69(3):778-783; discussion 783-774.
38. David TE, Feindel CM, Webb GD, Colman JM, Armstrong S, Maganti M. Aortic valve preservation in patients with aortic root aneurysm: results of the reimplantation technique. *Ann Thorac Surg.* 2007;83(2):S732-S735; discussion S785-S790.
39. Crawford ES, Coselli JS, Svensson LG, Safi HJ, Hess KR. Diffuse aneurysmal disease (chronic aortic dissection, Marfan, and mega aorta syndromes) and multiple aneurysms. Treatment by subtotal and total aortic replacement emphasizing the elephant trunk operation. *Ann Surg.* 1990;211(5):521-527.
40. Bavaria J, Vallabhajosyula P, Moeller P, Szeto W, Desai N, Pochettino A. Hybrid approaches in the treatment of aortic arch aneurysms: postoperative and midterm outcomes. *J Thorac Cardiovasc Surg.* 2013;145 (suppl 3):S85-S90.
41. Okita Y, Okada K, Omura A, et al. Surgical techniques of total arch replacement using selective antegrade cerebral perfusion. *Ann Cardiothorac Surg.* 2013;2(2):222-228.
42. Ghincea CV, Anderson DA, Ikeno Y, et al. Utility of neuromonitoring in hypothermic circulatory arrest cases for early detection of stroke: listening through the noise. *J Thorac Cardiovasc Surg.* 2020;S0022-5223(20):30455.
43. Sundt TM 3rd, Orszulak TA, Cook DJ, Schaff HV. Improving results of open arch replacement. *Ann Thorac Surg.* 2008;86(3):787-796; discussion 787-796.
44. Ueda Y, Miki S, Kusuhara K, et al. Surgical treatment of the aneurysm or dissection involving the ascending aorta and aortic arch using circulatory arrest and retrograde perfusion. *J Cardiovasc Surg (Torino).* 1990;31(5):553-558.
45. Englum BR, He X, Gulack BC, et al. Hypothermia and cerebral protection strategies in aortic arch surgery: a comparative effectiveness analysis from the sts adult cardiac surgery database. *Eur J Cardiothorac Surg.* 2017;52(3):492-498.
46. Bachet J, Guilmet D, Goudot B, et al. Antegrade cerebral perfusion with cold blood: a 13-year experience. *Ann Thorac Surg.* 1999;67(6):1874-1878; discussion 1891-1874.
47. Tanaka A, Safi HJ, Estrera AL. Current strategies of spinal cord protection during thoracoabdominal aortic surgery. *Gen Thorac Cardiovasc Surg.* 2018;66(6):307-314.
48. Afifi RO, Sandhu HK, Zaidi ST, et al. Intercostal artery management in thoracoabdominal aortic surgery: to reattach or not to reattach? *J Thorac Cardiovasc Surg.* 2018;155(4):1372-1378.e1371.
49. Ghincea CV, Ikeno Y, Aftab M, Reece TB. Spinal cord protection for thoracic aortic surgery: bench to bedside. *Semin Thorac Cardiovasc Surg.* 2019;31(4):713-720.
50. Svensson LG, Crawford ES, Hess KR, Coselli JS, Safi HJ. Variables predictive of outcome in 832 patients undergoing repairs of the descending thoracic aorta. *Chest.* 1993;104(4):1248-1253.
51. Coselli JS, LeMaire SA, Preventza O, et al. Outcomes of 3309 thoracoabdominal aortic aneurysm repairs. *J Thorac Cardiovasc Surg.* 2016;151(5):1323-1338.
52. Izgi C, Newsome S, Alpendurada F, et al. External aortic root support to prevent aortic dilatation in patients with Marfan syndrome. *J Am Coll Cardiol.* 2018;72(10):1095-1105. doi:10.1016/j.jacc.2018.06.053

CHAPTER 90

PERIPHERAL ARTERIAL SURGERY

Michael C. Siah, Gerardo Gonzalez-Guardiola, Khalil Chamseddin, James A. Walker, and Melissa L. Kirkwood

INTRODUCTION

Epidemiology

Peripheral arterial disease (PAD) is the chronic manifestation of atherosclerosis in the lower extremity vasculature. Its incidence continues to increase worldwide, with current epidemiologic estimates approaching 200 million people.[1] In the United States alone, 8 to 12 million Americans are estimated to be affected by PAD.[2] The domestic and global prevalence of PAD is expected to continue increasing as populations continue to age and the prevalence of diabetes grows. The burden caused by PAD has resulted in burgeoning health care costs associated with its care and the management of its complications.

PAD represents a disease process that markedly impairs the quality of patients' lives and is the primary cause of major amputation in the United States. Patients with PAD often suffer from high rates of cardiovascular death, myocardial infarction (MI), and stroke. It is generally uncommon among younger populations, as its prevalence is less than 5% in individuals less than 50 years of age. Its incidence increases with age, as it is prevalent in 12% to 15% of individuals over 65 years old and approaches 20% in individuals over 80 years of age.[2]

Risk Factors

PAD shares many of the same risk factors of atherosclerotic conditions affecting other vascular beds, namely the coronary and cerebrovascular arteries. The traditional risk factors for the development of PAD include increased age, gender, cigarette smoking, diabetes, hypertension, dyslipidemia, obesity, alcohol consumption, chronic kidney disease, race/ethnicity, and genetic factors. Additional risk factors include socioeconomic status, autoimmune diseases, and hyperhomocysteinemia.

PATHOGENESIS

PAD primarily occurs as a result of systemic processes. Endothelial dysfunction with atherosclerotic risk factors initiates an inflammatory pathway leading to PAD. Chronic endothelial injury from reactive oxygen species, cigarette toxins, and proinflammatory cytokines leads to increased endothelial dysfunction and permeability. Oxidized low-density lipoprotein (LDL), endothelial growth factors, and chemotactic agents recruit macrophages and promote vascular smooth muscle cell growth. Macrophages migrate into the subendothelial space and aggregate oxidized LDL, which results in foam cell formation. The activated macrophages create a positive feedback loop stimulating vascular smooth muscle cells, which eventually distort the overlying endothelium and arterial lumen. Production of matrix metalloproteinases, platelet-derived growth factor, interleukin-1, transforming growth factor-beta and tumor necrosis factor-alpha contributes to plaque formation and stabilization.

CLINICAL PRESENTATION

Common Signs and Symptoms

The spectrum of PAD can be differentiated into three distinct categories: asymptomatic disease, intermittent claudication (IC), and critical limb threatening ischemia (CLTI). The largest portion of patients with PAD are asymptomatic. Both IC and CLTI are much less common; however, they often represent the primary indication for referral to a vascular specialist for treatment.

IC is a clinical syndrome resulting in symptoms such as cramping, aching, or fatigue in the lower extremity. The symptoms are typically reproducible at certain walking distances and are completely relieved with cessation of the provocative activity. In more advanced PAD, such as those presenting with CLTI, patients endorse symptoms of constant pain at rest and develop ulceration, gangrene, or wounds that fail to heal. Location of the symptoms along the lower extremity may assist in identifying the level of arterial obstruction that is classified as aortoiliac, femoropopliteal, or infrapopliteal disease.

Physical Examination Findings

The initial approach to the physical examination in a patient with PAD requires a well-documented history and physical examination, with focus on the presence and quality of peripheral perfusion. Examination of the extremities is the most critical component of the physical examination from the vascular perspective. In patients with aortoiliac occlusive disease, the constellation of thigh and buttock claudication, impotence, and absent femoral pulses is known as Leriche syndrome.

A proper physical examination begins with inspection for skin changes, edema, atrophied muscles, nonhealing ulcers, and rubor. The pulse examination should identify presence, absence, or diminished pulses at the common femoral artery, popliteal artery, anterior tibial, posterior tibial, peroneal, and dorsalis pedis arteries while comparing to the contralateral extremity. Diminished femoral pulses or bilateral symptoms may be indicative of aortoiliac occlusive disease. In patients with nonpalpable pulses, Doppler auscultation may assist in the examination. The absence of a palpable pedal pulse generally suggests inadequate perfusion to allow for wound healing. The presence or absence of palpable peripheral pulses provides a general anatomic distribution of areas of atherosclerotic disease on a macroscopic level; however, a simple examination may not reflect the degree of perfusion in the local area of tissue loss.

Differential Diagnosis

The differential diagnosis of vascular disease encompasses pathologies that cause leg pain. Typically, those include neurogenic (spine disease), venous, joint, and other musculoskeletal disorders.

DIAGNOSIS

In addition to the history and physical examination, noninvasive vascular studies assist in objectively quantifying the degree of PAD. The ankle-brachial index (ABI) is the calculated ratio of the highest ankle systolic pressure divided by the highest brachial artery systolic pressure, with normal value considered as 1.0 to 1.4. A value between 0.4 and 0.9 is considered mild to moderate PAD corresponding to IC, whereas an ABI below 0.4 is associated with severe PAD, which may manifest as rest pain and tissue loss. The 2015 Society of Vascular Surgery (SVS) and 2016 American Heart Association/American College of Cardiology (AHA/ACC) guidelines recommend resting ABI to establish the diagnosis in patients with a history and physical examination suggestive of PAD.[3,4] In patients with abnormal ABI (<0.90) and lifestyle limiting symptoms despite guideline-directed medical treatment, further diagnostic imaging is recommended. Individuals with symptoms consistent with PAD and an ABI between 0.90 and 1.40 are recommended to undergo exercise ABI testing. With exercise treadmill ABI, the resting baseline ABI is taken, and the patient then walks on a treadmill at ~2 mph with 12° inclination for 20 minutes or until forced to stop because of symptoms. Postexercise ABI measurements are taken. A 20% decrease in ABI from baseline, a 30 mm Hg drop in ankle systolic pressure, or more than 3 minutes to recovery of baseline ankle systolic pressure is indicative of PAD.[5] With ABI greater than 1.40, the value may be falsely elevated because of the increased cuff pressure needed to occlude the vessels in patients with extensively calcified vessels. This more commonly affects diabetics and patients with renal failure. An ABI above 1.4 in a patient with blunted waveforms, and nonpalpable pedal pulses should be suggestive of calcified vessels.

Other noninvasive studies include toe digital pressures, segmental pressures along the lower extremities, and pulse volume recordings. Digital toe pressures and toe-brachial index (TBI) are most useful in patients with falsely elevated ABI because of calcified tibial disease. A TBI below 0.70 is indicative of PAD. Additionally, a systolic toe pressure less than 40 mm Hg is indicative of inability to heal wounds. AHA/ACC guidelines recommend TBI measurements as the next diagnostic step when the ABI is greater than 1.40.[4]

Segmental pressures use cuff pressures to measure the systolic pressure at various levels along the lower extremity. A decrease of 20 mm Hg across any level indicates a hemodynamically significant disease at that level, which may assist in localizing the area of obstruction. Similar to segmental pressures, pulse volume recordings obtain arterial waveforms at several levels along the lower extremity to identify the level of arterial disease. Distal to the diseased segments, the waveform becomes dampened with a decrease in amplitude or slope of the upstroke. Example waveforms are displayed in **Figure 90.1**.

In chronic arterial disease, noninvasive imaging techniques with anatomic data—including duplex ultrasound, magnetic resonance angiography (MRA) and computed tomography angiography (CTA)—have largely replaced catheter angiography for most patients and allow accurate assessment of disease distribution. The hemodynamic significance of a stenosis demonstrated by these techniques can be further evaluated with targeted duplex ultrasound or catheter angiography. The 2015 SVS guidelines recommend use of anatomic imaging studies such as duplex ultrasonography, CTA, or MRA only in patients being considered for revascularization. In our practice, we usually obtain preoperative CTA to guide interventions if there is a clinical indication of CLTI.[3] **Table 90.1** lists the various diagnostic tools.

Adjunct laboratory studies are aimed at assessing systemic risk factors. This should include a complete blood count, fasting blood glucose, hemoglobin A_{1c}, serum creatinine, and lipid panel.

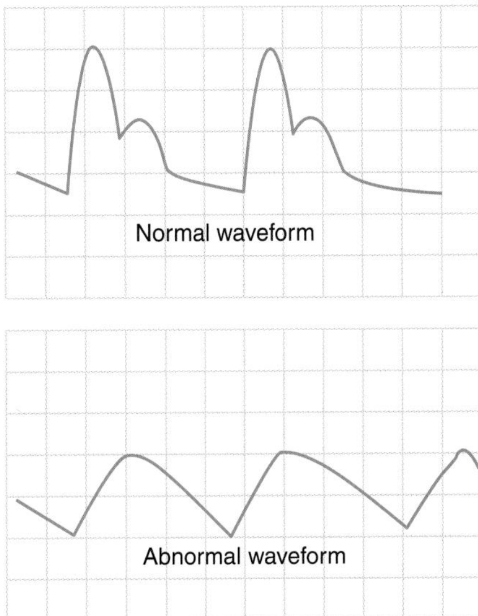

FIGURE 90.1 Pulse volume recording showing a decrease in amplitude and slope of the upstroke distal to the diseased segment.

TABLE 90.1 Diagnostic Studies for PAD

Diagnostic Modality	Sensitivity/Specificity	Limitations/Drawbacks	Guideline Recommendation SVS 2017
Ankle-brachial index (ABI)	Sensitivity 79%-95% Specificity > 95%	Falsely elevated with tibial calcification, not used for localization, screening tool	**Class IA:** first-line test to diagnose PAD in patients with consistent signs, symptoms, and risk factors. For ABI > 0.9 and symptoms of claudication, exercise ABI recommended
Duplex ultrasonography	Detect > 50% stenosis aortoiliac: sensitivity 86%, specificity 97% fem-pop: sensitivity 80%, specificity 96% infragenicular: sensitivity 83%; specificity 84%	Operator dependent, body habitus	**Class IB:** recommended in symptomatic patients being considered for revascularization
Segmental pressures/ Pulse volume recordings	No data	Falsely elevated with extensive collaterals, no assessment of profunda femoris or nonaxial vessels, limited with multilevel disease	**Class IIC:** recommended in symptomatic patients being considered for revascularization to quantify arterial disease and localize level of disease
CTA/MRA	CTA: sensitivity 93%, specificity 95% MRA: sensitivity 95%, specificity 95%	Limited evaluation of small-caliber vessels, extensive calcification, radiation exposure, nephrotoxicity, no assessment of hemodynamics	**Class IB:** recommended in symptomatic patients being considered for revascularization
Catheter angiography	Sensitivity 100%	Invasive, motion artifact, two-dimensional, access site complications, nephrotoxic	

CTA, computed tomography angiography; fem-pop, femoropopliteal; MRA, magnetic resonance angiogram; PAD, peripheral arterial disease; SVS, Society of Vascular Surgery 2017.

MANAGEMENT OF PERIPHERAL ARTERIAL DISEASE

Medical Approach

PAD is a systemic disease caused by multiple cardiovascular risk factors. Thus, managing these comorbidities is critical to the optimal treatment of these patients. Effective medical management of hypertension, hyperlipidemia, diabetes mellitus, smoking, and chronic kidney disease is essential. Medical management should be aimed at risk factor reduction and preventative lifestyle modification. The aggressive pharmacologic treatment of risk factors has been shown to benefit patients with symptomatic PAD; however, they have not shown significant benefit in asymptomatic patients when treated similarly.[6] The SVS guidelines provide Class IA evidence for smoking cessation interventions and patient education as primary management in asymptomatic patients.[3]

Antihypertensive treatment has been shown to reduce the risk of MI, stroke, heart failure, and cardiovascular death in patients with symptomatic PAD.[7] Treatment of hypertension should aim at a systolic blood pressure less than 140 mm Hg and diastolic pressure less than 90 mm Hg. For individuals with diabetes or chronic kidney disease, the blood pressure goal should be less than 130/80 mm Hg. Recommended agents for first-line therapy include angiotensin-converting enzyme (ACE) inhibitors. In 2000, the Heart Outcomes Prevention Evaluations (HOPE) study found that ramipril significantly reduced the risk of cardiovascular deaths in high-risk patients (relative risk 0.74, $P < .01$).[8] Caution should be used in prescribing ACE inhibitors to patients with renal artery stenosis.

Similar to hypertension, treatment of hyperlipidemia significantly reduces cardiovascular morbidity in PAD.[9] Recent guidelines recommend statin therapy based on estimation of 10-year cardiovascular risk. Because the 10-year cardiovascular risk in PAD patients is greater than 7.5%, statin treatment is indicated.[10] Management of hyperlipidemia includes moderate or high-intensity statin therapy to maintain LDL less than 100 mg/dL and less than 70 mg/dL in higher risk individuals.

In patients with diabetes mellitus, treatment should aim at achieving a hemoglobin A_{1c} level less than 7.0%. Diabetic patients with PAD are at higher risk for limb loss because of neuropathy leading to undiagnosed wounds and hyperglycemia predisposing to infections.

For patients with diagnosed PAD, guidelines recommend long-term antiplatelet therapy with a single agent.[4] Dual antiplatelet therapy is not recommended in the absence of another indication, such as postangioplasty or stent placement. Clopidogrel is an acceptable alternative to aspirin (75-325 mg daily) for patients with symptomatic PAD. In the 1996 randomized controlled trial (RCT) of Clopidogrel versus Aspirin in Patients at Risk of Ischemic Events (CAPRIE), clopidogrel use was associated with a 8.7% relative risk reduction in ischemic stroke, MI, and vascular death when compared to aspirin, with a similar safety profile.[11]

Smoking cessation significantly reduces risk for limb loss in patients with PAD. A multidisciplinary approach to assess the patients' willingness to quit, utilize nicotine replacement therapy with medications such as bupropion and varenicline, and participate in behavioral modification programs are key in successful smoking cessation. Bupropion has a 15% to 35% abstinence rate at 12 months in conjunction with nicotine replacement therapy, whereas varenicline has a success rate of 23% at 1 year.[12,13]

In addition to risk factor modification, in patients with IC a supervised exercise program is the first course of treatment. The AHA/ACC 2016 guidelines provide a high-level recommendation for supervised exercise program in the treatment of IC.[4] A 2012 Cochran Review of 22 RCTs comparing exercise therapy to placebo showed an increased maximal walking time (5 minutes) and pain-free walking distance with exercise; however, there was no change in ABI, mortality, or amputation rates. Routine low-intensity exercise programs allow for growth of collaterals, angiogenesis, augmented skeletal muscle efficiency, and improved microcirculation sensitivity to nitric oxide vasodilation.[14] For a successful exercise program, the patient should walk more than 30 minutes approximately three times per week for at least 12 weeks. Patients are instructed to walk until maximum pain is experienced at which point a short rest is allowed for symptom resolution, and the patient is then instructed to continue again. A routine 3-month follow-up should assess improvement of symptoms. In patients with no improvement or worsening of symptoms, a trial of phosphodiesterase inhibitors (cilostazol) with continuation of exercise therapy should be prescribed. Cilostazol and pentoxifylline are two U.S. Food and Drug Administration (FDA)-approved drugs for patients with IC. Cilostazol is contraindicated in patients with any level of heart failure. In an RCT comparing the effectiveness of 6-month treatment with cilostazol and pentoxifylline in 698 patients, the former increased maximal walking distance by 54% versus a 30% increase with pentoxifylline.[15] In the 2015 SVS guidelines, cilostazol 100 mg twice daily was recommended in patients with claudication without evidence of heart failure (Class IIA). For patients with contraindications to cilostazol, pentoxifylline 400 mg thrice daily is recommended (Class IIB).[3] Refer to **Table 90.2** for dosages and side effects of commonly prescribed medications.

Endovascular Management of Peripheral Arterial Disease

Since its inception in 1964, the endovascular management of PAD has grown to be a key treatment, allowing for less invasive management of both aortoiliac and infrainguinal pathology. Treatment of PAD in that time period, especially in the late 1990s to early 2000s, has undergone a significant shift, with endovascular surgery now far outnumbering open bypass procedures.[16,17] Endovascular therapy offers the benefit of lower perioperative morbidity, mortality, and cost, when compared to open arterial surgery, but with unclear long-term durability.[18]

Despite the prevalence of endovascular treatment of both CLTI and IC, there remains significant controversy in the role of endovascular modalities for the treatment of PAD, especially infrainguinal disease. High-quality RCTs are lacking, other than the Bypass Versus Angioplasty in Severe Ischaemia of the Leg (BASIL) study, which is now over 15 years old. This UK study compared initial bypass surgery to angioplasty in patients with severe limb ischemia and showed that for patients living less than 2 years, the angioplasty-first strategy reduced early morbidity and treatment cost. However, for individuals with longer life expectancy, the surgery-first strategy was associated with improvements in subsequent overall survival and amputation-free survival.[18]

Without high-quality evidence to guide treatment choices, the decision on treatment modality is based on the patient's overall health, estimated survival, surgeon's preference, and lesion morphology. The Trans-Atlantic Inter-Society Consensus (TASC II) guidelines, initially released in 2007, provide a framework based on lesion anatomy, to guide endovascular versus open arterial surgery. TASC A lesions—the least complex lesions—are recommended to undergo endovascular treatment, whereas TASC D lesions—the most complex—are best addressed with bypass surgery. Intermediate TASC B and C lesions may be addressed with either modality. This paradigm is now shifting, as noted by the supplement to TASC II in 2015, which now includes infrapopliteal lesions. Because of advances in endovascular techniques and technologies, endovascular strategies are now being used successfully to treat more complex TASC D lesions.[19]

The advent of drug-coated balloons (DCBs), drug-eluting stents (DESs), pedal and upper extremity access, advances in stent grafts, atherectomy, and hybrid procedures provides additional tools to the vascular surgeon. Pedal access, DCBs, DESs, and atherectomy are expanding therapeutic options in infrapopliteal disease, whereas hybrid procedures such as femoral endarterectomy with iliac stenting are expanding what can be achieved in the treatment of aortoiliac disease.

Three upcoming RCTs—BASIL-3, investigating DES versus DCB versus plain balloon angioplasty; BASIL-2 comparing vein bypass first versus best endovascular treatment first; and Best Surgical Therapy in Patients with Critical Limb Ischemia (BEST-CLI) comparing endovascular versus open arterial bypass—will provide further guidance on the role endovascular surgery occupies in PAD.

Aortoiliac Occlusive Disease

Patients' disease morphology and their overall health should be considered when deciding on the appropriate treatment plan. TASC II guidelines were developed to assist in the management of PAD.[20] Guidelines for aortoiliac disease state that lesions classified as TASC A should be treated preferentially with

TABLE 90.2 Medications Used for Peripheral Arterial Disease

Drugs	Dosage	Side Effects	Recommendation
Aspirin	75-325 mg daily	Rash, abdominal pain, tinnitus, bleeding, nausea	SVS Class IA AHA/ACC Class IA
Clopidogrel	75 mg daily	Bleeding, acute liver failure, aplastic anemia, agranulocytosis	SVS Class IB AHA/ACC Class IA
ACE inhibitor (ramipril)	10 mg daily	Dry cough, hyperkalemia, kidney failure, angioedema, pancreatitis	AHA/ACC Class IIA
Statin	Atorvastatin 40-80 mg daily (high intensity) Rosuvastatin 20-40 mg daily (high intensity)	Myopathy, new-onset diabetes, liver failure	SVS Class IA AHA/ACC Class IA
Cilostazol	100 mg twice daily	Fluid retention, headaches, abdominal pain, palpitations	SVS Class IIA AHA/ACC Class IA
Pentoxifylline	400 mg three times daily, titrate to 1800 mg daily	Nausea, headache, anxiety, insomnia	SVS Class IB

ACC, American Heart Association; ACE, angiotensin-converting enzyme; AHA, American College of Cardiology; SVS, Society of Vascular Surgery.

endovascular techniques, whereas lesions classified as TASC D should be treated preferentially with open arterial surgery. Unfortunately, the recommendations for TASC B or C lesions are less clear.

A meta-analysis of iliac occlusive disease showed stenting has superior results to angioplasty alone, with 4-year primary patency rates of 77% in IC and 67% in CLTI with stenting versus 68% in IC and 55% in CLTI with angioplasty.[21] Endovascular treatment of TASC A and B lesions are comparable to surgical aortofemoral bypass with limb salvage rates of 95% and 87% at 5 and 10 years, respectively.[22] When evaluating TASC B and C lesions, the overall patency is influenced by the outflow vessels. In a review by Timaran et al, the percutaneous and surgical treatment of these complex iliac lesions were compared. Although poor runoff was an independent risk factor for primary failure in both groups, iliac stenting showed inferior outcomes when compared to surgical revascularization.[23] Still, the use of stent grafting has emerged as a modality to treat TASC C and D lesions, especially when combined with femoral endarterectomy.[24,25]

Aortoiliac endovascular therapy is often used concomitantly with open surgical treatment in hybrid procedures. Indications for hybrid procedures include common femoral arterial stenosis more than 50%, in which open femoral endarterectomy is combined with iliac stenting, or when aortoiliac endovascular therapy is employed to provide sufficient inflow for distal surgical bypasses.

The approach for iliac artery endovascular revascularization includes contralateral, ipsilateral, or transbrachial arterial access. In our practice, we prefer to access the ipsilateral common femoral and cross the lesion in retrograde fashion. This approach provides excellent support for the delivery of angioplasty balloons and stents. In complete occlusion of the common iliac artery, a retrograde approach may lead to a subintimal dissection, whereas a contralateral approach may be more successful. Flush common iliac artery occlusions are often best addressed by upper extremity access, which allows greater support and decreases the likelihood of a dissection. In the setting of chronic total occlusion, reentry systems allow a lesion to be crossed in the subintimal plane, prior to reentering the true lumen. In the case of aortic bifurcation lesions, kissing iliac stents or kissing balloon angioplasty is utilized to protect the contralateral common iliac artery.

Infrainguinal Occlusive Disease

A TASC classification for infrainguinal occlusive disease assists in determining which treatment modality might be better suited for revascularization. Again, the TASC group recommends that type A lesions be treated with endovascular intervention, type D lesions be treated with surgery, and types B and C lesions be treated with either, depending on the patient characteristics. Our approach to lower extremity endovascular revascularization is typically via a contralateral femoral access, ipsilateral femoral or pedal access, transbrachial or radial approach. Pedal access allows for retrograde access of difficult to treat lesions and pedal lesions and has been shown to both increase the rate of wound healing and decrease the time to wound healing.[26] Interventions for lower extremity interventions include angioplasty, stenting, and atherectomy with varying degrees of patency. Additionally, DCB and DES further add to treatment modalities. The patency of percutaneous transluminal angioplasty (PTA) of a short femoropopliteal lesion is 70% to 80% at 1 year.[27] Patency rates for femoropopliteal stent implantation are affected by the stents used, the clinical characteristics, and morphology/length of the lesion. Advances in stent technology may offer improved results with higher radial strength and flexibility, but RCTs comparing these stent platforms are needed. For example, a Japanese trial found covered stent grafts effective in treating long-segment superficial femoral arterial lesions (>10 cm) with a primary patency of 88% to 92%, but was predominantly in patients with IC.[28] The patency for infrapopliteal balloon angioplasty is much less established and results are assessed by evaluating limb salvage. The 2-year limb salvage rate is 74% with angioplasty.[29] Data to support stent placement in the tibial arteries are insufficient, but these interventions may salvage unsuccessful tibial angioplasty. Atherectomy is used to treat severe femoropopliteal and tibial disease, but data from the Vascular Quality Initiative (VQI) show that long-term adverse outcomes occur more frequently after atherectomy than after other revascularization procedures.[30] The 5-year rate of major adverse limb events was 38% in patients receiving atherectomy versus 33% for PTA and 32% for stenting. Importantly, atherectomy was used to treat IC in 43% of the cases in this study. This finding puts into question the utility of atherectomy for PAD. In our practice, we employ atherectomy techniques for limb salvage and perhaps this should be an indication for this technique. Thus, further investigation into the indications of atherectomy is warranted.

In tibial and pedal arterial disease, angiosome (ie, an anatomic unit of tissue consisting of skin, subcutaneous tissue, fascia, muscle, and bone fed by a source artery and drained by specific veins)—targeted revascularization, though often discussed, has not shown consistent benefit in wound healing. When intervening on PAD, the possibility of the patient requiring repeat revascularization after their primary intervention should be considered. Current data are conflicting on whether previous endovascular intervention leads to worse outcomes in secondary surgical bypass, but repeat revascularization options should be considered when planning a patient's initial intervention.

Surgical Management of Peripheral Arterial Disease

In general, open surgical reconstruction for occlusive disease is never indicated in asymptomatic patients. The approach to management of patients with IC and CLI is nuanced and is oftentimes predicated on the anatomic distribution of the occlusive disease. Additionally, the physiologic state of the patient and the urgency of the intervention also influence surgical decision-making in any patient with PAD.

The introduction and advancement of endovascular therapies has changed the historical treatment algorithm in the management of PAD. Once a patient is identified to be a candidate for revascularization, therapy selection is tailored to a patient's specific needs. Considerations between selecting open and endovascular therapy are based upon a host of factors including the anatomic location of the occlusive disease, patient comorbidities, extent of tissue loss, history of previous interventions, and overall risk of anesthesia.

The surgeon has several fundamental techniques at their disposal for the management of PAD, namely endarterectomy and bypass.

Endarterectomy

Endarterectomy involves the removal of atherosclerotic plaque from an arterial segment by creating a plane between the plaque and media. Following plaque removal, the arteries are either closed primarily or, more commonly, closed with a patch (prosthetic or biologic) to prevent restenosis over time. Endarterectomy is typically reserved for larger vessels, namely the aorta, common iliac, external iliac, common femoral, deep femoral, and superficial femoral arteries. The success and durability of angioplasty and stenting in the aortoiliac system has largely been responsible for the abandonment of endarterectomy to be performed in these locations, as isolated endarterectomy is typically reserved for the femoral vessels. Femoral endarterectomy and profundaplasty remain durable therapies and, additionally, can be performed in conjunction with retrograde iliac stenting.

Surgical Arterial Bypass

Surgical arterial bypass provides a versatile therapy for patients, as it allows for revascularization anywhere along the length of lower extremity vasculature. The critical components of a successful bypass require minimally diseased inflow, suitable conduit (autogenous vs prosthetic), and patent outflow. The great saphenous vein represents the ideal conduit for any infrainguinal revascularization. Single-segment great saphenous vein has been shown to be superior to all other conduits with regard to primary and primary assisted bypass patency. Unfortunately, only 40% of patients have great saphenous vein suitable for use as a bypass conduit.

The selection of appropriate surgical revascularization of PAD is based on the clinical presentation and anatomic distribution of occlusive disease. Classically, PAD is differentiated into three anatomic locations: aortoiliac, femoropopliteal, or infrageniculate. Typically, patients with IC have a single level of disease; however, in patients with CLTI, multiple levels are generally affected and all need to be reconstructed to achieve adequate perfusion for limb salvage.

Aortoiliac Occlusive Disease

The surgical management of aortoiliac occlusive disease has been performed for the last 70 years. This can be performed via a direct or extra-anatomic bypass reconstruction. The aortobifemoral bypass is a direct reconstruction performed by attaching a bifurcated graft from the infrarenal abdominal aorta to bilateral common femoral arteries. The aorta is exposed via either a midline abdominal incision or a retroperitoneal incision. Bilateral femoral artery exposure is performed by groin incisions. Compared to percutaneous alternatives, open arterial reconstruction boasts 5-year patency approaching 90% in most series, whether performed for IC or CLTI. Aortobifemoral bypass is a major operation and is associated with major and minor complications approaching 15% to 30%. Major adverse cardiac events occur in less than 5% of patients and pulmonary complications occur in less than 7% of patients. Less commonly, renal failure, wound complications, and postoperative hemorrhage may occur.

Extra-anatomic reconstruction of aortoiliac occlusive disease is typically performed in patients with extensive comorbid conditions like severe coronary artery disease, heart failure, advanced pulmonary disease, renal failure, and hostile abdomens, all of which increase the risk of traditional direct revascularization. These techniques include femorofemoral bypass and axillofemoral bypass. Compared to aortobifemoral bypass, these interventions are less morbid; however, they are also less durable and generally reserved for patients with CLTI.

Infrainguinal Occlusive Disease—Open Arterial Bypass

Open arterial bypass is an effective and durable intervention for the management of femoropopliteal and infrageniculate arterial disease. Presently, the conduit of choice remains the great saphenous vein. In patients without suitable great saphenous veins, prosthetic bypasses can be performed; however, the patency rates associated with these bypasses are inferior. Revascularization with bypass of tibiopedal arterial disease also is durable therapy for selected patients. A variety of reports demonstrate 5-year patency data for vein bypasses more than 80%. Early complications after infrainguinal bypass are uncommon, with edema, wound complications, graft occlusion, and perioperative MI occurring in less than 15% of patients. In the long term, vein graft stenosis occurs in 40% of vein bypasses within 18 months. As a result, all bypasses should undergo duplex ultrasonography surveillance to identify threatened bypasses prior to occlusion.

SPECIAL CONSIDERATIONS

Hybrid procedures typically consist of a surgical bypass combined with either angioplasty or stenting to optimize graft inflow or outflow. The order of these procedures requires careful consideration, and the endovascular component is usually performed first to avoid compromising the inflow or outflow to a newly constructed graft by balloon inflation or hemostatic maneuvers. A dedicated hybrid room is the optimal environment, but satisfactory results can be obtained with a fluoroscopy-compatible operating room table and portable image intensifier with digital subtraction vascular processing software.

FOLLOW-UP PATENT CARE

Surveillance duplex ultrasonography following lower extremity revascularization can identify threatened open or endovascular revascularizations. A technical defect, intimal hyperplasia, and recurrent atherosclerosis are the main causes of restenosis following any revascularization procedure. Preemptive identification of narrowing following a revascularization procedure may help to preserve the primary patency of the intervention. Recurrent leg symptoms and/or a significant decrease in the ABI (0.15 or more) detects a failing bypass in only 50% of cases.

Identification of a restenosis in a vascular reconstruction prior to its occlusion allows for early intervention and repair of the narrowed segment. Duplex ultrasonography criteria have been developed to identify the restenosis arterial reconstruction: (a) a segment or bypass graft with a focal peak systolic velocity of greater than 300 cm/s and (b) low velocities throughout the segment or graft (<40-45 cm/s). In our practice we perform surveillance duplex ultrasonography at 1 month, every 3 months in the first year postprocedure, and every 6 to 12 months thereafter.

RESEARCH AND FUTURE DIRECTIONS

BASIL Trial

The BASIL trial compared the outcomes of 452 patients presenting to UK centers with severe limb ischemia. Patients were randomized to either a surgery-first (n = 228) or an angioplasty-first (n = 224) strategy. The primary endpoint was survival free from amputation for the trial limb. Trial duration was 5.5 years, with follow-up ending when the endpoints of death or above-ankle amputation of the trial leg were reached. At follow-up completion:

- 248 patients (55%) were alive without amputation of the trial leg
- 38 (8%) were alive following amputation
- 130 patients (29%) were dead without amputation

A surgery-first strategy was associated with a higher rate of early morbidity (57% vs 41%). Six-month amputation-free survival was not significantly different between the treatment groups, and health-related quality of life was similar. At 2 years, surgery was associated with a reduced risk of future amputation or death. A surgery-first strategy increased the hospital costs by about one-third. These results indicate that there is scope to substantially improve the medical treatment of risk factors. For patients with a short life expectancy, an angioplasty-first strategy reduced early morbidity and treatment cost, but for relatively fit patients expected to live beyond 2 years, a surgery-first strategy was more durable and carried a reduced reintervention rate, possibly outweighing the initial costs and increased short-term morbidity.[18]

BEST-CLI

BEST-CLI is an ongoing international research study aimed at figuring out the best treatment for patients with PAD. It is anticipated that the outcomes will lead to the best treatment and revascularization options available for CLI patients.[31]

Technology

As mentioned previously, balloon angioplasty, stenting, and atherectomy are primary endovascular treatment options for PAD. However, balloon angioplasty and bare metal stenting are limited by the high rate of restenosis of up to 50% within the first 12 months. Restenosis can be caused by stent fracture, negative vascular remodeling, vessel recoil and neointimal hyperplasia.[32,33] Development of new technology, including DCB and DES, aims to deliver antiproliferative pharmacology into the vessel wall to limit neointimal hyperplasia and prolong primary patency. Currently, the most studied DCB is paclitaxel-coated balloons. Local delivery of the agent allows for precise application into the vessel wall with long-term retention and limited downstream or systemic effects. Paclitaxel binds the beta subunit of tubulin preventing cellular division and ultimately limiting hyperplasia. The IN.PACT SFA trial followed 331 subjects comparing DCB to balloon angioplasty PTA for femoropopliteal lesions. The 36 months primary patency was 70% versus 45% for DCB and balloon angioplasty, respectively.[34] Similarly the multicenter LEVANT II study randomized patients with femoropopliteal disease trial to balloon angioplasty or the Lutonix paclitaxel-coated balloon (Bard, Covington, GA). At 1 year patients treated with DCB had higher primary patency by Doppler studies compared to balloon angioplasty (74% vs 59% respectively).[35] These studies show improved patency in the femoropopliteal segments with DCB treatment. Future studies will need to address varying doses and different compound excipients to optimize drug delivery.

Similar to DCB, DES aims to limit neointimal hyperplasia. DESs—coated with paclitaxel, sirolimus, or everolimus—have proven to be safe and effective in coronary interventions with reduced reintervention rates compared to bare metal stents. The Zilver PTX (Cook Medical, Bloomington, IN) is one of the available paclitaxel-eluting nitinol stents. The 5-year follow-up data comparing Zilver PTX DCB versus bare metal stenting for femoropopliteal disease showed improved primary patency (72% vs 53%, respectively) as well as increased freedom from target lesions revascularization (85% vs 72%, respectively).[36] For infrapopliteal disease, the ACHILLES study was an RCT comparing sirolimus DES to balloon angioplasty. At 1 year DES had better patency (75% vs 57%) with no significant difference in mortality or amputation rates.[37] These studies have demonstrated the efficacy of DCB and DES in prolonging the effects of vascular interventions.

Future research and technologic development to improve durability of vascular interventions are currently underway. Nanofiber delivery of nitric oxide to prevent intimal hyperplasia in treated vessels is a potential novel treatment currently under investigation.[38]

KEY POINTS

- ✔ The incidence of PAD is increasing worldwide and affects 12% to 15% of individuals over 65 years old and approaches 20% in individuals over 80 years of age.
- ✔ Similar to other atherosclerotic conditions, risk factors include increased age, cigarette smoking, diabetes, hypertension, dyslipidemia, obesity, alcohol consumption, and chronic kidney disease.
- ✔ Symptomatically, PAD ranges from asymptomatic, to IC, to CLTI with rest pain and tissue loss.
- ✔ ABI less than 0.9 is consistent with PAD, but the ABI can be falsely elevated in patients with diabetes mellitus or chronic kidney disease.
- ✔ Postexercise ABI, toe pressures, CTA, MRA, and duplex ultrasound are included in the diagnostic algorithm.
- ✔ For IC, initial management should be medical with smoking cessation, antiplatelet therapy, statin therapy, comorbidity optimization, and exercise programs.
- ✔ Surgical options for PAD include endovascular and open arterial bypass, with the ongoing BASIL-2, BASIL-3, and BEST-CLI investigating endovascular versus bypass first.
- ✔ New endovascular technologies such as DES, DCB, and atherectomy are being developed and studied for benefit versus risk to the patient.
- ✔ Patients with PAD often require multiple interventions in their lifetime and continued surveillance to identify threatened open or endovascular revascularizations.

REFERENCES

1. Fowkes FG, Rudan D, Rudan I, et al. Comparison of global estimates of prevalence and risk factors for peripheral artery disease in 2000 and 2010: a systematic review and analysis. *Lancet.* 2013;382(9901):1329-1340.
2. Allison MA, Ho E, Denenberg JO, et al. Ethnic-specific prevalence of peripheral arterial disease in the United States. *Am J Prev Med.* 2007;32(4):328-333.
3. Conte MS, Pomposelli FB. Society for Vascular Surgery Practice guidelines for atherosclerotic occlusive disease of the lower extremities management of asymptomatic disease and claudication. Introduction. *J Vasc Surg.* 2015;61(3 Suppl):1S.
4. Gerhard-Herman MD, Gornik HL, Barrett C, et al. 2016 AHA/ACC Guideline on the management of patients with lower extremity peripheral artery disease: executive summary: a report of the American College of Cardiology/American Heart Association Task Force on Clinical Practice Guidelines. *J Am Coll Cardiol.* 2017;69(11):1465-1508.
5. Ted Kohler DS. *Rutherford's Vascular Surgery.* Elsevier Saunders; 2014.
6. Fowkes FG, Price JF, Stewart MCW, et al. Aspirin for prevention of cardiovascular events in a general population screened for a low ankle brachial index: a randomized controlled trial. *JAMA.* 2010;303(9):841-848.
7. Psaty BM, Smith NL, Siscovick DS, et al. Health outcomes associated with antihypertensive therapies used as first-line agents. A systematic review and meta-analysis. *JAMA.* 1997;277(9):739-745.
8. Sleight P. The HOPE Study (Heart Outcomes Prevention Evaluation). *J Renin Angiotensin Aldosterone Syst.* 2000;1(1):18-20.
9. Heart Protection Study Collaborative Group. MRC/BHF Heart Protection Study of cholesterol lowering with simvastatin in 20,536 high-risk individuals: a randomised placebo-controlled trial. *Lancet.* 2002;360(9326):7-22.
10. Cheng AY, Leiter LA. Implications of recent clinical trials for the National Cholesterol Education Program Adult Treatment Panel III guidelines. *Curr Opin Cardiol.* 2006;21(4):400-404.
11. CAPRIE Steering Committee. A randomised, blinded, trial of clopidogrel versus aspirin in patients at risk of ischaemic events (CAPRIE). *Lancet.* 1996;348(9038):1329-1339.
12. Jorenby DE, Leischow SJ, Nides MA, et al. A controlled trial of sustained-release bupropion, a nicotine patch, or both for smoking cessation. *N Engl J Med.* 1999;340(9):685-691.
13. Gonzales D, Rennard SI, Nides M, et al. Varenicline, an alpha4beta2 nicotinic acetylcholine receptor partial agonist, vs sustained-release bupropion and placebo for smoking cessation: a randomized controlled trial. *JAMA.* 2006;296(1):47-55.

14. Watson L, Lane R, Harwood A, Leng GC. Exercise for intermittent claudication. *Cochrane Database Syst Rev.* 2008(4):CD000990.
15. Dawson DL, Cutler BS, Hiatt WR, et al. A comparison of cilostazol and pentoxifylline for treating intermittent claudication. *Am J Med.* 2000;109(7):523-530.
16. Goodney PP, Beck AW, Nagle J, Welch HG, Zwolak RM. National trends in lower extremity bypass surgery, endovascular interventions, and major amputations. *J Vasc Surg.* 2009;50(1):54-60.
17. Rowe VL, Lee W, Weaver FA, Etzioni D. Patterns of treatment for peripheral arterial disease in the United States: 1996-2005. *J Vasc Surg.* 2009;49(4):910-917.
18. Adam DJ, Beard JD, Cleveland T, et al. Bypass versus angioplasty in severe ischaemia of the leg (BASIL): multicentre, randomised controlled trial. *Lancet.* 2005;366(9501):1925-1934.
19. TASC Steering Committee, Jaff MR, White CJ, Hiatt WR, et al. An update on methods for revascularization and expansion of the TASC lesion classification to include below-the-knee arteries: a supplement to the inter-society consensus for the management of peripheral arterial disease (TASC II). *Ann Vasc Dis.* 2015;8(4):343-357.
20. Norgren L, Hiatt WR, Dormandy JA, et al. Inter-society consensus for the management of peripheral arterial disease (TASC II). *J Vasc Surg.* 2007;45(Suppl S):S5-S67.
21. Bosch JL, Hunink MG. Meta-analysis of the results of percutaneous transluminal angioplasty and stent placement for aortoiliac occlusive disease. *Radiology.* 1997;204(1):87-96.
22. Galaria II, Mark GD. Percutaneous transluminal revascularization for iliac occlusive disease: long-term outcomes in TransAtlantic Inter-Society Consensus A and B lesions. *Ann Vasc Surg.* 2005;19(3):352-360.
23. Timaran CH, Prault TL, Stevens SL, Freeman MB, Goldman MH. Iliac artery stenting versus surgical reconstruction for TASC (TransAtlantic Inter-Society Consensus) type B and type C iliac lesions. *J Vasc Surg.* 2003;38(2):272-278.
24. Rzucidlo EM, Powell RJ, Zwolak RM, et al. Early results of stent-grafting to treat diffuse aortoiliac occlusive disease. *J Vasc Surg.* 2003;37(6):1175-1180.
25. Psacharopulo D, Ferrero E, Ferri M, et al. Increasing efficacy of endovascular recanalization with covered stent graft for TransAtlantic Inter-Society Consensus II D aortoiliac complex occlusion. *J Vasc Surg.* 2015;62(5):1219-1226.
26. Nakama T, Watanabe N, Haraguchi T, et al. Clinical outcomes of pedal artery angioplasty for patients with ischemic wounds: results from the multicenter RENDEZVOUS registry. *J Am Coll Cardiol Intv.* 2017;10(1):79-90.
27. Muradin GS, Bosch JL, Stijnen T, Hunink MG. Balloon dilation and stent implantation for treatment of femoropopliteal arterial disease: meta-analysis. *Radiology.* 2001;221(1):137-145.
28. Ohki T, Kichikawa K, Yokoi H, et al. Outcomes of the Japanese multicenter Viabahn trial of endovascular stent grafting for superficial femoral artery lesions. *J Vasc Surg.* 2017;66(1):130-142.
29. Kandarpa K, Becker GJ, Hunink MG, et al. Transcatheter interventions for the treatment of peripheral atherosclerotic lesions: part I. *J Vasc Interv Radiol.* 2001;12(6):683-695.
30. Ramkumar N, Martinez-Camblor P, Columbo JA, Osborne NH, Goodney PP, O'Malley AJ. Adverse events after atherectomy: analyzing long-term outcomes of endovascular lower extremity revascularization techniques. *J Am Heart Assoc.* 2019;8(12):e012081.
31. Farber A, Rosenfield K, Siami FS, Strong M, Menard M. The BEST-CLI trial is nearing the finish line and promises to be worth the wait. *J Vasc Surg.* 2019;69(2):470.e472-481.e472.
32. Lindquist J, Schramm K. Drug-eluting balloons and drug-eluting stents in the treatment of peripheral vascular disease. *Semin Intervent Radiol.* 2018;35(5):443-452.
33. Mohapatra A, Saadeddin Z, Bertges DJ, et al. Nationwide trends in drug-coated balloon and drug-eluting stent utilization in the femoropopliteal arteries. *J Vasc Surg.* 2020;71(2):560-566.
34. Schneider PA, Laird JR, Tepe G, et al. Treatment effect of drug-coated balloons is durable to 3 years in the femoropopliteal arteries: long-term results of the IN.PACT SFA randomized trial. *Circ Cardiovasc Interv.* 2018;11(1):e005891.
35. Rosenfield K, Jaff MR, White CJ, et al. Trial of a paclitaxel-coated balloon for femoropopliteal artery disease. *N Engl J Med.* 2015;373(2):145-153.
36. Dake MD, Ansel GM, Jaff MR, et al. Durable clinical effectiveness with paclitaxel-eluting stents in the femoropopliteal artery: 5-year results of the zilver PTX randomized trial. *Circulation.* 2016;133(15):1472-1483; discussion 1483.
37. Scheinert D, Katsanos K, Zeller T, et al. A prospective randomized multicenter comparison of balloon angioplasty and infrapopliteal stenting with the sirolimus-eluting stent in patients with ischemic peripheral arterial disease: 1-year results from the ACHILLES trial. *J Am Coll Cardiol.* 2012;60(22):2290-2295.
38. Kapadia MR, Chow LW, Tsihlis ND, et al. Nitric oxide and nanotechnology: a novel approach to inhibit neointimal hyperplasia. *J Vasc Surg.* 2008;47(1):173-182.

CHAPTER 91

CAROTID ARTERY REVASCULARIZATION

Fatemeh Malekpour, Gerardo Gonzalez-Guardiola, Sooyeon Kim, and Melissa L. Kirkwood

INTRODUCTION

Although the stroke rate among the aging U.S. population has declined over the last decade, stroke remains one of the leading causes of morbidity and mortality in this country. Approximately 795,000 people suffer a stroke each year; in 140,000 of these cases, it results in mortality. In addition, there are roughly 7 million stroke survivors with varying degrees of disability.[1] The socioeconomic impact of cerebrovascular accidents (CVAs) has been well-documented. The annual economic burden of stroke is approximately US$34 billion.[1] Thus, prevention is the most important aspect of cerebrovascular care.

Approximately 70% of CVAs are caused by ischemia, the majority of which originate from extracranial atherosclerosis leading to shower emboli.[1] Other sources of cerebral ischemia include lacunar stroke owing to occlusion of the small perforating arteries (eg, lenticulostriate, thalamoperforating, and pontine perforating) as well as cardioembolic stroke frequently associated with atrial fibrillation or advanced left ventricular dysfunction. Equipped with the knowledge of both medical management and surgical therapies for extracranial cerebrovascular diseases, vascular surgeons are integral members of the health care team.

PATHOGENESIS

Cardiovascular risk factors, such as advanced age, obesity, diabetes mellitus, and hypertension, have been linked to the development of atherosclerosis. These atherosclerotic plaques are subject to constant high-shear stress within this stenotic environment. This leads to macrophage infiltration and lysis, chronic inflammation, plaque ulceration, neovascularization with intraplaque hemorrhage, and thrombus formation. Such progressive changes result in further luminal narrowing, plaque rupture, or occlusion. Ruptured plaques then recruit platelets and procoagulants, such as plasminogen activator inhibitor-1 and tissue factor, leading to thrombus formation and subsequent embolization. Carotid plaque ulceration and thrombus are more prevalent in symptomatic carotid stenosis.[2]

Atherosclerosis at the carotid bifurcation is the most common source of emboli (38%), followed by cerebral arteries (33%), proximal vertebral arteries (20%), and branch vessels of the aortic arch (9%).[3] About 50% of patients with transient ischemic attacks (TIAs) have hemodynamically significant carotid stenosis.[4]

CLINICAL PRESENTATION

Asymptomatic Carotid Disease

Patients with significant cardiovascular risk factors are at increased risks of developing carotid artery stenosis. Routinely associated physical examination findings, such as carotid bruits, are neither sensitive nor specific for detecting significant carotid artery stenosis. Carotid bruits may be present in approximately 5% of the general population over 50 years of age regardless of the atherosclerotic burden of the carotid artery.[5] Only 23% of bruits are found to be associated with hemodynamically significant stenosis.[5] Therefore, a carotid Doppler ultrasound is the initial diagnostic modality of choice for the workup of carotid artery disease.

Although routine screening of carotid arteries in the general population is not recommended, when carotid stenosis is detected in asymptomatic patients, about 10% to 15% may progress to severe carotid stenosis (>70%), warranting intervention.[6] Surveillance with serial carotid duplex examinations and cardiovascular risk modifications are important in these patients.

Symptomatic Carotid Stenosis

Symptoms indicative of thromboembolic events from the carotid artery or anterior cerebral circulation include hemiparesis, hemianesthesia, transient monocular blindness, or aphasia. Prompt diagnosis and treatment should be a priority when the patients present with such neurologic deficits.

Transient Ischemic Attack

TIA is defined as acute neurologic symptoms lasting less than 24 hours with no irreversible neurologic sequelae. TIAs can present with isolated motor, ocular, or language deficits or a combination. However, isolated sensory symptoms in only part of one extremity or face can be a diagnostic dilemma especially in the absence of motor, visual, or language deficits. In patients who experience TIAs, the risk of early stroke is 4% at 1 month and 30% to 50% at 5 years.[7,8]

Cerebrovascular Accident

CVA is defined as neurologic symptoms lasting longer than 24 hours with imaging evidence of cerebral infarction. Although advanced age is an important risk factor for cardiovascular morbidity, 31% of first strokes occur in patients younger than 65 years.[1] Within 5 years after the initial stroke,

5% to 20% of these younger patients will experience a fatal recurrent CVA.[1] The mortality association is even more pronounced in older patients. Approximately one in three patients aged ≥75 years will succumb to death within 1 year after their first stroke, and 50% to 70% within 5 years.[1]

Crescendo Transient Ischemic Attack

A phenomenon in which TIAs occur in increasing frequency while maintaining the complete recovery of neurologic symptoms between events.

Stroke-In-Evolution

There is no resolution of symptoms, but rather they wax and wane indicating ongoing neuron ischemia at risk for infarction.

Transient Monocular Blindness (Amaurosis Fugax)

Amaurosis fugax is classically described as a "shade coming down over the eye" that lasts for seconds to minutes secondary to thromboembolism to the ophthalmic artery, the terminal branch of the internal carotid artery. In 25% of the patients with symptomatic carotid disease, such visual disturbances are the presenting symptom. Amaurosis fugax is the most common ocular manifestation, but transient hemianopias and other subtle visual field defects may also occur. Following amaurosis fugax, the risk of stroke was thought to be about 10% per year, but the risk of stroke in patients with confirmed retinal artery occlusion was found to be less than 1% annually according to new studies.[9]

Jaw Claudication

Although uncommon, symptoms of jaw claudication with eating may occur because of poor perfusion of the masseter muscle from the stenotic external carotid artery (ECA). This can be seen in severe carotid artery atherosclerosis.

Aphasia

Aphasia denotes language disturbances and more commonly involves the left carotid circulation as Broca area is typically located in the left frontal operculum with Wernicke area in the left posterior superior temporal gyrus.

DIAGNOSIS

According to the 2016 American College of Radiology (ACR) Appropriateness Criteria, imaging is indicated in asymptomatic patients with significant cerebrovascular risk factors or a carotid bruit on physical examination.[10] In this setting, ultrasound, computed tomography (CT), or magnetic resonance imaging (MRI) can be utilized for initial evaluation. However, in symptomatic patients, cross-sectional imaging is preferred.

Ultrasound

Advantages of this modality include ease of access, low cost, high accuracy, low risk, and ability to evaluate hemodynamics. Limitations of this modality, as opposed to cross-sectional imaging, include the inability to assess arch vessel origins and intracranial vasculature and its operator variability.

The ACR, American Institute of Ultrasound in Medicine (AIUM), Society for Pediatric Radiology (SPR), and Society of Radiologists in Ultrasound (SRU) published joint recommendations for technique performing an ultrasound of the extracranial arteries.[11] Briefly, the examination should include grayscale imaging (B-mode), color Doppler imaging, and spectral Doppler velocity measurements. The study should interrogate the entire course of the common carotid arteries, carotid bulbs, internal carotid arteries, vertebral arteries, and ECA origins. One should describe plaque morphology including composition and intima-media thickness; it is thought that noncalcified plaque may be at increased risk for thromboembolism. It should document the specific location of plaques at areas of increased velocity concerning stenosis with associated post-stenotic turbulence.[12] The internal carotid artery end-diastolic velocity (ICA EDV), peak systolic velocity (PSV), and internal carotid artery to common carotid artery PSV ratio (ICA/CCA PSV) are useful adjuncts to quantify the severity of the disease.[12] These are particularly useful when evaluating persons with heart failure, as their absolute velocities will be decreased in this condition, thereby making ICA/CCA ratios a more reliable metric. The ultrasound characteristics in assessing carotid artery stenosis are described in **Tables 91.1** and **91.2**.

A stenosis ≥50% is considered significant in symptomatic patients for evaluation for surgery. For asymptomatic disease, greater than or equal to 70% is widely accepted as a threshold for repair (see **Figure 91.1A,B**).

Computed Tomography

CT has proven an invaluable tool for procedural planning. Advantages of CT include ease of access; high accuracy; specific description of the location; composition and length of lesions; anatomic variants; and detection of incidental comorbidities such as coronary artery disease, chronic obstructive pulmonary disease, vasculitis/vasculopathy, prior cerebral infarct, or cerebral aneurysm. Disadvantages include a modest dose of ionizing radiation, iodinated contrast with a risk of contrast-induced nephropathy, and potential for allergic reactions. Additionally, although CT may quantify the degree of stenosis, it cannot infer whether the lesion is hemodynamically significant.

CT angiography is obtained from the aortic arch to the level of the Circle of Willis. Stenoses are generally described according to the North American Symptomatic Carotid Endarterectomy Trial (NASCET) criteria as defined by the luminal diameter at an area of stenosis (A) relative to an immediately adjacent segment of the normal artery (B) using the following equation: $(B - A)/(B) \times 100$.

Magnetic Resonance Imaging

Magnetic resonance imaging (MRI) is becoming increasingly utilized in preprocedural evaluation. Advantages are similar to CT and include high accuracy and detection of anatomic variants and incidental comorbidities. Additionally, novel vessel wall imaging sequences are able to further characterize lesions such as dissection, intramural hematoma, or ulcerated plaques. Vessel wall imaging MRI is particularly valuable in patients with vasculitis, such as Takayasu or giant cell arteritis. Disadvantages are many and include increased length of

TABLE 91.1 Modified Washington Duplex Criteria

Grade	Stenosis	PSV (cm/s)	EDV (cm/s)	Flow Characteristics
A	Normal	<125		Normal with no plaque
B	1%-15%	<125		Normal with plaque or minimal spectral broadening
C	16%-49%	<125		Marked spectral broadening
D	50%-79%	>125	<140	Marked spectral broadening
D+	80%-99%	>125	>140	Marked spectral broadening
E	Occluded	No flow	No flow	No flow

EDV, end-diastolic velocity; PSV, peak systolic velocity.
Adapted with permission from Rasmussen TE, Clouse WD, Tonnessen BH. *Handbook of Patient Care in Vascular Diseases.* 6th ed. Philadelphia, PA: Wolters Kluwer; 2018. Table 12.1.

TABLE 91.2 Society of Radiologists in Ultrasound Consensus Criteria

	Primary Parameters		Additional Parameters	
Degree of Stenosis (%)	ICA PSV (cm/s)	Plaque Estimate (%)	ICA/CCA PSV Ratio	ICA EDV (cm/s)
Normal	<125	None	<2.0	<40
<50	<125	<50	<2.0	<40
50-69	125-230	≥50	2.0-4.0	40-100
≥70 but less than near occlusion	>230	≥50	>4.0	>100
Near occlusion	High, low, or undetectable	Visible	Variable	Variable
Total occlusion	Undetectable	Visible, no detectable lumen	Not applicable	Not applicable

CCA, common carotid artery; EDV, end-diastolic velocity; ICA, internal carotid artery; Plaque estimate (diameter reduction) with grayscale and color Doppler US; PSV, peak systolic velocity.
Adapted with permission from Rasmussen TE, Clouse WD, Tonnessen BH. *Handbook of Patient Care in Vascular Diseases.* 6th ed. Philadelphia, PA: Wolters Kluwer; 2018. Table 12.1.

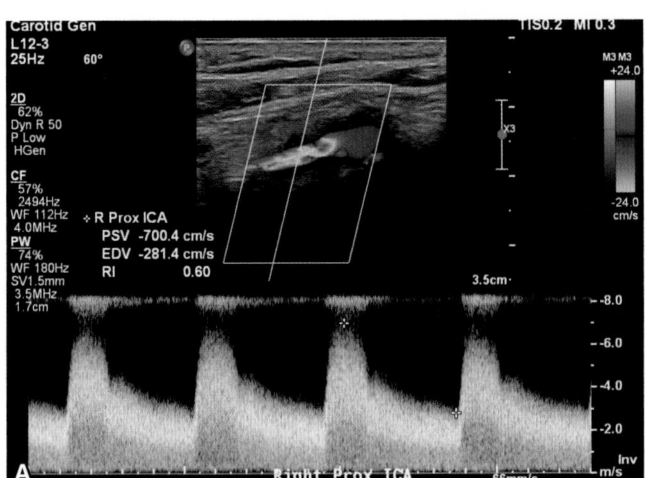

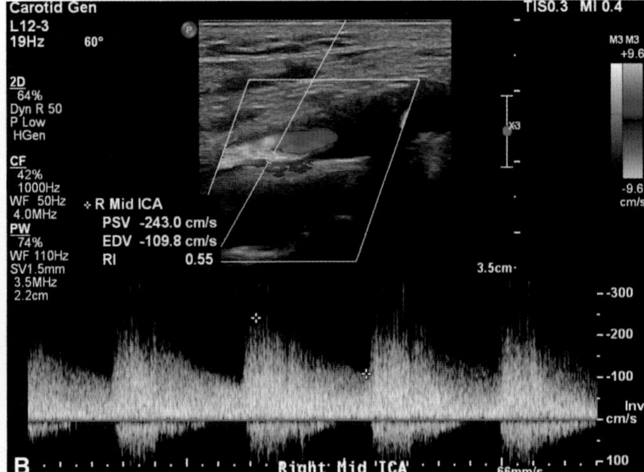

FIGURE 91.1 Carotid Doppler ultrasound demonstrating 70% to 99% stenosis with increased peak systolic velocity and end-diastolic velocity, post-stenotic turbulence, and a visible plaque in the proximal internal carotid artery. Panel A shows velocities in proximal right internal carotid artery and Panel B shows velocities in middle right internal carotid artery. (Courtesy of UT Southwestern Medical Center Vascular lab, Dallas, TX.)

examination, which can be prohibitive in persons with claustrophobia, altered mental status, or inability to lay flat; susceptibility artifact from metallic hardware such as prior stents or spinal fusion; or MRI-unsafe hardware such as pacemakers or some aneurysm clips. Additionally, use of gadolinium contrast is associated with a small risk of allergic reaction and risk of nephrogenic systemic fibrosis. However, this can be readily circumvented with noncontrast time-of-flight angiography. Description of lesions is also performed according to the NASCET criteria.

Arteriography

Although invasive, there are several situations where arteriography may improve diagnostic confidence such as with nondiagnostic or discordant noninvasive imaging results. The stroke risk associated with cerebrovascular arteriography is 1%. Access site and other complications can occur in up to 3% of patients.

MANAGEMENT OF THE PATIENT WITH CAROTID ARTERY STENOSIS

The primary goal in treating carotid artery stenosis is risk reduction and stroke prevention: by maximum medical therapy, endovascular therapy, or surgery. Regardless of the modality, a thorough understanding of the natural history of the disease is essential to formulating a rational and effective treatment strategy. Currently, the mainstay of management of extracranial cerebrovascular diseases includes medical management using antiplatelet and lipid-lowering agents as well as smoking cessation, carotid endarterectomy (CEA), carotid angioplasty and stenting (CAS), and transcarotid artery revascularization (TCAR) (see **Algorithm 91.1**).

Medical Management

Medical management is the cornerstone of all treatments of extracranial carotid disease. All patients should begin medical optimization of their comorbidities. Antihypertensives should be considered to maintain blood pressure less than 140/90 mm Hg.[1] Screening for diabetes or obstructive sleep apnea is recommended in this high-risk population. Initiation of a statin with a goal low-density lipoprotein cholesterol of less than 100 mg/dL is recommended.[1] Lifestyle modifications, including smoking cessation, diet, and exercise, are also essential.

In the setting of acute ischemic stroke, thrombolysis with tissue plasminogen activator (tPA) within 3 hours of symptom onset has been shown to improve survival in carefully selected patients.[13] In addition, as a mode of primary prevention of myocardial infarction (MI), antiplatelet therapy with aspirin (75-325 mg/day) is generally recommended. For secondary prevention of ischemic stroke, antiplatelet monotherapy with aspirin or clopidogrel (75 mg daily) is strongly recommended over anticoagulation.[1] In select symptomatic patients with severe carotid stenosis, dual antiplatelet therapy (DAPT) with aspirin and clopidogrel for 3 months is a reasonable consideration.[14] However, for those who are already on oral anticoagulation for indications such as atrial fibrillation or prosthetic heart valves, adding an antiplatelet agent may have a limited

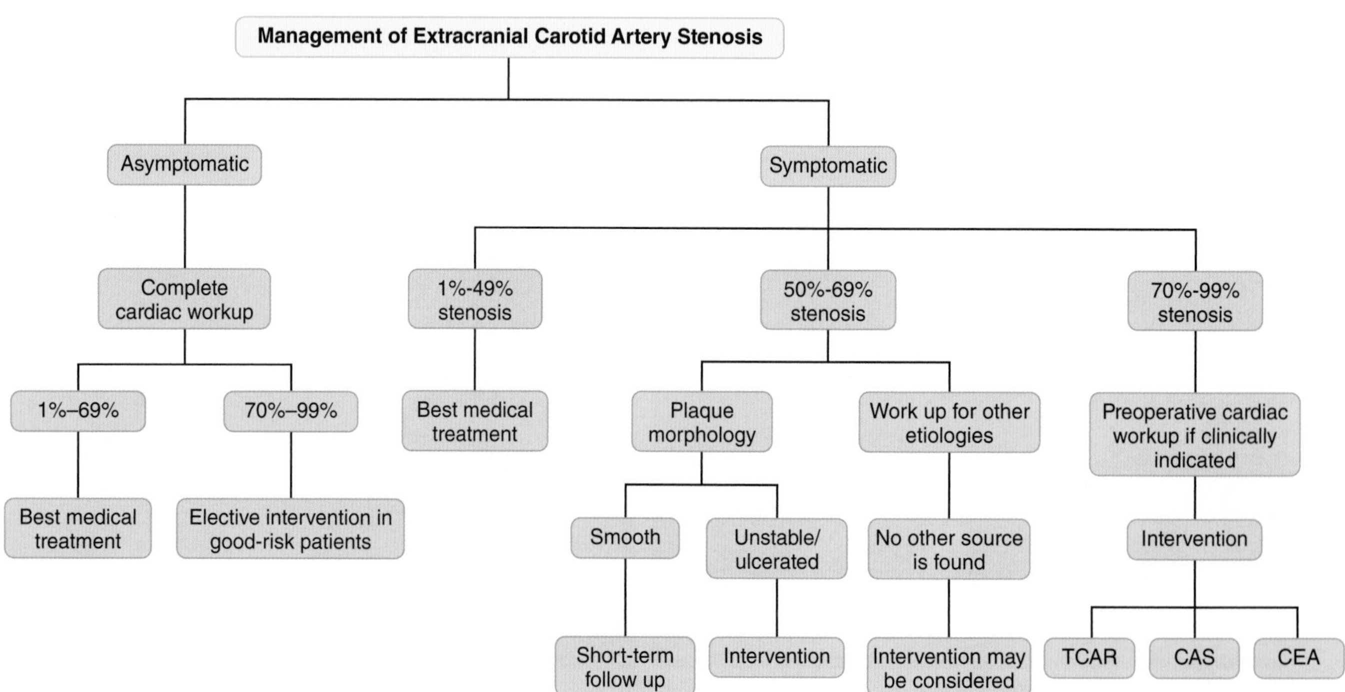

ALGORITHM 91.1 Approach to management of extracranial carotid artery stenosis. CAS, carotid artery stenting; CEA, carotid endarterectomy; TCAR, transcarotid revascularization.

benefit except for select cases in which unstable angina or coronary artery stenting is factored.[14] Compared to warfarin, newer oral anticoagulants, such as dabigatran, may have a lower risk of intracranial hemorrhage, emerging as a more favorable option for many.[15] Select medications commonly used in the management of extracranial carotid disease are described in **Tables 91.3**.

Stroke Risk Stratification

The major determinants of patient management in extracranial carotid artery disease are symptomatic status and degree of luminal stenosis. In addition, the plaque morphology, presence of contralateral stenosis, and evidence of silent emboli are factored into consideration. In the 1990s, several randomized clinical trials (RCTs) were performed to evaluate the outcomes of carotid artery interventions. Although these well-known RCTs have become the foundation for many of our clinical decisions, there are still several aspects of patient management for which we do not yet have the complete answers.

Symptomatic Patients

Both the NASCET and European Carotid Surgery Trial (ECST) enrolled patients with symptomatic carotid disease and demonstrated significantly increased risk of major stroke or mortality in the medical arms compared to the intervention arms.[16,17] NASCET showed symptomatic patients with >70% stenosis benefited from CEA, with a 29% relative risk reduction of stroke or death in 5 years.[16]

The highest risk of stroke is in the first month following TIA or minor stroke presentation. In one study, the risk of stroke was 2.8% within 30 days and 5.1% within 1 year.[8] Natural history studies, such as the Asymptomatic Carotid Stenosis and the Risk of Stroke Study (ACSRS), revealed that prior stroke or even contralateral TIA was an independent predictor of stroke.[18]

Asymptomatic Patients

A similar advantage in carotid revascularization was also shown in an asymptomatic population in the Asymptomatic Carotid Atherosclerosis Study (ACAS) trial and Asymptomatic Carotid Surgery Trial (ACST).[19,20] ACAS compared medical management with CEA in asymptomatic patients with >60% stenosis and demonstrated a lower 5-year stroke and death rate for CEA at 5.1% compared to medical therapy at 11%.[19]

Currently, the Carotid Revascularization and Medical Management for Asymptomatic Carotid Stenosis (CREST-2) trial is underway to determine the best modality for primary stroke prevention in patients with asymptomatic carotid stenosis. This study compares intensive medical management without carotid revascularization to CEA and CAS and is estimated to be completed by 2022. The outcomes of CREST-2 may help refine our treatment strategies in this asymptomatic population.

Degree of Stenosis

The degree of stenosis has a positive correlation with stroke risk.[16,17] In the ECST trial, the risk of major stroke at 6 years of follow-up in medically managed patients was 12% in patients with mild stenosis, 16% with moderate stenosis, and 26% with severe stenosis.[17] Similarly, in the ACSRS trial studying asymptomatic patients, the risk of major stroke at a mean follow-up of 48 months was 3% in patients with moderate stenosis and 6% with severe stenosis.[18]

SECTION 7

TABLE 91.3 Common Medications Used in Management of Extracranial Carotid Disease

Statin Agents	High-Intensity Dose (LDL Reduction > 50%)	Moderate-Intensity Dose (LDL Reduction 30%-50%)	Adverse Reaction
Atorvastatin	40-80 mg QD	10-20 mg QD	Muscle toxicity Hepatic impairment
Rosuvastatin	20-40 mg QD	5-10 mg QD	
Simvastatin	—	20-40 mg QD	
Antiplatelet Agents	**Dose**	**Adverse Reaction**	
Aspirin	75-325 mg QD	Upper gastrointestinal bleeding	
Clopidogrel	75 mg QD	Epistaxis, bruises	
Direct Oral Anticoagulants	**Dose**	**Adverse Reaction**	
Apixaban	2.5-5 mg BID	Nausea, no dosage adjustment needed unless ≥80 years and weight ≤60 kg, then reduce dose to 2.5 mg twice daily	
Dabigatran	110-150 mg BID	Dyspepsia/gastritis, no need for renal/hepatic dosage adjustment	
Rivaroxaban	15-20 mg QD	Wound secretion, back/abdominal pain, avoid in renal or hepatic impairment with coagulopathy	

BID, twice daily; LDL, low-density lipoprotein; QD, once daily.

Plaque Character and Progression

Giannoukas et al showed that larger plaques are less fibrotic, more lipid-laden, and contain more inflammatory cells and intraplaque hemorrhage.[21] Patients with plaque progression from less than 50% stenosis to more than 50% have increased odds of CVA by 1.68, especially if they progress to more than 80% stenosis.[22] There is a correlation between carotid plaque progression and major adverse cardiovascular events (MACE), stroke and cardiovascular deaths.[23] The plaque echogenic scale has been shown to be related to the symptomatic status of the plaque.[24]

Contralateral Disease

Contralateral carotid artery occlusion might increase the risk of stroke in patients with significant carotid stenosis.[25] The degree of collateral circulation, completeness of the circle of Willis, and vertebral artery disease all play roles in assessing the risk of future stroke.

Evidence of Clinically Silent Emboli

Although evidence of silent cerebral emboli seen on imaging may help predict the risk of future neurologic events, their absence does not imply minimal future symptoms in a patient with significant carotid artery disease.

Patient Selection for Carotid Intervention

When evaluating a patient for possible CEA, CAS, or TCAR, the following factors should be taken into consideration:

Life Expectancy

Patients with carotid artery disease often are advanced in age and have other cardiovascular comorbidities including coronary artery disease and chronic kidney disease, among others. As such, nonstroke-related mortality in this demographic is substantial. In the ECST trial, all-cause mortality during an average 6-year follow-up was 27%.[17] For this reason, one should carefully evaluate not only the perioperative risk but also life expectancy when considering a possible intervention. Asymptomatic patients, in particular, should have a life expectancy of at least 3 to 5 years to incur meaningful cerebrovascular risk reduction benefits from a carotid intervention.

Age

NASCET, ECST, and ACAS excluded octogenarians. ACST enrolled patients up to 91 years old, but the number of patients above 80 was too small for statistical analysis.[20] The Carotid Revascularization and Endarterectomy versus Stenting Trial (CREST) and the Stent-Protected Angioplasty versus Carotid Endarterectomy (SPACE) trial demonstrated an increased risk of stroke and mortality in older patients undergoing CAS compared to CEA, irrespective of symptomatic status.[26,27] Several other analyses from the National Inpatient Sample (NIS) and Vascular Quality Initiative (VQI) registries also showed increased periprocedural stroke rates in older patients (over 65-70 years of age) undergoing CAS compared to CEA.[28,29] This might be attributable to more unfavorable anatomy, such as tortuous aortic arch and great vessels as well as plaque instability, and decreased cerebrovascular reserve in older patients.

Sex

A smaller diameter of the carotid arteries in women has been proposed as a possible reason for more strokes in women than men following CEA. However, in many major trials, only a minority of the participants were women, and routine patching of the carotid artery was not the standard of care at the time of these trials, which might explain the difference in outcomes. Nonetheless, CEA was shown to be beneficial in symptomatic women with severe stenosis in both NASCET and ECST.[16,17] The CREST trial suggested a higher risk of stroke and/or death in women undergoing CAS versus CEA (5.5% vs 2.2%; $P = .01$), especially in the symptomatic subgroup.[26] However, a meta-analysis of three European RCTs showed no significant increase in stroke risk among women treated with CAS versus CEA.[30]

Given the unclear influence of sex on perioperative morbidity and mortality after CAS versus CEA, the consensus recommendations for choice of revascularization in women are thus similar to those in men: CAS is only selectively preferred in symptomatic women with unfavorable neck anatomy owing to a prior operation, irradiation, or prior cranial nerve injury and/or lesions above the level of the second cervical vertebral body (C2) or near the clavicle.[31]

Functional Status

Patients with an impaired functional status, severe dementia, or significant hemispheric neurologic deficits are unlikely to benefit from any carotid intervention. Perioperative cardiac events are associated with late mortality, thus warranting a preoperative cardiac evaluation. As both CEA and CAS procedures could be done under regional or local anesthesia, the perioperative morbidity caused by pulmonary disease is minimal unless there is active disease. Renal insufficiency is an independent risk factor for subsequent strokes.[1] It is also associated with increased incidence of complications after CEA and CAS.[18] Therefore, there is no consensus regarding the procedure of choice in this frail group of patients.

Contralateral Carotid Occlusion. There is a statistically significant albeit small increase in periprocedural stroke rates in patients with contralateral carotid occlusion who undergo CEA. This effect was not seen in those with contralateral carotid occlusion who underwent CAS.[32]

Timing of Intervention

CEA has proven beneficial in decreasing the risk of secondary stroke in symptomatic patients if performed within 7 days of initial symptoms; analogous data are conflicting regarding CAS.[33] Larger prospective studies focused on timing are needed to address the challenge of timing of CAS following TIA.

Asymptomatic Patients

Based on both the CREST and the Stenting and Angioplasty with Protection in Patients at High Risk for Endarterectomy (SAPPHIRE) trials, CAS outcomes are equivalent to CEA when performed by experienced interventionalists in properly selected asymptomatic patients. Nonetheless, based on recent studies, the best medical therapy may have similar results in many asymptomatic patients, especially those with recurrent stenosis and short life expectancy.[34] The ongoing CREST-2 trial is designed to answer the question of whether CAS is recommended in asymptomatic patients with severe carotid stenosis.

Combined Coronary and Carotid Disease

The sequence and choice of treatment are challenging in patients with significant carotid disease and comorbid coronary artery disease. An analysis of NIS data demonstrated a higher risk of perioperative stroke in patients undergoing CEA plus coronary artery bypass grafting (CABG) compared to staged CAS prior to CABG (odds ratio [OR], 1.62; CI: 1.1-2.5; $P = .02$) whereas in-hospital mortality was similar (5.2% vs 5.4%).[35] One meta-analysis showed a 9.1% rate of 30-day stroke and/or death in CAS plus CABG patients, but many of these patients had only asymptomatic carotid disease. One factor to consider in decision-making is the increased risk of major bleeding with cardiac surgery in patients following CAS on DAPT.

Choice of Intervention

Outcomes following CEA are more favorable compared to CAS in symptomatic patients, especially when performed within the first week of symptoms. However, in patients with difficult surgical neck anatomy such as presence of tracheostomy, contralateral nerve palsy, prior neck radiation, or with lesions close to the clavicle or above the level of C2 vertebral body, CAS is preferred to CEA. Several studies showed similar stroke risks in this group of patients after CEA or CAS, but higher incidence of cranial nerve injury after CEA.

On the other hand, there are several anatomic constraints before CAS is pursued. Although the CREST study did not find a correlation between CAS outcomes and other "high-risk" anatomic features—such as lesion length, eccentric or ulcerated lesions, degree of stenosis, procedural time—these results should be interpreted with caution as the current literature reports mixed results: a systemic review still identified these aforementioned anatomic features to be correlated with increased risks.[26,36]

Based on the Endarterectomy versus Angioplasty in Patients with Symptomatic Severe Carotid Stenosis (EVA-3S) trial, patients with ICA-CCA angulation $\geq 60°$ and/or target ICA lesions of $\geq$10 mm in length may have a higher risk of stroke and/or death after CAS.[37] Heavy circumferential calcification of the ICA can result in underexpansion and recoiling of the lesion, and distal ICA tortuosity can cause flow-limiting angulation following stent deployment. Although type III aortic arch was not associated with increased perioperative morbidity and mortality in the EVA-3S study, type II to III arch types are technically more challenging for the operators. Extensive aortic wall irregularities with multiple atheromas, a so-called shaggy aorta, and severe aortic calcification also increase the complexity of CAS, with the former sometimes considered a relative contraindication to CAS owing to the risk of emboli. Lipid-rich plaques, lesions longer than 15 mm, fresh thrombus, and nearly occlusive highly calcified lesions are associated with worse outcomes after CAS.[38] TCAR is an alternative stenting technique that allows the operators to bypass such sources of emboli, with emerging evidence of very low periprocedural stroke rate.

CAROTID ENDARTERECTOMY

Preoperative

When performing CEA, we recommend prescribing an antiplatelet agent (aspirin) throughout the perioperative period and continuing it indefinitely afterward. If the patient has been on DAPT, such as the combination of aspirin and clopidogrel, one should discontinue clopidogrel 5 days prior to surgery if feasible. If necessary, CEA can be performed while on DAPT, but there are significantly higher rates of postoperative hematoma.

Intraoperative

Adequate hydration is essential. Preoperative intravenous antibiotics are given within 30 to 60 minutes prior to skin incision. The operation may be performed under a cervical block alone in a well-tolerating, awake patient, and this facilitates direct neurological monitoring throughout the entirety of the case. However, should patient factors, such as anxiety or claustrophobia, prevent an awake procedure, general anesthesia with some form of neuromonitoring and/or protection (eg, electroencephalogram [EEG], stump pressures, or shunting) is used. Although routine shunting may be utilized by some surgeons, selective shunting is also accepted when the EEG changes or inadequate stump pressures are noted intraoperatively.

Surgical Technique: Carotid Endarterectomy

The incision is fashioned along the length of the sternocleidomastoid muscle, and the muscle and internal jugular vein are mobilized laterally to isolate the carotid artery. This usually requires ligation of the facial vein when present as it crosses over the carotid artery. The CCA is mobilized proximally to the atheromatous lesion. Often, the ICA and the ECA are dissected and controlled prior to manipulation of the carotid bulb to avoid the dreaded complication of distal embolization and subsequent stroke. When mobilizing the ICA, particular care must be taken to avoid injury to the hypoglossal nerve and the vagus nerve. Prior to vascular clamping, systemic heparin is given (80 U/kg). Once the vessels are controlled, the dissection is carried around the carotid bifurcation; it may be necessary to inject a local anesthetic in the area to block the nerve to the carotid body to prevent reflex bradycardia. After a longitudinal arteriotomy is made over the carotid bifurcation and carried distally into the ICA, endarterectomy is performed by separating the atheromatous plaque from the adventitia until healthy intima is encountered. A smooth, feathered edge is created to transition from the endarterectomized adventitial plane to the healthy intima distally. Any free-floating edges are tacked down with sutures lest they become a nidus for thrombus formation. The arteriotomy is typically repaired via a bovine patch angioplasty closure. Flow is established first to the ECA and then to the ICA to minimize embolization risk. Intraoperative carotid duplex is routinely performed at this time to identify any technical errors or residual disease. Once technical success is confirmed, the neck is closed in layers.

Complications: Carotid Endarterectomy

Immediate and delayed postoperative neurologic deficits should be recognized promptly and warrant a return to the operating room for interrogation and correction of any technical error. One of the most common postoperative problems after CEA is hemodynamic instability, which occurs about 20% of the time.[39] Patients who were hypertensive preoperatively are more likely to have severe postoperative hypertension. The incidence of neurologic deficits and death is significantly higher in these patients. The authors thus maintain postoperative systolic blood pressure in a range between 100 and 150 mm Hg. Neck hematomas may cause airway obstruction or dysphagia, often requiring an emergent return to the operating room for evacuation. One of the earliest signs of a developing hematoma is the inability to manage oral secretions. Varying degrees of nerve dysfunction may be seen, but the cranial nerve deficit occurs 3% of the time.[40] The more common finding is a marginal mandibular branch of the facial nerve paresis from a traction injury, which is usually self-limiting, resolving in 2 to 6 months. Albeit less frequent, late complications of CEA may also occur. With routine surveillance, recurrent carotid stenosis is seen in 10% of patients in the first year.[41] This tends to be more common in women and active smokers. The risk of a future stroke in this asymptomatic group appears to be low.[41]

CAROTID ARTERY STENTING

Since the first percutaneous carotid artery angioplasties in 1977 and 1980 and the first balloon-expandable stent deployment in carotid artery in 1989, technique and device design have evolved dramatically.[42,43] The catalyst for advancement was driven by the high rate of adverse events, including extrinsic compression of the first-generation stents.[44] By 1990, embolic protection devices (EPDs) were in widespread use during CAS.[45] Although CAS is faster and simpler than CEA, the major disadvantage is the increased risk of periprocedural stroke.[46] With the current data, CAS and CEA may be equivalent only in a carefully selected group of patients and operators.

Intraprocedural

Patients will require anticoagulation intraoperatively (unfractionated heparin 70-100 U/kg) with a goal activated clotting time of 250 to 300 seconds; heparin is rarely reversed at the completion of the procedure. One could alternatively prescribe bivalirudin especially in those with a heparin allergy. In case of hypotension and bradycardia during balloon angioplasty, 0.4 to 1.0 mg of intravenous atropine may be administered. Aggressive intravenous volume expansion, additional atropine, or vasopressors (intravenous phenylephrine 1-10 μg/kg/min or dopamine 5-15 μg/kg/min) may be needed in refractory hypotension. Intraoperative blood pressure control is essential: maintenance of systolic blood pressure below 180 mm Hg is necessary to decrease the risk of intracranial hemorrhage. In case of severe and persistent ICA vasospasm upon EPD retrieval, nitroglycerin is administered directly into the ICA.

Periprocedural

DAPT is given preoperatively. This includes aspirin 75 to 325 mg/daily and clopidogrel 75 mg/daily, starting at least 4 days prior to the procedure. An alternative is a loading dose of clopidogrel 300 to 600 mg, 4 to 6 hours prior to the procedure. Ticlopidine 250 mg twice daily may be used as an alternative in patients who are intolerant to clopidogrel. Most centers continue DAPT for 4 weeks after CAS. Longer duration of treatment is suggested in patients who are at high risk for restenosis or cardiovascular events. Otherwise, 75 to 100 mg/daily of aspirin is sufficient for long-term treatment. Available recommendations suggest prescribing statins early prior to CAS and monitoring liver function and creatine kinase.

Surgical Technique: Carotid Artery Stenting

Imaging and physiologic monitors should be readily available to continuously assess the patient. Patient alertness, speech, and motor function are also evaluated regularly: for instance, by asking the patient to answer simple questions and squeeze a plastic toy in the contralateral hand. Transcranial Doppler (TCD) could be used as an adjunctive monitoring technique.

Transfemoral Access

A 6F to 9F introducer access sheath is used in retrograde fashion via the common femoral artery.

Transcervical Access

This has been largely replaced by the TCAR method. A short CCA precludes transcervical access.

Transbrachial/Transradial Access

In case of aortoiliac occlusive disease or difficult access to the CCA, such as with a type III arch, a 6F guiding catheter may be used via the upper extremity.

Target Lesion Access

It is critical to establish a stable system in the proximal CCA. The system should be irrigated regularly, and the side port should be connected to blood pressure monitoring. Either a sheath-based or a guiding catheter-based platform could be used. In the sheath-based method, after selecting the ECA, a 6F 90-cm sheath is advanced over an exchange-length stiff 0.035-inch guidewire and positioned in the distal CCA, with care taken not to cross the bulb. In the guiding catheter-based platform, a 6F or 7F preshaped guiding catheter (eg, vertebral multipurpose curve or reversed-angle Vitek catheter) is positioned at the CCA level for the entire procedure. This method obviates the need for exchange wires and catheters. Adding a high-support 0.014-inch "buddy wire" and placing it in the ECA could add stability to this platform.

Arteriography

Obtaining anteroposterior and lateral views of the lesion, ECA, ICA, and intracranial vessels are required. Sometimes additional oblique views are obtained for better separation of the ECA and ICA.

Delivery System

Full angiographic views help in decision-making regarding EPD use. Distal filters are deployed into the ICA below the petrous segment. This should be kept in view during the entire procedure. Advancement of the device could cause dissection and spasm in the intracranial carotid artery. In severe stenosis, predilation with a 2.5- or 4-mm balloon with low inflation pressure (4-6 atmospheres) is recommended. Road mapping is used for stent deployment, and the stent is placed across the bulb in most cases as it is typically part of the disease. The distal CCA is used to size the stent, with a diameter range of 7 to 10 mm and a length of 3 to 4 cm. The stent can be cylindrical or tapered. Dilation after stent placement might be necessary especially in heavily calcified lesions. The balloon should be inflated only inside the stent. Completion angiogram with high magnification is necessary before retrieval of the EPD. In case of spasm, watchful waiting and direct injection of small doses of nitroglycerin (100-200 μg) are recommended. The interventionalist should attempt to use less than 60 mL of contrast. Heparin is generally not reversed, and access-site hemostasis is achieved by manual compression or a closure device.

Embolic Protection Device Selection

Most interventionalists favor employment of EPD for reducing periprocedural stroke in patients undergoing CAS. In a meta-analysis of 12,263 protected and 11,198 unprotected CAS, the relative risk of stroke was decreased in protected CAS (OR: 0.62; 95% CI: 0.54-0.72).[47] The three main EPD types are distal filters, distal occlusion balloons, and proximal protection devices with flow stasis (Mo.Ma system) or reversal. The last type gave rise to the TCAR protection mechanism discussed later.

Stent Selection

Carotid stent models are self-expandable stents, made of stainless steel (cobalt alloy) or nitinol (nickel-titanium alloy) which permits sufficient flexibility and scaffolding. A rigid stent in tortuous anatomy would be susceptible to a distal kink, and lack of adequate scaffolding may result in plaque protrusion through the stent struts. In closed-cell stents, all stent struts are interconnected, whereas that is not the case in open-cell stents. Open-cell stents are preferred in tortuous anatomy as they are more conformable. More studies are required to compare outcomes in closed- versus open-cell stents.

Complications: Carotid Artery Stenting

Neurologic. Neurologic complications are among the most feared risks and need to be addressed immediately if possible. Mild spasm of the carotid artery can be treated with nitroglycerin (200 μg) or observed until resolution. If a filled filter is flow limiting, it should be slowly closed and carefully withdrawn. In case of flow-limiting dissection, further stenting might be needed. Acute in-stent thrombosis requires immediate stent removal and endarterectomy. Neuro-rescue techniques might be necessary in case of visible distal embolization. If there is a developing focal neurologic deficit during CAS, without any obvious cause, it is recommended to complete the procedure and reassess the patient after retrieving the catheters.

Intracranial hemorrhage is a devastating but rare (<1%) complication, and the data regarding its prevalence in CAS versus CEA are controversial. It is generally thought to be more likely following CAS in patients with symptomatic disease, nearly occlusive carotid stenosis, hypertension, and contralateral carotid occlusion or severe disease.

Cardiovascular. Although the risk of periprocedural MI in CAS was half that of CEA in several trials such as EVA-3S, The International Carotid Stenting Study (ICSS), and CREST, different definitions of MI were used in the studies comparing CAS with CEA. In patients with congestive heart failure, the osmotic load of contrast during CAS may precipitate an exacerbation.

Severe bradycardia and hypotension from distension of the carotid bulb during CAS are seen frequently but rarely cause ischemia. Hypertension occurs in up to half of the patients who undergo CAS but is generally transient. Fluid resuscitation is the mainstay of prevention and treatment, with atropine or methoxamine infusion as needed for refractory cases.

Local and Other Complication. Access-site arterial occlusion and hemorrhage occur in up to 5% of patients after CAS. More uncommon complications included retroperitoneal hemorrhage, infection, pseudoaneurysm, and arteriovenous fistula. Most of these complications are self-limiting and rarely in need of blood transfusion (2%-3%).

TRANSCAROTID ARTERY REVASCULARIZATION

TCAR (Silk Road Medical Inc., Sunnyvale, CA) is one of the most novel techniques developed for carotid intervention (**Figure 91.2A,B**). The main benefits of TCAR include achieving endovascular carotid revascularization while maintaining outcomes comparable to those of CEA by avoiding aortic arch and carotid ostial manipulation.

Procedure Details

An incision is made at the base of the neck to achieve proximal control of CCA. This is followed by percutaneous access of the common femoral vein (CFV) in either groin. A specially designed short sheath is inserted into the proximal CCA, with particular care to avoid carotid bulb and ICA manipulation. Then the CCA and CFV are connected using the flow reversal system with a built-in filter. This flow reversal system takes advantage of the natural pressure gradient created temporarily by linking the carotid artery and femoral vein in which a retrograde flow from the ICA toward the CFV is established. As antegrade flow toward the ICA is diminished, it significantly decreases the risk of distal embolization. The rest of the procedure is very similar to CAS, including angiographic

SECTION 7

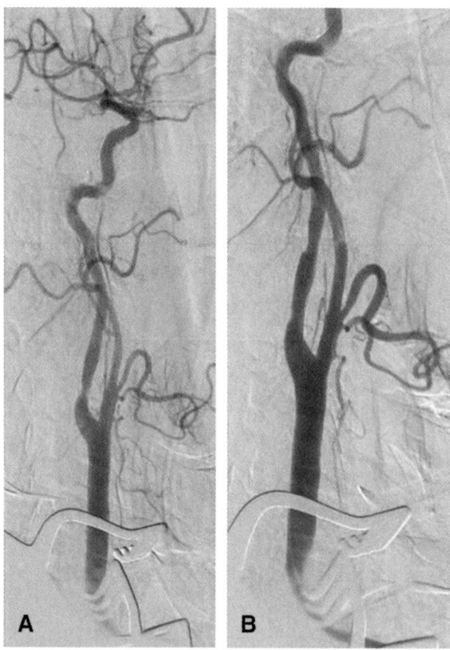

FIGURE 91.2 **(A,B)** Carotid artery stenosis treated by transcarotid arterial revascularization: **(A)** before and **(B)** after stent deployment. (Courtesy of UT Southwestern Medical Center, Dallas, Texas.)

confirmation of the lesion, crossing the lesion, predilation, and stent delivery. The delivery system and stents are all on short shafts as access is in the neck. Patients should be on statin and DAPT for 5 days preceding TCAR or receive a loading dose of clopidogrel and aspirin before the procedure.

Short-Term Outcomes and Ongoing Trials

By 2016, the Safety and Efficacy Study for Reverse Flow Used During Carotid Artery Stenting Procedure (ROADSTER) trial enrolled 216 patients and demonstrated an overall stroke rate of 1.4%.[48] The subsequent ROADSTER 2 study evaluated 632 patients who underwent TCAR across 42 sites with an overall stroke rate of 0.8%.[49] Furthermore, in a VQI analysis comparing the outcomes between TCAR and CAS, even with the increased burden of medical comorbidities, the TCAR cohort demonstrated half the risk of in-hospital TIA, stroke, or death while maintaining similar overall composite stroke and/or mortality rates.[50] However, further RCTs are needed to confirm these results.

FOLLOW-UP PATIENT CARE

For asymptomatic patients with moderate stenosis (50%-69%), a repeat duplex should be obtained every 6 months for 1 year. If unchanged, then annual surveillance is recommended. Should the patients develop any neurological signs in the interim, urgent stroke evaluation must ensue. In patients with lower perioperative risk for carotid revascularization, asymptomatic carotid stenosis with severe stenosis (70%-99%) should be further evaluated with CT angiography (CTA) of head and neck for preoperative preparation.

Within the first 3 months following CEA or CAS, a baseline duplex is routinely obtained. Afterward, a surveillance ultrasound is performed every 6 months for the first 2 years, annually thereafter for 5 years, and every 2 years for the life of the patient. In select high-risk patients, such as those after redo-CEA or in-stent restenosis; or with diabetes, prior cervical radiation, or heavy calcification, a closer follow-up is recommended. In these patients, one should repeat ultrasound every 6 months until stability is established and annually thereafter for the life of the patient.

KEY POINTS

- ✔ Besides a thorough history and physical examination of the patients with carotid artery stenosis, Doppler ultrasound and other imaging modalities play a major role in patient management and follow-up.
- ✔ Symptomatic status is the single most important factor in counseling, decision-making, and timing of treatment.
- ✔ Best medical therapy should be offered to all patients irrespective of symptomatic status or further intervention required.
- ✔ Carotid plaque morphology, contralateral carotid artery disease, intracranial atherosclerotic disease, combined coronary and carotid disease, unfavorable neck anatomy, and prior neck surgeries are considered in determining the choice of intervention.
- ✔ TCAR is the latest development in the armamentarium of carotid interventions with promising short- and mid-term results and a short learning curve. RCTs for further evaluation of its outcomes are ongoing.

REFERENCES

1. Benjamin EJ, Blaha MJ, Chiuve SE, et al. Heart disease and stroke statistics-2017 update: a report from the American Heart Association. *Circulation.* 2017;135(10):e146-e603.
2. Fisher M, Paganini-Hill A, Martin A, et al. Carotid plaque pathology: thrombosis, ulceration, and stroke pathogenesis. *Stroke.* 2005;36(2):253-257.
3. Ersoy H, Watts R, Sanelli P, et al. Atherosclerotic disease distribution in carotid and vertebrobasilar arteries: clinical experience in 100 patients undergoing fluoro-triggered 3D Gd-MRA. *J Magn Reson Imaging.* 2003;17(5):545-558.
4. Louridas G, Junaid A. Management of carotid artery stenosis. Update for family physicians. *Can Fam Physician.* 2005;51:984-989.
5. Park JH, Razuk A, Saad PF, et al. Carotid stenosis: what is the high-risk population? *Clinics (Sao Paulo).* 2012;67(8):865-870.
6. Lanzino G, Rabinstein AA, Brown RD Jr. Treatment of carotid artery stenosis: medical therapy, surgery, or stenting? *Mayo Clinic Proc.* 2009;84(4):362-368.
7. Modan B, Wagener DK. Some epidemiological aspects of stroke: mortality/morbidity trends, age, sex, race, socioeconomic status. *Stroke.* 1992;23(9):1230-1236.
8. Amarenco P, Lavallée PC, Labreuche J, et al. One-year risk of stroke after transient ischemic attack or minor stroke. *N Engl J Med.* 2016;374(16):1533-1542.

9. Laczynski DJ, Gallop J, Lyden SP, et al. Retinal artery occlusion does not portend an increased risk of stroke. *J Vasc Surg.* 2020;72:198-203.
10. Salmela MB, Mortazavi S, Jagadeesan BD, et al. ACR appropriateness criteria(®) cerebrovascular disease. *J Am Coll Radiol.* 2017;14(5s):S34-S61.
11. ACS Committee. AIUM-ACR-SPR-SRU practice parameter for the performance and interpretation of a diagnostic ultrasound examination of the extracranial head and neck. *J Ultrasound Med.* 2018;37(11):E6-E12.
12. Grant EG, Benson CB, Moneta GL, et al. Carotid artery stenosis: gray-scale and Doppler US diagnosis: Society of Radiologists in Ultrasound Consensus Conference. *Radiology.* 2003;229(2):340-346.
13. Lees KR, Bluhmki E, von Kummer R, et al. Time to treatment with intravenous alteplase and outcome in stroke: an updated pooled analysis of ECASS, ATLANTIS, NINDS, and EPITHET trials. *Lancet.* 2010;375(9727):1695-1703.
14. Meschia JF, Bushnell C, Boden-Albala B, et al. Guidelines for the primary prevention of stroke: a statement for healthcare professionals from the American Heart Association/American Stroke Association. *Stroke.* 2014;45(12):3754-3832.
15. Connolly SJ, Ezekowitz MD, Yusuf S, et al. Dabigatran versus warfarin in patients with atrial fibrillation. *N Engl J Med.* 2009;361(12):1139-1151.
16. Barnett HJM, Taylor DW, Haynes RB, et al. Beneficial effect of carotid endarterectomy in symptomatic patients with high-grade carotid stenosis. *N Engl J Med.* 1991;325(7):445-453.
17. European Carotid Surgery Trial Group. Randomised trial of endarterectomy for recently symptomatic carotid stenosis: final results of the MRC European Carotid Surgery Trial (ECST*). Lancet.* 1998;351(9113):1379-1387.
18. Nicolaides AN, Kakkos SK, Kyriacou E, et al. Asymptomatic internal carotid artery stenosis and cerebrovascular risk stratification. *J Vasc Surg.* 2010;52(6):1486-1496.e1481-1485.
19. Walker MD, Marler JR, Goldstein M, et al. Endarterectomy for asymptomatic carotid artery stenosis. *JAMA.* 1995;273(18):1421-1428.
20. Halliday A, Mansfield A, Marro J, et al. Prevention of disabling and fatal strokes by successful carotid endarterectomy in patients without recent neurological symptoms: randomised controlled trial. *Lancet.* 2004;363(9420):1491-1502.
21. Giannoukas AD, Sfyroeras GS, Griffin M, Saleptsis V, Antoniou GA, Nicolaides AN. Association of plaque echostructure and cardiovascular risk factors with symptomatic carotid artery disease. *J Cardiovasc Surg (Torino).* 2009;38(4):357-364.
22. Bertges DJ, Muluk V, Whittle J, Kelley M, MacPherson DS, Muluk SC. Relevance of carotid stenosis progression as a predictor of ischemic neurological outcomes. *Arch Intern Med.* 2003;163(19):2285-2289.
23. Sabeti S, Schlager O, Exner M, et al. Progression of carotid stenosis detected by duplex ultrasonography predicts adverse outcomes in cardiovascular high-risk patients. *Stroke.* 2007;38(11):2887-2894.
24. Nicolaides AN, Kakkos SK, Griffin M, et al. Effect of image normalization on carotid plaque classification and the risk of ipsilateral hemispheric ischemic events: results from the asymptomatic carotid stenosis and risk of stroke study. *Vascular.* 2005;13(4):211-221.
25. Inzitari D, Eliasziw M, Gates P, et al. The causes and risk of stroke in patients with asymptomatic internal-carotid-artery stenosis. North American Symptomatic Carotid Endarterectomy Trial Collaborators. *N Engl J Med.* 2000;342(23):1693-1700.
26. Voeks JH, Howard G, Roubin GS, et al. Age and outcomes after carotid stenting and endarterectomy: the carotid revascularization endarterectomy versus stenting trial. *Stroke.* 2011;42(12):3484-3490.
27. Ringleb PA, Allenberg J, Bruckmann H, et al. 30 day results from the SPACE trial of stent-protected angioplasty versus carotid endarterectomy in symptomatic patients: a randomised non-inferiority trial. *Lancet.* 2006;368(9543):1239-1247.
28. Khatri R, Chaudhry SA, Vazquez G, et al. Age differential between outcomes of carotid angioplasty and stent placement and carotid endarterectomy in general practice. *J Vasc Surg.* 2012;55(1):72-78.
29. Jim J, Rubin BG, Ricotta JJ 2nd, Kenwood CT, Siami FS, Sicard GA. Society for Vascular Surgery (SVS) Vascular Registry evaluation of comparative effectiveness of carotid revascularization procedures stratified by Medicare age. *J Vasc Surg.* 2012;55(5):1313-1320; discussion 1321.
30. Brown MM, Raine R. Should sex influence the choice between carotid stenting and carotid endarterectomy? *Lancet Neurol.* 2011;10(6):494-497.
31. De Rango P, Brown MM, Leys D, et al. Management of carotid stenosis in women: consensus document. *Neurology.* 2013;80(24):2258-2268.
32. Ricotta JJ 2nd, Upchurch GR Jr., Landis GS, et al. The influence of contralateral occlusion on results of carotid interventions from the Society for Vascular Surgery Vascular Registry. *J Vasc Surg.* 2014;60(4):958-965.
33. Rantner B, Goebel G, Bonati LH, Ringleb PA, Mas JL, Fraedrich G. The risk of carotid artery stenting compared with carotid endarterectomy is greatest in patients treated within 7 days of symptoms. *J Vasc Surg.* 2013;57(3):619-626.e612; discussion 625-616.
34. Brott TG, Halperin JL, Abbara S, et al. 2011 ASA/ACCF/AHA/AANN/AANS/ACR/ASNR/CNS/SAIP/SCAI/SIR/SNIS/SVM/SVS Guideline on the management of patients with extracranial carotid and vertebral artery disease: executive summary: a report of the American College of Cardiology Foundation/American Heart Association Task Force on Practice Guidelines, and the American Stroke Association, American Association of Neuroscience Nurses, American Association of Neurological Surgeons, American College of Radiology, American Society of Neuroradiology, Congress of Neurological Surgeons, Society of Atherosclerosis Imaging and Prevention, Society for Cardiovascular Angiography and Interventions, Society of Interventional Radiology, Society of NeuroInterventional Surgery, Society for Vascular Medicine, and Society for Vascular Surgery. *J Am Coll Cardiol.* 2011;57(8):1002-1044.
35. Timaran CH, Rosero EB, Smith ST, Valentine RJ, Modrall JG, Clagett GP. Trends and outcomes of concurrent carotid revascularization and coronary bypass. *J Vasc Surg.* 2008;48(2):355-360; discussion 360-351.
36. Khan M, Qureshi AI. Factors associated with increased rates of post-procedural stroke or death following carotid artery stent placement: a systematic review. *J Vasc Interv Neurol.* 2014;7(1):11-20.
37. Naggara O, Touze E, Beyssen B, et al. Anatomical and technical factors associated with stroke or death during carotid angioplasty and stenting: results from the endarterectomy versus angioplasty in patients with symptomatic severe carotid stenosis (EVA-3S) trial and systematic review. *Stroke.* 2011;42(2):380-388.
38. Setacci C, Chisci E, Setacci F, Iacoponi F, de Donato G, Rossi A. Siena carotid artery stenting score: a risk modelling study for individual patients. *Stroke.* 2010;41(6):1259-1265.
39. Bove EL, Fry WJ, Gross WS, Stanley JC. Hypotension and hypertension as consequences of baroreceptor dysfunction following carotid endarterectomy. *Surgery.* 1979;85(6):633-637.
40. Dasenbrock HH, Smith TR, Gormley WB, et al. Predictive score of adverse events after carotid endarterectomy: the NSQIP Registry Carotid Endarterectomy Scale. *J Am Heart Assoc.* 2019;8(21):e013412.
41. Frericks H, Kievit J, van Baalen JM, van Bockel JH. Carotid recurrent stenosis and risk of ipsilateral stroke: a systematic review of the literature. *Stroke.* 1998;29(1):244-250.
42. Mathias K. A new catheter system for percutaneous transluminal angioplasty (PTA) of carotid artery stenoses. *Fortschr Med.* 1977;95(15):1007-1011.
43. Kerber CW, Cromwell LD, Loehden OL. Catheter dilatation of proximal carotid stenosis during distal bifurcation endarterectomy. *AJNR Am J Neuroradiol.* 1980;1(4):348-349.
44. Roubin GS, New G, Iyer SS, et al. Immediate and late clinical outcomes of carotid artery stenting in patients with symptomatic and asymptomatic carotid artery stenosis: a 5-year prospective analysis. *Circulation.* 2001;103(4):532-537.
45. Theron J, Courtheoux P, Alachkar F, Bouvard G, Maiza D. New triple coaxial catheter system for carotid angioplasty with cerebral protection. *AJNR Am J Neuroradiol.* 1990;11(5):869-874; discussion 875-867.
46. Meier P, Knapp G, Tamhane U, Chaturvedi S, Gurm HS. Short term and intermediate term comparison of endarterectomy versus stenting for carotid artery stenosis: systematic review and meta-analysis of randomised controlled clinical trials. *BMJ.* 2010;340:c467.

47. Garg N, Karagiorgos N, Pisimisis GT, et al. Cerebral protection devices reduce periprocedural strokes during carotid angioplasty and stenting: a systematic review of the current literature. *J Endovasc Ther.* 2009;16(4):412-427.
48. Kwolek CJ, Jaff MR, Leal JI, et al. Results of the ROADSTER multicenter trial of transcarotid stenting with dynamic flow reversal. *J Vasc Surg.* 2015;62(5):1227-1234.
49. King AH, Kumins NH, Foteh MI, Jim J, Apple JM, Kashyap VS. The learning curve of transcarotid artery revascularization. *J Vasc Surg.* 2019;70(2):516-521.
50. Malas MB, Dakour-Aridi H, Wang GJ, et al. Transcarotid artery revascularization versus transfemoral carotid artery stenting in the Society for Vascular Surgery Vascular Quality Initiative. *J Vasc Surg.* 2019;69(1):92.e102-103.e102.

CHAPTER 92

TRANSPLANTATION AND LONG-TERM IMPLANTABLE MECHANICAL CIRCULATORY SUPPORT

Ryan J. Vela and Matthias Peltz

INTRODUCTION

Over 250,000 patients suffer from advanced heart failure (HF) in the United States.[1] These patients are either severely symptomatic on or failing guideline-directed heart failure medical therapy (GDMT) and merit consideration for *advanced heart failure therapies*—a term that refers to fully implantable mechanical circulatory support devices and cardiac transplantation. Prognosis in this patient population is poor, with an estimated 5-year survival of 20%.[2] Outcomes for patients on inotropes are particularly dismal, ranging from 6% to 50% survival at 1 year.[3,4]

Since Alexis Carrel first developed the surgical techniques essential for cardiac transplantation and performed the first heterotopic heart transplant in a dog in 1905,[5] progress in cardiac transplantation and mechanical circulatory support of the failing heart have often proceeded in parallel, in part because circulatory support is considered essential for both procedures. Whereas Carrel and Lindbergh received much of the early recognition, largely unknown in the West, Demikhov in 1937 described the first use of a total artificial heart to support the canine circulation and later, in 1951, the first orthotopic heart transplantation in the same animal model.[6,7] In the United States, Shumway and Lower developed the surgical technique and explored the immunologic mechanisms that laid the foundation for human heart transplantation.[8] It was left to Christiaan Barnard to perform the first human heart transplant on Louis Washkansky on December 3, 1967.[9] Despite early enthusiasm, initial outcomes were dismal, with only 20% of patients surviving 1 year. It became apparent that, although a number of skilled surgeons could perform the technical aspects of cardiac transplantation, the understanding of immunobiology and rejection was limited, leading to the demise of many recipients. For the next decade, transplantation was performed only at a handful of specialty centers where outcomes gradually improved. It was the discovery of cyclosporine and steroid-sparing immunosuppression protocols that led to more widespread adoption of cardiac transplantation and established it as the gold standard therapy for patients with end-stage cardiac disease.[10]

Even before the first human heart transplant, the development of cardiopulmonary bypass established the basis for cardiac support devices. The first ventricular assist device (VAD) for human use was created by Domingo Liotta in 1962. This paracorporeal device was implanted in 1963 to support a patient in cardiogenic shock following a complicated aortic valve replacement. Unfortunately, the patient did not survive.[11] Undeterred, Liotta and DeBakey in 1966 were able to successfully support a patient while awaiting cardiac recovery after the patient failed to wean off cardiopulmonary bypass during a mitral valve operation.[12] The first human total artificial heart implant was performed by Liotta and Denton Cooley in 1969 to support a patient while awaiting a donor heart.[13]

Technologies continued to evolve and by the 1980s, multiple left ventricular assist device (LVAD) platforms were available to bridge patients to cardiac transplantation.[14] In 1994, the implantable HeartMate VE LVAS™ by Thoratec Corporation (Pleasanton, CA) gained U.S. Food and Drug Administration (FDA) approval as a bridge to transplantation device (www.accessdata.fda.gov/scripts/cdrh/cfdocs/cfpma/pma.cfm?id=P920014). Although early VADs were initially intended to support patients while waiting for a donor organ, it became apparent that as technology continued to improve and systems became fully implantable, VADs could potentially also be considered as therapy for patients ineligible for transplantation, so-called destination therapy. This benefit was demonstrated in the landmark Randomized Evaluation of Mechanical Assistance for the Treatment of Congestive Heart Failure (REMATCH) trial comparing the HeartMate XVE™ LVAD by Thoratec to inotrope therapy.[15] Improved outcomes in the device group led to FDA approval in 2002 and Centers for Medicare & Medicaid Services (CMS) approval in 2003 for patients who were otherwise ineligible for transplantation, ushering in the modern era of advanced therapies for the failing heart. This pneumatic pump device was placed intra-abdominally and typically failed by 18 to 24 months, needing replacement. It was not until the introduction of continuous flow devices that potential indefinite support of patients became a possibility. The HeartMate II™ device by then Thoratec, Inc. (now Abbott, Abbott Park, IL), an axillary flow pump, proved to be vastly superior to its predecessor[16] and to this day remains the most frequently implanted device. Although smaller than the HeartMate XVE, it still required the development of a preperitoneal pocket to place the pump. Device technology has continued to evolve and the two most frequently implanted devices, the HeartWare™ HVAD™ (Medtronic, Minneapolis, MN) and HeartMate 3™ (Abbott, Abbott Park, IL), are both placed intrapericardially. These centrifugal flow devices also no longer have any contact surfaces between the impeller and the device housing, and blood is propelled in a near frictionless manner. The HVAD impeller is levitated by hydrostatic forces and magnetically powered whereas the HeartMate 3 is fully magnetically levitated.[17,18] As VAD technology and clinical experience managing these patients have evolved, outcomes have improved. However, Medtronic recently stopped the global sale and distribution of the HeartWare™ HVAD™ system because of an increased risk of neurologic adverse events and mortality associated with the internal pump and the potential for the internal pump to stop, with delay or failure to restart. See **Table 92.1** for outcomes from selected LVAD-related clinical studies.

INDICATIONS

The decision to pursue either transplantation or VADs is complex and depends on the disease etiology, symptoms, prognosis, overall candidacy, and availability of other treatment options. Although consideration of support in the setting of cardiogenic shock—characterized by failure to wean off inotropic support or need for temporary mechanical support—seems obvious, indications for their use in the ambulatory setting are frequently not considered even though guidelines for referral to an HF program are well established. These criteria include recurrent admissions for decompensated HF or intolerance of GDMT.[4] HF risk models, such as the Seattle Heart Failure Model, provide additional guidance for decision-making.[19] Evaluations for advanced HF therapies require a multidisciplinary approach with consideration of the candidate's comorbidities, social and financial support. These are discussed in detail in chapter 65.

Some patients with ischemic, valvular, congenital, or other structural heart diseases may be candidates for conventional high-risk cardiac surgery or transcatheter therapies. Expected procedural and long-term survival from these procedures is important for guidance in patients that may be candidates for multiple therapeutic options. Predictive models may be important tools to determine the optimal therapy for these patients as suggested by Yoon et al in their ischemic cardiomyopathy population.[20] Perioperative mortality for heart transplantation and LVADs is <5% for most cases and long-term median survival after cardiac transplantation exceeds 10 years for the majority of patients.[21] Long-term outcomes after LVAD implantation continue to improve, and although these remain inferior to transplantation, intermediate-term results are approaching survival after transplantation.[22] A reasonable approach to these patients is to consider advanced HF therapies when the predicted operative risk and 1-year survival of other interventions are worse than the expected outcomes from advanced therapies. At our program, we frequently perform at least a limited evaluation for cardiac transplantation and LVAD to be available as rescue therapy if cardiac complications from high-risk surgery or transcatheter interventions arise. See **Algorithm 92.1**.

Advanced HF therapies are typically considered only for patients with severe HF symptoms, New York Heart

TABLE 92.1 Survival After Left Ventricular Assist Device Implantation in Selected Clinical Studies

Study	Implant Dates	Devices	Indication	1-Year Survival	2-Year Survival
REMATCH[15]	1998-2001	HeartMate XVE	DT	52% HeartMate XVE 25% medical therapy	23% HeartMate XVE 8% medical therapy
HeartMate II[16]	2005-2007	HeartMate XVE HeartMate II	DT	55% HeartMate XVE 68% HeartMate II	24% HeartMate XVE 58% HeartMate II
ENDURANCE[17]	2010-2012	HeartMate II HVAD	DT	NA	67.6% HeartMate II 60.2% HVAD
ENDURANCE Supplemental[49]	2013-2015	HeartMate II HVAD	DT	82.2% HeartMate II 83.1% HVAD	NA
MOMENTUM 3[19]	2014-2016	HeartMate II HeartMate III	DT/BTT	84.1% HeartMate II 86.6% HeartMate III	76.7% HeartMate II 79.0% HeartMate III
LATERAL[38]	2015-2016	HVAD	BTT	89% HVAD	87% HVAD
2019 STS INTERMACS Annual Report[22]	2014-2018	HVAD HeartMate II HeartMate III	DT/BTT	81% HVAD 82% HeartMate II 87% HeartMate III	72% HVAD 72% HeartMate II 84% HeartMate III

BTT, bridge to transplantation; DT, destination therapy; HVAD, HeartWare ventricular assist device; STS, Society Thoracic Surgery.
Survival after left ventricular assist device (LVAD) implantation has improved over time. These benefits seem to be in part related to advances in technology. However, improvements in device management and understanding of LVAD physiology are equally important as demonstrated by improved outcomes for the same devices in more contemporary studies. The INTERMACS annual report only includes patients not enrolled in investigational studies and affirms that "real-world" results are similar to outcomes of patients enrolled in clinical trials. Device type was inferred from definitions used in this study.

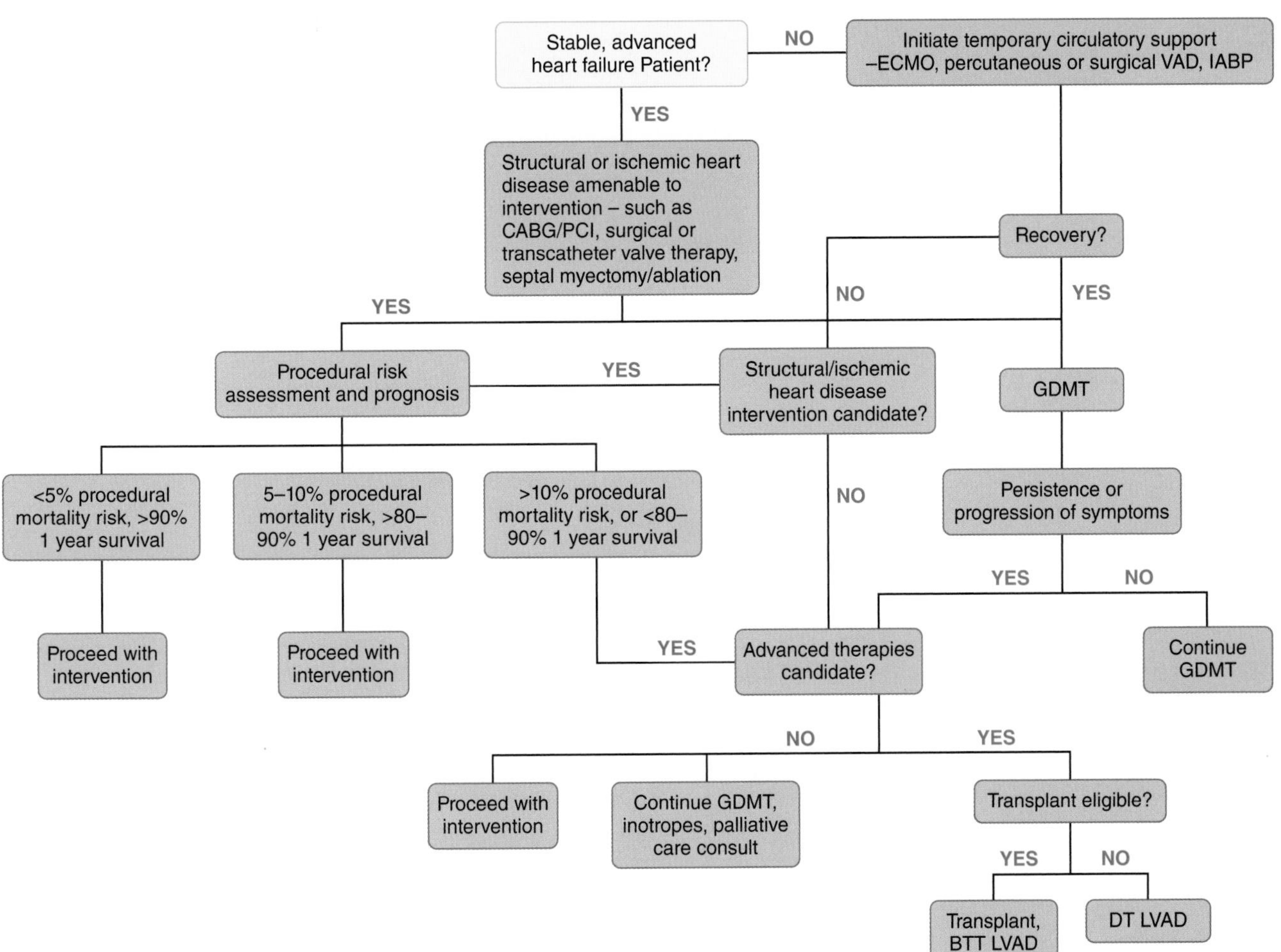

ALGORITHM 92.1 Surgical decision-making in advanced heart failure patients. Patient stability on presentation is the most immediate concern when evaluating a candidate for advanced heart failure therapies or other interventions. INTERMACS class 1 and 2 patients are usually too unstable to be considered for high-risk coronary artery bypass grafting, valve surgery, or transcatheter interventions. These patients often benefit from temporary circulatory support to stabilize them and reassess their candidacy. INTERMACS class 3 to 7 patients are by definition hemodynamically stable and can be evaluated for various treatment options. Decision-making for candidates with underlying coronary or structural heart disease is often based on the anticipated perioperative risk and subsequent outcomes. Patients with a procedural risk and expected 1-year survival better or similar to transplantation or LVAD placement should undergo these procedures preferentially. Transplantation or LVAD implantation may be preferable for high-risk cases if the patient is otherwise deemed a candidate and agrees to move forward. Patients who are not deemed suitable for advanced therapies candidates should be offered high-risk surgery or transcatheter therapies. BTT, bridge to transplantation; CABG, coronary artery bypass grafting; DT, destination therapy; ECMO, extracorporeal membrane oxygenation; GDMT, guideline-directed medical therapy; IABP, intraaortic ballon pump; LVAD, left ventricular assist device; PCI, percutaneous coronary intervention; VAD, ventricular assist device.

Association (NYHA) classes IIIB or IV. With the advent of durable VADs, advanced HF categories have been subdivided further by the Interagency Registry for Mechanically Assisted Circulatory Support (INTERMACS) Classification (see **Table 92.2**). The vast majority of patients treated with advanced HF therapies fall into categories 1 to 4 whereas the benefits of either cardiac transplantation or LVADs are less well established for higher INTERMACS classifications. The recent, nonrandomized Risk Assessment and Comparative Effectiveness of Left Ventricular Assist Device and Medical Management (ROADMAP) study compared the HeartMate 2™ to optimal medical management in INTERMACS class 4 to 7 patients.[23] Although symptom control and HF admissions were improved with device therapy, complications were increased and survival was not different in the intention-to-treat analysis.

Candidacy for device therapy involves an extensive multidisciplinary approach. This includes not only a thorough medical evaluation but also determination of adequate financial and social support to ensure long-term success of these interventions. Current decision-making for advanced therapy candidates is dependent on whether patients are eligible for cardiac transplantation or not. Transplantation is inherently limited by the availability of acceptable donor organs, and listing is reserved for the most suitable candidates.

Many other patients may be reasonable VAD candidates even if they are declined for cardiac transplantation. The

TABLE 92.2 INTERMACS Classification

NYHA Class	Heart Failure Stage	INTERMACS Profile	INTERMACS Profile Description
4	D	1	Critical cardiogenic shock—"crash and burn" patient characterized by hypotension requiring escalating vasoactive infusion requirement, organ malperfusion, lactic acidosis
4	D	2	Progressive decline on inotropic support as demonstrated by increasing dose requirements, refractory volume overload, malnutrition, and worsening end-organ perfusion
4	D	3	Inotrope dependent—patient either hospitalized or at home with stable end-organ perfusion and volume status
4	D	4	Resting symptoms—describes a patient with heart failure symptoms at rest and with activities of daily living that increase even with minimal activity. Patients typically are congested with difficulty to manage volume status and often intolerant of GDMT.
3b	C	5	Exertion intolerant—patients are comfortable at rest and with activities of daily living around the house but become symptomatic with minimal increases in activity and are mostly homebound.
3b	C	6	Exertion limited—patients who are comfortable at home and with basic activities outside the house. Patients may have experienced recent deteriorations and are intolerant of minor exertions such as grocery shopping.
3	C	7	Stable patient who can perform typical daily activities both within and outside the home environment with no recent decompensations but develops symptoms with moderate increases in activity.

Modifiers:
INTERMACS, Interagency Registry for Mechanically Assisted Circulatory Support; GDMT, guideline-directed heart failure medical therapy; NYHA, New York Heart Association.
TCS—Temporary Circulatory Support—modifier applies to hospitalized patients with profiles 1 to 3 that are maintained on a temporary mechanical circulatory support device, such as intra-aortic balloon pump, percutaneous or surgical ventricular assist device, or extracorporeal membrane oxygenation.
A—Arrhythmia—can apply to any INTERMACS profile for patients with frequent, symptomatic arrhythmias affecting the patient's clinical course, including frequent implantable cardiodefibrillator shocks are needed for cardioversion.
FF—Frequent Flyer—this modifier includes patients with frequent heart failure exacerbation admissions (two within 3 months or three in 6 months) and applies to nonhospitalized profile 3 and profiles 4 to 6 patients.

majority of patients are implanted as destination therapy, with that number increasing in the United States with the introduction of the new heart allocation system that has deprioritized bridge to transplantation VAD.[22] A small percentage of LVADs are placed as a bridge to recovery, usually in patients with more recent onset of symptoms. Although uncommon, excellent results have been obtained at some centers with this strategy.[24]

In the United States, until recently, CMS had different eligibility criteria for LVAD bridge to transplantation and destination therapy candidates. However, uniform patient eligibility criteria for implantation have now been established. These include inotrope dependence or cardiac index less than 2.2 L/min/m^2 while not on inotropes and meeting one of the following: (a) are on GDMT for at least 45 of the preceding 60 days and are failing to respond or (b) have advanced HF for at least 14 days and are dependent on an intra-aortic balloon pump or similar temporary mechanical circulatory support for at least 7 days (https://www.cms.gov/medicare-coverage-database/details/nca-proposed-decision-memo.aspx?NCAId=298).

ANATOMIC CONSIDERATIONS

Cardiac Transplantation

Orthotopic heart transplantation requires establishing connections between the donor and recipient system venous drainage, pulmonary artery, left atrium or pulmonary venous return, and finally the donor and recipient aortas. The main differences in implant techniques for most cases involve the systemic and pulmonary venous connections and are described later. Patients with congenital heart disease presenting for transplantation may have significant anatomic variations that require extensive pulmonary arterial reconstruction, modification of venous connections, or aortic reconstruction.[25]

Ventricular Assist Device Implantation

Current LVADs are almost always placed with the device inflow cannula inserted through the left ventricular apex. The outflow graft is then positioned along the diaphragm and then right atrium and sewn onto the proximal ascending aorta. For patients with prior cardiac surgery, preoperative imaging is important to assess the safety of sternal reentry and the presence of bypass grafts, for example. Alternate outflow access sites, such as the descending thoracic aorta, axillary, or innominate arteries can be used if prior cardiac surgery, such as presence of multiple bypass grafts, or unfavorable ascending aorta anatomy is noted on preoperative imaging and precludes an ascending aortic anastomosis.[26]

FUNDAMENTALS OF ADVANCED HEART FAILURE THERAPIES

Except for acute presentations, candidates for advanced therapies have typically undergone a rigorous cardiac evaluation to assess the etiology of their cardiomyopathy. Testing typically includes echocardiography, right and left heart catheterization, and cardiopulmonary exercise testing. The presence of significant valvular disease is of particular importance for LVAD therapy.

Additionally, evaluation of important noncardiac disease includes age-appropriate preventative screening (ie, colonoscopy, mammography, Pap smear, prostate-specific antigen testing) as well as imaging of the brain, chest, and abdomen to assess for noncardiac disease that may affect advanced therapies eligibility. Specific surgical considerations include prior cardiac operations. Although these are rare contraindications, knowledge of prior procedures can facilitate safe performance of the reoperation. Prior operative reports should be obtained whenever possible to guide surgical planning. Evaluation for suitable peripheral cannulation sites should be performed for high-risk reoperative cases.

CLINICAL APPLICATIONS

Orthotopic Heart Transplantation

The organ allocation system in the United States has underwent revision in October 2018 from a three- to six-tier system that further prioritizes the most critically ill patients on the waiting list (see **Table 92.3**). This change has led to increased use of temporary support devices and a reduction in the number of LVADs performed for bridge to transplantation as an indication.[22] Donor selection is dependent on both donor- and recipient-related variables. Important donor-related factors include age, height and weight, findings on cardiac diagnostic

SECTION 7

TABLE 92.3 Abbreviated Summary of Donor Heart Allocation in the United States

Heart Allocation Status	Eligibility Criteria (Duration of Status Prior to Downgrading or Need for Recertification)
1 (prior Status 1A)	1. Patients meeting hemodynamic criteria on: Extracorporeal membrane oxygenation (7 days) Nondischargeable surgically implanted biventricular support devices (14 days) 2. Life-threatening arrhythmias on a mechanical circulatory support device not considered candidates for ablative procedures (14 days)
2 (prior Status 1A)	1. Patients meeting hemodynamic criteria on: Intra-aortic balloon pump support (14 days) Percutaneous ventricular assist device (14 days) 2. Nondischargeable surgically implanted ventricular assist device (14 days) 3. Total artificial heart, right ventricular assist device, biventricular assist devices, ventricular assist device in single ventricle patients (14 days) 4. Mechanical circulatory device malfunction with imminent risk of device failure or inadequate circulatory support (14 days) 5. Refractory ventricular tachycardia/fibrillation not amenable to ablation (14 days)
3 (prior Status 1A)	1. Patients meeting hemodynamic criteria on high dose, single or multiple inotropes with intensive care unit hemodynamic monitoring (14 days) 2. Left ventricular assist device on discretionary 30-day status three times 3. Mechanical circulatory device with complications (14 days unless otherwise specified): Device or intracardiac thrombus Device infection (14-90 days depending on indication) Right heart failure Hemolysis Mucosal bleeding (14-90 days depending on indication) Aortic insufficiency (90 days) 4. Temporary support devices no longer meeting hemodynamic criteria justifying Status 1 or 2 criteria (14 days)

(*Continued*)

TABLE 92.3 Abbreviated Summary of Donor Heart Allocation in the United States (*Continued*)

Heart Allocation Status	Eligibility Criteria (Duration of Status Prior to Downgrading or Need for Recertification)
4 (prior Status 1B)	1. Dischargeable left ventricular assist device patient without discretionary 30-day time (90 days) 2. Single inotrope-dependent patients meeting hemodynamic criteria (90 days) 3. Adult congenital heart disease patients (90 days) 4. Ischemic heart disease with refractory angina (90 days) 5. Amyloidosis, restrictive or hypertrophic cardiomyopathy (90 days) 6. Repeat transplant candidates (90 days)
5 (prior Status 2)	Multivisceral transplant candidates not eligible for a higher priority status (180 days)
6 (prior Status 2)	All other candidates (180 days)

Summarized from Organ Procurement and Transplantation Network Policies. Policy 6: Allocation of Hearts and Heart-Lungs. https://optn.transplant.hrsa.gov/media/1200/optn_policies.pdf

studies, expected ischemic time, among others. The interaction of donor age and ischemic time is additive and of particular importance to avoid primary graft dysfunction.[27] Similarly, "undersizing" is better tolerated with younger donors: if the donor is of younger age, increasing recipient-donor weight difference does not result in increased death.[28] Oversizing is usually not an issue for patients with a dilated cardiomyopathy though this is a more important factor for candidates with hypertrophic or restrictive cardiomyopathies, for example. The Heart Transplant Sizing App is available to compare estimated donor and recipient heart mass (https://heart-transplant-sizing.app/) and further guide donor selection.

Cardiac transplantation is performed via a median sternotomy. Arterial cannulation, depending on the reentry risk or available aortic length, is either central in the distal ascending aorta or proximal aortic arch, or peripheral using femoral or axillary cannulation or both. Bicaval cannulation is instituted for venous drainage. In redo operations, we frequently perform the inferior vena cava cannulation peripherally to aid in the performance of the inferior vena cava anastomosis. After cardiopulmonary bypass is established, vena cavae are occluded, the aorta is cross-clamped, and the recipient cardiectomy is completed. At the same time, the donor heart is inspected for damage during the procurement and any cardiac pathology. A patent foramen ovale, if present, is closed—either at the recovery or implanting facility.[29] The donor heart is then brought to the surgical field. There are currently three different techniques for implantation of the donor heart: biatrial technique, bicaval technique, and total heart transplantation. These differ primarily in the construction of systemic and/or pulmonary venous drainage. The pulmonary artery and aortic anastomoses are the same among all three techniques.[25]

The left atrial or pulmonary venous anastomosis, as the most posterior and inaccessible structure, is performed first. The subsequent order of connections can vary. To minimize the donor ischemic time, the aortic anastomosis can be completed next, followed by cross-clamp removal and reperfusion of the organ. The disadvantage of this sequence is that the remainder of the structures are sutured while the heart is beating in a variably bloody surgical field. Except for when the anticipated donor ischemic time is prolonged, after completing the left atrial anastomosis, we construct the posterior row of the pulmonary artery, followed by the aortic and inferior vena cava reconstruction. The cross-clamp is then removed, and the anterior portion of the pulmonary artery and then the superior vena cava anastomoses are completed on the beating heart while the patient is rewarmed and the organ is reperfused.

The biatrial technique originally developed by Lowery and Shumway involves excision of the recipient heart retaining sizable left and right atrial cuffs. The left and right atrial connections are completed followed by the aortic and pulmonary artery anastomoses. The main advantage of this technique is its relative simplicity and shortened ischemic times. It also avoids the risk of anastomotic complications related to separate caval and pulmonary venous connections.

Since 2004, the bicaval technique has been favored in the United States.[30] Recipient cardiectomy for bicaval transplantation requires separate division of the recipient superior and inferior vena cavae and recovery of adequate donor tissue to anastomose both these structures. Whereas implantation times are slightly increased, bicaval transplantation seems to offer a number of benefits, including fewer arrhythmias, reduced tricuspid regurgitation, decreased need for pacemaker, and slightly increased perioperative and long-term survival.[30,31] Technical differences between the biatrial and bicaval techniques are illustrated in **Figure 92.1A,B**.

The total heart transplant procedure is performed in very few centers and retains almost no residual native recipient heart tissue. Recipient explantation leaves only a small left atrial cuff encompassing the right and left pulmonary veins. Donor heart procurement requires modification if donor lungs are also recovered. For the other two techniques usually, only a donor left atrial cuff anterior to the pulmonary veins, along with the left atrial appendage, is retrieved. For the total heart transplant method, the heart must be recovered with the entire left atrium except for similar-sized pulmonary vein cuffs. Implantation then begins by connecting the separate right and left pulmonary vein cuffs to the donor heart. The remainder of the procedure

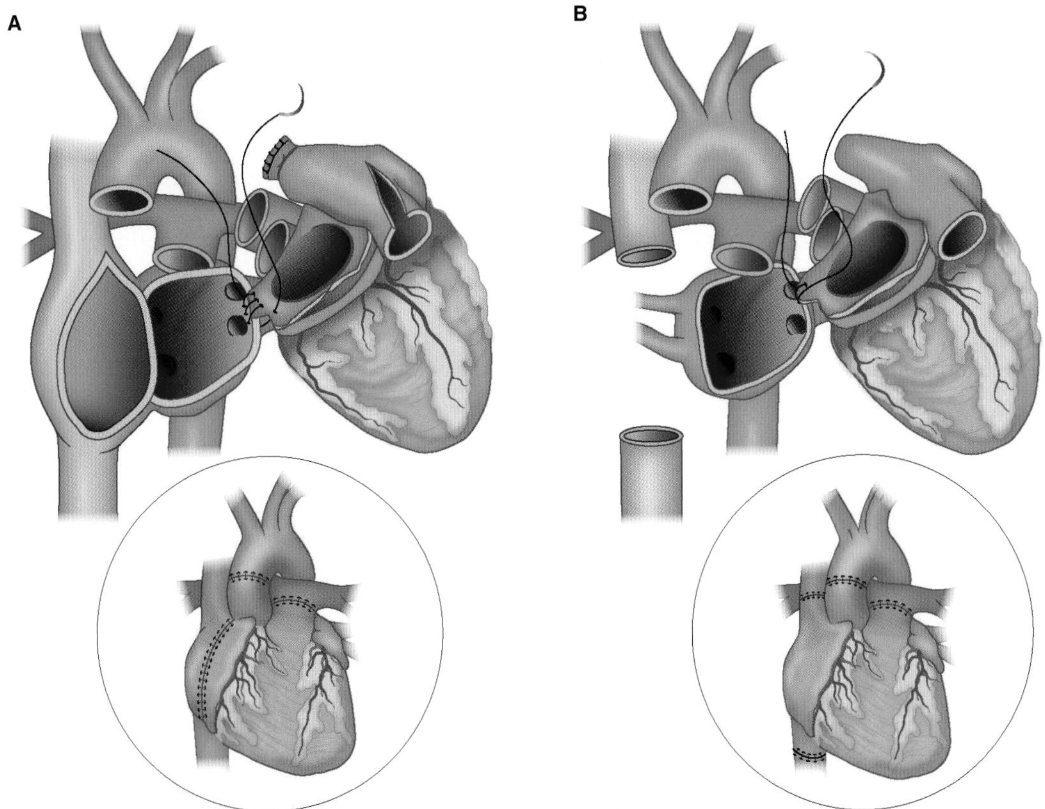

FIGURE 92.1 **(A,B)** Heart transplantation techniques. The two main heart implantation methods are the biatrial **(A)** and bicaval **(B)** techniques. The recipient cardiectomy differs mainly in the division of the left atrium and systemic venous return. Inset images below each technique demonstrate the completed appearance after implantation. In the biatrial technique, the recipient's right atrium is incised anterior to the superior and inferior vena cavae. Superiorly, the incision is carried onto the dome of the left atrium, extended just posterior to the left atrial appendage and anterior to the left superior pulmonary vein. The interatrial septum is divided, and the incision extended onto the inferior left atrium and directed anterior to the inferior left pulmonary vein connecting with the superior incision to complete division of the atria. The aorta and pulmonary artery are then divided proximally. A special aspect of preparing the donor organ is an incision directed from the inferior vena cava extending onto the right atrium to prepare for the right atrial anastomosis. In the bicaval technique, the recipient superior vena cava is transected at the atriocaval junction. The inferior vena cava division is best performed leaving a generous right atrial cuff to avoid retraction, particularly of the posterior wall. The left atrium is incised anterior to the right-sided pulmonary veins after dissection of Sondergaard groove. Left atrial division is completed by extending the incision superiorly and inferiorly as described for the biatrial technique. The donor organ does not usually require specific additional preparation for the bicaval technique.

otherwise is the same as the bicaval technique. No consistent benefits have been demonstrated with this technique.[30]

Heterotopic Cardiac Transplantation

Heterotopic transplantation is rarely performed in the current era. It allows implantation of the donor organ in parallel with the native organ to augment cardiac output, manage severe pulmonary hypertension, or accommodate a significant donor-recipient size mismatch. With the advent of VADs and improvements in immunosuppression, its use has faded. Implantation can be performed both in an isolated left ventricular and in a biventricular support configuration. The procedure is usually performed through a median sternotomy. The right pleura and pericardium are opened widely to eventually accommodate the donor heart. Bypass is initiated as for orthotopic techniques. The native heart is arrested with cardioplegia. Explantation of the donor organ is as described for the complete orthotopic technique. The left atrial anastomosis again is constructed first by creating a left atriotomy along Sondergaard groove and then sewing the left pulmonary vein cuff to it. The right cuff is oversewn. The cross-clamp can be removed at this point. In the biventricular configuration, an extended connection is created between the donor and recipient's right atria from the lateral superior vena cava onto the right atrium in a side-to-side fashion. An end-to-side aortic anastomosis is constructed after application of a side-biting aortic clamp. Finally, the donor's pulmonary artery is connected to the recipient's main pulmonary artery. This typically requires a graft to achieve adequate length. For isolated left ventricular support, implantation is as previously described except that the donor pulmonary artery is anastomosed to the recipient's right atrium to provide coronary sinus drainage.[32]

Combined Heart-Lung Transplantation

Heart-lung transplantation is now a relatively uncommon operation with only about 50 cases reported to the International Society for Heart and Lung Transplantation (ISHLT) Registry annually over the last several years.[33] Indications for combined heart-lung transplant can be owing to primary pulmonary disease, cardiac causes, or mixed etiologies.[34] Lung disease–based indications usually are related to pulmonary hypertension. Unfortunately, these patients often have right HF that either results in a prohibitive perioperative mortality risk or is anticipated not to reverse in the postoperative period. A range of corrected and uncorrected congenital cardiopulmonary abnormalities may also require heart-lung transplantation, such as untreated ventricular septal defects or atrial septal defects leading to pulmonary hypertension and eventually Eisenmenger syndrome, systemic or single ventricular failure associated pulmonary hypertension, or extensive pulmonary vascular abnormalities either primary or related to surgical correction. Chronic left HF of any etiology can induce secondary pulmonary hypertension that is either irreversible or expected to regress slowly, posing an undue risk to the donor's right ventricle in the perioperative period.

Although increased mortality is observed with a pulmonary vascular resistance as low as 2.5 Wood units,[35] combined heart-lung transplant is typically not considered unless the pulmonary vascular resistance, in the absence of reversibility, exceeds 5 to 6 Wood units or the transpulmonary gradient is over 15 to 20 mm Hg.[34] In many cases of elevated pulmonary vascular resistance caused by left ventricular failure, LVAD implantation can reverse pulmonary hypertension over time and allow for heart transplantation alone.

Recovery of the donor organs is similar to that of a heart-lung block without separation of the individual organs. Most of the trachea is recovered, along with the aortic arch and donor innominate veins depending on the need for excess length or need for vascular reconstructions.[29]

Heart-lung transplantation is performed through a median sternotomy. The pericardium is incised posterior to the phrenic nerves bilaterally to allow for the passage of the donor lungs into their respective hemithorax. Venting is performed through the left atrial appendage and this site is later oversewn. We perform explantation of the heart, right and left lungs separately and divide the trachea just proximal to the carina, taking care not to disturb the adjacent blood supply. The donor heart-lung block is brought to the surgical field, and lungs are passed into their respective pleural space posterior to the retrophrenic pericardial incision. The tracheal anastomosis is then completed connecting the distal donor and recipient tracheas. We prefer a telescoping technique that in our experience reduces airway complications. Next, the aortic anastomosis is completed, followed by the inferior and then superior vena cava or alternatively, a right atrial anastomosis as described for the biatrial orthotopic technique.[25]

Left Ventricular Assist Device Implantation

LVAD implantation involves a connection of the device inflow cannula usually through the left ventricular apex. Blood is subsequently delivered by the pump via an outflow graft that is most often sewn to the ascending aorta to provide systemic blood flow. Alternative connections, such as the axillary artery or descending thoracic aorta, can be considered if ascending aortic access is considered unfavorable because of either prior operations or calcifications that may affect device performance.[26] Device implantation is typically performed with the assistance of cardiopulmonary bypass though it can be performed entirely or partially off bypass. Additional procedures at the time of LVAD implant usually require the use of cardiopulmonary bypass and in some cases, cardioplegic arrest. There is no clear consensus whether significant mitral or tricuspid regurgitation should be addressed at the time of device implantation and whether practice patterns differ among centers.[36] More than mild aortic insufficiency should be addressed at the time of implantation by either bioprosthetic aortic valve replacement or oversewing the valve, especially in destination therapy patients.[37] Likewise, the presence of a mechanical aortic valve requires either patching of the valve or replacement with a bioprosthesis. Atrial-level shunts are closed. Coronary artery bypass is rarely performed and represents only about 5% of concurrent procedures.[36] The vast majority of devices are still being implanted using a full sternotomy for access to the left ventricle and aorta. Sternal-sparing approaches, however, are increasingly utilized. With this technique, a left anterior thoracotomy is used to approach the left ventricular apex. The outflow graft is then anastomosed to the ascending aorta by either a partial upper sternotomy or a second interspace right anterior thoracotomy.[26,38] Potential benefits of these techniques include reduced length of stay, earlier return to physical activity, fewer bleeding complications, and less severe right ventricular dysfunction.[38] See **Figure 92.2A,B**.

Right and Biventricular Assist Device Implantation

VADs are rarely deployed for isolated right ventricular failure. Although a temporary right ventricular assist device (RVAD) may be required owing to perioperative right ventricular failure, these devices are not intended for permanent support. The HeartMate 3™ system can be implanted in a right ventricular configuration either for isolated right ventricular or biventricular support. Biventricular devices may be implanted simultaneously at the time of the original operation or later owing to failure to wean off temporary right ventricular mechanical support, prolonged inotrope dependence, or even late right ventricular failure. Inflow can be via either the right ventricle or the right atrium. Teflon felt disks are often used to ensure unobstructed inflow into the device.[39] The outflow graft is anastomosed to the pulmonary artery. Downsizing of the graft may be required because of lower resistance of the pulmonary vasculature. Outcomes after biventricular assist device implantation are substantially worse compared to isolated LVAD mainly because of a much higher perioperative mortality risk in these critically ill patients and RVAD thrombosis-related complications.[40] A chest x-ray of a patient with biventricular devices is shown in **Figure 92.3**.

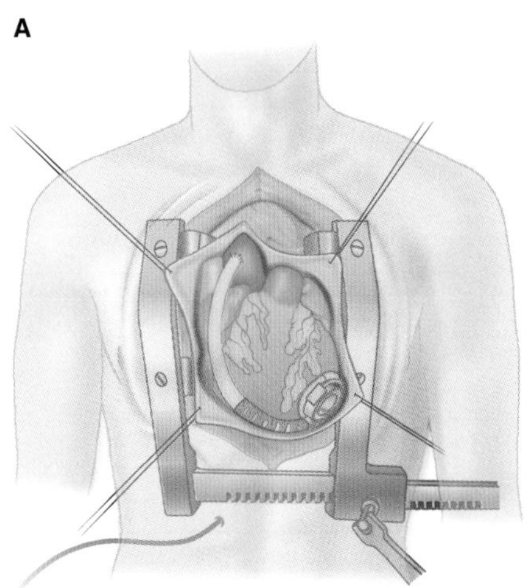

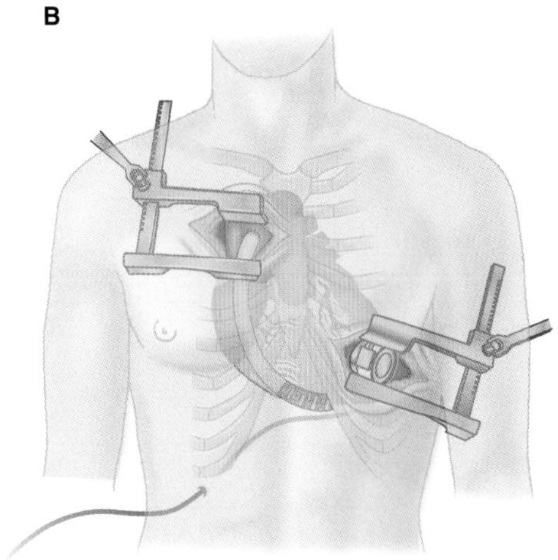

FIGURE 92.2 **(A,B)** Left ventricular assist device implantation. Left ventricular assist device implantation can be performed by a standard sternotomy **(A)** or sternal-sparing technique **(B)**. Usually, the first step involves securing the device sewing ring to the left ventricular apex. For sternotomy implants, the apex is mobilized to the surgical field using a number of surgical sponges. With the sternal-sparing technique, a left anterior thoracotomy is performed overlying the apex, usually the 5th or 6th interspace. Simultaneously, aortic exposure is obtained typically through a 2nd interspace right anterior thoracotomy as shown in view **(B)**. Computer tomography localization is useful for planning both exposures. Alternatively, the aorta can be approached via partial upper sternotomy that is "T'd" or "J'd" off into the appropriate interspace. Ultrasound guidance can then be used for more direct localization of the apex. Although the surgical field is more restricted, this approach provides direct access to the apex. The apex is then cored. Trabeculations are resected. The pump is inserted, directed toward the mitral valve, and secured to the sewing ring. If not previously completed, the outflow graft is now connected to the pump. With the sternotomy approach, the graft is then passed along the diaphragmatic surface and along the right atrium, oriented to minimize the risk of injury to the graft during reentry, particularly for transplant candidates. With the sternal-sparing technique, the graft is passed from the apex to the aortic exposure incision using a long clamp, taking care to maintain its orientation. We then turn the device on to its neutral speed setting to measure the outflow graft length while occluding the distal conduit. For both techniques, a partial occluding clamp is then applied to the proximal ascending aorta and the outflow graft anastomosis is constructed, completing the implantation.

SECTION 7

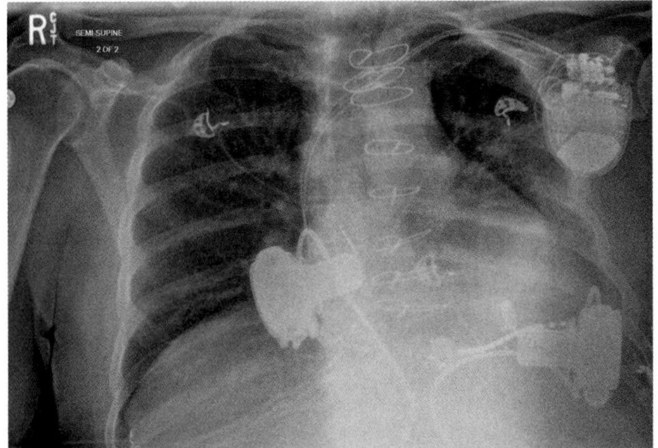

FIGURE 92.3 Chest x-ray of a biventricular assist device patient. This radiograph shows a patient supported with right and left ventricular HeartWare™ HVAD™ devices. The left-sided device is in the typical left ventricular apical location with the inflow cannula directed at the mitral valve. The right ventricular device was inserted into the right atrium with multiple Teflon felt spacers to position the inflow cannula well within the chamber to avoid suction events.

Total Artificial Heart

Total artificial heart is another therapeutic option for patients with biventricular failure. The only total artificial heart available in the United States at this point is by SynCardia Systems, LLC (Tucson, AZ). It is usually reserved as a bridge to transplantation device and, although a portable driver is available, patients are typically maintained on this technology while hospitalized awaiting a suitable donor. Implantation involves removal of both ventricles. Inflow cuffs to the two atrioventricular valves and respective grafts to the aorta and pulmonary artery are sewn. These are connected to the pneumatically powered pulmonary and systemic ventricles. Drivelines are passed through upper abdominal wall incisions and connected to the driver.[13] The CARMAT total artificial heart (CARMAT SA, Vélizy-Villacoublay, France) is current undergoing pivotal studies in Europe and in the process of initiating clinical studies in the United States. This device is intended to be a long-term support, fully dischargeable platform.[41] Additionally, both the HeartMate 3™ and HeartWare™ HVAD™ devices have been used in a total artificial heart configuration.[39,42] Outcomes of these therapies are compared in **Table 92.4**.

TABLE 92.4 Contemporary Outcomes After Adult Primary Transplantation and Durable Mechanical Circulatory Support Implantation

		Survival (%)				
Source	**Therapy**	**30-Day**	**1-Year**	**3-Year**	**5-Year**	**10-Year**
UNOS/SRTR[21]	Heart transplant	97.0	91.7	86.0	72	53
ISHLT[47]	Heart transplant	93.0	86.0	80.2	74.9	58.1
ISHLT[33]	Heart-lung transplant	83.7	70.0	58.7	54.5	40.0
INTERMACS	LVAD	95.4	86.7	65.2	42.7	NA
INTERMACS	TAH	91.3	43.8	30.3	18.2 (4 year)	NA
INTERMACS	BIVAD	86.7	64.1	39.5	32.3	NA

UNOS/SRTR—30-day, 1-year, and 3-year survival reflect outcomes in the United States from the January 2021 United Network for Organ Sharing/Scientific Registry of Transplant Recipients data. 5- and 10-year data were obtained from Suarez-Pierre et al and are unadjusted for the era.
ISHLT—International Society for Heart and Lung transplantation heart and combined heart-lung transplantation survival data were obtained from the 2019 Annual Report and are reported as the most recent available era for each data point.
INTERMACS—Mechanical circulatory support outcomes were obtained from the Society of Thoracic Surgery/INTERMACS Quarter 3 2020 Quality Assurance Report. 30-day and 1-year survival reflect data from the recent implant section of the report whereas 3- to 5-year data reflect outcomes of the most recent cohort of the full registry analysis.
BIVAD, biventricular assist device; LVAD, left ventricular assist device; TAH, total artificial heart.

LIMITATIONS OF ADVANCED HEART FAILURE THERAPIES

Cardiac Transplantation

The major limitation for cardiac transplantation is the limited donor supply. In 2018, a record number of 3443 transplants were performed in the United States. However, 3756 patients were added to the waitlist as the number of new candidates continued to exceed the number of available donors.[43] And, despite the recent increase in the number of heart transplants performed, this still only represents a small fraction of the number of patients with advanced HF.[1] Nearly 70% of all potential cardiac donors are declined by transplant centers for a number of reasons, including quality concerns, predicted ischemic times, or size.[44] Recent advances in preservation techniques, such as machine perfusion, have been used to recover higher risk donors and even organs from donors after circulatory determination of death and will hopefully lead to significant further increases in organ donor availability.[6]

Ventricular Assist Device Therapy

VAD therapy is not really resource-limited, but a thorough evaluation is essential to ensure a patient's limitation is primarily cardiac and not owing to other comorbidities that may lead to an undesirable postoperative outcome. Aside from other common surgical complications, such as bleeding, right ventricular failure is the most immediate concern in the perioperative period. This is manifest as a prolonged need for nitric oxide, need for inotropes (greater 14 days) and, in its severest form, need for temporary right ventricular assist device (RVAD). Multiple risk models, such as the University of Michigan RV Risk Score, the Pennsylvania RVAD Risk Score, and the European Registry for Patients with Mechanical Circulatory Support (EUROMACS) Score, have been developed to predict which patients are more likely to experience perioperative right ventricular failure. These models include indices of right ventricular function, for example, central venous pressure, pulmonary capillary wedge pressure, right ventricular stroke work index, pulmonary artery pulsatility index, severity of right ventricular dysfunction, and tricuspid regurgitation, along with patient-related physiologic data such as measures of renal and hepatic function and INTERMACS class.[45]

One- and 2-year survival after LVAD implantation are approaching outcomes from cardiac transplantation, but serious complications are frequent. LVAD trial results therefore often report a composite end point that includes survival free of disabling stroke or reoperation to replace or remove a malfunctioning device. Additional common major complications after LVAD implantation include gastrointestinal bleeding and device-related infections. Complication risks are highest in the first year after implantation, and the number of complications experienced seems to predict the likelihood of events in subsequent years, ranging from just over 20% per year for patients with event-free 1-year survival to nearly 40% per year in patients that experienced multiple adverse events in the first year after implantation.[46]

SPECIAL CONSIDERATIONS AND CONTRAINDICATIONS

Transplantation

In medically acceptable candidates, there are few absolute surgical contraindications to cardiac transplantation. Extensive vascular calcifications, most commonly in the ascending aorta and arch but at times within the atria, particularly in patients with underlying kidney disease, may affect the construction of anastomoses between the donor and recipient. Although these are sometimes prohibitive, often modifications of the implant technique, such as utilization of hypothermic circulatory arrest or replacement of the affected segment with a synthetic graft, will allow for implantation of the allograft. An increasing number of patients are presenting with multi-organ system disease that complicates decision-making even when cardiac disease dominates the clinical picture. Combined heart-kidney and to a lesser extend heart-liver transplants are being performed with increasing frequency.[47] Although implantation of a donor liver immediately follows the completion of the heart transplant, timing of a kidney transplant can be variable, often depending on factors related to the function of the transplanted heart. When the cardiac allograft is functioning well and bleeding is not a concern, implantation of the donor kidney can be performed in the same setting. More often, we monitor the patient for a few hours in the intensive care unit before proceeding with the kidney transplant. Occasionally, in the setting of significant cardiac allograft dysfunction, the donor kidney can be machine perfused to allow for the extension of the kidney ischemic interval for as long as 48 to 72 hours while the donor heart recovers.

Ventricular Assist Device Therapy

The presence of the external driveline, controller, and batteries continue to be the most significant factors accounting for the lack of patient acceptance of the therapy. Anticoagulation is mandatory for ventricular support devices. And thus, patients with contraindications to anticoagulation are not typically considered for device implantation. Vascular or cardiac calcifications are similarly problematic for durable mechanical circulatory support. End-stage renal disease or advanced chronic kidney disease present particular challenges for patients considered for destination therapy. Outcomes in these patients are poor, and while some patients are candidates for peritoneal dialysis, identifying hemodialysis centers accepting VAD patients is difficult and often excludes these patients from candidacy when they are not candidates for combined heart-kidney transplantation.[48]

FOLLOW-UP PATIENT CARE

Both heart transplant patients and VAD patients undergoing sternotomies require adherence to sternal precautions postoperatively. Early mobilization after LVAD implantation or cardiac transplantation is encouraged. Cardiac rehabilitation is typically started after discharge. Time to full recovery and clearance from all activity restrictions is usually later for transplant patients owing to delayed wound healing from immunosuppression. Patients undergoing sternal-sparing VAD implantation have an earlier return to normal activities and few if any activity restrictions after discharge once they no longer require narcotics for pain control.

Anticoagulation protocols after VAD implantation vary among centers and by device. Long-term anticoagulation consists of warfarin (target international normalized ratio [INR] 2-3) and aspirin (81-325 mg daily). Although many programs start heparin early after implantation once chest tube drainage is at an acceptable level, we favor early initiation of warfarin (evening of surgery) and aspirin (postoperative day 1) and delay heparin until postoperative day 3 if the INR is not at 1.8 or higher by that point. For currently used centrifugal flow devices, blood pressure is maintained below 85 to 90 mm Hg.[18,49] Guideline-directed medical therapy is restarted gradually depending on the patient's hemodynamics and weaning of inotropic support. LVAD education and driveline management are initiated in the intensive care unit and assume a greater focus as the patient progresses to the telemetry ward and approaches discharge. Long-term medical management and surveillance of transplant and VAD patients are beyond the scope of this chapter and are discussed in detail elsewhere.

RESEARCH AND FUTURE DIRECTIONS

Many donor hearts rejected for transplantation are declined largely owing to concerns about inadequate preservation. Both normothermic and hypothermic perfusion technologies are being explored to improve preservation of donor hearts, recover marginal donor organs, and even transplant organs from donors after circulatory determination of death. Additionally, research in xenotransplantation, organogenesis—either *de novo* or by repopulation of decellularized scaffolds—is ongoing and can potentially provide an unlimited pool of organs.[6]

VAD technology continues to evolve. Hemocompatibility-related complications are improving but continue to be a major source of device-related morbidity and mortality. The presence of the external driveline is the main impediment to acceptance of the technology and adversely impacts the patients' perceived quality of life. Development of rechargeable, internal batteries and transcutaneous energy transfer is critical to address these issues and is a major priority of device manufacturers. Although current devices now can almost always be placed intrapericardially, further reduction of size will provide additional flexibility in device placement and facilitate less invasive implant techniques. Incorporation of Wi-Fi and Bluetooth technology is being introduced to allow for improved remote monitoring and adjusting device parameters.[50]

KEY POINTS

- ✔ Understand clinical criteria that warrant consideration for referral to an advanced HF therapies program.
- ✔ Patients considered for high-risk cardiac interventions may benefit from a proactive advanced therapies evaluation to assess candidacy for transplantation or LVAD.
- ✔ Heart transplantation offers the best long-term survival for eligible advanced HF therapy patients.
- ✔ Donor selection criteria are evolving, and advancements in preservation techniques are expanding the suitable donor pool for cardiac transplantation.
- ✔ VAD technologies continue to improve, and short to intermediate outcomes are approaching results of heart transplantation.
- ✔ As technologies continue to evolve and durable mechanical circulatory support systems become fully implantable, patients will have treatment choices with similar outcomes and quality of life.

REFERENCES

1. Chaudry SP, Stewart GC. Advanced heart failure—prevalence, natural history, and prognosis. *Heart Fail Clin.* 2016;12:323-333.
2. Ammar KA, Jacobsen SJ, Mahoney DW, et al. Prevalence and prognostic significance of HF stages. Application of the American College of Cardiology/American Heart Association Heart Failure Staging Criteria in the Community. *Circulation.* 2007;115:1563-1570.
3. Gorodeski EZ, Chu EC, Reese JR, et al. Prognosis on chronic dobutamine or milrinone infusions for stage D heart failure. *Circ Heart Fail.* 2009;2:320-324.
4. Fang J, Ewald GA, Allen LA. Advanced (stage D) heart failure: a statement from the Heart Failure Society of America Guidelines Committee. *J Card Fail.* 2015;21(6):519-534.
5. Carrel A, Guthrie CC. The transplantation of veins and organs. *Am J Med.* 1905;10:1101.
6. Vela R, Jessen ME, Peltz M. Ice, ice, maybe? Is it time to ditch the igloo cooler? Benefits of machine perfusion preservation of donor hearts. *Artif Organs.* 2020;44:220-227.
7. Matskeplishvili S. Vladimir Petrovich Demikhov (1916-1998): a pioneer of transplantation ahead of his time, who lived out the end of his life as an unknown and in poor circumstances. *Eur Heart J.* 2017;38(46):3406-3410.
8. Fann JI, Baumgartner WA. Historical perspectives of The American Association for Thoracic Surgery: Norman E. Shumway, Jr (1923-2006*). J Thorac Cardiovasc Surg.* 2011;142:1299-1302.
9. Barnard CN. A human cardiac transplantation. *S Afr Med J.* 1967,30:1271-1274.
10. Wilhelm MJ, Ruschitzka F, Flammer AJ, et al. Fiftieth anniversary of the first heart transplantation in Switzerland in the context of the worldwide history of heart transplantation. *Swiss Med Wkly.* 2020;150:w20192. doi:10.4414/smw.2020.20192
11. Liotta D, Hall CW, Henly WS, et al. Prolonged assisted circulation during and after cardiac or aortic surgery: prolonged partial left ventricular bypass by means of intracorporeal circulation. *Am J Cardiol.* 1963;12:399-405.
12. Terzi A. Mechanical circulatory support: 60 years of evolving knowledge. *Int J Artif Organs.* 2019;42(5):215-225.
13. Cook JA, Shah KB, Quader MA, et al. The total artificial heart. *J Thorac Dis.* 2015;7(12):2172-2180.
14. Pennington DG, McBride LR, Peigh PS, et al. Eight years' experience with bridging to cardiac transplantations. *J Thorac Cardiovasc Surg.* 1994;107:472-481.
15. Rose EA, Gelijns A, Moskowitz AJ, et al. Long-term use of a ventricular assist device for end-stage heart failure. *N Engl J Med.* 2001;345:1435-1443.
16. Slaughter MS, Rogers JG, Milano CA, et al. Advanced heart failure treated with continuous-flow left ventricular assist device. *N Engl J Med.* 2009;261:2241-2251.
17. Rogers JG, Pagani FD, Tatooles AJ, et al. Intrapericardial left ventricular assist device for advanced heart failure. *N Engl J Med.* 2017;376:451-460.
18. Mehra MR, Uriel N, Naka Y, at al. A fully magnetically levitated left ventricular assist device—final report. *N Engl J Med.* 2019;380(17):1618-1627.
19. Michaels A, Cowger J. Patient selection for destination LVAD therapy: predicting success in the short and long term. *Curr Heart Fail Rep.* 2019;16:140-149.
20. Yoon DY, Smedira NG, Nowicki ER, et al. Decision support in surgical management of ischemic cardiomyopathy. *J Thorac Cardiovasc Surg.* 2010;139:283-293.
21. Suarez-Pierre A, Lui C, Zhou X, et al. Long-term survival after heart transplantation: a population-based nested case-control study. *Ann Thorac Surg.* 2020;111:889-898.
22. Teuteberg JJ, Cleveland JC, Cowger J, et al. The society of thoracic surgeons intermacs 2019 annual report: the changing landscape of devices and indications. *Ann Thorac Surg.* 2020;109:649-660.
23. Starling RC, Estep JD, Horstmanshof DA, et al. Risk assessment and comparative effectiveness of left ventricular assist device and medical management in ambulatory heart failure patients. *J Am Coll Cardiol.* 2015;66(16):1747-1761.
24. Selzman CH, Madden JL, Healy AH, et al. Bridge to removal: a paradigm shift for left ventricular assist device therapy. *Ann Thorac Surg.* 2015;99:360-367.
25. Craig JM, Lee S, Vlahakes GJ, et al. Heart transplantation procedure and surgical technique. In: Kirklin AD, Knechtle SJ, Larsen CP, et al., eds. *Textbook of Organ Transplantation.* 1st ed. John Wiley & Sons; 2014:657-666.
26. Maltais S, Danter MR, Haglund NA, et al. Nonsternotomy approaches for left ventricular assist device implantation. *Op Tech Thorac Cardiovasc Surg.* 2014;19:276-291.
27. Lund LH, Khush KK, Cherikh WS, et al. The registry of the International Society for Heart and Lung Transplantation: thirty-fourth adult heart transplantation report—2017; focus theme: allograft ischemic time. *J Heart Lung Transplant.* 2017;36:1037-1046.
28. Stehlik J, Feldman DS, Brown RN, et al. Interactions among donor characteristics influence post-transplant survival: a multi-institutional analysis. *J Heart Lung Transplant.* 2010;29:291-298.
29. Sharma A, Peltz M, Wait M, et al. The conduct of thoracic organ procurement. *Asian Cardiovasc Thorac Ann.* 2020;28(3):158-167.
30. Davies RR, Russo MJ, Morgan JA, et al. Standard versus bicaval techniques for orthotopic heart transplantation: an analysis of the United Network for Organ Sharing database. *J Thorac Cardiovasc Surg.* 2010;140:700-708.
31. Zijderhand CF, Veen KM, Caliskan K, et al. Biatrial versus bicaval orthotopic heart transplantation: a systematic review and meta-analysis. *Ann Thorac Surg.* 2020;110:684-691.
32. Kadner A, Chen RH, Adams DH. Heterotopic heart transplantation: experimental development and clinical experience. *Europ J Cardiothorac Surg.* 2000;17:474-481.
33. Chambers DC, Cherikh WS, Harhay MO, et al. The International Thoracic Organ Transplant Registry of the International Society for Heart and Lung Transplantation: thirty-sixth adult lung and heart-lung transplantation report—2019; Focus theme: donor and recipient size match. *J Heart Lung Transplant.* 2019;30:1042-1055.
34. Pasupneti S, Dhillon G, Reitz B, et al. Combined heart lung transplantation: an updated review of the current literature. *Transplantation.* 2017;1010:2297-2302.
35. Vakil K, Duval S, Sharma A, et al. Impact of pre-transplant pulmonary hypertension on survival after heart transplantation: a UNOS registry analysis. *Int J Cardiol.* 2014;176:595-599.
36. John R, Naka Y, Park SJ, et al. Impact of concurrent surgical valve procedures in patients receiving continuous-flow devices. *J Thorac Cardiovasc Surg.* 2014;147:581-589.
37. Maltais S, Haglund NA, Davis ME, et al. Outcomes after concomitant procedures with left ventricular assist device implantation: implications by device type and indication. *ASAIO J.* 2016;62:403-409.
38. McGee E, Danter M, Strueber M, et al. Evaluation of a lateral thoracotomy implant approach for a centrifugal-flow left ventricular assist device: the LATERAL clinical trial. *J Heart Lung Transplant.* 2019;38:344-351.
39. Milano CA, Schroder J, Daneshmand M. Total artificial heart replacement with 2 centrifugal blood pumps. *Op Tech Thorac Cardiovasc Surg.* 2016:20:306-321.
40. Shah P, Ha R, Singh R, et al Multicenter experience with durable biventricular assist devices. *J Heart Lung Transplant.* 2018;37:1093-1101.
41. Latrémouille C, Carpentier A, Leprince P, et al. A bioprosthetic total artificial heart for end-stage heart failure: results from a pilot study. *J Heart Lung Transplant.* 2018;37:33-37.
42. Hanke JS, Dogan G, Haverich A, et al. Implantation of two HeartMate3s in the setting of a Total Artificial Heart. *Op Tech Thorac Cardiovasc Surg.* 2021;26:67-80.
43. Colvin M, Smith JM, Hadley N, et al. OPTN/SRTR 2018 Annual data report: heart. *Am J Transplant.* 2020;20:340-426.
44. Israni AK, Zaun D, Hadley N, et al. OPTN/SRTR 2018 Annual data report: deceased organ donation. *Am J Transplant.* 2020:20(S1):509-541.

45. Sert DE, Karahan M, Aygun E, et al. Prediction of right ventricular failure after continuous flow left ventricular assist device implantation. *J Card Surg.* 2020;35:2965-2973.
46. Michelis KC, Zhong L, Peltz M, et al. Dynamic forecasts of survival for patients living with destination left ventricular assist devices: insights from INTERMACS. *J Am Heart Assoc.* 2020;9:e016203. doi: 10.1161/JAHA.119.016203
47. Khush KK, Cherikh WS, Chambers DC, et al. The International Thoracic Organ Transplant Registry of the International Society for Heart and Lung Transplantation: thirty-sixth heart transplantation report—2019; focus theme: donor and recipient size match. *J Heart Lung Transplant.* 2019;28:1056-1066.
48. Thomas SS, Zern EK, D'Alessandro DA. The renal challenge with left ventricular assist device therapy—when enough is enough. *JAMA Intern Med.* 2017;178:210-211.
49. Milano CA, Rogers JG, Tatooles AJ, et al. HVAD: the ENDURANCE supplemental trial. *J Am Coll Cardiol HF.* 2018;6:792-802.
50. Han JJ, Acker MA, Atluri P. Left ventricular assist devices synergistic model between technology and medicine. *Circulation.* 2018;138:2841-2851.

SECTION 7

CHAPTER 93

SURGICAL APPROACHES FOR COMMON CONGENITAL HEART DISEASES

Timothy J. Pirolli, Ryan R. Davies, Camille L. Hancock Friesen, and Robert D. B. Jaquiss

INTRODUCTION AND BACKGROUND

Congenital malformations of the cardiovascular system occur in approximately 1% of live births and are the most common type of birth defect.[1] With advances in fetal imaging, an increasing fraction of congenital heart disease (CHD) cases are diagnosed in utero, and this is especially true for approximately 20% of CHD cases, which may require intervention in the first few months of life.[2] For patients not diagnosed prenatally, the institution of mandatory screening of neonates by pulse oximetry has significantly increased the detection of cyanotic CHD cases in a timely fashion.[3] The remainder of CHD cases are identified during the evaluation of a cardiac murmur, as part of the investigation of unexplained hypertension, during the screening of asymptomatic populations, or occasionally incidentally.

In the majority of cases, the etiology of CHD remains obscure, and only 20% to 30% of cases have an identifiable genetic cause.[4] Copy number variants, single nucleotide variants, and aneuploidy have all been identified in patients with CHD. There are a few well-known examples of aneuploidy strongly associated with CHD, including Down syndrome (trisomy 21), Edwards syndrome (trisomy 18), Patau syndrome (trisomy 13), and Turner syndrome (45, X karyotype). As genetic analyses become more ubiquitous and sophisticated, it seems certain that many more genetic causes for CHD will be discovered.

Given the protean forms which CHD may take, the modes of presentation are not surprisingly widely varied. Perhaps, the most dramatic form of presentation is the neonate with systemic blood flow dependent on patency of the ductus arteriosus. If such patients are undiagnosed, normal ductal closure is associated with the rapid development of shock due to inadequate systemic blood flow. An example of such an anomaly is hypoplastic left heart syndrome (HLHS). In analogous fashion, patients with "ductal-dependent" pulmonary blood flow present with profound cyanosis as the ductus closes, as might be seen in a patient with tetralogy of Fallot (TOF) with severe pulmonary valve hypoplasia or atresia. Less urgent and dramatic manifestations of CHD are seen in children with large left-to-right shunts, such as a ventricular septal defect (VSD), who present with more subtle findings such as tachypnea and diaphoresis with feeding, and associated poor weight gain. Other patients have no signs or symptoms and may be detected when a chest radiograph or other diagnostic test is performed, and the cardiovascular anomaly is incidentally identified.

Regardless of the anomaly, the most common initial diagnostic modality is transthoracic echocardiography, which is quite frequently definitive in diagnosis and in guiding treatment. However, in a number of cases, anatomic and physiologic information derived from the echocardiogram may be augmented by cardiac catheterization, which permits accurate calculation of pulmonary and systemic resistances as well as the magnitude of any left-to-right or right-to-left shunt. In addition, direct measurement of intravascular or intracavitary pressures and gradients can be achieved at catheterization. Advanced three-dimensional imaging with cardiac computed tomography (CT) or cardiac magnetic resonance imaging (MRI) is increasingly undertaken and may facilitate "virtual reality" or three-dimensional printing to permit planning of patient-specific interventions.

The first definitive treatments for CHD were surgical and were accomplished without the use of cardiopulmonary bypass, which had not yet been invented. Beginning in the middle of the last century, surgeons developed techniques to effectively treat simple anomalies such as patent ductus arteriosus (PDA) and coarctation of the aorta.[5,6] The next step was the provision of palliative operations to provide additional pulmonary blood flow to children with cyanotic heart disease.[7] With Gibbons' proof-of-concept with a practical cardiopulmonary bypass machine, the era of open-heart surgery began.[8] In the ensuing decades, advances in care, equipment, and knowledge permitted surgical solutions for virtually any congenital cardiac malformation.[9] More recently, sophisticated and less-invasive catheter-based solutions have been introduced and become standard of care, particularly for the "simpler" congenital malformations.

Because the spectrum of congenital heart disease is so broad and varied, well beyond the scope of this chapter, in the following sections, we will describe considerations relevant for three important forms of CHD. Each will exemplify an important physiologic abnormality: left-to-right shunting illustrated by VSD, cyanotic CHD as seen in TOF, and univentricular circulation as seen in HLHS. These discussions are of necessity somewhat condensed and simplified, and the interested reader is referred to any of a number of excellent textbooks in congenital cardiology and cardiac surgery.

VENTRICULAR SEPTAL DEFECTS

INTRODUCTION

Ventricular septal defects are the most common congenital cardiac defect, with the possible exception of bicuspid aortic valve, and manifest in a variety of sizes and locations in the ventricular septum. Isolated VSDs account for approximately 20% to 30% of all congenital cardiac defects and occur in approximately 1 to 2 per 1000 live births. VSDs are classified by their anatomic location and various classification schemes exist to describe the same anatomic defect. A recent international effort to create a unified classification scheme for VSD nomenclature has resulted in four major categories (perimembranous, inlet VSD, trabecular muscular, and outlet VSD) and various subcategories based on specific location and malalignment of adjacent structures (**Table 93.1**).[10] However, this classification scheme has not been universally adopted, and thus it is critical to have a knowledge of the various synonyms to allow for familiarity. The relative location of each type of VSD is depicted in **Figure 93.1**.

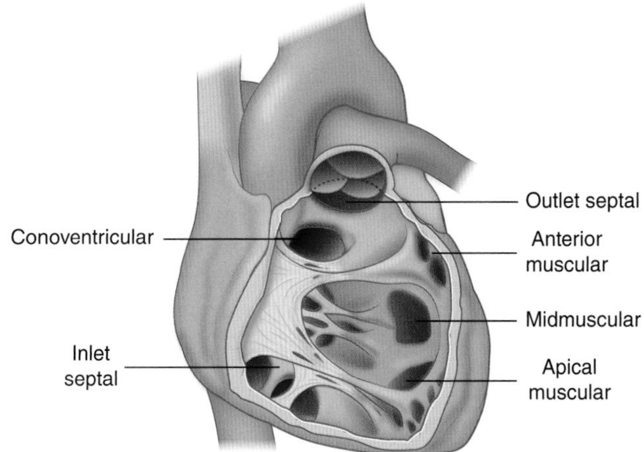

FIGURE 93.1 In this idealized view of the ventricular septum, the right ventricular free wall has been removed and the locations of various types of ventricular septal defect are demonstrated.

Pathogenesis

The pathophysiology of a VSD is dependent upon the size of the defect and the relative ratio of the systemic vascular resistance (SVR) to the pulmonary vascular resistance (PVR). The left-to-right shunting of blood is the result of the higher-pressured left ventricle forcing blood through the VSD to the low-pressured right ventricle due to the increased SVR after birth. As the PVR continues to drop in the days and weeks after birth, there will be increased left-to-right shunting across the VSD. Conversely, the shunting may decrease as the size of the VSD becomes smaller with time.

There is no universally accepted classification scheme for VSD size. Clinically, VSDs are often labeled as "small," "medium," and "large." These definitions are variable depending on the size of the patient, but typically in infants small VSDs are considered less than 4 mm in diameter, medium are 4 to 6 mm in diameter and large are greater than 6 mm in diameter.

TABLE 93.1 Common Nomenclature for Ventricular Septal Defect

International Society for Nomenclature of Pediatric and Congenital Heart Disease Scheme Classification	Common Alternate Nomenclature
Perimembranous	Perimembranous, membranous, subaortic, infra-cristal, conoventricular
Inlet	Atrioventricular canal type
Trabecular muscular	Muscular (anterior, apical, mid, multiple, postero-inferior)
Outlet	Supracristal, subpulmonary, conal, intraconal

The degree of shunting may be calculated by cardiac catheterization or MRI as pulmonic to systemic blood flow ratio (Qp:Qs). VSDs with a small shunt (Qp:Qs $<$ 1.5:1) are considered the most common ($>$50% of VSDs). VSDs with a moderate shunt (Qp:Qs of 1.5-2.3:1) typically result in mild-moderately increased right ventricular and pulmonary arterial pressures, as well as signs and symptoms of congestive heart failure. Large defects (Qp:Qs $>$ 2.3:1) have unrestrictive shunts with minimal pressure gradient between the two ventricles. This equalization (or near-equalization) of ventricular pressures can lead to left ventricular dilation and increased end-diastolic pressures, resulting in increased left atrial pressures, pulmonary venous pressures, and progressive symptoms of heart failure. Echocardiography can estimate the degree of shunting by measuring the pressure gradient across the VSD, but it does not give a precise Qp:Qs.

Clinical Features: Ventricular Septal Defect

The clinical presentation of a VSD is dependent upon the degree of shunting, the age of the patient, and associated congenital heart defects. The increased left-to-right shunting can result in pulmonary congestion from excessive circulation, leading to tachypnea. The increased demands on the left ventricle to maintain systemic cardiac output as blood is shunting across the VSD can lead to high-output failure and subsequent failure to thrive. Any increased demands for cardiac output (such as systemic illness, feeding, anemia, or other stressors on the body) can exacerbate this pathophysiology and associated symptoms.

Infants with moderate or larger VSDs may present with symptoms such as poor feeding, increased respiratory effort, poor weight gain, and tachycardia in the first month or two of life after PVR has declined. Smaller VSDs may be clinically silent until they are discovered later in life, even in adulthood. The discovery of an incidental murmur or symptoms from increased aortic regurgitation, development of right ventricular outflow obstruction from hypertrophy of infundibular muscles or, rarely, endocarditis may be the inciting event for discovery of a VSD later in life.

Diagnosis: Ventricular Septal Defect

Cardiac auscultation will uncover a systolic murmur, which varies in intensity and location due to the size and anatomy of the VSD. Larger VSDs may also exhibit a diastolic rumble (due to increased flow across the mitral valve) or palpable thrill over the precordium. The initial workup for a VSD often includes the following studies:

Electrocardiogram

Findings on electrocardiogram (EKG) are variable and nonspecific for VSDs. Evidence of left ventricular hypertrophy (increased voltage in leads II, III, aVF, V5, and V6) may be manifested in larger defects due to increased left ventricular workload over time. Evidence of right ventricular hypertrophy (right axis deviation, dominant R wave in V1, dominant S wave in V5 or V6, and QRS duration <120 ms) may be evident in patients with increased PVR. Patients with small VSDs often have normal EKGs.

Chest X-Ray

Patients with small VSDs often have normal-appearing chest x-rays. Larger VSDs with increased left-to-right shunting may have increased vascular markings and cardiomegaly.

Echocardiography

Two-dimensional transthoracic echocardiography is the gold standard for diagnosis. A thorough echocardiogram is critical for identifying the location, size, and number of VSDs; assessing ventricular function; and diagnosing associated congenital heart lesions. Three-dimensional and transesophageal echocardiography may more clearly delineate the VSD anatomy, if warranted.

Other Studies

For well defined, isolated VSDs, further workup is typically not warranted. If there are specific anatomic concerns beyond the VSDs or if there is a need for more hemodynamic data, cardiac catheterization or cardiac MRI may be considered.

MANAGEMENT OF VSD

Medical Management

The goals of medical management of young patients diagnosed with VSDs are directed toward standard therapies for congestive heart failure and to minimize the risk of failure to thrive. Stressors for patients with significant shunts, such as viral infection, may result in acute worsening of symptoms. Frequent monitoring by the cardiologist is necessary to adjust medical regimens and to decide upon timing of surgery.

Timing of Surgery

There is no simple algorithm for timing of surgery for infants with VSDs. Patients with symptoms despite maximal medical therapy, such as frequent hospitalizations or failure to thrive, warrant referral to surgery. Patients with estimated pulmonary artery pressures greater than half-systemic or continued enlargement of left-sided cardiac structures likely warrant surgical closure of their VSD. Patients with smaller VSDs who are asymptomatic may be monitored for spontaneous closure. The presence of associated congenital defects, development of a double-chambered right ventricle, or worsening aortic insufficiency may also be indications for surgery. In patients with suprasystemic pulmonary hypertension, VSD closure is contraindicated.

In patients with unrepaired VSDs who survive until adulthood, pulmonary vascular disease may develop leading to right-to-left shunting (Eisenmenger syndrome) and cyanosis due to chronic elevations of pressure and flow across the VSD.[11] These patients are typically inoperable. The American Heart Association (AHA)/American College of Cardiology (ACC) released an evidence based, expert consensus guideline algorithm for surgical closure of VSDs in adults (**Algorithm 93.1**).

Surgical Approach

Regardless of the location of the VSD, the standard approach for repair is via median sternotomy, although some surgeons may opt for a lower partial sternotomy or right thoracotomy. Patients are placed on cardiopulmonary bypass via bicaval cannulation, often with venting of the left heart via the right superior pulmonary vein. Mild to moderate systemic hypothermia is utilized. In rare circumstances, such as in very small infants, deep hypothermic circulatory arrest may be employed. Myocardial preservation is performed with a cardioplegic diastolic arrest of the heart with aortic cross-clamping. Caval snares are placed and secured to create as bloodless of a surgical field as possible. The options for visualization and approach to repair each type of VSD are dependent upon location and size of the defect(s).

Surgical Approach to Perimembranous VSD or Inlet VSD

With the proximity of the perimembranous or inlet (and many muscular) VSD to the tricuspid valve, the best approach is transatrial with visualization through the tricuspid valve. After the arrest of the heart, the right atrium is opened parallel to the atrioventricular groove. Knowledge of the anatomy within the right atrium is crucial to avoid injuring the conduction system during the repair (**Figure 93.2**).

With reflection of the anterior and septal leaflets of the tricuspid valve, the margins of the VSD are noted. Primary suture closure of VSDs is not recommended due to the risk of dehiscence, thus a patch of material of the surgeon's choice (such as autologous pericardium, treated bovine pericardium, Dacron, Gore-Tex) must be cut to size. Occasionally, the septal tricuspid valve leaflet may need to be divided or detached from the annulus to visualize the edges of the defect. The patch is then secured to the rims of the VSD with a continuous or interrupted technique utilizing a polypropylene or small braided pledgeted suture, taking care to avoid injuring the aortic valve, tricuspid valve, and conduction system (**Figure 93.3**). Care

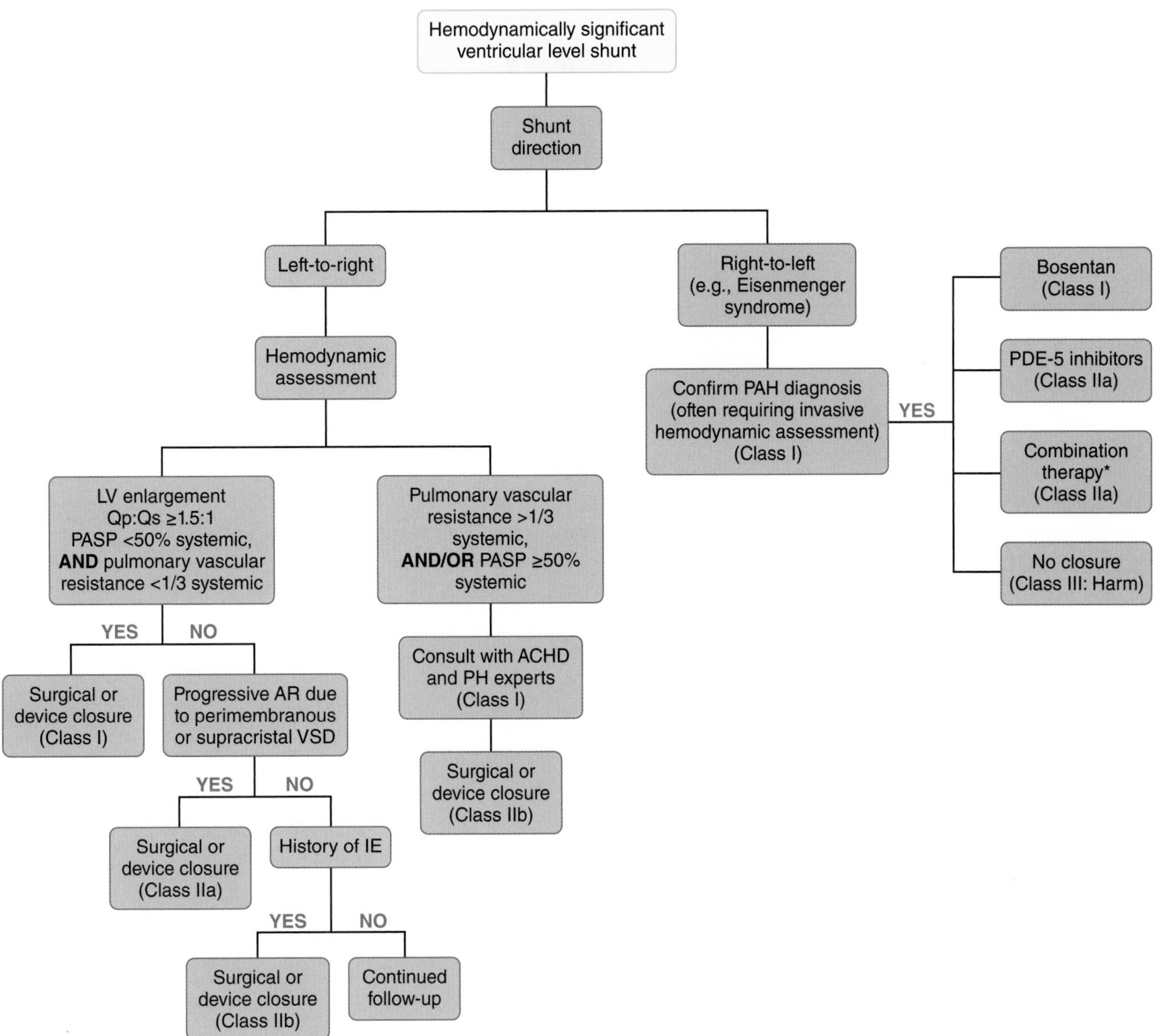

ALGORITHM 93.1 Management for hemodynamically significant VSD in adults.[17] Critical decisions are based on echocardiography and cardiac catheterization. ACHD, adult congenital heart disease; AR, aortic regurgitation; IE, infective endocarditis; LV, left ventricle; PAH, pulmonary artery hypertension; PASP, pulmonary artery systolic pressure; PDE, phosphodiesterase; PH, pulmonary hypertension; Qp:Qs, pulmonary to systemic blood flow; VSD, ventricular septal defect

should be taken to weave around chordal tissue appropriately to avoid ensnaring the chords and creating tricuspid regurgitation. Often, sutures are passed through the tricuspid annulus and buttressed with pledgets or a strip of patch material. The superior aspect of the defect near the aortic valve is most vulnerable to leaving a residual defect. The conduction system follows a course along the inferior margin of a perimembranous or inlet VSD; thus, superficial bites (or bites 3-5 mm away from the margin of the defect) are critical to prevent heart block (Figure 93.3).[12]

After repair of the VSD, the tricuspid valve should be tested for insufficiency with insufflation of saline into the right ventricular cavity. Commissuroplasty sutures between the anterior and septal or septal and posterior leaflets may need to be placed to decrease tricuspid regurgitation. In rare cases, a right ventriculotomy may be required to visualize the entirety of the defect for closure.

Surgical Approach to Supracristal Ventricular Septal Defect

Due to the position of the supracristal VSD inferior to the pulmonary valve, the ideal approach is transpulmonary. Once the heart is arrested, a transverse (or longitudinal) incision is created in the main pulmonary artery, taking care not to injure the pulmonary valve leaflets. Retraction of the leaflets laterally exposes the edges of the defect. The aortic valve may be visible through the VSD (and may prolapse through the defect) and care must be taken to avoid injuring the aortic valve with the suture needle during closure. As mentioned, patch material includes fresh (or glutaraldehyde treated) autologous pericardium, a modified

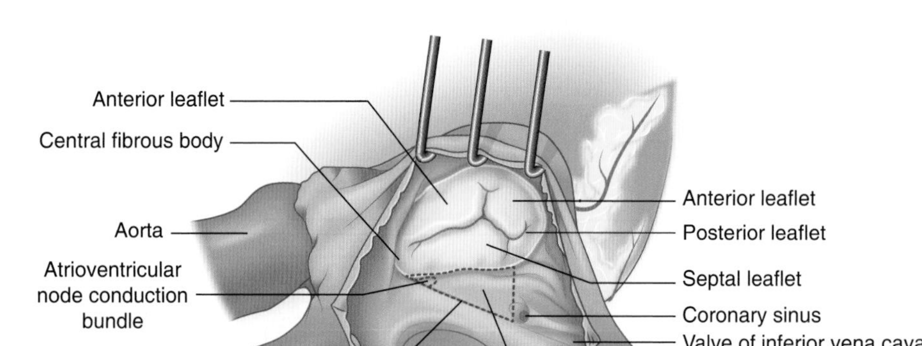

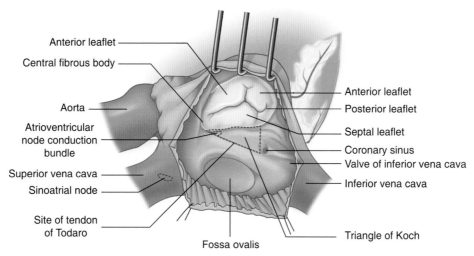

FIGURE 93.2 Surgical anatomy of the right atrium with special attention to the triangle of Koch.[13] The surgeon's view from right atriotomy with demonstration of relevant landmarks to be considered when performing closure of a ventricular septal defect.

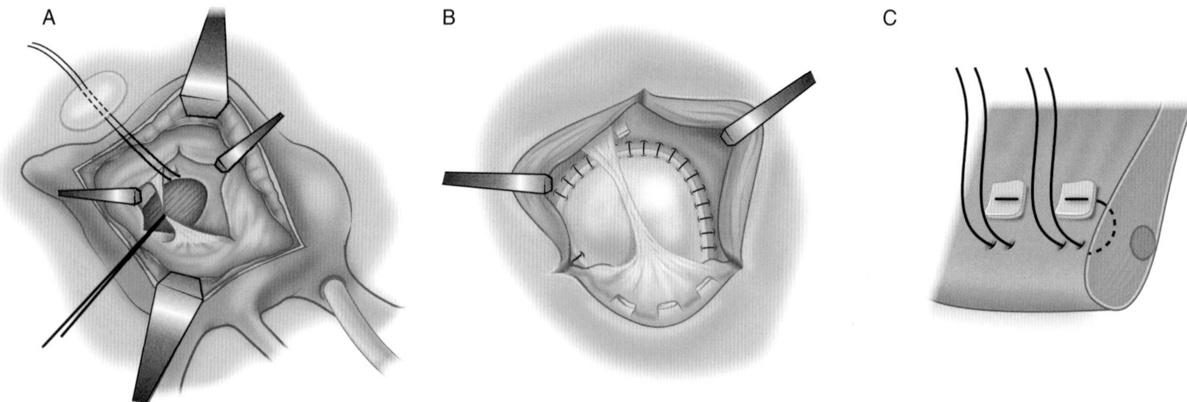

FIGURE 93.3 (A–C) Patch closure of a perimembranous ventricular septal defect. **View A:** Via a right atriotomy, the leaflets of the tricuspid valve are retracted, and a double-armed pledgeted suture is placed at the "12 o'clock" position, on the right ventricular aspect of the crest of the muscular component of the ventricular septal defect. The patch is lowered into position, and the suture tied. The arms of the suture are run clockwise and counterclockwise in a continuous fashion. With the patch thus secured to the muscular rim of the ventricular septal defect, additional interrupted pledgeted sutures are placed to secure the patch to the tricuspid annulus, with the pledgets on the right atrial aspect. The original running sutures are tied to the adjacent interrupted suture. **View B:** The completed repair is demonstrated. **View C:** Alternatively, as opposed to a running suture technique, interrupted sutures may be used on the muscular component as well. The concept of placing the sutures on the right ventricular aspect of the septum is emphasized in this schematic view with the position of the conduction tissues indicated by the dark circle. Note that the suture patch avoids injury to this vulnerable tissue.

bovine pericardium, or a synthetic patch material such as Dacron. However, a Dacron patch should be avoided in this scenario as the Dacron may heal to the ventricular aspect of the pulmonary valve leaflets, resulting in pulmonary insufficiency. The patch is secured to the inferior margin of the defect with a continuous or interrupted technique until the pulmonary valve leaflets are encountered. Then, sutures must be passed through the base of the leaflets, taking care not to injure the pulmonary valve or the adjacent aortic valve. Sutures are passed through the patch and secured (**Figure 93.4**).[13]

Surgical Approach to Muscular Ventricular Septal Defects (Including Interventional)

Many muscular VSDs may be repaired via the transatrial approach as described earlier. In select cases of large apical muscular defects, a right ventriculotomy may be necessary to close the defect. Select muscular VSDs may also be closed in the catheterization laboratory or in the operating room via a hybrid technique with a transcatheter technique.

Transcatheter closure of VSDs was first reported in 1988 and advancement in the technology has allowed for expanded

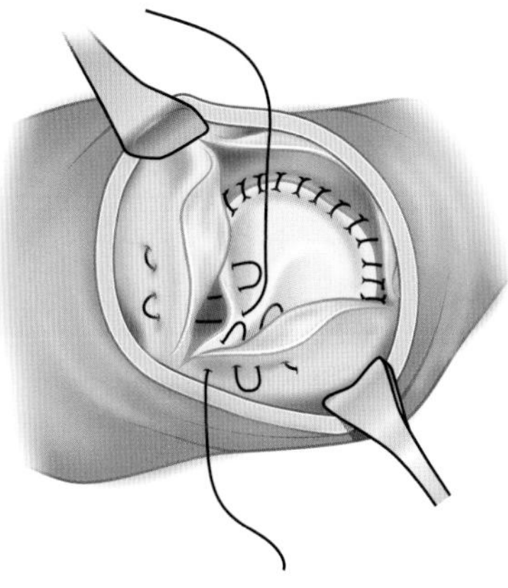

FIGURE 93.4 Transpulmonary patch repair of supracristal VSD. The repair of a supracristal VSD is accomplished via an incision in the anterior wall of the main pulmonary artery. The cusps of the pulmonary valve are retracted to expose the lower rim of the VSD. The patch is then secured to the lower rim with a continuous suture as shown. The upper portion of the patch is then secured to the "hinge point" of the two pulmonary valve cusps as shown.

use since that time. Although this topic is beyond the scope of this section, it should be noted that transcatheter closure of congenital perimembranous and muscular VSDs has been reported with improving outcomes. Risks of this procedure include conduction abnormalities, residual shunt, aortic valve distortion, hemolysis, device embolization, and endocarditis.[14]

For young patients with multiple, typically muscular, VSDs (known as a "swiss-cheese" ventricular septum), repair may be unfeasible. Placement of a pulmonary artery band to limit left-to-right shunting and minimize congestive heart failure may be the first-line treatment to allow for growth and future decision-making.

SURGICAL RESULTS

Surgical closure of isolated VSDs carries a less than 1% mortality risk according to the Society of Thoracic Surgeons (STS) Congenital Heart Surgery Database.[15] Complete heart block occurs in 1% to 3% of patients but is increasingly rare for repair of isolated VSDs. Due to the common use of intraoperative transesophageal echocardiogram, significant residual VSDs (>3 mm) that require re-operation are rare. Small residual VSDs are well-tolerated and often close on their own with time.[16] There is a small risk of development of a double-chambered right ventricle in patients with a small residual VSD postoperatively, although the frequency of this is unknown.

FOLLOW-UP PATIENT CARE

For patients with repaired VSDs, the need for any additional or ongoing medical or surgical intervention is extraordinarily unlikely. Early routine postoperative follow-up is necessary, but once through the acute convalescence, a patient with repaired VSD should not require an additional intervention. Antibiotic prophylaxis for infective endocarditis is recommended for patients with residual shunts after VSD repair.

FUTURE DIRECTIONS

Surgical closure of VSDs is the gold standard for therapy. Some surgeons advocate for the utilization of smaller incisions (ie, ministernotomy, right thoracotomy, video-assisted thoracoscopic surgery) for surgical repair with comparable results. The expanded role of transcatheter (or hybrid) closure of VSDs continues to be explored, despite higher rates of heart block.

TETRALOGY OF FALLOT

INTRODUCTION

Cyanotic heart lesions have been classically taught in medical school as the four "T's"; transposition of the great arteries, truncus arteriosus, total anomalous pulmonary venous return, and TOF. Of these, TOF is by far the most common. TOF spans a wide range of physiology, clinical presentation, and management. One thing, all TOF patients share is the ongoing hazard for morbidity and mortality, making it one of the complex congenital cardiac pathologies that mandate life-long surveillance.[17] Management and timing of intervention in TOF depends on which end of the pathophysiologic spectrum the patient lies and the philosophical approach to neonatal management chosen by the heart program, which is caring for the child. The mild end of the spectrum, which is sometimes referred to as a "pink TOF," is one in which the VSD is the dominant feature, and there is minimal right ventricular outflow obstruction. The other end of the spectrum, or "blue TOF," is composed of infants with right ventricular outflow tract obstruction as the dominant manifestation. At the "blue" end of the spectrum, patients may have such compromised antegrade pulmonary blood flow that the infant presents with symptomatic hypoxic crisis in the neonatal period as the PDA constricts and antegrade pulmonary blood flow proves insufficient. Cyanosis may also evolve over time from very mild to more severe as right ventricular outflow tract obstruction progresses. This progressive cyanosis occurs when there is sufficient obstruction to beget a vicious cycle of progressive right ventricular hypertrophy followed by increased outflow tract obstruction and reduced pulmonary blood flow.

As a result of the wide range of pathophysiology, intervention may be required urgently or emergently in the neonatal period or may be scheduled electively at 4 to 6 months of age like any other VSD. Management modalities include (a) emergency stenting of the PDA; (b) modified Blalock-Taussig-Thomas (BTT) shunt in a staged repair; (c) neonatal complete repair; and (d) valve-sparing pulmonary arterioplasty with VSD repair in the older infant. The heterogeneity of presentation in the TOF population explains the plentiful debate with regards to optimal timing and strategy of management. For a high-level review of some of the issues encountered in studying outcomes in surgically repaired TOF in neonates, the reader is referred to a recent commentary.[18]

PATHOGENESIS/EMBRYOLOGY

One of the more conceptually intuitive descriptions of the embryology and subsequent anatomy of TOF has been proposed by the Van Praaghs of Children's Hospital Boston.[19] In their view, the four cardinal anatomic features of TOF (VSD, right ventricular outflow tract (RVOT) obstruction, right ventricular hypertrophy, and aortic override) arise from one problem, namely underdevelopment of the conus. They have thus suggested that this pathology is a monology, rather than a tetralogy. The single developmental issue to which the clinical features of TOF is attributed is hypoplasia of the conus (also called the infundibulum), which is the cylinder of muscle in which the pulmonary valve sits. With underdevelopment of the conus—the muscle which normally grows large enough to contribute a portion of the interventricular septum—there is a void left, or a "conal ventriculoseptal defect," which is characterized by anterior displacement of the remnant septum as viewed on a parasternal long-axis echocardiogram. The hypoplastic conus creates a narrow passage, thus RVOT obstruction; the narrowing may involve any or all of three levels of the outflow tract including the subpulmonary region, the pulmonary valve itself, or the main pulmonary artery. The large conal VSD is unrestrictive and thus the right ventricle functions at the same pressure as the left ventricle resulting in right ventricular hypertrophy. The underdeveloped conus fails to "push" the aorta back into normal anatomic location over the left ventricle resulting in aortic override of the interventricular septum, seen best in short-axis imaging on the echocardiogram.

TOF may be associated with chromosomal abnormalities, notably 22q11 in DiGeorge syndrome. TOF may also be associated with other cardiac pathology (additional VSDs, atrial septal defect, PDA complete atrioventricular canal defect). TOF/absent pulmonary valve results from a different set of embryologic conditions and will not be discussed in this presentation. The anatomic substrate, as described earlier, results in fixed obstruction, but there is also an element of dynamic obstruction which may develop into a self-perpetuating loop of obstruction resulting in right ventricular hypertrophy and worsening obstruction.

CLINICAL PRESENTATION, SIGNS AND SYMPTOMS, DIFFERENTIAL DIAGNOSIS

Patients may present anywhere on the spectrum between primarily VSD physiology all the way to primarily obstruction to pulmonary blood flow. Patients who present with primarily VSD physiology will be clinically well until PVR decreases to 4 to 6 postnatal weeks, at which time left-to-right shunt will escalate and, like any other large VSD, the infant will present with signs and symptoms of congestive heart failure, including poor weight gain (failure to thrive), diaphoresis with feeds, tachypnea, and a murmur. At the other end of the spectrum, there will be neonates who experience profound cyanosis with ductal closing (so-called ductal-dependent pulmonary circulation). Some parents and caregivers are able to provide a history of hypercyanotic spells or "tet spells" that the infant or child will manifest with agitation resulting in significant desaturation. The classic description of a tet spell is that the child will self-resolve the episode by a Valsalva maneuver (typically described by a child squatting) to increase SVR. It is thought that the "spell" is equivalent to a spasm in the muscular obstruction of the RVOT, exaggerating the right-to-left shunt, which in turn can be overcome by a corresponding increase in SVR (**Figure 93.5**).

In the middle of the spectrum, the patient may behave like a patient with a VSD who has undergone pulmonary artery banding; that is the cumulative degree of right ventricular outflow tract obstruction may be sufficient to prevent excessive pulmonary blood flow, but not so severe as to provoke spells of severe cyanosis. Neonates who have ductal-dependence are a discrete population. Such patients may undergo primary neonatal repair or palliative staged repair, with an initial procedure to increase pulmonary blood flow (placement of a modified BT shunt, placement of a stent in the PDA, or placement of a stent in the right ventricular outflow tract).

DIAGNOSIS: TETRALOGY OF FALLOT

Transthoracic echocardiography is the diagnostic modality of choice and is generally sufficient for preoperative assessment. Standard views reveal the degree of right ventricular outflow obstruction and the degree of involvement of the pulmonary annulus and valve leaflets. Echocardiography is also the modality of choice for assessing the presence of a PDA, as well as

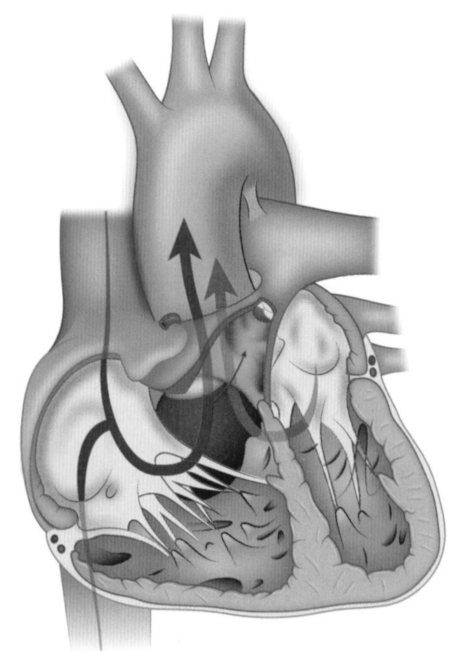

FIGURE 93.5 Depiction of blood flow during a "tet spell." The already obstructed right ventricular outflow tract has become abruptly narrower, forcing more right-to-left shunting, diverting deoxygenated ("blue") blood into the aorta and increasing systemic cyanosis. In extreme cases, the right ventricular outflow tract may be nearly obliterated during such a spell.

the size of the main and branch pulmonary arteries. It is often possible to determine from the echocardiogram the likelihood of sparing of the valve (avoiding the placement of an incision and augmenting patch across the pulmonary infundibulum—so call "transannular patch"—with associated pulmonary valvar insufficiency). This is based on indexing the diameter of the pulmonary annulus to the patient's body surface area and comparing that to a normative population. This is reported as the z score of the pulmonary annulus and is analogous to standard deviation. If the z score is less than or equal to −3, there is little likelihood of sparing the pulmonary annulus, whereas at z score greater than or equal to −1, it is likely that it will be possible to spare the annulus and a functional pulmonary valve will likely result. The only time a cardiac catheterization is required is (a) uncertainty about coronary anatomy (which can also be gleaned from cardiac CT or MRI)—if there is concern for an aberrantly oriented coronary that would preclude a transannular approach (given that around 30% of patients will be managed with a transannular patch); or (b) stenting of the PDA or right ventricular outflow tract are planned as the initial intervention in a staged repair. CT scan is routinely required for planning a ductal intervention to characterize the diameter, length, and course of the ductus as well as its orientation at the aortic origin and at the pulmonary artery insertion, as these are all elements considered by the interventional cardiologist in determining appropriate candidacy for ductal stenting.

MANAGEMENT: TETRALOGY OF FALLOT

The balance to be struck in TOF is to minimize the risk of serious cyanotic cardiovascular collapse and at the same time optimize the likelihood of sparing the pulmonary valve. Given this is a life-long disease, the long-term goal of sparing as much structurally and functionally normal right ventricular muscle as possible is part of the challenge that must inform the management strategy.

Medical Approach

Medical management is indicated in patients who have either acute or subacute declining oxygen saturation coincident with increasing right ventricular outflow tract gradients. The history or witnessed hypercyanotic spell is an indication of dynamic and dangerous compromise to pulmonary blood flow that carries a significant risk of mortality. In some patients with milder degrees of RVOT obstruction and intermittent desaturation, oral propranolol is used to reduce the heart rate (increasing ventricular stroke volume) and to diminish the force of contraction of the right ventricle. While propranolol may reduce the dynamic component of right ventricular outflow tract obstruction, it will have little effect on the fixed anatomic gradient. Such a strategy may allow the patient to be managed conservatively for a number of additional days-to-weeks to stabilize or to reach the optimal 3 to 4 months of age when the risk of intervention is lower. Occasionally neonates or infants present with life-threatening desaturation that may not fully respond to conservative measures. In an emergent situation, treatment is, in order, sedation, supplemental oxygen followed by intubation and paralysis. Barring resolution and stabilization, emergent mechanical circulatory support or emergent placement of a systemic-to-pulmonary artery shunt or stent may be required.

Interventional Approaches

Surgical approaches to palliation and repair are well established, and interventional catheterization approaches are emerging, which will be described separately. The history of surgical repair of TOF has followed the general course of pediatric cardiac surgery. In the early 1990s, palliative shunts were performed until patients were 12 months of age, at which time a definitive repair was performed. While the most important consideration at the time of the corrective surgery is the relief of RVOT obstruction, preservation of the pulmonary valve mechanism is ideal if it is possible to do so, and is often successful when the pulmonary annulus is larger than a z score of −2.[20] So-called "valve sparing" or "annulus sparing" techniques include surgical valvotomy, individual infundibular resection with or without patching, and main pulmonary artery incision and patching without breaching the annulus.[21] Introduction of the transannular patch, with an incision that spans the infundibulum, annulus, and main pulmonary artery, was associated with being able to perform "definitive" repair at an earlier age and smaller infant size. This approach gained significant traction,[22] but there was a recognition that there was a threshold of 4 months of age whereby earlier repair (i.e., neonatal repair) was associated with higher rates of mortality (**Figure 93.6**).

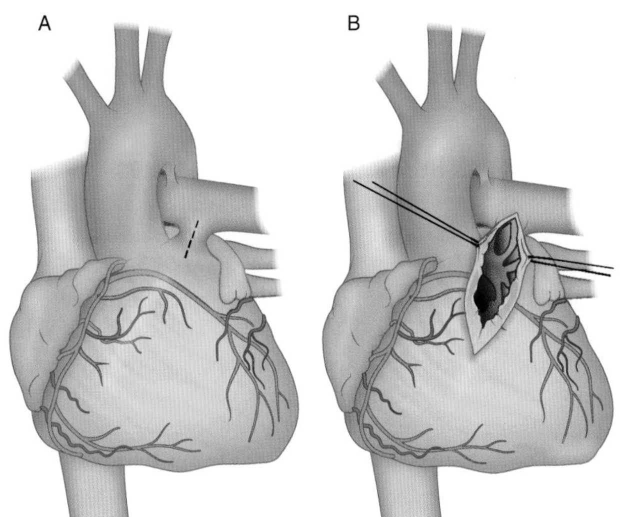

FIGURE 93.6 **(A,B)** Depiction of approach to a transannular patch. Significant variability exists in the extent to which the incision extends both above the annulus into the main pulmonary artery and proximal into the right ventricular outflow tract. The optimal incision is sufficient to reduce the right ventricular pressure to less than 50% systemic but leaves some "gating" of the outflow tract.

In general, elective repair is now performed in infants under 1 year of age (and most North American centers would operate electively under 8 months of age) with a surgical mortality risk of 2% to 3%.[23] The approach to neonatal intervention remains an area of considerable debate, although a recent review, which includes an unspecified number of ductal stented patients suggests that staged versus complete repair in the neonatal period is associated with improved early survival.[24] Review of large registry datasets allows us to reflect on treatment strategies and outcomes that surpass the immediate perioperative period, an important consideration in TOF with its lifetime and ongoing risk. Transplant and mortality-free survival were reported by Smith et al. from a multicenter database.[25] This report identified that after the early postoperative mortality risk, there is a continuous hazard for transplant or death, with the dominant long-term risk attributable to the presence of a genetic condition. Over time there has been little change in the repair strategy chosen, which argues that the choice of repair is likely dictated by the anatomic/pathophysiologic substrate of the patient even though proving this is difficult given there is no gold standard for grading the anatomic or physiologic "severity of TOF" before intervention.[26] In a single-center review of the surgical treatment of symptomatic neonates, the only predictor of annulus preservation was the size of the pulmonary annulus at the time of the first postnatal echocardiogram.[27] In a multicenter comparison of staged versus primary repair, a study that included percutaneous stenting, early mortality, and neonatal morbidity was lower in the staged group, but cumulative morbidity and reinterventions favored the primary repair group.[28] The approach must be optimized for individual patients, with the lens that the immediate requirement is adequate right ventricular pressure unloading. The next most important consideration in early management is to leave the right ventricular outflow as "protected" as possible; if that means sparing the annulus, so much the better.

Percutaneous Interventional Approaches

Percutaneous interventional options include PDA stenting and RVOT obstruction stenting.[29,30] Glatz et al report a multicenter study comparing PDA stents and BTT shunt (systemic-to-pulmonary artery shunt) for varying diagnoses, which share in common ductal-dependent pulmonary blood flow.[31] This study showed that the intensive care unit length of stay was half as long for the PDA-stented patients compared to the BTT shunt patients and the pulmonary arteries were 20% larger at the time of definitive repair in the PDA versus BTT shunt patients. However, PDA stent placement is not a panacea, as it is not uniformly applicable due to technical issues related to ductal anatomic variation. PDA stenting induces competitive diastolic flow like any systemic-to-pulmonary artery shunt. Likewise, RVOT obstruction stents that cross the pulmonary valve preclude valve preservation. Furthermore, depending on where they are deployed, removal of the stent may necessitate a large transannular incision and may impact the tricuspid valve. There may be some patients that might otherwise have had preservation of a borderline valve that subsequently required a transannular patch due to the presence of a stent in the right ventricular outflow tract obstruction.[32]

SPECIAL ISSUES, CONTROVERSIES, EMERGING THERAPIES: TETRALOGY OF FALLOT

Controversy remains as to whether staged or neonatal repair is the optimal approach for a symptomatic neonate, a matter which awaits a prospective randomized multicenter trial. As more percutaneous valve products become available, valve deployment into the transannular patched RVOT obstruction will become an option where currently they are not.

FOLLOW-UP PATIENT CARE: TETRALOGY OF FALLOT

TOF is considered a "complex" congenital heart diagnosis that requires regular long-term follow up because of the ongoing hazard for right ventricular dysfunction, pulmonary valve dysfunction, arrhythmias, and mortality.[17] Late issues primarily center around right ventricular function, which may have been subjected to long periods of hypertension/pressure overload and thus may develop restrictive physiology. Likewise, right ventricular function may be compromised by long periods of volume overload (because of systemic-to-pulmonary artery shunt or transannular patch with free pulmonic regurgitation), which then may lead to right ventricular dilation and decompensation. After establishing a threshold right ventricular volume (expressed as end-diastolic volume indexed to body surface area; 170 mL/m^2) that can be predicted to be associated with improved outcome following pulmonary valve replacement,[33] there has been little exploration with regards to optimal timing of pulmonary valve replacement to optimize long-term right ventricular function[34] but the weight of opinion is toward earlier valve replacement. Percutaneous pulmonary valve replacement has emerged over the past two decades as an interval option that is feasible for patients who have a nonpatulous right ventricular outflow tract obstruction. Consensus guidelines recommend either percutaneous or surgical pulmonary valve replacement are indicated for symptomatic patients with moderate or worse pulmonary regurgitation and asymptomatic patients with moderate or worse pulmonary regurgitation with ventricular enlargement or impaired right ventricular systolic function.[17]

RESEARCH AND FUTURE DIRECTIONS

As with all congenital heart malformations, there is intense activity exploring the genetic contributions to the development of TOF. If trials can be arranged, optimum management of the cyanotic neonate may become standardized. The role of percutaneous intervention seems certain to increase for both the small unrepaired patient and the older patient with a dysfunctional right ventricular outflow tract obstruction (residual obstruction, pulmonary valvar insufficiency, or both).

SINGLE VENTRICLE—HYPOPLASTIC LEFT HEART SYNDROME

INTRODUCTION

In some patients with CHD, ductal patency may be required to maintain systemic cardiac output. As with many congenital cardiac diagnoses, lesions resulting in ductal-dependent systemic blood flow occur on a spectrum. They may require intervention to correct obstruction of systemic output at a single level, more complex interventions to address multilevel obstruction, or require single ventricle palliation. HLHS represents the most severe end of the spectrum, where the underdevelopment of the left ventricular outflow tract and aortic valve along with hypoplasia of the left ventricle and mitral valve result in a heart that is incapable (even after surgical or catheter-based interventions) of supporting systemic cardiac output. In these patients, a single ventricle palliation strategy is employed. The complexity of both the surgical palliation and the fragility of the physiology of the resultant circulatory arrangement in HLHS make it one of the most challenging lesions to manage effectively.

HLHS has a prevalence rate of approximately 2 cases per 10,000 live births in the United States and represents 1.4% to 4.1% of all CHD cases.[35,36] Without surgical treatment, mortality exceeds 90% within the first year of life. The series of surgical operations successfully pioneered by Norwood and colleagues at Boston Children's Hospital has enabled significantly improved survival, but mortality within the first year remains above 25%.[37]

PATHOGENESIS AND EMBRYOLOGY: HLHS

The etiology of HLHS is complex, likely involving both genetic components and abnormal cardiac development related to altered *in utero* physiology. The genetics of HLHS do not follow Mendelian inheritance patterns, but first-degree relatives of patients with left heart obstructive lesions have a higher risk (10%-15%) of similar left-sided lesions.[38] A range of genetic syndromes and specific genetic mutations have been associated with HLHS. In addition, epigenetic phenomena may provide a link between environmental influences and abnormal DNA methylation resulting in altered cardiac development.[39]

Normal development of cardiac chambers is thought to be at least partially dependent on blood flow through those chambers.[40] A variety of anatomic lesions (mitral stenosis/atresia, aortic valve stenosis/atresia, aortic coarctation) resulting in *in utero* obstruction to systemic blood flow may thus result in hypoplasia of the systemic left ventricle. Left ventricular outflow obstruction, with the resultant alterations in left ventricular compliance and loss of preload through the foramen ovale, results in left ventricular hypoplasia. Thus, the final anatomy in patients with HLHS is likely dependent on a combination of underlying genetic defects, epigenetic factors, developmental physiology, and intrinsic abnormalities of the myocardium. The relative contribution of each of these factors remains uncertain and probably contributes to the wide spectrum of anatomic lesions.

CLINICAL PRESENTATION AND CLINICAL SIGNS

Among patients presenting in the postnatal period, clinical signs will vary depending on the degree of left heart obstruction, the degree of ductal patency, and the presence of obstructed pulmonary venous return. Patients with an intact atrial septum or other forms of obstructed pulmonary venous return will often present with severe cyanosis immediately at birth. In contrast, those with widely open atrial septum and a PDA may appear normal in the first days of life. Congenital cardiac screening with lower extremity oxygen saturations should identify most patients with HLHS, even before ductal closure.[41] In those not diagnosed at birth, the postnatal decrease in PVR and closing ductus arteriosus result in deterioration, with excessive pulmonary blood flow at the expense of diminishing systemic perfusion. Physical examination is marked by poor peripheral pulses. Chest radiograph and electrocardiogram are usually nondiagnostic. In the current era, approximately 50% of patients will be diagnosed during the prenatal period.[42] This has multiple advantages, permitting prenatal family counseling, delivery planning, and early initiation of prostaglandins to eliminate a period of hypoperfusion and cardiogenic shock. If the diagnosis of an intact atrial septum or restrictive atrial septum is suspected, appropriate preparation for immediate postnatal intervention can be put in place.

Anatomy: Left Heart Obstructive Lesions

Left heart obstructive lesions represent a spectrum of abnormalities with hypoplasia of the aortic valve and left ventricular outflow tract as well as varying degrees of left ventricular and mitral valve hypoplasia. Anatomic variants are generally classified by the patency of the aortic and mitral valves, in part because these have important prognostic implications.[43,44] Aortic atresia is present in approximately 50% of patients with left heart obstructive lesions (**Table 93.2**). Milder versions of HLHS form a continuum with critical aortic stenosis. Consequently, in some cases, the decision for univentricular palliation or biventricular repair may be difficult.

Anatomic features include a hypoplastic aorta (mean ascending aortic diameter of 3.2 mm), a variably hypoplastic aortic arch and, most commonly (75%), a significant coarctation. The coarctation may involve circumferential ductal tissue, which may affect the type of arch reconstruction. Abnormalities of the tricuspid valve and resulting insufficiency are common. Among patients with the aortic atresia/mitral stenosis subtype, ventriculo-coronary connections may be present along with subendocardial fibroelastosis resulting from subendocardial ischemia due to high left ventricular end-diastolic pressures. These patients are often considered to be at increased risk for mortality following the Norwood procedure. The atrial septum may be highly restrictive or intact in up to 10% of patients, and this portends poorer postoperative survival.

TABLE 93.2 Frequency of Anatomic Variants of Left Heart Obstructive Lesions

Inflow and Outflow Anatomy	Frequency	Aortic Anatomy	Frequency
Aortic atresia/mitral atresia (AA/MA)	35%	Aortic atresia	63%
Aortic atresia/mitral stenosis (AA/MS)	37%		
Aortic stenosis/mitral atresia (AS/MA)	5%	Aortic stenosis	37%
Aortic stenosis/mitral stenosis (AS/MS)	12%		
Other variants (Double outlet right ventricle/MA, etc.)	11%		
Other Anatomic Features			
Obstructed pulmonary venous return	3.5%		
Total anomalous pulmonary venous return	1.6%		

Derived on data from Bartram U, Grnenfelder JA. Causes of death after the modified Norwood procedure: a study of 122 postmortem cases. *Ann Thorac Surg.* 1997;64:1795-1802 and Tweddell JS, Sleeper LA, Ohye RG, et al. Intermediate-term mortality and cardiac transplantation in infants with single-ventricle lesions: risk factors and their interaction with shunt type. *J Thorac Cardiovasc Surg.* 2012;144:152.e2-159.e2.

DIAGNOSIS: HLHS

Echocardiography forms the mainstay of the diagnostic evaluation of patients with HLHS. Evaluation should include a detailed anatomic assessment with a particular focus on factors influencing early management. Early identification of an intact or highly restrictive atrial septum is important both for prognostic purposes and to guide urgent or emergent balloon septostomy where appropriate. Other features delineated on echocardiography with the potential to impact treatment strategy and outcomes include the size of the ascending aorta, the aortic arch branching pattern, the function and anatomy of the tricuspid and pulmonary valves, ventricular function, pulmonary venous connections and flow, and the presence of ventriculo-coronary connections. Catheterization is rarely required.

MANAGEMENT: HYPOPLASTIC LEFT HEART SYNDROME

Medical Approach

There is no long-term medical therapy for patients with HLHS. However, the use of prostaglandin is critical to maintenance of ductal patency following birth (or following presentation in those with a postnatal diagnosis). Since its initial description by Olley and colleagues in 1976, prostaglandin E (PGE) has been the mainstay of medical therapies to maintain ductal patency.[45] However, side effects associated with its use include apnea, pulmonary vasodilatation, and compromised gastrointestinal perfusion.[46] Importantly, the side effects are dose dependent, so the lowest dose necessary to maintain ductal patency should be used. In most patients, a dose of 0.01 μg/kg/min should be adequate. Early initiation of PGE among patients with suspected HLHS is critical to minimizing the risk of shock and myocardial ischemia with resultant poorer long-term outcomes.

Beyond the critical aspect of maintaining ductal patency, early perinatal medical management of children with HLHS should be directed at balancing systemic and pulmonary blood flow. The relative blood flow to each compartment will depend on the relative systemic and pulmonary vascular resistances. Potential strategies for manipulating pulmonary blood flow include inhaled respiratory gases and intravenous infusions. Oxygen is a pulmonary vasodilator, while hypercarbia is a potent pulmonary vasoconstrictor. Systemic vasodilators may be used in some patients, especially those with systemic atrioventricular valve regurgitation.

Percutaneous Intervention Approaches

Although completely percutaneous approaches to the management of HLHS are not possible, transcatheter interventions are commonly used in both the initial management of patients with HLHS and in long-term maintenance of optimal physiology. As noted earlier, patients with a highly restrictive or intact atrial septum may benefit from immediate postnatal balloon atrial septostomy. Although a life-saving procedure, patients with obstructed pulmonary venous drainage may have significant fetal pulmonary vascular changes that result in poorer prognosis, even with immediate postnatal decompression.

Hybrid approaches to the early management of HLHS may be used either as a routine palliation strategy or as a rescue intervention in high-risk neonates, to "stage" them to conventional palliation. These approaches include placement of bilateral pulmonary artery bands with stent placement into the ductus to maintain unobstructed systemic cardiac output (**Figure 93.7**). This approach was first reported by Gibbs et al in 1993.[47] By moving the complex cardiac surgical procedure farther away from the vulnerable neonatal period, it was hoped that the hybrid approach would both increase survival and improve neurodevelopmental outcomes.

Unfortunately, despite an increasing number of hybrid procedures being performed, an attendant improvement in

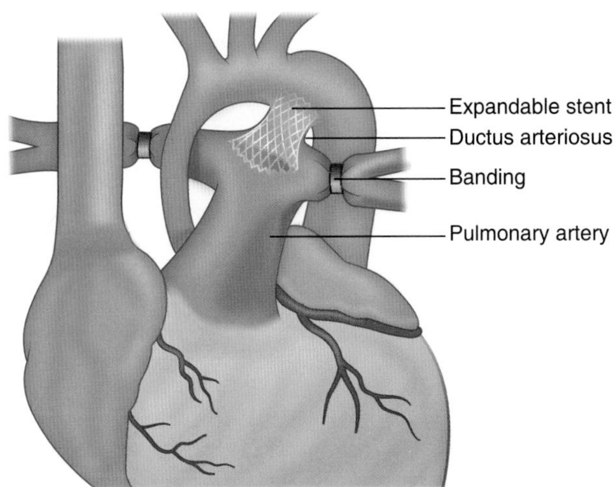

FIGURE 93.7 Hybrid approach to stage 1 palliation includes the application of bilateral pulmonary artery bands and placement of an expandable stent into the ductus arteriosus.

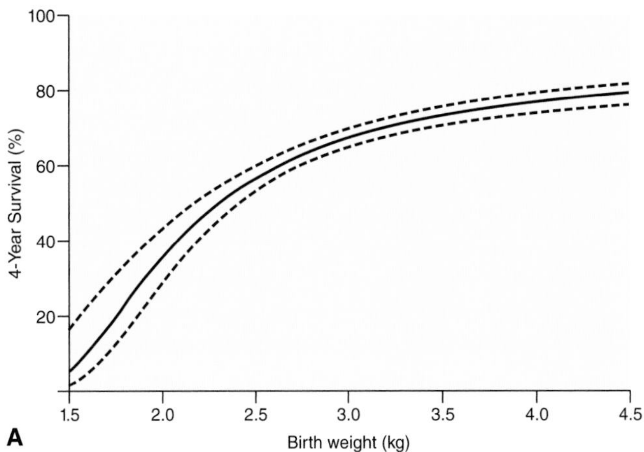

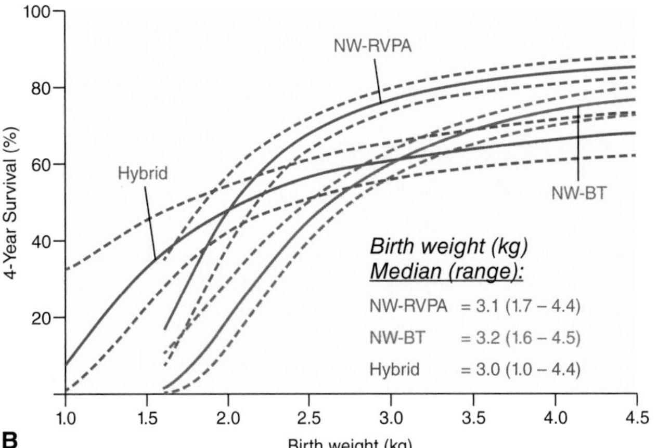

FIGURE 93.8 Outcomes following first stage palliation for patients with hypoplastic left heart syndrome based on birth weight and type of palliation. Lower birth weight is strongly predictive of poor long-term survival. Among the smallest patients, there may be a slight benefit of hybrid procedures over Blalock-Taussig shunts, but this is not true when compared to the right ventricle to pulmonary artery conduit. NW-BT, Norwood operation with a modified Blalock-Taussig shunt; NW-RVPA, Norwood operation with a right ventricle-to-pulmonary artery conduit. (Reprinted from Wilder TJ, McCrindle BW, Hickey EJ, et al.; Congenital Heart Surgeons' Society. Is a hybrid strategy a lower-risk alternative to stage 1 Norwood operation? *J Thorac Cardiovasc Surg.* 2017;153(1):163-172.e6. Copyright © 2016 by The American Association for Thoracic Surgery. With permission.)

outcomes has not been observed.[48] The hybrid procedure has been unable to mitigate the risk associated with several aspects of HLHS palliation (**Figure 93.8**).[49,50]

Despite interval growth before definitive surgical palliation, patients with low birth weight remain at high risk for mortality. The risk of mortality remains high in patients with aortic atresia, likely due to the ongoing risk of myocardial ischemia due to coronary perfusion that is dependent on retrograde arch flow. Finally, banding of the branch pulmonary arteries results in a higher rate of pulmonary artery interventions, which may impact subsequent outcomes following second-stage palliation.[51] While the routine use of hybrid palliation for all HLHS patients is uncommon, the use of hybrid palliation to rescue high-risk neonates, especially those in cardiogenic shock following postnatal presentation, or to bridge patients to transplantation is used at many institutions.[52,53]

Surgical Approaches: Staged Surgical Palliation

Stage 1 Palliation: Norwood Procedure

Successful palliation was first described by Norwood and colleagues in 1983.[37,38] While modifications and technical refinements to the procedure have resulted in better outcomes over time, the goals of initial palliation of HLHS remain unchanged: (1) unobstructed systemic outflow with unrestricted coronary blood flow, (2) unobstructed pulmonary venous return, and (3) controlled pulmonary blood flow. Relief of systemic outflow tract obstruction includes a combination of arch reconstruction (to relieve arch obstruction and treat coarctation) and anastomosis of the pulmonary artery and aorta (to provide unobstructed outflow from the right ventricle to the reconstructed aorta). An atrial septectomy is routinely performed to ensure unobstructed pulmonary venous return into the systemic right ventricle.

Establishment of controlled pulmonary blood flow is commonly accomplished using one of two techniques: a modified BTT shunt or a Sano right ventricle to pulmonary artery conduit.[36] The modified BTT shunt is constructed using a polytetrafluoroethylene (PTFE) tube connecting the innominate artery to the ipsilateral branch pulmonary artery. The Sano shunt uses a larger PTFE tube to connect the right ventricle to the main pulmonary artery, which has the advantage of eliminating diastolic runoff into the pulmonary arteries from the systemic circulation. This runoff contributes to decreased coronary perfusion and may make patients with a modified BTT shunt more susceptible to ischemia and clinical deterioration, particularly in the early

SECTION 7

postoperative period when an elevated diastolic pressure and poor systolic function may follow a long procedure on cardiopulmonary bypass. The primary disadvantage of the Sano shunt is the potential impact of a ventriculotomy on long-term cardiac function.

A multicenter randomized study, the Single Ventricle Reconstruction (SVR) trial, was performed to determine whether one approach had better outcomes.[36] Long-term follow-up is ongoing, but no significant difference has been observed in overall transplant-free survival between the two approaches at current follow-up. Subgroup analysis, however, does suggest that patients with aortic atresia (who may be particularly at risk for coronary ischemia) benefit from the use of a right ventricle to pulmonary artery conduit.[44] In addition, there appears to be an early survival advantage and improved overall survival (including transplants) with the right ventricle to pulmonary artery conduit. However, surgeon and institutional familiarity with the chosen strategy, rather than the particular strategy chosen, may be most important to achieving optimal outcomes.

Surgical Technique: Norwood Procedure

The Norwood procedure is performed via a median sternotomy. Initial dissection focuses on exposing the aortic arch and its branches, as well as the pulmonary arteries and ductus arteriosus. Multiple strategies for cardiopulmonary bypass and organ perfusion during the procedure have been advocated, with none having demonstrated clear superiority. While deep hypothermic circulatory arrest was traditionally employed for the entire arch reconstruction, its use is becoming less common. More commonly, selective cerebral perfusion (at a range of temperatures) is maintained by cannulating the innominate artery (either directly or with a "chimney" graft). Some surgeons advocate using an additional arterial cannula in the descending aorta to limit the risk of acute kidney injury.[53]

Following initiation of bypass and cooling to an appropriate temperature, the main pulmonary artery is divided proximal to its bifurcation. The opening on the distal side is then closed with a patch. The PDA is ligated, and proximal descending aorta is mobilized. The atrial septectomy is then performed, usually through the purse string for right atrial cannulation. At this point, either selective antegrade cerebral perfusion or deep hypothermic circulatory arrest may be used to complete the arch anastomosis. The techniques of an interdigitating arch anastomosis, described by Burkhart and colleagues in Toronto and subsequently by Tweddell and colleagues in Wisconsin, appear to have among the lowest rates of intervention (**Figure 93.9**).[54,55]

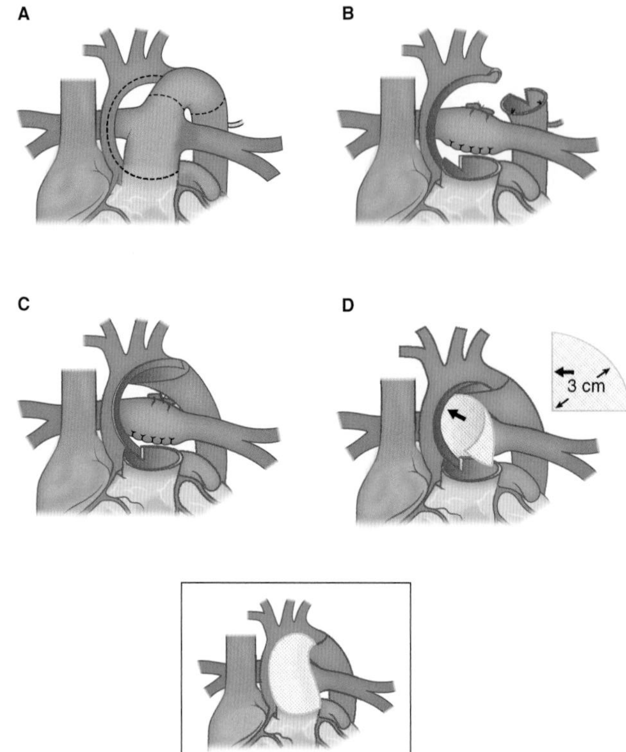

FIGURE 93.9 **(A–D)** and inset coarctectomy combined with an interdigitating arch reconstruction. **(A)** Preoperative anatomy. Dotted lines indicate the areas to be incised. **(B)** The aortic isthmus is divided, and all ductal tissue is excised. The undersurface of the arch is incised, and this incision is carried down the medial aspect of the ascending aorta. Cutbacks are performed in the posterior left lateral aspect of the proximal descending aorta and the pulmonary root leftward of the commissure that is adjacent to the ascending aorta. **(C)** Large interdigitating tissue-to-tissue connection is created between the open distal arch and the descending aorta. The descending aorta can be brought as far proximally as the distal ascending aorta. Finally, the adjacent points of the ascending aorta and pulmonary root cutback are sutured together. **(D)** Patch of homograft material is used to complete the arch reconstruction and neoascending aorta. A flat piece of homograft material is used that is in the shape of a quarter of a circle with a radius of 3 cm. The straight edge of the graft (open arrow) is sutured to the inner curvature, and the curved outer edge of the patch is sutured to the outer curvature. The patch is tailored as the suture-line transitions to the pulmonary root. Although a large portion of the original patch may be trimmed away, the 3-cm radius ensures that the neoascending aorta will be without obstruction because this corresponds to the circumference of the typical pulmonary root of the typical patient undergoing the Norwood Procedure. The final reconstruction is shown in the inset.

However, other options—including attempts at completely autologous reconstruction using a direct pulmonary artery to aortic arch anastomosis—have also been suggested. Key technical aspects of the arch reconstruction include ensuring an open descending aortic anastomosis, achieving a smoothly curved arch, and ensuring patent coronary flow at the proximal end of the amalgamated great vessels. Especially, in the case of aortic atresia, where all coronary flow will be retrograde from the amalgamated great vessels and the ascending aorta is often 2 to 3 mm in diameter, meticulous attention to the site of amalgamation is critical avoiding coronary inflow obstruction.

After completing the arch reconstruction, the modified BTT shunt or the Sano is performed to complete the surgical procedure (**Figure 93.10**).

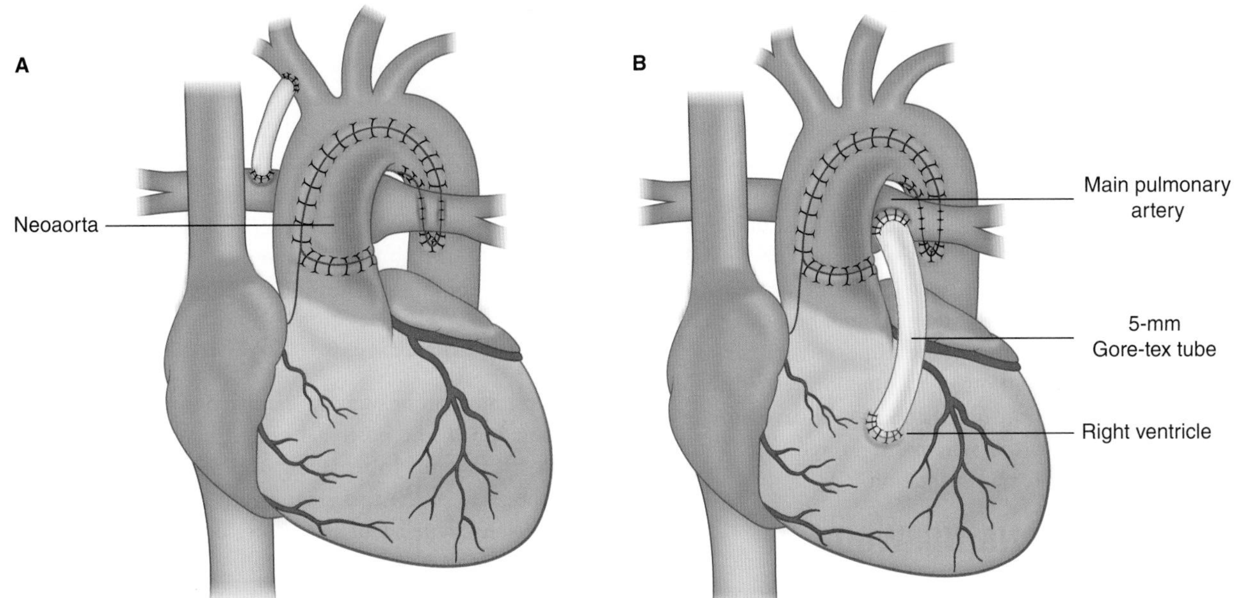

FIGURE 93.10 **(A)** Completed Norwood procedure with a modified Blalock-Taussig-Thomas shunt from the innominate artery to the right pulmonary artery. (Note that the shunt is temporarily clipped before coming off bypass as shown.) **(B)** Alternative pulmonary blood flow provided through a Sano type right ventricle to pulmonary artery conduit.

For placement of a modified BTT shunt, the "chimney" on the innominate artery is often used; this requires recannulation into the patch-augmented neoaortic root. Several techniques for performance of the Sano shunt have been described. The shunt may be placed either to the left or right of the neoaortic root, although placement to the right appears to result in a lower need for interventions. A ringed PTFE graft is commonly used. The distal anastomosis to the pulmonary artery may be constructed into the patch used to close the main pulmonary artery orifice or into native pulmonary artery tissue. Proximally, "dunking" of the ringed graft may have advantages over the larger ventriculotomy necessary to prevent proximal conduit obstruction where dunking is not used.[56] Following completion of the shunt and rewarming, the patient is weaned from cardiopulmonary bypass.

Perioperative Management. Appropriate preoperative management is critical to achieving optimal outcomes with the Norwood procedure. With the advent of PGE infusion, patients should be stabilized and malperfusion resolved before undergoing stage 1 palliation. Hybrid approaches to control pulmonary blood flow may be useful adjuncts when patients present in shock. Postoperatively, management is directed at maintaining systemic cardiac output and optimizing pulmonary function. Increased SVR is common in the postoperative period, and afterload reduction is necessary to control pulmonary blood and optimize systemic cardiac output.[57]

Interstage Period. The interstage period between stage 1 palliation and creation of a superior cavopulmonary connection remains a high-risk period. Factors contributing to this high-risk period include volume loading resulting from a parallel circulation, hypoxia present due to complete mixing, the potential for diastolic runoff, and low coronary perfusion pressure, as well as the deleterious consequences of residual or recurrent lesions including arch obstruction, atrioventricular valve regurgitation, pulmonary artery distortion, obstruction to shunt flow, arrhythmias, and restrictive atrial communication or obstructed pulmonary venous return. Outcomes have improved with comprehensive home monitoring programs, which assist with early identification of patients at risk.

Outcomes: Norwood Procedure. Mortality before second-stage palliation ranges from 5% to 30%.[58,59] In-hospital mortality for the Norwood procedure in the STS database is approximately 15%. Risk factors for mortality include prematurity, low birth weight, extracardiac anomalies, and genetic syndromes, as well as anatomic and physiologic factors such as atrioventricular valve regurgitation, a history of an intact atrial septum, or ventricular dysfunction. Some of these patients may be better managed with early referral to transplantation, especially where risk factors would be eliminated or treated by transplantation (eg, atrioventricular valve regurgitation).

Follow-Up Patient Care and Subsequent Palliation

Second-stage palliation of HLHS is performed following normalization of PVR. At this point, the stage 1 aortopulmonary shunt or right ventricle to pulmonary artery conduit is taken down and the superior caval blood flow is connected to the pulmonary artery through either a bidirectional Glenn anastomosis or a hemi-Fontan. This is usually best performed between 4 and 6 months of age. Creation of a superior cavopulmonary connection results in volume unloading and raises diastolic pressures. This results in improved circulatory stability and entry into a lower risk phase. Subsequent palliation with a Fontan completion creating a total cavopulmonary connection is most commonly performed between 2 and 4 years of age. This results in improved oxygen levels, but at the cost of increased venous pressures within the abdominal compartment. Likely primarily as a result of these increased pressures, patients with a Fontan circulation commonly develop mild hepatic and renal dysfunction, which may progress over time. Fontan failure may occur as the result of end-organ dysfunction related to high venous pressures, anatomic obstruction to the cavopulmonary pathways, or failure of the systemic right ventricle. Patients may go on to need heart transplantation.

FUTURE DIRECTIONS: NORWOOD PROCEDURE

Despite extraordinary advances since Norwood's first successful palliation, mortality for staged palliation remains high. Even successful palliation results in long-term challenges and a high risk of end-organ injury and eventual failure.[62] Better understanding risk factors for poor outcomes and improved prediction of failure of the later stages of palliation are important to improving the long-term prognosis of these patients. Eventually, the use of mechanical circulatory support may become the final stage of palliation, as improvements in ventricular assist devices make long-term "biventricular" support of these patients possible.

KEY POINTS

Ventricular Septal Defect

- ✔ Understanding both the location/rims of the VSD, as well as the anatomy of the surrounding structures (valves, conduction system) is critical to minimize the risk of iatrogenic injury.
- ✔ Small residual defects (<2 mm on echo) are often clinically insignificant and well-tolerated and may close on their own with time.
- ✔ Taking shallow suture bites (so that the needle is still visible) through the endocardium on the right ventricle is the optimal technique to avoid heart block during a VSD repair.

Tetralogy of Fallot

- ✔ Patients that are experiencing desaturation as the presenting symptomatology should be immediately referred to a center with pediatric cardiac surgical backup/coverage.
- ✔ Differentiating a hypercyanotic spell from less concerning episodes of cyanosis in infants with neonates should be approached carefully. It is preferable to "over diagnose" than "under diagnose" hypercyanotic spells.
- ✔ Pulmonary valve replacement is a common intervention required in adults with repaired TOF. Close collaboration between surgical and catheterization lab/intervention teams provides the optimal forum for decision-making and support for intervention.
- ✔ Familiarity with the AHA/ACC consensus guidelines for the common adult CHD pathologies is worthwhile for the less commonly encountered pathologies.

Hypoplastic Left Heart Syndrome

- ✔ Optimization of systemic cardiac output and end-organ function in the postnatal period before surgical palliation is essential to achieving optimal outcomes.
- ✔ The goals of the first stage palliation in HLHS remain unchanged: relief of left ventricular outflow tract and aortic arch obstruction, ensuring unrestricted pulmonary venous flow into the right atrium, and provision of controlled pulmonary blood flow.
- ✔ The interdigitating arch anastomosis appears to have the best long-term outcomes.
- ✔ By augmenting systemic cardiac output and limiting excessive pulmonary circulation, afterload reduction plays a key role in early postoperative management.
- ✔ The time period between first- and second-stage palliation remains a period of high-mortality risk and requires close follow-up and early evaluation of signs of residual or recurrent lesions.

REFERENCES

1. van der Linde D, Konings EE, Slager MA, et al. Birth prevalence of congenital heart disease worldwide: a systematic review and meta-analysis. *J Am Coll Cardiol.* 2011;58(21):2241-2247.
2. Holland BJ, Myers JA, Woods CR Jr. Prenatal diagnosis of critical congenital heart disease reduces risk of death from cardiovascular compromise prior to planned neonatal cardiac surgery: a meta-analysis. *Ultrasound Obstet Gynecol.* 2015;45(6):631-638.
3. Menahem S, Sehgal A, Meagher S. Early detection of significant congenital heart disease: the contribution of fetal cardiac ultrasound and newborn pulse oximetry screening. *J Paediatr Child Health.* 2021;57(3):323-327.
4. Nees SN, Chung WK. The genetics of isolated congenital heart disease. *Am J Med Genet C Semin Med Genet.* 2020;184(1):97-106.
5. Gross RE, Hubbard JP. Surgical ligation of a patent ductus arteriosus. Report of first successful case. *J Am Med Assoc.* 1939;112:729-731.
6. Crafoord D, Nyhlin G. Congenital coarctation of the aorta and its surgical management. *J Thorac Surg.* 1945;14:347-361.
7. Blalock A, Taussig HB. The surgical treatment of malformations of the heart in which there is pulmonary stenosis or atresia. *J Am Med Assoc.* 1945;132:189-202.
8. Gibbon JH Jr. Application of a mechanical heart and lung apparatus to cardiac surgery. *Minn Med.* 1954;37:171-180.
9. Cohn LH. Fifty years of open-heart surgery. *Circulation.* 2003;107(17):2168-2170.

10. Lopez L, Houyel L, Colan SD, et al. Classification of ventricular septal defects for the eleventh iteration of the international classification of diseases-striving for consensus: a report from the International Society for Nomenclature of Paediatric and Congenital Heart Disease. *Ann Thorac Surg*. 2018;106(5):1578-1589.
11. Penny DJ, Vick GW 3rd. Ventricular septal defect. *Lancet*. 2011;377(9771):1103-1112.
12. Fuller S. Ventricular septal defects. In: Kaiser LR, Kron IL, Spray TL, eds. *Mastery of Cardiothoracic Surgery*. 3rd ed. Wolters Kluwer; 2014:829-837.
13. Ardehali A, Chen JM. Ventricular septal defect. In: *Khonsari's Cardiac Surgery: Safeguards and Pitfalls in Operative Technique*. 5th ed. Wolters Kluwer; 2017:262-270.
14. Morray BH. Ventricular septal defect closure devices, techniques, and outcomes. *Interv Cardiol Clin*. 2019;8(1):1-10.
15. Jacobs JP, Mayer JE Jr, Pasquali SK, et al. The society of thoracic surgeons congenital heart surgery database: 2019 update on outcomes and quality. *Ann Thorac Surg*. 2019;107(3):691-704.
16. Bibevski S, Ruzmetov M, Mendoza L, et al. The destiny of postoperative residual ventricular septal defects after surgical repair in infants and children. *World J Pediatr Congenit Heart Surg*. 2020;11(4):438-443.
17. Stout KK, Daniels CJ, Aboulhosn JA, et al. 2018 AHA/ACC Guideline for the management of adults with congenital heart disease: a report of the American College of Cardiology/American Heart Association Task Force on Clinical Practice Guidelines. *Circulation*. 2019;139(14):e698-e800.
18. Jaquiss J. Commentary: precision surgery for cyanotic neonatal patients with tetralogy. *J Thorac Cardiovasc Surg*. 2020;159:1477-1478.
19. Van Praagh R. The first Stella Van Praagh Memorial Lecture: the history and anatomy of tetralogy of Fallot. *Sem Thorac Cardiovasc Surg*. 2009;12:19-38.
20. Vida VL, Guariento A, Zucchetta F, et al. Preservation of the pulmonary valve during early repair of tetralogy of Fallot: surgical techniques. *Semin Thorac Cardiovasc Surg Pediatr Card Surg Ann*. 2016;19:75-81.
21. Bacha EA, Scheule AM, Zurakowski D, et al. Lont-term results after early primary repair of tetralogy of Fallot. *J Thorac Cardiovasc Surg*. 2001;122:154-161.
22. VanArsdell GS, Maharaj GS, Tom J, et al. What is the optimal age for repair of tetralogy of Fallot? *Circulation*. 2000;102:Iii-123-129.
23. Al Habib HF, Jacops JP, Mavroudis C, et al. Contemporary patterns of management of tetralogy of Fallot: data from the Society of Thoracic Surgeons Database. *Ann Thorac Surg*. 2010;90:813-819; discussion 819-20.
24. Salva JJ, Faerber JA, Juang Y-SV, et al. 2-year outcomes after complete or staged procedure for tetralogy of Fallot in neonates. *J Am Coll Cardiol*. 2019;74:1570-1579.
25. Smith CA, McCracken C, Thomas AS, et al. Long-term outcomes of tetralogy of Fallot: a study from the Pediatric Cardiac Care Consortium. *JAMA Cardiol*. 2019;4:34-41. doi: 10.1001/jamamcardio.2018.4255
26. Hancock Friesen CL, Jaquiss RDB. Is the die cast by surgeon's choice or patient's anatomy? Late outcomes in tetralogy of Fallot. Invited Commentary. *Can J Cardiol*. 2021;37:184-185. doi: 04/2020;10.1016/j.cjca.2020.03.039
27. Jeon B, Kim D-H, Kwon BS, Choi ES, Park CS, Yun T-J. Surgical treatment of tetralogy of Fallot in symptomatic neonates and young infants. *J Thorac Cardiovasc Surg*. 2020;159:1466-1476.
28. Goldstein BH, Petit CJ, Qureshi AM, et al. Comparison of management strategies for neonates with symptomatic tetralogy of Fallot. *J Am Coll Cardiol*. 2021;77:1093-1106.
29. Sandoval JP, Chaturvedi RR, Benson L, et al. Right ventricular outflow tract stenting in tetralogy of Fallot infants with risk factors for early primary repair. *Circ Cardiovasc Intervent*. 2016;9:e003979.
30. Quandt D, Ramchandani B, Stickley J, et al. Stenting of the right ventricular outflow tract promotes better pulmonary arterial growth compared with modified Blalock-Taussig shunt palliation in tetralogy of Fallot-type lesions. *J Am Coll Cardiol Intervent*. 2017;10:1774-1784.
31. Glatz AC, Petit CJ, Goldstein BH, et al. Comparison between patent ductus arteriosus stent and modified Blalock-Taussig shunt as palliation for infants with ductal-dependent pulmonary blood flow: insights from the Congenital Catheterization Research Collaborative. *Circulation*. 2019;137:589-601.
32. VanArsdell GS, Levi DS. Neonatal tetralogy staged versus complete repair: is it time to rethink neonatal tetralogy? Editorial comment. *J Am Coll Cardiol*. 2019;74:1580-1581.
33. Therrien J, Siu SC, McLaughlin PR, et al. Pulmonary valve replacement in adults late after repair of tetralogy of Fallot: are we operating too late? *J Am Coll Cardiol*. 2000;36:1670-1675.
34. Mongeon F-P, Ali WB, Khairy P, et al. Pulmonary valve replacement for pulmonary regurgitation in adults with tetralogy of Fallot: a meta-analysis. A report for the writing committee of the 2019 update of the Canadian Cardiovascular Society Guidelines for the management of adults with congenital heart disease. *Can J Cardiol*. 2019;35:1772-1783.
35. Parker SE, Mai CT, Canfield MA, et al.; and National Birth Defects Prevention Network. Updated National Birth Prevalence estimates for selected birth defects in the United States, 2004-2006. *Birth Defects Res A Clin Mol Teratol*. 2010;88:1008-1016.
36. Ohye RG, Sleeper LA, Mahony L, et al. Comparison of shunt types in the Norwood procedure for single-ventricle lesions. *N Engl J Med*. 2010;362:1980-1992.
37. Norwood WI, Lang P, Hansen DD. Physiologic repair of aortic atresia-hypoplastic left heart syndrome. *N Engl J Med*. 1983;308:23-26.
38. Brenner JI, Berg KA, Schneider DS, Clark EB, Boughman JA. Cardiac malformations in relatives of infants with hypoplastic left-heart syndrome. *Am J Dis Child*. 1989;143:1492-1494.
39. Radhakrishna U, Albayrak S, Alpay-Savasan Z, et al. Genome-wide DNA methylation analysis and epigenetic variations associated with congenital aortic valve stenosis (AVS). *PLos One*. 2016;11:e0154010.
40. Hornberger LK, Sanders SP, Rein AJ, Spevak PJ, Parness IA, Colan SD. Left heart obstructive lesions and left ventricular growth in the midtrimester fetus. A longitudinal study. *Circulation*. 1995;92:1531-1538.
41. de-Wahl Granelli A, Wennergren M, Sandberg K, et al. Impact of pulse oximetry screening on the detection of duct dependent congenital heart disease: a Swedish prospective screening study in 39,821 newborns. *BMJ*. 2009;338:a3037.
42. Ailes EC, Gilboa SM, Riehle-Colarusso T, et al.; National Birth Defects Prevention Study. Prenatal diagnosis of nonsyndromic congenital heart defects. *Prenat Diagn*. 2014;34:214-222.
43. Bartram U, Grnenfelder JA. Causes of death after the modified Norwood procedure: a study of 122 postmortem cases. *Ann Thorac Surg*. 1997;64:1795-1802.
44. Tweddell JS, Sleeper LA, Ohye RG, et al. Intermediate-term mortality and cardiac transplantation in infants with single-ventricle lesions: risk factors and their interaction with shunt type. *J Thorac Cardiovasc Surg*. 2012;144:152.e2-159.e2.
45. Olley PM, Coceani F, Bodach E. E-type prostaglandins: a new emergency therapy for certain cyanotic congenital heart malformations. *Circulation*. 1976;53:728-731.
46. McElhinney DB, Hedrick HL, Bush DM, et al. Necrotizing enterocolitis in neonates with congenital heart disease: risk factors and outcomes. *Pediatrics*. 2000;106:1080-1087.
47. Gibbs JL, Wren C, Watterson KG, Hunter S, Hamilton JRL. Stenting of the arterial duct combined with banding of the pulmonary arteries and atrial septectomy or septostomy: a new approach to palliation for the hypoplastic left heart syndrome. *Br Heart J*. 1993;69:551-555.
48. Galantowicz M, Cheatham JP, Phillips A, et al. Hybrid approach for hypoplastic left heart syndrome: intermediate results after the learning curve. *Ann Thorac Surg*. 2008;85:2063-2071.
49. Davies RR, Radtke W, Bhat MA, Baffa JM, Woodford E, Pizarro C. Hybrid palliation for critical systemic outflow obstruction: neither rapid stage 1 Norwood nor comprehensive stage 2 mitigate consequences of early risk factors. *J Thorac Cardiovasc Surg*. 2015;149:182-191.
50. Wilder TJ, McCrindle BW, Hickey EJ, et al.; Congenital Heart Surgeons' Society. Is a hybrid strategy a lower-risk alternative to stage 1 Norwood operation? *J Thorac Cardiovasc Surg*. 2017;153:163.e6-172.e6.
51. Davies RR, Radtke WA, Klenk D, Pizarro C. Bilateral pulmonary arterial banding results in an increased need for subsequent pulmonary artery interventions. *J Thorac Cardiovasc Surg*. 2014;147:706-712.

52. Karamlou T, Overman D, Hill KD, et al. Stage 1 hybrid palliation for hypoplastic left heart syndrome-assessment of contemporary patterns of use: an analysis of The Society of Thoracic Surgeons Congenital Heart Surgery Database. *J Thorac Cardiovasc Surg*. 2015;149:195.e1-202.e1.
53. Hammel JM, Deptula JJ, Karamlou T, Wedemeyer E, Abdullah I, Duncan KF. Newborn aortic arch reconstruction with descending aortic cannulation improves postoperative renal function. *Ann Thorac Surg*. 2013;96:1721-1726.
54. Lamers LJ, Frommelt PC, Mussatto KA, Jaquiss RDB, Mitchell ME, Tweddell JS. Coarctectomy combined with an interdigitating arch reconstruction results in a lower incidence of recurrent arch obstruction after the Norwood procedure than coarctectomy alone. *J Thorac Cardiovasc Surg*. 2012;143:1098-1102.
55. Burkhart HM, Ashburn DA, Konstantinov IE, et al. Interdigitating arch reconstruction eliminates recurrent coarctation after the Norwood procedure. *J Thorac Cardiovasc Surg*. 2005;130:61-65.
56. Baird CW, Myers PO, Borisuk M, Pigula FA, Emani SM. Ring-reinforced Sano conduit at Norwood stage I reduces proximal conduit obstruction. *Ann Thorac Surg*. 2015;99:171-179.
57. Tweddell JS, Hoffman GM, Fedderly RT, et al. Phenoxybenzamine improves systemic oxygen delivery after the Norwood procedure. *Ann Thorac Surg*. 1999;67:161-167; discussion 167-8.
58. Ghanayem NS, Allen KR, Tabbutt S, et al. Interstage mortality after the Norwood procedure: results of the multicenter Single Ventricle Reconstruction trial. *J Thorac Cardiovasc Surg*. 2012;144:896-906.
59. Tweddell JS, Hoffman GM, Mussatto KA, et al. Improved survival of patients undergoing palliation of hypoplastic left heart syndrome: lessons learned from 115 consecutive patients. *Circulation*. 2002;106:I82-I89.

CHAPTER 94

CHEST WALL INFECTIONS FOLLOWING OPEN HEART SURGERY

Michael A. Wait

INTRODUCTION

Epidemiology

The majority of coronary artery bypass grafting (CABG) and valvular repair or replacement operations are performed through a median sternotomy incision. This procedure was first reported in the journal *Lancet* in 1897[1] by the British surgeon Herbert Meyrick Nelson Milton at the Kasr El Aini Hospital in Cairo for the treatment of tuberculous lymphadenopathy; later, it was reintroduced by Ormand Julian in 1957 to replace the more painful and disfiguring bilateral anterior thoracotomy for open heart surgery and then in 1964 for CABG.[2] The two most catastrophic complications of the median sternotomy soon followed—dehiscence and deep sternal wound infection (DSWI) with mediastinitis.[3] Indeed, Milton's second patient suffered fatal sternotomy dehiscence. The overall incidence of deep sternotomy wound infection or dehiscence is relatively uncommon, ranging from 0.1% to 5%. Oakley et al provided a review in 1996 in which centers reported incidences from 0.1% to 2%. The National Nosocomial Infection Surveillance (NNIS) system of the Centers for Disease Control and Prevention (CDC) in 1997 reported a sternal infection rate of 3.7%. More recently, the Society of Thoracic Surgeons (STS) Databank, a prospective registry, which has recorded outcome events of over 6 million cardiac surgical procedures since 1989, reports a DSWI incidence of 0.4%.[4]

The morbidity and mortality rate of DSWI is substantial. Mortality rates for DSWI as high as 30% have been reported[5] and are dependent upon the virulence of the infecting agent, patient comorbidities, and treatment modality used to effect healing of such an infection. DSWI morbidity includes suffering, chronic debility, reoperation, prolonged hospital stay (9-20 days), and cost.[6] Patients with DSWI experience on average an additional hospital cost of $20,000 in the first year in 1999 dollars; infected patients who died experienced an additional $60,547 more than those who survived. In 2008, an effort to control hospital costs and compel physicians to prevent DSWI was initiated by the Centers for Medicare & Medicaid Services (CMMS); acting in concert with the Deficit Reduction Act of 2006, CMMS established a list of hospital-acquired conditions (HAC) which, when acquired during hospitalization (ie, not present on admission), do not qualify the facility for additional payment (http://www.cms.gov/HospitalAcqCond/downloads/HACFactsheet.pdf).

Mediastinitis following CABG is one of the 12 listed HACs in this government action.

Risk Factors

Risk factors associated with a deep sternotomy wound infection can be categorized as occurring in the preoperative,[7,8] intraoperative, and postoperative phase of care; risk factors can also be considered modifiable and unmodifiable (**Table 94.1**).

Preoperative risk factors are primarily those related to patient conditions and comorbidities. Operative factors that contribute to wound infection are listed in Table 94.1. Antibiotic prophylaxis is proven to prevent surgical site infections. However, the timing of antibiotic prophylaxis more than 60 minutes before incision or more than 30 minutes after incision and variance of antibiotic choice to a nonrecommended prophylaxis agent is associated with DSWI. Use of bone wax as a topical hemostatic agent on the sternal bone marrow, intra-aortic balloon pump use, indiscriminate use of the Bovie electrocautery device, undrained fluid collections (especially blood), cardiopulmonary bypass time, total operative time, and operation in addition to CABG—such as a valve-CABG procedure—also contribute to the risk of DSWI.[8] Postoperative factors include the following: shock, need for a postop tracheostomy, poorly controlled hyperglycemia.

Interest was generated from the observation that patients who were on statin agents experienced fewer wound infections. Although the preoperative administration of statins has been demonstrated in cohort studies to reduce the incidence of all infections, they were not specifically linked to a statistically significant reduction in specific infections, such as DSWI.[9]

Blood transfusion following cardiac surgery has also been associated with increased infection risk,[10] which was not mitigated by the use of leukocyte-depleted blood products.[11] A tiered-level effect was observed in a study published by Murphy et al[12]; in a stepwise fashion, the infection rate was 3.9% in patients receiving up to 2 units of packed red blood cells, 6.9% for those receiving 3 to 5 units, and as high as 22% in those receiving 6 units of blood or more. Logistic regression analysis showed that the most significant predictor of infection was transfusion amount; the increased risk of infection was postulated to be related to transfusion-mediated immunomodulation. Relevant to blood transfusions, the independent effect of preoperative anemia has been evaluated but not demonstrated to directly affect the rate of sternal wound complications.[13]

TABLE 94.1 Patient and Operative Risk Factors Influencing Surgical Site Infections

Patient Risk Factors	Operative Risk Factors

• Age
• Septicemia
• Smoking/chronic obstructive pulmonary disease
• Peripheral vascular disease
• Obesity
• Diabetes, elevated hemoglobin A1c
• Chronic kidney disease
• End-stage renal disease on dialysis
• Chronic desquamating skin conditions (eczema, psoriasis)
• Connective tissue disease
• Presence of a colostomy
• Malnutrition
• Immunosuppression
• Prolonged mechanical ventilation
	• Skin Prep
	  • skin antisepsis
	  • skin shaving versus clipping
	• Duration of surgery
	• Antimicrobial prophylaxis, timing
	• Operating room and instrument antisepsis
	• Sterile technique break
	• Glycemic control
	• Surgical technique
	  • hemostasis, bleeding, transfusion
	  • dead space obliteration
	  • tissue trauma
	  • internal thoracic artery skeletonization vs pedicled
	  • bone marrow hemostatic agent

Hemoglobin A1c influences the risk of developing a wound infection. A single-center study from UT Southwestern Medical Center demonstrated that every 1% increase in preoperative hemoglobin A1c is associated with a 13% relative risk increase for a wound infection.[14] In addition, perioperative glycemic control—independent of hemoglobin A1c—influences the incidence of sternotomy wound infections and mediastinitis.[15]

The effect of single versus bilateral internal thoracic artery harvesting on the incidence of severe sternal wound complications has been extensively studied. In the Arterial Revascularization Trial,[16] patients were randomly assigned to undergo single ($N = 1554$) versus bilateral ($N = 1548$) internal thoracic artery grafting during CABG procedures; 23% of patients enrolled were diabetic. Although not a primary end-point of this trial, sternal wound complications (1.9% vs 3.5% in the single versus bilateral graft group, respectively) and sternal wound reconstruction (0.6% vs 2.0% in the single versus bilateral graft group, respectively) were not statistically different.

PATHOGENESIS

Infectious sternotomy incision complications can be classified as superficial or deep according to the STS guidelines and the 1988 CDC definitions for nosocomial infections[17]; superficial wound infections (SWI) are those limited to the epidermis, dermis, and superficial subcutaneous adipose. Additionally, SWI must include at least one of the following:

1. purulent drainage is present;
2. an organism is isolated from the incision;
3. at least one of the following symptoms is present: tenderness, swelling, redness, or heat;
4. the incision is opened by a surgeon; or
5. diagnosis is made by the surgeon or attending physician.

Infections involving the pectoralis fascia, sternal wires, sternal bone, or mediastinum collectively represent deep sternal wound infections (DSWI). DSWI must satisfy at least one of the following criteria:

1. an organism is isolated from a culture of mediastinal fluid or tissue;
2. evidence of mediastinitis is seen during operation or by histopathologic examination;
3. one of the following is present; fever greater than 38 °C, chest pain, sternal instability, *and* there is either purulent drainage from the mediastinum or an organism isolated from blood culture or culture of drainage of the mediastinal area. If organisms from common skin flora (coagulase-negative Staphylococci, diphtheroids, *Bacillus* species, *Propionibacterium* species) were isolated, two positive cultures with the same strain are required.[17]

SWI are more common than DSWI and can be adequately treated with local wound care, oral or parenteral antibiotics, and limited wound debridement. If during debridement of an infected sternotomy incision, the sternal wires become exposed, by definition it is classified as a DSWI.

Sternotomy wound infections more commonly follow CABG procedures than valve procedures, suggesting that the use of the internal thoracic artery causes devascularization of the ipsilateral hemisternum, which contributes to wound separation and necrosis, and subsequently progresses to a DSWI. Foreign bodies such as bone marrow wax are widely held to be a major contributory operative factor leading to DSWI. Bone wax is a hydrophobic derivative of petroleum by way of paraffin oil, combined with sterilized *Cera Alba* (the common honeybee) wax, and is used as a bone marrow hemostatic agent during sternotomy incisions for open heart surgery. Bone wax as a hemostatic agent works by mechanical occlusion of transected vessels in cancellous bone. Although highly efficacious, bone wax nonetheless behaves as a foreign body.[18]

The morbidity and mortality rate of patients who suffer DSWI is considerably higher than in those patients who do not experience DSWI; Tewarie et al reported a 20% mortality rate with infection (vs 0% without),[19] and Levi et al reported a 30% mortality rate for DSWI, which occurred in 0.67% of their study population.[5] Hospital length of stay was extended by 12 to 18 days for those cases which occurred during the same index hospitalization as the open heart procedure.[20]

The microbiology of DSWI is predominantly but not exclusively bacterial; *Staphylococcus aureus, Staphylococcus epidermidis,* and α-hemolytic Streptococcus continue to predominate, with Gram-negative aerobic and anaerobic bacteria contributing to a lesser extent.[21] Predominant anaerobes include *Prevotella* sp., *Porphyromonas* sp., *Peptostreptococcus* sp., *Propiobacter* sp., and *Bacteroides fragilis.* From a study by Ford et al, a higher proportion of Gram-negative bacteria (75% of cases) and fungal (9%) relative to Gram-positive bacteria (16%) were seen in patients whose only identifiable risk factor was prolonged intubation, mechanical ventilation, nasogastric suction, and time to enteral nutrition.[22] They concluded that gut translocation as a consequence of disuse was the major contributing factor in those infections.

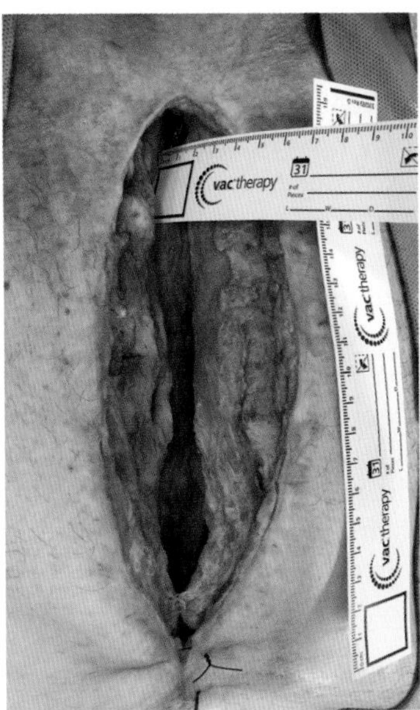

FIGURE 94.1 Median sternotomy incision demonstrating deep sternal wound infection. *Candida albicans* and *Corynebacterium striatum* were isolated on deep wound culture.

CLINICAL PRESENTATION

Common Signs and Symptoms

Common symptoms of DSWI are subjective fever, chills, anorexia, malaise, and wound drainage, which may be experienced as serous, sanguineous, or purulent. Sternal instability manifest by the sensation of positional sternal motion of each hemisterna relative to the other can occur. Signs of DSWI with dehiscence include objective fever, wound edge separation with purulent drainage, cellulitis, wound erythema, and subcutaneous abscess formation (**Figure 94.1**).

Major exsanguinating bleeding can be a sign of extension of the infection into the pericardium with the erosion of the mediastinal infection into arterial or vein grafts, the ascending aorta, or right ventricle. Distraction of sternal edges which have become densely adherent to the surface of the right ventricle can occur simultaneously with an acute increase in right ventricular pressure as occurs in coughing, sneezing, and vomiting. This causes a shear force, which exceeds the tensile strength of the inflamed heart. Sharp sternal edges, bone fragments, and fractured sternal wires can contribute to the injury by causing laceration of the right ventricle.[23]

Differential Diagnosis

The main differential diagnosis is distinguishing superficial from deep infection, and either of these conditions from aseptic fat necrosis or a sterile soft tissue or sternal dehiscence.[17] The presence of fever, pain out of proportion to the exam, purulent drainage, and cultures from the incisional wound or blood will usually suffice to make a secure differential diagnosis. When these clinical measures do not suffice, then the clinical suspicion of a DSWI can be established by the results of a radionuclide scintigraphy. With this technique, 99mTc-hexamethylene-propylene amine oxime HMPAO-labeled leukocytes are infused and the patient is scanned at 4 and 20 hours postinfusion. The diagnosis is established by the finding of tracer-avid uptake in the mediastinum in the proper clinical setting. The major benefit of this test is the high negative predictive value (~100%)[24] such that a negative test essentially rules out the presence of an infection.

MANAGEMENT OF STERNOTOMY WOUND INFECTION

The best practice management of sternotomy wound infection or sternal dehiscence has its basis in prevention. The basis of surgical prophylaxis of DSWI has well established: disinfectant skin preparation, surgical site electric clipping, iodine-impregnated adhesive skin barriers (eg, Ioban: 3M; St. Paul, MN, USA), adequate drainage of subcutaneous and substernal fluid collections, meticulous surgical hemostasis, strict perioperative and preoperative glycemic control, prophylactic antibiotics, and proper sternal closure.[18,25-28] With regard to topical skin disinfectant use, the addition of chlorhexidine (a longer-acting disinfectant that extends to 48 hours) to topical isopropyl alcohol was demonstrated to reduce mediastinitis from 4.2% to 1.9% ($P = .0002$).[27] Antibiotic prophylaxis can take the form of intranasal mupirocin, intravenous antibiotics, and locally delivered antibiotic therapy. Intravenous cefuroxime or cefazolin are the antibiotics recommended for prophylaxis according to the published STS guidelines[25] for those patients who are not cephalosporin allergic; the addition of the vancomycin to standard beta-lactam coverage in patients at a high risk of staphylococcal infection is also an STS guideline recommendation. Since *Staphylococcus* aureus is the most common (80%) microorganism isolated from SWI and DSWI, the demonstration of colonization of the anterior nasal vestibule becomes an important factor in infection prophylaxis. One study showed that 10.8% of *S. aureus* carriers developed sternal wound infection (90% of which were due to *S. aureus*) compared with only 1.8% wound infection rate in noncarriers (47% of which were due to *S. aureus*).[29] Nasal application of the antistaphylococcal bactericidal topical antibiotic mupirocin (2% mupirocin in a polyethylene glycol base) can clear methicillin-sensitive and methicillin-resistant *Staphylococcus*. However, in a randomized, placebo-controlled trial, prophylactic intranasal mupirocin administered to *S. aureus* carriers did not reduce the rates of overall surgical site infections by *S. aureus*.[30]

Although nonsternotomy approaches to cardiac surgery have emerged, the median sternotomy approach is the most utilized incision for CABG and valve repair or replacement surgery. Proper sternal closure follows four basic orthopedic principles, which date back into the 1950s:

1. anatomic fracture reduction and fixation to restore anatomical relationships
2. stable fixation
3. preservation of blood supply to the bone and surrounding soft tissue
4. early active mobilization of the patient

Sternotomy closure usually involves the placement of stainless steel nonbraided cerclage wires, which oppose the right and left hemisternal haves so that bony symphysis and neo-osteogenesis can occur (**Table 94.2**). Variations in the surgical technique of cerclage wire placement (simple single wires, double wires, alternative configuration [figure-of-eight, basket], braided stainless steel cables) have been studied as well as alternatives to sternal cerclage wires (broad plastic bands [Sternal ZipFix; Synthes CMF, West Chester, PA, USA], titanium plates with cortical screws, interlocking talon claw devices, wire-reinforced sternal cleat). The COSTA study[31] was a randomized trial that compared two closure techniques in patients at risk for an adverse sternal outcome following sternotomy. The techniques compared were standard stainless steel cerclage wires (N = 168) versus the Sternal Talon (Gebruder Martin GmbH & Co. KG-KLS Martin Group, Tuttlingen, Germany; N = 170). The 30-day primary endpoint of mediastinitis or sternal instability was similar for both techniques (4.7% vs 6.2%, respectively). A randomized trial comparing cerclage wires to rigid plate fixation (SternaLock blu; Zimmer Biomet, Jacksonville, FL, USA) in a modestly elevated-risk population demonstrated significantly improved radiographic evidence of sternal osteosynthesis and healing but no difference in SWI or DSWI.[32]

The addition of a depot formulation of local-delivery antibiotic was systematically evaluated in the Sternal Wound Infection and Other Postoperative End Points (SWIPE-1) trial of 1502 US patients with diabetes, high body mass index, or both undergoing cardiac surgery.[26] In these individuals at high risk of infection, the use of two gentamicin-collagen sponges compared with no intervention did not reduce the 90-day sternal wound infection rate or total infection rate. In a retrospective study, the application of vancomycin paste to the sternal edges of patients undergoing cardiac operations was not associated with a reduced risk of DSWI.[33]

The avoidance of bone marrow wax is an important contributing factor in the prevention of DSWI and sternal dehiscence. Nonunion of the sternum occurs in 2% to 8% of patients who undergo trans-sternal cardiac surgery; sterile fibrous nonunion without concomitant infection occurs in 0.5% to 5% of sternotomy cases. Bone wax, used as a topical hemostatic agent in sternal bone marrow, induces inflammation, fibrosis, foreign body reaction, and impairs osteoblast migration and normal wound healing; it is resistant to biodegradation by macrophages and retards osteoconductive capacity of bone.[8] Two other bone marrow hemostatic agents have been reviewed and compared with bone wax relevant to wound complications. Ostene (Ceremed, Inc., Los Angeles, CA, USA) is a water-soluble alkylene oxide copolymer with mechanical properties and hemostatic action similar to bone wax, but it is biodegradable and completely removed from the bone surface within 48 hours.[34] Boneseal (Terumo Cardiovascular Systems; Ann Arbor, MI, USA) is a composite of hydroxyapatite and polylactic acid also with wax-like physical properties; it was found to promote

TABLE 94.2 Surgical Techniques of Sternal Closure

Type	Manufacturer's Products

• Surgical stainless steel wires
  • simple single
  • double wires
• Alternative configuration
  • figure-of-eight
  • basket
	• A&E Medical™ Single wire sternum Sutures: A&E Medical, Farmingdale, NJ, USA
	• A&E Medical™ DoubleWire™ Sternum Sutures: A&E Medical, Farmingdale, NJ, USA

Braided stainless steel cables	Pioneer Surgical Technology, Marquette, MI, USA
Plastic bands	Sternal ZipFix: Synthes CMF, West Chester, PA, USA
Titanium plates with cortical screws	SternaLock Blue: Zimmer Biomet, Warsaw, IN, USA
Rachet interlocking claw	Sternal Talon: KLS Martin, Jacksonville, FL, USA
Wire-reinforced sternal cleat	AcuTie: Acumed, Hillsboro, OR, USA

neo-osteogenesis. A prospective randomized trial comparing Boneseal and Ostene in cardiothoracic surgery is ongoing.[35]

One of the commonly cited risk factors for a DSWI is the relative amount of tissue hypoxia that occurs in a sternotomy incision, which undergoes closure. By virtue of internal thoracic artery harvesting, the sternal edge loses significant blood supply, especially if injudicious use of electrocautery is utilized on the periosteum, and if bone wax is used as a marrow hemostatic agent. The thin coagulum of blood between the halves of the sternal marrow also contributes to a healing wound with low-tissue oxygenation. Hyperbaric oxygen has been used to treat refractory infected wounds, especially following radiation therapy, where wound hypoxia is a major contributing factor. Thus, there is a theoretical basis for its use in medically refractory DSWI, where adjunctive surgical options are either not available or not advisable. However, the level of evidence supporting hyperbaric oxygen use is only anecdotal, and presently, it can only be considered on a compassionate use basis.[36]

Negative pressure wound therapy is a topically applied vacuum dressing therapy, a relatively new adjunctive therapy in the prevention and management of DSWI. Negative pressure wound therapy reduces wound edema and exudates, decreases time to definitive closure, stimulates fibroblast proliferation and angiogenesis, and improves parasternal blood flow after internal mammary artery harvesting. Intact incisional wound vacuum dressings have an undefined role in the prophylactic prevention of a sternotomy wound infection in at-risk individuals, especially those with poorly controlled diabetes, obesity, and metabolic syndrome. To date, no randomized trials of negative pressure wound therapy in sternotomy infection prophylaxis or treatment have been published.

SURGICAL APPROACH

The surgical considerations of treating DSWI are focused on debridement of devitalized infected tissue, drainage of purulent fluid collections, and secondary soft tissue reconstruction of the resulting defect. Primary closure of debrided wounds—with or without local advancement of musculocutaneous or fasciocutaneous flaps—over paired drainage tubes, which allow continuous local irrigation of antibiotics[38] or antiseptic agents (dilute Povidone iodine 0.05%) has been successfully utilized in wounds where sternal bone stock is discovered to be largely preserved.[5] Myoplasty or musculocutaneous flaps have been successfully utilized, based on major vascular pedicles or myocutaneous perforators, in situations where major pedicles (ie, internal thoracic artery for pectoral or rectus muscle flaps) have been sacrificed.[39]

Devitalized infected tissue should be completely and radically resected in an excisional sharp debridement fashion. Phlegmonous, nonsuppurative inflamed infected tissue can be safely managed with intravenous antibiotics and careful, longitudinal observation. A phlegmon may represent cellulitis, which can favorably respond to antibiotic therapy alone; alternatively, a phlegmon may progress onto suppurative or necrotic tissue, which will require additional sharp excisional debridement.

Reconstructive surgical procedures following radical resection of devitalized infection serve the dual purpose of tissue transfer of well-vascularized soft tissue that can deliver antibiotics to an open wound as well as provision of immediate soft tissue coverage and skin barrier function. Closed incisional wound vacuum dressings (Prevena) have been used as prophylactic therapy for at-risk patients (primarily diabetes and obesity) and following myoplasty techniques to remove fluid collections that impair wound healing; one study reported a 24% absolute risk reduction in overall adverse wound-related events postoperatively with the use of an incisional wound vacuum dressing.[40] Negative pressure wound therapy utilizes a polyurethane foam sponge with pore sizes of 400 to 600 [illegible]m sealed air-tight with a transparent acrylic adhesive drape, which is changed every 48 to 72 hours.[37] Continuous negative pressure allows wound edge migration toward the midline and facilitates wound closure (**Figure 94.1**).

Surgical coordination between the cardiothoracic surgeon and the plastic/reconstructive surgeon is essential in the management of complex poststernotomy wound. The plastic/reconstructive surgeon is seminal in the curative management of wounds, which have large residual soft tissue defects following debridement procedures and in the management of chronically colonized wounds that have failed previous simpler attempts at wound closure. Plastic surgical technique options for the repair of large wound defect reconstruction include using the pectoralis, latissimus, serratus, and rectus myoplasty flaps and transdiaphragmatic omentoplasty. Compared with simple wound packing, radical debridement of sternal bone and costal cartilages, and soft tissue reconstruction with pectoralis and rectus myoplasty or omentoplasty flaps results in a marked decrease in mortality (50% vs 10%, respectively).[20] More recently, it was observed that routine radical sternectomy and coastal chondrectomy are unnecessary in many cases and techniques to preserve much of the bony sternum had equally good outcomes in terms of infection cure rates.

Pectoralis myoplasty is a useful, local option that utilizes chest wall muscles that can be accessed through the same incision as for the index open heart surgery. Commonly, the left internal thoracic artery (ITA) has been harvested for revascularization of the left anterior descending, or other, coronary artery; according to the STS Database, the left ITA is utilized in 99% of first-time coronary bypass operations. Conversely, the use of the right ITA is much lower; currently, only approximately 5% of first-time CABG procedures use both the left and the right ITAs as vascular conduits. The pectoral muscle receives blood flow from the ipsilateral ITA or the thoracoacromial artery musculocutaneous perforators if the ipsilateral ITA has been used as a vascular conduit. Operatively, the pectoralis major muscle is mobilized from the humeral head attachment and from the pectoralis minor and shifted medially to provide midline coverage. However, standard pectoralis advancement flaps suffer from the disadvantage, of providing insufficient wound coverage for the lower third of the sternum. A bipedicled approach—using the right rectus abdominis flap with blood supply from the intact right ITA and the left pectoralis myoplasty flap supplied by the thoracoacromial artery—has been commonly used to relieve this situation.[41]

SECTION 7

The most challenging lower-third sternotomy wound defects occur in patients where both right and left ITAs have been harvested for bypass conduit or have otherwise been injured by the necrotizing infection process or by a soft tissue debridement procedure. In that circumstance, an intercostal artery-supported vertical rectus myocutaneous flap based on segmental intercostal artery perforators can be utilized. In this technique, the deep and superficial inferior epigastric artery and vein are ligated. Segmental intercostal vessels mature and dilate, collateralizing with the lower remnants of the ITA and inferior epigastric artery (**Figure 94.2A**). A paddle of skin and fascia is rotated vertically into the lower sternal defect at a later date based on these perforators. The musculofascial defect in the abdominal wall is closed with a de-epithelialized porcine xenograft, and the abdominal wall skin defect is closed with adjacent skin transfer, which is usually plentiful (**Figure 94.2B**).

Other plastic surgical techniques to provide coverage for the lower-third sternal wounds include latissimus dorsi muscle combined with a fasciocutaneous extension flap, free vastus lateralis muscle flap with skin grafting, and omentoplasty.

Omentoplasty represents another technique, where well-vascularized tissue (ie, the greater omentum) can be a useful treatment option for patients whose pectoralis muscle mass is inadequate or inappropriate for use (**Figures 94.3** and **94.4**). The greater omentum possesses angiogenic factors, such as vascular endothelial growth factor (VEGF), which make it an ideal tissue for transfer into wounds that may be suffering from local tissue hypoxia. The greater omentum can be harvested laparoscopically based on the vascular supply from the right and left gastroepiploic artery through the vascular Arc of Barkow (**Figure 94.5**).[42] Operatively, this requires mobilization of the omentum from the greater curvature of the stomach and release from the taenia omentalis of the transverse colon. This large mass of omentum is then tunneled into the sternotomy wound through a relatively small defect in the anterior central tendon of the diaphragm, loose enough to allow for adequate venous drainage. Unlike the pectoralis flaps which can be mobilized as musculocutaneous units with skin coverage, the omentum requires separate skin coverage; usually, this is by the way of fasciocutaneous skin advancement from the chest wall, or from split-thickness skin graft applications.

Comparisons between the more rigorous operative procedures (pectoralis, latissimus, or rectus myoplasty) and the simpler omentoplasty have been reported. Nonrandomized, single-center reports have indicated superior results with pectoralis myoplasty techniques more than omentoplasty in terms of overall mortality but not recurrent mediastinitis, in the absence of sternal bone necrosis.[43]

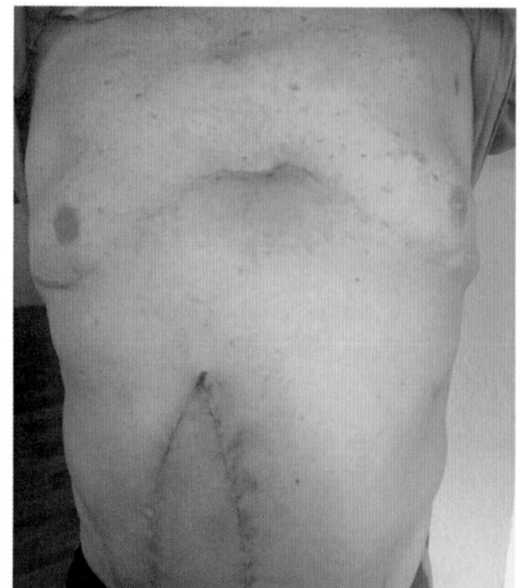

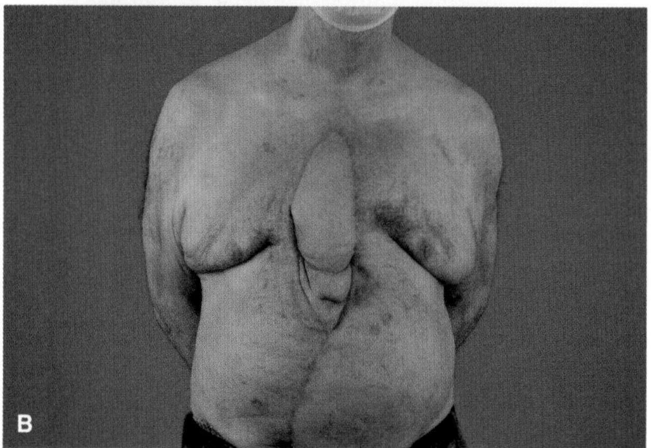

FIGURE 94.2 **A**. Delayed vertical rectus abdominus muscle (VRAM) flap, stage 1: isolation of fasciocutaneous skin paddle, ligation of deep, and superficial inferior epigastric artery and vein, and maturation of intercostal perforator collaterals to superficial epigastric artery. **B**. Vertical rectus abdominis musculocutaneous (VRAM) flap stage 2; transposition of pedicled paddle flap following full-thickness resection of infected sternum.

SPECIAL CONSIDERATIONS (INCLUDING EMERGING THERAPIES)

The concept that rigid chest wall reconstruction is advantageous over nonrigid reconstruction, by allowing for return to more unlimited and unrestricted postoperative physical activity has gained attraction in recent publications. One major concern is the addition of complexity to an already complex operation, and the introduction of a foreign body into a wound that is either heavily colonized with bacteria or frankly infected; another concern is cost. However, the introduction of rigid chest wall reconstruction as an adjunct to soft tissue reconstruction following conservative wound debridement for mediastinitis and DSWI has emerged as an achievable goal[28] and represents the current horizon for research into future surgical outcomes studies.

FOLLOW-UP PATIENT CARE

Longitudinal patient follow-up is highly recommended for any patient who has suffered a deep sternotomy wound infection. Late recurrences are not uncommon, and often require the coordinated efforts of a multidisciplinary team of cardiothoracic surgeons, plastic/reconstructive surgeons, infectious disease specialists, endocrinologists for control of diabetes, and rehabilitation expertise.

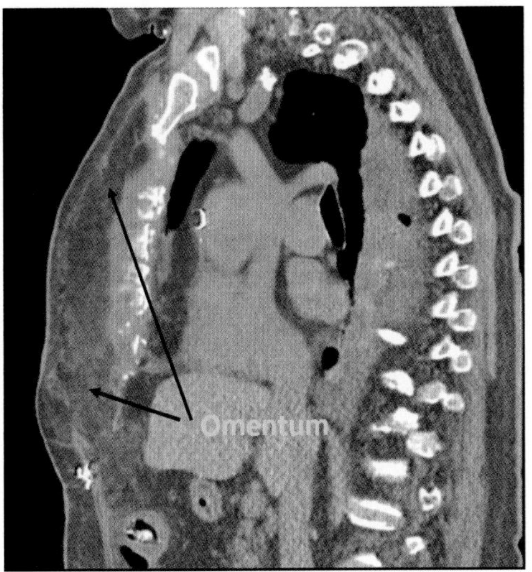

FIGURE 94.3 CT scan (sagittal view) of omentoplasty.

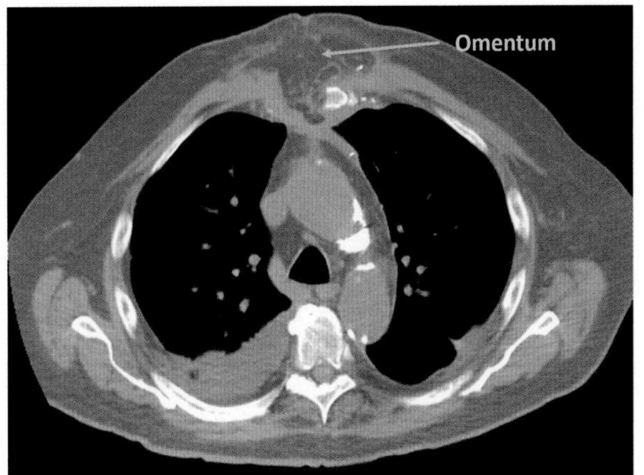

FIGURE 94.4 CT scan (axial view) of omentoplasty.

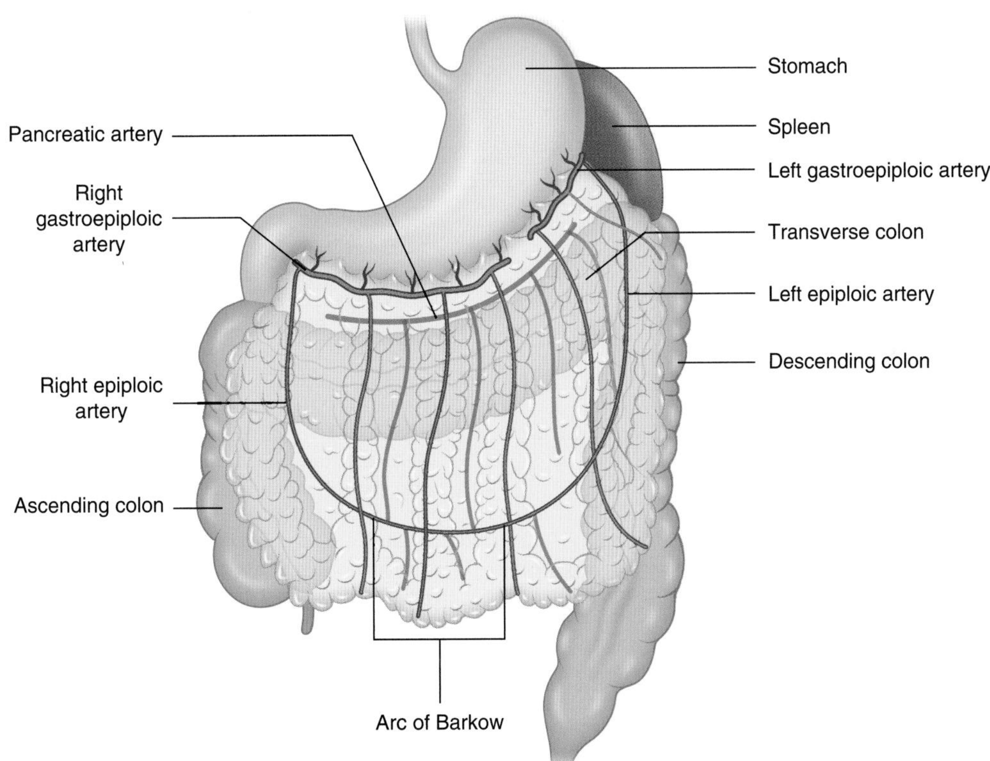

FIGURE 94.5 The greater omentum can be harvested laparoscopically based on the vascular supply from the right and left gastroepiploic arteries through the vascular Arc of Barkow.

RESEARCH AND FUTURE DIRECTIONS

The future research frontiers will revolve around risk modification, such as with improved longitudinal glycemic control in diabetic patients to achieve hemoglobin A1c levels in the 6% range. Other frontiers will involve infectious disease consultants to develop novel antibiotic coverage to deal with the rising incidence of antibiotic-resistant bacteria. Soft tissue transfer techniques continue to develop, with the focus on delayed harvesting of vascularized pedicle grafts in 2-stage procedures for wound coverage. The role of rigid bony thorax reconstruction will continue, with the aim of adding "functional" recovery to the goals of microbiologic eradication of infection and soft tissue open wound coverage.

KEY POINTS

- ✔ Rigid adherence to antibiotic prophylaxis guidelines is essential to minimizing sternal infections.
- ✔ Health care providers should provide a thorough preoperative evaluation and risk-factor modification of patients who must undergo a trans-sternal cardiac procedure.
- ✔ Consideration should be given for nonsternotomy minimally invasive approaches to patients whose anatomy and physiology reserves allow for it.
- ✔ Meticulous surgical technique is critical with the emphasis on:
  - limited electrocautery
  - use of alternative, noncautery energy sources
  - superb surgical hemostasis
  - blood product conservation
  - use of nonbone wax marrow hemostatic agents
  - rigid sternal apposition
  - sternal healing precautions
- ✔ Early recognition of superficial and deep sternal wound complications is important to allow early intervention.
- ✔ For patients with DSWI, preferred treatment includes limited radical debridement, use of temporary wound vacuum tissue coverage followed by nonrigid reconstruction using local tissue transfer (ie, pectus myoplasty) when appropriate and remote tissue transfer (ie, vertical rectus abdominis, omentoplasty) when required.

REFERENCES

1. Milton H. Mediastinal surgery. *Lancet.* 1897;1:872-875.
2. Julian OC, Lopez-Belio M, Dye W, et al. Median sternal incision in intracardiac surgery with extracorporeal circulation: a general evaluation of its use in heart surgery. *Surgery.* 1957;42:753-761.
3. Oakley R, El M, Wright J. Postoperative mediastinitis: classification and management. *Ann Thorac Surg.* 1996;61:1030-1036.
4. Edwards F, Engelman R, Houck P, et al. The Society of Thoracic Surgeons practice guideline series: antibiotic prophylaxis in cardiac surgery, Part I: Duration. *Ann Thorac Surg.* 2006;81(1):397-404.
5. Levi N, Olsen PS. Primary closure of deep sternal wound infection following open heart surgery; a safe operation? *J Cardiovasc Surg.* 2000;41(2):241-245.
6. Hollenbeak C, Murphy D, Koenig S, et al. The clinical and economic impact of deep chest surgical site infections following coronary artery bypass graft surgery. *Chest.* 2000;118:397-402.
7. Minakata K, Bando K, Tanaka R, et al. Preoperative chronic kidney disease as a strong predictor of postoperative infection and mortality after coronary artery bypass grafting. *Circulation.* 2014.78(9):2225-2231.
8. Wang J, Luo X, Jin X, et al. Effects of preoperative HbA1c levels on the postoperative outcomes of coronary artery disease surgical treatment in patients with diabetes mellitus and nondiabetic patients: a systematic review and meta-analysis. *J Diabetes Res.* 2020:3547491-93.
9. Coleman C, Lucek D, Hammond J, White CM. Preoperative statins and infectious complications following cardiac surgery. *Curr Med Res Opin.* 2007;12(8):1783-1790.
10. Rogers M, Blumberg N, Saint SK, et al. Allogeneic blood transfusions explain increased mortality in women after coronary artery bypass graft surgery. *Am Heart J.* 2006;152(6):1028-1034.
11. Sharma A, Slaughter T, Clements FM, et al. Association of leukocyte-depleted blood transfusions with infectious complications after cardiac surgery. *Surg Infect.* 2002;3(2):127-133.
12. Murphy P, Connery C, Hicks GL, Blumberg N. Homologous blood transfusion as a risk factor for postoperative infection after coronary artery bypass graft operations. *J Thorac Cardiovasc Surg.* 1992;104(4):1092-1099;
13. Kulier A, Levin J, Moser R, et al. Impact of preoperative anemia on outcome in patients undergoing coronary artery bypass graft surgery. *Circulation.* 2007;116:471-479.
14. Kong S, Peltz M, Pruszynski J, et al. Effect of HbA1c on post-operative outcomes after on-pump CABG. Presented at the 13th Annual Academic Surgical Congress, Jacksonville, FL, January 30-February 1, 2018 [Abstract 44.05]. https://www.asc-abstracts.org/abs2018/44-05-effect-of-hba1c-on-post-operative-outcomes-after-on-pump-cabg/
15. Guvener M, Pasaoglu I, Demircin M, et al. Perioperative hyperglycemia is a strong correlate of postoperative infection in type II diabetic patients after coronary artery bypass grafting. *Endocr J.* 2002;49(5):531-537.
16. Taggart D, Benedetto U, Gerry S, et al. Bilateral versus single internal thoracic artery grafts at 10-years. *N Engl J Med.* 2019;380:437-446.
17. Garner J, Jarvis W, Emori TG, Horan TC, Hughes J. CDC definitions for nosocomial infections, 1988. *Am J Infect Control.* 1988;16:128-140.
18. Goh SSC. Post-sternotomy mediastinitis in the modern era. *J Card Surg.* 2017;32(9):556-566.
19. Tewarie L, Zayat R, Haefner H, et al. Does percutaneous dilatational tracheostomy increase the incidence of sternal wound infection—a single center retrospective of 4100 cases. *J Cardiothorac Surg.* 2015;10:155.
20. Jones G, Jurkiewicz MJ, Bostwick J, et al. Management of the infected median sternotomy wound with muscle flaps. The Emory 20-year experience. *Ann Surg.* 1997;225(6):766-776.
21. Brook I, Frazier EH. Microbiology of mediastinitis. *Arch Intern Med.* 1996;156(3):333-336.
22. Ford E, Baisden C, Matteson ML, Picone A. Sepsis after coronary bypass grafting: evidence for loss of the gut mucosal barrier. *Ann Thorac Surg.* 1991;52(3):514-517.
23. Weyrauch D, Kemp W, Koponen M. Right ventricle rupture after open heart surgery. *Am J Forensic Med Pathol.* 2020;4:35-39.
24. Rouzet F, de Labriolle-Vaylet C, Trouillet J-L, et al. Diagnostic value of 99mTc-HMPAO-labeled leukocyte scintigraphy in suspicion of post-sternotomy mediastinitis relapse. *J Nucl Cardiol.* 2015;22(1):123-129.
25. Engelman R, Shahian D, Shemin R, et al. The Society of Thoracic Surgeons practice guideline series: antibiotic prophylaxis in cardiac surgery, part II: antibiotic choice. *Ann Thorac Surg.* 2007;83(4):1569-1576.
26. Bennett-Guerrero E, Ferguson TB, Lin M, et al. Effect of an implantable gentamicin-collagen sponge on sternal wound infections following cardiac surgery: a randomized trial. *JAMA.* 2010;304(7):755-762. doi:10.1001/jama.2010.1152
27. Madej T, Plotze K, Birkner C, Jatzwauk L, Klaus M, Waldow T. Reducing mediastinitis after sternotomy with combined chlorhexidine-isopropyl alcohol skin disinfection: analysis of 3,000 patients. *Surg Infect.* 2016;17(5):552-556.
28. Vos R, Jongbloed L, Sonker U, Kloppenburg GTL. Titanium plate fixation versus conventional closure for sternal dehiscence after cardiac surgery. *Thorac Cardiovasc Surg.* 2017;65(4):338-342.
29. Konvalinka A, Errett L, Fong IW. Impact of treating Staphylococcus aureus nasal carriers on wound infections in cardiac surgery. *J Hosp Infect.* 2006 Oct;64(2):162-8
30. Konvalinka A, Errett L, Fong IW. Impact of treating Staphylococcus aureus nasal carriers on wound infections in cardiac surgery. *J Hosp Infect.* 2006;64:162-168.
31. Leinberger T, Heilman C, Sorg S, et al. The COSTA study: sternal closure in high-risk patients—a prospective randomized multicenter trial. *Thorac Cardiovasc Surg.* 2018;66(6):508-516
32. Allen K, Thourani V, Naka Y, et al. Randomized, multicenter trial comparing sternotomy closure with rigid plate fixation to wire cerclage. *J Thorac Cardiovasc Surg.* 2017;153:888-896.

33. Lander H, Ejiofor J, McGurk S, Tsuyoshi K, Shekar P, Body S. Vancomycin Paste does not reduce the incidence of deep sternal wound infection after cardiac operations. *Ann Thorac Surg.* 2017;103(2):497-503
34. Vestergaard R, Nielsen P, Terp KA, Søballe K, Hanisokma J. Effects of hemostatic material on sternal healing after cardiac surgery. *Ann Thorac Surg.* 2014;97:153-160.
35. Tham T, Roberts K, Shanahan J, Burban J, Constantino P. Analysis of bone healing with a novel bone wax substitute compared with bone wax in a porcine bone defect model. *Future Sci OA.* 2018;4:FSO326. doi:10.4155/fsoa-2018-0004
36. Mills C, Bryson P. The role of hyperbaric oxygen therapy in the treatment of sternal wound infection. *Eur J Cardiothorac Surg.* 2006;30:153-159.
37. Atkins Z, Kistler J, Kistler J, Hurley K, Hughes GC, Wolf W. Does negative pressure wound therapy have a role in preventing poststernotomy wound complications? *Surg Innov.* 2009;16:140-146.
38. Bryant L, Spencer F, Trinkle J. Treatment of median sternotomy infection by mediastinal irrigation with an antibiotic solution. *Ann Surg.* 1969;169:914-920.
39. Chou E, Tai Y, Chen H-C, Chen K-T, et al. Simple and reliable way in sternal wound coverage-tripedicle pectoralis major myocutaneous flap. *Microsurgery.* 2008;28(6):441-446.
40. Lo Torto F, Monfirecola A, Kaciulyte J, et al. Preliminary result with incisional negative pressure wound therapy and pectoralis major muscle flap for median sternotomy wound infections in a high-risk patient population. *Int Wound J.* 2017;14(6):1335-1339.
41. Chou C, Tasi M, Sheen Y-T, et al. Endoscope-assisted pectoralis major-rectus abdominis bipedicle muscle flap for the treatment of poststernotomy mediastinitis. *Ann Plast Surg.* 2016;76:S28-S34.
42. Bruzoni M, Steinberg G, Dutta S. Laparoscopic harvesting of omental pedicle flap for cerebral revascularization in children with moyamoya disease. *J Pediatr Surg.* 2016;51:592-597.
43. Tewarie L, Moza A, Khattab MA, Autschbach R, Zayat R. Effective combination of different surgical strategies for deep sternal wound infection and mediastinitis. *Ann Thorac Cardiovasc Surg.* 2019;25(2):102-110.

SECTION 8

PREVENTIVE CARDIOLOGY

SECTION EDITOR: Michael Blaha

CHAPTER 95

PATHOPHYSIOLOGY OF ATHEROSCLEROSIS

Marcio Sommer Bittencourt, Giuliano Generoso, and Raul D. Santos

INTRODUCTION

Atherosclerosis, a term proposed by Marchand in 1904[1] as an update from *arteriosclerosis* used by Lobstein in 1829,[2] is the formation of fibrofatty lesions in the arterial wall. The word "atherosclerosis" is derived from the Greek word *atheros*, which means gruel. It describes the cheesy substance that exudes from the plaques on sectioning. The first suggestion that the cheesy substance was cholesterol came in 1910 when the German chemist Adolf Windaus found that plaques from human aortas contained 25-fold more cholesterol than normal aortas. Concomitantly, the "atherogenic diet" theory originated from Russian animal experiments performed during 1908 to 1913 by Anistchkow, and atherosclerotic disease was linked to lipid metabolism.[3,4] These findings supported the mid-20th century epidemiologic studies—the Seven Country Study[5] and Framingham Heart Study[6]—that observed an association between blood cholesterol levels and incidence of atherosclerosis-related cardiovascular outcomes. Subsequently, our understanding of mechanisms involved in atherogenesis has advanced rapidly with the advent of cell biology and knowledge about the inflammatory and immune responses involved in plaque formation and progression.

Atherosclerosis is the primary etiology for a broad spectrum of clinical manifestations of cardiovascular diseases (CVDs) that comprise ischemic heart disease, cerebrovascular disease, and peripheral artery disease. As the leading cause of death worldwide for over 80 years, ongoing research focusing on the metabolic pathways and risk factors associated with atherosclerosis has led to new pharmacologic and nonpharmacologic strategies for prevention and treatment.

STAGES OF PLAQUE FORMATION

The natural history of the atherogenic process can best be understood from the perspective of the stages of plaque formation: initiation, progression, stability, and plaque vulnerability (**Figure 95.1**).

Initiation of Atherosclerosis

Endothelial dysfunction is a critical feature in the onset of atherogenesis. The endothelium is in direct contact with, and reacts to, various mechanical and molecular stimuli to maintain hemostasis, inflammation, and vascular tone. Endothelial injury may be caused by several factors (listed in **Table 95.1**), particularly in regions of the vessel subject to low shear stress and altered blood flow.[7] These insults lead to a rise in angiotensin II, reduced nitric oxide (NO) production, and increase in the expression of superoxide dismutase, which compromise the integrity of the endothelial barrier. The reduced NO concentration is unable to inhibit the nuclear factor kappa-light chain enhancer of activated B cells (NF-kB) pathway, which leads to endothelial cell activation. Activated cells increase expression of cytokines (monocyte chemoattractant protein-1 and interleukin-8), monocyte adherence proteins (P-selectin, vascular cell adhesion protein-1, intercellular adhesion molecule-1), and proinflammatory receptors (toll-like receptor-2). The loss of endothelial integrity allows direct contact between blood constituents and the arterial intima—the site of atheroma development—and concomitant activation of endothelial cells results in a proinflammatory and prothrombotic environment (Figure 95.1).

Once endothelial damage has occurred, retention and accumulation of *cholesterol-loaded atherogenic lipoproteins* (ie, low-density lipoproteins [LDL], remnants of very low-density lipoproteins [VLDLs] and chylomicrons, and lipoprotein (a) [Lp(a)]) in the subendothelial space occur. Their accumulation in the intima further promotes endothelial dysfunction and triggers *inflammation*, which is the pivotal step for the development of fatty streak and the progression of atheroma. Both native and modified lipoproteins (ie, through oxidation and glycation) can trigger an immune response that participates in atherogenesis.[8] Inflammatory signals induce endothelium activation, expression of adhesion molecules, and chemoattractants that promote recruitment of monocytes into the subendothelial space, as well as other immune cells, including regulatory T cells, T helper dendritic cells (Th-1), and mast cells.

Once in the intima, monocytes are activated to become macrophages that internalize and degrade the proatherogenic lipoproteins retained in the subendothelial space. This amplifies and perpetuates the expression of inflammatory mediators. Following lipoprotein phagocytosis, free cholesterol is released and transported to the endoplasmic reticulum to be esterified and stored as cholesteryl ester in lipid droplets in the cytoplasm, thereby forming *foam cells*. In an attempt to reduce the formation and progression of foam cells, free cholesterol is cleared from macrophage cytoplasm by three major metabolic pathways—ATP-binding cassette subfamily G member 1,

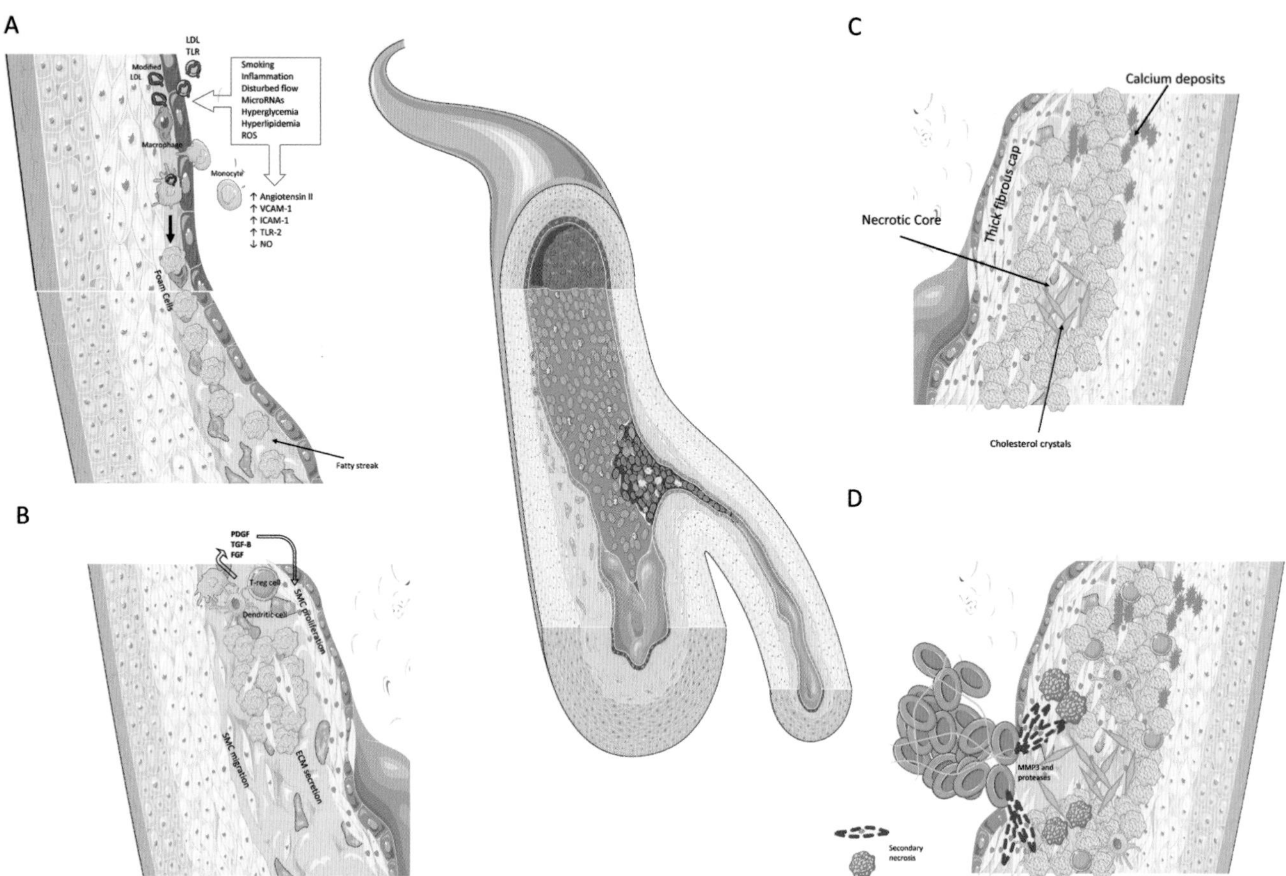

FIGURE 95.1 Pathophysiology of atherosclerosis. The figure is divided into four steps in the atherogenic process and its characteristics: **(A)** *initiation*: endothelial activation, subendothelial apoB-containing lipoprotein retention and fatty streak formation; **(B)** *progression*: migration and proliferation of smooth muscle cells, extracellular matrix secretion, and plaque development; **(C)** *stability*: a developed thick fibrous cap, formation of the necrotic core and calcification; **(D)** *vulnerable plaque/rupture*: progression of necrotic core because of secondary necrosis, release of oxidation products, MMP-3, proteinases and inflammatory mediators, thinning of the fibrous cap promotion, and plaque rupture. ECM, extracellular matrix; FGF, fibroblast growth factor; ICAM, intercellular adhesion molecule; LDL, low-density lipoprotein cholesterol; MMP3, matrix metalloproteinase 3; NO, nitric oxide; PDGF, platelet-derived growth factor; ROS, reactive oxygen species; SMC, smooth muscle cell; TGF-β, transforming growth factor beta; TLR, toll-like receptor; VCAM, vascular cell adhesion molecule.

scavenger receptor class B type I, and aqueous diffusion—and captured by native, cholesterol-poor high-density lipoproteins (HDLs) in the reverse cholesterol transport process.

Progression of Atherosclerotic Plaque

Inflammatory mediators released by macrophages (such as platelet-derived growth factor) stimulate the migration and proliferation of *smooth muscle cells* from the media to the intima layer. This is a crucial stage in the development of atheroma, as the presence of smooth muscle cells envisages plaque progression and a lower likelihood of plaque regression. Smooth muscle cells confer plaque stability, as they are the primary source of elastin, proteoglycans, and collagen, components of the extracellular matrix that make up the fibrous cap and protect against its rupture. HDL particles reduce the inflammatory response via mechanisms not related to cholesterol efflux such as antioxidative effects, decreasing expression of endothelial adhesion molecules, and reducing thrombosis.

The continuous accumulation of atherogenic lipoproteins in the intima, their modification and phagocytosis by both macrophages and metaplastic smooth muscle cells results in plaque volume growth. Finally, the progressive increase in intracellular free cholesterol levels, especially in the endoplasmic reticulum, may trigger apoptosis.

Plaque Stability

As the volume of cells in the atheromatous plaque increases, the vessel undergoes positive remodeling because of an increase in the internal elastic lamina area, which attenuates obstruction of the vessel lumen (ie, increasing the external diameter of the vessel to allow preservation of the arterial flow). This effect—termed the Glagov phenomenon—is the result of accumulation of macrophages that express matrix metalloproteinases (MMPs) like MMP-2, MMP-9, and MMP-13 that digest extracellular matrix proteins. Meanwhile, apoptosis of macrophages leads to their clearance from the plaque interior.

TABLE 95.1 Causes of Endothelial Damage

Causes	Mechanisms Involved
Diabetes mellitus	• ↑ Oxidative stress • eNOS uncoupling • ↑ AGE products
Hyperlipidemia	• ↓Response to acetylcholine • ↑Degradation of NO by ROS • Oxidation of LDL
Hypertension	• ↑ Mechanical stress on endothelial cells • Activation of renin-angiotensin-aldosterone pathway • ↑ Endothelin generation
Age	• ↓ Expression and activity of eNOS and NO • Increased ROS production
Smoking	• ↑ Oxidative stress • ↑ Inflammatory biomarkers
Obesity	• Impaired endothelium-dependent vasodilation • ↑ Vasoconstrictor activity of ET-1 • ↑ Prostanoid-mediated vasoconstriction • ↑ Inflammatory activation
Chronic inflammation	• Lectin-like oxidized LDL • Leukocyte adherence and migration (through TNF-α and IL-1 pathway) • ↑ Adhesion molecules (ie, VCAM and ICAM)

AGE, advanced glycation end; eNOS, endothelial nitric oxide synthase; ET-1, endothelin-1; ICAM, intercellular adhesion molecule; IL-1, interleukin 1; LDL, low-density lipoprotein cholesterol; NO, nitric oxide; ROS, reactive oxygen species; TNF-α, tumor necrosis factor alpha; VCAM, vascular cell adhesion molecule.

However, with atheroma progression, the process of clearing dead cells and associated cellular debris (called efferocytosis) becomes dysfunctional, thereby accumulation of cellular debris and deposition of cholesterol crystals contribute to the formation of the necrotic core. Smooth muscle cell migration and proliferation continue, building additional cell layers that result in a thick fibrous cap that covers the necrotic core. This cover protects the plaque against rupture and its consequent core exposure to prothrombotic factors.

Another factor involved in plaque stabilization is the development of vascular calcifications. This is an active process that resembles the process of bone mineralization. During plaque progression, some regions develop foci of calcium deposits, but this process is not uniform. Although microcalcifications in the fibrous cap may generate instability and predispose to plaque rupture initially, the evolution to extensive organized, structured calcifications may lead to lower risk of thrombotic events because of biomechanical stability.

Vulnerable Plaque, Plaque Rupture, and Erosion

Plaque vulnerability is the result of a continuous inflammatory insult associated with the development of the lipid core that increases the risk of plaque rupture, and it may develop in different stages of plaque progression. The progression of the necrotic core leads to the exposure of inflammatory and cytoplasmic oxidative components that cause necrosis of neighboring cells. This results in the release of oxidation products, cytokines, and inflammatory mediators that lead to degradation of extracellular matrix, reduction of collagen production, and death of smooth muscle cells. Moreover, the released metalloproteinases (such as MMP-3) promote the *thinning of the fibrous cap*, a fundamental alteration for atheroma complications. Such changes facilitate plaque rupture. The plaque content (ie, greater lipid area, concentration of cholesterol esters, and number of macrophages) correlates with the propensity for plaque rupture.

Once the plaque surface is breached, there is exposure of the necrotic core to procoagulant factors and blood platelets. As dysfunctional endothelium has reduced capacity to prevent clot formation and promote fibrinolysis, the plaque disruption triggers thrombus formation and, consequently, acute cardiovascular events.

In patients taking lipid-lowering therapies, the progression of plaque vulnerability may have different pathophysiologic features, such as plaque erosion and ulceration rather than plaque rupture. In advanced stages of atherosclerosis, apoptosis and consequent desquamation of endothelial cells occur, configuring areas of *plaque erosion* that, in contrast with plaque ruptures, contain few inflammatory cells, abundant extracellular matrix, and neutrophil extracellular traps.[9] The result is the organization of a less occlusive "white" thrombus with plaque erosion, which is more likely to be associated with the clinical presentation of a non-ST-segment elevation myocardial infarction.

EPIDEMIOLOGY

The peak incidence of atherosclerotic CVD deaths occurred in the 1960s and has since dropped steadily because of multiple efforts. Nevertheless, since the 1930s, mortality from heart disease and stroke has been the most prevalent cause of deaths every year in the United States[10,11] (**Figure 95.2**).

Despite the progressive decline in the incidence of heart disease deaths in the United States over the last 50 years, the economic impact of CVD is still alarming, with about $1 billion per day (2% of growth domestic product) in direct and indirect costs. In the United States, heart disease has an economic impact of $218 billion annually, whereas stroke costs about $45 billion and other peripheral vascular diseases cost $30 billion each year.[11] By 2035, direct costs of all CVD may exceed $750 billion, with more than half in hospital spending and $350 billion in productivity losses. Although there has been a reduction in CVD death for all ethnicities, the incidence in African Americans is still higher than in non-Hispanic whites and twice as high as in Hispanics.[12]

Although atherosclerotic CVD mortality rates continue to decline in high-income countries, this reduction is far less prominent in low- and middle-income countries that accounted for about 75% of the 15.2 million people who died of heart disease and stroke worldwide in 2016. These countries

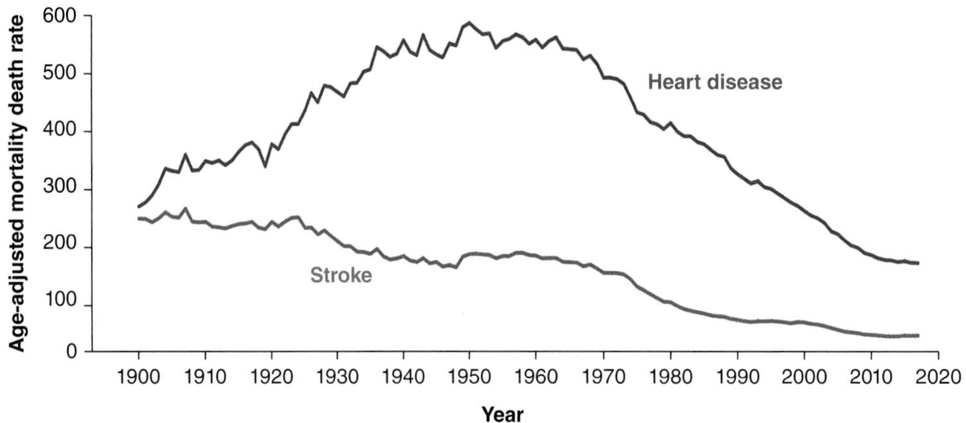

FIGURE 95.2 Temporal trend of the incidence of cardiovascular disease and stroke in the United States (1900-2017). (Data from National Center for Health Statistics. https://www.cdc.gov/nchs/data-visualization/mortality-trends/index.htm)

account for 86% of the premature CVD deaths worldwide, resulting in cumulative losses of US$7 trillion from 2013 until 2020.[13]

RISK FACTORS FOR ATHEROSCLEROSIS

Although most of the data associating risk factors with the development and progression of atherosclerosis are derived from epidemiologic studies, experimental and clinical data provide additional information on the mechanisms linking risk factors with the atherosclerotic process. However, atherosclerosis risk factors are often clustered together and have overlapping pathophysiologic pathways, which limit the potential to decompose the effects.

Age is a nonmodifiable independent risk factor for the development of atherosclerotic CVD, even after adjusting for other risk factors. Although there is a direct impact of aging, it is also a marker of the duration of exposure to other risk factors.

Dyslipidemia is the cornerstone of the atherogenic process, playing an important role in all stages of atheroma formation. Elevations in plasma apolipoprotein B–containing lipids are associated with an increased risk of atherosclerosis, and high plasma concentrations of LDL-cholesterol, Lp(a), and triglyceride-rich lipoprotein remnants have a direct association with atherosclerosis.

Experimental studies have shown the role of LDL in atherosclerotic plaque development. However, the well-established evidence that *LDL-cholesterol* has a causal relationship with the development of atherosclerosis comes from large genetic and population studies, such as from Mendelian randomization observations, but most importantly from clinical trials of LDL-cholesterol lowering medications. A reduction of 39 mg/dL (1 mmol/L) in LDL-C is associated with 22% and 32% lower risk of major atherosclerotic cardiovascular events, respectively, at 5 and 12 years.

HDL particles exert a series of antiatherogenic mechanisms like reverse cholesterol transport with reduction of cholesterol content in macrophages and anti-inflammatory, antithrombotic and antiproliferative properties. Epidemiologic studies have found an independent association of reduced plasma *HDL-cholesterol* levels with atherosclerotic events. However, genetic and intervention studies have failed to show a causal association of low plasma HDL-cholesterol concentration with atherosclerosis. In most situations, low plasma HDL-cholesterol levels persist as an important biomarker risk, though there is an increasing debate about whether HDL-cholesterol is a risk factor or a bystander in the development of atherosclerosis.

The complex metabolism of *triglycerides* and their relationship with fasting and postprandial states makes their association with atherosclerosis controversial. However, there is a growing interest in *triglyceride-rich lipoproteins*, especially their remnants, as a modifiable risk factor because they enter the subintima of blood vessels. Triglyceride-rich lipoproteins have been associated with an increased risk of atherosclerosis in epidemiologic as well as in Mendelian randomization studies where genes that reduce concentrations of triglyceride-rich lipoproteins (as VLDL and its remnants triglycerides) are associated with lower risk of atherosclerotic CVD. Triglyceride-depleted remnants of chylomicrons and VLDL may induce atherosclerosis by their relatively elevated cholesterol content rather than triglyceride content per se. However, the addition of triglycerides in those particles may increase oxidative stress and inflammation and play a role in atherogenesis. Excess triglycerides in lipoproteins also reduce antiatherogenic properties of HDL particles and lead to the formation of small dense LDL particles that are more prone to oxidation. In the REDUCE-IT study, the reduction of triglycerides with the use of icosapent ethyl led to a reduction in cardiovascular events. However, because triglyceride reduction only partially explains the results, there is still debate over whether triglyceride reduction per se prevents atherosclerotic cardiovascular events.

Lp(a) is an LDL-modified low-density atherogenic particle that contains apolipoprotein(a) in its structure and whose serum levels are highly dependent on heredity. Lp(a) may increase the risk of developing atherosclerosis not only because of its elevated cholesterol content but also by proinflammatory and prothrombotic effects. There is strong independent association of elevated Lp(a) with coronary heart disease and stroke as well as calcific degenerative aortic stenosis in observational, Mendelian randomization, and genome-wide association studies. However, the lack of adequate standardized biochemical tests—which reduces reliability of Lp(a) measurement in clinical practice—and the absence of therapies to reduce plasma Lp(a) concentration limit the use of this biomarker in clinical practice. Recent advances in therapy with a potent antisense oligonucleotide for apo(a) may change this scenario. Future implications of Lp(a) are discussed in "Research and Future Developments" section.

Hypertension is an important risk factor for atherosclerotic diseases and other diseases such as heart failure, atrial fibrillation, aortic dissection, and renal failure and is an important risk factor for atherosclerotic diseases.[14] Higher blood pressure levels directly correlate with subclinical atherosclerosis progression, CVD, and mortality. Hypertension contributes to the atherosclerotic process in several ways: (1) effecting structural changes in the arterial wall by triggering increases in medial thickness via smooth muscle cell proliferation and accumulation of extracellular matrix protein; (2) endothelial dysfunction driven by generation of reactive oxygen specimens and activation of the renin-angiotensin-aldosterone system; and (3) sympathetic nervous system imbalance, which also results in the proliferation of smooth muscle cells and endothelial dysfunction.

Smoking is a significant causal factor for atherosclerosis. The role of smoking in atherogenesis is attributed to its impact on oxidative stress, vascular inflammation, platelet aggregation, coagulation, vascular dysfunction, and lipid profile impairment.[15] As the deleterious effects may be partially reversed after smoking cessation, antitobacco strategies are among the most cost-effective interventions in preventing atherosclerotic disease.[16]

Diabetes mellitus is another major risk factor for atherosclerosis. Nearly 800 million people worldwide have diabetes or impaired glucose tolerance. Characterized as a chronic disease by high blood glucose levels and insulin resistance, diabetes contributes to micro- and macrovascular structural changes that double the risk of ischemic heart disease, stroke, and peripheral arterial disease. The main mechanisms associated with hyperglycemia that participate in atherogenesis are: (1) production of reactive oxygen species; (2) formation of advanced glycation end products with activation of their receptor axis; (3) vascular damage caused by polyol (ie, sorbitol) pathway metabolites; (4) activation of the diacylglycerol-protein kinase C pathway, which regulates endothelial permeability, extracellular matrix synthesis/turnover, cell growth, angiogenesis, cytokine activation, and leukocyte adhesion; and (5) chronic vascular inflammation.

Sedentary lifestyle, one of the four major modifiable risk factors for atherosclerotic CVD, is defined as the time spent on activities while one is in a seated, reclined, or lying posture involving low levels of energy expenditure (such as sitting, driving, watching television). Prolonged sitting time (>8 hours/day) is associated with CVD mortality, despite the time spent practicing physical activity.

The role of *obesity* in atherogenesis goes beyond overlap with other risk factors, because subcutaneous and visceral fat accumulation lead to subclinical inflammation through adipokines. These adipocyte-released cytokines induce insulin resistance, endothelial dysfunction, hypercoagulability, and systemic inflammation.[17] Obesity must be viewed as a severe pandemic: nearly 2 billion adults worldwide are obese or overweight, and the prevalence of childhood obesity has increased 10-fold over the past four decades.

An *unhealthy diet* is another modifiable risk factor for atherosclerotic CVD. Several dietary features are associated with other risk factors, such as dyslipidemia and hypertension. However, some aspects of diet are independently associated with the development of atherosclerosis. In particular, high amounts of saturated fatty acids and carbohydrates are associated with atherogenesis. They may drive atherogenic dyslipidemia (ie, increased visceral adiposity, hepatic triglyceride, de novo lipogenesis, plasma apoB, and small dense LDL particles) and contribute to overweight/obesity and insulin resistance. Conversely, some dietary habits reduce the risk of atherosclerotic CVD, such as those that replace saturated fats with polyunsaturated fatty acids, plant-based foods, healthy oils, and healthy (ie, nonsugar-sweetened) beverages. The Mediterranean-style and DASH (Dietary Approaches to Stop Hypertension) diets are endorsed by the American Heart Association.[18,19]

PATHOGENESIS

Atherosclerosis progresses slowly, over decades, and is asymptomatic until plaque progression leads to luminal reduction that causes impairment of blood flow to the affected territory. The disease can be restricted to a single vessel or a few segments initially, but as the disease progresses, it becomes systemic, involving multiple arterial territories such as lower extremities, carotid arteries, and coronary arteries, among others. In each territory, the symptomatic presentation depends on the disease progression: if a slowly progressing plaque leads to a gradual, steady blood flow reduction, progressive symptoms associated with stress conditions or exercise are expected. However, if a vulnerable plaque ruptures or if a plaque erosion or ulcer develops, the presentation can be of acute, intense ischemic symptoms of the affected territory (**Figure 95.3**).

CLINICAL PRESENTATION

Common Signs and Symptoms

Atherosclerosis is virtually ubiquitous in middle age to older individuals, though the vast majority of cases are asymptomatic, because most have only non–flow-limiting disease. When present, symptoms are usually associated with the reduction of blood flow according to the affected organ as detailed in Figure 95.3.

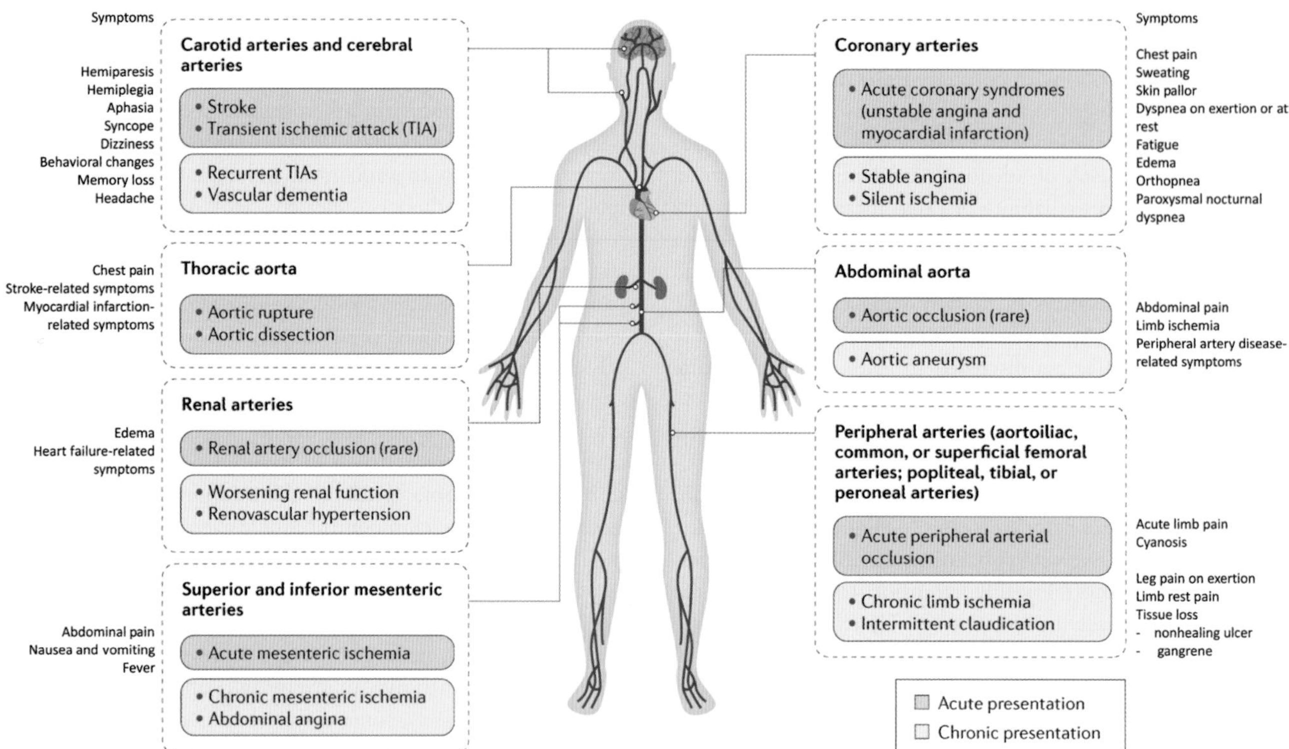

FIGURE 95.3 Clinical manifestations of atherosclerosis. (Adapted from Libby P, Buring JE, Badimon L, et al. Atherosclerosis. *Nat Rev Dis Primers.* 2019;5(1):56.)

Differential Diagnosis

Although the list of potential etiologies in the differential diagnosis of atherosclerosis is variable according to the territory involved, there are usually other causes of ischemia and reduced blood flow to that territory. As a general rule, this includes diseases such as vascular dissection, vasculitis, vasoconstriction, and arterial thromboembolism. Also, as the development of atherosclerosis is systemic, specific nonvascular diseases of each affected organ must be considered (such as the differential diagnosis of dementia).

DIAGNOSIS

Because of the insidious nature of plaque development, most individuals with atherosclerosis remain asymptomatic for decades. In this context, imaging tests can identify, directly or indirectly, the presence of atherosclerosis in the arterial beds long before the onset of symptoms. As there is a high prevalence of the atherosclerotic disease in the population, not every individual benefits from additional testing for the presence of atherosclerosis if asymptomatic. However, specific populations may benefit from screening for early diagnosis. In general, most cardiology societies recommend the use of a clinical risk score to stratify the risk of asymptomatic individuals and define the use of preventative therapies, such as aspirin or statins as well as nonpharmacologic interventions. However, for selected patients, additional tools such as imaging may be used to further stratify risk.

The *coronary artery calcium (CAC) score* measured by a non-contrast cardiac computed tomography scan is a useful risk stratification tool. After estimation of the cardiovascular risk (as discussed in Chapter 97), the CAC score may improve risk prediction and help shared decision-making on the need for pharmacologic interventions to reduce risk. Those who have no coronary calcium (CAC 0) show an extremely low incidence of cardiovascular outcomes and would have limited benefit from pharmacologic treatment. Conversely, a more extensive calcification (CAC >100 Agatston units) supports statin initiation even in individuals considered to be at low risk based on clinical factors. Additionally, evidence of atherosclerosis (such as CAC or plaque detected on carotid ultrasound or cardiac computed tomography angiography) may be useful to motivate patient engagement, changes in healthy lifestyle, and increased adherence to pharmacologic treatment if necessary. A list of imaging tests that can identify atherosclerosis and assess the impact of arterial lumen narrowing is presented in **Table 95.2.**

MANAGEMENT OF ATHEROSCLEROSIS

Medical Approach

Universal recommendations include nonpharmacologic interventions initially that modify risk factors: healthy diet, weight loss, smoking cessation, physical activity, blood pressure management, cholesterol control, and reducing glycemia. More details on these interventions are presented in Chapter 98.

TABLE 95.2 Diagnostic Imaging Tests to Identify Atherosclerosis

Test	Use in Clinical Practice	Limitations
Noninvasive imaging tests		
Ultrasonography/Doppler	• Abdominal aorta • Lower extremity arteries • Carotid arteries • Extra- and intracranial arteries	• Cannot assess smaller-caliber and nonsuperficial vessels
Computed tomography angiography	Virtually all vascular territories	• Radiation exposure • Iodinated contrast agent use
Magnetic resonance imaging	• Thoracic and abdominal aorta • Carotid arteries • Extra- and intracranial arteries	• Limited territories • Long study time • Loud noises and confined space • Cannot be performed in the presence of certain metallic biomedical devices or foreign bodies
Positron emission tomography/computed tomography (PET/CT)	• Research protocols to date • Evaluate plaque metabolism	• Radiation exposure • Limited to large-caliber arteries
Invasive imaging tests		
Invasive angiography	Virtually all vascular territories	• Radiation exposure • Iodinated contrast agent use • There is no direct plaque visualization
Intravascular ultrasonography	• Coronary arteries (selected)	• Radiation exposure • Iodinated contrast agent use (during catheterization procedure) • Limited availability
Optical coherence tomography	• Coronary arteries (selected)	• Radiation exposure • Iodinated contrast agent use (during catheterization procedure) • Limited availability

Pharmacologic Approach

Beyond lifestyle changes, pharmacologic treatment of risk factors is also crucial to reducing the progression of atherosclerosis. Antihypertensive drugs, statins, other lipid-lowering medications like monoclonal proprotein convertase subtilisin/kexin type 9 (PCSK9) inhibitors, and some antidiabetic medications are associated with a reduction of cardiovascular events in the asymptomatic population. Furthermore, patients who are symptomatic or in need of secondary prevention (ie, treatment after cardiovascular outcomes) may benefit from aspirin and other antiplatelet agent use, though their use in primary prevention is more controversial.

Percutaneous Interventions and Surgical Approach

Once there is hemodynamic or clinical evidence of atherosclerosis, interventions can (1) expand the lumen of the artery affected by the atheroma plaque (such as with percutaneous transluminal angioplasty) or (2) surgically construct a bypass around the lesion, delivering blood flow distal to the stenosis. However, there are no current indications of these procedures in asymptomatic individuals. The detailed indications for those procedures for symptomatic individuals are presented in other chapters.

FOLLOW-UP PATIENT CARE

Atherosclerosis is a slowly progressing chronic condition. Patient monitoring and follow-up are essentially directed toward risk factor management and lifestyle modifications. In primary prevention, medical management is guided according to the patient's cardiovascular risk stratification. When the patient has manifested atherosclerotic disease, monitoring tends to be closer, with stricter clinical goals.

RESEARCH AND FUTURE DIRECTIONS

The recent in-depth understanding of the role of inflammation and its metabolic pathways in atherogenesis have led to several studies of anti-inflammatory agents. A randomized clinical trial with canakinumab—a human anti-interleukin-1β monoclonal antibody—showed a 15% reduction in composite cardiovascular outcomes in the secondary prevention setting.[20] Another study using colchicine, an inexpensive anti-inflammatory agent, also found fewer ischemic cardiovascular events than with placebo for secondary prevention of cardiovascular events.[21] However, neither of the two is currently recommended for the treatment of atherosclerosis.

Another recently discovered marker of atherosclerotic risk is clonal hematopoiesis of indeterminate potential (CHIP).[22] Although the mechanism by which it causes acceleration in atherogenesis remains uncertain, there may be a deregulation in the expression of inflammatory genes, as CHIP mutations show an increase in the expression of proinflammatory genes (ie, interleukins 1 and 6). Also, there is an increased formation of extracellular neutrophil traps with pro-oxidant, proteolytic, and prothrombotic factors implicated in thrombosis and acute coronary events.[23] Despite the recent interest in CHIP as an additional potential pathway leading to atherosclerosis, no current therapies related to it are available.

For the management of dyslipidemia, several new drugs have been tested, such as bempedoic acid in reducing serum LDL-cholesterol[24]; the antisense agent AKCEA-APO(a)-L_{Rx} (pelacarsen) in the reduction of Lp(a) levels[25]; and inclisiran, a small interfering RNA that inhibits translation of the PCSK9 (NCT03399370, clinicaltrials.gov). Two antisense oligonucleotides, volanesorsen[26] and IONIS-ANGPTL3-L_{Rx},[27] are being tested to reduce triglycerides and triglyceride-rich lipoproteins.

KEY POINTS

- ✔ Atherosclerosis is a main agent of CVD, the leading cause of death worldwide.
- ✔ The stages of atherogenesis are initiation, progression, stability, and plaque vulnerability.
- ✔ Endothelial dysfunction is the critical initial occurrence that triggers atherogenesis.
- ✔ The known risk factors include age, dyslipidemia, hypertension, smoking, diabetes mellitus, sedentary lifestyle, unhealthy diet, and obesity.
- ✔ The role of noninvasive imaging tests is increasing in the atherosclerotic disease diagnosis.
- ✔ Therapeutic approach comprises behavior changes, pharmacologic treatment of risk factors, and, when it generates clinical repercussions, anatomic intervention.
- ✔ Recent discoveries about the triggers of inflammation, CHIP, and molecular inhibition of some lipoprotein synthesis will lead to future pharmacologic treatment.

REFERENCES

1. Marchand F. Über arteriosklerose (athero-sklerose) [On atherosclerosis (athero-sclerosis)]. *Verhandl D Kongr F Inn Med.* 1904;21:23-59.
2. Lobstein JF. *Traité d'anatomie pathologique (Textbook of pathologic anatomy).* Vol 2. 1833.
3. Anitschkow N, Chalatow S. Ueber experimentelle Cholesterinsteatose und ihre Bedeutung fuer die Entstehung einiger pathologischer Prozesse. *Zentrbl Allg Pathol Anat.* 1913;24:1-9 On experimental cholesterin steatosis and its significance in the origin of some pathological processes by N. Anitschkow and S. Chalatow, translated by Mary Z. Pelias, 1913. Arteriosclerosis 3, 178-182 (1983).
4. Ignatowski AC. Influence of animal food on the organism of rabbits. *Peterb Izviest Imp Voyenno-Med.* 1908;16:154-173.
5. Verschuren WM, Jacobs DR, Bloemberg BP, et al. Serum total cholesterol and long-term coronary heart disease mortality in different cultures. Twenty-five-year follow-up of the seven countries study. *JAMA.* 1995;274(2):131-136.
6. Kannel WB, Dawber TR, Thomas HE, Mcnamara PM. Comparison of serum lipids in the prediction of coronary heart disease. Framingham Study indicates that cholesterol level and blood pressure are major factors in coronary heart disease; effect of obesity and cigarette smoking also noted. *R I Med J.* 1965;48:243-250.
7. Gimbrone MA, García-Cardeña G. Endothelial cell dysfunction and the pathobiology of atherosclerosis. *Circ Res.* 2016;118(4):620-636.
8. Gisterå A, Hansson GK. The immunology of atherosclerosis. *Nat Rev Nephrol.* 2017;13(6):368-380.
9. Quillard T, Franck G, Mawson T, Folco E, Libby P. Mechanisms of erosion of atherosclerotic plaques. *Curr Opin Lipidol.* 2017;28(5):434-441.
10. Herrington W, Lacey B, Sherliker P, Armitage J, Lewington S. Epidemiology of atherosclerosis and the potential to reduce the global burden of atherothrombotic disease. *Circ Res.* 2016;118(4):535-546.
11. Virani SS, Alonso A, Benjamin EJ, et al. Heart disease and stroke statistics—2020 update: a report from the American Heart Association. *Circulation.* Published March 3, 2020. Accessed March 8, 2020. 141(9):e139-e596. https://www.ahajournals.org/doi/10.1161/CIR.0000000000000757
12. Benjamin EJ, Muntner P, Alonso A, et al. Heart disease and stroke statistics—2019 update: a report from the American Heart Association. *Circulation.* Published March 5, 2019. Accessed January 19, 2020. 139(10):e56-e528.. https://www.ahajournals.org/doi/10.1161/CIR.0000000000000659
13. World Health Organization. Global action plan for the prevention and control of noncommunicable diseases: 2013-2020. Published 2013. Accessed January 19, 2020. http://apps.who.int/iris/bitstream/10665/94384/1/9789241506236_eng.pdf
14. Lim SS, Vos T, Flaxman AD, et al. A comparative risk assessment of burden of disease and injury attributable to 67 risk factors and risk factor clusters in 21 regions, 1990-2010: a systematic analysis for the Global Burden of Disease Study 2010. *The Lancet.* 2012;380(9859):2224-2260.
15. Siasos G, Tsigkou V, Kokkou E, et al. Smoking and atherosclerosis: mechanisms of disease and new therapeutic approaches. *Curr Med Chem.* 2014;21(34):3936-3948.
16. Libby P, Buring JE, Badimon L, et al. Atherosclerosis. *Nat Rev Dis Primer.* 2019;5(1):56.
17. Rocha VZ, Libby P. Obesity, inflammation, and atherosclerosis. *Nat Rev Cardiol.* 2009;6(6):399-409.
18. Estruch R, Ros E, Salas-Salvadó J, et al. Primary prevention of cardiovascular disease with a mediterranean diet supplemented with extra-virgin olive oil or nuts. *N Engl J Med.* 2018;378(25):e34.
19. Siri-Tarino PW, Krauss RM. Diet, lipids, and cardiovascular disease. *Curr Opin Lipidol.* 2016;27(4):323-328.
20. Ridker PM, Everett BM, Thuren T, et al. Antiinflammatory therapy with canakinumab for atherosclerotic disease. *N Engl J Med.* 2017;377(12):1119-1131.
21. Tardif J-C, Kouz S, Waters DD, et al. Efficacy and safety of low-dose colchicine after myocardial infarction. *N Engl J Med.* 2019;381(26):2497-2505.
22. Jaiswal S, Natarajan P, Silver AJ, et al. Clonal hematopoiesis and risk of atherosclerotic cardiovascular disease. *N Engl J Med.* 2017;377(2):111-121.
23. Libby P, Ebert BL. CHIP (Clonal Hematopoiesis of Indeterminate Potential): potent and newly recognized contributor to cardiovascular risk. *Circulation.* 2018;138(7):666-668.

24. Laufs U, Banach M, Mancini GBJ, et al. Efficacy and safety of bempedoic acid in patients with hypercholesterolemia and statin intolerance. *J Am Heart Assoc.* 2019;8(7):e011662.
25. Tsimikas S, Karwatowska-Prokopczuk E, Gouni-Berthold I, et al. Lipoprotein(a) reduction in persons with cardiovascular disease. *N Engl J Med.* 2020;382(3):244-255.
26. Witztum JL, Gaudet D, Freedman SD, et al. Volanesorsen and triglyceride levels in familial chylomicronemia syndrome. *N Engl J Med.* 2019;381(6):531-542.
27. Graham MJ, Lee RG, Brandt TA, et al. Cardiovascular and metabolic effects of *ANGPTL3* antisense oligonucleotides. *N Engl J Med.* 2017;377(3):222-232.

CHAPTER 96

CARDIOVASCULAR DISEASE RISK ASSESSMENT IN CLINICAL PRACTICE

Miguel Cainzos-Achirica, Karan Kapoor, Tanuja Rajan, and Roger S. Blumenthal

INTRODUCTION

Cardiovascular disease (CVD) is one of the leading causes of death worldwide, and atherosclerotic cardiovascular disease (ASCVD) accounts for a large proportion of those deaths.[1,2] ASCVD is also a leading cause of morbidity, disability, potential years of life lost, and health care expenditure. Effective prevention remains crucial to reduce the burden of ASCVD throughout the world.

Strategies for the primary prevention of ASCVD can be directed (1) at the population level or (2) to individuals who are apparently healthy but at high risk of developing ASCVD. Whereas the population at large would benefit from avoiding harmful practices (ie, restricting access to tobacco products and sugary beverages) and encouraging healthy practices (ie, increasing community access to healthy foods and exercise facilities), medications for primary prevention (ie, statins, aspirin, etc) should be restricted to individuals who are most likely to benefit. For the latter, accurate identification of individuals at increased ASCVD risk is crucial.[3] In this chapter, we discuss the current state of ASCVD risk assessment, review tools widely used to estimate risk and inform prevention efforts, and present relevant guidance from the American College of Cardiology and the American Heart Association (ACC/AHA).[4,5] Alternative approaches presented in recent guidelines from the European Society of Cardiology and the European Atherosclerosis Society (ESC/EAS) are also considered.[6] Novel risk assessment approaches for secondary ASCVD prevention are also presented.

Clinical risk scores predicting a person's 10-year risk of having an ASCVD event remain the cornerstone of risk assessment in primary prevention. Although Pooled Cohort Equations (PCE) and Systematic Coronary Risk Evaluation (SCORE) are currently the major tools for clinical risk assessment, other 10-year scores are also available and may be valuable in certain contexts. Risk communication tools and scores aimed at predicting additional cardiovascular outcomes may help enhance patient adherence to the recommended prevention plan and may be particularly valuable in young adults.

Despite numerous advantages, clinical risk scores also have important limitations, and the CAC score improves risk assessment when management is uncertain. Also, characteristics associated with an increased ASCVD risk at the group level can be incorporated into clinic–patient discussions to "enhance" or "modify" risk assessment. Novel risk assessment tools are becoming available for patients with established ASCVD. These may facilitate further refining the matching of therapy intensity to risk. ASCVD risk assessment remains an active area of research, particularly for imaging techniques—such as CCTA—and genetic tools. These discoveries will hopefully result in improved, timelier primary prevention of ASCVD among apparently healthy individuals at relatively high risk for future events.

BASIC CONCEPTS AND TARGET POPULATIONS IN ASCVD RISK ASSESSMENT AND MANAGEMENT

Primary and *secondary* prevention are the emphasis of relevant clinical practice guidelines, including the 2018 AHA/ACC/Multi-Society Guidelines on the Management of Blood Cholesterol,[4] the 2019 ACC/AHA Guidelines on the Primary Prevention of Cardiovascular Disease,[5] and the 2019 ESC/EAS Guidelines for the Management of Dyslipidaemias.[6]

Atherosclerotic Cardiovascular Disease Risk Assessment in Primary Prevention

Primary prevention focuses on individuals with no known ASCVD (ie, without myocardial infarction [MI], angina, stroke, transient ischemic attack, or claudication). These individuals may have subclinical atherosclerotic disease, but at the time of risk assessment it will not have caused cardiovascular symptoms. ASCVD risk assessment attempts to stratify these individuals according to their probability of having an event in subsequent years.

Traditional ASCVD risk factor evaluation (ie, presence of hypertension, hyperlipidemia, diabetes, obesity, smoking status, exercise regimen, etc) is recommended every 4 to 6 years starting at age 20 years, and with this a 30-year risk estimate can be calculated up to age 59. In the United States, routine risk estimation for primary prevention is recommended between ages 40 and 75. In Europe, risk factor screening for ASCVD risk stratification purposes is recommended in men older than 40 years, and in women older than 50 years of age or who are postmenopausal.

Atherosclerotic Cardiovascular Disease Risk Assessment in Secondary Prevention Patients

Secondary prevention aims to reduce morbidity and mortality in patients with clinically overt ASCVD. The 2019 ESC/EAS guidelines provide validated tools that allow estimating 10-year and lifetime risk in secondary prevention patients.

CLINICAL RISK SCORES FOR PRIMARY ASCVD PREVENTION

Clinical risk scores estimate an individual's probability of developing an ASCVD event over a given period of time (eg, 10 years). These estimates are derived using data from cohorts of persons similar to those undergoing risk assessment, and they generate population-based probabilities—expressed as a percentage—that can then be applied to the individual patient by the clinician. These scores are typically stratified into categories (eg, low, intermediate, or high risk) that inform clinicians as to the proper primary preventive intervention (eg, none, lifestyle interventions alone, or lifestyle interventions plus pharmacotherapy).

Risk Scores for 10-Year Atherosclerotic Cardiovascular Disease Risk Assessment

U.S. and European guidelines recommend using clinical risk scores as the first step in primary prevention care (**Algorithms 96.1** and **96.2**).[4-8] The current standard is to use tools that predict the 10-year risk of developing an ASCVD event (ie, coronary heart disease [CHD] events or stroke).

The Pooled Cohort Equations (PCE). Since 2013, the ACC/AHA recommend using the PCE to predict 10-year risk of fatal and nonfatal ASCVD events.[4,5,9] The PCE were developed using data from five major U.S. cohort studies and include separate equations for non-Hispanic White and African American adults. For other racial/ethnic groups, the equations for non-Hispanic Whites are recommended, although the guidelines stress that these estimates should be interpreted cautiously. Using the PCE and the associated risk categories, individuals are classified as being at low (≥5%), borderline (5% to <7.5%), intermediate (7.5% to <20%), or high (≥20%) risk of a fatal/nonfatal ASCVD event over 10 years.

The Systematic Coronary Risk Evaluation (SCORE) charts. The ESC/EAS recommend using the SCORE charts and the associated online calculator (HeartScore[10]) to predict an individual's 10-year risk of a fatal ASCVD event.[6] For an approximation of the 10-year risk of fatal and nonfatal ASCVD events, the SCORE risk is multiplied by three. Separate equations are available for men and women as well as for high ASCVD risk (eg, Russia) and low ASCVD risk (eg, Spain) countries; locally recalibrated equations are encouraged when

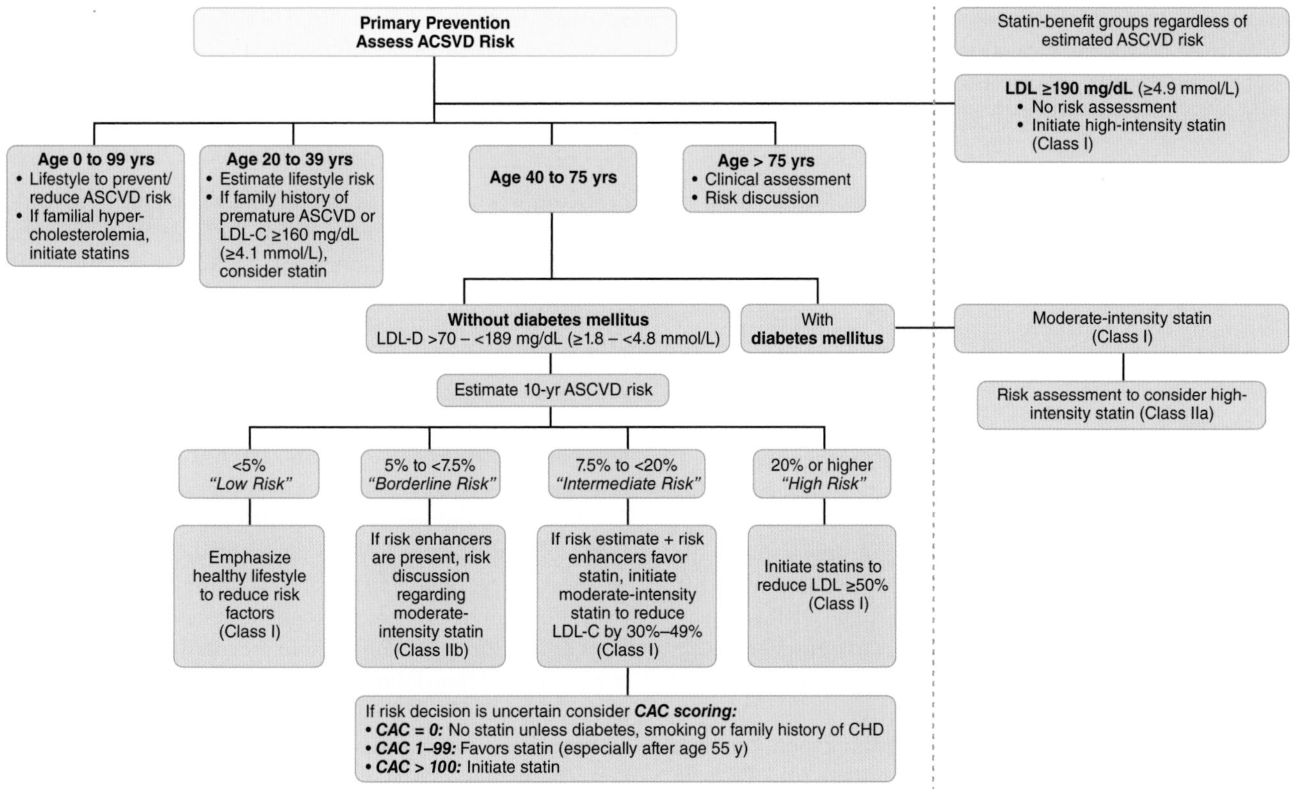

ALGORITHM 96.1 Risk assessment algorithm recommended in 2018/2019 ACC/AHA Guidelines. ACC/AHA, American College of Cardiology/American Heart Association; ASCVD, atherosclerotic cardiovascular disease; CAC, coronary artery calcium; LDL-C, low density lipoprotein cholesterol. ASCVD, atherosclerotic cardiovascular disease; CHD, coronary heart disease; LDL, low-density lipoprotein, LDL-C, low-density lipoprotein-cholesterol; CAC, xxxxx. (Reprinted with permission from 2018 AHA/ACC/AACVPR/AAPA/ABC/ACPM/ADA/AGS/APhA/ASPC/NLA/PCNA Guideline on the Management of Blood Cholesterol: A Report of the American College of Cardiology/American Heart Association Task Force on Clinical Practice Guidelines. *Circulation.* 2018;139(25):e1082-e1143. Copyright © 2018 American Heart Association, Inc.)

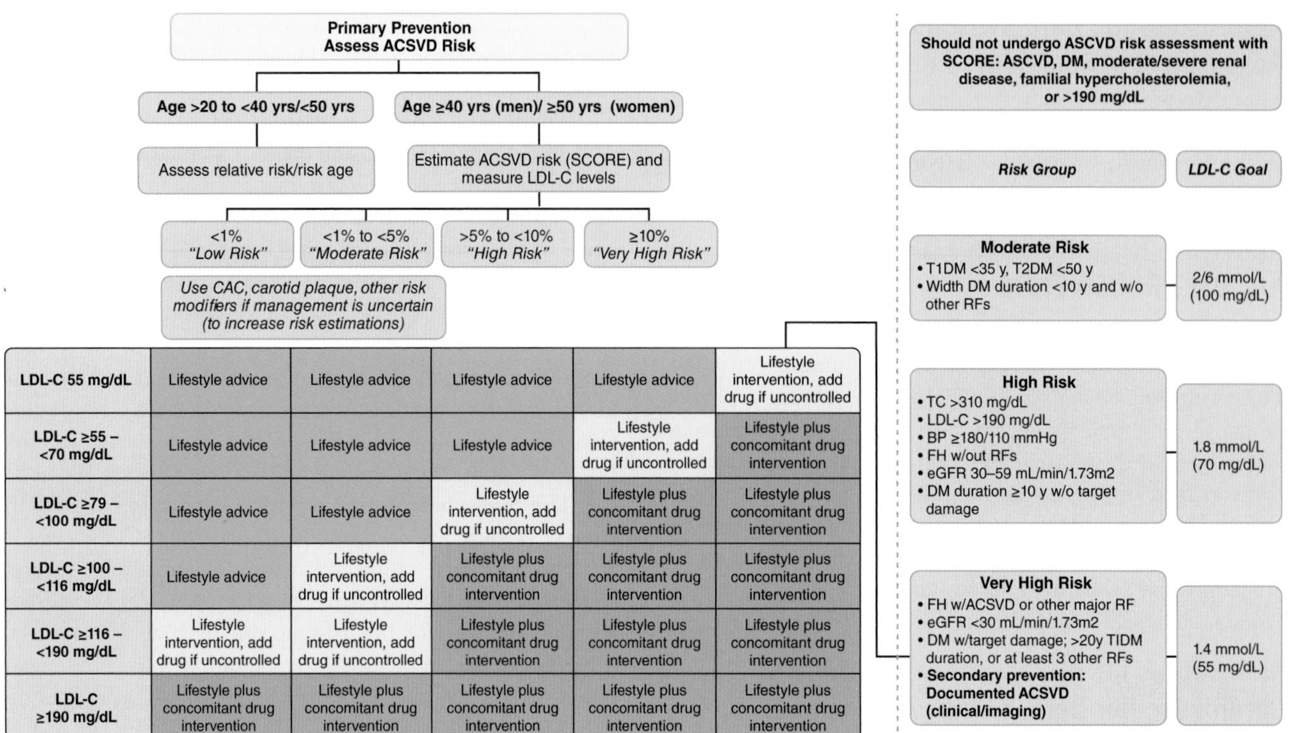

	<1%	<1% to <5%	>5% to <10%	≥10%	
LDL-C 55 mg/dL	Lifestyle advice	Lifestyle advice	Lifestyle advice	Lifestyle advice	Lifestyle intervention, add drug if uncontrolled
LDL-C ≥55 – <70 mg/dL	Lifestyle advice	Lifestyle advice	Lifestyle advice	Lifestyle intervention, add drug if uncontrolled	Lifestyle plus concomitant drug intervention
LDL-C ≥79 – <100 mg/dL	Lifestyle advice	Lifestyle advice	Lifestyle intervention, add drug if uncontrolled	Lifestyle plus concomitant drug intervention	Lifestyle plus concomitant drug intervention
LDL-C ≥100 – <116 mg/dL	Lifestyle advice	Lifestyle intervention, add drug if uncontrolled	Lifestyle plus concomitant drug intervention	Lifestyle plus concomitant drug intervention	Lifestyle plus concomitant drug intervention
LDL-C ≥116 – <190 mg/dL	Lifestyle intervention, add drug if uncontrolled	Lifestyle intervention, add drug if uncontrolled	Lifestyle plus concomitant drug intervention	Lifestyle plus concomitant drug intervention	Lifestyle plus concomitant drug intervention
LDL-C ≥190 mg/dL	Lifestyle plus concomitant drug intervention	Lifestyle plus concomitant drug intervention	Lifestyle plus concomitant drug intervention	Lifestyle plus concomitant drug intervention	Lifestyle plus concomitant drug intervention

ALGORITHM 96.2 Risk assessment algorithm recommended in the 2019 ESC/EAS Guidelines. ASCVD, atherosclerotic cardiovascular disease; BP, blood pressure; CAC, coronary artery calcium; DM, diabetes mellitus; eGFR, estimated glomerular filtration rate; FH, familial hypercholesterolemia; LDL-C, low density lipoprotein cholesterol; RF, risk factor(s); SCORE, Systematic Coronary Risk Evaluation; T1DM, type 1 diabetes mellitus; T2DM, type 2 diabetes mellitus; TC, total cholesterol. (Data from Mach F, Baigent C, Catapano AL, et al. 2019 ESC/EAS Guidelines for the management of dyslipidaemias: lipid modification to reduce cardiovascular risk. *Eur Heart J.* 2020;41(1):111-188.)

available. Using SCORE, individuals are classified as being at low (<1%), moderate (1% to <5%), high (5% to<10%), and very high (≥10%) 10-year risk of a fatal ASCVD event.

PCE versus SCORE. Both the PCE and SCORE use similar input information, although the online HeartScore calculator used in the latter includes additional characteristics. **Table 96.1** compares the landmark PCE and the SCORE scoring systems in detail.

Other 10-year ASCVD/CHD risk scores. The QRISK-3 was developed in the United Kingdom using database health care information from millions of British men and women, and accounts for race/ethnicity, country of origin, and additional risk factors such as atrial fibrillation (a strong risk factor for stroke) and inflammatory conditions.[11] The QRISK-3 may be more appropriate than the SCORE charts in some British populations (eg, in those of South Asian ancestry).

The Multi-Ethnic Study of Atherosclerosis (MESA) CHD Risk Score was developed in 2015 using more contemporary, multiethnic data than that used to derive the PCE. It accounts for family history of CVD, the coronary artery calcium (CAC) score, and also provides estimations for Hispanics and Chinese Americans.[12] The score is available as both a web-based and mobile application-based tool. More recently, the Astronaut Cardiovascular Health and Risk Modification (Astro-CHARM) score, which also incorporates CAC as a predictor, was developed to predict ASCVD events in individuals between 45 and 65 years of age[13] (**Table 96.2**). Finally, local validated risk calculators are available in many countries.

Scores for specific subgroups and patient populations. The ESC/EAS guidelines also include guidance for the use of primary prevention risk scoring tools for specific patient subgroups, such as the SCORE "O.P." in elderly individuals and the ADVANCE risk score and the DIAL model in patients with diabetes.[6] The U-PREVENT website[14] is a helpful online resource that helps identify the most appropriate score for each specific patient.

Strengths and weaknesses of 10-year ASCVD risk scoring. Convenience is a key advantage of the 10-year risk assessment using clinical risk scores, as most of the risk score calculators can be easily accessed online at no cost. In addition, most of them are parsimonious and use input information that is typically generated during a routine medical visit or that is already recorded in the patient's medical record. Conversely, 10-year risk scores also have important limitations. Risk discrimination and calibration issues have been noted, especially when scores used data from cohorts recruited 30 to 40 years ago to estimate risk in more contemporary, healthier populations.[15] To ameliorate this, in the 2018 and 2019 ACC/AHA guidelines, the intermediate risk category was defined with a broader range (10-year estimated risk ranging from 7.5% to <20%), than in the prior iterate (5% to <7.5%). This expanded the

TABLE 96.1 Characteristics of the Pooled Cohort Equations and the Systematic Coronary Risk Evaluation Charts for 10-Year ASCVD Risk Assessment

Feature	Pooled Cohort Equations	SCORE
Supporting scientific societies	ACC/AHA/Multi-Society	ESC/EAS
Derivation cohorts	Framingham (original and offspring), ARIC, CARDIA, and CHS	12 European cohorts
Year of introduction	2013	2003
Input variables	Age, sex, race, diabetes mellitus, total cholesterol, HDL cholesterol, systolic and diastolic blood pressure, antihypertensive medication use, smoking	Age, sex, total cholesterol, HDL cholesterol, systolic blood pressure, smoking; separate equations for high- and low-risk European countries; additional variables used by the online HeartScore
Timeframe of risk predictions	10 years	10 years
Outcome	Fatal and nonfatal hard ASCVD events	Fatal ASCVD events
Associated risk groups	Low (<5%), Borderline (≥5% to <7.5%), Intermediate (≥7.5% to <20%), and High (≥20%) 10-year risk	Low (<1%), moderate (≥1% to <5%), high (≥5% to <10%), and very high (≥10%) 10-year risk
Recalibration	Challenging due to inclusion of nonfatal outcomes; not performed since original development in 2013	Easier owing to inclusion only of fatal events; recalibration since 2003 done periodically; locally calibrated scores available in many European countries

ACC, American College of Cardiology; AHA, American Heart Association; ARIC, Atherosclerosis Risk in Communities; ASCVD, atherosclerotic cardiovascular disease; CARDIA, Coronary Artery Risk Development in Young Adults; CHS, Cardiovascular Health Study; EAS, European Atherosclerosis Society; ESC, European Society of Cardiology; HDL, high density lipoprotein; SCORE, Systematic Coronary Risk Evaluation.

population for a more personalized risk assessment.[4,5] Also, most clinical risk scores emphasize chronologic age, which results in most young adults receiving low-risk estimations and most elderly persons high-risk estimations regardless of their actual burden of preventable risk factors. This may result in the underdetection of high-risk young adults and in the overtreatment of healthy elderly individuals. Other key challenges include the difficulty to communicate 10-year probabilities derived from population-level data to individual patients in a meaningful way,[16] as well as the lack of risk information provided by these tools beyond the 10-year time horizon.

Other Approaches for Clinical Risk Assessment Using Risk Scores

Risk communication tools. Tools have been developed aimed at improving patients' understanding of their estimated risk and their adherence to the recommended interventions. These approaches include estimation of 30-year ASCVD risk and the "risk age" included in the ESC/EAS guidelines.[6] The latter communicates risk in terms of a person's biologic age (as compared to their chronologic age) and contrasts a person's risk to that of an older (or younger) person of the same sex with optimal risk factors. Similar tools had also been previously developed in the Framingham study (the so-called heart age) and in MESA (the so-called arterial age[17]). These tools are particularly relevant in younger patients, in whom 10-year risk estimations will often fail to communicate the lifetime risk associated with risk factors; for them, biologic age and "life-course" perspectives may be more compelling.[18]

Risk scores for other cardiovascular endpoints. Besides ASCVD, prediction and prevention of other related cardiovascular endpoints have gained attention as means to improve patient motivation and adherence to recommended interventions. For example, the 2019 PCE to Prevent Heart Failure (PCP-HF) predicts the probability of incident heart failure (HF) in apparently healthy individuals.[19] Other, more comprehensive 10-year risk scores have been developed that include not only ASCVD and HF but also additional cardiovascular endpoints such as peripheral arterial disease. An example is the 2008 Framingham 10-year General CVD Risk Profile Algorithm, although it needs to be updated.[20]

IMAGING TOOLS IN PRIMARY PREVENTION SETTINGS

Atherosclerotic plaque is the result of an individual's susceptibility and cumulative exposure to established and unknown cardiovascular risk factors. Epidemiologic studies have demonstrated that atherosclerotic plaque in the coronary, carotid, and other arteries is strongly and independently associated with incident ASCVD events.[21] Accordingly, visualizing the presence (or absence) of plaque in relevant vascular territories can improve risk estimation beyond clinical risk scores (**Figure 96.1**).

TABLE 96.2 Characteristics of Other Key Current Risk Scoring Systems for Primary ASCVD Prevention

Feature	MESA CHD Risk Score	Astro-CHARM	QRISK3
Country	United States	United States	United Kingdom
Derivation cohorts	MESA	MESA, DHS, and PACC	Very large, real-world U.K. primary care population
Racial/ethnic/ national groups	Non-Hispanic Whites, non-Hispanic Blacks, Hispanics, Chinese Americans (all in the United States)		Nine groups: White or non-stated, Indian, Pakistani, Bangladeshi, Chinese, Other Asian, Black Caribbean, Black African, Other
Input variables	Age, sex, race/ethnicity (four groups), CAC, total cholesterol, HDL cholesterol, SBP, smoking, diabetes, lipid-lowering medication, antihypertensive medication use, family history	Age, sex, race/ethnicity (four groups), CAC, total cholesterol, HDL cholesterol, SBP, smoking, diabetes, antihypertensive medication use, hsCRP, family history	Age, sex, ethnicity, national origin, postcode, smoking, diabetes, family history, atrial fibrillation, antihypertensive medication use, rheumatoid arthritis, total cholesterol:HDL cholesterol, SBP, BMI, CKD, systemic lupus erythematosus, corticosteroid use, migraine, severe mental illness, atypical antipsychotics, ED
Outcome	Hard CHD events plus revascularization only if prior or concurrent adjudicated angina	Hard ASCVD events	Hard ASCVD events plus transient ischemic attack
Derivation cohorts more contemporary than PCE/SCORE	Yes	Yes	Yes
Incorporates family history into risk assessment	Yes	Yes	Yes
Incorporates CAC into risk assessment	Yes	Yes	No

ASCVD, atherosclerotic cardiovascular disease; BMI, body mass index; CAC, Coronary artery calcium; CHD, coronary heart disease; CKD, chronic kidney disease; DHS, Dallas Heart Study; ED, erectile dysfunction; HDL, high density lipoprotein; hsCRP, high-sensitivity C-reactive protein; MESA, Multi-Ethnic Study of Atherosclerosis; PACC, Prospective Army Coronary Calcium Project; PCE, Pooled Cohort Equation; SBP, systolic blood pressure; SCORE, Systematic Coronary Risk Evaluation; U.K., United Kingdom.

The Coronary Artery Calcium Score

Among currently available cardiovascular imaging techniques, the CAC score is the best tool for enhanced 10-year ASCVD risk estimation.[4-6,22] The original CAC score derived by Drs. Arthur Agatston and Warren Janowitz in 1990[23] is obtained using noncontrast computed tomography.

Association With Events During Follow-Up and Prognostic Value Beyond Traditional Risk Factors

In MESA, a multiethnic prospective cohort study of U.S. adults free of CVD, all 6,814 participants underwent CAC scoring at the baseline study visit. Baseline CAC burden was independently associated with incident events after more than 10 years of follow-up, and CAC also demonstrated incremental prognostic value beyond traditional risk factors at predicting future events.[24]

MESA helped establish the prognostic value of a zero CAC score (ie, no calcium), which is associated with very low rates of incident CVD and particularly CHD events, even among individuals at high estimated risk or with a high burden of risk factors.[25] Conversely, higher CAC scores are associated with higher rates of events,[26] exceeding the traditional definitions of a coronary artery disease risk equivalent. Other population-based CAC studies from the United States and Europe are consistent with those from MESA.

Interpretation of Coronary Artery Calcium Scores in Clinical Practice: Combining Absolute and Relative Scores

Although absolute scores are easy to communicate and have demonstrated associations with events in a number of studies, relative scores based on percentiles of CAC score distributions across age, sex, and race/ethnicity can help interpret a score in a more nuanced manner, particularly among individuals at age extremes. This can be used to inform physician–patient discussions, particularly for motivating young patients with low—but non-zero—absolute scores.

Coronary Artery Calcium in Primary Prevention Guidelines

CAC has garnered increasing prominence in both the U.S. and European primary prevention risk assessment and management guidelines (**Table 96.3**). Specifically, the 2018 and 2019 ACC/AHA Guidelines[4,5] both recommend consideration of

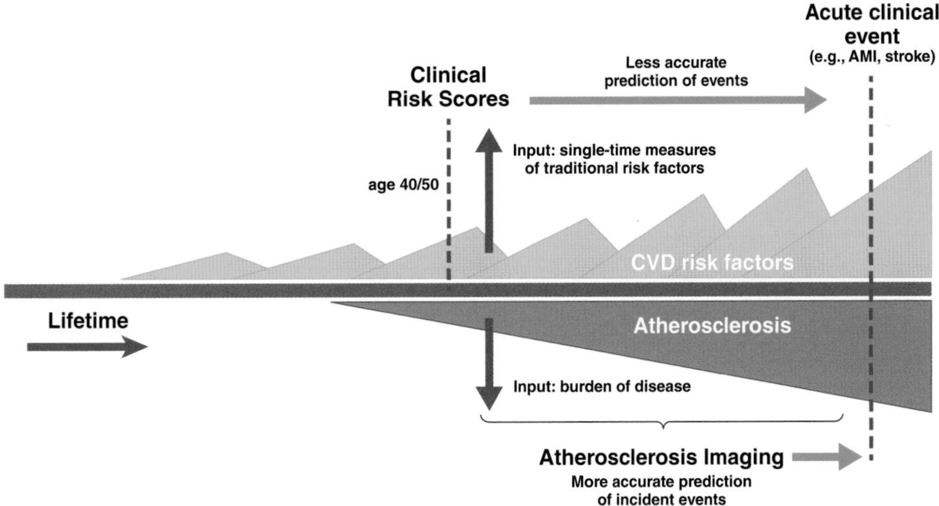

FIGURE 96.1 Risk assessment paradigms: clinical risk scores and atherosclerosis imaging. *Atherosclerotic imaging for identification and quantification of plaque can substantially improve risk stratification beyond clinical risk scores by directly identifying the disease process.* AMI, acute myocardial infarction; CVD, cardiovascular disease. (Adapted by permission from Springer: Cainzos-Achirica M, Di Carlo PA, Handy CE, et al. Coronary Artery Calcium Score: the "Mammogram" of the Heart? *Curr Cardiol Rep.* 2018;20(9):70. Copyright © 2018 Springer Nature.)

CAC scoring in borderline- (5% to <7.5% estimated 10-year risk) and intermediate-risk (7.5% to <20% estimated 10-year risk) individuals in whom the decision to initiate statin therapy is uncertain, to reclassify risk either upward (high CAC scores) or downward (CAC score of zero; class IIa, level of evidence [LOE] B). The 2019 ESC/EAS Guidelines also recommend consideration of a high CAC score as a risk modifier to be used to increase risk predictions,[6] while not mentioning the prognostic implications of a CAC score of zero.

Carotid Ultrasound Imaging

Carotid ultrasound imaging has garnered interest as a noninvasive atherosclerosis assessment by measurement of carotid plaque and carotid intima-media thickness (CIMT). A meta-analysis of 14 population-based cohorts demonstrated a 9% increase in future ASCVD risk for each 0.1-mm increase in CIMT thickness. However, that same analysis reported no clinically meaningful incremental prognostic benefit of CIMT beyond conventional risk factors. As such, neither the 2013 or 2018 Risk Assessment Guidelines nor the 2019 ACC/AHA Primary Prevention Guidelines endorses carotid ultrasound for routine risk assessment.[4,5,27]

The 2019 ESC guidelines do, however, put forth a Class IIa, LOE B for the assessment of arterial (carotid and/or femoral) plaque burden via arterial ultrasonography as a potential risk modifier in individuals at low or intermediate risk. The primary basis of this recommendation stems from a study using a novel, research-grade 3-dimensional carotid ultrasound to study carotid plaque burden, a more specific metric of atherosclerosis than CIMT. The net reclassification significantly improved with either carotid plaque burden (0.23) or CAC (0.25), and major adverse cardiovascular events (MACE) rates increased with higher levels of both.[28] The authors deemed the two modalities to be complementary: however, CAC is more widely available and reproducible than the research ultrasound technology. In addition, although a CAC score of zero is a strong negative risk marker, absence of carotid plaque is not nearly as powerful. Overall, whereas the evidence for both CIMT and carotid plaque assessment is substantially weaker than for CAC, selective assessment of plaque burden may still be relevant in select younger individuals in whom existing coronary plaque has not yet calcified.[29]

Cardiac Computed Tomographic Angiography

The ability of cardiac computed tomographic angiography (CCTA) to detect noncalcified plaque makes it an attractive test for potential ASCVD risk assessment.[30] However, studies on the added prognostic value of CCTA beyond traditional risk factors for risk assessment are scarce. Consequently, no societal body recommends using CCTA in *asymptomatic* individuals for risk assessment.

OTHER PROPOSED TESTS FOR FURTHER RISK ASSESSMENT IN PRIMARY ASCVD PREVENTION

In addition to atherosclerosis imaging techniques, other tests have been proposed as potential tools for risk assessment in primary prevention settings. Examples include measures of arterial function and stiffness, such as brachial flow-mediated dilation or pulse wave velocity, and circulating biomarkers such as troponins or natriuretic peptides. In general, the evidence demonstrating an added prognostic value of any of these tests beyond traditional risk factors is limited; for most of them, studies have demonstrated a clear superiority of CAC as the preferred test for further risk stratification.[31,32] Thus, neither U.S. nor European guidelines recommend these tests to guide routine preventive care.

TABLE 96.3 Summary of Major Guidelines and Expert Consensus Documents on Use of CAC for Risk Assessment in Asymptomatic Primary Prevention Individuals

Guideline/Statement	Summary of Recommendations on CAC for Risk Assessment	COR/LOE
2013 ACC/AHA Risk Assessment Guideline	If, after quantitative risk assessment using traditional risk factors, a risk-based treatment decision is uncertain, assessment of one or more of the following—family history, hsCRP, CAC, or ABI—may be considered to inform treatment decision-making	COR IIb, LOE: B
	Support revising risk assessment upward: CAC score ≥300 Agatston units or ≥75th percentile for age, sex, and ethnicity; no recommendations for CAC score of zero	
2017 Expert Consensus from the Society of Cardiovascular Computed Tomography	It is appropriate to perform CAC testing in the context of shared decision-making for asymptomatic individuals without clinical ASCVD who are 40-75 years of age and (a) in the 5% to <20% 10-year ASCVD risk group or (b) selectively in the <5% ASCVD risk group, such as those with a family history of premature coronary artery disease	N/A
2018 AHA/ACC/Multi-Society Cholesterol and 2019 ACC/AHA Primary Prevention Guidelines	In adults at intermediate risk (7.5% to <20% 10-year ASCVD risk) or selected adults at borderline risk (5% to <7.5% 10-year ASCVD risk) if risk-based decisions for preventive interventions (eg, statin therapy) remain uncertain, it is reasonable to measure a CAC score to guide clinician–patient risk discussion.	COR IIa, LOE: B
	In adults at intermediate risk (7.5% to <20% 10-year ASCVD risk) or selected adults at borderline risk (5% to <7.5% 10-year ASCVD risk) in whom a CAC score is measured for the purpose of making a treatment decision, and: If the CAC is zero, it is reasonable to withhold statin therapy and reassess in 5-10 years, as long as diabetes, family history of premature CHD, cigarette smoking are absent If CAC score is 1-99, it is reasonable to initiate statin therapy for patients ≥55 years; If CAC score is ≥100 or in the 75th percentile or higher, it is reasonable to initiate statin therapy.	COR IIa, LOE: B
2019 ESC/EAS Guideline for the Management of Dyslipidaemia	CAC assessment should be considered as a risk modifier in cardiovascular risk assessment of asymptomatic individuals at low or moderate risk	COR IIa, LOE: B

ABI, ankle-brachial index; ACC/AHA, American College of Cardiology/American Heart Association; ASCVD, atherosclerotic cardiovascular disease; CAC, coronary artery calcium; CHD, coronary heart disease; COR, class of recommendation; ESC/EAS, European Society of Cardiology/European Atherosclerosis Society; hsCRP, high sensitivity C-reactive protein; LOE, level of evidence.

RISK-ENHANCING FACTORS AND RISK MODIFIERS

Demographic and clinical features associated with a higher average ASCVD risk at the group level[4-6] are labelled "risk-enhancing factors" in the ACC/AHA guidelines[4,5] and "risk modifiers" by the ESC/EAS.[6] These include a family history of CHD/ASCVD, South Asian ancestry, increased circulating levels of lipoprotein[a], and chronic kidney disease, among other characteristics (**Table 96.4**). Because the increased risk associated with these features is not captured by most traditional risk scores, guidelines recommend considering them in addition to 10-year risk scoring. Typically, their presence should be used to make a stronger case for statin therapy initiation in individuals estimated to be at borderline or intermediate risk according to the PCE/SCORE in whom risk management with pharmacotherapy is unclear.

Although these characteristics are associated with an increased risk at the group level as compared to the general population, significant risk heterogeneity exists across individual persons with these characteristics.[33] For this reason, it has been proposed that aggressive pharmacotherapy may not be necessarily beneficial—at least on a 10-year time horizon—in all of these individuals, and that selective use of imaging tools such as CAC scanning may allow for a more personalized risk stratification and preventive therapy allocation.

RISK ASSESSMENT IN SPECIAL POPULATIONS

Women

Other subgroups have specific characteristics that also need to be taken into consideration for risk assessment. Several women's health features associated with an increased ASCVD risk, such as a history of premature menopause,[34] are included among the risk-enhancing characteristics listed in the ACC/AHA guidelines. In addition, some risk underestimation has been observed with traditional 10-year risk scores in young women.[35] Also, currently available scores may fail to capture

TABLE 96.4 Risk-Enhancing Factors and Risk Modifiers Included in Relevant 2018/2019 ACC/AHA and the 2019 ESC/EAS Guidelines

Risk-Enhancing Factors *2018 Multi-Society Guideline on the Management of Cholesterol and 2019 ACC/AHA Guideline on the Primary Prevention of ASCVD*	**Risk Modifiers** *2019 ESC/EAS Guidelines for the Management of Dyslipidaemias*
Family history of premature ASCVD	Family history of premature CVD
Primary hypercholesterolemia (LDL-C ≥ 160 mg/dL)	
Metabolic syndrome	
	Obesity and central obesity
Chronic kidney disease	Chronic kidney disease
Chronic inflammatory conditions (rheumatoid arthritis, advanced psoriasis, systemic lupus erythematosus, HIV infection)	Chronic immune-mediated inflammatory disorders; treatment for HIV infection
History of premature menopause and history of pregnancy-associated conditions that increase later ASCVD risk such as preeclampsia	
High-risk race/ethnicity (eg, South Asian ancestry, Native American)	
Persistently elevated primary hypertriglyceridemia (≥175 mg/dL, nonfasting)	Increased triglycerides
High-sensitivity C-reactive protein ≥2.0 mg/L	Increased high-sensitivity C-reactive protein
Lp(a) ≥50 mg/dL or ≥125 nmol/L	Extreme Lp(a) elevation; Lp(a) should be considered in selected patients with a family history of premature CVD and for reclassification in people who are borderline between moderate and high risk
ApoB ≥130 mg/dL	Increased ApoB
Ankle-brachial index <0.9	Ankle-brachial index <0.9 or >1.4
	Presence of albuminuria
CAC score not listed as a risk-enhancing factor	CAC score >100
	Presence of carotid or femoral plaque
	Social deprivation
	Physical inactivity
	Psychosocial stress including vital exhaustion
	Major psychiatric disorders
	Atrial fibrillation
	Left ventricular hypertrophy
	Obstructive sleep apnea
	Nonalcoholic fatty liver disease

ACC, American College of Cardiology; AHA, American Heart Association; ApoB, apolipoprotein B; ASCVD, atherosclerotic cardiovascular disease events; CAC, coronary artery calcium; CVD, cardiovascular disease; EAS, European Atherosclerosis Society; ESC, European Society of Cardiology; HIV, human immunodeficiency virus; LDL-C, low density lipoprotein cholesterol; Lp(a), lipoprotein a.

any potential adverse health effects resulting from the full incorporation of women into the job market (eg, increased levels of stress, workplace conflicts) that has taken place in recent decades in many countries.[36]

Under 40 years age group and over 75 years (elderly)

Risk estimation with 10-year risk scores in both young men and women is limited by the fact that most scores are not intended to be used in individuals younger than 40 years of age, and that low chronologic age generally results in low 10-year risk estimations. However, aggressive preventive interventions at early ages are likely to result in very large lifetime risk improvements,[37] and, therefore, are reasonable in young adults at highest relative ASCVD risk.

Lack of availability of ad hoc 10-year ASCVD risk scores above age 75 years is also an issue. In elderly individuals, risk scores will typically provide high-risk estimations, even among individuals free of modifiable risk factors. Although statin therapy will likely be beneficial in most of these individuals, pharmacologic side effects are considered to be more frequent at older ages, and so are drug–drug interactions, particularly among patients treated with multiple pharmacotherapies. Also, long-term reduction of ASCVD risk may not be a priority for some older patients. Consequently, individualization of management recommendations and incorporation of patient preferences will be particularly important in older persons.

Low Socioeconomic Status

Persons of low socioeconomic status are known to be particularly vulnerable to ASCVD.[38] Efforts should be made to minimize barriers and ensure access of these individuals to standard risk assessment approaches. Information on risk estimations and on proposed management plans should be adapted to their level of health literacy to ensure an effective risk communication and maximize patient adherence.

TOOLS FOR ASCVD RISK ASSESSMENT IN SECONDARY PREVENTION PATIENTS

The Second Manifestations of Arterial Disease (SMART) calculator provides 10-year estimations of the risk of a MI, stroke, or cardiovascular death in patients with a variety of previous ASCVD (ie, coronary artery disease, peripheral artery disease, abdominal aortic aneurysm, and polyvascular disease).[14] The SMART REACH (REduction of Atherothrombosis for Continued Health) calculator accounts for additional features and provides lifetime risk estimations as well as descriptions of the potential lifetime risk reductions that can be achieved with specific secondary prevention therapies.[14] These tools allow matching intensity of therapy to risk after an ASCVD event, potentially informing clinician–patient discussions and shared decision-making. This information may result in the further upward titration of statin therapy and/or addition of ezetimibe and, in the future, the addition of more expensive supplemental therapies such as PCSK9 inhibitors or high-dose icosapent ethyl, among others.

CLINICIAN–PATIENT RISK DISCUSSIONS AND SHARED DECISION-MAKING

Clinical primary prevention guidelines summarize recommendations for best ASCVD primary preventive care. Nevertheless, these documents also stress the importance of clinician–patient risk discussions and of shared decision-making when defining risk assessment and management plans for each individual patient.[4-6] Implementation of general recommendations should therefore be adapted to their preferences, expectations, and resources. In highly motivated individuals, further testing or incorporation of risk enhancers to the discussion may not be as relevant, because therapy will be initiated in most borderline/intermediate risk cases. On the other hand, in less motivated patients, clinical scoring using additional tools beyond 10-year scores, image testing such as CAC, and incorporation of risk-enhancing features should be considered to improve patient awareness. Still, once comprehensive risk information has been provided, the patient will have the last word, and the management and follow-up plan has to be consistent with their informed, autonomous decisions. However, reassessment of the patient's preferences should be pursued in subsequent visits, particularly among individuals at high estimated risk and reluctant to start risk-modifying therapy.

CHALLENGES, EVIDENCE GAPS, AND FUTURE DIRECTIONS

Dissemination efforts are needed to improve the implementation of current guideline recommendations as part of routine primary prevention care. Currently available clinical risk scores, such as the PCE and SCORE, will need to be further improved through recalibration and use of data from more contemporary, multiethnic cohorts with broader age ranges. Development of clinical risk scores for low-income areas as well as in developing countries will be a crucial step toward improving ASCVD prevention in regions where it is a major public health threat. Of note, the World Health Organization has recently released revised CVD risk charts to estimate risk in 21 global regions.[39]

Randomized trials have demonstrated that use of clinical risk scores improves risk factor management and reduce estimated risk during follow-up without causing harm.[40] Conversely, studies demonstrating the impact on outcomes of using risk-enhancing factors or atherosclerosis imaging tests to guide therapy allocation are not available. Trials of CAC and CCTA-based paradigms in primary prevention will assess their potential benefits as compared to clinical risk scoring alone. Should a benefit be demonstrated, access and adequate reimbursement of such tests in individuals most likely to benefit from them will need to be facilitated.

Research will also yield a better understanding of the potential value that polygenic risk scores—incorporating information on genetic polymorphisms associated with an increased ASCVD risk—have for improving risk prediction. These tools may be particularly useful for the detection of high genetic risk at early ages, thereby identifying individuals who may benefit from early, aggressive preventive interventions.

KEY POINTS

- ✔ Clinical risk scores predicting a person's 10-year risk of experiencing an ASCVD event remain the cornerstone of risk assessment in primary prevention in both the United States and Europe.
- ✔ The PCE and the SCORE charts are currently the major tools for clinical risk assessment, but other 10-year

risk scores are available and may be valuable in certain contexts.
- ✔ Clinical risk scores have important limitations, and atherosclerosis imaging by way of CAC score further refines risk assessment when management is uncertain.
- ✔ Risk communication tools and scores aimed at predicting additional outcomes may help enhance patient adherence to the recommended preventive therapies and may be particularly valuable in young adulthood.
- ✔ ASCVD risk assessment remains a very active area of research with particular focus on advanced imaging techniques such as CCTA and novel genetic-based risk assessment tools such as polygenic risk scores that may help identify those who may benefit from early, aggressive, and novel preventive interventions.

REFERENCES

1. Benjamin EJ, Muntner P, Alonso A, et al. heart disease and stroke statistics-2019 update: a report from the American Heart Association. *Circulation*. 2019;139:e56-e528.
2. European Heart Network. European cardiovascular disease statistics 2017. http://www.ehnheart.org/cvd-statistics.html
3. Zheng SL, Roddick AJ. Association of aspirin use for primary prevention with cardiovascular events and bleeding events: a systematic review and meta-analysis. *JAMA*. 2019;321:277-287.
4. Grundy SM, Stone NJ, Bailey AL, et al. 2018 ACC/AHA/AACVPR/AAPA/ABC/ACPM/ADA/AGS/APhA/ASPC/NLA/PCNA guideline on the management of blood cholesterol: a report of the American College of Cardiology/American Heart Association Task Force on Clinical Practice Guidelines. *J Am Coll Cardiol*. 2019;73:e285-e350.
5. Arnett DK, Blumenthal RS, Albert MA, et al. 2019 ACC/AHA guideline on the primary prevention of cardiovascular disease: a report of the American College of Cardiology/American Heart Association Task Force on Clinical Practice Guidelines. *J Am Coll Cardiol*. 2019;74:1376-1414.
6. Mach F, Baigent C, Catapano AL, et al. 2019 ESC/EAS guidelines for the management of dyslipidaemias: lipid modification to reduce cardiovascular risk. *Eur Heart J*. 2020;41(1):111-188.
7. Whelton PK, Carey RM, Aronow WS, et al. 2017 ACC/AHA/AAPA/ABC/ACPM/AGS/APhA/ASH/ASPC/NMA/PCNA guideline for the prevention, detection, evaluation, and management of high blood pressure in adults: a report of the American College of Cardiology/American Heart Association Task Force on Clinical Practice Guidelines. *J Am Coll Cardiol*. 2018;71:e127-e248.
8. American Heart Association Coronary Risk Handbook. *Estimating Risk of Coronary Heart Disease in Daily Practice*. American Heart Association; 1973:1-50.
9. Goff DC Jr, Lloyd-Jones DM, Bennett G, et al. 2013 ACC/AHA guideline on the assessment of cardiovascular risk: a report of the American College of Cardiology/American Heart Association Task Force on Practice Guidelines. *Circulation*. 2014;129:S49-S73.
10. European Association of Preventive Cardiology. HeartScore. http://www.heartscore.org/en_GB/
11. Hippisley-Cox J, Coupland C, Brindle P. Development and validation of QRISK3 risk prediction algorithms to estimate future risk of cardiovascular disease: prospective cohort study. *BMJ*. 2017;357:j2099.
12. McClelland RL, Jorgensen NW, Budoff M, et al. 10-year coronary heart disease risk prediction using coronary artery calcium and traditional risk factors: derivation in the MESA (Multi-Ethnic Study of Atherosclerosis) with validation in the HNR (Heinz Nixdorf Recall) study and the DHS (Dallas Heart Study). *J Am Coll Cardiol*. 2015;66:1643-1653.
13. Khera A, Budoff MJ, O'Donnell CJ, et al. Astronaut Cardiovascular Health and Risk Modification (Astro-CHARM) coronary calcium atherosclerotic cardiovascular disease risk calculator. *Circulation*. 2018;138:1819-1827.
14. U-Prevent. https://www.u-prevent.com/en-GB
15. DeFilippis AP, Young R, Carrubba CJ, et al. An analysis of calibration and discrimination among multiple cardiovascular risk scores in a modern multiethnic cohort. *Ann Intern Med*. 2015;162:266-275.
16. McEvoy JW, Diamond GA, Detrano RC, et al. Risk and the physics of clinical prediction. *Am J Cardiol*. 2014;113:1429-1435.
17. McClelland RL, Nasir K, Budoff M, et al. Arterial age as a function of coronary artery calcium (from the multi-ethnic study of atherosclerosis [MESA]). *Am J Cardiol*. 2009;103:59-63.
18. Karmali KN, Lloyd-Jones DM. Adding a life-course perspective to cardiovascular-risk communication. *Nat Rev Cardiol*. 2013;10:111.
19. Khan SS, Ning H, Shah SJ, et al. 10-year risk equations for incident heart failure in the general population. *J Am Coll Cardiol*. 2019;73:2388-2397.
20. D'Agostino RB Sr, Vasan RS, Pencina MJ, et al. General cardiovascular risk profile for use in primary care: the Framingham Heart Study. *Circulation*. 2008;117:743-753.
21. Erbel R, Budoff M. Improvement of cardiovascular risk prediction using coronary imaging: subclinical atherosclerosis: the memory of lifetime risk factor exposure. *Eur Heart J*. 2012;33:1201-1213.
22. Greenland P, Blaha MJ, Budoff MJ, et al. Coronary calcium score and cardiovascular risk. *J Am Coll Cardiol*. 2018;72:434-447.
23. Agatston AS, Janowitz WR, Hildner FJ, et al. Quantification of coronary artery calcium using ultrafast computed tomography. *J Am Coll Cardiol*. 1990;15:827-832.
24. Polonsky TS, McClelland RL, Jorgensen NW, et al. Coronary artery calcium score and risk classification for coronary heart disease prediction. *JAMA*. 2010;303:1610-1616.
25. Nasir K, Bittencourt MS, Blaha MJ, et al. Implications of coronary artery calcium testing among statin candidates according to American College of Cardiology/American Heart Association cholesterol management guidelines: MESA (Multi-Ethnic Study of Atherosclerosis). *J Am Coll Cardiol*. 2015;66:1657-1668.
26. Detrano R, Guerci AD, Carr JJ, et al. Coronary calcium as a predictor of coronary events in four racial or ethnic groups. *N Engl J Med*. 2008;358:1336-1345.
27. Lloyd-Jones DM, Braun LT, Ndumele CE, et al. Use of risk assessment tools to guide decision-making in the primary prevention of atherosclerotic cardiovascular disease: a special report from the American Heart Association and American College of Cardiology. *Circulation*. 2019;139:e1162-e1177.
28. Mortensen MB, Fuster V, Muntendam P, et al. Negative risk markers for cardiovascular events in the elderly. *J Am Coll Cardiol*. 2019;74:1-11.
29. Oren A, Vos LE, Uiterwaal CS, et al. Cardiovascular risk factors and increased carotid intima-media thickness in healthy young adults: the Atherosclerosis Risk in Young Adults (ARYA) study. *Arch Intern Med*. 2003;163:1787-1792.
30. NIH/US National Library of Medicine. Scottish Computed Tomography of the HEART Trial (SCOT-HEART). Accessed April 10, 2017. https://clinicaltrials.gov/ct2/show/NCT01149590
31. Yeboah J, McClelland RL, Polonsky TS, et al. Comparison of novel risk markers for improvement in cardiovascular risk assessment in intermediate-risk individuals. *JAMA*. 2012;308:788-795.
32. Blaha MJ, Cainzos-Achirica M, Greenland P, et al. Role of coronary artery calcium score of zero and other negative risk markers for cardiovascular disease: the Multi-Ethnic Study of Atherosclerosis (MESA). *Circulation*. 2016;133:849-858.
33. Dzaye O, Dudum R, Reiter-Brennan C, et al. Coronary artery calcium scoring for individualized cardiovascular risk estimation in important patient subpopulations after the 2019 AHA/ACC primary prevention guidelines. *Prog Cardiovasc Dis*. 2019;62(5):423-430. doi: 10.1016/j.pcad.2019.10.007.
34. Honigberg MC, Zekavat SM, Aragam K, et al. Association of premature natural and surgical menopause with incident cardiovascular disease [published online ahead of print, 2019 Nov 18]. *JAMA*. 2019;e1919191.

35. Michos ED, Nasir K, Braunstein JB, et al. Framingham risk equation underestimates subclinical atherosclerosis risk in asymptomatic women. *Atherosclerosis*. 2006;184:201-206.
36. Xu T, Magnusson Hanson LL, Lange T, et al. Workplace bullying and workplace violence as risk factors for cardiovascular disease: a multi-cohort study. *Eur Heart J*. 2019;40:1124-1134.
37. Luirink IK, Wiegman A, Kusters DM, et al. 20-year follow-up of statins in children with familial hypercholesterolemia. *N Engl J Med*. 2019;381:1547-1556.
38. Link BG, Phelan J. Social conditions as fundamental causes of disease. *J Health Soc Behav* 1995;35:80-94.
39. WHO CVD Risk Chart Working Group. World Health Organization cardiovascular disease risk charts: revised models to estimate risk in 21 global regions. *Lancet Glob Health*. 2019;7:e1332-e1345.
40. Karmali KN, Persell SD, Perel P, et al. Risk scoring for the primary prevention of cardiovascular disease. *Cochrane Database Syst Rev*. 2017;3(3):CD006887.

CHAPTER 97

LIFESTYLE IMPLEMENTATION FOR CARDIOVASCULAR DISEASE PREVENTION: A FOCUS ON SMOKING CESSATION, DIET, AND PHYSICAL ACTIVITY

Oluwaseun E. Fashanu, Gowtham R. Grandhi, and Erin D. Michos

INTRODUCTION

Cardiovascular disease (CVD) remains the leading cause of morbidity and mortality in the United States and the world despite large public health and healthcare expenditures.[1] Despite several advancements in pharmacologic management of CVD and the use of such therapies (eg, statins) in primary prevention, there remains an excess risk of incident CVD and CVD-related mortality, which may be partly attributed to patients' poor lifestyle choices. Promotion of a healthy lifestyle throughout one's life span is the foundation for all preventive efforts. Previous declines in CVD morbidity and mortality of decades past now appear to be blunted, likely in part because of unfavorable lifestyle behaviors. This led the American Heart Association (AHA) in 2010 to release their 2020 impact goals aimed at improving the cardiovascular (CV) health of all Americans by 20% while reducing deaths attributable to CVD by 20%.[2] Although CVD mortality in the United States declined during the years 2000-2011, it then plateaued during 2011-2014 and ceased to decline altogether from 2013 to 2015.[1,3] Furthermore, CVD mortality has risen among younger adults, particularly middle-aged women.[3,4] This worrisome trend reflects the rise in the rates of obesity, diabetes, and physical inactivity in the United States and worldwide during this same period.[1]

Poor lifestyle choices such as cigarette use, unhealthy diet, obesity, and physical inactivity adversely impact the CV health of individuals.[1] Promoting and establishing a healthy lifestyle can reduce the development of CVD risk factors in the first place (primordial prevention), delay the onset of CVD among individuals with risk factors (primary prevention), and prevent recurrent events among those with established clinical CVD (secondary prevention).

In an attempt to achieve their aforementioned 2020 impact goal, the AHA developed the concept of the "Life's Simple 7," defined by seven modifiable metrics that contribute to CV health, namely, the behavioral factors of smoking, diet, physical activity, and body mass index (BMI) and the health-related factors of blood pressure (BP), glucose, and cholesterol control.[2] Optimal CV health is defined as the presence of ideal levels at least 5 of the seven metrics: not smoking/smoking cessation for more than 12 months, having a heart-healthy diet, optimal physical activity levels, BMI less than 25 kg/m^2, BP less than 120/80 mmHg, glucose less than 100 mg/dL, total cholesterol less than 200 mg/dL in adults without the use of medications, and the absence of clinical CVD.[2] Based on recent data, none of the U.S. adult population met ideal levels of all seven metrics, with only 5% meeting six ideal metrics, and approximately 41% having two or less.[1] Several studies have shown an inverse dose-response association between having increasing numbers of these ideal metrics with CVD, non-CV diseases, and all-cause mortality.[5-7] A 2017 meta-analysis by Guo et al., consisting of thirteen prospective cohort studies and 198,126 participants, showed that having the highest number of ideal CV health metrics was associated with a lower risk of CVD (relative risk [RR] 0.22, 95% confidence interval [CI] 0.11, 0.42), CVD mortality (0.30 [0.18, 0.51]), and all-cause mortality (0.54 [0.41, 0.69]).[7] Similarly, each increase in ideal CV health metric was associated with a 19% lower risk of CVD mortality and 11% lower risk of all-cause mortality.[7]

This chapter presents lifestyle interventions for CVD prevention, with a particular focus on three metrics of the Life's Simple 7: smoking cessation, diet, and physical activity. Such underaddressed lifestyle changes will need to become a greater focus in managing and improving CV health globally.

SMOKING

Smoking leads to oxidative stress, increased sympathetic activation, endothelial dysfunction and injury, inflammation, and hypercoagulable states, conferring increased atherogenesis and thrombosis risk with resultant CVD.[8] Smoking cessation reduces the risk of CVD morbidity and mortality, as well as all-cause mortality, compared to continued smoking.[9] There has been a decline in the proportion of U.S. adults who smoke in recent years.[1] Nevertheless, in 2019, about 34.1 million—representing 14.0% of U.S. adult population—continued to smoke cigarettes, similar to estimates from 2018.[10,11] Despite the known deleterious effects of smoking, including pulmonary disease, CVD, and cancer, tobacco users continue to do so partly because of the addictive nature of nicotine, the active substance in tobacco. Cigarette smoking remains the leading cause of preventable disease and mortality in the United States according to the 2020 U.S. Surgeon General report and has been the focus of public health interventions in recent times.[9] Exposure to secondhand smoke also has its health consequences.[1] There is no safe level of smoking. Smoking even just one cigarette daily confers nearly half the risk of coronary heart disease (CHD) and stroke as smoking 20 cigarettes daily.[12]

Although smoking cessation decreases CVD risk, former smokers still have higher risk than never smokers.[13] The effects of smoking cessation on CHD risk reduce by half after the first year of quitting and equates that of never smokers after about 15 years of quitting. For stroke reduction, this takes about 5 to 15 years to equate the risk of never smokers.[9] Cigarette smoking worsens atherosclerosis and is associated with subclinical atherosclerosis markers, including ankle-brachial index, carotid intima-media thickness, and coronary artery calcification (CAC).[14] Though smoking cessation may slow the progression of subclinical atherosclerosis, it does not appear to be able to reverse it. Hence, the importance of avoiding cigarette use altogether if possible.

Cessation Advice/Treatment

Despite the proven benefits of smoking cessation, advice to quit by clinicians and prescriptions given for smoking cessation pharmacotherapies remain suboptimal.[15] In a nationally representative U.S. survey, the proportion of smokers who reported receiving physician advice to quit smoking was 60% in 2006 to 2007 and only modestly increased to 65% by 2014 to 2015.[15] As outlined in the 2019 American College of Cardiology (ACC)/AHA Guideline for the Primary Prevention of CVD, tobacco use should be assessed at every healthcare visit and individuals who smoke be counseled to quit (Class of Recommendation [COR] I, *Level of Evidence* [LOE] *A*).[16] As little as 3 minutes of assessment and counseling at each visit is recommended. One approach that has been shown to be effective is the Five A's method: Ask, Advise, Attempt, Assist, and Arrange (**Table 97.1**). Several modifications of the Five A's approach such as AAC (Ask, Advise, Connect) and AAR (Ask, Advise, Refer) may also be effective.

A variety of U.S. Food and Drug Administration–approved tobacco cessation pharmacotherapy, five nicotine replacement therapies (NRTs) and two non-nicotine oral medications (**Table 97.2**), and behavioral interventions are available

TABLE 97.1 Five A's Approach to Counseling Against Tobacco Use

Ask	All patients should be **asked** about tobacco use.
Advise	Tobacco users should be **advised** to quit.
Assess	Readiness to quit should be **assessed** at every visit.
Assist	Provide counseling, pharmacotherapy, and referrals to **assist** with quitting.
Arrange	**Arrange** follow-up contacts for those willing to quit and readdress quitting at follow-up in those unwilling to quit.

TABLE 97.2 U.S. Food and Drug Administration–Approved Pharmacotherapies for Smoking Cessation

Nicotine replacement therapies (NRTs)	Gum	No more than 24 gums or 20 lozenges daily. If smoking occurs ≤30 minutes after waking start with 4 mg, otherwise use 2 mg
	Lozenge	
	Nasal spray	No more than 40 sprays daily
	Oral inhaler	No more than 16 cartridges daily (10 mg per cartridge)
	Patch	7 mg, 14 mg, or 21 mg Use 21 mg patch if smokes ≥10 cigarettes daily
Non-nicotine oral medications	Sustained-release bupropion	150 mg titrated up to 300 mg daily May be used in combination with other NRTs
	Varenicline	0.5 mg titrated up to 1 mg daily

to help with quitting.[16] A combination of both counseling and pharmacotherapy is recommended to maximize the success of quitting in nonpregnant individuals. Data on the safety of NRT in pregnant or breastfeeding mothers are limited, so NRT should be used with caution. A report by the U.S. Preventive Services Task Force found mixed results concerning the risk of preterm delivery and mean birth weight among pregnant individuals using NRT. Some studies showed a lower risk of preterm delivery and higher mean birth weight, whereas others did not find any associations.[17] Nevertheless, cessation counseling advice remains crucial. Individualized short text messaging on cessation and web-based interventions have been shown to be effective. Public policies impact smoking cessation at the population level. Interventions such as the introduction of Tobacco 21 laws, which increases the age of being able to purchase cigarettes from 18 to 21 years, smoking policies such as the smoke-free indoor laws, tobacco education campaigns, cessation advise from healthcare providers, and the provision of quit lines (ie, free coaching over the phone) are effective.

Electronic Nicotine Delivery Systems

Electronic nicotine delivery systems (ENDS), also known as electronic cigarettes, e-cigarettes, or vape pens, are devices that produce aerosolized nicotine, flavored liquid, and solvents inhaled by users. They are usually battery operated, and they have become more popular among U.S. youths (most especially the flavored brands). Given the relatively new introduction of electronic cigarettes since 2007 to the United States and multiple varieties, the long-term effects on CV health are not well established. However, there is concern about the potential harmful effects of metals, such as lead and arsenic, as well as the unregulated amounts of nicotine (ranging for 0 mg/mL to as high as 59 mg/mL) these devices expose to users.[18,19] There is also an increased risk of nicotine addiction and progression to traditional cigarettes with electronic cigarette use, making their increased uptake among youths and never smokers concerning. According to a Centers for Disease Control and Prevention report, there was a 49% and 78% increase in electronic cigarette use among middle and high school students, respectively, between 2017 and 2018, partly eliminating prior progress made in the decline in use of tobacco products in these groups.[20]

Electronic cigarettes have been touted as a substitute for combustible cigarette cessation; however, substantial evidence for this is lacking. Five trials (n = 3117) reported inconsistent findings on the effectiveness of electronic cigarettes on smoking cessation at 6 to 12 months among smokers when compared with placebo or NRT, and none suggested higher rates of serious adverse events.[17]

Electronic cigarette use also adds to the dilemma of dual use of tobacco products. Dual use of tobacco products is the concurrent use of traditional cigarettes with other tobacco-containing products such as cigars, pipes, hookah, tobacco leaves, snuff, and electronic cigarettes. In 2013 to 2014, electronic cigarettes in addition to traditional cigarettes seemed to be the more common combination among young and adult dual users based on the Population Assessment of Tobacco and Health study.[21] It is therefore essential that healthcare providers ascertain electronic cigarette use in addition to traditional cigarettes during clinic visits while counseling against quitting.

NUTRITION AND DIET

Dietary Guidelines

Diet is recognized as one of the most important determinants of overall health, and as such, dietary guidelines for the purposes of heart disease prevention have been in place and evolving since the 1970s in the United States.[22] Suboptimal diet has been associated with nearly 50% of death secondary to heart diseases, stroke, and type 2 diabetes and shown to affect health regardless of age, sex, and sociodemographic characters.[23,24] The 2019 ACC/AHA Guideline for the Primary Prevention of CVD endorses (1) increased consumption of vegetables, fruits, legumes, and whole grains; (2) moderate consumption of vegetable oil, nuts, seafood, low-fat dairy, and lean meats; and (3) avoiding or restricting processed meats, saturated fats, trans-fats, salt, refined carbohydrates, and sugar-sweetened beverages (**Table 97.3**).[16,25] Additionally, it recommends plant-based and Mediterranean diets that share similarities, such as a high intake of fiber, antioxidants, vitamins, minerals, polyphenols, and monounsaturated and polyunsaturated fatty acids; and low intake of salt, refined sugar, carbohydrates with high glycemic load, and saturated and trans-fats.

Macronutrient Approaches to Optimize Health

Dietary Carbohydrates and Sugars

Dietary carbohydrates are the main source of energy. Whole grains are unprocessed and are a good source of fiber and micronutrients in contrast to refined grains that lack the outer layers of the edible kernel. Consumption of whole grains such as whole grain bread, oatmeal, breakfast cereal, brown rice, unrefined maize and sorghum is associated with greater risk reduction of CVD and all-cause mortality when compared to minimal benefit with refined grain such as white bread, white rice, and refined breakfast cereal. Most importantly, studies have shown a dose-response benefit in CVD risk and all-cause mortality with whole grain consumption.[26,27]

Supplementary sugars (other than naturally occurring sugars in milk and fruits) such as corn syrup, raw or brown sugar, and honey are often added to foods and beverages when processed or packaged. A majority of the added sugars are obtained from sugar-sweetened beverages (sodas, fruit drinks, energy/sports drinks), candy, cakes, and sweetened dairy products. Yang et al. reported a significant association between CVD mortality and increased added sugar consumption, with a 2.75-fold increase in hazard ratio (HR) for CVD deaths among individuals with greater than 25% of daily calorie consumption from added sugars when compared with individuals with less than 10% of daily calorie consumption.[28] Therefore, the ACC/AHA, the European Society of Cardiology, and the U.S. Departments of Agriculture and Health and Human Services dietary guidelines emphasize whole grain consumption and minimizing refined sugars and added sugars.[16,25,29,30]

Dietary Fats

Dietary fat comprises unsaturated fat, saturated fat, and *trans*-fat. Similar to carbohydrates, different fats have been found to have differential association with CVD and all-cause mortality. Unsaturated fats, which include monounsaturated

TABLE 97.3 Components of Heart-Healthy Diet

High	Moderation	Caution	Restrict
Leafy vegetables, fruits, whole grains, legumes	Vegetable oils, nuts, seeds, seafood, low-fat dairy, lean meat, coffee	Animal fat, refined grains, fruit juices, tinned fruits	Sodium, added sugar, processed and red meat, saturated and *trans*-fats

and polyunsaturated fatty acids, are predominantly found in vegetable oils, seeds, nuts, olives, and fish. These are often referred to as "healthy fats" because they are associated with reduced CVD risk and overall mortality, whereas *trans*- and saturated fats—primarily found in animal fats such as fatty meats, milk, and processed foods like margarine, butter, and cheese—have been associated with increased risk of most CV outcomes.

Using combined data from two large prospective cohort studies of 126,233 participants with a follow-up of over 25 years, Wang et al. demonstrated lower mortality with monounsaturated (HR 0.89 [0.84, 0.94]) and polyunsaturated fats (HR 0.81 [0.78, 0.84]).[31] Conversely, *trans*-fats had the highest total mortality (HR 1.13 [1.07, 1.18]) closely followed by saturated fats (HR 1.08 [1.03, 1.14]). Additionally, Wang et al. demonstrated that substituting saturated and *trans*-fats with unsaturated fats resulted in significant reduction in mortality, particularly with polyunsaturated fatty acids. Thus, the 2019 ACC/AHA Primary Prevention Guideline recommends replacing saturated fat with dietary monounsaturated and polyunsaturated fats to reduce atherosclerotic CVD risk (COR IIa, LOE B—Non-randomized) and that *trans*-fats should be avoided (COR III—harm, LOE B—Nonrandomized).[16]

Dietary Protein

The source of protein (plant vs. animal) has been shown to have varying association with CVD and all-cause mortality. This has been explored among longitudinal studies performed in the United States (n = 131,342) and Japan (n = 70,696), which showed that intake of plant protein was associated with a significant decrease in all-cause and CVD mortality, whereas consumption of animal protein was associated with an increased CVD mortality.[32,33] Furthermore, replacing 3% of energy with plant protein in place of processed red meat protein was associated with a 34% to 46% reduction in HR for all-cause mortality and when substituted for unprocessed red meat protein it was associated with a 42% reduction in HR for CVD mortality.[32,33] These data support the current recommendation for dietary protein to be obtained from lean meat, fish, and vegetable sources and to avoid processed meats.[16]

Dietary Patterns and Cardiovascular Health

The DASH Diet

The DASH (Dietary Approaches to Stop Hypertension) diet—which is rich in fruits, vegetables, and low-fat dairy foods and has reduced amounts of saturated fats, total fats, and cholesterol—was proposed in 1997 as a lifestyle intervention independent of medication to control hypertension. Individuals who consumed the DASH diet were found to have a significant reduction in BP, particularly among those with hypertension (11.4 and 5.5 mm Hg reduction in systolic and diastolic BP, respectively).[34] These results were confirmed by the DASH-Sodium trial, which also demonstrated a dose-related inverse association between BP and sodium intake.[35] In addition to reduction in BP, the DASH diet has been associated with reduction in low-density lipoprotein cholesterol (LDL-C) level (11.6 mg/dL) and estimated CV risk.[34,36] Therefore, U.S. Departments of Agriculture and Health and Human Services have recognized the DASH diet as an ideal eating plan, which has been further endorsed by the AHA.[16,25,30]

In a recent meta-analysis evaluating the association of DASH dietary pattern and cardiometabolic outcomes, Chiavaroli et al. found a 20% reduction in CHD incidence and 18% reduction in diabetes mellitus incidence, in addition to an improvement in BP, lipids, and glycemic control.[37]

The Mediterranean Diet

Fewer CVD-related deaths in the Mediterranean countries such as Greece, Spain, and Italy, when compared to United States and northern Europe, has kindled interest in their dietary habits. The Mediterranean diet, based on the dietary habits of these countries, is typically rich in vegetables, whole grains, fruits, nuts/seeds, legumes, and olive oil, along with a moderate consumption of seafood, poultry, and low-fat dairy. Although both the Mediterranean and the DASH diets are similar—including restricting red meat and saturated fats intake—the Mediterranean diet places a larger emphasis on dairy consumption in comparison to the DASH diet.

The Mediterranean diet is associated with a significantly lower CVD incidence and CVD/all-cause mortality.[38] The benefits of this diet were noted in 1999 in the Lyon Diet Heart Study, which explored the effect of the Mediterranean diet among individuals with myocardial infarction (MI) on secondary CVD prevention. The study reported a significant reduction in major adverse cardiac events: 54% and 72% reduction in all-cause mortality and nonfatal MI/cardiac mortality, respectively.[39] For primary prevention, the PREDIMED (Prevención con Dieta Mediterránea) randomized clinical trial demonstrated a 31% lower risk of MI, stroke, and CVD mortality among those assigned the Mediterranean diet plus extra-virgin olive oil, and a 28% lower risk for Mediterranean diet plus nuts, when compared to low-fat diet.[40] This study complements a prior study that demonstrated a 33% and 25% reduction in CHD and all-cause mortality, respectively, among those who consume the Mediterranean diet.[38]

The Vegetarian Diet

The vegetarian diet constitutes a wide variety of dietary patterns that are predominantly plant based, which limit or exclude foods from animal source such as meat, poultry, and seafood. Some vegetarian diets include eggs and/or dairy products, whereas the vegan diet is completely plant based and excludes all animal products. Studies have consistently shown that a vegetarian diet is associated with decreased CVD and diabetes risk and many other health benefits such as reducing systolic BP, improving cholesterol levels, and weight loss.[41] Although most studies have demonstrated health benefits among those who consume a vegetarian diet, data suggest a wide variation in the strength of association to CVD risk benefits.[41] Though a vegetarian diet emphasizes a diet rich in healthy plant foods, it is often misinterpreted as simply the absence of meat. Because the nutritional quality of plant foods varies considerably, the overall quality of a vegetarian diet could have different association with CVD and diabetes risk.

Satija et al., using a pooled sample of 209,298 participants from three prospective study cohorts, explored the relationship between diets and CHD incidence. They categorized diets into healthy plant foods (predominantly vegetables, fruits, whole grains, legumes, nuts, and oils), less healthy plant foods (refined grains, potatoes, desserts, and juices/sugar-sweetened beverages), and animal foods (dairy, eggs, seafood, meat, and animal fat).[42] They demonstrated that increased consumption of healthy plant foods is inversely associated with CVD risk, with 25% lower incidence of CHD. In contrast, an increased consumption of less healthy plant foods was directly associated with CHD incidence (32% higher incidence). Interestingly, individuals who predominantly consumed animal foods had a lower incidence of CHD when compared with those who consumed less healthy plant foods, though both diets had an increased CHD incidence compared to healthy plant foods.[42] Similar results were demonstrated with the incidence of type 2 diabetes mellitus, with a 34% lower incidence among individuals with a healthy plant food diet and 16% higher incidence among those with a less healthy plant diet.[43] Additionally, Kwok et al. demonstrated that consumption of canned fruit was associated with a 14% increased all-cause mortality, likely because of the added sugar/syrups.[27] Hence, it is important to remember not all vegetarian diets are healthy and to consider the quality of plant foods. Healthcare providers should be cautious while providing recommendations for vegetarian diets, with an emphasis on consumption of whole grain, vegetables, fresh fruit, nuts, legumes, and healthier oils in addition to restricting refined grains, sugar-sweetened beverages, and canned fruits and products with added sugar.

Emerging Dietary Trends

Interest in other dietary patterns has emerged, such as intermittent fasting diet and low-carbohydrate, high-fat diets (ketogenic diet and paleolithic diet). The evidence for these diets affecting total mortality, weight loss, and CV health is ambiguous and limited. Therefore, prospective studies with large sample size and long follow-up duration are crucial to recognize (or refute) the potential benefits of these diets before they can be safely recommended. Because of the lack of strength of evidence on impacting CV events, these diets are not supported by any major guidelines.

Comparison of Diets

In sum, there are several dietary patterns (such as DASH, Mediterranean, and healthy vegetarian diet) that are consistent with heart health and CVD prevention.[22] Although there are some subtle differences among them, these healthy dietary patterns are more alike than dissimilar. The 2019 ACC/AHA Guideline recommends a diet that emphasizes intake of vegetables, fruits, legumes, nuts, whole grains, and fish to decrease CVD risk factors (COR I, LOE B—Randomized).[16] Regardless of specific dietary pattern, experts are largely in agreement to avoid ultra-processed foods that have been linked to increased risk of CVD and mortality.[44,45] Ultra-processed foods unfortunately tend to be highly palatable, leading to increased calorie consumption and weight gain.[46] Ultra-processed foods are typically of high energy density, with low fiber and micronutrients, and high amounts of added sugars, sodium, saturated fats, and chemical additives.

Importance of Nutrition Counseling

Nutrition counseling plays a crucial role in primordial, primary, and secondary prevention of CVD. Although randomized clinical trials would provide the best evidence to shape guidelines for nutritional interventions, these trials are challenging to conduct given limitations with blinding and adherence to the intervention and the length of follow-up time needed to assess hard clinical outcomes. Thus, most of the evidence base for dietary recommendations come from epidemiologic studies, which have methodologic challenges—such as ascertainment bias and residual confounding from other lifestyle factors—which can promote erroneous causal inferences.[22,47] Rapidly evolving nutrition science and dietary recommendations, in addition to the conflicting messages from the food industries and media, are confusing to the general public. Therefore, physicians and healthcare providers play a critical role in counseling patients to bring awareness regarding evidence-based current dietary recommendations, caution about novel diets without scientific evidence, and address false beliefs. It is crucial for physicians to be well informed on nutritional topics to provide effective nutrition counseling to the patients during clinical visits.

Aggarwal et al. demonstrated that although 72% of the physicians believed they had provided effective counseling, only 21% of the patients thought they had gained beneficial information, as the physicians focused on the pathophysiology of the disease.[48] Pallazola et al. have provided guidance to the clinicians on best ways to advise patients on evidence-based heart-healthy diets during clinic visits[49]: patient-centered interviews to assess their knowledge of nutrition, patient's commitment to change, affordability to alter and maintain a healthy lifestyle, cultural background, limitations in consuming specific diets, and patient's goal are important factors to consider in successful counseling.

PHYSICAL ACTIVITY AND EXERCISE

A large proportion of the U.S. population, about half, remain inactive or do not achieve the recommended level of physical activity according to the 2018 Physical Activity Guidelines Advisory Committee Scientific Report.[50] Physical activity and exercise have long been recognized as being important to overall well-being. Physical activity affects various aspects of human health and functioning, including fitness, mental health, reduced risk of some cancer types as well as improved CV health. Increasing physical activity has been identified as a low-cost intervention that could reduce the burden of CVD, premature mortality, and economic burden of disease globally.[51,52]

Physical activity is defined as any movement of the skeletal muscle resulting in energy expenditure, usually measured in metabolic equivalents (METs), whereas "exercise" is a structured and repetitive activity performed to maintain or improve fitness and/or health. The guidelines focus on increasing total physical activity per week from any combination of activities, and not specifically just exercise. Physical activity exerts an independent effect on CV health, even independently of associations with CVD risk factors such as hypertension, obesity, and dyslipidemia. Physical activity can be classified based on the intensity and subsequent energy expenditure to include light- (1.6-2.9 METs), moderate- (3.0-5.9 METs), and vigorous-intensity (≥6 METs) activities (**Table 97.4**).

The 2019 ACC/AHA Guideline on the Primary Prevention of CVD recommends that adults be routinely counseled about optimization of a physically active lifestyle (COR I, LOE B—Randomized).[16] In some CVD risk groups, behavioral counseling has been shown to foster physical activity.[53] The 2019 ACC/AHA and the 2018 Physical Activity Guidelines both recommend that individuals get at least a cumulative of 150 minutes of moderate-intensity or 75 minutes of vigorous-intensity aerobic physical activity weekly or an equivalent combination (COR I, LOE B—Nonrandomized).[16,25,50] This is equivalent to performing 500 to 1000 MET-minutes per week of aerobic activity excluding muscle-strengthening activities. The CV benefits of these physical activity levels have been shown to increase in a dose-response manner, with 300 minutes of moderate or 150 minutes of vigorous-intensity physical activity or an equivalent combination of both providing additional benefit.[54] The 2018 Physical Activity Guideline additionally recommends to perform at least twice-weekly muscle-strengthening activity.[50]

Furthermore, any physical activity, even at levels lower than the minimum recommended amount, is associated with a significantly lower risk of CHD compared to being inactive.[54] Thus, the 2019 ACC/AHA Guideline states that for adults who are unable to meet the minimum recommended physical activity amounts, engaging in some moderate-to-vigorous physical activity, even if less than recommended, is beneficial for CVD risk reduction (COR IIA, LOE B—Nonrandomized).[16] Although prior guidelines recommended moderate-to-vigorous physical activity to be conducted in at least 10-minute increments (ie, "bouts"), the newer U.S. recommendations no longer set a minimum prescribed time for physical activity for a single session, as all activity counts toward the total weekly physical activity goals.[16,50]

Sedentary Behavior

Sedentary behavior includes low-energy-expenditure activities requiring 1.5 METS or less, such as sitting, lying, or being in a reclined position. Standing is, however, not considered to be a sedentary behavior even though it requires 1.5 METS or less.[16] Though being sedentary and being physically active may appear to represent opposite spectrums, individuals tend to spend their wake time performing a mixture. For example, an individual can attain the recommended duration of moderate- to vigorous-intensity physical activity weekly but still be engaged in a sedentary lifestyle for most of their awake state. However, sedentary behavior is independently associated with a higher CVD risk and poorer CV health outcomes even after accounting for baseline physical activity,[55] although the risk conferred by sedentary behavior is less among those with higher physical activity levels.[56] The 2019 ACC/AHA Primary Prevention Guideline states that decreasing sedentary behavior is a reasonable strategy to reduce CVD risk (COR IIb, LOE C—Limited Data)[16] and attempts should be made to substitute sedentary activities with other physical activity types, even with light-intensity activity. In general, the more physically active an individual is, the better, and all adults should be encouraged to move and reduce sedentary activities.

Benefits of Physical Activity Relating to CVD and Its Risk Factors

The adjusted population attributable fraction for CVD mortality because of inadequate physical activity was shown to be 11.9% (1.3%, 22.3%) in the National Health and Nutrition Examination Survey (NHANES).[57] Physical activity, irrespective of the amount, has been shown to reduce CVD-related mortality and all-cause mortality in the general population. A recent study by Saint-Maurice et al. including 315,059 men and women enrolled in the National Institutes of Health–AARP Diet and Health Study showed that participants who maintained higher levels of self-reported leisure-time physical activity compared to those who were inactive consistently throughout adulthood had a 42% and 36% lower risk of CVD-related mortality (HR 0.58 [0.53, 0.64]) and all-cause mortality (HR 0.64 [0.60 to 0.68]), respectively.[58] Similarly, less active participants who later increased their activity level had some improved CVD-related and all-cause mortality benefit.[58] Furthermore, a prospective epidemiology study by Florido et al. in the Atherosclerosis Risk in Communities

TABLE 97.4 Intensities of Physical Activity

Intensity	Sedentary behavior	Light	Moderate	Vigorous
METs	≤1.5	1.6-2.9	3.0-5.9	≥6
Examples	Sitting, watching TV, lying, driving	Leisure walking (≤2 mph), light household chores, cooking	Walking briskly (3-4 mph), vacuuming, recreational swimming, tennis (doubles)	Jogging, running, swimming laps, tennis (single), heavy gardening, mowing grass, snow shoveling

METs, metabolic equivalents; mph, miles per hour; TV, television.

Study showed that participants achieving the recommended physical activity levels were 16% less likely to have CVD events compared to those with poor physical activity levels after accounting for a number of CVD risk factors (HR 0.84 [0.74, 0.94]).[59]

Physical activity lowers BP levels in individuals who are normotensive and among those who have elevated BP, and reduces the risk of hypertension. Hypertensive individuals tend to get the greatest BP reductions with physical activity compared to normotensive individuals. On average, aerobic moderate-to vigorous-intensity physical activity reduces systolic BP 2 to 4 mmHg in individuals who are normotensive and 5 to 8 mm Hg in those who are hypertensive.[16] A diastolic reduction of 1 to 4 mm Hg may also be seen.[60] In a meta-analysis by Liu et al., meeting the recommended physical activity level was associated with a lower risk of hypertension (RR 0.94 [0.92, 0.97]) compared to inactive individuals, with increased benefit at higher amounts of physical activity.[61]

Insulin sensitivity and glucose uptake are improved in physically active individuals and this may help prevent, reduce the risk, or delay the onset of type 2 diabetes. In individuals with diabetes, moderate-to-vigorous activity improves glycemic control and reduces hemoglobin A1c levels. A 2015 meta-analysis showed that all levels of physical activity are associated with reduced risk of type 2 diabetes in an inverse manner.[62] Similarly, the risk of CVD mortality is reduced in individuals with diabetes who are physically active. A reduction in LDL-C and non–high-density lipoprotein cholesterol of 3 to 6 mg/dL and 6 mg/dL, respectively, may be seen in individuals who participate in aerobic moderate- to vigorous-intensity physical activity. Associations with high-density lipoprotein cholesterol and triglyceride levels are inconsistent.[60] Maintenance of an ideal BMI reduces the risk of CVD. Reduction in excessive weight gain and risk of being overweight and obese are all benefits of moderate- to vigorous-intensity physical activity.[16] Performing more than 150 minutes of physical activity provides more benefit.

SPECIAL CONSIDERATIONS

Children and Adolescents

The 2018 Physical Activity Guideline recommends that children and adolescents perform at least 60 minutes of moderate- to vigorous-intensity physical activity daily including muscle and bone strengthening physical activity.[50] Based on the 2017 Youth Risk Behavior Surveillance, only 46.5% of students reported having 60 minutes or more of physical activity for at least 5 days in a week.[63] A smaller number, 26%, reported meeting the AHA and federal guideline goal of 60 minutes or more per day every day.[63] Screen time on mobile phones, games, television, and computers may contribute to less physical activity. In fact, according to the 2017 Youth Risk Behavior Surveillance, 43% of students reported spending an average of 3 hours or more per day using the computer for activity not related to school work or playing video or computer games.[63] Replacing screen time with physical activity or incorporating physical activity into screen time may be helpful. A meta-analysis on the impact of Pokémon Go mobile-augmented reality game on physical activity found an increase in the amount of daily steps taken (1,446 steps [953 to 1,939]) and less sedentary behavior among game players.[64] However, the sustainability of such practices is unknown, and more research maybe needed to guide future recommendations.

Pregnancy

Physically active healthy pregnant women have better pregnancy outcomes, including reduced weight gain and lower risk of gestational diabetes. Exercise should be performed under the supervision of a healthcare provider. The 2018 Physical Activity Guideline recommends that pregnant women get at least 150 minutes of moderate-intensity physical activity weekly.[50] Women who were already meeting the adult recommendations prior to becoming pregnant should continue if they are able.

Chronic Medical Conditions and Functional Disability

The impact of chronic medical conditions that may limit physical activity, such as osteoarthritis, should not be overlooked. Although it may be reasonably difficult to attain the recommended level of weekly activity, individuals with these functional disabilities should be encouraged to explore other activity types or exercise routines that may be better suited for them. For example, an individual with knee osteoarthritis may be encouraged to participate in swimming rather that jogging, running, or jumping. Individuals with low activity levels still tend to benefit from increasing levels of physical activity. This also highlights the need for providers to take into consideration the other comorbidities of individuals before prescribing an exercise routine.

LIFESTYLE COUNSELING IN CLINICAL PRACTICE

The ABCDE approach to primary prevention of CVD is a useful framework to organize prevention recommendations in clinical setting and can be applied to both primary and secondary prevention (**Table 97.5**). It is reasonable to address each, or some, section of it at each contact with a healthcare provider using a shared decision-making and team-based approach.[16] Scheduling regular patient follow-up, motivational interviewing, goal setting, establishing methods for self-monitoring, providing feedback, and a combination of any of the listed strategies (all COR I; LOE *A*) have been shown to improve adopting and maintaining healthy lifestyle choices.

CHALLENGES, EVIDENCE GAPS, AND FUTURE DIRECTIONS

Implementation of lifestyle changes such as smoking cessation, consumption of heart-healthy diet, and increasing physical activity largely borders on the availability of

TABLE 97.5 ABCDE of Primary Prevention

A	**A**ssess risk	Use PCE or similar risk tool to estimate 10-year ASCVD risk for adults aged 40-75 years and lifetime risk estimation for those aged 20-59 years. Consider other risk-enhancing factors and selective use of CAC when appropriate to guide risk-based decision for pharmacotherapy.
A	**A**spirin	Low-dose aspirin may be considered for select individuals for primary prevention if at high risk for ASCVD and low risk of bleeding
B	**B**lood pressure	Maintain blood pressure <130/80 mm Hg. Lifestyle and nonpharmacologic interventions for everyone. Pharmacotherapy should be added to lifestyle for blood pressures ≥130/80 mm Hg for higher risk individuals and ≥140/90 mm Hg for lower risk individuals.
C	**C**holesterol	Heart-healthy diet, physical activity, and initiation of lipid-lowering therapy when appropriate based on ASCVD risk
C	**C**igarette Cessation	Using pharmacology and behavioral interventions
D	**D**iet/weight	Heart-healthy diet, caloric restriction, and physical activity
D	**D**iabetes prevention/ management	Employ lifestyle management. Maintain hemoglobin A1c goals. Use GLP-1 agonist and SGLT-2 inhibitors that have been shown to reduce ASCVD events and mortality when appropriate.
E	**E**xercise	≥150 minutes of moderate-intensity or 75 minutes of vigorous-intensity aerobic physical activity weekly and more than twice-weekly muscle-strengthening activity.

ASCVD, atherosclerotic cardiovascular disease; CAC, coronary artery calcium; GLP, glucagon-like peptide; PCE, pooled cohort equations; SGLT, sodium-glucose cotransporter.

optimal environmental and social factors such as safer neighborhoods, eradication of poverty, availability of infrastructure such as biking lanes and parks, providing fresh fruits, and reduction of food deserts (ie, social determinants of health).[16] The introduction of policies that facilitate individuals to engage and maintain these healthy life changes is also encouraged.

Future research is still needed to help provide insight on some aspects of lifestyle choices as it impacts CV health. For example, the impact of e-cigarette use on the primordial, primary, and secondary prevention of CV health needs further study. The use of NRTs and non-nicotine oral medications such as bupropion and varenicline for smoking cessation in pregnant women is not well established. The impact of light-intensity physical activity on CV health as well as the sustainability of using modern technology such as wearable devices maintaining physical activity remains uncertain.

KEY POINTS

- ✔ Primordial, primary, and secondary prevention strategies remain essential to improving CV health and reducing CVD risk at all levels.
- ✔ Tobacco use, including electronic cigarette, should be assessed at every healthcare visit, and individuals who use tobacco products should be counseled to quit.
- ✔ Five NRTs and two non-nicotine oral medications have been approved by the U.S. Food and Drug Administration for smoking cessation. Combination with behavioral interventions increases the chances of successfully quitting.
- ✔ The use of electronic cigarettes for cigarette cessation requires further study, and their long-term CVD effects remain unknown.
- ✔ The DASH, Mediterranean, and vegetarian diets have CV benefits.
- ✔ Increased consumption of vegetables, fruits, legumes, and whole grains is recommended.
- ✔ Moderate consumption of seafood, lean meats, low-fat dairy products, nuts, and vegetable oil while restricting processed meats, saturated fats, trans-fats, salt, refined carbohydrates, and sugar-sweetened beverages is recommended.
- ✔ Not all vegetarian diets are the same or healthy.
- ✔ Limited evidence is available on the CV benefits of intermittent fasting diet, ketogenic diet, and paleolithic diet.
- ✔ A cumulative of 150 minutes of moderate-intensity or 75 minutes of vigorous-intensity aerobic physical activity weekly or a combination of both and at least twice-weekly muscle-strengthening activity is recommended.
- ✔ Bouts of any duration of moderate- to vigorous-intensity physical activity are beneficial.
- ✔ Individuals with functional limitations should still be encouraged to participate in some form of physical activity levels more suited to their ability.
- ✔ There is an inverse dose-response function between increasing physical activity levels and CVD risk.
- ✔ We recommend that some components, if not all, of the ABCDE of primary prevention of CVD be addressed during individual contact with healthcare providers and be reemphasized at subsequent visits to build some level of accountability.

REFERENCES

1. Virani SS, Alonso A, Benjamin EJ, et al. Heart disease and stroke statistics-2020 update: a report from the American Heart Association. *Circulation*. 2020;141:e139-e596.
2. Lloyd-Jones DM, Hong Y, Labarthe D, et al. Defining and setting national goals for cardiovascular health promotion and disease reduction. *Circulation*. 2010;121:586-613.
3. Khan SU, Yedlapati SH, Lone AN, et al. A comparative analysis of premature heart disease- and cancer-related mortality in women in the USA, 1999-2018. *Eur Heart J Qual Care Clin Outcomes*. 2021;qcaa099.
4. Curtin SC. Trends in cancer and heart disease death rates among adults aged 45-64: United States, 1999-2017. *Natl Vital Stat Rep*. 2019;68:1-8.
5. Ogunmoroti O, Oni E, Michos ED, et al. Life's simple 7 and incident heart failure: the multi-ethnic study of atherosclerosis. *J Am Heart Assoc*. 2017;6(6):e005180.
6. Ogunmoroti O, Allen NB, Cushman M, et al. Association between life's simple 7 and noncardiovascular disease: the multi-ethnic study of atherosclerosis. *J Am Heart Assoc*. 2016;5 (10):e003954.
7. Guo L, Zhang S. Association between ideal cardiovascular health metrics and risk of cardiovascular events or mortality: a meta-analysis of prospective studies. *Clin Cardiol*. 2017;40:1339-1346.
8. Tibuakuu M, Kianoush S, DeFilippis AP, et al. Usefulness of lipoprotein-associated phospholipase A2 activity and c-reactive protein in identifying high-risk smokers for atherosclerotic cardiovascular disease (from the Atherosclerosis Risk in Communities Study). *Am J Cardiol*. 2018;121:1056-1064.
9. U.S. Department of Health and Human Services. Smoking cessation: a report of the surgeon general. 2020. Accessed March 17, 2020. https://www.hhs.gov/sites/default/files/2020-cessation-sgr-full-report.pdf
10. Creamer MR, Wang TW, Babb S, et al. Tobacco product use and cessation indicators among adults—United States, 2018. *MMWR Morb Mortal Wkly Rep*. 2019;68:1013-1019.
11. Cornelius ME, Wang TW, Jamal A, Loretan CG, Neff LJ. Tobacco Product Use Among Adults - United States, 2019. *MMWR Morb Mortal Wkly Rep*. 2020;69:1736-1742.
12. Hackshaw A, Morris JK, Boniface S, Tang J-L, Milenković D. Low cigarette consumption and risk of coronary heart disease and stroke: meta-analysis of 141 cohort studies in 55 study reports. *BMJ*. 2018;360:j5855.
13. Duncan MS, Freiberg MS, Greevy RA Jr, Kundu S, Vasan RS, Tindle HA. Association of smoking cessation with subsequent risk of cardiovascular disease. *JAMA*. 2019;322:642-650.
14. McEvoy JW, Nasir K, DeFilippis AP, et al. Relationship of cigarette smoking with inflammation and subclinical vascular disease: the Multi-Ethnic Study of Atherosclerosis. *Arterioscler Thromb Vasc Biol*. 2015;35:1002-1010.
15. Tibuakuu M, Okunrintemi V, Jirru E, et al. National trends in cessation counseling, prescription medication use, and associated costs among US adult cigarette smokers. *JAMA Netw Open*. 2019;2:e194585.
16. Arnett DK, Blumenthal RS, Albert MA, et al. 2019 ACC/AHA Guideline on the primary prevention of cardiovascular disease: a report of the American College of Cardiology/American Heart Association Task Force on Clinical Practice Guidelines. *Circulation*. 2019;140:e596-e646.
17. Patnode CD, Henderson JT, Coppola EL, Melnikow J, Durbin S, Thomas RG. Interventions for tobacco cessation in adults, including pregnant persons: updated evidence report and systematic review for the US Preventive Services Task Force. *JAMA*. 2021;325:280-298.
18. Olmedo P, Goessler W, Tanda S, et al. Metal concentrations in e-cigarette liquid and aerosol samples: the contribution of metallic coils. *Environ Health Perspect*. 2018;126:027010.
19. Jackler RK, Ramamurthi D. Nicotine arms race: JUUL and the high-nicotine product market. *Tob Control*. 2019;28:623-628.
20. Gentzke AS, Creamer M, Cullen KA, et al. Vital signs: tobacco product use among middle and high school students—United States, 2011-2018. *MMWR Morb Mortal Wkly Rep*. 2019;68:157-164.
21. Kasza KA, Ambrose BK, Conway KP, et al. Tobacco-product use by adults and youths in the United States in 2013 and 2014. *N Engl J Med*. 2017;376:342-353.
22. Fischer NM, Pallazola VA, Xun H, Cainzos-Achirica M, Michos ED. The evolution of the heart-healthy diet for vascular health: a walk through time. *Vasc Med*. 2020;25(2):184-193. doi:10.1177/1358863X19901287
23. Micha R, Peñalvo JL, Cudhea F, Imamura F, Rehm CD, Mozaffarian D. Association between dietary factors and mortality from heart disease, stroke, and type 2 diabetes in the United States. *JAMA*. 2017;317:912-924.
24. Global Burden of Disease Collaborators. Health effects of dietary risks in 195 countries, 1990-2017: a systematic analysis for the Global Burden of Disease Study 2017. *Lancet*. 2019;393:1958-1972.
25. Ferraro RA, Fischer NM, Xun H, Michos ED. Nutrition and physical activity recommendations from the United States and European cardiovascular guidelines: a comparative review. *Curr Opin Cardiol*. 2020;35:508-516.
26. Aune D, Keum N, Giovannucci E, et al. Whole grain consumption and risk of cardiovascular disease, cancer, and all cause and cause specific mortality: systematic review and dose-response meta-analysis of prospective studies. *BMJ*. 2016;353:i2716.
27. Kwok CS, Gulati M, Michos ED, et al. Dietary components and risk of cardiovascular disease and all-cause mortality: a review of evidence from meta-analyses. *Eur J Prev Cardiol*. 2019;26:1415-1429.
28. Yang Q, Zhang Z, Gregg EW, Flanders WD, Merritt R, Hu FB. Added sugar intake and cardiovascular diseases mortality among US adults. *JAMA Intern Med*. 2014;174:516-524.
29. Piepoli MF, Abreu A, Albus C, et al. Update on cardiovascular prevention in clinical practice: A position paper of the European Association of Preventive Cardiology of the European Society of Cardiology. *Eur J Prev Cardiol*. 2020;27:181-205.
30. U.S. Department of Agriculture and U.S. Department of Health and Human Services. *Dietary Guidelines for Americans, 2020-2025*. 9th Edition. December 2020. Available at DietaryGuidelines.gov.
31. Wang DD, Li Y, Chiuve SE, et al. Association of specific dietary fats with total and cause-specific mortality. *JAMA Intern Med*. 2016;176:1134-1145.
32. Budhathoki S, Sawada N, Iwasaki M, et al. Association of animal and plant protein intake with all-cause and cause-specific mortality in a Japanese Cohort. *JAMA Intern Med*. 2019;179:1509-1518.
33. Song M, Fung TT, Hu FB, et al. Association of animal and plant protein intake with all-cause and cause-specific mortality. *JAMA Intern Med*. 2016;176:1453-1463.
34. Appel LJ, Moore TJ, Obarzanek E, et al. A clinical trial of the effects of dietary patterns on blood pressure. DASH Collaborative Research Group. *N Engl J Med*. 1997;336:1117-1124.
35. Sacks FM, Svetkey LP, Vollmer WM, et al. Effects on blood pressure of reduced dietary sodium and the Dietary Approaches to Stop Hypertension (DASH) diet. DASH-Sodium Collaborative Research Group. *N Engl J Med*. 2001;344:3-10.
36. Appel LJ, Sacks FM, Carey VJ, et al. Effects of protein, monounsaturated fat, and carbohydrate intake on blood pressure and serum lipids: results of the OmniHeart randomized trial. *JAMA*. 2005;294:2455-2464.
37. Chiavaroli L, Viguiliouk E, Nishi SK, et al. DASH dietary pattern and cardiometabolic outcomes: an umbrella review of systematic reviews and meta-analyses. *Nutrients*. 2019;11:338.
38. Trichopoulou A, Costacou T, Bamia C, Trichopoulos D. Adherence to a mediterranean diet and survival in a Greek population. *N Engl J Med*. 2003;348:2599-2608.
39. de Lorgeril M, Salen P, Martin JL, Monjaud I, Delaye J, Mamelle N. Mediterranean diet, traditional risk factors, and the rate of cardiovascular complications after myocardial infarction: final report of the Lyon Diet Heart Study. *Circulation*. 1999;99:779-785.
40. Estruch R, Ros E, Salas-Salvado J, et al. Primary prevention of cardiovascular disease with a mediterranean diet supplemented with extra-virgin olive oil or nuts. *N Engl J Med*. 2018;378:e34.

41. Kwok CS, Umar S, Myint PK, Mamas MA, Loke YK. Vegetarian diet, Seventh Day Adventists and risk of cardiovascular mortality: a systematic review and meta-analysis. *Int J Cardiol.* 2014;176:680-686.
42. Satija A, Bhupathiraju SN, Spiegelman D, et al. Healthful and unhealthful plant-based diets and the risk of coronary heart disease in U.S. adults. *J Am Coll Cardiol.* 2017;70:411-422.
43. Satija A, Bhupathiraju SN, Rimm EB, et al. Plant-based dietary patterns and incidence of type 2 diabetes in US Men and Women: results from three prospective cohort studies. *PLoS Med.* 2016;13:e1002039.
44. Rico-Campa A, Martinez-Gonzalez MA, Alvarez-Alvarez I, et al. Association between consumption of ultra-processed foods and all cause mortality: SUN prospective cohort study. *BMJ.* 2019;365:11949.
45. Srour B, Fezeu LK, Kesse-Guyot E, et al. Ultra-processed food intake and risk of cardiovascular disease: prospective cohort study (NutriNet-Sante). *BMJ.* 2019;365:11451.
46. Hall KD, Ayuketah A, Brychta R, et al. Ultra-processed diets cause excess calorie intake and weight gain: an inpatient randomized controlled trial of ad libitum food intake. *Cell Metab.* 2019;30:226.
47. Cainzos-Achirica M, Bilal U, Kapoor K, et al. Methodological issues in nutritional epidemiology research—sorting through the confusion. *Curr Cardiovasc Risk Rep.* 2018;12:4.
48. Aggarwal M, Devries S, Freeman AM, et al. The deficit of nutrition education of physicians. *Am J Med.* 2018;131:339-345.
49. Pallazola VA, Davis DM, Whelton SP, et al. A clinician's guide to healthy eating for cardiovascular disease prevention. *Mayo Clin Proc Innov Qual Outcomes.* 2019;3:251-267.
50. Piercy KL, Troiano RP, Ballard RM, et al. The physical activity guidelines for Americans. *JAMA.* 2018;320:2020-2028.
51. Lear SA, Hu W, Rangarajan S, et al. The effect of physical activity on mortality and cardiovascular disease in 130,000 people from 17 high-income, middle-income, and low-income countries: the PURE study. *Lancet.* 2017;390:2643-2654.
52. Ding D, Lawson KD, Kolbe-Alexander TL, et al. The economic burden of physical inactivity: a global analysis of major non-communicable diseases. *Lancet.* 2016;388:1311-1324.
53. U.S. Preventive Services Task Force. Behavioral counseling interventions to promote a healthy diet and physical activity for cardiovascular disease prevention in adults with cardiovascular risk factors: US preventive services task force recommendation statement. *JAMA.* 2020;324:2069-2075.
54. Sattelmair J, Pertman J, Ding EL, Kohl HW 3rd, Haskell W, Lee IM. Dose response between physical activity and risk of coronary heart disease: a meta-analysis. *Circulation.* 2011;124:789-795.
55. Biswas A, Oh PI, Faulkner GE, et al. Sedentary time and its association with risk for disease incidence, mortality, and hospitalization in adults: a systematic review and meta-analysis. *Ann Intern Med.* 2015;162:123-132.
56. Ekelund U, Steene-Johannessen J, Brown WJ, et al. Does physical activity attenuate, or even eliminate, the detrimental association of sitting time with mortality? A harmonised meta-analysis of data from more than 1 million men and women. *Lancet.* 2016;388:1302-1310.
57. Yang Q, Cogswell ME, Flanders WD, et al. Trends in cardiovascular health metrics and associations with all-cause and CVD mortality among US adults. *JAMA.* 2012;307:1273-1283.
58. Saint-Maurice PF, Coughlan D, Kelly SP, et al. Association of leisure-time physical activity across the adult life course with all-cause and cause-specific mortality. *JAMA Netw Open.* 2019;2:e190355.
59. Florido R, Zhao D, Ndumele CE, et al. Physical activity, parental history of premature coronary heart disease, and incident atherosclerotic cardiovascular disease in the Atherosclerosis Risk in Communities (ARIC) Study. *J Am Heart Assoc.* 2016;5:e003505.
60. Eckel Robert H, Jakicic John M, Ard Jamy D, et al. 2013 AHA/ACC Guideline on lifestyle management to reduce cardiovascular risk. *Circulation.* 2014;129:S76-S99.
61. Liu X, Zhang D, Liu Y, et al. Dose-response association between physical activity and incident hypertension: a systematic review and meta-analysis of cohort studies. *Hypertension.* 2017;69:813-820.
62. Aune D, Norat T, Leitzmann M, Tonstad S, Vatten LJ. Physical activity and the risk of type 2 diabetes: a systematic review and dose-response meta-analysis. *Eur J Epidemiol.* 2015;30:529-542.
63. Kann L, McManus T, Harris WA, et al. Youth risk behavior surveillance—United States, 2017. *MMWR Surveill Summ.* 2018;67:1-114.
64. Khamzina M, Parab KV, An R, Bullard T, Grigsby-Toussaint DS. Impact of Pokémon go on physical activity: a systematic review and meta-analysis. *Am J Prev Med.* 2020;58:270-282.

CHAPTER 98

DIABETES AND CARDIOMETABOLIC MEDICINE

Cara Reiter-Brennan, Omar Dzaye, and Michael J. Blaha

INTRODUCTION

Epidemiology

In the United States, an estimated one-third of the population will develop type 2 diabetes mellitus (T2DM) over the course of their lifetimes. T2DM, in turn, predisposes to cardiovascular disease.[1] Diabetes is one of the leading causes of death worldwide (30%) and cardiovascular disease (CVD)-related deaths account for 70% of all deaths among diabetic patients. T2DM is the most common form of diabetes (>90%), whereas type 1 diabetes mellitus (T1DM) makes up 5% of all diabetic patients[2] (**Table 98.1**).

Risk Factors

The prevalence of T1DM is increased in patients with autoimmune diseases such as Hashimoto thyroiditis, type A gastritis, celiac disease, and adrenal dysfunction. Patients who are human leukocyte antigen (HLA)-DR3 and HLA-DR4 positive have a higher risk of developing T1DM.[3]

T2DM is strongly associated with metabolic syndrome (MetSyn), which is characterized by insulin resistance (IR). Older age, little physical activity, and obesity (especially high waist-to-hip ratio) all increase the risk of diabetes. Diabetes prevalence is higher in women with previous gestational diabetes mellitus (GDM) and in patients with hypertension or dyslipidemias. Individuals identifying with certain ethnic groups (African American, American, Hispanic/Latino, and American Asian) are also at higher risk of developing diabetes. Genetic disposition is more common in T2DM than in T1DM, with family history being a strong independent risk factor for T2DM.[4]

PATHOGENESIS

Type 1 Diabetes Mellitus

Current research suggests that T1DM is caused by an autoimmune response, often triggered by a viral infection. The most common antibodies found in T1DM patients are anti–glutamic acid decarboxylase (anti-GAD) antibodies, which target GAD, an enzyme found in the pancreatic cell. These promote the destruction of insulin-producing β-cells in the pancreas, ultimately resulting in absolute insulin deficiency.

T1DM develops because of absolute insulin deficiency as a result of autoimmune β-cell destruction. Without insulin, glucose cannot be absorbed into muscle and adipose tissue. Glycosuria leads to polyurea and hypovolemia, which in turn can cause polydipsia. Decrease of total body water facilitates loss of electrolytes and patients present with hypovolemia, hypokalemia, and hypomagnesemia. As a result, patients experience fatigue, weakness, and muscle cramps. In addition, insulin

TABLE 98.1 Differential Diagnosis of Type 1 and Type 2 Diabetes Mellitus

	Type 1 Diabetes Mellitus	Type 2 Diabetes Mellitus
Proportion of all diabetic cases (%)	5%	95%
Pathogenesis	Absolute insulin deficiency	Relative insulin deficiency and insulin resistance
Genetics	Human leukocyte antigen (HLA) association	No HLA association, but strong genetic disposition
Age of onset	Primarily childhood and adolescence	Predominantly >40 years of age, but rising incidence among youths <20 years of age (4.8% per year increase among individuals <20 years)[6]
Associated with poor lifestyle	No	Yes
Weight	Thin or normal weight	Obese
Ketoacidosis incidence	High	Low
Therapy	Insulin required	Lifestyle -< antidiabetic medication -> insulin

deficiency can lead to a catabolic state, promoting muscle wasting. Hyperglycemia may cause osmotic swelling of the lens, which presents itself as blurred vision. Patients with T1DM often experience weight loss because of the catabolic state.

Type 2 Diabetes Mellitus

T2DM is primarily caused by the defect of insulin secretion from β-cells in the context of increased insulin demand from IR. The condition is made worse by disordered gluconeogenesis, altered skeletal muscle metabolism, and glucotoxicity, resulting in further β-cell decline. Obesity, particularly visceral adiposity, is a strong risk factor for T2DM. Abdominal adipose tissue is metabolically active and is regarded as the primary contributor to worsening IR[5] (**Figure 98.1**).

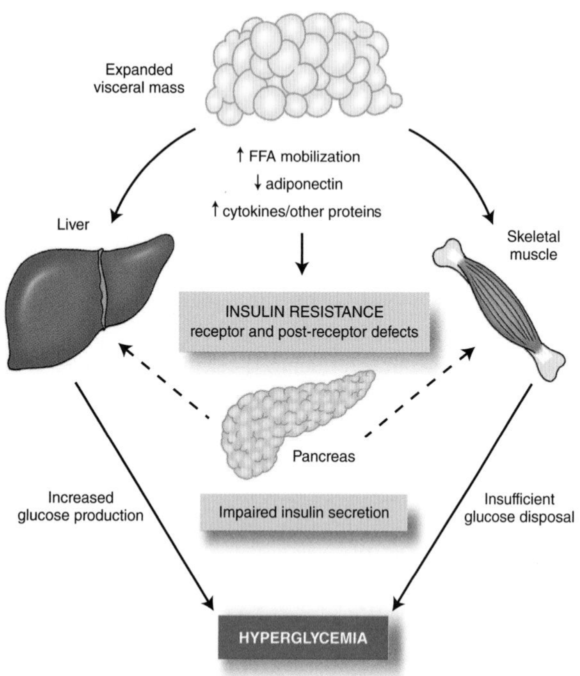

FIGURE 98.1 Pathogenesis of type 2 diabetes mellitus (T2DM). Pathogenesis of obesity-related T2DM. The expanded visceral fat mass in upper body obesity elaborates several factors that contribute to tissue insulin resistance. These include an increase in circulating free (nonesterified) fatty acids (FFAs) and other cytokines and proteins that inhibit insulin action, as well as a decrease in factors that enhance insulin signaling, such as adiponectin. These changes result in a block to insulin action in liver and skeletal muscle at the level of the insulin receptor and at postreceptor signaling sites, resulting in a failure of insulin to suppress hepatic glucose production and to promote glucose uptake into muscle. The resulting hyperglycemia is normally countered by increased insulin secretion by pancreatic β-cells. In persons with T2DM, the combination of resistance to insulin action and a genetically determined impairment of the β-cell response to hyperglycemia results in hyperglycemia, and T2DM ensues. (Reprinted with permission from Rubin R, Strayer DS, Rubin E. *Rubin's Pathology: Clinicopathologic foundations of medicine.* 6th ed. Philadelphia, PA: Wolters Kluwer Health/Lippincott Williams & Wilkins; 2011. Figure 22.5.)

Most patients present with no or few of the classic symptoms (polyuria, polydipsia, nocturia, blurred vision, and weight loss) and only hyperglycemia identified during routine laboratory testing prompts the diagnosis. Adults with T2DM rarely show signs of hyperosmolar hyperglycemia, a state marked by obtundation, hyperglycemia, and dehydration. Diabetic ketoacidosis (DKA) is also very uncommon but may occur with severe infections like pneumonia or urinary tract infections, or during inadequate insulin therapy.

Common Signs and Symptoms

T1DM is characterized by a sudden onset of disease. Up to 25% of initial presentations of T1DM may be DKA. In comparison, microvascular or macrovascular DM complications may be the first clinical signs in patients with T2DM.

Typical Symptoms of Diabetes

- Polyuria
- Polydipsia
- Polyphagia
- Fatigue
- Calf cramps
- Visual impairment (blurred vision)
- Disturbed wound healing
- Pruritus
- Weight loss (T1DM)
- Benign acanthosis nigricans (T2DM)

DIAGNOSIS

Algorithm 98.1 presents the criteria used to diagnose diabetes mellitus: fasting plasma glucose (FPG) levels, 2-hour plasma glucose (2h-PG) levels during an oral glucose tolerance test (OGTT), elevated glycated hemoglobin A1c (HbA1c) levels, or elevated random plasma glucose (RPG) levels in patients with hyperglycemia, or a hyperglycemic crisis. If hyperglycemia is not certain, diabetes can be diagnosed by two abnormal test results from the same sample or two separate test samples. If test results are at the margin of cutoff points, clinicians should observe patients closely and follow up with tests in 3 to 6 months.

In comparison to 2h-PG and FPG, HbA1c has multiple advantages, such as not requiring fasting, greater preanalytic stability, and less day-to-day variations because of illness or other stress factors. However, limitations of HbA1c include lower sensitivity of HbA1c at selected cutoff points and poor correlations between glucose levels and HbA1c levels in select patients. For instance, data from the National Health and Nutritional Examination Survey (NHANES) showed that using the threshold of 6.5% or more (48 mmol/dL), HbA1c only diagnosed 30% of diabetes compared to using collective measures of 2-h PG, FPG, and HbA1c.[7] In addition, clinicians should be aware of other conditions affecting hemoglobin glycation, such as HIV treatment, age, race/ethnicity, pregnancy, hemoglobinopathies/anemia, and genetic factors.[8]

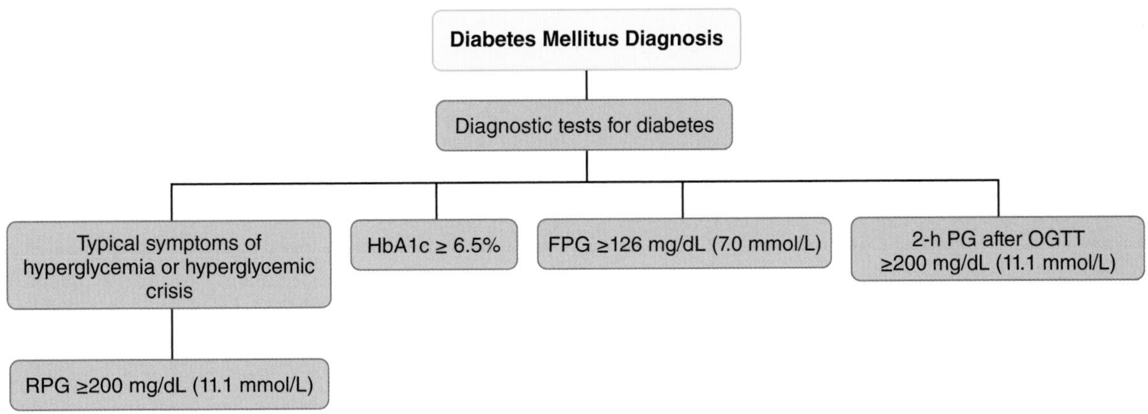

*FPG and PG levels are minimum of 8 hours of no caloric intake

ALGORITHM 98.1 Diabetes diagnosis. Possible testing modalities for diabetes include measuring fasting plasma glucose (FPG) levels, 2-hour plasma glucose (PG) levels during an oral glucose tolerance test (OGTT), elevated glycated hemoglobin A1c (HbA1C) levels or elevated random plasma glucose (RPG) levels.

MANAGEMENT OF PATIENTS WITH DIABETES

Lifestyle Intervention

Particularly for patients with T2DM, lifestyle intervention is effective in delaying onset and diabetes complications. Evidence from multiple randomized controlled trials suggests that lifestyle intervention can significantly reduce progression of MetSyn to overt T2DM. In the Diabetes Prevention Program[9] nondiabetic subjects who were randomly assigned to participate in an intensive lifestyle modification program were given metformin or a placebo for a mean of 2.8 years. Lifestyle modification programs consisted of healthy, low-calorie, and low-fat diet and 150 min of weekly moderate-intensity exercise in order to achieve a body weight reduction of at least 7%. In this randomized controlled trial, intensive lifestyle intervention was more effective than metformin in delaying the onset of T2DM, and both were more effective than placebo in preventing new T2DM. Modeled after the intervention in the Diabetes Prevention Program, the ADA/EASD 2019 Standards of Care suggest 7% weight loss and 150 min of moderate-intensity physical activity per week, in addition to healthy low-calorie eating patterns.

Glycemic Control

Improved glycemic control reduces progression and, in some instances, even reverses microvascular complications in patients with DM. However, these benefits have to be balanced with the risks of hypoglycemia and cardiovascular effects. Three major outcome trials ACCORD,[20] ADVANCE,[8] and VADT[21] randomizing over 23,000 patients with follow-up of 3 to 5 years compared the cardiovascular effects of intensive glycemic control versus standard care. The trials did not report cardiovascular benefits of tight glycemic control. ACCORD was terminated prematurely after observing increased mortality in individuals of the very intense glycemic control arm (1.41% vs 1.14% per year; 257 vs 203 deaths over a mean 3.5 years of follow-up; hazard ratio [HR] 1.22 [95% confidence interval (CI) 1.01-1.46]).[20] In all trials, severe hypoglycemia was more common in the intensive glycemic control group. As hypoglycemia is strongly associated with cardiovascular events and mortality, guidelines advocate for wariness of hypoglycemia and not persist in accomplishing euglycemia in individuals where HbA1c targets cannot be safely achieved.[18] In response to the complexity of adequate glycemic control, the 2019 ADA/EASD Standards of Medical Care emphasize the importance of shared decision-making to incorporate the distinct characteristics and preferences of each patient to induce optimal glycemic control.[18] In general, for nonpregnant adults, a general target of less than 7% HbA1c is still recommendable. In patients without CVD and long life expectancy, or only treated with lifestyle therapy or metformin, a more stringent HbA1c target (<6.5%) is suitable to prevent microvascular complications. HbA1c levels of 8% are acceptable in patients with short life expectancy, serious comorbidities, or inadequate self-management.[8]

General Therapeutic Plan According to Guidelines

Type 1 Diabetes Mellitus

Multiple daily injections of either basal or prandial insulin should be the main treatment strategy for patients with T1DM. Alternatively, subcutaneous administration through an insulin pump is equally safe and effective. To reduce hypoglycemia risk, rapid-acting insulin analogs are recommended. Education on matching insulin dosage with carbohydrate intake, preprandial glucose levels, and physical exercise is essential for patients starting insulin therapy.

Type 2 Diabetes Mellitus

The 2019 ADA/EASD Standards of Medical Care recommend an individualized approach to pharmacologic therapy of DM.

SECTION 8

When choosing the optimal antidiabetes medication, key comorbidities (atherosclerotic cardiovascular disease [ASCVD], heart failure [HF], and chronic kidney disease [CKD]), effect on body weight, side effects, risk of hypoglycemia, cost, and patient preference should be taken into account (**Algorithm 98.2**). Although traditionally metformin has been the first-line agent for all patients diagnosed with T2DM, the new 2019 ESC guidelines recommend sodium-glucose cotransporter-2 (SGLT-2) inhibitors or glucagon-like peptide-1 receptor agonist (GLP1-RA) monotherapy to metformin-naïve patients with ASCVD or high CVD risk.[10] (**e-Figure 98.1**) In such patients, if HbA1c target is not reached, metformin can be added. For patients at low CVD risk, metformin should still be the first choice and initiated at the time of diagnosis. If adequate glycemic control is not achieved after 3 months and patients do not have ASCVD or CKD, a combination of metformin with any of the following drugs is possible: SGLT-2 inhibitors, dipeptidyl peptidase 4 (DPP-4) inhibitors, GLP1-RAs, sulfonylureas, or thiazolidinediones (TZDs). Insulin is no longer considered part of initial therapy and should only be used if lifestyle intervention and other antidiabetic medications did not have the desired effect. In the absence of comorbidities, the decision of antidiabetic medications should be based on side effects and patient-specific factors. Multiple large randomized controlled studies have demonstrated the statistically significant cardiovascular benefits of SGLT-2 inhibitors and GLP1-RAs for patients with T2DM. In such cardiovascular outcome trials (CVOTs), SGLT-2 inhibitors demonstrated reduction in HF and CKD and thus should be prescribed in patients at increased risk of HF or CKD if estimated glomerular filtration rate (eGFR) is adequate. Specifically, evidence from CVOTs demonstrated reduction of HF incidence and CKD progression for canagliflozin, dapagliflozin, and empagliflozin. If eGFR is not acceptable or SGLT-2 inhibitors are not tolerated, clinicians should subscribe GLP1-RAs that demonstrated reduction of ASCVD events. GLP1-RAs are currently the most effective antidiabetic agents for weight loss and should be preferred when need for obesity treatment predominates.[11] GLP1-RAs are also a viable alternative for patients with high ASCVD risk. Currently, weekly injections with semaglutide and dulaglutide are preferred.[12] Worsening of glycemic control in T2DM contributes to progressive β-cell apoptosis during the course of the disease.[13] GLP1-RA may preserve β-cell function and thereby play a particularly important role early on in the disease process.[14,15] TZDs should be avoided in patients with HF. DPP-4 inhibitors are no longer considered first-line drugs because of the risk of HF associated with some agents and only modest reduction of HbA1c levels. As a result of the complete or almost-complete absence of β-cell function in patients with T1DM, insulin therapy is essential. For patients with T2DM however, insulin is a method of last resort and should only be introduced if treatment goals are not met with lifestyle modification and other antidiabetic medications. Because of the risk of hypoglycemia as well as weight gain, insulin should be avoided as long as possible in patients with T2DM. In addition, cost of insulin has been rising and may pose a significant burden for patients, contributing to therapy nonadherence.[16]

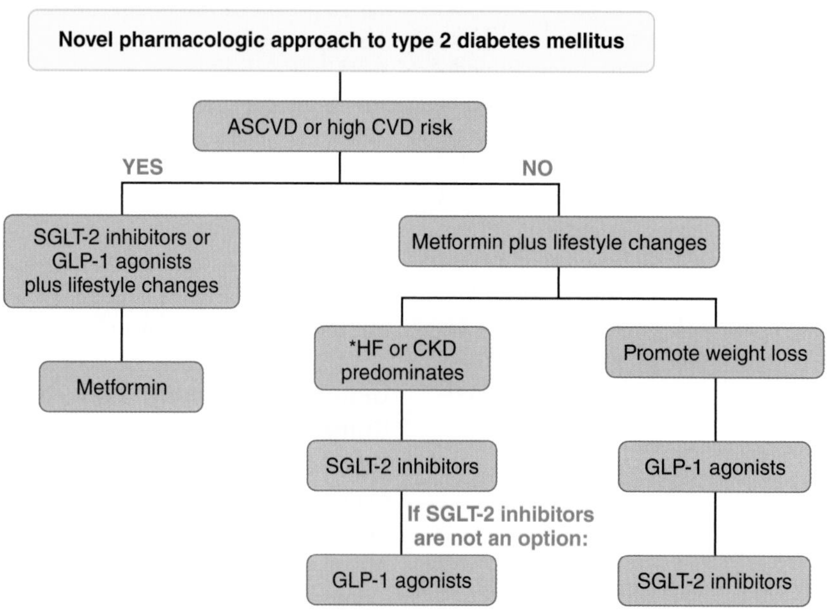

ALGORITHM 98.2 Novel pharmacologic approach to type 2 diabetes mellitus (T2DM). The 2019 ADA/EASD Standards of Medical Care recommend an individualized approach to pharmacologic therapy of diabetes mellitus. Cardiovascular comorbidities (ASCVD, HF, and CKD), body weight, side effects, risk of hypoglycemia, cost, and patient preference should be taken into account. SGLT-2 inhibitors should be preferred if HF or CKD predominates, whereas GLP-1 receptor agonists are the good agents to promote weight loss. ASCVD, atherosclerotic cardiovascular disease; CKD, chronic kidney disease; CVD, cardiovascular disease; GLP-1, glucagon-like peptide-1; HF, heart failure; SGLT-2, sodium-glucose cotransporter-2.

Pharmacologic Therapy for Type 1 Diabetes Mellitus

Insulin

For patients with T1DM, multiple daily injections or use of a subcutaneous insulin pump is the safest as well as the most effective method of insulin administration. In general, insulin doses range from 0.4 to 1.0 units/kg/day, with higher doses necessary during pregnancy, illness, and puberty.

Drug Interactions or Major Restrictions. A major disadvantage of insulin therapy is risk of hypoglycemia (**Table 98.2**). The 2019 ADA/EASD 2019 Standards of Care recommend rapid-acting insulin analogs to reduce risk of hypoglycemia in individuals with T1DM.[8] Insulin dosage may be increased when subscribed with diuretics,[17] steroids, and oral contraceptives, as these agents inhibit insulin release and elevate peripheral IR. Clinicians should also be aware of reducing insulin dosage in patients with renal impairment, as insulin clearance is compromised. Inhaled insulins are not recommended for patients diagnosed with asthma, chronic obstructive pulmonary disease, or other chronic lung diseases.[8]

Noninsulin Therapy Type 1 Diabetes Mellitus

Oral and injectable noninsulins for T1DM are still being studied for their effectiveness in adjunction to insulin treatment. Studies have demonstrated small reductions in body weight

TABLE 98.2 Dosage and Side Effects of Antidiabetics

Class	Dosage	Side Effects
Metformin	500-100 mg once to twice daily orally	Lactic acidosis Gastrointestinal effects Vitamin B12 deficiency
Sulfonylureas	Glimepiride 2-4 mg once daily orally, titrate in 1-2 mg increments, max 8 mg once daily Glipizide initial 2.5-5 mg once daily orally and titrate in 2.5-5 mg increments, max 40 mg once daily Glyburide initial 2.5-5 mg once daily orally, titrate in 2.5 mg increments, max 20 mg once daily	Weight gain Hypoglycemia
DPP-4 inhibitors	Linagliptin 5 mg once daily orally Sitagliptin 100 mg once daily orally Saxagliptin 5 mg once daily orally Alogliptin 25 mg once daily orally	Gastrointestinal effects Pancreatitis ?Heart failure
SGLT-2 inhibitors (e-Figure 98.2)	Dapagliflozin 5-10 mg once daily orally Empagliflozin 10-25 mg once daily orally Canagliflozin 100-300 mg once daily orally Ertugliflozin 5-15 mg once daily orally	Genital yeast infections and urinary tract infections
GLP-1 receptor agonists (e-Figure 98.3)	Exenatide initial 5 µg twice daily subcutaneous, maintenance dose after 1 month 10 µg twice daily subcutaneous Exenatide XR initial dose 2 mg subcutaneous once weekly Liraglutide initial 0.6 mg once daily subcutaneous, maintenance dose 1.2-1.8 mg once daily subcutaneous Dulaglutide initial dose 0.75 mg once weekly subcutaneous, and maintenance dose 0.75-1.5 mg once weekly subcutaneous Semaglutide initial 0.25 mg once weekly subcutaneous, and maintenance dose 0.5-1 mg once weekly subcutaneous. Semaglutide initial 3 mg once daily and maintenance dose 7-14 mg/day Lixisenatide initial dose 10 µg once daily subcutaneous for two weeks, maintenance dose 20 µg once daily subcutaneous.	Gastrointestinal effects ?Pancreatitis FDA black box: thyroid c-cell tumors
Thiazolidinediones (e-Figure 98.4)	Pioglitazone 15-45 mg once daily orally	Heart failure Weight gain Bladder cancer (pioglitazone) Bone fractures ↑LDL-C (rosiglitazone)
Insulin	Please refer to the most recent ADA Standards of Care guidelines for the current insulin initiation and titration recommendations	Weight gain Hypoglycemia

ADA, American Diabetic Association DPP-4, dipeptidyl peptidase 4; FDA, Food and Drug Administration; GLP, glucagon-like peptide; LDL-C, low-density lipoprotein cholesterol; SGLT-2, sodium-glucose cotransporter-2.

with GLP1-RAs.[18] There is evidence that metformin reduces insulin dosage and improves weight loss in T1DM patients, but more longitudinal trials are required.[19] SGLT-2 inhibitors reduced weight and improved glycemic control compared to insulin alone but were also associated with higher rate of ketoacidosis.[20] Currently, the antihyperglycemic pramlintide is the only antidiabetic agent approved for T1DM patients.

Pharmacologic Therapy for Type 2 Diabetes Mellitus

Cardiovascular Outcome Trials

In response to range of evidence suggesting that some diabetic drugs might pose risks to cardiovascular safety, in 2008, the U.S. Food and Drug Administration (FDA) published guidance for industry designing trials to adequately assess CVD risk of antidiabetic agents used in the treatment of T2DM.[21] Thereafter, there was an explosion of trials designed to assess noninferiority of experimental treatment versus placebo for three-point major adverse cardiovascular events (MACE; cardiovascular death, nonfatal myocardial infarction [MI], and nonfatal stroke) or four-point MACE (cardiovascular death, nonfatal MI, nonfatal stroke, hospitalization for unstable angina).[21] In response to these post-2008 CVOTs, there has been an unprecedented boom in our understanding of diabetes treatment, which has led to a paradigm shift toward drugs that are proven to reduce cardiovascular risk. The FDA has now approved label changes to antidiabetic agents to lower the risk of MACE (liraglutide,[22] canagliflozin,[23] semaglutide,[24] dulaglutide), cardiovascular death (empagliflozin[25]) and HF (dapagliflozin[26]). Based on the results of the CREDENCE trial, canagliflozin is approved to prevent renal failure among patients with T2DM and diabetic kidney disease. *Please refer to the E-Book for more detail on the respective CVOTs.*

Drugs That Lower Cardiovascular Disease Risk

Metformin. Metformin is the historical standard of care to promote glycemic control in patients with T2DM, as it can promote weight reduction (2-3%), has no harmful effects on the cardiovascular system, and may benefit patients with HF.[27]

- **Glycemic control.** For patients with low ASCVD risk where lifestyle intervention is insufficient, metformin should be prescribed because of its glycemic efficacy in the absence of side effects seen with other glucose-lowering agents.
- **Weight Loss.** Study participants in the Diabetes Prevention Program reduced 2.06% ± 5.65% of their body weight while taking metformin, whereas the placebo group only lost 0.02% ± 5.52% of body weight ($P < 0.001$).[28]
- **Cardiovascular outcomes.** A number of smaller studies, even though controversial, suggest a cardiovascular benefit of metformin for primary prevention in patients with new diagnosis of T2DM without CVD. A meta-analysis of 25 observational studies and 179 trials demonstrated that in comparison to sulfonylureas, there was lower cardiovascular mortality for metformin.[29] Data from the UK Prospective Diabetes Study (UKPDS) showed that in patients without CVD and newly diagnosed with T2DM, metformin reduced MI by 39%, coronary death by 50%, and stroke by 41%.[30]
- **Interactions or major restrictions.** Metformin works synergistically when administered together with SGLT-2 inhibitors, as well as with GLP1-RAs. Evidence suggests that the combination of SGLT-2 inhibitors and GLP1-RAs with metformin reduces arterial stiffness in T1DM and improves endothelial dysfunction in individuals with T2DM.[31-33] Metformin is contraindicated at eGFR < 30.[8]

Sodium-Glucose Cotransporter-2 Inhibitors. SGLT-2 inhibitors demonstrate high glycemic efficacy and cardiovascular benefits. For patients with HF and CKD, the addition of SGLT-2 inhibitors is recommended.[8]

In comparison to other antidiabetics, SGLT-2 inhibitors particularly demonstrated the reduction of HF-related endpoints and prevention of progression of kidney disease in patients with T2DM.[10,34] SGLT-2 inhibitors should not be started in patients with eGFR <60 mL/min/1.73 m^2 and stopped at eGFR <45 mL/min/1.73 m^2.

Glucagon-Like Peptide 1 Receptor Agonists. GLP1-RAs demonstrate high efficacy to reduce hyperglycemia as well as cardiovascular benefits, are associated with marked weight loss, and show few severe side effects. Agents can be administered by daily or weekly injections, or in tablet form (semaglutide).

- **Glycemic control.** In a meta-analysis of 17 trials, GLP1-RAs reduced HbA1c levels by approximately 1% compared to placebo.[11] Evidence even suggests that GLP1-RAs may be a reasonable alternative to insulin, as GLP1-RAs have similar glycemic efficacy but lower risks of hypoglycemia and weight gain.[35]
- **Cardiovascular outcomes.** The cardiovascular effects of GLP1-RAs were observed in six large CVOT trials, but only four of the trials (LEADER, SUSTAIN-6, REWIND, HARMONY OUTCOMES) significantly reduced the risk of major cardiovascular events (**e-Table 98.1**). Current European and American guidelines emphasize that liraglutide has the strongest evidence for cardiovascular benefit.[8,10]
- **Weight loss.** Weight loss associated with GLP1-RAs may explain some of the cardiovascular benefits. A meta-analysis of 17 trials demonstrated that GLP1-RAs were associated with approximately 1.5 to 2.5 kg of weight loss over 30 weeks, compared to placebo or an active comparator (Insulin glargine, DPP-4 inhibitor, TZD, sulfonylurea).[11] Compared to placebo, semaglutide was associated with an even greater weight loss of 13.8% and 11.6% body weight for 0.4 mg and 0.2 mg, respectively.[36]

Drugs That Do Not Lower Cardiovascular Disease Risk

Dipeptidyl Peptidase 4 Inhibitors. DPP-4 inhibitors are chemically derived oral antidiabetics and are competitive inhibitors of DPP-4.

- **Glycemic control.** DPP-4 inhibitors have moderate glycemic efficacy and are inferior to GLP1-RAs and had no advantage over sulfonylureas in meta-analysis.[37]

- **Cardiovascular effects.** No cardiovascular benefit was observed in CVOTs of DPP-4 inhibitors (**e-Table 98.1**). However, higher risk for hospitalization from HF was observed for saxagliptin[38] and alogliptin.[39] Observed risk was higher for saxagliptin than for alogliptin. Consequently, current 2019 ESC guidelines do not recommend saxagliptin for patients with T2DM and HF.[10]
- **Drug interactions and major restrictions**. Compared to monotherapy, combination therapy of DPP-4 inhibitors and sulfonylureas increases the risk of hypoglycemia by 50%.[40]

Thiazolidinediones. TZDs are a class of oral antidiabetics made up of the two agents, pioglitazone and rosiglitazone (since withdrawn from the market). TZDs have a high glucose efficacy and improve insulin sensitivity. Although they are inexpensive and have atherosclerotic benefits, they are not first-choice agents on account of serious safety concerns, such as weight gain,[41] fracture risk,[42] HF,[43,44] and incidences of bladder cancer.[45]

- **Glycemic control**. TZDs have high glycemic efficacy without excessive risk of hypoglycemia.[46]
- **Cardiovascular outcomes (benefits and risks)**. Although pioglitazone (Actos) was found to increase chronic heart failure (CHF), it is also associated with decreased mortality, MI, and stroke.[47] For instance, in PROACTIVE (Prospective Pioglitazone Clinical Trial in Macrovascular Events), pioglitazone nonsignificantly reduced the risk of the composite primary endpoint (death from any cause, nonfatal MI, coronary revascularization, or revascularization of the leg) compared to placebo.[44] The ADA/EASD 2019 Standards of Care as well as the 2019 ESC guidelines do not recommend TZDs with symptomatic HF.[8,10] These recommendations are based on results of two large outcome trials, ProACTIVE[44] and DREAM (Diabetes Reduction Assessment With Ramipril and Rosiglitazone Medication),[43] which demonstrated relatively increased risk of HF. Possibly fluid retention, an important side effect of TZDs, explains the association of TZDs with HF.
- **Drug interactions or major restrictions.** Glitazones are metabolized by cytochrome P450. Clinicians should be aware that combination therapy of rifampicin and TZDs increases the area under the curve (AUC), whereas simultaneous subscription with gemfibrozil increases AUC by almost threefold.[48,49] Glitazones cause fluid retention and are not recommended for patients with renal impairment.[50]

Sulfonylureas. Sulfonylureas are an orally administered, inexpensive drug with a high glucose-lowering efficacy. However, these benefits have to be balanced with high risk of hypoglycemia and weight gain.

- **Glycemic control**. Because of their direct insulinotropic effect, sulfonylureas have a very high glycemic efficacy. For instance, sulfonylureas lowered HbA1c by 1.51% compared to placebo, by 0.46% compared to insulin, and by 1.62% compared to other glucose-lowering agents (mean baseline HbA1c varied from 4.6% to 13.6% between the individual trials).[51]
- **Cardiovascular effect**. Although sulfonylureas more effectively reduce cardiovascular risk than only lifestyle intervention, they are less effective than metformin.[52] Since the 1960s, there is an ongoing debate regarding cardiovascular safety of sulfonylureas because of a study from the University Group Diabetes Program (UGDP), which observed a high incidence of cardiovascular mortality in individuals subscribed tolbutamide.[53] However, recent studies have affirmed the cardiovascular safety of sulfonylureas.[54]
- **Drug restrictions or major interactions**. Special care should be taken prescribing sulfonylureas to patients who may be more prone to hypoglycemic episodes, such as elderly patients or individuals with impaired renal function.[55-57] The ADA/EASD 2019 Standards of Care recommends short-acting sulfonylureas like gliclazide, in favor of long-acting agents, as these have a lower risk of hypoglycemic events.[58] Hypoglycemia risk may be enhanced by interaction with drugs utilizing CYP2C9 substrates, such as anti-inflammatory drugs.[59]

Insulin. After unsuccessful oral or GLP1-RA therapy, insulin is the only remaining therapeutic option in patients with T2DM. If patients show signs of catabolism like weight loss, hyperglycemia, HbA1c levels greater than 10%/86 mmol/mol or blood glucose levels are over 300 mg/dL/16.7 mmol/L, insulin can be prescribed.[8]

Insulin can reduce HbA1c levels up to 4.9% in patients with T2DM.[60] Therapy intensification through the addition of insulin to oral agents offers many benefits. A study comparing monotherapy to combination therapy, that is, patients receiving metformin as well as insulin, demonstrated significantly more reduction in HbA1c levels than in individuals administered only insulin. The study also demonstrated that individuals in the insulin-metformin group showed fewer incidences of hypoglycemia and gained less weight.[61] Combination of insulin with other oral agents such as TZDs and sulfonylureas showed similar metabolic benefits.[62] Addition of oral agents to insulin can lower required insulin dose up to 62%.[62]

SECTION 8

FOLLOW-UP CARE AND RESEARCH AND FUTURE DIRECTIONS

Microvascular Complications

Microvascular complications of DM include diabetic kidney disease, retinopathy, neuropathy, and peripheral vascular disease. Although each of these requires separate screening and management plans, optimizing glucose controls was shown to slow the progression of all types of microvascular complications. The landmark trial, UKPDS, including over 7600 subjects with T2DM and a median follow-up of 10 years, demonstrated that the microvascular complication rate was reduced by 25% in the intensive treatment arm (median HbA1c 7.0%) compared to the control treatment arm (median HbA1c 7.9%).[63]

Macrovascular Complications

ASCVD is the leading cause of morbidity and mortality in patients with DM.[64] In addition, individuals with DM are at risk of suffering from HF. Evidence suggests that rates for hospitalization from HF are twofold higher in patients with DM.[65]

Risk Assessment

Both major current DM guidelines, the 2019 guidelines by the American College of Cardiology and the American Heart Association (ACC/AHA) and the 2019 ADA/EASD Standards of Medical Care, endorse the sex-specific pooled cohort equation (PCE) to calculate the 10-year risk of first atherosclerotic cardiovascular disease (10-year ASCVD). For patients at intermediate cardiovascular risk (7.5%-20%) where preventive therapy plan is unclear, coronary artery calcium (CAC) may be useful. The CAC score is calculated from a noncontrast cardiac-gated computed tomography scan of the heart and measures the total atherosclerotic burden of a lifetime exposure of measured and unmeasured cardiovascular risk factors.[66] Evidence suggests that CAC is superior in predicting coronary heart disease and CVD events than traditional risk factors.[67]

Risk-Enhancing Factors

Guidelines additionally recommend annual evaluation of patients' diabetes-specific cardiovascular risk factors in order to accurately evaluate CVD risk. In clinical practice, it is recommended to assess the duration of DM, age of onset, and presence of any comorbid cardiometabolic risk factors (including presence of MetSyn).

Hypoglycemia

A major limiting factor of the treatment of T1DM and T2DM is the risk of hypoglycemic events. Episodes of hypoglycemia promote platelet aggregation,[68] inflammation,[69] endothelial dysfunction,[70] and proarrhythmogenic processes,[71] increasing the risk of adverse cardiovascular events. Clinicians should be aware of the individual risks of hypoglycemia of different glucose-lowering drugs (**e-Table 98.2**). Newer oral antidiabetics such as SGLT-2 inhibitors, GLP1-RAs, and DPP-4 inhibitors are associated with an extremely low risk or even reduce the risk of hypoglycemia.

Cardiac Surgery and Glycemic Control

Stress-induced hyperglycemia affects up to 40% of patients after cardiac surgery, irrespective of diabetes status, and is associated with higher in-hospital mortality and morbidity.[72,73] However, moderate glycemic control is sufficient to improve outcomes as tight glycemic control (<140 mg/dL) during cardiac surgery was associated with increased complications.[74] A perioperative blood glucose level of more than 150 and less than 180 mg/dL sustained through a continuous intravenous infusion pump for cardiac surgery patients with diabetes is recommended.[75] During the intensive care unit (ICU) stay, similarly, a blood glucose level between 150 and 180 mg/dL should be maintained for patients with and without diabetes.[75]

KEY POINTS

- ✔ T2DM is for most patients strongly driven by lifestyle. Treatment always begins with low-carbohydrate/low-glycemic-index diet principles, weight loss, and increased physical activity.
- ✔ DM treatment approach can be further refined through the consideration of ASCVD status, use of the 10-year ASCVD risk calculator, and CAC as risk in DM remains heterogeneous. Nearly all DM patients would benefit from statins as cardiovascular preventive therapy.
- ✔ When choosing pharmacologic treatment, consideration of the following key patient factors is important: (1) comorbidities (eg, ASCVD, CKD, or HF), (2) hypoglycemia risk, (3) effects on body weight, (4) side effects, (5) costs, and (6) patient preferences. Insulin as part of early care in T2DM is generally no longer recommended.
- ✔ For patients with established ASCVD, SGLT-2 inhibitors and GLP1-RAs lower risk of cardiovascular events.
- ✔ Patients with HF or are at high risk of HF should be subscribed SGLT-2 inhibitors, whereas TZDs and DPP-4 inhibitors are not recommended.
- ✔ GLP1-RAs are recommended for weight loss in patients with T2DM and are good options early in the natural history of atherosclerosis development.
- ✔ SGLT-2 inhibitors were shown to reduce CKD progression in patients with T2DM.
- ✔ Episodes of hypoglycemia pose significant risks to cardiovascular health and should be avoided. SGLT-2 inhibitors as well as GLP1-RAs are associated with low incidences of hypoglycemic episodes.
- ✔ Innovation in treatments and improved glycemic control have led to an increased life expectancy of patients with T1DM, but also posits patients at high risk for CVD. Clinicians should be aware and manage cardiovascular risk of patients with T1DM.

REFERENCES

1. Haffner S, Letho S, Ronnemaa T, Pyorala K, Laakson M. Mortality from coronary heart disease in subjects with and without type 2 diabetes and in nondiabetic subjects with and without prior myocardial infarction. *N Engl J Med.* 1998;339(4):229-234.
2. IDF Diabetes Atlas. Demographic and geographic outline. Published 2019. Accessed December 5, 2019. https://diabetesatlas.org/en/sections/demographic-and-geographic-outline.html
3. Noble JA, Valdes AM. Genetics of the HLA region in the prediction of type 1 diabetes. *Curr Diab Rep.* 2011;11(6):533-542. doi:10.1007/s11892-011-0223-x
4. Scott RA, Langenberg C, Sharp SJ, et al. The link between family history and risk of type 2 diabetes is not explained by anthropometric, lifestyle or genetic risk factors: the EPIC-InterAct study. *Diabetologia.* 2013;56(1):60-69. doi:10.1007/s00125-012-2715-x
5. Alberti KGMM, Zimmet P, Shaw J. The metabolic syndrome—A new worldwide definition. *Lancet.* 2005;366(9491):1059-1062. doi:10.1016/S0140-6736(05)67402-8
6. Centers for Disease Control and Prevention. Rates of new diagnosed cases of type 1 and type 2 diabetes continue to rise among children, teens.

Accessed July 15, 2020. https://www.cdc.gov/diabetes/research/reports/children-diabetes-rates-rise.html

7. Cowie CC, Rust KF, Byrd-Holt DD, et al. Prevalence of diabetes and high risk for diabetes using A1C criteria in the U.S. population in 1988-2006. *Diabetes Care.* 2010;33(3):562-568. doi:10.2337/dc09-1524
8. American Diabetes Association. Standards of medical care in diabetes-2019. *Diabetes Care.* 2019;42(suppl 1). doi:10.2337/dc19-Sint01
9. Knowler WC, Barrett-Connor E, Fowler SE, et al. Reduction in the incidence of type 2 diabetes with lifestyle intervention or metformin. *N Engl J Med.* 2002;346(6):393-403. doi:10.1056/NEJMoa012512
10. Cosentino F, Grant PJ, Aboyans V, et al. 2019 ESC Guidelines on diabetes, pre-diabetes, and cardiovascular diseases developed in collaboration with the EASD. *Eur Heart J.* 2019:1-69. doi:10.1093/eurheartj/ehz486
11. Shyangdan DS, Royle P, Clar C, Sharma P, Waugh N, Snaith A. Glucagon-like peptide analogues for type 2 diabetes mellitus. *Cochrane Database Syst Rev.* 2011;2011(10):CD006423. doi:10.1002/14651858.CD006423.pub2
12. Dave CV, Schneeweiss S, Wexler DJ, Brill G, Patorno E. Trends in clinical characteristics and prescribing preferences for SGLT2 inhibitors and GLP-1 receptor agonists, 2013-2018. *Diabetes Care.* 2020;43(4):921-924. doi:10.2337/dc19-1943
13. American Diabetemore Association. U.K. Prospective diabetes study 16: overview of 6 years' therapy of type II diabetes: a progressive disease. *Diabetes.* 1995;44(11):1249-1258. doi:10.2337/diabetes.44.11.1249
14. Van Raalte DH, Bunck MC, Smits MM, et al. Exenatide improves β-cell function up to 3 years of treatment in patients with type 2 diabetes: a randomised controlled trial. *Eur J Endocrinol.* 2016;175(4):345-352. doi:10.1530/EJE-16-0286
15. Leibowitz G, Cahn A, Bhatt DL, et al. Impact of treatment with saxagliptin on glycaemic stability and β-cell function in the SAVOR-TIMI 53 study. *Diabetes Obes Metab.* 2015;17(5):487-494. doi:10.1111/dom.12445
16. Cefalu WT, Dawes DE, Gavlak G, et al. Insulin access and affordability working group: conclusions and recommendations. *Diabetes Care.* 2018;41(6):1299-1311. doi:10.2337/dci18-0019
17. Salvetti A, Ghiadoni L. Thiazide diuretics in the treatment of hypertension: an update. *J Am Soc Nephrol.* 2006;17(4 suppl 2):S25-S29. doi:10.1681/ASN.2005121329
18. Holman RR, Coleman RL, Chan JCN, et al. Effects of acarbose on cardiovascular and diabetes outcomes in patients with coronary heart disease and impaired glucose tolerance (ACE): a randomised, double-blind, placebo-controlled trial. *Lancet Diabetes Endocrinol.* 2017;5(11):877-886. doi:10.1016/S2213-8587(17)30309-1
19. Vella S, Buetow L, Royle P, Livingstone S, Colhoun HM, Petrie JR. The use of metformin in type 1 diabetes: a systematic review of efficacy. *Diabetologia.* 2010;53(5):809-820. doi:10.1007/s00125-009-1636-9
20. Henry RR, Thakkar P, Tong C, Polidori D, Alba M. Efficacy and safety of canagliflozin, a sodium-glucose cotransporter 2 inhibitor, as add-on to insulin in patients with type 1 diabetes. *Diabetes Care.* 2015;38(12):2258-2265 doi:10.2337/dc15-1730
21. U.S. Department of Health and Human Services; Food and Drug Administration; Center for Drug Evaluation and Research (CDER). Guidance for industry diabetes mellitus-evaluating cardiovascular risk in new antidiabetic therapies to treat type 2 diabetes. 2008. Accessed July 2, 2019. https://www.fda.gov/media/71297/download
22. Marso SP, Daniels GH, Brown-Frandsen K, et al. Liraglutide and cardiovascular outcomes in type 2 diabetes. *N Engl J Med.* 2016;375(4):311-322. doi:10.1056/NEJMoa1603827
23. Neal B, Perkovic V, Mahaffey KW, et al. Canagliflozin and cardiovascular and renal events in type 2 diabetes. *N Engl J Med.* 2017;377(7):644-657. doi:10.1056/NEJMoa1611925
24. U.S. Food and Drug Administration. FDA approves Ozempic® for cardiovascular risk reduction in adults with type 2 diabetes and known heart disease, updates Rybelsus® label. Accessed July 15, 2020. https://www.prnewswire.com/news-releases/fda-approves-ozempic-for-cardiovascular-risk-reduction-in-adults-with-type-2-diabetes-and-known-heart-disease-updates-rybelsus-label-300988672.html
25. Zinman B, Wanner C, Lachin JM, et al. Empagliflozin, cardiovascular outcomes, and mortality in type 2 diabetes. *N Engl J Med.* 2015;373(22):2117-2128. doi:10.1056/NEJMoa1504720
26. U.S. Food and Drug Administration. FDA approves new treatment for a type of heart failure. Published 2020. Accessed July 15, 2020. https://www.fda.gov/news-events/press-announcements/fda-approves-new-treatment-type-heart-failure
27. Eurich DT, McAlister FA, Blackburn DF, et al. Benefits and harms of antidiabetic agents in patients with diabetes and heart failure: systematic review. *Br Med J.* 2007;335(7618):497. doi:10.1136/bmj.39314.620174.80
28. Bray GA, Edelstein SL, Crandall JP, et al. Long-term safety, tolerability, and weight loss associated with metformin in the Diabetes Prevention Program outcomes study. *Diabetes Care.* 2012;35(4):731-737. doi:10.2337/dc11-1299
29. Maruthur NM, Tseng E, Hutfless S, et al. Diabetes medications as monotherapy or metformin-based combination therapy for type 2 diabetes: a systematic review and meta-analysis. *Ann Intern Med.* 2016;164(11):740-751. doi:10.7326/M15-2650
30. Turner R. Effect of intensive blood-glucose control with metformin on complications in overweight patients with type 2 diabetes (UKPDS 34). *Lancet.* 1998;352(9131):854-865. doi:10.1016/S0140-6736(98)07037-8
31. Lunder M, Janić M, Japelj M, Juretič A, Janež A, Šabovič M. Empagliflozin on top of metformin treatment improves arterial function in patients with type 1 diabetes mellitus Clinical trial registration NCT03639545 NCT. *Cardiovasc Diabetol.* 2018;17(1):153. doi:10.1186/s12933-018-0797-6
32. Dore FJ, Domingues CC, Ahmadi N, et al. The synergistic effects of saxagliptin and metformin on CD34+ endothelial progenitor cells in early type 2 diabetes patients: a randomized clinical trial. *Cardiovasc Diabetol.* 2018;17(1):65. doi:10.1186/s12933-018-0709-9
33. Ke J, Liu Y, Yang J, et al. Synergistic effects of metformin with liraglutide against endothelial dysfunction through GLP-1 receptor and PKA signalling pathway. *Sci Rep.* 2017;7(1):1-11. doi:10.1038/srep41085
34. Perkovic V, Jardine MJ, Neal B, et al. Canagliflozin and renal outcomes in type 2 diabetes and nephropathy. *N Engl J Med.* 2019;380(24):2295-2306. doi:10.1056/NEJMoa1811744
35. Levin PA, Nguyen H, Wittbrodt ET, Kim SC. Glucagon-like peptide-1 receptor agonists: a systematic review of comparative effectiveness research. *Diabetes, Metab Syndr Obes Targets Ther.* 2017;10:123-139. doi:10.2147/DMSO.S130834
36. O'Neil PM, Birkenfeld AL, McGowan B, et al. Efficacy and safety of semaglutide compared with liraglutide and placebo for weight loss in patients with obesity: a randomised, double-blind, placebo and active controlled, dose-ranging, phase 2 trial. *Lancet.* 2018;392(10148):637-649. doi:10.1016/S0140-6736(18)31773-2
37. Karagiannis T, Paschos P, Paletas K, Matthews DR, Tsapas A. Dipeptidyl peptidase-4 inhibitors for treatment of type 2 diabetes mellitus in the clinical setting: systematic review and meta-analysis. *BMJ.* 2012;344:e1369. doi:10.1136/bmj.e1369
38. Scirica BM, Bhatt DL, Braunwald E, et al. Saxagliptin and cardiovascular outcomes in patients with type 2 diabetes mellitus. *N Engl J Med.* 2013;369(14):1317-1326. doi:10.1056/NEJMoa1307684
39. Zannad F, Cannon CP, Cushman WC, et al. Heart failure and mortality outcomes in patients with type 2 diabetes taking alogliptin versus placebo in EXAMINE: a multicentre, randomised, double-blind trial. *Lancet.* 2015;385(9982):2067-2076. doi:10.1016/S0140-6736(14)62225-X
40. Salvo F, Moore N, Arnaudl M, et al. Addition of dipeptidyl peptidase-4 inhibitors to sulphonylureas and risk of hypoglycaemia: systematic review and meta-analysis. *BMJ.* 2016;353:i2231. doi:10.1136/bmj.i2231
41. Kernan WN, Viscoli CM, Furie KL, et al. Pioglitazone after ischemic stroke or transient ischemic attack. *N Engl J Med.* 2016;374(14):1321-1331. doi:10.1056/NEJMoa1506930
42. Bilik D, McEwen LN, Brown MB, et al. Thiazolidinediones and fractures: evidence from translating research into action for diabetes. *J Clin Endocrinol Metab.* 2010;95(10):4560-4565. doi:10.1210/jc.2009-2638
43. DREAM Trial Investigators, Dagenais GR, Gerstein HC, et al. Effects of ramipril and rosiglitazone on cardiovascular and renal outcomes in people with impaired glucose tolerance or impaired fasting glucose: results of the Diabetes REduction Assessment with ramipril and rosiglitazone Medication (DREAM) trial. *Diabetes Care.* 2008;31(5):1007-1014. doi:10.2337/dc07-1868

44. Dormandy JA, Charbonnel B, Eckland DJ, et al. Secondary prevention of macrovascular events in patients with type 2 diabetes in the PROactive Study (PROspective pioglitAzone Clinical Trial In macroVascular Events): a randomised controlled trial. *Lancet.* 2005;366(9493):1279-1289. doi:10.1016/S0140-6736(05)67528-9
45. U.S. Food and Drug Administration. FDA Drug Safety Communication: Updated FDA review concludes that use of type 2 diabetes medicine pioglitazone may be linked to an increased risk of bladder cancer. Published 2016. Accessed June 30, 2019. https://www.fda.gov/drugs/drug-safety-and-availability/fda-drug-safety-communication-updated-fda-review-concludes-use-type-2-diabetes-medicine-pioglitazone
46. Bron M, Marynchenko M, Yang H, Yu AP, Wu EQ. Hypoglycemia, treatment discontinuation, and costs in patients with type 2 diabetes mellitus on oral antidiabetic drugs. *Postgrad Med.* 2012;124(1):124-132. doi:10.3810/pgm.2012.01.2525
47. Lincoff AM, Wolski K, Nicholls SJ, Nissen SE. Pioglitazone and risk of cardiovascular events in patients with type 2 diabetes mellitus: a meta-analysis of randomized trials. *J Am Med Assoc.* 2007;298(10):1180-1188. doi:10.1001/jama.298.10.1180
48. Niemi M, Backman JT, Neuvonen PJ. Effects of trimethoprim and rifampin on the pharmacokinetics of the cytochrome P450 2C8 substrate rosiglitazone. *Clin Pharmacol Ther.* 2004;76(3):239-249. doi:10.1016/j.clpt.2004.05.001
49. Niemi M, Backman JT, Granfors M, Laitila J, Neuvonen M, Neuvonen PJ. Gemfibrozil considerably increases the plasma concentrations of rosiglitazone. *Diabetologia.* 2003;46(10):1319-1323. doi:10.1007/s00125-003-1181-x
50. Armstrong C. ADA updates standards of medical care for patients with diabetes mellitus. *Am Fam Physician.* 2017;95(1):40-43. Accessed June 13, 2019. http://www.ncbi.nlm.nih.gov/pubmed/28075100
51. Hirst JA, Farmer AJ, Dyar A, Lung TWC, Stevens RJ. Estimating the effect of sulfonylurea on HbA1c in diabetes: a systematic review and meta-analysis. *Diabetologia.* 2013;56(5):973-984. doi:10.1007/s00125-013-2856-6
52. Bain S, Druyts E, Balijepalli C, et al. Cardiovascular events and all-cause mortality associated with sulphonylureas compared with other antihyperglycaemic drugs: a Bayesian meta-analysis of survival data. *Diabetes Obes Metab.* 2017;19(3):329-335. doi:10.1111/dom.12821
53. Meinert CL, Knatterud GL, Prout TE, Klimt CR. A study of the effects of hypoglycemic agents on vascular complications in patients with adult-onset diabetes. II. Mortality results. *Diabetes.* 1970;19:(suppl):789-830.
54. Boehringer Ingelheim and Eli Lilly and Company. Boehringer Ingelheim and Lilly announce the CAROLINA cardiovascular outcome trial of Tradjenta met its primary endpoint of non-inferiority compared with glimepiride. Published 2019. Accessed August 10, 2019. https://www.boehringer-ingelheim.us/press-release/boehringer-ingelheim-and-lilly-announce-carolina-cardiovascular-outcome-trial
55. Holstein A, Plaschke A, Egberts EH. Lower incidence of severe hypoglycaemia in patients with type 2 diabetes treated with glimepiride versus glibenclamide. *Diabetes Metab Res Rev.* 2001;17(6):467-473. doi:10.1002/dmrr.235
56. Van Dalem J, Brouwers MCGJ, Stehouwer CDA, et al. Risk of hypoglycaemia in users of sulphonylureas compared with metformin in relation to renal function and sulphonylurea metabolite group: population based cohort study. *BMJ.* 2016;354:i3625. doi:10.1136/bmj.i3625
57. Thorpe CT, Gellad WF, Good CB, et al. Tight glycemic control and use of hypoglycemic medications in older veterans with type 2 diabetes and comorbid dementia. *Diabetes Care.* 2015;38(4):588-595. doi:10.2337/dc14-0599
58. Douros A, Yin H, Yu OHY, Filion KB, Azoulay L, Suissa S. Pharmacologic differences of sulfonylureas and the risk of adverse cardiovascular and hypoglycemic events. *Diabetes Care.* 2017;40(11):1506-1513. doi:10.2337/dc17-0595
59. Parekh TM, Raji M, Lin Y-L, Tan A, Kuo Y-F, Goodwin JS. Hypoglycemia after antimicrobial drug prescription for older patients using sulfonylureas. *JAMA Intern Med.* 2014;174(10):1605. doi:10.1001/jamainternmed.2014.3293
60. Lingvay I, Kaloyanova PF, Adams-Huet B, Salinas K, Raskin P. Insulin as initial therapy in type 2 diabetes. *J Investig Med.* 2007;55(2):62-68. doi:10.2310/6650.2007.06036
61. Avilés-Santa L, Sinding J, Raskin P. Effects of metformin in patients with poorly controlled, insulin-treated type 2 diabetes mellitus. *Ann Intern Med.* 1999;131(3):182. doi:10.7326/0003-4819-131-3-199908030-00004
62. Yki-Järvinen H. Combination therapies with insulin in type 2 diabetes. *Diabetes Care.* 2001;24(4):758-767. doi:10.2337/diacare.24.4.758
63. UK Prospective Diabetes Study (UKPDS) Group. Intensive blood-glucose control with sulphonylureas or insulin compared with conventional treatment and risk of complications in patients with type 2 diabetes (UKPDS 33). *Lancet.* 1998;352(9131):837-853. doi:10.1016/S0140-6736(98)07019-6
64. Americam Diabetis Association. Economic costs of diabetes in the U.S. in 2017. *Diabetes Care.* 2018;41(5):917-928. doi:10.2337/DCI18-0007
65. McAllister DA, Read SH, Kerssens J, et al. Incidence of hospitalization for heart failure and case-fatality among 3.25 million people with and without diabetes mellitus. *Circulation.* 2018;138(24):2774-2786. doi:10.1161/CIRCULATIONAHA.118.034986
66. Blaha MJ, Silverman MG, Budoff MJ. Is there a role for coronary artery calcium scoring for management of asymptomatic patients at risk for coronary artery disease? *Circ Cardiovasc Imaging.* 2014;7(2):398-408. doi:10.1161/CIRCIMAGING.113.000341
67. McClelland RL, Jorgensen NW, Budoff M, et al. 10-year coronary heart disease risk prediction using coronary artery calcium and traditional risk factors derivation in the MESA (Multi-Ethnic Study of Atherosclerosis) with validation in the HNR (Heinz Nixdorf Recall) study and the DHS (Dallas Heart Study). *J Am Coll Cardiol.* 2015;66(15):1643-1653. doi:10.1016/j.jacc.2015.08.035
68. Angiolillo DJ, Fernandez-Ortiz A, Bernardo E, et al. Platelet function profiles in patients with type 2 diabetes and coronary artery disease on combined aspirin and clopidogrel treatment. *Diabetes.* 2005;54(8):2430-2435. doi:10.2337/diabetes.54.8.2430
69. Jin WL, Azuma K, Mita T, et al. Repetitive hypoglycaemia increases serum adrenaline and induces monocyte adhesion to the endothelium in rat thoracic aorta. *Diabetologia.* 2011;54(7):1921-1929. doi:10.1007/s00125-011-2141-5
70. Sommerfield AJ, Wilkinson IB, Webb DJ, Frier BM. Vessel wall stiffness in type 1 diabetes and the central hemodynamic effects of acute hypoglycemia. *Am J Physiol Metab.* 2007;293(5):E1274-E1279. doi:10.1152/ajpendo.00114.2007
71. Stahn A, Pistrosch F, Ganz X, et al. Relationship between hypoglycemic episodes and ventricular arrhythmias in patients with type 2 diabetes and cardiovascular diseases: silent hypoglycemias and silent arrhythmias. *Diabetes Care.* 2014;37(2):516-520. doi:10.2337/dc13-0600
72. Gelijns AC, Moskowitz AJ, Acker MA, et al. Management practices and major infections after cardiac surgery. *J Am Coll Cardiol.* 2014;64(4):372-381. doi:10.1016/j.jacc.2014.04.052
73. Ascione R, Rogers CA, Rajakaruna C, Angelini GD. Inadequate blood glucose control is associated with in-hospital mortality and morbidity in diabetic and nondiabetic patients undergoing cardiac surgery. *Circulation.* 2008;118(2):113-123. doi:10.1161/CIRCULATIONAHA.107.706416
74. Umpierrez G, Cardona S, Pasquel F, et al. Randomized controlled trial of intensive versus conservative glucose control in patients undergoing coronary artery bypass graft surgery: GLUCOCABG trial. *Diabetes Care.* 2015;38(9):1665-1672. doi:10.2337/dc15-0303
75. Sousa-Uva M, Head SJ, Milojevic M, et al. 2017 EACTS Guidelines on perioperative medication in adult cardiac surgery. *Eur J Cardiothoracic Surg.* 2018;53(1):5-33. doi:10.1093/ejcts/ezx314

CHAPTER 99

LIPID DISORDERS

Bibin Varghese, Renato Quispe, and Seth S. Martin

INTRODUCTION

Lipid disorders play a critical role in the development of atherosclerotic cardiovascular disease (ASCVD), including coronary heart disease (CHD), stroke, and peripheral vascular disease (PVD).[1] A wealth of evidence has confirmed the proportional, causal relationship between low-density lipoprotein cholesterol (LDL-C) and development of atherosclerosis and ASCVD.[2-5] One of the cornerstone therapies in preventive cardiology recommended by the current guidelines worldwide is pharmacologic LDL-C lowering with statin agents[6] and non-statin LDL-C lowering agents, in particular ezetimibe[7] and proprotein convertase subtilisin/kexin type 9 (PCSK9) inhibitors.[8,9] Despite the progress made in primary and secondary prevention with lipid-lowering therapies, further work in this field remains because ASCVD continues to be a leading cause of morbidity and mortality worldwide.[3,4]

This chapter provides an overview of the epidemiology, risk factors, pathogenesis, clinical presentation, diagnosis, and management of lipid disorders because they pertain to clinical practice.

Epidemiology

More than 12% of the U.S. population (29 million) have total cholesterol (TC) levels greater than 240 mg/dL[10] and 7% of U.S. adolescents (ages 6-19) have high cholesterol. In addition, only 55% (43 million) of the patients eligible for lipid-lowering therapy are currently taking it. Although there has been a substantial reduction in average TC levels in the United States over the past decades with lipid-lowering therapies, TC levels still remain the highest in North America and Europe.[11,12]

Risk Factors

Nonmodifiable risk factors such as age, sex, and ethnicity (ie, South Asian ancestry) are associated with dyslipidemia. Modifiable risk factors linked to dyslipidemia include obesity, blood glucose control, diet, and sedentary lifestyle.[5] Finally, secondary causes of lipid disorders including diabetes mellitus, hypothyroidism, medications, chronic kidney disease, nephrotic syndrome, cirrhosis, inflammatory diseases (ie, rheumatoid arthritis, psoriasis, human immunodeficiency virus [HIV] infection), premature menopause, and preeclampsia should be considered in the right clinical context as contributors to dyslipidemia.[3,4]

PATHOGENESIS

Lipids are hydrophobic molecules that play essential roles in the formation of lipid bilayers, energy storage, bile formation, and production of steroid hormones that are essential for the normal functioning of the human body.[2,13] Owing to their hydrophobic nature, lipids need to be transported in serum from sites of origin to target tissues via lipoproteins. Lipoproteins are complex macromolecules with the exterior, hydrophilic portions (free cholesterol, phospholipids, apolipoproteins) enveloping interior, hydrophobic components (such as triglycerides [TGs] and cholesterol esters). Lipoproteins are classified by size, density, lipid composition, and surface apolipoproteins. Examples of lipoproteins include chylomicrons, chylomicron remnants, very low-density lipoprotein (VLDL), intermediate-density lipoprotein (IDL), LDL, lipoprotein(a) (Lp(a)), and high-density lipoprotein (HDL) (**Figure 99.1** and **Table 99.1**).

The exogenous pathway for lipid transport begins in intestinal epithelial cells where fatty acids, the breakdown product of TG, and cholesterol are absorbed.[2,13] The fatty acids and cholesterol that are absorbed into intestinal epithelial cells are repackaged into apoB-48–containing TG-rich chylomicrons. These chylomicrons enter the circulation and are broken down by lipoprotein lipase (LPL) found on endothelial cells. The free fatty acids released by breakdown of TG within chylomicrons are either rapidly taken up by nearby tissues (such as muscle or adipose tissue) for energy or transported via lipid binding proteins to the liver for repackaging into VLDL.

The remnant chylomicron particles formed after interaction with LPL undergo reuptake in the liver via apolipoprotein E found on the surface of the remnant particles. As part of the endogenous pathway, the liver produces VLDL, a TG-rich lipoprotein that is smaller than a chylomicron, to transport TG to peripheral tissues to provide energy independent of dietary intake or food availability (**Figure 99.2**). As opposed to apoB-48 seen on the surface of chylomicrons, each VLDL has one apoB-100 protein on its surface that is recognized by the LDL receptor. Once VLDL particles are secreted by the liver, they also acquire apoC and apoE, at least in part, from HDL. VLDL particles are then broken down in the periphery by LPL. Formed after TG breakdown, VLDL remnants (and the previously mentioned chylomicron remnants) also undergo lipid and protein exchanges with HDL. The remnant particles shed apoC while keeping apoE, and exchange TG for cholesterol

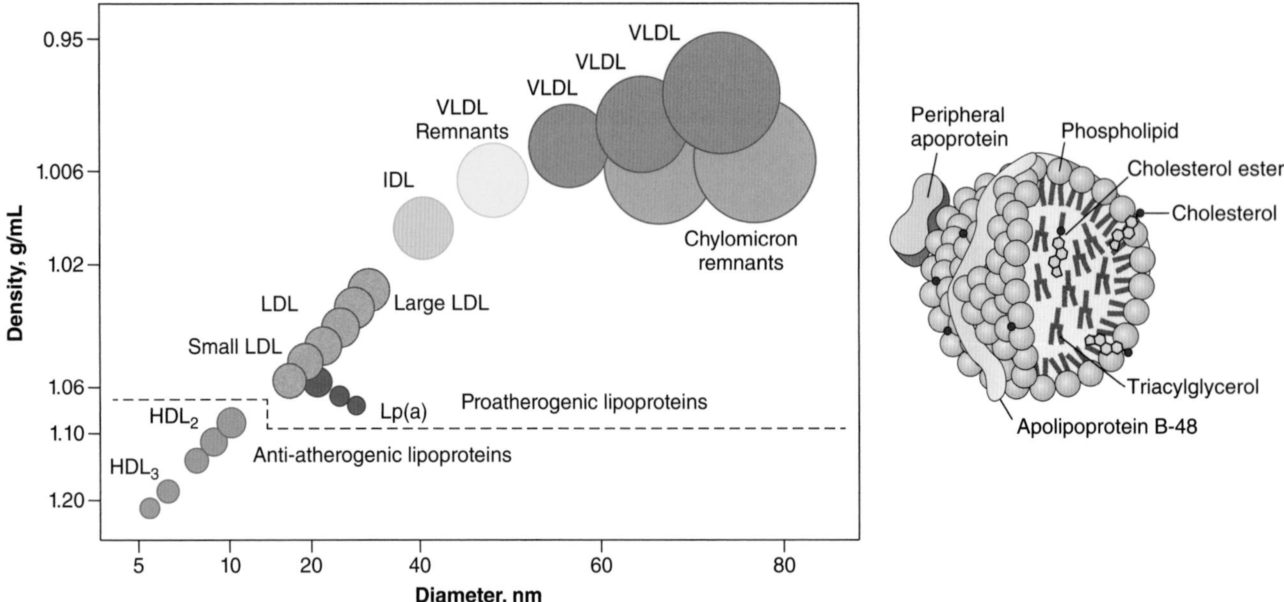

FIGURE 99.1 The lipoprotein classes are based on size, density, lipid composition, and surface apolipoproteins. Each of the lipoproteins plays an essential role in lipid metabolism and homeostasis. HDL, high-density lipoproteins; IDL, intermediate-density lipoprotein; Lp(a), lipoprotein(a); LDL, low-density lipoprotein; VLDL, very low-density lipoprotein.

TABLE 99.1 Characteristics of Lipoproteins

Lipoproteins	Density (g/mL)	Size (nm)	Protein (%)	Predominant lipids	Primary Apolipoprotein(s)
Lipoprotein(a) (Lp(a))	1.055-1.085	25	30-50	Cholesterol	B100, apoA
High-density lipoprotein (HDL)	1.063-1.210	~6-10	40-55	Cholesterol phospholipids	A-I, A-II
Low-density lipoprotein (LDL)	1.019-1.063	20-25	25	Cholesterol	B-100
Intermediate-density lipoprotein (IDL)	1.006-1.019	25-30	18	Triglyceride, cholesterol	B-100, apoE
Very low-density lipoprotein (VLDL)	<1.006	40-50	10	Triglycerides	B-100
Chylomicron remnants	0.95-1.006	30-80	~3-5	Triglycerides, cholesterol	ApoB48, apoE
Chylomicrons	<0.595	100-1000	~1-2	Triglycerides	ApoB48

ester with HDL via cholesterol ester transfer protein (CETP). This exchange of apolipoproteins, TG, and cholesterol ester serves to set the metabolic fate of the remnant particles and also helps transport cholesterol from HDL to VLDL remnants so that it can be processed by the liver as part of the reverse cholesterol transport pathway. The VLDL remnant particle, now relatively richer in cholesterol, is called IDL. IDL particles either undergo liver uptake via complex apoE-receptor interactions or undergo further breakdown via hepatic lipase to form LDL.

Because LDL is formed after TG breakdown, these particles are depleted in TG and relatively rich in cholesterol esters. LDL can be considered the "garbage product" of lipid metabolism. Although LDL has been classically considered as responsible for transporting cholesterol ester throughout the body, modern clinical evidence is reframing our understanding of the importance of this function. Specifically, patients treated with statins, ezetimibe, and PCSK9 inhibitors to maintain LDL cholesterol concentrations near-zero do not suffer adverse nonvascular effects.[6,14] After transport of the cholesterol ester to peripheral tissues, the LDL particles are uptaken by the LDL receptor on the hepatocyte via the single apoB on the surface of LDL. Once bound to the LDL receptor, clathrin-mediated endocytosis occurs, and the complex is degraded in the lysosome, releasing free cholesterol within the cell. The LDL receptor can then either be recycled back to the surface of the hepatocyte for further reuptake of LDL or it can be bound by the chaperone PCSK9, which pushes the LDL receptor toward a degradation pathway, thereby preventing recycling of the LDL receptor. The balance between the intrinsic rate of synthesis of hepatic LDL and the rate of uptake of LDL by its receptor is what determines the overall LDL particle number and LDL concentration within plasma.

LDL-C is a large component of the guideline recommendations for risk assessment and management of ASCVD.[3,4] It has the longest half-life relative to other lipoproteins and typically constitutes greater than 90% of circulating atherogenic lipoproteins.[15] In the presence of endothelial injury and

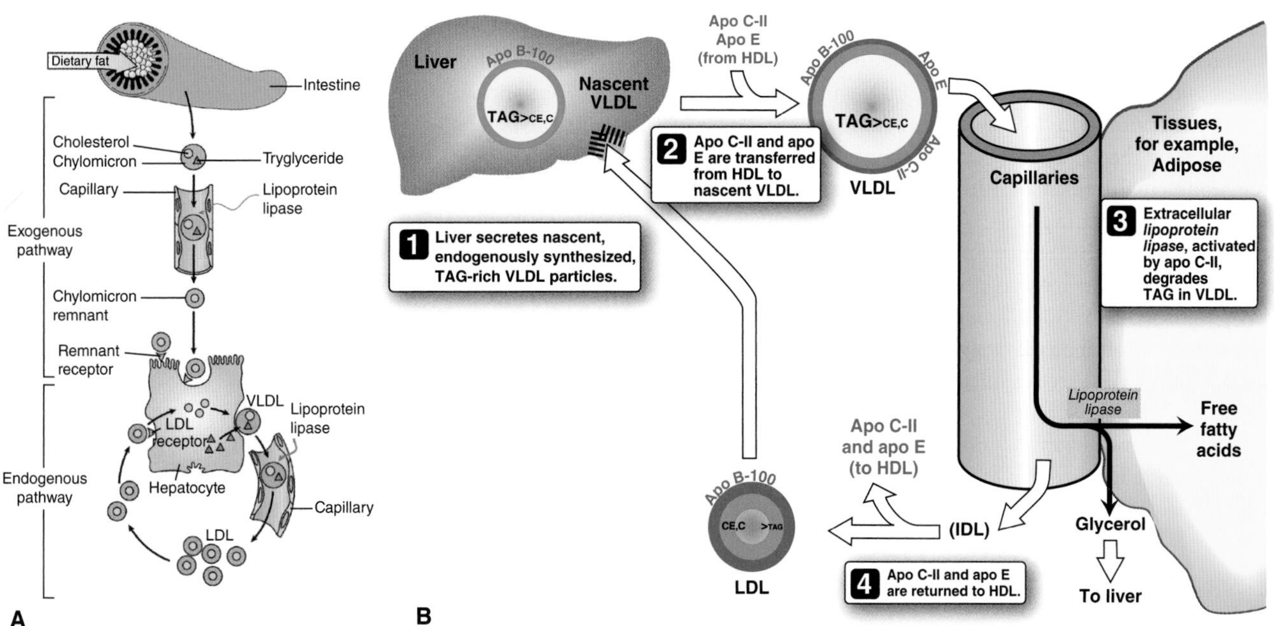

FIGURE 99.2 Lipid metabolism begins with exogenous dietary intake of triglycerides (TGs) and cholesterol-rich foods that are metabolized, absorbed, and repackaged into chylomicrons in intestinal epithelial cells. These particles are secreted into the lymphatic system and enter the circulation. The liver also produces endogenous triacylglycerol (TAG-rich) very low-density lipoprotein (VLDL) particles that transport TG and cholesterol to target tissues. Lipoprotein lipase (LPL) found on endothelial cells breaks down TG from chylomicrons and VLDL. Once the TGs are processed, lipid and apolipoprotein exchanges occur with high-density lipoprotein (HDL), which results in the formation of remnant particles. Remnant chylomicron particles are taken up by the liver. After TG breakdown and HDL exchanges, VLDL remnant particles are called intermediate density lipoprotein (IDL). The IDL particles are either taken up by the liver or undergo reaction with hepatic lipase and further lipid exchanges with HDL to form low-density lipoprotein (LDL). (A, Adapted with permission from Rubin E, Farber JL. *Pathology*. 3rd ed. Philadelphia, PA: Lippincott Williams & Wilkins; 1999. Figure 10.18.; B, Adapted with permission from Harvey RA, Ferrier DR. Lippincott Illustrated Reviews: *Biochemistry*. 5th ed. Philadelphia, PA: Wolters Kluwer Health/Lippincott Williams & Wilkins; 2010. Figure 18.17.)

increased oxidative stress, the LDL particles in circulation enter the endothelial lumen, and the single apoB particle on the surface of LDL becomes modified because of oxidative stress that leads to the cascade of events, causing foam cell formation and development of atherosclerosis.[16]

To date, most guidelines emphasize the significance of LDL-C concentration in preventive cardiology.[3,4] The reason for its prominence in guidelines is the wealth of clinical trial evidence for the benefit of pharmacotherapies that specifically target LDL-C. However, other broader measures of atherogenic cholesterol and lipoprotein burden may provide complementary information, such as non-HDL-C (estimated as TC minus HDL-C). Although both LDL-C and non-HDL-C are fundamentally cholesterol-based measures, it is postulated that the circulating concentration of atherogenic *particles* that come into contact with the lumen of the endothelium can be independently associated with risk in the setting of discordance between *cholesterol* and *particle* measures.[15] Because each of the atherogenic lipoproteins (LDL, VLDL, and IDL) have one apoB particle, levels of apoB are more closely correlated to particle numbers in circulation than to cholesterol-based measures.[17] Nevertheless, often the measures are highly correlated. However, in the case of discordance, apoB levels are more closely associated with ASCVD risk compared to LDL-C or non-HDL-C in cross-sectional and prospective observational studies and Bayesian analysis of statin trials.[15]

High-Density Lipoprotein-C

Levels of HDL-C have extensively been considered as a risk marker for atherosclerosis. HDL participates in reverse cholesterol transport, exerts anti-inflammatory roles, and prevents lipoprotein oxidation.[18] However, Mendelian randomization and genetic epidemiologic studies have not been able to demonstrate a causal relationship between HDL-C levels and atherosclerosis.[19,20]

Triglyceride-Rich Lipoproteins

Triglyceride -rich lipoproteins (TGRL), such as chylomicrons and VLDL, are typically increased in the postprandial state, and their metabolism leads to increased formation of remnant lipoproteins such as chylomicron remnants, VLDL remnants, and IDL remnant particles. Recently, clinical studies and Mendelian randomization studies have shown that these TGRLs and remnant particles are associated with ASCVD independent of LDL-C levels.[21]

Lipoprotein(a)

Lp(a) is an independent risk factor in the development of aortic stenosis and a predictor of cardiovascular risk.[22] Lp(a) is an LDL-like particle with the apoB covalently bound to apolipoprotein(a) via a single disulfide bond. The atherogenic potential of Lp(a) may be caused by its LDL-like domain and the prothrombotic effects of its inactive, plasminogen-like protease domain on apolipoprotein(a).[23] In addition, Lp(a) binds strongly to oxidized lipoproteins, which may explain how Lp(a) is independently associated with calcific aortic stenosis, CHD, and PVD, even in patients with normal LDL-C levels.[22] Lp(a) levels are primarily determined by the Lp(a) gene locus without significant dietary or environmental influences. Although medications that lower Lp(a) such as niacin and PCSK9 inhibitors provide only a modest 20% to 30% reduction in Lp(a) concentration, Mendelian randomization studies have suggested that the clinical benefit is likely proportional to absolute reduction in Lp(a) concentration. Lp(a) reduction of approximately 99 mg/dL is required to reduce the risk of CHD to a similar magnitude achieved by lowering LDL-C by approximately 40 mg/dL (1 mmol/L).[24] The advent of antisense oligonucleotide therapy is an exciting area of research because it has shown mean reductions in Lp(a) levels of approximately 80%.[23,25,26]

CLINICAL PRESENTATION

Most patients with dyslipoproteinemias are asymptomatic. Severe manifestations of lipid disorders such as familial hyperchylomicronemia in which TG concentrations are severely elevated because of the number of circulating chylomicrons can lead to limited blood flow to the pancreas and can present as recurrent bouts of pancreatitis. Other inheritable lipid disorders such as familial hypercholesterolemia (FH; type IIa) can present with corneal arcus and cutaneous manifestations such as xanthomas and xanthelasmas. Unfortunately, owing to the asymptomatic nature of dyslipoproteinemias, they can go unrecognized until they initially manifest as CHD, stroke, and PVD. Therefore, in patients with known risk factors, screening for dyslipoproteinemias is crucial for primary prevention of cardiovascular events[3,4] (**Algorithm 99.1**).

Differential Diagnosis

Often patients with lipid disorders present as part of the metabolic syndrome with modifiable risk factors that contribute to their overall cardiovascular risk. In these patients, secondary causes such as obesity, insulin resistance, diabetes, and hypothyroidism should be considered as secondary etiologies for dyslipidemia. Other risk-enhancing variables such as medications, history of preeclampsia, early menopause, inflammatory disorders (rheumatoid arthritis, psoriasis, HIV), South Asian ancestry, chronic kidney disease, persistently elevated

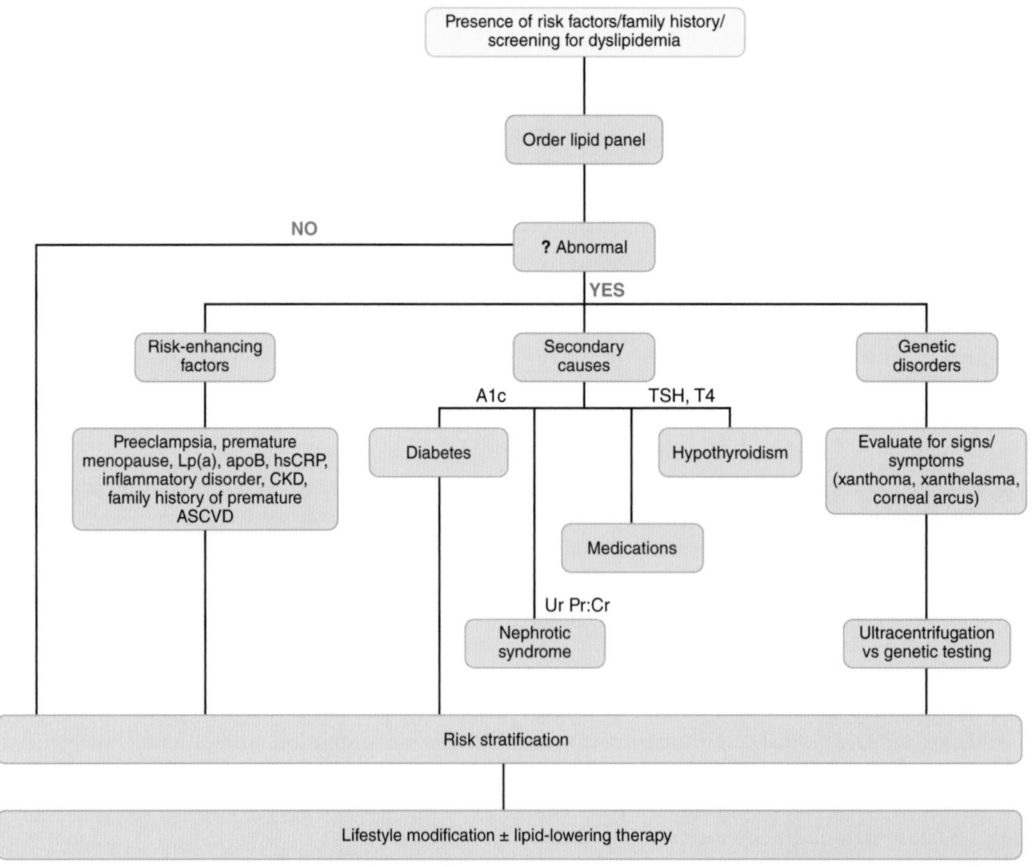

ALGORITHM 99.1 The diagnostic approach to dyslipidemia begins with a standard lipid panel. If the lipid panel returns abnormal results, genetic consideration, secondary causes, and risk-enhancing factors should be considered as part of the comprehensive approach for dyslipidemia risk stratification. A1c, glycated hemoglobin; apoB, apolipoprotein B; ASCVD, atherosclerotic cardiovascular disease; CKD, chronic kidney disease; hsCRP, high-sensitivity C-reactive protein; Lp(a), lipoprotein(a); TSH, thyroid-stimulating hormone; T4, free T4; Ur Pr:Cr, urine protein–creatinine ratio. Adapted from ACC/AHA guidelines.[3,4]

TG levels, low arterial-brachial index, elevated high-sensitivity C-reactive protein (hsCRP), elevated Lp(a), or apoB[5] should be considered in the evaluation of dyslipidemia on the basis of the clinical syndrome. A strong family history of premature CHD or cardiovascular disease, or other unique presenting signs/symptoms such as recurrent bouts of pancreatitis, or cutaneous manifestations (corneal arcus, tendon xanthomas, and xanthelasmas) should raise concern for an inheritable lipid disorder. The information about secondary causes of lipid disorders (mediations, renal disorders, inflammatory disorders, and genetic disorders) are discussed in the Supplementary Appendix.

DIAGNOSIS

The primary diagnostic modality in the evaluation of lipid disorders is a traditional lipid panel. The Friedewald equation—LDL-C = (TC) – (HDL-C) – (TG/5 in mg/dL)—was initially used to calculate LDL-C where TG/5 was used to estimate VLDL-C with the presumption that TG:VLDL-C ratio was approximately 5. However, the Friedewald equation is inaccurate when LDL-C is less than 70 mg/dL and in cases of hypertriglyceridemia (TG >400 mg/dL) because the TG:VLDL-C ratio varies significantly across a range of TG and TC levels. The Martin/Hopkins equation allows for more accurate calculation of LDL-C than does the Friedewald equation, even at LDL-C less than 70 mg/dL and TG greater than or equal to 150 mg/dL.[27,28] Use of this more accurate equation reduces discordance between LDL-C, non-HDL-C, and apoB, and can inform better clinical decisions on initiation of lipid lowering therapy.[29]

Once lipid abnormalities have been established via a lipid panel, secondary evaluation with plasma thyroid-stimulating hormone, hemoglobin A_{1c}, metabolic panel, and urine protein/Cr ratio may provide additional information. Measurement of Lp(a) and apoB should both be considered if the clinician feels comfortable with their interpretation and use and believes they may change clinical management. However, it should be noted that neither measure is standardized across laboratories, and, therefore, their accuracy is less certain.

ApoB may be considered especially useful in cases of mixed hyperlipidemia to help differentiate type III hyperlipidemia from other dyslipidemias.[3] An apoB-based algorithm has been suggested as a way to identify and distinguish the inheritable apoB dyslipoproteinemias using TC, TG, and apoB (**Algorithm 99.2**). This approach can be followed up with confirmatory ultracentrifugation analysis or genetic testing, as needed.[30]

Lipid abnormalities should be placed in the context of overall cardiovascular risk. In patients without preexisting cardiovascular disease, the risk of having a first ASCVD event over the next 10 years can be estimated using the pooled cohort equation. On the basis of current American College of Cardiology/American Heart Association (ACC/AHA) guidelines, apart from patients who are already known to benefit

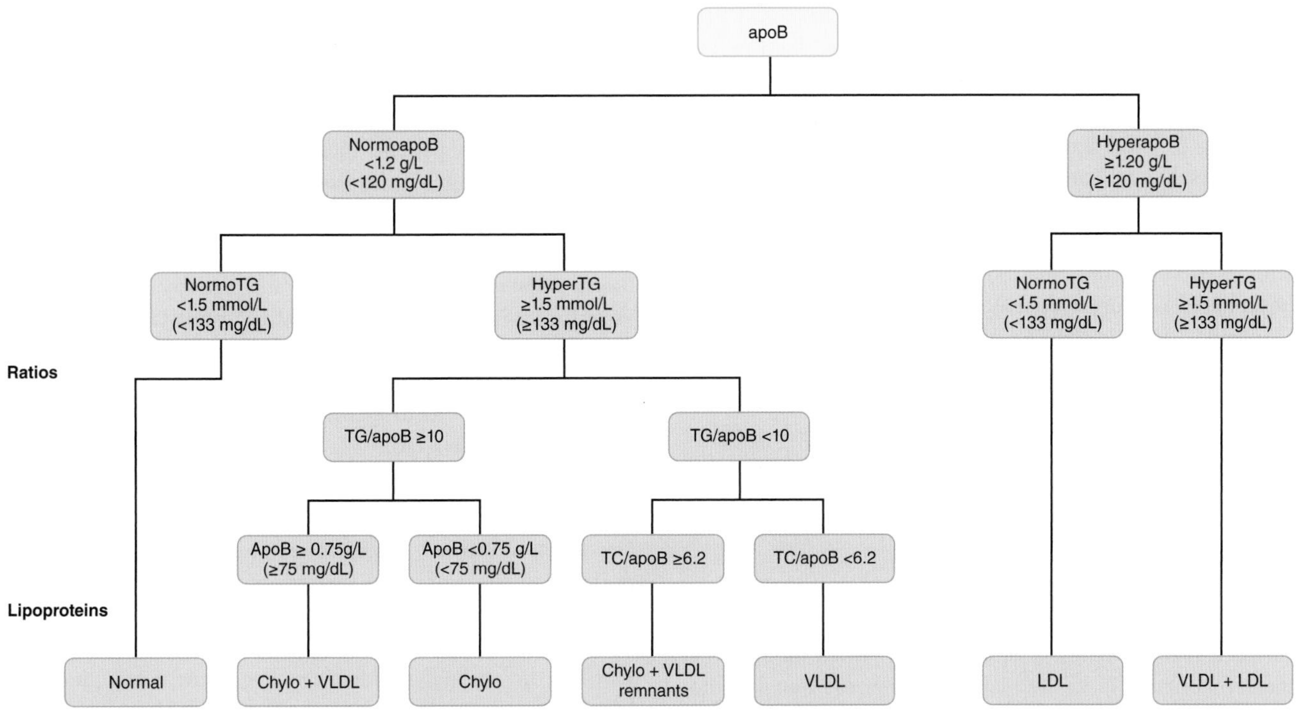

ALGORITHM 99.2 The apoB algorithm allows screening for the familial dyslipoproteinemias using apoB, TG, and TC levels. ApoB, apolipoprotein B; Chylo, chylomicron; LDL, low-density lipoprotein; TC, total cholesterol; TG, triglyceride; VLDL, very low-density lipoprotein. (Data from Sniderman AD, Thanassoulis G, Glavinovic T, et al. Apolipoprotein B Particles and Cardiovascular Disease: A Narrative Review. *JAMA Cardiol.* 2019; 4(12): 1287–1295.)

from statin therapy (ie, those with LDL-C ≥190 mg/dL or age 40-75 years with diabetes and LDL-C ≥70 mg/dL), ASCVD risk scores can help risk stratify patients into low- (<5%), borderline (5%-7.5%), intermediate- (7.5%-20%), and high-risk (>20%) categories for consideration of initiation of lipid-lowering therapy. Other risk-enhancing factors such as history of preeclampsia, early menopause, inflammatory disorders (rheumatoid arthritis, psoriasis, and HIV), South Asian ancestry, chronic kidney disease, persistently elevated TG levels, low ankle-brachial index, elevated hsCRP, and elevated Lp(a) or apoB should be taken into consideration when deciding on initiation of lipid-lowering therapy.[3-5]

Coronary artery calcium (CAC) score can also be considered as a measure of subclinical atherosclerosis.[5] The CAC score can be especially helpful in restratifying borderline and intermediate-risk category patients into high- or low-risk categories. A CAC score greater than 99 Agatston units or greater than 75th percentile for age, sex, and race serves as thresholds for initiation of lipid-lowering therapy. If CAC is 0, the risk of ASCVD over 10 years is generally less than 7.5% and, therefore, statin therapy can be deferred. However, special considerations, such as cigarette smoking, secondary causes of dyslipoproteinemias, and familial lipid disorders—such as FH or type III hyperlipidemia—should also be considered before deferring initiation of therapy.

MANAGEMENT OF THE PATIENT WITH LIPID DISORDER

Diet and Lifestyle Changes

Lifestyle modifications have beneficial effects on lipid parameters, with a potential to reduce cardiovascular risk by 50%.[31] Lifestyle interventions include dietary changes, weight loss, increasing physical activity, maintaining stable normal blood glucose levels, and smoking cessation. A diet rich in vegetables, fruits, whole grains, legumes, nuts, and soluble fiber with reduction in red meat consumption may lower plasma cholesterol levels up to 10%, and replacing saturated fats with polyunsaturated fats may reduce ASCVD by approximately 30%. Guidelines support the use of the Mediterranean diet and the Dietary Approaches to Stop Hypertension (DASH) diet as heart-healthy dietary choices.[5] Dietary changes and at least 150 minutes of moderate-intensity exercise a week promote weight loss, which can lead to lower TG levels and improved lipid parameters.[3,4]

Medications

Most treatment options focus on lowering plasma LDL-C concentration, with more recent guidelines recommending that "lower is better" because studies have supported the idea that further reduction in LDL-C safely provides additional cardiovascular risk reduction (**Table 99.2**).

Statins

Statins are the first-line pharmacotherapy to lower LDL-C levels. They competitively inhibit beta-hydroxy beta-methylbutyryl-coenzyme A (HMG-CoA) reductase, the rate-limiting enzyme in cholesterol synthesis, which leads to decreased production of cholesterol and increased clearance of LDL-C from the circulation as a result of expression of more LDL receptors on the surface of hepatocytes.

A recent meta-analysis showed that for every 1 mmol/L (~40 mg/dL) reduction in LDL-C with statin therapy, the risk of cardiovascular events decreased by 22%, and all-cause mortality decreased by 10%.[32] A consistent relative risk reduction in vascular events per unit change in LDL-C has been shown even in patients with normal LDL-C levels (<70 mg/dL).[33] However, the greatest benefactors of LDL-C lowering therapy are patients with higher baseline LDL-C levels,[34] consistent with the concept that benefit is proportional to the absolute lowering of the LDL-C concentration.

The benefit of statin therapy is also higher in patients with higher absolute risk, and hence the importance of assessment of risk factors and subclinical atherosclerosis imaging in primary prevention. In secondary prevention, the risk of future cardiovascular events is considered high, so guidelines recommend targeting greater than 50% reduction in LDL-C with maximally tolerated statin therapy. If LDL-C remains greater than or equal to 70 mg/dL at maximally tolerated statin doses, the addition of non-statin therapy (see subsequent text) can be considered to further lower LDL-C and, subsequently, cardiovascular risk.[3] Although statin therapy has been shown to reduce LDL-C, non-HDL-C, and apoB levels, it is ineffective in lowering Lp(a); indeed, an approximately linear relationship between Lp(a) levels and cardiovascular risk has been reported in patients on statin therapy.[35] For patients older than 75 years of age, there is established evidence of beneficial effects of statin therapy in secondary prevention, but less so for primary prevention.[36] Guidelines recommend continuing high-intensity statin therapy for patients older than 75 years of age if well tolerated, or modifying the dose to achieve moderate-intensity statin therapy to minimize adverse effects depending on clinical judgment.

Dosing of Statins. High-intensity statin therapy includes atorvastatin (Lipitor®) 40 to 80 mg/day, or rosuvastatin (Crestor®) 20 to 40 mg/day. Moderate-intensity statin therapy includes atorvastatin 10 to 20 mg/day, rosuvastatin 5 to 10 mg/day, fluvastatin (Lescol®) 20 to 80 mg/day, lovastatin (Mevacor®) 20 to 80 mg/day, pravastatin (Pravachol®) 20 to 40 mg/day, simvastatin (Zocor®) 10 to 40 mg/day, and pitavastatin (Livalo®) 2 to 4 mg/day.

Side Effects of Statins. Myalgias are the most commonly reported side effect of statin therapy, but causality is often unclear and not associated with elevated plasma creatine kinase levels. Statin intolerance is a major concern because statins are first-line therapy in dyslipidemia management, with significant benefits that outweigh the potential risks. If there are initial concerns of statin-induced myalgias, a plasma creatine kinase level should be checked, and, if normal, dose adjustments of the statin should be attempted. If the patient cannot tolerate the lowest possible dose, an alternative statin should be trialed.

TABLE 99.2 Lipid Medications

Medication (Class)	Dosage (Orally, Unless Otherwise Indicate)	Therapeutic Use	LDL-C or TG Lowering	Clinical Benefit (Studies)	Side Effects
Statins	High-intensity statin therapy: Atorvastatin 40-80 mg once daily Rosuvastatin 20-40 mg once daily ---------------------------------- *Moderate-intensity statin therapy:* Atorvastatin 10-20 mg once daily Rosuvastatin 5-10 mg once daily Fluvastatin 20-80 mg once daily Lovastatin 20-80 mg once daily Pravastatin 20-40 mg once daily	First-line agent for primary or secondary ASCVD prevention	>50% ↓ LDL-C ---------- 20%-55% ↓ LDL-C	↓ Risk (22%) for CV events ↓ 10% All-cause mortality [46]	Myalgias, myopathy, liver injury, increased risk of diabetes
Inhibitors of cholesterol absorption	Ezetimibe 10 mg once daily	Add-on therapy to statins for patients at high risk who do not meet LDL-C goal (LDL-C <70 mg/dL) and patients with statin intolerance	15%-20% ↓ LDL-C	↓ Relative risk (6%) for recurrent CV events in patients with ASCVD No large double-blind trial of ezetimibe monotherapy [5,38,52]	Gastrointestinal discomfort including diarrhea
PCSK9 inhibitors	Alirocumab 75-150 mg subcutaneously every 2 weeks or 300 mg every 4 weeks Evolocumab 140 mg subcutaneously every 2 weeks or 420 mg every 4 weeks	Third-line agent after statins and ezetimibe to achieve LDL-C goal (LDL-C <70 mg/dL) in patients with ASCVD or hypercholesterolemia	40%-65% ↓ LDL-C when added to statin ± ezetimibe	↓ Risk (~15%) for CV events in patients with stable atherosclerotic disease and those with clinical ASCVD No clear mortality benefit [53]	Injection site reactions
n-3 Long-chain fatty acids	Icosapent ethyl (Vascepa) 4 g once daily	Possible use in high-risk patients on statin therapy with TG 150-500 mg/dL	*No* LDL-C lowering; 20%-30% TG ↓	↓ Relative risk (25%) for CV events in patients on statin therapy at goal LDL-C levels [8]	Diarrhea, sore throat, joint pain
Bile acid sequestrants	Colesevelam 3750 mg once daily or 1875 mg twice daily Cholestyramine 3750 mg once daily or 1875 mg twice daily Colestipol 3750 mg once daily or 1875 mg twice daily	Fourth-line agent if not achieving LDL-C goal despite maximally tolerated lipid-lowering therapy	15%-20% LDL-C ↓	Possible ↓ risk (5%) for CV events [57] No trial evaluating benefit as add-on to statin therapy	Constipation, GI upset, possible increase in TG levels
Fibrates	Fenofibrate 50-160 mg once daily Gemfibrozil 600 mg twice daily	Third-line agent if TG > 500 mg/dL despite maximally tolerated TG-lowering therapies	40%-50% TG ↓	Possible ↓ risk (16%) for CV events No clear mortality benefit [56]	Muscle injury, cholelithiasis
Niacin	Niacin 500-2000 mg once daily	Usually not recommended because of lack of benefit, side effect profile, and more beneficial alternative therapies	15%-25% TG ↓ 10%-20% LDL-C ↓	No reduction in mortality or CV events [55]	Flushing, nausea, pruritus, transaminitis, gout, hyperglycemia

ASCVD, atherosclerotic cardiovascular disease;CV, cardiovascular; GI; gastrointestinal; LDL-C, low-density lipoprotein cholesterol; PCSK9, proprotein convertase subtilisin/kexin type 9; TG, triglyceride.

If the patient is still intolerant, there should be further review into other medications or medical conditions that cause myalgias. If no alternative explanation is found, statin therapy could be discontinued, but, after shared decision-making with the patient, a plan to rechallenge with statin therapy should be considered in the future.

With statin therapy, there is a low risk of muscle injury (<0.1%), rhabdomyolysis (<0.1%), liver injury (0.001%), and a slightly increased incidence of diabetes (0.2% per year). There have been no clear relationships between statin use and increased incidence of cancer[37] or impaired cognition.

Ezetimibe

Ezetimibe blocks the Niemann-Pick C1-like 1 cholesterol transfer protein that functions in absorption of dietary cholesterol and its enterohepatic circulation. The IMPROVE-IT trial demonstrated that combination ezetimibe and simvastatin compared to simvastatin alone showed a greater LDL-C reduction (54 mg/dL vs 70 mg/dL, respectively) from a baseline LDL-C less than 125 mg/dL, which resulted in a 6% relative risk reduction in recurrent cardiovascular events.[7] In an open-label, randomized study evaluating the use of ezetimibe in patients 75 years or older with elevated LDL-C and no history of coronary artery disease, ezetimibe monotherapy reduced the incidence of cardiovascular events, although there was no difference in the incidence of all-cause mortality.[38] Therefore, current guidelines recommend the addition of ezetimibe to maximally tolerated statin therapy in patients who need additional LDL-C lowering.[3] Although the effect on LDL-C is modest in the 18% to 20% range, this effect is equivalent roughly to what would be observed after doubling a statin dose three times.

Side Effects of Ezetimibe. Ezetimibe is generally well tolerated, but can cause gastrointestinal symptoms such as abdominal fullness, bloating, and diarrhea because of the malabsorptive effects of the drug. Muscle symptoms are also sometimes reported.

Proprotein Convertase Subtilisin/Kexin Type 9 Inhibitors

PCSK9 is an enzyme that binds to the LDL receptor to activate the receptor degradation pathway. PCSK9 inhibitors inactivate this enzyme and promote LDL receptor expression on the surface of the hepatocyte, which increases LDL-C clearance from the circulation. Two PCSK9 inhibitors are currently approved by the U.S. Food and Drug Administration (FDA) for use in the United States: evolocumab (Repatha®) and alirocumab (Praluent®).

In patients on maximally tolerated lipid-lowering therapy, PCSK9 inhibitors yield an approximately 60% reduction in LDL-C and also lowers Lp(a) by approximately 25%.[8,9] In the Further Cardiovascular Outcomes Research With PCSK9 Inhibition in Subjects With Elevated Risk (FOURIER) trial of patients with LDL-C greater than or equal to_70 mg/dL and stable atherosclerotic disease, the addition of PCSK9 inhibition to goal-directed therapy showed a 15% relative reduction in cardiovascular events.[8] The patients who benefited most from therapy were those at greatest cardiovascular risk, including those with PVD, recurrent myocardial infarction (MI), or elevated Lp(a). In the Evaluation of Cardiovascular Outcomes After an Acute Coronary Syndrome During Treatment With Alirocumab trial (ODYSSEY OUTCOMES) trial including patients with LDL-C greater than or equal to 70 mg/dL and a recent acute coronary syndrome, treatment with a PCSK9 inhibitor resulted in a similar relative risk reduction in cardiovascular events. A meta-analysis has shown that in patients receiving maximally tolerated statin therapy and/or ezetimibe, the addition of PCSK9 inhibition therapy further reduces the rates of MI, stroke, and coronary revascularization. Although no reduction in all-cause or cardiovascular mortality was demonstrated with the addition of PCSK9 inhibitor therapy,[39] the trials were not designed to assess this outcome given their short (<3 years) duration. With evidence suggesting a benefit with greater absolute reductions in LDL-C, the ability of PCSK9 inhibitor therapy to lower LDL-C concentration to 0 to 10 mg/dL is of interest. Although studies have shown no safety concerns with very low LDL-C over 2 to 3 years of follow-up,[14] longer term outcome studies are still needed to confirm safety. Reassuringly, individuals born with genetically low LDL-C due to PCKS9 inhibition do not show any untoward effects.

Side Effects of Proprotein Convertase Subtilisin/Kexin Type 9 Inhibitors. PCSK9 inhibitors are monoclonal antibodies injected subcutaneously every other week, and are generally well tolerated. The main side effect is a rash at the injection site. There are no other adverse effects that are typically seen with PCSK9 inhibitor therapy. However, cost and administrative barriers appear to be the greatest limiting variables preventing widespread clinical use.

N-3 Fatty Acids

Long-chain n-3 polyunsaturated fatty acids, such as eicosapentaenoic acid and docosahexaenoic acid, reduce TG levels by decreasing the production of VLDL, and increasing the rate of VLDL clearance. In the Reduction of Cardiovascular Events with Icosapent Ethyl–Intervention (REDUCE-IT) trial, patients with hypertriglyceridemia (135-500 mg/dL) and LDL-C levels that were controlled with statin therapy showed a 25% relative risk reduction in cardiovascular outcomes when treated with 4 g/day of icosapent ethyl (Vascepa®), a highly purified form of eicosapentaenoic acid. The substantial benefits noted with icosapent ethyl exceed the anticipated benefits from TG level reduction (~20%) and indicate that it may have alternative cardioprotective mechanisms that require further investigation.[40]

Side Effects. The primary listed side effects of icosapent ethyl include limited mobility because of joint or muscle stiffness, bleeding, and atrial fibrillation.

Percutaneous Intervention Approaches to Lowering Cholesterol

Lipoprotein apheresis, or extracorporeal removal of plasma cholesterol, is a treatment that significantly lowers levels of LDL-C (60%-80%), Lp(a) (70%), and other apoB lipoproteins. However, the procedure is laborious, time consuming, expensive, and, as such, is a treatment of last resort for patients who are refractory to medical therapy. For patients with heterozygous FH, lipoprotein apheresis produces an additional 54% reduction in LDL-C on top of alirocumab (a PCSK9 inhibitor), as observed in the Study of Alirocumab in Patients With Heterozygous Familial Hypercholesterolemia Undergoing Low-density Lipoprotein (LDL) Apheresis Therapy (ODYSSEY ESCAPE) trial.[41] However, the effect was less pronounced in homozygous FH in the Trial Assessing Long Term USe of PCSK9 Inhibition in Subjects With Genetic LDL Disorders (TAUSSIG) study, where combination therapy resulted in a 23% reduction in LDL-C owing to the low level of hepatic LDL receptors present in homozygous FH. Current guidelines recommend treatment with lipid apheresis in patients with homozygous FH with LDL-C greater than or equal to 500 mg/dL on maximal drug therapy, or high-risk patients with heterozygous

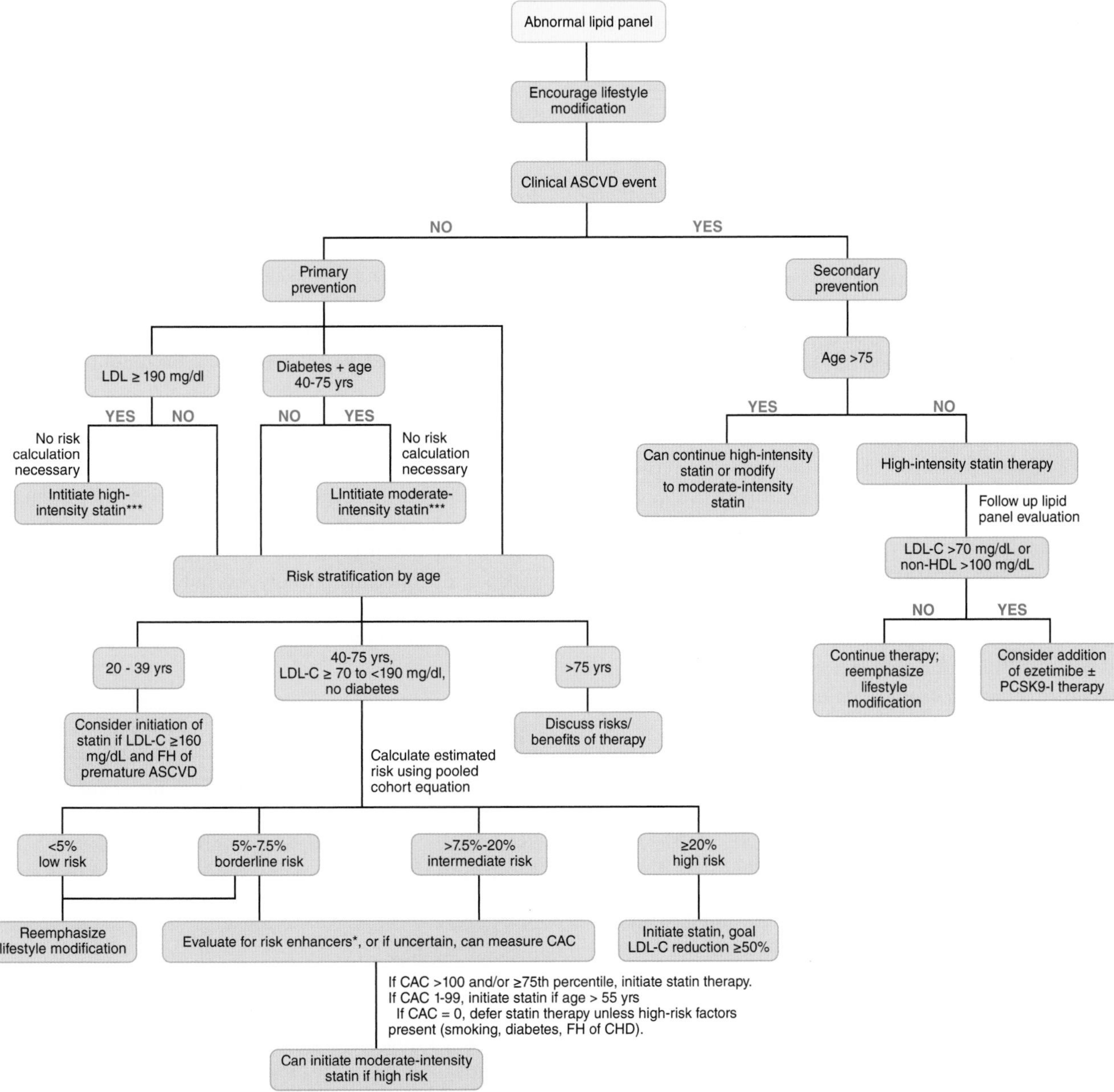

ALGORITHM 99.3 Approach to management of dyslipoproteinemias. Management of dyslipidemia generally falls in the realm of primary and secondary prevention. In secondary prevention, lipid-lowering therapies are used to reach target LDL-C levels. In primary prevention, lipid-lowering therapies can be prescribed as defined by high-risk features such as LDL-C greater than or equal to 190 mg/dL, diabetes, or risk stratification based on the pooled cohort equation. The CAC score can help restratify intermediate-risk patients within the pooled cohort equation into low- or high-risk categories to help determine whether they would benefit from lipid-lowering therapies. Some data from ACC/AHA guidelines figures. ASCVD, atherosclerotic cardiovascular disease; CAC, coronary artery calcium; CHD, coronary heart disease; FH, family history; LDL-C, low-density lipoprotein cholesterol; non-HDL-C, non–high-density lipoprotein cholesterol.[3,4]

FH with LDL-C levels greater than or equal to 160 mg/dL.[41] A new FDA "Group C" criterion has lowered the LDL-C threshold for secondary prevention from LDL-C greater than or equal to 160 mg/dL to greater than or equal to 100 mg/dL.

Surgical Approach

Gastric bypass serves as an efficient, cost-conscious, long-term surgical treatment option for obese patients with dyslipidemia and other cardiovascular risk factors. A study evaluating metabolic outcomes 12 years after gastric bypass showed that patients who undergo weight loss surgery have sustained weight loss (~57 lb), improved lipid parameters, better glycemic control, and lower blood pressure[42] compared to those who did not. In addition, bariatric surgery lowers the rate of cardiovascular events (MI and stroke) and all-cause mortality.[43] However, the nonnegligible operative and postoperative complications of bariatric surgery such as dysrhythmia, venous thromboembolism, wound infections, and treatment failure must be carefully taken into consideration before performing bariatric surgery.

SPECIAL CONSIDERATIONS AND EMERGING THERAPIES

Special Considerations

The recommendations provided in this chapter are based primarily on the ACC/AHA guidelines. Alternative guidelines such as the U.S. Preventive Services Task Force, the Department of Veterans Affairs, the National Lipid Association, the American Association of Clinical Endocrinologists, the European Society of Cardiology-European Atherosclerosis Society, and the Canadian Cardiovascular Society differ in terms of 10-year risk estimation, cutoff points for initiation of statin therapy, intensity of statin recommended, and LDL-C treatment thresholds.

Emerging Therapies

Inclisiran is a small interfering RNA that degrades PCSK9 messenger RNA and prevents PCSK9 synthesis. Phase 2 studies have shown dose-dependent 45% to 50% reductions in LDL-C levels with the added benefit of lower dose frequency requirements (ie, dosed initially, again at 3 months, and then once every 6 months) than with PCSK9 monoclonal antibody therapy. The A Randomized Trial Assessing the Effects of Inclisiran on Clinical Outcomes Among People With Cardiovascular Disease (ORION)-4 study, a 15,000-patient outcomes trial led by researchers at the University of Oxford in collaboration with the Thrombolysis in Myocardial Infarction (TIMI) Study group, is investigating whether the addition of inclisiran to guideline-directed medical therapy lowers the risk of major adverse cardiovascular events (coronary heart disease death, MI, stroke, or urgent revascularization) in patients with ASCVD. Bempedoic acid (Nexletol®) is an adenosine triphosphate (ATP) citrate lyase inhibitor that acts upstream of HMG-CoA reductase to upregulate the LDL receptor by reducing cholesterol synthesis. In patients already on maximally tolerated statin therapy with or without additional lipid-lowering therapy, bempedoic acid may reduce LDL-C an additional 18%.[44] The FDA considers bempedoic acid a first-in-class medication and approved it for the treatment of hypercholesterolemia in combination with diet and the highest tolerated statin therapy in adults with heterozygous FH or established ASCVD who require additional lowering of LDL-C. AKCEA-APO(a)-Lrx is an antisense oligonucleotide drug that targets Lp(a) with the ability to reduce Lp(a) levels by up to 80%.[23] Evaluation of the effects of targeted therapy against angiopoietin-like 3 (ANGPTL3), an inhibitor of LPL, which leads to reductions in TG and LDL-C levels, is currently under way. The impact of each of these novel therapies on cardiovascular outcomes are areas of active research.[5]

FOLLOW-UP PATIENT CARE

Guidelines recommend repeating lipid panels every 1 to 3 months after initiation or changes in lipid-lowering therapy to evaluate adherence, side effects, and the extent of LDL-C reduction. Once medication adherence and adequate medication effect is established, yearly lipid panels for routine assessment is recommended.

RESEARCH AND FUTURE DIRECTIONS

Research into novel therapeutics provides an exciting avenue in dyslipidemia management. However, as health care transitions into the realm of personalized medicine, and the link between genetics, dyslipidemia phenotypes, and cardiovascular risk is strengthened, research into individualized therapy based on genotype will become essential.

KEY POINTS

- ✔ Assessment for dyslipidemia early in life is essential because most patients are asymptomatic.
- ✔ The diagnosis of genetic lipid disorders, such as FH, is frequently missed in routine practice and must be specifically sought through careful personal and family history, as well as physical examination (eg, looking for cutaneous xanthomas).
- ✔ Involving members of the care team, such as nutritionists, to assist patients in lifestyle changes is helpful in a time-constrained health care delivery system.
- ✔ Patients who initially cannot tolerate statin therapy often respond to dose adjustments or switching to alternative statin therapy.
- ✔ Ezetimibe and PCSK9 inhibitors are valuable additions to statin therapy in high-risk patients needing additional LDL-C lowering and are well tolerated.
- ✔ Patients with hypertriglyceridemia should be considered for icosapent ethyl therapy.

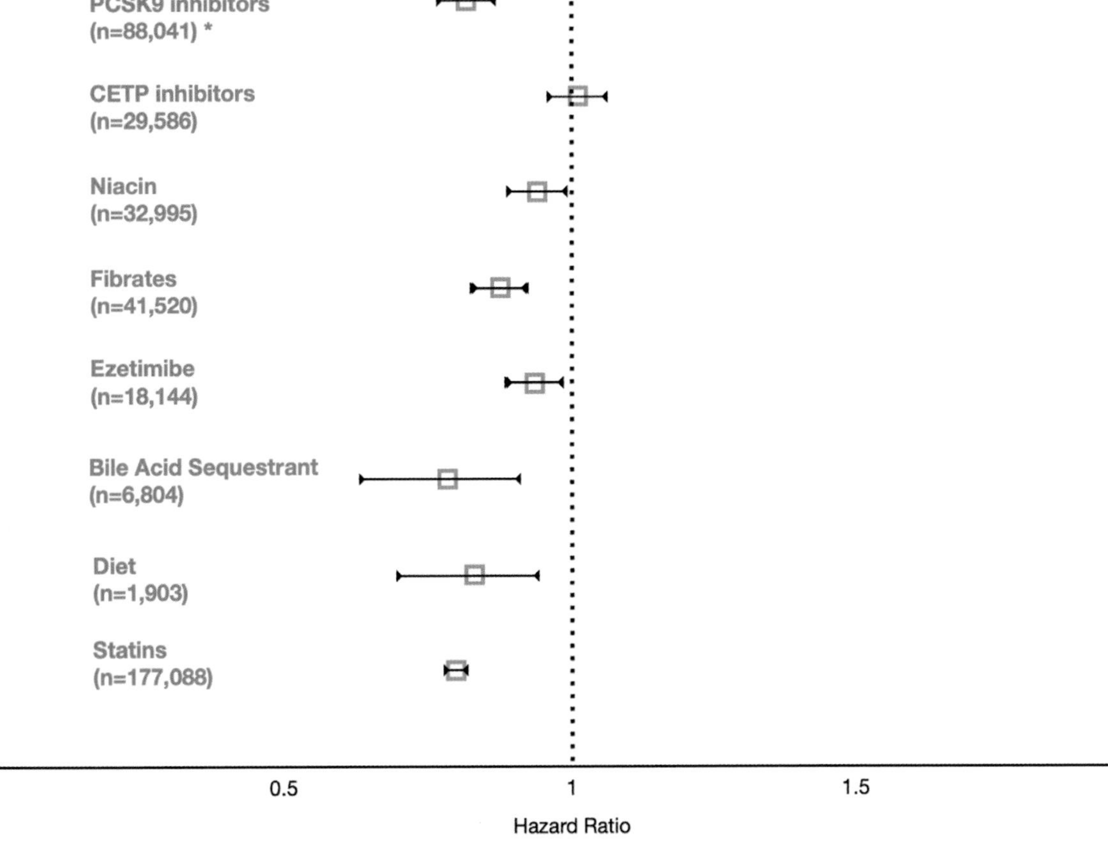

FIGURE 99.3 Clinical trial data showing relative risk reduction is proportional to low-density lipoprotein cholesterol (LDL-C) lowering. Hazard Ratios obtained from Silverman MG, Ference BA, Im K, et al. Association between lowering LDL-C and cardiovascular risk reduction among different therapeutic interventions: a systematic review and meta-analysis[32]. *JAMA*. 2016;316(12):1289-1297.
* Odds ratios were reported for Major Adverse Cardiovascular Events. AlTurki A, Marafi M, Dawas A, et al. Meta-analysis of randomized controlled trials assessing the impact of proprotein convertase subtilisin/kexin type 9 antibodies on mortality and cardiovascular outcomes[39]. *Am J Cardiol*. 2019;124(12):1869-1875.

REFERENCES

1. Yusuf S, Joseph P, Rangarajan S, et al. Modifiable risk factors, cardiovascular disease, and mortality in 155 722 individuals from 21 high-income, middle-income, and low-income countries (PURE): a prospective cohort study. *Lancet*. 2020;395(10226):795-808. doi:10.1016/S0140-6736(19)32008-2
2. Genest J, Libby P. Lipoprotein disorders and cardiovascular disease. In: Mann D, Zipes D, Libby P, et al., eds. *Braunwald's Heart Disease: A Textbook of Cardiovascular Medicine*. Elsevier; 2019:960-982.
3. Grundy SM, Stone NJ, Bailey AL, et al. 2018 AHA/ACC/AACVPR/AAPA/ABC/ACPM/ADA/AGS/APhA/ASPC/NLA/PCNA Guideline on the management of blood cholesterol. *J Am Coll Cardiol*. 2019;73:e285-e350.
4. Arnett DK, Blumenthal RS, Albert MA, et al. 2019 ACC/AHA guideline on the primary prevention of cardiovascular disease: executive summary: a report of the American College of Cardiology/American Heart Association Task Force on Clinical Practice Guidelines. *J Am Coll Cardiol*. 2019;74:1376-1414.
5. Michos ED, McEvoy JW, Blumenthal RS. Lipid management for the prevention of atherosclerotic cardiovascular disease. *N Engl J Med*. 2019;381:1557-1567.
6. Mihaylova B, Emberson J, Blackwell L, et al. The effects of lowering LDL cholesterol with statin therapy in people at low risk of vascular disease: meta-analysis of individual data from 27 randomised trials. *Lancet*. 2012;380:581-590.
7. Cannon CP. Blazing MA, Giugliano RP, et al. Ezetimibe added to statin therapy after acute coronary syndromes. *N Engl J Med*. 2015;372:2387-2397.
8. Sabatine MS, Giugliano RP, Keech AC, et al. Evolocumab and clinical outcomes in patients with cardiovascular disease. *N Engl J Med*. 2017;376:1713-1722.
9. Schwartz GG, Steg PG, Starek M, et al. Alirocumab and cardiovascular outcomes after acute coronary syndrome. *N Engl J Med*. 2018;379:2097-2107.
10. Centers for Disease Control and Prevention. High Cholesterol Facts. 2019. https://www.cdc.gov/cholesterol/facts.htm
11. Perak AM, Ning H, Kit BK, et al. Trends in levels of lipids and apolipoprotein B in US youths aged 6 to 19 years, 1999-2016. *JAMA*. 2019;321:1895-1905.
12. Rosinger A, Carroll MD, Lacher D, Ogden C. Trends in total cholesterol, triglycerides, and low-density lipoprotein in US adults, 1999-2014. *JAMA Cardiol*. 2017;2:339-341.
13. Feingold KR, Grunfeld C. Introduction to Lipids and Lipoproteins. In: Feingold KR, Anawalt B, Boyce A, Chrousos G, de Herder W, Dhatariya

K, eds. *Endotext.* MDText.com, Inc.; 2000. Accessed November 6, 2019. http://www.ncbi.nlm.nih.gov/books/NBK305896/
14. Giugliano RP, Pedersen TR, Park J-G, et al. Clinical efficacy and safety of achieving very low LDL-cholesterol concentrations with the PCSK9 inhibitor evolocumab: a prespecified secondary analysis of the FOURIER trial. *Lancet.* 2017;390:1962-1971.
15. Barter PJ, Ballantyne CM, Carmena R, et al. Apo B versus cholesterol in estimating cardiovascular risk and in guiding therapy: report of the thirty-person/ten-country panel. *J Intern Med.* 2006;259:247-258.
16. Kattoor AJ, Pothineni NVK, Palagiri D, Mehta JL. Oxidative stress in atherosclerosis. *Curr Atheroscler Rep.* 2017;19:42.
17. Sniderman AD, Thanassoulis G, Glavinovic T, et al. Apolipoprotein B particles and cardiovascular disease: a narrative review. *JAMA Cardiol.* 2019;4(12):1287-1295. doi:10.1001/jamacardio.2019.3780
18. Landmesser U. Coronary artery disease: HDL and coronary heart disease—novel insights. *Nat Rev Cardiol.* 2014;11:559-560.
19. Chiesa ST, Charakida M. High-density lipoprotein function and dysfunction in health and disease. *Cardiovasc Drugs Ther.* 2019;33:207-219.
20. Musunuru K, Kathiresan S. Surprises from genetic analyses of lipid risk factors for atherosclerosis. *Circ Res.* 2016;118:579-585.
21. Tada H, Nohara A, Inazu A, Mabuchi H, Kawashiri M-A. Remnant lipoproteins and atherosclerotic cardiovascular disease. *Clin Chim Acta.* 2019;490:1-5.
22. Thanassoulis G, Campbell CY, Owens DS, et al. Genetic associations with valvular calcification and aortic stenosis. *N Engl J Med.* 2013:368:503-512.
23. Tsimikas S, Karwatowska-Prokopczuk E, Gouni-Berthold I, et al. Lipoprotein(a) reduction in persons with cardiovascular disease. *N Engl J Med.* 2020;382:244-255.
24. Burgess S, Ference BA, Staley JR, et al. Association of LPA variants with risk of coronary disease and the implications for lipoprotein(a)-lowering therapies: a mendelian randomization analysis. *JAMA Cardiol.* 2018;3:619-627.
25. Tsimikas S. A test in context: lipoprotein(a): diagnosis, prognosis, controversies, and emerging therapies. *J Am Coll Cardiol.* 2017;69:692-711.
26. Tsimikas S. Potential causality and emerging medical therapies for lipoprotein(a) and its associated oxidized phospholipids in calcific aortic valve stenosis. *Circ Res.* 2019;124:405-415.
27. Martin SS, Blaha MJ, Elshazly MB, et al. Comparison of a novel method vs the Friedewald equation for estimating low-density lipoprotein cholesterol levels from the standard lipid profile. *JAMA.* 2013;310:2061-2068.
28. Quispe R, Hendrani A, Elshazly MB, et al. Accuracy of low-density lipoprotein cholesterol estimation at very low levels. *BMC Med.* 2017;15:83.
29. Sathiyakumar V, Park J, Quispe R, et al. Impact of novel low-density lipoprotein-cholesterol assessment on the utility of secondary non-high-density lipoprotein-C and apolipoprotein B targets in selected worldwide dyslipidemia guidelines. *Circulation.* 2018;138:244-254.
30. Sniderman A, Couture P, de Graaf J. Diagnosis and treatment of apolipoprotein B dyslipoproteinemias. *Nat Rev Endocrinol.* 2010;6:335-346.
31. Khera AV, Emdin CA, Drake I, et al. Genetic risk, adherence to a healthy lifestyle, and coronary disease. *N Engl J Med.* 2016;375:2349-2358.
32. Silverman MG, Ference BA, Im K, et al. Association between lowering LDL-C and cardiovascular risk reduction among different therapeutic interventions: a systematic review and meta-analysis. *JAMA.* 2016;316:1289-1297.
33. Sabatine MS, Wiviott SD, Im K, Murphy SA, Giugliano RP. Efficacy and safety of further lowering of low-density lipoprotein cholesterol in patients starting with very low levels: a meta-analysis. *JAMA Cardiol.* 2018;3:823-828.
34. Navarese EP, Robinson JG, Kowalewski M, et al. Association between baseline LDL-C level and total and cardiovascular mortality after LDL-C lowering: a systematic review and meta-analysis. *JAMA.* 2018;319:1566-1579.
35. Willeit P, Ridker PM, Nestel PJ, et al. Baseline and on-statin treatment lipoprotein(a) levels for prediction of cardiovascular events: individual patient-data meta-analysis of statin outcome trials. *Lancet.* 2018;392:1311-1320.
36. Cholesterol Treatment Trialists' Collaboration. Efficacy and safety of statin therapy in older people: a meta-analysis of individual participant data from 28 randomised controlled trials. *Lancet.* 2019;393:407-415.
37. Zaleska M, Mozenska O, Bil J. Statins use and cancer: an update. *Future Oncol.* 2018;14:1497-1509.
38. Ouchi Y, Sasaki J, Arai H, et al. Ezetimibe lipid-lowering trial on prevention of atherosclerotic cardiovascular disease in 75 or older (EWTOPIA 75): a randomized, controlled trial. *Circulation.* 2019;140:992-1003.
39. AlTurki A, Marafi M, Dawas A, et al. Meta-analysis of randomized controlled trials assessing the impact of proprotein convertase subtilisin/kexin type 9 antibodies on mortality and cardiovascular outcomes. *Am J Cardiol.* 2019;124:12. doi:10.1016/j.amjcard.2019.09.011
40. Bhatt DL, Steg PG, Miller M, et al. Cardiovascular risk reduction with icosapent ethyl for hypertriglyceridemia. *N Engl J Med.* 2019;380:11-22.
41. Thompson G, Parhofer KG. Current role of lipoprotein apheresis. *Curr Atheroscler Rep.* 2019;21:26.
42. Adams TD, Davidson LE, Litwin SE, et al. Weight and metabolic outcomes 12 years after gastric bypass. *N Engl J Med.* 2017;377:1143-1155.
43. Kuno T, Tanimoto E, Morita S, Shimada YJ. Effects of bariatric surgery on cardiovascular disease: a concise update of recent advances. *Front Cardiovasc Med.* 2019;6:94.
44. Ray KK, Bays HE, Catapano AL, et al. Safety and efficacy of bempedoic acid to reduce LDL cholesterol. *N Engl J Med.* 2019;380(11):1022-1032. doi:10.1056/NEJMoa1803917

CHAPTER 100

HYPERTENSION

Amal Abdellatif,* Mohamed B. Elshazly,* Parag H. Joshi, and John W. McEvoy
* Joint First Authors (Contributed Equally)

INTRODUCTION

Epidemiology

Hypertension (HTN) is one of the most common reasons for primary health care visits and prescription of chronic medications.[1] Hypertension directly increases the risk for premature death owing to cardiovascular diseases (CVD), including coronary artery disease (CAD), heart failure (HF), ischemic stroke, intracerebral hemorrhage,[2] kidney disease, and retinal vascular disease. Consequently, high blood pressure (BP) is the major global contributor to all-cause morbidity and mortality, resulting in an estimated 10.4 million deaths and 218 million disability-adjusted life years (DALYs) in 2017.[3]

By lowering the diagnostic threshold of HTN, the 2017 American College of Cardiology/American Heart Association (ACC/AHA) HTN clinical practice guidelines have significant global epidemiologic and clinical implications. Implementing these guideline recommendations renders 46% of U.S. adults as hypertensive, translating to 103.3 million hypertensive Americans.[4] Further, 53% of U.S. adults already on antihypertensive medication are considered undertreated by the new guidelines.[4] The resultant boost in the global prevalence of HTN from 26% to 31% translated to at least 1.8 billion hypertensive individuals worldwide.[5]

Hypertension is more prevalent in older populations, and in non-Hispanic Blacks compared to Hispanics and non-Hispanic Whites.[6] Because of the progressive loss of arterial elasticity, systolic blood pressure (SBP) consistently increases with advancing age, whereas diastolic blood pressure (DBP) peaks at the fifth decade before gradually decreasing in both sexes.[7]

Risk Factors

Careful risk factor assessment of the patient is of chief importance because it guides the treatment approach and dictates the need for and intensity of pharmacotherapy, or the lack thereof. Modifiable risk factors for essential (primary) HTN include obesity; physical inactivity; diets rich in sodium, saturated fats, and trans fats; excessive consumption of alcohol and tobacco, diabetes mellitus, psychosocial stress, and obstructive sleep apnea. Nonmodifiable risk factors include family history (genetic susceptibility), advancing age, black race, male sex (especially below the age of 65 years), and chronic kidney disease (CKD). All hypertensive patients should have their CVD risk factor profile assessed, so that they can be managed and advised accordingly. A separate discussion on HTN in the context of other CVD risk factors follows under the sub section "Cardiovascular Risk-Based Treatment Approach."

PATHOGENESIS

The pathogenesis of HTN is multifactorial and poorly understood. BP is a function of several dynamic factors including vascular tone and elasticity, cardiac output, blood volume, blood viscosity, vascular reactivity, and hormonal effects. The interplay of genetics, inflammation, sympathetic activation, environmental factors, and psychosocial elements also contributes to the complex pathogenesis of HTN.

Genetic Link

Genetic studies on HTN suggest distinct heritability patterns of primary (essential) and secondary HTN. Primary HTN tends to be associated with numerous common genetic variants or loci (also known as single nucleotide polymorphisms, SNPs), which have been identified through genome-wide association studies.[8] The distinct loci that independently influence BP impart a cumulative risk to the development of primary HTN; the number of risk alleles present proportionally raises the risk of disease. However, the heritability of HTN is only partially explained by the presence of such SNPs. Along with these SNPs, certain environmental factors like age, body mass index, sex, and salt consumption can modify the probability of HTN development.[9]

In contrast to the polygenic contributions to primary HTN, linkage analysis in family-based studies has shown the association of monogenic mutations with the development of secondary HTN. Thus far, 13 genes have been identified that lead to the development of familial hypertensive syndromes including classes of familial hyperaldosteronism and congenital adrenal hyperplasia.

Immunologic Role

Evidence supports an immunologic role in the pathogenesis of HTN through the overactivation of T cells that trigger a downstream cascade of inflammatory mediators augmenting the physiologic hypertensive response.[10]

Psychosocial Stressors

A role for psychosocial stressors has also been proposed in contributing to the development of HTN. Observational studies demonstrate a greater risk for incident HTN in patients with a heightened cortisol response to stressful events relative to patients with a lower response.[11]

CLINICAL PRESENTATION

Definitions and Guidelines

The relevance of HTN to CV mortality is a function of the correlation between BP levels and CVD risk as established in multiple observational studies and randomized controlled trials (RCTs).[12] Based on this large body of evidence, the 2017 ACC/AHA HTN clinical practice guidelines[13] provide more stringent definitions for HTN than previous versions, with the recommendation to assign the higher stage when SBP and DBP on office BP readings are discordant:

Normal BP	SBP <120 mm Hg and DBP <80 mm Hg
Elevated BP	SBP 120-129 mm Hg and DBP <80 mm Hg
Stage 1 HTN	SBP 130-139 mm Hg or DBP 80-89 mm Hg
Stage 2 HTN	SBP ≥140 mm Hg or DBP ≥90 mm Hg

The European Society of Cardiology (ESC) and National Institute for Health and Care Excellence (NICE) guidelines endorse the following definitions[14,15]:

Stage 1 HTN	SBP ≥140 mm Hg or DBP ≥90 mm Hg
Stage 2 HTN	SBP/DBP ≥150/95 mm Hg (NICE); SBP/DBP ≥160/100 mm Hg (ESC)

Accurate Blood Pressure Measurement

Accurate BP measurement is critical for the diagnosis and management of HTN. The diagnosis of HTN entails a multistep process, where BP measurements are obtained at two or more timepoints and settings in order to ensure the accuracy of readings and evaluate for less obvious diagnoses like white coat and masked HTN. Equivalent thresholds for HTN diagnosis within various measurement settings are outlined in **Table 100.1**.

A number of BP measurement methods are currently available and adopted with varying degrees based on cost, availability, reliability, and appropriateness as deemed by clinical judgment. The following is a brief discussion on the individual merits and limitations of these methods.

Ambulatory Blood Pressure Monitoring

The use of ambulatory BP monitoring (ABPM) is increasing in clinical practice based on a growing body of evidence supporting its superiority over both office-based and, perhaps also, home measurements.[15,16] ABPM helps confirm the diagnosis of HTN, establishes otherwise hard-to-elicit diagnoses such as white coat or masked HTN, results in more reliable treatment decisions, and provides additional prognostic information.

ABPM is performed using automated portable devices that automatically measure BP every 15 to 30 minutes during the day and every 30 to 60 minutes during sleep over 24 to 48-hour intervals.[15] The minimum number of recordings needed over a 24-hour period to get an accurate average BP is 10 recordings during waking hours and 5 recordings during sleep; however, European guidelines recommend 20 recordings during the awake period and 7 during sleep for a more accurate assessment.[15,17] Daytime, nighttime, and 24-hour averages are then calculated using these measurements and are used to make a diagnosis of HTN based on certain equivalent thresholds (**Table 100.1**).

Although the use of ABPM is not widely recommended for routine screening purposes, its primary utility is in cases of diagnostic uncertainty between office-based and home BP measurements. Patients who persistently have elevated office readings that average greater than 130/80 mm Hg and reliable home BP readings that average less than 130/80 mm Hg are said to have white coat HTN,[13] thought to be because of anxiety in part and an exaggerated sympathetic response. White coat HTN should be confirmed with multiple readings on different visits and out-of-office measurements, ideally with ABPM. If confirmed, patients with white coat HTN should be monitored annually with ABPM or home BP monitoring (HBPM) to detect progression to sustained HTN.[13] The recommendation for continued monitoring stems from observational studies suggesting that untreated white coat HTN places patients at a greater all-cause and CVD risk relative to normotension.[18] In addition, patients with white coat HTN are at an increased risk of developing sustained HTN over a 10-year period relative to their normotensive counterparts.[18] The utility of ABPM in the context of white coat HTN is also evident in patients with apparently resistant HTN whose otherwise appropriate response to pharmacotherapy at home could be unrecognized because of their white coat effect in the clinical setting.[15]

On the other hand, patients with persistently normal office BP readings who have hypertensive ambulatory measurements have a phenotype called *masked HTN*.[13] Detected on clinical studies that compared office BP measurement to ABPM or HBPM, masked HTN has a prevalence of 15% to 30% in subjects deemed normotensive by office measurements.[19] Like white coat HTN, masked HTN has been associated with an increased risk of CVD mortality and conversion to sustained HTN.[19] Accordingly, patients meeting target BPs yet suspected of having masked HTN should have ABPM or HBPM to assess its presence. These include those with mildly elevated office readings (ie, 120-129 mm Hg) who have already undergone lifestyle interventions, patients at increased CVD risk, and patients with target organ damage/remodeling like coronary heart disease, left ventricular hypertrophy, or CKD.[13,15]

TABLE 100.1 Hypertension Diagnosis Thresholds of Different Modalities as per ACC/AHA Practice Guidelines and European Society of Hypertension Practice Guidelines

Blood Pressure Thresholds as per the 2017 ACC/AHA HTN Clinical Practice Guidelines

	Clinic (SBP/DBP)	Home BP Monitoring (SBP/DBP)	Daytime Ambulatory BP Monitoring (SBP/DBP)	Nighttime Ambulatory BP Monitoring (SBP/DBP)	24-Hour Ambulatory BP Monitoring (SBP/DBP)
HTN diagnosis	≥130/80 mm Hg	≥130/80 mm Hg	≥130/80 mm Hg	≥110/65 mm Hg	≥125/75 mm Hg
White coat HTN	≥130/80 mm Hg	<130/80 mm Hg	<130/80 mm Hg	<110/65 mm Hg	<125/75 mm Hg
Masked HTN; untreated patients	120-129/<80 mm Hg	≥130/80 mm Hg	≥130/80 mm Hg	≥110/65 mm Hg	≥125/75 mm Hg
Masked uncontrolled HTN; treated patients	<130/80 mm Hg	≥130/80 mm Hg	≥130/80 mm Hg	≥110/65 mm Hg	≥125/75 mm Hg

BP Thresholds as per the European Society of Cardiology Practice Guidelines for HTN

	Clinic (SBP/DBP)	Home BP Monitoring (SBP/DBP)	Daytime Ambulatory BP Monitoring (SBP/DBP)	Nighttime Ambulatory BP Monitoring (SBP/DBP)	24-Hour Ambulatory BP Monitoring (SBP/DBP)
HTN diagnosis	≥140/90 mm Hg	≥135/85 mm Hg	≥135/85 mm Hg	≥120/70 mm Hg	≥130/80 mm Hg
White coat HTN	≥140/90 mm Hg	<135/85 mm Hg	<135/85 mm Hg	<120/70 mm Hg	<130/80 mm Hg
Masked HTN; untreated patients	<140/90 mm Hg	>135/85 mm Hg	>135/85 mm Hg	>120/70 mm Hg	>130/80 mm Hg
Masked uncontrolled HTN; treated patients	<140/90 mm Hg	≥135/85 mm Hg	≥135/85 mm Hg	≥120/70 mm Hg	≥130/80 mm Hg

DBP, diastolic blood pressure; HTN, hypertension; SBP, systolic blood pressure.
ACC/AHA Guidelines adapted from Whelton PK, Carey RM, Aronow WS, et al. 2017 ACC/AHA/AAPA/ABC/ACPM/AGS/APhA/ASH/ASPC/NMA/PCNA Guideline for the Prevention, Detection, Evaluation, and Management of High Blood Pressure in Adults: A Report of the American College of Cardiology/American Heart Association Task Force on Clinical Practice Guidelines. *J Am Coll Cardiol.* 2018;71(19):e127-e248. Copyright © 2018 by the American College of Cardiology Foundation. With permission; ESC/ESH Guidelines from Williams B, Mancia G, Spiering W, et al. 2018 ESC/ESH Guidelines for the management of arterial hypertension. *Eur Heart J.* 2018; 39(33): 3021-3104.

Another indication for the use of ABPM is to make more informed treatment decisions. In a trial comparing the treatment benefit derived from BP-lowering therapy when informed based on traditional office monitoring versus ABPM, fewer patients needed multidrug therapy and more patients were able to stop treatment altogether after the white coat effect was evident with ABPM.[15] Moreover, ABPM has the advantage of exposing alterations in BP that harbor unfavorable long-term cardiovascular effects like the early morning BP surge[a] and nocturnal HTN, also referred to as "nondipping." Because nocturnal BP is expected to decrease by at least 10% relative to daytime BP,[15] nondipping (defined as an overnight BP decrease <10% the daytime value) is a harbinger of CVD complications.[15] ABPM can theoretically be utilized to better time the administration of antihypertensives in nocturnal HTN[20] and in modifying medication dose and half-life in patients with early morning surge to better manage their BP.

ABPM, although considered the gold standard in diagnosing HTN, is yet to be more widely implemented in clinical practice in many countries. The US Centers for Medicare & Medicaid Services (CMS) recently proposed to pay for expanded use of ABPM for detection of suspected white coat HTN and masked HTN.[21] A systematic review conducted by the U.S. Preventive Services Task Force led to a recent endorsement of ABPM for clinical use.[22] Although ABPM is widely used in many European countries, these two developments may increase its use in the United States. Cost, availability, and lack of awareness regarding its potential benefits are factors that contribute to the suboptimal use of ABPM, making HBPM the next best available alternative.

Home Blood Pressure Monitoring

HBPM has become a popular modality of BP monitoring, providing valuable information that aids in the diagnosis of HTN and titration of antihypertensive treatment. Being a reliable, affordable, and convenient alternative to ABPM, its use is relatively more widespread. A meta-analysis demonstrated greater mean BP reductions when using HBPM over office-based BP, with the former achieving average BP reduction of 8/4 mm Hg more than the latter.[23] Like ABPM, HBPM is useful to identify subtle entities like white coat HTN and masked HTN. Indeed, HBPM may offer better prognostic information than ABPM.[16]

[a]Defined as the difference between the mean SBP 2 hours after awakening and the lowest SBP during sleep.

Current guidelines recommend using automated, oscillometric devices rather than traditional auscultatory devices that present challenges for patients to use properly.[13] Two readings—at least one minute apart—are recommended in the morning prior to medications as well as in the evening before dinner. At least 12 recordings over the course of a week are suggested for evaluation by the physician. A diagnosis of HTN, per American guidelines, is then made if the average of these readings is greater than or equal to 130/80 mm Hg.[13]

Patients should be educated and trained on proper performance with automated machines. See **e-Figure 100.1** for patient instructions for HBPM. This includes instructions to rest for at least 5 minutes prior to recording their BP, during which time they should sit with their back straight and supported, while laying their arm on a flat surface and keeping their legs uncrossed and feet flat on the floor. Patients should also be advised to avoid any caffeinated drinks, smoking, or exercise at least 30 minutes prior to taking their BP. In addition, the devices should be brought intermittently to the clinician's office so that their accuracy can be ascertained by the clinician through checking their readings against those of a mercury sphygmomanometer.

Office-Based Blood Pressure Measurement

Office-based BP measurement should only be used for screening purposes as initial readings are not typically reflective of true BP levels due to the white coat effect or other factors (ie, drugs, caffeine, anxiety, and physical exertion, etc) affecting the patient's instantaneous BP. Elevated readings on initial screening (ie, ≥130/80 mm Hg) should prompt confirmation through out-of-office measurement via HBPM or ABPM, unless the patient presents with BP greater than or equal to 160/100 mm Hg with evidence of target organ damage (ie, CKD or hypertensive retinopathy), which warrants immediate treatment.

Office BP measurement should be performed in accordance with the guidelines outlined in **e-Table 100.1** regarding the patient's posture and **e-Table 100.2** regarding the appropriateness of the cuff size, while also noting the timing of the measurement with respect to BP medications and the details of auscultatory technique. An average of two or more office readings taken on two or more occasions should be used to estimate the patient's BP.

Automated oscillometric BP measurement devices have become commonplace in clinical practice for their superior reliability relative to auscultatory devices and because they yield readings that are closer to daytime ambulatory readings, especially when BP is recorded with the patient unattended by a physician in a quiet room.[24] Because the automated oscillometric devices can also take multiple readings in one setting, the mean BP measurement can help to diminish the white coat effect.[24]

CLINICAL PRESENTATION

Signs and Symptoms

The initial evaluation of a patient with suspected or confirmed HTN should aim to do the following:

- Elicit other modifiable CVD risk factors: cigarette smoking, secondhand smoking, unhealthy diet, physical inactivity, obesity, dyslipidemia, diabetes mellitus[13]
- Ascertain the extent of target organ damage (if any)
- Identify red flags for secondary HTN
- Estimate a prognosis based on CVD risk factors

Table 100.2 includes elements in the history, physical examination, and laboratory tests that are important to consider in the evaluation of the hypertensive patient.

DIAGNOSIS

Primary Hypertension

Primary (or essential) HTN exists when no underlying secondary cause for elevated BP is present. Making the diagnosis of primary HTN entails obtaining accurate BP measurements on two or more occasions. Whether the BP values are obtained at the clinic or at home via HBPM,

1. the clinician must ensure the correct measurement technique is followed, and
2. an average of two or more separate readings are to be recorded on two or more different occasions in order to be used for clinical decision-making.

Diagnostic thresholds for HTN are listed in Table 100.1. **Algorithm 100.1** indicates steps that should be undertaken if the patient has an elevated BP on the initial office screening test. **Algorithm 100.2: Recommendations for treatment and follow-up after initial hypertension diagnosis** summarizes the recommended timeline of patient follow-up and treatment after initial diagnosis.

Secondary Hypertension

More extensive diagnostic testing for the hypertensive patient depends on the presence of features suggesting secondary HTN or resistant HTN (ie, failure to respond to therapies). See **Algorithm 100.3** Evaluation/screening for secondary hypertension. Unlike primary HTN, secondary HTN arises owing to an underlying specific etiology whose selective treatment leads to partial or complete restoration of normal BP. Common and uncommon causes of secondary HTN are presented in **Table 100.3** along with their respective clinical indications and screening tests. Clinical examination findings that should provoke screening for secondary HTN are shown in **Algorithm 100.3**.

Drug-resistant HTN is typically defined as systolic BP greater than or equal to 140 mm Hg despite adherence to at least three maximally tolerated doses of antihypertensives from complementary classes, including a diuretic at an appropriate dose, or when four or more medications are required to control SBP.[13]

MANAGEMENT OF THE PATIENT WITH HYPERTENSION

The management approach to HTN is a function of the diagnosis and clinical judgment. The process of treatment entails regular follow-up and multiple evaluations to refine the therapeutic approach to best meet the patient's needs and optimize BP control. Although some patients can afford to undergo a stepwise approach that solely starts with lifestyle

TABLE 100.2 Evaluation of the Hypertensive Patient: History, Physical Examination, and Laboratory Testing

History	Physical Examination	Laboratory Tests
• Duration of HTN, previous pharmacotherapy, dose and frequency, medication compliance • Other CVD risk factors: smoking, diabetes, CHD, dyslipidemia, lifestyle, diet • Medication history (eg, NSAIDs, steroids, sympathomimetics, cyclosporine) that raise concern for induced HTN • Family history of HTN, premature CVD death, renal disease, diabetes, pheochromocytoma • Obstructive sleep apnea: snoring at night, morning headaches, daytime somnolence • Symptoms of target organ damage: blurry vision, headaches, claudication, chest pain, dyspnea, neurologic deficits • Symptoms related to 2° HTN: episodic flushing, sweating, tachycardia, palpitations, proximal muscle weakness, skin thinning, flank pain • Psychosocial stress • Socioeconomic level • Sexual dysfunction	• General appearance: body habitus, muscle bulk, fat distribution, skin lesions • Fundoscopy: retinal hemorrhages, papilledema, cotton wool spots, arteriolar narrowing, and AV nicking • Neck: thyroid and carotids • Heart: palpation and auscultation • Lungs: rales/rhonchi • Abdomen: flank mass • Extremities: edema, peripheral pulses, femoral pulses, BP in all extremities • Vascular: bruits, standing BP • Neurologic assessment: orientation, focal weakness, sensory deficits, visual acuity	• CBC • Complete metabolic panel, including calcium • Serum creatinine, eGFR • Fasting glucose • Lipid profile • Urinalysis • TSH • ECG • 10-year ASCVD risk score • Patient with diabetes or CKD? If yes, check albumin-creatinine ratio and urinanalysis • Echocardiogram to assess for LVH in select cases (eg, patient known to have structural heart disease, symptoms suggestive of impending/deteriorating heart failure) • Other laboratory tests specific to secondary HTN (see following section)

ASCVD, atherosclerotic cardiovascular disease; BP, blood pressure; CBC, complete blood count; CKD, chronic kidney disease; CHD, coronary heart disease; CVD, cardiovascular disease; ECG, electrocardiogram; eGFR, estimated glomerular filtration rate; HTN, hypertension; LVH, left ventricular hypertrophy; NSAIDs, Nonsteroidal anti-inflammatory drugs; TSH, thyroid stimulating hormone.

interventions, others are initially recommended pharmacologic treatment. The advent of percutaneous and surgical approaches has also opened an avenue for the special management of select cases of HTN. The following section notes the use of CVD risk in allocating treatment intensity and discusses the available treatment options from the least to the most invasive.

Cardiovascular Risk-Based Treatment Approach

Owing to the role of HTN in the morbidity and mortality of CVD, there has been a growing tendency to consider cardiovascular risk factors in their entirety—rather than an isolated BP threshold—when allocating antihypertensive therapy. Data from RCTs show that BP-lowering treatment, when administered based on baseline CVD risk—as opposed to specific SBP thresholds—leads to the treatment of fewer patients and prevents more cardiovascular events for the same number of patients treated (lower number-needed-to-treat).[25]

The merit of this personalized risk-based treatment approach is evident in multiple meta-analyses showing that, although the relative risk reduction achieved per unit reduction of SBP is consistent across different levels of baseline CVD risk, the absolute risk reduction derived is greater for higher baseline absolute risk.[26]

Two landmark clinical trials—Systolic Blood Pressure Intervention Trial (SPRINT) and Heart Outcomes Prevention Evaluation-3 (HOPE-3)[27,28]—demonstrated the potential advantages of using CVD risk to triage intensity of BP therapies. In the HOPE-3 study of intermediate-risk patients without baseline CVD, a 6 mm Hg SBP reduction with candesartan and hydrochlorothiazide was not associated with significant benefit. Conversely, the SPRINT study of high-risk patients found significant reduction in all-cause CVD and HF events with intensive SBP lowering to less than 120 mm Hg (that resulted in an average 14.8 mm Hg SBP reduction).

The 2017 Hypertension Clinical Practice guidelines[13] recommended the initiation or intensification of antihypertensive treatment for stage 1 HTN patients who belong to one of five high-risk categories: age 65 years or more, diabetes, CKD, clinical atherosclerotic cardiovascular disease (ASCVD), or a 10-year Pooled Cohort Equation (PCE) estimated ASCVD risk greater than or equal to 10%. Patients with stage 2 HTN are also recommended for pharmacologic treatment, which is sought to achieve a BP target of less than 130/80 mm Hg in all treatment candidates. Thus, it is imperative that hypertensive patients be screened and managed for traditional CVD risk factors, in addition to being assessed for their 10-year CVD risk based on sex- and race-specific PCEs.

The global prevalence of HTN has notably increased in the wake of the most recent HTN guidelines from the United States,[4] generating a need for a more reliable means of allocating therapy. As a result, certain novel risk markers have been investigated with regard to their capacity to further inform cardiovascular risk assessment, even beyond traditional risk factors. Such markers include coronary artery calcium (CAC) and

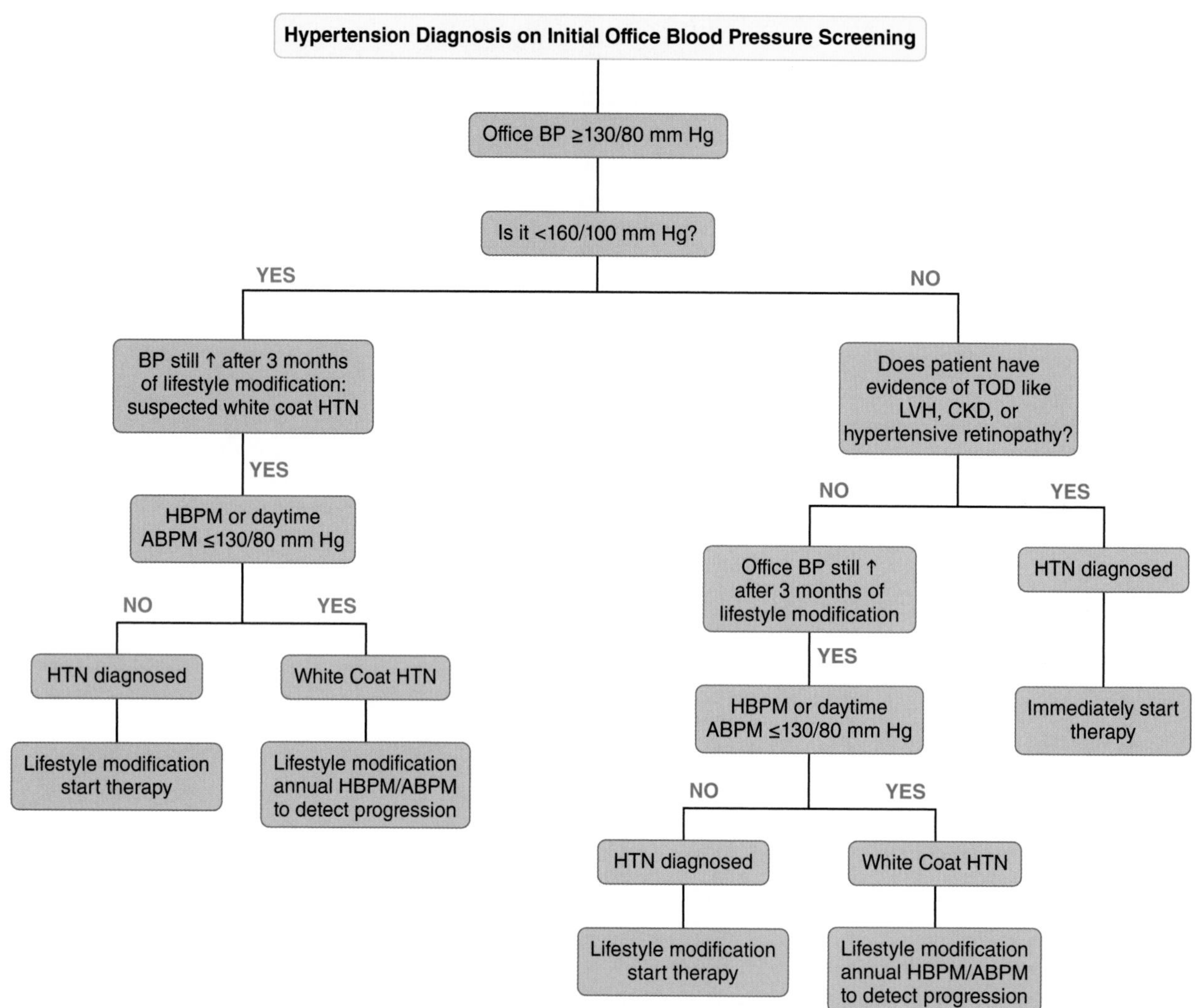

ALGORITHM 100.1 Hypertension diagnosis on initial office blood pressure screening. ABPM, ambulatory blood pressure monitoring; BP, blood pressure; CKD, chronic kidney disease; HBPM, home blood pressure monitoring; HTN, hypertension; LVH, left ventricular hypertrophy; TOD, target organ damage. (Adapted from Whelton PK, Carey RM, Aronow WS, et al. 2017 ACC/AHA/AAPA/ABC/ACPM/AGS/APhA/ASH/ASPC/NMA/PCNA Guideline for the Prevention, Detection, Evaluation, and Management of High Blood Pressure in Adults: A Report of the American College of Cardiology/American Heart Association Task Force on Clinical Practice Guidelines. *J Am Coll Cardiol.* 2018;71(19):e127-e248. Copyright © 2018 by the American College of Cardiology Foundation. With permission.)

myocardial biomarkers (ie, high-sensitivity cardiac troponin T and N-terminal pro B-type natriuretic peptide [NT-proBNP]).

CAC—measured with non-contrast computerized tomographic (CT) scans—is a powerful marker of subclinical atherosclerosis.[29] Its "power of zero," or its negative predictive value, bears a special advantage in asymptomatic, intermediate-risk patients where a score of zero (ie, no coronary calcium detected) can permit a focus on healthy diet and lifestyle, whereas a higher score can rather support administration of preventive medications.[30]

Observational studies have suggested the utility of CAC in risk stratifying patients across different BP thresholds satisfying both old and new definitions of HTN stages.[31,32] Higher CAC strata were consistently associated with increased incidence of CVD events independent of other risk factors and greater expected benefit from more intensive BP treatment.[31,32] Likewise, asymptomatic patients with abnormally elevated troponin T and NT-proBNP were more likely to develop incident CVD events irrespective of other risk factors and are estimated to attain higher absolute benefit from more intensive BP treatment.[33] Currently, these markers are not yet formally recommended as "risk-enhancers" in the current U.S. HTN guidelines and, therefore, are not ready for routine clinical practice.

Lifestyle Interventions

Nonpharmacologic therapy, also dubbed lifestyle intervention, is the foundation of therapy for all patients with elevated BP or a formal diagnosis of HTN. Several behavioral strategies have been associated with a significant BP reduction[13]:

- **Weight loss**. Every 1-kilogram reduction of body weight is expected to induce an approximately 1 mm Hg drop in BP. In particular, weight loss can lead to significant BP reduction in obese patients, independent of level of exercise,

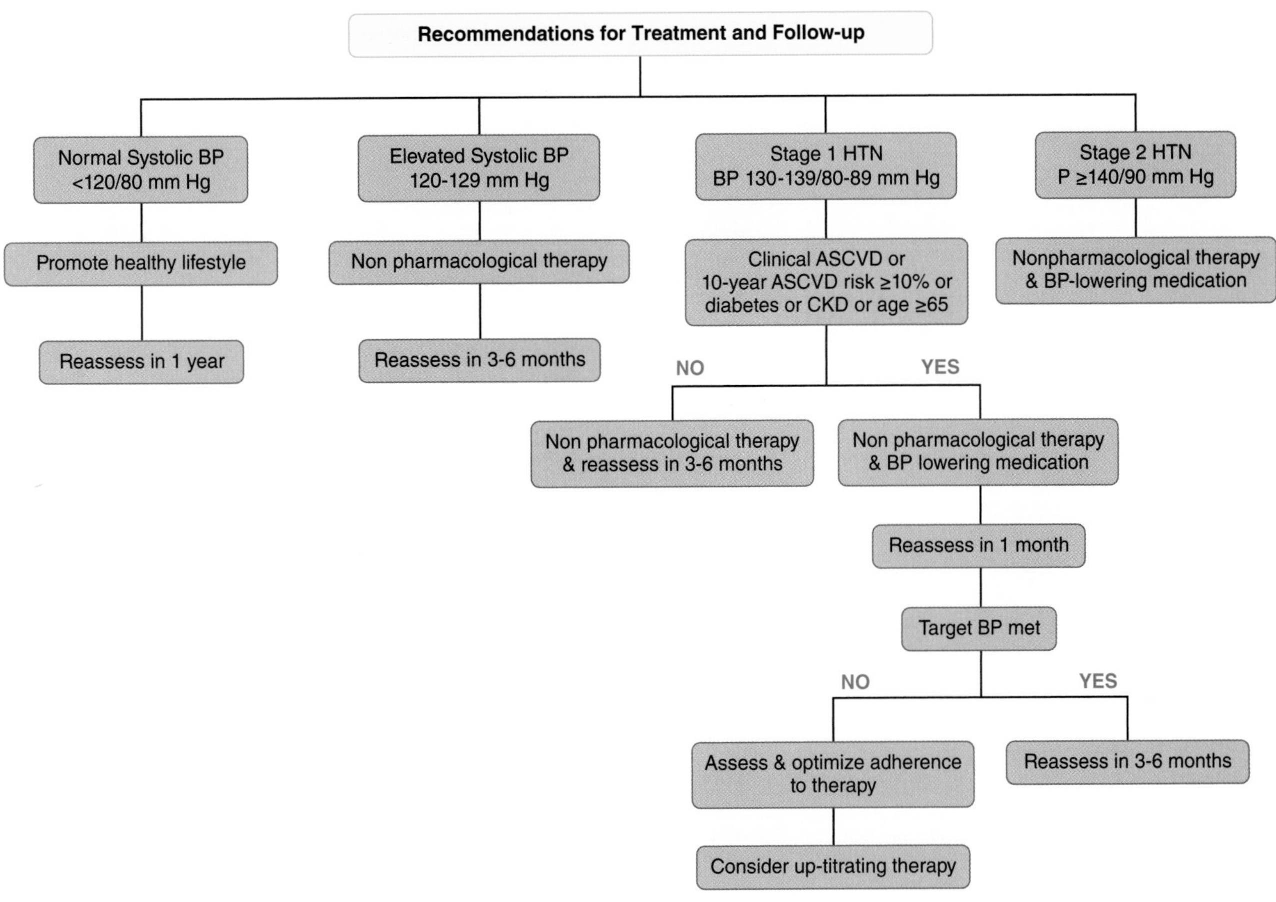

ALGORITHM 100.2 Recommendations for treatment and follow-up after initial hypertension diagnosis. ASCVD, atherosclerotic cardiovascular disease; BP, blood pressure; CKD, chronic kidney disease; HTN, hypertension. (Adapted from Whelton PK, Carey RM, Aronow WS, et al. 2017 ACC/AHA/AAPA/ABC/ACPM/AGS/APhA/ASH/ASPC/NMA/PCNA Guideline for the Prevention, Detection, Evaluation, and Management of High Blood Pressure in Adults: A Report of the American College of Cardiology/American Heart Association Task Force on Clinical Practice Guidelines. *J Am Coll Cardiol.* 2018;71(19):e127-e248. Copyright © 2018 by the American College of Cardiology Foundation. With permission.)

achieving on average an approximate 5 mm Hg SBP drop in most hypertensive subjects.

- **DASH diet.** The Dietary Approaches to Stop Hypertension (DASH) dietary pattern—which is rich in fruits, vegetables, whole grains, low-fat products, and reduced content of overall saturated fat—may be the most effective of all strategies, potentially achieving an approximate 11 mm Hg SBP drop in hypertensive patients.
- **Reduction in dietary sodium intake.** While optimal daily sodium consumption is less than 1500 mg, a daily target of less than 1000 mg is capable of inducing a drop of 5 to 6 mm Hg in SBP of hypertensive patients.
- **Enhancement of dietary potassium intake.** Consumption of a potassium-rich diet containing 3500 to 5000 mg/day can achieve around 4 mm Hg reduction in SBP in hypertensive patients, though care should be taken among patients with kidney disease.
- **Physical activity.** Aerobic, dynamic resistance, and isometric resistance exercise can bring about approximate BP reductions of 5 to 8 mm Hg, 4 mm Hg, and 5 mmHg, respectively, in hypertensive patients.
- **Moderate alcohol consumption.** In individuals who drink alcohol, reduction of daily consumption to two or fewer daily drinks in men and one or less daily drink in women can attain a 4 mm Hg SBP reduction in hypertensive patients.

Patients without an indication for the prompt initiation of antihypertensive therapy (ie, stage 2 HTN) should be advised to abide by the therapeutic lifestyle interventions mentioned above. If the patient's BP remains above the treatment target despite adopting a healthier lifestyle, pharmacotherapy should then be added to their treatment regimen.

Blood Pressure Treatment Targets

The 2017 ACC/AHA HTN guidelines recommended a universal BP treatment goal of less than 130/80 mm Hg for all patients with confirmed HTN who are deemed eligible for pharmacologic therapy regardless of age or concurrent comorbidities.[13] While it included trial data such as from SPRINT, the meta-analysis from which such a stringently unified BP treatment goal was derived had its own set of limitations like not being prospectively planned—therefore introducing

SECTION 8

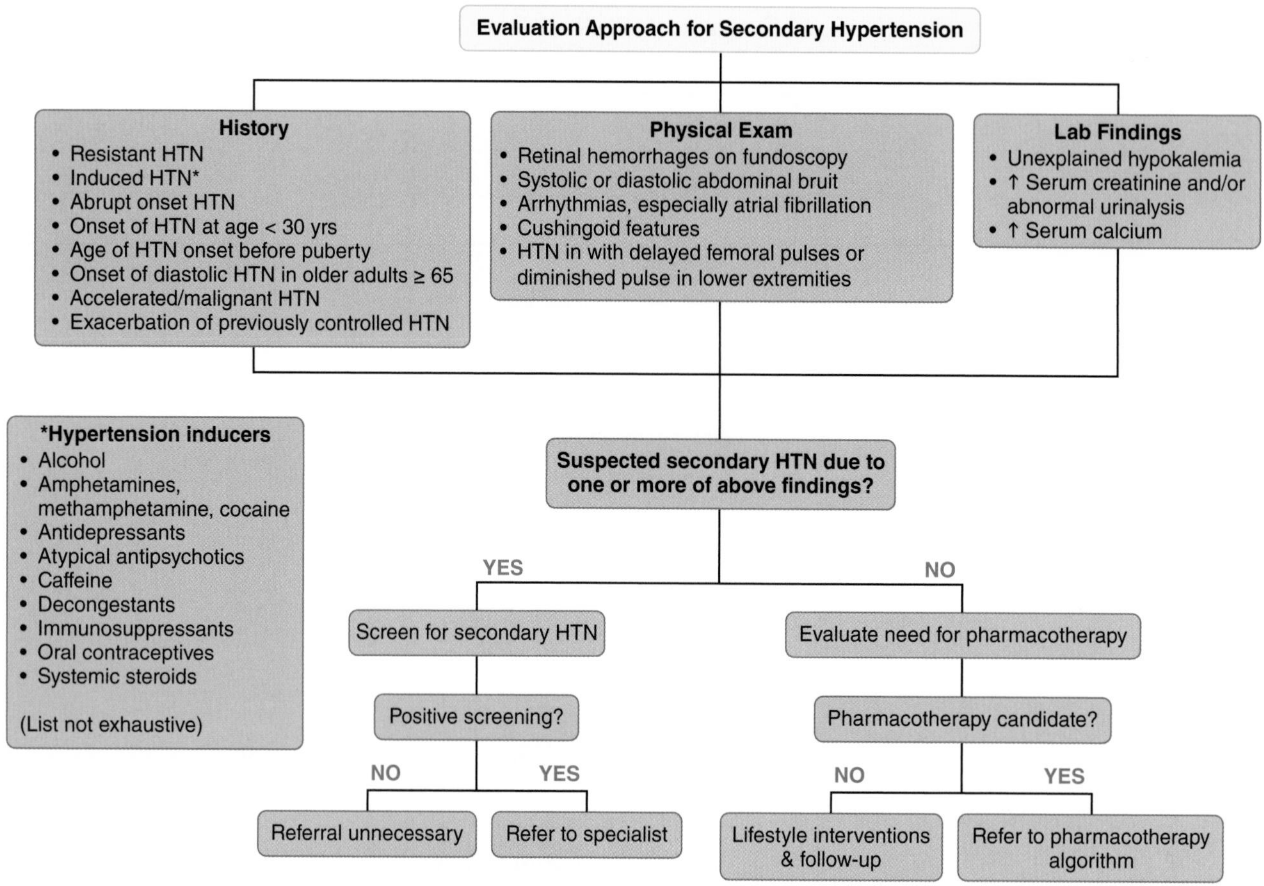

ALGORITHM 100.3 Evaluation/screening for secondary hypertension. BP, blood pressure; HTN, hypertension. *Hypertension inducers.

reporting bias—and lacking strong statistical evidence and a sufficiently large effect size. In addition, inconsistent reporting and description of adverse events—like hypotension and fractures—in the participant RCTs rendered those safety events unaccounted for in the systematic review. These limitations, among others, have called into question the robustness of the class I level of evidence B-R (assigned for RCTs) designated to the SBP treatment goal by the authors of the guidelines. Nonetheless, we believe the totality of data do justify a lower systolic goal of 130 mm Hg, though the diastolic goal of 80 mm Hg (vs the older goal of 90 mm Hg) is more questionable.

The above ACC/AHA BP treatment goal is in contrast to more conservative targets that were adopted by the subsequent European guidelines, particularly among specific patient subpopulations, namely, older patients and patients with CKD. The 2018 ESC/European Society of Hypertension (ESH) guidelines recommend a BP treatment target of 130 to 139/70 to 79 mm Hg in adults who are older than 65 years of age.[15] Acknowledging the difference between chronologic and biologic age, the authors of the 2018 European guidelines note that only the latter dictates the frailty and functionality level of the patient.[15] They contend that most patients who were enrolled in studies that endorsed more intensive BP control for individuals older than 65 years—like Hypertension in the Very Elderly Trial (HYVET) and SPRINT—were active and living independently; therefore, they are not representative of the entire population of elderly patients.[15] Another reason to carefully interpret the results of the SPRINT trial (which targeted a systolic BP of below 120 mm Hg) is its use of unattended automated office BP measurement as opposed to conventional office BP measurement employed in previous RCTs, which potentially eliminated the white coat effect and generated lower readings.[15] Accordingly, the European guidelines suggest a rather cautious treatment target for older patients in order to avoid the adverse events associated with pharmacotherapy in such a vulnerable population.

Similarly, the latest European guidelines opt for a BP treatment target of 130 to 139/70 to 79 mm Hg for patients with CKD, arguing against the presence of sufficient evidence to justify treatment to lower BP targets.[15] Although the European guidelines recommend a BP threshold greater than 140/90 mm Hg for the initiation of BP-lowering therapy in diabetic patients, they endorse treating to a target less than 130/80 mm Hg as recommended by the American guidelines,[13,15] but only if treatment is well tolerated. Of important note, both the aforementioned guidelines strongly recommend BP treatment targets of less than 130/80 mm Hg—if tolerated—in high-risk patients as dictated by the designated CVD risk scores, including patients with CAD and stroke/transient ischemic attack (TIA).[13,15]

TABLE 100.3 Common and Uncommon Causes of Secondary Hypertension: Clinical Indications, Clinical Findings, and Diagnostic Tests

Disorder or Condition	Prevalence	Clinical Indications	Physical Examination	Screening Tests	Additional/Confirmatory Tests
Common Causes of Secondary Hypertension					
Renal parenchymal disease	1%-2%	Urinary tract infections; obstruction, hematuria; urinary frequency and nocturia; analgesic (NSAID) abuse; family history of polycystic kidney disease; elevated serum creatinine; abnormal urinalysis	Abdominal mass (polycystic kidney disease) Skin pallor	Renal ultrasound	Tests to evaluate cause of renal disease
Renovascular disease	5%-34%	Resistant HTN; HTN of abrupt onset or worsening or increasingly difficult to control; moderate to severe HTN in a patient with diffuse athero-sclerosis and asymmetry in renal size; early onset HTN, especially in women (fibromuscular hyperplasia); onset of HTN with BP >160/100 mm Hg after age 55 years	• Abdominal systolic-diastolic bruit • Bruits over other arteries (carotid, femoral)	• Renal Duplex Doppler ultrasound • Magnetic Resonance Angiogram (MRA) • Abdominal CT	Bilateral selective renal intra-arterial angiography
Primary aldosteronism	8%-20%	Resistant HTN; HTN with hypokalemia (spontaneous or diuretic induced); muscle cramps or weakness; incidentally discovered adrenal mass; family history of early onset HTN or stroke	• Arrhythmias (with hypokalemia), especially atrial fibrillation	Plasma aldosterone-renin ratio under standardized conditions (correction of hypokalemia and withdrawal of aldosterone antagonists and other interfering medications for 4-6 weeks)	• Oral sodium loading test (with 24-h urine aldosterone) • Intravenous saline infusion test with plasma aldosterone at 4 hours of infusion • Adrenal CT scan • Adrenal vein sampling
Obstructive sleep apnea	25%-50%	Resistant HTN; snoring; fitful sleep; breathing pauses during sleep; daytime sleepiness	• Obesity • Mallampati class III-IV (visual assessment of distance from the tongue base to the roof of the mouth • Loss of normal nocturnal BP fall	• Berlin Questionnaire • Epworth Sleepiness Score • Overnight oximetry	Polysomnography

(*Continued*)

TABLE 100.3 Common and Uncommon Causes of Secondary Hypertension: Clinical Indications, Clinical Findings, and Diagnostic Tests (*Continued*)

Disorder/ Condition	Prevalence	Clinical Indications	Physical Examination	Screening Tests	Additional/Confirmatory Tests
Drug or alcohol induced	2%-4%	Sodium-containing antacids; caffeine; nicotine (smoking); alcohol; NSAIDs; oral contraceptives; cyclosporine or tacrolimus; sympathomimetics (decongestants, anorectics); cocaine, amphetamines and other illicit drugs; neuropsychiatric agents; erythropoiesis-stimulating agents; clonidine withdrawal; herbal agents (Ma Huang, ephedra)	• Fine tremor • Tachycardia • Sweating (cocaine, ephedrine, monoamine oxidase inhibitors) • Acute abdominal pain (cocaine)	Urinary drug screen (illicit drugs)	Response to withdrawal of suspected agent
Uncommon Causes of Secondary Hypertension					
Disorder/ Condition	**Prevalence**	**Clinical Indications**	**Physical Examination**	**Screening Tests**	**Additional/Confirmatory Tests**
Pheochromocytoma/ paraganglioma	0.1%-0.6%	Resistant HTN; paroxysmal HTN or crisis superimposed on sustained HTN; "spells," BP lability, headache, sweating, palpitations, pallor; positive family history of pheochromocytoma/ paraganglioma; adrenal incidentaloma	• Skin stigmata of neurofibromatosis (café au lait spots neurofibromas) • Orthostatic hypotension	24-hour urinary fractionated metanephrines or plasma metanephrines under standard conditions (supine position with in-dwelling IV cannula)	CT or MRI scan of abdomen/pelvis
Cushing syndrome	<0.1%	Rapid weight gain, especially with central distribution; proximal muscle weakness; depression; hyperglycemia	• Central obesity • "Moon facies" • Dorsal and supraclavicular fat pads • Wide (1 cm) violaceous striae • Hirsutism	Overnight 1 mg dexamethasone suppression test	24-hour urinary free cortisol excretion (preferably multiple); midnight salivary cortisol
Hypothyroidism	<1%	Dry skin; cold intolerance; constipation; hoarseness; weight gain	Delayed ankle reflex; periorbital puffiness; coarse skin; cold skin; slow movement; goiter	• Thyroid-stimulating hormone • Free thyroxine	None
Hyperthyroidism	<1%	Warm, moist skin; heat intolerance; nervousness; tremulousness; insomnia; weight loss; diarrhea; proximal muscle weakness	Lid lag; new tremor of the outstretched hands; warm, moist skin	• Thyroid-stimulating hormone • Free thyroxine	Radioactive iodine uptake and scan

Aortic coarctation (undiagnosed or repaired)	0.1%	Young patient (<30 years of age) with HTN or young adult with bicuspid aortic valve	• BP higher in upper extremities than in lower • Absent femoral pulses • Continuous murmur over patient's back, chest, or abdominal bruit • Left thoracotomy scar (postoperative)	Echocardiogram	Thoracic and abdominal CT angiogram or MRA
Primary hyperparathyroidism	Rare	Hypercalcemia	Usually none	Serum calcium	Serum parathyroid hormone
Congenital adrenal hyperplasia	Rare	HTN and hypokalemia; virilization (11-beta-hydroxylase deficiency [11-beta-OH]); incomplete masculinization in males and primary amenorrhea in females (17-alpha-hydroxylase deficiency [17-alpha-OH])	Signs of virilization (11-beta-OH) or incomplete masculinization (17-alpha-OH)	HTN and hypokalemia with low or normal aldosterone and renin	11-beta-OH: elevated deoxycorticosterone (DOC), 11-deoxycortisol, and androgens 17- alpha-OH; decreased androgens and estrogen; elevated deoxycorticosterone and corticosterone
Mineralocorticoid excess syndromes other than primary aldosteronism	Rare	Early onset HTN; resistant HTN; hypokalemia or hyperkalemia	Arrhythmias (with hypokalemia)	Low plasma aldosterone and renin	Urinary cortisol metabolites; genetic testing
Acromegaly	Rare	Acral features, enlarging shoe, glove, or hat size; headache, visual disturbances; diabetes mellitus	• Acral features • Large hands and feet • Frontal bossing	Serum growth hormone $\geq$1 ng/mL during oral glucose load	Elevated age- and sex-matched IGF-1 level; MRI scan of the pituitary

BP, blood pressure; CT, computerized tomography; HTN, hypertension; IGF, insulinlike growth factor; MRA, magnetic resonance angiography; MRI, magnetic resonance imaging; NSAIDS, nonsteroidal anti-inflammatory drugs.
Reprinted from Whelton PK, Carey RM, Aronow WS, et al. 2017 ACC/AHA/AAPA/ABC/ACPM/AGS/APhA/ASH/ASPC/NMA/PCNA Guideline for the Prevention, Detection, Evaluation, and Management of High Blood Pressure in Adults: A Report of the American College of Cardiology/American Heart Association Task Force on Clinical Practice Guidelines. *J Am Coll Cardiol.* 2018;71(19):e127-e248.

ACC/AHA	ESC/ESH	
Target <130/80 mm Hg for • All stage 2 hypertensive patients • Stage 1 hypertensive patients who – have clinical CVD or ASCVD risk score ≥10% – have diabetes mellitus – have CKD – are ≥65 years	**Target <130/80 mm Hg for hypertensive patients who** • are aged 18-65 • have diabetes • have CAD • have stroke/TIA	**Target of 130-139/70-79 mm Hg for hypertensive patients who** • have CKD • are ≥65 years

Pharmacotherapy

An important general principle regarding the efficacy of antihypertensive pharmacotherapy is that the main determinant of benefit derived from treatment is the magnitude of BP reduction, rather than the choice of individual drug(s) or therapeutic agent(s).[26] This principle has been largely corroborated through multiple large RCTs demonstrating that the same amount of BP reduction achieved by various drug classes yielded equivalent cardiovascular benefits.[b] Indeed, owing to the similar efficacy of different antihypertensive drug classes, they typically achieve a similar reduction in BP by the end of the drug titration phase in 40% to 50% of patients,[34] notwithstanding the possibility of interindividual variability.

Specific classes are recommended for initial monotherapy as long as the candidates do not have stage 2 HTN nor exceed their target BP by 20/10 mm Hg. These drugs include the following[13]:

- Thiazide diuretics
- Angiotensin converting enzyme (ACE) inhibitors/angiotensin II receptor blockers (ARBs)
- Calcium channel blockers (CCBs)

The drug of choice for initial monotherapy usually involves one of the drugs mentioned above, unless there are compelling indications for other drug classes that confer a special therapeutic advantage to a subset of patients (see **e-Table 100.3**). For example, non-dihydropyridine CCBs or beta blockers are better options for patients with atrial fibrillation for rate control. Similarly, beta blockers confer a survival advantage for patients with HF with reduced ejection fraction (HFrEF) and patients with a prior myocardial infarction (particularly if within the previous 5 years).

In patients who are most likely to require combination drug therapy to adequately control BP (ie, their SBP is 20 mm Hg or more above goal), it is still reasonable to start monotherapy with either a long-acting ACE inhibitor/ARB or a long-acting dihydropyridine CCB, because the second class can be added if its use is warranted. This dual combination therapy approach is supported by the ACCOMPLISH trial.[35] It is worthwhile noting the inherent risk of hyperkalemia associated with ACE inhibitors/ARBs, especially in patients with CKD or taking potassium-sparing drugs. They also pose a risk of acute renal failure in patients with bilateral renal artery stenosis. Also in favor of starting with CCBs is the fact that these agents do not interfere with aldosterone-renin ratio tests that are commonly used in secondary hypertension workups, whereas ACE inhibitors/ARBs do interfere. **See Algorithm 100.4 Antihypertensive Pharmacotherapy decision-making: monotherapy (stage 1) versus combination (stage 2).**

Alternatively, a thiazide diuretic can be used for initial monotherapy. The Antihypertensive and Lipid-Lowering Treatment to Prevent Heart Attack Trial (ALLHAT) study provides the only RCT-derived evidence of the benefit of a specific thiazide drug in reducing adverse cardiovascular effects, making chlorthalidone the preferred drug among its class.[13,36] Indapamide and hydrochlorothiazide are two other thiazides commonly used in clinical practice. Thiazide-like diuretics come with potential metabolic complications like hypokalemia, hyponatremia, glucose intolerance, and hyperuricemia; therefore, they should ideally be avoided in patients susceptible to such metabolic derangements. In addition, chlorthalidone and indapamide have a longer duration of action compared to hydrochlorothiazide, potentially leading to better nocturnal BP control.

Specific ethnic and age groups tend to demonstrate better responses to certain drug classes. For example, black patients and older adults (ie, ≥60 years) may respond better to thiazide diuretics or CCBs, and therefore are recommended to start monotherapy with one of these classes should they bear no special indications otherwise for other drug classes.[13,37] On the other hand, younger patients (ie, <50 years) tend to respond better to ACE inhibitors or ARBs and beta blockers (although the latter group is only recommended in the presence of a special indication).[38]

If monotherapy is not achieving adequate BP control of less than 130/80 mm Hg in a patient with stage 1 HTN, then the dosage should be up-titrated or a drug of a different class should be added to the treatment regimen.[13] It is important to understand that the highest BP reduction will be achieved at half the standard dose designated for a certain drug: each additional sequential dose increase will only further incur a modest BP reduction in SBP and DBP, while increasing the risk for adverse effects. For example, if an average SBP unit reduction of 7 mm Hg is achieved by half the standard dose of a drug, average reductions of 9 mm Hg and 10 mm Hg might be sequentially achieved with a standard dose and twice the standard dose, respectively.[39] Over time, many patients need more than one drug to maintain BP control.

[b]Two prominent exceptions are the ACCOMPLISH and ALLHAT trials. In ACCOMPLISH, the combination of amlodipine plus benazepril was associated with a lower incidence of CVD-related mortality compared to hydrochlorothiazide plus benazepril despite having an on-treatment SBP that was only 1 mm Hg lower. By contrast, in ALLHAT, chlorthalidone resulted in lower mean SBPs compared to amlodipine, lisinopril, and doxazosin, yet four drugs had the same frequency of primary outcome (composite of fatal CHD or fatal MI) at mean follow-up of 4 years.

TABLE 100.4 Dosage, Frequency, and Side Effects for Primary and Secondary Antihypertensive Medications. *Adapted from ACC/AHA Hypertension Clinical Practice Guidelines*[13]

Class	Drug	Usual Dose, Range (mg/day)[a]	Daily Frequency	Comments
First-Line Antihypertensive Agents				
Thiazide or thiazide-type diuretics	Chlorthalidone	12.5-25	1	Chlorthalidone is preferred on the basis of prolonged half-life and proven trial reduction of CVD. Monitor for hyponatremia, hypokalemia, hyperuricemia, and hypercalcemia. Use with caution in patients with history of acute gout unless patient is on uric acid–lowering therapy.
	Hydrochlorothiazide	25-50	1	
	Indapamide	1.25-2.5	1	
	Metolazone	2.5-5	1	
Angiotensin converting enzyme (ACE) inhibitors	Benazepril	10-40	1 or 2	Do not use in combination with ARBs or direct renin inhibitor. There is an increased risk of hyperkalemia, especially in patients with CKD or on potassium supplements or potassium-sparing drugs. There is a risk of acute renal failure in patients with severe bilateral renal artery stenosis. Do not use if patient has history of angioedema with ACE inhibitors. Avoid in pregnancy.
	Captopril	12.5-150	2 or 3	
	Enalapril	5-40	1 or 2	
	Fosinopril	10-40	1	
	Lisinopril	10-40	1	
	Moexipril	7.5-30	1 or 2	
	Perindopril	4-16	1	
	Quinapril	10-80	1 or 2	
	Ramipril	2.5-20	1 or 2	
	Trandolapril	1-4	1	
Angiotensin receptor blockers (ARBs)	Azilsartan	40-80	1	Do not use in combination with ACE inhibitors or direct renin inhibitor. There is an increased risk of hyperkalemia, especially in patients with CKD or on potassium supplements or potassium-sparing drugs. There is a risk of acute renal failure in patients with severe bilateral renal artery stenosis. Do not use if patient has history of angioedema with ARBs. Patients with a history of angioedema with an ACE inhibitor can receive an ARB 6 weeks after ACE inhibitor is discontinued. Avoid in pregnancy.
	Candesartan	8-32	1	
	Eprosartan	600-800	1 or 2	
	Irbesartan	150-300	1	
	Losartan	50-100	1 or 2	
	Olmesartan	20-40	1	
	Telmisartan	20-80	1	
	Valsartan	80-320	1	
Calcium channel blockers (CCB)—dihydropyridines	Amlodipine	2.5-10	1	Avoid use in patients with heart failure owing to reduced ejection fraction; amlodipine or felodipine may be used if required. Associated with dose-related pedal edema, which is more common in women than men.
	Felodipine	2.5-10	1	
	Isradipine	5-10	2	
	Nicardipine SR	60-120	2	
	Nifedipine LA	30-90	1	
	Nisoldipine	17-34	1	
Calcium channel blockers (CCB)—non-dihydropyridines	Diltiazem ER	120-360	1	Avoid routine use with beta blockers in patients with first degree or advanced heart block. Do not use in patients with heart failure owing to reduced ejection fraction. There are drug interactions with diltiazem and verapamil (*CYP3A4* major substrate and moderate inhibitor).
	Verapamil IR	120-360	3	
	Verapamil SR	120-360	1 or 2	
	Verapamil ER (delayed onset)	100-300	1 (in the evening)	

(*Continued*)

SECTION 8

TABLE 100.4 Dosage, Frequency, and Side Effects for Primary and Secondary Antihypertensive Medications. *Adapted from ACC/AHA Hypertension Clinical Practice Guidelines*[13] (*Continued*)

Class	Drug	Usual Dose, Range (mg/day)[a]	Daily Frequency	Comments
Second-Line Antihypertensive Agents				
Diuretics—loop	Bumetanide	0.5-2	2	
	Furosemide	20-80	2	
	Torsemide	5-10	1	
Diuretics—potassium sparing	Amiloride	5-10	1 or 2	
	Triamterene	50-100	1 or 2	
Diuretics—aldosterone antagonists	Eplerenone	50-100	1 or 2	
	Spironolactone	25-100	1	
Beta blockers—cardioselective	Atenolol	25-100	2	
	Betaxolol	5-20	1	
	Bisoprolol	2.5-10	1	
	Metoprolol tartrate	100-200	2	
	Metoprolol succinate	50-200	1	
Beta blockers—cardioselective and vasodilatory	Nebivolol	5-40	1	
Beta blockers—noncardioselective	Nadolol	40-120	1	
	Propranolol IR	80-160	2	
	Propranolol LA	80-160	1	
Beta blockers—intrinsic sympathomimetic activity	Acebutolol	200-800	2	
	Penbutolol	10-40	1	
	Pindolol	10-60	2	
Beta blockers—combined alpha- and beta-receptor	Carvedilol	12.5-50	2	
	Carvedilol phosphate	20-80	1	
	Labetalol	200-800	2	
Direct renin inhibitor	Aliskiren	150-300	1	
Alpha 1 blockers	Doxazosin	1-16	1	
	Prazosin	2-20	2 or 3	
	Terazosin	1-20	1 or 2	
Central alpha 2 agonist and other centrally acting drugs	Clonidine oral	0.1-0.8	2	
	Clonidine patch	0.1-0.3	1 weekly	
	Methyldopa	250-1000	2	
	Guanfacine	0.5-2	1	
Direct vasodilators	Hydralazine	100-200	2 or 3	
	Minoxidil	5-100	1	

[a]Dosages may vary from those listed in the FDA-approved labeling.

Reprinted from Whelton PK, Carey RM, Aronow WS, et al. 2017 ACC/AHA/AAPA/ABC/ACPM/AGS/APhA/ASH/ASPC/NMA/PCNA Guideline for the Prevention, Detection, Evaluation, and Management of High Blood Pressure in Adults: A Report of the American College of Cardiology/American Heart Association Task Force on Clinical Practice Guidelines. *J Am Coll Cardiol.* 2018;71(19):e127-e248.

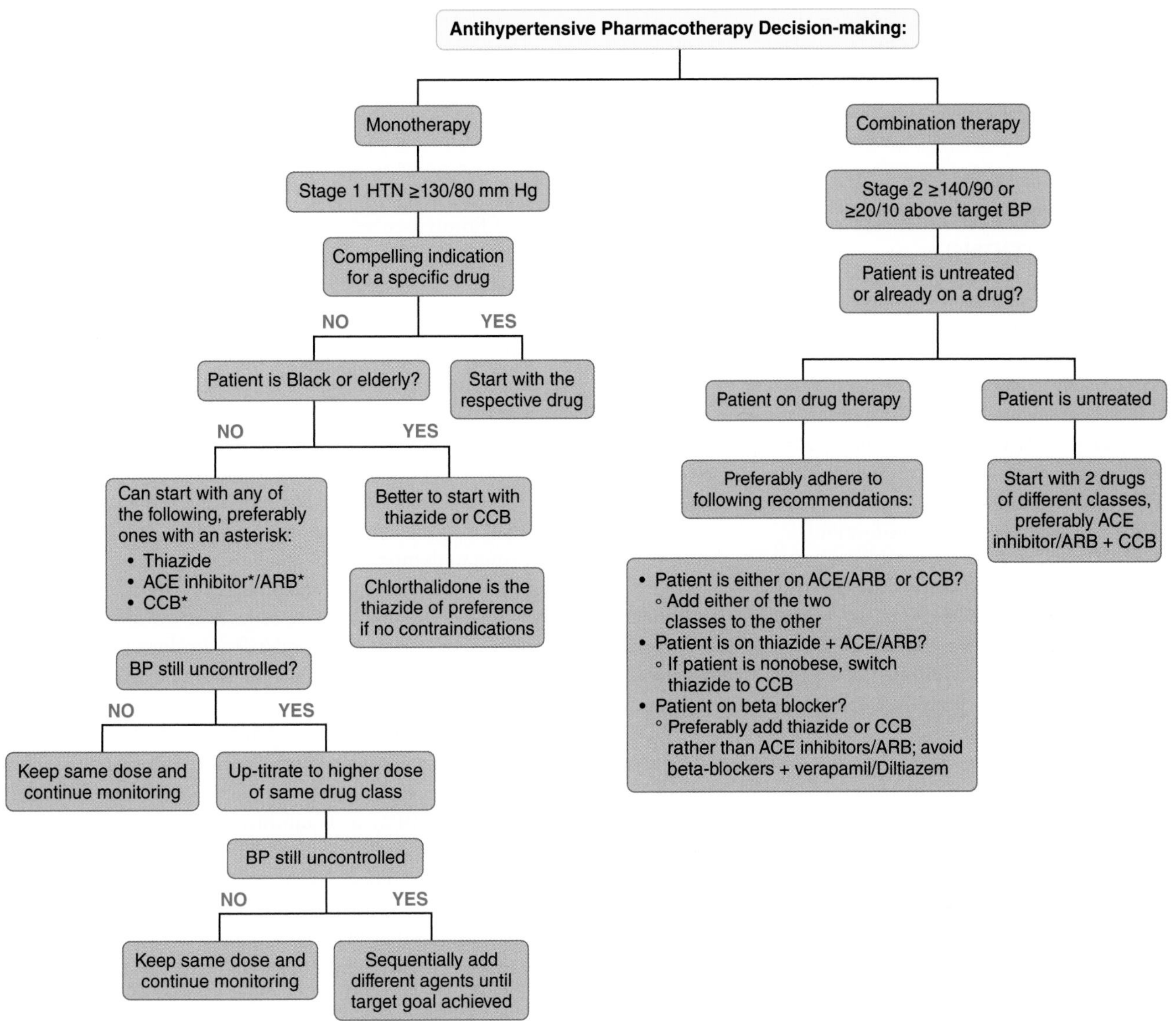

ALGORITHM 100.4 Pharmacotherapy decision-making: monotherapy (stage 1) versus combination (stage 2). ACE, angiotensin converting enzyme; ARB, angiotensin receptor blocker; BP, blood pressure; CCB, calcium channel blocker; HTN, hypertension.

Therefore, only a one-step up-titration in a single drug class is recommended, after which the introduction of a different class allows for the most benefit. Such a stepwise process ensures maximizing treatment benefit while minimizing potential side effects. In the case of dual or triple therapy, the use of combination pills rather than single pills is recommended in order to promote patient compliance and adherence to medication.[13] For patients who are already on an ACE inhibitor or an ARB, the addition of either drug to the other imparts a potential harm and is to be avoided. Instead, other classes like CCB or thiazides should be considered.

Initial combination therapy candidates include (1) patients with stage 2 HTN, and (2) patients whose BP is more than 20/10 mm Hg above treatment goal.[13] Orthostatic measurements should be taken before multidrug therapy is initiated. Combination therapy with long-acting ACE/ARB and either a long-acting dihydropyridine CCB or a thiazide may be considered, with the recognition that the thiazide-based treatment possibly gives less cardiovascular protection in patients of normal weight than patients who are obese, but the CCB-based therapy is equally effective across BMI subgroups and thus offers superior cardiovascular protection in nonobese hypertension. Accordingly, a combination of a long-acting ACE inhibitor/ARB and a thiazide is recommended for patients who are obese, whereas an ACE inhibitor/ARB + CCB is recommended for patients who are nonobese who are achieving suboptimal control with a thiazide.[40]

Other key considerations with combination therapy are the best drug options to be added to a beta blocker: thiazide diuretics or dihydropyridine CCBs. As previously noted, hypertensive patients on a beta blocker should have a compelling indication that warrants its use (ie, HF, atrial fibrillation, prior MI, etc). ACE inhibitors/ARBs are not ideal in patients treated with a beta blocker because the latter reduces downstream angiotensin II production. In addition, beta blockers should be judiciously used with non-dihydropyridine CCBs like verapamil and diltiazem for their cardiac depressant effect that can induce HF in individuals with reduced cardiac function and heart block or bradycardia in those with conduction system disease.

SURGICAL APPROACH AND SPECIAL CONSIDERATIONS

Resistant HTN—defined as systolic BP greater than or equal to 140 mm Hg despite adherence to at least three maximally tolerated doses of antihypertensive medications from complementary classes, including a diuretic, or when SBP is controlled on four or more medications—is prevalent in 13% of patients with HTN.[13] Although several novel antihypertensive drug therapies are in development, the high prevalence of resistant HTN calls for exploring novel therapeutic means of lowering BP beyond antihypertensive medications.

Renal Artery Revascularization

Renal artery stenosis (RAS) is a relatively uncommon secondary cause of resistant HTN estimated at 2% to 5% and is mostly caused by atherosclerotic disease (90%). Other nonatherosclerotic etiologies include fibromuscular dysplasia and large-vessel arteritis, such as Takayasu's.

When RAS is present, it is important to first determine whether it is the cause of the resistant HTN or whether it is an unrelated finding. This requires careful assessment of the patient's clinical presentation and accurate estimation of the severity of stenosis (ie, percent luminal diameter narrowing and unilateral vs bilateral involvement). An additional clue to the diagnosis of RAS-induced resistant HTN is an elevated plasma renin level.

For symptomatic RAS, several observational studies showed that percutaneous renal artery angioplasty and/or stenting significantly reduced BP in patients with resistant HTN, particularly those with aorto-ostial lesions.[41] However, three recent RCTs (STAR, ASTRAL, and CORAL) demonstrated no significant effect of percutaneous revascularization on progression of CKD or BP reduction compared to guideline-directed medical therapy in patients with atherosclerotic RAS.[42] Unfortunately, design flaws (ie, variability in inclusion and exclusion criteria, variable outcome definitions, and inadequate severity of stenosis with many patients having <70% stenosis) have raised concerns about the certainty of their results.[41] Therefore, the 2017 ACC/AHA HTN clinical practice guidelines provide a IIb recommendation for renal artery angioplasty and/or stent placement in patients with refractory HTN, worsening renal function, and/or intractable heart failure.[13] A class IIb recommendation is also provided for revascularization of patients with nonatherosclerotic RAS.

Surgical revascularization has a higher complication rate than percutaneous revascularization and may be considered in patients who fail endovascular therapy, those with specific anatomic considerations such as multiple small renal arteries (<4 mm) or early primary branching of the main renal artery, or those who undergo aortic reconstruction near the renal arteries for other indications. In those with RAS because of fibromuscular dysplasia, surgery can also be considered in branch RAS and renal arteries with extensive intimal fibroplasia.[43]

Renal Sympathetic Denervation

Overactivation of the sympathetic nervous system plays a major role in HTN. Older studies showed that surgical sympathectomy was an effective means of lowering BP in patients with resistant HTN. However, profound orthostatic hypotension was very common, and the procedure was abandoned.[44]

In the recent era of catheter ablation, preliminary data from nonrandomized and randomized unblinded studies showed that catheter-based radiofrequency or ultrasound renal artery ablation results in large reductions in office BP measurements and a relatively good safety profile. This led to its rapid and widespread adoption in clinical practice in more than 80 countries by 2014.[45] However, during that same year, the largest, randomized sham-controlled trial to date (SYMPLICITY-HTN-3), which enrolled 535 patients, failed to demonstrate a significant reduction in office-based BP measurement and ABPM at 6 months for renal artery denervation.[46] There was no difference in safety endpoints in the sham or treated groups. These results, corroborated by further trials,[47] led to reduced enthusiasm for renal artery denervation in patients with resistant HTN.

However, in 2017 and 2018, two smaller, sham-controlled trials showed that renal artery denervation using improved technology resulted in modest reduction in BP at 3 months in patients not taking antihypertensive medications.[48,49] A third trial in patients taking antihypertensive medications showed a modest 6-month reduction in office and 24-hour ambulatory BP with renal artery denervation compared with sham.[50] Of note, patients in this trial had modest resistant HTN (mean SBP 164.6 mm Hg) compared to those enrolled in SYMPLICITY-HTN-3 (mean SBP 179.7 mm Hg) and were treated with a multielectrode catheter that allowed for more circumferential denervation in the main renal artery and its branches. Although these trials using novel catheter ablation techniques show promise and a good safety profile, the BP reduction was modest (approximately 7 mm Hg). Larger sham-controlled clinical trials are needed to verify these potential benefits and safety profile, and outline appropriate use criteria for this procedure.

Two more surgical approaches that are currently being investigated for the treatment of resistant HTN are

[c]Based on post hoc analysis from ACCOMPLISH, revealing that the superiority of the amlodipine-based regimen was mostly pronounced in patients who were nonobese.

baroreflex activation therapy and arteriovenous anastomosis. Baroreflex activation therapy involves stimulating the carotid sinus baroreceptors in patients through the surgical or endovascular implantation of an activation device,[51] with the latter approach raising fewer safety concerns. Arteriovenous anastomosis reduces BP through the percutaneous implantation of a device that creates an anatomic channel shunting large volumes of arterial blood into the high capacitance venous system.[52] Randomized clinical outcome trials are yet to inform clinical practice of the efficacy and safety profiles of both modalities.

FOLLOW-UP PATIENT CARE

Follow-up patient care after initiating antihypertensive drug therapy is very important for monitoring for patient compliance, disease progression, and effectiveness of therapy. The 2017 ACC/AHA HTN clinical practice guidelines recommend monthly follow-up visits for patients initiated on a new or adjusted regimen until BP control is achieved, though follow-up every three months might be more practical in many settings. BP values used for monitoring BP control should ideally be obtained via ABPM or HBPM as previously discussed. Other systematic strategies for improving the follow-up care of hypertensive patients include implementing team-based care that involves multiple professionals like primary health care clinicians, cardiologists, dieticians, and social workers.[13] Telehealth technology, aimed at sharing BP and other medical data between patients and health care providers, is also recommended.[13] Such technology has proven advantageous in terms of achieving significant BP reductions with titration of therapy, especially in high-risk patients.

RESEARCH AND FUTURE DIRECTIONS

Future research is needed to develop better means of BP measurement, risk-based allocation of therapy, and management of resistant HTN. The benefits of out-of-office BP measurement have been well established in confirming (or contradicting) office readings, teasing out unapparent diagnoses, and informing therapeutic decisions. However, more information is needed regarding the relationship of measurements obtained from these devices to CVD outcomes so that more refined definitions of HTN severity and nuanced categorization of hypertensive entities—like masked and nocturnal HTN—can be construed.[16] The following topics are some examples of areas of innovation in the field of HTN that will likely impact future care.

Wearable "Smart" Blood Pressure Devices

Developing more convenient, affordable, and reliable means of BP monitoring such as inexpensive and smart wearables has been a recent focus. In 2018 and 2019, the FDA approved two wearable devices for BP measurement. The oscillometric smart wristwatch developed by Omron and known as the HeartGuide watch[53] uses a flexible synthetic inflatable cuff to measure BP intermittently including during sleeping hours. The other device is a cuffless smart watch developed by Biobeat that utilizes photoplethysmography green light technology to measure BP.[54] Other devices are currently in development and/or pending FDA review.

Wearable devices are, at present, predominantly used by young adults, particularly healthy ones, who choose to track their personalized physical activity and biometric data. Unfortunately, the price of most of these wearables is currently prohibitive for individuals with low socioeconomic status, who would probably benefit most from early screening for HTN. These devices can be used for the long-term management of patients with chronic HTN as a more convenient alternative to present-day 24-hour ABPM devices.[16] Validation studies for accuracy of these devices in diverse populations across the range of BP is necessary in order to assess their benefit for early detection and management of HTN.

Patient Risk Factor Subsets

The optimal treatment approach to certain subsets of patients has yet to be answered through large-scale trials. For example, whether more intensive BP control in young patients with diabetes can prevent early decline in renal function or target organ damage is unknown. By extension, more information about the CVD implications of target organ damage might inform whether its detection should spur more aggressive BP management. Furthermore, optimizing the selection of treatment candidates should be a subject of more research. Emerging evidence on the utility of CAC and cardiac biomarkers in predicting individuals with the highest absolute CVD risk even beyond traditional risk factors merits utilizing their prognostic value, while continuing to research further means of risk assessment.

Resistant Hypertension Procedure-Based Therapies

Resistant HTN should continue to drive research targeted at developing more potent management strategies as well as refining the currently available surgical modalities. After failing to achieve efficacy endpoints, the largest sham-controlled renal denervation clinical trial has rather prompted more complete renal ablation and better selection of procedure candidates in subsequent studies. Accordingly, novel ablation techniques should be studied in large, sham-controlled trials to better assess and quantify the benefits derived from this technique. Moreover, other techniques—like baroreflex activation therapy—should be further explored with regard to efficacy and safety.

Health Care Disparities in Certain Populations

Diminishing disparities in the quality of health care across gender, socioeconomic levels, and ages should be a priority. Providing incentives to health care providers and IT solutions to better monitor outcomes and shrink practice variability may prove beneficial.[13] Additional efforts should be invested in devising and implementing BP control interventions that target underprivileged patient populations. For example, involving HTN-trained clinical pharmacists in checking the BP of Black patients in barbershops and prescribing them antihypertensive medications accordingly has achieved significant BP reductions when compared to isolated lifestyle-modification education by barbers.[55]

Cost Effectiveness of Antihypertensive Medications

Clinicians should continue refining their approach to administering antihypertensive medications to achieve higher cost effectiveness. For example, the use of fixed, low-dose combination pills or "polypills" has consistently proven more effective in lowering BP when compared to either monotherapy or stepped-care approach,[56] although additional follow-up is needed to ascertain the long-term efficacy and tolerability of such a regimen.[57] In addition, new methods to measure drug compliance and therapeutic levels of antihypertensives may help identify noncompliant individuals and improve the management of resistant HTN (ie, avoid unnecessary escalations of therapy, investigations, and invasive procedures). Clinicians should also consider evidence on the diurnal variations of BP and antihypertensive medications.[20] In the Hygia Chronotherapy randomized clinical trial,[20] administering antihypertensive medications at bedtime—as opposed to upon awakening—achieved superior daytime and sleep-time BP control and was associated with less adverse CVD events. Further research is necessary to confirm the utility of nocturnal dosing.

Genetics

The applications of genomics, transcriptomics, epigenetics, and proteomics can be employed in investigating data from observational studies to gain better insights into the long-term effects of BP-lowering therapy as well as potential indicators of BP rise.[13]

KEY POINTS

- ✔ Accurate BP measurement is essential to diagnosing HTN. Office-based BP measurement should only be used for screening purposes, whereas ABPM and HBPM should be used to establish the diagnosis and monitor response to treatment.
- ✔ A careful history, physical examination, and basic laboratory tests should be performed during the patient's initial assessment. History of resistant HTN or other findings suggestive of secondary HTN warrant screening the patient accordingly.
- ✔ Hypertensive patients should be screened and managed for traditional CVD risk factors. Global CVD risk informs absolute treatment benefit when added to isolated BP thresholds.
- ✔ As per 2017 ACC/AHA HTN clinical practice guidelines, pharmacotherapy candidates include those with (1) stage 1 HTN and age greater than or equal to 65, diabetes, CKD, clinical ASCVD, or a 10-year PCE estimated risk score greater than or equal to 10%, and (2) stage 2 HTN.
- ✔ Implementing healthy lifestyle interventions is the first step in the management of HTN, after which pharmacotherapy is initiated if BP remains above treatment target.
- ✔ Initial combination therapy candidates include (1) patients with stage 2 HTN, and (2) patients whose BP is greater than 20/10 mm Hg above treatment goal. Fixed, low-dose combination pills are more effective in lowering BP than monotherapy or a stepped-care approach.
- ✔ Percutaneous renal artery angioplasty and/or stent placement, as well as surgical revascularization, are surgical options for the treatment of secondary HTN owing to renal artery stenosis. The efficacy and safety of radiofrequency-based renal denervation and other novel techniques for the treatment of resistant HTN is yet to be fully established.

REFERENCES

1. Yoon SS, Gu Q, Nwankwo T, et al. Trends in blood pressure among adults with hypertension: United States, 2003 to 2012. *Hypertension.* 2015;65(1):54-61.
2. Rapsomaniki E, Timmis A, George J, et al. Blood pressure and incidence of twelve cardiovascular diseases: lifetime risks, healthy life-years lost, and age-specific associations in 1·25 million people. *Lancet.* 2014;383(9932):1899-1911.
3. Stanaway JD, Afshin A, Gakidou E, et al. Global, regional, and national comparative risk assessment of 84 behavioural, environmental and occupational, and metabolic risks or clusters of risks for 195 countries and territories, 1990-2017: a systematic analysis for the Global Burden of Disease Study 2017. *Lancet.* 2018;392(10159):1923-1994.
4. Muntner P, Carey RM, Gidding S, et al. Potential US population impact of the 2017 ACC/AHA high blood pressure guideline. *Circulation.* 2018;137(2):109-118.
5. Mills KT, Bundy JD, Kelly TN, et al. Global disparities of hypertension prevalence and control: a systematic analysis of population-based studies from 90 countries. *Circulation.* 2016;134(6):441-450.
6. Egan BM, Zhao Y, Axon RN. US trends in prevalence, awareness, treatment, and control of hypertension, 1988-2008. *JAMA.* 2010;303(20):2043-2050.
7. Cheng S, Xanthakis V, Sullivan LM, et al. Blood pressure tracking over the adult life course: patterns and correlates in the Framingham heart study. *Hypertension.* 2012;60(6):1393-1399.
8. Ehret GB, Munroe PB, Rice KM, et al. Genetic variants in novel pathways influence blood pressure and cardiovascular disease risk. *Nature.* 2011;478(7367):103.
9. Simino J, Shi G, Bis JC, et al. Gene-age interactions in blood pressure regulation: a large-scale investigation with the CHARGE, Global Bpgen, and ICBP Consortia. *Am J Hum Genet.* 2014;95(1):24-38.
10. Madhur MS, Lob HE, McCann LA, et al. Interleukin 17 promotes angiotensin II–induced hypertension and vascular dysfunction. *Hypertension.* 2010;55(2):500-507.
11. Hamer M, Steptoe A. Cortisol responses to mental stress and incident hypertension in healthy men and women. *J Clin Endocrinol Metab.* 2012;97(1):E29-E34.
12. Lewington S, Clarke R, Qizilbash N, Peto R, Collins R, Prospective Studies Collaboration. Age-specific relevance of usual blood pressure to vascular mortality: a meta-analysis of individual data for one million adults in 61 prospective studies. *Lancet.* 2002;360(9349):1903-1913.
13. Whelton PK, Carey RM, Aronow WS, et al. 2017 ACC/AHA/AAPA/ABC/ACPM/AGS/APhA/ASH/ASPC/NMA/PCNA Guideline for the prevention, detection, evaluation, and management of high blood

pressure in adults: a report of the American College of Cardiology/American Heart Association Task Force on Clinical Practice Guidelines. *J Am Coll Cardiol.* 2018;71:e127-e248.
14. National Institute for Health and Care Excellence. Hypertension in adults: diagnosis and management. Clinical guideline [CG127]. Published August 24, 2011. https://www.Nice.Org.uk/guidance/cg127
15. Williams B, Mancia G, Spiering W, et al. 2018 ESC/ESH Guidelines for the management of arterial hypertension. *Eur Heart J.* 2018;39(33): 3021-3104.
16. Schwartz JE, Muntner P, Kronish IM, et al. Reliability of office, home, and ambulatory blood pressure measurements and correlation with left ventricular mass. *J Am Coll Cardiol.* 2020;76(25):2911-2922.
17. Shimbo D, Abdalla M, Falzon L, et al. Role of ambulatory and home blood pressure monitoring in clinical practice: a narrative review. *Ann Intern Med.* 2015;163(9):691-700.
18. Mancia G, Bombelli M, Brambilla G, et al. Long-term prognostic value of white coat hypertension: an insight from diagnostic use of both ambulatory and home blood pressure measurements. *Hypertension.* 2013;62(1):168-174.
19. Peacock J, Diaz KM, Viera AJ, et al. Unmasking masked hypertension: prevalence, clinical implications, diagnosis, correlates and future directions. *J Hum Hypertens.* 2014;28(9):521-528.
20. Hermida RC, Crespo JJ, Domínguez-Sardiña M, et al. Bedtime hypertension treatment improves cardiovascular risk reduction: the Hygia Chronotherapy Trial. *Eur Heart J.* 2020;41(48):4565-4576.
21. Jensen TS, Chin J, Ashby L, et al. Proposed decision memo for Ambulatory Blood Pressure Monitoring (ABPM). Centers for Medicare & Medicaid Services. Published April 9, 2019. Accessed June 20, 2019. https://www.cms.gov/medicare-coverage-database/details/nca-proposed-decision-memo.aspx?NCAId=294
22. U.S. Preventive Services Task Force. Final recommendation statement: high blood pressure in adults: screening. Published October 13, 2015. Accessed January 30, 2020. https://www.uspreventiveservicestaskforce.org/Page/Document/RecommendationStatementFinal/high-blood-pressure-in-adults-screening
23. Uhlig K, Patel K, Ip S, et al. Self-measured blood pressure monitoring in the management of hypertension: a systematic review and meta-analysis. *Ann Intern Med.* 2013;159(3):185-194.
24. Roerecke M, Kaczorowski J, Myers MG. Comparing automated office blood pressure readings with other methods of blood pressure measurement for identifying patients with possible hypertension: a systematic review and meta-analysis. *JAMA Intern Med.* 2019;179(3):351-362.
25. Karmali KN, Lloyd-Jones DM, Van der Leeuw J, et al. Blood pressure-lowering treatment strategies based on cardiovascular risk versus blood pressure: a meta-analysis of individual participant data. *PLoS Med.* 2018;15(3):e1002538.
26. Ettehad D, Emdin CA, Kiran A, et al. Blood pressure lowering for prevention of cardiovascular disease and death: a systematic review and meta-analysis. *Lancet.* 2016;387(10022):957-967.
27. Lonn EM, Bosch J, Jaramillo PL, et al. Blood-pressure lowering in intermediate-risk persons without cardiovascular disease. *N Engl J Med.* 2016;374(21):2009-2020.
28. Wright JT Jr, Williamson JD, Whelton PK, et al. A randomized trial of intensive versus standard blood-pressure control. *N Engl J Med.* 2015;373:2103-2116.
29. Blaha MJ, Silverman MG, Budoff MJ. Is there a role for coronary artery calcium scoring for management of asymptomatic patients at risk for coronary artery disease? Clinical risk scores are not sufficient to define primary prevention treatment strategies among asymptomatic patients. *Circ Cardiovasc Imaging.* 2014;7:398-408.
30. Blaha MJ, Cainzos-Achirica M, Greenland P, et al. Role of coronary artery calcium score of zero and other negative risk markers for cardiovascular disease: the Multi-Ethnic Study of Atherosclerosis (MESA). *Circulation.* 2016;133:849-858.
31. McEvoy JW, Martin SS, Dardari ZA, et al. Coronary artery calcium to guide a personalized risk-based approach to initiation and intensification of antihypertensive therapy. *Circulation.* 2017;135:153-165.
32. Elshazly MB, Abdellatif A, Dargham SR, et al. Role of Coronary Artery and Thoracic Aortic Calcium as Risk Modifiers to Guide Antihypertensive Therapy in Stage 1 Hypertension (From the Multiethnic Study of Atherosclerosis). *Am J Cardiol.* 2020;126:45-55.
33. Pandey A, Patel KV, Vongpatanasin W, et al. Incorporation of biomarkers into risk assessment for allocation of antihypertensive medication according to the 2017 ACC/AHA High Blood Pressure Guideline: a pooled cohort analysis. *Circulation* 2019;140(25):2076-2088.
34. Materson BJ, Reda DJ, Cushman WC, et al. Single-drug therapy for hypertension in men—a comparison of six antihypertensive agents with placebo. *N Engl J Med.* 1993;328(13):914-921.
35. Jamerson K, Weber MA, Bakris GL, et al. Benazepril plus amlodipine or hydrochlorothiazide for hypertension in high-risk patients. *N Engl J Med.* 2008;359(23):2417-2428.
36. Furberg CD, Wright JT, Davis BR, et al. Major outcomes in high-risk hypertensive patients randomized to angiotensin-converting enzyme inhibitor or calcium channel blocker vs diuretic: the Antihypertensive and Lipid-Lowering Treatment to Prevent Heart Attack Trial (ALLHAT). *J Am Med Assoc.* 2002;288(23):2981-2997.
37. Morgan TO, Anderson AI, Maclnnis RJ. ACE inhibitors, beta-blockers, calcium blockers, and diuretics for the control of systolic hypertension. *Am J Hypertens.* 2001;14(3):241-247.
38. Dickerson JEC, Hingorani AD, Ashby MJ, et al. Optimisation of antihypertensive treatment by crossover rotation of four major classes. *Lancet.* 1999;353(9169):2008-2013.
39. Law MR, Morris JK, Wald NJ. Use of blood pressure lowering drugs in the prevention of cardiovascular disease: meta-analysis of 147 randomised trials in the context of expectations from prospective epidemiological studies. *BMJ.* 2009;338:b1665.
40. Weber MA, Jamerson K, Bakris GL, et al. Effects of body size and hypertension treatments on cardiovascular event rates: subanalysis of the ACCOMPLISH randomized controlled trial. *Lancet.* 2013;381(9866): 537-545.
41. Prince M, Gupta A, Bob-Manuel T, Tafur J. Renal revascularization in resistant hypertension. *Prog Cardiovasc Dis.* 2019;63(1):58-63.
42. Kalra PA, Moss JG, Baigent C, et al. Revascularization versus Medical Therapy for Renal-Artery Stenosis. *N Engl J Med.* 2009;361(20): 1953-1962.
43. Hirsch AT, Haskal ZJ, Hertzer NR, et al. ACC/AHA 2005 Practice Guidelines for the management of patients with peripheral arterial disease (lower extremity, renal, mesenteric, and abdominal aortic) a collaborative report from the American Association for Vascular Surgery/Society for Vascular Surgery, Society for Cardiovascular Angiography and Interventions, Society for Vascular Medicine and Biology, Society of Interventional Radiology, and the ACC/AHA Task Force on Practice Guidelines (Writing Committee to Develop Guidelines for the Management of Patients With Peripheral Arterial Disease). *Circulation.* 2006;113(11): e463-e654.
44. Smithwick RH, Thompson JE. Splanchnicectomy for essential hypertension: results in 1,266 cases. *J Am Med Assoc.* 1953;152(16):1501-1504.
45. Thukkani AK, Bhatt DL. Renal denervation therapy for hypertension. *Circulation.* 2013;128(20):2251-2254.
46. Bhatt DL, Kandzari DE, O'Neill WW, et al. A controlled trial of renal denervation for resistant hypertension. *N Engl J Med.* 2014;370(15): 1393-1401.
47. Mathiassen ON, Vase H, Bech JN, et al. Renal denervation in treatment-resistant essential hypertension. A randomized, SHAM-controlled, double-blinded 24-h blood pressure-based trial. *J Hypertens.* 2016;34(8):1639.
48. Townsend RR, Mahfoud F, Kandzari DE, et al. Catheter-based renal denervation in patients with uncontrolled hypertension in the absence of antihypertensive medications (SPYRAL HTN-OFF MED): a randomised, sham-controlled, proof-of-concept trial. *Lancet.* 2017;390(10108): 2160-2170.
49. Azizi M, Schmieder RE, Mahfoud F, et al. Endovascular ultrasound renal denervation to treat hypertension (RADIANCE-HTN SOLO): a multicentre, international, single-blind, randomised, sham-controlled trial. *Lancet.* 2018;391(10137):2335-2345.

50. Kandzari DE, Böhm M, Mahfoud F, et al. Effect of renal denervation on blood pressure in the presence of antihypertensive drugs: 6-month efficacy and safety results from the SPYRAL HTN-ON MED proof-of-concept randomised trial. *Lancet.* 2018;391(10137):2346-2355.
51. Heusser K, Tank J, Engeli S, et al. Carotid baroreceptor stimulation, sympathetic activity, baroreflex function, and blood pressure in hypertensive patients. *Hypertension.* 2010;55(3):619-626.
52. Burchell AE, Lobo MD, Sulke N, et al. Arteriovenous anastomosis: is this the way to control hypertension? *Hypertension.* 2014;64(1):6-12.
53. MobiHealthNews. Omron's smartwatch blood pressure monitor cleared by FDA, launches in January. *MobiHealthNews.* Published December 20, 2018. Accessed March 1, 2020. https://www.mobihealthnews.com/content/omrons-smartwatch-blood-pressure-monitor-cleared-fda-launches-january
54. Hale C. FDA clears "cuffless" blood pressure tracking smartwatch from Biobeat. *Fierce Biotech.* Published August 27, 2019. https://www.fiercebiotech.com/medtech/fda-clears-cuffless-blood-pressure-tracking-smartwatch-from-biobeat
55. Victor RG, Lynch K, Li N, et al. A cluster-randomized trial of blood-pressure reduction in black barbershops. *N Engl J Med.* 2018;378(14):1291-1301.
56. Webster R, Salam A, Asita de Silva H, et al. Fixed low-dose triple combination antihypertensive medication vs usual care for blood pressure control in patients with mild to moderate hypertension in Sri Lanka: a randomized clinical trial. *JAMA.* 2018;320(6):566-579.
57. Chobanian AV, Bakris GL, Black HR, et al. The seventh report of the Joint National Committee on prevention, detection, evaluation, and treatment of high blood pressure: the JNC 7 report. *JAMA.* 2003;289(19):2560-2572.

CARDIAC REHABILITATION

Tamara Beth Horwich, Amir Behzad Rabbani, James S. Lee, and Arash B. Nayeri

INTRODUCTION

Cardiac rehabilitation (CR) is recognized as an essential component of the treatment and secondary prevention of coronary heart disease, and more recently has also become a vital part of treatment for heart failure with reduced ejection fraction (HFrEF). Cardiovascular disease is the number one cause of death in the United States; furthermore, approximately 20% of patients with myocardial infarction (MI) suffer an additional MI in the ensuing 5 years. CR programs improve quality of life (QoL) in patients with cardiovascular disease and also reduce cardiovascular mortality, hospitalizations, and events by approximately 25% in patients with coronary heart disease.[1]

CR programs were initially developed in the 1960s in response to seminal research demonstrating that exercise training significantly improved aerobic capacity and, conversely, inactivity and bed rest led to rapid deterioration of cardiovascular performance. Thus, physical activity restriction and bed rest, which had been standard of care post-MI since the 1930s, was realized to be a harmful treatment strategy.[2,3] Thus, early CR programs focused on medically supervised aerobic exercise training. CR programs have now evolved to include components such as nutritional counseling, stress management, psychological support, and education regarding risk factor reduction and treatment adherence (**Figure 101.1**). Thus, modern multidisciplinary CR programs are individualized and personalized to optimize not only physical health but also the psychological and social functioning of participants with various forms of cardiovascular disease.[4]

Much remains to be done with regard to modifiable risk factors and health behaviors in the U.S. population. Obesity

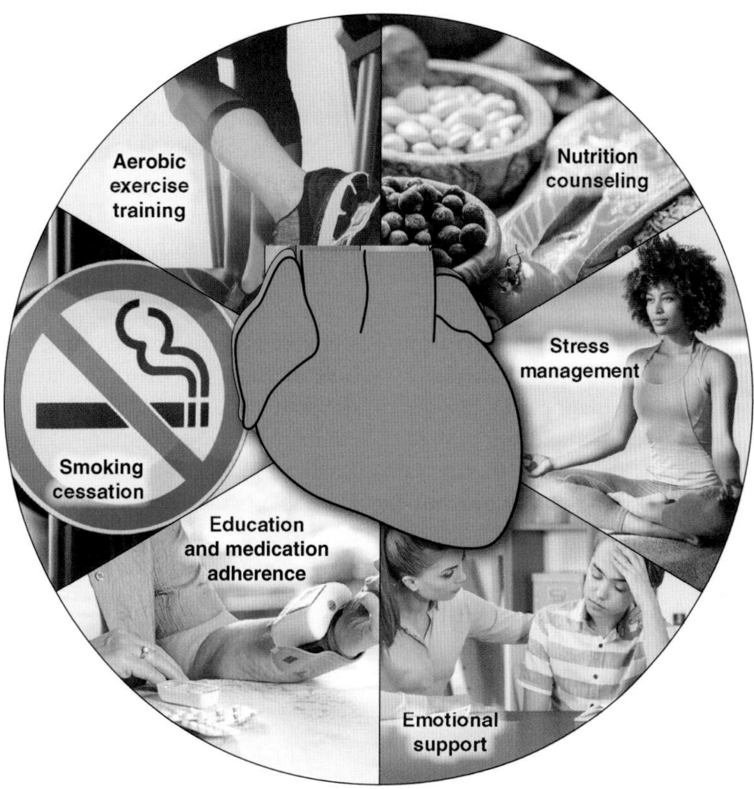

FIGURE 101.1 The core components of cardiac rehabilitation programs.

and metabolic syndrome are present in up to 35% of adults. Nearly 60% of adults in the United States are not regularly physically active, and less than 20% to 25% of adults get the 150 minutes/week of aerobic activity recommended by the American Heart Association (AHA).[5] Adequate fruit and vegetable intake (both of which lower the risk for heart disease and stroke) is seen in only 13% and 9% of the U.S. population, respectively, according to national surveys. Thus, the importance and relevance of CR in the treatment and prevention of cardiovascular disease is clearly evident. This chapter aims to define and describe components and types of CR, outline its indications and contraindications, as well as uncover its limitations and point in the direction of future research and development.

INDICATIONS FOR CARDIAC REHABILITATION

Coronary Artery Disease

CR programs have become a standardized and essential secondary prevention tool for patients with coronary artery disease (CAD). Over time, indications have expanded from patients following acute MI and post–coronary artery bypass graft to patients who have undergone percutaneous coronary intervention and those with stable CAD with angina pectoris. Identification of physical inactivity as a major CAD risk factor has led CR to become a class I recommendation in this patient population.[6] CAD is the predominant diagnosis of patients in CR programs across the United States. Multiple trials and meta-analyses have established the important role of CR as a therapy for patients with CAD.

Peripheral Artery Disease

In the United States, there are an estimated 8.5 million patients with peripheral arterial disease (PAD), resulting in significant morbidity, mortality, and impairment in QoL.[7] PAD can result in claudication, which is defined as fatigue, discomfort, cramping, or pain of vascular origin in the muscles of the lower extremities that is induced by exercise and relieved by rest (usually within 10 minutes). Structured exercise therapies have been established as an important component of care for patients with PAD. Favorable data from multiple randomized controlled trials have established supervised exercise therapy as a class I recommendation and first-line treatment for intermittent claudication.[8,9]

The role of supervised exercise therapy compared with lower extremity revascularization has been studied in the CLEVER (Claudication: Exercise Versus Endoluminal Revascularization) trial, randomizing patients with symptomatic aortoiliac disease to either supervised exercise therapy or endovascular stenting. The trial showed comparable outcomes at 6 and 18 months between supervised exercise therapy and revascularization, while both were superior to medical therapy alone.[9] The ERASE (Endovascular Revascularization and Supervised Exercise) trial randomized study subjects to either supervised exercise therapy alone or in combination with endovascular therapy. At 1 year, both groups showed improvement in walking times and QoL inventories; however, the combined supervised exercise therapy and endovascular arm showed greater improvement as compared to the supervised exercise therapy alone.[10] The body of evidence collectively supports the Class I indication to offer supervised exercise therapy to patients with intermittent claudication, either as stand-alone treatment or in combination with an endovascular strategy.

Postvalve Surgery

The evidence supporting the benefits of CR after valve surgery is less robust than the evidence for CR in coronary heart disease. A 2016 systematic review of exercise-based CR for adults after heart valve surgery found only two randomized controlled trials (total $n = 148$).[11] An improvement in exercise capacity was noted in the exercise groups, but no effect on other outcomes was found, likely because of the small numbers. A cohort study published in 2019 analyzed Medicare patients undergoing valve surgery in 2014 followed through 2015; this analysis found that CR was associated with a significant reduction in hospitalizations and a 4% absolute reduction in mortality in the 1 year following surgery.

A growing number of patients are undergoing transcatheter aortic valve replacement (TAVR) rather than surgical aortic valve replacement. A retrospective data review and small pilot study of CR in post-TAVR patients demonstrated improved QoL and exercise capacity[12]

Heart Failure and Heart Transplant

The HF-ACTION (Heart Failure: A Controlled Trial Investigating Outcomes of Exercise Training) trial, which studied 2331 patients with HFrEF, showed that aerobic exercise training significantly improved QoL and produced a modest, but nonsignificant improvement in the primary outcome of death and/or hospitalization for heart failure.[13] In another study of patients with chronic heart failure with severe systolic dysfunction, there was no excess of death and minimal nonfatal major cardiovascular events in the exercise group compared to control group.[14] Hence, in 2014, the Centers for Medicare & Medicaid Services (CMS) started covering CR for stable patients with chronic HFrEF and ongoing symptoms despite optimal medical therapy for the treatment of congestive heart failure.

Exercise training in heart failure with preserved ejection fraction (HFpEF) has also been shown to be a safe therapy that may improve exercise capacity, cardiorespiratory fitness, and QoL,[15] but it is not routinely covered for reimbursement at the time of this printing.

Although many orthotopic heart transplantation patients participate in CR, there are limited data behind the use of CR for these patients. The 2007 and 2011 statements from the

AHA on CR and the 2010 International Society of Heart and Lung Transplantation Guidelines recommend exercise training both prior to and after orthotopic heart transplantation, with formal CR as tolerated.

FUNDAMENTALS OF CARDIAC REHABILITATION

Table 101.1 shows the fundamental activities of the four phases of CR.

Supervised Exercise Therapy for Peripheral Arterial Disease

Supervised exercise therapy or intermittent claudication consists of a graded treadmill protocol spanning 36 sessions over 3 months, taking place usually in a hospital or outpatient facility directly supervised by qualified health care providers. Patients are asked to grade their claudication symptoms (Table 101.2) in a regular interval (eg, every 30 seconds), with documentation of claudication onset time and maximum walking times. Several standardized graded treadmill protocols can be used.[16-18] All protocols incorporate graded treadmill therapy that starts at a 2 mph walk at 0% grade and increases at a regular interval while monitoring claudication severity.

TABLE 101.1 Traditional Cardiac Rehabilitation Program Components

Phase I—INPATIENT supervised
Duration: 1-2 days during hospitalization
Historically involved early progressive mobilization for basic activities of daily living and self-care, but because of shorter hospital stays mainly consists of education on disease and recovery process, introductory counseling on prevention and treatment strategies, and follow-up planning to transition to outpatient phase II.
Phase II—OUTPATIENT supervised
Duration: Three 1-hour sessions per week, up to 36 sessions over 12 weeks
Medically supervised comprehensive secondary prevention treatment plan involving monitored exercise with training, psychosocial counseling, and educational programs for cardiovascular disease and nutrition with risk factor modification including smoking, hypertension, diabetes, cholesterol, and obesity. Main component of exercise prescription involves aerobic training with preferred duration of 30-45 min and intensity of 40%-80% of peak oxygen consumption, 65%-80% of maximal heart rate, 40%-80% heart rate reserve, or targeting a score of 11 through 16 on a Borg Rating of Perceived Exertion Scale.[36] Strength training and stretching are also incorporated into exercise component.
Phase III—OUTPATIENT supervised
Duration: 3-6 months
Extended independent, medically supervised exercise program emphasizing risk factor and behavior modification to support long-term maintenance of lifestyle and medication adherence to maintain optimum cardiovascular health
Phase IV—OUTPATIENT nonsupervised
Duration: indefinite
Independent maintenance exercise at home and in the community applying principles acquired throughout program.

TABLE 101.2 Claudication Pain Scale

Claudication Pain Scale
1—No Pain or Discomfort
2—Onset of Pain or Discomfort
3—Mild Pain or Discomfort
4—Moderate Pain or Discomfort
5—Severe Pain or Discomfort

Intensive Cardiac Rehabilitation

In 2010, CMS announced that Medicare would cover a new benefit category: Intensive CR. Intensive CR was defined as a CR program that would meet more frequently or for more hours and potentially employ a more rigorous program of lifestyle modification. Two intensive CR programs were initially approved by CMS—Dr. Dean Ornish's Program for Reversing Heart Disease and the Pritikin Program—with a third program, the Benson-Henry Institute Cardiac Wellness Program, added in 2014. Intensive CR is approved for all the same medical diagnoses as traditional CR, except PAD.

The Pritikin program is present at over 50 locations in the United States, and its approach has three pillars: safe and effective exercise, a healthy eating plan, and a healthy mindset. The Pritikin healthy eating plan encourages consumption of fruits, vegetables, whole grains, legumes, nonfat dairy, fish, and other lean proteins such as skinless white-meat poultry while absolutely avoiding foods rich in saturated fats—such as butter, fatty meats, and cheese—and processed meats.

The Ornish program, offered in over 15 U.S. states, is divided into four areas of lifestyle therapy that are given equal emphasis: nutrition, stress management, physical fitness, and group support sessions led by a medical health professional. The Ornish diet focuses on plant-based whole foods, particularly vegetables and fruits, restricts all meat including fish and chicken, and allows a small amount of nonfat dairy, with an overall 10% of calories coming from fat. The Lifestyle Heart Trial was a randomized controlled trial of the Ornish intensive lifestyle program (n = 28) versus no intervention (n = 20). The intervention group had reduction in angina, cholesterol levels, blood pressure, and weight, as well as a decrease in the average percentage coronary diameter stenosis by quantitative angiography versus Mild progression in the usual care/no intervention group.[19]

EXPECTED BENEFITS AND OUTCOMES OF CARDIAC REHABILITATION

Coronary Heart Disease

In numerous randomized clinical trials and meta-analyses, exercise-based CR programs have been well-demonstrated in coronary heart disease patients (ie, those with previous MI, coronary artery bypass graft or percutaneous coronary intervention or who have angina pectoris, or CAD) to reduce cardiovascular mortality by approximately 25% and to reduce hospital admissions by approximately 20% at 12 months follow-up, but overall mortality, MI, and risk of revascularization are unchanged. Furthermore, CR has consistently been demonstrated to improve health-related QoL.[1] **Table 101.3** summarizes additional expected beneficial outcomes of CR.

Heart Failure and Heart Transplant Outcomes

The largest trial to date demonstrating the efficacy of aerobic exercise training in HFrEF patients is the previously mentioned HF-ACTION study.[20] In a substudy of HF-ACTION, supervised exercise was associated with reduction in cardiovascular mortality and heart failure hospitalization in addition to a positive effect on QoL. There was an inverse association between the volume of exercise and adverse clinical events, and even moderate exercise levels (3-7 MET-hours per week) were of clinical benefit .[21]

In patients with HFpEF, a meta-analysis of the utility of exercise training indicated improved exercise capacity and QoL following CR.[22]

Aerobic exercise–based CR programs have also been associated with modest improvement in exercise capacity[23] and significant reduction in hospitalization rates[24] following orthotopic heart transplant. Additional evidence links CR participation with reduced mortality following heart transplantation.[25]

TABLE 101.3 Effect of Cardiac Rehabilitation on Cardiovascular Risk Factors

Obesity: Many patients entering cardiac rehabilitation are obese based on body mass index. Behavioral interventions and exercise regimens have been shown to lead to weight loss.[37]

Hypertension: Although the results are mixed, some studies suggest a modest improvement in blood pressure with cardiac rehabilitation.[38]

Diabetes Mellitus: The use of intensified comprehensive cardiac rehabilitation aimed at improving risk factor control in patients with type II diabetes mellitus or prediabetes can lead to significant reductions in hemoglobin A1C and other risk factors for cardiovascular disease (DANSUK study).[38]

Dyslipidemia: Participation in cardiac rehabilitation can improve lipid profiles, with a particular reduction in low-density lipoprotein cholesterol.[39] There are data also citing improvements in high-density lipoprotein cholesterol, particularly in women participants of cardiac rehabilitation.[40]

Tobacco Use: Participation in cardiac rehabilitation can lead to reductions in tobacco use, particularly in patients without depression and those with lower aggregate medical comorbidity.[41]

Depression and Anxiety: Exercise-based cardiac rehabilitation often results in reduced symptoms of depression, anxiety, and hostility.[42]

Intensive versus Traditional CR Outcomes

Excellent outcomes are associated with both traditional CR as well as intensive CR in terms of secondary prevention of CAD. Intensive CR has shown similar if not improved changes in cardiovascular risk factors compared to traditional CR. Reductions in cardiovascular risk factors such as blood pressure, cholesterol, blood sugar, and body mass index (BMI) have been documented for CMS-approved intensive CR programs.[26] **Figures 101.2 and 101.3** compare selected laboratory and anthropometric changes after intensive CR versus traditional CR at a single university center.[27] On multivariable regression analysis, the intensive cardiac rehab (ICR) program was the only variable significantly linked to reduction in body fat mass and visceral adiposity as measured by bioelectrical impedance.[27]

CONTRAINDICATIONS TO CARDIAC REHABILITATION

CR, as a medically supervised and physician-directed therapy, is exceedingly safe in the modern era, with a low occurrence of major cardiovascular events, in the range of 1 in 50,000 to 120,000 participants, with fatalities reported in 2 out of 1.5 million participants. The exercise portion of CR is contraindicated in patients with conditions that elevate the risk for adverse events during exercise, including the following: unstable angina; New York Heart Association (NYHA) Class IV heart failure; uncontrolled tachyarrhythmias or bradyarrhythmias; severe, symptomatic aortic or mitral stenosis; severe pulmonary hypertension myocarditis; recent systemic or pulmonary emboli; and uncontrolled hypertension at rest (systolic >200 mm Hg and/or diastolic >110 mm Hg).[28]

Supervised exercise therapy is well tolerated among patients with intermittent claudication with an excellent safety profile. However, supervised exercise therapy is contraindicated in patients suspected of having critical limb ischemia, such as patients with rest pain, nonhealing wounds, or gangrene.

LIMITATIONS OF CARDIAC REHABILITATION

Up to 80% of patients who are eligible for CR and have guideline-recommended diagnoses for CR do not get referred to CR. Furthermore, up to 48% of patients referred to CR after MI do not participate. Multiple challenges and barriers contribute to low participation of patients in CR programs.

Healthcare Access and Socioeconomic Disparities in the United States

Patient factors (gender, age, ethnicity, lack of health insurance, low socioeconomic status, low education, low health literacy or perceived need, language, cultural beliefs, work-related factors, limited social support, and home responsibilities), medical factors (complex comorbidities), and health care system factors (lack of referral, inefficient referral or follow-up process, support from referring physicians, patient-provider relationship, reimbursement, and program availability and characteristics)

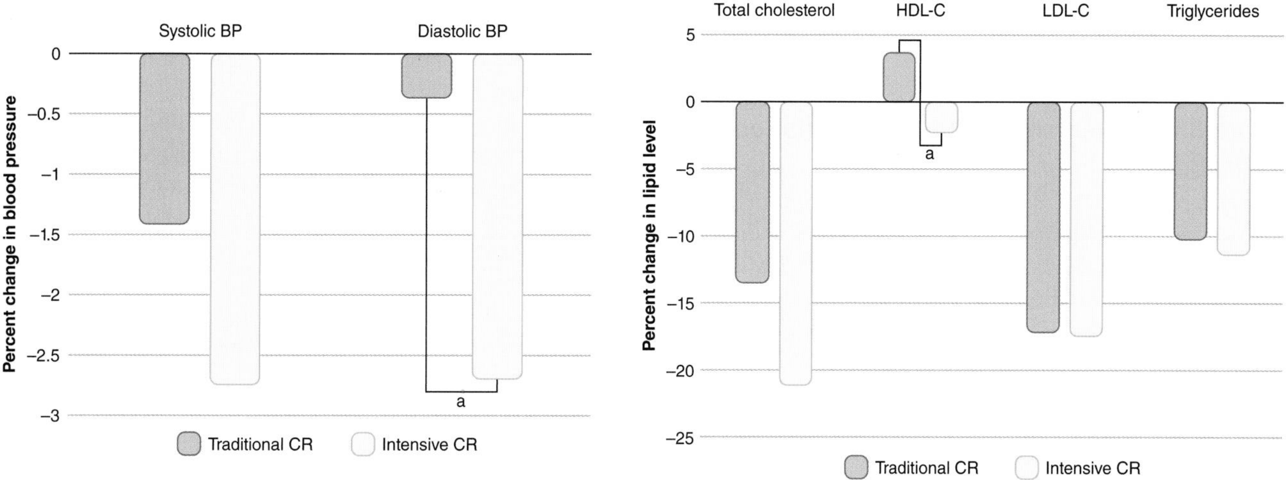

FIGURE 101.2 Cardiovascular risk factor changes during cardiac rehabilitation (CR). The left panel shows a greater decrease in systolic and diastolic blood pressure (BP) in the intensive CR group. The right panel compares changes in lipid levels in the traditional versus intensive CR group. [a]$P < .05$. HDL-C, high-density lipoprotein cholesterol; LDL-C, low-density lipoprotein cholesterol. (Reprinted with permission from Mirman AM, Nardoni NR, Chen AY, et al. Body Composition Changes During Traditional Versus Intensive Cardiac Rehabilitation in Coronary Artery Disease. *J Cardiopulm Rehabil Prev.* 2020;40(6):388-393.)

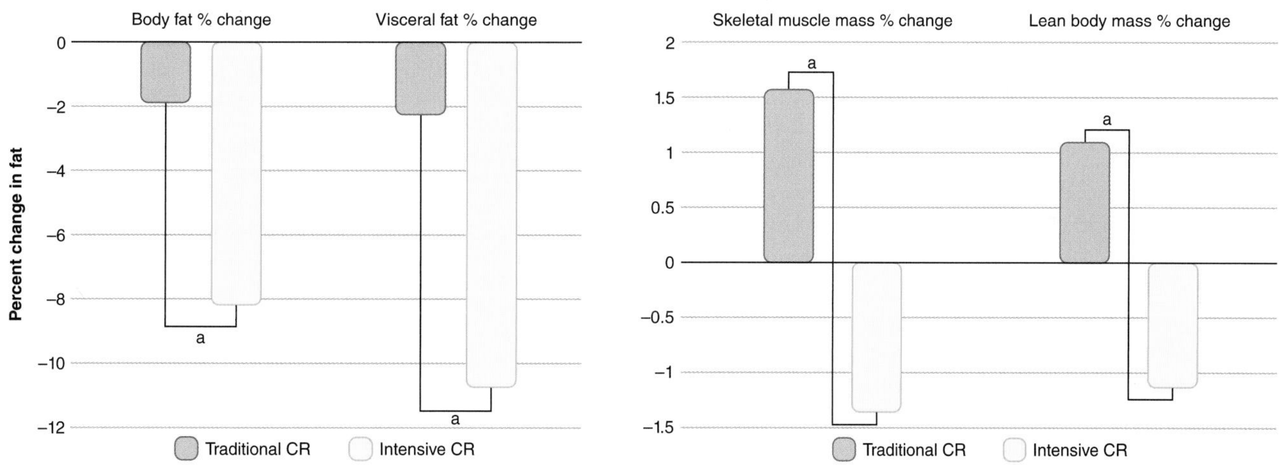

FIGURE 101.3 Body composition changes during cardiac rehabilitation (CR). The figure displays the percent changes observed in body fat, visceral adipose tissue, lean body mass, and skeletal muscle mass during the intensive and traditional CR programs. [a]$P < .05$. (Reprinted with permission from Mirman AM, Nardoni NR, Chen AY, et al. Body Composition Changes During Traditional Versus Intensive Cardiac Rehabilitation in Coronary Artery Disease. *J Cardiopulm Rehabil Prev.* 2020;40(6):388-393.)

comprise issues that still need to be addressed in order to increase participation in CR.[29,30]

Geographic variations in CR participation were shown through a comprehensive analysis of Medicare beneficiaries, which revealed the highest use states were concentrated in the North Central region of the United States with a greater than fourfold higher utilization rate in comparison to that in Southern states.[31] A 2018 study showed a wide variance of participation across states, from 3% to 42% in Medicare and 1% to 48% in Veterans Affairs populations.[32]

National analyses have historically reported underutilization of CR, which have ranged from 14% to 35%.[31,33] An updated observational study from 2020 revealed 24% of eligible Medicare beneficiaries participated in CR, with numbers decreasing with increasing age, female gender, Hispanic (37% less likely), non-Hispanic black (30% less likely), and Asian female populations. The study also noted only 27% of patients completed a full course of CR; participation was highest with a cardiac procedure–based qualifying diagnosis (35%) as opposed to those without a procedure (7%).[34] Despite the ongoing efforts to improve referral and patient participation in CR, the number of missed opportunities to improve long-term health outcomes remains significant.

Strategies to Improve Cardiac Rehabilitation Utilization

Strategies to improve CR utilization require a comprehensive analysis of the geographic area, patient population, and unique challenges that are faced by the health care delivery system. Automating the referral process, improving professional training, increasing patient and physician education, identifying and risk-stratifying eligible patients, and formalizing an integrated approach with the patient's support system and outpatient health care providers are necessary to improve patient participation and adherence. Current health care organizations are struggling to keep up with demand and balance available resources, which may allow for expansion of the role of modern technology (social media, telemedicine, and digital devices), implementation of home-based CR, and utilization of community resources through partnerships to develop hybrid programs.[29]

Home-based Cardiac Rehabilitation

Although the majority of CR in the United States is carried out at hospitals and medical centers, there is a growing number of centers offering CR remotely; patients participate from home or other remote settings and interact with CR providers virtually. Home-based CR was not reimbursed by CMS until September 2020, when both CR and intensive CR were provisionally added to the list of CMS-approved telehealth services in response to the COVID-19 pandemic.

Potential advantages of virtual CR include (1) overcoming logistic barriers such as travel time and transportation; (2) increasing the capacity of centers to enroll patients by eliminating the need for on-campus space; (3) decreasing waiting lists for CR programs; and (4) allowing for privacy and/or personalization of treatment via telehealth. Potential disadvantages include (1) less social interaction; (2) less patient accountability; (3) need for exercise space/equipment at home; and (4) concern for safety in high-risk patients.

In a recent review of studies, home-based CR had similar outcomes to traditional, hospital-based CR in terms of 1-year mortality, need for revascularization, improvement in exercise capacity and QoL, adherence to the program, and safety in low- to moderate-risk patients.[35]

KEY POINTS

- ✔ CR is a safe, effective, and integral part of the secondary prevention of cardiovascular diseases, including coronary heart disease, HFrEF, postcardiac valve surgery, and postorthotopic heart transplantation. For these indications, CR is reimbursed by CMS and most commercial insurers.
- ✔ CR is exceedingly safe in the modern era, with a low occurrence of major cardiovascular events, in the range of 1 in 50,000 to 120,000 participants, with fatalities reported as 2 out of 1.5 million participants.
- ✔ In patients with coronary heart disease, CR improves QoL and reduces cardiovascular mortality and cardiovascular hospitalizations by approximately 25%.
- ✔ Supervised exercise therapy in combination with medical therapy is an effective treatment for PAD with intermittent claudication, either as stand-alone or in conjunction with revascularization.
- ✔ Intensive CR programs offer additional hours of therapy (up to 72 hours) as well as more rigorous lifestyle modification in areas such as nutrition and psychological support and are now reimbursable through CMS and other insurers.
- ✔ CR is underutilized in the United States, with reports of only 14% to 35% of eligible patients enrolling in a program; underutilization is particularly high in women, minority populations, and underserved populations.
- ✔ Significant efforts to improve uptake and adherence to CR are critically important to boost the health and well-being of patients with cardiovascular or PAD.

REFERENCES

1. Anderson L, Thompson DR, Oldridge N, et al. Exercise-based cardiac rehabilitation for coronary heart disease. *Cochrane Database Syst Rev.* 2016; 2016(1):CD001800.
2. Mitchell JH, Levine BD, McGuire DK. The Dallas bed rest and training study. *Circulation.* 2019;140(16):1293-1295.
3. Saltin B, Blomqvist G, Mitchell JH, Johnson RL Jr, Wildenthal K, Chapman CB. Response to exercise after bed rest and after training. *Circulation.* 1968;38(suppl 5):VII1-VII78.
4. Horwich TB, Fonarow GC. Should i participate in a cardiac rehabilitation program? *JAMA Cardiol.* 2018;3(11):1136.
5. Menezes AR, Lavie CJ, Milani RV, Forman DE, King M, Williams MA. Cardiac rehabilitation in the United States. *Prog Cardiovasc Dis.* 2014; 56(5):522-529.
6. Thompson PD, Buchner D, Pina IL, et al. Exercise and physical activity in the prevention and treatment of atherosclerotic cardiovascular disease: a statement from the Council on Clinical Cardiology (Subcommittee on Exercise, Rehabilitation, and Prevention) and the Council on Nutrition, Physical Activity, and Metabolism (Subcommittee on Physical Activity). *Circulation.* 2003;107(24):3109-3116.
7. Mozaffarian D, Benjamin EJ, Go AS, et al. Heart disease and stroke statistics-2016 update: a report from the American Heart Association. *Circulation.* 2016;133(4):e38-e360.
8. Gerhard-Herman MD, Gornik HL, Barrett C, et al. 2016 AHA/ACC Guideline on the management of patients with lower extremity peripheral artery disease: executive summary. *Vasc Med.* 2017;22(3):NP1-NP43.
9. Murphy TP, Cutlip DE, Regensteiner JG, et al. Supervised exercise versus primary stenting for claudication resulting from aortoiliac peripheral artery disease: six-month outcomes from the claudication: exercise versus endoluminal revascularization (CLEVER) study. *Circulation.* 2012; 125(1):130-139.
10. Fakhry F, Spronk S, van der Laan L, et al. Endovascular revascularization and supervised exercise for peripheral artery disease and intermittent claudication: a randomized clinical trial. *JAMA.* 2015;314(18):1936-1944.
11. Patel DK, Duncan MS, Shah AS, et al. Association of cardiac rehabilitation with decreased hospitalization and mortality risk after cardiac valve surgery. *JAMA Cardiol.* 2019;4(12):1250-1259.

12. Pressler A, Christle JW, Lechner B, et al. Exercise training improves exercise capacity and quality of life after transcatheter aortic valve implantation: a randomized pilot trial. *Am Heart J.* 2016;182:44-53.
13. Flynn KE, Piña IL, Whellan DJ, et al. Effects of exercise training on health status in patients with chronic heart failure: HF-ACTION randomized controlled trial. *JAMA.* 2009;301(14):1451-1459.
14. Keteyian SJ, Isaac D, Thadani U, et al. Safety of symptom-limited cardiopulmonary exercise testing in patients with chronic heart failure due to severe left ventricular systolic dysfunction. *Am Heart J.* 2009;158(4): S72-S77.
15. Leggio M, Fusco A, Loreti C, et al. Effects of exercise training in heart failure with preserved ejection fraction: an updated systematic literature review. *Heart Fail Rev.* 2020;25(5):703-711.
16. Gardner AW, Skinner JS, Cantwell BW, Smith LK, Diethrich EB. Relationship between foot transcutaneous oxygen tension and ankle systolic blood pressure at rest and following exercise. *Angiology.* 1991;42(6):481-490.
17. Hiatt WR, Regensteiner JG, Hargarten ME, Wolfel EE, Brass EP. Benefit of exercise conditioning for patients with peripheral arterial disease. *Circulation.* 1990;81(2):602-609.
18. Treat-Jacobson D, Bronas UG, Leon AS. Efficacy of arm-ergometry versus treadmill exercise training to improve walking distance in patients with claudication. *Vasc Med.* 2009;14(3):203-213.
19. Ornish D, Brown SE, Scherwitz LW, et al. Can lifestyle changes reverse coronary heart disease? The Lifestyle Heart Trial. *Lancet.* 1990;336(8708): 129-133.
20. O'Connor CM, Whellan DJ, Lee KL, et al. Efficacy and safety of exercise training in patients with chronic heart failure: HF-ACTION randomized controlled trial. *JAMA.* 2009;301(14):1439-1450.
21. Keteyian SJ, Leifer ES, Houston-Miller N, et al. Relation between volume of exercise and clinical outcomes in patients with heart failure. *J Am Coll Cardiol.* 2012;60(19):1899-1905.
22. Pandey A, Parashar A, Kumbhani DJ, et al. Exercise training in patients with heart failure and preserved ejection fraction: meta-analysis of randomized control trials. *Circ Heart Fail.* 2015;8(1):33-40.
23. Anderson L, Nguyen TT, Dall CH, Burgess L, Bridges C, Taylor RS. Exercise-based cardiac rehabilitation in heart transplant recipients. *Cochrane Database Syst Rev.* 2017;4(4):CD012264.
24. Bachmann JM, Shah AS, Duncan MS, et al. Cardiac rehabilitation and readmissions after heart transplantation. *J Heart Lung Transplant.* 2018; 37(4):467-476.
25. Rosenbaum AN, Kremers WK, Schirger JA, et al. Association between early cardiac rehabilitation and long-term survival in cardiac transplant recipients. *Mayo Clin Proc.* 2016;91(2):149-156.
26. Freeman AM, Taub PR, Lo HC, Ornish D. Intensive cardiac rehabilitation: an underutilized resource. *Curr Cardiol Rep.* 2019;21(4):19.
27. Mirman AM, Nardoni NR, Chen AY, Horwich TB. Body composition changes during traditional versus intensive cardiac rehabilitation in coronary artery disease. *J Cardiopulm Rehabil Prev.* 2020;40(6):388-393.
28. Leon AS, Franklin BA, Costa F, et al. Cardiac rehabilitation and secondary prevention of coronary heart disease: an American Heart Association scientific statement from the Council on Clinical Cardiology (Subcommittee on Exercise, Cardiac Rehabilitation, and Prevention) and the Council on Nutrition, Physical Activity, and Metabolism (Subcommittee on Physical Activity), in collaboration with the American association of Cardiovascular and Pulmonary Rehabilitation. *Circulation.* 2005;111(3): 369-376.
29. Balady GJ, Ades PA, Bittner VA, et al. Referral, enrollment, and delivery of cardiac rehabilitation/secondary prevention programs at clinical centers and beyond: a presidential advisory from the American Heart Association. *Circulation.* 2011;124(25):2951-2960.
30. Sandesara PB, Lambert CT, Gordon NF, et al. Cardiac rehabilitation and risk reduction: time to "rebrand and reinvigorate". *J Am Coll Cardiol.* 2015;65(4):389-395.
31. Suaya JA, Shepard DS, Normand SL, Ades PA, Prottas J, Stason WB. Use of cardiac rehabilitation by Medicare beneficiaries after myocardial infarction or coronary bypass surgery. *Circulation.* 2007;116(15):1653-1662.
32. Beatty AL, Truong M, Schopfer DW, Shen H, Bachmann JM, Whooley MA. Geographic variation in cardiac rehabilitation participation in medicare and veterans affairs populations: opportunity for improvement. *Circulation.* 2018;137(18):1899-1908.
33. Centers for Disease Control and Prevention. Receipt of outpatient cardiac rehabilitation among heart attack survivors—United States, 2005. *MMWR Morb Mortal Wkly Rep.* 2008;57(4):89-94.
34. Ritchey MD, Maresh S, McNeely J, et al. Tracking cardiac rehabilitation participation and completion among medicare beneficiaries to inform the efforts of a national initiative. *Circ Cardiovasc Qual Outcomes.* 2020;13(1):e005902.
35. Thomas RJ, Beatty AL, Beckie TM, et al. Home-based cardiac rehabilitation: a scientific statement from the American Association of Cardiovascular and Pulmonary Rehabilitation, The American Heart Association, and the American College of Cardiology. *Circulation.* 2019;140(1):e69-e89.
36. Fletcher GF, Ades PA, Kligfield P, et al. Exercise standards for testing and training: a scientific statement from the American Heart Association. *Circulation.* 2013;128(8):873-934.
37. Savage PD, Lee M, Harvey-Berino J, Brochu M, Ades PA. Weight reduction in the cardiac rehabilitation setting. *J Cardiopulm Rehabil.* 2002; 22(3):154-160.
38. Soja AMB, Zwisler A-DO, Frederiksen M, et al. Use of intensified comprehensive cardiac rehabilitation to improve risk factor control in patients with type 2 diabetes mellitus or impaired glucose tolerance—the randomized DANish StUdy of impaired glucose metabolism in the settings of cardiac rehabilitation (DANSUK) study. *Am Heart J.* 2007;153(4):621-628.
39. Schwaab B, Zeymer U, Jannowitz C, Pittrow D, Gitt A. Improvement of low-density lipoprotein cholesterol target achievement rates through cardiac rehabilitation for patients after ST elevation myocardial infarction or non-ST elevation myocardial infarction in Germany: results of the PATIENT CARE registry. *Eur J Prev Cardiol.* 2019;26(3):249-258.
40. Savage PD, Brochu M, Ades PA. Gender alters the high-density lipoprotein cholesterol response to cardiac rehabilitation. *J Cardiopulm Rehabil.* 2004;24(4):248-254.
41. Salman A, Doherty P. Predictors of quitting smoking in cardiac rehabilitation. *J Clin Med.* 2020;9(8):2612.
42. Tu RH, Zeng ZY, Zhong GQ, et al. Effects of exercise training on depression in patients with heart failure: a systematic review and meta-analysis of randomized controlled trials. *Eur J Heart Fail.* 2014;16(7):749-757.

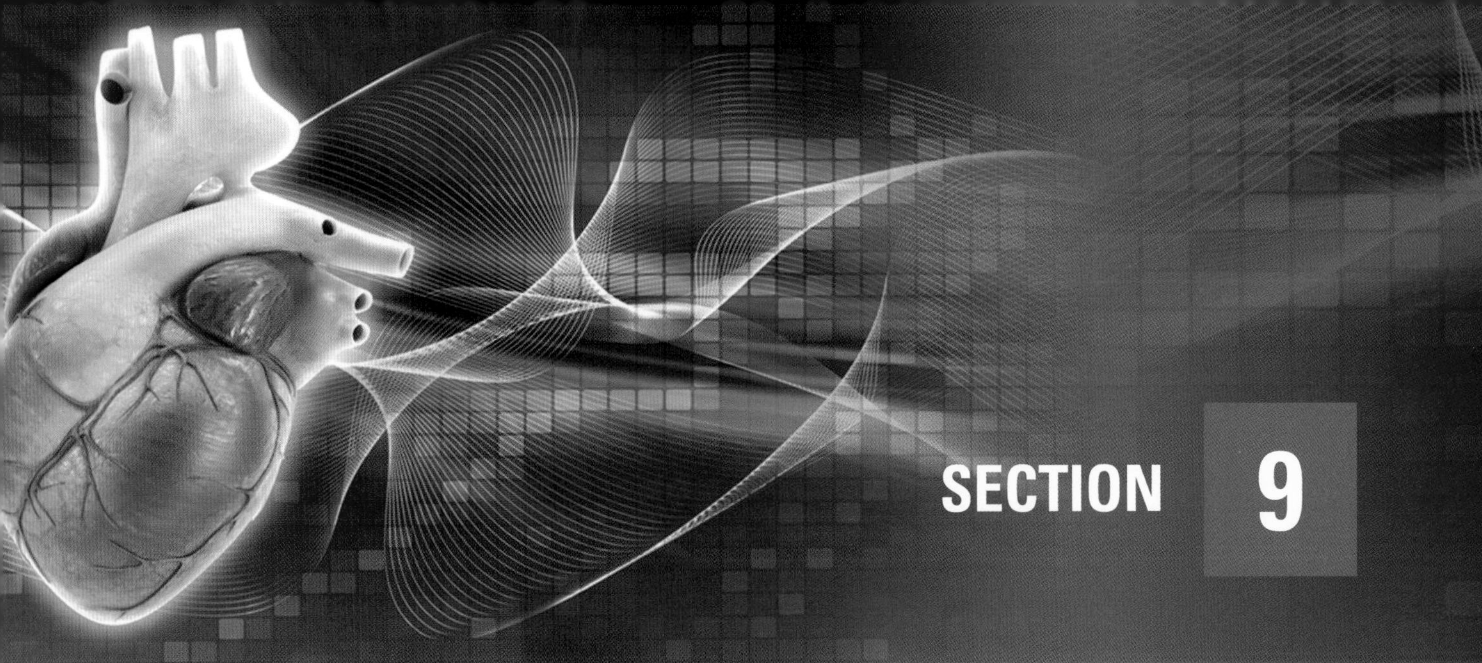

ADULT CONGENITAL HEART DISEASE

SECTION EDITOR: Karen K. Stout

CHAPTER 102

ANATOMIC AND PHYSIOLOGIC CLASSIFICATION OF CONGENITAL HEART DISEASE

David S. Majdalany and Francois Marcotte

INTRODUCTION AND CLASSIFICATIONS

Congenital heart diseases (CHD) comprise abnormalities in the cardiac anatomy that disrupt venous drainage, septation, and sequences of the cardiac segments, as well as valvular and great vessel function. The first comprehensive volume on congenital cardiac defects dates back to 1866, when Thomas B. Peacock published *Malformations of the Human Heart.* Subsequently, Maude Abbott's *Atlas of Congenital Heart Disease* correlated the clinical and pathologic findings of the congenital cardiac defects.[1,2] After the successful ligation of a patent ductus arteriosus (PDA) by Robert E Gross, in 1938, and further advancement in surgical palliation and repair of CHD, it became important to understand the nature and effects of a cardiac defect. The advent of multimodality imaging techniques and cardiac catheterization facilitated the early and accurate diagnosis of CHD.[3]

A number of classifications of CHD have been proposed, most notably the segmental approach described by Stella Van Praagh and the sequential approach described by Robert Anderson.[4,5] Both classifications aim at simplifying the complexity of CHD by dividing complexity to conquer, one level at time, in accordance with the cardiac segments identifiable during embryology. In the Van Praagh nomenclature, the sidedness (situs) of the atria, ventricles, and great vessels are determined separately; moreover, each congenital heart abnormality is assigned a 3-letter notation in parentheses. Atrial sidedness may be solitus (S), ambiguous (A), or inversus (I). Ventricular sidedness is either D-loop or solitus (S), L-loop or inversus (L), or ambiguous (X). The sidedness of the great vessels can either be solitus (S), inversus (I), D-transposition (D), L-transposition (L), or ambiguous (A). For example TGA (S,L,L) would correspond to congenitally corrected transposition of the great vessels. In this chapter, the Andersonian approach would be followed.

Normal cardiac anatomy consists of three segments: the atria, the ventricles, and the great vessels. The segments are divided into a right and a left component and arranged such that deoxygenated blood is routed to the lungs through the pulmonary artery (PA) and oxygenated blood is circulated systemically through the aorta.[6] The atrioventricular valves join the atria and the ventricles, whereas the semilunar valves serve as the connectors between the ventricles and the great vessels. For proper diagnosis of CHD, it is essential to identify the distinguishing features of the right- and left-sided structures.

CARDIAC POSITION AND AXIS

The first step in cardiac anatomic assessment is defining the heart location in the chest as well as the direction of the cardiac apex (**Figure 102.1A**). Normally, the heart is positioned in the left chest, which is referred to as levoposition. It can be altered by other associated CHD and abnormalities in the neighboring (ie, spine, lung, or diaphragmatic) structures. Dextroposition refers to the rightward shift of the heart, whereas midline shift is referred to as mesoposition.

The orientation of the base to the apex of the heart is referred to as the axis (**Figure 102.1B**). Normally, the heart is oriented inferiorly and to the left, and this is referred to as levocardia (left-sided). Dextrocardia (right-sided) refers to the orientation of the heart inferiorly and to the right, whereas mesocardia refers to the vertical and midline orientation of the heart.[7,8]

MORPHOLOGY OF THE CARDIAC SEGMENTS

Atria

The atrium is a receiving chamber lying between the systemic or pulmonary veins and the atrioventricular valves. Each atrium has a venous component, a vestibule, an appendage, and an atrial septum. The morphologic right atrium (RA) is characterized by connections to the vena cava and coronary sinus, a large pyramidal atrial appendage, numerous pectinate muscles, the crista terminalis, which is a muscular band that separates the pectinate portion from the rest of the atrium, and the limbus of the fossa ovalis (**Figure 102.2A**). On the other hand, the morphologic left atrium (LA) features a hook-shaped appendage, which may be multilobed, smooth walls with limited pectinate muscles, the valve of the fossa ovalis, pulmonary venous drainage, and the lack of a crista terminalis.[7,9]

Atrioventricular Valves

The atrioventricular valves (AV) connect the atria and the ventricles and separate them electrically. These valves travel with their respective ventricle. Hence, the mitral valve connects to the morphologic left ventricle (LV), whereas the tricuspid valve connects to the morphologic right ventricle (RV). A

A

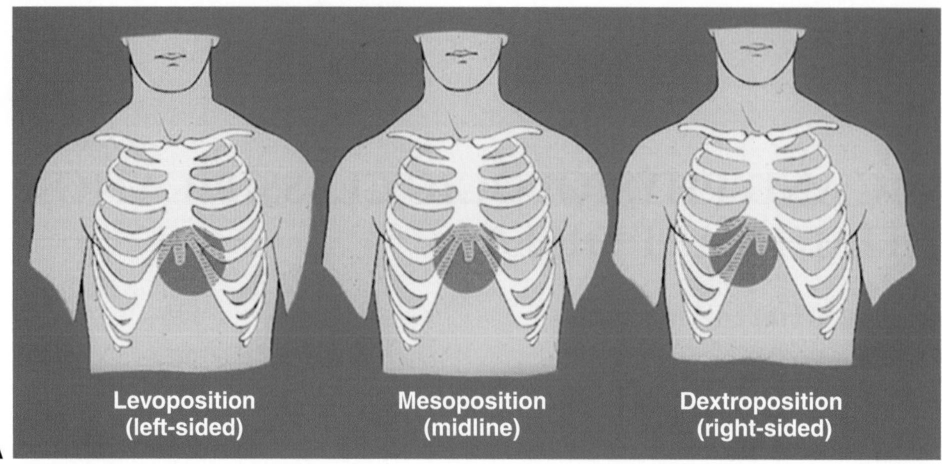

B

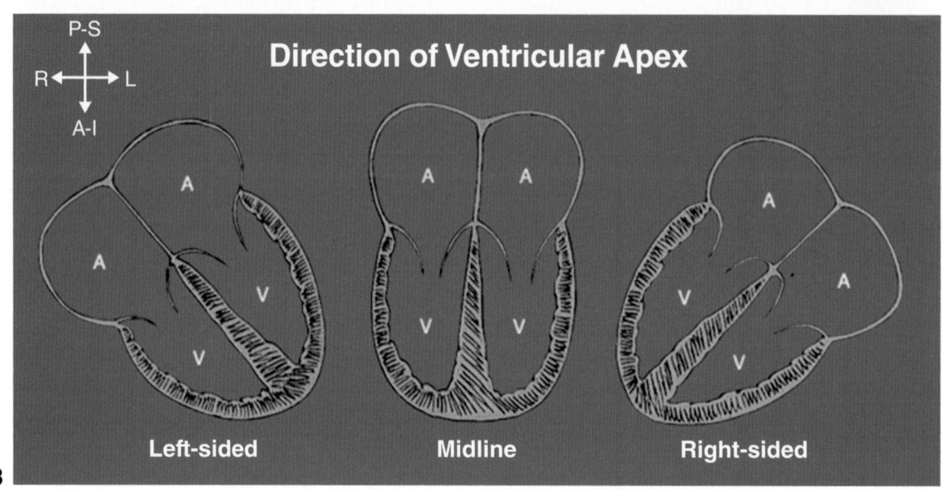

FIGURE 102.1 **(A)** Location of the heart: left-sided, midline, or right-sided. Cardiac position is determined only by the overall location of the heart relative to the anatomic midline (top). It has no relationship to the internal organization of the cardiac structures. If the majority of the heart is to the left, then the heart is in levoposition (left-sided). Conversely, if most of the heart is to the right of the midline, then we refer to the patient as having dextroposition (right-sided). When the heart is located centrally in the chest, the patient is said to have meso- or midline position. **(B)** Direction of ventricular apex. Determination of the cardiac axis requires knowledge of the internal arrangement of the heart. It refers to the right to left direction of the so-called base-to-apex axis. The apex of the heart is the ventricular apex, and the base is at the great artery origin(s). The normal base-to-apex axis is directed inferiorly and to the left (bottom right). This orientation is referred to as levocardia (left-sided). When the heart is vertically oriented and in the midline, the apex is directly inferior to the base. This situation is illustrated by the central diagram and is referred to as mesocardiac (midline). The diagram on the bottom right illustrates the concept of dextrocardia (right-sided), where the cardiac apex is inferior and to the right relative to the base. A, atrium; A-I, anterior-inferior; L, left; P-S, posterior-superior; R, right; V, ventricle. (Modified with permission from Eidem BW, O'Leary PW, Cetta F. *Echocardiography in Pediatric and Adult Congenital Heart Disease*. 2nd ed. Philadelphia, PA: Wolters Kluwer; 2014. Figure 2.10.)

very important landmark that can help distinguish the AV is the crux of the heart, where the ring of the tricuspid valve is more apically attached to the ventricular septum relative to the mitral valve annulus. Moreover, the tricuspid valve is associated with septal chordal attachments and separation from the semilunar valve by collar of muscle—the infundibulum—in contrast to the direct continuity of the mitral valve with the semilunar valve.[7]

Ventricles

Normal ventricles are characterized by three components: inlet, trabecular, and outlet regions, with no discrete boundaries between these parts. The inlet region includes the AV valve, its apparatus, and papillary muscles. The trabecular region extends from the papillary muscles to the apex, whereas the outlet portion leads toward the great vessels. The morphologic RV is typically crescent shaped and thin walled with coarse trabeculations and a moderator band. It is characterized by low septal insertion of the tricuspid valve with its septal chordal attachments and the presence of an infundibulum with resultant discontinuity between the tricuspid valve and the semilunar valve. The morphologic LV is typically circular and thick-walled in short axis. It features fine apical trabeculations, more basal ("higher") septal insertion of the mitral valve, which lacks

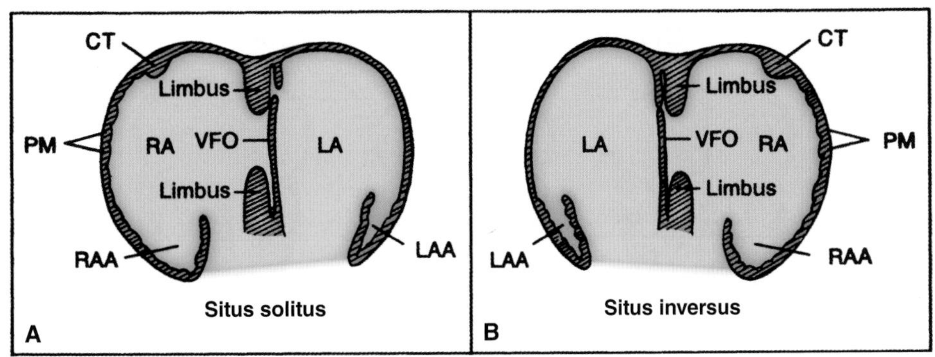

FIGURE 102.2 Cardiac-sidedness. **(A)** In *situs solitus,* the morphologic right and left atria are located in their proper side. The right and left atria are differentiated by their features. The right atrium has a large pyramidal atrial appendage, numerous pectinate muscles, the crista terminalis, and the limbus of the fossa ovalis. The morphologic LA features a hook-shaped appendage, smooth walls with limited pectinate muscles, the valve of the fossa ovalis, pulmonary venous drainage, and the lack of a crista terminalis. **(B)** *Situs inversus* is the mirror image of *situs solitus,* with the reversed position of the atria and lungs. CT, crista terminalis; LA, left atrium; LAA, left atrial appendage; PM, pectinate muscles; RA, right atrium; RAA, right atrial appendage; VFO, valve of the fossa ovalis. (Reprinted with permission from Allen HD, Driscoll DJ, Shaddy RE, et al. *Moss & Adams' Heart Disease in Infants, Children, and Adolescents: Including the Fetus and Young Adult.* 8th ed. Philadelphia, PA: Wolters Kluwer Health/ Lippincott Williams & Wilkins; 2012. Figure 2.3.)

septal chordal attachments, and continuity between the mitral and semilunar valves. In the setting of a hypoplastic ventricle where anatomic features can be difficult to discern or are absent, the rudimentary ventricle that is positioned along the anterosuperior surface of the heart is typically the morphologic RV, whereas a small chamber that occupies the postero-inferior aspect of the heart is typically the morphologic LV.[7,9]

Great Arteries

As the semilunar valves are normally fairly identical and trileaflet, the aorta and the PA are recognized by the branching patterns. The aorta typically arches to the left, traveling over the left bronchus, and gives rise to the coronary arteries as well as the head, neck, and upper extremity arteries before becoming the descending thoracic aorta. In contrast, a right aortic arch crosses over the right bronchus and is typically associated with mirror-imaging of the brachiocephalic arterial branching. The PA is recognized by its bifurcation into right and left branch PAs.[7,9]

SEQUENTIAL SEGMENTAL ANALYSIS

Cardiac Sidedness

The first step is to determine the venous return and the atrial arrangement. In *situs solitus,* the morphologic right and left atria are located in their proper side (Figure 102.2A). The superior and inferior vena cavae empty into the RA, whereas the pulmonary veins drain into the LA. Moreover, the lungs and bronchi are concordant with the trilobed right lung and short bronchus on the right side and the bilobed lung and long bronchus on the left side. *Situs inversus* is the mirror image of *situs solitus,* with the reversed position of the atria and lungs (Figure 102.2B).[6,7]

In some cases, there is no laterality, and thus the situs is ambiguous, with both atria and lungs exhibiting atriopulmonary isomerism, and this may be associated with polysplenia and asplenia syndromes with disordered arrangement of the abdominal organs (visceral heterotaxy). In right isomerism, both atria show a right morphology and imply missed development of the left morphology and are associated with asplenia, with total anomalous pulmonary venous return noted frequently. In left isomerism, both atria show a left morphology and are associated with polysplenia and an interrupted inferior vena cava with the azygous vein continuation draining into the superior vena cava.[6-9]

Atrioventricular Connections

Once atrial situs is established, the atrioventricular connections should be analyzed. AV connections can be biventricular, univentricular, or ambiguous. Ambiguous AV connections occur in the setting of right or left cardiac isomerism. Biventricular connections occur when each atrium is connected with one ventricle and can be further subdivided into concordant or discordant variants. Concordant AV junction refers to the appropriate atrium connecting to its morphologically appropriate ventricle. Discordant AV junction occurs when the RA connects to the LV and the LA connects to the RV—that is, ventricular inversion or L-looped ventricles (**Figure 102.3A**).[7]

Univentricular AV connections are characterized by both atria mostly (>75%) connecting to only one ventricle through two common or discrete AV valves. There are three patterns of univentricular AV connections: double-inlet ventricle, where two AV valves are present; single-inlet ventricle, where there is one AV valve; and common-inlet ventricle, where a common AV valve connects both atria to only one ventricle (**Figure 102.3B**). The main ventricular chamber in univentricular AV connections can either be of left, right, or indeterminate morphology. Moreover, the dominant ventricle is always associated with a rudimentary second ventricle—rudimentary morphologic RVs are typically found anterosuperiorly, whereas rudimentary morphologic LVs are located inferiorly.[6-9]

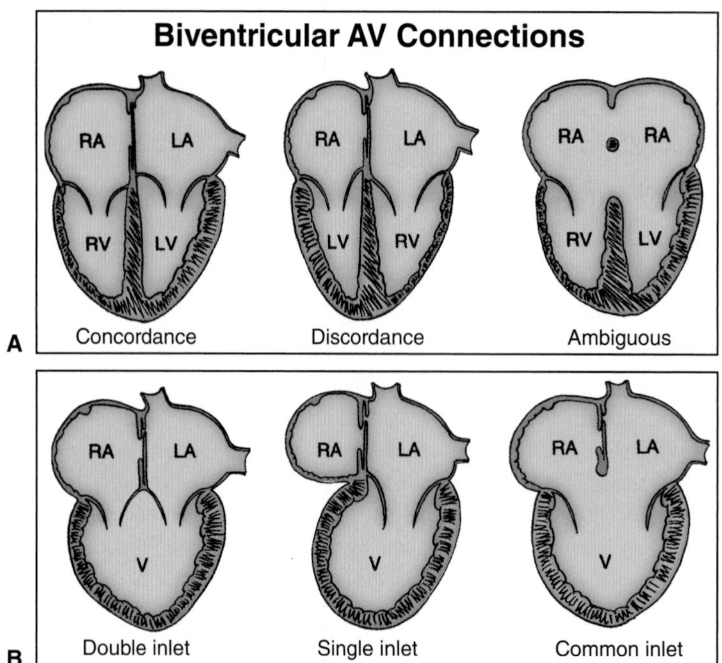

FIGURE 102.3 **(A)** Types of biventricular atrioventricular (AV) connections. The left panel refers to the normal connection that is consistent with AV concordance, where the morphologic right atrium (RA) connects to the morphologic right ventricle (RV) and the morphologic light atrium (LA) connects to the morphologic left ventricle (LV). The middle panel showcases AV discordance, where the morphologic RA connects to the morphologic LV and the morphologic LA connects to the morphologic RV. The septal insertion of the AV valves on the septum aids in the distinction between concordant and discordant AV connections. The panel on the right showcases the ambiguous AV connections, where the atrial septum is absent, the atria appear anatomically similar, and a common AV valve with no attachments to the ventricular septum. **(B)** Types of univentricular AV connections. These connections are described based on the type and number of the AV valve(s) that are related to the dominant ventricle. The left panel shows the double-inlet univentricular AV connection, where two separate atria with their own AV valves connect to a single ventricle. The middle panel shows the single-inlet univentricular AV connection, where there is atresia of one of the AV valves (either tricuspid or mitral valves). The diagram is an example of tricuspid atresia. The right panel showcases the common-inlet univentricular AV connection, where a common AV valve serves as a single-inlet/outlet from/into both atria and a single functional ventricular chamber. This can occur in the heterotaxy syndromes. (Modified with permission from Allen HD. *Moss & Adams' Heart Disease in Infants, Children, and Adolescents, Including the Fetus and Young Adult.* ©Wolters Kluwer Health and Pharma; 2016. Figure 7.14.)

The morphology of the AV valves can affect the type of AV connection. The AV valves can be atretic, common as in the case of complete atrial septal defect (ASD), straddling, or overriding. A straddling valve is characterized by the valvular apparatus inserting into the contralateral ventricle across the ventricular septum. An overriding valve refers to biventricular emptying of an AV valve and is associated with a malalignment of the atrial and ventricular septa. The degree of override determines the type of AV connection, with the valve being assigned to the ventricle receiving its larger part.[5,7]

Ventriculoarterial Connections

There are several types of ventricular arterial (VA) connections: concordant, discordant, double-outlet, single, or common outlet (**Figure 102.4**). Concordant VA connections imply that the morphologic RV gives rise to the PA, and the morphologic LV gives rise to the aorta. Discordant VA connections, which are consistent with transposition of the great vessels, are characterized by the aorta arising from the morphologic RV and a left ventricular origin of the PA. In the setting of AV concordance and VA discordance, the malformation is referred to as complete transposition of the great vessels, whereas AV and VA discordance refers to congenitally corrected transposition of the great vessels.[6-9]

Double-outlet VA connections are characterized by one arterial trunk and more than half of the other arterial trunk arising from one ventricle. This form of connection includes double-outlet LV, double-outlet RV, and most cases of Tetralogy of Fallot.[6,7]

A **single outlet VA** connection occurs when there is single patent great artery, as in the case of pulmonary atresia or aortic atresia. Moreover, a common outlet VA connection is characterized by undivided aortic and pulmonary roots, which is characteristic of truncus arteriosus.[6-9]

Just like AV valves, the morphology of the semilunar valves should be defined because they can be imperforate, regurgitant, stenotic, dysplastic, common, or overriding.

Describing the spatial relationship of the great arteries is another important anatomic assessment. The aorta is

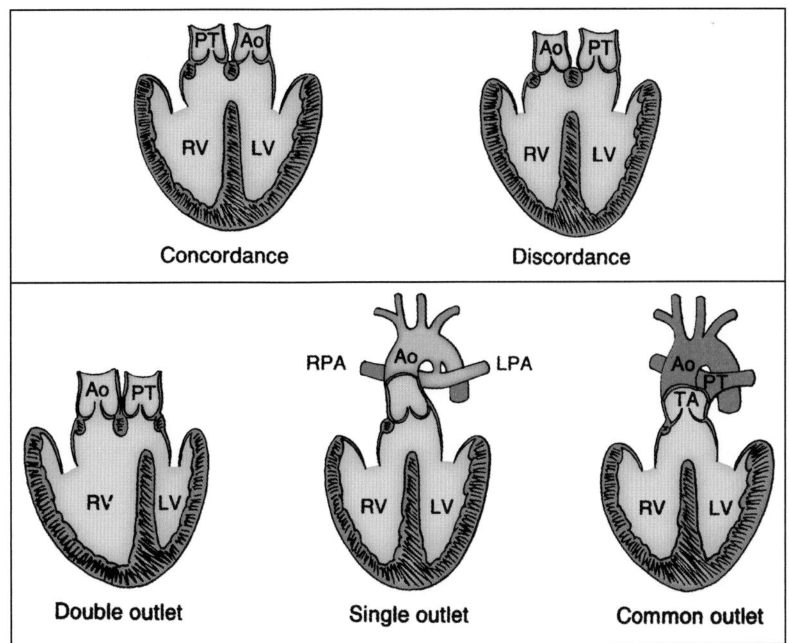

FIGURE 102.4 The five possible ventricular-arterial (VA) connections are shown schematically. Upper panel: Concordance indicates the normal state, and discordance is synonymous with transposition of the great arteries. Lower panel: There are three other possible connections: double outlet, which usually involves a right ventricle (RV); single outlet, which includes pulmonary atresia with ventricular septal defect; and common outlet, which represents truncus arteriosus (TA). Ao, aorta; LV, left ventricle; LPA, left pulmonary artery; PT, pulmonary trunk; RPA, right pulmonary artery. (Modified with permission from Allen HD. *Moss & Adams' Heart Disease in Infants, Children, and Adolescents: Including the Fetus and Young Adult.* 9th ed. Philadelphia, PA: Wolters Kluwer; 2016. Figure 7.16.)

generally described relative to the PA and is normally situated posterior and to the right of the PA. Both great vessels ascend in a spiral relationship. For the majority of CHD, the aortic position is normal or can be dextroposed, right lateral, right anterior, or left anterior. A left anterior aorta is typically encountered in double-inlet LV or congenitally corrected transposition of the great vessels, whereas a right anterior aorta is seen in complete transposition of the great vessels (often called D-TGA).

Finally, the morphology of the outflow tracts should be examined. Normally, the RV is associated with a muscular infundibulum, whereas there is continuity between the mitral and the aortic valves in the LV. Both outflow tracts can be muscular infundibulum, as is typically noted in double-outlet RV.[7,9]

Assessment of Associated Lesions

The final step of the segmental analysis is a thorough assessment of associated lesions that will impact the physiologic squeal and clinical presentations. Abnormalities involving the venous connections, atrial and ventricular septa, coronary arteries, and the aortic arch should be defined.[9]

After the cardiac anatomy is defined, it is vital to understand and discern the physiologic consequences that guide the subsequent management and proper medical, percutaneous, or surgical intervention.

PHYSIOLOGIC CLASSIFICATION OF CONGENITAL HEART DISEASE: CYANOTIC AND ACYANOTIC LESIONS

Congenital cardiac malformations affect the heart's ability to pump and separate blood from the systemic and pulmonary circulations. A clinically easily recognizable sign of heart disease is cyanosis, a bluish skin or mucosal discoloration resulting from oxyhemoglobin desaturation from the passage of deoxygenated blood into the arterial circulation. Cyanosis generally requires two conditions: first, the presence of a communication or shunt between the systemic and pulmonary circulation, at any level, and, second, the presence of a pressure gradient favorable to the passage of deoxygenated blood into the arterial circulation from obstruction to normal pulmonary blood flow.[10] This occurs either in the presence of a mechanical obstruction decreasing pulmonary blood flow or from increased pulmonary flow leading to a cascade of compensatory modifications that limit pulmonary blood flow and result in increased pulmonary pressures as coined by Victor Eisenmenger.[11] The presence or absence of cyanosis is a dichotomous characteristic to which the segmental or sequential approach can be grafted to provide a physiologic classification of CHD, proceeding from the systemic venous return through the right heart, the pulmonary circulation, the left heart, and the aorta. **Table 102.1** provides a list of the acyanotic lesions, whereas **Table 102.2** covers the cyanotic lesions.

TABLE 102.1 Acyanotic Lesions

Level	Right Heart Lesions	Left Heart Lesions
Venous	Persistent left SVC draining through coronary sinus to RA Interrupted IVC with azygos continuation	Partial anomalous pulmonary venous return to the SVC, IVC, or RA
Atrial	Atrial septal defect	Cor triatriatum
Atrioventricular	Atrioventricular septal defect (partial or complete)	Mitral stenosis (annular, valvular, parachute mitral valve)
Ventricular	Ventricular septal defect Double-chambered RV or infundibular stenosis	Discrete subaortic stenosis
Semilunar valves	Pulmonary stenosis	Congenital aortic stenosis/bicuspid/unicuspid or quadricuspid aortic valve
Great arteries	Supravalvular pulmonary stenosis Pulmonary artery sling Aortopulmonary window Patent ductus arteriosus Truncus arteriosus	Supravalvular aortic stenosis Coarctation of the aorta

IVC, inferior vena cava; RA, right atrium; RV, right ventricle; SVC, superior vena cava.

TABLE 102.2 Cyanotic Lesions

Level	Normal/Reduced Pulmonary Blood Flow	Increased Pulmonary Blood Flow
Venous	Anomalous SVC or IVC venous return to LA	Total anomalous pulmonary venous return to the RA
Atrio-ventricular	Tricuspid atresia with VA concordance and pulmonary stenosis Ebstein anomaly with atrial septal defect	Tricuspid atresia or double-inlet ventricle with VA discordance
Ventricular		Hypoplastic left heart syndrome
Semilunar valves	Pulmonary atresia with intact ventricular septum	Pulmonary atresia with VSD
Great arteries	Tetralogy of Fallot Double-outlet RV with pulmonary stenosis Classic or congenitally corrected transposition of the great vessels with pulmonary stenosis	Classic transposition of the great arteries with or without VSD

AV, atrioventricular; IVC, inferior vena cava; LA, left atrium; RA, right atrium; RV, right ventricle; SVC, superior vena cava; VA, ventriculoarterial; VSD, ventricular septal defect.

Acyanotic Congenital Heart Lesions

Acyanotic variants of systemic venous return include persistent left superior caval vein and interrupted inferior caval vein with azygos continuation. Pre-tricuspid shunts such as partial anomalous pulmonary venous return to the systemic veins or RA and interatrial shunts like ASD lead to the passage of oxygenated blood into the subpulmonary circulation under diastolic pressures and do not usually cause cyanosis, unless total anomalous pulmonary venous connection to the RA or caval veins occurs, necessitating an intracardiac shunt for initial survival.

Atrioventricular (AV) septal defects affect the crux or center of the heart at the usual insertion points of the AV valves. They may be partial (between the atria or ASD, between the ventricles or ventricular septal defect [VSD]) or complete between the atria and ventricles. Posttricuspid shunts such as complete AV septal defects, VSDs, aortopulmonary (AP) window, common arterial trunk (truncus arteriosus), or PDA lead to the passage of blood from the LV or aorta to the pulmonary artery (PA) under high pressure difference. If large or nonrestrictive, they lead to pulmonary overcirculation and vascular damage that triggers a cascade of cellular and proliferative events described by Heath & Edwards (intimal and medial hypertrophy, thrombosis and formation of neovascularization), causing eventual PA flow obstruction and a rise in central PA pressures that leads to a reversal of flow across the shunt known as the Eisenmenger syndrome. Obstructive right heart lesions like double-chambered RV or infundibular or pulmonary stenosis (PS) do not usually cause cyanosis, unless associated with a shunt situated upstream (ex. ASD). Significant pulmonary outflow tract or pulmonary arterial obstruction protects the pulmonary circulation against Eisenmenger syndrome if the shunt is situated upstream. A PA sling is an entity where the left PA originates from the right PA and may cause a vascular ring with bronchial obstruction as it passes leftward.

Obstructive or regurgitant left heart lesions are another group of acyanotic lesions that place hemodynamic load on the postcapillary circulation, sometimes leading to increased hydrostatic pressures and cardiogenic pulmonary edema and secondary pulmonary hypertension. Cor triatriatum is an obstructive midleft atrial membrane resulting from insufficient posterior left atrial wall resorption during fusion of the pulmonary venous buds to the primitive LA. Congenital mitral stenosis results from either annular and leaflet or subvalvular apparatus (parachute mitral valve) maldevelopment. Left ventricular (LV) outflow tract obstructions such as discrete subaortic stenosis, congenital aortic stenosis, bicuspid aortic valve, supravalvular aortic stenosis, and coarctation of the aorta complete the picture of obstructive acyanotic left heart congenital cardiovascular lesions that place a hemodynamic afterload on the LV. Aortic arch anomalies like aberrant subclavian vessels and double aortic arch may produce vascular rings around the trachea and esophagus from anomalous arterial course (Table 102.2).

Cyanotic Congenital Heart Lesions with Decreased Pulmonary Blood Flow

Anomalies in this category present the combination of a shunt lesion and an obstruction to pulmonary blood flow, protecting the cardiovascular circulation from Eisenmenger syndrome.[11] Anomalies in tricuspid valve leaflet migration during cardiac development such as those described by Wilhelm Ebstein lead to caudal septal and posterior leaflet displacement with variable degrees of tethering to the ventricular wall and tricuspid insufficiency or stenosis, which, in the presence of a patent foramen ovale (PFO) or ASD, lead to right to left shunting.[12] Complete tricuspid atresia requires an ASD, because complete obstruction to the RV is present with right ventricular hypoplasia, typically with subpulmonary stenosis and/or PS and ventriculoarterial (VA) concordance (the hypoplastic RV is connected to the PA, and the LV is connected to the aorta). Tetralogy of Fallot results from anterior malalignment of the conal septum and aortic root, leading to pulmonary outflow tract compression with variable degrees of hypoplasia, PS, and VSD. The RV is thus challenged by pulmonary outflow obstruction and exposure to systemic pressures with diminished pulmonary flow and compensated by free wall RV hypertrophy. Left-sided abnormalities causing cyanosis are rare but include partial anomalous (typically superior caval) systemic venous return to the LA.

Cyanotic Congenital Heart Lesions with Increased Pulmonary Blood Flow

Anomalies in this category present the combination of a large, typically posttricuspid shunt lesion without impedance to pulmonary blood flow, leading to pulmonary overcirculation and to Eisenmenger syndrome. Total anomalous pulmonary venous return leads to increased pulmonary blood flow because both systemic and pulmonary venous return are ultimately directed to the RA. Because no pulmonary venous return directly enters the LA, the interatrial septum must remain patent, conducting a mixture of oxygenated and deoxygenated blood from the pulmonary and caval veins into the systemic circulation. A **double-inlet ventricle** receives two AV valves carrying both systemic and pulmonary venous returns in the presence of an ASD because the RV is not connected directly to either AV valve. Double-inlet ventricle typically occurs with VA discordance or transposition of the great vessels with little impedance to pulmonary flow. Occasionally, tricuspid atresia can occur with VA discordance and typically little pulmonary outflow obstruction, also resulting in pulmonary overcirculation. In double-inlet LV and tricuspid atresia with VA discordance, the hypoplastic RV is a small subaortic chamber separated from the LV by a VSD (also called bulboventricular foramen), whereas the LV is connected to the PA. Pulmonary valve atresia is another cyanotic condition that may occur with or without associated VSD. The pulmonary circulation is palliated either by pulmonary arteries arising from the aorta (truncus arteriosus) or by hyperdevelopment of the bronchial circulation in the form of aortopulmonary collateral arteries. If uncorrected, these will cause cyanosis and increased pulmonary blood flow with rapid development of pulmonary hypertension.

Transposition of the great arteries (TGA) is a generally cyanotic condition with two major subtypes described: classic (or complete or D-TGA) and congenitally corrected. In classic TGA, there is AV concordance (the RA is connected to the RV, and the LA is connected to the LV) with VA discordance (the RV is connected to the aorta, and the LV is connected to the PA). Because deoxygenated blood is directed to the aorta and oxygenated blood to the PA, survival is dependent on the presence of an intra- or extracardiac shunt to enable some oxygenated blood to gain access to the systemic circulation, usually leading to pulmonary overcirculation (especially if a VSD or PDA is present), unless significant pulmonary valve stenosis is present.

Congenitally corrected TGA may be either cyanotic or acyanotic depending on associated lesions and is discussed separately. Left-sided abnormalities causing cyanosis and pulmonary overcirculation include, most notably, hypoplastic left heart syndrome, a condition incompatible with life where the LV and aorta are severely hypoplastic and the systemic and pulmonary circulation are dependent on the RV and, respectively, the ductus arteriosus and pulmonary arteries.

Cyanotic Congenital Heart Lesions That May Present Decreased or Increased Pulmonary Blood Flow

Double-outlet RV is another conotruncal abnormality where both great vessels arise from the RV with a VSD as sole exit from the LV. As the systemic venous return is directed to the RV, communication to both great vessels causes deoxygenated blood to have access to the aorta and cause cyanosis. In the absence of pulmonary outflow tract obstruction with the VSD lying immediately below the aortic valve, the physiology is similar to a VSD (with increased pulmonary blood flow), but if subpulmonary stenosis or PS is present, it resembles Tetralogy of Fallot (cyanotic with reduced pulmonary blood flow). In patients with a subpulmonary VSD, the physiology resembles classic TGA with pulmonary overcirculation unless PS is present with reduced pulmonary blood flow.

Congenital Heart Lesions That May Be Cyanotic or Acyanotic

Congenitally corrected transposition of the great arteries (CCTGA) is characterized by AV discordance (the RA is connected to a right-sided morphologic LV, and the LA is connected to a left-sided morphologic RV) with VA discordance (the right-sided LV is connected to the PA, and the left-sided RV is connected to the aorta). This arrangement ensures systemic venous blood is directed to the PA and pulmonary venous blood to the aorta, and hence the congenital correction. It is often associated with cardiac malrotation and mesocardia (midline heart) or dextrocardia (rightward heart). If no VSD or PS is present, the condition is acyanotic, may be associated with Ebstein-like abnormality of the left-sided tricuspid valve and regurgitation. If an isolated VSD is present, the condition resembles a simple VSD and depends on defect size to cause pulmonary arterial damage, and if isolated severe PS, the condition resembles a simple PS. If severe PS and VSD are present, cyanosis with decreased pulmonary blood flow ensues.

KEY POINTS

- ✔ The advancement in the diagnosis and intervention of CHD necessitated the understanding of the nature and effects of a cardiac defect. The advent of multimodality imaging techniques and cardiac catheterization facilitated the early and accurate diagnosis of CHD.
- ✔ Sequential segmental analysis of the heart facilitates the evaluation of the patient with suspected congenital cardiac anomalies and facilitates the anatomic classification of CHD.
- ✔ The heart can be divided into three levels: atria, ventricles, and the great vessels. Systematically, right-sided and left-sided structures at each level are assessed based on their positions, morphology, their connections to proximal and distal segments, and associated abnormalities such as shunts or obstruction.
- ✔ After the cardiac anatomy is defined, it is vital to understand and discern the physiologic consequences that guide the subsequent management.
- ✔ The physiologic classification of CHD can be based on the presence or absence of cyanosis. Cyanotic cardiac abnormalities can be associated with either increased pulmonary blood flow or decreased pulmonary blood flow.

REFERENCES

1. Rosenblum R. A classification of congenital heart disease: a physiologic approach. *Am J Cardiol.* 1963;12:126-128.
2. Abbot M. *Atlas of Congenital Heart Disease.* 1st ed. McGill-Queen's University Press; 2006.
3. Sauvage LR, Mansfield PB, Stamm SJ. Physiologic classification of congenital heart disease. *AORN J.* 1973;18(1):61-83.
4. Van Praagh R. The segmental approach to diagnosis in congenital heart disease. In: Bergsma D, ed. *Birth Defects Original Article Series. Vol. VIII, No 5. The National Foundation-March of Dimes.* Williams and Wilkins; 1972:4-23.
5. Anderson RH, Wilcox BR. How should we optimally describe complex congenitally malformed hearts? *Ann Thorac Surg.* 1996;62:710-716.
6. Thiene G, Frescura C. Anatomical and pathophysiological classification of congenital heart disease. *Cardiovasc Pathol.* 2010;19(5):259-274.
7. Allen HD, Shaddy RE, Penny DJ, et al. *Moss & Adams' Heart Disease in Infants, Children, and Adolescents, Including the Fetus and Young Adult.* 9th ed. Wolters Kluwer; 2016.
8. Eidem BW, O'Leary PW, Cetta F. *Echocardiography in Pediatric and Adult Congenital Heart Disease.* 2nd ed. Wolters Kluwer; 2015.
9. Gatzoulis MA, Webb GD, Daubeney PE. *Diagnosis and Management of Adult Congenital Heart Disease.* 3rd ed. Elsevier; 2018.
10. Wood P. The Eisenmenger syndrome or pulmonary hypertension with reversed central shunt. *Br Med J.* 1958;2:755-762.
11. Eisenmenger V. Inborn defects of ventricular partition of heart. *Z Klin Med.* 1897;32(suppl 1):1-28.
12. Ebstein W. On a very rare case of insufficiency of the tricuspid valve cause by a severe congenital malformation of the same. *Arch F Anat Physiol Wissensch Med Leipz.* 1866:238. translated by Scheiebler GL, Gravenstein JS, Van Mierop LHS. *Am J Cardiol.* 1968;22:867.

CHAPTER 103

EVALUATION OF SUSPECTED AND KNOWN ADULT CONGENITAL HEART DISEASE

Andrew R. Pistner and Anitra W. Romfh

INTRODUCTION

Epidemiology

Congenital heart disease (CHD) is the most common birth defect. The prevalence of CHD varies between 4 and 10 cases per 100 births and eventually 6 per 1000 in the adult population.[1,2] In one study, adult congenital heart disease (ACHD) was found to be slightly more prevalent in women than in men.[1] In addition, shunt lesions such as atrial septal defect (ASD), ventricular septal defect (VSD), patent ductus arteriosus (PDA), or atrioventricular (AV) septal defects were found to be more common in women. In contrast, transposition of the great arteries (complete and congenitally corrected) and aortic coarctation are more commonly found in men.[2]

With the increasing success of surgical and medical treatment of CHD in the pediatric age group, more patients with CHD are living to adulthood. More than 1.4 million adults are living with CHD, and this number is expected to increase with this shift in prevalence from children to adults.

Risk Factors

Various risk factors increase the probability of CHD such as patient genetics, maternal characteristics, and prenatal exposures. Much of the data describing these risk factors come from retrospective, population-based studies. The association between these risk factors and CHD is nonspecific in relation to the individual defects.

The presence of maternal CHD is associated with an increased risk of CHD in their offspring estimated at 4% to 5%.[3] The risk to offspring varies significantly among the cardiac defects but is at least twice as great when compared to mothers without CHD.[3] Maternal diabetes is associated with an increased risk of CHD in their offspring.[4] Pregestational diabetes mellitus is associated with an increased risk of conotruncal defects, D-transposition of the great arteries, AV septal defects, heterotaxy syndromes, and single ventricle physiology.[4-6] The risk of CHD is greater in offspring of women with preexisting diabetes compared to those who develop gestational diabetes.[6] In the National Birth Defects Prevention Study, tobacco use in the periconceptional period and first trimester of pregnancy was associated with an increased risk of right-sided obstructive cardiac defects as well as both ASDs and VSDs.[7] Maternal use of certain medications in the periconceptional period and first trimester of pregnancy has also been associated with an increased risk of CHD; folic acid antagonists, such as methotrexate, are associated with a twofold increase in CHD [4]. The association between maternal lithium use and Ebstein anomaly in the fetus was described in the early 1970s,[8] and more contemporary studies continue to show an increased risk ratio of 2.6.[9]

Genetic Syndromes

Various syndromic and nonsyndromic abnormalities are associated with CHD. With advances in genetic testing, diagnosis of these conditions in the pediatric period has become more common. However, patients with more subtle phenotypes of these syndromes may elude diagnosis into adulthood. The recognition of the features of these syndromes and their associated conditions provides direction in the evaluation of suspected CHD.

SYNDROMES ASSOCIATED WITH CONGENITAL HEART DISEASE

Down syndrome is the most common chromosomal abnormality associated with CHD and is most frequently caused by trisomy 21. Patients with this condition have facial dysmorphism, short stature, and cognitive defects. CHD is found in 40% to 50% of patients with Down syndrome, with the most common defects being AV septal defects, VSD, and ASD. Tetralogy of Fallot and PDA are seen more rarely. The adult patient with Down syndrome needs screening for comorbidities including sleep apnea, hypothyroidism, diabetes mellitus, and obesity which exacerbate cardiac disease. Evidence-based guidelines on the medical management of the adult with Down syndrome have recently been published.[10]

Turner syndrome is caused by a complete or partial absence of one of the X chromosomes and only affects females. Features of this syndrome include short stature, primary ovarian insufficiency, and a webbed neck. Cardiac manifestations of Turner syndrome include coarctation of the aorta and bicuspid aortic valve. Care of these patients benefits from a multidisciplinary approach with close involvement of cardiologists, endocrinologists, and gynecologists.[11]

DiGeorge syndrome is characterized by deficiency or absence of the thymus and or parathyroid gland, craniofacial defects, and cardiac defects. Ninety percent of patients with DiGeorge syndrome have a microdeletion of chromosome 22. The most common defects seen with 22q11 deletion include tetralogy of Fallot, interrupted aortic arch type B, truncus arteriosus, conoventricular VSDs, and other aortic arch abnormalities.[12] Mild cognitive impairment and neuropsychiatric disease including schizophrenia are commonly seen in adult patients with DiGeorge syndrome and should be screened for as part of their care for early intervention and prevention of gaps in care.[13] Given the autosomal dominant pattern of inheritance, women with suspected DiGeorge syndrome should be offered genetic testing in their preconception counseling visits.

Williams syndrome is an autosomal dominant condition caused by the deficiency of elastin and LIM kinase with a phenotypic presentation consisting of cardiac defects, infantile hypercalcemia, skeletal and kidney abnormalities, cognitive defects, and a "social personality." CHD occurs in approximately 75% of children with Williams syndrome, and the most frequent defect is supravalvar aortic stenosis, often with concomitant coronary artery abnormalities; pulmonary artery stenosis is the second most common cardiovascular abnormality. Ninety percent of patients present with a microdeletion of chromosome 7q11.23. Cognitive performance declines earlier in patients with Williams syndrome compared with the general population,[14] and this should be kept in mind with the adult patient.

Alagille syndrome is also an autosomal dominant condition and has features of cholestasis, skeletal and facial abnormalities along with cardiac defects such as peripheral pulmonary artery hypoplasia/atresia, tetralogy of Fallot, pulmonary stenosis, ASD, and VSD and is often associated with mutations in the *JAG1* gene. Adult patients with Alagille syndrome require a multidisciplinary approach, given that liver disease and nutrition are significantly impacted.

Noonan syndrome patients often present with short stature, facial dysmorphism, webbed neck, and chest deformity. Associated CHD includes valvar pulmonic stenosis, AV septal defect, aortic coarctation, and hypertrophic cardiomyopathy. The majority of Noonan cases are owing to mutations in the protein tyrosine phosphatase nonreceptor type 11 (*PTPN11*) gene.

The last major genetic syndrome associated with CHD is **Holt-Oram syndrome**, an autosomal dominant syndrome consisting of upper extremity defects (often hypoplastic or absent thumb) along with cardiac abnormalities such as an ASD or VSD. This syndrome is commonly caused by mutations in the T-box 5 (TBX5) transcription factor.[12]

The **VACTERL** association is the clinical description of various combinations of six conditions (supplying the acronym): vertebral defects, anal atresia, cardiac defects, tracheoesophageal fistula, renal anomalies, and limb anomalies. Cardiac anomalies are common in the VACTERL association relative to the other components, with VSDs being the most common cardiac defect.[15] Unlike the conditions described above, the genetics and causative etiology are not well understood at this time.

CLINICAL PRESENTATION

Patient History

The details of a patient's initial diagnosis and treatment of CHD may be provided by the patient or a parent and collateral history is key, as patients themselves may not know or recall the decision-making regarding childhood surgeries. It is important to elicit exercise tolerance from childhood and adolescent activities (ie, physical education, sports) with respect to peers. This is key in both the undiagnosed patient who may be referred for suspected disease in adulthood (such as an ASD) and in the patient with known CHD to bring out a gradual change that has occurred as a result of a previously dormant lesion. One of the most important "stress tests" in adulthood for women is the tolerance of pregnancy and provides clues as to the impact of a specific lesion on functional status.

In addition, obtaining the operative reports from the originating institution may provide a wealth of details regarding both the patient's initial presentation and the intracardiac anatomy that influenced one surgical procedure over another. The past often informs the future, and these details are essential in planning subsequent surgical and percutaneous interventions. Of note, female patient records will often require searching under a maiden name if a name change has occurred in adulthood through marriage, for example.

Physical Examination

Vital Signs

Vital signs can provide clues to underlying CHD and alert to alterations in cardiac physiology of those with known CHD. For example, a resting heart rate at the upper limit of normal in an atriopulmonary Fontan patient may heighten suspicion of an arrhythmia despite the seemingly "slow" rate, given the intra-atrial conduction delay. Baseline oximetry is an important measure, and additional measurement of pulse oximetry with ambulation provides information regarding latent ventilation/perfusion mismatch.

Four-Limb Blood Pressure

Measurement of blood pressure is part of the routine physical examination for patients with both acquired and CHD. In patients with known or suspected CHD, measurement of blood pressure in both arms, and at least one—but preferably both—leg provides a noninvasive assessment of the presence of aortic and peripheral arterial pathology. The systolic blood pressure should not differ more than 10 mm Hg between both arms. The presence of a greater arm blood pressure differential may be seen in left subclavian artery stenosis and aortic coarctation that is proximal to the left subclavian artery. Similarly, blood pressure in the lower extremities should be greater than that in the upper extremities owing to pulse wave amplification. Should the lower extremity blood pressure be lower by 20 mm Hg or more, the presence of aortic coarctation or restenosis after repair of coarctation should be suspected.[16] With the increased use of percutaneous procedures for the treatment of CHD and repeated femoral arterial access, the presence of a unilateral (usually right-sided) decreased blood pressure in a leg raises the possibility of femoral artery stenosis.

Inspection

Cyanosis is an abnormal blue discoloration of the skin and mucosa. Physiologically, cyanosis is the result of an increased absolute amount of deoxygenated hemoglobin present at the level of the capillaries. As such, the presence of cyanosis is dependent on the hemoglobin concentration (ie, a patient with increased hemoglobin may have a greater amount of deoxygenated hemoglobin compared to a patient with anemia).[17] As such, cyanosis in anemic patients may elude the examiner. Central cyanosis is most easily appreciated in the gums and mucosa of the mouth where there is dense capillary structure, whereas peripheral manifestations may only be seen through clubbing. Digital clubbing is the focal swelling of the distal phalanx resulting from the growth of connective tissue.[18] Clubbing can be the result of long-standing cyanosis but is also seen in other etiologies including malignancy, pulmonary disease, infection, inflammatory disease, and certain genetic conditions. Differential cyanosis (normal saturation of the upper extremity with lower saturation in the lower extremity) should raise the suspicion for a PDA with Eisenmenger physiology and in these patients, a toe saturation should be part of the routine examination.

Visualization of the jugular venous wave in the neck provides an estimation of the right atrial filling pressures and is a useful tool in evaluating suspected or known CHD, with a few caveats. In those patients with large and compliant right atrium, such as that seen in Ebstein anomaly, the pressure generated through the cardiac cycle may not be well transferred into the internal jugular veins. Similarly, the presence of stenosis between the internal jugular vein and the right atrium may also affect the appearance of the jugular venous pulse or may give clues to superior vena cava syndrome owing to systemic baffle obstruction in a patient with known complete transposition repaired by the atrial switch procedure. These patients may appear normal when seated upright on the exam table but may display a plethora of the head and neck when lying supine.

The presence of a pectus deformity of the chest may be seen in patients with CHD. Pectus excavatum or carinatum may be observed. There is also an increased incidence of scoliosis in patients with CHD.[19] Early literature indicated that scoliosis was more prevalent in cyanotic forms of CHD,[20] but the etiology is multifactorial.[21] In addition, chest asymmetry with a left parasternal bulge may indicate a right ventricular pressure or volume condition prior to maturation of the ribs.[22]

The presence of surgical scars provides a road map to the patient's previous surgeries. A median sternotomy is used in most CHD surgical procedures, and the presence of a right thoracotomy is commonly used in a right-sided Blalock-Thomas-Taussig (BTT) shunt. A left thoracotomy may indicate repair of coarctation of the aorta or that a left BTT shunt was performed in a patient with a right aortic arch.[26] Of note, both a BTT shunt and coarctation repaired by subclavian flap have been associated with ipsilateral Horner syndrome, so a careful neurologic examination must be documented once a thoracotomy scar is found.[23,24] In addition, accompanying growth asymmetry or restriction may be seen on the same side as the thoracotomy scar. A clamshell incision may have been employed with more complex cardiopulmonary lesions for improved exposure.[25] With advances in percutaneous treatments, some patients may not have scars aside from those related to vascular access. It is important to note areas of prior vascular cutdown as this may negatively impact future percutaneous access. (See **Figure 103.1.**)

Palpation

Palpation of the chest reveals the point of maximal impulse, which is associated with the apex of the ventricles. This can be used to identify cardiac position within the left or right hemithorax in addition to other examination maneuvers. In patients with levocardia, the point of maximal impulse is located approximately at the fifth intercostal space, along the midclavicular line.[27] The intensity, location, size, and duration of the point of maximal impulse may help identify cardiomegaly, as in other cardiology patients. Palpation of the parasternal area may reveal a precordial impulse that is variably referred to as a heave, lift, or thrust which suggests the presence of right ventricular pressure or volume overload.[28] In patients with pulmonary hypertension with an enlarged pulmonary artery, a "tap" may be felt near the left midclavicular line near the second interspace.

Palpation of the upper abdomen identifies the position of the liver, which may be helpful in the heterotaxy patient with the recognition that the liver may occupy a position other than the right upper quadrant. The presence of hepatomegaly and tenderness with palpation indicates congestion of the liver. Pulsatility may also be seen in this scenario when there is concomitant tricuspid valve disease (either regurgitation or stenosis). If known cirrhosis is present, such as in a Fontan patient, one should palpate for the presence of splenomegaly, which would be indicative of portal hypertension.

Peripheral pulses may be abnormal in patients with CHD. For example, a diminished or absent brachial or radial pulse suggests a previous ipsilateral classic BTT shunt or subclavian flap repair of aortic coarctation. In this situation, if blood pressure is taken on the ipsilateral side of the scar, it may be notably low owing to collateralization. As such, patients should be educated to instruct medical providers to avoid blood pressure cuff measurement and arterial lines in this arm. The presence of a radio-femoral or brachio-femoral delay is critical in evaluating a patient with suspected coarctation of the aorta or re-stenosis following repair of this condition, because the presence of collateral vessels in a chronic coarctation may mask an upper to lower blood pressure gradient. In patients with severe native coarctation of the aorta, the dorsalis pedis and posterior tibialis pulses may be diminished and only detectable with the use of a Doppler probe.

Auscultation

Auscultation is a central part of the cardiac examination. The traditional four locations of cardiac auscultation must be adapted to the location and orientation of the heart within the

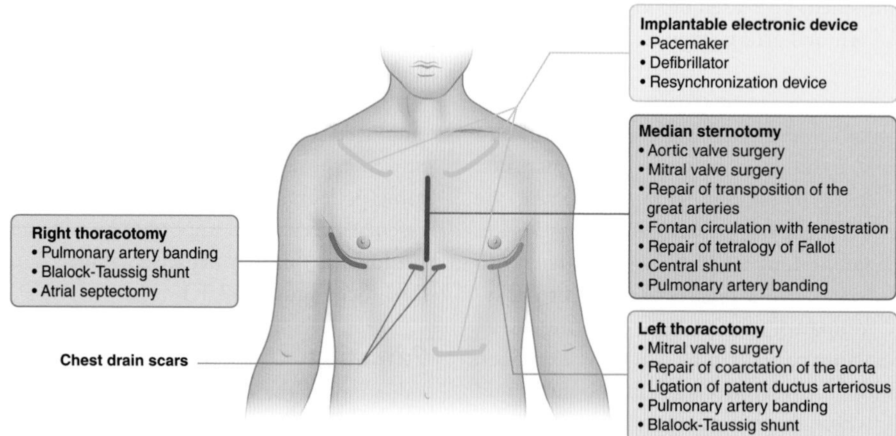

FIGURE 103.1 Recognizing past heart surgery. (Redrawn from Pandya B, Cullen S, Walker F. Congenital heart disease in adults. *BMJ.* 2016;354:i3905.)

chest in patients with CHD. As such, the presence of "distant heart sounds" near the left fifth intercostal space at the midclavicular line may actually be the result of dextrocardia, and heart sounds should be auscultated on the right chest instead.

The first heart sound (S1) corresponds to the closure of the mitral and tricuspid valves. S1 intensity is increased in mitral stenosis and high cardiac output states such as anemia and pregnancy. Decreased intensity of S1 is seen in first-degree AV block, and a variable S1 intensity is seen in complete heart block and atrial fibrillation. The presence of a mechanical valve will produce a high-frequency and characteristically "crisp" closure sound. If the mechanical valve is in the mitral position, valve closure occurs with S1, and in the aortic position, the crisp closure sound should occur with the second heart sound (S2). Decreased intensity in the closing sound or "muffling" of the closing sound is associated with valve thrombosis.

S2 corresponds to the closure of the aortic and pulmonic valves. The pulmonic component (P2) of S2 may be loud in patients with pulmonary hypertension. However, in patients with transposition of the great arteries, with the aorta lying anterior to the pulmonary artery and thus more proximal to the chest wall, a prominent aortic component (A2) of S2 will be heard. With normal AV conduction, physiologic splitting of S2 occurs with the A2 occurring prior P2. The splitting of S2 increases with inspiration related to prolonged right ventricular ejection owing to increased venous return and increased right ventricular volume. A widely split S2 occurs with an increased interval between A2 and P2 when there is a delayed or prolonged right ventricular ejection phase such as seen in right bundle branch block or pulmonary stenosis, respectively. The interval between A2 and P2 increases with inspiration as it does in physiologic splitting but is not eliminated with expiration. In fixed splitting of S2, the A2-P2 interval does not change with inspiration or expiration. This finding is commonly seen in unrepaired ASD. In these patients, P2 is delayed owing to the increased volume load of the right ventricle caused by left-to-right shunting. With diastolic pressure equalization, however, inspiration does not further augment right ventricular filling resulting in a "fixed" A2-P2 interval.[29] Conversely, a paradoxical or reverse splitting of S2 occurs where there is delayed closure of the aortic valve, as seen in the left bundle branch block and aortic stenosis.

The principles and interpretation of cardiac murmurs in normal anatomy apply in CHD. The difference in auscultation in a patient with CHD is to keep in mind concomitant or associated lesions. In addition, new or unexpected murmurs should prompt an evaluation for endocarditis. Common midsystolic murmurs in patients with normally related great arteries include pulmonary stenosis heard best at the left second and third interspaces with radiation to the interscapular area and aortic stenosis heard best at the right second interspace with radiation to the neck.

Common holosystolic murmurs include tricuspid and mitral regurgitation, heard best at the left sternal border and left apex, respectively. These murmurs may change locations and intensity in a patient with congenitally corrected transposition, for example, where L-looped ventricles displace systemic tricuspid regurgitation laterally to the left, and the murmur sounds harsher than traditional mitral regurgitation. Pressure-restrictive VSDs exhibit a harsh, holosystolic murmur as flow goes from a high- to low-pressure chamber. Keeping in mind "the company it keeps," concomitant aortic regurgitation may indicate that the VSD is supracristal, owing to prolapse of an aortic valve cusp. The presence of a continuous murmur in the setting of a patient with a known membranous VSD may alert the clinician to the presence of a concomitant ruptured sinus of Valsalva aneurysm. Another type of continuous murmur in an ACHD patient is a small or moderate-sized unrepaired PDA with normal vascular resistance and radiation to the back. The back can also be an important site of auscultation for aortopulmonary collaterals in the patient with tetralogy of Fallot and pulmonary atresia.

Common diastolic murmurs include aortic and pulmonary regurgitation, heard best at the left lower sternal border. A common "to and fro" murmur in a tetralogy of Fallot patient repaired by transannular patch with severe pulmonary regurgitation may consist of a loud, mid-peaking systolic murmur at the left upper sternal border (the "to" component) followed by a short, diastolic murmur in diastole (the "fro" component). After bioprosthetic pulmonary valve placement, in contrast, the murmur changes to a mid-systolic murmur heard best at the left upper sternal border (indicative of flow through the bioprosthetic valve) followed by a prosthetic P2 closure sound with silence in diastole.

DIAGNOSTIC TESTING

Chest X-Ray

Despite the growing use of cross-sectional imaging such as computed tomography (CT) and cardiac magnetic resonance (CMR) imaging, the chest x-ray (CXR) continues to provide helpful clues in the diagnosis of CHD. The CXR is also a quick and cost-efficient imaging modality that delivers a low amount of ionizing radiation. Careful evaluation of the cardiac silhouette provides supportive evidence of certain underlying conditions. The filling of the retrosternal space on the lateral radiograph suggests right ventricular dilation. Congenitally corrected transposition of the great arteries demonstrates a narrow vascular pedicle with an "absent" aortic knob owing to the anterior-posterior relationship of the great vessels. Diagnosis of the scimitar syndrome, or partial anomalous venous return of the right pulmonary veins via the inferior vena cava, originates from the curvilinear opacity of the anomalous veins on frontal radiographs.

The CXR also provides information about cardiac physiology. The presence of increased pulmonary vascularity may indicate excessive pulmonary circulation from left-to-right shunting. Prominent pulmonary artery size may be seen generally in CHD, especially in conotruncal lesions or in a patient with post-stenotic dilatation owing to pulmonary stenosis or a prior pulmonary artery band. Increased pulmonary artery size may also be seen with distal pruning of the pulmonary vascular bed in patients with pulmonary hypertension. Pulmonary edema may be seen in systolic heart failure or mitral valve disease, but may also be seen with diastolic heart failure such as in Shone complex.

Aortic size may also be enlarged generally in conotruncal lesions as well as in aortopathy such as that owing to the bicuspid aortic valve. Native coarctation presenting in adulthood may have the classic "3-sign" on CXR (dilatation of the aortic arch and left subclavian artery, indentation at the coarctation site, and post-stenotic dilatation of the descending aorta) along with notching of the underside of the ribs resulting from chronic collateral blood flow via the intercostal arteries.

Electrocardiography

The electrocardiogram (ECG) in CHD is often abnormal, but the features of the ECG follow usual patterns for the different forms of CHD. Some of these patterns exist only in the native disease, some resolve following surgical repair, and others only emerge following surgical repair.[30] A baseline ECG is useful for comparison in the patient who develops new symptoms owing to the increased incidence of arrhythmias in CHD related to the underlying defect and associated surgical repairs. Congenitally corrected transposition of the great arteries is associated with a 2% annual incidence of complete heart block,[31] and transposition of the great arteries following atrial switch repair demonstrates an increased incidence of sinus node dysfunction. The ECG of a transannular repair of tetralogy of Fallot frequently shows a right bundle branch block. Increased duration of the QRS interval (>180 ms) in these patients is associated with an increased risk of arrhythmia and sudden cardiac death.[32] The atriotomies and ventriculotomies used in the surgical repair of CHD create a substrate with myocardial scarring for intra-atrial reentrant tachycardia and ventricular tachycardias, respectively. (See **Table 103.1**.)

Echocardiography

Transthoracic echocardiography (TTE) remains the first-line imaging modality for the initial and serial evaluation of CHD. TTE has both excellent spatial and temporal resolution for visualization of small mobile structures such as valves. The use of Doppler provides a noninvasive hemodynamic assessment of both native and repaired CHD. In addition to the standard echocardiographic views (parasternal long axis, parasternal short axis, apical, and subcostal), additional imaging obtained from nonstandard transducer probe placement may be necessary in patients with abnormal situs or other abnormal cardiac orientation. The suprasternal notch view provides visualization of superior thoracic structures including the aortic arch and is particularly helpful in the evaluation of coarctation of the aorta and PDA. In addition, this window is useful for the interrogation of flow from the superior vena cava to the pulmonary artery (Glenn) in a patient with a Fontan. The high parasternal window provides visualization of more anterior thoracic structures such as right ventricular to pulmonary artery conduits. Owing to its anterior location, TTE is the preferred imaging modality for these structures. In addition, imaging of the descending aorta from the subcostal plane is helpful with severe aortic regurgitation or a hemodynamically significant PDA in which pulmonary vascular disease has not yet occurred. The use of sweeps is also helpful in delineating the spatial relationship of structures in patients with CHD. In some patients with chest wall deformities—such as pectus excavatum or with limited acoustic windows following sternotomy—TTE may generate inadequate images for evaluation. In these cases, transesophageal echocardiograph (TEE) is an alternative. Intraoperative TEE is recommended in the surgical repair of CHD and has utility in certain percutaneous structural interventions as well.[33]

Cardiac Magnetic Resonance Imaging

CMR imaging demonstrates cardiac and extra-cardiac vascular anatomy noninvasively and without the use of ionizing radiation. This can be particularly useful in those patients for whom

TABLE 103.1 Typical ECG Features in Adults With Common Forms of CHD

Congenital Diagnosis	Rhythm	PR Interval	QRS Axis	QRS Configuration	Atrial Enlargement	Ventricular Hypertrophy	Particularities
Secundum atrial septal defect	NSR; ↑ IART/AF with age	1° AVB 6%-19%	0°-180°; RAD; LAD in Holt-Oram or LAHB	rSr′ or rsR′ with RBBBi > RBBBc	RAE 35%	Uncommon	"Crochetage pattern"
Ventricular septal defect	NSR; PVCs	Normal or mild ↑; 1° AVB 10%	RAD with BVH; LAD 3%-15%	Normal or rsr′; possible RBBB	Possible RAE ± LAE	BVH 23%-61%; RVH with Eisenmenger	Katz-Wachtel phenomenon
AV canal defect	NSR; PVCs 30%	1° AVB >50%	Mod to extreme LAD; Normal with atypical	rSr′ or rsR′	Possible LAE	Uncommon in partial; BVH in complete; RVH with Eisenmenger	Inferoposteriorly displaced AVN
Patent ductus arteriosus	NSR; ↑ IART/AF with age	↑ PR 10%-20%	Normal	Deep S V_1, tall R V_5 and V_6	LAE with moderate PDA	Uncommon	Often either clinically silent or Eisenmenger
Pulmonary stenosis	NSR	Normal	Normal if mild; RAD with moderate/severe	Normal; severity	Possible RAE	RVH; severity correlates with R:S in V_1 and V_6	Axis deviation correlates with RVP
Aortic coarctation	NSR	Normal	Normal or LAD	Normal	Possible LAE	LVH, especially by voltage criteria	Persistent RVH rare beyond infancy
Ebstein anomaly	NSR; possible EAR, SVT; AF/IART 40%	1° AVB common; short if WPW	Normal or LAD	Low-amplitude multiphasic atypical RBBB	RAE with Himalayan P waves	Diminutive RV	Accessory pathway common; Q II, III, aVF, and V_1-V_4
Surgically repaired TOF	NSR; PVCs; IART 10%; VT 12%	Normal or mild ↑	Normal or RAD; LAD 5%-10%	RBBB 90%	Peaked P waves; RAE possible	RVH possible if RVOT obstruction or PHT	QRS duration ± QTd predictive of VT/SCD
L-TGA	NSR	1° AVB >50%; AVB 2% per year	LAD	Absence of septal q; Q in III, aVF, and right precordium	Not if no associated defects	Not if no associated defects	Anterior AVN; Positive T precordial; WPW with Ebstein
D-TGA/intra-atrial baffle	Sinus bradycardia 60%; EAR; junctional; IART 25%	Normal	RAD	Absence of q, small r, deep S in left precordium	Possible RAE	RVH; diminutive LV	Possible AVB if VSD or TV surgery
UVH with Fontan	Sinus brady 15%; EAR; junctional; IART >50%	Normal in TA; 1° AVB in DILV	LAD in single RV, TA, single LV with noninverted outlet	Variable; ↑↑ R and S amplitudes in limb and precordial leads	RAE in TA	RVH with single RV; possible LVH with single LV	Absent sinus node in LAI; AV block with L-loop or AVCD

TABLE 103.1 Typical ECG Features in Adults With Common Forms of CHD (*Continued*)

Congenital Diagnosis	Rhythm	PR Interval	QRS Axis	QRS Configuration	Atrial Enlargement	Ventricular Hypertrophy	Particularities
Dextrocardia	NSR; P-wave axis 105°-165° with situs inversus	Normal	RAD	Inverse depolarization and repolarization	Not with situs inversus	LVH: tall R V_1-V_2; RVH: deep Q, small R V_1 and tall R right lateral	Situs solitus: normal P-wave axis and severe CHD
ALCAPA	NSR	Normal	Possible LAD	Pathologic anterolateral-lat Q waves; possible anteroseptal Q waves	Possible LAE	Selective hypertrophy of posterobasal LV	Possible ischemia

AF, atrial fibrillation; ALCAPA, anomalous left coronary artery from the pulmonary artery; AVB, atrioventricular block; AVCD, atrioventricular canal defect; AVN, AV node; BVH, biventricular hypertrophy; CHD, congenital heart disease; DILV, double-inlet left ventricle; EAR, ectopic atrial rhythm; IART, intra-atrial reentrant tachycardia; LAD, left-axis deviation; LAE, left atrial enlargement; LAHB, left anterior hemiblock; LAI, left atrial isomerism; LV, left ventricle; LVH, left ventricular hypertrophy; NSR, normal sinus rhythm; PDA, patent ductus arteriosus; PHT, pulmonary hypertension; QTd, QT duration; RAD, right-axis deviation; RAE, right atrial enlargement; PVC, premature ventricular contraction; RBBB, right bundle branch block (c = complete; i = incomplete); RV, right ventricle; RVH, right ventricular hypertrophy; RVOT, right ventricular outflow tract; RVP, right ventricular pressure; SCD, sudden cardiac death; SVT, supraventricular tachycardia; TA, tricuspid atresia; TGA, transposition of the great arteries; TOF, tetralogy of Fallot; TV, tricuspid valve; UVH, univentricular heart; VSD, ventricular septal defect; VT, ventricular tachycardia; WPW, Wolff-Parkinson-White syndrome.

Reprinted with permission from Khairy P, Marelli AJ. Clinical use of electrocardiography in adults with congenital heart disease. *Circulation.* 2007;116(23):2734-2746.

echocardiography provides inadequate image quality because of limited acoustic windows related to chest anatomy or post-surgical changes or when evaluating deep intrathoracic structures not amendable to echocardiography. Image acquisition for CMR is typically longer than most noninvasive imaging modalities. Claustrophobia, patient motion, inability to perform breath-holding maneuvers, and contraindications to contrast agents (ie, gadolinium) may preclude the use of CMR. The presence of implanted metallic devices such as clips, stents, pacemaker generator and leads, and prosthetic valve material causes magnetic susceptibility artifact leading to local signal distortion, which may affect image quality.

Advances in CMR data acquisition and processing now allow generation of a large amount of physiologic data in a single study. Cine imaging with the use of ECG gating provides visualization of cardiac structures throughout the cardiac cycle and can be used to calculate chamber volume, mass, and systolic function, as well as cardiac output. Phase and four-dimensional velocity mapping can be used to accurately estimate valvular velocities, flow, and shunts. In CHD with multiple shunts, CMR imaging can evaluate both the absolute and relative flow of each individual shunt to better inform surgical planning. Tissue characterization and evaluation of myocardial fibrosis can be performed with parametric mapping and delayed contrast imaging.

Cardiovascular Computed Tomography

Cardiovascular computed tomography (CCT) is a cross-sectional imaging modality in those patients with either contraindication to CMR or imaging artifacts leading to suboptimal image quality. As the heart is a dynamic structure and moves throughout the cardiac cycle, the use of ECG gating—where images are acquired or processed only during certain portions of the cardiac cycle—is necessary to improve spatial resolution and reduce motion artifact. CCT also has excellent spatial resolution that makes it particularly well suited for characterization of small vascular structures such as coronary arteries. Advances in CCT technology and processing now permit accurate quantification of chamber size, mass, and function.[34] The timing of image acquisition relative to transit of contrast is important in opacification of the pulmonary arteries in a Fontan circulation, where intravenous contrast flows passively from the arm injection site to the superior vena cava and pulmonary arteries. This may lead to the errant diagnosis of pulmonary embolus.

The downside of ionizing radiation, however, is that it is associated with increased incidence of malignancy later in life. Over the lifetime, patients with CHD often undergo multiple procedures that expose them to ionizing radiation. Retrospective studies have identified an increased incidence of malignancy in patients with ACHD, and cumulative exposure to ionizing radiation was independently associated with malignancy.[35]

Cardiac Catheterization

Cardiac catheterization remains the gold standard method of evaluation of hemodynamics in patients with CHD. Angiography during cardiac catheterization also provides selective visualization of vascular structures along with pressure gradients. Wedge angiograms demonstrate the lack of distal arborization of pulmonary vasculature when pulmonary vascular disease is suspected. Use of a long cine loop with angiography is useful when pulmonary arteriovenous malformations are suspected in order to bring out the rapid return of contrast to the systemic side of the heart via the pulmonary veins. When combined with TEE, cardiac catheterization can be helpful in locating and closing baffle leaks in patients with atrial switch repair of D-transposition of the great arteries. Transcatheter pulmonary valve replacement is becoming an increasingly common alternative to surgical valve replacement. Lastly, cardiac catheterization and percutaneous intervention can be useful to occlude veno-venous or aortopulmonary collaterals.

Cardiopulmonary Exercise Testing

Patients with CHD have lower exercise capacity when compared to healthy controls, even for simple forms of CHD.[36] Thus, patient estimates of functional capacity do not always correlate well with objective measurements of aerobic capacity.[37] Patients with ACHD acclimatize to their reduced aerobic capacity from a young age and experience their limited functional capacity as "normal." In one study comparing older patients with acquired heart disease and heart failure to younger patients with ACHD, aerobic capacity was similar for each New York Heart Association functional class.[36] Exercise limitations in ACHD can be from several potential causes including ventricular or valvular dysfunction, ventilation-perfusion mismatch, restrictive lung disease, or desaturation. Cardiopulmonary exercise testing (CPET) provides an objective measurement of aerobic capacity and helps identify the etiology of exercise limitation. There are disease-specific reference values for exercise parameters allowing comparison of patients with similar anatomy.[38] CPET also provides prognostic value in that reduced aerobic capacity and inadequate heart rate reserve have been associated with increased mortality in CHD.[39] When CPET is paired with imaging such as echocardiography, it may be useful for bringing out the functional impact of lesions such as left ventricular outflow tract obstruction or pulmonary stenosis. Lastly, regular exercise testing forms the basis for an exercise prescription to give guidance on physical activity within the confines of their disease. Many ACHD patients have been exercise-restricted in youth, so using patient-centered decision-making to form an exercise prescription empowers the incorporation of physical activity into daily life.

KEY POINTS

- ✔ As children with CHD become adults, the outcome variable shifts from growth to that of functional status.
- ✔ Adult presentations of cardiac-associated genetic syndromes differ greatly from the neonatal descriptions, so understanding the implications in adulthood is key.
- ✔ When bringing in a new patient into the practice, the patient provides the history of present illness, but it is often the parents or caregivers who supply key details of the past medical history.
- ✔ Surgical scars are the patient's "road map" and should be thoroughly reconciled with the list of prior surgeries or complications of surgery.
- ✔ Every effort should be made to obtain prior operative reports that provide primary source data on initial anatomy and surgical details.
- ✔ Beware of taking blood pressure in the arm on the same side as a lateral thoracotomy (the presence of an ipsilateral scar can signify collateral blood flow is supplying the arm and may not be reflective of central blood pressure).
- ✔ Look for associated Horner syndrome or growth restriction when a thoracotomy scar is present.
- ✔ Patients with heterotaxy syndrome may have atypical positioning of their heart, requiring atypical assessments (like auscultation of the heart sounds on the right side of the chest with dextrocardia).
- ✔ Auscultation of murmurs in patient with ACHD should be done from the mindset of "the company it keeps" such that if you identify a murmur from one lesion look for the presence of other associated lesions.
- ✔ New or worsening murmurs may signify endocarditis, given the higher incidence of endocarditis in the ACHD population.
- ✔ In addition to the typical workup for pulmonary valve endocarditis (such as TTE or TEE), gated computed tomography angiography (CTA) is often a useful tool, given the anterior position of the valve.
- ✔ Patients with ACHD adapt to limitations lifelong, and thus objective exercise testing is an important benchmark. Regular follow-up testing is useful for following a lesion against the benchmark.
- ✔ ACHD patient estimates of functional capacity do not always correlate with objective measurements of aerobic capacity.
- ✔ Postoperatively, it is important to repeat cross-sectional imaging and an exercise test to serve as the "new baseline" going forward.

REFERENCES

1. Khan A, Gurvitz M. Epidemiology of ACHD: what has changed and what is changing? *Prog Cardiovasc Dis.* 2018;61(3-4):275-281.
2. Marelli, A. Trajectories of care in congenital heart disease—the long arm of disease in the womb. *J Intern Med.* 2020;288(4):390-399.
3. Cowan JR, Ware SM. Genetics and genetic testing in congenital heart disease. *Clin Perinatol.* 2015;42(2):373-393, ix.
4. Jenkins KJ, Correa A, Feinstein JA, et al. Noninherited risk factors and congenital cardiovascular defects: current knowledge: a scientific statement from the American Heart Association Council on Cardiovascular Disease in the Young: endorsed by the American Academy of Pediatrics. *Circulation.* 2007;115(23):2995-3014.
5. Becerra JE, Khoury MJ, Cordero JF, Erickson JD. Diabetes mellitus during pregnancy and the risks for specific birth defects: a population-based case-control study. *Pediatrics.* 1990;85(1):1-9.
6. Tinker SC, Gilboa SM, Moore CA, et al. Specific birth defects in pregnancies of women with diabetes: National Birth Defects Prevention Study, 1997-2011. *Am J Obstet Gynecol.* 2020;222(2):176 e1-176 e11.

7. Malik S, Cleves MA, Honein MA, et al. Maternal smoking and congenital heart defects. *Pediatrics*. 2008;121(4):e810-e816.
8. Nora JJ, Nora AH, Toews WH. Lithium, Ebstein's anomaly, and other congenital heart defects. *Lancet*. 1974;304(7880):594-595.
9. Patorno E, Huybrechts KF, Bateman BT, et al. Lithium use in pregnancy and the risk of cardiac malformations. *N Engl J Med*. 2017;376(23):2245-2254.
10. Tsou AY, Bulova P, Capone G, et al. Medical care of adults with down syndrome: a clinical guideline. *JAMA*. 2020;324(15):1543-1556.
11. Shah S, Nguyen HH, Vincent AJ. Care of the adult woman with Turner syndrome. *Climacteric*. 2018;21(5):428-436.
12. Pierpont ME, Brueckner M, Chung WK, et al. Genetic basis for congenital heart disease: revisited: a scientific statement from the American Heart Association. *Circulation*. 2018;138(21):e653-e711.
13. Fung WL, Butcher NJ, Costain G, et al. Practical guidelines for managing adults with 22q11.2 deletion syndrome. *Genet Med*. 2015;17(8):599-609.
14. Sauna-Aho O, Bjelogrlic-Laakso N, Sirén A, Kangasmäki V, Arvio M. Cognition in adults with Williams syndrome-A 20-year follow-up study. *Mol Genet Genomic Med*. 2019;7(6):e695.
15. Husain M, Dutra-Clarke M, Lemieux B, et al. Phenotypic diversity of patients diagnosed with VACTERL association. *Am J Med Genet A*. 2018;176(9):1830-1837.
16. Hager A, Kanz S, Kaemmerer H, Schreiber C, Hess J. Coarctation Long-term Assessment (COALA): significance of arterial hypertension in a cohort of 404 patients up to 27 years after surgical repair of isolated coarctation of the aorta, even in the absence of restenosis and prosthetic material. *J Thorac Cardiovasc Surg*. 2007;134(3):738-745.
17. McGee S. (Ed.) Cyanosis. *Evidence-Based Physical Diagnosis*. Elsevier; 2018:69-72.e1.
18. Myers KA, Farquhar DR. The rational clinical examination. Does this patient have clubbing? *JAMA*. 2001;286(3):341-347.
19. Kawakami N, Mimatsu K, Deguchi M, Kato F, Maki S. Scoliosis and congenital heart disease. *Spine (Phila Pa 1976)*. 1995;20(11):1252-1255; discussion 1256.
20. Luke MJ, McDonnell EJ. Congenital heart disease and scoliosis. *J Pediatr*. 1968;73(5):725-733.
21. Farley FA, Phillips WA, Herzenberg JE, Rosenthal A, Hensinger RN Natural history of scoliosis in congenital heart disease. *J Pediatr Orthop*. 1991;11(1):42-47.
22. Allen HD, Shaddy RE. Penny D, et al. *Moss and Adams' Heart Disease in Infants, Children, and Adolescents: Including the Fetus and Young Adult*. 9th ed. Wolters Kluwer; 2016.
23. Baudet E, al-Qudah A. Late results of the subclavian flap repair of coarctation in infancy. *J Cardiovasc Surg (Torino)*. 1989;30(3):445-449.
24. Marbarger JP Jr, Sandza JG Jr, Hartmann AF Jr, Weldon CS. Blalock-taussig anastomosis: the preferred shunt in infants and newborns. *Circulation*. 1978;58(3 Pt 2):I73-177.
25. Luciani G. The clamshell approach for the surgical treatment of complex cardiopulmonary pathology in infants and children. *Eur J Cardio-Thorac Surg*. 1997;11(2):298-306.
26. Pandya B, Cullen S, Walker F. Congenital heart disease in adults. *BMJ*. 2016;354:i3905.
27. Mann DL., Zipes DP, Libby P., et al. *Braunwald's Heart Disease: A Textbook of Cardiovascular Medicine*. 2015.
28. Hurst JW, Blackard E. Inspection and palpation of pulsations on the front of the chest. *Am Heart J*. 1958;56(2):159-164.
29. Perloff JK, Harvey WP. Mechanisms of fixed splitting of the second heart sound. *Circulation*. 1958;18(5):998-1009.
30. Khairy P, Van Hare GF, Balaji S, et al. PACES/HRS Expert Consensus Statement on the Recognition and Management of Arrhythmias in Adult Congenital Heart Disease: developed in partnership between the Pediatric and Congenital Electrophysiology Society (PACES) and the Heart Rhythm Society (HRS). Endorsed by the governing bodies of PACES, HRS, the American College of Cardiology (ACC), the American Heart Association (AHA), the European Heart Rhythm Association (EHRA), the Canadian Heart Rhythm Society (CHRS), and the International Society for Adult Congenital Heart Disease (ISACHD). *Heart Rhythm*. 2014;11(10):e102-e165.
31. Huhta JC, Maloney JD, Ritter DG, Ilstrup DM, Feldt RH. Complete atrioventricular block in patients with atrioventricular discordance. *Circulation*. 1983;67(6):1374-1377.
32. Gatzoulis MA, Balaji S, Webber SA, et al. Risk factors for arrhythmia and sudden cardiac death late after repair of tetralogy of Fallot: a multicentre study. *Lancet*, 2000;356(9234):975-981.
33. Stout KK, Daniels CJ, Aboulhosn JA, et al. 2018 AHA/ACC Guideline for the management of adults with congenital heart disease: a report of the American College of Cardiology/American Heart Association Task Force on Clinical Practice Guidelines. *J Am Coll Cardiol*, 2019;73(12):e81-e192.
34. Greupner J, Zimmermann E, Grohmann A, et al. Head-to-head comparison of left ventricular function assessment with 64-row computed tomography, biplane left cineventriculography, and both 2- and 3-dimensional transthoracic echocardiography: comparison with magnetic resonance imaging as the reference standard. *J Am Coll Cardiol*. 2012;59(21):1897-1907.
35. Cohen S, Liu A, Gurvitz M, et al. Exposure to low-dose ionizing radiation from cardiac procedures and malignancy risk in adults with congenital heart disease. *Circulation*. 2018;37(13):1334-1345.
36. Diller GP, Dimopoulos K, Okonko D, et al. Exercise intolerance in adult congenital heart disease: comparative severity, correlates, and prognostic implication. *Circulation*. 2005;112(6):828-835.
37. Gratz A, Hess J, Hager A. Self-estimated physical functioning poorly predicts actual exercise capacity in adolescents and adults with congenital heart disease. *Eur Heart J*. 2009;30(4):497-504.
38. Kempny A, Dimopoulos K, Uebing A, et al. Reference values for exercise limitations among adults with congenital heart disease. Relation to activities of daily life--single centre experience and review of published data. *Eur Heart J*. 2012;33(11):1386-1396.
39. Inuzuka R, Diller G-P, Borgia F, et al. Comprehensive use of cardiopulmonary exercise testing identifies adults with congenital heart disease at increased mortality risk in the medium term. *Circulation*. 2012;125(2):250-259.

CHAPTER 104

PREGNANCY AND REPRODUCTIVE HEALTH IN ADULT CONGENITAL HEART DISEASE

Evan F. Shalen and Abigail D. Khan

INTRODUCTION

Innovations in the treatment of congenital heart disease (CHD) have greatly improved survival, leading to a dramatic increase in the size of the population of adults with CHD (ACHD).[1] CHD is now the most prevalent type of heart disease in pregnant women worldwide.[2] Reproductive health issues are of paramount importance as the CHD population ages into adulthood, and counseling about contraception and pregnancy is the cornerstone of ACHD care.[3]

ACHD comprises a diverse group of disorders with a wide range of expected clinical outcomes. The diversity of the underlying conditions and the changing nature of the surgical approach to ACHD have resulted in significant heterogeneity in pregnancy risk. Similarly, the risks associated with contraception and assisted reproductive strategies vary, presenting a challenge to those delivering care to this population. In this chapter, we provide an overview of ACHD pregnancy risk and address reproductive-related care for both men and women with ACHD.

PATHOGENESIS

An understanding of the hemodynamic changes of pregnancy is critical to the management of pregnant ACHD patients. The major cardiovascular changes associated with normal pregnancy are as follows:

- An increase in the circulating plasma volume that begins by 6 weeks of gestation and peaks at 50% of baseline by 32 weeks.
- A decrease in systemic vascular resistance and blood pressure.
- An approximately 20% increase in heart rate.
- Ventricular remodeling, leading to increased left ventricular (LV) end-diastolic volume with preserved LV ejection fraction (LVEF) and increased stroke volume, resulting in a 30% to 50% increase in cardiac output.
- In active labor, 300 to 500 mL of blood is returned to the central circulation with each contraction, and cardiac output increases by 50%.
- The decreased preload associated with the performance of the Valsalva maneuver during pushing results in a decrease in cardiac output in some patients.

CLINICAL PRESENTATION

Most cases of CHD are known prior to pregnancy. In rare cases, the physiologic changes of pregnancy and/or the increased intensity of medical care yields a new diagnosis of CHD. The clinical presentation is variable; however, women can present with murmurs, arrhythmias, or dyspnea and peripheral edema.

DIAGNOSIS

Echocardiography

Echocardiography is the first-line diagnostic tool in pregnancy, carrying a high sensitivity and specificity with no documented adverse fetal effects. It provides both anatomic and hemodynamic information. It is generally possible to obtain adequate transthoracic images in pregnant patients. If not, transesophageal echocardiography can usually be safely performed, but the risks of the associated sedation should be discussed with the patient and obstetric and anesthesia teams. Noncontrast magnetic resonance imaging (MRI) is an option for those with poor acoustic echocardiographic windows. Ultrasound-enhancing agents are not typically used in pregnancy, because their risk is unknown. Saline contrast is assumed to be safe in pregnancy, but it has not been systematically studied.

Computed Tomography

The elevated heart rate associated with pregnancy can be a limiting factor in the acquisition of gated cardiac imaging. Consideration of cardiac Computed Tomography (CT) in pregnancy should include discussion with a radiologist about the expected radiation dose to the fetus and also with an obstetrician to help define the fetal risk. The typical fetal radiation dose from maternal chest imaging is low, although there is known association between in utero radiation exposure and childhood malignancy at higher levels of exposure.[4] Assessment of the blood-tissue interface and intravascular and vascular structures is enhanced with intravenous contrast. Low osmolar agents cross the placenta but have not been associated with fetal injury.[4]

Magnetic Resonance Imaging

MRI provides detailed imaging of the heart and central vasculature and is considered safe in pregnancy.[4] There appears to be no appreciable effect on offspring after first trimester maternal MRI exposure.[5] Gadolinium contrast agents are generally avoided as they are classified as category C (ie, animal reproduction studies have shown an adverse effect on the fetus, and there are no adequate and well-controlled studies in humans) by the Food and Drug Administration (FDA).[4]

Cardiac Catheterization

Invasive angiography and hemodynamic assessment are essential in the evaluation of some pregnant patients. Radiation exposure to the fetus should be minimized.[4]

Exercise Testing

Abnormal chronotropic response to stress testing either before pregnancy or in the first trimester is a predictor of adverse pregnancy events in women with CHD.[6] Stress testing to assess expected maternal response to pregnancy or to rule out cardiac ischemia is appropriate in selected patients, but the anticipated diagnostic benefits need to be weighed against the risks of the test. In general, submaximal exercise stress testing is safe in pregnancy.

MANAGEMENT OF THE PATIENT WITH ADULT CONGENITAL HEART DISEASE

Overview of Risk Stratification of Pregnant Women With Congenital Heart Disease

There are three commonly used risk scoring systems for pregnant women with CHD, each of which has unique strengths and limitations, and the information that they provide should be viewed as complementary to information gleaned from smaller, lesion-specific cohorts.

Cardiac Disease in Pregnancy Study II (CARPREG II) Risk Score

The Cardiac Disease in Pregnancy (CARPREG II) score was developed in a cohort of 1938 women with various types of heart disease[7] and identified 10 predictors of maternal cardiac events (**Table 104.1**). This score is easy to calculate, applies to women with and without CHD, and is appealing to clinicians and patients because it yields a user-friendly percentage risk. How the CARPREG II score performs in real-world cohorts has yet to be determined.

ZAHARA (Zwangerschap bij vrouwen met een Aangeboren HARtAfwijking-II [translated as "Pregnancy in Women with CHD II Risk Index"]) Risk Score

The ZAHARA score was developed in a large retrospective European cohort of women with CHD and identified eight factors associated with maternal cardiac complications (Table 104.1).[8] Like CARPREG, ZAHARA calculates a percentage predicted risk but is less commonly used in the United States. While some risk markers are common to both CARPREG and ZAHARA, there are important differences, likely related to study methodology and the characteristics of the study populations.

TABLE 104.1 Predictors of Pregnancy Risk in the CARPREG II and ZAHARA Studies

CARPREG II	ZAHARA
Prior cardiac events or arrhythmias Higher NYHA class[a] or cyanosis Mechanical valve High-risk left-sided valve disease/LVOT obstruction[b]	
Ventricular dysfunction[c]	Cardiac medications before pregnancy
Pulmonary hypertension[d]	≥ Moderate systemic atrioventricular valve regurgitation
Coronary artery disease	≥ Moderate pulmonary valve regurgitation
High-risk aortopathy[e]	–
No prior cardiac intervention	–
Late pregnancy assessment[f]	–

Note: Merged cells indicate risk factors that are common to both scores.
LVOT, left ventricular outflow tract obstruction; NYHA, New York Heart Association.
[a]CARPREG II: Baseline NYHA III-IV status, ZAHARA= NYHA prior to pregnancy >II.
[b]CARPREG II: aortic valve area <1.5 cm^2, subaortic gradient >30 mm Hg, mitral valve area <2 cm^2, or moderate to severe mitral regurgitation, ZAHARA: Peak aortic gradient >50 mm Hg or aortic valve area <1.0 cm^2.
[c]Left ventricular ejection fraction <55%.
[d]Right ventricular systolic pressure ≥50 mm Hg in the absence of right ventricular outflow obstruction.
[e]Marfan syndrome, bicuspid aortic valve with aortic diameter >45 mm, Loeys-Dietz syndrome, vascular Ehlers-Danlos syndrome or prior aortic dissection or pseudoaneurysm.
[f]First antenatal visit after 20 weeks' gestation.
Adapted from Silversides CK, Grewal J, Mason J, et al. Pregnancy outcomes in women with heart disease: the CARPREG II study. *J Am Coll Cardiol.* 2018;71:2419-2430; Drenthen W, Boersma E, Balci A, et al. Predictors of pregnancy complications in women with congenital heart disease. *Eur Heart J.* 2010;31:2124-2132.

World Health Organization Classification

The World Health Organization (WHO) classification is a qualitative scoring system that incorporates anatomic and physiologic features (**Table 104.2**).[9] The WHO score performs well as a predictor of maternal, obstetric, and fetal events and has a higher discriminative ability than the CARPREG or ZAHARA scores.[2,10] The WHO classification is the tool endorsed by major society guidelines.[9,11]

Risk Stratification by Defect Complexity

Simple Defects

Simple defects include small and uncomplicated atrial and ventricular septal defects (ASD, VSD); patent ductus arteriosus; mild pulmonic stenosis; and repaired ASD, VSD, and anomalous pulmonary venous return. These defects are associated with a minimally increased risk in pregnancy (Table 104.2).

TABLE 104.2 Modified WHO Classification of Maternal Cardiovascular Risk

WHO Class	Associated Risk	Lesion
I	No detectable increased risk of maternal mortality and no/mild increase in morbidity.	**Uncomplicated, small, or mild:** Pulmonary stenosis PDA Mitral valve prolapse **Repaired simple lesions** ASD or VSD PDA Anomalous pulmonary venous drainage **Isolated ectopic beats**
II	Small increased risk of maternal mortality or moderate increase in morbidity.	Unoperated ASD or VSD Repaired tetralogy of Fallot Most arrhythmias
II or III	May fall into higher or lower risk classification based on additional patient factors.	Mild left ventricular impairment Hypertrophic cardiomyopathy Native or tissue valvular heart disease not considered class I or IV Marfan syndrome without aortic dilation Bicuspid aortic valve aortopathy with aorta diameter < 45 mm Repaired coarctation
III	Significantly increased risk of maternal mortality or severe morbidity.	Mechanical valve Systemic right ventricle Fontan circulation Unrepaired cyanotic heart disease Other complex CHD Marfan syndrome with aortic diameter 40-45 mm Bicuspid aortopathy with aortic diameter 45-50 mm
IV	Extremely high risk of maternal mortality or severe morbidity; pregnancy contraindicated.	Pulmonary arterial hypertension Severe systemic ventricular dysfunction Peripartum cardiomyopathy with any residual left ventricular dysfunction Severe mitral stenosis Severe symptomatic aortic stenosis Marfan syndrome with aortic diameter >45 mm Bicuspid aortopathy with aortic diameter >50 mm Severe native aortic coarctation

ASD, atrial septal defect; CHD, congenital heart disease; PDA, patent ductus arteriosus VSD, ventricular septal defect.
Data from Regitz-Zagrosek V, Blomstrom Lundqvist C, Borghi C, et al. ESC Guidelines on the management of cardiovascular diseases during pregnancy: The task force on the management of cardiovascular diseases during pregnancy of the European Society of Cardiology (ESC). *Eur Heart J.* 2011;32(24):3147-3197 and Jastrow N, Meyer P, Khairy P, et al. Prediction of complications in pregnant women with cardiac diseases referred to a tertiary center. *Int J Cardiol.* 2011;151(2):209-213.

Paradoxical embolus is a concern for those with persistent intracardiac shunts, and avoidance of venous stasis with compression stockings and early ambulation after delivery is recommended.

Moderate Complexity Congenital Heart Disease

Preconception counseling is strongly recommended for patients with moderate complexity CHD, and pregnant patients need to be followed by a cardiologist with CHD experience and a high-risk obstetrician. Preconception imaging is useful for risk stratification and hemodynamic optimization, whereas those at elevated risk of arrhythmias should have ambulatory rhythm monitoring. In some cases, exercise testing is helpful to predict cardiac events.[6]

Vaginal delivery is preferred unless there is an obstetric indication for cesarean section. Rare exceptions include those with decompensated heart failure or significantly impaired LV function, severe aortic enlargement, and/or ongoing poorly tolerated arrhythmias. A multidisciplinary delivery plan, including a discussion of the location and mode of delivery and the need for cardiac monitoring, is recommended.

Moderate and Large Unrepaired Atrial Septal Defects. Most moderate and large unrepaired ASD are WHO Class II (Table 104.2), although pregnancy is contraindicated if there is severe pulmonary arterial hypertension (WHO Class IV). Preconception cardiac MRI can be helpful to accurately size the right ventricle (RV), define the shunt fraction, and determine whether there is partial anomalous pulmonary venous return. Hemodynamically significant ASDs should be closed prior to pregnancy.[3]

Unrepaired ASD is associated with an increased risk of arterial thromboembolism, and strategies to reduce the risk of venous stasis are recommended. Women with unrepaired ASD can also develop atrial arrhythmias. Whereas those with large shunts and associated RV enlargement and/or dysfunction are theoretically at higher risk of volume overload, clinical heart failure is rare.[12]

Tetralogy of Fallot. Most women with repaired Tetralogy of Fallot (TOF) tolerate pregnancy well, with a reported maternal cardiac event rate of 7% or less.[13,14] Heart failure and arrhythmias occur more frequently in women with RV dysfunction and/or moderate to severe pulmonary regurgitation.[15] Overall complication rates are low, even in those with significant pulmonary stenosis or regurgitation.[16,17]

Baseline assessment of pregnant women with TOF should include an echocardiogram, primarily to evaluate the RV and the degree of pulmonary regurgitation. Clinical follow-up every trimester is recommended, and a third trimester echocardiogram is useful, especially if there is a change in clinical status.[11] Pulmonary valve replacement prior to pregnancy should be considered in symptomatic patients with RV enlargement and severe pulmonary regurgitation.[11]

Aortic Coarctation. Severe native coarctation is a WHO Class IV lesion and requires repair before pregnancy.[9] Women with repaired coarctation tolerate pregnancy with a low risk of heart failure or arrhythmia.[12] There is an increased risk of hypertensive disorders of pregnancy, partly related to preexisting chronic hypertension.[18] Preconception evaluation includes cross-sectional imaging of the aorta, if not recently performed, as well as upper and lower extremity blood pressures. Those who are found to have hemodynamically significant residual coarctation should undergo evaluation for intervention.

Ebstein Anomaly of the Tricuspid Valve. Adults with Ebstein anomaly are at risk for tricuspid regurgitation, RV dysfunction, cyanosis related to shunting through an ASD, and arrhythmias.[19] Heart failure (3%), arrhythmias (4%), and worsening cyanosis are described complications of pregnancy; however, those without preexisting cyanosis and/or heart failure typically tolerate pregnancy well.[12,20] Paradoxical embolism is a concern in the setting of an ASD. Prophylactic closure of a small ASD or patent foramen ovale is not indicated.[11]

Preconception evaluation includes an assessment of RV size and function and the degree of tricuspid regurgitation, either by echocardiography or by cardiac MRI. A Holter monitor is reasonable to assess for arrhythmias. In those with an atrial shunt, exercise testing is helpful to assess for exercise-induced cyanosis. The frequency of follow-up in pregnancy is dictated by clinical status.

Atrioventricular Septal Defects. Most atrioventricular septal defects patients without residual valve disease or left ventricular outflow tract obstruction (LVOTO) tolerate pregnancy well. Prepregnancy surgery should be considered in those with symptomatic residual disease. A 10% rate of arrhythmias has been reported, with a risk of heart failure of 1%.[12] Deterioration in New York Heart Association (NYHA) functional class is relatively common and may persist after pregnancy.[21] There is a high rate of offspring atrioventricular septal defects (**Table 104.3**).[22]

The frequency of prenatal follow-up and imaging depends on the clinical status. In those at risk for paradoxical embolization, measures to prevent venous stasis are recommended.

Isolated Pulmonary Valve Stenosis. Preconception assessment includes echocardiography to define the severity of the stenosis with cardiac catheterization for confirmation if stenosis is severe. Relief of stenosis is recommended prior to pregnancy if the peak transvalvular gradient is greater than 64 mm Hg.[11] Interestingly, whereas maternal cardiac complications such as heart failure and arrhythmia are rare, hypertensive disorders of pregnancy may be more common.[23] In patients with severe stenosis who develop symptoms in pregnancy, balloon valvuloplasty may be considered.

Congenital Aortic Valve Disease. The most common cause of congenital aortic valve disease is a bicuspid valve. Women with

TABLE 104.3 Risk of Offspring Inheritance by Congenital Heart Disease (CHD) Lesion

CHD Lesion	Father Affected (%)	Mother Affected (%)
Atrial septal defect	1.5-3.5	4-6
Atrioventricular septal defect	1-4.5	11.5-14
Ventricular septal defect	2-3.5	6-10
Aortic stenosis	3-4	8-18
Pulmonic stenosis	2-3.5	4-6.5
Tetralogy of Fallot	1.5	2-2.5
Aortic coarctation	2-3	4-6.5
Patent ductus arteriosus	2-2.5	3.5-4
Hypoplastic left heart syndrome	21	
D-transposition of the great arteries	2	
L-transposition of the great arteries	3-5	
Ebstein anomaly	Unknown	6

Merged cells indicate offspring risk irrespective of parental gender. (Reprinted from Cowan JR, Ware SM. Genetics and genetic testing in congenital heart disease. *Clin Perinatol.* 2015;42(2):373-393. Copyright © 2015 Elsevier. With permission.)

aortic valve dysfunction in the setting of other forms of CHD are at higher risk for complications and need a comprehensive review of their anatomy and physiology.

Aortic regurgitation is well tolerated in the absence of ventricular dysfunction or heart failure. Women who meet criteria for valve replacement prior to pregnancy should receive counseling about the risks and benefits of prepregnancy surgery, including a discussion of the impact of valve type on subsequent pregnancy risk.[24] The outcomes of aortic stenosis in pregnancy depend on severity. Mild aortic stenosis is well tolerated, whereas those with severe aortic stenosis have an 18% risk of heart failure and a 3% risk of arrhythmia.[25] Maternal mortality was not observed in a large contemporary cohort but has been described historically.[25]

Preconception evaluation includes assessment of aortic stenosis/regurgitation severity and LV function by echocardiography. Exercise testing is useful to evaluate exercise capacity and blood pressure response. Those with severe symptomatic aortic stenosis, inducible symptoms on exercise testing, LVEF less than 50%, or a drop in blood pressure with exercise should undergo prepregnancy surgery.[11]

Pregnant women with moderate or more severe aortic stenosis warrant close monitoring with serial echocardiography. Valve gradients increase in pregnancy owing to high flow, and differentiating pathologic symptoms from those of normal pregnancy can be challenging. Those with symptomatic stenosis benefit from activity restriction, treatment with diuretics, and, in some cases, percutaneous balloon valvuloplasty or transcatheter aortic valve replacement.[26] Those who are not candidates for a percutaneous procedure need consideration of early delivery with surgical valve replacement thereafter. In severe symptomatic aortic stenosis, cesarean delivery is preferred and should occur in the cardiac operating room.

The risk of aortic dissection is higher in pregnancy and the postpartum period in those with bicuspid aortic valve-associated aortopathy.[27] Women with a bicuspid aortic valve need a preconception assessment of aortic dimension, with serial monitoring during pregnancy if the aorta is enlarged. Prepregnancy aortic surgery is recommended when the aortic diameter is greater than 50 mm.[11]

Congenital Mitral Valve Disease. Most of the data regarding mitral stenosis in pregnancy relates to those with rheumatic disease. Moderate and severe mitral stenoses are associated with significantly increased risk, and prepregnancy intervention should be pursued in many cases. In women who become pregnant, arrhythmias occur in 20% to 30% and heart failure in more than 50%, although mortality is rare.[28]

Pregnant women with moderate or more severe mitral stenosis should be monitored closely. Echocardiographic gradients increase in pregnancy owing to increased cardiac output, and stenosis severity should be graded by pressure half-time and/or direct planimetry. Beta-blocker therapy is beneficial to maximize diastolic filling time. Anticoagulation is indicated in patients at high risk for thrombosis ($\geq$ moderate mitral stenosis, left atrial spontaneous echocardiographic contrast, left atrial area $\geq$40 mL/m^2) or with known atrial fibrillation.

Mitral regurgitation is better tolerated in pregnancy than mitral stenosis, because the decreased afterload of the pregnant state decreases the regurgitant volume. Preconception evaluation includes an assessment of the severity of the regurgitation and measurement of LV function by echocardiogram or MRI. Those with symptoms and/or significant LV systolic dysfunction or dilation should undergo prepregnancy intervention because they are at high risk for heart failure.[29]

Complex Congenital Heart Disease

Patients with complex CHD should receive care at an ACHD center. Pregnancy is contraindicated in those with severe pulmonary hypertension or severe systemic ventricular dysfunction, regardless of the underlying lesion. A detailed multidisciplinary delivery plan is required, with attention to location and mode of delivery and potential anesthesia risks.

Fontan Palliation. Adult Fontan patients are at risk for ventricular dysfunction, valvular regurgitation, arrhythmias, thrombosis, and hepatic dysfunction. The lack of a subpulmonic pumping chamber results in decreased cardiac output and venous congestion, and oxygen saturation can be reduced in the presence of venovenous collaterals or a Fontan fenestration. An impaired exercise capacity is nearly universal,[30] and it is thus not surprising that women have difficulty tolerating the obligate increases in heart rate, stroke volume, and plasma volume of pregnancy.

The proper selection of Fontan patients for pregnancy is essential. Those with a history of ventricular dysfunction, cyanosis, and thromboembolic events are particularly high risk and merit a discussion of alternatives to pregnancy. Preconception review should include an assessment of ventricular function and valvular regurgitation, measurement of oxygen saturation at rest and with exercise, screening for arrhythmias, and an assessment of liver function.[3,9]

In a recent publication including 255 pregnancies in 133 women after the Fontan, the live birth rate was 45%.[31] The most common cause of pregnancy loss was spontaneous miscarriage, occurring in 45% of pregnancies. Premature delivery occurred in 59%. There were no reported maternal mortalities, but two women had pulmonary embolism. The most common cardiac complications were supraventricular arrhythmias (8.4%) and heart failure (3.9%). Obstetric bleeding occurred in 25%, perhaps related to frequent use of antiplatelet and anticoagulant medications.[31] The need for anticoagulation in Fontan pregnancy is controversial, with some advocating for it in all and others advocating an individualized approach.[9,31,32]

Regional anesthesia is recommended with careful attention to the risk of hypotension in a preload-dependent physiology. Fluid repletion may be required to maintain preload, but care must be taken to avoid precipitating volume overload. Many patients will be able to deliver without invasive monitoring on a labor and delivery floor. Vaginal delivery is preferred unless a cesarean section is required for obstetric indications. A shortened second stage is typically recommended.[9] Fontan patients are especially vulnerable to decompensation in the face of postpartum fluid shifts and need to be monitored for the first few days after delivery.

Systemic Right Ventricle. D-transposition of the great arteries (D-TGA) with a surgical atrial switch and L-transposition of the great arteries (L-TGA, or congenitally corrected transposition) are the most common lesions associated with a systemic RV. Common D-TGA complications include sinus node dysfunction and arrhythmias, baffle obstruction, RV dysfunction, and systemic tricuspid regurgitation. L-TGA patients face many of the same risks but also have a higher incidence of heart block and concomitant lesions such as pulmonic stenosis. In both groups, the systemic RV functions as an inferior systemic pump to the LV owing to its different morphology and geometry.

Proper patient selection for pregnancy is critical. Preconception review includes assessment of ventricular function and valvular regurgitation, measurement of resting and exercise oxygen saturation, and screening for arrhythmias. Those with significant RV dysfunction and/or mechanical valves are an especially high-risk group, and a discussion of alternatives to pregnancy is appropriate. Cardiac MRI is indicated for quantification of RV function in the absence of contraindications. Exercise testing is helpful to predict adverse outcomes.[6]

The physiologic limitations of the systemic RV are unmasked by pregnancy, resulting in a high risk of arrhythmias, heart failure, and worsening tricuspid regurgitation. The reported cardiac complication rate is 10% to 40% after atrial switch[33,34] and 16% to 26% in L-TGA.[35,36] The most common complications are supraventricular arrhythmias and heart failure. Mortality is rare. An irreversible decline in RV function can occur.[33,34]

Echocardiographic surveillance each trimester is reasonable given the risk of deterioration in RV function. Many women can deliver on a labor and delivery floor with cardiac monitoring.[9] Those with heart failure or active arrhythmias may require delivery in an intensive care unit. Vaginal delivery with a facilitated second stage is preferred unless a cesarean section is required for obstetric indications, and regional anesthesia is recommended.[9,11] Close monitoring for hemodynamic decompensation in the face of postpartum fluid shifts is recommended.

D-transposition of the Great Arteries After the Arterial Switch Operation. A growing population of women with a history of an ASO is becoming pregnant.[37] ASO patients have a systemic LV as opposed to a systemic RV, making them better suited physiologically for the demands of pregnancy. It should be noted that the available literature to date includes a young population of pregnant women. Whether or not pregnancy risk after the ASO will increase as women age has yet to be determined.[38]

The assessment of the ASO patient prior to pregnancy should include an evaluation of ventricular function, valvular regurgitation, and functional capacity. ASO patients can develop neo-aortic root dilatation, aortic regurgitation, myocardial ischemia, and pulmonary artery stenosis. An anatomic evaluation of coronary artery patency is recommended for adult ASO patients and should be undertaken prior to pregnancy.[3] Cardiac stress testing can be useful to evaluate chest pain.

The complication rate in ASO pregnancy is low.[37,38] Vaginal delivery is preferred unless there is an obstetric indication for a cesarean section. A facilitated second stage is not required for most patients with uncomplicated pregnancies. Given a risk of atrial arrhythmias, telemetry monitoring in labor may be prudent.

Cyanosis. Cyanosis has been shown to be associated with a high risk of adverse maternal and fetal outcomes.[7,8,39] Cyanotic patients who are contemplating pregnancy should receive detailed counseling at an ACHD center with an eye toward identifying any correctable sources of cyanosis prior to pregnancy. Pregnancy is contraindicated in Eisenmenger syndrome.[9]

Mechanical Valves. Pregnant women with mechanical valves are at high risk for complications.[40] A detailed discussion of the risks and benefits of anticoagulation strategies is outside the scope of this chapter, but can be found elsewhere.[9,11] Women with mechanical valves should receive preconception counseling taking into account the underlying cardiac lesion, the type and location of the valve, the cardiac function, and the type of anticoagulation that is planned during the pregnancy. Importantly, women of childbearing age who are undergoing valve replacement should be counseled about the potential risks of a mechanical valve in the event of a pregnancy.[24]

Major maternal complications of pregnancy include valve thrombosis, heart failure, arrhythmia, and bleeding. The risk of valve thrombosis during pregnancy depends on the type of valve, the position (with increased risk in mitral prostheses as compared to aortic), and the mode of anticoagulation. Thrombosis risk is lowest when warfarin is used throughout pregnancy (3.9%) and highest with unfractionated heparin (UFH, 9.2%).[41] Low molecular weight heparin (LMWH) is of intermediate risk assuming that there is dose adjustment according to anti-Xa levels.[11] A recent international registry-based study reported an overall valve thrombosis rate of 4.7%.[40] Although vitamin K antagonist (VKA) therapy is the safest for the mother, it is associated with embryopathy and increased rates of miscarriage and fetal death.[40] Guidelines suggest that continuation of VKAs in pregnancy can be considered when the required dose of VKA is low.[11]

Anticoagulation is associated with an increased risk of miscarriage and hemorrhage, but it is unclear whether one regimen is better than another in this regard.[40] Women on VKAs must be switched to a shorter acting anticoagulant during the third trimester so that it can easily be stopped prior to delivery. There is no consensus on the optimal timing or whether hospitalization with UFH or outpatient management with LMWH is preferred. The timing of resumption of anticoagulation after delivery depends on the mode of delivery and the presence of delivery-related complications.

Heart failure is a common complication in those with mechanical heart valves, affecting approximately 8% of pregnancies.[40] Maternal death occurs in 1% to 2% of mechanical valve pregnancies.[40]

Heart Failure. Pregnancy is contraindicated in those with an LVEF of less than 30% or NYHA Class III-IV symptoms

(Table 104.2). The risks of pregnancy, including the potential for an irreversible decline in ventricular function, should be discussed. Patients at high risk should have a preconception assessment by a heart failure/transplant specialist. Those with a history of peripartum cardiomyopathy need specific counseling that is outside the scope of this chapter.[42]

Medications should be reviewed for fetotoxicity. Angiotensin converting enzyme inhibitors, angiotensin receptor blockers, and aldosterone antagonists need to be stopped, ideally with monitoring for decompensation prior to pregnancy. Most beta-blockers, diuretics, and hydralazine and isosorbide dinitrate can be used during pregnancy.[9]

Women with heart failure require close follow-up with monitoring of cardiac function by echocardiography. A multidisciplinary delivery plan should be developed in consultation with a heart failure/transplant specialist and a high-risk obstetrician. Delivery at a center with ventricular assist device and heart transplantation services should be strongly considered.

Arrhythmia. Supraventricular and ventricular arrhythmias are common during pregnancy in women with CHD. Many, such as ectopic beats, are benign, whereas others are clinically signficant.[43] Bradyarrhythmias are relatively uncommon in pregnancy but can be an indication for a pacemaker if symptomatic. In women with documented arrhythmias prior to pregnancy, early electrophysiology consultation may be useful.

Management of Cardiac Events in Pregnancy

Heart Failure. Hypertensive disorders, early postpartum fluid shifts, and intravenous fluid use can all precipitate heart failure in the peripartum period. Judicious use of fluids and monitoring of volume status are recommended in those with moderate and complex CHD. A normal N-terminal probrain natriuretic protein (NT-proBNP) has been shown to predict a low risk of cardiac events in pregnancy in those with CHD, and this test can be useful in differentiating heart failure from the physiologic changes of pregnancy.[44]

Acute heart failure is managed with diuretics, although aggressive diuresis and resultant intravascular hypovolemia can impair placental blood flow.[9] The safety profile of inotropes in pregnancy is undefined. Close involvement of a high-risk obstetrician is required in such patients, because some will require early delivery. Cesarean section with recovery in the intensive care unit is recommended for women with refractory heart failure.

Heart failure may worsen in the early postpartum period owing to ongoing fluid shifts. The breastfeeding compatibility of heart failure medications should be discussed with obstetrics. In general, captopril, enalapril, and most beta-blockers are compatible with lactation.[9]

Arrhythmia. Unstable arrhythmias are treated with direct current cardioversion, which is considered safe in pregnancy, because fetal exposure to current is minimal.[43] Fetal monitoring is recommended during and after cardioversion. Adenosine is not known to be associated with fetal adverse events and can be used for suspected supraventricular tachycardia. Intravenous metoprolol may also be used. Calcium channel blockers and digoxin are considered relatively safe, although listed as pregnancy category C drugs.[9]

Decision-making regarding the use of antiarrhythmic therapy in pregnancy is complex. Sotalol is the only oral Class I or III antiarrhythmic listed as category B.[9] Intravenous lidocaine can be used safely and is also category B, although its use is not recommended during delivery.[9] The risks and benefits of using other agents should be weighed carefully.

Contraception, Assisted Reproduction, and Genetics

Contraception. Contraception should be discussed with all female patients of childbearing age, with referral to a family planning specialist if needed. ACHD providers should document any restrictions on mode of contraception in the medical chart to facilitate ongoing care. A detailed review of contraceptive strategies is outside the scope of this chapter but has been covered elsewhere.[45,46]

The major concerns of the ACHD provider in relation to contraception include (1) the failure rate, with a preference for long-acting highly effective methods, (2) the ease of compliance, and (3) the cardiovascular risks. There is limited data regarding contraceptive risks in CHD.[45] The primary theoretical risk, aside from contraceptive failure resulting in unplanned pregnancy, is related to the use of estrogen in women at risk for thrombosis. Significant systemic ventricular dysfunction, history of atrial fibrillation or flutter, pulmonary hypertension, mechanical valves and Fontan palliation all predispose to thrombosis and are contraindications to estrogen administration. Individuals with other CHD lesions of great complexity may also be at a higher risk of thrombosis.

Highly effective, long-acting, non-estrogen containing contraceptive methods include intrauterine devices (IUDs), implants, and surgical sterilization. IUDs are the preferred nonpermanent form of contraception for most women with high-risk cardiac conditions.[46] Endocarditis after IUD placement, once considered to be a risk in some patients, is unlikely, and antibiotic prophylaxis is not required. A vagal response to IUD placement can occur and can be problematic in patients with severe pulmonary hypertension or Fontan physiology. These patients are not candidates for IUD placement in an office setting.

Assisted Reproduction. Limited data suggests that CHD patients may be at higher risk for amenorrhea and other menstrual cycle abnormalities, especially those with cyanotic CHD and Fontan physiology,[47] and questions about the safety of fertility treatments are becoming increasingly common.[48] Few CHD-specific data are available. Women who wish to undergo fertility treatments should be cared for at a center at which both CHD and high-risk obstetric care is available in addition to reproductive endocrinology. Detailed counseling about the risks of fertility treatment and of pregnancy should be provided prior to commencing treatment. Women with WHO Class IV disease should be encouraged to pursue alternatives to pregnancy, such as surrogacy using an egg donor or adoption.

There are several important considerations for cardiologists evaluating CHD patients prior to fertility treatment. First, invasive procedures involving cervical manipulation and pain may be poorly tolerated in women with complex disease such as a Fontan repair. These should be performed with cardiac monitoring and in consultation with an anesthesiologist with knowledge of CHD physiology. Second, the risk of stopping anticoagulation for procedures needs to be evaluated in light of individual patient factors. Third, the adverse outcomes of fertility treatment should be considered, mainly ovarian hyperstimulation syndrome and multiple pregnancy. Close collaboration between the cardiologist and reproductive endocrinologist is required to determine an individualized treatment plan to minimize patient risk.

Genetics. The offspring of individuals with CHD are at higher risk for CHD.[22] The incidence in nonsyndromic CHD varies from 1% to 14%, depending on the type of defect and which parent is affected (Table 104.3). The incidence is higher in those with an underlying genetic syndrome such as DiGeorge, Williams, or Holt-Oram. All CHD patients contemplating pregnancy should be counseled about the risk of offspring CHD. Preconception evaluation by medical genetics is reasonable in ACHD patients with suspected syndromic CHD.

Male Reproductive Health

Although sexual activity does not pose risks to male patients with CHD beyond those associated with physical activity, men with CHD report significant anxiety surrounding sex and erectile dysfunction. Male sexual dysfunction is associated with depression and low quality of life, and sexual health should be proactively discussed.[3]

FOLLOW-UP PATIENT CARE

All patients should leave obstetric care with a defined contraceptive plan and a referral for ongoing cardiac care, which for the majority involves follow-up at an ACHD center. Recommended lesion-specific follow-up intervals can be found elsewhere.[3]

RESEARCH AND FUTURE DIRECTIONS

There are significant knowledge gaps regarding CHD pregnancy management. Further research is needed to understand the impact of management strategies on maternal and fetal outcomes. Emerging data from multicenter registries such as Registry of Pregnancy and Cardiac disease (ROPAC) and the newly formed Heart Outcomes in Pregnancy Expectations (HOPE) registry should provide a nuanced perspective on contemporary pregnancy management, with the ultimate goal of defining a standard for high-quality pregnancy care in this complex population.[2,49]

KEY POINTS

- ✔ All women with CHD of childbearing age should receive counseling about their contraception and pregnancy risk profile.
- ✔ A labor plan is useful for all patients, including the following:
  - Anticipated risks
  - Delivery mode/location
  - Need for telemetry
  - Need for intravenous filter
  - Anticoagulation plan
  - Contraindications to commonly used obstetric medications
  - Need for cardiac testing
  - Intake/output goal
  - Whom to call in the event of a cardiac emergency.
- ✔ Estrogen is contraindicated in systemic ventricular dysfunction, atrial fibrillation, pulmonary hypertension, mechanical valves, and the Fontan palliation.
- ✔ The risk of offspring CHD in patients with CHD is on average 3% to 5%.
- ✔ Regurgitant lesions are generally well tolerated in pregnancy unless there is coexisting symptomatic heart failure or ventricular dysfunction.
- ✔ Beta-blockers, with the exception of atenolol, are generally safe in pregnancy.

REFERENCES

1. Khairy P, Ionescu-Ittu R, Mackie AS, et al. Changing mortality in congenital heart disease. *J Am Coll Cardiol.* 2010;56:1149-1157.
2. Roos-Hesselink JW, Ruys TP, Stein JI, et al. Outcome of pregnancy in patients with structural or ischaemic heart disease: results of a registry of the European Society of Cardiology. *Eur Heart J.* 2013;34:657-665.
3. Stout KK, Daniels CJ, Aboulhosn JA, et al. 2018 AHA/ACC Guideline for the management of adults with congenital heart disease: executive summary: a report of the American College of Cardiology/American Heart Association task force on clinical practice guidelines. *J Am Coll Cardiol.* 2019;73:1494-1563.
4. Committee on Obstetric Practice. Committee opinion no. 723: Guidelines for diagnostic imaging during pregnancy and lactation. *Obstet Gynecol.* 2017;130:e210-e216.
5. Ray JG, Vermeulen MJ, Bharatha A, et al. Association between MRI exposure during pregnancy and fetal and childhood outcomes. *JAMA.* 2016;316:952-961.
6. Lui GK, Silversides CK, Khairy P, et al. Heart rate response during exercise and pregnancy outcome in women with congenital heart disease. *Circulation.* 2011;123:242-248.
7. Silversides CK, Grewal J, Mason J, et al. Pregnancy outcomes in women with heart disease: the CARPREG II study. *J Am Coll Cardiol.* 2018;71:2419-2430.
8. Drenthen W, Boersma E, Balci A, et al. Predictors of pregnancy complications in women with congenital heart disease. *Eur Heart J.* 2010;31:2124-2132.
9. Canobbio MM, Warnes CA, Aboulhosn J, et al. Management of pregnancy in patients with complex congenital heart disease: a scientific statement for healthcare professionals from the American Heart Association. *Circulation.* 2017;135:e50-e87.
10. Balci A, Sollie-Szarynska KM, van der Bijl AG, et al. Prospective validation and assessment of cardiovascular and offspring risk models for pregnant women with congenital heart disease. *Heart.* 2014;100:1373-1381.
11. Regitz-Zagrosek V, Blomstrom Lundqvist C, Borghi C, et al. ESC Guidelines on the management of cardiovascular diseases during pregnancy: the task force on the management of cardiovascular diseases during pregnancy of the European Society of Cardiology. *Eur Heart J.* 2011;32:3147-3197.

12. Drenthen W, Pieper PG, Roos-Hesselink JW, et al. Outcome of pregnancy in women with congenital heart disease: a literature review. *J Am Coll Cardiol.* 2007;49:2303-2311.
13. Veldtman GR, Connolly HM, Grogan M, et al. Outcomes of pregnancy in women with tetralogy of Fallot. *J Am Coll Cardiol.* 2004;44:174-180.
14. Pedersen LM, Pedersen TA, Ravn HB, et al. Outcomes of pregnancy in women with tetralogy of Fallot. *Cardiol Young.* 2008;18:423-429.
15. Khairy P, Ouyang DW, Fernandes SM, et al. Pregnancy outcomes in women with congenital heart disease. *Circulation.* 2006;113:517-524.
16. Romeo JLR, Takkenberg JJM, Roos-Hesselink JW, et al. Outcomes of pregnancy after right ventricular outflow tract reconstruction with an allograft conduit. *J Am Coll Cardiol.* 2018;71:2656-2665.
17. Egbe AC, El-Harasis M, Miranda WR, et al. Outcomes of pregnancy in patients with prior right ventricular outflow interventions. *J Am Heart Assoc.* 2019;8:e011730.
18. Vriend JW, Drenthen W, Pieper PG, et al. Outcome of pregnancy in patients after repair of aortic coarctation. *Eur Heart J.* 2005;26:2173-2178.
19. Connolly HM, Warnes CA. Ebstein's anomaly: outcome of pregnancy. *J Am Coll Cardiol.* 1994;23:1194-1198.
20. Kanoh M, Inai K, Shinohara T, et al. Influence of pregnancy on cardiac function and hemodynamics in women with Ebstein's anomaly. *Acta Obstet Gynecol Scand.* 2018;97:1025-1031.
21. Drenthen W, Pieper PG, van der Tuuk K, et al. Cardiac complications relating to pregnancy and recurrence of disease in the offspring of women with atrioventricular septal defects. *Eur Heart J.* 2005;26:2581-2587.
22. Pierpont ME, Brueckner M, Chung WK, et al. Genetic basis for congenital heart disease: revisited: a scientific statement from the American Heart Association. *Circulation.* 2018;138:e653-e711.
23. Drenthen W, Pieper PG, Roos-Hesselink JW, et al. Non-cardiac complications during pregnancy in women with isolated congenital pulmonary valvar stenosis. *Heart.* 2006;92:1838-1843.
24. Nishimura RA, Otto CM, Bonow RO, et al. 2014 AHA/ACC Guideline for the management of patients with valvular heart disease: executive summary. *Circulation.* 2014;129:2440-2492.
25. Orwat S, Diller GP, van Hagen IM, et al. Risk of pregnancy in moderate and severe aortic stenosis: from the Multinational ROPAC Registry. *J Am Coll Cardiol.* 2016;68:1727-1737.
26. Hodson R, Kirker E, Swanson J, et al. Transcatheter aortic valve replacement during pregnancy. *Circ Cardiovasc Interv.* 2016;9:1-8.
27. Wanga S, Silversides C, Dore A, et al. Pregnancy and thoracic aortic disease: managing the risks. *Can J Cardiol.* 2016;32:78-85.
28. Hameed A, Karaalp IS, Tummala PP, et al. The effect of valvular heart disease on maternal and fetal outcome of pregnancy. *J Am Coll Cardiol.* 2001;37:893-899.
29. Lesniak-Sobelga A, Tracz W, KostKiewicz M, Podolec P, Pasowicz M. Clinical and echocardiographic assessment of pregnant women with valvular heart diseases—maternal and fetal outcome. *Int J Cardiol.* 2004;94:15-23.
30. Diller GP, Dimopoulos K, Okonko D, et al. Exercise intolerance in adult congenital heart disease: comparative severity, correlates, and prognostic implication. *Circulation.* 2005;112:828-835.
31. Garcia Ropero A, Baskar S, Roos Hesselink JW, et al. Pregnancy in women with a Fontan circulation: a systematic review of the literature. *Circ Cardiovasc Qual Outcomes.* 2018;11:e004575.
32. Gouton M, Nizard J, Patel M, et al. Maternal and fetal outcomes of pregnancy with Fontan circulation: a multicentric observational study. *Int J Cardiol.* 2015;187:84-89.
33. Metz TD, Jackson GM, Yetman AT. Pregnancy outcomes in women who have undergone an atrial switch repair for congenital D-transposition of the great arteries. *Am J Obstet Gynecol.* 2011;205:273.e271-275.
34. Guedes A, Mercier LA, Leduc L, et al. Impact of pregnancy on the systemic right ventricle after a Mustard operation for transposition of the great arteries. *J Am Coll Cardiol.* 2004;44:433-437.
35. Kowalik E, Klisiewicz A, Biernacka EK, et al. Pregnancy and long-term cardiovascular outcomes in women with congenitally corrected transposition of the great arteries. *Int J Gynaecol Obstet.* 2014;125:154-157.
36. Therrien J, Barnes I, Somerville J. Outcome of pregnancy in patients with congenitally corrected transposition of the great arteries. *Am J Cardiol.* 1999;84:820-824.
37. Stoll VM, Drury NE, Thorne S, et al. Pregnancy outcomes in women with transposition of the great arteries after an arterial switch operation. *JAMA Cardiol.* 2018;3:1119-1122.
38. Horiuchi C, Kamiya CA, Ohuchi H, et al. Pregnancy outcomes and mid-term prognosis in women after arterial switch operation for dextro-transposition of the great arteries—tertiary hospital experiences and review of literature. *J Cardiol.* 2019;73:247-254.
39. Sliwa K, Baris L, Sinning C, et al. Pregnant women with uncorrected congenital heart disease: heart failure and mortality. *JACC Heart Fail.* 2020;8(2):100-110.
40. van Hagen IM, Roos-Hesselink JW, Ruys TP, et al. Pregnancy in women with a mechanical heart valve: data of the European Society of Cardiology registry of pregnancy and cardiac disease. *Circulation.* 2015;132:132-142.
41. Chan WS, Anand S, Ginsberg JS. Anticoagulation of pregnant women with mechanical heart valves: a systematic review of the literature. *Arch Intern Med.* 2000;160:191-196.
42. Bauersachs J, Konig T, van der Meer P, et al. Pathophysiology, diagnosis and management of peripartum cardiomyopathy: a position statement from the heart failure association of the European Society of Cardiology study group on peripartum cardiomyopathy. *Eur J Heart Fail.* 2019;21:827-843.
43. Knotts RJ, Garan H. Cardiac arrhythmias in pregnancy. *Semin Perinatol.* 2014;38:285-288.
44. Kampman MA, Balci A, van Veldhuisen DJ, et al. N-terminal pro-b-type natriuretic peptide predicts cardiovascular complications in pregnant women with congenital heart disease. *Eur Heart J.* 2014;35:708-715.
45. Abarbanell G, Tepper NK, Farr SL. Safety of contraceptive use among women with congenital heart disease: a systematic review. *Congenit Heart Dis.* 2019;14:331-340.
46. Moussa HN, Rajapreyar I. ACOG practice bulletin no. 212: pregnancy and heart disease. *Obstet Gynecol.* 2019;134:881-882.
47. Drenthen W, Hoendermis ES, Moons P, et al. Menstrual cycle and its disorders in women with congenital heart disease. *Congenit Heart Dis.* 2008;3:277-283.
48. Cauldwell M, Patel RR, Steer PJ, et al. Managing subfertility in patients with heart disease: what are the choices? *Am Heart J.* 2017;187:29-36.
49. Grodzinsky A, Florio K, Spertus JA, et al. Maternal mortality in the United States and the hope registry. *Curr Treat Options Cardiovasc Med.* 2019;21:42.

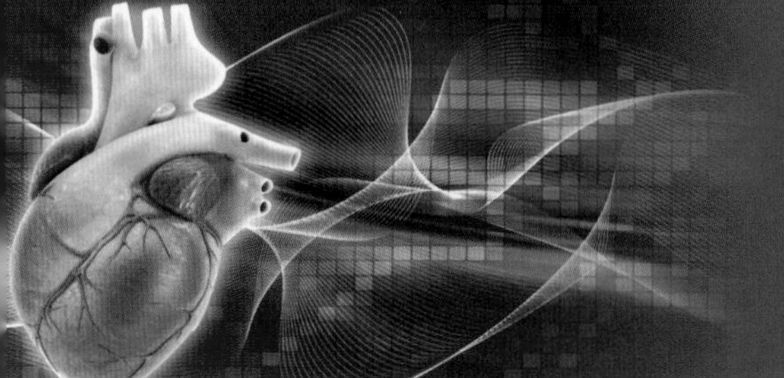

CHAPTER 105

PHARMACOLOGIC THERAPY FOR ADULT CONGENITAL HEART DISEASE

Dan G. Halpern, Rebecca Pinnelas, and Frank Cecchin

INTRODUCTION

As survival of congenital heart disease patients continues to improve, the role of pharmacologic therapy is pivotal in the care of adults with congenital heart disease (ACHD), complementing surgical, and interventional therapies. Wide-ranging pathology, underpowered trials, reliance on retrospective studies, and science extrapolated from acquired cardiovascular disease literature challenges the field. However, newly published evidence-based guidelines, together with growing research alliances and large international registries, help standardize care and improve outcomes.[1-3]

Initiation of chronic multidrug therapy at a young age raises long-term concerns. Polypharmacy, including noncardiac medications, is twice as prevalent among ACHD patients compared with the general population. Additionally, chronic multidrug therapy has been associated with a fourfold increased risk of mortality and adverse drug events, only in part explained by the congenital heart disease.[4] Therefore, prescribing clinicians should judiciously weigh the strength of the evidence in favor of pharmacologic therapy against potential long-term drug side effects. This chapter provides an overview of medical therapies recommended and used for the most common congenital heart pathologies Table 105.3. Individuals with acquired heart disease or risk factors for such should be treated according to American College of Cardiology (ACC)/ American Heart Association (AHA) guidelines.

PHARMACOKINETICS OF DRUGS IN ADULTS WITH CONGENITAL HEART DISEASE

Hemodynamic changes secondary to congenital heart disease may have profound effects on the pharmacokinetics of drugs, requiring dosing considerations and adjustments. Renal function may be attenuated by reduced cardiac output, renal venous congestion, and cyanosis. Hepatic congestion and fibrosis—as may occur in the setting of Fontan palliation for single ventricle or right-sided heart failure—may also affect the metabolism of drugs. Additionally, hepatitis C infection is a common finding in congenital patients treated with blood transfusions before 1992 and may lead to early cirrhosis. Protein-losing enteropathy in patients with Fontan circulation causes delayed drug absorption and hypoalbuminemia, which increases the free fraction of protein-bound medications.

Right-to-left shunting may affect physiologic first-pass metabolism and drug concentration. In an animal model of right-to-left shunting, administration of lidocaine bypassed the drug's first-pass metabolism within the lung, which resulted in a doubling of its peak arterial concentration and neurotoxicity at two-thirds of the traditional dose.[5] Conversely, prodrugs metabolized in the liver may actually have reduced drug concentrations with right-to-left shunting.

The basic tenets of medication administration in congenital heart patients include initiation of low dosages with careful and gradual increase of the dose based on hemodynamic response and side effects. Progressive dosing should be based on changing hemodynamics and routine hepatic and renal laboratory work. As some medications may increase the risk of arrhythmia, event monitors (with multiweek monitoring capabilities) are useful in identifying arrhythmia during and after medication titration.

MEDICAL MANAGEMENT OF ARRHYTHMIA

Arrhythmia is the leading cause of hospital admissions in the ACHD population (see **Table 105.1**). The basis for this high-arrhythmic load is a combination of cardiac developmental abnormalities and lifelong accumulation of arrhythmic substrate. Congenital heart disease is often associated with conduction system anomalies like accessory pathways and maldevelopment of the sinus and atrioventricular nodes. Additionally, the structure of the cardiac anomaly—such as the conal septum in tetralogy of Fallot (TOF)—may contribute to the genesis of ventricular tachycardia. Accumulation of multiple sutures or surgical scar lines, cyanosis, pressure, and volume-overloaded myocardium also contribute to the arrhythmia substrate in those with ACHD.[6] Not surprisingly, the burden of arrhythmia is directly proportional to the complexity of the cardiac lesion and the number of prior corrective cardiac surgeries. Suture lines, scarring, and fibrosis create anatomic barriers, which aid in propagation of the arrhythmic wavefront. While many of these arrhythmias can be successfully treated with a catheter or surgical ablation, long-term antiarrhythmic drug therapy is commonly used adjunctively since some mechanisms can be only modified and not completely cured. There is no role for drug treatment of chronic bradyarrhythmia, which can only be effectively treated with cardiac pacing.

TABLE 105.1 Arrhythmia Treatment Considerations in Congenital Heart Disease

- New-onset tachyarrhythmia should prompt a hemodynamic assessment.
- CHA_2DS_2-VASc score may underestimate thromboembolism risk in ACHD population with minimal cardiovascular risk factors.
- Low threshold for anticoagulation for tachyarrhythmia is recommended, especially in complex lesions (ie, single ventricle post-Fontan).
- Avoid AV nodal blocking agents in WPW (associated with Ebstein anomaly and L-TGA).
- Sinus node dysfunction and complete heart block are common in D-TGA postatrial switch and L-TGA, respectively.
- Consider early electrical cardioversion for tachyarrhythmia, as antiarrhythmic drug therapy often ineffective and not well tolerated.
- Radiofrequency ablation of common CHD-related tachyarrhythmias is frequently curative.
- Antiarrhythmic drug therapy for SVT according to CHD complexity: for simple and moderate lesions (ASD, VSD, repaired TOF) without significant ventricular dysfunction use Class IC agent (eg, flecainide, propafenone); for complex lesions (single ventricle post-Fontan) use Class III agent (eg, amiodarone, sotalol).
- Antiarrhythmic drug therapy for ventricular arrhythmia: beta-blockers and Class III agents. Placement of AICD according to guidelines
- High-risk for SCD: single ventricle post-Fontan, Eisenmenger syndrome, repaired TOF and Ebstein anomaly
- QRS duration >180 ms is associated with SCD in repaired TOF (QRS duration correlates with the degree of RV dysfunction).
- Class Ia and III agents are associated with QT interval prolongation.

ACHD, adult congenital heart disease; AICD, automatic implantable cardioverter defibrillator; ASD, atrial septal defect; AV, atrioventricular; CHD, congenital heart disease; ms, milliseconds; RV, right ventricle; SCD, sudden cardiac death; SVT, supraventricular tachycardia; TGA, transposition of the great arteries; TOF, tetralogy of Fallot; VSD, ventricular septal defect; WPW, Wolff-Parkinson-White.

Data derived from Stout KK, Daniels CJ, Aboulhosn JA, et al. 2018 AHA/ACC Guideline for the management of adults with congenital heart disease: executive summary: a report of the American College of Cardiology/American Heart Association Task Force on Clinical Practice Guidelines. *J Am Coll Cardiol.* 2019;73:1494-1563 and Helmut Baumgartner H, De Backer, J, Babu-Narayan SV, et al. ESC Scientific document group, 2020 ESC Guidelines for the management of adult congenital heart disease: The Task Force for the management of adult congenital heart disease of the European Society of Cardiology (ESC). Endorsed by: Association for European Paediatric and Congenital Cardiology (AEPC), International Society for Adult Congenital Heart Disease (ISACHD). *Eur Heart J.* 2021;42(6):563-645.

Pharmacotherapy for Atrial Tachyarrhythmia

Pharmacotherapy recommendations for atrial tachyarrhythmia not only take into consideration the congenital heart lesion complexity but should also consider additional factors such as coexisting sinus node dysfunction, impaired atrioventricular (AV) nodal conduction, systemic or subpulmonary ventricular dysfunction, associated therapies, child-bearing potential, and acquired comorbidities.[7] Simple and moderate complexity lesions such as atrial septal defect (ASD), ventricular septal defect (VSD), Ebstein anomaly, and TOF may be treated with Class IC antiarrhythmic agents (eg, flecainide and propafenone) if ventricular dysfunction is absent. Complex lesions with arrhythmias, such as single ventricles with Fontan palliation or cyanotic congenital heart disease, are treated with Class III antiarrhythmic agents (eg, amiodarone and sotalol). Specific considerations and dosing strategies vary among the different congenital lesions and antiarrhythmic drugs. Consultation with an electrophysiologist who has expertise with congenital heart disease is highly recommended.

Class IC antiarrhythmic drugs may have proarrhythmic effects in patients with structural heart disease and should not be used in the presence of hepatic dysfunction, prolonged PR interval (>250 ms), coronary artery disease, or moderately to severely depressed systolic dysfunction of a systemic or subpulmonary ventricle. In addition, Class IC antiarrhythmic agents can organize atrial fibrillation into a rapid atrial flutter (eg, with 1:1 conduction), thus requiring concomitant use of an AV nodal blocking agent.

Class III antiarrhythmic agents are associated with QTc prolongation, which could be challenging to assess in the setting of a significantly prolonged QRS complex in many ACHD patients. One strategy of correcting the QT interval in the setting of intraventricular conduction delay is to use the following equation: QTc (corrected) $= (QT-(QRS-120))/RR^{0.5}$.[8]

Mixed data regarding the proarrhythmic potential of sotalol exist; therefore, it is considered a second-line therapy. General guidelines for atrial fibrillation support the use of sotalol (Class IIa indication) for maintenance of sinus rhythm in patients with little or no heart disease, baseline QT interval less than 460 ms, normal serum electrolytes, creatinine clearance greater than 40 mL/min, and absence of risk factors associated with Class III antiarrhythmic drug-related proarrhythmia. Holter monitoring and stress testing are recommended after achieving the sotalol loading dose to rule out proarrhythmia. A recent large retrospective analysis showed that sotalol was safe and effective in low dosages in the ACHD population, but it was associated with significant bradycardia in the Fontan population.[9] Amiodarone has multiple toxicities (cardiac, lung, liver, thyroid, skin, eyes, and central nervous system) as well as multiple drug interactions. Amiodarone requires pulmonary toxicity monitoring (baseline chest x-ray and pulmonary function tests, then annual chest x-ray) together with frequent liver and thyroid function testing before initiation of therapy and then every 3 to 6 months thereafter. Dose reduction of digoxin and warfarin is required when administered concomitantly with amiodarone. When using antiarrhythmic drugs, it is always important to reassess the effects of sinus node function and AV node function. Bradycardia is a side effect of treatment with beta-blockers, calcium channel blockers, and Class III antiarrhythmic drugs. If their use is essential, permanent pacing may be needed to achieve effective antiarrhythmic drug dosages.

Arrhythmia-Specific Considerations

Intra-atrial reentrant tachycardia or "incisional tachycardia" is the most common tachyarrhythmia observed in ACHD patients. It can be a component of typical atrial flutter (peritricuspid valve reentry) or unrelated. The circuit propagates around right-atrial atriotomy incisions, scars from chronic fibrosis, ASD patches, and other anatomic barriers. It is often resistant to primary antiarrhythmic drug therapy and may require rate-controlling agents and chronic anticoagulation. Radiofrequency ablation may be curative as a primary treatment.

Accessory pathways or Wolff-Parkinson-White (WPW) syndrome is highly prevalent in Ebstein anomaly and congenitally corrected transposition of the great arteries (L-TGA). Radiofrequency catheter ablation of the accessory pathway is mainstay treatment. Treatment of supraventricular tachycardia (SVT) episodes in patients with WPW depends on the directionality of the circuit. Orthodromic AV reciprocating tachycardia (AVRT), appearing as a narrow complex tachycardia in which antegrade conduction occurs through the AV node with retrograde conduction through the accessory pathway. It is treated with vagal maneuvers or AV nodal blocking agents (ie, adenosine, beta-blockers, and calcium blockers) for acute termination, and beta-blockers for chronic treatment. Antidromic AVRT, in which antegrade conduction occurs through the accessory pathway with retrograde conduction through the AV node, appears as a wide complex tachycardia and is treated acutely with intravenous procainamide infusion. Atrial flutter or fibrillation in the setting of WPW syndrome should be treated with cardioversion, intravenous procainamide, or intravenous ibutilide. AV nodal blocking agents are contraindicated in antidromic AVRT and WPW syndrome with atrial fibrillation, as they may increase conduction through the accessory pathway. Thus, when unsure of the arrhythmic diagnosis, it may be safer to initially use procainamide.

Atrial fibrillation increases in prevalence with age and is observed in left-sided cardiac lesions such as congenital mitral stenosis, subaortic membrane, and aortic stenosis. Given the importance of maintaining sinus rhythm and preserving the "atrial kick" in patients with congenital heart disease, ablation therapy should be strongly considered as Class IC and III antiarrhythmic drugs have limited efficacy.

Anticoagulation is advised for patients with atrial tachyarrhythmia to reduce the thromboembolic risk. There is a lower threshold for full anticoagulation in the congenital heart disease population than predicted with the application of the CHA_2DS_2-VASc, as the ACHD population is younger and commonly lacks the traditional cardiovascular risk factors (eg, diabetes, hypertension, coronary artery disease).

Ventricular arrhythmia and the risk of sudden cardiac death (SCD) increase with age and congenital heart lesion complexity. Risk factors for SCD include prior SVT, increased QRS duration, and diminished systemic/subpulmonary ventricular function.[10] The highest risk congenital cardiac lesions include single ventricles palliated with a Fontan circuit, Eisenmenger syndrome, repaired TOF, and Ebstein anomaly. Other lesions at increased risk of ventricular arrhythmia and SCD include uncorrected transposition of the great arteries (d-TGA) with surgical atrial switch and L-TGA in which the right ventricle is the systemic ventricle. It is reasonable to prescribe beta-blockers to patients with d-TGA postatrial switch and intra-atrial reentrant tachycardia to protect against ventricular arrhythmias and SCD.[7] The relationship between QRS duration and its association with SCD (eg, QRS > 180 ms in repaired TOF) is regarded as an indirect assessment of right ventricular dysfunction for which surgical repair (eg, pulmonary valve replacement in TOF) may offer hemodynamic relief. However, it is unclear whether these surgical repairs eliminate the future arrhythmic risk. Drug therapy for ventricular arrhythmias in these patients includes beta-blockers and Class III antiarrhythmic drugs—with amiodarone being the mainstay—typically used in conjunction with an automatic implantable cardioverter defibrillator (AICD) device according to practice guidelines. Antiarrhythmic drugs may be helpful in reducing recurrent AICD discharges, and radiofrequency ablation of ventricular arrhythmia has also shown promise.

Importantly, while medical and invasive options for treating arrhythmias are available, new arrhythmias in the ACHD population should prompt an assessment of hemodynamics and new structural disease.

ANTICOAGULATION AND ANTIPLATELET THERAPY

ACHD may require anticoagulation or antiplatelet therapy for a variety of reasons, including risk or evidence of thromboembolism, atrial arrhythmia, ventricular dysfunction, mechanical valve replacement, and temporarily after shunt closure.[1] Atrial fibrillation, Fontan circulation, and CHA_2DS_2-VASc score greater than or equal to 1 are the most common reasons ACHD patients receive systemic anticoagulation.[11]

Per ACC/AHA 2020 guidelines, patients with bioprosthetic valves should receive aspirin lifelong if there is not an indication for other anticoagulation. Aspirin combined with vitamin K antagonists (VKA, ie, warfarin) is a IIb recommendation for mechanical valves.[12] The role of aspirin in the prevention of endocarditis or its embolic complications has not been established,[13] yet animal models suggest aspirin may inhibit fibrin and microthrombi formation that are the initial nidus for vegetations.[14]

Antiplatelet therapy is prescribed for the first 6 months after device closure of an intracardiac defect (eg, ASD, patent foramen ovale [PFO], VSD, and patent ductus arteriosus [PDA]) (see **Table 105.2**). A retrospective analysis of 789 patients who underwent device closure and were treated with aspirin, 100 mg, showed no major bleeding, low-device thrombosis risk (ASD 0% and PFO 0.2%), and stroke (0.4%), suggesting safety and effectiveness of low-dose aspirin in this group.[15] Low-dose aspirin is also commonly given for unrepaired shunt lesions for the prevention of paradoxic emboli, particularly during pregnancy and with known right-to-left shunting. It is not, however, safe in patients with Eisenmenger syndrome.

As the use of non-vitamin K oral anticoagulants (NOACs) increases in the general cardiology population, there has also

TABLE 105.2 Shunt Lesions Treatment Considerations

- Aspirin use for the first 6 months after the closure of a shunt and commonly used for right-to-left shunts
- Shunt closure is feasible when there is a left-to-right shunt with pulmonary vascular resistance <1/3 systemic vascular resistance or pulmonary artery systolic pressure <50% systemic and contraindicated when there is right-to-left shunting. Borderline cases are discussed elsewhere.
- Infective endocarditis prophylaxis for the first 6 months after the closure of a shunt

Data derived from Stout KK, Daniels CJ, Aboulhosn JA, et al. 2018 AHA/ACC Guideline for the management of adults with congenital heart disease: executive summary: a report of the American College of Cardiology/American Heart Association Task Force on Clinical Practice Guidelines. *J Am Coll Cardiol.* 2019;73:1494-1563 and Helmut Baumgartner H, De Backer, J, Babu-Narayan SV, et al. ESC Scientific document group, 2020 ESC Guidelines for the management of adult congenital heart disease: The Task Force for the management of adult congenital heart disease of the European Society of Cardiology (ESC). Endorsed by: Association for European Paediatric and Congenital Cardiology (AEPC), International Society for Adult Congenital Heart Disease (ISACHD). *Eur Heart J.* 2021;42(6):563-645.

been interest in their use in ACHD patients. In the recent prospective international NOTE (Nonvitamin K Oral anticoagulants for Thromboembolic prevention in patients with CHD), registry of 530 ACHD patients with the mostly moderate and complex disease treated with NOACs, an annual 1% thromboembolic and 1.1% major bleeding rate was noted, suggesting that the drugs were safe and effective across a range of CHD.[16] The choice of NOAC in the ACHD population may vary with the patient's renal function, liver function, and potential for drug-to-drug interactions.

Fontan palliation patients are at particularly high risk of thrombotic and embolic complications due to a low flow state, frequent presence of shunting, hepatic impairment, and coagulation abnormalities.[17] A Class I (LOE C) recommendation is made for warfarin in adults with Fontan palliation if they have a history of current thrombus, prior venous thromboembolism, atrial arrhythmia, and no contraindication to systemic anticoagulation. Fontan patients with significant veno-veno collaterals or residual right-to-left shunting may be considered for oral anticoagulation or antiplatelet therapy (ie, a Class IIb recommendation).[1] Studies evaluating warfarin versus aspirin in the Fontan population have shown mixed results. In one study of 210 Fontan patients followed for a median of 8.5 years after surgery, those who did not receive either aspirin or warfarin had a significantly higher risk of thromboembolic events, with no difference in events between the agents.[18] In another study of 278 patients with Fontan palliation, warfarin was associated with a lower risk of thromboembolic complications compared with antiplatelet therapy alone.[17] A single-center study summarizing 30 years of experience with 431 post-Fontan patients showed that warfarin was not superior to aspirin for preventing thromboembolic events, but it was associated with a higher bleeding rate.[19] NOAC use in the Fontan population is under investigation.[20]

In ACHD patients with pulmonary hypertension, anticoagulation should be cautiously used for thromboembolic or arrhythmic indications, recognizing that pulmonary arterial hemorrhage and rupture are major causes of morbidity, especially in Eisenmenger syndrome. In a retrospective cohort study of Eisenmenger syndrome patients, there was no difference in long-term survival between those who received anticoagulation and those who did not; however, bleeding complications occurred much more frequently in those who received anticoagulation (16% vs 0%, respectively).[21]

MEDICAL MANAGEMENT OF HEART FAILURE

Heart failure remains the primary cause of morbidity and mortality among ACHD patients (see **Table 105.3**). It is imperative to rule out correctable lesions (eg, valve disease, obstructive muscle bundles, and conduit stenosis) and treat reversible etiologies (eg, coronary artery disease, arrhythmias, hypertension, thyroid disease, and toxins). Neurohormonal blockade therapy with renin-angiotensin-aldosterone system inhibitors or beta-adrenergic blockers may be considered, but the extent to which such therapy benefits ACHD patients with heart failure is unknown.[1] The etiologies of heart failure in ACHD patients may differ from those with traditional left ventricular (LV) systolic dysfunction; however, there may be some similarities in neurohormonal activation pathways. ACHD patients with biventricular anatomy and systemic LV dysfunction (ie, usual anatomy) can be medically managed as per standard heart failure guidelines. Optimal pharmacologic therapy for the biventricular heart with a systemic right ventricle (RV) or single ventricle is undefined.

Biventricular Physiology With a Systemic Left Ventricular and Right Ventricular Dysfunction

Medical treatment options for systolic RV failure are scarce and include diuretic therapy and inotropes for acute failure. Correction of mechanical lesions causing volume overload (eg, repaired TOF with pulmonary regurgitation) or pressure overload (eg, pulmonary stenosis, double-chamber right ventricle) should improve RV loading conditions and function long term. RV failure in the setting of pulmonary hypertension should focus on pulmonary vasodilators, inotropic support, and diuretics. Digoxin is routinely used in the pediatric congenital heart patient for RV inotropic support, yet its efficacy for the treatment of RV failure in the adult is unknown. Digoxin modestly increased cardiac output in a small study of patients with RV failure and pulmonary hypertension.[22] Neurohormonal blockade with ramipril[23] or beta-blocker[24] does not appear to improve RV function in repaired TOF patients.

Biventricular Physiology With a Systemic Right Ventricle

The use of neurohormonal blockade in patients with a systemic RV (ie, d-TGA postatrial switch or L-TGA) has been

TABLE 105.3 Heart Failure Treatment Considerations in Congenital Heart Disease

- Correction of hemodynamically significant lesions should be attempted in conjunction with medical therapy.
- Systemic LV dysfunction (usual anatomy) is managed as per standard heart failure guidelines.
- Benefit of neurohormonal blockade in systemic RV heart failure (d-TGA postatrial switch and L-TGA) remains uncertain.
- ACE inhibitor treatment in d-TGA postatrial switch can cause orthostatic hypotension due to noncompliant atria and should be up-titrated cautiously.
- Beta-blockade can cause significant bradycardia in d-TGA postatrial switch and L-TGA (1%-2%/year complete heart block development).
- Diuretic therapy in single ventricle post-Fontan should be managed carefully as overdiuresis may cause hypotension.
- NOACs are being studied and are probably a safe option for Fontan-related thromboembolic disease.
- Sildenafil in the Fontan patient may improve exercise tolerance.

ACE, angiotensin-converting enzyme; LV, left ventricle; NOAC, non-vitamin K oral anticoagulants; RV, right ventricle; TGA, transposition of the great arteries.
Data derived from Stout KK, Daniels CJ, Aboulhosn JA, et al. 2018 AHA/ACC Guideline for the management of adults with congenital heart disease: executive summary: a report of the American College of Cardiology/American Heart Association Task Force on Clinical Practice Guidelines. *J Am Coll Cardiol.* 2019;73:1494-1563 and Yang H, Veldtman GR, Bouma BJ, et al. Non-vitamin K antagonist oral anticoagulants in adults with a Fontan circulation: are they safe. *Open Heart.* 2019;6:e000985.

incompletely studied, and the application of heart failure therapy should be used with caution. If utilized in patients with d-TGA postatrial switch, angiotensin-converting enzyme (ACE) inhibitors should be initiated at low doses with incremental up-titration as orthostatic hypotension may occur as a result of the noncompliant atria[42]. A systematic review and meta-analysis of six randomized controlled trials that assessed outcomes in systemic RV patients receiving ACE inhibitors, angiotensin-receptor blockers (ARBs), or aldosterone antagonists[25] showed their use was not associated with improvement in peak oxygen consumption, exercise capacity, RV dimensions, or RV systolic function.[25,26]

Randomized trials with beta-blockers for heart failure in systemic RV are not available. Although an observational study of patients with d-TGA postatrial switch and RV dysfunction treated with beta-blockers showed improvement in NYHA functional class compared with those who did not receive such therapy.[27] Beta-blockers should be used with caution due to the risk of bradyarrhythmias and heart block, especially in L-TGA patients in whom the annual risk of complete heart block is 1% to 2% per year.

Given the aforementioned data, the updated ACHD guidelines concluded that the benefit of neurohormonal blockade for patients with systemic RVs remains uncertain.[1]

Consideration of tricuspid valve replacement is recommended in patients with L-TGA and significant tricuspid regurgitation with early RV dysfunction (systemic RV ejection fraction $< 40\%$), as primary tricuspid valve disease, is common and plays a major role in systemic RV failure. In contrast, tricuspid regurgitation in d-TGA postatrial switch is mostly functional and secondary to the myopathy, which renders surgical repair of the valve less beneficial.

Other therapies for systemic RV failure include cardiac resynchronization therapy and, in the advanced disease state, ventricular assist devices and cardiac transplantation.

Single Ventricle Post-Fontan Palliation

Single ventricles palliated with a Fontan circulation lack a pulsatile subpulmonic chamber, thereby causing increased systemic venous pressures, passive flow entering the pulmonary circulation, and a chronic low-cardiac output state.

In the adult Fontan population, the use of neurohormonal blockade is empiric and lacks evidence. Despite the common use of ACE inhibitors in adult Fontan patients, no randomized studies have been performed in this population. In a randomized trial of pediatric Fontan patients, enalapril did not improve ventricular function or outcome (death or transplant) compared with placebo.[28] Reviews of this topic have found little compelling evidence for ACE inhibitor use; however, there may be a theoretical benefit with ACE inhibitor usage later in adulthood when afterload has started to increase.[29] Beta-blockade in single ventricle physiology is also controversial. In a randomized, placebo-controlled study of children with systolic heart failure, which included Fontan patients, no difference in clinical outcomes was observed in those taking carvedilol.[30]

Sildenafil, a phosphodiesterase type-5 inhibitor used as a pulmonary vasodilator, is hypothesized to improve pulmonary blood flow in the Fontan circuit by decreasing the pulmonary vascular resistance and subsequently augmenting the LV preload. In a meta-analysis of 381 Fontan patients, sildenafil improved functional class, 6-minute walk testing, and maximal oxygen consumption with a reduction in mean pulmonary pressures. However, no mortality benefit has yet been shown from this intervention.[31] There is controversy as to whether sildenafil should be initiated in patients with normal pulmonary vascular resistance.

Diuretic therapy is used for the relief of peripheral edema and chronic systemic venous congestion; however, in the setting of chronically reduced LV preload, overdiuresis may cause a reduction in cardiac output and hypotension.

Heparin, budesonide, and diuretics are the mainstay treatment for protein-losing enteropathy. This complication in the Fontan patient stems from excessively elevated systemic venous pressures and lymphatic congestion. It manifests as a malabsorption syndrome with hypoalbuminemia, diarrhea, and anasarca. Protein-losing enteropathy marks an advanced stage of the disease and warrants heart or heart-liver transplantation listing.

Sacubitril-Valsartan

Experience with sacubitril-valsartan in the ACHD population is limited and mixed. In a cohort of five patients with a variety of repaired congenital lesions who were previously able to tolerate ACE inhibitor or ARB therapy, all patients had improvement in functional class after 6 months of therapy with sacubitril-valsartan.[32,33] In a larger group of 23 patients (52% with systemic RV), no change in functional status with treatment was observed over a median follow-up of 7 months; however, there was a significant increase in creatinine and development of hypotension.

MANAGEMENT OF CYANOSIS

Chronic cyanosis persisting into adulthood predominantly indicates right-to-left shunting or complex anatomy with blood mixing (see **Table 105.4**). Chronic hypoxemia and cyanosis have physiologic effects on numerous organs and require a multisystem approach. Common manifestations of cyanosis include clubbing (osteoarthropathy), recurrent infections, platelet dysfunction, propensity for both bleeding and thrombosis, hyperuricemia and urate nephropathy, hypoventilation with decreased pulmonary diffusion capacity, and coronary artery ectasia. Interestingly, paragangliomas and pheochromocytomas are reported to be more prevalent in the cyanotic state.[34] Glomerular disease, proteinuria, and reduction in glomerular filtration rate should be anticipated and may require medication dose adjustments.

Drugs that reduce systemic vascular resistance (eg, calcium blockers, alpha-adrenergic blockers, ACE inhibitors) increase right-to-left shunting and exacerbate cyanosis. The same considerations apply when administrating anesthetic agents; propofol reduces systemic vascular resistance and increases right-to-left shunting as compared to ketamine in the pediatric population with shunts.[35] Deairing intravenous lines and the use of intravenous filters are imperative in the care of the cyanotic patient with right-to-left shunting. Hot tubs and saunas with extreme heat may also reduce systemic vascular resistance and worsen cyanosis and should be avoided. Therapies that could suppress the hypoxia-mediated drive such as opiates, narcotics, or excessive oxygen should be used with caution.

Given the increased risk of infections and in particular endocarditis with cyanosis, unrepaired, or partially repaired cyanotic congenital heart patients should receive prophylactic antibiotic therapy before dental procedures. New headaches or neurologic symptoms should prompt a high suspicion for brain abscesses. Influenza and pneumococcal vaccination should be current.

Increased erythropoietin production in the cyanotic state leads to secondary erythrocytosis and polycythemia, hyperviscosity, and iron deficiency anemia. A "normal" range hemoglobin concentration suggests relative anemia in the cyanotic patient. Iron deficiency is associated with worsening anemia, increased risk of neurologic events and myocardial ischemia and should be promptly corrected. There is no data to support routine phlebotomy for stroke prevention in the patient with polycythemia. In fact, phlebotomy results in worsening iron deficiency anemia, decreased oxygen capacity, and increased risk of stroke. Current practice focuses on symptoms of hyperviscosity such as headaches, fatigue, anorexia, visual changes, and neurologic symptoms. Symptoms commonly appear when hemoglobin or hematocrit are greater than 21 g/dL or 65%, respectively. Preventing dehydration is key in managing hyperviscosity syndrome, and thus hydration and diuretic dose reduction should be the initial steps in its treatment. For intractable hyperviscosity symptoms, phlebotomy may be performed by removing 400 to 500 mL of blood over 30 to 45 minutes followed by isovolume replacement with isotonic saline or reduced salt preparations if heart failure is a concern.

TABLE 105.4 Cyanosis Management

- Meticulous de-airing of intravenous access
- Avoid vasodilators that increase right-to-left shunting by reducing systemic vascular resistance
- Higher risk of both thrombosis and bleeding. Anticoagulation only with clear indications (eg, thrombosis or tachyarrhythmia)
- Higher risk of infection: consider infective endocarditis prophylaxis
- Headache or new neurologic symptoms may be a clue for brain abscess
- Ensure updated vaccination (ie, influenza, pneumococcus)
- Normal hemoglobin/hematocrit level in a cyanotic patient should be interpreted as anemia (iron deficiency anemia is common).
- Hyperviscosity syndrome: Initially attempt hydration and diuretic dose reduction. Phlebotomy is reserved for significant hyperviscosity symptoms.
- Supplemental oxygen for comfort, night-time use, during air travel, exercise, and with concomitant parenchymal lung disease
- Anesthesia performed by providers with expertise caring for ACHD patient
- Caution with therapies that suppress the hypoxia-mediated drive such as opiates, narcotics, and excessive oxygen
- Follow uric acid levels and treat hyperuricemia with allopurinol

ACHD, adult congenital heart disease.

Data derived from Stout KK, Daniels CJ, Aboulhosn JA, et al. 2018 AHA/ACC Guideline for the management of adults with congenital heart disease: executive summary: a report of the American College of Cardiology/American Heart Association Task Force on Clinical Practice Guidelines. *J Am Coll Cardiol.* 2019;73:1494-1563 and Helmut Baumgartner H, De Backer, J, Babu-Narayan SV, et al. ESC Scientific document group, 2020 ESC Guidelines for the management of adult congenital heart disease: The Task Force for the management of adult congenital heart disease of the European Society of Cardiology (ESC). Endorsed by: Association for European Paediatric and Congenital Cardiology (AEPC), International Society for Adult Congenital Heart Disease (ISACHD). *Eur Heart J.* 2021;42(6):563-645.

Hyperuricemia and gout are highly prevalent in the setting of increased cell turnover, diuretic use, renal insufficiency (which reduces urate excretion), and cyanosis. Allopurinol is used for the prevention of gout and colchicine for the acute attacks.

In the cyanotic patient, abnormalities in platelet function, coagulation, and fibrinolysis cause a relative hypercoagulable state as well as an increased risk of bleeding, especially in the setting of pulmonary hypertension. Thus, anticoagulation should only be used for clear thromboembolic or arrhythmic indications. Coagulation parameters in patients with elevated hematocrit (>55%) require laboratory adjustments to account for the reduced plasma volume.[1]

INFECTIVE ENDOCARDITIS

Infective endocarditis affects less than 1% of the ACHD population primarily targeting prosthetic valves, prosthetic material, residual shunts, and complex anatomy (see **Table 105.5**). Yet, the incidence is still significantly higher compared to the general population, with estimates of up to 30 times more events.[36] Prosthetic valves and valved conduits carry the highest risk of infection, which may explain why lesions such as pulmonary atresia with VSD, double outlet right ventricle, and TOF—which often need pulmonary valve replacement—carry the highest risk.[36] Concern for higher rates of endocarditis following transcutaneous pulmonary valve replacement is an ongoing debate. Other high-risk conditions include single ventricles and left-sided heart lesions. Native pulmonary valve disease and ASDs seem to have a lower propensity for infection.

Guidelines recommend dental prophylaxis for unrepaired cyanotic lesions, prosthetic heart valves, during the first 6 months after implantation of nonvalve prosthetics or surgical repair of lesions, residual shunt/jets adjacent to prosthetic material, history of infective endocarditis, and postheart transplantation. Prior ACHD guidelines recommended prophylaxis before vaginal deliveries in women with prosthetic valves.[37] Prophylaxis consists of antibiotic coverage of the common pathogens—*Streptococci* and *Staphylococci*—and includes amoxicillin 2 g taken an hour before the dental procedure and clindamycin 600 mg or azithromycin/clarithromycin 500 mg in cases of penicillin allergies. For patients with a history of infective endocarditis, a tailored approach is recommended based on prior speciation of organisms. Education regarding dental hygiene and biannual dental care is paramount in the routine care of ACHD patients.

CONTRACEPTION

Women with ACHD should receive prepregnancy counseling including guidance on safe and appropriate options for contraception, as cardiovascular disease portends increased risk of complications and death during pregnancy (see **Table 105.6**). In one cross-sectional survey, more than half of women with ACHD had not received contraceptive and reproductive

TABLE 105.5 Infective Endocarditis Prophylaxis Indications

- Prior endocarditis
- Prosthetic valves/prosthetic material for valve repair
- Unrepaired/palliated cyanotic CHD (ie, shunts/conduits)
- Repaired CHD with prosthetic material in the first 6 months after the procedure
- Repaired CHD with residual defect at site or adjacent to site of prosthetic patch or device
- Before vaginal delivery for patients with prosthetic valves or unrepaired/palliated cyanotic ACHD

ACHD, adult congenital heart disease; CHD, congenital heart disease.
Data derived from Stout KK, Daniels CJ, Aboulhosn JA, et al. 2018 AHA/ACC Guideline for the management of adults with congenital heart disease: executive summary: a report of the American College of Cardiology/American Heart Association Task Force on Clinical Practice Guidelines. *J Am Coll Cardiol.* 2019;73:1494-1563 and Warnes CA, Williams RG, Bashore TM, et al. ACC/AHA 2008 guidelines for the management of adults with congenital heart disease: a report of the American College of Cardiology/American Heart Association Task Force on Practice Guidelines (Writing Committee to Develop Guidelines on the Management of Adults With Congenital Heart Disease). Developed in Collaboration With the American Society of Echocardiography, Heart Rhythm Society, International Society for Adult Congenital Heart Disease, Society for Cardiovascular Angiography and Interventions, and Society of Thoracic Surgeons. *J Am Coll Cardiol.* 2008;52:e143-e263.

TABLE 105.6 Contraception in Congenital Heart Disease

- Absolute contraindications for pregnancy: Eisenmenger syndrome, pulmonary arterial hypertension, complex cyanotic heart disease, markedly diminished systemic ventricular function, severe mitral and aortic valve disease, and aortic enlargement
- Contraindication for estrogen-based contraception: prior thrombotic events, cyanosis, Fontan physiology, pulmonary hypertension, and mechanical valves
- Progestin-only preparations carry lower risk of thrombosis. Progesterone-based IUD and subdermal preparations are highly effective contraception.
- Contraindications to progestin-only preparations: history or suspected breast cancer, undiagnosed abnormal uterine bleeding, liver cirrhosis, tumor or acute disease, and suspected pregnancy.

IUD, intrauterine device.
Data derived from Stout KK, Daniels CJ, Aboulhosn JA, et al. 2018 AHA/ACC Guideline for the management of adults with congenital heart disease: executive summary: a report of the American College of Cardiology/American Heart Association Task Force on Clinical Practice Guidelines. *J Am Coll Cardiol.* 2019;73:1494-1563 and Thorne S, MacGregor A, Nelson-Piercy C. Risks of contraception and pregnancy in heart disease. *Heart.* 2006;92:1520-1525.

counseling related to their cardiac condition.[38] In another group of ACHD women of child-bearing age, 45% of pregnancies that occurred were unexpected.[39] High-risk congenital lesions in which pregnancy is contraindicated include Eisenmenger syndrome, pulmonary arterial hypertension, complex cyanotic heart disease, markedly diminished systemic ventricular function, severe mitral and aortic valve disease, and aortic enlargement (>45 mm in Marfan disease and >50 mm in bicuspid aortic valve disease). Pregnancy considerations and treatment in women with congenital heart disease are discussed elsewhere.[40]

Contraception safety in ACHD varies by underlying cardiac condition and options for treatment include hormonal (combined estrogen/progesterone and progesterone-only), intrauterine devices (IUDs), and barrier methods. The 2018 ACHD guidelines include a Class III recommendation warning of potential harm of estrogen-containing contraceptives in women who are at high risk of thromboembolic events, including those with prior thrombotic events, cyanosis, Fontan physiology, pulmonary artery hypertension, and mechanical valves.[1] Progestin-only preparations are safe and effective for high-risk ACHD women.[21,41] Subdermal progesterone implants and IUDs containing progesterone are highly effective and improve contraception compliance. They hold a minor but acceptable risk of thrombosis. Side effects include abnormal uterine bleeding, weight gain and fluid retention, acne, and depressed mood. Contraindications to progestin-only preparations include history or suspected breast cancer, undiagnosed abnormal uterine bleeding, acute liver disease, tumor or cirrhosis, and suspected pregnancy. The combination of bosentan (a dual endothelin receptor antagonist) and progesterone may reduce the efficacy of contraception, and increased international normalized ratio (INR) monitoring may be required with warfarin therapy when progestin-only preparations are used due to interactions with warfarin. Endocarditis prophylaxis should be considered before IUD placement in appropriate patients.

FUTURE DIRECTIONS

While medication use in the ACHD population historically was primarily supportive, the role of pharmacologic therapy in ACHD continues to expand as a result of advances in medical therapy, improved life expectancy through surgery and interventions, and the expansion of evidence-based literature of medication use in this population. International initiatives promoting multicenter evaluation of drug therapy are needed to address the care of a predominantly young population of adults with lifelong medical needs.

ACKNOWLEDGMENTS

The authors acknowledge Jodi Feinberg, NP for her valuable input.

KEY POINTS

- ✔ New tachyarrhythmia or heart failure syndrome should prompt an anatomic and hemodynamic assessment.
- ✔ Correction of hemodynamically significant lesions should be attempted in conjunction with medical therapy.
- ✔ Long-term treatment of tachyarrhythmia in the congenital heart patient commonly requires both an antiarrhythmic agent in conjunction with ablative procedures.
- ✔ Lower threshold for full anticoagulation in the congenital heart disease patient as commonly used models (eg, CHA_2DS_2-VASc) do not address the younger age of the population or its structural complexity.
- ✔ The role of neurohormonal blockade in treating systemic right ventricles and single ventricles is uncertain.
- ✔ Diuretic therapy in the palliated single ventricle patient (ie, Fontan) should be carefully monitored as overdiuresis may prompt further decrease in cardiac output.
- ✔ Every young woman with congenital heart disease should have an elaborate discussion about contraception and pregnancy risk.

REFERENCES

1. Stout KK, Daniels CJ, Aboulhosn JA, et al. 2018 AHA/ACC Guideline for the management of adults with congenital heart disease: executive summary: a report of the American College of Cardiology/American Heart Association Task Force on Clinical Practice Guidelines. *J Am Coll Cardiol.* 2019;73:1494-1563.
2. Helmut Baumgartner H, De Backer, J, Babu-Narayan SV, et al. ESC Scientific document group, 2020 ESC Guidelines for the management of adult congenital heart disease: The Task Force for the management of adult congenital heart disease of the European Society of Cardiology (ESC). Endorsed by: Association for European Paediatric and Congenital Cardiology (AEPC), International Society for Adult Congenital Heart Disease (ISACHD). *Eur Heart J.* 2021;42(6):563-645.
3. Mylotte D, Pilote L, Ionescu-Ittu R, et al. Specialized adult congenital heart disease care: the impact of policy on mortality. *Circulation.* 2014;129:1804-1812.
4. Woudstra OI, Kuijpers JM, Meijboom FJ, et al. High burden of drug therapy in adult congenital heart disease: polypharmacy as marker of morbidity and mortality. *Eur Heart J Cardiovasc Pharmacother.* 2019;5: 216-225.
5. Bokesch PM, Castaneda AR, Ziemer G, Wilson JM. The influence of a right-to-left cardiac shunt on lidocaine pharmacokinetics. *Anesthesiology.* 1987;67:739-744.
6. Walsh EP, Cecchin F. Arrhythmias in adult patients with congenital heart disease. *Circulation.* 2007;115:534-545.
7. Khairy P, Van Hare GF, Balaji S, et al. PACES/HRS expert consensus statement on the recognition and management of arrhythmias in adult congenital heart disease: developed in partnership between the Pediatric and Congenital Electrophysiology Society (PACES) and the Heart Rhythm Society (HRS). Endorsed by the governing bodies of PACES, HRS, the American College of Cardiology (ACC), the American Heart Association (AHA), the European Heart Rhythm Association (EHRA), the Canadian Heart Rhythm Society (CHRS), and the International Society for Adult Congenital Heart Disease (ISACHD). *Can J Cardiol.* 2014;30:e1-e63.
8. Patel P, Borovskiy Y, Deo R. Qtcc, a novel method for correcting Qt interval for Qrs duration, predicts all-cause mortality. *J Am Coll Cardiol.* 2015;65:A336-A336.
9. Moore BM, Cordina RL, McGuire MA, Celermajer DS. Efficacy and adverse effects of sotalol in adults with congenital heart disease. *Int J Cardiol.* 2019;274:74-79.
10. Koyak Z, Harris L, de Groot JR, et al. Sudden cardiac death in adult congenital heart disease. *Circulation.* 2012;126:1944-1954.

11. Yang H, Heidendael JF, de Groot JR, et al. Oral anticoagulant therapy in adults with congenital heart disease and atrial arrhythmias: implementation of guidelines. *Int J Cardiol.* 2018;257:67-74.
12. Catherine MO, Rick AN, Robert OB, et al. 2020 ACC/AHA Guideline for the management of patients with valvular heart disease: a report of the American College of Cardiology/American Heart Association Joint Committee on Clinical Practice Guidelines. *Circulation.* 2021;143:e72-e82.
13. Chan KL, Dumesnil JG, Cujec B, et al. A randomized trial of aspirin on the risk of embolic events in patients with infective endocarditis. *J Am Coll Cardiol.* 2003;42:775-780.
14. Veloso TR, Que YA, Chaouch A, et al. Prophylaxis of experimental endocarditis with antiplatelet and antithrombin agents: a role for long-term prevention of infective endocarditis in humans? *J Infect Dis.* 2015;211:72-79.
15. Rigatelli G, Zuin M, Dell'Avvocata F, Roncon L, Vassilev D, Nghia N. Light anti-thrombotic regimen for prevention of device thrombosis and/or thrombotic complications after interatrial shunts device-based closure. *Eur J Intern Med.* 2020;74:42-48.
16. Yang H, Bouma BJ, Dimopoulos K, et al. Non-vitamin K antagonist oral anticoagulants (NOACs) for thromboembolic prevention, are they safe in congenital heart disease? Results of a worldwide study. *Int J Cardiol.* 2020;299:123-130.
17. Egbe AC, Connolly HM, McLeod CJ, et al. Thrombotic and embolic complications associated with atrial arrhythmia after fontan operation: role of prophylactic therapy. *J Am Coll Cardiol.* 2016;68:1312-1319.
18. Potter BJ, Leong-Sit P, Fernandes SM, et al. Effect of aspirin and warfarin therapy on thromboembolic events in patients with univentricular hearts and Fontan palliation. *Int J Cardiol.* 2013;168:3940-3943.
19. Al-Jazairi AS, Al Alshaykh HA, Di Salvo G, De Vol EB, Alhalees ZY. Assessment of late thromboembolic complications post-fontan procedure in relation to different antithrombotic regimens: 30-years' follow-up experience. *Ann Pharmacother.* 2019;53:786-793.
20. Yang H, Veldtman GR, Bouma BJ, et al. Non-vitamin K antagonist oral anticoagulants in adults with a Fontan circulation: are they safe. *Open Heart.* 2019;6:e000985.
21. Abarbanell G, Tepper NK, Farr SL. Safety of contraceptive use among women with congenital heart disease: a systematic review. *Congenit Heart Dis.* 2019;14:331-340.
22. Rich S, Seidlitz M, Dodin E, et al. The short-term effects of digoxin in patients with right ventricular dysfunction from pulmonary hypertension. *Chest.* 1998;114:787-792.
23. Babu-Narayan SV, Uebing A, Davlouros PA, et al. Randomised trial of ramipril in repaired tetralogy of Fallot and pulmonary regurgitation: the APPROPRIATE study (Ace inhibitors for Potential PRevention Of the deleterious effects of Pulmonary Regurgitation In Adults with repaired TEtralogy of Fallot). *Int J Cardiol.* 2012;154:299-305.
24. Norozi K, Bahlmann J, Raab B, et al. A prospective, randomized, double-blind, placebo controlled trial of beta-blockade in patients who have undergone surgical correction of tetralogy of Fallot. *Cardiol Young.* 2007;17:372-379.
25. Zaragoza-Macias E, Zaidi AN, Dendukuri N, Marelli A. Medical therapy for systemic right ventricles: a systematic review (part 1) for the 2018 AHA/ACC Guideline for the Management of Adults With Congenital Heart Disease: a report of the American College of Cardiology/American Heart Association Task Force on Clinical Practice Guidelines. *Circulation.* 2019;139:e801-e813.
26. van der Bom T, Winter MM, Bouma BJ, et al. Effect of valsartan on systemic right ventricular function: a double-blind, randomized, placebo-controlled pilot trial. *Circulation.* 2013;127:322-330.
27. Doughan AR, McConnell ME, Book WM. Effect of beta blockers (carvedilol or metoprolol XL) in patients with transposition of great arteries and dysfunction of the systemic right ventricle. *Am J Cardiol.* 2007;99:704-706.
28. Hsu DT, Zak V, Mahony L, et al. Enalapril in infants with single ventricle: results of a multicenter randomized trial. *Circulation.* 2010;122:333-340.
29. Vonder Muhll I, Liu P, Webb G. Applying standard therapies to new targets: the use of ACE inhibitors and B-blockers for heart failure in adults with congenital heart disease. *Int J Cardiol.* 2004;97 Suppl 1:25-33.
30. Shaddy RE, Boucek MM, Hsu DT, et al. Carvedilol for children and adolescents with heart failure: a randomized controlled trial. *JAMA.* 2007;298:1171-1179.
31. Wang W, Hu X, Liao W, et al. The efficacy and safety of pulmonary vasodilators in patients with Fontan circulation: a meta-analysis of randomized controlled trials. *Pulm Circ.* 2019;9:2045894018790450.
32. Appadurai V, Thoreau J, Malpas T, Nicolae M. Sacubitril/Valsartan in adult congenital heart disease patients with chronic heart failure—a single centre case series and call for an international registry. *Heart Lung Circ.* 2020;29:137-141.
33. Maurer SJ, Pujol Salvador C, Schiele S, Hager A, Ewert P, Tutarel O. Sacubitril/valsartan for heart failure in adults with complex congenital heart disease. *Int J Cardiol.* 2020;300:137-140.
34. Opotowsky AR, Moko LE, Ginns J, et al. Pheochromocytoma and paraganglioma in cyanotic congenital heart disease. *J Clin Endocrinol Metab.* 2015;100:1325-1334.
35. Oklu E, Bulutcu FS, Yalcin Y, Ozbek U, Cakali E, Bayindir O. Which anesthetic agent alters the hemodynamic status during pediatric catheterization? Comparison of propofol versus ketamine. *J Cardiothorac Vasc Anesth.* 2003;17:686-690.
36. Kuijpers JM, Koolbergen DR, Groenink M, et al. Incidence, risk factors, and predictors of infective endocarditis in adult congenital heart disease: focus on the use of prosthetic material. *Eur Heart J.* 2017;38:2048-2056.
37. Warnes CA, Williams RG, Bashore TM, et al. ACC/AHA 2008 guidelines for the management of adults with congenital heart disease: a report of the American College of Cardiology/American Heart Association Task Force on Practice Guidelines (Writing Committee to Develop Guidelines on the Management of Adults With Congenital Heart Disease). Developed in Collaboration With the American Society of Echocardiography, Heart Rhythm Society, International Society for Adult Congenital Heart Disease, Society for Cardiovascular Angiography and Interventions, and Society of Thoracic Surgeons. *J Am Coll Cardiol.* 2008;52:e143-e263.
38. Hinze A, Kutty S, Sayles H, Sandene EK, Meza J, Kugler JD. Reproductive and contraceptive counseling received by adult women with congenital heart disease: a risk-based analysis. *Congenit Heart Dis.* 2013;8:20-31.
39. Lindley KJ, Madden T, Cahill AG, Ludbrook PA, Billadello JJ. Contraceptive use and unintended pregnancy in women with congenital heart disease. *Obstet Gynecol.* 2015;126:363-369.
40. Thorne S, MacGregor A, Nelson-Piercy C. Risks of contraception and pregnancy in heart disease. *Heart.* 2006;92:1520-1525.
41. Pijuan-Domenech A, Baro-Marine F, Rojas-Torrijos M, et al. Usefulness of progesterone-only components for contraception in patients with congenital heart disease. *Am J Cardiol.* 2013;112:590-593.
42. Tutarel O, Meyer GP, Bertram H, Wessel A, Schieffer B, Westhoff-Bleck M. Safety and efficiency of chronic ACE inhibition in symptomatic heart failure patients with a systemic right ventricle. *Int J Cardiol.* 2012;154:14-16.

CHAPTER 106

SHUNT LESIONS

Zachary L. Steinberg, Mathias Possner and Yonatan Buber

INTRODUCTION

Shunt lesions comprise a wide variety of anatomic abnormalities resulting in abnormal blood flow between cardiac chambers and great vessels. A shunt is labeled as "left-to-right" when oxygenated blood passes through a communication and mixes with deoxygenated blood. Left-to-right shunts do not result in hypoxemia and may therefore go unnoticed for an extended period of time. But an increase in pressure and volume through the cardiac chambers and pulmonary vasculature through which the shunted blood passes may result in significant and occasionally irreversible physiologic perturbations. Conversely, a shunt is labeled as "right-to-left" when deoxygenated blood passes through a communication and mixes with oxygenated blood. Right-to-left shunts may result in significant hypoxemia and are often diagnosed early in life owing to overt cyanosis. Most right-to-left shunts occur in response to a constellation of intracardiac abnormalities and are only rarely found as a result of a single isolated anatomic lesion.

This chapter reviews the anatomy, physiology, and management of some of the more common, isolated congenital and iatrogenic shunt lesions. As a rule, shunt physiology dictates treatment indications; however, shunt anatomy dictates treatment options. The remainder of this chapter is organized by the anatomic location of each shunt.

ATRIAL SEPTAL DEFECTS

EPIDEMIOLOGY AND PATHOGENESIS

Atrial septal defects (ASDs) include a group of abnormalities that result in a communication between the right and left atria. They are among the most common of all congenital heart defects with a prevalence of 1.6 per 1000 births worldwide.[1] In the absence of additional pathology, ASDs result in a left-to-right shunt. Although almost uniformly these shunts occur at low pressure owing to relatively passive blood flow between two low-pressure chambers, the long-standing volume load on the right atrium, right ventricle, and pulmonary artery vasculature may lead to atrial arrhythmias, right-sided chamber enlargement and dysfunction, and, rarely pulmonary arteriolar hypertension.[2]

There are several types of ASDs, each resulting from a unique developmental abnormality (**Figure 106.1**). Most

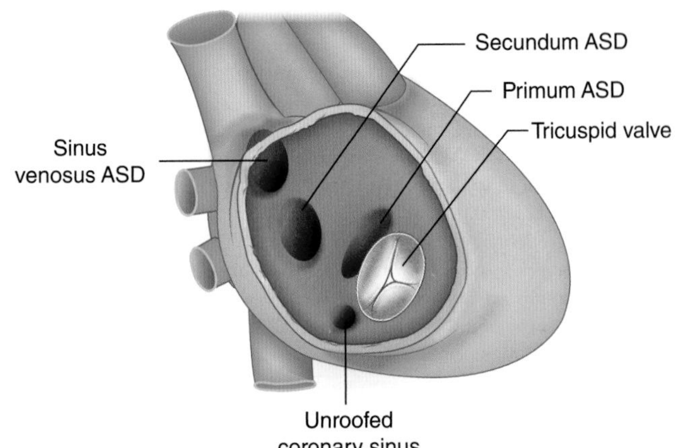

FIGURE 106.1 Atrial septal defect anatomy. ASD, atrial septal defect.

commonly encountered are secundum ASDs, which are located within the fossa ovalis, resulting from defects within the septum primum. Secundum defects vary greatly in size and shunt volume. Primum ASDs result from incomplete septation at the crux of the heart where the atrioventricular (AV) valves and atrial and ventricular septa meet and are part of a larger constellation of abnormalities known as endocardial cushion defects or AV septal abnormalities. These lesions, by definition, involve abnormalities of the developing AV valves and are often associated with ventricular septal defects (VSDs). As such, treatment indications and considerations for primum ASDs are described in a separate section (see section "Atrioventricular Septal Defects"). Sinus venosus ASDs are located superiorly at the junction of the superior vena cava (SVC) and the roof of the right atrium. These defects result from a deficiency in the development of the wall that normally separates the right pulmonary veins from the SVC and are accompanied by a posterosuperior ASD.[3] Thus, the definition of a sinus venosus ASD includes abnormal pulmonary venous return and typically results in a significant left-to-right shunt. The least common of all ASDs, an unroofed coronary sinus, results from a deficiency of the septal tissue surrounding the ostium of the coronary sinus, creating a communication between the atria.

CLINICAL PRESENTATION AND DIAGNOSIS: ATRIAL SEPTAL DEFECTS

A substantial proportion of adult patients with an undiagnosed ASD have minimal to no recognizable symptoms. When present, the most common symptom is mild to modest exertional dyspnea. Frequently, it is only after an ASD is repaired that long-standing exertional intolerance is realized in retrospect. In the presence of large shunts or advanced age, symptoms of congestive heart failure may manifest. ASDs are also associated with early-onset atrial arrhythmias, and younger patients presenting with new-onset atrial fibrillation should prompt further evaluation for structural cardiac abnormalities.

Physical examination findings are often unremarkable; however, cardiac auscultation may reveal subtle signs of excessive pulmonary blood flow. A fixed split S2 may be heard throughout the respiratory cycle, and a pulmonary systolic flow murmur may be present over the second intercostal space. In rare cases, a loud and palpable P2, jugular venous distension, or dependent edema may be present as a sign of either significant pulmonary hypertension or right ventricular dysfunction.

An electrocardiogram (ECG) may reveal evidence of right atrial enlargement and a right bundle branch block with or without right axis deviation. Septum primum defects are the exception with a right bundle branch block associated with left axis deviation. Sinus venosus defects may show an ectopic atrial rhythm (ie, negative P waves in the inferior ECG leads). Transthoracic echocardiography (TTE) typically establishes the diagnosis demonstrating evidence of flow between the atria on color Doppler; however, transesophageal echocardiography (TEE) provides a more comprehensive assessment of defect anatomy. Sinus venosus defects and associated abnormal pulmonary venous return are frequently difficult to visualize in an adult by TTE imaging. A significantly dilated right ventricle without identifiable intracardiac pathology by TTE should raise concerns for this diagnosis and prompt further evaluation with either a TEE or cross-sectional imaging. Cross-sectional imaging with either cardiac magnetic resonance (CMR) imaging or a cardiac computed tomographic angiogram (CCTA) provides an excellent assessment of sinus venosus anatomy and the number and location of anomalous pulmonary venous drainage. Both CMR and CCTA are useful adjuncts in other types of ASDs and offer accurate assessment of chamber size, presence of additional abnormalities, and, in the case of CMR, an estimate of the shunt magnitude.

Cardiac catheterization can aid in the diagnosis by confirming the presence of a shunt. Often, direct passage of a catheter through the defect is possible, helping to identify shunt location. Additionally, cardiac catheterization provides important hemodynamic information regarding intracardiac filling pressures, shunt magnitude, and pulmonary vascular resistance, all of which may influence treatment decisions.

MANAGEMENT: ATRIAL SEPTAL DEFECTS

ASD closure is recommended in the presence of impaired functional capacity, right atrial or ventricular enlargement, right ventricular dysfunction, or paradoxical embolism (**Algorithm 106.1**). Closure is not recommended and possibly harmful in the presence

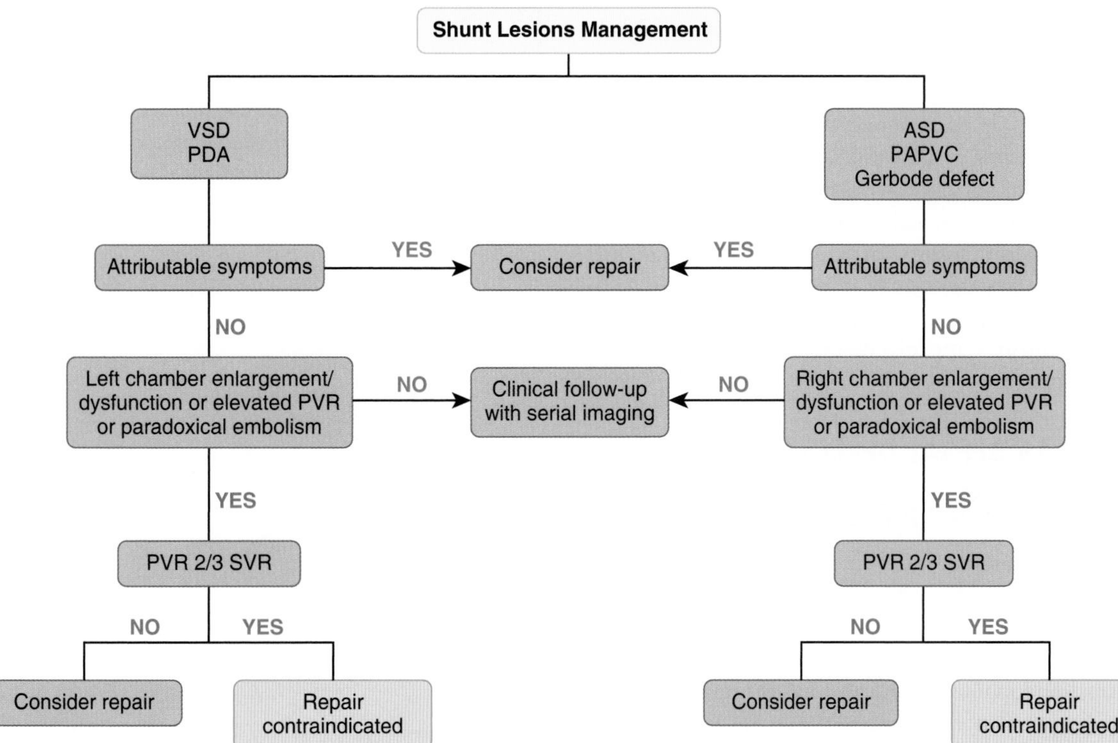

ALGORITHM 106.1 Shunt lesions management. ASD, atrial septal defect; PAPVC, partial anomalous pulmonary venous connection; PDA, patent ductus arteriosus; PVR, pulmonary vascular resistance; SVR, systemic vascular resistance; VSD, ventricular septal defect.

of significant pulmonary vascular resistance at greater than one-half to two-thirds systemic levels.[4] These patients should be co-managed with a pulmonary hypertension specialist.

Both surgical and transcatheter techniques exist for ASD closure; however, not all ASDs allow for transcatheter closure at present. Transcatheter ASD closure is the treatment of choice for secundum ASDs when anatomically feasible. In the presence of adequate circumferential tissue, device closure of secundum ASDs has a high rate of success at low risk.[5] Device embolization is infrequent and often successfully managed in the cardiac catheterization laboratory.[6] Device erosion is a life-threatening complication often requiring urgent surgical intervention. This rare complication remains poorly understood and, while associated with ASD rim tissue deficiency, no single identifiable subpopulation is recognized to be at substantially elevated risk to warrant contraindication of device closure.[7]

Surgery remains the mainstay of therapy for individuals with primum ASDs, sinus venosus defects, and unroofed coronary sinuses; however, new transcatheter techniques are emerging for the treatment of a subpopulation of sinus venosus lesions.[8] Surgical ASD closure remains an effective option for those with contraindications to transcatheter closure with very low mortality and an excellent long-term prognosis.[5,9] In general, patients with an indication for ASD closure who are not eligible for transcatheter occlusion should be referred for surgery.

FOLLOW-UP PATIENT CARE: ATRIAL SEPTAL DEFECTS

Lifelong follow-up is typically recommended regardless of whether the ASD has been treated. Post ASD device closure, patients should receive intermittent imaging follow-up within the first year to evaluate for device malposition, residual shunting, and erosion. Long-term follow-up is recommended following device and surgical closure every 3 to 5 years with an ECG and TTE imaging to assess for new-onset atrial arrhythmias, residual shunting, right ventricular size and function, pulmonary artery pressures, and, in the case of device closure, late erosion.[4] Patients in whom ASD closure has not been pursued, long-term follow-up every 3 to 5 years with either TTE or cross-sectional imaging is recommended in the absence of chamber enlargement, ventricular dysfunction, or elevated pulmonary artery pressures.

VENTRICULAR SEPTAL DEFECTS

EPIDEMIOLOGY AND PATHOGENESIS

VSDs are open communications in the interventricular septum, which result in a shunt between the left and right ventricles. They are the most common congenital heart defects worldwide with a prevalence of 2.6 per 1000 births,[1] although many are small and spontaneously close during somatic growth, such that the prevalence of isolated VSDs in adulthood is much lower.[10] VSDs are often isolated lesions but commonly occur as part of a constellation of defects such as in the case of atrioventricular septal defects (AVSDs), tetralogy of Fallot, and transposition of the great arteries.

In the absence of additional pathology, VSDs result in left-to-right shunting. The magnitude of shunting and clinical presentation widely vary and are predominantly dictated by the size of the defect. Large VSDs expose the pulmonary vascular bed to substantial volume and pressure. If left untreated, they almost always result in irreversible pulmonary arteriolar hypertension and, ultimately, reversal of the shunt (so-called Eisenmenger syndrome). Moderate-sized VSDs are often pressure restrictive, protecting the pulmonary vasculature from excessive pressure overload, but permit substantial shunted blow flow through the pulmonary vasculature and into the left heart, resulting in left-sided chamber enlargement and dysfunction and, occasionally, slowly progressive pulmonary arteriolar hypertension. Small-sized VSDs are both pressure and volume restrictive and are typically tolerated for many years without hemodynamic perturbations. However, the presence of a long-standing, high-velocity jet may result in adverse sequelae including right ventricular outflow tract hypertrophy and obstruction (ie, double outlet right ventricle), progressive aortic insufficiency, and endocarditis.

VSDs are classified based on their location within the interventricular septum although a well-defined nomenclature remains a topic of ongoing debate. In general, there are four major VSD classifications: perimembranous, muscular, conoventricular (also referred to as supracristal, juxtaarterial, subarterial, subpulmonic, or infundibular), and inlet VSDs **(Figure 106.2)**.

Perimembranous VSDs are located in the membranous ventricular septum and are the most common of all VSDs. Perimembranous VSDs are often congenital in etiology but may also result iatrogenically (eg, postaortic valve replacement). Muscular VSDs may be present anywhere within the muscular portion of the interventricular septum and can be found as a single defect or in multiples. Like perimembranous defects, muscular VSDs are most frequently congenital in etiology, although acquired muscular VSDs are a well-recognized

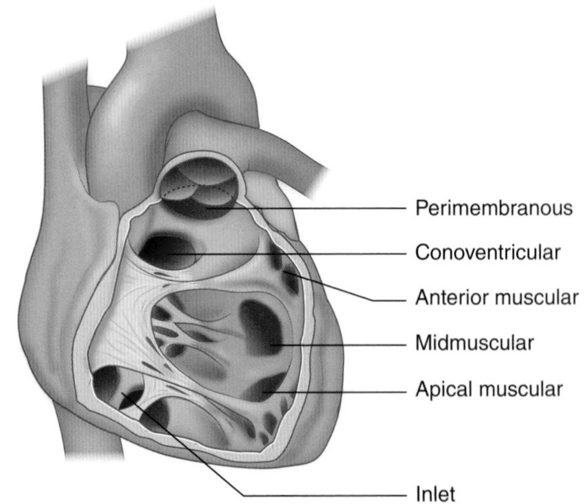

FIGURE 106.2 Ventricular septal defect anatomy.

complication of myocardial infarction (ie, postinfarct VSD) or surgical intervention (eg, postseptal myectomy). Conoventricular defects, located within the subpulmonary infundibulum, do not exist in isolation but rather as one of a constellation of defects in more complex congenital heart disease.[11] Inlet VSDs result from developmental abnormalities within the endocardial cushion and are associated with atrial and AV valve abnormalities (see section "Atrioventricular Septal Defects").

CLINICAL PRESENTATION AND DIAGNOSIS: VENTRICULAR SEPTAL DEFECT

The clinical presentation of a VSD depends on the size of the defect, the duration of the shunt, and the presence or absence of associated cardiac lesions. Individuals with small volume and pressure-restrictive VSDs (pulmonary to systemic blood flow ratio [Qp:Qs] < 1.5:1) often remain asymptomatic. Those with moderately sized VSDs (Qp:Qs 1.5-2:1) may develop symptoms of exertional intolerance and congestive heart failure. A long-standing volume load within the pulmonary circulation may lead to irreversible pulmonary arteriolar hypertension in select cases. Individuals with large VSDs are typically quite symptomatic with significantly reduced functional capacity and symptoms of congestive heart failure owing to excessive pulmonary circulation. If large VSDs are left untreated, rising pulmonary arteriolar hypertension often results in significant hypoxia caused by shunt reversal (right-to-left) known as Eisenmenger syndrome.

Cardiac auscultation typically reveals a harsh, holosystolic murmur heard throughout the precordium, but often loudest along the left sternal border. Even small VSDs may be heard clearly and, as such, the vast majority of VSDs are diagnosed in childhood. In patients with larger shunts, a widely split S2 throughout the respiratory cycle may be heard. In those with advanced pulmonary vascular disease, the murmur may disappear and a palpable P2 and cyanosis be present.

The diagnosis of a VSD is typically confirmed by TTE. Color Doppler usually locates the defect, identifies shunt direction, and aids in defect size assessment (Figure 106.1). Continuous-wave Doppler is useful for assessing VSD restriction and estimating pulmonary artery systolic pressures. TTE imaging is also important in assessing for left-sided chamber enlargement and dysfunction, right ventricular outflow tract obstruction, and evolving aortic valve regurgitation (**Table 106.1**). Cross-sectional imaging with CCTA or CMR aids in anatomic assessment of the defect and provides an accurate assessment of chamber size. CMR has the added benefit of quantifying shunt magnitude and aortic regurgitation.

TABLE 106.1 Echocardiographic Assessment of Patients With a Ventricular Septal Defect

Location and size of VSD	• Perimembranous VSD: Located in the membranous septum. Best visualized in the parasternal long-axis view. In a parasternal short-axis view below the aortic valve, the defect is typically located at 11 o'clock. • Muscular VSD: Located in the muscular septum, oftentimes occurs as multiple lesions. Color Doppler has a higher sensitivity than 2-dimensional echocardiography in the detection of small muscular VSDs. • Conoventricular VSD: Located in the right ventricular outflow tract portion of the ventricular septum. Shunts are typically visualized in the parasternal short-axis just below the aortic valve with shunt flow directed into the right ventricular outflow tract at 1 o'clock. • Inlet VSD: Part of atrioventricular septal defects. The defect is best visualized in the apical four-chamber view, adjacent to the mitral and tricuspid valve.
Flow direction and pressure gradient	• In small, restrictive VSDs, peak velocity can be used to estimate right ventricular pressures: RVSP = systolic blood pressure − 4 × (peak flow velocity across VSD)^2. • The flow pattern is important for the evaluation of left-to-right, bidirectional, or right-to-left shunt.
Left atrial and ventricular size	• Hemodynamically significant shunts result in dilation of the left atrium and ventricle.
Left ventricular function	• Left ventricular systolic function typically is preserved. • Left ventricular dysfunction can occur because of aortic regurgitation or after VSD closure in patients with prolonged left ventricular volume overload.
Aortic valve	• Because of the Venturi effect, aortic valve cusps may prolapse into the VSD resulting in progressive aortic valve regurgitation.
Tricuspid valve	• Tricuspid valve leaflet tissue may prolapse into the VSD, providing either a partial or complete seal of the defect.
Right ventricle	• Small, restrictive VSDs may promote muscle bundle hypertrophy resulting in partitioning of the right ventricular chamber (also known as a double-chambered right ventricle) and subpulmonic stenosis. • Right ventricular dysfunction may result from severe pulmonary hypertension in patients with excessive pulmonary circulation.
Pulmonary pressures	• Estimation of pulmonary artery systolic pressures via tricuspid regurgitation or VSD peak velocities is important for the detection of pulmonary hypertension.

RVSP, right ventricular systolic pressure; VSD, ventricular septal defect.

Cardiac catheterization may aid in the diagnosis by revealing the location of the defect via sequential oximetry (ie, shunt run) or ventriculography, and by quantifying the magnitude of the shunt. Invasive hemodynamics also provide important information on intracardiac filling pressures, pulmonary vascular resistance, and systemic cardiac output.

MANAGEMENT: VENTRICULAR SEPTAL DEFECT

The vast majority of patients who present with moderate- to large-sized VSDs in childhood will undergo early repair because of symptoms of excessive pulmonary circulation and/or left-sided chamber enlargement and/or left ventricular dysfunction (Algorithm 106.1). Thus, the majority of untreated VSDs in the adult population are smaller, pressure restricted lesions. On rare occasions, adults present with untreated, long-standing moderate- to large-sized VSD. Careful assessment of the pulmonary vasculature is paramount in determining candidacy for VSD closure. Closure is not recommended in the presence of severely elevated pulmonary vascular resistance,[4] and these patients should be comanaged by a pulmonary hypertension specialist. In patients with pressure-restrictive defects, indications for VSD closure hinge on the presence of symptoms, left-sided chamber enlargement, and additional sequelae such as aortic regurgitation, right ventricular outflow tract obstruction, and a history of endocarditis.

Both surgical and transcatheter options for VSD occlusion exist. Device closure is often pursued in patients with muscular VSDs and is highly successful in carefully selected patients with a low rate of complications.[12] Device closure may also be undertaken in patients with perimembranous VSDs; however, historically, this procedure has resulted in a high incidence of complete heart block.[12] Recent advances in device technology demonstrate a much lower risk of permanent heart block[13]; however, no devoted perimembranous VSD closure device is currently available in the United States.

In patients with contraindications for transcatheter VSD occlusion, surgical repair should be pursued. Surgical VSD repair is highly successful and carries a very low morbidity and mortality.[14] Although the type of repair is dictated by defect location and size, typically surgical patch closure with either autologous or synthetic patch material is performed, avoiding ventriculotomy when possible. In patients with VSD associated defects, such as right ventricular outflow tract obstruction or aortic valve prolapse and regurgitation, surgical repair of all defects is sought.

FOLLOW-UP PATIENT CARE

Lifelong follow-up for patients with VSDs is recommended regardless of whether it has been treated. In the absence of additional pathology, long-term follow-up after device or surgical closure is recommended every 3 years with an ECG and TTE imaging to assess for heart block, residual shunting, ventricular enlargement or dysfunction, and rising pulmonary artery pressures. In the absence of VSD hemodynamic or structural sequelae, long-term follow-up for patients in whom VSD closure has not been pursued is recommended every 3 years with either TTE or cross-sectional imaging.

ATRIOVENTRICULAR SEPTAL DEFECTS

EPIDEMIOLOGY AND PATHOGENESIS

AVSDs, alternatively referred to as AV canal or endocardial cushion defects, are a group of lesions that involve the AV junction, where the interatrial septum, the interventricular septum, and the AV valves meet. AVSDs carry a prevalence of 0.19 per 1000 births,[1] with a much higher incidence in individuals with trisomy 21.[10] AVSDs may also be present in heterotaxy syndrome, where a loss of sidedness leads to improper cardiac septation.

AVSDs are generally classified as partial, transitional (ie, incomplete), or complete (**Figure 106.3**). Partial AVSDs are characterized by the presence of a primum ASD. Defects that include both a primum ASD and a small, pressure-restrictive VSD are termed transitional. A complete AVSD includes a primum ASD and a large, unrestrictive VSD. Regardless of class, the hallmark of an AVSD is the presence of a common AV valve, which may sometimes appear as two distinct valves

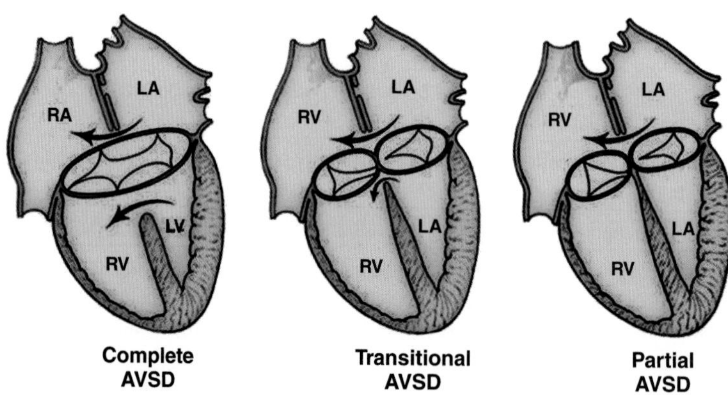

FIGURE 106.3 Atrioventricular septal defect anatomy. AVSD, atrioventricular septal defect; LA, left atrium; LV, left ventricle; RA, right atrium; RV, right ventricle.

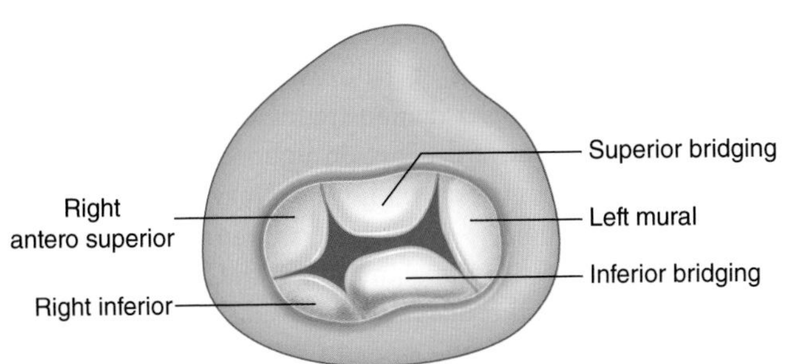

FIGURE 106.4 Common atrioventricular valve morphology.

in the absence of a VSD. The common valve consists of five leaflets: superior (anterior) and inferior (posterior) bridging leaflets that override the interventricular septum, a left mural leaflet, a right anterosuperior, and a right inferior leaflet (**Figure 106.4**). Abnormalities of the papillary muscles and chordal attachments may also be present.

The hemodynamic implications of AVSDs depend on the underlying anatomy. Complete AVSDs may present in a manner similar to unrestricted VSDs with pressure and volume overload predominantly affecting the pulmonary vasculature and left-sided cardiac chambers and early symptoms of excessive pulmonary circulation and heart failure. Partial and transitional AVSDs behave more similarly to ASDs with right-sided chamber enlargement and slowly progressive exertional symptoms. Two commonly associated intracardiac lesions include left-sided AV valve regurgitation and left ventricular outflow tract obstruction. Valve regurgitation, when present, typically occurs at the commissure between the superior and inferior bridging leaflets (frequently referred to as a "cleft") due to insufficient chordal support of the rudimentary leaflets.[15] Left ventricular outflow tract obstruction may result from anterior displacement of the common AV valve resulting in an elongated and hypoplastic outflow tract. Anomalous chordal attachments to the basal left ventricular septum may also contribute to this obstructive physiology. The AV node is shifted posteriorly and inferiorly in individuals with AVSDs leading to an elongated His bundle and leaving the conduction system vulnerable to injury during surgical repair.

CLINICAL PRESENTATION AND DIAGNOSIS: ATRIOVENTRICULAR SEPTAL DEFECT

Often, the diagnosis of an AVSD is made early in life. However, on occasion, patients with partial defects may escape detection and present later in life when either chronic right-sided volume overload or worsening AV valve regurgitation becomes clinically evident. Those with complete AVSDs typically manifest symptoms of excessive pulmonary circulation and heart failure during childhood if left untreated. When significant AV valve pathology or left ventricular outflow tract obstruction accompanies AV septal defects, marked symptoms of heart failure are often present.

Physical examination findings are variable and depend on the underlying anatomy and pathology. A holosystolic murmur is often present along the left sternal border in the presence of a VSD, and an apical holosystolic murmur may be heard when significant left-sided AV valve regurgitation is present. In those with partial AVSDs, examination findings are similar to those with other types of ASDs.

The classic ECG pattern for AVSDs includes first degree AV block, a right bundle branch block, and left axis deviation. TTE is the imaging modality of choice and frequently provides an accurate assessment of shunt location(s), valvular pathology, and outflow tract patency. The hallmark finding by TTE is a single AV valve with the absence of apical placement of the tricuspid valve annular plane, regardless of the presence of a VSD. TTE imaging should include a complete assessment of biventricular size and function, bilateral AV valve morphology and function with identification of chordal attachments, left ventricular outflow tract morphology, and an estimate of pulmonary artery pressures. Cross-sectional imaging with either CCTA or CMR may also be useful for further assessment of septal, left ventricular outflow tract, and chordal anatomy. CMR has the added benefit of quantifying AV valve regurgitation and shunt magnitude.

Cardiac catheterization may be of additional utility to quantify shunt magnitude, pulmonary vascular resistance, and ventricular filling pressures. Left ventriculography can be useful in identifying the size and location of a VSD and may reveal evidence of an elongated left ventricular outflow tract, also referred to as a "gooseneck" deformity.

MANAGEMENT: ATRIOVENTRICULAR SEPTAL DEFECT

Surgical repair is recommended for most AVSDs with rare exceptions in cases of minimal shunting and normal AV valve function. Recommendations for surgical intervention are similar to the indications for ASD and VSD repair and are largely dictated by the physiologic effects of volume and/or pressure loading on the cardiac chambers and pulmonary vasculature. The goal of surgical repair is to address all hemodynamically significant lesions including complete cardiac septation, AV valve repair when regurgitant, and relief of outflow tract obstruction when present.[16,17] When very large VSDs are present or when major chordae are anomalously connected to the ventricular septum, cardiac septation may not be possible. In these rare cases, palliation with a total cavopulmonary anastomosis (ie, Fontan procedure) may be necessary.

Although many individuals receive a durable repair, complete AV conduction block and progressive left-sided AV valve regurgitation may develop as a result of, or in spite of, surgical intervention leading to significant long-term morbidity.[18,19] Those with progressive left-sided AV valve regurgitation may require subsequent surgical interventions culminating in valve replacement.[20,21]

FOLLOW-UP PATIENT CARE: ATRIOVENTRICULAR SEPTAL DEFECT

Following AVSD repair, patients should be evaluated for residual AV valve regurgitation and the presence of atrial arrhythmias or conduction abnormalities. Patients who receive complete septation with little to no residual AV valve regurgitation, no outflow tract obstruction, and no conduction abnormalities may be followed up every 2 to 3 years with TTEs and ECGs. The risk of complete heart block and worsening AV valve regurgitation remains increased even years following surgical repair and must remain high on the differential in patients presenting with new-onset or progressive exertional intolerance. Patients with residual valve disease or outflow tract obstruction should be followed up annually with imaging.

PATENT DUCTUS ARTERIOSUS

EPIDEMIOLOGY AND PATHOGENESIS

Vital in normal fetal circulation, the ductus arteriosus shunts blood away from the developing lungs and into the descending aorta. Following birth and spontaneous respiration, if the ductus fails to close, the shunt changes direction with aortic blood flow now crossing the patent ductus arteriosus (PDA) and entering the pulmonary circulation.

PDAs are among the more commonly encountered isolated congenital heart defects, with a prevalence of 0.87 per 1000 births worldwide[1]; however, many remain small and may ultimately spontaneously close during early childhood. The degree of left-to-right shunting through a PDA is dependent on vessel size and length, with larger unrestricted lesions leading to left-sided cardiac chamber enlargement and dysfunction if left untreated. Ultimately, the substantial pulmonary vasculature pressure and volume load lead to irreversible pulmonary vascular disease. Smaller, pressure-restrictive shunts may still lead to a volume load, which may result in left-sided chamber enlargement and dysfunction and a slowly rising pulmonary artery vascular resistance.

CLINICAL PRESENTATION AND DIAGNOSIS: PATENT DUCTUS ARTERIOSUS

Moderate- to large-sized PDAs are typically diagnosed in early childhood either because of the presence of a murmur on routine examination or the development of symptoms caused by excessive pulmonary circulation. The vast majority of PDAs diagnosed in adulthood are small, pressure-restrictive shunts. Small PDAs are usually tolerated well with minimal symptoms either at rest or with exertion. However, chronic volume overload may ultimately result in left-sided chamber enlargement, atrial arrhythmias, ventricular dysfunction, and rising pulmonary arteriolar hypertension. When audible, a continuous systolic murmur followed by a diastolic murmur (ie, a continuous "machinery" murmur) can be heard within the second intercostal space and posterior thorax just medial to the left scapula.

An ECG is often unremarkable although left atrial enlargement may be present. A TTE will typically identify the lesion with color Doppler demonstrating aortic diastolic flow directed retrograde toward the main pulmonary artery in the parasternal short-axis window. PDA flow may also be appreciated originating from the distal aortic arch in the suprasternal notch window. Cross-sectional imaging with CMR and CCTA aids in confirming the diagnosis, assessing left-sided chamber dimensions, and, in the case of CMR, quantifying shunt magnitude.

Cardiac catheterization can help confirm the diagnosis with serial oximetry and passage of a wire or catheter across the PDA. Catheterization may be of additional use in assessing left-sided filling pressures, pulmonary vascular resistance, and systemic cardiac output. Shunt quantification via oximetry is notoriously unreliable because of unequal shunt distribution within the branch pulmonary arteries and absence of a distal mixing chamber from which to sample a mixed pulmonary artery oxygen saturation. Thus, CMR tends to provide a more accurate assessment of shunt magnitude.

MANAGEMENT: PATENT DUCTUS ARTERIOSUS

Shunt occlusion is indicated in patients with symptoms, evidence of left-sided chamber enlargement, or a history of pulmonary artery endocarditis (Algorithm 106.1).[4] The vast majority of PDAs are amenable to transcatheter closure. Multiple devices exist for transcatheter PDA closure allowing for a high likelihood of success, regardless of PDA size or shape,[22] and with rare long-term sequelae. For patients in whom transcatheter closure is either contraindicated or not feasible, surgical ligation is recommended.

FOLLOW-UP PATIENT CARE: PATENT DUCTUS ARTERIOSUS

Follow-up post-PDA occlusion, in the absence of chamber enlargement, dysfunction, or elevated pulmonary vascular resistance, is minimal. If the early postocclusion course remains uncomplicated, patients may be discharged from clinic within a year of PDA closure. For patients in whom PDA closure has not been pursued, long-term follow-up every 3 years with TTE or cross-sectional imaging is recommended.[4]

PARTIAL ANOMALOUS PULMONARY VENOUS CONNECTION

EPIDEMIOLOGY AND PATHOGENESIS

Partial anomalous pulmonary venous connection (PAPVC) occurs when at least one, but not all of the pulmonary veins anomalously drain into a chamber or vessel other than the left atrium. The most common sites of anomalous connections are to the SVC, the inferior vena cava, the innominate vein, and the right atrium. When all of the pulmonary veins anomalously connect to a venous structure or the right side of the heart, it is termed total anomalous pulmonary venous connection (TAPVC), which is typically diagnosed and surgically repaired in infancy.

PAPVC is a relatively rare condition with a reported incidence between 0.16% and 0.7%,[23,24] but the true prevalence remains unknown as many individuals with a single anomalous pulmonary venous connection remain asymptomatic and go undiagnosed. Anomalous connections of the right-sided pulmonary veins are 10 times more common than the left-sided pulmonary veins.[25]

There are several anatomic constellations in which PAPVC can occur. The most common consists of a connection between the right upper pulmonary vein (with or without the right middle pulmonary vein) to the SVC, a defect that is often associated with a superior sinus venosus defect (see section "Atrial Septal Defects"). Alternatively, all three right-sided pulmonary veins may be connected to the inferior vena cava via a large communicating vein (ie, "scimitar vein"). Connection of left pulmonary veins to either the innominate vein or the coronary sinus may also occur but are less common.

When present in isolation, PAPVC results in a left-to-right shunt leading to a volume load within the right-sided cardiac chambers in a manner similar to ASDs. When only one pulmonary vein is anomalously connected to the systemic venous circulation, a modest-sized shunt results often of minimal hemodynamic significance. When several pulmonary veins are anomalously connected, or when found in conjunction with lesions such as sinus venosus ASDs, the volume load may be much more significant leading to right-sided chamber enlargement, atrial arrhythmias, right ventricular dysfunction, and rising pulmonary vascular resistance.

CLINICAL PRESENTATION AND DIAGNOSIS: PARTIAL ANOMALOUS PULMONARY VENOUS CONNECTION

Patients with isolated PAPVC present in a similar manner to those with ASDs, often with little to no symptoms. However, a minority of affected individuals may develop more pronounced symptoms of volume overload, atrial arrhythmias, and ventricular dysfunction.

Physical examination and ECG findings are similar to those in patients with ASDs and are often subtle if present. TTE imaging may suggest the underlying pathology, but anomalous pulmonary venous connections are rarely visualized in adults. An enlarged and volume overloaded right ventricle may be the only evidence of an abnormality in an otherwise structurally normal heart. TEE imaging, on the other hand, is very useful in identifying left atrial pulmonary venous connections and high SVC imaging may demonstrate anomalous connections. Both CCTA and CMR are the gold standard imaging modality for identifying PAPVC and accurately assess right ventricular size and function.

Cardiac catheterization may help in confirming a diagnosis by identifying the shunt location via oximetry. A catheter may be passed into the anomalous vein to confirm its presence or, alternatively, pulmonary angiography may be performed with delayed acquisition to identify the location of pulmonary venous drainage. Invasive hemodynamics also provides important information regarding intracardiac filling pressures, shunt magnitude, and pulmonary vascular resistance, all of which may influence treatment decisions.

MANAGEMENT: PAPVC

In general, repair is recommended in the presence of symptoms, right ventricular enlargement or dysfunction, or rising pulmonary vascular resistance (Algorithm 106.1). Similar to patients with ASDs, surgical correction is not recommended in individuals with PAPVC and severely elevated pulmonary vascular resistance one-half to two-thirds systemic levels.[4]

Treatment options are largely limited to surgery for PAPVC repair. Single vein repair may be achieved by direct anastomosis of the vein to the left atrium. Other techniques are sometimes employed when anomalous veins are remote from the left atrium. When draining high into the SVC, SVC ligation above the anomalous connection may be performed with tunneling of the lower SVC, and with it the anomalous pulmonary venous flow, through a surgically created ASD. The high SVC is then anastomosed to the right atrial appendage. An isolated scimitar vein may be surgically repaired by pulmonary vein ligation from the inferior vena cava with direct anastomosis to the left atrium, or by tunneling a baffle from the anomalous vein, through the inferior vena cava, and across a surgically created ASD.[26]

FOLLOW-UP PATIENT CARE: PARTIAL ANOMALOUS PULMONARY VENOUS CONNECTION

Following repair, patients should be evaluated for symptom resolution and new-onset atrial arrhythmias or conduction disturbances. The risk of atrial arrhythmias, although low, remains higher in patients with PAPVC than in the general population. Conduction disturbances are a recognized complication of operative intervention, and their frequency depends on the type of repair.[27] Echocardiographic or cross-sectional imaging is recommended within 1 to 6 months postoperatively to evaluate for the presence of a residual shunt, normalization of right ventricular size and function, and pulmonary pressures. Pulmonary vein stenosis is a rare complication of surgical repair, which may present with a persistent cough or hemoptysis and should prompt further evaluation with either CCTA or CMR.

GERBODE DEFECT

A Gerbode defect is a rare cardiac septation defect in which the left ventricle directly communicates with the right atrium (**Figure 106.5**). These defects account for approximately 0.08% of all congenital intracardiac shunts and are often acquired as a complication of surgical intervention in the region of the AV junction (eg, VSD, ASD, and AV valve interventions).[28] Hemodynamically, Gerbode defects are similar to ASDs and PAPVC in that their volume load may result in right-sided chamber enlargement and dysfunction.

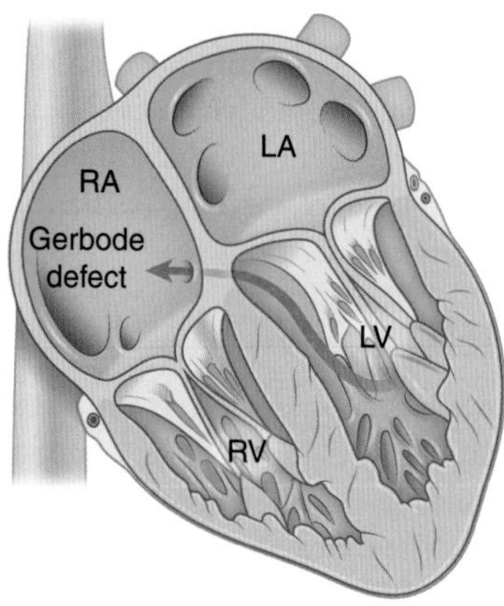

FIGURE 106.5 Gerbode defect anatomy. LA, left atrium; LV, left ventricle; RA, right atrium; RV, right ventricle.

Physical examination is often notable for a harsh, holosystolic murmur along the sternal border, akin to a VSD. TTE imaging is often very useful in identifying the lesion, quantitating the pressure gradient, and assessing right-sided chamber size and function. However, on occasion, it may be difficult to distinguish between a Gerbode defect and a ruptured sinus of Valsalva. TTE, CCTA, and CMR may be helpful in further defining the anatomy.

Indications and contraindications for repair are similar to that of other ASDs (**Algorithm 106.1**). Although no specific transcatheter closure device is available for this lesion, a variety of septal closure devices and vascular plugs have been demonstrated to be a safe and effective treatment strategy, although care must be taken to avoid interfering with AV valve function and AV nodal conduction.[29] Surgical repair often involves patch closure from the right atrial side to prevent recurrence and avoid conduction abnormalities.[30]

CORONARY ARTERY FISTULA

Coronary artery fistulae are abnormal connections between the coronary arteries and a cardiac chamber or great vessel. Although the vast majority of cases are congenital in etiology, fistulous tracts may enlarge over time leading to an increase in shunt magnitude. Rarer causes of these fistulae include external trauma and complications from percutaneous coronary intervention, cardiac surgery, or endomyocardial biopsy. Congenital coronary fistulae typically drain into low-pressure compartments such as the right atrium, right ventricle, or pulmonary arteries, resulting in a left-to-right shunt.[31] Although many of these lesions tend to be hemodynamically insignificant, larger shunts may result in chamber enlargement and increased pulmonary artery pressures. Coronary steal is another well-recognized sequela of coronary fistulae, with preferential blood flow into the low-pressure chamber resulting in downstream myocardial ischemia.

The large majority of coronary fistulae require no intervention with minimal to no long-term follow-up. However, patients with larger fistulae should receive intermittent evaluation for the development of chamber enlargement, heart failure, pulmonary hypertension, and signs or symptoms of myocardial ischemia. If present, fistula occlusion should be considered. Transcatheter occlusion is the preferred treatment modality and can be accomplished using a number of available devices including coils, umbrella devices, detachable balloons, and vascular plugs.[32] When transcatheter occlusion is contraindicated, surgical ligation of the fistula should be considered.

SURGICAL SHUNTS

Surgical shunts are most commonly utilized in the presence of complex congenital heart disease resulting in pulmonary under circulation. The goal of the shunt is to increase pulmonary blood flow while minimizing exposure of the pulmonary vasculature to excessive pressure. Rarely are these shunts utilized as a definitive repair but rather provide a temporary solution to hypoxemia in early childhood, increasing the success of a more definitive repair later in life. However, on occasion, these shunts are left in place and may continue to serve as a major source of pulmonary blood flow. **Figure 106.6** provides a basic reference for surgical shunt anatomy.

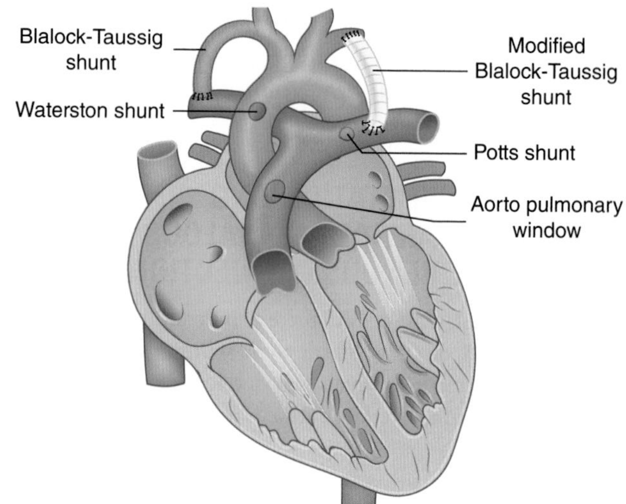

FIGURE 106.6 Surgical shunt anatomy. The Blalock-Taussig shunt is created by anastomosing the subclavian artery to the pulmonary artery. A modified Blalock-Taussig shunt connects the subclavian artery and pulmonary artery using a tube graft. Aortopulmonary windows, Waterston shunts, and Potts shunts are created by creating a communication between the pulmonary artery and the aorta. An aortopulmonary window connects the posterior main pulmonary artery with the anterior ascending aorta. A Waterston shunt connects the posterior ascending aorta with the anterior right pulmonary artery. A Potts shunt connects the posterior left pulmonary artery with the anterior descending aorta.

KEY POINTS

- ✔ Shunt lesions comprise a wide variety of anatomic abnormalities cardiac chambers and great vessels.
- ✔ Cardiac catheterization can aid in the diagnosis by confirming the presence of a shunt.
- ✔ Surgical shunts are most commonly utilized in the presence of complex congenital heart disease resulting in pulmonary under circulation.
- ✔ Regular follow up is indicated in all patients with shunts.

REFERENCES

1. van der Linde D, Konings EE, Slager MA, et al. Birth prevalence of congenital heart disease worldwide: a systematic review and meta-analysis. *J Am Coll Cardiol.* 2011;58:2241-2247.
2. Konstantinides S, Geibel A, Olschewski M, et al. A comparison of surgical and medical therapy for atrial septal defect in adults. *N Engl J Med.* 1995;333:469-473.
3. Van Praagh S, Carrera ME, Sanders SP, Mayer JE, Van Praagh R. Sinus venosus defects: unroofing of the right pulmonary veins—anatomic and echocardiographic findings and surgical treatment. *Am Heart J.* 1994;128:365-379.
4. Stout KK, Daniels CJ, Aboulhosn JA, et al. 2018 AHA/ACC Guideline for the management of adults with congenital heart disease: a report of the American College of Cardiology/American Heart Association Task Force on Clinical Practice Guidelines. *J Am Coll Cardiol.* 2019;73:e81-e192.
5. Du ZD, Hijazi ZM, Kleinman CS, Silverman NH, Larntz K. Comparison between transcatheter and surgical closure of secundum atrial septal defect in children and adults: results of a multicenter nonrandomized trial. *J Am Coll Cardiol.* 2002;39:1836-1844.
6. Levi DS, Moore JW. Embolization and retrieval of the Amplatzer septal occluder. *Catheter Cardiovasc Interv.* 2004;61:543-547.
7. Oyen N, Diaz LJ, Leirgul E, et al. Prepregnancy diabetes and offspring risk of congenital heart disease: a nationwide cohort study. *Circulation.* 2016;133:2243-2253.
8. Riahi M, Velasco Forte MN, Byrne N, et al. Early experience of transcatheter correction of superior sinus venosus atrial septal defect with partial anomalous pulmonary venous drainage. *EuroIntervention.* 2018; 14:868-876.
9. Roos-Hesselink JW, Meijboom FJ, Spitaels SE, et al. Excellent survival and low incidence of arrhythmias, stroke and heart failure long-term after surgical ASD closure at young age. A prospective follow-up study of 21-33 years. *Eur Heart J.* 2003;24:190-197.
10. Warnes CA, Liberthson R, Danielson GK, et al. Task force 1: the changing profile of congenital heart disease in adult life. *J Am Coll Cardiol.* 2001;37:1170-1175.
11. Wernovsky G, Anderson RH, Kumar K, et al. *Anderson's Pediatric Cardiology.* 4th ed. Elsevier; 2020.
12. Carminati M, Butera G, Chessa M, et al. Transcatheter closure of congenital ventricular septal defects: results of the European Registry. *Eur Heart J.* 2007;28:2361-2368.
13. Haas NA, Kock L, Bertram H, et al. Interventional VSD-closure with the Nit-Occlud® Lê VSD-Coil in 110 patients: early and midterm results of the EUREVECO-Registry. *Pediatr Cardiol.* 2017;38:215-227.
14. Mongeon FP, Burkhart HM, Ammash NM, et al. Indications and outcomes of surgical closure of ventricular septal defect in adults. *JACC Cardiovasc Interv.* 2010;3:290-297.
15. Kanani M, Elliott M, Cook A, Juraszek A, Devine W, Anderson RH. Late incompetence of the left atrioventricular valve after repair of atrioventricular septal defects: the morphologic perspective. *J Thorac Cardiovasc Surg.* 2006;132:640-646, 646.e1-3.
16. Hoohenkerk GJ, Bruggemans EF, Rijlaarsdam M, Schoof PH, Koolbergen DR, Hazekamp MG. More than 30 years' experience with surgical correction of atrioventricular septal defects. *Ann Thorac Surg.* 2010;90:1554-1561.
17. El-Najdawi EK, Driscoll DJ, Puga FJ, et al. Operation for partial atrioventricular septal defect: a forty-year review. *J Thorac Cardiovasc Surg.* 2000;119:880-889; discussion 889-890.
18. Bakhtiary F, Takacs J, Cho MY, et al. Long-term results after repair of complete atrioventricular septal defect with two-patch technique. *Ann Thorac Surg.* 2010;89:1239-1243.
19. Lacour-Gayet F, Bonnet N, Piot D, et al. Surgical management of atrio ventricular septal defects with normal caryotype. *Eur J Cardiothorac Surg.* 1997;11:466-472.
20. Backer CL, Stewart RD, Bailliard F, Kelle AM, Webb CL, Mavroudis C. Complete atrioventricular canal: comparison of modified single-patch technique with two-patch technique. *Ann Thorac Surg.* 2007;84: 2038-2046.
21. Monro JL, Alexiou C, Salmon AP, Keeton BR. Reoperations and survival after primary repair of congenital heart defects in children. *J Thorac Cardiovasc Surg.* 2003;126:511-520.
22. Jin M, Liang YM, Wang XF, et al. A retrospective study of 1,526 cases of transcatheter occlusion of patent ductus arteriosus. *Chin Med J.* 2015;128:2284-2289.
23. Healey JE Jr. An anatomic survey of anomalous pulmonary veins: their clinical significance. *J Thorac Surg.* 1952;23:433-444.
24. Haramati LB, Moche IE, Rivera VT, et al. Computed tomography of partial anomalous pulmonary venous connection in adults. *J Comput Assist Tomogr.* 2003;27:743-749.
25. Snellen HA, van Ingen HC, Hoefsmit EC. Patterns of anomalous pulmonary venous drainage. *Circulation.* 1968;38:45-63.
26. Fragata J, Magalhaes M, Baquero L, Trigo C, Pinto F, Fragata I. Partial anomalous pulmonary venous connections: surgical management. *World J Pediatr Congenit Heart Surg.* 2013;4:44-49.
27. Said SM, Burkhart HM, Schaff HV, et al. Single-patch, 2-patch, and caval division techniques for repair of partial anomalous pulmonary venous connections: does it matter? *J Thorac Cardiovasc Surg.* 2012;143:896-903.
28. Al-Hay AA, MacNeill SJ, Yacoub M, Shore DF, Shinebourne EA. Complete atrioventricular septal defect, Down syndrome, and surgical outcome: risk factors. *Ann Thorac Surg.* 2003;75:412-421.
29. Prifti E, Ademaj F, Baboci A, Demiraj A. Acquired Gerbode defect following endocarditis of the tricuspid valve: a case report and literature review. *J Cardiothorac Surg.* 2015;10:115.
30. Kelle AM, Young L, Kaushal S, Duffy CE, Anderson RH, Backer CL. The Gerbode defect: the significance of a left ventricular to right atrial shunt. *Cardiol Young.* 2009;19(suppl 2):96-99.
31. Qureshi SA. Coronary arterial fistulas. *Orphanet J Rare Dis.* 2006;1:51.
32. Mangukia CV. Coronary artery fistula. *Ann Thorac Surg.* 2012;93:2084-2092.

CHAPTER 107

LEFT-SIDED OBSTRUCTIVE LESIONS

Lauren Andrade and Yuli Y. Kim

INTRODUCTION

Left-sided obstructive lesions encompass a number of congenital heart defects affecting the mitral valve, left ventricular outflow tract, aortic valve, and aorta. Hypoplastic left heart syndrome and its variants are not addressed in this chapter.

Epidemiology

Left-sided obstructive lesions generally have a male predominance, and studies have reported familial clustering.[1] The *NOTCH-1* gene has been linked to the bicuspid aortic valve (BAV), aortic stenosis, and hypoplastic left heart syndrome.[2] A small study (38 probands) of family members of patients with hypoplastic left heart syndrome demonstrated that 19% of family members had congenital heart disease; of those, 72% were also left-sided obstructive lesions.[3] In general, left-sided lesions are associated with one another and often occur together.

Bicuspid Aortic Valve and Valvar Aortic Stenosis

The majority of aortic stenosis occurs at the valvar level (70%). BAV is the most common congenital cardiac defect and is found in approximately 1% of the population.[2] Males are more commonly affected with a 1.5:1 to 3:1 ratio over females.[4] BAV disease is also considered an aortopathy manifest as dilated aortic root and/or ascending aorta with increased risk of aortic dissection is approximately 8.4-fold higher than the general population.[5] Other associated lesions occur in ~20% including ventricular septal defect (VSD), patent ductus arteriosus (PDA), and aortic coarctation.[6] BAV has genetic, familial, and spontaneous occurrences. There are specific genetic syndromes, including Turner syndrome and Jacobsen syndrome, that are linked to BAV as well as coarctation of the aorta (CoA).[2] Approximately 10% of first-degree family members of those with BAV are found to have BAV as well; for this reason, American Heart Association (AHA)/American College of Cardiology (ACC) guidelines state it is reasonable (Class IIa) to screen all first-degree relatives of those with BAV.[7]

Subvalvular Aortic Stenosis

Subvalvular aortic stenosis comprises 10% to 20% of aortic stenosis and, like valvar aortic stenosis, has a male predominance of 2:1 to 3:1.[8] This lesion is associated with other cardiac lesions about half the time, including atrioventricular septal defect, VSD, aortic coarctation, valvar aortic stenosis, and mitral valve abnormalities.[8] Unlike other forms of aortic stenosis, subvalvular stenosis is not seen in neonates and is thus felt to most likely be an acquired lesion.[9]

Supravalvular Aortic Stenosis

Supravalvular stenosis is rare, accounting for 0.5% of all congenital heart disease and the remaining ~10% of aortic stenosis that is not valvar or subvalvular.[10] Half of patients with this lesion have Williams syndrome,[11] which is associated with developmental delay, characteristic facial features, and peripheral pulmonary stenosis. Patients with Williams syndrome have a defect in the elastin gene (7q11.23), which has an autosomal dominant inheritance pattern.[12]

Coarctation of the Aorta

CoA is a narrowing of the proximal descending aorta and/or distal aortic arch that obstructs blood flow to the body. This lesion is fairly common, accounting for 4% to 6% of all congenital heart diseases with a male predominance of 1.5:1.[4] It is primarily thought to be sporadic but, like all left-sided lesions, does exhibit familial clustering. In addition, ~5% to 15% of patients with Turner syndrome have CoA, which should be screened for in this population.[13] Patients with CoA often have other cardiac lesions including hypoplasia of the aortic arch, VSD, atrial septal defect (ASD), mitral valve disease, and BAV in 60% to 70%.[4]

Mitral Stenosis

Congenital mitral stenosis is rare and only accounts for 0.6% of congenital heart disease, with a male predominance of 1.5:1.[14] Supravalvular mitral stenosis, such as a membranous ring, is almost always associated with mitral valve stenosis. The complex of a supramitral ring, parachute mitral valve (all chordal attachments return to one papillary muscle), subvalvular aortic stenosis, and coarctation of the aorta is called *Shone complex* and again highlights the association between different left-sided obstructive lesions, although the complete constellation of lesions is not common.[15] Because congenital mitral stenosis and parachute mitral valve are rare and there is a high association with other defects, patients with these lesions warrant further evaluation.[7]

PATHOGENESIS

Bicuspid Aortic Valve and Valvar Aortic Stenosis

BAV occurs when, instead of the normal configuration of three cusps, two are partially or completely fused. The most common orientation is fusion of the right and left cusps, followed by right and noncoronary, and least commonly left and noncoronary cusps.[16] BAV may or may not have raphe and may simply have two cusps with either a horizontal or vertical orientation.

Unicuspid valves can also exist in which there are two sites of leaflet fusion or partial fusion, leaving a slit-like or *keyhole* like opening (**Figure 107.1**). Independent of the valve itself, there can also be annular hypoplasia in the setting of otherwise normal cusps leading to stenosis at the valvar level.

BAV stenosis occurs more frequently than BAV regurgitation. There is significant variability in the rate of valve disease progression in BAV, but nearly all affected patients develop calcification and some degree of valve dysfunction in the long-term. This is thought to be caused by shear stress and turbulent flow across the abnormal valve which promotes inflammation and myxomatous change, and stimulates osteogenic factors that lead to calcification.[17] Those that tend to have more asymmetric cusps and with right and noncoronary fusion may develop calcification at a faster rate.[16]

The physiologic result of significant valvar aortic stenosis is elevated afterload against which the left ventricle (LV) must work. In response to this afterload, the LV hypertrophies to maintain wall stress at a constant, even in cases of severe stenosis leading to (1) diastolic dysfunction with elevated left ventricular filling pressures and (2) increased myocardial oxygen demand. Mismatch between coronary perfusion and myocardial oxygen demand can result in subendocardial ischemia and infarction. The subendocardium and papillary muscles are vulnerable to decreased perfusion, particularly with exercise. Holter monitoring has revealed ventricular dysrhythmias which, in combination with increased myocardial oxygen demand, can lead to sudden death.[18]

Subvalvular Aortic Stenosis

Subvalvular aortic stenosis typically consists of either a membranous circumferential ring or a fibrous ridge of tissue in the left ventricular outflow tract below the aortic valve (**Figure 107.2**) comprising collagen, myocytes, and elastin.[19] The tissue may also have attachments to the mitral valve and its subvalvular apparatus or the aortic valve. Mitral valve abnormalities are associated with subvalvular aortic stenosis as well, including attachment of a papillary muscle to the interventricular septum or aortic leaflet, accessory mitral valve tissue, and muscularization of the subaortic portion of the anterior leaflet. Because this appears to be an acquired lesion, proposed mechanisms of development include abnormal endothelium and shear stress from congenital abnormalities in the left ventricular outflow tract.[20] The resulting physiology is similar to that outlined above in valvar aortic stenosis, with significant stenosis leading to elevated afterload and potential for left ventricular hypertrophy and dysfunction. In general, subvalvular aortic stenosis is progressive but the rate of progression is variable and can be stable for many years.[21] Aortic valve regurgitation can result from turbulent flow in the presence of a subaortic membrane or ridge.[22]

Supravalvular Aortic Stenosis

Supravalvular aortic stenosis develops just above the aortic valve and is related to abnormally thick, hypertrophied tissue consistent with the genetic abnormality of the elastin gene found in Williams syndrome. The most frequent site of stenosis occurs at the sinotubular junction, but it can also occur across the entire ascending aorta and transverse arch. Because of the proximity of the aortic valve cusp attachments to the sinotubular junction, these may also be thickened. Aside from the issues regarding coronary perfusion and myocardial demand mismatch noted above, patients with supravalvular aortic stenosis have additional risk factors for coronary ischemia. The coronary ostia, being located near or below the thickened sinotubular junction and just above abnormal aortic cusp attachments, can themselves be stenosed. Furthermore, narrowing distal to the coronaries not only exposes the coronary arteries to hypertension but also limits diastolic flow and perfusion, which could contribute to ischemia and sudden death.[23] Death in patients

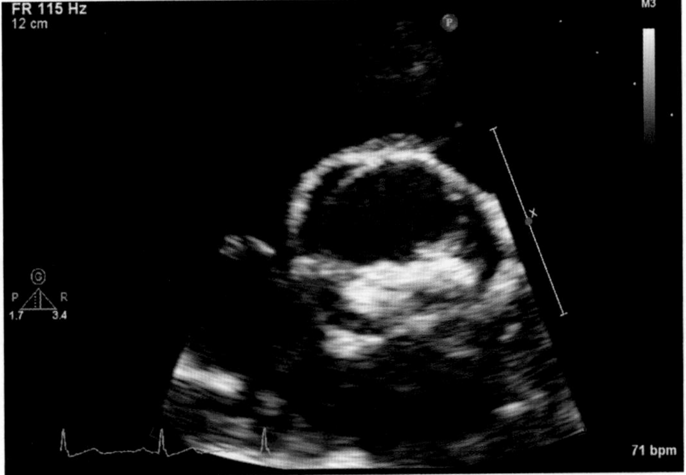

FIGURE 107.1 Transthoracic echocardiogram of a unicuspid aortic valve in the parasternal short-axis view.

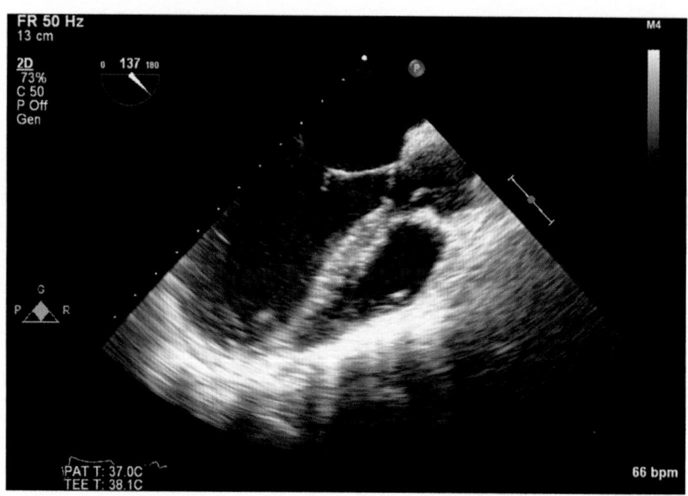

FIGURE 107.2 Transesophageal echocardiogram of a subaortic membrane, seen in the left ventricular outflow tract below the aortic valve.

with supravalvular aortic stenosis undergoing cardiac catheterization procedures has been reported, likely because of anesthesia and the resultant drop in diastolic blood pressure, as well as catheter manipulation near the coronaries.[24]

Coarctation of the Aorta

CoA occurs when there is either discrete or long segment narrowing of the aortic arch or proximal descending aorta. The most common site for discrete coarctation is at the isthmus, the insertion site of the PDA that is present in fetal and early neonatal circulation. There are two common theories as to how coarctation develops. One theory proposes that the ductal tissue present in the PDA is also present in a larger portion of aortic tissue and, therefore, creates a discrete narrowing as this ductal tissue constricts and the PDA closes shortly after birth.[25] The other prevailing theory is that a state of low flow across the aortic arch in utero leads to poor growth and development of the aortic arch.[26] Both theories may be accurate in that discrete coarctations seem more likely to be explained by the ductal tissue theory whereas a longer segment of narrowing across the arch may be more likely to occur in a *low-flow* state.

When severe, patients can develop significant collateral vessels including the intercostal, internal mammary, and scapular arteries in order to provide flow to the body, bypassing the area of coarctation. The fixed obstruction can lead to otherwise similar problems seen in aortic stenosis including left ventricular hypertrophy and dysfunction over time. Hypertension also develops as the blood vessels to the head and neck are typically proximal to the obstruction and thus exposed to high pressure. The lower body, including the kidneys and mesentery, however, gets less perfusion pressure. The renin-angiotensin-aldosterone system is therefore stimulated to retain fluid and increase blood pressure, further propagating elevated pressures proximal to the obstruction.[27]

An inherent vascular tissue abnormality is also likely present in patients with coarctation. The pathophysiology of the aorta in coarctation is notable for endothelial dysfunction and abnormal elastic properties even after repair.[28] Patients with CoA have also been found to have a higher rate of intracranial aneurysms (10%) than the general population,[29] thus supporting the concept of CoA as a diffuse arteriopathy.

Mitral Stenosis

Mitral stenosis can arise from a valve, or region above the valve, that is dysplastic. Mitral valve dysplasia typically involves thickened leaflets, a loss of interchordal space, and abnormalities of the papillary muscles. Parachute mitral valve is a specific type of dysplastic valve in which the mitral valve chordae all insert on a single papillary muscle, resulting in a *parachute* type of appearance that may or may not result in mitral stenosis. In supravalvular mitral stenosis, a membrane starts at the level of the mitral valve annulus, differentiating it from cor triatriatum which is a membrane located above the atrial appendage. A supramitral ring is another form of supravalvular mitral stenosis that can be circumferential and can extend to the mitral valve. As a result of obstruction to mitral inflow, the left atrial pressures may be elevated, depending on the degree of narrowing. This can lead to elevated pulmonary artery pressures, pulmonary edema, and ultimately elevated right heart pressures in cases of severe stenosis.

CLINICAL PRESENTATION

Bicuspid Aortic Valve and Valvar Aortic Stenosis

Many patients with BAV remain asymptomatic for many years. They may be referred for a murmur prior to the development of symptoms which include exertional angina, easy fatiguability, heart failure symptoms, syncope, or even sudden death.[6,30] Adults with severe aortic stenosis can remain asymptomatic despite this degree of disease. One study demonstrated that only 10% of patients with a gradient of >80 mm Hg had symptoms of angina.[31] Those with higher gradients are more likely to have symptoms, need intervention sooner, or experience death sooner than those with a relatively mild stenosis earlier in life.[32] Patients with BAV also may present with aortic dilatation or dissection.

The physical examination may show an increased apical cardiac impulse, a presystolic tap of a forceful atrial contraction, and a palpable thrill in the suprasternal notch or precordium in cases of moderate-severe stenosis. The second heart sound may be single owing to prolonged ejection time across the aortic valve and in very severe cases, there may be paradoxical splitting (A2 occurring after P2). There may be an S4 in patients with severe stenosis and diastolic dysfunction. There is typically an early systolic ejection click (loudest at the left sternal border and apex). A click and a suprasternal notch thrill are highly suggestive that stenosis is valvar as opposed to subvalvular or supravalvular. The classic crescendo-decrescendo murmur is usually loudest at the right upper sternal border that peaks later as severity increases and radiates to the carotids. There may be a delayed and/or diminished carotid upstroke.

Subvalvular Aortic Stenosis

Subvalvular aortic stenosis may also be asymptomatic and present with a murmur. It could also be discovered on follow-up for another lesion such as CoA, VSD, or atrioventricular canal defect. Symptoms similar to that of valvar aortic stenosis with fatigue, heart failure symptoms, syncope, or angina may develop as stenosis progresses. The systolic murmur is usually loudest at the left midsternal border and radiates to the upper sternal border and suprasternal notch. There is not usually a systolic ejection click unless there is a coexistent BAV. If there is associated aortic regurgitation, a diastolic murmur at the left sternal border may also be heard.

Supravalvular Aortic Stenosis

Supravalvular aortic stenosis may be asymptomatic or may be found owing to a history of Williams syndrome or a murmur heard on examination. Symptoms may be similar to valvar aortic stenosis, with special concern in patients with angina and syncope, given the additional risks for coronary ischemia. There will be a murmur similar to valvar aortic stenosis, located at the right sternal border and radiating to the suprasternal notch and the carotids but without a preceding systolic ejection click.

Coarctation of the Aorta

The hallmark of presentation is typically asymptomatic hypertension. However, if there is severe hypertension, patients can present with headache, epistaxis, heart failure, or even aortic dissection. Patients may also experience claudication because of poor perfusion of their lower extremities. Unrepaired, the average age of death for those with CoA is 35 years, with cause of death including heart failure, aortic dissection, endarteritis, endocarditis, myocardial infarction, and intracranial hemorrhage.[33] The prevalence of stroke in contemporary CoA patients is not well-described, but these patients experience hemorrhagic and ischemic stroke at a significantly younger age compared to the general population.[34] The association of intracranial aneurysm and CoA is thought to be related to either developmental abnormalities of the arterial wall or pathologic changes as a result of mechanical forces attributable to hypertension.[35] Vascular abnormalities including vertebral artery hypoplasia and incomplete posterior circle of Willis are associated with increased cerebral vascular resistance. There is a significantly higher prevalence of both of these cerebral vascular abnormalities in CoA patients compared to the general population and is an independent risk factor for hypertension in this population, highlighting another potential mechanism linking stroke and hypertension in CoA.[36]

On examination, lower extremity pulses may be decreased, delayed, or absent. There may also be a systolic murmur heard at the left upper chest under the clavicle radiating to the back representing turbulent flow across the area of narrowing. Cuff blood pressures can reveal lower blood pressure in the legs and hypertension in the arms. This may be variable depending upon the location of CoA in relation to the subclavian arteries. If distal to both the left and right subclavian arteries, as is typical, both arms will be hypertensive. However, if there is an anomalous subclavian artery or the coarctation is proximal to one of the subclavian takeoffs, then one arm or both may have blood pressure similar to those in the legs. There may also be continuous murmurs associated with collateral vessels.

Mitral Stenosis

Mitral stenosis may be largely asymptomatic depending on the degree of obstruction. Patients can present with symptoms of heart failure including dyspnea on exertion, orthopnea, and exercise intolerance, or new-onset atrial fibrillation. On examination, there may be a mid-diastolic and late diastolic murmur, usually low-pitched. There may also be a prominent S2 from pulmonary hypertension.

DIAGNOSIS

Electrocardiogram

The electrocardiogram (EKG) in aortic stenosis may demonstrate voltage for left ventricular hypertrophy, ST depressions, or T wave inversion in left precordial leads. These findings may be present in valvar, subvalvular, and supravalvular aortic stenosis as well as CoA as they primarily represent left ventricular hypertrophy and strain. Mitral stenosis may show evidence of left atrial enlargement or, in the setting of elevated pulmonary pressures, right ventricular hypertrophy, right axis deviation, and right ventricular strain.

Chest X-Ray

The chest x-ray in aortic stenosis may reveal a rounded apex from left ventricular hypertrophy, cardiomegaly, posterior displacement of the cardiac silhouette, left atrial enlargement, and valvar calcification. A dilated aorta is also sometimes present and may be apparent as widening of the mediastinal silhouette, an enlarged aortic knob, and displacement of the trachea. In those with long-standing unrepaired coarctation, there may be pre- and post-coarctation dilation of the aorta, creating the "3" appearance on the posterior-anterior chest x-ray as well as notching of the inferior surface of the ribs—usually, the fourth to eighth ribs are involved—from intercostal collateral vessel development. The chest x-ray in mitral stenosis may demonstrate a *straightening* of the left heart border, which results from underfilling of the LV and aorta in isolated mitral stenosis. If there is a significant elevation in left atrial and pulmonary pressures, then there may be pulmonary venous congestion and splaying of the carina as a result of a dilated left atrium.

Echocardiogram

Echocardiography is the mainstay of diagnosis in congenital heart disease and will typically be the initial diagnostic test of choice, given its accessibility, lack of radiation exposure, and high degree of sensitivity and specificity.

In evaluation of BAV by transthoracic echo (TTE), there may be thickening and doming of the valve and it may have a *fish-mouth* appearance *en face*. The mean Doppler gradient correlates well with the peak-to-peak gradient by cardiac catheterization and is thus used to grade aortic stenosis. The ACC/AHA guidelines grade aortic stenosis as mild when the mean transvalvular gradient is <25 mm Hg, moderate when the mean gradient is 25 to 40 mm Hg, and severe when the mean gradient >40 mm Hg.[37] This is only applicable with normal ventricular function and absence of additional defects such as a VSD, which could lead to underestimation of the transvalvular gradient as this can act as a left ventricular pressure *pop-off*. Higher contractility and stroke volume as well as a faster heart rate at a given stroke volume will also increase the transvalvular gradient.

In evaluating for subvalvular and supravalvular aortic stenosis, two-dimensional TTE imaging from multiple views can help delineate the nature of obstruction and color Doppler interrogation can help determine where flow acceleration starts. Use of pulsed-wave Doppler at multiple locations along the left ventricular outflow tract can determine the location of the obstruction.

Classic TTE findings of CoA include narrowing at the aortic isthmus with a *posterior shelf* and a downwardly displaced left subclavian artery. With Doppler interrogation, there is aliasing across the area of narrowing and continuation of forward flow in diastole, which can appear as two distinct populations of flow on the tracing. The abdominal aorta may show dampened pulsations and upstroke as well as continuation of forward flow in diastole from the continuous collateral flow.

The mitral valve can be imaged from multiple views to evaluate for thickening, leaflet excursion, and the subvalvular apparatus including the papillary muscles. If there is one papillary muscle or a predominant papillary muscle and limited space between them, this raises suspicion for an abnormally functioning mitral valve. The mean inflow gradient obtained by continuous-wave Doppler interrogation should be used to evaluate for the degree of stenosis.

Transesophageal echocardiography can be particularly useful for visualizing cardiac structures not well seen by TTE. This includes subaortic membranes and subaortic stenosis and details regarding the structure of an aortic valve or mitral valve, which can help determine if it is amenable to repair (or requires replacement).

Cardiac Catheterization

Catheterization is no longer a primary modality for diagnosis but is still utilized in complex lesions, when a noninvasive modality cannot sufficiently estimate a *true gradient* across an area of stenosis or if there are multiple levels of obstruction. In valvar aortic stenosis, the pressure in the LV and the aorta above the valve can be obtained to determine the peak-to-peak gradient. Similarly, this can be done by pullback across the left ventricular outflow tract, supravalvular region, or CoA.

In patients with supravalvular aortic stenosis, cardiac catheterization can carry excess risk. In the setting of coronary ostial stenosis, catheter manipulation at the coronary origins combined with effects of anesthesia places these patients at risk for ischemia and periprocedural cardiac arrest.

For isolated mitral stenosis, cardiac catheterization is not required as the mean inflow gradient by echocardiography is acceptable and correlates well with the catheterization-derived transmitral gradient. Cardiac catheterization can be useful if there are associated lesions such as a VSD in order to determine how much of the inflow gradient is caused by excess left-sided flow as opposed to the mitral valve stenosis.

Cardiac Magnetic Resonance Imaging and Computed Tomography

Cardiac magnetic resonance imaging (MRI) and computed tomography (CT) are typically reserved for more clear visualization of lesions that are not well seen by echocardiography. Valvar aortic stenosis does not usually require MRI or CT for diagnosis but may be helpful to follow a dilated ascending aorta in the case of BAV. Subvalvular and supravalvular aortic stenosis may be better visualized by MRI or CT. For supravalvular aortic stenosis, coronaries can also be evaluated by CT. CoA is particularly well-suited for CT or MR assessment especially in patients with more complex anatomies and those with poor acoustic windows (**Figure 107.3**). They are the imaging modalities of choice after repair to monitor for the development of re-coarctation or development of an aneurysm.

MANAGEMENT

Medical Approach

There is no medical therapy that will alter the progression of aortic valve disease, subvalvular aortic stenosis, supravalvular aortic stenosis, CoA, or mitral stenosis. Lipid-lowering agents have been trialed without meaningful impact on calcific aortic valve changes.[38] In patients with supravalvular aortic stenosis and associated coronary involvement, appropriate risk factor management for coronary atherosclerosis is recommended. Guideline-directed medical therapy of blood pressure control is warranted in those with CoA who are hypertensive.[39] When combining resting blood pressure, ambulatory blood pressure monitoring, and exercise testing, systemic hypertension has

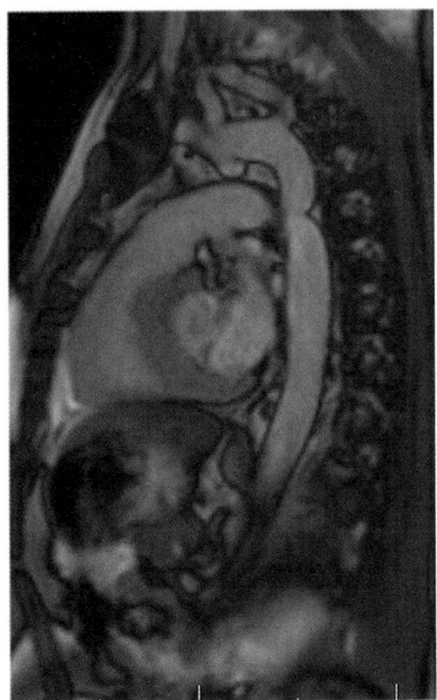

FIGURE 107.3 Sagittal MRI of coarctation of the aorta. MRI, magnetic resonance imaging.

been reported in as many as 70% of patients following coarctation repair.[40] Mitral stenosis may present with heart failure symptoms and in this case, diuretic therapy may be useful to improve symptoms of pulmonary edema. In addition, adequate heart rate control can result in a lower inflow gradient and can lengthen diastole, allowing for more filling of the LV, so therapy such as a β-blocker may be of benefit.

Percutaneous Intervention

Bicuspid Aortic Valve and Valvar Aortic Stenosis

Treatment is invasive for significant aortic stenosis with timing of intervention dependent on symptoms or sequelae of aortic stenosis impacting left ventricular function. Development of symptoms or an abnormal blood pressure response to exercise is also helpful in risk stratification. Guidelines for aortic valve intervention are outlined in **Table 107.1**. For valvar aortic stenosis, there is a role for catheter-based intervention in younger patients who may not have significant calcification or aortic regurgitation.[41] The 2018 ACC/AHA Guideline for the Management of Adults with Congenital Heart Disease states that young patients (generally under 25 years) with relatively mobile and minimally calcified aortic valves are candidates for balloon valvuloplasty. Patients who are older with more highly calcified and poorly mobile valves are at higher risk of developing significant aortic regurgitation if treated with balloon valvuloplasty.[42]

Transcatheter aortic valve replacement (TAVR) is being performed routinely in older patients with aortic stenosis and at high surgical risk with the expansion of indications now into the more moderate and lower risk surgical candidates,[43]

TABLE 107.1 AHA/ACC Guidelines for Intervention in Bicuspid Aortic Valve and Aortic Stenosis

AHA/ACC Recommendation	Class/LOE
AVR is recommended for symptomatic patients with severe high-gradient AS who have symptoms by history or on exercise testing.	I/B
AVR is recommended for asymptomatic patients with severe AS and LVEF <50%.	I/B
AVR is indicated for patients with severe AS when undergoing other cardiac surgery.	I/B
AVR is reasonable for asymptomatic patients with very severe AS (aortic velocity ≥5.0 m/s) and low surgical risk.	IIa/B
AVR is reasonable in asymptomatic patients with severe AS and decreased exercise tolerance or an exercise fall in blood pressure.	IIa/B
AVR is reasonable in symptomatic patients with low-flow/low-gradient severe AS with reduced LVEF with a low-dose dobutamine stress study that shows an aortic velocity ≥4.0 m/s (or mean pressure gradient ≥40 mm Hg) with a valve area ≤1.0 cm^2 at any dobutamine dose.	IIa/B
AVR is reasonable in symptomatic patients who have low-flow/low-gradient severe AS who are normotensive and have an LVEF ≥50% if clinical, hemodynamic, and anatomic data support valve obstruction as the most likely cause of symptoms.	IIa/C
AVR is reasonable for patients with moderate AS (aortic velocity 3.0-3.9 m/s) who are undergoing other cardiac surgery.	IIa/C
AVR may be considered for asymptomatic patients with severe AS and rapid disease progression and low surgical risk.	IIb/C
In adults with BAV, AS, and a noncalcified valve with no more than mild AR meeting indications for intervention per GDMT, it may be reasonable to treat with balloon valvuloplasty.	IIb/B

AHA/ACC, American Heart Association/American College of Cardiology; AR, aortic regurgitation; AS, aortic stenosis; AVR, aortic valve replacement; BAV, bicuspid aortic valve; GDMT, guideline-directed medical therapy; LOE, level of evidence; LVEF, left ventricular ejection fraction.

Reprinted from Nishimura RA, Otto CM, Bonow RO, et al.; American College of Cardiology/American Heart Association Task Force on Practice Guidelines. 2014 AHA/ACC guideline for the management of patients with valvular heart disease: a report of the American College of Cardiology/American Heart Association Task Force on Practice Guidelines. *J Am Coll Cardiol*. 2014;63(22):e57-e185. Copyright © 2014 American Heart Association, Inc., and the American College of Cardiology Foundation; Stout KK, Daniels CJ, Aboulhosn JA, et al. 2018 AHA/ACC Guideline for the Management of Adults With Congenital Heart Disease: Executive Summary: A Report of the American College of Cardiology/American Heart Association Task Force on Clinical Practice Guidelines. *J Am Coll Cardiol*. 2019;73(12):1494-1563. Copyright © 2019 by the American College of Cardiology Foundation. With permission.

but it has not yet been routinely performed or indicated in the younger congenital aortic stenosis population.

Subvalvular Aortic Stenosis, Supravalvular Aortic Stenosis, and Mitral Stenosis

In contrast to valvar aortic stenosis, subvalvular aortic stenosis does not respond to balloon dilation, and definitive therapy consists of surgical correction. Similarly, surgical repair is the procedure of choice for supravalvular aortic stenosis because of the proximity of the obstruction to the coronary arteries. In general, patients with congenital mitral valve stenosis will require surgery when they meet the criteria for intervention.

Coarctation of the Aorta

Intervention (surgical or catheter-based stenting) is recommended in cases of hypertension, and evidence of significant coarctation either by imaging or identifying a gradient of >20 mm Hg via cuff blood pressure, catheterization, or Doppler gradient. If there is evidence of left ventricular dysfunction, a lower gradient can be accepted as a reason for intervention.[7] Catheter-based intervention on coarctation using either covered or uncovered stents across the coarctation site is considered standard of care for those with amenable anatomy. Determining which patients are candidates for catheter-based versus surgical intervention depends upon the proximity of the coarctation to any neck vessels or the need to enlarge a more significant segment of a hypoplastic aortic arch. Stents can potentially cover and *jail* the origins of head and neck vessels, and therefore surgical repair may be preferred. Risks of stent placement include stent fracture, stent migration, and aneurysm formation. Imaging with CT or MR is utilized to screen for the development of these findings.[44] The COAST II (Covered Cheatham-Platinum Stents for Prevention or Treatment of Aortic Wall Injury Associated with Coarctation of the Aorta Trial) trial demonstrated an average decrease in coarctation gradient from 27 to 4 mm Hg with few resultant injuries to the aortic wall, reinforcing the safety and efficacy of catheter intervention for coarctation.[45] If surgical repair or stent placement is not feasible, balloon angioplasty of the coarctation (native or recurrent) is reasonable.[7]

Surgical Approach

Bicuspid Aortic Valve and Valvar Aortic Stenosis

Multiple types of surgical intervention can be performed for aortic stenosis. Surgical valvotomy in which the valve cusps are thinned and fusions are incised can be an effective method, although some valves are too dysplastic to be candidates for this procedure. This has the advantage of simply modifying the existing valve tissue without replacing the valve; however, it does expose the patient to a surgical procedure. Aortic valve replacement is often necessary. Replacement options include bioprosthetic valves, which do not require long-term anticoagulation but have a shorter life span compared to mechanical valves that are durable but require lifelong anticoagulation. The decision on which type of valve will be used is often a discussion between the surgeon and patient—considering the patient's age and lifestyle—and is beyond the scope of this chapter.

An alternative is the Ross procedure, which moves the native pulmonary valve into the aortic position and places a right ventricle to the pulmonary artery valved conduit for pulmonary blood flow. Advantages include no need for systemic anticoagulation and growth of the neo-aortic valve with somatic size but long-term issues require lifelong surveillance. Finally, for patients with a small aortic valve annulus, techniques to enlarge the annulus itself such as the Manouguian or Nicks procedure may be required to seat an appropriately sized prosthesis or the Konno operation to enlarge the left ventricular outflow tract and subvalvular area, which is often combined with the Ross procedure. Guidelines for aortic valve intervention are listed in Table 107.1.

Subvalvular Aortic Stenosis

Surgical resection of a discrete subaortic membrane, removal of a subaortic ridge of tissue, or removal of muscle in the left ventricular outflow tract causing narrowing is the standard of care, when intervention is indicated. In cases with a narrow, tunnel-like left ventricular outflow tract or small aortic annular more substantial muscle, resection may be warranted, including the Konno procedure, which is mentioned above. Subvalvular aortic stenosis surgery carries a 10% to 15% risk of heart block.[46] Guidelines for subvalvular aortic stenosis intervention are outlined in **Table 107.2**.

Supravalvular Aortic Stenosis

Surgical relief of the supravalvular stenosis is the intervention of choice. Multiple surgical techniques can be used including patching across the noncoronary sinus, patch across both the noncoronary and right coronary sinuses, and patches into all three sinuses (Brom technique).[47] If there are coronary concerns, these are addressed with either enlargement of the ostia or bypass grafting. As supravalvular aortic stenosis is rare, limited data are available on long-term outcomes, but it appears that recurrence is uncommon.[47] Patients with supravalvular aortic stenosis and evidence of coronary ischemia should have coronary-specific imaging performed and consideration of revascularization if appropriate.[7] Guidelines for supravalvular aortic stenosis intervention are outlined in Table 107.2.

Coarctation of the Aorta

Surgical coarctation repair may be undertaken when the patient's anatomy precludes catheter-based stent placement. Repair may be achieved by end-to-end anastomosis with the removal of the coarctation segment, by a subclavian flap repair in which tissue from the left subclavian artery is used to enlarge the area of the coarctation (and the subclavian is sacrificed), by a graft bypassing the area of coarctation, or there may be a patch repair across the area of coarctation. If the coarctation is discrete, the repair may be performed via a lateral thoracotomy, which provides adequate exposure. However, if there is a longer segment of arch hypoplasia, a median sternotomy approach may be undertaken to enable this segment to be enlarged.

TABLE 107.2 AHA/ACC Guidelines for Intervention in Subvalvular and Supravalvular Aortic Stenosis

AHA/ACC Recommendation	Class/ LOE
Surgical intervention is recommended for adults with subvalvular AS, a maximum gradient ≥ 50 mm Hg and symptoms attributable to the subvalvular AS.	I/C
Surgical intervention is recommended for adults with subvalvular AS and < 50 mm Hg maximum gradient and heart failure or ischemic symptoms, and/or LV systolic dysfunction attributable to subvalvular AS.	I/C
Surgical repair is recommended for adults with supravalvular AS (discrete or diffuse) and symptoms or decreased LV systolic function deemed secondary to aortic obstruction.	I/B
Coronary artery revascularization is recommended in symptomatic adults with supravalvular aortic stenosis and coronary ostial stenosis.	I/C
Surgical intervention may be considered for asymptomatic adults with subvalvular AS and at least mild AR and a maximum gradient ≥ 50 mm Hg to prevent the progression of AR.	IIb/C

AHA/ACC, American Heart Association/American College of Cardiology; AR, aortic regurgitation; AS, aortic stenosis; LOE, level of evidence; LV, left ventricular.
Reprinted from Stout KK, Daniels CJ, Aboulhosn JA, et al. 2018 AHA/ACC Guideline for the Management of Adults With Congenital Heart Disease: Executive Summary: A Report of the American College of Cardiology/American Heart Association Task Force on Clinical Practice Guidelines. *J Am Coll Cardiol.* 2019;73(12):1494-1563. Copyright © 2019 by the American College of Cardiology Foundation. With permission.

Mitral Stenosis

Indications for mitral valve intervention in congenital mitral stenosis include severe symptoms and severe stenosis defined by valve area <1.5 cm^2.[37] The severity and type of mitral valve abnormalities will determine what type of surgery needs to be undertaken. Surgery may involve fenestration of fused chordae, division of a single papillary muscle, or removal of accessory subvalvular tissue. If a supramitral ring exists, then excision of the membrane will be performed. If the valve and its supporting apparatus are too dysplastic to be repaired, then mitral valve replacement is often necessary, with similar considerations in valve choice as in the aortic position.

SPECIAL CONSIDERATIONS

As TAVRs become more routine, the target population is also broadening, now with evidence for performing TAVR in a low-risk population with senile calcific aortic stenosis.[48] In BAV, there are concerns regarding TAVR causing annulus rupture, paravalvar leak, and risk of heart block; however, these risks may be lower with newer generation devices.[49] Indications for TAVR in the congenital aortic stenosis population have not been established. These catheter-based valves will help avoid multiple re-do sternotomies; however, as with all bioprosthetic valves, they will require replacement over the course of several years, and there is a limit to how many valve-in-valve procedures are feasible. This will be an important consideration moving forward in the treatment of congenital aortic stenosis, particularly in a young population.

FOLLOW-UP PATIENT CARE

Follow-up care is dependent on the specific lesion as well as the severity of that lesion. In general, follow-up care involves clinic visit with an adult congenital heart disease provider, imaging (echocardiography, cardiac CT, or cardiac MRI), EKG, and intermittent exercise testing. Most left-sided obstructive lesions are well imaged by TTE alone; however, patients with repaired coarctation, dilated ascending aorta in the setting of BAV, and supravalvular aortic stenosis warrant interval cardiac CT or MRI. More rigorous blood pressure monitoring, including exercise testing as well as ambulatory blood pressure monitoring, may also be performed in patients with CoA owing to their higher risk of hypertension, even following successful repair. Based on studies demonstrating an increased risk of intracranial aneurysm formation in patients with CoA, screening for intracranial aneurysms with magnetic resonance angiography or CT angiography may be reasonable.[7] Coronary artery imaging is particularly important in supravalvular aortic stenosis. Recurrence rate of subaortic membrane is ~20%[50] and merits lifelong follow-up. The guidelines for follow-up in each of the conditions are detailed in **Tables 107.3** and **107.4**.

TABLE 107.3 Follow-Up for Aortic Stenosis

Follow-up for Aortic Stenosis
Exercise testing is reasonable to assess physiologic changes with exercise and to confirm the absence of symptoms in asymptomatic patients with a calcified aortic valve and an aortic velocity >4.0 m/s or mean pressure gradient >40 mm Hg
Progressive Class B • TTE every 3-5 years (mild severity, Vmax 2.0-2.9 m/s) • TTE every 1-2 years (moderate severity, Vmax 3.0-3.9 m/s)
Severe Class C • TTE every 6-12 months (Vmax ≥4.0 m/s)
Aortic dilation >4.5 cm • Image every 12 months (TTE, MRI, or CT)

CT, computed tomography; MRI, magnetic resonance imaging; TTE, transthoracic echocardiography; and Vmax, maximum velocity.
Reprinted from Stout KK, Daniels CJ, Aboulhosn JA, et al. 2018 AHA/ACC Guideline for the Management of Adults With Congenital Heart Disease: Executive Summary: A Report of the American College of Cardiology/American Heart Association Task Force on Clinical Practice Guidelines. *J Am Coll Cardiol.* 2019;73(12):1494-1563. Copyright © 2019 by the American College of Cardiology Foundation; Nishimura RA, Otto CM, Bonow RO, et al.; American College of Cardiology/American Heart Association Task Force on Practice Guidelines. 2014 AHA/ACC guideline for the management of patients with valvular heart disease: a report of the American College of Cardiology/American Heart Association Task Force on Practice Guidelines. *J Am Coll Cardiol.* 2014;63(22):e57-e185. Copyright © 2014 American Heart Association, Inc., and the American College of Cardiology Foundation. With permission.

TABLE 107.4 Follow-Up for Subaortic Stenosis, Supravalvular Aortic Stenosis Mitral Stenosis, and Coarctation of the Aorta

Physiologic Stage	Subvalvular Aortic Stenosis	Supravalvular Aortic Stenosis	Mitral Stenosis	Coarctation of the Aorta
Stage A[e]	Clinic visit, EKG, and TTE every 2 years Exercise test[a] as needed	Clinic visit, EKG, and TTE[b] every 2 years Cardiac CT[d] or MRI[c] every 36-60 months Exercise test[a] as needed	Clinic visit, EKG, TTE every 2 years Exercise test[a] as needed	Clinic visit, EKG, TTE[b] every 2 years Cardiac CT[d] or MRI[c] every 36-60 months Exercise test every 3 years
Stage B[e]	Clinic visit, EKG, TTE, and exercise test[a] every 2 years	Clinic visit, EKG, and TTE[b] every 2 years Cardiac CT[d] or MRI[c] every 36-60 months Exercise test[a] every 2 years	Clinic visit, EKG and TTE and exercise test[a] every 2 years	Clinic visit, EKG, and TTE[b] every 2 years Cardiac CT[d] or MRI[c] every 36-60 months Exercise test every 2 years
Stage C[e]	Clinic visit every 6-12 months EKG and TTE every 12 months Exercise test[a] every 2 years	Clinic visits every 6-12 months EKG and TTE[b] every 12 months Cardiac CT[d] or MRI[c] every 36-60 months Exercise test[a] every 2 years	Clinic visit every 6-12 months EKG and TTE every year Exercise test every[a] 2 years	Clinic visit every 6-12 months EKG and TTE[b] every year Cardiac CT[d] or MRI[c] every 1-2 years Exercise test every 2 years
Stage D[e]	Clinic visit every 3-6 months EKG, TTE, and exercise test[a] every 12 months	Clinic visits every 3-6 months EKG and TTE[b] every 12 months Cardiac CT[d] or MRI[c] every 36-60 months Exercise test[a] every 12 months	Clinic visit every 3-6 months EKG, TTE, and exercise test[a] every year	Clinic visit every 3-6 months EKG and TTE[b] every year Cardiac CT[d] or MRI[c] every 1-2 years Exercise test every year
Other	Stress testing for adults with left ventricular outflow tract obstruction to determine exercise capacity, symptoms, EKG changes, or arrhythmias may be reasonable in the presence of otherwise equivocal indications for intervention	Aortic imaging using TTE[b], TEE, cardiac MRI[c], or CTA[d] is recommended in adults with Williams syndrome or patients suspected of having supravalvular aortic stenosis	NA	Initial and follow-up aortic imaging using cardiac MRI[c] or CTA[d] is recommended Resting blood pressure should be measured in the upper and lower extremities Ambulatory blood pressure monitoring can be useful for the diagnosis and management of hypertension Screening for intracranial aneurysms by magnetic resonance angiography or CTA may be reasonable Exercise testing to evaluate for exercise-induced hypertension may be reasonable

CT, computed tomography; CTA, computed tomographic angiography; EKG, electrocardiogram; MRI, magnetic resonance imaging; NA, not applicable; TEE, transesophageal echocardiogram; TTE, transthoracic echocardiogram.

[a] Exercise test is 6-minute walk test or cardiopulmonary exercise test (CPET), depending on the clinical indication.

[b] Routine TTE may be unnecessary in a year when cardiac magnetic resonance imaging (CMR) is performed unless clinical indications warrant otherwise.

[c] CMR may be indicated for assessment of aortic anatomy. Baseline study is recommended with periodic follow-up CMR, with frequency of repeat imaging determined by anatomic and physiologic findings.

[d] If CCT cardiac CT is used instead of CMR imaging, the frequency should be weighed against radiation exposure. See Physiologic Stage listing below.

[e] Physiologic Stage A includes New York Heart Association (NYHA) functional class (FC) I symptoms, no hemodynamic or anatomic sequelae, no arrhythmias, normal exercise capacity, normal renal/hepatic/pulmonary function. Stage B includes NYHA FC II symptoms, mild hemodynamic sequelae (mild aortic enlargement, mild ventricular enlargement, mild ventricular dysfunction), mild valvular disease, trivial or small shunt (not hemodynamically significant), arrhythmia not requiring treatment, abnormal objective cardiac limitation to exercise. Stage C includes NYHA FC III symptoms, significant (moderate or greater) valvular disease; moderate or greater ventricular dysfunction (systemic, pulmonic, or both), moderate aortic enlargement, venous or arterial stenosis, mild or moderate hypoxemia/cyanosis, hemodynamically significant shunt, arrhythmias controlled with treatment, pulmonary hypertension (less than severe), end-organ dysfunction responsive to therapy. Stage D includes NYHA FC IV symptoms, severe aortic enlargement, arrhythmias refractory to treatment, severe hypoxemia (almost always associated with cyanosis), severe pulmonary hypertension, Eisenmenger syndrome, refractory end-organ dysfunction.

Data from Stout KK, Daniels CJ, Aboulhosn JA, et al. 2018 AHA/ACC Guideline for the Management of Adults With Congenital Heart Disease: Executive Summary: A Report of the American College of Cardiology/American Heart Association Task Force on Clinical Practice Guidelines. *J Am Coll Cardiol.* 2019;73(12):1494-1563.

RESEARCH AND FUTURE DIRECTIONS

The genetic contribution to congenital heart disease is an active area of research and may help to predict severity and inheritance patterns. Left-sided obstructive lesions appear to have a strong familial component, and additional studies will further elucidate this complex spectrum of disease.

KEY POINTS

- ✔ Patients with aortic stenosis presenting with angina or syncope require emergent evaluation as they are at risk for sudden death owing to ischemia and arrhythmia.
- ✔ Young patients with refractory hypertension deserve a thorough physical examination to evaluate for CoA.
- ✔ Patients with BAV should be screened for CoA and vice versa.
- ✔ Exercise testing can be helpful in risk-stratifying patients with left-sided obstructive lesions who have severe stenosis but are asymptomatic.
- ✔ Supravalvular aortic stenosis is rare, but when it is present poses a risk for coronary involvement, warranting additional coronary imaging.
- ✔ Subvalvular aortic stenosis is an acquired condition that should be evaluated in patients with risk factors such as abnormal left ventricular outflow tract anatomy.

REFERENCES

1. McBride KL, Marengo L, Canfield M, Langlois P, Fixler D, Belmont JW. Epidemiology of noncomplex left ventricular outflow tract obstruction malformations (aortic valve stenosis, coarctation of the aorta, hypoplastic left heart syndrome) in Texas, 1999-2001. *Birth Defects Res A Clin Mol Teratol.* 2005;73(8):555-561.
2. Pierpont ME, Brueckner M, Chung WK, et al. Genetic basis for congenital heart disease: revisited: a scientific statement from the American Heart Association. *Circulation.* 2018;138(21):e653-e711.
3. Loffredo CA, Chokkalingam A, Sill AM, et al. Prevalence of congenital cardiovascular malformations among relatives of infants with hypoplastic left heart, coarctation of the aorta, and d-transposition of the great arteries. *Am J Med Genet A.* 2004;124A(3):225-230.
4. Aboulhosn J, Child JS. Left ventricular outflow obstruction: subaortic stenosis, bicuspid aortic valve, supravalvar aortic stenosis, and coarctation of the aorta. *Circulation.* 2006;114(22):2412-2422.
5. Michelena HI, Khanna AD, Mahoney D, et al. Incidence of aortic complications in patients with bicuspid aortic valves. *JAMA.* 2011;306(10):1104-1112.
6. Braunwald E, Goldblatt A, Aygen MM, Rockoff SD, Morrow AG. Congenital aortic stenosis. I. Clinical and hemodynamic findings in 100 patients. II. Surgical treatment and the results of operation. *Circulation.* 1963;27:426-462.
7. Stout KK, Daniels CJ, Aboulhosn JA, et al. AHA/ACC guideline for the management of adults with congenital heart disease: executive summary: a report of the American College of Cardiology/American Heart Association Task Force on clinical practice guidelines. *J Am Coll Cardiol.* 2019;73:1494-1563.
8. Newfeld EA, Muster AJ, Paul MH, Idriss FS, Riker WL. Discrete subvalvular aortic stenosis in childhood. Study of 51 patients. *Am J Cardiol.* 1976;38(1):53-61.
9. Vogt J, Dische R, Rupprath G, de Vivie ER, Kotthoff S, Kececioglu D. Fixed subaortic stenosis: an acquired secondary obstruction? A twenty-seven year experience with 168 patients. *Thorac Cardiovasc Surg.* 1989;37(4):199-206.
10. Ewart AK, Morris CA, Ensing GJ, et al. A human vascular disorder, supravalvular aortic stenosis, maps to chromosome 7. *Proc Natl Acad Sci U S A.* 1993;90(8):3226-3230.
11. Williams JC, Barratt-Boyes BG, Lowe JB. Supravalvular aortic stenosis. *Circulation.* 1961;24:1311-1318.
12. Nickerson E, Greenberg F, Keating MT, McCaskill C, Shaffer LG. Deletions of the elastin gene at 7q11.23 occur in approximately 90% of patients with Williams syndrome. *Am J Hum Genet.* 1995;56(5):1156-1161.
13. Wong SC, Burgess T, Cheung M, Zacharin M. The prevalence of turner syndrome in girls presenting with coarctation of the aorta. *J Pediatr.* 2014;164(2):259-263.
14. Collins-Nakai RL, Rosenthal A, Castaneda AR, Bernhard WF, Nadas AS. Congenital mitral stenosis. A review of 20 years' experience. *Circulation.* 1977;56(6):1039-1047.
15. Shone JD, Sellers RD, Anderson RC, Adams P, Lillehei CW, Edwards JE. The developmental complex of "parachute mitral valve," supravalvular ring of left atrium, subaortic stenosis, and coarctation of aorta. *Am J Cardiol.* 1963;11:714-725.
16. Sabet HY, Edwards WD, Tazelaar HD, Daly RC. Congenitally bicuspid aortic valves: a surgical pathology study of 542 cases (1991 through 1996) and a literature review of 2,715 additional cases. *Mayo Clin Proc.* 1999;74(1):14-26.
17. Rajamannan NM, Subramaniam M, Rickard D, et al. Human aortic valve calcification is associated with an osteoblast phenotype. *Circulation.* 2003;107(17):2181-2184.
18. Wolfe RR, Driscoll DJ, Gersony WM, et al. Arrhythmias in patients with valvar aortic stenosis, valvar pulmonary stenosis, and ventricular septal defect. Results of 24-hour ECG monitoring. *Circulation.* 1993;87(2 suppl):I89-I101.
19. Ferrans VJ, Muna WF, Jones M, Roberts WC. Ultrastructure of the fibrous ring in patient with discrete subaortic stenosis. *Lab Invest.* 1978;39(1):30-40.
20. Cape EG, Vanauker MD, Sigfússon G, Tacy TA, del Nido PJ. Potential role of mechanical stress in the etiology of pediatric heart disease: septal shear stress in subaortic stenosis. *J Am Coll Cardiol.* 1997;30(1):247-254.
21. Oliver JM, Gonzβlez A, Gallego P, Sβnchez-Recalde A, Benito F, Mesa JM. Discrete subaortic stenosis in adults: increased prevalence and slow rate of progression of the obstruction and aortic regurgitation. *J Am Coll Cardiol.* 2001;38(3):835-842.
22. Wright GB, Keane JF, Nadas AS, Bernhard WF, Castaneda AR. Fixed subaortic stenosis in the young: medical and surgical course in 83 patients. *Am J Cardiol.* 1983;52(7):830-835.
23. Vincent WR, Buckberg GD, Hoffman JI. Left ventricular subendocardial ischemia in severe valvar and supravalvar aortic stenosis. A common mechanism. *Circulation.* 1974;49(2):326-333.
24. Abu-Sultaneh S, Gondim MJ, Alexy RD, Mastropietro CW. Sudden cardiac death associated with cardiac catheterization in Williams syndrome: a case report and review of literature. *Cardiol Young.* 2019:1-5.
25. Russell GA, Berry PJ, Watterson K, Dhasmana JP, Wisheart JD. Patterns of ductal tissue in coarctation of the aorta in the first three months of life. *J Thorac Cardiovasc Surg.* 1991;102(4):596-601.
26. Rudolph AM, Heymann MA, Spitznas U. Hemodynamic considerations in the development of narrowing of the aorta. *Am J Cardiol.* 1972;30(5):514-525.
27. Alpert BS, Bain HH, Balfe JW, Kidd BS, Olley PM. Role of the renin-angiotensin-aldosterone system in hypertensive children with coarctation of the aorta. *Am J Cardiol.* 1979;43(4):828-834.
28. de Divitiis M, Pilla C, Kattenhorn M, et al. Vascular dysfunction after repair of coarctation of the aorta: impact of early surgery. *Circulation.* 2001;104(12 suppl 1):I165-I170.
29. Connolly HM, Huston J, Brown RD, Warnes CA, Ammash NM, Tajik AJ. Intracranial aneurysms in patients with coarctation of the aorta: a prospective magnetic resonance angiographic study of 100 patients. *Mayo Clin Proc.* 2003;78(12):1491-1499.

30. Taniguchi T, Morimoto T, Shiomi H, et al. Sudden death in patients with severe aortic stenosis: observations from the current as registry. *J Am Heart Assoc.* 2018;7(11): e008397.
31. Wagner HR, Weidman WH, Ellison RC, Miettinen OS. Indirect assessment of severity in aortic stenosis. *Circulation.* 1977;56(1 suppl):I20-I23.
32. Otto CM, Burwash IG, Legget ME, et al. Prospective study of asymptomatic valvular aortic stenosis. Clinical, echocardiographic, and exercise predictors of outcome. *Circulation.* 1997;95(9):2262-2270.
33. Jenkins NP, Ward C. Coarctation of the aorta: natural history and outcome after surgical treatment. *QJM.* 1999;92(7):365-371.
34. Pickard SS, Gauvreau K, Gurvitz M, et al. Stroke in adults with coarctation of the aorta: a National Population-Based Study. *J Am Heart Assoc.* 2018;7(11):e009072.
35. Singh PK, Marzo A, Staicu C, et al. The effects of aortic coarctation on cerebral hemodynamics and its importance in the etiopathogenesis of intracranial aneurysms. *J Vasc Interv Neurol.* 2010;3(1):17-30.
36. Rodrigues JCL, Jaring MFR, Werndle MC, et al. Repaired coarctation of the aorta, persistent arterial hypertension and the selfish brain. *J Cardiovasc Magn Reson.* 2019;21(1):68.
37. Nishimura RA, Otto CM, Bonow RO, et al. AHA/ACC guideline for the management of patients with valvular heart disease: a report of the American College of Cardiology/American Heart Association Task Force on practice guidelines. *J Thorac Cardiovasc Surg.* 2014;148(1):e1-e132.
38. Parolari A, Tremoli E, Cavallotti L, et al. Do statins improve outcomes and delay the progression of non-rheumatic calcific aortic stenosis? *Heart.* 2011;97(7):523-529.
39. Hager A, Kanz S, Kaemmerer H, Schreiber C, Hess J. Coarctation Long-term Assessment (COALA): significance of arterial hypertension in a cohort of 404 patients up to 27 years after surgical repair of isolated coarctation of the aorta, even in the absence of restenosis and prosthetic material. *J Thorac Cardiovasc Surg.* 2007;134(3):738-745.
40. Canniffe C, Ou P, Walsh K, Bonnet D, Celermajer D. Hypertension after repair of aortic coarctation—a systematic review. *Int J Cardiol.* 2013;167(6):2456-2461.
41. Arora S, Strassle PD, Ramm CJ, et al. Transcatheter versus surgical aortic valve replacement in patients with lower surgical risk scores: a systematic review and meta-analysis of early outcomes. *Heart Lung Circ.* 2017;26(8):840-845.
42. Fleisher LA, Fleischmann KE, Auerbach AD, et al. ACC/AHA guideline on perioperative cardiovascular evaluation and management of patients undergoing noncardiac surgery: a report of the American College of Cardiology/American Heart Association Task Force on practice guidelines. *J Am Coll Cardiol.* 2014;64(22):e77-e137.
43. Garg A, Rao SV, Visveswaran G, et al. Transcatheter aortic valve replacement versus surgical valve replacement in low-intermediate surgical risk patients: a systematic review and meta-analysis. *J Invasive Cardiol.* 2017;29(6):209-216.
44. Qureshi AM, McElhinney DB, Lock JE, Landzberg MJ, Lang P, Marshall AC. Acute and intermediate outcomes, and evaluation of injury to the aortic wall, as based on 15 years experience of implanting stents to treat aortic coarctation. *Cardiol Young.* 2007;17(3):307-318.
45. Taggart NW, Minahan M, Cabalka AK, et al. Immediate outcomes of covered stent placement for treatment or prevention of aortic wall injury associated with coarctation of the aorta (COAST II). *JACC Cardiovasc Interv.* 2016;9(5):484-493.
46. Parry AJ, Kovalchin JP, Suda K, et al. Resection of subaortic stenosis; can a more aggressive approach be justified? *Eur J Cardiothorac Surg.* 1999;15(5):631-638.
47. Hazekamp MG, Kappetein AP, Schoof PH, et al. Brom's three-patch technique for repair of supravalvular aortic stenosis. *J Thorac Cardiovasc Surg.* 1999;118(2):252-258.
48. Tam DY, Vo TX, Wijeysundera HC, et al. Transcatheter vs surgical aortic valve replacement for aortic stenosis in low-intermediate risk patients: a meta-analysis. *Can J Cardiol.* 2017;33(9):1171-1179.
49. Yoon SH, Bleiziffer S, De Backer O, et al. Outcomes in transcatheter aortic valve replacement for Bicuspid versus Tricuspid aortic valve stenosis. *J Am Coll Cardiol.* 2017;69(21):2579-2589.
50. Anderson BR, Tingo JE, Glickstein JS, Chai PJ, Bacha EA, Torres AJ. When is it better to wait? Surgical timing and recurrence risk for children undergoing repair of subaortic stenosis. *Pediatr Cardiol.* 2017;38(6):1106-1114.

CHAPTER 108

RIGHT-SIDED LESIONS

Margaret M. Fuchs, C. Charles Jain, and Heidi M. Connolly

INTRODUCTION

The normal right ventricle (RV) has three components: the inlet (including tricuspid valve, chordae tendineae, and papillary muscles), the trabeculated apical portion, and the infundibulum or outflow tract. Under typical conditions, the right heart receives the systemic venous return and pumps to the low-impedance pulmonary vascular bed.[1] In the absence of a shunt lesion, the RV has identical output to the left ventricle but pumps at one-sixth of the left ventricular pressure. Right-sided congenital heart disease involving the tricuspid valve, RV outflow tract, or RV chamber itself can disrupt the normal hemodynamics. Valve regurgitation leads to volume overload and compensatory right heart chamber dilation. Obstruction of flow through the outflow tract results in high RV pressure and compensatory hypertrophy of the myocardium. Because of ventricular interdependence (related to the shared interventricular septum and constraining pericardium, among other factors), pressure or volume overload of the RV can impact the function and morphology of the left ventricle.[1]

Obstruction of blood flow out of the RV can occur proximal to the pulmonic valve, at the pulmonic valve, or distal to the pulmonic valve. These lesions may occur in isolation or in combination. It is important to identify the location and nature of the obstruction, which in some cases may require multiple imaging modalities.[2] After percutaneous or surgical relief of pulmonary valve obstruction, pulmonary regurgitation (PR) is the most common complication and requires close surveillance for adverse impact on the RV.

DOUBLE-CHAMBERED RIGHT VENTRICLE

A double-chambered right ventricle (DCRV) is defined as obstruction of blood flow at or within the sub-infundibular ventricle. It consists of a high-pressure proximal chamber and a low-pressure distal chamber.

DCRV is a rare congenital anomaly seen in approximately 0.5% to 2.0% of all congenital heart disease cases.[3] Some cases of DCRV may be secondary, related to compensatory muscular hypertrophy from a pressure-loading lesion, and therefore the true incidence of primary DCRV (muscular hypertrophy with no clear other cause) may be lower.[4] To date, there is no genetic mutation that has been associated with DCRV.

PATHOGENESIS AND ASSOCIATED DEFECTS

The obstruction in DCRV can be due to thickened trabeculations, anomalous muscle tissue, or an aberrant and hypertrophied moderator band (ie, septomarginal trabeculation).[3] Fibromuscular thickening of the infundibulum alone is often referred to as subvalvular pulmonic stenosis (PS). This may be a form of DCRV or secondary to pressure overload of the RV, as described earlier. DCRV is commonly associated with other congenital heart defects. Isolated DCRV is almost always associated with a membranous ventricular septal defect, often small. In addition, DCRV is associated with tetralogy of Fallot, Ebstein anomaly, and double outlet RV.[5]

CLINICAL PRESENTATION

Adults with DCRV can present with dyspnea, syncope, angina, and exertional intolerance. On examination, a holosystolic murmur is present along the lower left sternal border. Given the RV hypertrophy, an RV heave may be appreciable as well as a thrill.

Differential Diagnosis: Other causes of intraventricular obstruction to blood flow include muscle hypertrophy at the infundibulum, which can occur in PS as well as hypertrophic cardiomyopathy.

DIAGNOSIS

Identifying the level of obstruction in right-sided obstructive lesions can be challenging by physical examination.[2] The electrocardiogram (ECG) may reveal RV hypertrophy. Transthoracic echocardiography typically demonstrates obstructive muscle bands that are thickest and most identifiable during systole and are best seen on subcostal or parasternal short-axis imaging. However, DCRV can easily be missed by transthoracic echocardiography, with one series reporting a diagnostic sensitivity of only 15.6%.[5] Transesophageal echocardiography, cardiac magnetic resonance imaging (MRI), and cardiac catheterization with ventriculography (**Figure 108.1**) can be very helpful as well, particularly for nondiagnostic transthoracic echocardiography cases.[6,7]

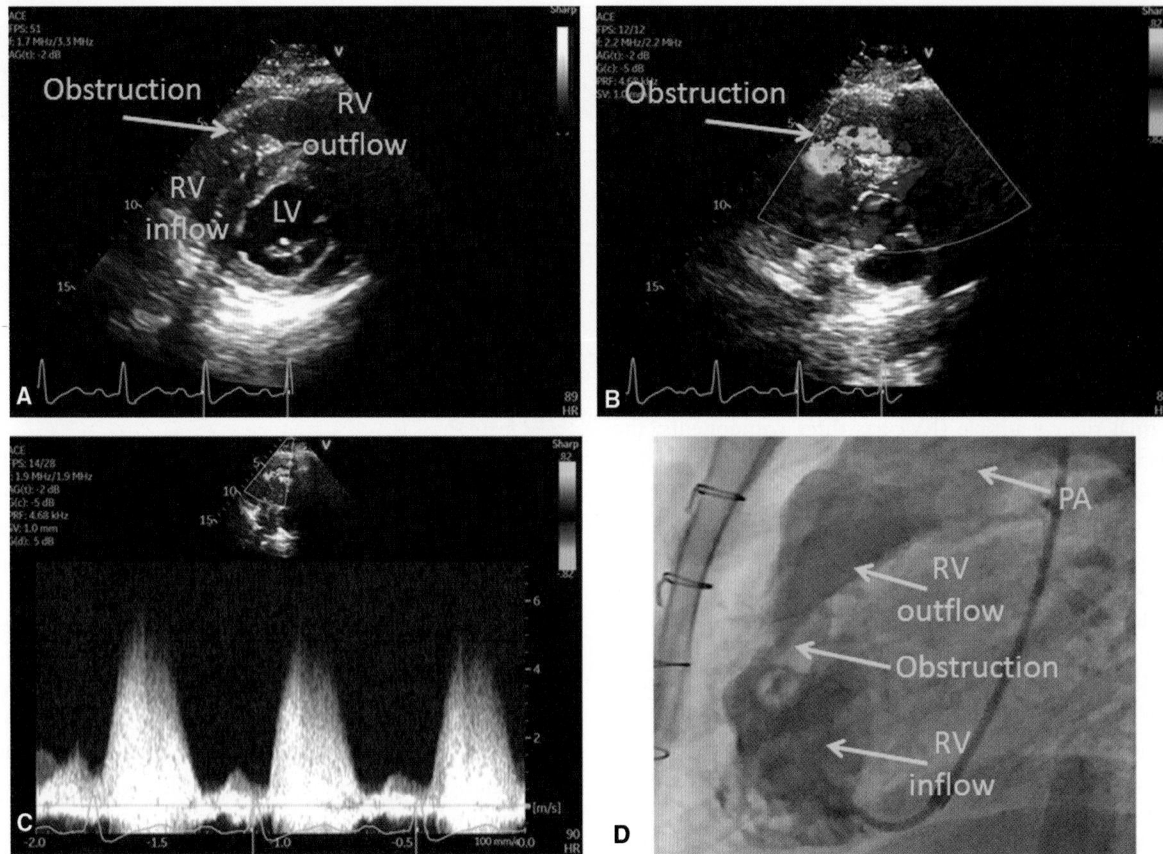

FIGURE 108.1 **(A,B)** Imaging in double-chambered right ventricle. Panels **(A and B)** Two-dimensional (panel **A**) and color Doppler transthoracic echocardiography (panel **B**) showing typical findings of right ventricular (RV) obstruction in a double-chamber RV (parasternal short-axis view). **(C)** Continuous-wave Doppler through that region of narrowing demonstrates severe RV obstruction with a maximal instantaneous pressure gradient >64 mm Hg. **(D)** Analogous findings to panel **(A)** can be seen on a lateral view during RV angiography (systolic frame) in the same patient. LV, left ventricle; PA, pulmonary artery.

MANAGEMENT: DOUBLE-CHAMBERED RIGHT VENTRICLE

Indications for intervention on DCRV include (a) moderate or greater obstruction (defined as peak velocity >3 m/s by Doppler echocardiography) with symptoms of heart failure, (b) exercise intolerance, or (c) severe asymptomatic obstruction (peak velocity >4 m/s by Doppler echocardiography).[8] Medical therapy has not been demonstrated to be beneficial. Although balloon valvotomy has been reported, its efficacy in most patients is yet to be established.[9] Surgical repair typically involves a transatrial or transventricular approach. Postoperatively, clinicians must be wary of conduction system disease, particularly right bundle branch block as the right bundle branch runs in the septomarginal trabecula and moderator band. Surgical resection by an experienced congenital surgeon tends to be definitive with excellent long-term results.[10,11]

VALVULAR PULMONARY STENOSIS

Valvular PS is a common congenital anomaly. Mild-to-moderate cases may be diagnosed for the first time in adulthood when a murmur is auscultated. Additionally, severe PS treated during childhood has excellent long-term survival, and therefore many adult patients born with PS now require long-term follow-up.[12,13] Three types of valvular PS occur: dome-type, dysplastic, and unicuspid/bicuspid pulmonic valves (**Table 108.1**).

Valvular PS makes up almost 90% of congenital RV outflow tract abnormalities.[14] The dome-type valve is the most common type of congenital pulmonic valve abnormality. Although there is no identified genetic abnormality, there does appear to be a chance of inheritance (<5%). Pulmonary valve dysplasia is commonly associated with Noonan syndrome and chromosome 12 mutation, with an autosomal dominant inheritance with variable penetrance.[15] Unicuspid, bicuspid, or quadricuspid pulmonic valves are rare, and bicuspid valves may be associated with tetralogy of Fallot. Any of the valve morphologies may also have associated pulmonic regurgitation, though stenosis is more typical.

CLINICAL PRESENTATION: VALVULAR PULMONARY STENOSIS

Ongoing pressure overload to the RV can cause hypertrophy and fibrosis, which may cause right-sided diastolic and

TABLE 108.1 Types of Pulmonary Valve Stenosis

Appearance	Morphology	Pulmonary Artery Dilation	Associated Abnormalities
Dome type	Narrow, "fish mouth"-like opening without proper raphe or commissures. Has preserved leaflet motion. Does not tend to have significant calcification.	Common, particularly of the main and left pulmonary artery	None
Dysplastic	Exuberantly thickened leaflets with limited mobility	Possible, though more commonly associated with hypoplastic pulmonary annulus and proximal pulmonary trunk	Genetic syndromes, particularly Noonan
Unicuspid or bicuspid	May be thickened with reduced mobility	Uncommon/unknown	Tetralogy of Fallot, transposition of the great arteries

eventually systolic dysfunction. Thus, patients with PS can present with right-sided heart failure or exertional symptoms (eg, dyspnea, syncope, chest pain) related to inadequate pulmonary blood flow with exertion and possibly RV ischemia. Examination findings depend on the severity of the stenosis. In severe disease, a prominent "A" wave in the jugular venous pulse is common. An RV heave is commonly present on cardiac palpation. Heart sounds are notable for an ejection click that decreases in intensity with inspiration and as PS progresses, and may no longer be audible as it moves closer to S1. Wide splitting of S2 will reflect the prolonged pulmonic ejection time. A right-sided S4 is expected in those with a prominent "A" wave in the jugular venous pressure. The systolic ejection murmur peak moves later in systole as severity progresses. Cyanosis can be observed when significant PS occurs in the setting of atrial septal defect or patent foramen ovale, related to high right atrial pressure and right-to-left atrial shunting.

Differential Diagnosis: Other causes of RV outflow tract obstruction should be considered.

DIAGNOSIS: VALVULAR PULMONARY STENOSIS

ECG in advanced disease (RV systolic pressure >60 mm Hg) will demonstrate RV hypertrophy, right atrial enlargement, and right axis deviation. Chest x-ray often reveals findings of preferential flow into the left pulmonary artery (PA) including increased vascular fullness in the left lung and dilation of main and left PAs (often referred to as "witch's nose," **Figure 108.2**). These findings are more common in dome-type valvular PS compared to valve dysplasia.

When PS is identified, it is critical to assess the severity of obstruction; this is typically done by Doppler echocardiography. PS is considered mild when the peak gradient is <36 mm Hg, moderate with peak gradient 36 to 64 mm Hg, and severe with peak gradient >64 mm Hg or mean gradient >35 mm Hg in the setting of normal RV function. In addition to quantifying the degree of stenosis, assessment of the degree of regurgitation (if present) is necessary, as this has therapeutic implications (see below).

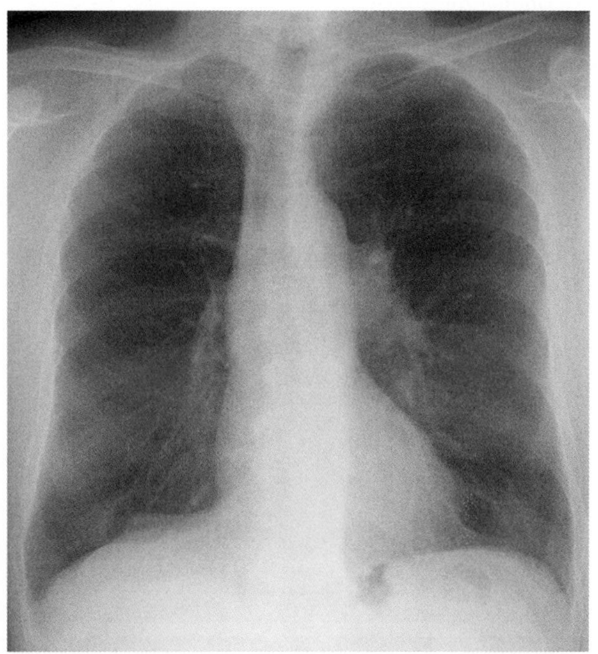

FIGURE 108.2 Chest x-ray in pulmonic stenosis. Chest radiography highlighting multiple features seen in patients with congenital pulmonic stenosis. There is evidence of right atrial and right ventricular enlargement. In addition, the main and left pulmonary arteries are enlarged. Note the absence of an enlarged left atrium or left ventricle, as well as relatively radiolucent lung fields.

Echocardiography

Transthoracic echocardiography is usually sufficient to define the morphology and severity of PS. Doppler echocardiography has been demonstrated to have good correlation with invasive hemodynamic assessment for the majority of patients.[16,17] In addition to assessing the pulmonary valve itself, PA dilation is often present and should be described. The RV peak systolic pressure can be estimated with continuous-wave Doppler of the tricuspid regurgitation jet. The PR jet (using the end-PR velocity) is used to estimate PA diastolic pressure. Patients with elevated RV systolic pressure often exhibit systolic ventricular septal flattening and RV hypertrophy (**Figure 108.3A-D**). Because isolated PS is a pressure-loading lesion, the ventricle does not tend to dilate, and, therefore, functional tricuspid regurgitation is not expected. Transesophageal echocardiography does not offer clear advantages over transthoracic echocardiography for evaluation of the pulmonic valve in most patients.

Cross-Sectional Imaging

Cardiac computed tomography (CT) and MRI are typically not required in the evaluation of PS, but can be used to clarify valve morphology if transthoracic echocardiographic imaging is limited. Cardiac CT angiography is commonly used to assess the coronary artery anatomy prior to planned surgical or transcatheter intervention. This is particularly important if transcatheter pulmonary valve-in-valve replacement is planned, as compression can occur if a coronary artery lies too close to the valve landing zone.

Catheterization

In patients with very severe PS and/or significant PR, echocardiographic Doppler evaluation may be less accurate than catheterization.[17] In these cases, invasive hemodynamic assessment with right heart catheterization can be beneficial to assess the RV pressure, degree of PS, and any branch PA stenosis. Angiography at the time of right heart catheterization can be used to assess RV size, function, and PA anatomy.

MANAGEMENT: VALVULAR PULMONARY STENOSIS

Medical Therapy and Surveillance

Patients with mild PS do not tend to have progression of valve disease. For these patients, follow-up every 3 to 5 years with examination, ECG, echocardiogram, and selective exercise testing is reasonable.[8] Moderate PS has a variable course, with some patients exhibiting progression and some patients demonstrating stable valve gradients over time. Follow-up every 1 to 2 years with the same cardiac testing is appropriate. Patients with severe PS should be considered for transcatheter or surgical intervention, as described next.

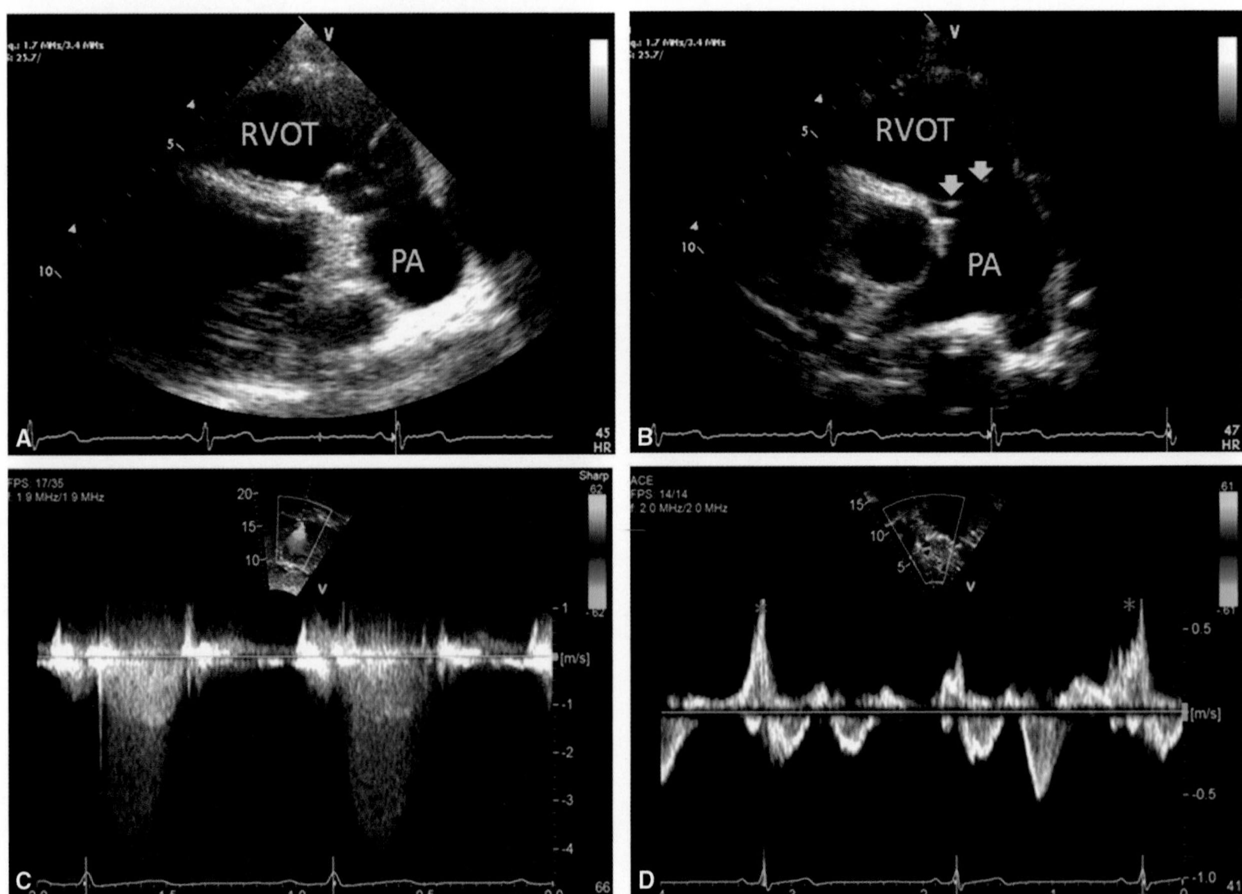

FIGURE 108.3 Transthoracic echocardiographic findings in pulmonic stenosis. **(A)** Modified parasternal short-axis view in a patient with dome-type pulmonic stenosis demonstrates mild cusp thickening. **(B)** Note the typical doming (arrows) of the cusps in this systolic frame from the same patient. **(C)** Continuous-wave Doppler through the pulmonic valve demonstrates findings consistent with moderate-severe pulmonic valve stenosis with a peak velocity of nearly 4 m/s, suggesting a peak gradient ≥60 mm Hg. **(D)** Hepatic vein pulsed-wave Doppler consistent with a noncompliant RV as suggested by a large atrial reversal (red asterisk). PA, pulmonary artery; RVOT, right ventricular outflow tract.

Percutaneous or Surgical Intervention

Since the 1980s, the treatment of choice for isolated PS has been percutaneous balloon valvuloplasty. Symptomatic patients with moderate or severe PS should be referred for percutaneous balloon valvuloplasty.[8] Other indications for balloon valvuloplasty are cyanosis related to atrial-level shunt and severe PS in the asymptomatic patient.[8] Patients who should be considered for primary surgical intervention include those with greater than moderate PR, a hypoplastic pulmonary annulus, subvalvular PS, or supravalvular PS. Traditionally, dysplastic pulmonic valves do not respond as well to percutaneous intervention as the more common dome-shaped pulmonary valves, but balloon valvuloplasty may still be appropriate as first-line therapy in select patients. Surgical intervention is recommended for those patients in whom balloon valvuloplasty failed to resolve symptoms/obstruction or for those who need other interventions such as tricuspid valve repair, surgical therapies for atrial arrhythmias, shunt closure, or left-sided interventions. Surgical management of PS can involve balloon valvuloplasty, valvotomy, or pulmonic valve replacement.[8]

SPECIAL CONSIDERATIONS: PREGNANCY

In patients who are pregnant, isolated PS tends to be well tolerated, even if severe. The mother tends to do very well, though the neonates tend to have higher rates of premature delivery and perinatal mortality (4.1%).[18] Percutaneous balloon valvuloplasty during pregnancy can reduce neonatal risk.

SUPRAVALVULAR PULMONARY STENOSIS

Supravalvular PS involves narrowing of the main or branch PA. It can occur in isolation, in association with RV outflow tract stenosis, or in the setting of a genetic abnormality associated with multiple other cardiac defects. In those with prior surgery, it can also occur at sites of prior interventions (eg, PA banding; Blalock-Thomas-Taussig, Potts, or Waterston shunts; or Jatene arterial switch/post-Lecompte maneuver).[19] Native peripheral PA stenosis occurs infrequently in congenital heart disease, and the incidence of postsurgical peripheral PA stenosis is not well defined.[20]

PATHOGENESIS AND ASSOCIATED DEFECTS

Native isolated peripheral PA stenosis is commonly seen either at the main PA bifurcation or in the left PA at the site of the closed ductus arteriosus. Postsurgical peripheral PA stenosis occurs as a complication of scarring at takedown sites of prior palliative shunts or surgical corrective procedures.

Isolated peripheral PA stenosis is frequently associated with ventricular septal defect. There are multiple genetic syndromes associated with peripheral PA stenosis including Alagille syndrome, Keutel syndrome, Williams syndrome, LEOPARD syndrome, Noonan syndrome, and congenital rubella. Peripheral PA stenosis can also occur in the setting of tetralogy of Fallot.

CLINICAL PRESENTATION: SUPRAVALVULAR PULMONARY STENOSIS

Patients with peripheral PA stenosis present similarly to valvular PS with dyspnea on exertion, right-sided heart failure, and exertional light-headedness. Examination may demonstrate a systolic or even continuous murmur. There will also be evidence of RV hypertension on examination, similar to findings in valvular PS.

DIAGNOSIS: SUPRAVALVULAR PULMONARY STENOSIS

ECG has no specific findings other than RV hypertrophy. Chest x-ray may show a relatively small vascular pedicle as well as increased lucency in the lung fields if the stenosis is unilateral. Transthoracic echocardiography may raise suspicion for increased pressures in the main PA, though two-dimensional (2D) visualization of the PAs can be challenging, especially in adult patients. Parasternal imaging with color flow and continuous-wave Doppler is the most helpful for identifying peripheral PA stenosis on echocardiography. Cross-sectional imaging with CT or MRI is generally required in the evaluation of peripheral PA stenosis.[21] In addition, direct measurement of pressure gradients in the catheterization lab can be very helpful to simultaneously assess the severity of stenosis and identify its precise location with pulmonary angiography (**Figure 108.4**).

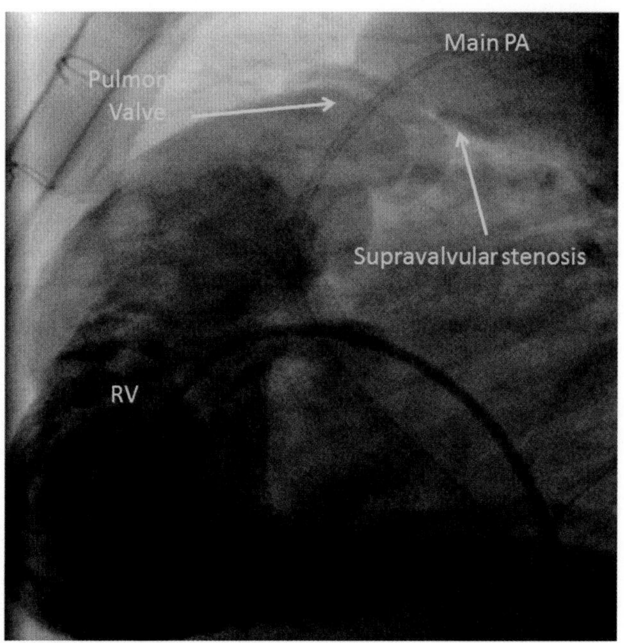

FIGURE 108.4 Right ventricular angiography in supravalvular pulmonic stenosis. Lateral view from right ventricular (RV) angiography in a 50-year-old male with tetralogy of Fallot status post repair. He had a bicuspid pulmonic valve with severe stenosis along with severe supravalvular stenosis of the main pulmonary artery (PA) just distal to the pulmonic valve.

MANAGEMENT: SUPRAVALVULAR PULMONARY STENOSIS

Intervention of peripheral PA stenosis is warranted for any symptomatic patient, those with decreased pulmonary blood flow, or those with significantly elevated RV pressures on echocardiography or catheterization. Those patients with PA stenoses that are not significant should continue to be monitored every 3 to 5 years with interval cross-sectional imaging in addition to ECG, chest x-ray, transthoracic echocardiography, and exercise testing. In a patient with severe obstruction, percutaneous peripheral intervention is the first step. Percutaneous balloon angioplasty, sometimes with stent placement, is commonly performed for branch PA stenosis. After percutaneous intervention, patients require close follow-up; up to a quarter will require repeat intervention for recurrent stenosis.[8]

PULMONARY ATRESIA WITH INTACT VENTRICULAR SEPTUM

Pulmonary atresia with intact ventricular septum is characterized by complete obstruction of flow through the RV outflow tract, often with RV and tricuspid valve hypoplasia.

Pulmonary atresia with intact ventricular septum is rare, estimated to occur in 4 to 5 per 100,000 live births,[22] and has no known genetic or gender association.[23]

PATHOGENESIS

Pulmonary atresia with intact ventricular septum is primarily defined by complete obstruction of flow through the RV outflow tract. Membranous atresia, related to atretic pulmonary valve and small annulus, occurs in 75% of cases, whereas the remaining 25% have muscular atresia, or obliteration of the muscular infundibulum.[22]

Right Ventricle

RV hypoplasia is present in the majority of cases, though there are a wide variety of RV morphologies possible.[24] Most commonly, all three portions of the normal RV are present with relative hypoplasia of each. About one-third of cases are characterized by overgrowth of the trabecular RV (termed a "bipartite" ventricle with only inlet and infundibulum) and a minority of cases are "unipartite" with muscular obliteration of the trabecular and infundibular portions.[22] At the other end of the spectrum, significant RV dilation can occur, in one series representing 4% of cases, and is usually associated with severe tricuspid regurgitation.[22]

Tricuspid Valve

RV hypoplasia is generally associated with a small tricuspid annulus and dysplastic tricuspid valve with abnormal papillary muscles and chordal attachments.[24] RV dilation is typically associated with tricuspid regurgitation. Ebstein-like malformation of the tricuspid valve has been estimated to occur in approximately 10% of cases.[22]

Coronary Arteries

Abnormalities of the coronary circulation are common in pulmonary atresia with intact ventricular septum and can contribute to morbidity and mortality in some patients.[23] Suprasystemic RV pressure pushes blood from the RV into vascular channels, consisting of intertrabecular spaces with thick, fibroelastic walls.[24] In some cases, these channels form major fistulous connections and communicate with the epicardial coronary circulation.[23] In the most severe form, epicardial coronary blood flow is at least partially dependent on flow from the RV to the coronary, termed "RV-dependent coronary circulation."[25] Stenosis or atresia of the proximal coronary artery is occasionally observed in these patients and, when present, leads to chronically deoxygenated coronary blood supply from the RV, in some cases contributing to long-term biventricular dysfunction.[25,26] Additionally, surgical RV decompression in a patient with RV-dependent coronary circulation can result in peri- or postoperative myocardial infarction because of abrupt decrease in coronary perfusion.[25]

PATHOPHYSIOLOGY

Given complete obstruction of flow through the RV outflow tract, and the lack of a ventricular septal defect, the only means of blood emptying from the right heart is across an atrial septal defect or patent foramen ovale. In some patients, there is also a lesser degree of connection to the systemic circulation via RV channels into the coronary arteries. After birth, a child with pulmonary atresia and intact ventricular septum is dependent on the ductus arteriosus to provide pulmonary blood flow until surgical management can be undertaken.

CLINICAL PRESENTATION: PULMONARY ATRESIA WITH INTACT VENTRICULAR SEPTUM

Pulmonary atresia with intact ventricular septum most commonly presents either during fetal life on routine fetal ultrasound or shortly after birth. Neonates will present with cyanosis and can have rapid clinical deterioration if the ductus arteriosus closes, eliminating all pulmonary blood flow. Patients surviving to adulthood with pulmonary atresia with intact ventricular septum have invariably undergone surgical palliation to establish pulmonary blood flow.

Common Signs and Symptoms

Adult patients frequently report reduced exercise capacity, particularly those with RV hypoplasia and a biventricular repair.[27] Additional signs and symptoms include cyanosis, heart failure, and rhythm disturbance, depending on the type of surgical palliation performed. Atrial arrhythmias occur in up to 80% of adult survivors of pulmonary atresia with intact ventricular septum.[28]

Differential Diagnosis: Pulmonary atresia with intact ventricular septum should be distinguished from other forms of RV outflow tract obstruction, including pulmonary atresia with ventricular septal defect, PS, tetralogy of Fallot, and tricuspid atresia.

DIAGNOSIS: PULMONARY ATRESIA WITH INTACT VENTRICULAR SEPTUM

The diagnosis of pulmonary atresia with intact ventricular septum is made by echocardiography, either prenatally with the use of fetal echocardiography or postnatally in the first few days after birth. At diagnosis, echocardiographic evaluation should include assessment of RV size, tricuspid annular dimension, presence of atrial septal defect, degree of atrial-level shunt, and presence of coronary anomaly (focusing on proximal coronary artery origins and any continuous flow, suggesting connection to the RV). Calculation of the tricuspid valve Z score (number of standard deviations from the normal population mean, indexed to body surface area) and assessment of the degree of RV hypoplasia are important metrics in determining the optimal surgical repair,[23] with implications for management in early infancy as well as long-term adult sequelae. After repair, features that distinguish pulmonary atresia with intact ventricular septum from other right-sided congenital cardiac disorders include the intact septum, tricuspid valve dysplasia, and a high prevalence of restrictive RV filling.

MANAGEMENT: PULMONARY ATRESIA WITH INTACT VENTRICULAR SEPTUM

Initial Surgical Palliation

The initial surgical management of infants with pulmonary atresia with intact ventricular septum depends on the anatomic features, as detailed earlier. Infants with relatively normal RV size (defined as tricuspid valve Z score > -2.5 and a tripartite RV) are candidates for biventricular repair, typically with RV outflow tract reconstruction. Those with moderate RV hypoplasia (bipartite ventricle, tricuspid valve Z score -2.5 to 4.5) are frequently managed with a one and half (1.5) ventricle repair, involving bidirectional cavopulmonary anastomosis (ie, closing any atrial communications, enlarging the RV outflow tract, and diversion of the superior vena caval blood to the PAs so that the small RV is tasked with pumping only the venous return from the inferior vena cava and not the entire cardiac output). Those with the most severe RV hypoplasia, with unipartite ventricles and Z score < -4.5, are managed with single ventricle palliation (Fontan vs surgical shunt) or transplant.[29]

Medical Therapy and Surveillance

Survivors of pulmonary atresia with intact ventricular septum require lifelong follow-up in a center with expertise in caring for patients with complex congenital heart disease. These patients commonly require reintervention and management of atrial arrhythmias.[8] Clinical follow-up is recommended annually, with concurrent ECG, echocardiogram, and cross-sectional imaging in select cases. Consideration should be given to annual ambulatory ECG monitoring to screen for rhythm disturbances.

Echocardiographic assessment of these patients should focus on anticipated sequelae of the individual's surgical palliation. In patients with biventricular repair, assessment of biventricular function is important, as well as detection of valve or conduit lesions of hemodynamic significance. Restrictive RV physiology, identified in some cases by diastolic forward flow through the pulmonary valve, is frequently observed in patients with biventricular repair and has been associated with greater myocardial fibrosis on cardiac MRI.[30] In patients with an RV-PA conduit, cardiac CT and MRI can also provide complementary information about conduit patency and PA anatomy. When there is concern about conduit function, cardiac catheterization is indicated to obtain direct measurement of RV and PA pressures.[8] Patients with single ventricle or surgical shunt palliation have a number of unique imaging considerations that are further discussed elsewhere in the text.

Atrial arrhythmias are common in patients with palliated pulmonary atresia with intact ventricular septum. In one series, atrial arrhythmias occurred in 80% of adult patients with all types of surgical palliation, including 75% of patients with biventricular repair.[28] Because of the high incidence of atrial arrhythmias, it has been suggested that all adult patients with pulmonary atresia with intact ventricular septum be considered for therapeutic anticoagulation therapy, unless contraindicated.[28] Ventricular arrhythmias occurred in 15% of patients in the same series (25% of biventricular repair patients).[28] Implantable cardioverter defibrillator (ICD) therapy is indicated for survivors of cardiac arrest, patients with sustained ventricular tachycardia, or patients with left ventricular ejection fraction $\leq 35\%$ with class II or III heart failure; there are no definitive guidelines for the use of primary prevention ICD in this population, and clinical judgment should be exercised.[31]

Surgical Reintervention

Surgical reintervention is anticipated in nearly all patients with palliated pulmonary atresia with intact ventricular septum. The management of patients with Fontan palliation and surgical shunts is reviewed elsewhere in the textbook. Patients with biventricular repair commonly require RV-PA conduit replacement, replacement of the tricuspid and/or pulmonary valves, and RV outflow tract reconstruction. PR is very common but compensatory RV dilation is often absent, related to restrictive RV physiology.[28] The timing of reintervention for severe PR should therefore be based on the patient's symptoms of exercise intolerance or heart failure. Reintervention on an RV-PA conduit is indicated when the patient demonstrates severe symptomatic obstruction or asymptomatic obstruction with reduced exercise capacity, or with progressive RV dilation or dysfunction.[8] The onset of a new cardiac arrhythmia should prompt careful evaluation of valve and conduit function, as deteriorating hemodynamics can be the inciting factor for the development of rhythm disturbances.

Percutaneous Interventions

In select patients, transcatheter interventions can be considered, most commonly conduit stenting and percutaneous pulmonary valve replacement. Transcatheter therapies have high procedural success with low mortality rate and are a good management option in patients with anatomy amenable to percutaneous intervention. Prior to percutaneous conduit therapy, coronary artery compression testing should be performed, as coronary compression has been observed in 5% to 6% of patients having conduit balloon angioplasty or stenting.[8]

SPECIAL CONSIDERATIONS—PREGNANCY IN PULMONARY ATRESIA WITH INTACT VENTRICULAR SEPTUM

Pregnancy outcomes in patients with biventricular repair of pulmonary atresia with intact ventricular septum have been evaluated in one small case series of five pregnancies. Minor cardiac arrhythmias were observed during two pregnancies and did not require medical intervention.[32] Two pregnancies were complicated by progressive PR, ultimately requiring valve replacement in the postpartum period.[32] Patients with severe PS or PR are at risk for developing heart failure or arrhythmias and should be followed regularly for these complications during pregnancy. Because of the complexity of the congenital cardiac defect, all patients with repaired or palliated pulmonary atresia with intact ventricular septum should be seen at a multidisciplinary care center before and during pregnancy, and the frequency of follow-up should be individualized.[33] Symptomatic right heart failure during pregnancy can be managed with diuretics and bed rest. Severe, symptomatic PS may warrant balloon valvuloplasty during pregnancy.[33]

EBSTEIN ANOMALY

Ebstein anomaly is a rare form of congenital heart disease involving primarily the tricuspid valve and RV. It has a wide spectrum of anatomic involvement and clinical presentation.

Ebstein anomaly is estimated to occur at a rate of 0.17 to 0.72 per 10,000 live births and has no correlation with gender or race.[34,35] An association with maternal age and multiple gestation pregnancy has been observed in some epidemiologic series, but not in others.[34-36] Antenatal exposure to lithium has historically been believed to be a cause of Ebstein anomaly[37]; however, the impact of lithium exposure has more recently been challenged.[38] A possible genetic link to left ventricular noncompaction has been identified in some patients, with observed mutations in genes encoding sarcomere proteins, including MYH7 and alpha-tropomyosin.[39,40] Most cases of Ebstein anomaly, however, are without identifiable genetic explanation.

PATHOGENESIS

Ebstein anomaly is primarily characterized by abnormalities of both the tricuspid valve and the RV. There is a wide spectrum of tricuspid valve anatomic derangements possible, and attention to valve morphology is critical to optimally plan surgical intervention and patient management.

Tricuspid Valve

The tricuspid valve leaflets in Ebstein anomaly demonstrate varying degrees of failure of delamination, or failure to separate from the underlying myocardium, leaving them adherent/tethered to the RV.[41] The septal and posterior leaflets are most severely affected, sometimes with very little functional tissue present.[41] The anterior leaflet is typically large and sail-like or tethered by fibrous tissue with direct insertion to a papillary muscle or the myocardium, thereby limiting mobility.[41,42] Fenestrations are often present in the anterior leaflet, contributing to tricuspid regurgitation.[43] The annular attachment of the septal and posterior leaflets is displaced apically and the functional tricuspid valve orifice is thereby shifted anteroapically toward the RV outflow tract.[41,42] In most cases, there is severe tricuspid regurgitation related to inability of the abnormal tricuspid leaflets to effectively coapt.[41] Rarely, excessive attachment of the anterior leaflet directly to the myocardium results in tricuspid stenosis or even an imperforate tricuspid valve.[42]

Right Ventricle

Displacement of the tricuspid valve results in two portions of the RV. The inlet RV, located between the anatomic (nondisplaced) tricuspid annulus and the functional RV, is referred to as the "atrialized" RV.[42] This portion tends to become very dilated and often dyskinetic, with pathologic specimens revealing fibrosis and sometimes absence of muscular tissue.[41,42] The functional RV is small and sometimes contains only the RV outflow tract.[41] Though it retains contractile function it is inherently myopathic and tends to become enlarged with declining function over time.[44] In the setting of severe RV enlargement, the ventricular septum can be pushed leftward with abnormal septal motion, which may contribute to impairment of left ventricular function.[41]

Associated Defects

The most common associated congenital anomaly is an atrial septal defect, both secundum type and patent foramen ovale, occurring in more than 80% of patients.[45] Ventricular septal defects and PS are also observed.[45] Left heart disease of some form occurs in up to 40% of patients,[46] including left ventricular noncompaction, abnormalities of left ventricular systolic or diastolic function, and left-sided valve disease.[46] Accessory conduction pathways occur in 5% to 25% of patients with Ebstein anomaly,[47] and Wolff-Parkinson-White syndrome is more commonly associated with Ebstein anomaly than any other form of congenital heart disease.[48]

CLINICAL PRESENTATION: EBSTEIN ANOMALY

Adults with a new diagnosis of Ebstein anomaly commonly present with palpitations.[49] Some adult patients report symptoms of right heart failure, including dyspnea, fatigue, and lower extremity edema.[41] Exercise intolerance can occur because of reduced RV function and severe tricuspid regurgitation resulting in low cardiac output, or related to exercise-induced cyanosis from right-to-left shunting across the atrial septum. Paradoxical embolism through an atrial septal defect or patent foramen ovale can also occur, especially in the setting of severe tricuspid regurgitation, and present as stroke or transient ischemic attack, brain abscess, or myocardial infarction.[50]

On physical examination, the jugular venous pulse is typically normal despite the presence of severe tricuspid regurgitation, related to the very large right atrium and atrialized RV accommodating tricuspid regurgitation without raising right atrial pressure.[51] Additionally, despite significant RV enlargement, the parasternal impulse of the RV is typically quite subtle.[51] By auscultation, the first heart sound is usually split with delayed tricuspid valve closure (T1). T1 is typically loud, related to increased tension in the anterior leaflet as it reaches its fully closed position; this is often referred to as the "sail sound."[52,53] If the anterior leaflet is very mobile, there can be multiple closure sounds with associated systolic ejection clicks.[41] The second heart sound is widely split because of right bundle branch block. The holosystolic murmur of tricuspid regurgitation is often very soft or absent in adults because of rapid equalization of pressure across the tricuspid valve.

Differential Diagnosis

Congenital tricuspid dysplasia results in abnormally formed leaflets and tricuspid valve dysfunction, but lacks the apical displacement, leaflet tethering, and myopathy of Ebstein anomaly. Tricuspid valve prolapse, tricuspid valve vegetations, and carcinoid heart disease can result in severe tricuspid regurgitation but will similarly not demonstrate the other features described earlier. Other forms of RV myopathy, including arrhythmogenic RV cardiomyopathy and Uhl anomaly, will have a morphologically normal tricuspid valve with regurgitation only if annular dilation has developed.

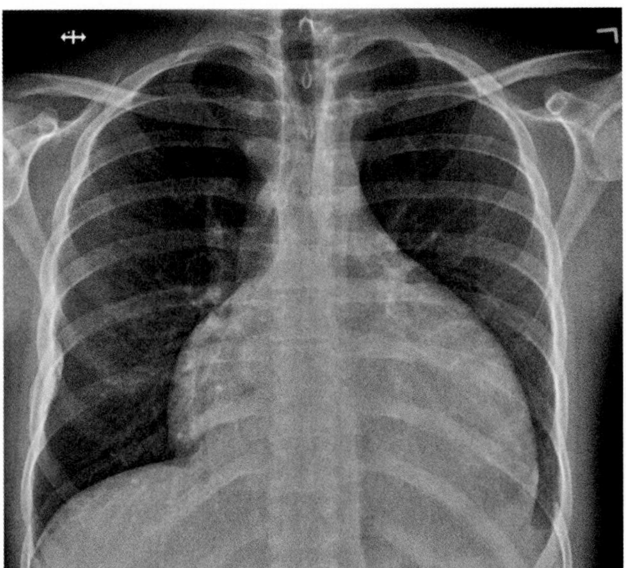

FIGURE 108.5 Chest x-ray of a 19-year-old male with Ebstein anomaly demonstrating marked cardiomegaly with clear lung fields and subtle aortic shadow.

DIAGNOSIS: EBSTEIN ANOMALY

The diagnosis of Ebstein anomaly should be suspected in a patient with typical signs and symptoms, as detailed earlier. The chest x-ray may demonstrate marked cardiomegaly and narrow vascular pedicle[51,53] (**Figure 108.5**). The ECG often reveals right atrial enlargement (so-called "Himalayan P waves"[51]), right bundle branch block, PR segment prolongation, and low-voltage QRS in the right-sided chest leads. Supraventricular tachycardia and atrial arrhythmias are common. When suspected, the diagnosis of Ebstein anomaly requires demonstration of apical displacement of the tricuspid septal leaflet. Calculation of the "displacement index" involves measuring the distance between the anterior mitral and septal tricuspid hinge points, which is then indexed to body surface area (**Figure 108.6**). A displacement index >8 mm/m^2 has been demonstrated to be a sensitive predictor of Ebstein anomaly.[54] Apical displacement is most commonly identified by echocardiogram using the apical four-chamber view, but can also be assessed using cardiac MRI and CT.

Echocardiography

Transthoracic echocardiography is the test of choice for the evaluation of a patient with suspected Ebstein anomaly. Echocardiography can confirm the diagnosis, assess the severity of disease, and identify other associated anomalies. Leaflet morphology should be assessed in detail. Leaflet tethering, defined as three or more attachments to the ventricular wall that impede leaflet motion, is expected and usually affects the septal and posterior leaflets more than the anterior leaflet.[44,55] Multiple

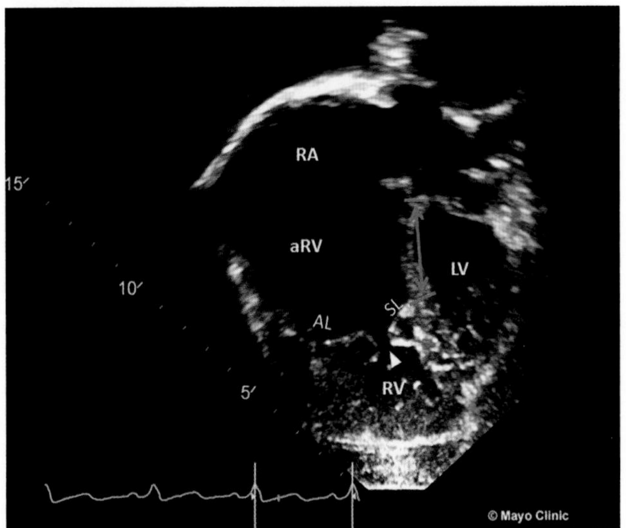

FIGURE 108.6 Transthoracic echocardiographic images from a patient with Ebstein anomaly. Apical four-chamber view (apex down format) in systole showing severe right heart enlargement, apical displacement of the tricuspid septal leaflet (SL) (red arrow), tethering of the tricuspid anterior leaflet (AL), and coaptation defect (arrowhead). aRV, atrialized right ventricle; LV, left ventricle; RA, right atrium; RV, right ventricle.

imaging windows are typically required to completely assess the valve anatomy. The anterior and septal leaflets are often best viewed in the apical four-chamber view (**Figure 108.6**), whereas the posterior leaflet may be better assessed using a parasternal RV inflow view or short-axis view.[44] Multiple jets of tricuspid regurgitation are expected related to malcoaptation and leaflet fenestration. Traditional methods of quantification are of limited utility because of multiple, complex jets of regurgitation.[53] Optimal evaluation, therefore, involves comprehensive 2D assessment of valve structure, color Doppler interrogation of visualized coaptation defects, and semi-quantitative grading of all regurgitant jets.[44]

The size and function of the RV should be assessed with echocardiography. The myopathic atrialized RV typically appears dilated, thin, and dysfunctional.[44] Qualitative visual assessment of the ventricular size (relative to the left ventricle) and function is generally employed. Associated anomalies, including atrial septal defect and patent foramen ovale, should be sought by echocardiography. If imaging is suboptimal, agitated saline can be used to detect the presence of a right-to-left atrial-level shunt.[56]

Cardiac Magnetic Resonance Imaging and Computed Tomography

The data obtained from cardiac MRI in patients with Ebstein anomaly are complementary to the echocardiographic assessment, and both modalities are often appropriate to evaluate these patients. Cardiac MRI can more easily quantify right heart size and function and, in some patients, can better demonstrate the posterior tricuspid leaflet.[57] Echocardiography remains the test of choice, however, to evaluate the degree of tricuspid regurgitation and to identify other associated cardiac anomalies.[44] For patients who cannot undergo MRI, cardiac CT can be utilized to assess ventricular volumes and ejection fraction.[44] It is also useful for the preoperative assessment of the coronary arteries.

MANAGEMENT: EBSTEIN ANOMALY

Patient management involves monitoring over time as well as consideration of surgical intervention and arrhythmia treatment, depending on the individual patient's course.

Medical Therapy and Surveillance

Adult patients with Ebstein anomaly should be seen in an adult congenital heart disease clinic, with assessment for possible symptomatic tricuspid regurgitation, right heart failure, cyanosis, and arrhythmia. Testing should include pulse oximetry, ECG, echocardiogram, and exercise test. Patients with moderate or greater functional limitation should have annual Holter or another prolonged rhythm monitor for surveillance of atrial and ventricular arrhythmias. It may be appropriate for patients with no or mild cardiac symptoms to be tested every 2 to 3 years. Exercise testing can provide an objective measure of functional capacity[8] and is especially helpful in adult patients with no reported symptoms. Exercise-induced desaturation may be demonstrated in the presence of a right-to-left shunt and can be a cause of exertional limitation. Cardiac MRI may be helpful every 1 to 2 years in patients with functional impairment, and every 3 to 5 years in patients with no or mild symptoms.[8]

Medical therapy does not have a prominent role in the management of patients with Ebstein anomaly; those patients with symptoms should be referred for surgical intervention. Despite the high prevalence of RV dysfunction and not-infrequent associated left ventricular dysfunction, there are no studies to date supporting the use of traditional heart failure medications in Ebstein anomaly.[58] Diuretics can be used to manage heart failure with volume overload prior to surgery, or if the patient is not a surgical candidate. Pharmacologic management of rhythm disturbances can be considered.

Patients with a history of unexplained syncope, documented supraventricular tachycardia (excluding atrial fibrillation), sustained ventricular tachycardia, or ventricular preexcitation should be seen by an electrophysiologist with experience with congenital heart disease and may benefit from an electrophysiologic study to assess for the presence of accessory pathway or atrial arrhythmias.[31] Pathway ablation, if required, is ideally performed prior to tricuspid valve surgery. The preoperative identification of atrial fibrillation or flutter allows for operative planning of surgical atrial ablation. Sudden death has increasingly been recognized as a threat to this patient population, with risk factors including prior ventricular tachycardia, heart failure, syncope, and PS.[59] Some patients should be considered for primary prevention ICD implantation.

Surgical Management: Ebstein Anomaly

Surgery is recommended for adults with Ebstein anomaly who have significant tricuspid regurgitation as well as one of the following: worsening exercise capacity, right heart failure symptoms, and progressive RV dysfunction. Surgery can also be considered in the setting of progressive RV enlargement, cyanosis from right-to-left shunt, paradoxical embolism, and atrial arrhythmia.[8] Tricuspid valve repair is the goal of operative intervention where possible.[43] Repair is optimally performed using the "cone reconstruction," which involves mobilizing the septal and posterior leaflet tissue as well as the anterior leaflet, creating a 360° cone that is reattached at the true annulus.[43,60] If present, atrial septal defect or patent foramen ovale should be closed at the time of operative intervention to address the risk of paradoxical embolism. If repair is not possible because of severe anatomic derangement of the tricuspid valve or patient comorbidities, tricuspid valve replacement should be performed. Bioprosthetic valves have demonstrated good durability in this patient population and are favored over mechanical prosthesis, with similar operation-free survival and better 20-year survival.[61,62] In the setting of severe RV dilation and dysfunction, a 1.5 ventricle repair with creation of a bidirectional cavopulmonary shunt can be considered to "offload" the RV. Although uncommon in Ebstein anomaly, pulmonary hypertension should be excluded with hemodynamic catheterization prior to cavopulmonary shunt creation, especially in patients in whom left ventricular diastolic dysfunction is suspected.[43]

Percutaneous Interventions: Ebstein Anomaly

In most cases, an atrial septal defect or patent foramen ovale should be addressed surgically at the time of tricuspid valve intervention. Uncommonly, a patient with Ebstein anomaly will have only mild tricuspid regurgitation but prominent right-to-left shunting across the atrial septum at rest or with exercise. In this case, percutaneous device closure of the atrial septal defect or patent foramen ovale can be considered. Studies have demonstrated that this is feasible and safe, and that most patients have improvement in exertional capacity.[63,64] In the setting of significant RV dysfunction, careful hemodynamic assessment with balloon test occlusion is required to ensure that shunt closure will be tolerated.[63]

In patients who have tricuspid bioprosthesis dysfunction, percutaneous valve-in-valve implantation can be considered in place of surgical valve replacement. An international multicenter registry of 81 Ebstein patients undergoing valve-in-valve replacement (either Sapien or Melody valve) demonstrated successful deployment in all patients with no procedural mortality.[65] Notably, there was a 5% rate of both acute valve thrombosis and endocarditis (most common in Melody valves, with eight patients requiring reintervention [percutaneous or surgical] to address valve dysfunction). There was no statistically significant difference between either type of valve implanted or anticoagulation strategy for those patients who developed valve dysfunction compared to those who did not. The long-term outcomes in this cohort of patients are not yet known.

SPECIAL CONSIDERATIONS—PREGNANCY IN EBSTEIN ANOMALY

Pregnancy is generally well tolerated in Ebstein anomaly. The inability to augment cardiac output in the setting of RV systolic dysfunction and tricuspid regurgitation predisposes patients with Ebstein anomaly to right heart failure, especially in the third trimester of pregnancy.[33] Arrhythmias can occur, driven by the underlying predisposition as well as hemodynamic and hormonal changes.[66] In patients with atrial-level shunt, cyanosis can occur or worsen and contribute to symptomatic limitation as well as fetal growth restriction.[33] Paradoxical embolism is a concern given enhanced hypercoagulability during pregnancy and reduced mobility during pregnancy or after delivery. Preterm delivery is more common compared to the general population, and maternal cyanosis is known to contribute to low fetal birth weight and mortality.[18,67] There is an increased risk of congenital heart disease in the fetus when the mother has Ebstein anomaly, observed to be 4% to 6% depending on the series.[18,68] Fetal echocardiogram is recommended around 20 weeks of pregnancy.[8]

FOLLOW-UP PATIENT CARE

There is significant heterogeneity in the clinical course of patients with right-sided congenital cardiac lesions. For example, patients with mild pulmonary valve stenosis may never require intervention. Long-term survival for patients with prior intervention for pulmonary valve stenosis is excellent; however, recurrent stenosis can occur and severe pulmonic regurgitation is common.[69] Pulmonary valve replacement is indicated for symptomatic patients and in select asymptomatic patients with marked RV dilation or dysfunction.[8]

Supravalvular PS can recur, particularly when the PAs are affected. Patients with pulmonary atresia with intact ventricular septum are subject to restrictive right heart physiology and often require recurrent interventions for both pulmonary and tricuspid valve disease.

Lifelong follow-up is indicated for patients with unrepaired or repaired Ebstein anomaly given the high lifetime likelihood of arrhythmias and right heart failure. Reintervention or advanced heart rhythm or heart failure therapies are often needed in patients with repaired Ebstein anomaly because the RV rarely returns to normal even with successful intervention, thus close follow-up is required to assess for changes over time.

RESEARCH AND FUTURE DIRECTIONS

There are many unknown issues in the care of patients with right-sided congenital heart disease, some of which include:

- Assessment of RV physiology and response to hemodynamic insults is actively being investigated by multiple modalities; this may impact our management of patients with right-sided congenital cardiac lesions.
- The optimal management of patients with DCRV, including ideal timing of intervention, particularly for the asymptomatic patient has yet to be established.
- The natural history of PA/intact ventricular septum reaching adulthood is still poorly understood and the optimal timing and type of interventions is unknown.
- The ideal timing of intervention in patients with asymptomatic severe tricuspid regurgitation related to Ebstein anomaly is unknown. Percutaneous valve intervention options are being performed more commonly and potentially altering the course of disease as patients may have longer intervals between reoperations.
- Cardiac surgery can be performed at a much lower risk than in prior decades, and this all amounts to potentially longer life expectancy for patients with right-sided lesions.

KEY POINTS

- ✔ The right heart is responsible for transporting systemic venous return to the low-impedance pulmonary vascular bed.
- ✔ Right-sided congenital heart disease can disrupt normal flow to the PAs, leading to right heart dilation and/or hypertrophy.
- ✔ Multiple right-sided lesions may occur together, and clinicians must consider the summative effects on the RV.
- ✔ Comprehensive assessment of the right heart with multiple imaging modalities is frequently required.
- ✔ Surgical or percutaneous intervention should be considered in symptomatic patients or in the setting of progressive RV dilation or dysfunction.

REFERENCES

1. Haddad F, Hunt SA, Rosenthal DN, Murphy DJ. Right ventricular function in cardiovascular disease, part I: anatomy, physiology, aging, and functional assessment of the right ventricle. *Circulation.* 2008;117(11):1436-1448.
2. Kirklin JW, Connolly DC, Ellis FH Jr, Burchell HB, Edwards JE, Wood EH. Problems in the diagnosis and surgical treatment of pulmonic stenosis with intact ventricular septum. *Circulation.* 1953;8(6):849-863.
3. Loukas M, Housman B, Blaak C, Kralovic S, Tubbs RS, Anderson RH. Double-chambered right ventricle: a review. *Cardiovasc Pathol.* 2013;22(6):417-423.
4. Maron BJ, Ferrans VJ, White RI Jr. Unusual evolution of acquired infundibular stenosis in patients with ventricular septal defect. Clinical and morphologic observations. *Circulation.* 1973;48(5):1092-1103.
5. Hoffman P, Wojcik AW, Rozanski J, et al. The role of echocardiography in diagnosing double chambered right ventricle in adults. *Heart.* 2004;90(7):789-793.
6. Singh NK, Karn JP, Gupt A, Senthil S. Double chambered right ventricle with ventricular septal defect presenting in adulthood. *J Assoc Physicians India.* 2011;59:451-453.
7. Miranda WR, Egbe A, Hagler DJ, Connolly HM. Double-chambered right ventricle in adults: Invasive and noninvasive hemodynamic considerations. *Int J Cardiol Congenital Heart Disease.* 2021;3:100115.
8. Stout KK, Daniels CJ, Aboulhosn JA, et al. 2018 AHA/ACC Guideline for the management of adults with congenital heart disease: a report of the American College of Cardiology/American Heart Association Task Force on Clinical Practice Guidelines. *J Am Coll Cardiol.* 2019;73(12):e81-e192.
9. Cil E, Saraclar M, Ozkutlu S, et al. Double-chambered right ventricle: experience with 52 cases. *Int J Cardiol.* 1995;50(1):19-29.
10. Baumstark A, Fellows KE, Rosenthal A. Combined double chambered right ventricle and discrete subaortic stenosis. *Circulation.* 1978;57(2):299-303.
11. Telagh R, Alexi-Meskishvili V, Hetzer R, Lange PE, Berger F, Abdul-Khaliq H. Initial clinical manifestations and mid-and long-term results after surgical repair of double-chambered right ventricle in children and adults. *Cardiol Young.* 2008;18(3):268-274.
12. Stephensen SS, Sigfusson G, Eiriksson H, et al. Congenital cardiac malformations in Iceland from 1990 through 1999. *Cardiol Young.* 2004;14(4):396-401.
13. Samanek M, Slavik Z, Zborilova B, Hrobonova V, Voriskova M, Skovranek J. Prevalence, treatment, and outcome of heart disease in live-born children: a prospective analysis of 91,823 live-born children. *Pediatr Cardiol.* 1989;10(4):205-211.
14. Garson A, Bricker JT, McNamara DG. *The Science and Practice of Pediatric Cardiology.* Lea & Febiger; 1990.
15. Bashore TM. Adult congenital heart disease: right ventricular outflow tract lesions. *Circulation.* 2007;115(14):1933-1947.
16. Lima CO, Sahn DJ, Valdes-Cruz LM, et al. Noninvasive prediction of transvalvular pressure gradient in patients with pulmonary stenosis by quantitative two-dimensional echocardiographic Doppler studies. *Circulation.* 1983;67(4):866-871.
17. Rao PS. Doppler ultrasound in the prediction of transvalvar pressure gradients in patients with valvar pulmonary stenosis. *Int J Cardiol.* 1987;15(2):195-203.
18. Drenthen W, Pieper PG, Roos-Hesselink JW, et al. Outcome of pregnancy in women with congenital heart disease: a literature review. *J Am Coll Cardiol.* 2007;49(24):2303-2311.
19. Fathallah M, Krasuski RA. Pulmonic valve disease: review of pathology and current treatment options. *Curr Cardiol Rep.* 2017;19(11):108.
20. Trivedi KR, Benson LN. Interventional strategies in the management of peripheral pulmonary artery stenosis. *J Interv Cardiol.* 2003;16(2):171-188.
21. Zucker EJ. Cross-sectional imaging of congenital pulmonary artery anomalies. *Int J Cardiovasc Imaging.* 2019;35(8):1535-1548.
22. Daubeney PEF, Delany DJ, Anderson RH, et al. Pulmonary atresia with intact ventricular septum. *J Am Coll Cardiol.* 2002;39(10):1670-1679.
23. Shinebourne EA, Rigby ML, Carvalho JS. Pulmonary atresia with intact ventricular septum: from fetus to adult: congenital heart disease. *Heart.* 2008;94(10):1350-1357.
24. Perloff JK, Marelli AJ. Pulmonary atresia with intact ventricular septum. In: Perloff JK, Marelli AJ, eds. *Perloff's Clinical Recognition of Congenital Heart Disease.* Vol Sixth Edition. Elsevier Saunders; 2012:429-438.
25. Giglia TM, Mandell VS, Connor AR, Mayer JE, Lock JE. Diagnosis and management of right ventricle-dependent coronary circulation in pulmonary atresia with intact ventricular septum. *Circulation.* 1992;86(5):1516-1528.
26. Calder AL, Co EE, Sage MD. Coronary arterial abnormalities in pulmonary atresia with intact ventricular septum. *Am J Cardiol.* 1987; 59(5):436-442.
27. Karamlou T, Poynter JA, Walters HL 3rd, et al. Long-term functional health status and exercise test variables for patients with pulmonary atresia with intact ventricular septum: a Congenital Heart Surgeons Society study. *J Thorac Cardiovasc Surg.* 2013;145(4):1018.e1013-1027.e1013.
28. John AS, Warnes CA. Clinical outcomes of adult survivors of pulmonary atresia with intact ventricular septum. *Int J Cardiol.* 2012;161(1):13-17.
29. Chikkabyrappa SM, Loomba RS, Tretter JT. Pulmonary atresia with an intact ventricular septum: preoperative physiology, imaging, and management. *Semin Cardiothorac Vasc Anesth.* 2018;22(3):245-255.
30. Liang X, Lam WWM, Cheung EWY, Wu AKP, Wong SJ, Cheung Y. Restrictive right ventricular physiology and right ventricular fibrosis as assessed by cardiac magnetic resonance and exercise capacity after biventricular repair of pulmonary atresia and intact ventricular septum. *Clin Cardiol.* 2010;33(2):104-110.
31. Khairy P, Van Hare GF, Balaji S, et al. PACES/HRS Expert Consensus Statement on the Recognition and Management of Arrhythmias in Adult Congenital Heart Disease: developed in partnership between the Pediatric and Congenital Electrophysiology Society (PACES) and the Heart Rhythm Society (HRS). Endorsed by the governing bodies of PACES, HRS, the American College of Cardiology (ACC), the American Heart Association (AHA), the European Heart Rhythm Association (EHRA), the Canadian Heart Rhythm Society (CHRS), and the International Society for Adult Congenital Heart Disease (ISACHD). *Heart Rhythm.* 2014;11(10):e102-e165.
32. Drenthen W, Pieper PG, Roos-Hesselink JW, et al. Fertility, pregnancy, and delivery after biventricular repair for pulmonary atresia with an intact ventricular septum. *Am J Cardiol.* 2006;98(2):259-261.
33. Regitz-Zagrosek V, Roos-Hesselink JW, Bauersachs J, et al. 2018 ESC Guidelines for the management of cardiovascular diseases during pregnancy. *Eur Heart J.* 2018;39(34):3165-3241.
34. Pradat P, Francannet C, Harris JA, Robert E. The epidemiology of cardiovascular defects, part I: a study based on data from three large registries of congenital malformations. *Pediatr Cardiol.* 2003;24(3):195-221.
35. Lupo PJ, Langlois PH, Mitchell LE. Epidemiology of Ebstein anomaly: prevalence and patterns in Texas, 1999-2005. *Am J Med Genet A.* 2011;155A(5):1007-1014.
36. Correa-Villasenor A, Ferencz C, Neill CA, Wilson PD, Boughman JA; Group TB-WIS. Ebstein's malformation of the tricuspid valve: genetic and environmental factors. *Teratology.* 1994;50:137-147.
37. Nora JJ, Nora AH, Toews WH. Letter: lithium, Ebstein's anomaly, and other congenital heart defects. *Lancet.* 1974;304(7880):594-595.
38. Diav-Citrin O, Shechtman S, Tahover E, et al. Pregnancy outcome following in utero exposure to lithium: a prospective, comparative, observational study. *Am J Psychiatry.* 2014;171(7):785-794.
39. van Engelen K, Postma AV, van de Meerakker JB, et al. Ebstein's anomaly may be caused by mutations in the sarcomere protein gene MYH7. *Neth Heart J.* 2013;21(3):113-117.
40. Kelle AM, Bentley SJ, Rohena LO, Cabalka AK, Olson TM. Ebstein anomaly, left ventricular non-compaction, and early onset heart failure associated with a de novo alpha-tropomyosin gene mutation. *Am J Med Genet A.* 2016;170(8):2186-2190.
41. Dearani JA, Mora BN, Nelson TJ, Haile DT, O'Leary PW. Ebstein anomaly review: what's now, what's next? *Expert Rev Cardiovasc Ther.* 2015;13(10):1101-1109.

42. Anderson KR, Zuberbuhler JR, Anderson RH, Becker AE, Lie JT. Morphologic spectrum of Ebstein's anomaly of the heart: a review. *Mayo Clin Proc.* 1979;54:174-180.
43. Holst KA, Connolly HM, Dearani JA. Ebstein's anomaly. *Methodist Debakey Cardiovasc J.* 2019;15(2):138-144.
44. Qureshi MY, O'Leary PW, Connolly HM. Cardiac imaging in Ebstein anomaly. *Trends Cardiovasc Med.* 2018;28(6):403-409.
45. Brown ML, Dearani JA, Danielson GK, et al. The outcomes of operations for 539 patients with Ebstein anomaly. *J Thorac Cardiovasc Surg.* 2008;135(5):1120-1136, 1136.e1121-1127.
46. Attenhofer Jost CH, Connolly HM, O'Leary PW, Warnes CA, Tajik AJ, Seward JB. Left heart lesions in patients with Ebstein anomaly. *Mayo Clin Proc.* 2005;80(3):361-368.
47. Hebe J. Ebstein's anomaly in adults. Arrhythmias: diagnosis and therapeutic approach. *Thorac Cardiovasc Surg.* 2000;48(4):214-219.
48. Khositseth A, Danielson GK, Dearani JA, Munger TM, Porter CJ. Supraventricular tachyarrhythmias in Ebstein anomaly: management and outcome. *J Thorac Cardiovasc Surg.* 2004;128(6):826-833.
49. Attie F, Rosas M, Rijlaarsdam M, et al. The adult patient with Ebstein anomaly: outcome in 72 unoperated patients. *Medicine.* 2000;79(1):27-36.
50. Attenhofer Jost CH, Connolly HM, Scott CG, Burkhart HM, Ammash NM, Dearani JA. Increased risk of possible paradoxical embolic events in adults with Ebstein anomaly and severe tricuspid regurgitation. *Congenit Heart Dis.* 2014;9:30-37.
51. Warnes CA, Williams RG, Bashore TM, et al. ACC/AHA 2008 Guidelines for the management of adults with congenital heart disease: a report of the American College of Cardiology/American Heart Association Task Force on Practice Guidelines (writing committee to develop guidelines on the management of adults with congenital heart disease). *Circulation.* 2008;118(23):e714-e833.
52. Crews TL, Pridie RB, Benham R, Leatham A. Auscultatory and phonocardiographic findings in Ebstein's anomaly: correlation of first heart sound with ultrasonic records of tricuspid valve movement. *Br Heart J.* 1972;34:681-687.
53. Perloff JK, Marelli AJ. Ebstein's anomaly of the tricuspid valve. In: Perloff JK, Marelli AJ, eds. *Clinical Recognition of Congenital Heart Disease.* 6th ed. Saunders; 2012:176-195.
54. Shiina A, Seward JB, Edwards WD, Hagler DJ, Tajik AJ. Two-dimensional echocardiographic spectrum of Ebstein's anomaly: detailed anatomic assessment. *J Am Coll Cardiol.* 1984;3(2):356-370.
55. Roberson DA, Silverman NH. Ebstein's anomaly: echocardiographic and clinical features in the fetus and neonate. *J Am Coll Cardiol.* 1989;14(5):1300-1307.
56. Saric M, Armour AC, Arnaout MS, et al. Guidelines for the use of echocardiography in the evaluation of a cardiac source of embolism. *J Am Soc Echocardiogr.* 2016;29(1):1-42.
57. Attenhofer Jost CH, Edmister WD, Julsrud PR, et al. Prospective comparison of echocardiography versus cardiac magnetic resonance imaging in patients with Ebstein's anomaly. *Int J Cardiovasc Imaging.* 2012;28(5):1147-1159.
58. Stout KK, Broberg CS, Book WM, et al. Chronic heart failure in congenital heart disease: a scientific statement from the American Heart Association. *Circulation.* 2016;133(8):770-801.
59. Attenhofer Jost CH, Tan NY, Hassan A, et al. Sudden death in patients with Ebstein anomaly. *Eur Heart J.* 2018;39(21):1970-1977.
60. da Silva JP, Baumgratz JF, da Fonseca L, et al. The cone reconstruction of the tricuspid valve in Ebstein's anomaly. The operation: early and midterm results. *J Thorac Cardiovasc Surg.* 2007;133(1):215-223.
61. Kiziltan HT, Theodoro DA, Warnes CA, O'Leary PW, Anderson BJ, Danielson GK. Late results of bioprosthetic tricuspid valve replacement in Ebstein's anomaly. *Ann Thorac Surg.* 1998;66:1539-1545.
62. Brown ML, Dearani JA, Danielson GK, et al. Comparison of the outcome of porcine bioprosthetic versus mechanical prosthetic replacement of the tricuspid valve in the Ebstein anomaly. *Am J Cardiol.* 2009;103(4):555-561.
63. Jategaonkar SR, Scholtz W, Horstkotte D, Kececioglu D, Haas NA. Interventional closure of atrial septal defects in adult patients with Ebstein's anomaly. *Congenit Heart Dis.* 2011;6:374-381.
64. Silva M, Teixeira A, Menezes I, et al. Percutaneous closure of atrial right-to-left shunt in patients with Ebstein's anomaly of the tricuspid valve. *EuroIntervention.* 2012;8(1):94-97.
65. Taggart NW, Cabalka AK, Eicken A, et al. Outcomes of transcatheter tricuspid valve-in-valve implantation in patients with Ebstein anomaly. *Am J Cardiol.* 2018;121(2):262-268.
66. Kounis NG, Zavras GM, Papadaki PJ, Soufras GD, Kitrou MP, Poulos EA. Pregnancy-induced increase of supraventricular arrhythmias in Wolff-Parkinson-White syndrome. *Clin Cardiol.* 1995;18(3):137-140.
67. Connolly HM, Warnes CA. Ebstein's anomaly: outcome of pregnancy. *J Am Coll Cardiol.* 1994;23(5):1194-1198.
68. Brown ML, Dearani JA, Danielson GK, et al. Functional status after operation for Ebstein anomaly: the Mayo Clinic experience. *J Am Coll Cardiol.* 2008;52(6):460-466.
69. Earing MG, Connolly HM, Dearani JA, Ammash NM, Grogan M, Warnes CA. Long-term follow-up of patients after surgical treatment for isolated pulmonary valve stenosis. *Mayo Clin Proc.* 2005;80(7):871-876.

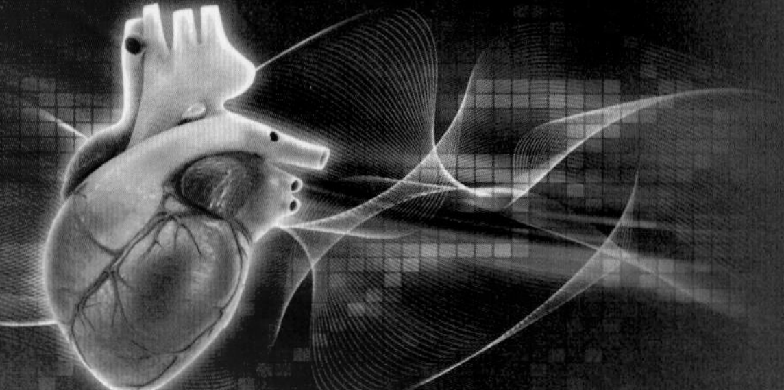

CHAPTER 109

COMPLEX LESIONS

Jeannette Lin, Prashanth Venkatesh, and Weiyi Tan

INTRODUCTION

Congenital heart defects and surgical palliations included in this chapter are considered "complex" congenital heart defects[1] and include D-transposition of the great arteries (D-TGA), congenitally corrected transposition of the great arteries (cc-TGA), hypoplastic left ventricle (LV) syndrome and the Fontan circulation, truncus arteriosus, and double outlet right ventricle (DORV). This diverse group of defects typically require complex surgical repairs and result in significant residual physiologic or anatomic abnormalities. Care of the patient with complex congenital heart disease (CHD) thus requires knowledge of the initial congenital cardiac diagnosis, as well as the surgical history and the anticipated sequelae and residual hemodynamic abnormalities. Advances in surgical and transcatheter interventions continue to modify morbidity and mortality for this patient population, and ongoing research is warranted to understand long-term survival with contemporary approaches in pediatric and adult congenital cardiac care.

D-TRANSPOSITION OF THE GREAT ARTERIES

D-TGA is a cyanotic congenital heart defect that accounts for 4% to 7% of all CHD, with a prevalence of 2.9 per 10,000 live births.[2] Because of the failure of the aorticopulmonary septum to spiral around its longitudinal axis during the first trimester in utero, the connections of the great vessels to the ventricles are discordant, with the aorta arising from the morphologic right ventricle (RV) and the pulmonary artery (PA) arising from the morphologic LV. The pulmonary and systemic circulations exist in parallel, resulting in neonatal cyanosis. Patients with this diagnosis require surgical repair to survive to adulthood. Most patients born in developed countries prior to the late 1980s to early 1990s underwent an atrial switch repair, whereas most patients born in the early 1990s or later underwent an arterial switch repair.

D-TGA AFTER ATRIAL SWITCH REPAIR

The atrial switch repair involves creation of intracardiac baffles to divert deoxygenated blood from the inferior vena cava (IVC) and superior vena cava (SVC) across the mitral valve into the subpulmonary LV, and oxygenated blood from the pulmonary veins across the tricuspid valve into the subaortic RV. This reestablishes a circulation in series and corrects cyanosis, albeit at the cost of retaining a systemic RV **(Figure 109.1)**.

CLINICAL PRESENTATION

Patients with D-TGA and atrial switch typically have normal growth and development, but have limited exercise capacity compared with their peers. Over time, chronic pressure overload of the systemic RV leads to RV systolic and diastolic dysfunction, which typically presents in the fourth to fifth decades of life as congestive heart failure. Furthermore, functional tricuspid regurgitation from RV dilation may exacerbate these symptoms.

Patients who have undergone the atrial switch are prone to arrhythmias, which affect 60% of patients by 20 years after atrial switch. Sinus node dysfunction is the most common cause of bradyarrhythmia presumably because of scarring related to the superior portion of the atrial redirection. Atrioventricular (AV) nodal dysfunction may also occur. Supraventricular tachyarrhythmias are very common, because of extensive intra-atrial scar.[2]

The intracardiac baffles may become obstructed or may develop baffle leaks. Obstruction of the SVC limb of the baffle mimics SVC syndrome with edema of the head and upper extremities. Obstruction of the IVC limb may result in hepatic congestion, abdominal bloating, early satiety, and lower extremity edema. Baffle leaks result in atrial-level shunting, typically "left-to-right" from the pulmonary venous atrium into the systemic venous atrium. As with all atrial-level shunts, this may increase the risk of paradoxical embolism. Large baffle leaks may cause volume loading of the subpulmonic LV and heart failure symptoms.

DIAGNOSTIC EVALUATION

Suspected arrhythmias should be evaluated with ambulatory electrocardiographic (ECG) monitoring. Transthoracic echocardiography (TTE) is useful to monitor valve and ventricular function and for surveillance of outflow tract obstruction, baffle leaks, or baffle stenosis. Transesophageal echocardiography (TEE) is superior to TTE for visualization of the baffles. Cardiac magnetic resonance imaging (CMRI) is an excellent tool for evaluation of RV size and function, baffle stenoses, and baffle leaks, particularly when combined with four-dimensional (4D) flow imaging. Computed tomography (CT) scans are a reasonable

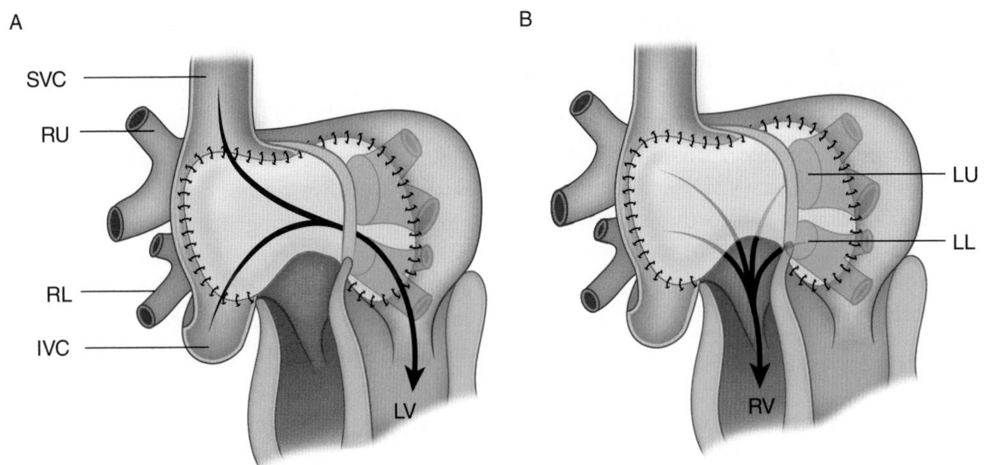

FIGURE 109.1 The atrial switch operation. **A**. A baffle directs blood from the SVC and IVC across the MV into the subpulmonary left ventricle. **B**. The pulmonary venous return is directed across the TV into the subaortic right ventricle. IVC, inferior vena cava; LL, left lower pulmonary vein; LU, left upper pulmonary vein; LV, left ventricle; RL, right lower pulmonary veins; RU, right upper pulmonary veins; RV, right ventricle; SVC, superior vena cava.

alternative to CMRI, particularly if patients have implantable devices that are not compatible with CMRI. CT scans have high spatial resolution and are useful in identifying baffle stenoses.

MANAGEMENT: D-TGA AFTER ATRIAL SWITCH REPAIR

Bradyarrhythmias necessitate permanent pacemaker in a median of 10% of patients.[2] Atrial arrhythmias after atrial switch can be malignant and predispose to sudden cardiac death.[2] An upfront rhythm control strategy, with antiarrhythmic therapy and/or catheter ablation, is hence preferred.[3]

Pharmacotherapy for systemic RV dysfunction currently lacks robust evidence and is not recommended by current guidelines,[3] though β-blockers may offer protection against appropriate implantable cardioverter-defibrillator (ICD) shocks,[4] and angiotensin-converting enzyme (ACE) inhibitors or angiotensin receptor blockers (ARBs) should be considered for patients with diabetes or hypertension.

Percutaneous baffle interventions such as angioplasty, stenting, and plugging of leaks have periprocedural success rates of 90% to 95%[5] and are preferred over surgical reoperation, where mortality can be as high as 26%.[6]

D-TGA AFTER ARTERIAL SWITCH OPERATION

The arterial switch operation involves translocation of the aorta and PA to the opposite root via supravalvar anastomoses. The coronary arteries are translocated and reimplanted along with islands of pericoronary sinus tissue ("buttons"), whereas the PA is moved anterior to the aorta via the Lecompte maneuver.[7]

In contrast to atrial switch repairs, following arterial switch operation the LV is the systemic ventricle. This confers a better long-term survival (>95%) after 25 years, making the arterial switch operation the current standard of care for D-TGA repair.[8]

CLINICAL PRESENTATION

The most common complications after arterial switch operation are supravalvar PA stenosis from anastomotic scarring or stretching of the branch PAs, and progressive dilation of the neoaorta with consequent neoaortic valvular regurgitation. Neoaortic stenosis and AV block are less common.[7,8] Ostial stenosis from the reimplanted coronary buttons may occur, and symptoms of angina, heart failure, or ventricular arrhythmias should prompt evaluation of the coronary arteries.[7]

DIAGNOSTIC EVALUATION

TTE, CMRI, and cardiac CT can define great vessel dilation/stenosis as well as ventricular and valvular function. Exercise testing, cardiac CT, and invasive angiography are useful if coronary stenosis is suspected. Baseline imaging of the coronary arteries as adult is recommended.[1]

MANAGEMENT: D-TGA AFTER ARTERIAL SWITCH OPERATION

Transcatheter balloon angioplasty and stenting is preferred over surgery for treating PA stenosis.[7,8] Severe neoaortic valvular regurgitation is usually accompanied by significant neoaortic dilation and is managed with surgical valve replacement with concomitant aortic grafting.[8] Coronary stenting and aortocoronary bypass grafting are management options for coronary artery stenosis.[3,7]

D-TGA WITH VENTRICULAR SEPTAL DEFECT AND PULMONIC STENOSIS AFTER RASTELLI OPERATION

The Rastelli operation is used as anatomic repair for D-TGA with concomitant ventricular septal defect (VSD) and pulmonary stenosis. Left ventricular outflow is baffled through the VSD into the aorta, and a valved conduit made of biologic or synthetic material directs blood from the RV to the PA, often with the proximal anastomosis on the RV free wall (**Figure 109.2**).

CLINICAL PRESENTATION

The mean life span of a RV-PA conduit in an adult is 10 to 15 years, with significant stenosis or regurgitation necessitating reoperation in 80% of patients by 20 years.[3,9] Obstruction and leak of the LV-aorta baffle can cause heart failure, whereas arrhythmias occur because of ventricular scarring from surgery. Conduit endocarditis can occur, especially in bovine xenografts.[10]

DIAGNOSTIC EVALUATION

Although TTE is valuable to evaluate biventricular function and pressures, the RV-PA conduit is often not well seen with this imaging modality. CMRI or cardiac CT is useful for conduit visualization and accurate quantification of RV size and function, which helps inform the decision to intervene on the conduit.

MANAGEMENT

Conduit degeneration is preferably managed via transcatheter pulmonary valve replacement with concomitant conduit angioplasty and stenting if indicated, though the conduit may need surgical replacement if this approach fails.[3,9] Percutaneous approaches are also preferred for baffle complications. Arrhythmias may necessitate pharmacotherapy, pacemakers, ICDs, and/or catheter ablation.

CONGENITALLY CORRECTED TRANSPOSITION OF THE GREAT ARTERIES

In cc-TGA or L-TGA, the great arteries are transposed, but there is concomitant ventricular inversion that reestablishes the two circulations in series, thus "correcting" the problem of cyanosis caused by the transposed great vessels (**Figure 109.3**). Although the circulation is physiologically normal, the RV serves as the systemic ventricle and the LV as the subpulmonary ventricle in this anatomy.

CLINICAL PRESENTATION

Patients are usually not cyanotic and are sometimes diagnosed in adulthood, either incidentally or for evaluation of a murmur or heart failure symptoms. Systemic RV failure develops

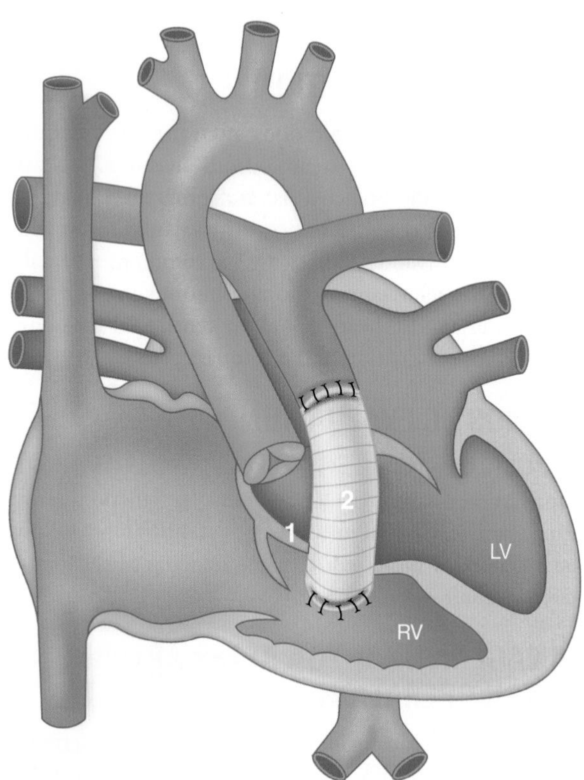

FIGURE 109.2 Rastelli operation. An interventricular tunnel directs blood from the LV to the aorta (labeled 1). The native pulmonary valve is oversewn, and a valved conduit directs flow from the RV to the pulmonary artery (labeled 2). LV, left ventricle; RV, right ventricle.

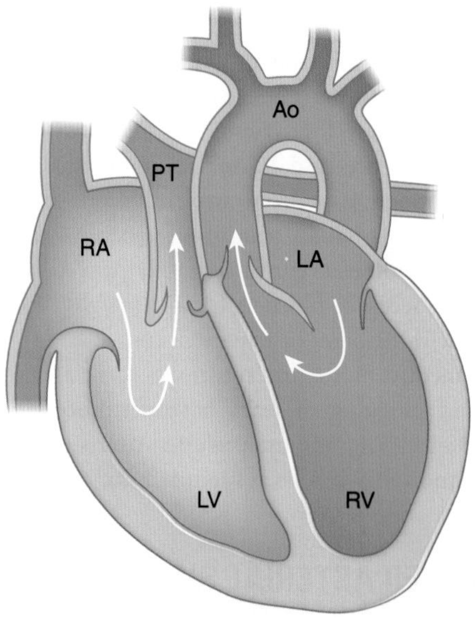

FIGURE 109.3 Congenitally corrected transposition of the great arteries. Systemic venous return to the RA flows across the mitral valve into the LV and then pulmonary artery. Pulmonary venous return flows across the tricuspid valve to the RV and Ao. Ao, aorta; LA, left atrium; LV, left ventricle; PT, pulmonary artery trunk; RA, right atrium; RV, right ventricle.

in up to 67% of patients by age 40, whereas over 50% develop significant tricuspid regurgitation because of Ebstein-like malformation of the tricuspid valve or functional tricuspid regurgitation.[11] Also, abnormal anterior displacement of the AV node confers a 2% annual risk of premature AV block,[12] which may be the presenting symptom leading to the diagnosis of cc-TGA in adulthood.

DIAGNOSTIC EVALUATION

TTE establishes the diagnosis of cc-TGA in adults and delineates ventricular and valvular function. CMRI is useful for quantification of RV (systemic ventricle) function, whereas ambulatory ECG monitors may reveal transient AV block in symptomatic patients.

MANAGEMENT: CONGENITALLY CORRECTED TRANSPOSITION OF THE GREAT ARTERIES

Common interventions in cc-TGA patients include pacemaker implantation (45% of patients with cc-TGA) and surgical tricuspid valve replacement for tricuspid regurgitation.[3,11] Valve replacement for tricuspid regurgitation has better outcomes than surgical repair, but must be done before RV (systemic ventricle) failure develops.[13] Transcatheter technologies for AV valve regurgitation may be useful in TGA patients, particularly if surgical risk is prohibitive because of systemic RV dysfunction.[14] Transplantation may be considered for severe RV systolic and/or diastolic failure refractory to medical management.

Patients with severe systemic RV dysfunction may benefit from ICD therapy for primary sudden cardiac death prevention, though current selection criteria lack robust evidence.[15] Advances in multimodality imaging for procedural planning and guidance can improve success rates of these interventions.

FONTAN CIRCULATION

PATHOGENESIS

In CHD, the goal of surgical repair is to establish a biventricular circulation whenever possible, with two circuits in series: one atrium and ventricle receives systemic venous return and pumps it forward to the pulmonary circulation, whereas a second atrium and ventricle receives pulmonary venous return and pumps it forward to the systemic circulation. In some congenital heart defects, the cardiac anatomy prohibits separation of the systemic and venous circulations. For example, in mitral atresia with a hypoplastic LV, or tricuspid or pulmonary atresia with a hypoplastic RV, the hypoplastic ventricle is too small to accommodate normal cardiac output, and attempting to partition the ventricles would result in severely elevated filling pressures within the hypoplastic ventricle and poor cardiac output. In other cases, such as unbalanced AV canal, the AV subvalvar apparatus may straddle the ventricular septum and prevent partitioning of the AV valve into left and right orifices. In such patients, the Fontan procedure allows for separation of the systemic venous and arterial circulations by redirecting flow from the systemic veins directly to the PA. In the absence of a subpulmonary ventricle, blood is propelled forward through the pulmonary circulation by negative intrathoracic pressure with inspiration. The pulmonary venous flow then returns to the dominant ventricle, which serves as the systemic ventricle pumping oxygenated blood to the aorta.

Fontan surgery was first described by Fontan and Baudet[16] in 1971 and has since undergone several revisions (**Figure 109.4A-C**). The classic Fontan involves anastomosis of the right atrial appendage to the main PA, and it was widely performed from the 1970s until the early 1990s. Because of right atrial dilation and the resultant risk of right atrial thrombus and arrhythmias, the classic Fontan was replaced by the lateral tunnel and extracardiac Fontan surgery in the early 1990s. In the lateral tunnel Fontan, synthetic material creates a tunnel within the right atrium, diverting blood from the IVC to the right PA. In the extracardiac Fontan, a tube constructed of synthetic material (ie, Gore-Tex) is used to direct IVC flow to the underside of the PA. This tube lays outside of the cardiac chambers, and thus is described as extracardiac; its main advantage over the lateral tunnel Fontan is the absence of suture lines within the atrium, and thus potentially decreased risk of atrial arrhythmias.

Prior to undergoing the Fontan surgery, patients may have had additional palliative procedures as neonates to allow for unobstructed pulmonary venous return (ie, repair of total anomalous pulmonary venous return), to ensure adequate mixing of systemic and pulmonary venous circulation (ie, atrial septectomy or septostomy), or to increase pulmonary blood flow (ie, ductus arteriosus stenting or modified Blalock-Taussig shunt). The modified Blalock-Taussig-Thomas shunt (**Figure 109.5**) is a small tube connecting the subclavian artery to the ipsilateral PA. In the single-ventricle patient, this shunt brings partially oxygenated blood from the aorta to the PA. It is typically performed in the first weeks of life, when pulmonary vascular resistance is still high. Between 3 and 6 months of life, a bidirectional Glenn shunt (SVC to ipsilateral PA, **Figure 109.6**) is typically performed, redirecting blood from the SVC to the PAs. The Fontan is subsequently completed when IVC flow is redirected to the PAs, either with a lateral tunnel or extracardiac conduit in the modern era.

CLINICAL PRESENTATION, COMPLICATIONS, AND TREATMENT

Adults with a Fontan palliation may have a broad spectrum of presentations. As deoxygenated blood now flows passively to the PAs without the usual intervening RA and RV, the pressure in the SVC and IVC is necessarily slightly higher than the mean pulmonary pressure. Thus, in a patient with a normal mean PA pressure of 10 to 15 mm Hg, the pressure in the Fontan pathway (RA, lateral tunnel, or extracardiac conduit), SVC, and IVC is typically 12 to 18 mm Hg.

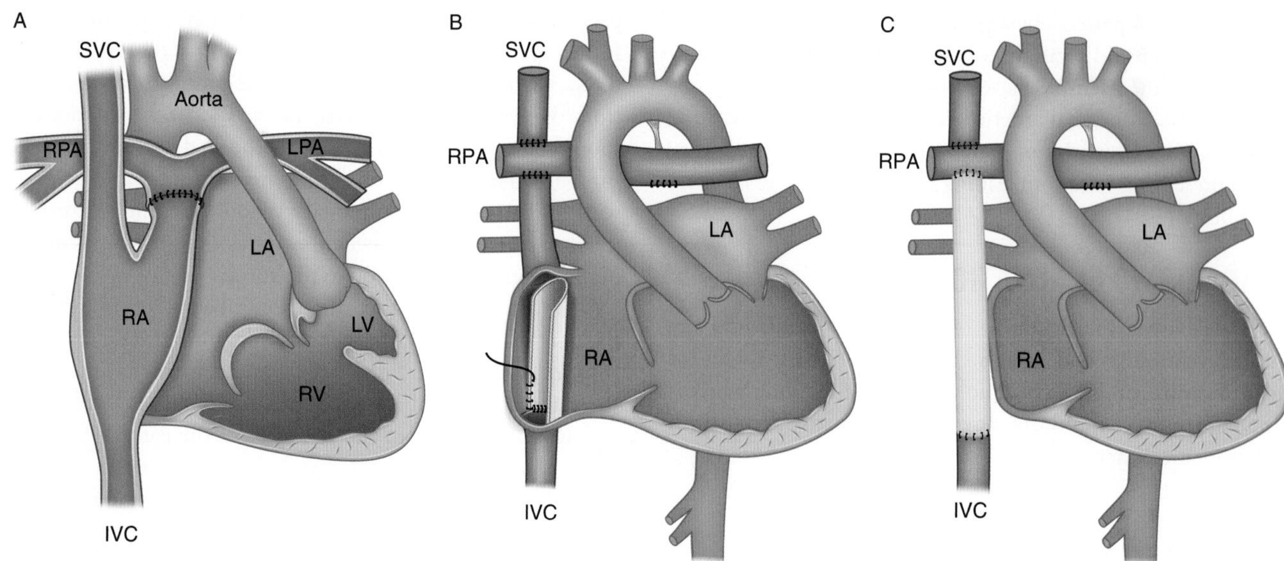

FIGURE 109.4 Variations of Fontan. **A**. The modified classic Fontan. **B**. The lateral tunnel Fontan. **C**. The extracardiac Fontan. LA, left atrium; LV, left ventricle; LPA, left pulmonary artery; IVC, inferior vena cava; RPA, right pulmonary artery; RV, right ventricle; SVC, superior vena cava.

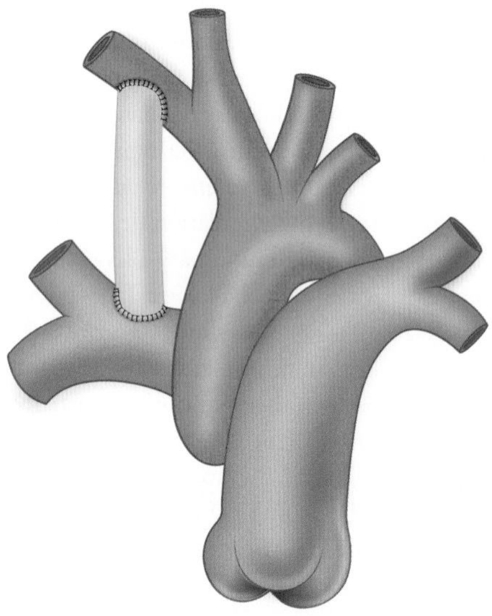

FIGURE 109.5 Modified Blalock-Taussig-Thomas shunt, with an interposition graft connecting the subclavian artery to the pulmonary artery.

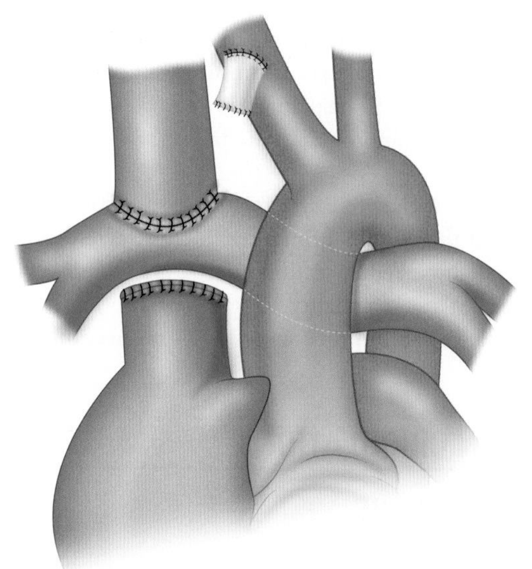

FIGURE 109.6 Bilateral Glenn shunt, an end-to-side anastomosis of the divided superior vena cava to the pulmonary artery.

Surveillance protocols for the stable adult Fontan patient should be performed with an understanding of the long-term sequelae of the Fontan circulation, and with the goal of early identification of problems that may increase morbidity or mortality (**Table 109.1**). In particular, any obstruction or increased resistance along the pathway of deoxygenated blood from the systemic veins to the pulmonary venous atrium will increase pressures in the Fontan and/or systemic veins and decrease ventricular preload. Examples include stenosis in the Fontan conduit or tunnel, PA or pulmonary vein stenosis, pulmonary vascular

TABLE 109.1 Studies for Surveillance of the Stable Adult Fontan Patient

Test/Study	Evaluation
Transthoracic echocardiogram	Ventricular systolic and diastolic function, atrioventricular valve stenosis/regurgitation, outflow tract obstruction, aortic valve regurgitation, Fontan baffle leaks/fenestration, Glenn shunt patency
CMRI or CT	Fontan baffle leaks/fenestration/thrombus, pulmonary artery stenosis, pulmonary vein stenosis
Laboratory studies, including assessment of liver function	Renal and liver function, coagulation studies, complete blood count including platelets
Liver imaging (ultrasonography, CT, MRI)	Liver parenchyma for monitoring for fibrosis, cirrhosis, hepatocellular carcinoma
Cardiac catheterization	Hemodynamics, oxygenation, cardiac function, pulmonary vascular resistance, venovenous collaterals, pulmonary arteriovenous malformations, arteriopulmonary collaterals

CMRI, cardiac magnetic resonance imaging; CT, computed tomography; MRI, magnetic resonance imaging.

disease, and competitive flow from aortopulmonary collaterals. Similarly, conditions that increase pressure in the LA—mitral valve stenosis or regurgitation, LV systolic or diastolic dysfunction, or LV outflow tract obstruction—will similarly increase Fontan pressures as the elevated LA pressure is transmitted to the Fontan circuit via the pulmonary veins and PAs.

Congestive Hepatopathy and Protein-Losing Enteropathy

Chronic elevation in systemic venous pressure leads to congestive hepatopathy. After the first decade of life with a Fontan circulation, most patients develop at least mild hepatic fibrosis, and some may develop cirrhosis after several decades of chronic hepatic congestion, often referred to as "Fontan-associated liver disease" (FALD). Hepatocellular carcinoma is reported in Fontan patients with cirrhosis, and screening protocols incorporate efforts at early diagnosis.[17] Lower extremity varicose veins from chronic venous hypertension are also common, and skin changes from venous stasis may also occur. Protein-losing enteropathy is another known complication and is diagnosed with a 24-hour stool α-1 antitrypsin test. Though the etiology of protein-losing enteropathy is not well understood, contributing factors include poor cardiac output, venous congestion, and lymphatic dysfunction.[18] Treatment for protein-losing enteropathy includes oral budesonide[19] and albumin infusions to offset protein loss and maintain intravascular oncotic pressure.

Atrial Arrhythmias and Thromboembolic Events

Severe dilation of the RA in patients with the modified RA-PA Fontan increases the risk of atrial arrhythmias, and the low-flow state increases the risk of thrombus formation. In patients with the lateral tunnel or extracardiac Fontan, the risk of thrombus formation is lower than those with a RA-PA Fontan, but it persists because of the low-flow state associated with all Fontan circuits. As thrombus can obstruct flow in the Fontan or PAs and be life-threatening, anticoagulation with a vitamin K antagonist or antiplatelet therapy may be considered with Fontan palliation to prevent thrombus formation.[1] Anticoagulation is recommended for patients with Fontan palliation with a history of thromboembolic events and those with a history of arrhythmias.[1] Atrial arrhythmias, even at relatively low heart rates, are poorly tolerated in patients with Fontan palliation, because they are preload dependent and cannot easily increase cardiac output. Restoration of sinus rhythm with antiarrhythmics or direct current cardioversion should be undertaken promptly upon identification of the arrhythmia, even when the patient appears relatively stable. Electrophysiology study and ablation should be considered in patients with atrial arrhythmias and, if undertaken, should be performed by electrophysiologists experienced in the care of CHD and Fontan patients. Surgical treatment with Fontan revision and Maze procedure may also be considered.

"Failing Fontan"

"Failing Fontan" physiology is characterized by declining functional capacity refractory to medical management and because of nonmodifiable factors. For example, patients with (1) ascites because of increased IVC pressures from a stenosis in the Fontan pathway; (2) protein-losing enteropathy that does not improve with medical management; (3) arrhythmias refractory to medical therapy and/or ablation; or (4) severe systolic or diastolic dysfunction on optimal medical management would all be considered with a "failing Fontan." Heart transplantation has been performed successfully for patients with failing Fontan physiology, though some patients with advanced liver disease may require combined heart-liver transplant.[20] Ventricular assist devices in patients with single-ventricle physiology is an area of active research[21] but not currently in widespread clinical use.

HYPOPLASTIC LEFT VENTRICLE SYNDROME

Hypoplastic left heart syndrome is a rare congenital heart defect, occurring in approximately 0.02% to 0.04% of live births in the Canada and the United States.[22,23] With surgical advancements in the 1980s and 1990s, 50% to 70% of patients with hypoplastic left heart syndrome are now surviving to 5 years of age, and many patients are expected to reach adulthood.[24] Traditional staged palliation consists of three stages:

1. Stage I, birth: Norwood procedure, typically involving disconnecting the right/left PA from the native main PA, atrial septectomy, anastomosis of the main PA and the hypoplastic native aortic arch to create a neoaorta, aortic arch augmentation, and a modified Blalock-Taussig or Sano shunt (from the RV to the pulmonary circulation);
2. Stage 2, 4 to 6 months of age: Glenn shunt;
3. Stage 3, 18 to 48 months of age: Fontan completion with a lateral tunnel or extracardiac conduit.

Alternatively, a hybrid approach has also been used to try to reduce mortality in frail neonates[25]:

1. Stage 1, birth: hybrid procedure, involving PA banding, maintaining patency of the ductus arteriosus with stenting or prostaglandin infusion, and balloon atrial septostomy or surgical atrial septectomy;
2. Stage 2, 3 to 8 months: Norwood-type palliation with reconstruction of the aortic arch and Glenn shunt;
3. Stage 3, 18 to 48 months of age: Fontan completion with a lateral tunnel or extracardiac conduit.

FOLLOW-UP PATIENT CARE

Patients with hypoplastic left heart syndrome who survive to adulthood have typically undergone Fontan completion and should be monitored similarly to other patients with Fontan palliation (previous section). Unlike some patients with Fontan palliation whose single ventricle is a morphologic LV and thus more likely to succeed as a systemic ventricle, patients with hypoplastic left heart syndrome have a morphologic RV as their systemic ventricle and are thus more likely to develop systolic and diastolic dysfunction and resultant failing Fontan physiology.[26] In addition, surveillance CT or MRI of the neoaorta and reconstructed aortic arch is recommended because of the risk of neoaorta dilation and aortic arch obstruction.

TRUNCUS ARTERIOSUS

PATHOGENESIS

Truncus arteriosus, also known as common arterial trunk, is a rare cyanotic congenital cardiac defect, occurring in 0.6 to 1.4 per 10,000 live births.[27] Truncus arteriosus is strongly associated with DiGeorge syndrome (22q11.2 deletion syndrome), which is characterized by specific facial features, variable immunodeficiency, and developmental delay. Prior to the development of surgical techniques to palliate and subsequently repair this defect, survival was very poor. Surgical repair was first performed successfully in 1962,[28] and subsequent refinement of the technique and material used for the right ventricular to PA conduit led to improved survival.[29,30]

Truncus arteriosus results from failure of the common arterial trunk to separate into the PA and the aorta in fetal life. Instead of separate aortic and pulmonary valves, there is a single truncal valve, which may be bicuspid, tricuspid, or quadricuspid. Instead of a separate main PA and aorta, there is a single large vessel, the truncus arteriosus, which functions as an aorta. The branch PAs in turn arise from the aorta. The right and left PAs may arise (1) from a "main PA" off the aorta (type I); (2) from separate but closely spaced ostia in the aorta (type II); (3) remotely from one another in the ascending aorta (type III); or (4) from the descending thoracic aorta (type IV). A VSD is typically present that is usually large and nonrestrictive, and the truncus arteriosus overrides the ventricular septum in 70% to 80% of cases, allowing for outflow from both ventricles into the truncus arteriosus.

CLINICAL PRESENTATION

Repair of truncus arteriosus is typically undertaken in the first 3 to 4 months of life and requires a Rastelli procedure (see section on D-TGA with VSD). This includes closure of the VSD, separation of the PAs from the aorta, reconstruction of the PA when needed, and placement of a valved conduit between the RV and the PA. As the child grows, he/she will outgrow the valved conduit and will require a reoperation to place a new, larger conduit. Patients will commonly undergo two to three surgeries prior to reaching adulthood.

Presentation of the adult with truncus arteriosus depends on the ventricular function and status of the RV-PA conduit and truncal valve. RV diastolic and systolic dysfunction is common because of pressure overload and multiple surgeries in childhood as they necessitate conduit replacement. Heart failure may develop because of RV systolic and/or diastolic dysfunction, as well as truncal/aortic valve regurgitation.

DIAGNOSTIC EVALUATION

Adults with truncus arteriosus should have routine surveillance of the RV-PA conduit for stenosis and/or regurgitation. As the RV-PA conduit often lies directly behind the sternum, it is often difficult to image satisfactorily by TTE, though gradients can often be obtained from the subcostal short-axis view. Periodic cross-sectional imaging with a CMRI is recommended to evaluate for conduit stenosis and regurgitation when the conduit is not optimally visualized by TTE. An ECG-gated CT scan may also define conduit stenosis with excellent spatial resolution, but does not provide information about flow through the valve or regurgitation. The truncal/aortic valve leaflets may be myxomatous, and truncal valves are associated most commonly with regurgitation. Severe truncal valve regurgitation may require valve replacement. Less frequently, the truncal valve may be stenotic.

Management: Truncus Arteriosus

Transcatheter pulmonary valve implantation is recommended for severe symptomatic conduit stenosis and/or regurgitation[38], though surgical conduit replacement is still often required in adults if the RV-PA conduit is felt to be too small to allow satisfactory reduction in the gradient with transcatheter pulmonary valve implantation or in cases of endocarditis. Patients with repaired truncus arteriosus, particularly those with DiGeorge syndrome, should be encouraged to maintain excellent dental hygiene in order to mitigate the risk of endocarditis. Antibiotics for prevention of infective endocarditis should be prescribed prior to dental procedures in patients with repaired truncus arteriosus, because of the presence of a prosthetic valve.

DOUBLE OUTLET RIGHT VENTRICLE

PATHOGENESIS

DORV comprises a group of morphologic variations that share the same abnormal ventriculoarterial alignment, where both great vessels arise either entirely or predominantly from the RV.[31] Although it initially seems like a straightforward diagnosis, the group of patients with a diagnosis of DORV is very heterogeneous, their clinical presentation can range from severe cyanosis at birth requiring a single-ventricle palliation to the occasional patient who survives into adulthood without repair. This section will aim to highlight the common presentation of the varying types of patients with DORV and the subsequent testing and management required for optimal care for this complex group.

DORV is an uncommon congenital heart defect, with an estimated incidence of 0.127 per 1000 live births,[27] and accounts for 0.5% to 1.5% of all congenital heart defects.[32] Although it is associated with some genetic defects, such as trisomy 13 and 18,[33] it is mainly a sporadic disease with no racial or sexual predisposition.[34] The varying number of phenotypes associated with the diagnosis of DORV suggests a multifactorial etiology.

Abnormalities of neural crest cell migration, outflow tract development, and ventricular septation in early fetal development (before 12 weeks of life) are thought to contribute to the pathology of DORV.[33] DORV is almost always associated with a VSD.[35] Because of the heterogeneous morphologic variations of DORV, which lead to a wide array of physiologic/hemodynamic states, it is useful to classify the variations of DORV based on the location of the VSD and its relationship to the semilunar valves (Figure 109.7).[36] It is also important

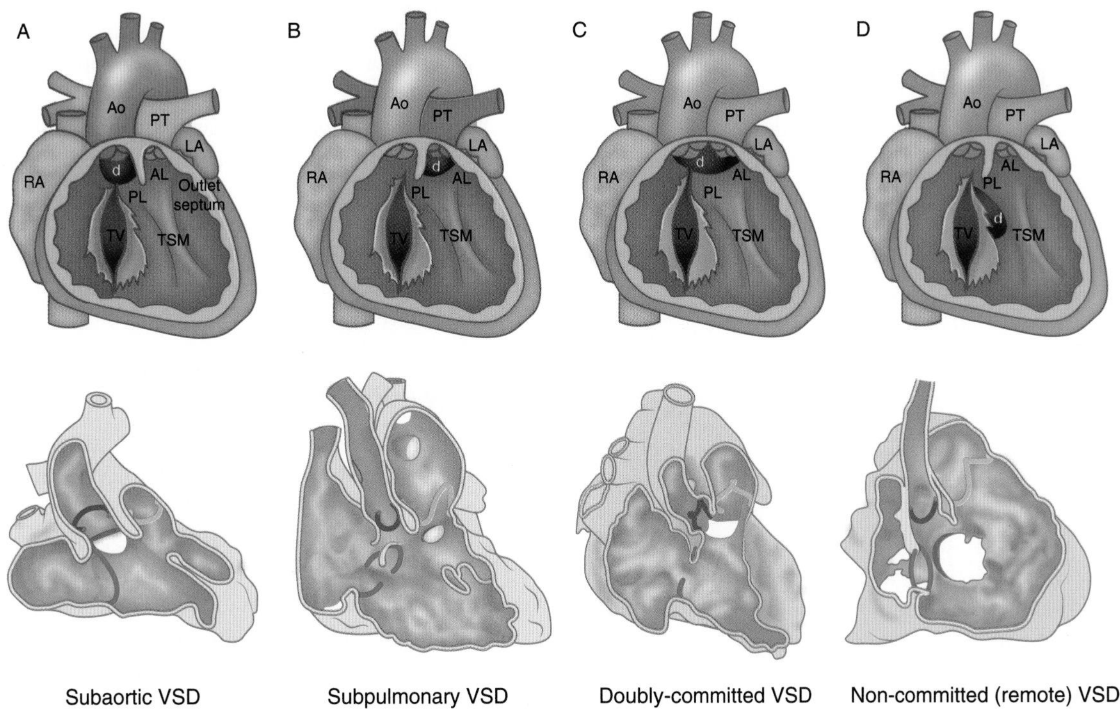

FIGURE 109.7 Different type of VSDs in double outlet right ventricle. The subaortic **(A)**, subpulmonary **(B)**, and doubly committed **(C)** VSDs classically involve the outlet part of the septum and therefore are cradled between the anterior and posterior limbs of the TSM. The classic noncommitted or remote VSD **(D)** involves the inlet part of the ventricular septum behind and below the posterior limb of the TSM. AL, anterior limb; Ao, aorta; d, ventricular septal defect; LA, left atrium; PL, posterior limb; PT, pulmonary trunk; RA, right atrium; TSM, trabecula septomarginalis; TV, tricuspid valve; VSD, ventricular septal defect.

to understand the spatial relationship of the great arteries, the infundibular morphology, and other cardiac lesions, such as outflow tract obstruction, AV valve abnormalities, ventricular hypoplasia and malposition, and coronary artery patterns. All of these features play a role in determining the physiology of an individual with DORV and the subsequent surgical repair that they will ultimately receive.

Some of the common pathophysiologic variants include DORV with:

- **VSD physiology** (ie, increased pulmonary blood flow). This DORV variant represents about 25% of cases and usually presents with heart failure.[32]
- **Tetralogy of Fallot physiology** (ie, balanced pulmonary blood flow). This variant represents about 66% of cases.[32] Patients with this type of DORV may be difficult to differentiate from patients with tetralogy of Fallot.
- **TGA physiology** (ie, transposition physiology with separate parallel circuits, or Taussig-Bing anomaly). These patients present early in life with cyanosis and heart failure.
- **Single-ventricle physiology** (ie, cyanosis with a functional single ventricle). Patients with a remote VSD, mitral atresia, or significant ventricular hypoplasia are examples of this type of DORV.

CLINICAL PRESENTATION

Very few patients survive to adulthood without corrective surgery. Patients with DORV usually present in infancy and can receive a variety of LV to the aorta, to more complex surgeries like an arterial switch with a patch redirecting flow from the LV to the neoaortic valve.[32,37] For those with single-ventricle physiology, complex multistage procedures to create a Fontan single-ventricle palliation may be necessary.

Because most patients with DORV have had surgical repair, the clinical presentation usually relates to the residual defects or sequelae from their surgeries. Patients can suffer from VSD patch leak, outflow obstruction (either aortic or pulmonary), semilunar valve regurgitation, AV valve stenosis or regurgitation, ventricular dysfunction, or arrhythmias. Patients can present with chest pain, heart failure, stroke, dyspnea, palpitations, syncope, or endocarditis. Unrepaired patients can present with cyanosis and signs of heart failure, or with pulmonary hypertension and Eisenmenger syndrome.[34]

DIAGNOSTIC EVALUATION

The workhorse diagnostic modality is the echocardiogram (either transthoracic or transesophageal). This imaging modality allows for assessment of ventricular function, valvular function, baffle leaks, and conduit patency. In patients with more complex anatomy—such as those with single-ventricle repairs or complex tunneled baffles—cardiac MRI or ECG-gated CT angiography is necessary. Sometimes a cardiac catheterization is helpful as a diagnostic (and therapeutic) tool, especially when trying to definitively assess the hemodynamics and anatomy of a patient with DORV. If there is a concern for an arrhythmia or conduction abnormality, an ECG or an ambulatory rhythm monitor is recommended. When patients present with functional complaints, such as shortness of breath with exertion, a stress echocardiogram can help unmask issues like heart block, outflow tract obstruction, or coronary artery disease.

MANAGEMENT: DOUBLE OUTLET RIGHT VENTRICLE

Standard guideline-directed medical therapy is indicated for those who present with heart failure. For those with arrhythmias, antiarrhythmic drugs are routinely used, but should be prescribed with the guidance of an electrophysiologist familiar with CHD.

With the advent of transcatheter valve replacement, patients with surgically repaired DORV with conduit or outflow tract obstruction/regurgitation are undergoing percutaneous valve replacements when possible. Percutaneous closure of residual VSD baffle leaks has been reported as well.[39]

Surgical reoperation is sometimes necessary for aortic valve disease, residual ventricular-level shunting or conduit obstruction or regurgitation not amenable to transcatheter pulmonary valve replacement. Heart transplantation may be considered in patients with ventricular dysfunction who have failed medical management.[40]

With the development of new therapies like the angiotensin-neprilysin inhibitors for heart failure,[41] and the transcatheter edge-to-edge clips for valvular regurgitation,[41] the medical and percutaneous options for patients with DORV are expanding. Many adult patients with DORV are benefiting from new medical therapies and advances in percutaneous interventions in order to stave off surgery.

FOLLOW-UP PATIENT CARE

Follow-up care should be lifelong. Overall survival at 15 years was 96% for patients with "simple" DORV lesions and 90% for those with "complex" lesions in one study, and freedom from reoperation was 72%.[40] Patients are at risk for developing LV outflow tract obstruction[42] and conduction problems requiring pacemaker implantation.[40] These patients need to continue lifelong follow-up with an adult congenital disease specialist who can manage the intricacies and nuances of care for this heterogeneous group of patients.[3]

With better imaging techniques, such as 4D MRI,[43] and three-dimensional printing technology,[44] surgeons are now better equipped to plan the surgical repair for patients with complex DORV. In the future, the use of virtual reality may help surgeons practice surgeries and guide providers in deciding who gets a biventricular or a single-ventricle repair. Newer medications for heart failure, as well as more durable prosthetic valves with improved percutaneous delivery systems, will also be important for the future care of patients with DORV.

KEY POINTS

- ✔ Understanding common sequelae of complex congenital heart defects requires an understanding of patients' native anatomy and surgical repair.
- ✔ Although echocardiogram remains the imaging modality for patients with complex CHD, advanced imaging with CMRI and cardiac CT is essential for evaluation of anatomy that is not well visualized by echocardiography, including complex baffles.
- ✔ DORV is a single diagnosis with many variations, depending on the location of the VSD and great arteries.
- ✔ Patients with Fontan palliation typically develop liver fibrosis and may develop cirrhosis. Ongoing surveillance for liver disease is essential.
- ✔ Advances in surgical and transcatheter interventions have resulted in improved survival for this patient population.

REFERENCES

1. Stout KK, Daniels CJ, Aboulhosn JA, et al. 2018 AHA/ACC Guideline for the management of adults with congenital heart disease: executive summary: a report of the American College of Cardiology/American Heart Association Task Force on Clinical Practice Guidelines. *J Am Coll Cardiol.* 2019;73(12):1494-1563.
2. Liu Y, Chen S, Zuhlke L, et al. Global birth prevalence of congenital heart defects 1970-2017: updated systematic review and meta-analysis of 260 studies. *Int J Epidemiol.* 2019;48(2):455-463.
3. Stout KK, Daniels CJ, Aboulhosn JA, et al. 2018 AHA/ACC Guideline for the management of adults with congenital heart disease: a report of the American College of Cardiology/American Heart Association Task Force on Clinical Practice Guidelines. *J Am Coll Cardiol.* 2019;73(12):e81-e192.
4. Khairy P, Harris L, Landzberg MJ, et al. Sudden death and defibrillators in transposition of the great arteries with intra-atrial baffles: a multicenter study. *Circ Arrhythm Electrophysiol.* 2008;1(4):250-257.
5. Bradley EA, Cai A, Cheatham SL, et al. Mustard baffle obstruction and leak - How successful are percutaneous interventions in adults? *Prog Pediatr Cardiol.* 2015;39(2 Pt B):157-163.
6. Khairy P, Landzberg MJ, Lambert J, O'Donnell CP. Long-term outcomes after the atrial switch for surgical correction of transposition: a meta-analysis comparing the Mustard and Senning procedures. *Cardiol Young.* 2004;14(3):284-292.
7. Kirzner J, Pirmohamed A, Ginns J, Singh HS. Long-term management of the arterial switch patient. *Curr Cardiol Rep.* 2018;20(8):68.
8. Khairy P, Clair M, Fernandes SM, et al. Cardiovascular outcomes after the arterial switch operation for D-transposition of the great arteries. *Circulation.* 2013;127(3):331-339.
9. Dearani JA, Danielson GK, Puga FJ, Mair DD, Schleck CD. Late results of the Rastelli operation for transposition of the great arteries. *Semin Thorac Cardiovasc Surg Pediatr Card Surg Annu.* 2001;4:3-15.
10. Mery CM, Guzman-Pruneda FA, De Leon LE, et al. Risk factors for development of endocarditis and reintervention in patients undergoing right ventricle to pulmonary artery valved conduit placement. *J Thorac Cardiovasc Surg.* 2016;151(2):432-439, 441.e1-2.
11. Graham TP Jr, Bernard YD, Mellen BG, et al. Long-term outcome in congenitally corrected transposition of the great arteries: a multi-institutional study. *J Am Coll Cardiol.* 2000;36(1):255-261.
12. Huhta JC, Maloney JD, Ritter DG, Ilstrup DM, Feldt RH. Complete atrioventricular block in patients with atrioventricular discordance. *Circulation.* 1983;67(6):1374-1377.
13. Deng L, Xu J, Tang Y, Sun H, Liu S, Song Y. Long-term outcomes of tricuspid valve surgery in patients with congenitally corrected transposition of the great arteries. *J Am Heart Assoc.* 2018;7(6).
14. Picard F, Tadros VX, Asgar AW. From tricuspid to double orifice morphology: percutaneous tricuspid regurgitation repair with the MitraClip device in congenitally corrected-transposition of great arteries. *Catheter Cardiovasc Interv.* 2017;90(3):432-436.
15. Venkatesh P, Evans AT, Maw AM, et al. Predictors of late mortality in D-transposition of the great arteries after atrial switch repair: systematic review and meta-analysis. *J Am Heart Assoc.* 2019;8(21):e012932.
16. Fontan F, Baudet E. Surgical repair of tricuspid atresia. *Thorax.* 1971;26(3):240-248.
17. Egbe AC, Poterucha JT, Warnes CA, et al. Hepatocellular carcinoma after fontan operation: multicenter case series. *Circulation.* 2018;138(7):746-748.
18. Rychik J. Protein-losing enteropathy after Fontan operation. *Congenit Heart Dis.* 2007;2(5):288-300.
19. Thacker D, Patel A, Dodds K, Goldberg DJ, Semeao E, Rychik J. Use of oral budesonide in the management of protein-losing enteropathy after the Fontan operation. *Ann Thorac Surg.* 2010;89(3):837-842.
20. Reardon LC, DePasquale EC, Tarabay J, et al. Heart and heart-liver transplantation in adults with failing Fontan physiology. *Clin Transplant.* 2018;32(8):e13329.
21. Miller JR, Lancaster TS, Callahan C, Abarbanell AM, Eghtesady P. An overview of mechanical circulatory support in single-ventricle patients. *Transl Pediatr.* 2018;7(2):151-161.
22. Report of the New England Regional Infant Cardiac Program. *Pediatrics.* 1980;65(2 Pt 2):375-461.
23. Samanek M, Slavik Z, Zborilova B, Hrobonova V, Voriskova M, Skovranek J. Prevalence, treatment, and outcome of heart disease in live-born children: a prospective analysis of 91,823 live-born children. *Pediatr Cardiol.* 1989;10(4):205-211.
24. Hirsch JC, Ohye RG, Devaney EJ, Goldberg CS, Bove EL. The lateral tunnel Fontan procedure for hypoplastic left heart syndrome: results of 100 consecutive patients. *Pediatr Cardiol.* 2007;28(6):426-432.
25. Caldarone CA, Benson L, Holtby H, Li J, Redington AN, Van Arsdell GS. Initial experience with hybrid palliation for neonates with single-ventricle physiology. *Ann Thorac Surg.* 2007;84(4):1294-1300.
26. Erikssen G, Aboulhosn J, Lin J, et al. Survival in patients with univentricular hearts: the impact of right versus left ventricular morphology. *Open Heart.* 2018;5(2):e000902.
27. Hoffman JIE, Kaplan S. The incidence of congenital heart disease. *J Am Coll Card.* 2002;39(12):1890-1900.
28. Behrendt DM, Kirsh MM, Stern A, Sigmann J, Perry B, Sloan H. The surgical therapy for pulmonary artery—right ventricular discontinuity. *Ann Thorac Surg.* 1974;18(2):122-137.
29. McGoon DC, Rastelli GC, Ongley PA. An operation for the correction of truncus arteriosus. *JAMA.* 1968;205(2):69-73.
30. Mavroudis C, Jonas RA, Bove EL. Personal glimpses into the evolution of truncus arteriosus repair. *World J Pediatr Congenit Heart Surg.* 2015;6(2):226-238.
31. Tchervenkov CI, Walters HL, Chu VF. Congenital Heart Surgery Nomenclature and Database Project: double outlet left ventricle. *Ann Thorac Surg.* 2000;69(99):264-269.
32. da Cruz EM, Ivy D, Jaggers J. *Pediatric and Congenital Cardiology, Cardiac Surgery and Intensive Care.* Springer; 2014:3572.
33. Lopez L, Geva T. Double-outlet ventricle. In: Lai WW, Mertens LL, Cohen MS, et al., eds. *Echocardiography in Pediatric and Congenital Heart Disease: From Fetus to Adult.* 2nd ed. Wiley-Blackwell; 2016:466-488.
34. Hugh D, David J, Robert E, Timothy F. Chapter 53 Double-Outlet Right Ventricle and Double-Outlet Left Ventricle Double-Outlet Right Ventricle Position of the Ventricular Septal Defect. Moss and Adams. 2008:1-56.
35. Ebadi A, Spicer DE, Backer CL, Fricker FJ, Anderson RH. Double-outlet right ventricle revisited. *J Thorac Cardiovasc Surg.* 2017;154(2):598-604.
36. Lev M, Bharati S, Meng CC, Liberthson RR, Paul MH, Idriss F. A concept of double-outlet right ventricle. *J Thorac Cardiovasc Surg.* 1972;64(2):271-281.

37. Freedom RM, Yoo SJ. Double-outlet right ventricle: Pathology and angiocardiography. *Semin Thorac Cardiovasc Surg Pediatr Card Surg Annu.* 2000;3:3-19.
38. Jones TK, Rome JJ, Armstrong AK, et al. Transcatheter pulmonary valve replacement reduces tricuspid regurgitation in patients with right ventricular volume/pressure overload. *J Am Coll Cardiol.* 2016;68(14):1525-1535.
39. Mortera C, Prada F, Rissech M, Bartrons J, Mayol J, Caffarena JM. Percutaneous closure of ventricular septal defect with an Amplatzer device. *Rev Esp Cardiol.* 2004;57(5):466-471.
40. Brown JW, Ruzmetov M, Okada Y, Vijay P, Turrentine MW. Surgical results in patients with double outlet right ventricle: a 20-year experience. *Ann Thorac Surg.* 2001;72(5):1630-1635.
41. McMurray JJV, Packer M, Desai AS, et al. Angiotensin-neprilysin inhibition versus enalapril in heart failure. *N Engl J Med.* 2014;371(11):993-1004.
42. Li S, Ma K, Hu S, et al. Surgical outcomes of 380 patients with double outlet right ventricle who underwent biventricular repair. *J Thorac Cardiovasc Surg.* 2014;148(3):817-824.
43. Skinner G, Durairaj S, Shebani SO. 20 Multimodality 4D imaging and modelling for complex double outlet right ventricles. *Heart.* 2017;103(suppl 3):A10-A11.
44. Yim D, Dragulescu A, Ide H, et al. Essential modifiers of double outlet right ventricle: revisit with endocardial surface images and 3-dimensional print models. *Circ Cardiovasc Imaging.* 2018;11(3):1-9.

CHAPTER 110

PULMONARY ARTERIAL HYPERTENSION ASSOCIATED WITH CONGENITAL HEART DISEASE

Nils Patrick Nickel, Richard A. Lange, Christine Bui, and Anitra W. Romfh

CLASSIFICATION OF PULMONARY HYPERTENSION IN CONGENITAL HEART DISEASE

Pulmonary hypertension (PH) is a heterogeneous hemodynamic and pathophysiologic disorder, characterized by an increased mean pulmonary arterial pressure (mPAP > 20 mm Hg).[1] PH can be caused by a variety of cardiovascular and respiratory conditions. The correct classification of PH is paramount because the various types differ significantly in their prognosis and clinical management. A framework focused on a hemodynamic definition in conjunction with a pathophysiologic and clinical classification helps identify patients who most likely benefit from targeted therapy.

Using the hemodynamic information, PH can be divided into three categories: precapillary, postcapillary, and combined pre- and postcapillary PH. The hemodynamic features of each category are displayed in Table 110.1. Precapillary PH shows evidence of increased pulmonary vascular resistance in the absence of increased pulmonary venous or left-sided filling pressures. Postcapillary PH is defined by elevated left-sided filling pressures and normal pulmonary vascular resistance. Combined post- and precapillary PH is present in patients with pulmonary venous congestion and elevated pulmonary vascular resistance out of proportion to the elevated pulmonary venous pressure.

The clinical classification of PH is designed to categorize clinical conditions associated with PH based on similar pathophysiologic mechanisms, clinical presentation, hemodynamic characteristics, and therapeutic management. A comprehensive and simplified version of the clinical classification of PH in children and adults is presented in Table 110.2, with PH divided into five different groups, according to underlying cause and pathophysiology. In the patient with congenital heart disease (CHD), PH may be owing to (1) pulmonary arterial hypertension (PAH, Group 1), so-called PAH-CHD, which is precapillary; (2) left heart dysfunction resulting in postcapillary PH (Group 2), as seen in valvular heart disease, congenital or acquired left heart inflow or outflow tract obstruction, cardiomyopathies, and pulmonary vein stenosis; or (3) complex cardiac conditions with PH owing to unclear or multifactorial (Group 5) such as complex congenital abnormalities in the pulmonary vasculature or single ventricle physiology.[1]

Because of the remarkable heterogeneity, PAH-CHD (Group 1) is further classified into clinical and anatomic-physiologic categories. PAH-CHD clinical categories include patients with simple operable and inoperable CHD, subgrouped as those with (1) Eisenmenger physiology; (2) PAH and left-to-right shunts; (3) PAH thought to be incidental to their CHD; and (4) postoperative/closed defects. The features of each of these are shown in Table 110.3. The anatomic-pathophysiologic classification of PAH-CHD differentiates between type, dimension, and direction of the shunt. The type of shunts is divided between pre-, post-tricuspid, or combined shunts and complex defects such as truncus arteriosus or transposition of the great arteries (TGA). The dimension of the shunt is defined by hemodynamic and anatomic parameters.

Epidemiology of PAH in CHD

The overall prevalence of PAH in adult patients over the entire CHD spectrum is reported to range from 3% to 10%.[2] PAH is most common in patients with Eisenmenger syndrome and left-to-right shunts (ie, ventricular septal defects [VSD], atrial septal defects [ASD], and patent ductus arteriosus [PDA]). Patients with isolated pre-tricuspid defects rarely develop severe PAH. Increased blood flow, pressure, and shear stress in the pulmonary circulation over time contribute to the development of PAH in CHD. It is therefore not surprising that the prevalence of PAH increases with age.[2] Furthermore, the size of the defect, gender, and genetic factors also play a role in the development of PAH in CHD patients.[3] The lifetime risk for PAH after CHD repair increases over time and ranges from 4% to over 15%, depending on the cardiac defect. Based on registry data, 7% to 37% of group 1 PAH is attributable to CHD.[4-6]

Outcomes of Patients With PAH-CHD

The presence of PAH has a significant impact on survival in patients with CHD.[7] However, with continuous improvements in clinical management and new therapies, outcomes in adults with PAH-CHD have improved over recent years.[8] In general, the outcome of PAH-CHD is associated with the size and the anatomy of the defect. Patients with the most complex defects (TGA, complete atrioventricular septal defect, Fontan, Eisenmenger physiology) have the lowest survival rates among CHD

TABLE 110.1 Hemodynamic Classification of Pulmonary Hypertension (With Clinical Group Correlation)

Classification	mPAP	PCWP	PVR and/or DPG[a]	Clinical Groups
Precapillary PH	>20 mm Hg	≤15 mm Hg	PVR ≥ 3 WU	1, 3, 4, 5
Postcapillary PH	>20 mm Hg	>15 mm Hg	PVR < 3 WU and/or DPG < 7 mmHg	2 and 5
Combined pre- and postcapillary PH	>20 mm Hg	>15 mm Hg	PVR ≥ 3 WU and/or DPG ≥ 7 mmHg	2 and 5

Note: Group 1: Pulmonary arterial hypertension associated with congenital heart disease; group 2: PH owing to left heart disease; group 3: PH owing to lung diseases and/or hypoxia; group 4: PH owing to pulmonary artery obstructions; group 5: PH with unclear and/or multifactorial mechanisms.

DPG, diastolic pressure gradient; mPAP, mean pulmonary artery pressure; PH, pulmonary hypertension; PCWP, pulmonary capillary wedge pressure; PVR, pulmonary vascular resistance; WU, Wood units.

[a]Diastolic pressure gradient (DPG) between pulmonary artery diastolic pressure and mean PCWP.

TABLE 110.2 Clinical Classification of Pulmonary Hypertension (With Congenital Heart Disease–Associated Pulmonary Hypertension Highlighted)

1 Pulmonary arterial hypertension (PAH)
- 1.1 Idiopathic PAH
- 1.2 Heritable PAH
- 1.3 Drug- and toxin-induced PAH
- 1.4 PAH associated with:
  - 1.4.1 Connective tissue disease
  - 1.4.2 HIV infection
  - 1.4.3 Portal hypertension
  - 1.4.4 *Congenital heart disease*
  - 1.4.5 Schistosomiasis
- 1.5 PAH long-term responders to calcium channel blockers
- 1.6 PAH with overt features of venous/capillaries (PVOD/PCH) involvement
- 1.7 Persistent PH of the newborn syndrome

2 PH owing to left heart disease
- 2.1 PH owing to heart failure with preserved LVEF
- 2.2 PH owing to heart failure with reduced LVEF
- 2.3 Valvular heart disease
- 2.4 *Congenital/acquired cardiovascular conditions leading to postcapillary PH*

3 PH caused by lung diseases and/or hypoxia
- 3.1 Obstructive lung disease
- 3.2 Restrictive lung disease
- 3.3 Other lung diseases with mixed restrictive/obstructive pattern
- 3.4 Hypoxia without lung disease
- 3.5 Developmental lung disorders

4 PH owing to pulmonary artery obstructions
- 4.1 Chronic thromboembolic PH
- 4.2 Other pulmonary artery obstructions

5 PH with unclear and/or multifactorial mechanisms
- 5.1 Hematologic disorders
- 5.2 Systemic and metabolic disorders
- 5.3 Others
- 5.4 *Complex congenital heart disease*

LVEF, left ventricular ejection fraction; PCH, pulmonary capillary hypertension; PH, pulmonary hypertension; PVOD, pulmonary vascular obstructive disease.

Some data from Galiè N, Humbert M, Vachiery JL, et al.; ESC Scientific Document Group. 2015 ESC/ERS Guidelines for the diagnosis and treatment of pulmonary hypertension: The Joint Task Force for the Diagnosis and Treatment of Pulmonary Hypertension of the European Society of Cardiology (ESC) and the European Respiratory Society (ERS): Endorsed by: Association for European Paediatric and Congenital Cardiology (AEPC), International Society for Heart and Lung Transplantation (ISHLT). *Eur Heart J.* 2016;37(1):67-119.

patients.[7] The underlying CHD anatomy is also an important parameter influencing PAH-CHD outcome, and there are key differences in adaptation of the right ventricle to pulmonary vascular remodeling. Patients with congenital post-tricuspid shunts have significant alterations in pulmonary blood flow and pressure early in life that can lead to the accelerated development of pulmonary vascular disease.[9] In these patients, the right ventricle is primed to sustain a higher afterload compared to other types of PAH patients, possibly owing to retention of a favorable neonatal right-heart phenotype.[10] In addition, the presence of an open shunt may act as a "pop-off," allowing decompression of the subpulmonary ventricle at the expense of cyanosis.[11] This is in line with the observation that patients with isolated pre-tricuspid shunts usually develop PAH later in life, and the development of severe PAH or Eisenmenger syndrome in these patients is associated with worse survival compared to PAH that occurs with post-tricuspid or complex lesions.[12] Many patients with pre-tricuspid PAH-CHD are thought to have an underlying pulmonary vascular disease process independent from the CHD.

In contrast to other forms of PAH, patients with PAH-CHD have the highest survival, with a 7-year survival rate of 67%, compared to 49% in patients with idiopathic PAH or 35% in those with connective tissue disease–associated PAH.[13] These findings are consistent with other PAH cohorts.[8,14]

PATHOGENESIS OF PULMONARY VASCULAR DISEASE IN CHD

Increased blood flow and circumferential stretch are "sensed" by vascular cells and lead to activation of transcription factors and altered gene expression, resulting in vascular remodeling.[15] Changes in vascular cell proliferation and migration, as well as dysregulated production of vasoactive mediators and their receptors, have been described in patients with PAH-CHD.[16] Remodeling of the pulmonary circulation can result in pulmonary vasodilation, constriction, vessel obliteration, or the development of arteriovenous malformations. These structural changes are influenced by local factors, blood flow, pressure, genetics, and hepatic venous return. Angiograms in children with CHD reveal that increased pulmonary blood flow in the

TABLE 110.3 Clinical Classification of Pulmonary Arterial Hypertension Associated With Congenital Heart Disease[a]

Classification	Definition	Features
Eisenmenger syndrome	Includes all large intra- and extra-cardiac defects which begin as left-to-right shunts and progress to severe elevation of PVR and reversal (right-to-left) or bidirectional shunting	Cyanosis, secondary erythrocytosis, gout, and multiple organ involvement
PAH associated with prevalent left-to-right shunts • Correctable[b] • Noncorrectable)	Includes moderate to large defects, PVR is mildly to moderately increased, left-to-right shunting is still prevalent	Cyanosis at rest is not a feature
PAH with small/coincidental defects	Marked elevation in PVR in the presence of small cardiac defects (ie, VSD < 1 cm or ASD < 2 cm[c]), which themselves do not account for the development of elevated PVR	Clinical picture is very similar to idiopathic PAH. Closing the defects is contraindicated
PAH after defect correction	Congenital heart disease is repaired, but PAH persists immediately after correction or recurs/develops months or years after correction	No significant postoperative hemodynamic lesions

ASD, atrial septal defect; PAH, pulmonary arterial hypertension; PVR, pulmonary vascular resistance; VSD, ventricular septal defect.
[a]Group 1.4.4 from **Table 110.2**.
[b]With surgery or percutaneous procedure.
[c]Size applies to adult patients.

absence of increased pressure or resistance is associated with enlarged proximal pulmonary arteries and veins but no signs of remodeling when compared to normal angiograms.[17] In patients with increased pulmonary blood flow and increased pressure, the pulmonary arteries are enlarged and tortuous. In patients with markedly elevated pulmonary pressure and increased resistance, abrupt termination of dilated and tortuous arteries and a diminished capillary blush are observed, indicating vessel obliteration or loss. This corresponds to the finding that PAH-CHD patients with the most severe PAH show evidence of distal pulmonary artery obliteration and loss on lung biopsy.[18]

Many studies since the 1950s have described the histopathologic changes in PAH-CHD: intimal and medial hypertrophy, muscularization of distal pulmonary arteries, in situ thrombosis, plexiform lesions, and perivascular inflammation are common features.[19] A more recent study showed that PAH-CHD lungs demonstrate the same features of pulmonary vascular remodeling as seen in patients with idiopathic PAH (muscular remodeling, extracellular matrix proliferation, plexiform lesions), independent of the underlying CHD defect. Recent and organized thrombi and perivascular inflammation are also common in both groups.[20]

Genetic factors are increasingly recognized as contributors to pulmonary vascular remodeling, although there is increasing evidence that the genetics of PAH-CHD differs from other forms of adult PAH. For instance, mutations in the bone-morphogenetic receptor 2 are found in 60% of patients with hereditable PAH,[21] but in less than 10% of children and 15% of adults with PAH-CHD.[22] Conversely, a mutation in the *SOX17* (SRY-related HMG-box17) gene was identified in 7% of PAH-CHD but only in 0.4% of adult PAH patients.[23] Hence, some patients with CHD are likely to be at increased risk for the development of pulmonary vascular disease in the setting of increased blood flow and shear stress.

CLINICAL PRESENTATION

Signs and Symptoms

The signs and symptoms of PH are nonspecific and related to progressive right ventricular dysfunction and heart failure or anatomical changes of the pulmonary circulation. The most common symptoms reported by patients with PAH-CHD are dyspnea, fatigue, light-headedness, syncope, chest pain, and hemoptysis. The pathogenesis of dyspnea in patients with PAH is multifactorial; hypoxemia, ventilation-perfusion mismatch, and reduced cardiac output likely play a role. Fatigue, light-headedness, and syncope can be direct consequences of reduced cardiac output and/or hypoxia. Additionally, patients with PAH exhibit reduced cerebrovascular reactivity to blood pCO_2 levels and a blunted increase in cerebral blood flow during exercise, thus increasing the risk for syncope.[24] Chest pain can be caused by myocardial ischemia of the hypertrophied and hypoperfused right ventricle or compression of the left main coronary artery by a dilated pulmonary trunk.[25]

Some symptoms can be caused directly by anatomical changes in the pulmonary circulation. Hemoptysis in patients with PAH-CHD can be the direct result of remodeling of the pulmonary vasculature, such as hypertrophied bronchial arteries and shunts between pulmonary arteries, veins, and bronchial circulation.[26] Wheezing and hoarseness can result from massive dilation of the pulmonary arteries compressing the large airways and recurrent laryngeal nerve (Ortner syndrome). Venous congestion and hypoperfusion from right-heart failure are commonly associated with organ dysfunction such as congestive hepatopathy, renal dysfunction, and myopathy.

Physical Examination

On physical examination, signs of PAH include a right ventricular lift, a wide split S2 with a prominent pulmonic component of the second heart sound, a pansystolic murmur of tricuspid regurgitation that increases in intensity with inspiration (Carvallo sign), elevated jugular venous pressure, and lower extremity edema. Genetic syndromes are commonly associated with PAH-CHD and can have specific physical examination features, as seen in Down syndrome.

Cyanosis—the bluish discoloration of mucus membranes or skin caused by an increased amount of deoxygenated blood (usually when systemic arterial saturation <85%)—is common in PAH-CHD. Peripheral cyanosis results from low cardiac output and peripheral vasoconstriction or venous congestion. Central cyanosis is seen in patients with right-to-left shunting from severe PAH (Eisenmenger), intrapulmonary shunting, or other complex CHD without significant PAH.[27] Differential cyanosis refers to cyanosis that only affects the lower extremities (ie, upper extremities are spared) and can be seen in patients with Eisenmenger syndrome owing to a large PDA. In reverse differential cyanosis—which can be seen in TGA with PDA and elevated pulmonary vascular resistance—the arms are more cyanotic than the legs.[28] Hypertrophic osteoarthropathy or clubbing can be observed in patients with long-standing tissue hypoxemia and cyanosis. Clubbing is characterized by enlargement of the anteroposterior and lateral diameter of the nail owing to the proliferation of connective tissue between the nail matrix and the distal phalanx. Clubbing and cyanosis are not specific to PAH and can be seen in any cardiopulmonary disease that is associated with tissue hypoxemia.

Differential Diagnosis

The differential diagnosis for a patient with CHD and suspected PH is broad because presenting signs and symptoms are usually nonspecific. Dyspnea, fatigue, and chest pain need to be thoroughly evaluated and cardiac, pulmonary, hematologic, and metabolic causes need to be considered. Because the prevalence of PAH in patients with CHD is high, extensive hemodynamic evaluation with an echocardiogram and/or right-heart catheterization is usually recommended in these patients to determine whether symptoms are related to progressive heart failure or other underlying causes such as concomitant lung disease, liver disease, or thromboembolic disorder. If PH is suspected, alternative causes should be evaluated, such as collagen vascular diseases, HIV infection, or liver disease with portal hypertension. Echocardiography can be helpful to evaluate concomitant left heart or valvular disease. Pulmonary function testing (PFT) is recommended to rule out obstructive or restrictive lung disease. Ventilation-perfusion scanning of the lung is recommended to evaluate chronic thromboembolic disease that can be missed on contrast computed tomography (CT) scans (**Algorithms 110.1 and 110.2**).

DIAGNOSIS

History and Physical Examination Findings

The history and physical examinations (described above) provide important initial information in patients with CHD and suspected PAH. PAH can develop at any age of a CHD patient's life. In some cases, PAH develops independently of the cardiac defect or after its repair in the absence of significant hemodynamic impairment.[29] Besides a detailed cardiac history about the anatomical defect and its hemodynamics, it is important to obtain detailed information about the duration and onset of symptoms, comorbidities (lung disease, obstructive sleep apnea, connective tissue disease, social history [ie, drugs toxins, HIV]), and family history.

Electrocardiogram

Electrocardiographic changes are more common in advanced PH, but a normal electrocardiogram (ECG) does not rule out PAH. Common ECG abnormalities include P-pulmonale (tall P-wave in lead II), right axis deviation, right bundle branch block, and right ventricular hypertrophy.[30]

ECG changes do not correlate well with clinical parameters such as exercise capacity or 6-minute walk distance. However, certain ECG features carry prognostic information. Increasing amplitude of the P-wave in lead II over time is associated with a 2.8-fold increased risk of death over 6 years.[31] Supraventricular arrhythmias, such as sinus tachycardia, atrial flutter, and fibrillation are common, with an estimated prevalence of 15% to 27% in patients with advanced disease (New York Heart Association [NYHA] Class III-IV heart failure symptoms).[32] Atrial arrhythmias may limit cardiac output, and atrial flutter and fibrillation are associated with worse outcomes in PAH.[33] Prolongation of the QRS complex and ventricular arrhythmias are rare in PAH patients but associated with severe disease and poor outcome.[34]

Chest Radiograph

Most patients with PAH have an abnormal chest radiograph (CXR); however, a normal CXR does not exclude PAH. There is no correlation between the extent of abnormalities seen on CXR and hemodynamic or clinical parameters.[35] Common findings on CXR in patients with PAH are central pulmonary artery dilation with attenuation of peripheral pulmonary blood vessels (pruning) and right atrial and ventricular enlargement.[36] Hilar artery enlargement is common in PAH. The normal diameter of the right interlobar pulmonary artery is around 15 mm in women and 16 mm in men.[37] The transverse diameter of the left interlobar pulmonary artery is difficult to appreciate in the posteroanterior view. Evaluation of the pulmonary artery to vein ratio may help to distinguish between pulmonary arterial and pulmonary venous hypertension. Calcification of the pulmonary arteries may be seen in severe cases of PAH, such as Eisenmenger syndrome. The CXR can also be indicative of underlying CHD, suggesting location and anatomy of the defect and other causes of PH, such as interstitial lung disease, emphysema, chest wall deformities.

Computer Tomography

CT of the chest is a pivotal part of the diagnostic workup of patients with PH. The most commonly used CT modalities are contrast and high-resolution scanning. Contrast CT allows

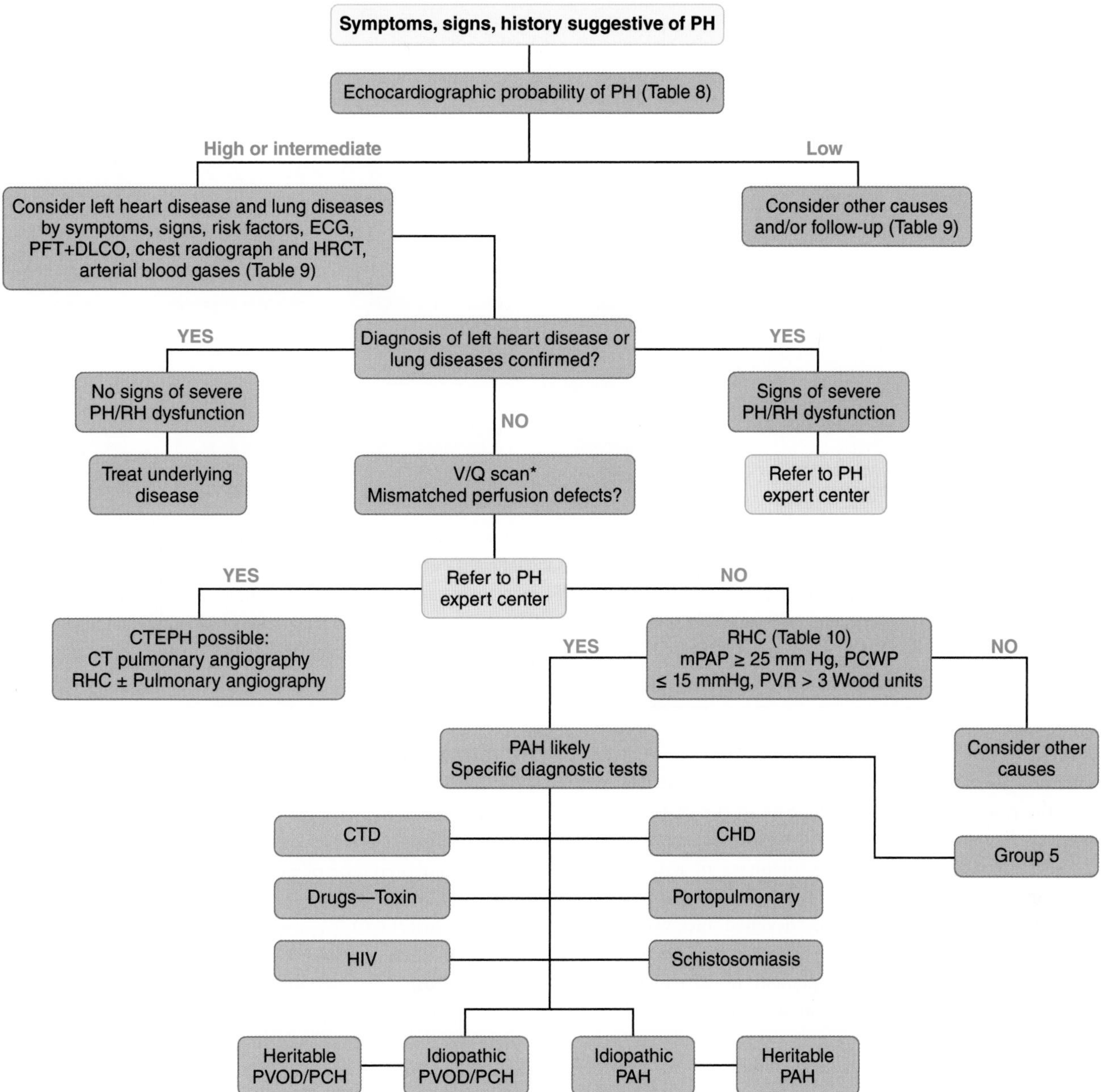

ALGORITHM 110.1 Diagnostic algorithm of PAH. CHD, congenital heart diseases; CT, computed tomography; CTD, connective tissue disease; CTEPH, chronic thromboembolic pulmonary hypertension; DLCO, carbon monoxide diffusing capacity; ECG, electrocardiogram; HIV, human immunodeficiency virus; HRCT, high resolution CT; mPAP, mean pulmonary arterial pressure; PAH, pulmonary arterial hypertension; PCWP, pulmonary capillary wedge pressure; PFT, pulmonary function tests; PH, pulmonary hypertension; PVOD/PCH, pulmonary veno-occlusive disease or pulmonary capillary hemangiomatosis; PVR, pulmonary vascular resistance; RHC, right heart catheterization; RV, right ventricular; V/Q ventilation/perfusion. *CT pulmonary angiography alone may miss diagnosis of chronic thromboembolic pulmonary hypertension. (From Galiè N, Humbert M, Vachiery JL, et al.; ESC Scientific Document Group. 2015 ESC/ERS Guidelines for the diagnosis and treatment of pulmonary hypertension: The Joint Task Force for the Diagnosis and Treatment of Pulmonary Hypertension of the European Society of Cardiology (ESC) and the European Respiratory Society (ERS): Endorsed by: Association for European Paediatric and Congenital Cardiology (AEPC), International Society for Heart and Lung Transplantation (ISHLT). *Eur Heart J.* 2016;37(1):67-119. Reproduced by permission of European Society of Cardiology & European Respiratory Society.)

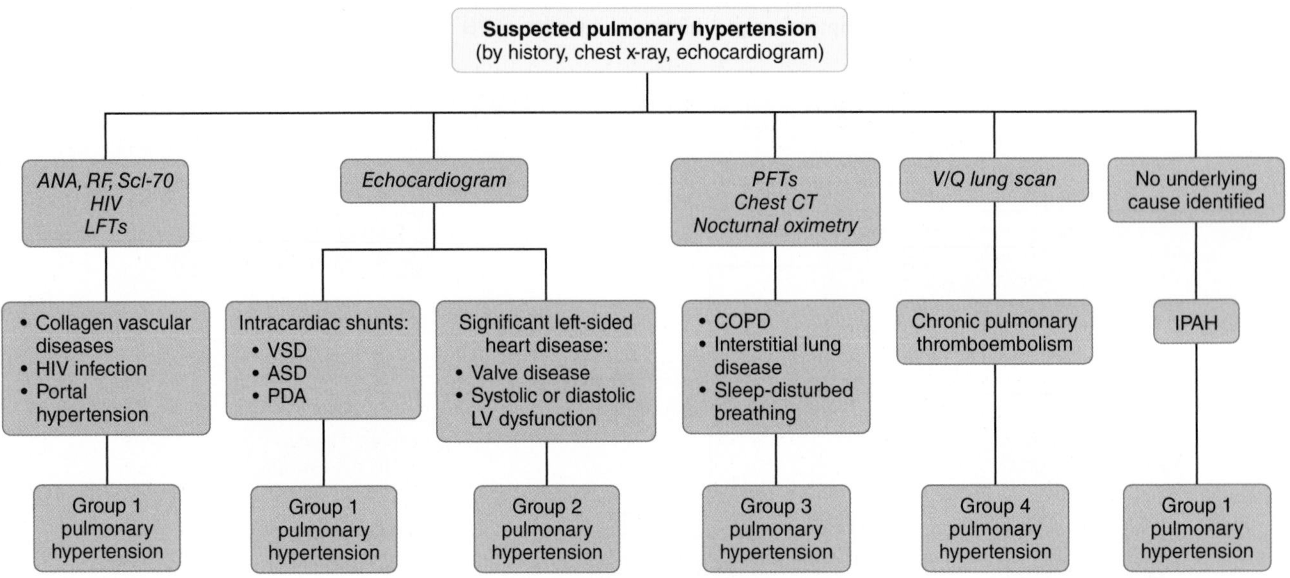

ALGORITHM 110.2 Suspected pulmonary hypertension algorithm. ANA, antinuclear antibodies; ASD, atrial septal defects; COPD, chronic obstructive pulmonary disease; CT, computed tomography; HIV, human immunodeficiency virus; IPAH, idiopathic pulmonary arterial hypertension; LV, left ventricular; LFT, liver function tests; PDA, patent ductus arteriosus; PFT, pulmonary function tests; RF, rheumatoid factor; Scl-70, Serum anti-topoisomerase antibody; V/Q, ventilation/perfusion; VSD, ventricular septal defects. (Republished with permission of McGraw Hill LLC from Kasper DL, Fauci AS, Hauser SL, eds., et al. *Harrison's Manual of Medicine.* 19th ed. New York, NY: McGraw-Hill, 2016:699-704; permission conveyed through Copyright Clearance Center, Inc.)

assessment of the pulmonary vasculature and right ventricle. Enlargement of the pulmonary artery or right ventricle may suggest the existence of PH. An increase in the main pulmonary artery diameter above 29 mm is highly suggestive of PH, as is the main PA:ascending aorta diameter or a segmental artery:bronchus ratio of less than 1.[38] An elevated right ventricle:left ventricular volume ratio, deviated intraventricular septum, and contrast regurgitation into the hepatic veins are common features of PH.[39] Enlargement of left-sided heart chambers is a marker of PH associated with left heart disease (Group 2 PH).[40]

Contrast CT scanning is also important to evaluate chronic thromboembolic pulmonary hypertension (CTEPH) (Group 4 PH). Although ventilation-perfusion (V/Q) scan is the gold standard, multidetector CT scanning is noninferior to V/Q scanning for diagnosis of CTEPH.[41]

Calcification of the pulmonary arteries observed on a noncontrast CT was initially thought to be a feature of severe PAH in patients with Eisenmenger syndrome.[39] More recently, it was shown that pulmonary artery calcification can be seen in patients with other forms of PAH and is associated with poor outcome.[42] Noncontrast CT may help narrow the diagnosis of PH, especially if underlying lung disease, such as interstitial lung disease, chronic obstructive lung disease, scleroderma, and sarcoidosis is suspected. The presence of interlobular septal thickening, centrilobular ground-glass opacities, and lymphadenopathy on CT should raise suspicion to consider PH mimics such as pulmonary venous obstructive disease and pulmonary capillary hemangiomatosis.[39]

Pulmonary Function Testing

PFT findings in patients with PAH are nonspecific: obstructive and restrictive defects have been described.[43,44] Reduction in diffusing capacity of carbon monoxide (DLCO) is an independent predictor of poor outcome and associated with poor functional capacity in patients with PAH.[45] However, reduction in DLCO is commonly seen in patients with other conditions such as parenchymal lung disease (emphysema, interstitial lung disease) and pulmonary vascular obstructive disease. Polysomnography is recommended in patients in whom sleep-disordered breathing, such as sleep apnea, is suspected. Nocturnal hypoxemia is highly prevalent in patients with PAH (up to 80%).[46] Vice versa, the prevalence of PH in sleep-disordered breathing is estimated to range between 17% and 34%.[47]

Echocardiography

Transthoracic echocardiography (TTE) is a useful screening tool for PH and allows assessment of the right heart and hemodynamics over time. TTE can be especially useful in identifying undiagnosed CHD patients. Echocardiographic signs suggestive of PH are increased right ventricular size (right:left ventricle basal diameter ratio >1), flattening of the interventricular septum in systole and/or diastole, inferior vena caval diameter >21 mm with decreased inspiratory collapse (<50%), and right atrial end-systolic area >18 cm^2.[48]

Many other useful echocardiographic measurements can be obtained in patients with PH and CHD. Right ventricular systolic pressure is derived from the peak tricuspid regurgitation velocity using continuous-wave Doppler. However, peak tricuspid regurgitation velocity can significantly underestimate or overestimate right ventricular systolic pressure and cannot be used to exclude a diagnosis of PH or stratify its severity. Right atrial pressure can be estimated based on inferior vena cava diameter and collapsibility. TTE can help in evaluating the cause of PH, especially in PAH-CHD, where the location and anatomy of a cardiac defect can be characterized. Longitudinal assessment of right ventricular function has important prognostic value, and several TTE parameters have been shown to correlate with functional class, 6-minute walk distance, and survival in PAH.[49] Similarly, right-heart functional parameters (ie, tricuspid annular plane systolic excursion, right ventricular effective systolic to diastolic duration, right atrial area, right atrial to left atrial ratio) predict outcome in patients with Eisenmenger physiology.[50]

MANAGEMENT OF PATIENTS WITH PAH-CHD

Medical therapies for PAH have evolved substantially over the last decades. PAH-targeted therapies now consist of multiple inhaled, oral, subcutaneous, or intravenous therapies targeting the phosphodiesterase, guanylate cyclase, and endothelin or prostacyclin pathways (**Algorithm 110.3**). Other treatment targets are currently under investigation.

Growing evidence exists that PAH-targeted therapy can be beneficial in PAH-CHD. PAH patients with an inadequate response to one therapy may have functional improvement when switched to an alternative class of medications that affect different targets in the same signaling pathway.[51]

However, the PAH-CHD patient population is challenging to treat owing to the heterogeneity and complexity of their cardiac lesions. Few randomized, controlled trials have investigated the effects of PAH-targeted therapy in prespecified PAH-CHD populations. With most clinical trials of targeted therapy, patients with PAH-CHD represented a minority of the overall patient population studied. Consequently, the results of these clinical trials should not be extrapolated broadly to the PAH-CHD population. However, PAH patients with coincidental small CHD and patients with PAH after shunt correction are thought to be pathophysiologic similar to patients with idiopathic PAH. It is therefore recommended to treat these patients according to current PAH guidelines.

Prostacyclins

One aim of PAH-targeted therapy is to improve hemodynamic and functional parameters associated with poor outcomes. Subcutaneous treprostinil—a prostacyclin vasodilator—has been shown in a randomized trial to improve exercise capacity, dyspnea, right-heart hemodynamics, and quality of life in PH patients, of whom 23% had PAH-CHD.[52] An oral prostacyclin analog, beraprost, was studied in a randomized trial in which 18% of the study population had PAH-CHD.[53] Improvement in 6-minute walk distance after 12 weeks of treatment was only observed in patients with idiopathic PAH, not in patients with PAH-CHD or other forms of PAH. Of note, patients with PAH-CHD received lower doses of beraprost, compared to patients with idiopathic pulmonary arterial hypertension (IPAH). A randomized, placebo-controlled trial with oral treprostinil monotherapy for 12 weeks that included patients with PAH-CHD (6% in the verum, and 4% in the placebo group) was associated with improved exercise capacity.[54] In a small nonrandomized controlled trial, subcutaneous treprostinil as an add-on to bosentan therapy was studied in adult patients with advanced PAH-CHD.[55] Addition of treprostinil was associated with improved 6-minute walking distance, functional capacity, and hemodynamics.

Endothelin Receptor Antagonists

Bosentan has been studied in a randomized, double-blind, placebo-controlled trial (BREATHE-5) in 54 patients with Eisenmenger syndrome; patients with PDA and complex CHD were excluded. Compared with placebo, bosentan therapy was associated with improved right-heart hemodynamics and increased exercise capacity[56] with the positive effects maintained for up to 40 weeks. Conversely, the Macitentan in Eisenmenger Syndrome to Restore Exercise Capacity (MAESTRO) study[57] did not show improvement in exercise capacity or functional class with macitentan versus placebo. Although both are endothelin receptor antagonists (ERAs), it is not entirely clear why bosentan but not macitentan was associated with improved exercise capacity and hemodynamics in patients with Eisenmenger syndrome. Different patient populations and affinities for endothelial receptor types A and B might have contributed to different effects on pulmonary vascular dilatation. Of note, another study showed that macitentan significantly reduced morbidity and mortality among patients with PAH in a dose-dependent manner; however, only 8% of these patients had repaired CHD and none had Eisenmenger syndrome.[58]

Phosphodiesterase-5 Inhibitors

Sildenafil, a short-acting phosphodiesterase-5 inhibitor (PDE-5I), was studied in a randomized controlled trial (RCT) that included 10 patients with Eisenmenger syndrome and was associated with improved exercise capacity, functional status, and right-heart hemodynamics.[59] Tadalafil, a long-acting PDE-5I, was studied in adult patients with PAH[60] or Eisenmenger syndrome.[61] It improved right-heart hemodynamics, functional class, exercise capacity and oxygen saturation, and decreased time to clinical worsening.

Guanylate Cyclase Stimulator

Riociguat, a guanylate cyclase stimulator, was assessed in a randomized trial that included patients with PAH-CHD (8% of the total patient population) and was found to improve right-heart hemodynamics, exercise capacity, and functional capacity and reduce time to clinical worsening.[62] A subsequent post hoc subgroup analysis including only PAH-CHD patients

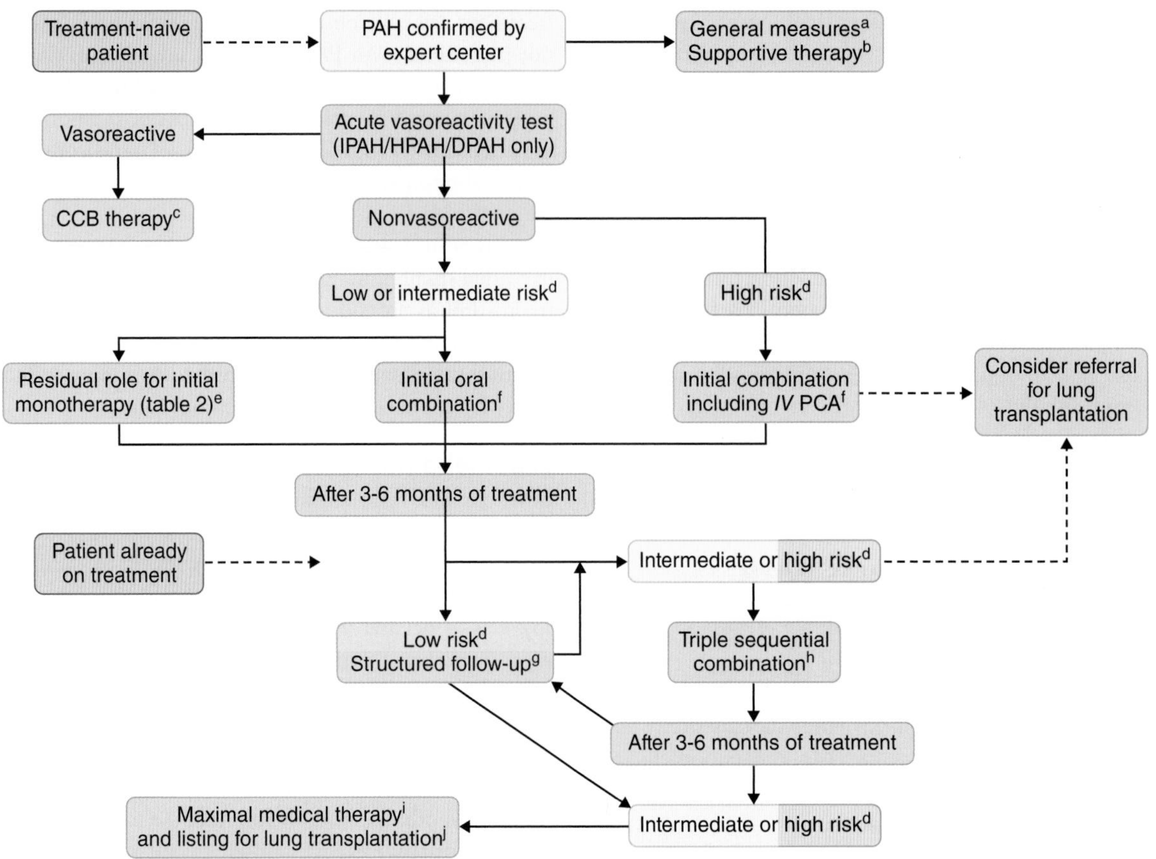

ALGORITHM 110.3 Treatment algorithm. CCB, calcium channel blocker; DPAH, drug-induced pulmonary arterial hypertension; HPAH, heritable pulmonary arterial hypertension; IPAH, idiopathic pulmonary arterial hypertension; PAH, pulmonary arterial hypertension; PCA, prostacyclin analogue; PH, pulmonary hypertension.

a: avoidance of pregnancy; regular healthcare maintenance; psychosocial support; supervised exercise training, in-flight O2 supplementation; in elective surgeries epidural rather than general anesthesia
b: diuretic treatment in patients with signs of RV failure; continuous long-term supplemental O2 if PaO2<60mmHg; oral anti-coagulants may be considered in patients with IPAH, HPAH, and DPAH; correction of anemia and/or iron status may be considered; use of angiotensin-2 receptor antagonists, beta-blockers and ivabradine is not recommended in patients with PAH unless required by co-morbidities
c: high dose of calcium channel blocker therapy is recommended in patients with IPAH, HPAH, DPAH who are responders to acute vaso-reactivity testing
d: see 2015 ESC/ERS PH guidelines Table 13
e: 2015 ESC/ERS PH guidelines Table 19
f: 2015 ESC/ERS PH guidelines Table 20
g: 2015 ESC/ERS PH guidelines Table 14
h: 2015 ESC/ERS PH guidelines Table 21
i: maximal medical therapy is considered triple combination therapy including parenteral therapy
j: 2015 ESC/ERS PH guidelines Table 22.

(From Galiè N, Channick RN, Frantz RP, et al. Risk stratification and medical therapy of pulmonary arterial hypertension. *Eur Respir J.* 2019;53(1):1801889. doi: 10.1183/13993003.01889-2018. Reproduced with permission of the © ERS 2021.)

from the same study confirmed the beneficial effects of Riociguat in this patient population.[63]

Combination Therapy

Current guidelines support upfront combination/dual therapy for patients with PAH. However, few patients with PAH-CHD were enrolled in the studies confirming the benefits of initial combination therapy. Hence, initial upfront combination therapy cannot be recommended for PAH-CHD patients.[64]

In patients with PAH treated with an ERA or PDE5-I, the addition of oral treprostinil did not improve exercise capacity.[65] In this study, only 6% of the patients had PAH-CHD. An RCT in Eisenmenger syndrome patients showed improved oxygen saturation when sildenafil (a PDE-5I) was added to bosentan (an ERA); however, it did not improve walking distance, functional class, or hemodynamics.[66] The addition of bosentan to sildenafil was studied in a randomized placebo-controlled trial including 20 adult patients (6% of the total study population) with PAH-CHD 2 years after repair.[67] The addition of bosentan was associated with improved 6-minute walking distance and decreased levels of NT-proBNP, but not with time to clinical worsening or mortality after 16 weeks. An RCT studying the effect of adding tadalafil to the ERA ambrisentan in clinically stable patients—including 6% of PAH-CHD after repair—found improvements in exercise capacity with combination therapy, with fewer patients experiencing clinical worsening during the 16-week study period.[68]

Two retrospective studies found beneficial effects of PAH-targeted therapy—mono or combination therapy—on exercise oxygen saturation and survival in patients with Eisenmenger syndrome.[8,69] Multiple smaller, nonrandomized trials of combination therapy in patients with Eisenmenger syndrome have provided mixed results in regard to 6-minute walk distance, functional class, biomarker levels, and hemodynamics.[70]

EISENMENGER SYNDROME

Eisenmenger syndrome occurs when a long-standing left-to-right cardiac shunt caused by a congenital heart defect (ie, VSD, PDA, aortopulmonary window, or less commonly ASD) leads to excessive pulmonary circulation and vascular damage that triggers a cascade of cellular and proliferative responses (ie, intimal and medial hypertrophy, thrombosis and formation of neovascularization), resulting in PH with systemic-level pulmonary arterial pressures, high pulmonary vascular resistance (>10 Wood units), and reversal of the shunt into a cyanotic right-to-left shunt.[71]

Presentation

Most patients with Eisenmenger syndrome have impaired exercise tolerance and exertional dyspnea. Palpitations are common and most often result from atrial fibrillation or flutter. As erythrocytosis (caused by arterial desaturation) develops, symptoms of hyperviscosity (visual disturbances, fatigue, headache, dizziness, and paresthesias) can appear. Patients with Eisenmenger syndrome can experience hemoptysis, bleeding complications, cerebrovascular accidents, brain abscess, syncope, and sudden death.

Examination

Patients with Eisenmenger syndrome typically have central cyanosis, digital clubbing, a right parasternal heave (owing to right ventricular hypertrophy), and a prominent pulmonic component of the second heart sound. The murmur caused by a VSD, PDA, or ASD disappears when Eisenmenger syndrome develops.

Imaging Studies

The chest x-ray often reveals normal heart size, prominent central pulmonary arteries, and diminished vascular markings (pruning) of the peripheral vessels. On TTE, evidence of right ventricular pressure overload and PH is present. The underlying cardiac defect can usually be visualized, although shunting across the defect may be difficult to demonstrate by Doppler because of the low jet velocity. If TTE is nondiagnostic, CMRI may demonstrate the magnitude and direction of the cardiac shunt and systolic function of the ventricles.

SPECIAL CONSIDERATIONS

Care of these patients requires attention to hyperviscosity, noncardiac procedures, contraception, paradoxical emboli, endocarditis prophylaxis, systemic vasodilatation, and stroke prevention.

Hyperviscosity

Phlebotomy with isovolumic replacement should be performed in patients with moderate or severe symptoms of hyperviscosity; however, it should not be performed in asymptomatic or mildly symptomatic patients regardless of the hematocrit. Repeated phlebotomy can result in iron deficiency, which can worsen the symptoms of hyperviscosity, because iron-deficient erythrocytes are less deformable than iron-replete ones. Anticoagulants and antiplatelet agents should be avoided because they exacerbate the hemorrhagic diathesis.

Noncardiac Surgery

Patients with Eisenmenger syndrome who are undergoing noncardiac surgery require meticulous management of anesthesia, with attention to maintenance of systemic vascular resistance, minimization of blood loss, and intravascular volume depletion, and prevention of iatrogenic paradoxical embolization. In preparation for noncardiac surgery, prophylactic phlebotomy (usually of 1-2 units of blood, with isovolumic replacement) is recommended for patients with a hematocrit greater than 65% to reduce the likelihood of perioperative hemorrhagic and thrombotic complications. Laparoscopic surgery using carbon dioxide for insufflation can cause the serum pH to decrease, which in turn constricts the pulmonary vasculature and can worsen right-to-left shunting.

Pregnancy and Contraception

Pregnancy is contraindicated for women with Eisenmenger syndrome, given the high risk of maternal mortality. One study demonstrated a 65% incidence of cardiac events, 48% incidence of heart failure, and 10% maternal mortality rate in pregnant Eisenmenger syndrome patients. Appropriate contraception should be recommended to patients of childbearing age. Progestin-only contraceptive methods are preferable, as estrogen is prothrombotic and may facilitate microthrombi in the pulmonary vasculature and worsening PAH. Patients may inquire about egg retrieval and surrogacy; however, prothrombotic risks are associated with the high levels of estrogen administration required for egg retrieval. In this situation, donor egg options or adoption may provide safer avenues for family planning.

Paradoxical Emboli

When venous lines are placed in the patient with Eisenmenger syndrome, air, thrombus, or bacteria may travel directly to the arterial circulation without the protective barrier of the lungs as a result of the right-to-left shunting. Vigilance with any peripheral or central venous access is paramount to prevent air embolism; in-line, bubble filters may provide a false sense of security.

Endocarditis

Endocarditis prophylaxis for regular dental cleaning and procedures in these patients is crucial. A high index of suspicion for endocarditis must be present in evaluating an Eisenmenger patient presenting with stroke, brain abscess, fever, or weight loss, for example.

Systemic Vasodilation

Medications that lower the systemic vascular resistance (ie, anesthetics, angiotensin-converting enzyme [ACE] inhibitors, or other medications to reduce afterload) can worsen right-to-left shunting. In addition, vigorous physical exercise can decrease systemic vascular resistance, increasing the shunt and worsening cyanosis. Patients should be counseled to avoid strenuous physical activity, particularly those with high isometric demands.

Stroke

Advanced pulmonary vasodilator therapies that require a chronic indwelling line carry a high risk of clot formation and associated strokes. If a patient requires a pacemaker or defibrillator, epicardial leads are essential. Iron deficiency is associated with an increased risk of stroke in patients with Eisenmenger syndrome because iron-deficient erythrocytes are less deformable than normal erythrocytes, and this lack of deformability can worsen hyperviscosity. Hence, iron deficiency should be treated appropriately in these patients. In addition, diuretic use can induce hemoconcentration and predispose to hyperviscosity syndrome. The routine use of antiplatelet agents or anticoagulation is not recommended as it exposes the patient to an increased risk of life-threatening bleeding without reducing the risk of stroke.

Prognosis

Although some patients with Eisenmenger syndrome expire during childhood or young adulthood, a sizable proportion survives to middle and old age. Compared to patients who develop PAH with a structurally normal heart, the Eisenmenger population had their heart defect throughout life, thus potentially facilitating adaptation of the right ventricle to pressure overload at an early age. Consequently, the survival among patients with Eisenmenger is better than for patients with idiopathic PAH. When death occurs, it is usually sudden, presumably caused by arrhythmias, but some patients die of heart failure, hemoptysis, brain abscess, or stroke. Predictors of death include patient age, pre-tricuspid location of the shunt (ie, ASD), lower oxygen saturation at rest, absence of sinus rhythm, low functional status (ie, NYHA, 6-minute walk test, or oxygen saturation with exercise), right ventricular function, conduction system disease (QRS duration ≥120 ms), and use of advanced therapy (ie, pulmonary arterial vasodilators).

Treatment

Supplemental oxygen and phlebotomy are often widely administered. However, studies show that oxygen therapy has neither short nor long-term beneficial effects, and repeated phlebotomies often lead to anemia, worsened exercise impairment, reduced quality of life, and an increased risk of thromboembolic events.

Pulmonary vasoactive disease targeting therapies (ie, ERAs, PDE-5I, or prostacyclin analog) are commonly prescribed (see **Table 110.4** for details). Multiple studies have shown these agents improve functional capacity, systemic arterial oxygen saturation, and pulmonary hemodynamics in patients with Eisenmenger syndrome. However, whether pulmonary vasoactive therapies improve their survival is unclear. Two retrospective, observational studies reported survival benefits in patients with Eisenmenger syndrome receiving advanced therapy compared to advanced therapy-naive patients. However, no prospective or randomized, controlled studies have confirmed this benefit. Hence, there is no convincing data or consensus that pharmacologic therapy improves the survival of patients with Eisenmenger syndrome.

Bosentan—an endothelin receptor antagonist—is currently the only pulmonary vasodilator with a Class I indication for Eisenmenger syndrome; however, experiences with other ERAs and with PDE-5I (ie, sildenafil and tadalafil) show favorable functional and hemodynamic results. Intravenous epoprostenol (a prostacyclin analog) has been used but is generally avoided owing to the risk of paradoxical embolism associated with indwelling central lines.

To date, the only definitive treatment for Eisenmenger syndrome is lung transplantation (in combination with shunt closure) or heart-lung transplantation. Patients with Eisenmenger syndrome appear to have a better posttransplantation prognosis than patients with idiopathic PAH or other types of CHD. Nevertheless, the paucity of donor organs and low survival rates post transplantation (ie, overall 1-year, 5-year, 10-year, and 15-year survival rates 84%, 70%, 56%, and 41%, respectively)[4] highlight the need for identification of patients most likely to benefit from transplantation.

FOLLOW-UP PATIENT CARE

Patients with Eisenmenger syndrome need to be followed regularly by a specialist in adult CHD as well as by a PH specialist.[72] In some instances, this may be the same physician.

Patients with Eisenmenger syndrome with symptomatic pulmonary vascular disease are categorized as physiologic stage D by the American College of Cardiology/American Heart Association (ACC/AHA) adult CHD management guideline, which suggests follow-up every 3 to 6 months with an appropriate adult CHD specialist. ECGs and echocardiograms should

TABLE 110.4 Selected Clinical Trials in – CHD-PAH and Eisenmenger (CHD only)

Class	Drug	Route of Administration	Typical Dose Range	Side Effects	Monitor
Endothelin Receptor Antagonist	Ambrisentan	Oral	5-10mg daily	Headache, flushing, peripheral edema, nasopharyngitis, pulmonary and peripheral edema	Anemia, liver dysfunction. Negative pregnancy test prior to and during treatment.
	Bosentan	Oral	62.mg twice daily, titrate up to 125mg twice daily		
	Macitentan	Oral	10mg daily		

Clinical Trials

Title	Trial Design	Population	PAH-targeted therapy	Main Findings
Evaluation of Macitentan in patients with Eisenmenger Syndrome results from the randomized, controlled MAESTRO Study, 2019	RCT, double-blind, placebo controlled, multi-center	226 patients with Eisenmenger syndrome aged ≥12 years (ES ASD, VSD, complex, Down syndrome)	16-week of macitentan 10 mg once daily, background PAH therapy was allowed	No △ in exercise capacity ↓NT-proBNP ↓PVR (in hemodynamic substudy with 39 patients)
Bosentan therapy in patients with Eisenmenger Syndrome: a multicenter, double-blind, randomized, placebo-controlled study, 2006[1]	RCT, double-blind, placebo controlled, multi-center	54 children and adults with ES, ASD>2cm, VSD>1cm; complex CHD were excluded	16 weeks of 62.5 – 125mg Bosentan twice daily	↓PVR, mPAP ↑6mwd No Δ in SpO2 ↑6mwd maintained after 24 weeks open label
Bosentan for the treatment of pulmonary arterial hypertension associated with congenital cardiac disease, 2006[2]	Retrospective, multi-center study	23 adult pts with ES due to ASD, VSD, PDA, Tetralogy of Fallot; 7 patients had corrective surgery	6 months of 62.5- 125mg of Bosentan twice daily; 5 patients were transitioned from treprostinil and 1 from beraprost to Bosentan	↑WHO-FC ↑SpO2 ↓in Hb ↑6mwd (on those not on previous PAH therapy) No clinical deterioration in patients transitioned form Treprostinil or Beraprost to Bosentan No Δ in liver function
Impact of bosentan on exercise capacity in adults after the Fontan procedure: a randomized controlled trial, 2013	prospective, multi-center randomized open label trial	42 adult patients with Fontan circulation, 74% increased BNP	6 month of Bosentan 125mg twice daily, one group started Bosentan after 3 month Majority FC I-II	No △ in exercise capacity, NYHA-FC, NT-proBNP, peak VO2, ventricular morphology No reported △ in liver enzymes, 1 patient with anemia
Bosentan improves exercise capacity in adolescents and adults after Fontan operation The TEMPO, 2014	RCT, double-blind, placebo controlled, multi-center	75 pts, Fontan physiology, normal NT-proBNP	14 weeks of bosentan 62.5 mg twice daily for 2 weeks, followed by 125 mg twice daily for 12 weeks	↑Peak VO2 ↑exercise capacity ↑NYHA-fC ↑NT-proBNP No △ in liver enzymes, or ↓in Hb

(*Continued*)

TABLE 110.4 Selected Clinical Trials in – CHD-PAH and Eisenmenger (CHD only) (*Continued*)

Title	Trial Design	Population	PAH-targeted therapy	Main Findings
Bosentan for the treatment of pulmonary arterial hypertension associated with congenital cardiac disease, 20062	Retrospective multi-center study	23 adult pts with ES due to ASD, VSD, PDA, Tetralogy of Fallot; 7 patients had corrective surgery	6 months of 62.5- 125mg of Bosentan twice daily; 5 pts were transitioned from treprostinil and 1 from beraprost to Bosentan	↑WHO-FC ↑SpO2 ↓in Hb ↑6mwd (on those not on previous PAH therapy) No clinical deterioration in patients transitioned form Treprostinil or Beraprost to Bosentan No Δ in liver function
Initial experience with Bosentan therapy in patients with the Eisenmenger Syndrome, 2004[3]	Single center, retrospective	9 adult patients with ES (ASD, VSD, tetralogy of fallot)	62.5 to 125mg of Bosentan twice daily for 5 to 14 month (median follow up 9.5 month)	↓WHO-FC ↓SpO2 No Δ in liver function or Hb levels
Ambrisentan for pulmonary arterial hypertension due to congenital heart disease, 2011	Single center, retrospective	17 patients with ASD, VSD, repaired and unrepaired, Down-syndrome	Ambrisentan at 5 to 10mg daily, follow-up after 3,9,12 month	↑exercise capacity No△ in resting or SaO2 or exercise SaO2, No Δ in Hb
Long-term efficacy of Bosentan in treatment of pulmonary arterial hypertension in children, 2010[4]	Single center, retrospective	31 Children post CHD repair (), 28 with ES, 20 with down syndrome	1-3 years of 15 – 125mg Bosentan twice daily; other PAH therapies were allowed	↑6mwd only after one year No Δ in PVR, mPAP (only available in 19 patients) One pt with ↑ liver enzymes One pt with ES developed hypotension
Early experience of Macitentan for pulmonary arterial hypertension in adult congenital heart disease, 2017	Single center, prospective, non-randomized, partially cross over from PDE5i or Bosentan	15 patients with ASD, VSD, PDA, repaired and unrepaired	Not reported	↑6mwd ↓WHO-FC ↑SpO2 No Δ in liver function
From bosentan to macitentan for pulmonary arterial hypertension and adult congenital heart disease: Further improvement? 2016	Multi center, prospective observational study	40 adult patients, 75% ES, ASD, VSD, complex defects, repaired and unrepaired	6 month of Macitentan (dose not reported), after switching form Bosentan (24h washout period)	↓ WHO-FC ↓ NT-pro-BNP ↑ TAPSE No Δ in 6mwd No Δ in liver function

Class	Drug	Route of Administration	Typical Dose Range	Side Effects	Monitor
PDE-5 Inhibitor	Sildenafil	Oral	5-100mg 3 times daily	Hypotension, Flushing, dyspepsia, diarrhea, priapism	—
	Tadalafil	Oral	10-40mg daily		—

Clinical Trials

Title	Trial Design	Population	PAH-targeted therapy	Main Findings
Clinical efficacy of phosphodiesterase-5 inhibitor Tadalafil in Eisenmenger Syndrome— a randomized, placebo-controlled, double-blind crossover study, 2011	RCT double blind, cross-over, single center	28 adult ES patients, ASD, VSD, 1 patient with aorto-pulmonary window, no data on repair status	6 weeks of Tadalafil 40 mg daily, followed by cross-over after a washout period of 2 weeks	↑exercise capacity, ↓NYHA-FC, ↑SpO2 ↓PVR

TABLE 110.4 Selected Clinical Trials in – CHD-PAH and Eisenmenger (CHD only) (*Continued*)

Title	Trial Design	Population	PAH-targeted therapy	Main Findings
Effect of sildenafil on hemodynamic response to exercise and exercise capacity in Fontan patients, 2008	Prospective randomized, single center	27pts with fontan circulation	Baseline exercise test, 0.7 mg/kg body weight oral dose of sildenafil citrate (25 to 50mg) or no treatment one hour before second exercise test	↑ exercise capacity, ↑pulmonary blood flow ↑CI No Δ in SaO2
Impact of oral Sildenafil on exercise performance in children and young adults after the Fontan operation: a randomized, double-blind, placebo-controlled, crossover trial, 2011	double-blind, placebo-controlled, crossover trial	28 children and adult patients with Fontan circulation	6 weeks of Sildenafil 20mg 3 times daily	↑ventilatory efficiency ↑VO2 in subgroup with elevated BNP No serious adverse events reported
Oral sildenafil treatment for Eisenmenger syndrome: a prospective, open-label, multicenter study, 2011	Prospective open-label, multicenter	84 adult ES ASD, VSD, PDA	12 month Sildenafil 20mg 3 times daily	↑exercise capacity, ↑resting SpO2, ↓mPAP, ↓PVR
The efficacy and safety of Sildenafil in patients with pulmonary arterial hypertension associated with the different types of congenital heart disease, 2011	prospective, open label, multi-center trial	55 pts with CHD ASD, VSD, PDA	12-weeks of Sildenafil 25mg 3 times daily	↑ exercise capacity ↓PVR No Δ in SVR ↑SpO2 (ASD group only)
Quality of life and functional capacity can be improved in patients with Eisenmenger syndrome with oral sildenafil therapy, 2010	Prospective open-label, single center	12 pts with ES, VSD, truncus arteriosus, TPGA, ASD, PDA, pulmonary atresia with VSD	3 month of Sildenfil 20mg 3 times daily	↑QoL ↓NYHA-FC ↑exercise capacity
Effects of chronic sildenafil in patients with Eisenmenger syndrome versus idiopathic pulmonary arterial hypertension, 2006	prospective open-label study	7 adult patients with ES (ASD, VSD	6 month Sildenafil, starting at 25 mg 12 hourly and increasing to 25 mg to 50mg 8 hourly as tolerated	↑NYHA-FC, ↑PBF ↓ mPAP ↓PVR ↓cyanosis
Role of oral sildenafil in severe pulmonary arterial hypertension: clinical efficacy and dose response relationship, 2006	non-randomized and non-placebo-controlled prospective study	21 ES (children and adults), ASD, VSD, PDA, ASD-VSD	10 weeks of Sildenfail 12.5mg 3 times daily, up titrated every 2weeks to max tolerated dose. Mean maximum dose achieved was 276.1±62.2 mg/day (range 75–300 mg/day).	↑NYHA-FC ↑ exercise capacity ↓PVR ↑CI ↑SpO2 Minimal side effects
Phosphodiesterase-5 inhibitor in Eisenmenger Syndrome a preliminary observational study, 2006	Observational	16 adult patients with ES ASD, VSD, PDA	Single dose of Tadalafil 1mg/kg up to 40mg 90 minutes before second hemodynamic assessment, the same dose was then continued daily for 12 weeks, and the patients were restudied	↑SpO2 ↑ NYHA-FC ↑exercise capacity ↓PVR No significant side effects

(*Continued*)

TABLE 110.4 Selected Clinical Trials in – CHD-PAH and Eisenmenger (CHD only) (*Continued*)

Title	Trial Design	Population	PAH-targeted therapy	Main Findings
A randomized, placebo-controlled, double-blind, crossover study to evaluate the efficacy of oral sildenafil therapy in severe pulmonary artery hypertension, 2006	Single center, randomized, double blind placebo-controlled crossover	10 patients with Eisenmenger	6 weeks of sildenafil 25mg 3 times daily if <30kg 50 mg 3 times daily if >30kg	↑6mwd ↓mPAP ↓WHO-FC ↑exercise duration No △ in systemic blood pressure
Impact of Sildenafil on survival of patients with Eisenmenger Syndrome, 2013	Single center observational	121 Adult patients with Eisenmenger (ASD, VSD, complex defects), 29 received Sildenafil	3-4 month of Sildenafil, dose not specified	↑6mwd ↓Hb ↓mPAP, PVR, HR ↑Survival (only in patients with WHO-FC I or II)

Class	Drug	Route of Administration	Typical Dose Range	Side Effects	Monitor
Guanylate Cyclase Stimulator	Riociguat	Oral	1.5-2.5mg 3 times daily	Headache, dizziness, nausea	Concomitant use with a PDE-5i carries risk of hypotension/death. Negative pregnancy test prior to and during treatment.

Clinical Trials

Title	Trial Design	Population	PAH-targeted therapy	Main Findings
Riociguat for pulmonary arterial hypertension associated with congenital heart disease, 2015	Post hoc subgroup analysis of the multi center randomized placebo controlled study (from PATENT1 and 2)	35 adult patients with CHD post repair (ASD, VSD, PDA)	12 weeks to 2 years of 1.5mg or 2.5mg of Riociguat	↑6mwd ↓WHO-FC ↓PVR ↓NT-pro-BNP Benefits sustained at 2 years

Class	Drug	Route of Administration	Typical Dose Range	Side Effects	Monitor
Synthetic Prostacyclin	Epoprostenol	IV	1-40+ ng/kg/min	Headache, jaw pain, nasopharyngitis, flushing, rash, arthralgias, nausea, vomiting, diarrhea, bleeding Subcutaneous or intravenous injection infusion site pain and infection	—
Prostacyclin Analogues	Iloprost	Inhaled	2.5-5yg 6 to 9 times daily		—
	Treprostinil	IV, subcutaneous, oral, inhaled	IV: 1-100+ ng/kg/min SQ: 1.25-100+ ng/kg/min Oral: 0.25-16mg twice daily Inhaled: 6yg 3-9 four times per day		Liver and kidney dysfunction
	Beraprost	Oral	—		—
	Selexipag	Oral	—		Liver function

TABLE 110.4 Selected Clinical Trials in – CHD-PAH and Eisenmenger (CHD only) (*Continued*)

Clinical Trials				
Title	**Trial Design**	**Population**	**PAH-targeted therapy**	**Main Findings**
Effects of inhaled Iloprost on congenital heart disease with Eisenmenger Syndrome, 2012	retrospective nonrandomized	12 adult patients with ES (VSD, ASD, ASD+VSD, PDA)	Inhaled Iloprost 10µg/dose six-times per day followed up to six month	↑ exercise capacity ↑NYHA-FC ↑SpO2 ↓mPAP (trend)
Effects of Inhaled Iloprost on exercise capacity, quality of life, and cardiac function in patients with pulmonary arterial hypertension secondary to congenital heart disease (the Eisenmenger Syndrome) (from the EIGER study), 2013	prospective, multicenter, single-arm trial, no placebo	13 adult patients with pts (univentricular heart, PDA, ASD, VSD, repaired and unrepaired	24 weeks of inhaled Iloprost at 2.5yg twice daily, up titrated to 4-6 times daily if tolerated (11 out of 13 achieved target dose of 10yg/day)	↑6mwd ↑QoL No sig △ TTE, NT-pro-BNP, SBP, Hb
Long-term Prostacyclin for pulmonary hypertension with associated congenital heart defects, 1999	Prospective, multicenter, no placebo	13 pts with PH ES ASD VSD, TPGA, PDA, papvr, aorto-pulmonary window	24 weeks of inhaled Iloprost from 2.5µg – 10µg 4-6 times per day	↑exercise capacity ↑Qol ↑RV myocardial performance index No △ in mPAP or PVR
Usefulness of epoprostenol therapy in the severely ill adolescent/adult with Eisenmenger physiology, 2003	Single-center, retrospective	8 adult and adolescent patients with Eisenmenger (ASD, VSD, PDA, complex defects), repaired and unrepaired.	3 month of intravenous epoprostenol at 7 to 20ng/kg/min	↑6mwd ↓WHO-FC ↑SpO2 ↓Hb ↓PVR
Long-term effects of continuous prostacyclin therapy in adults with pulmonary hypertension associated with congenital heart disease, 2013	Single-center, retrospective	9 adult patients with ASD, TGA, pre- and post-repair	One year of Prostacyclin therapy. 4 patients on IV Epoprostenol (22 – 32ng/kg/min), 2 patients on IV treprostinil (76- 82ng/kg/min), 2 patients on SC treprostinil (56- 76ng/kg/min), 3 patients on additional PDE5i	↓mPAP, No △ in PVR or CO, WHO-FC, SBP, NT-pro-BNP, ↑PA% ↑METs ↓GFR
Subcutaneous treprostinil in congenital heart disease-related pulmonary arterial hypertension, 2017	Three-center observational cohort study	32 adult patients with ASD, VSD, pulmonary atresia, complex defect, pre- and post-repair 22 with ES	6-12 month of SC treprostinil (average dose 17-31ng/kg/min) 6 patients on combination therapy with ERA and PDE5i	↑6mwd ↓WHO-FC ↓BNP ↑SpO2 (in ES) ↓mPAP ↓PVR ↑CO

(*Continued*)

TABLE 110.4 Selected Clinical Trials in – CHD-PAH and Eisenmenger (CHD only) (*Continued*)

Title	Trial Design	Population	PAH-targeted therapy	Main Findings
Effects of long-term iloprost treatment on right ventricular function in patients with Eisenmenger syndrome, 2016	Prospective multicenter, single arm study	11 adult patients with ES (VSD, PDA, ASD, Tetralogy of Fallot) 1 pt post-surgical repair	48 weeks of inhaled Iloprost from 2.5µg – 5µg 6-9 times per day as tolerated	↓mPAP, PVR ↑6mwd ↑TAPSE ↑SaO2 ↓WHO-FC ↓NT-pro-BNP No △ in Hb, SBP, GFR

Combination therapy

Title	Trial Design	Population	PAH-targeted therapy	Main Findings
Bosentan–sildenafil association in patients with congenital heart disease-related pulmonary arterial hypertension and Eisenmenger physiology, 2010	Single-center, open-label, singe arm, not placebo controlled	32 adult patients, 28 with Eisenmenger (VSD, AVC, ASD, single ventricle), unoperated.	6 month of Sildenafil 20mg 3 times daily, all patients were on Bosentan background therapy (62.5mg to 125mg twice daily)	↑6mwd ↓WHO-FC ↑SpO2 ↓NT-pro-BNP ↓PVR
Combination therapy with bosentan and sildenafil in Eisenmenger syndrome: a randomized, placebo-controlled, double-blinded trial, 2010	Single-center, RCT, placebo-controlled, cross over study	21 patients with Eisenmenger (Aorto-pulmonary window, VSD, ASD)	Bosentan 62.5mg twice daily for two weeks than 125mg twice daily, after 12 weeks randomized to Sildenafil 25m 3 times daily for two weeks than 50mg 3 times daily for 10 weeks or placebo.	Bosentan mono: ↑6mwd ↑pulmonary blood flow Sildenafil add on: No △ in 6mwd or hemodynamics ↑ SpO2 at rest
The effects of parenteral prostacyclin therapy as add-on treatment to oral compounds in Eisenmenger syndrome, 2019	Multi-center, retrospective cohort study	28 adult patients with Eisenmnenger (ASD, VSD)	All patients were on baseline PDE5i and ERA therapy, median follow up of 27 after SC or IV Epoprostenol at a median dose of 40ng/kg/min was added	↑ 6mwd ↓WHO-FC ↓NT-pro-BNP ↓mPAP, PVR, RAP No △ in SBP or SpO2
Improved survival among patients with eisenmenger syndrome receiving advanced therapy for pulmonary arterial hypertension, 2010	Retrospective, single center	229 adult patients with ES Repaired, unrepaired Pre-tricuspid Post-tricuspid Complex	Median follow up of 4 years of: ERA PDE5i Epoprostenol Combi (ERA+PDE5i)	↓mortality if on PAH therapy Improved hemodynamics (no details)
Pulmonary vasodilator therapy is associated with greater survival in eisenmenger syndrome, 2017	Multi-center, retrospective cohort study	253 adult patients with ES (ASD, VSD, PDA, complex lesions)	Median follow up of 9 years of : Bosentan + Sildenafil Macitentan + Sildenafil Macitentan + Tadalafil Selexipag + Prostacyclin Selexipag + Macitentan + Prostacyclin 50% combination therapy	↓mortality if on PAH therapy

TABLE 110.4 Selected Clinical Trials in – CHD-PAH and Eisenmenger (CHD only) (*Continued*)

Title	Trial Design	Population	PAH-targeted therapy	Main Findings
Effect of dual pulmonary vasodilator therapy in pulmonary arterial hypertension associated with congenital heart disease: a retrospective analysis, 2016[5]	Single center, retrospective study	30 adult patients with ASD, VSD, complex CHD, 3 with down syndrome	Mean treatment duration was 2.5 years with 62.5mg to 125mg Bosentan; if lack of clinical improvement or clinical worsening 25mg Sildenafil TWICE DAILY/3 times daily (up- titration possible) was added	↑6mwd Adding Sildenafil prevented further clinical deterioration in exercise capacity, but not 6mwd Bosentan was less effective in improving 6mwd in pts with Down syndrome

↑, increase; ↓, decrease; Δ, change; 6mwd, six-minute walking distance; ASD, atrial septal defect; AVC, atrioventricular canal; BID, twice a day; CHD, congenital heart disease; CI, cardiac index; CO, cardiac output; ERA, endothelin receptor antagonist; ES, Eisenmenger syndrome; GFR, glomerular filtration rate; Hb, hemoglobin; HR, heart rate; IV, intravenous; kg, kilograms; mcg, microgram; mg, milligram; METs, metabolic equivalents; mPAP, mean pulmonary artery pressure; ng, nanogram; NT-proBNP, n-terminal pro b-type natriuretic peptide; PAH, pulmonary arterial hypertension; PAPVR, partial anomalous pulmonary venous return; PBF, pulmonary blood flow; PDA, patent ductus arteriosus; PDE5i, phosphodiesterase 5 inhibitor; PVR, pulmonary vascular resistance; QoL, quality of life; RCT, randomized controlled trial; SaO_2, arterial oxygen content; SBP, systolic blood pressure; SC, subcutaneous; SVR, systemic vascular resistance; TAPSE, tricuspid annular plane systolic excursion; TGA, transposition of the great arteries; TID, three times per day; TTE, transthoracic echocardiogram; VO_2, maximum oxygen uptake; VSD, ventricular septal defect; WHO-FC, World Health Organization functional class.

be obtained at least annually, with an exercise test every 6 to 12 months.[72] We recommend that cross-sectional imaging—such as CMRI—be obtained approximately every 2 years or sooner if serial imaging is used to trend shunt flow. Cardiac catheterization should be obtained as clinically indicated, particularly if hemodynamics such as calculation of pulmonary vascular resistance or pulmonic and systemic blood flows are needed. The 6-minute walk test has traditionally been used to evaluate functional capacity in patients with Eisenmenger syndrome and is more commonly used than cardiopulmonary exercise testing, owing to its ease of administration and its traditional use in patients with other types of PAH. We suggest obtaining a 6-minute walk test prior to initiating vasodilator therapy and every 3 to 6 months afterward.

Owing to the often terminal nature of Eisenmenger syndrome, it is crucial for providers to provide adequate symptom management, and to facilitate timely discussions about patients' goals and values at the end of life. Palliative care can be involved for symptom management and to facilitate these discussions. Decisions about life-sustaining support and heart-lung transplantation eligibility are ideally made in the outpatient setting prior to a sudden clinical decompensation.

RESEARCH AND FUTURE DEVELOPMENTS

The current mainstay of PAH-targeted therapy is the pulmonary vasodilator. However, the pathobiology of PAH is complex and incompletely understood. Dysregulated pathways in PAH include transforming growth factor/bone-morphogenetic protein signaling, DNA damage, cellular growth factors, dysregulated metabolism, altered estrogen signaling, and inflammation. It is possible that the same pathways are dysregulated in patients with Eisenmenger syndrome. Many new treatment targets are currently under investigation to target bone-morphogenetic protein receptor signaling (FK506, sotatercept), ion channels (KCNK3), aquaporin, and neutrophil elastase (elafin).[73]

KEY POINTS

- ✔ Avoid routine phlebotomy and consider rehydration as the first line for hyperviscosity syndrome.
- ✔ Identify and treat iron deficiency with expeditious reassessment of the hematocrit in case there is a brisk, erythrocytic response to therapy.
- ✔ Tricuspid valve jet velocity in the setting of a large VSD, PDA, or aortopulmonary window may simply reflect systemic velocity and is not useful for estimating pulmonary artery pressures.
- ✔ Avoid indwelling leads or catheters owing to the risk of systemic embolization in the patient with Eisenmenger syndrome.
- ✔ Endocarditis prophylaxis is important with routine dental care.
- ✔ Renal function may be poorer than estimated by serum creatinine in the setting of cyanosis.
- ✔ In patients with Eisenmenger syndrome, vigilance to prevent air embolism is key with intravenous catheters even if an in-line air bubble filter is present.
- ✔ Avoid medications that reduce systemic vascular resistance in patients with Eisenmenger syndrome, as they increase right-to-left shunting and cyanosis.

REFERENCES

1. Simonneau G, Montani D, Celermajer DS, et al. Haemodynamic definitions and updated clinical classification of pulmonary hypertension. *Eur Respir J.* 2019;53(1):1801913. doi:10.1183/13993003.01913-2018
2. van Riel AC, Schuuring MJ, van Hessen ID, et al. Contemporary prevalence of pulmonary arterial hypertension in adult congenital heart disease following the updated clinical classification. *Int J Cardiol.* 2014;174:299-305. doi:10.1016/j.ijcard.2014.04.072
3. Lowe BS, Therrien J, Ionescu-Ittu R, et al. Diagnosis of pulmonary hypertension in the congenital heart disease adult population impact on outcomes. *J Am Coll Cardiol.* 2011;58:538-546. doi:10.1016/j.jacc.2011.03.033
4. Badesch DB, Raskob GE, Elliott CG, et al. Pulmonary arterial hypertension: baseline characteristics from the REVEAL Registry. *Chest.* 2010;137:376-387. doi:10.1378/chest.09-1140
5. Hoeper MM, Huscher D, Ghofrani HA, et al. Elderly patients diagnosed with idiopathic pulmonary arterial hypertension: results from the COMPERA registry. *Int J Cardiol.* 2013;168:871-880. doi:10.1016/j.ijcard.2012.10.026
6. Kopec G, Kurzyna M, Mroczek E, et al. Characterization of patients with pulmonary arterial hypertension: data from the Polish Registry of Pulmonary Hypertension (BNP-PL). *J Clin Med.* 2020;9(1):173. doi:10.3390/jcm9010173
7. Diller GP, Kempny A, Alonso-Gonzalez R, et al. Survival prospects and circumstances of death in contemporary adult congenital heart disease patients under follow-up at a large tertiary centre. *Circulation.* 2015;132:2118-2125. doi:10.1161/CIRCULATIONAHA.115.017202
8. Dimopoulos K, Inuzuka R, Goletto S, et al. Improved survival among patients with Eisenmenger syndrome receiving advanced therapy for pulmonary arterial hypertension. *Circulation.* 2010;121:20-25. doi:10.1161/CIRCULATIONAHA.109.883876
9. Dickinson MG, Bartelds B, Borgdorff MA, et al. The role of disturbed blood flow in the development of pulmonary arterial hypertension: lessons from preclinical animal models. *Am J Physiol Lung Cell Mol Physiol.* 2013;305:L1-L14. doi:10.1152/ajplung.00031.2013
10. Hopkins WE. The remarkable right ventricle of patients with Eisenmenger syndrome. *Coron Artery Dis.* 2005;16:19-25. doi:10.1097/00019501-200502000-00004
11. Budts W. Eisenmenger syndrome: medical prevention and management strategies. *Expert Opin Pharmacother.* 2005;6:2047-2060. doi:10.1517/14656566.6.12.2047
12. Kempny A, Hjortshoj CS, Gu H, et al. Predictors of death in contemporary adult patients with Eisenmenger syndrome: a multicenter study. *Circulation.* 2017;135:1432-1440. doi:10.1161/CIRCULATIONAHA.116.023033
13. Benza RL, Miller DP, Gomberg-Maitland M, et al. Predicting survival in pulmonary arterial hypertension: insights from the Registry to Evaluate Early and Long-Term Pulmonary Arterial Hypertension Disease Management (REVEAL). *Circulation.* 2010;122:164-172. doi:10.1161/CIRCULATIONAHA.109.898122
14. Manes A, Palazzini M, Leci E, et al. Current era survival of patients with pulmonary arterial hypertension associated with congenital heart disease: a comparison between clinical subgroups. *Eur Heart J.* 2014;35:716-724. doi:10.1093/eurheartj/eht072
15. Gupta V, Tonelli AR, Krasuski RA. Congenital heart disease and pulmonary hypertension. *Heart Fail Clin.* 2012;8:427-445. doi:10.1016/j.hfc.2012.04.002
16. Papamichalis M, Xanthopoulos A, Papamichalis P, et al. Adult congenital heart disease with pulmonary arterial hypertension: mechanisms and management. *Heart Fail Rev.* 2020;25:773-794. doi:10.1007/s10741-019-09847-5
17. Nihill MR, McNamara DG. Magnification pulmonary wedge angiography in the evaluation of children with congenital heart disease and pulmonary hypertension. *Circulation.* 1978;58:1094-1106. doi:10.1161/01.cir.58.6.1094
18. Rabinovitch M, Haworth SG, Castaneda AR, et al. Lung biopsy in congenital heart disease: a morphometric approach to pulmonary vascular disease. *Circulation.* 1978;58:1107-1122. doi:10.1161/01.cir.58.6.1107
19. Heath D, Edwards JE. The pathology of hypertensive pulmonary vascular disease; a description of six grades of structural changes in the pulmonary arteries with special reference to congenital cardiac septal defects. *Circulation.* 1958;18:533-547. doi:10.1161/01.cir.18.4.533
20. Stacher E, Graham BB, Hunt JM, et al. Modern age pathology of pulmonary arterial hypertension. *Am J Respir Crit Care Med.* 2012;186:261-272. doi:10.1164/rccm.201201-0164OC
21. Austin ED, Loyd JE. The genetics of pulmonary arterial hypertension. *Circ Res.* 2014;115:189-202. doi:10.1161/CIRCRESAHA.115.303404
22. Roberts KE, McElroy JJ, Wong WP, et al. BMPR2 mutations in pulmonary arterial hypertension with congenital heart disease. *Eur Respir J.* 2004;24:371-374. doi:10.1183/09031936.04.00018604
23. Zhu N, Welch CL, Wang J, et al. Rare variants in SOX17 are associated with pulmonary arterial hypertension with congenital heart disease. *Genome Med.* 2018;10:56. doi:10.1186/s13073-018-0566-x
24. Malenfant S, Brassard P, Paquette M, et al. Compromised cerebrovascular regulation and cerebral oxygenation in pulmonary arterial hypertension. *J Am Heart Assoc.* 2017;6(10):e006126. doi:10.1161/JAHA.117.006126
25. de Jesus Perez VA, Haddad F, Vagelos RH, et al. Angina associated with left main coronary artery compression in pulmonary hypertension. *J Heart Lung Transplant.* 2009;28:527-530. doi:10.1016/j.healun.2008.12.008
26. Dorfmuller P, Gunther S, Ghigna MR, et al. Microvascular disease in chronic thromboembolic pulmonary hypertension: a role for pulmonary veins and systemic vasculature. *Eur Respir J.* 2014;44:1275-1288. doi:10.1183/09031936.00169113
27. Ossa Galvis MM, Bhakta RT, Tarmahomed A, et al. *Cyanotic heart disease. StatPearls [Internet].* StatPearls Publishing; 2021.
28. Pahal P, Goyal A. *Central and peripheral cyanosis. StatPearls [Internet].* StatPearls Publishing; 2021.
29. Galie N, Humbert M, Vachiery JL, et al. 2015 ESC/ERS Guidelines for the diagnosis and treatment of pulmonary hypertension: The Joint Task Force for the Diagnosis and Treatment of Pulmonary Hypertension of the European Society of Cardiology (ESC) and the European Respiratory Society (ERS): Endorsed by: Association for European Paediatric and Congenital Cardiology (AEPC), International Society for Heart and Lung Transplantation (ISHLT). *Eur Heart J.* 2016;37:67-119. doi:10.1093/eurheartj/ehv317
30. Sun PY, Jiang X, Gomberg-Maitland M, et al. Prolonged QRS duration: a new predictor of adverse outcome in idiopathic pulmonary arterial hypertension. *Chest.* 2012;141:374-380. doi:10.1378/chest.10-3331
31. Bossone E, Paciocco G, Iarussi D, et al. The prognostic role of the ECG in primary pulmonary hypertension. *Chest.* 2002;121:513-518. doi:10.1378/chest.121.2.513
32. Drakopoulou M, Nashat H, Kempny A, et al. Arrhythmias in adult patients with congenital heart disease and pulmonary arterial hypertension. *Heart.* 2018;104:1963-1969. doi:10.1136/heartjnl-2017-312881
33. Olsson KM, Nickel NP, Tongers J, et al. Atrial flutter and fibrillation in patients with pulmonary hypertension. *Int J Cardiol.* 2013;167:2300-2305. doi:10.1016/j.ijcard.2012.06.024
34. Rich JD, Thenappan T, Freed B, et al. QTc prolongation is associated with impaired right ventricular function and predicts mortality in pulmonary hypertension. *Int J Cardiol.* 2013;167:669-676. doi:10.1016/j.ijcard.2012.03.071
35. Galie N, Humbert M, Vachiery JL, et al. 2015 ESC/ERS Guidelines for the diagnosis and treatment of pulmonary hypertension: The Joint Task Force for the Diagnosis and Treatment of Pulmonary Hypertension of the European Society of Cardiology (ESC) and the European Respiratory Society (ERS): Endorsed by: Association for European Paediatric and Congenital Cardiology (AEPC), International Society for Heart and Lung Transplantation (ISHLT). *Eur Respir J.* 2015;46:903-975. doi:10.1183/13993003.01032-2015
36. Pena E, Dennie C, Veinot J, et al. Pulmonary hypertension: how the radiologist can help. *Radiographics.* 2012;32:9-32. doi:10.1148/rg.321105232

37. Chang CH. The normal roentgenographic measurement of the right descending pulmonary artery in 1,085 cases and its clinical application. II. Clinical application of the measurement of the right descending pulmonary artery in the radiological diagnosis of pulmonary hypertensions from various causes. *Nagoya J Med Sci.* 1965;28:67-80.
38. Shen Y, Wan C, Tian P, et al. CT-base pulmonary artery measurement in the detection of pulmonary hypertension: a meta-analysis and systematic review. *Medicine (Baltimore).* 2014;93:e256. doi:10.1097/MD.0000000000000256
39. Rajaram S, Swift AJ, Condliffe R, et al. CT features of pulmonary arterial hypertension and its major subtypes: a systematic CT evaluation of 292 patients from the ASPIRE Registry. *Thorax.* 2015;70:382-387. doi:10.1136/thoraxjnl-2014-206088
40. Aviram G, Rozenbaum Z, Ziv-Baran T, et al. Identification of pulmonary hypertension caused by left-sided heart disease (World Health Organization Group 2) based on cardiac chamber volumes derived from Chest CT imaging. *Chest.* 2017;152:792-799. doi:10.1016/j.chest.2017.04.184
41. Remy-Jardin M, Ryerson CJ, Schiebler ML, et al. Imaging of pulmonary hypertension in adults: a position paper from the Fleischner Society. *Eur Respir J.* 2021;57(1):2004455. doi:10.1183/13993003.04455-2020
42. Tanguay VF, Babin C, Giardetti G, et al. Enhanced pulmonary artery radiodensity in pulmonary arterial hypertension: a sign of early calcification? *Am J Respir Crit Care Med.* 2019;199:799-802. doi:10.1164/rccm.201806-1027LE
43. Meyer FJ, Ewert R, Hoeper MM, et al. Peripheral airway obstruction in primary pulmonary hypertension. *Thorax.* 2002;57:473-476. doi:10.1136/thorax.57.6.473
44. Sun XG, Hansen JE, Oudiz RJ, et al. Pulmonary function in primary pulmonary hypertension. *J Am Coll Cardiol.* 2003;41:1028-1035. doi:10.1016/s0735-1097(02)02964-9
45. Stadler S, Mergenthaler N, Lange TJ. The prognostic value of DLCO and pulmonary blood flow in patients with pulmonary hypertension. *Pulm Circ.* 2019;9:2045894019894531. doi:10.1177/2045894019894531
46. Jilwan FN, Escourrou P, Garcia G, et al. High occurrence of hypoxemic sleep respiratory disorders in precapillary pulmonary hypertension and mechanisms. *Chest.* 2013;143:47-55. doi:10.1378/chest.11-3124
47. Sajkov D and McEvoy RD. Obstructive sleep apnea and pulmonary hypertension. *Prog Cardiovasc Dis.* 2009;51:363-370. doi:10.1016/j.pcad.2008.06.001
48. Rudski LG, Lai WW, Afilalo J, et al. Guidelines for the echocardiographic assessment of the right heart in adults: a report from the American Society of Echocardiography endorsed by the European Association of Echocardiography, a registered branch of the European Society of Cardiology, and the Canadian Society of Echocardiography. *J Am Soc Echocardiogr.* 2010;23:685-713; quiz 786-688. doi:10.1016/j.echo.2010.05.010
49. Forfia PR, Fisher MR, Mathai SC, et al. Tricuspid annular displacement predicts survival in pulmonary hypertension. *Am J Respir Crit Care Med.* 2006;174:1034-1041. doi:10.1164/rccm.200604-547OC
50. Moceri P, Dimopoulos K, Liodakis E, et al. Echocardiographic predictors of outcome in Eisenmenger syndrome. *Circulation.* 2012;126:1461-1468. doi:10.1161/CIRCULATIONAHA.112.091421
51. Hoeper MM, Simonneau G, Corris PA, et al. RESPITE: switching to riociguat in pulmonary arterial hypertension patients with inadequate response to phosphodiesterase-5 inhibitors. *Eur Respir J.* 2017;50(3):1602425. doi:10.1183/13993003.02425-2016
52. Simonneau G, Barst RJ, Galie N, et al. Continuous subcutaneous infusion of treprostinil, a prostacyclin analogue, in patients with pulmonary arterial hypertension: a double-blind, randomized, placebo-controlled trial. *Am J Respir Crit Care Med.* 2002;165:800-804. doi:10.1164/ajrccm.165.6.2106079
53. Galiè N, Humbert M, Vachiéry J-L, et al. Effects of beraprost sodium, an oral prostacyclin analogue, in patients with pulmonary arterial hypertension: a randomized, double-blind, placebo-controlled trial. *J Am Coll Cardiol.* 2002;39:1496-1502. doi:10.1016/s0735-1097(02)01786-2
54. Jing ZC, Parikh K, Pulido T, et al. Efficacy and safety of oral treprostinil monotherapy for the treatment of pulmonary arterial hypertension: a randomized, controlled trial. *Circulation.* 2013;127:624-633. doi:10.1161/CIRCULATIONAHA.112.124388
55. Skoro-Sajer N, Gerges C, Balint OH, et al. Subcutaneous treprostinil in congenital heart disease-related pulmonary arterial hypertension. *Heart.* 2018;104:1195-1199. doi:10.1136/heartjnl-2017-312143
56. Galie N, Beghetti M, Gatzoulis MA, et al. Bosentan therapy in patients with Eisenmenger syndrome: a multicenter, double-blind, randomized, placebo-controlled study. *Circulation.* 2006;114:48-54. doi:10.1161/CIRCULATIONAHA.106.630715
57. Gatzoulis MA, Landzberg M, Beghetti M, et al. Evaluation of macitentan in patients with Eisenmenger syndrome. *Circulation.* 2019;139:51-63. doi:10.1161/CIRCULATIONAHA.118.033575
58. Pulido T, Adzerikho I, Channick RN, et al. Macitentan and morbidity and mortality in pulmonary arterial hypertension. *N Engl J Med.* 2013;369:809-818. doi:10.1056/NEJMoa1213917
59. Singh TP, Rohit M, Grover A, et al. A randomized, placebo-controlled, double-blind, crossover study to evaluate the efficacy of oral sildenafil therapy in severe pulmonary artery hypertension. *Am Heart J.* 2006;151:851.e851-855. doi:10.1016/j.ahj.2005.09.006
60. Galie N, Brundage BH, Ghofrani HA, et al. Tadalafil therapy for pulmonary arterial hypertension. *Circulation.* 2009;119:2894-2903. doi:10.1161/CIRCULATIONAHA.108.839274
61. Mukhopadhyay S, Nathani S, Yusuf J, et al. Clinical efficacy of phosphodiesterase-5 inhibitor tadalafil in Eisenmenger syndrome—a randomized, placebo-controlled, double-blind crossover study. *Congenit Heart Dis.* 2011;6:424-431. doi:10.1111/j.1747-0803.2011.00561.x
62. Ghofrani HA, Galie N, Grimminger F, et al. Riociguat for the treatment of pulmonary arterial hypertension. *N Engl J Med.* 2013;369:330-340. doi:10.1056/NEJMoa1209655
63. Rosenkranz S, Ghofrani HA, Beghetti M, et al. Riociguat for pulmonary arterial hypertension associated with congenital heart disease. *Heart.* 2015;101:1792-1799. doi:10.1136/heartjnl-2015-307832
64. Galie N, Channick RN, Frantz RP, et al. Risk stratification and medical therapy of pulmonary arterial hypertension. *Eur Respir J.* 2019;53. doi:10.1183/13993003.01889-2018
65. Tapson VF, Torres F, Kermeen F, et al. Oral treprostinil for the treatment of pulmonary arterial hypertension in patients on background endothelin receptor antagonist and/or phosphodiesterase type 5 inhibitor therapy (the FREEDOM-C study): a randomized controlled trial. *Chest.* 2012;142:1383-1390. doi:10.1378/chest.11-2212
66. Iversen K, Jensen AS, Jensen TV, et al. Combination therapy with bosentan and sildenafil in Eisenmenger syndrome: a randomized, placebo-controlled, double-blinded trial. *Eur Heart J.* 2010;31:1124-1131. doi:10.1093/eurheartj/ehq011
67. McLaughlin V, Channick RN, Ghofrani HA, et al. Bosentan added to sildenafil therapy in patients with pulmonary arterial hypertension. *Eur Respir J.* 2015;46:405-413. doi:10.1183/13993003.02044-2014
68. Zhuang Y, Jiang B, Gao H, et al. Randomized study of adding tadalafil to existing ambrisentan in pulmonary arterial hypertension. *Hypertens Res.* 2014;37:507-512. doi:10.1038/hr.2014.28
69. Diller GP, Alonso-Gonzalez R, Dimopoulos K, et al. Disease targeting therapies in patients with Eisenmenger syndrome: response to treatment and long-term efficiency. *Int J Cardiol.* 2013;167:840-847. doi:10.1016/j.ijcard.2012.02.007
70. Condliffe R, Clift P, Dimopoulos K, et al. Management dilemmas in pulmonary arterial hypertension associated with congenital heart disease. *Pulm Circ.* 2018;8:2045894018792501. doi:10.1177/2045894018792501
71. Wood P. The Eisenmenger syndrome or pulmonary hypertension with reversed central shunt. *Br Med J.* 1958;2:755-762. doi:10.1136/bmj.2.5099.755
72. Stout KK, Daniels CJ, Aboulhosn JA, et al. 2018 AHA/ACC Guideline for the management of adults with congenital heart disease: executive summary: a report of the American College of Cardiology/American Heart Association Task Force on Clinical Practice Guidelines. *Circulation.* 2019;139:e637-e697. doi:10.1161/CIR.0000000000000602

73. Sitbon O, Gomberg-Maitland M, Granton J, et al. Clinical trial design and new therapies for pulmonary arterial hypertension. *Eur Respir J*. 2019;53(1):1801908. doi:10.1183/13993003.01908-2018
74. Galie N, Beghetti M, Gatzoulis MA, et al. Bosentan therapy in patients with Eisenmenger syndrome: a multicenter, double-blind, randomized, placebo-controlled study. *Circulation* 2006; 114: 48-54. 2006/06/28. DOI: 10.1161/CIRCULATIONAHA.106.630715.
75. Kotlyar E, Sy R, Keogh AM, et al. Bosentan for the treatment of pulmonary arterial hypertension associated with congenital cardiac disease. *Cardiol Young* 2006; 16: 268-274. 2006/05/27. DOI: 10.1017/S1047951106000114.
76. Christensen DD, McConnell ME, Book WM, et al. Initial experience with bosentan therapy in patients with the Eisenmenger syndrome. *Am J Cardiol* 2004; 94: 261-263. 2004/07/13. DOI: 10.1016/j.amjcard.2004.03.081.
77. Hislop AA, Moledina S, Foster H, et al. Long-term efficacy of bosentan in treatment of pulmonary arterial hypertension in children. *Eur Respir J* 2011; 38: 70-77. 2010/12/24. DOI: 10.1183/09031936.00053510.
78. Monfredi O, Heward E, Griffiths L, et al. Effect of dual pulmonary vasodilator therapy in pulmonary arterial hypertension associated with congenital heart disease: a retrospective analysis. *Open Heart* 2016; 3: e000399. 2016/04/22. DOI: 10.1136/openhrt-2016-000399.

CHAPTER 111

NONCARDIAC SURGERY IN THOSE WITH ADULT CONGENITAL HEART DISEASE

Dana Irrer and Joseph D. Kay

INTRODUCTION

Advances in surgical and medical treatments for children with congenital heart disease (CHD) have led to a steady increase in the number of adults with congenital heart disease (ACHD).[1] The combination of late sequela from the congenital cardiac defects, progressive noncardiac comorbidities (sometimes related to their congenital cardiac defects), and gaps in surveillance cardiac care places many of these patients at higher risk for anesthesia and noncardiac surgery than the general population.[2-13]

Although most noncardiac procedures can be performed without significant risk, minor procedures generally considered low risk in the general population may be associated with a higher risk in certain ACHD patients.[7] Patients with complex congenital cardiac lesions such as moderate to severe pulmonary hypertension or Eisenmenger syndrome have a high risk for adverse outcomes during noncardiac surgery, with mortality ranging from 4% to 10%.[3,14,15] Those with Fontan palliation for single-ventricle anatomy have also been shown to have a higher than normal complication rate, with rates as high as 31%.[8] Up to 48% of adverse outcomes may have been modifiable and are attributed to inadequate understanding of CHD physiology.[13]

In general, patients with CHD are at increased risk for hypotension, respiratory failure, acute kidney disease, pneumonia, and thromboembolic events.[16] Surgical risk relates to the complexity of CHD, the type of surgical procedure, urgency of the intervention, and availability of trained specialists and resources. Additionally, procedures in ACHD patients are associated with longer length of stays and higher hospital charges than patients with CHD across a spectrum of noncardiac procedures.[7,17] Thus, the ACHD population has unique preoperative imaging recommendations and perioperative monitoring considerations compared to the general population.

Guidelines have been established for perioperative cardiovascular evaluation and management of patients undergoing noncardiac surgery in the general population.[18] However, these guidelines have been developed primarily from evidence gathered from adults with acquired heart disease. Although recommendations may generally apply to most patients with CHD, these evaluation and management strategies are insufficient to adequately risk stratify many in this complex and heterogeneous group. Specifically, the guidelines do not account for the variable nonischemic mechanisms for ventricular dysfunction and arrhythmia seen in the ACHD population.[19] More recently, the American Heart Association (AHA) released a scientific statement on the diagnosis and management of noncardiac complications in ACHD patients and outlined the preoperative assessment of these patients before noncardiac surgery.[17]

In addition to the unique management concerns posted by complex congenital heart physiology, ACHD patients often have multi-organ involvement placing them at increased risk for perioperative complications.[5,6] These include lung and airway abnormalities, pulmonary hypertension, coagulopathy, neurocognitive deficits, mood disorders, liver and renal disease, immunodeficiency, infection risk, genetic syndromes, and malignancy. This increased incidence of comorbid disease requires additional scrutiny during preoperative assessment and perioperative management.

Cardiac Risk Stratification

Perioperative cardiovascular risk assessment for the general population is outlined in the "2014 ACC/AHA Guideline on Perioperative Cardiovascular Evaluation and Management of Patients Undergoing Noncardiac Surgery."[18] Although the principles outlined in these guidelines are helpful in assessing risks for the ACHD population as well, they fall short of identifying many specific risk factors present in this population based on surgical history. Compared to patients with acquired heart disease, ACHD patients have increased operative risk owing to nonischemic ventricular dysfunction and a higher incidence of pulmonary hypertension, residual intracardiac shunts, arrhythmia, and multi-organ dysfunction.[20-22] To date, there is not a specific tool in use for cardiac risk assessment with invasive procedures specific to ACHD patients, largely owing to the heterogeneity of the population. Hence, a stepwise, meticulous approach to perioperative cardiac assessment in ACHD was developed to guide workup and management (**Algorithm 111.1**).[17] Factors associated with perioperative mortality and morbidity in this population include cyanosis, congestive heart failure, poor general health, older age, pulmonary hypertension, operations on the respiratory and nervous systems, complex CHD, and urgent or emergent procedures.[10]

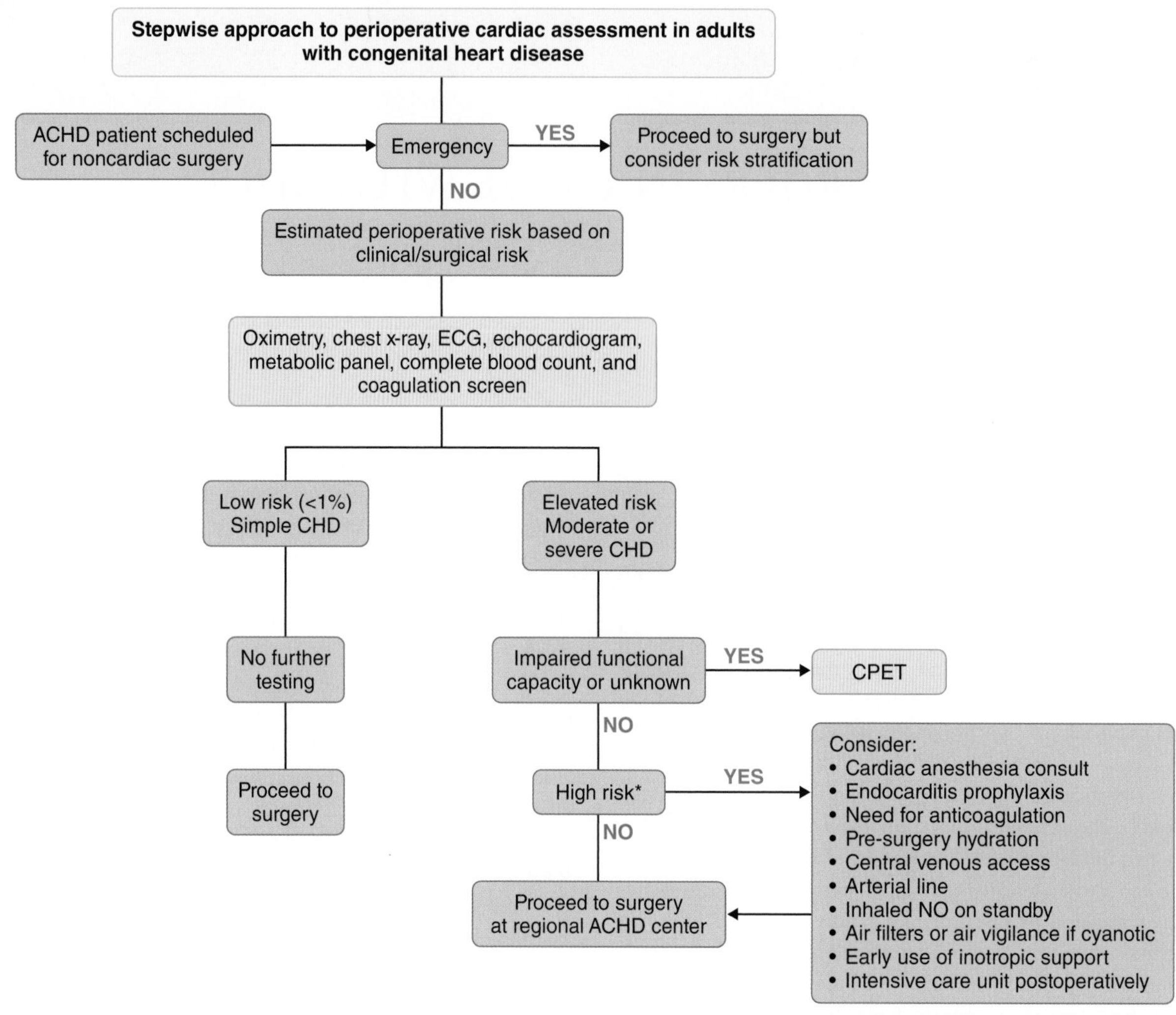

ALGORITHM 111.1 Stepwise approach to perioperative cardiac assessment in adults with congenital heart disease. ACHD, adult congenital heart disease; CHD, congenital heart disease; CPET, cardiopulmonary exercise testing; ECG, electrocardiogram; NO, nitric oxide. (Reprinted with permission from Lui GK, Saidi A, Bhatt AB, et al.; American Heart Association Adult Congenital Heart Disease Committee of the Council on Clinical Cardiology and Council on Cardiovascular Disease in the Young; Council on Cardiovascular Radiology and Intervention; and Council on Quality of Care and Outcomes Research. Diagnosis and Management of Noncardiac Complications in Adults With Congenital Heart Disease: A Scientific Statement From the American Heart Association. *Circulation.* 2017;136(20):e348-e392. Copyright © 2017 American Heart Association, Inc.)

PREOPERATIVE EVALUATION AND CONSIDERATIONS

Whenever possible, a comprehensive preoperative assessment by an ACHD expert is recommended for all ACHD patients undergoing noncardiac surgery in order to anticipate and prevent complications. Up to 48% of adverse outcomes in this population may be attributed to lack of adequate knowledge of CHD, previous treatments, and current physiology, and up to 40% of overall adverse events of noncardiac surgeries in ACHD patients are owing to inadequate preoperative assessment.[13] Current AHA and American College of Cardiology (ACC) guidelines outline the frequency of routine follow-up and preoperative evaluation based on both the anatomic complexity (A) and physiologic class (P) of the congenital heart lesion. According to expert consensus, even adult patients with "simple" CHD—such as a small or repaired atrial or ventricular septal defect, or mild pulmonic stenosis—should have at least a onetime follow-up with an ACHD cardiologist or possibly every 3 to 5 years or more as determined by the physiologic stage.[19]

Cardiologists with expertise in ACHD have extensive experience with this heterogeneous population, leading to better anticipation and identification of long-term complications related to underlying disease and interventions. Prior to undergoing any elective surgery, ACHD AP classification should be ascertained and providers should ensure patients are following guidelines regarding ACHD outpatient follow-up and outpatient testing including electrocardiography, echocardiography, functional testing, and cross-sectional imaging. Lapses in adult congenital cardiology care are unfortunately common and should be identified as they are associated with higher morbidity in the ACHD population.[23] Working with an adult congenital cardiologist, physiologic stage should be optimized prior to any invasive procedure.[3,7,13,24]

Location of Care

Ideally, noncardiac surgery risk stratification for ACHD patients should take place well before the planned elective surgical procedure. Those considered at increased risk for cardiovascular complications with surgery should have their elective procedures performed in an ACHD facility with the availability of cardiac and noncardiac subspecialists who are familiar with the management of this patient population. The 2018 ACC/AHA ACHD guidelines outline key personnel and services recommended for ACHD accreditation.[19] This includes ACHD board-certified or eligible cardiologists including those trained in electrophysiology, interventional cardiology, heart failure, congenital cardiac imaging, congenital cardiac surgery, cardiac anesthesiologists with CHD expertise, as well as knowledgeable subspecialty care including high-risk obstetrics, pulmonary hypertension, genetics, hepatology, pulmonology, nephrology, infectious disease, neurology, and mental health. Patients with moderate and complex CHD have better outcomes when cared for by an integrated multidisciplinary team. Improved survival has similarly been demonstrated when patients are managed at regional CHD centers.[25] This is related to several nuances in ACHD patients best addressed by cardiologists, anesthesiologists, and subspecialists with experience in ACHD care.

In reality, up to 74% of noncardiac surgeries in the ACHD population take place at non-ACHD centers.[26] Although this may be appropriate for many of these patients with simple congenital lesions with normal to near-normal functional capacity (ACHD AP classification 1A and 1B), patients should at least have preoperative consultation by an ACHD cardiologist, given the potential for long-term complications. Even simple congenital defects such as small ventricular septal defect can cause progressive changes leading to the development of right or left ventricular outflow tract narrowing, which could significantly increase anesthetic risk. In more complex cardiac lesions, remote practice locations and emergent procedures may preclude transfer prior to noncardiac surgery. In these situations, collaboration with a knowledgeable multidisciplinary ACHD team should be sought out early. ACHD cardiologists also frequently need to assist in the coordination of care between adult and pediatric trained providers with varied experience in adult congenital cardiology care. If the ACHD patient is managed in a pediatric center, access to adult subspecialty care is essential and may require formalized relationships between centers.[27] Similarly, patients cared for in adult centers should be done so in conjunction with an ACHD cardiologist.

History

A complete understanding of the patient's native congenital cardiac defect(s) and cardiac surgical history is critical prior to any elective procedure. Often, this proves difficult, as old records may be difficult to obtain or be incomplete. History obtained from the patient or family members may be inaccurate or misleading. Accurate knowledge of prior surgical interventions can be important for perioperative monitoring. Common examples encountered in most ACHD centers are patients with a history of the placement of classic Blalock-Thomas-Taussig shunts. For this procedure, the cardiac surgeon ligates the subclavian artery on the side of the lateral thoracotomy and attaches this in an end-to-side fashion to the ipsilateral branch pulmonary artery to augment pulmonary flow when the child was cyanotic. This procedure allows the cyanotic child to grow to a larger size when a complete operative repair can be performed at a lower risk. These patients should not have blood pressure measured in the affected arm, as this will not reflect central aortic pressure resulting in inappropriate perioperative fluid or vasoactive medication use. Many centers also perform subclavian patch repair for operative repair of coarctation of the aorta. In these cases, the left subclavian artery is ligated, and the proximal segment of the vessel is used to augment the aortic repair. Hence, for these patients, blood pressure needs to be measured on the right arm. A history of prior heart surgery alone carries a higher risk of morbidity and mortality during noncardiac surgery compared to peers.[7] Knowledge of native anatomy and interventions predicts long-term complications and guides preoperative screening.

Physical Examination

A detailed physical examination is particularly important in this population in gauging operative risk and providing perioperative monitoring. Skin assessment including evidence of prior sternotomy or thoracotomy scar may provide valuable information regarding prior interventions, which may have implications for intraoperative monitoring. As outlined above, right or left thoracotomy scars may indicate surgically sacrificed subclavian arteries in the setting of classic Blalock-Thomas-Taussig shunt or subclavian flap repair of aortic coarctation. Blood pressure and pulse assessment in all four limbs may also aid in this determination and guide which are inappropriate for invasive or noninvasive monitoring or line placement. Additionally, a discrepancy in upper and lower extremity blood pressure or radio-femoral delay in pulse may indicate recurrent stenosis in those with prior aortic coarctation repair. Hence, these patients may be at particularly high risk for decreased renal perfusion during periods of hypotension if the anesthesia team is relying on upper extremity blood pressure alone. All patients should have pulse oximetry testing. Cardiac auscultation may indicate severity of disease as valvar and ventricular dysfunction may decline over time related to underlying disease or prior repair or palliation. This may need to be addressed prior to general anesthesia or surgical intervention. As mentioned elsewhere, patients with CHD often have long-term multisystem complications related to their underlying disease or intervention, and care should be taken to complete a thorough physical examination.

Functional Assessment

Assessment of functional capacity is a key metric in determining perioperative risk.[18,28] To this end, the physiologic stage component of the ACHD AP classification system is valuable in determining surgical risk. It should be noted, however, that many patients with CHD have adapted to a lifelong decrease in functional capacity and will overestimate their physical capabilities and self-limit or avoid activities that exceed their physiologic limits. These individuals will often subjectively report normal or unchanged functional capacity. Hence, formal cardiopulmonary exercise testing or a 6-minute walk test provides an objective measurement of functional capacity.[29] Given a higher incidence of baseline reduced functional capacity compared to age-matched controls, this testing played a more important role in risk stratification for the ACHD population compared with the general population.[17] Reference values have been established for more frequent congenital lesions and postoperative physiology such as tetralogy of Fallot, aortic coarctation, Fontan and atrial or arterial switch procedures.[30] Although this compares the person's functional capacity to others with similar cardiac defects, to date the ACHD community has not developed a validated risk score for different surgical procedures.

Arrhythmia Assessment

Arrhythmias are common in the ACHD population and reoccurrences can worsen or become exacerbated by the stress of surgery or certain anesthetic agents. Up to 50% of ACHD patients will have some type of rhythm disturbance in the perioperative period.[31] Arrhythmias increase in prevalence as adults with CHD age and, along with heart failure, is the leading cause of death.[32] Factors contributing to the overall arrhythmia risk in this population include a congenitally displaced or malformed conduction system, abnormal hemodynamics from valvar disease, shunt physiology or chamber enlargement, primary myocardial disease, genetic influences, hypoxic tissue injury, and residual or postoperative sequelae including scar or direct damage to the conduction system.[33]

An electrocardiogram is recommended for all ACHD patients prior to noncardiac surgery. Findings such as a right bundle branch block are common in patients after ventricular septal defect closure, and preoperative electrocardiograms should be compared to prior baseline studies. Significant changes from baseline or additional findings—such as ventricular preexcitation, heart block, or ectopy—may prompt further evaluation in the form of ambulatory cardiac rhythm monitoring or exercise testing. A history of palpitations, unexplained syncope, sustained ventricular tachycardia, atrial fibrillation, or heart block should also prompt further preoperative ambulatory monitoring or exercise testing. A select few patients may benefit from an electrophysiology study and medical or interventional rhythm optimization prior to undergoing nonurgent surgery.[31] Providers should also exercise caution when holding beta-blocker or calcium channel blockers prior to noncardiac surgery, as these may be employed for antiarrhythmic effects in addition to their role in long-term heart failure management.

Specific congenital lesions or surgical interventions carry a long-term risk for heart block. Examples include individuals with congenitally corrected transposition (double discordance or L-transposition of the great arteries) or extensive ventricular septal defect repair. As such, many patients with CHD have epicardial or transvenous pacing systems and implanted cardioverter defibrillators which require preoperative assessment and reprogramming.[31] This is particularly important as electrocautery may interfere with device function leading to unnecessary shocks or far-field sensing of the pacemaker lead, leading to inappropriate pacemaker inhibition in someone who may be pacemaker dependent. Therefore, a clear understanding of the severity of the conduction system issues is critical, and preoperative programming of the device for surgery or utilization of a magnet over the device is needed.

Antiplatelet and Anticoagulation Therapy

Antiplatelet and anticoagulation therapy play an important role in stroke prevention for many ACHD patients. Indications for chronic therapy include reduction of systemic embolization in those with atrial arrhythmias or prior thromboembolism, residual shunt, or prosthetic valve or other material. The risk of withholding these should be determined for each type of noncardiac surgery and indication for use. In general, the 2014 guidelines for perioperative cardiovascular evaluation for the general population in regard to antiplatelet therapy and anticoagulation can be applied.[18] Patients with mechanical aortic or atrioventricular valves on Coumadin may require bridging anticoagulation before the surgery in order to reduce the bleeding risk at the time of surgery. This is particularly important in those patients with additional risk factors for thromboembolism including atrial fibrillation, prior stroke, systemic ventricular dysfunction, hypercoagulable state, or some older generation prosthetic valves with a less favorable thrombosis profile.[18] It should also be noted that many ACHD patients, particularly those with Fontan physiology, may be predisposed to both bleeding and thrombosis related to low cardiac output states, stasis of blood flow, and liver disease.[34] Hence, the surgical team needs to be prepared to address excessive bleeding for even straightforward surgeries such as appendectomy or cholecystectomy.

Vitamin K, fresh frozen plasma, and prothrombin complex concentrate can be used in the setting of emergent surgery and hemorrhage. In general, patients with arrhythmias, residual shunts, or bioprosthetic valves without risk factors may have vitamin K antagonist and antiplatelet therapy discontinued 4 to 5 days prior to a planned surgery based on the surgical bleeding risk. Newer anticoagulants, such as direct thrombin or Xa inhibitors, should be discontinued at least 48 hours prior to surgery when possible. Current ACC/AHA guidelines recommend intraoperative monitoring of activated partial thromboplastin time for dabigatran and prothrombin time for apixaban and rivaroxaban. Anticoagulation should be reinitiated as soon as considered safe in the setting of possible postoperative bleeding.[18]

Preoperative Testing

For nonemergent surgery, preoperative testing for ACHD patients should include pulse oximetry, electrocardiogram, and chest x-ray. For patients with at least moderate or complex adult congenital cardiac lesions, additional testing should include echocardiography, complete metabolic panel, complete blood count, and coagulation screen. Additional considerations are outlined below.

Laboratory Workup

In addition to routine laboratory tests, kidney and liver function testing should be performed on most ACHD patients prior to undergoing noncardiac surgery, given the high prevalence of multisystem disease in this population.[17] Plasma natriuretic protein levels may also help determine underlying ventricular dysfunction and fluid status. Complete blood count and iron studies are also commonly indicated in this population, and it should be noted that those with chronic hypoxemia may demonstrate either erythrocytosis or a relative iron deficiency anemia despite hemoglobin measuring in the normal to elevated range. Those with chronic cyanosis may benefit from iron supplementation to optimize tissue oxygen delivery prior to elective procedures. Hepatitis C testing is indicated for all who had cardiac surgery prior to 1992, in the era before routine screening of blood products. The prevalence of hepatitis C in the CHD population is as high as 9%.[35]

Imaging

Current ACHD guidelines recommend the frequency of echocardiography and cross-sectional imaging based on both the type of lesion and physiologic stage of the disease. For example, a patient with a history of Ebstein anomaly with normal tricuspid valve function, normal right ventricular function, and no history of arrhythmia (ACHD AP physiologic stage A) is recommended to have cardiac magnetic resonance or computed tomographic imaging every 5 years, whereas a patient with associated asymptomatic but moderate or severe valve disease (ACHD AP physiologic stage C) should have cross-sectional imaging performed at least every 1 to 2 years.[19] Prior to undergoing noncardiac surgery, ACHD patients should be at least up-to-date on recommended testing intervals. Beyond this, preoperative imaging may reveal underlying physiology or anatomy pertinent to surgical monitoring and management. Patients with a particularly high incidence of venous abnormalities that may make central venous access more difficult include those with heterotaxy syndromes, Mustard or Senning atrial switch procedures for complete transposition of the great vessels, or a Glenn shunt. Similarly, many congenital patients have had recurrent catheterizations or indwelling lines, which may contribute to femoral vessel occlusion limiting options for access. Assessment of vascular anatomy should be assessed prior to surgical procedures when central venous access may be needed.

EVALUATION FOR ACQUIRED CARDIAC DISEASE/CORONARY ARTERY DISEASE

No clear guidelines exist for preoperative assessment for coronary artery disease prior to noncardiac surgery in the ACHD population. Most centers utilize ACC/AHA guidelines, which advocate for coronary angiography or computed tomographic imaging prior to surgery in those with progressive angina or other objective evidence of ischemia, or decreased ventricular function.[18] Although this may identify coronary disease in the congenital population, these recommendations may not fully capture the risk for coronary artery disease or related perioperative complications. Overall, coronary artery disease is not a leading cause of death in the CHD population, but some congenital heart lesions does increase the risk for coronary artery disease. These include those with associated coronary anomalies, coarctation of the aorta (with secondary long-term hypertension), or those with a history of coronary manipulation, such as in the Ross procedure or arterial switch operation.[36] In contrast, those with a history of complex disease including single-ventricle palliation have an overall lower burden of coronary artery disease compared to the general population. Regardless, knowledge of an individual patient's coronary artery anatomy may be important prior to any surgical intervention for those at higher risk.

Heart Failure

Heart failure is the leading cause of hospital admission and death in the ACHD population.[37] In addition to common causes of heart failure in the aging general population, these patients are likely to suffer from obstructive lesions, valvar insufficiency, or intracardiac shunts that may lead to pressure or volume-loaded ventricles. Many CHD lesions result in a right ventricle that is not suited to long-term systemic hemodynamic stress. Importantly, as discussed previously, many patients with CHD have acclimated to cardiac dysfunction and may report few symptoms of functional limitations related to peers, thus making the preoperative physical examination and screening even more important in this population. Unfortunately, it remains unclear how many of those with heart failure and complex ACHD lesions (such as those with systemic right ventricles or those post-Fontan palliation) respond to medical therapy proven beneficial for heart failure in the absence of ACHD.

Pulmonary Hypertension

The prevalence of pulmonary hypertension in the ACHD has been reported to range from 2.5% to 5.8% with particular risk factors being previous aortic to pulmonary shunts and older age.[20,22] These individuals carry perioperative mortality of up to 10%.[3] For those at risk, preoperative assessment with functional testing, echocardiographic screening, and cardiac catheterization is particularly important. Those with near or supra-systemic pulmonary pressures should avoid elective surgical interventions where able, and if undergoing any procedure, should be optimized on pulmonary vasodilator support under careful management by a cardiac anesthesia team with inhaled nitric oxide or IV prostacyclins on hand.[15]

Noncardiac Pathology

Impairment of multiple organ systems is seen in many ACHD survivors, particularly in those with moderate to high complex lesions and those with older age at repair. These can contribute to increased perioperative complications. A history of prior cardiac surgery—independent of long-term noncardiac sequelae—and each specific lesion has long-term effects on several different body systems.

Lung

Pulmonary disease related to an underlying cardiac disease process can complicate perioperative management. For example, 44% to 56% of adults who underwent heart surgery in childhood have restrictive lung disease compared to 9% in the general population.[38] This is more likely in those who have undergone multiple sternotomies (ie, tetralogy of Fallot and Fontan palliation). Additionally, higher incidences of obesity, abnormal pulmonary development, and drug toxicity from medications such as amiodarone may also contribute to decreased lung function.[17] This has important implications for ventilator management and extubation in the perioperative period. Other complex cardiac lesions such as heterotaxy syndromes frequently have associated ciliary dyskinesia, which may predispose to postoperative pneumonia or prolonged ventilation.[39] Pulmonary function testing may be indicated prior to noncardiac intervention, as decreased forced vital capacity, which is common in the tetralogy of Fallot population, may be an independent predictor of hospitalization and death.[40] This is particularly important for those who have moderate or more impairment seen on previous cardiopulmonary testing.

Kidney

Chronic kidney disease is seen in 30% to 50% of ACHD patients, particularly in those with chronic hypoxemia and hypertension.[41] Up to half of Fontan patients living into their late 20s have renal dysfunction.[42] This can predispose to acute perioperative kidney injury and residual moderate to severe renal dysfunction and carries a fivefold increase in 6-year mortality.[13]

Liver

For those with Fontan physiology, the combination of chronic hypoxemia early in life, followed by chronically elevated hepatic venous pressure leads to hepatic congestion with hepatic fibrosis, cirrhosis, and a higher risk of developing hepatocellular carcinoma.[43] On screening laboratory tests, 94% of Fontan patients have elevated liver function tests.[44] The downstream effects of liver failure—such as varices, ascites, or coagulopathies—impact airway management, healing, and surgical bleeding.

Advanced Directive and Consent

CHD patients are at higher risk for developmental delay, mental health disorders, impaired executive functioning, and cerebral vascular disease both early and late in life.[45] This is multifactorial in etiology, compounded by the high prevalence of genetic syndromes, cyanosis, birth prematurity, and early exposure to cardiopulmonary bypass and/or extracorporeal membrane oxygenation.[46] Traditional risk factors for stroke, such as hypertension, heart failure, intracardiac shunt, and arrhythmias, are more prevalent in the ACHD population and further predispose them to cognitive dysfunction.[45] A discussion of advanced directives, goals of care, and identification of surrogate medical decision-makers prior to surgery is particularly important in these individuals who have variable executive functioning and increased morbidity and mortality associated with noncardiac surgery. Although many patients with severe cognitive impairment may require a guardian to assist with or perform consent, most ACHD patients are decisional but may have difficulties assessing risks and benefits related to procedures and postoperative compliance with treatment plans.

A checklist was developed as part of the 2018 AHA/ACC guidelines for the management of ACHD patients undergoing noncardiac surgery (**Table 111.1**),[19] which outlines preoperative workup, factors associated with perioperative morbidity and mortality, and intraoperative planning.

PERIOPERATIVE SPECIAL CONCERNS AND MANAGEMENT

Anesthesia

In addition to regular precautions being employed during noncardiac surgery, additional considerations are necessary for the ACHD population undergoing surgery/anesthesia. An anesthesia team knowledgeable in complex cardiology and cardiac physiology is necessary.[11] This should include the following[16]:

- Indications for endocarditis prophylaxis;
- Perioperative fluid management/hydration plan;
- Pacemaker/implantable cardioverter-defibrillator reprograming;
- Plan for hemodynamic monitoring and vascular access;
- Need for filters (to trap air bubbles) on intravenous lines in the setting of intra- or extracardiac shunts;
- Need for pulmonary vasodilators; and
- Early use and indications for inotropic support.

Anesthetic management in complex CHD poses unique challenges. In Fontan physiology, for example, care must be taken to avoid hypercarbia and acidosis, which can elevate pulmonary pressures and severely limit passive blood flow to the lungs and cardiac output. In the setting of a fenestration, elevated pulmonary pressures may exacerbate right-to-left shunting and hypoxemia, meaning inhaled nitric oxide must be readily available for pulmonary vasodilation. Fluid status can be particularly delicate as neither volume overload nor hypovolemia is tolerated well in the patient with a single ventricle. Similarly, high airway and intrathoracic pressure reduce central venous return and thus pulmonary blood flow, leading to low cardiac output. Hypothermia, metabolic acidosis, hypercarbia, and hypovolemia are also poorly tolerated in Eisenmenger syndrome because of worsening right-to-left shunting. When the balance of pulmonary and systemic vascular resistance has drastic effects on either end-organ perfusion or oxygenation, this guides vasoactive medication use, particularly in the setting of hypoxemia. Patients with right-to-left intracardiac shunts are also at risk for stroke related to paradoxical embolization, and care must be taken to secure IV filters on all lines to reduce the risk of systemic air embolism. Patients with supravalvar aortic stenosis can suffer significant myocardial ischemia on induction because they require elevated aortic root pressure to maintain coronary perfusion. Additionally, many ACHD patients

TABLE 111.1 ACHD Management Issues for Noncardiac Surgery

Clarify CHD diagnosis
- Clarify prior procedures, residua, sequelae, and current status, including ACHD AP classification
- Be aware that history obtained from only the patient and family may be faulty or incomplete
- Obtain and review old records to ensure accurate understanding of past procedures and clinical course
- Complete additional investigations required to define ACHD AP classification
- Develop management strategies to minimize risk and optimize the outcome

Factors associated with increased risk of perioperative morbidity and mortality:
- Cyanosis
- Congestive HF
- Poor general health
- Younger age
- Pulmonary hypertension
- Operations on respiratory and nervous systems
- Complex CHD
- Urgent/emergency procedures

Issues to consider:
- Endocarditis prophylaxis
- Complications related to underlying hemodynamics
- Abnormal venous and/or arterial anatomy affecting venous and arterial access
- Persistent shunts
- Valvular disease
- Arrhythmias, including bradyarrhythmias
- Erythrocytosis
- Pulmonary vascular disease
- Meticulous line care (also consider air filters for intravenous lines) to reduce risk of paradoxical embolus in patients who are cyanotic because of right-to-left shunts
- Adjustment of anticoagulant volume in tubes for some blood work in cyanotic patients
- Prevention of venous thrombosis
- Monitoring of renal and liver functions
- Periprocedure anticoagulation
- Possible need for nonconventional drug dosing
- Increased prevalence of hepatitis C infection because of prior procedures and remote blood transfusions
- Developmental disability

ACHD, adult congenital heart disease; AP, anatomic and physiologic; CHD, congenital heart disease; HF, heart failure.

suffer from limited options for vascular access owing to vessel occlusion or ligation related to recurrent catheterization, indwelling lines, and surgical intervention. Thus, knowledge of lesion-specific complications is important to perioperative anesthesia management for the ACHD population.

Endocarditis Prophylaxis

The 2007 AHA guidelines can help identify patients who may benefit from endocarditis prophylaxis.[47] In general, those with prosthetic heart valves, prior history of endocarditis, history of unrepaired cyanotic CHD including palliative shunts or conduits, history of CHD repaired with prosthetic material for the first 6 months post-procedure, or presence of residual defects after repair require prophylaxis. Of note, most gastrointestinal and genitourinary tract procedures are no longer believed to be at increased risk for bacteremia leading to endocarditis; hence, they no longer require antibiotic prophylaxis. Providers should reference guidelines regarding both indications by procedure and choice of antibiotic therapy, particularly in the setting of antibiotic allergy.

Vascular Access and Intraoperative Monitoring

ACHD patients often have limited options for vascular access related to a history of multiple prior catheterizations, indwelling lines, surgical ligation of vessels, or abnormal systemic venous return. A detailed cardiac history and review of available or necessary imaging data should be performed prior to noncardiac surgery. This will guide options for intraoperative monitoring and vascular access, particularly if the patient may require urgent or emergent central venous access or mechanical circulatory support. Options for invasive or noninvasive blood pressure monitoring might similarly be limited as patients with recurrent aortic coarctation, history of subclavian flap aortic coarctation repair, classic Blalock-Thomas-Taussig shunt, aberrant aortic arch vessel anatomy, or peripheral arterial stenosis related to previous interventions may have arm pressure measurements that differ substantially from central aortic pressure. Measurement of blood pressure in these affected limbs can lead to inappropriate fluid resuscitation and/or vasoactive medication management. Care should also be taken to place filters on all intravenous lines and monitor closely for air bubbles for all patients with intra-or extracardiac shunts to limit the possibility of paradoxical embolism and stroke. Although invasive hemodynamic monitoring may be useful during higher risk cases, one should be aware of potential complications related to their use. Pulmonary arterial catheters can trigger arrhythmias and microthrombi formation with the potential for embolism. Central venous catheters are also prothrombotic and may pose a further risk for paradoxical embolus. Risks and benefits of monitoring and access must be weighed thoughtfully in this population.

Electrophysiology Device Management

Many ACHD patients have an implantable cardiac defibrillator or pacemaker. Knowledge of the type of device, location, underlying heart rhythm, effect of a magnet placed over device, and whether the device requires reprogramming is key to perioperative management. Many of these patients have epicardial leads attached to devices placed subcutaneously in the abdominal wall, which may be predisposed to damage or infection in the setting of abdominal surgery. Depending on the location of the surgical field related to the device, electrocautery may lead to inappropriate implantable cardioverter-defibrillator device shocks or pacemaker inhibition during a procedure. Use of a magnet over the device to either inhibit implantable cardioverter-defibrillator device function or revert a pacemaker to an asynchronous mode may be necessary during a procedure but may also affect cardiac output during a case. Patients may also be at increased risk for malignant arrhythmias based on their underlying cardiac disease, and automated external defibrillators and antiarrhythmic medications should be available for use if necessary.

Fluid Management

Patients with shunt physiology require thoughtful consideration of agents used for induction and maintenance of anesthesia, as abrupt reduction in systemic vascular resistance may have significant hemodynamic consequences. Hypotension from peripheral vasodilation can result in increased right-to-left shunting and decreased oxygen delivery.[13] Often, these patients and others who are dependent on preload for pulmonary and systemic blood flow are admitted the evening prior to cardiac surgery for intravenous fluid administration, particularly if they will have a prolonged period without oral intake. Similarly, an increase in intrathoracic or abdominal pressure during a case may decrease systemic venous return and cardiac output. Pulse oximetry and arterial line monitoring are likely necessary for these higher risk patients, and central access may provide central venous pressure monitoring and a route for rapid fluid resuscitation. Optimization of fluid and respiratory status with close monitoring is necessary prior to any planned procedure, regardless of the complexity of cardiac disease.[3,7,13,24]

Saturation

Knowledge of baseline O_2 saturation is necessary as many patients with complex cardiac anatomy may have low baseline oxygen saturations. A rise in saturation in shunted patients may lead to excessive pulmonary blood flow at the expense of systemic blood flow, particularly in the setting of hypertension or pulmonary vasodilator therapies. Even in Fontan patients without a fenestration, baseline saturations may frequently be below 90% related to venous collaterals. Hence, careful understanding of the individual's baseline is critical.

Laparoscopic Procedures

Additional considerations for laparoscopic procedures should be undertaken in patients with Fontan physiology. Although intra-abdominal pressures less than 15 mm Hg are typically tolerated well in two ventricle circulations, this can be poorly tolerated in the Fontan population for prolonged periods of time related to reduced central venous return, pulmonary perfusion, and cardiac output. Care should be taken to monitor and limit intra-abdominal pressures to less than 10 mm Hg.[48]

POSTOPERATIVE PATIENT CARE

Follow-up after noncardiac surgery should be scheduled according to ACA/AHA ACHD guidelines or more frequently after noncardiac surgery based on expected fluid shifts, medication changes, or anticoagulation needs on a patient-by-patient basis.

Up to half of the perioperative adverse events occur in the period after surgery.[13] Hemodynamic compromise related to fluid shifts with intraoperative fluid resuscitation, arrhythmias, pulmonary edema, bleeding with anticoagulation management, deep venous or other thrombosis often occurs in this postoperative period.[3,10] Hence, intensive care unit (ICU) level monitoring may be needed for select high-risk patients postoperatively.[17] Patients with Eisenmenger syndrome, in particular, require at least 12 to 24 hours of monitoring in ICU-level care after noncardiac surgery because of changes in pulmonary vascular and systemic resistance after sedation. Intravenous lines with filters to prevent air embolism should remain in place for those at risk for paradoxical embolism, and lines should be removed when able to reduce infection and thromboembolism risk. The electrophysiology team should also be notified to reprogram any device as indicated. Reinitiation of anticoagulation and/or antiplatelet therapy should be based on the relative risk of bleeding versus thrombosis. In those at high risk for thrombosis, early ambulation and pneumatic compression devices should be employed, and heparin or oral anticoagulation should be restarted as soon as deemed safe from acute bleeding by the surgical team. Those who do not require bridging therapy or who are at lower risk of thrombosis may resume therapy several days after the procedure.

HIGHEST RISK PATIENTS AND SPECIAL CONSIDERATIONS

Fontan Palliation

The anesthesia team needs to pay extra attention to avoid physiologic conditions which increase pulmonary vascular resistance and carefully monitor for such conditions. These include even mild hypercarbia and acidosis, and maintenance of adequate preload. Higher supplemental oxygen can be utilized for pulmonary vasodilator effects, which, along with inhaled nitric oxide, may help treat low cardiac output in these patients. Those with Fontan physiology are also intolerant of high intrathoracic pressures. Hence, prolonged positive pressure ventilation and elevated intrathoracic and intra-abdominal pressures have a much more profound effect on reducing systemic venous return and pulmonary blood flow compared to patients with two ventricle physiology. Additional respiratory considerations include a likely history of restrictive lung disease related to recurrent sternotomy and possible thoracotomies over the course of staged palliation. Many Fontan patients will also have persistent hypoxemia related to veno-venous collateral formation and obligate right-to-left shunting or the presence of fenestrations. This increases the risk for erythrocytosis and paradoxical embolism. Because of the negative effects on systemic venous return, it is recommended to maintain intra-abdominal pressures less than 10 mm Hg during laparoscopic procedures. Arterial line monitoring with central access should be employed for monitoring and fluid resuscitation.[48] Neuraxial anesthesia is felt to be generally safe in Fontan patients but may complicate anticoagulation as indicated.[49]

Fontan palliation has several multisystem consequences that may increase risk related to noncardiac surgery; 71% of adults develop at least one major complication within 20 years of their Fontan operation, including atrial arrhythmias, thrombosis, Fontan failure, transplant, or death.[50] The kidney, lungs, liver, lymphatic system, brain, and peripheral vasculature are almost universally affected, and current guidelines for the routine monitoring of Fontan patients should be utilized, particularly as much of the dysfunction can remain asymptomatic for years.[34] As a result, the rate of perioperative complication in Fontan patients with noncardiac undergoing anesthesia is high, with up to 31% reporting complications.[8]

Eisenmenger Syndrome and Severe Pulmonary Hypertension

Patients with Eisenmenger syndrome have multisystem organ changes that lead to increased surgical morbidity and mortality. These are attributed to chronic cyanosis, fluid shifts, and bleeding risk. Increased risk related to surgical bleeding is attributed to collateralization of blood vessels, platelet dysfunction, and alterations in the clotting cascade. Although routine phlebotomy has fallen out of favor, preoperative isovolumic phlebotomy targeting a hematocrit less than 65% reduces blood viscosity and intraoperative bleeding risk. Oftentimes, blood removed with phlebotomy may be auto transfused during surgery.[51] Patients with Eisenmenger do not tolerate intraoperative hypothermia, metabolic acidosis, hypercarbia, and hypovolemia because of their effect on pulmonary and systemic vascular resistance, which increase right-to-left shunting. Although invasive hemodynamic monitoring is often useful during surgery, one should be aware of potential complications related to its use. Pulmonary arterial catheters can trigger arrhythmias and microthrombi formation with potential for systemic or pulmonary embolism. Central venous catheters are also prothrombotic and may pose a further risk for paradoxical embolus. Risks and benefits of monitoring and access must be weighed thoughtfully in this population. Patients with Eisenmenger should be monitored in an ICU setting for 12 to 24 hours after noncardiac surgery, given acute changes in pulmonary and systemic resistance.[17] Patients with Eisenmenger also require endocarditis prophylaxis.[47] Additional complications in this population affecting surgical risk include arrhythmia related to right heart enlargement, cyanotic kidney disease, airway compression, hemoptysis, and gastrointestinal bleeding.[16]

RESEARCH AND FUTURE DEVELOPMENTS

Although the population of adults with CHD is growing rapidly, the number of patients with a specific lesion or surgical intervention remains small. Given this heterogeneity in the ACHD population, ongoing collaboration with multicenter studies and large multinational databases are needed to better risk stratify and manage these patients undergoing noncardiac surgeries. A second major hurdle affecting care is the unmet needs for providers specializing in the care for ACHD. With the introduction of adult congenital cardiology comprehensive care center accreditation, an accredited training fellowship and research collaboratives such as the Alliance for Adult Research in Congenital Cardiology (AARCC) should be encouraged. As the number of accredited centers, board-certified ACHD providers, and workgroups increases, a larger proportion of the population in ACHD can contribute to stronger evidence-based management to improve perioperative management.

KEY POINTS

- ✔ Noncardiac surgery in the ACHD population should be performed when possible in regional, accredited centers of excellence.
- ✔ At a minimum, ACHD patients undergoing noncardiac surgery should be managed by a cardiologist and a multidisciplinary team familiar with ACHD.
- ✔ Knowledge of native anatomy, prior surgical or catheter-based interventions, and physiologic class dictates preoperative screening, risk assessment, and perioperative management.
- ✔ A discussion of advanced directives, goals of care, and identification of surrogate medical decision-makers prior to surgery is particularly important in individuals with ACHD who have variable executive functioning and increased morbidity and mortality associated with noncardiac surgery.
- ✔ Ongoing research collaboration is needed to guide future evidence-based care surrounding noncardiac surgery in the ACHD population.

REFERENCES

1. Gilboa SM, Devine OJ, Kucik JE, et al. Congenital heart defects in the United States: estimating the magnitude of the affected population in 2010. *Circulation.* 2016;134(2):101–109.
2. Agarwal S, Sud K, Menon V. Nationwide hospitalization trends in adult congenital heart disease across 2003-2012. *J Am Heart Assoc.* 2016;5(1): e002330.
3. Ammash NM, Connolly HM, Abel MD, Warnes CA. Noncardiac surgery in Eisenmenger syndrome. *J Am Coll Cardiol.* 1999;33(1):222–227.
4. Bhatt AB, Rajabali A, He W, Benavidez OJ. High resource use among adult congenital heart surgery admissions in adult hospitals: risk factors and association with death and comorbidities. *Congenit Heart Dis.* 2015;10(1):13–20.
5. Billett J, Cowie MR, Gatzoulis MA, Vonder Muhll IF, Majeed A. Comorbidity, healthcare utilisation and process of care measures in patients with congenital heart disease in the UK: cross-sectional, population-based study with case-control analysis. *Heart.* 2008;94(9):1194–1199.
6. Marelli AJ, Mackie AS, Ionescu-Ittu R, Rahme E, Pilote L. Congenital heart disease in the general population: changing prevalence and age distribution. *Circulation.* 2007;115(2):163–172.
7. Maxwell BG, Wong JK, Kin C, Lobato RL. Perioperative outcomes of major noncardiac surgery in adults with congenital heart disease. *Anesthesiology.* 2013;119(4):762–769.
8. Rabbitts JA, Groenewald CB, Mauermann WJ, et al. Outcomes of general anesthesia for noncardiac surgery in a series of patients with Fontan palliation. *Paediatr Anaesth.* 2013;23(2):180–187.

9. Rodriguez FH 3rd, Moodie DS, Parekh DR, et al. Outcomes of heart failure-related hospitalization in adults with congenital heart disease in the United States. *Congenit Heart Dis.* 2013;8(6):513–519.
10. Warner MA, Lunn RJ, O'Leary PW, Schroeder DR. Outcomes of noncardiac surgical procedures in children and adults with congenital heart disease. Mayo Perioperative Outcomes Group. *Mayo Clin Proc.* 1998;73(8):728–734.
11. Christensen RE, Gholami AS, Reynolds PI, Malviya S. Anaesthetic management and outcomes after noncardiac surgery in patients with hypoplastic left heart syndrome: a retrospective review. *Eur J Anaesthesiol.* 2012;29(9):425–430.
12. Mott AR, Fraser CD Jr, McKenzie ED, et al. Perioperative care of the adult with congenital heart disease in a free-standing tertiary pediatric facility. *Pediatr Cardiol.* 2002;23(6):624–630.
13. Maxwell BG, Posner KL, Wong JK, et al. Factors contributing to adverse perioperative events in adults with congenital heart disease: a structured analysis of cases from the closed claims project. *Congenit Heart Dis.* 2015;10(1):21–29.
14. Bennett JM, Ehrenfeld JM, Markham L, Eagle SS. Anesthetic management and outcomes for patients with pulmonary hypertension and intracardiac shunts and Eisenmenger syndrome: a review of institutional experience. *J Clin Anesth.* 2014;26(4):286–293.
15. Raines DE, Liberthson RR, Murray JR. Anesthetic management and outcome following noncardiac surgery in nonparturients with Eisenmenger's physiology. *J Clin Anesth.* 1996;8(5):341–347.
16. Gerardin JF, Earing MG. Preoperative evaluation of adult congenital heart disease patients for non-cardiac surgery. *Curr Cardiol Rep.* 2018;20(9):76.
17. Lui GK, Saidi A, Bhatt AB, et al. Diagnosis and management of noncardiac complications in adults with congenital heart disease: a scientific statement from the American Heart Association. *Circulation.* 2017;136(20):e348-e392.
18. Fleisher LA, Fleischmann KE, Auerbach AD, et al. 2014 ACC/AHA guideline on perioperative cardiovascular evaluation and management of patients undergoing noncardiac surgery: a report of the American College of Cardiology/American Heart Association Task Force on practice guidelines. *J Am Coll Cardiol.* 2014;64(22):e77-e137.
19. Stout KK, Daniels CJ, Aboulhosn JA, et al. 2018 AHA/ACC Guideline for the management of adults with congenital heart disease: executive summary: a report of the American College of Cardiology/American Heart Association Task Force on Clinical Practice Guidelines. *Circulation.* 2019;139(14):e637-e697.
20. Lowe BS, Therrien J, Ionescu-Ittu R, Pilote L, Martucci G, Marelli AJ. Diagnosis of pulmonary hypertension in the congenital heart disease adult population impact on outcomes. *J Am Coll Cardiol.* 2011;58(5):538–546.
21. van Riel ACMG, Blok IM, Zwinderman AH, et al. Lifetime risk of pulmonary hypertension for all patients after shunt closure. *J Am Coll Cardiol.* 2015;66(9):1084–1086.
22. van Riel ACMG, Schuuring MJ, Ivan Hessen D, et al. Contemporary prevalence of pulmonary arterial hypertension in adult congenital heart disease following the updated clinical classification. *Int J Cardiol.* 2014;174(2):299–305.
23. Yeung E, Kay J, Roosevelt GE, Brandon M, Yetman AT. Lapse of care as a predictor for morbidity in adults with congenital heart disease. *Int J Cardiol.* 2008;125(1):62–65.
24. Maxwell BG, Wong JK, Lobato RL. Perioperative morbidity and mortality after noncardiac surgery in young adults with congenital or early acquired heart disease: a retrospective cohort analysis of the National Surgical Quality Improvement Program database. *Am Surg.* 2014;80(4):321–326.
25. Mylotte D, Pilote L, Ionescu-Ittu R, et al. Specialized adult congenital heart disease care: the impact of policy on mortality. *Circulation.* 2014;129(18):1804–1812.
26. Maxwell BG, Maxwell TG, Wong JK. Decentralization of care for adults with congenital heart disease in the United States: a geographic analysis of outpatient surgery. *PLoS One.* 2014;9(9):e106730.
27. Ermis P, Dietzman T, Franklin W, Kim J, Moodie D, Parekh D. Cardiac resource utilization in adults at a freestanding children's hospital. *Congenit Heart Dis.* 2014;9(3):178–186.
28. Fleisher LA, Eagle KA. Clinical practice. Lowering cardiac risk in noncardiac surgery. *N Engl J Med.* 2001;345(23):1677–1682.
29. Mantegazza V, Apostolo A, Hager A. Cardiopulmonary exercise testing in adult congenital heart disease. *Ann Am Thorac Soc.* 2017;14(suppl_1):S93-S101.
30. Kempny A, Dimopoulos K, Uebing A, et al. Reference values for exercise limitations among adults with congenital heart disease. Relation to activities of daily life—single centre experience and review of published data. *Eur Heart J.* 2012;33(11):1386–1396.
31. Khairy P, Van Hare GF, Balaji S, et al. PACES/HRS Expert Consensus Statement on the Recognition and Management of Arrhythmias in Adult Congenital Heart Disease: developed in partnership between the Pediatric and Congenital Electrophysiology Society (PACES) and the Heart Rhythm Society (HRS). Endorsed by the governing bodies of PACES, HRS, the American College of Cardiology (ACC), the American Heart Association (AHA), the European Heart Rhythm Association (EHRA), the Canadian Heart Rhythm Society (CHRS), and the International Society for Adult Congenital Heart Disease (ISACHD*). Heart Rhythm.* 2014;11(10):e102-e165.
32. Verheugt CL, Uiterwaal CSPM, van der Velde ET, et al. Mortality in adult congenital heart disease. *Eur Heart J.* 2010;31(10):1220–1229.
33. Khairy P, Dore A, Talajic M, et al. Arrhythmias in adult congenital heart disease. *Expert Rev Cardiovasc Ther.* 2006;4(1):83–95.
34. Rychik J, Atz AM, Celermajer DS, et al. Evaluation and management of the child and adult with Fontan circulation: a scientific statement from the American Heart Association. *Circulation.* 2019;CIR0000000000000696.
35. Wang A, Book WM, McConnell M, Lyle T, Rodby K, Mahle WT. Prevalence of hepatitis C infection in adult patients who underwent congenital heart surgery prior to screening in 1992. *Am J Cardiol.* 2007;100(8):1307–1309. doi:10.1016/j.amjcard.2007.05.059
36. Bhatt AB, Foster E, Kuehl K, et al. Congenital heart disease in the older adult: a scientific statement from the American Heart Association. *Circulation.* 2015;131(21):1884–1931.
37. Stout KK, Broberg CS, Book WM, et al. Chronic heart failure in congenital heart disease: a scientific statement from the American Heart Association. *Circulation.* 2016;133(8):770–801.
38. Ginde S, Bartz PJ, Hill GD, et al. Restrictive lung disease is an independent predictor of exercise intolerance in the adult with congenital heart disease. *Congenit Heart Dis.* 2013;8(3):246–254.
39. Harden B, Tian X, Giese R, et al. Increased postoperative respiratory complications in heterotaxy congenital heart disease patients with respiratory ciliary dysfunction. *J Thorac Cardiovasc Surg.* 2014;147(4):1291–1298.e2.
40. Cohen KE, Buelow MW, Dixon J, et al. Forced vital capacity predicts morbidity and mortality in adults with repaired tetralogy of Fallot. *Congenit Heart Dis.* 2017;12(4):435–440.
41. Morgan C, Al-Aklabi M, Garcia Guerra G. Chronic kidney disease in congenital heart disease patients: a narrative review of evidence. *Can J Kidney Health Dis.* 2015;2:27.
42. Sharma S, Ruebner RL, Furth SL, Dodds KM, Rychik J, Goldberg DJ. Assessment of kidney function in survivors following Fontan palliation. *Congenit Heart Dis.* 2016;11(6):630–636.
43. Daniels CJ, Bradley EA, Landzberg MJ, et al. Fontan-associated liver disease: Proceedings from the American College of Cardiology Stakeholders Meeting, October 1 to 2, 2015, Washington DC. *J Am Coll Cardiol.* 2017;70(25):3173–3194.
44. Wu FM, Kogon B, Earing MG, et al. Liver health in adults with Fontan circulation: a multicenter cross-sectional study. *J Thorac Cardiovasc Surg.* 2017;153(3):656–664.
45. Marelli A, Miller SP, Marino BS, Jefferson AL, Newburger JW. Brain in congenital heart disease across the lifespan: the cumulative burden of injury. *Circulation.* 2016;133(20):1951–1962.
46. Marino BS, Lipkin PH, Newburger JW, et al. Neurodevelopmental outcomes in children with congenital heart disease: evaluation and management: a scientific statement from the American Heart Association. *Circulation.* 2012;126(9):1143–1172.

47. Wilson W, Taubert KA, Gewitz M, et al. Prevention of infective endocarditis: guidelines from the American Heart Association: a guideline from the American Heart Association Rheumatic Fever, Endocarditis and Kawasaki Disease Committee, Council on Cardiovascular Disease in the Young, and the Council on Clinical Cardiology, Council on Cardiovascular Surgery and Anesthesia, and the Quality of Care and Outcomes Research Interdisciplinary Working Group. *J Am Dent Assoc.* 2007;138(6):739–745, 747-760.
48. McClain CD, McGowan FX, Kovatsis PG. Laparoscopic surgery in a patient with Fontan physiology. *Anesth Analg.* 2006;103(4):856–858.
49. Tiouririne M, de Souza DG, Beers KT, Yemen TA. Anesthetic management of parturients with a Fontan circulation: a review of published case reports. *Semin Cardiothorac Vasc Anesth.* 2015;19(3):203–209.
50. d'Udekem Y, Iyengar AJ, Galati JC, et al. Redefining expectations of long-term survival after the Fontan procedure: twenty-five years of follow-up from the entire population of Australia and New Zealand. *Circulation.* 2014;130(11 suppl 1):S32-S38.
51. Baum VC, Perloff JK. Anesthetic implications of adults with congenital heart disease. *Anesth Analg.* 1993;76(6):1342–1358.

INDEX

Note: Page numbers followed by *f* and *t* followed by figures and tables.

F

I

N

O

P

S

U

V

W

X

Y

Z